# PSYCHIATRY
## SECOND EDITION

•TASMAN
•KAY
•LIEBERMAN

# PSYCHIATRY
## SECOND EDITION

## VOLUME 2

Edited by
*Allan Tasman*
Professor and Chair
Department of Psychiatry and Behavioral Sciences
University of Louisville School of Medicine
Louisville, Kentucky
USA

*Jerald Kay*
Professor and Chair
Department of Psychiatry
Wright State University School of Medicine
Dayton, Ohio
USA

*Jeffrey A. Lieberman*
Thad and Alice Eure Distinguished Professor of Psychiatry,
Pharmacology, and Radiology
Vice-Chairman for Research and Scientific Affairs Department of Psychiatry
Director, Mental Health and Neuroscience Clinical Research Center
University of North Carolina School of Medicine
Chapel Hill, North Carolina
USA

JOHN WILEY & SONS, LTD

*Other Wiley Editorial Offices*

John Wiley & Sons, Inc., 111 River Street, Hoboken, NJ 07030, USA

Jossey-Bass, 989 Market Street, San Francisco, CA 94103-1741, USA

Wiley-VCH Verlag GmbH, Boschstr. 12, D-69469 Weinheim, Germany

John Wiley & Sons Australia, Ltd., 33 Park Road, Milton, Queensland 4064, Australia

John Wiley & Sons (Asia) Pte Ltd., 2 Clementi Loop #02-01, Jin Xing Distripark, Singapore 129809

John Wiley & Sons Canada, Ltd., 22 Worcester Road, Etobicoke, Ontario, Canada M9W 1L1

Wiley also publishes its books in a variety of electronic formats. Some content that appears in print may not be
available in electronic books.

*British Library Cataloguing in Publication Data*

A catalogue record for this book is available from the British Library

ISBN 0 471 52177 9

Typeset in 9.5/11pt Times by Kolam Information Services Pvt. Ltd, Pondicherry, India
Printed and bound in Great Britain by William Clowes Ltd, Beccles, Suffolk
This book is printed on acid-free paper responsibly manufactured from sustainable forestry
in which at least two trees are planted for each one used for paper production.

# Dedications

*With love and thanks to Cathy, Joshua,*
*David, and Sarah, and to my parents, Goodie*
*and Zelda, for your love and support.*

**Allan**

*To my wife Rena, to my children Sarah,*
*Rachel, and Jonathan, and to my mother*
*Miriam, for their enduring love and support.*

**Jerry**

*To my father Howard (RIP) and*
*mother Ruth who inspired me;*
*and to my wife Rosemarie*
*and sons Jonathan and Jeremy who*
*supported me then and now.*

**Jeffrey**

# List of Contributors

**Henry David Abraham**
Massachusetts General Hospital
Harvard Medical School
175 Bedford Street
Lexington, MA 2420
USA

**Sonia Ancoli-Israel**
Department of Psychiatry, 116a
VA San Diego Healthcare System
3350 La Jolla Village Drive
San Diego, CA 92161
USA

**Jules Angst**
Zurich University
Psychiatric Hospital
P.O. Box 68
Zurich, 8029
Switzerland

**Martin M. Antony**
Anxiety Treatment and Research Centre
St. Joseph's Hospital
50 Charlton Avenue East
Hamilton, Ontario L8N 4A6
Canada

**Anri Aoba**
Department of Neuropsychiatry
St. Marianna University School
    of Medicine
2-16-1, Sugao
Maiyamae-ku
Kawasaki, Kanagawa 216-8511
Japan

**Gordon J. G. Asmundson**
Faculty of Kinesiology and Health Studies
University of Regina
Saskatchewan S4S 0A2
Canada

**Thomas F Babor**
University of Connecticut Health Center
Department of Community Medicine
    and Health Care
263 Farmington Avenue
MC-6325
Farmington, CT 06030-2103
USA

**Mark S. Bauer**
Mental Health and Behavioral Sciences
    Service
Providence VA Medical Center-116R
830 Chalkstone Avenue
Providence RI, 02908-4799
USA

**William R Beardslee**
Department of Psychiatry
Children's Hospital, Judge Baker
    Children's Center
3 Blackfan Circle
Boston, Massachusetts 2115
USA

**Jean C. Beckham**
Clinical Psychologist, PTSD Clinical
    Team
Duke University Medical Center,
Department of Psychiatry and
    Behavioral Sciences
DVAMC, 116B
Durham, NC 27705
USA

**Alan S. Bellack**
Department of Psychiatry
University of Maryland School of
    Medicine
737 W. Lombard Street, Room 551
Baltimore, MD 21201
USA

**David Bienenfeld**
Department of Psychiatry
Wright State University
School of Medicine
Dayton, OH 45401-0927
USA

**Lester Blumberg**
Department of Mental Health
25 Staniford Street
Boston, MA 2114
USA

**Robert J. Boland**
Department of Psychiatry and Human
    Behavior
Brown University
Butler Hospital
345 Blackstone Road
Providence, RI 2906
USA

**Neil W. Boris**
Department of Psychiatry and
    Neurology
Tidewater Building TB-52
Tulane University School of Medicine
1440 Canal Street
New Orleans, LA 70112-2715
USA

**Olga Brawman-Mintzer**
Department of Psychiatry
Medical University of South Carolina
5900 Core Rd Suite 203
N. Charleston, SC 29406
USA

**Alan Breier**
Leader, Zyprexa Product Team
Eli Lilly and Company
Lilly Corporate Center
Indianapolis, IN 46285
USA

**Evelyn Bromet**
SUNY
Department of Psychiatry
159 Putnam Hall
Stony Brook, NY 11794-8790
USA

**Richard P. Brown**
86 Sherry Lane
Kingston, NY 12401
USA

**Gerard E. Bruder**
Department of Biopsychology
New York State Psychiatric Institute,
Box 50
1051 Riverside Drive
New York, NY 10032
USA

**Deborah L. Cabaniss**
903 Park Avenue
New York, NY 10021
USA

**Arvid Carlsson**
Department of Pharmacology
University of Göteborg
Box 431
Göteborg SE 405 30
Sweden

**Kenneth Certa**
Jefferson Medical College
Department of Psychiatry
1000 Sansom St.
Philadelphia, PA 19107
USA

**Irene Chatoor**
Children's National Medical Center
Department of Psychiatry
111 Michigan Avenue, N.W.
Washington, DC 20010
USA

**Leslie Citrome**
Department of Psychiatry
Nathan Kline Institute
140 Old Orangeburg Road
Orangeburg, NY 10962
USA

**John F. Clarkin**
Weill Medical College at Cornell
 University
USA

**Keith H. Claypoole**
5493 Makaloa Street
Kapaa, HI 96746
USA

**Robert B. Clyman**
Kempe Children's Center
Department of Pediatrics
University of Colorado Health
 Sciences Center
1825 Marion St.
Denver, CO. 80218
USA

**Edwin H. Cook**
Department of Psychiatry
The University of Chicago
5841 S. Maryland Ave.
Chicago, IL 60637
USA

**Rees Cosgrove**
Director, Cingulotomy Assessment Unit
Attending Neurosurgeon
Massachusetts General Hospital
Boston, MA
USA

**Francine Cournos**
New York State Psychiatric Institute
Box 112
1051 Riverside Drive
New York, NY 10032
USA

**Linda W. Craighead**
Department of Psychology
University of Colorado
Boulder, CO
USA

**W. Edward Craighead**
Department of Psychology
D244 Muenzinger Building
University of Colorado
Boulder, CO 80309-0345
USA

**Jonathan R. T. Davidson**
Duke University Medical Center
Department of Psychiatry and
 Behavioral Sciences
Box 3812
Durham, NC 27710
USA

**Kenneth L. Davis**
Mount Sinai School of Medicine
Box 1230
1 Gustave L. Levy Place
New York, NY 10029
USA

**Karon Dawkins**
Department of Psychiatry
University of North Carolina School
 of Medicine
10522 Neurosciences Hospital
Chapel Hill, NC 27599-7160
USA

**Lynette C. Daws**
Department of Psychiatry
The University of Texas Health
 Science Center
San Antonio, TX
USA

**Joel E. Dimsdale**
Department of Psychiatry
UCSD School of Medicine
Mailcode 0804
9500 Gilman Drive
La Jolla, CA 92093-0804
USA

**Christian R. Dolder**
Department of Psychiatry
University of California
VA San Diego Healthcare System
3350 La Jolla Village Drive (116A-1)
San Diego, CA 92161
USA

**Darin D. Dougherty**
Department of Psychiatry
Massachusetts General Hospital-East
CNY 9132, Bldg. 149, 13th Street
Charleston, MA 2129
USA

**Ken Duckworth**
Deputy Commissioner for Clinical and
 Professional Services
Department of Mental Health
25 Staniford Street
Boston, MA 2114
USA

**Gary E. Duncan**
Department of Psychiatry
University of North Carolina at Chapel
 Hill
350A Taylor Hall, CB# 7090
Chapel Hill, NC 27599
USA

**Jane L. Eisen**
Department of Psychiatry and Human
 Behavior
Brown University School of Medicine
Box G-BH
Providence, Rhode Island 02912-G-BH
USA

**Stuart Eisendrath**
Department of Psychiatry
University of California
401 Parnassus Avenue
Box 0984
San Francisco, CA 94143-0984
USA

**Rif S. El-Mallekh**
Department of Psychiatry
University of Louisville School of
 Medicine
Louisville, KY 40292
USA

**Karen M. Emberger**
Duke University Medical Center
Durham, NC
USA

**Richard S. Epstein**
10401 Old Georgetown Road
Suite 400
Bethesda, MD 20814
USA

**Milton Erman**
Pacific Sleep Medicine Services
9834 Genesee Avenue, Suite 328
La Jolla, CA 92037-1223
USA

**Eugene W. Farber**
Department of Psychiatry and
 Behavioral Sciences
Emory University School of Medicine
 Grady Health System
1440 Clifton Road
Atlanta, GA 30322
USA

**Jan A. Fawcett**
Department of Psychiatry
Rush-Prebyterian-St. Luke's Medical
 Center
Chicago, IL
USA

**Jacqueline Maus Feldman**
Department of Psychiatry and
  Behavioral Neurobiology
University of Alabama at Birmingham
4-CCB 908 20th Street South
Birmingham, AL 35294
USA

**Alan Felix**
Department of Psychiatry
Columbia University
USA

**Susan J. Fiester**
35 Wisconsin Circle Suite 345
Chevy Chase, MD 20815-7015
USA

**Michael B. First**
Columbia University College of
  Physicians and Surgeons
New York State Psychiatric Institute
Box 121
New York, NY 10032
USA

**W. Wolfgang Fleischhacker**
Department of Biological Psychiatry
Innsbruck University Clinics
Anichstr. 35
Innsbruck A-6020
Austria

**Anne Fleming**
Department of Psychiatry
University of California
San Francisco, CA 94143-0984
USA

**Alan Frazer**
The University of Texas Health Science
  Center
Department of Pharmacology-7764
7703 Floyd Curl Drive – MC 7764
San Antonio, TX 78229-3900
USA

**Robert Freedman**
Department of Psychiatry
University of Colorado Health Sciences
  Center
Denver, CO 80262
USA

**Marlene P. Freeman**
Department of Psychiatry
University of Arizona
1501 North Campbell Avenue
P.O. Box 245002
Tucson, AZ 85724-5002
USA

**Edward S. Friedman**
Department of Psychiatry
University of Pittsburgh Medical Center
Pittsburgh, PA
USA

**Robert L. Frierson**
Department of Psychiatry
University of Louisville School of
  Medicine
Louisville, KY 40292
USA

**Paul J. Fudala**
Philadelphia Veterans Affairs Medical
  Center
Philadelphia, PA
USA

**Andrew C. Furman**
Emory University Psychoanalytic
  Institute
1256 Briarcliff Road, Suite 154
Atlanta, GA 30306
USA

**Genevieve Garratt**
Department of Psychology
University of Kansas
Lawrence, KS 66045
USA

**Pablo V. Gejman**
Schizophrenia Genetics Research
  Program
The University of Chicago
Jules F. Knapp Medical Research
  Center
924 East 57th Street, Room R-010
Chicago, IL 60637
USA

**Alan J. Gelenberg**
Department of Psychiatry
University of Arizona
1501 North Campbell Avenue
P.O. Box 245002
Tucson, AZ 85724-5002
USA

**Patricia L. Gerbarg**
86 Sherry Lane
Kingston, NY 12401
USA

**J. Christian Gillin**
Department of Psychiatry
University of California, San Diego
VA San Diego Healthcare System
  (116a)
3350 La Jolla Village Drive
La Jolla, CA 92161
USA

**Ira D. Glick**
Stanford University School of Medicine
401 Quarry Road, Suite 2122
Stanford, CA 94305
USA

**Robert N. Golden**
Department of Psychiatry
University of North Carolina School
  of Medicine
10501 Neurosciences Hospital
Chapel Hill, NC 27599-7160
USA

**Stephen M. Goldfinger**
Department of Psychiatry
SUNY HSCB
450 Clarkson Avenue
Brooklyn, NY 11203
USA

**Robert S. Goldman**
Clinical Director
Alzheimer Disease Management Team
Pfizer Pharmaceutical, Inc.
235 E. 42nd Street, 235/10/44
New York, NY 10017
USA

**Reed D. Goldstein**
950 Haverford Road
Suite 302
Bryn Mawr, PA 19010-3850
USA

**Michael D. Greenberg**
Rand Cooperation
Los Angeles
USA

**Laurence L. Greenhill**
Department of Clinical Psychiatry
Columbia University
College of Physicians and Surgeons
NY NYSPI-Unit 78
1051 Riverside Dr.
New York, NY 10032
USA

**Stanley I. Greenspan**
7201 Glenbrook Road
Bethesda, MD 20814
USA

**James L. Griffith**
Department of Psychiatry and
  Behavioral Sciences
Burns Building 8-408
The George Washington University
  Medical Center
2150 Pennsylvania Ave., N.W.
Washington, DC 20037
USA

**Roland R. Griffiths**
Department of Psychiatry and
  Behavioral Sciences
Johns Hopkins University School
  of Medicine
5510 Nathan Shock Drive
Baltimore, MD 21224
USA

**Amanda J. Gruber**
Department of Psychiatry
Harvard Medical School
Biological Psychiatry Laboratory
McLean Hospital
115 Mill Street
Belmont, MA 2478
USA

**Alan M. Gruenberg**
950 Haverford Road
Suite 302
Bryn Mawr, PA 19010-3850
USA

**Barry Gurland**
Stroud Center
Twr 3-30F
100 Haven Ave
New York, NY 10032
USA

**Jaswant Guzder**
Child Day Treatment Program
Department of Psychiatry
Sir Mortimer B Davis Jewish General
    Hospital
4333 Cote Ste Catherine Rd.
Montreal, Quebec H3T 1E4
Canada

**Jeffrey M. Halperin**
Department of Psychiatry and
    Department of Psychology
Queens College
65-30 Kissena Blvd.
Flushing, NY 11367
USA

**John Halpern**
Department of Psychiatry
McLean Hospital
USA

**Vahram Haroutunian**
Department of Psychiatry
Mount Sinai School of Medicine
1 Gustave L. Levy Place
New York, NY 10029
USA

**Michael E. Henry**
McLean Hospital
Harvard Medical School
Belmont, MA
USA

**Carlos A. Hernandez Avila**
University of Connecticut Health Center
Department of Psychiatry
263 Farmington Avenue, MC-2103
Farmington, CT 06030-2103
USA

**Ralph E. Hoffman**
Assistant Medical Director
Yale-New Haven Psychiatric Hospital
20 York Street LV 108
New Haven, CT 6504
USA

**Michael Hogan**
Director, Ohio Department of Mental
    Health
8th Floor Rhodes Tower
30 East Broad Street
Columbus, OH 43215-3430
USA

**Stephen S. Ilardi**
Department of Psychology
University of Kansas
Lawrence, KS 66045
USA

**G. Eric Jarvis**
Faculty Lecturer, Department of
    Psychiatry
Sir Mortimer B Davis – Jewish General
    Hospital
4333 Cote Ste Catherine Rd.
Montreal, Quebec H3T 1E4
Canada

**Michael A. Jenike**
Department of Psychiatry
Massachusetts General Hospital
East Bldg. 149, 13th Street
Charlestown, MA 2129
USA

**Dilip V. Jeste**
Department of Psychiatry
University of California
VA San Diego Healthcare System
3350 La Jolla Village Drive (116A-1)
San Diego, CA 92161
USA

**Charles Y. Jin**
Department of Psychiatry
Albert Einstein College of Medicine
1300 Morris Park Avenue
Bronx, NY 10461
USA

**Michael Kahn**
Beth Israel Deaconess Medical Center
1 Deaconess Road
Boston, MA 2215
USA

**Peter Kalivas**
Department of Physiology and
    Neuroscience
Medical University of South Carolina
173 Ashley Avenue – Suite 403
P.O. Box 250510
Charleston, SC 29425
USA

**Marshall Kapp**
Office of Geriatric Medicine and
    Gerontology
Wright State University School of
    Medicine
124 J FA White Health Center
3640 Colonial Glen Highway
Dayton, OH 45435
USA

**Nadine J. Kaslow**
Department of Psychiatry and
    Behavioral Sciences
Emory University School of Medicine
Grady Health System
1440 Clifton Road
Atlanta, GA 30322
USA

**Jerald Kay**
Department of Psychiatry
Wright State University School of
    Medicine
Dayton, OH 45401-0927
USA

**Rena L. Kay**
Department of Psychiatry
Wright State University School of
    Medicine
Dayton, OH 45401-0927
USA

**Richard S. E. Keefe**
Department of Psychiatry
Duke University Medical Center
Box 3270
Durham, NC 27710
USA

**Martin B. Keller**
Department of Psychiatry and Human
    Behavior
Brown University
Butler Hospital
345 Blackstone Road
Providence, RI 2906
USA

**Laurence J. Kirmayer**
Culture and Mental Health Research Unit
Institute of Community and Family
    Psychiatry
Sir Mortimer B. Davis – Jewish General
    Hospital
4333 Chemin de la Cote Ste Catherine
Montréal, Québec H3T 1E4
Canada

**William M. Klykylo**
Department of Psychiatry
Wright State University School of
  Medicine
P.O. Box 927
Dayton, OH 45401-0927
USA

**Robert Kohn**
Department of Psychiatry and Human
  Behavior
Brown University
Butler Hospital
345 Blackstone Blvd.
Providence, RI 2906
USA

**Thomas R. Kosten**
VA Connecticut Healthcare System
Department of Psychiatry 151D
950 Campbell Avenue, Bldg. 35
West Haven, CT 6516
USA

**Henry R. Kranzler**
University of Connecticut Health Center
Department of Psychiatry
263 Farmington Avenue, MC-2103
Farmington, CT 06030-6325
USA

**Anthony-Samuel LaMantia**
Department of Cell and Molecular
  Physiology
University of North Carolina at Chapel
  Hill
51 Medical Sciences Research Building
CB# 7545
Chapel Hill, NC 27599-7545
USA

**Harriet P. Lefley**
Department of Psychiatry D-29
University of Miami School of Medicine
P.O. Box 016960
Miami, FL 33101-6960
USA

**James L. Levenson**
Consultation/Liaison Psychiatry
West Hospital
1200 E. Broad Street, 8th Floor, North
  Wing
Richmond, VA 23219
USA

**Bennett L. Leventhal**
Department of Psychiatry
The University of Chicago
5841 S. Maryland Ave.
Chicago, IL 60637
USA

**Stephen B. Levine**
23230 Chagrin Blvd Suite #350
Beachwood, OH 44122-5402
USA

**Steven T. Levy**
Department of Psychiatry and
  Behavioral Sciences
Emory University School of Medicine
Grady Health System
1440 Clifton Road
Atlanta, GA 30322
USA

**Roberto Lewis-Fernández**
New York State Psychiatric Institute
Unit 69
1051 Riverside Drive
New York, NY 10032
USA

**Jeffrey A. Lieberman**
Department of Psychiatry
University of North Carolina
School of Medicine, CB# 7160
Chapel Hill, NC 27599-7160
USA

**Keh-Ming Lin**
Research Center on the Psychobiology
  of Ethnicity
Harbor-UCLA Research Institute
1124 W. Carson Street, B-4 South
Torrance, CA 90502
USA

**Margaret T. Lin**
Department of Psychiatry
Harbor-UCLA Research Institute
1124 W. Carson Street, B-4 South
Torrance, CA 90502
USA

**Walter Ling**
Drug Abuse Sciences, Inc.
25954 Eden Landing Road
Hayward, CA 94545-3616
USA

**Joyce H. Lowinson**
Albert Einstein College of Medicine and
  Rockefeller University
USA

**Christopher P. Lucas**
Department of Child Psychiatry
Columbia University
1051 Riverside Drive, Box Unit #78
New York, NY 10032
USA

**Bruce R. Lydiard**
Southeast Health Consultants, Inc.
1 Poston Road, Suite 150
Charleston, SC 29407
USA

**Rachel E. Maddux**
Department of Psychiatry
School of Medicine
University of California, San Diego
8950 Villa La Jolla Drive, Suite 2243
La Jolla, CA 92037
USA

**Mario Maj**
Institute of Psychiatry
University of Naples
Largo Madonna delle Grazie
Naples 1-80138
Italy

**José R. Maldonado**
Department of Psychiatry and
  Behavioral Sciences
Stanford University School of Medicine
401 Quarry Road, Office #2317
Stanford, CA 94305-5718
USA

**Mehul V. Mankad**
Department of Psychiatry and
  Behavioral Sciences
Box 3173/3837
Duke University Medical Center
Durham, NC 27710
USA

**J. John Mann**
Department of Neuroscience
New York State Psychiatric Institute
1051 Riverside Drive
Box 42
New York, NY 10032
USA

**John March**
Division of Child and Adolescent
  Psychiatry
Department of Psychiatry and
  Behavioral Sciences
Duke University Medical Center
Box 3527
Durham, NC 27710
USA

**Stephen R. Marder**
Psychiatric Services 116A
West Los Angeles VA Medical Center
11301 Wilshire Blvd.
Los Angeles, CA 90073
USA

**John C. Markowitz**
Cornell University Medical College
525 East 68th Street
Room 1322, Box #197
New York, NY 10021
USA

**Brian Martis**
Department of Psychiatry
Obsessive Compulsive Disorder Clinic
  and Research Clinic
University of Illinois at Chicago
Chicago, IL
USA

**Randi E. McCabe**
Anxiety Treatment and Research Centre
St. Joseph's Hospital
50 Charlton Avenue East
Hamilton, Ontario L8N 4A6
Canada

**Elinore F. McCance-Katz**
Department of Psychiatry
Box 98019
Medical College of Virginia
Richmond, VA 23298
USA

**Krista McFarland**
Department of Physiology and
   Neuroscience
Medical University of South Carolina
Charleston, SC 29425
USA

**Thomas H. McGlashan**
Yale Psychiatric Research
P.O. Box 208098
New Haven CT 06520-8098
USA

**Laura F. McNicholas**
Philadelphia Veterans Affairs Medical
   Center
Behavioral Health, 7E
39th & Woodland Aves
Philadelphia, PA 19104
USA

**Hunter McQuiston**
Projects Renewal, Inc.
200 Varick Street
New York, NY 10014
USA

**Arthur T. Meyerson**
200 E. 32nd Street Apt 15B
New York, NY 10016-6306
USA

**Juan E. Mezzich**
Mount Sinai School of Medicine
5th Avenue and 100th Street
Box 1093
New York, NY 10029-6574
USA

**David J. Miklowitz**
Department of Psychology
University of Colorado
CB345
Boulder, CO 80309
USA

**Robyn R. Miller**
Department of Psychiatry
Wright State University
School of Medicine
Dayton, OH
USA

**Kenneth Minkoff**
12 Jefferson Drive
Acton, MA 1720
USA

**John Misiaszek**
Department of Psychiatry
University of Arizona
1501 North Campbell Avenue
P.O. Box 245002
Tucson, AZ 85724-5002
USA

**Akira Miyake**
Department of Psychology
University of Colorado
Boulder, CO
USA

**Seiya Miyamoto**
Department of Neuropsychiatry
St. Marianna University School of
   Medicine
2-16-1, Sugao
Maiyamae-ku
Kawasaki, Kanagawa 216-8511
Japan

**Paul C. Mohl**
Department of Psychiatry
University of Texas Southwest Medical
   Center at Dallas
5323 Harry Hines Blvd.
Dallas, TX 75390-9070
USA

**Jeannine Monnier**
Medical University of South Carolina
Department of Psychiatry
5900 Core Rd Suite 203
N. Charleston, SC 29406
USA

**David P. Moore**
Central Hospital
LaGrange Road
Louisville, KY 40223
USA

**David A. Morilak**
Department of Pharmacology
The University of Texas Health Science
   Center
San Antonio, TX
USA

**Ann Kerr Morrison**
Wright State University
Department of Psychiatry
Dayton, OH 45435
USA

**Scott E. Moseman**
Western Psychiatric Institute and Clinic
3811 O'Hara Street
Pittsburgh, PA 15213
USA

**David A. Mrazek**
Department of Psychiatry and
   Psychology
Mayo Clinic
200 First Street SW
Rochester, MN 55905
USA

**Stephanie Mullins**
Morehead State University
Psychology Department
601 Ginger Hall
Morehead, KY 40351
USA

**Philip R. Muskin**
Columbia Presbyterian Medical Center
W. 168th Street
Box 427
New York, NY 10032
USA

**Jeffrey H. Newcorn**
Department of Psychiatry
Mount Sinai Hospital
Box 1230
1 Gustave L. Levy Place
New York, NY 10029
USA

**Ahmed Okasha**
Institute of Psychiatry
Ain Shams University
3, Shawarby Street
Kasr El Nil, Cairo
Egypt

**John M. Oldham**
New York State Psychiatric Institute
1051 Riverside Drive
New York, NY 10024
USA

**Michael J. Owen**
University of Wales College of Medicine
Department of Psychological Medicine
   and Medical Genetics
Tenovus Building
Heath Park
Cardiff CF14 4XN
UK

**Thomas Owley**
Department of Psychiatry
The University of Chicago
5841 S. Maryland Ave.
Chicago, IL 60637
USA

**Jayendra K. Patel**
Department of Psychiatry
University of Massachusetts Medical
   School
361 Plantation Street
Worcester, MA 1605
USA

**Michele T. Pato**
Center for Psychiatric and Molecular
 Genetics Institute for Human
 Performance
SUNY Upstate Medical University
750 East Adams Street
Syracuse, NY 13210
USA

**Teri Pearlstein**
Behavioral Health
Women and Infants Hospital
101 Dudley Street
Providence, RI 02905-2499
USA

**Katharine A. Phillips**
Butler Hospital
345 Blackstone Boulevard
Providence, RI 2906
USA

**Debra A. Pinals**
Department of Psychiatry
University of Massachusetts Medical
 School
55 Lake Avenue North
Worcester, MA 1655
USA

**Joseph Piven**
University of North Carolina at Chapel
 Hill School of Medicine
Department of Psychiatry
7011 Neurosciences Hospital, CB# 3365
Chapel Hill, NC 27599
USA

**Harrison G. Pope, Jr.**
Department of Psychiatry
Harvard Medical School
Biological Psychiatry Laboratory
McLean Hospital
115 Mill Street
Belmont, MA 2478
USA

**Mark H. Rapaport**
Department of Psychiatry
University of California, San Diego
8950 Villa La Jolla Drive, Suite 2243
La Jolla, CA 92037
USA

**Scott L. Rauch**
Department of Psychiatry
Massachusetts General Hospital-East
CNY 9132, Bldg. 149, 13th Street
Charleston, MA 2129
USA

**Michelle B. Riba**
Department of Psychiatry
University of Michigan Medical School
M4101 MSI Box 0624
1301 Catherine Road
Ann Arbor, MI 48109
USA

**Mark A. Riddle**
Department of Psychiatry and
 Behavioral Sciences
John Hopkins Hospital, CMSC 346
600 North Wolfe Street
Baltimore, MD 21287
USA

**Eva Ritvo**
Department of Psychiatry and
 Behavioral Sciences
University of Miami/Jackson Memorial
 Medical Center
Mental Health Hospital Center
1695 N.W. 9th Avenue, 3rd Floor
Miami, FL 33101
USA

**Barbara M. Rohland**
Department of Psychiatry
1400 Wallace Blvd
Amarillo, TX 79106
USA

**Neil Rosenberg**
2800 Tenth Avenue North
Billings, MT 59101
USA

**Erik Roskes**
Forensic Treatment
Springfield Hospital Center
6655 Sykesville Road
Sykesville, MD 21784
USA

**Cecile Rousseau**
McGill University
Montreal Children's Hospital
4018 St. Catherine St. West
Montreal, QC H3Z 1P2
Canada

**Matthew V. Rudorfer**
Division of Services and Intervention
 Research
National Institute of Mental Health,
NIH Neuroscience Center, Room 7160
6001 Executive Blvd, MSC 9635
Bethesda, MD 20892-9635
USA

**Maria Angeles Ruiperez**
Profesora Titular de Psicopatologica
Universitat Jaume I
Departamneto Psicologia Basica
Clinicay Psicobiologia
Campus de Borriol
12080 Castellon
Spain

**Harold A. Sackeim**
Department of Biological Psychiatry
New York State Psychiatric Institute
1051 Riverside Dr.
Unit 126
New York, NY 10032
USA

**Alan R. Sanders**
Department of Psychiatry
The University of Chicago
Chicago, IL 60637
USA

**David Schaffer**
Irving Philips Professor of Child
 Psychiatry
Columbia University
NYS Psychiatric Institute
1051 Riverside Drive
Unit 78
New York, NY 10032
USA

**Michael S. Scheeringa**
Department of Psychiatry and
 Neurology
Tidewater Building TB-52
Tulane University School of Medicine
1440 Canal Street
New Orleans, LA 70112-2715
USA

**Lon S. Schneider**
Department of Psychiatry and
 Behavioral Sciences
University of Southern California School
 of Medicine
Monroe Community Hospital
1975 Zonal Avenue, KAM 400
Los Angeles, CA 90033
USA

**John E. Schowalter**
Yale Child Study
P.O. Box 7900
New Haven, CT 06520-7900
USA

**Kurt P. Schulz**
Department of Psychiatry
Mount Sinai School of Medicine
Box 1230
1 Gustave L. Levy Place
New York, NY 10029
USA

**Ronald E. See**
Department of Physiology and
  Neuroscience
Medical University of South Carolina
Charleston, SC 29425
USA

**Larry J. Seidman**
Director, Neuropsychology Laboratory
Massachusetts Mental Health Center
74 Fenwood Road
Boston, MA 2115
USA

**Richard I. Shader**
Pharmacology and Experimental
  Therapeutics
Tufts University School of Medicine
136 Harrison Avenue
Boston, MA 2111
USA

**David Shaffer**
Department of Child Psychiatry
Columbia University
1051 Riverside Drive
Box #78
New York, NY 10032
USA

**Theodore Shapiro**
Department of Psychiatry
Cornell University Medical College
525 E. 68th Street
Box 140
New York, NY 10021
USA

**Vanshdeep Sharma**
Department of Psychiatry
Mount Sinai School of Medicine
Box 1230
1 Gustave L. Levy Place
New York, NY 10029
USA

**Charles W. Sharp**
Division of Neuroscience and Behavioral
  Research, NIDA
6001 Executive Boulevard
Room 4282 MSC 9555
Bethesda, MD 20892-9555
USA

**Leo Sher**
Department of Neuroscience
New York State Psychiatric Institute
Box 42
1051 Riverside Drive, Suite 2917
New York, NY 10032
USA

**Erin Shockey**
New York State Psychiatric Institute
New York, NY 10032
USA

**John Shuster**
Department of Psychiatry
UAB Center for Palliative Care
18 14th Street South
Birmingham, AL 35294
USA

**Edward K. Silberman**
Thomas Jefferson University
Jefferson Medical College of
  Pennsylvania
1025 Walnut Street
Curtis Building, Room 327G
Philadelphia, PA 19107
USA

**J. Arturo Silva**
P.O. Box 20928
San Jose, CA 95160
USA

**Larry B. Silver**
6286 Montrose Rd
Rockville, MD 20852
USA

**Daphne Simeon**
Psychiatry Box 1229
Mount Sinai Hospital
1 Gustave Levy Place
New York, NY 10029
USA

**Malini Singh**
St. Vincent's Hospital and Medical
  Center
New York, NY
USA

**Andrew E. Skodol**
New York State Psychiatric Institute
Box 121
1051 Riverside Drive
New York, NY 10032
USA

**Phil Skolnik**
Dov Pharmaceuticals
Continental Plaza
433 Hackensack Avenue
Hackensack, NJ 7601
USA

**Mark A. Slater**
Vice President, Clinical Research
  and Physician Services
Sharp HealthCare
8695 Spectrum Center Court
San Diego, CA 92123
USA

**Lois Slovik**
Department of Psychiatry
Massachusetts General Hospital and
  Harvard Medical School
Boston, MA 2114
USA

**Irma C. Smet**
University of Michigan Medical Center
Ann Arbour, MI
USA

**David E. Smith**
Drug Abuse Sciences, Inc.
25954 Eden Landing Road
Hayward, CA 94545-3816
USA

**Michael W. Smith**
Department of Psychiatry
Harbor-UCLA Research Institute
1124 W. Carson Street
B-4 South Torrance, CA 90502
USA

**Phyllis Solomon**
School of Social Work
University of Pennsylvania
3701 Locust Walk
Philidelphia, PA 19104
USA

**Douglas A. Songer**
Department of Psychiatry
Wright State University School of
  Medicine
Dayton, OH 45401-0927
USA

**Stephen M. Sonnenberg**
Department of Psychiatry
Uniformed Services University of the
  Health Sciences
4301 Jones Bridge Road
Bethesda, MD 20814
USA

**David Spiegel**
Department of Psychiatry and
  Behavioral Sciences
Stanford University
School of Medicine
401 Quarry Road
Stanford, CA 94305-5718
USA

**Brian Stafford**
Department of Psychiatry
Tidewater Building TB-52
Tulane University School of Medicine
1440 Canal Street
New Orleans, LA 70112-2715
USA

**Andrew Steptoe**
British Heart Foundation
Royal Free and University College
  Medical School
Department of Epidemiology and Public
  Health
Gower St. Campus
1-19 Torrington Place
London WC1E 6BT
UK

**Michael Stone**
Apt. 114
225 Central Park W.
New York, NY 10024
USA

**Walter N. Stone**
Department of Psychiatry
University of Cincinnati
311 Albert Sabin Way
Cincinnati, OH 45229
USA

**Eric C. Strain**
Department of Psychiatry and
    Behavioral Sciences
Johns Hopkins University School
    of Medicine
5510 Nathan Shock Drive
Baltimore, MD 21224
USA

**James J. Strain**
Box 1230
Mount Sinai/NYU Medical Center/
    Health Service
1 Gustave L. Levy Place
New York, NY 10029
USA

**Scott Stroup**
Department of Psychiatry
University of North Carolina at
    Chapel Hill
Chapel Hill, NC
USA

**Ezra S. Susser**
Department of Epidemiology
Columbia University
USA

**Holly A. Swartz**
Western Psychiatric Institute and Clinic
3811 O'Hara Street
Pittsburgh, PA 15213
USA

**Marvin S. Swartz**
Division of Social and Community
    Psychiatry
Department of Psychiatry and
    Behavioral Sciences
Duke University, Box 3173
Durham, NC 27710
USA

**Ludwik S. Szymanski**
53 W Boulevard Rd
Newton Center, MA 2159
USA

**Carol A. Tamminga**
Maryland Psychiatric Research Center
University of Maryland School of
    Medicine
P.O. Box 21247
Baltimore, MD 21228
USA

**Pierre N. Tariot**
Department of Psychiatry
University of Rochester School of
    Medicine
435 Henrietta Road
Rochester, NY 14620
USA

**Steven Taylor**
Department of Psychiatry
2255 Westbrook Mall,
University of British Columbia
Vancouver, BC V6T 2A1
Canada

**Michael E. Thase**
Department of Psychiatry
Thomas Detre Hall of the Western
    Psychiatric Institute and Clinic
University of Pittsburgh
3811 O'Hara Street
Pittsburgh, PA 15213-2593
USA

**Mauricio Tohen**
Lilly Corporate Center
DC 1758
Indianapolis, IN 46285
USA

**Martha C. Tompson**
Department of Psychology
Boston University
648 Beacon Street, 4th Floor
Boston, MA 2215
USA

**Kenneth E. Towbin**
Mood and Anxiety Disorders Program
    (MAP)
National Institute of Mental Health
    (NIMH)
Building 10 Rm 3S228A
9000 Rockville Pike
Bethesda, MD 20892-1279
USA

**Gary J. Tucker**
9429 45th Avenue, NE
Seattle, WA 98115
USA

**Jane A. Ungemack**
University of Connecticut Health Center
Department of Community Medicine
    and Health Care
263 Farmington Avenue, MC-6325
Farmington, CT 06030-6325
USA

**Amy M. Ursano**
Department of Psychiatry
UNC Chapel Hill
Chapel Hill, NC
USA

**Robert J. Ursano**
Department of Psychiatry
Uniformed Services University of the
    Health Sciences
4301 Jones Bridge Road
Bethesda, MD 20814
USA

**George Vaillant**
c/o Brigham and Women's Hospital
75 Francis Street
Boston, Massachusetts 2115
USA

**Susan C. Vaughan**
25 West 81st Street, Suite 1C
New York, NY 10024
USA

**Jan Volavka**
Department of Psychiatry
Nathan Kline Institute
140 Old Orangeburg Road
Orangeburg, NY 10962
USA

**John T. Walkup**
Department of Psychiatry and
    Behavioral Sciences
John Hopkins Hospital, CMSC 314
600 North Wolfe Street
Baltimore, MD 21287
USA

**B. Timothy Walsh**
NYSPI Unit 98
Room 2306
1051 Riverside Drive
New York, NY 10032
USA

**Philip S. Wang**
Division of Pharmacoepidemiology and
    Pharmacoeconomics
Brigham and Women's Hospital
    Harvard Medical School
221 Longwood Ave., Ste. 341
Boston, MA 2115
USA

**Anne L. Weickgenant**
Research Psychologist
San Diego VA Medical Center
3350 La Jolla Village Drive
San Diego, CA 92161
USA

**Daniel S. Weiss**
Department of Psychiatry
University of California San Francisco
    School of Medicine
Box 0984, LPPI Box F 181
San Francisco, CA 94143
USA

**Donald R. Wesson**
28 Sereno Circle
Oakland, CA 94619
USA

**Thomas A. Widiger**
115 Kastle Hall
Department of Psychology
University of Kentucky
Lexington, Kentucky 40506-0044
USA

**Serena Wieder**
The Washington School of Psychiatry
5028 Wisconsin Avenue, NW
Suite 400
Washington, DC 20016-4118
USA

**Maija Wilska**
Developmental Pediatrician and Chief
    Physician (Retired)
Rinnekoti Foundation
Espoo
Finland

**Ronald M. Winchel**
666 W End Ave Ste 1D
New York, NY 10025-7357
USA

**George E. Woody**
Treatment Research Institute
University of Pennsylvania/Phil a.
    VAMC
600 Public Ledger Building
150 South Independence Mall (W)
Philadelphia, PA 19106
USA

**Jesse H. Wright**
Department of Psychiatry and
    Behavioral Science
Norton Psychiatric Clinic
Louisville, KY
USA

**Yoram Yovell**
Moshav Bet Nekofa 61
D.N. North Judea 90830
Israel

**Sean H. Yutzy**
University of New Mexico
Health Sciences Center
Department of Psychiatry
Family Practice Building
2400 Tucker, N.E.
Albuquerque, NM 87131-5326
USA

**Charles H Zeanah**
Department of Psychiatry
University School of Medicine
1440 Canal Street
New Orleans, LA 70112-2715
USA

**Douglas Ziedonis**
Department of Psychiatry
Robert Wood Johnson Medical School
Room D349, 675 Hoes Lane
Piscataway, NJ 8854
USA

**Stephen R. Zukin**
Johns Hopkins University
School of Medicine
601 North Caroline Street
Room 3245, Nuclear Medicine
Baltimore, MD 21287-0807
USA

**Ilana Zylberman**
St. Luke's Division
411 W. 114 Street
New York, NY 10025
USA

# *Preface to First Edition*

This is an exciting time in the field of psychiatry. Scientific progress has expanded the diagnostic and therapeutic capabilities of psychiatry at the same time that psychiatry has begun to play a larger role in the delivery of care to a wider population, both in mental health and in primary care settings. Psychiatry at the end of the 20th century plays an important role among the medical specialties.

The physician-patient relationship provides the framework for quality psychiatric practice. The skilled clinician must acquire a breadth and depth of knowledge and skills in the conduct of the clinical interaction with the patient. To succeed in this relationship, the psychiatrist must have an understanding of normal developmental processes across the life cycle (physiological, psychological, and social) and how these processes are manifested in behavior and mental functions. The psychiatrist must also be expert in the identification and evaluation of the signs and symptoms of abnormal behavior and mental processes and be able to classify them among the defined clinical syndromes that constitute the psychiatric nosology.

To arrive at a meaningful clinical assessment, one must understand the etiology and pathophysiology of the illness along with the contributions of the patient's individual environmental and sociocultural experiences. Furthermore, the psychiatrist must have a command of the range of therapeutic options for any given condition, including comparative benefits and risks, and must weigh the special factors that can influence the course of treatment such as medical comorbidity and constitutional, sociocultural, and situational factors.

The view of psychiatric practice just described forms the framework for *Psychiatry*. Section I, Approaches to the Patient, describes the importance of therapeutic listening and the development of the skills and knowledge necessary to assess and manage the interpersonal context in which psychiatric treatment occurs. Section II, A Developmental Perspective on Normal Domains of Mental and Behavioral Function, provides a review of normal development from a variety of perspectives across the life cycle. Section III, Scientific Foundations of Psychiatry, follows with a review of the scientific knowledge on which our understanding of behavior and mental functions, as well as psychopathology, is based.

Because we believe that good clinical practice must be based on comprehensive and sophisticated clinical assessment, Section IV, Manifestations of Psychiatric Illness, provides a detailed review of clinical assessment. What logically follows in Section V, which constitutes the heart

of *Psychiatry*, is the discussion of psychiatric disorders. This section, which follows the nosology of the *Diagnostic and Statistical Manual of Mental Disorders*, Fourth Edition, differs from that found in other textbooks by the depth of the discussion of the clinical management of patients with each of these disorders. Unlike other texts, we have included substantial information on practical management; descriptions of common problems in management, including the treatment of refractory conditions; and discussions of typical issues that arise in the physician-patient relationship as treatment progresses.

The chapters in Section VI, Therapeutics, reflect our view that psychiatrists must be knowledgeable about a wide range of treatment options that include both somatic and psychotherapeutic interventions. The final section of the book, Section VII, Special Clinical Settings and Problems, reflects our belief that the sociocultural context within which the patient lives is a central aspect of the treatment process. Thus, we have included discussions of legal issues, reimbursement systems, ethical standards, the role of peer support and consumer advocacy, and the development of innovative non-hospital-based treatment programs.

Because no one should practice psychiatry without an appreciation of how the current knowledge base and treatment modalities have evolved historically, Appendix I, A Brief History of Psychiatry, provides a highly readable and scholarly review of the history of modern psychiatry. Because lifelong learning and the acquisition of new knowledge and skills are essential to optimal clinical practice, Appendix II, Research Methodology and Statistics, and Appendix III, Continued Professional Development, provide valuable information needed to assess the scientific worth of newly published literature in the field.

In a book with the depth and breadth of *Psychiatry*, a number of editorial decisions had to be made regarding the inclusion or omission of specific material and how information should be organized and presented. To make *Psychiatry* "user friendly," we have liberally used tables, charts, and illustrations to highlight key information. For example, clinical vignettes throughout the text are highlighted by a standard graphic element. Thus, an individual wishing to focus on the clinical aspects of psychiatry can do so by searching for the clinical vignettes located throughout the book. Whenever possible, we have used diagnostic and treatment decision trees to help both the novice and the experienced clinician arrive at a more rational method for making these clinical decisions. This reinforces the emphasis on clinical management issues in the section on disorders (Section V). Also, each chapter is extensively referenced so that the interested reader can use the information from any chapter for further exploration of a topic.

For hundreds of years, modern medicine has struggled to understand the interactions of the mind and body. A review of medical history of the last several centuries reveals that this problem was resolved in Western cultures by splitting the functions of the mind and the body. In recent decades, as a result of substantial research advances, this approach has begun to change. We come down clearly on the side of those who believe that such a split not only is undesirable but also does not reflect the true state of human life. Thus, we have made every possible attempt to integrate the information in this book within a biopsychosocial framework. Along with the emergence of neurobiology as a discipline, social psychiatry has evolved in recent decades as we have become more aware that the unique social and cultural background of each individual patient can influence the development and manifestations of illness, the physician-patient relationship, the response to treatment, and long-term management. Rather than relegate these issues to a specific chapter, we have chosen to integrate them throughout the entire book.

We envision that *Psychiatry* will have multiple uses. Clinicians at all levels of experience, from the medical student who wishes a quick review to the experienced clinician who wishes to delve into a particular psychiatric topic, will find that the structure and format of *Psychiatry* are conducive to meeting a variety of needs. Health care professionals in other fields of medicine who must recognize or treat psychiatric illness will also find much useful information here.

*Psychiatry* is the centerpiece of a series of works that will provide a comprehensive program for psychiatric learning. Companion texts will include a review and self-assessment referenced to *Psychiatry*, a behavioral sciences text for medical students that offers a distillation of key information that every physician in training must have, a pocket guide for ready reference in the clinical setting, and a book that focuses on the pharmacological aspects of psychiatric practice.

*Psychiatry* has been enriched by the contributions of literally hundreds of individuals. Our section editors did an outstanding job both in helping to select chapter authors and in developing the specific format and content of each section. Although editing a multiple-authored text such as *Psychiatry* is a complex and challenging task, our work was made considerably easier by the uniform excellence of our authors' chapters and the diligence of our section editors in helping to mold first drafts into final products.

In addition to the scholarly aspects of the text, a work of this magnitude cannot be produced without the strong and ongoing support of a large number of individuals responsible for its production. Each of us has had experience in editing other books, but never have we received such sustained and outstanding editorial support. Particular thanks go to Judy Fletcher, who approached Allan Tasman with her original idea for this book. Judy's accomplishments include not only successfully nurturing *Psychiatry* to fruition but also nurturing a baby daughter in the process. Judy was unfailingly available and helpful to us. Once the material reached the production stage, Les Hoeltzel, our developmental editor, did yeoman's work. A master of persuasion, Les shepherded the manuscripts through the production process into a finished textbook. Joanie Milnes, in Les' office, was consistently helpful and available.

Joan Lucas, in Allan Tasman's office, deserves our everlasting gratitude for her ability to keep track of hundreds of details and thousands of pages of manuscript and to maintain contact among three editors, seven section editors, and more than 100 chapter authors. Her level of organizational skill is matched only by her diplomatic skill in teasing delayed material from reluctant authors. Judy Yanko, in Jerry Kay's office, was also invaluable in sustaining our efforts. Maureen Ward, in Jeff Lieberman's office in New York (before he moved to North Carolina), efficiently and patiently coaxed, catalogued, and transferred dozens of chapters during the course of this project.

Most important, this work could not have been accomplished without strong support and encouragement from our families. With understanding and good humor, our spouses and children endured many hours of evening and weekend time devoted to work on *Psychiatry* that in other circumstances would have been devoted to them.

ALLAN TASMAN, MD

JERALD KAY, MD

JEFFREY A. LIEBERMAN, MD

# Preface to this Edition

When we undertook the development of the first edition of *Psychiatry*, our goal was to produce the highest quality textbook of general psychiatry; one that would provide a valuable resource to mental health clinicians, trainees, and students in a scholarly yet creative and accessible format. We have been very gratified by the response to the first edition of this textbook from colleagues, students, and reviewers who have found our book to be a comprehensive and valued reference. As we have watched the book's acceptance in both academic and clinical psychiatry settings, we have also been mindful of the march of science and the expanding knowledge base in our field. Thus, it became clear to us that between the successful reception of the first edition and the accelerated rate of scientific progress in psychiatry and neuroscience, it was time to plan for a second edition.

While this new edition maintains the same basic structure and philosophy on which the first edition was based, some significant changes have also been made. We maintain the emphasis on approaching the patient, and his/her diagnosis and treatment, from a biopsychosocial perspective, informed by an understanding of normal and pathological development, and complemented by an in-depth knowledge of the structure and function of the central nervous system. Moreover, we retain the focus on the centrality of the doctor–patient relationship in understanding our patients.

Because global scientific and medical communications are ever improving, we have expanded the book's scope to make it more international in its perspective. We have increased the emphasis on understanding how the cultural and ethnic background of our patients influences human development, disease expression and the nature of the doctor–patient relationship, and we have expanded our discussion of diagnostic and treatment variations around the world. Such additions are reflected by contributions from new authors and editors, with additional chapters, and new material within chapters. Additionally, the second edition contains 20 new chapters and extensive revisions of all chapters, reflecting all relevant clinical and scientific developments that have occurred since the first edition. With the benefit of an accelerated production process, we have been able to include many of the most important advances and references from 2002.

Once again, *Psychiatry* has benefited from the contributions of an incredibly scholarly and eminent group of authors and editors. The daunting task of producing this work was facilitated by their diligence and scholarship.

The publication of the second edition marks a new relationship with John Wiley & Sons, Ltd. Many individuals at Wiley have devoted themselves to helping produce and market the highest quality work, in particular Charlotte Brabants, Layla Paggetti, Amelia Bennett, and Andrew Spong. Charlotte, our editor, has been enthusiastic about the potential for the second edition since our first conversation, and that enthusiasm, paired with her skill and perseverance, has played an important role in bringing this work to fruition. Amelia has done sterling work to ensure that this edition has been produced with the highest standards of quality and on schedule. Just as with the first edition, we have also had tremendous help in our home institutions. Joan Lucas in Allan Tasman's office, Edward Depp in Jerry Kay's office, and Janice Linn and Tim McElwee in Jeff Lieberman's office all deserve credit for the quality and timeliness of this edition.

As before, this work could not have been completed without strong support and encouragement from our families. Though most of our children are now away from home, those remaining at home, and our spouses, deserve our thanks for their understanding as we took time to produce this work, time which otherwise would have been devoted to them.

ALLAN TASMAN, MD

JERALD KAY, MD

JEFFREY A. LIEBERMAN, MD

# Table of Contents

# Volume 2

# 62 Schizophrenia and Other Psychoses

Jayendra K. Patel
Debra A. Pinals
Alan Breier

Schizophrenia is the most severe and debilitating mental illness, and it has long been the focus of medical, scientific, and societal attention. The term *schizophrenia* is relatively new to our vocabulary, yet chronic psychotic illnesses have most likely been in existence throughout civilized times. The words used historically to describe psychotic symptoms included madness, folie, insanity, and dementia. They depict a constellation of symptoms that have been poorly understood and shrouded in mystery and fear. Even in the 21st century, the layperson's conception of schizophrenia is influenced by these early beliefs. It is only with our modern understanding of the pathophysiology and manifestations of this debilitating illness that the stigmata associated with schizophrenia can be overcome.

## Historical Overview

In prehistoric times, aberrant behavior was ascribed to magic and religious notions of evil forces that invaded and inhabited a human body. Many cultures treated deviant behavior with the practice of trephination, one of the earliest surgical procedures known (Figure 62–1). Trephining was performed by boring a hole into the skull of a living person to free the evil spirits. Trephined skulls have been found in Peruvian ruins and in parts of Africa, where the procedure is still performed. In primitive cultures, shamans, who were seen as healers and spiritual leaders, sought to extricate the negative powers from the body with medicinal herbs or ritual chanting and dancing. Interestingly, those who were considered shamans or spiritual healers were often mentally ill themselves. Later, hallucinations and delusions were attributed to the work of the devil or witchcraft. Those found guilty of such sins could be burned at the stake, leading to the unfortunate death of many people who most likely were suffering from severe mental illnesses.

Despite these prevailing religious and spiritual views of mental illness, scientific theory, and medical hypotheses were also considered. In ancient Greece, Hippocrates (1950) explained aberrant behavior and madness by relating it to internal imbalances of the four body humors. He stated that our emotions, both joyous and sorrowful, come from the brain. He went further to posit that when a brain is diseased, madness may ensue. Galen (1963), a prominent physician in the 1st century AD, also attributed mental illness to the disturbances of the humors, a theory he had derived from Hippocrates. He expanded on the Hippocratic and Aristotelian notion of mania and melancholia and described abnormalities in emotion and thought as a result of spirits and temperature alterations in the brain. Furthermore, he believed mental illnesses could be broken down into subtypes including aspects of paranoia and despair.

In the 18th century, Philippe Pinel, a prominent French physician, was one in a growing list of predecessors who believed that mental illness was a disease of the central nervous system and one that could be caused by hereditary or environmental factors (Weiner 1992). In his work with the mentally ill, he was known for his compassionate treatment of patients. He believed that patients would benefit from being properly clothed and nourished and that, except

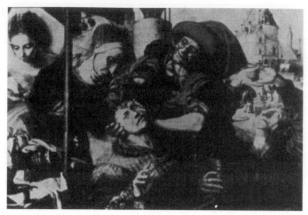

**Figure 62–1** *Extraction of the stone of madness by Saunders Memessen (1500? to 1566). (Source: Kales A, Kales AD, Vela-Beuno A, et al. [1990] Schizophrenia: Historical perspectives. In Recent Advances in Schizophrenia, Kales A, Stefanio CN, and Talbott JR [eds]. Springer-Verlag, New York, p. 5. Copyright 1990 Museo del Prado, Madrid.)*

in the most extreme circumstances, their chains should be removed, allowing them freedom within the hospital grounds. He offered instruction in how to handle patients who were potentially violent, with humane techniques that are used to this day. Pinel ended the common practice of viewing patients publicly for entertainment purposes. He implemented these humane changes in two French hospitals, Bicêtre and the Salpêtrière. Pinel was one of the early nosologists who categorized mental illness into subgroups and identified patients who had disturbances of intellect, emotion, or will. He also divided patients into those who had continuous symptoms and those who had signs of "intermittent madness" (Weiner 1992). These early concepts paved the way to our 20th century conceptualization of schizophrenia.

## Modern Concept of Schizophrenia

Our modern understanding of schizophrenia can begin with a look back to the 19th century. Although there were several influential contributors to early psychiatric nosology, there are a few leaders in psychiatry who are thought to have laid the foundation for current diagnostic criteria. To understand how the most recent diagnostic guidelines have been developed, one must place them in their historical context.

Emil Kraepelin (1856–1926) was a German psychiatrist who devoted his life's work to the task of describing and characterizing the symptoms his patients manifested. From these observations, he concluded that not all mental patients suffered from the same disease. He was one of the first to distinguish manic–depressive psychoses from other chronic psychotic illnesses (Kraepelin and Barclay 1919). Among the great contributions to the field of psychiatry are his insightful descriptions of the clinical presentation and course of these illnesses.

In naming the chronic illness he saw, Kraepelin borrowed from the French psychiatrist Benedict Augustin Morel, who in the 1850s had used the term *démence précoce* to describe a previously normal young boy who suddenly manifested symptoms of mental deterioration (Arieti 1955). Kraepelin, with a slightly different conception of

the symptom presentation, used the Latin of Morel's term to label the more chronic illness "dementia praecox." In contrast to Morel, Kraepelin emphasized the outcome of the illness in his descriptions. He believed that dementia praecox was characterized by early onset of symptoms followed by a progressive course culminating in dementia. Later he came to believe that not all patients with dementia praecox ended up in a demented state and a few even recovered. Kraepelin observed, however, that a common theme for these patients was that they experienced a withdrawn state with concomitant hallucinations or bizarre delusions with no impairment of consciousness, sensorium, or memory.

For Kraepelin, the description of the symptoms was of paramount importance, and he published a detailed account of his patients' symptoms in a monograph entitled *Dementia Praecox and Paraphrenia*. He divided patients into three subtypes—hebephrenic, catatonic, and paranoid—and later described paraphrenia as being a separate clinical entity resembling paranoia with either systematized or nonsystematized beliefs and not characterized by the deterioration of personality as in dementia praecox.

Eugen Bleuler (1857–1939) was a Swiss psychiatrist who is known, among other things, for coining the term schizophrenia. Although erroneously defined by lay people as multiple personality disorder, this term means literally "splitting of the mind." Bleuler used the word to capture his belief that this mental illness was one in which different aspects of the psyche were split, which resulted in the classical symptoms he went on to describe. In his paper entitled "Dementia praecox and the group of schizophrenias," he put forth his theory that schizophrenia consisted of not just one illness with one etiological basis but a heterogeneous group of illnesses with distinguishing characteristics and clinical courses (Bleuler 1950). He differed from Kraepelin in believing that these illnesses were not as often characterized by an early onset and a terminal dementia. Bleuler expanded and modified earlier Kraepelinian concepts including the subdivisions of diagnoses and included the category of simple schizophrenia, which was eventually also adopted by Kraepelin.

Perhaps one of his most important contributions was his emphasis on the content of symptom presentation. To Bleuler all patients had at least one fundamental or primary symptom, but other accessory or secondary symptoms were also manifested clinically. Bleuler's "four As," as they are now commonly called, consisted of primary symptoms: profound ambivalence, a looseness of associations, disturbance of affect (either excitation or withdrawal), and autism, which he described as living in an internal, unrealistic world, separated from normal social interaction. Bleuler attempted to describe negativism, which he thought was not only a result of motor disturbance but also had psychic meaning. His writings incorporated both Jungian and Freudian ideas in understanding the significance of these symptoms (Hoenig 1983). Although his symptom descriptions are not used in their entirety in modern diagnostic classification systems because of their limited specificity, the remnants of these descriptions can be seen in the *Diagnostic and Statistical Manual of Mental Disorders*, Fourth Edition (DSM-IV) (American Psychiatric Association 1994).

Kurt Schneider (1887–1967) has probably contributed to our current diagnostic classifications more than any other person. Schneider studied both Kraepelin's and Bleuler's ideas during his psychiatric training in Germany (Hoenig 1983). From his reading and his own clinical experience, he formulated a list of symptoms that he believed could be identified in his schizophrenia patients.

Without positing etiological theories, he described symptoms of first and second rank, based on which were most likely to be found in a patient with schizophrenia. According to Schneider, the diagnosis of schizophrenia was appropriate if the patient experienced just one first-rank symptom; the second-rank symptoms, although common in schizophrenia, were not as specific. His first-rank symptoms included delusions of thoughts being broadcast; feelings of an external force inserting thoughts or withdrawing them from the mind; thought interference; and the sensation of forces influencing behavior, will, or body functions. The first-rank symptoms also include specific hallucinatory experiences, such as hearing voices, often two or more, commenting on the patient's behavior or criticizing the patient. The second-rank symptoms included paranoia, affective extremes, apathy or absence of emotions, and any hallucinatory experience other than those already described. Schneider's description of these symptoms paved the way to modern diagnostic criteria used today.

## Diagnosis

### Evolution of Structured Diagnostic Criteria for Schizophrenia

A specific "operationalized" set of diagnostic criteria was first brought to light in a paper published by Feighner and colleagues (1972) of the St. Louis group. They presented a list of symptoms and signs that provided a reliable system for differentiating diagnostic groups. The St. Louis group emphasized the pattern and the duration of symptoms (requiring 6 months of symptoms to reach a diagnosis of schizophrenia) without regard to the etiology of the illness being observed. Feighner's group proposed that a set of consistent diagnostic criteria would facilitate and improve on research and clinical treatment of patients.

The research diagnostic criteria (RDC) were developed to improve diagnostic reliability in research, borrowing many of the concepts from the Feighner criteria and Schneiderian tradition. Unlike the Feighner criteria, the RDC diagnosis of schizophrenia does not require 6 months of active symptoms. Instead, schizophrenia is divided into three groups, based on temporal distinctions: acute (lasting 2 weeks–6 months); intermediate, that is, subacute or subchronic (lasting 6 months–2 years); and chronic (illness present for at least 2 years). This set of criteria excludes patients with a clear mood syndrome and assigns them to either an affective disorder or a schizoaffective disorder. For a diagnosis of schizophrenia, patients must have experienced two of nine symptoms listed, including delusions, thought disorder, hallucinations, or catatonic behavior. Many of these symptoms are derived directly from Schneiderian concepts. Diagnoses are assigned a degree of certainty (probable or definite) and are considered primary or secondary, based on the chronological presentation of con-

comitant illnesses. The RDC have remained essentially unchanged as other diagnostic classification system have been modified and revised, which allows homogeneously defined groups of patients to be compared over time.

Structured diagnostic aids made up of standardized questions were developed to increase the reliability of diagnostic assessments. Wing's Present State Examination (PSE) is an example. Like Schneider's description of first- and second-rank symptoms, it consists of a checklist of experiences covering a period of 1 month before the interview. This particular symptom algorithm has been widely used and validated around the world since its inception in 1970. The PSE was influential in the development of the RDC and, moreover, the structured interview that can be used with the RDC, the Schedule for Affective Disorders and Schizophrenia (SADS) (Endicott and Spitzer 1978). Specifically, the SADS is a comprehensive list of questions that correspond to specific symptoms. The SADS and the RDC are similar to the PSE in their emphasis on the length of time in which symptoms are present and in the presence of psychosis, which are required for the diagnosis of schizophrenia.

The diagnostic schemata of the PSE, the Feighner criteria, and the RDC also had a profound impact on the development of the most commonly used guideline for psychiatric nosology in the US, the *Diagnostic and Statistical Manual of Mental Disorders* (DSM), established by the American Psychiatric Association. This manual has gone through several revisions. DSM-I and DSM-II, now of more historical interest, postulated a somewhat broad, glossary-like definition of schizophrenia. Later versions have relied on field trials and consensus diagnoses of collaborating specialists to narrow the definition, making this manual an important resource for researchers, clinicians, politicians, attorneys, patients, family members, and even third-party payers.

DSM-III, developed in the 1970s and published by the American Psychiatric Association in 1980, viewed schizophrenia much more narrowly, and for the first time in the DSM specific criteria were required for a diagnosis of schizophrenia. These included a minimal duration of symptoms, at least 6 months, which had also been a requirement in the Feighner criteria. This decision stemmed from a debate about whether shorter (less than 6 months) psychotic episodes that resolved quickly were considered the same disease entity as the more chronic and unremitting type of illness (Astrup and Noreik 1966). In addition, DSM-III diagnostic criteria placed emphasis on the more easily validated Schneiderian concepts and included a multiaxial system of diagnosis.

The revised edition of DSM-III (DSM-III-R) was published in 1987. It was arranged similarly to its predecessor, that is, with a lettered list of criteria, broken down into numbered lists of specific symptoms. It incorporated some important changes, including the exclusion of transient psychosis by adding a 1-week minimal presence of symptoms in criteria A, unless these symptoms were eliminated by treatment during that period. DSM-III-R also eliminated the maximal age at onset (45 years) for schizophrenia. This major modification was based on a lack of compelling data supporting an age restriction. In fact, since this change was implemented, several studies have demonstrated that the index episode of schizophrenia can occur at any age (Rabins et al. 1984, Lacro et al. 1993, Castle and Murray 1993, Howard et al. 2000). Along the same lines, onset in childhood was considered, and wording was changed to allow for the possibility of differential prognoses.

## Diagnostic and Statistical Manual of Mental Disorders, Fourth Edition

The current edition, DSM-IV, was released in 1994, to coincide with the publication of the *International Statistical Classification of Diseases and Related Health Problems*, 10th Revision (ICD-10), which was published by the World Health Organization in 1992. Many of the changes allow greater consistency between these two widely used classification systems. In DSM-IV the issue of brief psychotic episodes was revisited, and the minimal duration of active symptoms was extended from 1 week to 1 month, much as in ICD-10. With a slight swing of the pendulum back toward a Bleulerian conceptualization, criterion A now places greater emphasis on negative symptoms, including avolition, flattened affect, and alogia. The rest of the

specific criteria, including criterion A and the criteria for the residual and prodromal syndromes, have been simplified from earlier versions.

In DSM-IV, criterion A of schizophrenia includes delusions, hallucinations, disorganized speech, disorganized or catatonic behavior, and negative symptoms. Two or more of these symptoms are required during the active phase of the illness. However, if the patient describes bizarre delusions or auditory hallucinations consisting of a voice commenting on the patient's behavior or voices conversing, only one of these symptoms is required to reach the diagnosis. It is important to distinguish negative symptoms, which are often difficult to appreciate, from the myriad factors that may contribute to the severity and serious morbidity associated with schizophrenia. Patients who are not motivated to attend to their personal hygiene or suffer from alogia and a flattened affect are sadly at a disadvantage in society. The addition of negative symptoms as a separate criterion in DSM-IV recognizes the prominence of these symptoms in patients with schizophrenia.

---

### DSM-IV-TR Criteria 295.xx

#### Schizophrenia

A. *Characteristic symptoms*: Two (or more) of the following, each present for a significant portion of time during a 1-month period (or less if successfully treated):

   (1) delusions

   (2) hallucinations

   (3) disorganized speech (e.g., frequent derailment or incoherence)

   (4) grossly disorganized or catatonic behavior

   (5) negative symptoms, i.e., affective flattening, alogia, or avolition

**Note:** Only one criterion A symptom is required if delusions are bizarre or hallucinations consist of a voice keeping up a running commentary on the person's behavior or thoughts, or two or more voices conversing with each other.

B. *Social/occupational dysfunction*: For a significant portion of the time since the onset of the disturbance, one or more major areas of functioning such as work, interpersonal relations, or self-care are markedly below the level achieved prior to the onset (or when the onset is in childhood or adolescence, failure to achieve expected level of interpersonal, academic, or occupational achievement).

C. *Duration*: Continuous signs of the disturbance persist for at least 6 months. This 6-month period must include at least 1 month of symptoms (or less if

successfully treated) that meet criterion A (i.e., active-phase symptoms) and may include periods of prodromal or residual symptoms. During these prodromal or residual periods, the signs of the disturbance may be manifested by only negative symptoms or two or more symptoms listed in criterion A present in an attenuated form (e.g., odd beliefs, unusual perceptual experiences).

D. *Schizoaffective and mood disorder exclusion*: Schizoaffective disorder and mood disorder with psychotic features have been ruled out because either (1) no major depressive, manic, or mixed episodes have occurred concurrently with the active-phase symptoms; or (2) if mood episodes have occurred during active-phase symptoms, their total duration has been brief relative to the duration of the active and residual periods.

E. *Substance/general medical condition exclusion*: The disturbance is not due to the direct physiological effects of a substance (e.g., a drug of abuse, a medication) or a general medical condition.

F. *Relationship to a pervasive developmental disorder*: If there is a history of autistic disorder or another pervasive developmental disorder, the additional diagnosis of schizophrenia is made only if prominent delusions or hallucinations are also present for at least a month (or less if successfully treated).

---

Reprinted with permission from the Diagnostic and Statistical Manual of Mental Disorders, Fourth Edition, Text Revision. Copyright 2000 American Psychiatric Association.

Criterion B addresses loss of social and occupational functioning, not exclusively because of any one of the items in criterion A. Patients may have difficulties maintaining employment, relationships, or academic achievements. If the illness presents at an early age, rather than as a degeneration or reversal of function, there may be a break from continued academic and social gains that are developmentally appropriate so that the person never achieves what had been expected.

Criterion C eliminates patients with less than 6 months of continued disturbance and again requires at least 1 month of the symptoms from criterion A. Criterion C allows prodromal and residual periods to include only negative symptoms or a less severely manifested version of the other symptoms of the A criteria.

Criterion D excludes patients who have a more compelling mood aspect of their illness and therefore their symptoms might instead meet criteria for schizoaffective disorder or a mood disorder. Both of these restrictions force a narrower view of the diagnosis of schizophrenia, which lessens the tendency of psychiatrists to overdiagnose schizophrenia.

Criterion E clarifies the fact that patients with schizophrenia are not suffering from other medical illnesses or the physiological effects of substances that might mimic the symptoms of schizophrenia. Finally, criterion F acknowledges that schizophrenia can be diagnosed in patients with autistic disorder or developmental disorder, as long as there have been prominent delusions or hallucinations that have lasted at least 1 month.

## DSM-IV Subtypes of Schizophrenia

In DSM-IV, schizophrenia has been divided into clinical subtypes, based on field trials of the reliability of symptom clusters. The subtypes are divided by the most prominent symptoms, although it is acknowledged that the specific subtype may exist simultaneously with or change over the course of the illness. DSM-IV also initiates an optional dimensional descriptor, which allows the condition to be characterized by the presence or absence of a psychotic, disorganized, or negative symptom dimension over the entire course of the illness.

### Paranoid Type

---

**DSM-IV-TR Criteria** 295.30

**Paranoid Type**

A type of schizophrenia in which the following criteria are met:

A. Preoccupation with one or more delusions or frequent auditory hallucinations.

B. None of the following is prominent: disorganized speech, disorganized or catatonic behavior, or flat or inappropriate affect.

---

Reprinted with permission from the Diagnostic and Statistical Manual of Mental Disorders, Fourth Edition, Text Revision. Copyright 2000 American Psychiatric Association.

In DSM-IV, paranoid-type schizophrenia is marked by hallucinations or delusions in the presence of a clear sensorium and unchanged cognition. Disorganized speech, disorganized behavior, and flat or inappropriate affect are not present to any significant degree. The delusions (usually of a persecutory or grandiose nature) and the hallucinations most often revolve around a particular theme or themes. Because of their delusions, these patients may attempt to keep the interviewer at bay, and thus they may appear hostile or angry during an interview. This type of schizophrenia may have a later age of onset and a better prognosis than the other subtypes.

### Disorganized Type

---

**DSM-IV-TR Criteria** 295.10

**Disorganized Type**

A type of schizophrenia in which the following criteria are met:

A. All of the following are prominent:

(1) disorganized speech

(2) disorganized behavior

(3) flat or inappropriate affect

B. The criteria are not met for catatonic type.

---

Reprinted with permission from the Diagnostic and Statistical Manual of Mental Disorders, Fourth Edition, Text Revision. Copyright 2000 American Psychiatric Association.

Disorganized schizophrenia, historically referred to as hebephrenic schizophrenia, presents with the hallmark symptoms of disorganized speech and/or behavior, along with flat or inappropriate (incongruent) affect. Any delusions or hallucinations, if present, also tend to be disorganized and are not related to a single theme. Furthermore, these patients would not be classified as having catatonic schizophrenia. These patients in general have more severe deficits on neuropsychological tests. According to DSM-IV, these patients tend to have an earlier age at onset, an unremitting course, and a poor prognosis.

### Catatonic Type

Catatonic schizophrenia has unique features that distinguish it from other subtypes of schizophrenia in DSM-IV for Catatonic Schizophrenia. During the acute phase of this illness, patients may demonstrate marked negativism or mutism, profound psychomotor retardation or severe psychomotor agitation, echolalia (repetition of words or phrases in a nonsensical manner), echopraxia (mimicking the behaviors of others), or bizarreness of voluntary movements and mannerisms. Some patients demonstrate a waxy flexibility, which is seen when a limb is repositioned on examination and remains in that position as if the patient were made of wax. Patients with catatonic stupor must be protected against bodily harm resulting from the profound psychomotor retardation. They may remain in the same

**Catatonic Type**

A type of schizophrenia in which the clinical picture is dominated by at least two of the following:

(1) motoric immobility as evidenced by catalepsy (including waxy flexibility) or stupor

(2) excessive motor activity (that is apparently purposeless and not influenced by external stimuli)

(3) extreme negativism (an apparently motiveless resistance to all instructions or maintenance of a rigid posture against attempts to be moved) or mutism

(4) peculiarities of voluntary movement as evidenced by posturing (voluntary assumption of inappropriate or bizarre postures), stereotyped movements, prominent mannerisms, or prominent grimacing

(5) echolalia or echopraxia

position for weeks at a time. Because of extreme mutism or agitation, patients may not be able to report any difficulties. Some patients may experience extreme psychomotor agitation, with grimacing and bizarre postures. These patients may require careful monitoring to safeguard them from injury or deterioration in nutritional status or fluid balance.

## Undifferentiated Type

There is no hallmark symptom of undifferentiated schizophrenia; thus, it is the subtype that meets the criterion A for schizophrenia but does not fit the profile for paranoid, disorganized, or catatonic schizophrenia.

**Undifferentiated Type**

A type of schizophrenia in which symptoms that meet criterion A are present, but the criteria are not met for the paranoid, disorganized, or catatonic type.

## Residual Type

The diagnosis of residual schizophrenia, according to DSM-IV, is appropriately used when there is a past history of an acute episode of schizophrenia but at the time of

**Residual Type**

A type of schizophrenia in which the following criteria are met:

A. Absence of prominent delusions, hallucinations, disorganized speech, and grossly disorganized or catatonic behavior.

B. There is continuing evidence of the disturbance, as indicated by the presence of negative symptoms or two or more symptoms listed in criterion A for schizophrenia, present in an attenuated form (e.g., odd beliefs, unusual perceptual experiences).

presentation the patient does not manifest any of the associated psychotic or positive symptoms. However, there is continued evidence of schizophrenia manifested in either negative symptoms or low-grade symptoms of criterion A. These may include odd behavior, some abnormalities of thought processes, or delusions or hallucinations that exist in a minimal form. This type of schizophrenia has an unpredictable, variable course.

## Cross-Cultural Definitions

Any diagnostic classification algorithm for an illness such as schizophrenia is necessarily limiting in its applicability to people of different cultures. Although its use allows some communication between mental health professionals internationally, there are bound to be distinct culturally acceptable definitions that may be more useful on a clinical level for a specific group of people. The ICD, now in its 10th revision, was developed by the World Health Organization to provide a means of collecting data regarding morbidity and mortality associated with health problems around the world. The chapter on mental illness, developed around the same time as DSM-IV, is easily understandable for those who are familiar with Western thinking. Yet the field of cross-cultural psychiatry is expanding. There is increased awareness of the need to work with patients within their own culturally diverse backgrounds. The classification schemes specific to local regions are often based on historical, religious, and traditional thinking unique to each setting.

As an example, psychiatric classification schemes in French-speaking countries utilize the nosological guidelines published by the Institut National de la Santé et de la Recherche Médicale (INSERM; National Institute of Health and Medical Research). According to this classification algorithm, an important distinction is made between transitory delusional states (*bouffée délirante*) and chronic delusional states, which are further subdivided into chronic interpretive psychosis, chronic hallucinatory psychosis, and chronic imaginative psychosis (Pichot 1990). This has led to some confusion for those who are familiar with the ICD and DSM systems. The different perceptions of schizophrenia are seen epidemiologically, and it is thought that in France, schizophrenia is diagnosed much less frequently than in the US. The discrepancy is based on historical differences between the French and German Kraepelinian concepts, which has led to marked differences between the French classifications and those in the US. However, the French distinctions have contributed in part to the establishment of a distinct diagnostic classification for patients who have been symptomatic for briefer periods, as in schizophreniform psychosis (Pichot 1990). This is not to say that there are cultural differences in psychotic symptoms among the French as compared to those seen in the US. Rather, the diagnostic classification schemes differ. Chinese psychiatric nosology and treatments, based on a history dating back 3,000 years, are quite different from those in DSM-IV and represent another example of cultural diagnostic differences. The original Chinese notions of mental illness were based, as in Western culture, on philosophy and religion. As Chinese medicine evolved, so did psychiatric concepts. The Chinese philosophy of yin and yang, or the opposing forces within all people, predominates in the interpretation of psychiatric symptoms (Wig 1990). Other psychiatric traditions are based on mythological stories that have been passed from generation to generation.

One must avoid imposing Western definitions of psychosis on non-Western societies. Psychosis and delusions, by definition, must be beliefs or experiences that are incongruent with those of the patient's social or cultural background. An example of the difficulties in sorting through these matters is *koro*, which is the belief that one's genitals are shrinking into one's abdomen, based on Chinese mythology involving a fear of death. Although this is generally rare, there have been epidemics involving entire communities who have suffered from this condition. By Western standards, someone presenting with this symptom could be considered to have a psychotic or delusional disorder and even possibly be given a diagnosis of schizophrenia. A Western psychiatrist might fail to recognize that in some parts of Asia, this is within culture-bound limits and would be the equivalent of a neurosis as opposed to a psychosis.

In New Zealand, the Maori are well integrated with their European neighbors. While working in Westernized jobs, however, most continue to hold firmly to their Maori traditions. The differences in religious beliefs can lead to difficult questions for mental health professionals, most of whom are of European descent. For example, Maoris who believe their relationship to the gods is unique, that they have been given special powers and messages from the gods to protect the Marae, or tribal community meeting place, may be within cultural norms and thus not meet any criteria for schizophrenia. In this context, the New Zealand government has long supported cross-cultural respect and communication and has created positions for cultural liaison specialists. These experts in Maori traditions are available to mental health teams to aid in decisions regarding diagnosis and treatment within a cultural context.

To determine where culture-bound beliefs end and delusions or inappropriate behaviors begin in a multicultural world is clearly not possible using only a written algorithm such as DSM-IV. A critical step toward sound cross-cultural clinical care is developing an awareness of and a respect for diversity. Utilizing the expertise of persons familiar with a specific culture allows appropriate diagnosis and treatment of schizophrenia worldwide.

## Epidemiology

### World Health Organization Studies
Three major studies conducted by the World Health Organization (WHO) have provided clinicians and researchers with invaluable information regarding the epidemiology of schizophrenia. By utilizing consistent diagnostic criteria, having large sample sizes across several countries of diverse cultures and development, and including follow-up data, the WHO has collected a significant data set from which we can derive epidemiological information.

The first of these studies is known as the International Pilot Study of Schizophrenia and was conducted from 1969 to 1977. This study assessed 1,202 patients across nine countries (Taiwan, Colombia, Czechoslovakia, Denmark, India, Nigeria, UK, US, and former USSR) utilizing Wing's Present State Examination, which was translated and back-translated to ensure consistency in diagnostic assessment across languages. A second major study, the Assessment and Reduction of Psychiatric Disability, examined social adjustment in 520 individuals with schizophrenia in seven countries: Bulgaria, Federal Republic of Germany, Netherlands, Sudan, Switzerland, Turkey, and Yugoslavia. From 1978 to 1986, the Determinants of Outcome of Severe Mental Disorders studied 1,379 patients in 10 countries who had sought help for mental illness and were diagnosed with probable schizophrenia (Jablensky et al. 1988). All three of these studies included long-term follow-up with assessments of the initial cohort for a period of up to 10 years. Although these studies were conducted with large sample sizes in different cultural settings, the methodology was consistent, with diagnostic assessments made by trained professionals, enhancing the reliability and validity of the conclusions.

### Epidemiological Catchment Area Program
One of the most comprehensive epidemiological undertaking in the US to date, the Epidemiological Catchment Area (ECA) program was planned as a result of a need for comprehensive data that would answer questions regarding the prevalence of mental disorders that could be utilized to implement services for those in need. Funded by the National Institute of Mental Health, the ECA program began in 1978 as a multisite program designed primarily to determine accurate prevalence rates of specific mental illnesses (Robins et al. 1984). Structured diagnostic interviews were administered to a population of almost 20,000 people residing in designated areas, and the corresponding DSM-III diagnoses were registered in a central data set.

### Epidemiological Findings: Incidence and Prevalence
The incidence of schizophrenia is defined as the number of new cases in a given population, usually per 1,000 persons, during a specific period of time (1 year by convention). In an illness with an insidious onset, such as schizophrenia, accurate incidence rates can be difficult to determine. Incidence rates are often calculated from first hospital

admission data, which may not correspond to the time when the illness first presented. Incidence rates can also be calculated from retrospective interviews or chart reviews, which may misrepresent accurate incidence rates because of imperfect charting, unreliable historical information given by patients and their families, and nonvalidated retrospective diagnoses. In any case, the incidence varies depending on the methods and the diagnostic criteria used. For example, the US–UK study is often cited as an example of epidemiological variation based on different diagnostic criteria (Kramer 1969). This study, conducted in the 1960s, found a lower incidence of schizophrenia in the UK than in the US. It is now widely accepted that this difference was found because a broader definition of schizophrenia was being used in the US, and it did not reflect true differences in the incidence of schizophrenia in each country.

The data obtained from the WHO studies are important in part because the same diagnostic criteria were used in all countries studied. According to the results of the International Pilot Study of Schizophrenia, schizophrenia is found in all cultures and the incidence rates per 1,000 people annually ranged from 0.15 in Denmark to 0.42 in India (WHO 1973). This finding is corroborated by a review of the literature, in which the incidence of schizophrenia across 13 studies representing seven countries is found to range between 0.11 (UK) and 0.54 (US) per 1,000 people per year (Eaton 1985). Small variations in these incidence rates, because they are so low, have little meaning epidemiologically. Furthermore, the range of incidence rates for schizophrenia decreases significantly when consistent, tightly defined diagnostic criteria are employed. It is reassuring that when investigators replicated studies using the design of the WHO 10-country study, results similar to the original study were reported from India (Rajkumar et al. 1993), UK (McNaught et al. 1997, Brewin et al. 1997), and Barbados (Hickling and Rodgers-Johnson 1995, Mahy et al. 1999).

Because schizophrenia is a chronic illness, the incidence rates must, by definition, be much lower than the prevalence rates. Prevalence is defined as the number of cases present in a specified population at a given time or time interval (e.g., at a specific point in time, during a time period, or over a lifetime). Lifetime prevalence represents the proportion of persons who have ever had the illness at a given time.

Lifetime prevalence rates of schizophrenia, based on the ECA data, were approximately 1% (range across three sites, 1–1.9%) (Robins et al. 1984). Point prevalence rates based on International Pilot Study of Schizophrenia data showed no significant differences across study centers: schizophrenia was found universally with relatively equal frequencies in a wide variety of cultures. Eaton's review of the literature showed a range of point prevalence between 0.6 and 8.3 cases of schizophrenia per 1,000 persons in the population. The rate of schizophrenia per 1,000 persons fell within a similar range when looking at lifetime prevalence, point prevalence and period prevalence, which Eaton hypothesized was related to the fact that schizophrenia is a chronic but not fatal illness (Eaton 1985). In an update of Eaton's review, it was noted that methodological differences may have partly accounted for statistical outliers in studies examining the incidence and prevalence of schizophrenia in different countries regardless of the type of

prevalence (Eaton 1991). Specific studies of smaller populations, such as Helgason's study of Iceland, found a 0.9% morbidity risk (which approximates point prevalence rates) of schizophrenia (Helgason 1964). This study has been highlighted because it examined 99% of patients in a closed population and supports the findings of the larger studies such as the ECA study.

Interestingly, smaller studies have found specific populations with either a higher or a lower prevalence of schizophrenia (Jablensky 1986, Hare 1987, Hovatta 1997). For example, a higher rate of schizophrenia has been found in a specific community in the north of Sweden, in northeastern Finland (Lehtinen 1996), in northwestern Croatia, and in western Ireland. Lower rates of schizophrenia have been found in, for example, parts of Tonga, Papua New Guinea, Taiwan, and Micronesia. In the US, schizophrenia was almost nonexistent in the Hutterite community, a Protestant sect living in South Dakota. Epidemiologists generally agree that these communities may represent aberrant findings. However, if these differences in prevalence rates are accurate, several theories have been offered as explanations, including genetic preloading, differences in diet, or even differences in factors such as maternal age (Hare 1987). A suggestion has been raised that there might a decline in the incidence of schizophrenia (Bojholm and Stromgren 1989) but the evidence so far is inconsistent and conflicting (Jeffreys et al. 1997, Brewin et al. 1997). This issue awaits further clarification.

## Sociodemographical Characteristics

### Age

One of the major changes from DSM-III to DSM-III-R was the abolition of the requirement for onset of symptoms before age 45 years for the diagnosis of schizophrenia. This led to more universal acceptance of the phenomenon of late-onset schizophrenia. DSM-IV retained the revision made in DSM-III-R, and ICD-10 now includes paraphrenia (a term originally used by Kraepelin to signify a diagnosis distinct from dementia praecox in that the patients did not experience a deterioration) in a list of subtypes of schizophrenia instead of an independent diagnosis. Late paraphrenia subsequently came into favor to describe a paranoid delusional disorder with an onset usually after age 60 years. These changes in nomenclature and accepted nosological criteria have greatly affected epidemiological studies of schizophrenia and age at onset.

An investigation of late-onset schizophrenia found that 28% of patients had the onset of illness after age 44 years and 12% after age 63 years, based on 470 chart reviews of patients who had sought psychiatric help during a period of 20 years (Castle and Murray 1993). Other studies have demonstrated that 23% of schizophrenia patients had an onset after their forties (Lacro et al. 1993). The 1-year prevalence rate for schizophrenia in patients between 45 and 64 years of age was found to be 0.6% according to the ECA study (Kieth et al. 1991). Furthermore, in a study of patients with onset after the age of 44 years, the majority of patients had symptoms that met all the criteria for schizophrenia found in DSM-III except for the age requirement, lending support to the need to discard the maximal age at onset limitation of DSM-III (Rabins et al. 1984). Thus, although the majority of patients have an early age at onset, a certain subgroup of patients may have a disturbance that meets all the criteria of schizophrenia with onset in their forties or later.

The phenomenology of late-onset compared with early-onset schizophrenia may be distinct, with later-onset cases having a higher level of premorbid social functioning and exhibiting paranoid delusions and hallucinations more often than formal thought disorder, disorganization, and negative symptoms (Howard et al. 1994, Almeida et al. 1995, Jeste et al. 1995). Studies have also shown a high comorbid risk of sensory deficits, such as loss of hearing or vision, in patients with late-onset schizophrenia (Pearlson et al. 1989). Specifically, late-onset patients are more likely to report visual, tactile, and olfactory hallucinations and are less likely to display affective flattening or blunting (Jeste et al. 1995, Howard et al. 2000). For individuals over 65 years age, community prevalence estimates range from 0.1 to 0.5% (Copeland et al. 1998, Castle and Murray 1993). One of the most robust finding among the late-onset cases is the higher prevalence seen in women (Howard et al. 1994, Almeida et al. 1995, Castle and Murray 1993, Howard et al. 2000). This does not appear to be due to sex differences in seeking care, societal role expectations (Hambrecht et al. 1992), or delay between emergence of symptoms and service contact (Riecher et al. 1989). The International Late-onset Schizophrenia group has suggested a new classification system of *late-onset schizophrenia* (onset after the age of 40 years) and a *very late onset schizophrenia-like psychosis* (onset after age 60) (Howard et al. 2000). Future studies will clarify how meaningful these categories are.

## Sex

A large body of data suggests that although men and women have an equivalent lifetime risk, the age at onset varies with sex. Although some sites showed different prevalence rates of schizophrenia in men and women, the overall prevalence rates, as reported in the ECA survey, did not differ significantly between sexes (Bourdon et al. 1992). However, there is strong evidence that onset of schizophrenia is on average 3.5 to 6 years earlier in men than in women (Flor-Henry 1985, Hafner 2000, Riecher-Rossler and Hafner 2000). The WHO 10-country study observed this phenomenon in most cultures studied (Jablensky et al. 1992). Therefore, incidence and prevalence rates of schizophrenia across sexes may vary according to age. Interestingly, in some cultural populations (e.g., West Ireland, Micronesia) the ratio of prevalence of schizophrenia for men could be as high as 2:1 (Kendler and Walsh 1995, Myles-Worsley et al. 1999).

Many studies have used criteria for schizophrenia that require onset before the age of 45 years, which also has accounted for some of the discrepancy in findings. There is undoubtedly a subgroup of patients who have a later onset of illness (after age 45 years), and this subgroup is made up predominantly of women (Flor-Henry 1985, Loranger 1984, Howard 2000, Almeida et al. 1995). Among these female schizophrenia patients, there is a higher incidence of comorbid affective symptoms (Flor-Henry 1985, Loranger 1984). When the effects of gender, premorbid personality, marital status, and family history of psychosis on the age at onset were removed in a reanalysis of WHO 10-country study data, there was a significant attenuation of the sex differences (Jablensky and Cole 1997).

## Race

The ECA data have shown that there is no significant difference in the prevalence of schizophrenia between black and white persons when corrected for age, sex, socioeconomic status, and marital status (Robins and Regier 1991). This finding is significant because it refutes prior studies that have shown the prevalence of schizophrenia to be much greater in the black population than in the white population. Adebimpe (1994) proposed several factors, including racial differences in help-seeking behavior, research populations, commitment status, and treatment, as explanations for some of these discrepancies. Efforts are being made to correct for some of these issues so that the epidemiological variables and heterogeneity of schizophrenia can be better understood in terms of race, whether black, white, Asian, or any other.

## Marital Status and Fertility

A study of marriage and fertility rates of individuals with schizophrenia compared with the general population showed that on average, by the age of 45 years, three times as many of those with schizophrenia as of the general population are still unmarried (40% of men and 30% of women with schizophrenia are still single by age 45) (Slater et al. 1971). Studies have also shown that fertility rates are lower in patients with schizophrenia compared with the general population (Vogel 1979). These observations may be related, and further investigation of the role of premorbid function, negative symptoms, and fertility rates, including rates among unmarried patients, is warranted. With the advent of the newer and more effective antipsychotic medications, and their increased use in first episode patients, it is possible that we may witness improved fertility and marriage rates in patients with schizophrenia.

## Socioeconomic Status

For many years, epidemiological studies revealed a higher incidence and prevalence of schizophrenia in groups with lower socioeconomic status (Mishler and Scotch 1963). With these findings came the hypothesis that lower social class could be considered a plausible risk factor for schizophrenia, possibly because of a higher risk of obstetrical complications, poorer nutrition, increased exposure to environmental toxins or infectious disease, or exposure to greater life stressors. In the past half century, studies have found that the actual incidence of schizophrenia does not vary with social class, based on first admission rates, adoption studies, and a series of studies examining the social class of the fathers of people with schizophrenia (Goldberg and Morrison 1963, Noreik and Odegard 1967).

When these findings did not validate the original theory, it became clear that lower socioeconomic status was more a result than a cause of schizophrenia. This led to the acceptance of the downward drift hypothesis, which stated that because of the nature of schizophrenic symptoms, people who develop schizophrenia are unable to attain employment and positions in society that would allow them to achieve a higher social status (Myerson 1940). Thus, these patients drift down the socioeconomic ladder, and because of the illness itself they may become dependent on society for their well-being.

## Immigration

Epidemiological studies of immigrant populations in the early part of the 20th century led to the supposition that the stress of immigration increased the risk for psychosis (Odegard 1932). However, further investigations of acculturation as a risk factor for schizophrenia have yielded mixed results (Eaton 1985). The opposite idea, that having a mental illness increased the likelihood of emigrating, has also been reviewed (Hare 1987, Eaton 1985). At this time, there is no conclusive evidence that emigration increases the risk of schizophrenia. Furthermore, immigration screening has become more rigorous since the earlier studies, and legal immigrants may therefore be less likely to have an increased risk for developing schizophrenia (Rosenthal et al. 1974).

The remarkably high incidence and prevalence rates of schizophrenia observed in second-generation Afro-Caribbean, and Suriname and Dutch Antilles migrants to the UK and Netherlands respectively are baffling. These findings have been replicated and data from 17 studies show a wide range of relative risk from 1.7 to 13.2 (Eaton and Harrison 2000). Diagnostic bias, misclassification (Sharpley et al. 2001), or biological risk factors (Hutchinson 1997, Selton et al. 1998) do not account for these findings. Thus, environmental risk factor(s), currently unknown, have been proposed to underlie this phenomena. The relationship between migration and schizophrenia is complex and needs further clarification (Bhugra 2000).

## Industrialization

With the increasing presence of the mentally ill on the streets of modern urban locations, the question has often been raised of whether urban life, or industrialized society, is a risk factor for the development of schizophrenia. In fact, there seems to be data suggesting that people in urban areas have a higher relative risk for schizophrenia than those in rural areas (Torrey 1980, Eaton 1974, Mortensen et al. 1999, Allardyce et al. 2001). Torrey and colleagues (1997) reanalyzed the US 1880 census data and found that urban residence was associated with a higher risk for psychosis. Marcelis and colleagues (1998) analyzed all first admissions for schizophrenia and other psychosis in Holland between 1942 and 1978 by place of birth and found a statistically significant relationship between size of urban areas and incidence of schizophrenia, affective, and other psychosis. Furthermore, in the WHO follow-up studies of the International Pilot Study of Schizophrenia, there was a significant difference in the course of schizophrenia between industrialized and developing nations, with individuals with schizophrenia in developing countries having a less severe and less chronic course of the illness (WHO 1979, Waxler 1979).

Various explanations for these discrepancies have been postulated (Cooper and Sartorius 1977). For example, in industrialized areas the family structure may impose more social stresses on the ill relative, who is often unable to work and perform by society's standards, whereas in developing countries the family structure may be protective, with other relatives supporting the ill relative. Another possible explanation is a selection factor in developing countries resulting from the higher infant mortality in nonindustrialized societies. According to this hypothesis, children in less developed countries who would be at risk for schizophrenia would not be as likely to survive, thus skewing the prevalence rates of schizophrenia in these areas (Cooper and Sartorius 1977). However, some suggest that this risk factor of increase incidence of psychosis in urban areas is more ecological then genetic (Jablensky 2000). Further investigation is needed to provide definitive answers as to why schizophrenia may have a higher prevalence and more severe course in industrialized nations.

## Season of Birth and Onset

That season of birth differs between individuals with schizophrenia and the general population has by now gained wide acceptance. This factor has been studied in the 20th century, with the predominant view that the birth rate of people with schizophrenia is highest in late winter (Jablensky 1986, Hare 1987, Eaton 1985). Torrey and colleagues (1997) confirmed this, reviewing approximately 250 studies and concluding that there is an excess of schizophrenia births during winter. In fact, there is approximately a 5 to 8% greater likelihood for individuals with schizophrenia to be born during winter months compared with the general population. This higher incidence of winter births has been found in both hemispheres, offering further evidence that this phenomenon is related to the colder months rather than specific calendar months.

It is clear that even though only a small proportion of all those with schizophrenia are born during winter months, the deviation from the seasonality of birth of the general population (the number of general births peaks in the spring) is a striking phenomenon. This finding is not unique to schizophrenia, and differences in seasonality of birth have been described for mania (Hare 1983), diabetes mellitus (Christy et al. 1982), Down syndrome, congenital hip dislocation, and certain cardiovascular malformations (Jongblet et al. 1982). It is therefore debatable whether this observation has etiological significance unique to schizophrenia.

Season of onset has also been considered in epidemiological investigations of schizophrenia. A preponderance of data dating back to the early 1800s indicates that the summer season is associated with a higher incidence of the onset of symptoms. Suicide rates also vary according to season, with a spring peak, indicating that the interaction of environment and psychopathology may be of some significance (Silverman 1968).

## Morbidity and Mortality

The economic costs of schizophrenia have been estimated to be six times the costs of myocardial infarction (Andrews 1985). The WHO has estimated that mental illness accounts for as much as two-fifths of all disability funding in the US (Jablensky et al. 1980). Amongst the homeless in New York City, a significant percentage of cost of hospital admissions were associated with schizophrenia patients (Salit et al. 1998). In the US, the cost of schizophrenia in 1994 was $44.9 billion and rising (Rice 1999). In the UK, 5.4% of total national health service inpatient costs were attributed to schizophrenia. When all services were combined together, approximately £2.6 billion were spent annually taking care of schizophrenia patients (Knapp 1997). In Australia, it is estimated that schizophrenia costs approximately $3 billion for treatment and due to lost productivity (Mowry and Nancarrow 2001). Much of the cost of schizophrenia is due to the high morbidity of this chronic illness. Premorbid deficits, cognitive deficits, and negative symptoms account for much of the disability (Johnstone et al. 1979). Also, schizophrenia patients with more severe courses may require repeated hospitalizations and may not be capable of maintaining independent living or stable employment.

The mortality rate of schizophrenia is estimated to be twice that of the general population. Approximately 10% of the mortality is secondary to suicide (Hare 1987). Young male patients with schizophrenia are most likely to complete suicide attempts, especially early in their illness (Drake et al. 1985, Breier and Astrachan 1984). Degree of social isolation, agitation, depression, a sense of hopelessness, a history of prior suicide attempts, and recent loss may be associated with increased risk of suicide among schizophrenia patients (Breier and Astrachan 1984). There is also some evidence that an increased number of relapses, rehospitalizations, and discharges lead to an increased risk of suicide. There have been observations that suicide rates of schizophrenia patients may be increasing in the era of shorter hospital stays and community treatment (Drake et al. 1985). However, with the advent of the novel antipsychotic medications and especially with clozapine use, it is possible that this risk of suicide may even out or decrease due to their possible protective effects against suicide (Meltzer and Okayli 1995). Other factors leading to increased mortality rates in schizophrenia patients include an increased incidence of accidents as well as a more frequent association with other medical illnesses (including cardiovascular disease), comorbid substance abuse, a general neglect of health, an increased rate of damaging behaviors such as smoking and poor diet, decreased access to health services and depression (Vieweg et al. 1995, Ruschena et al. 1998, Harris and Barraclough 1998, Ameddeo et al. 1995, Musselman et al. 1998, Schulz et al. 2000, Allebech et al. 1986, Zarate and Patel 2001).

## Comorbidity with Other Illnesses

Schizophrenia is associated with an increased frequency of tuberculosis (not accounted for by institutionalization), celiac disease, myxedema, and arteriosclerotic heart disease (Baldwin 1979, Hare 1987, Eaton 1985, Jablensky 1986, Harris and Barraclough 1998, Musselman et al. 1998, Schulz et al. 2000). Patients who present with atypical psychoses have been noted to have an increased risk of ankylosing spondylitis and uroarthritis, which may indicate a relationship between the histocompatibility complex and schizophrenia (Jablensky 1986, Osterberg 1978).

Along these lines, there is a strikingly decreased risk for rheumatoid arthritis among patients with schizophrenia (Jablensky 1986, Eaton 1985). Many of the studies supporting this observation were conducted before the use of phenothiazines, which eliminates any potential protective role of neuroleptics (Eaton 1985). It has been postulated that further investigation of this link may yield significant genetic or biological markers for both diseases.

Such studies of potential biological markers have yielded some interesting findings. Illnesses such as rheumatoid arthritis and ankylosing spondilitis are autoimmune disorders that are associated with human leukocyte antigens (HLA). The associated risks for these disorders and schizophrenia have led to speculation that some subgroup of patients with schizophrenia may be manifesting symptoms related to an autoimmune process. For example, studies have shown that there may be an association between HLA and types of schizophrenia (Ganguli et al. 1993, Zamani et al. 1994). In one recent study, the HLA frequency was increased for HLA A10, A11, and A29 and decreased for HLA A2 in patients with schizophrenia (Ozcan et al. 1996). Thus, although the presence of HLA is not universal among persons with schizophrenia, further investigation into this area may point to alternative hypothesis regarding etiology and treatment of a certain population of patients with schizophrenia.

Reversing the association, there are numerous medical illnesses with symptoms similar to those of schizophrenia (Jablensky 1986, Davison and Bagley 1969). Among examples of these, the most common neurological disorder appearing clinically similar to schizophrenia is epilepsy (Flor-Henry 1983), particularly of the temporal lobe. Other medical illnesses with symptoms similar to those of schizophrenia include basal ganglia calcifications and acute intermittent porphyria (Propping 1983). Imbalances of endocrine function as well as certain infectious diseases can present with symptoms that mimic schizophrenic psychosis. Further investigation of these illnesses may lead to a greater understanding of the pathophysiology of schizophrenia.

## Etiology

The cause of schizophrenia is currently not known. However, fast-paced developments in neuroscience combined with advances in psychiatric research have resulted in increased optimism about discovering the cause(s) and delineating the pathophysiology of this mysterious illness. A leading view is that schizophrenia may be heterogeneous with respect to etiology. Thus, multiple causative mechanisms may give rise to distinct disease subtypes. If this is true, it is important for psychiatric researchers to differentiate the homogeneous subtypes of this illness. Moreover, it has been proposed that more than one causative mechanism might interact (the so-called double-hit hypothesis) to cause the illness in some individuals. In this section, the main etiological theories of schizophrenia are examined.

## Genetics

Schizophrenia represents a daunting challenge for genetic researchers for several reasons: the paucity of extended multigenerational family histories containing large numbers of affected individuals; the possibility of genetic heterogeneity, such as more than one phenotype or more than one genetic variant; and a lack of agreement on the mode of transmission. Following genetic modeling of epidemiological data and the results of several genome screens for susceptibility genes, it appears that the probability of schizophrenia being a single gene disorder is unlikely. The probability that several genes of large effects may confer vulnerability to schizophrenia is diminishing too. Thus, the focus has shifted to multiple genes of small to moderate effects which may compound their effects through interactions with each other and with other nongenetic risk factors. (see Mowry and Nancarrow 2001 for more discussion). Despite these formidable obstacles, enormous progress has been made in search of genetic basis for schizophrenia. Moreover, the proteins expressed by the genes (proteome) are equally important in understanding the working of the cells being studied. Thus, genomics or the study of how genes control normal neuronal function is now moving on to proteomics or the study of different proteins expressed by the genome (Stahl 2000).

## Family Prevalence Studies

Wide agreement now exists that the rate of schizophrenia among first-degree family members of persons with schizophrenia is higher than in control families. The chance of occurrence is approximately 10 times greater among these individuals than in individuals with no first-degree relatives with schizophrenia (Kendler and Diehl 1993). There is approximately 6 times and 2 times greater chance of developing schizophrenia in second- and third-degree relatives of individuals with schizophrenia (Tsuang et al. 2001). In addition, the higher prevalence of schizophrenia spectrum disorders among family members of individuals with schizophrenia, such as schizoaffective disorder and schizoid and schizotypal personality disorders, provides support for a common genetic basis for this family of schizophrenia-like illnesses. Different studies have provided evidence for and against an increased prevalence of other psychotic disorders and nonpsychotic affective illnesses among relatives of persons with schizophrenia.

## Adoption Studies

Adoption studies constitute a powerful experimental strategy for examining the role of genetic versus environmental factors. In these studies, the rates of schizophrenia are compared in relatives of adoptees with and without schizophrenia. Danish adoption studies conducted in the 1960s and 1970s provided compelling evidence that adoptees with schizophrenia had higher rates of schizophrenia in their first-degree relatives than control adoptees (Kety et al. 1968, Kety 1987). A reanalysis of these data in the late 1980s confirmed the original finding that biological relatives of schizophrenia adoptees had significantly higher rates of schizophrenia (4.1%) than biological relatives of nonschizophrenia (control) adoptees (0.5%).

In Finland, a large study of adopted-away offspring of mothers with schizophrenia found that significantly more offspring of mothers with schizophrenia themselves developed schizophrenia (9.1%) than did control offspring (1.1%) (Tienari 1991). An interesting aspect of the Finnish study was the examination of family environment in the adoptive families. A relationship was found between a disruptive family environment and occurrence of schizophrenia in adoptees. This suggests that environmental factors might play a role in the manifestation of the illness in genetically susceptible individuals. However, the study did not make clear whether the schizophrenia adoptee caused the disruptive home environment or the disruptive environment contributed to the manifestation of the illness. Longitudinal assessment of environmental conditions throughout childhood before the onset of illness will be important in resolving this issue.

Several methodological issues are important in interpreting the data from adoption studies, including the diagnostic status of biological fathers and levels of psychopathology in adoptive families. Additional factors to consider are the intrauterine environment, birth complications, and length of time from birth to adoptive placement.

## Twin Studies

Another approach to examining genetic contributions to schizophrenia involves concordance studies of dizygotic (nonidentical) and monozygotic (identical) twin pairs. Available data indicate that the concordance of schizophrenia among dizygotic twins is approximately 8 to 12%. This is much greater than the 1% rate found in the general population and comparable to the rate of concordance of schizophrenia among first-degree siblings. The concordance of schizophrenia among monozygotic twins is approximately 50% (Kendler and Diehl 1993). Even though the high rate of concordance among monozygotic twin pairs is compelling evidence for genetic contributions, the fact that it is not higher than 50% suggests a role for additional, perhaps nongenetic, factors in the etiology of schizophrenia. Moreover, although monozygotic twins share the same genetic information, it is possible for a mutation to occur in one member of the twin pair and not the other. Birth order of twin pairs and different intrauterine effects are other factors to consider. An attractive and robust experimental design is provided by adoption away of monozygotic twin pairs, which effectively combines the strengths of both adoption and twin methodologies. The number of sets of adopted-away, monozygotic twin pairs affected with schizophrenia is relatively small. However, data available on the limited number of pairs meeting these criteria support the strong concordance of schizophrenia in monozygotic twins.

## Linkage and Association Studies

There was tremendous enthusiasm and hope riding on the two promising approaches to identify the faulty gene(s) responsible for schizophrenia: *linkage studies* and *association studies*. Linkage studies use polymorphic genetic markers to attempt to identify statistical agreement (known as a logarithm of the odds score) between the presence of the marker and illness in families under investigation. The human genome project has established a set of markers for the entire human genome that will make it possible to scan the entire genome for schizophrenia linkage. It should be noted that genetic markers mark a segment of DNA presumably where the gene of interest resides; they do not necessarily identify mutant genes themselves. Once linkage is established, the second stage of work begins, which entails searching the identified segment of DNA for the faulty gene. However, the linkage studies have a limited power to detect susceptibility genes of small effect, a most likely scenario in complex disease genetics such as schizophrenia. This can be overcome by association studies (Lichtermann et al. 2000).

Association studies actually use the candidate genes themselves and test the highly specific hypothesis that a mutation in the candidate gene occurs at a greater rate in the population of interest (in this case schizophrenia patients) than in nonaffected control populations. More recently, family based samples such as *trios* (consisting of the affected person and both parents, if available), are collected to avoid population stratification. The results have so far been equivocal. Serotonin 5-HT$_{2A}$ receptor gene and dopamine D$_3$ receptor gene are weakly associated with schizophrenia susceptibility (O'Donnell et al. 1999). The NMDA receptor holds promise based on animal models (Mohn et al. 1999). One limitation of this approach is that it is all or none; that is, the candidate gene either is or is not associated with the illness.

The Human Genome Project with its 3 billion base pairs and approximately 35,000 genes has ushered us into the "Genomic Era." However, systematic genome scans done recently have not resulted in strong evidence for linkage to any chromosomal region. Regions currently attracting most support are 6p (Schizophrenia Collaborative Linkage Group 1996), 6q (Cao et al. 1997, Levinson et al. 1998), 8p (Pulver et al. 1995, Schizophrenia Collaborative Linkage Group 1996), 13q (Blouin et al. 1998, Levinson et al. 2000), 3p (Schizophrenia Collaborative Linkage Group 1996), 22q (Gill et al. 1996, Moises et al. 1995), 5q (Levinson 1991), and 10p (Levinson et al. 2000, Faraone et al. 1998, Straub et al. 1998).

Velocardiofacial syndrome (VCFS) is associated with small interstitial deletions of chromosome 22q11 and a high rate of psychiatric comorbidity specifically schizophrenia. This has generated enormous interest in this disorder especially because of evidence suggesting that the migration of mesencephalic and cardiac neural crest cells may be associated with pathogenesis of midfacial and cardiac abnormalities; similarities of this process to the neurodevelopment theory of schizophrenia has raised interesting speculations (Murphy et al. 1999, Chow et al. 1994).

Studies focused on 15q14 (Freedman et al. 1997, 2001, Kaufman et al. 1998) have shown some interesting findings especially considering its location close to the gene for nicotinic receptors, a system possibly involved with aspects of cognition. Ongoing and future studies will clarify the relevance of these findings.

At the time of this writing, no genetic linkage or association related to schizophrenia has been discovered. There have been reports of suggestive linkages but there has been a failure to replicate these findings. It has become painfully clear that the replication studies are, in many ways, more important to establishing linkage than the initial report. Genes that have been found not to be associated with schizophrenia include the dopamine D$_2$ and D$_4$ genes.

The initial enthusiasm for these strategies has waned some as no gene has yet been isolated for schizophrenia or bipolar disorder. According to Merikangas (2002), the impediments that limited the success of linkage and association studies are etiologic and phenotypic heterogeneity of schizophrenia, lack of power, and high false positive rates. Thus, newer approaches such as multi-investigator collaborative studies to increase the power have already been implemented.

Meanwhile, modern functional genomic approaches such as DNA microarrays, based on the principles of nucleic acid hybridization, can check a tissue sample for presence of thousands of genes simultaneously. For example, Mirnics and colleagues (2000) employed cDNA microarrays and compared transcriptomes in schizophrenia and matched control subjects and found that only a few gene groups consistently differed between subjects and controls. In all subjects with schizophrenia, the most changed gene group was related to *presynaptic group secretory function* (PSYN) gene group and in particular the "mechanics" of neurotransmitter release. Thus, Mirnics and colleagues (2000) postulate that, as the most affected genes in the PSYN group varied across study subjects (suggesting that the illness has "distinct molecular signatures"), schizophrenia, therefore, may involve a combination of different sequence-related polygenic susceptibility factors and physiological adaptations that lead to impairment of the signaling between neurons. They find additional support for their hypothesis from reports of reduced expression of regulator of G-protein signaling 4 (RGS4) in individuals with schizophrenia. In the brain, RGS4 is one of the 20 or more RGS family members that serve as GTPase-activating proteins (GAPs), which reduce response duration of postsynaptic neurons after the release of presynaptic neurotransmitters that bind to G-protein coupled receptors. Thus, Mirnics and colleagues (2001) suggest that the deficits in PSYN and RGS4 expression may produce synaptic changes with pathophysiologic consequences relevant to schizophrenia.

Weinberger and colleagues (2001) suggest that the gene that encodes the postsynaptic enzyme catechol-*o*-methyl transferase (COMT) is preferentially involved in the metabolism of dopamine in frontal lobe. Dopamine is hypothesized to underlie aspects of cognition in frontal lobe such as information processing. Based on animal studies, family-based association studies, and fMRI studies in schizophrenia patients and general population, Weinberger and colleagues propose an interesting hypothesis that the COMT genotype with valenine allele (val/val type) may increase the risk of developing schizophrenia due to its effect on dopamine-mediated prefrontal information processing. Clearly, faster, innovative, and sophisticated techniques have ushered genetic research into a new era with a renewed promise to explore genetic basis of mental illnesses.

Researchers are urgently searching for schizophrenia phenotypes for subgroups or dimensions that may define etiologically or genetically distinct subtypes. Similarly, the field is yearning for *endophenotypes* with simpler architecture than schizophrenia to possibly guide to newer leads in research (Mowry and Nancarrow 2001). Latent genetically influenced traits, which may be related only indirectly to the classic disease symptoms defined in major classification systems are known as "endophenotypes" (Gottesman 1997). They reflect an underlying susceptibility to the disease phenotype (or some form of it). In schizophrenia we are interested in endophenotypes that are measurable by neurophysiological or neuropsychological means. Crucial characteristics of any endophenotype include the fact that it can be measured before the explicit onset of the illness, and that it represents the genetic liability of nonaffected relatives of probands with the disorder. For example, in genetically complex disorder such as schizophrenia, could separate genetic loci contribute to distinct aspects of the illness phenotype (e.g., evoked potentials, aspects of cognition, etc.)?

Multinational studies are underway using *simple tandem-repeat polymorphic* (STRP) markers genome screen technology to detect genes of small to moderate effect. Also large scale *single-nucleotide polymorphism* (SNP) analysis will allow genome screen of extremely small densities. Thus, advances in proteomics and genomics provide more powerful approaches to identify gene products involved in schizophrenia pathogenesis.

## Viral Hypotheses

The suggestion that psychotic illnesses may be related to an infectious process has a long history. Jean Etienne Esquirol in 1845 noted that some forms of psychotic illness followed "epidemic" illness patterns. In the early part of this century, Karl Menninger observed an association between the onset of schizophrenia and influenza epidemics. In addition, it has long been known that clinical features of viral encephalitis may include psychosis and other features resembling those of schizophrenia.

Two lines of evidence that have provoked the most interest in the possibility that viral infections are causative of schizophrenia are an increase in birth during influenza epidemics of individuals who subsequently develop schizophrenia and an increase in winter births among patients with schizophrenia because of the higher rate of viral infections in winter months. Mednick and colleagues (1988) reported a strong association between pregnancies during the 1957 influenza epidemic in Helsinki, Finland, and subsequent development of schizophrenia. Moreover, it was learned that the relationship between viral exposure and schizophrenia appears strongest when exposure occurred during the second trimester of pregnancy. This is of interest because the second trimester is a critical period for cortical and limbic development. It was therefore reasoned that second-trimester viral exposure might disrupt neuronal development in key areas of the brain, such as the hippocampus and prefrontal cortex, that have been implicated in this illness. In fact, there is some experimental evidence from animal models that viral exposure to these regions in the developing brain produces neuropathological changes resembling those observed in some postmortem studies of schizophrenia. However, reanalysis of previous data failed to detect significant association between *in utero* exposure to influenza epidemics and schizophrenia (Grech et al. 1997, Selten et al. 1998). Similarly, data from Australia failed to find an association between six influenza epidemics and schizophrenia (Morgan et al. 1997). These and other negative results (Crow and Done 1992) have raised serious questions about this theory. Interestingly, in the North Finland birth cohort, a significant association was found with laboratory confirmed diagnosis of viral infection, especially Coxsackie B5 meningitis in the neonatal period and risk of schizophrenia later on (Rantakallio et al. 1997).

Several studies have demonstrated an excess of winter births among patients with schizophrenia. Although statistically significant, the association between winter births and schizophrenia appears relatively small, occurring in less than 10% of cases. Thus, season of birth remains an interesting (and unresolved) research issue but has little use as a risk factor for the illness from a clinical perspective.

Exposure to influenza *in utero* and excess winter births are interesting although indirect lines of evidence for a viral cause of schizophrenia. To date, there has been no direct confirmation for any viral agent causing this illness, such as viral isolates or consistent findings of specific viral antibodies. Advances in neurovirology, however, are providing new insights into the role of viruses in brain diseases, leading to new hypotheses about schizophrenia. One area involves the search for neurotropic retroviruses. For example, Borna virus is a naturally occurring neurotropic agent in horses and sheep. The development of a serological assay method to detect antibodies for Borna virus led to the discovery that its hosts also include humans and that it has relative tropism for the hippocampus. Moreover, its clinical manifestations range from asymptomatic infection to profound behavioral abnormalities that resemble some aspects of schizophrenia. An association between deficit symptoms, Borna virus antibodies and summer birth excess has been reported (Waltrip et al. 1997). There is now an active research effort to determine whether Borna and other neurotropic viruses are more common in schizophrenia.

## Immune Dysfunction

Several research groups are exploring the possibility that schizophrenia may be associated with impaired immune function including alterations in autoimmunity (Muller and Ackenheil 1998). Anticardiolipin antibody and antinuclear antibody, two autoantibodies that are used as markers of autoimmune vulnerability, have been shown to be increased in patients with schizophrenia in some but not all studies of this illness. Specific histocompatibility antigens (human leukocyte antigens) have also been linked to several autoimmune diseases and have been investigated in schizophrenia with conflicting results (Miyanaga et al. 1984). Two other markers relevant to autoimmune function, impaired T lymphocyte proliferative response to the mitogen phytohemagglutinin and impaired interleukin-2 production, have shown more consistent alterations in patients with schizophrenia than in control populations (Coffey et al. 1983). Some of the most intriguing work in this area is focused on finding autoantibodies to brain tissue. Recent reports of atypical antipsychotic medications having immunomodulatory effects (Muller et al. 1997, Lin et al. 1998) and selective COX-2 inhibitor (a new type of nonsteroidal antiinflammatory drug used as a pain killer) having positive effects on schizophrenia symptoms are interesting and provide yet another avenue of research in understanding the complexity of schizophrenia (Muller et al. 2002).

## Birth Complications

Numerous studies have reported a higher rate of pregnancy and birth complications in patients with schizophrenia than in control populations (Jones et al. 1998, Dalman et al. 1999, Preti et al. 2000, McNeil et al. 1994, Cannon et al. 2002). The complication rates vary widely among studies, probably because of the inherent difficulties in obtaining reliable and valid retrospective data in this area. In one study, two-thirds of schizophrenia patients and less than one-third of control subjects had histories of obstetrical complications. Hypoxia is one possible result of pregnancy and birth complications that has been shown to disrupt brain development. The hippocampus and some neocortical regions are particularly sensitive to shortfalls in oxygen. Thus, one proposed mechanism for a role of pregnancy and birth complications in the cause of schizophrenia involves hypoxia-mediated damage to these areas. While some investigators agree with this theory (Geddes et al. 1999, Rosso et al. 2000, Zornberg 2000), others do not (McCreadie et al. 1994, Byrne et al. 2000, Kendell et al. 2000). Interestingly, some studies suggest that the rate of obstetric complications are higher in early-onset schizophrenia (Verdoux et al. 1997, Smith et al. 1998, Rosso et al. 2000), occur more often in males, in people with prominent negative symptoms, and no family history of schizophrenia (Cantor-Graae et al. 1994, McNeil 1995, Verdoux et al. 1997, Smith 1998, Rosso et al. 2000, Kotlicka-Antczak et al. 2001).

A meta-analysis of data involving 854 individuals from 11 research groups (Verdoux et al. 1997) suggest that the relationship between birth complications and age at onset tend to be linear and may indicate a causal effect. Jones and colleagues (1998), using North Finland birth cohort involving 11,017 patients reported a sevenfold excess among schizophrenia patients of perinatal brain injury. In a recent historical and meta-analytic review by Cannon and colleagues (2002), complications of pregnancy, abnormal fetal growth and development and complications of delivery were significantly associated with developing schizophrenia but the effect sizes were generally small with odds ratios of less than 2. They elaborate current methodological shortcomings and suggest need for newer and better approaches to inform our understanding of these important associations.

## Pathophysiology

Whereas *etiology* refers to the cause of an illness, *pathophysiology* refers to the abnormal processes that mediate the clinical manifestation of the illness. As was the case with etiology, the brain processes that give rise to schizophrenia are currently not known. However, rapidly converging bodies of neuroanatomical and neurochemical data appear to be closing in on defining the pathophysiology of this illness. In this section, these data are reviewed.

### Neuroanatomical Theories

The brains of patients with psychotic illnesses have been examined for hundreds of years. At the end of the 19th century, Alzheimer described loss of cortical neurons in patients with dementia precox. In 1915 Southard noted cerebral atrophy in patients. Although these early reports were suggestive of a brain lesion in schizophrenia, only recently have the investigative tools become available to probe the human brain in enough detail to confirm cerebral abnormalities in this illness.

Advances in *in vivo* brain imaging and postmortem methodology have provided powerful new tools for neuroanatomical investigations of this illness. *In vivo* structural brain analysis began in earnest with computed tomography (CT), which provided the most compelling evidence for morphological abnormalities in this illness. CT has been replaced by magnetic resonance imaging (MRI) for mor-

phological studies because of its superior anatomical resolution (1 mm or less in-plane resolution), ability to provide true volumetric and three-dimensional analysis of even minute brain regions, tissue segmentation capability and because it involves no radiation exposure. Positron emission tomography (PET), single-photon emission computed tomography (SPECT), functional MRI (fMRI), and MR spectroscopy (MRS) are imaging tools used to assess the functional and neurochemical activity of specific brain regions. Diffusion Tensor Imaging (DTI) and Line Scan Diffusion Imaging (LSDI) are newer MRI approaches that can provide sophisticated information on the orientation and integrity of neuron fibers *in vivo*. Advances in postmortem methodology include rapid access to brains after death, well-matched control groups, controls for neuroleptic exposure including studies of neuroleptic-naive populations, and application of new molecular biological techniques. The following is an examination of the brain structures most often implicated in the pathophysiology of schizophrenia.

### Enlarged Ventricles

The ventricles are the fluid-filled spaces in the center of the brain. The most consistent morphological finding in the literature of schizophrenia is enlarged ventricles which has been confirmed by a large number of CT and MRI studies (Pahl et al. 1990, Wolkin et al. 1998, McCarley et al. 1999, Henn and Braus 1999). The effect size of ventriculomegaly has been reported to be 0.7 (Raz and Raz 1990). Seventy-nine percent of the well designed studies report enlargement of lateral ventricles (Henn and Braus 1999). CT studies have tended to use ventricle–brain ratios to assess lateral ventricular size, and MRI studies have used more sophisticated quantifications. Lawrie and Abukmeil (1998), in a review report approximately 40% difference in volume between schizophrenia patients and controls across all volumetric MRI studies. It should be noted that although the ventricular increases are statistically significant, the ventricles are not grossly enlarged in most cases. In fact, radiologists most often read CT and MRI scans of patients with schizophrenia as normal. In addition, most studies of ventricular size demonstrate overlap between patients and normal control subjects, indicating that many patients have ventricles in the normal range. Nonetheless, enlargement of the ventricles is the first consistently reported finding confirming a brain abnormality in schizophrenia.

The pathophysiological significance of larger than normal ventricles is unclear (Lawrie and Abukmeil 1998). There have been reports that enlarged ventricles may be more prominent in more severely ill patients and related to poor response to neuroleptic medication, although these findings have not been consistently replicated. Ventricular enlargement, particularly third ventricle and temporal horn enlargement, has been found in first-episode patients with schizophrenia, which suggests that it is not secondary to chronic neuroleptic exposure or a progressive disease process. However, frontal horn enlargement is usually seen in chronic cases, suggesting possible progressive changes following onset of the illness (Bilder et al. 1994). Enlarged ventricles are most likely a secondary manifestation of brain atrophy or some other process resulting in either focal or generalized reductions in brain mass. Indeed,

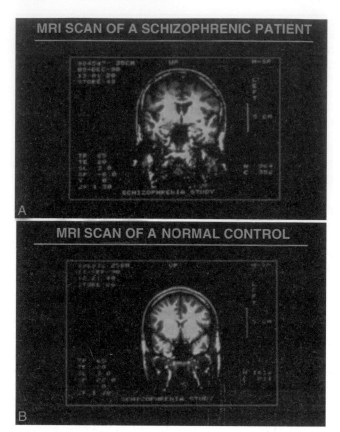

**Figure 62–2** *CT scans of a schizophrenic patient* (A) *and a healthy volunteer* (B). *Note enlarged ventricular spaces and brain atrophy in the scan of the patient with schizophrenia.*

there have been many reports of brain atrophy and reduced mass in the illness (Figure 62–2). Enlarged ventricles have also been reported in first-degree relatives of subjects with schizophrenia (Cannon et al. 1998, Seidman et al. 1997) and in persons suffering from schizotypal personality disorder (Buchsbaum et al. 1997) raising interesting speculations of whether ventriculomegaly may be an indicator of neurodevelopmental risk for schizophrenia (Lencz et al. 2001).

## Limbic System

The limbic structures that have been implicated in schizophrenia are the hippocampus, entorhinal cortex, anterior cingulate, and amygdala. These structures have important functions for memory (hippocampus), attention (anterior cingulate), and emotional expression and social affiliation (amygdala). The entorhinal cortex serves as a "way station" between hippocampus and neocortex in that neurotransmissions between these regions synapse in the entorhinal cortex. The entorhinal cortex, hippocampus, and other components of the parahippocampal gyrus are often considered "mesiotemporal" structures because of their close anatomical and functional relationship.

There are more reports of abnormalities in hippocampal and related mesiotemporal structures than other limbic structures in schizophrenia. In fact, mesiotemporal pathology is consistently found in studies of schizophrenia and mesiotemporal structures are leading candidates for the neuroanatomical site of this illness (Goldstein et al. 1999, Wright et al. 1999). This region has been implicated by

converging brain imaging and postmortem lines of evidence. One of the most consistent MRI morphological findings is reduction in size of the hippocampus (Breier et al. 1992). In addition, more than 25 postmortem studies have reported morphological and cytoarchitectural abnormalities in this structure. The findings have included reduced size and cellular number (Benes et al. 1998), white matter reductions, and abnormal cell arrangement. Nelson and colleagues (1998), conclude from a meta-analysis of 18 studies that there is a bilateral reduction of approximately 4% hippocampal volume in schizophrenia. However, reduced hippocampal volume is not reported by all studies (Harrison 1999, Maier et al. 2000). In another review, Lawrie and Abukmeil (1998) reported approximately 6% reduction in amygdala hippocampal complex. Reduction in the volume of amygdala is reported by some but not all (Altshuler et al. 1998). In a very interesting preliminary report from Australia, subjects who went on to develop schizophrenia had larger left hippocampal volumes compared to controls at baseline (during the prodrome) with subsequent reduction in volume after the onset of schizophrenia (Pantelis et al. 1999).

The anterior cingulate has been implicated in schizophrenia largely because of postmortem findings of reduced gamma-aminobutyric acid (GABA) interneurons (Benes et al. 1991). In addition, functional imaging studies have demonstrated altered metabolic activity both at rest and during selective attention tasks in the anterior cingulate in patients with schizophrenia (Baker 1997, Carter et al. 1997, Erkwoh et al. 1997, Fletcher 1999, Haznedar et al. 1997). Data from many studies suggest possible neurodevelopmental abnormalities in anterior cingulate in patients with schizophrenia (Benes 2000, Harrison 1999, Honer et al. 1997, Kalus et al. 1999). Bouras and colleagues (2001) reported mean total and laminar cortical thickness as well as mean pyramidal neuron size were significantly decreased in the dorsal and subgenual parts of anterior cingulate in schizophrenia patients. Thirty-one studies evaluated one or more of the medial temporal lobe structures—hippocampus, amygdala, parahippocampal gyrus, entorhinal cortex—with 77% reporting positive findings; this is one of the higher percentages of abnormalities reported in all regions of interest throughout the brain.

## Prefrontal Cortex

The prefrontal cortex is the most anterior portion of the neocortex, sitting behind the forehead. It has evolved through lower species to become one of the largest regions of the human brain, constituting approximately one-third of the cortex. It is responsible for some of the most sophisticated human functions. It contains a heteromodal association area that is responsible for integrating information from all other cortical areas as well as from several subcortical regions for the execution of purposeful behavior. Among its specific functions are working memory, which involves the temporary storage (seconds to minutes) of information, attention, and suppression of interference from internal and external sources. The most inferior portion of the prefrontal cortex, termed the orbital frontal cortex, is involved in emotional expression. Given its unique role, it is not surprising that the prefrontal cortex has been considered in the etiology of schizophrenia.

Indeed, several lines of evidence have implicated the prefrontal cortex in schizophrenia. CT studies have provided evidence for prefrontal atrophy, and some, although not all, MRI studies have found evidence for decreased volume of this structure (Breier et al. 1992, Andreasen et al. 1986, McCarley et al. 1999). One of the earliest observations from functional imaging studies of schizophrenia was reduced perfusion of the frontal lobes (Ingvar and Franzen 1974). This finding was subsequently replicated by several PET studies suggesting decreased frontal glucose utilization and blood flow, which came to be known as *hypofrontality*. Subsequent functional imaging studies provided further support for hypofrontality by demonstrating that patients with schizophrenia failed to activate their frontal lobes to the same degree as normal control subjects when performing frontal cognitive tasks (Weinberger and Berman 1988, Weinberger and Berman 1996, Kindermann et al. 1997). This finding has been questioned because patients with schizophrenia typically perform poorly in many cognitive paradigms, so it is unclear whether their lack of frontal activation is a primary frontal deficit or secondary to poor cognitive task performance related to factors such as lack of motivation, inattention, or cognitive impairment stemming from nonfrontal regions. Auditory hallucinations were found to be associated with increases in Broca's area, a portion of the frontal cortex responsible for language production (McGuire et al. 1993). This finding was of interest because it supported a hypothesis that auditory hallucinations were a form of abnormal "inner speech."

MRI studies employing diffusion tensor imaging have reported changes suggestive of an abnormality in white matter connectivity possibly due to reduced myelination of fiber tracts in patients with schizophrenia (Lim et al. 1999, Buchsbaum et al. 1998). Magnetic resonance spectroscopy (MRS) studies have reported reduced levels of neuronal membrane constituents (phosphomonoesters) and/or increased levels of their breakdown products (phosphodiesters) in patients with schizophrenia, primarily in the frontal cortex (Keshavan et al. 2000). Such abnormalities have been observed in treatment-naive first episode patients (Stanley et al. 1995) and have been correlated with trait-like negative symptoms and neurocognitive performance (Shioiri et al. 1994, Deicken et al. 1995).

Though sometimes contradictory, the neuroimaging studies consistently report abnormalities in orbitofrontal region; often, these abnormalities tend to correlate with severity of schizophrenia symptomatology, show gender differences in relation to spatial localization and the gray matter deficits may be more wide spread in chronic, as compared to medication-naive first episode patients (Lencz et al. 2001, Szeszko et al. 1999). Additional support for prefrontal cortical involvement in schizophrenia comes from postmortem studies with a range of findings. There have been reports of reduced cortical thickness, loss of pyramidal cells, malformed cellular architecture, loss of GABA interneurons, and evidence of failed neuronal migration. The Stanley Foundation Neuropathology Consortium is reported to be "the most extensively characterized collection of pathological specimens from patients with major mental illnesses" (Knable et al. 2001). Their exploratory analyses of prefrontal cortex from patients suffering from schizophrenia, bipolar disorder, and depression compared with samples from normal controls found the largest number of abnormalities in schizophrenia with an overlap with bipolar disorder. A majority of the abnormalities represented a decline in function suggesting a widespread failure of gene expression. Specifically, abnormalities involving the glycoprotein *Reelin* were observed in schizophrenia, a finding reported previously by other postmortem studies also (Impagnatiello et al. 1998, Guidotti 2000). *Reelin*, an extracellular matrix glycoprotein secreted from different GABAergic interneurons during development and adult life, may be important for the transcription of specific genes necessary for synaptic plasticity and morphological changes associated with learning. Future studies will clarify the role of *Reelin* in the pathology of schizophrenia.

Thus, a substantial body of evidence is converging on prefrontal cortex as a site of pathophysiology in schizophrenia (Bunney and Bunney 2000, Weinberger et al. 2001). The genetics of the prefrontal neurons, the cortical circuits and its underlying neurochemistry in the brains of individuals with schizophrenia is one the most intensely investigated area.

## Temporal Lobe

The superior temporal gyrus is involved in auditory processing and, with parts of the inferior parietal cortex, is a heteromodal association area that includes Wernicke's area, a language center. Because of the important role it plays in audition, it was hypothesized to be involved in auditory hallucinations. Indeed, MRI studies have found the superior temporal gyrus to be reduced in size in schizophrenia and have found a significant relationship between these reductions and the presence of auditory hallucinations (Barta et al. 1990). Similarly, Wernicke's area, which is involved in the conception and organization of speech, has been hypothesized to mediate the thought disorder of schizophrenia, particularly conceptual disorganization. Support for this hypothesis comes from a report of a patient with vascular and other lesions of this region that produce Wernicke's aphasia, a disruption in the organization of speech that resembles the thought disorder of schizophrenia. MRI studies have found a relationship between morphological abnormalities in this region and conceptual disorganization in schizophrenia (Shenton et al. 1992). McCarley and colleagues (1999) reviewed 118 MRI studies published from 1988 to 1998; 62% of the 37 studies of whole temporal lobe showed volume reduction and/or abnormal asymmetry. Of the 15 studies surveyed, 80% showed abnormalities in superior temporal gyrus, the *highest* percentage of any cortical region of interest. This difference appears to be largely due to gray matter. Most studies, including those involving first episode patients (Hirayasu et al. 1998), report abnormalities in *planum temporale* (area related to language) with specific reductions of left posterior superior temporal gyrus gray matter. According to the authors, the higher percentage of abnormalities in specifically defined regions of interest of medial temporal lobe and superior temporal gyrus suggests a nondiffuse distribution of temporal lobe structural changes.

## Other Neocortical Regions

There are positive as well as negative reports of both parietal and occipital lobes showing differences between patients with schizophrenia and healthy controls. Abnormalities involving cerebellum have been reported too. At present, the significance of these findings are not clear (McCarley et al. 1999).

## Striatum

The striatum, consisting of the caudate, putamen, globus pallidus, substantia nigra, and accumbens, is an output center for the cortex and has been traditionally thought to have a primary role in the execution of motor programs. Subsequent studies have demonstrated an important cognitive role for this structure as well. Moreover, in primary diseases of the striatum, such as Parkinson's and Huntington's diseases, clinical manifestations include psychosis and other schizophrenia type behavior, which has contributed to interest in this region in the pathophysiology of schizophrenia.

Two related bodies of data are most frequently cited regarding the role of the striatum in schizophrenia; these concern the mechanism of antipsychotic drugs and postmortem studies of altered dopamine $D_2$ receptor numbers. The dorsal striatum (caudate and putamen) is the site of the vast majority of $D_2$ receptors in brain. All effective antipsychotic drugs antagonize this receptor and thus, by extrapolation, it was reasoned that this region might be central to the pathophysiology of schizophrenia (Creese et al. 1975). Moreover, the most consistent postmortem finding in the schizophrenia literature is an increased density of striatal $D_2$ receptors. However, neuroleptic exposure causes up-regulation of $D_2$ receptors, which may account for this postmortem finding. A current view of the antipsychotic mechanism is that the dorsal striatum is involved in mediating the extrapyramidal side effects of antipsychotic medications and, based on rodent studies of antipsychotic drug mechanisms, the ventral striatum (nucleus accumbens) may be involved in antipsychotic efficacy. Thus, attention has shifted toward the possible role of the accumbens in mediating the psychosis of schizophrenia.

Several MRI studies have found an increased volume of the caudate, putamen, and globus pallidus in schizophrenia (Breier et al. 1992, Elkashef et al. 1994). In all cases, the patients included in these studies had exposure to typical neuroleptic treatment, which raised the possibility that striatal enlargement may be secondary to neuroleptic exposure. In a longitudinal study of neuroleptic-naive patients who were subsequently treated with typical neuroleptics, it was found that striatal size was not enlarged before antipsychotic drug treatment but increased after neuroleptic exposure, which supports the notion that (typical) neuroleptics may account for this consistent morphological finding (Chakos et al. 1994). This was further confirmed when increased size of caudate nucleus following long-term antipsychotic exposure normalized after switching to clozapine, an atypical antipsychotic drug which has significantly less activity in the striatal region (Chakos et al. 1995).

## Thalamus

The thalamus is a nucleus that receives subcortical input and outputs it to the cortex. One theory posits that the thalamus provides a filtering function for sensory input to the cortex. A deficit in thalamic filtering was proposed to account in part for the experiential phenomena of being overwhelmed by sensory stimuli reported by many patients with schizophrenia. Preclinical studies have demonstrated that antipsychotic drugs modulate thalamic input to the cortex, which has been offered as a model for antipsychotic drug action. Several MRI studies have reported reduced volume (Andreasen et al. 1994, Gur et al. 1998, Dasari et al. 1999, Hazlett et al. 1999) and functional abnormalities (Buchsbaum and Hazlett 1998, Hazlett et al. 1999) of thalamus in patients with schizophrenia. Postmortem studies have also found cell loss and reductions in tissue volume in thalamic nuclei. This thalamic tissue reduction is considered as a possible evidence of abnormal circuitry linking the cortex, thalamus, and cerebellum (Andreasen 1997).

## Neural Circuits

Because of the large number of different neuroanatomical findings in studies of schizophrenia and the appreciation that brain function involves integration of several brain regions, current thinking about the neuroanatomy of this illness is centered on neural circuits. Thus, investigators are attempting to examine the integrity of a variety of cortical–cortical and cortical–subcortical neural networks that function together to execute behavioral programs. It is conceivable that an isolated lesion anywhere in a neural circuit could result in dysfunction of the entire network, and therefore spurious conclusions could be drawn by investigating only one component of a neural network. Evidence suggests that schizophrenia may be associated with a decrease in synaptic connectivity of the dorsal prefrontal cortex though this is not reported by all studies. McGlashan and Hoffman (2000) have proposed the Developmentally Reduced Synaptic Connectivity (DRSC) model which proposes that cortical gray matter deficits may arise from either reduced baseline synaptic density due to genetic and/or perinatal factors, or excessive pruning of synapses during adolescence and early adulthood or both. Margolis and colleagues (1994) propose that there could be graded apoptosis rather than a necrotic fulminant process. Apoptosis is a form of cell death that occurs in many neurodegenerative disorders in which intra- or extracellular physiologic events trigger a programmed sequence of cellular actions resulting in cell destruction and evacuation (Bresden 1995). According to Goldman-Rakic and Selemon (1997), there is regionally specific decreased neuronal size in cortical layer III with cytoplasmic atrophy and generally reduced neuropil. The reduced size and increased density of neurons or glia and decreased cortical thickness suggest that cell processes and synaptic connections are reduced in schizophrenia. This is consistent with reports of decreased concentrations of synaptic proteins (e.g., synaptophysin). These cell processes and synapses could be lost as a consequence of a neurochemically mediated (through dopamine and or glutamate) synaptic apoptosis that would compromise cell function and alter brain morphology without, however, producing serious cell injury (and thus inducing glial reactions). However, McCarley and colleagues (1999) suggest that the main neural abnormality in schizophrenia involves neural connectivity (dendrite/neuropil/gray matter changes) rather than the number of neurons or network size. They suggest that a "failure of inhibition" on the cellular level is present in schizophrenia and may be linked to a "failure of inhibition" at the cognitive level. According to Lafargue and

Brasic (2000) abnormalities involving the temporolimbic–prefrontal cerebral circuitry is postulated to underlie the organizational and memory deficits commonly observed in schizophrenia patients. Furthermore, as reviewed by these authors, a possible insult or injury to the mechanism of GABAergic and glutamatergic influence during early corticogenesis may largely contribute to the later manifestation of clinical schizophrenia. Malfunction of the cooperating sensory systems of excitation and inhibition during the early stages of development of the brain could result in the failure of "pioneer neurons" to properly differentiate and migrate to their appropriate cerebral locations. Consequently the later migrating projection neurons may fail to reach or invade their preselected area-specific brain sites. A disturbance of the proper GABAergic and glutamatergic influences would upset NMDA mechanisms and normal cortical development. If such disturbance is actively occurring from the onset of cerebral ontogeny, the affected individual may suffer from the signs and symptoms observed in schizophrenia. A challenge for the future is developing new approaches to examining the brain as an integrated and highly interactive system. An unanswered question is whether the morphological differences reflect hypoplasia (failure to develop) or atrophy (shrinkage).

## Electrophysiology

Electroencephalogram (EEG) records the electrical activity of brain, which may reflect the mental functions carried out by the neurons possibly in "real time." However, the precise localization of this event in the specific brain region is poor. When EEG activity from repeated presentations of a specific stimulus is summed across trials, some potentials related to the specific processing of the target stimulus can be extracted from the EEG and are referred as *event-related potentials* (ERPs).

The P300 ERP, a positive deflection occurring approximately 300 milliseconds after the introduction of a stimulus, is regarded as a putative biological marker of risk for schizophrenia (Fricdman 1994, Bharath et al. 2000, Blackwood 2000). The P300 amplitudes are smaller in patients with schizophrenia and is one of the most replicated electrophysiological findings (Bruder 1999, Ford et al. 1999, McCarley et al. 1997). The P300 ERP is often elicited with an oddball paradigm, wherein two stimuli are presented in a random series such that one of them occurs relatively infrequently and subjects are instructed to respond to the infrequent target stimulus (Polich and Herbst 2000). Though the exact neural location of the normal P300 generation are uncertain (Halgren et al. 1995, McCarthy et al. 1997), it is thought that discriminating the target from a standard stimulus should involve frontal lobe. If the neuroelectric events that underlie P300 generation are related to an interaction between frontal lobe and hippocampal/temporal–parietal function (Knight 1996, Knight 1997, Kirino et al. 2000, Demiralp et al. 2001), disease states that affect frontal and temporal/parietal lobe function should also affect P300 measures. This hypothesis has been supported by findings of smaller P300 amplitudes over left temporal scalp locations relative to the homologous right temporal locations for patients with schizophrenia compared to controls (O'Donnell et al. 1999, McCarley et al. 1993).

Remarkably, reductions in the left posterior superior temporal gyrus gray matter volume (using MRI) correlated with the reduction in the temporal P300 amplitude in chronic and first episode schizophrenia (McCarley et al. 1993, 2002). Even though the magnitude of P300 component differences between patients with schizophrenia and control subjects is highly reliable across individual studies (Jeon and Polich 2001), variation for the group effect size is systematically associated with disease definition, stimulus parameters, task conditions, and recording methods (Polich 1998).

N400 is a negative deflection in the ERP occurring approximately 400 milliseconds after introduction of a stimulus, whose latency is thought to reflect the speed of linguistic operations related to semantic search (Van Petten and Kutas 1990). Abnormalities in the N400 amplitude in schizophrenia have been reported (Niznikiewicz et al. 1997, Nestor et al. 1997, Mathalon et al. 2002). Investigators suggest that individuals with schizophrenia do not use the context of the preceding portion of the sentence and fill-in responses to phrases based on the immediately preceding word rather than the whole sentence or passage.

Investigations using newer probes such as atypical antipsychotic agents and their effects on ERPs are interesting; clozapine, in a small sample using a double blind paradigm, improved the amplitude of the P300 but chlorpromazine did not (Patel et al. 2001). Thus, future studies promise interesting information in this area.

## Neurochemical Theories

### Dopamine

Dopamine is the most extensively investigated neurotransmitter system in schizophrenia. In 1973 it was proposed that schizophrenia is related to hyperactivity of dopamine (Matthysee 1973). This proposition became the dominant pathophysiological hypothesis for the next 15 years. Its strongest support came from the fact that all commercially available antipsychotic agents have antagonistic effects on the dopamine $D_2$ receptor in relation to their clinical potencies (Creese et al. 1975). In addition, dopamine agonists, such as amphetamine and methylphenidate, exacerbate psychotic symptoms in a subgroup of patients with schizophrenia. Moreover, as noted earlier, the most consistently reported postmortem finding in the literature of schizophrenia is elevated $D_2$ receptors in the striatum.

The dopamine hyperactivity hypothesis and the primacy of $D_2$ antagonism for antipsychotic drug action were seriously questioned largely because of the advent of clozapine, an atypical antipsychotic drug. Clozapine has proved to be the most efficacious treatment for chronic schizophrenia and yet it has one of the lowest levels of $D_2$ occupancy of all antipsychotic drugs. *In vivo* brain imaging studies demonstrated that clozapine $D_2$ occupancy levels were as low as 20% more than 12 hours after the last dose of medication in patients deriving excellent antipsychotic efficacy (compared with more than 80% $D_2$ occupancy for haloperidol) (Farde et al. 1988, 1989, 1990, 1992) (Figure 62–3). This started an extensive search for explanations underlying the extraordinary efficacy of clozapine. However, new information from PET studies has once again highlighted the central role that the dopaminergic system

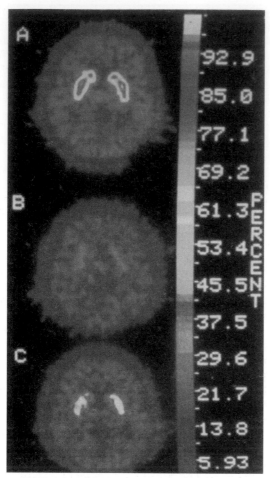

**Figure 62–3** $[^{11}C]$*Raclopride labeling of $D_2$ receptors in the striatum.* (A) *Medication-free healthy control subject.* (B) *Patient treated with 4 mg of haloperidol.* (C) *Patient treated with 500 mg of clozapine.* ( *Source: Farde L, Wiesel FA, Halldin C, et al. [1988] Central $D_2$-dopamine receptor occupancy in schizophrenic patients treated with antipsychotic drugs. Arch Gen Psychiatr 45, 71–76. Copyright 1988 American Medical Association.*) ( *See Color Plate VIII.*)

plays in treatment of psychosis. The typical and atypical antipsychotics are effective only when their $D_2$ receptor occupancy exceeds 65%, reinforcing the importance of $D_2$ antagonism in producing antipsychotic effects. However, an important difference between typical and atypical antipsychotics is in their affinity for the $D_2$ receptors. Medications like clozapine attach loosely to and dissociate rapidly from the dopamine $D_2$ receptors compared to typical antipsychotic agents (like haloperidol) which have strong affinity for and bind tightly to these receptors. Thus, Kapur and Seeman propose that this fast dissociation from the $D_2$ receptors and the low receptor affinity may explain the atypicality of clozapine (for more details see "mechanism of action of atypical antipsychotic drugs" on p. 1175).

Five subtypes of dopamine receptor have now been discovered, $D_1$, $D_2$, $D_3$, $D_4$, and $D_5$, and interest in dopamine receptors other than the $D_2$ receptor has arisen. Reduced levels of $D_1$-like dopamine receptors in the prefrontal cortex of patients with schizophrenia including in those never exposed to antipsychotic agents have been reported. The $D_1$ receptors are expressed predominantly by pyramidal neurons on their dendritic spines, where they possibly modulate glutamate-mediated inputs to these neurons—inputs that mainly come from other pyramidal and thalamic neurons. Thus the reduced $D_1$-like receptors seen in the prefrontal cortex of schizophrenia patients may underlie aspects of cognitive dysfunction and severity of negative symptoms (Nestler 1997).

There was hope that $D_4$ receptor could be a possible pathophysiological candidate for schizophrenia as clozapine was initially reported to have differential affinity for this receptor (van Tol et al. 1991). Contrary to initial expectations, $D_4$ receptors do not uniquely distinguish atypical antipsychotic medications from typical ones (Seeman et al. 1997, Tarazi 2000). Short-term clinical trials involving a limited range of doses of at least two drugs with high $D_4$ potency failed to show antipsychotic effects (Kramer et al. 1997, Truffinet et al. 1999).

Clinical trials of dopamine agonists have resulted in improvements in the negative symptoms of schizophrenia. A new model of dopamine dysfunction was proposed which stated that deficits in dopamine, perhaps in the prefrontal cortex, may result in negative symptoms and that concomitant dopamine dysregulation in the striatum, perhaps related to faulty presynaptic control of dopamine release, may be involved in positive symptoms. This bidirectional model is under investigation.

The DA hypothesis of schizophrenia has been critical in guiding schizophrenia research for several decades. Until recently, a main shortcoming of this hypothesis was absence of direct evidence linking DA dysfunction to schizophrenia. Sophisticated *in vivo* techniques have provided fascinating data directly implicating dopamine in developing psychosis. When the synthesis of dopamine in the brain was measured using PET scan following administration of radiolabeled fluro-L-DOPA, a dopamine precursor, an increase in dopamine was observed in drug-naïve schizophrenia patients compared to age matched controls (Hietala et al. 1994, Dao-Costellano et al. 1997, Lindstrom et al. 1999). Similarly, dopamine release in the basal ganglia was elevated in drug-naïve schizophrenia patients compared to age matched controls when measured by PET and SPECT scans following an amphetamine challenge. This dopamine elevation correlated to the induction of positive symptoms of schizophrenia (Laruelle et al. 1996, Breier et al. 1997, Abi-Dargham et al. 1998). Furthermore, SPECT studies using alpha-methyltyrosine showed that unchallenged release of dopamine was elevated in schizophrenia patients compared to controls (Laruelle et al. 1996). Arvid Carlsson, the Nobel Laureate, and his colleagues (2001), whose work led to the original dopamine hypothesis, appreciate the significance of this data but observe that a wide scatter exists with some values of dopamine release being within normal range in patients with schizophrenia. They suggest that these findings may reflect heterogeneity where dopamine dysfunction may be limited to a subgroup of patients with schizophrenia. Furthermore, the observation that the elevated dopamine release correlates with a good clinical response to antipsychotic medications leads Carlsson and colleagues to suggest that DA release may be state dependent such that studies done in acute conditions may yield different results then in chronic remitted patient. However, it is also becoming clear that dopamine works closely with serotonin, glutamate, and other systems such that changes in one system affects the balance of the other systems too (see later).

## Serotonin

Interest in serotonin as a pathophysiological candidate in schizophrenia arose in the 1950s with the discovery that the hallucinogen lysergic acid diethylamide (LSD) had primary effects on serotonin neurotransmission. Several studies were conducted to characterize its behavioral profile to determine whether LSD psychosis was a suitable model of schizophrenia. Indeed, LSD produces some features of schizophrenia, including a profound psychotic state, distractibility, social withdrawal, referential thinking, and delusions. However, the most prominent feature of LSD psychosis is visual hallucinations, and auditory hallucinations are exceedingly rare. Visual hallucinations are quite rare among patients with schizophrenia and auditory hallucinations are among the most common symptoms of the illness. Thus, because of the failure to mimic key features of schizophrenia and the growing interest in dopamine at that time, enthusiasm for serotonin's involvement in the pathophysiology of schizophrenia waned for some time (Breier 1995).

Clozapine has a relatively high affinity for specific serotonin (5-hydroxytryptamine [5-HT]) receptors (5-HT$_{2A}$ and 5-HT$_{2C}$) and risperidone, has even greater serotonin antagonistic properties (Schotte et al. 1996). Clozapine, risperidone, olanzapine, quetiapine, and ziprasidone, the novel antipsychotic agents, have a greater ratio of serotonin 5-HT$_{2A}$ to dopamine D$_2$ binding affinity. This has led to the hypothesis that the balance between serotonin and dopamine may be altered in schizophrenia (Meltzer et al. 1989c). Serotonin 5-HT$_{2A}$ (and other serotonin) receptor occupancy by the antipsychotic drugs, depending on the areas of the brain involved, could be associated with improvement in cognition, depression, and D$_2$ receptor mediated EPS (Kasper et al. 1999).

In addition to the renewed interest in serotonin because of the action of new antipsychotic drugs, several postmortem studies have found elevations of serotonin and its metabolites in the striatum of patients with schizophrenia. Again, as was the case with striatal D$_2$ receptors, previous neuroleptic exposure may have contributed to this finding. Another common finding is decreased 5-HT$_{2A}$ receptor densities in prefrontal cortex. Several postmortem studies (Gurevich and Joyce 1997, Burnet et al. 1997) and a recent *in vivo* PET study (Tauscher et al. 2002) have shown elevation of 5-HT$_{1A}$ receptor density in the cortex of patients with schizophrenia. The relevance of these findings are not clear. Some, but not all investigators, have reported that the partial serotoninergic agonist *m*-chlorophenylpiperazine causes psychotic exacerbations in patients with schizophrenia but has no psychosis-inducing properties in normal control subjects.

There has been an explosion of new information about the structure and function of 5-HT receptors (Breier 1995). To date, 15 serotonin receptor subtypes have been identified. Two receptors, 5-HT$_6$ and 5-HT$_7$, have been proposed as candidates for atypical drug action and are therefore reasonable targets for pathophysiological studies of schizophrenia. It is clear that the field is in the early stages of understanding the possible involvement of serotonin in schizophrenia.

## Glutamate and *N*-Methyl-D-aspartate Receptor

Glutamate is a major brain excitatory amino acid neurotransmitter and is critically involved in learning, memory, and brain development. There are five excitatory amino acid receptors in brain: *N*-methyl-D-aspartate (NMDA), AMPA, kainate, metabotropic, and L-AP-4. Interest in glutamate and the NMDA receptor in schizophrenia arose because of the similarity between phencyclidine (PCP) psychosis and the psychosis of schizophrenia. PCP is a noncompetitive antagonist of the NMDA receptor and produces a psychotic state that includes conceptual disorganization, auditory hallucinations, delusions, and negative symptoms. PCP produces more symptoms that are similar to those of schizophrenia than most other pharmacological agents. It should be noted that PCP produces behaviors that are not commonly seen in schizophrenia as well, including spatial and temporal distortion, dreamlike states, and violence. Other findings that support a hypoglutamatergic function in schizophrenia are decreased glutamate levels in cerebrospinal fluid and increased NMDA receptor number and decreased glutamate binding in neocortex in postmortem studies.

PCP and other highly potent NMDA receptor antagonists, such as MK-801, cause neuronal damage and therefore are not used as research tools in clinical populations. However, ketamine, a widely used dissociative anesthetic, is another noncompetitive NMDA antagonist and, at subanesthetic doses, produces a PCP-like psychosis resembling schizophrenia (Krystal et al. 1994, Tamminga 1999). In a PET study of healthy volunteers, subanesthetic ketamine administration produced a robust psychotic state and focal activation of the prefrontal cortex, suggesting that prefrontal NMDA receptors may mediate this schizophrenia-like behavioral syndrome. The Glutamate hypothesis of schizophrenia is one of the most active areas of research currently. Postmortem studies have reported alterations in NMDA recept or expression in certain brain areas of patients with schizophrenia (Gao et al. 2000). NMDA receptor is reported to play a critical role in guiding axons to their final destination during neurodevelopment. Also, abnormalities with glutamate transmission is reported in many areas of the brain such as frontal cortex, hippocampus, limbic cortex, striatum, and thalamus. Moreover, there are changes reported in the gene expression also in these areas. In animal models of NMDA receptor antagonists, atypical antipsychotic agents are more effective in ameliorating symptoms (Gainetdinov et al. 2001). Thus, hypoglutamatergia in schizophrenia may have very important downstream modulatory effects on catecholaminergic neurotransmission and play a critical role during neurodevelopment. It also plays an important role in synaptic pruning and underlies important aspects of neurocognition.

## GABA

GABA is the major inhibitory neurotransmitter in brain. Support for GABA's involvement in schizophrenia comes from two lines of investigation. First, clinical trials have demonstrated that benzodiazepines, administered both in conjunction with antipsychotic drugs and as the sole treatment, are effective at reducing symptoms in subgroups of schizophrenia patients (Wolkowitz and Pickar 1991). Benzodiazepines are agonists at GABA$_A$ receptors. Second, postmortem studies have found a deficit in GABA interneurons in the anterior cingulum and prefrontal cortex and decreased GABA uptake sites in hippocampus (Benes et al. 1991). GABAergic neurons are especially vulnerable to glucocorticoid hormones and also to glutamatergic excitotoxicity.

## Peptides

Several peptides have been hypothesized to play a pathophysiological role in schizophrenia. Interest in neurotensin arose because of the discovery that it is colocalized in some dopaminergic neurons and acts as a neuromodulator of this and other neurotransmitters. In preclinical studies, neurotensin was found to have effects that resembled those of antipsychotic drugs (Kasckow and Nemeroff 1991, Binder et al. 2001) and antipsychotic drugs cause increases in neurotensin levels in rat brain (Bisette et al. 1988). In addition, schizophrenia patients were found to have lower cerebrospinal fluid neurotensin levels than healthy control subjects and other patients with neuropsychiatric disorders. Another peptide with neuromodulatory actions that was found to be colocalized with dopamine and was therefore of interest in relation to schizophrenia is cholecystokinin. Unlike the case of neurotensin, however, there has been a lack of consistent data from postmortem and cerebrospinal fluid studies of patients with schizophrenia. Moreover, a clinical trial of CCK-8, a cholecystokinin analogue, has failed to demonstrate antipsychotic efficacy (Montgomery and Green 1988). Other peptides that are under consideration for a pathophysiological role in schizophrenia are somatostatin, dynorphin, substance P, and neuropeptide Y.

## Norepinephrine

Heightened noradrenergic function has been implicated in psychotic relapse in subgroups of schizophrenia patients (van Kammen et al. 1990). In addition, clozapine, but not other neuroleptic drugs, consistently produces increases in central and peripheral indices of noradrenergic function, and one study found a significant relationship between increases in plasma norepinephrine and improvement in positive symptoms (Breier et al. 1994) (Figure 62–4).

## The Biochemical Theory

Carlsson and colleagues (2001) provide a multineurotransmitter theory of schizophrenia which improves upon previous biochemical theories of schizophrenia. Accumulating evidence suggests that hyperdopaminergia in schizophrenia is probably secondary to some other phenomena. The data involving glutamatergic system suggests that NMDA receptor antagonism enhances the spontaneous and amphetamine-induced release of dopamine and thus raises the possibility that *hypoglutamatergia* could be related to the

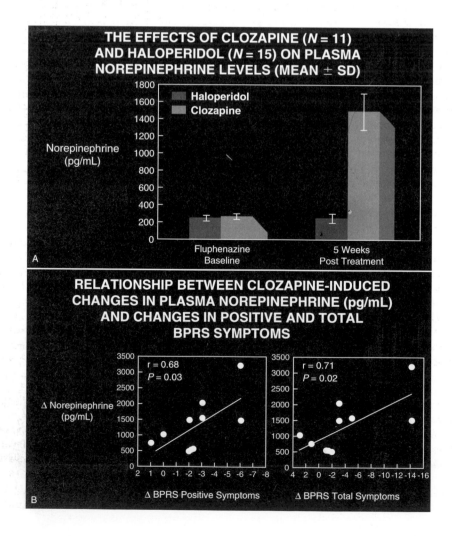

**Figure 62–4** (A) *Fivefold increase in plasma norepinephrine in patients with schizophrenia treated with clozapine for 5 weeks.* (B) *Significant relationship between improvement in symptoms and increases in plasma norepinephrine with clozapine. (Source: Breier A, Buchanan RW, Waltrip RW, et al. [1994] The effect of clozapine on plasma norepinephrine: Relationship to clinical efficacy. Neuropsychopharmacology 10, 1–7. Copyright 1994 American College of Neuropsychopharmacology. Reprinted with permission from Elsevier Science.)*

*hyperdopaminergia*. Carlsson and colleagues (2001) propose that psychotogenesis depends on an interaction between dopamine and glutamate pathways projecting to the striatum from the lower brain stem and cortex respectively. These neurotransmitters are predominantly antagonistic to each other, the former being inhibitory and the latter stimulatory when acting on striatal GABAergic projection neurons. These GABAergic neurons belong to striatothalamic pathways, which exert an inhibitory action on thalamocortical glutamatergic neurons, thereby filtering off part of the sensory input to the thalamus to protect the cortex from a sensory overload and hyperarousal. Hyperactivity of dopamine or hypofunction of the corticostriatal glutamate pathway should reduce this protective influence and could thus lead to confusion or psychosis. As a result, the indirect striatothalamic pathways have an inhibitory influence on the thalamus with the corresponding direct pathways exerting an opposite and excitatory influence. Both pathways are controlled by glutamatergic corticostriatal pathways enabling the cortex to regulate the thalamic gating in opposite directions. Thus, according to Carlsson and colleagues (2001), they appear to serve as *brakes* and *accelerators*.

It has been suggested that the activity of the direct pathways is predominantly phasic and of the indirect pathways is mainly tonic. This difference could have important consequences for a different responsiveness of the direct and indirect pathways to drugs. Thus the NMDA receptor antagonists are behavioral stimulants. AMPA receptor antagonists act in the same direction as NMDA antagonists in some and opposite direction in other experiments. Thus, the two most important animal models of psychosis are those induced by hyperfunction of dopamine and hypofunction of glutamate. The relationship between glutamate and serotonin is very important and interesting. Serotonin appears to play a more important role than dopamine in the behavioral stimulation induced by hypoglutamatergia. In two models of psychosis, haloperidol is quite powerful in alleviating the hyperdopaminergic stimulation induced by amphetamine but is least efficacious in the hypoglutamatergic behavioral stimulation induced by MK-801. However, M100907, a selective serotonin 5-HT$_{2A}$ antagonist is clearly more powerful in counteracting MK-801 than amphetamine-induced stimulation. These observations indicate that serotonin may play a more prominent role than dopamine in the behavioral stimulation induced by hypoglutamatergia. Schizophrenia is a syndrome of heterogeneous etiology and pathology. If one neurotransmitter is disturbed, it will inevitably have an impact on other neurotransmitters (Carlsson et al. 2001).

## Neurodevelopmental Versus Neurodegenerative Disease Processes

Neurodevelopmental hypotheses of schizophrenia posit that a disruption in normal development causes the illness (Weinberger 1987, Cannon et al. 2000). Thus, the "lesion" occurs well before the onset of the illness and interacts with maturation events such as neuronal precursor, glial proliferation and migration; axonal and dendritic proliferation; myelination of axons; programmed cell death and synaptic pruning (Lieberman 1999a); and is in all likelihood a nonprogressive disease process (Lewis 1997). Support for the neurodevelopment hypothesis includes the fact that the

majority of patients with schizophrenia do not have a course of illness marked by progressive deterioration such as found in dementias. In addition, brain morphological abnormalities commonly found in this illness, such as enlarged ventricles and reduced mesolimbic structures, do not appear to be progressive and, in fact, are present at the onset of the illness. Moreover, gliosis, which occurs during active pathological processes as part of the cellular reparative process in mature brains, is not commonly found in postmortem studies of schizophrenia.

That illness onset typically occurs in the teenage years and early twenties, as opposed to earlier in life when the proposed pathogenic insult occurs, has been explained by the fact that brain regions implicated in this illness, such as prefrontal cortex, are still undergoing myelination during the adolescent years and are therefore not fully functional until that time. Thus, an early lesion involving this region could remain silent until adolescence, when its normal functional capacity is expected to be realized. However, these assumptions have been questioned based on the MRI findings of changes in the volume of brain areas in patients with schizophrenia over a period of time (Woods 1998, Lieberman 1999b). As reviewed by Weinberger and McClure (2002), this has generated interest in the "neurodegenerative hypothesis" of schizophrenia as originally proposed by Kraepelin and others. However, based on the evidence available thus far, they suggest that it is unlikely that the MRI changes imply neurodegeneration. The argument is supported by the contradictory findings of clinical improvement in patients in the face of progressive changes in MRI. Furthermore, the magnitude of the changes suggested by some of the MRI studies are large enough to be observed in neurodegenerative diseases like Alzheimer's without the postmortem evidence of neurodegeneration. Thus, Weinberger and McClure caution against overinterpretation of the MRI data without converging information from other areas. They suggest that there may be other possible explanations for these findings including physiological variations, neuroadaptation, and so on. Newer and more sophisticated techniques will help interpret MRI data more coherently.

## Clinical Manifestations and Phenomenology

The idea that schizophrenia can be divided into subgroups has been explored since the illness was first described. Attempts to subdivide schizophrenia have been based on multiple factors including symptom patterns, as in paranoid versus nonparanoid or reactive versus process schizophrenia, or outcome, such as the good versus poor prognosis subtypes. Biological and clinical factors, including platelet monoamine oxidase activity, amphetamine induction of psychosis, neurological soft signs, and perinatal complications, have also been considered in subgrouping this complex illness, although these classifications have generally not withstood the test of time as valid means of subdividing schizophrenia.

### Positive and Negative Symptoms

There has been an emphasis on positive and negative symptom clusters in some schizophrenia patients. Positive and negative symptoms were first described by Sir John Russell Reynolds, a British neurologist who had worked with epileptic patients. In 1857, in a presentation to a division of the London Medical Society, he proposed that physical signs could manifest themselves in positive and negative forms (Berrios 1985). The prominent neurologist Hughlings-Jackson (Jackson 1987) expanded on Reynolds' statement by positing that negative symptoms could be thought of in terms of an upper motor neuron deficit that leads to the lower motor neuron hyperactivity, which he identified as a positive symptom. By definition, then, both negative and positive symptoms would be found in the same individual and there would be a causative relationship between them. In the psychiatric literature, positive symptoms have come to mean those that are actively expressed, such as hallucinations, thought disorder, delusions, and bizarre behavior, whereas negative symptoms reflect deficit states such as avolition, flattened affect, and alogia.

How these distinct symptom patterns are related in schizophrenia remains unresolved. Bleuler had conceptualized fundamental and accessory symptoms, and Schneider had divided symptoms into those of first and second rank, but neither specifically addressed positive and negative symptom subdivisions. Strauss and colleagues (1974) considered positive and negative symptoms as distinct symptom patterns associated with clinical course over time, with negative symptoms being more associated with poor long-term outcome. Subsequent hypotheses considered positive and negative symptoms to be either two end points of a spectrum of symptoms or a single disease process in which either the positive or negative symptoms are primary and the other symptoms become a secondary response.

That schizophrenia could be divided into a two-syndrome concept was put forth by Crow (1980) of the Clinical Research Center at Northwick Park Hospital in England. According to his theory, type I schizophrenia patients are those who present, often more acutely, with a predominantly positive symptom profile and who have a good response to neuroleptics. In contrast, type II schizophrenia patients are those who have a more chronic illness, more frequent evidence of intellectual impairment and enlarged ventricular size and cortical atrophy as seen on CT or MRI scans, a poorer response to neuroleptics, and predominantly negative symptoms. Crow further postulated that type I schizophrenia may be secondary to a hyperdopaminergic state, whereas type II disease may be due to structural abnormality of the brain.

The idea that positive and negative symptoms may be overlapping end points along a single continuum of biological and clinical manifestations has been described by Andreasen and colleagues (1982). In their study of 52 schizophrenia patients, they found that negative symptoms correlated with the presence of ventricular enlargement and that patients with small ventricles were more likely to manifest positive symptoms. In a separate report, Andreasen and Olsen (1982) posited that negative and positive symptoms reflect opposite extremes of a spectrum and that a mixed symptom pattern can exist and may be present 30% of the time. Others have suggested that although the positive and negative characteristics may be part of a continuum, they may not be related to the presence or absence of structural brain abnormalities; rather, there may be a relationship between the symptom pattern and outcome, depending on the clinical course.

A categorical scheme for differentiation of so-called primary and secondary negative symptoms was developed by Carpenter and colleagues (1985). This distinction is based in part on the fact that negative symptoms are not pathognomonic of schizophrenia. The negative symptoms that can be seen in a number of other illnesses, including depression and medical illness, and as a result of positive symptoms themselves or the side effects of medication, particularly extrapyramidal symptoms, are considered "secondary." The negative symptoms that are a core element of schizophrenia are deemed "primary" or "deficit" symptoms. This distinction enables further exploration of outcome variables and the heterogeneity of this illness and in many ways aids treatment decisions.

Because positive and negative symptoms may be seen differently by individual psychiatrists, valid psychometric scales have become important clinical and research tools. The Brief Psychiatric Rating Scale (BPRS) (Overall and Gorham 1961), for example, includes subscales for positive and negative symptoms, as does the Positive and Negative Syndrome Scale (PANSS) for schizophrenia (Kay et al. 1988). Others have more broadly defined negative symptoms. Crow (1985) proposed the use of a narrow definition, that is, flattened affect and poverty of speech, for negative symptoms, and Andreasen (1981) supported a broader definition in the widely used Scale for the Assessment of Negative Symptoms (SANS). This psychometric scale includes categories of alogia and flattened affect as well as items such as anhedonia, asociality, avolition, apathy, and deficits in attention.

Structured Clinical Interview for DSM-IV (SCID) is a semi-structured diagnostic interview designed to be administered by an experienced clinician. Though primarily used in research, a user-friendly clinician version (SCID-CV) is also available (First et al. 1996). It is a very helpful instrument for systematic evaluation in psychiatric patients.

## Symptom Cluster Analysis

Although the dichotomous positive–negative distinction has gained clinical and research recognition, several reports suggest that this division is incomplete. Much of the current interest in understanding the heterogeneity of schizophrenia has involved a more detailed look at the symptoms of schizophrenia. Sophisticated statistical techniques utilize factor analysis to reduce data to elucidate clusters of symptoms that are most likely to group together or be found independently.

An application of this approach found that there are three, rather than two, symptom dimensions that better subdivide schizophrenia. Correlational relationships between symptoms reveal that positive symptoms can be divided into two distinct groups. The first includes psychotic symptoms such as hallucinations and delusions, and the second includes symptoms of disorganization, consisting of thought disorder, bizarre behavior, and inappropriate affect. A third group is that of negative symptoms. Although these patterns of symptoms may be seen in different proportions in individuals and may change over time, they can be shown to have distinct clinical courses and may be related to independent neuropsychological deficits in a given individual (Andreasen et al. 1995).

In a 2-year follow-up study of these different symptom patterns, negative symptoms were found to remain stable and the other two dimensions were found to have a more fluctuating pattern (Arndt et al. 1995). This study found that the three symptom dimensions changed independently.

An earlier report supporting three distinct symptom dimensions came from a study of neuropsychological and neurological findings in relation to schizophrenic symptoms (Liddle 1987). In this study, patients with a predominantly negative symptom dimension were shown to have cognitive deficits related to the frontal lobe, as were patients with thought disorder and inappropriate affect, but the specific deficits appeared to be related to different regions of the frontal lobe. Furthermore, patients who presented primarily with delusions and hallucinations appeared to have neuropsychological deficits associated with the temporal lobe.

Further investigation is warranted to understand the role of these three symptom dimensions in the onset, course, and treatment of schizophrenia. In addition, this factor analytical division of schizophrenic symptoms must be evaluated to understand their relationship to genetic and neurochemical mechanisms.

## Cognitive Impairment

In an attempt to describe schizophrenia in a way that was different from prevailing psychodynamic principles of the day, McGhie and Chapman (1961) reported that schizophrenia patients demonstrated profound deficits in selective attention. This idea had also been described earlier by both Kraepelin (1919) and Bleuler (1950). At present, there is a growing body of literature supporting this observation. By now it is widely accepted that schizophrenia patients experience neuropsychological deficits that can be characterized by difficulties with attention, information processing, executive function, learning, and memory, which leads to a generalized performance deficit. Typically, there is a wide variance with some aspects of performance being more impaired then others. Interestingly, a small subgroup of the patients have cognitive functioning within the normal range (Palmer et al. 1997). Most patients with schizophrenia have only modest reductions in their IQs with an average of 90 (Frith et al. 1991, Kremen et al. 2001), and about 0.67 standard deviation below that of the general population. In contrast, their performance is usually worse (Heaton et al. 1994) even in first episode patients (Gold et al. 1999, Riley et al. 2000). Usually patients with schizophrenia underperform relative to estimates of their premorbid functioning (Harvey 2001). Cognitive impairments involving verbal learning, verbal delayed recall, working memory, vigilance and executive functioning have a significant negative impact on social and occupational functioning (Green 1996, Harvey et al. 1998). Two meta-analysis of 24 and 9 studies respectively suggest that treatment with novel antipsychotic agents improve cognitive function compared to typical antipsychotic agents (Keefe et al. 1999, Harvey 2001).

The degree of cognitive deficit appears to be more strongly associated with severity of negative symptoms, symptoms of disorganization, and adaptive dysfunction (Tollefson et al. 1997, Beasley et al. 1996) then with positive symptoms (Blin et al. 1996). Verbal fluency is severely impaired in patients with psychotic disorders and the use of atypical antipsychotic medications results in significant improvement (Keefe et al. 1999, Velligan and Miller 1999). Motor functions (e.g., reaction time, motor and graphomotor speed) improve with clozapine, olanzapine, and risperidone (Myer-Lindenberg et al. 1997, Gallhoffer et al. 1996, Purdon et al. 2000). Olanzapine improves motor functions more than either haloperidol or risperidone (Purdon et al. 2000). Furthermore, motor functions are related to outcome, underscoring the importance of this domain. The symbol–digit and digit–symbol tests have been among the most responsive tests to atypical antipsychotic treatment (Keefe et al. 1999).

As a test of executive function, performance on the Wisconsin Card Sorting Test (WCST) improves with clozapine, risperidone, and olanzapine, although many negative findings have been reported (Meltzer and McGurk 1999). In Wisconsin Card Sorting Test, subjects sort a series of stimulus cards by matching them to four "key cards" that differ by form, color, and number. Successful performance on the WCST depends upon learning how to sort the cards and how to switch the sorting strategy when appropriate, since the "correct" sorting strategy changes after 10 consecutive correct responses.

Though the novel antipsychotic agents appear to have beneficial effects on cognition, much work still remains to eliminate biases; also, effect sizes of these improvements are modest (Harvey and Keefe 2001).

## Information Processing and Attention

The term *information processing* is used to describe the process of taking information and encoding it in such a way that it can be understood and recalled when appropriately cued. This construct is related to neural circuits and a stepwise logical spread of neurochemical messages, which may be impaired in schizophrenia. *Attention*, simply defined, is the ability to focus on a stimulus, either through conscious effort or passively. These two constructs are interrelated, and our understanding of their composite parts has increased in complexity in the past few decades.

Measures of attention were developed from the idea that patients with schizophrenia cannot block out unimportant stimuli in the way that those without schizophrenia can. This phenomenon has come to be called *gating*. Gating is usually seen, for example, when a weak stimulus is delivered before a real stimulus. Normally, the first stimulus would dampen or eliminate the response to the second. Two measures to assess gating function in patients with schizophrenia are the P50 event-related potential (related to sensory gating) and pre-pulse inhibition of the startle response (related to sensorimotor gating). As an example of these measures, the P50 event-related potential examines responses to auditory stimuli, and the amplitude of the P50 is indicative of a response change between two stimuli. The amplitude reduction of the P50 response from a first auditory click to a second auditory click is known as P50 suppression. Data suggests that patients with schizophrenia have significantly lower than normal levels of P50 suppression (Light and Braff 2001, Braff and Geyer 1990).

Specific methods employed in the assessment of information processing and attention are numerous and have been reviewed (Braff 1993). The general principles behind each technique are related. Continuous performance tasks (Rosvold et al. 1956), for example, are tests of attention in which the subject must isolate a specific stimulus among repeated distractor stimuli. The stimulus can be in any sensory modality, such as a tone or a letter flashed on a screen. Another test of information processing is prepulse inhibition, which is the inhibition of a startle response by a weaker warning stimulus. Event-related potentials measure electrical brain activity after some sort of stimulus such as an auditory click.

Other information-processing measurements reported to be abnormal in some schizophrenia patients have included the skin conduction orienting response (Bernstein 1987). This test involves habituation to a stimulus applied to the skin. Eye-tracking abnormalities such as smooth pursuit eye movements have also been found to be abnormal in schizophrenia patients (Holzman 1987).

In general, patients with schizophrenia have impairments in information processing, especially when they are exposed to increasing demands on their attentional capabilities, such as under timed conditions or in stressful situations. Therefore, these deficits not only are viewed as trait linked (i.e., a manifestation of the illness itself) but may be compounded when state linked (i.e., when there are increases in symptoms) (Sacuzzo and Braff 1981). The trait-linked disturbances in neuropsychological parameters are seen in those at high risk for developing schizophrenia, those who have schizophrenia, and relatives who appear clinically unaffected, which may indicate a genetic vulnerability (Braff 1993, Cannon et al. 1994).

Many of these tests of attention and information processing have been associated with specific symptoms and neuropsychological impairment in schizophrenia. For example, one study showed that impaired prepulse inhibition was related to increased perseveration on neuropsychological tests of higher executive function (Butler et al. 1991). Others have shown that deficits in attention and information processing may be associated with positive and/or negative symptoms (Strauss 1993). Specifically, deficits in visual processing and motor function (as seen with continuous performance tasks) have been linked to negative symptoms (Nuechterlein et al. 1986), whereas positive symptoms seem to be related to auditory-processing dysfunction (Green and Walker 1986).

Interestingly, abnormalities in these tests of information processing are not induced by typical neuroleptic agents and, moreover, these medications may partially ameliorate the deficits (Spohn et al. 1977, Medalia et al. 1988). Attention has been reported to improve with risperidone (Stip and Lussier, 1996, Rossi et al. 1997, Kern et al. 1998), clozapine (Zahn et al. 1994, Grace et al. 1996), olanzapine (Purdon et al. 2001, Meltzer and McGurk 1999), and quetiapine (Sax et al. 1998). Investigations of the role of novel antipsychotic agents in improving these abnormalities in very large samples and with head-to-head comparisons to each other are under way (CATIE Study/NIMH 1999). Because these deficits are seen more frequently in individuals with schizophrenia, their relatives, and those at risk of developing schizophrenia, the application of information-processing and sophisticated attention techniques may lead to more information about the heritability and genetics of schizophrenia. Further investigation

regarding their correlation with specific symptom clusters, the effects of antipsychotic medications, and the relationship of these deficits to specific brain regions studied with PET and functional MRI should enhance our understanding of the neurocircuitry involved in these impairments.

## Learning and Memory

Although there are generally no consistent gross deficits of memory in schizophrenia patients, close examination of certain aspects of learning and memory has revealed striking abnormalities. Schizophrenia patients have been shown to be poorer in recall of word lists if the words are not grouped into categories (Koh 1978). Furthermore, unlike normal control subjects, schizophrenia patients do not seem to show an improvement in memory when asked to recall words with latent positive emotional meaning (Koh 1978). These findings have been attributed to poor cognitive organization in schizophrenia patients (Harvey et al. 1986).

Others have reported that patients with chronic schizophrenia had impairment in new learning and short-term memory but not remote memory (Calev et al. 1987), possibly indicating temporal–hippocampal dysfunction (Saykin et al. 1991). These may be more likely in patients with a poor premorbid course (Calev and Monk 1982) and ventricular enlargement (Golden et al. 1980). In addition, in a long-term follow-up study of schizophrenia patients, those with memory impairment had a poorer outcome in terms of social and occupational function (Tsuang 1982).

Typical neuroleptic medications have not been shown to affect memory (Calev 1984), unlike anticholinergic medications, which may decrease memory performance (Frith 1984, Zachariah et al. 2000). Despite these findings, some questions regarding the role of chronicity and (typical) neuroleptic exposure in memory impairment has remained. It appears, however, that these deficits are inherent to schizophrenia itself, as impairment in verbal memory has been demonstrated even in neuroleptic-naive first-episode schizophrenia patients (Saykin et al. 1994). Data from nine small sample studies did not suggest that atypical antipsychotic medication significantly improved verbal memory (Keefe et al. 1999). However, two recent small studies suggest that quetiapine may improve verbal memory (Velligan and Miller 1999, Purdon et al. 2000).

Working memory is a cognitive system that stores and processes information needed for planning and reasoning for a brief duration. Some cognitive scientists refer to short-term memory as working memory. Working memory consists of verbal and visual memory subsystems with a central principle that manipulates and coordinates information stored in the two systems for problem solving, planning and organizing activities. Separate areas of the prefrontal cortex may underlie different aspects of the working memory. The workspace used for such memory is capacity-limited. Patients with schizophrenia have significant dysfunction in this area and are unable to change an ineffective strategy (i.e., shift sets) even when feedback is provided (Stirling et al. 1997, Goldberg et al. 1998). This dysfunction occurs (albeit at a lower level) even in subjects with higher intelligence (Pantelis et al. 1999). Conventional antipsychotics do not appear to impair or improve working memory in patients with schizophrenia (Goldberg and Weinberger 1996). There is limited evidence to support clozapine's role in enhancing working memory (Galletly et al. 1997, Hagger et al. 1993, Lee et al. 1994, Grace et al. 1996). Risperidone may improve aspects of working memory functions (Green et al. 1997, Rossi et al. 1997, Meltzer and McGurk 1999). Studies involving evaluation of working memory using neuroimaging, pharmacological models of schizophrenia, and neurochemical function should further our understanding of this manifestation of schizophrenia.

## Differential Diagnosis

Making an accurate diagnosis of schizophrenia requires high levels of clinical acumen, extensive knowledge of schizophrenia, and sophisticated application of the principles of differential diagnosis. It is unfortunately common for patients with psychotic disorders to be misdiagnosed and consequently treated inappropriately. The importance of accurate diagnosis is underlined by an emerging database indicating that early detection and prompt pharmacological intervention may improve the long-term prognosis of the illness.

## Mental Status Examination

There is no specific laboratory test, neuroimaging study, or clinical presentation of a patient that yields a definitive diagnosis of schizophrenia. Schizophrenia can present with a wide variety of symptoms, and a longitudinal history of symptoms and comorbid clinical variables such as medical illness and a history of substance abuse are necessary before a diagnosis can be considered. The Mental Status Examination, much like the physical examination, is an additional clinical tool that aids the psychiatrist in generating a differential diagnosis and appropriate treatment recommendations.

### Appearance

Although a disheveled look is not pathognomonic for schizophrenia, patients with this disorder often present, especially acutely, with a disordered appearance. The description of a patient's appearance is an objective verbal sketch, much like the description of a heart murmur, that can uniquely identify a particular patient.

A person with schizophrenia often has difficulty attending to activities of daily living, either because of negative symptoms (apathy, social withdrawal, or motor retardation) or because of the presence of positive symptoms, such as psychosis, disorganization, or catatonia, that interfere with the ability to maintain personal hygiene. Also, schizophrenia patients often present with odd or inappropriate attire, such as a coat and hat worn during the summer or dark sunglasses worn during an interview. It is generally thought that the inappropriate dress is a manifestation of symptoms such as disorganization or paranoid ideation. It should be noted that some patients present quite neatly groomed. Thus appearance is noted but is not diagnostic.

### Attitude

Individuals with schizophrenia may be friendly and cooperative, or they may be hostile, annoyed, and defensive during an interview. The latter may be secondary to paranoid symptoms, which can make patients quite cautious and guarded in their responses to questions.

### Behavior

Schizophrenic patients can have bizarre mannerisms or stereotyped movements that can make them look unusual. Patients with catatonia can stay in one position for weeks, even to the point of causing serious physical damage to their body; for example, a patient who stands in one place for days may develop stress fractures, peripheral edema, and even pulmonary emboli. Patients with catatonia may have waxy flexibility, maintaining a position after someone else has moved them into it. Patients with catatonic excitement exhibit odd posturing or purposeless, repetitive, and often strange movements.

Behaviors seen in schizophrenia patients include choreoathetoid movements, which may be related to neuroleptic exposure but have been reported in patients even before neuroleptic use. Other behaviors or movement disorders may be seen as parkinsonian features, such as a shuffling gait or a pill-rolling tremor.

Psychomotor retardation may be present and may be a manifestation of catatonia or negative symptoms. On close observation, it is usually characterized, in this group of patients, as a lack of motor movements rather than slowed movements.

Patients may present with agitation, ranging from minimal to extreme. This agitation is often seen in the acute state and may require immediate pharmacotherapy. However, agitation may be secondary to neuroleptic medications, as in akathisia, which is felt as an internal restlessness making it difficult for the person to sit still. Akathisia can manifest itself in limb shaking, pacing, or frequent shifting of position. Severely agitated patients may be unresponsive to verbal limits and may require measures to ensure their safety and the safety of others around them.

### Eye Contact

Paranoid patients may look hypervigilant, scanning a room or glancing suspiciously at an interviewer. Psychotic patients may make poor eye contact, looking away, or appear to stare vacuously at the interviewer, making a conversational connection seem distant. Characteristic responding to internal stimuli is seen when a patient appears to look toward a voice or an auditory hallucination, which the patient may hear. A nystagmus may also be observed. This clinical finding has a large differential diagnosis, including Wernicke–Korsakoff syndrome; alcohol, barbiturate, or phenytoin intoxication; viral labyrinthitis; or brain stem syndromes including infarctions or multiple sclerosis (Adams and Victor 1989).

### Speech

In a Mental Status Examination, one usually comments on the rate, tone, and volume of a patient's speech, as well as any distinct dysarthrias that may be present. Pressured speech is usually thought of in conjunction with mania; however, it can be seen in schizophrenia patients, particularly on acute presentation. This is often difficult to assess, as it may be a normal variant or a cultural phenomenon, because some languages are spoken faster than others.

Tone refers to prosody, or the natural singsong quality of speech. Negative symptoms may include a lack of prosody, resulting in monotonous speech. Furthermore, odd tones may be consistent with neurological disorders or bizarre behavior.

Speech volume is important for a number of reasons. Loud speech can be a measure of agitation, it can occur in conjunction with psychosis, or it could even be an indication of hearing loss. Speech that is soft may be an indication of guardedness or anxiety.

Dysarthrias are notable because they can be idiopathic and long-standing, or they can be an indication of neurological disturbance. In patients who have been exposed to neuroleptics, orobuccal tardive dyskinesia should be considered when there is evidence of slurred speech.

## Mood and Affect

Affect, which is the observer's objective view of the patient's emotional state, is often constricted or flat in patients with schizophrenia. In fact, this is one of the hallmark negative symptoms. Flattened affect may also be a manifestation of pseudoparkinsonism, an extrapyramidal side effect of typical neuroleptics.

Inappropriate affect is commonly seen in patients with more predominant positive symptoms. A smile or a laugh while relating a sad tale is an example. Patients with catatonic excitement or hebephrenia may have bizarre presentations or affective lability, laughing and crying out of context with the situation. Emotional reactivity must alert the clinician to the possibility of neurological impairment as well, as in the case of pseudobulbar palsy (Adams and Victor 1989).

Mood is based on a patient's subjective report of how he or she feels, emotionally, at the time of the interview. It is not uncommon for patients with schizophrenia to be depressed (especially patients with history of higher premorbid functioning who may have some insight into the losses they are facing) or to be indifferent, with seemingly no emotional awareness of their situation.

## Thought Process

Because actual thoughts cannot be measured, thought processes are assessed by extrapolation from the organization of speech. Thought disorders can be more or less obvious, and a trained listener, much like a cardiologist who listens for heart murmurs or a neurologist who detects aphasias, is one who appreciates the normal logical pattern of flow of words and ideas in speech and can thus sense abnormalities.

There are many different versions of thought disorders: lack of logical connections of ideas (looseness of associations); shift of the original theme because of weak connections of ideas (tangentiality); overinclusiveness to the point of loss of the theme (circumstantiality); use of words and phrases with no relation to grammatical rules (word salad); repetition of words spoken by others (echolalia); use of sounds of other words, such as "yellow bellow, who is this fellow?" (clang associations); use of made-up words (neologisms); and repetition of a particular word or phrase, such as "this and that, this and that" (perseveration).

Other thought disorders are part of a constellation of negative symptoms. Examples would be thoughts that appear to stop abruptly, either because of interruption by an auditory hallucination or because the thought is lost (thought blocking); absence of thoughts (paucity of thought content); and a delayed response to questions (increased latency of response).

## Thought Content

Although not necessarily present in every patient, characteristic symptoms of schizophrenia include the belief that outside forces control a person's thought or actions. A patient might report that others can insert thoughts into her or his head (thought insertion), broadcast them to others (thought broadcasting), or take thoughts away (thought withdrawal). Other delusions, or fixed false beliefs, may also be prominent. Patients may describe ideas of reference, which is the phenomenon of feeling that some external event or report relates to oneself specifically; for example, a patient may infer special meaning from an image seen on television or a broadcast heard on the radio.

Paranoid ideation may be manifested as general suspiciousness or frank, well-systematized delusions. The themes may be considered bizarre, such as feeling convinced that aliens are sending signals through wires in the patient's ear, or nonbizarre, such as being watched by the Central Intelligence Agency or believing that one's spouse is having an affair. These symptoms can be quite debilitating and lead to a great deal of personal loss, which patients may not understand because the ideas are so real to them.

Patients with schizophrenia commonly express an abundance of vague somatic concerns, and a particular patient might develop a delusion around a real physiological abnormality. Therefore, somatic symptoms should be evaluated appropriately in their clinical context without automatically dismissing them as psychotic. Preoccupations and obsessions are also seen commonly in this population, and certain patients have comorbid obsessive–compulsive disorder.

The mortality rate for suicide in schizophrenia is approximately 10% (Hare 1987, Drake et al. 1985). It is therefore imperative to evaluate a patient for both suicidal and homicidal ideation. Patients of all diagnoses, and particularly schizophrenia, may not spontaneously articulate suicidal or homicidal ideation and must therefore be asked directly about such feelings. Moreover, psychotic patients may feel compelled by an auditory hallucination telling them to hurt themselves.

## Perceptions

Perceptual disturbances involve illusions and hallucinations. Hallucinations may be olfactory, tactile, gustatory, visual, or auditory, although hallucinations of the auditory type are more typical of schizophrenia. Hallucinations in the other sensory modalities are more commonly seen in other medical or substance-induced conditions. Auditory hallucinations can resemble sounds, background noise, or human voices. Auditory hallucinations that consist of a running dialogue between two or more voices or a commentary on the patient's behavior are typical of schizophrenia. These hallucinations are distinct from verbalized thoughts that most humans experience. They are often described as originating from outside the patient's head, as if they were emanating from the walls or the radiators in the room. Less commonly, a patient with schizophrenia describes illusions or misperceptions of a real stimulus, such as seeing demons in a shadow.

## Consciousness and Orientation

One of the observations that struck Kraepelin in his first descriptions of dementia praecox was that patients did not have clouding of consciousness. Patients with schizophrenia most likely have a clear sensorium unless there is some comorbid medical illness or substance-related phenomenon. A schizophrenia patient may be disoriented, but this could be a result of inattentiveness to details or distraction secondary to psychotic preoccupation. In fact, there is some literature suggesting that a subgroup of patients may present as disoriented to temporal relations such as the date or their own age (Crow 1986).

## Attention and Concentration

Studies utilizing continuous performance task paradigms have demonstrated repeatedly that schizophrenia patients have pervasive deficits in attention in both acute and residual phases (Walker 1981, Straube and Oades 1992). On a Mental Status Examination, these deficits may present themselves as the inability to perform mental exercises, such as spelling the word "earth" backward or serial subtractions.

## Memory

Careful assessment of memory in patients with schizophrenia may yield some deficits. Acquisition of new information, immediate recall, and recent and remote memory may be impaired in some individuals. Furthermore, answers to questions regarding memory may lead to idiosyncratic responses related to delusions, thought disorder, or other overriding symptoms of the illness. In general, schizophrenia patients do not show gross deficits of memory such as may be seen in patients with dementia or head trauma (Adams and Victor 1989, Straube and Oades 1992).

## Fund of Knowledge

Schizophrenia is not the equivalent of mental retardation, although these syndromes can coexist in some patients. Patients with schizophrenia generally experience a slight shift in intellectual functioning after the onset of their illness, yet they typically demonstrate a fund of knowledge consistent with their premorbid level. Schizophrenia patients manifest a characteristic discrepancy on standardized tests of intelligence, with the nonverbal scores being lower than the verbal scores (Straube and Oades 1992). Furthermore, some reports suggest that patients who have been chronically hospitalized or those with some cerebral atrophy may evidence diminished intellectual function (Johnstone et al. 1978).

## Abstraction

A classical aberration of mental function in a patient with schizophrenia involves the inability to utilize abstract reasoning, which is similar to metaphorical thinking, or the ability to conceptualize ideas beyond their literal meaning. For example, when the patient is asked what brought him or her to the hospital, a typical answer might be "an ambulance." On a Mental Status Examination, this concrete thinking is best elicited by asking a patient to interpret a proverb or state the similarities between two objects. For example, "a rolling stone gathers no moss" may mean, to the patient with schizophrenia, that "if a stone just stays in one place, the moss won't be able to collect." More profound difficulties in abstraction and executive function, often seen in schizophrenia, such as inability to shift cognitive focus or set, may be assessed by neuropsychological tests.

## Judgment and Insight

Individuals suffering from schizophrenia often display a lack of insight regarding their illness. Whether it is a reflection of a negative symptom, such as apathy, or a constricted display of emotion, patients often appear to be emotionally disconnected from their illness and may even deny that anything is wrong. Poor judgment, which is also characteristic and may be related to lack of insight, may lead to potentially dangerous behavior. For example, a patient walking barefoot in the snow because of the feeling that her or his shoes could be traced by surveillance cameras would be displaying both poor judgment and poor insight. On a formal Mental Status Examination, judgment is commonly assessed by asking patients what they would do if they saw a fire in a movie theater or if they saw a stamped, addressed envelope on the street. Insight can be ascertained by asking patients about their understanding of why they are being evaluated by a psychiatrist or why they are receiving a certain medication.

## Physical Examination

Although there are no pathognomonic physical signs of schizophrenia, some patients have neurological "soft" signs on physical examination. The neurological deficits include nonspecific abnormalities in reflexes, coordination (as seen in gait and finger-to-nose tests), graphesthesia (recognition of patterns marked out on the palm), and stereognosis (recognition of three-dimensional pictures). Other neurological findings include odd or awkward movements (possibly correlated with thought disorder), alterations in muscle tone, an increased blink rate, a slower habituation of the blink response to repetitive glabellar tap, and an abnormal pupillary response (Straube and Oades 1992).

The exact etiology of these abnormalities is unknown, but they have historically been associated with minimal brain dysfunction and may be more likely in patients with poor premorbid functioning and a chronic course (Straube and Oades 1992). These neurological abnormalities have been seen in neuroleptic-naive patients as well as those with exposure to traditional antipsychotic medication. Overall, the literature suggests that these findings may be associated with the disease itself, although further research is needed to determine the role of neuroleptic exposure in the manifestation of neurological signs and the extent to which schizophrenia is itself associated with neurological abnormalities (Johnstone and Owens 1981).

Neuroophthalmological investigations have shown that patients with schizophrenia have abnormalities in voluntary saccadic eye movements (rapid eye movement toward a stationary object) as well as in smooth pursuit eye movements. The influence of attention and distraction, neuroleptic exposure, and the specificity of smooth pursuit eye movements for schizophrenia have raised criticisms of this area of study, and further investigation is necessary to determine its potential as a putative genetic marker for schizophrenia.

## Other Conditions That Resemble Schizophrenia

### Schizoaffective Disorder

Possibly the most difficult diagnostic dilemma in cases in which a patient has both psychotic symptoms and affective symptoms is in the differentiation between schizophrenia and schizoaffective disorder. The term schizoaffective disorder was first coined by Kasanin (1933). Since then, there has been some controversy regarding this diagnostic entity. It has been included in studies of both affective disorder and schizophrenia and has at times been considered part of a continuum between the two, which has contributed to some of the diagnostic confusion.

In DSM-IV, schizoaffective disorder is treated as a unique clinical syndrome. A patient with schizoaffective disorder must have an uninterrupted period of illness during which, at some time, they have symptoms that meet the diagnostic criteria for a major depressive episode, manic episode, or a mixed episode concurrently with the diagnostic criteria for the active phase of schizophrenia (criteria A for schizophrenia). Additionally, *the patient must have had delusions or hallucinations for at least 2 weeks in the absence of prominent mood disorder symptoms*

---

**DSM-IV-TR Criteria** 295.70

**Schizoaffective Disorder**

A. An uninterrupted period of illness during which, at some time, there is either a major depressive episode, a manic episode, or a mixed episode concurrent with symptoms that meet criterion A for schizophrenia.

**Note:** The major depressive episode must include criterion A1: depressed mood.

B. During the same period of illness, there have been delusions or hallucinations for at least 2 weeks in the absence of prominent mood symptoms.

C. Symptoms that meet criteria for a mood episode are present for a substantial portion of the total duration of the active and residual periods of the illness.

D. The disturbance is not due to the direct physiological effects of a substance (e.g., a drug of abuse, a medication) or a general medical condition.

*Specify* type:

**Bipolar type:** if the disturbance includes a manic or a mixed episode (or a manic or a mixed episode and major depressive episodes)

**Depressive type:** if the disturbance only includes major depressive episodes

---

Reprinted with permission from the Diagnostic and Statistical Manual of Mental Disorders, Fourth Edition, Text Revision. Copyright 2000 American Psychiatric Association.

---

during the same period of illness. The mood disorder symptoms must be present for a substantial part of the active and residual psychotic period. The essential features of schizoaffective disorder must occur within a single uninterrupted period of illness where the "period of illness" refers to the period of active or residual symptoms of psychotic illness and this can last for years and decades. The total duration of psychotic symptoms must be at least 1 month to meet the criteria A for schizophrenia and thus, the minimum duration of a schizoaffective episode is also 1 month.

The criteria for major depressive episode requires a minimum duration of 2 weeks of either depressed mood or markedly diminished interest or pleasure. As the symptoms of loss of pleasure or interest commonly occur in nonaffective psychotic disorders, to meet the criteria for schizoaffective disorder criteria A, the major depressive episode must include pervasive depressed mood. Presence of markedly diminished interest or pleasure is not sufficient to make a diagnosis as it is possible that these symptoms may occur with other conditions too.

### Brief Psychotic Disorder and Schizophreniform Disorder

The distinctions among brief psychotic disorder, schizophreniform disorder, and schizophrenia are based on duration of active symptoms. As discussed earlier, DSM-III adopted a 6-month rule from the St. Louis group criteria. DSM-IV has maintained the requirement of 6 months of active, prodromal, and/or residual symptoms for a diagnosis of schizophrenia. Brief psychotic disorder is a transient psychotic state, not caused by medical conditions or substance use, that lasts for at least 1 day and up to 1 month. Schizophreniform disorder falls in between and requires symptoms for at least 1 month and not exceeding 6 months, with no requirement for loss of functioning.

---

**DSM-IV-TR Criteria** 298.8

**Brief Psychotic Disorder**

A. Presence of one (or more) of the following symptoms:

  (1) delusions

  (2) hallucinations

  (3) disorganized speech (e.g., frequent derailment or incoherence)

  (4) grossly disorganized or catatonic behavior

**Note:** Do not include a symptom if it is a culturally sanctioned response pattern.

B. Duration of an episode of the disturbance is at least 1 day but less than 1 month, with eventual full return to premorbid level of functioning.

C. The disturbance is not better accounted for by a mood disorder with psychotic features, schizoaffective disorder, or schizophrenia and is not due to the direct physiological effects of a substance (e.g., a drug of abuse, a medication) or a general medical condition.

*Specify* if:

**With marked stressor(s)** (brief reactive psychosis): if symptoms occur shortly after and apparently in response to events that, singly or together, would be markedly stressful to almost anyone in similar circumstances in the person's culture

**Without marked stressor(s):** if psychotic symptoms do *not* occur shortly after, or are not apparently in response to events that, singly or together, would be markedly stressful to almost anyone in similar circumstances in the person's culture

**With postpartum onset:** if onset within 4 weeks postpartum

Reprinted with permission from the Diagnostic and Statistical Manual of Mental Disorders, Fourth Edition, Text Revision. Copyright 2000 American Psychiatric Association.

### DSM-IV-TR Criteria 295.40

**Schizophreniform Disorder**

A. Criteria A, D, and E of schizophrenia are met.

B. An episode of the disorder (including prodromal, active, and residual phases) lasts at least 1 month but less than 6 months. (When the diagnosis must be made without waiting for recovery, it should be qualified as "provisional.")

*Specify* if:

**Without good prognostic features**

**With good prognostic features:** as evidenced by two (or more) of the following:

   (1) onset of prominent psychotic symptoms within 4 weeks of the first noticeable change in usual behavior or functioning

   (2) confusion or perplexity at the height of the psychotic episode

   (3) good premorbid social and occupational functioning

   (4) absence of blunted or flat affect

Reprinted with permission from the Diagnostic and Statistical Manual of Mental Disorders, Fourth Edition, Text Revision. Copyright 2000 American Psychiatric Association.

## Delusional Disorder

If the delusions that a patient describes are not bizarre (e.g., examples of bizarre delusions include the belief that an outside force or person has taken over one's body or that radio signals are being sent through the caps in one's teeth),

### DSM-IV-TR Criteria 297.1

**Delusional Disorder**

A. Nonbizarre delusions (i.e., involving situations that occur in real life, such as being followed, poisoned, infected, loved at a distance, or deceived by spouse or lover, or having a disease) of at least 1 month's duration.

B. Criterion A for schizophrenia has never been met. **Note:** Tactile and olfactory hallucinations may be present in delusional disorder if they are related to the delusional theme.

C. Apart from the impact of the delusion(s) or its ramifications, functioning is not markedly impaired and behavior is not obviously odd or bizarre.

D. If mood episodes have occurred concurrently with delusions, their total duration has been brief relative to the duration of the delusional periods.

E. The disturbance is not due to the direct physiological effects of a substance (e.g., a drug of abuse, a medication) or a general medical condition.

*Specify* type (the following types are assigned based on the predominant delusional theme):

**Erotomanic type:** delusions that another person, usually of higher status, is in love with the individual

**Grandiose type:** delusions of inflated worth, power, knowledge, identity, or special relationship to a deity or famous person

**Jealous type:** delusions that the individual's sexual partner is unfaithful

**Persecutory type:** delusions that the person (or someone to whom the person is close) is being malevolently treated in some way

**Somatic type:** delusions that the person has some physical defect or general medical condition

**Mixed type:** delusions characteristic of more than one of the above types but no one theme predominates

**Unspecified type**

Reprinted with permission from the Diagnostic and Statistical Manual of Mental Disorders, Fourth Edition, Text Revision. Copyright 2000 American Psychiatric Association.

it is wise to consider delusional disorder in the differential diagnosis. Delusional disorder is usually characterized by specific types of false fixed beliefs such as erotomanic, grandiose, jealous, persecutory, or somatic types. Delusional disorder, unlike schizophrenia, is not associated with a marked social impairment or odd behavior. Moreover, patients with delusional disorder do not experience hallucinations or typically have negative symptoms.

## Affective Disorder with Psychotic Features

If the patient experiences psychotic symptoms solely during times when affective symptoms are present, the diagnosis is more likely to be mood disorder with psychotic features. If the mood disturbance involves both manic and depressive episodes, the diagnosis is bipolar disorder. According to DSM-IV, affective disorders that are seen in patients with schizophrenia may fall in the category depressive disorder not otherwise specified or bipolar disorder not otherwise specified.

## Substance-Related Conditions

Psychotic disorders, delirium, and dementia that are caused by substance use, in DSM-IV, are distinguished from schizophrenia by virtue of the fact that there is clear-cut evidence of substance use leading to symptoms. Examples of psychotomimetic properties of substances include a PCP psychosis that can resemble schizophrenia clinically, chronic alcohol intoxication (Korsakoff's psychosis), and chronic amphetamine administration, which can lead to paranoid states. Therefore, patients who have symptoms that meet criterion A of schizophrenia in the presence of substance use must be reevaluated after a significant period away from the suspected substance, and proper toxicology screens must be performed to rule out recent substance abuse.

## General Medical Conditions

General medical conditions ranging from vitamin $B_{12}$ deficiency to Cushing's syndrome have been associated with a clinical presentation resembling that of schizophrenia. Because the prognosis for the associated medical condition is better than that for schizophrenia and the stigma attached to schizophrenia is significant, it is imperative to provide patients with a thorough medical work-up before giving a diagnosis of schizophrenia. This includes a physical examination; laboratory analyses including thyroid function tests, syphilis screening, and folate and vitamin $B_{12}$ levels; a CT or MRI scan; and a lumbar puncture when indicated in new-onset cases.

## Course of Illness

The most influential model for the long-term course of schizophrenia was proposed by Kraepelin. Inherent in the term dementia praecox was the view that the course of this illness was similar to that of the dementias in that they were progressive with worsening over time. This downhill trajectory had profound clinical and research implications throughout the century. For example, if patients with

schizophrenia recovered or even had a prolonged remission, it was generally considered that they had been erroneously diagnosed. Indeed, even in DSM-III, patients with schizophrenia were described as rarely recovering. Moreover, pathophysiological theories were influenced by this model in that disease processes that were progressive were given strong consideration.

The Kraepelinian model for this illness went essentially unchallenged for more than 50 years until well-designed epidemiological studies of schizophrenia were conducted. In long-term follow-up studies of 20 years or more, surprisingly favorable outcomes were observed: between 40 and 66% of patients had either recovered or were only mildly impaired at follow-up (Table 62–1). In the Vermont Longitudinal Study of Schizophrenia (Harding et al. 1987a, 1987b), 269 backward patients who were chronically institutionalized in the 1950s were followed up an average of 32 years later. The patients who met rigorously applied retrospective DSM-III diagnostic criteria for schizophrenia disorder ($N = 118$) during their index admission in the 1950s were found on follow-up to have outcomes that varied widely; 82% were not hospitalized in the year of the follow-up, 68% displayed slight or no symptoms, 81% were able to meet their own basic needs, and more than 60% had good social functioning. Thus, these data indicate that the long-term outcome of schizophrenia is heterogeneous, with substantially larger numbers of patients having better outcomes than would have been predicted by the Kraepelinian model.

Based on current epidemiological data, a new model of the natural course of schizophrenia has been proposed (Breier et al. 1991). This model has three phases: an early phase marked by deterioration from premorbid levels of functioning; a middle phase characterized by a prolonged period of little change termed the stabilization phase; and the last period, which incorporates the long-term outcome data just cited, which is called the improving phase (Figure 62–5).

## First Episode Schizophrenia

An enormous clinical and research effort is directed internationally towards patients in very early stages of their illness and especially during their first psychotic break with a focus on early and effective intervention. First episode provides a unique opportunity to intervene early and effectively and possibly change the course of illness. It is well known that there is a delay of 1 to 2 years on an average between onset of psychosis and starting of treatment (Lieberman and Fenton 2000). This duration of

| Table 62–1 | Long-Term Follow-up Studies of Schizophrenia | | | |
|---|---|---|---|---|
| Study | Location | Length of Follow-up (mean, year) | Sample Size (N) | Recovered or Significantly Improved (%) |
| DeSisto et al. (1992) | Maine | 36 | 117 | 45 |
| Harding et al. (1987) | Vermont | 32 | 82 | 67 |
| Tsuang et al. (1979) | Iowa | 35 | 186 | 46 |
| Huber et al. (1982) | Bonn | 22 | 502 | 57 |
| Ciompi et al. (1982) | Lausanne | 37 | 289 | 53 |
| Bleuler (1987) | Zurich | 23 | 208 | 53 |

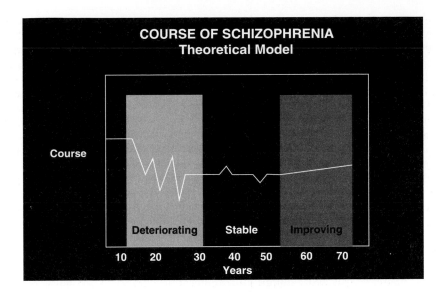

**Figure 62–5** *Model of the lifelong course of illness for schizophrenia. (Source: Breier A, Schreiber JL, Dyer J, et al. [1991] National Institute of Mental Health longitudinal study of chronic schizophrenia: Prognosis and prediction of outcome. Arch Gen Psychiatr 48, 239–246. Copyright 1991 American Medical Association.)*

untreated psychosis (DUP) is recognized by many though not all as an important indicator of subsequent clinical outcome (Norman 2001, Larsen et al. 2000). Larsen and colleagues (2000) examined 1-year outcome in 43 first episode patients and at 1-year follow-up 56% were in remission, 26% were still psychotic and 18% suffered multiple relapses. Both longer DUP and poor premorbid functioning predicted more negative symptoms and poor global functioning. DUP remained a strong predictor of outcome even after controlling for premorbid functioning. Clinical deterioration appears to be correlated with the duration of psychosis and number of episodes of psychosis (Wyatt 1991). The deterioration usually occurs during the first 5 years after onset and then stabilize at a level where they have persistent symptoms and are impaired in their social and vocational function. After that point additional exacerbation may occur but they are not usually associated with further deterioration (Lieberman 1999a).

Long-term studies of schizophrenia suggest that negative symptoms tend to be less common and less severe in the early stages of the illness but increase in prevalence and severity in the later stages. Positive symptoms such as delusions and hallucinations are more common earlier on while thought disorganization, inappropriate affect, and motor symptoms occur more commonly in the later stages of illness (McGlashan and Fenton 1993, Fenton and McGlashan 1994). A possible decline in the prevalence of the hebephrenic and catatonic subtypes of schizophrenia may be attributed to effective treatment and possible arrest of the progression of illness (Wyatt 1991). Thus with effective treatment, and with long-term compliance it is possible to produce favorable outcomes.

Following onset of the illness, patients experience substantial decline in cognitive functions from their premorbid levels (Saykin et al. 1994). However, it is unclear whether, after the first episode, there is further cognitive decline due to the illness. Some studies even suggest a slight and gradual improvement (Gur et al. 1998). Increased number of episodes and the longer duration of untreated psychosis are associated with greater cognitive dysfunction (Waddington 1995, 1997).

Patients with first episode psychosis usually have excellent clinical response to antipsychotic treatment early in their course of illness when compared to chronic multi-episode patients. *Effective and early intervention does help achieve clinical remission and good outcome* (Lieberman et al. 1993, Robinson et al. 1999). Some suggest that atypical antipsychotic medication should be used preferentially in the treatment of first episode patients with psychotic disorders (Lieberman 1996) as they are a highly treatment responsive group, and may be best able to optimize the outcome. In addition, first episode patients are sensitive to side effects, especially extrapyramidal and weight gain side effects. They require lower doses of medication to achieve therapeutic responses. The issue of treatment adherence is of critical importance in first episode patients. Although these patients respond very well with 1 year remission rates of greater than 80%, the 1-year attrition rates are as high as 60%. This important issue undermines management of first episode patients during this critical period of their illness.

## Treatment

It could be argued that the successful treatment of schizophrenia requires a greater level of clinical knowledge and sophistication than the treatment of most other psychiatric and medical illnesses. It begins with the formation of a therapeutic psychiatrist–patient relationship and must combine the latest developments in pharmacological and psychosocial therapeutics and interventions.

### Psychiatrist–Patient Relationship

The psychiatrist–patient relationship is the foundation for treating patients with schizophrenia. Because of the clinical manifestations of the illness, the formation of this relationship is often difficult. Paranoid delusions may lead to mistrust of the psychiatrist. Conceptual disorganization and cognitive impairment make it difficult for patients to attend to what the psychiatrist is saying and to follow even the simplest directions. Negative symptoms result in lack of emotional expression and social withdrawal, which can be demoralizing for the psychiatrist who is attempting to "connect" with the patient.

It is important for the psychiatrist to understand the ways in which the psychopathology of the illness affects the therapeutic relationship. The psychiatrist should provide constancy to the patient, which helps "anchor" patients in their turbulent world. The qualities of the relationship should include consistency, acceptance, appropriate levels of warmth that respect the patient's needs for titrating emotional intensity, nonintrusiveness, and, most important, caring. "Old-fashioned" family doctors who know their patients well, are easily approachable, have a matter-of-fact style, attend to a broad range of needs, and are available and willing to reach out during crises provide a useful model for the psychiatrist–patient relationship in the treatment of schizophrenia.

## Psychopharmacological Treatment

### Background
One hundred years ago, Philippe Pinel changed the philosophy of treating the mentally ill when he unchained patients and provided them with well-balanced diets in the hope that these interventions would ameliorate their symptoms (Weiner 1992). Attempts to treat these patients medically included interventions such as insulin shock, dialysis, and frontal lobotomies. These methods appeared effective at times, yet it was clear that something else was needed to help the poorly understood symptoms of schizophrenia.

Although chlorpromazine had been around since the late 1800s, it was not until 1952 that it was first used to treat psychosis. The seminal work of Delay and Deniker (1952) provided a pharmacological strategy that would forever change the face of schizophrenia. The implementation of chlorpromazine became the turning point for psychopharmacology. Patients who had been institutionalized for years were able to receive treatment as outpatients and live in community settings. The road was paved for the deinstitutionalization movement, and scientific understanding of the pathophysiology of schizophrenia burgeoned.

The discovery of chlorpromazine led to the development of other phenothiazines and new classes of antipsychotic medications, now totaling 11 different classes available in the US today. The word neuroleptic, literally "nerve cutting," was used to describe the tranquilizing effects of these medications. The enormous efforts to understand the mechanism of action of typical antipsychotics uncovered the intimate association of dopamine $D_2$ receptor blockade to the antipsychotic effects. This formed the basis of the hypothesis suggesting that symptoms of schizophrenia were possibly related to the hyperactivity of the (mesolimbic and mesocortical) dopaminergic systems in the brain. Antipsychotics developed subsequent to chlorpromazine such as haloperidol, thiothixene, and so on, were modeled on the (misguided) belief that induction of EPS was an integral part of having an antipsychotic efficacy. Over the years another belief developed that all antipsychotics were similar in their efficacy and varied only in their side effects. However, clozapine challenged these beliefs by being significantly superior in efficacy then the existing antipsychotics and having minimal to no EPS! This started the era of antipsychotic agents being referred to as either "typical" (conventional or traditional) or "atypical" (or novel) antipsychotic drugs. If chlorpromazine started the first revolution in the psychopharmacological treatment of schizophrenia, then clozapine ushered in the second and more profound revolution whose impact is felt beyond schizophrenia and its full extent is yet to be realized. Moreover, clozapine has invigorated the psychopharmacology of schizophrenia and rekindled one of the most ambitious searches for new antipsychotic compounds by the pharmaceutical industry. Following approval of clozapine in 1990, FDA has already approved four novel antipsychotics—risperidone (Risperdal® 1994), olanzapine (Zyprexa® 1996), quetiapine (Seroquel® 1997) and ziprasidone (Geodon® 2001)—and is on the verge of approving two more, a remarkable progress indeed.

### Clozapine and the Novel Antipsychotic Agents
Though clozapine, a dibenzodiazepine compound, was approved for use in the US in 1990, it had been available in European markets during the 1970s but had been found to be associated with agranulocytosis, a potentially fatal side effect, which led to its removal from clinical trials. The need for improved treatment of schizophrenia, particularly for patients who do not respond to traditional neuroleptics, generated interest in resuming investigations of clozapine's clinical efficacy.

Double–blind, controlled studies demonstrated the superior clinical efficacy of clozapine compared with standard neuroleptics, without the associated extrapyramidal symptoms (Kane et al. 1988, Breier et al. 1994). It is clearly superior to traditional neuroleptics for psychosis. A summary of the US studies of patients with chronic and treatment-resistant schizophrenia suggests that approximately 50% of patients derive a better response from clozapine than from traditional neuroleptics (Table 62–2). Its effect on negative symptoms is somewhat controversial and has started an intense and a passionate debate as to whether the efficacy of the medication is with primary or secondary negative symptoms or both (Meltzer 1995, Carpenter et al. 1995). There is substantial evidence that clozapine decreases relapses, improves stability in the community, and diminishes suicidal behavior. There have also been reports that clozapine may cause a gradual reduction in preexisting tardive dyskinesia (Tamminga et al. 1994).

Unfortunately, clozapine is associated with agranulocytosis, and because of this risk, it requires weekly white blood cell testing. Approximately 0.8% of patients taking clozapine and receiving weekly white blood cell monitoring develop agranulocytosis. Women and the elderly are at higher risk than other groups (Alvir et al. 1993). The period of highest risk is the first 6 months of treatment. These data has led to monitoring of white cell counts less frequently after first 6 months to every other week if a person has a history of white cell counts within normal range in the preceding 6 months. Current guidelines state that the medication must be held back if the total white blood cell count is 3,000/mm³ or less or if the absolute polymorphonuclear cell count is 1,500/mm³ or less. Patients who stop clozapine treatment continue to require blood monitoring for at least 4 weeks after the last dose according to current guidelines. Other side effects of clozapine include orthostatic hypotension, tachycardia, sialorrhea, sedation, elevated temperature, and weight gain (Baldessarini and Frankenburg 1991). Furthermore, clozapine can lower the seizure thresh-

| Table 62–2 | Clozapine Responder Rates in Chronic Schizophrenia: US Studies | | | |
|---|---|---|---|---|
| Study | Number of Inpatients | Illness Severity | Trial Duration | Responders (%) |
| Kane (1988) | 126 | ++++ | 6 wk | 30 |
| Meltzer (1990) | 51 | +++ | 6 mo | 61 |
| Conley (1992) | 25 | ++++ | 1 yr | 60 |
| Wilson (1992) | 37 | ++++ | 6 mo | 62 |
| Breier (1993) | 30 | ++ | 1 yr | 60 |
| Zito (1993) | 152 | ++++ | 1 yr | 43 |
| Pickar (1994) | 40 | +++ | 4 mo | 50 |

old in a dose-dependent fashion, with a higher risk of seizures seen particularly at doses greater than 600 mg/day.

Clozapine has an affinity for dopamine receptors ($D_1$, $D_2$, $D_3$, $D_4$, and $D_5$), serotonin receptors (5-$HT_{2A}$, 5-$HT_{2C}$, 5-$HT_6$, and 5-$HT_7$), alpha-1- and alpha-2-adrenergic receptors, nicotinic and muscarinic cholinergic receptors and $H_1$ histaminergic receptors. As clozapine has a relatively shorter half-life, it is usually administered twice a day.

The superior antipsychotic efficacy of clozapine has inspired an abundance of research in the field of modern psychopharmacology for the treatment of schizophrenia. Clozapine and the other novel compounds have an array of biochemical profiles, with affinities to dopaminergic, serotoninergic, and noradrenergic receptors (Figure 62–6 [see Color Plate VIII]). Research on the atypical antipsychotic compounds has led to a greater understanding of the biochemical effects of antipsychotic agents, leaving the basic dopamine hypothesis of schizophrenia insufficient to explain schizophrenic symptoms. Clozapine shows selectivity for mesolimbic neurons and does not increase the prolactin level. Binding studies have shown it to be a relatively weak $D_1$ and $D_2$ antagonist, compared with traditional neuroleptics (Farde et al. 1989). Clozapine shares the property of higher serotonin 5-$HT_{2A}$ to dopamine $D_2$ blockade ratio reported to impart atypicality. The noradrenergic system may also have a role in the mechanism of action of clozapine (Breier 1994). Clozapine, but not traditional neuroleptics, causes up to fivefold increases in plasma norepinephrine. Moreover, these increases in norepinephrine correlated with clinical response.

Following clozapine, risperidone was the first novel antipsychotic medication approved by FDA in 1994. Risperidone is currently the most prescribed novel antipsychotic medication. Risperidone is a benzisoxazol compound with a high affinity for 5-$HT_{2A}$ and $D_2$ receptors and has a high serotonin dopamine receptor antagonism ratio. It has high affinity for alpha-1-adrenergic and $H_1$ histaminergic receptors and moderate affinity for alpha-2-adrenergic receptors. Risperidone is devoid of significant activity against the cholinergic system and the $D_1$ receptors. The efficacy of this medication is equal to that of other first-line atypical antipsychotic agents (Marder and Meibach 1994, Peuskens 1995) and is well tolerated and can be given once or twice a day. It is available in a liquid form as well. The most common side effects reported are drowsiness, orthostatic hypotension, lightheadedness, anxiety, akathisia, constipation, nausea, nasal congestion, prolactin elevation, and weight gain. At doses above 6 mg/day EPS can become a significant issue. The risk of tardive dyskinesia at the regular therapeutic doses is low.

Olanzapine, a thienobenzodiazepine compound approved in 1996, is the second most prescribed novel antipsychotic agent. It has antagonistic effects at dopamine $D_1$ through $D_5$ receptors and serotonin 5-$HT_{2A}$, 5-$HT_{2C}$, and

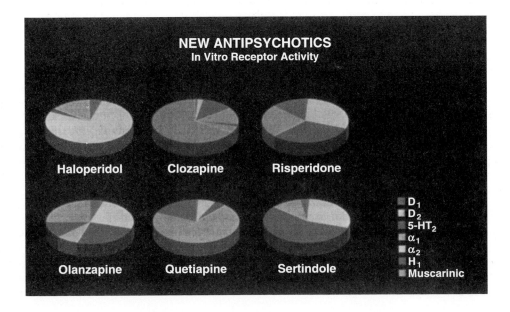

**Figure 62–6** *In vitro receptor affinity of new antipsychotic agents. (See Color Plate VIII.)*

5-HT$_6$ receptors. The antiserotonergic activity is more potent than the antidopaminergic one. It also has affinity for alpha-1-adrenergic, M$_1$ muscarinic acetylcholinergic and H$_1$ histaminergic receptors. It differs from clozapine by not having high affinity for the 5-HT$_7$, alpha-2-adrenergic, and other cholinergic receptors (Bymaster et al. 1999). It has significant efficacy against positive and negative symptoms and also improves cognitive functions (Beasley et al. 1997). EPS is minimal when used in the therapeutic range with the exception of mild akathisia. As the compound has a long half-life, it is used once a day and as it is well tolerated, it can be started at a higher dose or rapidly titrated to the most effective dose. It is available as a rapidly disintegrating wafer form (Zyprexa Zydis), which dissolves immediately in the mouth. An intramuscular form has also been approved by FDA. The major side effects of olanzapine include weight gain, sedation, dry mouth, nausea, lightheadedness, orthostatic hypotension, dizziness, constipation, headache, akathisia, and transient elevation of hepatic transaminases. The risk of tardive dyskinesia and NMS is low (Tollefson et al. 1997, Tran et al. 1997). Though used as a once-a-day medication, it is often administered twice a day with the average dose of 15 to 20 mg/day. However, doses higher than 20 mg/day are often used clinically and are thus being evaluated in clinical trials (Volavka et al. 2002, Lindenmayer et al. 2001, CATIE Study/NIMH 1999).

Quetiapine, a dibenzothiazepine compound approved in 1997, has a greater affinity for serotonin 5-HT$_2$ receptors than for dopamine D$_2$ receptors; it has considerable activity at dopamine D$_1$, D$_5$, D$_3$, D$_4$, serotonin 5-HT$_{1A}$, and alpha-1-, alpha-2-adrenergic receptors. Unlike clozapine, it lacks affinity for the muscarinic cholinergic receptors. It is usually administered twice a day due to a short half-life. Quetiapine is as effective as typical agents and also appears to improve cognitive function. Among 2,035 patients enrolled in seven controlled studies, quetiapine at all doses used did not have an EPS rate greater than placebo. This is in contrast to olanzapine, risperidone, and ziprasidone, where there were dose related effects on EPS levels. The rate of treatment emergent EPS was very low even in high at-risk populations

such as adolescent, parkinsonian patients with psychosis, and geriatric patients. There was no elevation of prolactin (Kasper and Muller-Spahn 2001). Major side effects include somnolence, postural hypotension, dizziness, agitation, dry mouth, and weight gain (Small et al. 1997). Akathisia occurs on rare occasions. The package insert warns about developing lenticular opacity or cataracts and advises periodic eye examination based on data from animal studies. However, recent data suggest that this risk may be minimal.

Ziprasidone, approved by FDA in 2001, has the strongest 5-HT$_{2A}$ receptor binding relative to D$_2$ binding amongst the atypical agents currently in use. Interestingly, ziprasidone has 5-HT$_{1A}$ agonist and 5-HT$_{1D}$ antagonist properties with a high affinity for 5-HT$_{1A}$, 5-HT$_{2C}$, and 5-HT$_{1D}$ receptors. As it does not interact with many other neurotransmitter systems, it does not cause anticholinergic side effects and produces little orthostatic hypotension and relatively little sedation. Just like some antidepressants, ziprasidone blocks presynaptic reuptake of serotonin and norepinephrine. Ziprasidone has a relatively short half-life and thus it should be administered twice a day and along with food for best absorption. Ziprasidone is not completely dependent on CYP3A4 system for metabolism, thus inhibitors of the cytochrome system do not significantly change the blood levels. Data for efficacy, side effects and dosing comes from a number of studies (Keck et al. 1998, Daniel et al. 1999, Goff et al. 1998, Arato et al. 1998). Ziprasidone at doses between 80 and 160 mg/day is probably the most effective for treating symptoms of schizophrenia. To assess the cardiac risk of ziprasidone and other antipsychotic agents, Pfizer and FDA designed a landmark study to evaluate the cardiac safety of the antipsychotic agents, given at high doses alone and with a known metabolic inhibitor in a randomized study involving patients with schizophrenia. This was done to replicate the possible worst-case scenario (overdose or dangerous combination treatment) in the real world. All antipsychotic agents studied caused some degree of QTc prolongation. Oral form of haloperidol was associated with the least and thioridazine with the greatest change (Figure 62–7). Major side effects

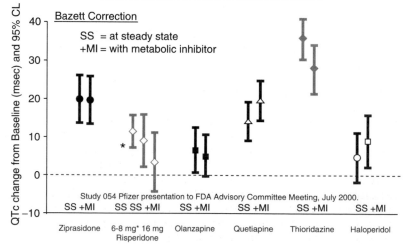

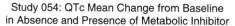

**Figure 62–7** *Study 054 was an open-label, parallel-group study in patients with schizophrenia to assess the effect of oral doses of ziprasidone, risperidone, olanzapine, quetiapine, thioridazine and haloperidol on the QT interval of the EKG. EKGs were measured to correspond to $T_{max}$ of the given drug. There were 25 patients per group. The highest dose for each drug was reached based on US package insert. For Risperidone two different doses were used based on common practice of using lower than approved doses. Later in the study, a CYP 450 metabolism inhibitor was coadministered and EKGs were obtained. QTc was calculated using Bazett's correction. Data from this study resulted in "black box" warning from FDA for mesoridazine and thioridazine. (FDA Psychopharmacological Drugs Advisory Committee: Briefing documents for ziprasidone, July 2000.) (Source: Pfizer Pharmaceuticals and www.fda.gov/ohrms/dockets/ac/00/backgrd/361961a.pdf.)*

reported with the use of ziprasidone are somnolence, nausea, insomnia, dyspepsia, and prolongation of QTc interval. Dizziness, weakness, nasal discharge, orthostatic hypotension, and tachycardia occur less commonly.

Ziprasidone should not be used in combination with other drugs that cause *significant* prolongation of the QTc interval. It is also contraindicated for patients with a known history of significant QTc prolongation, recent myocardial infarction, or symptomatic heart failure. Ziprasidone has low EPS potential, does not elevate prolactin levels, and causes approximately 1 lb weight gain in short term studies (Allison et al. 1999).

At present, with respect to efficacy, it does not appear that any one of the novel antipsychotic agents (except clozapine) is better than another one in treating schizophrenia. The randomized controlled trials suggest that, on average, these antipsychotic agents are each associated with 20% improvement in symptoms. However, clozapine is the only new antipsychotic agent that is more effective than haloperidol in managing treatment resistant schizophrenia (Kane et al. 1988, 2001). Unfortunately, its potential for treatment-emergent agranulocytosis, seizures, and the new warning of myocarditis, precludes its use as a first line agent for schizophrenia (Miller 2000). A major difference amongst the newer antipsychotic agents is the side effect profile and its effect on the overall quality of life of the patient.

**Acute Treatment.** Until recently, the typical antipsychotics were the mainstay of the treatment for acute episodes of psychosis. In last few years, the use of novel antipsychotics has surpassed the use of typical ones in the management of acute phase symptoms of schizophrenia, except for the use of parenteral and liquid forms of antipsychotics where typical antipsychotic agents still hold an upper hand. However, this trend will most likely change once the injectable preparations of the novel antipsychotics enter the market starting with olanzapine (already approved by FDA) (Brier et al. 2002) and followed by ziprasidone and aripiprazole. The primary goal of acute treatment is the amelioration of any behavioral disturbances that would put the patient or others at risk of harm. Acute symptom presentation or relapses are heralded by the recurrence of positive symptoms, including delusions, hallucinations, disorganized speech or behavior, severe negative symptoms, or catatonia. Quite frequently, a relapse is a result of antipsychotic discontinuation, and resumption of antipsychotic treatment aids in the resolution of symptoms. There is a high degree of variability in response rates among individuals. When treatment is initiated, improvement in clinical symptoms can be seen over hours, days, or weeks of treatment.

Studies have shown that although typical neuroleptics are undoubtedly effective, a significant percentage (between 20 and 40%) of patients show only a poor or partial response to traditional agents (Cole et al. 1964, Kane 1987). Furthermore, there is no convincing evidence that one typical antipsychotic is more efficacious as an antipsychotic than any other, although a given individual may respond better to a specific drug. Once an informed choice has been made between using a novel or typical antipsychotic medication by the patient and the clinician, selection of a specific antipsychotic agent should be based on efficacy,

side effect profile, history of prior response (or nonresponse) to a specific agent, or history of response of a family member to a certain antipsychotic agent. (For a pharmacotherapy decision tree based on Texas Medication Algorithm Project, see Figure 62–8.) Amongst the typical antipsychotic medications, low-potency, more sedating agents, such as chlorpromazine, were long thought to be more effective for agitated patients, yet there are no consistent data proving that high-potency agents are not equally useful in this context. The low-potency antipsychotics, however, are more associated with orthostatic hypotension and lowered seizure threshold and are often not as well tolerated at higher doses. Higher potency neuroleptics, such as haloperidol and fluphenazine, are safely used at higher doses and are effective in reducing psychotic agitation and psychosis itself. However, they are more likely to cause EPS than the low potency agents.

The efficacy of novel antipsychotic drugs on positive and negative symptoms is comparable to or even better than the typical antipsychotic drugs (Robinson et al. 1999, Arvantis and Miller 1997, Beasley et al. 1997, Peuskens and Link 1997, Small et al. 1997, Tollefson et al. 1997, Borison et al. 1996, Fabre et al. 1995, Marder and Meibach 1994, Ceskova and Svestka 1993, Chouinard et al. 1993, Hoyberg et al. 1993, Lieberman et al. 1993, Chakos et al. 2001, Geddes et al. 2000). The significantly low potential to cause EPS or dystonic reaction and thus the decreased long-term consequences of TD has made the novel agents more tolerable and acceptable in acute treatment of schizophrenia. Other significant advantages adding to the popularity of novel antipsychotics include their beneficial impact on mood symptoms, suicidal risk, and cognition. The selection of the first line treatment with novel antipsychotic (and occasionally typical antipsychotic agent) also depends on the circumstances under which the medications are started, for example, extremely agitated or catatonic patients would require intramuscular preparation of the antipsychotic agents which would limit the choice. Except for clozapine, which is not considered first line treatment because of substantial and potentially life threatening side effects, there is no convincing data supporting the preference of one atypical over the other. However, if the patient does not respond to one, a trial with another atypical antipsychotic is reasonable and may produce response.

Once the decision is made to use an antipsychotic agent, an appropriate dose must be selected. Initially, higher doses or repeated dosing may be helpful in preventing grossly psychotic and agitated patients from doing harm. In general, there is no clear evidence that higher doses of neuroleptics (more than 2,000 mg chlorpromazine equivalents per day) have any advantage over standard doses (400–600 chlorpromazine equivalents per day) (Kane 1987).

In an open trial, 80 schizophrenia inpatients were assigned to receive haloperidol at a dose of 5, 10, or 20 mg/day for 4 weeks (Van Putten et al. 1990). In this study, the patients receiving the highest dose of haloperidol initially demonstrated the most effective treatment of psychotic symptoms, but they were later found to have a higher incidence of EPS and emotional withdrawal. In a 6-week double-blind randomized study of 31 nonchronic treatment-refractory schizophrenia patients, standard doses of fluphenazine (20 mg/day) led to greater clinical

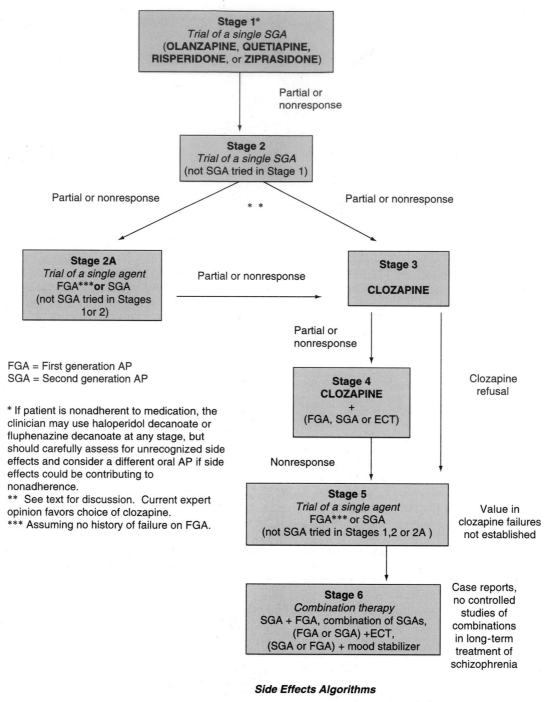

**Stage 1***
*Trial of a single SGA*
(**OLANZAPINE, QUETIAPINE, RISPERIDONE**, or **ZIPRASIDONE**)

Partial or nonresponse

**Stage 2**
*Trial of a single SGA*
(not SGA tried in Stage 1)

Partial or nonresponse        * *        Partial or nonresponse

**Stage 2A**
*Trial of a single agent*
FGA***or SGA
(not SGA tried in Stages 1or 2)

Partial or nonresponse →

**Stage 3**
**CLOZAPINE**

Partial or nonresponse

Clozapine refusal

**Stage 4**
**CLOZAPINE**
+
(FGA, SGA or ECT)

Nonresponse

FGA = First generation AP
SGA = Second generation AP

* If patient is nonadherent to medication, the clinician may use haloperidol decanoate or fluphenazine decanoate at any stage, but should carefully assess for unrecognized side effects and consider a different oral AP if side effects could be contributing to nonadherence.
** See text for discussion. Current expert opinion favors choice of clozapine.
*** Assuming no history of failure on FGA.

**Stage 5**
*Trial of a single agent*
FGA*** or SGA
(not SGA tried in Stages 1,2 or 2A )

Value in clozapine failures not established

**Stage 6**
*Combination therapy*
SGA + FGA, combination of SGAs,
(FGA or SGA) +ECT,
(SGA or FGA) + mood stabilizer

Case reports, no controlled studies of combinations in long-term treatment of schizophrenia

***Side Effects Algorithms***

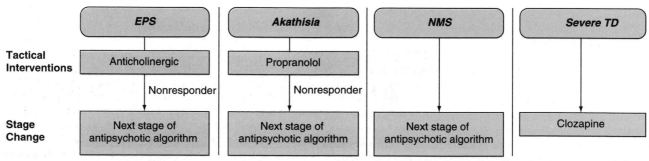

|  | *EPS* | *Akathisia* | *NMS* | *Severe TD* |
|---|---|---|---|---|
| **Tactical Interventions** | Anticholinergic | Propranolol |  |  |
|  | ↓ Nonresponder | ↓ Nonresponder | ↓ | ↓ |
| **Stage Change** | Next stage of antipsychotic algorithm | Next stage of antipsychotic algorithm | Next stage of antipsychotic algorithm | Clozapine |

*Continues*

**Coexisting Symptoms Algorithms**

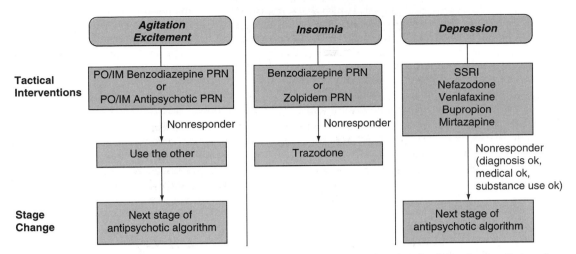

**Figure 62–8** *Selecting antipsychotic treatment using Texas Medication Algorithm for Schizophrenia. Choice of antipsychotic (AP) should be guided by considering the clinical characteristics of the patient and the efficacy and side effect profiles of the medication. Any stage(s) can be skipped depending on the clinical picture or history of antipsychotic failures. Texas Medication Algorithm Project for choosing antipsychotic treatment, managing side-effects and coexisting symptoms. This Project is a public-academic collaborative effort to develop, implement, and evaluate medication treatment algorithms for public sector patients. For more information or to view the most current version of the algorithm visit* www.mhmr.state.tx.us/centraloffice/medicaldirector/tmaptoc.html )

improvement than very high doses (up to 120 mg/day) (Quitkin et al. 1975). EPS seemed to account in part for the poorer response rate in the group treated with the higher doses. In general, the studies indicated that doses of high-potency neuroleptics such as haloperidol can be maintained at a total of 10 mg/day in an acute setting, and that there is no generalizable benefit of using higher doses. Early adjuvant treatment with anticholinergic medication may facilitate compliance with medication by decreasing intolerable side effects.

Some patients who are extremely agitated or aggressive may benefit from concomitant administration of high-potency benzodiazepines such as lorazepam, at 1 to 2 mg, until they are stable. Benzodiazepines rapidly decrease anxiety, calm the person, and help with sedation to break the cycle of agitation. They also help decrease agitation due to akathisia. The use of these medications should be limited to the acute stages of the illness to prevent tachyphylaxis and dependency. Benzodiazepines are quite beneficial in treatment of catatonic or mute patients but the results are only temporary though of enough duration to help with body functions and nutrition.

**Maintenance Treatment.** There is by now a great deal of evidence from long-term follow-up studies that patients have a higher risk of relapse and exacerbations if not maintained with adequate antipsychotic regimens (Hogarty et al. 1974, Davis 1975). Noncompliance with medication, possibly because of intolerable neuroleptic side effects, may contribute to increased relapse rates. In a double-blind, placebo-controlled study of relapse rates, 50% of patients in a research ward demonstrated clinically significant exacerbation of their symptoms within

3 weeks of stopping neuroleptic treatment (Pickar and Pinals 1995). Furthermore, in a comprehensive review of the literature on neuroleptic withdrawal examining 4,365 subjects, 53.2% of patients withdrawn from neuroleptics relapsed, compared with 15.6% of control subjects who were maintained with neuroleptic treatment (Gilbert et al. 1995). The length of follow-up was related to the risk of relapse. Unfortunately, in this review there were no clear demographical or clinical characteristics that consistently predicted relapse. Others have estimated that two-thirds of patients relapse after 9 to 12 months without neuroleptic medication, compared with 10 to 30% who relapse when *typical* neuroleptics are maintained (Straube and Oades 1992). Long-term outcome studies showed that persistent symptoms that do not respond to standard neuroleptic therapy are associated with a greater risk of rehospitalization (Breier et al. 1991). Nonpharmacological interventions may help decrease relapse rates (discussed later).

Long-term treatment of schizophrenia is a complex issue. It is clear that the majority of patients require maintenance medication. Some patients do well with stable doses of neuroleptics for years without any exacerbations. However, many patients who are maintained with a stable neuroleptic dose have episodic breakthroughs of their psychotic symptoms. In a study by Hogarty and associates (1974), 374 schizophrenia patients were followed up for 2 years after hospitalization and randomized to receive placebo alone, placebo and sociotherapy, chlorpromazine alone, or chlorpromazine and sociotherapy. In this study, the placebo-only group had a relapse rate that was almost twice that of the chlorpromazine-treated group. Unfortunately, the difficulty in tolerating neuroleptic side effects often results in noncompliance with medication. Furthermore, intensive case management and rehabilitation counseling did prevent relapse but only after a delayed period. Sociotherapy and drug treatment were found to have additive effects in preventing relapse.

Given the findings of Hogarty and colleagues, it would be prudent to assess patients for medication compliance when signs of relapse are suspected. Prodromal cues may be present before an exacerbation of psychotic symptoms. For example, any recent change in sleep, attention to activities of daily living, or disorganization may be a warning sign of an impending increase in psychosis.

With the increase use of novel antipsychotics it is widely anticipated that compliance will improve proportionately due to significantly less neurological side effects and possible beneficial effects on negative symptoms and neurocognition. In a landmark study comparing risperidone to haloperidol for effects on maintenance treatment, at the end of 1 year, patients taking risperidone were significantly better clinically, more patients were compliant with it and fewer patients had relapses. In this double blind prospective study, 397 stable outpatients were randomized to receive either risperidone or haloperidol for a minimum of 1 year. The Kaplan-Meier estimate of the risk of relapse at the end of study was 34% for the risperidone group and 60% for the haloperidol group. Early discontinuation of treatment for any reason was more frequent among haloperidol treated patients. Risperidone group had greater reductions in the mean severity of both psychotic symptoms and extrapyramidal side effects than those in the haloperidol group (Csernansky et al. 2002). This led to an FDA indication for its use in maintenance treatment. Olanzapine, at 5 to 15 mg/day has been reported to be superior to placebo and olanzapine 1 mg/day in preventing relapses in a 1-year double-blind study (Dellva et al. 1997). Long-term use of quetiapine and ziprasidone are also reported to have significant beneficial effects. The data from treatment with clozapine suggest its significant superiority compared to other treatments. In the treatment refractory patients, long-term randomized trials found significant reduction in rehospitalization (Essock et al. 1996, Rosenheck et al. 1997) and suicide rates (Meltzer and Okayli 1995).

For patients for whom compliance is a problem, long acting, depot neuroleptics are available in the US for both fluphenazine and haloperidol. The antipsychotic drug is esterified in an oily solution which is injected every 1 to 6 weeks to circumvent the need for daily oral antipsychotic medications in most cases (although some patients benefit from adjuvant oral medication). This form of medication delivery guarantees that the medication is in the system of the person taking it and eliminates the need to monitor daily compliance. This alternative should be considered if noncompliance with oral agents has led to relapses and rehospitalization. With these patients, maintenance treatment using long-acting preparations should begin as early as possible (Barnes and Curson 1994). In a meta analysis done by Adams and colleagues (2001), 3,348 patients were randomized in trials of fluphenazine decanoate. The study attrition rates were remarkably low at only 14% of those randomized compared to 40 to 60% in trials of oral atypical

antipsychotic agents (Thornley and Adams 1998). Depot antipsychotic drugs are effective maintenance therapy for patients with schizophrenia. However, currently we only have esters of typical antipsychotic agents and thus the significantly elevated risk of bothersome neurological side effects is an unfortunate limitation to their use. Fortunately, novel antipsychotic depot preparations are currently being investigated.

Many studies have investigated appropriate maintenance doses of standard antipsychotics. Effective maintenance treatment is defined as that which prevents or minimizes the risks of symptom exacerbation and subsequent morbidity. A series of interesting dose-finding studies were performed by Kane and colleagues (1983, 1985) to determine the minimal dosage required to prevent relapse and to reduce the risk of extrapyramidal symptoms and tardive dyskinesia. This group found that the relapse rate (56%) of patients treated with lower doses of fluphenazine decanoate (1.25–5 mg every 2 weeks) was significantly greater than the relapse rate (14%) of patients receiving standard doses (12.5–50 mg every 2 weeks). Other investigators have found that this low dosage range may appear to prevent relapse for a certain period (Marder et al. 1984) but fails to do so if patients are followed up for more than 1 year (Marder et al. 1987). Unfortunately, no specific dosage reliably prevents relapse, and there is no way to predict future relapse. This is true for the novel antipsychotic agents as well.

Plasma drug levels and their correlation with clinical response have also been considered in determining dosage requirements. However, the results remain controversial. Some studies have found that levels that were in excess of a certain therapeutic window led to an exacerbation of symptoms (Kane 1987). There is no strong evidence with which to sort out whether this finding was indeed a result of higher plasma levels, secondary to higher dosing for treatment-resistant patients, or due to the fact that the side effects associated with higher doses of neuroleptics may mimic exacerbations of the primary illness (Kane 1987). At this time, plasma drug levels are not recommended for dosage determination. They are clinically useful, however, for confirming compliance with medication and may provide information regarding toxicity or altered metabolism.

## Depression and Schizophrenia

Symptoms of depression occur in a substantial percentage of schizophrenia patients with a wide range of 7 to 75% and a modal rate of 25% and is associated with poor outcome, impaired functioning, suffering, higher rates of relapse or rehospitalization, and suicide (Heila et al. 1997, Siris 2000, Addington et al. 2002). It is important to distinguish depression as a symptom or as a syndrome when it occurs. There is an important overlap of symptoms of depression with the negative symptoms. Differentiating these states can sometimes be difficult especially in patients who lack the interpersonal communication skills to articulate their internal subjective states well. A link between typical antipsychotic use and depression has been suggested with some considering depression to be a form of medication induced akinesia. Many patients have a reaction of disappointment, a sense of loss or powerlessness, or awareness of psychotic symptoms or psychological deficits that contributes to depression (Lysaker et al. 1995). Depression in schizophrenia is heterogeneous and requires careful diagnostic clarification. DSM-IV suggests that the term "Postpsychotic depression" be used to describe depression that occurs at any time after a psychotic episode of schizophrenia, even after a prolonged interval. The atypical antipsychotic medications, with less potential to cause motor side effects and different mechanisms of action at receptor levels, themselves may contribute substantially towards a decrease in the rate of depression. Moreover, the atypical antipsychotic medications appear to be superior to standard neuroleptics in treatment of negative symptoms (Tandon et al. 1997, Borison et al. 1996, Beasley et al. 1996, Buchanan 1995, Franz et al. 1997). The clear advantage of atypical antipsychotic medications over the typical ones in treatment of psychosis itself can possibly further decrease the rate of depression. The impact of clozapine on the rate of suicide is significantly superior compared to the conventional agents (Meltzer and Okayli 1995). However, a large number of patients still end up with a depression that will require treatment with an antidepressant.

**Risks and Side Effects of Typical Neuroleptics.** Extrapyramidal symptoms are side effects of typical antipsychotic medications that include dystonias, oculogyric crisis, pseudoparkinsonism, akinesia, and akathisia. They are referred to collectively as extrapyramidal symptoms or EPS because they are mediated at least in part by dopaminergic transmission in the extrapyramidal system. Prevalence rates vary among the different types of extrapyramidal symptoms. When present, they can be uncomfortable for the patient and a reason for noncompliance.

Dystonias are involuntary muscular spasms that can be brief or sustained, involving any muscle group. They can occur with even a single dose of medication (Ayd 1961). When they develop suddenly, these spasms can be quite frightening to the patient and potentially dangerous, as in the case of laryngeal dystonias. They are more likely to be seen in young patients. Studies differ as to whether the prevalence is higher in males (Boyer et al. 1987) or females (Chakos et al. 1992). Prevalence rates for dystonias secondary to typical neuroleptic exposure range from 2 to 20% (Marsden et al. 1986).

Pseudoparkinsonism and akinesia are characterized by muscular rigidity, tremor, and bradykinesia, much as in Parkinson's disease. On examination patients typically have masked facies, cogwheel rigidity, slowing, and decreased arm swing with a shuffling gait. This condition is reported to be more prevalent than the dystonias, presenting with a frequency ranging from 15% (Ayd 1961, Marsden et al. 1986) to 35% (Chakos et al. 1992).

Akathisia is more common, affecting more than 20% of patients taking neuroleptic medications (Ayd 1961, Marsden et al. 1986). This clinical entity presents as motor restlessness or an internal sense of restlessness. Often patients experiencing akathisia are unable to sit still during an interview. Akathisia is difficult to differentiate from agitation. The tendency to treat agitation with neuroleptics may exacerbate akathisia, making treatment decisions challenging.

Treatment of EPS can be difficult but usually involves administration of anticholinergic medications. Some advocate the use of prophylactic anticholinergic agents when beginning typical neuroleptic treatment to decrease the incidence of EPS. This option may be appropriate, but it should be used with caution, considering the side effects associated with anticholinergic agents (Levinson 1991) and their potential for abuse (Land et al. 1991).

Treatment of acute dystonic reactions usually involves acute intramuscular administration of either an anticholinergic or diphenhydramine. Akathisia may not respond to anticholinergic medications. Both neuroleptic dosage reduction and the use of beta blocking agents such as propranolol have been found to be efficacious in the treatment of akathisia.

Nonextrapyramidal side effects of the typical antipsychotic agents include those that are secondary to blockade of muscarinic, histaminic, and alpha-adrenergic receptors. These side effects, which are more commonly seen with the low-potency neuroleptics, include sedation, tachycardia, and anticholinergic side effects such as urinary hesitancy or retention, blurred vision, or constipation. Other nonextrapyramidal side effects include some cardiac conduction disturbances, retinal changes, sexual dysfunction, weight gain, lowered seizure threshold, and a risk of agranulocytosis.

Neuroleptic malignant syndrome (NMS) is a relatively rare but serious phenomenon seen in approximately 1% of patients taking neuroleptics (Dickey 1991). It can be fatal in 15% of cases if not properly recognized and treated (Levinson 1991, Dickey 1991). Because the symptoms of NMS may reflect multiple etiologies, making diagnosis difficult, Levenson (Levenson 1985) has proposed clinical guidelines. According to Levenson, three major or two major and four minor manifestations are indicative of a high probability of NMS. Major manifestations of NMS comprise fever, rigidity, and increased creatine kinase levels, and minor manifestations include tachycardia, abnormal blood pressure, tachypnea, altered consciousness, diaphoresis, and leukocytosis. Others do not subscribe to the major-minor manifestation distinctions. In general, NMS is considered to be a constellation of symptoms that usually develops during 1 to 3 days. Although its pathogenesis is poorly understood, it has been associated with all antidopaminergic neuroleptic agents and presents at any time during treatment. It must be distinguished from other clinical entities, including lethal catatonia and malignant hyperthermia (Dickey 1991).

The mainstay of treatment is cessation of neuroleptic treatment and supportive care, including intravenous hydration, reversal of fever with antipyretics and cooling blankets, and careful monitoring of vital signs because of the risk of cardiac and respiratory disturbance. Rhabdomyolysis is one of the most serious sequelae of NMS; it can lead to renal failure unless patients are well hydrated (Levenson 1985). In some cases, dantrolene and bromocriptine have been reported to be effective pharmacological treatments (Granato et al. 1983). Though quite rare, NMS has been reported even with the use of novel antipsychotic agents. The decision to rechallenge the patient with neuroleptics after an episode of NMS must be made with caution.

One of the major risks of neuroleptic treatment with the traditional antipsychotic agents is that of tardive dyskinesia, a potentially irreversible syndrome of involuntary choreoathetoid movements and chronic dystonias associated with long-term neuroleptic exposure. These buccal, orofacial, truncal, or limb movements can be exacerbated by anxiety and disappear during sleep. They can present with a range of severity, from subtle tongue movements to truncal twisting and pelvic thrusting movements and even possible respiratory dyskinesias. The prevalence rates for this syndrome range from less than 10 to more than 50% (American Psychiatric Association Task Force 1980), but it is generally accepted that the risk increases 3 to 5% per year for each year the patient is treated with typical neuroleptics (Kane et al. 1988). Older age is a considerable risk factor for tardive dyskinesia, and there is some evidence that women are at increased risk for the development of this condition (American Psychiatric Association Task Force 1980). Of note, a withdrawal dyskinesia that resembles tardive dyskinesia may appear on cessation of the neuroleptic. The specific mechanism involved in tardive dyskinesia remains unclear, although supersensitivity of dopaminergic receptors has been implicated.

All patients receiving traditional neuroleptic treatment should be monitored regularly for any signs of a movement disorder. DSM-IV now includes a diagnosis of neuroleptic-induced tardive dyskinesia. If tardive dyskinesia is suspected, the benefits of antipsychotic treatment must be carefully weighed against the risk of tardive dyskinesia. This should be discussed with the patient, and the antipsychotic should be removed if clinically feasible or at least maintained at the lowest possible dose that provides antipsychotic effect. This would also be an indication to switch to the novel antipsychotic agents with significantly reduced risk of TD or in the case of clozapine no risk of TD. In many instances, clozapine (and possibly quetiapine or olanzapine) may be the best treatment that can be offered for the TD itself (Tamminga et al. 1994). Unfortunately, there is no specific treatment of tardive dyskinesia, although some investigators have proposed the use of adrenergic agents such as clonidine, calcium channel blockers, vitamin E, benzodiazepines, valproic acid, or reserpine to reduce the spontaneous movements (American Psychiatric Association Task Force 1980).

Sudden death in psychiatric patients treated with typical antipsychotic drugs has been reported for a long time (Hollister and Kosek 1965). Sudden cardiac deaths probably occur from prolongation of the ventricular action potential duration represented as the QT interval (or QTc when corrected for heart rate) on the electrocardiogram resulting in a polymorphic ventricular tachycardia termed *torsades de pointes* that can degenerate into ventricular fibrillation (Tamargo 2000). The incidence of *torsades de pointes* is unknown and the specific duration of the QTc interval at which the risk of an adverse cardiac event is greatest has not been established. QTc prolongation alone does not appear to explain *torsades de pointes*; several other risk factors must be present simultaneously with QT prolongation before *torsades de pointes* occur. These risk factors may include hypokalemia, hypomagnesemia, hypocalcemia, bradycardia, preexisting cardiac diseases (life-threatening arrhythmias, cardiac hypertrophy, heart failure, and congenital QT syndrome), female gender, advancing age, baseline QTc interval of more than 460 m/sec and a long list of medications (Tamargo 2000). In some instances, *torsades de pointes* may be associated with an increase in drug plasma concentrations (e.g., combination with drugs that inhibit the cytochrome P450 systems) (Tamargo 2000, Yap and Camm 2000). Thus, the increase in polypharmacy in psychiatry is especially of concern (Frye et al. 2000). The frequency of ECG abnormalities in patients treated with antipsychotic drugs is unclear (Warner et al. 1996, Mehtonen et al. 1991, Reilly et al. 2000). QTc prolongation has been reported with virtually all antipsychotic drugs (Thomas 1994, Cohen et al. 2000, Czekalla et al. 2001). QTc prolongation by more than two standard deviations was reported in 8% of psychiatric patients treated with antipsychotics and especially in those receiving thioridazine (Reilly et al. 2000, Ray et al. 2001). Of the typical antipsychotic drugs, haloperidol, chlorpromazine, trifluoperazine, mesoridazine, prochlorperazine, droperidol, and fluphenazine have all been reported to cause QTc prolongation and *torsades de pointes*, but thioridazine may be the worst offender (Buckely et al. 1995, Haverkamp et al. 2000, Ray et al. 2001). Pimozide, another typical antipsychotic, has also been associated with QTc prolongation, *torsades de pointes* and deaths (Committee on Safety of Medicines and Medicines Control Agency 1995). A reevaluation by the FDA of the cardiac safety parameters of thioridazine, mesoridazine, and droperidol resulted in a black box warning due to significant QTc prolongation. Thus, it is important to monitor QTc interval in the high-risk population to prevent this rare, but potentially fatal side effect.

## Side Effects of Novel Antipsychotic Agents

One of the most significant advantages of the newer antipsychotic agent is the relatively less risk of developing EPS and TD. However, treatment emergent substantial weight gain is a harbinger for long-term health consequences and frequently an important reason for noncompliance with medication. According to a meta-analysis done by Allison and colleagues (1999), clozapine and olanzapine are associated with a weight gain of about 10 lb over 10 weeks and ziprasidone was among the agents with the lowest weight gain at an average of 1 lb over the same period. Risperidone and quetiapine are intermediate with approximately 5 lb (see Figure 62–9). Patients with schizophrenia, independent of the use of antipsychotic agents are at higher risk of developing diabetes mellitus relative to the general population (Fucetola et al. 1999, Dixon et al. 2000, Thakore et al. 2002). The data from Patient Outcome Research Team (PORT) suggest that the rate of diabetes mellitus and obesity amongst patients with major mental illness was substantially higher even before the advent of the novel antipsychotic drugs. This was more so in women and nonwhite population (Dixon et al. 2000). Thakore and colleagues (2002) investigated visceral fat distribution in drug-naïve and drug-free patients with schizophrenia. Compared to controls, patients with schizophrenia had central obesity and signficantly higher levels of plasma cortisol. Thus patients with schizophrenia are at a higher risk to develop major medical problems even before they are exposed to antipsychotic medications. However,

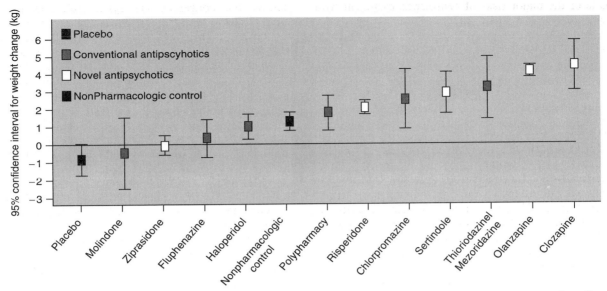

**Figure 62–9** *Ninety-five percent confidence intervals for weight changes after 10 weeks of standard drug doses, estimated from a random effects model. (Source: Allison DB, Mentore JL, Heo M, et al. [1999] Antipsychotic-induced weight gain: A comprehensive research synthesis. Am J Psychiatr 156, 1686–1696. Copyright 1999 American Psychiatric Association; http://ajp.psychiatryonline.org. Reprinted by permission.)*

this risk has been exacerbated with the introduction of the novel antipsychotic agents as seen by the dramatic rise in number of published cases and reports of significant hyperglycemia associated with the use of these medications, particularly olanzapine and clozapine (Masand 2000, Wirshing et al. 1998, Henderson et al. 2000, Hagg et al. 1998, Newcomer et al. 2002) and a few reports with quetiapine (Procyshyn et al. 2000) and risperidone (Haupt and Newcomer 2001). The risk of antipsychotic-induced weight gain and secondary diabetes with clozapine and olanzapine may result from changes in glucose metabolism and insulin resistance induced by these agents. In approximately 40% of the cases of hyperglycemia, insulin resistance appears to occur even in absence of significant weight gain raising some interesting questions about how these medications may interact with the insulin-glycemic control (e.g. Wirshing et al. 1998, Hagg et al. 1998, Newcomer et al. 2002). Unfortunately, in the case of clozapine, the risk of developing abnormal glucose and diabetes mellitus appears to be cumulative over the years as reported by Henderson and colleagues (2000) (see Figure 62–10). There are no effective countermeasures available to help with weight gain and hyperglycemia. The substantial increased risk to the health of patients with schizophrenia due to these effects is worrisome and an important shortcoming of these efficacious and important medications.

Amongst the novel agents, risperidone, due to its potent dopamine $D_2$ blockade, remove the inhibitory dopaminergic tone in the tuberoinfundibular neurons resulting in significant increase in prolactin levels. This increase in prolactin is significantly more than usually seen with the typical antipsychotic agents. It is likely that the serotonin system is also involved along with dopamine in raising the prolactin levels. Clozapine and quetiapine on the other hand, are less potent at the $D_2$ receptors and thus are unlikely to cause prolactin elevations. In some individuals, these elevations of prolactin lead to amenorrhea, galactorrhea, gynecomastia, and may

possibly decrease bone mineral density. Ziprasidone and olanzapine, within the therapeutic dose range do not cause significant increases in prolactin levels.

Cases of sudden death while receiving clozapine therapy (in physically healthy young adults with schizophrenia) from myocarditis and cardiomyopathy (Kilian et al. 1999, Modai et al. 2000, Grenade et al. 2001) led to a black box warning from FDA (www.FDA.gov 2002).

## Treatment Resistance and Negative Symptoms

The concept of treatment resistance has entered into common clinical judgment with the burgeoning interest in atypical antipsychotics, particularly clozapine. Treatment resistance was originally defined for research purposes (Kane et al. 1988). Patients who had failed to respond to or could not tolerate adequate trials of standard

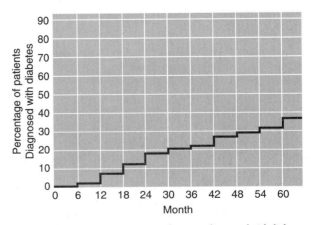

**Figure 62–10** *Cumulative percentage of patients diagnosed with diabetes mellitus (N=30) over a 60-month period among 82 patients receiving clozapine. (Source: Henderson DC, Cagliero E, Gray C, et al. [2000] Clozapine, diabetes mellitus, weight gain and lipid abnormalities: A five-year naturalistic study. Am J Psychiatr 157, 975–981. Copyright 2000 American Psychiatric Association; http://ajp.psychiatryonline.org. Reprinted by permission.)*

neuroleptics from three different biochemical classes and who had a clinically significant psychopathology rating based on the Brief Psychiatric Rating Scale qualified as treatment resistant. However, this research definition did not necessarily encompass patients who, by clinical standards, would meet the definition of treatment resistance. Marder and Van Putten (1988) suggested that backward schizophrenic patients, who are severely symptomatic or with severe tardive dyskinesia or extrapyramidal symptoms, especially those with suboptimal responses to traditional agents, should be eligible for a trial of the atypical antipsychotic agent clozapine. One might also think of clinical treatment resistance as seen in patients who had an early age of illness onset with subsequent repeated hospitalizations and neuroleptic trials and who cannot achieve a level of social and occupational function commensurate with their age and level of education.

The concept of treatment resistance has undergone significant modification in recent years and is reviewed by Conley and Kelly (2001). The original concept of treatment refractory applied to the use of typical antipsychotic agents. With the advent of the novel agents, which are generally more effective than the traditional ones, the patient should fail at least one novel antipsychotic agent before initiating a trial of clozapine mainly to avoid its side effects. The definition of the duration of a drug trial has also evolved over the years. It is increasingly appreciated that a 4 to 6 weeks duration of treatment with an antipsychotic agent at therapeutic doses can be considered an adequate trial. The recommended dosing has also undergone changes. The original recommendation considered a trial of 1,000 mg equivalent of chlorpromazine as a necessary minimum requirement but this threshold is now reduced to 400 to 600 mg/day equivalent based on the knowledge that these doses block enough dopamine $D_2$ receptors with higher doses providing no additional benefit. Thus, a 4 to 6 week trial of 400 to 600 mg of chlorpromazine equivalent is accepted as an adequate antipsychotic trial.

In treatment refractory patients, typical antipsychotic use results in less than 5% response rate (Kane et al. 1988). Clozapine is the only antipsychotic drug proven more efficacious in rigorously defined treatment refractory groups. Chakos and colleagues (2001) did a meta-analysis of 12 controlled studies involving 1,916 patients. Seven studies involved clozapine. The data showed that treatment resistant schizophrenia patients had more favorable outcomes when treated with clozapine rather than a typical antipsychotic agent. However, monitoring of blood counts and fear of its side effects makes it one of most underused effective treatment for schizophrenia.

There is a dearth of good clinical data that indicates how effective risperidone is in this group. In one well-controlled double-blind study, risperidone was more effective and better tolerated than haloperidol though the efficacy was not comparable to clozapine (Wirshing et al. 1999). Two other studies have compared risperidone to clozapine in refractory patients and showed the efficacy of risperidone to be similar to clozapine but, the definition used of "treatment refractory" status and the study design are either not comparable or have limitations (Klieser et al. 1995, Bondolfi et al. 1998). From these and other open label-studies, risperidone clearly appears to be superior to typical anti-

psychotics in treatment refractory patients but does not appear to be as efficacious as clozapine.

Olanzapine has been reported to have better outcome than haloperidol in the treatment-resistant schizophrenia group from a double-blind study (Breier and Hamilton 1999). However, when olanzapine was compared to chlorpromazine in a treatment refractory group using a double-blind study design, the outcome with olanzapine was not comparable to what is typically seen with the use of clozapine (Conley et al. 1998). When patients refractory to olanzapine in this trial were subsequently treated with clozapine, the response rate was similar to what is seen with the use of clozapine in treatment-refractory group. Similar findings were reported from an open label study of olanzapine in a treatment refractory group (Sanders and Mossman 1999). Thus, it appears that though olanzapine was better than standard treatment it was not as efficacious as clozapine for treatment refractory patients. However, these studies were conducted using the standard doses of olanzapine. Recent studies using higher doses of olanzapine up to 50 mg/day appear to be better and comparable to clozapine in efficacy (Volavka et al. 2002, Lindenmayer et al. 2001, Tollefson et al. 2001) suggesting that the treatment refractory group may need higher doses of olanzapine to have a meaningful outcome.

Negative symptoms, such as apathy, amotivational syndrome, flattened affect, and alogia, are often the most problematic for patients with schizophrenia, accounting for much of the morbidity associated with this illness. In addition, these symptoms are often the most difficult to treat and do not respond well to traditional neuroleptics. The atypical antipsychotic agents are more effective against the negative symptoms than the typical agents (Kane et al. 1988, Chouinard et al. 1993, Tollefson et al. 1997). However, the magnitude of the effect of these compounds on primary negative symptoms is not clear. Clearly, one of the goals of psychopharmacological research is to develop new antipsychotic agents with low associated risk, a more effective treatment for negative and cognitive symptoms, a further reduction in positive symptoms, and an improvement in long-term relapse rate for patients with chronic schizophrenia.

## Augmentation of Typical Neuroleptics

When a patient has shown an inadequate response to traditional neuroleptic agents from different classes and there a good reason for not switching to a novel antipsychotic drug, other strategies may be necessary to ameliorate residual symptoms. Adding a different type of psychotropic medication may augment the neuroleptic response in some individuals. Several neuroleptic augmentation strategies have been studied, including the addition of beta-blockers, thyrotropin-releasing hormone, clonidine, and valproic acid, with mixed results (Meltzer 1992). Carbamazepine was initially shown to be effective when added to neuroleptic treatment for schizophrenic patients with electroencephalographic abnormalities and violent outbursts (Hakola and Laulumaa 1982). Later investigation showed that carbamazepine provided adjunctive amelioration of psychotic and affective symptoms when combined with neuroleptics (Klein et al. 1984). Another study reported a significant antipsychotic effect of the addition of carbamazepine to neuroleptics in only one of six treatment-resistant patients (Herrera et al.

1987). However, the group as a whole improved significantly in terms of anxiety, withdrawal, and depression.

Lithium has been evaluated extensively for its efficacy as an additional treatment of schizophrenia (Meltzer 1992, Delva and Letemendia 1982). In one study, lithium seemed to improve psychotic symptoms of patients who had not adequately responded to neuroleptics alone (Small et al. 1975). Although lithium does not seem to affect positive or negative symptoms specifically, it may be beneficial for patients who present at the depressed end of the spectrum (Meltzer 1992).

The use of benzodiazepines as augmenting agents in the treatment of schizophrenia has also been extensively studied (Meltzer 1992, Wolkowitz et al. 1990). There may be some patients who show improvement in psychotic symptoms, and others who show improvement in negative symptoms. Interestingly, there has been a suggestion that the triazolobenzodiazepines may be more effective than other types of benzodiazepines in augmenting the neuroleptic response (Wolkowitz et al. 1990).

Antidepressant medications have also been considered in the treatment of depression associated with schizophrenia. Although there is some evidence that typical neuroleptics themselves cause depression (Galdi 1983), there undoubtedly are schizophrenic patients who have primary depressive symptoms. Negative symptoms are often difficult to distinguish from depression (both have features of amotivation, apathy, and social withdrawal), but those that are secondary to depression may respond to the addition of an antidepressant to the patient's medication regimen (Carpenter et al. 1985). One study reported that fluoxetine as an adjuvant agent was effective in treating both positive and negative symptoms in patients (Goff et al. 1990), although other reports of selective serotonin reuptake inhibitors have been less encouraging. In a separate study, tranylcypromine combined with a typical neuroleptic agent was shown to be helpful in treating negative symptoms (Bucci 1987).

Others have hypothesized a more specific role of the noradrenergic system in the treatment of schizophrenia. For example, Litman and colleagues (1993) noted the improvement of patients with chronic schizophrenia given idazoxan, a highly selective alpha-2-antagonist, in combination with fluphenazine. Levodopa and D-amphetamine have also been used to enhance treatment of negative symptoms (Meltzer 1992). Although this may be promising, these treatments are associated with the risk of exacerbation of positive symptoms and must therefore be used with caution.

The use of electroconvulsive therapy with concomitant neuroleptic treatment has also been evaluated (Salzman 1980). With electroconvulsive therapy as an adjuvant treatment, it appears the patient may improve initially, but relapse is likely. However, patients with comorbid affective symptoms may have some increased benefit (Meltzer 1992). In general, however, this option should be considered only if the patient is not a candidate for a trial with an atypical antipsychotic agent and only if the patient has severe persistent symptoms.

When agonists of the glycine site of the NMDA receptor were added to typical antipsychotic agents in a placebo-controlled study, significant improvement were reported in negative symptoms and aspects of cognitive functioning (Heresco-Levy et al. 1999). D-cycloserine, a partial agonist at the glycine site produced a selective improvement of negative symptoms at 6 weeks (Goff et al. 1999). Augmentation with another endogenous full agonist, D-serine was associated with significant improvement in negative, positive, and cognitive symptoms when added to conventional agents in an 8-week trial (Tsai et al. 1998).

## Mechanism of Action of the Atypical Antipsychotic Agents

A higher ratio of the serotonin 5-HT$_{2A}$ receptor to dopamine D$_2$ receptor blockade is reported to predict *atypicality*. This, along with other data, formed the basis of the *serotonin–dopamine hypothesis* that explains the possible mechanism of action underlying the efficacy of the atypical antipsychotics (Meltzer et al. 1989c, Meltzer 1995). However, studies using PET paradigm failed to detect differences in the serotonin receptor affinities between typical and atypical antipsychotics. Moreover, atypical antipsychotic agents produce high 5-HT$_{2A}$ receptor occupancy at doses that are not sufficient to produce antipsychotic effects. This has raised some questions about the importance of 5-HT$_{2A}$ blockade for a drug to be either atypical or have antipsychotic efficacy (Kapur and Seeman 2001, Kapur and Remington 2001). Though the typical antipsychotics, compared to the atypical ones, show a much higher affinity for the D$_2$ receptors, both are effective only when their D$_2$ receptor occupancy exceeds 65%, suggesting that D$_2$ antagonism is important in producing antipsychotic effects. Thus, some suggest that the major difference between typical and atypical antipsychotic medications may lie in their affinity for the D$_2$ receptor. *Affinity* is the ratio of the rate at which the drug moves *off* of and *on* to the receptor. Interestingly, Seeman and colleagues found that 99% of the difference in affinity of the antipsychotic was driven by differences in their K$_{off}$ at the D$_2$ receptor. Difference in the K$_{on}$ did not account for any significant differences in affinity. Thus, PET studies suggest that all antipsychotics (typical as well as atypical) attach to the D$_2$ receptor with a similar rate constant but differ in how fast they come off of the receptor. Thus, Kapur and Seeman (2001) propose that this relationship between fast K$_{off}$ and low receptor affinity of the antipsychotic drug for dopamine D$_2$ receptor may explain atypicality. Furthermore, *in vivo*, antipsychotic agents modulate dopaminergic transmission and compete with endogenous dopamine. Thus, drugs with fast K$_{off}$ (e.g., clozapine, quetiapine, etc.) modulate dopamine transmission differently from drugs with a slow K$_{off}$ (e.g., haloperidol). For example, clozapine reaches equilibrium and goes on to and off of the receptors significantly faster than haloperidol. When the concentration of endogenous dopamine rises physiologically, drugs like clozapine decrease their D$_2$ occupancy much faster and accommodate to natural surges of dopamine more readily then haloperidol (Kapur and Seeman 2001).

Clinically, a significant difference between the typical and the atypical antipsychotic medications is the extent to which EPS occurs during treatment with therapeutic doses of antipsychotic drugs. PET studies suggest that the threshold for clinical antipsychotic response is lower than that of

A

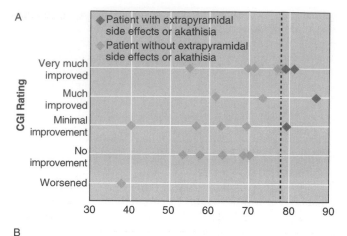

B

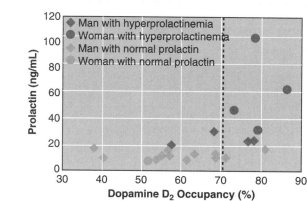

**Figure 62–11** *Relation of dopamine $D_2$ occupancy to CGI-rated clinical response* (A) *and prolactin level* (B) *among patients with first-episode schizophrenia receiving haloperidol. Dotted line in part A indicates 78% $D_2$ occupancy, which was associated with a significantly greater likelihood of extrapyramidal side effects or akathisia. Dotted line in part B indicates 72% $D_2$ occupancy, which was associated with a significantly greater likelihood of hyperprolactinemia. (Source: Kapur S, Zipursky R, Jones C, et al. [2000] Relationship between $D_2$ occupancy, clinical response, and side effects: A double-blind PET study of first-episode schizophrenia. Am J Psychiatr 157, 514–520. Copyright 2000 American Psychiatric Association; http://ajp. psychiatryonline.org. Reprinted by permission.)*

developing EPS and can be separated based on $D_2$ receptor occupancy (Farde et al. 1992, Nordstrom and Farde 1998). Specifically, $D_2$ occupancy of 65% or more significantly predicted clinical response, while $D_2$ occupancy of 78% or above significantly predicted EPS. Similarly, $D_2$ occupancy of 72% or higher resulted in prolactin elevation (Kapur et al. 1996, 2000) (Figure 62–11). Risperidone and olanzapine achieve strong antipsychotic activity only at doses that occupy 65% or more $D_2$ receptors, which is similar to haloperidol (Nordstrom and Farde 1998) (Figure 62–12). On the other hand, although clozapine and quetiapine show less than 60% $D_2$ occupancy 12 hours after drug administration (Seeman and Tallerico 1999) these differences partly reflect a fast decline in $D_2$ occupancy. For example, quetiapine showed 60 and 20% $D_2$ occupancy 2 and 12 hours after receiving the medication. Similarly, clozapine showed 71% $D_2$ occupancy 1 to 2 hours after dose administration with a decline to 55% at 12 hours and 26% at 24 hours. It appears that both typical and atypical antipsychotics block sufficient number of $D_2$ receptors to achieve antipsychotic effect but differ in the kinetics of receptor occupancy.

It has been proposed that $5-HT_{2A}$ occupancy exerts an attenuating effect on the $D_2$ related EPS. Antipsychotic agents, both typical and atypical, give rise to EPS only when they exceed 78 to 80% $D_2$ occupancy; and when they do so, concomitant $5-HT_{2A}$ blockade does not appear to offer protection from these. Since clozapine and quetiapine never exceed this threshold of $D_2$ occupancy, they do not give rise to EPS. Since olanzapine and risperidone exceed this threshold in a dose dependent fashion, they give rise to EPS also in a dose-dependent fashion.

Efforts to produce antipsychotic effects without effective $D_2$ blockade have generally been unsuccessful; for example, drugs that act only on $5-HT_2$ (MDL-100907), $D_4$ (L-745, 850), $5-HT_2$ and $D_4$ (fananserin), and dopamine $D_1$ receptors (SCH-23390) failed to show significant antipsychotic effects in clinical trials. These data have led Seeman and colleagues to propose that low $D_2$ receptor affinity and binding affinity contribute meaningfully towards atypicality without additional blockade of serotonin $5-HT_2$ receptors, a position that lacks universal agreement. The role of serotonin and $5-HT_{2A}$ receptors appears to be complex in schizophrenia and it's treatment. Preclinical and clinical data suggest serotonin $5-HT_{2A}$ receptor blockade is an important property of an atypical antipsychotic drug. The role of other serotonin and dopamine receptor subtypes along with the alpha-1-adrenergic and glutamate and other receptors awaits further clarification.

## New Directions

Psychopharmacological research has focused on developing compounds with unique combinations of effects at these different neurotransmitter sites. Future strategies for the treatment of schizophrenia are based on novel constructs of its pathophysiology.

One area of interest involves the glutamatergic system. Glutamate, the major excitatory neurotransmitter in the brain, is implicated in information processing and memory, functions that are impaired in schizophrenia. PCP, an NMDA antagonist, causes a syndrome with symptoms clinically similar to those of schizophrenia. These observations have led to the hypothesis that the glutamatergic NMDA receptor is involved in the pathophysiology of schizophrenia (Javitt and Zukin 1990). Investigation of compounds that alter NMDA receptor activity is under way to learn more about the clinical significance of this neurotransmitter system.

In another area of drug development, researchers are studying G proteins, ubiquitous proteins found on cell membranes, where they play a critical role in second-messenger systems. These proteins have been found to be related to dopamine receptors in schizophrenic patients and to be involved in the mechanism of action of lithium in the treatment of bipolar disorder (Manji and Lenox 1994). Advanced genetic technology using techniques that could lead to altered receptor function "upstream" is also being explored. Given the enhanced understanding of influential biochemical, genetic, and neurodevelopmental interactions, there is promise of developing treatment strategies that would provide a more effective, safe means of amelioriating both the positive and negative symptoms of schizophrenia.

There is tremendous interest in early identification of potential subjects who may go on to develop schizophrenia.

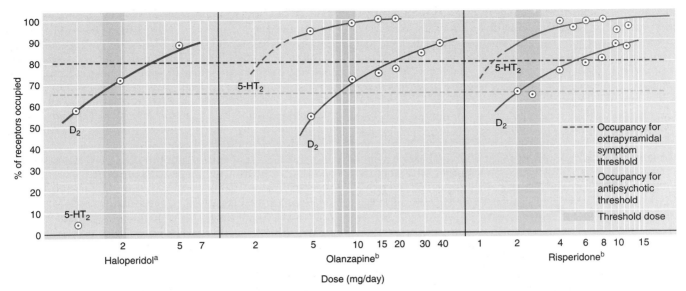

**Figure 62–12** *Relation of threshold for clinical response to occupancy of dopamine $D_2$ and serotonin $5\text{-}HT_2$ receptors for haloperidol, olanzapine, and risperidone. [a]Threshold for response to haloperidol is 65% (1.5–2.1 mg/day); [b]Olanzapine (7.5–10 mg/day) and risperidone (2 mg/day) also reach their thresholds of effectiveness only when their $D_2$ occupancy reaches 65%, despite the fact that haloperidol has a negligible effect at the $5\text{-}HT_2$ receptor and olanzapine and risperidone show high $5\text{-}HT_2$ occupancy. (Source: Kapur S and Seeman P[2001] Does fast dissociation from the dopamine $D_2$ receptor explain the action of atypical antipsychotics? A new hypothesis. Am J Psychiatr 158, 360–369. Copyright 2001 American Psychiatric Association; http://ajp.psychiatryonline.org. Reprinted by permission.)*

Attempts are underway to understand possible role for use of various treatment interventions before the onset of psychosis such that there can either be delay in onset of psychosis and possible change in the course of illness for the better.

## Nonpharmacological Treatment of Schizophrenia

### Background
Although psychopharmacological intervention has proved to be the foundation on which the treatment of schizophrenia depends, other approaches to the management of these patients serve a critical function. Studies have shown repeatedly that symptoms of schizophrenia have not only a genetic component but also an environmental aspect, and interactions with family and within the community can alter the course of the illness.

For many years, a dichotomous view of treatment options was tenaciously debated as dynamic psychiatry was challenged by developments in the neurosciences. A more unified view is now accepted, as it has become clear that psychopharmacological treatment strategies are most efficacious if combined with some type of psychosocial intervention and vice versa. It can be said that because of the chronic nature of schizophrenia, one or more treatments may be required throughout the illness and they are likely to have to be modified as symptoms change over time.

### Psychosocial Rehabilitation
Bachrach has defined psychosocial rehabilitation as "a therapeutic approach that encourages a mentally ill person to develop his or her fullest capacities through learning and environmental supports" (Bachrach 2000). According to the author, the rehabilitation process should appreciate the unique life circumstances of each person and respond to the individual's special needs while promoting both the treatment of the illness and the reduction of its attendant disabilities. The treatment should be provided in the context of the individual's unique environment taking into account social support network, access to transportation, housing, work opportunities, and so on. Rehabilitation should exploit the patient's strengths and improve his/her competencies. Ultimately, rehabilitation should focus on the positive concept of restoring hope to those who have suffered major setbacks in functional capacity and their self-esteem due to major mental illness. To have this hope grounded in reality, it requires promoting acceptance of one's illness and the limitations that come with it. While work offers the ultimate in sense of achievement and mastery, it must be defined more broadly for the mentally ill and should include prevocational and nonvocational activities along with independent employment. It is extremely important that work is individualized to the talents, skills, and abilities of the individual concerned. However, psychosocial rehabilitation has to transcend work to encompass medical, social, and recreational themes. Psychosocial treatment's basic principle is to provide comprehensive care through active involvement of the patient in his or her own treatment. Thus, it is important that a holding environment be created where patients can safely express their wishes, aspirations, frustrations, and reservations such that they ultimately mold the rehabilitation plan. Clearly, to achieve these goals, the intervention has to be ongoing.

Given the chronicity of the illness, the process of rehabilitation must be enduring to encounter future stresses and challenges. These goals cannot be achieved without a stable relationship between the patient and rehabilitation counselor, which is central to an effective treatment and positive outcome. Thus, psychosocial rehabilitation is intimately connected to the biological intervention and forms a core component of the biopsychosocial approach to the treatment of schizophrenia. In the real world, programs often deviate from the aforementioned principles and end up putting excessive and unrealistic expectations on patients, thus achieving exactly the opposite of the intended values of the program (see Bachrach 2000 for more details).

## Psychodynamic Approach

Many attempts have been made to understand the psychodynamic implications and meaning of schizophrenic symptoms. To mention all of the contributors who laid the foundations of psychodynamic theory is beyond the scope of this work. However, several names are important to put this vast field into historical perspective. Adolph Meyer (1866–1950), for example, contributed to our appreciation of a longitudinal, rather than a cross-sectional, perspective of the patient. He was one of the first to consider that maladjustment early on may have some influence on later psychotic development (Arieti 1955). In his work with patients, Sigmund Freud (1855–1939) thought that schizophrenia was an illness that represented a regression and a subsequent turning away from social supports because of unresolved conflicts. He observed that these patients had difficulties in developing transference, which was a necessary step to effective analysis. Freud concluded that schizophrenic patients could not benefit from this treatment (Gabbard 1990). Carl Jung (1875–1960) concentrated specifically on the psychotic content, looking for symbolic meaning through word association tests while working with schizophrenia patients at the Bergozoli Hospital in Switzerland. He believed that humans shared images and mythological symbols or archetypes through a collective unconscious, which was reflected in the psychotic processes of the schizophrenic (Arieti 1955). Harry Stack Sullivan (1892–1949) focused his life's work on interpersonal therapy with schizophrenic patients. He thought that even the most severe schizophrenic patient was capable of a relational attachment (Arieti 1955, Gabbard 1990).

Psychotherapeutic technique held promise for many years as a potential for unraveling the mystery of individuals' symptoms, with the hope of improvement in course and symptoms and even cure. Based on derivations of the classical analytical school, symptoms of schizophrenia were thought of in terms of conflict and defense mechanisms. For example, when paranoid patients believe they are being preyed on, they are projecting onto others their own internal, unconscious wish to kill. Thus, unconscious conflicts became manifest as psychotic symptoms. To the psychodynamic therapist then, affectively laden material elicits an increase in thought disorder or psychotic responses, as it touches on the patient's unconscious feelings. These conceptualizations of schizophrenia influenced early work with these patients.

Although the psychodynamic understanding of intrapsychic events has been of historical interest, the application of traditional psychodynamic principles as primary treatment modalities is not recommended. One of the first studies that compared outcomes between medication-treated patients and psychotherapy-treated patients was conducted at the Camarillo State Hospital in 1968. This study found that the group of patients who received neuroleptic medica-tion showed greater improvement than those who received psychotherapy alone (May 1968). Subsequent studies have replicated these findings even when different types of therapy are examined. Evidence suggests that insight-oriented individual psychotherapy may not be as helpful for patients with schizophrenia as supportive, goal-directed individual therapy combined with medication treatment and social skills training.

## Individual Psychotherapy

Individual therapy in a nontraditional sense can begin on meeting a patient. Even the briefest of normalizing contacts with an agitated, acutely psychotic patient can have therapeutic value. Psychodynamic interpretations are not helpful during the acute stages of the illness and may actually agitate the patient further. The psychiatrist using individual psychotherapy should focus on forming and maintaining a therapeutic alliance (which is also a necessary part of psychopharmacological treatment) (Frank and Gunderson 1990) and providing a safe environment in which the patient is able to discuss symptoms openly. A sound psychotherapist provides clear structure about the therapeutic relationship and helps the patient to focus on personal goals.

Often, a patient is not aware of or does not have insight into the fact that some beliefs are part of a specific symptom. A psychotherapist helps a patient to check whether his or her reality coincides with that of the therapist. The therapeutic intervention then becomes a frank discussion of what schizophrenia is and how symptoms may feel to the patient. This objectifying of psychotic or negative symptoms can prove of enormous value in allowing the patient to feel more in control of the illness. A good analogy is to diabetic patients, who know they have a medical illness and are educated about the symptoms associated with exacerbation. Just as these patients can check blood glucose levels, schizophrenia patients can discuss with a therapist their sleep patterns, their interpersonal relationships, and their internal thoughts, which may lead to earlier detection of relapses.

Schizophrenia often strikes just as a person is leaving adolescence and entering young adulthood. The higher the premorbid level of social adjustment and functioning, the more devastating and confusing the onset of symptoms becomes. Young male patients with a high level of premorbid function are at increased risk of suicide, presumably in part because of the tremendous loss they face (Drake et al. 1985). These feelings can continue for years, with schizophrenia patients feeling isolated and robbed of a normal life. Therefore, a component of individual work (which can also be achieved to some degree in a group setting) with these patients is a focus on the impact schizophrenia has had on their lives. Helping patients to grieve for these losses is an important process that may ultimately help them achieve a better quality of life.

## Group Psychotherapy

Acutely psychotic patients do not benefit from group interaction. In fact, a quiet place with decreased social contact is most useful until medications have controlled acute symptoms (Kanas et al. 1980). It is common in inpatient settings to slowly integrate patients into the ward community only as they appear less agitated and are able to remain in good behavioral control with improvement in psychotic symptoms. As their condition improves, inpatient group therapy prepares patients for interpersonal interactions in a controlled setting. After discharge, patients may benefit from day treatment programs and outpatient groups, which provide ongoing care for patients living in the community.

Because one of the most difficult challenges of schizophrenia is the inherent deficits in relatedness, group therapy is an important means of gathering patients together and providing them with a forum for mutual support. Insight-oriented groups may be disorganizing for patients with schizophrenia, but task-oriented, supportive groups provide structure and a decreased sense of isolation for this population of patients. Keeping group focus on structured topics, such as daily needs or getting the most out of community services, is useful for these patients (Gabbard 1990). In the era of community treatment and brief hospitalizations, many patients are being seen in medication groups, which they attend regularly to discuss any side effects or problems and to get prescriptions.

## Psychoeducational Treatment

One of the inherent deficits from which schizophrenia patients suffer is an inability to engage appropriately in social or occupational activities. This debilitating effect is often a lasting feature of the illness, despite adequate psychopharmacological intervention. This disability often isolates patients and makes it difficult for them to advocate appropriate social support or community services. Furthermore, studies have found that there is a correlation between poor social functioning and incidence of relapse (Linn et al. 1980). One of the challenges of this area of study is the great deal of variability in individual patients. However, standardized measures have been developed to ascertain objective ratings of social deficits. These assessments have become important tools in the determination of effective nonpharmacological treatment strategies.

The literature suggests that schizophrenia patients can benefit from social skills training (Wallace et al. 1980, Brady 1984). This model is based on the idea that the course of schizophrenia is, in part, a product of the environment, which is inherently stressful because of the social deficits from which these patients suffer. The hypothesis is that if patients are able to monitor and reduce their stress, they could potentially decrease their risk of relapse.

For this intervention to be successful, patients must be aware of and set their own goals. Goals such as medication management, activities of daily living, and dealing with a roommate are achievable examples. Social skills and deficits can be assessed by patients' self-report, observation of behavioral patterns by trained professionals, or a measurement of physiological responses to specific situations (e.g., increased pulse when asking someone to dinner). Patients can then begin behavioral training in which appropriate social responses are shaped with the help of instructors.

One example of such a program, discussed by Liberman and colleagues (1985), is a highly structured curriculum that includes a training manual, audiovisual aids, and role-playing exercises. Behaviors are broken down into small bits, such as learning how to maintain eye contact, monitor vocal volume, or ameliorate body language. The modules are learned one at a time, with role playing, home-

work, and feedback provided to the participants. In several studies, Liberman and coworkers (1986) have shown that patients who were treated with social skills training and medication spent less time hospitalized, with fewer relapses than those treated with holistic health measures (e.g., yoga, stress management) on 2-year follow-up. Research such as this in the field of social skills training is growing as the inherent deficits in information processing, executive function, and interpersonal skills are further elucidated.

Earlier studies have suggested that educational interventions influence both knowledge and drug use errors. Similarly, patient education improves compliance. Merinder (2000) reviewed patient education in seven randomized trials, four naturalistic studies and eight studies with mixed samples. The author concludes that knowledge and compliance can be improved by the interventions used and in some circumstances, relapse and symptomatology can be partly influenced. The didactic format influences knowledge more readily while interventions with behavioral contents influence compliance. Patient education programs tend to use more didactic interactive format, enabling a more thorough negotiation of illness attitudes.

**Social Skills Training.** In large number of patients, deficits in social competence persist despite antipsychotic treatment. These deficits can lead to social distress whereas social competence can alleviate distress related to social discomfort. The "token economy" programs with operant conditioning paradigms were used in past to discourage undesirable behavior. However, nowadays there are better ways to deal with these behaviors. Paradigms using instruction, modeling, role-playing, and positive reinforcement are helpful. Controlled studies suggest that schizophrenia patients are able to acquire lasting social skills after attending such programs and apply these skills to everyday life. Besides reducing anxiety, social skills training also improve level of social activity and foster new social contacts. This in turn improves the quality of life and significantly shortens duration of inpatient care. However, their impact on symptom resolution and relapse rates is unclear.

**Cognitive Remediation.** Patients with schizophrenia generally demonstrate poor performance in various aspects of information processing. Cognitive dysfunction can be a rate-limiting factor in learning and social functioning. Additionally, impaired information processing can lead to increased susceptibility to stress and thus to an increase risk of relapse. Practice appears to improve some of the cognitive dysfunction. Remediation of cognitive dysfunctions with social skills training has been reported to have positive impact. Mojtabai and colleagues (1998) performed a comprehensive meta-analysis of 106 controlled studies that were published between 1966 and 1994. They found that various types of cognitive behavioral therapies were particularly effective. Social skills training program, cognitive training program to improve neurocognitive functioning, and cognitive behavioral therapy approaches are oriented towards coping with symptoms, the disorder and everyday problems.

**Cognitive Adaptation Training.** Cognitive adaptation training (CAT) is a novel approach to improve adaptive functioning and compensate for the cognitive impairments associated with schizophrenia. A thorough functional needs assessment is done to measure current adaptive functioning. Besides measuring adaptive functioning and quantifying apathy and disinhibition, a neurocognitive assessment using tests to measure executive function, attention, verbal and visual memory, and visual organization is also completed. Treatment plans are adapted to the patient's level of functioning, which includes patient's level of apathy. Interventions include removal of distracting stimuli, use of reminders such as checklists, signs, and labels. In a randomized trial, 45 patients were randomized to a standard medication plus CAT group; standard medication follow-up group and a control group which included standard medication plus a condition designed to control for therapist time. At 9 months there was a significant improvement in positive and negative symptoms in the CAT group compared with the two other groups, namely follow-up group and control group of standard medication plus controlled therapist time. The most consistent improvement was in favor of CAT group and involved motivation as measured by rating instruments. The GAF scores also differed significantly between the groups. The relapse rates for CAT, control, and follow-up groups were significantly different (13.33, 67.67, and 33.33%, respectively) (Velligan et al. 2000).

## Family Therapy

A large body of literature explores the role of familial interactions and the clinical course of schizophrenia. Many of these studies have examined the outcome of schizophrenia in relation to the degree of expressed emotion (EE) in family members. EE is generally defined as excessive criticism and overinvolvement of relatives. Schizophrenia patients have been found to have a higher risk of relapse if their relatives have high EE levels. Clearly, a patient's disturbing symptoms at the time of relapse may affect the level of criticism and overinvolvement of family members, but evidence suggests that preexisting increased EE levels in relatives predict increased risk of schizophrenic relapse and that interventions that decrease EE levels can decrease relapse rates.

Specifically, studies have demonstrated effective strategies to lowering the risk of relapse with the use of family intervention and measurements of EE levels (Leff et al. 1982, Falloon et al. 1982, 1985, Hogarty et al. 1986). For example, in a study by Falloon and colleagues (1982, 1985), 36 patients were randomly assigned to one of two treatment groups. One group received family therapy, the other individual therapy. In both groups the patients were maintained with appropriate neuroleptic doses. Family therapy was done in the home, with a focus on education about schizophrenia and ways in which families could achieve lowered stress levels and improved problem-solving skills. Specific problem-solving mechanisms were rehearsed and modeled by trained therapists. The individual treatment was supportive psychotherapy for the patient, which was conducted at the clinic. At the end of 9 months, family therapy was found to be a more effective means of preventing relapse (one relapsed out of 18) than individual therapy (eight relapsed out of 19). Moreover, the advantages of the family therapy persisted after a second year of less intensive follow-up (Falloon et al. 1985).

Hogarty and colleagues (1986) examined the effectiveness of neuroleptics alone, neuroleptics plus psycho-educational family treatment (based on addressing EE levels), social skills training for neuroleptic-treated patients with schizophrenia, and the combination of all three. Perhaps not surprisingly, they found a decreased relapse rate in the patients treated with medication and family therapy as well as in the group treated with neuroleptic and social skills training. The combination of the treatments had an additive effect and was far superior to medication treatment alone.

A controlled investigation of the effects of social intervention was also conducted (Leff 1982). Patients were divided into groups, one that received routine outpatient treatment and one that underwent social intervention. In this study, one of the social interventions included reducing the time patients spent with their high-EE relatives. In addition, families received psychoeducational lectures about schizophrenia and its natural course and symptoms. Patients with schizophrenia received neuroleptics throughout the study. Relatives participated in group sessions that addressed coping mechanisms and familial interaction. As in the other studies, the patients who received the social interventions had a fivefold decrease in relapse rates that was sustained after 2-year follow-up.

Barbato and D'Avanzo (2000) critically reviewed family interventions in 25 randomized studies involving 1744 patients. Though the studies suffer from methodological limitations, the efficacy of family intervention on relapse rate is fairly well supported. This efficacy was particularly evident when contrasted with low quality or uncontrolled individual treatments. The addition of family intervention to standard treatment of schizophrenia has a positive impact on outcome to a moderate extent. Family intervention effectively reduces the short-term risk of clinical relapse after remission from an acute episode. There is evidence of effect on patient's mental state and social functioning, or on any family-related variables. The elements common to most effective interventions are inclusion of the patient in at least some phases of the treatment, long duration, and information and education about the illness provided within a supportive framework. There is sufficient data only for male chronic patients living with high EE parents. Evidence is limited for recent onset patients, women, and people in different family arrangements and families with low EE. Research in family intervention is still a growing field. Thus, at present it is unclear if the effect seen with family therapy is due to family treatment or more intensive care.

Leff (2000) concluded from his review that family interventions reduced relapse rates by one half over the first year of combined treatment with medications and family therapy. Medications and family therapy augment each other. Psychoeducation by itself is not enough. It also seems that multiple family groups are more efficacious then single family sessions. Attempts are being made to generalize training of mental health workers in effectively implementing these strategies.

Based on these findings, it is clear that there is a significant interaction between the level of emotional involvement and criticism of relatives of probands with schizophrenia and the outcome of their illness. Identifying the causative factors in familial stressors and educating involved family members about schizophrenia lead to long-term benefits for patients.

Future work in this field must examine these interactions with an understanding of modern sociological and biological advances in genetics, looking at trait carriers, social skills assessments, positive and negative symptoms, and medication management with the novel antipsychotic agents.

## Case Management

Assertive Community Treatment (ACT) is a community care model with a caseload per worker of 15 patients or less in contrast to standard case management (SCM) with a caseload of 30 to 35 patients. Intensive clinical case management (ICCM) differs from ACT by the case manager not sharing the caseload. In the ACT model, most services are provided in the community rather than in the office; the caseloads are shared across clinicians rather than individual separate caseloads. These are time unlimited services provided directly by the ACT team and not brokered out and 24-hour coverage is provided. Research on the ACT model confirms that it is successful in making patients comply with treatment and leads to less inpatient admissions. ACT also improves housing conditions (fewer homeless patients, more patients in stable housing), employment, quality of life, and patient satisfaction. No clear differences between ACT and standard or intensive clinical case management are reported with mental condition, social functioning, self-esteem, or number of deaths.

## Combining Pharmacological and Psychosocial Treatments

The combination of pharmacological and psychosocial interventions in schizophrenia can have complex interactions. For example, psychotherapies improve medication compliance on one hand but are more effective in the presence of antipsychotic treatment. Family psychoeducation has been reported to decrease the level of expressed emotion in the family resulting in better social adjustment and a need for lower dose of antipsychotic medications. Marder and colleagues (1996), found in their study that pharmacological and psychosocial treatments affect different outcome dimensions. Medications affect relapse risk whereas skills training affect social adjustment. The VA cooperative study by Rosenheck and colleagues (1998), found that patients who received clozapine were more likely to participate in these treatments and led to improved quality of life. The qualitative differences in the interactions between the newer antipsychotic agents and psychotherapy suggest a hopeful trend of better utilization of psychosocial treatments (Marder 2000).

## Self-Directed Treatment

Groups such as the National Alliance for Mentally Ill (NAMI) and the Manic–Depressive Association offer tremendous resources to psychiatric patients and their relatives. They provide newsletters, neighborhood meetings, and support groups to interested persons. These nonprofessional self-help measures may feel less threatening to patients and their families and provide an important adjunct to professional settings.

Structured self-help clubs have also been effective means of bolstering patients' social, occupational, and living skills. The Fountain House was the first such club aimed at social rehabilitation (Beard 1982). Patients who are involved are called members of the club, giving them a sense of belonging to a group. They are always made to feel welcome, useful, and productive members of the club community.

The clubhouse model has expanded to provide services such as transitional employment programs, apartment programs, outreach programs, and medication management and consultation services, to name a few. A self-supportive rehabilitation program for mentally ill patients is an important option for many schizophrenic patients who might otherwise feel isolated and out of reach.

## Stigma

Though tremendous progress has occurred in understanding and treatment of schizophrenia, stigmatizing attitudes still prevail (Crisp et al. 2000); in a survey, schizophrenia elicited the most negative opinions and over 70% of those questioned thought that schizophrenia patients were dangerous and unpredictable. Thus, stigma surrounding schizophrenia can cause people suffering from the illness to develop low self-esteem, disrupt personal relationships, and decrease employment opportunities (Penn et al. 1994). The World Psychiatric Association (WPA), has initiated an international program aimed at developing tools to fight stigma and discrimination (Sharma 2001).

---

**Clinical Vignette 1**

Mr. A first sought psychiatric help at the age of 19 years. During his first year of college he had a difficult adjustment. He had never had close friends, but at school he felt isolated from his family. Although he had always been a good student, averaging As and Bs in high school, he was unable to achieve the same level of academic performance. He became increasingly distressed by his sense of isolation and his inability to maintain an adequate grade point average. Around the middle of his first year of college he saw a psychiatrist, who thought he was having an adjustment reaction to his new surroundings. He was not given medication at the time but was referred for supportive psychotherapy. After two appointments with his therapist, he decided it was not helpful.

Shortly thereafter, he began to feel that the other students were staring at him and laughing at him behind his back. Then he began to feel as if they were playing tricks on him, sending secret messages to him over the radio to torment him. This experience lasted over 6 months. He also began hearing two voices, which he did not recognize. These voices would comment on his behavior and criticize his actions. They began to tell him to stay out of his dormitory room at night. The voices also warned him that the dormitory food was poisoned. One night, he was picked up by police for loitering and was brought to an emergency department.

The emergency department psychiatrist saw him as a disheveled, unshaven man who was agitated during the interview, pacing across the examining room. He was wearing dark sunglasses, although it was the middle of the night, and he said he did not want the examiner to read his mind by looking into his eyes, so he kept the sunglasses on throughout the interview. His speech was of normal rate and prosody, although there were long pauses in some of his responses. He was able to respond to questions clearly, and his thought processes were logical, although he repeatedly spoke angrily as if responding to voices. He did say that the voices had been telling him to kill himself for the past two nights, although he said he was trying not to listen to them. The patient showed only some difficulty in concentration on a cognitive examination. His judgment was fair in that he recognized his need for some help, but he showed no insight into his symptoms.

The psychiatrist felt that the patient was potentially dangerous to himself because of the command auditory hallucinations and required hospitalization. Mr. A did not agree to come into the hospital, and the psychiatrist sought involuntary hospitalization through appropriate procedures. In the hospital, the patient was initially quite agitated, requiring intramuscular haloperidol and lorazepam. Almost immediately his behavior calmed, and he was able to agree to hospitalization and treatment. He was treated with risperidone, and the dose was titrated up to 3 mg/day by mouth at bedtime. After 1 week with this medication regimen, he began to experience a decrease in his auditory hallucinations and paranoid ideation. He was sleeping better and was no longer concerned about the foods he was eating.

Clinical Vignette 2

Ms. T, a 31-year-old woman, came to the US in her early twenties to study at a local university. Her family had sent her overseas after her mother was taken into a local psychiatric hospital in her native country. She had difficulty relating to her American classmates but was able to learn English and complete her coursework successfully. After graduation, she found a position working for a small company. Initially, she was punctual for work and her appearance was professional, although eccentric. Ms. T rarely socialized with her coworkers and generally spent her time alone. Several months after a prolonged visit from her previously estranged parents, she was notably more anxious. It became increasingly difficult for her to work closely with others. Ms. T gradually began to appear more disheveled and, at times, malodorous. Her supervisor grew concerned as she began to arrive late to work and seemed disorganized about her responsibilities. Her coworkers noted her bizarre behavior over several months. She began expressing concern about alien forces that would hide messages on her desk. She arrived at work one morning, speaking in rhymes that were partly in her native language and gesturing oddly, explaining that the day had arrived when the aliens would present themselves. Her concerned supervisor saw that she was unable to be shaken from this strange behavior and escorted her to a nearby emergency department for an evaluation.

The emergency department psychiatrist immediately made arrangements for admission, as Ms. T was not able to care for herself at that time. Results of her laboratory tests and physical examination were all within normal limits, and there was no evidence of substance abuse. Her brain MRI scan was also normal. With no identifiable organic cause, more than 1 month of active symptoms, and a 6-month prodromal period, Ms. T was given a presumptive diagnosis of schizophrenia, undifferentiated type.

In the hospital, she was given trifluoperazine at 10 mg twice daily. Her odd mannerisms gradually abated. In addition, her worries about the alien forces and her thought processes seemed to clear over the next few weeks. As her symptoms abated, she was able to participate in the structured group activities while in the hospital.

Eventually, Ms. T was moved to a day program. Her treatment team and Ms. T worked together and planned for her to move out of her apartment and into a psychiatric halfway house. She was not able to return to work, but during the next 6 months she adjusted well to participating in activities at her day program, helping in the clerical office. In the following 10 years, she was hospitalized three times because of noncompliance with medications. After her medication was changed to haloperidol decanoate, Ms. T remained stable and compliant with monthly appointments. Two years later, during her regular neurological examination looking for evidence of movement disorder, she exhibited mild tardive dyskinesia, which appeared to increase over time. On further evaluation, Ms. T had developed sustained insight into her illness and formed a strong alliance with her caseworker. After discussions with the patient and her team, a decision was made to switch her from haloperidol decanoate to oral olanzapine. The dose was titrated up to olanzapine 20 mg/day given at bedtime with weekly monitoring of compliance. She tolerated the switch well with further improvement in her clinical symptoms including symptoms of depression. One year later, her symptoms of tardive dyskinesia were in remission as well.

## OTHER PSYCHOSES

### Schizoaffective Disorder

Kraepelin's landmark classification at the dawn of the 20th century could not accurately classify those patients who manifested both psychotic (schizophrenia-like) and affective symptoms and had a better course of illness then schizophrenia (Kraepelin 1919). It was Kasanin (1933), who coined the term *schizoaffective disorder* to describe some of these patients. However, over the decades, these patients were often classified as having atypical schizophrenia, good prognosis schizophrenia, remitting schizophrenia, or cycloid psychosis. Inherent within these diagnoses was the implication that they shared similarities to schizophrenia and also appeared to have a relatively better course of illness. With the advent of effective treatment of bipolar disorder with lithium salts, some of these patients started responding to lithium, and the term schizoaffective disorder gained further momentum and evolved in the direction of bipolar disorder. Unfortunately, this lack of diagnostic clarity has plagued the diagnosis of schizoaffective disorder such that there is much that is unknown about the illness.

### Epidemiology

As discussed earlier, the diagnosis of schizoaffective disorder has undergone numerous changes through the decades making it difficult to get reliable epidemiology information. When data was pooled together from various clinical studies, approximately 2 to 29% of those patients diagnosed to have mental illness at the time of the study were suffering from schizoaffective disorder with women having a higher prevalence (Keck et al. 2001). This could possibly be explained by a higher rate of depression in women. Relatives of women suffering from schizoaffective disorder have a higher rate of schizophrenia and depressive disorders compared to relatives of male schizoaffective subjects. The estimated lifetime prevalence of schizoaffective disorder is possibly in the range of 0.5 to 0.8%. In the inpatient settings of New York State psychiatric hospitals, approximately 19% of 6,000 patients had a diagnosis of schizoaffective disorder (Levinson et al. 1999).

## Gender and Age

The depressive type of schizoaffective disorder appears to be more common in older people while the bipolar type probably occurs more commonly in younger adults. The higher prevalence of the disorder in women appears to occur particularly amongst those who are married. As in schizophrenia, the age of onset for women is later than that for men. Depression tends to occur more commonly in women.

## Etiology

The etiology of schizoaffective disorder is unknown. There is a dearth of data relating to this illness. Studies involving families of schizoaffective probands suggest that they have significantly higher rates of relatives with mood disorder than families of schizophrenia probands. It is possible that some of the same environmental theories that apply to schizophrenia and bipolar disorder may also apply to schizoaffective disorder.

Over the years, the concept of schizoaffective disorder has evolved such that many view it as either a type of schizophrenia or a type of mood disorder. Evans and colleagues (1999) suggest that schizoaffective disorder represents a variant of schizophrenia in terms of clinical symptoms, family history and treatment. Moreover, in their study and others', schizophrenia patients did not differ from schizoaffective ones on cognitive impairment (Bornstein et al. 1990, Beatty et al. 1993). Williams and associates (1987) suggest that the disorder represents a variant of either schizophrenia or mood disorder while others consider it to be on a continuum of illness intermediate between schizophrenia or mood disorder (Taylor 1992, Kendler et al. 1995a). Lapierre's (1994) opinion is that schizoaffective disorder represents a phenotypic variation of either schizophrenia or mood disorder and over the long term becomes a subtype of either one. Alternatively, some view schizoaffective disorder as the simultaneous expression of schizophrenia and a mood disorder. However, Kendler and colleagues (1995b) observe that schizoaffective patients differ significantly from both schizophrenia and mood disorder patients. Specifically, schizoaffective patients have more affective symptoms, fewer negative symptoms and a better course and outcome than schizophrenia. Bertelsen and Gottesman (1995) reviewed the literature relevant to genetic predisposition to schizoaffective disorder. Though variable, the results generally suggest that schizoaffective disorder is either a phenotypic variation or an expression of a genetic interform between schizophrenia and mood disorder, a position similar to Kendler. However, the possibility that schizoaffective disorder is distinct from schizophrenia and mood disorders is not supported by the observations that only a small percentage of the relatives of schizoaffective disorder probands have schizoaffective disorder.

It is most likely that schizoaffective disorder is a heterogeneous condition that includes all of the possibilities mentioned above. Thus, depending on the type of schizoaffective disorder studied an increased prevalence of either schizophrenia or mood disorders may be found in their relatives. As a group, patients with schizoaffective disorder have a prognosis intermediate between mood disorders and schizophrenia. Thus, on an average they have a better course than those suffering from schizophrenia, respond to mood stabilizers more often and tend to have a relatively nondeteriorating course.

## Diagnosis

Schizoaffective disorder criteria have evolved over the years and undergone major changes. According to the DSM-IV, a patient with schizoaffective disorder must have an uninterrupted period of illness during which, at some time, they meet the diagnostic criteria for a major depressive episode, manic episode, or a mixed episode concurrently with the diagnostic criteria for the active phase of schizophrenia (criteria A for schizophrenia). Additionally, "the patient must have had delusions or hallucinations for at least 2 weeks in the absence of prominent mood disorder symptoms" during the same period of illness. The mood disorder symptoms must be present for a substantial part of the active and residual psychotic period. The essential features of schizoaffective disorder must occur within a single uninterrupted period of illness where the "period of illness" refers to the period of active or residual symptoms of psychotic illness and this can last for years and decades. The total duration of psychotic symptoms must be at least 1 month to meet the criteria A for schizophrenia and thus, the minimum duration of a schizoaffective episode is also 1 month.

The criteria for major depressive episode requires a minimum duration of 2 weeks of either depressed mood or markedly diminished interest or pleasure. As the symptoms of loss of pleasure or interest commonly occur in nonaffective psychotic disorders, to meet the criteria for schizoaffective disorder criteria A, the major depressive episode must include pervasive depressed mood. Presence of markedly diminished interest or pleasure is not sufficient to make a diagnosis as it is possible that these symptoms may occur with other conditions too.

The DSM-IV diagnosis of schizoaffective disorder can be further classified as schizoaffective disorder *bipolar type* or schizoaffective disorder *depressive type*. For a person to be classified as having the bipolar subtype he/she must have a disorder that includes a manic or mixed episode with or without a history of major depressive episodes. Otherwise the person is classified as having depressive subtype having had symptoms that meet the criteria for a major depressive episode with no history of having had mania or mixed state.

## Clinical Features

The clinical signs and symptoms of schizoaffective disorder include all the signs and symptoms of schizophrenia, and a manic episode and/or a major depressive episode. The schizophrenia and mood symptoms may occur together or in an alternate sequence. The clinical course can vary from one of exacerbations and remissions to that of a long-term deterioration. Presence of mood-incongruent psychotic features—where the psychotic content of hallucinations or delusions is not consistent with the prevailing mood—more likely indicate a poor prognosis.

## Differential Diagnosis

The possible differential diagnosis consists of bipolar disorder with psychotic features, major depressive disorder with psychotic features, and schizophrenia. Clearly, substance induced states and symptoms caused by coexisting medical conditions should be carefully ruled out. All conditions listed in differential diagnosis of schizophrenia, bipolar disorder, and major depressive disorder should be considered including but not limited to those patients undergoing treatment with steroids, those abusing substances such as PCP and medical conditions such as temporal lobe epilepsy. In circumstances where there is ambiguity, it may be prudent to delay making a final diagnosis until the most acute symptoms of psychosis have subsided and time is allowed to establish a course of illness and collect collateral information.

## Course and Prognosis

Due to the evolving nature of the diagnosis and limited studies done thus far, much remains unknown. However, to the extent that this illness has symptoms from both a major mood disorder and schizophrenia, theoretically one can confer a relatively better prognosis then schizophrenia and a relatively poorer prognosis then bipolar disorder. In one study where DSM-III and DSM-IV patients with schizoaffective disorder were followed for 8 years, the outcome of these patients more closely resembled schizophrenia then mood disorder with psychosis. Some data indicate that patients with a diagnosis of schizoaffective disorder bipolar type have a 2 to 5 years course similar to that of bipolar disorder, while patients diagnosed to have schizoaffective disorder depressive type have a course similar to schizophrenia on outcome measures such as occupational and social functioning after the index episode (Grossman et al. 1991). Regardless of the subtype, the following variables are harbingers of a poor prognosis:

(a) a poor premorbid history
(b) an insidious onset
(c) absence of precipitating factors
(d) a predominance of psychotic symptoms, especially deficit or negative ones
(e) an early age of onset
(f) an unremitting course, and
(g) a family history of schizophrenia.

The corollary would be that the opposite of each of these characteristics would suggest a better prognosis. Interestingly, the presence or the absence of Schneiderian first-rank symptoms does not seem to predict the course of illness. The incidence of suicide in patients with schizoaffective disorder is at least 10%. Some data indicate that the suicidal behavior may be more common in women then men.

In a small sample comparing 27 schizoaffective disorder with 27 bipolar disorder patients, first rank symptoms and mood-incongruent psychosis did not differ between the two groups (Strakowski et al. 1999). Over 70% of the sample included unemployed or unskilled laborers. A few studies have reported that low socioeconomic status is a strong predictor of poor outcome (Strakowski et al. 1998, 1999).

In one study, 82% of those patients who were suffering from a first episode of schizoaffective disorder and had recovered, experienced psychotic relapse within 5 years. These patients had high rates of second and third relapses despite careful monitoring. Medication discontinuations in first episode patients who are stable for 1 year substantially increase relapse risks. Aside from medication status, premorbid social adjustment was the only predictor of relapse in their study. Poor adaptation to school and premorbid social isolation predicted initial relapse independent of medication status. Thus, like schizophrenia, the risk of relapse is diminished by antipsychotic maintenance treatment (Robinson et al. 1999).

## Treatment

With the shifting definitions of schizoaffective disorder, evaluating the treatment of schizoaffective disorder is not easy. Mood stabilizers, antidepressants, and antipsychotic medications clearly have a role in management of these patients. The presenting symptoms, their duration and intensity, and patient choices need to be incorporated into deciding what treatment(s) to choose.

## Antipsychotic Medications

Atypical antipsychotic medications are reported to be more effective than the typical ones in the treatment of schizoaffective disorder (Levinson et al. 1999, Keck et al. 1999). They appear to have a more broad-spectrum effects then the typical agents. Optimizing antipsychotic treatment, especially with the novel agents is more likely to be effective than the routine use of adjunctive antidepressants or mood stabilizers. However, when indicated, the use of antidepressants is well supported in schizoaffective patients who present with a full depressive syndrome after stabilization of psychosis.

Olanzapine is effective against symptoms of psychosis, mania, and depression. Tollefson and colleagues (1997) studied 300 patients with schizoaffective disorder bipolar type, one of the largest studies of its kind in schizoaffective disorder, and reported that olanzapine was significantly superior to haloperidol in treating affective and psychotic symptoms.

Ziprasidone was studied in 115 hospitalized patients with acute episode of schizoaffective disorder using a double blind randomized design. Ziprasidone was significantly superior to placebo and was well tolerated (Keck et al. 2001). Ziprasidone also has significant antidepressant effects at doses of 120 to 160 mg/day.

Vieta and colleagues (2001) studied 102 schizoaffective disorder bipolar type patients where risperidone was added to their existing regimen of mood stabilizers in the absence of an antipsychotic agent. Risperidone had significant clinical efficacy and a favorable safety profile when combined with mood stabilizers in patients with schizoaffective disorders. The response rate was comparatively better than what is typically observed in schizophrenia studies (Keck et al. 1999). Hillert and associates (1992) also reported that treatment with risperidone reduced both psychotic and mood symptoms in patients with schizoaffective disorder depressed type. However, Janicak and colleagues (2001), in a small sample, did not find significant differences between haloperidol and risperidone in a short-term 6-week double-blind randomized study. However, risperidone produced significantly greater responders in the patients with severe depression and also improved the sleep factor. Moreover, risperidone did not exacerbate manic symptoms, a prevailing concern at the time when this study was conducted. Furthermore, the risperidone group had less EPS compared to haloperidol. Efficacy of clozapine in schizoaffective disorder has been reported in several short term studies or chart reviews (Naber et al. 1989, Banov et al. 1994). Clozapine monotherapy has been reported to be effective in treatment up to 16 months in a small sample (Zarate et al. 1995). Presence of affective symptoms predicted good response to clozapine (Cassano et al. 1997). When clozapine use was compared in treatment refractory schizophrenia, bipolar disorder, and schizoaffective disorder the outcomes were significantly better in bipolar disorder and schizoaffective disorder (Banov et al. 1994, Zarate et al. 1995, Green et al. 2000, Ciapparelli et al. 2000). Persistent and enduring improvement with clozapine lasting 1 to 2 years have been reported (Ciapparelli et al. 2000). Clozapine also helps decrease suicidality (Ciapparelli et al. 2000, Meltzer 1998). Thus, clozapine use may be beneficial in treatment refractory schizoaffective disorder as it has both mood stabilizing and antipsychotic properties, a substantial advantage.

### Mood Stabilizers

Two small open label studies suggest that valproic acid is effective in treating the manic symptoms associated with schizoaffective disorder, bipolar type (Puzynski and Klosiewicz 1984, Emrich et al. 1985) with 65.2% reduction in manic episodes in 5 patients after 29 to 51 months. Similar results were reported by Hayes (1989) where 79% of the patients reported improvement after 1-year treatment with valproic acid. Bogan and associates (2000) also reported 75% improvement in Clinical Global Impression scale in a small sample.

Three double-blind, parallel-group studies examined the efficacy of lithium carbonate in schizoaffective mania. One study found that chlorpromazine alone was as effective as the combination of chlorpromazine and lithium. Another study, with a small sample found that the combination of lithium and haloperidol was more effective than haloperidol itself in patients with predominantly affective symptoms compared to those with predominantly psychotic symptoms. Reports of carbamazepine use is sparse and difficult to draw conclusions from. Lamotrigine was also reported to be useful in 3 cases of schizoaffective disorder (Erfurth et al. 1998).

**Antidepressants.** The novel antipsychotic agents are often efficacious against depression in patients who suffer from both depression and psychosis negating the need for routine use of antidepressants. However, there are patients who remain depressed even with optimal antipsychotic and mood stabilizer treatment. SSRIs are widely used in patients who present with schizoaffective disorder with depression. If the SSRIs and newer antidepressants do not show efficacy, tricyclic antidepressants do have a role. Interestingly, chlorpromazine in combination with amitriptyline was reported to be as effective as chlorpromazine alone. Many studies suggest that addition of antidepressants helps in effective treatment of depression in schizoaffective disorder. Occasionally, antidepressants may worsen the course. For patients suffering from depression where they are not responding adequately and are at risk for suicide, ECT is an effective alternative.

**Psychosocial Treatment.** To the extent that schizoaffective disorder shares symptoms with schizophrenia, most of the psychosocial treatments used in the treatment of schizophrenia are likely to be useful in the treatment of schizoaffective disorder. Specifically, patients benefit from individual supportive therapy, family therapy, group therapy, cognitive–behavioral therapy, and social skills training. Many patients would be suitable candidates for assertive community therapy (ACT). Depending on the level of recovery, some of the patients may need rehabilitation services to assist them with either developing skills for some form of employment or assistance to maintain a job. Family members benefit from support groups such as NAMI or MDA groups.

---

Clinical Vignette 3

Ms. Jones is a 29-year-old married woman with two children. She reported having problems with her sleep 9 months after the birth of her second child as marking the beginning of her illness. She was erratic, irritable, and gradually declined in her functioning. Her family noticed that she was unable to care for herself and her children. She was paranoid, suspicious of her neighbors, and felt that they were spying on her. She isolated herself in the house. Soon she was also noted to have euphoric mood with racing thoughts and grandiose delusions of being a very powerful person endowed with gifts from god. She was barely sleeping, only a few hours a day. After approximately 6 weeks of this behavior, she was brought to hospital after she got into a verbal altercation with her neighbor. There was no history of any medical problems, medication use, or any drug abuse. She was admitted to the hospital, started on valproic acid, and the dose was titrated up to 1,500 mg/day with blood levels of 80. Her symptoms of mania resolved within 2 weeks and she was discharged. However, on the follow-up visit, she reported being suspicious of her neighbor and felt that she was being watched. Her husband reported that patient kept the shades down on the side where the neighbors lived. She was started on ziprasidone 20 mg (QTc interval within normal range) twice a day and the dose was increased to 120 mg/day. Her symptoms resolved completely at the next visit. One year later, she was doing well on monotherapy of ziprasidone 120 mg/day and had started working part time.

## Brief Psychotic Disorder

Brief psychotic disorder is defined by DSM-IV-TR as a psychotic disorder that lasts more than 1 day and less than a month. Moreover, the disorder may develop in response to severe psychosocial stressors or group of stressors.

European and Scandinavian countries have traditionally diagnosed this type of psychosis as *psychogenic psychoses*, *reactive psychosis*, or *brief reactive psychosis*. Some have also referred to this condition as *hysterical psychosis*. These terms are probably more commonly used in Scandinavian countries due to Langfeldt and Leonhard's contributions to the classification of psychosis that does not have a course like schizophrenia. In the US, brief reactive psychosis was formally included as a diagnostic category in DSM-III. Subsequently it has undergone a change in its name to *brief psychotic disorder*.

## Epidemiology

This illness is not uncommon, but, unfortunately, reliable estimates of the incidence, prevalence, sex ratio, and average age of onset are not available. It is believed that this disorder is more common among young people with occasional cases involving older people. This disorder may be seen more commonly in patients from low socioeconomic classes and in those with personality disorders such as histrionic, paranoid, schizotypal, narcissistic, and borderline. Though immigrants and people who have experienced major disasters are reported to be at a higher risk, well-controlled studies have failed to show this.

## Etiology

As with other psychotic illnesses, this condition appears to be heterogeneous; clearly, more research is necessary. The development of psychosis is an important indication of severity of this illness and may suggest either a breakdown of or inadequate coping mechanisms.

## Diagnosis

The DSM-IV diagnostic criteria specify the presence of at least one clear psychotic symptom lasting a minimum of 1 day to a maximum of 1 month. Furthermore, DSM-IV allows the specification of two additional features: the presence or the absence of one or more marked stressors and a postpartum onset. DSM-IV describes a continuum of diagnosis for psychotic disorder based primarily on duration of the symptoms. Once the duration criteria are met, other conditions such as etiological medical illnesses and substance-induced psychosis need to be excluded. In those cases where the duration of psychosis lasts more than 1 month, appropriate diagnosis to be considered are other psychotic conditions based on reevaluation of the clinical features, duration of psychosis, and presence of mood symptoms.

## Clinical Features

People suffering from this disorder usually present with an acute onset, manifest at least one major symptom of psychosis, and do not always include the entire symptom constellation seen in schizophrenia. Affective symptoms, confusion, and impaired attention may be more common in brief psychotic disorders than in chronic psychotic conditions. Some of the characteristic symptoms include emotional lability, outlandish behavior, screaming or muteness, and impaired memory for recent events. Some of the symptoms suggest a diagnosis of *delirium* and may warrant a more complete medical workup. The symptom patterns include acute paranoid reactions, reactive confusions, excitations, and depressions. In French psychiatry, *Bouffee delirante* is similar to brief psychotic disorder.

## Precipitating Stressors

The precipitating stressors most commonly encountered are major life events that would cause any person significant emotional turmoil. Such events include the death of a close family member or severe accidents. Rarely, it could be accumulation of many smaller stresses.

## Differential Diagnosis

Although the classical presentation may be short in duration and associated with stressors, a thorough and careful evaluation is necessary. Additional information is critical to rule out other major psychotic conditions as temporal association of stressors to the acute manifestation of symptoms may be coincidental and thus misleading. Other conditions to be ruled out include psychotic disorder due to a general medical condition, substance-induced psychosis, factitious disorder with predominantly psychological signs and symptoms, and malingering. Patients with epilepsy and delirium may also present with similar symptoms. Additional conditions to be considered are dissociative identity disorder and psychotic episodes associated with borderline and schizotypal personality disorder that may last for less than a day.

## Course and Prognosis

As defined by DSM-IV, the duration of the disorder is less than 1 month. Nonetheless, the development of such a significant psychiatric disorder may indicate a patient's mental vulnerability. An unknown percentage of patients who are first classified as having brief psychotic disorder later display chronic psychiatric syndromes such as schizophrenia and bipolar disorder. Patients with brief psychotic disorders generally have good prognosis, and European studies indicate that 50 to 80% of all patients have no further major psychiatric problems.

The length of the acute and residual symptoms is often just a few days. Occasionally, depressive symptoms follow the resolution of the psychosis. Suicide is a concern during both the psychotic phase and the postpsychotic depressive phase. Indicators of good prognosis are good premorbid adjustment, few premorbid schizoid traits, severe precipitating stressors, sudden onset of symptoms, confusion and perplexity during psychosis, little affective blunting, short duration of symptoms, and absence of family history of schizophrenia.

## Treatment

These patients may require short-term hospitalizations for a comprehensive evaluation and safety. Antipsychotic drugs are often most useful along with benzodiazepines. Long-term use of medication is often not necessary and should be avoided. If maintenance medications are necessary, the diagnoses may need to be revised. Clearly, the newer antipsychotic agents have a better neurological side effect profile and would be preferred over the typical agents.

Psychotherapy is necessary to help the person reintegrate the experience of psychosis and possibly the precipitating trauma. Individual, family, and group therapies may be necessary in some individuals. Many patients need help to cope with the loss of self-esteem and confidence.

---

Clinical Vignette 4

A 35-year-old recently separated immigrant woman was brought to the emergency room in an acutely agitated state with auditory hallucinations and confusion. She immigrated to the US 2 years ago to join her husband of 5 years. They separated 3 months ago; she lost her job a month later and had to bear significant financial hardship. Her father was medically ill and passed away unexpectedly 6 weeks previously. According to people close to her, she started having symptoms approximately 7 days before her admission. She was reported to be restless, pacing, and preoccupied with the recent stressors. On various occasions, her speech was tangential or incoherent. Her mood was labile and she appeared to be perplexed at times. Her attention and concentration was poor. She was paranoid of her husband (family members denied him being a threat to her) and often felt that her deceased father was communicating with her. She had passive suicidal thoughts. She was often upset about being hospitalized and demanded release from the hospital. She would get quite angry and throw tantrums if her request for discharge was denied. There was no history of alcohol or drug use. She was in good physical health. There was no history of similar or other episodes.

Admission work up was essentially normal. The urine toxicology screen, pregnancy test, and EEG were normal. Following admission, she was started on a low dose of benzodiazepine and an atypical antipsychotic agent. Her symptoms of agitation and psychosis responded rapidly within 1 week. Individual and group therapy sessions were very helpful in addressing her recent stressors and providing emotional support. Family therapy was offered but the patient and her family rejected it. With the help of individual and group therapy, she was able to develop some coping skills. Following discharge, she continued to respond to the low dose antipsychotic treatment and other therapies. She was not having any symptoms of psychosis and was able to deal with her stressors better. Approximately 3 weeks after discharge, though her stressors continued, she was responding well to the treatment, reached her baseline functioning, but due to significant weight gain and sedation, she decided to discontinue her medication. Six months later, she has continued with psychotherapy and group therapy, and has maintained her baseline functioning.

## Schizophreniform Disorder

Gabriel Langfeldt (1939) suggested the term *Schizophreni-form Disorder* in 1937 for a heterogeneous group of patients characterized by the similarity of their symptoms to those of schizophrenia albeit with a good clinical outcome. Langfeldt observed that those patients whose diagnosis was questionable as schizophrenia had a much better outcome than those whose diagnosis was confirmed as schizophrenia; these patients were thus classified as having schizophreniform psychosis. Langfeldt also noted that these patients often had good premorbid adjustment, an abrupt onset of symptoms, frequent presence of psychosocial stressor(s), and a good prognosis.

## Epidemiology

Little is known about the incidence, prevalence, and sex ratio of schizophreniform disorder (Poulton et al. 2000). A strong linear relationship has been reported between self-reported psychotic symptoms in childhood at age 11 years and subsequent development of adult schizophreniform disorder. Those children with strong symptoms were 16 times more likely to have a schizophreniform diagnosis by age 26 years compared to control group. Forty-two percent of those who developed schizophreniform psychosis by age 26 years in the cohort had reported 1 or more psychotic symptoms at age 11 years. Interestingly, these psychotic symptoms which appeared at age 11 years did not predict mania or depression at age 26 years (Poulton 2000). Over the years, schizophreniform psychosis has moved much closer to the diagnosis of schizophrenia. ECA studies indicate prevalence of 0.2% lifetime prevalence and 1-year prevalence of 0.1%.

## Family History

Several studies suggest that the relatives of patients with schizophreniform psychosis are at a high risk of having psychiatric disorders. The relatives of patients with schizophreniform psychosis are more likely to have mood disorders than are the relatives of patients with schizophrenia. In addition, the relatives of patients with schizophreniform disorder are more likely to have a diagnosis of a psychotic mood disorder than are the relatives of patients with bipolar disorders.

## Etiology

Schizophreniform psychosis, similar to other psychosis, is probably heterogeneous and due to an unknown cause. In general, some patients have a disorder similar to schizophrenia, whereas others have a disorder similar to mood disorders. Some data, however, indicate a close relation to schizophrenia. Several studies have shown that patients with schizophreniform disorder, as a group, have more affective symptoms (especially mania) and a better outcome than do patients with schizophrenia. In addition, the increased presence of mood disorders in the relatives of patients with schizophreniform disorder indicates a relation to mood disorders. Thus, the biological and epidemiological data are most consistent with the hypothesis that the current diagnostic category defines a group of patients, some of whom have a disorder similar to schizophrenia and others similar to a mood disorder.

## Brain Imaging

As in schizophrenia, a relative activation deficit in the inferior prefrontal region of the brain while the patient is performing Wisconsin Card Sorting Test is reported. One study showed that the deficit was limited to the left hemisphere indicating a similarity to schizophrenia. More studies are needed to determine the long-term course which is often variable and sometimes similar to schizophrenia but more often a shortened course quite different from schizophrenia. Some data indicate that patients with schizophreniform disorder may have enlarged ventricles, as seen on CT scans and MRI, while other data indicate that unlike the enlargement seen in schizophrenia, the ventricular enlargement in schizophreniform disorder is not correlated with outcome measures or other biological measures.

## Other Biological Measures

Although brain-imaging studies suggest a similarity between schizophreniform disorder and schizophrenia, one study of electrodermal activity has indicated a difference. Patients with schizophrenia born during the winter and spring months had hyporesponsive skin conductances, but this association was absent in patients with schizophreniform disorder. Though the significance of this one study would be difficult to interpret, the results do suggest caution in assuming similarity between patients with schizophrenia and those with schizophreniform disorder. Data from a study of eye tracking in the two groups also indicate that there are differences on some biological measures between schizophrenia and schizophreniform psychosis.

## Diagnosis

Schizophreniform disorder shares a majority of the DSM-IV-TR diagnostic features with schizophrenia (see diagnostic criteria on p. 1161) except the following two criteria: (a) the total duration of the illness which includes the prodrome, active, and residual phases is at least 1 month but less than 6 months in duration; (b) though impairment in social and occupational functioning may occur during the illness, it is not required or necessary. Thus, the duration of more than 1 month eliminates brief psychotic disorder as a possible diagnosis; if the illness lasts or has lasted for more than 6 months, the diagnosis has to be reevaluated for other possible conditions including schizophrenia. Therefore, the diagnosis of schizophreniform disorder is intermediate between brief psychotic disorder and schizophrenia. Hence, those patients whose duration of episode lasted more than a month and less than 6 months, and have recovered would be diagnosed as having schizophreniform disorder. On the other hand those patients who have not recovered from an episode, which is less than 6 months but more than one month in duration, and are likely to have schizophrenia would be diagnosed to have schizophreniform disorder until the 6 months criteria is met for schizophrenia. The diagnosis of 'provisional' schizophreniform disorder is made while the clinician monitors the evolving course of the illness, waits for the symptoms to resolve, or when the clinician cannot obtain a reliable history from a patient about the duration of the symptoms.

## Specifiers for Prognostic Features

The DSM-IV has specifiers for the presence or absence of good prognostic features. These features include a rapid onset (within 4 weeks) of prominent psychotic symptoms, presence of (psychogenic) confusion or perplexity at the height of the psychotic episode, good premorbid adjustment as evidenced by social and occupational functioning, and the absence of deficit symptoms such as blunted or flat affect.

## Clinical Features

The clinical signs and symptoms and the Mental Status Examination of the patient with schizophreniform disorder are often similar to those with schizophrenia, but the presence of affective symptoms usually predict a favorable course. Alternatively, a flat or blunted affect may predict an unfavorable course.

## Differential Diagnosis

This is similar to schizophrenia. Psychotic disorder caused by a general medical condition and substance-induced psychotic disorder must be ruled out. General medical conditions to be considered are HIV infection, temporal lobe epilepsy, CNS tumors, and cerebrovascular disease, all of which can also be associated with relatively short-lived psychotic episodes. The increasing number of reports of psychosis associated with the use of anabolic steroids by young men who are attempting to build up their muscles to perform better in athletic activities require careful history. Factitious disorder with predominantly psychological signs and symptoms and malingering may need to be ruled out in some instances.

## Course and Prognosis

This is, as anticipated, variable. The DSM IV specifiers 'with good prognostic features' and 'without good prognostic features' though helpful in guiding the clinician, require further validation. However, confusion or perplexity at the height of the psychotic episode is the feature best correlated with good outcome. Also, the shorter the period of illness, the better the prognosis is likely to be. There is a significant risk of suicide in these patients. Postpsychotic depression is quite likely and should be addressed in psychotherapy. Psychotherapy may help speed the recovery and improve the prognosis. By definition, schizophreniform disorder resolves within 6 months with a return to baseline mental functioning.

## Treatment

Hospitalization is often necessary and allows for effective assessment, treatment, and supervision of a patient's behavior. The psychotic symptoms, usually treated with a 3- to 6-month course of antipsychotic drugs, respond more rapidly than in patients with schizophrenia. One study found that 75% of the patients with schizophreniform psychosis compared to 20% of those with schizophrenia responded to antipsychotic agents within 8 days. ECT may be indicated for some patients, especially those with marked catatonic features or depression. If a patient has recurrent episodes, trials of lithium carbonate, valproic acid, or carbamazepine may be warranted for prophylaxis. Psychotherapy is usually necessary to help patients integrate the psychotic experience into their understanding of their minds, brains, and lives.

---

Clinical Vignette 5

Mr. A is a 25-year-old married white male who was brought to the emergency room by his family with complaints of paranoid thinking, agitation, auditory hallucinations, and insomnia. His family noticed that he was anxious, withdrawn, and had difficulty sleeping through the night 6 weeks previously. He reported to his wife that he was being harassed by his coworkers and felt that they were plotting against him. Mr. A reported hearing voices of a man and a woman with derogatory content. He did not leave the house for prolonged periods and complained of being under surveillance. He became quite agitated when his wife tried to have him visit a psychiatrist. When his family attempted to intervene, he threatened assault towards his brother. He did not report any precipitating factors except for a well-deserved promotion 6 months ago and his wife becoming pregnant 3 months ago. He was physically healthy and was not taking any medications. There was no past history of head injury or a seizure disorder. He did not consume any alcohol or drugs in the last 12 months. There was a history of occasional marijuana and alcohol use many years ago. He reported that his father had suffered from depression and was effectively treated for the same. He was described as a reliable and good worker and was with his current employer for 4 years. He had a few friends and was well adjusted with his wife. His admission laboratory workup and a head CT scan were within normal range, and his urine toxicology screen did not reveal any drugs. An atypical antipsychotic agent was initiated with benzodiazepines as needed for agitation, anxiety, and insomnia. He received individual and group therapy during the inpatient stay. He improved rapidly and was discharged 10 days later. He tolerated the medication well except for mild weight gain. He continued with individual therapy and had a few family counseling sessions. The patient decided to gradually discontinue his antipsychotic medications after 3 months of recovery. After one and a half years, he continues to work for the same firm, is back to his baseline, and does not have any residual symptoms.

## Delusional Disorder

Delusional disorder refers to a group of disorders, the chief feature of which is the presence of *nonbizarre* delusions. People suffering from this illness do not regard themselves as mentally ill and actively oppose psychiatric referral. Because they may experience little impairment, they generally remain outside hospital settings, appearing reclusive, eccentric, or odd, rather than ill. They are more likely to have contacts with professionals such as lawyers and other medical specialists for health concerns. The current shift in diagnosis from *paranoid* to *delusional* helps avoid the ambiguity around the term 'paranoid.' This also emphasizes that other delusions besides the paranoid ones are included in this diagnosis. It is important to understand the definition of nonbizarre delusion so as to reach an unambiguous diagnosis. Nonbizarre delusions typically involve situations or circumstances that can occur in real life (e.g., being followed, infected, or deceived by a lover) and are believable.

## Diagnostic Criteria

According to DSM-IV-TR, the diagnosis of delusional disorder can be made when a person exhibits nonbizarre delusions of at least 1 month's duration that cannot be attributed to other psychiatric disorders. Nonbizarre delusions must be about phenomena that, although not real, are within the realm of being possible. In general, the patient's delusions are well systematized and have been logically developed. If the person experiences auditory or visual hallucinations, they are not prominent except for tactile or olfactory hallucinations where they are tied in to the delusion (e.g., a person who believes that he emits a foul odor might experience an olfactory hallucination of that odor). The person's behavioral and emotional responses to the delusions appear to be appropriate. Usually the person's functioning and personality are well preserved and show minimal deterioration if at all.

## Epidemiology

Though the existence of delusional disorder has been known for a long time, relatively little is known about the demographics, incidence, and prevalence. Unfortunately, people suffering from this illness function reasonably well in the community and lack insight resulting in minimal or no contact with the mental health system. However, the crude incidence is roughly 0.7 to 3.0 per 100,000 with a more frequent occurrence in females. Some have associated this condition with widowhood, celibacy, and history of substance abuse. In one study, 1.2% of 4,144 consecutively attending subjects in an outpatient clinic were diagnosed to have delusional disorder. Half of the subjects were diagnosed to have *persecutory* type of delusional disorder. Females suffering from this disorder were significantly older than males. In a retrospective study from China, 0.83% of 10,418 outpatients met DSM-IV criteria of delusional disorder with equal gender distribution. The age range was 17 to 86 years with an average age of 42 ± 15 years. Women were significantly older then men at age of onset (46 versus 38.7). The mean duration of symptom onset to first psychiatry visit was 2.4 years and did not differ significantly between the sexes. Auditory hallucinations were reported in 11.6%, tactile hallucinations in 5.8%, visual hallucinations in 2.3%, and olfactory hallucinations in 2.3%. The delusional disorder subtypes were persecutory type 70.9%, mixed 14%, jealous 8.1%, somatic 2.3%, unspecified 2.1%, erotomanic 1.2%, and grandiose 1.2% (Hsiao 1999). Kendler (1982) reported a prevalence of 0.24 to 0.3% with a sex ratio of female to male of 1.18:1. Yamada and associates (1998) reported a 3:1 female to male ratio among their patients from Japan. Hwu and colleagues (1989) reported the lifetime prevalence of 0.48% in cities, 0.67% in townships, and 0.33% in rural villages. The gender ratios were not significantly different in their studies. Someya and colleagues (1987) reported that persecutory type of delusional disorder was more common (64%) followed by jealous type at (19%) in their cohort. Yamada and associates (1998) reported that persecutory type was most common at 51% followed by somatic type at 27.5% and jealous type at 13.7%. Both Yamada's and Hsiao's group did not find significant differences in the frequency of subtypes of delusional disorder between the sexes. Depressive symptomatology was present in 43% of the patients at their first visit (Hsiao et al. 1999). Higher frequency of depression has been reported by others (Marino et al. 1993) at 50.7%. Both, depression before the onset of delusions and after the onset of delusions have been reported (Marino et al. 1993, Chiu et al. 1990). The subgroup of patients who have hallucinations may have a poorer outcome depending on the intensity of the hallucinations (Serretti et al. 1999).

## History

The classical description of paranoia by Karl Ludwig Kahlbaum in 1863 paved the way for classification of paranoia. Kraepelin struggled with the concept of paranoia and his thinking finally evolved to define paranoia as an uncommon, insidious, chronic illness characterized by a fixed delusional system, an absence of hallucination, and a lack of deterioration of personality. Bleuler, on the other hand, viewed paranoia as a rare and milder version of schizophrenia and was not comfortable with a separate diagnosis. Freud used the autobiography of Daniel Paul Schreber, a jurist, and interpreted how unconscious homosexual tendencies were defended against by denial and projection in the form of delusions of persecution. His case study laid the basis for the psychodynamic understanding of paranoia.

## Etiology

Etiology of the delusional disorder is unknown. Risk factors associated with the disorder include advanced age, sensory impairment/isolation, family history, social isolation, personality features (e.g. unusual interpersonal sensitivity), and recent immigration. Some have reported higher association of delusional disorder with widowhood, celibacy, and history of substance abuse. Age of onset is later than schizophrenia and earlier in men compared to women.

## Subtypes

### Persecutory Type

This is the most common form of delusional disorder (Yamada et al. 1998). Here the person affected believes that he or she is being followed, spied on, poisoned or drugged, harassed, or conspired against. The person affected may get preoccupied by small slights that can become incorporated into the delusional system. These individuals may resort to legal actions to remedy perceived injustice. Individuals suffering from these delusions often become resentful and angry with a potential to get violent against those believed to be against them.

### Jealous Type

Individuals with this subtype have the delusional belief that their spouses/lovers are unfaithful. This is often wrongly inferred from small bits of benign evidence which is used to justify the delusion. Delusions of infidelity have also been called *conjugal paranoia*. The term *Othello syndrome* has been used to describe morbid jealousy. This delusion usually affects men, with no history of prior psychiatric problems. The condition is difficult to treat and may diminish only on separation, divorce, or death of the spouse. Marked jealousy (pathological jealousy or morbid jealousy) is a symptom of many disorders including schizophrenia and not unique to delusional disorder. Jealousy is a powerful emotion and when it occurs in delusional disorder or as part of another condition, it can be potentially dangerous and has been associated with violence including suicidal and homicidal behavior.

### Erotomanic Type

These patients have delusions of secret lovers. Most frequently, the patient is a woman, though men are also susceptible to these delusions. The patient believes that a suitor, usually more socially prominent than herself, is in love with her. This can become central focus of the patient's existence and the onset can be sudden. Erotomania is also referred to as *de Clerambault's syndrome*. Again, these delusions can occur as part of other disorders too. Generally women (but not exclusively so), unattractive in appearance, working at a lower-level jobs, who lead withdrawn, lonely single lives with few sexual contacts are reported to be more prone to develop this condition. They select lovers who are substantially different from them. They exhibit what has been called paradoxical conduct, the delusional phenomenon of interpreting all denials of love no matter how clear as secret affirmations of love. Separation from the love object may be the only satisfactory means of intervention. When it affects men, it can manifest with more aggressive and possibly violent pursuit of love. Thus, such people are often in

forensic system. The object of aggression is often companions or protectors of the love object who are viewed as trying to come between the lovers. However, resentment and rage in response to an absence of reaction from all forms of love communication may escalate to a point that the love object may be in danger too.

Approximately 10% of stalkers have a primary diagnosis of erotomania (Meloy 1996). Menezies and colleagues (1995) conducted the first predictive study of violence among erotomanic males and found that serious antisocial behavior (a criminal history) unrelated to the delusion and concurrent multiple objects of fixations discriminated between the dangerous and the nondangerous men. In a review by Meloy (1996), if violence occurred the object of love was target at least 80% of the time. The next most likely target was a third party perceived as impeding access to the object. He referred to this latter behavior as *triangulation*. Triangulation when present in jealousy, whether delusional or not, is motivated by a perceived competition for the love object (Meloy 1999).

### Somatic Type

Delusional disorder with somatic delusions has been called *monosymptomatic hypochondriacal psychosis*. This disorder differs from other conditions with hypochondriacal symptoms in degree of reality impairment. Munro (1988, 1991) has described the largest series of cases and has used content of delusions to define three main types:

***Delusions of Infestations (Including Parasitosis).*** Delusional parasitosis is one of the most common presentations of monohypochondriacal psychosis, which occurs in absence of other psychiatric illness (Munro 1982). In one study involving 52 patients, 88% of the cases were above 45 years of age (Bhatia et al. 2000). The prevalence of this condition is unknown (Berrios 1985). There appears to be a higher incidence of illness among middle-aged and elderly individuals. In the study mentioned above, 65% of the patients were females (Bhatia et al. 2000). This is similar to some reports but not all. The onset is insidious and chronic (Lyell 1983).

*Matchbox sign* describes the common phenomenon that occurred not so long ago in patients suffering from this condition. During their clinic visit, the patient would present with peeled skin, and other substances connected to delusional thinking in an empty old-fashioned matchbox as evidence that they were infested with insects (Lancet 1983, Morris 1991). Delusional parasitosis has been described in association with many physical illnesses such as vitamin $B_{12}$ deficiency, pellagra, neurosyphilis, multiple sclerosis, thalamic dysfunction, hypophyseal tumors, diabetes mellitus, severe renal disease, hepatitis, hypothyroidism, mediastinal lymphoma, and leprosy. Use of cocaine and presence of dementia has also been reported.

Psychogenic parasitosis was also known as Ekbom's syndrome before being referred to as *delusional parasitosis*. Females experienced this disorder twice as often as males. Entomologists, pest control specialists, and dermatologists had often seen the patient before seen by a psychiatrist. All investigators have been impressed by the concurrent medical illnesses associated with this condition. Others have attempted to distinguish between delusional and nondelusional aspects of presentation to establish clearer diagnosis and thus management.

***Delusions of Dymorphophobia.*** This condition includes delusions such as of misshapenness, personal ugliness, or exaggerated size of body parts.

***Delusions of Foul Body Odors or Halitosis.*** This is also called *olfactory reference syndrome*.

The frequency of these conditions is low, but they may be under diagnosed because patients present to dermatologists, plastic surgeons, and infectious disease specialists more often than to psychiatrists. Patients with these conditions do respond to pimozide, a typical antipsychotic medication and also to SSRIs. Usually prognosis is poor without treatment. It affects both sexes equally. Suicide apparently motivated by anguish is not uncommon.

## Grandiose Type

This is also referred to as *megalomania*. In this subtype, the central theme of the delusion is the grandiosity of having made some important discovery or having great talent. Sometimes there may be a religious theme to the delusional thinking such that the person believes that he or she has a special message from god.

## Mixed Type

This subtype is reserved for those with two or more delusional themes. However, it should be used only where it is difficult to clearly discern one theme of delusion.

## Unspecified Type

This subtype is used for cases in which the predominant delusion cannot be subtyped within the above mentioned categories. A possible example is certain delusions of misidentification, for example, *Capgras's syndrome*, named after the French psychiatrist who described the 'illusions of doubles.' The delusion here is the belief that a familiar person has been replaced by an imposter. A variant of this is *Fregoli's syndrome* where the delusion is that the persecutors or familiar persons can assume the guise of strangers and the very rare delusion that familiar persons could change themselves into other persons at will (intermetamorphosis). Each disorder is not only a rare delusion but is highly associated with other conditions such as schizophrenia and dementia.

## Course and Prognosis

Though the onset can occur in adolescence, generally it begins from middle to late adulthood with variable patterns of course, including lifelong disorder in some cases. Delusional disorder does not lead to severe impairment or change in personality, but rather to a gradual, progressive involvement with the delusional concern. Suicide has often been associated with this disorder. The base rate of spontaneous recovery may not be as low as previously thought, especially because only the more severely afflicted are referred for psychiatric treatment. Retterstol (Retterstol and Opjordsmoen 1991, Retterstol 1970) has provided much information on this. The more chronic forms of the illness tend to have their onset early in the fifth decade. Onset is acute in nearly two-thirds of the cases and gradual in the remainder. In almost half of the cases the delusion disappears at follow-up, improves in 10%, and is unchanged in 31%. In the more acute forms of the illness, the age of onset is in the fourth decade, a lasting remission occurs in over half of the patients and a pattern of chronicity develops in only 10%; a relapsing course has been observed in 37%. Thus, the more acute and earlier the onset of the illness, the more favorable the prognosis. The presence of precipitating factors, married status and female gender are associated with better outcome. The persistence of delusional thinking is most favorable for cases with persecutory delusions and somewhat less favorable for delusions of grandeur and jealousy. However, the outcome in terms of overall functioning appears somewhat more favorable for the jealous subtype.

## Comorbidity

Depression occurs frequently and is often an independent disorder in these patients.

## Treatment

Though generally considered resistant to treatment and interventions, the management is focused on managing the morbidity of the disorder by reducing the impact of the delusion on the patient's (and family's) life. However, in recent years the outlook has become less pessimistic or restricted in planning effective treatment for these conditions. An effective and therapeutic clinician–patient relationship is important but difficult to establish.

### Somatic Treatment

Overall, treatment results suggest that 80.8% of cases recover either fully or partially. Pimozide, the most frequently reported treatment produced full remission in 68.5% and partial recovery in 22.4% ($N = 143$). There are reports of treatment with other typical antipsychotic agents with variable success in small number of subjects. SSRIs have been used and reported to be helpful. The newer atypical antipsychotic agents have been used in small number of cases with success but the data is anecdotal. Bhatia and colleagues (2000) report that pimozide, fluoxetine, and amitriptyline were used in their study with pimozide showing good response.

### Psychosocial Treatment

As mentioned earlier, developing a therapeutic relationship is very important and yet significantly difficult, and requires frank and supportive attitude. Supportive therapy is very helpful in dealing with emotions of anxiety and dysphoria generated because of delusional thinking. Cognitive therapy, when accepted and implemented, is helpful. Confrontation

---

**Clinical Vignette 6**

***Delusional Disorder—Somatic Type***

Ms. K is a 32-year-old woman who presented to a dermatology clinic with complaints of "bugs" infecting her fingers, lips, scalp, ears, nose, face, and genitals for the last 3 months. She believed that her husband was the source of infection as she had observed him frequently scratching his scalp. However, she stated her husband feels that "it (her condition) is all in her head." She noticed others scratching while around her and believed that they had become infested by her presence. She brought multiple samples of the "bugs" in plastic bags.

On physical examination, there were multiple superficial excoriations over her nose, forehead, ears, scalp, jaw, and upper trunk. The dermatologist believed that the patient was suffering from psychogenic parasitosis and reassured Ms. K that her symptoms would be taken seriously and that an entomologist would evaluate her samples. She was prescribed fluocinolone for scalp inflammation, and asked to return to clinic with her husband in 1 week.

Ms. K returned to the clinic with her husband, frantically claiming that "things were falling off" of her and that she always saw "red dots" at the outset of her symptoms. She denied pruritus, scratching, or seeing "bugs." Her speech was pressured and she was crying. She was upset at her husband for blaming her symptoms on "nerves." On examination, she demonstrated numerous, crusted bloody excoriations, and her pubis was shaved smooth. Her husband was also examined, and no suspicious lesions were noted. The dermatologist spoke to the husband and patient both alone and together. Her husband had excellent insight. Ms. K was reassured and asked to await the results from the entomologist. The entomologist's report contained skin debris and some incidental insect parts (*Cullicoides* species, which are not associated with dermatoses). Ms. K continued to worsen over the next several clinic visits, despite reassurance by the dermatologist. She also continued to bring in numerous samples and frequently stated that she believed that her husband is the "root of the problem." She was delusional and displayed poor insight. She refused psychiatric help but agreed to 50 mg intramuscular haloperidol decanoate. The dermatologist was hoping to control symptoms enough to allow psychiatric referral. She improved remarkably following injection and her skin was nearly clear. She did not feel that she was causing others to scratch around her. She also stopped bringing in samples of bugs. Though she demonstrated limited insight, she still felt that her illness was not due to psychiatric issues. She questioned taking medications when "all this started with my husband." Pimozide was started at 2 mg/day with a plan to gradually increase the dose upwards. Ms. K continued to show improvement in her symptoms but her insight had not improved much so her dose was doubled to 4 mg/day. Six weeks after starting pimozide, Ms. K's progress halted. She continued to state that her husband was scratching her scalp, which she believed to be the root of the problem. The dermatologist emphasized the success of haloperidol decanoate therapy and recommended it once more, but the patient refused it. Ms. K was instructed to increase the dose of pimozide to 6 mg/day. Numerous phone conversations over the next several weeks revealed that she was probably noncompliant with the prescribed oral medications. She reported a different dosage each conversation and was unable to give the name of her pharmacy on several occasions, nor could she describe the pills. Her delusions and complaints about her husband persisted. Meanwhile, she had seen another physician who treated her with lindane for pediculosis. She finally agreed to visit the psychosomatic clinic. She was seen by a psychiatrist and was diagnosed to have delusional disorder, somatic type. There were no symptoms of mania or

depression noted. The anxiety and sleep disturbances associated with delusional thinking were treated with clonazepam. Four days later, Ms. K paged the dermatologist stating that she was much worse and needed to be seen immediately. She presented to the clinic with her hair matted down with calamine lotion, numerous superficial erosions, and various exogenous particles in her hair, but no parasites or nits were seen. There were serious concerns about her compliance. She refused the haloperidol decanoate injections due to side effects but agreed to visit the psychosomatic clinic again. She became quite erratic with her dermatology and psychosomatic clinic visits. She continued to have delusional thinking and other symptoms. After missing several clinic visits and with possible erratic compliance, she presented to the psychosomatic clinic with symptoms of anxiety and depression. As she was refusing haloperidol and was noncompliant with pimozide, she was switched to olanzapine 5 mg/day. During subsequent visits her husband reported past history of bouts of depression with neurovegetative symptoms possibly meeting the diagnosis of major depressive disorder with psychotic features. Her dose of olanzapine was meanwhile increased to 20 mg/day. She was started on an antidepressant the dose of which was gradually increased. Laboratory examinations for thyroid function tests, folate, and other chemistries were within normal range.

Unfortunately, Ms. K did not comply with medication recommendations, continued to seek the source of infestation, and resisted recommendations for either intramuscular (IM) medications or an inpatient admission. She was lost to follow-up. The last call for the patient came from her veterinarian. The patient had repeatedly brought her dog into the veterinarian's office, requesting evaluation of her pet for parasites, though the dog was not infested. The veterinarian was encouraged to refer the patient back to the psychosomatics clinic, but no further visits ensued.

*Source: Adapted with permission from Slaughter JR et al. (1998). Copyright 1998 American Psychiatric Publishing.*

Clinical Vignette 7

### *Delusional Disorder—Jealous Type*

A 35-year-old male janitor was admitted to a psychiatric hospital after violating a restraining order brought by his wife. The patient firmly believed (contrary to the facts in this case) that his wife was having an affair with someone for the last few years. He reported that he had often noticed his wife speaking softly and pleasantly with someone on the phone and would stop the conversation as soon as he entered the house. His attempts to trace the call were futile, further confirming his suspicion. He had noticed that his side of the bed was often ruffled as if someone had slept on it. He had also noticed that the bedroom window was on occasion open even when he had made sure that it was locked when he left for his night shift. His wife reported that she had caught him sniffing her undergarments and looking for evidence of recent sexual activity. When his wife confronted him, he angrily accused her of infidelity. Her attempts to reassure him by explaining the alleged evidence of infidelity made him even more suspicious. He started having his house under surveillance to detect the alleged lover. When no unusual activity was noticed, he concluded that she had become cautious.

He surprised her on a few occasions by coming home earlier then anticipated, and her not opening the door immediately resulted in further accusations and verbal arguments. He also went to her workplace unannounced. When his wife told him that he was losing his mind and reading too much into benign actions and events, he became infuriated and they had their first physical altercation resulting in police intervention. She refused to press charges the first time but when she was assaulted again, she brought a restraining order against him. She moved in with her mother. He started spying on her activities at her mother's place and confronted her at her work place with allegations of having an affair with someone there. She called the police when he assumed a threatening posture towards her resulting in his arrest and subsequent admission to a hospital by court order. He vehemently denied having any psychiatric illness, became very angry with his wife blaming her for his plight, and remained preoccupied with his wife's alleged infidelity. The psychiatrist interviewed the patient and his wife separately and other family members. A diagnosis of delusional disorder, jealous type was reached and he was started on an atypical antipsychotic medication after much discussion about the alternatives to refusal of treatment. The patient's agitation and the intensity of the delusional thinking decreased but he remained convinced that his wife was having an affair with someone. The patient lacked insight into his illness. His wife started divorce proceedings, which was yet another proof of her scheme to get him out of the way so that she can marry her alleged lover. Following treatment with an antipsychotic agent and individual therapy, though the patient still believed that his wife did have an affair, he did not have thoughts of pursuing or hurting her.

of the delusional thinking usually does not work and can further alienate the patient.

## Shared Psychotic Disorder

Shared psychotic disorder is a rare disorder, which is also referred to as *shared paranoid disorder, induced psychotic disorder, folie a deux,* and *double insanity.* Jules Baillarger, in 1860, first described the syndrome and called it *folie a communiquee,* while Lasegue and Falret, in 1877, first described *folie a deux.* In this disorder, the transfer of delusions takes place from one person to another. Both persons are closely associated for a long time and typically live together in relative social isolation. In its more common form, *folie imposee,* the individual who first has the delusion is often chronically ill and typically is the influential member of the close relationship with another individual, who is more suggestible and who develops the delusion too. The second individual is frequently less intelligent, more gullible, more passive, or more lacking in self-esteem than the primary case. If the two people involved are separated, the second individual may abandon the delusion. However, this is not seen consistently. Other forms of shared psychotic disorder reported are *folie simultanee,* where similar delusional systems develop independently in two closely associated people. Occasionally more than two individuals are involved (e.g. *folie a trois, quatre, cinq;* also *folie a famille*) but such cases are very rare. The most common dyadic relationships who develop this disorder are sister–

sister, husband–wife, and mother–child. Almost all cases involve members of a single family.

### Epidemiology
More than 95% of all cases of shared psychotic disorder involve two members of the same family. About a third of the cases involve two sisters, another one-third involve husband and wife or a mother and her child. The dominant person is usually affected by schizophrenia or a similar psychotic disorder. In 25% of all cases, the submissive person is usually affected with physical disabilities such as deafness, cerebrovascular diseases, or other disability that increases the submissive person's dependence on the dominant person. This condition is more common in people from low socioeconomic groups and in women.

### Etiology
There is some data that suggest that people suffering from shared psychotic disorder may have a family history of schizophrenia. The dominant person suffering from this illness often has schizophrenia or a related psychotic illness. The dominant person is usually older, more intelligent, better educated, and has stronger personality traits than the submissive person, who is usually dependent on the dominant person. The affected individuals usually live together or have an extremely close personal relationship, associated with shared life experiences, common needs and hopes, and often, a deep emotional rapport with each other. The relationship between the people involved is usually somewhat or completely isolated from external societal cultural inputs. The submissive person may be predisposed to a mental disorder and may have a history of a personality disorder with dependent or suggestible qualities as well as a history of depression, suspiciousness, and social isolation. The dominant person's psychotic symptoms may develop in the submissive person through the process of identification. By adopting the psychotic symptoms of the dominant person, the submissive person gains acceptance by the other.

### Diagnosis
An important feature in the diagnosis is that the person with shared psychotic disorder does not have a preexisting psychotic disorder. The delusions arise in the context of a close relationship with a person who suffers from delusional thinking and resolve on separation from that person.

### Clinical Features
The key symptom of shared psychosis is the unquestioning acceptance of another person's delusions. The delusions themselves are often in the realm of possibility and usually not as bizarre as those seen in patients with schizophrenia. The content of the delusion is often persecutory or hypochondriacal. Symptoms of a coexisting personality disorder may be present, but signs and symptoms that meet criteria for schizophrenia, mood disorders, and delusional disorder are absent. The patient may have ideation about suicide or pacts about homicide; clinicians must elicit this information during the interview.

### Differential Diagnosis
Malingering, factitious disorder with predominantly psychological sign and symptoms, psychotic disorder due to a

general medical condition, and substance-induced psychotic disorder must be considered.

## Course and Prognosis

Though separation of submissive person from the dominant person should resolve the psychosis, this probably occurs only in 10 to 40 % of the cases. Unfortunately, when these individuals are discharged from hospital, they usually move back together.

## Treatment

The initial step in treatment is to separate the affected person from the source of the delusions, the dominant individual. Antipsychotic agents may be used if the symptoms have not abated in a week after separation. Psychotherapy with the nondelusional members of the patient's family should be undertaken, and psychotherapy with both the patient and the person sharing the delusion may be indicated later in the course of treatment. To prevent redevelopment of the syndrome the family may need family therapy and social support to modify the family dynamics and to prevent redevelopment of the syndrome. Steps to decrease the social isolation may also help prevent the syndrome from reemerging.

---

### Clinical Vignette 8

*Folie a Quatre*

Four members of a large Nigerian family presented with shared persecutory and religious delusions. The first to exhibit symptoms and therefore the presumptive inducer was a 25-year-old midwife (LM) with a 5-year history of persecutory delusions exacerbated in the year before presentation when her family refused to allow her marriage plans. She had become increasingly suspicious and accused others of being witches threatening her family. Attempts to help her with herbal medicines prescribed by a traditional healer, confirmed her delusions of being poisoned. She ate and slept little, and become socially isolated. She also became increasingly argumentative, verbally and physically aggressive, and preoccupied with religious observances. She was well dressed and covered her head with a white veil to signify purity. She held a Bible in her hand and gave "greeting in Jesus' name." Although calm and coherent, she frowned throughout the interview. She accused her relatives of planning with evil forces to eliminate her. She admitted seeing visions of her brother being anointed by the Holy Spirit.

Her brother (DM), older sister (TM) and 15-year-old niece (NM, TM's daughter) all gathered with other members of the family to pray for her. These three were subsequently noticed to be expressing the same persecutory and religious ideation. Their mother and other family members were extremely concerned to find appropriate treatment for the four. DM had worked intermittently as a schoolteacher and his presentation was very similar to LM. He also believed that his mother and older brother were witches who had collaborated with his wife to kill him by taking him to the traditional healer. He was argumentative, irrational but coherent, and expressed the belief that forces were pulling blood from his legs and other relatives were plotting to kill him. Both TM and NM expressed the same delusional thinking that others were planning to kill them all.

All four were admitted to their local psychiatric hospital but DM and LM failed to improve and were transferred to

another hospital. Following their transfer, TM and NM made rapid recoveries and were discharged. DM and LM required higher doses of conventional antipsychotic agents and were commenced on depot injections. Attempts were made to separate LM from her brother. Despite this, they continued to meet and prayed incessantly together. They continued to express their shared persecutory beliefs, but after about 3 weeks of treatment their mental state had begun to improve and the pair spent less time together. After 8 weeks both were well enough for discharge and outpatient follow-up on depot medication. LM was subsequently able to return to work and DM enrolled for a course in a theological college.

*Source: Adapted with permission from Mela M et al. (1997). Copyright 1997 Elsevier Science, B.V.*

---

### Clinical Vignette 9

*Folie Simultanee*

Twin A, a 30-year-old white female who had no previous psychiatric problems, was admitted to a psychiatric ward following a serious suicide attempt. Six months before admission, twin A and her husband found a sperm-filled condom in their bathroom after returning from an evening out. They were concerned that their baby-sitter had sexually abused their children, although there was no visible evidence.

Shortly thereafter, twin B, who lived in a neighboring city, sent twin A information on ritualistic sexual abuse by satanic cults. The twins then began meeting together and reading literature on satanic worship and ritualistic sexual abuse by satanic cults. Over time, the twins gradually reduced their social activities except for a few specific meetings. They attended support groups for parents of ritualistically sexually abused children and were convinced that increasingly more people were involved in satanic cults. Within the month before admission, they believed that the satanic cult involved their husbands, family members, neighborhood, church, and the police department. They believed that their children were forced to drink urine and to witness child sacrifice. They also believed that the children were ongoing victims of ritualistic sexual abuse and torture by means of having their feet dipped in hot water.

Several days before admission, the twins met together to view a four-part television series on satanic worship. This resulted in further "hysteria" between the two and the creation of a suicide pact. The evening prior to admission, twin B was brought for evaluation at the hospital. When twin A learned that twin B was at the hospital, she believed that the satanists had abducted her. This prompted a suicide attempt with her partially severing her carotid artery. She experienced a massive hemorrhage, requiring 10 units of packed red blood cells before surgical repair.

Following stabilization, twin A was transferred to the inpatient ward and information was obtained through interviews with the twins and multiple family members. There was no evidence of mood disorders, substance abuse problems, or hallucinations in either twin. Both twins maintained the same delusional system at approximately the same intensity without one being dominant.

*Source: Adapted with permission from White TG (1995). Copyright 1995 Canadian Psychiatric Association.*

## Comparison of DSM-IV/ICD-10 Diagnostic Criteria

The ICD-10 and DSM-IV-TR criteria sets for schizophrenia are similar in many important ways although not identical. The ICD-10 Diagnostic Criteria for Research provide two ways to satisfy the criteria for schizophrenia: having one Schneiderian first-rank symptom or having at least two of the other characteristic symptoms (hallucinations accompanied by delusions, thought disorder, catatonic symptoms, and negative symptoms). In contrast to DSM-IV-TR which requires 6 months of symptoms (including prodromal, active, and residual phases), the ICD-10 definition of schizophrenia requires only a 1-month duration thereby encompassing the DSM-IV-TR diagnostic categories of both schizophrenia and schizophreniform disorder. Thus, cases of DSM-IV-TR schizophreniform disorder are diagnosed in ICD-10 as schizophrenia.

The DSM-IV-TR and ICD-10 definitions of schizoaffective disorder differ with regard to the relationship of the schizoaffective disorder category with the category mood disorder with psychotic features. In DSM-IV-TR, the differentiation depends on the temporal relationship between the mood and psychotic symptoms (i.e., mood disorder with psychotic features is diagnosed whenever the psychotic symptoms occur only in the presence of a mood episode, regardless of the characteristics of the psychotic symptoms). In contrast, the ICD-10 definition of schizoaffective disorder is much broader. It includes situations in which certain specified psychotic symptoms (i.e., thought echo, insertion, withdrawal, or broadcasting; delusions of control or passivity; voices giving a running commentary; disorganized speech, catatonic behavior) occur even if they are confined to a mood episode. Therefore, many cases of DSM-IV-TR mood disorder with mood-incongruent psychotic features would be considered to be schizoaffective disorder in ICD-10. Furthermore, the ICD-10 definition suggests that there should be an "approximate balance between the number, severity, and duration of the schizophrenic and affective symptoms." For delusional disorder, the ICD-10 Diagnostic Criteria for Research specify a minimum 3-month duration in contrast to the 1-month minimum duration in DSM-IV-TR.

In contrast to the single DSM-IV-TR category brief psychotic disorder, ICD-10 has a much more complex way of handling brief psychotic disorders. It includes criteria sets for four specific brief psychotic disorders that differ based on types of symptoms (i.e., with or without symptoms of schizophrenia) and course (i.e., whether they change rapidly or not). Furthermore, the maximum duration of these brief psychotic episodes varies depending on the type of symptoms (i.e., 1 month for schizophrenia-like symptoms and 3 months for predominantly delusional). In contrast, DSM-IV-TR has a single criteria set and a maximum 1-month duration.

Finally, the ICD-10 and DSM-IV-TR definitions of shared psychotic disorder are almost identical.

## References

Abi-Dargham A, Gil R, Krystal J, et al. (1998) Increased striatal dopamine transmission in schizophrenia: Confirmation in a second cohort. Am J Psychiatr 155, 761–767.

Adams CE, Fenton MK, Quraishi S, et al. (2001) Systematic meta-review of depot antipsychotic drugs for people with schizophrenia. Br J Psychiatr 179, 290–299.

Adams RD and Victor M (1989) Principles of Neurology, 4th ed. McGraw-Hill, New York.

Adebimpe VR (1994) Race, racism and epidemiological surveys. Hosp Comm Psychiatr 45, 27–31.

Addington DD, Azorin JM, Falloon IRH, et al. (2002) Clinical issues related to depression in schizophrenia: An international survey of psychiatrists. Acta Psychiatr Scand 105, 189–195.

Allardyce J, Boydell J, Van Os J, et al. (2001) Comparison of the incidence of schizophrenia in rural Dumfries and Galloway and urban Camberwell. Br J Psychiatr 179, 335–339.

Allebech P, Varia A, and Wistedt B (1986) Suicide and violent death among patients with schizophrenia. Acta Psychiatr Scand 74, 43–49.

Allison DB, Mentore JL, Heo M, et al. (1999) Antipsychotic-induced weight gain: A comprehensive research synthesis. Am J Psychiatr 156, 1686–1696.

Almeida O, Howards R, Levy R, et al. (1995) Psychotic states rising in late life (late paraphrenia): Psychopathology and nosology. Br J Psychiatr 166, 205–214.

Altshuler LL, Bartzokis G, Grieder T, et al. (1998) Amygdala enlargement in bipolar disorder and hippocampal reduction in schizophrenia: An MRI study demonstrating neuroanatomic specificity. Arch Gen Psychiatr 55, 663–664.

Alvir JM, Lieberman JA, Safferman AZ, et al. (1993) Clozapine-induced agranulocytosis: Incidence and risk factors in the United States. N Engl J Med 329, 162–167.

Ameddeo F, Bisoffi G, Bonizzato P, et al. (1995) Mortality among patients with psychiatric illness: A ten-year case register study in an area with community-based system of care. Br J Psychiatr 166, 783–788.

American Psychiatric Association (1994) Diagnostic and Statistical Manual of Mental Disorders, 4th ed. APA, Washington DC.

American Psychiatric Association (APA) Task Force (1980) Task force on late neurological effects of antipsychotic drugs: Tardive dyskinesia. Am J Psychiatr 137, 1163–1172.

Andreasen NC (1981) Scale for the Assessment of Negative Symptoms (SANS). University of Iowa, Iowa City, IA.

Andreasen NC (1997) The role of the thalamus in schizophrenia. Can J Psychiatr 42, 27–33.

Andreasen NC and Olsen SA (1982) Negative vs. positive schizophrenia: Definition and validation. Arch Gen Psychiatr 39, 789–794.

Andreasen NC, Arndt S, Alliger R, et al. (1995) Symptoms of schizophrenia: Methods, meanings and mechanisms. Arch Gen Psychiatr 52, 341–351.

Andreasen NC, Arndt S, Swayze V, et al. (1994) Thalamic abnormalities in schizophrenia visualized through magnetic resonance image averaging. Science 266, 294–298

Andreasen NC, Nasrallah HA, Dunn VD, et al. (1986) Structural abnormalities in the frontal system in schizophrenia: A magnetic resonance imaging study. Arch Gen Psychiatr 43, 135–144.

Andreasen NC, Olsen SA, Dennert JW, et al. (1982) Ventricular enlargement in schizophrenia: Relationship to positive and negative symptoms. Am J Psychiatr 139, 297–302.

Andrews G, Hall W, Goldstein G, et al. (1985) The economic costs of schizophrenia: Implications for public policy. Arch Gen Psychiatr 42, 537–543.

Arato M, O'Conner R, Bradbury JE, et al. (1998) Ziprasidone in the long-term treatment of negative symptoms and prevention of exacerbation of schizophrenia. Eur Psychiatr 13(Supp 4), 303.

Aravantis LA and Miller BG (1997) Multiple fixed doses of "Seroquel" (quetiapine) in patients with acute exacerbation of schizophrenia: A comparison with haloperidol and placebo. The Seroquel Trial 13 Study Group. Biol Psychiatr 42, 233–246.

Arieti S (1955) Interpretation of Schizophrenia. Robert Brunner, New York.

Arndt S, Andreasen NC, Flaum M, et al. (1995) A longitudinal study of symptom dimensions in schizophrenia. Prediction and patterns of change. Arch Gen Psychiatr 52, 341–351.

Astrup C and Noreik K (1966) Functional Psychoses: Diagnostic and Prognostic Models. Springfield.

Ayd FJ (1961) A survey of drug induced extrapyramidal reactions. JAMA 175, 1054–1061.

Bachrach LL (2000) Psychosocial rehabilitation and psychiatry in the treatment of schizophrenia: What are the boundaries? Acta psychiatr Scand 102(Suppl 407), 6–10.

Baker SC, Frith CD, and Dolan RJ (1997) The interaction between mood and cognitive function studied with PET. Psychol Med 27, 565–578.

Baldessarini RJ and Frankenburg FR (1991) Clozapine: A novel antipsychotic agent. N Engl J Med 324, 746–754.

Baldwin JA (1979) Schizophrenia and physical disease. Psychol Med 9, 611–618.

Barbato A and D'Avanzo B (2000) Family interventions in schizophrenia and related disorders: A critical review of clinical trials. Acta Psychiatr Scand 102, 81–97.

Barta PE, Pearlson GD, Powers RE, et al. (1990) Auditory hallucinations and smaller superior temporal gyral volume in schizophrenia. Am J Psychiatr 147, 1457–1462.

Banov MD, Zarate CA Jr., Tohen M, et al. (1994) Clozapine therapy in refractory affective disorders: Polarity predicts response in long-term follow-up. J Clin Psychiatr 55, 411–414.

Barnes TR and Curson DA (1994) Long-term depot antipsychotics. A risk-benefit assessment. Drug Safety 10, 464–479.

Beard JH, Propst RN, and Malamud TJ (1982) The Fountain House model of psychiatric rehabilitation. Psychosoc Rehabil J 5, 47–53.

Beasley CM Jr., Hamilton SH, Crawford AM, et al. (1997) Olanzapine versus haloperidol: Acute phase results of the international double-blind olanzapine trial. Eur Neuropsychopharmacol 7, 125–137.

Beasley CM Jr., Tollefson G, Tran P, et al. (1996) Olanzapine versus placebo and haloperidol: Acute phase results of the North American double-blind olanzapine trial. Neuropsychopharmacology 14, 111–123.

Beatty WW, Jocic Z, Monson N, et al. (1993) Memory and frontal lobe dysfunction in schizophrenia and schizoaffective disorder. J Nerv Ment Dis 181, 448–453.

Benes FM (2000) Emerging principles of altered neural circuitry in schizophrenia. Brain Res Brain Res Rev 31, 251–269.

Benes FM, Kwok EW, Vincent MS, et al. (1998) A reduction of nonpyramidal cells in sector CA2 of schizophrenics and manic depressives. Biol Psychiatr 44, 88–97.

Benes FM, McSparren J, Bird ED, et al. (1991) Deficits in small interneurons in prefrontal and cingulate cortices of schizophrenic and schizoaffective patients. Arch Gen Psychiatr 48, 996–1001.

Bernstein AS (1987) Orienting response research in schizophrenia: Where we have come and where we might go. Schizophr Bull 13, 623–641.

Berrios GE (1985) Positive and negative symptoms and Jackson. A conceptual history. Arch Gen Psychiatr 42, 95–97.

Bertelsen A and Gottesman II (1995) Schizoaffective psychoses: Genetical clues to classification. Am J Med Genet 60, 7–11.

Bharath S, Gangadhar BN, and Janakiramaiah N (2000) P300 in family studies of schizophrenia: Review and critique. Int J Psychophysiol 38, 43–54.

Bhatia MS, Jagawat T, and Choudhary S (2000) Delusional Parasitosis: A clinical profile. Int J Psychiatr Med 30, 83–91.

Bhugra D (2000) Migration and schizophrenia. Acta Psychiatr Scand, 102(Suppl 407), 68–73.

Bilder RM, Bogerts B, Wu H, et al. (1994) Independence of morphological markers in schizophrenia. Biol Psychiatr 35, 730.

Binder EB, Kinkead B, Owens MJ, et al. (2001) The role of neurotensin in the pathophysiology of schizophrenia and the mechanism of action of antipsychotic drugs. Biol Psychiatr 50, 856–872.

Bisette G, Dole K, Johnson M, et al. (1988) Antipsychotic drugs increase neurotensin concentrations after destruction of dopamine neurons by 6–OHDA. Soc Neurosci Abstr 14, 1211.

Blackwood D (2000) P300, a state and a trait marker in schizophrenia. Lancet 355, 771–772.

Bleuler E and Zinkin J (trans) (1950) Dementia Praecox or the Group of Schizophrenics. International Universities Press, New York.

Blin O, Azorin JM, and Bouhours P (1996) Antipsychotic and anxiolytic properties of risperidone, haloperidol, and methotrimeprazine in schizophrenic patients. J Clin Psychopharmacol 16, 38–44.

Blouin JL, Dombroski BA, Nath SK, et al. (1998) Schizophrenia susceptibility loci on chromosomes 13q32 and 8p21. Nat Genet 20, 70–73.

Bogan AM, Brown ES, and Suppes T (2000) Efficacy of Divalproex therapy for schizoaffective disorder. J Clin Psychopharmacol 20, 520–522.

Bojholm S and Stromgren E (1989) Prevalence of schizophrenia on the island of Bornholm in 1935 and in 1983. Acta Psychiatr Scand 79(Suppl 348), 157–166.

Bondolfi G, Dufour H, Patris M, et al. (1998) Risperidone versus clozapine in treatment-resistant chronic schizophrenia: A randomized double-blind study. Am J Psychiatr 155, 499–504.

Borison RL, Aravantis LA, and Miller BG (1996) ICI 204,636, an atypical antipsychotic: Efficacy and safety in a multicenter, placebo-controlled trial in patients with schizophrenia. US Seroquel Study Group. J Clin Psychopharm 16, 158–169.

Bornstein RA, Nasrallah HA, Olson SC, et al. (1990) Neuropsychological deficit in schizophrenic subtypes: Paranoid, nonparanoid, and schizoaffective subgroups. Psychiatr Res 31, 15–24.

Bouras C, Kovari E, Hof PR, et al. (2001) Anterior cingulate cortex pathology in schizophrenia and bipolar disorder. Acta Neuropathol 102, 373–379.

Bourdon KH, Rae DS, Lacke BZ, et al. (1992) Estimating the prevalence of mental disorders in US adults from the Epidemiological Catchment Area survey. Pub Health Rep 107, 663–668.

Boyer WF, Bakalar NH, and Lake CR (1987) Anticholinergic prophylaxis of acute haloperidol-induced acute dystonic reactions. J Clin Psychopharmacol 7, 164–166.

Brady JP (1984) Social skills training for psychiatric patients. I: Concepts, methods, and clinical results. Am J Psychiatr 141, 333–340.

Braff DL (1993) Information processing and attention dysfunctions in schizophrenia. Schizophr Bull 19, 233–259.

Braff DL and Geyer MA (1990) Sensorimotor gating and schizophrenia: Human and animal model studies. Arch Gen Psychiatr 47, 181–188.

Bredesen DE (1995) Neural apoptosis. Ann Neurol 38, 839–851.

Breier A (1994) Clozapine and noradrenergic function: Support for a novel hypothesis for superior efficacy. J Clin Psychiatr 55, 122–125.

Breier A (1995) Serotonin, schizophrenia and antipsychotic drug action. Schizophr Res 14, 187–202.

Breier A and Astrachan BM (1984) Characterization of schizophrenic patients who commit suicide. Am J Psychiatr 141, 610–611.

Breier A and Hamilton SH (1999) Comparative efficacy of olanzapine and haloperidol for patients with treatment-resistant schizophrenia. Biol Psychiatr 45(4), 403–411.

Breier A, Buchanan RW, Elkashef A, et al. (1992) Brain morphology and schizophrenia: An MRI study of limbic, prefrontal cortex and caudate structures. Arch Gen Psychiatr 49, 921–926.

Breier A, Buchanan RW, Waltrip RW, et al. (1994) The effect of clozapine on plasma norepinephrine: Relationship to clinical efficacy. Neuropsychopharmacology 10, 1–7.

Breier A, Meehan K, Birkett M, et al. (2002) A double-blind, placebo-controlled dose-response comparison of intramuscular olanzapine and haloperidol in the treatment of acute agitation in schizophrenia. Arch Gen Psychiatr 59, 441–448.

Breier A, Schreiber JL, Dyer J, et al. (1991) National Institute of Mental Health longitudinal study of chronic schizophrenia: Prognosis and prediction of outcome. Arch Gen Psychiatr 48, 239–246.

Breier A, Su T-P, Saunders R, et al. (1997) Schizophrenia is associated with elevated amphetamine-induced synaptic dopamine concentrations: Evidence from a novel positron emission tomography method. Proc Natl Acad Sci USA 94, 2569–2574.

Brewin J, Cantwell R, Dalkin T, et al. (1997) Incidence of schizophrenia in Nottingham. Br J Psychiatry 171, 140–144.

Bruder G, Kayser J, Tenke C, et al. (1999) Left temporal lobe dysfunction in schizophrenia: Event-related potential and behavioral evidence from phonetic and tonal dichotic listening tasks. Arch Gen Psychiatr 56, 267–276.

Bucci L (1987) The negative symptoms of schizophrenia and the monoamine oxidase inhibitors. Psychopharmacology 91, 104–108.

Buchanan RW (1995) Clozapine: Efficacy and safety. Schizophr Bull 21, 579–591.

Buchsbaum MS and Hazlett E (1998) Positron emission tomography studies of abnormal glucose metabolism in schizophrenia. Schizophr Bull 24, 343–364.

Buchsbaum MS, Tang CY, Peled S, et al. (1998) MRI white matter diffusion anisotropy and PET metabolic rate in schizophrenia. Neuroreport 9, 425–430.

Buchsbaum MS, Yang S, Hazlett E, et al. (1997) Ventricular volume and asymmetry in schizotypal personality disorder and schizophrenia assessed with magnetic resonance imaging. Schizophr Res 27, 45–53.

Buckley NA, Whyte IM, and Dawson AH (1995) Cardiotoxicity more common in thioridazine overdose than with other neuroleptics. J Toxicol Clin Toxicol 33, 199–204.

Bunney WE and Bunney BG (2000) Evidence for a compromised dorsolateral prefrontal cortical parallel circuit in schizophrenia. Brain Res Brain Res Rev 31, 138–146.

Burnet PW, Eastwood SL, and Harrison PJ (1997) [3H]WAY-100635 for 5-HT$_{1A}$ receptor autoradiography in human brain: A comparison with

[3H]8-OH-DPAT and demonstration of increased binding in the frontal cortex in schizophrenia. Neurochem Int 30, 565–574.

Butler RW, Jenkins MA, Geyer MA, et al. (1991) Wisconsin Card Sorting deficits and diminished sensorimotor gating in a discrete subgroup of schizophrenic patients. In Advances in Neuropsychiatry and Psychopharmacology: Schizophrenia Research, Vol. 1, Tamminga CA and Schulz SC (eds). Raven Press, New York, pp. 163–168.

Bymaster F, Perry KW, Nelson DL, et al. (1999) Olanzapine: A basic science update. Br J Psychiatr 174(Suppl 37), 36–40.

Byrne M, Browne R, Mulryan N, et al. (2000) Labor and delivery complications and schizophrenia: Case control study using ccontemporaneous labour ward records. Br J Psychiatr 176, 531–536.

Calev A (1984) Recalled recognition in mildly disturbed schizophrenics: The use of matched tasks. Psychol Med 14, 425–429.

Calev A and Monk AF (1982) Verbal memory tasks showing no deficit in schizophrenia—fact or artefact? Br J Psychiatr 141, 528–530.

Calev A, Berlin H, and Lerer B (1987) Remote and recent memory in long-hospitalized chronic schizophrenics. Biol Psychiatr 22, 79–85.

Cannon M, Jones PB, and Murray RM (2002) Obstetric complications and schizophrenia: Historical and meta-analytic review. Am J Psychiatr 159, 1080–1092.

Cannon TD, Rosso IM, Hollister JM, et al. (2000) A prospective cohort study of genetic and perinatal influences in the etiology of schizophrenia. Schizophr Bull 26, 249–256.

Cannon TD, van Erp TG, Huttunen M, et al. (1998) Regional gray matter, white matter, and cerebrospinal fluid distributions in schizophrenic patients, their siblings, and controls. Arch Gen Psychiatr 55, 1084–1091.

Cannon TD, Zorilla LE, and Shtasel D (1994) Neuropsychological function in siblings discordant for schizophrenia and healthy volunteers. Arch Gen Psychiatr 51, 651–661.

Cantor-Graae E, McNeil TF, Sjostrom K, et al. (1994) Obstetrics complications and their relationship to other etiological risk factors in schizophrenia: A case-control study. J Nerv Ment Dis 182, 645–650.

Cao Q, Martinez M, Zhang J, et al. (1997) Suggestive evidence for a schizophrenia susceptibility locus on chromosome 6q and a confirmation in an independent series of pedigrees. Genomics 43, 1–8.

Carlsson A, Waters N, Holm-Waters S, et al. (2001) Interactions between monoamines glutamate, and GABA in schizophrenia: New evidence. Annu Rev Pharmacol Toxicol 41, 237–260.

Castle DJ and Murray RM (1993) The epidemiology of late-onset schizophrenia. Schizophr Bull 19, 691–700.

Carpenter WT, Heinrichs DS, and Alphs LD (1985) Treatment of negative symptoms. Schizophr Bull 11, 440–452.

Carpenter WT Jr., Conley RR, Buchanan RW, et al. (1995) Patient response and resource management: Another view of clozapine treatment of schizophrenia. Am J Psychiatr 152, 827–832.

Carter CS, Mintun M, Nichols T, et al. (1997) Anterior cingulate gyrus dysfunction and selective attention deficits in schizophrenia: [$^{15}$O]H$_2$0 PET study during single-trial Stroop task performance. Am J Psychiatr 154, 1670–1675.

CATIE (1999) (Clinical Antipsychotic Trials of Intervention Effectiveness) funded by National Institute of Mental Health and coordinated by University of North Carolina at Chapel Hill (www.nih.nimh.gov; www.catie.unc.edu).

Ceskova E and Svestka J (1993) Double-blind comparison of risperidone and haloperidol in schizophrenic and schizoaffective psychoses. Pharmacopsychiatry 26, 121–124.

Chakos MH, Lieberman JA, Alvir J, et al. (1995) Caudate nuclei volumes in schizophrenic patients treated with typical antipsychotics or clozapine. Lancet 345, 456–457.

Chakos MH, Lieberman JA, Bilder RM, et al. (1994) Increase in caudate nuclei volumes of first-episode schizophrenic patients taking antipsychotic drugs. Am J Psychiatr 151, 1430–1436.

Chakos MH, Lieberman JA, Hoffman E, et al. (2001) Effectiveness of second-generation antipsychotics in patients with treatment-resistant schizophrenia: A review and meta-analysis of randomized trials. Am J Psychiatr 158, 518–526.

Chakos MH, Mayerhoff DI, Loebel AD, et al. (1992) Incidence and correlates of acute extrapyramidal symptoms in first episode of schizophrenia. Psychopharmacol Bull 28, 81–86.

Chiu S, McFarlane AH, and Dobson N (1990) The treatment of nondelusional psychosis associated with depression. Br J Psychiatr 156, 112–115.

Chouinard G, Jones B, Remington G, et al. (1993) A Canadian multicenter placebo-controlled study of fixed doses of risperidone and haloperidol in the treatment of chronic schizophrenic patients. J Clin Psychopharmacol 13, 25–40.

Chow EWC, Bassett AS, and Weksberg R (1994) Velo-cardio-facial syndrome and psychotic disorders: Implications for psychiatric genetics. Am J Med Genet 54, 107–112.

Christy M, Christau B, Molbak AG, et al. (1982) Diabetes and month of birth (Letter). Lancet 2, 216.

Ciapparelli A, Dell'Osso L, Pini S, et al. (2000) Clozapine for treatment-refractory schizophrenia, schizoaffective disorder, and psychotic bipolar disorder: A 24-month naturalistic study. J Clin Psychiatr 61, 329–334.

Coffey CE, Sullivan JL, and Rice JR (1983) T lymphocytes in schizophrenia. Biol Psychiatr 18, 113–119.

Cohen HW, Gibson G, and Alderman MH (2000) Excess risk of myocardial infarction in patients treated with antidepressant medications: Association with use of tricyclic agents. Am J Med 108, 2–8.

Cole JO, Klerman GL, and Goldberg SC (1964) Phenothiazine treatment in acute schizophrenia. Arch Gen Psychiatr 10, 246–261.

Conley RR and Kelly DL (2001) Management of treatment resistance in schizophrenia. Biol Psychiatr 50, 898–911.

Conley RR, Tamminga CA, Bartko JJ, et al. (1998) Olanzapine compared with chlorpromazine in treatment-resistant schizophrenia. Am J Psychiatr 155(7), 914–920.

Committee on Safety of Medicines and Medicines Control Agency (1995) Cardiac arrhythmias with pimozide (Orap). Curr Prob Pharmacovigil 21, 1.

Cooper JE and Sartorius N (1977) Cultural and temporal variations in schizophrenia: A speculation on the importance of industrialization. Br J Psychiatr 130, 50–55.

Copeland JRM, Dewey ME, Scott A, et al. (1998) Schizophrenia and delusional disorder in older age: Community prevalence, incidence, comorbidity, and outcome. Schizophr Bull 24, 153–161.

Creese I, Burt DR, and Snyder SH (1975) Dopamine receptor binding predicts clinical and pharmacological potencies of antischizophrenic drugs. Science 192, 481–483.

Crisp A, Gelder M, Rix S, et al. (2000) Stigmatization of people with mental illness. Br J Psychiatr 177, 4–7.

Crow TJ (1980) Molecular pathology of schizophrenia: More than one disease process? Br Med J 280, 66–68.

Crow TJ (1985) The two-syndrome concept: Origins and current status. Schizophr Bull 11, 471–486.

Crow TJ (1986) Temporal disorientation in chronic schizophrenia. The implications of an "organic" psychological impairment for the concept of functional psychosis. In Contemporary Issues in Schizophrenia, Kerr TA and Snaith RP (eds). Gaskall, Royal College of Psychiatrists, London, pp. 168–174.

Crow TJ and Done DJ (1992) Prenatal influenza does not cause schizophrenia. Br J Psychiatr 161, 390–393.

Csernansky JG, Mahmoud R, Brenner R, et al. (2002) A comparison of risperidone and haloperidol for the prevention of relapse in patients with schizophrenia. N Engl J Med 346, 16–22.

Czekalla J, Beasley CM Jr., Dellva MA, et al. (2001) Analysis of the QTc interval during olanzapine treatment of patients with schizophrenia and related psychosis. J Clin Psychiatr 62, 191–198.

Dalman C, Allebech P, Cullberg J, et al. (1999) Obstetric complications and the risk of schizophrenia: A longitudinal study of a national birth cohort. Arch Gen Psychiatr 56, 234–240.

Daniel DG, Zimbaroff DL, Potkin SG, et al. (1999) Ziprasidone 80 mg/day and 160 mg/day in acute exacerbation of schizophrenia and schizoaffective disorder: A 6-week placebo-controlled trial. Neuropsychopharmacology 20, 491–505.

Dao-Costellano MH, Paillere-Martinot ML, Hantraye P, et al. (1997) Presynaptic dopaminergic function in the striatum of schizophrenic patients. Schizophr Res 23, 167–174.

Dasari M, Friedman L, Jesberger J, et al. (1999) A magnetic resonance imaging study of thalamic area in adolescent patients with either schizophrenia or bipolar disorder as compared to healthy controls. Psychiatr Res 91, 155–162.

Davis JM (1975) Overview: Maintenance therapy in psychiatry-I. Schizophrenia. Am J Psychiatr 132, 1237–1245.

Davison K and Bagley CR (1969) Schizophrenia-like psychoses associated with organic disorders of the central nervous system: A review of the literature. In Current Problems in Neuropsychiatry, Herrington RN (ed).

Headley Brothers, Ashford, Kent, UK, pp. 113–184. Br J Psychiatr Special Publication 4.

Deicken RF, Merrin EL, Floyd TC, et al. (1995) Correlation between left frontal phospholipids and Wisconsin Card Sort Test performance in schizophrenia. Schizophr Res 14, 177–181.

Delay J and Deniker P (1952) Trente-huit cas de psychoses traités par la cure prolongée et continué de 4560 RP. LeCongres des Al et Neurol. de Langue Fr. In Comptes Rendu du Congrès. Masson et Cie, Paris.

Dellva MA, Tran P, Tollefson GD, et al. (1997) Standard olanzapine versus placebo and ineffective-dose olanzapine in the maintenance treatment of schizophrenia. Psychiatr Serv 48, 1571–1577.

Delva NJ and Letemendia FJJ (1982) Lithium treatment in schizophrenia and schizoaffective disorders. Br J Psychiatr 141, 387–400.

Demiralp T, Ademoglu A, Comerchero M, et al. (2001) Wavelet analysis of P3a and P3b. Brain Topogr 13, 251–267.

Dickey W (1991) The neuroleptic malignant syndrome. Prog Neurobiol 36, 425–436.

Dixon L, Weiden P, Delahanty J, et al. (2000) Prevalence and correlates of diabetes in national schizophrenia samples. Schizophr Bull 26, 903–912.

Drake RE, Gates C, Whitaker A, et al. (1985) Suicide among schizophrenics: A review. Compr Psychiatr 26, 90–100.

Eaton WW (1974) Residence, social class and schizophrenia. J Health Soc Behav 15, 289–299.

Eaton WW (1985) Epidemiology of schizophrenia. Epidemiol Rev 7, 105–126.

Eaton WW (1991) Update on the epidemiology of schizophrenia. Epidemiol Rev 13, 320–328.

Eaton WW and Harrison G (2000) Ethnic disadvantage and schizophrenia. Acta Psychiatr Scand 1102(Suppl 407), 38–43.

Elkashef AM, Buchannan RW, Gellad F, et al. (1994) Basal ganglia pathology in schizophrenia and tardive dyskinesia: An MRI quantitative study. Am J Psychiatr 151, 752–755.

Emrich HM, Dose M, and von Zerssen D (1985) The use of sodium divalproex, carbamazepine and oxycarbazepine in patients with affective disorders. J Affect Disord 8, 243–250.

Endicott J and Spitzer RL (1978) A diagnostic interview: The Schedule for Affective Disorders and Schizophrenia (SADS). Arch Gen Psychiatr 35, 837–844.

Erfurth A, Walden J, and Grunze H (1998) Lamotrigine in the treatment of schizoaffective disorder. Neuropsychobiology 38, 204–205.

Erkwoh R, Sabri O, Steinmeyer EM, et al. (1997) Psychopathological and SPECT findings in never-treated schizophrenia. Acta Psychiatr Scand 96, 51–57.

Essock SM, Hargreaves WA, Covell NH, et al. (1996) Clozapine's effectiveness for patients in state hospitals: Results from a randomized trial. Psychopharmacol Bull 32, 683–697.

Evans JD, Heaton RK, Paulsen JS, et al. (1999) Schizoaffective disorder: A form of schizophrenia or affective disorder? J Clin Psychiatr 60, 874–882.

Fabre LFJ, Aravantis L, Pultz J, et al. (1995) ICI 204,636, a novel atypical antipsychotic: Early indication of safety and efficacy in patients with chronic and subchronic schizophrenia. Clin Ther 17, 366–378.

Falloon IRH, Boyd JL, McGill CW, et al. (1982) Family management in the prevention of exacerbations of schizophrenia: A controlled study. N Engl J Med 306, 1437–1440.

Falloon IRH, Boyd JL, McGill CW, et al. (1985) Family management in the prevention of morbidity of schizophrenia: Clinical outcome of a two-year longitudinal study. Arch Gen Psychiatr 42, 887–896.

Faraone SV, Matise T, Svrakic D, et al. (1998) Genome scan of European-American schizophrenia pedigrees: Results of the NIMH genetics initiative and millennium consortium. Am J Med Genet 81, 290–295.

Farde L, Nordstrom AL, Wiesel FA, et al. (1992) PET-analysis of central $D_1$ and $D_2$ dopamine receptor occupancy in patients treated with classical neuroleptics and clozapine-relation to extrapyramidal side effects. Arch Gen Psychiatr 49, 538–544.

Farde L, Wiesel FA, Halldin C, et al. (1988) Central $D_2$-dopamine receptor occupancy in schizophrenic patients treated with antipsychotic drugs. Arch Gen Psychiatr 45, 71–76.

Farde L, Wiesel FA, Nordstrom AL, et al. (1989) $D_1$ and $D_2$ dopamine receptor occupancy during treatment with conventional and atypical neuroleptics. Psychopharmacology 99, S28–S29.

Farde L, Wiesel FA, Stone-Elander S, et al. (1990) $D_2$ dopamine receptors in neuroleptic-naive schizophrenic patients: A positron emission tomography study with [$^{11}$C] raclopride. Arch Gen Psychiatr 47, 213–219.

Feighner JP, Robins E, Guze SB, et al. (1972) Diagnostic criteria for use in psychiatric research. Arch Gen Psychiatr 26, 57–63.

Fenton WS and McGlashan TM (1994) Antecedents, symptom progression, and long-term outcome of the deficit syndrome in schizophrenia. Am J Psychiatr 151, 351–356.

First M, Spitzer R, Gibbon M, et al. (1996) Structured Clinical Interview for Axis I Disorders—Clinician Version. Biometrics Research, New York State Psychiatric Institute, New York.

Fletcher P, McKenna PJ, Friston KJ, et al. (1999) Abnormal cingulate modulation of fronto-temporal connectivity in schizophrenia. Neuroimage 9(3), 337–342.

Flor-Henry P (1983) Cerebral Basis of Psychopathology. John Wright, Boston.

Flor-Henry P (1985) Schizophrenia: Sex differences. Can J Psychiatr 30, 319–322.

Ford JM, Mathalon DH, Marsh L, et al. (1999) P300 amplitude is related to clinical state in severely and moderately ill patients with schizophrenia. Biol Psychiatr 46, 94–101.

Frank AF and Gunderson JG (1990) The role of the therapeutic alliance in the treatment of schizophrenia: Relationship to course and outcome. Arch Gen Psychiatr 47, 228–236.

Franz M, Lis S, Pluddemann K, et al. (1997) Conventional versus atypical neuroleptics: Subjective quality of life in schizophrenic patients. Br J Psychiatr 170, 422–425.

Freedman R, Coon H, Myles-Worsley M, et al. (1997) Linkage of a neurophysiological deficit in schizophrenia to a chromosome 15 locus. Proc Natl Acad Sci USA 94, 587–592.

Freedman R, Leonard S, Gault J, et al. (2001) Linkage disequilibrium for schizophrenia at the chromosome 15q13–14 locus of the alpha-7-nicotinic acetylcholine receptor subunit gene (CHRNA7). Am J Med Genet 105, 20–22.

Frith CD (1984) Schizophrenia, memory and anticholinergic drugs. J Abnormal Psychol 93, 339–341.

Frith CD, Leary J, Cahill C, et al. (1991) Performance on psychological tests. Demographic and clinical correlates of the results of these tests. Br J Psychiatr (Suppl) 13, 26–29.

Frye MA, Ketter TA, Leverich GS, et al. (2000) The increasing use of polypharmacotherapy for refractory mood disorder: 22 years of study. J Clin Psychiatr 61, 9–15.

Fucetola R, Newcomer JW, Craft S, et al. (1999) Age- and dose-dependent glucose-induced increases in memory and attention in schizophrenia. Psychiatr Res 88, 1–13.

Gabbard GO (1990) Psychodynamic Psychiatry in Clinical Practice. American Psychiatric Press, Washington DC.

Gainetdinov RR, Mohn AR, and Caron MG (2001) Genetic animal models: Focus on schizophrenia. Trends Neurosci 24, 527–533.

Galdi J (1983) The causality of depression in schizophrenia. Br J Psychiatr 142, 621–625.

Galen and Harkins PW (trans) (1963) On the Passions and Errors of the Soul. Ohio State University Press, Columbus, OH.

Galletly CA, Clark RC, McFarlane AC, et al. (1997) The relationship between changes in symptoms ratings, neuropsychological test performance, and quality of life in schizophrenic patients treated with clozapine. Psychiatr Res 72, 161–166.

Gallhoffer B, Bauer U, Lis S, et al. (1996) Cognitive dysfunction in schizophrenia: Comparison of treatment with atypical antipsychotic agents and conventional neuroleptic drugs. Eur Neuropsychopharmacol 6, 13–20.

Ganguli R, Brar JS, Roy Chengappa KN, et al. (1993) Autoimmunity in schizophrenia: A review of recent findings. Ann Med 25, 489–496.

Gao XM, Sakai K, Roberts RC, et al. (2000) Ionotropic glutamate receptors and expression of N-methyl-D-aspartate receptor subunits in subregions of human hippocampus: Effects of schizophrenia. Am J Psychiatr 157, 1141–1149.

Geddes J, Freemantle N, Harrison P, et al. (2000) Atypical antipsychotics in the treatment of schizophrenia: Systematic overview and meta-regression analysis. Br Med J 321, 1371–1376.

Geddes JR, Verdoux H, Takei N, et al. (1999) Schizophrenia and complications of pregnancy and labor: An individual-patient data meta-analysis. Schiophr Bull 25, 413–423.

Gilbert PL, Harris MJ, McAdams LA, et al. (1995) Neuroleptic withdrawal in schizophrenic patients: A review of the literature. Arch Gen Psychiatr 52, 173–188.

Gill M, Vallada H, Collier D, et al. (1996) A combined analysis of $D_2S278$ marker alleles in affected sib-pairs: Support for a susceptibility locus for schizophrenia at chromosome 22q12. Schizophrenia Collaborative Linkage Group (Chromosome 22). Am J Med Genet 67, 40–45.

Goff DC, Brotman AW, Waites M, et al. (1990) Trial of fluoxetine added to neuroleptics for treatment-resistant schizophrenic patients. Am J Psychiatr 147, 492–494.

Goff DC, Posever T, Herz L, et al. (1998) An exploratory haloperidol-controlled dose-finding study of ziprasidone in hospitalized patients with schizophrenia or schizoaffective disorder. J Clin Psychopharmacol 18, 296–304.

Goff DC, Tsai G, Levitt J, et al. (1999) A placebo-controlled crossover trial of D-cycloserine added to conventional neuroleptics in patients with schizophrenia. Arch Gen Psychiatr 56, 21–27.

Gold S, Arndt S, Nopoulos P, et al. (1999) Longitudinal study of cognitive function in first-episode and recent-onset schizophrenia. Am J Psychiatr 156, 1342–1348.

Goldberg EM and Morrison SL (1963) Schizophrenia and social class. Br J Psychiatr 109, 785–802.

Goldberg TE and Weinberger DR (1996) Effects of neuroleptic medications on the cognition of patients with schizophrenia: A review of recent studies. J Clin Psychiatr 57, 62–65.

Goldberg TE, Patterson K, Taqqu Y, et al. (1998) Capacity limitations in short-term memory in schizophrenia. Psychol Med 28, 665–673.

Golden CJ, Moses SJA, Zelazowski R, et al. (1980) Cerebral ventricular size and neuropsychological impairment in young chronic schizophrenics. Arch Gen Psychiatr 37, 619–623.

Goldman-Rakic PS and Selemon LD (1997) Functional and anatomical aspects of prefrontal pathology in schizophrenia. Schizophr Bull 23, 437–458.

Goldstein JM, Goodman JM, Seidman LJ, et al. (1999) Cortical abnormalities in schizophrenia identified by structural magnetic resonance imaging. Arch Gen Psychiatr 56, 537–547.

Gottesman II (1997) Twins: En route to QTLs for cognition. Science 276, 1522–1523.

Grace J, Bellus SP, Raulin ML, et al. (1996) Long-term impact of clozapine and psychosocial treatment on psychiatric symptoms and cognitive functioning. Psychiatr Serv 4, 41–45.

Granato JF, Stern BJ, Ringel A, et al. (1983) Neuroleptic malignant syndrome: Successful treatment with dantrolene and bromocriptine. Ann Neurol 14, 89–90.

Grech A, Takei N, and Murray RM (1997) Maternal exposure to influenza and paranoid schizophrenia. Schizophr Res 26(2–3), 121–125.

Green AI, Tohen M, Patel JK, et al. (2000) Clozapine in treatment refractory psychotic mania. Am J Psychiatr 157, 982–986.

Green M and Walker E (1986) Attentional performance in positive and negative-symptom schizophrenia. J Nerv Ment Dis 174, 203–213.

Green MF (1996) What are the functional consequences of neurocognitive deficits in schizophrenia? Am J Psychiatr 153, 321–330.

Green MF, Marshall BD, Wirshing WC, et al. (1997) Does risperidone improve verbal working memory in treatment-resistant schizophrenia? Am J Psychiatr 154, 799–804.

Grenade LL, Graham D, and Trontell A (2001) Myocarditis and cardiomyopathy associated with clozapine use in the United States. New Engl J Med 345, 224.

Grossman LS, Harrow M, Goldberg JF, et al. (1991) Outcome of schizoaffective disorder at two long-term follow-ups: Comparisons with outcome of schizophrenia and affective disorders. Am J Psychiatr 148, 1359.

Guidotti A, Auta J, Davis JM, et al. (2000) Decrease in reelin and glutamic acid decarboxylase 67 (GAD67) expression in schizophrenia and bipolar disorder: A postmortem brain study. Arch Gen Psychiatr 57, 1061–1069.

Gur RE, Cowell P, Turetsky BI, et al. (1998) A follow-up MRI study of schizophrenia: Relationship of neuroanatomic changes with clinical and neurobehavioral measures. Arch gen Psychiatr 55, 145–152.

Gurevich EV and Joyce JN (1997) Alterations in the cortical serotonergic system in schizophrenia: A postmortem study. Biol Psychiatr 42, 529–545.

Hafner H (2000) Onset and early course as determinants of the further course of schizophrenia. Acta Psychiatr Scand 102(Suppl) 407, 44–48.

Hagg S, Joelsson L, Mjorndal T, et al. (1998) Prevalence of diabetes and impaired glucose tolerance in patients treated with clozapine compared with patients treated with conventional depot neuroleptic medications. J Clin Psychiatr 59, 294–299.

Hagger RK, Buckley P, Kenny JT, et al. (1993) Improvement in cognitive functions and psychiatric symptoms in treatment-refractory schizophrenic patients receiving clozapine. Biol Psychiatr 34, 702–712.

Hakola HPA and Laulumaa VA (1982) Carbamazepine in treatment of violent schizophrenics (Letter). Lancet 1, 1358.

Halgren E, Baudena P, Clarke J, et al. (1995) Intracerebral potentials to rare target and distractor auditory and visual stimuli II. Medial, lateral, and posterior temporal lobe. Electroencephelogr Clin Neurophysiol 94, 229–250.

Hambrecht M, Maurer K, Hafner H, et al. (1992) Transnational stability of gender differences in schizophrenia? An analysis based on the WHO study on determinants of outcome of severe mental disorders. Eur Arch Psychiatr Clin Neurosci 242, 6–12.

Harding CM, Brooks GW, Ashikaga T, et al. (1987a) The Vermont longitudinal study of persons with severe mental illness. I. Methodology, study sample, and overall status 32 years later. Am J Psychiatr 144, 718–726.

Harding CM, Brooks GW, Ashikaga T, et al. (1987b) The Vermont longitudinal study of persons with severe mental illness II. Long-term outcome of subjects who retrospectively met DSM-III criteria for schizophrenia. Am J Psychiatr 144, 727–735.

Hare EH (1983) Epidemiological evidence for a viral factor in the aetiology of the functional psychoses. Adv Biol Psychiatr 12, 52.

Hare EH (1987) Epidemiology of schizophrenia and affective psychoses. Br Med Bull 43, 514–530.

Harris EC and Barraclough B (1998) Excess mortality of mental disorder. Br J Psychiatr 173, 11–33.

Harrison PJ (1999) The neuropathology of schizophrenia: A critical review of the data and their interpretation. Brain 122, 593–624.

Harvey PD (2001) Abbreviated cognitive assessment in schizophrenia: Recent data on feasibility. J Adv Schizophr Brain Res 3, 73–78.

Harvey PD and Keefe RSE (2001) Studies of cognitive change in patients with schizophrenia following novel antipsychotic treatment. Am J Psychiatr 158, 176–184.

Harvey PD, Earle-Boyer EA, Wielgus MS, et al. (1986) Encoding memory and thought disorder in schizophrenia and mania. Schizophr Bull 12, 252–261.

Harvey PD, Howanitz E, Parrella M, et al. (1998) Symptoms, cognitive functioning, and adaptive skills in geriatric patients with lifelong schizophrenia: A comparison across treatment sites. Am J Psychiatr 155, 1080–1086.

Haupt DW and Newcomer JW (2001) Risperidone-associated diabetic ketoacidosis. Psychosomatics 42, 279–280.

Haverkamp W, Breithardt G, Camm AJ, et al. (2000) The potential for QT prolongation and proarrhythmia by non-antiarrhythmic drugs: Clinical and regulatory implications. Report on a Policy Conference of the European Society of Cardiology. Cardiovasc Res 47, 219–233.

Hayes SG (1989) Long-term use of valproate in primary psychiatric disorders. J Clin Psychiatr 50(Suppl 3), 35–39.

Hazlett EA, Buchsbaum MS, Byne W, et al. (1999) Three-dimensional analysis with MRI and PET of the size, shape and function of the thalamus in the schizophrenia spectrum. Am J Psychiatr 156, 1190–1199.

Haznedar MM, Buchsbaum MS, Luu C, et al. (1997) Decreased anterior cingulate gyrus metabolic rate in schizophrenia. Am J Psychiatr 154, 682–684.

Heaton RK, Paulsen JS, McAdams LA, et al. (1994) Neuropsychological deficits in schizophrenics relationship to age, chronicity and dementia. Arch Gen Psychiatr 51, 469–476.

Heila H, Isometsa ET, Henriksson MM, et al. (1997) Suicide and schizophrenia: A nationwide psychological autopsy study on age- and sex-specific clinical characteristics of 92 suicide victims with schizophrenia. Am J Psychiatr 154, 1235–1242.

Helgason T (1964) Epidemiology of mental disorders in Iceland. Acta Psychiatr Scand 40(Suppl), 173.

Henderson DC, Cagliero E, Gray C, et al. (2000) Clozapine, diabetes mellitus, weight gain and lipid abnormalities: A five-year naturalistic study. Am J Psychiatr 157, 975–981.

Henn FA and Braus DF (1999) Structural neuroimaging in schizophrenia: An integrative view of neuromorphology. Eur Arch Psychiatr Clin Neurosci 249(Suppl 4) IV/48–IV/56.

Heresco-Levy U, Javitt DC, Ermilov M, et al. (1999) Efficacy of high-dose glycine in the treatment of enduring negative symptoms of schizophrenia. Arch Gen Psychiatr 56, 29–36.

Herrera JM, Sramek JJ, and Costa JF (1987) Efficacy of adjunctive carbamazepine in the treatment of chronic schizophrenia. Drug Intel Clin Pharm 21, 355–358.

Hickling F and Rodgers-Johnson P (1995) The incidence of first contact schizophrenia in Jamaica. Br J Psychiatr 167, 474–481.

Hietala E, Syvalaht K, Vuorio K, et al. (1994) Striatal dopamine receptor characteristics in neuroleptic-naïve schizophrenic patients studied with positron emission tomography. Arch Gen Psychiatr 51, 116–123.

Hillert A, Maier W, Wetzel H, et al. (1992) Risperidone in the treatment of disorders with a combined psychotic and depressive syndrome: A functional approach. Pharmacopsychiatry 25, 213–217.

Hippocrates (1950) The Medical Works of Hippocrates. Blackwell Scientific, Oxford.

Hirayasu Y, Shenton ME, Salisbury DF, et al. (1998) Lower left temporal lobe MRI volumes in patients with first-episode schizophrenia compared with psychotic patients with first-episode affective disorder and normal subjects. Am J Psychiatr 155, 1384–1391.

Hoenig J (1983) The concept of schizophrenia: Kraepelin-Bleuler-Schneider. Br J Psychiatr 142, 547–556.

Hogarty GE, Anderson CM, Reiss DJ, et al. (1986) Family psychoeducation, social skills training, and maintenance chemotherapy in the aftercare treatment of schizophrenia. I. One-year effects of a controlled study on relapse and expressed emotion. Arch Gen Psychiatr 43, 633–642.

Hogarty GE, Goldberg SC, Scholler NR, et al. (1974) Drugs and sociotherapy in the aftercare of schizophrenia patients. Arch Gen Psychiatr 31, 603–608.

Hollister LE and Kosek JC (1965) Sudden death during treatment with phenothiazine derivatives. JAMA 192, 1035–1038.

Holzman PS (1987) Recent studies of psychophysiology in schizophrenia. Schizophr Bull 13, 49–76.

Honer WG, Falkai P, Young C, et al. (1997) Cingulate cortex synaptic terminal proteins and neural cell adhesion molecule in schizophrenia. Neuroscience 78, 99–110.

Hovatta I, Terwilliger JD, Lichtermann D, et al. (1997) Schizophrenia in the genetic isolate of Finland. Am J Med Genet Neuropsychiatr Genet 74, 353–360.

Howard R, Almeida OP, and Levy R (1994) Phenomenology, demography and diagnosis in late paraphrenia. Psychol Med 24, 397–410.

Howard R, Rabins PV, Seeman MV, et al. (2000) Late-onset schizophrenia and very-late-onset schizophrenia-like psychosis: An international consensus. Am J Psychiatr 157, 172–178.

Hoyberg OJ, Fensbo C, Remvig J, et al. (1993) Risperidone versus pepehnazine in the treatment of chronic schizophrenic patients with acute exacerbations. Acta Psychiatr Scand 88, 395–402.

Hsiao MC, Liu CY, Yang YY, et al. (1999) Delusional disorder: Retrospective analysis of 86 Chinese outpatients. Psychiatr Clin Neurosci 53, 673–676.

Hutchinson G, Takei N, Bhugra D, et al. (1997) Increased rate of psychosis among African-Caribbeans in Britain is not due to an excess of pregnancy and birth complications. Br J Psychiatr 171, 145–147.

Hwu HG, Yeh EK, and Chang LY (1989) Prevalence of psychiatric disorders in Taiwan defined by the Chinese Diagnostic Interview Schedule. Acta Psychiatr Scand 79, 136–147.

Impagnatiello F, Guidotti A, Pesold C, et al. (1998) A decrease of reelin expression as a putative vulnerability factor in schizophrenia. Proc Natl Acad Sci USA 95, 15718–15723.

Ingvar DH and Franzen G (1974) Abnormalities of cerebral blood flow distribution in patients with chronic schizophrenia. Acta Psychiatr Scand 50, 425–462.

Jablensky A (1986) Epidemiology of schizophrenia: A European perspective. Schizophr Bull 12, 52–73.

Jablensky A (2000) Epidemiology of schizophrenia: The global burden of disease and disability. Eur Arch Psychiatr Clin Neurosci 250, 274–285.

Jablensky A and Cole SW (1997) Is the earlier age at onset of schizophrenia in males a confounded finding? Results from a cross-cultural investigation. Br J Psychiatr 170, 234–240.

Jablensky A, Sartorius N, Ernberg G, et al. (1988) Schizophrenia: Manifestation, Incidence and Course in Different Cultures. World Health Organization, Geneva.

Jablensky A, Sartorius N, Ernberg G, et al. (1992) Schizophrenia: Manifestations, Incidence and Course in Different Cultures. A World Health Organization Ten-Country Study. Psychological Medicine Monograph (Suppl 20). Cambridge University Press, Cambridge.

Jablensky A, Schwarz R, and Tomov T (1980) WHO collaborative study on impairments and disabilities associated with schizophrenic disorders. Acta Psychiatr Scand 62(Suppl 285), 152–163.

Jackson JH (1987) Remarks on evolution and dissolution of the nervous system. J Ment Sci 33, 25–48.

Janicak PG, Keck PE Jr., Davis JM, et al. (2001) A double-blind, randomized, prospective evaluation of the efficacy and safety of risperidone versus haloperidol in the treatment of schizoaffective disorder. J Clin Psychopharm 21, 360–368.

Javitt DC and Zukin SR (1990) The role of excitatory amino acids in neuropsychiatric illness. J Neuropsychiatr Clin Neurosci 2, 44–52.

Jeffreys SE, Harvey CA, McNaught AS, et al. (1997) The Hampstead Schizophrenia Survey 1991. I: Prevalence and service use comparisons in an inner London health authority, 1986–1991. Br J Psychiatr 170, 301–306.

Jeon YW and Polich J (2001) P300 asymmetry in schizophrenia: A meta-analysis. Psychiatr Res, 104, 61–74.

Jeste DV, Harris MJ, Krull A, et al. (1995) Clinical and neuropsychological characteristics of patients with late-onset schizophrenia. Am J Psychiatr 152, 722–730.

Jeste DV, Harris MJ, Krull J, et al. (1997) Clinical and neuropsychological characteristics of patients with late-onset schizohrenia. Am J Psychiatr 152, 722–730.

Johnstone EC and Owens DGC (1981) Neurological changes in a population of patients with chronic schizophrenia and their relationship to physical treatment. Acta Psychiatr Scand 63(Suppl 291), 103–110.

Johnstone EC, Crow TJ, Frith CD, et al. (1978) The dementia of dementia praecox. Acta Psychiatr Scand 57, 305–324.

Johnstone EC, Frith CD, Gold A, et al. (1979) The outcome of severe acute schizophrenic illnesses after one year. Br J Psychiatr 134, 28–33.

Jones PB, Rantakallio P, Hartikainen AL, et al. (1998) Schizophrenia as a long-term outcome of pregnancy, delivery, and perinatal complications: A 28-year follow-up of the 1966 North Finland general population birth cohort. Am J Psychiatr 155, 355–364.

Jongbloet PH, Mulder A, and Hamers AJ (1982) Seasonality of preovulatory nondisjunction and the etiology of Down syndrome. A European collaborative study. Hum Genet 62, 134–138.

Kales A, Kales AD, Vela-Beuno A, et al. (1990) Schizophrenia: Historical perspectives. In Recent Advances in Schizophrenia, Kales A, Stefanio CN, and Talbott JR (eds). Springer-Verlag, New York, p. 5.

Kalus P, Senitz D, Lauer M, et al. (1999) Inhibitory catridge synapses in the anterior cingulate cortex of schizophrenics. J Neural Transm 106, 763–771.

Kanas N, Rogers M, Dreth E, et al. (1980) The effectiveness of group psychotherapy during the first three weeks of hospitalization: A controlled study. J Nerv Ment Dis 168, 487–492.

Kane JM (1987) Treatment of schizophrenia. Schizophr Bull 13, 133–156.

Kane JM, Marder SR, Schooler NR, et al. (2001) Clozapine and haloperidol in moderately refractory schizophrenia: A 6-month randomized and double-blind comparison. Arch Gen Psychiatr 58, 965–972.

Kane JM, Rifkin A, Woerner MG, et al. (1983) Low-dose neuroleptic treatment of outpatient schizophrenics. Arch Gen Psychiatr 40, 893–896.

Kane JM, Rifkin A, Woerner MG, et al. (1985) High-dose versus low-dose strategies in the treatment of schizophrenia. Psychopharmacol Bull 21, 533–537.

Kane JM, Woerner M, and Lieberman J (1988) Tardive dyskinesia: Prevalence, incidence and risk factors. J Clin Psychopharmacol 8, 525–565.

Kapur S and Remington G (2001) Dopamine $D_2$ receptors and their role in atypical antipsychotic action: Still necessary and may even be sufficient. Biol Psychiatr 50, 873–883.

Kapur S and Seeman P (2001) Does fast dissociation from the dopamine $D_2$ receptor explain the action of atypical antipsychotics? A new hypothesis. Am J Psychiatr 158, 360–369.

Kapur S, Remington G, Jones C, et al. (1996) The $D_2$ occupancy with low-dose haloperidol treatment: A PET study. Am J Psychiatr 153, 948–950.

Kapur S, Zipursky R, Jones C, et al. (2000) Relationship between $D_2$ occupancy, clinical response, and side effects: A double-blind PET study of first-episode schizophrenia. Am J Psychiatr 157, 514–520.

Kasanin J (1933) The acute schizoaffective psychoses. Am J Psychiatr 13, 97–126.

Kasckow J and Nemeroff C (1991) The neurobiology of neurotensin: Focus on neurotensin-dopamine interactions. Regul Peptides 36, 153–164.

Kasper S and Muller-Spahn F (2001) Review of quetiapine and its clinical applications in schizophrenia. Expert Opin Pharmacother 1, 783–801.

Kasper S, Tauscher J, Kufferle B, et al. (1999) Dopamine- and serotonin-receptors in schizophrenia: Results of imaging-studies and implications for pharmacotherapy in schizophrenia. Eur Arch Psychiatr Clin Neurosci 249(Suppl 4), IV/83–IV/89.

Kay SR, Opler LA, and Lindemayer JP (1988) Reliability and validity of the positive and negative syndrome scale for schizophrenics. Psychiatr Res 23, 99–110.

Keck P Jr., Buffenstein A, Ferguson J, et al. (1998) Ziprasidone 40 and 120 mg/day in the acute exacerbation of schizophrenia and schizoaffective disorder: A 4-week placebo-controlled trial. Psychopharmacology 140, 173–184.

Keck PE, McElroy SL, and Strakowski SM (1999) Schizoaffective disorder: Role of atypical antipsychotic. Schizophr Res 35(Suppl), 121–125.

Keck PE Jr., Reeves K, Harrigan E, et al. (2001) Ziprasidone in the short-term treatment of patients with schizoaffective disorder: Results from two double-blind, placebo-controlled, multicenter studies. J Clin Psychopharmacol 21, 27–35.

Keefe RS, Perkins D, Silva SG, et al. (1999) The effects of atypical antipsychotic drugs on neurocognitive impairment in schizophrenia. Schizophr Bull 25, 201–222.

Keith SJ, Regier DA, and Rae DS (1991) Schizophrenic disorders. In Psychiatric Disorders in America, Robins LN and Regier DA (eds). Free Press, New York, pp. 33–52.

Kendell RE, McInneny K, Jusczak E, et al. (2000) Obstetric complications and schizophrenia: Two case-control studies based on structured obstetric records. Br J Psychiatr 174, 516–522.

Kendler KS (1982) Demography of paranoid psychosis (delusional disorder): A review and comparison with schizophrenia and affective illness. Arch Gen Psychiatr 39, 890–902.

Kendler KS and Diehl SR (1993) The genetics of schizophrenia: A current, genetic-epidemiologic perspective. Schizophr Bull 19, 261–285.

Kendler KS and Walsh D (1995) Gender and schizophrenia. Results of an epidemiologically-based family study. Br J Psychiatr 167, 184–192.

Kendler KS, McGuire M, Gruenberg AM, et al. (1995b) Examining the validity of DSM-III-R schizoaffective disorder and its putative subtypes in the Roscommon family study. Am J Psychiatr 152, 755–764.

Kendler KS, Neale MC, and Walsh D (1995a) Evaluating the spectrum concept of schizophrenia in the Roscommon family study. Am J Psychiatr 152, 749–754.

Kern RS, Green MF, Marshall BD Jr., et al. (1998) Risperidone versus haloperidol on reaction time, manual dexterity, and motor learning in treatment-resistant schizophrenia patients. Biol Psychiatr 44, 726–732.

Keshavan MS, Stanley JA, and Pettegrew JW (2000) Magnetic resonance spectroscopy in schizophrenia: Methodological issues and findings Part II. Biol Psychiatr 48, 369–380.

Kety SS (1987) The significance of genetic factors in the etiology of schizophrenia: Results from the national study of adoptees in Denmark. J Psychiatr Res 21, 423–429.

Kety SS, Rosenthal D, Wender PH, et al. (1968) The types and prevalence of mental illness in the biological and adoptive families of adopted schizophrenics. J Psychiatr Res 6, 345–362.

Kilian JG, Kerr K, Lawrence C, et al. (1999) Myocarditis and cardiomyopathy associated with clozapine. Lancet 354, 1841–1845.

Kindermann SS, Karimi A, Symonds L, et al. (1997) Review of functional magnetic resonance imaging in schizophrenia. Schizophr Res 27, 143–156.

Kirino E, Belger A, Goldman-Rakic P, et al. (2000) Prefrontal activation evoked by infrequent target and novel stimuli in a visual target detection task: An event-related functional magnetic resonance study. J Neurosci 20, 6612–6618.

Klein E, Beutal E, Lerer B, et al. (1984) Carbamazepine and haloperidol versus placebo and haloperidol in excited psychosis: A controlled study. Arch Gen Psychiatr 41, 165–170.

Klieser E, Lehmann E, Kinzler E, et al. (1995) Randomized, double-blind, controlled trial of risperidone versus clozapine in patients with chronic schizophrenia. J Clin Psychopharmacol 1(Suppl 1), 45S–51S.

Knable MB, Torrey EF, Webster MJ, et al. (2001) Multivariate analysis of prefrontal cortical data from the Stanley Foundation Neuropathology Consortium. Brain Res Bull 55, 651–659.

Knapp M (1997) Costs of schizophrenia. Br J Psychiatr 171, 509–518.

Knight RT (1996) Contribution of human hippocampal region to novelty detection. Nature 383, 256–259.

Knight RT (1997) Distributed cortical network for visual attention. J Cogn Neurosci 9, 75–91.

Koh SD (1978) Remembering of verbal materials by schizophrenic young adults. In Language and Cognition in Schizophrenia, Schwartz S (ed). Lawrence Erlbaum, Hillsdale, NJ.

Kotlicka-Antczak M, Gmitrowicz A, Sobow TM, et al. (2001) Obstetric complications and Apgar score in early-onset schizophrenic patients with prominent positive and prominent negative symptoms. J Psychiatr Res 35, 249–257.

Kraepelin E and Barclay RM (trans) (1919) Dementia Praecox and Paraphrenia, Robertson GM (ed). E & S Livingstone, Edinburgh.

Krlmen WS, Seidman LJ, Faraone SV, et al. (2001) Intelligence quotient and neuropsychological profiles in patients with schizophrenia and in normal volunteers. Biol Psychiatr 50, 453–462.

Kramer M (1969) Cross-national study of diagnosis of the mental disorders: Origin of the problem. Am J Psychiatr 10(Suppl), 1–11.

Kramer MS, Last B, Getson A, et al. (1997) The effects of a selective $D_4$ dopamine receptor antagonist (L-745,870) in acutely psychotic inpatients with schizophrenia. $D_4$ Dopamine Antagonist Group. Arch Gen Psychiatr 54, 567–572.

Krystal JH, Karper LP, Siebyl JP, et al. (1994) Subanesthetic effects of the noncompetitive NMDA antagonist, ketamine, in humans, psychotomimetic, perceptual, cognitive, and neuroendocrine responses. Arch Gen Psychiatr 51, 199–214.

Lacro JP, Harris MJ, and Jeste DV (1993) Late life psychosis. Int J Geriatr Psychiatr 8, 49–57.

Lafargue T and Brasic J (2000) Neurodevelopmental hypothesis of schizophrenia: A central sensory disturbance. Med Hypotheses 55, 314–318.

Lancet (1983) The matchbox sign. Lancet 1, 26.

Land W, Pinsky D, and Salzman C (1991) Psychopharmacology: Abuse and misuse of anticholinergic medications. Hosp Comm Psychiatr 42, 580–581.

Langfeldt G (1939) The Schizophreniform States. Oxford University Press, London.

Lapierre YD (1994) Schizophrenia and manic depression: Separate illnesses or a continuum? Can J Psychiatr 39, S59–S64.

Larsen TR, Moe LC, Vibe-Hansen L, et al. (2000) Premorbid functioning versus duration of untreated psychosis in 1-year outcome in first-episode psychosis. Schizophr Res 45, 1–9.

Laruelle M, Abi-Dargham A, van Dyck CH, et al. (1996) Single photon emission computerized tomography imaging of amphetamine-induced dopamine release in drug-free schizophrenic subjects. Proc Natl Acad Sci USA 20, 9235–9240.

Lawrie SM and Abukmeil SS (1998) Brain abnormality in schizophrenia: A systematic and quantitive review of volumetric magnetic resonance imaging studies. Br J Psychiatr 172, 110–120.

Lee MA, Thompson PA, and Meltzer HY (1994) Effects of clozapine on cognitive function in schizophrenia. J Clin Psychiatr 55, 82–87.

Leff J (2000) Family work for schizophrenia: Practical application. Acta Psychiatr Scand, 102(Suppl 407), 78–82.

Leff J, Kuipers L, Berkowitz R, et al. (1982) A controlled trial of social intervention in the families of schizophrenic patients. Br J Psychiatr 141, 121–134.

Lehtinen V (1996) The epidemiology of mental disorders in Finland. Nord J Psychiatr 50(Suppl 36), 25–30.

Lencz T, Bilder RM, and Cornblatt B (2001) The timing of neurodevelopmental abnormality in schizophrenia: An integrative review of the neuroimaging literature. CNS Spectrums 6, 233–255.

Levenson JL (1985) Neuroleptic malignant syndrome. Am J Psychiatr 142, 1137–1145.

Levinson DF (1991) Pharmacologic treatment of schizophrenia. Clin Ther 13, 326–352.

Levinson DF, Holmans P, Straub RE, et al. (2000) Multicenter linkage of schizophrenia candidate region of chromosomes 5q, 6q, 10p, and 13q: Schizophrenia linkage collaborative group III. Am J Hum Genet 67, 652–663.

Levinson DF, Mahtani MM, Nancarrow DJ, et al. (1998) Genome scan of schizophrenia. Am J Psychiatr 155, 741–750.

Levinson DF, Umapathy C, and Musthaq M (1999) Treatment of schizoaffective disorder and schizophrenia with mood symptoms. Am J Psychiatr 156, 1138–1148.

Lewis DA (1997) Development of the prefrontal cortex during adolescence: Insights into vulnerable neural circuits in schizophrenia. Neuropsychopharamcology 16, 358–398.

Lieberman JA (1996) Atypical antipsychotic drugs as a first-line treatment of schizophrenia: A rationale and hypothesis. J Clin Psychiatr 57(Suppl 11), 68–71.

Lieberman JA (1999a) Is schizophrenia a neurodegenerative disorder? A clinical and neurobiological perspective. Biol Psychiatr 46, 729–739.

Lieberman JA (1999b) Searching for the neuropathology of schizophrenia: Neuroimaging strategies and findings. Am J Psychiatr 156, 1133–1136.

Lieberman JA and Fenton W (2000) Delayed detection of psychosis: Causes, consequences, and effect on public health. Am J Psychiatr 157, 1727–1730.

Lieberman JA, Darlene J, Geisler S, et al. (1993) Time course and biologic correlates of treatment response in first-episode schizophrenia. Arch Gen Psychiatr 50, 369–376.

Lieberman JA, Jody D, Geisler S, et al. (1993) Time course and biologic correlates of treatment response in first-episode schizophrenia. Arch Gen Psychiatr 50, 369–376.

Liberman RP, Massel HK, Mosk MD, et al. (1985) Social skills training for chronic mental patients. Hosp Comm Psychiatr 36, 396–403.

Liberman RP, Mueser KT, and Wallace CJ (1986) Social skills training for schizophrenic individuals at risk for relapse. Am J Psychiatr 143, 523–526.

Lichtermann D, Karbe E, and Maier W (2000) The genetic epidemiology of schizophrenia and of schizophrenia spectrum disorders. Eur Arch Psychiatr Clin Neurosci 250, 304–310.

Liddle PF (1987) Schizophrenic syndromes, cognitive performance and neurological dysfunction. Psychol Med 17, 49–57.

Light GA and Braff DL (2001) Measuring P50 suppression and prepulse inhibition in a single recording session. Am J Psychiatr 158, 2066–2068.

Lim KO, Hedehus M, Moseley M, et al. (1999) Compromised white matter tract integrity in schizophrenia inferred from diffusion tensor imaging. Arch Gen Psychiatr 56, 367–374.

Lin A, Kenis G, Bignotti S, et al. (1998) The inflammatory response system in treatment-resistant schizophrenia: Increased serum interleukin-6. Schizophr Res 32, 9–15.

Lindenmayer JP, Volavka J, Lieberman J, et al. (2001) Olanzapine for schizophrenia refractory to typical and atypical antipsychotics: An open-label prospective trial. J Clin Psychopharm 21, 448–453.

Lindstrom L, Gefvert O, Hogberg G, et al. (1999) Increased dopamine synthesis rate in medial prefrontal cortex and striatum in schizophrenia indicated by L(-beta-11C) DOPA and PET. Biol Psychiatr 46, 681–688.

Linn MW, Klett J, and Caffey FM (1980) Foster home characteristics and psychiatric patient outcome. Arch Gen Psychiatr 37, 129–132.

Litman RE, Hong WW, Weissman EM, et al. (1993) Idazoxan, an $a_2$ antagonist, augments fluphenazine in schizophrenic patients: A pilot study. J Clin Psychopharmacol 13, 264–267.

Loranger AW (1984) Sex difference in age at onset of schizophrenia. Arch Gen Psychiatr 41, 157–161.

Lyell A (1983) Delusions of parasitosis. Br J Psychiatr 108, 485–499.

Lysaker PH, Bell MD, Bioty SM, et al. (1995) The frequency of associations between positive and negative symptoms and dysphoria in schizophrenia. Compr Psychiatr 36, 113–117.

Mahy C, Mallet R, Leff J, et al. (1999) First contact incidence rate of schizophrenia in Barbados. Br J Psychiatr 175, 28–33.

Maier M, Mellers J, Toone B, et al. (2000) Schizophrenia, temporal lobe epilepsy and psychosis: An in vivo magnetic resonance spectroscopy and imaging study of the hippocampus/amygdala complex. Psychol Med 30(3), 571–581.

Manschreck TC (1996) Delusional disorder: The recongnition and management of paranoia. J Clin Psychiatr 57(Suppl 3), 32–38.

Marcelis M, Navarro-Mateu F, Murray R, et al. (1998) Urbanization and psychosis: Study of 1942–1978 birth cohorts in The Netherlands. Psychol Med 28, 871–879.

Marder SR (2000) Integrating pharmacological and psychosocial treatments for schizophrenia. Acta Psychiatr Scand 102(Suppl 407), 87–90.

Marder SR and Meibach RC (1994) Risperidone in the treatment of schizophrenia. Am J Psychiatr 151, 825–835.

Marder SR and Van Patten T (1988) Who should receive clozapine? Arch Gen Psychiatr 45, 865–867.

Marder SR, Van Patten T, Mintz J, et al. (1984) Costs and benefits of two doses of fluphenazine. Arch Gen Psychiatr 41, 1025–1029.

Marder SR, Van Patten T, Mintz J, et al. (1987) Low- and conventional-dose maintenance therapy with fluphenazine decanoate: Two-year outcome. Arch Gen Psychiatr 44, 518–521.

Marder SR, Wirshing W, Mintz J, et al. (1996) Two-year outcome of social skills training and group psychotherapy for outpatients with schizophrenia. Am J Psychiatr 153, 1585–1592.

Margolis RL, Chuang DM, and Post RM (1994) Programmed cell death: Implications for neuropsychiatric disorders. Biol Psychiatr 35, 946–956.

Marino C, Nobile M, Bellodi L, et al. (1993) Delusional disorder and mood disorder: Can they coexist? Psychopathology 26, 53–61.

Marsden CD, Mindham RHS, and Mackay AVP (1986) Extrapyramidal movement disorders produced by antipsychotic drugs. In The Psychopharmacology and Treatment of Schizophrenia, Bradley PB and Hirsch SR (eds). Oxford University Press, Oxford.

Masand PS (2000) Weight gain associated with psychotropics. Expert Opin Psychopharmacol 1, 377–389.

Mathalon DH, Faustman WO, and Ford JM (2002) N400 and automatic semanting processing abnormalities in patients with schizophrenia. Arch Gen Psychiatr 59, 641–648.

Matthysse S (1973) Antipsychotic drug actins: A clue to a neuropathology of schizophrenia? Fed Proc 32, 200–205.

May PRA (1968) Treatment of Schizophrenia: A Comparative Study of Five Treatment Methods. Science House, New York.

McCarley RW, O'Donnell BF, Niznikiewicz MA, et al. (1997) Update on electrophysiology in schizophrenia. Int Rev Psychiatr 9, 373–386.

McCarley RW, Salisbury DF, Hirayasu Y, et al. (2002). Association between smaller left posterior superior temporal gyrus volume on magnetic resonance imaging and smaller left temporal P300 amplitude in first-episode schizophrenia. Arch Gen Psychiatr 59, 321–331.

McCarley RW, Shenton ME, O'Donnell BF, et al. (1993) Auditory P300 abnormalities and left posterior temporal gyrus reduction in schizophrenia. Arch Gen Psychiatr 50, 190–197.

McCarley RW, Wible CG, Frumin M, et al. (1999) MRI anatomy of schizophrenia. Biol Psychiatr 45, 1099–1119.

McCarthy G, Luby M, Gore J, et al. (1997) Infrequent events transiently activate human prefrontal and parietal cortex as measured by functional MRI. J Neurophysiol 77, 1630–1634.

McCredie RG, Connolly MA, Williamson DJ, et al. (1994) The Nithsdale Schizophrenia Surveys. XII: "Neurodevelopmental" schizophrenia: A search for clinical correlates and putative aetiological factors. Br J Psychiatr 165, 340–346.

McGhie A and Chapman J (1961) Disorders of attention and perception in early schizophrenia. Br J Med Psychol 34, 103–116.

McGlashan TH and Fenton WS (1993) Subtype progression and pathophysiologic deterioration in early schizophrenia. Schizophr Bull 19, 71–84.

McGlashan TH and Hoffman RE (2000) Schizophrenia as a disorder of developmentally reduced synaptic connectivity. Arch Gen Psychiatr 57, 637–648.

McGuire PK, Shah GMS, and Murray RM (1993) Increased blood flow in Broca's area during auditory hallucinations in schizophrenia. Lancet 324, 703–706.

McNaught A, Jeffreys SE, Harvey CA, et al. (1997) The Hampstead Schizophrenia Survey 1991. II Incidence and migration in inner London. Br J Psychiatr 170, 307–311.

McNeil TF (1995) Perinatal risk factors and schizophrenia: Selective review and methodological concerns. Epidemiol Rev 17, 107–112.

McNeil TF, Kaij L, Torrey EF, et al. (1994) Obstetric complications in histories of monozygotic twins discordant and concordant for schizophrenia. Acta Psychiatr Scand 89, 196–204.

Medalia A, Gold JM, and Merriam A (1988) The effects of neuroleptics in neuropsychological test results of schizophrenics. Arch Clin Neuropsychol 3, 249–271.

Mednick SA, Machon RA, Huttunen MO, et al. (1988) Adult schizophrenia following prenatal exposure to an influenza epidemic. Arch Gen Psychiatr 45, 189–192.

Mehtonen O-P, Aranko K, Malkonen L, et al. (1991) A survey of sudden death associated with the use of antipsychotic or antidepressant drugs: 49 cases in Finland. Acta Psychiatr Scand 84, 58–64.

Mela M, Obenbe A, and Farmer AE (1997) Folie a Quatre in a large Nigerian sub-ship. Schizophr Res 23, 91–93.

Meloy JR (1996) Stalking (obsessional following): A review of some preliminary studies. Aggr Viol Behav 1, 147–162.

Meloy JR (1999) Case report: Erotomania, triangulation, and homicide. J Forens Sci 44, 421–424.

Meltzer HY (1989a) Duration of a clozapine trial in neuroleptic-resistant schizophrenia. Arch Gen Psychiatr 46, 672.

Meltzer HY (1989b) The role of serotonin in antipsychotic drug action. Neuropsychopharmacology 21(Supp 2), 106S–115S.

Meltzer HY (1992) Treatment of the neuroleptic–nonresponsive schizophrenic patient. Schizophr Bull 18, 515–542.

Meltzer HY (1995) Clozapine: Is another view valid? Am J Psychiatr 821–825.

Meltzer HY (1998) Suicide in schizophrenia: Risk factors and clozapine treatment. J Clin Psychiatr 59(Suppl 3) 15–20.

Meltzer HY and McGurk SR (1999) The effects of clozapine, risperidone, and olanzapine on cognitive function in schizophrenia. Schizophr Bull 25, 233–255.

Meltzer HY and Okayli G (1995) The reduction of suicidality during clozapine treatment in neuroleptic-resistant schizophrenia: Impact on risk-benefit assessment. Am J Psychiatr 152, 183–190.

Meltzer HY, Matsubara S, and Lee JC (1989c) The ratios of serotonin-2 and dopamine-2 affinities differentiate atypical and typical antipsychotic drugs. Psychopharmacol Bull 25, 390–392.

Menzies R, Federoff J, Green C, et al. (1995) Prediction of dangerous behavior in male erotomania. Br J Psychiatr 166, 529–536.

Merikangas K (2002) Genetic epidemiology: Bringing genetics to the population—the NAPE Lecture 2001. Acta Psychiatr Scand 105, 3–13.

Merinder LB (2000) Patient education in schizophrenia: A review. Acta Psychiatr Scand 102, 98–106.

Mirnics K, Middleton FA, Lewis DA, et al. (2001) Analysis of complex brain disorders with gene expression microarrays: Schizophrenia as a disease of the synapse. Trends Neurosci 24, 479–486.

Mirnics K, Middleton FA, Marquez A, et al. (2000) Molecular characterization of schizophrenia viewed by microarray analysis of gene expression in prefrontal cortex. Neuron 28, 53–67.

Mishler EG and Scotch NA (1963) Sociocultural factors in the epidemiology of schizophrenia: A review. Psychiatry 26, 315–351.

Miyanaga K, Machiyama T, and Juji T (1984) Schizophrenic disorders and HLA-DR antigens. Biol Psychiatr 19, 121–129.

Modai I, Hirschmann S, Rava A, et al. (2000) Sudden death in patients receiving clozapine treatment: A preliminary investigation. J Clin Psychopharmacol 20, 325–327.

Mohn AR, Gainetdinov RR, Caron MG, et al. (1999) Mice with reduced NMDA receptor expression display behaviors related to schizophrenia. Cell 98, 427–436.

Moises HW, Yang L, Kristbjarnarson H, et al. (1995) An international two-stage genome-wide search for schizophrenia. Am J Hum Genet 34, 630–649.

Montgomery SA and Green M (1988) The use of cholecystokinin in schizophrenia: A review. Psychol Med 18, 593–603.

Morgan V, Castle D, Page A, et al. (1997) Influenza epidemics and incidence of schizophrenia, affective disorders and mental retardation in Western Australia: No evidence of major effect. Schizophr Res 26, 25–39.

Morris M (1991) Delusional parasitosis. Br J Psychiatr 159, 83–87.

Mortensen PB, Pederson CB, Westergaard T, et al. (1999) Effects of family history and place and season of birth on the risk factors for schizophrenia. N Engl J Med 340, 603–608.

Motjabai R, Nicholson RA, and Carpenter PN (1998) Role of psychosocial treatments in management of schizophrenia: A meta-analytic review of controlled outcome studies. Schizophr Bull 24, 569–587.

Mowry BJ and Nancarrow DJ (2001) Molecular genetics of schizophrenia: Proceedings of the Australian Neuroscience Society Symposium. Clin Exp Pharmacol Physiol 28, 66–69.

Muller N and Ackenheil M (1998) Psychoneuroimmunology and the cytokine action in the CNS: Implications for psychiatric disorders. Prog Neuropsychopharmacol Biol Psychiatr 22, 1–33.

Muller N, Empel M, Riedel M, et al. (1997) Neuroleptic treatment increases soluble IL-2 receptors and decreases soluble IL-6 receptors in schizophrenia. Eur Arch Psychiatry Clin Neurosci 247, 308–313.

Muller N, Riedel M, Scheppach C, et al. (2002) Beneficial antipsychotic effects of Celecoxib add-on therapy compared to risperidone alone in schizophrenia. Am J Psychiatr 159, 1029–1034.

Munro A (1982) Paranoia revisited. Br J Psychiatr 141, 344–349.

Munro A (1988) Monosymptomatic hypochondriacal psychosis. Br J Psychiatr 153(Suppl 2), 37–40.

Munro A (1991) Phenomenologic aspects of monodelusional disorders. Br J Psychiatr 159(Suppl 14), 62–64.

Murphy KC, Jones LA, and Owen MJ (1999) High rates of schizophrenia in adults with velocardio-facial syndrome. Arch Gen Psychiatr 56, 940–945.

Musselman DL, Evans DL, and Nemeroff CB (1998) The relationship of depression to cardiovascular disease: Epidemiology, biology, and treatment. Arch Gen Psychiatr 55, 580–592.

Myer-Lindenberg A, Gruppe H, Bauer U, et al. (1997) Improvement of cognitive function in schizophrenic patients receiving clozapine or zotepine: Results from a double-blind study. Pharmacopsychiatr 30, 35–42.

Myerson A (1940) Review: Mental disorders in urban areas. Am J Psychiatr 96, 995–997.

Myles-Worsley M, Coon H, Tiobech J, et al. (1999) Genetic epidemiological study of schizophrenia in Palau, Micronesia: Prevalence and familiality. Am J Med Genet 88, 4–10.

Naber D, Leppig M, Grohmann R, et al. (1989) Efficacy and adverse effects of clozapine in the treatment of schizophrenia and tardive dyskinesia: A retrospective study of 387 patients. Psychopharmacology (Berl) 99, 73–76.

Nelson MD, Saykin AJ, Flashman LA, et al. (1998) Hippocampal volume reduction in schizophrenia as assessed by magnetic resonance imaging: A meta-analytic study. Arch Gen Psychiatr 55, 433–440.

Nestler EJ (1997) Schizophrenia: An emerging pathophysiology. Nature 385, 578–579.

Nestor PG, Kimble MO, O'Donnell BF, et al. (1997) Aberrant semantic activation in schizophrenia: A neurophysiological study. Am J Psychiatr 157, 640–646.

Newcomer JW, Haupt DW, Fucetola R, et al. (2002) Abnormalities in glucose regulation during antipsychotic treatment of schizophrenia. Arch Gen Psychiatr 59, 337–345.

Niznikiewicz MA, O'Donnell BF, Nestor PG, et al. (1997) ERP assessment of visual and auditory language processing in schizophrenia. J Abnorm Psychol 106, 85–94.

Nordstrom Al and Farde L (1998) Plasma prolactin and central $D_2$ receptor occupancy in antipsychotic drug-treated patients. J Clin Psychopharmacol 18, 305–310.

Noreik K and Odegard O (1967) Age at onset of schizophrenia in relation to socio-economic factors. Br J Soc Psychiatr 1, 243–249.

Norman RM and Malla AK (2001) Duration of untreated psychosis: A critical examination of the concept and its importance. Psychol Med 31, 381–400.

Nuechterlein KH, Edell WS, Norris M, et al. (1986) Attentional vulnerability indicators, thought disorder and negative symptoms. Schizophr Bull 12, 408–426.

Odegard O (1932) Emigration and insanity: A study of mental disease among the Norwegian-born population of Minnesota. Acta Psychiatr Neurol Scand 7(Suppl 4), 1–206.

O'Donnell BF, McCarley RW, Potts GF, et al. (1999) Identification of neural circuits underlying P300 abnormalities in schizophrenia. Psychophysiology 36(3), 253–257.

Osterberg E (1978) Schizophrenia and rheumatic disease. Acta Psychiatr Scand 58, 339–359.

Overall JE and Gorham DE (1961) The Brief Psychiatric Rating Scale. Psychol Rep 10, 799–812.

Ozcan ME, Taskin R, Banoglu R, et al. (1996) HLA antigens in schizophrenia and mood disorders. Biol Psychiatr 39, 891–895.

Pahl JJ, Swayze VW, and Andreasen NC (1990) Diagnostic advances in anatomical and functional brain imaging in schizophrenia. In Recent Advances in Schizophrenia, Kales A, Stefanis CN, and Talbott J (eds). Springer-Verlag, New York, pp. 163–189.

Palmer BW, Heaton RK, Paulsen JS, et al. (1997) Is it possible to be schizophrenic yet neuropsychologically normal? Neuropsychology 11, 437–446.

Pantelis C, Barber FZ, Barbes TR, et al. (1999) Comparison of set-shifting ability in patients with chronic schizophrenia and frontal lobe damage. Schizophr Res 37, 251–270.

Patel JK, Niznikiewicz MA, Shafa R, et al. (2001) Clozapine enhances P300 amplitude in patients with schizophrenia (Abstract). Schizophr Res 49(Suppl), 255.

Pearlson GP, Kreger L, Rabins PW, et al. (1989) A chart review study of late-onset and early-onset schizophrenia. Am J Psychiatr 146, 1568–1574.

Penn D, Guynan R, Daily T, et al. (1994) Dispelling the stigma of schizophrenia, what sort of information is best? Schizophr Bull 20, 1393–1395.

Peuskens J (1995) Risperidone in the treatment of patients with chronic schizophrenia: A multinational, multicentre, double-blind, parallel-group study versus haloperidol. Br J Psychiatr 166, 712–726.

Peuskens J and Link CG (1997) A comparison of quetiapine and chlorpromazine in the treatment of schizophrenia. Acta Psychiatr Scand 96, 265–273.

Pichot P (1990) The diagnosis and classification of mental disorders in the French-speaking countries: Background, current values and comparisons with other classifications. In Sources and Traditions of Classification in Psychiatry, Sartorius N, Jablensky A, Regier DA, et al. (eds). Hognefe & Huber, Toronto, pp. 7–35.

Pickar D and Pinals D (1995) Drug-free symptoms in schizophrenia. Presented at the 34th Annual Meeting of the American College of Neuropsychopharmacology, San Juan, PR.

Polich J (1998) P300 clinical utility and control of variability. J Clin Neurophysiol 15, 14–33.

Polich J and Herbst KL (2000) P300 as a clinical assay: Rationale, evaluation, and findings. Int J Psychophysiol 38, 3–19.

Poulton R, Caspi A, Moffitt TE, et al. (2000) Children's self-reported psychotic symptoms and adult schizophreniform disorder: A 15-year longitudinal study. Arch Gen Psychiatr 57, 1053–1058.

Preti A, Cardascia L, Zen T, et al. (2000) Risk for obstetric complications and schizophrenia. Psychiatr Res 96, 127–139.

Procyshyn RM, Pande S, and Tse G (2000) New-onset diabetes mellitus associated with quetiapine. Can J Psychiatr 45, 668–669.

Propping P (1983) Genetic disorders presenting as "schizophrenia": Karl Bonhoeffer's early view of the psychoses in the light of medical genetics. Hum Genet 65, 1–10.

Pulver AE, Lasseter VK, Kasch L, et al. (1995) Schizophrenia: A genome scan targets chromosomes 3p and 8p as potential sites of susceptibility genes. Am J Med Genet 60, 252–260.

Purdon SE, Jones BDW, Stip E, et al. (2000) Neuropsychological change in early phase schizophrenia during 12 months of treatment with olanzapine, risperidone, or haloperidol. Arch Gen Psychiatr 57, 249–258.

Puzynski S and Klosiewicz L (1984) Divalproex amide in the treatment of affective and schizoaffective disorders. J Affect Disord 6, 115–121.

Quitkin AF, Rifkin A, and Klein DF (1975) Very high doses vs. standard dosage fluphenazine in schizophrenia. Arch Gen Psychiatr 32, 1276–1281.

Rabins P, Pauker S, and Thomas J (1984) Can schizophrenia begin after age 44? Compr Psychiatr 25, 290–293.

Rajkumar S, Padmavati R, Thara R, et al. (1993) Incidence of schizophrenia in an urban community in Madras. Indian J Psychiatr 35, 18–21.

Rantakallio P, Jones P, Moring J, et al. (1997) Association between central nervous system infections during childhood and adult onset schizophrenia and other psychoses: A 28-year follow-up. Int J Epidemiol 26, 837–843.

Ray WA, Meredith S, Thapa PB, et al. (2001) Antipsychotics and the risk of sudden cardiac death. Arch Gen Psychiatr 58, 1161–1167.

Raz S and Raz N (1990) Structural brain abnormalities in the major psychoses: A quantitative review of the evidence from computerized imaging. Psychol Bull 108, 93–108.

Rice DP (1999) The economic impact of schizophrenia. J Clin Psychiatr 60(Suppl 1), 4–6.

Riecher A, Maurer K, Loffler W, et al. (1989) Schizophrenia: A disease of single young males? Preliminary results from an investigation on a representative cohort admitted to hospital for the first time. Eur Arch Psychiatr Neurosci 239, 210–212.

Riecher-Rossler A and Hafner H (2000) Gender aspects in schizophrenia: Bridging the border between social and biological psychiatry. Acta Psychiatr Scand 102(Suppl 407), 58–62.

Riley JG, Ayis SA, Ferrier IN, et al. (2000) QTc-interval abnormalities and psychotropic drug therapy in psychiatric patients. Lancet 355, 1048–1052.

Retterstol N (1970) Prognosis in Paranoid Psychoses. Charles Thomas, Springfield, IL.

Retterstol N and Opjordsmoen S (1991) Fatherhood, impending or newly established, precipitating delusional disorders: Long-term course and outcome. Psychopathology 24, 232.

Robins LN and Regier DA (eds) (1991) Psychiatric Disorders in America: The Epidemiologic Catchment Area Study. Free Press, New York.

Robins LN, Helzer JE, Weissman MM, et al. (1984) Lifetime prevalence of specific psychiatric disorders in 3 sites. Arch Gen Psychiatr 41, 949–958.

Robinson D, Woerner MG, Alvir JMJ, et al. (1999) Predictors of relapse following response from a first episode of schizophrenia or schizoaffective disorder. Arch Gen Psychiatr 56, 241–247.

Rosenheck R, Cramer J, Xu W, et al. (1997) A comparison of clozapine and haloperidol in hospitalized patients with refractory schizophrenia: Department of Veterans Affairs Cooperative Study Group on clozapine in refractory schizophrenia. N Engl J Med 337, 809–815.

Rosenheck R, Teckett J, Peters J, et al. (1998) Does participation in psychosocial treatment augment the benefit of clozapine? Arch Gen Psychiatr 55, 618–625.

Rosenthal D, Goldberg I, Jacobsen B, et al. (1974) Migration, heredity, and schizophrenia. Psychiatry 37, 321–329.

Rossi A, Mancini F, Stratta P, et al. (1997) Risperidone, negative symptoms and cognitive deficit in schizophrenia: An open study. Acta Psychiatr Scand 95, 40–43.

Rosso IM, Cannon TD, Huttunen T, et al. (2000) Obstetric risk factors for early-onset schizophrenia in a Finnish birth cohort. Am J Psychiatr 157, 801–807.

Rosvold HE, Mirsky AF, Sarasan I, et al. (1956) A continuous performance test of brain damage. J Cogn Psychol 20, 343–350.

Ruschena D, Mullen PE, Burgess P, et al. (1998) Sudden death in psychiatric patients. Br J Psychiatr 172, 331–336.

Sacuzzo DP and Braff DL (1981) Early information processing deficit in schizophrenia: New findings using RDC, schizophrenic subgroups and manic controls. Arch Gen Psychiatr 38, 175–179.

Salit SA, Kuhn EM, Hartz AJ, et al. (1998) Hospitalization costs associated with homelessness in New York City. N Engl J Med 338, 1734–1740.

Salzman C (1980) The use of ECT in the treatment of schizophrenia. Am J Psychiatr 137, 1032–1041.

Sanders RD and Mossman D (1999) An open trial of olanzapine in patients with treatment-refractory psychoses. J Clin Psychopharmacol 19, 62–66.

Sax KW, Strakowski SM, and Keck PEJ (1998) Attentional improvement following quetiapine fumarate treatment in schizophrenia. Schizophr Res 33, 151–155.

Saykin AJ, Gur RC, Gur RE, et al. (1991) Neuropsychological function in schizophrenia: Selective impairment in memory and learning. Arch Gen Psychiatr 48, 618–624.

Saykin AJ, Shtasel DL, Gur RE, et al. (1994) Neuropsychological deficits in neuroleptic-naive patients with first episode schizophrenia. Arch Gen Psychiatr 51, 124–131.

Schizophrenia Collaborative Linkage Group for Chromosomes 3, 6, and 8 (1996) Additional support for schizophrenia linkage on chromosomes 6 and 8: A multicenter study. Am J Med Gene 67, 580–594.

Schotte A, Janssen PF, Gommeren W, et al. (1996) Risperidone compared with new and reference antipsychotic drugs: In vitro and in vivo receptor binding. Psychopharmacology (Berl) 124, 57–73.

Schulz R, Beach SR, Ives DG, et al. (2000) Association between depression and mortality in older adults: The cardiovascular health study. Arch Intern Med 160, 1761–1768.

Seeman P and Tallerico T (1999) Rapid release of antipsychotic drugs from dopamine $D_2$ receptors: An explanation for low receptors occupancy and rapid clinical relapse upon withdrawl of clozapine or quetiapine. Am J Psychiatr 156, 876–884.

Seeman P, Corbett R, and Van Tol HH (1997) Atypical neuroleptics have low affinity for dopamine $D_2$ receptors or are selective for $D_4$ receptors. Neuropsychopharmacology 16(2), 93–110.

Seidman LJ, Faraone SV, Goldstein JM, et al. (1997) Reduced subcortical brain volumes in nonpsychotic siblings of schizophrenic patients: A pilot magnetic resonance imaging study. Am J Med Genet 74, 507–514.

Selten JP, Slaets JPJ, and Kahn R (1998) Prenatal exposure to influenza and schizophrenia in Surinamese and Dutch Antillean immigrants to The Netherlands. Schizophr Res 30, 101–103.

Serretti A, Lattuada E, Cusin C, et al. (1999) Factor analysis of delusional disorder symptomatology. Compr Psychiatr 40, 143–147.

Sharma T (2001) Schizophrenia in the UK—A mark of shame? J Adv Schizophr Brain Res 3, 70–73.

Sharpley MS, Hutchinson G, Murray RM, et al. (2001) Understanding the excess of psychosis among the African-Caribbean population in England. Br J Psychiatr 178, S60–S68.

Shenton ME, Kikinis R, Jolesz FA, et al. (1992) Abnormalities of the left temporal lobe and thought disorder in schizophrenia: A quantitative magnetic resonance imaging study. N Engl J Med 327, 604–611.

Shioiri T, Kato T, Inubushi T, et al. (1994) Correlations of phosphomo-noesters measured by phosphorus-31 magnetic resonance spectroscopy in frontal lobes and negative symptoms in schizophrenia. Psychiatr Res 55, 223–235.

Silverman C (1968) The epidemiology of depression: A review. Am J Psychiatr 124, 883–891.

Siris SG (2000) Depression in schizophrenia: Perspective in the era of "atypical" antipsychotic agents. Am J Psychiatr 157, 1379–1389.

Slater E, Hare EH, and Price JS (1971) Marriage and fertility of psychiatric patients compared with national data. Soc Biol 18(Suppl), S60–S73.

Slaughter JR, Zanol K, Rezvani H, et al. (1998) Psychogenic parasitosis. A case series and literature review. Psychosomatics 39, 491–500.

Small JG, Hirsch SR, Aravantis LA, et al. (1997) Quetiapine in patients with schizophrenia: A high- and low-dose double-blind comparison with placebo. Arch Gen Psychiatr 54, 549–557.

Small JG, Kellamus JJ, Milstein V, et al. (1975) A placebo controlled study of lithium combined with neuroleptics in chronic schizophrenic patients. Am J Psychiatr 132, 1315–1317.

Smith GN, Kopala LC, Lapointe JS, et al. (1998) Obstetric complications, treatment response and brain morphology in adult onset and early-onset males with schizophrenia. Psychol Med 28, 645–653.

Someya T, Masui A, Takahashi S, et al. (1987) Classification of paranoid disorders: A survey of 144 cases. Jpn J Psychiatr Neurol 41, 162–163.

Spohn HE, Lacoursiere RB, Thompson K, et al. (1977) Phenothiazine effects on psychological and psycho-physiological dysfunction in chronic schizophrenia. Arch Gen Psychiatr 34, 633–644.

Stahl SM (2000) New drug discovery in the postgenomic era: From genomics to proteomics. J Clin Psychiatr 61, 894–895.

Stanley JA, Williamson PC, Drost DJ, et al. (1995) An in vivo study of the prefrontal cortex of schizophrenic patients at different stages of illness via phosphorus magnetic resonance spectroscopy. Arch Gen Psychiatr 52, 399–406.

Stip E and Lussier I (1996) The effect of risperidone on cognition in patients with schizophrenia. Can J Psychiatr 41, 35–40.

Stirling JD, Hellewell JS, and Hewitt J (1997) Verbal memory impairment in schizophrenia: No sparing of short-term recall. Schizophr Res 25, 85–95.

Straub RE, MacLean CJ, Martin RB, et al. (1998) A schizophrenia locus may be located in region 10p15 p11. Am J Med Genet 81, 296–301.

Straube ER and Oades RD (1992) Schizophrenia: Empirical Research and Findings. Academic Press, San Diego, CA.

Strauss JS, Carpenter WT Jr., and Bartko JJ (1974) The diagnosis and understanding of schizophrenia. Part III. Speculations on the processes that underlie schizophrenic symptoms and signs. Schizophr Bull 11, 61–69.

Strauss ME (1993) Relations of symptoms to cognitive deficits in schizophrenia. Schizophr Bull 19, 215–231.

Strakowski SM, Keck PE, McElroy SL, et al. (1998) Twelve-month outcome following a first hospitalization for affective psychosis. Arch Gen Psychiatr 55, 49–55.

Strakowski SM, Keck PE, Sax KW, et al. (1999) Twelve-month outcome of patients with DSM-III-R schizoaffective disorder: Comparisons to matched patients with bipolar disorder. Schizophr Res 35, 167–174.

Szeszko PR, Bilder RM, Lencz T, et al. (1999) Investigation of frontal lobe subregions in first-episode schizophrenia. Psychiatr Res 90, 1–15.

Tamargo J (2000) Drug-induced torsades de pointes: From molecular biology to bedside. Jpn J Pharmacol 83, 1–19.

Tamminga CA (1999) Glutamatergic aspects of schizophrenia. Br J Psychiatr 174(Suppl 37), 12–15.

Tamminga CA, Thaker GK, Moran M, et al. (1994) Clozapine in tardive dyskinesia: Observations from human and animal model studies. J Clin Psychiatr 55, 102–106.

Tandon R, Harrigan E, and Zorn SH (1997) Ziprasidone: A novel antipsychotic with unique pharmacology and therapeutic potential. J Serotonin Res 4, 159–177.

Tarazi FI and Baldessarini RJ (2000) Dopamine $D_4$ receptors: Neuropsy-chiatric Implications. TEN 2, 54–58.

Tauscher J, Kapur S, Verhoeff NPLG, et al. (2002) Brain serotonin 5-HT$_{1A}$ receptor binding in schizophrenia measured by PET and [$^{11}$C]WAY-100635. Arch Gen Psychiatr 59, 514–520.

Taylor MA (1992) Are schizophrenia and affective disorder related? A selective literature review. Am J Psychiatr 149, 22–32.

Thakore JH, Mann JN, Vlahos I, et al. (2002) Increased visceral fat distribution in drug-naïve and drug-free patients with schizophrenia. Int J Obstet Rel Metab Disord 26, 137–141.

Thomas SHL (1994) Drugs, QT interval abnormalities and ventricular arrhythmias. Adverse Drug React Toxicol Rev 13, 77–102.

Thornley B and Adams CE (1998) Content and quality of 2000 controlled trials in schizophrenia over 50 years. Br Med J 317, 1181–1184.

Tienari P (1991) Interaction between genetic vulnerability and family environment: The Finnish adoptive family study of schizophrenia. Acta Psychiatr Scand 84, 460–465.

Tollefson GD, Beasley CM Jr., Tran PV, et al. (1997) Olanzapine versus haloperidol in the treatment of schizophrenia and schizoaffective and schizophreniform disorders: Results of an international collaborative trial. Am J Psychiatr 154, 457–465.

Tollefson GD, Birkett MA, Kiesler GM, et al. (2001) Double-blind comparison of olanzapine vs. clozapine in schizophrenic patients clinically eligible for treatment with clozapine. Biol Psychiatr 49(1), 52–63.

Torrey EF (1980) Schizophrenia and Civilization. Aronson, New York.

Torrey EF, Bowler AE, and Clark K (1997) Urban birth and residence as risk factors for psychoses: An analysis of 1880 data. Schizophr Res 25, 169–176.

Tran PV, Dellva MA, Tollefson GD, et al. (1997) Extrapyramidal symptoms and tolerability of olanzapine versus haloperidol in the acute treatment of schizophrenia. J Clin Psychiatr 58, 205–211.

Truffinet P, Tamminga CA, Fabre LF, et al. (1999) A placebo-controlled study of the $D_4$/5-HT$_{2A}$ antagonist fananserin in the treatment of schizophrenia. Am J Psychiatr, 156, 419–425.

Tsai GE, Yang P, Chung LC, et al. (1998) D-Serine added to antipsychotics for the treatment of schizophrenia. Biol Psychiatr 44, 1081–1089.

Tsuang MT (1982) Memory deficit and long-term outcome in schizo-phrenia: A preliminary study. Psychiatr Res 6, 355–360.

Tsuang MT, Stone WS, and Faraone SV (2001) Genes, environment and schizophrenia. Br J Psychiatr 178(Suppl 40), S18–S24.

van Kammen DP, Peters J, Yao J, et al. (1990) Norepinephrine in acute exacerbations of chronic schizophrenia. Arch Gen Psychiatr 47, 161–168.

Van Petten C and Kutas M (1990) Interactions between sentence context and word frequency in event-related brain potentials. Mem Cogn 18(4), 380–393.

Van Putten T, Marder SR, and Mintz J (1990) A controlled dose comparison of haloperidol in newly admitted schizophrenic patients. Arch Gen Psychiatr 47, 754–758.

van Tol HHM, Pounzow JR, Guan HC, et al. (1991) Cloning of the gene for a human $D_4$ receptor with high affinity for the antipsychotic clozapine. Nature 350, 610–614.

Velligan DI and Miller AL (1999) Cognitive dysfunction in schizophrenia and its importance to outcome: The place of atypical antipsychotic in treatment. J Clin Psychiatr 60(Suppl 23), 25–28.

Velligan DI, Bow-Thomas CC, Huntzinger C, et al. (2000) Randomized controlled trial of the use of compensatory strategies to enhance adaptive functioning in outpatients with schizophrenia. Am J Psychiatr 157, 1317–1323.

Verdoux H, Geddes JR, Takei N, et al. (1997) Obstetric complications and age at onset in schizophrenia: An international collaborative meta-analysis of individual patient data. Am J Psychiatr 154, 1220–1227.

Vieta E, Herraiz M, Fernandez A, et al. (2001) Efficacy and safety of risperidone in the treatment of schizoaffective disorder: Initial results from a large, multicenter surveillance study. J Clin Psychiatr 62, 623–630.

Vieweg V, Levenson J, Pandurangi A, et al. (1995) Medical disorders in the schizophrenic patients. Int J Psychiatr Med 25, 137–172.

Vogel HP (1979) Fertility and sibship size in a psychiatric patient population: A comparison with national census data. Acta Psychiatr Scand 60, 48–50.

Volavka J, Czobar P, Sheitman B, et al. (2002) Clozapine, olanzapine, risperidone, and haloperidol in the treatment of patients with chronic schizophrenia and schizoaffective disorder. Am J Psychiatr 159, 255–262.

Waddington JL, Scully PJ, and O'Callighan E (1997) The new anti-psychotics, and their potential for early intervention in schizophrenia. Schizophr Res 28, 215–222.

Waddington JL, Youssef HA, and Kinsella A (1995) Sequential cross-sectional and 10-year prospective study of severe negative symptoms in relation to duration of initially untreated psychosis in chronic schizo-phrenia. Psychol Med 25, 849–857.

Walker E (1981) Attentional and neuromotor functions of schizophrenics, schizoaffectives, and patients with other affective disorders. Arch Gen Psychiatr 38, 1355–1358.

Wallace CJ, Nelson CJ, Liberman RP, et al. (1980) A review and critique of social skills training with schizophrenic patients. Schizophr Bull 6, 42–63.

Waltrip RW, Buchanan RW, Carpenter WT, et al. (1997) Borna disease virus antibodies and the deficit syndrome of schizophrenia. Schizophr Res 23, 253–257.

Warner JP, Barnes TRE, and Henry JA (1996) Electrocardiographic changes in patients receiving neuroleptic medication. Acta Psychiatr Scand 93, 311–313.

Waxler NE (1979) Is outcome for schizophrenia better in nonindustrial societies? The case of Sri Lanka. J Nerv Ment Dis 167, 144–158.

Weinberger DR (1987) Implications of normal brain development for the pathogenesis of schizophrenia. Arch Gen Psychiatr 44, 660–669.

Weinberger DR and Berman KF (1988) Speculation of the meaning of cerebral metabolic "hypofrontality" in schizophrenia. Schizophr Bull 14, 157–168.

Weinberger DR and Berman KF (1996) Prefrontal function in schizophrenia: confounds and controversies. Philos T Roy Soc B 351, 1495–1503.

Weinberger DR and McClure RK (2002) Neurotoxicity, neuroplasticity, and MRI morphometry: What is happening in the schizophrenic brain? Arch Gen Psychiatr 59, 553–558.

Weinberger DR, Egan MF, Bertolino A, et al. (2001) Prefrontal neurons and the genetics of schizophrenia. Biol Psychiatr 50, 825–844.

Weiner DB (1992) Philippe Pinel's memoir on madness. Am J Psychiatr 149, 725–732.

White TG (1995) Folie Simultanee in monozygotic twins. Can J Psychiatr 40, 418–420.

Wig NN (1990) The Third World perspective on psychiatric diagnosis and classification. In Sources and Traditions of Classification in Psychiatry, Sartorius N, Jablensky A, Regier DA, et al. (eds). Hognefe & Huber, Toronto, pp. 181–210.

Williams PV and McGlashan TH (1987) Schizoaffective psychosis, I: Comparative long-term outcome. Arch Gen Psychiatr 44, 130–137.

Wirshing DA, Marshall BD Jr., Green MF, et al. (1999) Risperidone in treatment-refractory schizophrenia. Am J Psychiatr 156(9), 1374–1379.

Wirshing DA, Spellberg BJ, Erhart SM, et al. (1998) Novel antipsychotics and new onset diabetes. Biol Psychiatr 44, 778–783.

Wolkin A, Rusinek H, Vaid G, et al. (1998) Structural magnetic resonance image averaging in schizophrenia. Am J Psychiatr 155, 1064–1073.

Wolkowitz OM and Pickar D (1991) Benzodiazepines in the treatment of schizophrenia: A review and reappraisal. Am J Psychiatr 148, 714–726.

Wolkowitz OM, Rapaport MH, and Pickar D (1990) Benzediazepine augmentation of neuroleptics. In The Neuroleptic-Nonresponsive Patient: Characterization and Treatment, Angrist B and Schulz SC (eds). American Psychiatric Press, Washington DC, pp. 87–108.

Woods BT (1998) Is schizophrenia a progressive neurodevelopmental disorder? Toward a unitary pathogenetic mechanism. Am J Psychiatr 155, 1661–1670.

World Health Organization (1973) Report of the International Pilot Study of Schizophrenia, Vol. 1. World Health Organization, Geneva.

World Health Organization (1979) Schizophrenia: An International Follow-up Study. John Wiley, New York.

Wright IC, Sharma T, Ellison ZR, et al. (1999) Supra-regional brain systems and the neuropathology of schizophrenia. Cereb Cortex 9, 366–378.

Wyatt RJ (1991) Neuroleptics and the natural course of schizophrenia. Schizophr Bull 17, 325–351.

Yamada N, Nakajima S, and Noguchi T (1998) Age at onset of delusional disorder is dependent on the delusional theme. Acta Psychiatr Scand 97, 122–124.

Yap YG and Camm J (2000) Risk of Torsades de pointes with noncardiac drugs. Br Med J 320, 1158–1159.

Zachariah E, Kumari V, Mehrotra R, et al. (2000) Effects of 10 mg oral procyclidine administration on memory functions in healthy human subjects. Schizophr Res 41, 278.

Zahn TP, Pickar D, and Haier RJ (1994) Effects of clozapine, fluphenazine, and placebo on reaction time measures of attention and sensory dominance in schizophrenia. Schizophr Res 13, 133–144.

Zamani MG, De Hert M, Spaepen M, et al. (1994) Study of the possible association of HLA class II, $CD_4$ and $CD_3$ polymorphisms with schizophrenia. Am J Med Genet 54, 372–377.

Zarate CA Jr. and Patel JK (2001) Sudden cardiac death and antipsychotic drugs: Do we know enough? (Commentary). Arch Gen Psychiatr 58, 1168–1171.

Zarate CA Jr., Tohen M, Banov MD, et al. (1995) Is clozapine a mood stabilizer? J Clin Psychiatr 56, 108–112.

Zornberg GL, Buka SL, and Tsuang MT (2000) Hypoxic-ischemia-related fetal/neonatal complications and risk of schizophrenia and other nonaffective psychoses: A 19-year longitudinal study. Am J Psychiatr 157, 196–202.

# 63 • •● Mood Disorders: Depression

Alan M. Gruenberg
Reed D. Goldstein

Major Depressive Episode
Dysthymic Disorder

## Introduction

Major depressive disorder (MDD), dysthymic disorder (DD), depressive disorder not otherwise specified (DDNOS) are the group of clinical conditions in the *Diagnostic and Statistical Manual of Mental Disorders*, Fourth Edition (DSM-IV) (American Psychiatric Association 1994) characterized by depressive symptomatology. These conditions specifically exclude a history of manic, mixed or hypomanic episodes, and are not due to the physiologic effects of substances of abuse, other medications, or toxins. This chapter reviews the descriptive characteristics, epidemiology, etiology and pathophysiology, course and natural history, and treatment of these conditions. This chapter addresses each of these disorders separately. However, in the longitudinal course, an individual may suffer from both DD and MDD, referred to as double depression (Keller and Shapiro 1982). In addition, some of the diagnostic criteria are shared between DD and MDD. All of these depressive disorders require prospective observation because subsequent symptoms, such as mania or psychosis, can result in an eventual change in diagnosis. Reevaluation of the diagnosis also may be required upon further elaboration of the history. For example, when an episode of depression remits and is subsequently followed by a manic episode, the diagnosis is changed from MDD to bipolar disorder. When DD evolves into MDD, and the patient subsequently develops a hypomanic episode, rediagnosis of the condition to bipolar II disorder is required. When an episode of MDD remits, and is followed by the occurrence of psychosis which dominates the clinical presentation, a rediagnosis of schizophrenia or schizoaffective disorder may be required. When the clinical history reveals significant trauma during childhood, an episode of MDD may be concurrent with a diagnosis of posttraumatic stress disorder (PTSD). Given these caveats, this chapter will emphasize the importance of prospective and careful naturalistic observation to understand the clinical heterogeneity of depressive disorders.

## Definition

The depressive disorders are characterized by lifelong vulnerability to episodes of disease, involving depressed mood or loss of interest and pleasure in activities. Individuals may demonstrate ongoing potential for cycling of mood from euthymia to depression to recovery and sometimes to hypomania or mania. When individuals cycle to hypomania or mania, then a diagnosis of bipolar II (in the case of hypomania) or bipolar I (in the case of mania) is made. When the mood disorder is severe, assessment for psychosis is essential.

In most definitions of depression, a distinction is drawn between a feeling state of dejection, sadness, or unhappiness, which may be brief in duration, and a clinical syndrome characterized by persistent sadness, profound discouragement, or despair which persists two weeks or more and is associated with a change from previous functioning. This clinical syndrome invariably involves alterations in mood experienced by an individual as a feeling of sadness, irritability, dejection, despair, or loss of interest or pleasure. Associated neurovegetative or biological signs of depression include impairment in sleep, appetite, energy level, libido, and psychomotor activity. Beck (1973) emphasizes cognitive manifestations of the depressive syndrome, including distortions about oneself, one's experience in the world and the future, accompanied by self-blame and indecision. These core symptoms of depression are evident in children or adolescents with MDD although the depressed mood may be manifested by irritability or social withdrawal. Older adults may show a preponderance of somatic preoccupation and memory impairment in association with the signs of MDD. The current DSM-IV-TR criteria (A) for MDD are noted below:

**DSM-IV-TR Criteria** 296.xx

**Major Depressive Episode**

A. Five (or more) of the following symptoms have been present during the same 2-week period and represent a change from previous functioning; at least one of the symptoms is either (1) depressed mood or (2) loss of interest or pleasure.

**Note:** Do not include symptoms that are clearly due to a general medical condition, or mood-incongruent delusions or hallucinations.

(1) Depressed mood most of the day, as indicated by either subjective report (e.g., feels sad or empty) or observation made by others (e.g., appears tearful). **Note:** In children and adolescents, can be irritable mood.

(2) Markedly diminished interest or pleasure in all, or almost all, activities most of the day, nearly every day (as indicated by either subjective account or observation made by others).

(3) Significant weight loss when not dieting or weight gain (e.g., a change of more than 5% of body weight in a month), or decrease or increase in appetite nearly every day. **Note:** In children, consider failure to make expected weight gains.

(4) Insomnia or hypersomnia nearly every day.

(5) Psychomotor agitation or retardation nearly every day (observable by others, not merely subjective feelings of restlessness or being slowed down).

(6) Fatigue or loss of energy nearly every day.

(7) Feelings of worthlessness or excessive or inappropriate guilt (which may be delusional) nearly every day (not merely self-reproach or guilt about being sick).

(8) Diminished ability to think or concentrate, or indecisiveness, nearly every day (either by subjective account or as observed by others).

(9) Recurrent thoughts of death (not just fear of dying), recurrent suicidal ideation without a specific plan, or a suicide attempt or a specific plan for committing suicide.

B. The symptoms do not meet criteria for a mixed episode.

C. The symptoms cause clinically significant distress or impairment in social, occupational, or other important areas of functioning.

D. The symptoms are not due to the direct physiological effects of a substance (e.g., a drug of abuse, a medication) or a general medical condition (e.g., hypothyroidism).

E. The symptoms are not better accounted for by bereavement, i.e., after the loss of a loved one, the symptoms persist for longer than 2 months or are characterized by marked functional impairment, morbid preoccupation with worthlessness, suicidal ideation, psychotic symptoms, or psychomotor retardation.

Reprinted with permission from the Diagnostic and Statistical Manual of Mental Disorders, Fourth Edition, Text Revision. Copyright 2000 American Psychiatric Association.

## History

Depressive disorders have plagued mankind since the earliest documentation of human experience. Jackson (1986) describes the history of these clinical syndromes in detail. The earliest references, from ancient Greek descriptions of depression, refer to a syndrome of melancholia, which translated from Greek means black bile (Jackson 1986). In humoral theory, "black bile" was considered as an etiologic factor in melancholia. The Greek tradition also referred to melancholic temperament, which is comparable to our current understanding of early-onset DD and depressive personality. During the late 19th and early 20th century, phenomenologists increasingly used the term *mental depression* to refer to the clinical syndrome of melancholia. Kraepelin (1921) described mood as dejected, gloomy, and hopeless in the depressed phase of manic depressive insanity and withdrawn and irritable in paranoia. Kraepelin identified several depressive states including simple retardation, motor retardation with delusions and hallucinations, and stupor as part of manic depressive insanity. He further distinguished depression which represents one pole of manic depressive insanity from melancholia which involves depression with fear, agitation, self-accusation, persecution, and hypochondriacal symptoms.

Our current perspective on the spectrum of depressive experiences stems from these important observations. The use of the term melancholia to refer to the depressive syndrome became less common as depression and manic–depressive disease were used more frequently in the early 20th century. In the *Diagnostic and Statistical Manual of Mental Disorders,* Second Edition (DSM-II) (American Psychiatric Association 1968), the term involutional melancholia denoted an episode of severe depression associated with menopause. Currently, the specifier with melancholic features is applied to the diagnosis of MDD if it is associated with a profound loss of interest and lack of reactivity to favorable external events. Other symptoms characteristic of melancholia include a distinct quality to the depressive mood characterized by marked worsening in the morning, early morning awakening, psychomotor retardation or agitation, significant anorexia and excessive guilt. These melancholic features are noted as a modifier of MDD in DSM-III, DSM-III-R, and in DSM-IV (American Psychiatric Association 1980, 1987, 1994).

## Suicidal Phenomena

Our current definitions of MDD emphasize suicidal ideation, thoughts of death, and suicide attempts as a cardinal criterion symptom of the disorder. Suicidality is the feature of depressive disorder that poses substantial risk of mortality in the disease. Prevention of suicide, more than any other treatment goal, requires immediate intervention and may require hospitalization. The risk for subsequent completed suicide for an individual hospitalized for an episode of severe MDD is estimated to be 15% (Coryell et al. 1982).

## Epidemiology

### Prevalence and Incidence

The prevalence and incidence data on MDD vary to some degree due to methodological differences, nature of interview format, geographic location, and setting of sample. Large scale epidemiologic studies of mood disorders began in earnest in the early 1950s, culminating with a reanalysis of the NIMH epidemiologic catchment area (ECA) (Weissman et al. 1988b) study (probability sample of over 18,000 adults in five US communities) and more recently, results from the National Comorbidity Survey (NCS) (Kessler et al. 1994).

Across epidemiologic studies, MDD is found to be a common psychiatric disorder. The lifetime risk for MDD in community samples vary from 10 to 25% for women and 5 to 12% for men (American Psychiatric Association 2000). The point prevalence of MDD for adults in community samples has varied from 5 to 9% for women and from 2 to 3 % for men (American Psychiatric Association 2000). While the incidence rates of MDD in prepubertal boys and girls are equal, women over the course of their lifetime are 2 to 3 times more likely to have MDD after puberty (Kornstein 1997). Whereas a strong relationship exists between low social class and schizophrenia, a weaker but nevertheless meaningful relationship may exist between low income status and the occurrence of MDD (Blazer et al. 1994). Analyses of the ECA data indicated that the lowest income group manifested twice the risk of MDD than the highest income group while the NCS concluded that individuals with low socioeconomic status demonstrate higher risk for MDD than individuals who are economically well-off. The rates of MDD may also be influenced by childhood adversity including severe physical abuse, sexual abuse, neglect and poor care (Harkness and Monroe 2002). The NCS identified the risk factors associated with having MDD comorbid with another mental disorder as opposed to MDD alone. These risk factors include: younger age, lower level of education, and lower income.

### Lifetime Risk and Lifetime Prevalence

Lifetime risk refers to the proportion of individuals being studied who would go on to develop the disorder during their lifetime. Estimates of lifetime risk of MDD in community samples vary from 20 to 25% for women and 7 to 12%

for men (Depression Guideline Panel 1993a). Lifetime prevalence refers to those individuals who, up to the time of assessment, have had symptoms that met diagnostic criteria at some point in their lives. The NCS estimated overall lifetime prevalence of MDD as 17.1%. The estimated prevalence was twice as high in females than males. The ECA study and NCS identified higher lifetime prevalence in younger age groups consistent with the birth cohort effect and possible recall bias.

### Point Prevalence

Point prevalence or current prevalence refers to the proportion of the individuals that have the disorder being studied at a designated time (Boyd and Weismann 1981). The specific point prevalence of MDD in community samples has ranged from 5 to 9% for women and 2 to 3% for men. The current point prevalence estimates in the NCS were 4.9%. The point prevalence of MDD in primary care outpatient settings ranges from 4.8 to 8.6% (Depression Guideline Panel 1993a). In hospitalized patients for all medical conditions, more than 14% had MDD (Feldman et al. 1987).

### Children and Adolescents

For preschool children, the point prevalence is thought to be of 0.8% (Depression Guideline Panel 1993a). Point prevalences of major and minor depressive disorder of 1.8 and 2.5%, respectively, were found in a sample of 9-year-old children from the general population, based upon the use of a semistructured diagnostic instrument (Kashani et al. 1983). A semistructured diagnostic instrument was used to find a 4.7% point prevalence rate of major depression in a community sample of 150 adolescents. Those adolescents diagnosed with MDD had symptoms that met criteria for dysthymia as well. A point prevalence rate of 3.3% was found for dysthymia (Kashani et al. 1987). Weller and Weller (1990) have shown the prevalence of MDD in clinical samples of children and adolescents to be 58% in educational clinics, 28% in outpatient psychiatric clinics, and 40 to 60% in psychiatric hospitals. By comparison, a prevalence of 7% is found in hospitalized pediatric patients. Emslie et al. (1990) assessed depressive symptoms by self-report in a large sample of high school students of mixed ethnic background in an urban school district. They found that hispanic females reported more severe depression whereas white males reported the least severe scores of depression. For males and females, African-Americans and hispanics reported significantly more depression than whites. Female gender, being behind in school, and non-white ethnicity predicted higher self-report scores of depressive symptoms.

### Older Adult

Weissman and colleagues (1991) found a 1% prevalence of MDD in adults 65 years and older who lived in the community. The data indicate that a lower lifetime prevalence of MDD was found in the oldest age group ($\geq$ age 65) in comparison to younger age groups. Women manifest an increased prevalence of MDD in comparison to men and no significant differences were found across racial or ethnic groups. However, other community samples of older adults were found to have a high prevalence (8–15%) of clinically significant depressive symptoms (but not a formal diagnosis of MDD). In a recent Stockholm group, the frequency of MDD was 5.9% and the rate of DD was 8.3% (Forsell et al. 1994).

In comparison to community settings, higher prevalence rates for MDD are found in treatment settings for older adults: 11% in hospitals, 5% in outpatient non-psychiatric clinics, and 12% in long-term care settings (Blazer 1994). There is also a higher prevalence rate in treatment settings of clinically significant depression that is not severe enough to warrant a formal diagnosis of MDD: 25% prevalence in hospitals (Koenig et al. 1988) and 30.5% in long-term care facilities (Parmelee et al. 1989).

## Birth Cohort

Klerman and Weissman (1989) as well as The Cross-National Collaborative Group (1992) called attention to a changing rate of MDD for recent birth cohorts found in: North America, Puerto Rico, Western Europe, Middle East, Asia, and the Pacific Rim. Specifically, earlier age of onset and increased rate of depression occur in individuals born in more recent decades. Historical, social, economic, or biological events most likely account for the variability in rate of depression noted in different countries included in the study. However, an overall increase in the rate of depression was noted across many of the geographic locations.

Older adults continue to manifest a higher suicide rate than in younger age groups. However, suicide rates have increased in younger age groups as the changing rate of MDD is observed in younger cohorts. In keeping with the birth cohort effect, recurrences of MDD in late life may become a significant health concern as the population ages.

## Risk Factors

Familiarity with risk factors for MDD may help the clinician recognize or diagnose this common and serious psychiatric illness. Accordingly, The Depression Guideline Panel (1993a) enumerated ten primary risk factors for depression:

(1) History of prior episodes of depression
(2) Family history of depressive disorder especially in first-degree relatives
(3) History of suicide attempts
(4) Female gender
(5) Age of onset before age 40
(6) Postpartum period
(7) Comorbid medical illness
(8) Absence of social support
(9) Negative, stressful life events
(10) Active alcohol or substance abuse.

In the NCS, 4.9% of subjects were diagnosed as having a current episode of MDD. Of the subjects with depression, 43.7% had noncomorbid depression while 56.3% had comorbid conditions. This distribution of comorbid versus noncomorbid conditions is consistent with other reports of community and clinical samples examining the extent of co-occurrence. In the NCS, certain risk factors, including: (1) younger age, (2) lower level of education, and (3) lower income, were more associated with comorbid depression than noncomorbid depression.

## Comorbidity Patterns: General Medical Conditions

Whereas a 4 to 5% current prevalence rate of MDD exists in community samples, symptoms of depression are found in 12 to 36% of patients with a general medical condition (Depression Guideline Panel 1993). The rate of depression may be higher in patients with a specific medical condition. MDD is identified as an independent condition and calls for specific treatment when it occurs in the presence of a general medical condition.

The Depression Guideline Panel (1993a) includes four possible relationships between depression and a general medical condition: (1) depression is biologically caused by the general medical condition, (2) an individual who carries a genetic vulnerability to MDD manifests the onset of depression triggered by the general medical condition, (3) depression is psychologically caused by the general medical condition, and (4) no causal relationship exists between the general medical condition and mood disorder. The first two cases warrant initial treatment directed at the general medical disorder. Treatment is advocated for persistent depression upon stabilization of the general medical condition. When the general medical condition causes depression, specific treatment for the former condition is optimized, while psychiatric management, education, and antidepressant medication are administered to treat the depression. In cases where the two conditions are not etiologically related, appropriate treatment is indicated for each disorder.

## Stroke

Some poststroke patients manifest depression due to cerebrovascular disease related to cerebral infarction in left frontal and left subcortical brain regions. Mood disorder due to cerebrovascular disease is diagnosed when an individual manifests a recent stroke and has significant symptoms of depression. A point prevalence of mood disorder due to cerebrovascular disease in poststroke patients between 10 and 27% has been documented, with an average duration of depression lasting approximately 1 year (Depression Guideline Panel 1993). Case reports of mood disorder due to cerebrovascular disease in poststroke patients suggest poor treatment compliance, irritability, and personality change (Ross and Rush 1981).

## Dementia

According to DSM-IV-TR, when symptoms of clinically significant depressed mood accompany dementia of the Alzheimer's Type, and in the clinician's judgment, the depression is due to the direct physiological effects of the Alzheimer's disease, mood disorder due to Alzheimer's disease is diagnosed. When dementia consistent with cerebrovascular disease leads to prominent cognitive deficits, focal neurological signs and symptoms, significant impairment in functioning as well as predominant depressed mood, vascular dementia with depressed mood is diagnosed. The distinction between depressive disorders and dementing disorders is often complicated because depression and dementia commonly co-occur. Treatment of co-occurring depressive features may relieve symptoms and improve overall quality of life.

## Parkinson's Disease

Fifty percent of patients with Parkinson's disease experience a MDD during the course of the illness. When depression occurs in this context, one diagnoses mood disorder due to Parkinson's disease. Active treatment of the depressive disorder may result in improvement in the signs and symptoms of depression without alleviation of the involuntary movement disorder or cognitive changes associated with subcortical brain disease. The underlying etiology of associated dementia and depressive disorder in Parkinson's disease appears to involve physiologic changes in subcortical brain regions.

## Diabetes

It is estimated that the prevalence of depression in treated patients with diabetes is three times as frequent than in the general population. Further, there is no difference in the prevalence rate of depression in patients with insulin-dependent diabetes mellitus (Type I) in comparison to patients with noninsulin-dependent mellitus (Type II). The symptomatic presentation of MDD in patients with diabetes is similar to patients without diabetes. Consequently, full assessment of and treatment for MDD is recommended in patients who become depressed during the course of diabetes (Depression Guideline Panel 1993a). The relatively high point prevalence rate may be due to higher detection rate in this treated population, having a chronic illness, as well as metabolic and endocrine factors.

## Coronary Artery Disease

When MDD is present, increased morbidity and mortality is reported in postmyocardial infarction patients as well as in patients having coronary artery disease without myocardial infarction (MI). Therefore, treatment of MDD in patients with coronary artery disease is indicated. Prevalence estimates of MDD in postmyocardial infarction range from 40 to 65%. Over a 15-month period, patients 55 years or older who had mood disorder evidenced a mortality rate four times higher than expected, and coronary heart disease or stroke accounted for 63% of the deaths (Depression Guideline Panel 1993a). Depression may promote poor adherence to cardiac rehabilitation and worse outcome. During the first year following MI, depression is considered to be associated with a three- to fourfold increase in subsequent cardiovascular morbidity and mortality. Depression in patients with coronary artery disease is associated with more social problems, functional impairment, and increased health care utilization (Musselman et al. 1998). Recent studies of erectile dysfunction, cardiovascular disease, and depression demonstrate that all three conditions share many of the same risk factors (Goldstein 2000).

## Cancer

MDD occurs in 25% of patients with cancer at some time during the illness. MDD should be assessed and treated as an independent disorder. The intense reaction in patients diagnosed with cancer may lead to dysphoria and sadness without evolving a full syndrome of MDD. The consulting psychiatrist must evaluate the patient's response to chemotherapy, side effects of the treatment, and medication interactions in the overall assessment of the patient. Among patients with cancer, MDD is typically characterized by heightened distress, impaired functioning, and decreased capacity to adhere to treatment. Treating comorbid MDD with psychotherapy or pharmacotherapy may improve the overall outcome in patients with cancer and mitigate complications of MDD.

## Chronic Fatigue Syndrome

Lifetime rates of MDD in patients with chronic fatigue syndrome range from 46 to 75%. Comorbid anxiety and somatization disorders are also common in patients with chronic fatigue. According to the Centers for Disease Control (CDC) criteria, the diagnosis of chronic fatigue syndrome is excluded in patients whose symptoms meet criteria for a formal psychiatric disorder, such as MDD or DD. Patients whose symptoms meet criteria for both a mood disorder and chronic fatigue syndrome should be maximally treated for the mood disorder with appropriate pharmacotherapy and cognitive–behavioral psychotherapy (Depression Guideline Panel 1993a). The etiological relationship between mood disorder and chronic fatigue syndrome is unclear.

## Fibromyalgia

In comparison to other general medical conditions, little is known about the relationship between fibromyalgia and MDD. Two studies (Alfici et al. 1989, Hudson et al. 1985) have found higher lifetime rates of major mood disorder in fibromyalgia patients in comparison to rheumatoid arthritis patients.

## Depression Due to Medications

If MDD is judged to be a direct physiologic effect of a medication, then substance induced mood disorder is diagnosed. Medications reported to cause depression involve several drugs from the associated groups listed in Table 63–1.

Among antihypertensive treatment, beta-adrenergic blockers have been studied regarding the risk of depression. No significant differences are found between individuals treated with beta blockers and those treated with other antihypertensives regarding the propensity to develop depressive symptoms. Lethargy is the most common side effect reported. No significant depressive complications are reported with calcium channel blockers or angiotensin converting enzyme (ACE) inhibitors.

Hormonal treatments, such as corticosteroids and anabolic steroids, can elicit depression, mania, or psychosis. Oral contraceptives require monitoring regarding the possible precipitation of depressive symptoms.

Because patients with seizure disorders and Parkinson's disease are at high risk for concomitant MDD, it is difficult to establish a link between anticonvulsant or anti-Parkinsonian treatment and the precipitation of depression. Nevertheless, patients require close monitoring and evaluation for evolution of depressive symptomatology.

| Table 63–1 | Medications Associated with Depression | |
|---|---|---|

| Cardiovascular Drugs | Hormones | Psychotropics |
|---|---|---|
| Methyldopa | Oral contraceptives | Benzodiazepines |
| Reserpine | Corticotropin and glucocorticoids | Neuroleptics |
| Propranolol | Anabolic steroids | |
| Guanethidine | | |
| Clonidine | | |
| Thiazide diuretics | | |
| Digitalis | | |
| **Anticancer Agents** | **Anti-inflammatory and Anti-infective Agents** | **Others** |
| Cycloserine | Nonsteroidal antiinflammatory agents | Cocaine (withdrawal) |
| | Ethambutol | Amphetamines (withdrawal) |
| | Disulfiram | Levodopa |
| | Sulfonamides | Cimetidine |
| | Baclofen | Ranitidine |
| | Metoclopramide | |

## Comorbidity Patterns: Other Clinical Psychiatric Disorders

More than 40% of patients with MDD have additional symptoms that meet criteria during their lifetime for one or more additional psychiatric disorders (Sargeant et al. 1990). In a recent community sample, assessing both pure and comorbid MDD based upon findings from the NCS, the current prevalence of major depression was 4.9% (Blazer et al. 1994). Of the sample with current MDD, 56.3% also had another psychiatric disorder. The expression "comorbidity" comes from general medicine and denotes distinct but coexisting conditions. The multiaxial format of DSM-IV requires delineation of multiple diagnoses on Axis I (clinical psychiatric syndromes), if present and specification of co-occurring syndromes on Axis I and II (personality disorders). The presence of a comorbid psychiatric disorder may alter the course of major mood disorder in a dramatic fashion and is identified as a primary risk factor for poor treatment response. Therefore, proper assessment, preferably with the use of a semistructured diagnostic instruments, additional informants, and longitudinal observation, will identify comorbid conditions. In addition, specific guidelines are available to inform decision-making regarding which illness (MDD or other psychiatric disorder) becomes the initial focus of treatment (Depression Guideline Panel 1993a).

### Alcohol/Drug Dependence

Results of family and twin studies in a population-based female sample are consistent with a modest correlation of the liability between alcohol dependence and MDD (Kendler et al. 1993a). It is common for individuals with alcohol dependence to evidence signs of depression or MDD, but alcoholism is not thought to be a common consequence of mood disorder. Between 10 and 30% of patients with alcoholism manifest depression (Petty 1992), whereas alcoholism is thought to occur in under 5% of depressed patients (Depression Guideline Panel 1993a).

Depressed women are more likely to self-medicate their mood disorder with alcohol than are depressed men (Depression Guideline Panel 1993a). The effect of comorbid alcoholism on the course of major mood disorder is unclear. Some evidence suggests that remission of depression occurs within the first month of sobriety (Brown and Schuckit 1988, Dorus et al. 1987). The effect of comorbid depression requires further attention in relation to the course of drug dependence. Drug dependence is often associated with major mood disorder and the presence of associated comorbid personality disorder.

### Anxiety Disorders

The co-occurrence of symptoms of anxiety and depression is very common. Kendler et al. (1986) found very high genetic correlations between MDD and generalized anxiety disorder in contrast to a modest overlap between phobic disorders and MDD. Anxiety symptoms commonly appear in depressive syndromes and MDD is frequently comorbid with anxiety disorders. From a longitudinal perspective, either symptom constellation can be a precursor to the development of the other disorder. The combination of anxiety and depression predicts greater severity and impairment than the presence of each syndrome in isolation (Depression Guideline Panel 1993a). The association of severe panic and MDD is one of the predictors of suicidal risk. The clinician is advised to assess for symptoms of each disorder and to obtain a thorough family history. Patients with anxiety disorders often experience prior episodes of MDD or have relatives who suffer from mood disorder.

Ten to 20% of outpatients with MDD evidence comorbid panic disorder while 30 to 40% of depressed outpatients have had symptoms that met criteria for generalized anxiety disorder during the course of the mood disorder. In both cases, the anxiety disorder has preceded the major mood disorder about 50% of the time. An increased incidence of MDD is noted in patients with anxiety disorders who are followed over time. For example, Munjack and Moss (1981) found that 91% of their agoraphobic patients manifested a MDD within a 3-year period. MDD is a commonly manifested clinical outcome of a chronic anxiety state (Akiskal 1990).

The clinician is advised to evaluate three factors in order to determine treatment approaches when MDD co-occurs with panic disorder or social phobia: (1) the patient's family history, (2) the constellation of symptoms that were first evident in the current episode, and (3) the symptoms that cause the patient the most distress.

Recovery is less likely and symptomatology more severe in patients with comorbid MDD and panic disorder than in cases with a single diagnosis. Lifetime suicide rate is twice as high for patients with comorbid panic disorder and MDD than in panic disorder alone. It is imperative to assess for the presence of mood disorder and suicidality in patients who present with symptoms of anxiety.

## Obsessive–Compulsive Disorder

The occurrence of symptoms of depression is very common in patients with obsessive–compulsive disorder (OCD), although full symptom criteria may not be reached to warrant a formal diagnosis of MDD. Ten to 30% of patients with OCD have mood symptoms that meet full criteria for MDD. The relationship between OCD and schizophrenia is less clear. Patients with OCD are at increased risk to develop MDD but not schizophrenia (Goodwin and Jamison 1990). It is important to distinguish between obsessive–compulsive personality features which can accompany and are exacerbated during an episode of depression and OCD itself. Symptoms of depression often diminish with successful initial treatment of OCD, since biological treatments typically involve use of selective serotonergic antidepressant medications such as clomipramine, fluoxetine, or fluvoxamine.

## Posttraumatic Stress Disorder

Individuals with PTSD often experience co-occurring depressive disorders, anxiety disorders, and substance use disorders. The range of reported rates of concurrent depressive disorder in patients with PTSD is 30 to 50% (Bleich et al. 1997, Kessler et al. 1995) Many of the symptoms of PTSD overlap with signs and symptoms of depression such that both PTSD and MDD can be considered to be the result of traumatic events. In addition, depressive disorder may be associated with worse outcome in individuals with co-occurring PTSD (Shalev et al. 1998).

## Somatization Disorder

It is common for patients with MDD to experience somatic symptoms including pain, although the intensity and frequency of the somatic complaints and the range of body systems affected do not usually meet criteria for somatization disorder. Patients who have mood symptoms that meet criteria for MDD evidence more complaints of pain, experience more physical, interpersonal, and occupational limitations, and perceive their overall health as worse than patients with chronic medical illness (Wells et al. 1989). The clinician should carefully evaluate for the presence of MDD in cases where the patient reports unexplained pain. Typically, pain complaints are relieved upon successful treatment of the MDD. However, somatoform disorders, as outlined in DSM-IV, may be associated with demoralization and depression.

## Eating Disorders

There are little data available regarding prevalence of eating disorders in patients with MDD. However, 33 to 50% of patients with anorexia nervosa or bulimia nervosa experience a comorbid mood disorder. Between 50 and 75% of patients with an eating disorder have a history of a MDD over a lifetime. Initial treatment is aimed at the eating disorder. If depression continues after proper nourishment has been reestablished in anorexia nervosa, treatment is directed at the primary mood disorder.

## Personality Disorders

High rates of personality disorders are found in depressed inpatients and outpatients. Most studies report a rate of co-occurrence between 30 and 40% in outpatients and 50 to 60% in inpatient samples (Shea et al. 1992). Sixty-three percent of our sample of acutely ill patients (mostly inpatients) with a MDD were assigned at least one Axis II diagnosis on the basis of a semistructured diagnostic instrument (Gruenberg et al. 1993). Several studies have found that patients with comorbid MDD and personality disorder evidence an earlier age of onset for the first episode of depression, increased severity of depressive symptoms, more episodes, longer duration of episodes, poorer response to both pharmacotherapy and psychotherapy, and increased risk for self-injury (Black et al. 1988, Charney et al. 1981, Ionescu and Popescu 1989, Pfohl et al. 1984, Shea et al. 1987).

A particular relationship is noted for comorbid MDD and borderline personality disorder (BPD). In a general psychiatric population, depressed patients show an estimated rate of 6% for co-occurring BPD (Depression Guideline Panel 1993). The link between BPD and MDD remains controversial. Gunderson and Phillips (1991) offered four possible relationships regarding the coexistence of MDD and BPD: (1) depression is primary and produces the symptoms of BPD, (2) BPD is primary and produces the symptoms of MDD, (3) MDD and BPD coexist but are unrelated, and (4) both disorders have nonspecific overlapping sources. For each hypothesis, the authors evaluated evidence from six areas: (1) comorbidity, (2) phenomenology, (3) family prevalence, (4) drug response, (5) biological factors, and (6) pathogenesis and outcome. The authors concluded that the evidence supports the notion that MDD and BPD coexist as independent disorders.

## Grief and Bereavement

Depressive symptoms associated with normal grieving usually begin within 2 to 3 weeks of the loss and resolve spontaneously over 6 to 8 weeks. If full symptom criteria for MDD persist for more than 2 months beyond the death of a loved one, then an episode of MDD can be diagnosed. Specific treatment for a major depressive episode such as short-term psychotherapy focusing on unresolved grief or pharmacotherapy is indicated.

## Etiology and Pathophysiology

Depressive disorders are common and recurrent, and associated with substantial psychosocial dysfunction as well as excess morbidity and mortality. Greater understanding of the underlying etiology and pathophysiology of MDD is the focus of genetic, neurobiologic, and psychosocial investigation.

## Integration of Genetic and Environmental Theories

Unipolar or nonbipolar MDD has been demonstrated to cluster in the first-degree relatives of patients with depression. The observation that MDD is familial, however, does not address whether the familial aggregation may be due to genetic or familial environmental factors. Multiple risk factors for MDD have been reported including gender, early parental loss, parental separation, rearing patterns, trauma and abuse, personality factors, prior major depression, low social class, and stressful recent life events (Kendler et al. 1993b). While familial aggregation is largely due to genetic factors, those environmental risk factors not shared by relatives are clearly important in etiology.

Behavioral genetics involves the search for genetic transmission or mechanisms associated with environmental or cultural transmission of psychiatric disorders. An understanding of the genetic liability to MDD will likely not yield identification of a single dominant gene responsible for this disorder because of substantial clinical heterogeneity, and probable genetic heterogeneity.

Twin studies provide methods for separating genetic and environmental contributions to the aggregation of depressive disorders in families. Several twin studies of MDD ascertained in clinical settings have reported higher concordance rates in monozygotic (MZ) than in dizygotic (DZ) twins, consistent with evidence of genetic liability to depression. A community-based twin study of major depression has confirmed the role of genetic factors in liability to adult depressive symptomatology (Kendler et al. 1992).

Kendler and colleagues (1992) estimated a 33 to 45 % genetic liability to depression in women, depending on the criteria used to diagnose MDD. Moreover, a moderate role for individual specific environmental experiences was demonstrated to influence the risk for depression. A subsequent report on the prediction of major depression in women demonstrated an important etiologic role for the combination of genetic factors and specific individual environmental experiences in influencing vulnerability to depression. Given the estimated heritability in MDD, converging evidence supports the important role of environmental experiences in the etiology of major depression (Brown and Harris 1978). Kendler's work emphasizes individual specific life events including recent personal stressors rather than those that are shared by other family members.

Only one of three adoption studies of depression show significant clustering of unipolar disorder in biological relatives of adoptees with major depression, highlighting the significance of both genetic and environmental sources of the liability to depression. In the Danish Adoption Study of unipolar disorder, significantly higher rates of depression were found in the biological relatives of hospitalized adopted probands with depressive disorder compared to the biological relatives of control adoptees. No increased rate of depression was found in the adoptive-relatives of proband versus control adoptees, however (Wender et al. 1986). The US adoption study demonstrated increased risk of depression in adoptees with a positive family history of depression in biological relatives, but this was short of statistical significance (Cadoret et al. 1990). Kendler and colleagues (1992) call for further research to examine the vulnerability within generations (the focus of twin studies) versus across generations (the focus of adoption studies).

The genetics of depressive temperament, a characterologic trait which may be predisposing to MDD, has not been the focus of empirical investigation. Family studies of clinical depression in childhood and adolescence demonstrate that early-onset depression, including depression in childhood, is more familial and likely to be associated with greater genetic liability (Orvaschel 1990).

All attempts to develop integrated etiologic models of depression have identified multiple psychosocial risk factors. In particular, female gender, limited social support, dependent, self-critical, and neurotic personality traits, and stressful life events appear to influence the vulnerability to MDD. Whether specific life events are as important later in the course of MDD as in the precipitation of initial episodes is the subject of ongoing investigation. Post (1992) argued that negative, stressful life events are associated with the initial or second episode of recurrent MDD whereas neurobiological factors are most relevant with subsequent recurrent episodes. Post asserted that sensitization to stressors and episodes may become encoded at the level of gene expression, underscoring the role of neurobiological factors in the progression of the illness.

Since genetic factors are operative in the etiology of MDD and prior depressive episodes place an individual at risk for future depression, indirect genetic factors operate in the vulnerability to lifetime risk. In summary, clinical and genetic epidemiologic studies suggest that MDD is a multifactorial disorder influenced by several genetic and environmental risk factors. The effectiveness of the individual's social support network in association with successful treatment may protect the individual from the vulnerability to recurrent MDD.

## Neurobiological Theories

Biological mechanisms associated with the clinical syndrome of MDD emerge from animal models of depression and clinical research in humans informed by the contributions of neurochemistry and molecular biology. Animal models of depression in which typical antidepressant pharmacologic treatments reverse depression have substantiated the biological aspects of the depressive syndrome. In these animal models of depression, monkeys separated from their mothers show despair (Harlow and Harlow 1962). Antidepressant medications reverse these syndromes, and neurochemical changes associated with these interventions provide evidence for a direct pharmacologic effect of antidepressant treatment (McKinney 1988).

Nevertheless, the complex interrelation and interdependence of neurochemical systems involving critical neurotransmitters, synaptic regulation, nerve cell mediation and modulation, neuropeptides, and neuroendocrine systems are poorly understood. In the past four decades, explorations of these mechanisms have focused on simpler hypotheses derived from clinical observations of drug effects. The interaction of these multiple systems has been difficult to investigate in the laboratory.

In the early 1950s, the use of reserpine in hypertensive patients, leading to depression in up to 15% of these individuals, predicted the association of amine depletion and MDD. This amine depletion effect of antihypertensives associated with the initial efficacy of monoamine oxidase inhibitors in depression contributed to the emerging hypothesis that catecholamine deficit was etiologic in major depression (Schildkraut 1965). The pharmacologic bridge asserted that clinical action of antidepressant drugs provided evidence supporting neurochemical hypotheses of MDD. Monamine oxidase inhibitors (MAOIs) blocked the enzymatic metabolism of norepinephrine, dopamine, and serotonin, furthering evidence of catecholamine activity in MDD. Therapeutic benefits of tricyclic antidepressants (TCAs) and their pharmacologic activity provided further impetus to the biological hypotheses, which currently prevail. The development of selective serotonin reuptake inhibitors (SSRIs) which are effective treatments in MDD lends further support to the serotonergic hypotheses in MDD. The antidepressant–receptor activity reported by Goodwin and Jamison (1990) includes down-regulation (decreasing the number) of postsynaptic beta-adrenergic receptors while enhancing response to serotonergic and alpha-adrenergic stimulation.

Studies of neurotransmitters such as norepinephrine (NE), serotonin (5-HT), dopamine (DA), gamma-amino butyric acid (GABA), and acetylcholine (ACh) as well as their metabolites including 3-methoxy-4-hydroxyphenylglycol (MHPG), 5-hydroxyindoleacetic acid (5-HIAA), dihydroxyphenyl acetic acid (DOPAC), vanillyl mandelic acid (VMA), and homovanillic acid (HVA) have been studied extensively in patients with MDD, bipolar disorder, and controls. There are no consistent neurochemical findings distinguishing the two clinical syndromes (Goodwin and Jamison 1990). However, certain aspects of the depressive syndrome do appear to be significantly associated with certain neurotransmitter metabolite observations. The principal metabolite of serotonin, 5-HIAA, has been examined in postmortem studies of depressed patients including suicide victims and deaths unrelated to suicide. Decreased cerebrospinal fluid 5-HIAA is present in those depressed patients who have committed suicide (Goodwin and Jamison 1990). The data suggest that serotonergic system dysregulation is associated with suicide and associated impulsivity and aggressivity. Studies examining the principal metabolite of norepinephrine and dopamine, MHPG and HVA respectively, do not demonstrate consistent findings in relation to suicide or other clinical subtyping. In addition to cerebrospinal fluid studies, many observations of urinary and plasma levels of catecholamine metabolites have been performed in MDD. These studies do not provide consistent support for a straightforward catecholamine excess/deficit hypothesis of MDD.

Recent studies challenging the simpler paradigm of catecholamine deficit or excess in depression have focused upon neurotransmitter modulation of nerve cell regulation as well as effects of neurotransmitter systems on receptor sensitivity. Additional studies show that patients with depression as well as those who have died by suicide are reported to have lower levels of the serotonin transporter (SERT) than in control subjects (Owens and Nemeroff 1998). As the pharmacology of the neurotransmitters and receptors is further explicated, receptor changes leading to effects on second messenger systems and the generation of new proteins affecting gene expression will become the focus of the neurobiology of MDD.

## Sleep Studies and Biological Rhythm Disturbances

Specific abnormalities in sleep and circadian rhythms are among the most consistent findings in biological psychiatry. Clinical observations of insomnia and hypersomnia are commonly noted as a central feature of depressive disorder. Polysomnography (PSG) demonstrates that the progression of sleep from nonrapid eye movement (non-REM) stages 1 to 4 to rapid eye movement (REM) sleep is disrupted in MDD. EEG recordings demonstrate a shorter than normal onset of REM sleep termed reduced or shortened REM latency. The frequency of eye movements during REM sleep is greater, termed increased REM density. During the sleep laboratory evaluation, increased awakening during sleep leads to the reduction in total sleep time in MDD. Non-REM abnormalities include prolonged sleep latency, increased wakefulness, decreased arousal threshold, and early morning awakening (Kupfer and Thase 1983). Rush and colleagues (1986a) and Giles and colleagues (1989) have suggested that sleep EEG parameters are more trait-like and that some sleep EEG alterations may precede the onset of clinical depression.

Biological rhythm abnormalities include advances in the timing of daily rhythms such as REM sleep, cortisol, and body temperature. Endogenous processes within a day (approximately 25 hours) are *circadian rhythms*. Episodic recurrences of the illness over days, months, or years are called *infradian rhythms* (a period of more than a day). *Ultradian rhythms* are oscillations that occur more than once daily and occur at the cellular and neurohormonal level (Goodwin and Jamison 1990). Mechanisms which explain the alterations in oscillation of biological rhythms in depression are not well delineated. Clearly, homeostatic regulation of cellular, biochemical, and psychological phenomenon is necessary to maintain euthymia. The phase advance of a "strong oscillator" leading to depression has been suggested by Wehr and colleagues (1979). Seasonal variation in mood disorders represents the effect of change in light and temperature on the individual's biological vulnerability to depression. Treatments involving light manipulation have begun to address the impact of seasonal change on those individuals vulnerable to depression with seasonal pattern.

## Neurohormonal Theories

The contribution of endocrine system alterations in depression has been examined extensively in biological studies. Both hypothyroidism and hypercortisolism may result in depression.

### Hypothalamic–Pituitary–Thyroid Axis

Hypothalamic–pituitary–thyroid (HPT) axis abnormalities are commonly seen in patients with bipolar disorder. Thyroid hormone has been used in antidepressant augmentation as well as in modulation of rapid cycling bipolar disorder (Bauer and Whydrow 1990, Goodwin et al. 1982). Neurotransmitters regulate hypothalamic functioning and initiate release of thyrotropin-releasing hormone (TRH) into the portal circulation. TRH is transported to the pituitary causing release of thyroid-stimulating hormone (TSH). TSH modulates synthesis and release of $T_3$ and $T_4$.

Thyroid studies in depression are not conclusive. There are more reports of slightly increased peripheral $T_4$ in major depression than low $T_4$. Some patients have mild or "subclinical" hypothyroidism as reflected in slight TSH abnormalities and associated antithyroid antibodies. The TRH stimulation test has provided suggestive findings: (1) blunted TSH response to TRH occurs in approximately 30% of depressed patients, (2) a possible bipolar/unipolar difference has been reported with bipolar depression showing an augmented TSH response while unipolar depression shows a blunted response (Goodwin and Jamison 1990), and (3) CSF TRH is found to be raised in some patients with depression, possibly responsible for the blunted response of TSH to TRH, and lower levels of circulating $T_3$ and $T_4$. One implication of the suggested bipolar–unipolar distinction is that bipolar depressed patients may demonstrate a false hypothyroidism, when their TSH response is consistent with the underlying bipolar disorder. Effective treatment of the bipolar disorder may reverse the TSH abnormality.

## Hypothalamic–Pituitary–Adrenal Axis

The hypothalamic–pituitary–adrenal axis (HPA) has been the subject of intensive investigation as well. The observation of elevated cortisol secretion from the adrenal glands has been replicated consistently in patients with major depression. Corticotropin-releasing factor (CRF) is the hypothalamic hormone that regulates pituitary secretion of corticotropin (ACTH). CRF activity is influenced by multiple neurotransmitters such as 5HT, NE, ACh, and GABA. ACTH binds to cells in the adrenal cortex producing release of glucocorticoids, particularly cortisol. Cortisol inhibits secretion of ACTH at the anterior pituitary and CRF at the hypothalamus. Measurements of 24-hour urinary cortisol, cortisol in the CSF, and cortisol following dexamethasone suppression suggested increased cortisol secretion in MDD. The dexamethasone suppression test (DST) performed by offering dexamethasone at 11PM followed by serum cortisol at 8AM, 4PM, and 11PM, is an neuroendocrine probe that demonstrated adrenocortical hyperactivity in melancholia (Carroll et al. 1981). DST nonsuppression usually normalizes with recovery from depression. Persistent nonsuppression is associated with early relapse of MDD (Greden et al. 1983).

Increased secretion of CRF may explain the hypercortisolemia in MDD and the HPA axis overactivity. Nemeroff and colleagues (1984) demonstrated increased CSF concentrations of CRF in patients with depression compared to individuals with other psychiatric disorders and control subjects. Another suggestion of HPA axis hyperactivity is the observation of adrenal gland hypertrophy in MDD patients (Nemeroff et al. 1992).

One of the most consistent findings in biological studies of MDD is hypercortisolism, which likely results from state-dependent influences involving stress, neurotransmitter dysregulation, and associated effects on HPA activity. CRF antagonists are currently being investigated to treat depression (Holsber 1999).

## Intracellular Abnormalities

A number of intracellular changes, which involve alterations in cellular second-messenger systems and ion channels, are postulated to occur in depression. These may involve changes in guanine triphosphate binding proteins, G-proteins on the receptor (Manji 1992), cyclic adenosine monophosphate (cAMP) regulation (Duman 1998), reduced

protein kinase activity (Shelton et al. 1996), and brain-derived neurotrophic factors (BDNF) (Post and Weiss 1998). Stress itself has been associated with lowered levels of BDNF, which leaves cells vulnerable to neurotoxic effects of stress. Antidepressants as well as electroconvulsive therapy increase BDNF. BDNF has been found to increase functioning of serotonin (Duman 1998, Duman et al. 1997).

## Psychosocial Theories

A number of psychosocial mechanisms have been implicated in the etiology and pathophysiology of MDD. Modern psychological explanations of depression emerged in the latter part of the 19th century and represented a shift from humoral theory. Concurrently, the longitudinal, observational, and descriptive perspectives emphasized by Kraepelin coincided with development of psychoanalytic and psychological approaches to depression.

## Psychoanalytic Theory

Introduced by Freud (1957) and Abraham (1927), psychoanalytic theory addressed the role of libidinal drives and their management. In Freud's early work, depression and melancholia were forms of "actual neuroses," in contrast to "psychoneuroses." Freud asserted that periodic depression and melancholia appeared in combination with severe anxiety. He emphasized the common ground between neurasthenia and melancholia, noting that neurasthenic symptoms characterized by prominent anxiety were often accompanied by depression. This observation set the stage for psychiatry's current focus on comorbid syndromal clinical presentations. Conditions in which panic states lead to severe depression are found to be more refractory and associated with worse outcome. Those depressive states which emerge acutely with less associated anxiety are more likely to be depressed phases of bipolar disorder.

Freud and Abraham emphasized the connection between mourning and melancholia, through the introjection and identification with an ambivalently-experienced lost object. The melancholic patient experiences a loss of self-esteem with associated hopelessness and helplessness, prominent guilt, and self-denigration. In psychoanalytic theory, this results from internally directed anger. Anger or aggression associated with ambivalence is turned against the self, leading to the depressive experience. Both introjection and internalization of negative aspects of the lost object plague the depressed patient (Freud 1957).

Abraham argued that subtler forms of loss in the child's early development predispose the person to later episodes of depression in the face of disappointment and loss. This vulnerability follows the child's experience of both early loss as well as early traumatic experiences. Self-psychologists have described the effects of loss and trauma on the development of a coherent self experience. Psychoanalysts after Freud also focused on early attachment difficulties and the impact of separation and loss which predisposes the individual to later depression experience (Bowlby 1980). Bibring (1953) described loss of self-esteem which arose from conflicts between one's expectations (ego ideal) and one's reality.

## Behavioral Theory

In the behavioral perspective, an overgeneralized depressive response to loss of social support is observed. The individual's social environment no longer provides reinforcement to the individual, and the depressed patient feels increasingly isolated and unsupported. The lack of social support appears to be one of the strongest factors in promoting vulnerability to depression (Skinner 1953).

The experience of depression elicits negative responses from others, including rejection from spouses, children, and other important individuals. In the social context, the persistence of depression, according to Coyne (1976), is associated with the continuing experience of negative responses from others over time. Behavioral treatments which involve social skills training and self-monitoring of mood attempt to alleviate behavioral consequences of depressive disorder. Lewinsohn (1974) suggested that individuals with depression have social skill deficits that make it difficult to obtain reinforcement from the social environment.

## Cognitive Theory

The cognitive or cognitive–behavioral perspective originally developed by Beck (1976) emphasizes a set of dysfunctional attitudes, cognitions, and images associated with depressive symptomatology. The cognitive–behavioral theory is the most empirically examined psychosocial theory in relation to the management and treatment of the depressed patient. In Beck's cognitive theory, cognitive distortions cause depression and are associated with maintenance of the disorder. The "cognitive triad" involves negative views of one's self, one's world and current situation, and the future. The cognitive theory delineates the importance of cognitive distortions, the "cognitive triad," and a conception of negative self-image which is called negative self schemas.

The cognitive perspective is elaborated further by learned helplessness models, and hopelessness theory (Abramson 1989, Seligman 1975). In hopelessness theory, "depressogenic attributional style" leads individuals to regard stressful events as permanent rather than temporary, and affecting most of one's life rather than a specific aspect of one's life. Certain attributional styles lead to personal or internal, rather than global or external, explanations of the depressive disorder. The cognitive perspective as well as contributions from the helplessness–hopelessness models formed an empirical basis for CBT, initially developed by Beck and colleagues (1973). In CBT, education, behavioral assignments, and cognitive retraining form the active components of the psychotherapy (Beck et al. 1979). This cognitive therapy has been demonstrated to be an effective short-term psychotherapy for depression (DeRubeis et al. 1990).

## Interpersonal Theory

Another current therapy called interpersonal therapy derives from a focus on difficulties in current interpersonal functioning. The relationship between psychological health and one's interpersonal environment has received substantial attention since 1940. Adolf Meyer articulated that psychological impairment was a consequence of difficulty adapting to the environment. Interpersonal approaches to the treatment of psychiatric disorders are described by Harry Stack Sullivan, and Frieda Fromm-Reichmann as well. These authors highlighted the importance of one's current experience, functioning in social roles, interpersonal relationships, and adaptation to stress and environmental change (Klerman et al. 1984).

The current iteration of the interpersonal approach is reflected in the development of a specific treatment for depression termed interpersonal psychotherapy of depression (IPT). IPT involves a formal diagnostic assessment, inventory of important current and past relationships, and definition of the current problem area. In IPT, four areas of focus that could relate to depressive symptoms are: (1) grief, (2) interpersonal role disputes, (3) role transitions, and (4) interpersonal deficits.

## Social Rhythm Theory

An attempt at integration of biological and psychosocial theories of depression has focused on the disruption of biological rhythms associated with psychosocial stressors.

The loss of "social zeitgebers" has been proposed as a link between biological and psychosocial formulations (Ehlers 1988). The social zeitgebers theory suggests that social relationships, interpersonal continuity, and work tasks entrain biological rhythms. Disruptions of social rhythms due to loss of relationships interfere with biological rhythms that maintain homeostasis. This disruption leads to changes in neurobiological processes including alterations in neurotransmitter functions, neuroendocrine regulation, and neurophysiologic control of sleep/wake cycle and other normal circadian oscillations.

## Diagnosis and Differential Diagnosis

The detection of depression in both primary care settings and mental health settings requires the presence of mood disturbance or loss of interest and pleasure in activities for 2 weeks or more accompanied by at least four other symptoms of depression. There are problems in differential diagnosis because depressive experiences vary from individual to individual. MDD is sometimes called unipolar depression or recurrent unipolar depression because the depressive episodes tend to recur in a lifetime. DD is characterized by at least 2 years of depressed mood accompanied by two or three depressive symptoms which falls short of threshold criteria for a major depressive episode. Depressive disorder not otherwise specified (DDNOS) includes a set of conditions which do not meet criteria for MDD, DD, or adjustment disorder with depressed mood. These syndromes include premenstrual dysphoric disorder, minor depressive disorder, recurrent brief depressive disorder, and postpsychotic depressive disorder occurring during the residual phase of schizophrenia. In DSM-IV, two other depressive disorders are diagnosed based upon etiology and include mood disorder due to a general medical condition and substance-induced mood disorder.

The core symptoms comprising a major depressive episode are illustrated in the DSM-IV criteria. Each symptom is critical to evaluate in a patient with depressive symptomatology since each represents one of the essential features of a major depressive episode. Their persistence for much of the day, nearly every day for at least 2 weeks, is the criterion for diagnosis. The clinical syndrome is associated with significant psychological distress or impairment in psychosocial or work functioning.

The clinical observation of mood reveals variations in presentation. An individual may have depressed symptomatology and experience typical sadness. Another individual may deny sadness and experience internal agitation and dysphoria. Another individual with depression may experience no feelings at all, and the depressed mood is inferred from the degree of psychological pain that is exhibited. Some individuals experience irritability, frustration, somatic preoccupation, and the sensation of being numb.

An equally important aspect of the depressive experience involves loss of interest or pleasure, when an individual feels no sense of enjoyment in activities which were previously considered pleasurable. There is associated reduction in all drives including energy and alteration in sleep, interest in food, and interest in sexual activity.

A common experience of insomnia or hypersomnia is noted in individuals with persistent depression. Observations of psychomotor activity include profound psychomotor retardation leading to stupor in more severe cases or alternatively significant agitation leading to inability to sit still and profound pacing in agitated forms of depression.

The complaint of guilt or guilty preoccupation is a common aspect of the depressive syndrome. Delusional forms of guilt are a common presentation of depressive disorder with psychotic features.

The loss of ability to concentrate, to focus attention, and to make decisions is a particularly distressing symptom for individuals. One may experience a loss of memory which simulates dementia. Loss of concentration is reflected in an inability to perform both complicated and more simple tasks. The loss of ability to perform in school may be a symptom of MDD in children, and memory difficulties in the older adult may be mistaken for a primary dementia. In some older adults, a depressive episode with memory difficulties occurs in the early phase of an evolving dementia.

The most common psychiatric syndrome associated with thoughts of death, suicidal ideation, or completed suicide is MDD. The experience of hopelessness is commonly associated with suicidal ideation. The preoccupation with suicide in MDD requires that the assessment always includes careful monitoring of suicidality.

## Subtyping of MDD

The current subtyping of MDD is based on severity, cross-sectional features, and course features.

## Severity

The rating of severity is based on a clinical judgment of the number of criteria present, the severity of the symptomatology, and the degree of functional distress. The ratings of current severity are classified as mild, moderate, severe without psychotic features, severe with psychotic features, in partial remission, or in full remission. The definition of "mild" refers to a episode results in only mild impairment in occupational or psychosocial functioning or mild disability. "Moderate" implies a level of severity which is intermediate between mild and severe and is associated with moderate impairment in psychosocial functioning. The definition of "severe" describes an episode which meets several symptoms in excess of those required to make a diagnosis of major depressive episode and is associated with marked impairment in occupational or psychosocial functioning and definite disability characterized by inability to work or perform basic social functions. Severe with psychotic features indicates the presence of delusions or hallucinations which occur in the context of the major depressive

episode. Since the introduction of DSM-III, the categories of mood-congruent versus mood-incongruent psychotic features are made in the context of a psychotic depressive disorder. When the content of delusions or hallucinations is consistent with depressive themes, a mood-congruent psychotic diagnosis is made. When the psychotic features are not related to depressive themes or include symptoms such as thought insertion, broadcast, or withdrawal, the modifier of mood-incongruent psychotic features is used. A recent review has suggested that mood-incongruent psychosis in MDD is associated with a poorer prognosis (Kendler 1991). For depression with psychotic features, whether they are mood-congruent or mood-incongruent, antipsychotic medication in combination with antidepressant medication or electroconvulsive therapy (ECT) is required to treat the disorder.

Partial remission indicates that the episode no longer meets full criteria for major depressive episode but that some symptoms are still present or the period of remission has been less than 2 months. In full remission, the individual has no significant symptoms of depression for a period of at least 2 months.

## Cross-sectional Features

The assessment of cross-sectional features involves the presence or absence of catatonic, melancholic, or atypical features during an episode of depression. The specifier with catatonic features is used when profound psychomotor retardation, prominent mutism, echolalia, echopraxia, or stupor dominate the clinical picture. The presentation of catatonia requires a differential diagnosis which includes schizophrenia, catatonic type, bipolar I disorder, catatonic disorder due to a general medical condition, medication-induced movement disorder leading to catatonic features, or neuroleptic malignant syndrome.

The specifier with melancholic features is applied when the depressive episode is characterized by profound loss of interest or pleasure in activities and lack of reactivity to external events as well as usual pleasurable stimuli. In addition, at least three of the following melancholic features must be present: depression is typically worse in the morning, early morning awakening, psychomotor change with marked retardation or agitation, significant weight loss, or profound and excessive guilt. MDD with melancholic features is particularly important to diagnose because of the prediction that it is more likely to respond to somatic treatment including electroconvulsive therapy. Individuals with melancholic features experience more recurrence of MDD. The findings of hypercortisolism following dexamethasone as well as reduced REM latency is associated with the melancholic subtype of MDD (Rush et al. 1991).

Finally, the category of MDD with atypical features was previously called "atypical depression." This syndrome is characterized by prominent mood reactivity in which there is excessive responsiveness of mood to external events and at least two of the following associated features: increased appetite or weight gain, hypersomnia, leaden paralysis (a feeling of profound anergia or heavy feeling), and interpersonal hypersensitivity (rejection sensitivity). Depressive episodes with atypical features are also common in individuals with bipolar I or II disorder as well as seasonal affective disorder.

## Course Features

MDD is diagnosed with certain course features such as postpartum onset, seasonal pattern, recurrent, chronic, and with or without full interepisode recovery. Depression with onset in the postpartum period has been the subject of increasing attention in psychiatric consultation to obstetrics and gynecology. The presence of a MDD may occur from 2 weeks to 12 months after delivery, beyond the usual duration of postpartum "blues" (3–7 days). Postpartum blues are brief episodes of labile mood and tearfulness which occur in 50 to 80% of women within 5 days of delivery. However, depression is seen in 10 to 20% of women after childbirth (Miller 2002), which is higher than rates of depression found in matched controls. There is greater vulnerability in women with prior episodes of major mood disorder particularly bipolar disorder, and there is a high risk of recurrence with subsequent deliveries after an MDD with postpartum onset. The postpartum onset episodes can present either with or without psychosis. Postpartum psychotic episodes occur in 0.1 to 0.2% of deliveries. Depression in postpartum psychosis is associated with prominent guilt and may involve individuals with a prior history of bipolar I disorder. If an episode of postpartum psychosis occurs, there is a high risk of recurrence with subsequent deliveries. Heightened attention to identification of postpartum episodes is required because of potential risk of morbidity and mortality to mother and newborn child.

The specifier with seasonal pattern is diagnosed when episodes of MDD occur regularly in fall and winter seasons and subsequently remit during spring and summer. When the pattern of onset and remission occurs for the last 2 years, one diagnoses an MDD with seasonal pattern. Often, this pattern is characterized by atypical features including low energy, hypersomnia, weight gain, and carbohydrate craving. Although the predominant pattern is fall–winter depression, a minority of individuals show the reverse seasonal pattern with spring–summer depression. Specific forms of light therapy with 2500 lux exposure has been shown to be effective in MDD with seasonal pattern (Whirz-Justice 1993). Because seasonal depression has clinical features which are similar to atypical features, the risk of a possible bipolar II disorder must be considered since atypical features are more common in depressive episodes occurring as part of bipolar II. These individuals when exposed to antidepressant medication or bright light therapy may evolve a switch into hypomanic or manic episode.

Clinical and scientific attention to the course of MDD focuses upon the depiction of longitudinal course. Life charting of MDD involves the use of several course specifiers. Each episode is denoted with or without full recovery. MDD manifests either a single or recurrent pattern of episodes. Remission of depression requires a 2-month interval in which the criteria are not met for a major depressive episode. The specifier chronic MDD involves the persistence of a major depressive episode continually, satisfying full MDD criteria for at least 2 years.

## Depression in Children and Adolescents

In prepubertal children, MDD occurs equally among boys and girls (Depression Guideline Panel 1993a). MDD in childhood is considered to have high recurrence rates with up to 70% recurrence in 5 years. After puberty, girls experience an increased rate of depression as compared to boys. There is increased risk of depressive disorder in children and adolescence when one or more of the parents are depressed. The earlier the age of onset of depression, the higher the familiar loading. In addition, a number of childhood psychosocial risk factors have been identified to be associated with juvenile-onset MDD. These risk factors include: more perinatal insults, motor skill abnormalities, instability in caregivers, and psychopathology in the first-degree relatives (Jafee et al. 2002). Adolescent-onset depression often takes on a more chronic course associated with dysthymic symptoms. In adolescence, MDD appears to be associated with greater fatigue, worthlessness, and more prominent vegetative signs while DD has more prominent changes in mood, irritability, anger, and hopelessness. The signs and symptoms used for diagnosis in children and adolescents are identical to those used for diagnosis in adults. The sequelae of depression in children and adolescents is often characterized by disruption in school performance, social withdrawal, increased behavioral disruption, and substance abuse. Differential diagnosis among children and adolescents with MDD include behavioral disorders such as conduct disorder, attention deficit hyperactivity disorder, and bipolar disorder.

Later-onset MDD in adolescents is also associated with decline in school performance, social withdrawal, or disruptive behavior. The critical differential diagnostic consideration in adolescents with MDD is the misdiagnosis of depression when the clinical presentation will evolve into a diagnosis of bipolar disorder. When depression occurs during adolescence, it often heralds a severe disorder with recurrent course and a family history of MDD is often noted. An additional psychosocial risk factor in later-onset depression in adolescence is childhood sexual abuse.

In a community sample of adolescents, ages 14 to 18 years, onset of MDD was associated with female gender and suicidal ideation. The mean age of onset for the first episode of MDD was 14.9 years. Episodes of MDD were relatively longer in adolescents who had onset before the age of 15 (Lewinsohn et al. 1994).

## Major Depressive Disorder in the Older Adult

Older adults with depression often experience cognitive impairment as part of the clinical syndrome. Symptoms of depression may simulate dementia with concentration difficulties, memory loss, and distractibility. Commonly, MDD and dementia co-occur. It is less frequent that findings of dementia are fully explained on the basis of depression (pseudodementia). The prevalence of MDD in older adults residing in nursing homes is estimated to be approximately 30% (Depression Guideline Panel 1993a). MDD in the elderly often co-occurs in the presence of medical conditions which complicates the treatment for both the depression and the primary medical condition. Careful evaluation of medications may also reveal explanations for associated symptoms of depression. Older adults with first onset of depression must be carefully evaluated for co-occurring medical conditions. Among the common disorders to be considered are silent cerebral ischemic events, undiagnosed cancer, or complications of metabolic conditions such as adult-onset diabetes mellitus and thyroid dysfunction.

## Depression in Ethnic Groups

In working with individuals of different ethnic groups, the language which expresses depressive symptomatology varies. Nonwestern cultural expressions emphasize somatic complaints more prominently than psychological complaints. Depending on the particular ethnic group understanding the specific "language of depression" is important, because the prevalence estimates cross-culturally do not appear to differ significantly from those reported in the US.

## Assessment

The assessment of MDD involves the specific identification of 5 of 9 criterion symptoms which would constitute a diagnosis of MDD. A careful general medical assessment to ascertain the presence of an etiologic general medical condition is required. After the assessment for general medical conditions, one examines the individual for the presence of alcohol or drug dependence. Then the clinician is required to assess retrospectively the occurrence of prior episodes of mood disorder, either depression or mania. It is necessary to examine for other comorbid psychiatric disorders as well. Depressive illnesses are very common and recurrent, but an individual with MDD may or may not recall prior episodes. It is therefore essential to interview a significant other in addition to the patient to identify prior manic, hypomanic, or prior depressive episodes. Family inquiry allows one to elicit the family history of addiction, anxiety, depressive disorder, mania, psychosis, trauma, or neurologic disorders in first-degree relatives.

To assess risk for suicide, one inquires about the presence of active suicidal ideation in relation to the current episode of depression and a history of prior suicide attempts. The occurrence of significant life events such as separation, divorce, and death of significant others may precipitate the episode. It is also necessary to review onsets of other medical conditions which may precipitate a new episode of depression. When alcohol or other drug use co-occurs with such significant life events, the risk of suicidal behavior during an episode of depression increases. The presence of a recent suicide attempt may suggest the need for immediate hospitalization and treatment.

### General Medical Assessment

The individual who presents for outpatient or hospital treatment for a primary depressive disorder will require general medical examination including a physical examination and laboratory testing to rule out an associated medical condition. Clinical assessment, including the cognitive mental status examination, will direct the extent of the general medical examination.

Laboratory studies in the management of the individual with MDD includes complete blood count with differential, electrolytes, chemical screening for renal and liver function, as well as thyroid function studies. More detailed evaluation will depend upon the nature of the clinical presentation as well as neuropsychological examination. These studies may identify cerebral vulnerability factors that would complicate the treatment for MDD.

When clinical signs suggest cognitive disruption or cognitive impairment, the clinician may also consider administering neuropsychological tests or conducting more focused neurologic examination to explore cognitive, behavioral, and neurologic correlates of brain function. Neuropsychological assessment may help to clarify the relative contribution of depression or another disease process to the patient's clinical presentation. Further, neuropsychological assessment will provide a functional analysis of the patient's cognitive and behavioral strengths and limitations. Neurological examination may reveal minor neurological abnormalities suggesting early neurodevelopmental vulnerability.

### Psychodiagnostic Assessment

Traditional psychological testing may complement structured diagnostic instruments developed to ascertain the presence or absence of depressive disorders according to DSM-IV criteria. Psychological testing such as the Rorschach Inkblot Test are sensitive to the degree of affective lability, intensity of suicidality and impulse control in individuals with depression. In addition, inventories are commonly used in outpatient and inpatient settings to establish scores of clinical severity of depressive symptoms. Self-administered scales include the Beck Depression Inventory (Beck et al. 1961), the Zung Self-Rating Depression Scale (Zung 1965), and the Inventory for Depressive Symptomatology (self-report) (Rush et al. 1987). Psychiatrist-administered scales used for assessment of depressive symptoms include the Hamilton Rating Scale for Depression (Hamilton 1960), the Montgomery Asberg Depression Rating Scale (Montgomery and Asberg 1979), and the Inventory for Depressive Symptomatology (psychiatrist rated) (Rush et al. 1986). Structured diagnostic interviews that have been developed to confirm major psychiatric syndromes include the present state examination (Wing et al. 1967), the schedule for affective disorders and schizophrenia (SADS) (Endicott and Spitzer 1978), and structured clinical interview for DSM-IV Axis I disorders (SCID-I) (First et al. 1994). The use of these structured diagnostic interviews reliably predicts the presence of an MDD. It is essential to recognize that a cross-sectional assessment is only one component of the total assessment. Corroborative family data and longitudinal assessment and reassessment of mood disorder symptoms are crucial in following the natural history and course of MDD.

## Course and Natural History

### Clinical Course

In order to document onset of depressive phases as well as periods of remission, psychiatrists must pay careful attention to clinical course. Improvements in assessment procedures, including structured interview guides for the assessment of depression as well as rating scales for depression, will promote better attention to course and natural history of MDD. Long-term studies of depression must incorporate information on recovery, recurrence and chronicity.

### Age of Onset

The mean age of onset of major depression is 27 years of age (Weissman et al. 1988b), although an individual can experience the onset of MDD at any age.

### Natural History of Episodes

New symptoms of MDD often develop over several to several weeks. Early manifestations of an episode of

MDD include anxiety, sleeplessness, worry, and rumination prior to the experience of overt depression. Over a lifetime, the presence of one major depressive episode is associated with a 50% chance of a recurrent episode (Thase 1990). A history of two episodes is associated with a 70 to 80% risk of a future episode. Three or more episodes are associated with extremely high rates of recurrence (National Institute of Mental Health Consensus Development Conference Statement 1985). Because the majority of cases of MDD recur, continuation treatment and ongoing education regarding warning signs of relapse or recurrence are essential in ongoing clinical care. In an MDD when single episode recurs, a change in diagnosis to MDD recurrent is necessitated.

In comparison to individuals who develop a single episode (many of whom return to premorbid functioning), individuals with recurrent episodes of depression are at greater risk to manifest bipolar disorder (Depression Guideline Panel 1993a). Individuals who experience several recurrent episodes of depression may develop a hypomanic or manic episode requiring rediagnosis to bipolar disorder. In children and adolescents, the transformation of a diagnosis of depression to a diagnosis of bipolar disorder is higher. Approximately 40% of adolescents who are depressed, evolve a bipolar course. Because bipolar disorder is initiated with a depressive episode in at 4 of 5 cases (Goodwin and Jamison 1990), it is important to identify those patients who are most likely to develop a bipolar disorder. Therefore, the clinician is confronted with significant diagnostic and treatment challenges when called upon to evaluate a patient, particularly an adolescent, who presents with depression and has no previous history of mania. Several risk factors have been identified (Akiskal 1983, Goodwin and Jamison 1990), which predict when a first episode of MDD will evolve into bipolar disorder: (1) the first episode of depression emerges during adolescence, (2) the depression is severe and includes psychotic features; (3) psychomotor retardation and hypersomnia are present, (4) a family history of bipolar disorder exists, particularly across two to three generations, and (5) the patient experiences hypomania induced by antidepressant medication.

Recurrent MDD requires longitudinal observation because of its highly variable course. Generally, complete remission of an episode of MDD heralds a return to premorbid levels of social, occupational, and interpersonal functioning. Therefore, the goal of treatment is a focus on achieving full remission of depressive symptoms and recovery. Untreated episodes of depression last 6 to 24 months (Goodwin and Jamison 1990). Symptom remission and a return to premorbid level of functioning characterize approximately 66% of depressed patients (Depression Guideline Panel 1993a). By comparison, roughly 5 to 10% of patients continue to experience a full episode of depression for greater than 2 years and approximately 20 to 25% of patients experience partial recovery between episodes. Furthermore, 25% of patients manifest "double depression," characterized by the development of MDD superimposed upon a mild, chronic depression (DD) (Keller and Shapiro 1982). Patients with double depression often demonstrate poor interepisode recovery. Four characteristics are seen in a partial remission of an episode (Depression Guideline Panel 1993a): (1) increased likelihood of a subsequent epi-

sode, (2) partial interepisode recovery following subsequent episodes, (3) longer-term treatment may be required, and (4) treatment with a combination of pharmacotherapy and psychotherapy may be indicated.

Follow-up naturalistic studies have indicated that 40.3% of individuals with MDD carry the same diagnosis 1 year later, 2.6% evidence DD, 16.7% manifest incomplete recovery, and 40.5% do not meet criteria for MDD (Depression Guideline Panel 1993a). Keller and colleagues (1992) highlight the potential for chronicity in MDD. A 5-year follow-up study indicated that 50% of 431 patients showed recovery by 6 months but 12% of the sample continued to be depressed for the entire 5-year period. The authors noted that inadequate treatment may have contributed to chronicity.

## Definitions of Remission, Relapse, Recovery, and Recurrence

The precise nature of severity and duration of phases during the natural course of MDD has not been empirically demonstrated in longitudinal, prospective studies. Further, Prien and colleagues (1991) pointed to considerable inconsistency in the way published articles defined concepts relating to changes in the clinical course of MDD. In response, Frank and colleagues (1991) suggested provisional operational criteria, based upon their conceptual scheme of change points during the natural course of unipolar MDD. Important change points heretofore used without clear distinction, which pertain to the natural course of recurrent unipolar depression, include: remission, recovery, relapse, and recurrence. The authors based their proposed criteria upon several principles: measurable phenomena such as symptom severity, observed clinical course, and temporal focus (i.e., applicable to single or recurrent episodes). Definitions of remission, recovery, relapse, and recurrence proposed by Frank and colleagues are illustrated in Table 63–2.

## Factors Affecting Recurrence and Outcome

Poor outcome and likelihood of recurrent episodes is associated with comorbid conditions such as personality disorder, active substance or alcohol abuse, organicity, or medical illness. Recurrence and outcome may be affected by the rapidity of clinical intervention. Inadequate treatment (e.g., insufficient dosing or duration of pharmacotherapy) contributes to poor outcome, including chronic MDD.

| Table 63–2 | Proposed Definitions of Remission, Recovery, Relapse, and Recurrence |
|---|---|
| Remission | A period in which the individual is asymptomatic. Does not meet syndromal criteria for MDD, and has no more than minimal symptoms; in clinical practice, this remission extends from 2 to 9 mo. |
| Recovery | A remission that lasts more than 9 mo without relapse after appropriate treatment. |
| Relapse | A return of symptoms meeting criteria for a full syndrome of an episode of MDD that occurs during a period of remission but before recovery. |
| Recurrence | A manifestation of a new episode of MDD that occurs during recovery. |

Several authors have asserted that early treatment intervention in an episode of MDD is considered to be somewhat more effective than later intervention in an episode (Kupfer et al. 1989).

## Prognosis

MDD must be viewed as a serious medical illness. Although depression is treatable, the prognosis for an individual diagnosed with MDD involves important implications regarding morbidity, social functioning, and mortality.

### Morbidity

Patients with MDD report health difficulties and actively use health services. Studies have indicated that as many as 23% of depressed patients report health difficulties severe enough to keep them bedridden (Wells et al. 1988). A community sample of patients with MDD demonstrated increased health care utilization in comparison to patients in the general medical setting (Regier et al. 1988). The Medical Outcomes Study (Wells et al. 1989) examined role functioning, social functioning, and number of days in bed secondary to poor health, and compared the degree of impact of depression and other chronic medical conditions. Depression was associated with more impairment in occupational and interpersonal functioning, and more days in bed, in comparison to several common medical illnesses.

Patients with MDD were shown to be as functionally impaired as patients with serious, chronic medical conditions as well (Katon et al. 1990). Patients with MDD in a clinical sample evidence severely impaired occupational functioning, such as loss of work time (Wells et al. 1989). Further, long-term diminished activity has been shown to characterize a community sample of depressed patients (Wells et al. 1988).

### Mortality

A significant relationship exists between MDD and mortality, characterized by suicide and accidents (Wells 1985). Therefore, an accurate diagnosis of MDD, early appropriate intervention, and specific assessment of suicidality is essential. Fifteen percent of patients with MDD who require hospitalization due to severe depression will die by committing suicide (Coryell et al. 1982). Approximately 10% of patients with MDD who attempt suicide will eventually succeed in killing themselves. Roughly 50% of individuals who have successfully committed suicide carried a primary depressive diagnosis (Barklage 1991).

Fawcett and colleagues (1990) looked at factors associated with suicide at different time points during the course of depression. Factors associated with suicide 1 year after assessment included severe anhedonia, insomnia, concentration difficulties, and comorbid panic attacks or substance abuse. Factors associated with suicide at 1 to 5 years after the assessment included prior suicide attempts, suicidal ideation, and hopelessness.

Patients with MDD who were admitted to nursing homes were found to have a 59% greater likelihood of death within the first year of admission in comparison to nondepressed admissions. The ECA study indicated that patients with MDD 55 years of age and older evidence a mortality rate over the next 15 months four times higher than nondepressed controls matched for age.

The occurrence of MDD in patients who previously have been hospitalized following MI is demonstrated as an independent risk factor for mortality at 6 months (Frasure-Smith et al. 1993). The consequences of MDD were at the very least commensurate with that of left ventricular dysfunction and history of past MI.

## Goals of Treatment

The goals of treatment in MDD are full remission of symptoms of depression with restoration of optimal work and social functioning. During the course of treatment ongoing education of the individual and family regarding remission, relapse, and recurrence is critical. This education alerts both those affected by the illness and their families to the early signs of relapse and can assist in prevention of recurrence. Improved social and work functioning following an episode of depression is an important associated goal of treatment. Many studies have demonstrated the benefit of depression-specific psychotherapy as an important aspect of maintaining remission and improving work and social functioning. The establishment of a collaborative working relationship among the patient, family and psychiatrist is an essential aspect of recovery. The data which demonstrate efficacy in psychiatric management and treatment infers that a collaborative relationship is present.

## Phases of Treatment

All psychiatric treatment whether pharmacotherapy or psychotherapy or the integration of pharmacotherapy and psychotherapy, first requires a well-established diagnostic formulation in order to achieve optimal response to treatment. As the diagnostic process is undertaken an ongoing therapeutic alliance must be established. In the treatment of MDD an understanding of the clinical history of each individual's distress is necessary. As the clinical history is elicited the appropriate target signs and symptoms of MDD are obtained and the patient is educated as to the nature of the symptom patterns which represent his or her unique form of depressive disorder.

The phases of treatment include:

1. An acute phase directed at reduction and elimination of depressive signs and symptoms, and active restoration of psychosocial and work functioning.
2. A continuation phase directed at prevention of relapse and reduction of recurrence through ongoing education, pharmacotherapy, and depression-specific psychotherapy.
3. A maintenance phase of treatment directed at prevention of future episodes of depression based upon the patient's personal history of relapse and recurrence.

Acute phase treatment may involve all interventions that are directed toward decreasing signs and symptoms of depression and maintaining the individual's capacity to work and interact with others in a manner consistent with premorbid levels of social and work functioning. The acute phase treatments may include supportive psychotherapy focusing on resolution of current disputes. A form of supportive therapy may be combined with recommendations for pharmacotherapy. The standard pharmacotherapies which are available for treatment of depression have increased dramatically in the past 2 decades. In mild to moderate depressive disorder, more depression-specific forms of psychotherapy have been established including cognitive–behavioral psychotherapy, interpersonal psychotherapy, or short-term dynamic psychotherapy. In these forms of psychotherapy, which have been studied to address mild to moderate nonbipolar depressive disorder, the focus of the psychotherapy is very clearly explicated to the patient before the initiation of the psychotherapy. For severe depressive disorder with melancholic or psychotic features, these specific forms of short-term psychotherapy may not be as effective as focused pharmacotherapy. Pharmacotherapy in these conditions is associated with more rapid treatment response than is psychotherapy. During the acute phase of treatment for depressive disorder the optimal treatment should result in resolution of depressive signs and symptoms anytime between week 8 and week 16 of treatment. If resolution of depressive signs and symptoms does not occur during the first 2 to 4 months then the initial diagnostic formulation must be reviewed and alternative treatment strategies must be introduced. Some of the factors associated with lack of complete treatment response include the presence of co-occurring personality disorders, concurrent alcohol or substance abuse, a poor therapeutic alliance leading to lack of adherence to treatment recommendations, and persistent or unfavorable side effects of treatment.

When acute phase treatment does lead to remission of signs and symptoms, then the next phase of treatment begins. This phase of treatment is termed continuation treatment and its goal is prevention of relapse. It is often necessary to maintain ongoing pharmacotherapy for 6 to 12 months after an acute episode of depression during this continuation phase, because there is substantial vulnerability to relapse if medication treatment is prematurely interrupted. During the continuation phase ongoing psychotherapy may be particularly important to address residual symptoms of depression, and to alert the individual to a depressive response to subsequent traumatic circumstances, as well as ongoing clinical interaction with significant others is required in order to address persisting interpersonal conflicts, and may promote even more complete recovery from the depressive episode. The continuation phase of treatment typically lasts 9 to 12 months to minimize the risk of recurrent episode. If this represents the initial episode of depression, then medication treatment may be carefully withdrawn at the end of the continuation phase. However, if this represents a history of recurrence of depression (particularly two or more episodes in the preceding 3 years), maintenance treatment may well be recommended. In addition, maintenance treatment is recommended if two prior episodes have occurred within one's lifetime.

Maintenance treatment of MDD is focused on prevention of future episodes of depression, after a recent recurrence of MDD and a prior history of two or more episodes of MDD. Often the maintenance phase of treatment involves ongoing treatment with antidepressants or alternatively mood-stabilizing treatment (particularly lithium carbonate), or a combination to sustain recovery from depression. When there is early onset (adolescent onset) of depressive symptoms with associated psychosocial impairment, then ongoing maintenance treatment along with rehabilitative psychotherapy may be most critical. During maintenance treatment, continuing education of the patient and family, identification of prodromal symptoms, and continuing efforts at work and psychosocial rehabilitation are indicated. Often the trials of maintenance pharmacotherapy in depression demonstrate the preventive benefit of maintenance medication. In the most often quoted study, recurrence rates of 20 to 25% were found in individuals maintained with full dose of imipramine, while the recurrence rate was 80 to 100% in those patients treated with placebo. The advantage of ongoing maintenance medicine has also been demonstrated at 5 to 10 years. With tricyclic antidepressants, maintenance medication is likely more effective at full dose rather than lower doses. Limited data exists as to the dosing of SSRIs or other types of antidepressants in maintenance treatment.

## Site of Treatment
The site of treatment for MDD is based upon the severity of the acute episode and the psychiatrist's judgment of the individual's potential for suicide. Individuals with mild to moderate depression are often treated in primary care or psychiatry office settings. Acute phase pharmacotherapy involving antidepressant medication is often initiated by a primary care physician. However, the overall longitudinal care of MDD in primary care is the subject of increasing attention. Typically, individuals do not receive treatment for long enough periods and there is limited attention to the domains of social or work functioning. The referral to a psychiatrist may include a request for more expertise regarding medication as well as the need for depression-specific psychotherapy. In addition, there has been a lack of focused attention to the role of integrated psychotherapy and pharmacotherapy in primary care. Inpatient treatment for depression is recommended when there is an immediate risk for suicide or recent suicide attempt. In these settings safety of the individual is the primary concern and often more intensive treatments including electroconvulsive therapy may be initiated. When there are comorbid general medical conditions and psychiatric disorders, inpatient psychiatric hospitalization may be useful to stabilize both the general medical condition as well as the associated psychiatric disorder.

## General Approaches to Treatment
Initiation of treatment follows a careful psychiatric diagnostic interview. Assessment of the longitudinal clinical history must rule out bipolar disorder, comorbid PTSD, other anxiety disorders, and personality disorder. A completed mental status examination is used to rule out associated psychosis or marked cognitive disruption. When these procedures are conducted empathically, the beginning of a favorable therapeutic alliance is established. In all circumstances an effective therapeutic alliance facilitates recovery from MDD.

## Pharmacotherapy and Other Somatic Treatment
Treatment during the acute phase with medication is highly efficacious in reducing signs and symptoms of MDD.

Antidepressant medication has the most specific effect on reduction of symptoms and is often associated with improved psychosocial functioning. When symptoms of depression are mild to moderate, a course of depression-specific psychotherapy without medicine may also be effective. If symptoms of depression are moderate to severe, acute phase treatment with medications is often indicated. A wide variety of antidepressant medications have been documented as effective in moderate to severe MDD.

The range of treatments available in the US has included the tricyclic antidepressants available since the 1960s, monoamine oxidase inhibitors (MAOIs) available since the late 1950s, heterocyclic antidepressants available since the 1970s, and between 1989 and until the present newer SSRIs have been available. In addition, antidepressants with both serotonergic and noradrenergic activity or

noradrenergic activity alone have become available in the 1990s. Clearly, clinical trials comparing the efficacy of newer treatments with standard tricyclic antidepressants have shown equal efficacy with improvement in overall tolerance to side effects with newer treatments.

Antidepressant medications which are currently available for acute treatment of MDD are listed in the associated table (Table 63–3).

Choice of treatment with a specific antidepressant treatment in a given clinical situation is based on prior treatment response to medication, consideration of potential side effects, history of response in first-degree relatives to medicines, and the associated presence of co-occurring psychiatric disorders that may lead to a more specific choice of antidepressant treatment. Table 63–4 illustrates an algorithm developed for pharmacotherapy of MDD which in-

| Table 63–3 | Antidepressant Medications | | | | | | |
|---|---|---|---|---|---|---|---|
| **Category** | | | **Side Effects** | | | | |
| Trade Name | Compound | Usual Therapeutic Dose (mg) | Sedation | Hypotension (Decreased Blood Pressure) | Anticholinergic (i.e., Dry Mouth Constipation) | Cardiac (Slowed Heart Rate) | |
| Tricyclics | | | | | | | |
| Tertiary Amines | | | | | | | |
| Anafranil | Clomipramine | 150–300 | High | High | High | Yes | |
| Elavil | Amitriptyline | 150–300 | High | High | High | Yes | |
| Sinequan | Doxepin | 150–300 | High | Moderate | Moderate | Yes | |
| Surmontil | Trimipramine | 150–300 | High | Moderate | Moderate | Yes | |
| Tofranil | Imipramine | 150–300 | Moderate | High | Moderate | Yes | |
| Secondary Amines | | | | | | | |
| Norpramine | Desipramine | 100–300 | Low | High | Low | Yes | |
| Pamelor | Nortriptyline | 50–150 | Moderate | Low | Low | Yes | |
| Vivactil | Protriptyline | 20–60 | Low | Low | High | Yes | |
| Monoamine Oxidase Inhibitors | | | | | | | |
| Marplan | Isocarboxazid | 30–60 | Low | Moderate | Low | Low | |
| Nardil | Phenelzine | 45–90 | Low | Moderate | Low | Low | |
| Parnate | Tranylcypromine | 30–90 | Low | Moderate | Low | Low | |
| Atypical Agents | | | | | | | |
| Asendin | Amoxapine | 200–300 | Low | Moderate | Low | Yes | |
| Desyrel | Trazodone | 300–600 | High | High | Minimal | Low | |
| Ludiomil | Maprotiline | 150–200 | Moderate | Moderate | Low | Low | |
| Wellbutrin | Bupropion | 150–450 | Minimal | Low | Minimal | Yes | |
| Selective Serotonin Reuptake Inhibitors | | | | | | | |
| Paxil | Paroxetine | 20–50 | Low | Minimal | Minimal | Low | |
| Prozac | Fluoxetine | 20–100 | Minimal | Minimal | Minimal | Low | |
| Zoloft | Sertraline | 50–300 | Minimal | Minimal | Minimal | Low | |
| Luvox | Fluvoxamine | 150–400 | Low | Low | Low | Low | |
| Celexa | Citalopram | 20–50 | Minimal | None | None | Minimal | |
| Lexapro | Escitalopram | 10–30 | Minimal | None | None | Minimal | |
| Serotonin/ Norepinephrine Reuptake Inhibitors | | | | | | | |
| Effexor | Venlafaxine | 75–450 | Low | None | None | Minimal | |
| Serotonin Transport Blocker and Antagonist | | | | | | | |
| Serzone | Nefazadone | 200–600 | Minimal | Low | Minimal | Minimal | |
| Alpha-2-Adrenergic Antagonist | | | | | | | |
| Remeron | Mirtazapine | 30–60 | Moderate | Low | Minimal | Minimal | |

## Table 63–4  Pharmacotherapy Algorithm in Major Depressive Disorder

### Major Depressive Disorder, Single or Recurrent Episode, with Psychotic Features

Begin effective monotherapy with bupropion SR, citalopram, escitalopram, fluoxetine, nefazodone, paroxetine, sertraline, or venlafaxine XR (augment with lithium carbonate 600–900 mg).

or

Begin effective monotherapy with alternative antidepressant from list above (augment with bupropion SR, mirtazepine, or tricyclic antidepressant, either nortriptyline or desipramine, recognizing important drug interactions.

If ineffective, consider tranylcypromine, augmented with lithium carbonate, if necessary, for anergic features.

or

Consider phenelzine, augmented with lithium carbonate, if necessary, for anxious, dependent, and phobic features.

Augment with atypical antipsychotics for agitation, rumination, or suspicion.

or

Offer electroconvulsive therapy to remission (ECT).

### Major Depressive Disorder, Single or Recurrent Episode, with Psychotic Features

Begin typical or atypical antipsychotic to adequate doses in order to interrupt delusional features, augmented with SSRI, venlafaxine XR, or tricyclic antidepressants, either nortriptyline or desipramine, recognizing important drug interactions.

or

Begin amoxapine as alternative.

or

Begin electroconvulsive therapy as alternative, in context of immediate suicide risk, physical deterioration, or prior response to electroconvulsive therapy.

### Major Depressive Disorder with Atypical Features

Begin SSRI starting at low dose to minimize early side effects.

or

Begin MAOI, either phenelzine or tranylcypromine, to therapeutic doses.

### Major Depressive Disorder with Catatonic Features

Begin lorazepam 1–3 mg/d, to interrupt catatonic symptoms; evaluate for presence of psychotic features or longitudinal history of bipolar disorder.

Add antipsychotic medication to therapeutic doses or lithium carbonate to therapeutic doses, if bipolar or schizoaffective disorder emerges from the longitudinal history.

---

cludes a staged trial of newer medications (because of their superior side effect profiles) followed by treatments with older medicines available for the treatment of MDD. The ultimate goal of pharmacotherapy is complete remission of symptoms during a standard 6- to 12-week course of treatment.

## Selective Serotonin Reuptake Inhibitors

The most commonly prescribed antidepressant medicines in the past 10 years are SSRIs. They are selectively active at serotonergic neurochemical pathways and are effective in mild to moderate nonbipolar depression. They may also be particularly effective in MDD with atypical features as well as DD. Often these treatments are well tolerated and involve single daily dosing for MDD. Because of selective serotonergic activity, these treatments have also been demonstrated to be effective with co-occurring OCD, panic disorder, generalized anxiety disorder, PTSD, premenstrual dysphoric disorder, bulimia nervosa, social anxiety disorder, as well as MDD. They tend to be reasonably well tolerated in individuals with comorbid medical conditions. There are particular medication-specific interactions based on inhibition of cytochrome P-450 liver enzyme systems which require attention if an individual is taking other medications for primary medical conditions or associated psychiatric conditions. The currently available SSRIs in the US include fluoxetine (Prozac), paroxetine (Paxil), sertraline (Zoloft), fluvoxamine (Luvox), and citalopram (Celexa).

## Other Newer Antidepressants

In addition to SSRIs, greater attention has been brought to medicines with dual noradrenergic and serotonergic pathways including venlafaxine (Effexor XR) which has become available in both immediate release (IR) and extended release (XR) formulations. In addition, an alpha-2-adrenergic agonist, mirtazapine (Remeron) has become available, as well as a serotonin transport blocker and antagonist nefazodone (Serzone). Recent concerns about hepatic complications associated with nefazodone has required liver function monitoring. A predominantly noradrenergic and dopaminergic agonist, bupropion (Welbutrin), is also available in an immediate release and sustained release (SR) preparation.

## Tricyclic Antidepressants in Individuals with Severe MDD Including Melancholic Features

Tricyclic antidepressants have been best studied in individuals with MDD with melancholic features and with psychotic features. The combination of typical antipsychotic pharmacotherapy in association with tricyclic antidepressants has been recommended. The side effect profile of tricyclic antidepressants has included moderate to severe sedation, anticholinergic effects including constipation and cardiac effects which has made these medicines less popular in typical primary care or psychiatric practice. Nevertheless, the secondary amines which are metabolites of imipramine and amitriptyline, specifically desipramine and nortriptyline, have continued to be useful agents in more refractory depression.

## Monoamine Oxidase Inhibitors

There continues to be a role for the use of MAOIs in patients with MDD with atypical features. These agents particularly may be useful in intervention in depressive episodes with atypical features, characterized by prominent mood reactivity, reverse neurovegetative symptom patterns (i.e., overeating and oversleeping), and marked interpersonal rejection sensitivity. MAOIs continue to have a significant role in treatment of comorbid panic disorder, social phobia, and agoraphobia if individuals are not responsive to SSRIs. The ongoing prescription of phenelzine

(Nardil) or tranylcypromine (Parnate) requires continued education of the patient regarding standard food interactions involving tyramine as well as specific drug–drug interactions involving sympathomimetic medications. These cautions regarding diet and drug interaction makes MAO inhibitors less attractive to primary care physicians and most psychiatrists. However, they continue to be effective treatments which may be useful in depression with atypical features as well as anergic bipolar depression.

## Therapeutic Blood Levels

Although therapeutic blood level monitoring in the treatment of MDD may have a role in future treatments, the only group of medicines where there has been reliable assessment of blood levels are the tricyclic antidepressants. Because tricyclic antidepressants have significant drug–drug interactions with certain SSRIs there continues to be a need for therapeutic blood monitoring particularly with nortriptyline and desipramine.

## General Pharmacotherapy Recommendations

Increasingly, a trial of one class of antidepressants may be associated with incomplete response leading to a question of augmenting a treatment with another medicine versus switching from one medicine to another within the same class or to a different class altogether. Augmentation strategies with other medications, including adding lithium carbonate and other antidepressants, particularly those with a different mechanism of action, atypical antipsychotics, thyroid and stimulants, have been the focus of a number of reviews of treatment resistance (Thase and Rush 1995). A staging system for treatment resistant depression (TRD) has been proposed and ranges from failure to respond to a single agent (Stage 1) to failure of multiple treatments and electroconvulsive therapy (Stage 5) as shown in Table 63–5.

## Clinical Management

All of the antidepressant medications used in the treatment of MDD must be prescribed in the context of an overall clinical psychiatric relationship characterized by supportive interaction with the patient and family and ongoing education about the nature of the disorder and its treatment. Clinical management optimally involves careful monitoring of symptoms using standardized instruments and careful

| Table 63–5 | Staging Criteria for Treatment Resistant Depression |
|---|---|
| Stage | Description |
| 1. | Failure of at least one adequate trial of an antidepressant |
| 2. | Stage 1 resistance plus failure of adequate trial of an antidepressant from a distinctly different class than in Stage 1 |
| 3. | Stage 2 resistance plus failure of an adequate trial of a tricyclic antidepressant (TCA) |
| 4. | Stage 3 resistance plus failure of an adequate trial of a monoamine oxidase inhibitor (MAOI) |
| 5. | Stage 4 resistance plus failure of a course of bilateral electroconvulsive therapy (ECT). |

attention to side effects of medication in order to promote treatment adherence. Outpatient visits, which may be scheduled weekly at the outset of treatment, and subsequently biweekly encouragement and sustain collaborative treatment relationships. These office consultations allow the psychiatrist to make dosage adjustments as indicated, monitor side effects, and measure clinical response to treatment.

For the majority of individuals with MDD, a course of 6 to 8 weeks of acute treatment with weekly outpatient visits is indicated. Subsequent office visits may be scheduled every 2 to 4 weeks during the continuation phase of treatment. Appropriate adjustments of dose are determined by the psychiatrist as indicated by best clinical judgments of medication effect. The dose of an SSRI may be adjusted every 3 days on the basis of telephone contact and follow-up visits may be scheduled every 7 to 10 days. Similarly, the adjustment of dosing of tricyclic antidepressants and MAOIs must be attended to carefully in the first 2 to 3 weeks of treatment. Optimal dosing ranges of SSRIs, tricyclics, and MAOIs are noted in Table 63–3. Because of the early anxiety, agitation, and occasional insomnia associated with SSRIs, somewhat lower doses may be initiated early in the course before achieving the typical standard therapeutic dose.

Incomplete response, which entails the failure to respond to acute treatment with an antidepressant medication at 6 to 8 weeks, requires reassessment of diagnosis and determination of adequacy of dosing. Ongoing substance abuse, associated general medical condition or concurrent psychiatric disorder may partially explain a lack of complete response. If substance dependence is present, a full substance-free interval (preferably 4 weeks or longer) with appropriate detoxification and rehabilitation may be indicated. If a reassessment discloses an associated psychiatric disorder, then more specific treatment of that associated disorder, whether it be bipolar disorder or concurrent post-traumatic disorder, is necessary. If the reassessment suggests an associated comorbid personality disorder, then appropriate and more specialized psychotherapy may be necessary in order to achieve a complete response to treatment. As indicated before, if the MDD has psychotic features, then antipsychotic pharmacotherapy to adequate doses must be initiated prior to initiating a course of standard tricyclic antidepressants or a combined serotonin norepinephrine uptake inhibitor such as venlafaxine (Effexor). If MDD is associated with severe personality disorder (e.g., borderline personality disorder), then adjunctive psychotherapy and low dose antipsychotic medications may be necessary. If the patient has severe melancholic, delusional, or catatonic features, a course of electroconvulsive therapy may be necessary to achieve remission of symptoms.

There is also evidence that continuation of treatment beyond 6 to 12 weeks may convert some partial responders to responders if drug treatment is increased to full doses. This time allows for evaluation of the role of focused psychotherapy to address residual interpersonal disputes, loss or grief, or ongoing social deficits. The associated augmentation strategies to standard treatments include lithium carbonate augmentation, tricyclic antidepressant augmentation of SSRIs, thyroid hormone augmentation, and bupropion augmentation of SSRIs.

## Electroconvulsive Therapy

Electroconvulsive therapy (ECT) remains an effective treatment in patients with severe MDD and those individuals with psychotic MDD. Many patients who have responded to electroconvulsive therapy do not respond to pharmacotherapy. There is increased need for understanding the role of maintenance electroconvulsive therapy in those individuals who respond to electroconvulsive therapy because ongoing pharmacotherapy does not always prevent recurrence of depression after ECT is successful. ECT can be particularly useful in interrupting acute suicidality for those patients who may require rapid resolution of symptoms. ECT may be indicated in older adults when lack of self-care and weight loss may represent a greater risk. The most common side effect associated with electroconvulsive therapy is amnesia for the period of treatment. There is no consistent evidence to suggest chronic cognitive or memory impairment as a result of ECT.

## Other Somatic Treatments

Light therapy investigators have continued to demonstrate benefit in individuals with seasonal MDD by providing greater than 2500 lux light therapy for 1 to 2 hours/day. Many of these patients experience recurrent winter depression in the context of a recurrent MDD or bipolar II disorder. Bright light exposure has been associated with favorable response within 4 to 7 days. As with electroconvulsive therapy, light therapy is best prescribed by specialists who have experience in its use and can appropriately evaluate the indication for light therapy and monitor carefully the response to treatment.

Ongoing investigation of alternative brain stimulation techniques have been the subject of recent investigation. The use of a powerful magnet to provide transcranial magnetic stimulation has been the subject of several open trials. It is not yet determined whether the repetitive transcranial magnetic stimulation demonstrates its effectiveness through reduction of inhibitory neurotransmission or other mechanisms (George et al. 1999).

In addition, open clinical trials of vagus nerve stimulation (VNS) which has been found to be effective in epilepsy has been the subject of attention in refractory MDD. Several sites of investigation have begun to reveal positive effects at 9 months using VNS implantation (Rush et al. 2000). This procedure requires the implantation of a stimulating device in the chest with the capacity to stimulate the vagus nerve at regular intervals through the course of the day.

## Psychosocial Treatment

The past decade has also led to the development of more specific depression-based treatment for MDD. These treatments have included supportive psychiatric management techniques during pharmacotherapy, interpersonal psychotherapy, cognitive–behavioral therapy, brief dynamic psychotherapy, and marital and family therapy.

## Psychiatric Management and Supportive Psychotherapy

Psychiatric management and supportive psychotherapy is the standard in psychiatric office practice. The psychiatrist focuses on establishing a positive therapeutic relationship in the course of diagnosis and initiation of treatment of depression. The psychiatrist is attentive to all signs and symptoms of the disorder with particular attention to suicidality. The psychiatrist provides ongoing education, collaboration with the patient, and supportive feedback to the patient regarding ongoing response and prognosis. The supportive psychotherapeutic management of depression facilitates the ongoing pharmacologic response. Brief supportive psychotherapy in individuals with mild to moderate depression is indicated to improve medication compliance, to facilitate reduction of active depressive signs and symptoms, and to provide education regarding relapse and recurrence.

## Interpersonal Psychotherapy

Interpersonal psychotherapy in outpatients with nonbipolar MDD has been demonstrated to be effective in acute treatment trials. Interpersonal psychotherapy of depression addresses four areas of current interpersonal difficulties:

1. Interpersonal loss or grieving
2. Role transitions
3. Interpersonal disputes
4. Social deficits.

This type of treatment, like other psychotherapies for depression, also involves education about the nature of MDD and the relationship between symptoms of depressive disorder and current interpersonal difficulties.

Prior studies demonstrated efficacy of interpersonal psychotherapy for outpatients with depression. Interpersonal psychotherapy, cognitive–behavioral psychotherapy, and medication treatment were comparable on several outcome measures and superior to placebo. (Elkin et al. 1989, Hollon et al. 1992). Medication treatment was associated with the most rapid response and was superior to both interpersonal psychotherapy and cognitive–behavioral therapy in more severely depressed patients. Continuation studies with interpersonal psychotherapy (Thase et al. 1997) offered monthly, as well as during maintenance treatment, have demonstrated response in prevention of recurrence, and was superior to placebo treatment. Those patients who received ongoing interpersonal psychotherapy and medication had the longest intervals without recurrence of depressive symptoms.

## Cognitive–Behavioral Therapy

Cognitive–behavioral therapy for depression is a form of treatment aimed at symptom reduction through the identification and correction of cognitive distortions. These involve negative views of the self, one's current world, and the future. Several controlled studies have demonstrated the efficacy of cognitive therapy in resolution of MDD in adults (Depression Guideline Panel 1993b). Cognitive–behavioral therapy as well as interpersonal psychotherapy was somewhat less effective than medication treatment in moderate to severe MDD. However, other investigators (Hollon et al. 1992) have suggested a relatively equal response to cognitive–behavioral therapy and medication in more severely depressed outpatients.

## Brief Dynamic Psychotherapy

Brief dynamic psychotherapy addresses current conflicts as manifestations of difficulty in early attachment and disruption of early object relationships. Brief dynamic psychotherapy was not specifically designed for treatment of MDD and is currently the subject of ongoing studies as well as controlled clinical trials in comparison with medication treatment. The results of these trials will allow us to address the appropriate role of brief dynamic psychotherapy in outpatients with mild to moderate depression. In addition, it will be important to understand whether dynamic psychotherapy may address demoralization or response to traumatic circumstances.

## Marital and Family Therapy

It has been difficult to assess the specific efficacy of marital or family therapy in individuals with MDD based on current studies to date. There is substantial evidence that marital distress is a major event associated with the development of a depressive episode. Marital discord often will persist after the remission of depression and subsequent relapses are frequently associated with disruptions of marital relationships. There has been a single study (O'Leary and Beach 1990) focusing on efficacy of behaviorally oriented marital therapy in reducing symptoms of depression. There has been no controlled clinical trial of marital therapy in relation to other treatments for promoting the resolution of depressive signs and symptoms. Both acute and continuation phase treatment of MDD will require ongoing attention to marital and family issues to prevent recurrence of depression.

## Factors Influencing Treatment Response

There are a number of factors which influence ultimate treatment response in MDD including patient characteristics, diagnostic issues, comorbidity, treatment-related complications including side effects, and demographic factors. Reevaluation of diagnosis, comorbidity, and the physician–patient relationship itself is often critical.

### Suicide Risk

Patients with MDD are often at increased risk for suicide. Suicidal risk assessment is especially indicated as patients begin to recover from depression with increased energy and simultaneous continued despair. Persistent suicidal ideation coupled with increased energy can often lead to impulsive suicidal acts. The careful attention to the physician–patient relationship can mediate suicidal urges through availability and accessibility. Outpatients and inpatients with MDD and melancholic features will often require antidepressant therapy addressing multiple neurotransmitter systems, or ECT as well.

### Psychotic Features

MDD with psychotic features requires careful assessment to rule out comorbid psychiatric conditions. The combined treatment with antipsychotic as well as antidepressant medication is indicated. In addition, electroconvulsive therapy is an effective intervention in psychotic depression and may be considered as a first line alternative.

### Catatonic Features

MDD with catatonic features can be associated with significant morbidity due to the individual's refusal to eat or drink. Active treatment with a benzodiazepine such as lorazepam 1 to 3 mg daily may offer short-term treatment response. Subsequent treatment with lithium alone or in association with antidepressants may be indicated given the possible link between catatonic features and bipolar vulnerability (Hawkins et al. 1995). If psychosis is associated with catatonia, then atypical antipsychotic medication or a course of electroconvulsive therapy may be indicated as well (Bush et al. 1996).

### Atypical Features

Atypical features are associated with significant comorbid anxiety disorders, reverse neurovegetative symptoms such as hypersomnia, increased appetite, and weight gain as well as fatigue and leaden paralysis. SSRIs are likely to be effective in individuals with MDD with atypical features as well as MAOIs. Conversely, tricyclic antidepressants, in particular, are unlikely to be effective in such individuals.

### Severity

Individuals with mild to moderate depression may be effectively treated with psychotherapy, pharmacotherapy, or the combination. Individuals with severe MDD often require somatic intervention with antidepressant medication or electroconvulsive therapy.

### Recurrence

Because MDD is a recurrent disorder, current treatment guidelines (Hirschfeld 1994) suggest maintenance antidepressant treatment at full therapeutic doses if there is a history of more than two prior episodes of MDD.

### History of Hypomania or Mania

Any of the antidepressant treatments including medication, electroconvulsive therapy, light therapy, or newer somatic interventions may induce hypomania or mania in individuals who are vulnerable to bipolar disorder. Individuals who may have a family history of bipolar disorder should be carefully evaluated for treatment with lithium carbonate or other anticonvulsant mood stabilizers before antidepressant treatment because they are at particular risk for antidepressant-induced mania. Attention to this history of prior hypomania or mania as well as family history may promote treatment response if such individuals have mood stabilizing treatment offered initially.

## Comorbid Psychiatric Disorders with Major Depressive Disorder

### Alcohol or Substance Dependence

The comorbidity of MDD and alcohol or other substance dependence requires careful attention to both diagnoses. The first priority in treatment is abstinence from alcohol or substance use. Co-occurring addiction will complicate depressive disorders and increases risk for suicide. If detoxification from alcohol or other substance abuse is required, this should be undertaken before initiation of any somatic antidepressant therapy. Individuals who have a family history of depression or bipolar disorder are likely to require early initiation of appropriate mood disorder treatment following detoxification.

### Obsessive–Compulsive Disorder
In individuals with OCD, lifetime risk of MDD approaches 70%. The use of higher dose SSRI treatment is often indicated to treat both conditions. Alternatively, the tricyclic antidepressant, clomipramine (Anafranil), may be effective for those individuals with both OCD and MDD who do not respond to SSRIs.

### Panic Disorder
Lifetime risk of MDD approaches 50% in individuals with panic disorder. Because many of the SSRI and other antidepressants are effective treatments to treat panic as well as depression, these treatments have gained increasing popularity. One may continue to prescribe short-term courses of benzodiazepines, including lorazepam or clonazepam to alleviate acute symptoms of panic as low doses of antidepressant treatments are introduced into the treatment for comorbid panic and MDD. In addition, MAOIs continue to be effective treatments for both panic and MDD.

### Generalized Anxiety Disorder
Lifetime risk of MDD in individuals with generalized anxiety disorder (GAD) approaches 40%. New studies demonstrating efficacy of venlafaxine (Effexor) as well as paroxetine (Paxil) make these effective interventions in situations in which an individual has both MDD and GAD.

### Posttraumatic Stress Disorder
An essential feature of PTSD is the vulnerability to the development of MDD. Recent studies (Friedman 1998) demonstrate effectiveness in treating the core symptoms of PTSD as well as MDD. In addition, specific psychotherapy which addresses the core aspects of PTSD may be appropriate in individuals with comorbid PTSD and MDD in order to minimize the vulnerability to depression because of persistent PTSD symptomatology (Foa et al. 1999).

### Cognitive Impairment
When cognitive impairment is due to depressive disorder (as in "pseudodementia"), active treatment of depression may minimize associated cognitive difficulties. Many seniors evolve mild cognitive impairment and depression as early signs of dementia. Nevertheless, when MDD is mild it requires specific antidepressant treatment, or when severe or psychotic, electroconvulsive therapy.

### Dysthymic Disorder
The exacerbation of a persistent or chronic DD into a more severe depressive episode is termed "double depression". Many treatments for MDD are also useful in DD. It is likely that SSRIs, newer antidepressants as well as tricyclic antidepressants are effective for both DD and MDD. Specific forms of psychotherapy which are cognitive–behavioral have been investigated as effective in addressing poor inter-episode recovery from MDD associated with DD.

### Personality Disorder
Increasing evidence of the co-occurrence of MDD with personality disorder with rates up to 40 to 50% in outpatient clinics suggests incomplete response to antidepressants alone (Shea et al. 1992). Specific psychotherapy treatments which focus on maladaptive personality traits may facilitate the ongoing response to antidepressant pharmacotherapy.

## General Medical Conditions Co-occurring with Major Depressive Disorder

### Asthma
Ongoing attention to pharmacotherapy of individuals with asthma relates to the use of bronchodilators and steroid inhalers for asthma. These may complicate associated anxiety and depression and must be addressed carefully in consideration of appropriate antidepressant therapy. Generally, SSRIs and newer antidepressants appear to be well tolerated with typical asthma treatments.

### Cardiac History
SSRIs, newer mixed noradrenergic and serotonergic reuptake inhibitors, bupropion, and ECT are likely to be safe treatments for patients with cardiac disease (Glassman et al. 2002).

### Epilepsy
In individuals with epilepsy and MDD, adjunctive antidepressant medications, particularly SSRIs and bupropion are well tolerated in combination with most anticonvulsant treatments.

### Glaucoma
Previously, tricyclic antidepressants with anticholinergic properties were known to precipitate acute angle closure glaucoma in vulnerable patients. The effect on intraocular pressure is benign with newer antidepressant treatments.

### Hypertension
Many older antihypertensive treatments including reserpine and alpha methyldopa were reported to precipitate depression. Fatigue, lethargy, and possible depression were associated with beta-adrenergic blockers. Newer antihypertensive drugs including angiotensin converting enzyme inhibitors (ACEI) and calcium channel blockers have fewer side effects and are tolerated well in combination with standard antidepressant treatments.

### Parkinson's Disease
There is prominent co-occurrence of MDD with Parkinson's disease. The prescription of low dose SSRIs, bupropion, and mixed noradrenergic serotonergic reuptake inhibitors may be helpful in the management of comorbid MDD and Parkinson's disease without risk of worsening the underlying movement disorder or promoting psychosis.

## Demographic and Sociocultural Factors in Treatment

### Children
It is increasingly important to identify children at risk for MDD. There have been insufficient controlled studies of pharmacotherapy or psychotherapy in children with MDD. However, early studies of SSRIs appear promising in terms of overall treatment efficacy in children with MDD.

## Adolescents

Adolescent-onset depression with psychotic features may be an early predictor of bipolar course. Adolescent-onset depression, therefore, must be carefully diagnosed, ruling out a bipolar history in the family and assessing evidence for mixed hypomanic or manic states in the prepubertal or pubertal period (Geller and Luby 1997). The appropriate prescription of lithium carbonate in those individuals with bipolar vulnerability must precede antidepressant pharmacotherapy. Alternatively, early studies suggest the role for standard SSRIs in adolescents with nonbipolar depression (Emslie et al. 1997, Keller et al. 2001).

## Older Adults

MDD in older adults is often characterized by more prominent somatic signs and cognitive impairment. It is important to diagnose and treat depression to minimize associated morbidity and mortality. Standard SSRI pharmacotherapy is likely to be associated with demonstrated efficacy as is depression-specific psychotherapy assuming the level of depression is mild to moderate.

## Gender

Because of substantial hormonal changes associated with the onset of menses, pregnancy and delivery, and menopause, hormonal effects must be part of the standard assessment of depression. Woman may be at somewhat higher risk for depression at these critical intervals of hormonal change. Standard antidepressant pharmacotherapy as well as depression-specific psychotherapy appear to be equally effective in both men and women. Both men and women require careful attention to sexual side effects of antidepressant pharmacotherapy in the course of the longitudinal management.

### Refractory Major Depressive Disorder

A staging system for treatment-resistant depression (TRD) has been proposed and ranges from failure to respond to a single agent (Stage 1) to failure of multiple treatments and electroconvulsive therapy (Stage 5; Thase and Rush 1995), and is presented in Table 63–5. The term refractory depression has been proposed to describe patients who have Stage 5 treatment-resistant depression (Thase and Rush 1995).

Refractory MDD or Stage 5 in this table is estimated to occur in up to 20% of patients (Thase and Howland 1994). A larger percentage of patients with MDD, up to 30%, may show only partial improvement. The concept of treatment-resistant depression or refractory depression describes this lack of response to a number of clinical trials using optimal dosing and duration of antidepressant medication. One must typically offer the patient a rational series of treatment trials using optimal dosing and duration of each antidepressant. Many individuals consider a patient refractory if a course of three, four, or five treatments is offered without substantial clinical response. The standard approach to the management of refractory depression includes increasing the antidepressant dose and monitoring for a full 8 to 12 week course augmenting the treatment with several augmentation strategies using an adequate combination of antidepressant drug treatment and psychotherapy and switching to alternative somatic treatments including ECT when indicated.

Refractory MDD is ameliorated in the context of a caring and collaborative treatment relationship based on a favorable therapeutic alliance. Patients sometimes will undermine treatment through their own persistent use of substances such as alcohol or lack of adherence to specific pharmacotherapy recommendations. In this context the attention to the therapeutic alliance is particularly critical. In assessing an individual with refractory symptoms, pharmacologic factors including pharmacokinetic considerations, drug–drug interactions, and extreme sensitivity to antidepressant drugs must be considered.

Despite many alternative strategies, substantial morbidity and occasional mortality are associated with refractory MDD. In addition, careful attention to psychosocial factors associated with refractoriness is critical. These psychosocial factors include early childhood adversity and abuse, early family dysfunction, increased neuroticism, and marked disruption in the development of a stable sense of self.

## DYSTHYMIC DISORDER

### Definition

Dysthymic disorder is defined by the presence of chronic depressive symptoms most of the day, more days than not, for at least 2 years. While chronic depressive conditions were traditionally conceptualized as characterological and amenable to psychotherapy and resistant to pharmacotherapy, recent pharmacologic trials of antidepressants as well as depression-specific psychotherapy have demonstrated effectiveness in the overall treatment of DD. Both focused interpersonal and variations of cognitive–behavioral psychotherapy have demonstrated response in dysthymia. Individuals with DD have a substantial risk for the development of MDD. This highlights the importance of early assessment and treatment to minimize subsequent long-term complications.

If signs and symptoms of DD follow a MDD, then a diagnosis of MDD, in partial remission, is made. A diagnosis of DD can be made if the individual develops full remission of MDD for 6 months and subsequently develops signs and symptoms of DD which then last a minimum of 2 years. In contrast, the diagnosis of chronic MDD is made when an episode of MDD meets full criteria for MDD continuously for at least 2 years. If DD has been present for at least 2 years in adults (or 1 year in children and adolescents) and is subsequently followed by a superimposed MDD, then both DD and MDD are diagnosed, which is often referred to as "double depression." The following specifiers apply to DD as noted in DSM-IV:

1. Early onset—if the onset of dysthymic symptoms occurs before age 21
2. Late onset—if the onset of dysthymic symptoms occurs at age 21 or older, and with atypical features.

Atypical features refer to a pattern of symptoms which include mood reactivity and two of the additional atypical symptoms (i.e., weight gain or increased appetite, hypersomnia, leaden paralysis, or interpersonal rejection sensitivity). Early-onset DD is usually associated with subsequent

## DSM-IV-TR Criteria 300.4

**Dysthymic Disorder**

A. Depressed mood for most of the day, for more days than not, as indicated either by subjective account or by observation by others, for at least 2 years. **Note:** In children and adolescents, mood can be irritable and duration must be at least 1 year.

B. Presence, while depressed, of two (or more) of the following:

   (1) poor appetite or overeating

   (2) insomnia or hypersomnia

   (3) low energy or fatigue

   (4) low self-esteem

   (5) poor concentration or difficulty making decisions

   (6) feelings of hopelessness

C. During the 2-year period (1 year for children or adolescents) of the disturbance, the person has never been without the symptoms in criteria A and B for more than 2 months at a time.

D. No major depressive episode has been present during the first 2 years of the disturbance (1 year for children and adolescents); i.e., the disturbance is not better accounted for by chronic major depressive disorder or major depressive disorder, in partial remission.

**Note:** There may have been a previous major depressive episode provided there was a full remission (no significant signs or symptoms for 2 months) before development of the dysthymic disorder. In addition, after the initial 2 years (1 year in children or adolescents) of dysthymic disorder, there may be superimposed episodes of major depressive disorder, in which case both diagnoses may be given when the criteria are met for a major depressive episode.

E. There has never been a manic episode, a mixed episode, or a hypomanic episode, and criteria have never been met for cyclothymic disorder.

F. The disturbance does not occur exclusively during the course of a chronic psychotic disorder, such as schizophrenia or delusional disorder.

G. The symptoms are not due to the direct physiological effects of a substance (e.g., a drug of abuse, a medication) or a general medical condition (e.g., hypothyroidism).

H. The symptoms cause clinically significant distress or impairment in social, occupational, or other important areas of functioning.

*Specify* if:

**Early onset:** if onset is before age 21 years

**Late onset:** if onset is age 21 years or older

*Specify*
(for most recent 2 years of dysthymic disorder):

**With atypical features**

Reprinted with permission from the Diagnostic and Statistical Manual of Mental Disorders, Fourth Edition, Text Revision. Copyright 2000 American Psychiatric Association.

episodes of MDD. DD with atypical features may herald a bipolar I or II course.

Ongoing studies have not completely clarified the distinction between DD and depressive personality disorder. Depressive temperaments may predispose an individual to a condition within the spectrum of Axis I mood disorders. However, it may not be specifically associated with MDD. This depressive temperament may also be associated with vulnerability to bipolar disorder.

### Epidemiology

A lifetime prevalence of 4.1% for women and 2.2% for men was reported for DD (Weissman et al. 1988a). In adults, DD is more common in women than in men. In children DD occurs equally in both sexes. Across both women and men, DD has a 2.5% 12-month prevalence (Kessler et al. 1994).

### Comorbidity Patterns

Individuals with early-onset DD are at substantial risk for development of other psychiatric conditions including alcohol or substance dependence, MDD, and personality dis-orders. Up to 15% of patients with DD may also have a substance use pattern that meets criteria for comorbid alcohol or substance dependence diagnosis. The most common associated personality disorders include mixed, dependent, and borderline personality (Marin et al. 1993). Childhood and adolescent-onset DD is associated with a substantial risk for later occurrence of both MDD and bipolar disorder.

### Etiology and Pathophysiology

### Biological Findings

Sleep abnormalities demonstrate reduced REM latency, increased REM density, reduced slow wave sleep, and impaired sleep continuity in 25 to 50% of individuals with DD. There are minimal data on cortisol or thyroid abnormalities in individuals with DD. Other neurobiological studies have not yielded consistent results.

### Diagnosis and Differential Diagnosis

The diagnosis of DD cannot be made, if depressive symptoms occur during the course of a nonaffective psychosis such as schizophrenia, schizoaffective disorder, or delusional disorder. Diagnosis of depressive disorder NOS is made if there are symptoms which meet criteria for MDD during the residual phase of a psychotic disorder. If DD is determined to be etiologically related to a chronic medical condition, then one diagnoses secondary mood disorder due to a general medical condition. If substance dependence is judged to be the etiologic factor, then a substance-induced mood disorder is diagnosed. Individuals with DD often have co-occurring personality disorders and in these situations separate diagnoses on Axis I and II are made.

## Course and Natural History

Dysthymic disorder often begins in late childhood or early adolescence and by definition takes a chronic course. The risk for development of MDD among children who have DD is significant because childhood onset of DD is an early marker for recurrent mood disorder, both recurrent MDD and bipolar disorder.

The course of DD suggests impairment in functional status including social and occupational and physical functioning. Patients who have both DD and MDD have more severe functional impairment. Untreated DD contributes to significant occupational and financial burden. There is substantial reduction in activity, more days spent in bed, more complaints of poor general medical health, and more disability days than reported in the general population.

## Goals and Approaches to Treatment

The treatment goals in DD are similar to those in MDD. They include full remission of symptoms and full psychosocial recovery. Many individuals who have been enrolled in clinical trials for MDD have an associated history of DD. Recent randomized controlled trials of pharmacotherapy (Keller et al. 2000) and cognitive–behavior therapy suggest a favorable response to active treatments. The most favorable response occurred in those individuals treated with both active medication and specific cognitive–behavioral treatments.

## DEPRESSIVE DISORDER NOT OTHERWISE SPECIFIED

Depressive disorder NOS refers to a variety of conditions listed in DSM-IV that are distinguished from MDD, DD, adjustment disorder with depressed mood, or adjustment disorder with mixed anxiety and depressed mood. These conditions involve a large number of depressed individuals who do not meet formal criteria for MDD or DD. In the ECA study, 11% of subjects had DD NOS. In a primary care outpatient sample, the prevalence of DD NOS was 8.4 to 9.7%. DD NOS is associated with impairment in overall functioning and general health (Wells et al. 1989). Among the conditions listed as occurring within this category are premenstrual dysphoric disorder, minor depressive disorder, recurrent brief depressive disorder, postpsychotic depressive disorder of schizophrenia, and depressive episode superimposed on delusional disorder or other psychotic disorder.

## Premenstrual Dysphoric Disorder

Premenstrual DD is characterized by depressed mood, marked anxiety, affective lability, and decreased interest in activities, experienced during the last week of the luteal phase which remits during the follicular phase of the menstrual cycle. This pattern occurs for most months of the year. The severity of symptoms is comparable to MDD, but the duration is briefer by definition. The symptoms disappear with the onset of menses. Current criteria emphasize the disturbance in mood as well as impairment in social functioning associated with premenstrual DD. Current assessments require that the typical cyclical patterns be confirmed by at least 2 months of prospective daily ratings. Premenstrual DD often worsens with increasing age, but then diminishes at menopause. Premenstrual DD appears to respond to standard SSRI treatments including fluoxetine (Prozac) as well as sertraline (Zoloft) but may not respond to other types of antidepressants, such as bupropion. This responsiveness to SSRIs suggests a premenstrual serotonergic hypoactivity which may account for the premenstrual dysphoric symptomatology (Eriksson et al. 2002). For a more detailed discussion of premenstrual DD, see Chapter 65.

## Minor Depressive Disorder

Minor depressive disorder is characterized by episodes lasting 2 weeks and characterized by at least two but fewer than five depressive symptoms. Minor depressive disorder is also associated with less psychosocial impairment than MDD. The prevalence of minor depressive disorder reported in primary care settings ranges from 3.4 to 4.7%. A number of general medical conditions have been associated with minor depressive disorder including stroke, cancer, and diabetes. Maier and colleagues (1992) report increased symptoms of minor depressive disorder in families in which a proband with MDD is present. In the differential diagnosis of minor depressive disorder, one must consider adjustment disorder with depressed mood and other experiences of sadness that may be part of grieving. Because of frequent co-occurrence with general medical condition, one must rule out a secondary mood disorder due to a general medical condition.

Minor depressive disorder tends to begin in late adolescence and probably affects men and women equally. Minor depressive disorder is often associated with greater impairment of routine activities in older adults. Consultation psychiatrists should pay careful attention to depressive symptoms in association with medical illness in order to establish the impact of depressive disorder on the overall course and recovery from general medical conditions (Cassem 1990).

## Recurrent Brief Depressive Disorder

Recurrent brief depressive disorder refers to brief episodes of recurrent depressive symptoms that last for at least 2 days but less than 2 weeks and meet full criteria (except duration) for MDD. These episodes typically occur monthly for 12 months, but are not specifically related to menstrual cycles. These depressive episodes typically cause clinically significant distress and impairment in social and occupational functioning. In some individuals, RBDD is associated with a high degree of suicidality (Maier et al. 1997).

Associated clinical features may include comorbid substance dependence or anxiety disorders. By definition, recurrent brief depressive episodes are not associated with menstrual cycles and are equally common among men as women.

Up to 12 to 20% of first-degree relatives of patients with recurrent brief depressive disorder have MDD. Ongoing research focusing on familial aggregation and associated comorbid conditions is important. It will be particularly important to address its association with personality characteristics and the overlap between personality disorder and the syndrome of RBDD.

## Mixed Anxiety–Depressive Disorder

The syndrome of mixed anxiety–depressive disorder is commonly diagnosed in outpatient medical practices internationally and it is included as a disorder in ICD-10. It is typically associated with dysphoric mood lasting at least 1 month and at least four associated clinical symptoms which are derived from both symptoms associated with MDD, DD, panic disorder, and generalized anxiety disorder. These symptom characteristics include: difficulty concentrating or mind going blank; sleep disturbance characterized by difficulty falling or staying asleep or restless; unsatisfying sleep; fatigue or low energy; irritability; worry;

being easily moved to tears; hypervigilance; anticipating the worst; hopelessness and pessimism about the future; and low self-esteem or feelings of worthlessness. The symptoms cause significant impairment in social and occupational functioning or other aspects of functioning. These symptoms must not be due to the direct physiologic effects of a substance or a general medical condition. Finally, the symptoms are present in the absence of criteria being met for MDD, DD, panic disorder, or generalized anxiety disorder. The presence of these common mixed anxious and depressive symptoms is estimated to range from 1 to 2% in primary care settings.

## Postpsychotic Depressive Disorder of Schizophrenia

The diagnosis of postpsychotic depressive disorder of schizophrenia is intended to cover depressive episodes occurring during the residual phase of schizophrenia. In the residual phase there may be associated negative symptoms which can be difficult to differentiate from mood symptoms. The diagnosis should be made only if the full criteria

---

**Clinical Vignette 1**

Ms. A is a 36-year-old married woman with a history of prepubertal-onset MDD. Marked depressive symptoms in childhood included social withdrawal, fatigue, and suicidal preoccupation. Early treatment interventions included family psychotherapy, individual psychotherapy, day treatment, and tricyclic antidepressant treatment. However, the patient did not recover and hospitalization was required during early adolescence. After a 1-month hospitalization the patient experienced moderate amelioration of symptoms and completed high school. College work was initiated, but it was not completed because of recurrent MDD superimposed on DD (double depression). Multiple courses of antidepressants after tricyclic antidepressants included tranylcypromine (Parnate) augmented with lithium carbonate, bupropion (Wellbutrin), and SSRIs as they became available. Moderate symptom remission was achieved with high dose fluoxetine (Prozac). The patient was able to marry, but under conditions of subsequent separation and divorce recurrent depression ensued. Subsequently, electroconvulsive therapy demonstrated modest treatment response. The patient subsequently developed more sustained recovery from symptoms from high doses of venlafaxine (Effexor XR), which was augmented by atypical antipsychotic pharmacotherapy.

Continuing psychotherapy monitoring mood-related symptom exacerbation and associated responses to stress has promoted optimal treatment response. In this case, the longitudinal care of a patient, who experienced early-onset MDD, superimposed on DD, and associated mixed personality pathology ultimately required maintenance antidepressant pharmacotherapy augmented with atypical antipsychotic pharmacotherapy and active cognitive–behavioral and interpersonal psychotherapy to promote remission of symptoms and optimal psychosocial functioning.

---

**Clinical Vignette 2**

Mr. D is a 70-year-old married man with recurrences of severe MDD. Despite prior exposures to newer antidepressant pharmacotherapy as well as outpatient electroconvulsive therapy, there was minimal response. The patient had experienced classic melancholic symptoms of depression including agitation, anhedonia, insomnia, guilt, and weight loss. Because of persistent melancholic features and lack of response to electroconvulsive therapy, the patient and family developed secondary hopelessness about any response to treatment. A review of the family history suggested that the patient's father had depression of later onset and that his mother had postpartum depression with subsequent well intervals, until later recurrence of depressive symptoms. MDD with melancholic features was diagnosed, but there was a suggestive history of bipolar history in the extended family. During the third recurrence and most severe episode of depression, pretreatment with lithium carbonate at low to moderate doses, was begun. Subsequent exposure to standard tricyclic antidepressant treatment for melancholic symptoms led to a gradual amelioration of insomnia, agitation, and anorexia during the initial 3 weeks of treatment. Focused psychotherapy addressing his transition from working to retirement, grieving over the loss of both parents, and his children's transition from home was undertaken simultaneously. By 6 weeks, mood, guilt, and associated depressive symptomatology were improved. Continued presence of anxiety and early morning distress lasting 1 to 2 hours persisted despite general resolution of the depressive symptoms. Because of the severity and longstanding nature of the depressive syndrome, maintenance treatment with lithium carbonate 600 mg daily and full dose tricyclic antidepressant was continued. During this time the patient was able to return to full psychosocial functioning in retirement and make a substantial contribution in a number of volunteer efforts in the community. MDD, even when seemingly refractory to electroconvulsive therapy, is often amenable to appropriate full dose pharmacotherapy, targeted psychotherapy, and ongoing maintenance psychiatric management.

are met for a major depressive episode and if the symptoms are not due to substance abuse, akinesia, or other antipsychotic medication effects.

Features associated with the development of a postpsychotic depressive episode include limited social support, the impact of prior hospitalization, or the trauma of having a major mental illness. It is estimated that up to 25% of individuals with schizophrenia experience postpsychotic depressive disorder. There is no significant age of onset difference between men and women. Individuals who have a family history of MDD may be at higher risk for postpsychotic depression. Treatment studies have demonstrated the efficacy of standard antidepressive medication in the postpsychotic depressive disorder of schizophrenia.

## References

Abraham K (1927) Notes on the psychoanalytic investigation and treatment of manic–depressive insanity and allied conditions. In Selected Papers on Psychoanalysis, Institute of Psychoanalysis (eds). Hogarth Press, London, pp. 418–502.

Abramson LY, Metalsky GI, and Alloy LB (1989) Hopelessness depression: A theory-based subtype of depression. Psychol Rev 96, 358–372.

Alfici S, Sigal M, and Landau M (1989) Primary fibromyalgia syndrome—a variant of depressive disorder? Psychother Psychosom 51, 156–161.

Akiskal HS (1990) Toward a clinical understanding of the relationship of anxiety and depressive disorders. In Comorbidity of Mood and Anxiety Disorders, Maser JD and Cloninger CR (eds). American Psychiatric Press, Washington DC, pp. 597–607.

Akiskal HS (1983) Dysthymic disorder: Psychopathology of proposed chronic depressive subtypes. Am J Psychiatr 140, 11–20.

American Psychiatric Association (1968) Diagnostic and Statistical Manual of Mental Disorders, 2nd ed. APA, Washington DC.

American Psychiatric Association (1980) Diagnostic and Statistical Manual of Mental Disorders, 3rd ed. APA, Washington DC.

American Psychiatric Association (1987) Diagnostic and Statistical Manual of Mental Disorders, 3rd ed. Rev. APA, Washington DC.

American Psychiatric Association (1994) Diagnostic and Statistical Manual of Mental Disorders, 4th ed. APA, Washington DC.

American Psychiatric Association (2000) Diagnostic and Statistical Manual of Mental Disorders, 4th ed. Text Rev. APA, Washington DC.

Barklage NE (1991) Evaluation and management of the suicidal patient. Emerg Care Q 7, 9–17.

Bauer MS and Whydrow PC (1990) Rapid cycling bipolar affective disorder, II: Treatment of refractory rapid cycling with high dose levothyroxine: A preliminary study. Arch Gen Psychiatr 47, 435–440.

Beck AT (1973) The Diagnosis and Management of Depression. University of Pennsylvania Press, Philadelphia.

Beck AT (1976) Cognitive Therapy and the Emotional Disorders. International Universities Press, New York.

Beck AT, Rush AJ, and Shaw BF (1979) Cognitive Therapy of Depression. Guilford Press, New York.

Beck AT, Ward C, Mendelson M, et al. (1961) An inventory for measuring depression. Arch Gen Psychiatr 4, 53–63.

Bibring E (1953) The mechanism of depression. In Affective Disorders: Psychoanalytic Contributions to their Study, Greenacre P (ed). International Universities Press, New York.

Black DW, Bell S, and Hulbert J (1988) The importance of axis II in patients with major depression: A controlled study. J Affect Disord 14, 115–122.

Blazer DG (1994) Epidemiology of late-life depression. In Diagnosis and Treatment Depression in Late Life: Results of the NIH Consensus Development Conference, Schneider LS, Reynolds CF, Lebowityz BD, et al. (eds). American Psychiatric Press, Washington DC, pp. 9–19.

Blazer DG, Kessler RC, and McGonagle KA (1994) The prevalence and distribution of major depression in a national community sample: The national comorbidity survey. Am J Psychiatr 151, 979–986.

Bleich A, Koslowsky M, and Dolev A (1997) Posttraumatic stress disorder and depression. Br J Psychiatr 170, 479–482.

Bowlby J (1980) Attachment and Loss, Vol. 3: Loss: Sadness and Depression. Basic Books, New York.

Boyd JH and Weismann (1981) Epidemiology of affective disorders. Arch Gen Psychiatr 38, 1039–1046.

Brown GW and Harris T (1978) Social Origins of Depression: A Study of Psychiatric Disorder in Women. Free Press, New York.

Brown SA and Schuckit MA (1988) Changes in depression among abstinent alcoholics. J Stud Alcohol 49, 412–417.

Bush G, Fink M, Petrides G, et al. (1996) Catatonia, II: Treatment with lorazepam and electroconvulsive therapy. Acta Psychiatr Scand 93, 137–143.

Cadoret RD, O'Gorman TW, and Haywood E (1990) Genetic and environmental factors in major depression. J Affect Disord 19, 23–29.

Cassem EH (1990) Depression and anxiety secondary to medical illness. Psychiatr Clin N Am 13, 597–612.

Carroll BJ, Feinberg M, and Greden JR (1981) A specific laboratory test for the diagnosis of melancholia. Arch Gen Psychiatr 38, 15–22.

Charney DS, Nelson JC, and Quinlan DM (1981) Personality traits and disorder in depression. Am J Psychiatr 138, 1601–1604.

Coryell WR, Noyes R, and Clancy J (1982) Excess mortality in panic disorder: A comparison with primary unipolar depression. Arch Gen Psychiatr 39, 701–703.

Coyne JC (1976) Toward an interactional description of depression. Psychiatry 39, 28–40.

Cross-National Collaborative Group (1992) The changing rate of major depression: Cross-national comparisons. J Am Med Assoc 268, 3098–3105.

Depression Guideline Panel (1993a) Depression in Primary Care: Vol. 1. Detection and Diagnosis, Clinical Practice Guideline, No. 5. (April) U.S. Department of Health and Human Services, Public Health Agency, Agency for Health Care and Policy Research, AHCPR Publication No. 93-0550.

Depression Guideline Panel (1993b) Depression in Primary Care: Vol. 2. Treatment of Major Depression, Clinical Practice Guideline, No. 5. (April) U.S. Department of Health and Human Services, Public Health Agency, Agency for Health Care and Policy Research, AHCPR Publication No. 93-0551.

DeRubeis RJ, Hollon SD, Grove WM, et al. (1990) How does cognitive therapy work? Cognitive change and symptom change in cognitive therapy and pharmacotherapy for depression. J Consult Clin Psychiatr 58(6), 862–869.

Dorus W, Kennedy J, and Gibbons RD (1987) Symptoms and diagnosis of depression in alcoholics. Alcohol: Clin Exp Res 11, 150–154.

Duman RS (1998) Novel therapeutic approaches beyond the serotonin receptor. Biol Psychiatr 44, 324–335.

Duman RS, Heminger GR, and Nestler EJ (1997) A molecular and cellular theory of depression. Arch Gen Psychiatr 54, 597–606.

Ehlers CL, Frank E, and Kupfer DJ (1988) Social zeitgebers and biological rhythms. Arch Gen Psychiatr 45, 948–952.

Elkin I, Shea TM, and Watkins JT (1989) National Institute of Mental Health Treatment of Depression Collaborative Research Program. Arch Gen Psychiatr 46, 971–982.

Endicott J and Spitzer RL (1978) A diagnostic interview: The schedule for affective disorders and schizophrenia. Arch Gen Psychiatr 35, 837–844.

Emslie GE, Weinberg WA, and Rush JA (1990) Depressive symptoms by self-report in adolescent: Phase I of the development of a questionnaire for depression by self-report. J Child Neurol 5, 114–121.

Emslie GJ, Rush AJ, and Weiberg WA (1997) A double-blind, randomized placebo-controlled trial of fluoxetine in children and adolescents with depression. Arch Gen Psychiatr 54, 1031–1037.

Eriksson E, Andersch B, Ho HP, et al. (2002) Diagnosis and treatment of premenstrual dysphoria. J Clin Psychiatr 63(Suppl 7), 16–23.

Fawcett J, Scheftner WA, and Fogg L (1990) Time-related predictors of suicide in major affective disorder. Am J Psychiatr 147, 1189–1194.

Feldman E, Hawton MR, and Arden M (1987) Psychiatric disorder in medical inpatients. Q J Med 63, 405–412.

First MB, Spitzer RL, Gibbon M, et al. (1994) Structured Clinical Interview for Axis I DSM-IV disorders—Patient Edition (SCID-I/P, Version 2.0). Biometrics Research Department, New York State Psychiatric Institute, New York.

Foa EB, Davidson JRT, and Frances A (1999) The expert consensus guideline series: Treatment of posttraumatic stress disorder. J Clin Psychiatr 60(Suppl 16), 4–76.

Forsell Y, Jorm AF, and Wonblad B (1994) Association of age, sex, cognitive dysfunction and disability with major depressive symptoms in an elderly sample. Am J Psychiatr 11, 1600–1604.

Frank E, Prien RG, and Jarrett RB (1991) Conceptualization and rationale for consensus definitions of terms in major depressive disorder: Remission, recovery, relapse and recurrence. Arch Gen Psychiatr 48, 851–855.

Frasure-Smith N, Lesperance F, and Talajic M (1993) Depression following myocardial infarction: Impact on 6-month survival. J Am Med Assoc 270, 1819–1825.

Freud S (1957) Morning and melancholia. In The Standard Edition of the Complete Psychological Works of Sigmund Freud, Vol. 14. Strachey J (trans-ed). Hogarth Press, London, pp. 237–258.

Friedman MJ (1998) Current and future drug treatment for posttraumatic stress disorder patients. Psychiatr Ann 28, 461–468.

Geller B and Luby J (1997) Child and adolescent bipolar disorder: A review of the past 10 years. J Am Acad Child Adolesc Psychiatr 36, 1168–1176.

George MS, Lisanby SH, and Sakeim HA (1999) Applications in neuropsychiatry. Arch Gen Psychiatr 56, 300–311.

Giles DE, Jarret RB, and Roff HP (1989) Clinical predictors of recurrence in depression. Am J Psychiatr 146, 764–767.

Glassman AH, O'Connor CM, Califf RM, et al. (2002) Sertraline treatment of major depression in patients with acute mi or unstable angina. J Am Med Assoc 288, 701–707.

Goldstein I (2000) The mutually reinforcing triad of depressive symptoms, cardiovascular disease and erectile dysfunction. Am J Cardiol 86(2A), 41F–45F.

Goodwin FK and Jamison KR (1990) Manic–Depressive Illness. Oxford University Press, New York.

Goodwin FK, Prange AJ, and Post RM (1982) Potentiation of antidepressant effects by L-triodothyconine in tricyclic nonresponders. Am J Psychiatr 139, 34–38.

Greden JR, Gardner R, and King D (1983) Dexamethasone suppression tests in antidepressant treatment of melancholia. Arch Gen Psychiatr 40, 493–500.

Gruenberg AM, Goldstein RD, and Bruss GS (1993) Co-occurrence of major mood disorder and personality disorder. Poster presented at Third International Congress on the Disorders of Personality, Cambridge, Massachusetts.

Gunderson JG and Phillips KA (1991) A current view of the interface between borderline personality disorder and depression. Am J Psychiatr 148, 967–975.

Hamilton M (1960) A rating scale for depression. J Neurol Neurosurg Psychiatr 23, 56–62.

Harkness KL and Monroe SM (2002) Childhood adversity and the endogenous versus nonendogenous distinction in women with major depression. Am J Psychiatr 159, 387–393.

Harlow HF and Harlow HF (1962) Social deprivation in monkeys. Sci Am 207, 136–146.

Hawkins JM, Archer KJ, Strakowski SM, et al. (1995) Somatic treatments of catatonia. Int J Psychiatr Med 25, 345–369.

Hirschfeld RMA (1994) Guidelines for the long-term treatment of depression. J Clin Psychiatr 55(Suppl), 61–69.

Hollon SD, DeRubeis RJ, and Evans MD (1992) Cognitive therapy and pharmacotherapy for depression: Singly and in combination. Arch Gen Psychiatr 49, 774–781.

Holsber F (1999) The rationale for corticotropin-releasing hormone receptor (CRH-R) antagonists to treat depression and anxiety. J Psychiatr Res 33, 181–214.

Hudson JI, Hudson MS, and Pliner LF (1985) Fibromyalgia and major affective disorder: A controlled phenomenology and family history study. Am J Psychiatr 142, 441–446.

Ionescu R and Popescu C (1989) Personality disorders in students with depressive pathology. Neurol Psychiatr (Bucur) 27, 45–55.

Jackson SW (1986) Melancholia and Depression. Yale University Press, New Haven.

Jaffee SR, Moffitt TE, Caspi A, et al. (2002) Differences in early childhood risk factors for juvenile-onset and adult-onset depression. Arch Gen Psychiatr 59, 215–222.

Kashani JH, Carlson GA, and Beck NC (1987) Depression, depressive symptoms, and depressed mood among a community sample of adolescents. Am J Psychiatr 144, 931–934.

Kashani JH, McGee RO, and Clarkson SE (1983) Depression in a sample of 9-year old children. Arch Gen Psychiatr 40, 1217–1223.

Katon W, vonKorff M, and Lin E (1990) Distressed high utilizers of medical care: DSM-III-R diagnoses and treatment needs. Gen Hosp Psychiatr 12, 355–362.

Keller M and Shapiro RW (1982) "Double depression": Superimposition of acute depressive episodes on chronic depressive disorders. Am J Psychiatr 139, 438–442.

Keller MB, Lavori PW, and Mueller JI (1992) Time to recovery, chronicity and levels of psychopathology in major depression: A 5-year prospective follow-up of 431 subjects. Arch Gen Psychiatr 49, 809–816.

Keller MB, McCullough JP, Klein DN, et al. (2000) A comparison of nefazodone, cognitive behavioral analysis system of psychotherapy and their combination for the treatment of chronic depression. New Engl J Med 342, 1462–1470.

Keller MB, Ryan ND, and Birmaher B (2001) Efficacy of paroxetine in the treatment of adolescent major depression: A randomized controlled trial. J Am Acad Child Adolesc Psychiatr 40, 762–772.

Kendler KS, Heath AC, Martin AG, et al. (1986) Symptoms of anxiety and symptoms of depression: Same genes, different environments? Arch Gen Psychiatr 44, 451–457.

Kendler KS, Heath AC, and Neale AC (1993a) Alcoholism and major depression in women: A twin study of the causes of comorbidity. Arch Gen Psychiatr 50, 690–698.

Kendler KS, Kessler RC, and Neale MC (1993b) The prediction of major depression in women: Toward an integrated etiologic model. Am J Psychiatr 150, 1139–1147.

Kendler KS, Neale MC, and Kessler RC (1992) A population-based twin study of major depression in women. Arch Gen Psychiatr 49, 257–266.

Kendler KS (1991) Mood-incongruent psychotic affective illness: An historical and empirical review. Arch Gen Psychiatr 48, 362–369.

Kessler RC, McGonagle KA, and Zhao S (1994) Lifetime and 12-month prevalence of DSM-III-R psychiatric disorders in United States. Arch Gen Psychiatr 51, 8–19.

Kessler RC, Somega A, and Bromet E (1995) Posttraumatic stress disorder in the National Comorbidity Survey. Arch Gen Psychiatr 52, 1048–1060.

Klerman GI and Weissman MM (1989) Increasing rates of depression. J Am Med Assoc 261, 2229–2235.

Klerman GI, Weissman MM, Rounsaville BJ, et al. (1984) Interpersonal Psychotherapy of Depression. Basic Books, New York.

Koenig HG, Meador KG, and Cohen HJ (1988) Depression in elderly hospitalized patients with medical illness. Arch Intern Med 148, 1929–1936.

Kornstein SG (1997) Gender differences in depression: Implications for treatment. J Clin Psychiatr 58(Suppl 15), 12–18.

Kraepelin E (1921) Manic–Depressive Insanity and Paranoia, Barday RM (trans), Robertson OM (ed). Livingstone, Edinburgh.

Kupfer DJ and Thase ME (1983) The use of the sleep laboratory in the diagnosis of affective disorders. Psychiatr Clin N Am 6, 3–25.

Kupfer DJ, Frank E, and Perel JM (1989) The advantage of early treatment intervention in recurrent depression. Arch Gen Psychiatr 46, 771–775.

Lewinsohn PM (1974) A behavioral approach to depression. In The Psychology of Depression: Contemporary Theory and Research, Friedman RJ and Katz MM (eds). John Wiley, New York.

Lewinsohn PM, Clarke GN, and Seely JR (1994) Major Depression in community adolescents: Age at onset, episode duration, and time to recurrence. J Am Acad Child Adolesc Psychiatr 33, 809–818.

Lewinsohn PM, Sullivan JM, and Grossup SJ (1980) Changing reinforcing events: An approach to the treatment of depression. Psychother: Theor Res Pract 47, 322–334.

Maier W, Gansicke M, and Weiffenbach O (1997) The relationship between major and subthreshold variants of unipolar depression. J Affect Disord 45, 41–51.

Maier W, Lichteimann D, and Minges J (1992) The risk of minor depression in families of probands with major depression: Sex differences and familiarity. Eur Arch Psychiatr Clin Neurosci 242, 89–92.

Manji HK (1992) G proteins: Implications for psychiatry. Am J Psychiatr 149, 756–760.

Marin DB, Kocsis JH, and Frances AJ (1993) Personality disorders in dysthymia. J Pers Disord 7, 223–231.

McKinney WT (1988) Models of Mental Disorders: A New Comparative Psychiatry. Plenum Medical Book Company, New York.

Miller LJ (2002) Postpartum depression. J Am Med Assoc 287(6), 762–765.

Montgomery SA and Asberg MC (1979) A new depression scale designed to be sensitive to change. Br J Psychiatr 134, 382–389.

Munjack DJ and Moss HB (1981) Affective disorder and alcoholism. Arch Gen Psychiatr 38, 869–871.

Musselman DL, Evans DL, and Nemeroff CB (1998) The relationship of depression to cardiovascular disease. Arch Gen Psychiatr 55, 580–592.

Nemeroff CB, Krishnan KRR, and Reed D (1992) Adrenal gland enlargement in major depression: A computed tomography study. Arch Gen Psychiatr 49, 384–387.

Nemeroff CB, Widerlov E, and Bisatte G (1984) Elevated concentrations of CSF corticotropin-releasing factor-like immunoreactivity in depressed patients. Science 226, 1342–1344.

National Institute of Mental Health Consensus Development Conference Statement (1985) Mood disorders: Pharmacologic prevention of recurrences. Am J Psychiatr 142, 469–476.

O'Leary KD and Beach SRH (1990) Marital therapy: A viable treatment for depression and marital discord. Am J Psychiatr 147, 183–186.

Orvaschel H (1990) Early onset psychiatric disorder in high risk children and increased familial morbidity. J Am Acad Child Adolesc Psychiatr 29, 184–188.

Owens MJ and Nemeroff CB (1998) The serotonin transporter and depression. Depress Anx 8(Suppl 1), 5–12.

Parmelee PA, Katz IR, and Lawton MP (1989) Depression among institutionalized aged: Assessment and prevalence estimation. J Gerontol 44(1), M22–M29.

Petty F (1992) The depressed alcoholic: Clinical features and medical management. Gen Hosp Psychiatr 14, 458–464.

Pfohl B, Stangl D, and Zimmerman M (1984) The implications of DSM-III personality disorders for patients with major depression. J Affect Disord 7, 309–318.

Post RM (1992) Transduction of psychosocial stress into the neurobiology of recurrent affective disorder. Am J Psychiatr 149, 999–1010.

Post RM and Weiss SRB (1998) Sensitization and kindling phenomena in mood, anxiety and obsessive–compulsive disorders: The role of serotonergic mechanisms in illness progression. Biol Psychiatr 44, 193–206.

Prien RF, Carpenter LL, and Kupfer DJ (1991) The definition and operational criteria for treatment outcome of major depressive disorder. Arch Gen Psychiatr 48, 796–800.

Regier DA, Boyd JH, and Burke JD Jr. (1988) One-month prevalence of mental disorders in the United States: Based on five epidemiologic catchment area sites. Arch Gen Psychiatr 145, 1351–1357.

Ross ED and Rush AJ (1981) Diagnosis and neuroanatomical correlates of depression in brain-damaged patients: Implications for a neurology of depression. Arch Gen Psychiatr 38, 1344–1354.

Rush AJ, Cain JW, and Raese J (1991) Neurobiological bases for psychiatric disorders. In Comprehensive Neurology, Rosenberg RN (ed). Raven Press, New York, pp. 555–603.

Rush AJ, Erman MK, and Giles DE (1986a) Polysomnographic findings in recently drug-free and clinically remitted depressed patients. Arch Gen Psychiatr 43, 878–884.

Rush AJ, George MS, and Sackeim HA (2000) Vagus nerve stimulation (VNS) for treatment-resistant depressions: A multicenter study. Biol Psychiatr 47, 276–286.

Rush AJ, Giles GE, and Schlesser MA (1986b) The inventory for depressive symptomatology (IDS): Preliminary finding. Psychiatr Res 18, 65–87.

Rush AJ, Hiser W, and Giles DE (1987) A comparison of self-reported versus clinician-rated symptoms in depression. J Clin Res 48, 246–248.

Sargeant JK, Bruce ML, and Florio LP (1990) Factors associated with 1-year outcome of major depression in the community. Arch Gen Psychiatr 47, 519–526.

Schildkraut JJ (1965) The catecholamine hypothesis of affective disorders: A review of supporting evidence. Am J Psychiatr 122, 509–522.

Seligman MEP (1975) Helplessness: On Depression, Development and Death. WH Freeman, San Franciso.

Shalev AY, Feedman S, and Peri T (1998) Posttraumatic stress disorder and depression. Am J Psychiatr 155, 630–637.

Shea MT, Glass DR, Pilkonis PA, et al. (1987) Frequency and implications of personality disorders in a sample of depressed outpatients. J Pers Disord 1, 27–42.

Shea MT, Widiger TA, and Klein MH (1992) Comorbidity of personality disorders and depression: Implications for treatment. J Consult Clin Psychol 60, 857–868.

Shelton RC, Mainer DH, and Sulser F (1996) cAMP-dependent protein kinase activity in major depression. Am J Psychiatr 153, 1037–1042.

Skinner BF (1953) Science and Human Behavior. Free Press, New York.

Thase ME (1990) Relapse and recurrence in unipolar major depression: Short-term and long-term approaches. J Clin Psychiatr 51(Suppl 6), 51–57.

Thase ME and Howland RH (1994) Refractory depression: Relevance of psychosocial factors and therapies. Psychiatr Ann 24, 232–240.

Thase ME, Greenhouse JB, Frank E, et al. (1997) Treatment of major depression with psychotherapy or psychotherapy-pharmacotherapy combinations. Arch Gen Psychiatr 54, 1009–1015.

Thase ME and Rush AJ (1995) Treatment-resistant depression. In Psychopharmacology: The Fourth Generation of Progress, Bloom F and Kupfer DJ (eds). Raven Press, New York, pp. 1081–1097.

Wehr TA, Wirz-Justice A, and Goodwin FK (1979) Phase advance of the circadian sleep-wake cycle as an antidepressant. Science 206, 710–713.

Weissman MM, Bruce ML, and Leaf PJ (1991) Affective disorders. In Psychiatric Disorders in America, Robins LN and Regier DA (eds). Free Press, New York, pp. 53–80.

Weissman MM, Leaf PJ, and Bruce ML (1988a) The epidemiology of dysthymia in five communities: Rates, risks, comorbidity, and treatment. Am J Psychiatr 145, 815–819.

Weissman MM, Leaf PJ, and Tischler GL (1988b) Affective Disorders in five United States communities. Psychol Med 18, 141–153.

Weller EB and Weller RA (1990) Depressive disorders in children and adolescents. In Psychiatric Disorders in Children and Adolescents, Garfinkle BD, Carlson GA, and Weller EB (eds). WB Saunders, Philadelphia, pp. 3–20.

Wells KB (1985) Depression as a Tracer Condition for the National Study of Medical Care Outcomes-Background Review. Rand, Santa Montica.

Wells KB, Golding JM, and Burnam MA (1988) Psychiatric disorder and limitations in physical functioning in a sample of the Los Angeles general population. Am J Psychiatr 145, 712–717.

Wells KB, Stewart A, and Hays RD (1989) The functioning and well-being of depressed patients: Results from the medical outcomes study. J Am Med Assoc 262, 914–919.

Wender PH, Kety SS, and Rosenthal D (1986) Psychiatry disorders in the biological and adoptive families of adopted individuals with affective disorders. Arch Gen Psychiatr 46, 923–929.

Whirz-Justice A, Graw P, and Kraucht K (1993) Light therapy in seasonal affective disorder is independent of time of day or circadian phase. Arch Gen Psychiatr 50, 929–937.

Wing JK, Birley JLT, Cooper JE, et al. (1967) Reliability of a procedure for measuring and classifying "present psychiatric state." Br J Psychiatr 111, 499–515.

Zung WWK (1965) A self-rating depression scale. Arch Gen Psychiatr 12, 63–70.

# 64 Mood Disorders: Bipolar (Manic–Depressive) Disorders

Mark S. Bauer

Manic Disorder
Mixed Episode
Hypomanic Episode
Cyclothymic Disorder
Rapid-Cycling

## Definition

The cardinal symptoms of manic–depressive disorder are discrete periods of abnormal mood and activation that define depressive and manic or hypomanic episodes. Diagnosis of such episodes, as in almost all other diagnosis in psychiatry, is based exclusively on *phenomenology*, the descriptive appearance of the syndrome of interest. This is because there are few diagnoses for which the pathophysiology is known or for which valid and reliable diagnostic tests are available. This situation existed in most of medicine in the 19th century. For example, before the identification of the spirochete as the causative agent in syphilis, physicians actively debated the core characteristics and syndromal limits of general paresis. Definitional discussions ended for the most part when the causative agent was discovered and accurate laboratory testing was developed. Discussions of definition of mood disorders, including manic–depressive (bipolar) disorder, are at a similar stage as those of general paresis in the 19th century. Because we have neither clear pathophysiology nor accurate diagnostic tests to identify persons with a syndrome of interest, we base our diagnoses on phenomenology.

## Historical Background

During the past several years, as part of the development of the *Diagnostic and Statistical Manual of Mental Disorders*, Fourth Edition (DSM-IV) (American Psychiatric Association 1994a, 2000), an extensive effort has been made to review evidence to identify core characteristics and limits of the various psychiatric syndromes, including mood disorders. Of all psychiatric nosological systems, DSM-IV has had perhaps the highest standards for requiring scientific data for additions, deletions, or modifications of the various syndromes. A sample of these data can be found in the multivolume sourcebook for DSM-IV published as a companion to DSM-IV (Widiger et al. 1994–1997).

One may conceive of phenomenological data for the diagnosis of manic–depressive disorder as being of two types: *cross-sectional* and *longitudinal*. Cross-sectional data refer to descriptive aspects of a syndrome that occur at a particular point in time, such as the number and type of depressive symptoms that occur during an episode of depression. Longitudinal data refer to the course of symptoms over time, such as the timing, duration, and recurrence of depressive episodes. Both cross-sectional and longitudinal data are essential for the definition of mood disorders and the proper diagnosis of manic–depressive disorder. It is not infrequent that diagnostic errors occur when longitudinal data are neglected as the psychiatrist focuses solely on cross-sectional presentation: "This must be manic–depressive disorder because the patient appears manic at the present time," or "This cannot be manic–depressive disorder because the patient is depressed now."

Kraepelin's treatise *Manic–Depressive Insanity and Paranoia* (Kraepelin 1989, Berrios and Hauser 1988) is a classic in terms of both the importance of its scientific insights and the lucidity of its prose. It was a seminal work in the study of manic–depressive disorder precisely because of its emphasis on longitudinal as well as cross-sectional data. Kraepelin observed that patients who had symptoms of psychosis were of two main types: those whose illness followed a progressive downhill course and those whose illness remitted and recurred, frequently with return to their normal interepisode baseline. The former illness he termed *dementia praecox* "early dementia," which we now call schizophrenia. The latter he called manic–depressive psychosis. This latter group included almost all severe mood disorders, grouping together persons with severe depressive episodes regardless of whether they experienced mania as well. Thus, he utilized not only cross-sectional data (the occurrence of mood episodes) but also longitudinal data (the tendency of mood episodes to remit and recur) to separate mood disorders from schizophrenia.

Later, Leonhard and Berman (1957) proposed the distinction between manic–depressive, or bipolar disorder and pure depressive disorder, which has come to be called unipolar depression. Phenomenologically, he based this distinction on the occurrence of manic episodes in the former disorder but not in the latter, and supported this distinction by the observation that mania tended to occur more frequently in family members of patients with manic–depressive rather than unipolar disorder. This is an example of corroborating purely phenomenological distinctions with other types of empirical evidence, as was later codified in Robins and Guze's (1970) classic article on the definition of schizophrenia, which eventually served as the basis for evaluating most of the evidence for mood disorder validation for DSM-IV-TR.

This categorical approach to diagnosis, which clearly demarcates manic–depressive disorder from schizophrenia on the one hand and from unipolar depression on the other, is most successful when classic cases are considered. In reality, however, many borderline cases exist in which features of more than one syndrome exist and clear categorization is not possible. In recognition of this reality, Bleuler's classic *Textbook of Psychiatry* (Bleuler and Brill 1924) proposed that manic–depressive disorder and schizophrenia lie on a continuum that has no sharp border, with patients often exhibiting characteristics of both syndromes and evolving a course midway between the two. This syndrome is indeed not uncommon and has been recognized in the major diagnostic classification schemes as schizoaffective disorder (Levitt and Tsuang 1988, Blacker and Tsuang 1992).

The lineage of the atheoretical, phenomenological approach to diagnosis in the current DSM system certainly begins with the careful observations of Kraepelin and others. However, its most recent roots lie in the St. Louis or Feighner criteria (Feighner et al. 1972), which specified explicit phenomenological criteria for the identification of various psychiatric disorders. The St. Louis criteria and the closely related Research Diagnostic Criteria (Spitzer et al. 1978) served as the diagnostic systems for most clinical psychiatric research in the 1970s and early 1980s, providing a common language for description of patients among investigators and increasing comparability of diagnostic samples across various sites. This phenomenological "technology" diffused into clinical practice and was codified for clinical use by the third edition of the DSM and its revision (American Psychiatric Association 1980, 1987). Currently, the DSM-IV-TR and the closely related *International Statistical Classification of Diseases and Related Health Problems*, 10th Revision (ICD-10) (World Health Organization 1994) serve as the basis for the diagnosis of manic–depressive disorder both in clinical practice and in psychiatric research, although long-term psychiatric studies begun under the Research Diagnostic Criteria have continued to use that fairly comparable schema.

In the first edition of this textbook (Tasman et al. 1997), the disorders in this chapter were referred to as "Bipolar Disorders," yet this newer edition includes the older term "manic–depressive disorder." An increasing amount of data indicates that mania and hypomania do not typically take the classic, euphoric, optimistic form that appears to be the polar opposite of depression. Rather, hyperactivation appears to be the core symptom of mania and hypomania while mood itself is quite variable; dysphoria and depression rather than euphoric mood are the rule rather than the exception; and patients rate their quality of life during mania or hypomania as worse than or no better than normal, rather than being enhanced as commonly supposed. Thus the term *manic–depressive* is more accurate and less misleading than *bipolar*, which implies that the two characteristic mood states are somehow polar opposites (see assessment and differential diagnosis: phenomenology later in the chapter).

## Episodes as the Basis for Diagnosis of Manic–Depressive Disorder

The DSM-based definition of manic–depressive disorder is built on the identification of individual mood *episodes* (Table 64–1). DSM-IV criteria for individual mood episodes are summarized below for manic, mixed, and hypomanic episodes; criteria for major depressive episodes can be found in Chapter 93. Criteria for these episodes are reviewed in greater detail in the subsequent section on diagnosis. It is important to understand that the diagnosis of manic–depressive disorder derives from the occurrence of individual episodes over time. Persons who experience a manic, hypomanic, or mixed episode, virtually all of whom also have a history of one or more major depressive episodes (Winokur et al. 1969), are diagnosed with manic–depressive disorder. Those who experience major depressive and manic episodes are diagnosed with *bipolar I* disorder, and those with major depressive and hypomanic (milder manic) episodes are diagnosed with *bipolar II* disorder.

Not surprisingly, most data regarding manic–depressive disorder come from the study of the more severe end of the spectrum, primarily type I disorder. Throughout this chapter, data on manic–depressive disorder derive from

| Table 64–1 | Summary of Mood Episodes and Mood Disorders | |
|---|---|
| **Episode** | **Disorder** |
| Major depressive episode | Major depressive disorder, single episode |
| Major depressive episode + major depressive episode | Major depressive disorder, recurrent |
| Major depressive episode + manic/ mixed episode | Manic–depressive disorder, type I |
| Manic/mixed episode | Manic–depressive disorder, type I |
| Major depressive episode + hypomanic episode | Manic–depressive disorder, type II |
| Chronic subsyndromal depression | Dysthymic disorder |
| Chronic fluctuations between subsyndromal depression and hypomania | Cyclothymic disorder |

## DSM-IV-TR Criteria

**Manic Episode**

A. A distinct period of abnormally and persistently elevated, expansive, or irritable mood, lasting at least 1 week (or any duration if hospitalization is necessary).

B. During the period of mood disturbance, three (or more) of the following symptoms have persisted (four if the mood is only irritable) and have been present to a significant degree:

   (1) inflated self-esteem or grandiosity

   (2) decreased need for sleep (e.g., feels rested after only 3 hours of sleep)

   (3) more talkative than usual or pressure to keep talking

   (4) flight of ideas or subjective experience that thoughts are racing

   (5) distractibility (i.e., attention too easily drawn to unimportant or irrelevant external stimuli)

   (6) increase in goal-directed activity (either socially, at work or school, or sexually) or psychomotor agitation

   (7) excessive involvement in pleasurable activities that have a high potential for painful consequences (e.g., engaging in unrestrained buying sprees, sexual indiscretions, or foolish business investments)

C. The symptoms do not meet criteria for a mixed episode.

D. The mood disturbance is sufficiently severe to cause marked impairment in occupational functioning or in usual social activities or relationships with others, or to necessitate hospitalization to prevent harm to self or others, or there are psychotic features.

E. The symptoms are not due to the direct physiological effects of a substance (e.g., a drug of abuse, a medication, or other treatment) or a general medical condition (e.g., hyperthyroidism).

**Note:** Manic-like episodes that are clearly caused by somatic antidepressant treatment (e.g., medication, electroconvulsive therapy, light therapy) should not count toward a diagnosis of manic–depressive I disorder.

Reprinted with permission from the Diagnostic and Statistical Manual of Mental Disorders, Fourth Edition, Text Revision. Copyright 2000 American Psychiatric Association.

## DSM-IV-TR Criteria

**Mixed Episode**

A. The criteria are met both for a manic episode and for a major depressive episode (except for duration) nearly every day during at least a 1-week period.

B. The mood disturbance is sufficiently severe to cause marked impairment in occupational functioning or in usual social activities or relationships with others, or to necessitate hospitalization to prevent harm to self or others, or there are psychotic features.

C. The symptoms are not due to the direct physiological effects of a substance (e.g., a drug of abuse, a medication, or other treatment) or a general medical condition (e.g., hyperthyroidism).

**Note:** Mixed-like episodes that are clearly caused by somatic antidepressant treatment (e.g., medication, electroconvulsive therapy, light therapy) should not count toward a diagnosis of manic–depressive I disorder.

Reprinted with permission from the Diagnostic and Statistical Manual of Mental Disorders, Fourth Edition, Text Revision. Copyright 2000 American Psychiatric Association.

studies of type I disorder unless otherwise noted. DSM-IV-TR is the first version of the DSM series to include a specific category for bipolar II disorder. Previously, persons with depressive and hypomanic episodes were grouped under the broad "bipolar disorder not otherwise specified," which included a variety of unusual presentations. On the basis of evidence reviewed by Dunner (1993), the disorder was given separate categorical status.

This separation of type II from both type I and major depressive disorders was supported by several types of evidence. For instance, type II disorder occurs more frequently in families of persons with type II in comparison to families of persons with type I or major depressive disorder (Fieve et al. 1984, Coryell et al. 1984, Endicott et al. 1985). Study of the course over time of type II disorder indicated that persons with hypomania tended to have recurrent hypomanic episodes and did not convert into type I by developing mania (Coryell et al. 1995). In addition, persons with type II disorder may have more episodes over time than persons with type I (Dunner 1993), indicating that the course of type II differs from that of type I. However, biological differences between these manic–depressive types have not been reliably demonstrated (Dunner 1993).

Nonetheless, as outlined later, it should not be construed that manic–depressive disorder type II is in all respects milder than type I, although hypomania is by definition less severe than mania. Specifically, the social and occupational function and quality of life for persons with type II disorder are similar to those for persons with type I disorder.

Persons who experience subsyndromal manic–depressive mood fluctuations over an extended period

## DSM-IV-TR Criteria

### Hypomanic Episode

A. A distinct period of persistently elevated, expansive, or irritable mood, lasting throughout at least 4 days, that is clearly different from the usual nondepressed mood.

B. During the period of mood disturbance, three (or more) of the following symptoms have persisted (four if the mood is only irritable) and have been present to a significant degree:

(1) inflated self-esteem or grandiosity

(2) decreased need for sleep (e.g., feels rested after only 3 hours of sleep)

(3) more talkative than usual or pressure to keep talking

(4) flight of ideas or subjective experience that thoughts are racing

(5) distractibility (i.e., attention too easily drawn to unimportant or irrelevant external stimuli)

(6) increase in goal-directed activity (either socially, at work or school, or sexually) or psychomotor agitation

(7) excessive involvement in pleasurable activities that have a high potential for painful consequences (e.g., the person engages in unrestrained buying sprees, sexual indiscretions, or foolish business investments)

C. The episode is associated with an unequivocal change in functioning that is uncharacteristic of the person when not symptomatic.

D. The disturbance in mood and the change in functioning are observable by others.

E. The episode is not severe enough to cause marked impairment in social or occupational functioning, or to necessitate hospitalization, and there are no psychotic features.

F. The symptoms are not due to the direct physiological effects of a substance (e.g., a drug of abuse, a medication, or other treatment) or a general medical condition (e.g., hyperthyroidism).

**Note:** Hypomanic-like episodes that are clearly caused by somatic antidepressant treatment (e.g., medication, electroconvulsive therapy, light therapy) should not count toward a diagnosis of manic–depressive II disorder.

Reprinted with permission from the Diagnostic and Statistical Manual of Mental Disorders, Fourth Edition, Text Revision. Copyright 2000 American Psychiatric Association.

## DSM-IV-TR Criteria 301.13

### Cyclothymic Disorder

A. For at least 2 years, the presence of numerous periods with hypomanic symptoms and numerous periods with depressive symptoms that do not meet criteria for a major depressive episode.

**Note:** In children and adolescents, the duration must be at least 1 year.

B. During the above 2-year period (1 year in children and adolescents), the person has not been without the symptoms in criterion A for more than 2 months at a time.

C. No major depressive episode, manic episode, or mixed episode has been present during the first 2 years of the disturbance.

D. The symptoms in criterion A are not better accounted for by schizoaffective disorder and are not superimposed on schizophrenia, schizophreniform disorder, delusional disorder, or psychotic disorder not otherwise specified.

E. The symptoms are not due to the direct physiological effects of a substance (e.g., a drug of abuse, a medication) or a general medical condition (e.g., hyperthyroidism).

F. The symptoms cause clinically significant distress or impairment in social, occupational, or other important areas of functioning.

Reprinted with permission from the Diagnostic and Statistical Manual of Mental Disorders, Fourth Edition, Text Revision. Copyright 2000 American Psychiatric Association.

without major mood episodes are diagnosed with *cyclothymic disorder*. Much less is known about this milder disorder because afflicted persons present for medical attention less frequently than those with full-blown manic–depressive disorder. Cyclothymic disorder has been considered at various times a temperament, a personality disorder, and a disorder at the milder end of the manic–depressive spectrum (Akiskal 1981). Available data clearly indicate that cyclothymic disorder is related to the more severe manic–depressive disorders (Akiskal et al. 1977, Goodwin and Jamison 1990). However, it is not clear to what degree such categorical disorders may be related to underlying dimensional characteristics such as temperament (Akiskal and Akiskal 1988), however vaguely we presently define that construct.

### Etiology and Pathophysiology

Dichotomous thinking has characterized the debate over the last decades regarding the causes and pathological bases of manic–depressive disorder and mental disorders in general. At one time, psychological and biological paradigms were consistently presented as mutually exclusive. Similarly, dichotomous thinking based on nature (genes) and nurture (environment) as the cause of manic–depressive disorder has at times shaped the approach to the issues.

| Table 64-2 | Major Hypotheses of the Pathophysiological Basis of Manic–Depressive Disorder |
|---|---|

| Hypotheses | Key References* |
|---|---|
| **Neurotransmitter** | |
| Norepinephrine | Prange (1964) |
| | Schildkraut (1965) |
| | Bunney et al. (1972a, 1972b, 1972c) |
| Dopamine | Goodwin and Sack (1974) |
| | Crow and Deakin (1981) |
| Serotonin | Coppen et al. (1972) |
| | Goodwin and Jamison (1990) |
| Acetylcholine | Janowsky et al. (1973) |
| Second-messenger systems | Stahl (2000) |
| | Sassi and Soares (2002) |
| **Neuroendocrine** | |
| Various | Amsterdam et al. (1983) |
| Thyroid | Bauer and Whybrow (1990) |
| **Neuroanatomical** | Altshuler et al. (2000) |
| | Brambilla et al. (2001) |
| | Sassi and Soares (2002) |
| **Cell Degeneration** | Manji and Lenox (2000) |
| **Physiological** | |
| Membrane, electrolytes | Goodwin and Jamison (1990) |
| Biological rhythms, annual | Faedda et al. (1993) |
| Biological rhythms, circadian | *Wehr et al. (1982) |
| | Halaris (1987) |
| Kindling | Post et al. (1986a, 1986b) |
| **Psychosocial Hypotheses** | |
| Stress | Johnson and Roberts (1995) |
| | Ellicott et al. (1990) |
| | Leverich (1990) |
| Psychoanalytic factors | Fenichel (1945) |
| | Cooper (1985) |
| | Kahn (1993) |
| Integrative biopsychosocial hypotheses | Johnson and Roberts (1995) |
| | Hume et al. (1988) |

*The key references are either reviews or well-referenced primary data articles that will provide the reader with an entrance into the area.

However, it is clear from current data that no single paradigm can explain the occurrence, and variability in course and severity of manic–depressive disorder. Rather, a more integrative approach to understanding the causes of manic–depressive disorder is needed, one which recognizes the contributions of varying degrees of importance from several sources.

The various hypotheses regarding the basis of manic–depressive disorder are presented below as if they were separate and mutually exclusive proposals, with outline and key references provided in Table 64–2. However, our approach to understanding the likely causes of manic–depressive disorder is as reductionistic as it might appear. Rather, it derives from the statistical technique of logistic regression, albeit in a qualitative rather than quantitative fashion. That is, if the occurrence of manic–depressive disorder is the "dependent variable," there may be multiple "independent variables" that contribute to its occurrence. Some independent variables may have a very strong association (i.e., explain a large percentage of the variance), while

others may be less important in predicting the dependent variable. Moreover, several independent variables may themselves be associated with one another, rather than being mutually independent. Thus, in understanding studies on a putative cause of manic–depressive disorder one must keep in mind that there may be other causes that are not addressed in a particular study, but that may contribute nonetheless to the findings.

Further, in trying to understand the source of symptoms at a particular time in a particular person with manic–depressive disorder—which we all do as clinicians trying to treat individuals—we must keep in mind that there may be multiple sources that lead to the symptoms that we are trying to treat.

Thus, it is not likely that biological theories will explain all the pathology seen in manic–depressive disorder. Similarly, the effectiveness of medications such as lithium renders purely psychosocial theories untenable. An integrative *biopsychosocial* mindset will likely be the most successful approach to treatment, as Engel articulated for all illnesses, both medical and psychiatric (Engel 1977).

## Genetic and Congenital Hypotheses

Since the first edition of this textbook there has been a multitude of studies on the genetic basis of manic–depressive disorder, particularly those using new molecular biological tools. This research, including both molecular and more traditional studies, is well summarized in two recent reviews (Craddock and Jones 1999, Potash and DePaulo 2000).

Available evidence indicates that familial factors are important determinants of who will develop manic–depressive disorder. Numerous studies have shown that relatives of manic–depressive *probands* (identified cases) have higher rates of manic–depressive disorder than controls or unipolar probands (Table 64–3). Overall, rates of manic–depressive disorder in first-degree relatives (parents, siblings, children) of probands with manic–depressive disorder are elevated 5 to 10 times over rates found in the general population. In the latter group, the rates are 0.5 to 1.5%, while in the former group rates are 5 to 15% (Table 64–3).

Interestingly, rates of unipolar depression in first-degree relatives are about twofold elevated over those in the general population. Because of the rate of depression in

| Table 64-3 | Rates of Manic–Depressive Disorder in First-Degree Relatives |
|---|---|

| | Proband is: | | |
|---|---|---|---|
| Study | Manic–Depressive | Unipolar | Control |
| Taylor et al. (1980) | 4.8 | 4.1 | – |
| Baron et al. (1982) | 14.5 | 3.1 | – |
| Gershon et al. (1982) | 8.0 | 2.2 | 0.5 |
| Coryell et al. (1985) | 7.0 | 2.8 | – |
| Tsuang et al. (1985) | 3.9 | 2.2 | 0.2 |

the general population (5–20%), this means that a twofold increase is a rate of about 20%. Important for genetic counseling, this in turn means that the probability that a manic–depressive proband will have a unipolar child is greater than the probability that they will have a manic–depressive child (5–15% versus 20%); note that it is most likely that they will have neither (100 minus 25–35%).

Most genetic research has been done on manic–depressive type I disorder. However, manic–depressive type II also appears to have a familial component. Manic–depressive type II probands have more manic–depressive type I disorder and more manic–depressive type II disorder than unipolar depressives and less type I disorder than type I probands (Endicott et al. 1985, Simpson et al. 1993).

Familial occurrence does not differentiate between inborn and environmental factors. Familial aggregation could be due to sharing genetic material, nongenetic congenital factors (e.g., similar inherited or acquired intrauterine factors, or exposure to similar perinatal risk factors), or physiologic or psychological environmental factors.

Data from other types of studies indicate that at least part of this risk is due to biological, and likely genetic factors. Twin studies indicate that *monozygotic* twins (derived from a single egg and sperm and therefore having an identical genome) have higher concordance rates for manic–depressive disorder than do *dizygotic* twins (derived from fertilization of two eggs)—60 to 80% for monozygotic twins versus 20 to 30% for dizygotic twins (Price 1968, Bertelsen 1979). Further, one adoption study showed that rates of manic–depressive disorder in persons adopted away from their biological families are closer to those in the biological families than the adoptive families (Price 1968, Mendlewicz and Rainer 1977). Finally, linkage studies, as summarized later, have suggested that in certain families manic–depressive disorder may be linked to specific genes. On the other hand, studies of monozygotic twins also indicate that only 40 to 70% are concordant for manic–depressive disorder. Thus, although there is clearly a genetic component to this illness, genetics is not destiny. More complex explanations must be sought (DePaolo et al. 1989).

Several *genetic loci*, or locations on chromosomes, have been proposed (Craddock and Jones 1999, Potash and DePaulo 2000) but independent confirmations have been lacking. Overall, the number of families in which a single gene has been associated with manic–depressive disorder is small. Further, no single locus has been replicated in multiple studies. The disparity in these findings may have several explanations. First, of course, is that the findings are falsely positive due to chance or to methodological problems. Alternatively, different genes may produce manic–depressive phenotype in different families. Finally, some studies indicate that manic–depressive disorder is polygenic, rather than due to a single gene (Gershon et al. 1982). It is also likely that genes may confer susceptibility to the disorder without actually determining that the disorder occurs. That is, to have the disorder one must have both the gene and another factor. This other factor may be a genetic (polygenic inheritance), change to the genome (see later), or an environmental (intrauterine, postnatal physiologic, or psychosocial) stressor.

A related approach to investigating genetic contributions to manic–depressive disorder is to look for differences in genes that code for components of systems thought to be involved in the pathophysiology of the disorder. Chief among such candidate genes have been those responsible for dopamine and serotonin receptors, transporters, and metabolic enzymes (Potash and DePaulo 2000). The recent study by Mundo and coworkers (2001) is interesting in this regard. It showed that individuals who developed manic symptoms when treated with serotonin-active antidepressants had higher rates of the gene coding for a particular form of the serotonin transporter, compared to those similarly treated who did not develop manic symptoms. In addition, several studies have indicated that the gene coding for the norepinephrine-metabolizing enzyme catechol-*O*-methyl transferase (COMT) may be associated with the rapid cycling form of manic–depressive disorder (Lachman et al. 1996, Kirov et al. 1998, Papolos et al. 1998).

In addition, though, recent evidence raises the possibility that the expression of a psychiatric illness that is coded genetically may not be due simply to the presence or absence of specific genes, but rather to modifying pieces of DNA in close proximity to important genes. Specifically, small sections of DNA, three base-pairs in length (called *trinucleotide repeats*), appear to be overrepresented in genetic disorders with prominent psychiatric symptoms, including fragile X syndrome and Huntington's disease. The disproportionate number of trinucleotide repeats are hypothesized to be responsible for over- or underexpression of the candidate gene, ultimately leading to neuropsychiatric symptoms (Petronis and Kennedy 1995). Recent evidence indicates that this may also be the case for manic–depressive disorder (Lindblad et al. 1998)

There has been little exploration of nongenetic congenital factors that may be responsible for manic–depressive disorder, although it is reasonable to suppose that intrauterine or perinatal factors that produce brain injury may lead to manic–depressive mood syndromes, just as head trauma in adult life may lead to mood disorders as well as cognitive impairment. Finally, nonbiologic familial factors have also been considered as etiologic in classic psychoanalytic descriptions such as anger turned inward contributing to depression and mania being a defense against depression (Abraham 1927). More recent work on environmental factors in the development of manic–depressive disorder has focused on effects of stress on the expression of episodes in already established manic–depressive disorder rather than on the development of the disorder itself (Post 1992).

It is intriguing in this regard that trinucleotide repeats, may actually change over the postconceptual period (i.e., during development), leading to changes in gene expression (Petronis and Kennedy 1995). This is contrary to classical Mendelian genetic theory, which assumes that genetic material is allocated during conception and cell division followed by the playing out of a genetically derived script, impervious to the impact of environmental factors. In contrast, data on these unstable regions of DNA provides the basis for hypothesizing that environment may actually alter genetic expression and perhaps transmission on to the next generation.

## Neurotransmitter Hypotheses

A wide range of hypotheses have been put forward regarding the biological basis of manic–depressive and other mood disorders. The major hypotheses and their supporting evidence have been recounted in great detail in excellent and still reasonably current review by Goodwin and Jamison (1990). Stahl (2000) and Sassi and Soares (2002) have reviewed these issues in detail using the methodologies more recently available. To be specific, investigators have approached manic–depressive disorder from neurochemical, neuroendocrine, neuroanatomic, and neurophysiologic vantage points, in addition to the genetic and psychosocial orientations outlined above.

Each of these sets of methodologies has provided heuristically powerful conceptual models that have been tested, refined, and tested again. Each has something of value to contribute regarding the pathologic basis of manic–depressive disorder. Nonetheless we do not yet have data to indicate whether the disorder is basically a disorder of a particular neurotransmitter, a particular neuroanatomic locus, or a particular physiologic system. Integration of these hypotheses awaits development of new methodologies for clinical neurobiologic investigations.

By extension from studies of depression and the actions of antidepressant medications, several neurotransmitter hypotheses have been proposed. Predominant among these has been the catecholamine hypothesis, articulated with regard to depression, by Prange (1964) and by Schildkraut (1965). Deficiency of norepinephrine or its effects was postulated to cause depression. A series of studies by Bunney and coworkers (1972a, 1972b, 1972c) explicitly extended these observations to manic–depressive disorder, proposing that changes in catecholamine function were responsible for the switch to mania.

Dopamine, which has been a prominent focus of schizophrenia research but relatively neglected in affective disorders until recently, has received attention specifically in the study of mania. Dopamine may underlie several of the prominent features of mania, including psychosis (Goodwin and Sack 1974), alterations in activity level (Goodwin and Sack 1974), and reward mechanisms (Crow and Deakin 1981). More recently, demonstration of prominent dopaminergic effects of the antidepressants nomifensine and bupropion have served to generate more attention for the role of dopamine in mood disorders (Kapur and Mann 1992). Serotonin has received somewhat more consistent attention as a substrate of mood disorders, particularly in Europe (Coppen et al. 1972). Attention to serotonin in the US has increased recently when the relatively selective serotonin reuptake inhibitors fluoxetine, sertraline, and paroxetine were demonstrated to have antidepressant efficacy. A "permissive hypothesis" whereby serotonin alterations permit instability of catechol systems leading to manic and depressive episodes has been articulated in broad strokes by Goodwin and Jamison (1990, pp. 422–423) but has not been extensively developed.

Janowsky and coworkers (1973) proposed that acetylcholine deficits were associated with mania. As with the serotonin hypothesis, this posits that the cholinergic system also interacts with the catecholaminergic system to produce affective instability. Finally, recent evidence also suggests that plasma gamma-aminobutyric acid (GABA) may also be involved in the pathophysiology of manic–depressive disorder (Benes and Berretta 2001, Post et al. 1992, Petty et al. 1993, 1996).

## Second-Messenger System Hypotheses

Since the first edition of this book, much of the effort in investigating neurochemical systems involved in manic–depressive disorder has focused on the role of postreceptor intracellular mechanisms, known as second-messenger (and sometimes third- and fourth-messengers). This research is well summarized in the recent reviews by Stahl (2000) and by Sassi and Soares (2002).

When neurotransmitters bind to postsynaptic neuronal receptors, a series of intracellular events are initiated that are mediated by chemical systems linked to those receptors. So-called G-proteins link the receptors to second-messenger systems, which in turn are linked to protein kinases that control the synthesis and operation of cellular components (Sassi and Soares 2002).

The cyclic AMP and phosphatidyl inositol systems are the most extensively studied of these second-messenger systems. Recent data have generated substantial interest in the phosphatidyl inositol system as a possible mediator of the clinical effects of lithium in manic–depressive disorder, particularly since this second-messenger system is linked to subtypes of adrenergic, serotonergic, dopaminergic, and cholinergic neurotransmitter systems. Specifically, lithium at therapeutically relevant concentrations has been demonstrated to inhibit phosphatidyl inositol turnover in cultured cell lines and animal studies (el-Mallakh and Li 1993, Lenox and Watson 1994). In clinical studies, persons with manic–depressive disorder have demonstrated alterations in platelet phosphatidyl inositol levels (Brown et al. 1993) and responsiveness of neutrophil phosphoinositol accumulation (Greil et al. 1991). Cell lines derived from persons with manic–depressive disorder have been found to exhibit abnormalities of phosphatidyl inositol metabolism (Banks et al. 1990). In a magnetic resonance spectroscopy study of persons with manic–depressive disorder, phosphomonoester levels were found to be higher when in the manic state than in remission or in normal controls (Kato et al. 1994, Deicken et al. 1995).

## Neuroendocrine Hypotheses

Neuroendocrine hypotheses have sought to elucidate important mechanisms in the production and maintenance of symptoms rather than identify a specific etiologic agent in manic–depressive or other mood disorders. These hypotheses were developed from the literature on stress response in otherwise normal subjects (Mason 1975). Typical neuroendocrine studies investigate peripheral or cerebrospinal fluid abnormalities of a particular system in persons with mood disorders and in controls and propose that either the neuroendocrine system itself or the neurotransmitter system that controls the hormone is in some way linked to the pathophysiology of the mood disorder of interest. Perhaps the most complete battery of neuroendocrine assessments in manic–depressive disorder was conducted by Amsterdam and colleagues (1983). Taken together, the literature does not identify particular endocrine findings as characteristic of manic–depressive disorder.

Although neuroendocrine research has not been as "hot" an area as some others since the first edition of this book, the thyroid system continues to receive consistent attention from some researchers (Bauer and Whybrow 2001). The thyroid axis may be of particular relevance to the pathophysiology of mood disorders since it serves not only as a dependent variable that is studied as a function of mood (as most neuroendocrine systems have been), but because the thyroid axis has also been studied as an independent variable of some impact. Several studies have shown that thyroid hormone administration may actually ameliorate mood disorders in certain paradigms. Specifically, there is evidence that the thyroid hormone triiodothyronine ($T_3$) may speed the response of individuals with depression to antidepressant treatment and may convert nonresponders to responders (Joffe et al. 1993). Further, in the rapid cycling variant of manic–depressive disorder, evidence indicates that supplementation with high doses of the thyroid hormone thyroxine ($T_4$) may induce remission in persons who are refractory to standard pharmacotherapy (Bauer and Whybrow 1990). In both these types of studies, response to thyroid supplementation occur in subjects regardless of whether they had preexisting thyroid disease.

The mechanism for these effects has been the subject of much speculation. Various models posit that the brain is functionally hypothyroid either due to changes in hormone synthesis, transport, or metabolism, or due to increased demand; alternatively, other models propose that the brain has an excess of a thyroid-related substance, which administration of exogenous thyroid hormone diminishes (Bauer and Whybrow 1990, 2001, Joffe et al. 1993).

## Neuroanatomic Hypotheses

Two main types of studies have provided information on the possible neuroanatomic bases of manic–depressive disorder. In the first type, brains of persons with brain injuries who develop a phenomenologically manic–depressive picture have been analyzed, often neuropathologically, to determine sites of injury that may have produced the manic–depressive clinical picture. For example, lesions of the right side of the brain, particularly frontotemporal lesions, may be associated with manic-like syndromes (Starkstein et al. 1988).

In the second type of study, persons with manic–depressive disorder who do not have a known organic basis for their illness are studied either with *anatomic* (computerized tomography, magnetic resonance imaging [MRI]) or *functional* imaging (single photon or positron emission tomography, or functional MRI or spectroscopy [MRS]) to identify regions of abnormality.

Among anatomic studies, abnormalities of computerized tomography (Nasrallah et al. 1989, Strakowski et al. 1993a, 1993b) and subcortical (Jurjus et al. 1993a, Strakowski et al. 1993a, 1993b) MRI have demonstrated abnormalities in persons with manic–depressive disorder. However, not all findings have been replicated (Jurjus et al. 1993b) and the findings may not be specific for manic–depressive disorder. Further, the degree to which anatomic abnormalities reflect pathogenic factors, as opposed to end organ damage or effects of chronic medication usage, has yet to be established.

MRI studies have been an area of intense interest over the past several years, with particular interest in the size of the temporal lobes, limbic system, basal ganglia, ventricles, and total brain volume. Unfortunately, no consistent findings have emerged (Altshuler et al. 2000, Brambilla et al. 2001, Hauser et al. 2000, Sassi and Soares 2002).

Similarly, there has been substantial interest in quantitating and localizing so-called "$T_2$ hyperintensities" found in MRI studies of individuals with manic–depressive disorder. These phenomena, thought to represent increased water content of microregions of the brain, also occur in chronic medical illnesses such as hypertension and diabetes. Unfortunately, no consistency regarding prevalence or distribution in manic–depressive disorder has yet been demonstrated (Altshuler et al. 1995, Yildiz et al. 2001).

Among functional imaging studies, blood flow, glucose metabolism, and more recently functional MRI/MRS and neurotransmitter binding have been the major variables of interest. In studies using blood flow methodologies, frontal (Buchsbaum et al. 1986) and temporal (Post et al. 1987) cortical structures have been the site of abnormalities in manic–depressive disorder, while among subcortical areas the caudate has received the most attention (Baxter et al. 1985). Although no consistent evidence has emerged regarding a single neurotransmitter system or a single brain region, some promising results have recently emerged regarding serotonin 5-HT$_{1A}$ receptor levels in several brain regions (Drevets et al. 1999).

## Cell Degeneration and Neuroprotective Effects of Medications

One of the most exciting areas of recent research focuses on the possibility that lithium and perhaps certain anticonvulsants such as valproate may actually exert a *neuroprotective* effect in manic–depressive disorder. Evidence indicates that these agents may protect nerve cells by stimulating production of protective proteins or by stimulating nerve growth (Manji and Lenox 2000). Interestingly, there is some clinical evidence from MRI that lithium treatment may actually increase total brain gray matter, although this will of course require replication (Manji and Lenox 2000). Thus, it is possible that cellular degeneration, albeit not as virulent as in Alzheimer's, may play a role in manic–depressive disorder.

## Hypotheses Regarding Complex Physiologic Systems

Several complex systems, which for want of a better alternative are grouped together in this section as "physiologic" systems, have been postulated to play a pathogenic role in manic–depressive disorder. Classic theories of membrane and electrolyte balance (Goodwin and Jamison 1990, pp. 467–481) abnormalities have been extensively investigated in the past but appear, for the time being, to have passed out of favor. Two other hypotheses regarding complex systems have been of interest over the years: the biological rhythms and kindling theories.

### Biological Rhythms

Two types of data indicate that biological rhythms may play a role in the pathogenesis of manic–depressive disorder. First, there are a large number of observational studies that have demonstrated seasonal peaks in the onset of affective episodes or hospitalizations for mood disorders. For manic–depressive disorder, the predominant seasons appear to be spring and fall (Goodwin and Jamison 1990, Kamo et al. 1993), although other patterns may occur with some consistency across years (Faedda et al. 1993). Seasonal affective disorder in which persons become depressed and remit at specific, regular times of year, has been codified in DSM-IV by applying the course modifier "seasonal pattern" to recurrent mood disorders (Bauer and Dunner 1993). Although the relationship of seasonal affective disorder, particularly the winter depression variant, to manic–depressive disorder is not yet clear, there does appear to be some overlap. For instance, in most studies a large percentage of persons with seasonal affective disorder have manic–depressive disorder. In addition, the clinical picture of winter depression is similar to the hypersomnolent, anergic, hyperphagic depression common in manic–depressive disorder (Bauer and Dunner 1993). Further, treatment with bright light has been shown to be efficacious in winter depression (Terman et al. 1989) and also appears to be an effective antidepressant in nonseasonal manic–depressives treated in the winter (Deltito et al. 1991) and perhaps in the summer (Bauer 1993); bright light also appears to be capable of inducing manic symptoms as do other antidepressants (Bauer et al. 1994b).

The second type of data which may provide a mechanism for seasonal patterns is that persons with manic–depressive disorder often exhibit abnormalities of circadian or daily rhythms. Many rhythmic parameters have been studied in persons with manic–depressive and other mood disorders, with various abnormalities found regarding the *amplitude* (height of the rhythm) and *phase* (timing of the rhythm) (Halaris 1987). Among the most promising findings is that light sensitivity to suppression of the rhythmic hormone melatonin may be altered in persons with manic–depressive disorder (Lewy et al. 1980, 1985) and their relatives (Nurnberger et al. 1989).

One of the most prominent biological rhythms, sleep, has also been implicated in the pathogenesis of manic–depressive disorders. However, it should be noted that it is not clear whether it is the rhythmic aspects of sleep or its nonrhythmic, restorative components which are most relevant. One of the most striking findings in mania is the lack of need for sleep and there is evidence that sleep deprivation may be both antidepressant and promanic (Wehr et al. 1982). Thus further exploration of sleep disturbance in manic–depressive disorder, both as a dependent and an independent variable, is warranted.

### Kindling Models

The second major hypothesis involving complex physiologic systems proposes an analogy between the occurrence of episodes in manic–depressive disorder and seizures in animal models of epilepsy. Post and coworkers (1985, 1986a, 1986b) have proposed that an autonomous pattern of affective episodes in manic–depressive disorder may develop from increasing sensitization of an individual to stressors. This process was proposed to be similar to kindling in animals and humans, in which subthreshold convulsant stimuli can decrease the threshold for seizures and eventually lead to spontaneous seizures. An analogy was also drawn between mood episodes in manic–depressive

disorder and behavioral sensitization in animals, in which repeated exposure to pharmacological stimuli can decrease the threshold for specific behavioral responses.

There are several attractive aspects to this hypothesis. It is supported by the increased frequency of episodes over the course of manic–depressive disorder (Angst 1981) and the response of many persons with manic–depressive disorder to treatment with the anticonvulsants carbamazepine and valproate. However, the clinical data in support of this heuristically powerful conceptual paradigm are at this point quite limited (Bauer and Whybrow 1991). Thus it is not clear whether the increase in episode frequency sometimes seen is due to accumulating damage from prior episodes, or is simply the unfolding over time of what was destined from the beginning to be a malignant case of the illness.

### Stress and Manic–Depressive Disorder

The possible association of stressful life events and the onset of depression has generated substantial interest among researchers from various theoretical backgrounds (Brown et al. 1977, Brown 1989, Beck et al. 1979, Klerman et al. 1984, Perris 1984a, 1984b, 1984c, Paykel and Cooper 1992, Johnson and Roberts 1995). Most of the literature regarding analysis of the relationship between stressful life events and manic–depressive disorder has focused on the precipitation of episodes in established manic–depressive disorder rather than the onset of the disorder *de novo*.

Hall and coworkers (1977) in a prospective study of persons with manic–depressive type I disorder found no difference in life events among those who became manic, those who became depressed, and those who remained well; the only exception was a somewhat increased incidence of work difficulties in those who developed manic symptoms. In a prospective study, Sclare and Creed (1990) found no difference in events prior to and subsequent to admission for mania. In contrast, a retrospective study by Kennedy and coworkers (1983) reported an increased rate in adverse life events not directly related to illness in the 4 months preceding admission to the hospital for mania compared to 4 months after. In a prospective study, Hunt and coworkers (1992) found a severalfold increase in adverse life events the month prior to manic or depressive relapse, compared to baseline, without difference between manic and depressive relapses. In a prospective study, Ellicott and coworkers (1990) found that there were subgroups of persons with manic–depressive disorder who had varying thresholds of sensitivity to stress, and identified a significant association between stressful life events and the onset of mood disturbance. Of interest was that medication levels and compliance with treatment regimes did not account for any of the variance in outcome. Leverich (1990) also identified several factors, including stressful life events, associated with mood disturbance during the maintenance medication prophylaxis of mood disorders in general.

Thus, there are several studies that demonstrate a relationship between stressful life events and the onset of affective episodes in already established manic–depressive disorder. However, several studies failed to find meaningful associations. There are also several types of methodological problems that may make interpretation of the studies difficult, and comparison across studies impossible. Examples of such problems include recall bias in retrospective design, and in both retrospective and prospective studies sample heterogeneity, length of time window for identification of relevant events, definition of onset of mood episode, and choice of signal event (e.g., hospitalization versus onset of episode). Further, within prospective studies, differences in attribution and recall can be significantly different depending on whether a person is interviewed for life events prior to or after the index episode has commenced.

Thus it is likely that adverse life events are associated with mood episodes, particularly those episodes that are sufficiently severe to warrant hospitalization. In this respect such life events need to be attended to for clinical purposes. However, from a theoretical point of view it is not clear that such events actually play a pathogenic role.

## Psychosocial Hypotheses

The psychological theories of mood disorders are broad in scope, and have included psychoanalytic, interpersonal, and cognitive–behavioral. These theories propose that the symptoms of mood disorders are produced by psychological factors, with biological components playing at most a secondary role in the expression of symptoms. Unfortunately, the bulk of theory regarding the psychological basis of mood disorders concerns depression, with little attention as yet to mania or manic–depressive disorder.

Cognitive theory tenets regard depression as an affective response to negative beliefs (Beck et al. 1979, Rush and Hollon 1991). Attributions regarding events are based on unrealistically negative assumptions: that when bad things happen, they happen because of one's inadequacy, they will always happen, and similar bad things will happen in other situations. Relatively stable patterns of attribution develop relatively early in life, and misinterpretations of events and maladaptive responses are triggered by proximate events (Abramson et al. 1978, Seligman et al. 1979).

Comparatively, behavior theory views depression as a consequence of a low rate of response-contingent positive reinforcement. The goal of behavior therapy is to increase positive reinforcement by participation in pleasant activities or building assertive skills needed to elicit social rewards. The learned helplessness model (Seligman 1975) and behavioral therapy for depression (Lewinsohn 1974) testify to the merit of these theoretical strategies.

The interpersonal theory of depression, which serves as the theoretical basis for interpersonal psychotherapy (IPT) (Klerman et al. 1984, Weissman and Klerman 1991), builds on the work of Adolph Meyer and Harry Stack Sullivan, both of whom considered an individual's environment to play an important role in symptom development and protection from illness. Interpersonal theory proposes that depression develops most often in the context of adverse events, particularly interpersonal loss. IPT then aims at reducing symptoms by psychoeducation and subsequently by addressing problems in interpersonal relationships, primarily focusing on grief, role disputes, role transitions, and interpersonal deficits.

Psychoanalytic theories regarding depression are wideranging, with perhaps their most concise and elegant formulation in Freud's classic *Mourning and Melancholia*

(Freud 1924). Further development of his theories of depression are found throughout his *New Introductory Lectures in Psychoanalysis* (Freud 1933). For subsequent development of psychoanalytic theories of depression, the reader is referred in particular to Abraham (1927) and Fenichel (1945).

As with these other theories, psychoanalytic theory regarding mania has been much more limited than for depression. Theories focus on mania as a defense against underlying depression, which is not always completely successful. For instance, Dooley (1921) proposed that mania was a mechanism whereby one could ward off painful depressive thoughts. Schwartz (1961) suggested that mania, particularly its hyperactive and grandiose components, functioned as a defense against underlying emptiness and deprivation.

Fenichel (1945) also considered mania to be a response to depression. He proposed that in depression symptoms were caused by a battering superego punishing the self, while "...the triumphant character of mania arises from the release of energy hitherto bound in the depressive struggle and now seeking discharge." Nonetheless, he succinctly remarks later in a discussion of cyclicity in manic–depressive and other mood disorders: "...yet it is impossible to get rid of the impression that additional purely biological factors are involved."

More recent psychoanalytic theorists have emphasized the need for revision of traditional psychoanalytic theories in the face of accumulating evidence of a biological component to major mental illnesses, including manic–depressive disorder. It is also important to note that there is no consistent evidence that manic–depressive disorder is caused by or associated with personality disorders, as defined by the DSM system (Goodwin and Jamison 1990, pp. 281–317). However, some recent psychoanalytic clinicians have proposed that analytic treatment may be helpful in reducing stresses that may precipitate episodes (Kahn 1993).

It is worth quoting Cooper (1985) at length with regard to revisions in psychoanalytic thinking necessitated by the recognition of substantial biological components to the major mental illnesses:

> Most analytic treatment carries with it a strong implication that it is a major analytic task of the patient to accept responsibility for his actions. In the psychoanalytic view, this responsibility is nearly total.... However, it now seems likely that there are patients with depressive, anxious, and dysphoric states for whom the usual psychodynamic view of responsibility seems inappropriate.... There is a group of chronically depressed and anxious patients...whose mood regulation is vastly changed by antidepressant medication. The entry of these new molecules into their metabolism alters, tending to normalize, the way they see the world, the way they do battle with their superegos, the way they respond to object separation. It may be that we have been coconspirators with these patients in their need to construct a rational-seeming world in which they hold themselves unconsciously responsible for events.

## Psychobiological Hypotheses

Successful treatment of manic–depressive disorder with medications has made the biological basis of this disorder incontrovertible. Nonetheless, psychosocial factors may play prominent roles in the development of manic–depressive disorder and, once established, in its course. Several models that integrate psychological factors and biological mechanisms have been developed. These have been well reviewed recently by Johnson and Roberts (1995).

Several examples illustrate the diversity of these proposals. As described above, the kindling model proposes that discrete environmental stressors may be translated into enduring neurobiological changes that are responsible for mood episodes in manic–depressive disorder. Ehlers and coworkers (1988) have proposed that the regulation of biological rhythms in persons with manic–depressive disorder may be disrupted by changes in psychosocial events. Specifically, they propose that mood episodes cause disruptions in social rhythms (e.g., eating, sleeping, and other aspects of one's daily routine). They propose that these social rhythms are important regulators of biological circadian rhythms and without these regulators abnormalities of circadian develop, leading to the onset, worsening, or perpetuation of mood symptoms. Depue and colleagues (1985, Depue and Iacono 1989) have proposed that mood disordered individuals, including those with manic–depressive spectrum disorders, have deficits in the regulation of biological responses to stress. Thus, environmental stressors may cause disruptions of biological systems that cause mood symptoms in vulnerable individuals, even though similar stressors may not cause disruptions in those without mood disorders.

Hume and colleagues (1988) have proposed another stress-vulnerability model specifically for manic–depressive disorder in which the threshold for commencement of mood symptoms, particularly in manic–depressive disorder, is influenced by a combination of the "perception" one has of stressful life events and a vulnerable biochemical mood regulatory system. Thus, adverse life events, coupled with both psychological and biological vulnerability, are required to produce both the mood and the somatic symptoms of depression. Similar to cognitive theorists, Hume described attributions regarding the cause of adverse events, particularly one's control over events (Rotter 1966), as particularly important in producing the psychological vulnerability to depression and manic–depressive disorder. However, they do not describe specific mechanisms by which manic, as opposed to depressive, symptoms may be produced.

## Conclusions: The Biopsychosocial Approach

Numerous family genetic studies indicate that there is a hereditary biological component to manic–depressive disorder—yet the fact that only 40 to 70% of monozygotic twins are concordant for manic–depressive disorder indicates that genetics is not destiny. Most neurotransmitter systems and most neuroendocrine axes studied to date have shown some abnormalities in manic–depressive disorder—yet it is not clear to what degree these are individual in the pathogenesis of symptoms, and to what degree these findings reflect "downstream," or secondary changes. Each of the complex physiologic and psychosocial hypotheses are attractive heuristically—yet they have in most cases little supporting data and are notoriously difficult to test.

Absent certainty, we in our roles as treating clinicians and educators of individuals and families who suffer with manic–depressive disorder are best advised to take a nonreductionistic and biopsychosocial view of this illness, as initially articulated by Engel (1977). There are currently many promising leads, as there have been many promising leads in the past that turned cold. We know for certain that the illness is not fully genetically determined and is probably not fully explainable in biological terms. However, it is also beyond doubt, based on pharmacologic treatment studies that there is a biological component to the illness. Attention to the role of environmental, particularly psychosocial, factors is also quite likely important in modulating the course of the disease. Thus, the section on treatment later in the chapter deals with an equal level of attention to both pharmacologic and psychosocial interventions for manic–depressive disorder.

## Assessment and Differential Diagnosis

## Phenomenology

### Overview

Mood episodes are discrete periods of altered feeling, thought, and behavior. Typically they have a distinct onset and offset, beginning over days or weeks and eventually ending gradually after several weeks or months. As noted earlier, manic–depressive disorder is defined by the occurrence of depressive plus manic, hypomanic, or mixed episodes, or the occurrence of only manic or mixed episodes.

Major depressive episodes are defined by discrete periods of depressed or blue mood or loss of interest or pleasure in life that typically endures for weeks but must last for at least 2 weeks (see Chapter 93). These symptoms are often accompanied by changes in sleep, appetite, energy, cognition, and judgment. Depressive episodes in manic–depressive disorder are indistinguishable from those in major depressive disorder. About half of persons with manic–depressive disorder experience depressive episodes characterized by decreased sleep and appetite, whereas about half experience more "atypical" symptoms of increased sleep and appetite. Recall that the differential diagnosis between major depressive and manic–depressive disorders is made not by cross-sectional symptom analysis but by longitudinal course. The diagnostic decision tree for manic–depressive disorder is given in Figure 64–1.

Manic episodes are defined by discrete periods of abnormally elevated, expansive, or irritable mood accompanied by marked impairment in judgment and social and occupational function. These symptoms are frequently accompanied by unrealistic grandiosity, excess energy, and increases in goal-directed activity that frequently have a high potential for damaging consequences.

Hypomanic and manic symptoms may be identical, but hypomanic episodes are less severe. A person is "promoted" from hypomania to mania (type II to type I manic–depressive disorder) by the presence of one of three features: psychosis during the episode, sufficient severity to warrant hospitalization, or marked social or occupational role impairment. This is an imperfect set of criteria, however,

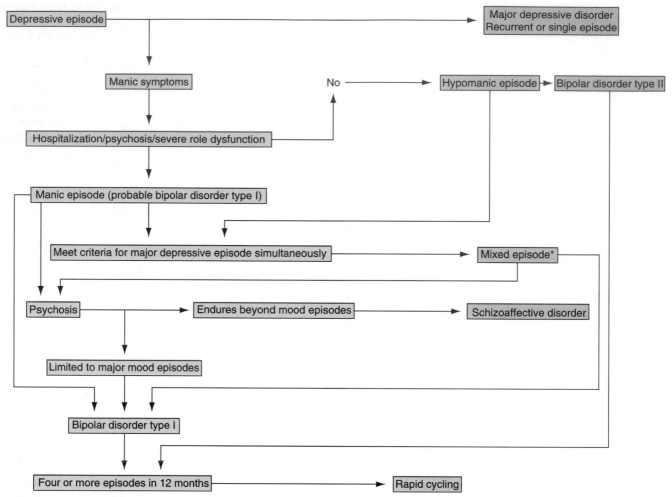

**Figure 64–1** *Diagnostic decision tree for manic–depressive disorder. The building blocks for a diagnosis of manic–depressive disorder are individual episodes and their characteristics, as summarized in Table 64–1. This decision tree helps the psychiatrist through the steps that lead to diagnosis of manic–depressive disorder and identification of its subtypes. *Does not apply to hypomanic episode as per DSM-IV. (Source: Bauer M, Whybrow P, Gyulai L, et al. [1994a] Testing definitions of dysphoric mania and hypomania: Prevalence, clinical characteristics, and interepisode stability. J Affect Disord 32, 201–211; McElroy S, Keck P, Pope H, et al. [1992] Clinical and research implications of the diagnosis of dysphoric or mixed mania or hypomania. Am J Psychiatr 149, 1633–1644.)*

because psychosis may or may not be an integral part of manic–depressive disorder (see below), because hospitalization may be due to social or personal factors or comorbidities not related to the disorder itself, and because the concept of marked role function impairment is not well operationalized (American Psychiatric Association 1994a, 2000). Overall, however, there is evidence that type II and type I manic–depressive disorders are separable (see the earlier section on episodes as the basis for diagnosis of manic–depressive disorder). From time to time, individual authors propose additional subtypes of manic–depressive disorder, but these are not formally or consistently recognized.

It is important to note that the phenomonologic differentiation between hypomania and mania is not as cut-and-dried as one would hope—and as many genetic and biological studies assume. Of the three characteristics by which one is "promoted" from hypomania to mania, only the presence of psychosis is firmly grounded in the characteristics of the individual. The other two characteristics, marked social or occupational role impairment or hospitalization, clearly have components that are primarily external

to the individual. If for instance, one individual has relatively mild manic symptoms but is living with a family who is unable to tolerate the behavior, she/he is more likely to be hospitalized. Similarly, the comorbid presence of a severe disorder is more likely to result in hospitalization and a "promotion" from type II to type I disorder. Contrarily, limited insurance benefits, or a more tolerant family increase the probability that a manic syndrome of a given severity will be managed without hospitalization and thus be diagnosed as "hypomania" rather than "mania." Genetic and biological investigators are thus well advised to keep these phenomenological issues in mind when designing studies—otherwise reifying what are psychosocial rather than genetic or biological distinctions may introduce unwarranted variability into their studies.

## A "Bipolar" Disorder?

Classically, mania has been considered to be the opposite of depression: manic individuals were said to be cheery, optimistic, and self-confident. Hence the name bipolar disorder. However, in most descriptive studies, substantial proportions of hypomanic and manic patients actually exhibit substantial dysphoric symptoms (Bauer et al. 1991, 1994a). Mixed episodes, defined as the simultaneous occurrence of full-blown manic and depressive episodes, are the most prominent example of dysphoria during mania. Although it may have been suggested that dysphoric mania may constitute a separate subtype of mania (McElroy et al. 1992), the inclusion of this additional dichotomy is premature, and it may be of more use scientifically and clinically to consider dysphoric symptoms dimensionally rather than categorically (Bauer et al. 1994b).

Further evidence that (hypo)mania is not the polar opposite of depression comes from investigation of self-reported quality of life in the various mood states of manic–depressive disorder (Vojta et al. 2001). Although classically thought to be a desirable state, patients with mania or hypomania rate their preference for that state as equal to or less than their preference for euthymia, with depression and mixed states being rated less preferable. The ratings of quality of life for (hypo)mania were normally rather than bimodally distributed. Thus, the rating was not the average of two disparate groups; rather, (hypo)mania appears simply not to be a desirable state.

## Additional Features: Psychosis and Rapid Cycling

Psychosis can occur in either pole of the disorder. If psychotic symptoms are limited to the major mood episode, the individual is considered to have manic–depressive disorder with psychotic features. On the other hand, if psychotic symptoms endure significantly into periods of normal mood, the diagnosis of schizoaffective disorder is made. For formal research diagnostic criteria and DSM definitions, 2 weeks of psychotic symptoms during normal mood is sufficient to convert a diagnosis of manic–depressive or major depressive disorder into schizoaffective disorder, because it is thought that such persons have a clinical course midway between individuals with mood disorders or schizophrenia. However, this cutoff point is fairly arbitrary, and its validity is not well established (Levitt and Tsuang 1988, Blacker and Tsuang 1992). For example, it may be that psychotic symptoms actually represent a separate, comorbid disorder, or they may be integral

### DSM-IV-TR Criteria

#### Rapid-Cycling Specifier

*Specify* if:

**With rapid cycling** (can be applied to manic–depressive I disorder or manic–depressive II disorder). At least four episodes of a mood disturbance in the previous 12 months that meet criteria for a major depressive, manic, mixed, or hypomanic episode.

**Note:** Episodes are demarcated by either partial or full remission for at least 2 months or a switch to an episode of opposite polarity (e.g., major depressive episode to manic episode).

features of severe manic–depressive disorder that simply take longer to resolve. Identification of pathophysiological and genetic bases of psychosis and of manic–depressive disorder will certainly help to resolve these issues.

Rapid cycling is defined by the occurrence of four or more mood episodes within 12 months. It should be noted that, despite the name, the episodes are not necessarily or even commonly truly cyclical; the diagnosis is based simply on episode counting (American Psychiatric Association 1994a). This subcategory is of significance because it predicts a relatively poorer outcome and worse response to lithium and other treatments (Bauer and Whybrow 1993, Bauer et al. 1994c). Although rapid cycling has been considered by some to be an "end stage" of the disorder, empirical evidence indicates that it may have its onset at any time during the disorder (Bauer and Whybrow 1991, 1993, Bauer et al. 1994c) and may come and go during the course of illness (Coryell et al. 1992). Several specific risk factors may be associated with rapid cycling, each of which may give clues to its pathophysiology. These include female gender, antidepressant use, and prior or current hypothyroidism (Bauer and Whybrow 1993, Bauer et al. 1994c).

## History, Physical Examination, and Laboratory Studies

Krauthammer and Klerman (1978) conceptualized secondary mania as mania occurring close on the heels of a specific known physiological insult, such as general medical illness or exposure to mania-inducing pharmacological agents. Strakowski and coworkers (1994) further suggested that there may also be general medical illnesses that appear unusually frequently during the course of primary manic–depressive disorder for various reasons but without actually inducing a manic state. Our concern here is with the former.

Although the diagnosis of manic–depressive disorder is made on the basis of phenomenology, there are several reasons to conduct a thorough medical history and physical examination. First, there are several general medical or substance-related causes of manic depression that, if treated, may lead to the resolution of the mood episode (see later). Similarly, mania may be the first sign of a general medical illness that will be progressive and serious in its own right. Second, medical evaluation is necessary before starting medications used in the treatment of manic–depressive disorder. Finally, for many patients with psychiatric illnesses, particularly chronic or severe illnesses, their first contact with medical care as an adult is during the psychiatric interview—often under inpatient or even involuntary conditions. Because psychiatric illness is clearly not *protective* against medical illnesses, and since even common general medical illnesses may never have been screened for in the past, a thorough medical history and physical examination are necessary parts of the basic care of patients.

Many textbooks recommend a history, physical examination, and laboratory testing for the routine evaluation of persons with mood disorders. Although the history and physical examination are commonsense medical procedures, the use of laboratory testing, particularly routine screening batteries, is supported by few data (Bauer et al. 1993, Agency for Health Care Policy and Research 1993). For instance, using screening for thyroid abnormalities in individuals presenting with depressed mood as an example, Briggs and coworkers (1993) found no evidence that the prevalence of thyroid disorders among ambulatory patients with depression exceeds that in the general population. It was therefore recommended to follow standard screening recommendations for the general population in individuals with depression.

The overall approach to evaluating persons with manic–depressive disorder for medical problems may be generalized as follows: Persons with psychiatric disorders, including manic–depressive disorder, should have regular screening for disease detection and health maintenance purposes as recommended for the general population. However, it should also be kept in mind that individuals with manic–depressive disorder, by virtue of having an often severe and disabling behavioral disorder, are less likely than the general population to have had adequate medical screening and treatment. Thus, special care must be made to ensure that health problems are not overlooked and that appropriate treatment or referral is effected. Unfortunately, it is the exception rather than the rule to have well-integrated medical and mental health systems, such as those found at the Department of Veterans affairs or certain staff model health maintenance organizations, so that the mental health provider can assume that some effort will need to be expended to ensure adequate care is delivered for individuals with manic–depressive disorder.

All newly identified psychiatric patients should undergo a history and if indicated a physical examination. If results of the history or physical examination reveal abnormalities, or if the psychiatric illness is associated with particular general medical conditions, more intensive testing is warranted. A clear example of the last situation is when a person with manic–depressive disorder who has extensive exposure to lithium presents for treatment; such persons, particularly the elderly, require laboratory testing for renal and thyroid abnormalities that can be caused by lithium treatment.

Which general medical illnesses may cause symptoms of manic–depressive disorder? Most medical illnesses that affect brain function have been described in case reports or small case series to cause one or another psychiatric syndrome. Several general medical illnesses have been associated with the development of manic–depressive disorder (Table 64–4), although none can be considered specific risk factors. Case reports or case series that propose that a putative causative medical illness is associated with manic–depressive disorder must be interpreted with caution. For

| Table 64–5 | Treatments and Drugs Commonly Associated with Mania | |
| --- | --- | --- |
| **Antidepressants** | | **Dopaminergic Agents** |
| Medications | | Levodopa |
| Bright visible spectrum light treatment | | |
| Electroconvulsant therapy | | |
| **Adrenergic Agents** | | **Drugs of Abuse** |
| Decongestants | | Alcohol |
| Bronchodilators | | Cocaine |
| Stimulants | | Hallucinogens |
| | | Amphetamines |
| | | Caffeine |
| **Other Agents** | | |
| Isoniazid | | |
| Corticosteroids | | |
| Anabolic steroids | | |
| Disulfiram | | |

instance, Josephson and MacKenzie (1979) described an association between hyperthyroidism and mania. However, almost all of these patients had additional factors that most likely contributed to the development of mania, such as a preexisting mood disorder due to a general medical condition or a prior history of mood disorders. Too much thyroid hormone in and of itself is not likely to cause mania (Bierwaltes and Ruff 1958). On the other hand, administration of medications has been observed frequently in clinical practice to be associated with the onset of mania, particularly in patients with preexisting depression. Such medications are listed in Table 64–5. Depressive symptoms may also be associated with certain medical conditions (Table 64–6) and medications or drugs (Table 64–7).

Some controversies have been hotly debated, particularly regarding the role of antidepressants in causing mania and rapid cycling (Prien et al. 1973b, Lewis and Winokur 1982, Wehr et al. 1993, Altshuler et al. 1995). Of particular importance to psychiatric practice, all efficacious antidepressant treatments have been suspected to cause the induction of mania, with the exception of lithium and the possible exception of psychotherapy. Occasionally when a new antidepressant is developed, hope is raised that it will be the agent that will not induce mania. Clinical experience has not borne out these early hopes. This caveat for antidepressants also includes nonpharmacological antidepressants such as light and electroconvulsive therapy (ECT). The latter effect is paradoxical, as ECT is also used successfully to treat mania.

## Age, Gender, and Cultural Issues in Diagnosis and Assessment

It is important to note that manic–depressive disorder is a worldwide problem. Worldwide, the Global Burden of Disease studies (Murray and Lopez 1996, 1997) estimate that in established market economies mental disorders account for 43% of the disability and 22% of the global burden (premature death plus life lived with disability) of all diseases. Manic–depressive disorder is among the top 10 of all dis-

| Table 64–4 | Medical Disorders Commonly Associated with Mania | |
| --- | --- | --- |
| **Neurologic Disorders** | | **Endocrine** |
| Stroke | | Hyperthyroidism (in those with preexisting manic–depressive disorder) |
| Head trauma | | Postpartum status |
| Dementia | | |
| Brain tumors | | |
| Infection (including HIV) | | |
| Multiple sclerosis | | |
| Huntington's disease | | |

| Table 64-6 | Medical Disorders Commonly Associated with Depression |
|---|---|

**Neurologic Disorders**

Stroke
Head trauma
Dementia
Brain tumors
Infection (including HIV)
Multiple sclerosis
Parkinson's disease
Huntington's disease

**Endocrine**

Addison's disease
Cushing's disease
Hypothyroidism
Hyperthyroidism
Postpartum status

**Cancers**

Pancreatic

**Metabolic**

$B_{12}$, folate deficiencies

*Any Medical Disease that Causes Significant
Loss of Function or Self-esteem*

| Table 64-7 | Treatments and Drugs Commonly Associated with Depression |
|---|---|

| High Blood Pressure Medications | Hormones |
|---|---|
| Alphamethyldopa | Corticosteroids |
| Clonidine | Oral contraceptives |
| | Anabolic steroids |
| **Ulcer Medications** | **Psychotropic Agents** |
| Cimetadine | Benzodiazepines |
| Ranitidine | Neuroleptics |
| **Drugs of Abuse** | |
| Alcohol | |
| Sedatives | |
| Amphetamine (withdrawal) | |
| Cocaine (withdrawal) | |
| Nicotine (withdrawal) | |

eases in terms of global burden worldwide, and fifth in terms of self-reported disability (Andrews et al. 1998).

There are no major differences in the manifestations of manic–depressive disorder across gender, age, or culture. However, women appear to be at higher risk for rapid cycling (Bauer and Whybrow 1993, Bauer et al. 1994c), dysphoria during mania (McElroy et al. 1992, Bauer et al. 1994a), and comorbid disorders (Strakowski et al. 1992, 1994). Note, however, that affective psychoses may be rela-

tively underdiagnosed, and schizophrenia overdiagnosed, in African-Americans compared to Caucasians (Strakowski et al. 1993c).

Among children and adolescents, the diagnosis of manic–depressive disorder is often complicated by less consistent mood and behavior baseline than occur in adults (Carlson and Kashani 1988). Little evidence is available regarding course and outcome in children. Available data indicate that, as with adults, mixed or cycling episodes predict more recurrences; unlike in adults, manic and mixed presentations may be associated with relatively shorter episodes compared with depressive presentations (Strober et al. 1995).

## Epidemiology

### Epidemiological Studies of Manic–Depressive Disorder

Epidemiological studies assess the *incidence* (onset frequency), *prevalence* (overall population load), and related characteristics in large samples of persons who are not preselected on the basis of presentation for clinical care. These studies are a valuable complement to clinic-based studies for several reasons. First, epidemiological studies avoid biases inherent in studying clinic-based samples. For example, clinical populations may underrepresent the milder (or most severe) variants of a disorder; further, willingness to request clinical care may be associated with sample characteristics that bias the sample in unknown ways. In addition, epidemiological studies may be helpful in determining overall population load for a particular disorder, which can be helpful in planning health services. On the other hand, the large sample size and required methodology for most epidemiological studies limit the extent to which any individual subject can be assessed. Smaller sample, higher intensity clinic-based samples serve as the basis for our most fine grained phenomenological data and virtually all of our neurobiological data.

Estimates of the lifetime risk for manic–depressive I disorder from epidemiological studies have ranged from 0.2 to 0.9% (Fremming 1951, Parsons 1965, James and Chapman 1975, Weissmann and Myers 1978, Helgason 1979). The Epidemiological Catchment Area (ECA) study found a lifetime prevalence rate of 1.2% for combined type I and type II variants (Weissmann et al. 1988); this agrees closely with the earlier study of Weissman and Myers (1978), which found 0.6% prevalence for each of the types individually. These rates are approximately tenfold greater than the prevalence rate for schizophrenia and about one-fifth that for major depressive disorder. Little is known regarding the prevalence of cyclothymic disorder.

Unlike major depressive disorder, manic–depressive disorder has an approximately equal gender distribution (Weissmann et al. 1988). Few consistent data are available regarding differences in prevalence across ethnic, cultural, or rural–urban settings. However, one of the more intriguing puzzles is the tendency of manic–depressive disorder to occur in higher socioeconomic strata than schizophrenia, which tends to aggregate in lower socioeconomic strata. Although many theories have been advanced to explain this phenomenon (Goodwin and Jamison 1990, pp. 169–174), no certain mechanism has been identified. However, several issues are clear. First, the finding is most likely not exclusively due to diagnostic bias (i.e., overdiagnosing persons of lower socioeconomic class with schizophrenia more frequently than manic–depressive disorder and the converse in persons of higher socioeconomic class). Second, the upward socioeconomic "drift" is not due to highly impaired patients "dragged" upward by higher functioning family members who are normal or who have adaptive subsyndromal manic–depressive spectrum characteristics; rather, patients themselves, at least those with type II disorder, are in many cases highly successful and occupy higher socioeconomic levels (Coryell et al. 1989). Third, the findings are not limited to the US but have been replicated in European samples as well (Lenzi et al. 1993).

Of particular interest in regard to the epidemiology of manic–depressive disorder is that the incidence of manic–depressive disorder (and depressive disorders) appears to have increased since the 1940s (Gershon et al. 1987). Reasons for this are not clear, although environmental factors, either physiological or psychosocial, may be responsible. For instance, exposure to increasingly severe social stressors, or the breakdown of cultural supports that may buffer stresses, may contribute; increases in exposure to putative environmental toxins might also be considered. In addition, in those families afflicted with manic–depressive disorder across generations, those in later generations tend to have earlier onset. This may be due to changes in genetic loading across generations or to environmental factors either within the family or in the wider environment (McInnis et al. 1993). Regardless of the cause, the increasing incidence and earlier onset of manic–depressive disorder indicate that this illness is not likely to decrease in importance as a clinical and public health issue.

## Comorbidity: The Occurrence of Manic–Depressive Disorder with Other Psychiatric Disorders

Alcohol and drug abuse and dependence represent the most consistently described and most clinically important psychiatric comorbidities with manic–depressive disorder. Whereas rates of alcohol abuse combined with alcohol dependence are from 3 to 13% in the general population, lifetime rates for alcohol dependence from ECA data indicate that they are greater than 30% in persons with manic–depressive I disorder (Regier et al. 1990). Further, ECA lifetime rates for drug dependence in individuals with manic–depressive I disorder are greater than 25% and rates for any substance abuse or dependence are above 60%. Comparable rates for alcohol, drug, or any substance abuse or dependence in major depressive disorder in ECA data are, respectively, 12, 11, and 27%. Thus, manic–depressive disorder represents an enriched sample for substance use disorders, with substantially greater rates than for the general population or even those with unipolar depression.

Recent data from the Stanley Foundation in Bipolar Research Network (McElroy et al. 2001) indicate substantially lower rates of substance use disorders (42% lifetime, 4% current), including lower rates of alcohol use disorders (33% lifetime, 2% current). However, it should be kept in mind that these rates derive from a sample that presents for care at specialty research sites that are predominantly private and/or academic centers.

The reasons for the co-occurrence of manic–depressive disorder and substance dependence are not clear. One hypothesis suggests that persons with manic–depressive disorder self-medicate with drugs or alcohol. According to this hypothesis, patients blunt the painful symptoms of depression with drugs (McLellan et al. 1985); similarly, they may heighten the manic energy with stimulants (Weiss et al. 1988). Contrarily, they may also use substances to decrease manic symptoms, particularly if the symptoms are predominantly irritable or dysphoric. Alternatively, chronic substance use may convert otherwise unipolar depression into manic–depressive disorder by inducing substance-induced manic episodes (according to DSM-IV, such persons would not be classified as having manic–depressive disorder but would be considered to have a substance-induced mood disorder) or by causing chronic central nervous system changes that change the course of the illness irreversibly, as Himmelhoch and colleagues (1976) proposed.

Finally, it is possible that some common genetic predisposition for mood instability is associated with both manic–depressive mood phenomenology and increased craving for substances, and the predominant phenotypic expression is then determined by other genetic or environmental factors. According to this hypothesis, some persons possessing the gene develop manic–depressive disorder, some develop substance dependence, and some develop both. Regardless of the mechanism, comorbid substance dependence represents an important clinical challenge for clinicians treating persons with manic–depressive disorder.

Lifetime anxiety disorders have been described in as many as 44% of individuals with manic–depressive disorder (McElroy et al. 2001). Other psychiatric comorbidities have been described in modest proportions of manic–depressive patients. Interestingly, data indicate that comorbidity may be higher in women with manic–depressive disorder than in men (Strakowski et al. 1992, 1994), which may contribute to the tendency for the female gender to be associated with more complex forms of manic–depressive disorder such as rapid cycling (Bauer and Whybrow 1993, Bauer et al. 1994c) and dysphoric mania (McElroy et al. 1992, Bauer et al. 1994a).

## Course

### Clinical Outcome, Functional Outcome, and Illness Costs

Traditionally, mental health research has focused on symptoms: how to quantitate them, what causes them, and how to reduce them. This orientation is sensible, as our professional goal is to reduce suffering, and this research orientation grows naturally out of the age-old dyadic patient–caregiver relationship. However, several developments in society at large, in biomedical treatment in general, and in mental health research in particular have led to an expansion of the purview for mental health research beyond simple symptom reduction to include understanding the impact of illness and its care on a patient's overall quality of life and how to make the best use of available resources (Stewart et al. 1989, National Institute of Mental Health 1992, Leaf 1993).

With this orientation, we can therefore conceptualize outcome in manic–depressive disorder according to three separate but interrelated domains: *clinical outcome, functional outcome,* and *illness costs.* Clinical outcome consists of parameters that measure the illness itself, such as symptom severity, episode number, and duration. Functional outcome consists of social and occupational status and subjective quality of life, areas of growing concern in both medical research (Stewart et al. 1989) and mental health research (Wells et al. 1989, Markowitz et al. 1989, Broadhead et al. 1990, National Institute of Mental Health 1992, Massion et al. 1993). Illness costs consist of both direct (treatment) costs and indirect illness costs, which include lost productivity, necessary nontreatment social supports, and nontreatment interventions such as jail and the legal system. Each domain is reviewed below.

## Clinical Outcome Studies

Manic–depressive disorder has its onset in most persons in adolescence and young adulthood, between the ages of 15 and 30. However, prepubertal mania and first-onset disease in the ninth decade of life are not unheard of. Once developed, multiple episodes are the rule. A review of the literature indicated that the majority of patients have four or more episodes in a lifetime (Goodwin and Jamison 1990). Among rapid-cycling patients, the basis for the diagnosis is four or more episodes in a year with an average of more than 50 lifetime episodes (Roy-Byrne et al. 1985). There is no typical pattern to episode recurrence, with some patients having isolated manic, hypomanic, or depressive episodes, others switching from one pole to the other in linked episodes, and still others switching continually from one pole to the other in quasi-cyclical fashion. However, even among rapid-cycling patients, episodes are rarely periodic. Rather, the pattern is more accurately described by chaotic dynamics (Angst 1981, Gottschalk et al. 1995).

Episode length typically ranges from 4 to 13 months, with depressive episodes typically longer than manic or hypomanic episodes (Goodwin and Jamison 1990, p. 40). Women appear to have more depressive relapses than manic ones, whereas men have a more even distribution (Angst 1978). Also women predominate among rapid-cycling patients, representing 70 to 90% in most studies (Bauer and Whybrow 1993, Bauer et al. 1994c).

Early estimations of outcome in manic–depressive disorder were by and large optimistic, based on two types of data. First, manic–depressive disorder had been separated from *dementia praecox* (schizophrenia) by Kraepelin (1989) on the basis of relatively favorable outcome in terms of remitting versus chronic course of psychosis. Subsequent comparative studies, up until the present day, have found manic–depressive disorder to have better outcome than schizophrenia in terms of many parameters, including chronicity of symptoms, severity of impairment, and social and occupational function (Lundquist 1945, Petterson 1977, Tsuang et al. 1979, Broctington et al. 1983, Williams and McGlashon 1987). Second, tremendous optimism accompanied the introduction of lithium treatment for manic–depressive disorder in the 1960s.

However, this relatively optimistic view, which derived primarily from experience in controlled clinical trials, contrasts with the overall guarded prognosis described by most longitudinal studies in the last 3 decades, which have been less controlled but more inclusive than formal clinical trials. In the early studies, 62% of manic–depressive patients had equivocal to poor outcome (Levinstein et al. 1966) and 45%

of manic patients were chronically ill 6 years after hospitalization (Bratfos and Haug 1968). Another study found only 14.3% to be "well in every way" (Winokur et al. 1969) and another later study found only 24% in "full remission" during follow-up (Tohen et al. 1990).

Although these studies include data from the prelithium era, more recent studies from the lithium era are not terribly reassuring. Approximately 20 to 40% of patients with manic–depressive disorder do not respond well to lithium (Prien and Gelenberg 1989), and that proportion may increase to as much as 80% for certain subgroups such as patients who experience rapid-cycling pattern (Dunner and Fieve 1974, Maj et al. 1989) or mixed manic and depressive episodes (Keller et al. 1986a). When assessed 1.5 years after index hospitalization, between 7 and 32% of manic–depressive patients remain chronically ill, depending on polarity of index episode (Keller et al. 1986a). Only 26% of one sample had good outcome after hospitalization for mania, whereas 40% had moderate and 34% had poor outcome (Harrow et al. 1990). The probability of remaining ill at 1, 2, 3, and 4 years after hospitalization for mania was, respectively, 51, 44, 33, and 28% (Tohen et al. 1990). Sixty percent of an ambulatory sample of manic–depressive patients had fair to poor outcome based on a global outcome score after 1-year follow-up (O'Connell et al. 1991).

Relatively little is known regarding clinical outcome in manic–depressive type II patients (Goodwin and Jamison 1990), although they appear to be at least as impaired in terms of relapse as manic–depressive type I patients. For instance, 70% of manic–depressive II patients followed up for 5 years experienced multiple relapses, whereas only 11% were episode free (Coryell et al. 1989).

Subsyndromal affective symptoms may remain in up to 13 to 34% (Harrow et al. 1990), and substantial interepisode morbidity may remain despite adequate treatment with lithium (Nilsson and Axelsson 1989). It is not clear whether such interepisode pathology represents incompletely resolved major affective episodes, medication side effects, demoralization due to functional impairment, or a combination of these factors (Welner et al. 1977, Nilsson and Axelsson 1989, Gitlin et al. 1989). It should be noted here that side effects are more than a trivial issue, as they may lead to medication discontinuation in 18 to 53%, a figure that is greater in lower socioeconomic classes (Goodwin and Jamison 1990). Thus, clinical outcome in manic–depressive disorder is heterogeneous, and lithium has not proved to be a panacea.

## Functional Outcome Studies

Substantial levels of functional impairment are also characteristic of manic–depressive disorder, even when major clinical indices have improved. The book-length study of manic–depressive patients in the prelithium era by Winokur and colleagues (1969) documented their sample's functional impairment in detail. For instance, 79% of those employed before their index episode lost their jobs during that episode. Among those with incomplete remission during follow-up, 73% had long-term decrements in occupational status. Even more striking, 25% of those with complete remissions or only infrequent episodes developed similar occupational decrements. In another early study, 60% had less than satisfactory social recovery (Hastings 1958).

In a study of persons with manic–depressive disorder treated at the National Institute of Mental Health (NIMH), only 41% had returned to their jobs at 3 years of follow-up, and 15% were totally unemployed. Forty-five percent had normal family and social function, 21% evidenced "complete social withdrawal," and 11% "complete family disruption" (Carlson et al. 1974). On global outcome assessment, 57% were judged recovered, 10% had intermittent episodes, and 28% were functionally impaired with moderate to severe affective symptoms. Dion and coworkers (1988) found that although 80% of their sample of manic–depressive patients became symptom free by 6 months after an index major affective episode, only 43% were employed and only 21% were employed at preepisode levels. Harrow and colleagues (1990) found at 1.7 years of prospective follow-up after an index manic episode that 23% of patients were continuously unemployed, with 36% underemployed in comparison to preepisode levels. Occupational function was significantly worse than in a comparison group of depressive patients without history of mania. In addition, 36% showed at least moderate impairment in social function. These deficits were unrelated to the presence of symptoms, with the exception of psychosis, which was associated with profound impairment. Tohen and coworkers (1990) found 28% of subjects unemployed after index hospitalization for mania. Bauwens and associates (1991) found that levels of functional disability correlated both with number of prior episodes and with residual interepisode psychopathology.

Five-year follow-up data from the NIMH Collaborative Program on the Psychobiology of Depression (Coryell et al. 1989) provide evidence that levels of impairment in manic–depressive type I and type II disorders are similar. This included similarly fair to very poor work (in 30 and 42% of patients with types I and II, respectively), marital (30 and 23%), social (45 and 45%), and recreational (45 and 48%) function; sense of satisfaction or contentment (57 and 62%); and overall social adjustment (68 and 62%). More recent analysis of that data set has revealed enduring deficits in educational and occupational status at 5 years of follow-up in a mixed group of manic–depressive and unipolar patients, even in those who were recovered for 2 years (Coryell et al. 1993). This led the authors to comment succinctly: "Follow-up studies have usually defined recovery as the absence of symptoms. The present findings show that this convention may result in an overly benign portrayal of outcome" (Coryell et al. 1993, pp. 726).

Much less is known about which characteristics predict functional deficits in manic–depressive disorder, an issue of some importance in identifying high-risk groups for particular attention. A recent review (Bauer and Whybrow 2001) indicates, surprisingly, that baseline demographic and functional outcome do not predict future functional outcome. However ongoing depressive symptoms, even to a mild degree, are strongly associated with ongoing functional deficits. The direction of causability is not clear, however. It is plausible that depressive symptoms render individuals less able to function in work and personal roles. It is equally plausible that unemployment, divorce, social isolation, and the like can cause or exacerbate depressive symptoms. In fact, both are likely. In any event, careful attention to functional deficits, depressive symp-

toms, and their interplay is important to optimizing care and hopefully outcome.

## Personal and Societal Costs of Manic–Depressive Disorder

Although there are as yet few available data regarding direct and indirect illness costs for manic–depressive disorder, the direct treatment costs of manic–depressive disorder are substantial. Among the major mental disorders, the rate of hospitalization for manic–depressive disorder is exceeded only by that for schizophrenia (Klerman et al. 1992). If one can extrapolate to manic–depressive patients from the data for aggregate mental illness costs (McGuire 1991), 55% of treatment costs derive from public sector services and 45% from the private sector.

It is also clear that substantial loss of productivity, in addition to personal suffering, may occur in manic–depressive disorder. In mental illness in general, functional impairment was responsible for 55% of the costs of nonaddictive mental illness in the US in 1986 (Rice et al. 1990). In 1955, the figure was 39% (Fein 1958). Although these figures are derived from different methodologies and assumptions and may not be directly comparable (McGuire 1991), both studies indicate that functional impairment accounts for a substantial component of mental illness costs. It is even more striking that the functional impairment may be responsible for as much as 75% of the costs of affective illness (Stoudemire et al. 1986). Specifically in manic–depressive disorder, evidence indicates that costs from lost productivity are substantial as well. For instance, 19% of persons with manic–depressive disorder attempt suicide at some time in their lives (Klerman et al. 1992), thus placing almost one-fifth of persons with manic–depressive disorder at high risk of loss of life through this one cause alone. Without adequate treatment, a person with manic–depressive disorder from age 25 years can expect to lose 14 years of effective major activity (e.g., work, school, family role function) and 9 years of life (US Department of Health, Education, and Welfare 1979). The indirect costs of this disorder are also high, because 15% of persons with manic–depressive disorder are unemployed for at least 5 consecutive years and more than 25% of those younger than age 65 years receive disability payments (Klerman 1992). Therefore, it stands to reason that treatments targeted at reducing functional impairment, as well as clinical outcome, can have a substantial impact on the burden of mental illness costs to society and quality of life for the individual and her or his family (National Institute of Mental Health 1992).

## Rating Scales

A plethora of rating scales is available for assessing manic and depressive symptoms, and associated features such as psychosis, functional status, and health care costs. For general information, the reader is referred to the recent compilations of rating scales by the APA (American Psychiatric Association Task Force for the Handbook of Psychiatric Measures 2000). For clinical usage, clinicians rating scales in general use for depression can also be used for depressive episodes in manic–depressive disorder. Most share in the shortcoming of tending to underrate hypersomnia, hyperphagia, and weight gain, "atypical" features that are common in manic–depressive disorder. Among mania scales, the Young Mania Rating Scale (Young et al. 1978, 1983) is well validated on outpatients as well as inpatients, and for hypomanic as well as manic episodes.

Self-report scales have the advantage of being brief (typically 5 minutes) and amenable to frequent, even daily, usage without undue burden. However, there have been questions about their reliability and validity, particularly in severely ill manic patients, although one instrument, the Internal State Scale (Bauer et al. 1991) has demonstrated reasonable psychometric properties across several replications (Cooke et al. 1996, Bauer et al. 2000).

## Treatment*

### General Considerations

Traditionally, treatment for manic–depressive disorder has been categorized as acute versus prophylaxis, or maintenance; that is, treatment geared toward resolution of a specific episode versus continued treatment to prevent further symptoms. Treatment can also be considered along several other lines (Table 64–8). For instance, interventions can be categorized as somatotherapy (pharmacotherapy, ECT, and light treatment) and psychotherapy. In addition, treatment can be categorized according to intensity. The division into inpatient versus outpatient treatment is becoming more and more blurred as partial or day hospital programs and intensive ambulatory treatment coupled with night hospital programs or respite beds become more popular.

In general, more structured treatment settings, such as full or partial hospitalization, are indicated if patients are likely to endanger self or others, if manic–depressive disorder is complicated by other medical or psychiatric illnesses that make ambulatory management particularly dangerous, or if more aggressive management is desired than is easily available on an ambulatory basis (e.g., intensive psychosocial intervention or rapid dosage titration of

| Table 64–8 | Classification Schemata for Manic–Depressive Disorder Treatment and Its Goals |
| --- | --- |

1. Acute versus maintenance
2. Somatic versus psychotherapeutic
3. The intensity-of-care continuum*
   A. Full hospitalization
   B. Partial or day hospitalization
   C. Night hospitalization or respite beds
   D. Ambulatory care
4. Categorization by goal
   A. Improve clinical outcome
   B. Improve functional outcome
   C. Improve host factors
     i. Illness management skills
     ii. Medical and psychiatric comorbidities

*Indications for increased intensity of care: danger to self or others; complicating medical or psychiatric comorbidities; aggressive medication titration; social factors that compromise treatment.

---

*For a complete discussion of this topic, see Bauer and McBride 2002; of how to use various psychopharmacologic agents, see Bauer 2003.

psychotropic agents). In addition, although it is frequently an afterthought in textbooks, social factors play an important role in the decision to hospitalize in the real world of clinical psychiatry. Such reasons may include lack of social support to ensure medication compliance during acute illness, social stresses aggravating symptoms and making treatment compliance difficult (e.g., manipulative or hostile living situation), or lack of transportation to accommodate frequent ambulatory appointments during acute illness. Unfortunately, it is sometimes the case, although less frequent in this era of managed care, that a person's insurance plan covers inpatient but not ambulatory mental health treatment, forcing expensive inpatient care when less costly, time-limited, intensive ambulatory care would suffice.

Finally, treatment can be categorized according to its goals. Following our conceptual approach from the previous section, treatment can be focused on improving clinical outcome (episodes and symptoms) or functional outcome (social and occupational function and health-related quality of life). Although this categorization appears straightforward, clinical practice reveals many subtleties. For instance, it is erroneous to assume that clinical outcome is the domain of pharmacotherapy and that functional outcome is the domain of psychotherapy. In actuality, most psychotherapies by design focus on improving symptoms. Likewise, pharmacotherapeutic stabilization of symptoms clearly contributes to improved role function. Further, treatments that improve one domain may cause decrements in another. For instance, effective maintenance treatment with lithium may come at the cost of hand tremor, which interfere with work function and causes embarrassment in social situations.

Balancing the costs and benefits of various specific treatments—and every somatic and psychotherapeutic treatment has both costs and benefits—requires active participation of the patients and, if available, the families (Bauer and McBride 2002). Compassionate psychoeducation and alliance building are integral goals of each form of treatment. In analogy to infectious disease treatment, attention to such host factors can often make the difference between success and failure of treatment.

### The "Efficacy–Effectiveness Gap"

Great optimism justifiably accompanied the introduction of lithium in the 1960s, with the drug projected to save society millions of dollars in direct and indirect treatment costs (Reifman and Wyatt 1980). However, there are reasons to be concerned that lithium has made much less of an impact than originally projected, and there is clear evidence that manic–depressive disorder remains a major health concern, even with the addition of anticonvulsants to our armamentarium.

For example, readmission rates for manic–depressive disorder may be as high as 90% during 2-year follow-up, with no difference between lithium-treated and nontreated patients (Markar and Mandar 1989). Overall, the impact of lithium "under ordinary clinical conditions" (Dickson and Kendall 1986) appears to be much less than would be expected from results of randomized clinical trials (Symonds and Williams 1981, Parker et al. 1985, Mander 1989).

How can these data be reconciled with early estimates projecting dramatic decreases in treatment costs due to the introduction of lithium? (Reifman and Wyatt 1980). Presumably, the medications themselves do not differ between controlled clinical trials and general clinical practice. If anything, the diffusion over time of the new pharmacological technology into general clinical practice might be expected to lead to further gains in illness management beyond those initially seen. The use of several anticonvulsants such as carbamazepine, valproic acid, and lamotrigine in the treatment of manic–depressive disorder holds promise for further improvement in outcome. For instance, these drugs may have *efficacy* in controlled clinical trials, but concerns regarding the *effectiveness* of lithium in clinical practice also apply to the use of these anticonvulsants.

What, then, are the sources of this *efficacy–effectiveness gap* (Institute of Medicine 1985) in the treatment of manic–depressive disorder? It is likely that the gap is in part due to the exclusion of "complicated" manic–depressive patients from clinical trials (e.g., those with substance abuse, personality disorders, or medical problems) and those unwilling to risk exposure to placebo. Although such exclusions are appropriate for establishing the efficacy of potential treatments, the exclusivity of structured clinical trials limits their relevance in the general clinical setting. For example, with regard to lithium, a review of cases from one academic center found that only a minority of patients were able to be maintained with lithium monotherapy in their practice (Sachs et al. 1994); although this may be an atypical treatment setting in that it is an academic center, many public sector clinics anecdotally report similar patterns.

Another likely contributor to the efficacy–effectiveness gap is variation in provider attributes such as attitudes and capabilities. For instance, it is well established that even at academic medical centers, the intensity of medication treatment for mood disorders is much less than that which experts consider optimal (Keller et al. 1986b). It is possible, then, that supporting providers with specific data regarding treatment options will aid in decreasing the efficacy–effectiveness gap. With this in mind, several organizations have developed clinical practice guideline to assist providers. Prominent clinical practice guidelines for manic–depressive disorder include those from the American Psychiatric Association (1994b), the Texas Department of Mental Health and Mental Retardation (Gilbert et al. 1998, Rush et al. 1999), the Canadian Psychiatric Association (Haslam et al. 1997), and a group of experts supported by unrestricted grants from the pharmaceutical industry (Kahn et al. 1997, Sachs et al. 2000).

It has also been recognized that the organization and orientation of caregiving systems may not optimally support and may even inhibit appropriate care, thereby contributing to the efficacy–effectiveness gap. These concerns have led medical and mental health researchers and clinicians to consider the organization of caregiving systems as an object of study in its own right. An area of developing research to address these issues focuses on development and evaluation of disease manage programs, similar to those for managing chronic medical illnesses such as diabetes or hypertension (Wagner et al. 1996, Von Korff et al. 1997). Such programs are typically organized around "collaborative practice" principles that focus on optimizing patient participation in treatment while reducing system- and provider-derived barriers (Bauer 2001a, Bauer et al. 1997, 2002, Simon et al. 2002).

## Somatotherapy

### Efficacious Agents for Various Phases of Manic–Depressive Disorder

The introduction of lithium for the treatment of manic–depressive disorder in the 1960s revolutionized management of the illness. Before that, manic–depressive disorder was managed with treatment targeted only toward resolution of individual episodes: antidepressants and ECT for depressive episodes and neuroleptics and occasionally ECT for mania. In contrast, not only did lithium provide an additional treatment for acute mania and depression in manic–depressive disorder, it was also demonstrated to have substantial prophylactic, or preventive, effects on both manic and depressive episodes. While additional information can be found on specific agents in other chapters of this textbook (Chapters 96 and 97), an overview of efficacy and side effect data is provided here. The reader is also referred to an extensive summary in the book by Bauer and McBride (2002).

Over the past 10 years medications have proliferated for the treatment of various phases of the disorder. The clinician must pick through an array of scientific data and marketing claims in order to choose the appropriate treatment. Two conceptual approaches help in this task.

First, available scientific data can be reviewed and evaluated according to the techniques of "evidence-based medicine." For instance, quantitative techniques such as meta-analysis provide numeric conclusions with regard to significance of similar interventions in diverse studies (Irwig et al. 1994). More qualitative techniques of evidence-based medicine (EBWG 1992, Chalmers 1993, ACC/AHA 1996) have been used in reviewing and summarizing treatment interventions in medicine and more recently in mental health. Briefly, these techniques consist of comprehensively identifying relevant data-based articles, summarizing their methods and conclusions, and then in a standardized fashion rating the scientific quality of the evidence based on the rigor of their methodology. In the 1980s, the US Agency for Healthcare Research and Quality (AHRQ) (formerly the Agency for Health Care Policy and Research; AHCPR) developed guidelines for the identification and treatment of depression in primary care using techniques of evidence-based medicine (AHCPR 1993). This basic system was adapted by the US Department of Veterans Affairs for developing their treatment guidelines for a wide variety of medical, surgical, and psychiatric disorders (VHA 1997, Bauer et al. 1999). Evidence-based techniques of one type or another also serve as the basis for guidelines from the American Psychiatric Association(1994b), the Canadian Psychiatric Association (Haslam et al. 1997), and the Texas Department of Mental Health and Mental Retardation (Gilbert et al. 1998, Rush et al. 1999); however, not all guidelines are evidence-based in this sense (Kahn et al. 1997, Sachs et al. 2000). We have found the evidence-based medicine approach useful to classify studies by quality of data in doing our reviews both of pharmacologic and psychotherapeutic interventions for manic–depressive dis-

| Table 64–9 | AHCPR/AHRQ Evidence Classification System* |
| --- | --- |
| Class A: | Randomized or other controlled trials<br>Examples: Randomized controlled trials of intervention versus waiting list control or no added treatment; other controlled trials with treatment assignment independent of subject characteristic, time of presentation, etc. |
| Class B: | Well-designed clinical studies<br>Examples: Open studies with a priori design and follow-up period of designated endpoint; pre/post mirror-image studies with "post" period designed a priori. |
| Class C: | Case series, case reports, retrospective chart reviews.<br>Examples: Prospectively gathered data on a series of patients followed in treatment; retrospective chart review after implementation of an intervention. |

*Source: Adapted from AHCPR (Agency for Health Care Policy and Research) (1993) Depression Panel Guideline Report. US Government Printing Office, Washington DC.

| Table 64–11 | Summary of Class A Efficacy Data for Treating the Various Phases of Manic–Depressive Disorder* (At Least 2 Placebo-Controlled Trials) | |
| --- | --- | --- |
| | Mania | Depression |
| Acute | Lithium<br>Carbamazepine<br>Valproate<br>Olanzapine<br>Verapamil | Lithium<br>Lamotrigine |
| Prophylaxis | Lithium | Lithium |

*Source: Summarized from Bauer MS and McBride L (2002) Structured group psychotherapy for manic–depressive disorder: The life goals program, 2nd ed. Springer-Verlag New York.

order. AHCPR/AHRQ system for evidence classification can be found in Table 64–9.

The second conceptual approach that we have found useful is to propose an explicit definition for the term "mood stabilizer" and evaluate the role of various medications against this definition. The US Food and Drug Administration (FDA) does not formally define the term, but it stands to reason that an agent would be optimally useful for treatment of manic–depressive disorder if it had efficacy in four roles: (a) treatment of acute manic symptoms, (b) treatment of acute depressive symptoms, (c) prophylaxis of manic symptoms, and (d) prophylaxis of depressive symptoms. This approach leads to the conceptual 2 × 2 table illustrated in Table 64–10. Agents used in manic–depressive disorder can be listed in any or all of the four boxes in the table in which they have proven efficacy, and according to this schema an agent may be categorized as a mood stabilizer if it can be listed as having efficacy in each of the four boxes.

We have reviewed the available peer-reviewed literature on treatment trials for four types in manic depressive disorder published in December 2001, as summarized in detail elsewhere (Bauer and McBride 2002). Following the FDA lead of considering an agent to have efficacy with at least two such positive trials, we have listed the agents according to the revised 2 × 2 table in Table 64–11. Complete analysis to date can be found in Bauer and McBride (2002).

As can be seen, at least two placebo-controlled Class A studies support the antimanic efficacy of lithium (Maggs 1963, Bunney et al. 1968, Goodwin et al. 1969, Stokes et al.

| Table 64–10 | Organizing Efficacy Evidence: The Mood Stabilizer 2 × 2 Table | |
| --- | --- | --- |
| | Mania | Depression |
| Acute | | |
| Prophylaxis | | |

1971), carbamazepine (Ballenger 1978, 1980), valproate (Emrich et al. 1980, Pope et al. 1991, Bowden et al. 1994), olanzapine (Tohen 1999, 2000), and verapamil (Giannini et al. 1984, Dubovsky 1986). There are additional Class A controlled trials (nonplacebo-controlled) that support efficacy for multiple older, typical neuroleptics as well as the benzodiazepines, lorazepam, and clonazepam.

In contrast to evidence regarding acute mania, evidence is scarce concerning efficacy of specific agents for acute depressive episodes. Most treatment is undertaken primarily by extension from treatment experience in unipolar depression. While a comprehensive discussion of evidence for efficacy of various antidepressants in unipolar depression is clearly beyond the scope of this chapter, it has been amply reviewed in several references (Gareri et al. 2000, Thase and Sachs 2000) including Chapter 97 in this book. Efficacy data from two or more Class A studies exist only for lithium (Fieve et al. 1968, Goodwin et al. 1969, 1972, Baron et al. 1975, Mendels 1976) and lamotrigine (Calabrese et al. 1999, Bowden et al. 1999). Support for the efficacy of valproate and carbamazepine in acute depressive episodes in manic–depressive disorder is notably lacking.

In reviewing studies of agents for the prophylaxis of manic or depressive symptoms, we discovered that most of the studies reported recurrence rates without distinguishing between manic and depressive symptoms. For instance, some studies reported such statistics as time-to-first-episode without specifying whether the first episode was manic or depressed. Other studies reported summary statistics for affective symptoms without separating manic or depressive symptoms. We found that when studies did report specific polarity of symptoms during recurrence, it was infrequent that they reported impact of treatment on recurrence of depressive symptoms. Far and away, the most placebo-controlled support for any prophylactic agent comes from studies of lithium (Baastrup and Schou 1967, Coppen et al. 1971, Cundall et al. 1972, Stallone et al. 1973, Prien et al. 1973a, 1973b, Fieve et al. 1976, Dunner et al. 1976) including studies of relapse prevention for depression (Fieve et al. 1976, Stallone et al. 1973, Kane et al. 1982), with support from controlled trials that are not placebo-controlled for carbamazepine and lamotrigine. The one prophylaxis study of valproate (Bowden et al. 2000) showed no difference from placebo (lithium was also found to be no different from placebo in this study, although the study was underpowered to make definitive conclusions about this comparison).

Thus, in summary, this standardized evidence-based review of available treatments for manic–depressive disorder indicates that, to date, only lithium fulfills the stringent definition of a mood stabilizer. It is hoped that additional agents soon take their place in the ranks based on high quality data.

It may be surprising that, given the paucity of data on treatment of acute depression and prophylaxis of manic–depressive disorder, we frequently encounter many other medications used chronically in this illness, sometimes as first-time agents, for instance, valproate, carbamazepine. Although neuroleptics have acute antimanic evidence, despite the fact that there is little evidence for prophylactic efficacy, they are often used chronically. This is because these agents are typically started during the course of an acute manic episode and clinicians are loathe to stop them and switch to a different agent such as lithium. In addition, many individuals have failed or have been intolerant of treatment with lithium and they are therefore treated using the "next best thing." This is not necessarily suboptimal treatment. However, it is important that the clinician recognize that data on long-term prophylactic efficacy is quite scanty for these agents—as it is for many other agents used in psychiatric practice.

Several additional issues in prophylaxis of manic–depressive disorder deserve comment. First, when is lifetime, or at least long-term, prophylaxis warranted? After one manic episode? One hypomanic episode? One depressive episode with a strong family history of manic–depressive disorder? There is insufficient empirical evidence with which to make strong recommendations, although a creative study by Zarin and Pass (1987) using computer-based modeling investigated tradeoffs of treatment versus observation based on costs and benefits of recurrence risks and drug side effects under several strategies. In clinical practice without clear guidelines, such decisions need to take into account the capability of the patient and family in reporting symptoms, rapidity of onset of episodes, episode severity, and associated morbidity. Clearly, the risks of a wait-and-see strategy would be different in a person who had a psychotic manic episode than in a person who had mild hypomania.

Second, can lithium ever be discontinued? Again, there are no solid data on which to base this decision. However, if lithium discontinuation is contemplated, there is evidence that rapid discontinuation (in less than 2 weeks) is more likely to result in relapse than slow taper (2–4 weeks), with relapse rates higher in type I than in type II patients (Faedda et al. 1993, Suppes et al. 1993). In type I patients, relapse rates for rapid discontinuation versus slow taper were, respectively, 96 and 73%, whereas in type II patients they were 91 and 33% (Faedda et al. 1993). There is some theoretical concern, based on a report of four patients, that patients in whom lithium has been discontinued may not be recaptured by resumption of lithium (Post et al. 1992), but these are preliminary observations on a sample from the NIMH that may not be representative of persons with manic–depressive disorder seen in general clinical practice.

Third, a set sequence of treatment for refractory manic–depressive disorder has yet to be established. In particular, persons with rapid cycling represent a treatment dilemma (Bauer 1994). Although antidepressants may induce rapid cycling, they often leave the person in a protracted, severe depression. Switching from one antimanic agent to another often results in resumption of cycling. Complex treatment strategies may be required, such as anticonvulsants plus lithium, combinations of anticonvulsants, or adjuvant treatment with high doses of the thyroid hormone thyroxine.

## A Simple Treatment Algorithm for Manic–Depressive Disorder

A treatment algorithm for refractory manic–depressive disorder, including strategies to deal with rapid cycling is found in Figure 64–2. It is derived from clinical practice guidelines from the USVA and, by design, primarily specifies drug classes rather than individual agents. The entry point for this algorithm is the occurrence of any major mood episode (depression, hypomania, mania, or mixed episode) in an unmedicated patient. Patients with recurrence on medications may enter the algorithm at the appropriate point along the flow diagram. For simplicity of presentation, only depressive and cycling outcomes are illustrated. This is because depressive episodes are more common than manic or hypomanic episodes, and all but the most refractory of the latter episodes are relatively easily treated by the addition (or resumption) of lithium or anticonvulsants or the use of neuroleptics, as summarized above.

## Balancing Beneficial and Unwanted Effects of Medications

All psychotropic medications have side effects. Some are actually desirable (e.g., sedation with some antidepressants in persons with prominent insomnia), and specific medications are often chosen on the basis of desired side effects. However, side effects usually represent factors that decrease a patient's quality of life and compromise compliance. Reviews of side effects of antidepressants and neuroleptics can be found in the chapters on depression and schizophrenia, respectively. It should be recalled in regard to antidepressants, however, that all can cause rapid cycling and mixed states in persons with manic–depressive disorder. These effects are not uncommonly encountered in clinical practice and should be watched for, even in persons taking mood-stabilizing agents.

Extensive reviews of side effects of the agents most commonly encountered in the treatment of manic–depressive disorder are available elsewhere in this text (Chapters 95, 96, and 97), in books by Bauer and colleagues (Bauer and McBride 2002, Bauer 2003), Hyman and coworkers (1995), Schatzberg and coworkers (1997), and Ellsworth and coworkers (2001). It is also worth noting that electronic references are also proliferating, both for the desktop computer (www.Medscape.com) and for hand-held devices (www. ePocrates.com). Several excellent review articles have summarized side effects of lithium (Gitlin et al. 1989, Goodwin and Jamison 1990, p. 701–709) and the various anticonvulsants (Swann 2001) including carbamazepine (Ketter and Post 1994), and sodium valproate (Keck et al. 1994), and lamotrigine (Botts and Raskind 1999) are also readily available.

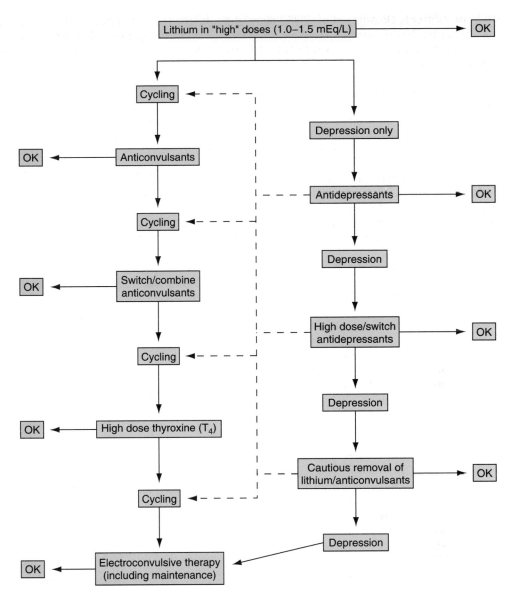

**Figure 64–2** *Treatment algorithm for manic–depressive disorder. (Source: Reprinted from Bauer MS [1994] Rapid cycling. In Anticonvulsants in Mood Disorders, Joffe RT and Calabrese JR [eds]. Marcel Dekker, New York, pp. 1–26.) Note: Refractory mania is relatively rare. This general algorithm addresses the more common clinical scenarios of depression and rapid cycling.*

A brief overview of the most frequent or important side effects of lithium, carbamazepine, and valproic acid can be found in Table 64–12a–c. Note that some side effects may be encountered at any serum level of the drug, even within the therapeutic range. Some side effects may be dose-related even within that range and may respond to dosage reduction. Others are more idiosyncratic and may need other management, as detailed in a subsequent section. Note that not all laboratory findings represent pathological processes that are associated with or presage morbidity for the patient; that is, not all are clinically significant.

Note also that the concept of the "therapeutic level" is not as straightforward as we would like to assume. The lower limit is usually established by the lowest level necessary for therapeutic effect, whereas the upper limit is set by the lowest level associated with regular, significant toxicity. This range is never established with complete precision. For some medications such as lithium, the therapeutic window is actually quite narrow, with toxic effects developing with some regularity after the upper limit of the therapeutic

range is surpassed and with serious toxicity developing at only modestly higher serum levels. As a further complication, for many persons the minimum level of lithium for good response may be substantially above the 0.5 to 0.8 mEq/L that is usually set as the lower therapeutic limit, but this is reached only at the cost of increased incidence of side effects (Gelenberg et al. 1989). On the other hand, experience with valproic acid, the upper limit of the therapeutic range for mood stabilization may actually be 125 mg/dL rather than the listed range of 100 mg/dL usually accepted for antiepileptic effect, and this level may be reached without undue side effects (Keck et al. 1994).

Thus, established therapeutic levels should be used as important guidelines, and exceeding therapeutic levels should be done only with careful monitoring. However, one must not be falsely reassured that reaching the lower level of a therapeutic range is equally effective for all patients, while taking with a grain of salt the upper limits of the therapeutic range in drugs with a wider therapeutic window.

| Table 64–12a | Side Effects of Lithium and Commonly Used Anticonvulsants, I: Life-Threatening | | |
|---|---|---|---|
| | At Therapeutic Levels | | At Toxic Levels |
| | Idiopathic | Dose-Related | Dose-Related |
| Lithium | | | Renal failure<br>Encephalopathy |
| CBZ | Agranulocytosis*<br>Aplastic anemia*<br>Stevens–Johnson* | | |
| VPA | Hepatic necrosis | Thrombocytopenia | Thrombocytopenia |
| LMT | Stevens–Johnson* | | |

*Typically during first 1–6 months of treatment.

| Table 64–12b | Side Effects of Lithium and Commonly Used Anticonvulsants, II: Clinically Significant Side Effects | | | |
|---|---|---|---|---|
| | Lithium | CBZ | VPA | LMT |
| Neurologic/muscular | Lethargy<br>Memory (anomia)<br>Tremor*<br>Myoclonus | Lethargy<br>Blurred vision<br><br>Ataxia* | Lethargy<br>Depression<br>Tremor*<br>Ataxia | Lethargy<br>Ataxia<br>Blurred vision<br>Headache |
| Endocrine/metabolic | Weight gain*<br>Hypothyroidism | | Weight gain* | |
| Cardiopulmonary | | | | |
| Hematologic | | | Thrombocytopenia | |
| Renal | Polyuria | | | |
| Hepatic | | Jaundice | Jaundice | |
| Gastrointestinal | Nausea*<br>Diarrhea* | Nausea* | Nausea* | Nausea* |
| Dermatologic | Maculopapular rash<br>Psoriasis<br>Acne | Maculopapular rash<br>Alopecia | Maculopapular rash | Maculopapular rash |
| Other | | | Back pain | |

*Most common reasons in our experience for noncompliance.

| Table 64–12c | Side Effects of Lithium and Commonly Used Anticonvulsants, III: Subclinical Laboratory Abnormalities | | | |
|---|---|---|---|---|
| | Lithium | CBZ | VPA | LMT |
| Neurologic/muscular | | | | |
| Endocrine/metabolic | Increased TSH | Decreased FTI | | |
| Cardiopulmonary | EKG T-wave depression | | | |
| Hematologic | Leukocytosis<br>(to 20,000) | Leukopenia | Thrombocytopenia<br>(OK > 20,000) | |
| Renal | Decreased<br>urine specific gravity, GFR | | | |
| Hepatic | | Increased LFTs | Increased LFTs | |

Another important issue to consider is drug–drug interactions, which may lead to side effects (see Bauer 2003 for a comprehensive review). Such interactions are often associated with increases in serum levels of the drug of interest. For example, addition of thiazide diuretics, or nonsteroidal anti-inflammatory agents, the latter available over the counter, is a common reason for increase in lithium level and development of toxicity. Drug–drug interactions for anticonvulsants have been reviewed in the references above. However, at other times the drug–drug interactions may not be reflected in an increased serum level if the main interaction is displacement of protein-bound drug. Because free drug concentrations are usually 1 to 10% of total serum drug, a displacement of even 50% of bound drug may be associated with negligible if any changes in total serum level. However, since both therapeutic and toxic effects are due to free, not bound, drug, unwanted side effects may develop despite total drug levels measured in the therapeutic range.

## Guiding Principles of Managing Side Effects

As noted previously, some side effects may be desirable. However, in many cases they are impediments to treatment, frequently of sufficient importance to lead to noncompliance (Jamison et al. 1979). As clinicians, however, we might reframe the noncompliance issue more appropriately as "insufficient provider–patient cost-benefit analysis." Stressing compliance when a person suffers from significant side effects is usually much less effective than working to set appropriate expectations of the patient and to find a regimen of minimal toxicity. Goodwin and Jamison's (1990, p. 672) point that managing side effects is as much psychotherapeutic as medical is well taken in this regard.

Nonetheless, the astute psychiatrist does have several strategies available to improve patients' tolerance of medications. First, dose reduction may be achieved without compromising efficacy in some patients. Some side effects, such as lithium-induced nausea, usually respond well to this, whereas others, such as lithium-induced memory loss, improve less reliably.

Second, simple changes in preparation may be helpful, such as using enteric-coated lithium. Uncoated valproic acid causes nausea so frequently that only the coated forms are routinely used; however, the pediatric "sprinkle" preparation may be of some benefit in persons with nausea even with enteric-coated valproic acid.

Third, changing the administration schedule may ameliorate side effects. Commonsense strategies such as taking nausea-inducing medications after a meal should not be overlooked. Single daily dosing of lithium, carbamazepine, or valproic acid may decrease daytime sedation without compromising efficacy. For more obscure reasons, single daily dosing of lithium appears to decrease polyuria quite effectively (Bowen et al. 1991).

Fourth, addition of medications to counteract side effects can sometimes be the only way to continue treatment. Addition of beta-blockers can reduce lithium- or valproic acid-induced tremors. Judicious use of thiazide diuretics, often in conjunction with potassium-sparing diuretics or potassium supplements, can reduce lithium-induced polyuria.

Finally, change to another drug may be the only alternative. This is clearly indicated in the case of serious allergic reactions. Polypharmacy should be avoided wherever possible.

## Psychotherapies

Since the first edition of this textbook, one of the fastest moving areas of research in manic–depressive disorder has been psychotherapy. It is important to note that psychotherapy has been studied almost exclusively in the context of ongoing medication management, rather than as a substitute for, or alternative to, medication treatment. Rather, psychotherapy has been utilized as an adjuvant treatment to optimize outcome in the illness. Psychotherapy has been viewed as having one or more of several roles in the management of the disorder.

Recall that both somatic therapies and psychotherapies to date have been predominantly oriented toward improving clinical outcome. Under this conceptualization psychotherapy has been thought to directly address symptoms, such as cognitive therapy for depressive symptoms. Less frequently has psychotherapy been developed with an explicit component geared toward addressing the functional deficits in manic–depressive disorder. However, functional outcome has often been measured in formal trials of various types of psychotherapy. A third conceptualization has been to use psychotherapy as a predominantly educative method to assist patients in participating more effectively in treatment. In this latter regard, treatment is geared toward improving "host factors," that is, those factors not directly due to the disease but that have an impact on its course or treatment, through education, support, and problem solving. Such host factors include illness management skills, which may be improved through psychoeducation and attention to building the therapeutic alliance. Basics of education are summarized in Table 64–13.

**Table 64–13  Basics of Education to Improve Disease Management Skills**

### 1. Principles

A. Gear education to educational, cultural, motivational factors of individuals and their families.
B. Include both knowledge about the disorder in general and exploration of the individual's specific form of illness and how it affects their own life.
C. Pay close attention to opportunities for destigmatization and demystification.
D. Emphasize the role of the person in treatment and his/her family as comanagers of the illness, including judging costs and benefits of specific treatment options according to the individual's priorities.

### 2. Components of Psychoeducation

A. The disorder
  a. Biological basis
    i. Genetic factors (especially for persons of childbearing age)
    ii. Possible brain mechanisms
  b. Environmental components
    i. Psychosocial factors
    ii. Physical environmental factors
  c. Course and outcome
    i. Prevalence
    ii. Episode types and patterns
    iii. Potential triggers for episodes
    iv. Comorbidities and complications
B. Treatment
  a. Somatic therapies: somatic and psychosocial
    i. Goals
    ii. Side effect recognition and management
    iii. Costs and benefits of individual treatment options
  b. Coping skills
    i. Recognition of early warning signs of relapse
    ii. Avoidance/management of triggers for episodes
    iii. Activation of adaptive coping behaviors and avoidance of maladaptive responses

| Table 64–14 | Patterns of Efficacy Across Psychotherapy Type and Outcome Domaina* | | |
|---|---|---|---|
| **Intervention** | **Clinical Outcome** | **Functional Outcome** | **Disease Management Skills** |
| Couples/partners | + Davenport et al. (1977) (C)<br>− Clarkin et al. (1998) (A) | + Davenport et al. (1977) (C)<br>+ Honig et al. (1997) (A/B)<br>+ Clarkin et al. (1998) (A) | + Van Gent (1991) (A)<br>− Clarkin et al. (1998) (A) |
| Group, interpersonal and/or psychoeducational | + Volkmar et al. (1981) (C)<br>+ Kripke and Robinson (1985) (C)<br>+ Van Gent (1988) (C)<br>+ Van Gent and Zwart (1993) (C)<br>+ Cerbone et al. (1992) (C)<br>+ Weiss et al. (2000) (B) | + Volkmar et al. (1981) (C)<br>+ Kripke and Robinson (1985) (C)<br>+ Cerbone et al. (1992) (C)<br>+ Bauer et al. (1998) (B) | + Van Gent et al. (1988) (C)<br>+ Van Gent and Zwart (1993) (C)<br>+ Cerbone et al. (1992) (C)<br>+ Bauer et al. (1998) (B)<br>− Weiss et al. (2000) (B) |
| Cognitive–behavioral | +/− Palmer and Williams (1995) (B)<br>+ Zaretsky et al. (1999) (B)<br>+ Lam et al. (2000) (A) | +/− Palmer and Williams (1995) (B)<br>+ Lam et al. (2000) (A) | +/− Cochran (1984) (A) |
| Family | + Clarkin et al. (1990) (A)<br>+ Retzer et al. (1991) (C)<br>+ Miklowitz et al. (1999) (A) | + Clarkin et al. (1990) (A) | − Miklowitz et al. (1999) (A) |
| Interpersonal/social rhythms | − Hlastala et al. (1997) (A)<br>− Frank et al. (1999) (A) | | |
| Individual psychoeducation | + Perry et al. (1999) (A) | + Perry et al. (1999) (A) | + Peet and Harvey (1991) (A) |
| Other/eclectic | + Benson (1975) (C) | | |

*Studies analyzed by type of intervention, positive (+), negative (−), or equivocal (+/−) impact on the outcome domain noted, and quality of evidence (A, B, or C). See text for detail.

An evidence-based review similar to that for somatotherapy has recently been done for psychotherapeutic interventions. This review (Bauer 2001b, Bauer and McBride 2002), also using the AHCPR/AHRQ evidence categorization scheme, identified five main types of psychotherapy that have been studied in manic–depressive disorder: couples–partners, group interpersonal or psychoeducative, cognitive–behavioral, family, and interpersonal and social-rhythms. As summarized in Table 64–14, couples–partners, cognitive–behavioral, and family methods all have some Class A data supporting a role in improving clinical outcome or functional outcome or the intermediate outcome variable of improving illness management skills. An additional finding in this review, which is quite striking, is the degree of convergent validity across interventions regarding agenda for disease management information and skills to be imparted. Specifically, imparting education, focusing on early warning symptoms and triggers of episodes, and developing detailed and patient-specific action plans are found across most of the other interventions as well. For instance, this core agenda is also an important part of such diverse approaches as the cognitive–behavioral interventions of Palmer and Williams (1995) and Lam and coworkers (2000); the psychoeducational interventions of Bauer and coworkers (1998), Perry and coworkers (1999), and Weiss and coworkers (2000); the interpersonal and social rhythms therapy (IPSRT) intervention of Frank and coworkers (1999); and the family intervention of Miklowitz and coworkers (1999). Whether or not the developers of these interventions came to this common agenda in isolation or as part of ongoing collaborations and discussions is less important than the impressive fact that the agenda has been identified and incorporated into each of these interventions. Thus, given the positive results most of these interventions with explicit disease management components (i.e., patient education, collaborative management strategies with the patient, inclusion of as wide a social support system as is available) have produced, it is likely that this basic approach will be critical. It will perhaps be more critical even than the specific type of intervention in which these disease management components are embedded.

## Special Features Influencing Treatment

### Treatment of Comorbid Disorders

As noted earlier, several reversible "organic" factors may cause mood episodes, either *de novo* or in the course of already established manic–depressive disorder. For instance, removal of pro-manic drugs, both illicit and prescribed, is advisable in the treatment of substance-induced manic episodes. Treatment of general medical conditions, such as hypothyroidism, that may complicate course or treatment is also important.

Several conceptual approaches, not always explicit, underlie the choice of approach to managing comorbid disorders. Psychiatrists may assume that the comorbid disorder is caused by manic–depressive disorder and consequently that treatment of the manic–depressive disorder will lead to resolution of the comorbidity. For instance, panic attacks might be considered a consequence of mood episodes, or alcohol use a means of self-medication of depressive symptoms or a function of increased appetitive drive due to mania. On the other hand, psychiatrists may assume that the mood instability of manic–depressive disorder is due to the comorbid illness. For instance, mood episodes may be thought to be due to alcohol or drug intoxication or withdrawal or to intrapsychic or psychophysiological effects of prior trauma.

The unfortunate truth is that we have few data available to support either approach. Even the temporal sequence of onsets (e.g., manic–depressive disorder preceding substance abuse or vice versa) provides little information and in fact may be misleading in planning treatment. The literature on alcohol dependence comorbidity, which is perhaps the most extensively studied of the comorbidities, provides no data with which to plan treatment strategy.

It stands to reason, however, that some type of *parallel* (simultaneous) treatment is preferable to *sequential* treatment (treating one disorder until resolution and then attending to the other), as the prognosis of manic–depressive disorder is worse when complicated by substance use (Himmelhoch et al. 1976, Himmelhoch 1979) and the course of alcoholism is worse when complicated by mood disorders (Rounsaville 1987). It is also likely that the highly confrontative approaches of some traditional substance dependence treatment programs will not likely serve the needs of often highly impaired depressed or manic persons. Some general principles of treatment of comorbid mood and substance use disorders have been summarized in a monograph from the federal Center for Substance Abuse Treatment (Ries 1994).

## Treatment of Manic–Depressive Disorder Across the Life Cycle

Although the somatotherapeutic and psychotherapeutic mainstays of treatment endure across the life cycle, several phases of life present particular challenges. There exist few data on treatment of manic–depressive disorder in childhood (Strober et al. 1995). Treatments are chosen by extension from the adult literature, with the one caveat that there have been rare cases of liver failure in conjunction with valproic acid use in children younger than 10 years of age who have been exposed to multiple anticonvulsants (Dreifuss 1989).

In pregnancy, there is some evidence that lithium may be teratogenic, associated with increased rates of cardiac abnormalities (Weinstein and Goldfield 1975), although more recent data indicate that this risk may be overestimated (Cohen et al. 1994). Valproic acid and perhaps carbamazepine (Robert and Guiband 1983, Delgado-Escueta and Janz 1992, Scolnik et al. 1994) have been associated with neural tube defects (Robert and Guiband 1983), leaving the neuroleptics, antidepressants, and ECT as the preferable management strategies during pregnancy, particularly during the first trimester. Specific treatment strategies have been reviewed elsewhere (Sitland-Marken et al. 1989). It should be kept in mind, however, that treatment decisions are based on *risk*, not *certainty*. Risk of fetal malformation, parental attitude toward raising children with birth defects, severity of illness, and ease of management with alternative therapies all need to be considered in conjunction with the woman and her partner.

Aging also presents certain treatment concerns. As discussed in Chapters 93 and 97, tricyclic antidepressants may be associated with clinically significant cardiac conduction abnormalities, hypotension, sedation, glaucoma, and urinary retention, particularly in the presence of prostatic hypertrophy. These are of even greater concern in the elderly. The risk of sedation due to neuroleptics and benzodiazepines and of hypotension due to low-potency neuroleptics can also particularly complicate treatment of elderly persons with manic–depressive disorder. Such side effects can cause far-reaching and serious complications, such as hip fracture (Ray et al. 1987), which is not infrequently the initial event in a cascade of complications that can be terminal.

By contrast, lithium, carbamazepine, and valproic acid are relatively well tolerated in the elderly once attention is given to the slower clearance of drugs in general in this population group. The risk of clinically significant renal toxicity with appropriately dosed lithium is not great (Schou 1988, Gitlin 1993, Kehoe 1994). Although glomerular filtration rate decreases with age in persons treated with lithium, the rate of decline does not appear to be accelerated by lithium treatment (Lokkegaard et al. 1985, Vaamonde et al. 1986). Nonetheless, careful monitoring of renal function is needed in the elderly.

In addition, increasing age is clearly a risk factor for hypothyroidism (Bauer et al. 1993), as is lithium use (Bauer et al. 1990). Thus, elderly persons taking lithium should be followed up carefully for decrements in thyroid function, although hypothyroidism is not an indication for lithium discontinuation but rather simply for thyroid hormone supplementation.

## Summary

Manic–depressive disorder is a recurrent, major mood disorder that, if untreated, may lead to substantial morbidity. Its occurence, course, and treatment are best understood in terms of Engel's biopsychosocial perspective. State-of-the-art treatment extends beyond simple symptom reduction. Attention to outcome across three domains should guide management. These domains are clinical outcome, functional outcome, and illness costs, all of which matter greatly to the patients we treat.

The mainstay of treatment is combined somatotherapy and psychotherapy in a collaborative practice approach. Lithium is currently the only agent to have placebo-controlled and Class A data to support the fourfold definition of a mood stabilizer. A number of other agents have demonstrated ability in one or more of these roles. Side effects to all these treatments are the rule rather than the exception and require active medical and psychotherapeutic management.

A variety of psychotherapeutic modalities has been demonstrated to be efficacious in manic–depressive disorder. Most of these share a common agenda of educating patients to be better at self-monitoring and self-management tasks. Attention to system factors that can inhibit or support effective care should not be neglected. The goal of structuring symptoms to support care is to implement joint decision making in a collaborative manner.

## Comparison of DSM-IV/ICD-10 Diagnostic Criteria

The ICD-10 item set for a manic episode contains nine items in contrast to the seven items in the DSM-IV-TR criteria set, the two additional items being marked sexual energy or indiscretions and loss of normal social inhibitions. However, the number of items required by ICD-10 Diagnostic Criteria for Research remains the same as the number in DSM-IV-TR (i.e., three items if mood is euphoric, four items if mood is irritable) which is likely to result in a more inclusive diagnosis of a manic episode in ICD-10. Furthermore, the duration of mixed episodes differ, with DSM-IV-TR requiring a duration of 1 week (as is the case for a manic episode), whereas the ICD-10 Diagnostic Criteria for Research require a duration of at least 2 weeks.

The criteria sets for hypomanic episode differ as well. The ICD-10 Diagnostic Criteria for Research contain several additional items (increased sexual energy and increased sociability) and does not include the DSM-IV-TR items inflated self-esteem and flight of ideas. Furthermore, ICD-10 does not require that the change in mood be observed by others.

Regarding the definition of bipolar I disorder, in addition to differences in the diagnostic criteria for a manic and major depressive episode, the ICD-10 definition of "Bipolar Affective Disorder" (i.e., any combination of hypomanic, manic, mixed, and depressive episodes) does not distinguish between bipolar I and bipolar II disorder (i.e., cases of DSM-IV-TR Bipolar II Disorder are diagnosed as Bipolar Affective Disorder in ICD-10). However, ICD-10 Diagnostic Criteria for Research does include diagnostic criteria for bipolar II in its appendix that is identical to the criteria set in DSM-IV-TR.

For cyclothymic disorder, the ICD-10 Diagnostic Criteria for Research provides list of symptoms that must be associated with the periods of depressed mood and hypomania which differ from the ICD-10 item sets for dysthymic disorder and hypomania. In contrast, the DSM-IV-TR definition of cyclothymic disorder.

## Acknowledgment

Portions of this chapter have been adapted with permission from Bauer MS and McBride L (2002) *Structured Group Psychotherapy for Manic–Depressive Disorder*, 2nd ed. Springer-Verlag, New York.

## References

Abraham K (1927) Notes on the psycho-analytical investigation and treatment of manic–depressive insanity and allied conditions (1911). In Selected Papers of Karl Abraham, M.D., Bryan D and Strachey A (trans). Hogarth Press, London, pp. 137–156.

Abramson L, Seligman M, and Teasdale J (1978) Learned helplessness in humans: Critique and reformulation. J Abnorm Psychol 87, 49–74.

ACC/AHA (American College of Cardiology/American Heart Association) (1996) Task force on practice guidelines ACC/AHA guidelines for the management of patients with acute myocardial infarction. J Am Coll Cardiol 28, 1328–1428.

AHCPR (Agency for Health Care Policy and Research) (1993) Depression Panel Guideline Report. US Government Printing Office, Washington DC.

Akiskal HS (1981) Subaffective disorders: Dysthymic, cyclothymic, and bipolar II disorders in the "borderline" realm. Psychiatr Clin N Am 4, 25–46.

Akiskal HS and Akiskal K (1988) Reassessing the prevalence of bipolar disorders: Clinical significance and artistic creativity. Psychiatr Psychobiol 3, 29S–36S.

Akiskal HS, Djenderedjian AH, Rosenthal RH, et al. (1977) Cyclothymic disorder: Validating criteria for inclusion in the bipolar affective group. Am J Psychiatr 134, 1227–1233.

Altshuler LL, Bartzokis G, Grieder T, et al. (2000) An MRI study of temporal lobe structures in men with bipolar disorder or schizophrenia. Biol Psychiatr 48(2), 147–162.

Altshuler LL, Curran J, Hauser P, et al. (1995) T2 hyperintensities in bipolar disorder: Magnetic resonance imaging comparison and literature meta-analysis. Am J Psychiatr 152(8), 1139–1144.

American Psychiatric Association (1980) Diagnostic and Statistical Manual of Mental Disorders, 3rd ed. APA, Washington DC.

American Psychiatric Association (1987) Diagnostic and Statistical Manual of Mental Disorders, 3rd ed., Rev. APA, Washington DC.

American Psychiatric Association (1994a) Diagnostic and Statistical Manual of Mental Disorders, 4th ed. APA, Washington DC.

American Psychiatric Association (1994b) Practice guideline for the treatment of persons with bipolar disorder. Am J Psychiatr 151(Suppl), 1–36.

American Psychiatric Association (2000) Diagnostic and Statistical Manual of Mental Disorders, 4th ed., Rev. APA, Washington DC.

American Psychiatric Association Task Force for the Handbook of Psychiatric Measures (2000) Handbook of Psychiatric Measures. APA, Washington DC.

Amsterdam JD, Winokur A, Lucki I, et al. (1983) A neuroendocrine test battery in bipolar patients and health subjects. Arch Gen Psychiatr 40, 515–521.

Andrews G, Sanderson K, and Beard J (1998) Burden of disease: Methods of calculating disability from mental disorder. Br J Psychiatr 173, 123–131.

Angst J (1978) The course of affective disorders: 2. Typology of bipolar manic–depressive illness. Arch Psychiatr Nervenkr 226, 65–73.

Angst J (1981) Course of affective disorders. In Handbook of Biological Psychiatry, van Praag (ed). Marcel Dekker, New York, pp. 225–242.

Baastrup P and Schou M (1967) Lithium as a prophylactic agent: Its effect against recurrent depression and manic–depressive psychosis. Arch Gen Psychiatr 16, 162–172.

Ballenger JC and Post RM (1978) Therapeutic effects of carbamazepine in affective illness: A preliminary report. Commun Psychopharmacol 2, 159–175.

Ballenger JC and Post RM (1980) Carbamazepine in manic–depressive illness: A new treatment. Am J Psychiatr 137(7), 782–790.

Banks R, Aiton J, Cramb G, et al. (1990) Incorporation of inositol into the phosphoinositides of lymphoblastoid cell lines established from bipolar manic–depressive patients. J Affect Disord 19, 1–8.

Baron M, Gershon ES, Rudy V, et al. (1975) Lithium carbonate response in depression. Arch Gen Psychiatr 32, 1107–1111.

Baron M, Gruen R, Asnis L, et al. (1982) Schizoaffective illness, schizophrenia, and affective disorders: Morbidity risk and genetic transmission. Acta Psychiatr Scand 65, 253–262.

Bauer M and Whybrow P (1990) Rapid cycling bipolar affective disorder II. Adjuvant treatment of refractory rapid cycling with high dose thyroxine. Arch Gen Psychiatr 47, 435–440.

Bauer M and Whybrow PC (2001) Thyroid hormone, neural tissue, and mood modulation. World J Biol Psychiatr 2, 59–69.

Bauer M, Halpern L, and Schriger D (1993) Screening depressives for causative medical illness: The example of thyroid function testing. I. Literature review, meta-analysis, and hypothesis generation. Depression 1, 210–219.

Bauer M, Whybrow P, and Winokur A (1990) Rapid cycling bipolar affective disorder I: Association with grade I hypothyroidism. Arch Gen Psychiatr 47, 427–432.

Bauer M, Whybrow P, Gyulai L, et al. (1994a) Testing definitions of dysphoric mania and hypomania: Prevalence, clinical characteristics, and inter-episode stability. J Affect Disord 32, 201–211.

Bauer MS (1993) Summertime bright-light treatment of bipolar major depressive episodes. Biol Psychiatr 33, 663–665.

Bauer MS (1994) Rapid cycling. In Anticonvulsants in Mood Disorders, Joffe RT and Calabrese JR (eds). Marcel Dekker, New York, pp. 1–26.

Bauer MS (2001a) The collaborative practice model for bipolar disorder: Design and implementation in a multisite randomized controlled trial. Bipolar Disord 3, 233–244.

Bauer MS (2001b) An evidence-based review of psychosocial interventions for bipolar disorder. Psychopharmacol Bull 35, 109–134.

Bauer MS (2003) Field Guide to Psychiatric Assessment and Treatment. Lippincott, Williams & Wilkins, Philadelphia.

Bauer MS and Dunner DL (1993) Validity of seasonal pattern as a modifier for recurrent mood disorders for DSM-IV. Compr Psychiatr 34, 159–170.

Bauer MS and McBride L (2002) Structured group psychotherapy for manic–depressive disorder: The life goals program, 2nd ed. Springer-Verlag, New York.

Bauer MS and Whybrow P (1993) Validity of rapid cycling as a modifier for bipolar disorder in DSM-IV. Depression 1, 11–19.

Bauer MS and Whybrow PC (1991) Rapid cycling bipolar disorder: Clinical features, treatment, and etiology. In Advances in Neuropsychiatry and Psychopharmacology, Vol. 2, Amsterdam JD (ed). Raven Press, New York, pp. 191–208.

Bauer MS, Calabrese J, Dunner DL, et al. (1994b) Multisite data reanalysis of the validity of rapid cycling as a course modifier for bipolar disorder in DSM–IV. Am J Psychiatr 151, 506–515.

Bauer MS, Callahan A, Jampala C, et al. (1999) Clinical practice guidelines for bipolar disorder from the Department of Veterans Affairs. J Clin Psychiatr 60, 9–21.

Bauer MS, Crits-Christoph P, Ball W, et al. (1991) Independent assessment of manic and depressive symptoms by self-rating scale: Characteristics and implications for the study of mania. Arch Gen Psychiatr 48, 807–812.

Bauer MS, Kurtz JW, Rubin LB, et al. (1994c) Mood and behavioral effects of four-week light treatment in winter depressives and controls. J Psychiatr Res 28, 135–145.

Bauer MS, McBride L, Chase C, et al. (1998) Manual-based group psychotherapy for bipolar disorder: A feasibility study. J Clin Psychiatr 59, 449–455.

Bauer MS, McBride L, Shea N, et al. (1997) Impact of an easy-access clinic-based program for bipolar disorder: Quantitative analysis of a demonstration project. Psychiatr Serv 48, 491–496.

Bauer MS, Vojta C, Kinosian B, et al. (2000) The Internal State Scale: Replication of its discriminating abilities in a multisite, public sector sample. Bipolar Disord 2, 340–346.

Bauer MS, Williford W, Dawson E, et al. (2002) Principles of effectiveness trials and their implementation in VA Cooperative Study #430, "Reducing the efficacy-effectiveness gap in bipolar disorder." J Affect Disord 67, 61–78.

Bauwens F, Tracy A, Pardoen D, et al. (1991) Social adjustment of remitted bipolar and unipolar outpatients. A comparison with age- and sex-matched controls. Br J Psychiatr 151, 239–244.

Baxter LR Jr., Phelps ME, Mazziotta JC, et al. (1985) Cerebral metabolic rates for glucose in mood disorders: Studies with positron emission tomography and fluorodeoxyglucose F 18. Arch Gen Psychiatr 42, 441–447.

Beck AT, Rush AJ, Shaw B, et al. (1979) Cognitive Therapy of Depression. Guilford Press, New York.

Benes FM and Berretta S (2001) GABAergic interneurons: Implications for understanding schizophrenia and bipolar disorder. Neuropsychopharmacology 25(1) (July), 1–27.

Benson R (1975) The forgotten treatment modality in bipolar illness: Psychotherapy. Dis Nerv Syst 36, 634–638.

Berrios G and Hauser R (1988) The early development of Kraepelin's ideas on classification: A conceptual history. Psychol Med 18, 813–821.

Bertelsen A (1979) A Danish twin study of manic–depressive disorders. In Origin, Prevention, and Treatment of Affective Disorders, Schou M and Stromgren E (eds). Academic Press, London, pp. 227–239.

Bierwaltes WH and Ruff GE (1958) Thyroxin and triiodothyronine in excessive dosage to euthyroid humans. Arch Intern Med 101, 569–576.

Blacker D and Tsuang M (1992) Contested boundaries of bipolar disorder and the limits of categorical diagnosis in psychiatry. Am J Psychiatr 149, 1473–1483.

Bleuler E and Brill AA (English ed) (1924) Textbook of Psychiatry, 4th German ed. Macmillan, New York.

Botts SR and Raskind J (1999) Gabapentin and lamotrigine in bipolar disorder. Am J Health-Syst Pharm 56, 1939–1944.

Bowden C, Brugger A, Swann A, et al. (1994) Efficacy of divalproex vs lithium and placebo in the treatment of mania. J Am Med Assoc 271, 918–924.

Bowden CL, Calabrese JR, McElroy SL, et al. (1999) The efficacy of Lamotrigine in rapid cycling and nonrapid cycling patients with bipolar disorder. Soc Biol Psych 45, 953–958.

Bowden CL, Calabrese JR, McElroy SL, et al. (2000) A randomized, placebo-controlled 12 month trial of divalproex and lithium in treatment of outpatients with bipolar I disorder. Arch Gen Psychiatr 57, 481–489.

Bowen RC, Groff P, and Groff E (1991) Less frequent lithium administration and lower urine volume. Am J Psychiatr 148, 189–192.

Brambilla P, Harenski K, Nicoletti M, et al. (2001) MRI study of posterior fossa structures and brain ventricles in bipolar patients. J Psychiatr Res 35(6) (Nov–Dec), 313–322.

Bratfos O and Haug J (1968) The course of manic–depressive psychosis. A follow-up investigation of 215 patients. Acta Psychiatr Neurol Scand 44, 89–112.

Briggs J, McBride L, Hagino O, et al. (1993) Screening depressives for causative medical illness: The example of thyroid function testing II. Hypothesis testing in ambulatory depressives. Depression 1, 220–224.

Broadhead WE, Blazer D, George L, et al. (1990) Depression, disability days, and days lost from work in a prospective epidemiologic survey. JAMA 264, 2524–2528.

Brockington IF, Hillier V, Francis A, et al. (1983) Definitions of mania: Concordance and prediction of outcome. Am J Psychiatr 140, 435–439.

Brown G (1989) Life events and measurement. In Life Events and Stress, Brown G and Harris T (eds). Guilford Press, New York, pp. 3–45.

Brown G, Harris T, and Copeland J (1977) Depression and loss. Br J Psychiatr 130, 1–18.

Brown A, Mallinger A, and Renbaum L (1993) Elevated platelet membrane phosphatidylinositol-4,5-bisphosphate in bipolar mania. Am J Psychiatr 150, 1252–1254.

Buchsbaum MS, Wu J, DeLisi LE, et al. (1986) Frontal cortex and basal ganglia metabolic rates assessed by positron emission tomography with [$^{18}$F]2-deoxyglucose in affective illness. J Affect Disord 10, 137–152.

Bunney WE, Goodwin FK, Davis JM, et al. (1968) A behavioral-biochemical study of lithium treatment. Am J Psychiatr 125(5), 91–104.

Bunney WE Jr., Goodwin FK, and Murphy DL (1972a) The "switch process" in manic–depressive illness III. Theoretical implications. Arch Gen Psychiatr 27, 312–317.

Bunney WE Jr., Goodwin FK, Murphy DL, et al. (1972b) The "switch process" in manic–depressive illness II. Relationship to catecholamines, REM sleep, and drugs. Arch Gen Psychiatr 27, 304–309.

Bunney WE Jr., Murphy D, Goodwin FK, et al. (1972c) The "switch process" in manic–depressive illness I. A systematic study of sequential behavior change. Arch Gen Psychiatr 27, 295–302.

Calabrese JR, Bowden CL, McElroy SL, et al. (1999) Spectrum of activity of lamotrigine in treatment-refractory bipolar disorder. Am J Psychiatr 156(7), 1019–1023.

Carlson GA and Kashani JH (1988) Phenomenology of major depression from childhood through adulthood: Analysis of three studies. Am J Psychiatr 145, 1222–1225.

Carlson G, Kotin J, Davenport Y, et al. (1974) Follow-up of 53 bipolar manic–depressive patients. Br J Psychiatr 124, 134–149.

Cerbone M, Mayo J, Cuthbertsone B, et al. (1992) Group therapy as an adjunct to medication in the management of bipolar disorder. Group 16, 174–187.

Chalmers I (1993) The Cochrane Collaboration: Preparing, maintaining, and disseminating systematic reviews of the effects of health care. Ann NY Acad Sci 703, 156–163.

Clarkin JF, Carpenter D, Hull J, et al. (1998) Effects of psychoeducational intervention for married patients with bipolar disorder and their spouses. Psychiatr Serv 49, 531–533.

Clarkin JF, Glick I, Haas G, et al. (1990) A randomized clinical trial of inpatient family intervention. V. Results for affective disorder. J Affect Disord 18, 17–28.

Cochran S (1984) Preventing medical noncompliance in the outpatient treatment of bipolar affective disorders. J Consult Clin Psychol 52, 873–878.

Cohen LS, Friedman JM, and Jefferson JW (1994) A reevaluation of risk of in utero exposure to lithium. JAMA 271, 146–150.

Cooke R, Kruger S, and Shugar G (1996) Comparative evaluation of two self-report mania rating scales. Biol Psychiatr 40, 279–283.

Cooper A (1985) Will neurobiology influence psychoanalysis? Am J Psychiatr 142, 1395–1402.

Coppen A, Noguera R, Bailey J, et al. (1971) Prophylactic lithium in affective disorders: Controlled trial. Lancet 2, 275–279.

Coppen A, Prange AJ Jr., Whybrow PC, et al. (1972) Abnormalities of indolamines in affective disorders. Arch Gen Psychiatr 26, 474–478.

Coryell W, Endicott J, and Keller M (1992) Rapidly cycling affective disorders: Demographics, diagnosis, family history, and course. Arch Gen Psychiatr 49, 126–131.

Coryell W, Endicott J, Andreasen N, et al. (1985) Bipolar I, bipolar II, and nonbipolar major depression among the relatives of affectively ill probands. Am J Psychiatr 142, 817–821.

Coryell W, Endicott J, Keller M, et al. (1989) Bipolar affective disorder and high achievement: A familial association. Am J Psychiatr 146, 983–988.

Coryell W, Endicott J, Maser J, et al. (1995) Long-term stability of polarity distinctions in affective disorders. Am J Psychiatr 152, 385–390.

Coryell W, Endicott J, Reich T, et al. (1984) A family study of bipolar II disorder. Br J Psychiatr 145, 49–54.

Coryell W, Keller M, Endicott J, et al. (1989) Bipolar II illness: Course and outcome over a five-year period. Psychol Med 19, 129–141.

Coryell W, Scheftner W, Keller M, et al. (1993) The enduring psychosocial consequences of mania and depression. Am J Psychiatr 150, 720–727.

Craddock N and Jones I (1999) Genetics of bipolar disorder. J Med Gener 36, 585–594.

Crow T and Deakin J (1981) Affective change and the mechanisms of reward and punishment: A neurochemical hypothesis. In Biological Psychiatry, Perris C, Struwe G, and Jansson B (eds). Elsevier, Amsterdam, pp. 536–541.

Cundall RL, Brooks PW, and Murray LG (1972) A controlled evaluation of lithium prophylaxis in affective disorders. Psychol Med 2, 308–311.

Davenport Y, Ebert M, Adland M, et al. (1977) Couples group therapy as an adjunct to lithium maintenance of the manic patient. Am J Orthopsychiatr 47, 495–502.

Deicken RF, Calabrese G, Merrin EL, et al. (1995) Asymmetry of temporal lobe phosphorous metabolism in schizophrenia: A 31 phosphorous magnetic resonance spectroscopic imaging study. Biol Psychiatr 38(5), (Sept 1) 279–286.

Delgado-Escueta A and Janz D (1992) Consensus guidelines: Preconception counseling, management, and care of the pregnant woman with epilepsy. Neurology 42(Suppl 5), 149–160.

Deltito J, Moline M, Pollak C, et al. (1991) Effects of phototherapy on nonseasonal unipolar and bipolar depressive spectrum disorders. J Affect Disord 23, 231–237.

DePaolo JR, Simpson SG, Folstein S, et al. (1989) The new genetics of bipolar affective disorder: Clinical implications. Clin Chem 35/7(B), B28–B32.

Depue R and Iacono W (1989) Neurobiological aspects of affective disorders. Ann Rev Psychol 40, 457–492.

Depue R, Kleinman R, Davis P, et al. (1985) The behavioral high-risk paradigm and bipolar disorder, VIII: Serum free cortisol in nonpatient cyclothymic subjects selected by the GBI. Am J Psychiatr 142, 175–181.

Dickson W and Kendell R (1986) Does maintenance lithium prevent recurrences of mania under ordinary clinical conditions? Psychol Med 16, 521–530.

Dion G, Tohen M, Anthony W, et al. (1988) Symptoms and functioning of patients with bipolar disorder six months after hospitalization. HOSP Comm Psychiatr 39, 652–657.

Dooley L (1921) A psychoanalytic study of manic depressive psychoses. Psychoanal Rev 8, 144–167.

Dreifuss FE (1989) Valproate toxicity. In Antiepileptic Drugs, 3rd ed, Levy R, Mattson RH, Meldrum B, et al. (eds). Raven Press, New York, pp. 643–651.

Drevets WC, Frank E, Price JC, et al. (1999) PET imaging of serotonin 1A receptor binding in depression. Biol Psychiatr 46(10), 1375–1387.

Dubovsky SL, Franks RD, Allen S, et al. (1986) Calcium antagonists in mania: A double-blind study of verapamil. Psychiatr Res 18, 309–320.

Dunner DL (1993) A review of the diagnostic status of "bipolar II" for the DSM-IV work group on mood disorders. Depression 1, 2–10.

Dunner DL and Fieve RR (1974) Clinical factors in lithium prophylaxis failure. Arch Gen Psychiatr 30, 229–233.

Dunner DL, Fleiss JL, and Fieve RR (1976) Lithium carbonate prophylaxis failure. Br J Psychiatr 129, 40–44.

EBWG (Evidence-Based Working Group) (1992) A new approach to teaching the practice of medicine. J Am Med Assoc 268, 2420–2425.

Ehlers C, Frank E, and Kupfer D (1988) Social zeitgebers and biological rhythms. Arch Gen Psychiatr 45, 948–952.

Ellicott A, Hammen C, Gitlin M, et al. (1990) Life events and the course of bipolar disorder. Am J Psychiatr 147(9), 1194–1198.

Ellsworth AJ, Witt DM, Dugdale DC, et al. (2001) Mosby's 2001–02 Medical Drug Reference. Mosby, St. Louis.

el-Mallakh R and Li R (1993) Is the $Na^+$-$K^+$-ATPase the link between phosphoinositide metabolism and bipolar disorder? Rev J Neuropsychiatr Clin Neurosci 5, 361–368.

Emrich HM, Zerssen DV, Kissling W, et al. (1980) Effect of sodium valproate on mania: The GABA-hypothesis of affective disorders. Arch Psychiatr Nervenkr 229, 1–16.

Endicott J, Nee J, Andreasen N, et al. (1985) Bipolar II: Combine or keep separate? J Affect Disord 8, 17–28.

Engel GL (1977) The need for a new medical model: A challenge for biomedicine. Science 129, 186–196.

Faedda GL, Tondo L, Baldessarrni RJ, et al. (1993) Outcome after rapid vs gradual discontinuation of lithium treatment in bipolar disorders. Arch Gen Psychiatr 50, 448–455.

Feighner JP, Robins E, Guze SB, et al. (1972) Diagnostic criteria for use in psychiatric research. Arch Gen Psychiatr 26, 57–63.

Fein R (1958) Economics of Mental Illness. Basic Books, New York.

Fenichel O (1945) The Psychoanalytic Theory of Neuroses. WW Norton, New York, p. 408.

Fieve R, Go R, Dunnere D, et al. (1984) Search for biological/genetic markers in a long-term epidemiological and morbid risk study of affective disorders. J Psychiatr Res 18, 425–445.

Fieve RR, Kumbaraci R, and Dunner DL (1976) Lithium prophylaxis of depression in bipolar I, bipolar II, and unipolar patients. Am J Psychiatr 133(8), 925–929.

Fieve RR, Platman SR, and Plutchik RR (1968) The use of lithium in affective disorders I: Acute endogenous depression. Am J Psychiatr 125, 487–491.

Frank E, Swartz H, Mallinger AG, et al. (1999) Adjunctive psychotherapy for bipolar disorder: Effects of changing treatment modality. J Abnorm Psychol 108, 579–587.

Fremming KH (1951) The Expectation of Mental Infirmity in a Sample of the Danish Population, No. 7, Occasional Papers in Eugenics. Cassell, London.

Freud S (1924) Mourning and Melancholia, Collected Papers, Vol. 4. Hogarth Press, London.

Freud S (1933) New introductory lectures on psychoanalysis. In Standard Edition, Vol. 22, Mosbacher E and Strachey J (trans). Basic Books, New York, Imago Publishing, London, pp. 3–182.

Gareri P, Falconi U, De Fazio P, et al. (2000) Conventional and new antidepressant drugs in the elderly. Prog Neurobiol 61(4) (July), 353–396.

Gelenberg AJ, Kane JM, Keller MB, et al. (1989) Comparison of standard and low serum levels of lithium for maintenance treatment of bipolar disorder. New Engl J Med 321, 1489–1493.

Gershon ES, Hamovit J, Guroff JJ, et al. (1982) A family study of schizoaffective, bipolar I, bipolar II, unipolar, and normal control probands. Arch Gen Psychiatr 39, 1157–1167.

Gershon ES, Hamovit JH, Guroff JJ, et al. (1987) Birth-cohort changes in manic and depressive disorders in relatives of bipolar and schizoaffective patients. Arch Gen Psychiatr 44, 314–319.

Giannini AJ, Houser WL, Loiselle RH, et al. (1984) Antimanic effects of verapamil. Am J Psychiatr 141(12), 1602–1603.

Gilbert D, Altshuler K, Rago W, et al. (1998) Texas medication algorithm project: Definitions, rationale, and methods to develop medication algorithms. J Clin Psychiatr 59, 345–351.

Gitlin M (1993) Lithium-induced renal insufficiency. J Clin Psychopharmacol 13, 276–279.

Gitlin M, Cochran S, and Jamison K (1989) Maintenance lithium treatment: Side effects and compliance. J Clin Psychiatr 50, 127–131.

Goodwin FK and Jamison KR (1990) Manic–Depressive Illness. Oxford University Press, New York, pp. 369–596.

Goodwin FK and Sack RL (1974) Behavioral effects of a new dopamine-beta-hydroxylase inhibitor (dusaric acid) in man. J Psychiatr Res 11, 211–217.

Goodwin FK, Murphy DL, and Bunney WF Jr. (1969) Lithium carbonate treatment in depression and mania: A longitudinal double-blind study. Arch Gen Psychiatr 21, 486–496.

Goodwin FK, Murphy DL, Dunner DL, et al. (1972) Lithium response in unipolar versus bipolar depression. Am J Psychiatr 129, 44–47.

Gottschalk A, Bauer M, and Whybrow P (1995) A chaotic attraction in bipolar disorder. Arch Gen Psychiatr 52, 947–959.

Greil W, Steber R, and vanCalker D (1991) The agonist-stimulated accumulation of inositol phosphates is attenuated in neutrophils from male patients under chronic lithium therapy. Biol Psychiatr 30, 443–451.

Halaris A (ed) (1987) Chronobiology and Psychiatric Disorders. Elsevier, New York.

Hall K, Dunner D, Zeller G, et al. (1977) Bipolar illness: A prospective study of life events. Compr Psychiatr 18, 497–502.

Harrow M, Goldberg J, Grossman L, et al. (1990) Outcome in manic disorders. A naturalistic follow-up study. Arch Gen Psychiatr 47, 665–671.

Haslam D, Kennedy S, Kusumakar V, et al. (1997) The treatment of bipolar disorder: Review of the literature, guidelines, and options. Can J Psychiatr 42, 67S–99S.

Hastings D (1958) Follow-up results in psychiatric illness. Am J Psychiatr 114, 1057–1066.

Hauser P, Matochik J, Altshuler LL, et al. (2000) MRI-based measurements of temporal lobe and ventricular structures in patients with bipolar I and bipolar II disorders. J Affect Disord 60(1) (Oct), 25–32.

Helgason T (1979) Epidemiological investigations concerning affective disorders. In Origin, Preventions, and Treatment of Affective Disorders, Schou M and Stromgren E (eds). Academic Press, London, pp. 241–255.

Himmelhoch J (1979) Mixed states, manic–depressive illness, and the nature of mood. Psychiatr Clin N Am 2, 449–459.

Himmelhoch J, Mulla D, Neil JF, et al. (1976) Incidence and significance of mixed affective states in a bipolar population. Arch Gen Psychiatr 33, 1062–1066.

Hlastala SA, Frank E, Mallinger AG, et al. (1997) Bipolar depression: An underestimated treatment challenge. Depress Anx 5, 73–83.

Honig A, Hofman A, Rozendaal N, et al. (1997) Psycho-education in bipolar disorder: Effect on expressed emotion. Psychiatr Res 72, 17–22.

Hume AJA, Barker PJ, Robertson W, et al. (1988) Manic–depressive psychosis: An alternative therapeutic model of nursing. J Adv Nursing 13, 93–98.

Hunt N, Bruce-Jones W, and Silverstone T (1992) Life events and relapse in bipolar affective disorder. J Affect Dis 25, 13–20.

Hyman SE, Arana JW, and Rosenbaum JF (1995) Handbook of Psychiatric Drug Therapy, 3rd ed. Little Brown, Boston.

Institute of Medicine (1985) Assessing Medical Technologies. National Academy Press, Washington DC.

Irwig L, Tosteson AN, Gatsonis C, et al. (1994) Guidelines for meta-analyses evaluating diagnostic tests. Ann Intern Med 120, 667–676.

James NM and Chapman CJ (1975) A genetic study of bipolar affective disorder. Br J Psychiatr 126, 449–456.

Jamison KR, Gerner RH, and Goodwin FK (1979) Patient and physician attitudes toward lithium: Relationship to compliance. Arch Gen Psychiatr 36, 866–869.

Janowsky DS, El-Yousef MK, Davis JM, et al. (1973) Parasympathetic suppression of manic symptoms by physostigmine. Arch Gen Psychiatr 28, 542–547.

Joffe R, Singer W, Levitt A, et al. (1993) A placebo-controlled comparison of lithium and triiodothyronine augmentation of tricyclic antidepressant in unipolar refractory affective depression. Arch Gen Psychiatr 50, 387 393.

Johnson S and Roberts JR (1995) Life events and bipolar disorder: Implications from biological theories. Psychol Bull 117, 434–449.

Josephson AM and MacKenzie TB (1979) Appearance of manic psychosis following rapid normalization of thyroid status. Am J Psychiatr 136, 846–847.

Jurjus GJ, Nasrallah HA, Brogan M, et al. (1993a) Developmental brain anomalies in schizophrenia and bipolar disorder: A controlled MRI study. J Neuropsychiatr Clin Neurosci 5, 375–378.

Jurjus GJ, Nasrallah HA, Olson SC, et al. (1993b) Cavum septum pellucidum in schizophrenia, affective disorder, and health controls: A magnetic resonance imaging study. Psychol Med 23, 319–322.

Kahn D, Docherty, Carpenter D, et al. (1997) Consensus methods in practice guideline development: A review and description of a new method. Psychopharmacol Bull 33, 631–639.

Kahn DA (1993) The use of psychodynamic psychotherapy in manic–depressive illness. J Am Acad Psychoanal 21(3), 441–455.

Kamo J, Shin-ichiro T, Susumo N, et al. (1993) Season and Mania. Jpn J Psychiatr Neurol 47(2), 473–474.

Kane JM, Quitkin FM, Rifkin A, et al. (1982) Lithium carbonate and imipramine in the prophylaxis of unipolar and bipolar II illness: A prospective, placebo-controlled comparison. Arch Gen Psychiatr 39(9) (Sept), 1065–1069.

Kapur S and Mann JJ (1992) Role of the dopaminergic system in depression. Biol Psychiatr 32, 1–17.

Kato T, Takahashi S, Shioiri T, et al. Reduction of brain phospphocreatine in bipolar II disorder detected by phosphorous-31 magnetic resonance spectroscopy. J Affect Disord 31, 125–133.

Keck PE, McElroy SL, and Bennett JA (1994) Pharmacology and pharmacokinetics of valproic acid. In Anticonvulsants in Mood Disorders, Joffe RT and Calabrese JR (eds). Marcel Dekker, New York, pp. 27–42.

Kehoe RF (1994) A cross-sectional study of glomerular function in 740 unselected lithium patients. Acta Psychiatr Scand 89, 68–71.

Keller M, Lavori P, Coryell W, et al. (1986a) Differential outcome of episodes of illness in bipolar patients: Pure manic, mixed/cycling, and pure depressive. JAMA 255, 3138–3142.

Keller M, Lavori P, Klerman G, et al. (1986b) Low levels and lack of predictors of somatotherapy and psychotherapy received by depressed patients. Arch Gen Psychiatr 43, 458–466.

Kennedy S, Thompson R, Stancer HC, et al. (1983) Life events precipitating mania. Br J Psychiatr 142, 398–403.

Ketter TA and Post RM (1994) Clinical pharmacology and pharmacokinetics of carbamazepine. In Anticonvulsants in Mood Disorders, Joffe RT and Calabrese JR (eds). Marcel Dekker, New York, pp. 147–188.

Kirov G, Murphy KC, Arranz MJ, et al. (1998) Low activity allele of catechol-O-methyltransferase gene associated with rapid cycling bipolar disorder. Mol Psychiatr 3(4), 342–345.

Klerman G, Olfson M, Leon A, et al. (1992) Measuring the need for mental health care. Health Affairs 11, 23–33. (Statistics from prepublication draft from Dr. A. Leon)

Klerman G, Weissman M, Rounsaville B, et al. (1984) Interpersonal Psychotherapy of Depression. Basic Books, New York.

Kraepelin E (1989) Manic–depressive insanity and paranoia. In Classics of Psychiatry and Behavioral Science, Barclay RM (trans) and Robertson GM (ed). Classics of Psychiatry and Behavioral Sciences Library Birmingham, AL. (Originally published in 1921, E&D Livingstone, Edinburgh.)

Krauthammer C and Klerman GL (1978) Secondary mania: Manic syndromes associated with antecedent physical illness or drugs. Arch Gen Psychiatr 35, 1333–1339.

Kripke DF and Robinson D (1985) Ten years with a lithium group. McLean Hosp J 10, 1–11.

Lachman HM, Morrow B, Shprintzen R, et al. (1996) Association of codon 108/158 catechol-O-methyltranferase gene polymorphism with the psychiatric manifestations of velocardia-facial syndrome. Am J Med Genet 67(5), 468–472.

Lam DH, Bright J, Jones S, et al. (2000) Cognitive therapy for bipolar illness—a pilot study of relapse prevention. Cogn Ther Res 24, 503–520.

Leaf A (1993) Preventive medicine for our ailing health care system. JAMA 269, 616–618.

Lenox R and Watson D (1994) Lithium and the brain: A psychopharmacological strategy to a molecular basis for manic–depressive illness (review). Clin Chem 40, L309–L314.

Lenzi A, Lazzerini F, Marazziti D, et al. (1993) Social class and mood disorders: Clinical features. Soc Psychiatr Epidemiol 28, 56–59.

Leonhard K and Berman R (trans) Robins E (ed) (1979) The Classification of Endogenous Psychoses, 5th ed. Irvington Publishers, New York. (Originally published in 1957, Aufteilung de Endogenen Psychosen. Akademie-Verlag, Berlin.)

Leverich M (1990) Factors associated with relapse during maintenance treatment of affective disorders. Int J Clin Psychopharmacol 5, 135–156.

Levinstein S, Klein D, and Pollack M (1966) Follow-up study of formerly hospitalized voluntary psychiatric patients: The first two years. Am J Psychiatr 122, 1102–1109.

Levitt J and Tsuang M (1988) The heterogeneity of schizoaffective disorders: Implications for treatment. Am J Psychiatr 145, 926–936.

Lewinsohn P (1974) A behavioral approach to depression. In The Psychology of Depression: Contemporary Theory and Research, Friedman R and Katz M (eds). John Wiley, New York, pp. 157–185.

Lewis JL and Winokur G (1982) The induction of mania: A natural history study with controls. Arch Gen Psychiatr 39, 303–306.

Lewy A, Nurnberger J, Wehr T, et al. (1985) Supersensitivity to light: Possible trait marker for manic–depressive illness. Am J Psychiatr 142, 725–727.

Lewy A, Wehr T, Goodwin F, et al. (1980) Light suppresses melatonin secretion in humans. Science 210, 1267–1269.

Lindblad K, Bylander PO, Zander C, et al. (1998) Mol Psychiatr 3(5), 405–410.

Lokkegaard H, Andersen N, and Henriksen H (1985) Renal function in 153 manic–depressive patients treated with lithium for more than five years. Acta Psychiatr Scand 71, 347–355.

Lundquist G (1945) Prognosis and course in manic–depressive psychosis. Acta Psychiatr Neurol Scand 35(Suppl), 1–96.

Maggs R (1963) Treatment of manic illness with lithium carbonate. Br J Psychiatr 150, 863–864.

Maj M, Pirozzi R, and Starace F (1989) Previous pattern of course of the illness as a predictor of response to lithium prophylaxis in bipolar illness. J Affect Disord 17, 237–241.

Mander A (1989) Diagnosis change, lithium use, and admissions for mania in Edinburgh. Acta Psychiatr Scand 80, 434–436.

Manji HK and Lenox RH (2000) Signaling: Cellular insights into the pathophysiology of bipolar disorder. Biol Psychiatr 15 48(6), 518–530.

Markar H and Mander A (1989) Efficacy of lithium prophylaxis in clinical practice. Br J Psychiatr 155, 496–500.

Markowitz J, Weissman M, Oulette R, et al. (1989) Quality of life in panic disorder. Arch Gen Psychiatr 46, 984–992.

Mason J (1975) Emotion as reflected in patterns of endocrine integration. In Emotions—Their Parameters and Measurement, Levi L (ed). Raven Press, New York, pp. 143–181.

Massion A, Warshaw M, and Keller M (1993) Quality of life and psychiatric morbidity in panic disorder and generalized anxiety disorder. Am J Psychiatr 150, 600–607.

McElroy S, Keck P, Pope H, et al. (1992) Clinical and research implications of the diagnosis of dysphoric or mixed mania or hypomania. Am J Psychiatr 149, 1633–1644.

McElroy SL, Altshuler LL, Suppes T, et al. (2001) Axis I psychiatric comorbidity and its relationship to historical illness variables in 288 patients with bipolar disorder. Am J Psychiatr 153(3), 420–426.

McGuire T (1991) Measuring the economic costs of schizophrenia. Schizophr Bull 17, 375–388.

McInnis MG, McMahon FJ, Chase GA, et al. (1993) Anticipation in bipolar affective disorder. Am J Hum Genet 53, 385–390.

McLellan AT, Childress AR, and Woody GE (1985) Drug abuse and psychiatric disorders: Role of drug choice. In Substance Abuse and Psychopathology, Alterman AI (ed). Plenum Press, New York, pp. 137–172.

Mendels J (1976) Lithium in the treatment of depression. Am J Psychiatr 133, 373–378.

Mendlewicz J and Rainer JD (1977) Adoption study supporting genetic transmission in manic–depressive illness. Nature 268, 327–329.

Miklowitz DJ, Simoneau TL, George EL, et al. (1999) Family-focused treatment of bipolar disorder: 1-year effects of a psychoeducational program in conjunction with pharmacotherapy. Biol Psychiatr 48, 582–592.

Mundo E, Walker M, Cate T, et al. (2001) The role of serotonin transporter protein gene in antidepressant-induced mania in bipolar disorder: Preliminary findings. Arch Gen Psychiatr 58(6), 539–544.

Murray CJL and Lopez AD (eds) (1996) The Global Burden of Disease: A Comprehensive Assessment of Mortality and Disability from Diseases, Injuries, and Risk Factors in 1990 and Projected to 2020. Harvard University Press, Cambridge, MA.

Murray CJL and Lopez AD (1997) Regional patterns of disability-free life expectancy and disability-adjusted life expectancy: Global Burden of Disease study. Lancet 349, 1347–1352.

Nasrallah H, Coffman J, and Olson S (1989) Structural brain imaging findings in affective disorders: An overview. J Neuropsychiatr Clin Neurosci 1, 21–26.

National Institute of Mental Health National Advisory Mental Health Council (1992) Caring for People with Severe Mental Disorders. A National Plan of Research to Improve Services. US Government Printing Office, DHHS publication ADM91-1762, Washington DC.

Nilsson A and Axelsson R (1989) Psychopathology during long-term lithium treatment of patients with major affective disorders: A prospective study. Acta Psychiatr Scand 80, 375–388.

Nurnberger J, Berrettini W, Tamarkin L, et al. (1989) Supersensitivity to melatonin suppression by light in young people at high risk for affective disorder: A preliminary report. Neuropsychopharmacol 1, 217–223.

O'Connell R, Mayo J, Flatow L, et al. (1991) Outcome of bipolar disorder on long-term treatment with lithium. Br J Psychiatr 159, 123–129.

Palmer AG and Williams H (1995) CBT in a group format for bipolar affective disorder. Behav Cogn Psychother 23, 153–168.

Papolos DF, Veit S, Faedda GL, et al. (1998) Ultra-rapid cycling bipolar disorder is associated with low activity catecholamine-O-methyltransferase allele. Mol Psychiatr 3(4), 346–349.

Parker G, O'Donnell M, and Walter S (1985) Changes in the diagnoses of the functional psychoses associated with the introduction of lithium. Br J Psychiatr 146, 377–382.

Parsons PL (1965) Mental health of Swansea's old folk. Br J Prev Soc Med 19, 43–47.

Paykel E and Cooper Z (1992) Life events and social stress. In Handbook of Affective Disorders, Paykel E (ed). Guilford Press, New York, pp. 149–170.

Peet M and Harvey NS 1991 Lithium maintenance: 1. A standard education programme for patients. Br J Psychiatr 158, 197–200.

Perris H (1984a) Life events and depression: Part 1. Effect of sex, age, and civil status. J Affect Dis 7, 11–24.

Perris H (1984b) Life events and depression: Part 2. Results in diagnostic subgroups and in relation to the recurrence of depression. J Affect Dis 7, 25–36.

Perris H (1984c) Life events and depression: Part 3. Relation to severity of the depressive syndrome. J Affect Dis 7, 37–44.

Perry A, Tarrier N, Morriss R, et al. (1999) Randomised controlled trial of efficacy of teaching patients with bipolar disorder to identify early symptoms of relapse and obtain treatment. Br Med J 318, 149–153.

Petronis A and Kennedy J (1995) Unstable genes—unstable mind? Am J Psychiatr 152, 164–172.

Petterson WU (1977) Manic–depressive illness: A clinical, social, and genetic study. Acta Psychiatr Scand (Suppl), 269.

Petty F, Kramer GL, Fulton M, et al. (1993) Low plasma GABA is a trait-like marker for bipolar illness. Neuropsychopharmacol 9, 125–132.

Petty F, Rush J, Davis J, et al. (1996) Plasma gaba predicts acute reponse to divalproex in mania. Biol Psychiatr 39, 278–284.

Pope H, McElroy S, Keck P, et al. (1991) Valproate in the treatment of acute mania. Arch Gen Psychiatr 48, 62–68.

Post R, Rubinow D, and Ballenger J (1985) Conditioning, sensitization, and kindling: Implications for the course of affective illness. In Neurobiology of Mood Disorders, Post R and Ballenger J (eds). Williams & Wilkins, Baltimore, pp. 432–466.

Post R, Rubinow D, and Ballenger J (1986a) Conditioning, sensitization, and the longitudinal course of affective illness. Br J Psychiatr 149, 191–201.

Post RM (1992) Transduction of psychosocial stress into the neurobiology of recurrent affective disorder. Am J Psychiatr 149, 999–1010.

Post RM, DeLisi LE, Holcomb HH, et al. (1987) Glucose utilization in the temporal cortex of affectively ill patients: Positron emission tomography. Biol Psychiatr 22, 545–553.

Post RM, Leverich GS, Altshuler L, et al. (1992) Lithium-discontinuation-induced refractoriness: Preliminary observations. Am J Psychiatr 149, 1727–1729.

Post RM, Uhde TW, Rubinow DR, et al. (1986b) Antimanic effects of carbamazepine: Mechanisms of action and implications for the biochemistry of manic–depressive illness. In Mania: New Research and Treatment, Swann A (ed). American Psychiatric Press, Washington DC, pp. 95–176.

Potash JB and DePaulo JR (2000) Searching high and low: A review of the genetics of bipolar disorder. Bipolar Disord 2, 8–26.

Prange AJ (1964) The pharmacology and biochemistry of depression. Dis Nerv Syst 25, 217–221.

Price J (1968) Neurotic and endogenous depression: A phylogenetic view. Br J Psychiatr 114, 119–120.

Prien R and Gelenberg A (1989) Alternatives to lithium for the preventive treatment of bipolar disorder. Am J Psychiatr 146, 840–848.

Prien R, Caffey E, and Klett CJ (1973a) Prophylactic efficacy of lithium carbonate in manic–depressive illness. Report of the Veterans Administration and National Institute of Mental Health Collaborative Study Group. Arch Gen Psychiatr 28, 337–341.

Prien RF, Klett CJ, and Caffey EM Jr. (1973b) Lithium carbonate and imipramine in prevention of affective episodes: A comparison in recurrent affective illness. Arch Gen Psychiatr 29, 420–425.

Ray WA, Griffin MR, Schaffner W, et al. (1987) Psychotropic drug use and the risk of hip fracture. New Engl J Med 316, 363–369.

Regier D, Farmer M, Rae D, et al. (1990) Comorbidity of mental disorders with alcohol and other drugs. Results from the Epidemiological Catchment Area (ECA) Study. JAMA 264, 2511–2518.

Reifman A and Wyatt RJ (1980) Lithium: A brake in the rising cost of mental illness. Arch Gen Psychiatr 37, 385–388.

Retzer A, Simon FB, Weber G, et al. (1991) A follow-up study of manic–depressive and schizoaffective psychoses after systemic family therapy. Fam Process 30, 139–153.

Rice D, Kelman S, Miller L, et al. (1990) The Economic Costs of Alcohol and Drug Abuse and Mental Illness: 1985 National Institute of Mental Health, DHHS publication (ADM) 90-1694, Rockville, MD.

Ries R (1994) Assessment and Treatment of Patients with Coexisting Mental Illness and Alcohol and Other Drug Abuse. National Institute of Mental Health, DHHS publication (ADM) 94-2078, Rockville, MD.

Robert E and Guiband P (1983) Maternal valproic acid and congenital neural tube defects. Lancet 2, 937.

Robins E and Guze SB (1970) Establishment of diagnostic validity in psychiatric illness: Its application to schizophrenia. Am J Psychiatr 126, 983–987.

Rotter J (1966) Generalized expectancies for internal versus external control of reinforcement. Psychol Monogr 80, 1–28.

Rounsaville BJ, Dolinsky ZS, Babor TF, et al. (1987) Psychopathology as a predictor of treatment outcome in alcoholics. Arch Gen Psychiatr 44, 505–513.

Roy-Byrne P, Post R, Uhde T, et al. (1985) The longitudinal course of recurrent affective illness: Life chart data from research patients at the NIMH. Acta Psychiatr Scand 71(Suppl 317), 3–34.

Rush AG, Rago WV, Crismon ML, et al. (1999) Medication treatment for the severely and persistently mentally ill: The Texas Medication Algorithm Project. J Clin Psychiatr 60, 284–291.

Rush AJ and Hollon S (1991) Depression. In Integrating Pharmacotherapy and Psychotherapy, Beitman B and Klerman G (eds). American Psychiatric Press, Washington DC, pp. 121–142.

Sachs G, Lafer B, Truman C, et al. (1994) Miracle, myth, and misunderstanding. Psychiatr Ann 24, 299–306.

Sachs G, Printz DJ, Kahn DA, et al. (2000) Medication Treatment of Bipolar Disorder 2000. McGraw-Hill Healthcare Information Programs, Minneapolis.

Sassi RB and Soares JC (2002) Neural circuitry and signaling in bipolar disorder. In Brain Circuitry in Psychiatry: Basic Science and Clinical Implications, Kaplan GB and Hammer RP (eds). American Psychiatric Press, pp. 179–200.

Schatzberg AF, Cole JO, and DeBattista C (1997) Manual of Clinical Psychopharmacology, 3rd ed. American Psychiatric Press, Washington DC.

Schildkraut J (1965) The catecholamine hypothesis of affective disorder: A review of supporting evidence. Am J Psychiatr 122, 509–522.

Schou M (1988) Effects of long-term lithium treatment on kidney function: An overview. J Psychiatr Res 22, 287–296.

Schwartz D (1961) Some suggestions for a unitary formulation of manic–depressive reactions. Psychiatry 24, 238–245.

Sclare P and Creed F (1990) Life events and the onset of mania. Br J Psychiatr 156, 508–514.

Scolnik D, Nulman I, and Rovet J (1994) Neurodevelopment of children exposed in utero to phenytoin and carbamazepine monotherapy. JAMA 271, 767–770.

Seligman M (1975) Helplessness: On Depression, Development, and Death. Freeman, San Francisco.

Seligman ME, Abramson LY, Semmel A, et al. (1979) Depressive attributional style. J Abnorm Psychol 88(3) (June), 242–247.

Simon GE, Ludman EJ, Unutzer J, et al. (2002) Design and implementation of a randomized trial evaluating systematic care for bipolar disorder. Bipolar Disord 4, 226–236.

Simpson SG, Folstein SE, Meyers DA, et al. (1993) Bipolar II: The most common bipolar phenotype? Am J Psychiatr 150, 901–903.

Sitland-Marken PA, Rickman LA, Wells BG, et al. (1989) Pharmacologic management of acute mania in pregnancy. J Clin Psychopharmacol 9, 78–87.

Spitzer RL, Endicott J, and Bobins E (1978) Research diagnostic criteria: Rationale and reliability. Arch Gen Psychiatr 35, 773–782.

Stahl SM (2000) Essential Psychopharmacology, 2nd ed. Ch. 5: Depression and bipolar disorders. Cambridge University Press, Cambridge, pp. 135–197.

Stallone F, Shelley E, Mendlewicz J, et al. (1973) The use of lithium in affective disorders III: A double-blind study of prophylaxis in bipolar illness. Am J Psychiatr 130(9), 1006–1010.

Starkstein SE, Boston JD, and Robinson RGG (1988) Mechanisms of mania after brain injury: 12 case reports and review of the literature. J Nerv Ment Dis 176, 87–100.

Stewart A, Greenfield S, Hays R, et al. (1989) Functional status and well-being of patients with chronic conditions. JAMA 262, 907–913.

Stokes PE, Shamoian CA, Stoll PM, et al. (1971) Efficacy of lithium as acute treatment of manic–depressive illness. Lancet 1, 1319–1325.

Stoudemire A, Frank R, Hedemark N, et al. (1986) The economic burden of depression. Gen Hosp Psychiatr 8, 387–394.

Strakowski SM, McElroy SL, Keck PE, et al. (1994) The co-occurrence of mania with medical and other psychiatric disorders. Int J Psychiatr Med 24, 305–328.

Strakowski SM, Shelton RC, and Kolbrener ML (1993c) The effects of race and comorbidity on clinical diagnosis in patients with psychosis. J Clin Psychiatr 54, 96–102.

Strakowski SM, Tohen M, Stoll AL, et al. (1992) Comorbidity in mania at first hospitalization. Am J Psychiatr 149, 554–556.

Strakowski SM, Wilson DR, Tohen M, et al. (1993a) Structural brain abnormalities in first-episode mania. Biol Psychiatr 33, 602–609.

Strakowski SM, Woods BT, and Tohen M (1993b) MRI subcortical signal hyperintensities in mania at first hospitalization. Biol Psychiatr 33, 204–206.

Strober M, Schmidt-Lackner S, Freeman R, et al. (1995) Recovery and relapse in adolescents with bipolar affective illness: A five-year naturalistic, prospective follow-up. J Am Acad Child Adolesc Psychiatr 34, 724–731.

Suppes T, Baldessarini RJ, Faedda GL, et al. (1993) Discontinuation of maintenance treatment in bipolar disorder: Risks and implications. Harv Rev Psychiatr 1, 131–144.

Swann AC (2001) Major system toxicities and side effects of anticonvulsants. J Clin Psychiatr 62(Suppl 14), 16–21.

Symonds R and Williams P (1981) Lithium and the changing incidence of mania. Psychol Med 11, 193–196.

Tasman A, Jay K, and Lieberman JA (1997) Psychiatry. WB Saunders, Philadelphia, PA.

Taylor MA, Abrams R, and Hayman MA (1980) The classification of affective disorders: A reassessment of the bipolar–unipolar dichotomy: A clinical, laboratory, and family study. J Affect Disord 2, 95–109.

Terman M, Terman J, Quitkin F, et al. (1989) Light therapy for seasonal affective disorder: A review of efficacy. Neuropsychopharmacology 2, 1–22.

Thase ME and Sachs GS (2000) Bipolar depression: Pharmacotherapy and related therapeutic strategies. Biol Psychiatr 48(6) (Sept 15), 558–572.

Tohen M, Jacobs TG, Grundy SL, et al. (2000) Efficacy of olanzapine in acute bipolar mania: A double-blind, placebo-controlled study. Arch Gen Psychiatr 57, 841–849.

Tohen M, Sanger TM, McElroy SL, et al. (1999) Olanzapine versus placebo in the treatment of acute mania. Am J Psychiatr 156(5), 702–709.

Tohen M, Waternaux C, and Tsuang M (1990) Outcome in mania: A 4-year prospective follow-up of 75 patients utilizing survival analysis. Arch Gen Psychiatr 47, 1106–1111.

Tsuang M, Woolson R, and Fleming J (1979) Long-term outcome of major psychoses. Arch Gen Psychiatr 36, 1295–1301.

Tsuang MT, Faraone SV, and Fleming JA (1985) Familial transmission of major affective disorders: Is there evidence supporting the distinction between unipolar and bipolar disorders? Br J Psychiatr 146, 268–271.

US Department of Health, Education, and Welfare Medical Practice Project (1979) A State-of-the-Science Report for the Office of the Assistant Secretary of the US Department of Health, Education, and Welfare, Policy Research, Baltimore.

Vaamonde C, Milian N, Magrinat G, et al. (1986) Longitudinal evaluation of glomerular filtration rate during long-term lithium therapy. Am J Kidney Dis 7, 213–216.

Van Gent E, Vida S, and Zwart F (1988) Group therapy in addition to lithium therapy in patients with bipolar disorders. Acta Psychiatr Belg 88, 405–418.

Van Gent EM and Zwart F (1991) Psychoeducation of partners of bipolar-manic patients. J Affect Disord 21, 15–18.

Van Gent EM and Zwart FM (1993) Five-year follow-up after educational group therapy added to lithium prophylaxis: Five years after group added to lithium. Depression 1, 225–226.

VHA (Veterans Health Administration) (1997) Clinical Guidelines for Management of Persons with Psychoses. Office of Performance Management, VHA Headquarters, Washington DC.

Vojta C, Kinosian B, Glick H, et al. (2001) Self-reported quality of life across mood states in bipolar disorder. Compr Psychiatr 42(3) (May–June), 190–195.

Volkmar F, Shakir S, Bacon S, et al. (1981) Group therapy in the management of manic–depressive illness. Am J Psychother 35, 226–234.

Von Korff M, Gruman J, Schaefer J, et al. (1997) Collaborative management of chronic illness. Ann Intern Med 127, 1097–1102.

Wagner EH, Austin BT, and Von Korff M (1996) Organizing care for patients with chronic illness. Milbank Q 74, 511–544.

Wehr T, Goodwin F, Wirz-Justice A, et al. (1982) 48-hour sleep–wake cycles in manic–depressive illness: Naturalistic observations and sleep deprivation experiments. Arch Gen Psychiatr 39, 559–565.

Wehr T, Murdock R, Persad E, et al. (1993) Can antidepressants induce rapid cycling? (letters). Arch Gen Psychiatr 50, 495–498.

Weinstein MR and Goldfield MD (1975) Cardiovascular malformations with lithium use during pregnancy. Am J Psychiatr 132, 529–531.

Weiss RD, Griffin ML, Greenfield SF, et al. (2000) Group therapy for patients with bipolar disorder and substance dependence: Results of a pilot study. J Clin Psychiatr 61, 361–367.

Weiss RD, Mirin SM, Griffin ML, et al. (1988) Psychopathology in cocaine abusers: Changing trends. J Nerv Ment Dis 176, 719–725.

Weissman M and Klerman G (1991) Interpersonal psychotherapy for depression. In Integrating Pharmacotherapy and Psychotherapy, Beitman B and Klerman G (eds). American Psychiatric Press, Washington DC, pp. 379–394.

Weissman MM and Myers JK (1978) Affective disorders in a US urban community: The use of research diagnostic criteria in an epidemiological survey. Arch Gen Psychiatr 35, 1304–1311.

Weissman MM, Leaf PJ, Tischler GL, et al. (1988) Affective disorders in five United States communities. Psychol Med 18, 141–153.

Wells K, Stewart A, Hays R, et al. (1989) The functioning and well-being of depressed patients. Results from the Medical Outcomes Study. JAMA 262, 914–919.

Welner A, Welner Z, and Leonard A (1977) Bipolar manic–depressive disorder: A reassessment of course and outcome. Compr Psychiatr 18, 327–332.

Widiger TA, Frances AJ, Pincus HA, et al. (eds) (1994–1997) DSM-IV Sourcebook, Vol. 1 and 2. American Psychiatric Association, Washington DC.

Williams P and McGlashan T (1987) Schizoaffective psychosis I. Comparative long-term outcome. Arch Gen Psychiatr 44, 130–137.

Winokur G, Clayton PJ, and Reich T (1969) Manic–Depressive Illness. CV Mosby, St. Louis.

World Health Organization (1994) International Statistical Classification of Diseases and Related Health Problems, 10th Rev. World Health Organization, Geneva.

Yildiz A, Sachs GS, Dorer DJ, et al. (2001) 31P Nuclear Magnetic Resonance Spectroscopy Findings in Bipolar Illness: A Meta-Analysis. Psychiatr Res 106 (3), 181–191.

Young RC, Biggs JT, Ziegler VE, et al. (1978) A rating scale for mania: Reliability, validity, and sensitivity. Br J Psychiatr 133, 429–435.

Young RC, Nysewander RW, and Schreiber MT (1983) Mania scale scores, signs, and symptoms in forty inpatients. J Clin Psychiatr 44, 98–100.

Zaretsky AE, Segal ZV, and Gemar M (1999) Cognitive therapy for bipolar depression: A pilot study. Can J Psychiatr 44, 491–494.

Zarin DA and Pass TM (1987) Lithium and the single episode: When to begin long-term prophylaxis for bipolar disorder. Med Care 25, S76–S84.

# 65 Mood Disorders: Premenstrual Dysphoric Disorder

Teri Pearlstein

## Premenstrual Dysphoric Disorder (PMDD)

## Definition

Premenstrual syndrome (PMS) is a combination of emotional, behavioral, and physical symptoms that occur in the premenstrual or luteal phase of the menstrual cycle. The term "premenstrual tension" appeared in the medical literature 70 years ago (Frank 1931) but widely accepted diagnostic criteria for PMS do not exist. Diagnostic criteria for PMS often require a minimum of one premenstrual symptom, such as the criteria proposed in the *American College of Obstetrics and Gynecology Practice Guidelines* (American College of Obstetrics and Gynecology 2000) or in the *International Classification of Diseases*, 10th Revision (World Health Organization 1993). Approximately 80% of women report at least mild premenstrual symptoms, 20 to 50% report moderate to severe premenstrual symptoms, and approximately 5% of women report severe symptoms for several days with impairment of role and social functioning (American Psychiatric Association 1994). The 5% of women with the severest form of PMS generally have symptoms that meet the diagnostic criteria for premenstrual dysphoric disorder (PMDD).

The diagnostic criteria for PMDD are listed in the appendix of DSM-IV (American Psychiatric Association 1994), and they are an updated version of the older DSM-III-R criteria for late luteal phase dysphoric disorder (American Psychiatric Association 1987). A clinician can indicate that a woman has symptoms that meet the diagnostic criteria for PMDD by using the DSM-IV diagnosis 311, depressive disorder not otherwise specified. To meet the PMDD criteria, at least five out of 11 possible symptoms must be present in the premenstrual phase; these symptoms should be absent shortly following the onset of menses; and at least one of the 5 symptoms must be depressed mood, anxiety, lability, or irritability. The PMDD criteria require that role functioning be impaired as a result of the premenstrual symptoms. The functional impairment reported by women with PMDD is similar in severity to the impairment reported in major depressive disorder and dysthymic disorder (Pearlstein et al. 2000). Unlike the functional impairment reported in depressive disorders, women with severe PMS and PMDD report more disruption in their relationships and parenting roles than in their work roles (Campbell et al. 1997, Hylan et al. 1999, Robinson and Swindle 2000).

The PMDD criteria require that a woman prospectively rate her emotional, behavioral, and physical symptoms over two menstrual cycles to confirm the diagnosis. Several studies have reported that retrospective reports of premenstrual symptoms may inaccurately identify the timing or amplify the severity of symptoms compared to prospective reporting (Schnurr et al. 1994). Charting two menstrual cycles is advantageous, since some women have variability of symptom severity from cycle to cycle due to factors such as seasonal worsening, or a woman might have the unusual presence of follicular phase psychological symptoms due to a transient stressor. Studies conducted over the past two decades have used different instruments for daily ratings and various scoring methods to measure the premenstrual increase of symptoms (Schnurr et al. 1994). More recent studies tend to utilize visual analog scales, or Likert scale daily rating forms such as the Daily Record of Severity of Problems (Endicott and Harrison 1990), with a scoring method that compares the average of symptom scores during the premenstrual days to the average of symptom scores postmenses.

A woman presenting with PMS should ideally bring to her clinician two cycles of an established daily rating form, or alternatively ratings of her most problematic symptoms, rated with anchor points ranging from "not present" to "severe." The clinician should review the daily ratings to confirm that the symptoms are in fact confined largely to the premenstrual phase, with the relative absence of symptoms in the follicular phase, and the clinician should also assess premenstrual functional impairment (Figure 65–1). Ratings that demonstrate follicular symptoms with increased symptom severity in the premenstrual phase suggest "premenstrual exacerbation" of an underlying disorder rather than PMDD. The DSM-IV-TR PMDD criteria state that the premenstrual symptoms should not be an exacerbation of an underlying disorder, but that PMDD could be superimposed on another disorder, like panic disorder. No formal guidelines exist for how to apply this criterion clinically.

**DSM-IV-TR Criteria**

## Diagnostic Criteria for PMDD

Research Criteria for Premenstrual Dysphoric Disorder

A. In most menstrual cycles during the past year, five (or more) of the following symptoms were present for most of the time during the last week of the luteal phase, began to remit within a few days after the onset of the follicular phase, and were absent in the week postmenses, with at least one of the symptoms being either (1), (2), (3), or (4):

  (1) markedly depressed mood, feelings of hopelessness, or self-deprecating thoughts

  (2) marked anxiety, tension, feelings of being "keyed up," or "on edge"

  (3) marked affective lability (e.g., feeling suddenly sad or tearful or increased sensitivity to rejection)

  (4) persistent and marked anger or irritability or increased interpersonal conflicts

  (5) decreased interest in usual activities (e.g., work, school, friends, hobbies)

  (6) subjective sense of difficulty in concentrating

  (7) lethargy, easy fatigability, or marked lack of energy

  (8) marked change in appetite, overeating, or specific food cravings

  (9) hypersomnia or insomnia

  (10) a subjective sense of being overwhelmed or out of control

  (11) other physical symptoms, such as breast tenderness or swelling, headaches, joint or muscle pain, a sensation of "bloating," weight gain

B. The disturbance markedly interferes with work or school or with usual social activities and relationships (e.g., avoidance of social activities, decreased productivity and efficiency at work or school).

C. The disturbance is not merely an exacerbation of the symptoms of another disorder such as major depressive disorder, panic disorder, dysthymic disorder, or a personality disorder (although it may be superimposed on any of these disorders).

D. Criteria A, B, and C must be confirmed by prospective daily ratings during at least two consecutive symptomatic cycles. (The diagnosis may be made provisionally prior to this confirmation).

## Differential Diagnosis

Depression and anxiety disorders are the most common Axis I psychiatric disorders that may be concurrent and exacerbated premenstrually, with less clear evidence for bipolar disorder, eating disorders, and substance abuse (Endicott 1994, Hendrick et al. 1996, Pearlstein and Stone 1998). Since most PMDD symptoms are affective or anxiety-related, "pure PMS" or PMDD is generally not diagnosed when an underlying depression or anxiety disorder is present; these women would be considered to have premenstrual exacerbation of their underlying depression or anxiety disorder. Personality disorders are not elevated in prevalence in women with PMDD (Critchlow et al. 2001), but women with PMDD and a personality disorder may demonstrate premenstrual phase amplification of personality dysfunction (Berlin et al. 2001). Schizophrenia may be an example of a disorder that does not have premenstrual exacerbation of psychotic symptoms but may have the superimposition of affective and anxiety symptoms of PMDD (Choi et al. 2001). The prevalence of premenstrually exacerbated disorders is unknown, but women with these conditions present frequently to their primary care clinician or gynecologist. Since most recent treatment studies have been conducted on women with PMS and PMDD without follicular symptomatology, this literature is not particularly informative on how to treat women with premenstrually exacerbated disorders. The general guideline is to treat the underlying disorder first and see if subsequent daily ratings suggest persistence of premenstrual symptoms that might meet criteria for PMDD.

Several medical conditions should also be considered when evaluating a woman with premenstrual complaints. Symptoms of endometriosis, polycystic ovary disease, thyroid disorders, disorders of the adrenal system, hyperprolactinemia, and panhypopituitarism may mimic symptoms of PMS. Several medical disorders may demonstrate a premenstrual increase in symptoms without accompanying emotional symptoms, such as migraines, asthma, epilepsy, irritable bowel syndrome, diabetes, allergies, and autoimmune disorders (Pearlstein and Stone 1998, Case and Reid 2001). It is presumed that the menstrual cycle fluctuations of gonadal hormones influence some of the symptoms of these medical conditions.

## Epidemiology

Irritability has been identified as the most common premenstrual symptom in US and European samples (Endicott et al. 1999, Angst et al. 2001). Studies examining age, menstrual cycle characteristics, cognitive attributions, socioeconomic variables, lifestyle variables, and number of children have not yielded consistent conclusions (Endicott et al. 1999, Steiner and Born 2000). Studies have suggested some genetic liability for PMS, but the overlap with genetic liability for major depression or personality characteristics has received mixed reports (Treloar et al. 2002). A polymorphism in the serotonin transporter promoter gene has been suggested in women who have both PMDD and seasonal affective disorder (Praschak-Rieder et al. 2002). Elevated lifetime prevalence of major depressive disorder in women with PMDD has been reported in several studies (Endicott 1994), as well as an elevated lifetime prevalence of postpartum depression (Critchlow et al. 2001). Even though

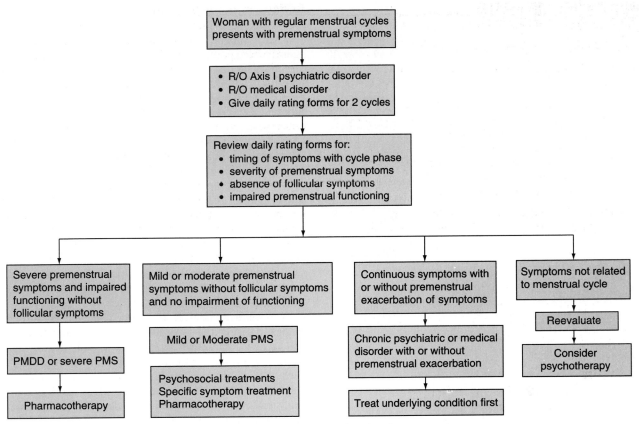

**Figure 65–1** *Diagnosis and initial treatment algorithm of premenstrual symptoms.*

premenstrual symptoms are described in women from menarche to menopause, it is unclear if symptoms remain stable or increase in severity with age (Endicott et al. 1999, Wittchen et al. 2002). PMS has been described in several countries and cultures and some cultures have a preponderance of somatic rather than emotional symptoms (Steiner and Born 2000).

## Etiology

There are several recent reviews of pathophysiologic hypotheses of PMS and PMDD and their evidence (Roca et al. 1996, Parry 1997, Yonkers 1997, Sundstrom et al. 1999, Steiner and Born 2000, Steiner and Pearlstein 2000). The majority of studies do not identify consistent abnormalities of hormones of the hypothalamic–pituitary–gonadal (HPG) axis, thyroid hormones, cortisol, prolactin, glucose, prostaglandins, vitamins, or electrolytes (Parry 1997). Decreased luteal phase peripheral beta-endorphin levels have been reported, but this may not reflect central opioid activity. Women with PMDD are more sensitive to the anxiolytic properties of carbon dioxide inhalation and lactate infusion, and increased adrenergic receptor binding may reflect abnormal noradrenergic function (Parry 1997, Sundstrom et al. 1999, Steiner and Born 2000). Women with PMDD have abnormal melatonin secretion and other circadian system abnormalities (Parry and Newton 2001).

Since abnormalities in the HPG axis have not been identified, it is thought that premenstrual symptoms may occur due to a differential sensitivity to mood-perturbing effects of gonadal steroid fluctuations in women with PMS and PMDD (Schmidt et al. 1998). It is probable that the etiology of the "differential sensitivity" is multifactorial. The specific neurotransmitter, neuroendocrine, and neurosteroid abnormalities in women with PMS and PMDD are not known, but serotonin, norepinephrine, gamma-aminobutyric acid (GABA), allopregnanolone (an anxiolytic metabolite of progesterone that acts at the $GABA_A$ receptor), and factors involved in calcium homeostasis are all possibly involved.

A large number of studies have reported abnormalities in the serotonin system in women with PMS and PMDD. These include abnormal levels of whole blood serotonin, serotonin platelet uptake, and platelet tritiated imipramine binding; abnormal responses to serotonergic probes such as L-tryptophan, buspirone, meta-chlorophenylpiperazaine and fenfluramine; and exacerbation of premenstrual symptoms after tryptophan depletion (Halbreich and Tworek 1993, Yonkers 1997, Sundstrom et al. 1999, Steiner and Pearlstein 2000, Parry 2001). Several studies have also suggested that women with PMDD have decreased luteal phase levels of GABA, abnormal allopregnanolone levels, and decreased sensitivity of the $GABA_A$ receptor as shown by flumazenil challenge, and the sedative and saccadic eye velocity responses to benzodiazepines (Sundstrom et al. 1999, Girdler et al. 2001). It is possible that the rapid efficacy of selective serotonin reuptake inhibitors (SSRIs) in PMDD may be due in part to their ability to increase allopregnanolone levels in the brain, thus enhancing GABA transmission as well as serotonin transmission (Guidotti and Costa 1998, Griffin and Mellon 1999).

Several factors that influence calcium and bone homeostasis fluctuate with the menstrual cycle and it is possible that some of these factors are abnormal in women with PMS and PMDD (Thys-Jacobs 2000). One study reported decreased bone mineral density in women with prospectively-confirmed PMS (Thys-Jacobs et al. 1995); however, a later study in women with PMDD failed to find decreased bone mineral density compared to controls (Halbreich and Kahn 2001). Thys-Jacobs and colleagues reported that women with PMS had reduced periovulatory calcium levels and elevated parathyroid hormone levels compared to controls, perhaps secondary to elevated pre-ovulatory estrogen levels, and these authors proposed that women with PMS may have a cyclical, transient secondary hyperparathyroidism (Thys-Jacobs and Alvir 1995). It has been reported that when calcium homeostasis is corrected in primary hyperparathyroidism, cerebrospinal fluid mono-amine metabolites normalize and affective symptoms are reduced (Joborn et al. 1991). It is possible that the administration of supplemental calcium normalizes the periovulatory fluctuations in calcium and parathyroid hormone, thus regulating calcium effects on neurotransmitter synthesis and release leading to symptom relief in women with PMS (Thys-Jacobs 2000).

## Treatment

### Antidepressant Treatment

The treatment studies of SSRIs in PMDD have suggested a similar efficacy rate to treatment studies of SSRIs in major depressive disorder, with 60 to 70% of women responding to SSRIs compared to approximately 30% of women responding to placebo. In general, the effective SSRI doses are similar to the doses recommended for the treatment of major depressive disorder (Figure 65–2). A review of 15 randomized controlled trials (RCTs) of SSRIs reported that women with severe PMS or PMDD were approximately seven times more likely to respond to SSRIs compared to placebo (Dimmock et al. 2000). This review included 12 trials with continuous (daily) dosing of fluoxetine (Stone et al. 1991, Wood et al. 1992, Menkes et al. 1993, Steiner et al. 1995, Ozeren et al. 1997, Pearlstein et al. 1997, Su et al. 1997), sertraline (Yonkers et al. 1997, Freeman et al. 1999), paroxetine (Eriksson et al. 1995), citalopram (Wikander et al. 1998), and fluvoxamine (Veeninga et al. 1990); and four trials with intermittent dosing (SSRI administered during the luteal phase only from ovulation to menses) of sertraline (Halbreich and Smoller 1997, Young et al. 1998, Jermain et al. 1999) and citalopram (Wikander et al. 1998). The efficacy of the continuous and intermittent dosing RCTs was equivalent (Dimmock et al. 2000).

Two of the reviewed RCTs with continuous dosing involved large samples. One RCT compared fluoxetine 20 mg, 60 mg, and placebo over 6 months in 277 women with PMS (Steiner et al. 1995). Fluoxetine 20 mg/day was better tolerated than 60 mg, although both dosages were more efficacious than placebo in reducing premenstrual emotional, behavioral, and physical symptoms. It was surprising that fluoxetine improved each physical symptom assessed and the mechanism by which SSRIs improve physical symptoms is not clear (Steiner et al. 2001). The other large RCT involved daily flexible-dose sertraline over 3 months, and the average dose of 110 mg/day was more effective than placebo in reducing premenstrual symptoms

(Yonkers et al. 1997) and improving psychosocial functioning in 243 women (Pearlstein et al. 2000).

Since this review, a large RCT has reported that fluoxetine 20 mg/day during the luteal phase only was superior to placebo in reducing premenstrual emotional and physical symptoms in 252 women with PMDD (Cohen et al. 2002). Fluoxetine 10 mg/day during the luteal phase only was superior to placebo in reducing emotional symptoms but not physical symptoms. The results of another large RCT suggested that sertraline 50 to 100 mg/day during the luteal phase only was superior to placebo for improving premenstrual emotional symptoms and impaired functioning, but not for premenstrual physical symptoms (Halbreich et al. in press). There have not been reports of discontinuation symptoms from these doses of fluoxetine and sertraline when abruptly stopped from the first day of menses. Weekly fluoxetine 90 mg administered 2 weeks and 1 week prior to the expected onset of menses in 257 women with PMDD has been reported to be superior to placebo in reducing premenstrual emotional symptoms and improving premenstrual functioning, but not in reducing premenstrual physical symptoms (Miner et al. 2002). There are no published studies to date of the efficacy of "symptom onset" dosing of SSRIs, that is, administering SSRIs the postovulatory day that premenstrual symptoms appear until menses. The efficacy of intermittent dosing, as well as the findings from most SSRI trials that efficacy is achieved by the first treatment cycle, has suggested a more rapid and different mechanism of action of SSRIs in PMDD compared to its effect in major depressive disorder, which typically takes 2 to 6 weeks. As discussed above, it has been hypothesized that the rapid improvement of premenstrual symptoms by SSRIs may be due to an increase in allopregnanolone levels.

A large RCT with daily dosing of venlafaxine, an antidepressant with both serotonergic and noradrenergic action, reported that an average dose of 130 mg/day reduced emotional and physical symptoms of PMDD in 157 women (Freeman et al. 2001c). Smaller RCTs have reported efficacy with clomipramine, a tricyclic antidepressant with largely serotonergic action, in daily dosing (Sundblad et al. 1992) and luteal phase dosing (Sundblad et al. 1993). The doses of clomipramine reported to be effective for PMS (25–75 mg q.d.) are lower than expected effective doses for major depressive disorder (see Figure 65–2). One RCT reported that nefazodone was not superior to placebo in PMS (Landen et al. 2001); however, increasing nefazodone in the luteal phase was reported to improve premenstrual exacerbation of major depressive disorder in a small cross-over study (Miller et al. 2002). Three RCTs have compared SSRIs to nonserotonergic antidepressants and placebo, and each has reported specific efficacy of the SSRI over placebo and the nonserotonergic antidepressant. A large study compared sertraline to desipramine and placebo (Freeman et al. 1999), and two smaller studies compared paroxetine to maprotiline and placebo (Eriksson et al. 1995), and fluoxetine to bupropion and placebo (Pearlstein et al. 1997). The selective superiority of serotonergic antidepressants for PMDD is compatible with the postulated serotonin dysfunction in PMDD.

Most SSRI trials have been 6 months or less in duration, so efficacy-based long-term treatment recommenda-

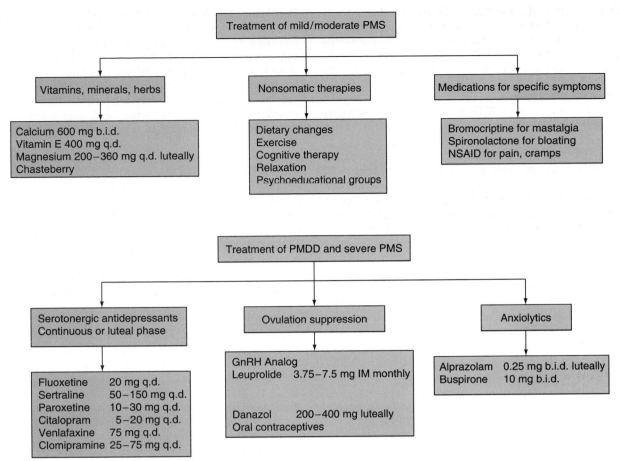

**Figure 65–2** *Treatment algorithm of premenstrual symptoms.*

tions do not exist. Clinically, many women note the recurrence of premenstrual symptoms after SSRI discontinuation and many clinicians treat women over a long period of time. As reviewed, a few open studies report maintenance of SSRI efficacy over a couple of years (Yonkers 1997). Studies are needed to identify whether or not some women develop tolerance to the SSRI and need a higher dose over time and whether or not some women stay in remission for a period of time following SSRI discontinuation.

## Ovulation Suppression Treatments

Gonadotropin releasing hormone (GnRH) agonists suppress ovulation by downregulating GnRH receptors in the hypothalamus, leading to decreased follicle-stimulating hormone and luteinizing hormone release from the pituitary, resulting in decreased estrogen and progesterone levels. GnRH agonists are administered parenterally (e.g., subcutaneous monthly injections of goserelin, intramuscular monthly injections of leuprolide, daily intranasal buserelin) (see Figure 65–2). Ten double-blind, placebo-controlled studies of GnRH agonists in PMS and PMDD have been published to date, and GnRH agonists are reported to be superior to placebo in 8 of these studies (Johnson 1998, Pearlstein and Steiner 2000). GnRH agonists lead to improvement in most emotional and physical premenstrual symptoms, with possible decreased efficacy for premenstrual dysphoria and severe premenstrual symptoms

(Brown et al. 1994), or for the exacerbation of chronic depression (Freeman et al. 1997). After relief of PMS is achieved with a GnRH agonist, "add-back" hormone strategies have been investigated due to the undesirable medical consequences of the hypoestrogenic state resulting from prolonged anovulation. As reviewed, the addition of estrogen and progesterone to goserelin (Leather et al. 1999) and leuprolide (Schmidt et al. 1998) led to the reappearance of mood and anxiety symptoms (Pearlstein and Steiner 2000). Since women with severe PMS and PMDD have an abnormal response to normal hormonal fluctuations (Schmidt et al. 1998), it is not surprising that women in these studies had the induction of mood and anxiety symptoms from the addition of gonadal steroids, reducing the benefit of the replacement strategy.

Danazol, a synthetic steroid, alleviates premenstrual symptoms when administered at 200 to 400 mg q.d. doses that induce anovulation (Hahn et al. 1995). A recent study with danazol 200 mg/day administered during the luteal phase only, not causing anovulation, reported that breast tenderness but not other premenstrual symptoms were reduced (O'Brien and Abukhalil 1999). Prolonged anovulation with estrogen and progesterone administered most of the cycle or oophorectomy are not common treatments, largely due to the medical risks from the prolonged hypoestrogenic state, leading to the same long-term health issues as with GnRH agonists. Oophorectomy should be reserved for women, with severe PMS and PMDD, unresponsive to antidepressants or hormonal treatment. In addition, the small literature with estrogen and progesterone administered most of the cycle has yielded mixed reports, (Johnson 1998, Epperson et al. 1999, Pearlstein and Steiner 2000).

## Oral Contraceptives

Even though oral contraceptives (OCs) are a commonly prescribed treatment for PMS (Campbell et al. 1997, Hylan et al. 1999), there is minimal literature endorsing its efficacy. Two older studies in samples with confirmed PMS did not report efficacy with monophasic or triphasic OCs (Backstrom et al. 1992, Graham and Sherwin 1992). Anecdotally, women report that oral contraceptives may benefit, worsen, or not affect their premenstrual symptoms. For example, a recent prospective study of women starting OC reported that 35% of women reported that an OC improved their PMS (by retrospective report), while 21% of women reported that the OC made their PMS worse, contributing to OC discontinuation (Sanders et al. 2001). As reviewed, the induction of dysphoria may be related to the type and dose of the progestin component, the androgenic properties of the progesterone, or to the estrogen/progestin ratio (Kahn and Halbreich 2001). A more recent RCT compared an oral contraceptive to placebo in 82 women with PMDD (Freeman et al. 2001a). Even though the OC containing ethinyl estradiol 30 μg and drospirenone 3 mg improved most premenstrual symptoms, due in large part to a placebo response rate of 40%, the OC was significantly more efficacious than placebo only in decreasing food cravings, increased appetite, and acne. Oral contraceptives have been reported to not alter the response to SSRIs in women with PMDD (Freeman et al. 2001b).

## Progesterone

The early assumption that PMS was due to a progesterone deficiency, which has never been substantiated, led to luteal phase progesterone being one of the earliest treatments of PMS in the literature. A recent systematic review of published double-blind placebo-controlled randomized studies of luteal phase progesterone (given as vaginal suppositories or oral micronized tablets) and progestogens reported that there was no clinically meaningful difference between all progesterone forms and placebo, although there was a small statistically significant superiority of progesterone over placebo (Wyatt et al. 2001). There was also a slight advantage for oral micronized progesterone and the authors postulated that this may be due to the increase in allopregnanolone levels derived from this form of progesterone. Another review of progesterone studies also concluded that progesterone was not superior to placebo in efficacy (Epperson et al. 1999).

## Other Medications

Alprazolam (administered during the luteal phase) has been reported to be superior to placebo in most studies (Smith et al. 1987, Harrison et al. 1990, Berger and Presser 1994, Freeman et al. 1995) but not all (Schmidt et al. 1993), and although it has a lower efficacy rate than SSRIs, it is effective for premenstrual emotional symptoms. Alprazolam should be tapered over the first few days of menses each cycle. An early (Rickels et al. 1989) and a more recent

(Landen et al. 2001) study of buspirone 25 mg/day during the luteal weeks indicate some efficacy. Spironolactone has been reported to decrease premenstrual emotional and physical symptoms (Wang et al. 1995). Bromocriptine has been reported to decrease premenstrual breast tenderness (Andersch 1983). Previous studies reporting efficacy that deserve further study include nonsteroidal anti-inflammatory drugs (Mira et al. 1986), doxycycline (Toth et al. 1988), naltrexone (Chuong et al. 1988) and atenolol (Rausch et al. 1988).

## Herbal Treatments

A comprehensive review of 27 RCTs of complementary and alternative treatments in women with PMS reported that no treatment could be recommended based on existent evidence (Stevinson and Ernst 2001). Since the review was published, a randomized controlled trial of agnus castus fruit (chasteberry) in 170 women with PMS reported that chasteberry was superior to placebo in reducing irritability, mood alteration, anger, headache, and breast fullness (Schellenberg 2001). However, the method of diagnosis of PMS in the subjects was not clear in this study. Two open studies with this herb in women with self-reported PMS have reported benefit on emotional and physical symptoms (Berger et al. 2000) and on breast pain (Loch et al. 2000). An open study in a small number of women with prospectively-confirmed PMS suggested efficacy of daily hypericum (Stevinson and Ernst 2000). A controlled study of *ginkgo biloba* indicated some efficacy for breast pain (Tamborini and Taurelle 1993). Reviews of studies of evening primrose oil have not suggested efficacy (Budeiri et al. 1996, Stevinson and Ernst 2001). One small RCT reported that homeopathic medicine was not superior to placebo in women with PMS (Chapman et al. 1994), while another small RCT reported that five different single-dose homeopathic treatments selected based on symptom profiles were superior to placebo in terms of reducing PMS (Yakir et al. 2001).

## Dietary Supplementation

The largest treatment study to date in women with PMS has been a comparison of calcium 600 mg b.i.d. to placebo (Thys-Jacobs et al. 1998). Calcium was reported to have a 48% efficacy rate for reducing the emotional and physical symptoms of the PMDD diagnostic criteria, except for fatigue and insomnia, compared to 30% for placebo. However, women with concurrent psychiatric illness were not clearly excluded, and other treatments except for analgesics were allowed. The efficacy of calcium was somewhat less in women who were also taking oral contraceptives. The results of this study were notable, and calcium deserves further study. There is a study reporting efficacy with tryptophan in PMDD, which has not been available in the US for a period of time (Steinberg et al. 1999).

Several early studies were conducted with vitamin $B_6$ for the treatment of PMS and a review of the early studies reported a lack of efficacy (Kleijnen et al. 1990). A recent meta-analysis of 9 controlled trials including 940 women with PMS indicated only weak support for vitamin $B_6$ (50–100 mg/day) in reducing premenstrual symptoms (Wyatt et al. 1999). Three small trials have suggested efficacy with magnesium (Facchinetti et al. 1991, Walker et al. 1998, De Souza et al. 2000). An early study suggested efficacy for vitamin E and deserves replication (London et al. 1987). Several trials have been conducted with multinutrients containing several vitamin and mineral components. As reviewed, results from these studies have been mixed and several of the supplements studied contained quantities of vitamins that exceeded daily recommended levels (Bendich 2000, Stevinson and Ernst 2001).

## Lifestyle Modifications and Psychosocial Treatments

Many lifestyle modifications and psychosocial treatments have been suggested for PMS. Lifestyle modifications are often suggested through self-help materials or in an individual or group psychoeducation format. A recent study reported that a weekly peer support and professional guidance group for four sessions was superior to waitlist control in terms of reducing premenstrual symptoms. The treatment consisted of diet and exercise regimens, self-monitoring and other cognitive techniques, and environment modification (Taylor 1999). Another study reported that a four-session group intervention over 18 weeks emphasizing diet, exercise, and a positive reframing of a woman's perceptions of her menstrual cycle experiences was superior to a control condition for reducing premenstrual symptoms (Morse 1999). Studies have not been conducted on individual lifestyle or psychosocial treatments to identify which components are most efficacious.

Dietary recommendations include decreased caffeine, frequent snacks or meals, reduction of refined sugar and artificial sweeteners, and increase in complex carbohydrates. As reviewed, premenstrual increased appetite and carbohydrate craving increases the availability of tryptophan in the brain, leading to increased serotonin synthesis (Pearlstein 1996). One controlled study reported that a drink containing simple and complex carbohydrates was superior to drinks that did not increase tryptophan availability for reducing premenstrual dysphoria, increased appetite, and decreased memory (Sayegh et al. 1995). Other than this study, there have been no published controlled trials of specific dietary regimens.

Exercise is likewise a frequently recommended treatment for PMS that has yet to be tested in a sample of women with prospectively-confirmed PMS or PMDD. As reviewed, negative effect and other premenstrual symptoms improve with regular exercise in women in general (Pearlstein 1996, Scully et al. 1998). It is not clear if aerobic exercise is superior to nonaerobic exercise in terms of symptom relief. Cognitive therapy (CT) is reported to be a promising treatment for PMS. Two studies in women with prospectively-confirmed PMS has reported superiority of individual CT over a waitlist control (Blake et al. 1998) and superiority of group CT over information-focused therapy for reducing symptoms (Christensen and Oei 1995). As reviewed, a few controlled studies conducted in women with less rigorously-defined PMS indicate further support for CT and some support for relaxation therapy (Pearlstein 1996).

## Other Treatments

Although results of studies of light therapy have been equivocal, a recent crossover study reported that evening bright light for two premenstrual weeks decreased depression and tension (Lam et al. 1999). As reviewed, both light therapy and sleep deprivation may decrease premenstrual dysphoria by correcting abnormal circadian rhythms found in women with PMDD (Parry and Newton 2001). Preliminary controlled studies with massage (Hernandez-Reif et al. 2000), reflexology (Oleson and Flocco 1993), chiropractic manipulation (Walsh and Polus 1999), and biofeedback (Van Zak 1994) have suggested positive efficacy. Acupuncture has not been studied systematically.

## Conclusion

Women with severe PMS and PMDD comprise a substantial proportion of menstruating women. These women have several symptomatic days each month that lead to disrupted relationships and decreased quality of life. Women presenting with premenstrual complaints need to prospectively rate their symptoms for two menstrual cycles to rule out the presence of a concurrent psychiatric or medical disorder. Once the diagnosis of severe PMS or PMDD is confirmed, SSRI medication is considered the first line treatment (American College of Obstetrics and Gynecology 2000, Altshuler et al. 2001). SSRI medication may be administered daily or intermittently (from ovulation to menses) to be effective. Nutritional approaches, exercise, and cognitive therapy may be appropriate as first treatments in mild cases, otherwise they should accompany medication treatment (Altshuler et al. 2001). Second line treatment options include changing to a second SSRI, gonadal hormone therapy (such as GnRH analogs or oral contraceptives), or adding adjunctive anxiolytics, calcium, or other medications targeted to specific symptoms (American College of Obstetrics and Gynecology 2000, Altshuler et al. 2001). Future studies are still needed for women with severe PMS and PMDD, such as to identify predictors for which women may benefit from hormonal strategies, to determine the optimal duration for medication treatment, and to determine whether or not some women may maintain remission following successful medication treatment.

---

**Clinical Vignette**

Ms. A is a 34-year-old married woman who presents to her gynecologist for her first annual exam since giving birth to her third child 6 months before. Ms. A had always noted 2 to 3 days of irritability, mood swings, and cravings for chocolate before her menses prior to conceiving her third child, but she did not feel that these symptoms had interfered with her functioning. Since her menses has resumed in the past year, Ms. A has noted 10 to 14 days of tension, lack of patience, yelling at her husband and children, feeling more sensitive and overwhelmed, low energy, feeling more clumsy, increased appetite and cravings for sweets, desire to be alone, abdominal bloating, and breast tenderness. Ms. A tells her gynecologist that now the symptoms are interfering with her quality of life and her functioning as a homemaker and she requests medication for her symptoms. Ms. A has an unremarkable psychiatric or medical history.

Ms. A is given a self-help pamphlet which details the recommended dietary, exercise, and lifestyle modifications. She is also encouraged to chart her most troublesome symptoms daily. The gynecologist discusses

## Comparison of DSM-IV/ICD-10 Diagnostic Criteria

Premenstrual Dysphoric Disorder is not included in ICD-10. A related condition "premenstrual tension syndrome" is included in Chapter 14 for diseases of the genitourinary system.

## References

Altshuler LL, Cohen LS, Moline ML, et al. (2001) The Expert Consensus Guideline Series. Treatment of depression in women. Postgrad Med 1–107.

American College of Obstetrics and Gynecology (2000) Premenstrual Syndrome. ACOG Practice Bulletin. American College of Obstetrics and Gynecology, Washington DC.

American Psychiatric Association (1987) Diagnostic and Statistical Manual of Mental Disorders, 3rd ed., Rev. APA, Washington DC.

American Psychiatric Association (1994) Diagnostic and Statistical Manual of Mental Disorders, 4th ed. APA, Washington DC.

Andersch B (1983) Bromocriptine and premenstrual symptoms: A survey of double-blind trials. Obstetr Gynecol Surv 38, 643–646.

Angst J, Sellaro R, Stolar M, et al. (2001) The epidemiology of perimenstrual psychological symptoms. Acta Psychiatr Scand 104, 110–116.

Backstrom T, Hansson-Malmstrom Y, Lindhe B-A, et al. (1992) Oral contraceptives in premenstrual syndrome: A randomized comparison of triphasic and monophasic preparations. Contraception 46, 253–268.

Bendich A (2000) The potential for dietary supplements to reduce premenstrual syndrome (PMS) symptoms. J Am College Nutr 19, 3–12.

Berger CP and Presser B (1994) Alprazolam in the treatment of two sub samples of patients with late luteal phase dysphoric disorder: A double-blind, placebo-controlled crossover study. Obstetr Gynecol 84, 379–385.

Berger D, Schaffner W, Schrader E, et al. (2000) Efficacy of Vitex agnus castus L. extract Ze 440 in patients with premenstrual syndrome (PMS). Arch Gynecol Obstetr 264, 150–153.

Berlin RE, Raju JD, Schmidt PJ, et al. (2001) Effects of the menstrual cycle on measures of personality in women with premenstrual syndrome: A preliminary study. J Clin Psychiatr 62, 337–342.

Blake F, Salkovskis P, Gath D, et al. (1998) Cognitive therapy for premenstrual syndrome: A controlled trial. J Psychosom Res 45, 307–318.

Brown CS, Ling FW, Andersen RN, et al. (1994) Efficacy of depot leuprolide in premenstrual syndrome: Effect of symptom severity and type in a controlled trial. Obstetr Gynecol 84, 779–786.

Budeiri D, Li Wan Po A, and Dornan JC (1996) Is evening primrose oil of value in the treatment of premenstrual syndrome? Control Clin Trials 17, 60–68.

Campbell EM, Peterkin D, O'Grady K, et al. (1997) Premenstrual symptoms in general practice patients. Prevalence and treatment. J Reprod Med 42, 637–646.

Case AM and Reid RL (2001) Menstrual cycle effects on common medical conditions. Compr Ther 27, 65–71.

Chapman EH, Angelica J, Spitalny G, et al. (1994) Results of a study of the homeopathic treatment of PMS. J Am Inst Homeo 87, 14–21.

Choi SH, Kang SB, and Joe SH (2001) Changes in premenstrual symptoms in women with schizophrenia: A prospective study. Psychosom Med 63, 822–829.

Christensen AP and Oei TP (1995) The efficacy of cognitive behaviour therapy in treating premenstrual dysphoric changes. J Affect Disord 33, 57–63.

Chuong CJ, Coulam CB, Bergstralh EJ, et al. (1988) Clinical trial of naltrexone in premenstrual syndrome. Obstetr Gynecol 72, 332–336.

Cohen LS, Miner C, Brown E, et al. (2002) Premenstrual daily fluoxetine for premenstrual dysphoric disorder: A placebo-controlled, clinical trial using computerized diaries. Obstetr Gynecol 100(3), 435–444.

Critchlow DG, Bond AJ, and Wingrove J (2001) Mood disorder history and personality assessment in premenstrual dysphoric disorder. J Clin Psychiatr 62, 688–693.

De Souza MC, Walker AF, Robinson PA, et al. (2000) A synergistic effect of a daily supplement for 1 month of 200 mg magnesium plus 50 mg vitamin B$_6$ for the relief of anxiety-related premenstrual symptoms: A randomized, double-blind, crossover study. J Women's Health Gender-Based Med 9, 131–139.

Dimmock PW, Wyatt KM, Jones PW, et al. (2000) Efficacy of selective serotonin reuptake inhibitors in premenstrual syndrome: A systematic review. Lancet 356, 1131–1136.

Endicott J (1994) Differential diagnoses and comorbidity. In Premenstrual Dysphorias. Myths and Realities, Gold JH and Severino SK (eds). American Psychiatric Press, Washington DC, pp. 3–17.

Endicott J and Harrison W (1990) Daily Rating of Severity of Problems Form. Department of Research Assessment and Training. New York State Psychiatric Institute, New York.

Endicott J, Amsterdam J, Eriksson E, et al. (1999) Is premenstrual dysphoric disorder a distinct clinical entity? J Women's Health Gender-Based Med 8, 663–679.

Epperson CN, Wisner KL, and Yamamoto B (1999) Gonadal steroids in the treatment of mood disorders. Psychosom Med 61, 676–697.

Eriksson E, Hedberg MA, Andersch B, et al. (1995) The serotonin reuptake inhibitor paroxetine is superior to the noradrenaline reuptake inhibitor maprotiline in the treatment of premenstrual syndrome. Neuropsychopharmacology 12, 167–176.

Facchinetti F, Borella P, Sances G, et al. (1991) Oral magnesium successfully relieves premenstrual mood changes. Obstetr Gynecol 78, 177–181.

Frank RT (1931) The hormonal causes of premenstrual tension. Arch Neurol Psychiatr 26, 1053–1057.

Freeman EW, Rickels K, Sondheimer SJ, et al. (1995) A double-blind trial of oral progesterone, alprazolam, and placebo in treatment of severe premenstrual syndrome. J Am Med Assoc 274, 51–57.

Freeman EW, Sondheimer SJ, and Rickels K (1997) Gonadotropin-releasing hormone agonist in the treatment of premenstrual symptoms with and without ongoing dysphoria: A controlled study. Psychopharmacol Bull 33, 303–309.

Freeman EW, Rickels K, Sondheimer SJ, et al. (1999) Differential response to antidepressants in women with premenstrual syndrome/premenstrual dysphoric disorder: A randomized controlled trial. Arch Gen Psychiatr 56, 932–939.

Freeman EW, Kroll R, Rapkin A, et al. (2001a) Evaluation of a unique oral contraceptive in the treatment of premenstrual dysphoric disorder. J Women's Health Gender-Based Med 10, 561–569.

Freeman EW, Rickels K, and Sondheimer SJ (2001b) Concurrent use of oral contraceptives with antidepressants for premenstrual syndromes. J Clin Psychopharmacol 21, 540–542.

Freeman EW, Rickels K, Yonkers KA, et al. (2001c) Venlafaxine in the treatment of premenstrual dysphoric disorder. Obstetr Gynecol 98, 737–744.

Girdler SS, Straneva PA, Light KC, et al. (2001) Allopregnanolone levels and reactivity to mental stress in premenstrual dysphoric disorder. Biol Psychiatr 49, 788–797.

Graham CA and Sherwin BB (1992) A prospective treatment study of premenstrual symptoms using a triphasic oral contraceptive. J Psychosom Res 36, 257–266.

Griffin LD and Mellon SH (1999) Selective serotonin reuptake inhibitors directly alter activity of neurosteroidogenic enzymes. Proc Natl Acad Sci US Am 96, 13512–13517.

Guidotti A and Costa E (1998) Can the antidysphoric and anxiolytic profiles of selective serotonin reuptake inhibitors be related to their ability to increase brain 3-alpha-, 5-alpha-tetrahydroprogesterone (allopregnanolone) availability? Biol Psychiatr 44, 865–873.

Hahn PM, Van Vugt DA, and Reid RL (1995) A randomized, placebo-controlled, crossover trial of danazol for the treatment of premenstrual syndrome. Psychoneuroendocrinology 20, 193–209.

Halbreich U and Tworek H (1993) Altered serotonergic activity in women with dysphoric premenstrual syndromes. Int J Psychiatr Med 23, 1–27.

Halbreich U and Kahn LS (2001) Are women with premenstrual dysphoric disorder prone to osteoporosis? Psychosom Med 63, 361–364.

Halbreich U and Smoller JW (1997) Intermittent luteal phase sertraline treatment of dysphoric premenstrual syndrome. J Clin Psychiatr 58, 399–402.

Halbreich U, Bergeron R, Yonkers KA, et al. (in press) Efficacy of intermittent, luteal phase sertraline treatment of premenstrual dysphoric disorder. Obstet Gynecol.

Harrison WM, Endicott J, and Nee J (1990) Treatment of premenstrual dysphoria with alprazolam. A controlled study. Arch Gen Psychiatr 47, 270–275.

Hendrick V, Altshuler LL, and Burt VK (1996) Course of psychiatric disorders across the menstrual cycle. Harv Rev Psychiatr 4, 200–207.

Hernandez-Reif M, Martinez A, Field T, et al. (2000) Premenstrual symptoms are relieved by massage therapy. J Psychosom Obstetr Gynaecol 21, 9–15.

Hylan TR, Sundell K, and Judge R (1999) The impact of premenstrual symptomatology on functioning and treatment-seeking behavior: Experience from the United States, United Kingdom, and France. J Women's Health Gender-Based Med 8, 1043–1052.

Jermain DM, Preece CK, Sykes RL, et al. (1999) Luteal phase sertraline treatment for premenstrual dysphoric disorder. Arch Fam Med 8, 328–332.

Joborn C, Hetta J, Niklasson F, et al. (1991) Cerebrospinal fluid calcium, parathyroid hormone, and monoamine and purine metabolites and the blood-brain barrier function in primary hyperparathyroidism. Psychoneuroendocrinology 16, 311–322.

Johnson SR (1998) Premenstrual syndrome therapy. Clin Obstet Gynecol 41, 405–421.

Kahn LS and Halbreich U (2001) Oral contraceptives and mood. Expert Opin Pharmacother 2, 1367–1382.

Kleijnen J, Ter Riet G, and Knipschild P (1990) Vitamin $B_6$ in the treatment of the premenstrual syndrome—a review. Br J Obstetr Gynaecol 97, 847–852.

Lam RW, Carter D, Misri S, et al. (1999) A controlled study of light therapy in women with late luteal phase dysphoric disorder. Psychiatr Res 86, 185–192.

Landen M, Eriksson O, Sundblad C, et al. (2001) Compounds with affinity for serotonergic receptors in the treatment of premenstrual dysphoria: A comparison of buspirone, nefazodone and placebo. Psychopharmacology 155, 292–298.

Leather AT, Studd JW, Watson NR, et al. (1999) The treatment of severe premenstrual syndrome with goserelin with and without 'add-back' estrogen therapy: A placebo-controlled study. Gynecol Endocrinol 13, 48–55.

Loch EG, Selle H, and Boblitz N (2000) Treatment of premenstrual syndrome with a phytopharmaceutical formulation containing Vitex agnus castus. J Women's Health Gender-Based Med 9, 315–320.

London RS, Murphy L, Kitlowski KE, et al. (1987) Efficacy of alpha-tocopherol in the treatment of the premenstrual syndrome. J Reprod Med 32, 400–404.

Menkes DB, Taghavi E, Mason PA, et al. (1993) Fluoxetine's spectrum of action in premenstrual syndrome. Int Clin Psychopharmacol 8, 95–102.

Miller MN, Miller BE, Chinouth R, et al. (2002) Increased premenstrual dosing of nefazodone relieves premenstrual magnification of depression. Depress Anx 15, 48–51.

Miner C, Brown E, McCray S, et al. (2002) Weekly luteal-phase dosing with enteric-coated fluoxetine 90 mg in premenstrual dysphoric disorder: A randomized, double-blind, placebo-controlled clinical trial. Clin Ther 24(3) (Mar), 417–433.

Mira M, McNeil D, Fraser IS, et al. (1986) Mefenamic acid in the treatment of premenstrual syndrome. Obstet Gynecol 68, 395–398.

Morse G (1999) Positively reframing perceptions of the menstrual cycle among women with premenstrual syndrome. J Obstetr Gynecol Neonatal Nurs 28, 165–174.

O'Brien PM and Abukhalil IE (1999) Randomized controlled trial of the management of premenstrual syndrome and premenstrual mastalgia using luteal phase-only danazol. Am J Obstetr Gynecol 180, 18–23.

Oleson T and Flocco W (1993) Randomized controlled study of premenstrual symptoms treated with ear, hand, and foot reflexology. Obstet Gynecol 82, 906–911.

Ozeren S, Corakci A, Yucesoy I, et al. (1997) Fluoxetine in the treatment of premenstrual syndrome. Eur J Obstetr Gynecol Reprod Biol 73, 167–170.

Parry BL (1997) Psychobiology of premenstrual dysphoric disorder. Sem Reprod Endocrinol 15, 55–68.

Parry BL (2001) The role of central serotonergic dysfunction in the aetiology of premenstrual dysphoric disorder: Therapeutic implications. CNS Drugs 15, 277–285.

Parry BL and Newton RP (2001) Chronobiological basis of female-specific mood disorders. Neuropsychopharmacology 25, S102–S108.

Pearlstein T (1996) Nonpharmacologic treatment of premenstrual syndrome. Psychiatr Ann 26, 590–594.

Pearlstein T and Stone AB (1998) Premenstrual syndrome. Psychiatr Clin N Am 21, 577–590.

Pearlstein T and Steiner M (2000) Nonantidepressant treatment of premenstrual syndrome. J Clin Psychiatr 61, 22–27.

Pearlstein TB, Halbreich U, Batzar ED, et al. (2000) Psychosocial functioning in women with premenstrual dysphoric disorder before and after treatment with sertraline or placebo. J Clin Psychiatr 61, 101–109.

Pearlstein TB, Stone AB, Lund SA, et al. (1997) Comparison of fluoxetine, bupropion, and placebo in the treatment of premenstrual dysphoric disorder. J Clin Psychopharmacol 17, 261–266.

Praschak-Rieder N, Willeit M, Winkler D, et al. (2002) Role of family history and 5-HTTLPR polymorphism in female seasonal affective disorder patients with and without premenstrual dysphoric disorder. Eur Neuropsychopharmacol 12, 129–134.

Rausch JL, Janowsky DS, Golshan S, et al. (1988) Atenolol treatment of late luteal phase dysphoric disorder. J Affect Disord 15, 141–147.

Rickels K, Freeman E, and Sondheimer S (1989) Buspirone in treatment of premenstrual syndrome. Lancet 1, 777.

Robinson RL and Swindle RW (2000) Premenstrual symptom severity: Impact on social functioning and treatment-seeking behaviors. J Women's Health Gender-Based Med 9, 757–768.

Roca CA, Schmidt PJ, Bloch M, et al. (1996) Implications of endocrine studies of premenstrual syndrome. Psychiatr Ann 26, 576–580.

Sanders SA, Graham CA, Bass JL, et al. (2001) A prospective study of the effects of oral contraceptives on sexuality and well-being and their relationship to discontinuation. Contraception 64, 51–58.

Sayegh R, Schiff I, Wurtman J, et al. (1995) The effect of a carbohydrate-rich beverage on mood, appetite, and cognitive function in women with premenstrual syndrome. Obstet Gynecol 86, 520–528.

Schellenberg R (2001) Treatment for the premenstrual syndrome with agnus castus fruit extract: Prospective, randomised, placebo-controlled study. Br Med J 322, 134–137.

Schmidt PJ, Grover GN, and Rubinow DR (1993) Alprazolam in the treatment of premenstrual syndrome. A double-blind, placebo-controlled trial. Arch Gen Psychiatr 50, 467–473.

Schmidt PJ, Nieman LK, Danaceau MA, et al. (1998) Differential behavioral effects of gonadal steroids in women with and in those without premenstrual syndrome. New Engl J Med 338, 209–216.

Schnurr PP, Hurt SW, and Stout AL (1994) Consequences of methodological decisions in the diagnosis of late luteal phase dysphoric disorder. In Premenstrual Dysphorias. Myths and Realities, Gold JH and Severino SK (eds). American Psychiatric Press, Washington DC, pp. 19–46.

Scully D, Kremer J, Meade MM, et al. (1998) Physical exercise and psychological well being: A critical review. Br J Sports Med 32, 111–120.

Smith S, Rinehart JS, Ruddock VE, et al. (1987) Treatment of premenstrual syndrome with alprazolam: Results of a double-blind, placebo-controlled, randomized crossover clinical trial. Obstet Gynecol 70, 37–43.

Steinberg S, Annable L, Young SN, et al. (1999) A placebo-controlled clinical trial of L-tryptophan in premenstrual dysphoria. Biol Psychiatr 45, 313–320.

Steiner M and Born L (2000) Advances in the diagnosis and treatment of premenstrual dysphoria. CNS Drugs 13, 287–304.

Steiner M and Pearlstein T (2000) Premenstrual dysphoria and the serotonin system: Pathophysiology and treatment. J Clin Psychiatr 61, 17–21.

Steiner M, Steinberg S, Stewart D, et al. (1995) Fluoxetine in the treatment of premenstrual dysphoria. Canadian Fluoxetine/Premenstrual Dysphoria Collaborative Study Group. New Engl J Med 332, 1529–1534.

Steiner M, Romano SJ, Babcock S, et al. (2001) The efficacy of fluoxetine in improving physical symptoms associated with premenstrual dysphoric disorder. Br J Obstetr Gynaecol 108, 462–468.

Stevinson C and Ernst E (2000) A pilot study of Hypericum perforatum for the treatment of premenstrual syndrome. Br J Obstetr Gynaecol 107, 870–876.

Stevinson C and Ernst E (2001) Complementary/alternative therapies for premenstrual syndrome: A systematic review of randomized controlled trials. Am J Obstetr Gynecol 185, 227–235.

Stone AB, Pearlstein TB, and Brown WA (1991) Fluoxetine in the treatment of late luteal phase dysphoric disorder. J Clin Psychiatr 52, 290–293.

Su TP, Schmidt PJ, Danaceau MA, et al. (1997) Fluoxetine in the treatment of premenstrual dysphoria. Neuropsychopharmacology 16, 346–356.

Sundblad C, Hedberg MA, and Eriksson E (1993) Clomipramine administered during the luteal phase reduces the symptoms of premenstrual syndrome: A placebo-controlled trial. Neuropsychopharmacology 9, 133–145.

Sundblad C, Modigh K, Andersch B, et al. (1992) Clomipramine effectively reduces premenstrual irritability and dysphoria: A placebo-controlled trial. Acta Psychiatr Scand 85, 39–47.

Sundstrom I, Backstrom T, Wang M, et al. (1999) Premenstrual syndrome, neuroactive steroids and the brain. Gynecol Endocrinol 13, 206–220.

Tamborini A and Taurelle R (1993) Value of standardized Ginkgo biloba extract (EGb 761) in the management of congestive symptoms of premenstrual syndrome. Rev Franc Gynecol Obstetr 88, 447–457.

Taylor D (1999) Effectiveness of professional–peer group treatment: Symptom management for women with PMS. Res Nurs Health 22, 496–511.

Thys-Jacobs S (2000) Micronutrients and the premenstrual syndrome: The case for calcium. J Am College Nutr 19, 220–227.

Thys-Jacobs S and Alvir JM (1995) Calcium-regulating hormones across the menstrual cycle: Evidence of a secondary hyperparathyroidism in women with PMS. J Clin Endocrinol Metab 80, 2227–2232.

Thys-Jacobs S, Silverton M, Alvir J, et al. (1995) Reduced bone mass in women with premenstrual syndrome. J Women's Health 4, 161–168.

Thys-Jacobs S, Starkey P, Bernstein D, et al. (1998) Calcium carbonate and the premenstrual syndrome: Effects on premenstrual and menstrual symptoms. Premenstrual Syndrome Study Group. Am J Obstetr Gynecol 179, 444–452.

Toth A, Lesser ML, Naus G, et al. (1988) Effect of doxycycline on premenstrual syndrome: A double-blind randomized clinical trial. J Intern Med Res 16, 270–279.

Treloar SA, Heath AC, and Martin NG (2002) Genetic and environmental influences on premenstrual symptoms in an Australian twin sample. Psychol Med 32, 25–38.

Van Zak DB (1994) Biofeedback treatments for premenstrual and premenstrual affective syndromes. Int J Psychosom 41, 53–60.

Veeninga AT, Westenberg HG, and Weusten JT (1990) Fluvoxamine in the treatment of menstrually related mood disorders. Psychopharmacology 102, 414–416.

Walker AF, De Souza MC, Vickers MF, et al. (1998) Magnesium supplementation alleviates premenstrual symptoms of fluid retention. J Women's Health 7, 1157–1165.

Walsh MJ and Polus BI (1999) A randomized, placebo-controlled clinical trial on the efficacy of chiropractic therapy on premenstrual syndrome. J Manip Physiol Ther 22, 582–585.

Wang M, Hammarback S, Lindhe BA, et al. (1995) Treatment of premenstrual syndrome by spironolactone: A double-blind, placebo-controlled study. Acta Obstetr Gynecol Scand 74, 803–808.

Wikander I, Sundblad C, Andersch B, et al. (1998) Citalopram in premenstrual dysphoria: Is intermittent treatment during luteal phases more effective than continuous medication throughout the menstrual cycle? J Clin Psychopharmacol 18, 390–398.

Wittchen HU, Becker E, Lieb R, et al. (2002) Prevalence, incidence and stability of premenstrual dysphoric disorder in the community. Psychol Med 32, 119–132.

Wood SH, Mortola JF, Chan YF, et al. (1992) Treatment of premenstrual syndrome with fluoxetine: A double-blind, placebo-controlled, crossover study. Obstetr Gynecol 80, 339–344.

World Health Organization (1993) International Classification of Diseases-10th Rev. World Health Organization, Geneva.

Wyatt K, Dimmock P, Jones P, et al. (2001) Efficacy of progesterone and progestogens in management of premenstrual syndrome: Systematic review. Br Med J 323, 776–780.

Wyatt KM, Dimmock PW, Jones PW, et al. (1999) Efficacy of vitamin $B_6$ in the treatment of premenstrual syndrome: Systematic review. Br Med J 318, 1375–1381.

Yakir M, Kreitler S, Brzezinski A, et al. (2001) Effects of homeopathic treatment in women with premenstrual syndrome: A pilot study. Br Homeo J 90, 148–153.

Yonkers KA (1997) Antidepressants in the treatment of premenstrual dysphoric disorder. J Clin Psychiatr 58, 4–10.

Yonkers KA, Halbreich U, Freeman E, et al. (1997) Symptomatic improvement of premenstrual dysphoric disorder with sertraline treatment. A randomized controlled trial. Sertraline Premenstrual Dysphoric Collaborative Study Group. J Am Med Assoc 278, 983–988.

Young SA, Hurt PH, Benedek DM, et al. (1998) Treatment of premenstrual dysphoric disorder with sertraline during the luteal phase: A randomized, double-blind, placebo-controlled crossover trial. J Clin Psychiatr 59, 76–80.

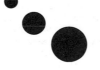

CHAPTER

# 66 Anxiety Disorders: Panic Disorder With and Without Agoraphobia

Gordon J.G. Asmundson
Steven Taylor

Panic Disorder with Agoraphobia
Panic Disorder without Agoraphobia

## Clinical Vignette

Sandra B. was a 20-year-old college student who presented to a student health clinic reporting recurrent panic attacks. Her first attack occurred seven months earlier while smoking marijuana at an end-of-term party. At the time she felt depersonalized, dizzy, short of breath, and her heart was beating wildly. Sandra had an overwhelming fear that she was going crazy. Friends took her to a nearby hospital emergency department where she was given a brief medical evaluation, reassured that she was simply experiencing anxiety and given a prescription for lorazepam. In the following months, Sandra continued to experience unexpected panic attacks and became increasingly convinced that she was losing control of her mind. Most of her panics occurred unexpectedly during the day, although they sometimes also occurred at night, wrenching her out of a deep sleep. Sandra began avoiding a variety of substances (e.g., alcohol, marijuana, coffee) and activities (e.g., aerobics classes) because they produced bodily sensations, such as palpitations and dizziness, that she feared. She believed that if these sensations became too intense then she might "tip over the edge" into insanity. Increasingly, Sandra also began to avoid shopping malls, lecture halls, and other public places for fear that she would have a panic attack and lose control. Whenever she contemplated entering these situations she became highly anxious and sometimes panicked if she actually entered them. As a result of avoiding lectures, her grades began to fall and she was at risk for failing her courses. She became increasingly depressed and, at times, contemplated suicide as a way of ending her misery. At the urging of a roommate she eventually sought help from the student health clinic.

## Definitions and Diagnostic Criteria

According to the *Diagnostic and Statistical Manual of Mental Disorders*, Fourth Edition, Text Revision (DSM-

IV-TR) (American Psychiatric Association 2000), panic disorder is defined by recurrent and unexpected panic attacks. At least one of these attacks must be followed by one month or more of

(1) persistent concern about having more attacks,
(2) worry about the implications or consequences of the attack, or
(3) changes to typical behavioral patterns (e.g., avoidance of work or school activities) as a result of the attack.

In addition, the panic attacks must not stem solely from the direct effects of illicit substance use, medication, or a general medical condition (e.g., hyperthyroidism, vestibular dysfunction) and are not better explained by another mental disorder (e.g., such as social phobia for attacks that occur only in social situations). A diagnosis of panic disorder with agoraphobia is warranted when the criteria for panic disorder are satisfied and accompanied by agoraphobia.

Although panic attacks are a cardinal feature of panic disorder and in combination with agoraphobia (i.e., anxiety about being in a place or a situation that is not easily escaped or where help is not easily accessible if panic occurs) are essential to a diagnosis of panic disorder with agoraphobia, the criteria sets for panic attacks and for agoraphobia are listed separately as standalone noncodable conditions that are referred to by the diagnostic criteria for panic disorder and agoraphobia without history of panic disorder. Notwithstanding, accurate diagnosis is difficult without a proficient understanding of these features. Tables 66–1 and 66–2 show the DSM-IV-TR criteria for panic attack and agoraphobia, respectively. While the criteria for agoraphobia are generally straightforward, panic attacks can be difficult to understand.

A number of investigations (Brown and Deagle 1992, Norton et al. 1999, Wilson et al. 1992) indicate that people report having what they consider to be a panic attack

1281

| Table 66–1 | Definition and Criteria for Panic Attack |
|---|---|

A panic attack is a discrete period of intense fear or discomfort in the absence of real danger that develops abruptly, reaches a peak within 10 min, and is accompanied by four (or more) of the following symptoms:

(1) palpitations, pounding heart, or accelerated heart rate
(2) sweating
(3) trembling or shaking
(4) sensations of shortness of breath or smothering
(5) feeling of choking
(6) chest pain or discomfort
(7) nausea or abdominal distress
(8) feeling dizzy, unsteady, light-headed, or faint
(9) derealization (feelings of unreality) or depersonalization (being detached from oneself)
(10) fear of losing control or going crazy
(11) fear of dying
(12) paresthesias (numbness or tingling sensations)
(13) chills or hot flushes

Adapted from American Psychiatric Association (2000) Diagnostic and Statistical Manual of Mental Disorders, 4th ed., Text Rev. American Psychiatric Association, Washington DC.

| Table 66–2 | Criteria for Agoraphobia |
|---|---|

A. Agoraphobia is characterized by anxiety about being in places or situations from which escape might be difficult (or embarrassing) or in which help may not be available in the event of having an unexpected or situationally predisposed panic attack or panic-like symptoms. Agoraphobic fears typically involve characteristic clusters of situations, such as being outside the home alone, being in a crowd, standing in a line, being on a bridge, or traveling in a motor vehicle.

B. The situations are avoided or are endured with marked distress or worry about having a panic attack or panic-like symptoms. Confronting situations is aided by the presence of a companion.

C. The anxiety or avoidance is not better accounted for by another mental disorder.

Adapted from American Psychiatric Association (2000) Diagnostic and Statistical Manual of Mental Disorders, 4th ed., Text Rev. American Psychiatric Association, Washington DC.

during or in association with actual physical threat (i.e., a true alarm situation). It is, however, important to distinguish between a fear reaction in response to actual threat and a panic attack. In an attempt to do so, the DSM-IV-TR has clarified that panic attacks occur "in the absence of real danger" (p. 430). Such attacks involve a paroxysmal occurrence of intense fear or discomfort accompanied by a minimum of 4 of the 13 symptoms shown in Table 66–1. The DSM-IV-TR recognizes three characteristic types of panic attacks, including those that are *unexpected* (i.e., not associated with an identifiable internal or external trigger and appear to occur "out of the blue"), *situationally bound* (i.e., almost invariably occur when exposed to a situational trigger or when anticipating it), and *situationally predisposed* (i.e., usually, but not necessarily, occur when exposed to a situational trigger or when anticipating it). The term *limited symptom attacks* is used to refer to panic-like episodes comprising fewer than four symptoms.

Although unexpected panic attacks are required for a diagnosis of panic disorder, not all panic attacks that occur in panic disorder are unexpected. The occurrence of unexpected attacks can wax and wane and over the developmental course of the disorder they tend to become situationally bound or predisposed. Moreover, unexpected panic attacks as well as those that are situationally bound or predisposed can occur in the context of other psychiatric disorders, including all of the other anxiety disorders (e.g., a person with social phobia might have an occasional unexpected panic attack without the other feature required to diagnose panic disorder; a dog phobic might panic whenever a large dog is encountered) (Barlow 1988) and some general medical conditions. A clear understanding of the distinction between types of panic attacks outlined in the DSM-IV-TR provides a foundation for diagnosis and differential diagnosis. As described by Taylor (2000), however, consideration of other characteristics of panic—including duration of attacks, frequency of attacks, number and intensity of symptoms, nature of catastrophic thinking, and mechanism responsible for termination of an attack—can be important in identifying exacerbating and controlling factors.

## Historical Overview

Descriptions of cases resembling agoraphobia date back thousands of years, appearing in the writings of Hippocrates and others. The term *agoraphobia* was, however, coined less than 150 years ago by Westphal (1871) to describe patients who seemingly experienced unexpected and situational panic attacks accompanied by anticipatory anxiety and functional incapacitation when walking the streets of their neighborhoods (Kuch and Swinson 1992). Westphal wrote that "it is not possible for them to walk across open spaces and through certain streets...they are troubled in their freedom and movement...they absolutely do not know the reasons for this fear...it comes by itself; a sudden occurrence, strange thing...[and] stimulation of alcohol makes it easier to overcome" (translated by Knapp and Schumacher 1988). Although this description alludes to a panic-like occurrence, Westphal did not make an association between panic attacks and agoraphobia. Freud (1894/1949), whose description of anxiety attacks holds many similarities (but also some notable differences) to contemporary descriptions of panic disorder, was the first to explicate this association. In describing agoraphobia, he specifically mentioned the role of panic, anticipatory anxiety, and escape concerns as central to the condition (Freud 1895/1949). Interestingly, the writings of both Westphal and Freud allude to mechanisms and processes that today comprise part of modern biological and psychological models of panic disorder. These models are discussed in detail in the sections that follow below.

Reference to panic-like symptoms can also be found in the writings about popular historical figures such as Darwin (Barloon and Noyes 1997) and in the cardiology literature. Some of the terms used in this literature began to appear in conjunction with DaCosta's work on Civil War soldiers (e.g., irritable heart, DaCosta's syndrome, soldiers heart) and subsequent observations of those participating in World War I and II (i.e., effort syndrome, neurocirculatory asthenia, cardiac neurosis). The early cardiology literature is replete with attempts to link panic-like symptoms to some form of cardiac pathology, most notably mitral valve prolapse. Research has for the most part failed to support this hypothesis (Shear et al. 1990, Sivaramakrishnan et al. 1994).

The origin of the panic disorder construct as a separate diagnostic entity was influenced by the work of a number of researchers but none so much as Donald Klein in the late 1950s and early 1960s (Klein 1964, 1980). Klein observed that contrary to expectation a subgroup of patients with anxiety neurosis did not improve on chlorpromazine (an antipsychotic sedative) and in some cases became worse. When he gave this subgroup imipramine, a new compound derived from modifications to chlorpromazine, marked improvements were observed. Prior to taking imipramine these patients unlike those who were responsive to chlorpromazine had been experiencing rapid rushes of terror, racing hearts, and other physical sensations, which prompted them to rush to the nurses station with reports that they were about to die. On the basis of this differential drug response, Klein concluded that imipramine was effective against these seemingly spontaneous episodes of panic and, importantly, that these attacks were distinct from other forms of anxiety. He also suggested that agoraphobia was a consequence of spontaneous panic attacks.

Due in large part to the pioneering work of Klein and his colleagues, anxiety neurosis was later divided in the *Diagnostic and Statistical Manual of Mental Disorders, Third Edition (DSM-III)* (American Psychiatric Association 1980) into generalized anxiety disorder and panic disorder. Diagnosis of panic disorder required a minimum of three panic attacks that were of sudden onset, involved at least 4 of 12 symptoms, and occurred within a three-week period. Phobic neurosis was divided into simple phobia, social phobia, and agoraphobia. Agoraphobia without panic attacks was considered to be conceptually distinct from agoraphobia with panic attacks.

The distinction between agoraphobia with and without panic was dropped in the *Diagnostic and Statistical Manual of Mental Disorders*, Third Edition, Revised (DSM-III-R) (American Psychiatric Association 1987). Despite evidence that it is rare (Noyes et al. 1986), at least in those who present for treatment (Wittchen et al. 1998), agoraphobia without a history of panic disorder remained a separate codable diagnosis. The DSM-III-R was restructured to include separate diagnoses for panic disorder without agoraphobia and panic disorder with agoraphobia. Diagnosis of panic disorder required (1) at least 4 panic attacks (of sudden onset and comprising at least four of 13 symptoms) in a four-week period or (2) one or more unexpected attacks followed by at least one month of persistent worry over subsequent attacks. Changes in the DSM-IV and DSM-IV-TR, as described above, involved removal of the criteria sets for panic attacks and agoraphobia from the criteria set for panic disorder and refinements to the definition of panic disorder necessitating both recurrent unexpected attacks and associated persistent worry or behavioral change.

## Prevalence and Course

The one-year prevalence for any panic attack, whether unexpected or situationally cued, is approximately 28% (Brown and Deagle 1992, Norton et al. 1992). Lifetime prevalence rates for unexpected panic attacks and agoraphobia are approximately 4 and 9%, respectively (Wittchen

---

**DSM-IV-TR Criteria** 300.21

### Panic Disorder with Agoraphobia

A. Both (1) and (2):

   (1) recurrent unexpected panic attacks

   (2) at least one of the attacks has been followed by one month (or more) of one (or more) of the following:

      (a) persistent concern about having additional attacks

      (b) worry about the implications of the attack or its consequences (e.g., losing control, having a heart attack, "going crazy")

B. The presence of agoraphobia.

C. The panic attacks are not due to the direct physiological effects of a substance (e.g., a drug of abuse, a medication) or a general medical condition (e.g., hyperthyroidism).

D. The panic attacks are not better accounted for by another mental disorder, such as social phobia (e.g., occurring on exposure to feared social situations), specific phobia (e.g., on exposure to a specific phobic situation), obsessive–compulsive disorder (e.g., on exposure to dirt in someone with an obsession about contamination), post-traumatic stress disorder (e.g., in response to stimuli associated with a severe stressor), or separation anxiety disorder (e.g., in response to being away from home or close relatives).

Reprinted with permission from the Diagnostic and Statistical Manual of Mental Disorders, Fourth Edition, Text Revision. Copyright 2000 American Psychiatric Association.

---

et al. 1998). Investigations of unexpected panic attacks in college student samples using self-report methodology have revealed similar rates, ranging from approximately 5% (Norton et al. 1986, Wilson et al. 1991) to 11% (Asmundson and Norton 1993).

The National Comorbidity Study (Eaton et al. 1994) has reported the lifetime prevalence of panic disorder (with or without agoraphobia) in the general population to be 3.5%. However, despite uncertainty as to the reason, this rate is somewhat of an anomaly in the literature. Most epidemiological studies, including those based on Epidemiologic Catchment Area and other data sources have consistently shown lifetime rates between 1 and 2% (Eaton et al. 1991, Reed and Wittchen 1998, Weissman et al. 1997). Weisman and colleagues (1997) have demonstrated that despite some minor variation lifetime prevalence rates are generally consistent around the world. One-year prevalence rates in the general community also vary slightly from lifetime rates, being between 0.2 and 1.7% (Weissman et al. 1997). In treatment seeking individuals, the prevalence of panic disorder is considerably higher. Approximately 10% of patients in mental health clinics and between 10

## DSM-IV-TR Criteria 300.21

### Panic Disorder Without Agoraphobia

A. Both (1) and (2):

    (1) recurrent unexpected panic attacks

    (2) at least one of the attacks has been followed by 1 month (or more) of one (or more) of the following:

        (a) persistent concern about having additional attacks

        (b) worry about the implications of the attack or its consequences (e.g., losing control, having a heart attack, "going crazy")

B. Absence of agoraphobia.

C. The panic attacks are not due to the direct physiological effects of a substance (e.g., a drug of abuse, a medication) or a general medical condition (e.g., hyperthyroidism).

D. The panic attacks are not better accounted for by another mental disorder, such as social phobia (e.g., occurring on exposure to feared social situations), specific phobia (e.g., on exposure to a specific phobic situation), obsessive–compulsive disorder (e.g., on exposure to dirt in someone with an obsession about contamination), post-traumatic stress disorder (e.g., in response to stimuli associated with a severe stressor), or separation anxiety disorder (e.g., in response to being away from home or close relatives).

Reprinted with permission from the Diagnostic and Statistical Manual of Mental Disorders, Fourth Edition, Text Revision. Copyright 2000 American Psychiatric Association.

| Table 66-3 | Epidemiology and Course of Panic Disorder With and Without Agoraphobia |
|---|---|
| Lifetime prevalence | |
|   Panic disorder | 1–2% |
|   Unexpected panic attack | 4–11% |
|   Agoraphobia | 9% |
| Age of onset | 15–30 yr (bimodally distributed) |
| Sex distribution | Females diagnosed slightly more than twice as often as men |
| Course | Typically chronic |
| 5-yr remission rate | 39% |

and 60% in various medical specialty clinics (e.g., cardiology, respiratory, vestibular) have panic disorder (Chignon et al. 1993, Rouillon 1997, Spinhoven et al. 1993, Stein et al. 1994). Panic disorder with agoraphobia is more common than panic disorder without agoraphobia in clinical samples (American Psychiatric Association 2000).

Age of onset for panic disorder is distributed bimodally, typically developing between 15 and 19 or 25 and 30 years (Ballenger and Fyer 1996). The clinical features of panic disorder such as number and severity of symptoms are much the same across the sexes (Oei et al. 1990). However, women are diagnosed with panic disorder more than twice as often as men (Weissman et al. 1997). Recent research indicates that women are more likely to have panic disorder with agoraphobia and that they are more likely to have recurrence of symptoms after remission of their panic attacks than are men (Yonkers et al. 1998). Men, on the other hand, are more likely to have panic disorder without agoraphobia (Yonkers et al. 1998) and are more likely to self medicate with alcohol than are women (Cox et al. 1993). The literature remains unclear as to why these sex differences exist but alludes to the possible role of biological and/or socialization factors (Bekker 1996, Yonkers 1994)

Panic disorder symptoms may wax and wane but, if left untreated, the typical course is chronic (Keller et al. 1994, Uhde et al. 1985). Data from a sample of patients assessed and treated through the Harvard/Brown Anxiety Disorders Research Program and followed prospectively over a 5-year period indicated remission rates in both men and women to be 39% (Yonkers et al. 1998). In general among those receiving tertiary treatment, approximately 30% of patients have symptoms that are in remission, 40 to 50% are improved but still have significant symptoms, and 20 to 30% are unimproved or worse at 6 to 10 years follow-up (American Psychiatric Association 2000). A summary of findings from studies of the prevalence and course of panic disorder is provided in Table 66–3.

### Costs of Panic Disorder

Panic disorder with or without agoraphobia is associated with impaired occupational and social functioning and poor overall quality of life (Katerndahl and Realini 1997, Leon et al. 1995). People with panic disorder, compared to people in the general population, report poorer physical health (Markowitz et al. 1989). Panic disorder is a leading reason for seeking emergency department consultations (Weissman 1991) and a leading cause for seeking mental health services, surpassing both schizophrenia and mood disorders (Boyd 1986). Panic disorder exceeds the economic costs associated with many other anxiety disorders such as social phobia, generalized anxiety disorder, and obsessive–compulsive disorder (Greenberg et al. 1999). The high medical costs are partly because panic disorder patients quite often present to their primary care physician or hospital emergency departments, thinking they are in imminent danger of dying or 'going crazy' (Katerndahl and Realini 1995). In these settings, patients may undergo a series of extensive medical tests before panic disorder is, if ever, finally diagnosed. Ruling out general medical conditions is good clinical practice but the process contributes substantially to the costs that panic disorder places on health care systems.

### Comorbidity

Lifetime comorbidity (i.e., the co-occurrence of two or more disorders at any point in a person's life, regardless

| Table 66–4 | Comorbidity Data |
|---|---|
| Lifetime comorbidity rate | > 90% |
| Common comorbid conditions | Other anxiety disorders |
| | Major depression |
| | Somatoform disorders |
| | Pain-related disorders |
| | Substance use disorders |
| | Personality disorders |

of whether or not they overlap) in panic disorder is common, with over 90% of community-dwelling and treatment seeking patients having had symptoms meeting diagnostic threshold for at least one other disorder (Robins et al. 1991). Comorbidity can pose considerable challenge to treatment. Below we provide a summary review of the conditions that most often co-occur with panic disorder (also see Table 66–4). The reader is referred to Taylor (2000) for detailed discussion of the various comorbidity models and how they account for the co-occurrence of other disorders with panic disorder.

## Other Anxiety Disorders

The rates of lifetime comorbidity between panic disorder and other anxiety disorders, although variable across epidemiological studies, are high. The most common comorbid anxiety disorders are social phobia and generalized anxiety disorder (15–30%) followed by specific phobia (2–20%), obsessive compulsive disorder (10%), and posttraumatic stress disorder (2–10%) (American Psychiatric Association 2000). To date, there are no studies that have reported comorbid panic disorder and acute stress disorder. The most parsimonious explanation of high comorbidity between panic disorder and the other anxiety disorders is that they share a common diathesis.

## Major Depressive Disorder

Epidemiological studies indicate that major depressive disorder occurs in up to 65% of patients with panic disorder at some point in their lives. In approximately two thirds of these cases, the symptoms of depression develop along with, or secondary to, panic disorder (American Psychiatric Association 2000; Kessler et al. 1998). However, since depression precedes panic disorder in the remaining third (Breier et al. 1984), depressive symptoms co-occurring with panic disorder cannot be considered simply as a demoralized response to paroxysms of anxiety. While the risk of developing secondary depression appears to be more closely associated with the severity of agoraphobia than with the severity or frequency of panic attacks, this may be a confound of misdiagnosing some behavioral manifestations of depression as agoraphobia (Taylor 2000). Panic disorder and depression do not appear to be identical disorders (Stein and Uhde 1990) and their co-occurrence may be due to a shared diathesis or mutual exacerbation of symptoms.

## Somatoform and Pain-Related Disorders

Somatoform and pain-related disorders are frequently comorbid with panic disorder. For example, hypochondria-

sis has been diagnosed in approximately 20% of panic disorder patients attending general medical clinics (Noyes et al. 1999) and in almost 50% of those attending anxiety disorders clinics (Noyes 2001). Acute and chronic musculoskeletal pain (i.e., pain that persists for six months or longer), respectively, are reported by approximately 85 and 40% of panic disorder patients attending anxiety disorders clinics (Asmundson et al. 2001). Irritable bowel syndrome, a condition characterized persistent abdominal pain and defecation difficulties, co-occurs in 17 to 41% of treatment seeking panic disorder patients (Lydiard et al. 1994; Noyes et al. 1990). Emerging evidence suggests that comorbidity between panic disorder and both somatoform and pain-related disorders may be best explained by a shared diathesis model (Asmundson and Taylor 1996, Asmundson et al. 2001).

## Substance Use Disorders

As illustrated in the case of Sandra B., panic disorder can be precipitated by the use of psychotropic drugs (Ballenger and Fyer 1996). Risk is higher with chronic use (Louie et al. 1996). Alcohol has been identified as playing a precipitating, maintaining, and aggravating role in panic disorder. The 6-month prevalence of alcohol abuse or dependence in panic disorder has been reported to be 40% in men and 13% in women (Leon et al. 1995). These rates are higher than those observed in people with other anxiety disorders and those with no anxiety disorder (Leon et al. 1995). Although alcohol problems have been reported to precede panic disorder in a majority of cases (Otto et al. 1992), most reports indicate that alcohol problems develop secondary to panic disorder, often as a means of self-medication (Bibb and Chambless 1986). Those having panic disorder with agoraphobia appear to be at greater risk for comorbid alcohol abuse or dependence than those without agoraphobia (Thyer et al. 1986).

## Personality Disorders

Lack of reliable assessment instruments for personality disorders as well as overlapping diagnostic criteria necessarily limit the degree of confidence in reports of comorbidity with panic disorder. Notwithstanding, 40 to 50% of panic disorder patients have been reported to qualify for one or more personality disorders (American Psychiatric Association 1998), a rate which exceeds that of 13% observed in community control samples (Diaferia et al. 1993). The most commonly reported co-occurring personality disorders are avoidant, dependant, and histrionic personality disorders (Chambless et al. 1992, Stein et al. 1993, Taylor and Lively 1995). These disorders do not co-occur uniquely with panic, also being common in patients with depression and other anxiety disorders (McNally 1994), and they often persist despite remission of panic symptoms (Mavissakalian and Hamann 1992). Reasons for comorbidity between panic and personality disorders remain unclear.

## Etiology

### Cognitive Models—The Vicious Cycle

There are several contemporary cognitive models of panic disorder which, for the most part, are based on variations of the "fear of anxiety" construct. Goldstein and Chambless (1978) proposed that fear of anxiety arises through the association of interoceptive cues with panic attacks. In other words, people with panic disorder are thought to learn to fear the recurrence of aversive panic episodes and thereby develop a fear of panic-related symptoms. Refuting the premise that fear of anxiety develops from the experience of panic attacks, Clark (1986) posited that panic attacks are the product of a tendency to *catastrophically misinterpret* autonomic arousal sensations that occur in the context of nonpathological anxiety (as well as physical illness, exercise, and ingestion of certain substances). Reiss and colleagues (Reiss 1999, Reiss and McNally 1985), incorporating components of the Goldstein and Chambless and Clark models, proposed that panic attacks arise as a consequence of both

(1) a predispositional tendency to catastrophically misinterpret and respond with fear to the benign arousal sensations, and
(2) a learned fear of anxiety that is maintained by the experience of panic episodes.

Most recently, Bouton, Mineka, and Barlow (2001) have described a variant of the original fear of anxiety model, suggesting that panic disorder develops when exposure to panic attacks conditions a person to respond with anticipatory anxiety (and sometimes with panic) to internal arousal and contextual cues. While each of these models has proven fruitful in research and treatment contexts, we focus below on the model of Clark (1986).

As described above, Clark (1986) proposes that panic attacks arise from the catastrophic misinterpretation of benign arousal sensations. To illustrate the cognitive processes proposed to underlie panic attacks, consider Sandra B.'s experience during one of her many attacks. In this instance, she had dizziness sensations stemming from influenza, perceived them as threatening, became aroused, misinterpreted the sensations as being indicative that she was losing her mind, became further aroused with increasing dizziness, had further thoughts of going mad, and spiraled into panic. This vicious cycle is shown in Figure 66–1.

The vicious cycle model makes several assumptions. First, while recognizing that initial panic attacks may be caused by other factors (e.g., drug-related autonomic surges), it assumes that people prone to panic disorder have an enduring tendency to catastrophically misinterpret benign arousal sensations. Second, it assumes that misinterpretations can occur at the conscious and unconscious level (Clark 1988). Third, the cycle can be entered into at any point. For example, the cycle can be initiated by a contextual trigger, such as influenza-related dizziness in the case of Sandra B., or simply by having catastrophic thoughts about bodily sensations. Fourth, physiological changes are viewed as one of several components in a process, rather than as a pathogenic mechanism.

Cognitive models can also account for agoraphobia. Agoraphobia has long been regarded as a product of operant conditioning (Marks 1987). As noted above, it most often develops as a consequence of panic attacks. These attacks typically occur in particular situations (e.g., when in line at a shopping mall, when driving) and motivate the person to avoid or escape these situations. The avoidance and escape behaviors are negatively reinforced by the reduction of aversive autonomic arousal and other anxiety-related sensations. Cognitive factors such as expectations that an attack will be imminent and harmful and that coping will be ineffective play a significant role by influencing and maintaining avoidance behavior (Taylor and Rachman 1994).

A growing body of literature supports the vicious cycle model. Thoughts of imminent catastrophe have been identified as triggers of panic attacks (Hibbert 1984). Patients with panic disorder relative to healthy and patient controls have been shown to be

(1) characterized by strategic and automatic information processing (i.e., memory, attention) biases for physical threat cues (Logan and Goetsch 1993, McNally 1996),
(2) more accurate, in some instances, at detecting body sensations (Ehlers and Breuer 1996),
(3) more likely to report fear of somatic sensations and beliefs in their harmful consequences (Taylor 1999), and
(4) more susceptible to the influence of instructional

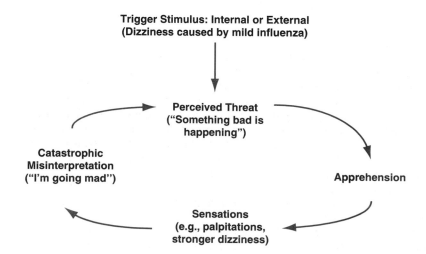

**Figure 66–1** *Application of the cognitive model to illustrate one of Sandra B.'s panic attacks.*

manipulations of control in response to pharmacological panic provocation challenges, panicking less often under the illusion of greater control in some (Rapee et al. 1986, Sanderson et al. 1989) but not all (Welkowitz et al. 1999) cases.

Research shows that treatments stemming from the cognitive model (reviewed later in this chapter) are effective.

## Biological Models

Evidence suggests that several neurotransmitter systems, involving neurotransmitters or neuromodulators such as serotonin, noradrenalin, adenosine, gamma-aminobutyric acid, and cholecystokinin-4, play a role in panic disorder (McNally 1994). Various brain structures in the limbic system and associated regions have also been implicated. Contemporary biological models of panic, beginning with the pioneering work of Klein (1980), have grown in number and complexity in recent years in an effort to integrate and explain these findings. Recent emphasis has focused on the amygdala, a limbic structure that appears to be involved in coordinating the different neurotransmitters involved in anxiety disorders (Goddard and Charney 1997). Today, there is no single, leading biological model of panic. However, there are a number of useful models that guide research and clinical practice (Gorman et al. 2000, Klein 1993). Among the most promising is the neuroanatomical hypothesis recently revised by Gorman and colleagues (2000). This hypothesis is useful for several reasons. First, it integrates a wide range of findings, including animal research and studies of humans. Second, it provides a unifying framework for understanding why panic disorder is associated with so many biological dysregularities such as abnormalities in neurotransmitter systems and irregularities on various indices of autonomic functioning (Abelson et al. 2001, Cohen et al. 2000, Wilhelm et al. 2001, Yeragani et al. 2000). Third, the model accounts for treatment-outcome data, which show that both pharmacological and psychological therapies are effective treatments for panic disorder (as reviewed later in this chapter).

## Neuroanatomical Hypothesis

Gorman and colleagues (2000) begin with the observation that there is a remarkable similarity between the physiological and behavioral consequences of panic attacks in humans and conditioned fear responses in animals. Similarities include autonomic arousal, fear evoked by specific cues (i.e., contextual fear), and avoidance of these cues. Animal research indicates that conditioned fear responses are mediated by a "fear network" in the brain, consisting of the amygdala and its afferent and efferent projections, particularly its connections with the hippocampus, medial prefrontal cortex, hypothalamus, and brainstem. Animal studies also show that activation of this network produces biological and behavioral reactions that are similar to those associated with panic attacks. Thus, Gorman and colleagues (2000) posit that a similar network is involved in panic disorder.

The fear network consists of a complex matrix of interconnections, implicating a number of brain structures and neurotransmitter systems. Sensory input passes through the anterior thalamus to the lateral nucleus of the amygdala. Input is then transferred to the central nucleus of the amygdala, which coordinates autonomic and behavioral responses (Davis 1992, LeDoux et al. 1988). Direct sensory input to the amygdala from brainstem structures and the sensory thalamus enables a rapid response to potentially threatening stimuli. The central nucleus of the amygdala projects to the following structures:

(1) the parabrachial nucleus, producing an increase in respiratory rate,
(2) the lateral nucleus of the hypothalamus, causing autonomic arousal and sympathetic discharge,
(3) the locus coeruleus, leading to an increase in norepinephrine and to increases in blood pressure, heart rate, and behavioral fear responses (e.g., freezing),
(4) the paraventricular nucleus of the hypothalamus, resulting in an increase in the release of adrenocorticoids, and
(5) the periaqueductal gray region, leading to avoidance behaviors (Davis 1992, LeDoux et al. 1988).

In addition, there are reciprocal connections between the amygdala and the sensory thalamus, prefrontal cortex, insula, and primary somatosensory cortex (de Olmos 1990).

According to Gorman and colleagues (2000), panic attacks arise from excessive activation of the fear network. In other words, the fear network becomes sensitized (conditioned) to respond to noxious stimuli such as internal (bodily sensations) and external (contexts or situations) that the person associates with panic. Sensitization of the network may be manifested by the strengthening of various projections from the central nucleus of the amygdala to brainstem sites (such as the locus ceruleus, periaqueductal gray region, and hypothalamus). The network could be over activated if brainstem inputs to the amygdala are dysregulated. However, autonomic activation (e.g., increased respiration and heart rate) and neuroendocrine activation (e.g., increased cortisol secretion) does not occur in all panic attacks. Moreover, a variety of biological agents with diverse physiological properties can trigger panic attacks in people with panic disorder (e.g., sodium lactate, yohimbine, $CO_2$, caffeine, cholecystokinin-4) (McNally 1994). It is, therefore, unlikely that a single brainstem dysregulation is responsible for panic or, in turn, that brainstem dysregulation is the only way of producing an overactive fear network (Gorman et al. 2000, McNally 1994).

Gorman and colleagues (2000) identify various other ways of activating the fear network. For example, the amygdala receives input from cortical regions involved in the processing and evaluation of sensory information. Therefore, a neurocognitive deficit in these cortico-amygdala pathways could result in the catastrophic misinterpretation of sensory information (i.e., misinterpretation of bodily sensations), leading to an inappropriate activation of the fear network. Notice that this pathway resembles the cognitive model of panic described earlier in this chapter. Thus, Gorman and colleagues (2000) model integrates the cognitive model and places it in a neuroanatomical context.

In addition to playing a role in panic disorder, the fear network is thought to play a role in other anxiety disorders and in mood disorders. This is consistent with the comorbidity between panic disorder and these disorders. Abnormalities in the fear network may vary from disorder to disorders. For example, the strength of various connections between components of the network may distinguish various disorders.

Medications, particularly selective serotonin reuptake inhibitors (SSRIs), are thought to desensitize the fear network. This may happen in a number of ways. SSRIs increase serotonergic transmission in the brain (Blier et al. 1987). Serotonergic neurons originate in the brainstem raphe and project throughout the central nervous system (Tork and Hornung 1990). Some of these projections have inhibitory influences. For example, the greater the activity in the raphe, the greater the inhibition of noradrenergic neurons in the locus ceruleus, resulting in a reduction of cardiovascular symptoms associated with panic attacks, such as tachycardia (Aston-Jones et al. 1991). Similarly, the greater the activity in the raphe, the greater inhibition in the periaqueductal gray region, resulting in a reduction in avoidance behavior (Viana et al. 1997). Increased serotonergic activity also may reduce hypothalamic release of corticotropin-releasing factor, thereby resulting in a reduction of cortisol (Brady et al. 1992) and a reduction in activity of the locus ceruleus (Butler et al. 1990), thereby leading to a reduction in fear. SSRIs may also directly inhibit activity of the lateral nucleus of the amygdala (Stutzman and LeDoux 1999). Thus, there appear to be several ways in which SSRIs could desensitize the fear network. Effective psychological therapies are thought to reduce contextual fear and catastrophic misinterpretations at the level of the medial prefrontal cortex and hippocampus.

Gorman and colleagues (2000) neuroanatomical hypothesis is elegant and comprehensive. However, it is a work in progress and will need to be modified as new findings emerge. Additional brain structures may need to be included in the fear network. For example, a growing body of research suggests that the bed nucleus of the stria terminalis (which is associated with the amygdala) plays an important role in fear (Rosen and Schulkin 1998) and, therefore, should also be included in the fear network.

### Environmental and Genetic Factors

The fear network is thought to be influenced by genetic factors and stressful life events, particularly events in early childhood (Gorman et al. 2000). The search for genetic markers and candidate genes for panic disorder has revealed several possible loci but, to date, none have been replicated across studies (van den Heuvel et al. 2000). Research with monozygotic and dizygotic twins show that panic disorder is moderately heritable, with 32 to 46% of variance in liability for panic being attributed to genetic factors (Kendler et al. 1993, Scherrer et al. 2000, van den Heuvel et al. 2000).

Vulnerability to panic disorder appears to result from a combination of disorder-specific and disorder-nonspecific factors (Kendler et al. 1995, Scherrer et al. 2000). The importance of nonspecific genetic factors is consistent with observation that panic disorder is often comorbid with other disorders. Twin studies suggest that nonspecific factors influence the vulnerability to several disorders, including panic disorder, bulimia nervosa, generalized anxiety

disorder, and alcohol dependence (Kendler et al. 1995, Scherrer et al. 2000). Genetic factors specific to panic disorder may be those that influence the tendency to catastrophically misinterpret bodily sensations. This cognitive tendency is a distinguishing feature of panic disorder, as described above. Recent twin research indicates that it is moderately heritable in women but not men (Jang et al. 1999). Thus, some specific genetic factors in panic disorder appear to be sex-linked.

Environmental events occurring during particular developmental phases such as separation from the primary caregiver during early childhood may activate the genes that modulate the fear network, thereby creating a vulnerability to panic disorder. Research suggests that later events, occurring during adolescence or early adulthood, then precipitate panic disorder in vulnerable individuals. These events may stress the individual at a psychological or physiological level. Events commonly associated with the onset of panic disorder include

(1) separation, loss, or illness of a significant other,
(2) being the victim of sexual assault or other forms of interpersonal violence,
(3) financial or occupational stressors, and
(4) intoxication with, or withdrawal from, a psychoactive substance such as marijuana, cocaine, or anesthetic (Taylor 2000).

### Dynamic Models

The most promising psychodynamic models for understanding panic disorder are those that focus specifically on this disorder. Rather than review all the models, we will summarize the model developed by the Cornell Panic-Anxiety Study Group (Milrod et al. 1997, Shear et al. 1993) because it has led to a promising treatment. According to the Cornell group, people at risk for panic disorder have (1) a neurophysiological vulnerability to panic attacks, and/or (2) multiple experiences of developmental trauma. These factors lead the child to become frightened of unfamiliar situations and to become excessively dependent on the primary caregiver to provide a sense of safety. The caregiver is unable to provide support always, so the child develops a fearful dependency. This leads, in turn, to the development of unconscious conflicts about dependency (independence versus reliance on others) and anger (expression versus inhibition). The dependency conflict is said to express itself in a number of ways. Some panic-vulnerable people are sensitive to separation and overly reliant on others, while others are sensitive to suffocation and overly reliant on a sense of independence. These conflicts can activate conscious or unconscious fantasies of catastrophic danger, which can trigger panic attacks. In addition, the conflicts evoke aversive emotions, such as anxiety, anger, and guilt. The otherwise benign arousal sensations accompanying these emotions can become the focus of "conscious as well as unconscious cognitive catastrophizing" (Shear et al. 1993, p. 862), thereby leading to panic attacks.

### Assessment

The most comprehensive and accurate diagnostic information emerges when the clinician uses open ended questions and empathic listening, combined with structured inquiry about specific events and symptoms (American Psychiatric Association 1995). Useful structured interviews include the *Structured Clinical Interview for DSM-IV* (SCID-IV) (First et al. 1996) and the *Anxiety Disorders Interview Schedule for DSM-IV* (ADIS-IV; Di Nardo et al. 1994). A complete assessment for panic disorder also includes a general medical evaluation (American Psychiatric Association 1995), consisting of a medical history, review of organ systems, physical examination, and blood tests. A general medical evaluation is important for identifying general medical conditions that mimic or exacerbate panic attacks or panic-like symptoms (e.g., seizure disorders, cardiac conditions, pheochromocytoma) (Goldberg 1988, Raj and Sheehan 1987). These disorders should be investigated and treated before contemplating a course of panic disorder treatment. It is also important to rule out the other anxiety disorders and major depressive disorder as primary factors in the person's panic attacks and avoidance prior to initiating treatment for panic disorder Figure 66-2.

Diagnostic information can be usefully supplemented by short self-report questionnaires to assess the severity of symptoms and other variables (Taylor 2000) The *Beck Depression Inventory* (Beck and Steer 1987) and *Beck Anxiety Inventory* (Beck and Steer 1993) are quick, reliable, and valid measures that can be administered at the start of each treatment session to assess the severity of past-week general anxiety and depression. The *Anxiety Sensitivity Index* (Peterson and Reiss 1992) is another useful short questionnaire that can be used to gauge the severity of the patient's fear of bodily sensations. Scores on this scale can be used to assess whether treatment is altering the patient's tendency to catastrophically misinterpret bodily sensations. This scale has good reliability and validity, is sensitive to treatment-related effects, and its posttreatment scores predict who is likely to relapse after panic treatment (Taylor 1999).

Another useful questionnaire to monitor treatment progress is the *Panic and Agoraphobia Scale* (Bandelow 1995). This 13-item scale was designed as a short, sensitive measure for treatment outcome studies. The patient is asked to rate the past-week frequency and/or severity of the following: (1) panic attacks, (2) agoraphobia, (3) anticipatory anxiety (i.e., worry about having an panic attack), (4) panic-related disability in various areas of functioning, and (5) worry about the health-related implications of panic (e.g., worry that panic attacks will lead to a heart attack). The Panic and Agoraphobia Scale has good reliability and validity and is sensitive in detecting treatment-related change (Bandelow et al. 1995, 1998). It has the advantage of providing a broad assessment of many features of panic disorder and agoraphobia. A limitation is that it does not distinguish between full and limited symptom panic attacks or among the types of panics (i.e., unexpected, situationally bound, situationally predisposed). When asked to recall their attacks, patients may have difficulty making these distinctions. Prospective (ongoing) monitoring is needed to provide this information.

To gain more detailed information on panic attacks, clinicians and clinical researchers are increasingly including some form of prospective monitoring in their assessment batteries (Shear and Maser 1994). The most widely used are the *panic attack records*. The patient is provided with a definition of a panic attack and then given a pad of panic attack records that can be readily carried in a purse or pocket. The patient is instructed to carry the records at all times and to complete one record (sheet) for each full-blown or limited symptom attack, soon after the attack occurs. Variants on the panic diaries developed by Barlow and colleagues (Barlow and Craske 1994, Rapee et al. 1990) are among the most informative and easy to use. A version is shown in Figure 66-3, which shows details of one of Sandra B.'s panic attacks. These records are then reviewed during treatment sessions to glean information about the links among beliefs, bodily sensations, and safety behaviors, and to assess treatment progress.

Sandra B. reported that the panic attack summarized in Figure 66-3 occurred when she was in a neighborhood supermarket. As she walked down the aisle she looked at the long rows of fluorescent lights and then began to feel mildly depersonalized (see Taylor, Chapter 4, for a discussion of the effects of fluorescent lighting and other environmental triggers of depersonalization). Upon noticing this sensation she began to increasingly worry that the depersonalization might become so intense that she would lose all contact with reality, to the point that she would be permanently insane. This greatly frightened her and led to an increase in the intensity of arousal sensations (as described in the cognitive model of panic). In an effort to reduce the intensity of the feared depersonalization she averted her gaze from the lights and began studying the list of ingredients on cereal boxes. This distracting safety behavior calmed her down and reduced the feared depersonalization to the point that she was able to make her way to the express checkout counter and leave with the grocery items she had collected.

Note that the panic attack record serves as a useful memory aid to help patients recall the details and circumstances of their panic attacks. This example shows how the panic attack record helped Sandra B. recall that she used distraction as a safety behavior. Armed with this information, the therapist could set up exposure exercises to help Sandra B. learn whether distraction was essential to protecting her from the effects of depersonalization.

## Treatment

There are a number of approaches that can be taken in treating panic disorder with and without agoraphobia. Both single and combined treatment modalities are presented in Figure 66-4.

## Pharmacotherapies

Controlled studies show that effective anti-panic medications include tricyclic antidepressants (e.g., imipramine), monoamine oxidase inhibitors (MAOIs; e.g., phenelzine), high-potency benzodiazepines (e.g., alprazolam), and SSRIs (e.g., fluvoxamine). These treatments have broadly similar efficacy, although there is some evidence that SSRIs tend to be most effective (Boyer 1995, Taylor 2000). The classes of medication differ in their side effects and their contraindications. Anticholinergic effects (e.g., blurred vision, dry mouth) are common problems with tricyclics. They are also contraindicated in patients with particular

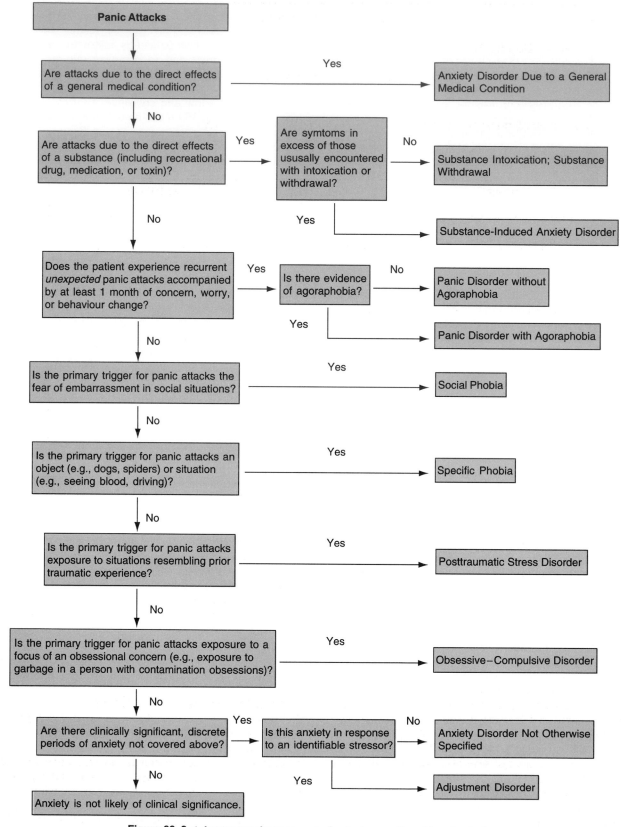

**Figure 66–2** *A decision tree for assessment of patients presenting with panic attacks.*

---

PANIC ATTACK RECORD

NAME:  **Sandra.B.**

DATE:  **Oct 2**          TIME:  **4pm**          DURATION (min):  **15**

WITH: SPOUSE _____          FRIEND _____          STRANGER _____          ALONE ✓

STRESSFUL SITUATION: YES / NO          EXPECTED: YES / NO

MAXIMUM ANXIETY (CIRCLE)

0 -------- 1 -------- 2 -------- 3 -------- 4 -------- 5 -------- 6 -------- 7 -------- 8
NONE                          MODERATE                          EXTREME

SENSATIONS (CHECK):

| | | | | | |
|---|---|---|---|---|---|
| POUNDING HEART | ✓ | SWEATING | ✓ | HOT/COLD FLASH | ✓ |
| TIGHT/PAINFUL CHEST | ✓ | CHOKING | ___ | FEAR OF DYING | ___ |
| BREATHLESS | ✓ | NAUSEA | ___ | FEAR OF GOING CRAZY | ✓ |
| DIZZY | ✓ | UNREALITY | ✓ | FEAR OF LOSING CONTROL | ✓ |
| TREMBLING | ___ | NUMB/TINGLE | ✓ | | |

THOUGHTS OR MENTAL IMAGES AT THE TIME (DESCRIBE):

**I'm losing contact with reality**

---

**Figure 66–3** *A completed panic attack record for Sandra B.*

comorbid cardiac disorders (Simon and Pollack 2000). Dietary restrictions (i.e., abstaining from foods containing tyramine) are a limitation of many MAOIs (Stein and Stahl 2000, Taylor 2000). Sedation, impaired motor coordination, and addiction are concerns with benzodiazepines (Barbone et al. 1998, Taylor 2000).

When efficacy and side effects are considered together, SSRIs emerge as the most promising drug treatments for panic disorder. However, even SSRIs have side effects, with the most problematic being a short-term increase in arousal-related sensations (Pohl et al. 1988). To overcome this problem, SSRIs can be started at a low dose (e.g., 5–10 mg/d for paroxetine; 12.5–25 mg/d for sertraline) and then increased gradually (e.g., up to 10–50 mg/d for paroxetine; up to 25–200 mg/d for sertraline). The choice of SSRI is determined on the basis of several factors, including side effects, patient preference, and the patient's history of responding (or not responding) to particular agents (Simon and Pollack 2000).

For drug refractory patients, or patients who are unable to tolerate SSRI side effects, combination medications are sometimes used. For example, SSRIs can be augmented with benzodiazepines (Uhlenhuth et al. 1999). The latter are used to dampen the side effects of SSRIs. Despite some positive preliminary reports supporting this strategy,

its value in the treatment of panic disorder remains to be properly evaluated. An alternative strategy is to change the patient's medication. Some of the newer, non-SSRI antidepressants could be considered, such as venlafaxine, nefazodone, buproprion, or gabapentin (Simon and Pollack 2000). A concern with using these newer medications to treat panic disorder is that there are few data to guide the clinician. Another approach to the drug refractory patient is to use a psychosocial treatment such as cognitive-behavioral therapy (CBT), as an alternative or adjunctive intervention.

## Cognitive–Behavioral Therapy

CBT treatment packages include a number of components, such as psychoeducation (e.g., information about the cognitive model of panic), breathing retraining, cognitive restructuring, relaxation exercises, interoceptive exposure, and situational exposure (Taylor 2000). Breathing retraining involves teaching the patient to breathe with the diaphragm rather than with the chest muscles. Cognitive restructuring focuses on challenging patient's beliefs about the dangerousness of bodily sensations (e.g., challenging the belief that palpitations lead to heart attacks).

Interoceptive exposure involves inducing feared bodily sensations to further teach patients that the sensations are harmless. For example, Sandra B.'s treatment involved

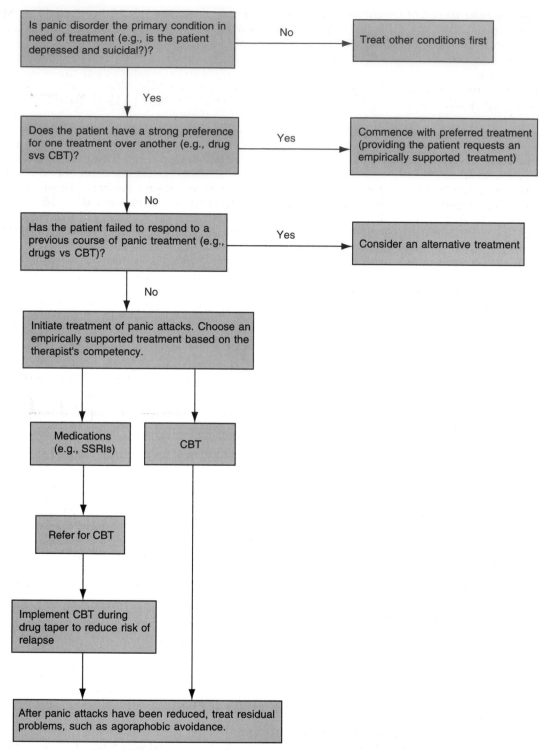

**Figure 66–4** *A decision tree for treating panic disorder and agoraphobic avoidance.*

interoceptive exposure exercises that induced depersonalization. Several tasks were used, including (1) staring at a ceiling fluorescent light for 1 minute, (2) staring at her reflection in the mirror for 2 minutes, and (3) staring at a spot on the wall for 3 minutes. Multiple tasks were used in order to promote the generalization of treatment effects (i.e., to help her learn that depersonalization was harmless regardless of how it arises).

Situational exposure involves activities that bring the patient into feared situations such as shopping malls, bridges, or tunnels. In Sandra B.'s case, situational and interoceptive exposure were combined. She was asked to visit a lighting store to spend time inspecting the various fluorescent lamps. Exposure exercises are often framed as "behavioral experiments" to test patients' beliefs about the catastrophic consequences of arousal-related sensations.

Sandra B.'s exposure exercises helped her test the belief that depersonalization leads to permanent insanity. The exercises were also used to help her test the alternative, non-catastrophic belief that depersonalization is an unpleasant but harmless experience.

A common practice in CBT is to encourage patients to refrain from engaging in safety behaviors. Prior to treatment, Sandra B. typically engaged in distraction whenever she was exposed to depersonalization-inducing stimuli such as fluorescent lights. The CBT therapist encouraged her to refrain from distraction so she could learn that depersonalization is harmless, even when it becomes intense. Evidence suggests that reducing safety behaviors improves treatment efficacy (Taylor 2000). Despite the advantages of exposure exercises, they are medically contraindicated in some cases. For example, a hyperventilation exercise would not be used in a patient with severe asthma (Taylor 2000).

A large body of evidence shows that CBT is effective in reducing panic attacks, agoraphobia, and associated symptoms such as depression (Taylor 2000). However, not all CBT interventions may be necessary. Interoceptive exposure, situational exposure, and cognitive restructuring are the most widely used and supported interventions. Several studies suggest that breathing retraining reduces panic frequency. However, recent research casts doubt about the importance of hyperventilation in producing panic attacks. This suggests that breathing retraining may only be useful for a minority of patients, for which chest breathing or hyperventilation plays a role in producing panic symptoms (Taylor 2001). Breathing retraining may be counterproductive if it prevents patients from learning that their catastrophic beliefs are unfounded. Given these concerns, breathing retraining should be used sparingly in the treatment of panic disorder. If used at all, the clinician should ensure that the patient understands that breathing exercises are used to remove unpleasant but harmless sensations. Interoceptive exposure and cognitive restructuring are important for helping patients learn that the sensations are not dangerous.

How effective is CBT compared to other therapies? A small but growing literature suggests that the efficacy of CBT is equal to or greater than that of alprazolam and imipramine at posttreatment (Barlow et al. 2000, Taylor 2000). Future research is needed to compare CBT to other pharmacotherapies, such as SSRIs. Preliminary evidence suggests that CBT is effective in treating patients who have failed to respond to pharmacotherapies (Otto et al. 1999, Pollack et al. 1994). Follow-up studies suggest that CBT is effective in the long term and is likely to be more effective than short-term pharmacological treatment. It is not known whether drug treatments would be as effective as CBT if patients remained on their medications. Any conclusions about the long-term efficacy of panic treatments are necessarily tentative because patients sometimes seek additional treatment during the follow-up interval.

## Other Psychosocial Interventions

Several other approaches have been used in the treatment of panic disorder, including psychodynamic psychotherapies (Milrod et al. 2000, Wiborg and Dahl 1996), hypnosis (e.g., Delmonte 1995, Stafrace 1994), Eye Movement Desensitization and Reprocessing (EMDR) (Shapiro 1995), and mindfulness meditation (Kabat-Zinn 1990, Miller et al. 1995). Support for these treatments is limited largely to case studies and uncontrolled trials. Controlled studies (Feske and Goldstein 1997), although few in number, indicate that hypnosis and EMDR are of limited value in treating panic disorder. When used to treat this disorder, these treatments may be no better than placebo (Taylor 2000). Interventions that look more promising are mindfulness meditation (Miller et al. 1995) and psychodynamic psychotherapies modified to specifically focus on panic symptoms (Milrod et al. 2000, Wiborg and Dahl 1996). However, none have been extensively evaluated as panic treatments and none have been compared to empirically supported treatments such as CBT or SSRIs.

## Combining CBT with Pharmacotherapies

### Simultaneous Treatments

Many clinicians believe the optimal treatment consists of drugs combined with some form of psychosocial intervention (Alexander 1991, Fahy et al. 1992, Marriott et al. 1989). This view arose from observations that even the most effective drugs and the most effective psychosocial interventions do not eliminate panic disorder in all cases. It was thought that combination treatments might be a way to improve treatment outcome. The available evidence provides mixed support for this view. Evidence suggests that the efficacy of CBT is not improved when it is combined with either diazepam or alprazolam (Hafner and Marks 1976, Riley et al. 1995, Wardle et al. 1994). In fact, some studies have found that the efficacy of situational exposure is *worsened* when alprazolam is added (Echeburúa et al. 1993, Marks et al. 1993).

Several studies have compared CBT to CBT combined with imipramine. These results have also been mixed. Adding imipramine in the range of 150–300 mg/day to either situational exposure or CBT sometimes improves treatment outcome in the short-term, provided that patients are able to tolerate the dose (Barlow et al. 2000, Taylor 2000). Any advantage of combined treatment tends to be lost at follow-up. Similarly, studies of combining CBT with SSRIs (fluvoxamine or paroxetine) have produced mixed results, with some studies finding the combination is no better than CBT alone (Sharp et al. 1996), others finding that the combination is most effective (de Beurs et al. 1995, Oehrberg et al. 1995), and yet others finding the combination to be most effective for some symptoms but not others (Stein et al. 2000). Methodological limitations of these studies might account for the inconsistent findings (Taylor 2000).

It remains unclear whether treatment outcome is enhanced by combining CBT with SSRIs. Neuroanatomical model (Gorman et al. 2000) with its dual emphasis on cortical and serotonergic mechanisms suggests that this combined treatment might be superior to CBT alone and to SSRIs alone. On the other hand, pharmacotherapies such as SSRIs might undermine the patient's confidence in implementing CBT, particularly if they attribute their gains to medications rather than to their own efforts at using the skills learned in CBT (Basoglu et al. 1994, Brown and Barlow 1995). Large, well-designed studies are needed to explore these important issues.

## Sequential Treatments

A more promising type of combined therapy is a sequential approach, where patients are treated with pharmacotherapy during the acute phase, and then are treated with CBT as the medication is phased out. Several studies have shown that adding CBT during the tapering period for alprazolam and clonazepam reduces the relapse rate associated with these drugs (Abelson and Curtis 1993, Bruce et al. 1999, Hegel et al. 1994, Otto et al. 1993, Spiegel et al. 1994). It remains to be demonstrated that CBT can reduce relapse when patients are tapered off other antipanic drugs such as SSRIs. However, there is no reason to expect that CBT would not be helpful in these cases.

## Conclusion

Panic disorder with or without agoraphobia is a common condition with a lifetime prevalence of approximately 2%. As in the case of Sandra B., panic disorder is often comorbid with major depressive disorder and also commonly co-occurs with other disorders such as anxiety disorders and substance-use disorders. Treatment planning typically begins with a thorough assessment, including a medical history, a structured diagnostic interview, and prospective monitoring of symptoms. Based on contemporary biological and cognitive-behavioral models, there are several treatment options that can be considered. These include various pharmacotherapies, particularly SSRIs, and psychosocial interventions that have proven effective in controlled trials. While mixed, there is evidence to suggest that treatments that combine SSRIs and CBT may be more effective than either treatment alone, at least in some symptom domains.

## Comparison of DSM-IV/ICD-10 Diagnostic Criteria

The ICD-10 Diagnostic Criteria for Research for a panic attack are identical to the DSM-IV-TR criteria set except that ICD-10 includes an additional item (i.e., dry mouth). In contrast to the DSM-IV-TR algorithm which does not give special weight to any particular symptom, the ICD-10 algorithm requires that at least one of the symptoms be palpitations, sweating, trembling, or dry mouth. Like DSM-IV-TR, ICD-10 requires recurrent panic attacks but, in contrast to DSM-IV-TR, it does not include a criterion requiring that the panic attacks be clinically significant.

The ICD-10 Diagnostic Criteria for Research for Agoraphobia differ markedly from the DSM-IV-TR criteria. The ICD-10 Diagnostic Criteria for Research specify that there be fear or avoidance of at least two of the following situations: crowds, public places, traveling alone, or traveling away from home. Furthermore, ICD-10 requires that at least two symptoms of anxiety (i.e., from the list of 14 panic symptoms) be present together on at least one occasion and that these anxiety symptoms be "restricted to, or predominate in, the feared situations or contemplation of the feared situations." In contrast, DSM-IV-TR Agoraphobia is defined in terms of "anxiety about being in places or situations from which escape might be difficult (or embarrassing) or in which help may not be available in the event of having an unexpected or situationally predisposed panic attack." No specific avoided situations or specific types of anxiety symptoms are required for a diagnosis.

## References

Abelson JL and Curtis GC (1993) Discontinuation of alprazolam after successful treatment of panic disorder: A naturalistic follow-up study. J Anx Disord 7, 107–117.

Abelson JL, Weg JG, Nesse RM, et al. (2001) Persistent respiratory irregularity in patients with panic disorder. Biol Psychiatr 49, 588–595.

Alexander PE (1991) Management of panic disorders. J Psychoactive Drugs 23, 329–333.

American Psychiatric Association (1980) Diagnostic and Statistical Manual of Mental Disorders, 3rd ed., American Psychiatric Association, Washington DC.

American Psychiatric Association (1987) Diagnostic and Statistical Manual of Mental Disorders, 3rd ed., Rev. American Psychiatric Association, Washington DC.

American Psychiatric Association (1994) Diagnostic and Statistical Manual of Mental Disorders, 4th ed. American Psychiatric Association, Washington DC.

American Psychiatric Association (1995) Practice guidelines for psychiatric evaluation of adults. Am J Psychiatr 152 (Nov Suppl), 63–80.

American Psychiatric Association (1998) Practice guidelines for the treatment of patients with panic disorder. Am J Psychiatr 155 (May Suppl), 1–34.

American Psychiatric Association (2000) Diagnostic and Statistical Manual of Mental Disorders 4th ed., Text Rev. American Psychiatric Association, Washington DC.

Asmundson GJG and Norton GR (1993) Anxiety sensitivity and spontaneous and cued panic attacks in college students. Behav Res Ther 31, 199–201.

Asmundson GJG and Taylor S (1996) Role of anxiety sensitivity in pain-related fear and avoidance. J Behav Med 19, 573–582.

Asmundson GJG, Wright KD, Taylor S, et al. (2001) Future directions and challenges in assessment, treatment, and investigation of health anxiety. In Health Anxiety: Clinical and Research Perspectives on Hypochondriasis and Related Disorders, Asmundson GJG, Taylor S and Cox BJ (eds). John Wiley, London, pp. 365–381.

Aston-Jones G, Akaoka H, Charlety P, et al. (1991) Serotonin selectivity attenuates glutamate-evoked activation of noradrenergic locus coeruleus neurons. J Neurosci 11, 760–769.

Ballenger JC and Fyer AJ (1996) Panic disorder and agoraphobia. In DSM-IV Sourcebook, Vol. 2, Widiger TA, Frances AJ, Pincus HA, et al. (eds). American Psychiatric Association, Washington DC, pp. 411–471.

Bandelow B (1995) Assessing the efficacy of treatments for panic disorder and agoraphobia. II. The panic and agoraphobia scale. Int Clin Psychopharmacol 10, 73–81.

Bandelow B, Brunner E, Broocks A, et al. (1998) The use of the panic and agoraphobia scale in a clinical trial. Psychiatr Res 77, 43–49.

Bandelow B, Hajak G, Holzrichter S, et al. (1995) Assessing the efficacy of treatments for panic disorder and agoraphobia. I. Methodological problems. Int Clin Psychopharmacol 10, 83–93.

Barbone F, McMahon AD, and Davey PG (1998) Association of road-traffic accidents with benzodiazepine use. Lancet 352, 1331–1336.

Barloon TJ and Noyes R (1997) Charles Darwin and panic disorder. J Am Med Assoc 277, 138–141.

Barlow DH (1988) Anxiety and Its Disorders. Guilford Press, New York.

Barlow DH and Craske MG (1994) Mastery of Your Anxiety and Panic II: Client Workbook. Psychological Corporation, San Antonio, TX.

Barlow DH, Gorman JM, Shear MK, et al. (2000) Cognitive–behavioral therapy, imipramine, or their combination for panic disorder: A randomized controlled trial. JAMA 283, 2529–2536.

Basoglu M, Marks IM, Kiliç C, et al. (1994) Alprazolam and exposure for panic disorder with agoraphobia: Attribution of improvement to medication predicts subsequent relapse. Br J Psychiatr 164, 652–659.

Beck AT and Steer RA (1987) Manual for the Revised Beck Depression Inventory. Psychological Corporation, San Antonio, TX.

Beck AT and Steer RA (1993) Manual for the Beck Anxiety Inventory. Psychological Corporation, San Antonio, TX.

Bekker MHJ (1996) Agoraphobia and gender: A review. Clin Psychol Rev 16, 129–146.

Bibb J and Chambless DL (1986) Alcohol use and abuse among diagnosed agoraphobics. Behav Res Ther 24, 49–58.

Blier P, DeMontigny C, and Chaput Y (1987) Modifications of the serotonin system by antidepressant treatments: Implications for the therapeutic response in major depression. J Clin Psychopharmacol 7, 24S–35S.

Bouton ME, Mineka S, and Barlow DH (2001) A modern learning theory perspective on the etiology of panic disorder. Psychol Rev 108, 4–32.

Boyd JH (1986) Use of mental health services for the treatment of panic disorder. Am J Psychiatr 143, 1569–1574.

Boyer W (1995) Serotonin uptake inhibitors are superior to imipramine and alprazolam in alleviating panic attacks: A meta-analysis. Int Clin Psychopharmacol 10, 45–49.

Brady LS, Gold PW, Herkenham M, et al. (1992) The antidepressants fluoxetine, idazoxan and phenelzine alter corticotropin-releasing hormone and tyrosine hydroxylase mRNA levels in the rat brain: Therapeutic implications. Brain Res 572, 117–125.

Breier A, Charney DS, and Heninger GR (1984) Major depression in patients with agoraphobia and panic disorder. Arch Gen Psychiatr 41, 1129–1135.

Brown TA and Barlow DH (1995) Long-term outcome in cognitive–behavioral treatment of panic disorder: Clinical predictors and alternative strategies for assessment. J Consult Clin Psychol 63, 754–765.

Brown TA, and Deagle EA (1992) Structured interview assessment of nonclinical panic. Behav Ther 23, 75–85.

Bruce TJ, Spiegel DA, and Hegel MT (1999) Cognitive–behavioral therapy helps prevent relapse and recurrence of panic disorder following alprazolam discontinuation: A long-term follow-up of the Peoria and Dartmouth studies. J Consult Clin Psychol 67, 151–156.

Butler PD, Weiss JM, Stout JC, et al. (1990) Corticotropin-releasing factor produces fear-enhancing and behavioral activating effects following infusion into the locus coeruleus. J Neurosci 10, 176–183.

Chambless DL, Renneberg B, Goldstein A, et al. (1992) MCMI-diagnosed personality disorders among agoraphobic outpatients: Prevalence and relationship to severity and treatment outcome. J Anx Disord 6, 193–211.

Chignon JM, Lepine JP, and Ades J (1993) Panic Disorder in Cardiac Outpatients. Am J Psychiatr 150, 780–785.

Clark DM (1986) A cognitive approach to panic. Behav Res Ther 24, 461–470.

Clark DM (1988) A cognitive model of panic attacks. In Panic: Psychological Perspectives, Rachman S and Maser JD (eds). Lawrence Erlbaum, Hillsdale, NJ, pp. 71–89.

Cohen H, Benjamin J, Geva AB, et al. (2000) Autonomic dysregulation in panic disorder and in posttraumatic stress disorder: Application of power spectrum analysis of heart rate variability at rest and in response to recollection of trauma or panic attacks. Psychiatr Res 96, 1–13.

Cox BJ, Swinson RP, Shulman ID, et al. (1993) Gender effects and alcohol use in panic disorder with agoraphobia. Behav Res Ther 31, 413–416.

Davis M (1992) The role of the amygdala in fear and anxiety. Annu Rev Neurosci 15, 353–375.

de Beurs E, van Balkom AJLM, Lange A, et al. (1995) Treatment of panic disorder with agoraphobia: Comparison of fluvoxamine, placebo, and psychological panic management combined with exposure and of exposure in vivo alone. Am J Psychiatr 152, 683–691.

Delmonte MM (1995) The use of hypnotic regression with panic disorder: A case report. Aust J Clin Hypnother Hypnosis 16, 69–73.

de Olmos J (1990) Amygdaloid nuclear gray complex. In The Human Nervous System Paxinos G (ed). Academic Press, San Diego, pp. 583–610.

Diaferia G, Sciuto G, Perna G, et al. (1993) DSM-III-R personality disorders and panic disorder. J Anx Disord 7, 153–161.

Di Nardo P, Brown TA, and Barlow DH (1994) Anxiety Disorders Interview Schedule for DSM-IV. Graywind, New York.

Eaton WW, Dryman A, and Weissman MM (1991) Panic and phobia: The diagnosis of panic disorder. In Psychiatric Disorders in America: The Epidemiologic Catchment Area Study, Robins LN and Reiger DA (eds). Free Press, New York, pp. 155–179.

Eaton WW, Kessler RC, Wittchen HU, et al. (1994) Panic and panic disorder in the United States. Am J Psychiatr 151, 413–420.

Echeburúa E, De Corral P, Bajos EG, et al. (1993) Interactions between self-exposure and alprazolam in the treatment of agoraphobia without current panic: An exploratory study. Behav Cogn Psychother 21, 219–238.

Ehlers A and Breuer P (1996) How good are patients with panic disorder at perceiving their heartbeats? Biol Psychol 42, 165–182.

Fahy TJ, O'Rourke D, Brophy J, et al. (1992) The Galway study of panic disorder I. Clomipramine and lofepramine in DSM-III-R panic disorder: A placebo-controlled trial. J Affect Disord 25, 63–76.

Feske U and Goldstein AJ (1997) Eye movement desensitization and reprocessing treatment for panic disorder: A controlled outcome and partial dismantling study. J Consult Clin Psychol 65, 1026–1035.

First MB, Spitzer RL, Gibbon M, et al. (1996) Structured Clinical Interview for DSM-IV Axis I—Patient. Biometrics Research Department, New York State Psychiatric Institute, New York.

Freud S (1894/1949) The justification for detaching from neurasthenia a particular syndrome: The 'anxiety neurosis'. In Collected Papers of Sigmund Freud, Vol. I, E Jones (ed). Hogarth Press, London, pp. 76–106.

Freud S (1895/1949) Obsessions and phobias: Their psychical determinants and aetiology. In Collected Papers of Sigmund Freud, Vol. I, E Jones (ed). Hogarth Press, London, pp. 128–137.

Goddard AW and Charney DS (1997) Toward an integrated neurobiology of panic disorder. J Clin Psychiatr 58(Suppl 2), 4–12.

Goldberg RJ (1988) Clinical presentations of panic-related disorders. J Anx Disord 2, 61–75.

Goldstein AJ and Chambless DL (1978) A reanalysis of agoraphobia. Behav Ther 9, 47–59.

Gorman J, Kent JM, Sullivan GM, et al. (2000) Neuroanatomical hypothesis of panic disorder, Rev. Am J Psychiatr 157, 493–505.

Greenberg PE, Sisitsky T, Kessler RC, et al. (1999) The economic burden of anxiety disorders in the 1990s. J Clin Psychiatr 60, 427–435.

Hafner RJ and Marks IM (1976) Exposure in vivo of agoraphobics: Contributions of diazepam, group exposure and anxiety evocation. Psychol Med 6, 71–88.

Hegel MT, Ravaris CL, and Ahles TA (1994) Combined cognitive–behavioral and time-limited alprazolam treatment of panic disorder. Behav Ther 25, 183–195.

Hibbert GA (1984) Ideational components of anxiety: Their origin and content. Br J Psychiatr 144, 618–624.

Jang KL, Stein MB, Taylor S, et al. (1999) Gender differences in the etiology of anxiety sensitivity: A twin study. J Gender Specific Med 2, 39–44.

Kabat-Zinn J (1990) Full Catastrophe Living. Delta, New York.

Katerndahl DA and Realini JP (1995) Where do panic attack sufferers seek care? J Fam Pract 40, 237–243.

Katerndahl DA and Realini JP (1997) Quality of life and panic-related work disability in subjects with infrequent panic and panic disorder. J Clin Psychiatr 58, 153–158.

Keller MB, Yonkers KA, Warshaw MG, et al. (1994) Remission and relapse in subjects with panic disorder and panic with agoraphobia. J Nerv Ment Disord 182, 290–296.

Kendler KS, Neale MC, Kessler RC, et al. (1993) Panic disorder in women: A population-based twin study. Psychol Med 23, 397–406.

Kendler KS, Walters EE, Neale MC, et al. (1995) The structure of the genetic and environmental risk factors for six major psychiatric disorders in women: Phobia, generalized anxiety disorder, panic disorder, bulimia, major depression and alcoholism. Arch Gen Psychiatr 52, 374–383.

Kessler RC, Stang PE, Wittchen H-U, et al. (1998) Lifetime panic-depression comorbidity in the National Comorbidity Survey. Arch Gen Psychiatr 55, 801–808.

Klein DF (1964) Delineation of two drug-responsive anxiety syndromes. Psychopharmacologia 5, 397–408.

Klein DF (1980) Anxiety reconceptualized. Compr Psychiatr 21, 411–427.

Klein DF (1993) False suffocation alarms, spontaneous panics, and related conditions: An integrative hypothesis. Arch Gen Psychiatr 50, 306–317.

Knapp TJ and schumacher MT (1988) Westphal's "Die agoraphobie" with Commentary: The Beginnings of Agoraphobia. University Press of America, New York, pp. 59–74.

Kuch K and Swinson RP (1992) Agoraphobia: What Westphal really said. Can J Psychiatr 37, 133–136.

LeDoux JE, Iwata J, Cicchetti P, et al. (1988) Different projections of the central amygdaloid nucleus mediate autonomic and behavioral correlates of conditioned fear. J Neurosci 8, 2517–2519.

Leon AC, Portera L, and Weissman MM (1995) The social costs of anxiety disorders. Br J Psychiatr 166(Suppl 27), 19–22.

Logan AC and Goetsch VL (1993) Attention to external threat cues in anxiety states. Clin Psychol Rev 13, 541–559.

Louie AK, Lannon RA, Ritzick EA, et al. (1996) Clinical features of cocaine-induced panic. Biol Psychiatr 40, 938–940.

Lydiard RB, Greenwald S, Weissman MM, et al. (1994) Panic disorder and gastrointestinal symptoms: Findings from the NIMH Epidemiologic Catchment Area project. Am J Psychiatr 151, 64–70.

Markowitz JS, Weissman MM, Ouellette R, et al. (1989) Quality of life in panic disorder. Arch Gen Psychiatr 46, 984–992.

Marks IM (1987) Fears, phobias, and rituals. Oxford University Press, New York.

Marks IM, Swinson RP, Basoglu M, et al. (1993) Alprazolam and exposure alone and combined in panic disorder with agoraphobia: A controlled study in London and Toronto. Br J Psychiatr 162, 776–787.

Marriott P, Judd F, Jefferys D, et al. (1989) Panic and phobic disorders. Part I: Problems associated with drug therapy. Curr Ther 107–121.

Mavissakalian M and Hamann MS (1992) DSM-III personality characteristics of panic Disorder with agoraphobia patients in stable remission. Compr Psychiatr 33, 305–309.

McNally RJ (1994) Panic Disorder: A Critical Analysis. Guilford Press, New York.

McNally RJ (1996) Cognitive bias in the anxiety disorders. In Nebraska symposium on motivation, 1995: Perspectives on anxiety, panic, and fear. Current Theory and Research in Motivation, Vol. 43. Hope DA (ed). University of Nebraska Press, Lincoln, pp. 211–250.

Miller JJ, Fletcher K, and Kabat-Zinn J (1995) Three-year follow-up and clinical implications of a mindfulness meditation-based stress reduction intervention in the treatment of anxiety disorders. Gen Hosp Psychiatr 17, 192–200.

Milrod BL, Busch FN, Cooper AM, et al. (1997) Manual of panic-focused psychodynamic psychotherapy. American Psychiatric Association, Washington, DC.

Milrod B, Busch F, Leon AC, et al. (2000) Open trial of psychodynamic psychotherapy for panic disorder: A pilot study. Am J Psychiatr 157, 1878–1880.

Norton GR, Cox BJ, and Malan J (1992) Nonclinical panickers: A critical review. Clin Psychol Rev 12, 121–139.

Norton GR, Dorward J, and Cox BJ (1986) Factors associated with panic attacks in nonclinical subjects. Behav Ther 17, 239–252.

Norton GR, Pidlubny SR, and Norton PJ (1999) Predicting panic attacks and related variables. Behav Ther 30, 319–330.

Noyes R Jr (2001) Hypochondriasis: Boundaries and comorbidities. In Health Anxiety: Clinical and Research Perspectives on Hypochondriasis and Related Conditions, Asmundson GJG, Taylor S, Cox BJ (eds). John Wiley, Chichester, UK, pp. 132–160.

Noyes R Jr, Cook B, Garvey M, et al. (1990) Reduction of gastrointestinal symptoms with treatment for panic disorder. Psychosomatics 31, 75–79.

Noyes R, Jr, Crowe RR, Harris EL, et al. (1986) Relationship between panic disorder and agoraphobia: A family study. Arch Gen Psychiatr 45, 423–428.

Oehrberg S, Christiansen PE, and Behnke K (1995) Paroxetine in the treatment of panic disorder: A randomized double-blind placebo-controlled study. Br J Psychiatr 167, 374–379.

Oei TPS, Wanstall K, and Evans L (1990) Sex differences in panic disorder and agoraphobia. J Anx Disord 4, 317–324.

Otto MW, Pollack MH, Penava SJ, et al. (1999) Group cognitive–behavior therapy for patients failing to respond to pharmacotherapy for panic disorder: A clinical case series. Behav Res Ther 37, 763–770.

Otto MW, Pollack MH, Sachs GS, et al. (1992) Alcohol dependence in panic disorder patients. J Psychiatr Res 26, 29–38.

Otto MW, Pollack MH, Sachs GS, et al. (1993) Discontinuation of benzodiazepine treatment: Efficacy of cognitive–behavior therapy for patients with panic disorder. Am J Psychiatr 150, 1485–1490.

Peterson RA and Reiss S (1992) Anxiety Sensitivity Index Manual, 2nd ed., International Diagnostic Systems, Worthington, OH.

Pohl R, Yergani V, Balon R, et al. (1988) The jitteriness syndrome in panic disorder patients treated with antidepressants. J Clin Psychiatr 49, 100–104.

Pollack MH, Otto MW, Kaspi SP, et al. (1994) Cognitive–behavior therapy for treatment-refractory panic disorder. J Clin Psychiatr 55, 200–205.

Raj A and Sheehan DV (1987) Medical evaluation of panic attacks. J Clin Psychiatr 48, 309–313.

Rapee RM, Craske MG, and Barlow DH (1990) Subject-described features of panic attacks using self-monitoring. J Anx Disord 4, 171–181.

Rapee R, Mattick R, and Murrell E (1986) Cognitive mediation in the affective component of spontaneous panic attacks. J Behav Ther Exp Psychiatr 17, 245–254.

Reiss S (1999) The sensitivity theory of aberrant motivation. In Anxiety Sensitivity: Theory, Research, and Treatment of the Fear of Anxiety, Taylor S (ed). Lawrence Erlbaum, Mahwah, NJ, pp. 35–58.

Reiss S and McNally RJ (1985) The expectancy model of fear. In Theoretical Issues in Behavior Therapy, Reiss S and Bootzin RR (eds). Academic Press, New York, pp. 107–121.

Reed V and Wittchen HU (1998) DSM-IV panic attacks and panic disorder in a community sample of adolescents and young adults: How specific are panic attacks? J Psychiatr Res 32, 335–345.

Riley WT, McCormick MGF, Simon EM, et al. (1995) Effects of alprazolam dose on the induction and habituation processes during behavioral panic induction treatment. J Anx Disord 9, 217–227.

Robins LN, Locke BZ, and Regier DA (1991) An overview of psychiatric disorders in America. In Psychiatric Disorders in America: The Epidemiologic Catchment Area Study, Robins LN and Reiger DA (eds). Free Press, New York, p. 328.

Rosen JB and Schulkin J (1998) From normal fear to pathological anxiety. Psychol Rev 105, 325–350.

Rouillon F (1997) Epidemiology of Panic Disorder. Human Psychopharmacol 12, S7–S12.

Sanderson WC, Rapee RM, and Barlow DH (1989) The influence of an illusion of control on panic attacks induced via inhalation of 5.5% carbon dioxide-enriched air. Arch Gen Psychiatr 46, 157–162.

Scherrer JF, True WR, Xian H, et al. (2000) Evidence for genetic influences common and specific to symptoms of generalized anxiety and panic. J Affect Disord 57, 25–35.

Shapiro F (1995) Eye Movement Desensitization and Reprocessing: Basic Principles, Protocols, and Procedures. Guilford Press, New York.

Sharp DM, Power KG, Simpson RJ, et al. (1996) Fluvoxamine, placebo, and cognitive–behaviour therapy used alone and in combination in the treatment of panic disorder and agoraphobia. J Anx Disord 10, 219–242.

Shear MK, Cooper AM, Klerman GL, et al. (1993) A psychodynamic model of panic disorder. Am J Psychiatr 150, 859–866.

Shear MK, Devereaux RB, and Kramer-Fox R (1990) Mitral valve prolapse and anxiety: How close is the association? In Behavior Aspects of Cardiovascular Disease, Shapiro A and Baum A (eds). Lawrence Erlbaum, Hillsdale, NJ, pp. 31–42.

Shear MK and Maser JD (1994) Standardized assessment for panic disorder research: A conference report. Arch Gen Psychiatr 51, 346–354.

Simon NM and Pollack MH (2000) The current status of the treatment of panic disorder: Pharmacotherapy and cognitive–behavioral therapy. Psychiatr Ann 30, 689–696.

Sivaramakrishnan K, Alexander PJ, and Saharsarnamam N (1994) Prevalence of panic disorder in mitral valve prolapse: A comparative study with a cardiac control group. Acta Psychiatr Scand 89, 59–61.

Spiegel DA, Bruce TJ, Gregg SF, et al. (1994) Does cognitive–behavior therapy assist slow-taper alprazolam discontinuation in panic disorder? Am J Psychiatr 151, 876–881.

Spinhoven P, Onstein EJ, Sterk PJ, et al. (1993) Hyperventilation and panic attacks in general hospital patients. Gen Hosp Psychiatr 15, 148–154.

Stafrace S (1994) Hypnosis in the treatment of panic disorder with agoraphobia. Aust J Clin Hypnosis 22, 73–86.

Stein DJ, Hollander E, and Skoder AE (1993) Anxiety disorders and personality disorders: A review. J Pers Disord 7, 87–104.

Stein DJ and Stahl S (2000) Serotonin and anxiety: Current models. Int Clin Psychopharmacol 15(Suppl 2), S1–S6.

Stein MB, Asmundson GJG, Ireland D, et al. (1994) Panic disorder in patients attending a clinic for vestibular disorders. Am J Psychiatr 151, 1697–1700.

Stein MB, Norton GR, Walker JR, et al. (2000) Do SSRIs enhance the efficacy of very brief cognitive–behavioral therapy for panic disorder? A pilot study. Psychiatr Res 94, 191–200.

Stein MB and Uhde TW (1990) Panic disorder and major depression: Lifetime relationship and biological markers. In Clinical Aspects of Panic Disorder, Ballenger JC (ed). John Wiley, New York, pp. 151–168.

Stutzman GE and LeDoux JE (1999) GABAergic antagonists block the inhibitory effects of serotonin in the lateral amygdala: A mechanism for modulation of sensory inputs related to fear conditioning. J Neurosci 19, RC8.

Taylor S (1999) Anxiety Sensitivity. Lawrence Erlbaum, Mahwah, NJ.

Taylor S (2000) Understanding and Treating Panic Disorder: Cognitive–Behavioral Approaches. John Wiley, New York.

Taylor S (2001) Breathing retraining in the treatment of panic disorder: Efficacy, caveats, and indications. Scand J Behav Ther 30, 1–8.

Taylor S and Livesley WJ (1995) The influence of personality on the clinical course of neurosis. Curr Opin Psychiatr 8, 93–97.

Taylor S and Rachman S (1994) Stimulus estimation and overprediction of fear. Br J Clin Psychol 33, 173–181.

Thyer BA, Parrish RT, Himle J, et al. (1986) Alcohol abuse among clinically anxious patients. Behav Res Ther 24, 357–359.

Tork I and Hornung J-P (1990) Raphe nuclei and the serotonergic system. In The Human Nervous System, Paxinos G (ed). Academic Press, San Diego, pp. 1001–1022.

Uhde TW, Boulenger JP, Roy-Byrne PP, et al. (1985) Longitudinal course of panic disorder: Clinical and biological considerations. Prog Neuro-Psychopharmacol Biol Psychiatr 9, 39–51.

Uhlenhuth EH, Balter MB, Ban TA, et al. (1999) International study of expert judgment on therapeutic use of benzodiazepines and other psychotherapeutic medications. IV. Treatments in recommendations for the pharmacotherapy of anxiety disorders. Depress Anx 9, 107–116.

van den Heuvel OA, van de Wetering BJM, Veltman DJ, et al. (2000) Genetic studies of panic disorder: A review. J Clin Psychiatr 61, 756–766.

Viana MB, Graeff FG, and Loschmann PA (1997) Kainate microinjection into the dorsal raphe nucleus induces 5-HT release in the amygdala and periaqueductal gray. Pharmacol Biochem Behav 58, 167–172.

Wardle J, Hayward P, Higgitt A, et al. (1994) Effects of concurrent diazepam treatment on the outcome of exposure therapy in agoraphobia. Behav Res Ther 32, 203–215.

Welkowitz LA, Papp L, Martinez J, et al. (1999) Instructional set and physiological response to $CO_2$ inhalation. Am J Psychiatr 156, 745–748.

Weissman MM (1991) Panic disorder: Impact on quality of life. J Clin Psychiatr 52, 6–9.

Weissman MM, Bland RC, Canino GJ, et al. (1997) The cross-national epidemiology of panic disorder. Arch Gen Psychiatr 54, 305–309.

Westphal CFO (1871) Die agoraphobia, eine neuropathische erscheinung. Arch Psychiatr Nervenkrankheiten 3, 138–161 and 219–221.

Wiborg IM and Dahl AA (1996) Does brief dynamic psychotherapy reduce the relapse rate of panic disorder? Arch Gen Psychiatr 53, 689–694.

Wilhelm FH, Trabert W, and Roth WT (2001) Physiological instability in panic disorder and generalized anxiety disorder. Biol Psychiatr 49, 596–605.

Wilson KG, Sandler LS, Asmundson GJG, et al. (1991) Effects of instructional set on self-reports of panic attacks. J Anx Disord 5, 43–63.

Wilson KG, Sandler LS, Asmundson GJG, et al. (1992) Panic attacks in the nonclinical population: An empirical approach to case identification. J Abnorm Psychol 101, 460–468.

Wittchen HU, Reed V, and Kessler RC (1998) The relationship of agoraphobia and panic in a community sample of adolescents and young adults. Arch Gen Psychiatr 55, 1017–1024.

Yeragani VK, Pohl R, Jampala VC, et al. (2000) Increased QT variability in patients with panic disorder and depression. Psychiatr Res 93, 225–235.

Yonkers KA (1994) Panic disorder in women. J Women's Health 3, 481–486.

Yonkers KA, Zlotnick C, Allsworth J, et al. (1998) Is the course of panic disorder the same in women and men? Am J Psychiatr 155, 596–602.

# 67 Anxiety Disorders: Social and Specific Phobias

Martin M. Antony
Randi E. McCabe

Social Phobia (Social Anxiety Disorder)
Specific Phobia

## Definition

The experience of fear and the related emotion of anxiety are universal and familiar to everyone. Fear exists in all cultures and appears to exist across species. Presumably, the purpose of fear is to protect an organism from immediate threat and to mobilize the body for quick action to avoid danger. Emotion theorists consider fear to be an alarm response that fires in the presence of imminent threat or danger. The function of the primarily noradrenergic mediated fear response is to facilitate immediate escape from threat (flight) or attack on the source of threat (fight) (Barlow 1991, 2002). Therefore, fear is often referred to as a fight-or-flight response (Cannon 1929). All the manifestations of fear are consistent with its protective function. For example, heart rate and breathing rate increase to meet the increased oxygen needs of the body, increased perspiration helps to cool the body to facilitate escape, and pupils dilate to enhance visual acuity.

Anxiety, on the other hand, is a future-oriented mood state in which the individual anticipates the possibility of threat and experiences a sense of uncontrollability focused on the upcoming negative event. In the *Diagnostic and Statistical Manual of Mental Disorders*, Fourth Edition, Text Revision (DSM-IV-TR) (American Psychiatric Association 2000), anxiety is defined as "the apprehensive anticipation of future danger or misfortune accompanied by a feeling of dysphoria or somatic symptoms of tension" (p. 820). If one were to put anxiety into words, one might say, "Something bad might happen soon. I am not sure I can cope with it but I have to be ready to try." Anxiety is primarily mediated by the gamma-aminobutyric acid-benzodiazepine system (Barlow 1991, 2002).

Despite evidence that fear and anxiety are mediated by different brain systems, anxiety and fear are related, which makes sense ethologically. Experiencing anxiety after encountering signals of impending danger seems to lower the threshold for fear which is triggered when danger actually occurs (e.g., being attacked by a mugger or almost being hit by an automobile). Anxiety leads to a shift in attention toward the source of danger so that individuals become more vigilant for relevant threat cues and therefore are more likely to experience fear in the face of perceived immediate threat.

Fear and anxiety are not always adaptive. At times, the responses can occur in the absence of any realistic threat or out of proportion to the actual danger. Almost everyone has situations that arouse anxiety and fear despite the fact that the actual risk is minimal. It is not unusual to become anxious before a job interview or a speech. Many individuals feel fearful when exposed to situations such as dental visits, seeing certain animals, or being at certain heights. For some people, these fears reach extreme levels and may cause significant distress or impairment in functioning. It is at this point that what we typically refer to as shyness and fearfulness might meet diagnostic criteria for social phobia or specific phobia, respectively (see DSM-IV-TR Criteria 300.23 and 300.29).

As discussed later, phobias are the most common of the anxiety disorders and among the most common of all mental disorders. However, despite the frequency with which phobias occur in the general population, they have tended to be relatively ignored by clinicians and researchers. In the case of social phobia, it was not until the publication of the *Diagnostic and Statistical Manual of Mental Disorders*, Third Edition (DSM-III) (American Psychiatric Association 1980) that the diagnostic category was created. The introduction of social phobia to the diagnostic nomenclature has led to a slow but steady increase in research on the disorder, so that social phobia has now become a more popular topic of study among researchers on anxiety disorders. In addition to being widespread, social phobia is associated with significant functional impairment. Individuals with social phobia experience impairment in their work, home, and social relationships (Antony et al. 1998b). Also, social phobia often presents comorbidly with other mental disorders. Despite the high prevalence rate and significant impairment, generalized social phobia is rarely diagnosed or treated in a primary care setting (Katzelnick et al. 2001). Katzelnick and colleagues (2001) found that only 0.5% of patients with generalized social phobia were accurately diagnosed even though over 44% had made a visit to a mental health specialist or had been prescribed antidepressants.

With respect to specific phobias, the lack of attention is probably due to several factors. First, many physicians and researchers may view specific phobias to be less severe than other disorders, therefore warranting less attention. In addition, few individuals with specific phobias present for treatment, and the ones who do seek help tend to differ from untreated individuals with phobias with respect to the number and types of specific phobias (Chapman et al. 1993). As with social phobia, there has been an increase in attention paid to specific phobias, along with increased recognition that these phobias can interfere seriously with an individual's ability to function. It is not unusual for flying phobias to lead individuals to refuse job promotions that involve travel or to avoid visiting distant family members. Likewise, individuals with insect phobias may avoid being outside during the summer.

In the DSM-IV-TR (American Psychiatric Association 2000), social phobia (also known as social anxiety disorder) is defined as a "marked and persistent fear of one or more social or performance situations in which the person is exposed to unfamiliar people or to possible scrutiny of others." Typical situations feared by individuals with social

phobia include meeting new people, interacting with others, attending parties or meetings, speaking formally, eating or writing in front of others, dealing with people in authority, and being assertive. Specific phobia is defined as a "marked and persistent fear that is excessive or unreasonable, cued by the presence or anticipation of a specific object or situation (e.g., flying, heights, animals, receiving an injection, seeing blood)."

The diagnostic criteria for specific and social phobias share many features. For both disorders, the phobic situation must almost invariably lead to an anxiety response (immediately, in the case of specific phobias), which may take the form of a panic attack. In addition, the individual must recognize that the fear is excessive or unreasonable (although this feature may be absent in children), avoid the phobic situation or endure it with intense distress, and experience marked distress or functional impairment as a result of the phobia. In the case of social phobia, the fear must not be related to another mental disorder or medical condition. For example, if an individual develops difficulties communicating after suffering a stroke, the fear must be unrelated to having other people notice one's problems in speaking. However, if the psychiatrist judges that social anxiety is substantially in excess of what most individuals with this disability would experience, a diagnosis of anxiety disorder not otherwise specified may be appropriate.

Finally, for both disorders the fear must not be better accounted for by another problem. For example, an

## DSM-IV-TR Criteria 300.23

### Social Phobia (Social Anxiety Disorder)

A. A marked and persistent fear of one or more social or performance situations in which the person is exposed to unfamiliar people or to possible scrutiny by others. The individual fears that he or she will act in a way (or show anxiety symptoms) that will be humiliating or embarrassing. **Note:** In children, there must be evidence of the capacity for age-appropriate social relationships with familiar people and the anxiety must occur in peer settings, not just in interactions with adults.

B. Exposure to the feared social situation almost invariably provokes anxiety, which may take the form of a situationally bound or situationally predisposed panic attack. **Note:** In children, the anxiety may be expressed by crying, tantrums, freezing, or shrinking away from social situations with unfamiliar people.

C. The person recognizes that the fear is excessive or unreasonable. **Note:** In children, this feature may be absent.

D. The feared social or performance situations are avoided or else are endured with intense anxiety or distress.

E. The avoidance, anxious anticipation, or distress in the feared social or performance situation(s)

interferes significantly with the person's normal routine, occupational (or academic) functioning, or social activities or relationships, or there is marked distress about having the phobia.

F. In individuals under age 18 years, the duration is at least 6 months.

G. The fear or avoidance is not due to the direct physiological effects of a substance (e.g., a drug of abuse, a medication) or a general medical condition and is not better accounted for by another mental disorder (e.g., panic disorder with or without agoraphobia, separation anxiety disorder, body dysmorphic disorder, a pervasive developmental disorder, or schizoid personality disorder).

H. If a general medical condition or another mental disorder is present, the fear in criterion A is unrelated to it, for example, the fear is not of stuttering, trembling in Parkinson's disease, exhibiting abnormal eating behavior in anorexia nervosa or bulimia nervosa.

*Specify* if:

**Generalized:** if the fears include most social situations (also consider the additional diagnosis of avoidant personality disorder)

Reprinted with permission from the Diagnostic and Statistical Manual of Mental Disorders, Fourth Edition, Text Revision. Copyright 2000 American Psychiatric Association.

**Specific Phobia**

A. Marked and persistent fear that is excessive or unreasonable, cued by the presence or anticipation of a specific object or situation (e.g., flying, heights, animals, receiving an injection, seeing blood).

B. Exposure to the phobic stimulus almost invariably provokes an immediate anxiety response, which may take the form of a situationally bound or situationally predisposed panic attack. **Note:** In children, the anxiety may be expressed by crying, tantrums, freezing, or clinging.

C. The person recognizes that the fear is excessive or unreasonable. **Note:** In children, this feature may be absent.

D. The phobic situation(s) is avoided or else is endured with intense anxiety or distress.

E. The avoidance, anxious anticipation, or distress in the feared situation(s) interferes significantly with the person's normal routine, occupational (or academic) functioning, or social activities or relationships, or there is marked distress about having the phobia.

F. In individuals under age 18 years, the duration is at least 6 months.

G. The anxiety, panic attacks, and phobic avoidance associated with the specific object or situation are not better accounted for by another mental disorder, such as obsessive–compulsive disorder (e.g., fear of dirt in someone with an obsession about contamination), posttraumatic stress disorder (e.g., avoidance of stimuli associated with a severe stressor), separation-anxiety disorder (e.g., avoidance of school), social phobia (e.g., avoidance of social situations because of fear of embarrassment), panic disorder with agoraphobia, or agoraphobia without history of panic disorder.

*Specify* type:

**Animal type**

**Natural environment type** (e.g., heights, storms, water)

**Blood-injection-injury type**

Situational type (e.g., airplanes, elevators, enclosed places)

**Other type** (e.g., fear of choking, vomiting, or contracting an illness; in children, fear of loud sounds or costumed characters)

individual with obsessive–compulsive disorder who fears contamination from contact with injections would not receive an additional diagnosis of specific phobia unless there were additional concerns about injections that were unrelated to contamination (e.g., fear of fainting during an injection, fear of pain from the needle). Each diagnosis has specifiers and subtypes to allow for the provision of more specific diagnostic information. For social phobia, the psychiatrist can specify whether the phobia is generalized (i.e., includes most social situations). For specific phobias, the psychiatrist can indicate which one of five types best describes the focus of the phobia: animal, natural environment, blood-injection-injury, situational, or other.

## Etiology and Pathophysiology

### Psychological Factors

#### Psychoanalytic Perspectives

Historically, the etiology of phobic disorders was typically explained from a psychoanalytic perspective. Freud postulated that phobias may often stem from an unresolved oedipal conflict. Specifically, incestuous sexual desire is proposed to lead to anxiety associated with being attacked and castrated. Although the defense mechanism of repression is typically used to protect the individual from experiencing the anxiety (and the underlying conflict), when repression is insufficient the ego must use additional defense mechan-

isms. In the case of individuals with phobias, Freud proposed that displacement of the anxiety to a less relevant object or situation occurs (such as a dog or some other animal), so that the feared object is used to symbolize the primary source of the conflict. Patients with phobias use avoidance to further escape the effects of the anxiety (Nemiah and Uhde 1989). Although Freud's theory was once influential, its impact on current thinking among researchers has waned. Rather, most current research on psychological factors in the development of phobias has tended to focus on conditioning and information-processing theories and their interaction with neurobiological processes.

### Learning and Conditioning Perspectives

Emotions are "contagious." That is, we learn to respond to stimuli, in part, by observing other people's responses and also by our own experiences in these situations. In other words, we come to fear dangerous situations easily. This is important from an ethological perspective because our ancestors who could learn to fear threatening objects or situations easily were more likely to survive and pass these genes to their offspring. This inherited tendency to learn to experience fear in particular situations is the basis of conditioning models of phobia development.

**Mowrer's Two-Stage Model.** The two-stage model of Mowrer (1939) was a precursor to current conditioning models for phobia development. According to Mowrer, the first stage in the development of fear involves a classical conditioning process by which a previously neutral stimulus is associated with an aversive stimulus so that the neutral stimulus becomes a trigger for fear. For example, a fear of dogs might develop after an individual is bitten (an aversive stimulus) by a dog (a neutral stimulus). Mowrer's second stage relies on operant conditioning principles to explain the maintenance of phobias. According to Mowrer, phobias are maintained by negative reinforcement resulting from avoidance of the phobic object. In other words, avoidance prevents the uncomfortable symptoms that occur when one is frightened and thereby maintains the desire to avoid the phobic object and situation.

Despite the research interest generated by Mowrer's model, the model suffers from several problems. First, many individuals report no specific conditioning experiences that trigger their phobias. In fact, many individuals report having fears despite never even having encountered the phobic situation, let alone having experienced a trauma in the phobic situation. Second, Mowrer's theory does not explain why many individuals experience traumas but never develop fears. For example, one study found that although traumatic events were reported to be the cause of fear among 56% of individuals with fears of dogs, 66% of non-fearful subjects reported a history of traumatic experiences with dogs that did not lead to the development of fear (Di Nardo et al. 1988).

**Rachman's Pathways to Fear Development.** In response to these and other concerns with Mowrer's model, Rachman (1977) proposed three pathways to the development of fear. The first of these is *direct conditioning*, which typically involves the experience of being hurt or frightened by the phobic object or situation. Examples include being involved in an automobile accident, being humiliated in front of a group, falling or almost falling from a high place, or fainting at the sight of blood. Rachman's second pathway is called *vicarious acquisition*, which involves witnessing some traumatic event or seeing someone behave fearfully in the presence of a phobic situation. For example, a child might develop a fear of snakes after seeing her father behave fearfully around snakes, or someone might develop a fear of public speaking after seeing another individual heckled by the audience during a presentation. For the third pathway, Rachman proposed that fears can develop through *informational and instructional pathways*. It is not surprising that individuals might develop flying phobias, given the frequency with which plane crashes are reported in the news. Similarly, a child might develop a fear of heights if his parents frequently warned him of the dangers of being near high places.

In addition to these pathways, Rachman acknowledged the role of biological constraints on the development of fear. Of particular relevance is the fact that fears are not randomly distributed. To explain this observation, Seligman (1971) proposed that organisms are predisposed to learn certain associations and not others. Seligman called his theory "preparedness" and hypothesized that individuals are "prepared" to develop some associations that lead to fear and not others. For example, an individual might be more likely to develop a fear of dogs after being bitten than to develop a fear of flowers after being pricked by a thorn.

Seligman proposed that these associations evolved through natural selection processes to facilitate survival.

Evidence for the theory of preparedness is mixed. Although some authors have concluded that the studies to date do not support preparedness (McNally 1987), it may be argued that these studies have not adequately tested the theory. Most studies examining preparedness have attempted to associate dangerous objects (e.g., snakes) and nondangerous objects (e.g., flowers) with an aversive electrical shock and have found few differences in the subsequent development of fear. However, preparedness predicts that some "associations" are more difficult to establish than others, not that some "objects" are more easily feared than others. The theory does not necessarily predict that shock should be more easily associated with snakes than with flowers. A more appropriate experiment might be to compare the effects of a minor snakebite to the effects of being pricked by a thorny flower on the development of fear of each object. In any event, there is now strong evidence that conditioning processes play an important role in the development of phobic disorders (Bouton et al. 2001).

Numerous studies have examined the prevalence of Rachman's three pathways to fear development, as illustrated in Table 67–1. Most of these studies have focused on the development of specific phobias, although a few studies included social phobia groups. The majority of studies have found support for the model, indicating that both direct and indirect forms of phobia acquisition occur frequently across a wide range of phobia types (McNally and Steketee 1985, Merckelbach and Muris 1997, Muris et al. 1997, Townend et al. 2000). However, numerous people report onsets that are unrelated to these pathways (e.g., "I have had this fear for as long as I can remember" or "I have always had this fear"). Overall, it appears that direct and indirect methods of fear development are relatively common, although the frequency of these onsets varies greatly across studies for a variety of reasons. First, studies have been inconsistent with respect to the populations studied (e.g., clinical groups, nonclinical subjects such as college students, individuals recruited through advertisements). In addition, some studies included mixed groups of patients with a given fear (e.g., flying fears can be due to a specific phobia of flying, claustrophobia, or agoraphobia). Third, studies differed in the ways in which each pathway was defined. For example, an onset that followed an unexpected panic attack was included among the traumatic onsets in some studies but not others. Finally, some studies allowed subjects to list multiple causes, whereas other studies had subjects rate only the primary cause.

In addition to methodological differences, the inconsistency across studies may be partly explained by the lack of reliability of retrospective self-report. More recent studies have examined onset of phobias in children and included parental interviews to avoid problems associated with retrospective report (Merckelbach and Muris 1997, Poulton et al. 1999).

Despite the prevalence of direct and indirect conditioning events and informational onsets, it appears that they are not the whole story. In fact, studies have begun to include normal comparison groups and have found that these events are equally common in individuals who do not

| Table 67–1 | Percentage of Individuals with Phobias Reporting Various Types of Onset* | | | |
|---|---|---|---|---|
| Study | Type of Fear | Direct Conditioning | Vicarious Conditioning | Information |
| McNally and Steketee (1985) | Animals | 23 | 0 | 4 |
| Menzies and Parker (2001) | Heights | 19 | 15 | 7 |
| Di Nardo et al. (1988) | Dogs | 56 | – | – |
| Merckelbach and Muris (1997) | Spiders | 23 | 15 | 4 |
| Merckelbach et al. (1992) | Spiders | 66 | 59 | 34 |
| Ehlers et al. (1994) | Driving | 36 | 12 | 16 |
| Merckelbach et al. (1996) | Spiders | 41 | 18 | 5 |
| Menzies and Clarke (1993b) | Heights | 18 | 20 | 8 |
| Öst (1991) | Blood | 49 | 26 | 7 |
| | Injection | 57 | 21 | 5 |
| Öst and Hugdahl (1985) | Blood | 46 | 32 | 9 |
| | Dentists | 69 | 12 | 6 |
| Kleinknecht (1994) | Blood-injury | 76 | 20 | 3 |
| Rimm et al. (1977) | Various | 36 | 7 | 9 |
| Hofmann et al. (1995a) | Public speaking | 89 | 57 | 54 |
| Muris et al. (1997) | Animals | 45 | 0 | 29 |
| | Medical | 44 | 0 | 11 |
| | Spiders | 42 | 0 | 13 |
| | Social (failure and criticism) | 50 | 0 | 0 |
| | All fears | 40 | 1 | 27 |
| Öst (1985) | Blood | 50 | 25 | 2 |
| | Animals | 50 | 22 | 20 |
| | Dentists | 66 | 16 | 0 |
| | Enclosed places | 68 | 7 | 13 |
| | Social | 56 | 16 | 3 |
| Antony (1994) | Heights | 20 | 0 | 0 |
| | Animals | 20 | 7 | 7 |
| | Blood-injections | 27 | 0 | 7 |
| | Driving | 33 | 13 | 13 |

*Figures are rounded off to the nearest percent.

have phobias (Hofmann et al. 1995, Menzies and Parker 2001, Merckelbach et al. 1992). Ultimately, to answer the question of how phobias begin, we must discover the variables that lead only certain individuals to develop phobias after experiencing conditioning events or receiving information that leads to fear. For example, several investigators have found that a tendency to feel "disgust" in response to certain stimuli may be important in the development of some animal phobias and blood phobias (Davey et al. 1993, Merckelbach et al. 1993, Page 1994, Sawchuk et al. 2000, Woody and Teachman 2000). In addition, heightened disgust sensitivity in parents has been found to predict fear of disgust-relevant animals (e.g., snakes, mice, slugs, and cockroaches) in children (de Jong et al. 1997).

Several other variables have also been suggested as mediating factors in the development of fear. Stress at the time of the event may make individuals more likely to react fearfully. In addition, previous and subsequent exposure to the phobic object may protect an individual from the development of a phobia. For example, someone who grew up around dogs may be less likely to develop a phobia after being bitten than someone who has spent little time around dogs. The context of the event may also influence the reaction. For example, being with another supportive individual at the time of the trauma may protect an individual from

developing fear. Finally, a number of individual difference variables such as perceived control, trait anxiety, and various personality factors may influence an individual's likelihood of developing a phobia after a conditioning event. In fact, there is evidence that personality factors and parenting styles may be especially relevant to the development of social phobia.

It has been proposed that a fourth nonassociative pathway be added to Rachman's three associative pathways to fear development (Poulton and Menzies 2002). Nonassociative fear models (Menzies and Clarke 1995) propose that a limited number of fears are not acquired by conditioning or other learning processes. Rather, these evolutionary adaptive fears are proposed to be innate or biologically determined. This is similar to preparedness theory, however, it maintains that fears are acquired through a learning or conditioning process and that some fears are more easily learned than others. According to Poulton and Menzies (2002), the nonassociative pathway to fear acquisition helps to explain a number of research findings that run counter to associative models of fear development including the nonrandom distribution of common fears, and the emergence of some fears without any prior specific associative learning experiences (i.e., direct conditioning, vicarious conditioning, or informational transmission).

**Personality Variables.** The work of Kagan and others (Kagan et al.1984, Rosenbaum et al. 1991) has suggested that as early as 18 months of age, children differ with respect to their tendency to interact with other individuals, toys, and objects. Although about 70% of children are somewhat exploratory in these situations, about 15% of children are extremely exploratory, and the remaining 15% are quite shy and withdrawn. The behavior exhibited by the shy and withdrawn children has been called "behavioral inhibition" and has been proposed to be a predisposing factor in the development of social phobia and other anxiety disorders (Turner et al. 1996). One study found that the prevalence of social phobia was significantly greater (17%; $N = 64$) in children with behavioral inhibition than without (5%; $N = 152$) (Biederman et al. 2001). In addition, compared with nonanxious individuals, patients with social phobia describe their parents as having (1) discouraged them from socializing, (2) placed undue importance on the opinions of others, and (3) used shame as a means of discipline (Bruch and Heimberg 1994). Other predictors of the development of social phobia include a childhood history of separation anxiety, self-consciousness or shyness in childhood and adolescence, and a low frequency of dating in adolescence (Bruch 1989, Bruch and Heimberg 1994).

Perfectionism is another personality variable that has been associated with social phobia (Antony et al. 1998a). Although several other anxiety disorders have also been associated with perfectionism, concern about making mistakes and a perception of having critical parents are highest among individuals with social phobia compared to individuals with other anxiety disorders (e.g., panic disorder, obsessive–compulsive disorder, or specific phobia).

**Cognitive Variables.** Numerous studies have examined the role of cognitive variables in social and specific phobias and have consistently found that individuals with these disorders exhibit attentional and attributional biases regarding the phobic object or situation. In studies of information processing, people with social and specific phobias devote more attention to threat-related information than do nonphobic individuals (Kindt and Brosschot 1999, Mattia et al. 1993). They also show perceptual and cognitive distortions consistent with their phobias (Jones and Menzies 2000, Pauli et al. 1998, Purdon et al. 2001, Rapee 1997, Roth et al. 2001). For example, individuals with snake or spider phobias tend to overestimate the degree of activity in the feared animal before treatment but not after treatment (Rachman and Cuk 1992). Likewise, people with social phobia tend to rate their own performance during public speaking more critically than do nonphobic control subjects (Rapee and Lim 1992). Furthermore, the discrepancy between self-ratings and observer ratings is greater for people with social phobia than control subjects (Norton and Hope 2001). In addition, individuals with social phobia tend to report more negative self-evaluative thoughts and underestimate their performance when interacting with others relative to nonanxious subjects (Stopa and Clark 1993). More recent research has found that compared to nonanxious individuals, individuals with social phobia are more likely to experience negative imagery and to take an observer's point of view (i.e., see themselves from an external perspective) when exposed to feared social situations

(Hackman et al. 1998, Wells and Papageorgiou 1999). Other research has found that social phobia is associated with impaired thought suppression affecting both social phobia-related stimuli as well as nonsocial phobia-related stimuli (Fehm and Margraf 2002). Although it is clear that cognitive biases exist in individuals with phobias and that attentional and attributional biases improve after effective treatment, it is not known whether the cognitive biases exhibited by patients contribute to the development of the fear or whether they are simply a manifestation of the fear.

## Genetic and Family Factors

Specific phobias and social phobia tend to run in families. It appears that being a first-degree relative of an individual with a specific phobia puts one at a greater risk for a specific phobia compared with first-degree relatives of never mentally ill controls (31% versus 11%). However, the particular phobia that is transmitted is usually different from that in the relative, although it is often from the same general type (e.g., animal, situational). Furthermore, relatives of people with specific phobias are not at increased risk for other types of anxiety disorders (including social phobia) or subclinical fears (Fyer et al. 1990). The heritability of blood and injection phobias may be even greater than that for other phobias. One study found that 61% of individuals with blood phobia and 29% of those with injection phobias reported having a first-degree relative with the same fear (Öst 1992). However, these findings should be interpreted with caution because relatives did not undergo independent interviews.

Findings for individuals with social phobia and their families show a similar pattern. In one study, 16% of first-degree relatives of subjects with social phobia had symptoms that met criteria for social phobia, whereas only 5% of first-degree relatives of never mentally ill control subjects had social phobia (Fyer et al. 1993). Furthermore, there is no increased risk among relatives of people with social phobia to develop other anxiety disorders. A more recent study found that in comparison to probands in a comparison group, the relative risk for generalized social phobia and avoidant personality disorder were tenfold for first-degree relatives of probands with social phobia (Stein et al. 1998).

Of course, the existence of a disorder in multiple family members does not necessarily imply genetic transmission. Family members often share learning experiences and other environmental factors. To establish a genetic relationship among family members with a particular disorder, twin studies, adoption studies, and molecular genetics studies are typically conducted. Currently, there are no adoption or molecular genetics studies of social or specific phobias, and twin studies have yielded conflicting results.

A twin study by Skre and colleagues (1993) found that although many of the anxiety disorders have a strong genetic component, in the case of specific and social phobias, environmental influences seem to be most important. In contrast, Andrews and colleagues (1990) found a genetic contribution to the development of neurotic traits and symptoms that may predispose individuals to develop anxiety disorders in general, but not a particular anxiety disorder. This study included individuals with social phobia but not specific phobias. Another twin study examining genetic transmission of both specific and social phobias found heritability estimates of 51% for social phobia, 47% for animal phobias, 59% for blood-injection-injury phobias, and 46% for situational phobias (Kendler et al. 1999). Consistent with previous research (Page and Martin 1998), individual-specific environmental influences (e.g., experiencing a traumatic event in the phobic situation) were found to be etiologically significant in the development of both social and specific phobias but family-specific environmental influences (e.g., shared environment) were not (Kendler et al. 1999). In another genetic study of specific and social phobias conducted by Kendler and colleagues (1992), both genetic and individual-specific environmental factors (e.g., phobia-specific traumatic event) were influential in the development of specific phobia whereas for social phobia, both genetic and nonspecific environmental factors have an etiological role.

Although there are conflicting findings on whether there is a general genetic factor (influencing risk for any anxiety disorder) or a specific genetic factor (influencing risk for specific anxiety disorders such as specific and social phobias), some general conclusions can be made. In the case of social phobia, there seems to be a moderate (based on the strength of the correlations from twin studies) disorder-specific genetic influence combined with specific and non-specific environmental influences. In the case of specific phobia, evidence supports a disorder-specific genetic contribution combined with disorder-specific environmental influences (e.g., traumatic conditioning experiences involving the phobic object or situation).

Although the nature of the genetic contribution has yet to be specified (a low threshold for alarm reactions or vasovagal responses is one possibility), specific and social phobias may be related to personality factors that have been found to be highly heritable. Two traits that may be relevant are neuroticism (or emotionality) and extroversion (or sociability) (Plomin 1989). Average heritability estimates for these traits are about 50% across a wide range of genetic studies. Emotionality probably predisposes individuals to develop a range of anxiety and mood disorders whereas sociability may be most relevant to social phobia. Furthermore, certain phobias may have other specific genetic contributions. Up to 70% of individuals with blood phobia report a history of fainting on exposure to blood (Öst 1992). It has been suggested that an inherited overactive baroreflex may contribute to the high rate of familial transmission of blood phobias (Adler et al. 1991).

## Other Biological Factors

In contrast to the situation with other anxiety disorders, little is known about the physiological correlates of specific and social phobias. Only a few studies have examined physiological correlates of specific phobia. Research examining brain activity during the experience of phobic fear using positron emission tomography has yielded inconsistent results (Rauch et al. 1995, Wik et al. 1997), with some studies finding changes in cerebral blood flow associated with viewing phobia-relevant scenes and some studies finding no differences in cerebral blood flow between participants with and without phobias. Specific phobia may have been of less interest to researchers because no effective pharmacological treatments exist for this disorder. However, effective drug treatments have been identified for

social phobia, leading to an increased interest in the biological factors underlying this disorder (Mathew et al. 2001).

Studies on the relationship between serotonin and social phobia have been mixed. Selective serotonin reuptake inhibitors (SSRIs) have been shown to be very effective in the treatment of social phobia. In addition, there is evidence of augmented cortisol response to fenfluramine in patients with social phobia, suggesting an association between social phobia and selective supersensitivity in the serotonergic system (Tancer et al. 1994/1995). However, there is research showing that [$^3$H] paroxetine binding (an indicator of serotonergic functioning) does not differ between social phobia patients and nonanxious controls (Stein et al. 1995).

There has also been some evidence to suggest a relationship between dopamine and social phobia. Unlike panic disorder, which responds well to a variety of tricyclic antidepressants and monoamine oxidase inhibitors (MAOIs) (Buigues and Vallejo 1987, Schweizer et al. 1993), social phobia tends to have a positive response to MAOIs and show little response to tricyclic antidepressants (Levin et al. 1989). Whereas tricyclic antidepressants tend to act on noradrenergic and serotonergic systems, MAOIs affect noradrenergic, serotonergic, and dopaminergic systems (Cooper et al. 1983). This finding has led some investigators to suggest that the dopamine system is primarily involved in social phobia (Levin et al. 1989), which would explain why biological challenges that appear to affect noradrenergic activity (e.g., sodium lactate infusion, carbon dioxide inhalation) have little effect on patients with social phobia, despite having panicogenic effects in patients with panic disorder (Rapee et al. 1992). The dopamine hypothesis is consistent with findings that dopamine metabolite levels correlate with measures of extroversion (King et al. 1986) as well as findings that mice bred to be timid have been shown to be deficient in brain dopamine concentration (Lewis et al. 1989). In addition, a neuroimaging study found that striatal dopamine reuptake site densities were significantly lower in patients with social phobia as compared to controls (Tiihonen et al. 1997).

With respect to neuroendocrine correlates in social phobia, studies of the hypothalamic–pituitary–thyroid and hypothalamic–pituitary–adrenal axes in social phobia have found few differences between patients with social phobia and control persons. For example, research has found that patients with social phobia and control subjects did not differ on tests of thyroid function (Tancer et al. 1990) or levels of urinary free cortisol (Potts et al. 1991). However, more recent studies have found evidence of cortisol differences associated with social anxiety. Some research has found that shy children have higher salivary cortisol than nonshy children (Schmidt et al. 1997). Other research has found that in comparison to control volunteers, social phobia patients exhibited dichotomies in the distribution and magnitude of their cortisol response to a speech task (social phobia-related stress task), but not a physical exercise task (nonsocial phobia-related stress task) (Furlan et al. 2001).

Recent imaging studies have found a number of differences between social phobia patients and controls. One study using functional magnetic resonance imaging (fMRI) found that conditioned aversive stimuli were associated with increased activation in the amygdala and hippocampus of social phobia patients, whereas decreased activation in these areas was observed in normal controls (Schneider et al. 1999). Other research using repeat proton magnetic resonance spectroscopy has found significant differences between social phobics and controls in cortical gray matter. Specifically, Tupler and colleagues (1997) found that social phobia is associated with specific choline and myoinositol abnormalities in cortical and subcortical gray areas of the brain. Another study using single photon emission computer tomography (SPECT) found that after an 8-week trial of citalopram there was significantly decreased activity in the anterior and lateral part of the left temporal cortex, the left cingulum, and the anterior, lateral, and posterior part of the left midfrontal cortex in a small ($N = 15$) sample of social phobia patients (Van der Linden et al. 2000a). Compared to treatment responders, treatment nonresponders had higher activity at baseline in the lateral left temporal cortex and the lateral left midfrontal regions. Further research is necessary to understand the significance of these imaging findings as well as their specificity to social phobia.

A few studies have examined patterns of brain activity associated with shyness. In a study on high and low shyness (anxious self-preoccupation and avoidance of social situations) and sociability (preference to be socially active and seek out social situations) in college students, Schmidt (1999) found that shyness was associated with greater relative right frontal EEG activity, whereas sociability was associated with greater relative left frontal EEG. In addition, Schmidt (1999) found the pattern of absolute EEG power in each frontal hemisphere differed for high shy/high social participants and high shy/low social participants.

Finally, there may be good reason to consider different underlying mechanisms in patients with performance-related phobias (e.g., public speaking) than in patients with generalized social phobia (i.e., those who fear most social situations). Individuals with performance-related phobias tend to show more autonomic reactivity (e.g., rapid heart beat) in the phobic situation than do patients with generalized social phobia (Levin et al. 1993). In addition, beta blockers such as atenolol may be useful for decreasing performance anxiety in normal individuals (Gorman and Gorman 1987), although they have little effect on patients with generalized social phobia (Liebowitz et al. 1992). These facts have led some investigators to suggest that adrenergic hyperactivity may be involved in performance anxiety but not in generalized social phobia (Levin et al. 1989). However, it should be noted that despite limited evidence for the use of beta blockers in normal groups (e.g., musicians with performance anxiety), their utility for treating patients with a diagnosis of social phobia (e.g., performance fears that lead to significant distress or impairment) has not been established.

## Assessment and Differential Diagnosis

## Assessment

### Special Issues in Psychiatric Examination and History

As is the case with most disorders, a comprehensive assessment is important in helping the psychiatrist to decide which treatment approach is most appropriate for a given patient. In the case of specific and social phobias, a thorough evaluation should include a structured or semistructured interview, self-report measures, and a behavioral assessment. Each of these measures provides different types of information that may be relevant to later treatment decisions. This section provides an overview of relevant assessment issues. Additional comprehensive reviews may be found in several recent volumes (Antony et al. 2001b, McCabe and Antony 2002).

During all parts of the initial evaluation, the psychiatrist should be sensitive to several issues. First, for many patients with phobias, even discussing the phobic object can provoke anxiety. For example, some patients with spider phobias experience panic attacks when they discuss spiders. Some patients with blood phobias faint when they discuss surgical procedures. Therefore, the psychiatrist should ask the patient whether discussing the phobic object or situation will provoke anxiety. If the interview is likely to be a source of stress, the psychiatrist should emphasize the importance of the information that is being collected, as well as the potential therapeutic value of discussing the feared object. As described in a later section, exposure to the feared stimulus is an essential component of the treatment of most specific phobias. Of course, the interviewer should use his or her judgment when deciding how much to push the patient in the first session. For treatment to be effective, establishing trust in the psychiatrist early in the course of treatment is essential.

With respect to social phobia, the assessment itself may be considered a phobic stimulus. Because individuals with social phobia fear the evaluation of others, a psychiatric interview may be especially frightening. Even completing self-report questionnaires in the waiting room may be difficult for patients who fear writing in front of others. The psychiatrist should be sensitive to this possibility and provide reassurance when appropriate.

### Structured and Semistructured Interviews

Although there are numerous structured and semistructured interviews available (Summerfeldt and Antony 2002), two of the most commonly used interviews for diagnosing anxiety disorders are the Anxiety Disorders Interview Schedule for DSM-IV (ADIS-IV) (Brown et al. 1994) and the Structured Clinical Interview for Axis I DSM-IV-TR Disorders-Patient Edition (SCID-I/P for DSM-IV-TR) (First et al. 2001). Current and lifetime diagnoses of specific phobia and social phobia based on the ADIS-IV have been shown to have good to excellent reliability for the specific phobia types and the generalized type of social phobia (Brown et al. 2001b). To date, there are few published studies on the psychometric properties of the SCID-I. One study (Zanarini et al. 2000) found that the reliability (both interrater and test–retest) for social phobia was in the fair to good range and the reliability for other Axis I disorders was also good. Previous versions of the SCID-I for the DSM-III-R have been shown to be reliable, especially for phobic disorders (Antony and Swinson 2000a, Summerfeldt and Antony 2002). Each interview has advantages and disadvantages. Although the SCID-I provides detailed assessment of a broader range of disorders relative to the ADIS-IV (including eating disorders and psychotic disorders), the ADIS-IV provides more detailed information on each of the anxiety disorders and, like the SCID-I, includes sections to provide DSM-IV diagnoses for the mood disorders and other disorders that are typically associated with the anxiety disorders (e.g., substance use and somatoform disorders). In addition, the ADIS-IV includes more questions to help differentiate specific and social phobias from other disorders with which they share features.

### Self-Report Measures

Numerous self-report measures have been created for the assessment of specific phobias and social anxiety. The main advantage of self-report measures is the time that they save for the psychiatrist. Relevant self-report measures are recommended before the clinical interview if possible. This will allow the interviewer to follow up specific responses during the interview. Measures can be administered again, periodically, to assess progress and outcome. It should be noted that questionnaire measures do not always correlate highly with performance on behavioral measures (Klieger and Franklin 1993). Furthermore, there is evidence that men are more likely than women to underestimate their fear on specific phobia measures (Pierce and Kirkpatrick 1992). The most common questionnaires used to screen for specific phobias are the various versions of the Fear Survey Schedule (Geer 1965, Wolpe and Lang 1964). In addition, a variety of measures exist to assess fear of specific objects and situations. For example, the Mutilation Questionnaire (Klorman et al. 1974) is among the most common tests for assessing fear of situations involving blood and medical procedures. Self-report measures for assessing both specific phobia and social anxiety are listed in Table 67–2. Detailed reviews of these and other measures are available (Antony et al. 2001b, McCabe and Antony 2002).

| Table 67–2 | Common Measures for Specific and Social Phobias |
|---|---|

#### Specific Phobia

Fear Survey Schedule (FSS) (Geer 1965, Wolpe and Lang 1964, 1969, 1977)
Fear Questionnaire (FQ) (Marks and Mathews 1979)
Fear of Flying Scale (FFS) (Haug et al. 1987)
Acrophobia Questionnaire (AQ) (Cohen 1977)
Mutilation Questionnaire (MQ) (Klorman et al. 1974)
Medical Fear Survey (MFS) (Kleinknecht et al. 1996)
Dental Anxiety Inventory (DAI) (Stouthard et al. 1993)
Claustrophobia Situations Questionnaire (CSQ) (Febbraro and Clum 1995)

#### Social Phobia

Social Phobia Inventory (SPIN) (Davidson 1998, Connor et al. 2000)
Mini-Social Phobia Inventory (Mini-SPIN) (Connor et al. 2001)
Social Phobia and Anxiety Inventory (SPAI) (Turner et al. 1989)
Social Interaction Anxiety Scale (SIAS) (Mattick and Clarke 1998)
Social Phobia Scale (SPS) (Mattick and Clarke 1998)
Brief Social Phobia Scale (BSPS) (Davidson et al. 1991b)
Liebowitz Social Phobia Scale (LSPS) (Liebowitz 1987)

### Behavioral Tests

Behavioral testing is an important part of any comprehensive evaluation for a phobic disorder. This is particularly the case if behavioral or cognitive–behavioral treatment will be used. Because most individuals with phobias avoid the objects and situations that they fear, patients may find it difficult to describe the subtle cues that affect their fear in the situation. In addition, it is not unusual for patients to misjudge the amount of fear that they typically experience in the phobic situation. A behavioral approach test can be useful for identifying specific fear triggers as well as for assessing the intensity of the patient's fear in the actual situation.

To conduct a behavioral approach test, patients should be instructed to enter the phobic situation for several minutes. For example, an individual with a snake phobia should be instructed to stand as close as possible to a live snake and note the specific cues that affect the fear (e.g., size of snake, color, movement) and the intensity of the fear (perhaps rating it on a 0–100-point scale). Patients should pay special attention to their physical sensations (e.g., palpitations, sweating, blushing), negative thoughts (e.g., "I will fall from this balcony"), and anxious coping strategies (e.g., escape, avoidance, distraction).

The behavioral approach test will help in the development of a specific treatment plan. However, before treatment patients will often be reluctant to enter the feared situation. If this is the case, the information collected during the behavioral approach test may be elicited during the early part of behavioral treatment.

### Differences in Sex, Cultural, and Developmental Presentation

**Sex Differences.** As mentioned earlier, specific phobias tend to be more common among women than men. This finding seems to be strongest for phobias from the animal type, whereas sex differences are smaller for height phobias and blood-injury-injection phobias. In addition, social phobia tends to be slightly more prevalent among women than men, although these differences are relatively small (Antony and Swinson 2000a).

There are several reasons why women may be more likely than men to report specific phobias. First, as discussed earlier, there is evidence that men tend to underreport their fear (Pierce and Kirkpatrick 1992). Also, women may be more likely than men to seek treatment for their difficulties, which would account for the fact that sex differences are often larger in treatment samples compared with epidemiological samples. In addition, as discussed later, sex ratios for phobias differ across cultures, which may be explained by cultural differences in treatment seeking. Finally, the sex difference in prevalence may reflect actual differences between men and women in susceptibility to develop phobias.

Women and men are taught to deal differently with typical phobic stimuli. Traditionally, boys more than girls are often encouraged to play with spiders and toy snakes and to engage in more adventurous activities (e.g., hiking in high places). In addition, women may have more role models for the development of fear than men do. Images of women standing on chairs when they see a mouse or running away from spiders are common in children's cartoons and other media, but men are rarely depicted as being frightened by these objects. Therefore, it is possible that in Western cultures women learn to fear certain situations more strongly than do men. Of course, it is difficult to know whether culture and the media are responsible for sex differences or simply reflect differences that exist for other reasons (e.g., different predisposing factors). It will be interesting to see whether sex ratios for phobias change as traditional gender roles continue to change.

One study examining sex differences and social phobia found significant gender differences in the presentation of social phobia (Turk et al. 1998). Whereas men were more fearful than women of urinating in public bathrooms and returning items to a store, women were more fearful than men of a number of situations including talking to people in authority, public speaking, being the center of attention, expressing disagreement, and throwing a party. Sex differences were not found in terms of comorbidity, social phobia subtypes, or duration of illness.

**Cultural Differences.** Little is known about cultural differences in specific and social phobias. Several reasons have been suggested for this lack of relevant data. First, individuals from minority cultures in the US tend to underuse traditional mental health facilities and are more likely than other groups to terminate treatment after one session (Sue 1990). When African-Americans seek mental health services, they may be more likely to present to a physician, minister, or community mental health clinic than a university hospital, which is where much of the research tends to take place (Neal and Turner 1991). In addition, certain minority groups may be less likely to participate in psychological research because of the negative ways in which research data have historically been used to affect government policies toward minority groups (Neal and Turner 1991).

Nevertheless, a few studies bear on the issue of cultural differences in phobias. For example, there is evidence from epidemiological studies that African-Americans are 1.5 to 3 times as likely as whites to report phobic disorders, even after controlling for education and socioeconomic status (Brown et al. 1990, Curtis et al. 1998, Warheit et al. 1975). Several explanations for this finding have been provided. For example, some of the fears reported by African-American individuals may reflect realistic concerns that were misdiagnosed as phobias. For example, African-American persons in inner city communities may have more realistic reasons to fear violence (Warheit et al. 1975). Furthermore, African-Americans experience more negative evaluation from others, and some of their social concerns may be realistic. Another possibility is that African-Americans experience more chronic stress than whites and therefore may be more susceptible to the development of phobias and other problems. Finally, there may be cultural differences in response biases on questionnaire measures of fear and during interviews (Brown et al. 1990).

Other research has found that specific phobias are more common among US-born Mexican-Americans than in US-born whites or immigrant Mexican-Americans, after controlling for sex, age, socioeconomic status, and various other variables (Karno et al. 1989, Vega et al. 1998). No group differences emerged for the prevalence of social phobia across these groups (Karno et al. 1989). Some of the factors mentioned (e.g., differences in stress and response biases) may explain the differences between whites and Mexican-Americans born in the US. In addition, it has been suggested that "selective migration" may account for the relatively low rate of phobias in immigrant Mexican-Americans. In other words, individuals with specific phobias may be less likely to emigrate.

A variety of studies have shown that specific phobias, social phobia, and related conditions exist across cultures. For example, in Japan, a condition exists called *taijin kyôfu* in which individuals have an "obsession of shame." This condition has much overlap with social phobia in that it is often accompanied by fears of blushing, having improper facial expressions in the presence of others, looking at others, shaking, and perspiring in front of others (Takahashi 1989). In addition, studies have identified individuals with social and specific phobias in a variety of other non-Western countries including Saudi Arabia (Chaleby 1987), India (Raguram and Bhide 1985), Japan (Kleinknecht et al. 1997), and other East Asian countries (Chang 1997, Lee and Oh 1999). Interestingly, in some other cultures, the sex ratio for phobias tends to be reversed. For example, in studies from Saudi Arabia and India, up to 80% of individuals reporting for treatment of phobias were male. Similarly, in Japan about 60% of patients with *taijin kyôfu* are male. In the case of phobias in India, it has been suggested that traditional gender roles may account for the difference in treatment seeking in Indian men and women (Raguram and Bhide 1985). Specifically, Indian women are often discouraged from leaving the house alone or conversing with others without the husband's permission. It is difficult to know how cultural expectations affect sex differences in phobias in other cultures.

Psychiatrists treating patients from different cultures should be aware of cultural differences in presentation and response to treatment. In a review of culture-specific strategies in counseling, Sue (1990) summarized data on cultural differences in verbal communication styles, proxemics (i.e., use of interpersonal space), nonverbal communication, and other verbal cues (e.g., tone and loudness). Many cues that a psychiatrist might use to aid in the diagnosis of social phobia in white Americans may not be useful for diagnosing the condition in other cultures. For example, although many psychiatrists interpret a lack of eye contact as indicating shyness or a lack of assertiveness, avoidance of eye contact among Japanese and Mexican-Americans is often viewed as a sign of respect, according to Sue (1990). In contrast to white Americans, Japanese are apparently more likely to view smiling as a sign of embarrassment or discomfort. Furthermore, cultural differences in tone and volume of speech may lead psychiatrists to misinterpret their patients. For example, whereas white Americans often are uncomfortable with silence in a conversation, British and Arab individuals may be more likely to use silence for privacy and other cultures use silence to indicate agreement among the parties or a sign of respect. In addition, Asian individuals have been reported to speak more quietly than white Americans, who in turn speak more quietly than those from Arab countries. Therefore, differences in the volume of speech should not be taken to imply differences in assertiveness or other indicators of social anxiety.

Treatment methods may have to be adapted for different cultures. For example, the direct style of many cognitive and behavioral therapists may be more likely to be perceived as rude or insensitive by individuals with certain cultural backgrounds than those with other backgrounds. It should be noted that individuals within a culture differ on these variables just as individuals across cultures differ. Therefore, although psychiatrists should be aware of cultural differences, these differences should not blind the psychiatrist to relevant factors that are unique to each individual patient.

**Developmental Differences.** Several studies have begun to look at the prevalence of phobias across the life span. Little is known about the prevalence of phobias among elderly persons, although there is some evidence that the prevalence of phobic disorders may decrease slightly after age 65 years (Eaton et al. 1991).

Among children, specific and social fears are common (Francis 1990, Straus and Last 1993). Because these fears may be transient, DSM-IV-TR has included a provision that social and specific phobias not be assigned in children unless they are present for more than 6 months. In addition, children may be less likely than adults to recognize that their phobia is excessive or unrealistic. The specific objects feared by children are often similar to those feared by adults, although children may be more likely to fear objects and situations that are not easily classified in the four main specific phobia types in DSM-IV-TR (e.g., balloons or costumed characters). In addition, children often report specific and social phobias having to do with school. Children with social phobia tend to avoid changing for gym class in front of others, eating in the cafeteria, or speaking in front of the class. They may stay home sick on days when frightening situations arise or may make frequent trips to the school nurse. Whereas some investigators have found that boys and girls are equally likely to present for treatment of phobias (Straus and Last 1993), others have found social phobia to be more common among girls than boys (Anderson et al. 1987). In one prospective study of childhood anxiety disorders, Last and colleagues (1996) found that almost 70% of children with a specific phobia were recovered over a 3- to 4-year period compared to a recovery rate of 86% for social phobia. Thus, almost a third of the clinical sample with specific phobia had symptoms that still met clinical criteria for specific phobia at the end of the follow-up period. This was the lowest recovery rate among the anxiety disorders that were studied. However, those in the clinical sample with specific phobia had the lowest rate of development of new psychiatric disorders (15%) compared to the other anxiety disorders studied (e.g., the rate of development for new psychiatric disorders was 22% for those in the clinical sample with social phobia).

## Diagnosis and Differential Diagnosis

Social anxiety is associated with a variety of DSM-IV disorders. Similarly, several disorders other than specific phobia are associated with fear and avoidance of circumscribed stimuli. Therefore, accurate diagnosis of specific and social phobias depends on a thorough understanding of the DSM-IV criteria and knowledge of how to distinguish these disorders from related conditions. Correct diagnosis depends on being able to evaluate the patient's focus of apprehension, reasons for avoidance, and range of situations feared.

Panic disorder with agoraphobia may easily be misdiagnosed as social phobia or a specific phobia (especially the situational type). For example, many patients with panic disorder avoid a variety of social situations because of anxiety about having others notice their symptoms. In addition, some individuals with panic disorder may avoid circumscribed situations, such as flying, despite reporting no other significant avoidance. Four variables should be considered in making the differential diagnosis: (1) type and number of panic attacks, (2) focus of apprehension, (3) number of situations avoided, and (4) level of intercurrent anxiety.

Patients with panic disorder experience unexpected panic attacks and heightened anxiety outside of the phobic situation, whereas those with specific and social phobias typically do not. In addition, individuals with panic disorder are more likely than those with specific and social phobias to report fear and avoidance of a broad range of situations typically associated with agoraphobia (e.g., flying, enclosed places, crowds, being alone, shopping malls). Finally, patients with panic disorder are typically concerned only about the possibility of panicking in the phobic situation or about the consequences of panicking (e.g., being embarrassed by one's panic symptoms). In contrast, individuals with specific and social phobias are usually concerned about other aspects of the situation as well (e.g., being hit by another driver, saying something foolish).

Consider two examples in which the differential diagnosis with panic disorder might be especially difficult. First, individuals with claustrophobia are typically extremely concerned about being unable to escape from the phobic situation as well as being unable to breathe in the situation. Therefore, like patients with panic disorder and agoraphobia, they usually report heightened anxiety about the possibility of panicking. The main variable to consider in such a case is the presence of panic attacks outside of claustrophobic situations. If panic attacks occur exclusively in enclosed places, a diagnosis of specific phobia might best describe the problem. In contrast, if the patient has unexpected or uncued panic attacks as well, a diagnosis of panic disorder might be more appropriate.

A second example is a patient who avoids a broad range of situations including shopping malls, supermarkets, walking on busy streets, and various social situations including parties, meetings, and public speaking. Without more information, this patient's problem might appear to meet criteria for social phobia, panic disorder with agoraphobia, or both diagnoses. As mentioned earlier, patients with panic disorder often avoid social situations because of anxiety about panicking in public. In addition, patients with social phobia might avoid situations that are typically avoided by individuals with agoraphobia for fear of seeing someone that they know or of being observed by strangers. To make the diagnosis in this case, it is necessary to assess the reasons for avoidance.

It may be difficult to distinguish among types of specific phobias. For example, is a bridge phobia best considered a situational type (i.e., driving) or a natural environment type (i.e., heights)? This decision should be based on the context of the bridge phobia. If the individual fears falling or fears other high places, a height phobia may be the appropriate diagnosis. In contrast, if bridges are one of many driving-related situations that the person fears, a driving phobia might be more appropriate.

Other diagnoses that should be considered before a diagnosis of specific phobia is assigned include posttraumatic stress disorder (PTSD) (if the fear follows a life-threatening trauma and is accompanied by other PTSD symptoms such as reexperiencing the trauma), obsessive–compulsive disorder (if the fear is related to an obsession, e.g., contamination), hypochondriasis (if the fear is related to a belief that he or she has some serious illness), separation-anxiety disorder (if the fear is of situations that might lead to separation from the family, for example, traveling on an airplane without one's parents), eating disorders (if the fear is of eating certain foods but not related to a fear of choking), and psychotic disorders (if the fear is related to a delusion).

Social phobia should not be diagnosed if the fear is related entirely to another disorder. For example, if an individual with obsessive–compulsive disorder avoids social situations only because of the embarrassment of having others notice her or his excessive hand washing, a diagnosis of social phobia would not be given. Furthermore, individuals with depression, schizoid personality disorder, or a pervasive developmental disorder may avoid social situations because of a lack of interest in spending time with others. To be considered social phobia, an individual must avoid these situations specifically because of anxiety about being evaluated negatively.

In the case of generalized social phobia, the diagnosis of avoidant personality disorder should be considered as well. Individuals with avoidant personality disorder tend to display more interpersonal sensitivity and have poorer social skills than social phobic patients without avoidant personality disorder (Turner et al. 1986). Furthermore, most studies suggest that the differences between avoidant personality disorder and social phobia are more quantitative than qualitative and that the former may simply be a more severe form of the latter (Widiger 1992). Therefore, most patients who meet criteria for avoidant personality disorder will meet criteria for social phobia as well.

Finally, social and specific phobias should be distinguished from normal states of fear and anxiety. Many individuals report mild fears of circumscribed situations or mild shyness in certain social situations. Others may report intense fears of public speaking or heights but insist that these situations rarely arise and that they have no interest in being in these situations. For the criteria for a specific or social phobia to be met, the individual must report significant distress about having the fear or must report significant impairment in functioning.

A variety of factors should be considered in deciding whether a patient's fear exceeds the threshold necessary for a diagnosis of specific or social phobia. To make the differential diagnosis between normal fears and clinical phobias, the psychiatrist should consider the extent of the individual's avoidance, the frequency with which the phobic stimulus is encountered, and the degree to which the individual is bothered by having the fear. For example, an individual who fears seeing snakes in the wild but who lives in the city, never encounters snakes, and never even thinks about snakes would probably not be diagnosed with a specific phobia. In contrast, when an individual's fear of snakes leads to avoidance of walking through parks, camping, swimming, and watching certain television programs, despite having an interest in doing these things, a diagnosis of specific phobia would be appropriate.

Similar factors should be considered in deciding at what point normal shyness reaches an intensity that warrants a diagnosis of social phobia. An individual who is somewhat quiet in groups or when meeting new people but does not avoid these situations and is not especially distressed by his or her shyness would probably not receive a diagnosis of social phobia. In contrast, an individual who frequently refuses invitations to socialize because of anxiety, quits a job because of anxiety about having to talk to customers, or is distressed about her or his social anxiety would be likely to receive a diagnosis of social phobia.

Diagnostic decision trees for social and specific phobias are presented in Figures 67–1 and 67–2.

## Specific Phobia Phenomenology and Subtypes

As discussed earlier, DSM-IV defines five main types of specific phobia: animal, natural environment, blood-injection-injury, situational, and other. These types were introduced on the basis of a series of reports to the DSM-IV Anxiety Disorders Work Group (Craske 1989, Curtis et al. 1990) showing that specific phobia types tend to differ on a variety of dimensions including age at onset, sex composition, patterns of covariation among phobias, focus of apprehension, timing and predictability of the phobic response, and type of physiological reaction during exposure to the phobic situation.

Although anxiety about physical sensations and the occurrence of panic is a feature typically associated with panic disorder, several studies have shown that panic-focused and symptom-focused apprehensions are not unique to panic disorder and agoraphobia. In fact, individuals with specific phobias score a full standard deviation above the mean for normal persons on the Anxiety Sensitivity Index (Reiss et al. 1986), a questionnaire that measures anxiety related to experiencing the physical sensations of fear. In other words, individuals with specific phobias tend to report anxiety about the sensations (e.g., racing heart, breathlessness, dizziness) typically associated with their fear. Also, there is evidence that in addition to fearing danger from the phobic object (e.g., a plane crash, being bitten by a dog) many individuals with specific phobias fear danger as a result of their reaction in the phobic situation (e.g., having a panic attack, losing control, being embarrassed) (Arntz et al. 1993, McNally and Steketee 1985). Also, the few relevant studies that have been conducted suggest that there may be differences in sensation-focused apprehension across specific phobia types.

Data are converging to indicate that individuals with phobias from the situational (e.g., claustrophobia) and blood-injury-injection types may be especially internally focused on their fear (Antony et al. 1997a, Hugdahl and Öst 1985). Whereas individuals with situational phobias

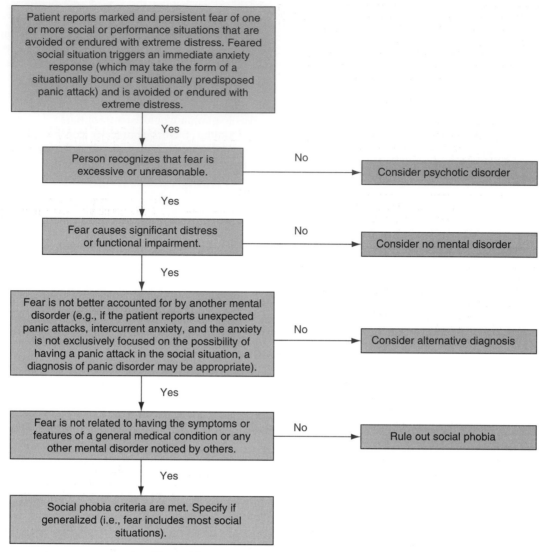

**Figure 67–1** *Diagnostic decision tree for social phobia.*

tend to fear the possible consequences of panic, those with blood-injury-injection phobias seem uniquely concerned about sensations that indicate that fainting is imminent (e.g., lightheadedness, hot flashes).

Specific phobia types may differ with respect to timing and predictability of the phobic response as well. One study based on retrospective self-reports found that individuals with phobias of driving, enclosed places, and blood-injury were more likely to report that their fear was delayed in the phobic situation than were those with animal phobias (Craske et al. 1993). These data suggest that delayed and unpredictable panic attacks may be more characteristic of situational phobias than of other phobia types, consistent with the argument that situational phobias share more features with agoraphobia than do other specific phobia types.

Perhaps the most consistent difference among specific phobia types is the tendency for individuals with blood-injury-injection phobias to report a history of fainting in the phobic situation. Although all phobia types are associated with panic attacks in the phobic situation, only

patients with blood and injection phobias report fainting (Antony et al. 1997b). Specifically, individuals with blood-injury-injection phobias experience a diphasic physiological response, which includes an initial increase in arousal followed by a sharp drop in heart rate and blood pressure that can lead to fainting. This response occurs at times in approximately 70% of people with blood phobias and 56% of those with injection phobias and seems to be unique to situations involving blood and medical procedures (Öst 1992). In other words, people who faint in these situations still show the usual type of response (i.e., increased arousal) in other situations that they fear. Disgust has been identified as a potential mediator of faintness associated with blood-injury-injection stimuli (Page in press).

The different responses experienced in different phobias have been explained from an evolutionary perspective. As mentioned earlier, the typical phobic responses of fear and panic are adaptive in that the increased arousal facilitates escape. In contrast, the most adaptive response during serious injury may be a drop in blood pressure to prevent excessive bleeding. It has been suggested that this

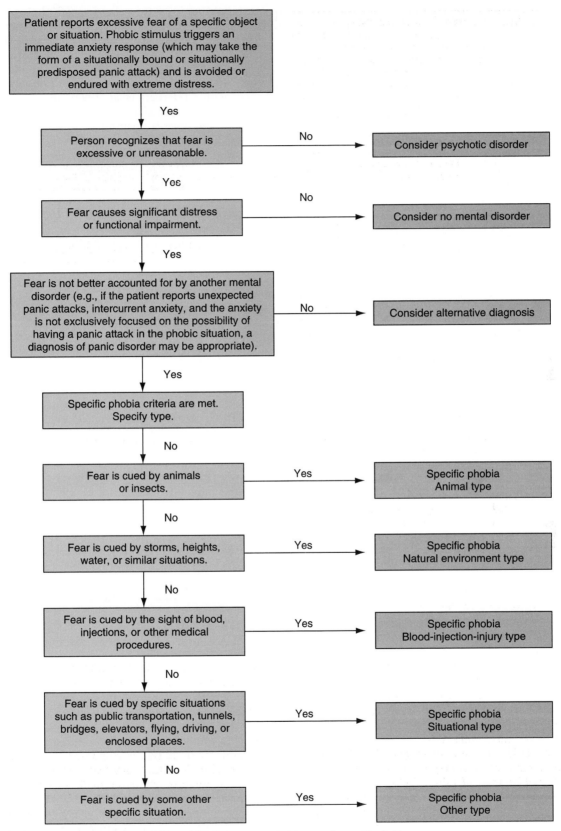

**Figure 67–2** *Diagnostic decision tree for specific phobia.*

response is mediated by an overactive sinoaortic baroreflex that is triggered by heightened arousal in situations involving blood or needles (Adler et al. 1991). Of course, in people with blood and injection phobias, the response is excessive and unwarranted, as there is typically no danger of excessive blood loss.

## Social Phobia Phenomenology and Subtypes

Many researchers in the area of social phobia tend to classify the disorder into two main subtypes. DSM-IV requires that diagnosticians specify whether a social phobia diagnosis is "generalized," or includes most social situations. In addition, a "discrete or circumscribed" subtype is often used by investigators to describe patients with only one domain of social anxiety, usually involving performance-related situations (e.g., public speaking).

Several studies have examined differences among these subtypes. Specifically, patients with generalized social phobias tend to be younger, less educated, and less likely to be employed than are patients with discrete social phobias. In addition, generalized social phobias are associated with more depression, anxiety, general distress, and concerns about negative evaluation from others (Heimberg et al. 1990, Turner et al. 1992). As discussed earlier, discrete social phobias appear to be associated with greater cardiac reactivity.

Heimberg and colleagues (1993a) have suggested that a third subtype, called "nongeneralized" social phobia, be added to describe patients who (1) may or may not have discrete social fears, (2) report significant anxiety in situations involving social interaction, and (3) have at least one social domain in which they do not experience significant anxiety. An example of an individual with nongeneralized social phobia would be a person who functions well at work but feels anxious when meeting new people at casual parties and other situations outside of work. Although the nongeneralized subtype was not adopted in DSM-IV, it has been evaluated in several research studies. In studies comparing generalized and nongeneralized social phobia, individuals with generalized social phobia tend to be more likely to have additional psychiatric diagnoses, poorer social skills, more functional impairment, poorer performance on a social interaction role play test, earlier age at onset, and more social avoidance than those with nongeneralized social phobia (Herbert et al. 1992). In addition, patients with generalized social phobia describe themselves as more shy and describe their families as more overprotective and less likely to socialize with others, compared to people with nongeneralized social phobia (Bruch and Heimberg 1994).

Several other methods of subtyping social phobia have been attempted as well (Holt et al. 1990, 1992). Overall, it appears that social phobia can take a variety of different forms. Further research is needed to determine if the DSM-IV method of classifying the subtypes of social phobia can be improved.

## Epidemiology and Comorbidity

### Prevalence and Incidence

As discussed earlier, phobias are among the most common psychiatric disorders. Findings based on large community samples from five sites in the Epidemiological Catchment Area (ECA) study (Eaton et al. 1991) yielded lifetime prevalence estimates of 11.25% for specific phobias and 2.73% for social phobia. Estimates from the National Comorbidity Survey (NCS) (Kessler et al. 1994) were consistent with previous findings on specific phobias: a lifetime prevalence of 11.30% in a sample of more than 8,000 individuals from across the US. Table 67–3 lists lifetime prevalence rates for particular specific fears and phobias based on findings of the NCS (Curtis et al. 1998), with phobias of animals and heights being the most frequently diagnosed specific phobias. For social phobia, data from the NCS indicate a lifetime prevalence rate of 13.3%, much higher than that in the previously reported ECA study. This

**Table 67–3**  **Lifetime Prevalence of Specific Fears with and without Specific Phobia**

| Specific Fear | Lifetime Fears[a] % | Lifetime Fears[a] s.e. | Lifetime Phobia Given Fear[b] % | Lifetime Phobia Given Fear[b] s.e. | Lifetime Phobia with Specific Fear In Total Sample[c] % | Lifetime Phobia with Specific Fear In Total Sample[c] s.e. |
|---|---|---|---|---|---|---|
| Height | 20.4 | 0.7 | 26.2 | 1.8 | 5.3 | 0.5 |
| Flying | 13.2 | 0.7 | 26.9 | 2.4 | 3.5 | 0.3 |
| Closed spaces | 11.9 | 0.6 | 35.1 | 2.5 | 4.2 | 0.4 |
| Being alone | 7.3 | 0.6 | 40.7 | 3.3 | 3.1 | 0.4 |
| Storms | 8.7 | 0.5 | 33.1 | 3.4 | 2.9 | 0.4 |
| Animals | 22.2 | 1.1 | 25.8 | 1.2 | 5.7 | 0.4 |
| Blood | 13.9 | 0.7 | 32.8 | 2.1 | 4.5 | 0.3 |
| Water | 9.4 | 0.6 | 35.8 | 2.8 | 3.4 | 0.3 |
| Any | 49.5 | 1.2 | 22.7 | 1.1 | 11.3 | 0.6 |

[a] Prevalence of lifetime fears in the total sample.

[b] Probability of specific phobia diagnosis in people endorsing each fear.

[c] Percentage of people in total sample with specific phobia and each lifetime fear (i.e., 5.3% of total sample have lifetime specific phobia and a height fear).

*Source*: Curtis GC, Magee WJ, Eaton WW, et al. (1998) Specific fears and phobias: Epidemiology and classification. Br J Psychiatr 173, 212–217. Copyright 1998 The British Journal of Psychiatry.

difference is likely due to methodological variations across the two studies (Antony and Swinson 2000a).

Results from epidemiological studies (Bourdon et al. 1988, Curtis et al. 1998) show that most specific phobias are more common in women than in men, although there are differences in sex ratio among phobia types. Specifically, the ratio of females to males is smaller for height phobias than for other specific phobia types. Among social phobia situations, sex differences are less pronounced than for most specific phobia types. In the NCS (Kessler et al. 1994), relatively small sex differences in social phobia prevalence were confirmed, with lifetime estimates of 11.1% for males and 15.5% for females. In addition, the relatively equal numbers of men and women with social phobia in epidemiological studies is consistent with findings from samples of individuals presenting for treatment (Hofmann and Barlow 2002, Marks 1985).

Most studies have found the mean age at onset of social phobia to be in the middle to late teens (Marks and Gelder 1966, Öst 1987, Thyer et al. 1985). However, other research has found a mean onset age of only 12.8 (Chartier et al. 1998). In one study on a sample of 200 adults with a primary diagnosis of social phobia, 80% of the sample reported onset of social phobia before age 18 (Otto et al. 2001). This is supported by research finding that social phobia is common in children and is diagnosed in a significant percentage of children referred to a specialty anxiety disorders clinic (Albano et al. 1995). A history of childhood anxiety has been associated with an earlier age of onset of social phobia as well as greater severity and comorbidity (Otto et al. 2001). Mean age at onset for specific phobias appears to differ depending on the type of phobia. Phobias of animals, blood, storms, and water tend to begin in early childhood (Curtis et al. 1990, Marks and Gelder 1966, Öst 1987), whereas phobias of heights tend to begin in the teens (Curtis et al. 1990), and phobias of the situational type (e.g., claustrophobia) begin even later, with mean ages at onset in the late teens to middle twenties (Curtis et al. 1990, Himle et al. 1989, Öst 1987).

## Comorbidity Patterns

The issue of comorbidity has received increasing attention in the years since the *Diagnostic and Statistical Manual of Mental Disorders*, Third Edition, Revised (DSM-III-R) (American Psychiatric Association 1987), was published. Before that time, the diagnostic decision rules in DSM-III were arranged hierarchically, such that having one diagnosis precluded the assignment of other diagnoses lower on the hierarchy. According to DSM-III-R and DSM-IV, patients may receive multiple diagnoses. The issue of comorbidity is important for several reasons. First, covariation among disorders provides valuable information about the nature of specific disorders as well as the utility of current diagnostic nomenclature. For example, high rates of co-occurrence between two disorders could reflect overlap in the definitions of two disorders (as may be the case with social phobia and avoidant personality disorder) or shared etiological pathways. In addition, comorbidity may have implications for treatment. For example, an individual with social phobia who abuses alcohol might be less likely to benefit from treatment for social phobia if the alcohol abuse affects compliance with the social phobia treatment.

## Specific Phobias

One of the variables considered by the DSM-IV Anxiety Disorders Work Group in its decision to classify specific phobias by types was the pattern of covariation observed among specific phobias within each of the four main types (Curtis et al. 1990). For example, about 70% of individuals with blood phobias tend to have injection phobias as well (Öst 1992). In addition, numerous factor analytical studies have found that blood-injection-injury phobias tend to cluster together as do animal phobias, natural environment phobias, and situational phobias (Arrindell 1980, Landy and Gaupp 1971, Liddell et al. 1991, Wilson and Priest 1968). In other words, having a phobia of one specific phobia type makes an individual more likely to have additional phobias of the same type than of other types. However, the clustering is not perfect; many studies show exceptions to this pattern (Curtis et al. 1998) and it has been argued that assigning specific phobias to types may not be diagnostically useful for a number of reasons (Antony et al. 1997b). The research on the classification of specific phobia types is inconsistent. For example, in several of these studies, height phobias tend to be associated with situational phobias (e.g., claustrophobia), despite height phobias being listed as an example of the natural environment type in DSM-IV (Muris et al. 1999). Furthermore, it is not always clear where a particular phobia should be assigned. Is a phobia of dentists an example of a blood-injection-injury phobia or does it fall into the "other" type? Finally, it has been argued (Antony et al. 1997b) that simply naming the phobia (e.g., specific phobia, choking) is more informative and clinically useful than using the type classification "specific phobia, other type."

Specific phobias tend to co-occur with other specific phobias. One study found that 76% of a sample of 915 individuals with a lifetime history of specific phobias had one or more co-occurring specific phobias (Curtis et al. 1998). This finding is consistent with research showing that individuals with specific phobias often report multiple fears on a fear survey (Hofmann et al. 1997). However, other research indicates that comorbid phobias may not be as prevalent (Fredrikson et al. 1996) and that numbers in previous studies may have been inflated by a lack of discrimination between multiple phobias and fears of multiple situations that are accounted for by a single phobia. A recent methodologically rigorous study found that 15% of patients with a principal diagnosis of specific phobia also met criteria for another type of specific phobia (Brown et al. 2001a).

In addition, specific phobias often co-occur with other DSM-IV disorders. A recent study found that 33% of patients presenting with a principal diagnosis of specific phobia had additional symptoms that met criteria for an Axis I anxiety or mood disorder (Brown et al. 2001a). However, compared with individuals who have other anxiety disorders, individuals with principal diagnoses of a specific phobia are less likely to have additional diagnoses. Rather, specific phobias typically occur on their own or as additional diagnoses of lesser severity than the principal diagnosis. For example, in one study, specific phobias occurred in about 27% of individuals with panic disorder and agoraphobia, in 16% of individuals with generalized anxiety disorder, and in 3 to 9% of individuals with other

DSM-III-R disorders (Moras et al. 1995). Other studies confirm that specific phobias are a frequently occurring additional diagnosis, particularly with other anxiety disorders (Curtis et al. 1998, Goisman et al. 1995). However, specific phobias tend to occur less frequently in the context of other disorders such as depression (Schatzberg et al. 1998) and alcohol use disorders (Lehman et al. 1998).

Whereas the above mentioned studies reflect "syndrome" comorbidity, one can also discuss comorbidity at the "symptom" level. In other words, one can examine the frequency with which specific fears are associated with disorders regardless of whether they meet criteria for specific phobia. One study examined the rate of subclinical specific phobias (i.e., those not meeting a clinical threshold for distress or functional impairment) in a sample of patients with anxiety disorders (Antony et al. 1994). In this study, specific fears were the most frequently assigned subclinical diagnoses, with 28% of these patients reporting subclinical fears. In fact, almost half of all subclinical diagnoses assigned were specific fears. In summary, it appears that specific phobias commonly occur as additional diagnoses, at both clinical and subclinical levels.

## Social Phobia

Social anxiety is a feature of many disorders. Individuals with panic disorder, obsessive–compulsive disorder, or eating disorders often avoid social situations because of the possibility of being judged negatively if their symptoms are noticed by others. However, to meet diagnostic criteria for social phobia, one's concerns must not be exclusively related to the symptoms of another disorder. With this criterion in mind, social phobia still tends to be associated with a variety of other DSM-IV disorders. Furthermore, unlike specific phobias, social phobia is frequently associated with additional disorders of lesser severity. One study conducted in two outpatient clinics in a managed care setting found a comorbidity rate of 43.6% in patients with generalized social phobia (Katzelnick et al. 2001). In another study, almost 60% of patients with social phobia had additional symptoms that met criteria for one or more additional diagnoses (Sanderson et al. 1990). The most frequently assigned additional diagnoses in this study were specific phobias (25%), dysthymia (21%), and panic disorder with agoraphobia (17%). The presence of comorbid mood disorders has been associated with a greater duration of social phobia as well as more severe impairment before and after cognitive–behavioral therapy (CBT) (Erwin et al. 2002). Other studies have found that panic disorder with or without agoraphobia, generalized anxiety disorder, major depressive disorder, and substance abuse are common additional diagnoses as well (Brown et al. 2001a, Mennin et al. 2000, Van Ameringen et al. 1991). In one prospective study, an estimated relative risk ratio of 2.30 for alcohol abuse or dependence was found in individuals with subclinical social phobia relative to individuals without social phobia or subclinical social fears, suggesting that individuals with subclinical social phobia were more than twice as likely to develop alcohol use disorders than were individuals without social phobia or subclinical social anxiety (Crum and Pratt 2001).

As an additional diagnosis, social phobia is often assigned in patients with panic disorder with agoraphobia, generalized anxiety disorder, obsessive–compulsive dis-

order, and major depressive disorder (Brown et al. 2001a). Social phobia is also common among patients with eating disorders (Schwalberg et al. 1992) and alcohol abuse (Riemann 1993) as well. When social phobia coexists with a mood disorder, substance abuse disorder, or another anxiety disorder, the social phobia tends to predate the other disorder (Van Ameringen et al. 1991). Treatment of these disorders should include components that address the social phobia when both disorders occur together.

## Course and Natural History

As discussed earlier, the mean age at onset of social phobia is in the middle teens. The age at onset of specific phobias varies depending on the phobia type, with phobias of animals, blood, storms, and water tending to begin in early childhood, phobias of heights beginning in the teens, and situational phobias beginning in the late teens to middle twenties. Although childhood fears are often transient (e.g., most children outgrow fear of the dark without treatment), fears that persist into adulthood usually have a chronic course unless treated.

Although many phobias begin after a traumatic event, many patients do not recall the specific onset of their fear, and few empirical data have examined the initial period after the fear onset. Clinically, however, some patients report a sudden onset of fear, whereas others report a more gradual onset. Studies examining the onset of phobias have tended to assess the onset of the *fear* rather than the onset of the *phobia* (i.e., the point at which the fear creates significant distress or functional impairment). A study by Antony and colleagues (1997b) suggests that the fear and phobia onset are often not the same. Patients with specific phobias of heights, animals, blood-injection, or driving were asked to estimate the earliest age at which they could recall having their fear and the earliest age at which they could recall experiencing distress or functional impairment due to their fear. As shown in Table 67–4, phobias began at an average of 9 years after the fear onset. Anecdotally, the types of factors leading to the transition from fear to phobia included gradual increases in the intensity of fear, additional traumatic events (e.g., panic attacks, car accidents), increased life stress, and changes in living situation (e.g., starting a job that requires exposure to heights). Similarly, it is not unusual for individuals with social phobia to report having been shy as children, although their anxiety may not have reached phobic proportions until later.

## Treatment

### Goals and Nature of Treatment

The main goal of treatment is to decrease fear and phobic avoidance to a level that no longer causes significant distress or functional impairment. In some cases, treatment includes strategies for improving specific skill deficits as well. For example, individuals with social phobia may lack adequate social skills and can sometimes benefit from social skills training. Likewise, some individuals with specific phobias of driving may have poor driving skills if their fear prevented them from learning how to drive properly. Typically, effective treatment for social phobia lasts several months, although treatment of discrete social phobias (e.g., public speaking) may take less time. Specific phobias can

| Table 67–4 | Mean Age of Onset (and Standard Deviations) for Specific Fears and Phobias and Agoraphobia | | | | | | |
|---|---|---|---|---|---|---|---|
| | | | Earliest Age of Recall (by Group) | | | | |
| | Heights (N = 15) | Animals (N = 15) | Blood-Injection (N = 15) | Driving (N = 15) | PDA (N = 15) | F | $\eta^2$ |
| Fear | 20.47[ac] | 10.80[ab] | 7.93[b] | 25.67[c] | 28.14[c] | 8.78*** | 0.34 |
| | (17.53) | (8.37) | (3.71) | (11.84) | (11.95) | | |
| Phobia | 34.13[a] | 20.00[bcd] | 14.50[b] | 32.20[acd] | 29.07[ac] | 6.95*** | 0.29 |
| | (16.36) | (10.21) | (8.30) | (12.49) | (11.52) | | |
| Difference | 13.66[a] | 9.2[ab] | 6.50[ab] | 6.53[ab] | 0.93[b] | 4.08** | 0.19 |
| | (11.66) | (10.64) | (7.53) | (8.17) | (1.73) | | |

*Note*: PDA, panic disorder with agoraphobia. "Fear" refers to the age at which the fear began for individuals with specific phobias or the age at which panic attacks began for individuals in the panic disorder with agoraphobia (PDA) group. "Phobia" refers to the age at which the fear began to cause significant distress or functional impairment for the specific phobia groups or the age at which the individuals with PDA met full criteria for the disorder. "Difference" was calculated by subtracting ages of onset for the *fear* from those for the *phobia*. Group means (across rows) sharing superscript letters do not differ at $P < 0.05$. **$P < 0.01$; ***$P < 0.001$. *Source*: Antony MM, Brown TA, and Barlow DH (1997b) Heterogeneity among specific phobia types in DSM-IV. Behav Res Ther 35, 1089–1100. Copyright 1997 Elsevier Science.

usually be treated relatively quickly. In fact, for certain phobias, the vast majority of individuals are able to achieve clinically significant, long-lasting improvement in as little as one session of behavioral treatment (Öst et al. 1991b, 1997a, 2001).

Effective treatments fall into one of two main categories: pharmacological treatment and CBT. Pharmacological treatments have been used effectively for treating social phobia, although it is generally accepted that they are of limited utility for treating specific phobias. In contrast, CBT has been used with success for the treatment of specific and social phobias. Despite the existence of effective treatments, fewer than half of those who seek treatment in an anxiety disorders specialty clinic have previously received evidence-based treatments for their social anxiety (Rowa et al. 2000). Tables 67–5 and 67–6 summarize various treatments for social and specific phobias.

## Pharmacotherapy

### Specific Phobia

As discussed earlier, pharmacotherapy is generally thought to be ineffective for specific phobias. However, little research has been conducted to assess the utility of medications for specific phobias, and it is not uncommon for phobic patients occasionally to be prescribed low dosages of benzodiazepines to be taken in the phobic situation (e.g., while flying). The few relevant studies that have been conducted have examined the use of benzodiazepines and beta blockers alone or in combination with behavioral treatments for specific phobias and in general have found that drugs do not contribute much to the treatment of specific phobias (Antony and Barlow 2002). However, one problem with the research to date is that it has not taken into account differences among specific phobia types. For example, claustrophobia and other phobias of the situational type appear to share more features with panic disorder than with the other specific phobia types (Antony et al. 1997a). Therefore, medications that are effective for panic disorder (e.g., imipramine, alprazolam) may prove

to be effective for situational phobias. Although there are few studies examining this hypothesis, preliminary data suggest that benzodiazepines may be helpful in the short term but lead to greater relapse in the long-term and possibly interfere with the therapeutic effects of exposure across sessions (Wilhelm and Roth 1996). For example, one study found that CBT and providing a benzodiazepine both led to fear reduction during dental surgery; however, whereas benzodiazepine treatment was associated with greater relapse during follow-up, CBT was associated with further improvements (Thom et al. 2000).

There have been very few controlled studies to date examining the effectiveness of antidepressants for specific phobia. One placebo-controlled, double-blind pilot study found that paroxetine was superior to placebo in reducing anxiety and fear levels in individuals with different types of specific phobia (Benjamin et al. 2000). There have also been several case study reports indicating the usefulness of selective serotonin reuptake inhibitors in the treatment of specific phobia. One single-case study found fluvoxamine to be effective in the treatment of a specific phobia of storms in an 11-year-old boy who also had depression, school phobia, and obsessive–compulsive symptoms (Balon 1999). Another single-case study found that fluoxetine led to a reduction in flying phobia in two patients being treated for depression.

### Social Phobia

In contrast to specific phobias, social phobia has been treated successfully with a variety of pharmacological interventions including SSRIs such as sertraline (Blomhoff et al. 2001, Van Ameringen et al. 2001), fluvoxamine (Stein et al. 1999, van Vliet et al. 1994) and paroxetine (Allgulander and Nilsson, 2001, Liebowitz et al. 2002, Stein et al. 1998), benzodiazepines such as clonazepam (Davidson et al. 1993) and alprazolam (Reich and Yates 1988), traditional monoamine oxidase inhibitors (MAOIs) such as phenelzine (Heimberg et al. 1998), and reversible inhibitors of monoamine oxidase A (RIMA) such as moclobemide (Versiani et al. 1992, 1996) and brofaromine (Lott et al. 1997).

| Table 67-5 | Treatments for Social Phobia | | |
|---|---|---|---|
| Treatment | Advantages | Disadvantages | Rating |
| Cognitive–behavioral therapy (CBT) (e.g., exposure, cognitive restructuring, social skills training, education) | Good treatment response<br>Brief course of treatment<br>Treatment gains maintained at follow-up<br>Considered first line | May lead to temporary increases in discomfort or fear. | ++++ |
| SSRIs (e.g., paroxetine, fluvoxamine, sertraline) | Good treatment response<br>Early response, relative to CBT<br>Broad spectrum efficacy for comorbid disorders (i.e., depression)<br>Lack of abuse potential<br>Considered first line | Side effects are common.<br>Cost is a factor.<br>May be a risk of relapse after discontinuation. | +++ |
| Moclobemide | Good treatment response in some studies<br>Fewer side effects than phenelzine<br>Considered second line | Side effects common.<br>Does not separate from placebo in some studies.<br>Potential exists for relapse after discontinuation. | ++ |
| Benzodiazepines (e.g., clonazepam, alprazolam) | Good treatment response<br>Considered adjunctive or second line | Side effects and withdrawal occur.<br>Potential for abuse.<br>Relapse after discontinuation is likely.<br>Does not treat certain comorbid conditions (i.e., depression). | ++ |
| MAOIs (e.g., phenelzine) | Good treatment response<br>Early response<br>Considered third line | Relatively high rate of adverse effects.<br>Dietary restrictions must be followed.<br>Numerous drug interactions.<br>Potential exists for relapse after discontinuation. | ++ |
| Gabapentin | Possibly beneficial<br>Considered third line | Side effects are common.<br>More research is needed. | ++ |
| β-blockers (e.g., atenolol) | Appears to be useful for "stage fright" in actors, musicians, and other performers | Drugs are not effective for generalized social phobia.<br>Benefits for discrete social phobias are questionable.<br>Side effects occur.<br>Potential exists for relapse after discontinuation. | + |

++++ First treatment of choice. Helpful for most patients, with few side effects. Good long-term benefits.

+++ Helpful for most patients. Potential for relapse after treatment is discontinued.

++ More controlled research needed, although preliminary studies suggest potential benefit OR research has been mixed.

+ Not especially effective for generalized social phobia.

Numerous controlled trials across a range of SSRIs including sertraline, fluvoxamine, and paroxetine have demonstrated their effectiveness in the treatment of social phobia, such that the SSRIs are currently considered the first-line medication treatment (for a meta-analysis of RCTs see Van der Linden et al. 2000b). Preliminary research indicates that paroxetine may be useful in the treatment of individuals with comorbid social phobia and alcohol use disorder (Randall et al. 2001). Due to their tolerability and efficacy, the SSRIs have been referred to as "the new gold standard" in pharmacological treatment for social phobia (Van Ameringen et al. 1999b, 2000). Uncontrolled open trials and case series studies with citalopram (Bouwer and Stein 1998, Simon et al. 2001) and fluoxetine (Perugi et al. 1994/1995) suggest that these SSRIs may also be beneficial in the treatment of social phobia. Another benefit of SSRIs is their broad spectrum efficacy for common comorbid disorders such as depression and panic disorder.

Treatment of social phobia with other antidepressants (e.g., imipramine, nefazodone, venlafaxine) has been studied in a number of uncontrolled open trials. One study on 15 patients did not support the efficacy of imipramine for social phobia (Simpson et al. 1998). A number of studies examining the nonselective antidepressant nefazodone found it to be effective in 66 to 70% of patients (Van Ameringen et al. 1999a). In addition, the serotonin and norepinephrine reuptake inhibitor venlafaxine has been found to be effective in reducing social phobia symptoms in two studies with small samples of patients, the majority of whom did not respond to SSRIs (Altamura et al. 1999, Kelsey 1995).

| Table 67-6 | Treatments for Specific Phobias | | |
|---|---|---|---|
| Treatment | Advantages | Disadvantages | Rating |
| *In vivo* exposure | Highly effective<br>Early response<br>Treatment gains maintained at follow-up | May lead to temporary increases in discomfort or fear. | ++++ |
| Applied tension | Highly effective for patients with blood-injection phobias who faint<br>Early response<br>Treatment gains maintained at follow-up | Treatment is relevant for a small percentage of patients with specific phobias. | +++ |
| Applied relaxation | May be effective for some patients | Treatment has not been extensively researched for specific phobias. | ++ |
| Cognitive therapy | May help to reduce anxiety about conducting exposure exercises | Treatment has not been extensively researched for specific phobias.<br>Treatment is probably not effective alone. | ++ |
| Benzodiazepines | May reduce anticipatory anxiety before patient enters phobic situation, and may reduce fear, particularly in situational specific phobias | Treatment has not been extensively researched for specific phobias.<br>Treatment is probably not effective alone, in many cases.<br>Side effects (e.g., sedation) occur.<br>Discontinuation of symptoms may undermine benefits of treatment. | ++ |
| SSRIs | May reduce panic sensations for individuals with situational phobias that are similar to panic disorder (e.g., claustrophobia) | Treatment has not been extensively researched for specific phobias.<br>There are a few studies (primarily case reports) with promising results.<br>Discontinuation of medication may result in a return of fear. | ++ |

++++ Treatment of choice. Effective for almost all patients.

+++ Very effective for a subset of patients.

++ May be helpful for some patients. More research needed.

Research on the use of anxiolytics for the treatment of social phobia have focused on high potency benzodiazepines (e.g., clonazepam, alprazolam) and the non-benzodiazepine buspirone. Several studies have examined the utility of clonazepam for treating social phobia. In a placebo-controlled study, Davidson and colleagues (1993) found that 78% of patients responded to clonazepam (mean dosage, 2.4 mg/day), whereas only 20% responded to placebo. One study comparing clonazepam to cognitive–behavioral group therapy found that patients in both conditions improved significantly and no differences between treatment conditions were observed aside from greater improvement in the clonazepam group at 12 weeks of treatment (Otto et al. 2000). These results confirmed findings from smaller open trials and case studies supporting the use of clonazepam for social phobia (mean dosages, 2.1–2.75 mg/day) (Davidson et al. 1991a, Munjack et al. 1990). In addition, uncontrolled pilot studies have suggested that alprazolam (mean dosage, 2.9 mg/day) (Lydiard et al. 1988, Reich and Yates 1988) may be effective for social phobia, although more controlled clinical trials are needed. The findings on buspirone are mixed. A number of controlled trials have found no significant advantage of buspirone over placebo (Clark and Agras

1991, van Vliet et al. 1997). This is in contrast to previous uncontrolled studies that found some benefit to buspirone (Munjack et al. 1991, Schneier et al. 1993).

Due to the potentially severe side effects of MAOIs as well as the necessity for certain dietary restrictions, they are not recommended as a first-line treatment. The findings from more recent trials involving RIMAs have been less encouraging than initial studies suggested. For example, a fixed dose study conducted over 12 weeks found that moclobemide did not have a significant benefit over placebo at five dosages ranging from 75 to 900 mg/day (Noyes et al. 1997). Other studies have also found poor responses to moclobemide (Oosterbaan et al. 2001, Schneier et al. 1998). Discontinuation of MAOIs and RIMAs have been associated with a tendency to relapse.

Research on beta blockers indicates that they are no better than placebo for most patients with generalized social phobia (Liebowitz et al. 1992). Although beta blockers have been used to treat individuals from nonpatient samples with heightened performance anxiety (e.g., people with public speaking anxiety, musicians with stage fright) (Hartley et al. 1983, James et al. 1983), their efficacy for treating individuals with discrete social phobia has not been established. Nevertheless, beta blockers are often prescribed for discrete performance-related social phobias.

Preliminary findings suggest that gabapentin, a medication typically used in the treatment of partial seizures, may be effective in the treatment of social phobia. A placebo-controlled trial found that patients taking gabapentin had significant reductions in social anxiety compared to the placebo group (Pande et al. 1999). However, more research is needed to confirm this finding.

## Psychosocial Treatments

### Specific Phobias

Numerous studies have shown that exposure-based treatments are effective for helping patients to overcome a variety of specific phobias including fears of blood (Öst et al. 1984, 1991a), injections (Öst 1989), dentists (Jerremalm et al. 1986, Moore and Brødsgaard 1994), spiders (Hellström and Öst 1995, Muris et al. 1998, Öst 1996a, Öst et al. 1991b, 1997b), snakes (Gauthier and Marshall 1977, Hepner and Cauthen 1975), rats (Foa et al. 1977), enclosed places (Craske et al. 1995, Öst et al. 1982), thunder and lightning (Öst 1978), water (Menzies and Clarke 1993a), flying (Beckham et al. 1990, Howard et al. 1983, Öst et al. 1997b), heights (Baker et al. 1973), choking (Greenberg et al. 1988, McNally 1986), and balloons (Houlihan et al. 1993).

Furthermore, the way in which exposure is conducted may make a difference. Exposure-based treatments can vary on a variety of dimensions including the degree of therapist involvement, duration and intensity of exposure, frequency and number of sessions, and the degree to which the feared situation is confronted in imagination versus in real life. In addition, because individuals with certain specific phobias often report a fear of panicking in the feared situation, investigators (Antony and Swinson 2000a) have suggested that adding various panic management strategies (e.g., cognitive restructuring, exposure to feared sensations) may help to increase the efficacy of behavioral treatments for specific phobias. It remains to be shown whether the addition of these strategies will improve the efficacy of treatments that include only exposure.

Several reviews have summarized the effects of the above mentioned variables on exposure-based treatments (Antony and Barlow 1998, 2002, Antony and Swinson 2000a). Although some studies have led to contradictory results, the following generalizations are more or less accepted by the majority of investigators. First, exposure seems to work best when sessions are spaced close together. Second, prolonged exposure seems to be more effective than exposure of shorter duration. Third, during exposure sessions, patients should be discouraged from engaging in subtle avoidance strategies (e.g., distraction) and overreliance on safety signals (e.g., being accompanied by one's spouse during exposure). Fourth, real-life exposure is more effective than exposure in imagination. Fifth, exposure with some degree of therapist involvement seems to be more effective than exposure that is exclusively conducted without the therapist present (Park et al. 2001). Exposure may be conducted gradually or quickly. Both approaches seem to work equally well, although patients may be more compliant with a gradual approach. Finally, in the case of

blood and injection phobias, the technique called applied muscle tension (Öst and Sterner 1987) should be considered as an alternative or addition to exposure therapy. Applied muscle tension involves having patients repeatedly tense their muscles, which leads to a temporary increase in blood pressure and prevents fainting upon exposure to blood or medical procedures.

Cognitive strategies have also been used either alone or in conjunction with exposure for treating specific phobias (Craske and Rowe 1997). The evidence suggests that the addition of cognitive strategies to exposure may provide added benefit (Craske et al. 1995) for some individuals. For a detailed guide to integrating cognitive strategies with exposure see Antony and Swinson (2000a).

Specific phobias are among the most treatable of the anxiety disorders (Figure 67–3). For example, in as little as one session of guided exposure lasting 2 to 3 hours, the majority of individuals with animal or injection phobias are judged much improved or completely recovered (Antony et al. 2001a, Öst 1989, Öst et al. 1997b). A recent study demonstrated that one session of exposure treatment was effective in the treatment of children and adolescents with various specific phobias (Öst et al. 2001). Moreover, exposure conducted with a parent present was equally effective as exposure treatment conducted alone (Öst et al. 2001). However, despite how straightforward the concept of exposure may seem, many subtle clinical issues can lead to problems in implementing exposure-based treatments. For example, although a patient might be compliant with therapist-assisted exposure practices, he or she may refuse to attempt exposure practices alone between sessions. In such cases, involving a spouse or other family member as a coach during practices at home may help. In addition, gradually increasing the distance between therapist and patient during the therapist-assisted exposures will help the patient to feel comfortable when practicing alone. However, to maintain the patient's trust and to maximize the effectiveness of behavioral interventions, it is important that exposure practices proceed in a predictable way, so that the patient is not surprised by unexpected events. Several self-help books and manuals for treating a range of specific phobias have been published in the past decade. Whereas some of these manuals were developed to be used with the assistance of a therapist (Bourne 1998, Antony et al. 1995, Craske et al. 1997), others were developed for self-administration (Brown 1996).

Recent developments in technology have started to have an impact on the treatment of specific phobias. Videotapes are commonly used to show feared stimuli to patients during exposure. Computer administered treatments have also been used (Smith et al. 1997). More recent is the use of virtual reality to expose patients to simulated situations that are more difficult to replicate *in vivo* such as flying (Kahan et al. 2000) and heights (Rothbaum et al. 1995). Emerging data on the effectiveness of virtual reality is encouraging (Rothbaum et al. 2000). However, other preliminary studies indicate that *in vivo* exposure is still superior (Dewis et al. 2001).

### Social Phobia

Empirically validated psychosocial interventions for social phobia have primarily come from a cognitive–behavioral perspective and include four main types of treatment:

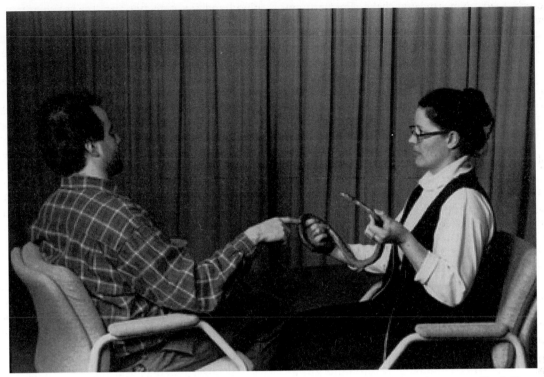

**Figure 67–3** *Predictable, prolonged exposure to the feared stimulus is the treatment of choice for most specific phobias.*

(1) exposure-based strategies, (2) cognitive therapy, (3) social skills training, and (4) applied relaxation (Antony and Swinson 2000a, Turk et al. 1999). Exposure-based treatments involve repeatedly approaching fear-provoking situations until they no longer elicit fear. Through repeated exposure, patients learn that their fearful predictions do not come true despite their having confronted the situation. Table 67–7 illustrates an example of an exposure hierarchy that might be used to structure a patient's exposure practices. An exposure hierarchy is a list of feared situations that are rank ordered by difficulty and used to guide exposure practices for phobic disorders including social phobia and specific phobia. The patient and therapist generate a list of situations that the patient finds anxiety provoking. Items are placed in descending order from most anxiety provoking to least anxiety provoking, and each item is rated with respect to how anxious the patient might be to practice the item. Exposure practices are designed to help the patient become more comfortable engaging in the activities from the hierarchy. Cognitive therapy helps patients identify and change anxious thoughts (e.g., "Others will think I am stupid if I participate in a conversation at work") by teaching them to consider alternative ways of interpreting situations and to examine the evidence for their anxious beliefs. Social skills training is designed to help patients to become more socially competent when they interact with others. Treatment strategies may include modeling, behavioral rehearsal, corrective feedback, social reinforcement, and homework assignments. Finally, applied relaxation has been studied primarily by Öst and colleagues (1984) and involves learning to relax one's muscles during rest, during

movement, and eventually in anxiety-provoking social situations.

Although these methods are presented as four distinct treatment approaches, there is often overlap among the various treatments. Social skills training typically requires exposure to the phobic situation so that new skills may be practiced (e.g., behavioral rehearsal). The same may be said of applied relaxation, which includes learning to conduct relaxation exercises in the phobic situation. In fact, most treatments for social phobia involve some type of exposure to anxiety-provoking social

| Table 67–7 | Exposure Hierarchy for Generalized Social Phobia | |
|---|---|---|
| Item | | Fear Rating (0–100) |
| Have a party and invite everyone from work. | | 99 |
| Go to work Christmas party for 1 h without drinking. | | 90 |
| Invite Cindy to have dinner and see a movie. | | 85 |
| Go for a job interview. | | 80 |
| Ask boss for a day off from work. | | 65 |
| Ask questions in a meeting at work. | | 65 |
| Eat lunch with coworkers. | | 60 |
| Talk to a stranger on the bus. | | 50 |
| Talk to cousin on the telephone for 10 min. | | 40 |
| Ask for directions at the gas station. | | 35 |

interactions and performance-related tasks. Furthermore, many cognitive–behavioral therapists treat patients using several different strategies delivered in a comprehensive package.

Studies demonstrating the efficacy of CBT for social phobia are too numerous to describe in detail, although several representative studies are reviewed here. In addition, studies that specifically compare cognitive–behavioral and medication treatments are described. For interested readers, more comprehensive reviews on CBT for social phobia have been written by Heimberg (2001) and Fresco and Heimberg (2001). Also, a clinical description of a cognitive–behavioral group treatment (CBGT) for social phobia is provided by Turk and colleagues (2001) and by Heimberg and Becker (2002).

Several studies have compared various cognitive–behavioral strategies and their combinations for treating social phobia. For example, Wlazlo and colleagues (1990) compared social skills training to exposure therapy conducted either individually or in groups. All three treatments led to significant improvements and there were no differences between treatments. However, exposure therapy conducted in groups tended to be more effective for the subset of patients with social skills deficits, most likely by enabling those individuals with deficits to develop their skills through exposure to social situations and interactions in the group. Mattick and Peters (1988) found that guided exposure was more effective when cognitive therapy was included than when exposure was conducted without cognitive therapy. Scholing and Emmelkamp (1993) failed to replicate this finding and found that treatment was equally effective when exposure was conducted alone, it followed several sessions of cognitive therapy, or was integrated with cognitive therapy from the first session.

Whereas these studies examined the use of specific cognitive–behavioral strategies, other studies have examined the use of comprehensive treatments that include several therapeutic components. For example, Turner and colleagues (1994) evaluated their multicomponent social phobia treatment that included education, social skills training, exposure, and programmed practice between sessions. All patients had the generalized subtype of social phobia and were judged to be severely disabled by their symptoms. On a comprehensive measure of end-state functioning, 85% of patients met moderate to high end-state functioning criteria by the end of treatment. Unfortunately, this study did not include a comparison treatment group.

Heimberg and colleagues (1990) compared supportive psychotherapy with a comprehensive CBGT package that included exposure to simulated and real social situations as well as cognitive restructuring for the treatment of social phobia. Although both groups improved on most measures, patients receiving CBGT were significantly more improved immediately after treatment and at 3- and 6-month follow-up. CBGT was more effective despite that patient ratings of treatment credibility and expectations for improvement were equal for both treatments. Patients receiving CBGT continued to be more improved at 5-year follow-up (Heimberg et al. 1993b), although only 41% of the original sample participated in the follow-up study, which limited the validity of these findings. Other research has confirmed

that cognitive–behavior therapy is superior to supportive therapy (Cottraux et al. 2000).

Heimberg and colleagues (1998) compared four treatments for social phobia: (1) CBGT, (2) phenelzine, (3) supportive psychotherapy, and (4) placebo. Overall, both phenelzine and CBGT were equally effective after 12 weeks of treatment and were significantly more effective than placebo or supportive psychotherapy. Phenelzine tended to work more quickly than CBGT and appeared to be more effective on a few measures. However, preliminary analyses of long-term outcome showed that after discontinuing treatment, patients receiving CBGT were more likely than patients who received phenelzine to maintain their gains, with approximately half of patients taking phenelzine relapsing, compared to none of the patients that responded to CBGT (Liebowitz et al. 1999).

In a randomized clinical trial comparing cognitive therapy to moclobemide for social phobia, Oosterbaan and colleagues (2001) found that cognitive therapy was significantly better than moclobemide, but not placebo, after 15 weeks of active treatment. After a 2-month follow-up period, cognitive therapy was significantly better than both moclobemide and placebo. In addition, treatment gains in the cognitive therapy group were maintained over a 15-month follow-up period.

A study by Haug and colleagues (2000) examined the effect of exposure therapy alone or in combination with sertraline for generalized social phobia in a primary care setting. Family physicians (FPs) were trained for 30 hours in assessment of social phobia and in the application of exposure therapy. FPs reported satisfaction with the training program and found that the exposure treatment was also useful for treating patients with other conditions. Although exposure therapy and sertraline were effective alone, the combination of exposure therapy and sertraline appeared to confer added benefit.

According to cognitive models of social phobia, one of the mechanisms by which CBT works is by causing a positive shift in an individual's self representation (e.g., decreased negative self-focused thoughts and increased task-focused thoughts and positive self-focused thoughts). Indeed, there is evidence that following CBT, individuals report significantly fewer negative self-focused thoughts (Hofmann 2000). Similarly, cognitive biases are reduced following successful pharmacotherapy treatment as well and are related to the degree of symptomatic improvement in both psychological and pharmacological treatments (McManus et al. 2000).

In summary, it seems clear that effective psychosocial treatments and medications for social phobia exist. Although both types of treatments appear to be equally effective, each has advantages and disadvantages. Medication treatments may work more quickly and are less time-consuming for the patient and therapist. In contrast, improvement after CBT appears to last longer. Due to medication side effects, CBT may be more appropriate for some individuals. More studies are needed to examine the efficacy of combined medication and psychosocial treatments for social phobia. A meta-analysis of 24 studies examining cognitive–behavioral and medication treatments for social phobia found that both treatments were more effective than control conditions (Gould et al. 1997). In this study, the

SSRIs and benzodiazepines tended to have the largest effect sizes among medications and treatments involving exposure either alone or with cognitive therapy had the largest effect sizes among CBT. Another meta-analytic study of 108 psychological and pharmacological treatment-outcome trials found that the pharmacotherapies (SSRIs, benzodiazepines, MAO inhibitors) were the most consistently effective treatments, with both SSRIs and benzodiazepine treatments equally effective and more effective than control groups (Fedoroff and Taylor 2001). Further, maintenance of treatment gains for CBT was moderate and continued during follow-up intervals. In comparison, it is not known the extent to which treatment gains for medication treatments are maintained following discontinuation. Recent reviews of the efficacy of pharmacological and cognitive–behavioral treatments suggest that successful treatments may involve medication, CBT, or a combination of both (Scott and Heimberg 2000). The detailed application of cognitive–behavioral therapy to social phobia is now available in self-help format (Antony and Swinson 2000b). Self-help manuals may be used on their own or as a valuable tool in conjunction with therapy.

Treatment decision trees for social and specific phobias are presented in Figures 67–4 and 67–5.

## Predictors of Treatment Outcome

Few studies have examined predictors of outcome for treatment of specific and social phobias. However, the few studies that do exist fall into two main categories. First, several investigators have attempted to match treatment strategies to specific characteristics of patients. Second, several studies have examined the relationship between individual differences (e.g., duration and severity of illness, personality factors) and response to treatment.

Öst and colleagues conducted a series of studies to investigate whether specific types of individuals might benefit from particular types of treatment. For example, Öst and colleagues (1982) identified a group of individuals with claustrophobia who were primarily *behavioral responders* (i.e., for whom avoidance was the principal mode of responding) and another who were primarily *physiological responders* (i.e., for whom the principal response was increased arousal in the phobic situation). In this study, behavioral responders benefited more from exposure than from applied relaxation, whereas physiological responders benefited most from applied relaxation. Similar findings were found for behavioral and physiological responders with social phobia (Öst et al. 1981). However, despite small differences in treatment efficacy for different types of patients, the majority of patients seem to do well with either type of behavioral treatment. Furthermore, many patients do not fall neatly into one category of responders but rather show features of both avoidance and physiological responding. Finally, several studies have failed to show differences in treatment efficacy for individuals with dental phobia (Jerremalm et al. 1986) and social phobia (Mersch et al. 1989) who have different response styles, which raises questions about the reliability of previous findings.

Heimberg and Juster (1995) reviewed some other predictors of response to CBT for social phobia. Subtype of social phobia seems to predict outcome (with generalized social phobia being associated with a worse treatment outcome than nongeneralized social phobia), but not when severity of symptoms is controlled. In other words, individuals with more severe symptoms before treatment can be expected to have more severe symptoms after treatment. With respect to comorbidity on outcome, findings have been mixed. Some research has found that the presence of comorbidity (additional personality, mood, or anxiety disorders) did not affect outcome following CBT for social phobia (Brown et al. 1995, Hofmann et al. 1995b, Van Velzen et al. 1997). However, other research has found that the presence of depression and avoidant personality traits were associated with a poorer outcome (Chambless et al. 1997, Scholing and Emmelkamp 1999).

Most pharmacological studies have failed to examine predictors of outcome. One exception was a study by Van Ameringen and colleagues (1993), who found that a shorter duration of symptoms and older age at onset were associated with more positive outcomes after treatment of social phobia with fluoxetine.

Several studies have examined characteristics of individual subjects that predict outcome in the behavioral treatment of specific phobias. Two studies have found that coping style predicts outcome. In one study, "monitors" (those who cope with fear by seeking fear-relevant information, e.g., scanning a room for spiders in the case of an individual with spider phobia) responded more poorly to behavioral treatment and relapsed more often compared with "blunters" (those who cope with fear by avoiding fear-relevant information, e.g., avoiding looking around for spiders for fear of seeing them) (Muris et al. 1993). However, another study led to opposite findings, with monitors responding most (Steketee et al. 1989). Finally, a study by Antony and colleagues from their Center (2001a) found no relationship between coping style and treatment outcome in a group of patients with spider phobia.

Other patient-related variables that may be associated with treatment outcome for specific phobias include symptom severity, level of generalized anxiety, and previous experience with the phobic stimulus. Specifically, patients with more severe height phobias have been shown to demonstrate greater change after treatment than did patients with less severe phobias (Baker et al. 1973), although that does not imply that their posttreatment symptoms are less severe. In addition, elevated generalized anxiety has been shown to be associated with poorer outcome in patients with height phobia (Baker et al. 1973). Moreover, extensive prior experience with flying has been shown to be associated with a worse outcome after behavioral treatment for flying phobia (Solyom et al. 1973). Despite these findings, other research examining potential predictors of outcome in the treatment of specific phobia (e.g., age of onset, duration of phobia, method of onset, family history, anxiety, depression, heart rate, severity, and blood pressure) failed to find a stable predictor of outcome (Hellström and Öst 1996).

It should be noted that none of these findings has been replicated and they should therefore be interpreted with caution. Much more research is needed to identify predictors of outcome with CBT and especially with pharmacological treatment. For example, little is known about the

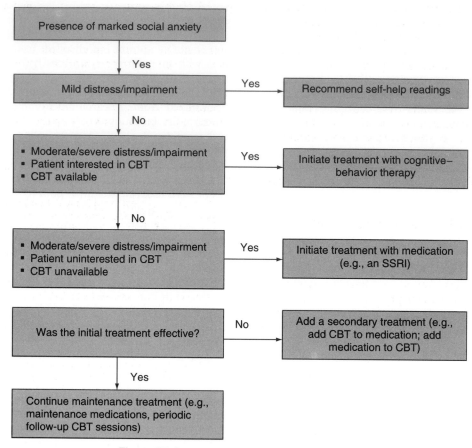

**Figure 67–4** *Treatment decision tree for social phobia.*

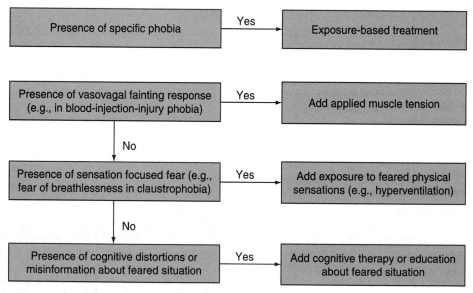

**Figure 67–5** *Treatment decision tree for specific phobia.*

effectiveness of treatments for specific and social phobias in special populations (e.g., elderly persons, culturally diverse groups). There has also been a lack of research on the impact of comorbidity on success of treatment with specific phobias.

## Relapse and Return of Fear

With respect to specific phobia, it is common for some return of fear to occur in the presence of the phobic stimulus (Craske 1999). Although relapse following treatment of a specific phobia is believed to be rare (Öst 1996b), one study found a considerable proportion of individuals experienced a clinically significant return of symptoms over an average 12-year follow-up period (Lipsitz et al. 1999). A number of variables have been identified that predict return of fear including distraction during exposure, a relatively quick reduction in fear during exposure (Rose and McGlynn 1997), a relatively slow reduction in fear during exposure (Rachman and Whittal 1989), higher initial heart rate (Craske and Rachman 1987), spacing of exposure sessions and the degree to which the exposure stimuli are varied (Rowe and Craske 1998a, 1998b), the tendency to overassociate fear-relevant stimuli with aversive outcomes (de Jong et al. 1995), and depression (Salkovskis and Mills 1994).

## Refractory Patients and Nonresponse to Initial Treatment

Several variables may lead to an initially poor treatment response. Anticipating potential difficulties will help increase treatment efficacy. Possible reasons for a worse outcome include poor compliance, poor motivation, and poor understanding of the treatment procedures. In addition, interpersonal issues and other possible conflicts may interfere with the successful treatment of specific and social phobias.

Patients fail to comply with treatment procedures for a variety of reasons. In the case of pharmacological treatments, patients may avoid taking medications because of side effects, lack of confidence in efficacy, or preference for an alternative type of treatment. If patients are not compliant with medications, the physician should attempt to identify the reasons for poor compliance and to suggest methods of increasing compliance or changing to another type of treatment.

In the case of CBT, common reasons for poor compliance are anxiety about conforming to treatment, lack of time, and lack of motivation to conduct the treatment properly. Because CBT requires patients to confront the situations they fear most, patients often feel extreme anxiety about participating in the treatment. Patients should be reassured that their anxiety is normal and that they will never be forced to do anything that they are unwilling to try. Furthermore, the difficulty of exposure tasks should be increased gradually to maximize treatment compliance. If patients do not have the time or motivation to conduct treatment as suggested, therapists should be willing to find ways to make the treatment more accessible to the patient. For example, involvement of a friend or relative of the patient as a coach may allow the patient to conduct more practices without the therapist's assistance. The therapist could also explore the possibility that the patient consider beginning treatment later, when more time is available.

Poor motivation can lead to poor compliance with the treatment procedures. If a patient's symptoms are not especially severe, the distress and impairment created by the disorder may not be enough to motivate the patient to take medications regularly or to confront the phobic situation in a systematic way. Furthermore, as a patient improves in treatment, she or he may experience a decrease in motivation. Patients should be encouraged to continue with treatment assignments even after improvement. More complete improvements may protect against a return of symptoms.

Finally, treatment procedures may be complicated for some patients. This is especially the case for CBT. Patients may fail to complete homework assignments (e.g., monitoring anxious cognitions) simply because the treatment rationale and the specifics of how to conduct the treatment procedures were not made clear. Therefore, therapists should continually assess the patient's understanding of the treatment procedures.

---

**Clinical Vignette 1 • Social Phobia**

Ms. K is a 29-year-old student who presented with social phobia. She reported being shy as a child and could remember pretending to be ill to stay home from school. As she got older, she met more children and by high school was quite comfortable with her friends at school. Meeting new people was still difficult, as was public speaking in class. Fortunately, neither situation came up often.

In college, Ms. K's problem became worse. Several of her classes required her to make presentations. In addition, because she lived off campus, she found it particularly difficult to meet friends. The few times she tried to talk to people in class, she felt as though she had nothing to say. Before long, she stopped trying. Ms. K did not avoid her class presentations at first. Rather, she tended to overprepare for them and tried to use overheads when possible because the dark room helped to decrease her anxiety. Still during presentations she could feel her heart pounding and she tended to have difficulty breathing. Her mouth became dry and she was sure that her classmates could see her shaking and perspiring.

After her first year of college, Ms. K began to avoid any class that required presentations. In addition, she found herself avoiding other situations in which people might notice her shaking. Specifically, she avoided writing in front of others, holding drinking glasses, and other situations that might focus other people's attention on her hands. She also avoided engaging in conversation with others and when people approached her, she tried to end the conversation as quickly as possible. In addition to fearing that others would notice her anxiety, Ms. K felt that others might see her as weak, unattractive, or foolish.

During a diagnostic interview, it was found that Ms. K was suffering from social phobia. She seemed bright and motivated, and it was decided that she might benefit from CBGT for social phobia. However, the patient initially rejected this option because of anxiety about participating in a group. Therefore, she started 10 mg of paroxetine and gradually increased the dosage to 50 mg. Because of difficulties due to sexual dysfunction, the dosage was decreased to 40 mg and her sexual symptoms subsided.

During a period of 6 weeks, Ms. K felt more comfortable around people and decided that she was willing to participate in a 12-session CBGT program. Treatment included a variety of components, including information about the nature of anxiety and social phobia, cognitive restructuring, role-play exposures to anxiety-provoking situations (e.g., group presentations), and homework assignments to enter feared situations. In addition, Ms. K practiced purposely shaking in front of others, until the symptom was no longer frightening to her. Over the course of the CBGT, Ms. K's medication was gradually discontinued.

---

**Clinical Vignette 1** *continued*

By the end of treatment, Ms. K was essentially symptom free and criteria for social phobia were no longer met. Furthermore, she had met several new friends and had enrolled in a few classes that required her to make presentations. Although she still became nervous before speaking in public, she looked forward to the presentations. She rarely experienced shaking in front of others and was no longer particularly concerned about shaking.

---

**Clinical Vignette 2 • Specific Phobia**

Mr. D, a 38-year-old attorney, presented for treatment of snake phobia. Growing up in New York City he rarely saw snakes, although he reported fearing toy snakes even as a child. In his late twenties, he relocated to a rural area where he encountered snakes every few weeks. Mr. D began to avoid entering his backyard and walking in his neighborhood, even with his family. Before he drove to work his wife checked the area around his car for snakes. His fear became worse over time so that even seeing a photograph of a snake induced a panic attack.

When Mr. D did see a snake he tended to have an intense panic attack, including breathlessness, dizziness, palpitations, and a feeling that he might lose control and embarrass himself. He was not sure how the fear developed, nor could he identify what bothered him about snakes, except perhaps something about their movement. Mr. D decided to move back to the city and had just put his house up for sale when he presented for treatment.

Mr. D had a specific phobia of snakes and reported no other significant problems with anxiety. Before he began behavioral treatment, a full assessment of his fear was conducted. A hierarchy of feared situations was generated ranging from moderately anxiety provoking tasks (e.g., looking at a photograph of a snake) to extremely difficult tasks (e.g., touching a snake). In addition, a behavioral approach test was conducted during which it was discovered that Mr. D could stand no closer than 10 feet from a live snake in an aquarium. In addition, during the behavioral approach test he became aware that his main anxious thought was that the snake would touch him and perhaps bite him. His fear tended to increase when the snake looked in his direction or moved in the aquarium.

Mr. D was treated during two sessions of therapist-assisted exposure, each lasting 120 minutes. During the sessions, he practiced the various tasks on his hierarchy and continued to do so even when his fear was overwhelming. Each step was first demonstrated by the therapist. By the end of two sessions, Mr. D was able to look at, touch, and hold a snake with minimal anxiety. At 1-month follow-up, he reported that he no longer avoided situations in which he might see snakes and had decided to continue living in his house.

## Comparison of DSM-IV/ICD-10 Diagnostic Criteria

The ICD-10 Diagnostic Criteria for Research for Social Phobia specify that at least two symptoms of anxiety (i.e., from the list of 14 panic symptoms) be present together on at least one occasion along with at least one of the following anxiety symptoms: blushing or shaking, fear of vomiting, and urgency or fear of micturition or defecation. Furthermore, these anxiety symptoms must be "restricted to, or predominated in, the feared situations or contemplation of the feared situations." In contrast, the DSM-IV criteria do not specify any particular types of anxiety symptoms nor is any restriction placed on whether anxiety can occur in situations other than social situations.

For specific phobia, the ICD-10 Diagnostic Criteria for Research also specify that the anxiety symptoms be "restricted to, or predominated in, the feared situations or contemplation of the feared situation." DSM-IV again does not impose any such restriction.

## References

Adler PSJ, France C, and Ditto B (1991) Baroreflex sensitivity at rest and during stress in individuals with a history of vasovagal syncope. J Psychosom Res 35, 1–7.

Albano AM, DiBartolo PM, Heimberg RG, et al. (1995) Children and adolescents: Assessment and treatment. In Social Phobia: Diagnosis, Assessment, and Treatment, Heimberg RG, Liebowitz MR, Hope DA, et al. (eds). Guilford Press, New York, pp. 387–425.

Allgulander C and Nilsson B (2001) A prospective study of 86 new patients with social anxiety disorder. Acta Psychiatr Scand 103, 447–452.

Altamura AC, Piolo R, Vitto M, et al. (1999) Venlafaxine in social phobia: A study in selective serotonin reuptake inhibitor nonresponders. Int Clin Psychopharmacol 14, 239–245.

American Psychiatric Association (1980) Diagnostic and Statistical Manual of Mental Disorders, 3rd ed. APA, Washington DC.

American Psychiatric Association (1987) Diagnostic and Statistical Manual of Mental Disorders, 3rd ed., Rev. APA, Washington DC.

American Psychiatric Association (2000) Diagnostic and Statistical Manual of Mental Disorders, 4th ed., Text Rev. APA, Washington DC.

Anderson JC, Williams S, McGee R, et al. (1987) DSM-III disorders in preadolescent children. Arch Gen Psychiatr 44, 69–76.

Andrews G, Stewart G, Allen R, et al. (1990) The genetics of six neurotic disorders: A twin study. J Affect Disord 19, 23–29.

Antony MM (1994) Heterogeneity among specific phobia types in DSM-IV. Unpublished doctoral dissertation. State University of New York, University at Albany, Albany, NY.

Antony MM and Barlow DH (1998) Specific phobia. In Handbook of Cognitive and Behavioural Treatments for Psychological Disorders, Caballo VE (ed). Pergamon, Oxford, UK, pp. 1–22.

Antony MM and Barlow DH (2002) Specific phobias. In Anxiety and Its Disorders: The Nature and Treatment of Anxiety and Panic, 2nd ed., Barlow DH (ed). Guilford Press, New York.

Antony MM and Swinson RP (2000a) Phobic Disorders and Panic in Adults: A Guide to Assessment and Treatment. American Psychological Association, Washington DC.

Antony MM and Swinson RP (2000b) Shyness and Social Anxiety Workbook: Proven Techniques for Overcoming Fears. New Harbinger, Oakland, CA.

Antony MM, Brown TA, and Barlow DH (1997a) Response to hyperventilation and 5.5% $CO_2$ inhalation of subjects with types of specific phobia, panic disorder, or no mental disorder. Am J Psychiatr 154, 1089–1095.

Antony MM, Brown TA, and Barlow DH (1997b) Heterogeneity among specific phobia types in DSM-IV. Behav Res Ther 35, 1089–1100.

Antony MM, Craske MG, and Barlow DH (1995) Mastery of Your Specific Phobia. The Psychological Corporation, San Antonio, TX.

Antony MM, McCabe RE, Leeuw I, et al. (2001a) Effect of exposure and coping style on in vivo exposure for specific phobia of spiders. Behav Res Ther 39, 1137–1150.

Antony MM, Moras K, Meadows EA, et al. (1994) The diagnostic significance of the functional impairment and subjective distress criterion: An illustration with the DSM-III-R anxiety disorders. J Psychopathol Behav Assess 16, 253–262.

Antony MM, Orsillo SM, and Roemer L (eds) (2001b) Practitioner's Guide to Empirically-Based Measures of Anxiety. Kluwer Academic/Plenum Publishers, New York.

Antony MM, Purdon CL, Huta V, et al. (1998a) Dimensions of perfectionism across the anxiety disorders. Behav Res Ther 36, 1143–1154.

Antony MM, Roth D, Swinson RP, et al. (1998b) Illness intrusiveness in individuals with panic disorder, obsessive–compulsive disorder, or social phobia. J Nerv Ment Dis 186, 311–315.

Arntz A, Lavy E, van den Berg G, et al. (1993) Negative beliefs of spider phobics: A psychometric evaluation of the Spider Phobia Beliefs Questionnaire. Adv Behav Res Ther 15, 257–277.

Arrindell WA (1980) Dimensional structure and psychopathology correlates of the Fear Survey Schedule (FSS-III) in a phobic population: A factorial definition of agoraphobia. Behav Res Ther 18, 229–242.

Baker BL, Cohen DC, and Saunders JT (1973) Self-directed desensitization for acrophobia. Behav Res Ther 11, 79–89.

Balon R (1999) Fluvoxamine for phobia of storms. Acta Psychiatr Scand 100, 244–246.

Barlow DH (1991) Disorders of emotion. Psychol Inq 2, 58–71.

Barlow DH (2002) Anxiety and Its Disorders: The Nature and Treatment of Anxiety and Panic, 2nd ed. Guilford Press, New York.

Beckham JC, Vrana SR, May JG, et al. (1990) Emotional processing and fear measurement synchrony as indicators of treatment outcome in fear of flying. J Behav Ther Exp Psychiatr 21, 153–162.

Benjamin J, Ben-Zion IZ, Karbofsky E, et al. (2000) Double-blind placebo-controlled pilot study of paroxetine for specific phobia. Psychopharmacology 149, 194–196.

Biederman J, Hirshfeld-Becker DR, Rosenbaum JF, et al. (2001) Further evidence of association between behavioral inhibition and social anxiety in children. Am J Psychiatr 158, 1673–1679.

Blomhoff S, Haug TT, Hellström K, et al. (2001) Randomised controlled general practice trial of sertraline, exposure therapy and combined treatment in generalised social phobia. Br J Psychiatr 179, 23–30.

Bourdon KH, Boyd JH, Rae DS, et al. (1988) Gender differences in phobias: Results of the ECA community survey. J Anx Disord 2, 227–241.

Bourne EJ (1998) Overcoming specific phobia: A hierarchy and exposure-based protocol for the treatment of all specific phobias (therapist protocol). New Harbinger, Oakland, CA.

Bouton ME, Mineka S, and Barlow DH (2001) A modern learning-theory perspective on the etiology of panic disorder. Psychol Rev 108, 4–32.

Bouwer C and Stein DJ (1998) Use of the selective serotonin reuptake inhibitor citalopram in the treatment of generalized social phobia. J Affect Disord 49, 79–82.

Brown D (1996) Flying Without Fear. New Harbinger, Oakland, CA.

Brown TA, Campbell LA, Lehman CL, et al. (2001a) Current and lifetime comorbidity of the DSM-IV anxiety and mood disorders in a large clinical sample. J Abnorm Psychol 110, 585–599.

Brown TA, Di Nardo PA, and Barlow DH (1994) Anxiety Disorders Interview Schedule for DSM-IV (ADIS-IV). The Psychological Corporation, San Antonio, TX.

Brown TA, Di Nardo PA, Lehman CL, et al. (2001b) Reliability of DSM-IV anxiety and mood disorders: Implications for the classification of emotional disorders. J Abnorm Psychol 110, 49–58.

Brown DR, Eaton WW, and Sussman L (1990) Racial differences in prevalence of phobic disorders. J Nerv Ment Dis 178, 434–441.

Brown EJ, Heimberg RG, and Juster HR (1995) Social phobia subtypes and avoidant personality disorder: Effect on severity of social phobia, impairment, and outcome of cognitive–behavioral treatment. Behav Ther 26, 467–486.

Bruch MA (1989) Familial and developmental antecedents of social phobia: Issues and findings. Clin Psychol Rev 9, 37–47.

Bruch MA and Heimberg RG (1994) Differences in perceptions of parental and personal characteristics between generalized and nongeneralized social phobics. J Anx Disord 8, 155–168.

Buigues J and Vallejo J (1987) Therapeutic response to phenelzine in patients with panic disorder and agoraphobia with panic attacks. J Clin Psychiatr 48, 55–59.

Cannon WB (1929) Bodily Changes in Pain, Hunger, Fear, and Rage, 2nd ed. Appleton-Century-Crofts, New York.

Chaleby K (1987) Social phobias in Saudis. Soc Psychiatr 22, 167–170.

Chambless DL, Tran GQ, and Glass CR (1997) Predictors of response to cognitive behavioral treatment for social phobia. J Anx Disord 11, 221–240.

Chang SC (1997) Social anxiety (phobia) and East Asian culture. Depress Anx 5, 115–120.

Chapman TF, Fyer AJ, Mannuzza S, et al. (1993) A comparison of treated and untreated simple phobia. Am J Psychiatr 150, 816–818.

Chartier MJ, Hazen AL, and Stein MB (1998) Lifetime patterns of social phobia: A retrospective study of the course of social phobia in a non-clinical population. Depress Anx 7, 113–121.

Clark DB and Agras WS (1991) The assessment and treatment of performance anxiety in musicians. Am J Psychiatr 148, 605–698.

Cohen DC (1977) Comparison of self-report and overt-behavioral procedures for assessing acrophobia. Behav Ther 8, 17–23.

Connor KM, Davidson JRT, Churchill LE, et al. (2000) Psychometric properties of the Social Phobia Inventory (SPIN): New self-rating scale. Br J Psychiatr 176, 379–386.

Connor KM, Kobak KA, Churchill LE, et al. (2001) Mini-SPIN: A brief screening assessment for generalized social anxiety disorder. Depress Anx 14, 137–140.

Cooper JR, Bloom FE, and Roth RH (1983) The Biochemical Basis of Neuropharmacology. Oxford University Press, New York.

Cottraux J, Note I, Albuisson E, et al. (2000) Cognitive behavior therapy versus supportive therapy in social phobia: A randomized controlled trial. Psychother Psychosom 69, 137–146.

Craske MG (1989) The Boundary Between Simple Phobia and Specific Phobia. Report to the DSM-IV Anxiety Disorders Work Group. Phobia and Anxiety Disorders Clinic, Albany, New York.

Craske MG (1999) Anxiety disorders: Psychological Approaches to Theory and Treatment. Westview Press, Boulder, CO.

Craske MG and Rachman SJ (1987) Return of fear: Perceived skill and heart rate responsivity. Br J Clin Psychol 26, 187–199.

Craske MG and Rowe MK (1997) A comparison of behavioral and cognitive treatments for phobias. In Phobias: A Handbook of Theory, Research, and Treatment, Davey GCL (ed). John Wiley, New York.

Craske MG, Antony MM, and Barlow DH (1997) Mastery of Your Specific Phobia: Therapist Guide. Psychological Corporation/Graywind Publications, San Antonio, TX.

Craske MG, Mohlman J, Yi J, et al. (1995) Treatment of claustrophobia and snake/spider phobias: Fear of arousal and fear of context. Behav Res Ther 33, 197–203.

Craske MG, Zarate R, Burton T, et al. (1993) Specific fears and panic attacks: A survey of clinical and nonclinical samples. J Anx Disord 7, 1–19.

Crum RM and Pratt LA (2001) Risk of heavy drinking and alcohol use disorders in social phobia: A prospective analysis. Am J Psychiatr 158, 1693–1700.

Curtis GC, Hill EM, and Lewis JA (1990) Heterogeneity of DSM-III-R Simple Phobia and the Simple Phobia/Agoraphobia Boundary: Evidence from the ECA Study. Report to the DSM-IV Anxiety Disorders Work Group. University of Michigan, Ann Arbor, MI.

Curtis GC, Magee WJ, Eaton WW, et al. (1998) Specific fears and phobias: Epidemiology and classification. Br J Psychiatr 173, 212–217.

Davey CL, Forster L, and Mayhew G (1993) Familial resemblances in disgust sensitivity and animal phobias. Behav Res Ther 31, 41–50.

Davidson JRT (1998) Social Phobia Inventory (SPIN). Unpublished scale. Duke University Medical School, Durham, NC.

Davidson JRT, Ford SM, Smith RD, et al. (1991a) Long-term treatment of social phobia with clonazepam. J Clin Psychiatr 52, 16–20.

Davidson JRT, Potts NLS, Richichi EA, et al. (1991b) The Brief Social Phobia Scale. J Clin Psychiatr 52, 48–51.

Davidson JRT, Potts N, Richichi E, et al. (1993) Treatment of social phobia with clonazepam and placebo. J Clin Psychopharmacol 13, 423–428.

de Jong PJ, Andrea H, and Muris P (1997) Spider phobia in children: Disgust and fear before and after treatment. Behav Res Ther 35, 559–562.

de Jong PJ, van den Hout M, and Merckelbach H (1995) Covariation bias and return of fear. Behav Res Ther 33, 211–213.

Dewis LM, Kirkby KC, Martin F, et al. (2001) Computer-aided vicarious exposure versus live graded exposure for spider phobia in children. J Behav Ther Exp Psychiatr 32, 17–27.

Di Nardo PA, Guzy LT, Jenkins JA, et al. (1988) Etiology and maintenance of dog fears. Behav Res Ther 26, 241–244.

Eaton WW, Dryman A, and Weissman MM (1991) Panic and phobia. In Psychiatric Disorders in America: The Epidemiologic Catchment Area Study, Robins LN and Regier DA (eds). Free Press, New York, pp. 155–179.

Ehlers A, Hofmann SG, Herda CA, et al. (1994) Clinical characteristics of driving phobia. J Anx Disord 8, 323–337.

Erwin BA, Heimberg RG, Juster H, et al. (2002) Comorbid anxiety and mood disorders among persons with social anxiety disorder. Behav Res Ther 40, 19–35.

Febbraro GAR and Clum GA (1995) A dimensional analysis of claustrophobia. J Psychopathol Behav Assess 17, 335–351.

Fedoroff IC and Taylor S (2001) Psychological and pharmacological treatments for social phobia: A meta-analysis. J Clin Psychopharmacol 21, 311–324.

Fehm L and Margraf J (2002) Thought suppression: Specificity in agoraphobia versus broad impairment in social phobia? Behav Res Ther 40, 57–66.

First MB, Spitzer RL, Gibbon M, et al. (2001) Structured Clinical Interview for DSM-IV-TR Axis I Disorders, Research Version, Patient Edition. (SCID-I/P). New York State Psychiatric Institute, Biometrics Research, New York.

Foa EB, Blau JS, Prout M, et al. (1977) Is horror a necessary component of flooding (implosion)? Behav Res Ther 15, 397–402.

Francis G (1990) Social phobia in childhood. In Handbook of Child and Adult Psychopathology: A Longitudinal Perspective, Hersen M and Last CG (eds). Pergamon Press, New York, pp. 163–168.

Fredrikson M, Annas P, Fischer H, et al. (1996) Gender and age differences in the prevalence of specific fears and phobias. Behav Res Ther 26, 241–244.

Fresco DM and Heimberg RG (2001) Empirically supported psychological treatments for social phobia. Psychiatr Ann 31, 489–496.

Furlan PM, DeMartinis N, Schweizer E, et al. (2001) Abnormal salivary cortisol levels in social phobic patients in response to acute psychological but not physical stress. Biol Psychiatr 50, 254–259.

Fyer AJ, Mannuzza S, Chapman TF, et al. (1993) A direct interview family study of social phobia. Arch Gen Psychiatr 50, 286–293.

Fyer AJ, Mannuzza S, Gallops MS, et al. (1990) Familial transmission of simple phobias and fears. Arch Gen Psychiatr 47, 252–256.

Gauthier J and Marshall WL (1977) The determination of optimal exposure to phobic stimuli in flooding therapy. Behav Res Ther 15, 403–410.

Geer JH (1965) The development of a scale to measure fear. Behav Res Ther 3, 45–53.

Goisman RM, Goldenberg I, Vasile RG, et al. (1995) Comorbidity of anxiety disorders in a multicenter anxiety study. Compr Psychiatr 36, 303–311.

Gorman JM and Gorman LK (1987) Drug treatment of social phobia. J Affect Disord 13, 183–192.

Gould RA, Buckminster S, Pollack MH, et al. (1997) Cognitive–behavioral and pharmacological treatment for social phobia: A meta-analysis. Clin Psychol Sci Pract 4, 291–306.

Greenberg DB, Stern TA, and Weilburg JB (1988) The fear of choking: Three successfully treated cases. Psychosomatics 29, 126–129.

Hackmann A, Surawy C, and Clark DM (1998) Seeing yourself through others' eyes: A study of spontaneously occurring images in social phobia. Behav Cogn Psychother 26, 3–12.

Hartley LR, Ungapen S, Dovie I, et al. (1983) The effect of beta-adrenergic blocking drugs on speakers' performance and memory. Br J Psychiatr 142, 512–517.

Haug T, Brenne L, Johnsen BH, et al. (1987) The three-systems analysis of fear of flying: A comparison of a consonant vs. a nonconsonant treatment method. Behav Res Ther 25, 187–194.

Haug TT, Hellstrom K, Blomhoff S, et al. (2000) The treatment of social phobia in general practice. Is exposure therapy feasible? Fam Pract 17, 114–118.

Heimberg RG (2001) Current status of psychotherapeutic interventions for social phobia. J Clin Psychiatr 62, 36–42.

Heimberg RG and Becker RE (2002) Cognitive–Behavioral Group Treatment for Social Phobia. Guilford Press, New York.

Heimberg RG and Juster HR (1995) Cognitive–behavioral treatments: Literature review. In Social Phobia: Diagnosis, Assessment, and Treatment, Heimberg RG, Liebowitz MR, Hope DA, et al. (eds). Guilford Press, New York, pp. 261–309.

Heimberg RG, Dodge CS, Hope DA, et al. (1990) Cognitive–behavioral group treatment for social phobia: Comparison with a credible placebo control. Cog Ther Res 14, 1–23.

Heimberg RG, Holt CS, Schneier FR, et al. (1993a) The issue of subtypes in the diagnosis of social phobia. J Anx Disord 7, 249–269.

Heimberg RG, Hope DA, Dodge CS, et al. (1990) DSM-III-R subtypes of social phobia: Comparison of generalized social phobics and public speaking phobics. J Nerv Ment Dis 173, 172–179.

Heimberg RG, Liebowitz MR, Hope DA, et al. (1998) Cognitive–behavioral group therapy vs. phenelzine therapy for social phobia: 12-week outcome. Arch Gen Psychiatr 55, 1133–1141.

Heimberg RG, Salzman DG, Holt CS, et al. (1993b) Cognitive–behavioral group treatment for social phobia: Effectiveness at five-year follow-up. Cogn Ther Res 17, 325–339.

Hellström K and Öst L-G (1995) One-session therapist directed exposure vs. two forms of manual directed self-exposure in the treatment of spider phobia. Behav Res Ther 33, 959–965.

Hellström K and Öst L-G (1996) Prediction of outcome in the treatment of specific phobia: A cross validation study. Behav Res Ther 34, 403–411.

Hepner A and Cauthen NR (1975) Effect of subject control and graduated exposure on snake phobias. J Consult Clin Psychol 43, 297–304.

Herbert JD, Hope DA, and Bellack AS (1992) Validity of the distinction between generalized social phobia and avoidant personality disorder. J Abnorm Psychol 101, 332–339.

Himle JA, McPhee K, Cameron OJ, et al. (1989) Simple phobia: Evidence for heterogeneity. Psychiatr Res 28, 25–30.

Hofmann SG (2000) Self-focused attention before and after treatment of social phobia. Behav Res Ther 37, 717–725.

Hofmann SG and Barlow DH (2002) Social phobia. In Anxiety and its Disorders: The Nature and Treatment of Anxiety and Panic, 2nd ed. Barlow DH (ed). Guilford Press, New York, pp. 454–476.

Hofmann SG, Ehlers A, and Roth WT (1995a) Conditioning theory: A model for the etiology of public speaking anxiety? Behav Res Ther 35, 567–571.

Hofmann SG, Lehman CL, and Barlow DH (1997) How specific are specific phobias? J Behav Ther Exp Psychiatr 28, 233–240.

Hofmann SG, Newman MG, Becker E, et al. (1995b) Social phobia with and without avoidant personality disorder: Preliminary behavior therapy outcome findings. J Anx Disord 9, 427–438.

Holt CS, Heimberg RG, Hope DA, et al. (1990) A search for situational features of social phobia: Clustering social situational anxiety. Presented at the Annual Meeting of the Association for Advancement of Behavior Therapy (Nov), San Francisco, CA.

Holt CS, Heimberg RG, Hope DA, et al. (1992) Situational domains of social phobia. J Anx Disord 6, 63–77.

Houlihan D, Schwartz C, Miltenberger R, et al. (1993) The rapid treatment of a young man's balloon (noise) phobia using in vivo flooding. J Behav Ther Exp Psychiatr 24, 233–240.

Howard WA, Murphy SM, and Clarke JC (1983) The nature and treatment of fear of flying: A controlled investigation. Behav Ther 14, 557–567.

Hugdahl K and Öst L-G (1985) Subjectively rated physiological and cognitive symptoms in six different clinical phobias. Pers Individ Diff 6, 175–188.

James IM, Burgoyne W, and Savage IT (1983) Effect of pindolol on stress-related disturbances of musical performance: Preliminary communication. J Roy Soc Med 76, 194–196.

Jerremalm A, Jansson L, and Öst L-G (1986) Individual response patterns and the effects of different behavioral methods in the treatment of dental phobia. Behav Res Ther 24, 587–596.

Jones MK and Menzies RG (2000) Danger expectancies, self-efficacy and insight in spider phobia. Behav Res Ther 38, 585–600.

Kagan J, Reznick JS, Clarke C, et al. (1984) Behavioral inhibition to the unfamiliar. Child Dev 55, 2212–2225.

Kahan M, Tanzer J, Darvin D, et al. (2000) Virtual reality-assisted cognitive-behavioral treatment for fear of flying: Acute treatment and follow-up. Cyber Psychol Behav 3, 387–392.

Karno M, Golding JM, Burnam MA, et al. (1989) Anxiety disorders among Mexican Americans and non-Hispanic whites in Los Angeles. J Nerv Ment Dis 177, 202–209.

Katzelnick DJ, Kobak KA, DeLeire T, et al. (2001) Impact of generalized social anxiety disorder in managed care. Am J Psychiatr 158, 1999–2007.

Kelsey JE (1995) Venlafaxine in social phobia. Psychopharmacol Bull 31, 767–771.

Kendler KS, Karkowski LM, and Prescott CA (1999) Fear and phobias: Reliability and heritability. Psychol Med 29, 539–553.

Kendler KS, Neale MC, Kessler RC, et al. (1992) The genetic epidemiology of phobias in women: The interrelationship of agoraphobia, social phobia, situational phobia, and simple phobia. Arch Gen Psychiatr 49, 273–281.

Kessler RC, McGonagle KA, Zhao S, et al. (1994) Lifetime and 12-month prevalence of DSM-III-R psychiatric disorders in the United States: Results from the National Comorbidity Survey. Arch Gen Psychiatr 51, 8–19.

Kindt M and Brosschot JF (1999) Cognitive bias in spider-phobic children: Comparison of a pictorial and a linguistic spider Stroop. J Psychopathol Behav Assess 21, 207–220.

King RJ, Mefford IN, and Wang C (1986) CSF dopamine levels correlate with extraversion in depressed patients. Psychiatr Res 19, 305–310.

Kleinknecht RA (1994) Acquisition of blood, injury, and needle fears and phobias. Behav Res Ther 32, 817–823.

Kleinknecht RA, Dinnel DL, Kleinknecht EE, et al. (1997) Cultural factors in social anxiety: A comparison of social phobia symptoms and Taijin Kyofusho. J Anx Disord 11, 157–177.

Kleinknecht RA, Thorndike RM, and Walls MM (1996) Factorial dimensions and correlates of blood, injury, injection and related medical fears: Cross validation of the Medical Fear Survey. Behav Res Ther 34, 323–331.

Klieger DM and Franklin ME (1993) Validity of the Fear Survey Schedule in phobia research: A laboratory test. J Psychopathol Behav Assess 15, 207–217.

Klorman R, Hastings J, Weerts T, et al. (1974) Psychometric description of some specific-fear questionnaires. Behav Ther 5, 401–409.

Landy FJ and Gaupp LA (1971) A factor analysis of the FSS-III. Behav Res Ther 9, 89–93.

Last CG, Perrin S, Hersen M, et al. (1996) A prospective study of childhood anxiety disorders. J Am Acad Child Adolesc Psychiatr 35, 1502–1510.

Lee SH and Oh KS (1999) Offensive type of social phobia: Cross-cultural perspectives. Int Med J 6, 271–279.

Lehman CL, Patterson MD, Brown TA, et al. (1998) Lifetime alcohol use disorders in patients with anxiety or mood disorders. Paper presented at the meeting of the Association for Advancement of Behavior Therapy (Nov), Washington DC.

Levin AP, Saoud JB, Strauman T, et al. (1993) Responses of "generalized" and "discrete" social phobics during public speaking. J Anx Disord 7, 207–221.

Levin AP, Schneier FR, and Liebowitz MR (1989) Social phobia: Biology and pharmacology. Clin Psychol Rev 9, 129–140.

Lewis MH, Gariepy J, and Devaud LL (1989) Dopamine and social behavior: A mouse model of 'timidity'. Presented at the meeting of the American College of Neuropsychopharmacology (Dec), Maui, HI.

Liddell A, Locker D, and Burman D (1991) Self-reported fears (FSS-II) of subjects aged 50 years and over. Behav Res Ther 29, 105–112.

Liebowitz MR (1987) Social phobia. Mod Prob Pharmacopsychiatr 22, 141–173.

Liebowitz MR, Heimberg RG, Schneier FR, et al. (1999) Cognitive–behavioral group therapy versus phenelzine in social phobia: Long term outcome. Depress Anx 10, 89–98.

Liebowitz MR, Schneier F, Campeas R, et al. (1992) Phenelzine vs. atenolol in social phobia: A placebo-controlled comparison. Arch Gen Psychiatr 49, 290–300.

Liebowitz MR, Stein MB, Tancer M, et al. (2002) A randomized, double-blind, fixed-dose comparison of paroxetine and placebo in the treatment of generalized social anxiety disorder. J Clin Psychiatr 63, 66–74.

Lipsitz JD, Mannuzza S, Klein DF, et al. (1999) Specific phobia 10–16 years after treatment. Depress Anx 10, 105–111.

Lott M, Greist JH, Jefferson JW, et al. (1997) Brofaromine for social phobia: A multicenter, placebo-controlled, double-blind study. J Clin Psychopharmacol 17, 255–260.

Lydiard RB, Laraia MT, Howell EF, et al. (1988) Alprazolam in the treatment of social phobia. J Clin Psychiatr 49, 17–19.

Marks IM (1985) Behavioral treatment of social phobia. Psychopharmacol Bull 21, 615–618.

Marks IM and Gelder MG (1966) Different ages of onset in varieties of phobia. Am J Psychiatr 123, 218–221.

Marks IM and Mathews AM (1979) Brief standard self-rating for phobic patients. Behav Res Ther 17, 263–267.

Mathew SJ, Coplan JD, and Gorman JM (2001) Neurobiological mechanisms of social anxiety disorder. Am J Psychiatr 158, 1558–1567.

Mattia JI, Heimberg RG, and Hope DA (1993) The revised Stroop color-naming task in social phobics. Behav Res Ther 31, 305–313.

Mattick RP and Clarke JC (1998) Development and validation of measures of social phobia scrutiny fear and social interaction anxiety. Behav Res Ther 36, 455–470.

Mattick RP and Peters L (1988) Treatment of severe social phobia: Effects of guided exposure with and without cognitive restructuring. J Consult Clin Psychol 56, 251–260.

McCabe RE and Antony MM (2002) Specific and social phobias. In Handbook of Assessment, Treatment Planning, and Outcome Evaluation: Empirically Supported Strategies for Psychological Disorders. Antony MM and Barlow DH (eds). Guilford Press, New York.

McManus F, Clark DM, and Hackmann A (2000) Specificity of cognitive biases in social phobia and their role in recovery. Behav Cogn Psychother 28, 201–209.

McNally RJ (1986) Behavioral treatment of choking phobia. J Behav Ther Exp Psychiatr 17, 185–188.

McNally RJ (1987) Preparedness and phobias: A review. Psychol Bull 101, 283–303.

McNally RJ and Steketee GS (1985) The etiology and maintenance of severe animal phobias. Behav Res Ther 23, 431–435.

Mennin DS, Heimberg RG, and MacAndrew SJ (2000) Comorbid generalized anxiety disorder in primary social phobia: Symptom severity, functional impairment, and treatment response. J Anx Disord 14, 325–343.

Menzies RG and Clarke JC (1993a) A comparison of in vivo and vicarious exposure in the treatment of childhood water phobia. Behav Res Ther 31, 9–15.

Menzies RG and Clarke JC (1993b) The etiology of fear of heights and its relationship to severity and individual response patterns. Behav Res Ther 31, 355–365.

Menzies RG and Clarke JC (1995) The etiology of phobias: A non-associative account. Clin Psychol Rev 15, 23–48.

Menzies RG and Parker L (2001) The origins of height fear: An evaluation of neoconditioning explanations. Behav Res Ther 39, 185–199.

Merckelbach H and Muris P (1997) The etiology of childhood spider phobia. Behav Res Ther 35, 1031–1034.

Merckelbach H, Arntz A, Arrindell WA, et al. (1992) Pathways to spider phobia. Behav Res Ther 30, 543–546.

Merckelbach H, de Jong PJ, Arntz A, et al. (1993) The role of evaluative learning and disgust sensitivity in the etiology and treatment of spider phobia. Adv Behav Res Ther 15, 243–255.

Merckelbach H, Muris P, and Schouten E (1996) Pathways to fear in spider phobic children. Behav Res Ther 34, 935–938.

Mersch PPA, Emmelkamp PMG, and Lips C (1989) Social phobia: Individual response patterns and the effects of behavioral and cognitive interventions. Behav Res Ther 27, 421–434.

Moore R and Brødsgaard I (1994) Group therapy compared with individual desensitization for dental anxiety. Comm Dent Oral Epidemiol 22, 258–262.

Moras K, Di Nardo PA, Brown TA, et al. (1995) Comorbidity, functional impairment, and depression among the DSM-III-R anxiety disorders. Unpublished manuscript, State University of New York, Albany, New York.

Mowrer OH (1939) Stimulus response theory of anxiety. Psychol Rev 46, 553–565.

Munjack DJ, Baltazar PL, Bohn PB, et al. (1990) Clonazepam in the treatment of social phobia: A pilot study. J Clin Psychiatr 51, 35–40.

Munjack DJ, Bruns J, Baltazar PL, et al. (1991) A pilot study of buspirone in the treatment of social phobia. J Anx Disord 5, 87–98.

Muris P, de Jong PJ, Merckelbach H, et al. (1993) Is exposure therapy outcome affected by a monitoring coping style? Adv Behav Res Ther 15, 291–300.

Muris P, Mayer B, and Merckelbach H (1998) Trait anxiety as a predictor of behaviour therapy outcome in spider phobia. Behav Cogn Psychother 26, 87–91.

Muris P, Merckelbach H, and Collaris R (1997) Common childhood fears and their origins. Behav Res Ther 35, 929–937.

Muris P, Schmidt H, and Merckelbach H (1999) The structure of specific phobia symptoms among children and adolescents. Behav Res Ther 37, 863–868.

Neal AM and Turner SM (1991) Anxiety disorders research with African-Americans: Current status. Psychol Bull 109, 400–410.

Nemiah JC and Uhde TW (1989) Phobic disorders. In Comprehensive Textbook of Psychiatry, Vol. 5, Kaplan HI and Sadock BJ (eds). Williams & Wilkins, Baltimore, pp. 972–984.

Norton PJ and Hope DA (2001) Kernels of truth or distorted perceptions: Self and observer ratings of social anxiety and performance. Behav Ther 32, 765–786.

Noyes R, Moroz G, Davidson JRT, et al. (1997) Moclobemide in social phobia: A controlled dose-response trial. J Clin Psychopharmacol 17, 247–254.

Oosterbaan DB, van Balkom AJLM, Spinoven P, et al. (2001) Cognitive therapy versus moclobemide in social phobia: A controlled study. Clin Psychol Psychother 8, 263–273.

Öst L-G (1978) Behavioral treatment of thunder and lightning phobias. Behav Res Ther 16, 197–207.

Öst L-G (1985) Ways of acquiring phobias and outcome of behavioral treatment. Behav Res Ther 23, 683–689.

Öst L-G (1987) Age of onset in different phobias. J Abnorm Psychol 96, 223–229.

Öst L-G (1989) One-session treatment for specific phobias. Behav Res Ther 27, 1–7.

Öst L-G (1991) Acquisition of blood and injection phobia and anxiety response patterns in clinical patients. Behav Res Ther 29, 323–332.

Öst L-G (1992) Blood and injection phobia: Background and cognitive, physiological, and behavioral variables. J Abnorm Psychol 101, 68–74.

Öst L-G (1996a) One-session group treatment for spider phobia. Behav Res Ther 34, 707–715.

Öst L-G (1996b) Long term effects of behavior therapy for specific phobia. In Long Term Treatments of the Anxiety Disorders, Mavissakalian MR and Prien RF (eds). American Psychiatric Press, Washington DC.

Öst L-G, and Hugdahl K (1985) Acquisition of blood and dental phobia and anxiety response patterns in clinical patients. Behav Res Ther 23, 27–34.

Öst L-G and Sterner U (1987) Applied tension: A specific behavioral method for treatment of blood phobia. Behav Res Ther 25, 25–29.

Öst L-G, Brandberg M, and Alm T (1997a) One versus five sessions of exposure in the treatment of flying phobia. Behav Res Ther 35, 987–996.

Öst L-G, Fellenius J, and Sterner U (1991a) Applied tension, exposure in vivo, and tension-only in the treatment of blood phobia. Behav Res Ther 29, 561–574.

Öst L-G, Ferebee I, and Furmark T (1997b) One-session group therapy of spider phobia: Direct versus indirect treatments. Behav Res Ther 35, 721–732.

Öst L-G, Jerremalm A, and Johansson J (1981) Individual response patterns and the effects of different behavioral methods in the treatment of social phobia. Behav Res Ther 19, 1–16.

Öst L-G, Johansson J, and Jerremalm A (1982) Individual response patterns and the effects of different behavioral methods in the treatment of claustrophobia. Behav Res Ther 20, 445–460.

Öst L-G, Lindahl I-L, Sterner U, et al. (1984) Exposure in vivo vs. applied relaxation in the treatment of blood phobia. Behav Res Ther 22, 205–216.

Öst L-G, Salkovskis PM, and Hellström K (1991b) One-session therapist directed exposure vs. self-exposure in the treatment of spider phobia. Behav Ther 22, 407–422.

Öst L-G, Svensson L, Hellström K, et al. (2001) One-session treatment of specific phobias in youths: A randomized clinical trial. J Consult Clin Psychol 69, 814–824.

Otto MW, Pollack MH, Gould RA, et al. (2000) A comparison of the efficacy of clonazepam and cognitive–behavioral group therapy for the treatment of social phobia. J Anx Disord 14, 345–358.

Otto MW, Pollack MH, Maki KM, et al. (2001) Childhood history of anxiety disorders among adults with social phobia: Rates, correlates, and comparisons with patients with panic disorder. Depress Anx 14, 209–213.

Page AC (1994) Blood-injury phobia. Clin Psychol Rev 14, 443–461.

Page AC (in press) The role of disgust in faintness elicited by blood and injection stimuli. J Anx Disord.

Page AC and Martin NG (1998) Testing a genetic structure of blood-injury-injection fears. Am J Med Genet 81, 377–384.

Pande AC, Davidson JR, Jefferson JW, et al. (1999) Treatment of social phobia with gabapentin: A placebo-controlled study. J Clin Psychopharmacol 19, 341–348.

Park J-M, Mataix-Cols D, Marks IM, et al. (2001) Two-year follow-up after a randomised controlled trial of self- and clinician-accompanied exposure for phobia/panic disorders. Br J Psychiatr 178, 543–548.

Pauli P, Wiedemann G, and Montoya P (1998) Covariation bias in flight phobics. J Anx Disord 12, 555–565.

Perugi G, Nassini S, Lenzi M, et al. (1994/1995) Treatment of social phobia with fluoxetine. Anxiety 1, 282–286.

Pierce KA and Kirkpatrick DR (1992) Do men lie on fear surveys? Behav Res Ther 30, 415–418.

Plomin R (1989) Environment and genes: Determinants of behavior. Am Psychol 44, 105–111.

Potts NLS, Davidson JRT, Krishnan KRR, et al. (1991) Levels of urinary free cortisol in social phobia. J Clin Psychiatr 52, 41–42.

Poulton R and Menzies RG (2002) Nonassociative fear acquisition: A review of the evidence from restrospective and longitudinal research. Behav Res Ther 40, 127–149.

Poulton R, Menzies RG, Craske MG, et al. (1999) Water trauma and swimming experiences up to age 9 and fear of water at age 18: A longitudinal study. Behav Res Ther 37, 39–48.

Purdon C, Antony MM, Monteiro S, et al. (2001) Social anxiety in college students. J Anx Disord 15, 203–215.

Rachman S (1977) The conditioning theory of fear-acquisition: A critical examination. Behav Res Ther 15, 375–387.

Rachman S and Cuk M (1992) Fearful distortions. Behav Res Ther 30, 583–589.

Rachman S and Whittal M (1989) The effect of an aversive event on the return of fear. Behav Res Ther 27, 513–520.

Raguram R and Bhide AV (1985) Patterns of phobic neurosis: A retrospective study. Br J Psychiatr 147, 557–560.

Randall CL, Johnson MR, Thevos AK, et al. (2001) Paroxetine for social anxiety disorder and alcohol use in dual-diagnosed patients. Depress Anx 14, 255–262.

Rapee RM (1997) Perceived threat and perceived control as predictors of the degree of fear in physical and social situations. J Anx Disord 11, 455–461.

Rapee RM and Lim L (1992) Discrepancy between self- and observer ratings of performance in social phobics. J Abnorm Psychol 101, 728–731.

Rapee RM, Brown TA, Antony MM, et al. (1992) Response to hyperventilation and inhalation of 5.5% carbon dioxide-enriched air across the DSM-III-R anxiety disorders. J Abnorm Psychol 101, 538–552.

Rauch SL, Savage CR, Alpert NM, et al. (1995) A positron emission tomographic study of simple phobic symptom provocation. Arch Gen Psychiatr 52, 20–28.

Reich J and Yates W (1988) A pilot study of treatment of social phobia with alprazolam. Am J Psychiatr 145, 590–594.

Reiss S, Peterson RA, Gursky DM, et al. (1986) Anxiety sensitivity, anxiety frequency, and the prediction of fearfulness. Behav Res Ther 24, 1–8.

Riemann BC (1993) The prevalence of anxiety disorders in alcoholics. Presented at the meeting of the Association for Advancement of Behavior Therapy (Nov), Boston, MA.

Rimm DC, Janda LH, Lancaster DW, et al. (1977) An exploratory investigation of the origin and maintenance of phobias. Behav Res Ther 15, 231–238.

Rose MP and McGlynn FD (1997) Toward a standard experiment for studying posttreatment return of fear. J Anx Disord 11, 263–277.

Rosenbaum JF, Biederman J, Hirshfeld DR, et al. (1991) Behavioral inhibition in children: A possible precursor to panic disorder or social phobia. J Clin Psychiatr 52, 5–9.

Roth D, Antony MM, and Swinson RP (2001) Interpretations for anxiety symptoms in social phobia. Behav Res Ther 39, 129–138.

Rothbaum BO, Hodges LF, Kooper R, et al. (1995) Effectiveness of computer-generated (virtual reality) graded exposure in the treatment of acrophobia. Am J Psychiatr 152, 626–628.

Rothbaum BO, Hodges LF, Smith S, et al. (2000) A controlled study of virtual reality exposure therapy for the fear of flying. J Consult Clin Psychol 68, 1020–1026.

Rowa K, Antony MM, Brar S, et al. (2000) Treatment histories of patients with three anxiety disorders. Depress Anx 12, 92–98.

Rowe MK and Craske MG (1998a) Effects of an expanding-spaced vs. massed exposure schedule on fear reduction and return of fear. Behav Res Ther 36, 701–717.

Rowe MK and Craske MG (1998b) Effects of varied-stimulus exposure training on fear reduction and return of fear. Behav Res Ther 36, 719–734.

Salkovskis PM and Mills I (1994) Induced mood, phobic responding and the return of fear. Behav Res Ther 32, 439–445.

Sanderson WC, Di Nardo PA, Rapee RM, et al. (1990) Syndrome comorbidity in patients diagnosed with a DSM-III-R anxiety disorder. J Abnorm Psychol 99, 308–312.

Sawchuk CN, Lohr JM, Tolin DF, et al. (2000) Disgust Sensitivity and contamination fears in spider and blood-injection-injury phobias. Behav Res Ther 38, 753–762.

Schatzberg AF, Samson JA, Rothschild AJ, et al. (1998) McLean Hospital Depression Research Facility: Early-onset phobic disorders and adult-onset major depression. Br J Psychiatr 173, 29–34.

Schmidt LA (1999) Frontal brain electrical activity in shyness and sociability. Psychol Sci 10, 316–320.

Schmidt LA, Fox NA, Rubin KH, et al. (1997) Behavioral and neuroendocrine responses in shy children. Dev Psychobiol 30, 127–140.

Schneider F, Weiss U, Kessler C, et al. (1999) Subcortical correlates of differential classical conditioning of aversive emotional reactions in social phobia. Biol Psychiatr 45, 863–871.

Schneier FR, Goetz D, Campeas R, et al. (1998) Placebo-controlled trial of moclobemide in social phobia. Br J Psychiatr 172, 70–77.

Schneier FR, Saoud JB, Campeas R, et al. (1993) Buspirone in social phobia. J Clin Psychopharmacol 13, 251–256.

Scholing A and Emmelkamp PMG (1993) Exposure with and without cognitive therapy for generalized social phobia: Effects of individual and group treatment. Behav Res Ther 31, 667–681.

Scholing A and Emmelkamp PMG (1999) Prediction of treatment outcome in social phobia: A cross-validation. Behav Res Ther 37, 659–670.

Schwalberg MD, Barlow DH, Alger SA, et al. (1992) Comparison of bulimics, obese binge eaters, social phobics and individuals with panic disorder on comorbidity across the DSM-III-R anxiety disorders. J Abnorm Psychol 101, 675–681.

Schweizer E, Rickels K, Weiss S, et al. (1993) Maintenance drug treatment of panic disorder: I. Results of a prospective, placebo-controlled comparison of alprazolam and imipramine. Arch Gen Psychiatr 50, 51–60.

Scott EL and Heimberg RG (2000) Social phobia: An update on treatment. Psychiatr Ann 30, 678–686.

Seligman MEP (1971) Phobias and preparedness. Behav Ther 2, 307–320.

Simon NM, Sharma SG, Worthington JJ, et al. (2001) Citalopram for social phobia: A clinical case series. Prog Neuro-Psychopharmacol Biol Psychiatr 25, 1469–1474.

Simpson HB, Schneier FR, Campeas RB, et al. (1998) Imipramine in the treatment of social phobia. J Clin Psychopharmacol 18, 132–135.

Skre I, Onstad S, Torgerson S, et al. (1993) A twin study of DSM-III-R anxiety disorders. Acta Psychiatr Scand 88, 85–92.

Smith KL, Kirkby KC, Montgomery IM, et al. (1997) Computer-delivered modeling of exposure for spider phobia: Relevant versus irrelevant exposure. J Anx Disord 11, 489–497.

Solyom L, Shugar R, Bryntwick S, et al. (1973) Treatment of fear of flying. Am J Psychiatr 130, 423–427.

Stein MB, Chartier MJ, Hazen AL, et al. (1998) A direct-interview family study of generalized social phobia. Am J Psychiatr 155, 90–97.

Stein MB, Delaney SM, Chartier MJ, et al. (1995) [³H] paroxetine binding to platelets of patients with social phobia: Comparison to patients with panic disorder and healthy volunteers. Biol Psychiatr 37, 224–228.

Stein MB, Fyer AJ, Davidson JRT, et al. (1999) Fluvoxamine treatment of social phobia (social anxiety disorder): A double-blind, placebo-controlled study. Am J Psychiatr 156, 756–760.

Stein MB, Liebowitz MR, Lydiard RB, et al. (1998) Paroxetine treatment of generalized social phobia (social anxiety disorder): A randomized controlled trial. J Am Med Assoc 380, 708–713.

Steketee G, Bransfield S, Miller SM, et al. (1989) The effect of information and coping style on the reduction of phobic anxiety during exposure. J Anx Disord 3, 69–85.

Stopa L and Clark DM (1993) Cognitive processes in social phobia. Behav Res Ther 31, 255–267.

Stouthard MEA, Mellenbergh GJ, and Hoogstraten J (1993) Assessment of dental anxiety: A facet approach. Anx Stress Coping 6, 89–105.

Straus CC and Last CG (1993) Social and simple phobias in children. J Anx Disord 7, 141–152.

Sue DW (1990) Culture-specific strategies in counseling: A conceptual framework. Prof Psychol Pract 21, 424–433.

Summerfeldt LJ and Antony MM (2002) Structured and semi-structured diagnostic interviews. In Handbook of Assessment, Treatment Planning, and Outcome Evaluation: Empirically Supported Strategies for Psychological Disorders, Antony MM and Barlow DH (eds). Guilford Press, New York.

Takahashi T (1989) Social phobia syndrome in Japan. Compr Psychiatr 30, 45–52.

Tancer ME, Mailman RB, Stein MB, et al. (1994/1995) Neuroendocrine responsivity to monoaminergic system probes in generalized social phobia. Anxiety 1, 216–223.

Tancer ME, Stein MB, Gelernter CS, et al. (1990) The hypothalamic-pituitary-thyroid axis in social phobia. Am J Psychiatr 147, 929–933.

Thom A, Sartory G, and Jöhren P (2000) Comparison between one-session psychological treatment and benzodiazepine in dental phobia. J Consult Clin Psychol 68, 378–387.

Thyer BA, Parrish RT, Curtis GC, et al. (1985) Ages of onset of DSM-III anxiety disorders. Compr Psychiatr 26, 113–121.

Tiihonen J, Kuikka J, Bergstrom K, et al. (1997) Dopamine reuptake site densities in patients with social phobia. Am J Psychiatr 154, 239–242.

Townend E, Dimigen G, and Fung D (2000) A clinical study of child dental anxiety. Behav Res Ther 38, 31–46.

Tupler LA, Davidson JRT, Smith RD, et al. (1997) A repeat proton magnetic resonance spectroscopy study in social phobia. Biol Psychiatr 42, 419–424.

Turk CL, Fresco DM, and Heimberg RG (1999) Social phobia: Cognitive behavior therapy. In Handbook of Comparative Treatments of Adult Disorders, 2nd ed., Hersen M and Bellack AS (eds). John Wiley, New York.

Turk CL, Heimberg RG, and Hope DA (2001) Social anxiety disorder. In Clinical Handbook of Psychological Disorders: A Step-by-Step Treatment Manual, 3rd ed., Barlow DH (ed). Guilford Press, New York.

Turk CL, Heimberg RG, Orsillo SM, et al. (1998) An investigation of gender differences in social phobia. J Anx Disord 12, 209–223.

Turner SM, Beidel DC, Cooley MR, et al. (1994) A multicomponent behavioral treatment for social phobia: Social effectiveness therapy. Behav Res Ther 32, 381–390.

Turner SM, Beidel DC, Dancu CV, et al. (1986) Psychopathology of social phobia and comparison with avoidant personality disorder. J Abnorm Psychol 95, 389–394.

Turner SM, Beidel DC, Dancu CV, et al. (1989) An empirically derived inventory to measure social fears and anxiety: The Social Phobia and Anxiety Inventory. Psychol Assess J Consult Clin Psychol 1, 35–40.

Turner SM, Beidel DC, and Townsley RM (1992) Social phobia: A comparison of specific and generalized subtype and avoidant personality disorder. J Abnorm Psychol 101, 326–331.

Turner SM, Beidel DC, and Wolff PL (1996) Is behavioral inhibition related to the anxiety disorders? Clin Psychol Rev 16, 157–172.

Van Ameringen M, Lane RG, Walker JR, et al. (2001) Sertraline treatment of generalized social phobia: A 20-week, double-blind, placebo-controlled study. Am J Psychiatr 158, 275–281.

Van Ameringen M, Mancini C, and Oakman JM (1999a) Nefazodone in social phobia. J Clin Psychiatr 60, 96–100.

Van Ameringen M, Mancini C, Oakman JM, et al. (1999b) Selective serotonin reuptake inhibitors in the treatment of social phobia: The emerging gold standard. CNS Drugs 11, 307–315.

Van Ameringen M, Mancini C, Oakman JM, et al. (2000) Selective serotonin reuptake inhibitors in the treatment of social phobia: First line treatment at the turn of the century. In Pharmacotherapy of Anxiety Disorders, Palmer KJ (ed). Adis International Publications, Hong Kong, pp. 17–30.

Van Ameringen M, Mancini C, and Streiner DL (1993) Fluoxetine efficacy in social phobia. J Clin Psychiatr 54, 27–32.

Van Ameringen M, Mancini C, Styan G, et al. (1991) Relationship of social phobia with other psychiatric illness. J Affect Disord 21, 93–99.

Van Der Linden G, Van Heerden B, Warwick J, et al. (2000a) Functional brain imaging and pharmacotherapy in social phobia: Single photon emission computed tomography before and after treatment with the selective serotonin reuptake inhibitor citalopram. Prog Neuro-Psychopharmacol Biol Psychiatr 24, 419–438.

Van der Linden GHH, Stein DJ, and van Balkom AJLM (2000b) The efficacy of the selective serotonin reuptake inhibitors for social anxiety disorder (social phobia): A meta-analysis of randomized controlled trials. Int Clin Psychopharmacol 15(Suppl 2), S15–S23.

Van Velzen CJM, Emmelkamp PMG, and Scholing A (1997) The impact of personality disorders on behavioral treatment for social phobia. Behav Res Ther 35, 889–900.

van Vliet IM, den Boer JA, and Westenberg HGM (1994) Psychopharmacological treatment of social phobia: A double-blind placebo-controlled study with fluvoxamine. Psychopharmacology 115, 128–134.

van Vliet IM, den Boer JA, Westenberg HGM, et al. (1997) Clinical effects of buspirone in social phobia: A double-blind placebo-controlled study. J Clin Psychiatr 58, 164–168.

Vega WA, Kolody B, Aguilar-Gaxiola S, et al. (1998) Lifetime prevalence of DSM-III-R psychiatric disorders among urban and rural Mexican Americans in California. Arch Gen Psychiatr 55, 771–778.

Versiani M, Nardi AE, Mundim FD, et al. (1992) Pharmacotherapy of social phobia: A controlled study with moclobemide and phenelzine. Br J Psychiatr 161, 353–360.

Versiani M, Nardi AE, Mundim FD, et al. (1996) The long-term treatment of social phobia with moclobemide. Int Clin Psychopharmacol 11(Suppl 3), 83–88.

Warheit GJ, Holzer CE, and Arey S (1975) Race and mental health: An epidemiological update. J Health Soc Behav 16, 243–256.

Wells A and Papageorgiou C (1999) The observer perspective: Biased imagery in social phobia, agoraphobia, and blood/injury phobia. Behav Res Ther 37, 653–658.

Widiger TA (1992) Generalized social phobia versus avoidant personality disorder: A commentary on three studies. J Abnorm Psychol 101, 340–343.

Wik G, Fredrikson M, and Fischer H (1997) Evidence of altered cerebral blood-flow relationships in acute phobia. Int J Neurosci 91, 253–263.

Wilhelm FH and Roth WT (1996) Acute and delayed effects of alprazolam on flight phobics during exposure. Paper presented at the meeting of the Association for Advancement of Behavior Therapy (Nov), New York.

Wilson GD and Priest HF (1968) The principal components of phobic stimuli. J Clin Psychol 24, 191.

Wlazlo Z, Schroeder-Hartwig K, Hand I, et al. (1990) Exposure in vivo vs. social skills training for social phobia: Long-term outcome and differential effects. Behav Res Ther 28, 181–193.

Wolpe J and Lang PJ (1964) A Fear Survey Schedule for use in behaviour therapy. Behav Res Ther 2, 27–30.

Wolpe J and Lang PJ (1969) Manual for the Fear Survey Schedule. Educational and Industrial Testing Service, San Diego, CA.

Wolpe J and Lang PJ (1977) Manual for the Fear Survey Schedule (revised). Educational and Industrial Testing Service, San Diego, CA.

Woody SR and Teachman BA (2000) Intersection of disgust and fear: Normative and pathological views. Clin Psychol Sci Pract 7, 291–311.

Zanarini MC, Skodol AE, Bender D, et al. (2000) The Collaborative Longitudinal Personality Disorders Study: Reliability of axis I and II diagnoses. J Pers Disord 14, 291–29.

# 68 Obsessive–Compulsive Disorder

Michele T. Pato
Jane L. Eisen
Katharine A. Phillips

Obsessive–Compulsive Disorder

## Definition and Overview

Obsessive–compulsive disorder (OCD) is an intriguing and often debilitating syndrome characterized by the presence of two distinct phenomena: obsessions and compulsions. Obsessions are intrusive, recurrent, unwanted ideas, thoughts, or impulses that are difficult to dismiss despite their disturbing nature. Compulsions are repetitive behaviors, either observable or mental, that are intended to reduce the anxiety engendered by obsessions. Both obsessions and compulsions have been described in a wide variety of psychiatric and neurological disorders (Jenike 1990). However, obsessions and compulsions that clearly interfere with functioning and/or cause significant distress are the hallmark of OCD.

Although OCD was originally considered rare, findings from the Epidemiologic Catchment Area (ECA) survey in 1984 demonstrated that OCD was 50 to 100 times more common than had been previously believed (Myers et al. 1984, Robins et al. 1984). With increasing recognition of OCD, both in the mental health field and in the media, many individuals with OCD have pursued treatment for this disorder. This has led to systematic investigation of clinical features such as symptom subtype, course, comorbidity, and the role of insight both descriptively and as mediators of treatment response.

These studies, conducted over the past 15 years, have greatly furthered our understanding of the clinical characteristics of this disorder. OCD is now considered a relatively common disorder that usually has its onset during puberty, although it may begin as early as age 2 years and infrequently begins after age 35 years. Women develop OCD slightly more often than men. Earlier studies found that the course of OCD is usually chronic, with symptom severity waxing and waning over time. However, those studies, which had a number of methodological limitations, were conducted prior to the availability of effective treatments for this disorder. More recent evidence suggests that some individuals have a more episodic and favorable course.

Several large studies have found that the most common obsession is contamination, and the most common compulsion is checking. However, most individuals with this disorder have multiple obsessions and compulsions over time. A number of psychiatric disorders cooccur with OCD, major depressive disorder being most frequent. Comorbidity with tic disorders is well established. That association plus a familial relationship between OCD and tic disorders has led to suggestions that tic-related OCD is a specific phenotype of OCD that is more closely related to tic disorders.

There has been considerable interest in the role of insight, or awareness, in OCD. An ability to recognize the senselessness of the obsessions and the ability to resist obsessional ideas have been considered fundamental components of OCD (Jaspers 1923, Lewis 1936). However, research findings during the past decade have demonstrated a continuum of insight in this disorder, which ranges from excellent (i.e., complete awareness of the senselessness of the content of the obsessions), through poor insight, to delusional thinking (i.e., the obsessions are held with delusional conviction) (Insel and Akiskal 1986, Eisen and Rasmussen 1993, Kozak and Foa 1994, Lelliot et al. 1988, Foa and Kozak 1995). To reflect these findings, the *Diagnostic and Statistical Manual of Mental Disorders*, Fourth Edition (DSM-IV) established a new OCD specifier—with poor insight—and also noted that, in cases of delusional OCD, an additional diagnosis of delusional disorder or psychotic disorder not otherwise specified may be appropriate (American Psychiatric Association 1994).

In this chapter we review the epidemiology, clinical features, differential diagnosis, etiology and pathophysiology, and treatment of OCD.

## Epidemiology

Since the 15th century, the psychiatric literature has contained striking descriptions of patients with debilitating obsessions and compulsions. Until the mid-1980s, however, OCD was considered extremely rare. This perception was based on studies from the 1950s and 1960s that examined the frequency of psychiatric diagnoses in inpatient and outpatient settings. The results of a large psychiatric epidemiological study, the national ECA survey, conducted

**Definition of Obsessive–Compulsive Disorder**

Either obsessions or compulsions:
*Obsessions as defined by (1), (2), (3), and (4):*

(1) recurrent and persistent thoughts, impulses, or images that are experienced, at some time during the disturbance, as intrusive and inappropriate and that cause marked anxiety or distress

(2) the thoughts, impulses, or images are not simply excessive worries about real-life problems

(3) the person attempts to ignore or suppress such thoughts, impulses, or images, or to neutralize them with some other thought or action

(4) the person recognizes that the obsessional thoughts, impulses, or images are a product of his or her own mind (not imposed from without as in thought insertion)

*Compulsions as defined by (1) and (2):*

(1) repetitive behaviors (e.g., hand washing, ordering, checking) or mental acts (e.g., praying, counting, repeating words silently) that the person feels driven to perform in response to an obsession, or according to rules that must be applied rigidly

(2) the behaviors or mental acts are aimed at preventing or reducing distress or preventing some dreaded event or situation; however, these behaviors or mental acts either are not connected in a realistic way with what they are designed to neutralize or prevent or are clearly excessive

At some point during the course of the disorder, the person has recognized that the obsessions or compulsions are excessive or unreasonable. Note: This does not apply to children.

The obsessions or compulsions cause marked distress, are time consuming (take more than 1 hour a day), or significantly interfere with the person's normal routine, occupational (or academic) functioning, or usual social activities or relationships.

If another Axis I disorder is present, the content of the obsessions or compulsions is not restricted to it (e.g., preoccupation with food in the presence of an eating disorder; hair pulling in the presence of trichotillomania; concern with appearance in the presence of body dysmorphic disorder; preoccupation with drugs in the presence of a substance use disorder; preoccupation with having a serious illness in the presence of hypochondriasis; preoccupation with sexual urges or fantasies in the presence of a paraphilia; or guilty ruminations in the presence of major depressive disorder).

The disturbance is not due to the direct physiological effects of a substance (e.g., a drug of abuse, a medication) or a general medical condition.

*Specify* if:

**With poor insight:** if, for most of the time during the current episode, the person does not recognize that the obsessions and compulsions are excessive or unreasonable

in the US in 1984, painted a different picture of OCD's prevalence. This study found that OCD was the fourth most common psychiatric disorder (after the phobias, substance use disorders, and major depressive disorder), with a prevalence of 1.6% over 6 months and a lifetime prevalence of 2.5% (Myers et al. 1984, Robins et al. 1984). Although the ECA survey has been criticized as overestimating OCD's prevalence (Stein et al. 1997) a subsequent study in the US and several epidemiological studies in other countries have supported its findings (Flament et al. 1988, Bland et al. 1988, Orley and Wing 1979, Zohar et al. 1992, Angst 1994, Yeh and Chang 1989). Using the same instrument as the ECA, studies have been done in diverse cultures, including Puerto Rico, Canada, Germany, Taiwan, New Zealand, and Korea, as part of the Cross National Collaborative Group (Weissman et al. 1994). The lifetime (range 1.9–2.5%) and annual (range 1.1–1.8%) prevalence rates of OCD were remarkably consistent across countries with the exception of Taiwan. The rates in Taiwan were substantially lower than in all the other sites, paralleling Taiwan's low rates of other psychiatric disorders.

## Clinical Features

## Demographic Characteristics

### Gender Distribution

Women appear to develop OCD slightly more frequently than do men. A pooled sample from two studies with a total of 991 subjects found that 52% of the subjects were women (Foa and Kozak 1995, Rasmussen and Eisen 1992). However, a study that assessed the presence of comorbid disorders characterized by psychosis (schizophrenia, delusional disorder) or psychosislike features (schizotypal personality disorder) in 475 patients with OCD found a different sex ratio. Fifty-six percent of the patients with OCD who did not have one of these comorbid disorders were women, whereas 85% of those with one of these comorbid disorders were men (Eisen and Rasmussen 1993).

A predominance of males has also been observed in child and adolescent OCD populations. In a study of 70 probands with OCD who were ages 6 to 18 years, 67% were males (Leonard et al. 1989). This finding may be due to the fact that males develop OCD at a younger age than do females.

## Marital Status

In a study of 250 subjects with OCD 52% were married, 43% were never married, and 5% were divorced (Rasmussen and Eisen 1992). The percentage of patients who had never married was significantly higher than that of age-matched controls. However, a study comparing marital status in probands with OCD and an age-matched group of patients with major depressive disorder found no significant differences between the two groups (Coryell 1981). Although marital status was not found to be a predictor of course in a number of follow-up studies, a recent prospective study of 107 subjects with OCD found that being married significantly increased the probability of partial remission, with married patients more than twice as likely to remit as unmarried ones (Steketee et al. 1999).

## Course and Natural History

### Age at Onset

Age at onset usually refers to the age when OCD symptoms (obsessions and compulsions) reach a severity level wherein they lead to impaired functioning or significant distress or are time-consuming (i.e., meet DSM-IV criteria for the disorder). Reported age at onset is usually during late adolescence. In one study drawn from an OCD clinic sample ($N = 560$), the onset for males occurred significantly earlier than for females ($19.5 \pm 9.2$ years versus $22.0 \pm 9.8$ years). In this study, 83% of patients experienced the onset of significant symptoms between ages 10 and 24 years, whereas less than 15% experienced onset after age 35 years (Rasmussen and Eisen 1998). People with OCD, however, usually describe the onset of minor symptoms in childhood, well before the onset of symptoms meeting full criteria for the disorder.

In several studies, earlier age at onset has been associated with an increased rate of OCD in first-degree relatives (Pauls et al. 1995, Nestadt et al. 2000). These data suggest that there is a familial type of OCD characterized by early onset. Age at onset of OCD may also be a predictor of course. The vast majority of patients report a gradual worsening of obsessions and compulsions prior to the onset of full-criteria OCD, which is followed by a chronic course (see later). However, Swedo and colleagues (1998) have described a subtype of OCD that begins before puberty and is characterized by an episodic course with intense exacerbations. Exacerbations of OCD symptoms in this subtype have been linked with Group A beta-hemolytic Streptococcal infections, which has led to the subtype designation of pediatric autoimmune neuropsychiatric disorders associated with streptococcal infections (PANDAS). In their study of 50 children with PANDAS, the average age of onset was 7.4 years. Whether the course of illness in patients with PANDAS continues to be episodic into adulthood, or, as is the case with postpubertal onset, tends to be chronic, is not known.

### Course of Illness

Earlier phenomenological and follow-up studies consistently showed the course of OCD to be continuous and chronic in which patients were rarely symptom free at follow-up (Ingram 1961, Kringlin 1965, Pollitt 1957, Lewis 1936, Lo 1967). However, these studies had a number of methodological limitations, including a lack of standardized criteria to determine the diagnosis, diagnoses based on chart review, a lack of structured interviews, a retrospective study design, and a lack of consensus on definitions of relapse, remission, and recovery. In keeping with the older literature, a more recent study showed that the course of OCD is usually waxing and waning—that is, once a patient acquires OCD, obsessions or compulsions, or both, are present continuously, with varying degrees of intensity over time. Relatively few patients had either a progressively deteriorating course or a truly episodic course (Rasmussen and Eisen 1991). Although this study had some methodological advantages over previous studies, it was not prospective, and the effect of treatment on the course of illness was not addressed.

A more recent 2-year naturalistic prospective study of 65 adults with OCD, in which the effect of treatment was assessed, supported earlier findings that OCD is usually chronic with fluctuations in symptom intensity but no lasting remission; it is notable that this course was most common even during an era when effective treatments were available. Although 50% of the subjects achieved partial remission in the first year of the study, the probability of subsequent relapse was 48%. Only 12% achieved full and sustained remission (Eisen et al. 1999). In contrast, a better outcome was found in a follow-up study of 144 people with OCD assessed in the 1950s and again in the 1990s (mean length of follow-up from illness onset was 47 years). Most subjects reported a significant decrease in OCD symptom severity, which varied from complete recovery (20%), to recovery with continued subclinical symptoms (28%), to continued OCD but with clear improvement (35%). Better outcome was associated with later age of onset and poorer social functioning at baseline (Skoog and Skoog 1999).

In a prospective study of children with OCD, the majority (52%) of the 25 patients had moderate to severe OCD in the 2- to 7-year follow-up period (Flament et al. 1990), which is consistent with the data on adults. A more recent prospective study of 54 children with OCD who were treated with clomipramine yielded a more hopeful picture of OCD's course. At 2 to 7 years after initial referral, 43 of these patients still had symptoms that met criteria for OCD, but 73% were considered much or very much improved, and 11% were completely asymptomatic (Leonard et al. 1993). This study suggested that appropriate somatic treatment may improve outcome only while the patient continues to receive this treatment (see later).

## Phenomenology

OCD's clinical presentation is characterized by phenomenological subtypes based on the content of the obsessions and corresponding compulsions. The list of subtypes in the Yale-Brown Obsessive–Compulsive Scale (Y-BOCS) (Table 68–1) was generated on the basis of clinical interviews with OCD patients in the 1980s (Goodman et al. 1989a). These subtypes are remarkably consistent with phenomenological descriptions in the psychiatric literature beginning with scrupulosity in the 15th century (Pitman 1994):

| Table 68-1 | Yale-Brown Obsessive–Compulsive Scale Symptom Checklist |
|---|---|

| | |
|---|---|
| Aggressive obsessions<br>　Fear might harm others<br>　Fear might harm self<br>　Violent or horrific images<br>　Fear of blurting out obsessions or insults<br>　Fear of doing something embarrassing<br>　Fear of acting on other impulses (e.g., robbing a bank, stealing groceries, overeating)<br>　Fear of being responsible for things going wrong (e.g., others will lose their job because of patient)<br>　Fear something terrible might happen (e.g., fire, burglary)<br>　Other<br>Contamination obsessions<br>　Concerns or disgust with bodily waste (e.g., urine, feces, saliva)<br>　Concern with dirt or germs<br>　Excessive concern with environmental contaminants (e.g., asbestos, radiation, toxic wastes)<br>　Excessive concern with household items (e.g., cleansers, solvents, pets)<br>　Concerned will become ill<br>　Concerned will become ill (aggressive)<br>　Other<br>Sexual obsessions<br>　Forbidden or perverse sexual thoughts, images, or impulses<br>　Content involves children<br>　Content involves animals<br>　Content involves incest<br>　Content involves homosexuality<br>　Sexual behavior toward others (aggressive)<br>　Other<br>Hoarding or collecting obsessions<br>Religious obsessions | Obsession with need for symmetry or exactness<br>Miscellaneous obsessions<br>　Need to know or remember<br>　Fear of saying certain things<br>　Fear of not saying things just right<br>　Intrusive (neutral) images<br>　Intrusive nonsense sounds, words, or music<br>　Other<br>Somatic obsession–compulsion<br>Cleaning or washing compulsions<br>　Excessive or ritualized hand washing<br>　Excessive or ritualized showering, bathing, brushing the teeth, or\grooming<br>　Involves cleaning of household items or inanimate objects<br>　Other measures to prevent contact with contaminants<br>Counting compulsions<br>Checking compulsions<br>　Checking that did not or will not harm others<br>　Checking that did not or will not harm self<br>　Checking that nothing terrible did or will happen<br>　Checking for contaminants<br>　Other<br>Repeating rituals<br>Ordering or arranging compulsions<br>Miscellaneous compulsions<br>　Mental rituals (other than checking or counting)<br>　Need to tell, ask, or confess<br>　Need to touch<br>Measures to prevent<br>　Harm to self<br>　Harm to others<br>　Terrible consequences<br>Other |

William of Oseney ... read two or three books of Religion and devotion very often ... (he) had read over those books 3 hours every day. In a short time he had read over those books three times more hellip; (He) began to think ... that now he was to spend 6 hours every day in reading those books, because he had now read them over six times. He presently considered that ... he must be tied to 12 hours every day (Hunter and Macalpine 1982).

The basic types of obsessions and compulsions seem to be consistent across cultures (Rasmussen and Eisen 1992). The most common obsession is fear of contamination, followed by pathological doubt, a need for symmetry, and aggressive obsessions (Figure 68–1). The most common compulsion is checking, which is followed by washing, symmetry, the need to ask or confess, and counting (Figure 68–2). Children with OCD present most commonly with washing compulsions, which are followed by repeating rituals (Swedo et al. 1989a).

Most patients have multiple obsessions and compulsions over time, with a particular fear or concern dominating the clinical picture at any one time. The presence of obsessions without compulsions, or compulsions without obsessions, is unusual. In the DSM-IV OCD field trial of 431 patients, only 2% had predominantly obsessions and 2% had predominantly compulsions; the remaining 96% endorsed both obsessions and compulsions (Foa and Kozak 1995). Patients who appear to have obsessions without compulsions frequently have unrecognized reassurance rituals or mental compulsions, such as repetitive, ritualized praying, in addition to their obsessions. Pure compulsions are also unusual in adults, although they do occur in children, especially in the young (e.g., 6 to 8 years of age; Swedo et al. 1989a). Most people have both mental and behavioral compulsions; in the DSM-IV field trial 79.5% reported having both mental and behavioral compulsions, 20.3% had behavioral compulsions only, and 0.2% had only mental compulsions.

The search for whether specific obsessions and compulsions have predictive value in terms of treatment response, biologic markers, or genetic transmission has not been particularly fruitful. There has been considerable interest in exploring whether certain clusters of obsessions and compulsions represent specific OCD phenotypes. A number of studies have addressed this question systematically using the Y-BOCS Symptom Checklist to identify groups of obsessions and compulsions that cluster together on factor analysis. Several studies have found between 3 and 5 such symptom dimensions: *symmetry/ordering, hoarding, contamination/cleaning, aggressive obsessions/*

Obsessive symptoms at admission

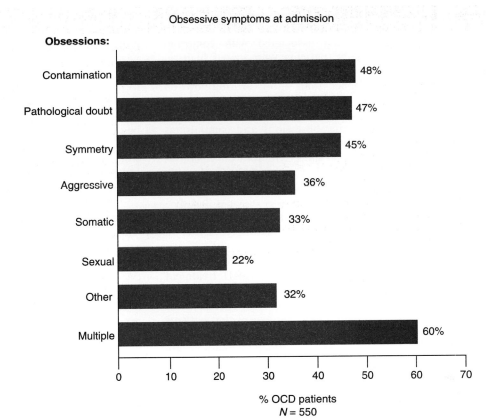

**Figure 68–1** *Obsessive symptoms at the time of initial evaluation in 550 patients with OCD.*

Compulsive symptoms at admission

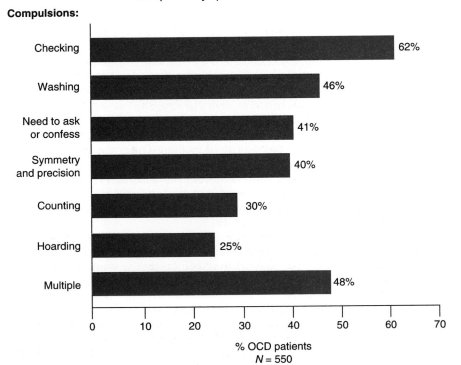

**Figure 68–2** *Compulsive symptoms at the time of initial evaluation in 550 patients.*

*checking*, and *sexual/religious obsessions* (Baer 1994, Leckman et al. 1997, Mataix-Cois et al. 1999). The symmetry dimension has been associated with comorbid tic disorder; in one study, patients who scored high on this dimension had a relative risk for chronic tic disorder that was 8.5 times higher than those scoring low on this factor (Leckman et al. 1997). It appears that these symptom dimensions are stable over time—that is, although a patient's specific obsessions and compulsions may change over time, new obsessions and compulsions that develop are often within the same symptom dimension as the previous symptoms (Mataix-Cois et al. 2002). A study using positron emission tomography to evaluate neural correlates of these symptom dimensions suggests that dysfunction in separate regions of the brain (e.g., striatum and prefrontal cortex) may mediate these factors (Rauch et al. 1998).

Data were analyzed from a number of placebo-controlled serotonin reuptake inhibitor (SRI) treatment studies to assess whether symptom factors or dimensions were associated with treatment response (Mataix-Cois et al. 1999). No clear pattern emerged except that patients with hoarding obsession had a significantly poorer response to SRIs. Whether these identified dimensions are associated with response to behavioral treatment, biological markers, or genetic transmission has yet to be investigated.

The following descriptions of some common obsessions and compulsions illustrate the clinical presentation of these symptoms. In some cases a particular symptom may belong to more than one "type" of obsessive or compulsive grouping. Thus it is often up to the clinician to decide which category to place a symptom so that it best describes the patient's symptoms overall; it may even be best to classify it in more than one category. For instance, a patient who has concerns about cancer may have hand washing as a compulsion related to her somatic obsession. If this is the only reason that she washes her hands, to avoid getting cancer, you might simply classify this as a somatic obsession with the accompanying compulsion. However if the patient also washes repeatedly to avoid contamination in general, not just for cancer, she would have both contamination and somatic obsessions and compulsions.

## Contamination

Contamination obsessions are the most frequently encountered obsessions in OCD. Such obsessions are usually characterized by a fear of dirt or germs. For example, a 38-year-old computer programmer was excessively preoccupied with the thought that her apartment would become dirty. She had never allowed a visitor into her apartment or worn a coat during the winter, because she feared that she would be unable to protect her apartment from dirt brought inside by either a visitor or a coat. To avoid contamination, she washed her clothes and showered immediately on entering her home.

Contamination fears may also involve toxins or environmental hazards (e.g., asbestos or lead) or bodily waste or secretions. Patients usually describe a feared consequence of contacting a contaminated object, such as spreading a disease or contracting an illness themselves. Occasionally, however, the fear is based not on a fear of disease but on a fear of

the sensory experience of not being clean. The content of the contamination obsession and the feared consequence commonly changes over time; for example, a fear of cancer may be replaced by a fear of a sexually transmitted disease.

Many patients with contamination fears use avoidance to prevent contact with contaminants, as is illustrated by a 58-year-old housewife who spent the entire day sitting in a chair to avoid touching anything in the house that might be dirty. In some cases, a specific feared object and associated avoidance become more generalized. For example, a woman with a fear of acquired immunodeficiency syndrome (AIDS) initially avoided anything that looked like dried blood but eventually avoided anything red.

Excessive washing is the compulsion most commonly associated with contamination obsessions. This behavior usually occurs after contact with the feared object; however, proximity to the feared stimulus is often sufficient to engender severe anxiety and washing compulsions, even though the contaminated object has not been touched. Most patients with washing compulsions perform these rituals in response to a fear of contamination, but these behaviors occasionally occur in response to a drive for perfection or a need for symmetry. Some patients, for example, repeatedly wash themselves in the shower until they feel "right" or must wash their right arm and then their left arm the same number of times.

## Need for Symmetry

Need for symmetry is a term that describes a drive to order or arrange things perfectly or to perform certain behaviors symmetrically or in a balanced way. Patients describe an urge to repeat motor acts until they achieve a "just right" feeling that the act has been completed perfectly. Patients with a prominent need for symmetry may have little anxiety but rather describe feeling unsettled or uneasy if they cannot repeat actions or order things to their satisfaction. In addition to a need for perfection, the drive to achieve balance or symmetry may be connected with magical thinking. For example, a 22-year-old college student felt compelled to walk across doorway thresholds exactly in the center to prevent something terrible from happening to his parents. The desire to "even up" or balance movements may be present in patients with tapping or touching rituals. Such a patient may, for example, feel that the right side of the chair must be tapped after the left side has been tapped. Such urges and behaviors are frequently seen in patients with comorbid tic disorders (Leckman et al. 1994), who may, for example, describe an urge to tic on the right side of their body after experiencing a tic on the left side.

Patients with a need for symmetry frequently present with obsessional slowness, taking hours to perform acts such as grooming or brushing their teeth. A 23-year-old cook spent 2 hours a day brushing his teeth in a symmetrical fashion and as a result developed gingival erosion. He reported being exquisitely aware of exactly how the toothbrush touched each surface of each tooth and of how he placed the toothbrush and cup down after finishing. He was unable to describe any obsession or fear about not performing this task adequately but rather felt unable to stop until he had brushed completely, despite warnings from his dentist about the harm he was causing.

## Somatic Obsessions

Patients with somatic obsessions are worried about the possibility that they have or will contract an illness or disease. In the past, the most common somatic obsessions consisted of fears of cancer or venereal diseases. However, a fear of developing AIDS has become increasingly common. Checking compulsions consisting of checking and rechecking the body part of concern, as well as reassurance seeking, are commonly associated with this fear. For example, a 29-year-old firefighter spent 3 hours a day examining his throat in the mirror and palpating his lymph nodes to determine whether he had throat cancer. He also repeatedly asked his wife whether she thought his throat looked normal. While it may be difficult to distinguish the somatic obsessions of OCD from those of hypochondriasis, there are several distinguishing features, which are discussed later in the chapter. Somatic obsessions are more easily distinguished from somatization disorder in which patients with somatic obsessions usually focus on one illness at a time and are not preoccupied with a diverse, apparently unrelated array of somatic symptoms.

## Sexual and Aggressive Obsessions

People with sexual or aggressive obsessions are plagued by fears that they might harm others or commit a sexually unacceptable act such as molestation. Often, they are fearful not only that they will commit a dreadful act in the future but also that they have already committed the act. Patients are usually horrified by the content of their obsessions and are reluctant to divulge them. It is striking that the content of these obsessions tends to consist of ideas that patients find particularly abhorrent. A 32-year-old librarian who wanted to be a good mother had intrusive thoughts of stabbing her daughter. The horror and revulsion that she experienced in response to this image is typical of patients' reactions to their aggressive and sexual thoughts.

Patients with these highly distressing obsessions frequently have checking and confession or reassurance rituals. They may report themselves to the police or repeatedly seek out priests to confess their imagined crimes. For example, a 63-year-old mother of five children and seven grandchildren felt compelled to confess to her priest that she might have had a sexual thought or feeling while drying herself after showering. A 29-year-old secretary constantly checked the local news to be certain that she had not murdered someone. An unsolved murder case caused her tremendous anxiety and led to extensive reassurance rituals.

## Pathological Doubt

Pathological doubt is a common feature of patients with OCD who have a variety of different obsessions and compulsions. Individuals with pathological doubt are plagued by the concern that, as a result of their carelessness, they will be responsible for a dire event. They may worry, for example, that they will start a fire because they neglected to turn off the stove before leaving the house. Although many patients report being fairly certain that they performed the act in question (e.g., locking the door, unplugging the hairdryer, paying the correct amount on a bill), they cannot dismiss the nagging doubt "What if?"

Such patients often describe doubting their own perceptions. A 42-year-old man felt incapable of throwing grocery bags away because he feared he might not have completely emptied them. Immediately after staring into an empty bag, he inevitably thought, "What if I missed something important in there?" A 33-year-old lawyer was unable to mail anything because she feared she had inadvertently placed written misinformation inside the envelope.

Excessive doubt and associated feelings of excessive responsibility frequently lead to checking rituals. For example, individuals may spend several hours checking their home before they leave. As with contamination obsessions, pathological doubt can lead to marked avoidance behavior. Some patients become housebound to avoid the responsibility of potentially leaving the house unlocked.

Pathological doubt is also embedded in the cognitive framework of a number of other obsessions. Patients with aggressive obsessions may be plagued by the doubt that they inadvertently harmed someone without knowing that they did so. For example, a young mother did not allow her children to have friends sleep at her house because she feared she might harm them during the night. Although she agreed that it was preposterous to think that she might commit a violent act without being aware of it, she nonetheless stated that she "did not want to take a chance," and she was unable to dismiss her nagging worry and doubt.

## Insight

An awareness of the senselessness or unreasonableness of obsessions (often referred to as insight) and the accompanying struggle against the obsessions (referred to as resistance) have generally been considered fundamental components of OCD (Jaspers 1923, Lewis 1936) and its diagnosis. Jaspers clearly emphasized this point in his description of obsessions:

> Compulsive thoughts, impulses, etc., should be confined to anxieties or impulses which can be experienced by the individual as an incessant preoccupation, though he is convinced of the *groundlessness* of the anxiety, the *senselessness* of the impulse and the *impossibility* of the notion. Thus compulsive events, strictly speaking, are all such events, the existence of which is strongly *resisted* by the individual in the first place and the content of which appears to him as *groundless, meaningless or relatively incomprehensible.*

However, during the past century there have been numerous descriptions of patients with OCD who are completely convinced of the reasonableness of their obsessions and need to perform compulsions. In 1986, Insel and Akiskal described several such patients and presented the hypothesis that patients with OCD have varying degrees of insight and resistance, with obsessive–compulsive psychosis at one extreme of a hypothesized continuum. They also noted a fluidity between neurotic (i.e., associated with insight) and psychotic states in these patients.

One study that investigated the range of insight in OCD used an interview that evaluated several insight-related parameters, including the fixity of beliefs underlying the obsession, bizarreness, resistance, and degree of control (Lelliott et al. 1988). The fixity dimension included several constructs: strength of the belief in the feared situation, how the patient thought others viewed the belief, and the patient's response to evidence that contradicted the belief. A full range of responses was found in the 43 patients assessed, which led the authors to conclude that good insight is not necessarily present and that insight spans a spectrum from good to absent (i.e., delusional thinking).

More recently, degree of insight in OCD was addressed during the DSM-IV field trial in which patients were asked if they feared consequences other than anxiety if they did not perform their compulsions (Foa and Kozak 1995). Fifty-eight percent believed that harmful consequences would occur. The degree of certainty that their obsessions were reasonable ranged across the entire spectrum of insight: 30% were uncertain whether they actually needed to perform their compulsions to avoid harm; however, 4% were certain, and 26% were mostly certain. Again, this finding supports the notion that patients with OCD do not always maintain good insight but rather have varying degrees of insight. Although patients may be aware that their obsessions are excessive—that is, recognizing that they spend too much time thinking about them—they may have little insight into the fact that the belief underlying their obsession (e.g., that they will get cancer from stepping on a chemically treated lawn) is senseless, unreasonable, or unrealistic.

To reflect these findings, DSM-IV established a new OCD specifier, with poor insight. This specifier applies to "an individual who, for most of the time in the current episode, does not recognize that the obsessions or compulsions are excessive or unreasonable." DSM-IV also acknowledges that the beliefs that underlie OCD obsessions can be delusional and notes that in such cases an additional diagnosis of delusional disorder or psychotic disorder not otherwise specified may be appropriate.

Despite these changes, there was no generally accepted, reliable, and valid method to assess degree of insight. To address the need for a scale that measures insight in OCD and other psychiatric disorders, Eisen and Phillips developed the Brown Assessment of Beliefs Scale, a semistructured clinician-administered interview with specific probes and anchors that measures various dimensions of delusionality (Eisen et al. 1998). Items assess dimensions such as conviction, perception of others' views of the belief, fixity, and insight (awareness that obsessions and compulsions are caused by a psychiatric illness). Combining data from a number of studies, 20 to 25% of individuals with OCD at some point during their illness are fairly convinced that their obsessions are realistic and that consequences other than anxiety would occur if they did not perform their compulsions. Nonetheless, most people with OCD are aware that other people think their symptoms are unrealistic and that the obsessions are caused by a psychiatric illness (Eisen et al. 1997a).

Whether insight is an important predictor of prognosis and treatment response is an intriguing issue that has received little investigation. The literature on insight as a predictor of response to behavioral therapy is conflicting;

several studies found that patients with poor insight or overvalued ideas did not respond as well to behavioral therapy as patients with good insight (Foa 1979, Foa et al. 1999). In contrast, another study found that patients with high conviction about their obsessions and the need to perform compulsions responded just as robustly to behavioral treatment as did patients with good insight (Lelliott et al. 1988). In the only study that has to our knowledge assessed whether insight predicts medication response, patients with poor insight at study baseline were just as likely to have response of OCD symptoms to open-label sertraline as those with good to excellent insight. In addition, insight improved with sertraline treatment during this 16-week study (Eisen et al. 2001).

More studies are needed to determine the effect of insight on treatment response. For example, to our knowledge no studies have assessed whether adding an antipsychotic to an SRI is more effective in patients with poor insight than in those with good insight. Studies that assess the impact of insight on compliance with and refusal of behavioral therapy are also needed.

## Comorbidity

OCD frequently occurs in association with other Axis I disorders. In a study of 100 patients with primary OCD, 67 had a lifetime history of major depressive disorder, and 31 had symptoms that met criteria for current major depressive disorder (Rasmussen and Eisen 1991). Although it may be difficult to distinguish a primary from a secondary diagnosis, some individuals with OCD view their depressive symptoms as occurring secondary to the demoralization and hopelessness accompanying their OCD and report that they would not be depressed if they did not have OCD. However, others view their major depressive symptoms as occurring independently of their OCD symptoms, which may be less severe when they cycle into an episode of major depression, because they feel too apathetic to be as concerned with their obsessions and too fatigued to perform compulsions. Conversely, OCD symptoms may intensify during depressive episodes.

Although findings have varied, the generally accepted frequency of tic disorders in patients with OCD is far higher than in the general population, with a rate of approximately 5 to 10% for Tourette's Disorder and 20% for any tic disorder (Leonard et al. 1992, Pitman et al. 1987). Conversely, patients with Tourette's disorder have a high rate of comorbid OCD, with 30 to 40% reporting obsessive–compulsive symptoms (Lees et al. 1984, Robertson et al. 1988). The likelihood of childhood onset of OCD is greater in this group, and the presence of tics is associated with more severe OCD symptoms in children (Leonard et al. 1992). There is an increased rate of both OCD and tic disorders in the first-degree relatives of OCD probands with a family lifetime history of tics (Pauls et al. 1995, Nestadt 2000), and an increased frequency of tic disorders in the first-degree relatives of OCD probands compared to controls (Grados et al. 2001). There are also phenomenologic observations that link OCD and tic disorders. Individuals with both OCD and tics have several features that distinguish them from individuals with OCD alone. They more frequently have symmetry, ordering and arranging, and hoarding compulsions (Leckman et al. 1994), and they more frequently try to attain a "just right" feeling (Miguel et al. 2000). These data strengthen the notion that tic disorders and OCD are highly related. In fact, it has been suggested that tic disorders are an alternative expression or phenotype of the familial OCD subtype (Grados et al. 2001).

Anxiety disorders frequently coexist with OCD, with relatively high lifetime rates of specific phobia (22%), social phobia (18%), and panic disorder (12%) in patients with OCD (Rasmussen and Eisen 1991). In one study, 17 of 100 subjects with OCD had a lifetime history of an eating disorder (Rasmussen and Eisen 1991). Conversely, in 93 subjects with an eating disorder, 37 had symptoms that met criteria for comorbid OCD (Rubenstein et al. 1992).

In another study, 14% (N = 67) of 475 OCD subjects had psychotic or psychoticlike symptoms (Eisen and Rasmussen 1993). These 67 subjects were quite heterogeneous: 18 (4% of the larger cohort) had comorbid schizophrenia, 8 (2%) had comorbid delusional disorder unrelated to OCD, and 14 (3%) had comorbid schizotypal personality disorder. In the remaining 27 patients (6% of the larger cohort), the only psychotic symptom was a delusional conviction about the reasonableness of the obsessions (i.e., delusional OCD, or OCD without insight). Of interest, the 27 subjects without insight were similar to the subjects without any psychotic symptoms (i.e., OCD with insight) in terms of epidemiological and clinical features, such as course of illness. In contrast, several studies of OCD and comorbid schizophrenia found that compared to subjects with OCD alone, those with comorbid schizophrenia have a worse prognosis in terms of long-term outcome (social relations, employment, psychopathology, and global functioning; Fenton and McGlashan 1986). Similarly, treatment studies of patients with OCD and comorbid schizotypal personality disorder have shown a poorer prognosis and poorer response to psychotropic medications for the comorbid group (Jenike et al. 1986). Thus, it appears important to differentiate OCD plus a comorbid psychotic disorder, which may have a relatively poor outcome, from delusional OCD, which may be more similar to OCD with insight and without comorbid psychosis.

Retrospective follow-up studies that have examined the subsequent development of schizophrenia in patients with OCD have had varying results, with rates ranging from 0.7% to as high as 12.3% (Pollitt 1957, Ingram 1961, Kringlin 1965, Lo 1967, Rosenberg 1968, Rudin 1953, Muller 1953, Welner et al. 1976). These studies are, however, methodologically limited in which none were prospective, diagnoses were made by chart review, and standardized diagnostic criteria were not used, which probably resulted in the inclusion of affective psychoses. In reviewing this literature, Goodwin and colleagues (1969) concluded that people with OCD were at no greater risk for developing schizophrenia than the general population.

Conversely, studies of patients with schizophrenia or schizoaffective disorder have found rates of OCD ranging from 8 to 46% (Eisen et al. 1997a, Porto et al. 1997, Berman et al. 1995). This strikingly large range is most likely due to the OCD criteria used (i.e., subclinical OCD symptoms versus OCD symptoms severe enough to cause significant impairment or distress). Regardless, it is clear that a significant number of people with schizophrenia have OCD symptoms which require assessment and may benefit from treatment.

The relationship between OCD and personality disorders, particularly obsessive–compulsive personality disorder (OCPD), has received considerable attention. Early observations noted the presence of OCPD traits in patients with OCD (Lewis 1936). Systematic studies have yielded inconsistent findings. In a study of 96 subjects with OCD that used the Structured Clinical Interview for DSM-III personality disorders (SCID), 36 had a personality disturbance that met criteria for one or more personality disorders (Baer et al. 1990). Dependent (N = 12), histrionic (N = 9), and obsessive–compulsive (N = 6) personality disorders were most frequent. However, a study that used the Diagnostic and Statistical Manual of Mental Disorders, Third Edition, Revised (DSM-III-R) criteria found that OCPD was present in 25 of 59 subjects with OCD; the higher rate of OCPD found with the DSM-III-R criteria may reflect changes in the criteria set between DSM-III and DSM-III-R. A recent study of the rate of OCPD in first-degree relatives of OCD probands found a similar frequency of OCPD in people with OCD. OCPD occurred in 32% of the probands and was twice as frequent in the relatives of OCD probands as in relatives of control probands (Samuels et al. 2000), suggesting that OCPD may share a common familial etiology with OCD.

Although personality disorders are considered to be stable over time, one study found that of 17 OCD patients with a personality disorder, 9 of the 10 treatment responders no longer met criteria for either avoidant or dependent personality disorder after successful pharmacotherapy, raising the question of whether these personality disorders actually represented a coping style in response to OCD (Ricciardi et al. 1992).

## Differential Diagnosis

OCD is sometimes difficult to distinguish from certain other disorders. Obsessions and compulsions may appear in the context of other syndromes, which can raise the question whether the obsessions and compulsions are a symptom of another disorder or whether both OCD and another disorder are present (see section on Comorbidity). A general guideline is that if the content of the obsessions is not limited to the focus of concern of another disorder (e.g., an appearance concern, as in body dysmorphic disorder, or food concerns, as in an eating disorder) and if the obsessions or compulsions are preoccupying as well as distressing or impairing, OCD should generally be diagnosed.

Diagnostic dilemmas may also arise when it is unclear whether certain thoughts are obsessions or whether, instead, they are ordinary worries, ruminations, overvalued ideas, or delusions. In a similar vein, questions may develop about whether certain behaviors constitute true compulsions or whether they should instead be conceptualized as impulses, tics, or addictive behaviors.

## Obsessive–Compulsive Disorder Versus Other Anxiety Disorders

Both OCD and the other anxiety disorders are characterized by the use of avoidance to manage anxiety. However, OCD is distinguished from these disorders by the presence of compulsions. For OCD patients with preoccupying fears or worries but no rituals, several other features may be useful in establishing the diagnosis of OCD. In social phobia and specific phobia, fears are circumscribed and related to specific triggers (in specific phobia) or social situations (in social phobia). Although circumscribed situations may initially trigger obsessions and compulsions in OCD, triggers in OCD become more generalized over time, unlike the triggers in social and specific phobias, in which the evoking situations remain circumscribed.

As many as 60% of people with OCD experience full-blown panic symptoms. However, unlike panic disorder, in which panic attacks occur spontaneously, panic symptoms occur in OCD only during exposure to specific feared triggers such as contaminated objects. The worries that are present in generalized anxiety disorder (GAD) are more ego syntonic and involve an exaggeration of ordinary concerns, whereas the obsessional thinking of OCD is more intrusive, is limited to a specific set of concerns (e.g., contamination, blasphemy), and usually has an irrational, senseless, or unreasonable quality. Also, whereas the worry of GAD is considered primarily thoughtlike in nature, obsessional symptoms may consist of thoughts, impulses, or images.

## Obsessive–Compulsive Disorder Versus Psychotic Disorders

One question is how to differentiate OCD from psychotic disorders such as schizophrenia and delusional disorder. Another question is how to distinguish OCD with insight from OCD without insight (delusional OCD). One distinguishing feature between OCD and the psychotic disorders is that the latter are not characterized by prominent ritualistic behaviors. If compulsions are present in a patient with prominent psychotic symptoms, the possibility of a comorbid OCD diagnosis should be considered. Furthermore, although schizophrenia may be characterized by obsessional thinking, other characteristic features of the disorder, such as prominent hallucinations or thought disorder, are also present. With regard to delusional disorder, paranoid and grandiose concerns are generally not considered to fall under the OCD rubric. However, some other types of delusional disorder, such as the somatic and jealous types, seem to bear a close resemblance to OCD and are not always easily distinguished from it. It will be interesting to see whether future research indicates that certain types of somatic delusional disorder (e.g., the delusional variant of hypochondriasis) and the jealous type of delusional disorder (also referred to as pathological jealousy) are actually variants of OCD.

The second issue noted above—how to distinguish OCD with insight from OCD without insight—is complex. As previously discussed, insight in OCD is increasingly being recognized as spanning a spectrum from good to poor to absent. Both clinical observations and research findings indicate that some individuals hold their obsessional concerns with delusional intensity and believe that their concerns are reasonable. In DSM-IV, delusional OCD may be double-coded as both OCD and delusional disorder or as both OCD and psychotic disorder not otherwise specified, in other words, patients with delusional OCD would receive both diagnoses. This double coding reflects the fact that it is unclear whether OCD with insight and OCD without insight constitute the same or different disorders. Further research using validated scales to assess insight in OCD is needed to shed light on this question.

## Obsessive–Compulsive Disorder Versus Impulse Control Disorders

Differential diagnosis questions have been raised with regard to kleptomania, trichotillomania, pathological gambling, and other disorders involving impulsive behaviors. Several features have been said to distinguish these disorders from OCD. For example, compulsions—unlike behaviors of the impulse control disorders—generally have no gratifying element, although they do diminish anxiety. In addition, the affective state that drives the behaviors associated with these disorders may differ. In OCD, fear is frequently the underlying drive that leads to compulsions, which, in turn, decrease anxiety. In the impulse control disorders, patients frequently describe heightened tension, but not fear, preceding an impulsive behavior. However, OCD and the impulse control disorders have some features in common (McElroy et al. 1993). Research is ongoing to explore the relationship between OCD and the impulse control disorders by examining similarities and differences in treatment response, biological markers, and familial transmission.

## Obsessive–Compulsive Disorder Versus Tourette's Disorder

Complex motor tics of Tourette's disorder may be difficult to distinguish from OCD compulsions. Both tics and compulsions are preceded by an intrusive urge and are followed by feelings of relief. However, OCD compulsions are usually preceded by both anxiety and obsessional concerns, whereas, in Tourette's disorder, the urge to perform a tic is not preceded by an obsessional fear. This distinction breaks down to some extent when considering the "just right" perceptions of some patients with OCD (Leckman et al. 1994). The "just right" perception refers to the need to perform a certain motor action, such as touching, tapping, checking, ordering, arranging, or counting, until it feels right. Determining when an action has been performed enough or perfectly may depend on tactile, visual, or auditory perceptions. In a study of patients with Tourette's disorder and OCD symptoms, most patients could distinguish between the mental urge to do something repeatedly until it felt right and a physical urge to perform a motor tic. However, it is sometimes difficult for psychiatrists to distinguish between complex tics and compulsions, especially when a patient has both disorders (Miguel et al. 1995).

## Obsessive–Compulsive Disorder Versus Hypochondriasis

Fears of illness that occur in OCD, referred to as somatic obsessions, may be difficult to distinguish from hypochondriasis. Usually, however, patients with somatic obsessions have other current or past classic OCD obsessions unrelated to illness concerns. Patients with OCD also often engage in classic OCD rituals, such as checking or reassurance seeking, in an attempt to diminish their illness concerns. Unlike patients with OCD, patients with hypochondriasis experience somatic and visceral sensations. Although insight and resistance have been used to distinguish OCD from hypochondriasis, with the concern in hypochondriasis being said to be egosyntonic (realistic and totally justified) and that of OCD to be egodystonic (unacceptable and undesirable thoughts, actions, or both), studies have demonstrated a range of insight in OCD. Attempting to differentiate these disorders by degree of insight or egosyntonicity may therefore be of limited usefulness.

## Obsessive–Compulsive Disorder Versus Body Dysmorphic Disorder

Body dysmorphic disorder (BDD), a preoccupation with an imagined or slight defect in appearance (e.g., thinning hair, facial scarring, or a large nose), has many similarities to OCD (Phillips 1991). Patients with BDD experience obsessional thinking about the supposed defect and usually engage in associated repetitive ritualistic behaviors, such as mirror checking and reassurance seeking. Preliminary evidence suggests that BDD also appears similar to OCD in terms of age of onset, course of illness, and other variables (Phillips et al. 1995). Nonetheless, emerging data suggest that there are some important differences between the two disorders (Phillips et al. 1998), and they are currently classified separately in DSM-IV. Insight, for example, is more frequently impaired in BDD than in OCD (Eisen et al. 1997b). If the content of a patient's obsessions involves a concern about a supposed defect in appearance, BDD, rather than OCD, is the diagnosis that should be given.

## Obsessive–Compulsive Disorder Versus Obsessive–Compulsive Personality Disorder

Obsessive–compulsive personality disorder is a lifelong maladaptive personality style characterized by perfectionism, excessive attention to detail, indecisiveness, rigidity, excessive devotion to work, restricted affect, lack of generosity, and hoarding. OCD and OCPD have historically been considered variants of the same disorder on a continuum of severity, with OCD viewed as the more severe manifestation of illness. Contrary to this notion, studies using structured interviews to establish diagnosis have found that not all patients with OCD also have OCPD. One reason for the perception that these disorders are linked lies in the frequency of several OCPD traits in patients with OCD. In one study, the majority of 114 patients with OCD had perfectionism and indecisiveness (82 and 70, respectively). In contrast, other OCPD traits, such as restricted affect, excessive devotion to work, and rigidity, were seen infrequently.

Although perfectionism and indecisiveness are relatively common traits in patients with OCD, the distinction between OCD and OCPD is important, and several guidelines may be useful in distinguishing them. Unlike OCPD, OCD is characterized by distressing, time-consuming egodystonic obsessions and repetitive rituals aimed at diminishing the distress engendered by obsessional thinking. One of the hallmarks that traditionally has been used to distinguish OCD from OCPD is that, in contrast, OCPD features are considered egosyntonic. In addition, as previously noted, the traits of restricted affect, excessive devotion to work, and rigidity are generally characteristic of OCPD but not OCD. Although useful, these guidelines are not absolute, and some patients defy easy categorization. Some

patients, for example, spend hours each day engaged in egosyntonic behaviors such as excessive cleaning; such patients may seek treatment not because they are disturbed by their behaviors but because the behaviors cause problems in functioning or family friction. It is unclear whether some of these patients should be diagnosed with OCPD or subthreshold OCD.

## Obsessive–Compulsive Spectrum Disorders

Certain disorders other than OCD—such as BDD, hypochondriasis, and eating disorders—are characterized by obsessional thinking and/or ritualistic behaviors. On the basis of these apparent similarities with OCD, the concept of OCD spectrum disorders has been developed. They have been defined as disorders that share features with OCD (Hollander 1993) and are posited to have "spectrum membership" on the basis of their similarities with OCD across multiple domains. These domains include not only symptoms but also treatment response, comorbidity, joint familial loading, sex ratio, age at onset, course, premorbid personality characteristics, and presumed cause. Cause is inferred from characteristics such as neurological deficits, response to biological challenges, biochemical indices, brain imaging patterns (functional and anatomical), and epidemiological risk factors. It is worth noting that there are currently no operational criteria for what constitutes an OCD spectrum disorder (Phillips et al. 1995; McElroy 1994); for example, in which of the preceding domains must similarities be documented, and how similar in each domain must the disorder be to OCD?

Disorders postulated to be OCD spectrum disorders include BDD, hypochondriasis, eating disorders, "grooming" disorders such as nail biting and trichotillomania, and the impulse disorders (Hollander 1993, Thiel et al. 1995; see Figure 68–3). Of interest is a recent study investigating the frequency of these disorders in first-degree relatives of people with OCD. BDD, hypochondriasis, any eating disorder (although not anorexia or bulimia individually), and

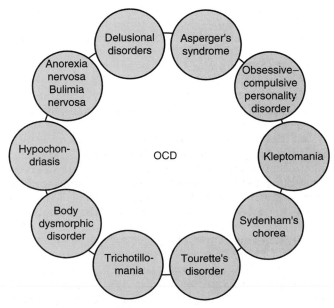

**Figure 68–3** *OCD spectrum disorders.*

grooming disorders (but not the impulse control disorders) were found more frequently in probands with OCD than in general population controls. In addition, BDD and grooming disorders (although not the other disorders) were significantly more common in the first-degree relatives of OCD probands than in relatives of controls (Bienvenu et al. 2000). This finding suggests that certain of the proposed OCD spectrum disorders may have a familial link to OCD. The relationship of these disorders with OCD is an area in which exciting research will be conducted in coming years.

## Etiology and Pathophysiology

A number of intriguing avenues have been investigated to determine the etiology and pathophysiology of OCD. Although our understanding of what causes this disorder has continued to grow, there is still much to learn. It is likely that OCD is caused by a complex interaction of factors rather than a single defect. However, for the purpose of clarity, these factors are described separately.

## Genetic Factors

A number of approaches have been used to evaluate the role of heredity in OCD. Twin studies have examined rates of concordant monozygotic twins versus discordant monozygotic twins with OCD. A review of this literature reveals a concordance rate of 63% in monozygotic twins (Rasmussen and Tsuang 1986). Although these studies have methodological limitations (e.g., a lack of a comparison group consisting of dizygotic twins), the data do support the notion that genetic factors are implicated in the expression of OCD. Given the concordance rate of less than 100% in monozygotic twins, it is clear that environment also plays a role in OCD's phenotypic expression.

A second approach to examining the role of genetics in OCD has been to investigate the rate of OCD in family members of OCD probands. A number of studies before 1988 found increased frequency of OCD in family members (McKeon and Murray 1987). However, it is difficult to interpret these findings because the studies were hampered by several methodological limitations, including a lack of direct assessment of family members and a lack of consistent OCD criteria, structured interviews, or a control group. Several subsequent studies that used considerably improved methodology (Pauls et al. 1995, Lenane et al. 1990, Fyer et al. 1993, Riddle et al. 1990, Black et al. 1992) interviewed first-degree relatives of adult OCD probands using structured interviews; a control group was used in two of these studies (Pauls et al. 1995, Black et al. 1992). Pauls and associates (1995), in their study of 446 first-degree relatives of 100 OCD probands, found that 10.3% of these subjects had full OCD, and 7.9% had subthreshold OCD. These rates were significantly higher than rates in control group relatives (1.9% had OCD, and 2% had subthreshold OCD). In two other family studies, an increased frequency of familial OCD was found in families in which the proband had an early age of OCD onset, before age 14 years (Bellodi et al. 1992) and 18 years (Nestadt et al. 2000).

Further evidence supporting familial transmission of OCD has been obtained by studying the frequency of OCD in relatives of patients with Gilles de la Tourette's Syndrome (TS). In a number of studies of TS patients, the frequency of obsessive–compulsive symptoms was much higher (40%) than that predicted by general population rates (Pauls et al. 1995). Family studies have similarly found higher rates of OCD symptoms among family members of TS patients (Pauls et al. 1986) as well as higher rates of Tourette's disorder and tics in first-degree relatives of children with OCD (Leonard et al. 1992). In addition, as previously noted, there are differences in the types of OCD symptoms seen in patients with TS plus OCD versus those with OCD alone. Moreover, it has been found that even among those OCD patients who do not have TS, if they share the TS/OCD symptom cluster (checking and ordering), they are more likely to have a positive family history for OCD. This may imply that there are distinct subtypes of OCD, some of which are familial and some of which are not (Eapen et al. 1997). Taken together, available data support familial transmission in some cases of OCD and suggest that genetic factors play an important role in its etiology, particularly in patients with comorbid tic disorder. Thus, in recent years a molecular genetics approach has begun to be applied to OCD, although there have been not significant findings to date. Segregation analysis, which would help to establish patterns of disease transmission, has revealed only that it is unlikely that OCD is a single gene disease (Pauls 1999). Association studies with candidate genes have focused mostly on the serotonin and dopamine systems, since medications treating OCD and TS are known to involve these systems. However, these studies have not yielded any significant consistently positive results (Nicolini et al. 1999, Pato et al. 2002). Nonetheless, as the technology improves and a better understanding of OCD's etiology and subtypes is gained, these genetics analyses could prove more fruitful.

## Neurobiological Factors

### Neuroanatomical Aspects

Brain imaging techniques have advanced the search for abnormalities in brain functioning and/or structure in patients with OCD. Numerous studies have now been done with both structural imaging—CT (computed tomography) and MRI (magnetic resonance imaging) (Szeszko et al. 1999, Robinson et al. 1995)—and functional imaging—PET (positron emission tomography), SPECT (single photon emission computed tomography), fMRI (functional magnetic resonance imaging), and MRS (magnetic resonance spectroscopy). These techniques have demonstrated abnormalities in OCD patients (Saxena et al. 1998, Cottraux and Gerard 1998). These abnormalities occur at rest and with symptom provocation (Rauch et al. 1994, Brieter et al. 1996), and they are "normalized" with effective treatment (Baxter et al. 1992, Benkelfat et al. 1990, Hoehn-Saric et al. 1991, Swedo et al. 1992).

While not all results are in agreement, a majority of these studies have implicated abnormalities in the orbitofrontal cortex, anterior cingulate cortex, and structures of the basal ganglia and thalamus. These structures are proposed to be linked in neuroanatomical circuits (Insel 1992, Baxter 1992). One well-articulated model by Saxena and colleagues (1998) proposes that OCD symptoms are mediated by hyperactivity in orbitofrontal–subcortical circuits, which might be due to an imbalance in tone between direct and indirect striato–pallidal pathways (Baxter et al. 1987,

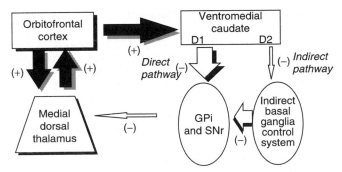

**Figure 68–4** *Model of OCD pathophysiology: Imbalance of direct >> indirect pathway "tone" in orbitofrontal–subcortical circuit. GPi = Globus Pallidus interna; SNr = Substantia Nigra. (Source: Saxena S, Brody AL, Schwartz JM, et al. [1998] Neuroimaging and frontal–subcortical circuitry in obsessive–compulsive disorder. Br J Psychiatr 173[Suppl 35], 26–37.)*

1988, Nordahl et al. 1989, Swedo et al. 1989b, Saxena et al. 1998) (see Figure 68–4). Some studies have implicated a preferential role for right anterolateral orbitofrontal cortex in both OCD symptoms and symptom response. This view has neurocognitive implications because studies of executive function in OCD patients have shown that patients have difficulty with alternation tasks and tasks that involve making choices (Gold et al. 1996, Cavedini et al. 2001, Gehring et al. 2000). A number of treatment studies (see later) with clomipramine, fluoxetine, paroxetine, and cognitive behavioral therapy (CBT) have shown a decrease in caudate glucose metabolism with successful treatment (Saxena et al. 1998).

Further indirect evidence implicating a role for basal ganglia dysfunction in OCD lies in the clinical relationship between neurological insults to the basal ganglia and the subsequent development of obsessions and compulsions. There is an association between OCD and Tourette's disorder, Sydenham's chorea, bilateral necrosis of the globus pallidus, and postencephalitic parkinsonian symptoms.

## Neurochemical Aspects

The hypothesis that OCD involves an abnormality in the serotonin neurotransmitter system has been called the serotonin hypothesis. Several different lines of investigation support this hypothesis: (1) therapeutic response of patients to chronic administration of medication, (2) measurements of central and peripheral neurotransmitter or metabolite concentration, and (3) pharmacologic challenge paradigms which measure behavioral and neuroendocrine effects produced by acute administration of selective pharmacologic agents (Pigott 1996).

All the evidence from treatment studies point to a role for serotonin and speak of a need for prolonged administration to see a positive effect. All of the antidepressants that effectively treat OCD affect serotonin (Greist et al. 1995b). These antidepressants are potent inhibitors of the presynaptic reuptake of serotonin (i.e., SRIs). Those antidepressants that primarily affect the noradrenergic system have not been found to have antiobsessional properties. Exactly how the SRIs improve OCD symptoms remains unclear; while the immediate action of these agents may be to increase serotonin in the synapse, they undoubtably cause a cascade of changes, both presynaptically and post-

synaptically. A number of studies have examined the relationship between SRI blood levels and improvement in OCD, with inconsistent results. One study found that clinical improvement correlated with blood levels of clomipramine (which specifically affects serotonin) but not desmethylclomipramine (an active metabolite of clomipramine that affects both noradrenergic and serotoninergic systems; Insel et al. 1983). However, this finding has not been consistently replicated (Thoren et al. 1980, Flament et al. 1987).

Decreased levels of cerebrospinal 5-hydroxyindoleacetic acid, a serotonin metabolite that is reduced with serotonin reuptake inhibition, have been correlated with clinical improvement after clomipramine treatment (Thoren et al. 1980). A decrease in platelet serotonin levels—an indirect measure of neuronal reuptake—has been highly correlated with clinical improvement with clomipramine ($r = 0.77$; Flament et al. 1987). These various studies—measures of plasma levels of SRIs, metabolite concentration, and serotonin platelet concentration—generally support the association between improvement of OCD with an SRI and acute alterations of serotonin in the brain and, in turn, support the serotonin hypothesis. Figure 68–5 shows a serotonin synapse with several of the possible sites of action for drugs that alter OCD symptoms.

Pharmacologic challenge studies constitute yet another line of evidence supporting the role of serotonin in the pathophysiology of OCD. The serotonin receptor partial agonist *m*-chlorophenylpiperazine has been shown to increase symptoms of OCD and anxiety in patients with OCD but to have no effect in normal control subjects (Zohar et al. 1987, Hollander et al. 1992). The increase in obsessions can be blocked with pretreatment by the serotonin receptor antagonist metergoline (Pigott et al. 1991) or by chronic treatment with clomipramine (Zohar et al 1988). However, results with *m*-chlorophenylpiperazine have been contradictory (Charney et al. 1988, Pigott et al. 1993), which may reflect methodological issues or the fact that this agent has complex effects on multiple receptors. Challenge studies with other serotonergic agents have not implicated serotonin in the pathophysiology of OCD. For example, no behavioral or neuroendocrine changes were found after administration of fenfluramine, a serotonin-releasing and reuptake-blocking agent (Hewlett and Martin 1993), or after administration of tryptophan, a serotonin precursor that increases serotonin synthesis (Barr et al. 1994), which differs from findings in depression (Delgado and Moreno 1998). It is unclear whether these negative findings are attributable to methodological limitations or constitute evidence against the serotonin hypothesis.

Although available data are not entirely consistent, on balance there is now substantial evidence implicating serotonin in the pathophysiology of OCD. However, the exact role of this neurotransmitter and whether it is involved in the etiology, or is instead part of a final common pathway, of this disorder remains unclear.

The role of the dopamine system in OCD's pathophysiology has also been investigated (Goodman et al. 1990). When added to the SRIs, dopamine antagonists (neuroleptic agents) decrease symptoms of OCD in patients with OCD and comorbid tics, as well as in patients with OCD and comorbid schizotypal personality disorder. It has been

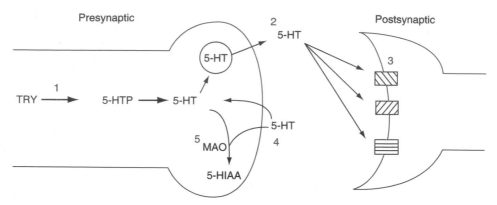

**Figure 68–5** *Diagram of a serotonin (5-HT) synapse describes several of the possible sites of action for drugs that alter OCD symptoms. At (1) the rate-limiting step in serotonin synthesis, L-tryptophan (TRY) is hydroxylated to 5-hydroxytryptophan (5-HTP). After serotonin is formed, it is sequestered into vesicles that are released at the presynaptic cell membrane (2). Fenfluramine increases this release. Once released, serotonin can interact with a number of different postsynaptic receptors (3). Several selective agonists (buspirone, m-chlorophenylpiperazine) have been developed to activate each of these serotonin receptor subtypes. Metergoline is a nonselective antagonist, blocking serotonin effects at each of these sites. The inactivation of serotonin is mediated by reuptake (4), the step inhibited by clomipramine, fluvoxamine, and fluoxetine. Finally (5), serotonin is either metabolized to its metabolite, 5-hydroxyindoleacetic acid (5-HIAA), by the enzyme monoamine oxidase (MAO), or recycled back into vesicles for release. (Source: Insel TR and Winslow JT [1990] Neurobiology of obsessive–compulsive disorder. In Obsessive–Compulsive Disorders: Theory and Management, 2nd ed, Jenike MA, Baer L, and Minichiello WE [eds]. Mosby Year Book, St. Louis, Missouri, p. 118.)*

hypothesized that some forms of OCD, particularly OCD plus Tourette's disorder, may involve an imbalance in activity between serotonergic and dopaminergic systems (Goodman et al. 1990a, Stein et al. 1997, Saxena et al. 1996, McDougle et al. 2000, Koran et al. 2000).

Given the complex interactions and overlap among monoaminergic and other receptors in the brain, it is likely that a number of neurotransmitters are involved in OCD's pathophysiology and etiology. Drawing from these rather conflicting results, Baumgarten and Grozdanovic (1998) propose that serotonergic projections from the mesotelencephalon may be secondarily involved in the disease process through primary derangements of orbitofronto/cingulostriatal projection systems, areas that have already been implicated in neuroimaging studies (see above and Figure 68–4). It is these orbitofronto/cingulo-striatal projections that are involved in adapting behavior to changing external demands and internal emotional status, a core problem in OCD, and which feed back onto the monoaminergic midbrain nuclei. Thus the effect of long-term treatment with SRIs is probably several: to change the ratio of dopamine to serotonin turnover, alter the gene expression of target neurons to stress-related neuropeptides, and decrease the sensitivity of subtypes of presynaptic serotonin auto- and heteroceptors belonging to the $5-HT_1$ receptor family. Ongoing research is expected to elucidate further the likely role of serotonin and the possible role of other neurotransmitters in OCD.

## Animal Models

Animal models may provide an important window on treatment efficacy and the influence of environmental and genetic factors in OCD. Because of the inherent difficulties in studying cognitive aspects of OCD (such as guilt, overresponsibility, and doubt) in animals, attention has focused on repetitive motor actions that are similar to compulsions. Ethologists have observed that when specific, goal-directed actions are thwarted, animals may substitute unrelated behaviors, known as displacement behaviors, which frequently involve digging, pecking, or grooming (Tinbergen 1953). These motor actions have several elements: they are triggered by conflict over territory or by frustration, they continue in a stereotyped fashion, and they are excessive and/or inappropriate to the context in which they are performed. Thus, they are similar to the compulsive behaviors of OCD. Pharmacologic challenges may provide further evidence to support the idea that displacement behaviors are useful analogues to OCD compulsions. Some preliminary evidence, for example, indicates that clomipramine diminishes grooming displacement behavior in rats, whereas treatment with an antidepressant that is not effective in combatting obsessional behavior (desipramine) does not (Winslow and Insel 1991).

Another animal model for OCD is acral lick disorder, in which dogs and cats groom themselves excessively, causing cutaneous lesions (Goldberger and Rapoport 1991). As in OCD, stress increases these excessive grooming behaviors. Of interest is the positive responsive of acral lick disorder to clomipramine, fluoxetine, and sertraline but not to placebo, which lends support to the hypothesis that this behavior represents an animal model of OCD (Rapoport et al. 1992).

Pitman (1991), in reviewing the OCD animal model literature, pointed out that a number of models implicate excessive dopaminergic activity in repetitive behaviors. For example, dopamine antagonists such as haloperidol decrease stereotyped behaviors in animals induced by amphetamine administration, stimulation, or stress. Others, like Dodman (1998) have pointed out that neostriatal structures (caudate nucleus and putamen) and limbic structures are important in habit learning and are also identified sites of dysfunction in OCD. If the previously described unbalanced neural circuitry model of OCD is correct, it could be postulated that in both humans and animals encrypted motor programming or cognitive/emotional programs in the basal ganglia and limbic regions could have abnormal feedback loops resulting in lack of knowledge about completion of a task or thought process, which is often the impetus for compulsive repetitive behavior (Dodman 1998). Animal models offer the advantage of accessibility and ease of manipulation for controlled trials and as such can play a valuable role in understanding OCD's etiology.

## Learning Theory

A model based on the psychological concept of conditioning has also been used to understand the development of obsessions and compulsions (Baer and Minichiello 1990). Compulsions, whether mental or observable, usually decrease the anxiety engendered by obsessional thoughts. Thus, if a person is preoccupied with fears of contamination from germs, repetitive hand washing usually decreases the anxiety caused by these fears. The compulsion becomes a conditioned response to anxiety. Because of the tension-reducing aspect of the compulsion, this learned behavior becomes reinforced and eventually fixed (Rachman and Hodgson 1980). Compulsions, in turn, actually reinforce anxiety because they prevent habituation from occurring; that is, by performing a compulsion, contact with the fear-evoking stimulus (e.g., dirt) is not maintained, and habituation (a decrease in fear associated with the stimulus) does not occur. Thus, the vicious circle linking obsessions and compulsions is maintained (Figure 68–6). This learning theory model of OCD has had a major influence on the way behavioral therapy is used in its treatment.

## Psychoanalytic Theory

Psychoanalytic theory is based on the concept that psychiatric symptoms have psychological meaning stemming from unconscious conflicts. In Freud's theory, themes of control, aggression, and autonomy are dominant during the anal period of development, which occurs during toilet training. Poorly resolved childhood struggles over control can result in conflicts over obedience and defiance. The unconscious conflict between passivity and aggression, or obedience and defiance, may lead to anxiety. The anxiety produced by these conflicts leads to the formation of obsessions and compulsions as well as the defenses of reaction formation, isolation, and undoing.

Much of the psychoanalytic literature on OCD does not distinguish between the phenomena observed in OCD (obsessions and compulsions) and the traits of OCPD (MacKinnon and Michels 1971). This distinction has relevance because of treatment implications. Although the clinical observations of earlier psychoanalysts, such as Freud's famous Ratman case (Freud 1963), reflect current clinical presentations of Axis I OCD, understanding symptoms from the psychoanalytic perspective have not yielded improvement in this disorder's symptoms. Conversely, char-

acterologic problems such as perfectionism, indecisiveness, and rigidity, seen in OCPD, may benefit from a psychoanalytic orientation that focuses on the meaning of these symptoms or traits; such traits have typically not responded well to medications alone, although further investigation of this question is needed.

Recent theory has attempted to integrate the biology of OCD with psychological models by proposing a phylogenetic model based on systems theory. In this model, behavioral inhibition and harm-assessment systems, which develop early in human phylogeny, are disrupted. This disruption can occur at a hierarchically primary level of biological organization, resulting in neurobiologic disturbance, or at a hierarchically higher level of organization, leading to psychological disturbances. Such a model can help to explain the diversity of symptoms seen in OCD, from the more primitive biologically based behaviors based on fight/flight and risk to more psychologically sophisticated behaviors involving morality and guilt. This model might also explain why neither biological or psychological treatments alone always lead to complete remission of symptoms (Cohen et al. 1997).

## Treatment

### General Considerations

Both pharmacologic and behavioral therapies have proved effective for OCD. The majority of controlled treatment trials have been performed with adults age 18 to 65 years. However, these therapies have been shown effective for patients of all ages. In general, children and the elderly tolerate most of these medications well. For children, lower doses are indicated because of lower body mass (Leonard et al. 1989, 1991, Flament et al. 1985). For instance, the recommended dose for clomipramine in children is up to 150 mg/day (3 mg/kg/day) versus 250 mg/day in adults. Use of lower doses should also be considered in the elderly because their decreased ability to metabolize medications can increase the risk of side effects and toxicity (Pato and Steketee 1997, Pato and Zohar 2001). Behavioral therapy has also been used successfully in all age groups, although when treating children with this modality it is usually advisable to use a parent as a cotherapist. A flowchart that outlines treatment options for OCD is shown in Figure 68–7.

In general, the goals of treatment are to reduce the frequency and intensity of symptoms as much as possible and to minimize the amount of interference the symptoms cause. It should be noted that few patients experience a cure or complete remission of symptoms. Instead, OCD should be viewed as a chronic illness with a waxing and waning course. Symptoms are often worse during times of psychosocial stress. Even when on medication, individuals with OCD are often upset when they experience even a mild symptom exacerbation, anticipating that their symptoms will revert to their worst, which is rarely the case. Anticipating with the patient that stress may make the symptoms worse can often be helpful in long-term treatment. Expert consensus guidelines, based on completion of a survey by 79 experts in the field, provide a reasonable approach to clinical practice in treating patients with OCD. However like any consensus report, based on clinical practice, not all of the

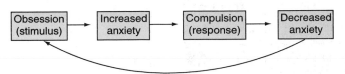

**Figure 68–6** *Learning theory of OCD.*

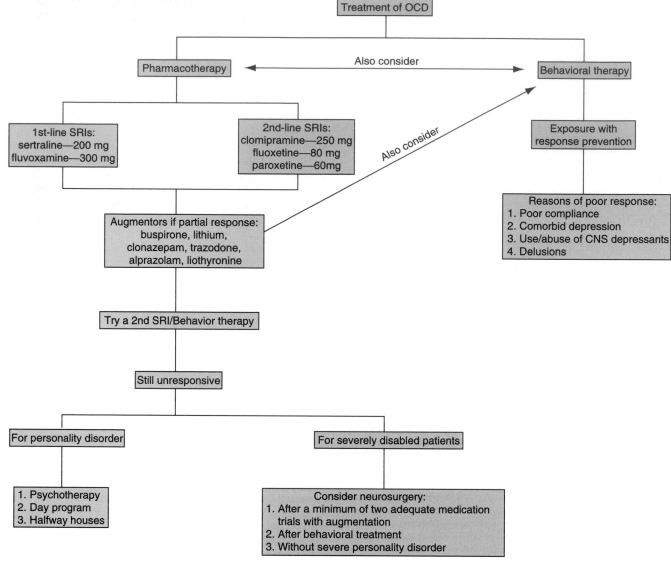

**Figure 68–7** *Flowchart of treatment options for OCD.*

recommendations are supported by empirical data (March et al. 1997). Further work in neurosurgical techniques, particularly less invasive approaches like gamma knife (Lippitz et al. 1999, Jenike 1998) and possibly transmagnetic stimulation may offer other options in the future for treating OCD (Greenberg et al. 1997) (see later).

## Pharmacological Treatments

The most extensively studied agents for OCD are medications that affect the serotonin system (see Figure 68–5). Many studies implicate the serotonin system in OCD's pathophysiology, although comparative studies also seem to implicate other neurotransmitter systems, including the dopaminergic system, in treatment response (Greist et al. 1995b, Goodman et al. 1990). The principal pharmacologic agents used to treat OCD are the SRIs, which include clomipramine, fluoxetine, fluvoxamine, sertraline, paroxetine, and citalopram.

Outcome measures in OCD treatment trials generally include the Yale-Brown Obsessive–Compulsive Scale (Y-BOCS; Goodman et al. 1989a,c), a reliable and valid 10-item, 40-point semi-structured instrument that assesses the severity of obsessions and rituals during the preceding week. Studies conducted since 1989 have generally used the Y-BOCS as one of the major outcome measures. Most studies have used Y-BOCS scores of 16 to 20 as a study entry criterion, although it has been argued that higher scores (e.g., 20–21) might reduce the increasing placebo response rates being obtained in OCD studies (Greist et al. 1995). Treatment response is generally considered to constitute at least a 25 to 35% reduction in OCD symptoms as measured by the Y-BOCS (Goodman et al. 1993). Another frequently used global outcome measure is the National Institute of Mental Health Global Obsessive–Compulsive Scale (NIMH-OC) (Pato et al. 1994) (Clinical Vignette 2).

### Clomipramine

The tricyclic antidepressant clomipramine is among the most extensively studied pharmacological agents in OCD. This drug is unique among the antiobsessional agents in which in addition to its potency as an SRI, it has significant affinity for noradrenergic, dopaminergic, muscarinic, and histaminic receptors. An extensive review of all double-blind trials of clomipramine in OCD is included in the 1991 report of The Clomipramine Collaborative Study Group (1991). The largest double-blind placebo-controlled trial of clomipramine in OCD was conducted by this group, with 520 patients at 21 sites. Both outcome measures, the Y-BOCS and the NIMH-OC, demonstrated a significant decrease in the severity of OCD symptoms in the group receiving clomipramine compared to the placebo group. Duration of treatment was 10 weeks, and the mean dose was approximately 200 mg/day, with 69% of patients taking 150 to 250 mg/day. About half (51–60%) of the patients receiving clomipramine experienced a 35% or greater reduction in symptoms as measured by the Y-BOCS, whereas only 7 to 7.5% of the placebo group had a similar response. The most common side effects were those typical of the tricyclic antidepressants, including dry mouth, dizziness, tremor, fatigue, somnolence, constipation, nausea, increased sweating, headache, mental cloudiness, and sexual dysfunction. Previous data have indicated that at doses of 300 mg/day or more, the risk of seizures is 2.1% (DeVeaugh-Geiss et al. 1989), but at doses of 250 mg/day or less, the risk of seizures is low (0.48%) and comparable to that of other tricyclic antidepressants. It is therefore recommended that doses of 250 mg/day or less be used. Elderly patients may be more prone to tricyclic side effects, such as orthostatic hypotension, constipation (which may lead to fecal impaction), forgetfulness, and mental cloudiness, which might be confused with dementia. Most of these side effects can be treated by simply lowering the dose, although the cardiac conduction effects of tricyclic antidepressants may preclude the use of clomipramine in patients with preexisting cardiac conduction problems, especially atrioventricular block.

Recent studies of IV clomipramine have been particularly promising because it seems to have a quicker onset of action and fewer side effects than the oral form, and it may be effective even in patients who do not respond to oral clomipramine. Oral clomipramine, like other SRIs, usually takes a minimum of 4 to 6 weeks to produce a clinically significant clinical response, but in at least one study by Koran, in which he used IV pulse dosing, patients showed a response within 4.5 days (Koran et al. 1997, Fallon et al. 1998). The reasons for this unique response are not fully understood, but it is postulated that the IV preparation avoids first-pass hepatoenteric metabolism, leading to increased bioavailability of the parent compound clomipramine. This in turn may play a role in rapidly desensitizing serotonergic receptors or initiating changes in postsynaptic serotonergic neurons. Although studies of IV clomipramine for obsessional states date as far back as 1973 (Walter 1973); this preparation is still not FDA-approved for clinical use in the US. Cardiac monitoring is recommended during the use of IV clomipramine.

## Fluoxetine

Fluoxetine (as well as fluvoxamine, sertraline, paroxetine, and citalopram) is often referred to as an selective serotonin reuptake inhibitor (SSRI) and sometimes as serotonin transport inhibitor (STI) (Greist et al. 1995b) because they have a far more potent effect on serotonergic than on noradrenergic or other neurotransmitter systems. Despite their different chemical structures, all of the SSRIs appear to have similar efficacy in treating OCD (Greist et al. 1995b).

Fluoxetine was first marketed in the US in 1987 for the treatment of depression, and was the first available SSRI in this country. Initially, on the basis of fluoxetine's selectivity for serotonin receptors, researchers were hopeful that this medication would be more efficacious than clomipramine, which has affinity for cholinergic, adrenergic, and histaminic receptors in addition to serotonergic ones (Rapoport et al. 1980). Although open trials (Turner et al. 1985, Jenike et al. 1989, Liebowitz et al. 1989, Levine et al. 1989) and fixed-dose double-blind trials (Wood et al. 1993, Tollefson et al. 1994b) have borne out the efficacy of fluoxetine for OCD, it has not been shown to be more effective than clomipramine (Greist et al. 1995b, Pigott et al. 1990).

The fixed-dose trials of fluoxetine are particularly noteworthy (Tollefson et al. 1994a, 1994b) because there are few published fixed-dose trials with any of the antiobsessional agents in OCD. Although these studies indicated that doses of 20, 40, and 60 mg/day were all effective when compared with placebo, there was a trend toward 60 mg/day being more effective. Some patients who did not respond at lower doses responded at higher doses, and others who responded at lower doses showed increased improvement at a higher dose (Wood et al. 1993, Tollefson et al. 1994a). In addition, patients maintained their improvement or experienced increased improvement during the 5- to 6-month follow-up period (Tollefson et al. 1994a, Levine et al. 1989).

Fluoxetine has fewer side effects than clomipramine, reflecting its more selective mechanism of action. The most common side effects are headache, nausea, insomnia, anorexia, dry mouth, somnolence, nervousness, tremor, and diarrhea. Side effects occur more frequently at higher doses (Tollefson et al. 1994b). Fluoxetine's long half-life, which is unique among the SRIs, is 2 to 4 days for the parent compound and 4 to 16 days for its active metabolite (Pato et al. 1991a, Devane 1994). This long half-life can be beneficial for patients who do not comply with treatment, because relatively high steady-state levels are maintained even when several doses are missed. However, the long half-life can present problems when switching or discontinuing fluoxetine, because 5 weeks or more may be required for the medication to be completely cleared from the body. Hence the added delay, 5 weeks rather than 2 weeks for the other SRIs, is required when switching from fluoxetine to an MAOI.

## Fluvoxamine

Fluvoxamine became available for the treatment of OCD in the US in 1995. It is a unicyclic agent which differs from the other SSRIs in that it does not have an active metabolite. A number of systematic blinded clinical trials, most of which were placebo-controlled, have demonstrated fluvoxamine's effectiveness in treating OCD (Goodman et al. 1989b, Jenike et al. 1990b, Mallya et al. 1992). An additional study found fluvoxamine to be more effective than the tricyclic agent desipramine (Goodman et al. 1990b). Similar to other OCD trials, 52% of patients in the fluvoxamine group improved, whereas few patients responded to desipramine or placebo. All of these trials, except for one, were 8 to 10 weeks in duration; in the one briefer study (Goodman et al. 1989b), which lasted only 6 weeks, five of the nine responders moved from a partial response to a full response after an additional 2 weeks of treatment. As has been demonstrated for the other SSRIs, relatively long treatment trials are indicated before concluding that an SSRI is ineffective in OCD.

The largest and most recent fluvoxamine study (reviewed in Goodman et al. 1997) was a 10-week multicenter double-blind placebo-controlled study of 320 patients. The mean dose of fluvoxamine was 249 mg/day. As in the other studies, the fluvoxamine-treated patients had a significant reduction in OCD symptoms; however, unlike most of the earlier medication trials there was a relatively high placebo response rate of 11%. One of the important conclusions from this study was that prior failure to respond to another SSRI was associated with a lower likelihood of responding to fluvoxamine. Nonetheless, six of 31 patients in whom a previous trial of clomipramine or fluoxetine had failed did respond to fluvoxamine. Lack of response at 4 and 6 weeks did not predict response at 10 weeks, and the authors concluded that a full 10 weeks of treatment was needed to assess treatment response. This is an interesting finding in light of more recent data (Strauss et al. 1997) from a small sample of 8 patients, which showed through the use of 19F magnetic resonance spectroscopy, that steady state drug levels in the brain are achieved more quickly (within 1 month) with fluvoxamine than fluoxetine (the only other SRI measured in this way to date). Clinically, seven of the eight patients in the Strauss study, responded within this 1-month period. Such an early onset of response has not been seen as consistently in the larger treatment trials, but these study techniques deserve further exploration.

All of the fluvoxamine studies showed a similar side effect profile, which included insomnia, nervousness, fatigue, somnolence, nausea, headache, and sexual dysfunction (Goodman et al. 1989b, 1990b, 1997, Jenike et al. 1990, Mallya et al. 1992). Insomnia and nervousness tended to occur early in treatment, whereas fatigue and somnolence occurred later. Overall, the medication was well tolerated, with only 10 to 15% of patients dropping out of treatment because of side effects.

## Sertraline

Sertraline is a naphthalenamine derivative with an active metabolite, *n*-desmethylsertraline. Findings from a multicenter fixed-dose placebo-controlled study of 325 patients showed that sertraline was significantly more effective than placebo, with efficacy similar to that demonstrated for fluoxetine and fluvoxamine in other studies (Greist et al. 1995a, 1995b). There was a trend towards 200 mg/day being more effective than 50 mg/day or 100 mg/day. Similar to other SSRI trials, the dropout rate from adverse side effects was only 10%. Typical side effects included nausea, headache, diarrhea, insomnia, and dry mouth.

A more recent study compared sertraline to the non-SRI antidepressant desipramine for patients with OCD and comorbid depression. Although these medications were similarly efficacious for depression, sertraline was more effective for OCD symptoms, supporting the use of an SRI-like sertraline rather than a norepinephrine reuptake inhibitor like desipramine in such patients. In addition, even though desipramine did improve depressive symptoms, a significantly greater number of patients treated with sertraline achieved remission from depression (Hoehn-Saric et al. 2000).

## Paroxetine

Paroxetine is another SSRI that differs in structure from those previously discussed. It is a phenylpiperidine compound that is marketed as an antidepressant and that, like sertraline, shows promise in the treatment of OCD. Results of a fixed-dose multicenter trial of 348 patients indicated that paroxetine is effective for OCD. As was suggested in the sertraline study, higher doses (40 or 60 mg/day) may be needed because 20 mg/day was no more effective than placebo (Wheadon et al. 1993). Paroxetine's efficacy, as noted below, is comparable to that of other SRIs (Zohar and Judge 1996). Side effects are similar to those of other SSRIs and include lethargy, dry mouth, nausea, insomnia, somnolence, tremor, sexual dysfunction, and decreased appetite. Reports of an acute discontinuation syndrome, which can include general malaise, asthenia, dizziness, vertigo, headache, myalgia, loss of appetite, nausea, diarrhea, and abdominal cramps, warrant a gradual reduction in dose if this medication is to be discontinued (Barr et al. 1994b, Bryois et al. 1998, Domeinguez and Goodrick 1995, Keuthen et al. 1994). Occasional patients may experience some of these symptoms even if their dose is delayed by only a few hours.

## Citalopram

Citalopram is the newest SSRI available for the treatment of OCD. A bicyclic phthaline derivative with S (active) and R (inactive) enantiomers, it is unique in its selectivity for serotonin reuptake compared to the other SRIs. It has few significant secondary binding properties, and its minimal effect on hepatic metabolism probably makes it safer to combine with other medications. A multicenter fixed-dose placebo-controlled trial with 401 patients showed that 52 to 65% of patients responded in the three dosage groups compared to a 37% response rate in the placebo group. While there was a trend for a higher dose to lead to a higher response rate, as with other SRIs, there was no statistical difference between the three doses used (20, 40, and 60 mg/day). Typical side effects included fatigue, sweating, dry mouth, ejaculation failure, nausea, and insomnia, although many patients habituated to these side effects in 4 to 6 weeks. Thus, citalopram is a good choice for OCD treatment because of its side effect profile and low probability of causing drug–drug interactions (Montgomery et al. 2001, Richter 2001).

## Other Agents

Most studies of other medications for OCD have consisted of only case reports or small samples. One small trial suggested that venlafaxine, a medication which, like clomipramine, inhibits reuptake of both serotonin and norepinephrine, may hold some promise (Zajecka et al. 1990). Buspirone, which has partial 5-hydroxytryptamine-1A serotonin agonist properties, was effective in one small blinded study in which it was compared with clomipramine (Pato et al. 1991b); However, buspirone was ineffective in a small open trial (Jenike and Baer 1988). Trazodone appeared effective in several open trials (Lydiard 1986, Hermesh et al. 1990) but not in a controlled study (Pigott et al. 1992a). Several reports have suggested that MAOIs may be effective (Jenike et al. 1983, Jenike 1981, Dominguez and Mestre 1994). However, a more recent controlled study found that phenelzine was less efficacious than fluoxetine for OCD, although a subgroup of patients with symmetry obsessions responded to phenelzine (Jenike et al. 1997). Clonazepam appeared promising in a comparative study with clomipramine (Hewlett et al. 1992). However, few of these agents have been promising enough to warrant large blinded efficacy trials.

## Which SRI to Choose?

The efficacy of each SRI—clomipramine, fluoxetine, fluvoxamine, sertraline, paroxetine, and citalopram—is supported by existing data. During the last 10 years at least seven head-to-head SRI comparison studies have been done, six of which compared clomipramine to fluoxetine (Pigott et al. 1990, Lopez-Ibor et al. 1996), fluvoxamine (Freedman et al. 1994, Koran et al 1996), paroxetine (Zohar and Judge 1996), or sertraline (Bisserbe et al. 1997); one study compared fluvoxamine to both paroxetine and citalopram (Mundo et al. 1997). Except for the Bisserbe study (1997), the sample sizes were small, usually with 10 to 30 patients per group. All of the studies found that the agents studied were equally efficacious, although they may have been underpowered to detect differences among medications.

However, several meta-analyses (Jenike et al. 1990a, Greist et al. 1995, Griest and Jefferson 1998) of OCD trials, which compared SRIs across large placebo-controlled multicenter trials, lend some support to the notion that clomipramine might be more effective than the more selective agents. In a four-way (clomipramine, fluoxetine, fluvoxamine, and sertraline) meta-analysis, effect sizes were computed by comparing the average change in Y-BOCS scores pooled over various studies with different medications (Griest et al. 1995b). Clomipramine led to the largest effect sizes. However, like most meta-analyses, these studies are flawed by factors that include variations in the study protocol, sample size, and the number of treatment-resistant and treatment-naïve subjects. Nonetheless, as Griest and colleagues (1995b) point out, these differences cannot explain the fact that the clomipramine trial had a lower drop out rate (12% overall) (Griest and Jefferson 1998, Greist et al. 1995b) than other trials, despite a higher rate of side effects (e.g., 97% for clomipramine versus 57% for fluoxetine [Jenike et al. 1990a]). In conclusion, these meta-analyses support a trial of clomipramine in all patients who do not respond to SRIs, even though clomipiramine tends to cause more side effects.

A number of studies have assessed predictors of medication response. Predictors of poor response include failure to respond to a previous SRI, early age of OCD onset, presence of schizotypal personality disorder, and presence of hoarding. However, not all studies have had consistent findings, and more investigation of this issues is needed using larger and more narrowly defined samples. (Goodman et al. 1997, Stein et al. 2001, Mataix-Cois et al., 1999, Baer and Jenike 1992, Ravizza et al. 1995, Ackerman et al. 1994, Alonso et al. 2001, Eisen et al. 2001, Erzegovesi et al. 2001).

It is worth noting that the SSRIs, via their effect on the liver cytochrome system, can inhibit the metabolism of certain other drugs. Fluoxetine can elevate blood levels of a variety of coadministered drugs, including tricyclic antidepressants (such as clomipramine), carbamazepine, phenytoin, and trazodone (Devane 1994). However, the other SSRIs (with the exception of citalopram) can theoretically cause similar elevations, although fewer reports on such interactions are currently available. Some clinicians have taken advantage of these interactions by carefully combining fluvoxamine with clomipramine in order to block clomipramine's metabolism to desmethylclomipramine; this in turn favors serotonin reuptake inhibition provided by the parent compound rather than the norepinephrine reuptake inhibition provided by the metabolite. However, caution should be used with this approach since the elevation in clomipramine levels, and perhaps other compounds, can be nonlinear and quickly lead to dangerous toxicity (Szegedi et al. 1996); at the very least, clomipramine levels should be carefully monitored.

All of the SSRIs are generally well tolerated, with a relatively low percentage of patients experiencing notable side effects or discontinuing them because of side effects. In addition, these compounds are unlikely to be lethal in overdose, except for clomipramine, which can lead to cardiac arrhythmias and death. All these agents can cause sexual side effects, ranging from anorgasmia to difficultly with ejaculatory function. However such symptoms are not readily volunteered by the patient, thus it is important to ask. Should such symptoms be experienced, conservative measures may include dosage reduction, transient drug holidays for a special weekend or occasion, or switching to another SRI since patients may not have the same degree of dysfunction with a different agent. However if the clinician feels that it is critical to continue to same agent, various treatments have been reported in the literature. Usually taken within a few hours of sexual activity, no one agent has been shown to work consistently. Among those that have been tried are, yohimbine, buspirone, cyproheptadine, buproprion, dextroamphetamine, methylphenidate, amantidine, nefazodone, to name a few (Jenike et al. 1998, pp. 506–508). (See Chapter 97 for further discussion of SRIs.) (Clinical Vignette 2).

## Assessing Treatment Resistance

Before concluding that a patient is treatment-resistant, the adequacy of previous treatment trials must be assessed (Goodman et al. 1993, Jenike 1993; see Table 68–2). In particular, it is critical to know both the duration and dose of every medication that has been used. Typically, patients who appear treatment-resistant have received an inadequate duration of treatment, which should be a minimum of 10 to 12 weeks, or an inadequate medication dose, which should be the maximum dose for any particular agent. Some psychiatrists consider patients truly treatment-resistant only if they have failed several adequate pharmacologic trials, including one with clomipramine, and several augmentation strategies including behavioral therapy (March et al. 1997). With this kind of aggressive treatment, 80 to 90% of patients usually experience some improvement, although few patients become symptom-free (Jenike 1993, Rasmussen et al. 1993).

| Table 68–2 | Things to Consider in Patients with Obsessive–Compulsive Disorder in Whom Initial Treatment Fails |
|---|---|

**Was the diagnosis correct?**

Is there an Axis II disorder, especially schizotypal or obsessive–compulsive personality disorder?

Are there comorbid diagnoses that could interfere with treatment response?

Is there a major depressive disorder?

Are there obsessive thoughts, overvalued ideas, or delusions?

**Was the pharmacotherapy trial adequate?**

Was a known effective agent used?

Was the dose adequate?

Was the duration of treatment long enough?

**Was behavioral therapy performed?**

Were an adequate number of sessions attended?

Did the patient comply with homework assignment?

Was there cognitive impairment inhibiting the ability to implement treatment?

Was there concurrent use of central nervous system depressants that affect ability to attend to evoked anxiety?

When inadequate treatment is not the reason for poor treatment response, it is important to assess the accuracy of the diagnosis. Schizotypal personality disorder, borderline personality disorder, avoidant personality disorder, and OCPD seem to be associated with poorer response to pharmacotherapy, particularly if the personality disorder is the primary diagnosis (Jenike et al. 1986, Goodman et al. 1993, Stein et al. 2001).

Behavioral therapy (see later) seems less effective in patients with comorbid major depressive disorder. Comorbid depression may inhibit the ability to learn and to habituate to anxiety (Jenike 1993). Initial pharmacotherapy sometimes improves depression, as well as OCD symptoms, and may increase the likelihood of success with behavioral treatment.

## Augmentation Strategies

If a patient has had only a partial response to an antiobsessional agent of adequate dose and duration, the next question is whether to change the SRI or add an augmenting agent. Current clinical practice suggests that if there is no response at all to an SRI, it may be best to change to another SRI. However, if there has been some response to treatment, an augmentation trial of at least 2 to 8 weeks may be warranted (Jenike 1993, Goodman et al. 1993, March et al. 1997, Griest and Jefferson 1998). No augmentation agent has been firmly established as efficacious. Although many augmentation agents appeared promising in open trials, they failed to be effective in more systematic trials (Goodman et al. 1993), although some of the later studies did not report response to the SRI alone, leaving unanswered the question of whether some augmentation strategies may be effective in partial SRI responders. Many questions about augmentation remain unanswered, including the optimal duration of augmentation, comparative efficacy of different agents, predictors of response, and mechanism of action (Jenike 1992, 1993). Nonethe-

less, these agents do help some patients significantly, and thus their systematic use should be considered (see Table 68–3).

In patients with severe symptoms or comorbid psychosis or tic disorder, pimozide 1 to 3 mg/day, haldol 2 to 10 mg/day, and other neuroleptic agents (risperdone 2–8 mg/day and olanzapine 2.5–10 mg/day) have been used with some success (Goodman et al. 1993, McDougle et al. 1990, 2000, Stein et al. 1997, Saxena et al. 1996, Koran et al. 2000). However, the use of a neuroleptic agent should be considered carefully in light of the risk of extrpyramidal symptoms and side effects such as weight gain, lethargy, and tardive dyskinesia. Thus, when a neuroleptic drug is used, target symptoms should be established before beginning treatment, and the medication discontinued within several months if target symptoms do not improve.

The use of lithium (300–600 mg/day) and buspirone (up to 60 mg/day) as augmentation agents has also been explored. Both agents looked promising in open trials (Jenike 1992, Jenike et al. 1991, Markovitz et al. 1990) but failed to be effective in more systematic trials (McDougle et al. 1991, 1993, Pigott et al. 1992). Augmentation with fenfluramine (up to 60 mg/day), clonazepam (up to 5 mg/day), clonidine (0.1–0.6 mg/day) and trazodone (100–200 mg/day), as well as the combination of clomipramine with any of the SSRIs, has had anecdotal success but has not been evaluated in methodologically rigorous studies (Rasmussen et al. 1993, Pigott et al. 1992). Some potential augmenting agents and their dosage ranges are presented in Table 68–3.

| Table 68–3 | Potential Augmenting Agents for Treatment-Resistant Obsessive–Compulsive Disorder |
|---|---|

| Augmenting Agent | Suggested Dosage Range* |
|---|---|
| Lithium | 300–600 mg/d† |
| Clonazepam | 1–3 mg/d |
| Tryptophan | 2–10 g/d‡ |
| Trazodone | 100–200 mg/d |
| Buspirone | 15–60 mg/d |
| Alprazolam | 0.5–2 mg/d |
| Methylphenidate | 10–30 mg/d |
| Haloperidol | 2–10 mg/d |
| Pimozide | 2–10 mg/d |
| Nifedipine | 10 mg t.i.d |
| Liothyronine sodium | 10–25 mg/d |
| Clonidine | 0.1–0.6 mg/d |
| Fenfluramine | Up to 60 mg/d |

*Add these to an ongoing trial of antidepressant medication. It should be noted that most of these dosages have not been tested with rigorous clinical trials but simply represent some of the reported doses tried in the current literature. Some would not recommend augmentation unless the initial treatment showed some response.

†*Use with caution*—there have been some reports of elevated lithium levels with ongoing fluoxetine treatment.

‡Because the use of l-tryptophan has been implicated in an increased incidence of eosinophilia, the authors advise against the prescribing and use of this agent until the issue is resolved.

*Source*: Jenike MA (1991) Management of patients with treatment-resistant obsessive–compulsive disorder. In Current Treatments of Obsessive–Compulsive Disorder, Pato MT and Zohar J (eds). American Psychiatric Press, Washington DC, p. 146.

## Behavioral Therapy

Behavioral therapy is effective for OCD both as a primary treatment and as an augmentation agent (Marks et al. 1988, 1980, Foa et al. 1985, Griest 1994). This form of therapy is based on the principle of exposure and response prevention. The patient is asked to endure, in a graduated manner, the anxiety that a specific obsessional fear provokes while refraining from compulsions that allay that anxiety. The principles behind the efficacy of behavioral treatment are explained to the patient in the following way. Although compulsions, either covert or overt, usually immediately relieve anxiety, this is only a short-term solution; the anxiety will ultimately return, requiring the performance of another compulsion. However, if the patient resists the anxiety and urge to ritualize, the anxiety will eventually decrease on its own (i.e., habituation will occur), and the need to perform the ritual will eventually disappear. Thus, behavioral therapy helps the patient habituate to the anxiety and extinguish the compulsions.

Compulsions, especially overt behaviors like washing rituals, are more successfully treated by behavioral therapy than are obsessions alone or covert rituals like mental checking. This is because covert rituals are harder to physically resist than are rituals like hand washing and checking a door. In fact, Jenike (1993) reported that washing rituals are the most amenable to behavioral treatment, followed by checking rituals and then mental rituals.

For rituals that do not constitute overt behaviors, techniques other than exposure and response prevention have been used in conjunction with exposure and response prevention. These approaches include imaginal flooding and thought stopping. In imaginal flooding, the anxiety provoked by the obsessions is evoked by continually repeating the thought, often with the help of a continuous-loop tape or the reading of a "script" composed by the patient and therapist, until the thought no longer provokes anxiety. In thought stopping, an compulsive mental ritual (e.g., continually repeating a short prayer in one's head) is stopped by simply shouting, making a loud noise, or snapping a rubber band on the wrist in an attempt to interrupt the thought.

In the early stages of treatment, a behavioral assessment is performed. During this assessment, the content, frequency, duration, amount of interference and distress, and attempts to resist or ignore the obsessions and compulsions are catalogued. An attempt is made to clarify the types of symptoms, any triggers that bring on the obsessions and compulsions, and the amount and type of avoidance used to deal with the symptoms. For instance, in the clinical vignette described later, the fact that Ms. Z stopped preparing meals to deal with her obsessional concerns about contamination was carefully documented. The patient, usually with the help of a therapist, then develops a hierarchy of situations according to the amount of anxiety they provoke. During treatment, patients gradually engage in the anxiety-provoking situations included in their hierarchy without performing anxiety-reducing rituals (see Clinical Vignette 1).

Behavioral therapy can be used with patients of any age and has been used in young children, often with the help of a parent as a cotherapist. However, systematic trials of behavioral treatment in children have not been performed.

More recently, behavioral therapy in a group setting has been explored and found as effective as, and perhaps even more effective than, individual behavioral treatment (Fals-Stewart et al. 1993, Van Noppen et al. 1998). The group seems to act as a catalyst for change by promoting group cohesion, support, and encouragement. Groups can include patients with different symptoms, though each has a personalized hierarchy, so that one patient can encourage another. Van Noppen and associates (1991) included family members in groups because families are often affected by the patient's rituals and often function as unwilling participants in rituals. As members of the group, family members not only gain knowledge and understanding about OCD but can be cotherapists at home for homework assignments.

Despite its efficacy, behavioral therapy has limitations. To begin with, about 15 to 25% of patients refuse to engage in behavioral treatment initially or drop out early in treatment because it is so anxiety-provoking (Griest 1994; see Figure 68–8). Behavioral treatment fails in another 25% of patients for a variety of other reasons (Griest 1994, Foa et al. 1983), including concomitant depression; the use of central nervous system depressants, which may inhibit the ability to habituate to anxiety; lack of insight; poor compliance with homework, resulting in inadequate exposure; and poor compliance on the part of the therapist in enforcing the behavioral paradigm (Griest 1994). Thus, overall, 50 to 70% of patients are helped by this form of therapy.

One of the issues that has emerged in treating OCD with CBT is the lack of trained therapists and the cost of repeated individual exposure sessions. Thus, in addition to developing group treatments which allow therapists to treat a number of patients simultaneously, researchers have begun to develop computer-guided behavior therapy. Several recent reports have shown that while this modality is not as effective as individual behavior therapy, it does allow for significant improvement in symptoms over a control condition like relaxation therapy (Greist et al. 2002).

Behavior therapy can be used as the sole treatment of OCD, particularly with patients whose contamination fears or somatic obsessions make them resistant to taking

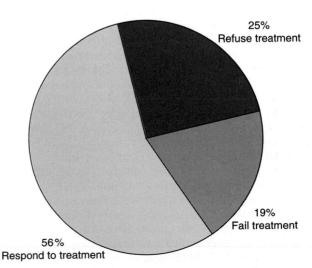

**Figure 68–8** *Diagram of behavioral therapy results.*

medications. Behavioral treatment is also a powerful adjunct to pharmacotherapy. Some research appears to indicate that combined treatment may be more effective than pharmacotherapy or behavioral therapy alone, although these findings are still preliminary (Marks et al. 1980, Cottraux et al. 1990, Foa 1994, Simpson et al. 1999). Some studies have even suggested that adding pharmacotherapy to behavior therapy may be particularly helpful in reducing obsessions while compulsions respond to behavior therapy (Hohagen et al. 1998, Direnfeld et al. 2000). From a clinical perspective, it may be useful to have patients begun treatment with medication to reduce the intensity of their symptoms or comorbid depressive symptoms if present; patients may then be more amenable to experiencing the anxiety that will be evoked by the behavioral challenges they perform (see Chapter 86 for further discussion).

Work by Baxter and colleagues (1992) has illustrated some interesting correlations between treatment response and changes in neuroanatomy and neurophysiology. These investigators studied two groups of nine patients each, with one group treated with medication only (fluoxetine up to 80 mg/day for 10 weeks) and the other group treated with individual behavioral therapy only (exposure and response prevention for 10 weeks). Positron emission tomography scans with $^{18}$F-fluorodeoxyglucose were performed on all patients before and after treatment. Compared with nonresponders and control subjects, responders in both the medication and the behavioral treatment groups showed a decrease in activity in the right head of the caudate nucleus. This finding seems to support the notion that both forms of treatment bring about similar changes in neurophysiology which lead to improvement in symptoms. These results also provide important theoretical links with the serotonin hypothesis described earlier in this chapter, as basal ganglion structures like the caudate nucleus have been postulated to mediate serotonin function (Rapoport and Wise 1988, Zohar and Insel 1987, Schwartz 1998).

## Psychotherapy

The use of psychotherapeutic techniques of either a psychoanalytic or a supportive nature has not been proved successful in treating the specific obsessions and compulsions that are a hallmark of OCD. However, the more characterological aspects that are part of obsessive–compulsive personality disorder may be helped by a more psychoanalytically oriented approach. As noted earlier, the defense mechanisms of reaction formation, isolation, and undoing, as well as a pervasive sense of doubt and need to be in control, are hallmarks of the obsessive–compulsive character. Salzman (1983) and MacKinnon and Michels (1971) have written elegantly on how to approach the maladaptive aspects of this character style in therapy. In essence, the patient must be encouraged to take risks and learn to feel comfortable with, or at least less anxious about, making mistakes and to accept anxiety as a natural and normal part of human experience. Techniques for meeting such goals in treatment may include the psychiatrist's being relatively active in therapy to ensure that the patient focuses on the present rather than getting lost in perfectly recounting the past, as well as the psychiatrist's being willing to take risks and present herself or himself as less than perfect.

## Neurosurgery

Occasionally, even after receiving adequate pharmacotherapy (including augmentation), adequate behavioral therapy, and a combination of behavioral therapy and pharmacotherapy, patients may still experience intractable OCD symptoms. Such patients may be candidates for neurosurgery. Although criteria for who should receive neurosurgery vary, it has been suggested that failure to respond to at least 5 years of systematic treatment is a reasonable criterion (Mindus and Jenike 1992). Frequently used criteria are the following: a minimum of two adequate medication trials with augmentation plus adequate behavioral therapy in the absence of severe personality disorder.

The procedures that have been most successful interrupt tracts involved in the serotonin system. The surgical procedures used—anterior capsulotomy, cingulotomy, and limbic leukotomy—all aim to interrupt the connection between the cortex and the basal ganglia and related structures. Current stereotactic surgical techniques involve the creation of precise lesions, which are often only 10 to 20 mm, to specific tracts. These procedures have often been done with radio-frequency heated electrodes and more recently with gamma knife techniques. Postsurgical risks have been minimized, and in some cases cognitive function and personality traits improve along with symptoms of OCD (Jenike 1998).

Data compiled from a number of small studies have yielded success rates of 25 to 84% with treatment (Mindus and Jenike 1992, Jenike 1998). However most samples are small, and the procedures have often differed in both lesion location and size, making it difficult to compare them. However, in a recent prospective long-term follow-up study, all 44 patients received the same procedure (cingulotomy), although some had single procedures and others multiple procedures (Dougherty et al. 2002). This study had several important findings. Clinical improvement occurred in 32 to 45% of patients, depending on the criteria used to rate full or partial response, and the average effect size was 1.27, comparable to that seen in pharmacologic trials (1.09–1.53). However, these changes were not immediately apparent postoperatively, and most patients were encouraged to engage in pharmacotherapy and/or behavior therapy postoperatively. The longitudinal follow-up component of the study, which was a mean duration of 32 months, allowed the researchers to assess the longer-term impact of the procedure in ways other studies could not. Of particular note, patients continued to show improvement for up to 29 months after surgery without receiving further procedures. As a result, the authors noted that the typical 6-month wait before deciding whether to repeat and extend the lesion may be too brief. In conclusion, neurosurgical treatments offer hope to some of the most severely ill and treatment-resistant patients and should therefore be considered. However, which surgical lesions are most effective in which patients still needs much more study (see Chapter 93 for further discussion).

## Issues in the Physician–Patient Relationship

Treatment for OCD is often effective, leading to at least some response in a majority of patients. However, treatment adherence is difficult for some patients, which may interfere with treatment efficacy. Short- and long-term compliance with treatment can be greatly facilitated by considering how the nature of the illness affects the treatment modalities used.

At the core of OCD are the concepts of obsessional doubt, risk aversion, and a need to feel in control of one's environment. These three concepts affect behavioral and pharmacological treatment. In the initial phases of behavioral treatment, it may be difficult to engage the patient in treatment because of his or her doubt that the treatment will be effective and an unwillingness to experience the anxiety that results from exposure to feared stimuli. Extra time often must be spent convincing patients of the potential efficacy of treatment and lack of serious side effects from behavioral treatment. Unlike pharmacological treatment, in which the side effects can be quantified in medical terms, the side effects that patients fear from behavioral treatment are related to their cognitive distortions. For instance, those with contamination fears may be thoroughly convinced that simply walking by an AIDS clinic will put them at risk of contracting AIDS or that simply using a public bathroom will give them a communicable disease. Thus, reassurance that this is not the case and that it is safe to engage in behavioral treatment may first involve playing out the catastrophic consequences in their mind or role-playing and discussing the irrational nature of the fear to the fullest extent possible.

When behavioral treatment is started, it is customary to develop a hierarchy of subjective units of distress, which rate particular events according to how much anxiety they produce. For some patients, the ability to develop this hierarchy and thereby obtain a sense of control over their fears, and the ability to begin with the least stressful challenges, can allow them to engage in behavioral treatment.

Similar concerns related to doubt, risk aversion, and control must also be addressed when pharmacological treatment is undertaken. In the initial treatment phases, the major task is getting the patient to engage in treatment. Patients with OCD, particularly those with contamination and somatic obsessions, often have numerous questions about medication safety and may be hesitant to take them. Patients with contamination and somatic obsessions may be more likely to engage in behavioral treatment initially.

Although it is important that patients have a thorough understanding of side effects, the psychiatrist should not be thorough to an obsessional degree. Many patients with OCD want a detailed understanding of every side effect and have difficulty differentiating which side effects are of concern and which are not. Thus, it is critical when discussing side effects to present an objective assessment of the relative frequency and severity of various side effects. It is important to emphasize that even though some of the rare side effects are more serious than the more common side effects, they are unlikely to occur. It is also worth keeping in mind that the patient's concerns about a particular side effect may be different from the psychiatrist's. Again, it may help to elicit the catastrophic fears that the patient has and address the irrational obsessional qualities of those fears.

The initial phase of treatment is often the most difficult. This has to do with both risk aversion and a need to be in control. With pharmacologic treatment, patients may occasionally experience an initial worsening of symptoms in addition to side effects. This can be terrifying to the patient and can lead to an abrupt discontinuation of the medication. Warning the patient before treatment that this might occur increases the patient's sense of control. Similarly, the antiobsessional effects of treatment often take 6 to 10 weeks to be seen and are often gradual in onset. This gradual response is usually delayed until after the patient experiences side effects. Thus, the early phase of treatment may need to focus on encouraging the patient to stay on medication despite side effects and no improvement. Side effects can often be framed as a good sign that the medication is being actively absorbed by the body. Again, preparing patients in advance helps them feel in control and able to continue treatment. The gradual onset of improvement, although in some cases frustrating, is also reassuring to patients who might feel out of control if improvement occurred too rapidly.

Unlike many patients with mood disorders, most patients with OCD do not have full recovery from their symptoms. Although the majority of patients, perhaps as many as 85%, experience some improvement, most tend to remain symptomatic to some degree (The Clomipramine Collaborative Study Group 1991, Jenike 1993, Rasmussen et al. 1993, Orloff et al. 1994). Nonetheless, symptom improvement of even 10 to 15% can have a dramatic effect on their lives.

## Duration and Discontinuation of Treatment

Little systematic research has been performed to guide decisions about continuation, maintenance, and discontinuation of treatment. The largest study of extended pharmacologic treatment involved fluoxetine (Tollefson et al. 1994b). In this study, 70 patients who had responded to fluoxetine and 198 patients who had not responded during an acute 13-week trial were given the opportunity to continue on medication for another 6 months. At the end of the 6 months, 74.3% of those who had responded initially experienced further improvement. In the nonresponder group, 91.7% experienced a decrease in symptoms when the medication dose was increased from the previous unsuccessful dose. Only 19% of patients ($N = 13$) experienced a significant worsening of symptoms during the follow-up period. Similar to previous reports on fluoxetine (Levine et al. 1989, Fontaine and Chouinard 1989, Frankel et al. 1990), this study suggested that symptom improvement was maintained over time. Even more important, further improvement occurred in responders with longer treatment and in nonresponders with continued treatment at higher doses.

In another study, 85 patients who had been treated with a variety of antiobsessional medications were followed up 1 to 3.5 years after initial treatment (Orloff et al. 1994). Ninety-four percent of the patients were still taking medication, and 87% had maintained previous gains or achieved further improvement. Thus, from a clinical point of view, it seems wise to continue medication for an extended period, perhaps for 6 months to a year after initiating treatment, because during this period improvement is maintained and some patients experience further improvement. Overall, this extended duration of treatment did not result in worsening side effects; in fact, in most cases patients habituated to side effects. In general, the most bothersome side effects that persist with SRI treatment appear to be fatigue, weight gain, and sexual dysfunction (Rasmussen et al. 1993).

In recent years a number of studies of long-term efficacy have emerged. One study that included a follow-up period of 2 years for 38 OCD patients on sertraline showed continued efficacy with fewer side effects with longer-term treatment (Rasmussen et al. 1997). Another study assessed a larger group of patients and attempted to answer important clinical questions not only about long-term efficacy but about the effects of medication discontinuation after 1 year of treatment (Koran et al. 2002). The latter is an important question because few studies of systematic discontinuation have been done, and in those that have been done relapse rates were quite high, above 90% (Pato et al. 1988, Leonard et al. 1991). This sertraline study (Koran et al. 2002) involved 223 patients who had been successfully treated with single-blind sertraline for 52 weeks who were then randomized in a double-blind manner to continue treatment for another 6 months or placebo. One-third of the patients in the placebo group relapsed; this was surprisingly lower than the percentage found in earlier studies. The authors offered several plausible explanations for this, which included the possibility that 1 year of effective treatment may provide sustained benefit for patients, and that patients may have engaged in self-directed behavior therapy, something that was not readily available at the time of the previous discontinuation studies. They also noted that while OCD symptom ratings did not worsen in the placebo-treated group as a whole, quality of life did significantly deteriorate. This finding points to the need for more sensitive measures of patient improvement and for further studies of long-term treatment efficacy.

Some preliminary data have suggested that in treatment responders it may be possible to decrease the dose of clomipramine over the longer term without subsequent relapse (Pato et al. 1990). Two studies have more systematically addressed this issue. In one study (Mundo et al. 1997), patients were treated with one-third or two-thirds of their effective doses of clomipramine or fluvoxamine, without experience a worsening of symptoms over 102 days. In another study (Ravizza et al 1996), doses of clomipramine, fluoxetine, or fluvoxamine were halved, without worsening of symptoms over the next 3 months. Thus it may be possible to decrease the SRI dose in longer-term treatment, although this important issue needs further investigation.

The data on discontinuation of behavioral therapy are also encouraging. In summarizing data from several 1- to 6-year follow-up studies of behavioral therapy, O'Sullivan and Marks (1991) noted that overall about 75% of patients continued to do well at follow-up. However, most studies also noted that few patients were symptom-free. One small study looked at the role of behavioral therapy in the context of medication discontinuation and was a bit less optimistic, finding that at least three of five patients who discontinued medication while receiving behavioral therapy had a relapse of symptoms requiring medication reinitiation (Baer et al. 1994). A larger clinical trial is currently assessing this issue.

## Conclusion

For many patients with OCD the illness is life long, starting in early childhood and extending into adulthood. It is often familial and accompanied by comorbid conditions including, depression, other anxiety disorders, Tourette's syndrome and even psychosis. However, with a combination of pharmacologic and behavioral treatment, at adequate dose and duration, patients can often have significant improvement in symptoms and overall function.

---

**Clinical Vignette 1 • Behavioral Therapy**

Ms. Z was a married woman in her late twenties whose primary OCD symptom consisted of severe contamination obsessions. She feared that she would contract cancer from various substances, such as detergents, chemical lawn treatments, foods, asbestos, gasoline, oil spills on beaches, and batteries. She also had aggressive obsessions that if she did not do certain things, harm would come to her family members. In response to these fears, Ms. Z washed more than 100 times per day, avoided situations that might lead to contamination, checked items repeatedly for evidence of contamination, and sought reassurance from others more than 50 times a day.

Ms. Z's symptoms dated back to age 8 years when she had aggressive obsessions and felt that she had to touch certain things in her room. Her life had been riddled with magical thinking; to combat fears of dying or to prevent bad things from happening to others, she had to open and close the refrigerator in a certain way, had to close lids a certain way, had to touch the floor, and had to touch both of her eyes. She kept most of these rituals hidden from others.

Around the time she became pregnant in her late twenties, Ms. Z's symptoms worsened. Her contamination fears heightened to the point that she avoided contact with family members and relatives who might be contaminated with cancer or contaminated because of where they lived. Her husband was drawn into her rituals, often giving her reassurance. She eventually stopped cooking because of her fears of insecticides, bacteria, and chemicals on food, and her son and husband ate meals at a relative's house.

At initial evaluation, Ms. Z spoke of the distress and impairment she experienced from her symptoms and her desire to stop her strange behavior. After a failed attempt of 6 months of insight-oriented psychotherapy, Ms. Z began combined behavioral therapy and pharmacotherapy consisting of clomipramine which was gradually increased from 50 to 250 mg/day (although it may appear obvious, it may be helpful to clarify that the clomipramine doses started low, perhaps 50 mg/day and was raised gradually to 250 mg).

Behavioral therapy was initially begun on an individual basis. During the first sessions, psychoeducation and exposure and response prevention techniques were discussed. One of the first homework assignments included keeping a daily record of how many times Ms. Z washed her hands. When she returned for the next session, she reported that the frequency had decreased; as she stated, "Knowing I had to write down when I had the urge prevented me from washing. Having to stop and think about why I was doing the ritual helped me to resist." (In 10% of patients, record keeping alone results in a decrease in target behaviors.) Sessions continued, with the therapist modeling exposure and response prevention. For example, the therapist asked

Ms. Z to join her in touching doorknobs, floors, shoes, batteries, paint chips, and plant soil while continually reassuring her, identifying the cancer fear as OCD, and pushing her to understand that her initial urge to avoid or wash could easily become a command if she did not challenge the feeling. After every session, a specific homework assignment was negotiated that Ms. Z could practice daily. She was instructed to call the therapist if she had trouble with the homework assignments. Ms. Z reported compliance with homework assignments as well as a decrease in anxiety, but she continued to experience severe fear of contamination.

Ms. Z then entered a 10-session behavioral therapy group that strengthened her confidence and encouraged her to participate in group exercises (touching objects and resisting washing). By allowing her to share her experiences with other group members, the group also validated her feelings of frustration and isolation. Independently, Ms. Z began to choose goals such as allowing her son to have a toy that she had taken away because it was "contaminated," resisting washing his hands, and making herself lunch for work.

However, it became apparent that as certain symptoms improved, Ms. Z continued to engage in many elaborate rituals at home. To address this problem, home visits were planned. While in the home, the therapist encouraged Ms. Z to touch and clean avoided articles of clothing, throw away rubber gloves that were used to prevent contamination, and even share feared contaminated foods like grapes and celery that Ms. Z had been avoiding because they could not be adequately washed or peeled.

Eventually, Ms. Z also enrolled with her husband in a second eight-session group behavioral treatment that included family members. This gave her husband the ability to observe participant modeling of exposure and response prevention with the support and validation of other family members.

During the next 18 to 24 months of treatment, Ms. Z began to set more challenging behavioral goals and decreased treatment from as many as three individual therapy sessions and two group and family behavioral group sessions per week to one individual behavioral session per week, with sustained improvement between sessions. She eventually contracted to cook meals, do laundry, and buy groceries and was able to have guests come to her house without experiencing excessive contamination concerns.

---

Clinical Vignette 2 • Pharmacotherapy

Ms. M was a 38-year-old married teacher who had experienced OCD symptoms since age 10 years. At that time, she had a need to reread sentences, as well as a need to check things like doors and faucets to guard against something bad happening. Her symptoms subsided somewhat during her teenage years but resurfaced during her early twenties. She sought treatment from a hypnotherapist in her late twenties and subsequently did relatively well, with only minimal symptoms, for the next 10 years. She noted, however, that during that time she continued to be a nervous person who worried about everything.

At the time of her initial visit, she reported a significant worsening of her OCD symptoms during the previous weeks. In particular, she began to have trouble driving her car. She often found herself retracing her route to ascertain

that she had not hit something or to pick up road debris that she was worried might get in her way. This behavior greatly lengthened her driving time and, as a result, Ms. M began to drive less and to avoid unnecessary trips like driving to stores to shop. As her symptoms worsened, she began to avoid driving at night because she worried that she would not see debris and other objects in the road. In addition, much to her chagrin, she began to involve her husband in her rituals by asking him to drive back with her to make sure that nothing was wrong. She also experienced increased checking behavior, for example, rechecking how she had written a check or retracing her steps at school to ascertain that she had not kicked something down the stairs. Overall, she estimated that her symptoms were moderately severe and taking about 3 hours per day. Ms. M had also begun to experience prominent neurovegetative symptoms of depression, including early morning awakening, decreased energy and initiative, psychomotor slowing, and a 10-pound weight loss.

Ms. M was entered in a 10-week placebo-controlled blinded clomipramine trial and received clomipramine 250 mg/day. Within 3 weeks of starting treatment, she began to show some signs of improvement. She reported less frequent episodes of driving back and less avoidance of driving to go shopping; however, she did not experience much change in other checking behaviors. After 5 to 6 weeks at 250 mg/day of clomipramine, Ms. M noted marked improvement (approximately 85%) in her symptoms. She had only transient episodes of needing to drive back, which lasted less than 5 minutes, and no avoidance of driving; her checking had also improved. She began to have some symptom-free days. Ms. M also had no depressive symptoms and experienced a general sense of well-being that was a significant improvement from her baseline. However, she began to complain of significant drowsiness and fatigue, despite adequate sleep, as well as dry mouth and tremor.

Within 10 weeks of beginning treatment, Ms. M was virtually free of OCD symptoms, experiencing only a few mild and transient episodes. Because she was at the end of the blinded medication period, her clomipramine dose was decreased from 250 to 150 mg/day. Within 1 week, she reported that she had started retracing her route while driving and had other symptoms of OCD that occupied about 1 hour per day. Her dose was increased to 200 mg/day, but in 1 week she called her physician to say that she was distressed because her OCD symptoms had interfered with her ability to pick up her child and that her symptoms had increased to 3 hours per day. Her clomipramine was increased to 250 mg/day. Within 8 weeks, Ms. M had returned to her previous level of good health. She was driving normally, was not checking or engaging in avoidance behavior, and had no obsessional fear of harm coming to others. Although on some days she experienced about 45 minutes of fleeting symptoms, on other days she was totally symptom-free. However, she was experiencing some side effects, such as dry mouth, tremor, weight gain, and fatigue. Her fatigue became marked to the point that she came home from her job as a school teacher exhausted and slept 16 hours a day on the weekend.

After 1 year at 250 mg/day of clomipramine, a taper was again attempted, and the medication was discontinued within a month. Before the taper, Ms. M's Y-BOCS score was 4 (out of a possible total score of 40), but after 2 weeks without medication it rose to 6, indicating an increased effort on her part to resist her obsessions and compulsions.

---

**Clinical Vignette 2** *continued*

After 7 weeks of not taking medication, her Y-BOCS score rose to 10, and after 15 weeks it rose to 16, indicating moderate symptom severity. She noted that she had 1 to 3 hours of obsessions and 1 hour of compulsions per day, with increasing effort needed to resist symptoms. In addition, she noted the return of her nervousness and tendency to worry. However, Ms. M also had a lessening of her fatigue and lost 5 of the 10 pounds she had gained on the medication.

The return of symptoms was distressing to Ms. M, and she decided to try another medication. Sertraline was begun, and after only 6 to 8 weeks of treatment, at 200 mg/day, she had a remission of all OCD symptoms and the return of a sense of well-being. She had no side effects. At 5 months of follow-up she remained symptom-free, and her Y-BOCS score had decreased to 1, with only 15 minutes of symptoms per week.

## Comparison of DSM-IV/ICD-10 Diagnostic Criteria

The ICD-10 Diagnostic Criteria for Research for Obsessive–Compulsive Disorder differentiate between obsessions and compulsions based on whether they are thoughts, ideas, or images (obsessions) or acts (compulsions). In contrast, DSM-IV-TR distinguishes between obsessions and compulsions based on whether the thought, idea, or image causes anxiety or distress or prevents or reduces it. Thus, in DSM-IV-TR, there can be cognitive compulsions which would be considered obsessions in ICD-10. In addition, ICD-10 sets a minimum duration of at least 2 weeks whereas DSM-IV-TR has no minimum duration.

## References

Ackerman D, Greenland S, Bystritsky A, et al. (1994) Predictors of treatment response in OCD: Multivariate analyses from multicenter trial of clomipramine. J Clin Psychopharmacol 14(4), 247–254.

Alonso P, Menchon JM, Pifarre J, et al. (2001) Long-term follow-up and predictors of clinical outcome in obsessive–compulsive patients treated with serotonin reuptake inhibitors and behavioral therapy. J Clin Psychiatr 62(7), 535–540.

American Psychiatric Association (1994) Diagnostic and Statistical Manual of Mental Disorders, 4th ed. American Psychiatric Association, Washington DC.

Angst A (1994) The epidemiology of obsessive–compulsive disorder. In Current Insights in Obsessive Compulsive Disorder, Hollander E, Zohar J, Marazziti D, et al. (eds). John Wiley, West Sussex, UK, pp. 93–104.

Baer L (1994) Factor analysis of symptom subtypes of obsessive–compulsive disorder and their relation to personality and tic disorders. J Clin Psychiatr 55, 18–23.

Baer L and Jenike M (1992) Personality disorders in OCD. Psychiatr Clin N Am 15(4), 803–812.

Baer L, Jenike MA, Ricciardi JN, et al. (1990) Standardized assessment of personality disorders in obsessive–compulsive disorder. Arch Gen Psychiatr 47, 826–830.

Baer L and Minichiello WE (1990) Behavior therapy for obsessive–compulsive disorder. In Obsessive–Compulsive Disorders: Theory and Management. Jenike MA, Baer L, and Minichiello WE (eds). Year Book Medical Publishers, St. Louis, Missouri.

Baer L, Ricciardi J, Keuthen W, et al. (1994) Discontinuation of obsessive–compulsive disorder medication with behavioral therapy (letter). Am J Psychiatr 151, 1842.

Barr LL, Goodman WK, McDougle LJ, et al. (1994) Tryptophan depletion in patients with obsessive–compulsive disorder who respond to serotonin reuptake inhibitors. Arch Gen Psychiatr 51, 309–317.

Barr LL, Goodman WK, and Price LH (1994b) Physical symptoms associated with paroxetine discontinuation (letter). Am J Psychiatr 151, 289.

Baumgarten HG and Grozdanovic Z (1998) Role of serotonin in obsessive–compulsive disorder. Br J Psychiatr 173(Suppl 35), 13–20.

Baxter LR (1992) Neuroimaging studies of obsessive–compulsive disorder. Psychiatr Clin N Am 15, 871–884.

Baxter LR, Phelps ME, Mazziotta JC, et al. (1987) Local cerebral glucose metabolic rates in obsessive–compulsive disorder. A comparison with rates in unipolar depression and in normal controls. Arch Gen Psychiatr 4, 211–218.

Baxter LR, Schwartz JM, Bergman KS, et al. (1992) Caudate glucose metabolic rate changes with both drug and behavior therapy for obsessive–compulsive disorder. Arch Gen Psychiatr 49, 681–689.

Baxter LR, Schwartz JM, Mazziotta JC, et al. (1988) Cerebral glucose metabolic rates in nondepressed patients with obsessive–compulsive disorder. Am J Psychiatr 145, 1560–1563.

Bellodi L, Sciuto G, Diaferia G, et al. (1992) Psychiatric disorders in the families of patients with obsessive–compulsive disorder. Psychiatr Res 42, 111–120.

Benkelfat C, Nordahl TE, Semple WE, et al. (1990) Local cerebral glucose metabolic rates in obsessive–compulsive disorder. Patients treated with clomipramine. Arch Gen Psychiatr 47, 840–848.

Berman I, Kalinowski, and Berman SM (1995) Obsessive and Compulsive Symptoms in Chronic Schizophrenia. Compr Psychiatr 36(1), 6–10.

Bienvenu OJ, Samuels JF, Riddle MA, et al. (2000) The relationship of obsessive–compulsive disorder to possible spectrum disorders: Results from a family study. Biol Psychiatr 48(4), 287–293.

Bisserbe JC, Lane RM, and Flament MF (1997). A double-blind comparison of sertraline and clomipramine in outpatients with obsessive–compulsive disorder. Eur Psychiatr 12, 82–93.

Black DW, Nayes R, Goldstein RB, et al. (1992) A family study of obsessive–compulsive disorder. Arch Gen Psychiatr 49, 362–368.

Bland RC, Newman SC, and Orn H (1988) Lifetime prevalence of psychiatric disorders in Edmonton. Acta Psychiatr Scand 77(Suppl), 33–42.

Brieter HC, Rauch SL, Kwong KK, et al. (1996) Functioning magnetic resonance imaging of symptoms provocation in obsessive–compulsive disorder. Arch Gen Psychiatr 49, 595–606.

Bryois C, Rubin C, Zbinden JD, et al. (1998) Withdrawal syndrome caused by selective serotonin reuptake inhibitors: Apropos of a case. Schweiz Rundsch Med Prax 87, 345–348.

Cavedini P, Cisima M, Riboldi G, et al. (2001 Aug) A neuropsychological study of dissociation in cortical and subcortical functioning in obsessive–compulsive disorder by Tower of Hanoi task. Brain Cogn 46(3), 357–63.

Charney D, Goodman W, Price L, et al. (1988) Serotonin function in obsessive–compulsive disorder. A comparison of the effects of tryptophan and m-chlorophenylpiperazine in patients and healthy subjects. Arch Gen Psychiatr 45, 177–185.

Cohen LJ, Stein D, and Galykner I (1997) Towards an intergration of psychological and biological models of obsessive–compulsive disorder: Phylogenetics considerations. CNS Spect 2(10), 26–44.

Coryell W (1981) Obsessive–compulsive disorder and primary unipolar depression: Comparisons of background, family history, course and mortality. J Nerv Ment Dis 169, 220–224.

Cottraux J and Gerard D (1998) Neuroimaging and neuroanatomical issues in obsessive–compulsive disorder; Toward and integrative model-perceived impulsivity. In Obsessive–Compulsive Disorder: Theory Research and Treatment, Richard P, Swinson, Martin M, et al. (eds). Guilford Press, New York, pp. 154–180.

Cottraux J, Mollard E, Bouvard M, et al. (1990) A controlled study of fluvoxamine and exposure in obsessive–compulsive disorder. Int Clin Psychopharmacol 5, 17–30.

Delgado PL and Moreno FA (1998) Different roles for serotonin in anti-obsessionl durg action and the pathophysiology of obsessive–compulsive disorder. Br J Psychiatr 173(Suppl 35), 21–25.

Devane CL (1994) Pharmacogenetics and drug metabolism of newer antidepressant agents. J Clin Psychiatr 55(Suppl), 38–45.

DeVeaugh-Geiss J, Landau P, and Katz R (1989) Treatment of obsessive–compulsive disorder with clomipramine. Psychiatr Ann 19, 97–101.

Direnfeld D, Pato MT, and Gunn S (2000) Behavior Therapy as Adjuvant Treatment in OCD. Poster presentation, at APA annual meeting, 14–18 May. Chicago, Illinois.

Dodman NH (1998) Veterinary models of obsessive–compulsive disorder. In Obsessive–Compulsive Disorders: Practical Management, Jenike M, Baer L, and Minichiello W (eds). Mosby, St. Louis, Missouri, pp. 318–334.

Dominguez RA, and Goodrick PJ (1995) Adverse events after abrupt discontinuation of paroxetine. Pharmacotherapy 15, 778–780.

Dominguez RA and Mestre SM (1994) Management of treatment-refractory obsessive–compulsive disorder patients. J Clin Psychiatr 55(Suppl), 86–92.

Dougherty DD, Laer L, Cosgrove GR, et al. (2002) Prospective long-term follow-up of 44 patients who received cingulotomy for treatment refractory obsessive–compulsive disorder. Am J Psychiatr 159, 269–275.

Eapen V, Robertson MM, Alsobrook JP, et al. (1997) Obsessive compulsive symptoms in Gilles de la Tourette's syndrome and obsessive compulsive disorder: Differences by diagnosis and family history. Am J Med Genet 74(4), 432–438.

Eisen JL and Rasmussen SA (1993) Obsessive–compulsive disorder with psychotic features. J Clin Psychiatr 54, 373–379.

Eisen JL, Beer DA, Pato MT, et al. (1997a) Obsessive–compulsive disorder in schizophrenia and schizoaffective disorders. Am J Psychiatr 154, 271–273.

Eisen JL, Goodman W, Keller MB, et al. (1999) Patterns of remission and relapse in OCD: A 2-year prospective study, J Clin Psychiatr 60, 346–351.

Eisen JL, Phillips KA, Beer DA, et al. (1998) The Brown assessment of beliefs scale: reliability and validity, Am J. Psychiatr 155, 102–108.

Eisen JL, Phillips KA, and Rasmussen SA (1997) Insight in body dysmorphic disorder versus OCD. New research program and abstracts, American Psychiatric Association, 150th Annual Meeting. American Psychiatric Association, San Diego, CA.

Eisen JL, Rasmussen SA, Phillips KA, et al. (2001) Insight and treatment outcome in obsessive–compulsive disorder. Compr Psychiatr 42(6), 494–497.

Erzegovesi S, Cavallini MC, Cavedini P, et al. (2001) Clinical predictors of drug response in obsessive–compulsive disorder. J Clin Psychopharmacol 21(5), 488–492.

Fallon BA, Liebowitz MR, and Campeas R, (1998) Inravenous clomipramine for obsessive–compulsive disorder refractory to oral clomipramine. Arch Gen Psychiatr 55, 918–924.

Fals-Stewart W, Marks AP, and Schafer J (1993) A comparison of behavioral group therapy and individual behavioral therapy in treating obsessive–compulsive disorder. J Nerv Ment Dis 18, 189–193.

Fenton WS and McGlashan TH (1986) The prognostic significance of obsessive–compulsive symptoms in schizophrenia. Am J Psychiatr 143, 437–441.

Flament MF, Koby E, Rapoport JL, et al. (1990) Childhood obsessive-compulsive disorder: A prospective follow-up study. J Child Psychol Psychiatr 31, 363–380.

Flament MF, Rapoport JL, Berg O, et al. (1985) Clomipramine treatment of childhood compulsive disorder. Arch Gen Psychiatr 42, 977–983.

Flament MF, Rapoport JL, Murphy DL, et al. (1987) Biochemical changes during clomipramine treatment of childhood obsessive–compulsive disorder. Arch Gen Psychiatr 44, 219–225.

Flament MF, Whitaker A, Rapoport JL, et al. (1988) Obsessive-compulsive disorder in adolescence: An epidemiologic study. J Am Acad Child Adolesc Psychiatr 27, 764–771.

Foa EB (1979) Failure in treating obsessive–compulsives. Behav Res Ther 17, 169–176.

Foa EB (1994) Recent findings in the efficacy of behavioral therapy and clomipramine for obsessive–compulsive disorder (OCD). Presented at the 14th National Conference of the Anxiety Disorders Association of America, 20 March, Santa Monica, CA.

Foa EB and Kozak MJ (1995) DSM-IV field trial: Obsessive–compulsive disorder. Am J Psychiatr 152, 90–96.

Foa EB, Abramowitz JS, Franklin ME, et al. (1999) Feared consequences, fixity of belief, and treatment outcome in patients with obsessive-compulsive disorder. Behav Ther 30, 717–724.

Foa EB, Grayson JB, Steketee GS, et al. (1983) Success and failure in the behavioral treatment of obsessive–compulsives. J Consult Clin Psychol 51, 287–297.

Foa EB, Steketee GS, and Ozarow BJ (1985) Behavior therapy with obsessive–compulsives: From theory to treatment. In Obsessive-Compulsive Disorder: Psychological and Pharmacological Treatment, Mavisskalian M, Turner SM, and Michelson L (eds). Plenum Press, New York, pp. 49–129.

Fontaine R and Chouinard G (1989) Fluoxetine in the long-term treatment of obsessive–compulsive disorder. Psychiatr Ann 19, 88–91.

Frankel A, Rosenthal J, Nezu A, et al. (1990) Efficacy of long-term treatment of obsessive–compulsive disorder. Mt Sinai J Med 57, 348–352.

Freedman CPL, Trimble MR, Deakin JFW, et al. (1994) Fluvoxamine versus clomipramine in the treatment of obsessive–compulsive disorder: A multicenter randomized double-blind paralellel group comparison. J Clin Psychiatr 55, 301–305.

Freud S (1963) An infantile neurosis. In The Standard Edition of the Complete Psychologic Works of Sigmund Freud, Vol. 17. Strachey J (trans-ed). Hogarth Press, London. Originally published in 1955.

Fyer A, Mannuzza S, Chapman TF, et al. (1993) Familial transmission of obsessive–compulsive disorder. Presented, at the First International Obsessive–Compulsive Disorder Conference, 12–13 March, Capri, Italy.

Gehring WJ, Himle J, and Nisenson LG (2000) Action-monitoring dysfuntion in obsessive–compulsive disorder. Psychol Sci 11(1), 1–6.

Goldberger E and Rapoport JL (1991) Canine acral lick dermatitis: Response to the anti-obsessional drug clomipramine. J Am Anim Hosp Assoc 27, 179–182.

Gold JM, Berman KF, Randolph C, et al. (1996) PET validation of novel prefrontal task: Delayed response alternation. Neuropsychology 10, 3–10.

Goodman WK, Ward H, Kablinger A, et al. (1997) Fluvoxamine in the treatment of obsessive–compulsive disorder and related conditions. J Clin Psychiatr 58, 32–49.

Goodman WK, McDougle CJ, Barr LC, et al. (1993) Biological approaches to treatment-resistant obsessive–compulsive disorder. J Clin Psychiatr 54(Suppl), 16–26.

Goodman WK, McDougle CJ, Lawrence HP, et al. (1990a) Beyond the serotonin hypothesis: A role for dopamine in some forms of obsessive–compulsive disorder. J Clin Psychopharmacol 51(Suppl), 36–43.

Goodman WK, Price LH, Delgado PL, et al. (1990b) Specificity of serotonin reuptake inhibitors in the treatment of obsessive–compulsive disorder. Arch Gen Psychiatr 47, 577–585.

Goodman WK, Price LH, Rasmussen SA, et al. (1989b) Efficacy of fluvoxamine in obsessive–compulsive disorder: A double-blind comparison with placebo. Arch Gen Psychiatr 46, 36–44.

Goodman WK, Price LH, Rasmussen SA, et al. (1989a) The Yale-Brown Obsessive–Compulsive Scale. Development, use, and reliability. Arch Gen Psychiatr 46, 1006–1011.

Goodman WK, Price LH, Rasmussen SA, et al. (1989) The Yale-Brown Obsessive–Compulsive Scale. I. Development, use, and reliability. Arch Gen Psychiatr 46(11) (Nov), 1006–1011.

Goodman WK, Price LH, Rasmussen SA, et al. (1989c) The Yale-Brown Obsessive–Compulsive Scale. II. Validity. Arch Gen Psychiatr 46, 1012–1016.

Goodwin DW, Guze SB, and Robbins E. (1969) Follow-up studies in obsessional neurosis Arch Gen Psychiatr 20, 182–187.

Grados MA, Riddle MA, Samuels JF, et al. (2001) The familial phenotype of obsessive–compulsive disorder in relation to tic disorders: The Hopkins OCD family study. Biol Psychiatr 50(8), 559–565.

Greenberg BD, George MS, Martin JD, et al. (1997) Effect of prefrontal repetitive transcranial magnetic stimulaton in obsessive–compulsive disorder: A preliminary study. Am J Psychiatr 154, 867–869.

Griest JH (1994) Behavior therapy for obsessive–compulsive disorder. J Clin Psychiatr 55(Suppl), 60–68.

Griest JH and Jefferson JW (1998) Pharmacotherapy for obsessive-compulsive disorder. Brit J Psychiatr 173(Suppl 35), 64–70.

Griest J, Chouinard G, DuBoff E, et al. (1995a) Double–blind parallel comparison of three dosages of sertraline and placebo in outpatients with obsessive–compulsive disorder. Arch Gen Psychiatr 52, 289–295.

Greist JH, Jefferson JW, Kobak KA, et al. (1995b) Efficacy and tolerability of serotonin transport inhibitors in obsessive–compulsive disorder. Arch Gen Psychiatr 52, 53–60.

Greist JH, Marks IM, Baer L, et al. (2002 Feb) Behavior therapy for obsessive–compulsive disorder guided by a computer or by a clinican compared with relaxation as a control. J Clin Psychiatr 63(2), 138–145.

Hermesh H, Aizenberg D, and Munitz H (1990) Trazodone treatment in clomipramine resistant obsessive–compulsive disorder. Clin Neuropharmacol 13, 322–328.

Hewlett WA and Martin K (1993) Fenfluramine challenges and serotonergic functioning in obsessive–compulsive disorder. Presented at the

First International Obsessive–Compulsive Disorder Congress, 12–13 March, Capri, Italy.

Hewlett WA, Vinogrador S, and Agrash S (1992) Clomipramine, clonazepam, and clonidine treatment of obsessive–compulsive disorder. J Clin Psychopharmacol 12, 420–430.

Hoehn-Saric R, Ninan P, Black DW, et al. (2000) Multicenter double-blind comparison of sertraline and desipramine for concurrent obsessive–compulsive and major depressive disorders. Arch Gen Psychiatr 57, 76–82.

Hoehn-Saric R, Pearlson G, Harris G, et al. (1991) Effects of fluoxetine on regional cerebral blood flow in obsessive–compulsive patients. Am J Psychiatr 148, 1243–1245.

Hohagen F, Winkelmann G, Rasche-Rauchle H, et al. (1998) Combination of behavior therapy with fluvoxamine in comparison with behaviour therapy and placebo. Brit J Psychiatr 173(Suppl 35), 71–78.

Hollander E, DeCaria C, Nitescu A, et al. (1992) Serotonergic function in obsessive–compulsive disorder: Behavioral and neuroendocrine responses to oral *m*-chlorophenylpiperazine and fenfluramine in patients and healthy volunteers. Arch Gen Psychiatr 49, 21–28.

Hollander E (1993) Introduction. In Obsessive–Compulsive Related Disorders, Hollander E (ed). American Psychiatric Press, Washington DC, pp. 1–16.

Hunter R and Macalpine I (1982) Three Hundred Years of Psychiatry 1535–1860: A History Presented in Selected English Texts. Hartsdale, Carlisle, NY, pp. 164–165.

Ingram JE (1961) Obsessional illness in mental health hospital patients. J Ment Sci 107, 382–402.

Insel TR (1992) Toward a neuroanatomy of obsessive–compulsive disorder. Arch Gen Psychiatr 49, 739–744.

Insel TR and Akiskal HS (1986) Obsessive–compulsive disorder with psychotic features: A phenomenological analysis. Am J Psychiatr 143, 1527–1533.

Insel T, Murphy D, Cohen R, et al. (1983) Obsessive–compulsive disorder: A double-blind study of clomipramine and clorgyline. Arch Gen Psychiatr 40, 605–612.

Insel TR and Winslow JT (1990) Neurobiology of obsessive–compulsive disorder. In Obsessive–Compulsive Disorders: Theory and Management, 2nd ed, Jenike MA, Baer L, and Minichiello WE (eds). Mosby Year Book, St. Louis, Missouri, p. 118.

Jaspers K (1923) Hoeing J and Hamilton MW (trans) (1963) General Psychopathology. University of Chicago Press, Chicago. (Originally published in 1923)

Jenike MA (1981) Rapid response of severe obsessive–compulsive disorder to tranylcypromine. Am J Psychiatr 138, 1249–1250.

Jenike MA (1990) Theories of etiology. In Obsessive–Compulsive Disorders: Theory and Management, Jenike MA, Baer L, Minichiello WE (eds). Mosby Year Book, St. Louis, Missouri.

Jenike MA (1991) Management of patients with treatment-resistant obsessive–compulsive disorder. In Current Treatments of Obsessive–Compulsive Disorder, Pato MT and Zohar J (eds). American Psychiatric Press, Washington DC, p. 146.

Jenike MA (1992) Pharmacologic treatment of obsessive–compulsive disorders. Psychiatr Clin N Am 15, 895–919.

Jenike MA (1993) Augmentation strategies for treatment-resistant obsessive–compulsive disorder. Harv Rev Psychiatr 1, 17–26.

Jenike MA (1998) Neurosurgical treatment of obsessive–compulsive disorder. Br J Psychiatr 173(Suppl 35), 79–90.

Jenike MA and Baer L (1988) Buspirone in obsessive–compulsive disorder: An open trial. Am J Psychiatr 145, 1285–1286.

Jenike MA, Butolph L, Baer L, et al. (1989) Open trial of fluoxetine in obsessive–compulsive disorder. Am J Psychiatr 146, 909–911.

Jenike MA, Baer L, and Buttolph L (1991) Buspirone augmentation of fluoxetine in patients with obsessive–compulsive disorder. J Clin Psychiatr 1, 13–14.

Jenike MA, Baer L, and Griest JH (1990a) Clomipramine versus fluoxetine in obsessive–compulsive disorder: A retrospective comparison of side effects and efficacy. J Clin Psychopharmacol 10, 122–124.

Jenike MA, Baer L, Minichiello WE, et al. (1986) Concomitant obsessive–compulsive disorder and schizotypal personality disorder. Am J Psychiatr 143, 530–532.

Jenike MA, Baer L, Minichiello WE, et al. (1997) Placebo-controlled trial of fluoxetine and phenelzine for obsessive–compulsive disorder. Am J Psychiatr 154, 1261–1264.

Jenike MA, Baer L, and Minichiello WE (1998) Obsessive–Compulsive Disorder: Practical Management. Mosby, St. Louis, Missouri.

Jenike MA, Hyman SE, Baer L, et al. (1990b) A controlled trial of fluvoxamine for obsessive–compulsive disorder: Implications for a serotonergic theory. Am J Psychiatr 147, 1209–1215.

Jenike MA, Surman OS, Cassem NH, et al. (1983) Monoamine oxidase inhibitors in obsessive–compulsive disorder. J Clin Psychiatr 44, 131–132.

Keuthen NJ, Cyr R, Ricciarde JA, et al. (1994) Medication withdrawal symptoms in obsessive–compulsive disorder patients treated with paroxetine (letter). J Clin Psychopharmacol 14, 206–207.

Koran LM, Hackett E, Rubin A, et al. (2002) Efficacy of sertraline in the long term treatment of obsessive–compulsive disorder. Am J Psychiatr 159, 88–95.

Koran LM, McElroy SL, Davison JRT, et al. (1996) Fluvoxamine versus clomipramine for obsessive–compulsive disorder: A double-blind comparison. J Clin Psychopharmacol 16, 121–129.

Koran LM, Ringold AL, and Elliot MA (2000) Olanzapine augmentation for treatment resistant obsessive–compulsive disorder. J Clin Psychiatr 61, 514–517.

Koran LM, Sallee FR, and Pallanti S (1997) Rapid benefit of intravenous pulse loading of clomipramine in obsessive–compulsive disorder. Am J Psychiatr 154, 396–401.

Kozak MJ and Foa EB (1994) Obsessions, overvalued ideas, and delusions in obsessive–compulsive disorder. Behav Res Ther 32, 343–353.

Kringlin E (1965) Obsessional neurotics: A long-term follow-up. Br J Psychiatr 111, 709–722.

Leckman JL, Walker DE, Goodman WK, et al. (1994) "Just right" perceptions associated with compulsive behavior in Tourette's syndrome. Am J Psychiatr 151, 675–680.

Leckman JF, Boardman J, Grice DE, et al. (1997) Symptoms of obsessive–compulsive disorder. Am J Psychiatr 154, 911–917.

Lees AJ, Robertson M, Trimble MR, et al. (1984) A clinical study of Gilles de la Tourette syndrome in the United Kingdom. J Neurol Neurosurg Psychiatr 47, 1–8.

Lelliot PT, Noshirvani HF, Basoglu M, et al. (1988) Obsessive–compulsive beliefs and treatment outcome. Psychol Med 18, 697–702.

Lenane MC, Swedo SE, Leonard H, et al. (1990) Psychiatric disorders in first-degree relatives of children and adolescents with obsessive–compulsive disorder. J Am Acad Child Adolesc Psychiatr 29, 407–412.

Leonard HL, Lenane MC, Swedo SE, et al. (1992) Tics and Tourette's disorder: A 2- to 7-year follow-up of 54 obsessive–compulsive children. Am J Psychiatr 149, 1244–1251.

Leonard HL, Swedo SE, Lenane MD, et al. (1991) A double-blind desipramine substitution during long-term clomipramine treatment in children and adolescents with obsessive–compulsive disorder. Arch Gen Psychiatr 48, 922–927.

Leonard HL, Swedo SE, Lenane MC, et al. (1993) A 2- to 7-year follow-up study of 54 obsessive–compulsive children and adolescents. Arch Gen Psychiatr 50, 429–439.

Leonard HL, Swedo SE, Rapoport JL, et al. (1989) Treatment of childhood obsessive–compulsive disorder with clomipramine and desipramine: A double-blind crossover comparison. Arch Gen Psychiatr 46, 1088–1092.

Levine R, Hoffman JS, Knepple ED, et al. (1989) Long-term fluoxetine treatment of a large number of obsessive–compulsive patients. J Clin Psychopharmacol 9, 281–283.

Lewis A (1936) Problems of obsessional illness. Proc R Soc Med 29, 325–336.

Liebowitz MR, Hollander E, Schneier F, et al. (1989) Fluoxetine treatment of obsessive–compulsive disorder: An open clinical trial. J Clin Psychopharmacol 9, 423–427.

Lippitz BE, Mindus P, Meyerson BA, et al. (1999 March) Lesion topography and outcome after thermocapsulotomy or gamma knife capsulotomy for obsessive–compulsive disorder: Relevance of the right hemisphere. Neurosurgery 44(3), 452–458; discussion 458–460.

Lo W (1967) A follow-up study of obsessional neurotics in Hong Kong Chinese. Br J Psychiatr 113, 823–832.

Lopez-Ibor JJ, Saiz J, Cottraux J, et al. (1996) Double-blind comparison of fluoxetine versus clomipramine in the treatment of obsessive–compulsive disorder. Eur neuropsychopharmacol 6, 111–118.

Lydiard RB (1986) Obsessive–compulsive disorder successfully treated with trazodone. Psychosomatics 27, 258–259.

MacKinnon RA and Michels R (1971) The obsessive patient. In The Psychiatric Interview in Clinical Practice, MacKinnon RA and Michels R (eds). WB Saunders, Philadelphia, pp. 89–109.

Mallya GK, White K, Waterman C, et al. (1992) Short- and long-term treatment of obsessive–compulsive disorder with fluvoxamine. Ann Clin Psychiatr 4, 77–80.

March JS, Frances A, Carpenter D, et al. (1997) The expert consensus guildline series: Treatment of obsessive–compulsive disorder. J Clin Psychiatr 58(suppl 4).

Markovitz PJ, Stagnos J, and Calabresa JR (1990) Buspirone augmentation of fluoxetine on obsessive–compulsive disorder. Am J Psychiatr 147, 798–800.

Marks I, Lelliot P, Basoglsu M, et al. (1988) Clomipramine, self exposure and therapist-added exposure in obsessive–compulsive ritualizers. Br J Psychiatr 152, 522–534.

Marks I, Stern A, Mawson D, et al. (1980) Clomipramine and exposure for obsessive–compulsive rituals. Br J Psychiatr 136, 1–25.

Mataix-Cois D, Rausch SL, Baer L, et al. (2002) Stability in Adult obsessive–compulsive disorder: Data from a naturalistic two-year follow-up study. Am J Psychiatr 159, 263–268.

Mataix-Cois D, Rausch SL, Manzo P, et al. (1999) Use of factor-analyzed symptom dimensions to predict outcome with serotonin reuptake inhibitors and placebo in the treatment of obsessive–compulsive disorder. Am J Psychiatr 156, 1409–1416.

McDougle CJ, Epperson CN, Pelton GH, et al. (2000) A double-blind, placebo-controlled study of risperdone addition in serotonin reuptake inhibitor refractory obsessive–compulsive disorder. Arch Gen Psychiatr 57, 794–801.

McDougle CJ, Goodman WK, Leckman JF, et al. (1993) Limited therapeutic effect of addition of buspirone in fluvoxamine refractory obsessive–compulsive disorder. Am J Psychiatr 150, 647–649.

McDougle CJ, Goodman WK, Price LH, et al. (1990) Neuroleptic addition in fluvoxamine refractory obsessive–compulsive disorder. Am J Psychiatr 147, 652–654.

McDougle CJ, Price LH, Goodman WK, et al. (1991) A controlled trial of lithium augmentation in fluvoxamine refractory obsessive–compulsive disorder: Lack of efficacy. J Clin Psychopharmacol 11, 175–184.

McElroy SL, Hudson JI, Phillips KA, et al. (1993) Clinical and theoretical implications of a possible link between obsessive–compulsive and impulse control disorders. Depression 1, 121–132.

McElroy SL, Phillips KA, and Keck PE Jr (1994) Obsessive–compulsive spectrum disorders. J Clin Psychiatr 55(Suppl), 33–51.

McKeon P and Murray R (1987) Familial aspects of obsessive–compulsive neurosis. Br J Psychiatr 51, 528–534.

Miguel DC, Do Rosario-Campos MC, Prado HS, et al. (2000) Sensory phenomena in obsessive–compulsive disorder and Tourette's disorder. J Clin Psychiatr 61(2), 150–156.

Miguel EC, Coffey BJ, Baer L, et al. (1995) Phenomenology of intentional behaviors in obsessive-compulsive disorder and Tourette's disorder. J Clin Psychiatr 56, 246–255.

Mindus P and Jenike MA (1992) Neurosurgical treatment of malignant obsessive–compulsive disorder. Psychiatr Clin N Am 15, 921–938.

Montgomery SA, Kasper S, Stein DL, et al. (2001 March) Citalopram 20 mg, 40 mg and 60 mg are all effective and well tolerated compared with placebo in obsessive–compulsive disorder. Int Clin Psychopharmacol 16(2), 75–86.

Muller C (1953) Der ubergong Zwangsnevrose in Schizphrenic im licht der Katamnese. Schweiz Arch Neurol Psychiatr 72, 218–225.

Mundo E, Bianchi L, and Bellodi L (1997) Efficacy of fluvoxamine, paroxetine and citalopram in the treatment of obsessive–compulsive disorder: A single-blind study. J Clin Psychopharmacol 17, 267–271.

Myers JK, Weissman MM, Tischler GL, et al. (1984) Six–month prevalence of psychiatric disorders in three communities, 1980 to 1982. Arch Gen Psychiatr 41, 949–958.

Nestadt G, Samuels J, Riddle M, et al. (2000) A family study of obsessive–compulsive disorder. Arch Gen Psychiatr 57, 358–363.

Nicolini H, Cruz C, Camarena B, et al. (1999) Understanding the genetic basis of obsessive–compulsive disorder. CNS Spect 4(5), 32–48.

Nordahl TE, Benkelfat C, Semple WE, et al. (1989) Cerebral glucose metabolic rates in obsessive–compulsive disorder. Neuropsychopharmacology 2, 23–28.

Orley J and Wing JK (1979) Psychiatric disorders in two African villages. Arch Gen Psychiatr 36, 513–520.

Orloff LM, Battle MA, Baer L, et al. (1994) Long-term follow-up of 85 patients with obsessive–compulsive disorder. Am J Psychiatr 151, 441–442.

O'Sullivan G and Marks I (1991) Follow-up studies of behavioral treatment of phobia and obsessive–compulsive neurosis. Psychiatr Ann 21, 368–373.

Pato MT and Steketee G (eds) (1997) OCD Across the Life Cycle in American Psychiatric Press: Review of Psychiatry, Vol. 16. American Psychiatric Press, Washington DC.

Pato MT and Zohar J (eds) (2001) Current Treatments of Obsessive–Compulsive Disorder. American Psychiatric Press, Washington DC.

Pato MT, Eisen JL, and Pato CN (1994) Rating scales for obsessive–compulsive disorder. In Current Insights in Obsessive–Compulsive Disorder, Hollander E, Zohar J, Marazziti D, et al. (eds). John Wiley, West Sussex, UK, pp. 77–92.

Pato MT, Hill JL, and Murphy DL (1990) What is the lowest therapeutically effective clomipramine dose in obsessive–compulsive disorder patients? Psychopharmacol Bull 26, 211–214.

Pato MT, Murphy DL, and DeVane CL (1991a) Sustained plasma concentrations of fluoxetine and/or norfluoxetine four and eight weeks after fluoxetine discontinuation. J Clin Psychopharmacol 11, 224–225.

Pato MT, Pato CP, and Pauls DL (2002) Recent findings in the genetics of OCD. J Clin Psychiatr 63(Suppl 6), 30–33.

Pato MT, Pigott TA, Hill JL, et al. (1991b) Controlled comparison of buspirone and clomipramine in obsessive–compulsive disorder. Am J Psychiatr 148, 127–129.

Pato MT, Zohar-Kadouch R, Zohar J, et al. (1988) Return of symptoms after discontinuation of clomipramine in patients with obsessive–compulsive disorder. Am J Psychiatr 145, 1521–1525.

Pauls DL (1999) Phenotypic variability in obsessive–compulsive disorder and its relationship to familial risk. CNS Spect 4(6), 57–61.

Pauls DL, Alsobrook MP, Goodman W, et al. (1995) A family study of obsessive–compulsive disorder. Am J Psychiatr 152, 76–84.

Pauls DL, Towbin KE, Leckman JF, et al. (1986) Gilles de la Tourette's syndrome and obsessive–compulsive disorder: Evidence supporting a genetic relationship. Arch Gen Psychiatr 43, 1180–1182.

Phillips KA (1991) Body dysmorphic disorder: The distress of imagined ugliness. Am J Psychiatr 148, 1138–1149.

Phillips KA, Gunderson CG, Mallya G, et al. (1994) A comparison study of body dysmorphic disorder and obsessive–compulsive disorder. Presented at the 33rd Annual Meeting of the American College of Neuropsychopharmacology, San Juan, Puerto Rico.

Phillips KA, McElroy SL, Hudson JI, et al. (1995) Body dysmorphic disorder: An OCD spectrum disorder, a form of affective spectrum disorder, or both? J Clin Psychiatr 56(Suppl), 41–51.

Pigott TA (1996) OCD: Where the serotonin selective story begins. J Clin Psychiatr 57(Suppl 6), 11–20.

Pigott TA, Hill JL, Grady TA, et al. (1993) A comparison of the behavioral effects of oral versus intravenous mCPP administration in OCD patients and the effect of metergoline prior to i.v. mCPP. Biol Psychiatr 33, 3–14.

Pigott TA, L'Hereux F, Hill JL, et al. (1992a) A double-blind study of adjuvant buspirone hydrochloride in clomipramine-treated patients with obsessive–compulsive disorder. J Clin Psychopharmacol 12, 11–18.

Pigott TA, Littenfer XF, Rubenstein CS, et al. (1992b) A double-blind, placebo-controlled study of trazodone in patients with obsessive–compulsive disorder. J Clin Psychopharmacol 12, 156–162.

Pigott TA, Pato MT, Bernstein SE, et al. (1990) Controlled comparison of clomipramine and fluoxetine in the treatment of obsessive–compulsive disorder. Arch Gen Psychiatr 47, 926–932.

Pigott TA, Zohar J, Hill JL, et al. (1991) Metergoline blocks the behavioral and neuroendocrine effects of orally administered m-chlorophenylpiperazine in patients with obsessive–compulsive disorder. Biol Psychiatr 29, 418–426.

Pitman RA (1994) Obsessive–compulsive disorder in western history. In Current Insights in Obsessive–Compulsive Disorder, Hollander E, Zohar J, Marazziti D, et al. (eds). John Wiley, West Sussex, UK, pp. 3–10.

Pitman RK (1991) Historical considerations. In Psychobiology of Obsessive–Compulsive Disorder, Zohar J, Insel T, and Rasmussen S (eds). Springer-Verlag, New York, pp. 1–12.

Pitman RK, Green RC, Jenike MA, et al. (1987) Clinical comparison of Tourette's disorder and obsessive–compulsive disorder. Am J Psychiatr 144, 1166–1171.

Pollitt JD (1957) Natural history of obsessional states. Br Med J 1, 194–198.

Porto L, Bermanzohn PC, and Pollack S, et al. (1997) A profile of obsessive–compulsive symptoms in schizophrenia. CNS Spect 2, 21–25.

Rachman SJ and Hodgson RJ (1980) Obsessions and Compulsions. Prentice-Hall, Englewood Cliffs, NJ.

Rapoport JL and Wise SP (1988) Obsessive–compulsive disorder: Is it a basal ganglion dysfunction? Psychopharmacol Bull 24, 380–384.

Rapoport J, Elkins R, and Mikkelsen E (1980) Clinical controlled trial of clomipramine in adolescents with obsessive–compulsive disorder. Psychopharmacol Bull 16, 61–65.

Rapoport JL, Ryland D, and Kriete M (1992) Drug treatment of canine acral lick: An animal model of obsessive–compulsive disorder. Arch Gen Psychiatr 49, 517–521.

Rasmussen SA and Eisen JL (1991) Phenomenology of obsessive–compulsive disorder. In Psychobiology of Obsessive–Compulsive Disorder, Insel J, Rasmussen S (eds). Springer-Verlag, New York, pp. 743–758.

Rasmussen SA and Eisen JL (1992) The epidemiology and clinical features of OCD. Psychiatr Clin N Am 15, 743–758.

Rasmussen SA and Eisen JL (1998) The Epidemiology and Clinical Features of Obsessive–Compulsive Disorder. In Obsessive–Compulsive Disorders: Practical Management, Jenike M, Baer L, and Minichiello W (eds). Mosby, St. Louis, Missouri.

Rasmussen SA and Tsuang MT (1986) Clinical characteristics and family history in DSM-III obsessive–compulsive disorder. Am J Psychiatr 143, 317–322.

Rasmussen SA, Eisen JL, and Pato MT (1993) Current issues in the pharmacologic management of obsessive–compulsive disorder. J Clin Psychiatr 54(Suppl), 4–9.

Rasmussen S, Hackett E, DuBoff E, et al. (1997) A 2-year study of sertraline in the treatment of obsessive–compulsive disorder. Int Clin Psychopharmacol 12(6), 309–316.

Rauch SL, Dougherty DD, Shin LM, et al. (1998) Neural correlates of factor-analyzed OCD symptom dimensions: A PET Study.

Rauch SL, Jenike MA, Alpert NM, et al. (1994) Regional cerebral blood flow measured during symptom provocation in obsessive–compulsive disorder using oxygen 15-labeled carbon dioxide and positron emission tomography. Arch Gen Psychiatr 51, 62–70.

Ravizza L, Barzega G, Bellino S, et al. (1995) Predictors of drug treatment response in obsessive–compulsive disorder. J Clin Psychiatr 56(8), 368–373.

Ravizza L, Barzega G, Bellino S, et al. (1996) Drug treatment of obsessive–compulsive disorder (OCD): Long-term trial with clomipramine and selective serotonin reuptake inhibitors (SSRIs). Psychopharmacol Bull 32(1), 167–173.

Ricciardi JN, Baer L, Jenike MA, et al. (1992) Changes in DSM-III-R axis II diagnoses following treatment of obsessive–compulsive disorder. Am J Psychiatr 149, 829–831.

Richter MA (2001) Citalopram in current treatments of obsessive–compulsive disorder, Pato MT, and Zohar J (eds). American Psychiatric Press, Washington DC, pp. 93–107.

Riddle MA, Schaill L, King R, et al. (1990) Obsessive–compulsive disorder in children and adolescents: Phenomenology and family history. J Am Acad Child Adolesc Psychiatr 29, 766–772.

Robertson MM, Trimble MR, and Lees AJ (1988) The psychopathology of the Gilles de la Tourette syndrome: A phenomenological analysis. Br J Psychiatr 152, 283–390.

Robins LN, Helzer JE, Weissman MM, et al. (1984) Lifetime prevalence of specific psychiatric disorders in three sites. Arch Gen Psychiatr 41, 958–967.

Robinson D, Wu H, Munne RA, et al. (1995) Reduced Caudate Nucleus Volume in obsessive–compulsive disorder. Arch Gen Psychiatr 52, 393–398.

Rosenberg CM (1968) Complications of obsessional neurosis. Br J Psychiatr 114, 447–478.

Rubenstein CS, Pigott TA, L'Heureux F, et al. (1992) A preliminary investigation of the lifetime prevalence of anorexia and bulimia nervosa in patients with obsessive–compulsive disorder. J Clin Psychiatr 53, 309–314.

Rudin E (1953) Ein Beitrag zur Frage der Zwangskrankheit. Arch Psychiatr Nervenkr 191, 14–54.

Salzman L (1983) Psychoanalytic therapy of the obsessional patient. Curr Psychiatr Ther 9, 53–59.

Samuels J, Nestadt G, and Bienvenu OJ (2000) Personality disorders and normal personality dimensions in obsessive–compulsive disorder. Br J Psychiatr 177, 457–462.

Savage C (1996) Neuropsychology of OCD: New findings and applications. J Clin Psychiatr 57, 498–500.

Saxena S, Brody AL, Schwartz JM, et al. (1998) Neuroimaging and frontal–subcortical circuitry in obsessive–compulsive disorder. Br J Psychiatr 173(Suppl 35), 26–37.

Saxena S, Wang D, Bystritsky A, et al. (1996) Risperdone Augmentation of SRI treatment for refractory obsessive–compulsive disorder. J Clin Psychiatr 57, 303–306.

Schwartz JH (1998) Neuroanatomical aspects of cognitive–behavioral therapy response in obsessive–compulsive disorder" an evolving perspective on brain and behavior. Br J Psychiatr 173(Suppl 35), 38–44.

Simpson HB, Gorfinkle KS, and Liebowitz MR (1999) Cognitive–behavioral therapy as an adjunct to serotonin reuptake inhibitors in obsessive–compulsive disorder: An open trial. J Clin Psychiatr 60, 584–590.

Skoog G and Skoog I (1999) A 40-year follow-up of patients with obsessive–compulsive disorder. Arch Gen Psychiatr 56, 121–127.

Stein DJ, Bouwer C, Hawkridge S, et al. (1997) Risperidone augmentation of serotonin reuptake inhibitors in obsessive–compulsive disorder and related disorders. J Clin Psychiatr 58, 119–122.

Stein DJ, Seedat S, Shapira NA, et al. (2001) Management of treatment-resistant obsessive–compulsive disorder. In Current Treatment of Obsessive–Compulsive Disorder, Pato MT, Zohar J (eds). American Psychiatric Press, Washington DC, pp. 221–237.

Stein MB, Fordee DR, Anderson G, et al. (1997) Obsessive–Compulsive disorder in the Community: An Epidemiologic survey with Clinical Reappraisal. Am J Psychiatr 154, 1120–1126.

Steketee G, Eisen JL, Dyke I, et al. (1999) Predictors of Course in Obsessive–Compulsive Disorder. Psychiatr Res 89, 229–238.

Strauss WL, Layton ME, Hayes CE, et al. (1997) 19F magnetic resonance spectroscopy investigation in vivo of acute and steady-state brain fluvoxamine levels in obsessive–compulsive disorder. Am J Psychiatr 54, 516–522.

Swedo SE, Leonard HL, Garvey M, et al. (1998) Pediatric autoimmune neuropsychiatric disorders associated with streptococcal infection: Clinical description of the first 50 cases. Am J Psychiatr 155, 264–271.

Swedo SE, Pietrini P, Leonard HL, et al. (1992) Cerebral glucose metabolism in childhood onset obsessive–compulsive disorder. Revisualization during pharmacology. Arch Gen Psychiatr 49, 690–694.

Swedo SE, Rapoport JL, Leonard H, et al. (1989a) Obsessive–compulsive disorder in children and adolescents: Clinical phenomenology of 70 consecutive cases. Arch Gen Psychiatr 46, 335–341.

Swedo SE, Schapiro MB, Grady CL, et al. (1989b) Cerebral glucose metabolism in childhood-onset obsessive–compulsive disorder. Arch Gen Psychiatr 46, 518–523.

Szegedi A, Wetzel H, Leal M, et al. (1996) Combination treatment with clomipramine and fluvoxamine: drug monitoring, safety and tolerability data. J Clin Psychiatr 57, 257–264.

Szeszko PR, Robinson D, Alvir JMJ, et al. (1999) Orbital frontal and amygdala volume reductions in obsessive–compulsive disorder. Arch Gen Psychiatr 56, 913–919.

The Clomipramine Collaborative Study Group (1991) Efficacy of clomipramine in OCD: Results of a multicenter double-blind trial. Arch Gen Psychiatr 48, 730–738.

Thiel A, Broocks A, Ohlmeier M, et al. (1995) Obsessive–compulsive disorder among patients with anorexia nervosa and bulimia nervosa. Am J Psychiatr 152, 72–75.

Thoren P, Asberg M, Bertilsson L, et al. (1980) Clomipramine treatment of obsessive–compulsive disorder. II. Biochemical aspects. Arch Gen Psychiatr 37, 1289–1294.

Tinbergen N (1953) Social Behaviour in Animals. Theissen, Chapman and Hall, London.

Tollefson GD, Birkett M, Koran L, et al. (1994a) Continuation treatment of OCD: Double-blind and open-label experience with fluoxetine. J Clin Psychiatr 55(Suppl), 69–76.

Tollefson GD, Rampey AH, Potvin JH, et al. (1994b) A multicenter investigation of fixed dose fluoxetine in the treatment of obsesssive–compulsive disorder. Arch Gen Psychiatr 51, 559–567.

Turner SM, Jacob RG, Beidel DC, et al. (1985) Fluoxetine treatment of obsessive–compulsive disorder. J Clin Psychopharmacol 5, 207–212.

Van Noppen BL, Rasmussen SA, McCartney L, et al. (1991) A multifamily group approach as an adjunct to treatment of obsessive–compulsive disorders. In Current Treatments of Obsessive–Compulsive Disorder, Pato MT and Zohar J (eds). American Psychiatric Press, Washington DC, pp. 115–134.

Van Noppen BL, Pato MT, Marsland R, et al. (1998) A time-limited behavioral group for treatment of obsessive–compulsive disorder. J Psychother Pract Res 7, 272–280.

Walter CS (1973) Clinical impression of treatment of obsessional states with intravenous clomipramine. J Int Med 1, 413–416.

Weissman MM, Bland RC, Canino GL, et al. (1994) The cross-national epidemiology of obsessive–compulsive disorder. J Clin Psychiatr 55, 5–10.

Welner A, Reich T, Robins E, et al. (1976) Obsessive compulsive neurosis: Record, follow-up and family studies. Compr Psychiatr 17, 527–539.

Wheadon D, Bushnell W, and Steiner M (1993) A fixed-dose comparison of 20, 40, or 60 mg paroxetine to placebo in the treatment of obsessive–compulsive disorder. Presented at the Annual Meeting of the American College of Neuropsychopharmacology Honolulu, Hawaii.

Winslow J and Insel T (1991) Neuroethological models of obssessive–compulsive disorder. In Psychobiology of Obsessive–Compulsive Disorder, Zohar J, Insel T, Rasmussen S (eds). Springer-Verlag, New York pp. 208–227.

Wood A, Tollefson GD, and Birkett M (1993) Pharmacotherapy of obsessive–compulsive disorder—experience with fluoxetine. Int Clin Psychopharmacol 8, 301–306.

Yeh EH and Chang L (1989) Prevalence of psychiatric disorders in Taiwan. Acta Psychiatr Scand 79, 136–147.

Zajecka JM, Fawcett J, and Guy C (1990) Co-existing major depression and obsessive–compulsive disorder treated with venlafaxine. J Clin Psychopharmacol 10, 152–153.

Zohar AH, Pauls DL, RatzoniG, et.al. (1997) Obsessive–Compulsive Disorder with and without tics in and epidemiologic sample of adolescents. Am J Psychiatr 154, 274–276.

Zohar AH, Ratoni G, Pauls DL, et al. (1992) An epidemiological study of obsessive–compulsive disorder and related disorders in Israeli adolescents. J Am Acad Child Adolesc Psychiatr 31, 1057–1061.

Zohar J and Insel TR (1987) Obsessive–compulsive disorder: Psychobiological approaches to diagnosis, treatment, and pathophysiology. Biol Psychiatr 22, 667–687.

Zohar J and Judge R (1996) Paroxetine versus clomipramine in the treatment of obsessive–complsive disorder. Br J Psychiatr 169, 468–474.

Zohar J, Insel TR, Zohar KR, et al. (1988) Serotonergic responsivity in obsessive–compulsive disorder. Effects of chronic clomipramine treatment. Arch Gen Psychiatr 45, 167–172.

Zohar J, Mueller E, Insel T, et al. (1987) Serotonergic responsivity in obsessive–compulsive disorder: Comparison of patients and healthy controls. Arch Gen Psychiatr 44, 946–951.

# 69 Anxiety Disorders: Traumatic Stress Disorders

Jean C. Beckham
Jonathan R.T. Davidson
John S. March

Posttraumatic Stress Disorder

Acute Stress Disorder

This chapter reviews posttraumatic stress disorders (PTSD), and the relatively new diagnosis of acute stress disorder (ASD). We provide definitions and summarize epidemiology, etiology, pathophysiology, diagnosis, differential diagnosis, and comorbidity. We also review the course and natural history of these disorders. Finally, we review overall goals of treatment and discuss specific treatment approaches and factors influencing response.

## POSTTRAUMATIC STRESS DISORDER

### Definition

PTSD is defined in the *Diagnostic and Statistical Manual of Mental Disorders*, Fourth Edition (DSM-IV) by six different criteria (American Psychiatric Association 1994, see pp. 427–429). First, the disorder arises in a person who has been exposed to a traumatic event in which he or she experienced, witnessed, or was confronted with actual or threatened death or serious injury or a threat to the physical integrity of self or others. Furthermore, the response must have involved intense fear, helplessness, or horror. In children, it is allowed that the response may take the form of disorganized or agitated behavior.

Second, there must have been at least one of five possible intrusive symptoms occurring as a result of exposure to the trauma, as exhibited in either dream activity or waking life. These include recollections, images, thoughts, or perceptions of the event, recurrent distressing dreams, acting as if the trauma were recurring, and intense psychological or physical distress on exposure to internal or external cues resembling the trauma. Allowance is made for a different set of reactions in children, in whom intrusive symptoms may take the form of repetitive play, frightening dreams without recognizable content, or reenactment of the trauma.

Third, persistent avoidance of stimuli associated with the trauma and numbing of general responsiveness must occur as exhibited by at least three of seven symptoms. Although grouped together as one criterion, it is likely that phobic avoidance, numbing, and withdrawal do not reflect the same underlying phenomenon.

Fourth, there must be at least two symptoms indicating the presence of increased arousal (i.e., difficulty sleeping, irritability or anger, difficulty concentrating, hypervigilance, or exaggerated startle response). Symptoms of PTSD should last at least 1 month, and it is necessary that the disturbances cause clinically significant distress or impairment in social, occupational, or other areas of functioning.

PTSD is considered to be "acute" if the duration of symptoms is between 1 and 3 months or "chronic" if it is 3 months or greater. If symptoms do not occur until at least 6 months have passed since the stressor, the delayed-onset subtype is given.

### Epidemiology

Community-based studies conducted in the US have documented a lifetime prevalence rate for PTSD of approximately 8% of the adult population (Kessler et al. 1995). General population female-to-male lifetime prevalence ratio is 2:1 (Breslau 2001). General population prevalence rates from other countries are unavailable. The highest rates of PTSD occurrence for particular traumatic exposures (occurring in one-third to three-fourths of those exposed) are among survivors of rape, military combat and captivity, graves registration (i.e., registering dead bodies through the morgue), and ethnically or politically motivated interment and genocide (Breslau 2001).

Epidemiological studies show that PTSD often remains chronic, with a significant number of people remaining symptomatic several years after the initial event. In support of this view are epidemiological data that show that recovery frequently does not occur. For example, the National Vietnam Veterans Readjustment study (Kulka et al. 1990) found lifetime and current prevalence rates of PTSD to be, respectively, 30.9 and 15.2% in men and 26.9 and 8.5% in women. In a population of rape victims, Kilpa-

## DSM-IV-TR Criteria 309.81

### Posttraumatic Stress Disorder

A. The person has been exposed to a traumatic event in which both of the following were present:

   (1) the person experienced, witnessed, or was confronted with an event or events that involved actual or threatened death or serious injury, or a threat to the physical integrity of self or others

   (2) the person's response involved intense fear, helplessness, or horror. **Note:** In children, this may be expressed instead by disorganized or agitated behavior

B. The traumatic event is persistently reexperienced in one (or more) of the following ways:

   (1) recurrent and intrusive distressing recollections of the event, including images, thoughts, or perceptions. **Note:** In young children, repetitive play may occur in which themes or aspects of the trauma are expressed

   (2) recurrent distressing dreams of the event. **Note:** In children, there may be frightening dreams without recognizable content

   (3) acting or feeling as if the traumatic event were recurring (includes a sense of reliving the experience, illusions, hallucinations, and dissociative flashback episodes, including those that occur on awakening or when intoxicated). **Note:** In young children, trauma-specific reenactment may occur

   (4) intense psychological distress at exposure to internal or external cues that symbolize or resemble an aspect of the traumatic event

   (5) physiological reactivity on exposure to internal or external cues that symbolize or resemble an aspect of the traumatic event

C. Persistent avoidance of stimuli associated with the trauma and numbing of general responsiveness (not present before the trauma), as indicated by three (or more) of the following:

   (1) efforts to avoid thoughts, feelings, or conversations associated with the trauma

   (2) efforts to avoid activities, places, or people that arouse recollections of the trauma

   (3) inability to recall an important aspect of the trauma

   (4) markedly diminished interest or participation in significant activities

   (5) feeling of detachment or estrangement from others

   (6) restricted range of affect (e.g., unable to have loving feelings)

   (7) sense of a foreshortened future (e.g., does not expect to have a career, marriage, children, or a normal life span)

D. Persistent symptoms of increased arousal (not present before the trauma), as indicated by two (or more) of the following:

   (1) difficulty falling or staying asleep

   (2) irritability or outbursts of anger

   (3) difficulty concentrating

   (4) hypervigilance

   (5) exaggerated startle response

E. Duration of the disturbance (symptoms in criteria B, C, and D) is more than 1 month.

F. The disturbance causes clinically significant distress or impairment in social, occupational, or other important areas of functioning.

*Specify* if:

**Acute:** if duration of symptoms is less than 3 months

**Chronic:** if duration of symptoms is 3 months or more

*Specify* if:

**With delayed onset:** if onset of symptoms is at least 6 months after the stressor

trick and colleagues (1987) found a lifetime prevalence rate of 75.8% and a current prevalence rate of 39.4%. In children, studies by Pynoos and associates (1987, 1993) revealed prevalence rates of 58.4% in children exposed to sniper attacks in the US and 70.2% in those exposed to an earthquake in Armenia. In two of the Epidemiological Catchment Area (ECA) sites, Davidson and coworkers (1991) and Helzer and others (1987) found that 47 and 33%, respectively, retained the diagnosis of PTSD for more than 1 year. Kessler and colleagues (1995) docu-

mented that one-third of those diagnosed with PTSD fail to recover even after many years. Therefore, chronicity of PTSD is not limited to the more severe treatment-seeking samples.

## Etiology and Pathophysiology

### The Event

PTSD is defined in terms of etiology as much as phenomenology. The disorder cannot exist unless the individual has been exposed to a traumatic event with a particular set of properties. Community-based epidemiological studies suggest that 70% of individuals will experience at least one traumatic event meeting criterion A(1)—see table description of PTSD over the course of their lifetime (Norris 1992). The relative severity of the traumatic event, predisposing factors, and peritraumatic environmental factors must all be considered in understanding the etiology of PTSD. In most instances, occurrence of the disorder represents the outcome of an interaction among these three groups of factors.

The likelihood of developing PTSD with regard to the nature of the event was reviewed by March (1993, 1990). A consistent relationship occurred between magnitude of stress exposure and risk of developing PTSD. This association held up in many different trauma populations in adults and children.

In the St. Louis ECA study, PTSD rates were three times higher in wounded Vietnam veterans than in non-wounded veterans (Hezler et al. 1987). In the North Carolina ECA study, PTSD was much more likely to occur in sexual assault victims who were physically injured than in those who were noninjured (Winfield et al. 1990). Other studies have shown similar results in Vietnam veterans (Kulka et al. 1990) and victims of a volcanic eruption (Shore et al. 1986). In children, effects of the stressor remain primary within and across a variety of settings. Pynoos and colleagues (1987, 1993) showed that physical proximity to the stressful event was linearly related to the risk of PTSD symptoms in two different populations. Saigh (1991) revealed that PTSD could arise in children from direct, witnessed, or verbal exposure. Aspects of the symptom picture vary with stressor-specific factors (Nader et al. 1991, Kendall-Tackett et al. 1993).

March (1993) concluded that besides the objective event characteristics—namely, actual or threatened death or injury or threat to physical integrity—cognitive and affective responses to the stressor are also important in determining the likelihood that PTSD will develop. In particular, the experience of intense fear, helplessness, or horror is a determinant of a person's likelihood to develop PTSD. The range of identified events that may be considered traumatic has increased, which is likely due to a change in definition from the DSM-III-R to the DSM-IV. In DSM-III-R, a traumatic event was considered to be an event "outside the range of human experience." This definition was modified in DSM-IV to indicate that a traumatic event is defined as an event that involves experiencing or witnessing actual or threatened death or serious injury or learning about an unexpected or violent death and having a response that involves intense fear, helplessness, or horror. There are medical/surgical events (Shalev 1990) such as a cancer diagnosis or open heart surgery that have been documented to meet criterion A (DSM-IV criteria for PTSD) in some individuals. Medical events that are witnessed may also be considered traumatic if the witness's response involves intense fear, helplessness, and horror. For example, the spouse of a patient with diabetes who witnessed multiple medically indicated amputations in the patient can consider it a traumatic event.

## Biological Factors

Identification of biological changes related to PTSD has provided hypotheses for understanding how some individuals develop PTSD in response to a traumatic event whereas others do not (Yehuda 2002). As summarized by Yehuda (2002), patients with chronic PTSD have increased circulating levels of norepinephrine (Yehuda et al. 1998) and increased reactivity of the alpha-2-adrenergic receptors (Southwick et al. 1993). These changes have been hypothesized to possibly account for some of the somatic symptoms that occur in individuals with PTSD. Neuroanatomical studies have implicated alterations in the amygdala and hippocampus in patients with PTSD (Rauch et al. 2000). Functional magnetic resonance imaging and positron-emission tomography have demonstrated increased reactivity of the amygdala and anterior paralimbic region to trauma-related stimuli (Lieberzon et al. 1999). Furthermore, in response to trauma-related stimuli, there is decreased reactivity of the anterior cingulate and orbitofrontal areas (Shin et al. 1999). These biological alterations suggest that there may be a neuroanatomical substrate for symptoms (intrusive recollections and other cognitive problems) that characterize PTSD (Schnuff et al. 2001, Vasterling et al. 1998). However, it is unknown whether these changes are preexisting, a result of traumatic exposure, or a result of having PTSD (Pitman 2001).

## Sympathetic Nervous System Alterations

A meta-analytic review found a positive association between the diagnosis of PTSD and basal cardiovascular activity (Yehuda et al. 1998). Particularly, individuals with a current PTSD diagnosis had higher resting heart rate relative to both trauma-exposed individuals without a PTSD diagnosis and nontrauma-exposed controls. An additional analysis revealed that differences were greatest in studies with the most chronic PTSD samples (Buckley and Kaloupek 2001). Along with increased 24-hour urinary catecholamines, results suggest increase in sympathetic tone (Pitman 1993). There has been repeated demonstration that there is heightened sympathetic arousal in PTSD patients when reexposed to the original trauma in controlled settings.

Although a conditioning model provides a viable explanation of the process through which trauma-related cues may generate the heightened physiological responses characteristic of PTSD, it does not explain why some individuals develop PTSD when exposed to traumatic events, while others do not. It has been hypothesized that differential susceptibility to developing PTSD might be attributable in part to individual differences in conditionability, such that some individuals more readily acquire and maintain a conditioned response compared with others, and thus may be more likely to develop PTSD after a traumatic event. A single recent study has provided support for this hypothesis, finding greater conditionability in individuals with PTSD (Orr et al. 2000). However, further study is needed to evaluate whether this conditionability is a precursor or consequence of PTSD.

There is evidence of brain dysfunction in individuals with PTSD as evidenced by abnormalities in evoked potentials. For example, as reported by Pitman and colleagues (1999), electroencephalographic event-related potential (ERP) response abnormalities in PTSD include reduced P2 amplitude at high stimulus intensities, impaired P1 habituation, and attenuated P3 amplitude to target auditory stimuli. Larger P3 and N1 amplitude responses and shorter P3 and N1 latencies have been reported in PTSD subjects in response to trauma-related stimuli. Based on a review of these studies (Pitman et al. 1999) these ERP findings suggest that PTSD patients have increased cortical inhibition to high-intensity stimuli, impairments in memory and concentration, auditory gating deficits and heightened selective attention to trauma-related stimuli. However, whether these processing abnormalities are a precursor or a result of PTSD awaits further study.

Further, there is some evidence that psychophysiological response to acute trauma exposure may predict the development of PTSD. Shalev and colleagues (1990) demonstrated that on arrival to the emergency department, regardless of whether PTSD ultimately developed, survivors of traumatic events showed elevated heart rates upon arrival to the emergency department, which at later assessment occasions, were normal. However, those who subsequently developed PTSD showed higher emergency department and 1-week heart rates than those who did not.

## Neuroendocrine Factors

The hypothalamic–pituitary–adrenal (HPA) axis has been the most extensively studied neuroendocrine system in PTSD, the findings of which were comprehensively reviewed by Yehuda and coworkers (1991). They summarized the principal findings as follows: reduced 24-hour urinary cortisol excretion, supersuppression of cortisol after low-dose dexamethasone administration, blunting of corticotropin in response to corticotropin-releasing hormone, and increased numbers of glucocorticoid receptors. Their interpretation of these findings suggested that chronic PTSD is accompanied by supersuppression of the emergency HPA response to acute stress. The authors speculated that this may result from the organism's attempt to protect itself from the potentially toxic effect of high levels of corticosteroids that might occur with repeated exposure to stress or from reminders of the trauma. In further support of the importance of HPA axis alteration in PTSD is the finding (Yehuda et al. 1991) that glucocorticoid receptor changes also correlate with the severity of PTSD symptoms, but not with the less specific anxiety and depressive symptoms measured on other rating scales. More recently, in a large sample of Vietnam veterans, combat-exposed veterans with current PTSD had lower cortisol compared to noncombat-exposed veterans without PTSD or combat-exposed veterans with lifetime PTSD but without current PTSD (Boscarino 1996).

Further evidence for abnormalities in neurotransmitter regulation comes from provocation studies conducted with Vietnam veterans. Administration of yohimbine, an alpha-2-adrenergic antagonist, provoked symptoms of PTSD in combat veterans who had PTSD as did the serotoninergic challenge with *m*-chlorophenylpiperazine. Of considerable interest is that there was no overlap between these two groups, suggesting some selectivity in the way in which neurotransmitter systems can be affected between individuals (Southwick et al. 1993, Krystal et al. 1989). Finally, evidence to support alteration of noradrenergic and serotoninergic pathways in PTSD comes from the clinical effects of medications that are selective for these neurotransmitter systems, as discussed later. The opioid system has also been investigated, but less extensively and without any consensus being obtained. One early study (Pitman et al. 1990) found the existence of a naloxone-reversible analgesia in combat veterans exposed to the reminders of the trauma.

## Sleep Studies

Studies support that there are two distinct, but possibly interrelated types of sleep complaints in individuals with PTSD: nightmares that replicate traumatic events and impairment in initiating and maintaining sleep (Neylan et al. 1998). Data further suggest that sleep problems in PTSD can also include excessive motor activity and awakenings with somatic anxiety symptoms (Inman et al. 1990, Mellman et al. 1995). There is support for these complaints using polysomnography (PSG) studies, particularly in reduced sleep time or efficiency, and increased awakenings in the PTSD patients (Mellman in press). There has also been documentation of PTSD subgroups that evidence breathing-related sleep disorders. Although most studies have involved combat veterans, more recent studies have included civilian PTSD populations (Krakow et al. 2001). Initial data indicate that for up to 2 months following exposure to trauma, development of PTSD is associated with a more fragmented rapid eye movement sleep (Mellman et al. 2001).

## Psychological Factors

### Behavioral Models

Conditioning theory has been helpful in explaining the process through which stimuli that are associated with a traumatic event can alone elicit intense emotional responses in individuals who have PTSD. Cues (i.e., conditioned stimuli) that are present at the time of the trauma (the unconditioned stimulus) become associated with the unconditioned emotional response (fear, helplessness, or horror). Following the traumatic event, these cues alone can then repeatedly elicit the strong emotional response. For example, a woman who has been raped (unconditioned stimulus) in a dark alley (conditioned stimulus) by a man (conditioned stimulus) and has an intense fear response (unconditioned response) may demonstrate a fear response (now the conditioned response) when she sees a dark alley (conditioned stimulus) or is in the presence of a man (conditioned stimulus). Avoidance behaviors develop to decrease anxiety associated with the conditioned stimuli. For example, the woman who has been raped may avoid going outside when it is dark and also avoid being in the company of men. Behavioral treatments using exposure principles require confrontation with the feared situation and may ultimately lead to reduction of anxiety (Solomon et al. 1992).

### Cognitive and Information Processing

Exposure to a severe or unexpected event may result in an inability to process and assimilate the experience adequately or to deal effectively with its impact. A period of prolonged, difficult, and often incomplete assimilation occurs. The experience is kept alive in active memory, intruding itself into awareness either during the day or at night. The pain of the unbidden experience is followed by active attempts to avoid reminders of the trauma. These intrusive and avoidance phases often alternate (Horowitz 1973).

Foa and Kozak (1986) proposed that fear can be considered a cognitive structure with three elements: stimulus, response, and meaning. To reduce fear, the fear memory must first be activated and then new information provided to modify the fear structure. Cognitive interventions can be used to recognize and change maladaptive cognitions and to replace interpretations of danger by realistic or safer interpretations, with the ultimate hope that the patient will integrate the new information into the fear structure, leading to a more realistic appraisal of the degree of danger.

## Genetic–Familial Factors

Connor and Davidson (1997) reviewed many of the complexities involved in studying familial risk factors of PTSD. From the available literature, which is based on male combat veterans, general population surveys and rape-trauma-related PTSD, there is evidence to suggest that anxiety and depression in families is a risk factor for PTSD (Davidson et al. 1998). A twin study of Vietnam veterans concordant and discordant for combat exposure has shown that a significant part of the variance is explained on the basis of genetic factors with respect to all three symptom clusters (i.e., intrusive, avoidant, and hyperarousal symptoms) (True et al. 1993). McLeod and colleagues (2001) examined the role of genetic and environmental influences on the relationship between combat exposure, posttraumatic stress disorder symptoms and alcohol use in 4,072 male–male twin pairs; the authors tested three hypotheses: (1) alcohol use and PTSD may share an environmental risk factor (i.e., combat) that increases the possibility that they will occur together; (2) the relationship between PTSD and alcohol problems is that one may develop as a consequence of the other; and (3) PTSD and alcohol problems occur together because of a shared vulnerability that increases risk for both disorders. Their analyses supported hypothesis (3); the same additive genetic influences that affect the level of combat exposure also include the level of alcohol use and level of PTSD symptoms. These findings are most consistent with the shared vulnerability hypothesis in which combat exposure, PTSD symptoms, and alcohol use are associated because some portion of the genes that influence vulnerability to combat also influence vulnerability to PTSD symptoms and alcohol consumption. It is important to note, however, that specific unique environmental factors the twins did not share were more important than genetic factors for combat exposure and PTSD symptoms, whereas environmental influences appeared about equally important as genetic influences on alcohol use. These results were consistent with previous findings by this group (McLeod et al. 2001). Overall, the evidence suggests that psychiatric history, both personal or in family members, increases the likelihood of being exposed to a trauma and of developing PTSD once exposed (True and Lyons 1999, Hidalgo and Davidson 2000).

King and colleagues (2001) have developed a congenital learned helplessness animal model in which rats genetically bred for learned helplessness behavior, exhibited physiologic symptoms of analgesia, learning deficits and

hyporesponsivity of the hypothalamic–pituitary–adrenal axis similar to those observed in humans with PTSD. Hypothalamic–pituitary–adrenal axis hypofunction, physiologic markers of increased arousal, and increased acoustic startle response are all potential PTSD-associated traits that might be susceptible to genetic analysis. However, the capacity of these traits to distinguish PTSD from non-PTSD patients and their familial pattern must be better defined before they can be employed in genetic studies.

## Other Factors

Although systematic research is scant, it may be that individuals exposed to repeated or continuous trauma, particularly of an interpersonal nature, may be more likely to develop PTSD. Trauma involving loss of community or support structures is likely to be particularly damaging. Because social support has been held to produce a buffering effect, lack of support might be considered an additional vulnerability factor. Women are at more risk than men for PTSD.

## Diagnosis

## Assessment and Diagnostic Features

The diagnosis of PTSD is based on a history of exposure to a traumatic stressor, the simultaneous appearance of three different symptom clusters, a minimal duration, and the existence of functional disturbance. Features of the disorder have been presented earlier in the chapter. To qualify as traumatic the event must have involved actual or threatened death or serious injury or a threat to the patient or others, and exposure to this event must arouse an intense affective response characterized by fear, helplessness, or horror. In children, disorganized or agitated behavior can be seen in lieu of an intense affective response. Symptomatically, there must be at least one of five possible intrusive-reexperiencing symptoms. These have the quality of obsessive, recurring, intrusive, and distressing recollections either in the form of imagery or thoughts, or in the form of recurrent distressing dreams. Intense psychological distress or physiological reactivity on exposure to either an external reminder or an internal reminder of the trauma can also occur. The flashback experience, or reliving of the event, is less common.

Symptom cluster C in the DSM-IV-TR criteria in actuality embodies two somewhat different psychopathologies—namely, phobic avoidance and numbing or withdrawal. The phobic avoidance is expressed either in (1) efforts to avoid thoughts and feelings, and conversations associated with the trauma or (2) in efforts to avoid activities places or people that arouse recollections of the trauma. (3) Psychogenic amnesia, a more dissociative symptom, also is in this symptom grouping, followed by (4) markedly diminished interest, (5) feeling detached or estranged, (6) having a restricted range of affect, and (7) having a sense of a foreshortened future. At least three of these seven symptoms must be present.

Hyperarousal symptoms, somewhat similar to those of generalized anxiety disorder, are also present in PTSD and at least one of five of the following symptoms is required: difficulty sleeping, irritability or anger, poor concentration, hypervigilance, and exaggerated startle response.

With regard to the symptoms as a whole, it is evident that they embody features of different psychiatric disorders, including obsessive–compulsive processes, generalized anxiety disorder, panic attacks, phobic avoidance, dissociation, and depression. Finally, it is necessary for symptoms to have lasted at least 1 month and for the disturbance to have caused clinically significant distress or impairment.

## Assessment and Differential Diagnosis

PTSD symptoms may overlap with symptoms of a number of other disorders in the DSM-IV. Both PTSD and adjustment disorder are etiologically related to stress exposure. PTSD may be distinguished from adjustment disorder by assessing whether the traumatic stress meets the severity criteria described earlier. Also, if there are an insufficient number of symptoms to qualify for the diagnosis, this might merit a diagnosis of adjustment disorder.

Specific phobia may arise after traumatic exposure. For example, after an automobile accident, victims may develop phobic avoidance of traveling, but without the intrusive or hyperarousal symptoms. In such cases, a diagnosis of specific phobia should be given instead of a diagnosis of PTSD.

The criteria set for generalized anxiety disorder include a list of six symptoms of hyperarousal, of which four are common to PTSD: being on edge, poor concentration, irritability, and sleep disturbance. PTSD requires the additional symptoms as described earlier, and the worry in PTSD is focused on concerns about reexperiencing the trauma. In contrast, the worry in generalized anxiety disorder is about a number of different situations and concerns. However, it is possible for the two conditions to coexist.

In obsessive–compulsive disorder, recurring and intrusive thoughts occur, but the patient recognizes these to be inappropriate and unrelated to any particular life experience. Obsessive–compulsive disorder is a common comorbid condition in PTSD and may develop with generalization (e.g., compulsive washing for months after a rape to reduce contamination feelings). It may also develop by activation of an underlying obsessive–compulsive disorder diathesis.

Autonomic hyperarousal is a cardinal part of panic attack, which may indicate a diagnosis of panic disorder. To distinguish between panic disorder and PTSD, the therapist needs to assess whether panic attacks are related to the trauma or reminders of the same (in which case they would be subsumed under a diagnosis of PTSD) or whether they occur unexpectedly and spontaneously (in which case a diagnosis of panic disorder would be justified).

Depression and PTSD share a significant overlap, including four of the criterion C cluster symptoms and three of the criterion D cluster symptoms. Thus, an individual who presents with reduced interest, estrangement, numbing, impaired concentration, insomnia, irritability, and sense of a foreshortened future may manifest either disorder. PTSD may give rise to depression as well, and it is possible for the two conditions to coexist. In a few instances, a patient with prior depression may be more vulnerable to developing PTSD. Reexperiencing symptoms are present only in PTSD.

Dissociative disorders also overlap with PTSD. In the early aftermath of serious trauma, the clinical picture may be predominantly one of the dissociative states (see the section on acute stress disorder [ASD]). ASD differs from PTSD in that the symptom pattern occurs within the first few days after exposure to the trauma, lasts no longer than 4 weeks, and is typically accompanied by prominent dissociative symptoms.

More rarely, PTSD must be distinguished from other disorders producing perceptual alterations, such as schizophrenia and other psychotic disorders, delirium, substance use disorders, and general medical conditions producing psychosis (e.g., brain tumors).

The differential diagnosis is important but, notwithstanding, PTSD is unlikely to occur in isolation. Psychiatric comorbidity is the rule rather than the exception, and a number of studies have demonstrated that, in both clinical and epidemiological populations (Davidson et al. 1991, Davidson et al. 1985), a wide range of disorders is likely to occur at an increased probability. These include major depressive disorder, all of the anxiety disorders, alcohol and substance use disorders, somatization disorder, and schizophrenia and schizophreniform disorder. A few studies have documented the course of comorbid conditions. For example, Shalev and colleagues (1990) have shown that major depressive disorder co-occurs with PTSD, but can take a separate course. Several researchers have provided evidence that comorbid substance abuse tends to be a consequence rather than a precursor of PTSD (Breslau et al. 1991, Bremmer et al. 1996).

## Assessment

PTSD assessment experts have suggested that the comprehensive evaluation of PTSD should include information from the individual, collaterals, psychometric indices (such as self-reported questionnaires), and a clinical interview (Keane et al. 1987). The standard for diagnosis in clinical research studies is to always use a structured clinical interview. The use of self-report instruments can be used to corroborate information obtained in the clinical interview, or can be used as a screening assessment for a clinical interview. All information would then be integrated on the basis of clinical judgment, especially if discrepancies existed. A number of structured interviews exist, along with other self-rating scales. The "gold standard" of clinical interviewing is the Clinician-Administered PTSD scale (Blake et al. 1990). Other instruments that have been used to evaluate PTSD are the Structured Clinical Interview for DSM-IV (Spitzer et al. 1989), the Diagnostic Interview Schedule (Robins et al. 1981), and the Structured Interview for PTSD (Davidson et al. 1989). Self-rated measures that can be used include self-rating psychometric assessments, such as the Davidson Trauma Scale (Davidson et al. 1997), the Short PTSD Rating Instrument (Connor and Davidson 2001) (SPRINT), the PTSD Checklist (Weathers et al. 1979), the PK scale (Keane et al. 1984) on the Minnesota Multiphasic Personality Inventory, the Mississippi Scale for Combat-Related PTSD (Keane et al. 1988), the Impact of Events Scale (Horowitz et al. 1979), and the PTSD Scale (Foa et al. 1993, 1995).

Structured interview and psychometric measures are also available for children with PTSD but are less well developed with regard to validity and reliability (Stallings and March in press). Nader and colleagues (1994) have developed a version of the Clinician-Administered PTSD

Scale for children and adolescents. This scale allows for current and lifetime diagnoses as well as the dimensional assessment of PTSD symptoms and related psychopathology. It has also been suggested (Costello 1989) that the use of additional measures such as the Conners Parent Rating Scale and Conners Teacher Rating Scale (Conners 1985) are important adjuncts to assess externalizing collateral symptoms, whereas the Children's Depression Inventory (Kovacs 1985) can be used to assess internalizing symptoms found in PTSD.

## Course and Natural History

Immediately following traumatic exposure, a high percentage of individuals develop a mixed symptom picture, which includes disorganized behavior, dissociative symptoms, psychomotor change, and sometimes, paranoia. The diagnosis of ASD (see pages 1372–1375 of this chapter) accounts for many of these reactions. These reactions are generally short-lived, although by 1 month the symptom picture often settles into a more classic PTSD presentation, such that after rape, for example, as many as 90% of individuals may qualify for the diagnosis of PTSD. Approximately 50% of people with PTSD recover, and approximately 50% develop a persistent, chronic form of the illness still present 1 year following the traumatic event.

The longitudinal course of PTSD is variable (Blank 1993). Permanent recovery occurs in some people, whereas others show a relatively unchanging course with only mild fluctuation. Still others show a more obvious fluctuation with intermittent periods of well-being and recurrences of major symptoms. In a limited number of cases, the passage of time does not bring a resolution of symptoms, and the patient's condition tends to deteriorate with age. Particular symptoms that have been noted to increase with time in many people include startle response, nightmares, irritability, and depression. Clinicians during World War II also observed that the existence of marked startle response and hypervigilance in the acute aftermath of exposure to combat often represented a comparatively poor prognostic sign. In children, PTSD can be, and often is, chronic and debilitating (Nader et al. 1990).

General medical conditions may occur as a direct consequence of the trauma (e.g., head injury, burns). In addition, chronic PTSD may be associated with increased rates of adverse physical outcomes, including musculoskeletal problems and cardiovascular morbidity (Beckham et al. 1997, Boscarino 1997, Schnurr and Jankowski 1999).

## Overall Goals of Treatment

General principles of treating PTSD involve explanation and destigmatization, which can be provided both to the patient and to family members. This often includes a description of the symptoms of PTSD and the way in which it can affect behaviors and relationships. Information can be given about general treatment principles, pointing out that sometimes cure is attainable but that at other times symptom containment is a more realistic treatment goal, particularly in chronic and severe PTSD. Regaining self-esteem and attaining greater control over impulses and affect are also desired in many instances. Information can be provided as to appropriate literature, local support groups and resources, and names and addresses of national advo-

cacy organizations. If the therapist attends to these important issues early in treatment, the patient is able to more readily build trust and also to appreciate that the therapist shows a good understanding both of the condition and of the patient.

PTSD is sometimes comparatively straightforward to treat and at other times it is more complicated. However, treatment by a mental health provider (rather than a primary care provider) is almost always indicated. The initial history taking can evoke strong affect to a greater degree than is customarily found in other disorders. In fact, it may take several interviews for the details to emerge. A sensitive yet persistent approach is needed on the part of the interviewer. During treatment, although the mental health care provider will clearly want to impart a sense of optimism to the patient, it is also a reflection of reality to point out early that recovery may be a slow process and that some symptoms (e.g., phobic avoidance, startle response) may persist. It is important for the mental health care provider to be comfortable in hearing and tolerating unpleasant affect and often horrifying stories. All these must take place in a noncritical and accepting manner. Specific treatment approaches include the use of pharmacotherapy, psychotherapy, anxiety management, and attention to the general issues described earlier.

## Pharmacotherapy

PTSD may be accompanied by enduring neurochemical and psychophysiological changes and can lead to substantial impairment and distress. Sometimes the intensity of symptoms is severe enough to preclude the effective use of trauma-focused psychotherapy. In these situations, the use of medication should not be delayed unnecessarily. Initial studies showed benefit for the tricyclic antidepressant and monoamine oxidase inhibitor medications. However, the selective serotonin reuptake inhibitors (SSRIs) have now replaced these as first-line agents, based upon evidence from several placebo-controlled trials. The main groups of medications relevant to the treatment of PTSD along with dose ranges and chief side effects are listed in Table 69–1. A suggested sequencing of treatment is outlined in Table 69–2.

Two double-blind clinical trials in more than 100 patients support the efficacy of amitriptyline and imipramine in combat veterans with PTSD (Frank et al. 1988, Davidson et al. 1990). In both studies, the medication was effective on intrusive PTSD symptoms and, to a weaker extent, on avoidant symptoms (Table 69–3). Of importance was that clinical efficacy occurred in patients who did not suffer from depressive illness, suggesting that the effect of tricyclic agents in PTSD is independent of antidepressant properties. In fact, Davidson and others (1993) found that response was inversely correlated with baseline depression level.

Phenelzine has been found to be effective in symptom reduction based on Kosten and colleagues (1991). Of note was the finding that avoidant symptoms improved to a much greater degree with phenelzine than with the tricyclic agents. However, the side effects of phenelzine limit its use to a third- or fourth-line drug to be used only when other, safer medications have failed to work. Several placebo-controlled trials have shown positive effects for the SSRI medications, including fluoxetine, sertraline (Davidson et al.

| Table 69–1 | Medications in Posttraumatic Stress Disorder: Dose Ranges and Side Effects | |
|---|---|---|
| Drug Category | Dose Range (mg/d) | Common or Problematical Side Effects |
| Antidepressants | | Gastrointestinal disturbance, sexual dysfunction, agitation |
| Selective serotonin reuptake inhibitors | | |
| Fluoxetine | 10–60 | |
| Fluvoxamine | 50–300 | |
| Sertraline | 50–200 | Insomnia |
| Paroxetine | 10–60 | Tiredness |
| Nefazodone | 50–600 | Headache, dry mouth, nausea |
| Tricyclic antidepressants | | Anticholinergic effects, cardiovascular symptoms, weight gain, sexual dysfunction, sedation (for all tricyclic antidepressants) |
| Amitriptyline | 50–300 | |
| Imipramine | 50–300 | |
| Monoamine oxidase inhibitors | | |
| Phenelzine | 15–90 | Weight gain, dizziness, sleep disturbance, sexual dysfunction, hypertensive reactions, hyperpyretic states |
| Anticonvulsants | | |
| Carbamazepine | 200–1500 | Hematological effects |
| Valproic acid | 125–2000 | Gastrointestinal disturbance, sedation |
| Lamotrigine | 50–200 | Rash, exfoliative dermatitis, Stevens–Johnson syndrome |
| Mood stabilizers | | |
| Lithium carbonate | 300–1200 | Gastrointestinal disturbance, polyuria, headache |
| Antiadrenergic drugs | | |
| Propranolol | 20–160 | Depression, hypertension, rebound hypertension |
| Clonidine | 0.1–0.4 | Memory problems, dizziness, tiredness |
| Prazosin | 2–10 | Dizziness, hypotension |
| Anxiolytics | 0.5–6 | |
| Benzodiazepines | | |
| Clonazepam | 0.5–6 | Sedation, memory problems, incoordination, dependence, withdrawal, rebound, disinhibition (for all benzodiazepines) |
| Alprazolam | 0.25–4 | |
| Diazepam | 2–40 | |
| Chlordiazepoxide | 5–40 | |
| Others | | |
| Azapirones | 5–60 | Agitation, gastrointestinal disturbance, headaches |
| Buspirone | | |
| Neuroleptics | | |
| Thioridazine | 25–300 | Extrapyramidal symptoms |
| Haloperidol | 0.5–4 | Sedation, anticholinergic effects |
| Others | | |

2001, Brady et al. 2000) and paroxetine (Marshall et al. 1998). Long-term use of sertraline is associated with a substantial reduction in relapse over a 15-month period (Frank et al. 1988). Data support positive effects for SSRI in men and women and in adults who have survived all major classes of trauma (e.g., combat, sexual violence, nonsexual violence, and accident). Each of these medications has broad-spectrum properties across the full symptom range of the disorder as well as improving function and, perhaps, resilience or stress-coping (Connor et al. 1999). They also support the benefit of SSRI in those with and without cormorbid major depression (Davidson et al. 2001, Brady et al. 2000, Marshall et al. 1998, Connor et al. 1999, van der Kolk et al. 1994, Davidson et al. in press).

There have been a number of open studies suggesting benefit of carbamazepine, propranolol, clonidine, and valproic acid. There have also been two negative double-blind placebo-controlled trials of desipramine and phenelzine (Davidson 1992); however, treatment length may have been too short because in the study by Davidson and associates (1990) it was not until week 8 that amitriptyline became superior to placebo.

At this point, the indications for antipsychotic and mood-stabilizing drugs are poorly defined, but clinical experience suggests that they continue to have a role in the pharmacologic treatment of PTSD. Antipsychotic medications can be useful in patients with poor impulse control or in those who manifest features of borderline personality disorder. Lithium and carbamazepine can also be useful in such patients but might benefit individuals who are subject to mood swings and angry or explosive outbursts. The appropriate role for the use of benzodiazepines is not well-defined. The antiphobic and antiarousal effects of the benzodiazepines should, in theory, be helpful in PTSD. However, withdrawal from short-acting benzodiazepines may also introduce an additional set of problems with intense symptom rebound. In patients who have a propensity to abuse alcohol and other substances, benzodiazepines are not recommended.

Overall, the antidepressants, mood stabilizers, and anticonvulsants are the medication groups that are generally considered primary for treating PTSD; beta-blockers, alpha-2-agonists, and anxiolytics have a less clearly defined place. Often, patients need a combination of drugs but polypharmacy should be utilized in a carefully planned fashion. Also, since the time course of response may be slow, it is advisable to persist with a particular course of action for at least 8 weeks before deciding that it has been unhelpful. It is possible that avoidance and numbing symptoms respond more effectively to SSRI drugs.

## Cognitive, Cognitive–Behavioral, and Behavioral Therapies

Despite theoretical differences, most schools of psychotherapy recognize that cognitively oriented approaches to the treatment of anxiety must include an element of exposure (Marks 1987). Because PTSD involves aberrant and voluntary programs for the avoidance of danger that are conditioned by real experience, correction of these "fear structures" requires exposure to ensure habituation. Although a range of possible PTSD interventions has recently been reviewed (Foa et al. 2000) including group therapy, cognitive–behavioral therapy, eye movement desensitization and reprocessing, and psychodynamic therapy, the preponderance of current evidence suggests that the primary effective component of PTSD treatment is prolonged exposure (Rothbaum et al. 2000). Prolonged exposure depends on the fact that anxiety will be extinguished in the absence of real threat, given a sufficient duration of exposure *in vivo* or in imagination to traumatic stimuli. In PTSD, the patient retells the traumatic experience as if it were happening again, until doing so becomes a pedestrian exercise and anxiety decreases. Between sessions, patients perform exposure homework, including listening to tapes of the flooding sessions and limited exposure *in vivo*. A review of 12 studies suggests that prolonged exposure is a component of the most well-controlled study designs and is associated with positive results (Rothbaum et al. 2000). However,

| Table 69–3 | Factors Associated with Good Response to Tricyclic Drug Therapy and Direct Therapeutic Exposure in Combat Veterans with Posttraumatic Stress Disorder | |
|---|---|---|
| | Pharmacotherapy | Psychotherapy |
| Older age | No effect | Yes |
| Lower level of trauma intensity | Yes | Yes |
| Fewer comorbid disorders | Yes | Yes |
| Low depression score | Yes | Yes |
| Low PTSD symptom severity score | Yes | Yes |
| Low anxiety symptom score | Yes | Yes |
| Low avoidance of trauma cues | Yes | Unknown |
| Low autonomic arousal | Yes | Unknown |
| Low neuroticism | Yes | Unknown |
| Good social adjustment | Unknown | Yes |

| Table 69–2 | Pharmacotherapy Steps for Posttraumatic Stress Disorder |
|---|---|
| **Step 1** | |
| Selective serotonin reuptake inhibitor (SSRI) Adjunctive medications: If prominent hyperarousal: benzodiazepine or buspirone If prominent mood liability or explosiveness: anticonvulsant or lithium If prominent dissociation: valproic acid If persistent insomnia: trazodone If psychotic: atypical antipsychotic | |
| **Step 2** | |
| If no response or intolerance to SSRI: Dual action antidepressant, e.g., mirtazapine, venlafaxine Adjunctive medications as above | |
| **Step 3** | |
| If no response to Step 1 or 2: Monoamine oxidase inhibitor Adjunctive medications as above | |
| **Step 4** | |
| Other useful drugs: Propranolol—hyperarousal Clonidine—startle response Neuroleptics—psychosis, poor impulse control | |

not every patient may be a candidate for exposure. Due to the high anxiety and temporarily increased symptoms associated with prolonged exposure, there are patients who will be reluctant to confront traumatic reminders. Patients in whom guilt or anger are primary emotional responses to the traumatic event (as opposed to anxiety) may not profit from prolonged exposure (Foa et al. 1995, Pitman et al. 1991). More empirical research is needed to evaluate how this efficacious treatment can be most effectively implemented in nonacademic settings. In addition, additional research is needed to identify methods to increase patient tolerability of the treatment.

Anxiety management techniques are designed to reduce anxiety by providing patients with better skills for controlling worry and fear. Among such techniques are muscle relaxation, thought stopping, control of breathing and diaphragmatic breathing, communication skills, guided self-dialogue, and stress inoculation training (SIT). Although these interventions have less empirical evidence regarding treatment efficacy for PTSD, generally the results are positive and further controlled evaluation across trauma population samples is needed.

Further, cognitive approaches to the treatment of PTSD have also gained empirical support (Resick and Schnicke 1992). A cognitive approach to treatment includes training patients in challenging problematic cognitions such as self-blame. In a recent comparison of cognitive therapy to imaginal exposure in the treatment of chronic PTSD, both treatments were associated with positive improvements at posttreatment and follow-up, with no differences in outcome between treatments (Tarrier et al. 1999). However, patients who received imaginal exposure were more likely to experience an increase in PTSD symptoms during the treatment course, and those who did were more likely to miss treatment sessions, rate the therapy as less credible, and be rated as less motivated by the therapist.

Other recent approaches have focused on efficaciously treating one aspect of PTSD symptomatology, such as anger (Yehuda 1999), nightmares (Krakow et al. 2001), or authority problems (Lubin and Johnson 2000). There has also been a recent report of positive results using interventions to target both PTSD and a comorbid disorder. For example, Triffleman and colleagues (1999) reported patient improvement using a group intervention to simultaneously treat co-occurring substance abuse and PTSD. Falsetti and colleagues (2001) have reported an intervention entitled multiple channel exposure therapy (M-CET) to treat comorbid panic attacks and PTSD.

In contrast to the treatment-efficacy literature for adults with PTSD, the child-focused PTSD literature is limited to open trials and case reports (Ruggiero et al. 2001). Treatment practices for childhood PTSD have recently been surveyed (Cohen et al. 2001). However, in their review of the current literature, Ruggiero and colleagues (2001) underscore that adult treatment approaches need to be empirically evaluated for use in children with PTSD.

As no single treatment for PTSD has been shown to be curative, patient characteristics, characterization of the nature and range of stress responses of trauma victims (McFarlane and Yehuda 2000), partial response (Taylor et al. 2001), treatment combinations, sequencing of treatment approaches, and further well-controlled investigations of current approaches are all important empirical topics to be addressed. For example, in patients unwilling to undergo exposure therapy, teaching of affect management skills may be helpful (Wolfsdorf and Zlotnick 2001).

## Psychodynamic Therapy

Psychodynamically based approaches emphasize the interpretation of the traumatic event as being a critical determinant of symptoms. Treatment is geared to alter attributions, usually by means of slow exposure and through confrontation and awareness of the negative affect that have been generated by the trauma. Conflictual meanings begin to appear, and it is the task of treatment to reinterpret the experience in a more realistic and adaptive fashion. During such treatment, it is important to ensure that the affect intensity is not overwhelming or disorganizing. Obviously, support needs to be provided throughout, and sometimes other treatment approaches are used adjunctively. Excessive and maladaptive behaviors such as avoidance, use of alcohol or work, or risk taking may occur as a means of coping with the experience and these need to be identified and addressed.

Using psychodynamic concepts, Horowitz (1973) developed a trauma-focused, time-limited, psychotherapeutic approach. Periods of intrusion are considered an attempt at mastery rather than a failure in defenses, whereas emotional numbness is seen as a result of defensive overcontrol. Overwhelmingly intrusive symptoms are counteracted by means of structuring, and avoidance and numbing are met with procedures to minimize such behavior. With this approach, as with any psychotherapeutic approach, the establishment of a safe therapeutic alliance is essential and medications are used sparingly. The goal of such trauma-focused therapy is to achieve an end point in which the trauma is meaningfully integrated into the survivor's life schema, with reduction of intensity and frequency of the intrusive and avoidant phases of PTSD. Although this approach awaits controlled testing, it aspires to reduce all aspects of PTSD symptoms.

Roth and Newman (1991) presented a conceptual framework for understanding the emotional impact of sexual trauma. The survivor must come to understand the affective impact of the event so that she or he is no longer preoccupied or driven by negative feelings or self-defeating behaviors. It is also important for the survivor to grapple with the meaning of the trauma so as to reach adaptive resolution. Preliminary studies utilizing this approach show promise of efficacy.

## Special Features Influencing Treatment

### Psychiatric Features

Several important issues of comorbidity need to be considered in the treatment of PTSD. These may suggest either a contraindication to a particular treatment or the need to first treat the comorbid state before embarking energetically on the PTSD problems. Thus, comorbid depression needs to be treated, as it is likely to interfere with the benefits of behavioral therapy or other psychotherapies. In fact, as mentioned earlier, in some instances guilt-bound issues may worsen with exposure. A suicidally depressive individual with PTSD needs to be adequately treated before dealing with issues of PTSD, which may in fact worsen suicidiality in some instances.

Occasionally, severe depression comorbid with PTSD may need to be treated with electroconvulsive therapy. Although this form of treatment has no proven place as a major intervention for PTSD per se, in comorbid cases it has been noted that PTSD symptoms may also abate when they are tied to the presence of depression. Davidson and Fairbank 1993 reported that amitriptyline is less likely to help combat veterans with PTSD if they have been exposed to more severe forms of combat trauma, and also if they have more severe symptoms of depression, anxiety, and PTSD. Antisocial and severe borderline personality disorder may be contraindications to various forms of psychotherapy and are unlikely to respond well to pharmacotherapy.

### General Medical Comorbidity

PTSD patients have been shown to have an increased risk of physical conditions, with particular conditions perhaps being more prevalent (gastrointestinal disease and cardiovascular disease) (Boscario 1997, Schnurr and Janowski 1999, Beckham et al. 1998). There is also evidence that chronic pain and PTSD are commonly associated, even when PTSD has not followed serious physical injury (Beckham et al. 1997).

### Demographical Features

It is not known to what extent sex or age is likely to determine treatment outcome. However, it is generally believed that lack of psychosocial supports can interfere with successful adaptation to trauma and response to treatment.

## Nonresponse to Treatment

A stepwise sequence of approaches may be used in the treatment of PTSD but it must be said that there are no definitive guidelines currently in place. As a result, the particular order in which treatments are considered varies based on individual circumstances. Also, no uniform definition exists as to what constitutes a good or poor response to treatment. In general, some symptoms of chronic PTSD persist, albeit at a considerably reduced level, in people who have undergone treatment. A summary of the limited information available for predicting response to pharmacotherapy and behavioral therapy in PTSD arising from combat trauma is given elsewhere (Davidson and Fairbank 1993).

Management problems are likely to occur as a result of both therapist-related factors and factors related to the patient. With regard to the therapist, it must be recognized that much of the material offered by the patient is charged with affect and, at times, may strain credibility and lead to high levels of doubt. The therapist may fall into the error of being unable to accept such an emotionally charged experience and thus rejecting or denying its validity. Equally, the therapist may fall into the error of overidentification with the patient such that impartiality is lost. It is important for therapists not to become overinvolved with rescue or to break down customary therapist–patient boundaries.

Although not unique to PTSD, powerful violent urges may arise in the patient during treatment, which may challenge the therapist's feeling of safety. Simple strategies, such as where the patient and therapist sit with respect to proximity of escape, merit attention. For example, a female therapist dealing with a highly hostile and threatening male patient would do well to be sure that she can exit the room quickly if necessary and not be trapped behind a desk with the patient having control of the exit. Another simple yet important issue calling for attention is whether there is an available alarm if the therapist is dealing regularly with violent or threatening patients.

With respect to the patient, there are times when decompensation occurs to such an extent that the provider will have to judge whether hospitalization is indicated. Denial of particularly painful issues can lead to avoidance of therapy and missed appointments. Similarly, the emergence of unpleasant or troubling side effects with medication may also lead to treatment discontinuation. At all times, it is advisable for the therapist to remind the patient that difficult issues will arise periodically and that, rather than the patient taking unilateral action to drop out of treatment, these issues are best discussed with the therapist, with the hope that they can be resolved and further treatment progress can be made.

At times, it is helpful to engage the spouse or significant family member in treatment because of the difficulties and stresses to which they may be subjected. Furthermore, they can provide information that might help the therapist to acquire a better grasp of the severity of symptoms as well as their effects on the lives of others. For example, sleeping partners can give a more graphic account of the nocturnal disturbances that may occur in symptomatic patients with PTSD. They may also provide important supplementary information as to the effects of poor impulse regulation or impaired memory or concentration on daytime behaviors in an individual.

Given that many patients with PTSD are receiving more than one treatment, coordination of effort between providers is important. At times, different philosophical persuasions may result in one provider being somewhat less supportive of another's efforts, a situation in which everybody loses. Mutual respect for each other's efforts is essential if optimal progress is to be made by the patient.

## Summary of Treatment

Whatever the type of treatment administered, a number of goals are common to all and can be summarized as follows: (1) to reduce intrusive symptoms; (2) to reduce avoidance symptoms; (3) to reduce numbing and withdrawal; (4) to dampen hyperarousal; (5) to reduce psychotic symptoms when present; and (6) to improve impulse control when this is a problem.

By reducing troublesome symptoms, a number of other important goals can also be accomplished as follows: (1) to develop the capacity to interpret events more realistically with respect to their threat content; (2) to improve interpersonal work and leisure functioning; (3) to promote self-esteem, trust, and feelings of safety; (4) to explore and clarify meanings attributed to the event; (5) to promote access to memories that have been dissociated or repressed when judged to be clinically appropriate; (6) to strengthen social support systems; and (7) to move from identification as a victim to that of a survivor.

The three major treatment approaches, pharmacotherapeutic, cognitive–behavioral, and psychodynamic, all emphasize different aspects of the problem. Pharmacotherapy targets the underlying neurobiological alterations found in PTSD and attempts to control symptoms so that the above treatment goals can be more effectively accomplished. Cognitive–behavioral treatments emphasize the phobic avoidance and counterproductive reenactments that often occur, along with the identification of faulty beliefs that arise owing to the trauma, and replace them with more adaptive beliefs, usually in association with direct therapeutic exposure. The psychodynamic approach emphasizes the associations that arise from the trauma experience and that lead to unconscious and conscious representations. Defense mechanisms that lead to lack of memory, and the contributions from early development, are also brought into play in psychodynamic therapy.

# ACUTE STRESS DISORDER

## Definition

It has long been recognized that clinically significant dissociative states are seen in the immediate aftermath of overwhelming trauma. In addition, many individuals may experience less clinically severe dissociative symptoms or alterations of attention and time sense. Because such syndromes, even when short-lasting, can produce major disruption of everyday activities, they may require clinical attention. During triage situations after a disaster, it can be important to recognize this clinical picture, which may require treatment intervention and which may also be predictive of later PTSD. As a result of these considerations, a decision was made to include in DSM-IV a new entity, acute stress disorder (ASD), grouped together with PTSD in the anxiety disorders section. Essentially, it

## DSM-IV-TR Criteria 308.3

### Acute Stress Disorder

A. The person has been exposed to a traumatic event in which both of the following were present:

(1) the person experienced, witnessed, or was confronted with an event or events that involved actual or threatened death or serious injury, or a threat to the physical integrity of self or others

(2) the person's response involved intense fear, helplessness, or horror

B. Either while experiencing or after experiencing the distressing event, the individual has three (or more) of the following dissociative symptoms:

(1) a subjective sense of numbing, detachment, or absence of emotional responsiveness

(2) a reduction in awareness of his or her surroundings (e.g., "being in a daze")

(3) derealization

(4) depersonalization

(5) dissociative amnesia (i.e., inability to recall an important aspect of the trauma)

C. The traumatic event is persistently reexperienced in at least one of the following ways: recurrent images, thoughts, dreams, illusions, flashback episodes, or a sense of reliving the experience; or distress on exposure to reminders of the traumatic event.

D. Marked avoidance of stimuli that arouse recollections of the trauma (e.g., thoughts, feelings, conversations, activities, places, people).

E. Marked symptoms of anxiety or increased arousal (e.g., difficulty sleeping, irritability, poor concentration, hypervigilance, exaggerated startle response, motor restlessness).

F. The disturbance causes clinically significant distress or impairment in social, occupational, or other important areas of functioning or impairs the individual's ability to pursue some necessary task, such as obtaining necessary assistance or mobilizing personal resources by telling family members about the traumatic experience.

G. The disturbance lasts for a minimum of 2 days and a maximum of 4 weeks and occurs within 4 weeks of the traumatic event.

H. The disturbance is not due to the direct physiological effects of a substance (e.g., a drug of abuse, a medication) or a general medical condition is not better accounted for by brief psychotic disorder, and is not merely an exacerbation of a preexisting Axis I or Axis II disorder.

Reprinted with permission from the Diagnostic and Statistical Manual of Mental Disorders, Fourth Edition, Text Revision. Copyright 2000 American Psychiatric Association.

represents the clinical features of PTSD along with conspicuous dissociative symptoms, of which at least three must be present. The possible dissociative symptoms in ASD are a subjective sense of numbing; detachment or absence of emotional response; reduced awareness of one's surroundings; derealization; depersonalization; and dissociative amnesia.

However, there is a lack of empirical evidence for some of the assumptions inherent in the conceptualization of ASD, and there has been a call for empirical evidence of acutely traumatized individuals to address these assumptions (Bryant and Harvey 1997). The current emphasis placed on acute dissociative responses may be flawed in that there are multiple pathways to PTSD, and most trauma survivors who display severe acute stress reactions without dissociation can develop PTSD (Harvey and Bryant 1999). Reviews of these conceptual issues have recently been published (Bryant and Harvey 1997, Marshall et al. 1999).

### Epidemiology

Little is known about the epidemiology of ASD as defined in DSM-IV, but after events such as rape and criminal assault, the clinical picture of acute PTSD is found in between 70 and 90% of individuals, although frequency of the particular dissociative symptoms is unknown. One problem of most postdisaster surveys is that they evaluate subjects at points several months or years after the event. This makes any meaningful assessment of acute stress syndromes difficult. One exception was the self-report-based assessment of morbidity 2 months after an earthquake in Ecuador, which found a 45% rate of caseness (being a clinical case), with most prominent symptoms being fear, nervousness, tenseness, worry, insomnia, and fatigue (Lima et al. 1989).

In a study by Koopman and colleagues (1994) of individuals who had been exposed to a firestorm, the participants showed a high incidence of dissociative symptoms, including time distortions, alterations in cognition and memory, and derealization. Most of these symptoms had lessened by a 4-month follow-up. A study by Bryan and Panasetis (2001) reported that 53% of participants reported panic attacks during their trauma, and those who had symptoms that met criteria for ASD reported more peritraumatic panic symptoms. These data suggest that peritraumatic panic may be related to subsequent PTSD.

Retrospective reports of acute stress symptoms should be interpreted cautiously because of the influence of current symptoms on recall of acute symptoms. In a longitudinal study evaluating report of acute stress symptoms at 1 month and 2 years posttrauma, at least one of the four ASD diagnostic clusters was recalled inaccurately by 75% of patients (Harvey and Bryant 2000).

## Etiology

Little is known about the etiology of ASD specifically, but it is likely that many of the same factors that apply to PTSD are relevant for ASD that is, trauma intensity, preexisting psychopathology, family and genetic vulnerability, abnormal personality, lack of social supports at the time of the trauma, and physical injury are all likely to increase vulnerability for ASD.

The role of acute arousal in the development of PTSD has been evaluated in one study (Bryant et al. 2000). Resting heart rate (HR) and ASD symptoms together were found to account for 36% of the variance in PTSD prediction (Bryant and Harvey 2000). Further, a formula using resting HR following the trauma exposure (HR > 90 beats/minute) and the diagnosis of ASD to predict PTSD development possessed strong sensitivity (88%) and specificity (85%) (Bryant et al. 2000).

## Diagnosis and Differential Diagnosis

ASD may need to be distinguished from several related disorders (Figure 69–1). Brief psychotic disorder may be a more appropriate diagnosis if the predominant symptoms are psychotic. It is possible that major depressive disorder can develop posttraumatically and that there may be some overlap with ASD, in which case both disorders are appropriately diagnosed. When ASD-like symptoms are caused by direct physiological perturbation, the symptoms may be more appropriately diagnosed with reference to the etiological agent. Thus, an ASD-like picture that develops secondary to head injury is more appropriately diagnosed as mental disorder due to a general medical condition, whereas a clinical picture related to substance use (e.g., alcohol intoxication) is appropriately diagnosed as substance-induced disorder. Substance-related ASD is confined to the period of intoxication or withdrawal. Head injury-induced ASD needs substantiating by evidence from the history, physical examination, and laboratory testing that the symptoms are a direct physiological consequence of head trauma. Recently, a self-report scale of ASD has been developed, the Acute Stress Disorder Scale (ASDS). The scale has demonstrated good test–retest reliability ($r = 0.94$), and in one sample (bushfire survivors), the ASDS predicted 91% of survivors who developed PTSD and 93% of those who did not (Bryant et al. 2000).

Because ASD by definition cannot last longer than 1 month, if the clinical picture persists, a diagnosis of PTSD is appropriate. Some increased symptoms are expected in the great majority of subjects after exposure to major stress. These remit in most cases and only reach the level of clinical diagnosis if they are prolonged, exceed a tolerable quality, or interfere with everyday function. Resolution may be more difficult if there has been previous psychiatric morbidity, subsequent stress, and lack of social support.

## Course and Natural History

Although data do not exist on the course and natural history of ASD as now defined, studies by Koopman and coworkers (1994) indicated that dissociative and cognitive symptoms, which are so common in the immediate wake of trauma, improve spontaneously with time. However, they also found that the likelihood of developing PTSD symptoms at 7-month follow-up was more strongly related to the occurrence of dissociative symptoms than to anxiety symptoms immediately after exposure to the trauma. However, other studies have questioned the dissociative criteria as critical for the prediction of later PTSD (Marshall et al. 1999, Brewin et al. 1999).

## Treatment

Lundin (1994) reviewed the treatment of acute traumatic stress states and pointed out the six general principles involved in administering any treatment immediately after trauma. These include principles of brevity, immediacy, centrality, expectancy, proximity, and simplicity. That is, treatment of acute trauma is generally aimed at being brief, provided immediately after the trauma whenever possible, administered in a centralized and coordinated fashion with the expectation of the person's return to normal function and as proximately as possible to the scene of the trauma, and not directed at any uncovering or explorative procedures but rather at maintaining a superficial, reintegrating approach.

People most highly at risk, and therefore perhaps most in need of treatment, are as follows: survivors with psychiatric disorders; traumatically bereaved people; children, especially when separated from their parents; individuals who are particularly dependent on psychosocial supports, such as the elderly, handicapped, and mentally retarded individuals; and traumatized survivors and body handlers.

Different components of treatment include providing information, psychological support, crisis intervention, and emotional first aid. Providing information about the trauma is important as it can enable the survivor to fully recognize and accept all the details of what happened. Information needs to be given in a way that conveys hope and the possibility that psychological pain and threat of loss may be coped with. Unrealistic hope needs to be balanced by the provision of realistic explanations as to what happened. Psychological support helps to strengthen coping mechanisms and promotes adaptive defenses. The survivor benefits if he or she recognizes the need to take responsibility for a successful outcome and is as actively involved with this as possible. Crisis intervention is often used after disasters and acts of violence or other serious traumas. It has been described by a number of investigators. Emotional first aid has been described by Caplan (1984) using the six principles presented earlier and is used to achieve any of the following: acceptance of feelings, symptoms, reality, and the need for help; recognition of psychologically distressing issues; identification of available resources; acceptance of responsibility and absence of blame; cultivation of an optimistic attitude; and efforts to resume activities of daily life as much as possible.

Civilian trauma survivors with ASD were found to engage in the cognitive strategies of punishment and worry more than survivors without ASD (Warda and Bryant 1998), and cognitive–behavioral therapy has been shown to reduce these strategies and increase the use of reappraisal and social control strategies (Bryant et al. 2001). However, the relation of these findings to the development of PTSD has not yet been determined.

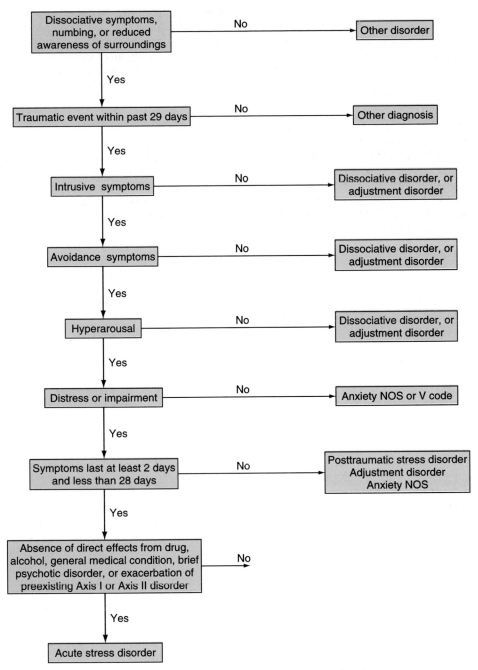

**Figure 69–1** *Diagnostic decision tree for acute stress disorder.*

There is little investigation as to whether early recognition and effective treatment of acute stress reactions prevent the development of PTSD, although it is safe to assume that they are likely to have beneficial effects in this regard. Nonetheless, as was recognized during World War II, rapid and effective treatment of acute combat stress did not always prevent veterans from developing subsequent chronicity. More recently, an intervention designed to prevent the development of PTSD and administered in the acute phase, critical incident stress debriefing (Mitchell and Everly 2000), has been found to be ineffective in preventing the development of PTSD (Carlier 2000, Carlier et al. 2000). However,

there has been an initial study with motor vehicle accident survivors that suggested exposure therapy and exposure therapy with anxiety management training may be effective in preventing PTSD (Bryant et al. 1999).

---

Clinical Vignette 1

Ben, a 9-year-old third-grader, developed PTSD when a drunken driver struck a car in which he was riding. Ben's mother was severely injured, and Ben broke his left arm and left lower leg. He recalled being extremely frightened as the car careened out of control, coming to rest upside down. However, his worst moments came when he saw the emergency helicopter taking his unconscious mother to the hospital. Ben believed that she was dead or would die and thought that he too might die without her there to help him.

Despite an excellent medical outcome and full recovery for both Ben and his mother, he developed characteristic PTSD symptoms, including intrusive images, dreams, and traumatic play; avoidance of being driven in cars and compulsive reassurance seeking; affective constriction; and mild hyperarousal. (Ben's mother had no memory of the event and was free of emotional sequelae). Because of significant disturbances in memory and concentration and worsening school performance, Ben's teacher entertained the possibility of attention-deficit hyperactivity disorder. However, the consulting psychologist, recognizing the absence of hyperactivity symptoms before age 7 and the relationship between Ben's school problems and the life-threatening accident, made the correct diagnosis of PTSD.

Treatment consisted of cognitive–behavioral psychotherapy, including psychoeducation, anxiety management training, and exposure. The family members and Ben's teacher were involved in all steps of the treatment program; Ben was symptom-free after 12 weekly treatment sessions and remained in remission 1 year later.

---

Clinical Vignette 2

Mr. R, a 34-year-old married man, was referred for medication management by his counselor. He had been healthy until a life-endangering airplane accident 2 years earlier, in which all passengers were killed except for him. He was still experiencing intrusive memories and reliving of the event when seen, despite having had helpful individual counseling. The events of the accident were engraved in his memory with much clarity, and he could not understand how he survived. He was physically injured, with a broken ankle, severe lacerations of his arm, and damage to his back and face. Whenever he saw a plane, he experienced a resurgence of symptoms, and he was unable to take airplane trips. Whenever he rode in an elevator, the sensation while ascending or descending reminded him of the incident, and he became upset. He experienced hundreds of nightmares relating to the accident, felt as if he were constantly waiting for something bad to happen, and often found it impossible to direct his attention and his mind away from trauma images and memories. He had become fearful of even going to sleep. There was a general reduction of interest in things, and many of his former hobbies no longer gave him any pleasure. He found doing his job to be extremely difficult and thought about quitting. He revisited the site of the accident on each anniversary.

The initial treatment plan recognized that he had already received helpful individual counseling, the focus of which had been on reliving and retelling the story, accepting the painful consequences, and dealing with feelings of guilt because of his survival. Although he recognized the usefulness of these approaches, the intensity of his symptoms continued to be distressing and troublesome. As a result, it was agreed to initiate treatment with sertraline (25 mg), increasing upward to 50 mg after a week, supplemented by clonazepam (0.25 mg) at night, largely to facilitate sleep and to reduce hyperarousal and startle

response. It was explained to Mr. R that the sertraline would be expected to help more with the intrusive and avoidant and numbing symptoms. He also completed two self-rating scales for PTSD, the Impact of Events Scale (IES) (Keane et al. 1988) and the Davidson Trauma Scale (DTS) (Davidson et al. 1997). The baseline IES score was 47 (range of scores is 0–88), and the baseline DTS score was 101 (range of scores is 0–136). After 5 weeks, the dose of sertraline was increased to 100 mg/day and the dose of clonazepam remained at 0.25 mg. By the sixth week, his symptom distress was much less, with an IES score of 22 and a DTS score of 49. In other words, there was a greater than 50% reduction of symptoms. On an everyday level, he noticed much less avoidance of going into situations reminding him of the trauma, reduced frequency and severity of nightmares and daytime recollections, and greater ability to focus on important tasks related to his work and family. However, he continued to describe persistent startle response.

Mr. R did not continue his individual therapy, feeling that he had maximal benefit after receiving this form of treatment for more than 1 year. He continued with his medication for another year and noticed improved ability to deal with situations that might have been extremely distressing to him, including being direct witness to a fatal traffic accident. He was still unable to take airplane trips. At one point during his medication management, he unilaterally opted to discontinue his medication without discussing it because of sexual difficulties, which were particularly vexing to him, as he and his wife were attempting to start a family. The use of cyproheptadine proved to be helpful in counteracting this side effect. He was also involved in litigation after the accident and recognized that it was going to be extremely protracted. The litigation also brought with it a whole new set of problems, in which he felt himself being put in the victim position. He acknowledged that, although much progress had been made and he was much more highly functional, "nothing is quick with this condition" and that he still had a number of symptoms. He was willing to consider the possibility of additional treatment focused on his fear of flying. He also recognized that when he had stopped his medicine, the symptoms came back with a vengeance, and at present he became more compliant in taking his antidepressant and anxiolytic medications.

## Comparison of DSM-IV/ICD-10 Diagnostic Criteria

The ICD-10 Diagnostic Criteria for Research for Posttraumatic Stress Disorder provides a different stressor criterion: a situation or event "of exceptionally threatening or catastrophic nature, which would be likely to cause pervasive distress in almost everyone" which is similar to the DSM-III-R definition of a traumatic stressor. DSM-IV-TR instead defines a traumatic stressor as "an event or events that involved actual or threatened death or serious injury, or a threat to the physical integrity of self or others." Furthermore, the ICD-10 diagnostic algorithm differs from that specified in DSM-IV-TR in that the DSM-IV criterion D (i.e., symptoms of increased arousal) is not required. In contrast to DSM-IV-TR which requires that the symptoms persist for more than one month, the ICD-10 Diagnostic Criteria for Research do not specify a minimum duration.

For acute stress disorder, the ICD-10 Diagnostic Criteria for Research differs in several ways from the DSM-IV-TR criteria: (1) primarily anxiety symptoms are included; (2) it is required that the onset of the symptoms be within 1 hour of the stressor; and (3) the symptoms must begin to diminish after not more than 8 hours (for transient stressors) or 48 hours (for extended stressors). In contrast to DSM-IV-TR, the ICD-10 Diagnostic Criteria for Research does not require dissociative symptoms or that the event be persistently reexperienced.

## References

American Psychiatric Association (1994) Diagnostic and Statistical Manual of Mental Disorders, 4th ed. APA, Washington DC.

Beckham JC, Crawford AL, Kirby AC, et al. (1997) Chronic posttraumatic stress disorder and chronic pain in Vietnam combat veterans. J Psychosom Res 43, 379–389.

Beckham JC, Moore SD, Feldman ME, et al. (1998) Self-report and physician-rated health in combat veterans with posttraumatic stress disorder. Am J Psychiatr 155, 1565–1569.

Blake DD, Weathers FW, Nagy LM, et al. (1990) A clinician rating scale for assessing current and lifetime PTSD: The CAPS-1. Behav Ther 13, 187–188.

Blank AS (1993) The longitudinal course of posttraumatic stress disorder. In Posttraumatic Stress Disorder: DSM-IV and Beyond, Foa EB (ed). American Psychiatric Press, Washington DC, pp. 3–22.

Boscarino JA (1996) Posttraumatic stress disorder, exposure to combat, and lower plasma cortisol among Vietnam veterans: Findings and clinical implications. J Consult Clin Psychol 64, 191–201.

Boscarino JA (1997) Diseases among men 20 years after exposure to severe stress: Implications for clinical research and medical care. Psychosom Med 59, 605–614.

Brady K, Pearlstein T, Asnis GM, et al. (2000) Efficacy and safety of sertraline treatment of posttraumatic stress disorder: A randomized controlled trial. J Am Med Assoc 283, 1837–1844.

Bremner JD, Southwick SM, Carnell A, et al. (1996) Chronic PTSD in Vietnam combat veterans: Course of illness and substance abuse. Am J Psychiatr 153, 369–375.

Breslau N (2001) The epidemiology of posttraumatic stress disorder: What is the extent of the problem? J Clin Psychiatr 62, 16–22.

Breslau N, Davis GC, Andreski P, et al. (1991) Traumatic events and posttraumatic stress disorder in an urban population of young adults. Arch Gen Psychiatr 48, 216–222.

Brewin CR, Andrews B, Rose S, et al. (1999) Acute stress disorder and posttraumatic stress disorder in victims of violent crimes. Am J Psychiatr 156, 360–366.

Bryant RA and Harvey AG (1997) Acute stress disorder: A critical review of diagnostic issues. Clin Psychol Rev 17, 757–773.

Bryant RA and Harvey AG (2000) Acute Stress Disorder: A Handbook of Theory, Assessment, and Treatment. American Psychological Association, Washington DC.

Bryant RA and Panasetis P (2001) Panic symptoms during trauma and acute stress disorder. Behav Res Ther 39, 961–966.

Bryant RA, Harvey AG, Guthrie R, et al. (2000) A prospective study of psychophysiological arousal, acute stress disorder, and posttraumatic stress disorder. J Abnorm Psychol 109, 341–344.

Bryant RA, Moulds M, and Guthrie R (2001) Cognitive strategies and the resolution of acute stress disorder. J Traum Stress 14, 213–219.

Bryant RA, Sackville T, Dang ST, et al. (1999) Treating acute stress disorder: An evaluation of cognitive behavior therapy and supportive counseling techniques. Am J Psychiatr 156, 1780–1786.

Buckley TC and Kaloupek DG (2001) A meta-analytic examination of basal cardiovascular activity in posttraumatic stress disorder. Psychosom Med 63, 585–594.

Caplan G (1984) Principles of Preventive Psychiatry. Basic Books, New York.

Carlier IV (2000) Critical incident stress debriefing. In International handbook of human response to trauma. The Plenum series on stress and coping, Yehuda R (ed). Kluwer Academic/Plenum Publishers, New York, pp. 379–387.

Carlier IV, Voerman AE, and Gersons BP (2000) The influence of occupational debriefing on posttraumatic stress symptomatology in traumatized police officers. Br J Med Psychol 73, 87–98.

Cohen JA, Mannarino AP, and Rogal S (2001) Treatment practices for childhood posttraumatic stress disorder. Child Abuse Neglect 25, 123–135.

Conners CK (1985) The Conners Rating Scales: Instruments for the Assessment of Childhood Psychopathology. Children's Hospital National Medical Center, Washington DC.

Connor KM and Davidson JRT (1997). Familial risk factors in posttraumatic stress disorder. Ann NY Acad 821, 35–51.

Connor KM and Davidson JRT (2001) SPRINT: A brief global assessment of posttraumatic stress disorder. Int Clin Psychopharmacol 16, 279–284.

Connor KM, Sutherland SM, Tupler LA, et al. (1999) Fluoxetine in posttraumatic stress disorder: Randomized double-blind study. Br J Psychiatr 175, 17–22.

Costello E (1989) Developments in child psychiatric epidemiology. J Am Acad Child Adolesc Psychiatr 29, 836–841.

Davidson JRT (1992) Drug therapy of posttraumatic stress disorder. Br J Psychiatr 160, 309–314.

Davidson JRT and Fairbank JA (1993) The epidemiology of posttraumatic stress disorder. In Posttraumatic Stress Disorder: DSM-IV and Beyond, Foa EB (ed). American Psychiatric Press, Washington DC, pp. 147–172.

Davidson JRT, Book SW, Colket JT, et al. (1997) Assessment of a new self-rating scale for posttraumatic stress disorder: The Davidson Trauma Scale. Psychol Med 27, 153–160.

Davidson JRT, Hughes GH, Blazer DG, et al. (1991) Posttraumatic stress disorder in the community: An epidemiologic study. Psychol Med 21, 713–721.

Davidson JRT, Kudler HS, Saunders WB, et al. (1993) Predictors of response to amitriptyline in PTSD. Am J Psychiatr 150, 1024–1029.

Davidson JRT, Kudler HS, Smith BD, et al. (1990) Treatment of posttraumatic stress disorder with amitriptyline and placebo. Arch Gen Psychiatr 47, 259–266.

Davidson JRT, Pearlstein T, Londborg P, et al. (2001) Efficacy of sertraline in preventing relapse of posttraumatic stress disorder: Results of a 28-week double-blind placebo-controlled study. Am J Psychiatr 158, 1974–1981.

Davidson JRT, Rothbaum BO, van der Kolk B, et al. (2001) Multicenter, double-blind comparison of sertraline and placebo in the treatment of posttraumatic stress disorder. Arch Gen Psychiatr 58, 485–492.

Davidson JRT, Smith RD, and Kudler HS (1989) Validity and reliability of the DSM-III criteria for posttraumatic stress disorder: Experience with a structured interview. J Nerv Ment Dis 177, 330–341.

Davidson JRT, Swartz M, Storck M, et al. (1985) A diagnostic and family study of posttraumatic stress disorder. Am J Psychiatr 142, 90–93.

Davidson JRT, Tupler LA, Wilson WH, et al. (1998) A family study of chronic posttraumatic stress disorder following rape trauma. J Psychiatr Res 32, 301–309.

Falsetti SA, Resnick HS, Davis J, et al. (2001) Treatment of posttraumatic stress disorder with comorbid panic attacks: Combining cognitive processing therapy with panic control treatment techniques. Group Dynamics 5, 252–260.

Foa EB and Kozak MJ (1986) Emotional processing of fear: Exposure to corrective information. Psychol Bull 99, 20–35.

Foa EB, Keane TM and Friedman MJ (2000) Effective treatments for PTSD: Practice Guidelines from the International Society for Traumatic Stress Studies. Guilford Press, New York.

Foa EB, Riggs DS, Dancu CV, et al. (1993) Reliability and validity of a brief instrument for assessing posttraumatic stress disorder. J Traum Stress 6, 459–473.

Foa EB, Riggs DS, Massie ED, et al. (1995) The impact of fear activation and anger on the efficacy of exposure treatment for posttraumatic stress disorder. Behav Ther 26, 487–499.

Frank JB, Giller ELJ, Kosten TB, et al. (1988) A randomized clinical trial of phenelzine and imipramine for posttraumatic stress disorder. Am J Psychiatr 145, 1289–1291.

Harvey AG and Bryant RA (1999) Dissociative symptoms in acute stress disorder. J Traum Stress 12, 573–680.

Harvey AG and Bryant RA (2000) Memory for acute stress disorder symptoms: A two year prospective study. J Nerv Ment Dis 188, 602–607.

Helzer JE, Robins LN, and McEnvoy L (1987) Posttraumatic stress disorder in the general population. New Eng J Med 317, 1630–1634.

Hidalgo RB and Davidson JRT (2000) Posttraumatic stress disorder: Epidemiology and health-related considerations. J Clin Psychiatr 61, 5–13.

Horowitz M, Wilner NR, and Alvarez W (1979) Impact of event scale: A measure of subjective distress. Psychosom Med 41, 209–218.

Horowitz MJ (1973) Phase-oriented treatment of stress response syndromes. Am J Psychother 27, 506–515.

Inman DJ, Silver SM, and Doghramji K (1990) Sleep disturbance in posttraumatic stress disorder: A comparison with non-PTSD insomnia. J Traum Stress 3, 429–437.

Keane TM, Caddell JM, and Taylor KL (1988) Mississippi Scale for Combat-Related Posttraumatic Stress Disorder. J Cons Clin Psychol 56, 85–90.

Keane TM, Malloy T, and Fairbank JA (1984) Empirical development of an MMPI subscale for the assessment of combat-related posttraumatic stress disorder. J Consult Clin Psychol 52, 888–891.

Keane TM, Wolfe J, and Taylor KL (1987) Posttraumatic stress disorder: Evidence of diagnostic validity and methods of psychological assessment. J Clin Psychol 43, 32–43.

Kendall-Tackett KA, Williams LM, and Finkelhor D (1993) Impact of sexual abuse on children: A review and synthesis of recent empirical studies. Psychol Bull 113, 164–180.

Kessler RC, Sonnega A, Bromet E, et al. (1995) Posttraumatic stress disorder in the National Comorbidity Survey. Arch Gen Psychiatr 52, 1048–1060.

Kilpatrick DB, Saunders BE, Veronen LJ, et al. (1987) Criminal Victimization: Lifetime prevalence, reporting to police, and psychological impact. Crime Delinquency 33, 479–489.

King JA, Abend S and Edwards E (2001) Genetic predisposition and the development of posttraumatic stress disorder in an animal model. Biol Psychiatr 50, 231–237.

Koopman C, Classen C, and Spiegel D (1994) Predictors of posttraumatic stress symptoms among survivors of the Oakland/Berkeley, California firestorm. Am J Psychiatr 151, 888–894.

Kosten TR, Frank JB, Dan E, et al. (1991) Pharmacotherapy for posttraumatic stress disorder using phenelzine or imipramine. J Nerv Ment Dis 179, 366–370.

Kovacs M (1985) The Children's Depression Inventory (CDI). Psychopharmacother Bull 21, 995–998.

Krakow B, Hollifield M, Johnston L, et al. (2001) Imagery rehearsal therapy for chronic nightmares in sexual assault survivors with posttraumatic stress disorder: A randomized control trial. J Am Med Assoc 286, 537–545.

Krakow B, Melendez D, Pederson B, et al. (2001) Complex insomnia: Insomnia and sleep-disordered breathing in a consecutive series of crime victims with nightmares and PTSD. Biol Psychiatr 49, 948–953.

Krystal JH, Kosten TB, Perry BD, et al. (1989) Neurobiological aspects of PTSD: Review of clinical and preclinical studies. Behav Ther 20, 177–198.

Kulka RA, Schlenger WE, Fairbank JA, et al. (1990) Trauma and the Vietnam War generation: Report of Findings from the National Vietnam Veterans Readjustment Study. Brunner/Mazel, New York.

Lieberzon I, Taylor SF, Amdur R, et al. (1999) Brain activation in PTSD in response to trauma-related stimuli. Biol Psychiatr 45, 817–826.

Lima BR, Chavez H, Samniego N, et al. (1989) Disaster severity and emotional disturbance: Implications for primary mental health care in developing countries. Acta Psychiatr Scand 79, 74–82.

Lubin H and Johnson DR (2000) Interactive psychoeducational group therapy in the treatment of authority problems in combat-related posttraumatic stress disorder. Int J Psychophysiol 50, 277–296.

Lundin T (1994) The treatment of acute trauma: Posttraumatic stress disorder prevention. Psychiatr Clin N Am 17, 385–391.

March JS (1990) The nosology of posttraumatic stress disorder. J Anx Disord 4, 61–82.

March JS (1993) What constitutes a stressor? In Posttraumatic Stress Disorder: DSM-IV and Beyond. Foa EB (ed). American Psychiatric Press, Washington DC, pp. 37–54.

Marks IM (1987) Fears, Phobias, and Rituals. Oxford University Press, New York.

Marshall RD, Schneier FR, Fallon BA, et al. (1998) An open trial of paroxetine in patients with noncombat related, chronic posttraumatic stress disorder. J Clin Psychopharmacol 18, 10–18.

Marshall RD, Spitzer R, and Liebowitz MR (1999) Review and critique of the new DSM-IV diagnosis of acute stress disorder. Am J Psychiatr 156, 1677–1688.

McFarlane AC and Yehuda R (2000) Clinical treatment of posttraumatic stress disorder: Conceptual challenges raised by recent research. Austral New Zeal J Psychiatr 34, 940–953.

McLeod DS, Koenen KC, Meyer JM, et al. (2001) Genetic and environmental influences on the relationship among combat exposure, posttraumatic stress disorder symptoms, and alcohol use. J Traum Stress 14, 259–275.

Mellman TA (2002) Anxiety disorders and sleep. In Sleep Medicine, Lee-Chiong TL, Sateia MJ, and Carskadon MA (eds). Hanley & Belfus, Philadelphia.

Mellman T, David D, Bustamante V, et al. (2001) Dreams in the acute aftermath of trauma and their relationship to posttraumatic stress disorder. J Traum Stress 14, 234–241.

Mellman T, Kulick-Bell R, Ashlock LE, et al. (1995) Sleep events among veterans with combat-related posttraumatic stress disorder. Am J Psychiatr 152, 110–115.

Mitchell JT and Everly GS (2000) Critical incident stress management and critical incident stress debriefings: Evolution, effects, and outcomes. In Psychological Debriefing: Theory, Practice, and Evidence. Wilson JP (ed). Cambridge University Press, New York, pp. 71–90.

Nader K, Blake DD, Kriegler J, et al. (1994) Clinician Administered PTSD Scale for Children (CAPS-C). Current and Lifetime Diagnosis Version and Instruction Manual. UCLA Neuropsychiatric Institute and National Center for PTSD.

Nader K, Pynoos RS, Fairbanks L, et al. (1990) Children's PTSD reactions one year after a sniper attack at their school. Am J Psychiatr 147, 1526–1530.

Nader K, Stuber M, and Pynoos RS (1991) Posttraumatic stress reactions in preschool children with catastrophic illness: Assessment needs. Compr Ment Health Care 1, 223–239.

Neylan TC, Marmar CR, Metzler TJ, et al. (1998) Sleep disturbances from a nationally representative sample of male Vietnam veterans. Am J Psychiatr 155, 929–933.

Norris FH (1992) Epidemiology of Trauma: Frequency and impact of different potentially traumatic events on different demographic events. J Consult Clin Psychol 60, 409–418.

Orr SP, Metzger LJ, Lasko NB, et al. (2000) De novo conditioning in trauma-exposed individuals with and without posttraumatic stress disorder. J Abnorm Psychol 109, 290–298.

Pitman RK (1993) Biological Findings in posttraumatic stress disorder: Implications for DSM-IV classification. In Posttraumatic Stress Disorder: DSM-IV and Beyond, Foa EB (ed). American Psychiatric Press, Washington DC.

Pitman RK (2001) Hippocampal diminution in PTSD: More (or less?) than meets the eye. Hippocampus 11, 73–74.

Pitman RK, Altman B, Greenwald E, et al. (1991) Psychiatric complications during flooding therapy for posttraumatic stress disorder. J Clin Psychiatr 52, 17–20.

Pitman RK, Orr SP, Shalev A, et al. (1999) Psychophysiologic alterations in posttraumatic stress disorder. Sem Clin Neuropsychiatr 4, 234–241.

Pitman RK, van der Kolk BA, Orr SP, et al. (1990) Naloxone-reversible analgesic response to combat-related stimuli in posttraumatic stress disorder: A pilot study. Arch Gen Psychiatr 47, 541–544.

Pynoos RS, Frederick CJ, Nader K, et al. (1987) Life threat and posttraumatic stress in school-age children. Arch Gen Psychiatr 44, 1057–1063.

Pynoos RS, Goenjian A, Tashjian M, et al. (1993) Posttraumatic stress reactions in children after the 1988 American earthquake. Br J Med Psychol 163, 239–247.

Rauch SL, Whalen PJ, Shin LM, et al. (2000) Exaggerated amygdala response to masked facial stimuli in posttraumatic stress disorder: A functional MRI study. Biol Psychiatr 47, 769–776.

Resick PA and Schnicke MK (1992) Cognitive processing therapy for sexual assault victims. J Cons Clin Psychol 60, 748–756.

Robins LN, Helzer JE, Croughlan JL, et al. (1981) NIMH Diagnostic Interview Schedule. National Institute of Mental Health, Rockville, MD.

Roth S and Newman E (1991) The process of coping with sexual trauma. J Traum Stress 4, 279–297.

Rothbaum BO, Meadows EA, Resick PA, et al. (2000) Cognitive-behavioral therapy. In Effective Treatments for PTSD: Practice Guidelines from the International Society for Traumatic Stress Studies. Friedman MJ (ed). Guilford Press, New York, pp. 320–325.

Ruggiero KJ, Morris TL, and Scotti JR (2001) Treatment for children with posttraumatic stress disorder: Current status and future directions. Clin Psychol-Sci Pract 8, 210–227.

Saigh PA (1991) The development of posttraumatic stress disorder following four different types of traumatization. Behav Res Ther 29, 213–216.

Schnuff N, Neylan TC, Lenoci MA, et al. (2001) Decreased hippocampal N-acetylaspartate in the absence of atrophy in posttraumatic stress disorder. Biol Psychiatr 50, 952–959.

Schnurr PP and Jankowski MK (1999) Physical health and posttraumatic stress disorder: Review and synthesis. Sem Clin Neuropsychiatr 4, 295–304.

Shalev A, Bleich A, and Ursano RJ (1990) Posttraumatic stress disorder: Somatic comorbidity and effort tolerance. Psychosom 31, 197–203.

Shin LM, McNally RJ, Kosslyn SM, et al. (1999) Regional cerebral blood flow during script-driven imagery in childhood sexual abuse-related PTSD: A PET investigation. Am J Psychiatr 156, 575–584.

Shore J, Tatem E, and Vollmer W (1986) Evaluation of mental effects of disaster: Mount St Hellen's eruption. Am J Pub Health 76, 76–83.

Solomon SD, Gerrity ET, and Muff AM (1992) Efficacy of treatments for posttraumatic stress disorder: An empirical review. J Am Med Assoc 268, 633–638.

Southwick SM, Krystal JH, Morgan CA, et al. (1993) Abnormal noradrenergic function in posttraumatic stress disorder. Arch Gen Psychiatr 50, 266–274.

Spitzer R, Williams JBW, and Gibbon M (1989) Structured Clinical Interview for DSM-III-R. New York State Psychiatric Institute, New York.

Stallings P and March JS (1995) Assessment of anxiety in children and adolescents. In Anxiety Disorders in Children and Adolescents, March JS (ed). Guilford Press, New York.

Tarrier N, Pilgrim H, Sommerfield C, et al. (1999) A randomized trial of cognitive therapy and imaginal exposure in the treatment of chronic posttraumatic stress disorder. J Con Clin Psychol 67, 13–18.

Taylor S, Fedoroff IC, Koch WJ, et al. (2001) Posttraumatic stress disorder arising after road traffic collisions: Patterns of response to cognitive-behavioral therapy. J Consult Clin Psychol 69, 541–551.

Triffleman E, Carroll K, and Kellogg S (1999) Substance dependence posttraumatic stress disorder therapy: An integrated cognitive–behavioral approach. J Subst Abuse 17, 3–14.

True WR and Lyons MJ (1999) Genetic risk factors for PTSD: A twin study. In Risk Factors for Posttraumatic Stress Disorder, Yehuda R (ed). American Psychiatric Press, Washington DC, pp. 61–78.

True WR, Rice J, Eisen SA, et al. (1993) A twin study of genetic and environmental contributions to liability for posttraumatic stress symptoms. Arch Gen Psychiatr 50, 257–265.

van der Kolk B, Dreyfuss D, Michaels M, et al. (1994) Fluoxetine in posttraumatic stress disorder. J Clin Psychiatry 55, 517–522.

Vasterling JJ, Brailey K, Constans JI, et al. (1998) Attention and memory dysfunction in posttraumatic stress disorder. Neuropsychology 12, 125–133.

Warda G and Bryant RA (1998) Thought control strategies in acute stress disorder. Behav Res Ther 36, 1171–1175.

Weathers FW, Litz BT, Herman DS, et al. (1997) Three studies on the psychometric properties of the PTSD Checklist (PCL), submitted for review.

Winfield I, George LK, Swartz M, et al. (1990) Sexual assault and psychiatric disorders among a community sample of women. Am J Psychiatr 147, 335–341.

Wolfsdorf BA and Zlotnick C (2001) Affect management in group therapy for women with posttraumatic stress disorder and histories of childhood sexual abuse. J Clin Psychiatry 57, 169–181.

Yehuda R (1999) Managing anger and aggression in patients with posttraumatic stress disorder. J Clin Psychiatry 15, 33–37.

Yehuda R (2002) Posttraumatic stress disorder. New Engl J Med 346(2), 108–114.

Yehuda R, Giller ELJ, Southwick SM, et al. (1991) Hypothalamic-pituitary-adrenal dysfunction in posttraumatic stress disorder. Biol Psychiatr 30, 266–274.

Yehuda R, Siever LJ, Teicher MH, et al. (1998) Plasma norepinephrine and 3-methoxy-4-hydroxyphenylglycol concentrations and severity of depression in combat posttraumatic stress disorder and major depressive disorder. Biol Psychiatr 44, 56–63.

# 70 Anxiety Disorders: Generalized Anxiety Disorder

Jeannine Monnier
R. Bruce Lydiard
Olga Brawman-Mintzer

## Generalized Anxiety Disorder

## Definition

Generalized anxiety disorder (GAD) was first defined as a separate diagnostic entity in the *Diagnostic and Statistical Manual of Mental Disorders*, Third Edition (DSM-III) (American Psychiatric Association 1980). Prior to the introduction of DSM-III, patients with severe and chronic anxiety were given the diagnosis of anxiety neurosis, a term introduced by Freud over 100 years ago. The DSM-III definition of GAD required uncontrollable anxiety or worry that was not due to a particular life problem. This anxiety or worry needed to be excessive or unrealistic in relation to objective life circumstances and had to persist for 1 month or longer. In DSM-III, the diagnosis of GAD could not be assigned if patients met criteria for another mental disorder, thus obscuring the independent diagnostic status of GAD. These hierarchical exclusion rules were dropped in the revised DSM-III (DSM-III-R), allowing for the first time an independent diagnosis of GAD in addition to other mental disorders (American Psychiatric Association 1987), the only exception being that GAD could not be diagnosed if it occurred exclusively during a mood or psychotic disorder. Further, in the DSM-III-R definition, duration criterion was extended from 1 month to 6 months.

This general approach has been maintained in the *Diagnostic and Statistical Manual of Mental Disorders*, Fourth Edition (DSM-IV) (American Psychiatric Association 1994) where GAD is currently defined as excessive anxiety and worry (apprehensive expectation) occurring for a majority of days during at least a 6-month period, about a number of events or activities (such as work or school performance; see DSM-IV). In individuals with GAD, the anxiety and worry are accompanied by at least three of six somatic symptoms (only one accompanying symptom is required in children), which include restlessness or feeling keyed up or on edge, being easily fatigued, difficulty concentrating or mind going blank, irritability, muscle tension, and sleep disturbance. In addition, the affected individual has difficulty controlling his/her worry, and the anxiety, worry, or somatic symptoms cause clinically significant distress or impairment in social, occupational, and/or other important areas of functioning. Further, the GAD symptoms should not be due to the direct physiological effects of a substance such as drugs or alcohol or a general medical condition, and should not occur exclusively during a mood disorder, psychotic disorder, or pervasive developmental disorder.

Worry and anxiety are part of normal human behavior and it may be difficult to define a cutoff point distinguishing normal or trait anxiety (i.e., a relatively stable tendency to perceive various situations as threatening) from GAD. However, as described in the DSM-IV definition of GAD, individuals suffering from a "disorder" exhibit significant distress and impairment in functioning as a result of their anxiety symptoms.

## Etiology and Pathophysiology

Recent attention has been devoted to the investigation of biological correlates of GAD. In the following section, the authors review the existing information regarding the biological abnormalities in GAD.

## Family Studies

Family studies suggest a familial (and probably a genetic) basis for certain anxiety disorders such as panic disorder (Fyer et al. 1993). Genetic transmission of a disorder suggests that certain gene-encoded changes in proteins and the resulting biological abnormalities may play a role in the pathophysiology of specific disorders. Although there are numerous family and twin studies of "anxiety neurosis," only few investigators examined familiar patterns of GAD utilizing more recent DSM-III and DSM-III-R diagnostic criteria for GAD. Torgersen (1983) studied a sample of twins from Norway treated for psychiatric illness and found a concordance rate for DSM-III-defined GAD of 0% in monozygotic twins and 5% in dizygotic twins. Similarly, in an Australian twin study, Andrews and associates (1990) found no significant difference in concordance rates for DSM-III-defined GAD in monozygotic and dizygotic twins. In contrast, Noyes and associates (1987) studied 20 probands with DSM-III diagnosis of GAD who had no history of panic attacks and found significantly higher rates of GAD in relatives of patients with GAD compared with control subjects.

In a more recent study, Skre and collaborators (1993) examined 20 monozygotic and 29 dizygotic twins with DSM-III-R-defined GAD. They found GAD to be diagnosed in 22% of first-degree relatives of 33 probands with anxiety disorders. In the largest twin study to date which included 1,033 female twin pairs, Kendler and associates (1992a) found that genetic factors play a significant, but not overwhelming role in the etiology of GAD, with the heritability of GAD estimated at around 30% in comparison to 70% heritability in major depression. In addition, the authors found that the vulnerability to GAD and major depression is influenced by the same genetic factors (Kendler et al. 1992b).

Other studies have suggested that while genetic factors may predispose a person to GAD, unique and familial environmental factors play an important role in the development of GAD (Kendler et al. 1995, Scherrer et al. 2000). Others have found no support for the role of inheritance in GAD (Mendlewicz et al. 1993). Research in the area of molecular genetic studies of anxiety disorders has not yet added clarity to this debate (Jetty et al. 2001).

In summary, the available data suggest at most a modest genetic contribution to the etiology of GAD.

## Biological Studies

Relatively few studies have addressed issues regarding the biological aspects of GAD. Existing studies have focused on the evaluation of catecholamine and autonomic responses, neuroendocrine measures, sleep, neuroanatomical/neuroimaging studies, infusion studies, and evaluation of other neurotransmitter systems (Table 70–1).

## Catecholamine Function

Several studies suggest that healthy subjects under stress display increased levels of circulating catecholamines

---

### Generalized Anxiety Disorder

A. Excessive anxiety and worry (apprehensive expectation), occurring more days than not for at least 6 months, about a number of events or activities (such as work or school performance).

B. The person finds it difficult to control the worry.

C. The anxiety and worry are associated with three (or more) of the following six symptoms (with at least some symptoms present for more days than not for the past 6 months). **Note:** Only one item is required in children.

  (1) restlessness or feeling keyed up or on edge

  (2) being easily fatigued

  (3) difficulty concentrating or mind going blank

  (4) irritability

  (5) muscle tension

  (6) sleep disturbance (difficulty falling or staying asleep, or restless unsatisfying sleep)

D. The focus of anxiety and worry is not confined to features of an Axis I disorder, e.g., the anxiety or worry is not about having a panic attack (as in panic disorder), being embarrassed in public (as in social phobia), being contaminated (as in obsessive–compulsive disorder), being away from home or close relatives (as in separation anxiety disorder), gaining weight (as in anorexia nervosa), having multiple physical complaints (as in somatization disorder), or having a serious illness (as in hypochondriasis), and the anxiety and worry do not occur exclusively during posttraumatic stress disorder.

E. The anxiety, worry, or physical symptoms cause clinically significant distress or impairment in social, occupational, or other important areas of functioning.

F. The disturbance is not due to the direct physiological effects of a substance (e.g., a drug of abuse, a medication) or a general medical condition (e.g., hyperthyroidism) and does not occur exclusively during a mood disorder, a psychotic disorder, or a pervasive developmental disorder.

Reprinted with permission from the Diagnostic and Statistical Manual of Mental Disorders, Fourth Edition, Text Revision. Copyright 2000 American Psychiatric Association.

---

**Table 70–1  Generalized Anxiety Disorder: Biological Studies**

| Measure | Results |
|---|---|
| Catecholamine function | |
|   Plasma catecholamine levels | Negative |
|   Platelet $\alpha_2$-adrenoreceptor binding sites | Decreased |
|   Growth hormone response to clonidine stimulation | Blunted |
|   Yohimbine stimulation | Negative |
|   Levels of catecholamine degradation enzymes | Normal |
| Hypothalamic–pituitary–adrenal axis | |
|   Urinary free cortisol | Normal |
|   Dexamethasone suppression test | Nonsuppression |
|   Thyroid function | Normal |
| Autonomic function | |
|   Autonomic activity at rest | Normal |
|   Autonomic response to stress (skin conductance) | Lower |
| Challenge studies | |
|   Lactate infusion | Increased anxiety symptoms/not panic attacks |
| Neurotransmitter abnormalities | |
|   Benzodiazepine binding sites | Decreased |
|   Serotonergic activation via $m$-chlorophenylpiperazine administration | Anxiogenic |

(Rose 1984). Therefore, researchers hypothesized that abnormalities in catecholamine function may be a concomitant of pathological anxiety such as GAD. Some investigators have found that anxiety reactions may be associated with increases in plasma and urinary catecholamine levels. In an early study, Matthew and associates (1980) reported that patients with GAD had higher plasma catecholamine levels than normal comparison subjects. However, a second study by the same investigators failed to replicate these findings (Matthew et al. 1982). The authors concluded that the previous findings might have been related to the stress of venipuncture (the second study used an indwelling catheter to control for the effects of venipuncture). Another study which used an indwelling catheter instead of venipuncture failed to find differences in resting epinephrine and norepinephrine levels between GAD patients and controls (Munjack et al. 1990).

An alternate line of research exploring possible differences in adrenergic systems in GAD patients focused on the study of catecholamine receptors. Since then available techniques did not allow for direct assessment of brain adrenergic receptor function, researchers developed an indirect method for investigating brain neurochemical function by studying peripheral receptors on platelets and lymphocytes. However, data in GAD have been mixed and inconclusive. For example, some researchers found increased norepinephrine (NE) and free 3-methoxy-4-hydroxyphenylethelene glycol (MHPG) levels in GAD patients, and decreased presynaptic alpha-2-adrenoreceptors, while others failed to confirm these findings (Tiihonen et al. 1997). Abelson and colleagues (1991) found a blunted growth hormone response to clonidine (an alpha-2-adrenergic agonist) stimulation in GAD patients, suggesting a possible decrease in the sensitivity of alpha-2-adrenergic receptors in these patients. Charney and colleagues (1989) failed to find differences between GAD patients and controls in cardiovascular responses such as blood pressure and heart rate, self-rated anxiety, as well as in the levels of plasma MHPG and cortisol following yohimbine (alpha-2-antagonist) stimulation. Finally, studies exploring the metabolic pathways of catecholamines such as levels of enzymes responsible for the degradation of catecholamines (catechol-O-methyl transferase, dopamine-beta-hydroxylase, and monoamine oxidase) also failed to show differences between GAD patients and controls (Khan et al. 1986).

In summary, there is limited evidence for abnormalities in catecholamine function in GAD patients; however, current data do not support a strong association between abnormal catecholamine system function and GAD.

## Neuroendocrine Studies

Since increases in plasma cortisol levels have been shown to be a critical component of normal stress responses (Curtis et al. 1970), researchers hypothesized that plasma baseline cortisol levels may be elevated in patients with GAD. This hypothesis was not supported by studies measuring urinary free cortisol levels in GAD patients when compared with normal controls (Rosenbaum et al. 1983). However, these findings do not exclude the possibility of hypothalamic–pituitary–adrenal (HPA) axis dysfunction in patients with GAD. The test most commonly used to assess HPA function is the dexamethasone suppression test (DST). Indeed, some studies have shown a higher prevalence of an "escape" (nonsuppression) response in following dexamethasone administration (that was not attributable to the presence of depression) in GAD patients when compared to normal comparison subjects (Avery et al. 1985). These data indicate that there may be dysregulation of the HPA axis in these patients, as observed following dexamethasone suppression test, possibly associated with abnormal stress response in these individuals.

As psychiatric disorders have also been associated with thyroid abnormalities, Munjack and Palmer (1988) compared total serum thyroxine, free thyroxine index, triiodothyronine resin uptake, and thyroid-stimulating hormone in 52 patients with GAD, 41 patients with panic disorder, and 14 normal comparison subjects. The authors, however, found no difference in thyroid function between these groups.

## Psychophysiology: Autonomic Function

Consistent with the response pattern observed in HPA function studies are findings from studies evaluating peripheral markers of autonomic function such as electrodermal activity, skin conductance, respiration, and blood pressure. While these studies failed to demonstrate differences in measures of electrodermal activity, respiration, blood pressure, and heart interbeat interval at rest, researchers observed that female patients with GAD showed a significantly lower skin conductance response to stress provoking situations and a slower habituation to stress (Hoehn-Saric et al. 1989). These data suggest that patients with GAD may have weaker autonomic responses to stress as well as a more prolonged time to recovery.

## Sleep Studies

Although restless and decreased sleep are common complaints in GAD patients, there have been only a few polysomnographic studies in this patient population. There is some evidence suggesting that patients with GAD have a longer rapid eye movement (REM) latency, shorter REM duration, increased sleep onset latency, and less total sleep time compared with control subjects (Papadimitriou et al. 1988). These findings may differentiate patients with GAD from patients with depression, who show shorter REM latencies.

## Challenge Studies: Lactate Infusion

Challenge studies have become an increasingly important tool in the investigation of the phenomenology and biology of anxiety disorders. The interest in the lactate challenge model evolved from the observation that intravenous administration of sodium lactate provokes physiological and psychological symptoms of panic in patients with panic disorder at a significantly higher rate than in normal comparison subjects (Cowley et al. 1988). Cowley and associates (1988) evaluated the response of patients with GAD to the administration of sodium lactate. The authors found that patients with GAD without current or prior panic attacks demonstrated a lower rate of lactate-induced panic attacks than patients with panic disorder. However, they were significantly more likely to report increased anxiety symptoms than nonpsychiatric controls, suggesting some similarities with panic disorder.

## Neurotransmitter Abnormalities

Alterations in different neurotransmitter systems have been implicated in the pathophysiology of various anxiety disorders. It is generally accepted that anxiety disorders are not associated with abnormalities in only one neurotransmitter system; rather dynamic interactions among several different neurotransmitter systems are believed likely to underlie different anxiety states. Presently, there are data suggesting that the catecholamine (described earlier), serotonin, and GABA-benzodiazepine systems may be involved in the pathophysiology of anxiety disorders.

**GABA-Benzodiazepines.** Benzodiazepines have been the treatment of choice for many patients with GAD. They act at specific recognition sites in the brain, the benzodiazepine receptors, which are located in a subunit of a receptor for gamma-aminobutyric acid (GABA), the major inhibitory neurotransmitter in the brain. Several lines of evidence suggest that the GABA-benzodiazepine receptor complex may be involved in the mediation of anxiety responses. Studies with animals suggest a relationship between benzodiazepine receptors, and fear and anxiety. For example, studies examining response following exposure to stressful stimuli in animal models (e.g., cold swim) have shown a decrease in benzodiazepine receptor binding in the frontal cortex, hippocampus, and hypothalamus, which are areas related to fear and anxiety (Drugan et al. 1989). Models using gamma-2 knockout mice have shown a reduction in GABA$_A$ receptor clustering in the hippocampus and cerebral cortex along with behavioral inhibition to aversive stimuli and increased responsiveness in trace fear conditioning (Lesch 2001).

Research with humans also supports the role of benzodiazepine receptor problems in anxiety reactions (Dorow et al. 1987, Ferrarese et al. 1990, Rickels et al. 1988a, Rocca et al. 1998). The peripheral benzodiazepine receptors found on platelets and lymphocytes have been studied most extensively and studies suggest that there is a decrease in the number of benzodiazepine-binding sites on platelets and lymphocytes of patients with GAD (Rocca et al. 1998). Researchers have shown that low levels of peripheral lymphocyte benzodiazepine receptors are reversed with effective treatment. Following successful treatment with benzodiazepines, the number of binding sites increased (Ferrarese et al. 1990, Rocca et al. 1998). However, the peripheral benzodiazepine receptors are pharmacologically distinct from central benzodiazepine receptors, and, therefore, the significance of these results is unclear. Roy-Byrne and colleagues (1991), using the slowing of saccadic eye movements as a measure of central benzodiazepine effects, have shown a possible decrease in the sensitivity to diazepam in patients with GAD. This suggests that benzodiazepine receptors may be different in patients with GAD. Benzodiazepine-induced chemotaxis is also impaired in GAD patients but is not restored with diazepam treatment (Sacerdote et al. 1999).

**Serotonin.** Alterations in serotonergic (5-HT) neurotransmission have been implicated in the mediation of fear and anxiety responses in animal models (Ramboz et al. 1998,

Taylor et al. 1985) and in humans (Iny et al. 1994, Garvey et al. 1993, Garvey et al. 1995, Kahn et al. 1991). Specifically, researchers hypothesize that anxiety may represent dysregulated serotonergic activity in critical brain areas. For example, serotonin receptor 1A (5-HT$_{1A}$) knockout mice show behaviors consistent with increased anxiety (Ramboz et al. 1998). Further, there is evidence suggesting that the reduction of serotonergic neurotransmission in animals, achieved by lesions of the serotonin system or serotonin receptor blockade, has anxiolytic effects in animal models (Eison 1990). This hypothesis is further supported by the observation that many anxiolytic agents affect serotonergic neurotransmission (Gray 1988). Specifically, drugs that affect serotonergic activity, such as the serotonin (5-HT$_{1A}$) receptor agonists buspirone, ipsapirone, and gepirone decrease the firing of serotonergic neurons and exert antianxiety effects in GAD patients (Gray 1988). Finally, Germine et al. (1992) found that the administration of *m*-chlorophenylpiperazine (*m*CPP), a compound that activates the various serotonin receptors, causes greater anxiety responses in patients with GAD than in normals.

Given the available data, whether overactivity or underactivity of the 5-HT system is the mechanism for GAD development remains unclear (Jetty et al. 2001, Nutt 2001).

**Neuropeptides.** Neuropeptides may also play a role in the pathogenesis of GAD and other anxiety disorders. The cholecystokinin (CCK) system is one of the neuropeptides implicated in anxiety in animal models (Harro et al. 1993, Lydiard 1994, Woodruff and Hughes 1991). CCK, a highly abundant neurotransmitter in the brain, has also been implicated in anxiety in humans (Bradwejn and Koszycki 1992, Brawman-Mintzer et al. 1997, Kennedy et al. 1999, Adams et al. 1995, Goddard et al. 1999). CCK may be possibly involved in the pathophysiology of panic disorder and may also play a role in the biology of GAD (Lydiard 1994). Corticotropin-releasing factor (CRF), a major physiological regulator of adreno corticotropic hormone (ACTH), appears to be involved in stress and anxiety responses (Koob 1999, Chrousos and Gold 1992). Administration of CRF to various parts of animal brains has elicited anxiety and fear responses (e.g., suppression of exploratory behavior, shock-induced freezing) (Butler et al. 1990, Griebel 1999, Koob and Gold 1997). Interestingly, both these peptides are functionally antagonized by benzodiazepines.

Neuropeptide Y (Britton et al. 1997, Widerlov et al. 1988, Boulenger et al. 1996, Stein et al. 1996) and tachykinins (Beresford et al. 1995) may play a role in anxiety. Further, research has suggested that glutamate may play a role in anxiety in both animal models and human studies (Trullas et al. 1989, Miserendino et al. 1990, Moghaddam et al. 1994).

## Neuroanatomic Sites of Anxiety

Several potential neuroanatomic anxiogenic sites in the central nervous system (CNS) have been proposed based on brain imaging and neuroanatomic studies. The areas potentially involved in anxiety are the parts of the limbic system involving the hippocampus, prefrontal cortex, occipital lobes, basal ganglia and brain stem structures, specifically the locus coeruleus, nucleus paragigantocellularis, and periaqueductal gray (Gray 1988). These structures are rich in noradrenergic, GABAergic, and serotonergic receptors which are believed to be involved in the pathophysiology of different anxiety states such as GAD.

## Cerebral Blood Flow and Metabolism Studies

Only a few imaging studies in GAD have appeared in the literature. In one study, patients with GAD displayed decreases in cortical blood flow compared with control subjects. Significant negative correlations between state anxiety and cerebral blood flow in most brain regions were observed (Mathew et al. 1982). Wu and colleagues (1991) evaluated 18 patients who met DSM-III criteria for GAD using positron emission tomography (PET) measurements of cerebral glucose at "baseline" (during a passive viewing task), following a cognitive vigilance task designed to stimulate anxiety, and following treatment with benzodiazepines. They found a higher relative metabolic rate for GAD patients in parts of the occipital, temporal, frontal lobes, and cerebellum relative to normal control subjects during a passive viewing task. The authors also found a decrease in absolute basal ganglia metabolic activity in GAD patients. During the vigilance task, GAD patients showed a significant increase in relative basal ganglia metabolism. The authors did not find a global decrease in cortical metabolism, as had been predicted by blood flow studies. Finally, benzodiazepine treatment resulted in a significant decrease in glucose metabolism in cortical surface (especially in the occipital cortex), the limbic system, and basal ganglia compared with patients receiving placebo.

Using magnetic resonance imaging (MRI) and single photon emission tomography (SPET), Tiihonen and colleagues (1997) found that those with GAD had decreased benzodiazepine receptor binding in the left temporal pole as compared to matched healthy controls. In a study using functional MRI in GAD patients, Lorberbaum and colleagues (2001) found greater activity in the right cingulate, right medial prefrontal and orbitofrontal cortex, right temporal poles, and right dorsomedial thalamus, during periods of anticipatory anxiety, compared with rest periods, than matched control subjects. Further, only matched control subjects displayed increased activity in the medial prefrontal cortex.

In summary, the limited number of imaging studies to date in patients with GAD suggest changes in regional brain activity in this population.

## Psychological Mechanisms

### Cognitive–Behavioral Model

Psychological models, which emphasize the cognitive–behavioral processes involved in the onset and maintenance of GAD, have emerged in recent years. Individuals' thoughts and behaviors are thought to instigate and maintain episodes of anxiety. Such thoughts and behaviors may be triggered by life events. For example, Blazer and associates (1987) found evidence suggesting the importance of negative life events in the onset of GAD. Additionally, one's cognitive style may trigger anxiety.

In support of cognitive theories of GAD, anxious individuals with GAD were more likely to perceive ambiguous information as threatening and/or negative, and to perceive that they are more likely than others to experience threatening situations (Rapee 1991). Patients with GAD also pay more attention to the detection of potentially threatening information and incorporate this information into highly elaborate cognitive schemas, thus lowering their threshold for activation of an anxiety response (Josephs 1994). The threatening information then elicits anxious affect and the individual begins to worry in an attempt to further define the problem.

Barlow and colleagues also postulated that patients with GAD are likely to be characterized by a perception of lack of control over threatening events (Rapee 1991). In addition, the authors found that patients are likely to believe that they have little control over their emotions, especially their worrying, leading to further distress. It has been suggested that the interaction between perceived uncontrollability and a cognitive focus on negative/threatening stimuli may amplify the general worry to pathological levels (Rapee 1991). Finally, Borkovec and colleagues (1993) suggested that worrying may suppress emotional processing, and temporarily reduce anxiety. This may help maintain the pathological cognitive state (Rapee 1991).

In summary, cognitive–behavioral models of GAD have proposed useful alternatives to traditional psychodynamic models of anxiety. Cognitive–behavioral treatment strategies, designed to modify maladaptive thought patterns and behaviors, have gained acceptance as effective interventions in the treatment of GAD.

### Psychodynamic Theories

Psychodynamic theories offer a different view of the origins of anxiety disorders. In his initial explanation of the origin of anxiety (called toxic theory of anxiety), Freud stated that an abnormal amount of undischarged sexual energy (or libido) can manifest itself as anxiety (Josephs 1994). He believed that unexpressed/ungratified sexual wishes result in undischarged libido that is experienced subjectively as anxiety. Freud described various examples of unexpressed sexual urges such as sexual trauma (for example, activation of sexual urges following seduction in childhood), unhealthy sexual practices (such as coitus interruptus), and repression (when the threatening sexual urge or wish is banished from consciousness).

In his later work, Freud abandoned the toxic model, and developed another conceptual framework for the understanding of anxiety called the "signal theory of anxiety" (Josephs 1994). The concept of signal anxiety followed the development of Freud's structural model of the mind, which proposes three interacting psychological functions: ego (which mediates between the demands of primitive drives, the social and parental prohibitions, and reality), superego (representing the internalized parental and social prohibitions), and id (representing the primitive drives and urges) (Josephs 1994). Freud believed that anxiety serves as a signal to the ego of a threat (in the form of an unconscious drive or wish arising from the id), which, if enacted, may be dangerous to the ego, signaling the potential punishment by the superego or the external world. According to this model, the ego can activate defense mechanisms, such as repression, and prevent the actualization of the forbidden urge either by preventing the expression of the wish or by avoiding the life situations in which the wish might be potentially expressed. Ideally, repression into the unconscious (i.e., out of subject's awareness) should successfully contain the drives. However, if the defenses fail, one may experience symptomatic anxiety and other distressing psychological symptoms. Implicit in this model is the concept that the individuals themselves are not consciously aware of these processes. Therefore, the promotion of subjects' insight into unconscious conflicts and the uncovering of the unconscious origins of anxiety through interpretation and other techniques is the primary goal (and method) of the psychoanalytic treatment approach.

## Other Psychodynamic Theories

Sullivan developed a theory of anxiety based on the importance of interpersonal relationships (Josephs 1994). He viewed affects (such as anxiety) as forms of interpersonal communication. According to this model, anxiety communicates the sense of insecurity in interpersonal relationships. For example, a mother who is insecure in her role may communicate her insecurity to the infant when she is anxious in her child's presence. The child in turn identifies her anxiety and expresses anxious affect himself. Another approach to the understanding of the origins of anxiety was offered by object relations theorists such as Klein and Bowlby. They believed that anxiety reflects a fear of the loss of the nurturing object or fear of being hurt by the antagonistic object (Josephs 1994).

Finally, self psychology theorists, such as Kohut, believed that the individual strives to achieve and maintain an integrated, cohesive sense of self (Josephs 1994). Beginning in early age, the individual develops this sense of self through idealization of important others, such as important caregivers (called self-objects), and through a process of positive interaction with caregivers (called mirroring). He believed that inadequate provision of these experiences can lead to anxiety (fear of disintegration) and the loss of the cohesive self (Josephs 1994).

## Assessment and Differential Diagnosis

GAD patients frequently report that they have been anxious all their lives. Typically, they were moderately anxious during childhood, later developing full-blown GAD when their stress levels increased through activities such as attending college or starting to work. Some studies found that between 10 and 30% of patients with GAD report onset of their disorder before age (Hoehn-Saric et al. 1993). Patients with early onset of symptoms report experiencing significant anxiety and fears, social isolation, obsessionality, more academic difficulties, and disturbed home environment during their childhood. The social maladjustment and emotional overreactivity persist into adulthood. Epidemiological studies (Kendler et al. 1992a, Burke et al. 1991) and clinical studies (Barlow et al. 1986, Rogers et al. 1999) suggest that the onset of GAD typically begins between the late teens and late twenties. However, not all GAD patients have a lifelong history of excessive anxiety. Some patients develop their disorder at a later age, that is, in one's thirties or later. These patients frequently report identifiable, precipitating stressful events, specifically unexpected, negative, important events in the year preceding development of GAD (Blazer et al. 1987, Hoehn-Saric et al. 1993).

Patients with GAD experience chronic anxiety and tension. They find the worry as being uncontrollable. However, some patients intentionally initiate and maintain worry with an almost superstitious assumption that, by doing so, they can avert a negative event (Rapee 1991). Patients tend to worry predominantly about family, personal finances, work, and illness (Sanderson and Barlow 1990). They are also likely to report worrying over minor matters, such as making a slight social faux pas. The majority report being anxious for at least 50% of the time during an average day (Sanderson and Barlow 1990). In children and adolescents, the worries often revolve around the quality of their performance in school or other competitive areas (American Psychiatric Association 1994). They may also worry about potential catastrophic events. They are concerned with their own physical or mental imperfections or inadequacies, and typically require excessive reassurance (Bernstein and Borchardt 1991). They often appear shy, overcompliant, perfectionistic, and frequently describe multiple physical complaints (Bernstein and Borchardt 1991). They may have an unusually mature and serious manner and appear older than their actual age (Bernstein and Borchardt 1991). These children are often the eldest in small, competitive, achievement-oriented families (Bernstein and Borchardt 1991).

Individuals with GAD commonly complain of feeling tense, jumpy, and irritable. They have difficulty falling or staying asleep, and tire easily during the day (Brawman-Mintzer et al. 1993). Particularly distressing to patients is the difficulty in concentrating and collecting their thoughts (Brawman-Mintzer et al. 1993). Cognitions appear to play a central role in GAD, as well as other anxiety disorders. Patterns of cognitions, however, appear to be disorder-specific. When the frequency of anxiety, worry, or panic attacks among patients with GAD and panic disorder, as well as the severity of anxiety associated with each were examined (Breitholtz et al. 1999), 34% of GAD patients' cognitions were found to center on interpersonal conflict or the issue of acceptance by others, while only 1.4% of panic disorder patients reported such concerns. While patients with GAD also had exaggerated worries over relatively minor matters, panic disorder patients reported a significantly greater frequency of cognitions concerning physical dangers or catastrophes (e.g., accident, injury, death).

Patients may present complaining of muscular tension, especially in their neck and shoulders (Brawman-Mintzer et al. 1993). They may experience headaches, frequently described as frontal and occipital pressure or tension. They complain about sweaty palms, feel shaky and tremulous, complain of dryness of the mouth, and experience palpitations and difficulty breathing (Brawman-Mintzer et al. 1993). Patients may also experience gastrointestinal symptoms such as heartburn and epigastric fullness. Approximately 30% of patients experience severe gastrointestinal symptoms of irritable bowel syndrome (Tollefson et al. 1991). The physical complaints frequently lead patients to seek medical attention, and most will initially consult a primary care physician. Although they frequently complain of palpitations and difficulty breathing, studies suggest that patients with GAD do not differ from normal comparison subjects on measures of respiration and heart rate (Kollai and Kollai 1992). Patients with GAD may also present complaining of chest pain. Although chest pain is more frequently reported by patients with panic disorder, Carter and Maddock (1992) observed that 34% of patients with GAD without panic attacks experienced chest pain. They also found that these patients were predominantly males and many had undergone extensive cardiac evaluations that revealed no demonstrable cardiac pathology.

Special laboratory and diagnostic evaluation of patients with GAD may occasionally be required to exclude general medical conditions that mimic symptoms of generalized anxiety (see the section, Differential Diagnosis). An evaluation to identify these disorders includes a personal and family medical history, review of systems, and a careful physical examination including neurological examination. Laboratory evaluation should include an electrocardiogram, screening for abusable substances, urinalysis, complete blood count, serum electrolytes, liver and thyroid function tests, calcium, phosphorus, and blood urea nitrogen.

## Differential Diagnosis

### Psychiatric Conditions

Anxiety can be a prominent feature of many psychiatric disorders. In addition, the substantial overlap of symptoms between GAD and other psychiatric disorders such as major depressive disorder, often creates diagnostic and treatment dilemmas for the clinician and may complicate the difficult task of differential diagnosis and treatment planning. This section will highlight the major disorders that should be considered in the differential diagnosis of GAD (Figure 70–1).

### Major Depressive Disorder and Dysthymic Disorder

Several symptom profiles discriminate between major depressive disorder or dysthymic disorder and GAD (Brown et al. 1994). Patients with major depressive disorder exhibit higher rates of dysphoric mood, psychomotor retardation, suicidal ideation, guilt, hopelessness, and helplessness, as well as more work impairment than patients with GAD (Riskind et al. 1991). In contrast, patients with GAD show higher rates of somatic symptoms, specifically, muscle tension and autonomic symptoms (e.g., respiratory or cardiac complaints) than depressed patients.

### Panic Disorder With/Without Agoraphobia

Some researchers have suggested that GAD is attributable to panic disorder (Mennin et al. 1998). However, clear differences exist between GAD and panic disorder. For example, panic disorder is characterized by the presence of panic attacks; that is, recurrent, discrete episodes of intense anxiety or fear associated with a cluster of somatic symptoms reflecting autonomic hyperactivity such as rapid heartbeat, dizziness, numbness or tingling, trouble breathing or choking, and nausea or vomiting. In contrast, patients with GAD experience predominantly symptoms of muscle tension and vigilance such as fatigue, muscle soreness, insomnia, difficulty concentrating, restlessness, and irritability (Brawman-Mintzer et al. 1994). Patients with panic disorder tend to seek treatment earlier in life than patients with GAD (Noyes et al. 1992). Additionally, reports of types of worry differ between those diagnosed with GAD and those with panic disorder. For example, panic patients worry about having additional panic attacks, whereas GAD patients worry unrealistically about a number of everyday issues.

### Obsessive–Compulsive Disorder

Anxiety is part of the clinical picture of obsessive–compulsive disorder (OCD) and may be a central factor in initiating and maintaining obsessions and compulsions. Interestingly there are also some data suggesting that OCD and GAD may be related. For example, Black and associates (1992) found an increased prevalence of GAD among relatives of patients with OCD. However, several features distinguish the excessive worry that accompanies GAD from the obsessional thoughts of OCD. Obsessive thoughts are described as ego-dystonic intrusions that often take the form of urges, impulses, or images. They are often senseless and are frequently accompanied by time-consuming compulsions designed to reduce mounting anxiety. In contrast, the worries in GAD are about realistic concerns, such as health and finances.

### Other Anxiety Disorders

In phobic disorders, the anxiety is characteristically associated with a specific phobic object or situation that is frequently avoided by the patient. Such is the case with social anxiety disorder as well, in which the individual is afraid of or avoids situations in which he or she may be the focus of potential scrutiny by others. Anxiety is also a characteristic part of the presentation of posttraumatic stress disorder (PTSD) and acute stress disorder. However, unlike in GAD, the principal symptoms experienced in PTSD and acute stress disorder follow exposure to a traumatic event and are characterized by avoidance of reminders of the event and persistent reexperiencing of the traumatic event (American Psychiatric Association 1994). In addition, in contrast to GAD which must last at least 6 months, acute stress disorder does not persist for more than 4 weeks (American Psychiatric Association 1994). Finally, in adjustment disorders anxiety when present occurs in response to a specific life stressor or stressors and generally does not persist for more than 6 months (American Psychiatric Association 1994).

### Mixed Anxiety–Depressive Disorder

Many patients fail to meet criteria for either an anxiety or mood disorder. The DSM-IV appendix contains a research criteria set defining mixed anxiety–depressive disorder in individuals who have had four or more listed symptoms of anxiety or depression for a minimum of 4 weeks (American Psychiatric Association 1994). Treatment studies in this patient subgroup are currently underway.

### Normal Anxiety

As mentioned earlier, worry and anxiety are part of normal human behavior, and it may be difficult to define a cut off point distinguishing normal or trait anxiety (i.e., a relatively stable tendency to perceive various situations as threatening) from GAD. However, individuals suffering from a "disorder" exhibit significant distress and impairment in functioning as a result of their anxiety symptoms.

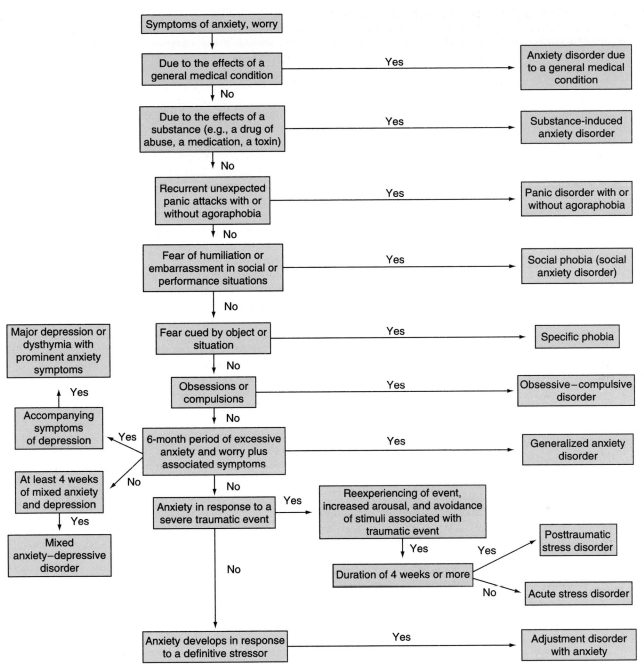

**Figure 70–1** *Diagnostic decision tree for GAD.*

In addition, several biological measures distinguish normal response to stress from responses accompanying GAD. For example, studies suggest that normal subjects under stress display a higher increase in autonomic symptoms of arousal such as skin conductance levels than subjects with GAD (Hoehn-Saric et al. 1989). In addition, they also display faster habituation to repeated stressful stimuli than subjects with GAD (Hoehn-Saric et al. 1989).

## Anxiety Disorder due to a General Medical Condition

Many general medical conditions may present with prominent anxiety symptoms. If not identified and properly addressed, these conditions may adversely affect the treatment outcome of the anxious patient. In this section we will highlight important medical conditions in the differential diagnosis of generalized anxiety (see Table 70–2).

## Cardiovascular Disorders

Patients with GAD may complain of palpitations, skipped heartbeats, and chest pain. In addition, many GAD patients, especially males, fear having an acute myocardial infarction and often present to the emergency room for evaluation. However, most patients with GAD without a concomitant cardiovascular disease do not experience

| Table 70–2 | Medical Conditions and Drugs That May Cause Anxiety |
|---|---|

| Endocrine Disorders | Cardiovascular and Circulatory Disorders |
|---|---|
| Addison's disease | Anemia |
| Cushing's syndrome | Congestive heart failure |
| Hyperparathyroidism | Coronary insufficiency |
| Hyperthyroidism | Dysrhythmia |
| Hypothyroidism | Hypovolemia |
| Carcinoid | Myocardial infarction |
| Pheochromocytoma | |
| **Drug Intoxication** | **Respiratory Disorders** |
| Anticonvulsants | Asthma |
| Antidepressants | Chronic obstructive |
| Antihistamines | pulmonary disease |
| Antihypertensive agents | Pulmonary embolism |
| Antiinflammatory agents | Pulmonary edema |
| Antiparkinsonian agents | |
| Caffeine | |
| Digitalis | |
| Sympathomimetics | |
| Thyroid supplements | |
| | **Immunological, Collagen, and Vascular Disorders** |
| **Substance Use Related** | |
| Cocaine | Systemic lupus erythematosus |
| Hallucinogens | Temporal arteritis |
| Amphetamines | |
| **Withdrawal Syndromes** | **Metabolic Conditions** |
| Alcohol | Acidosis |
| Narcotics | Acute intermittent porphyria |
| Sedatives–hypnotics | Electrolyte abnormalities |
| | Hypoglycemia |
| **Gastrointestinal Disorders** | **Neurological Disorders** |
| Peptic ulcer disease | Brain tumors |
| | Cerebral syphilis |
| | Cerebrovascular disorders |
| | Encephalopathies |
| | Epilepsy (especially temporal lobe epilepsy) |
| | Postconcussive syndrome |
| | Vertigo |
| | Akathisia |
| **Infectious Diseases** | |
| Miscellaneous viral and bacterial infections | |

severe chest pain. Following the controversial evidence suggesting an association between mitral valve prolapse (MVP) and panic disorder, researchers evaluated the prevalence of MVP in patients with GAD (Dager et al. 1986) and found no evidence of increased prevalence in patients with GAD. Nevertheless, patients with anxiety symptoms associated with unexplained chest pain should be evaluated for possible cardiovascular disease.

## Hyperthyroidism

Anxiety is a prominent feature of hyperthyroidism with some overlap in the symptomatology of thyrotoxicosis and GAD. Symptoms such as tachycardia, tremulousness, irritability, weakness, and fatigue are common to both disorders. In GAD, however, the peripheral manifestations of excessive concentrations of circulating thyroid hormones are absent, including symptoms such as weight loss, increased appetite, warm and moist skin, heat intolerance, and dyspnea on effort. Presence of goiter makes the diagnosis of hyperthyroidism likely; however, the absence of thyroid enlargement does not exclude it. Thus, confirmatory laboratory tests (free $T_4$, $T_3$, and TSH) assume significant diagnostic importance. In mild cases, laboratory tests may be within the upper limit of the normal range, in which case a thyroid releasing hormone stimulation test is indicated.

## Pheochromocytomas

Pheochromocytomas, also known as chromaffin tumors, produce, store, and secrete catecholamines. They are derived most often from the adrenal medulla, as well as the sympathetic ganglia, and occasionally from other sites. The clinical features of these tumors, most commonly hypertension and hypertensive paroxysms, are predominantly due to the release of catecholamines. Patients may also experience diaphoresis, tachycardia, chest pain, flushing, nausea and vomiting, headache, and significant apprehension. Although the clinical presentation frequently mimics spontaneous panic attacks, pheochromocytomas should also be considered in the differential diagnosis of GAD. The diagnosis of pheochromocytoma can be confirmed by increased levels of catecholamines (epinephrine and norepinephrine) or catecholamine metabolites (metanephrines and vanillylmandelic acid) in a 24-hour urine collection.

## Other Medical Conditions

Menopause is commonly referred to as the period that encompasses the transition between the reproductive years and beyond the last episode of menstrual bleeding. Frequently associated with significant anxiety, menopause should be considered in the differential diagnosis of GAD. However, other associated symptoms such as vasomotor instability, atrophy of urogenital epithelium and skin, and osteoporosis make the diagnosis of menopause probable. Another endocrinologic disorder, hyperparathyroidism, can present with anxiety symptoms, and the initial evaluation of serum calcium levels may be indicated. Finally, certain neurologic conditions such as complex partial seizures, intracranial tumors and strokes, and cerebral ischemic attacks may be associated with symptoms typically observed in anxiety disorders and may require appropriate evaluation.

## Substance-Induced Anxiety Disorder

Anxiety disorders can occur frequently in association with intoxication and withdrawal from several classes of substances (see Table 70–2). Excessive use of caffeine, especially in children and adolescents, may cause significant anxiety. Cocaine intoxication may be associated with anxiety, agitation, and hypervigilance. During cocaine withdrawal, patients may also present with prominent anxiety, irritability, insomnia, fatigue, depression, and cocaine craving. Adverse reaction to marijuana includes extreme anxiety that usually lasts less than 24 hours. Mild opioid withdrawal presents with symptoms of anxiety and dysphoria. However, accompanying symptoms such as elevated blood pressure, tachycardia, pupilary dilation, rhinorrhea, piloerection, and lacrimation are rare in patients with GAD.

The clinical phenomenology observed both in alcohol and sedative–hypnotic drug withdrawal and in GAD, although variable, may be highly similar. In both conditions, nervousness, tachycardia, tremulousness, sweating, nausea, and hyperventilation occur prominently. Additionally, the same drugs (i.e., benzodiazepines) can be used to treat anxiety symptoms, and some patients may use alcohol in an attempt to alleviate anxiety. Thus, the symptoms of an underlying anxiety disorder may be difficult to differentiate from the withdrawal symptoms associated with the use of benzodiazepines or alcohol.

The use of many commonly prescribed medications may produce side effects manifesting as anxiety (see Table 70–2). Such medications include sympathomimetics or other bronchodilators such as theophilline, anticholinergics, antiparkinsonian preparations, corticosteroids, thyroid supplements, oral contraceptives, antihypertensive, and cardiovascular medications such as digitalis, insulin (secondary to hypoglycemia), and antipsychotic and antidepressant medications. Finally, heavy metals and toxins such as organophosphates, paint, and insecticides may also cause anxiety symptoms.

## Epidemiology and Comorbidity

Despite the shifting diagnostic criteria affecting the prevalence studies, current data indicate that GAD is probably one of the more common psychiatric disorders. Breslau and Davis (1985) reported a lifetime prevalence of 45% for GAD, according to DSM-III diagnostic criteria. However, when these researchers used the more stringent criteria outlined in the DSM-III-R, which required a duration of 6 months, the prevalence rate dropped dramatically to 9%. The Epidemiologic Catchment Area Study (ECA) (Blazer et al. 1991), a five-center epidemiological study of the prevalence of psychiatric disorders in the US, reported a lifetime prevalence for DSM-III-defined GAD of 4.1 to 6.6% in the three sites that assessed for GAD. One of the most recent epidemiological surveys of DSM-III-R GAD was conducted as a part of the National Comorbidity Survey of psychiatric disorders in the US by Kessler and colleagues (Kessler et al. 1994, Wittchen et al. 1994). The composite international diagnostic interview, a structured psychiatric interview, was administered to a representative national sample and evaluated the prevalence of 14 DSM-III-R psychiatric disorders. Prevalence rates in the total sample ($N = 8,098$) were 1.6% for current GAD (defined as the most recent 6-month period of anxiety), 3.1% for 12-month GAD, and 5.1% for lifetime GAD, with lifetime prevalence higher in females (6.6%) than males (3.6%).

Studies examining DSM-IV GAD prevalence rates have been conducted outside the US. Wittchen and colleagues (1998) examined GAD in a sample of adolescents and adults in Munich, Germany and found a lifetime prevalence of 0.8% and a 12-month prevalence of 0.5%.

Bhagwanjee and colleagues (1998) examined rates of GAD in a sample from South Africa and found current prevalence of GAD in a sample of adults to be 3.7%. In another German sample, Carter and colleagues (2001) reported a 12-month prevalence rate of 1.5%.

GAD appears at even higher rates in clinical settings, particularly in primary care settings. For example, Shear and colleagues (1994) found prevalence rates of GAD, using DSM-III-R criteria, reported by patients at four primary care centers, to be twice as high as those reported in community samples (i.e., 10 versus 5.1%). Similarly, a collaborative study by the World Health Organization (WHO) across 15 international sites reported prevalence rates of GAD at approximately 8% in primary care settings (Maier et al. 2000, Sartorius et al. 1996).

Those with anxiety symptoms meeting criteria for GAD in the ECA study reported receiving more outpatient mental services during the previous year than those diagnosed with other psychiatric disorders (Blazer et al. 1991). Many of those with GAD in the National Comorbidity Survey sought professional help for GAD (66% of participants) and used medications to reduce their symptoms of GAD (44% of participants) (Wittchen et al. 1994). Over 80% of the GAD group in the Harvard/Brown Anxiety Disorders Research Program (HARP) data indicated that they received psychotherapy and/or pharmacotherapy (Yonkers et al. 1996).

Rates of GAD appear similar in special populations such as children and the elderly. GAD appears to be less prevalent in children than in adults. Data from the National Comorbidity Study indicate that for both lifetime and 12-month prevalence rates, GAD occurs at the lowest rate in younger ages and at the highest rate in older adults (Wittchen et al. 1994). Anderson and associates (1987) reported a 1-year prevalence rate of 2.9% for overanxious anxiety disorder, the DSM-III-R equivalent of GAD in children. In a community sample of 150 adolescents, Kashani and Orvaschel (1988) reported a 6-month prevalence rate of 7.3% for overanxious anxiety disorder. Finally, in a clinical setting the prevalence of childhood overanxious anxiety disorder was even higher, with up to 52% of the children seen having anxiety symptoms that met criteria for the disorder (Last et al. 1987). It should be mentioned that in DSM-IV, the diagnosis of childhood overanxious anxiety disorder was subsumed within the diagnosis of GAD. Epidemiological data on prevalence of GAD in childhood using DSM-IV criteria are currently lacking. In the elderly, GAD appears to account for the majority of anxiety disorders, with prevalence rates ranging from 0.7 to 7.3% (Beekman et al. 1998, Flint 1994).

Although it is unclear whether childhood GAD predisposes to the development of adult GAD or represents an early manifestation of adult GAD, these studies further suggest that generalized anxiety is highly prevalent both in the community and in the clinical population.

## GAD: Comorbidity With Other Disorders

The term comorbidity implies the co-occurrence of two or more psychiatric disorders in the same individual within a defined period of time. Due to the existence of hierarchical exclusionary rules present in diagnostic classification systems prior to the introduction of DSM-III-R in 1987, the evaluation of psychiatric comorbidity in GAD was not possible, and only recently has been routinely assessed. Despite different methodological approaches, the available studies report a high prevalence of psychiatric comorbidity in patients with GAD. For example, in some studies more than 90% of GAD patients had additional symptoms that fulfilled criteria for at least one or more concurrent disorders (range of 45–91%) (Sanderson and Barlow 1990, Brawman-Mintzer et al. 1993).

An examination of the relative frequencies of various comorbid diagnoses in patients with GAD obtained from the available studies reveals that other anxiety and mood disorders frequently complicate the course of GAD (Sanderson and Barlow 1990, Brawman-Mintzer et al. 1993, Wittchen et al. 1994, see diagnostic decision tree for GAD). Angst (1993) evaluated psychiatric comorbidity in a longitudinal epidemiological study in Zurich, Switzerland. Strong associations between GAD and major depression and between GAD and dysthymia were found, but a relatively low association with panic disorder was found. A high comorbidity of GAD with hypomania was also found. Further, the presence of comorbidity was associated with a high suicide attempt risk. In addition, individuals with comorbid disorders were treated more frequently and endorsed more work impairment than GAD patients without comorbid disorders.

Large epidemiological studies have reported similar findings. For example, the National Comorbidity Survey showed 90% of respondents with lifetime GAD had at least one other lifetime disorder and of those with current GAD, 66% had at least one other current disorder (Wittchen et al. 1994). The most common comorbidities (specifically that criteria for both disorders were met) were found for mood disorders (major depression and dysthymia), panic disorder, and (for current comorbidity only) agoraphobia. Other studies have also found that the highest comorbidities were with depressive disorders, and panic disorders (Sanderson and Barlow 1990, Brawman-Mintzer et al. 1993, Wittchen et al. 1994, Sartorius et al. 1996, Yonkers et al. 1996, Fifer et al. 1994, Pini et al. 1997, Starcevic et al. 1992).

GAD usually has an earlier onset than other anxiety and depressive disorders when comorbid disorders are present (Brown and Barlow 1992). Brawman-Mintzer and associates (1993) found that GAD had an onset before dysthymia and panic disorder, and after simple and social phobia. Further, onset of major depression seemed to follow the onset of anxiety. Similar findings have been reported by other investigators (Fava et al. 1992, Kessler et al. 2000, Massion et al. 1993).

As in adult GAD, childhood GAD (or overanxious anxiety disorder as it was earlier labeled) is also characterized by an unusual degree of comorbidity. Kashani and coworkers (1990) observed that over 50% of children with overanxious disorder had symptoms that met criteria for at least one additional psychiatric diagnosis. Among the most prevalent current comorbid diagnoses are social phobia (16–59%), simple phobia (21–55%), panic disorder (3–27%) and depression (8–39%). Furthermore, Masi and coworkers (1999) found, in those children and adolescents they sampled, that 87% had a comorbid disorder. In particular, high rates of separation anxiety, social anxiety, and depressive disorders were found.

Alcoholism also complicates the clinical course of GAD for some patients; however, the available literature suggests that the diagnosis of alcohol abuse is not as prevalent in GAD as in other anxiety disorders, and the pattern of abuse is often a brief and nonpersistent one (Brawman-Mintzer et al. 1993). GAD onset is usually later than that of the alcohol use disorder (Kushner et al. 1999). Personality disorders have been observed to co-occur in approximately 50% of patients with GAD (Emmanuel et al. 1992, Gasperini et al. 1990). For example, rates of GAD and personality disorders in clinical populations have ranged from 31 to 46% (Gasperini et al. 1990, Mauri et al. 1992, Mavissakalian et al. 1993, Sanderson et al. 1991, Starcevic et al. 1995). Cluster C personality disorders, specifically avoidant personality disorder, dependent personality disorder, and obsessive–compulsive personality disorder are common (Mauri et al. 1992, Mavissakalian et al. 1993). Interestingly, Cluster A personality traits, in particular suspiciousness and mistrust, may be prominent in GAD as well (Mavissakalian et al. 1993).

Comorbid GAD is associated with increased severity of comorbid disorders (Kessler 2000). Additionally, the presence of comorbid disorders in GAD patients is related to increased rates of negative outcomes such as disability, impairment, and cost of care (Angst 1993, Massion et al. 1993, Yonkers et al. 1996, Murphy et al. 1986, Noyes et al. 1980, Souetre et al. 1994). Rates of relapse for GAD patients with comorbid depression appear higher than in noncomorbid GAD patients (Yonkers et al. 1996). Further, comorbidity is also associated with greater treatment seeking (Bland et al. 1997). Data indicate that patients with comorbid GAD and depression may have poorer response to treatment than patients with either disorder only (Brown et al. 1996, Joffe et al. 1993).

In summary, the available data suggest that GAD is often accompanied by other concurrent psychiatric disorders, specifically anxiety and mood disorders. The presence of these comorbid conditions may reflect a more severe psychopathology, and may have important implications for the course, treatment response, and the prognosis of the primary disorder (Wittchen et al. 1994). Due to the high rates of comorbidity, some have suggested comorbid disorders should be better studied to further our understanding of GAD (Maser 1998).

## Course

Retrospective and prospective reports indicate that the typical course of GAD is chronic, nonremitting, and that it often persists for a decade or longer (Blazer et al. 1991, Angst and Vollrath 1991, Mancuso et al. 1993, Noyes et al. 1996). For example, Noyes and colleagues (1996) evaluated 112 patients with anxiety neuroses (a DSM-II term that is roughly equivalent to GAD) 4 to 9 years after the onset of the disorder and found that only 12% of the patients were symptom-free, while 48% had moderate to severe levels of anxiety symptoms. In addition, 25% of patients reported moderate to marked impairment in functioning. Rickels and colleagues (1986) reported that two-thirds of patients treated initially with diazepam relapsed within 1 year of discontinuation of treatment. Other studies utilizing criteria prior to the DSM-III-R for GAD found comparable levels of chronicity, with almost half the patients reporting moderate symptoms at follow-up (Yonkers et al. 2000). Mancuso and associates (1993) evaluated 44 patients with DSM-III-R-defined GAD approximately 16 months following discontinuation of successful treatment with the benzodiazepine adinazolam. The authors found that half of the subjects still had anxiety symptoms that met diagnostic criteria for GAD at follow-up. These patients also reported significant feelings of dissatisfaction, as well as impairment in job performance.

HARP, a prospective, naturalistic study of 711 adults with DSM-III-R anxiety disorders, recruited initially from psychiatric clinics and hospitals in the Boston Metropolitan area, indicated that only 15% of those with GAD at baseline experienced a full remission for 2 months or longer at any time during the first year after baseline, and only 25% had a full remission in the 2 years after baseline (Yonkers et al. 1996). Further, among patients who experienced full or partial remission, 27 and 39% respectively, experienced a full relapse during a 3-year follow-up period (Yonkers et al. 2000). Chronicity of GAD was also associated with cluster B and C personality disorders or a concurrent Axis I comorbidity (Mancuso et al. 1993, Yonkers et al. 2000). Wittchen and coworkers (1994) found that approximately 80% of subjects with GAD reported substantial interference with their life, a high degree of professional help-seeking, and a high prevalence of taking medications because of their GAD symptoms. The disability associated with GAD was found to be similar to that found in individuals with panic disorder or major depression (Kessler et al. 1999).

In summary, GAD appears to be a chronic and relapsing illness with significant morbidity. Additionally, patients experience significant distress and impairment in functioning. Thus, it appears that chronic/long-term treatment of this disorder may be required in many cases.

## Treatment Approaches

As mentioned before, GAD is a complex and variable condition. It is a chronic, relapsing illness, which means that most treatments do not cure the patient. Furthermore, it also suggests that when treatments are discontinued, symptoms may return. It follows that a thorough understanding of the long-term benefits and risks associated with the different treatments available is important. Thus, each case must be considered individually according to the severity and chronicity of the disorder, the severity of somatic symptoms, the presence of stressors, and the presence of specific personality traits. The clinician may also need to work with the patient to determine how much improvement is sufficient. For example, a reduction in disability may occur without a marked change in symptoms. Symptoms may persist but occur less frequently, or their intensity may be reduced. All these variations have important treatment implications, including decisions regarding the need for long-term treatment. Patients with milder forms of GAD may respond well to simple psychological interventions, and require no medication treatment. In more severe forms of GAD, it may become necessary to see the patient regularly and to provide both more specific psychological and pharmacological interventions. Figure 70–2 can be used as a guide to the treatment of GAD.

During the early (acute) phase of treatment, an attempt should be made to control the patient's symptomatology. It may take 3 to 6 months for an optimal response to be achieved. However, there may be a considerable variation in the length of the initial treatment phase. For example, clinical response to benzodiazepines occurs early in treatment. Response to other anxiolytic medications or to cognitive–behavioral treatment generally requires longer periods of time. During the maintenance phase, treatment gains are consolidated. Unfortunately, studies suggesting how long treatment should be continued are limited. Routinely, pharmacological treatment is continued for a total of 6 to 12 months before attempting to discontinue medications. Recent data indicate that "maintenance" psychotherapeutic treatments such as cognitive–behavioral therapy may be helpful in maintaining treatment gains in patients with anxiety disorders following the discontinuation of pharmacotherapy (Speigel et al. 1994). It is clear that many patients may experience chronic and continuous symptoms that require years of long-term treatment.

## Doctor–Patient Relationship

The vast majority of patients with GAD who present for treatment have been ill for many years and frequently have received a variety of treatments. Some patients have been sent to psychiatrists for treatment as a "last resort" in order to learn how to cope with their various ill-defined somatic and emotional complaints. Patients may feel shame and guilt over their inability to control symptoms. They are often demoralized and angry, and feel that their symptoms are not taken seriously. Thus, it is important to help the patient understand their illness and to conceptualize it as a health problem rather than a "personal weakness." Once the burden of perceived responsibility is lifted from the patient, and they believe that effective treatment of their illness is possible, a working alliance with the treating physician can begin. The treatment plan should be outlined clearly, and the patient cautioned that recovery may have a gradual, variable course. Finally, during the critical early stages of treatment, the clinician should make a special effort to be available in person or by phone to answer questions and provide support.

## Pharmacotherapy

Below, we will discuss the use of various anxiolytic agents in the treatment of GAD. Table 70–3 provides a summarization of this information.

### Benzodiazepines

Benzodiazepines are commonly used for the treatment of GAD and are still considered by some clinicians to be the first-line treatment for GAD (Uhlenhuth et al. 1999). Several controlled studies have demonstrated the efficacy of different benzodiazepines such as diazepam, chlordiazepoxide, and alprazolam in the treatment of GAD. The available placebo-controlled studies found that diazepam, alprazolam, and lorazepam were effective in the treatment of GAD (Cohn and Wilcox 1984, Cutler et al. 1993, Ellie and Lamontagne 1984, Laakmann et al. 1998, Rickels et al. 1983, Rickels et al. 1997, Ruiz 1983).

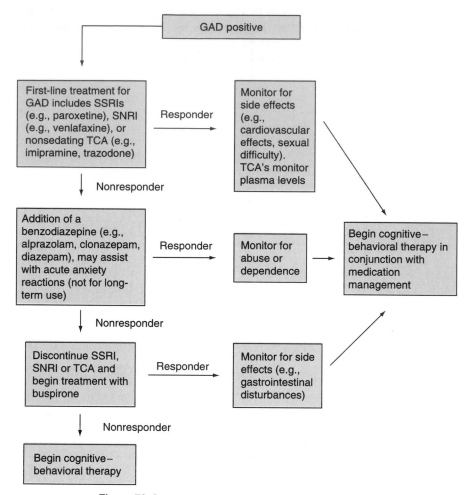

**Figure 70–2** *Generalized anxiety disorder treatment flowchart.*

The benzodiazepines have a broad spectrum of effects including sedation, muscle relaxation, anxiety reduction, and decreased physiologic arousal (e.g. palpitations, tremulousness, etc.). Interestingly, available studies indicate that benzodiazepines have the most pronounced effect on hypervigilance and somatic symptoms of GAD, but exhibited fewer effects on psychic symptoms such as dysphoria, interpersonal sensitivity, and obsessionality (Hoehn-Saric et al. 1988).

The main difference between individual benzodiazepines is potency and elimination half-life. These differences may have important treatment implications. For example, benzodiazepines with relatively short elimination half-lives such as alprazolam (range of 10–14 hours) may require dosing at least three to four times a day in order to avoid interdose symptom rebound. Conversely, the use of longer-acting compounds such as clonazepam (range of 20–50 hours) may minimize the risk of interdose symptom recurrence. In comparative studies of different benzodiazepines, alprazolam appeared to perform somewhat better than lorazepam. Cohn and Wilcox (1984) evaluated the efficacy of alprazolam and lorazepam in a double-blind, placebo-controlled trial in the treatment of GAD patients. Both alprazolam (at mean dose of 3.3 mg/day) and lorazepam (at mean dose of 5.1 mg/day) were significantly more effective than placebo in the treatment of psychic and somatic anxiety

symptoms; however, there was a trend for alprazolam to be more effective than lorazepam. Data from the HARP study indicate that the most frequently reported medication used by GAD patients was alprazolam (31%) followed by clonazepam (23%) (Yonkers et al. 1996).

Benzodiazepines exert their therapeutic effects quickly, often after a single dose. However, concern has emerged over the use of benzodiazepines, particularly long-term benzodiazepine use. Side effects of benzodiazepines, such as sedation, psychomotor impairment, and memory disruption were noted by treating clinicians, and confirmed in research studies (Lader 1999). Further, although it was suggested that the use pattern of benzodiazepines by patients with anxiety disorders may not represent abuse, addiction, or drug dependence as typically understood (Romach et al. 1995), the chronic use of benzodiazepines in the treatment of GAD has been increasingly discouraged in recent years (Ballenger et al. 2001).

When initiating treatment with benzodiazepines, it is helpful for patients to take an initial dose at home in the evening to see how it affects them. Gradual titration to an effective dose allows for limiting unwanted adverse effects. A final daily dosage of alprazolam between 2 and 4 mg/day, 1 and 2 mg/day for clonazepam, or 15 and 20 mg/day of diazepam, is usually sufficient for the majority of patients. Upon treatment discontinuation, it is important

| Table 70–3 | Anxiolytic Agents | | |
|---|---|---|---|
| Drug | Daily Dosage Range (mg) | Advantages | Disadvantages |
| Selective serotonin reuptake inhibitors | | Efficacy with GAD | Gastrointestinal side effects |
| Paroxetine | 20–40 | Efficacy with comorbid depression | Delayed onset |
| Fluoxetine | 20–60 | | Sexual side effects |
| Sertraline | 50–200 | | |
| Citalopram | 20–40 | Favorable side effects profile compared with TCAs | |
| Fluvoxamine | 100–300 | Easy dosing schedule | |
| Serotonergic and noradrenergic reuptake inhibitors | | | |
| Venlafaxine extended release (XR) | 75–225 | Efficacy with GAD Efficacy with comorbid depression | Gastrointestinal side effects Sexual side effects Potential for increased blood pressure |
| Benzodiazepines | | Rapid onset of action | Sedation |
| Alprazolam | 2–6 | Favorable side effects profile | Multiple doses for shorter acting agents |
| Clonazepam | 1–3 | | Physical dependence |
| Lorazepam | 4–10 | | Limited antidepressant effects |
| Diazepam | 15–20 | | Sexual side effects |
| Tricyclic antidepressants | | | |
| Imipramine | 75–300 | Once-daily dosage Efficacy with comorbid depression | Delayed onset Need for titration Activation Anticholinergic effects Orthostatic hypotension Weight gain Toxicity in overdose Sexual side effects |
| Atypical antidepressants | | | |
| Trazodone | 150–600 | Once-daily dosage Efficacy with comorbid depression Low anticholinergic effects | Delayed onset Orthostatic hypotension Weight gain Sexual side effects Priapism (rare) Sedation |
| Azapirones | | | |
| Buspirone | 30–60 | No withdrawal symptoms No physical dependence Favorable side effects profile | Multiple doses |

to consider appropriate taper in order to avoid withdrawal symptoms. Possible factors that may contribute to the severity of withdrawal and the ultimate outcome of benzodiazepine taper include the dosage, duration of treatment, the benzodiazepine elimination half-life and potency, and the rate of benzodiazepine taper (gradual versus abrupt). Additionally, patient factors such as premorbid personality features have been implicated. It appears that a taper rate of 25% per week is probably too rapid for many patients (Brawman-Mintzer and Lydiard 1994). We, therefore, recommend a slow benzodiazepine taper of at least 4 to 8 weeks, with the final 50% of the taper conducted even more gradually, with the patient decreasing by the lowest possible daily dose of the benzodiazepines during this period. We also recommend continuing to use divided doses of short to intermediate half-life benzodiazepines (alprazolam, lorazepam) during taper to minimize fluctuations in benzodiazepine levels over a 24-hour period, or using longer half-life benzodiazepines (such as clonazepam) which have the advantage of maintaining a once- or twice-daily dosing schedule.

## Tricyclic Antidepressants

Clinical trials conducted in the early 1990s have confirmed that tricyclic antidepressants (TCAs) may also be effective in the treatment of GAD (Brawman-Mintzer and Lydiard 1994). Rickels and colleagues (1993) completed a placebo-controlled study which compared imipramine, trazodone, and diazepam in GAD patients without comorbid depression or panic disorder. Data analysis revealed that the efficacy of imipramine and trazodone was comparable to diazepam. It should be noted that diazepam demonstrated greater efficacy than imipramine during the first 2 weeks of treatment with the greatest degree of response in the somatic and hyperarousal symptoms; however, imipramine and trazodone exhibited higher efficacy after 6 to 8 weeks of treatment with psychic symptoms of tension, apprehension, and worry being more responsive to the antidepressants. Wingerson et al. (1992) found that clomipramine was also effective in the treatment of patients with GAD. These studies, as well as other trials, suggest that TCAs may be especially effective in the treatment of psychic symptoms of GAD (Brawman-Mintzer and Lydiard 1994).

The relationship between plasma levels of TCAs and their anxiolytic efficacy in patients with GAD has not been studied. Until this relationship is clarified, decisions regarding the total daily doses and the monitoring of plasma levels should be based on the patient's treatment response and side effects profile. Further, due to potential jitteriness, restlessness, and agitation during the initial stages of treatment, we suggest that the initial dose of the TCAs in patients with GAD may need to be low (for example 10 mg/day of imipramine), and increased gradually.

Adverse effects commonly associated with the use of TCAs include anticholinergic effects (dry mouth, blurred vision, constipation), cardiovascular effects (orthostatic hypotension, slightly increased heart rate), sexual side effects, and weight gain (Lydiard et al. 1996). As mentioned, patients may also experience significant jitteriness, restlessness, and agitation during the initial stages of treatment. These side effects often limit the acceptability of TCAs by many patients. Potential toxicity in overdose has been of concern to clinicians as well. Due, in part, to the side effect profile, need for dose titration, and importantly the emergence of new and effective agents (as described below), the use of TCAs in the treatment of GAD has been reserved for those resistant to these newer agents.

## Serotonin Reuptake Inhibitors

Selective serotonin reuptake inhibitors (SSRIs) are rapidly becoming a key tool in the treatment of GAD. Recent estimates suggest that 19% of experts recommend the use of SSRIs as first-line treatment for GAD, reflecting a 15% increase in 5 years (Uhlenhuth et al. 1999). In the first controlled study examining the efficacy of SSRIs in the treatment of GAD, Rocca and colleagues (1997) conducted an 8-week, double-blind, treatment trial of paroxetine (at 20 mg/day), imipramine (mean dose of 75 mg/day), and 2'-chlordesmethyldiazepam (mean dose of 4.2 mg/day) in the treatment of 81 DSM-IV-diagnosed GAD patients. Both antidepressants were more effective in reducing psychic symptoms of anxiety (such as interpersonal sensitivity, anger and hostility) than the benzodiazepine treatment.

Recently, Bellew and colleagues (2000) presented the results of a large (566 subjects), double-blind, placebo-controlled fixed-dosage multicenter trial using paroxetine (at 20 mg and 40 mg per day) in the treatment of DSM-IV GAD patients. Those in the paroxetine group reported statistically significant reduction in total anxiety scores over those in the placebo group. Improvement in GAD symptoms was dose-dependent. In a placebo-controlled flexible-dose trial ($N = 324$), Pollack and colleagues (1997) found paroxetine in doses of 20 to 50 mg once daily to be effective in the treatment of patients with GAD, and that improvement was significant and typically occurred within the first 8 weeks of treatment. Based on these data, paroxetine was recently approved by the Food and Drug Administration (FDA) for the use in the treatment of GAD.

SSRIs are generally well tolerated. The most problematic side effect associated with SSRI use is interference with sexual function (e.g., delayed orgasm or abnormal ejaculation) in women and men (Michelson et al. 2000, Rosen et al. 1999). A variety of treatment strategies have been suggested for the management of SSRI-induced sexual dysfunction. Such strategies include waiting for tolerance to develop, dosage reduction, drug holidays, and various augmentation strategies with 5-hydroxytryptamine-2 (5-HT$_2$), 5-HT$_3$, and alpha-2-adrenergic receptor antagonists, 5-HT$_{1A}$ and dopamine receptor agonists, and phosphodiesterase (PDE5) enzyme inhibitors (Rosen et al. 1999).

## Serotonergic and Noradrenergic Reuptake Inhibitors

The antidepressant venlafaxine extended release (XR) is an inhibitor of both 5-HT and NE reuptake (SNRI). Several large, placebo-controlled trials have evaluated it in the treatment of patients with DSM-IV-diagnosed GAD. As a result, venlafaxine XR was the first antidepressant approved by the FDA for the treatment of GAD. Results from two short-term studies indicate that venlafaxine XR (75, 150, and 225 mg/day) was significantly more effective than placebo and superior to buspirone on certain anxiety measures (Sheehan 1999). A 6-month randomized, fixed-dose (37.5, 75, and 150 mg/day) study further supported the long-term efficacy of venlafaxine XR in the treatment of GAD at doses as low as 75 mg/day (Sheehan 1999). Three placebo-controlled studies have demonstrated the efficacy of venlafaxine XR in GAD, with both psychic and somatic symptoms of anxiety being controlled (Allgulander et al. 2001, Davidson et al. 1999, Gelenberg et al. 2000). A review of short- and long-term studies examining venlafaxine XR using measures of efficacy illustrated the usefulness of this SNRI in the treatment of GAD and in the prevention of relapse (Sheehan 2001). The adverse events for GAD patients treated with venlafaxine XR resembled those in depression trials. The most common adverse events included nausea, somnolence, dry mouth, dizziness, sweating, constipation, and anorexia.

## Other Antidepressants

As mentioned, Rickels and colleagues (1993) compared the efficacy of trazodone, imipramine, and diazepam in the treatment of patients with GAD. The authors found that both trazodone and imipramine had comparable efficacy to diazepam. In addition, trazodone and imipramine exhibited higher efficacy in the treatment of psychic symptoms such as tension, apprehension, and worry.

Nefazodone is a phenylpiperazine compound chemically related to trazodone. The efficacy of nefazodone in the treatment of GAD has been evaluated in one open-label trial (Hedges et al. 1996). Of the 15 study completers ($N = 21$), 12 were rated as overall much or very much improved following treatment with nefazodone. More research, however, is required to further define the potential of nefazodone in treating patients with GAD.

Several other psychotherapeutic agents have been tested in the treatment of individuals with GAD. For example, the alpha-2-adrenoreceptor antagonist mitrazapine, which is also a 5-HT$_2$, 5-HT$_3$, and H(1) receptors antagonist, has been evaluated as a potential anxiolytic in the treatment of patients with major depressive disorder and comorbid GAD in an 8-week, open-label study (Goodnick et al. 1999). Results suggest that this antidepressant may be useful in the treatment of anxiety symptoms.

## Azapirones

The azapirone group of drugs was introduced in response to concerns over chronic benzodiazepine use in subjects with anxiety symptoms. Buspirone hydrochloride, the only currently marketed azapirone, was the first nonbenzodiazepine anxiolytic agent approved for the treatment of persistent anxiety by FDA. Results have been mixed about the efficacy of buspirone over placebo and benzodiazepines (Spiegel et al. 1994, Pollack et al. 1997, Davidson et al. 1999, Delle Chiaie et al. 1995, Enklemann 1991, Rickels et al. 1988b, Rickels et al. 1982, Bohm et al. 1990, Goldberg and Finnerty 1979, Lader and Scotto 1998, Pecknold et al. 1989, Wheatley 1982). For example, in four placebo-controlled studies that compared buspirone to a standard benzodiazepine, two showed no benefit for diazepam and buspirone over placebo, and two showed no benefit for buspirone over placebo (Olajide and Lader 1987, Pecknold et al. 1985, Ross and Matas 1987). Benzodiazepines may also be slightly more effective than buspirone in the treatment of somatic symptoms of anxiety but no significant differences appear to exist between buspirone and benzodiazepines in measures of psychic anxiety (Rickels et al. 1997). Buspirone, however, may be more effective in the treatment of anger/hostility symptoms than benzodiazepines (Rickels et al. 1997).

Side effects most frequently associated with buspirone use included gastrointestinal system-related side effects, such as appetite disturbances and abdominal complaints, and dizziness. Prior use of benzodiazepines may adversely affect the therapeutic response to buspirone (Schweizer et al. 1986). DeMartinis and colleagues (2000) found that buspirone treatment was less effective for patients who had been taking benzodiazepines within 30 days of initiating buspirone treatment. Delle Chiaie and colleagues (1995) reported that a gradual 2-week taper of lorazepam with a simultaneous addition of buspirone for 6 weeks prevents the development of clinically significant rebound anxiety or benzodiazepine withdrawal. This approach was shown to provide clinically significant relief of anxiety symptoms in GAD patients previously treated with benzodiazepines for 8 to 14 weeks.

Perhaps the most significant problem with the use of buspirone has been that experts have advocated too low a dose to produce symptom reduction. In order to achieve optimal response, buspirone dosing in the range of at least 30 to 60 mg/day is currently recommended.

Although other azapirone drugs have been assessed in the treatment of GAD, their efficacy is yet unclear. Those compounds that have been most studied are gepirone and ipsapirone, both demonstrating potential efficacy in the treatment of GAD, albeit inconsistently and only with small effect size (Rickels et al. 1997, Cutler et al. 1994). Neither of these drugs is available in the US market.

## Other Agents

Hydroxyzine is a histamine-1 receptor blocker and a muscarinic receptor blocker. Recent controlled trials with the antihistamine have suggested that this compound may be effective in the acute treatment of GAD symptoms (Lader and Scotto 1998, Ferreri and Hantouche 1998). Finally, the potential use of the anticonvulsant gabapentin in the treatment of anxiety symptoms has also been suggested (Pollack et al. 2000).

## Nonpharmacological Treatments

Numerous studies have shown that psychological interventions are beneficial in the comprehensive management of anxiety disorders (Brown et al. 1993). However, data suggesting that specific psychotherapeutic techniques yield better results in the treatment of patients with GAD are inconclusive and more evidence is needed on the comparative efficacy and long-term effects of different psychological treatments.

In this section, we will outline the important nonpharmacological interventions in the treatment of GAD.

### Cognitive–Behavioral Therapy

In recent years specific cognitive–behavioral therapy (CBT) interventions for the treatment of patients with anxiety disorders have been developed. Components of CBT include teaching patients to identify and label irrational thoughts and to replace them with positive self-statements or modify them by challenging their veracity. The cognitive modification approaches are combined with behavioral treatments such as exposure or relaxation training. There is currently evidence suggesting that CBT may be more effective in the treatment of GAD than other psychotherapeutic interventions, such as behavioral therapy alone or nonspecific supportive therapy (Chambless and Gillis 1993). For example, Barlow and colleagues (1984) showed significant improvement in clinical ratings and measures of anxiety in patients with GAD treated with relaxation and CBT. A nontreatment (waiting list) control group remained unchanged. Six additional studies confirmed the efficacy of CBT compared with waiting list or pill placebo (Borkovec and Costello 1993). Further, Borkovec and colleagues (1993) observed that patients tend to maintain improvement following CBT over 6 to 12 months of follow-up.

CBT targeting intolerance of uncertainty, erroneous beliefs about worry, poor problem orientation, and cognitive avoidance demonstrated effectiveness at posttreatment (no change in the delayed treatment control group) 6- and 12-month follow-up, with 77% of the treatment group no longer having symptoms meeting criteria for a GAD diagnosis (Ladouceur et al. 2000). Cognitive therapy was also compared to analytic psychotherapy, and was found to be significantly more effective (Borkovec and Costello 1993). Overall, two-thirds in the cognitive therapy group achieved clinically significant improvements and cognitive therapy was associated with significant reductions in medication usage.

A meta-analytic review of controlled trials examining CBT and pharmacotherapy for GAD, which included 35 studies, demonstrated the robustness of CBT in the treatment of GAD (Gould et al. 1997). Overall, both modalities offered clear efficacy to patients, with the effect size for CBT not being statistically different from psychopharmacological approaches. CBT demonstrated greater effects in reducing depression and was associated with clear maintenance of treatment gains, whereas long-term efficacy of pharmacologic treatment was attenuated following medication discontinuation.

Barlow and colleagues (1986) developed a CBT approach to GAD which concentrates on the behavioral element of direct exposure to the contents of patients' worry and apprehension (i.e., a deconditioning strategy) in addition to relaxation techniques (progressive muscle relaxation) and cognitive restructuring. The authors found that this technique is effective in reducing anxiety symptoms in patients with GAD.

## Supportive Psychotherapy

Many patients with milder forms of GAD will benefit from simple psychological interventions such as supportive psychotherapy. They may experience lessening of anxiety when given the opportunity to discuss their difficulties with a supportive clinician and to become better informed about their illness. Thus, basic supportive techniques such as reassurance, clarification of patient concerns, direct suggestions, and advice are often effective in reducing anxiety symptoms.

## Relaxation and Biofeedback

Relaxation techniques such as progressive muscle relaxation and biofeedback have also been utilized in the treatment of patients with anxiety symptoms. Few controlled studies have examined their effectiveness. In a recent controlled study, Borkovec and Costello (1993) compared a comprehensive relaxation treatment and cognitive–behavioral therapy in the treatment of patients with DSM-III-R-defined GAD. The authors found that both treatments were equally effective and superior to a nonspecific supportive treatment intervention. Biofeedback was also found to be effective in the treatment of patients with GAD (Rice et al. 1993). It should be noted that relaxation may be associated with a paradoxical increase in anxiety and tension in patients with GAD. However, with repeated training, specifically in the context of cognitive–behavioral therapy (see the section on cognitive–behavioral therapy), this phenomenon may be used to achieve habituation and anxiety extinction.

## Psychodynamic Psychotherapy

The psychoanalytic literature offers a vast amount of clinical case report data supporting the efficacy of psychodynamic psychotherapies in the treatment of patients with anxiety disorders such as GAD. Unfortunately, controlled studies evaluating the efficacy of psychodynamic psychotherapies in the treatment of patients with GAD are not available. This section will highlight some of the important principles necessary for the understanding of the different psychodynamic treatment models.

First, it is important to note that the psychoanalytic theories view anxiety as an indicator of certain unconscious conflicts, rather than as a primary target symptom to be alleviated. It is, therefore, the clinician's task to use various techniques to help the patient uncover these unconscious conflicts. It is believed that the newly gained understanding of the underlying reasons for symptoms will have a therapeutic effect, thereby reducing anxiety. Through interpretation of previously unconscious conflicts and unconscious origins of anxiety, the patient will be able to utilize new insights and find more adaptive outlets or solutions to problems (Joseph 1994). Harry Stack Sullivan developed an alternative to Freud's classical model of anxiety (Joseph 1994). In his theory, anxiety reflects the failure to develop secure interpersonal interactions, such as an emphatic and secure mother–infant relationship. He believed that the

child learns to identify anxiety states in himself and significant others and develops protective defensive strategies which enable him to avoid experiencing anxiety. However, the defenses employed (termed security operations) are generally restrictive and may result in limiting the subject's interpersonal interactions. Therefore, the task of the therapist, according to Sullivan's model, is to trace the patterns of interpersonal interactions throughout the patient's developmental stages (rather than to uncover the unconscious drives), thereby promoting a more accurate perception of self and others and subsequently better social adaptation.

Another therapeutic approach to the treatment of anxiety symptoms was offered by object relation and self psychology theorists (Joseph 1994). They view anxiety as a result of the loss of or inadequate emotional relationships with significant others. Therefore, the primary focus of therapy shifts to emphasize the importance of the relationship to the therapist, who functions as an empathic object providing emotionally corrective experiences (Joseph 1994). For example, the patient may learn that an important person may be imperfect but still be trusted and nurturing.

Finally, most psychodynamically oriented therapists agree that the outcome of psychodynamic psychotherapy is determined by factors reflecting patient's maturity and strength. Specifically factors such as patient's capacity for introspection, intelligence, ability to relate to the therapist, and ability to bear painful feelings should be carefully evaluated.

## Long-term Management of Generalized Anxiety Disorder

As mentioned, GAD is a chronic, continuous condition in the majority of patients. Frequently beginning in adolescence or early adulthood, the course of GAD can persist for decades, with relatively low remission rates. The HARP data indicate that among the 164 GAD patients followed, only 15% had a full remission for 2 months or longer at any time during the first follow-up year, 25% had a full remission during the 2-year follow-up, and only 35% had a full remission after 5 years (Yonkers et al. 1996). In a 5-year follow-up study of 64 GAD patients, only 18% of GAD subjects achieved a full remission compared with 45% of panic disorder subjects (Woodman et al. 1999).

Despite these findings, less research has been conducted to assess the efficacy of chronic long-term anxiolytic therapy. To our knowledge, only three double-blind, controlled studies evaluating the long-term pharmacological treatment of GAD have been conducted (Brawman-Mintzer and Lydiard 1994). The first, a 1-year follow-up of patients who participated in a 6-month diazepam maintenance study, found that two-thirds of all patients relapsed within a 1-year period after diazepam discontinuation. In the second study, Rickels and others (Brawman-Mintzer et al. 1994) treated GAD patients for 6 months with buspirone or clorazepate, and reevaluated them after discontinuation at 6 and 40 months. The authors found that the improvement achieved in both treatment groups was sustained during the 6-month maintenance phase, with no need for an increase in medication intake, and no evidence of tolerance or abuse. At follow-up, approximately 60% of patients treated initially with clorazepate compared with 30% of patients treated initially with buspirone were experiencing at least moderate anxiety symptoms. Finally, in a recent study, Stocchi and colleagues (2001) found that many patients with GAD are not able to remain symptom-free for long periods without treatment. Therefore, a long-term therapy may be needed in many patients. Generally, the current recommendation for GAD treatment suggests a treatment period of approximately 1 year after response has been established prior to considering treatment discontinuation (Pollack 2001).

Stress management and problem-solving techniques along with specific psychotherapeutic approaches such as cognitive–behavioral therapy should be attempted in addition to medication treatment.

## Comorbidity and the Treatment of GAD

As mentioned previously, the available data suggest that GAD is often accompanied by other concurrent psychiatric disorders, specifically anxiety and mood disorders. The presence of these comorbid conditions may reflect more severe loading for psychopathology, and may have important implications on the course and treatment response of the primary disorder. In the National Comorbidity Survey, more patients with comorbidity experienced interference with daily activities than did patients with pure GAD (Wittchen et al. 1994). The presence of a comorbid anxiety disorder and major depressive disorder is frequently associated with a poorer overall outcome than for patients with a single psychiatric disorder (Kessler et al. 1999). Currently, there are treatment options that can target both GAD and major depressive disorder simultaneously. The use of SSRIs and the SNRI venlafaxine is recommended as the first-line treatment for comorbid GAD and depression (Pollack 2001, Howell et al. 2001).

Social anxiety disorder frequently complicates the course GAD. With the recent data indicating that the SSRIs such as sertraline and paroxetine are effective in the treatment of social anxiety disorder (MacQueen et al. 2001, Bourin et al. 2001), these agents may be useful in the treatment of comorbid social anxiety disorder and GAD. The benzodiazepines that have been established as effective in the treatment of patients with GAD also appear to be effective in the treatment of patients with social anxiety disorder (Brawman-Mintzer and Lydiard 1994). Thus, these agents (considering the caveats associated with their use described earlier) may have a therapeutic role in patients with GAD and coexisting social phobia. Finally patients with GAD and concurrent panic disorder or panic attacks may be effectively treated with SSRIs, TCAs, and benzodiazepines. However, buspirone is probably ineffective in the treatment of panic disorder (Brawman-Mintzer and Lydiard 1994).

Concurrent alcohol and substance abuse tend to confuse the clinical picture of GAD and can interfere with the therapeutic efforts. Additionally, symptoms associated with alcohol withdrawal or other sedative–hypnotics may mimic the underlying anxiety disorder. If a substance abuse problem exists, the clinician and the patient should take the necessary steps to discontinue the use of the abused substance. This may well include specific substance abuse treatment. Specifically, the need for detoxification should be assessed and discussed with the patient. Following cessation of substance abuse the patient's symptomatology should be reevaluated. The use of benzodiazepines in these patients may be contraindicated, and alternative treatments with SSRIs, SNRIs, TCAs, buspirone, or gabapentin may be needed.

## Treatment of GAD in the Elderly

To date, anxiety disorders in the elderly have received only limited attention. However, evaluation of the available epidemiological data suggests that GAD is highly prevalent in the geriatric population (prevalence rates ranging from 0.7 to 7.1%), accounting for the majority of anxiety disorder cases in this group (Flint 1994). Beckman and colleagues (1998) reported similar findings demonstrating that GAD was the most common of the pervasive late-life anxiety disorders. In the elderly, anxiety symptoms are often associated with depression, medical conditions, and cognitive dysfunction. Thus, a careful differential diagnosis to eliminate exogenous causes of anxiety and identification of other coexisting conditions is necessary. For example, treatment of medical illness, depression, or underlying dementia may reduce anxiety symptoms. Dose reductions or elimination of anxiety-inducing medications as well as reducing stressful life circumstances may also reduce anxiety symptoms. However, if these interventions are not effective in reducing anxiety, pharmacotherapy may be necessary. Several factors influencing pharmacologic treatment in the elderly should be considered. These factors include alterations in pharmacokinetics and pharmacodynamics of psychotropic drugs, primarily because of reduced hepatic clearing efficiency, alterations in the response of the central nervous system to drugs, such as changes in receptor sensitivity, and concurrent medical conditions that may alter drug effect, side effect profile, and toxicity (Salzman 1990). In this section we will outline specific guidelines for the use of the available anxiolytic medications in the elderly population.

Benzodiazepines can be effective in the treatment of anxiety symptoms. However, older patients are often sensitive to their effects. Adverse effects may include increased sedation, tendency to fall, psychomotor discoordination, and cognitive impairment (Salzman 1990). Older patients may become disinhibited by benzodiazepines and experience agitation and aggression. The administration of long-acting benzodiazepines such as diazepam and chlorazepate may result in increased accumulation of the drug predisposing the patient to these side effects (Salzman 1990). Conversely, the use of short half-life high potency benzodiazepines such as alprazolam may be associated with more severe withdrawal symptoms following rapid discontinuation (Salzman 1990). Because of these factors, benzodiazepines should be prescribed for the briefest period of time, at the lowest therapeutic dose, giving preference for the short half-life, low-potency benzodiazepines such as oxazepam. We recommend initiating treatment with oxazepam at low doses (10 mg t.i.d.), to be increased gradually, while carefully monitoring for the emergence of side effects.

Buspirone has been extensively used in the treatment of GAD symptoms. The lack of associated sedation, discoordination, and dependence with the use of busopirone makes its use in the elderly less problematic. However, additional research is needed to determine its long-term efficacy in the GAD elderly population. The average therapeutic doses of buspirone for elderly patients range from 5 to 20 mg/day.

The use of TCAs in the anxious elderly patient should be viewed in light of the side-effect profile of TCAs. Side effects commonly associated with the use of TCAs, such as the anticholinergic effects and orthostatic hypotension may be especially troublesome in these patients. We, therefore, recommend the use of TCAs with low anticholinergic and hypotensive effects such as desipramine and nortryptiline, starting at low doses (10 mg/day) that are raised slowly and gradually.

Finally, despite the widespread use of the newer antidepressant agents, specifically the SSRIs and the SNRIs in the treatment of adult GAD patients, very limited data exist regarding their use in the anxious elderly population. However preliminary evidence suggests that they can decrease symptoms, improve quality of life, and potentially promote healthier outcomes in geriatric patients who have comorbid anxiety and depression and/or comorbid mental and physical illness (Doraiswamy 2001). A potential drawback of venlafaxine in this population is the need to monitor for drug-induced blood pressure elevation in those taking the medication.

Most controlled studies examining CBT in older adults have focused on the treatment of GAD. This literature suggests that CBT is effective in the treatment of GAD in this population. For example, group-administrated CBT was found to be effective in reducing GAD and coexistent symptoms in older adults (Stanley et al. 1996). Initial results of another study examining CBT in older adults demonstrated reduction in anxiety and worry and increase in life satisfaction compared to a minimal contact group (Stanley et al. 1999). Gorenstein and coworkers (1999) presented preliminary data suggesting that combining CBT with medication was superior to medication management alone.

In conclusion, several agents may play an important role in the treatment of anxiety in the elderly. However, until more studies in the elderly GAD population are available, treatment choices should be guided by clinical judgment and specific factors relevant to this patient population, such as medical comorbidity and age-associated changes in the drug metabolism.

## Treatment of GAD in Adolescents and Children

The treatment of GAD in adolescents and children should be multifaceted, including psychotherapy for the patient, psychoeducation for the parents, and pharmacotherapy when other psychotherapeutic interventions have not produced satisfactory outcome. Kendall and colleagues have demonstrated the use of CBT in successfully treating GAD in children (Kendall 1994, Kendall et al. 1997). The addition of family anxiety management skills taught to parents appears to increase treatment success (Barrett et al. 1996).

Pharmacotherapy in children and adolescents differs from that of the adult population primarily because of the difference in the hepatic biotransformation and elimination of many psychotropic drugs that may require some adjustments in treatment regimen. Hepatic metabolic rate is faster in children and adolescents than in adults, reaching adult values around 15 years of age. Thus a particular milligram per kilogram (mg/kg) dose will yield a lower blood level in a child than in an adult, and higher mg/kg doses than based on those for adults may be necessary (Popper 1993). This applies for all liver-metabolized drugs, such as antidepressants, anxiolytics, anticonvulsants, and neuroleptics. In addition, the higher clearance of these drugs requires more frequent administration of medications (i.e., small divided doses rather than one large dose).

Over the years, a number of medications have been used in the treatment of childhood GAD (previously classified as overanxious anxiety disorder). Unfortunately, only a few studies have been conducted in children with overanxious anxiety disorder. Following positive results in an uncontrolled study of alprazolam, Simeon and associates (1992) conducted a double-blind, placebo-controlled trial in 21 children with overanxious anxiety disorder. They found that alprazolam showed only a trend towards more effectiveness than placebo; however, the relatively low doses (range of 0.5–1.5 mg/day) may have been subtherapeutic. In a double-blind, crossover trial, Graae and associates (1994) found no significant improvement relative to baseline for clonazepam or placebo. Given these limited findings and the reported occurrence of significant behavioral activation, other side effects, and their addictive potential, the use of benzodazepines to treat children with GAD is suspect.

The use of SSRIs in the treatment of GAD in children and adolescents appears promising; however, no controlled trials with large samples have been conducted. Three published reports of fluoxetine treatment for overanxious disorder indicate a reduction in anxiety with minimal side effects (Manassis and Hood 1998, Birmaher et al. 1994, Fairbanks et al. 1997). Fairbanks and colleagues (1997), in the most recent of these reports, conducted a 9-week open-label study of fluoxetine treatment for 16 outpatients (age: 9–18 years) with mixed anxiety disorders. The mean dosage of fluoxetine for children was 24 mg/day and for adolescents was 40 mg/day. One of the seven children with GAD in this study showed significant clinical improvement. Side effects were mild and transient, including drowsiness, sleep problems, decreased appetite, nausea, abdominal pain, and excitement.

Buspirone may also be effective in the treatment of GAD in children and adolescents. Kutcher and coworkers (1992) conducted a pilot study in children and adolescents with overanxious anxiety disorder. They reported that buspirone in doses ranging from 15 to 30 mg/day was effective in reducing anxiety following 6 weeks of continuous treatment. No controlled studies have been completed for the treatment of GAD in children to date. The authors recommended initiating treatment with buspirone at 5 mg/day (2.5 mg/day in children), and raising the dose gradually to an average of 20 to 30 mg/day (in three divided doses), not to exceed 60 mg/day. TCAs have not been studied in overanxious anxiety disorder. It should be noted that cardiovascular side effects may occur more frequently in children and adolescents than in adults, and preexisting conduction abnormalities may be associated with significant TCA effect on cardiac conduction. However, the clinical significance of TCA-induced changes in cardiac conduction is not clear. Recently, Biederman (1991) reported sudden death events in 3 children treated with desipramine. Although the exact role of the TCAs in these events is not clear, the clinician should carefully weigh the risks and benefits of treatment with TCAs in this patient population. Given this lack of efficacy data for GAD and the concern of significant cardiovascular side effects in children, TCAs should not be a first-line treatment in children and adolescents with GAD (Riddle et al. 1991).

## Treatment Resistance

Significant advances have been made in the past several years in the pharmacological treatment of GAD. There are now a number of effective pharmacological and nonpharmacological treatments available. However, the clinician is frequently faced with a patient whose anxiety symptomatology is not responding satisfactorily to the standard treatment. Different factors, such as inadequate length of treatment, low dose, and noncompliance may contribute to treatment failure in the management of patients with GAD. Pharmacologic treatment is often complicated by the occurrence of side effects, which may impair quality of life, deter clinicians from prescribing adequate doses, and contribute to noncompliance. For example, some antidepressants, including SSRIs, TCAs, and venlafaxine, are associated with activation, overstimulation, or "jitters" primarily during the initial stage of treatment (Gorman et al. 1987). When evaluating noncompliance, clinicians should also assess for akathisia (Lane 1998) and worsening of anxiety and hypomania or mania. Further, the presence of comorbid general medical and psychiatric conditions in GAD patients may be associated with nonresponse or lower response rates and should be carefully assessed during patient evaluation. Finally, the use of concurrent medications that can precipitate anxiety symptoms may affect the response to treatment.

When faced with treatment, clinician should evaluate whether an adequate treatment trial was complete. We believe that an attempt should be made to maintain the patient on medication for at least 6 weeks. Although there are no data suggesting that certain doses may be particularly effective in the treatment of GAD, it is advisable to titrate the medication up to maximally tolerated doses prior to discontinuing the medication for nonresponse. It is important to inquire about the presence of side effects such as sedation, anticholinergic effects, or sexual side effects, which may limit the attainment of a therapeutic dosage and reduce compliance. Additionally, many patients with GAD fear that they may become "drug-dependent" and thus avoid dose increases. Some estimate of the patient's compliance may be helpful in determining whether a treatment was adequate, as indicated by blood plasma levels or pill counts. Drug plasma levels may also be useful to identify patients who are rapid metabolizers. A careful evaluation for the presence of psychiatric comorbid conditions that may contribute to treatment refractoriness should follow. As mentioned, comorbidity which may reflect more severe loading for psychopathology is often associated with increased severity of illness and poorer response to treatment in comparison to patients with an uncomplicated (i.e., single) disorder. Thus, treatment strategies in GAD patients with a concurrent disorder may differ from those in an uncomplicated disorder, often requiring multiple drug therapy. The clinician should also be alert to the presence of underlying general medical conditions such as hyperthyroidism which may present with refractory anxiety, or conditions/medications which may alter the effects of treatment such as hepatic disease or medications (e.g., steroids) that affect hepatic clearance.

The use of psychotherapy, such as the cognitive–behavioral therapy, in conjunction with pharmacotherapy may also enhance response in the treatment-resistant patient. Finally, education and psychological support for patients and their families may help them to better understand and deal with their illness, especially during periods of increased stress, and consequently improve treatment outcome.

## Summary

In conclusion, GAD appears to be a chronic, frequently comorbid condition, often requiring long-term management. Benzodiazepines were, at one time, the first-line treatment choice for GAD. However, newer medication may offer more hope for those with GAD. SSRIs and SNRIs are promising new pharmocotherapies for GAD. Additionally, these treatments may be especially effective for patients presenting with depressive symptomatology. Further, buspirone and TCAs have been shown to be an important treatment alternative to benzodiazepines, and the TCAs may be especially effective in patients presenting with depressive symptomatology. Finally psychotherapy, specifically cognitive–behavioral therapy, is an additional treatment strategy, potentially effective in maintaining treatment gains. Further information is needed on long-term treatment, medication discontinuation and comparative efficacy of pharmacotherapies, psychotherapies, and combination in the treatment of uncomplicated and comorbid GAD.

Clinical Vignette 1

LS is a 36-year-old woman, who presented to a primary care physician complaining that she has difficulty falling and staying asleep. During the evaluation the patient described herself as a nervous and anxious person. She had married for the second time approximately 10 months earlier and started a new job as a director of a child care center shortly thereafter. With further prompting, she described recurrent worries that she may be fired from her new job and "plunge" into financial difficulties. This worry, although completely unfounded, occupied her much of the time, making it difficult for her to concentrate and preventing her from falling asleep at night. She stated that she wakes up often in the middle of the night worrying about her numerous obligations. She felt edgy and irritable, and described frequent arguments with her husband. She has also experienced significant muscle tension especially in her neck and shoulders and sought help from a chiropractor.

During the interview and examination the patient was restless, frequently changing her position. Her gestures were abrupt, her handshake was limp and cold, and she would sigh often. Careful physical examination and laboratory evaluation were within normal limits.

LS's history and physical evaluation supported the diagnosis of generalized anxiety disorder.

---

**Clinical Vignette 2**

RJ is a 27-year-old graduate student who presented to his primary care physician with complaints of recurrent frontal headaches. He asked his physician to order a CT scan or an MRI because he feared that this may be a sign of a serious and a life-threatening illness. However, the headaches appeared to worsen during times of stress, and abated when the patient was on vacation with a friend. During the interview the patient admitted that he is very worried about the quality of his research at the university, even though he had received consistently positive evaluations. He attributed the perceived academic difficulties to his forgetfulness and diminished ability to concentrate during the last 6 months. He also described feeling fatigued, as well as significant indigestion, abdominal pain associated with bouts of changes in bowel movements (alternating diarrhea and constipation).

For the past 6 months he had few social contacts because of his symptoms and his girlfriend demanded that he seek professional help. Following complete physical evaluation, including consultation with a gastroenterologist, a diagnosis of generalized anxiety disorder and irritable bowel syndrome was made.

## Comparison of DSM-IV/ICD-10 Diagnostic Criteria

The ICD-10 Diagnostic Criteria for Research specify that four symptoms from a list of 22 be present. In contrast, DSM-IV-TR requires three out of a list of six (of which five are included among the ICD-10 list of 22).

## References

Abelson JL, Glitz D, Cameron OG, et al. (1991) Blunted growth hormone response to clonidine in patients with generalized anxiety disorder. Arch Gen Psychiatr 48, 157–162.

Adams JB, Pyke RE, Costa J, et al. (1995) A double-blind, placebo-controlled study of a CCK-B receptor antagonist, CI-988, in patients with generalized anxiety disorder. J Clin Psychopharmacol 15(6), 428–434.

Allgulander C, Hackett D, and Salinas E (2001) Venlafaxine extended release (ER) in the treatment of generalized anxiety disorder. Br J Psychiatr 179, 15–22.

American Psychiatric Association (1980) Diagnostic and Statistical Manual of Mental Disorders, 3rd ed. APA, Washington DC.

American Psychiatric Association (1987) Diagnostic and Statistical Manual of Mental Disorders, 3rd ed. Rev. APA, Washington DC.

American Psychiatric Association (1994) Diagnostic and Statistical Manual of Mental Disorders, 4th ed. APA, Washington DC.

Anderson JC, Williams S, and McGee R (1987) DSM-III disorders in preadolescent children: Prevalence in a large sample from the general population. Arch Gen Psychiatr 44, 69–76.

Andrews G, Stewart S, Allen R, et al. (1990) The genetics of six neurotic disorders: A twin study. J Affect Disord 19, 23–29.

Angst J (1993) Comorbidity of anxiety, phobia, compulsion, and depression. Int J Clin Psychopharmacol 8(Suppl 1), 21–25.

Angst J and Vollrath M (1991) The natural history of anxiety disorder and generalized anxiety disorder. Acta Psychiatr Scand 141, 572–575.

Avery DH, Osgodd TB, Ishiki DM, et al. (1985) The DST in psychiatric outpatients with generalized anxiety disorder, panic disorder, or primary affective disorder. Am J Psychiatr 142, 844–848.

Ballenger JC, Davidson JRT, Lecrubier Y, et al. (2001) Consensus statement on generalized anxiety disorder from the international consensus group on depression and anxiety. J Clin Psychiatr 62(Suppl 11), 53–58.

Barlow DH, Blanchard RB, Vermilyea JB, et al. (1986) Generalized anxiety and generalized anxiety disorder: Description and reconceptualization. Am J Psychiatr 143, 40–44.

Barlow DH, Cohen AS, and Waddell MT (1984) Panic and generalized anxiety disorders: Nature and treatment. Behav Ther 15, 431–449.

Barrett PM, Dadds MR, and Rappe RM (1996) Family treatment of childhood anxiety: A controlled trial. J Consult Clin Psychol 64, 333–342.

Beekman ATF, Bremmer MA, Deeg DJH, et al. (1998) Anxiety disorders in later life: A report from the longitudinal aging study, Amsterdam. Int J Geriatr Psychiatr 13, 717–726.

Bellew KM, McCafferty JP, Iyengar M, et al. (2000) Paroxetine treatment of GAD: A double-blind, placebo-controlled trial. American Psychiatric Association 2000 Annual Meeting (May 13–18), Chicago, IL.

Beresford IJ, Sheldrick RL, Ball DI, et al. (1995) GR159897, a potent non-peptide antagonist at tachykinin NK2 receptors. Eur J Psychopharmacol 272(2–3), 241–248.

Bernstein GA and Borchardt CM (1991) Anxiety disorders of childhood and adolescence: A critical review. J Am Acad Child Adolesc Psychiatr 30(4), 519–532.

Bhagwanjee A, Parekh A, Paruk Z, et al. (1998) Prevalence of minor psychiatric disorders in an adult African rural community in South Africa. Psychol Med 28, 1137–1147.

Biederman J (1991) Sudden death in children treated with a tricyclic antidepressant—A commentary. Biol Ther Psychiatr Newslett 14, 1–4.

Birmaher B, Waterman GS, Ryan N, et al. (1994) Fluoxetine for childhood anxiety disorders. J Am Acad Child Adolesc Psychiatr 33, 993–999.

Black DW, Noyes R, Goldstein RB, et al. (1992) A family study of obsessive–compulsive disorder. Arch Gen Psychiatr 49, 362–368.

Bland RC, Newman SC, and Orn H (1997) Help-seeking for psychiatric disorders. Can J Psychiatr 42, 935–942.

Blazer D, Hughes D, and George LK (1987) Stressful life events and the onset of a generalized anxiety syndrome. Am J Psychiatr 144, 1178–1183.

Blazer DG, Hughes D, George LK, et al. (1991) Generalized anxiety disorder. In Psychiatric Disorders in America: The Epidemiologic Catchment Area Study, Robins LN and Regier DA (eds). Free Press, New York, pp. 180–203.

Bohm C, Placchi M, Stallone F, et al. (1990) A double-blind comparison of buspirone, clobazam, and placebo in patients with anxiety treated in a general practice setting. J Clin Psychopharmacol 10(Suppl 3), 38S–42S.

Borkovec TD and Costello E (1993) Efficacy of applied relaxation and cognitive–behavioral therapy in the treatment of generalized anxiety disorder. J Consult Clin Psychol 61(4), 611–619.

Boulenger JP, Jerabek I, Jolicoeur FB, et al. (1996) Elevated plasma levels of neuropeptide Y in patients with panic disorders. Am J Psychiatr 153(1), 114–116.

Bourin M, Chue P, and Guillon Y (2001) Paroxetine: A review. CNS Drug Rev 7(1), 25–47.

Bradwejn J and Koszycki D (1992) The cholecystokinin hypothesis of panic and anxiety disorders: A review. Ann NY Acad Sci 713, 273–282.

Brawman-Mintzer O and Lydiard RB (1994) Psychopharmacology of anxiety disorders. Psychiatr Clin N Am 1, 51–79.

Brawman-Mintzer O, Lydiard RB, Bradwejn J, et al. (1997) Effects of the cholecystokinin agonist pentagastrin in patients with generalized anxiety disorder. Am J Psychiatr 154(5), 700–702.

Brawman-Mintzer O, Lydiard RB, Crawford MM, et al. (1994) Somatic symptoms in generalized anxiety disorder with and without comorbid psychiatric disorders. Am J Psychiatr 151, 930–932.

Brawman-Mintzer O, Lydiard RB, Emmanuel N, et al. (1993) Psychiatric comorbidity in patients with generalized anxiety disorder. Am J Psychiatr 150, 1216–1218.

Breitholtz E, Johansson B, and Öst LG (1999) Cognitions in generalized anxiety disorder and panic disorder patients: A prospective approach. Behav Res Ther 37, 533–544.

Breslau N and Davis GC (1985) DSM-III Generalized anxiety disorder: An empirical investigation of more stringent criteria. Psychiatr Res 14, 231–238.

Britton KT, Southerland S, Van Uden E, et al. (1997) Anxiolytic activity of NPY receptor agonists in the conflict test. Psychopharmacology 132(1), 6–13.

Brown C, Schulberg HC, Madonia MJ, et al. (1996) Treatment outcomes for primary care patients with major depression and lifetime anxiety disorders. Am J Psychiatr 153, 1293–1300.

Brown TA and Barlow DH (1992) Comorbidity among anxiety disorders: Implications for treatment and DSM-IV. J Consult Clin Psychol 60, 835–855.

Brown TA, Barlow DH, and Liebowitz MR (1994) The empirical basis of generalized anxiety disorder. Am J Psychiatr 151(9), 1272–1280.

Brown TA, O'Leary D, and Barlow DH (1993) Generalized anxiety disorder. In Clinical Handbook of Psychological Disorders: A step-by-step Treatment Manual, Barlow DH (ed). Guilford Press, New York, pp. 137–188.

Burke KC, Burke JD Jr., Rae DS, et al. (1991) Comparing age at onset of major depression and other psychiatric disorders by birth cohorts in five US community populations. Arch Gen Psychiatr 48(9), 789–795.

Butler PD, Weiss JM, Stout JC, et al. (1990) Corticotropin-releasing factor produces fear-enhancing and behavioral activating effects following infusion into the locus coeruleus. J Neurosci 10(1), 176–183.

Carter CS and Maddock RJ (1992) Chest pain in generalized anxiety disorder. Int J Psychiatr Med 22(3), 291–298.

Carter RM, Wittchen HU, Pfister H, et al. (2001) One-year prevalence of sub-threshold and threshold DSM-IV generalized anxiety disorder in a nationally representative sample. Depress Anx 3, 78–88.

Chambless DL and Gillis MM (1993) Cognitive therapy of anxiety disorders. J Clin Consult Psychol 61(2), 248–260.

Charney DS, Woods SW, and Heninger GR (1989) Noradrenergic function in generalized anxiety disorder: Effects of yohimbine in healthy subjects and patients with generalized anxiety disorder. Psychiatr Res 27, 173–182.

Chrousos GP and Gold PW (1992) The concepts of stress and stress disorders. Overview of physical and behavioral homestasis. JAMA 267(9), 1244–1252.

Cohn JB and Wilcox CS (1984) Long-term comparison of alprazolam, lorazepam, and placebo in patients with an anxiety disorder. Psychopharmacology 4(2), 93–98.

Cowley DS, Dager SR, McClellan J, et al. (1988) Response to lactate infusion in generalized anxiety disorder. Biol Psychiatr 24, 409–414.

Curtis G, Fogel M, McEvoy D, et al. (1970) Urine and plasma corticosteroids, psychological tests, and effectiveness of psychological defenses. J Psychiatr Res 7, 237–247.

Cutler NR, Hesselink JM, and Sramek JJ (1994) A phase II multicenter dose-finding, efficacy, and safety trial of ipsapirone in outpatients with generalized anxiety disorder. Prog Neuro-psychopharmacol Biol Psychiatr 18(3), 447–463.

Cutler NR, Sramek JJ, Keppel Hesselink JM, et al. (1993) A double-blind, placebo-controlled study comparing the efficacy and safety of ipsapirone versus lorazepam in patients with generalized anxiety disorder: A prospective multicenter trial. J Clin Psychopharmacol 13(6), 429–437.

Dager SR, Comess KA, and Dunner DL (1986) Differentiation of anxious patients by two-dimensional echocardiographic evaluation of the mitral valve. Am J Psychiatr 143, 533–535.

Davidson JR, DuPont RL, Hedges D, et al. (1999) Efficacy, safety, and tolerability of venlafaxine extended release and busiprone in outpatients with generalized anxiety disorder. J Clin Psychiatr 60(8), 528–535.

Delle Chiaie R, Pancheri P, Casacchia M, et al. (1995) Assessment of the efficacy of buspirone in patients affected by generalized anxiety disorder, shifting buspirone from prior treatment with lorazepam: A placebo-controlled, double-blind study. J Clin Psychopharmacol 15(1), 12 19.

DeMartinis N, Rynn M, Rickels K, et al. (2000) Prior benzodiazepine use and buspirone response in the treatment of generalized anxiety disorder. J Clin Psychiatr 61(2), 91–94.

Doraiswamy PM (2001) Contemporary management of comorbid anxiety and depression in geriatric patients. J Clin Psychiatr 62(Suppl 12), 30–35.

Dorow R, Duka T, Holler L, et al. (1987) Clinical perspectives of beta-carbolines from first studies in humans. Brain Res Bull 19(3), 319–326.

Drugan RC, Skolnick P, Paul SM, et al. (1989) A pretest procedure reliably predicts performance in two animal models of inescapable stress. Pharmacol Biochem Behav 33(3), 649–654.

Eison MS (1990) Serotonin: A common neurobiologic substrate in anxiety and depression. J Clin Psychopharmacol 10, 26S–30S.

Ellie R and Lamontagne Y (1984) Alprazolam and diazepam in the treatment of generalized anxiety. J Clin Psychopharmacol 4(3), 125–129.

Emmanuel NP, Mintzer O, Lydiard RB, et al. (1992) Prevalence of personality disorders in general anxiety disorder. Presented at the 12th National Conference of the Anxiety Disorders Association of America, Houston, Texas.

Enklemann R (1991) Alprazolam versus buspirone in the treatment of outpatients with generalized anxiety disorder. Psychopharmacology 105(3), 428–432.

Fairbanks JM, Pine DS, Tancer NK, et al. (1997) Open fluoxetine treatment of mixed anxiety disorders in children and adolescents. J Child Adolesc Psychopharmacol 7, 17–29.

Fava GA, Grandi S, Rafanelli C, et al. (1992) Prodromal symptoms in panic disorder with agoraphobia: A replication study. J Affect Disord 26, 85–88.

Ferrarese C, Appollonio I, Frigo M, et al. (1990) Decreased density of benzodiazepine receptors in lymphocytes of anxious patients: Reversal after chronic diazepam treatment. Acta Psychiatr Scand 82(2), 169–173.

Ferreri M and Hantouche EG (1998) Recent clinical trials of hydroxyzine in generalized anxiety disorder. Acta Psychiatr Scand 98(Suppl 393), 102–108.

Fifer SK, Mathias SD, Patrick DL, et al. (1994) Untreated anxiety among primary care patients in a health maintenance organization. Arch Gen Psychiatr 51, 740–750.

Flint AJ (1994) Epidemiology and comorbidity of anxiety disorders in the elderly. Am J Psychiatr 151, 640–649.

Fyer AJ, Mannuzza S, Chapman TF, et al. (1993) A direct interview family study of social phobia. Arch Gen Psychiatr 50, 286–293.

Garvey MJ, Noyes R Jr., Woodman C, et al. (1993) A biological difference between panic disorder and generalized anxiety disorder. Biol Psychiatr 34(8), 572–575.

Garvey MJ, Noyes R Jr., Woodman C, et al. (1995) Relationship of generalized anxiety symptoms to urinary 5-hydroxyindoleacetic acid and vanillymandelic acid. Psychiatr Res 57(1), 1–5.

Gasperini M, Battaglia M, Diaferia G, et al. (1990) Personality features related to generalized anxiety disorder. Compr Psychiatr 31(4), 363–368.

Gelenberg AJ, Lydiard RB, Rudolph RL, et al. (2000) Efficacy of venlafaxine extended-release capsules in nondepressed outpatients with generalized anxiety disorder: A 6-month randomized controlled trial. JAMA 283, 3082–3088.

Germine M, Goddard AW, Woods SW, et al. (1992) Anger and anxiety responses to m-chlorophenylpiperazine in generalized anxiety disorder. Biol Psychiatr 32, 457–461.

Goddard AW, Woods SW, Money R, et al. (1999) Effects of the CCK antagonist CI-988 on responses to mCPP in generalized anxiety disorder. Psychiatr Res 85, 225–240.

Goldberg HL and Finnerty RJ (1979) The comparative efficacy of buspirone and diazepam in the treatment of anxiety. Am J Psychiatr 136(9), 1184–1187.

Goodnick PJ, Puig A, DeVane CL, et al. (1999) Mirtazapine in major depression with comorbid generalized anxiety disorder. J Clin Psychiatr 60, 446–448.

Gorenstein EE, Papp LA, and Kleber MS (1999) CBT for anxiety and anxiolytic drug dependence in later life: An interim report. In Assessment and Treatment of Anxiety in Late Life, Stanley MA (Chair). Symposium conducted at the meeting of the Association for the Advancement of Behavior Therapy, Toronto, Canada.

Gorman JM, Liebowitz MR, Flyer AJ, et al. (1987) An open trial of fluoxetine in the treatment of panic attacks. J Clin Psychopharmacol 7, 329–332.

Gould RA, Otto MA, Pollack MH, et al. (1997) Cognitive–behavioral and pharmacological treatment of generalized anxiety disorder: A preliminary meta-analysis. Behav Ther 28(2), 285–305.

Graae F, Milner J, Rizzotto L, et al. (1994) Clonazepam in childhood anxiety disorders. J Am Acad Child Adolesc Psychiatr 33, 372–376.

Gray JA (1988) The neuropsychological basis of anxiety. In Handbook of Anxiety Disorders, Last CG and Hersen M (eds). Pergamon Press, New York, pp. 10–37.

Griebel G (1999) Is there a future for neuropeptide receptor ligands in the treatment of anxiety disorders? Pharmacol Ther 82(1), 1–61.

Harro J, Vasar E, and Bradwejn J (1993) CCK in animal and human research on anxiety. TIPS 14, 244–249.

Hedges DW, Reimherr FW, Strong RE, et al. (1996) An open trial of nefazodone in adult patients with generalized anxiety disorder. Psychopharmacol Bull 32(4), 671–676.

Hoehn-Saric R, Hazlett RL, and McLeod DR (1993) Generalized anxiety disorder with early and late onset of anxiety symptoms. Compr Psychiatr 34(5), 291–298.

Hoehn-Saric R, McLeod DR, and Zimmerli WD (1988) Differential effects of alprazolam and imipramine in generalized anxiety disorder: Somatic versus psychic symptoms. J Clin Psychiatr 49, 293–301.

Hoehn-Saric R, McLeod DR, and Zimmerli WD (1989) Somatic manifestations in women with generalized anxiety disorder. Arch Gen Psychiatr 46, 1113–1119.

Howell HB, Brawman-Mintzer O, Monnier J, et al. (2001) Generalized anxiety disorder in women. Psychiatr Clin N Am 24(1) (Mar), 165–178.

Iny LJ, Pecknold J, Suranyi-Cadotte BE, et al. (1994) Studies of a neurochemical link between depression, anxiety, and stress from [3H]imipramine and [3H]paroxetine binding on human platelets. Biol Psychiatr 36(5), 281–291.

Jetty PV, Charney DS, and Goodard AW (2001) Neurobiology of generalized anxiety disorder. Psychiatr Clin N Am 24(1), 75–98.

Joffe RT, Bagby RM, and Levitt A (1993) Anxious and nonanxious depression. Am J Psychiatr 150(8), 1257–1258.

Josephs L (1994) Psychoanalytic and related interpretations. In Anxiety and Related Disorders. A Handbook, Wolman BB and Stricker G (eds). Wiley-Interscience, New York, pp. 11–29.

Kahn RS, Wetzler S, Asnis GM, et al. (1991) Pituitary hormone response to meta-chlorophenylpiperazine in panic disorder and healthy control subjects. Psychiatr Res 37(1), 25–34.

Kashani JH and Orvaschel H (1988) Anxiety disorders in mid-adolescence: A community sample. Am J Psychiatr 145, 960–964.

Kashani JH, Vaidya AF, and Soltys SM (1990) Correlates of anxiety in psychiatrically hospitalized children and their parents. Am J Psychiatr 147, 319–323.

Kendall PC (1994) Treating anxiety disorders in children: Results of a randomized clinical trial. J Consult Clin Psychol 62, 100–110.

Kendall PC, Flannery-Schroeder E, Panichelli-Mindel SM, et al. (1997) Therapy for youths with anxiety disorders: A second randomized clinical trial. J Consult Clin Psychol 65, 366–380.

Kendler KS, Neale MC, Kessler RC, et al. (1992a) Generalized anxiety disorder in women. Arch Gen Psychiatr 49, 267–272.

Kendler KS, Neale MC, Kessler RC, et al. (1992b) Major depression and generalized anxiety disorder. Arch Gen Psychiatr 49, 716–722.

Kendler KS, Walters EE, Neale MC, et al. (1995) The structure of the genetic and environmental risk factors for six major psychiatric disorders in women: Phobia, generalized anxiety disorder, panic disorder, bulimia, major depression, and alcoholism. Arch Gen Psychiatr 52(5), 374–383.

Kennedy JL, Bradwejn J, Koszycki D, et al. (1999) Investigation of cholestokinin system genes in panic disorder. Mol Psychiatr 4(3), 284–285.

Kessler RC (2000) The epidemiology of pure and comorbid generalized anxiety disorder: A review and evaluation of recent research. Acta Psychiatr Scand 406(Suppl), 7–13.

Kessler RC, DuPont RL, Berglund P, et al. (1999) Impairment in pure and comorbid generalized anxiety disorder and major depression at 12 months in two national surveys. Am J Psychiatr 156, 1915–1923.

Kessler RC, Keller MB, and Wittchen HU (2000) The epidemiology of generalized anxiety disorder. The Psychiatr Clin N Am 24(1), 19–40.

Kessler RC, McGonagle KA, Zhao S, et al. (1994) Lifetime and 12-month prevalence of DSM-III-R psychiatric disorders in the United States: Results from the National Comorbidity Survey. Arch Gen Psychiatr 51, 8–19.

Khan A, Lee E, Dager S, et al. (1986) Platelet MAO-B activity in anxiety and depression. Biol Psychiatr 21, 847–849.

Kollai M and Kollai B (1992) Cardiac vagal tone in generalized anxiety disorder. Br J Psychiatr 161, 831–835.

Koob GF (1999) Corticotropin-releasing factor, norepinephrine, and stress. Biol Psychiatr 46(9), 1167–1180.

Koob GF and Gold LH (1997) Molecular biological approaches in the behavioural pharmacology of anxiety and depression. Behav Pharmacol 8, 652.

Kushner MG, Sher KJ, and Erickson DJ (1999) Prospective analysis of the relationship between DSM-III anxiety disorders and alcohol use disorders. Am J Psychiatr 156(5), 723–732.

Kutcher SP, Reiter S, Gardner DM, et al. (1992) The pharmacotherapy of anxiety disorders in children and adolescents. Pediatr Psychopharmacol 15(1), 41–67.

Laakmann G, Schule C, Lorkowski G, et al. (1998) Buspirone and lorazepam in the treatment of generalized anxiety disorder in outpatients. Psychopharmacology 136(4), 357–366.

Lader M and Scotto JC (1998) A multicentre double-blind comparison of hydroxyzine, buspirone, and placebo in patients with generalized anxiety disorder. Psychopharmacology 139(4), 402–406.

Lader MH (1999) Limitations on the use of benzodiazepines in anxiety and insomnia: Are they justified? Eur Neuropsychopharmacol 9(Suppl 6), S399–S405.

Ladouceur R, Dugas MJ, Freeston MH, et al. (2000) Efficacy of a cognitive–behavioral treatment for generalized anxiety disorder: Evaluation in a controlled clinical trial. J Clin Consult Psychol 68(6), 957–964.

Lane RM (1998) SSRI-induces extrapyramidal side effects and akathisia: Implications for treatment. Psychopharmacology 12, 192–214.

Last CG, Hersen M, and Karzdin AE (1987) Comparison of DSM-III separation anxiety and overanxious disorders: Demographic characteristics and patterns of comorbidity. J Am Acad Child Adolesc Psychiatry 4, 527–531.

Lesch KP (2001) Genetic dissection of anxiety and related disorders. In Anxiety Disorders, Nutt D and Ballenger J (eds). Blackwell Science, Oxford.

Lorberbaum JP, Varon D, Brawman-Minzter O, et al. (2001) The functional neuroanatomy of anticipatory anxiety in healthy adults and patients with generalized anxiety disorder. Presented at the 21st National Conference of Anxiety Disorders Association of America, Atlanta.

Lydiard RB (1994) Neuropeptides and anxiety: Focus on cholecystokinin. Clin Chem 40, 315–318.

Lydiard RB, Brawman-Mintzer O, and Ballenger JC (1996) Recent developments in the psychopharmacology of anxiety disorders. J Consult Clin Psychol 64(4), 660–668.

MacQueen G, Born L, and Steiner M (2001) The selective serotonin reuptake inhibitor sertraline: Its profile and use in psychiatric disorders. CNS Drug Rev 7(1), 1–24.

Maier W, Gaeniscke M, Freyberger HJ, et al. (2000) Generalized anxiety disorder (ICD-10) in primary care from a cross-cultural perspective: A valid diagnostic entity? Acta Psychiatr Scand 101, 29–36.

Manassis K and Hood J (1998) Individual and familial predictors of impairment in childhood anxiety disorders. J Am Acad Child Adolesc Psychiatr 37, 428–434.

Mancuso DM, Townsend MH, and Mercante DE (1993) Long-term follow-up of generalized anxiety disorder. Compr Psychiatr 34, 441–446.

Maser JD (1998) Generalized anxiety disorder and its comorbidities: Disputes at the boundaries. Acta Psychiatr Scand 98(Suppl 393), 12–22.

Masi G, Mucci M, Favilla L, et al. (1999) Symptomatology and comorbidity of generalized anxiety disorder in children and adolescents. Compr Psychiatr 40, 210–215.

Massion AO, Warshaw MG, and Keller MB (1993) Quality of life and psychiatric morbidity in panic disorder and generalized anxiety disorder. Am J Psychiatr 150, 600–607.

Mathew RJ, Weinman ML, and Claghorn JL (1982b) Anxiety and cerebral blood flow. In The Biology of Anxiety, Mathew RJ (ed). Brunner/Mazel, New York.

Matthew RJ, Ho BT, Francis DJ, et al. (1982a) Catecholamines and anxiety. Acta Psychiatr Scand 65, 142–147.

Matthew RJ, Ho BT, Kralik P, et al. (1980) Catechol-O-methyltransferase and catecholamines in anxiety and relaxation. Psychiatr Res 3, 85–91.

Mauri M, Sarno N, Rossi VM, et al. (1992) Personality disorders associated with generalized anxiety, panic, and recurrent depressive disorders. J Pers Disord 6, 162–167.

Mavissakalian MR, Hamann MS, Abou Haidar S, et al. (1993) DSM-III personality disorders in generalized anxiety, panic/agoraphobia, and obsessive–compulsive disorders. Compr Psychiatr 34(4), 243–248.

Mendlewicz J, Papadimitriou G, and Wimotte J (1993) Family study of panic disorder: Comparison to generalized anxiety disorder, major depression, and normal subjects. Psychiatr Genet 3, 73–78.

Mennin D, Heimberg RG, and Jack MS (1998) Generalized anxiety disorder in primary social phobia: Functional and treatment implications. Presented at the 18th National Conference of Anxiety Disorders Association of America, Boston.

Michelson D, Bancroft J, Targum S, et al. (2000) Female sexual dysfunction associated with antidepressant administration: A randomized, placebo-controlled study of pharmacologic intervention. Am J Psychiatr 157, 239–243.

Miserendino MJ, Sananes CB, Melia KR, et al. (1990) Blocking of acquisition but not expression of conditioned fear-potentiated startle by NMDA antagonists in the amygdala. Nature 345(6277), 716–718.

Moghaddam B, Bolinao ML, Stein-Behrens B, et al. (1994) Glucocorticoids mediate the stress-induced extracellular accumulation of glutamate. Brain Res 655(1–2), 251–254.

Munjack DJ and Palmer R (1988) Thyroid hormones in panic disorder, panic disorder with agoraphobia and generalized anxiety disorder. J Clin Psychiatr 49, 229–231.

Munjack DJ, Baltazar PL, DeQuattro V, et al. (1990) Generalized anxiety disorder: Some biochemical aspects. Psychiatr Res 32, 35–43.

Murphy JM, Olivier DC, Sobol AM, et al. (1986) Diagnosis and outcome: Depression and anxiety in a general population. Psychol Med 16(1), 117–126.

Noyes R, Clancy J, Hoenk PR, et al. (1980) The prognosis of anxiety disorders. Arch Gen Psychiatr 37, 173–178.

Noyes R, Clarkson C, Crowe RR, et al. (1987) A family study of generalized anxiety disorder. Am J Psychiatr 144, 1019–1024.

Noyes R, Woodman C, Garvey MJ, et al. (1992) Generalized anxiety disorder vs. panic disorder. Distinguishing characteristics and patterns of comorbidity. J Nerv Ment Dis 180, 369–379.

Noyes R Jr., Holt CS, and Woodman CL (1996) Natural course of anxiety disorders. In Long-term Treatments of Anxiety Disorders, Mavissakalian MR and Prien RF (eds). American Psychiatric Press, Washington DC.

Nutt DJ (2001) Neurobiological mechanisms in generalized anxiety disorder. J Clin Psychiatr 62(Suppl 11), 22–27.

Olajide D and Lader M (1987) A comparison of buspirone, diazepam, and placebo in patients with chronic anxiety states. J Clin Psychopharmacol 7(3), 148–152.

Papadimitriou GN, Kerkhofs M, Kempenaers C, et al. (1988) EEG sleep studies in patients with generalized anxiety disorder. Psychiatr Res 26, 183–190.

Pecknold JC, Familamiri P, Chang H, et al. (1985) Buspirone: Anxiolytic? Prog Neuropsychopharmacol Biol Psychiatr 9(5–6), 639–642.

Pecknold JC, Matas M, Howarth BG, et al. (1989) Evaluation of buspirone as an antianxiety agent: Buspirone and diazepam vs. placebo. Can J Psychiatr 34(8), 766–771.

Pini S, Cassano GB, Simonini E, et al. (1997) Prevalence of anxiety disorders comorbidity in bipolar depression unipolar depression and dysthymia. J Affect Disord 42, 145–153.

Pollack J (2001) Optimizing pharmacotherapy of generalized anxiety disorder to achieve remission. Clin Psychiatr 19(Suppl), 20–25.

Pollack MH, Matthews J, and Scott EL (2000) Gabapentin as a potential treatment for anxiety disorders. Am J Psychiatr 155(7), 992–993.

Pollack MH, Worthington JJ, Manfro GG, et al. (1997) Abecarnil for the treatment of generalized anxiety disorder: A placebo-controlled comparison of two dosage ranges of abecarnil and buspirone. J Clin Psychiatr 58(Suppl 1), 19–23.

Popper CW (1993) Psychopharmacologic treatment of anxiety disorders in adolescents and children. J Clin Psychiatr 54(Suppl 5), 52–63.

Ramboz S, Oosting R, Amara DA, et al. (1998) Serotonin receptor 1A knockout: An animal model of anxiety-related disorder. Proc Natl Acad Sci USA 95(24), 14476–14481.

Rapee RM (1991) Generalized anxiety disorder: A review of clinical features and theoretical concepts. Clin Psychol Rev 11, 419–440.

Rice KM, Blanchard EB, and Purcell M (1993) Biofeedback treatments of generalized anxiety disorder: Preliminary results. Biofeedback Self-Reg 18(2), 93–104.

Rickels K, Case WG, and Schweizer E (1988a) The drug treatment of anxiety and panic disorder. Stress Med 4(4), 231–239.

Rickels K, Case WG, Downing RW, et al. (1986) One-year follow-up of anxious patients treated with diazepam. J Clin Psychopharmacol 6, 32–36.

Rickels K, Csanalosi I, Greisman P, et al. (1983) A controlled clinical trial of alprazolam for the treatment of anxiety. Am J Psychiatr 140(1), 82–85.

Rickels K, Downing R, Schweizer E, et al. (1993) Antidepressants for the treatment of generalized anxiety disorder. Arch Gen Psychiatr 50, 884–895.

Rickels K, Schweizer E, DeMartinis N, et al. (1997) Gepirone and diazepam in generalized anxiety disorder: A placebo-controlled trial. J Clin Psychopharmacol 17(4), 272–277.

Rickels K, Schweizer R, Csanalosi I, et al. (1988b) Long-term treatment of anxiety and risk of withdrawal. Prospective comparison of clorazepate and buspirone. Arch Gen Psychiatr 45(5), 444–450.

Rickels K, Weisman K, Norstad N, et al. (1982) Buspirone and diazepam in anxiety: A controlled study. J Clin Psychiatr 43(12 Pt 2), 81–86.

Riddle MA, Nelson JC, Kleinman CS, et al. (1991) Case study: Sudden death in children receiving Norpramin: A review of three reported cases and commentary. J Am Acad Child Adolesc Psychiatr 30, 104–108.

Riskind JH, Moore R, Harman B, et al. (1991) The relation of generalized anxiety disorder to depression in general and dysthymic disorder in particular. In Chronic Anxiety: Generalized Anxiety Disorder and Mixed Anxiety–Depression, Rapee RM and Barlow DH (eds). Guilford Press, New York.

Rocca P, Beoni AM, Eva C, et al. (1998) Peripheral benzodiazepine receptor messenger RNA is decreased in lymphocytes of generalized anxiety disorder patients. Biol Psychiatr 43(10), 767–773.

Rocca P, Fonzo V, Scotta M, et al. (1997) Paroxetine efficacy in the treatment of generalized anxiety disorder. Acta Psychiatr Scand 95, 444–450.

Rogers MP, Warshaw MG, Goisman RM, et al. (1999) Comparing primary and secondary generalized anxiety disorder in a long-term naturalistic study of anxiety disorder. Depress Anx 10, 1–7.

Romach M, Busto U, Somer G, et al. (1995) Clinical aspects of chronic use of alprazolam and lorazepam. Am J Psychiatr 152(8), 1161–1167.

Rose RM (1984) Overview of endocrinology of stress. In Neuroendocrinology and Psychiatric Disorders, Brown GM (ed). Raven Press, New York, pp. 95–122.

Rosen RC, Lane RM, and Menza M (1999) Effects of SSRIs on sexual function: A critical review. J Clin Psychopharmacol 19, 67–85.

Rosenbaum AH, Schatzberg AF, Jost FA, et al. (1983) Urinary free cortisol levels in anxiety. Psychosomatics 24, 835–837.

Ross CA and Matas M (1987) A clinical trial of buspirone and diazepam in the treatment of anxiety. J Clin Psychopharmacol 19, 67–85.

Roy-Byrne PP, Cowley DS, Hommer D, et al. (1991) Neuroendocrine effects of diazepam in panic and generalized anxiety disorders. Biol Psychiatr 30, 73–80.

Ruiz AT (1983) A double-blind study of alprazolam and lorazepam in the treatment of anxiety. J Clin Psychiatr 44(2), 60–62.

Sacerdote P, Panerai AE, Frattola L, et al. (1999) Benzodiazepine-induced chemotaxis is impaired in monocytes from patients with generalized anxiety disorder. Psychoneuroendocrinology 24(2), 243–249.

Salzman C (1990) Anxiety in the elderly: Treatment strategies. J Clin Psychiatr 51(Suppl 10), 18–21.

Sanderson WC and Barlow DH (1990) A description of patients diagnosed with DSM-III-R generalized anxiety disorder. J Nerv Ment Dis 178, 588–591.

Sanderson WC, Wetzler S, Beck AT, et al. (1991) Prevalence of personality disorders among patients with anxiety disorders. Psychiatr Res 51(2), 167–174.

Sartorius N, Ustun B, Lecrubier Y, et al. (1996) Depression comorbid with anxiety: Results from the WHO study on psychological disorders in primary health care. Br J Psychiatr 168(Suppl 30), 38–43.

Scherrer JF, True WR, Xian H, et al. (2000) Evidence for genetic influences common and specific to symptoms of generalized anxiety disorder and panic. J Affect Disord 57(1–3), 25–35.

Schweizer E, Rickels K, and Lucki I (1986) Resistance to the anxiety effect of buspirone in patients with a history of benzodiazepine use. New Engl J Med 314, 719–720.

Shear MK, Schulberg HC, and Madonia M (1994) Panic and generalized anxiety disorder in primary care. Paper presented at a meeting of the Association for Primary Care, Washington DC.

Sheehan DV (1999) Venlafaxine extended release (XR) in the treatment of generalized anxiety disorder. J Clin Psychiatr 60(Suppl 22), 23–28.

Sheehan DV (2001) Attaining remission in generalized anxiety disorder: Venlafaxine extended release comparative data. J Clin Psychiatr 62(9S), 26–31.

Simeon JG, Ferguson HB, and Knott V (1992) Clinical, cognitive, and neurophysiological effects of alprazolam in children and adolescents with overanxious and avoidant disorders. J Am Acad Child Adolesc Psychiatr 31, 29–33.

Skre I, Torgersen S, Lygren S, et al. (1993) A twin study of DSM-III-R anxiety disorders. Acta Psychiatr Scand 88, 85–92.

Souetre E, Lozet H, Cimarosti I, et al. (1994) Cost of anxiety disorders: Impact of comorbidity. J Psychosom Res 38(Suppl 1), 151–160.

Spiegel DA, Bruce TJ, Gregg SF, et al. (1994) Does cognitive–behavior therapy assist slow-taper alprazolam discontinuation in panic disorder. Am J Psychiatr 151, 876–881.

Stanley MA, Beck JG, and Glassco JD (1996) Treatment of generalized anxiety disorder in older adults: A preliminary comparison of cognitive–behavioral and supportive approaches. Behav Ther 27, 565–581.

Stanley MA, Beck JG, Novy DM, et al. (1999) Cognitive–behavioral treatment of generalized anxiety disorder in older adults. In Assessment and Treatment of Anxiety in Late Life, Stanley MA (Chair). Symposium conducted at the meeting of the Association for the Advancement of Behavior Therapy, Toronto, Canada.

Starcevic V, Uhlenhuth EH, and Fallon S (1995) The tridimensional personality questionnaire as an instrument for screening personality disorders: Use in patients with generalized anxiety disorder. J Pers Disord 9, 247–253.

Starcevic V, Uhlenhuth EH, Kellner R, et al. (1992) Matters of comorbidity and panic disorder and agoraphobia. Psychiatr Res 42, 171–183.

Stein MB, Hauger RL, Dhalla KS, et al. (1996) Plasma neuropeptide Y in anxiety disorders: Findings in panic disorder and social phobia. Psychiatr Res 59(3), 183–188.

Stocchi F, Jokinen R, and Lepola U (2001) Efficacy and tolerability of paroxetine for long-term treatment of generalized anxiety disorder. Presented at 2001 Annual Meeting of the American Psychiatric Association (May 5–10), New Orleans.

Taylor DP, Eison MS, Riblet LA, et al. (1985) Pharmacological and clinical effects of buspirone. Pharmacol Biochem Behav 23(4), 687–694.

Tiihonen J, Kuikka J, Rasanen P, et al. (1997) Cerebral benzodiazepine receptor binding and distribution in generalized anxiety disorder: A fractal analysis. Mol Psychiatr 2(6), 463–471.

Tollefson GD, Luxenberg M, Valentine R, et al. (1991) An open label trial of alprazolam in comorbid irritable bowel syndrome and generalized anxiety disorder. J Clin Psychiatr 52(12), 502–508.

Torgersen S (1983) Genetic factors in anxiety disorder. Arch Gen Psychiatr 40, 1085–1089.

Trullas RB, Jackson B, and Skolnick P (1989) Anxiolytic properties of 1-aminocyclopropanecarboxylic acid, a ligand at strychnine-insensitive glycine receptors. Pharmacol Biochem Behav 34(2), 313–316.

Uhlenhuth EH, Balter MB, Ban TA, et al. (1999) International study of expert judgement on therapeutic use of benzodiazepines and other psychotherapeutic medications: VI. Trends in recommendations for the pharmacotherapy of anxiety disorders, 1992–1997. Depress Anx 9, 107–116.

Wheatley D (1982) Buspirone: Multicenter efficacy study. J Clin Psychiatr 42, 92–94.

Widerlov E, Lindstrom LH, Wahlestedt C, et al. (1988) Neuropeptide Y and peptide YY as possible cerebrospinal fluid makers for major depression and schizophrenia, respectively. J Psychiatr Res 22(1), 69–79.

Wingerson D, Nguyen C, and Roy-Byrne PP (1992) Clomipramine treatment for generalized anxiety disorder. J Clin Psychopharmacol 12, 214–215.

Wittchen HU, Nelson CB, and Lachner G (1998) Prevalence of mental disorders and psychological impairments in adolescents and young adults. Psychol Med 28, 109–126.

Wittchen HU, Zhao S, Kessler RC, et al. (1994) DSM-III-R generalized anxiety disorder in the National Comorbidity Survey. Arch Gen Psychiatr 51, 355–364.

Woodman CL, Noyes R, Black DW, et al. (1999) A 5-year follow-up study of generalized anxiety disorder and panic disorder. J Nerv Ment Disord 187, 3–9.

Woodruff GN and Hughes J (1991) Cholecystokinin antagonists. Ann Rev Pharmacol Toxicol 31, 469–501.

Wu JC, Buchsbaum MS, Hershey TG, et al. (1991) PET in generalized anxiety disorder. Biol Psychiatr 29, 1181–1199.

Yonkers KA, Dyck IR, Warshaw M, et al. (2000) Factors predicting the clinical course of generalized anxiety disorder. Br J Psychiatr 176, 544–549.

Yonkers KA, Massion A, Warshaw M, et al. (1996) Phenomenology and course of generalized anxiety disorder. Br J Psychiatr 168, 308–313.

# 71 Somatoform Disorders

Sean H. Yutzy

Somatization Disorder
Undifferentiated Somatoform Disorder
Conversion Disorder
Pain Disorder
Hypochondriasis
Body Dysmorphic Disorder
Somatoform Disorder Not Otherwise Specified

## Definition

The somatoform disorders are a major diagnostic class in the *Diagnostic and Statistical Manual of Mental Disorders*, Fourth Edition, Text Revision (DSM-IV-TR) (American Psychiatric Association 2000) that groups together conditions characterized by physical symptoms suggestive of but not fully explained by a general medical condition or the direct effects of a substance. In this class, symptoms are not intentionally produced and are not attributable to another mental disorder. To warrant a diagnosis, symptoms must be clinically significant in terms of causing distress or impairment in important areas of functioning. As summarized in Table 71–1, the disorders included in this class are somatization disorder, undifferentiated somatoform disorder, conversion disorder, pain disorder, hypochondriasis, body dysmorphic disorder, and somatoform disorder not otherwise specified (NOS).

The somatoform disorders were first officially grouped together in the *Diagnostic and Statistical Manual of Mental Disorders*, Third Edition (DSM-III) (American Psychiatric Association 1980). The class was characterized by the presence of physical (somatic) symptoms that were not fully explained by physical conditions. In DSM-IV-TR, the phrase "general medical condition or the direct effects of a substance" corresponds to the "physical disorders" of DSM-III and the *Diagnostic and Statistical Manual of Mental Disorders*, Third Edition, Revised (DSM-III-R) (American Psychiatric Association 1987). By definition, a general medical condition includes any medical condition not considered mental or psychiatric. Substances include any drugs of abuse

The late Ronald L. Martin was the first author of this chapter in the first edition.

(including alcohol), medications, or toxins. By "direct effect" is meant the actual physiological effects of a substance, such as intoxication or withdrawal, rather than indirect effects, such as the psychosocial consequences of abuse or dependence. This cumbersome terminology was adopted to avoid the designation of certain conditions as physical, organic, or biological, which could be interpreted to imply that such factors did not contribute to conditions identified as mental, functional, or psychiatric. In essence, general medical condition refers to any nonpsychiatric medical condition, which includes any medical condition not listed in the mental disorders section of the *International Statistical Classification of Diseases and Related Health Problems*, 10th Revision (ICD-10) (World Health Organization 1992). Examples include virtually all infectious and parasitic, endocrine, nutritional, metabolic, immunity, and congenital disorders of any organ system (including the nervous system). DSM-III and DSM-III-R (American Psychiatric Association 1987) required that "no demonstrable organic findings or known physiologic mechanisms" be present, whereas DSM-IV specifies only that the physical symptoms not be *fully* accounted for by a general medical condition or the direct effects of a substance.

The somatoform disorders class was created for clinical utility, not on the basis of an assumed common etiology or mechanism. In DSM-IV-TR terms, it was designed to facilitate the differential diagnosis of conditions in which the first diagnostic concern is the need to "exclude occult general medical conditions or substance-induced etiologies for the bodily symptoms." As shown in Figure 71–1, only after such explanations are reasonably excluded should somatoform disorders be considered.

Many criticisms of the somatoform disorder category have been raised, and the disbanding of the class with re-

| Table 71–1 | DSM-IV Somatoform Disorders Criteria Indicating Changes from DSM-III-R* | | | |
|---|---|---|---|---|
| **DSM-IV Disorder** | **General Description** | **Temporal Requirements** | **Threshold for Diagnosis†** | **Exclusion Criteria‡** |
| Somatization disorder | "A history of many physical complaints" *Symptoms required: 4 pain, 2 nonpain gastrointestinal, 1 nonpain sexual or reproductive, and 1 pseudoneurological (conversion or dissociative)* *No exclusive list of symptoms* | Onset "...before age 30 years" "...occur for a period of several years" | "...result in treatment being sought or significant impairment in social, occupational, or other important areas of functioning" | "...cannot be fully explained by a known GMC or the DES" or "...when there is a related GMC... complaints or... impairment is in excess of ...expected" *"...not intentionally produced or feigned"* *No exclusion based on other mental disorder* |
| Undifferentiated somatoform disorder | "One or more physical complaints (e.g., fatigue, loss of appetite, gastrointestinal or urinary complaints)" | "...duration...at least 6 months" | *"...clinically significant distress or impairment in social, occupational, or other important areas of functioning"* | "...cannot be fully explained by a known GMC or the DES" or "...when there is a related GMC... complaints or... impairment is in excess of ...expected" *"...not intentionally produced or feigned"* "...not better accounted for by another mental disorder" |
| Conversion disorder | *"One or more symptoms or deficits affecting voluntary motor or sensory function that suggest a neurological or other GMC"* "Psychological factors judged...associated with the symptom... symptom is preceded by conflicts or other stressors" *Specify: "with motor symptom or deficit," "with sensory symptom or deficit," "with seizures or convulsions," or "with mixed presentation"* | No temporal requirements | *"...clinically significant distress or impairment in social, occupational, or other important areas of functioning or warrants medical evaluation"* | "...cannot be...fully explained by a GMC, or by the DES, or as a culturally sanctioned behavior or experience" "...not intentionally produced or feigned" "...not limited to pain or sexual dysfunction *...not exclusively... during the course of somatization disorder...not better accounted for by another mental disorder"* |
| Pain disorder | *"Pain in one or more anatomical sites is the predominant focus of the clinical presentation"* "Psychological factors ...judged... important role in onset, severity, exacerbation, or maintenance of the pain" *Code: "...with psychological factors," "...with both psychological factors and a GMC" ("...with a GMC" not a mental disorder)* | *"Specify if: acute: duration of less than 6 months" or "chronic: duration of 6 months or longer"* | *"...sufficient severity to warrant clinical attention"* "...clinically significant distress or impairment in social, occupational, or other important areas of functioning" | "...not intentionally produced or feigned" *"...not better accounted for by a mood, anxiety, or psychotic disorder ...not... dyspareunia"* |

*Continues*

**Table 71–1    DSM-IV Somatoform Disorders Criteria Indicating Changes from DSM-III-R*** *Continued*

| DSM-IV Disorder | General Description | Temporal Requirements | Threshold for Diagnosis† | Exclusion Criteria‡ |
|---|---|---|---|---|
| Hypochondriasis | "Preoccupation... fears of having, or ... idea ... one has, a serious disease based on ... misinterpretation of bodily symptoms" "... persists despite appropriate medical evaluation and reassurance" **"Specify if: with poor insight"** | "... duration ... at least 6 months" | "*... clinically significant distress or impairment in social, occupational, or other important areas of functioning*" | "... not of delusional intensity ... *not restricted to a circumscribed concern about appearance*" "*... not better accounted for by generalized anxiety disorder, obsessive compulsive disorder, panic disorder, a major depressive episode, separation anxiety, or another somatoform disorder*" |
| Body dysmorphic disorder | "Preoccupation with an imagined defect in appearance. If a slight physical anomaly ... concern is markedly excessive" | No temporal requirements | "*... clinically significant distress or impairment in social, occupational, or other important areas of functioning*" | *No exclusion for delusional disorder, somatic type* "... not better accounted for by another mental disorder (e.g., ... anorexia nervosa)" |
| Somatoform disorder not otherwise specified | "Disorders ... somatoform symptoms ... not meet criteria for any specific somatoform disorder" Examples: *pseudocyesis*, nonpsychotic hypochondriacal symptoms, unexplained physical complaints | Less than 6 months in duration (except for *pseudocyesis*) | | "... not meet criteria for any specific somatoform disorder" |

*Actual DSM-IV criteria wording is in quotation marks. Criteria substantively changed from DSM-III-R are in boldface and italicized. GMC, General medical condition, DES, direct effects of a substance. Although not specified in the criteria for each the DSM-IV text specifies that for all somatoform disorders:

†"the symptoms must cause clinically significant distress or impairment in social, occupational, or other areas of functioning;"

‡"the physical symptoms are not intentional (i.e., under voluntary control)," and "there is no diagnosable GMC to fully account for the physical symptoms."

*Source*: Reprinted from Martin RL (1995) DSM-IV changes for the somatoform disorders. Psychiatr Ann 25, 29–39, copyright 1995 Slack Publications.

assignment of various of the disorders to other classes has been considered (Hales 1996). As summarized by Murphy (1990), criticisms include contentions that because the category is delineated on the basis of presenting symptoms, it is "superficial"; that the individual disorders are not qualitatively distinct from one another or from "normality" and hence would be better described dimensionally rather than differentiated categorically; that the disorders are derived from hospital rather than community or primary care-based populations; and, perhaps the most serious challenge, that the grouping "gives the spurious impression of understanding." On the other hand, proponents maintain that the somatoform grouping represents a major advance over previous systems and that segregation of such disorders into a class has helped clarify the conceptualization of the "mind–body" distinction, promoted greater consistency in terminology, and led to better descriptive distinctions between specific disorders (Cloninger 1987, Cloninger and Yutzy 1993). Supporters contend that maintaining this diagnostic class will foster more generalizable and thereby more clinically applicable research, an intent that appears to be sup-

ported when the literature before and after DSM-III is compared (Martin 1996). In the end, DSM-IV left the class virtually intact from DSM-III-R.

A somatoform disorder category similar to the DSM-IV class is included in ICD-10, perhaps demonstrating growing international acceptance for the grouping (Martin 1995). The ICD-10 category differs from the DSM-IV class in that it requires "persistent requests for medical investigations" and resistance to consideration of "psychological causation" despite "repeated negative findings and reassurances by doctors that the symptoms have no physical basis." In DSM-IV, such elements are required only in hypochondriasis and body dysmorphic disorder. The ICD-10 grouping also encompasses different disorders: somatization disorder; undifferentiated somatoform disorder; hypochondriacal disorder (of which body dysmorphic disorder is a subtype); somatoform autonomic dysfunction (a disorder not included in DSM-IV-TR); persistent somatoform pain disorder; other somatoform disorders; and somatoform disorder, unspecified. Somatoform autonomic dysfunction approximates the psychophysiological

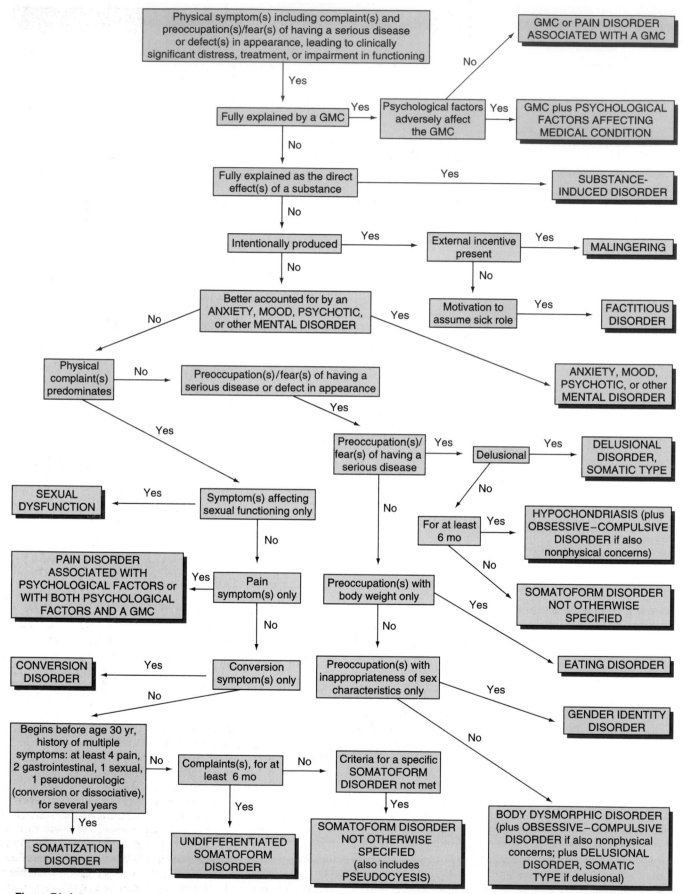

**Figure 71–1** *Somatic symptom diagnostic exploration and treatment algorithm. Differential diagnosis of clinically significant physical symptoms. Shadowed boxes represent diagnostic categories; GMC, General medical condition.*

"reactions" or "disorders" of the *Diagnostic and Statistical Manual of Mental Disorders*, First Edition (DSM-I) and the *Diagnostic and Statistical Manual of Mental Disorders*, Second Edition (DSM-II), respectively, encompassing syndromes involving organ systems under autonomic nervous system control. In the DSM-IV-TR, many such syndromes are included under psychological factors affecting medical condition. Conversion disorder is not included as a distinct somatoform disorder in ICD-10 but is subsumed under dissociative (conversion) disorder. Also of note, there is no ICD-10 condition corresponding to pain disorders specified as acute in DSM-IV; ICD-10 considers only persistent pain disorders.

The somatoform disorder concept should be distinguished from traditional concepts of "psychosomatic illness" and "somatization." The psychosomatic illnesses involved structural or physiological changes hypothesized as deriving from psychological factors. In the DSM-III, DSM-III-R, and DSM-IV somatoform disorders, such objective changes are generally not evident. The "classic" psychosomatic illnesses of Alexander (1950) included bronchial asthma, ulcerative colitis, thyrotoxicosis, essential hypertension, rheumatoid arthritis, neurodermatitis, and peptic ulcer. In DSM-IV, most of these illnesses would be diagnosed as a general medical condition on Axis III, and in some cases with an additional designation of psychological factors affecting medical condition on Axis I. By definition, the diagnosis of "psychological factors affecting medical condition" is not a psychiatric disorder, but it is included in DSM-IV in the section for other conditions that may be a focus of clinical attention; it involves the presence of one or more specific psychological or behavioral factors that adversely affect a general medical condition (see Chapter 80 for more information).

The descriptive use of the term "somatization" in somatization disorder is not to be confused with theories that generally postulate a somatic expression of psychological distress (Lipowski 1988, Kellner 1990, Malt 1991). Steckel (Steckel et al. 1943), who coined the term, defined somatization in 1943 as the process of a "bodily disorder" occurring as the expression of a "deep-seated neurosis." However, as argued by Kellner (1990), "empirical studies ... suggest that there is no single theory that can adequately explain somatization, which is not only multifactorially determined but is an exceedingly complex phenomenon." Furthermore, treatment strategies derived from somatization theories have not proven effective. For example, the postulation that patients with somatoform disorders are alexithymic, that is, are unable to process emotions and psychological conflicts verbally and therefore do so somatically, suggested that teaching such patients to "appreciate" and "verbalize" their emotions would circumvent the need to "somatize" them. Such treatment approaches have been ineffective (Cloninger 1987).

## Diagnosis and Differential Diagnosis

As shown in Figure 71–1, after it is determined that physical symptoms are not fully explained by a general medical condition or the direct effect of a substance, somatoform disorders must be differentiated from other mental conditions with physical symptoms.

In contrast to malingering and factitious disorder, symptoms in somatoform disorders are not under voluntary control, that is, they are not intentionally produced or feigned. Determination of intentionality may be difficult and must be inferred from the context in which symptoms present. Somatic symptoms may also be involved in disorders in other diagnostic classes. However, in such instances, the overriding focus is on the primary symptom complex (i.e., anxiety, mood, or psychotic symptoms) rather than the physical symptoms. In panic disorder and in generalized anxiety disorder, physical symptoms such as chest pain, shortness of breath, palpitations, sweating, and tremulousness may occur. However, such somatic symptoms occur only in the context of fear or anxious foreboding. In general, there is a lack of a consistent physical focus. In mood disorders (particularly major depressive disorder) and in schizophrenia and other psychotic disorders, somatic preoccupations, fears, and even delusions and false perceptions may be evident. In the mood disorders, these are generally mood congruent (e.g., "I'm so worthless not even my organs work anymore"), whereas in the psychoses, bizarre and mood-incongruent beliefs are typical (e.g., "Half of my brain was removed by psychic neurosurgery").

## Differentiation Among the Various Somatoform Disorders

Whereas it is assumed that the specific disorders in the somatoform grouping are heterogeneous in terms of pathogenesis and pathophysiology, they are also phenomenologically diverse (see Table 71–1 and Figure 71–1). In somatization disorder, undifferentiated somatoform disorder, conversion disorder, and pain disorder, the focus is on the physical complaints themselves, and thus on perceptions. In hypochondriasis and body dysmorphic disorder, emphasis is on physically related preoccupations or fears, and thus on cognitions. Somatization disorder and, to a lesser extent, undifferentiated somatoform disorder are characterized by multiple symptoms of different types; conversion disorder, pain disorder, hypochondriasis, and body dysmorphic disorder are defined on the basis of a single symptom or a few symptoms of a certain type (see Figure 71–1). Whereas somatization disorder, undifferentiated somatoform disorder, and hypochondriasis are, by definition, at least 6 months in duration, conversion disorder, pain disorder, body dysmorphic disorder, and somatoform disorder NOS may be of short duration as long as they are associated with clinically significant distress or impairment.

## Epidemiology

In view of the vicissitudes of diagnostic approaches and the recency of the current somatoform disorder grouping, it is not surprising that estimates of the frequency of this group of disorders in the general population as well as in clinical settings are inconsistent if not nonexistent. Yet, existing data seem to indicate that such problems are indeed common and account for a major proportion of clinical services, especially in primary care settings. A World Health Organization study reported ICD-10 diagnoses of hypochondriasis in nearly 1% and of somatization disorder in nearly 3% of patients in primary care clinics in 14 countries (Ormel et al. 1994). Another study using primary care sites found 14% of 1,000 patients to be suffering from some somatoform disorder: 8% with "multisomatoform disorder" (see the undifferentiated somatoform disorder section), 4% with somatoform disorder NOS, 2% with hypochondriasis, and 1% with somatoform pain disorder (Spitzer et al. 1994).

Considering prevalence in nonclinic, community populations, Escobar and coworkers (1989) reported that nearly 20% of community respondents in Puerto Rico and 4.4% of comparable non-Hispanic Los Angeles residents fulfilled criteria for an "abridged somatization disorder," a construct with a lower threshold than somatization disorder that would generally correspond to a DSM-IV-TR diagnosis of either undifferentiated somatoform disorder or somatoform disorder NOS. In the Epidemiological Catchment Area community study (Robins et al. 1984), a low estimate of the frequency of somatization disorder (0.06–0.6%) was reported. Methodological problems may have led to a falsely low rate, as discussed in the somatization disorder section. Other studies have estimated much greater frequency, at least among women (Table 71–2).

In consideration of the substantial frequency of somatoform disorders in nonpsychiatric settings, instruments have been designed to aid primary care physicians in diagnosing psychiatric conditions. The Primary Care Evalu-

| Table 71–2 | Epidemiology and Natural History of the Somatoform Disorders | | |
|---|---|---|---|
| Somatoform Disorder | Prevalence and Incidence | Age at Onset | Course and Progress |
| Somatization disorder | US women 0.2–2%; women/men = 10:1 | First symptoms by adolescence, full criteria met by mid-20s, not after 30 yr by definition | Chronic with fluctuations in severity<br>Most active in early adulthood<br>Full remissions rare |
| Undifferentiated somatoform disorder | "Abridged somatization disorder" type estimated as 11–15% of US adults, 20% in Puerto Rico<br>Preponderance of women in US but not Puerto Rico | Variable | Variable conversion disorder |
| Conversion disorder | Conversion symptoms common, as high as 25%<br>Treated conversion symptoms: 11–500 per 100,000<br>5–14% of general hospital admissions<br>5–24% of psychiatric outpatients<br>1–3% of psychiatric outpatient referrals<br>4% of neurological outpatient referrals<br>1% of neurological admissions | Late childhood to early adulthood, most before age 35 yr<br>If onset in middle or late life, neurological or general medical condition more likely | Individual conversion symptoms generally remit within days to weeks<br>Relapse within 1 yr in 20–25% |
| Pain disorder | 10–15% of US adults with work disability owing to back pain yearly<br>A predominant symptom in more than half of general hospital admissions<br>Present in as many as 38% of psychiatric admissions, 18% of psychiatric outpatients | Any age | Good if less than 6 mo in duration<br>Unemployment, personality disorder, potential for compensation, and habituation to addictive drugs associated with poorer prognosis |
| Hypochondriasis | Perhaps 4–9% in general medical settings, but unclear whether full syndrome criteria are met<br>Equal in both sexes | Early adulthood typical | 10% recovery, two-thirds a chronic but fluctuating course, 25% do poorly<br>Better prognosis if acute onset, absence of personality disorder, absence of secondary gain |
| Body dysmorphic disorder | Not routinely screened for in psychiatric or general population studies<br>Perhaps 2% of patients seeking corrective cosmetic surgery | Adolescence or early adulthood<br>Perhaps in women at menopause | Generally chronic, fluctuating severity<br>In a lifetime, multiple defects perceived<br>Incapacitating: one-third house-bound |
| Somatoform disorder NOS | Unknown | Variable | Variable |

ation of Mental Disorders (PRIME-MD) (Spitzer et al. 1994) includes somatoform items in its screening questionnaire and in its physician education guide. The DSM-IV Primary Care Edition (DSM-IV-PC) includes an "unexplained physical symptoms" algorithm among the nine it included to address the most common psychiatric symptom groups presenting in primary care settings (American Psychiatric Association 1995).

The epidemiology of the specific somatoform disorders is discussed individually in following sections.

## Treatment

Whereas specific somatoform disorders indicate specific treatment approaches, some general guidelines apply to the somatoform disorders as a whole (Figure 71–2 and Table 71–3). By reorganizing and synthesizing the recommendations of Stoudemire (1988) and Kellner (1991) into three goals and three general strategies, the therapeutic goals include (1) as an overriding goal, prevention of the adoption of the sick role and chronic invalidism; (2) minimization of unnecessary costs and complications by avoiding unwarranted hospitalizations, diagnostic and treatment procedures, and medications (especially those of an addictive potential); and (3) effective treatment of comorbid psychiatric disorders, such as depressive and anxiety syndromes. The three general treatment strategies include (1) consistent treatment, generally by the same physician, with careful coordination if multiple physicians are involved; (2) supportive office visits, scheduled at regular intervals rather than in response to symptoms; and (3) a gradual shift in focus from symptoms to an emphasis on personal and interpersonal problems.

## SOMATIZATION DISORDER

### Definition

As defined in DSM-IV, somatization disorder is a polysymptomatic somatoform disorder characterized by multiple recurring pains and gastrointestinal, sexual, and pseudoneurological symptoms occurring for a period of years with onset before age 30 years. The physical complaints are not intentionally produced and are not fully explained by a general medical condition or the direct effects of a substance. To warrant diagnosis, they must result in medical attention or significant impairment in social, occupational, or other important areas of functioning.

The concept and criteria for somatization disorder (historically referred to as hysteria or Briquet's syndrome) embraced by DSM-IV are the distillation of a long and convoluted struggle to describe this complex, multifaceted syndrome (Martin 1988). As reviewed by Veith (1965), the origins of the concept can be traced to descriptions in the medical literature of the pre-Hippocratic Egyptians, who

---

### DSM-IV-TR Criteria 300.81

#### Somatization Disorder

A. A history of many physical complaints beginning before age 30 years that occur over a period of several years and result in treatment being sought or significant impairment in social, occupational, or other important areas of functioning.

B. Each of the following criteria must have been met, with individual symptoms occurring at any time during the course of the disturbance:

  (1) *four pain symptoms*: a history of pain related to at least four different sites or functions (e.g., head, abdomen, back, joints, extremities, chest, rectum, during menstruation, during sexual intercourse, or during urination)

  (2) *two gastrointestinal symptoms*: a history of at least two gastrointestinal symptoms other than pain (e.g., nausea, bloating, vomiting other than during pregnancy, diarrhea, or intolerance of several different foods)

  (3) *one sexual symptom*: a history of at least one sexual or reproductive symptom other than pain (e.g., sexual indifference, erectile or ejaculatory dysfunction, irregular menses, excessive menstrual bleeding, vomiting throughout pregnancy)

  (4) *one pseudoneurological symptom*: a history of at least one symptom or deficit suggesting a neurological condition not limited to pain (conversion symptoms such as impaired coordination or balance, paralysis or localized weakness, difficulty swallowing or lump in throat, aphonia, urinary retention, hallucinations, loss of touch or pain sensation, double vision, blindness, deafness, seizures; dissociative symptoms such as amnesia; or loss of consciousness other than fainting)

C. Either (1) or (2):

  (1) after appropriate investigation, each of the symptoms in criterion B cannot be fully explained by a known general medical condition or the direct effects of a substance (e.g., a drug of abuse, a medication)

  (2) when there is a related general medical condition, the physical complaints or resulting social or occupational impairment is in excess of what would be expected from the history, physical examination, or laboratory findings

D. The symptoms are not intentionally produced or feigned (as in factitious disorder or malingering).

---

Reprinted with permission from the Diagnostic and Statistical Manual of Mental Disorders, Fourth Edition, Text Revision. Copyright 2000 American Psychiatric Association.

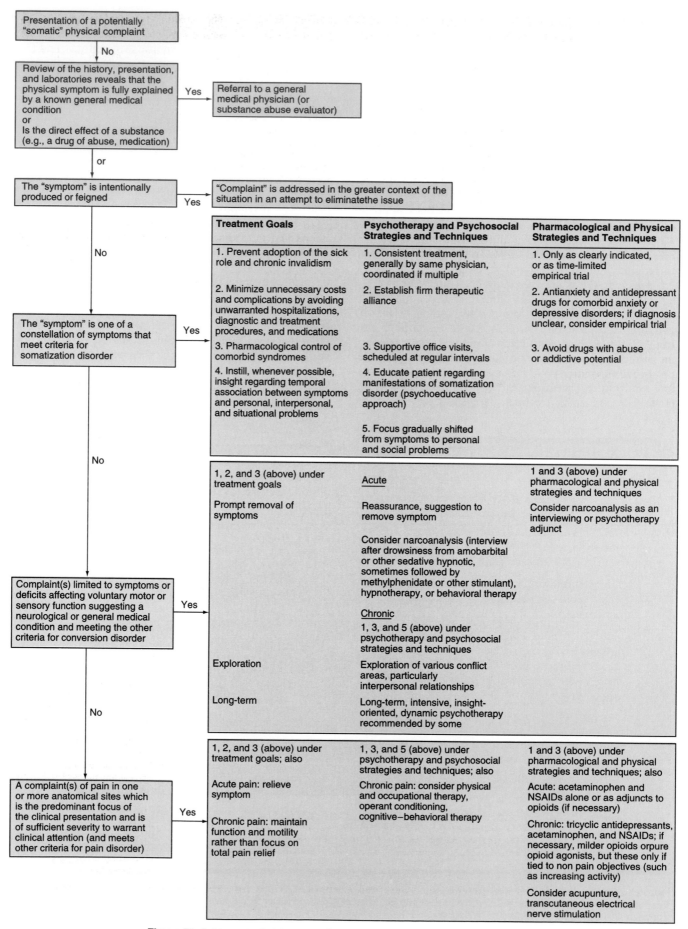

**Figure 71–2** *Diagnostic decision tree and treatment algorithm for Somatoform Disorders.*

| Table 71–3 | Treatment of DSM-IV-TR Somatoform Disorders | | |
|---|---|---|---|
| **Somatoform Disorder** | **Treatment Goals** | **Psychotherapy and Psychosocial Strategies and Techniques** | **Pharmacological and Physical Strategies and Techniques*** |
| Somatoform disorders, as a group | 1. Prevent adoption of the sick role and chronic invalidism<br>2. Minimize unnecessary costs and complications by avoiding unwarranted hospitalizations, diagnostic and treatment procedures, and medications<br>3. Pharmacological control of comorbid syndromes | 1. Consistent treatment, generally by same physician, coordinated if multiple<br>2. Supportive office visits, scheduled at regular intervals<br>3. Focus gradually shifted from symptoms to personal and social problems | 1. Only as clearly indicated, or as time-limited empirical trial<br>2. Avoid drugs with abuse or addictive potential |
| Somatization disorder | 1, 2, and 3; also<br>• Instill, whenever possible, insight regarding temporal association between symptoms and personal, interpersonal, and situational problems | 1, 2, and 3; also<br>• Establish firm therapeutic alliance<br>• Educate patient regarding manifestations of somatization disorder (psychoeducative approach)<br>• Consistent reassurance | 1 and 2, also<br>• Antianxiety and antidepressant drugs for comorbid anxiety or depressive disorders; if diagnosis unclear, consider empirical trial |
| Undifferentiated somatoform disorder | 1, 2, and 3 | 1, 2, and 3 | 1 and 2 |
| Conversion disorder | 1, 2, and 3; also<br>• Prompt removal of symptoms | Acute:<br>• Reassurance, suggestion to remove symptom<br>• Consider narcoanalysis (interview after drowsiness from amobarbital or other sedative–hypnotic, sometimes followed by methylphenidate or other stimulant), hypnotherapy, or behavioral therapy<br>Chronic:<br>1, 2, and 3<br>• Exploration of various conflict areas, particularly interpersonal relationships<br>• Long-term, intensive, insight-oriented dynamic psychotherapy recommended by some | 1 and 2; also<br>• Consider narcoanalysis as an interviewing or psychotherapy adjunct |
| Pain disorder | 1, 2, and 3; also<br>• Acute pain: Relieve symptom<br>• Chronic pain: Maintain function and motility rather than focus on total pain relief | 1, 2, and 3; also<br>• Chronic pain: Consider physical and occupational therapy, operant conditioning, cognitive–behavioral therapy | 1 and 2; also<br>• Acute: Acetaminophen and NSAIDs alone or as adjuncts to opioids (if necessary)<br>• Chronic: Tricyclic antidepressants, acetaminophen, and NSAIDs; if necessary, milder opioids or pure opioid agonists, but these only if tied to nonpain objectives (such as increasing activity)<br>• Consider acupuncture, transcutaneous electrical nerve stimulation |
| Hypochondriasis | 1, 2, and 3; also<br>• Pharmacological control of central syndrome itself | 1, 2, and 3; also<br>• Cognitive–behavioral therapy involving prevention of checking rituals and reassurance seeking | 2; also<br>• Attempt to decrease hypochondriacal symptoms with SSRIs at higher than antidepressant doses or clomipramine |

*Continues*

| Table 71–3 | Treatment of DSM-IV-TR Somatoform Disorders *Continued* | | |
| --- | --- | --- | --- |
| Somatoform Disorder | Treatment Goals | Psychotherapy and Psychosocial Strategies and Techniques | Pharmacological and Physical Strategies and Techniques* |
| Body dysmorphic disorder | 1, 2, and 3, especially avoiding corrective surgery; also • Pharmacological control of central syndrome itself | 1, 2, and 3; also • Cognitive–behavioral therapy involving prevention of checking rituals and reassurance seeking | 2; also • Attempt to decrease hypochondriacal symptoms with SSRIs at higher than antidepressant doses or clomipramine |
| Somatoform disorder NOS | 1, 2, and 3; also • Evaluate carefully for alternative general medical or other psychiatric disorder to which the symptoms can be attributed | 1, 2, and 3 | 1 and 2 |

*NSAIDs, Nonsteroidal antiinflammatory drugs; SSRIs, selective serotonin reuptake inhibitors.

attributed otherwise unexplained physical symptoms to peregrinations of the uterus; this hypothesis probably derived from observations that such presentations were predominantly seen in women with onset during the reproductive years. In the 5th century AD, the Hippocratic literature formalized the concept, adopting the term *hysteria* from the Greek word for uterus. In time, belief in a uterine cause was abandoned, but use of the term hysteria continued.

In the mid-19th century, Paul Briquet (1859) adopted the term hysteria for the syndrome he described in his monograph, *Traité Clinique et Thérapeutique à l'Hystérie*, as characterized by dramatic and excessive medical complaints without evidence of an organic cause. Ultimately, such a description would constitute the basis for somatization disorder, yet the medical complaint aspect of hysteria was overshadowed for many years by psychodynamic interpretations originating with observations by Breuer and Freud (1955). In fact, much of Freud's theory of the unconscious can be traced to his work with hysteria. According to psychodynamic theory, "psychic energy" was converted into physical symptoms, thereby the term *conversion*. Although conversion symptoms were eventually reserved for pseudoneurological complaints, the more general term somatization came to be used for any body symptoms explained as an expression of a neurosis (Lipowski 1988, Steckel et al. 1943).

In time, the physical complaint aspect of hysteria was de-emphasized, with increased attention to intrapsychic, personality, or characterological features of hysteria. Meanwhile, in lay usage, hysteria came to signify excessive or histrionic emotional displays regardless of whether physical symptoms were involved. By the 1950s, the meaning had become so diffuse that the term hysteria, as attacked by Chodoff and Lyons (1958), had at least five connotations, only one of which related to physical complaints.

In 1951, Purtell and colleagues (1951) resurrected Briquet's formulation of a syndrome characterized by multiple medically unexplained somatic complaints, adding a quantitative perspective that required a given number of symptoms from a specified list for a diagnosis. This approach was refined in 1962 by Perley and Guze (1962) and again in 1972 by Feighner and colleagues (1972), who included hysteria among the 13 psychiatric diagnoses "canonized" as sufficiently studied to be considered valid and reliable psychiatric disorders. As summarized by Barsky (1989), the validity, reliability, and internal consistency of the Feighner criteria for hysteria were supported in clinical, epidemiological, and follow-up studies. In particular, the syndrome was stable, with an 80 to 90% probability that 6 to 8 years after the diagnosis was made, the clinical picture would be essentially the same and no new medical or mental disorder would develop as an explanation for the original complaints.

Unfortunately, although feasible in research settings, the Feighner hysteria criteria were cumbersome clinically. Twenty-five medically unexplained symptoms from a specified list of 59 symptoms organized into 10 groups were required for a "definite" diagnosis, 20 for a "probable" diagnosis. Dissemination to different functions and organ systems was considered an essential aspect of the syndrome, a diagnosis requiring symptoms from 9 of the 10 groups.

DSM-I and DSM-II mentioned only conversion and dissociative reactions (hysterical neurosis: conversion and dissociative types in DSM-II), virtually ignoring a polysymptomatic disorder. ICD-9 listed somatization disorder and Briquet's disorder under other neurotic disorders. DSM-III recognized the need for inclusion of the syndrome characterized in the Feighner criteria but sought to make the diagnosis more usable. Somatization disorder was the term coined to escape the pejorative connotation of hysteria, yet avoiding the use of eponyms such as Briquet's syndrome. It also attempted to simplify the criteria of Feighner and colleagues by reducing the required number of symptoms to 14 in women and 12 (to prevent a possible sex bias) in men, from a list of 37 potential symptoms, and abolishing the group requirement. Whereas the Feighner criteria approach and its predecessors included anxiety and depressive symptoms, DSM-III did not, allowing diagnoses of comorbid anxiety and mood disorders. DSM-III-R incorporated minor changes, including elimination of the sex differential; it required 13 symptoms in both men and women and shortened the list of potential symptoms to 35.

Despite such efforts to simplify, the somatization disorder construct remained cumbersome, which undoubtedly contributed to underuse (Cloninger 1996). As a result, a new diagnostic algorithm was developed by Cloninger and colleagues from a reanalysis of an existing data set requiring four pain, two nonpain gastrointestinal, one sexual or reproductive, and one pseudoneurological symptom (either conversion or dissociative) (Cloninger and Yutzy 1993, Yutzy et al. 1992). In a multisite field trial study, these criteria were shown to identify a syndrome with good correspondence to hysteria as defined by Feighner and colleagues (because of demonstrated reliability and validity of the "diagnostic gold standard") (Yutzy et al. 1995), as well as with DSM-III and DSM-III-R criteria. The ICD-10 also includes somatization disorder within a somatoform disorder grouping. However, in addition to multiple unexplained somatic symptoms, ICD-10 requires "persistent refusal to accept medical reassurance that there is no adequate physical cause for the physical symptoms." Attributable in part to this requirement, DSM-IV, Feighner, DSM-III, and DSM-III-R criteria all showed poor agreement with the ICD-10 criteria in the multisite field trial (Yutzy et al. 1995).

It remains to be seen whether the DSM-IV diagnosis of somatization disorder will be used broadly and appropriately. Unresolved problems include that the term somatization disorder has acquired a pejorative connotation; a tendency to diagnose more readily treatable symptoms such as anxiety and depressive syndromes without considering the underlying illness; and that authorization and reimbursement for treatment of this chronic condition are often challenged or denied. It is relatively easier to obtain approval for an intervention on the basis of major depressive disorder, for example, than on the basis of a disorder that is much more likely to be poorly understood by case reviewers.

Thus, whereas somatization disorder as currently defined in DSM-IV is not entirely equivalent to the many previous definitions, it has a common conceptual core and appears to identify populations of patients similar to those defined by the Purtell–Robins, Perley–Guze, DSM-III, and DSM-III-R criteria. Thus, subsequent discussions in this chapter use the term somatization disorder, even in reviewing findings ascertained by these other various criteria.

## Epidemiology

In the US, somatization disorder is found predominantly in women, with a female/male ratio of approximately 10:1 (see Table 71–2). This ratio is not as large in some other cultures (e.g., in Greeks and Puerto Ricans). Thus, gender- and culture-specific rates are more meaningful than generalized figures. The lifetime prevalence of somatization disorder in US women has been estimated to be between 0.2 and 2%. The magnitude of this discrepancy is attributable, at least in part, to methodological differences. The Epidemiological Catchment Area study (Robins et al. 1984), the most recent large-scale general population study in the US to include an assessment for somatization disorder, found a lifetime risk of somatization disorder of only 0.2 to 0.3% in US women. However, this study may have underestimated the prevalence of somatization disorder because nonphysician interviewers were used. It is argued that it is difficult for lay interviewers to critically assess whether somatic symptoms are fully explained by physical conditions. As a result, they may more readily accept patients' general medical explanations of symptoms, resulting in fewer diagnoses of somatization disorder. With age and method of assessment taken into account, the lifetime risk for somatization disorder was estimated to be 2% in US women (Cloninger et al. 1975).

## Etiology and Pathophysiology

Many theories on the cause of somatization disorder have been proposed since the early uterine hypothesis was dismissed. Yet, etiology remains unknown. Psychodynamic hypotheses regarding the physical expression of unconscious conflict by conversion or somatization have been influential. Even Freud assumed a "constitutional diathesis," as had Charcot before him. Evidence exists for both biological and psychosocial contributions.

Somatization disorder has been shown to be familial. It is observed that in 10 to 20% of female relatives of patients affected by somatization disorder there is a lifetime risk in US women 10 to 20 times greater than that of the general population (Guze et al. 1986). Yet, aggregation in families may be attributable to both genetic and environmental factors. A cross-fostering study of a Swedish population demonstrated that genetic background and postnatal influences contribute to the risk of somatization disorder independently (Bohman et al. 1984, Cloninger et al. 1984). Of additional interest are observations that male relatives of patients with somatization disorder show increased rates of antisocial personality and alcoholism, suggesting an etiological link (Cloninger 1993).

Certain promising theories have focused on learning principles with possible organic underpinnings. Ford (1983) and later Quill (1985) postulated a social communication model based on learning theory to explain somatization disorder. Both hypothesized that individuals learn to somatize as a means of expressing their wants and needs and evoking care, nurturance, and support from family and caregivers. That different sex ratios may exist in different cultures suggests that such learning differs from culture to culture.

In the 1970s, impaired information-processing problems involving attention and memory were identified in experimental neuropsychological testing (Ludwig 1972, Bendefeldt et al. 1976). Such deficits may result in vague, nonspecific, and impressionistic description for experience. These may underlie a tendency for excessive somatic complaints and, together with tendencies for impulsiveness and monotony intolerance, may contribute to the often associated multiple personal and social problems (Cloninger 1993). In 1981, Flor-Henry and coworkers (1981) reported that the pattern of neuropsychological defects found in subjects with somatization disorder differed from that in normal control, schizophrenic, and psychotic depression comparison groups. Subjects with somatization disorder had greater bilateral, symmetrical patterns of frontal lobe dysfunction in comparison with normal control subjects and greater dominant hemisphere impairment than control and depressive subjects. Nondominant hemisphere dysfunction was also identified, with greater impairment in the anterior as opposed to posterior regions. However, subjects with somatization disorder had less nondominant hemisphere disorganization than schizophrenic subjects. Of interest, these findings were similar to findings in male patients with antisocial personality disorder, giving further support to an etiological link with this disorder.

## Diagnosis and Differential Diagnosis

As defined in DSM-IV, somatization disorder is characterized by multiple recurring physical symptoms and, as will be described, often multiple psychiatric complaints (Wetzel et al. 1994). Thus, it is not surprising that somatization disorder may present in a manner suggestive of multiple general medical and, although too often forgotten, psychiatric disorders (Table 71–4). Indeed, it can be said that an essential aspect of somatization disorder is its simulation of other syndromes. As described by Preskorn (1995),

"Briquet's syndrome (i.e., somatization disorder) is fundamentally a syndrome of apparent syndromes" (see Table 71–4). Thus, the first task in the diagnosis of somatization disorder is the exclusion of other suggested medical and psychiatric conditions.

To help in this, Cloninger (1986) identified three features that generally characterize somatization disorder but rarely general medical disorders. Slightly restated, these are (1) involvement of multiple organ systems, (2) early onset and chronic course without development of physical signs or structural abnormalities, and (3) absence of laboratory abnormalities characteristic of the suggested physical disorders (Table 71–5). Another way of characterizing the distinction is the "reverse funnel effect" (Pinta 1995, personal communication). With most general medical conditions, the process of investigation "funnels down" to fewer

---

| **Table 71–4** | **Somatoform Disorders: A Syndrome of Simulated Syndromes** | | |
|---|---|---|---|

| Symptom Examples | Examples of Simulated Neurological Conditions | Examples of Simulated Nonneurological General Medical Conditions | Examples of Simulated Psychiatric Conditions |
|---|---|---|---|
| Symptoms* of somatization disorder | | | |
| Pain | | | |
|   Headache | Migraine | Temporal arteritis | Pain disorder |
|   Abdomen | "Abdominal epilepsy" | Peptic ulcer disease | Pain disorder |
|   Back | Lumbosacral radiculopathy | Ruptured disk | Pain disorder |
|   Joints or extremities | | Fibromyalgia | Pain disorder |
|   Chest | | Angina | Panic disorder |
|   Menstruation, intercourse | | Endometriosis | Dyspareunia, vaginismus |
|   Urination | Neurogenic bladder | Urinary tract infection | |
| Gastrointestinal (nonpain) | | | |
|   Difficulty swallowing | Myasthenia gravis | Esophageal motility disorder | Eating disorder |
|   Nausea | Raised intracranial pressure | Meniere's disease | Eating disorder |
|   Bloating | | Galactase deficiency | Eating disorder |
|   Vomiting (nonpregnancy) | Raised intracranial pressure | | Eating disorder |
|   Diarrhea | | Irritable bowel syndrome | Eating disorder |
|   Intolerance to several foods | | Food allergy | Eating disorder |
| Sexual (nonpain) | | | |
|   Loss of interest | | | Major depressive episode |
|   Erectile–ejaculatory dysfunction | Diabetic neuropathy | Antihypertensive drug effect | |
|   Menorrhagia | | Leiomyofibroma | |
|   Vomiting throughout pregnancy | | Preeclampsia, eclampsia | |
| Pseudoneurological | | | |
|   Conversion | | | |
|     Sensory | Stroke (hemianesthesia) | | Schizophrenia/(hallucinations) |
|     Motor | Huntington's disease | Myopathy | Catatonia |
|     Seizures | Epilepsy | Electrolyte imbalance | Catatonia |
|     Mixed | Multiple sclerosis | Electrolyte imbalance | Catatonia |
|   Dissociative | | | |
|     Amnesia | Amnestic disorder | Anticholinergic drug effects | Dissociative identity disorder |
|     Loss of consciousness (nonfainting) | Coma | Metabolic encephalopathy | Catatonia |
| Symptoms* often associated with somatization disorder | | | |
|   Anxiety, panic | | Pheochromocytoma | Generalized anxiety and panic disorders |
|   Dysphoria, affective lability | Frontal lobe syndrome | Endocrinopathy | Major mood disorders |
|   Cluster B personality features | Frontal lobe syndrome | Acute intermittent porphyria | Brief psychotic disorder |

*All of these symptoms may be reported by patients with somatization disorder, without the clinical consistency and pathological findings to support the diagnosis of neurological, general medical, or psychiatric conditions separate from somatization disorder.

Developed in conjunction with Sheldon H. Preskorn.

| Table 71–5 | Discrimination of Somatization Disorder from General Medical Conditions |
|---|---|

| Features Suggesting Somatization Disorder | Features Suggesting a General Medical Condition |
|---|---|
| Involvement of multiple organ systems | Involvement of single or few organ systems |
| Early onset and chronic course without development of physical signs or structural abnormalities | If early onset and chronic course, development of physical signs and structural abnormalities |
| Absence of laboratory abnormalities characteristic of the suggested general medical condition | Laboratory abnormalities evident |

*Source*: Martin RL and Yutzy SH (1994) Somatoform disorders. In The American Psychiatric Press Textbook of Psychiatry, 2nd ed., Hales RE, Yudofsky SC, and Talbott JA (eds). American Psychiatric Press, Washington DC, p. 600.

and fewer specific diagnostic possibilities; in somatization disorder, the more extensive the investigation, the greater the number of suggested disorders.

Several general medical disorders may also fit this pattern and may be confused with somatization disorder. These include multiple sclerosis, other neuropathies, systemic lupus erythematosus, acute intermittent porphyria, other hepatic and hematopoietic porphyrias, hypercalcemia, certain chronic systemic infections such as brucellosis and trypanosomiasis, myopathies, and vasculitides. In general, such conditions begin with disseminated, nonspecific subjective symptoms and transient or equivocal physical signs or laboratory abnormalities.

Somatization disorder is characterized by excessive psychiatric as well as physical complaints (Wetzel et al. 1994). Thus, other psychiatric disorders, including anxiety and mood disorders and schizophrenia, may be suggested. Although no specific exclusion criteria regarding other psychiatric disorders are given, one must be careful in accepting "comorbidity" and critically evaluate whether suggested syndromes are truly additional syndromes or simply manifestations of somatization disorder (Preskorn 1995).

The overlap between somatization disorder and anxiety disorders may be a particular problem. Patients with somatization disorder frequently complain of many of the same somatic symptoms as patients with anxiety disorders, such as increased muscle tension, features of autonomic hyperactivity, and even discrete panic attacks. Likewise, anxiety disorder patients may report irrational disease concerns and such somatic complaints as those involving gastrointestinal function that are commonly seen in somatization disorder. However, patients with anxiety disorders neither typically report sexual and menstrual complaints or conversion or dissociative symptoms as in somatization disorder, nor do they have the associated histrionic presentation and personal, marital, and social maladjustment common in patients with somatization disorder (Cloninger 1993).

It must be remembered that an anxiety disorder may be comorbid with somatization disorder. Here, objective observation of the patient rather than reliance on the patient's report may facilitate an additional diagnosis. For example, patients with somatization disorder may report that they are presently overwhelmed by anxiety while speaking calmly or even cheerfully about their symptoms, or they may be redirectable while in the midst of a reported panic attack.

Mood disorders (in particular depression) frequently present with multiple somatic complaints, especially in certain cultures such as in India, where somatic but not mental complaints are acceptable. A longitudinal history identifying age at onset and course of illness may facilitate discrimination of a mood disorder from somatization disorder. In mood disorders, the age at onset of the somatic symptoms is generally later than in somatization disorder; their first appearance generally correlates discretely with the onset of mood symptoms, and a lengthy pattern of multiple recurring somatic complaints is not seen. Also, resolution of the underlying mood disorder will generally result in disappearance of the somatic complaints.

From the other perspective, patients with somatization disorder often present with depressive complaints. In somatization disorder, a thorough investigation will reveal a multitude of somatic as well as "depressive" symptoms. Interestingly, somatization disorder patients complaining of depression have been found to proffer greater depressive symptoms than individuals with major depression (DeSouza et al. 1988). As in anxiety disorders, major depressive episodes may occur in patients with somatization disorder and must be differentiated from the tendency to have multiple complaints, which is characteristic of somatization disorder. As with anxiety disorders, in considering comorbidity with a depressive disorder, the patient's reports should be corroborated by collateral information or by direct observation. Thus, the veracity of the self-report of overwhelming depression and suicidal ideation should be doubted if the patient appears cheerful and charming, at least at times, when interviewed, or if the patient is reported to be actively involved in social activities on an inpatient psychiatric service.

Schizophrenia may present with generally single but occasionally multiple unexplained somatic complaints. Interview usually uncovers psychotic symptoms such as delusions, hallucinations, or disorganized thought. In some cases, the underlying psychosis cannot be identified initially, but in time, schizophrenia will become manifest (Goodwin and Guze 1989). Hallucinations are included as examples of conversion symptoms in DSM-IV, as they were in the Purtell, Perley–Guze, and Feighner criteria, which may lead to diagnostic problems (Martin 1996). As discussed in the conversion disorder section, careful analysis of this symptom is warranted so that a misdiagnosis is not made, relegating a patient to long-term neuroleptic treatment on the basis of conversion hallucinations.

Patients with histrionic, borderline, and antisocial personality disorders frequently have an excess of somatic complaints, at times presenting with somatization disorder. Cloninger and Guze (1979) and Cloninger and colleagues (1975) have identified that antisocial personality disorder and somatization disorder cluster in individuals and within families and may share common causes. Dissociative phenomena, in particular dissociative identity disorder, are commonly associated with somatization disorder (Martin 1996). Because dissociative symptoms are included in the diagnostic criteria for somatization, a separate diagnosis of a dissociative disorder is not made if such symptoms occur only in the course of somatization disorder.

Unlike in hypochondriasis and body dysmorphic disorder, in which preoccupations and fears concerning the interpretation of symptoms predominate, the focus in somatization disorder is on the physical complaints themselves. Unlike in pain disorder and conversion disorder, multiple complaints of different types are reported; by definition in DSM-IV, the history is of pain in at least four sites or functions (e.g., pain with intercourse, pain in swallowing), at least two nonpain gastrointestinal symptoms, at least one nonpain sexual or reproductive symptom, and at least one conversion or dissociative (i.e., pseudoneurological) symptom.

Whereas criteria require the onset of symptoms before the age of 30 years, most patients will have had some symptoms at least by adolescence or early adulthood. Symptoms are often described in a dramatic yet imprecise way and may be reported inconsistently from interview to interview (Martin et al. 1979). The medical history is usually complicated with multiple medical investigations, procedures, and medication trials. If there have been symptoms for at least 6 months but the onset is later than at age 30 years, or if the required number and distribution of symptoms are not evident, undifferentiated somatoform disorder is diagnosed. If the duration has been less than 6 months, somatoform disorder NOS applies. In general, the greater the number and diversity of symptoms, and the longer they have been present without development of signs of an underlying general medical condition, the greater can be the confidence that a diagnosis of somatization disorder is correct.

## Course, Natural History, and Prognosis

Somatization disorder is rare in children younger than 9 years of age (Robins and O'Neal 1953) (see Table 71–2). Characteristic symptoms of somatization disorder usually begin during adolescence, and the criteria are met by the mid-twenties (Guze and Perley 1963). Somatization disorder is a chronic illness characterized by fluctuations in the frequency and diversity of symptoms (Guze et al. 1986). Full remissions occur rarely, if ever. Whereas the most active symptomatic phase is in early adulthood, aging does not appear to lead to total remission (Goodwin and Guze 1989). Pribor and colleagues (1994) found that women with somatization disorder older than 55 years did not differ from younger somatization patients in the number of somatic symptoms. Longitudinal follow-up studies have confirmed that 80 to 90% of patients initially diagnosed with somatization disorder will maintain a consistent clinical picture and be rediagnosed similarly after 6 to 8 years (Cloninger 1993, Cloninger et al. 1986). Women with somatization disorder seen in psychiatric settings are at increased risk for attempted suicide, although such attempts are usually unsuccessful and may reflect manipulative gestures more than intent to die (Martin et al. 1985). It is not clear whether such risk is true for patients with somatization disorder seen only in general medical settings.

## Treatment

First, a "management" rather than a "curative" strategy is recommended for somatization disorder. With the current absence of an identified definitive treatment, a modest, practical, empirical approach should be taken. This should include efforts to minimize distress and functional impairments associated with the multiple somatic complaints; to avoid unwarranted diagnostic and therapeutic procedures and medications; and to prevent potential complications including chronic invalidism and drug dependence.

In such regard, the general recommendations outlined for somatoform disorders should be followed (see Table 71–3). Consistent with these guidelines, Ford (1983) and Quill (1985) recommended that the patient be encouraged to see a single physician with an understanding of and, preferably, experience in treating somatization disorder. This helps limit the number of unnecessary evaluations and treatments. Both Smith and colleagues (1986) and Murphy (1982) advocated routine, brief, supportive office visits scheduled at regular intervals to provide reassurance and prevent patients from "needing to develop" symptoms to obtain care and attention. This "medical" management can well be provided by a primary care physician, perhaps with consultation with a psychiatrist. The study by Smith and colleagues (1986) demonstrated that such a regimen led to markedly decreased health care costs, with no apparent decrements in health or satisfaction of patients.

More ambitious goals have been proposed with the recommendation for multiple approaches including individual psychotherapy, nonfocused group therapy, and electroconvulsive therapy (Martin and Yutzy 1994). Whereas early observations indicated some promise with each of these approaches, studies have been generally uncontrolled and used small samples. Subsequent investigations have rarely attempted to replicate reported findings using sophisticated methodology.

Of note in the treatment of somatization disorder was the identification in 1935 by Luff and Garrod (1935) of a three-part approach. Scallett and coworkers (1976) subsequently endorsed this approach, which they called eclectic, recommending "reeducation, reassurance, and suggestion." This approach was further developed by multiple authors, such as Quill (1985), Cloninger (1986), Smith and colleagues (1986), and Murphy (1982), from whom three interrelated components emerge: (1) establishment of a strong physician–patient relationship or bond; (2) education of the patient regarding the nature of the psychiatric condition; and (3) provision of support and reassurance.

The first component, establishing a strong therapeutic bond, is important in the treatment of somatization disorder. Without it, it will be difficult for the patient to overcome skepticism deriving from past experience with many physicians and other therapists who "never seemed to help." In addition, trust must be strong enough to withstand the stress of withholding unwarranted diagnostic and therapeutic procedures that the patient may feel are indicated. The cornerstone of establishing a therapeutic relationship is laid when the psychiatrist indicates an understanding of the patient's pain and suffering, legitimizing the symptoms as real. This demonstrates a willingness to provide direct compassionate assistance. A full investigation of the medical and psychosocial histories, including extensive record review, will illustrate to patients the willingness of the psychiatrist to gain the fullest understanding of them and their plight. This also provides another opportunity to evaluate for the presence of an underlying medical disorder and to obtain a fuller picture of psychosocial difficulties that may relate temporally to somatic symptoms.

Only after the diagnosis has been clearly established and the therapeutic alliance is firmly in place can the psychiatrist confidently limit diagnostic evaluations and therapies to those performed on the basis of objective findings as opposed to merely subjective complaints. Of course, the psychiatrist should remain aware that patients with somatization disorder are still at risk for development of general medical illnesses so that a vigilant perspective should always be maintained.

The second component is education. This involves advising patients that they suffer from a "medically sanctioned illness," that is, a condition recognized by the medical community and one about which a good deal is known. Ultimately, it may be possible to introduce the concept of somatization disorder, which can be described in a positive light (i.e., the patient does not have a progressive, deteriorating, or potentially fatal medical disorder, and the patient is not "going crazy" but has a condition by which many symptoms will be experienced). A realistic discussion of prognosis and treatment options can then follow.

The third component is reassurance. Patients with somatization disorder often have control and insecurity issues, which often come to the forefront when they perceive that a particular physical complaint is not being adequately addressed. Explicit reassurance should be given that the appropriate inquiries and investigations are being performed and that the possibility of an underlying physical disorder as the explanation for symptoms is being reasonably considered.

In time, it may be appropriate to gradually shift emphasis away from somatic symptoms to consideration of personal and interpersonal issues. In some patients, it may be appropriate to posit a causal theory between somatic symptoms and "stress," that is, that there may be a temporal association between symptoms and personal, interpersonal, and even occupational problems. In patients for whom such "insight" is difficult, behavioral techniques may be useful.

Even following such therapeutic guidelines, patients with somatization disorder are often difficult to treat. Attention-seeking behavior, demands, and manipulation are common, necessitating firm limits and careful attention to boundary issues. This, again, is a management rather than a curative approach. Thus, such behaviors should generally be dealt with directively rather than interpreted to the patient.

## Pharmacological and Other Somatic Treatments

No effective somatic treatments for somatization disorder itself have been identified. In the 1960s, Wheatley (1962) reported that low doses of anxiolytic drugs provided symptom amelioration in double-blind clinical trials using general practitioners. He also noted that whereas chlordiazepoxide was recommended for reasons of effectiveness, preference by patients, safety, and symptom relief, the best results were obtained by optimistic physicians using low doses of any anxiolytic medication. Surprisingly little systematic study of the pharmacological management of somatization disorder has been done since.

Patients with somatization disorder may complain of anxiety and depression, suggesting readily treatable comorbid psychiatric disorders. As previously discussed, it is often difficult to distinguish actual comorbid conditions from aspects of somatoform disorder itself. Pharmacological interventions are likely to be helpful in the former but not in the latter. At times, such discrimination will be impossible, and an empirical trial of such treatments may be indicated. Patients with somatization disorder are often inconsistent and erratic in their use of medications. They will often report unusual side effects that may not be explained pharmacologically. This makes evaluation of treatment response difficult. In addition, drug dependence and suicide gestures and attempts are not uncommon.

---

Clinical Vignette 1

A 35-year-old, separated, employed woman was admitted to a psychiatric unit after presenting to the emergency department reporting suicidal feelings that followed a series of arguments with her most recent common-law husband. She reported having been depressed nearly continuously for the past 4 years but had never responded well to antidepressant medications, which often had an "opposite" effect on her. She endorsed virtually all symptoms of a major depressive episode as outlined in DSM-IV. However, she did not appear to be depressed in the interview. In addition to problems with depression, she reported problems with anxiety, complaining of episodes of shortness of breath, chest pain, palpitations, tremulousness, and a feeling of impending doom. At times, she would have prolonged periods with some or all of these symptoms. She reported that she had had a great number of medical problems, but "the doctors keep telling me there's nothing really wrong with me." She reported extreme headaches, "like a knife being stuck through the back of my head into my eye," as well as other headaches virtually every day; other pains including abdominal pain, associated at times with nausea and vomiting; periods of constipation, followed by diarrhea, which had resulted in evaluation for gallbladder and peptic ulcer disease with no significant findings; and pain "in all of my joints," but particularly in her knees and her back, that she said had been diagnosed as degenerative arthritis at age 27 years, yet no deformities had developed since. She had menstrual problems since menarche, with pain that put her to bed and excessive flow with "big, blue clots," which resolved only after a hysterectomy 2 years earlier at age 33 years. The mother of four, she reported a long history of sexual problems including pain with intercourse. She had been told that she had a "tipped uterus." Throughout her life, she was seldom orgasmic and had not enjoyed sex "for years." She reported episodes of blurred vision with "spots" in front of her eyes, which caused her to stop work. She would also have periods when she just could not hear anything, "like someone put their hands over my ears." She also reported periods of uncontrollable shaking and a feeling that she was losing control of her body, for which she had been evaluated for seizures. She reported that, at times, she had feared having some serious medical disease, but "with all the workups I have had, I am sure they would have found something by

Clinical Vignette 1 *continued*

now." She did relate that she found group therapy with "other people with problems like mine" beneficial.

The patient was diagnosed with somatization disorder and comorbid panic disorder. Panic attacks have ceased since institution of buspirone, but she continues to have multiple somatic complaints. After several months of weekly supportive psychotherapy emphasizing education and reassurance, she is beginning to acknowledge that it is unlikely that physical explanations for her symptoms will be identified. She is also showing progress in dealing more constructively with interpersonal and occupational issues.

## UNDIFFERENTIATED SOMATOFORM DISORDER

### Definition

As defined in DSM-IV, this category includes disturbances of at least 6 months' duration, with one or more unintentional, clinically significant, medically unexplained physical complaints (see Table 71–1). In a sense, it is a residual category, subsuming syndromes with somatic complaints that do not meet criteria for any of the "differentiated"

---

**DSM-IV-TR Criteria** 300.81

**Undifferentiated Somatoform Disorder**

A. One or more physical complaints (e.g., fatigue, loss of appetite, gastrointestinal or urinary complaints).

B. Either (1) or (2):

   (1) after appropriate investigation, the symptoms cannot be fully explained by a known general medical condition or the direct effects of a substance (e.g., a drug of abuse, a medication)

   (2) when there is a related general medical condition, the physical complaints or resulting social or occupational impairment is in excess of what would be expected from the history, physical examination, or laboratory findings

C. The symptoms cause clinically significant distress or impairment in social, occupational, or other important areas of functioning.

D. Duration of the disturbance is at least 6 months.

E. The disturbance is not better accounted for by another mental disorder (e.g., another somatoform disorder, sexual dysfunction, mood disorder, anxiety disorder, sleep disorder, or psychotic disorder).

F. The symptom is not intentionally produced or feigned (as in factitious disorder or malingering).

---

somatoform disorders yet are not better accounted for by any other mental disorder. On the other hand, it is a less residual category than somatoform disorder NOS, in that the disturbance must last at least 6 months (see Figure 71–1). Virtually any unintentional, medically unexplained physical symptoms causing clinically significant distress or impairment can be considered. In effect, this category serves to capture syndromes that resemble somatization disorder but do not meet full criteria.

The term undifferentiated somatoform disorder was introduced in 1987 with DSM-III-R, replacing the atypical somatoform disorder of DSM-III. However, the category has not been well used, not only by psychiatrists but also by primary care physicians for whom identification of such a syndrome could be useful. Terms that have been used in a similar manner include *subsyndromal*, *forme fruste*, or *abridged* somatization disorder (Kirmayer and Robbins 1991). Escobar and coworkers (1989), defining an abridged syndrome as requiring at least six significant unexplained somatic symptoms for women and four for men, argued that especially in primary care settings, such a condition was much more common than a full somatization disorder and it predicted disability and future use of medical services. This group also argued that this construct met many of the suggested requirements for validity as a psychiatric disorder, although adequate follow-up and family studies have not yet been done.

Due to this as well as the underuse of such a construct, perhaps attributable, at least in part, to the ambiguity of designation as undifferentiated, consideration was given to differentiating an abridged somatization syndrome as "multisomatoform disorder" in DSM-IV. However, owing to uncertainties about the nature of such an entity, especially as to overlap with other syndromes such as anxiety and depressive disorders, and because the few data available suggested a variable course (Cloninger 1996), unlike somatization disorder, such a syndrome was left under the undifferentiated somatoform disorder rubric in DSM-IV. A more specific designation could have proved misleading clinically, promoting a false sense of security, with a tendency to preclude efforts to uncover a general medical or substance-related explanation for symptoms or to identify another psychiatric condition better accounting for the symptoms.

The DSM-IV undifferentiated somatoform disorder category is little changed from DSM-III-R. General medical condition or the direct effects of a substance, as elsewhere in DSM-IV, replaces the "organic pathology" of DSM-III-R, and a threshold of requiring clinically significant distress or impairment was added. Exclusion occurs on the basis of symptoms not better accounted for by another mental disorder rather than by occurrence exclusively during the course of another mental disorder.

### Epidemiology

Some have argued that undifferentiated somatoform disorder is the most common somatoform disorder. Escobar and coworkers (1991), using an abridged somatization disorder construct requiring six somatic symptoms for women and four for men, reported that 11% of non-Hispanic US whites and Hispanics, 15% of US blacks, and 20% of Puerto Ricans in Puerto Rico fulfilled criteria. A preponderance of women was evident in all groups except the Puerto Rican sample (see Table 71–2). According to Escobar, such an abridged somatoform syndrome is 100 times more prevalent than a full somatization disorder.

## Etiology and Pathophysiology

Theories of etiology involving the concept of somatization have been posited by some. As reviewed by Kirmayer and Robbins (1991), somatization can be viewed as "a pattern of illness behavior by which bodily idioms of distress may serve as symbolic means of social regulation as well as protest or contestation." However, as previously discussed, such hypotheses have defied verification.

If it is assumed that undifferentiated somatoform disorder is simply an abridged form of somatization disorder, etiological theories reviewed under that diagnosis should apply. An intriguing research question is why the syndrome is fully expressed in some and only partially expressed in others.

## Diagnosis and Differential Diagnosis

In comparison to when the full criteria for the well-validated somatization disorder are met, exclusion of an as yet undiscovered general medical or substance-induced explanation for physical symptoms is far less certain when the less stringent criteria for undifferentiated somatoform disorder are met. Thus, the diagnosis of undifferentiated somatoform disorder should remain tentative, and new symptoms should be carefully investigated.

Because undifferentiated somatoform disorder represents somewhat of a residual category, the major diagnostic process, once occult general medical conditions and substance-induced explanations have been considered, is one of exclusion. As shown in Figure 71–1, whether the somatic symptoms are intentionally produced as in malingering and factitious disorder must be addressed. Here, motivation for external rewards (for malingering) and a pervasive intent to assume the sick role (for factitious disorder) must be assessed. The next consideration is whether the somatic symptoms are the manifestation of another psychiatric disorder. Anxiety and mood disorders commonly present with somatic symptoms; high rates of anxiety and major depressive disorders are reported in patients with somatic complaints attending family medicine clinics (Kirmayer et al. 1993). Of course, undifferentiated somatoform disorder could be diagnosed in addition to one of these disorders, so long as the symptoms are not accounted for by the other psychiatric disorder. Crucial in this determination is whether the symptoms are present during periods in which the anxiety or mood disorders are not actively present.

Next, other somatoform disorders must be considered. In general, undifferentiated somatoform disorders are characterized by unexplained somatic complaints; the most common according to Escobar and coworkers (Escobar et al. 1989) are female reproductive symptoms, excessive gas, abdominal pain, chest pain, joint pain, palpitations, and fainting, rather than preoccupations or fears as in hypochondriasis or body dysmorphic disorder. However, a patient with some manifestations of these two disorders but not meeting full criteria could conceivably receive a diagnosis of undifferentiated somatoform disorder. An example is a patient with recurrent yet shifting hypochondriacal concerns that do respond to medical reassurance. If symptoms are restricted to those affecting the domains of sexual dysfunction, pain, or pseudoneurological symptoms, and the specific criteria for a sexual dysfunction, pain disorder, and/or conversion disorder are met, the specific disorder or disorders should be diagnosed. If other types of symptoms or symptoms of more than one of these disorders have been present for at least 6 months, yet criteria for somatization disorder are not met, undifferentiated somatoform disorder should be diagnosed. By definition, undifferentiated somatoform disorder requires a duration of 6 months. If this criterion is not met, a diagnosis of somatoform disorder NOS should be considered.

Patients with an apparent undifferentiated somatoform disorder should be carefully evaluated for somatization disorder. Typically, patients with somatization disorder are inconsistent historians, at one evaluation reporting a large number of symptoms fulfilling criteria for the full syndrome, at another time endorsing fewer symptoms (Martin et al. 1979). In addition, with follow-up, additional symptoms may become evident, and criteria for somatization disorder will be satisfied. Patients with multiple somatic complaints not diagnosed with somatization disorder because of a reported onset later than 30 years of age may be inaccurately reporting a later age at onset. If the late age at onset is accurate, the patient should be carefully scrutinized for an occult general medical disorder.

In addition to the range of symptoms specified in the other somatoform disorders, patients complaining primarily of fatigue (chronic fatigue syndrome), bowel problems (irritable bowel syndrome), or multiple muscle aches/weakness (fibromylagia) can be considered for undifferentiated somatoform disorder. Substantial controversy exists regarding the etiology of such syndromes. Even if an explanation on the basis of a known pathophysiological mechanism cannot be established, many argue that the syndromes should be considered general medical conditions. However, for the time being, these syndromes could be considered in a highly tentative manner under the undifferentiated somatoform disorder rubric. Careful reconsideration of the psychiatric label should be undertaken at regular intervals if the symptoms persist. The psychiatrist should remain ever vigilant to the emergence of another general medical or psychiatric condition. Noteworthy is also the fact, when patients are diagnosed with chronic fatigue syndrome, careful evaluation procedures as recommended by an international study group should be followed (Fukuda et al. 1994).

## Course, Natural History, and Prognosis

As shown in Table 71–2, it appears that the course and prognosis of undifferentiated somatoform disorder are highly variable. This is not surprising, because the definition of this disorder allows a great deal of heterogeneity.

## Treatment

In view of the broad inclusion and minimal exclusion criteria for undifferentiated somatoform disorder, it is difficult to make treatment recommendations beyond the generic guidelines outlined for the somatoform disorders in general. More definitive recommendations await a more extensive empirical database. A substantial proportion of patients with undifferentiated somatoform disorders improve or recover with no formal therapy. However, appropriate psychotherapy and pharmacological intervention may accelerate the process.

Kellner (1991) outlined some recommendations for patients with symptoms of headache, fibromyalgia, and chronic fatigue syndrome, conditions that some would include under undifferentiated somatoform disorder. Generally recommended are brief psychotherapy of a supportive and educative nature. As with somatization disorder, the physician–patient relationship is of great importance. Judicious use of pharmacotherapy may be of benefit also, particularly if the somatoform syndrome is intertwined with an anxiety or depressive syndrome. Here, usual antianxiety and antidepressant medications are recommended. Patients with unexplained pains may benefit from pain management strategies as outlined in the pain disorder section.

---

**Clinical Vignette 2**

A 34-year-old woman was referred for psychiatric evaluation of "possible depression and anxiety" by her primary care physician. For at least the past 2 years, she complained of painful, prolonged menstruation with excessive flow, abdominal cramping even when not menstruating, fatigue, and headaches. Medical investigation including extensive blood work, gynecological examination, and gastrointestinal evaluations did not establish any objective findings. Despite her reports of excessive menstruation, she had never been anemic and had not lost any weight. Her headaches varied. Some were preceded by an aura and were associated with nausea, vomiting, and photophobia, but most were consistent with "tension headaches" and relieved by acetaminophen. When discussing her personal life, the patient became tearful. Although she remained married, she reported little support from her husband of 9 years who was dedicated to his work, spending excessive hours at the office and on the road, leaving the patient with much of the responsibility for the household and their three young children aged 8, 6, and 3 years. She felt that she could not tolerate the situation much longer. She was sad but thought that if her home situation improved, she would have hope. She felt exhausted from the time she awoke in the morning to when she went to bed, had some loss of appetite but no weight loss, remained interested in things, but "just didn't have the time." She reported trouble concentrating but attributed it to being interrupted every 5 minutes with some "kid problem." She felt down on herself and that she was "wasting all the potential I have" taking care of the home and her children. She denied any suicidal ideation but believed that "if I died everyone would see how much I do around here!" She denied feeling tense or anxious or any episodes of apprehension.

She had no prior history of psychiatric problems, and before the onset of her menstrual and abdominal problems, she had been in good health. However, on further exploration, she reported that she had a period in her teens when she had similar problems after breaking up with a boyfriend and experiencing some academic problems. She also later reported occasional miscellaneous medical problems for which she sought medical attention; these were generally associated with "something that was going around."

The psychiatric impression was (1) possible undifferentiated somatoform disorder but rule out depressive disorder NOS or dysthymic disorder; (2) rule out somatization disorder; although the patient's history as presently obtained did not fulfill criteria, it was noted that she was an inconsistent historian, and thus a thorough review of her medical records was indicated; (3) possible unidentified general medical condition; and (4) partner relational problem. Recommendations included that (1) the patient's home situation be assessed for possible redistribution of the work and responsibility load; (2) the patient and her husband be referred for marital counseling; (3) while the patient's psychiatric history was being further assessed, an antidepressant medication with a low sedation side effect profile should be started on a trial basis; and (4) the primary care physician should be advised to be vigilant for a possible unidentified underlying general medical condition, given the ambiguity of the patient's psychiatric status.

---

# CONVERSION DISORDER

## Definition

As defined in DSM-IV, conversion disorders are characterized by symptoms or deficits affecting voluntary motor or sensory function that suggest yet are not fully explained by a neurological or other general medical condition or the direct effects of a substance (see Table 71–1). The diagnosis is not made if the presentation is explained as a culturally sanctioned behavior or experience, such as bizarre behaviors resembling a seizure during a religious ceremony. Symptoms are not intentionally produced or feigned, that is, the person does not consciously contrive a symptom for external rewards, as in malingering, or for the intrapsychic rewards of assuming the sick role, as in factitious disorder.

Four subtypes with specific examples of symptoms are defined: with motor symptom or deficit (e.g., impaired coordination or balance, paralysis or localized weakness, difficulty swallowing or lump in throat, aphonia, and urinary retention); with sensory symptom or deficit (e.g., loss of touch or pain sensation, double vision, blindness, deafness, and hallucinations); with seizures or convulsions; and with mixed presentation (i.e., has symptoms of more than one of the other subtypes). The list of examples is also contained among the pseudoneurological symptoms listed in the diagnostic criteria for somatization disorder. Although determination is highly subjective and of questionable reliability and validity, association with psychological factors is required.

To a great extent, the concept of a conversion disorder derived from the work of neurologists such as Charcot, Breuer and Freud (1893–1895) in the late 19th and early 20th centuries and more recently of Ziegler and Paul (1954) and Marsden (1986). Conversion disorder was called conversion reaction in DSM-I and hysterical neurosis, conversion type in DSM-II. In both DSM-I and DSM-II, the conversion process was restricted to symptoms affecting

## DSM-IV-TR Criteria 300.11

**Conversion Disorder**

A. One or more symptoms or deficits affecting voluntary motor or sensory function that suggest a neurological or other general medical condition.

B. Psychological factors are judged to be associated with the symptom or deficit because the initiation or exacerbation of the symptom or deficit is preceded by conflicts or other stressors.

C. The symptom or deficit is not intentionally produced or feigned (as in factitious disorder or malingering).

D. The symptom or deficit cannot, after appropriate investigation, be fully explained by a general medical condition, or by the direct effects of a substance, or as a culturally sanctioned behavior or experience.

E. The symptom or deficit causes clinically significant distress or impairment in social, occupational, or other important areas of functioning or warrants medical evaluation.

F. The symptom or deficit is not limited to pain or sexual dysfunction, does not occur exclusively during the course of somatization disorder, and is not better accounted for by another mental disorder.

*Specify* type of symptom or deficit:

**With motor symptom or deficit** (e.g., impaired coordination or balance, paralysis or localized weakness, difficulty swallowing or lump in throat, aphonia, and urinary retention)

**With sensory symptom or deficit** (e.g., loss of touch or pain sensation, double vision, blindness, deafness, and hallucinations)

**With seizures or convulsions** (includes seizures or convulsions with voluntary sensory components)

**With mixed presentation** (if symptoms of more than one category are evident)

Reprinted with permission from the Diagnostic and Statistical Manual of Mental Disorders, Fourth Edition, Text Revision. Copyright 2000 American Psychiatric Association.

the voluntary motor and sensory nervous systems. Symptoms for which there was some physiological understanding (generally involving the autonomic nervous system) were subsumed under the psychophysiological disorders.

Unfortunately, conversion disorder or conversion hysteria came to be equated, at least by some, with hysteria, a term used by others to describe a more pervasive, chronic, and polysymptomatic disorder, denoted as somatization disorder in DSM-III, DSM-III-R, and DSM-IV. Whereas conversion symptoms are among its most dramatic symp-

toms, somatization disorder is characterized by multiple unexplained symptoms in many organ systems; in conversion disorder, even a single symptom affecting voluntary motor or sensory function may suffice. Such nosological inconsistencies have resulted in a great deal of confusion, both in research and in clinical practice.

To add to confusion, DSM-III and DSM-III-R used a broadened definition of conversion, including disorders characterized by symptoms involving any "loss or alteration in physical functioning suggesting a physical disorder," as long as the mechanism of conversion was evident, that is, the symptom was "an expression of a psychological conflict or need." Thus, disparate symptoms, including those involving primarily the autonomic or endocrine system, for example, "psychogenic" vomiting (assumedly expressing revulsion and disgust) and "pseudocyesis" (interpreted as representing unconscious conflict regarding pregnancy), were included as examples of conversion symptoms. In DSM-IV, conversion disorder was again restricted to symptoms affecting the voluntary motor and sensory systems. This change was consistent with the symptomatic, epidemiological, and prognostic differences between the pseudoneurological conversion symptoms and other types of symptoms involving "function."

The relationship of conversion disorder to the dissociative disorders warrants comment (Martin 1996). Long recognized as related, they were subsumed as subtypes of hysterical neurosis in DSM-II: conversion involving voluntary motor and sensory functioning, and dissociation affecting memory and identity. They are unified in one category in ICD-10: dissociative (conversion) disorders. DSM-IV retained the basic organization of DSM-III and, DSM-III-R, classifying conversion disorder with the somatoform disorders; the dissociative disorders compose their own major grouping. However, the DSM-IV-TR text acknowledges the symptomatic, epidemiological, and probable pathogenetic similarities between conversion and dissociative symptoms. Such symptoms have been attributed to similar psychological mechanisms, and they often occur in the same individual, sometimes during the same episode of illness. DSM-IV-TR does suggest that patients with conversion disorder be carefully scrutinized for dissociative symptoms.

Hallucinations are included among the sensory nervous symptoms in DSM-IV. Whereas the concept of conversion hallucinations has a long tradition (Martin 1996), DSM-III and DSM-III-R noted hallucinations as a manifestation of only two nonpsychotic disorders: posttraumatic stress disorder, in which a traumatic event is reexperienced; and multiple personality disorder (dissociative identity disorder in DSM-IV), wherein one or more personalities hear the voice of, talk with, or engage in activities with one or more of the other personalities. Inclusion of hallucinations as a conversion symptom was supported by the somatization disorder field trial, in which one third of a large sample of nonpsychotic women with evidence of unexplained somatic complaints reported a history of hallucinations. Among the 40% who had symptoms that met criteria for somatization disorder, more than half reported hallucinations (Martin 1995, unpublished data). Women with other conversion symptoms were more likely to report hallucinations than were those with no other conversion symptoms.

In general, conversion hallucinations (referred to by some as pseudohallucinations) differ in several ways from those in psychotic conditions. Conversion hallucinations typically occur in the absence of other psychotic symptoms, insight that the hallucinations are not real may be retained, and they often involve more than one sensory modality, whereas hallucinations in psychoses generally involve a single sensory modality, usually auditory. Conversion hallucinations also often have a naive, fantastic, or childish content, as if they are part of a fairy tale, and are described eagerly, sometimes even provocatively, as an interesting story (e.g., "I was driving downtown and a flying saucer flew over my car and I saw you [the psychiatrist] in a window and I heard your voice calling to me"). They often bear some understandable psychological purpose, although the patient may not be aware of intent. In the example given, the "sighting" was reported at the time that no further sessions were scheduled.

## Epidemiology

Vastly different estimates of the incidence and prevalence of conversion disorder have been reported. Much of this difference may be attributable to methodological differences from study to study, including the changing definition of conversion disorder, ascertainment procedures, and populations studied. General population estimates have generally been derived indirectly, extrapolating from clinic or hospital samples.

Conversion symptoms themselves may be common; it was reported that 25% of normal postpartum and medically ill women had a history of conversion symptoms at some time during their life (Cloninger 1993), yet in some instances, there may have been no resulting clinically significant distress or impairment. Lifetime prevalence rates of treated conversion symptoms in general populations are much more modest, ranging from 11 to 500 per 100,000 (Martin 1996) (see Table 71–2). About 5 to 24% of psychiatric outpatients, 5 to 14% of general hospital patients, and 1 to 3% of outpatient psychiatric referrals reported a history of conversion symptoms (Cloninger 1993, Ford and Folks 1985, Toone 1990), although their current treatment was not necessarily for conversion symptoms. A rate of nearly 4% of outpatient neurological referrals (Perkin 1989) and 1% of neurological admissions (Ziegler and Paul 1954) involved conversion disorder. In virtually all studies, an excess (to the extent of 2:1 to 10:1) of women reported conversion symptoms relative to men (Ljunberg 1957, Stefansson et al. 1976, Raskin et al. 1966). In part, this may relate to the simple fact that women seek medical evaluation more often than men do, but it is unlikely that this fully accounts for the sex difference. There is a predilection for lower socioeconomic status; less educated, less psychologically sophisticated, and rural populations are overrepresented (Veith 1965, Weinstein et al. 1969, Lazare 1981, Folks et al. 1984). Consistent with this, higher rates (nearly 10%) of outpatient psychiatric referrals are for conversion symptoms in "developing" countries (Stafanis et al. 1976). As countries develop, there may be a declining incidence in time, which may relate to increasing levels of education, and medical and psychological sophistication (Nandi et al. 1992).

## Etiology and Pathophysiology

The term conversion implies etiology because it is derived from a hypothesized mechanism of converting psychological conflicts into somatic symptoms, often symbolically (e.g., repressed rage is converted into paralysis of an arm that could be used to strike). A number of psychological factors have been promoted as part of such an etiological process, but evidence for their essential involvement is scanty at best. Theoretically, anxiety is reduced by keeping an internal conflict or need out of awareness by symbolic expression of an unconscious wish as a conversion symptom (primary gain). However, individuals with active conversion symptoms often continue to show marked anxiety, especially on psychological tests (Lader and Sartorious 1968, Mears and Horvath 1972). Symbolism is infrequently evident, and its evaluation involves highly inferential and unreliable judgments (Raskin et al. 1966). Overinterpretation of symbolism in persons with occult medical disorder may contribute to misdiagnosis. Secondary gain, whereby conversion symptoms allow avoidance of noxious activities or the procurement of otherwise unavailable support, may also occur in persons with medical conditions, who may take advantage of such benefits (Raskin et al. 1966, Watson and Buranen 1979).

Individuals with conversion disorder may show a lack of concern out of keeping with the nature or implications of the symptom (the so-called *la belle indifférence*). However, indifference to symptoms is not invariably present in conversion disorder (Lewis and Berman 1965) and is also seen in individuals with general medical conditions (Weinstein et al. 1969), on the basis of denial or stoicism (Pincus 1982). Conversion symptoms may present in a dramatic or histrionic fashion and may be highly suggestible. A dramatic presentation is also seen in distressed individuals with medical conditions. Even symptoms based on an underlying medical condition may respond to suggestion, at least temporarily (Gatfield and Guze 1962). In many instances, preexisting personality disorders (in particular histrionic personality disorder) are evident and may predispose to conversion disorder. Persons with conversion disorder may often have a history of disturbed sexuality (Lewis 1974) many (one-third) report a history of sexual abuse, especially incestuous. Thus, two-thirds may not report such a history. Individuals with conversion disorder are often reported to be the youngest or the youngest of a sex in sibling order, but this is not a consistent finding (Ziegler et al. 1960, Stephens and Kamp 1962).

If not directly etiological, many psychosocial factors have been suggested as predisposing to conversion disorder. At a minimum, many persons with conversion disorder are in chaotic domestic and occupational situations. As previously mentioned, individuals from rural backgrounds and those who are psychologically and medically unsophisticated appear to be predisposed, as are those with existing neurological disorders. In the last case, a tendency to conversion symptoms has been attributed to "modeling," that is, patients with neurological disorders are likely to have observed in others, as well as in themselves, various neurological symptoms, which they then may simulate as conversion symptoms.

Available data suggest a genetic contribution. Conversion symptoms are more frequent in relatives of individuals with conversion disorder (Toone 1990). In a nonblinded study, rates of conversion disorder were found to be elevated tenfold in female (fivefold in male) relatives of patients with conversion disorder (Ljunberg 1957). Accumulated data from available twin studies show 9 concordant and 33 discordant monozygotic pairs and no concordant but 43 discordant dizygotic pairs (Inouye 1972). Nongenetic familial factors, particularly incestuous childhood sexual abuse, may also be involved in some. Nearly one-third of individuals with medically unexplained seizures reported childhood sexual abuse, compared with less than 10% of those with complex partial epilepsy (Alper et al. 1993). Data looking specifically at abuse history in other well-defined conversion disorder cases are not available.

## Diagnosis and Differential Diagnosis

As shown in Figure 71–1, the first consideration is whether the conversion symptoms are explained on the basis of a general medical condition. Because conversion symptoms by definition affect voluntary motor or sensory function (thus pseudoneurological), neurological conditions are usually suggested, but other general medical conditions may be implicated as well. Neurologists are generally first consulted by primary care physicians for conversion symptoms; psychiatrists become involved only after neurological or general medical conditions have been reasonably excluded. Nonetheless, psychiatrists should have a good appreciation of the process of making such exclusions. More than 13% of actual neurological cases are diagnosed as functional before the elucidation of a neurological illness (Perkin 1989). Even after referral, vigilance for an emerging general medical condition should continue. A significant percentage—21 (Gatfield and Guze 1962) to 50 (Slater and Glithero 1965)—of patients diagnosed with conversion symptoms are found to have neurological illness on follow-up.

Apparent conversion symptoms mandate a thorough evaluation for possible underlying physical explanation. This evaluation must include a thorough medical history; physical (especially neurological) examination; and radiographical, blood, urine, and other tests as clinically indicated. Reliance should not be placed on determination of whether psychological factors explain the symptom. As reviewed by Cloninger (1987), such determinations are unreliable except, perhaps, in cases in which there is a clear and immediate temporal relationship between a psychosocial stressor and the symptom, or in cases in which similar situations led to conversion symptoms in the past. A history of previous conversion or other unexplained symptoms, particularly if somatization disorder is diagnosable, lessens the probability that an occult medical condition will be identified (Cloninger 1993). Although conversion symptoms may occur at any age, symptoms are most often first manifested in late adolescence or early adulthood. Conversion symptoms first occurring in middle age or later should increase suspicion of an occult physical illness.

Symptoms of many neurological illnesses may appear inconsistent with known neurophysiological or neuropathological processes, suggesting conversion and posing diagnostic problems. These illnesses include multiple sclerosis, in which blindness due to optic neuritis may initially present with normal fundi; myasthenia gravis, periodic par-

alysis, myoglobinuric myopathy, polymyositis, and other acquired myopathies, in which marked weakness in the presence of normal deep tendon reflexes may occur; and Guillain–Barré syndrome, in which early extremity weakness may be inconsistent (Cloninger 1993).

Complicating diagnosis is the fact that physical illness and conversion or other apparent psychiatric overlay are not mutually exclusive. Patients with physical illnesses that are incapacitating and frightening may appear to be exaggerating symptoms. Also, patients with actual neurological illness will also have "pseudo" symptoms. For example, patients with actual seizures may have pseudoseizures as well (Desai et al. 1982). Considering these observations, psychiatrists should avoid a rash and hasty diagnosis of conversion disorder when faced with symptoms that are difficult to interpret.

As with the other somatoform disorders, symptoms of conversion disorder are not intentionally produced, in distinction to malingering or factitious disorder. To a large part, this determination is based on assessment of the motivation for external rewards (as in malingering) or for the assumption of the sick role (as in factitious disorder). The setting is often an important consideration. For example, conversion-like symptoms are frequent in military or forensic settings, in which obvious potential rewards make malingering a serious consideration.

A diagnosis of conversion disorder should not be made if a conversion symptom is fully accounted for by a mood disorder or by schizophrenia (e.g., disordered motility as part of a catatonic syndrome of a psychotic mood disorder or schizophrenia). If the symptom is a hallucination, it must be remembered that the descriptors differentiating conversion from psychotic hallucinations should be seen only as rules of thumb. Differentiation should be based on a comprehensive assessment of the illness. In the case of hallucinations, posttraumatic stress disorder and dissociative identity disorder (multiple personality disorder) must also be excluded. If the conversion symptom cannot be fully accounted for by the other psychiatric illness, conversion disorder should be diagnosed in addition to the other disorder if it meets criteria (e.g., an episode of unexplained blindness in a patient with a major depressive episode). In hypochondriasis, neurological illness may be feared ("I have strange feelings in my head; it must be a brain tumor"), but the focus here is on preoccupation with fear of having the illness rather than on the symptom itself as in conversion disorder.

By definition, if symptoms are limited to sexual dysfunction or pain, conversion disorder is not diagnosed. Criteria for somatization disorder require multiple symptoms in multiple organ systems and functions, including symptoms affecting motor or sensory function (conversion symptoms) or memory or identity (dissociative symptoms). Thus, it would be superfluous to make an additional diagnosis of conversion disorder in the context of a somatization disorder.

A last consideration is whether the symptom is a culturally sanctioned behavior or experience. Conversion disorder should not be diagnosed if symptoms are clearly sanctioned or even expected, are appropriate to the sociocultural context, and are not associated with distress or impairment. Seizure-like episodes, such as those that occur in conjunction with certain religious ceremonies, and culturally expected responses, such as women "swooning" in response to excitement in Victorian times, qualify as examples of these symptoms.

## Course, Natural History, and Prognosis

Age at onset is typically from late childhood to early adulthood. Onset is rare before the age of 10 years (Maloney 1980) and after 35 years, but cases with an onset as late as the ninth decade have been reported (Weddington 1979). The likelihood of a neurological or other medical condition is increased when the age at onset is in middle or late life. Development is generally acute, but symptoms may develop gradually as well. The course of individual conversion symptoms is generally short; half (Folks et al. 1984) to nearly all (Carter 1949) symptoms remit by the time of hospital discharge. However, symptoms relapse within 1 year in one-fifth to one-fourth of patients. Typically, one symptom is present in a single episode, but multiple symptoms are generally involved longitudinally. Factors associated with good prognosis include acute onset, clearly identifiable precipitants, a short interval between onset and institution of treatment, and good intelligence (Toone 1990). Conversion blindness, aphonia, and paralysis are associated with relatively good prognosis, whereas patients with seizures and tremor do more poorly. Some patients diagnosed initially with conversion disorder will have a presentation that meets criteria for somatization disorder when they are observed longitudinally (Kent et al. 1995).

Individual conversion symptoms are generally self-limited and do not lead to physical changes or disabilities. Rarely, physical sequelae such as atrophy may occur. Marital and occupational problems are not as frequent in patients with conversion disorder as they are in those with somatization disorder (Tomasson et al. 1991, Coryell and House 1984). In a long-term follow-up study, excess mortality by unnatural causes was observed (Coryell and House 1984). However, the reason for this was unclear in that none of the deaths was by suicide.

## Treatment

Reports of the treatment of conversion disorder date from those of Charcot, which generally involved symptom removal by suggestion or hypnosis. Breuer and Freud, using such psychoanalytic techniques as free association and abreaction of repressed affects, had more ambitious objectives in their treatment of Anna O., including the resolution of unconscious conflicts. To date, whereas some recommend long-term, intensive, insight-oriented psychodynamic psychotherapy in pursuit of such goals (Ford 1995), most psychiatrists advocate a more pragmatic approach, especially for acute cases.

Therapeutic approaches vary according to whether the conversion symptom is acute or chronic. Whichever the case, direct confrontation is not recommended. Such a communication may cause a patient to feel even more isolated. An undiscovered physical illness may also underlie the presentation.

In acute cases, the most frequent initial aim is removal of the symptom. The pressure behind accomplishing this depends on the distress and disability associated with the symptom (Ford 1995). If the patient is not in great distress and the need to regain function is not immediate, a conservative approach of reassurance, relaxation, and suggestion is recommended (Ford 1983). With this technique, the patient is reassured that on the basis of evaluation the symptom will disappear completely and, in fact, is already beginning to do so. The patient can then be encouraged to ventilate about recent events and feelings, without any causal relationships being suggested. This is in contrast to attempts at abreaction, by which repressed material, particularly regarding a painful experience or a conflict, is brought back to consciousness.

If symptoms do not resolve with such conservative approaches, a number of other techniques for symptom resolution may be instituted. It does appear that prompt resolution of conversion symptoms is important because the duration of conversion symptoms is associated with a greater risk of recurrence and chronic disability (Cloninger 1993). The other techniques include narcoanalysis (e.g., amobarbital interview), hypnosis, and behavioral therapy (Ford 1995). In narcoanalysis, amobarbital or another sedative–hypnotic medication such as lorazepam is given intravenously to the point of drowsiness. Sometimes this is followed by administration of a stimulant medication, such as methamphetamine. The patient is then encouraged to discuss stressors and conflicts. This technique may be effective acutely, leading to at least temporary symptom relief as well as expansion of the information known about the patient. This technique has not been shown to be especially effective with more chronic conversion symptoms. In hypnotherapy, symptoms may be removed with the suggestion that the symptoms will gradually improve posthypnotically. Information regarding stressors and conflicts may be explored as well. Formal behavioral therapy, including relaxation training and even aversive therapy, has been proposed and reported by some to be effective. In addition, simply manipulating the environment to interrupt reinforcement of the conversion symptom is recommended.

Anecdotally, somatic treatments including phenothiazines, lithium, and electroconvulsive therapy have been reported effective. However, in many cases, this may be attributable to simple suggestion. In other cases, resolution of another psychiatric disorder, such as a psychotic disorder or a mood disorder, may have led to the symptom's removal. It should be evident from the preceding discussion that in acute conversion disorders, it may be not the particular technique but the influence of suggestion that is specifically associated with symptom relief. It is likely that in various rituals, such as exorcism and other religious ceremonies, immediate "cures" are based on suggestion. Suggestion seems to play a major role in the resolution of "mass hysteria," in which a group of individuals who believe that they have been exposed to some noxious influence such as a "toxin" or even a "spell" experience similar symptoms that do not appear to have any organic basis. Often, the epidemic can be contained if affected individuals are segregated. Simple announcements that no such factor has been identified and that symptoms experienced by the group have been linked to mass hysteria have been effective.

Thus far, this discussion has centered on acute treatment primarily for symptom removal. Longer-term approaches include strategies previously discussed for somatization disorder—a pragmatic, conservative approach involving support and exploration of various conflict areas, particularly of interpersonal relationships. A certain degree of insight may be attained, at least in terms of appreciating relationships between various conflicts and stressors and the development of symptoms. Others advocate long-term, intensive, insight-oriented dynamic psychotherapy.

---

### Clinical Vignette 3

A 47-year-old woman was referred for psychiatric consultation by her primary care physician at the recommendation of a neurologist. She had been admitted to the hospital 2 days earlier, after presenting with mild acidosis attributed to poor control of her insulin-dependent diabetes mellitus. She had become concerned that insulin was "making me fat" and had been taking it erratically for several weeks. On admission, she also complained of generalized muscle weakness, more pronounced on the left side, especially in the arm, and reported that she had had a "stroke" affecting the right side 1 year before, for which she was not hospitalized. On examination, the neurologist observed that the patient showed no atrophy or spasticity and that deep tendon reflexes were decreased but equal bilaterally. On testing of the left upper extremity, the patient was observed to show weakness in extending and flexing the arm against resistance, yet more careful examination revealed residual strength inconsistent with that shown in these tests. Her primary care physician reported some question of a stroke 1 year before, which was never clearly ascertained. A "hysterical component to the neurological symptoms" was considered. Nonetheless, diagnostic procedures were instituted, including magnetic resonance imaging. No abnormalities were seen by this test. Two days later, it was concluded that a stroke was improbable, and noting reports of depressed mood, the neurologist recommended psychiatric consultation.

When seen by the psychiatric consultant, she still complained of the weakness, although it was somewhat improved and not so clearly localized to the left side. She also mentioned that she had been depressed for several weeks before admission and that she had been treated with some success with fluoxetine in the past. She reported multiple conflicts concerning her living situation. She was living with her married son and felt that his wife resented her presence. She felt "trapped" in that she could not afford to live independently. Medical records indicated that diabetes mellitus had been diagnosed at age 36 years and was treated with oral hypoglycemic agents until age 41 years, when insulin became necessary for adequate control. The record also revealed several episodes of transient unexplained weakness as well as occasional problems with headaches and joint pain going back to age 26 years, with several mentions of temporal proximity of such symptoms to marital and occupational difficulties. Yet, criteria for somatization disorder were not fulfilled.

The psychiatrist's provisional diagnoses were (1) psychological factors affecting medical condition (noncompliance with insulin regimen); (2) conversion disorder, with motor symptom or deficit; and (3) possible major depressive disorder, recurrent. Treatment with sertraline, 50 mg at bedtime, was recommended. It was also suggested to the patient that her tests were now completed and that it was expected that her weakness would continue to improve. When the psychiatrist visited her the next day, she reported that her weakness was better and that she was also beginning to feel less depressed. The patient was encouraged to continue to see her primary care physician and to comply with his recommendations, and she was referred to social work for assistance with her living situation. Referral for outpatient psychiatric care was also recommended.

This clinical vignette illustrates several important aspects concerning the diagnosis, course, and treatment of conversion disorder. As is not uncommon, the patient does suffer from a medical illness to which many symptoms can ordinarily be attributed. However, the extent of her complaints, the lack of neuroanatomical verification, and inconsistencies of her report and the documented history suggested a possibility that her motor symptoms were not fully attributable to a general medical condition. This interpretation was supported by her past history of apparent conversion symptoms as well as some other somatic complaints. Although she was also complaining of depression, her history was vague, and her "response" to 1 day of treatment with an antidepressant drug was unlikely to be "pharmacological." Her motor symptoms were resolving with reassurance and suggestion, such that the short-term prognosis for her motor symptoms was good. However, her history of noncompliance with medical treatment, and multiple situational and interpersonal problems indicated the advisability of continued psychosocial if not psychiatric intervention.

## PAIN DISORDER

### Definition

The term pain disorder was new to DSM-IV. It replaced the DSM-III-R designation somatoform pain disorder. Because the disorder was already included in the somatoform grouping, somatoform was redundant. In addition, whereas the DSM-III-R somatoform pain disorder was more neutral than the DSM-III psychogenic pain disorder, it maintained differentiation between imaginary or exaggerated and real pain, following a dualistic dichotomy of separating mind and body. The matter of determining psychogenicity was always a problem (Williams and Spitzer 1982). As reviewed by Cloninger (1993), raters show only moderate agreement on such questions even when they are given the same information. Yet, both DSM-III psychogenic pain disorder and DSM-III-R somatoform pain disorder required that the pain not have an organic or pathophysiological explanation and that the complaint or impairment be greatly in excess of what would be expected from the physical findings.

As defined in DSM-IV, the essential feature of pain disorder is pain with which psychological factors "have an important role in the onset, severity, exacerbation, or maintenance" (see Table 71–1). Pain disorder is subtyped as pain disorder associated with psychological factors and pain disorder associated with both psychological factors and a general medical condition. The third possibility, pain disorder associated with a general medical condition, is not considered to be a mental disorder, because the requirement is not met that psychological factors play an important role. Thus, the DSM-IV concept of pain disorder as a mental

---

### Diagnostic Criteria for Pain Disorder

A. Pain in one or more anatomical sites is the predominant focus of the clinical presentation and is of sufficient severity to warrant clinical attention.

B. The pain causes clinically significant distress or impairment in social, occupational, or other important areas of functioning.

C. Psychological factors are judged to have an important role in the onset, severity, exacerbation, or maintenance of the pain.

D. The symptom or deficit is not intentionally produced or feigned (as in factitious disorder or malingering).

E. The pain is not better accounted for by a mood, anxiety, or psychotic disorder and does not meet criteria for dyspareunia.

*Code* as follows:

**307.80 Pain disorder associated with psychological factors:** Psychological factors are judged to have the major role in the onset, severity, exacerbation, or maintenance of the pain. (If a general medical condition is present, it does not have a major role in the onset, severity, exacerbation, or maintenance of the pain.) This type of pain disorder is not diagnosed if criteria are also met for somatization disorder.

*Specify* if:

**Acute:** Duration of less than 6 months

**Chronic:** Duration of 6 months or longer

**307.89 Pain disorder associated with both psychological factors and a general medical condition:** Both psychological factors and a general medical condition are judged to have important roles in the onset, severity, exacerbation, or maintenance of the pain. The associated general medical condition or anatomical site of the pain (see below) is coded on Axis III.

*Specify* if:

**Acute:** Duration of less than 6 months

**Chronic:** Duration of 6 months or longer

**Note:** The following is not considered to be a mental disorder and is included here to facilitate differential diagnosis.

**Pain disorder associated with a general medical condition:** A general medical condition has a major role in the onset, severity, exacerbation, or maintenance of the pain. (If psychological factors are present, they are not judged to have a major role in the onset, severity, exacerbation, or maintenance of the pain.) The diagnostic code for the pain is selected based on the associated general medical condition if one has been established or on the anatomical location of the pain if the underlying general medical condition is not yet clearly established—for example, low back (724.2), sciatic (724.3), pelvic (625.9), headache (784.0), facial (784.0), chest (786.50), joint (719.4), bone (733.90), abdominal (789.0), breast (611.71), renal (788.0), ear (388.70), eye (379.91), throat (784.1), tooth (525.9), and urinary (788.0).

---

disorder was broadened and allowed the psychiatrist much greater specificity in considering etiological factors and a more useful schema for differential diagnosis. The focus is placed on the presence of psychological factors rather than the exasperating determination of whether the pain is attributable to organic disease.

In addition, DSM-IV requires that pain be the predominant focus of the clinical presentation and that it cause clinically significant distress or impairment. Specifiers of acute (duration of less than 6 months) and chronic (duration of 6 months or longer) are provided. Both DSM-III and DSM-III-R required chronicity: prolonged in DSM-III, for at least 6 months in DSM-III-R. This left no place for clinically significant syndromes of recent onset or limited duration and undoubtedly contributed to the fact that DSM-III and DSM-III-R pain diagnoses were little used.

With the changes outlined, the DSM-IV-TR-defined pain disorder is compatible with current theories of pain and should be more clinically applicable.

### Epidemiology

Given the tortuous course of changing diagnostic criteria, only estimates can be made for the epidemiological parameters of pain disorder. As to pain itself, some empirical studies suggest that it is common. Perhaps as indirect evidence of this is the proliferation of pain clinics nationally. Of course, many patients attending these clinics fall into the category of pain disorder associated with a general medical condition, but undoubtedly, some also have involvement of psychological factors as required for a diagnosis of pain disorder as a mental disorder. The same would apply to the 10 to 15% of adults in the US in any given year who have work disability because of back pain (Osterweis et al. 1987). Pain has been found to be a predominant symptom in 75% of consecutive general medical patients, with 75% of these (thus 50% overall) judged as having no identifiable physical cause (King 1994). As reviewed by Stoudemire (1988), no apparent physical basis is found in 40 to 50% of patients presenting with nonspecific abdominal pain. At least half of such patients show major personality problems in addition, with such aberrations associated with poor outcome. Whereas primary care and other nonpsychiatric physicians probably see most pain patients, 38% of psychiatric inpatient admissions (Delaplaine et al. 1978) and 18% attending a psychiatric outpatient clinic (Chaturvedi 1987) report pain as a significant problem.

## Etiology and Pathophysiology

In considering the etiology of pain disorder, possible mechanisms of pain itself must be considered. As reviewed by King (1994), the definition of pain sanctioned by the International Association for the Study of Pain Subcommittee on Taxonomy is "an unpleasant sensory and emotional experience associated with actual or potential tissue damage." It goes on to acknowledge that pain is not simply "activity induced in the nociceptor and nociceptive pathways by a noxious stimulus" but "is always a psychological state. . . ." Thus, it accepts the hypothesis that pain involves psychological as well as physical factors.

Many theories of the etiology and pathophysiology of pain involving both biological and psychological factors have been proposed. It is known that a neuropathway descends from the cerebral cortex and medulla, which inhibits the firing of pain transmission neurons when it is activated (Cloninger 1993). This system is apparently mediated by the endogenous opiate-like compounds, endorphins, and by serotonin. Indeed, metabolites of both of these neurotransmitters may be reduced in the cerebrospinal fluid of chronic pain patients (von Knorring and Attkisson 1979).

The gate control theory developed by Melzack and Wall (1983), as reviewed by King (1994), links biological and psychological factors. It hypothesizes a gate-like mechanism involving the dorsal horn of the spinal cord by which large A-beta fibers as well as small A-delta and C fibers carry impulses from the periphery to the substantia gelatinosa and T-cells in the spinal cord. Activation of the large fibers inhibits, whereas activation of the small fibers facilitates transmission to the T-cells. In addition, impulses descending from the brain, influenced by cognitive processes, may either inhibit or facilitate transmission of pain impulses. Such a mechanism may explain how psychological processes affect pain perception.

By definition, both pain disorder associated with psychological factors and pain disorder associated with both psychological factors and a general medical condition involve psychological factors. In the case of the former, it is presumed that there is little contribution from general medical conditions; in the latter, both physical and psychological factors contribute. A plethora of not necessarily mutually exclusive theories has been proposed to explain how this takes place.

As reviewed by Cloninger (1993), psychological constructs involving learning theories, both operant and classical conditioning, may apply. In operant paradigms, pain-related complaints are reinforced by increased attention, relief from obligations, monetary compensation, and the pleasurable effects of analgesics. In classical conditioning, originally neutral settings such as a workplace or bedroom where pain was experienced come to evoke pain-related behavior. Social and cultural attitudes may also have effects. Patients with unexplained pain are more likely than others to have close relatives with chronic pain. Although findings have differed from study to study, ethnic differences may also have effects, such as greater pain tolerance in Irish and Anglo-Saxon groups in comparison to southern Mediterranean groups.

## Diagnosis and Differential Diagnosis

As shown in Figure 71–1, the diagnostic approach begins with assessment of whether the presentation is fully explained by a general medical condition. If not, it may be assumed that psychological factors play a major role. If it is judged that psychological factors do not play a major role, a diagnosis of pain disorder associated with a general medical condition may apply. As previously mentioned, this does not have a mental disorder code.

If psychological factors are involved, the first consideration is whether the pain is feigned. If so, either malingering or factitious disorder is diagnosed, depending on whether external incentives or assumption of the sick role is the motivation. Evidence of malingering includes consideration of external rewards relative to the chronology of the development and maintenance of the pain. In factitious disorder, a pattern of successive hospitalizations and medical evaluations is evident. Inconsistency in presentation, lack of correspondence to known anatomical pathways or disease patterns, and lack of associated sensory or motor function changes suggest malingering or factitious disorder, but pain disorder associated with psychological factors may show this pattern as well. The key question is whether the patient is experiencing rather than feigning the pain.

Determination of the relative contributions of psychological and general medical factors is difficult. Of course, careful assessment of the nature and severity of the potential underlying medical condition and the nature and degree of pain that would be expected should be made. Traditionally, the so-called conversion V or neurotic triad (consisting of elevation of the hypochondriasis and hysteria scales with a lower score on the depression scale) on the Minnesota Multiphasic Personality Inventory has been purported to indicate emotional indifference to the somatic concerns as might be expected if the symptom is attributable to psychological factors rather than organic disease. However, evidence indicates that this configuration may also occur as an adjustment to chronic illness.

A diagnosis of pain disorder requires that the pain be of sufficient severity to warrant clinical attention, that is, it causes clinically significant distress or impairment. A number of instruments have been developed to assess the degree of distress associated with the pain. Such measures include the numerical rating scale and visual analog scale as described by Scott and Huskisson (1976), the McGill Pain Questionnaire, and the West Haven-Yale Multidimensional Pain Inventory (Osterweis et al. 1987).

DSM-IV includes a number of exclusionary conventions. By definition, if pain is restricted to pain with sexual intercourse, the sexual disorder, dyspareunia, not pain disorder, is diagnosed. If pain occurs in the context of a mood, anxiety, or psychotic disorder, pain disorder is diagnosed only if it is an independent focus of clinical attention and is not better accounted for by the other disorder, a highly subjective judgment.

If pain occurs exclusively during the course of somatization disorder, pain disorder is not diagnosed because pain symptoms are part of the criteria for somatization disorder and are thereby subsumed under the more comprehensive diagnosis. Because somatization disorder is virtually a lifelong condition, this exclusion generally applies in someone with somatization disorder by history. Important here is that in addition to pain, somatization disorder involves multiple symptoms of the gastrointestinal system, the reproductive system, and the central and peripheral nervous systems; whereas in pain disorder, the focus is on pain symptoms only.

Specification of acute versus chronic pain disorder on the basis of whether the duration is less than or greater than 6 months is an important distinction. Whereas acute pain, in most cases, will be linked with physical disorders, when pain remains unexplained after 6 months, psychological factors are often involved (Cloninger 1993). However, the psychiatrist must remember that a significant minority (in one study 19%) of patients with chronic pain of no apparent physical origin will ultimately be found to have occult organic disease (Cloninger 1993).

In patients with unexplained pelvic pain, psychiatrists should be warned about cavalier conclusions regarding the absence of physical disease. With laparoscopy, a high frequency of occult organic disease has been identified in several studies. Thus, laparoscopy may be indicated in patients with pelvic pain. Electromyography may be helpful in distinguishing muscle contraction headaches. Failure to show coronary artery spasm with provocative procedures and failure to respond to nitroglycerin may be useful in distinguishing patients with pain disorder from those in whom the pain is attributable to coronary artery disease.

## Course, Natural History, and Prognosis

Given the heterogeneity of conditions subsumed under the pain disorder rubric, course and prognosis vary widely. The subtyping at 6 months is of significance. The prognosis for total remission is good for pain disorders of less than 6 months' duration. However, for syndromes of greater than 6 months' duration, chronicity is common. The site of the pain may be another factor. As described by Stoudemire and Sandhu (1987), certain anatomically differentiated pain syndromes can be distinguished, and each has its own characteristic pattern. These include syndromes characterized primarily by headache, facial pain, chest pain, abdominal pain, and pelvic pain. In such syndromes, symptoms tend to be recurrent, with relapses occurring in association with stress. A high rate of depression has been observed among patients with unexplained facial pain. Facial pain is often alleviated by antidepressant medication. This effect has been observed in both patients with depressive symptoms and those without.

Other factors affecting course and prognosis include associated psychiatric illness and external reinforcement. Employment at the outset of treatment predicts improvement (Martin 1995). Chronicity is more likely in the presence of certain personality diagnoses or traits, such as pronounced passivity and dependency. External reinforcement includes litigation involving potential financial compensation or disability. Continuation of the pain disorder may prove more lucrative than its resolution and return to work. Level of activity, which is generally associated with improvement, is discouraged by fears of losing compensation. Thus, although outright malingering may be rare (Leavitt and Sweet 1986), pain behaviors are often reinforced and maintained. Habituation with addictive drugs is associated with greater chronicity.

## Treatment

Treatment of pain overall has been well summarized by King (1994). An overriding guideline is that the psychiatrist not do anything that will actually perpetuate and even promote "pain-related behavior." Thus, a major goal is to encourage activity. Other guidelines include avoidance of sedative–antianxiety drugs, judicious use of analgesics on a fixed interval schedule so as not to reinforce pain-related behaviors, avoidance of opioids, and consideration of alternative treatment approaches such as relaxation therapy. Depression should be treated with appropriate antidepressant drugs, not sedative–antianxiety medications. The difficulties in managing pain disorder patients have resulted in the establishment of many clinics and programs especially designed for pain. Referral to such a service may be indicated. Intervention should best be provided early in the course of the syndrome, before pain-related behaviors become entrenched. Once continuing disability compensation is established, therapeutic efforts become much more difficult.

The preceding general guidelines apply whether or not a general medical basis for the pain is involved. Of course, if only pain disorder associated with psychological factors is involved, psychological management will be the mainstay. For patients with pain associated with general medical factors (not a mental disorder) in which psychological factors do not play a major role, efforts should be made to prevent the development of psychological problems in response to the resulting distress, isolation and loss of function, and iatrogenic effects such as exposure to potentially addicting drugs.

In acute pain, the major goal is to relieve the pain (Osterweis et al. 1987). Thus, pharmacological agents generally play a more significant role than in chronic syndromes. Whereas the risk of developing opioid dependence appears to be surprisingly low (4 per 12,000) among patients without a prior history of dependence (Porter and Jick 1980), nonopioid agents should be used whenever they can be expected to be effective. As discussed for chronic pain, these include particularly acetaminophen and the nonsteroidal antiinflammatory drugs (NSAIDs), of which aspirin is considered a member. Even if an opioid analgesic is employed, these drugs should be continued as adjuncts; often, they lessen the required dose of the opioid.

It is with the chronic syndromes that proper management is crucial to ease distress and prevent the development of additional problems. As advised by King (1994), the overriding goal is to maintain function, because total relief of the pain may not be possible. Physical and occupational therapy may play a major role. There may be resistance to the involvement of a psychiatrist as an indication that the pain is not seen as real. Such issues must first be resolved. An attempt should be made to ascertain the roles that psychological and general medical factors play in the maintenance of the pain.

A large variety of psychotherapies including individual, group, and family strategies have been employed. Two techniques that warrant special attention are operant conditioning and cognitive–behavioral therapy. In operant conditioning, the pattern of reinforcement of pain behavior by medication, attention, and excuse from responsibilities is to be interrupted and reinforcement shifted to usual daily activities. To assess the role of operant conditioning, it may be necessary to have patients keep a diary and to interview family members to identify any conditioning patterns. In cognitive–behavioral therapies, the goal is the identification and correction of attitudes, beliefs, and expectations. Biofeedback and relaxation techniques may be used to minimize muscle tension that may aggravate if not cause pain. Hypnosis may also be used to achieve muscle relaxation and to help the patient "dissociate" from the pain.

Pharmacological intervention may also be useful in chronic syndromes. Effort should be made to avoid opioids if possible. Agents to be tried first include antidepressants, acetaminophen, NSAIDs (including aspirin), and anticonvulsants such as carbamazepine. Antidepressants seem particularly useful for neuropathic pain, headache, facial pain, fibrositis, and arthritis (including rheumatoid arthritis). Analgesic action seems to be independent of antidepressant effects. Most work has been done with the tricyclic antidepressants; other classes, such as the monoamine oxidase inhibitors (MAOIs) and the selective serotonin reuptake inhibitors (SSRIs), may be effective as well. Although it was thought that the action is mediated by serotoninergic effects, agents such as desipramine with predominantly noradrenergic activity seem to be effective as well. NSAIDs, of which aspirin, ibuprofen, naproxen, and piroxicam are commonly used examples, may alleviate pain through inhibition of prostaglandin synthesis. Unfortunately, this effect may also contribute to side effects, such as aggravation of peptic or duodenal ulcers and interference with renal function. For patients unable to tolerate NSAIDs, acetaminophen should be tried.

If opioid analgesics are used, it is recommended that use be tied to objectives such as increasing level of activity rather than simply pain alleviation (King 1994). Milder opioids, such as codeine, oxycodone, and hydrocodone, should be implemented first. The once widely used propoxyphene has less analgesic effect than these drugs; it is not devoid of abuse potential as once thought and is not recommended. Pure opioid agonists such as morphine, methadone, and hydromorphone should be tried next. Meperidine, also in this class, is contraindicated for prolonged use because accumulation of the toxic metabolite, normeperidine, a cerebral irritant, may result in anxiety, psychosis, or seizures. Meperidine may also have a lethal interaction with MAOIs. There are no advantages to mixed opioid agonist–antagonists. The commonly used pentazocine should be avoided because it has abuse potential and psychotomimetic effects in some patients. It remains to be seen whether newer agents (buprenorphine, butonphanol, and nalbuphine) have lower abuse potential as claimed. Above all, psychiatrists should be judicious in the use of opioid analgesics, considering not only their abuse potential but their large number of side effects including constipation, nausea and vomiting, excessive sedation, and, in higher doses, respiratory depression that may be fatal (King 1994).

In addition to pharmacotherapy, a number of other "physical" techniques have been used, such as acupuncture and transcutaneous electrical nerve stimulation. These carry little risk of adverse effects or aggravation of the pain disorder. Other procedures such as trigger point injections, nerve blocks, and surgical ablation may be recommended if specifically indicated by an underlying general medical disorder.

As can be seen in the preceding discussion, the management of pain disorders is not monomodal. A great number of psychological and physical factors and interventions may be considered.

---

Clinical Vignette 4

A 60-year-old dentist was referred to a psychiatrist for an evaluation by an insurance company from which the patient was receiving $2,000 per month on the basis of disability resulting from "groin" pain. The pain began suddenly nearly 5 years before while he was working at his office. He described it as a burning pain most severe in his left scrotum and perianal area and radiating down his left leg. The pain was not aggravated by urination, defecation, sexual intercourse, or activity. Thus began a series of diagnostic and treatment procedures including a radical prostatectomy with vascular sparing, a partial colonectomy, a lumbar laminectomy, and intrathecal anesthetic injection of vertebral facets. Whereas objective indications for each surgery were present, including chronic prostatitis and seminal vesiculitis, diverticulitis and hemorrhagic dysplasia of the colon, and probable compression of a lumbar vertebra, none of these procedures appreciably relieved his pain. A working diagnosis of lumbosacral plexopathy was given by the neurologist who had assumed his care. The patient was receiving oxycodone (5 mg) and acetaminophen (325 mg) (Percocet) three to four times daily; naproxen (Naprosyn) (250 mg three times daily); and carbamazepine (Tegretol) (100 mg/day). The patient took medications religiously and never took more than prescribed. He reported that with this regimen, "the edge was taken off of the pain," but he did not have adequate relief. Yet, when attempts were made to discontinue the Percocet, "it became intolerable." After the onset of the pain, the patient was not able to maintain his practice, leaving it in the hands of his son who was also a dentist; "Even if I could stand the pain, I couldn't concentrate on my work well enough to do justice to my patients." He worked only occasionally, performing some simple procedures. "I wish I could return to work because I certainly can't support myself on my disability check. Besides, I'm like an adult hyperactive child. I need to stay busy."

At the time of the onset of the pain, the patient was in the midst of highly contested divorce settlement proceedings. The divorce from his wife of 12 years had resulted from the wife's long-standing infidelity, which had come as a total surprise to the patient when he discovered it. He previously divorced a wife of 26 years after she had become unfaithful. The patient had a successful dental practice. Throughout his life, he had been a hard worker, a workaholic, supporting himself through dental school; subsequently, he put his children through college and graduate or professional school. He had no history of alcohol or drug abuse. He had an episode of depression and "bizarre behavior" at the time of his first divorce, was hospitalized and treated with medications, but did not follow through with recommended outpatient care. With the current episode of pain, he also had a depressive syndrome, initially with ideas that other family members had been involved in a conspiracy with his wife and that he himself was being investigated by the Central Intelligence Agency. He was again briefly hospitalized and treated with haloperidol and fluoxetine; he was prescribed fluoxetine and lithium on discharge. For follow-up care, he chose an old professional friend as his psychiatrist, who maintained him with fluoxetine (20 mg/day) and saw the patient sporadically for supportive psychotherapy, which according to the patient "didn't amount to much." Lithium had been discontinued on the insistence of the patient, who reported that it made him "dopey." The patient now minimized the episode leading to hospitalization, saying that he was "upset and hurt" by his wife's infidelity. He reported that he still felt depressed but was much better. "Who wouldn't be depressed if they were in pain all the time and couldn't work!"

Psychiatric diagnoses included (1) pain disorder associated with psychological and general medical features and (2) major depressive disorder, recurrent, with psychotic features in the past. It was also concluded that the patient was disabled from performing the duties of his occupation. Recommendations included (1) that the patient be considered temporarily disabled and be given compensation; (2) referral to a regional pain clinic for more thorough evaluation of pain management; and (3) referral to a psychiatrist (preferably incorporated in the pain clinic referral) with whom the patient does not have a friendship such that objectivity could be maintained.

This clinical vignette illustrates a number of factors important in consideration of pain disorders. First, in this case, it is virtually impossible to dissect the pain complaint as either wholly physically or psychologically based. In all likelihood, the two are intertwined here. Malingering is unlikely. The patient, at least consciously, is motivated to return to work because of both interest and financial incentive. The level of disability compensation is not adequate to maintain his customary style of living. It does not appear that the patient is simply drug seeking, because he has no history of substance abuse and has never overused his opioid medication. Second, the patient fits one stereotype of a person vulnerable to a pain disorder, considering his strong work ethic and reluctance to see things on a psychological or emotional level. Third, despite many evaluations, it does not appear that the patient is yet receiving optimal pain management. He is continued on an opioid analgesic. Whereas treatment with an NSAID and carbamazepine may be appropriate, the carbamazepine is dosed such that it is unlikely to be at a therapeutic plasma level; and a tricyclic antidepressant, which would be the treatment of choice, has not been tried. Last, the psychiatrist is faced with the dilemma of either recommending disability compensation, which may work to reinforce the pain behavior and prolong it, or not recommending compensation to which the patient is legitimately entitled.

# HYPOCHONDRIASIS

## Definition

As defined in DSM-IV, the essential feature in hypochondriasis is preoccupation with fears or the idea of having a

---

**DSM-IV-TR Criteria** 300.7

## Hypochondriasis

A. Preoccupation with fears of having, or the idea that one has, a serious disease based on the person's misinterpretation of bodily symptoms.

B. The preoccupation persists despite appropriate medical evaluation and reassurance.

C. The belief in criterion A is not of delusional intensity (as in delusional disorder, somatic type) and is not restricted to a circumscribed concern about appearance (as in body dysmorphic disorder).

D. The preoccupation causes clinically significant distress or impairment in social, occupational, or other important areas of functioning.

E. The duration of the disturbance is at least 6 months.

F. The preoccupation is not better accounted for by generalized anxiety disorder, obsessive–compulsive disorder, panic disorder, a major depressive episode, separation anxiety, or another somatoform disorder.

*Specify* if:

**With poor insight:** If, for most of the time during the current episode, the person does not recognize that the concern about having a serious illness is excessive or unreasonable

Reprinted with permission from the Diagnostic and Statistical Manual of Mental Disorders, Fourth Edition, Text Revision. Copyright 2000 American Psychiatric Association.

serious disease based on the "misinterpretation of bodily symptoms." This is in contrast to somatization disorder, conversion disorder, and pain disorder, in which the symptoms themselves are the predominant focus (see Table 71–1). There was some debate in the development of DSM-IV as to whether it was necessary that a body complaint be present. On the basis of empirical data, however, it was determined that this requirement was a valid one and helped to distinguish the "disease conviction" of hypochondriasis from "disease fear" as in phobic disorder (Cote et al. 1996). Bodily symptoms may be interpreted broadly to include misinterpretation of normal body functions. In hypochondriasis, the preoccupation persists despite reassurance from physicians and the accumulation of evidence to the contrary. As in the other somatoform disorders, symptoms must result in clinically significant distress or impairment in important areas of functioning. The duration must be at least 6 months. Hypochondriasis is not diagnosed if the hypochondriacal concerns are better accounted for by another psychiatric disorder, such as major depressive episodes or various psychotic disorders with somatic delusions.

Clinical descriptions of a syndrome characterized by preoccupation with body function are found in the writings of the Hippocratic era (Stoudemire 1988). The Greeks attributed the syndrome to disturbances of viscera below the xiphoid cartilage (i.e., hypochondria). Even into the 19th century, hypochondriasis was applied specifically to somatic complaints below the diaphragm, rather than the topographically nonspecific concept of more recent usage (Cloninger 1993). As reviewed by Murphy (1990), Gillespie in 1928 encapsulated a concept of hypochondriasis consistent with the current concept, emphasizing preoccupation with a disease conviction "far in excess of what is justified," which showed "an indifference to the opinion of the environment, including irresponsiveness to persuasion." Gillespie considered hypochondriasis a discrete disease entity. DSM-I did not include hypochondriasis as a separate illness. Hypochondriacal preoccupation was mentioned as one of the malignant symptoms observed in psychotic but not reactive depression. DSM-II included hypochondriacal neurosis. In DSM-III, DSM-III-R, and DSM-IV, hypochondriasis is included as one of the somatoform disorders.

Throughout the modern period, there has been controversy as to whether hypochondriasis represented an independent, discrete disease entity as was proposed by Gillespie. Some maintain that hypochondriasis is virtually always secondary to another psychiatric disorder, usually depression (Kenyon 1976). A number of studies suggested that of the many patients with hypochondriacal complaints, few meet criteria for the full diagnosis (Barsky et al. 1993). Moreover, the lack of bimodality to the complaints suggests a continuum rather than a discrete entity (Noyes et al. 1993).

In the development of DSM-IV, owing to observations that the disease conviction resembled disease phobia or the incorrigible ideas of obsessive–compulsive disorder, placement of hypochondriasis with the anxiety disorders was considered (Cote et al. 1996). Similarly, a case can be made that disease conviction is on a continuum with somatic delusions of disease, suggesting inclusion with the delusional disorders. In the end, such considerations were resolved by keeping hypochondriasis with the somatoform disorders, defining it in terms of an idea that one already has a particular illness rather than fears of acquiring one to distinguish it from a disease phobia, and by excluding cases in which the idea was of delusional proportions to differentiate hypochondriasis from delusional disorder, somatic type.

## Epidemiology

Some degree of preoccupation with disease is apparently common. As reviewed by Kellner (1991), 10 to 20% of "normal" and 45% of "neurotic" persons have intermittent unfounded worries about illness, with 9% of patients doubting reassurances given by physicians. In another review, Kellner (1985) estimated that 50% of all patients attending physicians' offices "suffer either primary hypochondriacal symptoms or have minor somatic disorders with hypochondriacal overlay." How these relate to hypochondriasis as a disorder is difficult to assess because these estimates do not appear to distinguish between a focus on the symptoms themselves (as in somatization disorder) and preoccupation with the implications of the symptoms (as in hypochondriasis). The Epidemiological Catchment Area study (Robins et al. 1984) did not consider hypochondria-

sis. A 1965 study reported prevalence figures ranging from 3 to 13% in different cultures (Kenyon 1965), but it is not clear whether this represents a syndrome comparable to the current definition or just hypochondriacal symptoms. As already noted, many patients manifest some hypochondriacal symptoms as part of other psychiatric disorders, and others have transient hypochondriacal symptoms in response to stresses such as serious physical illness yet never fulfill the inclusion criteria for DSM-IV hypochondriasis. Assessment of the incidence and prevalence of hypochondriasis undoubtedly requires study of general or primary care rather than psychiatric populations, because patients with hypochondriasis are convinced that they suffer from some physical illness. To date, study of such populations suggests that 4 to 9% of patients in general medical settings suffer from hypochondriasis (Fallon et al. 1993).

It does appear that hypochondriasis is equally common in males and females. Data concerning socioeconomic class are conflicting.

## Etiology and Pathophysiology

Until recently, psychoanalytic hypotheses of etiology predominated. Freud hypothesized that hypochondriasis represented "the return of object libido onto the ego with cathexis of the body" (Viederman 1985). Subsequently, the cathexis to the body hypothesis was elaborated on to include interpretations involving disturbed object relations—displacement of repressed hostility to the body to communicate anger indirectly to others. Dynamic mechanisms involving masochism, guilt, conflicted dependency needs, and a need to suffer and be loved at the same time have also been suggested (Stoudemire 1988). The presence of such "narcissistic" mechanisms has been suggested as the reason that patients with hypochondriasis were "unanalyzable." Other psychological theories involve defense against feelings of low self-esteem and inadequacy, perceptual and cognitive abnormalities, and operant conditioning involving reinforcement for assumption of the sick role.

Biological theories have been suggested as well. Hypochondriacal ideas have been attributed to a hypervigilance to insult, including overperception of physical problems (Barsky and Klerman 1983). This has been posited in particular in reference to hypochondriasis as an aspect of depression or anxiety disorders. Hypochondriasis has been included by some in the posited obsessive–compulsive spectrum disorders along with obsessive–compulsive and body dysmorphic disorders, anorexia nervosa, Tourette's disorder, trichotillomania, pathological gambling, and other impulsive disorders (Hollender 1993). All these disorders involve repetitive thoughts or behaviors that patients are unable to delay or inhibit without great difficulty. Evidence for this clustering includes observations of clinical improvement with SSRIs such as fluoxetine even in nondepressed patients with hypochondriasis, body dysmorphic disorder, obsessive–compulsive disorder, and anorexia nervosa. Because such a response is not evident with non-SSRI antidepressants, some type of common serotonin dysregulation is suggested for these disorders.

## Diagnosis and Differential Diagnosis

As shown in Figure 71–1, the first step in approaching patients with distressing or impairing preoccupation with or fears of having a serious disease is to exclude the possibility of explanation on the basis of a general medical condition. Fears that may seem excessive may also occur in patients with general medical conditions with vague and subjective symptoms early in their disease course. These include neurological diseases, such as myasthenia gravis and multiple sclerosis; endocrine diseases; systemic diseases that affect several organ systems, such as systemic lupus erythematosus; and occult malignant neoplasms (Kellner 1991). The disease conviction of hypochondriasis may actually be less amenable to medical reassurance than the fears of patients, with general medical illnesses, who may at least temporally accept such encouragement. Hypochondriacal complaints are not often intentionally produced such that differentiation from malingering and factitious disorder is seldom a problem.

Exclusion is made if the preoccupation is better accounted for by another psychiatric disorder. DSM-IV lists generalized anxiety disorder, obsessive–compulsive disorder, panic disorder, a major depressive episode, separation anxiety, or another somatoform disorder as candidates. Chronology will be of utmost importance in such discriminations. Hypochondriacal concerns occurring exclusively during episodes of another disturbance, such as an anxiety or depressive disorder, do not warrant an additional diagnosis of hypochondriasis. The presence of other psychiatric symptoms will also be helpful. For example, a patient with hypochondriacal complaints as part of a major depressive episode will show other symptoms of depression, such as sleep and appetite disturbance, feelings of worthlessness, and self-reproach, although depressed elderly patients may deny sadness or other expressions of depressed mood. A confounding factor is that patients with hypochondriasis often have comorbid anxiety or depressive syndromes (Kenyon 1965). Again, characterizing the symptoms by chronology will be useful. Treatment trials may also have diagnostic significance. Depressed patients who are hypochondriacal may respond to non-SSRI antidepressant medications or electroconvulsive therapy (often necessary to reverse a depressive state of sufficient severity to lead to such profound symptoms), with resolution of the hypochondriacal as well as the depressive symptoms.

Hypochondriasis is differentiated from other somatoform disorders such as pain, conversion, and somatization disorders by its predominant feature of preoccupation with and fears of having an underlying illness based on the misinterpretation of body symptoms, rather than the physical symptoms themselves. Patients with these other somatoform disorders at times are concerned with the possibility of underlying illness, but this will generally be overshadowed by a focus on the symptoms themselves.

The next consideration is whether the belief is of delusional proportions. Patients with hypochondriasis, although preoccupied, generally acknowledge the possibility that their concerns are unfounded. Delusional patients do not. Somatic delusions of serious illness are seen in some cases of schizophrenia and in delusional disorder, somatic type. In general, patients with schizophrenia that have such delusions also show other signs of schizophrenia, such as disorganized speech, peculiarities of thought and behavior, hallucinations, and other delusions. Belief that an underlying illness is being caused by some bizarre process may

also be seen (e.g., "I'm trying not to defecate because it will cause my brain to turn to jelly"). Schizophrenic patients may also show improvement with neuroleptic treatment, at least in the "active" symptoms of their illness, under which somatic delusions are included.

Differentiation from delusional disorder, somatic type, may be more difficult. It is often a thin line between preoccupation and fear that is a conviction and that which is a delusion. Often, the distinction is made on the basis of whether the patient can consider the possibility that the conviction is erroneous. Yet, patients with hypochondriasis vary in the extent to which they can do this. DSM-IV acknowledges this by its inclusion of the specifier with poor insight. In the past, some argued that differentiation could be made on the basis of response to neuroleptics, especially pimozide; patients with delusional disorder, but not hypochondriasis, respond. Interestingly, there is now at least one report of successful treatment of a syndrome corresponding to delusional disorder, somatic type, in a nondepressed patient with the SSRI paroxetine (Brophy 1994). As with hypochondriasis, response was obtained only when the dose was raised beyond an antidepressant dose (to 60 mg/day).

If it is concluded that the preoccupations are not delusional, the next consideration is whether the duration requirement of 6 months has been met (see Figure 71–1). Syndromes of less than 6 months' duration are diagnosed under either somatoform disorder NOS or adjustment disorder if the symptoms are an abnormal response to a stressful life event. The reason to make such a distinction is to distinguish hypochondriasis from transient syndromes, the longitudinal course of which have been shown to be more variable, suggesting heterogeneity (Barsky et al. 1993).

Other diagnostic considerations include whether the preoccupations or fears are restricted to preoccupations with being overweight, as in anorexia nervosa; with the inappropriateness of one's sex characteristics, as in a gender identity disorder; or with defects in appearance, as in body dysmorphic disorder. The preoccupations of hypochondriasis resemble the obsessions, and the health checking and efforts to obtain reassurance resemble the compulsions of obsessive–compulsive disorder. However, if such manifestations are health centered only, obsessive–compulsive disorder is not diagnosed. If, on the other hand, nonhealth related obsessions and compulsions are present, obsessive–compulsive disorder may be diagnosed in addition to hypochondriasis.

## Course, Natural History, and Prognosis

Data are conflicting, but it appears that the most common age at onset is in early adulthood. Available data suggest that approximately 25% of patients with a diagnosis of hypochondriasis do poorly, 65% show a chronic but fluctuating course, and 10% recover. This pertains to the full syndrome. A much more variable course is seen in patients with just some hypochondriacal concerns. It appears that acute onset, absence of a personality disorder, and absence of secondary gain are favorable prognostically.

## Treatment

Until recently, it appeared that patients with hypochondriasis as a primary condition benefited, but only modestly, from psychiatric intervention. Patients referred early for psychiatric evaluation and treatment showed a slightly better prognosis than those continuing with only medical evaluations and treatments (Kellner 1983). Of course, the first step in treatment is getting the patient to a psychiatrist. Patients with hypochondriasis generally present initially to nonpsychiatric physicians and are often reluctant to see a psychiatrist. Referral should be done sensitively, with the referring physician stressing to the patient that his or her distress is real and that psychiatric evaluation will be a supplement to, not a replacement for, continued medical care.

Initially, the generic techniques outlined for the somatoform disorders in general should be followed. However, it has not been demonstrated that a specific psychotherapy for hypochondriasis is available. As reviewed by Fallon and colleagues (1993), dynamic psychotherapy is of minimal effectiveness; supportive–educative psychotherapy as described by Kellner (1991) is only somewhat helpful, and primarily for those with syndromes of less than 3 years' duration; and cognitive–behavioral therapy, especially response prevention of checking rituals and reassurance seeking, is of only moderate effectiveness at best. All of these techniques seem to lack definitive effects on hypochondriasis itself.

Until recently, this could be said of pharmacological approaches also. Pharmacotherapy of comorbid depressive or anxiety syndromes was often effective, and control of such syndromes aided in general management, yet hypochondriasis itself was not ameliorated. Although controlled trials are lacking, anecdotal and open-label studies suggest that serotoninergic agents such as clomipramine and the SSRI fluoxetine may be effective in ameliorating hypochondriasis. Similar effects are expected from the other SSRIs. Response to fluoxetine has been reported with doses recommended for obsessive–compulsive disorder, rather than usual antidepressant doses (i.e., 60–80 mg rather than 20–40 mg/day). Such pharmacotherapy is best combined with the generic psychotherapy recommendations for somatoform disorders, as well as with cognitive–behavioral techniques to disrupt the counterproductive checking and reassurance-seeking behaviors.

---

**Clinical Vignette 5**

A 26-year-old single man presented for psychiatric evaluation at the insistence of his job supervisor, who was concerned that the patient was not keeping up with his assignments at work. The patient reported that he could not concentrate on his work because for the past 4 years he had been constantly preoccupied with the thought that there was something seriously wrong with his arms resulting from a "strain" while he moved furniture. Although there was minimal pain associated, he was convinced that the problem would progress and he would lose the use of his arms. Multiple consultations with orthopedic surgeons and neurologists had not identified any underlying physical problem. He rejected physical therapy for fear that it would only aggravate the underlying problem. Physical activity involving his arms was avoided as much as possible. Not able to avoid driving to work, he wore a prosthesis that he

had constructed from various elastic bandages "to prevent any strain." He arrived at work early to be ensured a parking space that was easy to enter.

In addition to this preoccupation, he also feared that ulcerative colitis was developing. This began after his father died of a gastrointestinal hemorrhage when the patient was 16 years old. Initially diagnosed as possible ulcerative colitis, it was found at postmortem examination to be due to a ruptured abdominal aneurysm. The patient fully accepted this diagnosis, yet he could not stop thinking that he was at risk for ulcerative colitis despite multiple gastrointestinal evaluations that failed to find any signs of the illness in him. He adhered to a strict diet, avoiding any "roughage," and was concerned about "regularity." He would awaken every day 2 hours earlier than necessary to have enough time for a bowel movement before going to work. The slightest gastrointestinal sensation would aggravate his concern, and he would carefully examine his stool for any signs of blood or mucus. He reported that his work attendance was excellent but that most of the time he would just sit at his desk and move papers around to look busy while thinking about his health problems. "I have a civil service job and until now I got away with it." The patient had no prior psychiatric evaluations. For both of his health concerns, he was able to consider the possibility that there was no underlying physical cause, "but I can't stop thinking about them. What if all the doctors are wrong?"

The psychiatrist's diagnosis was hypochondriasis, with poor insight. The patient was to be further evaluated for a concurrent major depressive episode and also for nonhealth preoccupations that would suggest an additional diagnosis of obsessive–compulsive disorder. The psychiatrist's recommendations included (1) a trial of fluoxetine to be increased to 60 mg/day if tolerated; (2) supportive–educative psychotherapy to ensure compliance and for support; and (3) cognitive–behavioral therapy to reinforce use of his arms, to extinguish assumptions that he needed a special diet, and to reassure him that dire consequences would not occur if his bowel movements were not absolutely punctual.

This clinical vignette illustrates several important typical aspects of hypochondriasis. First, the onset of the disorder was early, in the late teens, with consolidation of symptoms by early adulthood. Second, a chronic course was observed, with some fluctuation in severity. The physical complaints themselves were minimal. It was the preoccupation with fears of underlying illness that predominated and led to distress and impairment.

## BODY DYSMORPHIC DISORDER

### Definition

As defined in DSM-IV, the essential feature of this disorder is preoccupation with an imagined defect in appearance or a markedly excessive concern with a minor anomaly. DSM-III-R dictated "in a normal-appearing person," but this phrase was eliminated from the definition as nonessential, redundant, and inaccurate. In body dysmorphic disorder, a person could be preoccupied with an imagined defect while she or he actually had some other anomaly and was not normal appearing. To exclude conditions with trivial or minor symptoms, the preoccupation must cause clinically significant distress or impairment. By definition, body dysmorphic disorder is not diagnosed if symptoms are limited to preoccupation with body weight, as in anorexia nervosa or bulimia nervosa, or to perceived inappropriateness of sex characteristics, as in gender identity disorder.

According to De Leon and coworkers (1989), preoccupations most often involve the nose, ears, face, or sexual organs. Common complaints include a diversity of imagined flaws of the face or head, including defects in the hair (e.g., too much or too little), skin (e.g., blemishes), and shape or symmetry of the face or facial features (e.g., nose is too large and deformed). However, any body part may be the focus, including genitals, breasts, buttocks, extremities, shoulders, and even overall body size.

Body dysmorphic disorder has been well described in the European and Japanese literature, generally designated dysmorphophobia, often under the rubric of the monosymptomatic hypochondriacal psychoses (Munro 1980). Until recently, it had been virtually ignored in the US literature as well as clinically. Such a disorder was not mentioned in DSM-I or DSM-II (Andreasen and Bardach 1977). Dysmorphophobia was included parenthetically as an example of an atypical somatoform disorder in DSM-III. It was renamed body dysmorphic disorder when included in DSM-III-R. This term was retained in DSM-IV and DSM-IV-TR. ICD-10 lists body dysmorphic disorder as a type of hypochondriacal disorder. Since inclusion in DSM-III, increased study has led to a better characterization of the disorder, which has promoted better detection clinically. Since 1996, it has been included in the Structured Clinical Interview for DSM-IV-Axis I disorders (SCID-I) (First et al. 1996) designed for research purposes. However, the clinical version of this instrument, the Structured Clinical Interview for DSM-IV-Clinical Version (SCID-CV) (First et al. 1997), only includes a single screening question and not the full criteria for the condition.

The definition of the disorder was reexamined for DSM-IV on several counts, but especially as to its relationship to other psychiatric disorders (Phillips and Hollander 1996). After much deliberation, it was determined that body dysmorphic disorder, although often comorbid with anxiety and mood disorders, was sufficiently discrete to be maintained as a separate disorder. As discussed in the differential diagnosis section, it can be distinguished from depressive disorders and from most anxiety disorders, although it resembles obsessive–compulsive disorder in phenomenology, course, and even response to treatment. It was also decided to keep it with the somatoform disorders grouping, although it does not share much with the other disorders in this grouping (with the exception of hypochondriasis), beyond the fact that affected patients are generally referred to psychiatrists from other physicians and that they also present with medically unexplained physical complaints (defects in appearance in body dysmorphic disorder).

In terms of its relationship to the psychotic disorders, DSM-IV dropped the DSM-III-R exclusionary rule that body dysmorphic disorder not be diagnosed if the preoccupation was of delusional intensity (i.e., the patient totally lacked insight or the ability to consider the possibility that the concern was unjustified). This exclusion remains in ICD-10. As De Leon and colleagues (1989) pointed out, it is extremely difficult to determine whether a dysmorphic concern is delusional in that with body dysmorphic disorder, a continuum exists from clearly nondelusional preoccupations to unequivocal delusions such that defining a discrete boundary between the two ends of the spectrum would be artificial. Furthermore, individual patients seem to move back and forth along this continuum. Support for rejecting the exclusion is preliminary evidence that dysmorphic preoccupations may respond to the same pharmacotherapy (SSRIs), regardless of whether the concerns are delusional (Hollander et al. 1993). Perhaps as a reflection of the state of knowledge at this point, both body dysmorphic disorder and delusional disorder, somatic type, can be diagnosed on the basis of the same symptoms, in the same individual, at the same time. Thus, the definition of body dysmorphic disorder differs from hypochondriasis, which is not diagnosed if hypochondriacal concerns are determined to be delusional.

## Epidemiology

Knowledge of such parameters is still incomplete. In general, patients with body dysmorphic disorder first present to nonpsychiatrists such as plastic surgeons, dermatologists, and internists because of the nature of their complaints and are not seen psychiatrically until they are referred (De Leon et al. 1989). Many resist or refuse referral because they do not see their problem as psychiatric; thus, study of psychiatric clinic populations may underestimate the prevalence of the disorder. It has been estimated that 2% of patients seeking corrective cosmetic surgery suffer from this disorder (Andreasen and Bardach 1977). Although women outnumber men in this population, it is not known whether this sex distribution holds true in the general population.

## Etiology and Pathophysiology

A number of sociological, psychological, and neurobiological theories have been proposed. Body dysmorphic disorder has been explained, at least in part, as an exaggerated incorporation of societal ideals of physical perfection and acceptance of cosmetic plastic surgery to attain such goals. A high frequency of insecure, sensitive, obsessional, schizoid, anxious, narcissistic, introverted, and hypochondriacal personality traits in body dysmorphic patients have been described (Phillips 1991). Various psychodynamic mechanisms and symbolic meanings of dysmorphic symptoms have been suggested (Phillips 1991), going back to Freud's case of the Wolfman who had dysmorphic preoccupations regarding his nose.

Some interesting neurobiological possibilities have emerged, particularly concerning observations that hypochondriasis, body dysmorphic disorder, and a number of other conditions involving compelling repetitive thoughts or behaviors may respond preferentially to SSRIs, not to other antidepressant drugs. An obsessive–compulsive spectrum disorders grouping, the pathological process of which is mediated by serotoninergic dysregulation, has been suggested. As further evidence, symptoms of body dysmorphic disorder as well as those of obsessive–compulsive disorder may be aggravated by the partial serotonin agonist *m*-chlorophenylpiperazine (Hollander et al. 1992).

## Diagnosis and Differential Diagnosis

The preoccupations of body dysmorphic disorder must first be differentiated from usual concerns with grooming and appearance. Attention to appearance and grooming is universal and socially sanctioned. However, diagnosis of body dysmorphic disorder requires that the preoccupation cause clinically significant distress or impairment. In addition, in body dysmorphic disorder, concerns focus on an imaginary or exaggerated defect, often of something, such as a small blemish, that would warrant scant attention even if it were present. Persons with histrionic personality disorder may be vain and excessively concerned with appearance. However, the focus in this disorder is on maintaining a good or even exceptional appearance, rather than preoccupation with a defect. Such concerns are probably unrelated to body dysmorphic disorder. In addition, by nature, the preoccupations in body dysmorphic disorder are essentially unamenable to reassurance from friends or family or consultation with physicians, cosmetologists, or other professionals.

Next, the possibility of an explanation by a general medical condition must be considered (see Figure 71–1). As mentioned, patients with this disorder often first present to plastic surgeons, oral surgeons, and others, seeking correction of defects. By the time a mental health professional is consulted, it has generally been ascertained that there is no physical basis for the degree of concern. As with other syndromes involving somatic preoccupations (or delusions), such as olfactory reference syndrome and delusional parasitosis (both included under delusional disorder, somatic type), occult medical disorders, such as an endocrine disturbance or a brain tumor, must be excluded.

In terms of explanation on the basis of another psychiatric disorder, there is little likelihood that symptoms of body dysmorphic disorder will be intentionally produced as in malingering or factitious disorder. Unlike in other somatoform disorders, such as pain, conversion, and somatization disorders, preoccupation with appearance predominates. Somatic preoccupations may occur as part of an anxiety or mood disorder. However, these preoccupations are generally not the predominant focus and lack the specificity of dysmorphic symptoms. Because patients with body dysmorphic disorder often become isolative, social phobia may be suspected. However, in social phobia, the person may feel self-conscious generally but will not focus on a specific imagined defect. Indeed, the two conditions may coexist, warranting both diagnoses. Diagnostic problems may present with the mood-congruent ruminations of major depression, which sometimes involve concern with an unattractive appearance in association with poor self-esteem. Such preoccupations generally lack the focus on a particular body part that is seen in body dysmorphic disorder. On the other hand, patients with body dysmorphic disorder commonly have dysphoric affects described by them variously as anxiety or depression. In some cases, these affects can be subsumed under body dysmorphic disorder; but in other instances, comorbid diagnoses of anxiety or mood disorders are warranted.

Differentiation from schizophrenia must also be made. At times, a dysmorphic concern will seem so unusual that such a psychosis may be considered. Furthermore, patients with this disorder may show ideas of reference in regard to defects in their appearance, which may lead to the consideration of schizophrenia. However, other bizarre delusions, particularly of persecution or grandiosity, and prominent hallucinations are not seen in body dysmorphic disorder. From the other perspective, schizophrenia with somatic delusions generally lacks the focus on a particular body part and defect. Also in schizophrenia, bizarre interpretations and explanations for symptoms are often present, such as "this blemish was a sign from Jesus that I am to protect the world from Satan." Other signs of schizophrenia, such as hallucinations and disorganization of thought, are also absent in body dysmorphic disorder. As previously mentioned, the preoccupations in body dysmorphic disorder appear to be on a continuum from full insight to delusional intensity whereby the patient cannot even consider the possibility that the preoccupation is groundless. In such instances, both body dysmorphic disorder and delusional disorder, somatic type, are to be diagnosed.

Body dysmorphic disorder is not to be diagnosed if the concern with appearance is better accounted for by another psychiatric disorder. Anorexia nervosa, in which there is dissatisfaction with body shape and size, is specifically mentioned in the criteria as an example of such an exclusion. DSM-III-R also mentioned transsexualism (gender identity disorder in DSM-IV) as such a disorder. Although not specifically mentioned in DSM-IV, if a preoccupation is limited to discomfort or a sense of inappropriateness of one's primary and secondary sex characteristics, coupled with a strong and persistent cross-gender identification, body dysmorphic disorder is not diagnosed.

The preoccupations of body dysmorphic disorder may resemble obsessions and ruminations as seen in obsessive–compulsive disorder. Unlike the obsessions of obsessive–compulsive disorder, the preoccupations of body dysmorphic disorder focus on concerns with appearance. Compulsions are limited to checking and investigating the perceived physical defect and attempting to obtain reassurance from others regarding it. Still, the phenomenology is similar, and the two disorders are often comorbid. If additional obsessions and compulsions not related to the defect are present, obsessive–compulsive disorder can be diagnosed in addition to body dysmorphic disorder.

## Course, Natural History, and Prognosis

Age at onset appears to peak in adolescence or early adulthood (Phillips 1991). Body dysmorphic disorder is generally a chronic condition, with a waxing and waning of intensity but rarely full remission (Phillips et al. 1993). In a lifetime, multiple preoccupations are typical; in one study, the average was four (Phillips et al. 1993). In some, the same preoccupation remains unchanged. In others, new perceived defects are added to the original ones. In others still, symptoms remit, only to be replaced by others. The disorder is often highly incapacitating, with many patients showing marked impairment in social and occupational activities. Perhaps a third becomes housebound. Most attribute their limitations to embarrassment concerning their perceived defect, but the attention and time-consuming nature of the preoccupations and attempts to investigate and rectify defects also contribute. The extent to which patients with body dysmorphic disorder receive surgery or medical treatments is unknown. Superimposed depressive episodes are common, as are suicidal ideation and suicide attempts. Actual suicide risk is unknown.

In view of the nature of the defects with which patients are preoccupied, it is not surprising that they are found most commonly among patients seeking cosmetic surgery. Preoccupations persist despite reassurance that there is no defect to surgically correct. Surgery or other corrective procedures rarely if ever lead to satisfaction and may even lead to greater distress with the perception of new defects attributed to the surgery.

## Treatment

First, the generic goals and treatments as outlined for the somatoform disorders overall should be instituted. These are beneficial in interrupting an unending procession of repeated evaluations and the possibility of needless surgery, which may lead to additional perceptions that surgery has resulted in further disfigurement.

Traditional insight-oriented therapies have not generally proved to be effective. Results with traditional behavioral techniques, such as systematic desensitization and exposure therapy, have been mixed. At least without amelioration with effective pharmacotherapy, the preoccupations do not extinguish as would be expected with phobias. A cognitive–behavioral approach similar to what was recommended for hypochondriasis may be more effective. This includes response prevention techniques whereby the patient is not permitted to repetitively check the perceived defect in mirrors. In addition, patients are advised not to seek reassurance from family and friends, and these persons are instructed not to respond to such inquiries. Some patients adopt such behaviors spontaneously, avoiding mirrors and other reflecting surfaces, refusing even to allude to their perceived defects to others. Such "self-techniques" may be encouraged and refined.

Biological treatments have long been used but until recently were of limited benefit to patients with body dysmorphic disorder. Approaches have included electroconvulsive therapy, tricyclic and MAOI antidepressants, and neuroleptics (particularly pimozide) (Andreasen and Bardach 1977). In most reports of positive response to tricyclic or MAOI antidepressant drugs, it is unclear whether response was truly in terms of the dysmorphic syndrome or simply represented improvement in comorbid depressive or anxiety syndromes. Response to neuroleptic treatment has been suggested as a diagnostic test to distinguish body dysmorphic disorder from delusional disorder, somatic type (Riding and Munro 1975). The delusional syndromes often respond to neuroleptics; body dysmorphic disorders, even when the body preoccupations are psychotic, generally do not. Pimozide has been singled out as a neuroleptic with specific effectiveness for somatic delusions, but this specificity does not appear to apply to body dysmorphic disorder.

An exception to this uninspiring picture is the observation of a possible preferential response to antidepressant drugs with serotonin reuptake blocking effects, such as clomipramine, or SSRIs, such as fluoxetine and fluvoxamine (Hollander et al. 1992). Phillips and coworkers (1993) reported that more than 50% of patients with body dysmorphic disorder showed a partial or complete remission with either clomipramine or fluoxetine, a response not predicted on the basis of coexisting major depressive or obsessive–compulsive disorder. As with hypochondriasis, effectiveness is generally achieved at levels recommended for obsessive–compulsive disorder rather than for depression (e.g., 60–80 mg rather than 20–40 mg/day of fluoxetine). The SSRIs appear to ameliorate delusional as well as nondelusional dysmorphic preoccupations. Successful augmentation of clomipramine or SSRI therapy has been suggested with buspirone, another drug with serotoninergic effects. Neuroleptics, particularly pimozide, may also be helpful adjuncts, particularly if delusions of reference are present. Little seems to be gained with the addition of anticonvulsants, or benzodiazepines to the SSRI therapy.

As yet, rigorous studies have not been conducted, but anecdotal observations and open-label studies show promise for effective treatment with SSRIs and other serotoninergic agents for this, until now, therapeutically exasperating disorder. If such approaches fulfill their initial promise, integrated approaches using pharmacotherapy and other modalities such as cognitive–behavioral therapy may provide effective treatment options.

---

Clinical Vignette 6

A 22-year-old single woman who lived with her parents was referred for psychiatric consultation because of preoccupations of 4 years that there was something wrong with the way her teeth were situated in her jaw. She could not specify what exactly was wrong but insisted that her teeth felt "funny" and at times would actually relocate, especially while she was eating. She spent "hours" each day in front of a mirror examining her teeth from various angles. With the exception of her parents, she had become essentially a recluse in that people avoided her because she would repeatedly ask their opinion as to whether they thought her teeth were abnormally placed. At one family function, she showed her mouth full of food to a relative, asking if her teeth could be seen moving, disgusting the relative, who insisted the parents arrange for a psychiatric evaluation. By the time of referral, she had received multiple dental, orthodontic, and oral surgery evaluations, none of which indicated any abnormality. Despite this, she was "absolutely sure" that there was something wrong with her teeth or mouth. She would not even consider hypothetically that her concerns were unfounded and might be the consequence of a misinterpretation or of a psychiatric disturbance. As described by her parents, their family physician had tried treatment with alprazolam ("to calm her down"), imipramine ("in case she's depressed and it might help any pain"), and low-dose haloperidol ("she might be schizophrenic").

The psychiatrist diagnosed body dysmorphic disorder and delusional disorder, somatic type. He recommended (1) continued psychiatric care with the institution of pharmacotherapy with sertraline, 50 mg/day to be increased to 150 mg as tolerated; (2) preventing the patient from self-checking by removing all mirrors from her living space; and (3) that no response be given to any questions about the appearance of her mouth or teeth. The patient was carefully advised that the last two measures were being instituted. The rationale was explained to reassure her that they were not being instituted punitively. The patient showed little comprehension of these explanations.

This clinical vignette illustrates several important aspects of body dysmorphic disorder. The age at onset of the disorder in this patient is typical at 18 years. Although her perception that her teeth were relocating was atypical, the locale of her preoccupation (the teeth) is fairly common. Her pattern of seeking reassurance from self-examination and soliciting the opinion of others is also common in these patients. The patient's actual physical complaints were minimal. She reported no pain and no actual physical discomfort in her mouth, it was "how they looked." The patient gave no evidence of even partial insight that her perceptions regarding her mouth and teeth were erroneous. Thus, she qualified for a diagnosis of delusional disorder, somatic type, as well as body dysmorphic disorder, as is allowed in the DSM-IV criteria. Last, the patient was appropriately prescribed an SSRI with the expectation of reaching a dose higher than that recommended for depression. Because this patient was also delusional, the neuroleptic pimozide was also considered as an adjunct. The behavioral manipulations of preventing self-checking and seeking reassurance from others were also recommended.

## SOMATOFORM DISORDER NOT OTHERWISE SPECIFIED

### Definition

Somatoform disorder NOS is the true residual category. By definition, disorders considered under this category are characterized by somatic symptoms, but criteria for any of the specific somatoform disorders are not met. Several examples are given, but syndromes potentially included under this category are not limited to these. Unlike for undifferentiated somatoform disorder, no minimal duration is required. This category was incorporated into DSM-III-R, replacing the DSM-III atypical somatoform disorder, a residual category requiring that physical symptoms and complaints not be explained on the basis of demonstrable organic findings or a known pathophysiological mechanism and that they were "apparently linked to psychological factors." The only example given was dysmorphophobia. DSM-III-R similarly

---

**DSM-IV-TR Criteria** 300.81

### Somatoform Disorder Not Otherwise Specified

This category includes disorders with somatoform symptoms that do not meet criteria for any specific somatoform disorder. Examples include:

1. Pseudocyesis: a false belief of being pregnant that is associated with objective signs of pregnancy, which may include abdominal enlargement (although the umbilicus does not become everted), reduced menstrual flow, amenorrhea, subjective sensation of fetal movement, nausea, breast engorgement and secretions, and labor pains at the expected date of delivery. Endocrine changes may be present, but the syndrome cannot be explained by a general medical condition that causes endocrine changes (e.g., a hormone-secreting tumor).

2. A disorder involving nonpsychotic hypochondriacal symptoms of less than 6 months' duration.

3. A disorder involving unexplained physical symptoms (e.g., fatigue or body weakness) of less than 6 months' duration that are not due to another mental disorder.

Reprinted with permission from the Diagnostic and Statistical Manual of Mental Disorders, Fourth Edition, Text Revision. Copyright 2000 American Psychiatric Association.

required that criteria for any specific somatoform or adjustment disorder with physical symptoms not be met. Examples given were nonpsychotic hypochondriacal symptoms and nonstress-related physical complaints of less than 6 months' duration. DSM-IV lists as examples pseudocyesis, disorders involving hypochondriacal complaints but of less than 6 months' duration, and disorders involving unexplained physical complaints such as fatigue or body weakness not due to another mental disorder and again of less than 6 months' duration. This last syndrome would seem to resemble neurasthenia of short duration, a syndrome with a long historical tradition with inclusion in DSM-II, ICD-9, and ICD-10. Neurasthenia was considered for inclusion as a separate DSM-IV somatoform disorder. Reasons that it was not included in DSM-IV include difficulties in delineating it from depressive and anxiety disorders and from other somatoform disorders. If included, neurasthenia could have become a clinical "wastebasket" that could facilitate premature closure of diagnostic inquiry, such that underlying general medical conditions as well as other mental disorders would more likely be overlooked.

Inclusion of pseudocyesis deserves special mention. This syndrome, not mentioned at all in DSM-II, was included in DSM-III and DSM-III-R as an example of a conversion symptom under the broadened definition of conversion, on the basis that it represented a somatic expression of a psychological conflict or need, in this case involving ambivalence toward pregnancy. The resulting conflict was resolved somatically as a false pregnancy, lessening anxiety (primary gain) and leading to unconsciously needed environmental support (secondary gain). With the restriction of conversion in DSM-IV to include only symptoms affecting voluntary motor and sensory function, pseudocyesis was excluded from the conversion disorder definition. In a sense, it is placed in the somatoform disorder NOS category for lack of a more appropriate place. Pseudocyesis is a reasonably discrete syndrome for which specific criteria as listed in DSM-IV can be delineated. These criteria were derived from a review of the existing literature (Lipowski 1988). However, given its rarity, it is not listed as a specified somatoform disorder. Whelan and Stewart (1990) reported six cases in 20 years of consulting to a unit in which 2,500 women delivered per year. It could also be described as a psychophysiological endocrine disorder. On the basis of a literature review (Lipowski 1988), in many cases, a neuroendocrine change accompanies and at times may antedate the false belief of pregnancy. This approaches inclusion as a medical condition, which would lend itself to consideration of psychological factors affecting medical condition. However, in most instances, a discrete general medical condition (such as a hormone-secreting tumor) cannot be identified.

## Diagnosis and Differential Diagnosis

As a residual category, somatoform disorder NOS is to be diagnosed after all other possibilities are excluded (see Figure 71–1). After it is determined that a syndrome with somatoform symptoms is not attributable to a nonsomatoform psychiatric disorder and does not meet criteria for any of the specific somatoform disorders (including, on the symptom-focused side, pain, conversion, and somatization disorders and, on the preoccupation-focused side, hypochondriasis or body dysmorphic disorder), the two diagnostic possibilities that remain are undifferentiated somatoform disorder and somatoform disorder NOS. Except in the case of pseudocyesis, these two are differentiated on the basis of whether the disturbance is of 6 months' duration. If symptoms last more than 6 months, undifferentiated somatoform disorder is diagnosed; if less than 6 months, somatoform disorder NOS.

---

Clinical Vignette 7

A 64-year-old man was referred for psychiatric consultation by a gastroenterologist because of the patient's uncompromising preoccupation of 4 months that he suffered from colon cancer. This fear developed after the patient underwent lower bowel radiography to evaluate complaints of constipation unimproved with dietary changes, stool softeners, and laxatives. He was allowed to view his radiographs, and he noted a "shadow" that he was convinced represented a cancer mass. The patient was reshown the film with explicit explanation. He was satisfied temporarily, but he soon became concerned that if it was not cancer, a rubber tube may have been left in his colon from the barium enema examination and, if left there, would eventually cause cancer. The patient could consider that his concern might be unfounded, yet "I just can't shake the idea that I have cancer." The patient had no other unusual ideas or prominent symptoms. He denied feeling sad and was not

worried about other things. He did feel that "this is draining all my energy" and had difficulty in concentrating on any of his usual interests or hobbies. He did not feel guilty about anything and was not contemplating suicide or wishing to be dead, but "I just know this thing is going to kill me!" He had no prior history of excessive health concerns and had never felt any need for psychiatric treatment.

The psychiatrist's diagnosis was (1) possible somatoform disorder NOS, consider hypochondriasis early in its course, but ruled out major depressive disorder or delusional disorder, somatic type, as alternative explanations; (2) ruled out occult general medical condition underlying his complaints: a gastrointestinal disorder with subtle symptoms and no objective findings; depressive disorder NOS; delusional disorder, somatic type; or mental disorder NOS due to a general medical condition. It was recommended that the patient be (1) thoroughly evaluated for a general medical condition, including endocrine studies, and (2) empirically started on an SSRI.

This clinical vignette illustrates an important aspect of somatoform disorder NOS. In using this diagnosis, the psychiatrist must remain cognizant that it is a residual category, and vigilance must be maintained for the emergence of a previously undetected general medical or psychiatric condition.

## CONCLUSION

As a group, the syndromes now subsumed under the rubric of somatoform disorders are relatively common and are associated with great direct and indirect costs to society. Yet, they have remained a "stepchild" of psychiatry, underdiagnosed and underresearched. Perhaps the first step in bringing these conditions into the light was the formalization of criteria and nomenclature and their aggregation into a group in DSM-III. This has allowed a practical approach to the differential diagnosis of conditions with physical symptoms suggestive of underlying general medical conditions (see Figure 71–1). Moreover, the definition of this group has been conducive to more coordinated research in which findings are more comparable from one investigation to another. With this, therapeutic direction is emerging, with some general guidelines for all of these disorders; some specific ways of managing patients with somatization disorder, undifferentiated somatoform disorder, and conversion disorder; and a more utilitarian approach to management of patients with pain disorders.

It appears that pharmacological inroads are being made in the treatment of hypochondriasis and body dysmorphic disorder in terms of the possible efficacy of SSRIs. This pharmacological "probe" suggests that these disorders may be more closely linked with the so-called obsessive–compulsive spectrum disorders (Hollender 1993) than with the other somatoform disorders, a linkage that may be reflected in future diagnostic systems. Even if this turns out to be the case, the somatoform disorder concept will have served its purpose in stimulating and making possible research leading to a better understanding and ultimately more effective treatments for these complex conditions.

Much work remains to be done before the knowledge concerning the somatoform disorders and their treatment catch up with the understanding of other groupings of psychiatric disorders.

## Comparison of DSM-IV/ICD-10 Diagnostic Criteria

The ICD-10 Diagnostic Criteria for Research for Somatization Disorder has both a different item set and algorithm. Six symptoms are required out of a list of 14 symptoms which are broken down into the following groups: 6 gastrointestinal symptoms, 2 cardiovascular symptoms, 3 genitourinary symptoms, and 3 "skin and pain" symptoms. It is specified that the symptoms occur in at least two groups. In contrast, DSM-IV-TR requires 4 pain symptoms, 2 gastrointestinal symptoms, 1 sexual symptom and 1 pseudoneurological symptom. Furthermore, the ICD-10 Diagnostic Criteria for Research specify that there must be "persistent refusal to accept medical reassurance that there is no adequate physical cause for the physical symptoms." DSM-IV-TR only requires that the symptoms result in treatment being sought or significant impairment in social, occupational, or other important areas of functioning and that the symptoms cannot be fully explained by a known general medical condition or substance. For Undifferentiated Somatoform Disorder, the ICD-10 Diagnostic Criteria for Research and the DSM-IV-TR criteria are almost identical.

Regarding conversion disorder, ICD-10 considers conversion a type of dissociative disorder and includes separate criteria sets for dissociative motor disorders, dissociative convulsions, and dissociative anesthesia and sensory loss in a section that also includes dissociative amnesia and dissociative fugue.

For pain disorder, the ICD-10 Diagnostic Criteria for Research require that the pain last at least 6 months and that it not be "explained adequately by evidence of a physiological process or a physical disorder." In contrast, DSM-IV-TR does not force the clinician to make this inherently impossible judgment and instead requires the contribution of psychological factors. Furthermore, DSM-IV-TR includes both acute (duration less than 6 months) and chronic pain (more than 6 months). This disorder is referred to in ICD-10 as "Persistent Somatoform Pain Disorder."

ICD-10 provides a single criteria set that applies to both the DSM-IV-TR categories of hypochondriasis and body dysmorphic disorder. The ICD-10 Diagnostic Criteria for Research for Hypochondriasis specifies that the belief is of a "maximum of two serious physical diseases" and requires that at least one be specifically named by the individual with the disorder. The DSM-IV-TR has no such requirement.

## References

Alexander F (1950) Psychosomatic Medicine. WW Norton, New York.
Alper K, Devinsky O, Vasquez B, et al. (1993) Nonepileptic seizures and childhood sexual and physical abuse. Neurology 43, 1950–1953.
American Psychiatric Association (1980) Diagnostic and Statistical Manual of Mental Disorders, 3rd ed. APA, Washington DC.
American Psychiatric Association (1987) Diagnostic and Statistical Manual of Mental Disorders, 3rd ed., Rev. APA, Washington DC.
American Psychiatric Association (2000) Diagnostic and Statistical Manual of Mental Disorders, 4th ed, Text Rev. APA, Washington DC.
American Psychiatric Association (1995) Diagnostic and Statistical Manual of Mental Disorders, 4th ed., Primary Care ed. APA, Washington DC.
Andreasen NC and Bardach J (1977) Dysmorphophobia: Symptom or disease? Am J Psychiatr 134, 673–676.
Barsky AJ (1989) Somatoform disorders. In Comprehensive Textbook of Psychiatry, Vol. 1, 5th ed., Kaplan HI and Sadock BJ (eds). Williams & Wilkins, Baltimore, pp. 1009–1027.
Barsky AJ and Klerman GL (1983) Overview: Hypochondriasis, bodily complaints, and somatic styles. Am J Psychiatr 140, 273–282.
Barsky AJ, Cleary PD, Sarnie MK, et al. (1993) The course of transient hypochondriasis. Am J Psychiatr 150, 484–488.
Bendefeldt F, Miller LL, and Ludwig AM (1976) Cognitive hysteria. Arch Gen Psychiatr 33, 1250–1254.
Bohman M, Cloninger CR, von Knorring A-L, et al. (1984) An adoption study of somatoform disorders. III. Cross-fostering analysis and genetic relationship to alcoholism and criminality. Arch Gen Psychiatr 41, 872–878.
Breuer J and Freud S (1955) Studies on hysteria. In The Standard Edition of the Complete Psychological Works of Sigmund Freud, Vol. 2, Strachey J (trans-ed). Hogarth Press, London. Originally published in 1893–1895.
Briquet P (1859) Traité Clinique et Thérapeutique à l'Hystérie. J-B Bailliére & Fils, Paris.
Brophy JJ (1994) Monosymptomatic hypochondriacal psychosis treated with paroxetine: A case report. Irish J Psychol Med 11, 21–22.
Carter AB (1949) The prognosis of certain hysterical symptoms. Br Med J 1, 1076–1079.
Chaturvedi SK (1987) Prevalence of chronic pain in psychiatric patients. Pain 19, 231–237.
Chodoff P and Lyons H (1958) Hysteria, the hysterical personality and "hysterical conversion." Am J Psychiatr 131, 734–740.
Cloninger CR (1986) Somatoform and dissociative disorders. In Medical Basis of Psychiatry, Winokur G and Clayton PJ (eds). WB Saunders, Philadelphia, pp. 123–151.
Cloninger CR (1987) Diagnosis of somatoform disorders: A critique of DSM-III. In Diagnosis and Classification in Psychiatry: A Critical Appraisal of DSM-III, Tischler GL (ed). Cambridge University Press, New York, pp. 243–259.
Cloninger CR (1993) Somatoform and dissociative disorders. In Medical Basis of Psychiatry, 2nd ed., Winokur G and Clayton PJ (eds). WB Saunders, Philadelphia, pp. 169–192.
Cloninger CR (1996) Somatization disorder. In DSM-IV Sourcebook, Vol. 2, Widiger TA, Frances AJ, Pincus HA, et al. (eds). American Psychiatric Association, Washington DC, pp. 885–892.
Cloninger CR and Guze SB (1979) Psychiatric illness and female criminality: The role of sociopathy and hysteria in the antisocial woman. Am J Psychiatr 127, 303–311.
Cloninger CR and Yutzy S (1993) Somatoform and dissociative disorders: A summary of changes for DSM-IV. In Current Psychiatric Therapy, Dunner DL (ed). WB Saunders, Philadelphia, pp. 310–313.
Cloninger CR, Martin RL, Guze SB, et al. (1986) A prospective follow-up and family study of somatization in men and women. Am J Psychiatr 143, 873–878.
Cloninger CR, Reich T, and Guze SB (1975) The multifactorial model of disease transmission. III. Familial relationship between sociopathy and hysteria (Briquet's syndrome). Br J Psychiatr 127, 23–32.
Cloninger CR, Sigvardsson S, von Knorring A-L, et al. (1984) An adoption study of somatoform disorders. II. Identification of two discrete somatoform disorders. Arch Gen Psychiatr 41, 863–871.
Coryell W and House D (1984) The validity of broadly defined hysteria and DSM-III conversion disorder: Outcome, family history, and mortality. J Clin Psychiatr 45, 252–256.
Cote G, O'Leary T, Barlow DH, et al. (1996) Hypochondriasis. In DSM-IV Sourcebook, Vol. 2, Widiger TA, Frances AJ, Pincus HA, et al. (eds). American Psychiatric Association, Washington DC, pp. 933–948.
De Leon J, Bott A, and Simpson G (1989) Dysmorphophobia: Body dysmorphic disorder or delusional disorder, somatic subtype? Compr Psychiatry 30, 457–472.
Delaplaine R, Ifabumuyi OI, Merskey H, et al. (1978) Significance of pain in psychiatric hospital patients. Pain 4, 143–152.
Desai BT, Porter RJ, and Penry K (1982) Psychogenic seizures. A study of 42 attacks in six patients, with intensive monitoring. Arch Neurol 39, 202–209.
DeSouza C, Othmer E, Gabrielli W, et al. (1988) Major depression and somatization disorder: The overlooked differential diagnosis. Psychiatr Ann 18, 340–348.
Escobar JI, Rubio-Stipec, Canino G, et al. (1989) Somatic Symptom Index (SSI): A new and abridged somatization construct: Prevalence and

epidemiological correlates in two large community samples. J Nerv Ment Dis 177, 140–146.

Escobar JI, Swartz M, Rubio-Stipec M, et al. (1991) Medically unexplained symptoms: Distribution, risk factors, and comorbidity. In Current Concepts of Somatization: Research and Clinical Perspectives, Kirmayer LJ and Robbins JM (eds). American Psychiatric Press, Washington DC, pp. 63–68.

Fallon BA, Klein BW, and Liebowitz MR (1993) Hypochondriasis: Treatment strategies. Psychiatr Ann 23, 374–381.

Feighner JP, Robins E, Guze SB, et al. (1972) Diagnostic criteria for use in psychiatric research. Arch Gen Psychiatr 26, 57–63.

First MB, Spitzer RL, Williams JBW, et al. (1996) Structured Clinical Interview for DSM-IV Axis I Disorders (SCID-I). New York State Psychiatric Institute, Biometrics Research, New York.

First MB, Spitzer RL, Williams JBW, et al. (1997) Structured Clinical Interview for DSM-IV—Clinical Version (SCID-CV). American Psychiatric Press, Washington DC.

Flor-Henry P, Fromm-Auch D, Tapper M, et al. (1981) A neuropsychological study of the stable syndrome of hysteria. Biol Psychiatr 16, 601–626.

Folks DG, Ford CV, and Regan WM (1984) Conversion symptoms in a general hospital. Psychosomatics 25, 285–295.

Ford CV and Folks DG (1985) Conversion disorders: An overview. Psychosomatics 26, 371–383.

Ford CV (1983) The Somatizing Disorders: Illness as a Way of Life. Elsevier Scientific, New York.

Ford CV (1995) Conversion disorder and somatoform disorder not otherwise specified. In Treatments of Psychiatric Disorders, Vol. 2, 2nd ed., Gabbard GO (ed). American Psychiatric Association, Washington DC, pp. 1735–1753.

Fukuda K, Straus SE, Hickie I, et al. (1994) The chronic fatigue syndrome: A comprehensive approach to its definition and study. Ann Intern Med 121, 953–959.

Gatfield PD and Guze SB (1962) Prognosis and differential diagnosis of conversion reactions (a follow-up study). Dis Nerv Syst 23, 1–8.

Goodwin DW and Guze SB (1989) Psychiatric Diagnosis, 4th ed., Oxford University Press, New York.

Guze SB and Perley MJ (1963) Observations on the natural history of hysteria. Am J Psychiatr 19, 960–965.

Guze SB, Cloninger CR, Martin RL, et al. (1986) A follow-up and family study of Briquet's syndrome. Br J Psychiatr 149, 17–23.

Guze SB, Cloninger CR, Martin RL, et al. (1986) A follow-up and family study of Briquet's syndrome. Br J Psychiatr 149, 17–23.

Hales RE (1996) Psychiatric system interface disorders (PSID). In DSM-IV Sourcebook, Vol. 2, Widiger TA, Frances AJ, Pincus HA, et al. (eds). American Psychiatric Association, Washington DC, pp. 871–884.

Hollander E, Cohen LJ, and Simeon D (1993) Body dysmorphic disorder. Psychiatr Ann 23, 359–364.

Hollander E, DeCaria CM, Nitescu A, et al. (1992) Serotonergic function in obsessive–compulsive disorder. Behavioral and neuroendocrine responses to oral m-chlorophenylpiperazine and fenfluramine in patients and healthy volunteers. Arch Gen Psychiatr 49, 21–28.

Hollender E (1993) Obsessive–compulsive spectrum disorders: An overview. Psychiatr Ann 23, 355–358.

Inouye E (1972) Genetic aspects of neurosis. Int J Ment Health 1, 176–189.

Kellner R (1983) The prognosis of treated hypochondriasis: A clinical study. Acta Psychiatr Scand 67, 69–79.

Kellner R (1985) Functional somatic symptoms and hypochondriasis. A survey of empirical studies. Arch Gen Psychiatr 42, 821–832.

Kellner R (1990) Somatization: Theories and research. J Nerv Ment Dis 178, 150–160.

Kellner R (1991) Psychosomatic Syndromes and Somatic Symptoms. American Psychiatric Press, Washington DC.

Kent D, Tomasson K, and Coryell W (1995) Course and outcome of conversion and somatization disorders: A four-year follow-up. Psychosomatics 36, 138–144.

Kenyon FE (1965) Hypochondriasis: A survey of some historical, clinical, and social aspects. Br J Psychiatr 138, 117–133.

Kenyon FE (1976) Hypochondriacal states. Br J Psychiatr 129, 1–14.

King SA (1994) Pain disorders. In The American Psychiatric Press Textbook of Psychiatry, 2nd ed., Hales RE, Yudofsky SC, and Talbott JA (eds). American Psychiatric Press, Washington DC, pp. 591–622.

Kirmayer LJ and Robbins JM (1991) Introduction: Concepts of somatization. In Current Concepts of Somatization: Research and Clinical

Perspectives, Kirmayer LJ and Robbins JM (eds). American Psychiatric Press, Washington DC, pp. 1–19.

Kirmayer LJ, Robbins JM, Dworkind M, et al. (1993) Somatization and the recognition of depression and anxiety in primary care. Am J Psychiatr 150, 734–741.

Lader M and Sartorious N (1968) Anxiety in patients with hysterical conversion symptoms. J Neurol Neurosurg Psychiatr 31, 490–495.

Lazare A (1981) Conversion symptoms. N Engl J Med 305, 745–748.

Leavitt F and Sweet JJ (1986) Characteristics and frequency of malingering among patients with low back pain. Pain 25, 357–374.

Lewis WC (1974) Hysteria: The consultant's dilemma: 20th century demonology, pejorative epithet, or useful diagnosis? Arch Gen Psychiatr 30, 145–151.

Lewis WC and Berman M (1965) Studies of conversion hysteria. I. Operational study of diagnosis. Arch Gen Psychiatr 13, 275–282.

Lipowski ZJ (1988) Somatization: The concept and its clinical application. Am J Psychiatr 145, 1358–1368.

Ljunberg L (1957) Hysteria: Clinical, prognostic and genetic study. Acta Psychiatr Scand 32(Suppl), 1–162.

Ludwig AM (1972) Hysteria. A neurobiological theory. Arch Gen Psychiatr 27, 771–777.

Luff MC and Garrod M (1935) The after-results of psychotherapy in 500 adult cases. Br Med J 2, 54–59.

Maloney MJ (1980) Diagnosing hysterical conversion disorders in children. J Pediatr 97, 1016–1020.

Malt UF (1991) Somatization: An old disorder in new bottles? Psychiatr Fenn 22, 1–13.

Marsden CD (1986) Hysteria—a neurologist's view. Psychol Med 16, 277–288.

Martin RL (1988) Problems in the diagnosis of somatization disorder: Effects on research and clinical practice. Psychiatr Ann 18, 357–362.

Martin RL (1995) DSM-IV changes for the somatoform disorders. Psychiatr Ann 25, 29–39.

Martin RL (1996) Conversion disorder, proposed autonomic arousal disorder, and pseudocyesis. In DSM-IV Sourcebook, Vol. 2, Widiger TA, Frances AJ, Pincus HA, et al. (eds). American Psychiatric Association, Washington DC, pp. 893–914.

Martin RL and Yutzy SH (1994) Somatoform disorders. In The American Psychiatric Press Textbook of Psychiatry, 2nd ed., Hales RE, Yudofsky SC, and Talbott JA (eds). American Psychiatric Press, Washington DC, pp. 591–622.

Martin RL, Cloninger CR, and Guze SB (1979) The evaluation of diagnostic concordance in follow-up studies, II: A blind prospective follow-up of female criminals. J Psychiatr Res 15, 107–125.

Martin RL, Cloninger CR, Guze SB, et al. (1985) Mortality in a follow-up of 500 psychiatric outpatients. Arch Gen Psychiatr 42, 58–66.

Mears R and Horvath TB (1972) "Acute" and "chronic" hysteria. Br J Psychiatr 121, 653–657.

Melzack R and Wall PD (1983) The Challenge of Pain. Basic Books, New York.

Munro A (1980) Monosymptomatic hypochondriacal psychosis. Br J Hosp Med 24, 34–38.

Murphy GE (1982) The clinical management of hysteria. JAMA 247, 2559–2564.

Murphy MR (1990) Classification of the somatoform disorders. In Somatization: Physical Symptoms and Psychological Illness, Bass C (ed). Blackwell Scientific, Oxford, UK, pp. 10–39.

Nandi DN, Banerjee G, Nandi S, et al. (1992) Is hysteria on the wane? A community survey in West Bengal, India. Br J Psychiatr 160, 87–91.

Noyes R, Kathol RG, and Fisher MM (1993) The validity of DSM-III-R hypochondriasis. Arch Gen Psychiatr 50, 961–970.

Ormel J, VonKorff M, Ustun B, et al. (1994) Common mental disorders and disability across cultures: Results from the WHO Collaborative Study on Psychological Problems in General Health Care. JAMA 272, 1741–1748.

Osterweis M, Kleinman A, Mechanic D (eds). (1987) Pain and Disability. National Academy Press, Washington DC.

Perkin GD (1989) An analysis of 7836 successive new outpatient referrals. J Neurol Neurosurg Psychiatr 52, 447–448.

Perley M and Guze SB (1962) Hysteria: The stability and usefulness of clinical criteria. A quantitative study based upon a 6–8 year follow-up of 39 patients. N Engl J Med 266, 421–426.

Phillips KA (1991) Body dysmorphic disorder: The distress of imagined ugliness. Am J Psychiatr 148, 1138–1149.

Phillips KA and Hollander E (1996) Body dysmorphic disorder. In DSM-IV Sourcebook, Vol. 2, Widiger TA, Frances AJ, Pincus HA, et al. (eds). American Psychiatric Association, Washington DC, 949–960.

Phillips KA, McElroy S, Keck PE, et al. (1993) Body dysmorphic disorder: 30 cases of imagined ugliness. Am J Psychiatr 150, 302–308.

Pincus J (1982) Hysteria presenting to a neurologist. In Hysteria, Roy A (ed). John Wiley, Chichester, UK, pp. 131–144.

Porter J and Jick H (1980) Addiction rare in patients treated with narcotics [letter]. N Engl J Med 302, 303.

Preskorn SH (1995) Beyond DSM-IV: What is the cart and what is the horse? Psychiatr Ann 25, 53–62.

Pribor EF, Smith DS, and Yutzy SH (1994) Somatization disorder in elderly patients. Am J Geriatr Psychiatr 2, 109–117.

Purtell JJ, Robins E, and Cohen ME (1951) Observations on clinical aspects of hysteria. A quantitative study of 50 hysteria patients and 156 control subjects. JAMA 146, 902–909.

Quill TE (1985) Somatization disorder. One of medicine's blind spots. JAMA 254, 3075–3079.

Raskin M, Talbott JA, and Meyerson AT (1966) Diagnosis of conversion reactions: Predictive value of psychiatric criteria. JAMA 197, 530–534.

Riding J and Munro A (1975) Pimozide in the treatment of monosymptomatic hypochondriacal psychosis. Acta Psychiatr Scand 52, 23–30.

Robins E and O'Neal P (1953) Clinical features of hysteria in children. Nerv Child 10, 246–271.

Robins LN, Helzer JE, Weissman MM, et al. (1984) Lifetime prevalence of specific psychiatric disorders in three sites. Arch Gen Psychiatr 41, 949–958.

Scallet A, Cloninger CR, and Othmer E (1976) The management of chronic hysteria: A review and double-blind trial of electrosleep and other relaxation methods. Dis Nerv Syst 37, 347–353.

Scott J and Huskisson EC (1976) Graphic representation of pain. Pain 2, 175–184.

Slater ETO and Glithero C (1965) A follow-up of patients diagnosed as suffering from "hysteria." J Psychosom Res 9, 9–13.

Smith GR Jr, Monson RA, and Ray DC (1986) Psychiatric consultation in somatization disorder. A randomized controlled study. N Engl J Med 314, 1407–1413.

Spitzer RL, Williams JBW, Kroenke K, et al. (1994) Utility of a new procedure for diagnosing mental disorders in primary care: The PRIME-MD 1000 Study. JAMA 272, 1749–1756.

Stafanis C, Markidis M, and Christodoulou G (1976) Observations on the evolution of the hysterical symptomatology. Br J Psychiatr 128, 269–275.

Steckel W, Paul E, and Paul C (trans) (1943) The Interpretation of Dreams: New Developments and Technique. Liveright, New York.

Stefansson JH, Messina JA, and Meyerowitz S (1976) Hysterical neurosis, conversion type: Clinical and epidemiological considerations. Acta Psychiatr Scand 59, 119–138.

Stephens JH and Kamp M (1962) On some aspects of hysteria: A clinical study. J Nerv Ment Dis 13, 275–282.

Stoudemire A and Sandhu J (1987) Psychogenic/idiopathic pain syndromes. Gen Hosp Psychiatr 9, 79–86.

Stoudemire GA (1988) Somatoform disorders, factitious disorders, and malingering. In Textbook of Psychiatry, Talbott JA, Hales RE, and Yudofsky SC (eds). American Psychiatric Press, Washington DC, pp. 533–556.

Tomasson K, Kent D, and Coryell W (1991) Somatization and conversion disorders: Comorbidity and demographics at presentation. Acta Psychiatr Scand 84, 288–293.

Toone BK (1990) Disorders of hysterical conversion. In Physical Symptoms and Psychological Illness, Bass C (ed). Blackwell Scientific Publications, London, pp. 207–234.

Veith I (1965) Hysteria: The History of a Disease. University of Chicago Press, Chicago.

Viederman M (1985) Somatoform and factitious disorders. In Psychiatry, Vol. 1, Cavenar JO (ed). JB Lippincott, Philadelphia, pp. 1–20.

von Knorring L and Attkisson CC (1979) Endorphins in CSF of chronic pain patients, in relation to augmenting–reducing response in visual averaged evoked response. Neuropsychobiology 5, 322–326.

Watson CG and Buranen C (1979) The frequency and identification of false positive conversion reactions. J Nerv Ment Dis 167, 243–247.

Weddington WW (1979) Conversion reaction in an 82-year-old man. J Nerv Ment Dis 167, 368–369.

Weinstein EA, Eck RA, and Lyerly OG (1969) Conversion hysteria in Appalachia. Psychiatr 32, 334–341.

Wetzel RD, Guze SB, Cloninger CR, et al. (1994) Briquet's syndrome (hysteria) is both a somatoform and a "psychoform" illness: An MMPI study. Psychosom Med 56, 564–569.

Wheatley D (1962) Evaluation of psychotherapeutic drugs in general practice. Psychopharmacol Bull 2, 25–32.

Whelan CI and Stewart DE (1990) Pseudocyesis—a review and report of six cases. Int J Psychiatr 20, 97–108.

Williams JBW and Spitzer RL (1982) Idiopathic pain disorder: Critique to pain-prone disorder and a proposal for a revision of the DSM-III category psychogenic pain disorder. J Nerv Ment Dis 170, 410–419.

World Health Organization (1992) The ICD-10 Classification of Mental and Behavioral Disorders Clinical Descriptions and Diagnostic Guidelines, 10th Rev., World Health Organization, Geneva.

Yutzy SH, Cloninger CR, Guze SB, et al. (1995) DSM-IV field trial: Testing a new proposal for somatization disorder. Am J Psychiatr 152, 97–101.

Yutzy SH, Pribor EF, Cloninger CR, et al. (1992) Reconsidering the criteria for somatization disorder. Hosp Comm Psychiatr 43, 1075–1076, 1149.

Ziegler DK and Paul N (1954) On the natural history of hysteria in women. Dis Nerv Syst 15, 3–8.

Ziegler FJ, Imboden JB, and Meyer E (1960) Contemporary conversion reactions: A clinical study. Am J Psychiatr 116, 901–910.

# 72 Factitious Disorders

Anne Fleming
Stuart Eisendrath

Factitious Disorders
Factitious Disorder Not Otherwise Specified
Factitious Disorder by Proxy

## Introduction

A patient with factitious disorder consciously induces or feigns illness in order to obtain a psychological benefit by being in the sick role. It is the conscious awareness of the production of symptoms that differentiates factitious disorder from the somatoform disorders in which the patient unconsciously produces symptoms for an unconscious psychological benefit. It is the underlying motivation to produce symptoms that separates factitious disorders from malingering. Patients who malinger consciously feign or induce illness in order to obtain some external benefit such as money, narcotics, or excuse from duties. While the distinctions among these disorders appear satisfyingly clear, in practice, patients often blur the boundaries. Patients with somatoform disorders will sometimes consciously exaggerate symptoms which they have unconsciously produced, and it is a rare patient who consciously creates illness and yet receives no external gain at all, be it disability benefits, excuse from work, or even food and shelter.

Talcott Parsons described the "sick role" in 1951 and noted that in our society there are four aspects of this role. First, the patient is not able to will himself or herself back to health but instead must "be taken care of." Second, the patient in the sick role must regard the sickness as undesirable and want to get better. Third, the sick patient is obliged to seek medical care and cooperate with his or her medical treatment. Finally, the sick patient is exempted from the normal responsibilities of his or her social role (Parsons 1951).

Patients with factitious disorder seek, often desperately, the sick role. They usually have little insight into the motivations of their behaviors but are still powerfully driven to appear ill to others. In many cases, they endanger their own health and life in search of this role. Patients with this disorder will often induce serious illness or undergo numerous unnecessary, invasive procedures. As most people avoid sickness, the actions of these patients appear to run counter to human nature. Also, since entry into the "sick role" requires that the sick person should try to get better, patients with factitious disorder must conceal the voluntary origin of their symptoms. The inexplicability of their actions combined with their deceptive behavior stir up both intense interest and intense (usually negative) countertransference in health care providers.

While physicians have known about the feigning of illness since at least ancient Greece (Feldman 2000), it is likely that Richard Asher's 1951 article in *Lancet* brought the concept of factitious illness into general medical knowledge. Asher coined the term *Munchausen's syndrome* referring to the Baron von Munchausen, a character in German literature who was known for greatly exaggerating the tales of his exploits. (The use of this term may be somewhat unfair to the baron. Apparently, Rudolf Raspe, his unauthorized biographer, may have greatly overstated both the Baron's exploits and his tendency to exaggerate [Guziec et al. 1994]). Asher described Munchausen's syndrome as severe, chronic factitious disorder combined with antisocial behavior including wandering from hospital to hospital (peregrination). However, his memorable term has often been used interchangeably with "factitious disorder" and incorrectly applied to patients with less severe forms of the disease.

Patients have been known to create or feign numerous illnesses, both acute and chronic, in all of the medical specialties. These illnesses can be either physical or psychological. It appears that the only limit is the creativity and knowledge of a given patient. In fact, there is at least one case report of a patient who feigned factitious disorder itself (Gurwith and Langston 1980). The patient claimed to have Munchausen's syndrome, to have undergone numerous unnecessary procedures and operations, and, as a result, to need immediate hospitalization. He displayed his abdomen, which appeared to have numerous surgical scars and hinted that searches of his hospital room would be fruitful. However, collateral information revealed that the physicians and hospitals he had reported had never treated the patient, and his "scars" washed off with soap and water. Patients with factitious disorder are often quite medically sophisticated. Even though acquired immune deficiency syndrome was not described until the early 1980s, the first factitious cases

**Factitious Disorder**

A. Intentional production or feigning of physical or psychological signs or symptoms.

B. The motivation for the behavior is to assume the sick role.

C. External incentives for the behavior (such as economic gain, avoiding legal responsibility, or improving physical well-being, as in malingering) are absent.

**Code based on type**

300.16 With Predominantly Psychological Signs and Symptoms: if psychological signs and symptoms predominate in the clinical presentation
300.19 With Predominantly Physical Signs and Symptoms: if physical signs and symptoms predominate in the clinical presentation
300.19 With Combined Psychological and Physical Signs and Symptoms: if both psychological and physical signs and symptoms are present and neither predominates in the clinical presentation

followed shortly thereafter, at least as early as 1986 (Miller et al. 1986).

## Definition

For a diagnosis of factitious disorder (see DSM-IV-TR criteria for factitious disorder) to be justified, a person must be intentionally producing illness; his or her motivation is to occupy the sick role, and there must not be external incentives for the behavior. The diagnosis is further subclassified, depending on whether the factitious symptoms are predominantly physical, psychological, or a combination. The DSM also includes a category (see DSM-IV-TR criteria for factitious disorder not otherwise specified) for patients with factitious symptoms who do not meet the listed criteria. The most common example of factitious disorder not otherwise specified is factitious disorder by proxy, in which the individual creates symptoms in another person, usually a dependent, in order to occupy the sick role. Patients who readily admit to inducing symptoms, such as self-mutilating patients, are not diagnosed with factitious disorder as they are not using their symptoms to occupy the sick role.

## Factitious Disorder with Predominantly Physical Signs and Symptoms

Patients with this subtype of factitious disorder present with physical signs and symptoms. The three main methods patients use to create illness are: (1) giving a false history, (2) faking clinical and laboratory findings, and (3) inducing

**Factitious Disorder Not Otherwise Specified**

This category includes disorders with factitious symptoms that do not meet the criteria for factitious disorder. An example of is factitious disorder by proxy: the intentional production or feigning of symptoms in another person who is under the individual's care for the purpose of indirectly assuming the sick role.

illness (e.g., by surreptitious medication use, inducing infection, or preventing wound healing) (Eisendrath 1994). There are reports of factitious illnesses in all of the medical specialties. Particularly common presentations include fever, self-induced infection, gastrointestinal symptoms, impaired wound healing, cancer, renal disease (especially hematuria and nephrolithiasis), endocrine diseases, anemia, bleeding disorders, and epilepsy (Wise and Ford 1999). True Munchausen's syndrome fits within this subclass and is the most severe form of the illness. According to the DSM-IV, patients with Munchausen's syndrome have chronic factitious disorder with physical signs and symptoms, and in addition, have a history of recurrent hospitalization, peregrination, and *pseudologia fantastica*—dramatic, untrue, and extremely improbable tales of their past experiences (American Psychiatric Association 2000).

Clinical Vignette 1

**Munchausen's Syndrome**

A 42-year-old man was brought in by ambulance from a public park after complaining of shortness of breath and collapsing. Onlookers called 911. In the emergency room, the patient complained of shortness of breath and chest pain. He reported that he had a history of multiple pulmonary emboli necessitating Greenfield filter placement. He seemed to be very familiar with the medical terminology and clinical findings in pulmonary emboli. The patient had an extensive workup including a high resolution CT scan, but all studies were normal. The medical team noted that the patient appeared to be holding his breath when his oxygen saturation was being measured, and in addition, was performing a Valsalva maneuver during his ECGs. The medical resident attempted to clarify the patient's history by obtaining collateral information. The hospitals contacted reported that the patient had presented numerous times with the same complaints, and there had been suspicion of a factitious disorder. The medical resident informed the patient of the conflicting information, at which point the patient became very angry and immediately left the hospital. He was lost to follow up.

## Factitious Disorder with Predominantly Psychological Signs and Symptoms

Another subtype of factitious disorder includes patients who present feigning psychological illness. They both report and mimic psychiatric symptoms. These patients can be particularly difficult to diagnose as psychiatric diagnosis depends greatly on the patient's report. There are reports of factitious psychosis, posttraumatic stress disorder, and bereavement (Pope et al. 1982, Sparr and Pankratz 1983, Snowdon et al. 1978). In addition, there are reports of psychological distress due to false claims of being a victim of stalking, rape, or sexual harassment (Pathe et al. 1999, Feldman et al. 1994, Feldman-Schorrig 1996), and these cases are often diagnosed with a factitious psychological disorder such as posttraumatic stress disorder. While patients with factitious psychological symptoms feign psychiatric illness, they also often suffer from true comorbid psychiatric disorders, particularly Axis II disorders and substance abuse (Pope et al. 1982, Popli et al. 1992). Case reports suggest that patients with psychological factitious disorder have a high rate of suicide and a poor prognosis (Eisendrath 2001, Pope et al. 1982, Popli et al. 1992). While Munchausen's syndrome is considered a subset of physical factitious disorder, there are case reports of patients presenting with psychological symptoms who also have some of the key features of Munchausen's (pathological lying, wandering, and recurrent hospitalizations) (Merrin et al. 1986, Popli et al. 1992).

---

Clinical Vignette 2

**Factitious Disorder with Psychological Features**

A 46-year-old man presented complaining of symptoms of posttraumatic stress disorder (PTSD). He reported intense flashbacks, numbing and avoidance, and irritability resulting from his experience as a combat veteran. He began intensive treatment for PTSD including support groups, individual therapy, and medication management. He was an extremely active participant in the support groups and would recount detailed horrors of his time in combat. A staff member verifying the patient's history learned the patient had served in the military but was not a combat veteran. The patient was confronted in a supportive manner, and he admitted that he had fabricated his history. It was recommended that the patient continue in psychiatric treatment, and he agreed to do so.

---

## Factitious Disorder with Combined Psychological and Physical Signs and Symptoms

DSM-III separated factitious disorder into two disorders, based on whether the symptoms were physical or psychological. However, case reports clarified that this distinction was often artificial (Merrin et al. 1986, Parker 1993). Some patients present with simultaneous psychological and physical factitious symptoms, and some patients move between physical and psychological presentations over time. For example, a patient who presented with factitious posttraumatic stress disorder was confronted about the nature of his symptoms and then began complaining of physical symptoms. DSM-IV was revised to account for patients who present with both psychological signs and symptoms, though this category of patients is the least well-studied.

## Factitious Disorder Not Otherwise Specified (Factitious Disorder by Proxy)

Some individuals pursue the sick role not by feigning illness in themselves, but instead by creating it in another person, usually someone dependent on the perpetrator. They seek the role of caring for an ill individual (the sick role by proxy). While the victim is usually a child, there are reports of victimization of elders and developmentally delayed adults. The veterinary literature even reports cases of factitious disorder by proxy in which the victim is a pet (Munro and Thrusfield 2001). Due to the unique characteristics of this disorder, it will be discussed in a separate section at the end of the chapter.

## Clinical Findings

Due to the inherently deceptive nature of patients with factitious disorder, the literature is largely confined to case reports and case series. It is likely that many patients with less severe forms of the disease escape detection, and their clinical characteristics might be quite different. In addition, the literature on factitious disorder with physical symptoms is much more extensive than the literature on the other subtypes. As a result, we will discuss the features of the factitious disorders as a whole, referring to specific characteristics of patients with psychological symptoms (either alone or accompanying physical symptoms) when they are known.

Numerous reports (Carney and Brown 1983, Reich and Gottfried 1983, Wise and Ford 1999) in the literature describe two different subclasses of factitious patients. The first type fits with the classic Munchausen's syndrome diagnosis: they have chronic factitious symptoms associated with antisocial traits, pathological lying, minimal social supports, wandering from hospital to hospital, and very poor work and relationship functioning. They are often very familiar with hospital procedure and use this knowledge to present dramatically during off-hours or at house officer transition times when the factitious nature of their symptoms is least likely to be discovered. Male patients compromise the majority of these cases. Patients with Munchausen's syndrome appear to have an extremely poor prognosis (Eisendrath 2001, Carney and Brown 1983). Fortunately, this most severe class of patients makes up the minority of factitious patients, probably fewer than 10%.

The second, and more typical, type of patient does not display pathological lying or wandering. Their recurrent presentations are usually within the same community, and they become well known within the local health care system. They often have stable social supports and employment, and a history of a medically related job. This larger class of factitious patients is mostly made up of women, and is more likely to accept psychiatric treatment and to show improvement. Plassmann (1994a) reviewed 1,070 cases of patients with factitious, but not Munchausen's disorder. He found that 78% of the patients were women and 58% had a medically related job. Finally, there are individuals who may have an episode of factitious disorder in reaction to a life stressor, but may return to premorbid functioning after the stressor is resolved (Goldstein 1998).

All types of factitious disease show a strong association with substance abuse (Kent 1994), as well as borderline and narcissistic personality disorders. In a case series by Ehlers and Plassman (1994), 9 of 18 patients had personality features that met criteria for borderline personality disorder, and another 6 of 18 had personality features that met criteria for narcissistic personality disorder. Factitious patients span a broad age range. Reports in the literature show patients ranging from 4 to 85 years (Croft and Jervis 1989, Davis and Small 1985). Of note, a 4-year-old patient with factitious disorder reported that he had been coached by his mother and may be better diagnosed as a victim of factitious disorder by proxy (Croft and Jervis 1989). The next youngest case found was 8 years old (Absolut de la Gastine et al. 1998, Libow 2000). Ethnicity is frequently not reported in case studies and series, so it is difficult to determine if there are any ethnic differences in the prevalence or presentation of factitious disorder.

## Diagnosis and Differential Diagnosis

The diagnosis of factitious disorder is made in several ways. Factitious disorder is occasionally diagnosed accidentally when the patient is discovered in the act of creating symptoms. A history of inconsistent or unexplainable signs and symptoms or failure to respond to appropriate treatment can prompt health care providers to probe for evidence of the disorder, as can evidence of peregrination or pathological lying. In some cases, it is a diagnosis of exclusion in an otherwise inexplicable case. The differential diagnosis of factitious disorder includes rare or complex physical illness, somatoform disorders, malingering, other psychiatric disorders, and substance abuse (McKane and Anderson 1997). It is especially important to rule out genuine physical illness since patients with factitious disorder often induce real physical illness. Furthermore, it is always important to remember the patients with factitious disorder are certainly not immune to the physical illnesses that plague the general population.

If there is suspicion of factitious disorder, confirmation can be difficult. Laboratory examination can confirm some factitious diagnoses such as exogenous insulin or thyroid hormone administration. Collateral information from family members or previous health care providers can also be extremely helpful. Factitious disorder with psychological signs and symptoms can be particularly difficult to diagnose, as so much of psychiatric diagnosis relies on the patient's report. However, there is some evidence that neuropsychological testing may be helpful in making the diagnosis. Both McCaffrey and Bellamy-Campbell (1989) and Fairbank and colleagues (1985) report the ability to detect over 90% of cases of factitious posttraumatic stress disorder using the MMPI. However, Perconte (Perconte and Goreczny 1990) was unsuccessful in attempting to replicate the findings. In addition, there is a report of MMPI test results being used to support a diagnosis of factitious disorder with psychological features in a woman thought to be feigning symptoms of multiple personality disorder (Coons 1993). See Figure 72–1.

## Epidemiology

The nature of factitious disorder makes it difficult to determine how common it is within the population. Patients attempt to conceal themselves, thereby artificially lowering the prevalence. The tendency of patients to present several

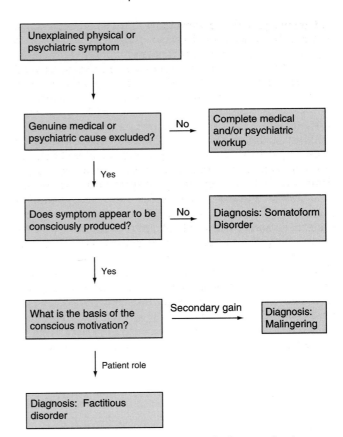

**Figure 72–1** *Diagnostic decision tree for factitious disorder.*

times at different facilities, however, may artificially raise the prevalence. Most estimates of the prevalence of the disease, therefore, rely on the number of factitious patients within a given inpatient population. Such attempts have generated estimates that 0.5 to 3% of medical and psychiatric inpatients suffer from factitious disorder. Of 1,288 patients referred for psychiatric consultation at a Toronto general hospital, 10 (0.8%) were diagnosed with factitious disorder. A prospective examination of all 1,538 patients hospitalized in a Berlin neurology department over 5 years found five (0.3%) cases of factitious disorder (Bauer and Boegner 1996). An examination of 506 patients with fever of unknown origin (FUO) revealed that 2.2% of the fevers were of factitious origin (Rumans and Vosti 1978), and a review of 199 Belgian patients with FUO found 7 of 199 (3.5%) to be factitious (Knockaert et al. 1992). A similar study of patients with FUO at the National Institutes of Health (NIH) revealed that 9.3% of the fevers were factitious (Aduan et al. 1979). The increased prevalence found at the NIH may be due to the fact that the study was undertaken in a more tertiary setting, and it is a reminder that the prevalence of factitious disorder likely varies widely depending on the population and the setting. Gault and colleagues (1988) examined 3,300 renal stones brought in by patients and found that 2.6% of these stones were mineral and felt to be submitted by factitious or malingering patients. There is much less data on the prevalence of factitious disorder with psychological features. A study of psychiatric inpatients showed a prevalence of 0.5% of admissions determined to be a result of a factitious psychological condition (Bhugra 1988). There are few data about the prevalence of factitious disorder in an outpatient population. Because factitious patients do not readily identify themselves in large community surveys, it is not currently possible to determine the prevalence of the disorder in the general population.

## Etiology

Both psychological and biological factors have been postulated to play a role in the etiology of factitious disorder. Although numerous case reports have generated speculation that factitious disorder may run in families, this could be explained by environmental factors, genetic factors, or both. The presence of central nervous system (CNS) abnormalities in some patients with factitious disorders have led some to hypothesize that underlying brain dysfunction contributes to factitious disorder. One review of factitious patients with *pseudologia fantastica* found CNS abnormalities (such as EEG abnormality, head injury, imaging abnormalities, or neurological findings) in 40% of the patients (King and Ford 1988). There have been case reports of MRI (Fenelon et al. 1991) and SPECT (Mountz et al. 1996) abnormalities, but it is unknown if these abnormalities were related to the disorder.

In addition, childhood developmental disturbances are thought to contribute to factitious disorder. Predisposing factors are thought to include (1) serious childhood illness or illness in a family member during childhood, especially if the illness was associated with attention and nurturing in an otherwise distant family, (2) past anger with the medical profession, (3) past significant relationship with a health care provider, and (4) factitious disorder in a parent (McKane and Anderson 1997).

Patients with factitious disorder create illness in pursuit of the sick role. For these patients, being in the sick role allows them to compensate for an underlying psychological deficit. Most authors identify several common psychodynamic motivations for factitious disorder (Feldman 2000, Eisendrath 2001, Guziec et al. 1994, Folks 1995, Hyler and Sussman 1981). First, patients with little sense of self may seek the sick role in order to provide a well-defined identity around which to structure themselves. Others may seek the sick role in order to meet dependency needs which have gone unmet elsewhere. As a patient, they receive the attention, caring, and nurturing of the health care environment and are relieved of many of their responsibilities. In addition, some patients may engage in factitious behaviors for masochistic reasons. They feel they deserve punishment for some forbidden feelings and thus they should suffer at the hands of their physicians. Other patients may be motivated by anger at physicians and dupe them in retaliation. Patients with a history of childhood illness or abuse may attempt to master past traumas by creating a situation over which they have control. Finally, some authors have speculated that some patients may be enacting suicidal wishes through their factitious behavior (Schoenfeld et al. 1987, Roy and Roy 1995).

## Treatment and Prognosis

The goals in treating patients with factitious disorder are twofold; first to minimize the damage done by the disorder to both the patient's own health and the health care system.

The second goal is to help patients recover, at least partially, from the disorder. These goals are furthered by treating comorbid medical illnesses, avoiding unnecessary procedures, encouraging patients to seek psychiatric treatment, and providing support for health care clinicians. Because the literature is based exclusively on case reports and series, determining treatment effectiveness is difficult. As mentioned before, patients with true Munchausen's syndrome (including antisocial traits, pathological lying, wandering, and poor social support) are felt to be refractory to treatment. While factitious disorder is extremely difficult to cure, effective techniques exist to minimize morbidity, and some patients are able to benefit greatly from psychiatric intervention.

The course of untreated factitious disorder is variable. While patients with factitious disorder commonly suffer a great deal of morbidity, fatal cases appear to be less common. One survey of 41 cases noted only one fatality, though many of the other cases were life-threatening (Reich and Gottfried 1983). However, patients with psychological signs and symptoms are reported to have a high rate of suicide and a poor prognosis (Pope et al. 1982, Popli et al. 1992).

Soon after Asher's (1951) article was published, many patients with factitious disorder were vigorously confronted once the nature of their illness was discovered. Unfortunately, most patients would deny their involvement and seek another provider who was unaware of their diagnosis (Eisendrath 2001). In addition, the idea of "blacklists" was proposed in order to aid detection of these patients. However, issues regarding patient confidentiality as well as concerns about cursory medical evaluations that might miss genuine physical illness prevented this idea from being adopted (Eisendrath 2001). Although aggressive confrontation is usually unsuccessful, supportive, nonpunitive confrontation may be helpful for some. In one case series, 33 patients were confronted with the factitious nature of their illness. While only 13 admitted feigning illness, most of the patients' illnesses subsequently improved, at least in the short term (Reich and Gottfried 1983).

Eisendrath suggested three alternatives to confrontation that he found effective. First is inexact interpretation, in which the psychiatrist interprets the psychodynamics thought to be underlying the patient's behavior without explicitly identifying the factitious behavior. He gave the example of a patient suspected of having factitious disorder who developed septicemia after her boyfriend proposed marriage. The consultant suggested that the patient might feel a need to punish herself when good things happened to her. She agreed, and soon after, admitted that she had injected a contaminant intravenously (Eisendrath 2001). The second technique is the therapeutic double-blind. The physician presents the patient with a new medical intervention to treat his or her illness. The patient is told that one possibility is that the patient's illness has a factitious origin, and that, if so, the treatment would not be expected to work while, if the illness is biological, the treatment will work and the patient will improve. The patient must decide to give up the factitious illness or admit it. A third technique is to provide the patient with a face-saving way, such as hypnosis or biofeedback, of giving up his or her symptoms without admitting that they are not genuine. Eisendrath (2001) points out that in emergent situations, there may not be time for nonconfrontational techniques, and more directly confrontational means may be necessary.

Another important component in the treatment of patients with factitious disorder is the coordination of health care among all providers. This allows for fewer unnecessary interventions, minimizes splitting among the health care team, and allows the health care team to vent and process the strong emotions that arise when caring for factitious patients. This decreases both the negative impact on the providers and the chance that anger will be acted out on the patient.

There are no clear data supporting the effectiveness of medications in treating factitious disorder. There is a case report of effective pimozide treatment in a patient thought to have delusional symptoms (Prior and Gordon 1997), as well as a case report of a factitious patient with comorbid depression improving when treated with an antidepressant in addition to intensive psychotherapy (Earle and Folks 1986).

While many patients with factitious disorder are hesitant to pursue psychiatric treatment, there are numerous case reports of successful treatment of the disorder with long-term psychotherapy. In many of these cases, the therapy lasted several years, including one patient who received treatment while imprisoned for over 10 years (Miller et al. 1985). Plassman reports a case series of 24 factitious patients. Twelve of these patients accepted psychotherapy and 10 continued with long-term treatment, lasting up to $4\frac{1}{2}$ years. He reports "significant, or at least marked, improvement" in those 10 patients (Plassmann 1994b). These case reports support the idea that treatment of patients with factitious disorder is not impossible, and these patients can improve. However, expectations must be realistic as improvement in the disorder itself can take several years. Techniques that target short-term reduction in the production of factitious symptoms can be effective more quickly. See Figure 72–2 for a treatment flowchart for factitious disorder.

## Ethical Considerations

Treating patients with factitious disorder often raises ethical questions including those regarding confidentiality, privacy, and medical decision-making, and it is important to be alert to these issues. Often, patients with factious disorder will want to keep their diagnosis confidential, even when to do so may harm the patient or others. For example, although a consulting physician may diagnose a patient with factitious disorder, the patient may refuse consent to reveal this information to the referring physician. If the consultant does inform the referring physician, she has violated the patient's confidentiality, but if she does not, the referring physician is likely to continue to treat the patient for the incorrect diagnosis. Dilemmas regarding patient privacy also arise with factitious patients. For example, hospital room searches could often help clarify the diagnosis or remove materials the patient is using to harm himself, but these searches also violate the patient's privacy. Dilemmas surrounding medical decision-making can arise when a patient with factitious disorder refuses treatment or requests potentially harmful treatments. It can often be difficult to resolve these ethical dilemmas. In general, even though the facti-

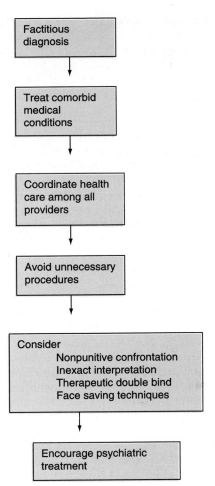

**Figure 72–2** *Treatment flowchart for factitious disorder.*

tious patient is deceptive within the doctor–patient relationship, the physician is not released from his or her responsibilities within that relationship, and the patient retains his or her rights of confidentiality, privacy, and autonomy. As with all patients, emergency situations require different ethical guidelines. Often, an ethics consultation can be very helpful in sorting through the difficult issues of patient care in the setting of factitious disorder.

## Factitious Disorder by Proxy

In factitious disorder by proxy, one person creates or feigns illness in another person, usually a child, though occasionally the victim is an elder or developmentally delayed adult. Factitious disorder by proxy is not defined as a specific disorder in DSM-IV but instead is listed under the "not otherwise specified" heading with research criteria included. While rare instances of fathers perpetrating factitious disorder by proxy have been reported (Meadow 1998), the perpetrator is usually the mother (Rosenburg 1987). Usually the victim is a preverbal child (McClure et al. 1996). While numerous symptoms have been reported, common presentations include apnea, seizures, and gastrointestinal problems. The mothers appear extremely caring and attentive when observed, but appear indifferent to the child when they are not aware of being observed (Eisendrath 2001).

## DSM-IV-TR Criteria

**Factitious Disorder by Proxy**

A. Intentional production of or feigning of physical or psychological signs or symptoms in another person who is under the individual's care.

B. The motivation for the perpetrator's behavior is to assume the sick role by proxy.

C. External incentives for the behavior (such as economic gain) are absent.

D. The behavior is no better accounted for by another mental disorder.

Reprinted with permission from the Diagnostic and Statistical Mannual of Mental Disorders, Fourth Edition, Text Revision. Copyright 2000 American Psychiatric Association.

As in factitious disorder, the exact prevalence of factitious disorder by proxy is unknown. There have been studies of the annual incidence of factitious disorder by proxy in the general population in both the UK and New Zealand. In New Zealand, the annual incidence of factitious disorder by proxy in children less than 16 years was found to be 2.0/100,000 (18 total cases) (Denny et al. 2001). In the UK the annual incidence in children under 16 was 0.5/100,000 (128 total cases) (McClure et al. 1996). As for the incidence within clinical populations, an Argentinean survey of 113 children with FUO found four (3.5%) cases of factitious fever (Chantada et al. 1994). A survey of 20,090 children brought in with apnea found 54 (0.27%) to be victims of factitious disorder by proxy (Kravitz and Willmott 1990). Finally, a review of children brought in for treatment of acute, life threatening episodes of diverse etiologies ranging from seizure disorders to electrolyte abnormalities found 1.5% to be factitious (Rahilly 1991). Factitious disorder by proxy appears to have a much higher mortality rate than self-inflicted factitious disorder. In Rosenberg's survey of 117 victims, there was a 9% mortality rate (Rosenberg 1987), and of the 54 victims of the disorder in the apnea survey, three index cases and five siblings were dead at follow-up (Kravitz and Wilmott 1990). More recently, McClure found that 8 of 128 index cases in the UK were fatal (6.25%) (McClure et al. 1996) while Denny reported no fatalities in 18 index cases (Denny et al. 2001).

The diagnosis of factitious disorder by proxy is usually made by having an index of suspicion in a child with unexplained illnesses. The diagnosis is supported if symptoms occur only in the parent's presence and resolve with separation. Covert video surveillance has been used to diagnose this condition, though it raises questions of invasion of privacy. In general, it has been felt that the welfare of the child overrides the parent's right to privacy.

As counterintuitive as it is to comprehend why anyone would induce illness in oneself, it can be even more difficult to understand inducing illness in one's own child. The perpetrator in factitious disorder by proxy appears to seek not the "sick role" but the "parent to the sick child" role. This role is similar to the sick role in that it provides structure, attention from others, caring, and relief from usual responsibilities. The parent also receives some psychological benefit from inducing illness in his or her child. Based on case reports, the parent often has a comorbid personality disorder and a history of family dysfunction (Bools et al. 1994).

## Treatment

Due to the high morbidity and mortality, treatment requires at least temporary separation from the parent and notification of local child protective agencies. The perpetrators often face criminal charges of child abuse. There is high psychiatric morbidity in the children—many go on to develop factitious disorder or other psychiatric illnesses themselves. Psychiatric intervention is necessary to ameliorate this morbidity as much as possible in these children (McGuire and Feldman 1989). There are some case reports of successful psychotherapeutic treatments of the parents in this disorder (Rand and Feldman 2001).

Clinical Vignette 3

**Factitious Disorder by Proxy**

A 6-month-old infant presented to the emergency room after a seizure. The family reported no significant past medical history. The infant was resuscitated. There was no evidence of infection, the patient had a normal blood glucose, and the urine toxicology screen was negative. After 5 hours, the child recovered. The infant presented again 5 days later with another seizure. The infant's blood glucose was low, and continued to fall below normal levels despite administration of dextrose. A blood insulin level was elevated and a c-peptide level suggested endogenous hyperinsulinism. The workup (including CT scan) was otherwise normal. Further history revealed that both grandmothers had Type II diabetes and took oral hypoglycemic agents. A blood test on the infant was positive for sulfonylurea. A case conference was held, and it was discovered that the mother's first child had been removed from the home due to charges of abuse. It was recommended that the infant be placed in foster care while the police investigated the case. (*Owen et al. 2000*).

## Summary

Patients with factitious disorder seek, often desperately, the sick role. Due to the nature of the disorder, the literature on factitious disorder is largely confined to case reports and case series, limiting the information available. Patients with factitious disorder present with a broad spectrum of signs and symptoms, and effective diagnosis often requires a high index of suspicion. The differential diagnosis of factitious disorder includes physical illness, somatoform disorders, malingering, psychiatric illness, and substance abuse. While factitious disorder is extremely difficult to cure, effective techniques exist to minimize morbidity, and some patients are able to benefit greatly from psychiatric intervention.

## Comparison of DSM-IV/ICD-10 Diagnostic Criteria

The ICD-10 Diagnostic Criteria for Research and the DSM-IV criteria sets are almost identical.

# References

Absolut de la Gastine G, Penniello MJ, Le Treust M, et al. (1998) Urinary calculi and Munchausen's syndrome. Arch Pediatr 5(5) (May), 517–520.

Aduan RP, Fauci AS, Dale DC, et al. (1979) Factitious fever and self-induced infection: A report of 32 cases and review of the literature. Ann Int Med 90(2) (Feb), 230–242.

American Psychiatric Association (2000) Diagnostic and Statistical Manual of Mental Disorders, 4th ed., Text Rev. APA, Washington DC.

Asher R (1951) Munchausen's syndrome. Lancet 1, 339–341.

Bauer M and Boegner F (1996) Neurological syndromes in factitious disorder. J Nerv Ment Dis 184(5) (May), 281–288.

Bhugra D (1988) Psychiatric Munchausen's syndrome. Literature review with case reports. Acta Psychiatr Scand 77(5) (May), 497–503.

Bools C, Neale B, and Meadow R (1994) Munchausen syndrome by proxy: A study of psychopathology. Child Ab Negl 18(9) (Sept), 773–788.

Carney MW and Brown JP (1983) Clinical features and motives among 42 artifactual illness patients. Br J Med Psychol 56 (Pt1) (May), 57–66.

Chantada G, Casak S, Plata JD, et al. (1994) Children with fever of unknown origin in Argentina: An analysis of 113 cases. Pediatr Infect Dis J 13(4) (Apr), 260–263.

Coons PM (1993) Use of the MMPI to distinguish genuine from factitious multiple personality disorder. Psychol Rep 73(2) (Oct), 401–402.

Croft RD and Jervis M (1989) Munchausen's syndrome in a 4-year-old. Arch Dis Child 64(5) (May), 740–741.

Davis JW and Small GW (1985). Munchausen's syndrome in an 85-year-old man. J Am Geriatr Soc 33(2) (Feb), 154–155

Denny SJ, Grant CC, and Pinnock R (2001) Epidemiology of Munchausen syndrome by proxy in New Zealand. J Paediatr Child Health 37(3) (June), 240–243.

Earle JR Jr and Folks DG (1986) Factitious disorder and coexisting depression: A report of successful psychiatric consultation and case management. Gen Hosp Psychiatr 8(6) (Nov), 448–450.

Ehlers W and Plassmann R (1994) Diagnosis of narcissistic self-esteem regulation in patients with factitious illness (Munchausen syndrome). Psychother Psychosom 62(1–2), 69–77.

Eisendrath SJ (1994) Factitious physical disorders. W J Med 160(2) (Feb), 177–179.

Eisendrath SJ (2001) Factitious disorders and malingering. In Treatment of Psychiatric Disorders, 3rd ed., Gabbard GO (ed). American Psychiatric Publishing, Washington DC, pp. 1825–1844.

Fairbank JA, McCaffrey RJ, and Keane TM (1985) Psychometric detection of fabricated symptoms of posttraumatic stress disorder. Am J Psychiatr 142(4) (Apr), 501–503.

Feldman MD, Ford CV, and Stone T (1994) Deceiving others/deceiving oneself: Four cases of factitious rape. S Med J 87(7) (July), 736–738.

Feldman-Schorrig S (1996) Factitious sexual harassment. Bull Am Acad Psychiatr Law 24(3), 387–392.

Feldman M (2000) Factitious disorders. In Comprehensive Textbook of Psychiatry, 7th ed., Sadock B and Sadock V (eds). Lippincott, Williams & Wilkins, Philadelphia, pp. 1533–1544.

Fenelon G, Mahieux F, Roullet E, et al. (1991) Munchausen's syndrome and abnormalities on magnetic resonance imaging of the brain. BMJ 302(6783) (Apr), 996–997.

Folks DG (1995) Munchausen's syndrome and other factitious disorders. Neurol Clin 13(2) (May), 267–281.

Gault MH, Campbell NR, and Aksu AE (1988) Spurious stones. Nephron 48(4), 274–279.

Goldstein AB (1998) Identification and classification of factitious disorders: An analysis of cases reported during a ten-year period. Int J Psychiatr Med 28(2), 221–241.

Gurwith M and Langston C (1980) Factitious Munchausen's syndrome. New Engl J Med 302(26) (June), 1483–1484.

Guziec J, Lazarus A, and Harding JJ (1994) Case of a 29-year-old nurse with factitious disorder. The utility of psychiatric intervention on a general medical floor. Gen Hosp Psychiatr 16(1) (Jan), 47–53.

Hyler SE and Sussman N (1981) Chronic factitious disorder with physical symptoms (the Munchausen syndrome). Psychiatr Clin N A 4(2) (Aug), 365–377.

Kent JD (1994) Munchausen's syndrome and substance abuse. J F Subs Abuse Treat 11(3) (May–June), 247–251.

King BH and Ford CV (1988) Pseudologia fantastica. Acta Psychiatr Scand 77(1) (Jan), 1–6.

Knockaert DC, Vanneste LJ, Vanneste SB, et al. (1992) Fever of unknown origin in the 1980s. An update of the diagnostic spectrum. Arch Int Med 152(1) (Jan), 51–55.

Kravitz RM and Wilmott RW (1990) Munchausen syndrome by proxy presenting as factitious apnea. Clin Pediatr (Phila) 29(10) (Oct), 587–592.

Libow JA (2000) Child and adolescent illness falsification. Pediatrics 105(2) (Feb), 336–342.

McCaffrey RJ and Bellamy-Campbell R (1989) Psychometric detection of fabricated symptoms of combat-related posttraumatic stress disorder: A systematic replication. J Clin Psychol 45(1) (Jan), 76–79.

McClure RJ, Davis PM, Meadow SR, et al. (1996) Epidemiology of Munchausen syndrome by proxy, nonaccidental poisoning, and non-accidental suffocation. Arch Dis Child 75(1) (July), 57–61.

McGuire TL and Feldman KW (1989) Psychologic morbidity of children subjected to Munchausen's syndrome by proxy. Pediatrics 83(2) (Feb), 289–292.

McKane JP and Anderson J (1997) Munchausen's syndrome: Rule breakers and risk takers. Br J Hosp Med 58(4) (Aug 207–Sep 2), 150–153.

Meadow R (1998) Munchausen syndrome by proxy abuse perpetrated by men. Arch Dis Child 78(3) (Mar), 210–216.

Merrin EL, Van Dyke C, Cohen S, et al. (1986) Dual factitious disorder. Gen Hosp Psychiatr 8(4) (July), 246–250.

Miller F, Weiden P, Sacks M, et al. (1986) Two cases of factitious acquired immune deficiency syndrome. Am J Psychiatr 143(11) (Nov), 1483.

Miller RD, Blancke FW, Doren DM, et al. (1985) The Munchausen patient in a forensic facility. Psychiatr Q 57(1) (Spring), 72–76.

Mountz JM, Parker PE, Liu HG, et al. (1996) Tc-99m HMPAO brain SPECT scanning in Munchausen syndrome. J Psychiatr Neurosci 21(1) (Jan), 49–52.

Munro HM and Thrusfield MV (2001) 'Battered pets': Munchausen's syndrome by proxy (factitious illness by proxy). J Small Animal Pract 42(8) (Aug), 385–389.

Owen L, Ellis M, and Shield J (2000) Deliberate sulphonylurea poisoning mimicking hyperinsulinaemia of infancy. Arch Dis Child 82(5) (May), 392–393.

Parker PE (1993) A case report of Munchausen syndrome with mixed psychological features. Psychosomatics 34(4) (July–Aug), 360–364.

Parsons T (1951) The Social Structure. Free Press, Glencoe, Illinois, pp 436–439.

Pathe M, Mullen PE, and Purcell R (1999) Stalking: False claims of victimisation. Br J Psychiatr 174 (Feb), 170–172.

Perconte ST and Goreczny AJ (1990) Failure to detect fabricated posttraumatic stress disorders with the use of the MMPI in a clinical population. Am J Psychiatr 147(8) (Aug), 1057–1060.

Plassmann R (1994a) Munchausen's syndrome and factitious diseases. Psychother Psychosom 62(1–2), 7–26.

Plassmann R (1994b) Inpatient and outpatient long-term psychotherapy of patients suffering from factitious disorders. Psychother Psychosom 62(1–2), 96–107.

Pope HG Jr, Jonas JM, and Jones B (1982) Factitious psychosis: Phenomenology, family history, and long-term outcome of nine patients. Am J Psychiatr 139(11) (Nov), 1480–1483.

Popli AP, Masand PS, and Dewan MJ (1992) Factitious disorders with psychological symptoms. J Clin Psychiatr 53(9) (Sept), 315–318.

Prior TI and Gordon A (1997) Treatment of factitious disorder with pimozide. Can J Psychiatr 42(5) (June), 532.

Rahilly PM (1991) The pneumographic and medical investigation of infants suffering apparent life threatening episodes. J Paediatr Child Health 27(6) (Dec), 349–353.

Rand DC and Feldman MD (2001) An explanatory model for Munchausen by proxy abuse. Int J Psychiatr Med 31(2), 113–126.

Reich P and Gottfried LA (1983) Factitious disorders in a teaching hospital. Ann Int Med 99(2) (Aug), 240–247.

Rosenberg DA (1987) Web of deceit: A literature review of Munchausen syndrome by proxy. Child Abuse Neglect 11(4), 547–563.

Roy M and Roy A (1995) Factitious hypoglycemia. An 11-year follow-up. Psychosomatics 36(1) (Jan–Feb), 64–65.

Rumans LW and Vosti KL (1978) Factitious and fraudulent fever. Am J Med 65(5) (Nov), 745–755.

Schoenfeld H, Margolin J, and Baum S (1987) Munchausen syndrome as a suicide equivalent: Abolition of syndrome by psychotherapy. Am J Psychother 41(4) (Oct), 604–612.

Snowdon J, Solomons R, and Druce H (1978) Feigned bereavement: Twelve cases. Brit J Psychiatr 133 (July), 15–19.

Sparr L and Pankratz LD (1983) Factitious posttraumatic stress disorder. Am J Psychiatr 140(8) (Aug), 1016–1019.

Wise MG and Ford CV (1999) Factitious disorders. Prim Care 26(2) (June), 315–326.

# 73 Dissociative Disorders

David Spiegel
José R. Maldonado

Dissociative Amnesia
Dissociative Fugue
Depersonalization Disorder
Dissociative Identity Disorder
Dissociative Trance Disorder
Acute Stress Disorder

Dissociative phenomena are best understood through the term *désagrégation* (disaggregation) originally given by Janet (1920). Events normally experienced as connected to one another on a smooth continuum are isolated from the other mental processes with which they would ordinarily be associated. The dissociative disorders are a disturbance in the organization of identity, memory, perception, or consciousness. When memories are separated from access to consciousness, the disorder is dissociative amnesia. Fragmentation of identity results in dissociative fugue or dissociative identity disorder (DID; formerly multiple personality disorder). Disintegrated perception is characteristic of depersonalization disorder. Dissociation of aspects of consciousness produces acute stress disorder and various dissociative trance and possession states. Numbing and amnesia are diagnostic components of post-traumatic stress disorder (PTSD). These dissociative and related disorders are more a disturbance in the organization or structure of mental contents than in the contents themselves. Memories in dissociative amnesia are not so much distorted or bizarre as they are segregated from one another. The identities lost in dissociative fugue or fragmented in DID are two-dimensional aspects of an overall personality structure. In this sense, patients with DID suffer not from having more than one personality but rather from having less than one personality. The problem involves information processing: the failure of integration of elements rather than the contents of the fragments.

The dissociative disorders have a long history in classical psychopathology, being the foundation on which Freud began his explorations of the unconscious (Breuer and Freud 1955) and Janet (1920) developed dissociation theory. Although much attention in psychiatry has shifted to diagnosis and treatment of mood, anxiety, and thought disorders, dissociative phenomena are sufficiently persistent and interesting that they have elicited growing attention

from both professionals and the public. There are at least four reasons for this:

(1) They are fascinating phenomena in and of themselves, involving the loss of or change in identity, or memory, or a feeling of detachment from extreme and traumatic physical events.
(2) Dissociative disorders seem to arise in response to traumatic stress.
(3) Dissociative disorders remain an area of psychopathology for which the best treatment is psychotherapy, although adjunctive pharmacological interventions can be helpful.
(4) Dissociation as a phenomenon has much to teach us about information processing in the brain.

## Development of the Concept

The French philosopher and psychologist Pierre Janet (1920) is credited with the initial description of the disorder, *désagrégation mentale*. The French term *désagrégation* carries with it a different nuance than the English translation, dissociation. It implies a separation of mental contents despite their general tendency to aggregate or be processed together. Janet described hysteria as "a malady of the personal synthesis" (Janet 1920, p. 332). The problem is a difficulty in integration rather than a proliferation of components of consciousness, memory, identity, or perception. Janet viewed dissociation as a purely pathological process.

Jean Martin Charcot (1890), the well-known neurologist and fellow countryman of Janet, was interested in hypnosis and taught the technique to Freud. He believed that even a normal process such as hypnosis, which could be used to access disaggregated mental contents, was itself evidence of dissociative pathology (*un état nerveux artificiel ou expérimental*, "an artificial or experimental nervous state" [Charcot 1890]). Charcot taught, for example, that once patients were cured of hysteria, they would no longer be hypnotizable. This clearly is not the case. Indeed, many normal individuals are highly hypnotizable (Hilgard 1965, Spiegel and Spiegel 1978).

The dissociative disorders might have been studied more intensively during the 20th century had not Janet's and Charcot's work been so thoroughly eclipsed by Freud's psychoanalytic theory, emphasizing as it did repression rather than dissociation. In his early writings with Breuer, Freud explored the unconscious through an examination of similar dissociative phenomena. Cases in the studies on hysteria (Breuer and Freud 1955), such as that of Anna O., clearly involved dissociation. Indeed, Anna O. had many symptoms suggestive of DID. The fragmentation of identity and memory, typical of such states, provided a natural stage for developing a theory involving the unconscious: the processing of information not readily available to consciousness. The vehicle they employed to explain this lack of integration was the concept of "hypnoid states." Breuer and Freud (1955) thought that dissociative symptoms could be attributed to the capacity to enter these hypnoid states, rather than the reverse, as Charcot had thought. To develop a more general theory of human psychopathology, Freud went on to study other kinds of patients, such as those with obsessive–compulsive disorder (Freud 1995) and schizophrenia (Freud 1958a). This shift in the population of patients he studied may well account for his increasing interest in repression rather than dissociation as a model of motivated forgetting. Much has been made of the fact that Freud abandoned the trauma theory of the etiology of the neuroses. What may have happened is that he abandoned the study of individuals for whom trauma could plausibly be applied as an etiological factor in their psychiatric disorder.

Hilgard (1977) developed a neodissociation theory that revived interest in Janetian psychology and dissociative psychopathology. He postulated divisions in mental structure that were horizontal rather than vertical, as was the case in Freud's archeological model. This model allowed for immediate access to consciousness of any of a variety of warded-off memories, which is not the case in Freud's system. In the dynamic unconscious model, repressed memories must first go through a process of transformation as they are accessed and lifted from the depths of the unconscious, for example, through the interpretation of dreams or slips of the tongue (Freud 1958b). In Hilgard's model, amnesia is a crucial mediating mechanism that creates barriers dividing one set of mental contents from another. Thus, flexible use of amnesia is conceptualized as a key defensive strategy. Therefore, reversal of amnesia is an important therapeutic tool.

Repression as a general model for keeping information out of conscious awareness differs from dissociation in four important ways:

(1) In repression, information is disguised as well as hidden. Dissociated information is stored in a discrete and untransformed manner, for example, as a memory of some element of a traumatic experience, whereas repressed information is usually disguised and fragmented. Even when repressed information becomes available to consciousness, its meaning is hidden, for example, in dreams or slips of the tongue.
(2) Retrieval of repressed information requires translation. Retrieval of dissociated information can often be direct. Techniques such as hypnosis can be used to access warded-off memories. By contrast, uncovering of repressed information often requires repeated recall trials through intense questioning, psychotherapy, or psychoanalysis with subsequent interpretation (i.e., of dreams).
(3) Repressed information is not discretely organized temporally. The information kept out of awareness in dissociation is often for a discrete and sharply delimited time, whereas repressed information may be for a type of encounter or experience scattered across times.
(4) Repression is less specifically tied to trauma. Dissociation seems to be elicited as a defense most commonly after episodes of physical trauma, whereas repression is in response to warded-off fears, wishes, and other dynamic conflicts.

Whether dissociation is a subtype of repression or vice versa, both are important methods for managing complex and affectively charged information. Given the complexity of human information processing, the synthesis of perception, cognition, and affect is a major task. Mental function is composed of a variety of reasonably autonomous subsystems involving a perception, memory storage and retrieval, intention, and action (Spiegel 1991, Rumelhart and McClelland 1986, Cohen and Servain-Schreiber 1992a, 1992b, Baars 1988). Indeed, the accomplishment of a sense of mental unity is an achievement, not a given (Spiegel 1990, Kihlstrom and Hoyt 1990). It is remarkable not that dissociative disorders occur at all, but rather that they do not occur more often.

Models of mental experience are presented in Table 73–1.

| Table 73–1 | Models of Mental Experience | |
|---|---|---|
| Mental Function | Dissociation | Repression |
| Organization | Horizontal | Vertical |
| Barriers | Amnesia | Dynamic conflict |
| Etiology | Trauma | Developmental conflict over unacceptable wishes |
| Nature of contents | Untransformed: traumatic memories | Disguised, primary process: dreams, slips |
| Means of access | Hypnosis | Interpretation |
| Treatment | Psychotherapy emphasizing access, control, and working through traumatic memories | Psychotherapy emphasizing interpretation, transference |

## Epidemiology

Dissociative disorders are not among the more common psychiatric illnesses but are not rare. Few good epidemiological studies have been performed. Some estimate the prevalence at only 1 per 10,000 in the population (Coons 1984), but far higher proportions are reported among psychiatric populations. In fact, the prevalence of the disorder seems to be associated to the specific population under study. For example, data from the general population suggest that the numbers are higher than initially described by Coons (Kluft 1991), as high as 1% (Ross 1991, Ross et al. 1991b, Vanderlinden et al. 1991). On the other hand, the data seem to indicate that the numbers are even higher in specialized inpatient populations, as high as 3% (Kluft 1991, Ross 1991, Ross et al. 1991a).

There has been a rise in reported cases, which may be attributed to greater awareness of the diagnosis among mental health professionals, to the availability of specific criteria, and to previous misdiagnosis of DID as schizophrenia or borderline personality disorder. Some experts attribute possible underdiagnosis to family disavowal of sexual and physical abuse. However, there is also controversy about possible overdiagnosis of the syndrome, while others propose that the increase is the result of hypnotic suggestion and inadequate handling by therapists (Brenner 1994, 1996, Frankel 1990, Ganaway 1989, 1995, McHugh 1995a, 1995b, Spanos et al. 1985, 1986). Individuals who most commonly have the disorder are highly hypnotizable and therefore especially sensitive to suggestion or cultural influences. Although psychiatrists' expectations amplified with hypnosis may account for some cases, they cannot account for many patients diagnosed without benefit of hypnosis or by "skeptical" psychiatrists.

Women make up the majority of cases, accounting for 90% of the cases or more, in some studies (Putnam et al. 1986, Coons et al. 1988, Schultz et al. 1989). Strangely, the most common dissociative disorder diagnosis falls into the "not otherwise specified" category, both in the US (Mezzich et al. 1989, Saxe et al. 1993) and in non-Western countries, where dissociative trance and possession trance are the most common dissociative disorder diagnoses (Adityanjee et al. 1989, Saxena and Prasad 1989). Dissociative disorders are ubiquitous around the world, although the structure of the symptoms varies across cultures (Adityanjee et al. 1989, Berger et al. 1994, Boe et al. 1993, Brown et al. 1999, Coons and Milstein 1986, Draijer and Langeland 1999, Eriksson and Lundin 1996, Friedl and Draijer 2000, Horen et al. 1995, Modestin et al. 1996, Putnam 1989, Ronquillo 1991, Sar et al. 2000, Wittkower 1970). Indeed, the symptomatology reflects cultural biases. In Western cultures, which emphasize the importance of the individual, dissociation often takes the form of dissociated elements of individual personality, while in Eastern cultures, which are more sociocentric, possession trance, in which patients feel themselves to be taken over by an outside entity or entities, is more common.

## Diagnostic Criteria and Treatment

There has been a section on the dissociative disorders in the *Diagnostic and Statistical Manual of Mental Disorders*, Third Edition (DSM-III) and its revised edition (DSM-III-R), as well as in the DSM-IV. We now review the diagnosis and

---

### DSM-IV-TR Criteria 308.12

**Dissociative Amnesia**

A. The predominant disturbance is one or more episodes of inability to recall important personal information, usually of a traumatic or stressful nature, that is too extensive to be explained by ordinary forgetfulness.

B. The disturbance does not occur exclusively during the course of dissociative identity disorder, dissociative fugue, posttraumatic stress disorder, acute stress disorder, or somatization disorder and is not due to the direct physiological effects of a substance (e.g., a drug of abuse, a medication) or a neurological or other general medical condition (e.g., amnestic disorder due to head trauma).

C. The symptoms cause clinically significant distress or impairment in social, occupational, or other important areas of functioning.

Reprinted with permission from the Diagnostic and Statistical Manual of Mental Disorders, Fourth Edition, Text Revision. Copyright 2000 American Psychiatric Association.

---

treatment of the dissociative disorders as defined in the DSM-IV-TR (American Psychiatric Association 2000).

## Dissociative Amnesia

This is the classical functional disorder of episodic memory. It does not involve procedural memory or problems in memory storage, as in Wernicke–Korsakoff syndrome. Furthermore, unlike dementing illnesses, dissociative amnesia is reversible (Janet 1920), for example, by using hypnosis or narcoanalysis. It has three primary characteristics:

(1) Type of memory lost: The memory loss is episodic. The first-person recollection of certain events, rather than knowledge of procedures, is lost.
(2) Temporal structure: The memory loss is for one or more discrete time periods, ranging from minutes to years. It is not vagueness or inefficient retrieval of memories but rather a dense unavailability of memories that were encoded and stored. Unlike the situation in amnestic disorders, for example, resulting from damage to the medial temporal lobe in surgery (the case of H.M. [Milner 1959]), in Wernicke–Korsakoff syndrome, or in Alzheimer's dementia, there is usually no difficulty in learning new episodic information. Thus, the amnesia of dissociative disorders is typically retrograde rather than anterograde (Loewenstein 1991). However, a dissociative syndrome of continuous difficulty in incorporating new information that mimics organic amnestic syndromes has been observed (Schacter 1995).
(3) Type of events forgotten: The memory loss is usually for events of a traumatic or stressful nature. This fact

has been noted in the language of the DSM-IV diagnostic criteria. In one study (Coons and Milstein 1986), the majority of cases involved child abuse (60%), but disavowed behaviors such as marital problems, sexual activity, suicide attempts, criminal activity, and the death of a relative have also been reported as precipitants.

Dissociative amnesia most frequently occurs after an episode of trauma, and its onset may be gradual or sudden.

---

**Clinical Vignette 1**

A 30-year-old woman was beaten and raped by a man who drove her home from a party. She had refused his request to enter her apartment, but he returned a few minutes later claiming that he had to make a phone call. He then sexually assaulted her. She screamed and struggled and called the police immediately afterward. He was arrested when he returned to retrieve some jewelry she had pulled off his neck during the struggle. She had not suffered a concussion but began to lose memory of the rape in the ensuing week. By the end of the week she had no memory of the rape but became listless and depressed. Her psychotherapist used hypnosis to help retrieve her memory, which she was gradually able to do. Her recollections were consistent with her physical injuries and reports of neighbors who heard her screams.

---

Dissociative amnesia occurs most often in the third and fourth decades of life (Coons and Milstein 1986, Ross 1989, Putnam 1989). It usually involves one episode, but multiple periods of lost memory are not uncommon (Coons and Milstein 1986). Comorbidity with conversion disorder, bulimia nervosa, alcohol abuse, and depression are common, and Axis II diagnoses of histrionic, dependent, or borderline personality disorders occur in a substantial minority of such patients (Coons and Milstein 1986).

The typical course of dissociative amnesia is described in Clinical Vignette 2.

---

**Clinical Vignette 2**

A 54-year-old man was involved in a motorcycle accident. He was wearing a helmet, which was damaged but did protect him during the accident. He was determined by the doctors in the emergency room to have suffered no significant head trauma. He did not lose consciousness, and he talked with a friend after the accident about it. However, he had no memory of the accident or of the 12 hours afterward. His first recollection was of a friend telling him, "You crashed my motorcycle." When he returned the next day to the hospital where he had been treated, he recognized a nurse as familiar, and she told him that he had been yelling when they treated his injured left knee. Yet this visit did not stimulate any direct recollection of his time in the hospital. He had recovered no memory of the accident a month later.

---

Such individuals typically demonstrate not vagueness or spotty memory but rather a loss of any episodic memory for a finite period. They may not initially be aware of the memory loss; that is, they do not remember that they do not remember. They often report being told that they have done or said things that they cannot remember.

Some individuals do suffer from episodes of selective amnesia, usually for specific traumatic incidents, which may be interwoven with periods of intact memory. In these cases, the amnesia is for a type of material remembered rather than for a discrete time period (Loewenstein 1991).

## Implicit Effects of Dissociated Memories

Although information is kept out of consciousness in dissociative amnesia, it may well exert an influence on consciousness: out of sight does not mean out of mind. For example, a rape victim with no conscious recollection of an assault nonetheless behaves like someone who has been sexually victimized. As noted in Clinical Vignette 1, such individuals often suffer detachment and demoralization, are unable to enjoy intimate relationships, and show hyperarousal to stimuli reminiscent of the trauma. This loss of explicit memory with retention of implicit knowledge is similar to priming in memory research. Individuals who have read a word in a list complete a word stem (a partial word such as "pre" for "present") more quickly if they have seen that word minutes or even hours earlier. This priming effect occurs despite the fact that they cannot consciously recall having read the word, or even the list in which it occurred. When asked in a free recall format to list the word they have seen, they cannot name it, yet they act as though they have seen it and do remember it. Similarly, individuals instructed in hypnosis to forget having seen a list of words nonetheless demonstrate priming effects of the hypnotically suppressed list (Kihlstrom 1987). It is the essence of dissociative amnesia that material kept out of conscious awareness is nonetheless active and may influence consciousness indirectly (Van der Hart 2001).

Individuals with dissociative amnesia generally do not suffer disturbances of identity, except to the extent that their identity is influenced by the warded-off memory. It is not uncommon for such individuals to develop depressive symptoms as well, especially when the amnesia occurs in the wake of a traumatic stressor.

## Treatment

### Psychotherapy

Often, patients suffering from dissociative amnesia experience spontaneous recovery when they are removed from the stressful or threatening situation, when they feel safe, and/or when exposed to personal cues from their past (i.e., home, pets, family members) (Kardiner and Spiegel 1947, Loewenstein 1991, Maldonado et al. 2000, Maldonado and Spiegel 2002, Reither and Stoudemire 1988). In cases where exposure to a safe environment is not enough to restore normal memory functioning, pharmacologically-facilitated interviews may prove useful (Baron and Nagy 1988, Naples and Hackett 1978, Perry and Jacobs 1982).

### Hypnosis

Most patients with dissociative disorder are highly hypnotizable on formal testing and are therefore easily able to make use of hypnotic techniques such as age regression (Spiegel and Spiegel 1978). Hypnosis can enable such patients to reorient temporally and therefore achieve access to otherwise dissociated and unavailable memories.

**Abreaction.** If there is traumatic content to the warded-off memory, patients may abreact, that is, express strong emotion as these memories are elicited. Such abreactions are rarely damaging in themselves but are not intrinsically therapeutic either. They may be experienced by the patient as a reinflicting of the traumatic stressor. Such patients need psychotherapeutic help in integrating these warded-off memories and the associated affect into consciousness, thereby gaining a sense of mastery over them.

**Screen Technique.** One technique that can help bring such memories into consciousness while modulating the affective response to them is a projective technique known as "the screen technique" (Spiegel 1981). While using hypnosis, such patients are taught to recall the traumatic event as if they were watching it on an imaginary movie or television screen. This technique is often helpful for individuals who are unable to remember the event as if it were occurring in the present, either because for some highly hypnotizable individuals that approach is too emotionally taxing or because others are not sufficiently hypnotizable to be able to engage in such hypnotic age regression. The screen can be employed to facilitate cognitive restructuring of the traumatic memory, for example, by picturing on the left side of the screen some component of the traumatic experience, and on the right side something they did to protect themselves or someone else during it. This makes the memory both more complex and more bearable.

A particularly useful feature of this technique is that it allows for the recollection of traumatic events without triggering an uncontrolled reliving of the trauma, as is the case of traumatic flashbacks. The screen technique provides a "controlled dissociation" between the psychological and somatic aspects of memory retrieval. Individuals can be put into self-hypnosis and instructed to get their body into a state of floating comfort and safety. They can do this by imagining that they are somewhere safe and comfortable: "Imagine that you are floating in a bath, a lake, a hot tub, or just floating in space." They are reminded that no matter what they see on the screen their bodies are safe and comfortable: "Do the work on your imaginary screen, not in your body." In this way the tendency for physiological arousal to accompany and intensify the working through of traumatic memories can be controlled, facilitating the psychotherapeutic work.

---
Clinical Vignette 3

A victim of a violent attempted rape had developed a selective amnesia for much of the physical struggle itself. She had suffered a basilar skull fracture, although she had not been rendered unconscious. She had a generalized seizure shortly after the assault. She initially sought help with hypnosis in an attempt to improve her recollection of the assailant's face.

She was instructed in the screen technique and used it to relive the assault. She remembered two things she had not previously recalled. One was that she recognized that he intended not merely to rape her but to kill her. On the other side of the screen she came to the realization that the assailant was surprised at how hard she was fighting with him. She became convinced that had she let him drag her into her apartment, she probably would not have survived. She was tearful and frightened as she recalled this aspect of the attack, which had been previously unavailable to consciousness.

She was then instructed to divide the imaginary screen in half, on the left side picturing an image of the viciousness and intensity of the assault on her and on the right side recognizing what she had done to protect herself. She was instructed to concentrate on these two aspects of the assault and then, when she was ready, to bring herself out of the state of self-hypnosis. She was told that she could use this as a self-hypnosis exercise to be employed several times a day, if she wished, as a means of putting her memories of the rape into perspective. This cognitive and emotional restructuring of the traumatic memories made them more bearable in consciousness.

Before this psychotherapy, she had blamed herself for having fought so hard that she was seriously injured. Afterward, she recognized that she may well have saved her life by fighting off the assailant so vigorously. This positive therapeutic outcome occurred despite the fact that she was unable to recall any new details about the assailant's physical appearance. Furthermore, she had brought into consciousness painful and frightening details of the attack involving recognition of the seriousness of the threat to her life. Seeing the seriousness of the danger, however, allowed her to acknowledge the magnitude of the threat and therefore give herself credit for the nature of her response to it.

---

The psychotherapy of dissociative amnesia involves accessing the dissociated memories, working through affectively loaded aspects of these memories, and supporting the patient through the process of integrating these memories into consciousness.

## Dissociative Fugue

Dissociative fugue combines failure of integration of certain aspects of personal memory with loss of customary identity and automatisms of motor behavior (American Psychiatric Association 2000). It involves one or more episodes of sudden, unexpected, purposeful travel away from home, coupled with an inability to recall portions or all of one's past, and a loss of identity or the assumption of a new identity. The onset is usually sudden, and it frequently occurs after a traumatic experience or bereavement. A single episode is not uncommon, and spontaneous remission of symptoms can occur without treatment.

It was originally thought that the assumption of a new identity, as in the classical case of the Reverend Ansel Bourne (James 1984), was typical of dissociative fugue. However, a review of the literature (Reither and Stoudemire 1988) shows that in the majority of cases there is loss of personal identity but no clear assumption of a new identity.

Many cases of dissociative fugue remit spontaneously. Again, hypnosis can be useful in accessing dissociated material. The case in Clinical Vignette 4 was reported by Spiegel and Spiegel (1978).

## DSM-IV-TR Criteria 308.13

### Dissociative Fugue

A. The predominant disturbance is sudden, unexpected travel away from home or one's customary place of work, with inability to recall one's past.

B. Confusion about personal identity or assumption of new identity (partial or complete).

C. The disturbance does not occur exclusively during the course of dissociative identity disorder and is not due to the direct physiological effects of a substance (e.g., a drug of abuse, a medication) or a general medical condition (e.g., temporal lobe epilepsy).

D. The symptoms cause clinically significant distress or impairment in social, occupational, or other important areas of functioning.

Reprinted with permission from the Diagnostic and Statistical Manual of Mental Disorders, Fourth Edition, Text Revision. Copyright 2000 American Psychiatric Association.

### Clinical Vignette 4

A woman who appeared dazed but physically unharmed was brought into an army hospital emergency department by the base guards because she had been found wandering nearby. She said that she did not know who she was, where she lived, or how she happened to be there. Initially, plans were made to admit her to the hospital for a full neurological and psychiatric evaluation. She proved to be highly hypnotizable, and hypnosis age regression was used to take her back to an earlier year. She then reported her name and that she lived some 500 miles away. The time was changed again to a period just before this apparent fugue episode. She reported having received unsigned letters from someone at that army base, where, it turned out, her husband was stationed. These letters suggested that her husband was having an affair. This had deeply upset her. She and her husband were reunited and reconciled, and the fugue episode ended.

Not infrequently, fugue episodes represent dissociated but purposeful activity.

### Clinical Vignette 5

A businessman found himself on a transatlantic flight from California to London without recollecting who he was or how he had gotten on the airplane. In later psychotherapy, exploring these fugue episodes, it was determined that he had had an extremely conflicted relationship with a successful but neglectful father. The father had recently died, leaving him financially well-off but emotionally ambivalent. He had spent his boyhood years in London and he recognized in therapy that the travel to London seemed to represent an unconscious attempt to revisit his childhood years and "set his father straight," something he had never been able to do while his father was alive. In this case the dissociative fugue was a form of pathological grief reaction.

Hypnosis can be helpful in treating dissociative fugue by accessing otherwise unavailable components of memory and identity. The approach used is similar to that for dissociative amnesia. Hypnotic age regression can be used as the framework for accessing information available at a previous time. Demonstrating to patients that such information can be made available to consciousness enhances their sense of control over this material and facilitates therapeutic working through of emotionally laden aspects of it.

### Clinical Vignette 6

A woman in a Veterans Administration hospital had lost all memory for the preceding 10 months and insisted that she was in another hospital where she had been the previous December. She proved on testing with the hypnotic induction profile (Spiegel and Spiegel 1978) to be highly hypnotizable (10 of 10 on the induction score). She was hypnotized with a simple rapid induction technique involving the following instruction: "On one, do one thing, look up. On two, do two things, slowly close your eyes and take a deep breath. On three, do three things, let the breath out, let your eyes relax but keep them closed, and let your body float. Then let one hand or the other float up into the air like a balloon and that is your signal to yourself that you are ready to concentrate."

When she did this, she was told that we would be changing times, counting backward in years, and that when her eyes opened she would be at an earlier time in her life. We agreed that when I touched her forehead, she would close her eyes and we would change times again. We then began counting several years back. When she opened her eyes, she spoke as though she were in a different location earlier in her life. She was reoriented to the time when she really was in the other psychiatric hospital in a different city, and she talked about that experience. She was then instructed to close her eyes again and count forward in months to the present month. She opened her eyes and was then properly oriented and had episodic memory for what had transpired in her life in recent months.

Once reorientation is established and the overt identity and memory loss of the fugue have been resolved, it is important to work through interpersonal or intrapsychic issues that underlie the dissociative defenses. Such individuals are often relatively unaware of their reactions to stress because they can so effectively dissociate them (Spiegel 1974). Thus, effective psychotherapy is anticipatory, helping patients to recognize and modify their tendency to set aside their own feelings in favor of those of others.

Patients with dissociative fugue may be helped with a psychotherapeutic approach that facilitates conscious integration of dissociated memories and motivations for behavior previously experienced as automatic and unwilled. It is often helpful to address current psychosocial stressors, such as marital conflict, with the involved individuals, as in the case of the woman found on the army base. To the extent that current psychosocial stress triggers fugue, resolution of that stress can help resolve it and reduce the likelihood of recurrence. Highly hypnotizable individuals prone to these extreme dissociative symptoms (Spiegel and Spiegel 1978, Spiegel 1974, Spiegel et al. 1988) often have great difficulty in asserting their own point of view in a personal relationship. Rather, they interact with others as though they were undergoing a spontaneous trance experience. One such individual described herself as a "disciple in search of a teacher." Psychotherapy can help such individuals recognize and modify their tendency to unthinking compliance with others and extreme sensitivity to rejection and disapproval.

In the past, medication facilitated interviews were used to reverse dissociative amnesia or fugue. However, such techniques offer no advantage over hypnosis and are not especially effective (Perry and Jacobs 1982). Not infrequently, the ceremony of injecting the drug elicits spontaneous hypnotic phenomena before the pharmacological effect is felt, and sedation, respiratory depression, and other side effects can be troublesome. It also promotes dependency on the therapist. On the contrary, when hypnosis is used, patients are trained on self-hypnotic techniques, promoting the use of hypnosis instead of spontaneous dissociation. This enhances the patients' level of control while enhancing a sense of mastery and self-control.

## Depersonalization Disorder

This dissociative disorder involves lack of integration of one or more components of perception. The essential feature of depersonalization disorder is the occurrence of persistent feelings of unreality, detachment, or estrangement from oneself or one's body, usually with the feeling that one is an outside observer of one's own mental processes (American Psychiatric Association 2000, Steinberg 1991). Individuals suffering depersonalization are distressed by it. They are aware of some distortion in their perceptual experience and therefore are not hallucinating or delusional. Affected individuals often fear that they are "going crazy." The symptom is not infrequently transient.

Derealization, in which affected individuals notice an altered perception of their surroundings, resulting in the world seeming unreal or dream-like, frequently occurs as well. Such individuals often ruminate anxiously about this symptom and are preoccupied with their own somatic and mental functioning.

Depersonalization frequently co-occurs with a variety of other symptoms, especially anxiety, panic, or phobic symptoms. It is often a symptom of PTSD and also occurs as a symptom of alcohol and drug abuse, as a side effect of the use of prescription medication, and during stress and sensory deprivation. The symptom of depersonalization is also commonly seen in the course of a number of other neurological and psychiatric disorders (Pies 1991). It is considered a disorder when it is a persistent and predominant symptom. The phenomenology of the disorder involves both the initial symptoms themselves and the reactive anxiety caused by them.

## Treatment

Depersonalization is most often transient and may remit without formal treatment. Recurrent or persistent deper-

> **DSM-IV-TR Criteria** 300.6
>
> **Depersonalization Disorder**
>
> A. Persistent or recurrent experiences of feeling detached from, and as if one is an outside observer of, one's mental processes or body (e.g., feeling like one is in a dream).
>
> B. During the depersonalization experience, reality testing remains intact.
>
> C. The depersonalization causes clinically significant distress or impairment in social, occupational, or other important areas of functioning.
>
> D. The depersonalization experience does not occur exclusively during the course of another mental disorder, such as schizophrenia, panic disorder, acute stress disorder, or another dissociative disorder, and is not due to the direct physiological effects of a substance (e.g., a drug of abuse, a medication) or a general medical condition (e.g., temporal lobe epilepsy).

Reprinted with permission from the Diagnostic and Statistical Manual of Mental Disorders, Fourth Edition, Text Revision. Copyright 2000 American Psychiatric Association.

sonalization should be thought of both as a symptom in itself and as a component of other syndromes requiring treatment, such as anxiety disorders and schizophrenia.

The symptom itself may respond to training in self-hypnosis. Paradoxically, induction or deliberate worsening of symptoms may provide relief by teaching a method of controlling them. For example, a hypnotic induction may induce transient depersonalization symptoms, such as a sense of detachment from part of the body, in such individuals. This is a useful exercise, in that by having a structure for inducing the symptoms, one provides the patient with a context for understanding and controlling them. They are presented as a spontaneous form of hypnotic dissociation that can be modified. Such individuals can be taught to induce a pleasant sense of floating lightness or heaviness in place of the anxiety-related somatic detachment. The use of an imaginary screen to picture problems in a way that detaches them from the typical somatic response is also helpful (Spiegel and Spiegel 1978). Other relaxation techniques such as systematic desensitization, progressive muscle relaxation, and biofeedback may also be of help. Psychotherapy aimed at working through emotional responses to any traumatic or other stressors that tend to elicit the depersonalization is also helpful.

---

Clinical Vignette 7

> A 54-year-old businesswoman was referred for evaluation of lifelong depersonalization symptoms, episodes characterized by a feeling of detachment, alternating with eruptions of uncharacteristic anger or childlike behavior. The episodes occurred more frequently after relationship problems or losses, dismissive or controlling treatment by

others, and especially around important family holidays, such as Thanksgiving and her birthday. She had a history of parental physical abuse early in life. She was tested with the Hypnotic Induction Profile and scored 8.5/10 points, indicating moderate to high hypnotizability. She was taught a self-hypnosis exercise in which she felt her body to be floating comfortably while she pictured herself in a pleasant outdoor scene. She was then able to experience an emotion of anger as she thought about her last episode of depersonalization, and made an association to an earlier episode of parental mistreatment. She was instructed to practice this self-hypnosis exercise three times a day, and observe if she felt a depersonalization episode coming on. Follow-up 3 weeks later indicated that there was a decrease in the number of spontaneous depersonalization episodes, and she found that she could use the self-hypnosis to identify and work through feelings that she had previously been unaware of or that had created difficulties for her. She was, for example, able to recognize a feeling of hurt and rejection at the close of a prior therapy, cry over it, and "move beyond" it. She saw the hypnosis exercise as a means of understanding previously alien feelings and working through them, while increasing her ability to induce relaxation and handle stress.

---

**DSM-IV-TR Criteria** 308.14

### Dissociative Identity Disorder

A. The presence of two or more distinct identities or personality states (each with its own relatively enduring pattern of perceiving, relating to, and thinking about the environment and self).

B. At least two of these identities or personality states recurrently take control of the person's behavior.

C. Inability to recall important personal information that is too extensive to be explained by ordinary forgetfulness.

D. The disturbance is not due to the direct physiological effects of a substance (e.g., blackouts or chaotic behavior during alcohol intoxication) or a general medical condition (e.g., complex partial seizures). **Note:** In children, the symptoms are not attributable to imaginary playmates or other fantasy play.

Reprinted with permission from the Diagnostic and Statistical Manual of Mental Disorders, Fourth Edition, Text Revision. Copyright 2000 American Psychiatric Association.

---

Pharmacological approaches involve balancing therapeutic benefit and risk. Antianxiety medications are most commonly used and may be helpful in reducing the amplification of depersonalization caused by anxiety. However, depersonalization and derealization are also side effects of antianxiety drugs, so their use should be carefully monitored. Increasing dosage, a standard technique when there is lack of therapeutic response, may also increase symptoms, leading to a spiral of increasing symptoms and drug dosage but without therapeutic benefit.

However, appropriate pharmacological treatment for comorbid disorders is an important part of treatment. Use of antianxiety medications for generalized anxiety or phobic disorders (Stein and Uhde 1989) or of antipsychotic medications (Nuller 1982) for psychotic disorders is often beneficial in conditions in which there is contributory comorbidity.

## Dissociative Identity Disorder (Multiple Personality Disorder)

Dissociative identity disorder is a rare but real disorder that is the most widely discussed of the dissociative disorders. It involves the "presence of two or more distinct identities or personality states (each with its own relatively enduring pattern of perceiving, relating to, and thinking about the environment and self)" (American Psychiatric Association 2000). The diagnostic criteria also require that "At least two of these identities or personality states recurrently take control of the person's behavior" (American Psychiatric Association 2000), and that there be amnesia: "Inability to recall important personal information that is too extensive to be explained by ordinary forgetfulness" (American Psychiatric Association 2000). It is a failure of integration of various aspects of identity and personality structure. Often different relationship styles (dependent versus assertive/aggressive) and mood states (depressed versus hostile)

segregate with different identities and personal memories. Such patients may be mystified by events that occurred in another "state," or by responses of others to them for behavior that occurred in a different "state." This fragmentation of personality often occurs in response to trauma in childhood, and is perceived by the patient as protective, allowing him or her to tolerate and partially evade chronic abuse. These patients thus view treatment ambivalently as an attempt to deprive them of a defense against attack. They also tend to see others as irrational and unfair, since response to one aspect of their personality frequently reflects experience with other aspects. One DID patient (prior to diagnosis) reported puzzlement about accusations by friends and acquaintances that she had made hostile comments for which she had no memory. She would find people angry at her for no reason. Thus their personality fragmentation renders them vulnerable to interpersonal problems yet gives them the belief that they are relatively protected from them.

### Prevalence

There are no convincing studies of the absolute prevalence of DID, although there is widespread agreement that the number of diagnosed cases has increased considerably in the US and some European countries in the past 2 decades (Boon and Draijer 1993). Two studies have estimated the prevalence as approximately 1% of psychiatric inpatients (Saxe et al. 1993, Ross et al. 1991a). Factors that may account for the increase in the number of true reported cases include (1) more general awareness of the diagnosis among mental health professionals, (2) the availability of specific diagnostic criteria starting with DSM-III, and (3) reduced misdiagnosis of DID as schizophrenia or borderline personality disorder.

Other authors attribute the increase in reported cases to social contagion, hypnotic suggestion, and misdiagnosis (Frankel 1990, Ganaway 1995, McHugh 1995a,

1995b, Spanos et al. 1986). Proponents of this point of view argue that these individuals are highly hypnotizable and therefore quite suggestible. They would therefore be especially vulnerable to direct or implicit hypnotic suggestion. They note that not infrequently a few specialist psychiatrists make the vast majority of diagnoses. However, it has been observed that the symptoms of patients diagnosed by specialists in dissociation do not differ from those of patients diagnosed by psychiatrists, psychologists, and physicians in more general practice who diagnose one or two cases a year. Furthermore, such patients have been noted to persist in presenting symptoms for an average of 6.5 years before attaining the diagnosis (Putnam 1985). They encounter many psychiatrists who are convinced that they do not have DID and that they have some other disorder, such as schizophrenia. Were they so easily suggestible, it seems likely that they would accept a suggestion that they have other disorders as well, such as schizophrenia or borderline personality disorder.

Nonetheless, because these patients are indeed highly hypnotizable and therefore suggestible (Spiegel 1974, Frischholz 1985), care must be taken in the manner in which the illness is presented to them. However, it is unlikely that the increased number of cases currently reported is accounted for by suggestion alone. Reduction in previous misdiagnosis and increased recognition of the prevalence and sequelae of physical and sexual abuse in childhood (Kluft 1984a, 1991, Frischholz 1985, Spiegel 1984, Terr 1991, Herman et al. 1989) are also reasonable explanations.

## Course

The disorder is more frequently recognized during childhood (Kluft 1984a) but typically emerges between adolescence and the third decade of life; it rarely presents as a new disorder after age 40 years, but there is often considerable delay between initial symptom presentation and diagnosis (Putnam et al. 1986).

Untreated, it is a chronic and recurrent disorder. It rarely remits spontaneously, but the symptoms may not be evident for certain time periods (Kluft 1985). DID has been called "a disease of hiddenness" (Schacter 1995). The dissociation itself hampers self-monitoring and accurate reporting of symptoms and history. Many patients with the disorder are not fully aware of the extent of their dissociative symptoms. They may be reluctant to bring up symptoms because of confusion or shame about the illness or because they encountered previous skepticism. Furthermore, because the majority of patients report histories of sexual and physical abuse (Kluft 1985, 1991, Coons and Milstein 1986, Spiegel 1984, Braun and Sachs 1985), the shame associated with that and fear of retribution may inhibit reporting of symptoms as well.

## Comorbidity

The major comorbid psychiatric illnesses are the depressive disorders, substance use disorders, and borderline personality disorder. Sexual, eating, and sleep disorders co-occur less commonly. Such patients frequently display self-mutilative-behavior, impulsiveness, and overvaluing and devaluing of relationships. Indeed, approximately a third of patients with DID have symptoms that fit criteria for borderline personality disorder as well. Such individuals are also more fre-

quently depressed (Horevitz and Braun 1984). Conversely, research shows dissociative symptoms in many patients with borderline personality disorder, especially those who report histories of physical and sexual abuse (Chu and Dill 1990, Ogata et al. 1990). Indeed, the impulsiveness, splitting, hostility, and fear of abandonment, frequently seen in certain personality states, are similar to the presentation of many patients with borderline personality disorder (Breuer and Freud 1955, pp. 706–710). Many such patients also have symptoms that meet criteria for PTSD, with intrusive flashbacks, recurrent dreams of physical and sexual abuse, avoidance of and loss of pleasure in usually pleasurable activities, and symptoms of hyperarousal, especially when exposed to reminders of childhood trauma (Breuer and Freud 1955, pp. 463–468, Kluft 1985, 1991, Spiegel and Cardeña 1990).

Thus, comorbidity is a complex issue. In addition, these patients are not infrequently misdiagnosed as having schizophrenia (Kluft 1987). This diagnostic confusion is understandable in that they have an apparent delusion that their bodies are occupied by more than one person. In addition, they frequently have auditory hallucinations when one personality state speaks to or comments on the activities of another. When misdiagnosed as schizophrenic, patients with DID are frequently given neuroleptics, which results in a poor therapeutic response and a flattening of affect, which tends to confirm the misdiagnosis (since flat affect is characteristic of schizophrenia).

Individuals with DID commonly report somatic or conversion symptoms (Ross et al. 1990) and other psychosomatic symptoms, such as migraine headaches (Spiegel 1987). Studies have shown that approximately a third of these patients have complex partial seizures (Schenk and Bear 1981), although later studies did not show seizure rates that high. Furthermore, the studies did not show substantial elevations in scores on Dissociative Experiences Scale in patients with complex partial seizures as compared with those of other neurological patients (Loewenstein and Putnam 1988). However, there is sufficient comorbidity that patients recently diagnosed with DID should be evaluated for the possibility of a seizure disorder.

## Psychological Testing

The diagnosis can be facilitated by psychological testing. Scales of trait dissociation have been developed (Bernstein and Putnam 1986, Ross 1989, Carlson et al. 1993), and patients with DID score extremely high on these scales, in contrast to normal populations and other groups of patients (Ross et al. 1990, Steinberg et al. 1990). Those with DID score far higher than normal individuals on standard measures of hypnotizability, whereas schizophrenic patients tend to have lower than normal scores or the absence of high hypnotizability (Spiegel et al. 1982, Spiegel and Fink 1979, Lavoie and Sabourin 1980, Pettinati 1982, Pettinati et al. 1990, Van der Hart and Spiegel 1993). Thus, there is comparatively little overlap in the hypnotizability scores of patients with schizophrenia and those with DID. Form level on the Rorschach test is usually within the normal range, but there are frequent emotionally dramatic responses, often involving mutilation (especially with the color cards) of a type that is often seen in histrionic personality disorder as well (Scroppo et al. 1998). Form level is an assessment of the match between the percept (what the subject reports seeing) and the inkblot structure. Good form level involves relatively little distortion of the image to match percept to inkblot. Good form level is useful in distinguishing patients with DID (formerly multiple personality disorder [American Psychiatric Association 1994]) from those with schizophrenia, who have poor form level.

## Treatment

### Psychotherapy

**Therapeutic Direction.** It is possible to help patients with DID gain control over the dissociative process underlying their symptoms in several ways (Maldonado et al. 2000, Maldonado and Spiegel 2002). The fundamental psychotherapeutic stance should involve meeting patients halfway, a form of structured empathy in which their experience of themselves as fragmented is acknowledged while the reality that the fundamental problem is a failure of integration of disparate memories and aspects of the self is kept in view. In this sense, such individuals suffer from having less than one personality rather than more than one. Therefore, the goal in therapy is to facilitate integration of disparate elements. This can be done in a variety of ways.

Secrets are frequently a problem with such patients, who attempt to use the psychiatrist to reinforce a dissociative strategy of withholding relevant information from certain personality states. Such patients often like to confide in the psychiatrist with the idea that the information is to be kept from other parts of the self, for example, traumatic memories or plans for self-destructive activities.

### Clinical Vignette 8

A 35-year-old woman with DID confided in her psychiatrist in one personality state that she planned to commit suicide. The psychiatrist noted that other parts of herself would be quite alarmed to learn of this plan and said that he planned to inform them. "You can't do that," she protested. "Why not?" inquired the psychiatrist. "Doctor-patient confidentiality," she replied. The psychiatrist was unmoved by this argument.

Clear limit setting and commitment on the part of the psychiatrist to helping all portions of the patient's personality structure learn about warded-off information are important. It is wise to clarify explicitly that the psychiatrist will not become involved in secret collusion. Furthermore, when important agreements are negotiated, such as commitments on the part of patients to seek medical help before acting on a thought to harm themselves or others, it is useful to discuss with the patients that this is an "all-points bulletin," requiring attention from all the relevant personality states. The excuse that certain personality states were "not aware" of the agreement should not be accepted.

**Hypnosis.** Hypnosis can be helpful in facilitating psychotherapy as well as establishing the diagnosis (Spiegel and Spiegel 1978, Braun 1984, Kluft 1982, Maldonado et al. 2000). First of all, the simple structure of hypnotic induction may elicit dissociative phenomena.

### Clinical Vignette 9

The Hypnotic Induction Profile (Spiegel and Spiegel 1978) was administered to a woman who had suffered hysterical pseudoseizures. In the middle of a routine induction her head suddenly turned to the side and she relived an episode, in which she had been abducted and sexually assaulted, with considerable affect as if it were happening in the present. This enabled her and the psychiatrist to reanalyze her symptoms as spontaneous dissociation, similar to the hypnotic state she had been in. The capacity to elicit such symptoms on command provides the first hint of the ability to control them. Most of these patients have the experience of being unable to stop dissociative symptoms but are often intrigued by the possibility of starting them. This carries with it the potential for changing or stopping them as well.

Hypnosis can be helpful in facilitating access to dissociated personalities. They may simply occur spontaneously during hypnotic induction, as in Clinical Vignette 9. An alternative strategy is to hypnotize the patient and use age regression to reorient to a time when a different personality state was manifest. An instruction later to change times back to the present usually elicits a return to the other personality state. This then becomes a means of teaching such an individual how to control the dissociative process.

Alternatively, entering the state of hypnosis may make it possible simply to address and elicit different identities or personality states. Patients can be taught a simple self-hypnosis exercise for this purpose. For example, the patient can be told to count to herself or himself from one to three, as was previously described in Clinical Vignette 6. After some formal exercises such as this, it is often possible to ask the patient to speak with a given alter personality, without the formal use of hypnosis. Merely asking to talk with a given identity usually suffices after a while.

**Memory Retrieval.** Because the loss of memory in DID is complex and chronic (Charcot 1890), its retrieval is likewise a more extended and integral part of the psychotherapeutic process. The therapy becomes an integrating experience of information sharing among disparate personality elements. Conceptualizing DID as a chronic PTSD, the psychotherapeutic strategy involves a focus on working through traumatic memories in addition to controlling the dissociation.

Controlled access to memories greatly facilitates psychotherapy. As with dissociative amnesia, a variety of strategies can be employed to help patients with DID break down amnesic barriers. Eliciting various identities or personality states can facilitate access to memories previously unavailable to consciousness. While so-called "pseudomemories" can occur (Charcot 1890), previously dissociated traumatic memories are often accurate (Janet 1920).

Once these memories of earlier traumatic experience have been brought into consciousness, it is crucial to help the patient work through the painful affect, inappropriate self-blame, and other reactions to these memories (Spiegel et al. 1982, Lindemann 1944). It may be useful to have patients visualize the memories rather than relive them as a means of making their intensity more manageable. It can also be useful to have patients divide the memories, for example, picturing on one side of an imaginary screen something an abuser did to them and on the other side how they tried to protect themselves from the abuse.

---

A young woman with DID remembered a particularly painful episode in hypnosis. When she was 12 years old her stepfather smoked a good deal of marijuana and then forced her to have oral sex with him. She recalled being repelled by what he was forcing her to do and then remembered that she gagged and vomited all over him. "I spoiled his fun. He threw me up against a wall but it did not bother me a bit because I knew I ruined it for him." She was instructed to picture on one side of the screen what he had done to her and on the other what she had done to him.

---

Such techniques can help make the traumatic memories more bearable by placing them in a broader perspective, one in which trauma victims can also identify adaptive aspects of their response to the trauma.

This and similar approaches can help these individuals work through traumatic memories, enabling them to bear them in consciousness and therefore reducing the need for dissociation as a means of keeping such memories and associated painful affect out of consciousness. Although these techniques can be helpful and often result in reduced fragmentation and integration (Spiegel 1984, 1986a, Kluft 1986), a number of complications can occur in the psychotherapy of these patients.

The therapeutic process can be thought of as a kind of grief work (Lindemann 1944) in which information retrieved from memory is reviewed, traumatic memories are put into perspective, and emotional expression is encouraged and worked through, thereby making it more possible to endure and disseminate the information as widely as possible among various parts of the patient's personality structure. Instructions to other alter personalities to "listen" while a given one is talking and reviewing previously dissociated material can be helpful.

**The Rule of Thirds.** The psychotherapy of DID can be a time-consuming and emotionally taxing process. The rule of thirds (Kluft 1991, Schacter 1995) is a helpful guideline. Spend the first third of the psychotherapy session assessing the patient's current mental state and life problems and defining a problem area that might benefit from retrieval into conscious memory and working through. Spend the second third of the session accessing and working through this memory. Allow a final third for helping the patient assimilate the information, regulate and modulate emotional responses, and discuss any responses to the psychiatrist and plans for the immediate future. The psychiatrist may resist doing this because the intense abreactive materials are often so compelling and interesting. The patient may also resist sharing information across personalities. Nonetheless, the psychiatrist can be helpful in imposing structure on often chaotic memories and identity states.

Given the intensity of the material that often emerges involving memories of sexual and physical abuse and sudden shifts in mental state accompanied by amnesia, the psychiatrist is called on to take a clear and structured role in managing the psychotherapy. Appropriate limits must be set concerning self-destructive or threatening behavior, agreements must be made regarding physical safety and treatment compliance, and other matters must be presented to the patient in such a way that dissociative ignorance is not an acceptable explanation for failure to live up to the agreements.

### Traumatic Transference

Transference applies with special meaning to patients who have been physically and sexually abused, especially in childhood. They have experienced individuals who are presumed to be caretakers acting instead in an exploitative and sometimes sadistic fashion. They thus expect similar betrayal from psychiatrists. Although their reality testing is good enough that they can perceive genuine caring, they often unconsciously expect psychiatrists to exploit them. They may experience working through of traumatic memories as a reinflicting of the trauma, with the psychiatrist taking sadistic pleasure in their suffering. They may expect excessive passivity on the part of the psychiatrist, identifying the psychiatrist with some uncaring family figure who knew that abuse was occurring but did little or nothing to stop it. It is important in managing the therapy to keep these issues in mind and make them frequent topics of discussion. This can diffuse, if not eliminate, such traumatic transference distortions of the therapeutic relationship (Spiegel 1988).

**Integration.** The ultimate goal of psychotherapy is integration of these multiple ego states. It is often the case that one or more of the personality states may exert considerable resistance to the process of integration, particularly early in the process of therapy. Also patients may experience efforts of integration as an attempt on the part of the therapist to "kill" personalities. These fears must be worked through and the patient needs to understand that the goal is to learn how to control the episodes of dissociation. This gives patients a sense of gradually being able to control their dissociative processes in order to work through the traumatic memories. In order to enhance mastery and control, the process of the psychotherapy must help patients minimize rather than reinforce the content of traumatic memories, which often involves reexperiencing a sense of helplessness in a symbolic reenactment of the trauma (Freud 1958a, Maldonado et al. 2000).

At the same time, the dissociative defense represents an internalization of the abusive people in the patient's past, a kind of identification with the aggressor, which makes the patient feel powerful rather than helpless. Setting aside the defense also means acknowledging and bearing the helplessness of having been victimized and working through the irrational self-blame that gave such individuals a fantasy of control over events during which they were helpless. Yet, difficult as it is, ultimately the goal of psychotherapy is mastery over the dissociative process, controlled access to dissociative states, integration of warded-off painful memories and material, and a more integrated continuum of identity, memory, and consciousness. Although there have been no controlled trials of the outcome of psychotherapy for this disorder, case series reports indicate a positive outcome in a majority of cases (Kluft 1984b, 1986, 1991).

| Table 73-2 | Stages of Therapy |
|---|---|
| **Stage** | **Technique** |
| Establishing treatment | Education, atmosphere of safety, instill confidence |
| Preliminary interventions | Confirm diagnosis, set limits, access dissociation with hypnosis |
| History gathering | Explore components of dissociative structure |
| Working through trauma | Grief work |
| Move toward integration | Enhance communication across dissociative states |
| Integration–resolution | Encourage development of integrated self |
| Learning coping skills | Help with life decisions and relationships |
| Solidification of gains | Transference examination |
| Follow-up | Maintenance |

*Source*: Kluft RP (1991) Multiple personality disorder. In American Psychiatric Press Review of Psychiatry, Vol. 10, Tasman A and Goldfinger SM (eds). American Psychiatric Press, Washington DC.

The stages of therapy are presented in Table 73–2.

## Psychopharmacology

As with other dissociative disorders, there is little evidence that psychoactive drugs are of great help in reversing dissociative symptoms (Maldonado et al. 2000). In the past, short-acting barbiturates such as sodium amobarbital were used intravenously to reverse functional amnesia, but this technique is no longer employed, largely because of poor results (Perry and Jacobs 1982). Research data provide no evidence suggesting that any medication regimen has any significant therapeutic effect on the dissociative process manifested by DID patients (Loewenstein 1991, Markowitz and Gill 1996, Putnam 1989). To date, pharmacological treatment has been limited to symptom control or the management of comorbid conditions (e.g., depression).

Of all available classes of psychotropic agents, antidepressants are the most useful class for the treatment of patients with DID. That is because patients suffering from dissociation frequently experience comorbid dysthymic or major depressive disorder. The newer agents—selective serotonin reuptake inhibitors (SSRIs)—are particularly useful, given their high level of effectiveness, low side effect profile, and even lower danger in overdose, compared with tricyclic antidepressants and monoamine oxidase inhibitors. Nevertheless, medication compliance may be a problem with dissociative patients because dissociated personality states may interfere with medication taking or may take the medication in an overdose attempt.

Benzodiazepines have mostly been used to facilitate recall by controlling secondary anxiety associated with retrieval of traumatic memories (i.e., medication facilitated interviews). Nevertheless, despite their short-term usefulness, CNS-depressant agents may cause sudden mental state transitions, which may in turn increase rather than decrease amnesic barriers. Therefore, as useful as they could be on short-term basis (i.e., acute management of a panic attack), the long term of these agents may, in fact, contribute rather than treat dissociative episodes.

There are several uses for anticonvulsant agents. We know that seizures disorders have a high rate of comorbidity with DID. Thus, anticonvulsant agents may help control the dissociation associated with epileptogenic activity. On the other hand, anticonvulsant agents have proven to be effective in the management of mood disorders, as well as the impulsiveness associated with personality disorders and brain injury. Also despite their effectiveness, these agents produce less amnestic side effects than the benzodiazepines and thus may be preferred. On the other hand, the need for closer monitoring due to potential toxicity, particularly in overdoses, makes their use less desirable than the newer SSRIs.

Of all pharmacological agents available, antipsychotics may be the less desirable. First, they are rarely useful in reducing dissociative symptoms. In fact, there have been reports of increased levels of dissociation and an increased incidence of side effects when used in patients suffering from dissociative disorders.

## Dissociative Trance Disorder

### Dissociative Trance

Dissociative trance disorder has been divided into two broad categories, dissociative trance and possession trance (American Psychiatric Association 2000). Dissociative trance phenomena are characterized by a sudden alteration in consciousness, not accompanied by distinct alternative identities. In this form the dissociative symptom involves an alteration in consciousness rather than identity. Also, in dissociative trance, the activities performed are rather simple, usually involving sudden collapse, immobilization, dizziness, shrieking, screaming, or crying. Memory is rarely affected, and if there is amnesia, it is fragmented.

Dissociative trance phenomena frequently involve sudden, extreme changes in sensory and motor control. A classic example is the *ataque de nervios*, prevalent in Latin American countries. For example, this phenomenon is estimated to have a 12% lifetime prevalence rate in Puerto Rico (Lewis-Fernandez 1994). A typical episode involves a sudden feeling of anxiety, followed by total body shakes, which may mimic convulsions. This is then followed by hyperventilation, unintelligible screaming, agitation, and often violent bodily movements. Often, this is followed by collapse and probably transient loss of consciousness. After the episode is over, subjects complain of fatigue and having been confused, although this behavior is dramatically different from classic postictal states. Some subjects may experience amnesia at least to some aspects of the event (Lewis-Fernandez 1994).

Other examples include *lata* and "falling out." Lata represents the Malay version of trance disorder. In these episodes, afflicted individuals usually experience a sudden vision, mostly of a threatening spirit. The observable behavior includes screaming or crying and physical manifestation of overtly violent behavior which often requires the sufferer to be physically restrained. Patients often report episodes of amnesia, but there is no clear possession by the offending spirit (Lewis-Fernandez 1994). On the other hand, "falling out" more commonly occurs among African-Americans in the southern US. Similarly to other trance episodes, the affected individual may enter a trance

## DSM-IV-TR Criteria

### Dissociative Trance Disorder

A. Either (1) or (2):

   (1) trance, i.e., temporary marked alteration in the state of consciousness or loss of customary sense of personal identity without replacement by an alternate identity, associated with at least one of the following:

   (a) narrowing of awareness of immediate surroundings, or unusually narrow and selective focusing on environmental stimuli

   (b) stereotyped behaviors or movements that are experienced as being beyond one's control

   (2) possession trance, a single or episodic alteration in the state of consciousness characterized by the replacement of customary sense of personal identity by a new identity. This is attributed to the influence of a spirit, power, deity, or other person, as evidenced by one (or more) of the following:

   (a) stereotyped and culturally determined behaviors or movements that are experienced as being controlled by the possessing agent

   (b) full or partial amnesia for the event

B. The trance or possession trance state is not accepted as a normal part of a collective cultural or religious practice.

C. The trance or possession trance state causes clinically significant distress or impairment in social, occupational, or other important areas of functioning.

D. The trance or possession trance state does not occur exclusively during the course of a psychotic disorder (including mood disorder with psychotic features and brief psychotic disorder) or dissociative identity disorder, and is not due to the direct physiological effects of a substance or a general medical condition.

Reprinted with permission from the Diagnostic and Statistical Manual of Mental Disorders, Fourth Edition, Text Revision. Copyright 2000 American Psychiatric Association.

state, followed by bodily collapse, the inability to see or speak, despite the fact that they are fully conscious. Temporary confusion may be observed, although subjects are not usually amnesic to what occurred during the episode (Lewis-Fernandez 1994).

### Possession Trance

In contrast to dissociative trance episodes, possession trance involves the assumption of a distinct alternative identity. The new identity is presumed to be that of a deity, ancestor, or spirit who has transiently taken possession of the subject's mind and body. Different from dissociative trance episodes, which are characterized by rather crude, simplistic, regressive-like behaviors, possession trance victims often exhibit rather complex behavior. During these episodes, subjects may, for example, express otherwise forbidden thoughts or needs, engage in unusually and uncharacteristic aggressive behavior (e.g., verbal or physical expressions of aggression), or may attempt to negotiate for change in family or social status. Also, in contrast to dissociative trance episodes, possession trance episodes often are followed by dense amnesia for a large portion of the episode during which the spirit identity was in control of the subject's behavior.

### Cultural Context

Dissociative-like phenomena have been described in virtually every culture (Lewis-Fernandez 1994, Katz 1982, Kirmayer 1994). Yet they appear to be more prevalent in the less heavily industrialized Second and Third World countries. Studies on the prevalence of dissociative disorders in India have suggested that the 1-year prevalence of dissociative trance disorder is approximately 3.5% of all psychiatric hospitalizations, making it a highly frequent mental disorder (Adityanjee et al. 1989, Saxena and Prasad 1989). Trance and possession syndromes are by far the most common type of dissociative disorders seen around the world. On the other hand, DID, which is relatively more common in the US, is virtually never diagnosed in underdeveloped countries. This difference in prevalence and distribution of dissociative disorder across different populations may be mediated by cultural, as well as biological factors. For example, Eastern culture is far more sociocentric than Western culture. Thus, being "possessed" by an outside entity would be more culturally comprehensible and acceptable in the East. On the other hand, an apparent proliferation of individual identities would fit better with the Western preoccupation with individualism. Nonetheless, the underlying dissociative mechanism inhibiting integration of perception, memory, and identity may suggest a common underlying mechanism amongst these dissociative syndromes.

Trance and possession episodes are usually understood as an idiom of distress and yet they are not viewed as normal. That is, they are not a generally accepted part of cultural and religious practice, which often does involve normal trance phenomena, such as trance dancing in the Balinese Hindu culture. Trance dancers enjoy the remarkable privilege of being the only portion of this socially rigid society able to elevate their social status. The way they are able to do that is by developing the ability to enter trance states. During these altered states of consciousness, which usually occur within the context of a socially acceptable ceremony setting, they dance over hot coals, hold a sword at their throat, or in other ways exhibit supernormal powers of concentration and physical prowess. The mechanism mediating these phenomena is not fully understood, but there is evidence of elevations in plasma noradrenaline, dopamine, and beta-endorphin among Balinese trance dancers during trance states. This form of trance is considered socially normal and even exalted.

By contrast, disordered trance and possession trance are viewed by the local community as an aberrant form of

| Table 73-3 | Characteristics of Dissociation in Western and Eastern Cultures | |
|---|---|---|
| Dissociative Phenomenon | Western | Eastern |
| Splitting of consciousness | Depersonalization | Dissociative trance |
| Splitting of identity | DID (multiple personality disorder): multiple internal identities | Possession trance: control by external identities |
| Splitting of memory | Dissociative amnesia | Secondary in dissociative trance, more common in possession trance |
| Loss of somatic control | Conversion disorder | Dissociative trance, e.g., *lata, ataque de nervios* |
| Treatment | Therapist induces dissociation in subject, often with hypnosis | Healer enters trance or dissociative state to take on offending spirit |

behavior that requires intervention. Such symptoms often arise in the context of family or social distress, for example, discomfort in a new family environment. Thus, cultural informants make it clear that people with dissociative trance disorder are abnormal.

Differences in culture clearly influence almost all mental disorders (Table 73–3). Delusional content of a schizophrenic patient is often dramatically different in a Hindu versus a Christian. Similarly, the manifestations of major depressive disorder may take a different form in China, where it looks more like what used to be called neurasthenia, where it may present with far more somatic symptoms, compared with predominantly guilty ruminations, seen in Western patients (Kleinman 1977). Similarly, variations in the form and presentation of the various dissociative disorders, depending on the population under study, only underscore the ubiquity of the mechanism of dissociation. The DSM-IV task force voted to include dissociative trance disorder in the appendix of the DSM-IV (American Psychiatric Association 2000) to stimulate further research on the question of whether it should be a separate Axis I disorder or whether it should be included as a subtype in the category of dissociative disorders not otherwise specified.

## Treatment

Treatment of these disorders varies from culture to culture. Rubbing the body with special potions, negotiating to change the affected person's social circumstances, and physical restraint are often used. Ceremonies to remove or appease the invading spirit are also employed.

## Dissociation and Trauma

One of the important developments in the modern understanding of dissociative disorders is the establishment of a clearer link between trauma and dissociation (Spiegel and Cardeña 1991, Spiegel and Spiegel 1978). Although the role of traumatic stress in eliciting dissociative symptoms was a part of Janet's early thinking (Van der Hart et al. 1989) as well as that of Breuer and Freud (1955), more attention was paid to the symptoms, developmental issues, and personality features than to the role of traumatic stressors themselves. Later work has examined in more detail the proximate role of trauma in eliciting dissociative symptoms.

Trauma can be understood as the experience of being made into an object, a thing, the victim of someone else's rage or of nature's indifference. Trauma represents the ultimate experience of helplessness: loss of control over one's own body. There is growing clinical evidence that dissociation occurs as a defense during traumatic experiences, constituting an attempt to maintain mental control at the moment when physical control has been lost (Spiegel et al. 1988, Putnam 1985, Kluft 1984a, Spiegel 1984). Many assault victims report floating above their body, feeling sorry for the person being assaulted beneath them. Patients, victims of childhood abuse, have reported "taking themselves elsewhere" where they could "safely play," by themselves or with imaginary friends, while their bodies were brutally abused by a perpetrator. In fact, there is evidence (Terr 1991) that children exposed to multiple traumas as opposed to single-blow traumas are more likely to use dissociative defense mechanisms, which include spontaneous trance episodes and amnesia.

As noted in the section on DID, there is an accumulating literature suggesting a connection between a history of childhood physical and sexual abuse and the development of dissociative symptoms (Coons and Milstein 1986, Kluft 1984a, 1985, Spiegel 1984). Similarly, dissociative symptoms have been found to be more prevalent in patients with Axis II disorders, such as borderline personality disorder, when there has been a history of childhood abuse (Herman et al. 1989, Chu and Dill 1990).

Another means of examining the putative connection between dissociation and trauma is to look at the prevalence of dissociative symptoms after recent trauma (Spiegel and Cardeña 1991). If it is indeed the case that trauma seems to elicit dissociative symptoms, they should be observable in the immediate aftermath of trauma. In the early literature examining responses to trauma, Lindemann (1944), studying the aftermath of the Coconut Grove fire, observed that the individuals who acted as though little or nothing had happened had an extremely poor long-term prognosis. These were individuals who had been injured or had lost loved ones. Indeed, it was the absence of posttraumatic symptoms in this group, compared with the agitation, dysphoria, and restlessness that typified the majority of survivors, that led him to formulate the normal process of acute grief.

Several subsequent researchers have observed that psychic numbing is a predictor of later PTSD symptoms. In fact, Solomon and Mikulincer (1988) observed that psychic numbing accounted for 20% of the variance in later PTSD symptoms among Israeli combat soldiers. Similarly, McFarlane (1986) found that numbing in response to the Ash Wednesday bush fires in Australia was a strong predictor of later posttraumatic symptoms.

Research on survivors of other life-threatening events, including hostage taking, indicated that more than half have experienced a sense of detachment, feelings of unreality (i.e., depersonalization), lack of emotions, hyperalertness, and automatic movements (Noyes and Kletti 1977, Madakasira and O'Brien 1987, Sloan 1988, Noyes and Slymen 1978–1979). Numbing, anhedonia, and an inability to feel deeply about anything were reported in about a third of the survivors of the Hyatt Regency skywalk collapse (Wilkinson 1983) and in a similar proportion of survivors of the North Sea oil rig disaster (Holen 1993). These findings are consistent with our studies of survivors of the Loma Prieta earthquake (Cardeña and Spiegel 1993). One quarter of this sample of normal students reported marked depersonalization during and immediately after the event.

Although these dissociative responses to traumatic stressors have been conceptualized as adaptive defenses to overwhelming situations, the thrust of the literature indicates that the presence of dissociative symptoms in the immediate aftermath of trauma is a strong predictor of the development of later PTSD (Solomon and Mikulincer 1988, McFarlane 1986, Freinkel et al. 1994, Koopman et al. 1994, Marmar et al. 1994, Birmes 2001). For example, victims of the Oakland-Berkeley firestorm who reported significant dissociative symptoms had suffered relatively greater exposure to the fire and also were more likely to have significant symptoms of PTSD 7 months later (Koopman et al. 1994). Similarly, Marmar and coworkers (1994) found that peritraumatic dissociation was a strong predictor of later PTSD symptoms among Vietnam veterans. Thus, physical trauma seems to elicit dissociation, perhaps in individuals who are prone to the use of this defense by virtue of either previous traumatic experience or a constitutional tendency to dissociate. This dissociative reaction may, in some cases, resolve quickly. However, in others it may become the matrix for later posttraumatic symptoms, such as dissociative amnesia for the traumatic episode. Indeed, more extreme dissociative disorders, such as DID, have been conceptualized as chronic PTSDs (Kluft 1984b, 1991, Spiegel 1984, 1986b). Recollection of trauma tends to have an off–on quality involving either intrusion or avoidance (Horowitz 1976), in which victims either intensively relive the trauma as though it were recurring or have difficulty remembering it (Madakasira and O'Brien 1987, Cardeña and Spiegel 1993, Christianson and Loftus 1987). Thus, physical trauma seems to elicit dissociative responses, which, in turn, predispose to the development of later PTSD, perhaps by reducing the likelihood of working through the traumatic experiences afterward.

## Acute Stress Disorder

As a result of this line of research, a new diagnostic category, acute stress disorder, was included in DSM-IV-TR (American Psychiatric Association 2000). There was an

---

### DSM-IV-TR Criteria 308.3

**Acute Stress Disorder**

A. The person has been exposed to a traumatic event in which both of the following have been present:

    (1) the person experienced, witnessed, or was confronted with an event or events that involved actual or threatened death or serious injury, or a threat to the physical integrity of self or others

    (2) the person's response involved intense fear, helplessness, or horror

B. Either while experiencing or after experiencing the distressing event, the individual has three (or more) of the following dissociative symptoms:

    (1) a subjective sense of numbing, detachment, or absence of emotional responsiveness

    (2) reduction in awareness of his or her surroundings (e.g., "being in a daze")

    (3) derealization

    (4) depersonalization

    (5) dissociative amnesia (i.e., inability to recall an important aspect of the trauma)

C. The traumatic event is persistently reexperienced in at least one of the following ways: recurrent images, thoughts, dreams, illusions, flashback episodes, or a sense of reliving the experience; or distress on exposure to reminders of the traumatic event.

D. Marked avoidance of stimuli that arouse recollections of the trauma (e.g., thoughts, feelings, conversations, activities, places, people).

E. Marked symptoms of anxiety or increased arousal (e.g., difficulty sleeping, irritability, poor concentration, hypervigilance, exaggerated startle response, motor restlessness).

F. The disturbance causes clinically significant distress or impairment in social, occupational, or other important areas of functioning or impairs the individual's ability to pursue some necessary task, such as obtaining necessary assistance or mobilizing personal resources by telling family members about the traumatic experience.

G. The disturbance lasts for a minimum of 2 days and a maximum of 4 weeks and occurs within 4 weeks of the traumatic event.

H. The disturbance is not due to the direct physiological effects of a substance (e.g., a drug of abuse, a medication) or a general medical condition, is not better accounted for by brief psychotic disorder, and is not merely an exacerbation of a preexisting Axis I or Axis II disorder.

---

acute stress reaction category in the *Diagnostic and Statistical Manual of Mental Disorders*, Second Edition (DSM-II), and the *International Classification of Diseases*, Ninth Revision (ICD-9) has a similar category. It was thought that the inclusion of this diagnosis would facilitate early detection and intervention and would also remedy a hole in the nosology: how to diagnose a substantial minority of victims of acute trauma who are quite symptomatic within the first month after the occurrence of the traumatic stressor.

Although acute stress disorder is classified among the anxiety disorders in DSM-IV-TR (American Psychiatric Association 2000), mention is made of it in this chapter because half of the symptoms of this disorder are dissociative in nature.

These diagnostic criteria would designate approximately a third of individuals exposed to serious trauma as symptomatic. Dissociative symptoms occurring at the time of the trauma are strongly predictive of later development of PTSD (Koopman et al. 1994, Marmar et al. 1994, Classen et al. 1993, Freud 1995) and are associated with higher cortisol levels during exposure to uncontrollable stress (Freud 1958a). Similarly, the occurrence of PTSD is predicted by intrusion, avoidance, and hyperarousal symptoms in the immediate aftermath of rape (Rothbaum and Foa 1993) and combat trauma (Blank 1993, Solomon et al. 1988). Although most individuals experiencing serious trauma are initially symptomatic, the majority recover without developing PTSD. Most studies demonstrate that 25% or less of those who experience serious trauma later become symptomatic.

This diagnostic category is useful not only for research on the normal and abnormal processes of adjusting to trauma, but also as a means of providing an important opportunity for early intervention, and thus, prevention of later psychopathology. Even though dissociation has a role at the time of trauma, if the defense persists too long it may interfere with the working through of traumatic material. Lindemann (1944) described the term *grief work*, referring to process needed to put traumatic experience into perspective and reduce the likelihood of later symptoms. In this context, psychotherapy, aimed at helping individuals acknowledge, bear, and put into perspective a traumatic experience shortly after the trauma, should be helpful in reducing the incidence of later PTSD.

## Theoretical and Research Issues: Models and Mechanisms of Dissociation

### Dissociation and Information Processing

Dissociation may seem like a historical aberration, a throwback to earlier and more primitive models of the mind. Yet these disorders are surprisingly congruent with information processing–based theories of mental function. For example, connectionist and parallel distributed processing models (Rumelhart and McClelland 1986) take a bottom-up rather than a top-down approach to cognitive organization. Traditional models emphasize a supraordinate structure in which broad categories of information structure the processing of specific examples of those categories, that is, the category "sweet" must exist to make sense of "sugar," "candy," and "jelly." In the parallel distributed processing models, subunits or neural nets process information through patterns of co-occurrence of input stimuli that lead to activation patterns in these neural nets, which produce pattern recognition. The output of one neuronal system becomes the input to another, thereby gradually building up integrated and complex patterns of activation and inhibition. A bottom-up processing model system has the advantage of accounting for the processing of vast amounts of information and the ability to recognize patterns with approximate information. Nevertheless, such models make the classification and integration of information problematical.

Information seems to be processed on the basis of the co-occurrence of patterns of activation rather than its appearance in a predefined category. Therefore, in parallel distributed processing system models, failures in integration of mental contents are theoretically likely to occur. Inappropriate but apparent similarities may appear when activation patterns are similar, and conversely, no two pieces of information are necessarily connected. There have been models created to explain psychotic, dissociative, and mood disorders, based on abnormal or defective neuronal association network patterns (Li and Spiegel 1992, Hoffman 1987). These neural models assumed that when there are problems with the processing of input information (a model for traumatic input), the brain is more likely to have difficulty achieving a coherent and balanced output. This could then lead to the development of dissociation of information and data manifested in the subject's inability to process smoothly all of the incoming information.

### Dissociation and Memory Systems

There are two broad categories of memory known as explicit and implicit (Schacter 1992), declarative and procedural (Squire 1987), or episodic and semantic (Tulving 1983). These two basic memory systems serve different functions. Explicit or episodic memory involves recall of personal experience identified with the self, for example, "I went dancing last night." The second type is known as implicit or procedural memory. This involves the execution of routine operations, such as driving a car, or typing on a keyboard. Most of these rather automatic operations could be carried out with little conscious awareness, but yet with a high degree of proficiency. These two types of memory seem to reside in different cerebral anatomical localizations. Episodic memory seems to be primarily associated with limbic system function, primarily involving the hippocampal formation and mamillary bodies. On the other hand, procedural memory appears to be a function of basal ganglia and cortical functioning (Kosslyn and Koenig 1992).

The fact that there are separate memory systems may account for certain types of dissociative phenomena (Spiegel et al. 1993). For example, the automaticity observed in certain types of dissociative disorders reflect the separation of self-identification associated with explicit memory from routine activity in implicit or procedural memory. It is thus not at all foreign to our mental processing to act in an automatic way devoid of explicit self-identification. Future research on the neurobiology of memory may well provide insights into the functional disintegration of memory, perception, identity, and consciousness seen in dissociative disorders (Zola-Morgan et al. 1982, Zola-Morgan and Squire 1985).

## Conclusion

The dissociative disorders constitute a challenging and fascinating spectrum of psychiatric illnesses. The failure of integration of memory, identity, perception, and consciousness seen in these disorders results in symptoms that illustrate fundamental problems in the organization of mental processes. Dissociative phenomena often occur during and after physical trauma but may also represent transient or chronic defensive patterns. Dissociative disorders are generally treatable and are a domain in which psychotherapy is a primary modality, although pharmacological treatment of comorbid conditions such as depression can be quite helpful. The dissociative disorders are ubiquitous around the world, although they take a variety of forms. They represent a fascinating diagnostic, therapeutic, and investigative challenge.

## Comparison of DSM-IV/ICD-10 Diagnostic Criteria

The ICD-10 Diagnostic Criteria for Research for dissociative amnesia specify that there be a "convincing association in time between the onset of symptoms of the disorder and stressful events, problems, or needs." In DSM-IV-TR, the criteria set notes that the forgotten information is usually of a stressful or traumatic nature.

For dissociative fugue, in contrast to DSM-IV-TR, the ICD-10 Diagnostic Criteria for Research specify "amnesia for the journey." Furthermore, in contrast to DSM-IV-TR, the ICD-10 Diagnostic Criteria for Research do not indicate that there is an inability to recall one's past during the fugue or that there be confusion about personal identity.

Dissociative identity disorder is included in ICD-10 as an example of an "other dissociative (conversion) disorder" under the rubric "multiple personality disorder." The ICD-10 Diagnostic Criteria for Research and the DSM-IV-TR criteria are almost identical.

Finally, ICD-10 has a single category "depersonalization–derealization syndrome" for presentations characterized by either depersonalization or derealization. In contrast, the DSM-IV-TR category includes only depersonalization and mentions derealization as an associated feature. Furthermore, unlike DSM-IV-TR which includes this category in the dissociative disorders section, ICD-10 includes the category within the "other neurotic disorders" grouping.

## References

Adityanjee R, Raju GSP, and Khandelwal SK (1989) Current status of multiple personality disorder in India. Am J Psychiatr 146, 1607–1610.

American Psychiatric Association (1994) Diagnostic and Statistical Manual of Mental Disorders, 4th ed. APA, Washington DC.

American Psychiatric Association (2000) Diagnostic and Statistical Manual of Mental Disorders, 4th ed., Text Rev. APA, Washington DC.

Baars BJ (1988) A Cognitive Theory of Consciousness. Cambridge University Press, New York.

Baron DA and Nagy R (1988) The amobarbital interview in a general hospital setting, friend or foe: A case report. Gen Hosp Psychiatr 10, 220–222.

Berger D, Saito S, Ono Y, et al. (1994) Dissociation and child abuse histories in an eating disorder cohort in Japan. Acta Psychiatr Scand 90, 274–280.

Bernstein EM and Putnam FW (1986) Development, reliability, and validity of a dissociation scale. J Nerv Ment Dis 174, 727–735.

Birmes P (2001) Peritraumatic dissociation, acute stress, and early posttraumatic stress disorder in victims of general crime. Can J Psychiatr – Rev Can Psychiatr 46, 649–651.

Blank A (1993) The longitudinal course of posttraumatic stress disorder. In Posttraumatic Stress Disorder: DSM-IV and Beyond, Davidson JRT and Foa EB (eds). American Psychiatric Press, Washington DC, pp. 3–22.

Boe T, Haslerud J, and Knudsen H (1993) Multiple personality: A phenomenon also in Norway? Tidsskr Nor Laegeforen 113, 3230–3232.

Boon S and Draijer N (1993) Multiple personality disorder in The Netherlands: A clinical investigation of 71 patients. Am J Psychiatr 150, 489–494.

Braun BG (1984) Uses of hypnosis with multiple personality. Psychiatr Ann 14, 34–40.

Braun BG and Sachs RG (1985) The development of multiple personality predisposing, precipitating, and perpetuating factors. In Childhood Antecedents of Multiple Personality, Kluft RP (ed). American Psychiatric Press, Washington DC, pp. 37–64.

Brenner I (1994) The dissociative character: A reconsideration of "multiple personality." J Am Psychoanal Assoc 42, 819–846.

Brenner I (1996) The characterological basis of multiple personality. Am J Psychother 50, 154–166.

Breuer J and Freud S (1955) Studies on hysteria. In The Standard Edition of the Complete Psychological Works of Sigmund Freud, Vol. 2, Strachey J (trans-ed). Hogarth Press, London, pp. 183–251. (Originally published in 1895)

Brown L, Russell J, Thornton C, et al. (1999) Dissociation, abuse and the eating disorders: Evidence from an Australian population. Austral NZ J Psychiatr 33(4), 521–528.

Cardeña E and Spiegel D (1993) Dissociative reactions to the San Francisco Bay Area earthquake of 1989. Am J Psychiatr 150, 474–478.

Carlson EB, Putnam FW, Ross CA, et al. (1993) Validity of the Dissociative Experiences Scale in screening for multiple personality disorder: A multicenter study. Am J Psychiatr 150, 1030–1036.

Charcot JM (1890) Oeuvres Complets de JM Charcot, Vol. 11. Lecrosnier et Babe, Paris.

Christianson SA and Loftus EF (1987) Memory for traumatic events. Appl Cogn Psychol 1, 225–239.

Chu JA and Dill DL (1990) Dissociative symptoms in relation to childhood physical and sexual abuse. Am J Psychiatr 147, 887–892.

Classen C, Koopman C, and Spiegel D (1993) Trauma and Dissociation. Bull Menninger Clin 57, 178–194.

Cohen JD and Servain-Schreiber D (1992a) A neural network model of disturbance in the processing of context in schizophrenia. Psychiatr Ann 22, 131–136.

Cohen JD and Servain-Schreiber D (1992b) Introduction to neural network mode in psychiatry. Psychiatr Ann 22, 113–118.

Coons PM (1984) The differential diagnosis of multiple personality. Psychiatr Clin N Am 12, 51–67.

Coons PM and Milstein V (1986) Psychosexual disturbances in multiple personality: Characteristics, etiology, treatment. J Clin Psychiatr 47, 106–110.

Coons PM, Bowman ES, and Milstein V (1988) Multiple personality disorder: A clinical investigation of 50 cases. J Nerv Ment Dis 176, 519–527.

Draijer N and Langeland W (1999) Childhood trauma and perceived parental dysfunction in the etiology of dissociative symptoms in psychiatric inpatients. Am J Psychiatr 156(3), 379–385.

Eriksson NG and Lundin T (1996) Early traumatic stress reactions among Swedish survivors of the Estonia disaster. Br J Psychiatr 169, 713–716.

Frankel FH (1990) Hypnotizability and dissociation. Am J Psychiatr 147, 823–829.

Freinkel A, Koopman C, and Spiegel D (1994) Dissociative symptoms in media eyewitnesses of execution. Am J Psychiatr 151(9), 1335–1339.

Freud S (1958a) Psycho-analytic notes on an autobiographical account of a case of paranoia (dementia paranoides). In The Standard Edition of the Complete Psychological Works of Sigmund Freud, Vol. 12, Strachey J (trans-ed). Hogarth Press, London, pp. 3–82. (Originally published in 1911)

Freud S (1958b) The interpretation of dreams. In The Standard Edition of the Complete Psychological Works of Sigmund Freud, Vol. 4 and 5, Strachey J (trans-ed). Hogarth Press, London. (Originally published in 1900)

Freud S (1995) Notes upon a case of obsessional neurosis. In The Standard Edition of the Complete Psychological Works of Sigmund Freud, Vol. 10, Strachey J (trans-ed). Hogarth Press, London, pp. 153–249. (Originally published in 1909)

Friedl MC and Draijer N (2000) Dissociative disorders in Dutch psychiatric inpatients. Am J Psychiatr 157(6), 1012–1013.

Frischholz EJ (1985) The relationship among dissociation, hypnosis, and child abuse in the development of multiple personality. In Childhood Antecedents of Multiple Personality, Kluft RP (ed). American Psychiatric Press, Washington DC, pp. 100–126.

Ganaway GK (1989) Historical versus narrative truth: Clarifying the role of exogenous trauma in the etiology of MPD and its variants. Dissociation 2, 205–220.

Ganaway GK (1995) Hypnosis, childhood trauma, and dissociative identity disorder: Toward an integrative theory. Int J Clin Exp Hypn 43, 127–144.

Herman JL, Perry JC, and Van der Kolk BA (1989) Childhood trauma in borderline personality disorder. Am J Psychiatr 146, 490–495.

Hilgard ER (1965) Hypnotic Susceptibility. Harcourt, Brace & World, New York.

Hilgard ER (1977) Divided Consciousness: Multiple Controls in Human Thought and Action. Wiley-Interscience, New York.

Hoffman RE (1987) Computer simulations of neural information processing and the schizophrenia/mania dichotomy. Arch Gen Psychiatr 44, 178–187.

Holen A (1993) The North Sea Oil Rig Disaster. Plenum Press, New York.

Horen SA, Leichner PP, and Lawson JS (1995) Prevalence of dissociative symptoms and disorders in an adult psychiatric inpatient population in Canada. Can J Psychiatr 40, 185–191.

Horevitz RP and Braun BG (1984) Are multiple personalities borderline? Psychiatr Clin N Am 7, 69–87.

Horowitz MJ (1976) Stress Response Syndromes. Jason Aronson, New York.

James W (1984) William James on Exceptional Mental States. The 1896 Lowell Lectures, Taylor E (ed). The University of Massachusetts Press, Amherst, MA.

Janet P (1920) The Major Symptoms of Hysteria. Macmillan, New York, p. 332.

Kardiner A and Spiegel H (1947) War, Stress, and Neurotic Illness. Hoeber, New York.

Katz R (1982) Boiling Energy: Community Healing Among the Kalahari Kung. Harvard University Press, Cambridge, MA.

Kihlstrom JF (1987) The cognitive unconscious. Science 237, 1445–1452.

Kihlstrom JF and Hoyt IP (1990) Repression, dissociation and hypnosis. In Repression and Dissociation: Implications for Personality Theory, Psychopathology, and Health, Singer JL (ed). University of Chicago Press, Chicago, pp. 181–208.

Kirmayer KJ (1994) Pacing the void: Social and cultural dimensions of dissociation. In Dissociation: Culture, Mind and Body, Spiegel D (ed). American Psychiatric Press, Washington DC, pp. 91–122.

Kleinman A (1977) Depression, somatization and the "new cross-cultural psychiatry." Soc Sci Med 11, 3–10.

Kluft RP (1982) Varieties of hypnotic intervention in the treatment of multiple personality. Am J Clin Hypn 24, 230–240.

Kluft RP (1984a) Multiple personality in childhood. Psychiatr Clin N Am 7, 121–134.

Kluft RP (1984b) Treatment of multiple personality disorder: A study of 33 cases. Psychiatr Clin N Am 7, 9–29.

Kluft RP (1985) The natural history of multiple personality disorder. In Childhood Antecedents of Multiple Personality, Kluft RP (ed). American Psychiatric Press, Washington DC, pp. 197–238.

Kluft RP (1986) Personality unification in multiple personality disorder: A follow-up study. In Treatment of Multiple Personality Disorder, Braun BG (ed). American Psychiatric Press, Washington DC, pp. 29–60.

Kluft RP (1987) First rank symptoms as diagnostic indicators of multiple personality disorder. Am J Psychiatr 144, 293–298.

Kluft RP (1991) Multiple personality disorder. In American Psychiatric Press Review of Psychiatry, Vol. 10, Tasman A and Goldfinger SM (eds). American Psychiatric Press, Washington DC, pp. 161–188.

Koopman C, Classen C, and Spiegel D (1994) Predictors of posttraumatic stress symptoms among Oakland-Berkeley firestorm survivors. Am J Psychiatr 151, 888–894.

Kosslyn SM and Koenig O (1992) Wet Mind: The New Cognitive Neuroscience. Free Press, New York.

Lavoie G and Sabourin M (1980) Hypnosis and schizophrenia: A review of experimental and clinical studies. In Handbook of Hypnosis and Psychosomatic Medicine, Burrows GD and Dennerstein L (eds). Elsevier/North-Holland Biomedical Press, New York, pp. 377–419.

Lewis-Fernandez (1994) Culture and dissociation: A comparison of ataque de nervios among Puerto Ricans and "possession syndrome" in India. In Dissociation: Culture, Mind and Body, Spiegel D (ed). American Psychiatric Press, Washington DC, pp. 123–167.

Li D and Spiegel D (1992) A neural network model of dissociative disorders. Psychiatr Ann 22, 144–147.

Lindemann E (1944) Symptomatology and management of acute grief. Am J Psychiatr 101, 141–148.

Loewenstein RJ (1991) Psychogenic amnesia and psychogenic fugue: A comprehensive review. In American Psychiatric Press Review of Psychiatry, Vol. 10, Tasman A and Goldfinger SM (eds). American Psychiatric Press, Washington DC, pp. 189–222.

Loewenstein RJ and Putnam FW (1988) A comparative study of dissociative symptoms in patients with complex partial seizures, multiple personality disorder, and posttraumatic stress disorder. Dissociation 1, 17–23.

Madakasira S and O'Brien K (1987) Acute posttraumatic stress disorder in victims of a natural disaster. J Nerv Ment Dis 175, 286–290.

Maldonado JR and Spiegel D (2002) Dissociative disorders. In Textbook of Psychiatry, 4th ed., Talbott JA and Yudosky S (eds). American Psychiatric Press, Washington DC. (In Press. Expected date of Publication: Summer 2002)

Maldonado JR, Butler LD, and Spiegel D (2000) Treatment of dissociative disorders. In Treatments That Work, Nathan P and Gorman JM (eds). Oxford University Press, New York, pp. 463–496.

Markowitz JS and Gill HS (1996) Pharmacotherapy of dissociative identity disorder. Ann Pharmacother 30, 1498–1499.

Marmar CR, Weiss DS, Schlenger WE, et al. (1994) Peritraumatic dissociation and posttraumatic stress in male Vietnam theater veterans. Am J Psychiatr 151, 902–907.

McFarlane AC (1986) Posttraumatic morbidity of a disaster. A study of cases presenting for psychiatric treatment. J Nerv Ment Dis 174, 4–14.

McHugh PR (1995a) Dissociative identity disorder as a socially constructed artifact. J Pract Psychiatr Behav Health 1, 158–166.

McHugh PR (1995b) Witches, multiple personalities, and other psychiatric artifacts. Nature Med 1, 110–114.

Mezzich JE, Fabrega H, Coffman GA, et al. (1989) DSM-III disorders in a large sample of psychiatric patients: Frequency and specificity of diagnoses. Am J Psychiatr 146, 212–219.

Milner B (1959) The memory defect in bilateral hippocampal lesions. Psychiatr Res Rep 11, 42–52.

Modestin J, Ebner G, Junghan M, et al. (1996) Dissociative experiences and dissociative disorders in acute psychiatric inpatients. Compr Psychiatr 37(5), 355–361.

Naples M and Hackett T (1978) The Amytal interview: History and current uses. Psychosomatics 19, 98–105.

Noyes R and Kletti R (1977) Depersonalization in response to life-threatening danger. Compr Psychiatr 18, 375–384.

Noyes R and Slymen DJ (1978–1979) The subjective response to life-threatening danger. Omega 9, 313–321.

Nuller YL (1982) Depersonalization: Symptoms, meaning, therapy. Acta Psychiatr Scand 66, 451–458.

Ogata S, Silk K, Goodrich S, et al. (1990) Childhood sexual and physical abuse in adult patients with borderline personality disorder. Am J Psychiatr 147, 1008–1013.

Perry JC and Jacobs DJ (1982) Overview: Clinical applications of the Amytal interview in psychiatry emergency settings. Am J Psychiatr 139, 552–559.

Pettinati HM (1982) Measuring hypnotizability in psychotic patients. Int J Clin Exp Hypn 30, 404–416.

Pettinati HM, Kogan LG, Evans FJ, et al. (1990) Hypnotizability of psychiatric inpatients according to two different scales. Am J Psychiatr 147, 69–75.

Pies R (1991) Depersonalization's many faces. Psychiatr Times 8(4), 27–28.

Putnam FW (1985) Dissociation as a response to extreme trauma. In Childhood Antecedents of Multiple Personality, Kluft RP (ed). American Psychiatric Press, Washington DC, pp. 65–97.

Putnam FW (1989) Diagnosis and Treatment of Multiple Personality Disorder. Guilford Press, New York.

Putnam FW, Guroff JJ, Silberman ED, et al. (1986) The clinical phenomenology of multiple personality disorder: Review of 100 recent cases. J Clin Psychiatr 47, 285–293.

Reither AM and Stoudemire A (1988) Psychogenic fugue states: A review. South Med J 81, 568–571.

Ronquillo EB (1991) The influence of "espiritismo" on a case of multiple personality disorder. Dissociation 4, 39–45.

Ross CA (1989) Multiple Personality Disorder: Diagnosis, Clinical Features, and Treatment. John Wiley, New York.

Ross CA (1991) Epidemiology of multiple personality disorder and dissociation. Psychiatr Clin North Am 14, 503–518.

Ross CA, Anderson G, Fleisher WP, et al. (1991a) The frequency of multiple personality disorder among psychiatry inpatients. Am J Psychiatr 148, 1717–1720.

Ross CA, Joshi S, and Currie R (1991b) Dissociative experiences in the general population: A factor analysis. Hosp Comm Psychiatr 42, 297–301.

Ross CA, Miller SD, Reagor P, et al. (1990) Structured interview data on 102 cases of multiple personality disorder from four centers. Am J Psychiatr 147, 596–601.

Rothbaum BO and Foa EB (1993) Subtypes of posttraumatic stress disorder and duration of symptoms. In Posttraumatic Stress Disorder: DSM-IV and Beyond, Davidson JRT and Foa ED (eds). American Psychiatric Press, Washington DC, pp. 23–35.

Rumelhart DE and McClelland JL (1986) Parallel Distributed Processing: Explorations in the Microstructure of Cognition. The MIT Press, Cambridge, MA.

Sar V, Tutkun H, Alyanak B, et al. (2000) Frequency of dissociative disorders among psychiatric outpatients in Turkey. Compr Psychiatr 41(3), 216–222.

Saxe GN, van der Kolk BA, Berkowitz R, et al. (1993) Dissociative disorders in psychiatric patients. Am J Psychiatr 150, 1037–1042.

Saxena S and Prasad K (1989) DSM-III subclassification of dissociative disorders applied to psychiatric outpatients in India. Am J Psychiatr 146, 261–262.

Schacter D (1992) Understanding implicit memory: A cognitive neuroscience approach. Am Psychol 47, 559–569.

Schacter DL (1995) Memory distortion: History and current status. In Memory Distortion: How Minds, Brains, and Societies Reconstruct the Past, Schacter DL (ed). Harvard University Press, Cambridge, MA, pp. 1–42.

Schenk L and Bear D (1981) Multiple personality and related dissociative phenomena in patients with temporal lobe epilepsy. Am J Psychiatr 138, 1311–1316.

Schultz R, Braun BG, and Kluft RP (1989) Multiple personality disorder: Phenomenology of selected variables in comparison to major depression. Dissociation 2, 45–51.

Scroppo JC, Drob SL, Weinberger JL, et al. (1998) Identifying dissociative identity disorder: A self-report and projective study. J Abnorm Psychol 107(2), 272–284.

Sloan P (1988) Posttraumatic stress in survivors of an airplane crash landing: A clinical and exploratory research intervention. J Traum Stress 1, 211–229.

Solomon Z and Mikulincer M (1988) Psychological sequelae of war: A two-year follow-up study of Israeli combat stress reaction (CSR) casualties. J Nerv Ment Dis 176, 264–269.

Solomon Z, Mikulincer M, and Bleich A (1988) Characteristic expressions of combat-related posttraumatic stress disorder among Israeli soldiers in the 1982 Lebanon war. Behav Med 14, 171–178.

Spanos NP, Weekes JR, and Bertrand LD (1985) Multiple personality: A social psychological perspective. J Abnorm Psychol 94, 362–376.

Spanos NP, Weekes JR, Menary E, et al. (1986) Hypnotic interview and age regression procedures in elicitation of multiple personality symptoms: A simulation study. Psychiatr 49, 298–311.

Spiegel D (1981) Vietnam grief work using hypnosis. Am J Clin Hypn 24, 33–40.

Spiegel D (1984) Multiple personality as a posttraumatic stress disorder. Psychiatr Clin N Am 7, 101–110.

Spiegel D (1986a) Dissociating damage. Am J Clin Hypn 29, 123–131.

Spiegel D (1986b) Dissociation, double binds, and posttraumatic stress in multiple personality disorder. In Treatment of Multiple Personality Disorder, Braun B (ed). American Psychiatric Press, Washington DC, pp. 61–77.

Spiegel D (1987) Chronic pain masks depression, multiple personality disorder. Hosp Comm Psychiatr 38, 933–935.

Spiegel D (1988) The treatment accorded those who treat patients with multiple personality disorder. J Nerv Ment Dis 176, 535–536.

Spiegel D (1990) Hypnosis, dissociation, and trauma: Hidden and overt observers. In Repression and Dissociation: Implications for Personality Theory, Psychopathology, and Health, Singer JL (ed). University of Chicago Press, Chicago, pp. 121–142.

Spiegel D (1991) Dissociation and trauma. In American Psychiatric Press Review of Psychiatry, Vol. 10, Tasman A and Goldfinger SM (eds). American Psychiatric Press, Washington DC, pp. 261–275.

Spiegel D, Cardeña E (1990) New uses of hypnosis in the treatment of posttraumatic stress disorder. J Clin Psychiatr 51(Suppl), 39–43.

Spiegel D and Cardeña E (1991) Disintegrated experience: The dissociative disorders revisited. J Abnorm Psychol 100, 366–378.

Spiegel D and Fink R (1979) Hysterical psychosis and hypnotizability. Am J Psychiatr 136, 777–781.

Spiegel D, Detrick D, and Frischholz EJ (1982) Hypnotizability and psychopathology. Am J Psychiatr 139, 431–437.

Spiegel D, Frischholz EJ, and Spira J (1993) Functional Disorders of Memory. In American Psychiatric Press Review of Psychiatry, Vol. 12, Oldham JM, Riba MB, and Tasman A (eds). American Psychiatric Press, Washington DC, pp. 747–782.

Spiegel D, Hunt T, and Dondershine H (1988) Dissociation and hypnotizability in posttraumatic stress disorder. Am J Psychiatr 145, 301–305.

Spiegel H (1974) The grade 5 syndrome: The highly hypnotizable person, Int J Clin Exp Hypn 22, 303–319.

Spiegel H and Spiegel D (1978) Trance and Treatment: Clinical Uses of Hypnosis. Basic Books, New York, pp. 13–14. Copyright 1978 HarperCollins Publishers. Reprinted 1987. American Psychiatric Press, Washington DC.

Squire LR (1987) Memory and Brain. Oxford University Press, New York.

Stein MB and Uhde TW (1989) Depersonalization disorder: Effects of caffeine and response to pharmacotherapy. Biol Psychiatr 26, 315–320.

Steinberg M (1991) The spectrum of depersonalization: Assessment and treatment. In American Psychiatric Press Review of Psychiatry, Vol. 10, Tasman A and Goldfinger SM (eds). American Psychiatric Press, Washington DC, pp. 223–247.

Steinberg M, Rounsaville B, and Ciucchetti D (1990) The structured clinical interview for DSM-III-R dissociative disorders: Preliminary report on a new diagnostic instrument. Am J Psychiatr 147, 76–81.

Terr LC (1991) Childhood traumas: An outline and overview. Am J Psychiatr 148, 10–20.

Tulving E (1983) Elements of Episodic Memory. Clarendon Press, Oxford.

Van der Hart O (2001) Generalized dissociative amnesia: Episodic, semantic and procedural memories lost and found. Austral NZ J Psychiatr 35, 589–600.

Van der Hart O and Spiegel D (1993) Hypnotic assessment and treatment of trauma-induced psychoses. Int J Clin Exp Hypn 41, 191–209.

Van der Hart O, Brown P, and Van der Kolk BA (1989) Pierre Janet's treatment of posttraumatic stress. J Traum Stress 2, 379–396.

Vanderlinden J, Van Dyck R, Vandereycken W, et al. (1991) Dissociative experiences in the general population of the Netherlands and Belgium: A study with the Dissociative Questionnaire (DIS-Q). Dissociation 4, 180–184.

Wilkinson CB (1983) Aftermath of a disaster: The collapse of the Hyatt Regency Hotel skywalks. Am J Psychiatr 140, 1130–1134.

Wittkower ED (1970) Transcultural psychiatry in the Caribbean: Past, present and future. Am J Psychiatr 127, 162–166.

Zola-Morgan S and Squire LR (1985) Medial temporal lesions in monkeys impair memory in a variety of tasks sensitive to human amnesia. Behav Neurosci 99, 22–34.

Zola-Morgan S, Squire LR, and Mishkin M (1982) The neuroanatomy of amnesia: Amygdala-hippocampus vs. temporal stem. Science 218, 1337–1339.

Stephen B. Levine

Hypoactive Sexual Desire Disorder
Sexual Aversion Disorder
Sexual Dysfunction Due to a General Medical Condition
Substance-Induced Sexual Dysfunction
Female Sexual Arousal Disorder
Male Erectile Disorder
Female Orgasmic Disorder
Male Orgasmic Disorder
Premature Ejaculation
Dyspareunia
Vaginismus
Sexual Dysfunction Not Otherwise Specified
Gender Identity Disorder
Gender Identity Disorder Not Otherwise Specified
Exhibitionism
Pedophilia
Voyeurism
Sexual Sadism
Frotteurism
Stalking
Fetishism
Transvestic Fetishism
Sexual Masochism
Paraphilia Not Otherwise Specified
Sexual Disorder Not Otherwise Specified

## Preface

A wide array of sexuality topics impact psychiatry. These topics range from those constituting a major social burden, such as teenage pregnancy, sex crimes, and sexually transmitted diseases, to those involving ethical and moral values, such as abortion, extramarital affairs, commercial sex industries, and crossing sexual boundaries with patients. They include those with a developmental or medical focus, such as sexual dysfunction or sexual dysfunction due to substance abuse or medical conditions, and those involving lifestyles, such as sexual minority status and drugs for sexual enhancement. There are also those that center on psychiatry's undisputed responsibility, such as psychotropic medication-induced sexual dysfunction and the sexual consequences of psychiatric illness. No discipline, no ideology, no religion, and certainly no textbook chapter is sufficient to fully understand and encompass the myriad expressions of human sexuality.

Psychiatry has known for almost a century that child development lays the foundation for a wide variety of adult sexual outcomes (Freud 1905). These are reflected in the variations of gender, orientation, intention, and ease of sexual expression with chosen partners. Psychiatry has also been long aware that the conduct of adolescent and adult sexual life is laden with concern, and sometimes anguish, in every person. In the last generation, we have acquired greater convictions about the profound public health implications of several sexual patterns. First came awareness of the high incidence of childhood sexual abuse and its long-term consequences. Then came the data showing that some psychiatrists and other trusted professionals engaged in genital intimacies with patients. Psychiatry responded by unambiguously clarifying our ethical standards. At about the same time the AIDS epidemic led to a greater awareness of the lives of homosexual and bisexual men. In the 1990s when the Internet usage grew without regulation, addictions to at-home pornography appeared. As the use of SSRIs became widespread, psychiatrists learned about their negative sexual impact. In 1998 an effective pill for erectile dysfunction created an explosion of media interest across the world. The Viagra story reminded us that sexual function is really important to people.

Psychiatry prides itself about being the only field that can comprehend the biopsychosocial aspects of illness. We understand that all sexual expression is simultaneously constituted by biological, psychological, and social forces. We also know that sexual disorders are a high prevalence, high incidence source of personal suffering (Spector and Carey 1990), affecting almost every person at some time in the life cycle. Sexual disorders often play a subtle role in the genesis of other psychiatric disorders as presented in Figure 74–1.

Patients assume their psychiatrists know about sexuality. Therapists can be helpful to many individuals and couples with these problems if they have an interest in the area, a comfort with the subject, and a modest fund of knowledge (Levine et al. 2003). Sometimes the help can be given quite efficiently. The assistance is often based on knowledge of the diverse origins of these problems (Kendler et al. 1995). To be able to treat a broad range of sexual disorders the psychiatrist needs to be diagnostically competent, skillful with medications, and willing to engage in psychotherapeutic processes. This chapter provides background information for these three goals.

## The Components of Sexuality

An adult's sexuality has seven components—gender identity, orientation, intention (what one wants to do with a partner's body and have done with one's body during sexual behavior), desire, arousal, orgasm, and emotional satisfaction (Levine 1989). The first three components constitute our sexual identity. The second three comprise our sexual function. The seventh, emotional satisfaction, is based on our personal reflections on the first six (Table 74–1). The DSM-IV-TR designates impairments of five of these components as pathologies. Variations in orientation and the failure to find ordinary sexual experience emotionally satisfying, although problems for some, are not designated as "disorders."

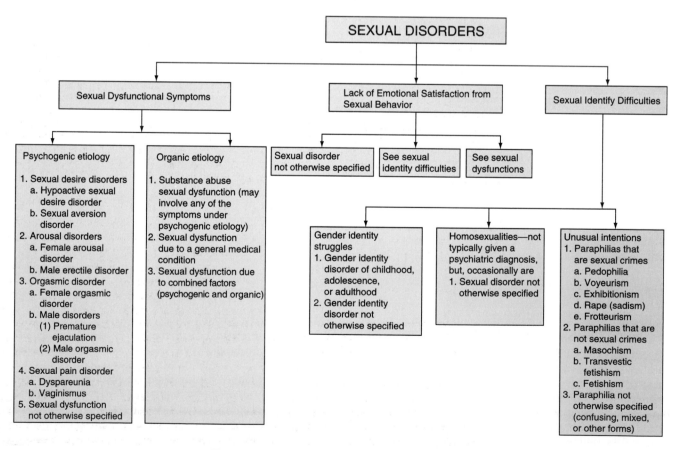

**Figure 74–1** *Diagnostic decision tree for sexual disorders.*

| Table 74-1 | Mechanisms of Sexual Equilibrium |
|---|---|

**I. Interplay of Each Person's Seven Sexual Components**

| Person A | | Person B |
|---|---|---|
| Gender identity | ⇄ | Gender identity |
| Orientation | ⇄ | Orientation |
| Intention | ⇄ | Intention |
| Desire | ⇄ | Desire |
| Arousal | ⇄ | Arousal |
| Orgasm | ⇄ | Orgasm |
| Emotional satisfaction | ⇄ | Emotional satisfaction |

**II. Regard That Each Person Has for the Partner's Component Characteristics**

Positive regard leads to:
   Increased sensual abandon,
   Positive attitudes toward self and partner, and
   Frequent sexual behavior
Negative regard leads to:
   Increased personal inhibition,
   Hostile critical attitudes toward self and partner, and
   Limited motivation to engage in partner sexual behavior

## Sexual Development Through the Life Cycle

While the psychological foundations for a healthy sexual life are laid down during childhood through parent–child relationships, each subsequent phase of life—adolescence, young adulthood, middle-life, and older age—has inherent developmental challenges and potentials. The normal tasks of sexual development at each phase provide the clinician with an understanding of age-related etiologies of sexual disorders (Levine 1992). Adolescent sexual troubles often reflect difficulties consolidating a personally acceptable sexual identity. Young adult dysfunctions often indicate the presence of psychological obstacles to growing comfortable as a sexual pleasure-seeking, pleasure-giving person while integrating sex into the larger context of human attachment. Middle-life disorders often represent failures to maintain psychological intimacy and to diplomatically negotiate tensions within an increasingly complex interpersonal relationship. The dysfunctions of older persons often represent failures to preserve sexual function in the face of biological assaults of menopause, aging, illness, medications, radiation, and surgery. Most etiologic factors can operate in another epoch as well. For instance, a young person's new indifference to sexual behavior may be due to an SSRI or an older person's new marriage may expose previously avoided personal discomfort with receiving and giving sexual pleasure.

## THE SEXUAL DYSFUNCTIONS

### Significance of Sexual Dysfunction

While sex is widely thought of as recreation, psychiatrists recognize it as an important means of establishing and reaffirming emotional attachments. Sexual competence—the ability to desire a partner, become aroused, and attain orgasm in a cooperative manner when together—is a valuable developmental accomplishment because it enables a person to experience the physical expressions and emotional complexities of love. Mutually pleasurable sexual behavior tends to recur far more often in couples than unilaterally satisfying behavior. Mutually pleasurable sexual behavior allows both partners to be comforted and stabilized by loving and feeling loved. The dysfunctions are symptomatic deficits in the quest for these widespread ideals: sexual competence, fun, and stabilization of the self.

### DSM-IV Diagnoses

DSM-IV specifies three criteria for each sexual dysfunction (American Psychiatric Association 1994). The first criterion describes the psychophysiologic impairment—for example, absence of sexual desire, arousal, or orgasm. The second and third criteria are the same for each impairment: the dysfunction causes marked distress or interpersonal difficulty and the dysfunction is not better accounted for by another Axis I diagnosis or not due exclusively to the direct physiological effects of a substance (e.g., a drug of abuse, a medication) or a general medical condition. Table 74–2 lists the first criterion of each of the twelve sexual dysfunction diagnoses. DSM-IV gives the clinician additional latitude for deciding when a person who meets the first criterion qualifies for a disorder. The doctor is asked to consider the effects of the individual's age, experience, ethnicity and cultural background, the degree of subjective distress, adequacy of sexual stimulation, and symptom frequency. No instructions are provided about how to exercise this judgment. In this way DSM-IV makes it clear that understanding sexual life requires more than counting symptoms; it requires judgment.

### Epidemiology

Numerous attempts to describe the prevalence of sexual dysfunction have been made in the previous 25 years. These range from attempts to define the frequency of a particular dysfunction, for instance male erectile disorder, to attempts to estimate the prevalence of a series of separate dysfunction—for example, desire, arousal, and orgasmic disorders of women. All such efforts quickly confront methodological influences of sampling, means of obtaining the information, definition of each dysfunction, purpose of the study, and perspective of its authors (Laumann and Michaels 2001). These data not surprisingly, therefore, demonstrate a range of prevalence depending on the problem studied. Gender identity disorders are relatively rare (> 1–2%). Lifelong sexual desire disorders among women may involve 15% but are less frequent among men. Acquired desire disorders among older individuals are probably three times as common. Perhaps more than half of women at age 55 years have recognized a deterioration in their sexual function. Perhaps 25% of women in their twenties have difficulty having orgasm and 33% of men less than age 40 claim to ejaculate too rapidly. The majority of men by age 70 years are likely to be having erection problems. The recent careful epidemiologic study, designed by sociologists, successfully generated a representative sample of the US (Laumann et al. 1994a). They interviewed men and women between age 18 and 59 years and found that sexual dysfunction is common, particularly among young women and older men. This is noteworthy for psychiatrists because our studies of sexual dysfunction caused by medications or acquired psychiatric disorders tend to assume that patients are generally functionally intact prior to becoming ill or taking medi-

**Table 74–2    Delineating Criteria of 12 Sexual Dysfunction Diagnoses**

| Sexual Desire Disorders | Sexual Arousal Disorders | Orgasmic Disorders | Sexual Pain Disorders |
|---|---|---|---|
| Hypoactive sexual desire disorder:<br><br>persistently or recurrently deficient (or absent) sexual fantasies and desire for sexual activity | Female sexual arousal disorder:<br><br>persistent or recurrent inability to attain, or to maintain until completion of the sexual activity, an adequate lubrication-swelling response of sexual excitement | Female orgasmic disorder:<br><br>persistent or recurrent delay in, or absence of, orgasm after a normal sexual excitement phase | Dyspareunia:<br><br>recurrent or persistent genital pain associated with sexual intercourse in either a male or a female |
| Sexual aversion disorder:<br><br>persistent or recurrent extreme aversion to, and avoidance of, all (or almost all) genital sexual contact with a sexual partner | Male erectile disorder:<br><br>persistent or recurrent inability to attain, or to maintain until completion of the sexual activity, an adequate erection | Male orgasmic disorder:<br><br>persistent or recurrent delay in, or absence of, orgasm after a normal sexual excitement phase during sexual activity<br><br>Premature ejaculation:<br><br>persistent or recurrent ejaculation with a minimal sexual stimulation before, on, or shortly after penetration and before the person wishes it | Vaginismus:<br><br>recurrent or persistent involuntary spasm of the musculature of the outer third of the vagina that interferes with sexual intercourse |
| Sexual Dysfunction Due to a General Medical Condition | Substance-Induced Sexual Dysfunction | Sexual Dysfunction Not Otherwise Specified | |
| any of the above-mentioned diagnoses must be judged to be exclusively due to the direct physiological effects of a medical condition | a sexual dysfunction that is fully explained by substance use in that it develops within a month of substance intoxication | for problems that do not meet the categories just described | |

cations. This assumption is not tenable based on a generation of epidemiologic studies.

## Sexual Equilibrium

Etiologic ideas about sexual dysfunction are a relatively simple conceptual challenge involving notions about the individual's psychology and his or her cultural expectations. In contrast, for couples, they involve two individual psychologies, their interpersonal impact on one another, and their cultures. The clinician must be wary when one coupled person is presented as having a sexual dysfunction and the partner is presented as "normal." Sexual dysfunction in a couple is a two-person problem in terms of immediate effects and often in terms of cause as well (Table 74–1). How a partner regards the sexual characteristics of the other is a subtle ingredient of sexual comfort, competence, and dysfunction. For instance, a young woman's new inability to attain orgasm with her husband may be traced to her embarrassment at sharing her excitation with him because she perceives him to be generally critical of her. Similarly, the origin of a husband's erectile dysfunction may be traced to the emergence of his wife's negative regard for him, which stemmed from something other than his sexual behavior. This *ordinary* connectivity of a couple's sexual function is referred to as the couple's sexual equilibrium (Levine 1998). The sexual equilibrium explains five observations:

1. Improvement and deterioration of sexual function can rapidly occur;
2. When a couple's nonsexual relationship is good, their sexual life may not be;
3. Individual psychotherapy is often insufficient to help coupled patients improve their sexual life;
4. A negative attitude from the partner can block improvement in a couple's sexual life regardless of the therapy format and therapist skill;
5. A conversation with a therapist who is attuned to the emotional meanings of a couple's interaction can shift a dysfunctional equilibrium back to mutually satisfying sexual behavior.

## The Problems of Sexual Desire

Sexual desire manifestations are diverse: erotic fantasies, sexual dreams, initiation of sexual behavior, receptivity to partner-initiated sexual behavior, masturbation, genital sensations, heightened responsivity to erotic environmental cues, and sincere statements about wanting to behave sexually. For most of the 20th century, these have been referred to as manifestations of libido. Psychiatrists spoke of libido as if it was a homogeneous instinctive force. Clinicians will find it far more useful to conceptualize that the diverse and changeable desire manifestations are produced by the intersection of three mental forces: drive (biology), motive (psychology), and wish (culture).

**Drive.** By only partially understood psychoneuroendocrine mechanisms, the preoptic area of the anterior-medial hypothalamus and the limbic system periodically produce sexual drive. Drive is recognized by genital tingling, heightened responsivity to erotic environmental cues, plans for self or partner sexual behavior, nocturnal orgasm, and increased erotic preoccupations. These are often spontaneous. Although people can become aroused and attain orgasm without evident drive, it propels the entire sexual psychophysiological process. Without drive, the sexual response system is far less efficient and capable. While men as a group seem to have significant more drive than women as a group, in both sexes, drive requires the presence of a modest amount of testosterone. Drive is frequently dampened by medications that act within the central nervous system, substances of abuse, psychiatric illness, systemic physical illness, despair, and aging. It is heightened by low doses of a few often-abused substances such as alcohol or amphetamine, manic mechanisms, falling in love, joy, and some dopaminergic compounds such as those used to treat Parkinson's disease.

**Motive.** The psychological aspect of desire is referred to as *motive* and is recognized by willingness to bring one's body to the partner for sexual behavior either through initiation or receptivity. Motive often directly stems from the person's perception of the context of the nonsexual and sexual relationship. Sexual desire diagnoses are often made in persons who have adequate drive manifestations. Most sexual desire problems in physically healthy adults are simply generated by one partner's *unwillingness* to engage in sexual behavior. This is often a secret, however. Sexual motives are originally programmed by social and cultural experiences. Children and adolescents acquire values, beliefs, expectations, and rules for sexual expression. Young people have to find a way to negotiate their way through the fact that their early motives to behave sexually frequently coexist with their motives *not* to engage in sexual behavior. Conflicted motives often persist throughout life but the reasons for the conflict evolve. A teenager possessed of considerable drive and motive to make love may inhibit all sexual activities because of moral considerations emanating from religious education or the sense that he or she is just not developmentally ready yet.

**Wish.** An 80-year-old man who had no drive manifestations and had avoided all sexual contact with his wife for a decade because he could not get an erection, passionately answered a doctor's query about his sexual desire, "Of course, I have sexual desire! I am a red-blooded American male! Why do you think I am here?" In fact, he was only speaking about his wish to be sexually capable now that an effective treatment for erectile problems existed. The doctor asked an imprecise question. The doctor should have separately explored his drive manifestations, his sexual motivation to exchange sexual pleasure with his wife in recent years, and his wish for sexual rejuvenation.

The appearance and disappearance of sexual desire is often enigmatic to a patient, but its ebb and flow result from the ever-changing intensities of its components, biological *drive*, psychological *motive*, and socially acquired concepts, *wish* (Table 74–3) (Levine 2002). In women, this interplay is generally more difficult to delineate because drive and motive are sometimes inseparable (Basson 2003).

| Table 74–3 | Three Interactive Components of Sexual Desire |
|---|---|

**Sexual Drive = Biological Component**

Evolves over time, decreasing with increasing age

Diminished by many psychotropic and antihypertensive medications

Manifested by the internally stimulated genital sensations and thoughts of sexual behavior that occur within a person's privacy

**Sexual Motivation = Psychological Component**

Highly contextual in terms of relationship status

The most socially and psychologically responsive of the three components

Evolves over time but not predictably

Manifested by a person's willingness to bring his or her body to a specific person for sexual behavior

**Sexual Wish = Social Component**

Expectations for sexual behavior based on membership in various subcultural groups such as family, religion, gender, region, and nation

These expectations begin as cognitions of what is right and wrong and what a person is entitled to sexually and are influenced by what people think others in their cohort are experiencing

Often clinically difficult to distinguish from motivation, which wishes influence

## Sexual Desire Diagnoses

Two official diagnoses are given to men and women whose desires for partner sexual behavior are deficient: hypoactive sexual desire disorder (HSDD) and sexual aversion disorder (SAD). The differences between the two revolve around the emotional intensity with which the patient avoids sexual behavior. When visceral anxiety, fear, or disgust is routinely felt as sexual behavior becomes a possibility, sexual aversion is diagnosed. HSDD is far more frequently encountered. It is present in at least twice as many women than men; female to male ratio for aversion is far higher (Kaplan 1987). Like all sexual dysfunctions, the desire diagnoses may be lifelong or may have been acquired after a period of ordinary fluctuations of sexual desire. Acquired disorders may be partner specific ("situational") or may occur with all subsequent partners ("generalized").

Clinical Vignette 1

A 51-year-old secretary explained that she had had a wonderful sexual life with her husband until she humorously asked whether he had ever had an affair during their 20-year marriage. He shocked her by confessing a past "insignificant" one. As she thought about this over a week, she became increasingly enraged and asked him to leave the home. Several weeks later, he came back after constant phone contact and in response to her coming down with a flu-like illness. When their sexual behavior resumed 2 months later, she became the "ice queen"—unable to stand his touches. Her aversion lasted 6 months. Four years later when she discovered that he was having an affair, she redeveloped her aversion, adding that she felt that he was raping her when he touched her and that she could not stand his saliva or semen. She did everything she could do to avoid

---

**DSM-IV-TR Criteria** 302.71

### Hypoactive Sexual Desire Disorder

A. Persistently or recurrently deficient (or absent) sexual fantasies and desire for sexual activity. The judgment of deficiency or absence is made by the clinician, taking into account factors that affect sexual functioning, such as age and the context of the person's life.

B. The disturbance causes marked distress or interpersonal difficulty.

C. The sexual dysfunction is not better accounted for by another Axis I disorder (except another sexual dysfunction) and is not due exclusively to the direct physiological effects of a substance (e.g., a drug of abuse, a medication) or a general medical condition.

*Specify* type:

**Lifelong type**

**Acquired type**

*Specify* type:

**Generalized type**

**Situational type**

*Specify:*

**Due to psychological factors**

**Due to combined factors**

---

---

**Clinical Vignette 1** *continued*

sex. Her second period of aversion lasted 4 years before she was referred from her gynecologist for psychotherapy. At this time, she saw no relationship between her discoveries of his infidelity and her sexual aversion state.

When the psychiatrist concludes that the patient's acquired generalized HSDD is either due to a medical condition, a medication, or a substance of abuse, the diagnosis is further elaborated to sexual dysfunction due to general medical condition (for instance, HSDD due to multiple sclerosis). The frequency of the specific etiologies are heavily dependent on the clinical setting. In oncology settings, medical causes occur in high frequency; in drug rehabilitation programs, methadone maintenance will be a common cause. In marital therapy clinics, anger and loss of respect for the partner, hidden incompatibility of sexual identity between the self and the partner because of covert homosexuality or paraphilia, an affair, or childhood sexual abuse will commonly be the basis. In general psychiatry settings, medication side effects will often be the top layer of several causes. When a major depression disorder is diagnosed, for instance, the desire disorder is often assumed to be a symptom

---

**DSM-IV-TR Criteria** 302.79

### Sexual Aversion Disorder

A. Persistent or recurrent extreme aversion to, and avoidance of, all (or almost all) genital sexual contact with a sexual partner.

B. The disturbance causes marked distress or interpersonal difficulty.

C. The sexual dysfunction is not better accounted for by another Axis I disorder (except another sexual dysfunction).

*Specify* type:

**Lifelong type**

**Acquired type**

*Specify* type:

**Generalized type**

**Situational type**

*Specify:*

**Due to psychological factors**

**Due to combined factors**

---

---

of the depression. This usually is incorrect. The desire disorder often preceded the decompensation into depression.

### From a Desire Diagnosis to Dynamics

Those with *lifelong* deficiencies of sexual desire are often perceived to be struggling with either: (1) sexual identity issues involving gender identity, orientation, or a paraphilia; (2) having failed to grow comfortable as a sexual person due to extremely conservative cultural backgrounds, developmental misfortunes, or abuses. Occasionally the etiology is enigmatic, raising the important question whether it is possible to never have any sexual drive manifestations on a biological basis. (Theoretically, the answer is yes.) Both acquired and lifelong desire disorders are often associated with past or chronic mood disorders. Disorders of desire are often listed as "of unknown etiology" (Rosen and Leiblum 1995), but clinicians should be skeptical of this idea because:

1. The patient may not tell the doctor the truth early in the relationship;
2. The patient may have strong defenses against knowing the truth;
3. The patient may not be able to speak freely in front of the partner;
4. The patient may not know what is occurring in the partner's life, despite being influenced negatively by it;
5. The doctor may not realize the usual causes of the problem;
6. The doctor may not believe in developmental influences on the organization of adult sexual function.

Chapter 74 • Sexual Disorders

## DSM-IV-TR Criteria

### Sexual Dysfunction due to ... *[Indicate the General Medical Condition]*

A. Clinically significant sexual dysfunction that results in marked distress or interpersonal difficulty predominates in the clinical picture.

B. There is evidence from the history, physical examination, or laboratory findings that the sexual dysfunction is fully explained by the direct physiological effects of a general medical condition.

C. The disturbance is not better accounted for by another mental disorder (e.g., major depressive disorder).

*Select* code and term based on the predominant sexual dysfunction:

**625.8   Female hypoactive sexual desire disorder due to** ... *[indicate the general medical condition]:* if deficient or absent, sexual desire is the predominant feature

**608.89   Male hypoactive sexual desire disorder due to** ... *[indicate the general medical condition]:* if deficient or absent, sexual desire is the predominant feature

**607.84   Male erectile disorder due to** ... *[indicate the general medical condition]:* if male erectile dysfunction is the predominant feature

**625.0   Female dyspareunia due to** ... *[indicate the general medical condition]:* if pain associated with intercourse is the predominant feature

**608.89   Male dyspareunia due to** ... *[indicate the general medical condition]:* if pain associated with intercourse is the predominant feature

**625.8   Other female sexual dysfunction due to** ... *[indicate the general medical condition]:* if some other feature is predominant (e.g., orgasmic disorder) or no feature predominates

**608.89   Other male sexual dysfunction due to** ... *[indicate the general medical condition]:* if some other feature is predominant (e.g., orgasmic disorder) or no feature predominates

**Coding note:** Include the name of the general medical condition on Axis I, e.g., 607.84 male erectile disorder due to diabetes mellitus; also code the general medical condition on Axis III.

Reprinted with permission from the Diagnostic and Statistical Manual of Mental Disorders, Fourth Edition, Text Revision. Copyright 2000 American Psychiatric Association.

Sexual aversion should strongly suggest three possibilities to the clinician:

1. that a remote traumatic experience is being relived by the partner's expression of interest in sexual behavior;

| Table 74–4 | Obstacles to Discovering the Psychological Contributants to a Sexual Desire Disorder |
|---|---|

**Obstacles That Reside in the Patient**

The patient may not tell the psychiatrist the truth about life circumstances

The patient may have strong defenses against knowing the truth

The patient may be unable to tell the truth in front of the partner

The patient may not actually know what is occurring in the partner's life, although she or he is reactive to it

**Obstacles That Reside in the Psychiatrist**

The psychiatrist may not realize the psychological factors that usually cause these problems

The psychiatrist may not believe that developmental influences can organize an adult sexual function such as sexual motivation

The psychiatrist may not like to deal with the murky complexity of nonbiological developmental and interpersonal issues when thinking about etiology

2. that without the symptom the patient feels powerless to say "no" to sexual advances;

3. the patient feels guilty about her own sexual behavior with another person.

The doctor's attention should focus on the patient's sexual development as a child, adolescent, and young adult when the aversion is lifelong, whereas when it is *acquired*, the focus of the history should be on the period immediately prior to the onset of the symptom.

Desire disorders require the clinician to think both in terms of development and personal meanings of sex to their individual patients (Table 74–4). Because all explanations are speculative, they should at least make compelling sense of the patients' life experiences. Some explanations are based on the influence of remote developmental processes. The term *madonna–whore complex* misleads us into thinking this is only a male pattern. The syndrome is manifested by normal sexual capacity with anyone but the fiancé or spouse. Freud interpreted this as a sign of incomplete resolution of the oedipal complex (Freud 1912). The man was thought to be unable to sexually desire his beloved because he had unconsciously made her into his mother. He withdrew his sexual interest from her to protect himself from symbolic incest. Some women are comparably unable to sexually enjoy their partners because they unconsciously confuse their beloved with their father. Another form can be seen among patients whose parents were grossly inadequate caregivers. When these men and women find a reliable, kind, supportive person to marry, they quickly discover a strong motive to avoid sexual behavior with their fiancé. The patient makes the partner into a good-enough parent, experiences anxiety as an unconscious threat of incest associated with the possibility of sex, and becomes skillful at avoiding sexual opportunities (Levine 1998b).

Most sexual desire disorders are difficult to quickly overcome. Brief treatment generally should not be undertaken. Serious individual or couple issues frequently underlie these diagnoses. They have to be afforded time to emerge and to be worked through. However, clinicians need not be pessimistic about all of these conditions. For

## DSM-IV-TR Criteria 292.89

**Substance-Induced Sexual Dysfunction**

A. Clinically significant sexual dysfunction that results in marked distress or interpersonal difficulty predominates in the clinical picture.

B. There is evidence from the history, physical examination, or laboratory findings that the sexual dysfunction is fully explained by substance use as manifested by either (1) or (2):

   (1) the symptoms in criterion A developed during, or within a month of, substance intoxication

   (2) medication use is etiologically related to the disturbance

C. The disturbance is not better accounted for by a sexual dysfunction that is not substance induced. Evidence that the symptoms are better accounted for by a sexual dysfunction that is not substance induced might include the following: the symptoms precede the onset of the substance use or dependence (or medication use); the symptoms persist for a substantial period of time (e.g., about a month) after the cessation of intoxication, or are substantially in excess of what would be expected given the type or amount of the substance used or the duration of use; or there is other evidence that suggests the existence of an independent non-substance-induced sexual dysfunction (e.g., a history of recurrent non-substance-related episodes).

**Note:** This diagnosis should be made instead of a diagnosis of substance intoxication only when the sexual dysfunction is in excess of that usually associated with the intoxication syndrome and when the dysfunction is sufficiently severe to warrant independent clinical attention.

*Code* [specific substance]-induced sexual dysfunction:

(291.8 Alcohol; 292.89 Amphetamine [or Amphetamine-like Substance]; 292.89 Cocaine; 292.89 Opioid; 292.89 Sedative, Hypnotic, or Anxiolytic; 292.89 Other [or Unknown] Substance)

*Specify* if:

**With impaired desire**

**With impaired arousal**

**With impaired orgasm**

**With sexual pain**

*Specify* if:

**With onset during intoxication:** if the criteria are met for intoxication with the substance and the symptoms develop during the intoxication syndrome

Reprinted with permission from the Diagnostic and Statistical Manual of Mental Disorders, Fourth Edition, Text Revision. Copyright 2000 American Psychiatric Association.

example, helping a couple resolve a marital dispute may return them to their usual normal sexual desire manifestations. For many individuals and couples, therapy assists the couple to more calmly accept the profound implications of continuing marital discord, infidelity, homosexuality, or other contributing factors. Some treatment failures lead to divorce and the creation of a relationship with a new partner. There is then no further sign of the desire problem. Problems rooted in early developmental experiences are particularly difficult to overcome. While DSM-IV asks the clinician to make many distinctions among the desire disorders, no follow-up study has been published in which either the subtypes (lifelong, acquired, situational, generalized) or etiologic organizers (relationship deterioration with and without extramarital affairs, sexual identity incompatibilities, parental, and medical) are separated into good and poor prognosis categories (O'Carroll 1991).

Developmental and identity matters are typically approached in long-term individual psychotherapy. In these sessions women often discuss the development of their femininity from adolescence to young womanhood, focusing on issues of body image, beauty, social worth to others, moral sensibilities, social awkwardness, and whether they consider themselves deserving of personal physical pleasure. Men often discuss similar issues in terms of masculinity.

Anger, loss of respect, marital discord, and extramarital affairs may be approached in either individual or con-joint formats. In either setting, patients often formulate the etiology as having fallen out of love with the partner. Those whose cultural backgrounds limit their ease in being a sexual person are often encouraged in educational and cultural experiences that might help them outgrow their earliest notions about what is proper sexual behavior.

### The Problems of Sexual Arousal

The emotion interchangeably referred to as sexual arousal or sexual excitement generates changes in respiration, pulse, and muscular tension as well as an increased blood flow to the genitals. Genital vasocongestion creates vaginal lubrication, clitoral tumescence, labial color changes, and penile erection, testicular elevation, and penile color changes (Masters and Johnson 1966). How arousal is centrally coordinated in either sex remains mysterious. During love-making, men and women do not necessarily maintain or progressively increase their arousal; rather often there is a fluctuating intensity of arousal which is reflected in variations in vaginal wetness and penile turgidity and nongenital signs of arousal.

### Female Sexual Arousal Disorder

The specificity and validity of this disorder is unclear. In women it is far more difficult to separate arousal and desire problems than in men. The perimenopausal period is now recognized as generating complaints about decreased drive, motivation, lubrication, and arousal in at least 35 to 50% of women (Dennerstein et al. 2000). However, it is unclear whether to label the problem as primarily of desire or arousal. It is assumed to be endocrine in origin even though estrogen, progesterone, and testosterone replacement do not reliably reverse the pattern. Even in younger regularly menstruating women, however, diminished motivation and dampened drive makes it difficult to sustain arousal. Many have called into question the accepted notions that desire necessarily precedes arousal and that they are separate physiological processes (Basson 2001). Female arousal disorder implies that drive and motivation are relatively intact although arousal is difficult. The disorder is usually an *acquired* diagnosis. Premenopausal women who have it focus on the lack of moisture in the vagina or their failure to be excited by the behaviors that previously reliably brought pleasure. They have drive and motive and wish, but enigmatically are unable to sustain arousal. Some mental factor arises to distract them from their excitement during lovemaking. Therapy is focused, therefore, on the meaning of what preoccupies them. This often involves the dynamics of their current individual or partnered life or the influence of their past relationships on their present. With therapy the diagnosis often is changed to a HSDD.

In peri- and postmenopausal women, arousal problems are more often focused on the body as a whole rather than just genital moisture deficiencies. Skin insensitivity, often a euphemism for decreased pleasure in response to oral and manual nipple, breast, and vulvar stimulation, is often initially treated as a symptom of "estrogen" deficiency. Early in the menopause, a small minority of women have an increase in drive due to changing testosterone–estrogen ratios. Yet, they may still subjectively experience arousal as different than it used to be. Therapy often focuses on the women's concerns about estrogen replacement and the consequences of menopause in terms of body image, attractiveness, fears of partner infidelity, loss of health and vigor, and aging.

Aging of the female arousal mechanisms, whether simply due to shifts in ovarian endocrine production or systemic aging mechanisms, occurs earlier than deterioration of orgasmic physiology. Women with decreasing arousal are often, therefore, still reliably orgasmic with the use of vaginal lubricants well into old age. Women who have been treated with chemotherapy for breast cancer are a particularly problematic group to offer assistance to for their new arousal problems. Fear of stimulating remaining cancerous cells makes systemic estrogen replacement contraindicated.

In 1999 a renewed interest in female arousal disorder sometimes casually called female sexual dysfunction (Berman and Goldstein 2001) surfaced in response to the efficacy of Viagra for men's arousal problems. It was reasoned that since the penis and clitoris are embryologic homologues with comparable adult histology, the drug would improve women's arousal. An open-labeled study concluded that Viagra was highly effective (Berman et al. 2001) but when placebo-controlled trials were concluded, the drug did not improve arousal any more than placebo (Basson et al. 2002).

Here is a relatively simple case of an acquired arousal disorder that was most likely a combination of perimeno-

## DSM-IV-TR Criteria 302.72

**Female Sexual Arousal Disorder**

A. Persistent or recurrent inability to attain, or to maintain until completion of the sexual activity, an adequate lubrication-swelling response of sexual excitement.

B. The disturbance causes marked distress or interpersonal difficulty.

C. The sexual dysfunction is not better accounted for by another Axis I disorder (except another sexual dysfunction) and is not due exclusively to the direct physiological effects of a substance (e.g., a drug of abuse, a medication) or a general medical condition.

*Specify* type:
**Lifelong type**
**Acquired type**

*Specify* type:
**Generalized type**
**Situational type**

*Specify:*
**Due to psychological factors**
**Due to combined factors**

Reprinted with permission from the Diagnostic and Statistical Manual of Mental Disorders, Fourth Edition, Text Revision. Copyright 2000 American Psychiatric Association.

pausal biological changes and more important psychological ones.

A regularly menstruating 50-year-old widow complained of difficulty with arousal with her new "good-enough" lover. She was motivated to behave sexually with him but something seemed to have happened to her since her husband developed a brain tumor and died and she spent 2 years without dating. Her body, which used to work well sexually, had ceased to be reliably sexually functional. She was intermittently vaginally dry despite using a lubricant, she had trouble sustaining excitement, and orgasm only occasionally occurred with great effort. She could masturbate efficiently when alone, but was not motivated to do it—"What good is it?" Not depressed clinically, she was baffled by her failure to adapt to her new situation. Her conversation wove together two themes: the unusually happy life she had with her husband who tragically died so young leaving her to grieve forever and her musings about the meaning of her new friend's wife's suicide. "Let's face, as nice as he is, he is no George."

## Male Erectile Disorder

The mechanisms of erection—the sequestering and maintaining arterial blood within the corpora cavernosa—are being elucidated by urological research. Their research has

## DSM-IV-TR Criteria 302.72

### Male Erectile Disorder

A. Persistent or recurrent inability to attain, or to maintain until completion of the sexual activity, an adequate erection.

B. The disturbance causes marked distress or interpersonal difficulty.

C. The erectile dysfunction is not better accounted for by another Axis I disorder (other than a sexual dysfunction) and is not due exclusively to the direct physiological effects of a substance (e.g., a drug of abuse, a medication) or a general medical condition.

*Specify* type:

**Lifelong type**

**Acquired type**

*Specify* type:

**Generalized type**

**Situational type**

*Specify:*

**Due to psychological factors**

**Due to combined factors**

Reprinted with permission from the Diagnostic and Statistical Manual of Mental Disorders, Fourth Edition, Text Revision. Copyright 2000 American Psychiatric Association.

At every age, *selectivity* of erectile failure is the single most important diagnostic feature of primary erectile dysfunction. Clinicians should inquire about the relative firmness and duration of erections under each of these circumstances: masturbation, sex other than intercourse, sex with other female or male partners, upon stimulation with explicit media materials, in the middle of the night, and upon awakening. If under some circumstances the erection is firm and lasting, the clinician can usually assume that the man's neural, endocrine, and vascular physiology is sufficiently normal and that the problem is psychogenic in origin. This is true even for men in their fifties and older. Clinicians often feel more certain about this diagnosis when no diseases thought to lead to erectile dysfunction are present (O'Keefe and Hunt 1995).

**Clinical Vignette 2**

A 35-year-old man who is potent reliably with his wife becomes sexually anxious when he attempts to have intercourse with a new partner. During foreplay with her, he has been lastingly erect. But when he attempts to penetrate he does so with a softening erection and it becomes a race between rapid ejaculation and loss of erection.
*Patient:* "What is going on here doctor?"
*Doctor:* "What is going on here?"
*Patient:* "I know there is nothing wrong with me physically."
*Doctor:* "Me, too. So why did you spend so much time with the urologist?"
*Patient:* "I guess I did not want to face what I am doing about my wife and children and my resentment of being confined by marriage."

led to a diminishing emphasis on "psychogenic impotence" diagnosis (Krane et al. 1989). Urologists may refer to male erectile disorders (ED) of a psychogenic origin as "adrenergic" ED, a reference to the preponderance of sympathetic tone on the corporal mechanisms that maintain flaccidity. Adrenergic dominance of the penile arterial tone is created by a mind that perceives the sexual context as a dangerous, frightening, or as unwanted.

The prevalence of ED rises dramatically in the sixth decade of life from less than 10 to 30%; it increases further during the seventh decade (Feldman et al. 1994). Aging, medical conditions such as diabetes, prostatic cancer, hypertension, and cardiovascular risk factors predict the most common pattern of ED due to a medical condition in this age group. While medication-induced, neurological, endocrine, metabolic, radiation, and surgical causes of erectile dysfunction also exist, in population studies diabetes, hypertension, smoking, lipid abnormalities, obesity, and lack of exercise are correlated with the progressive deterioration of erectile functioning in the sixth and seventh decades (Althof and Seftel 1995). These factors are thought to create a relative penile anoxemia which stimulates the conversion of corporal smooth muscle cells into fibrocytes. The gradual loss of elasticity of the corpora interferes with filling and sequestering of arterial blood (Carrier et al. 1993). Erections at first become unreliable and finally impossible to obtain or sustain.

Lifelong male ED typically is psychogenic and involves either a sexual identity dilemma—such as transvestism, gender identity disorder, a homoerotic orientation, a paraphilia, or another diagnosis that expresses the patient's fear of being sexually close to a partner. Sexual identity problems are often initially denied unless the clinician is nonjudgmental and thorough during the inquiry. However, obsessive–compulsive disorder, schizoid personality, a psychotic disorder, or severe character disorders may be present. Occasionally, a reasonably normal young man with an unusually persistent fear of sexual intercourse seeks attention. These good prognosis cases are sometimes informally referred to as anxious beginners (Table 74–5). With that exception, men with lifelong male arousal disorder (MAD), when taken into individual therapy are usually perceived as having a strong motive to avoid sexual behavior and while dysfunctional with a partner during much of their therapy might equally be diagnosed as having HSDD with normal drive but a motive to avoid partner sex. The prognosis with older men with lifelong erectile dysfunction is poor even with modern erectogenic agents. Long-term therapy, even if it does not enable regular intercourse, may enable more emotional and sexual closeness to a partner. Some reasonably masculine appearing men with mild gender identity problems can quickly become potent if they can reveal their need during sexual relationship to cross-

| Table 74–5 | What the Psychiatrist Should Expect to Encounter Among Men Who Have Never Been Able to Have Intercourse with a Woman |
|---|---|

### Unconventional Sexual Identity

Gender identity problem
  Wish to be a woman
  A history of cross-dressing in women's clothing in private and/or public
  Suspected by psychiatrist but information initially withheld
Homoeroticism
  Without sexual behavior with men
  With sexual behavior with men but not known to the female partner
  With sexual behavior with men and known to the female partner
Paraphilia
  One or more of a wide range of paraphilic patterns
  Preference for prepubertal or young adolescents often initially denied unless thoroughly, systematically, and nonjudgmentally questioned
  Compulsivity with or without obvious paraphilic imagery confined to masturbation with the help of pornographic images for stimulation

### Serious Character Disorders
(Men Have Strong Fear of Closeness to Women)

Obsessive–compulsive
Schizotypal
Schizoid
Avoidant
Past history of psychotic decompensation

### Anxious Beginners

Psychiatrically normal young men with inordinate anxiety and shyness that quickly respond to psychiatrist's encouragement and optimism and partner warmth and patience

dress (use a fetish article of clothing) to a partner who calmly accepts his requirement. However, most of these men have inordinate fears of sexually bonding to any woman and, in therapy, become preoccupied with basic developmental issues. Some of them marry and form companionate relationships that are rarely or never consummated.

In dramatic contrast, men with long-established good potency who have recently lost their erectile capacities with their partner—acquired psychogenic ED—have a far better prognosis (Table 74–6). They may be treated in individual or couples format, depending on the precipitants of the sexual problem and the status of their relationship with their partner. Many of these therapies become focused on resentments that have not been identified, discussed, and worked through by the couple. Such distressed couples are most efficiently helped in a conjoint format. When extramarital affairs are part of the relationship deterioration and cannot be discussed, most clinicians simply work with one spouse. Potency is frequently lost following a separation or divorce. Impaired potency after a spouse's death is either about unresolved grief or problems that exist prior to the wife's terminal illness. Men also often get worried about their potency when their financial or vocational lives

crumble, when they have a serious new physical illness such as a myocardial infarction or stroke, or when their wives become seriously ill. The esthetics of lovemaking require a context of reasonable physical health; when one spouse becomes chronically ill or disfigured by illness or surgery, either one of the couple may lose their willingness to be sexual. This may be reflected in impaired erections or sexual avoidance.

Regardless of the precipitating factors, men with arousal disorders have performance anxiety. They anticipate erectile failure before sex begins and vigilantly monitor their state of tumescence during sex (Masters and Johnson 1970). Performance anxiety is present in almost all impotent men. Performance anxiety is efficiently therapeutically addressed by identifying it to the patient and asking him to make love without trying intercourse on several occasions to demonstrate to himself how different lovemaking can feel for him when he is not risking failure. This enables many to relax, concentrate on sensation, and return to previous states of sensual abandon during lovemaking. This technique is known as *sensate focus*.

The psychological treatment of acquired arousal disorders is often highly satisfying for the professional because many of the men are anxious for help. Motivation to behave sexually is often present, fear can be allayed, and men can learn to appreciate the emotional complexity of their lives. They can be shown how their minds prevented intercourse until they could acknowledge what has been transpiring within and around them. Many recently separated men, for example, are grieving, angry, guilty, uncertain, and worried about their finances. Yet, they may propel themselves into a new relationship. Two characteristics seem to predispose to erectile problems at key life transitions: (1) The pursuit of the masculine standard that men ought to be able to perform intercourse with anyone, anywhere, under any circumstances; (2) The inability to readily grasp the nature and significance of his inner experiences. "Yes, my schizophrenic daughter became homeless in another city, my wife was depressed and began drinking to excess in response, and I had a financially costly affair with

| Table 74–6 | Apparent Precipitants of Recently Acquired Psychogenic Erectile Disorder and Their Associated Private Emotions* |
|---|---|

Deterioration of marital relationship: anger, guilt, disdain, sadness
Divorce: abandonment, anger, guilt, sadness, shame
Deterioration of personal or spousal health: sadness, anxiety, anger, shame
Death of spouse ("widower's impotence"): sadness, longing, guilt
Threat of or actual unemployment: anxiety, worthlessness, guilt, anger, shame
Financial reversal: shame, guilt, anxiety
Surreptitious extramarital affair: guilt
Reunited marriage after extramarital affair: shame, anxiety

*These short lists of simple emotions are a mere introduction to what transpires within the man's mind as a result of the meanings that the sexual behavior has for him. Although incomplete and oversimplified, they are listed to remind the psychiatrist that what the man feels about his life competes with sexual arousal during sexual behavior to generate the psychogenic erectile dysfunction.

| Table 74–7 | Pathogenesis Model for Acquired Erectile Dysfunction |
|---|---|

Functional cognitive predispositions
   A normal (or real, adequate, or competent) man is able to have intercourse with anyone under any circumstances
   Feelings are a womanly intrusion on my reason; I am disinterested and relatively unaware of them.
Precipitating events (see Table 74–6)
   ↓
One episode of erectile failure
   ↓
Performance anxiety
   ↓
Another episode of erectile failure
   ↓
More performance anxiety
   ↓
Decreased frequency of sexual initiation
   ↓
Changes in the sexual equilibrium
   ↓
Established pattern of impotence with partner

my secretary. What do these have to do with my loss of potency?" (Table 74–7).

Sildenafil revolutionized the treatment of erectile dysfunction in 1998. This phosphodiesterase type 5 inhibitor maintains corporal vasodilation by preventing the degradation of cGMP. Sexual arousal leads to the corporal secretion of nitric oxide which is converted by an enzyme into cGMP. Sildenafil is increasingly effective as the dose is increased from 25 to 50 up to 100 mg. The drug must not be used when any organic nitrate is being taken because it dangerously potentiates the hypotensive effect of the nitrates risking brain and myocardial infarction (Goldstein et al. 1998). Sildenafil is dramatically underutilized by psychiatrists.

Prior to sildenafil, urologists argued that most erectile dysfunction was organic in origin, but since the drug works at about the same rate regardless of the pretreatment etiology, most erectile dysfunction is now recognized to be of mixed—organic and psychosocial—origin (Lue 2000). Three conditions have unique response profiles: after prostatectomy the response rate is approximately 34%, among diabetics it is approximately 43%, and among the spinal cord injured, it is approximately 80%, the same rate seems to improve psychogenic ED. Other medical interventions are also effective in varying degrees for largely organic erectile dysfunction: vacuum pump, the intracavernosal injection of vasodilating substances, intraurethral aprostadil, the surgical implantation of a penile prostheses (Ohl 1994), and outside the US, sublingual apomorphine. Because sildenafil's rate of improving erections is significantly higher than the restoration of a mutually satisfactory sexual equilibrium (approximately 44%), psychological ED that persists after medication should be treated by a mental health professional (Pallas et al. 2000).

## Problems with Orgasm

### Female Orgasmic Disorder

The attainment of reasonably regular orgasms with a partner is a crucial personal developmental step for young women. This task of adult sexual development rests upon a subtle interplay of physiology, individual psychology, and culture. Reliable orgasmic attainment is usually highly valued by the woman and is often reflected in enhanced self-esteem, confidence in her femininity, relationship satisfaction, and the motive to continue to behave sexually.

Orgasm is the reflexive culmination of arousal. It is manifested by rhythmic vaginal wall contractions and the release of muscular tension and pelvic vasocongestion, accompanied by varying degrees of pleasurable body sensations. Its accomplishment requires: (1) the physiologic apparatus to augment and sustain arousal; (2) the psychological willingness to be swept away by excitement; and (3) tenacious focus on the required physical work of augmenting arousal. The diagnosis of female orgasmic disorder

---

**DSM-IV-TR Criteria** 302.73

**Female Orgasmic Disorder**

A. Persistent or recurrent delay in, or absence of, orgasm following a normal sexual excitement phase. Women exhibit wide variability in the type or intensity of stimulation that triggers orgasm. The diagnosis of female orgasmic disorder should be based on the clinician's judgment that the woman's orgasmic capacity is less than would be reasonable for her age, sexual experience, and the adequacy of sexual stimulation she receives.

B. The disturbance causes marked distress or interpersonal difficulty.

C. The orgasmic dysfunction is not better accounted for by another Axis I disorder (except another sexual dysfunction) and is not due exclusively to the direct physiological effects of a substance (e.g., a drug of abuse, a medication) or a general medical condition.

*Specify* type:
**Lifelong type**

**Acquired type**

*Specify* type:
**Generalized type**

**Situational type**

*Specify:*
**Due to psychological factors**

**Due to combined factors**

Reprinted with permission from the Diagnostic and Statistical Manual of Mental Disorders, Fourth Edition, Text Revision. Copyright 2000 American Psychiatric Association.

(FOD) is made when the woman's psychology persistently interferes with her body's natural progression through arousal.

Estimates of prevalence of both lifelong and acquired psychological FOD range from 10 to 30% (Laumann et al. 1994b). Some of this variability is due to the different definitions of anorgasmia. It remains a difficult scientific judgment, however, where to draw the line between dysfunction and normality—for example, is it normal to attain orgasms during one-third of partner sexual experiences? (Tiefer 1998). Few women are always orgasmic.

During most of the 20th century, psychoanalysts thought that almost 90% of women were orgasmically dysfunctional. Prior to 1970, the accepted concept of normality required a woman to be brought to orgasm by penile thrusting. Orgasmic fulfillment through solitary masturbation or partner manual or oral stimulation was viewed as signifying the presence of a neurotic obstacle to mature femininity. This paternalistic idea has weakened considerably in the last generation.

The biologic potential for orgasmic attainment is an inborn endowment of nearly all physically healthy women. The cultural and psychological factors that influence orgasmic attainment are usually fundamental to the etiology of FOD. Centuries-old beliefs that sexual knowledge, behavior, and sexual pleasure were not the prerogative of "good girls" powerfully affects some women's sexual adjustment. These beliefs cause young women to be uninformed about the location and role of their clitoris and ashamed of their erotic desires and sexual sensations. For women with FOD, modern concepts of equality of sexual expression are insufficient to overcome these traditional beliefs. These emotionally powerful beliefs often lay behind their classic dysfunctional pattern: the women can become aroused to a personal plateau beyond which they cannot progress; thereafter, their excitement dissipates. After numerous repetitions, they begin to lose motivation to participate in sex with their partner. They may eventually meet criteria for HSDD.

## Diagnosis

The doctor should know the answers to the following questions. Does the patient have orgasms under any of the following sexual circumstances: solitary masturbation, partner manual genital stimulation, oral–genital stimulation, vibratory stimulation, any other means? Does she have orgasms with a partner different than her significant other? How are they stimulated? Does a particular fantasy make orgasmic attainment easier or possible? Under what conditions has she ever been orgasmic? Has she had an orgasm during her sleep?

### Lifelong Varieties

The lifelong *generalized* variety of the disorder is recognized when a woman has never been able to attain orgasm alone or with a partner by any means, although she regularly is aroused. When a woman can only readily attain orgasm during masturbation, she is diagnosed as having a lifelong *situational* type. Women with any form of lifelong FOD more clearly have conflicts about personal sexual expression due to fear, guilt, ignorance, or obedience to tradition than those with the acquired variety. Women who can masturbate to orgasm often feel fear and embarrassment about sharing their private arousal with any other person.

### Acquired Varieties

The acquired varieties of this disorder are more common and are characterized by both complete anorgasmia, too-infrequent orgasms, and too-difficult orgasmic attainment. The most common cause of this problem are serotonergic compounds. Prospective studies of various antidepressants have demonstrated up to 70% incidence of this disorder among those treated with serotonergic antidepressants. Bupropion and nefazadone do not cause this problem (Segraves 1998). When medications are not the cause of an acquired FOD, the doctor needs to carefully assess the meaning of the changes in her life prior to the onset of the disorder. Some of these women are in the midst of making a transition to a new partner after many years in another relationship. Some seem to suffer from memories of earlier shame-ridden behaviors such as incest.

### Treatment

When a doctor applies a label of disorder to a relatively anorgasmic woman, the woman often privately interprets the diagnosis as meaning that she has a serious and difficult problem to overcome. Physicians need to be careful about this because some of these women are relatively easy to help. It must be realized that many women gradually undo the effects of their culture on their own and grow to be increasingly responsive sexually with time and growing trust of their partners. Clinicians can do many women a great service by offering education and reassurance. Giving an inhibited woman new-to-her information in an encouraging manner can subdue her anxiety and foster her optimism. On the other hand, some women with this disorder are profoundly entrenched in not being too excited and treatments fail. The ideal era to begin treatment is young adulthood (Killman et al. 1986).

Four formats are known to be of help. Individual therapy is the most commonly employed. In lifelong varieties of the disorder, therapy focuses on the cultural sources of sexual inhibition and how and when they impacted upon the patient. In the situational varieties, the therapist focuses on the meaning of the life changes that preceded the onset of the disorder. Group therapy is highly effective in helping women to reliably masturbate to orgasm and moderately effective in overcoming partner inhibition. It is typically done with college and graduate students in campus settings, not older women. Couple therapy may be useful to assist the couple with the subtleties of their sexual equilibrium. The personal and interpersonal dimensions of orgasmic attainment can be stressed. Often other issues then come to the fore that initially seemed to have little to do with orgasmic attainment. The most cost-effective treatment is bibliotherapy. Female orgasmic attainment has been widely written about in the popular press since the early 1970s. It is widely believed that these articles and books, which strongly encourage knowledge of her genital anatomy, masturbation, and active pursuit of orgasm, have enabled many women to grow more comfortable and competent in sexual expression.

---

**DSM-IV-TR Criteria** 302.74

**Male Orgasmic Disorder**

A. Persistent or recurrent delay in, or absence of, orgasm following a normal sexual excitement phase during sexual activity that the clinician, taking into account the person's age, judges to be adequate in focus, intensity, and duration.

B. The disturbance causes marked distress or interpersonal difficulty.

C. The orgasmic dysfunction is not better accounted for by another Axis I disorder (except another sexual dysfunction) and is not due exclusively to the direct physiological effects of a substance (e.g., a drug of abuse, a medication) or a general medical condition.

*Specify* type:

**Lifelong type**

**Acquired type**

*Specify* type:

**Generalized type**

**Situational type**

*Specify:*

**Due to psychological factors**

**Due to combined factors**

## Male Orgasmic Disorder

When a man can readily attain a lasting erection with a partner, yet is consistently unable to attain orgasm in the body of the partner, he is diagnosed with male orgasmic disorder (MOD). The disorder has three levels of severity: (1) the most common form is characterized by the *ability* to attain orgasm with a partner outside of her or his body, either through oral, manual, or personal masturbation; (2) the more severe form is characterized by the man's inability to ejaculate in his partner's presence; and (3) the rarest form is characterized by the inability to ejaculate when awake. The disorder is usually lifelong and not partner specific. These men cannot allow themselves to be swept away in arousal by another person. They are sexually vigilant to not allow themselves to be controlled by the partner's power to convey them to orgasm. This power would provide the partner with personal pleasure and the man with this disorder, while initially appearing to be a sexual superman, ultimately disappoints the partner. Their psychological dysfunction represents a capacity to use a mental mechanism which other men would love to possess in smaller degrees. Both the partners and the therapists of these men tend to describe them as controlling, unemotional, untrusting, hostile, obsessive–compulsive, or para-

noid. Some of these men get better with psychotherapy, others improve spontaneously with time, and, for others the dysfunction leads to the cessation of the aspiration for sex with a partner. One controlled study of patients with numerous sexual dysfunctions suggested that bupropion 300 to 450 mg/day may improve the capacity to ejaculate in a minority of patients. Another controlled study found that 150 mg/day was insufficient (Masand et al. 2001).

## Premature Ejaculation

Premature ejaculation is a high prevalence (25–40%) (Frank et al. 1978) disorder seen primarily in heterosexuals characterized by an untameably low threshold for the reflex sequence of orgasm. The problem, a physiological *efficiency* of sperm delivery, causes social and psychological distress. In failing to develop a sense of control over the timing of his orgasm in the vagina, the man fails to meet his standards of being a satisfying sexual partner. However, his partner does not explicitly or implicitly object, his rapidity is not likely to cause him to seek medical attention. The range of intravaginal containment times among self-diagnosed patients extends from immediately before or upon vaginal entry (rare), to less than a minute (usual), to less than the man and his partner desire (not infrequent). Time alone is a misleading indicator, however. The essence of the

---

**DSM-IV-TR Criteria** 302.75

**Premature Ejaculation**

A. Persistent or recurrent ejaculation with minimal sexual stimulation before, on, or shortly after penetration and before the person wishes it. The clinician must take into account factors that affect duration of the excitement phase, such as age, novelty of the sexual partner or situation, and recent frequency of sexual activity.

B. The disturbance causes marked distress or interpersonal difficulty.

C. The premature ejaculation is not due exclusively to the direct effects of a substance (e.g., withdrawal from opioids).

*Specify* type:

**Lifelong type**

**Acquired type**

*Specify* type:

**Generalized type**

**Situational type**

*Specify:*

**Due to psychological factors**

**Due to combined factors**

self-diagnosis is an emotionally unsatisfying sexual equilibrium apparently due to the man's inability to temper his arousal. Most men sometimes ejaculate before they wish to, but not persistently.

## Clinical Approach

The history should clarify the answers to following questions: Why is he seeking therapy now? Is the patient a sexual beginner or a beginner with a particular partner? Does he have inordinately high expectations for intravaginal containment time for a man his age and experience? Is he desperate about losing the partner because of the rapid ejaculation? Is the relationship in jeopardy for another reason? Does his partner have a sexual dysfunction? Does she have orgasms with him other than through intercourse? Is he requesting help in order to cover his infidelity? Is his partner now blaming the man's sexual inadequacy for her infidelity? Is his new symptom a reflection of his fear about having a serious physical problem during sex such as angina, a stroke, or another myocardial infarction? The answers will enable the doctor to classify the rapid ejaculation into an acquired or lifelong and specific or general pattern, to sense the larger context in which his sexual behavior is conducted, and to plan treatment.

Premature ejaculation reflects to the man's sense that his contribution to the sexual equilibrium is deficient. It implies that he considers that he is far behind most men in his vaginal containment time and that he wants to provide his partner with a better opportunity to be nurtured during lovemaking through prolonged intercourse. Typically, he aspires to "bring" his partner to orgasm during intercourse. If anxiety lowers the ejaculatory threshold and keeps it from its natural evolution to a higher level over time, then premature ejaculation is a self-perpetuating pattern. Premature ejaculation may last a lifetime.

## Therapy

There are three efficient approaches to this dysfunction. The first is simply to refuse to confirm the patient's self-diagnosis. Some anxious beginners, men with reasonable intravaginal containment times of 2 or more minutes, and those with exaggerated notions of sexual performance can be calmed down by a few visits. When they no longer think of themselves as dysfunctional their intravaginal containment times improve. The second is the use of serotonergic medications. In a study of 15 carefully selected stable couples, daily administration of clomipramine 25 and 50 mg increased intravaginal containment times on average of 249 and 517% over baseline observations (Althof et al. 1995). At these dosage levels, there were few side effects. Numerous similar reports testify to the fact that various serotonergic reuptake inhibitors can significantly lengthen the duration of intercourse (Waldinger et al. 1994). Clinicians need to determine with each patient whether the medication can be taken within hours or days of anticipated intercourse. Improvement is not sustained after medication is stopped. Serotonergic medications are the most common treatment of rapid ejaculation because they are so quickly effective in over 90% of men. The third approach is behaviorally-oriented sex therapy that trains the man to focus his attention on his penile sensations during vaginal containment and to signal his partner to cease movement or to apply a firm squeeze of the glans/shaft area to interrupt the escalation of arousal. This requires an increase in communication and full cooperation of the partner which in themselves can go a long way in improving their sexual equilibrium.

Rapid ejaculation in some men reflects mere inexperience; for others it is stubborn physiological efficiency; for others it reflects fear of personal harm, which is either related to physical illness or to unresolved fears of closeness to a woman; and yet for others it reflects a partnership with a profoundly inhibited blaming partner. If the psychodynamic question is asked of men with persistent rapid ejaculation "Why does this man want to finish intercourse so quickly?" the answers vary from, "It is not a relevant question!" to "I'm afraid of her!" to "I'm afraid of what will happen to me." For instance, a large percentage of men ejaculate quickly for the first months after a myocardial infarction.

The advantages of costlier couple psychotherapy are to allow the man and his partner to understand their lives better, to address both of their sexual anxieties, and to deal with other important nonsexual issues in their relationship. Effective psychotherapy allows the man to become positioned to continue the usual biological evolution that occurs during the life cycle from rapid ejaculation, which is true for many young men, to occasional difficulty in ejaculating, which is true for many men in their sixties.

## Sexual Pain Disorders

The clinician needs to consider a series of questions when dealing with a woman who reports painful intercourse. Does she have a known gynecologic abnormality which is generally associated with pain? Is there anything about her complaint of pain that indicates a remarkably low pain threshold? Does she now have an aversion to sexual intercourse? At what level of physical discomfort did she develop the aversion? Does her private view of her current relationship affect her willingness to be sexual and her experience of pain? Does her partner's sexual style cause her physical or mental discomfort—for example, is he overly aggressive or does he stimulate memories of former abuse? What has been the partner's response to her pain? What role does her anticipation of pain play in her experience of pain?

These clinical questions are typical biopsychosocial ones. Sex-limiting pain often is the result of the subtle interplay of personal and relational, cognitive and affective, and fundamental biological processes that are inherent in other human sexual struggles that operate to produce these confusing disorders (Meana and Binik 1994).

The DSM-IV presents dyspareunia and vaginismus as distinct entities. However, they have been viewed as inextricably connected in much of the modern sexuality literature—vaginismus is known to create dyspareunia and dyspareunia has been known to create vaginismus.

## Dyspareunia

### Terminology

Recurrent uncomfortable or painful intercourse in either gender is known as dyspareunia. Women's dyspareunia varies from discomfort at intromission, to severe unsparing pain during penile thrusting, to vaginal irritation following intercourse. In both sexes, recurring coital pain leads to inhibited arousal and sexual avoidance. "Dyspareunia" is used as both a symptom and a diagnosis. When coital pain is caused solely by defined physical pathology, dyspareunia due to a medical condition is diagnosed. When coital pain is due to vaginismus, insufficient lubrication, or other presumably psychogenic factors, dyspareunia not due to a medical condition diagnosis is made. Psychogenic etiologies may include a CNS pain perception problem raising the question, "What do we mean by psychogenic?" This arena's nomenclature will undoubtably change when a breakthrough in understanding the causes of coital pain occurs.

## Psychogenic Sources of Dyspareunia

Pain associated with intercourse may have purely subjective or psychologic origin. Couple dynamics are often relevant, but the pain may be seen as a means of not allowing painful memories of childhood sexual abuse into clear focus. Fear of or helplessness about negotiating interpersonal conflicts may eventually lead to pain becoming a solution for avoiding unwanted sexual behaviors. While physicians tend to assume that pain has unconscious origins, sometimes it is merely faked; more often the patient is quite aware of its developmental origins but is too embarrassed to quickly communicate it to the doctor.

---

### DSM-IV-TR Criteria 302.76

**Dyspareunia**

A. Recurrent or persistent genital pain associated with sexual intercourse in either a male or a female.

B. The disturbance causes marked distress or interpersonal difficulty.

C. The disturbance is not caused exclusively by vaginismus or lack of lubrication, is not better accounted for by another Axis I disorder (except another sexual dysfunction), and is not due exclusively to the direct physiological effects of a substance (e.g., a drug of abuse, a medication) or a general medical condition.

*Specify* type:

**Lifelong type**

**Acquired type**

*Specify* type:

**Generalized type**

**Situational type**

*Specify:*

**Due to psychological factors**

**Due to combined factors**

---

Personal psychological origins of painful intercourse pass through the common denominator of anxiety. Such anxiety may take the forms of dread of physical damage, worry about the psychological dependence that might result from physical union, fear of a first or another pregnancy, or a sexually transmitted disease. Intense anxiety, the psychological source of her pain, may lead to involuntary contraction of vaginal muscles which is the mechanical source of her pain. Thus, dyspareunia and vaginismus reinforce each other. Both situational and acquired dyspareunia may reflect a woman's conscious or unconscious motivation to avoid sex with a particular partner; it may be her only means to express her despair about their nonsexual relationship. *Lifelong* dyspareunia draws the clinicians attention to developmental experiences.

## Differential Diagnosis

Because the *symptom* dyspareunia is produced by numerous organic conditions, the psychiatrist should be certain that the patient has had a pelvic examination by a person equipped to assess a broad range of regional pathology (McKay 1992). Vulvovestibulitis is diagnosed by pain in response to cotton swab touching in a normal appearing vulvar vestibule. A fundamental question remains unanswered about this often devastating problem: "Is the disorder of local or central origin?" In these patients and some others, the pain can not be classified with certainty as a *symptom* or a *disorder*. Pain upon penile or digital insertion may be due to an intact hymen or remnants of the hymenal ring, vaginitis, cervicitis, episiotomy scars, endometriosis, fibroids, ovarian cysts, and so on. Postcoital dyspareunia often begins at orgasm when uterine contractions occur. Fibroids, endometriosis, and pelvic inflammatory disease should be considered. Postmenopausal pain, particularly if the woman has had many years without intercourse, is often a result of thinning of the vaginal mucosa, loss of elasticity of the labia and vaginal outlet, and decreased lubrication. Normal menopause, however, is often associated with mild pain due to inadequate lubrication (in both partners).

The brilliant younger daughter of an immigrant family who married an accomplished man of her age and educational attainment developed painful intercourse shortly after marriage. Each had refused parental wishes to arrange a marriage. Each family seemed quite pleased with this love union. Shortly after marriage, she had significant continuing pain on intercourse. They avoided sex. Her easy acceptance of this led the clinician to suspect and correctly diagnose a prolactin secreting pituitary tumor. When that was effectively treated with bromocriptine, they returned to intercourse only to find that she still had significant pain. They sought additional assistance because she was also despairing that she would never become pregnant. Her symptoms resolved in individual therapy after she spent several intense sessions discussing the shame of sexual molestation by her older sister. She could never bear to bring such news to her proud parents or her husband. She eventually did tell her husband.

Dyspareunia in men is usually due to a medical condition. Herpes, gonorrhea, prostatitis, and Peyronie's disease cause pain during intercourse. Remote trauma to the penis may cause penile chordee or bowing which makes intercourse mechanically difficult and sometimes painful. Pain experienced upon ejaculation can be a side effect of trazo-done.

## Vaginismus

Vaginismus is an involuntary spasm of the musculature of the outer third layer of the vagina which makes penile penetration difficult or impossible. The diagnosis is not made if an organic cause is known. Although a woman with vaginismus may wish to have intercourse, her symptom prevents the penis from entering her body. It is as though her vagina says, "No!" In lifelong vaginismus, the anticipation of pain at the first intercourse causes muscle spasm. Pain reinforces the fear and on occasion, the partner's response gives her good reason to dread a second opportunity to have intercourse. Early episodic vaginismus may be common among women, but most of the cases that are brought to medical attention are chronic. Lifelong vaginismus is relatively rare. The clinician needs to focus attention on what may have made the idea of intercourse so overwhelming to her: parental intrusiveness, sexual trauma, childhood genital injury, illnesses whose therapy involved orifice penetration, and surgery?

The woman with lifelong vaginismus not only has a history of unsuccessful attempts at penetration but displays an avoidance of finger and tampon penetration. The most dramatic aspect of her history, however, is her inability to endure a speculum examination of her vagina. Vaginismus is a phobia of vaginal entrance.

---

### DSM-IV-TR Criteria 302.51

**Vaginismus**

A. Recurrent or persistent involuntary spasm of the musculature of the outer third of the vagina that interferes with sexual intercourse.

B. The disturbance causes marked distress or interpersonal difficulty.

C. The disturbance is not better accounted for by another Axis I disorder (e.g., somatization disorder) and is not due exclusively to the direct physiological effects of a general medical condition.

*Specify* type:

**Lifelong type**

**Acquired type**

*Specify* type:

**Generalized type**

**Situational type**

*Specify:*

**Due to psychological factors**

**Due to combined factors**

Reprinted with permission from the Diagnostic and Statistical Manual of Mental Disorders, Fourth Edition, Text Revision. Copyright 2000 American Psychiatric Association.

## Treatment of Dyspareunia and Vaginismus

While vaginismus has the reputation of being readily treatable by gynecologists by pairing relaxation techniques with progressively larger vaginal dilators, the mental health professional typically approaches the problem differently. The psychiatric approach to both vaginismus and dyspareunia is attuned to the role that her symptom plays in her life. The therapy, therefore, does not begin with a cavalier, optimistic attempt to remove the symptom, which only frightens some patients. Rather, it begins with a patient exploration of the developmental and interpersonal meanings of the need for the symptom. "I wonder how this problem originally got started? Can you tell me a bit more about your life?" In the course of assisting women with these problems a variety of techniques may be utilized including relaxation techniques, sensate focus, dilatation, marital therapy, and medication. Short-term therapies should not be expected to have lasting good results because once the symptom is relieved, other problematic aspects of the patient's sexual equilibrium and nonsexual relationship often come into focus. Clinicians have developed an impression that women with a diagnosis of dyspareunia are particularly difficult to help permanently. However, this is a largely unstudied topic.

## Sexual Dysfunction Not Otherwise Specified

This diagnosis is reserved for circumstances that leave the doctor uncertain as to how to diagnose the patient. This may occur when the patient has too many fluctuating dysfunctional symptoms without a clear pattern of prominence of anyone of them. Sometimes the psychiatrist is unable to determine whether the dysfunction is the basic complaint or when the sexual complaints are secondary to marital dysfunction. At other times the etiology is the uncertain: psychogenic, due to a general medical condition, or substance-induced. When the patient does not emphasize the dysfunction as the problem but emphasizes instead the lack of emotional satisfaction from sex, the psychiatrist may temporarily provide this NOS diagnosis. It is usually possible to find a better dysfunction diagnosis after therapy begins.

## GENDER IDENTITY DISORDERS

The organization of a stable gender identity is the first component of sexual identity to emerge during childhood. The processes that enable this accomplishment are so subtle that when a daughter consistently acts as though she realizes that "I am a girl and that is all right," or when a son's behavior announces that "I am a boy and that is all right," families rarely even remember their children's confusion and behaviors to the contrary. Adolescent and adult gender problems are not rare. They are however commonly hidden from social view, sometimes long enough to developmentally evolve into other less dramatic forms of sexual identity.

### Early Forms

#### Extremely Feminine Young Boys

Although occasionally the parents of a feminine son have a convincing anecdote about persistent feminine interests dating from early in the second year of life, boyhood femininity is more typically only apparent by the third year. By the fourth year playmate preferences become obvious. Same-sex playmate preference is a typical characteristic of young children. Cross-gender–identified children consistently demonstrate the opposite sex playmate preference (Maccoby and Jacklin 1987). The avoidance of other boys has serious consequences in terms of social rejection and loneliness throughout the school years. The peer problems of feminine boys cause some of their behavioral and emotional problems which are in evidence by middle-to-late childhood (Zucker 1990). However, psychometric studies support clinical impressions that feminine boys have emotional problems even before peer relationships become a factor—that is, something more basic about being cross-gender–identified creates problems. Young feminine boys have been shown to be depressed and have difficulties with separation anxiety (Coates and Person 1985).

Speculations about the origin of boyhood femininity generally suggest converging cumulative forces. Any child's cross-gender identifications are likely to involve a host of factors: constitutional forces, problematic interactions with parents, problematic internal processing of life experiences, and family misfortune—financial, reproductive, physical disease, emotional illness, or death of vital persons. These factors are sometimes restated as temperament, disturbed family functioning, separation–individuation problems, and trauma.

Temperament is a dual phenomenon being both the child's predisposition to respond to the world in a certain way and the aspects of the child to which others respond. The common temperamental factors of feminine boys have been described as: a sense of body fragility and vulnerability that leads to the avoidance of rough-and-tumble play; timidity and fearfulness in the face of new situations; a vulnerability to separation and loss; an unusual capacity for positive emotional connection to others; an ability to imitate; sensitivities to sound, color, texture, odor, temperature, and pain (Coates et al. 1992).

The development of boyhood femininity *may* occur within the mind of the toddler in response to a loss of emotional availability of the nurturant mother. The child creates a maternal (feminine) self through imitation and fantasy in order to make up for the mother's emotional unavailability. This occurs beyond the family's awareness and is left in place by the family either ignoring what has transpired in the son or valuing it. The problem for the effeminate boy is that reality—the social expectations of other people—is unyielding on gender issues; the adaptive early life solution becomes progressively more maladaptive with time.

The answer to the question whether boyhood femininity is entirely constitutional, an adaptive solution, or due to a combination that includes some other process is not known. A few reports of femininity giving way to psychotherapeutic interventions with young boys and their families are of heuristic value but limited in follow-up duration (Zucker 1995).

Green prospectively studied a large well-matched group of feminine boys for over a decade and discovered that boyhood effeminacy was a frequent precursor of adolescent homoeroticism and homosexual behavior rather than gender identity disorders. He observed, as had others before, that without therapy feminine gender role behaviors give rise to more masculine behavioral styles as adolescence emerges (Green 1987).

## Masculine Girls: Tomboys

The masculinity of girls may become apparent as early as age 2 years. The number of girls brought to clinical attention for cross-gendered behaviors, self-statements, and aspirations is consistently less than boys by a factor of 1:5 at any age of childhood in Western countries (except Poland). It is not known whether this reflects a genuine difference in incidence of childhood gender disorders, cultural perceptions of femininity as a negative in boys versus the neutral-to-positive perception of boy-like behaviors in girls, the broader range of cross-gender expression permitted to girls but not to boys, or an intuitive understanding that cross-gender identity more accurately predicts homosexuality in boys than girls.

The distinction between tomboys and gender-disordered girls is often difficult to make. Tomboys are thought of as not as deeply unhappy about their femaleness, not as impossible to occasionally dress in stereotypic female clothing, and not thought to have a profound aversion to their girlish and future womanly physiologic transformations. Tomboys are able to enjoy some feminine activities along with their obvious pleasures in masculine-identified toys and games and the company of boys. Girls who are diagnosed as gender-disordered generally seem to have a relentless intensity about their masculine preoccupations and an insistence about their future. The onset of their cross-gendered identifications is early in life. Although most lesbians have a history of tomboyish behaviors, most tomboys develop a heterosexual orientation.

## The Subjectivity of a Well-Developed Gender Disorder

Children, teenagers, and adults exist who rue the day they were born to their biological sex and who long for the opportunity to simply live their lives in a manner befitting the other gender. They repudiate the possibility of finding happiness within the broad framework of roles given to members of their sex by their society. Their repudiation is not motivated by an intellectual attack on sexism, homophobia, or any other injustice imbedded in cultural mores. A gender-disordered person literally repudiates his or her body, repudiates the self in that body, and rejects performing roles expected of people with that body. It is a subtle, usually self-contained rebellion against the need of others to designate them in terms of their biological sex.

The repudiation and rebellion may first occur as a subjective internal drama of fantasy, as behavioral expression in play, or a preference for the company of others. Regardless of when and how it is displayed, the drama of the gender-disordered involves the relentless feeling that "life would be better—easier, fuller, more enjoyable—if I and others could experience me as a member of the opposite sex."

By mid-adolescence, the extremely gender-disordered have often envisioned the solution for their paralyzing self-consciousness: to live as a member of the opposite gender, to transform their bodies to the extent possible by modern medicine, and to be accepted by all others as the opposite sex. Most people with these cross-gender preoccupations, however, do not go beyond the fantasy or private cross-

## DSM-IV-TR Criteria

### Gender Identity Disorder

A. A strong and persistent cross-gender identification (not merely a desire for any perceived cultural advantages of being the other sex). In children, the disturbance is manifested by four (or more) of the following:

    (1) repeatedly stated desire to be, or insistence that he or she is, the other sex

    (2) in boys, preference for cross-dressing or simulating female attire; in girls, insistence on wearing only stereotypical masculine clothing

    (3) strong and persistent preferences for cross-sex roles in make-believe play or persistent fantasies of being the other sex

    (4) intense desire to participate in the stereotypical games and pastimes of the other sex

    (5) strong preference for playmates of the other sex

    In adolescents and adults, the disturbance is manifested by symptoms such as a stated desire to be the other sex, frequent passing as the other sex, desire to live or be treated as the other sex, or the conviction that he or she has the typical feelings and reactions of the other sex.

B. Persistent discomfort with his or her sex or sense of inappropriateness in the gender role of that sex.

    In children, the disturbance is manifested by any of the following: in boys, assertion that his penis or testes are disgusting or will disappear or assertion that it

would be better not to have a penis, or aversion toward rough-and-tumble play and rejection of male stereotypical toys, games, and activities; in girls, rejection of urinating in a sitting position, assertion that she has or will grow a penis, or assertion that she does not want to grow breasts or menstruate, or marked aversion toward normative feminine clothing.

    In adolescents and adults, the disturbance is manifested by symptoms such as preoccupation with getting rid of primary and secondary sex characteristics (e.g., request for hormones, surgery, or other procedures to physically alter sexual characteristics to simulate the other sex) or belief that he or she was born the wrong sex.

C. The disturbance is not concurrent with a physical intersex condition.

D. The disturbance causes clinically significant distress or impairment in social, occupational, or other important areas of functioning.

*Code* based on current age:

**302.6**   **Gender identity disorder in children**

**302.85**   **Gender identity disorder in adolescents or adults**

*Specify* (for sexually mature individuals):

**Sexually attracted to males**

**Sexually attracted to females**

**Sexually attracted to both**

**Sexually attracted to neither**

Reprinted with permission from the Diagnostic and Statistical Manual of Mental Disorders, Fourth Edition, Text Revision. Copyright 2000 American Psychiatric Association.

dressing. Those that do, eventually come to psychiatric attention. When a clinician is called in, the family has one set of hopes, the patient another. The clinician has many tasks, one of which is to mediate between the ambitions of the gender-disordered person and society and see what can be done to help the patient. Negative countertransference may steer the clinician to deal with the opportunity expeditiously: "Obviously the patient is sick, maybe psychotic, and needs help. I don't take care of people who do these things. Refer *it* out!" With a little supervisory encouragement to perform a thorough evaluation, therapists soon find that these patients possess many of the ordinary aspects of life and one unusual ambition—they often want to be the opposite sex so badly that they are willing to make it a priority over family, friends, vocation, and material acquisition.

### Diagnostic Criteria of Gender Identity Disorder

Adults who permanently change their bodies to deal with their gender dilemmas represent the far end of the spectrum

of adaptations to gender problems (Devor 1999). Even the lives of those who reject bodily change, however, have considerable pain because the images of a better gendered self may recur throughout life, becoming more powerful whenever life becomes strained or disappointing.

    The diagnosis of the extreme end of the gender identity disorder spectrum is clinically obvious. The challenging diagnostic task for clinicians is to suspect a gender problem and inquire about gender identity and its evolution in those whose manner suggest a unisexed or cross-gendered appearance, those with dissociative gender identity disorder (GID), severe forms of character pathology, and those who seem unusual in some undefinable manner.

    DSM-IV provides the clinician with two Axis I gender diagnoses. To qualify for the first, a patient of any age must meet four criteria.

**Criterion 1: Strong, Persistent Cross-Gender Identification.** Because young children may not verbalize enough about their inner experiences for the clinician to be certain that this criterion is met, at least four of five manifestations of cross-gender identification must be present: (1) repeat-edly stated desire to be, or insistence that he or she is, the opposite sex; (2) in boys, preference for cross-dressing or simulating female attire; in girls, insistence on wearing stereotypical masculine clothing; (3) strong and persistent preferences for cross-gender roles in fantasy play or persis-tent fantasies of being the opposite sex; (4) intense desire to participate in the games and pastimes of the opposite sex; (5) strong preference for playmates of the opposite sex.

In adolescence and adulthood, this criterion is fulfilled when the patient states the desire to be the opposite sex, has frequent social forays into appearing as the opposite sex, desires to live or be treated as the opposite sex, or has the conviction that his or her feelings and reactions are those typical of the opposite sex.

**Criterion 2: Persistent Discomfort with One's Gender or the Sense of Inappropriateness in a Gender Role.** This criterion is fulfilled in boys who assert that their penis or testicles are disgusting or will disappear or that it would be better not to have these organs; or who demonstrate an aversion toward rough-and-tumble play and rejection of male stereotypical toys, games, and activities. In girls, rejec-tion of urinating in a sitting position or assertion that they do not want to grow breasts or menstruate, or marked aversion towards normative feminine clothing fulfill this criterion.

Among adolescents and adults, this criterion is fulfilled by the patients' exhibiting the following characteristics: preoccupation with getting rid of primary and secondary sex characteristics; preoccupation with thoughts about hor-mones, surgery, or other alterations of the body to enhance the capacity to pass as a member of the opposite sex such as electrolysis for beard removal, cricoid cartilage shave to minimize the Adam's apple, breast augmentation; or pre-occupation with the belief that one was born into the wrong sex.

**Criterion 3: Not Due to an Intersex Condition.** In the vast majority of clinical circumstances the patient possesses normal genital anatomy and sexual physiology. When a patient with a gender identity disorder and an accompany-ing intersex condition such as congenital adrenal hyperpla-sia, an anomaly of the genitalia, or a chromosomal abnormality is encountered, the clinician will be uncertain whether the intersex condition is the cause of the GID. The clinician may either diagnose gender identity dis-order not otherwise specified (GIDNOS) or classify the patient as having a GID and list the physical factor on Axis III as a comorbid condition. The relationship be-tween GID and intersex conditions is controversial topic that may get clarified with further research being done in Germany.

**Criterion 4: Significant Distress and Impairment.** It is likely that many children, adolescents, and adults struggle for a while to consolidate their gender identity but eventu-ally find an adaptation that does not impair their capacities to function socially, academically, or vocationally as a member of their sex. These persons do *not* qualify for GID nor do those who simply are not stereotypic in how they portray their gender roles. Mental health professionals occasionally encounter parents who are disturbed by their adolescent child's gender roles. Parental distress is not the point of criterion 4; this criterion refers to patient distress.

## Diagnostic Criteria of Gender Identity Disorder Not Otherwise Specified (GIDNOS)

If an accurate community-based study of the gender-impaired could be conducted, most cases would be diag-nosed as GIDNOS. The diagnostician needs to understand that gender identity development is a dynamic evolutionary process and clinicians get to see people at crisis points in their lives. At any given time, although it is clear that the patient has some form of GID, it may not be that which is described in DSM-IV as GID. Here is one example: an adult female calls herself a "neuter." She wants her breasts removed because she hates to be perceived as a woman. For 2 years she has been exploring "neuterdom" and "I am definitely not interested in being a man!" If in 2 years, she evolves to meet criterion 1, her current GIDNOS diagnosis will change.

GIDNOS is a large category designed to be inclusive of those with unusual genders who do not clearly fit the criteria of GID. There is no implication that if a patient is labeled GIDNOS that his or her label cannot change in the future. GIDNOS would contain the many forms of trans-vestism—masculine-appearing boys and teenagers with per-sistent cross-dressing (former fetishistic transvestites) who are evolving toward GID, socially isolated men who want to become a woman shortly after their wives or mothers die (secondary transvestites) but express considerable ambiva-lence about the very matter they passionately desired at their last visit, extremely feminized homosexuals including those with careers as "drag queens" who seem to want to change their sex when depressed, and so on. GIDNOS would also capture men who want to be rid of their genitals with-out being feminized, unisexual females who imagine them-selves as males but who are terrified of any social expression of their masculine gender identity, hypermasculine lesbians in periodic turmoil over their gender, and those women who strongly identify with both male and female who lately want mastectomies. In using gender identity diagnoses, clinicians need to remember that extremely masculine women or ex-tremely feminine men are not to be dismissed as homosex-ual. "Lesbian" or "gay" is only a description of orientation. They are more aptly described as also cross-gendered.

Here is an example of the type of sexual identity prob-lem that would not be picked up in an epidemiologic survey. Some would call him a fetishistic transvestite.

---

Clinical Vignette 3

A couple married for 32 years sought help immediately after the wife unexpectedly returned home and discovered that her husband had been out in public dressed as a woman. She was certain that his public passing as a woman represented a worsening of his judgment. Thirty years before, he had revealed that he was sexually aroused by women's clothing and wanted to cross-dress for lovemaking. She adamantly refused to consider it. Since that incident, she never mentioned it again trying to act as though she was unaware of his "secret." Privately, she periodically worried that he was putting on her panty hose and bra to masturbate. Their sexual frequency declined after his initial request and, over the ensuing 20 years, she slowly developed an aversion to being touched by him. Sexual behavior ceased 10 years ago.

The 55-year-old masculine-appearing physical education teacher husband elected to enter individual therapy where he expressed his dilemma. He wanted to spare his wife pain. She believed that his "prurient" interest would go away if only he had more faith and prayed more, but he knew that nothing, including his fundamentalist religious patterns, diminished his periodic need to wear women's clothing. "If I tell her about my cross-dressing, she withdraws in anger. If I do not tell her about it, her imagination about how often I am doing it runs wild and she punishes me for cross-dressing that I don't do. If I stop cross-dressing, I deprive myself of unparalleled comfort and sumptuous pleasure and the desire eventually overtakes me. I lose either way. Should I honor my wife or my own identity?" His daily rate of masturbation has not changed much. He thinks he masturbates to cope with her refusal to have sexual behavior together. "My cross-dressing has actually kept me from having affairs with other women, thankfully."

People who qualify for GIDNOS often cause diagnostic uncertainty. In this case, three factors point to the paraphilia fetishistic transvestism as a diagnosis: his arousal to female clothing was reported to have increased over time, he cross-dresses without a well-developed feminine identity, and he masturbates daily. Let's now add to this description his wife's new diagnoses of advanced ovarian cancer. As he copes with this bad news and helps her with the painful process of dying, within his privacy is stirring his need to increase his social presentation as a woman, his fantasies of having genital reconstruction, and his recognition that his grief is balanced by his opportunity to live as a woman soon. If the psychiatrist sees him after his wife's death, GIDNOS might appear to be the new diagnosis. Fetishistic transvestism, GIDNOS, and GID can be evolutionary points in a person's life.

## The Relationship of Gender Identity Disorders to Orientation

The usual clarity of distinctions between heterosexual, bisexual, and homosexual orientations rests upon the assumption that the biological sex and psychological gender of the person and the partner are known. A woman who designates herself as a lesbian is understood to mean she is erotically attracted to other women. "Lesbian" loses its meaning if the woman says she feels she *is* a man and lives as one. She insists, "I am a heterosexual man; men are attracted to women as am I!" The baffled clinician may erroneously think, "You are a female therefore you are a lesbian!" DSM-IV suggests that adults with GIDs should be subgrouped according to which sex the patient is currently sexually attracted: males, females, both, or neither. This makes sense for most gender patients because it is their gender identity that is most important to them. Some are rigid about the sex of those to whom they are attracted because it supports their idea about their gender, others are bierotic and are not too concerned with their orientation, still others have not had enough experiences to overcome their uncertainty about their orientation. A few

gender patients find all partners too complicated and are only interested in themselves (Blanchard 1989).

## Treatment Options for the Gender Identity Disorders

The treatment of these conditions, although not as well-based on scientific evidence as some psychiatric disorders, has been carefully scrutinized by multidisciplinary committees of specialists within the Harry Benjamin International Gender Dysphoria Association for over 20 years. For more details in managing an individual patient, please consult its "Standards of Care" (Meyer et al. 2001). The treatment of any GID begins after a careful evaluation, including parents, other family members, spouses, psychometric testing, and occasionally physical and laboratory examination. The details will depend on age of the patient. It is possible, of course, to have a GID as well as mental retardation, a psychosis, dysthymia, severe character pathology, or any other psychiatric diagnosis (Table 74–8).

## Individual Psychotherapy

No one knows how to cure an adult's gender problem. People who have long lived with profound cross-gender identifications do not get insight—either behaviorally modified or medicated—and find that they subsequently have a conventional gender identity. Psychotherapy is useful, nonetheless (Lothstein et al. 1981). If the patient is able to trust a therapist, there can be much to talk about—family relationships are often painful, barriers to relationship intimacy are profound, work poses many difficult issues, and the patient has to make monumental decisions. The central one is, "How am I going to live my life? Should I go through with cross-gender living, hormone therapy, mastectomy, or

| Table 74–8 | Steps in Evaluation of the Profoundly Gender Disordered* |
|---|---|

Formal evaluation and diagnosis—gender identity disorder or gender identity disorder NOS. Can the patient be referred to a gender program? Is another treatable psychiatric or physical disorder present?

Individual psychotherapy within the gender program or with an interested professional. Do the diagnoses remain the same? If yes, does the patient consistently want to

    Discuss his (or her) situation but make no changes?

    Increase cross-dressing toward cross-living?

    Prepare the family for the real-life test?

    Obtain permission to proceed with hormones?

Approval for hormones from a gender committee or on written recommendation from the psychiatrist to an endocrinologist. Individual or group psychotherapy should continue.

Real-life test of living and working full time in the aspired-to gender role for at least 1 year. Does the patient want to continue to surgery?

Gender committee approval for surgery. Many patients have cosmetic surgery other than that listed with only ordinary patient–surgeon consent. This most often involves breast augmentation but may include numerous other attempts to improve ability to pass as opposite sex and be attractive.

    Men—genital reconstruction

    Women—mastectomy, hysterectomy, genital reconstruction

*Most patients will not complete all of these steps.

genital surgery?" The therapist can help the patient recognize the drawbacks and advantages of the various available options and to respect the initially unrecognized or unstated ambivalence. Completion of the gender transformation process usually takes longer than the patient desires, and the therapist can be an important source of support during and after these changes.

## Group Therapy

Group therapy for gender-disordered people has the advantages of allowing patients to know others with gender problems, of decreasing their social isolation, and of being among people who do not experience their cross-gender aspirations and their past behaviors as weird (Keller et al. 1982). Group members can provide help with grooming and more convincing public appearances. The success of these groups depends on the therapist's skills in patient selection and using the group process. Groups are generally only available in a few specialized treatment programs.

## "Real-Life Test"

Living in the aspired-to-gender role—working, relating, conducting the activities of daily living—is a vital process that enables one of three decisions: to abandon the quest, to simply live in this new role, or to proceed with breast or genital surgery (Peterson and Dickey 1995). Some clinicians use the real-life test as a criterion for recommending hormones but this varies because some patients' abilities to present themselves in a new way is definitely enhanced by prior administration of cross-sex hormones. The reason for the real-life test is to give the patient, who created a transsexual solution in fantasy, an opportunity to experience the solution in social reality. Passing the real-life test is expected to be associated with improved psychological function (Blanchard et al. 1985).

## Hormone Therapy

Ideally, hormones should be administered by endocrinologists who have a working relationship with a mental health team dealing with gender problems. The effects of administration of estrogen to a biological male are: breast development, testicular atrophy, decreased sexual drive, decreased semen volume and fertility, softening of skin, fat redistribution in a female pattern, and decrease in spontaneous erections. Breast development is often the highest concern to the patient. Because hair growth is not affected by estrogens, electrolysis is often used to remove beard growth. Side effects within recommended doses are minimal but hypertension, hyperglycemia, lipid abnormalities, thrombophlebitis, and hepatic dysfunction have been described. The most dramatic effect of hormones is on the sense of well-being. Patients report feeling calmer, happier knowing that their bodies are being demasculinized and feminized. All results derive from open-labeled studies.

The administration of androgen to females results in an increased sexual drive, clitoral tingling and growth, weight gain, and amenorrhea and hoarseness. An increase in muscle mass may be apparent if weight training is undertaken simultaneously. Hair growth depends on the patient's genetic potential. Androgens are administrated intramuscularly 200 to 300 mg/month and are generally safe. It is prudent, however, to periodically monitor hepatic, lipid,

and thyroid functioning. Most patients are delighted with their bodily changes, although some are disappointed that they remain short, wide-hipped, relatively hairless men with breasts that do not significantly regress.

## Surgical Therapy

Surgical intervention is the final external step. It should not occur without mental health professional's input, even when the patient provides a heart-felt convincing set of reasons to bypass the real-life test, hormones, and therapeutic relationship. Genital surgery is expensive, time-consuming, at times painful, and has frequent anatomic complications and functional disappointments. Surgery can be expected to add further improvements in the lives of patients (Mate-Cole et al. 1990)—more social activities with friends and family, more activity in sports, more partner sexual activity, and improved vocational status.

**Males.** Surgery consists of penectomy, orchiectomy, vaginoplasty, and fashioning of a labia. The procedures used for the creation of a neovagina have evolved over the years. Postoperatively, the patient must maintain the patency of the neovagina by initially constantly wearing and then periodically using a vaginal dilator. Vaginal stenosis or shortening is a frequent complication (McEwan et al. 1986). The quest for an unmistakable feminine shape leads many young adult patients to augmentation mammoplasty and the shaving of their cricoid cartilage.

**Females.** The creation of a male-appearing chest through mastectomies and contouring of the chest wall requires only a brief hospital stay. Patients are usually immediately delighted with their new-found freedom, but their fantasies of going shirtless are often not fulfilled due to the presence of two noticeable horizontal chest scars. The creation of a neophallus that can become erect, contain a functional urethra throughout its length (enabling urination while standing), and pass as an unremarkable penis in a locker room has been a significant surgical challenge. It is far from perfected (Gilbert et al. 1988). The surgery is, however, the most time-consuming, technically difficult, and expensive of all the sex reassignment procedures. Erection is made possible by a penile prosthesis. Many prudent patients consider themselves reassigned when they have a hysterectomy, oophorectomy, and mastectomy. Some just have a mastectomy. They find a partner who understands the situation and supports the idea of living with, and loving with, female genitals.

## THE PARAPHILIAS

A paraphilia is a disorder of intention, the final component of sexual identity to develop in children and adolescents. Intention refers to what individuals want to do with a sexual partner and what they want the partner to do with them during sexual behavior. Normally, the images and the behaviors of intention fall within ranges of peaceable mutuality. The disorders of intention are recognized by unusual eroticism (images) and often socially destructive behaviors such as sex with children, rape, exhibitionism, voyeurism, masochism, obscene phone calling, or sexual touching of strangers. While 5% of the diagnoses of paraphilia are given to women, etiologic speculations refer to male sexual identity development gone awry. This raises the important question about what happens to girls who have the same developmental misfortunes that are speculated to create male paraphilia (Beier 2000). Accounts of paraphilic behaviors have been in the nonmedical literatures for centuries, but they have been of psychiatric interest only since 1905 (Freud 1905). Freud thought of the paraphilias as deviations in the aim of the sexual instinct. He coined the term by combining the Greek words for "along the side" (*para*) and "love" (*philia*). In 1905, paraphilia denoted those fixed preferences for sexual behaviors that led to forms of orgasmic attainment other than the uniting of penis and vagina.

Now it is apparent that paraphilias occur among individuals of all orientations and among those with conventional and unconventional gender identities. A homosexual sadist is paraphilic only on the basis of sexual cruelty. A transsexual who desires to be beaten during arousal is paraphilic only on the basis of masochism.

## Three General Characteristics of the Paraphilias

### A Longstanding, Unusual, Highly-Arousing Erotic Preoccupation

Erotic intentions that are not longstanding, unusual, and highly arousing may be problematic in some way but they are *not* clearly paraphilic. The *sine qua non* of the diagnosis of paraphilia is unusual, often hostile, dehumanized eroticism which has preoccupied the patient for most of his adolescent and adult life. The paraphilic fantasy is often associated with this preoccupying arousal when it occurs in daydreams and masturbation reveries or is encountered in explicit films or magazines. The specific imagery varies from one paraphilic patient to the next, but both the imagined behavior and its implied relationship to the partner are unusual in that they are preoccupied with aggression. Images of rape, obscene phone calling, exhibitionism, and touching of strangers, for example, are rehearsals of victimization. In masochistic images, the aggression is directed at the self—for instance, autoerotic strangulation, slavery, torture, spanking. In others, the aggression is well-disguised as *love* of children or teenagers. In some, such as simple clothing fetishism, the aggression may be absent. Aggression is so apparent in most paraphilic content, however, that when none seems to exist, the clinician needs to wonder whether it is actually absent or being hidden from the doctor. Paraphilic fantasies often rely heavily upon the image of a partner who does not possess "personhood." Some imagery in fact has no pretense of a human partner at all; clothing, animals, or excretory products are the focus. Other themes such as preoccupation with feet or hair, combine both human and inanimate interests. Paraphilic images are usually devoid of any pretense of caring or human attachment. The hatred, anger, fear, vengeance, or worthlessness expressed in them require no familiarity with the partner. Paraphilic images are conscious—clearly known to the individual. They should not be confused with speculations about "unconscious" aggression or sadomasochism that some assume are part of all sexual behavior (Kernberg 1991). Clinicians should expect to occasionally see paraphilic patients whose preoccupations are not hostile to others.

An individual's paraphilic themes often change in intensity or seem to change in content from time to time. The stimuli for these changes often remain unclear. It is a moot point whether changes should be considered a shift to a different disorder, a new paraphilia, or a natural evolution of the basic problem. The shifts from imagining talking "dirty" on the phone in order to scare a woman to imagining raping can be considered an intensification of sadism. Switches between sadism and masochism or voyeurism and exhibitionism are common. Changes from voyeurism to pedophilia or from pedophilia to rape, however, raise the question whether a new disorder has developed. The most socially significant shifts are from erotic imagery to sexual behavior. In most instances, it is reasonable to consider that paraphilia is a basic developmental disorder in which particular erotic and sexual manifestations are shaped by the individuality of the person's history.

Most paraphilic adults can trace their fantasy themes to puberty and many can remember these images from earlier years. When adolescent rapists or incest offenders are evaluated, they often are able to report prepubertal aggressive erotic preoccupations. Men who report periodic paraphilic imagery interspersed with more usual eroticism have had their paraphilic themes from childhood or early adolescence. To make a diagnosis of paraphilia, the patient must evidence at least 6 months of the unusual erotic preoccupation. Duration is usually not in question, even among adolescents, however (Shaw 1999).

### Pressure to Act Out the Fantasy

To be paraphilic means that the erotic imagery exerts a pressure to play out the often imagined scene. In its milder forms, the pressure results merely in a preoccupation with a behavior. For instance, a man who prefers to be spoken to harshly and dominated by his wife during sex thinks about his masochistic images primarily around their sexual behaviors. He does not spend hours daydreaming of his erotic preferences. In its more intense forms, paraphilias create a *drivenness* to act out the fantasy in sexual behavior—usually in masturbation. Frequent masturbation, often more than once daily, continues long after adolescence. In the most severe situations, the need to attend to the fantasy and masturbate is so overpowering that life's ordinary activities cannot efficiently occur. Masturbation and sometimes partner-seeking behavior—such as finding a woman to shock through exhibiting an erection—is experienced as driven. The patient reports either that he cannot control his behavior or he controls it with such great effort that his work, study, parenting, and relationships are disrupted. This pressure to behave sexually often leads the man to believe he has a high sex drive. Some severe paraphilics describe their masturbation-to-orgasm frequencies as 10/day. Even when the patient's estimate of his frequency of orgasm strains credulity less, the return of sexual drive manifestations so soon after orgasm suggests that either something is wrong with the patients' sexual drive generator, their satiety mechanisms, or that their existential anxiety overpowers their other defense mechanisms.

Paraphilic men often report collecting and viewing pornography, visiting sexual book stores to see explicit videos or peep shows, frequenting prostitutes for their special sexual behaviors, downloading explicit images from the Internet, or extensively using telephone sex services or strip clubs. Victimization of others, the public health problem, is the least common form of sexual acting out but it is by no means rare (Abel et al. 1987). When the behavioral diagnosis of exhibitionism, pedophilia, or sadism is made, the clinician should assume that the numbers of victims far exceed the number stated in the criminal charges.

Two other conditions, compulsive sexual behavior and sexual addiction not part of the DSM-IV, are informally and synonymously used to refer to heterosexual and homosexual men and women who display an intense drivenness to behave sexually without paraphilic imagery. The personal, interpersonal, and medical consequences of paraphilic and nonparaphilic sexual compulsivity seem indistinguishable as do their usual psychiatric comorbidities: depression, anxiety disorders, substance abuse, and attention deficit disorders (Kafka and Prentky 1998).

## Partner Sexual Dysfunction

A severe sexual dysfunction involving desire, arousal, or orgasm with a partner, although not invariably present among paraphilics, often is (Pawlak 1991). The wives of paraphilics tell stories with these themes: "He is not interested in sex with me." "He never initiates." "He doesn't seem to enjoy our sexual life together except when...." "He is usually not potent." "Even when we do make love, he rarely ejaculates." Some paraphilic men however are able to function well without paraphilic fantasies but others are either able to primarily function when their partners are willing to meet their special requirements for arousal or when they fantasize about their paraphilic script (Abel 1989).

## Speculations About the Underlying Problem

Paraphilia has been considered in 15 somewhat different ways, depending on era, ideology, and region: (1) an impairment in the bonding function of sexuality; (2) a courtship disorder; (3) the erotic form of hatred motivated by the need for revenge for childhood trauma; (4) a fixation to childhood misunderstandings that women had penises and that men could lose theirs during sex (castration anxiety); (5) the unsuccessful repair of early life passive, helpless experiences with a terrifying, malignant, malicious preoedipal mother; (6) a strategy to stabilize a conventional masculine or feminine gender identity; (7) a strategy to deny the differences between the sexes and the generations of child and parent; (8) an outcome of childhood sexual abuse; (9) a consequence of far less than ideal parent–child relationships; (10) a soft neurological sign of a neural wiring defect; (11) a released behavior due to cerebral pathology—for example, temporal lobe dysfunction, or substance abuse; (12) the sexual face of an addiction disorder; (13) an unusual manifestation of an affective disorder; (14) an obsessive–compulsive spectrum disorder; (15) a defective self-system requiring a patch—that is, a sexual preoccupation—to shore up the private, carefully-hidden-from-others sense of inadequate subjective masculinity.

Whatever its ultimate etiologies and nature, the paraphilias are sexual identity disorders that generally make normal erotic and sexual loving unattainable. Culture asks us to have some image of attachment, some ability to neutralize anger toward others, some ability to contain the anxiety over closeness, and some psychological motive to simultaneously enhance the self and the partner through

sexual contact. Ordinary intentions aim for peaceable mutuality between real people; paraphilic ones aim at aggressive one-sidedness. This sexual identity disorder could be referred to as a disorder of self, specifically of that part of the self that maintains a sense of masculinity. Paraphilics often bear an enigmatic paradox between what they want to be and what they are. They often hunger for a behavior which feels uncontrollable or sick and which robs them of autonomy. This is why the behaviors are often thought of as addictions and are often associated with other forms of substance abuse, obsessive–compulsive phenomena, and affective symptoms. Relative to the dynamic fluctuations of sexual dysfunctions, intention disorders are tenacious throughout life.

## The Specific Paraphilias

## Criminal Sex Offending Behaviors

### Exhibitionism

Exhibitionism generally involves teenagers and men displaying their penises so that the witness will be shocked or (in the paraphilic's fantasy) sexually interested. They may or may not masturbate during or immediately following this act of victimization. This diagnosis is not usually made when a man is arrested for "public indecency" and his penile exposures are motivated to arrange homosexual contact in a public place generally unseen by heterosexuals. Penile display in parks is one way to make anonymous contact. The presence or absence of exhibitionistic imagery allows the clinician to make the distinction between paraphilia and homosexual courting.

### Pedophilia

Pedophilia is the most widely and intensely socially repudiated of the paraphilias. Pedophiles are men who erotically and romantically prefer children or young adolescents. They are grouped into categories depending upon their erotic preferences for boys or girls and for infant, young, or pubertal children. Some pedophiles have highly age- and sex-specific tastes, others are less discriminating. Since the diagnosis of pedophilia requires that over a period of at least 6 months, recurrent, intense sexually arousing fantasies, sexual urges, or behaviors involving sexual activity with a prepubescent child or children, the disorder should not be expected to be present in every person who is guilty of child molestation. Some intrafamilial child abuse occurs over a shorter time interval and results from combinations of deteriorated marriages, sexual deprivation, sociopathy, and substance abuse. Child molestation, whether paraphilic or not, is a crime, however. Child molesters show several patterns of erectile responses to visual stimulation in the laboratory. Some have their largest arousal to children of a specific age and others respond to both children and adults (Barbaree and Marshall 1989). Others respond with their greatest arousal to aggressive cues.

### Voyeurism

Men whose sexual life consist of watching homosexual or heterosexual videos in sexual book stores occasionally come to psychiatric attention after being charged with a crime following a police raid. They may or may not qualify for

## DSM-IV-TR Criteria 302.82

**Voyeurism**

A. Over a period of at least 6 months, recurrent, intense sexually arousing fantasies, sexual urges, or behaviors involving the act of observing an unsuspecting person who is naked, in the process of disrobing, or engaging in sexual activity.

B. The fantasies, sexual urges, or behaviors cause clinically significant distress or impairment in social, occupational, or other important areas of functioning.

Reprinted with permission from the Diagnostic and Statistical Manual of Mental Disorders, Fourth Edition, Text Revision. Copyright 2000 American Psychiatric Association.

this diagnosis. The voyeurs who are more problematic for society are those who watch women through windows or break into their dwellings for this purpose. Some of these crimes result in rape or nonsexual violence, but many are motivated by pure voyeuristic intent (which is subtly aggressive).

## Sexual Sadism

While rape is an extreme variety of sadism, paraphilic sadism is present only in a minority of rapists. It is defined by the rapist's prior use of erotic scripts that involve a partner's fear, pain, humiliation, and suffering. Rapists are highly dangerous men whose antisocial behaviors are generally thought to be unresponsive to ordinary psychiatric methods. Their violence potential often makes psychiatric therapy outside of institutions imprudent. Noncriminal paraphilic sadism—that is, arousal to images of harming another that has not crossed into the behavioral realm, can be treated in outpatient settings.

## DSM-IV-TR Criteria 302.84

**Sexual Sadism**

A. Over a period of at least 6 months, recurrent, intense sexually arousing fantasies, sexual urges, or behaviors involving acts (real, not simulated) in which the psychological or physical suffering (including humiliation) of the victim is sexually exciting to the person.

B. The fantasies, sexual urges, or behaviors cause clinically significant distress or impairment in social, occupational, or other important areas of functioning.

Reprinted with permission from the Diagnostic and Statistical Manual of Mental Disorders, Fourth Edition, Text Revision. Copyright 2000 American Psychiatric Association.

## DSM-IV-TR Criteria 302.89

**Frotteurism**

A. Over a period of at least 6 months, recurrent, intense sexually arousing fantasies, sexual urges, or behaviors involving touching and rubbing against a nonconsenting person.

B. The fantasies, sexual urges, or behaviors cause clinically significant distress or impairment in social, occupational, or other important areas of functioning.

Reprinted with permission from the Diagnostic and Statistical Manual of Mental Disorders, Fourth Edition, Text Revision. Copyright 2000 American Psychiatric Association.

### Frotteurism

Frotteurism, the need to touch and rub against nonconsenting persons, although delineated as a criminal act, is probably better understood as the most socially benign form of paraphilic sadism. Frotteurism often occurs in socially isolated men who become sexually driven to act out. They often are unaware of how frightening they can be.

### Stalking

Stalking is the latest erotic preoccupation to be criminalized. Forensic psychiatry has defined various motivations for arrested stalkers, including those who have made the transition from romantic to violent preoccupation with the victim. Stalking is particularly frightening because murder occasionally results. It is likely that stalking as a behavior is the product of further deterioration of an already compromised mind, although not necessarily a paraphilic one.

Clinical Vignette 4

A 43-year-old married policeman was incarcerated after evidence linked him to six rapes. Five years prior to his arrest, he described to his psychotherapist the adolescent beginning of lifelong eroticisation of stalking. He masturbated to images of following woman years before he began to incorporate rape into the scenario. He spent much of his leisure time selecting women visually, finding out about them, and following them. The vast majority of his "victims" were never aware of his stalking behaviors, but these behaviors fuelled his more than daily masturbation. He claimed and his wife confirmed that for most of their marriage he had no apparent sexual interest in her.

### Noncriminal Forms of Paraphilia

Because the individual manifestations of paraphilia depend on the particular individual life history of the affected, over forty paraphilic categories have been identified (Money 1986), although only a few are listed in the DSM-IV. Most of these are unusual means of attaining arousal during masturbation or consenting partner behaviors. Each of the themes identified below demonstrate a wide

## DSM-IV-TR Criteria 302.81

**Fetishism**

A. Over a period of at least 6 months, recurrent, intense sexually arousing fantasies, sexual urges, or behaviors involving the use of nonliving objects (e.g., female undergarments).

B. The fantasies, sexual urges, or behaviors cause clinically significant distress or impairment in social, occupational, or other important areas of functioning.

C. The fetish objects are not limited to articles of female clothing used in cross-dressing (as in transvestic fetishism) or devices designed for the purpose of tactile genital stimulation (e.g., a vibrator).

range of manifestations from the bizarre to the more "reasonable" and from the common to the unique. They often subtly combine elements of more than one paraphilia.

### Fetishism

Fetishism, the pairing of arousal with wearing or holding an article of clothing or inanimate object such as an inflatable doll, has a range of manifestations from infantilism in which a person dresses up in diapers to pretend he is a baby to the far more common use of a female undergarment for arousal purposes. Fetishism when confined to one garment for decades is classified as a paraphilia, but many cases involve more complex varieties of cross-dressing and overlap with gender identity disorders, usually GIDNOS. Fetishistic transvestism is the diagnosis used when it is apparent that the urges to use the clothing of the opposite sex is part of a larger mental preoccupation with that sex.

### Sexual Masochism

Sexual masochism is diagnosed over a range of behaviors from the sometimes fatal need to nearly asphyxiate oneself to the request to be spanked by the partner in order to be excited. Masochism may be the most commonly reported or acknowledged form of female paraphilia, although it is more common among men. Sadists and masochists sometimes find one another and work out arrangement to act out their fantasies and occasionally reverse roles.

### Paraphilia Not Otherwise Specified

Paraphilia not otherwise specified is a DSM-IV category for other endpoints of abnormal sexual development that lead to preoccupations with amputated body parts, feces, urine, sexualized enemas, and sex with animals.

### Treatment

Four general approaches are employed to treat the paraphilias. The treatments are not mutually exclusive, rather they are often multimodal in application.

## DSM-IV-TR Criteria 302.83

**Sexual Masochism**

A. Over a period of at least 6 months, recurrent, intense sexually arousing fantasies, sexual urges, or behaviors involving the act (real, not simulated) of being humiliated, beaten, bound, or otherwise made to suffer.

B. The fantasies, sexual urges, or behaviors cause clinically significant distress or impairment in social, occupational, or other important areas of functioning.

## DSM-IV-TR Criteria 302.03

**Transvestic Fetishism**

A. Over a period of at least 6 months, in a heterosexual male, recurrent intense sexually arousing fantasies, sexual urges, or behaviors involving cross-dressing.

B. The fantasies, sexual urges, or behaviors cause clinically significant distress or impairment in social, occupational, or other important areas of functioning.

*Specify* if:

**With gender dysphoria:** if the person has persistent discomfort with gender role or identity

### Evaluation Only

Evaluation only is often selected when the evaluator concludes that the paraphilia is benign in terms of society, the patient will be resistant to the other approaches, and does not suffer greatly in terms of social and vocational functioning in ways that might be improved. Often these are isolated men with private paraphilic sexual pleasures, such as telephone sex with a masochistic scenario.

### Psychotherapy

What constitutes psychotherapy for paraphilia heavily depends on the therapist training rather than strident declarations of treatment of choice. Little optimism exists that any form of therapy can permanently change the nature of a long established paraphilic erotic script, even among teenage sex offenders. Individual psychodynamic psychotherapy can be highly useful in diminishing paraphilic intensifications and gradually teaching the patient better management techniques of the situations that have triggered acting out. Well-described cognitive–behavioral interventions exist for interrupting paraphilic arousal via pairing masturbatory excitement with either aversive imagery or aversive stimuli. Comprehensive behavioral treatment involves social skills training, assertiveness training, and confrontation with the rationalizations that are used to minimize awareness of the victims of sexual crimes, and marital therapy (Abel 1995). The self-help movement has created 12-step programs for sexual addictions to which many individuals now belong. Group psychotherapy is offered by trained therapists as well. When the lives of paraphilics are illuminated in various therapies, it becomes apparent that the emotional pain of the patients is thought to be great; the sexual acting out is often perceived as a defense against recurrent unpleasant emotions from any source. These often, however, involve self-esteem and primitive anxiety.

## Medications

In the early 1980s, depo-medroxy-progesterone (Provera) was first used to treat those who were constantly masturbating, seeking out personally dangerous sexual outlets, or committing sex crimes. The weekly 400 to 600 mg injections often led to the men being able to work, study, or participate in activities that were previously beyond them because of concentration or attention difficulties (Gijs and Gooren 1996). In the late 1980s, the use of oral Provera, 20 to 120 mg/day led to similar results: the drug enabled these men to leave their former state in which their sexual needs took priority over other life demands—and they did not have depo-Provera's side effect profile: weight gain, hypertension, muscle cramps, and gynecomastia. Today, gonadotrophin-releasing blockers are occasionally used for this purpose (Kreuger and Kaplan 2001). The possible side effects are similar to oral Provera. Despite the fact that the clinical results are among the most powerful effected by any psychopharmacologic treatment, many psychiatrists cannot overcome their disinclination about giving a "female" hormone to a man or working with patients who victimize others sexually. Serotonergic agents are now more commonly used as a first line of treatment and their administration, of course, creates fewer countertransference obstacles (Risen and Althof 1995). While these studies are not as methodologically sophisticated as they need to be, the SSRIs are in widespread use for compulsive sexual behaviors and sexual obsessions. Their efficacy is the source of the speculation that some of the paraphilias may be an obsessive–compulsive spectrum disorder.

## External Controls

Sexual advantage-taking, whether it be by a paraphilic physician with his patients, by a pedophilic mentally retarded man in the neighborhood, or of a grandfather who has abused several generations of his offspring, can often be stopped by making it *impossible* for these behaviors to be *un*known to most people in his life. The doctor's staff can be told, the neighbors can know, the family can meet to discuss the current crisis and review who has been abused over the years and plan to never allow grandfather alone with any child in or outside the family. The concept of external control is taken over by the judicial system when sex crimes are highly repugnant or heinous. The offender is removed from society for punishment and the protection of the public. Increasing pressure exists to criminalize sexual advantage-taking by physicians who are even more susceptible to losing their medical licenses at least for several years.

Psychiatrists need to be realistic about the limitations of various therapeutic ventures. Sexual acting out may readily continue during therapy beyond the awareness of the therapist (Travin 1995). The more violent and destructive the paraphilic behavior to others, the less the therapist should risk ambulatory treatment. Since paraphilia occurs in patients with other psychiatric conditions, the psychiatrist needs to remain vigilant that the treatment program is comprehensive and does not lose sight of the paraphilia just because the depressive or compulsive symptoms are improved. Paraphilia may be improved by medications and psychotherapy but the clinician should expect that the intention disorder is the patient's lasting vulnerability.

## SEXUAL DISORDER NOT OTHERWISE SPECIFIED

If the clinician is uncertain about how to categorize a person's problem, it is more reasonable to use this diagnosis than one that does not encompass the range of the patient's suffering. Sexual disorder not otherwise specified can be used when the therapist perceives a dramatic interplay between issues of sexual identity and sexual dysfunction, or when "everything" seems to be amiss. DSM-IV-TR, however, encourages the clinician to make multiple sexual diagnoses involving, for instance, a gender identity disorder, a desire disorder, erectile, and orgasmic disorder.

DSM-IV-TR provides two examples when it would be appropriate to use the diagnosis sexual disorder NOS: (1) nonparaphilic compulsive sexual behaviors—that is, relentless pursuit of masturbatory or heterosexual or homosexual partner experiences without evidence of paraphilic imagery; (2) complicated or exaggerated struggles to manage homosexual urges. Despite the removal of homosexuality from the DSM in 1974 (Bayer 1981), men (particularly) and women still generate symptoms in their struggle to balance the demands of their homoeroticism with their ambitions to participate in conventional family life. This ongoing struggle can generate a variety of anxiety, depressive, compulsive, substance abusing, and suicidal states.

---

Clinical Vignette 5

A 45-year-old married, mustached, corporate middle manager, father of four sons ages 16 to 25 years, sought help for 3 years of consistent, and a decade of episodic, erectile dysfunction with his wife. He often failed to find their functional sexual behavior deeply satisfying. What concerned him more immediately however were his "addictions" to masturbation and watching homosexual pornography and his preoccupations with fellatio, anal receptive intercourse, and thoughts of having intercourse with women entertainers of different races. Ever since he arranged for a man to perform fellatio on him 3 years ago and he found it to be the most thrilling sex of his life, he has been unable to get homosexual imagery out of his mind. His masturbation dramatically increased (he began to masturbate at work) and he began having images of receiving anal penetration (sometimes accompanied by inserting his finger into his anus). He began cruising

Clinical Vignette 5 *continued*

bookstores looking for mustached, handsome, masculine men with whom to perform and receive fellatio. His participation in Sex and Love Addicts Anonymous meetings had become insincere; the stories he heard greatly excited him and he worried that his befriending others often just led to negotiations for sex. His sexual experiences with his wife now could only be maintained by the fantasy that he was with a man. He reported that a previous therapist after hearing about his periodic adolescent homoerotic fantasies and his 3 years of cruising told him during their first session, "Face it. You are simply gay." This greatly distressed the patient. When, during the second visit, he sensed that the therapist might have been trying to seduce him, he decided not to return.

Treatment with a serotonergic agent dramatically diminished his erotic preoccupations. After months of dramatic benefit from this "miracle," he began to periodically stop the medication so that his homoerotic thoughts would return and he could cruise for homosexual sex on business trips. His discussions in twice-monthly, half-hour therapy eventually led to more motivation to engage in sex with his wife and eventually his potency with her improved. He could not, however, dependably ejaculate in her vagina. He was able to masturbate to orgasm in her presence after he brought her to numerous orgasms during intercourse. He preferred not to recall his thwarted hunger for closeness to his mustached father, his two molestation experiences with a priest as a 16-year-old, and his feelings about his sons' emerging sexual expressions. When his and his wife's best male friend died from a malignancy within 6 weeks of initial diagnosis, he experienced an upsurge in compulsivity that kept him from thinking about his loss.

"I don't think I am simply gay. I don't like the gay lifestyle. I can't stand effeminacy in men! My good life with my family and in the corporation would be destroyed. I don't even think of me that way. I am some kind of bisexual. I just love homosexual sex. I want to suck and be sucked. I think it would be great to be screwed up the ass. But I'm too afraid of AIDS to do it. I'd like to screw a woman rock star or two, but that is probably not very likely." At various times, his mental state could accurately be described as largely depressed, anxious, paranoid, obsessive, compulsive, or dissociated. He feels dishonesty with his wife is the best policy even when she inquires whether he is a homosexual.

Here is an 8-year follow-up. Married still, a grandfather several times over, still working for the same corporation, he has come to recognize that he is far more homosexual than heterosexual, is disinterested in sex with his wife who still accuses him of being gay because of his sexual dysfunctions and his pleasures in travelling, and has had differential response to sildenafil. The drug barely works with his wife who also takes it, but it routinely enhances his sexual capacity with a man. He actually does not need it with a male partner but uses it with a sense of enhancement. Mustached men still excite him but he has sex with other men without disappointment. He loves anal sex and occasionally permits condomless contact. These invariably create months of obsession about getting AIDS and repeated HIV testing. "Let's face it," he recently told me, "I'm gay but I never want anyone in my family to ever discover it."

## FINAL THOUGHTS

A specific diagnosis like vaginismus or GIDNOS does not, per se, dictate the type and course of therapy. The clinician is called upon to weigh many factors in planning treatment. Accurate diagnosis is a vital first step but it quickly gives way to other, more artful considerations. "What factors set up this problem and what forces maintain it? What is the essence of this situation? What does this diagnosis mean in ordinary human terms? Can medication play a useful role? How am I to help? What am I to say? When and how should I say it?" These are essentially psychotherapy considerations. The sexual disorders challenge the doctor to integrate the advances of modern psychiatry with the traditions of less biologically-oriented psychiatry and the knowledge accumulating in forensic settings for the purpose of seeing if the patient's distress can be lastingly altered. In this challenge, clinical science inevitably gives way to clinical art. The art involves enabling the patient's distress to make sense so that the underlying struggle—the developmental task—can be successfully negotiated.

### Comparison of DSM-IV/ICD-10 Diagnostic Criteria

For hypoactive sexual desire disorder, the ICD-10 Diagnostic Criteria for Research and the DSM-IV-TR criteria are essentially identical except that ICD-10 specifies a minimum duration of at least 6 months (DSM-IV-TR has no minimum duration).

The ICD-10 Diagnostic Criteria for Research for Sexual Aversion Disorder differs from the DSM-IV-TR criteria in several ways. In contrast to DSM-IV-TR which restricts the condition to the aversion to, and avoidance of, sexual genital contact, ICD-10 also includes presentations characterized by sexual activity resulting in "strong negative feelings and an inability to experience any pleasure." Furthermore, ICD-10 excludes cases in which the aversion is due to performance anxiety. Finally, ICD-10 specifies a minimum duration of at least 6 month whereas DSM-IV-TR does not specify any minimum duration.

For female sexual arousal disorder and male erectile disorder, the ICD-10 Diagnostic Criteria for Research and the DSM-IV-TR criteria are essentially equivalent except that ICD-10 specifies a minimum duration of at least 6 months. ICD-10 includes a single category ("Failure of Genital Response") with two separate criteria sets by gender. In contrast, DSM-IV-TR includes tow separate categories.

For female and male orgasmic disorders, the ICD-10 Diagnostic Criteria for Research and the DSM-IV-TR criteria are essentially equivalent except that ICD-10 specifies a minimum duration of at least 6 months. In contrast to DSM-IV-TR which has male and female versions defined separately, ICD-10 has a single category that applies to both genders.

For premature ejaculation, the ICD-10 Diagnostic Criteria for Research and the DSM-IV-TR criteria are essentially equivalent except that ICD-10 specifies a minimum duration of at least 6 months. Similarly, the ICD-10 Diagnostic Criteria for Research and the DSM-IV-TR criteria for Dyspareunia and Vaginismus are essentially equivalent except that ICD-10 specifies a minimum duration of at least 6 months. Furthermore, these conditions are referred to in ICD-10 as "Nonorganic Dyspareunia" and "Nonorganic Vaginismus."

The definition of a paraphillia is essentially the same in DSM-IV-TR and ICD-10. However, ICD-10 does not include a separate category for Frotteurism and has a combined "Sadomasochism" category.

For gender identity disorder, ICD-10 defines three separate disorders: "Gender Identity Disorder of Childhood," "Dual-role Transvestism," and "Transsexualism" all of which are included under the single DSM-IV-TR category Gender Identity Disorder.

## References

Abel GG (1989) Paraphilias. In Comprehensive Textbook of Psychiatry, Vol. V, Kaplan and Sadock (eds). Williams & Wilkins, Baltimore, pp. 1069–1085.

Abel GG and Osborn CA (1995) Behavioral therapy treatment for sex offenders. In Sexual Deviation, 3rd ed., Rosen I (ed). Oxford University Press, London.

Abel GG, Becker JV, Mittelman MS, et al. (1987) Self-reported sex crimes of nonincarcerated paraphiliacs. J Interpers Viol 2, 3.

Althof SE and Seftel AD (1995) The evaluation and management of erectile dysfunction. Psychiatr Clin N Am 18(1), 177–192.

Althof SE, Levine SB, Corty E, et al. (1995) Double-blind crossover study of clomipramine for rapid ejaculation in 15 couples. J Clin Psychiatr 56(9), 402–407.

American Psychiatric Association (1994) Diagnostic and Statistical Manual, 4th ed. APA, Washington DC.

Barbaree HE and Marshall WL (1995) Erectile responses amongst heterosexual child molesters. Can J Behav Sci.

Basson R (2001) Using a different model for female sexual response to address women's problematic low sexual desire. J Sex Marit Ther 27, 395–403.

Basson R (2003) Women's difficulties with low desire and sexual avoidance. In Handbook of Clinical Sexuality for Mental Health Professionals, Levine SB, Risen CB, and Althof SE (eds). Brunner/Routledge, New York.

Basson R, McInnes R, Smith MD, et al. (2002) Efficacy and safety of sildenafil citrate in women with sexual dysfunction associated with female sexual arousal disorder. J Women's Health Gender-Based Stud 11(4), 367–377.

Bayer R (1981) Homosexuality and American Psychiatry: The Politics of Diagnosis. Basic Books, New York.

Beier KM (2000) Female analogies to perversion. J Sex Marit Ther 26, 79–91.

Berman JR and Goldstein I (2001) Female sexual dysfunction. Urol Clin N Am 28(2) (May), 405–416.

Berman JR, Berman LA, Lin H, et al. (2001) Effect of sildenafil on subjective and physiologic parameters of female sexual response in women with sexual arousal disorder. J Sex Marit Ther 27, 411–420.

Blanchard R (1989) The concept of autogynephilia and the typology of male gender dysphoria. J Nerv Ment Dis 177, 616–623.

Blanchard R, Steiner BW, and Clemmensen LH (1985) Gender dysphoria, gender reorientation, and the clinical management of transsexualism. J Consult Clin Psychol 53, 295–304.

Carrier S, Brock G, Kour NW, et al. (1993) Pathophysiology of erectile dysfunction. Urology 42(4), 468–481.

Coates S and Person E (1985) Extreme boyhood femininity: Isolated behavior or pervasive disorder? J Am Acad Child Psychiatr 24, 702–709.

Coates S, Friedman RC, and Wolfe S (1992) The etiology of boyhood gender identity disorder: A model for integrating psychodynamics, temperament, and development. Psychoanal Dialogues 1, 481–523.

Dennerstein L, Dudley EC, Hopper JL, et al. (2000) A prospective population-based study of menopausal symptoms. Obstet Gynecol 96(3) (Sep), 351–358.

Devor H (1999) FTM: Female to Male Transsexualism. Indiana University Press, Bloomington, Ind.

Feldman HA, Goldstein I, Hatzichristou DG, et al. (1994) Impotence and its medical and psychosocial correlates: Results of the Massachusetts male aging study. J Urol 151(1), 54–61.

Frank E, Anderson C, and Rubinstein D (1978) Frequency of sexual dysfunction in "normal" couples. New Engl J Med 299, 111–113.

Freud S (1905) Three essays on the theory of sexuality. In The Standard Edition of the Complete Works of Sigmund Freud, Strachy J (ed) (1953) Hogarth Press, London, pp. 125–243.

Freud S (1912) On the universal tendency to debasement in the sphere of love (Contributions to the Psychology of Love II). In Standard Edition of the Complete Works of Sigmund Freud, Vol. 11, Strachey L (ed). Hogarth Press, London, pp. 179–190.

Gijs L and Gooren L (1996) Hormonal and psychopharmacological interventions in the treatment of paraphilias: An update. J Sex Res 33, 273–290.

Gilbert DA, Winslow BH, Gilbert DM, et al. (1988) Transsexual surgery in the genetic female. Clin Plas Surg 15(3), 471–487.

Goldstein I, Lue TF, Padma-Nathan H, et al. (1998) Oral sildenafil in the treatment of erectile dysfunction. Sildenafil Study Group. N Engl J Med 338(20) (May), 1397–1404.

Green R (1987) "Sissy Boy Syndrome" and the Development of Male Homosexuality. Yale University Press, New Haven.

Kafka MP and Prentky RA (1998) Attention-deficit/hyperactivity disorder in males with paraphilia and paraphilia-related disorder: A comorbidity study. J Clin Psychiatr 59(7), 388–396.

Kaplan HS (1987) Sexual Aversion, Sexual Phobias, and Panic Disorder. Brunner/Mazel, New York.

Keller AC, Althof SE, and Lothstein LM (1982) Group psychotherapy with gender identity patients—a four year study. Am J Psychother 36, 223–228.

Kendler KS, Walters EE, Neale MC, et al. (1995) The structure of the genetic and environmental risk factors for six major psychiatric disorders in women. Arch Gen Psychiatr 52(5), 374–383.

Kernberg OF (1991) Aggression and love in the relationship of a couple. In Perversions and Near-Perversions in Clinical Practice: New Psychoanalytic Perspectives, Fogel GI and Myers WA (eds). Yale University Press, New Haven.

Killman PR, Mills KH, Caid C, et al. (1986) Treatment of secondary orgasmic dysfunction: An outcome study. Arch Sex Behav 15, 211–229.

Krane RJ, Goldstein I, and Saenz de Tejada I (1989) Impotence. New Engl J Med 321, 1648–1659.

Kreuger RB and Kaplan MS (2001) Depot-leuprolide acetate for treatment of paraphilias: A report of twelve cases. Arch Sex Behav 30(4), 409–422.

Laumann EO and Michael RT (eds) (2001) Sex, Love, and Health in America: Private Choices and Public Policies. University of Chicago Press, Chicago.

Laumann EO, Gagnon J, and Michael RT (1994a) Sex In America, University of Chicago Press, Chicago.

Laumann EO, Gagnon JH, Michael RT, et al. (1994b) The Social Organization of Sexuality. University of Chicago Press, Chicago.

Levine SB (1998a) The Nature of Love in Sexuality in Mid-Life. Kluwer Academic/Plenum Publishers, New York, pp. 1–22.

Levine SB (1998b) Sexuality in Midlife. Kluwer Academic/Plenum Publishers, New York.

Levine SB (1989) Sex Is Not Simple. Ohio Psychology Publications, Columbus.

Levine SB (1992) Sexual Life: A Clinician's Guide. Plenum Press, New York.

Levine SB (2002) Re-exploring the concept of sexual desire. J Sex Marit Ther 28(1), 39–51.

Levine SB, Risen CB, and Althof SE (eds) (2003) Handbook of Clinical Sexuality for Mental Health Professionals. Brunner/Routledge, New York.

Lothstein LM and Levine SB (1981) Expressive psychotherapy with gender dysphoric patients. Arch Gen Psychiatr 38, 924–929.

Lue TF (2000) Erectile dysfunction. N Engl J Med 342(24) (June 15), 1802–1813.

Maccoby EE and Jacklin CN (1987) Gender segregation in childhood. Adv Child Dev Behav 20, 239–287.

Masand PS, Ashton AK, Gupta S, et al. (2001) Sustained-release bupropion for selective serotonin reuptake inhibitor-induced sexual dysfunction: A randomized, double-blind, placebo-controlled, parallel-group study. Am J Psychiatr 158(5) (May), 805–807.

Masters WH and Johnson V (1966) Human Sexual Response. Little, Brown & Co, Boston.

Masters WH and Johnson V (1970) Human Sexual Inadequacy. Little, Brown & Co, Boston.

Mate-Kole C, Freschi M, and Robin A (1990) A controlled study of psychological and social change after surgical gender reassignment in selected male transsexuals. Br J Psychiatr 157, 261–264.

McEwan L, Ceber S, and Davis J (1986) Male-to-female surgical genital reassignment. In Transsexualism and Sex Reassignment, Walters WAW and Ross MJ (eds). Oxford University Press, New York.

McKay M (1992) Vulvodynia: Diagnostic patterns. Dermatol Clin N Am 10, 423–433.

Meana M and Binik YM (1994) Painful coitus: A review of female dyspareunia. J Nerv Ment Dis 182(5), 264–272.

Meyer W (Chairman), Bockting WO, Cohen-Kettenis P, et al. (2001) Harry Benjamin International Gender Dysphoria Association's The Standard of Care for Gender Identity Disorders, Sixth Version, 6th Rev. Symposion Publishing, Dusseldorf.

Money J (1986) Lovemaps: Clinical Concepts of Sexual/Erotic Health and Pathology, Paraphilia, and Gender Transpositions in Childhood, Adolescence, and Maturity. Irvington Publishers, New York.

O'Carroll R (1991) Sexual desire disorders: A review of controlled treatment studies. J Sex Res 28, 607–624.

Ohl DA (1994) Treatments for erectile dysfunction. In Sexual Dysfunction, Lechtenberg R and Ohl DA (eds). Philadelphia, pp. 292–361.

O'Keefe M and Hunt DK (1995) Assessment and treatment of impotence. Med Clin N Am 79(2), 415–434.

Pallas J, Levine SB, Althof SE, et al. (2000) A study using Viagra in a mental health practice. J Sex Marit Ther 26(1), 41–50.

Pawlak AE, Boulet JR, and Bradford JMW (1991) Discriminant analysis of a sexual-function inventory with intrafamilial and extrafamilial child molesters. Arch Sex Behav 20(1), 27–34.

Petersen ME and Dickey R (1995) Surgical sex reasssignment: A comparative survey of international centers. Arch Sex Behav 24(2), 135–156.

Risen CB and Althof SE (1995) A case of a paraphilia. In Case Studies in Sex Therapy, Rosen RC and Leiblum SR (eds). Guilford Press, New York.

Rosen RC and Leiblum SR (1995) Hypoactive sexual desire. Psychiatr Clin N Am 18(1) (Mar), 107–121.

Segraves RT (1998) Antidepressant-induced sexual dysfunction. J Clin Psychiatr 59(Suppl 4), 48–54.

Shaw J (ed) (1999) Sexual Aggression. American Psychiatric Press, Washington DC.

Spector IP and Carey MP (1990) Incidence and prevalence of the sexual dysfunctions: A critical review the empirical literature. Arch Sex Behav 19(4), 389–408.

Tiefer L (1998) A feminist critique of the sexual dysfunction nomenclature. Women Ther 7, 3–21.

Travin S (1995) Compulsive sexual behaviors. Psychiatr Clin N Am 18(1), 155–169.

Waldinger MD, Hengeveld MW, and Zwinderman AH (1994) Paroxetine treatment of premature ejaculation: A double-blind, randomized, placebo-controlled study. Am J Psychiatr 151(9), 1377–1379.

Zucker KJ (1990) Psychosocial and erotic development in cross-gender identified children. Can J Psychol 35(6), 487–495.

Zucker KJ (1995) Treatment of Cross-gender Identified Children. A presentation at the Society for Sexual Therapy and Research Meeting (Mar), New York.

# 75 ● ● Eating Disorders

B. Timothy Walsh

Anorexia Nervosa
Bulimia Nervosa

In the current psychiatric nomenclature of the *Diagnostic and Statistical Manual of Mental Disorders*, Fourth Edition (DSM-IV-TR), the eating disorders consist of two clearly defined syndromes: anorexia nervosa and bulimia nervosa. Many individuals presenting for treatment of an eating disorder (Figure 75–1) fail to meet formal criteria for either anorexia nervosa or bulimia nervosa, which raises an important theoretical and practical question: What is an eating disorder? Although this topic has received surprisingly little attention, it has been suggested that a working definition of an eating disorder might be "a persistent disturbance of eating behavior or behavior intended to control weight, which significantly impairs physical health or psychosocial functioning" (Fairburn and Walsh 2002). This definition clearly encompasses the recognized disorders, anorexia nervosa and bulimia nervosa. In addition, it provides a basis for viewing eating disorders as clinically significant problems that do not meet criteria for anorexia nervosa or bulimia nervosa. The term atypical eating disorder is often applied to such problems, even though the number of individuals suffering from them may well outnumber those with "typical" eating disorders. One example of an atypical eating disorder is that of women who are overly concerned about their weight, have dieted to a below-normal weight, but have not ceased menstruating and, therefore, do not meet full criteria for anorexia nervosa. Another is that of individuals who binge and vomit regularly, but at less than the twice-a-week frequency required for bulimia nervosa.

An additional example of a clinically important atypical eating disorder is the occurrence of frequent binge-eating that is not followed by the self-induced vomiting or other inappropriate attempts to compensate that are characteristic of bulimia nervosa. This disturbance, for which the name binge-eating disorder has been proposed (DSM-IV appendix B) (Yanovski 1993), is a common behavioral pattern among obese individuals who present for treatment at weight loss clinics.

At present, obesity is not considered an eating disorder. Obesity refers to an excess of body fat and is viewed as a general medical, not a psychiatric, condition. At this stage of our knowledge, obesity is conceived as an etiologi-cally heterogeneous condition. Obese individuals are at increased risk for a number of serious medical problems and are subject to significant social stigmatization and its psychological sequelae. However, the widely held assumption that obesity is the result of a psychiatric disorder in which eating is used as a coping mechanism for depression or anxiety has not been substantiated by empirical research. Studies of obese and normal-weight subjects from the general (nonpatient) population have found no more psychiatric disturbance in those who are overweight than in those who are of normal weight (Seidell and Thjhuis 2002). Therefore, it seems appropriate at present to describe as having an eating disorder only those obese individuals who manifest a clear behavioral abnormality that impairs health or psychosocial functioning.

## ANOREXIA NERVOSA

### History

The syndrome of anorexia nervosa was clearly recognized and, in fact, named in the late 19th century. Almost simultaneously, Sir William Gull in England and Charles Lasègue in France described series of cases of young women with impressive weight loss and psychological disturbance. Gull termed this illness "anorexia nervosa" and Lasègue—*anorexie hystérique*. The salient clinical features described more than 100 years ago are remarkably similar to those presented by patients in the opening years of the 21st century.

It is likely that cases of anorexia nervosa were also recognized well before the 19th century. In 1689, in a Treatise on Consumptions, Richard Morton (1689) described an 18-year-old girl with amenorrhea and self-imposed weight loss that he attributed to "a multitude of cares and passions of her mind"; this young woman eventually died of her illness, which Morton termed "nervous consumption" to emphasize its important psychological determinants. Bell (1985) has suggested that the fasting and asceticism of some medieval saints might today be viewed as manifestations of an eating disorder (Figure 75–2). Anorexia nervosa's long history suggests that although changing cultural norms for what is viewed as esthetically desirable may have played a role in increasing the frequency of anorexia

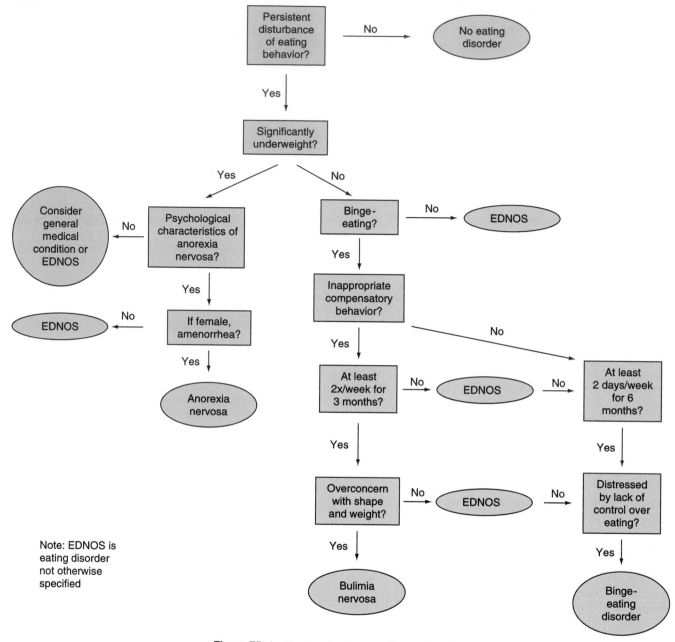

**Figure 75–1**   *Algorithm for diagnosis of eating disorders.*

nervosa, they do not fully explain the occurrence of the syndrome.

## Definition

The DSM-IV-TR criteria require the individual to be significantly underweight for age and height. Although it is not possible to set a single weight loss standard that applies equally to all individuals, DSM-IV-TR provides a benchmark of 85% of the weight considered normal for age and height as a guideline. Despite being of an abnormally low body weight, individuals with anorexia nervosa are intensely afraid of gaining weight and becoming fat, and remarkably, this fear typically intensifies as the weight falls.

DSM-IV-TR criterion C requires a disturbance in the person's judgment about his or her weight or shape. For example, despite being underweight, individuals with anorexia nervosa often view themselves or a part of their body as being too heavy. Typically, they deny the grave medical risks engendered by their semistarvation and place enormous psychological importance on whether they have gained or lost weight. For example, someone with anorexia nervosa may feel intensely distressed if her or his weight increases by half a pound. Finally, criterion D requires that women with anorexia nervosa be amenorrheic.

The DSM-IV-TR criteria for anorexia nervosa are generally consistent with recent definitions and descriptions of this illness. In addition, in DSM-IV-TR, a new subtyping scheme was introduced. DSM-IV-TR suggests that individuals with anorexia nervosa be classed as having one of two variants, either the binge-eating/purging type or the

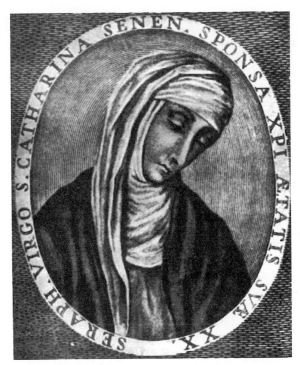

**Figure 75–2** *Engraving of St. Catherine of Siena, whose religious practices bore some resemblance to anorexia nervosa. (Source: Bedoyere MDL [1947] Catherine: Saint of Sienna. Hollis and Carter, London.)*

restricting type. Individuals with the restricting type of anorexia nervosa do not engage regularly in either binge-eating or purging and, compared with individuals with the binge-eating/purging form of the disorder, are not as likely to abuse alcohol and other drugs, exhibit less mood lability, and are less active sexually. There are also indications that the two subtypes may differ in their response to pharmacological intervention (Halmi et al. 1986).

## Epidemiology

Anorexia nervosa is a relatively rare illness. Even among high-risk groups, such as adolescent girls and young women, the prevalence of strictly defined anorexia nervosa is only about 0.5%. The prevalence rates of partial syndromes are substantially higher (Van Hoeken et al. 1998). Despite the infrequent occurrence of anorexia nervosa, most studies suggest that its incidence has increased significantly during the last 50 years, a phenomenon usually attributed to changes in cultural norms regarding desirable body shape and weight.

Anorexia nervosa usually affects women; the ratio of men to women is approximately 1:10 to 1:20. Anorexia nervosa occurs primarily in industrialized and affluent countries and some data suggest that even within those countries, anorexia nervosa is more common among the higher socioeconomic classes. Some occupations, such as ballet dancing and fashion modeling, appear to confer a particularly high risk for the development of anorexia nervosa. Thus, anorexia nervosa appears more likely to develop in an environment in which food is readily available but in which, for women, being thin is somehow equated with higher or special achievement.

---

**DSM-IV-TR Criteria** 307.1

**Anorexia Nervosa**

A. Refusal to maintain body weight at or above a minimally normal weight for age and height (e.g., weight loss leading to maintenance of body weight less than 85% of that expected; or failure to make expected weight gain during period of growth, leading to body weight less than 85% of that expected).

B. Intense fear of gaining weight or becoming fat, even though underweight.

C. Disturbance in the way in which one's body weight or shape is experienced, undue influence of body weight or shape on self-evaluation, or denial of the seriousness of the current low body weight.

D. In postmenarcheal females, amenorrhea, i.e., the absence of at least three consecutive menstrual cycles. (A woman is considered to have amenorrhea if her periods occur only following hormone, e.g., estrogen, administration.)

*Specify* type:

**Restricting type:** during the current episode of anorexia nervosa, the person has not regularly engaged in binge-eating or purging behavior (i.e., self-induced vomiting or the misuse of laxatives, diuretics, or enemas).

**Binge-eating/purging type:** during the current episode of anorexia nervosa, the person has regularly engaged in binge-eating or purging behavior (i.e., self-induced vomiting or the misuse of laxatives, diuretics, or enemas).

Reprinted with permission from the Diagnostic and Statistical Manual of Mental Disorders, Fourth Edition, Text Revision. Copyright 2000 American Psychiatric Association.

## Etiology

At present, the etiology of anorexia nervosa is fundamentally unknown. However, from several sources, such as the epidemiological data just reviewed, it is possible to identify risk factors whose presence increases the likelihood of anorexia nervosa. It is also possible to describe the course and complications of the syndrome and to suggest interactions between features of the disorder, for example, between malnutrition and psychiatric illness. Thus, as indicated in Figure 75–3, the difficulties that lead to the development of anorexia nervosa may be distinct from the forces that intensify the symptoms and perpetuate the illness once it has begun.

## Genetic and Twin Studies

Anorexia nervosa occurs more frequently in biological relatives of patients who present with the disorder. The prevalence rate of anorexia nervosa among sisters of patients is estimated to be approximately 6%; the morbid risk among other relatives ranges from 2 to 4%. Some evidence

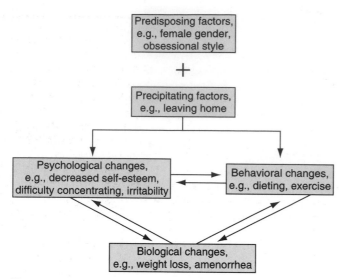

**Figure 75–3** *Schematic diagram illustrating how an interplay of factors may lead to the initiation and persistence of anorexia nervosa.*

for a genetic component in the etiology of anorexia nervosa comes from twin studies, which reported substantially higher concordance rates for monozygotic than for dizygotic twin pairs (Klump et al. 2001). However, conclusive data for genetic transmission of the disorder are not yet available.

## Family Studies

Individual psychiatric disorders in parents, dysfunctional family relationships, and impaired family interaction patterns have been implicated in the etiology of anorexia nervosa. Mothers of individuals with anorexia nervosa are often described as overprotective, intrusive, perfectionistic, and fearful of separation; fathers are described as withdrawn, passive, emotionally constricted, obsessional, moody, and ineffectual. Family systems theorists have suggested that impaired family interactions such as pathological enmeshment, rigidity, overprotectiveness, and difficulties confronting and resolving conflicts are central features of anorexic pathology (Minuchin et al. 1978). However, few empirical studies have been conducted to date, particularly studies that also examine psychiatrically or medically ill comparison groups. Therefore, the precise role of the family in the development and course of anorexia nervosa, although undoubtedly important, has not been clearly delineated.

## Psychosocial Factors

The increased prevalence of anorexia nervosa has been connected to the current emphasis in contemporary Western society on an unrealistically thin appearance in women (Hsu 1996). There is substantial evidence that a desire to be slim is common among middle- and upper-class white women and that this emphasis on slimness has increased significantly during the past several decades. In the US, anorexia nervosa develops much more frequently in white adolescents than in adolescents from other racial groups. It has been suggested that a variety of characteristics may protect African-American girls from having eating dis-

orders, including more acceptance of being overweight, more satisfaction with their body image, and less social pressure regarding weight (Striegel-Moore et al. 2000).

It has also been suggested that the emphasis of contemporary Western society on achievement and performance in women, which is a shift from the more traditional emphasis on deference, compliance, and unassertiveness, has left many young women vulnerable to the development of eating disorders such as anorexia nervosa. These multiple and contradictory role demands are embodied within the modern concept of a superwoman who performs all of the expected roles (e.g., is competent, ambitious, and achieving, yet also feminine, nurturing, and sexual) and, in addition, devotes considerable attention to her appearance (Gordon 1990).

## Psychodynamic Factors

Various psychoanalytic theories have been postulated (e.g., defense against fantasies of oral impregnation; underlying deficits in the development of object relations; deficits in self-structure), but such hypotheses are difficult to verify. Bruch (1973, 1982) suggested that anorexia nervosa stems from failures in early attachment, attempts to cope with underlying feelings of ineffectiveness and inadequacy, and an inability to meet the demands of adolescence and young adulthood. These ideas, as well as her conceptualization that the single-minded focus on losing weight in anorexia nervosa is the concrete manifestation of a struggle to achieve a sense of identity, purpose, specialness, and control, are compelling and clinically useful. Cognitive–behavioral theories emphasize the distortions and dysfunctional thoughts (e.g., dichotomous thinking) that may stem from various causal factors, all of which eventually focus on the belief that it is essential to be thin.

Although the existence of a specific predisposing personality style has not been conclusively documented, certain traits have commonly been reported among women with anorexia nervosa. Women hospitalized for anorexia nervosa have greater self-discipline, conscientiousness, and emotional caution than women hospitalized for bulimia nervosa and women with no eating disorders (Casper et al. 1992). In addition, even after they have recovered from their illness, women who have had anorexia nervosa tend to avoid risks and to exhibit high levels of caution in emotional expression and strong compliance with rules and moral standards (Srinivasagam et al. 1995).

## Developmental Factors

Because anorexia nervosa typically begins during adolescence, developmental issues are thought to play an important etiological role. Critical challenges at this time of life include the need to establish independence, a well-defined personal identity, fulfilling relationships, and clear values and principles to govern one's life. Family struggles, conflicts regarding sexuality, and pressures regarding increased heterosexual contact are also common. However, it is not clear that difficulties over these issues are more salient for individuals who will develop anorexia nervosa than for other adolescents. Depression has been implicated as a nonspecific risk factor, and higher levels of depressive symptoms as well as insecurity, anxiety, and self-consciousness have been documented in adolescent girls in comparison with adolescent boys. Similarly, the progression of physical and sexual maturation and the concomitant increase in women's percentage of body fat may have a substantial impact on the self-image of adolescent girls, particularly because the relationship between self-esteem and satisfaction with physical appearance and body characteristics is stronger in women than in men.

## Pathophysiology

An impressive array of physical disturbances has been documented in anorexia nervosa, and the physiological bases of many are understood (Walsh 2001) (Table 75–1). Most of these physical disturbances appear to be secondary consequences of starvation, and it is not clear whether or how the physiological disturbances described here contribute to the development and maintenance of the psychological and behavioral abnormalities characteristic of anorexia nervosa. The remainder of this section briefly describes the major physical abnormalities of anorexia nervosa and what is understood about their etiology.

The central nervous system is clearly affected. Computed tomography has demonstrated that individuals with anorexia nervosa have enlarged ventricles, an abnormality that improves with weight gain. The cerebrospinal fluid concentrations of a variety of neurotransmitters and their metabolites are altered in underweight patients with anorexia nervosa and tend to normalize as weight is restored. An intriguing exception may be the serotonin metabolite 5-hydroxyindoleacetic acid, which has been reported to be elevated in the cerebrospinal fluid of patients with anorexia nervosa after they have achieved a normal or near-normal weight. Kaye (1997) has suggested that the elevated 5-hydroxyindoleacetic acid levels may reflect a serotoninergic abnormality that is tied to the obsessional traits often observed in anorexia nervosa.

Some of the most striking physiological alterations in anorexia nervosa are those of the hypothalamic–pituitary–gonadal axis. In women, estrogen secretion from the ovaries is markedly reduced, accounting for the occurrence of amenorrhea. In analogous fashion, testosterone production is diminished in men with anorexia nervosa. The decrease in gonadal steroid production is due to a reduction in the pituitary's secretion of the gonadotropins luteinizing hormone and follicle-stimulating hormone, which in turn is secondary to diminished release of gonadotropin-releasing hormone from the hypothalamus. Therefore, the amenorrhea of anorexia nervosa is properly viewed as a type of hypothalamic amenorrhea. It is of interest that in a significant minority amenorrhea begins before substantial weight loss has occurred, suggesting that factors other than malnutrition, such as psychological distress, contribute significantly to the disruption of the reproductive endocrine system.

In an adult with anorexia nervosa, the status of the hypothalamic–pituitary–gonadal axis resembles that of a pubertal or prepubertal child—the secretion of estrogen or testosterone, of luteinizing hormone and follicle-stimulating hormone and of gonadotropin-releasing hormone is reduced. This endocrinological picture may be contrasted with that of postmenopausal women who have a similar reduction in estrogen secretion but who, unlike women with anorexia nervosa, show increased pituitary gonadotropin secretion. Furthermore, even the circadian patterns of luteinizing hormone and follicle-stimulating hormone secretion in adult women with anorexia nervosa closely resemble the patterns normally seen in pubertal and prepubertal girls (Figure 75–4). Although similar abnormalities are also seen in other forms of hypothalamic amenorrhea and are therefore not specific to anorexia nervosa, it is nonetheless striking that this syndrome is accompanied by a physiological arrest or regression of the reproductive endocrine system.

The functioning of other hormonal systems is also disrupted in anorexia nervosa, although typically not as profoundly as is the reproductive axis. Presumably as part of the metabolic response to semistarvation, the activity of the thyroid gland is reduced. Plasma thyroxine levels are somewhat diminished, but the plasma level of the pituitary hormone and thyroid-stimulating hormone is not elevated. The activity of the hypothalamic–pituitary–adrenal axis is increased, as indicated by elevated plasma levels of cortisol and by resistance to dexamethasone suppression. The regulation of vasopressin (antidiuretic hormone) secretion from the posterior pituitary is disturbed, contributing to the development of partial diabetes insipidus in some individuals.

Anorexia nervosa is often associated with the development of leukopenia and of a normochromic, normocytic anemia of mild to moderate severity. Surprisingly, leukopenia does not appear to result in a high vulnerability to infectious illnesses. Serum levels of liver enzymes are sometimes elevated, particularly during the early phases of refeeding, but the synthetic function of the liver is rarely

| Table 75–1 | Medical Problems Commonly Associated with Anorexia Nervosa |
|---|---|

Skin
  Lanugo
Cardiovascular system
  Hypotension
  Bradycardia
  Arrhythmias
Hematopoietic system
  Normochromic, normocytic anemia
  Leukopenia
    Diminished polymorphonuclear leukocytes
Fluid and electrolyte balance
  Elevated blood urea nitrogen and creatinine concentrations
  Hypokalemia
  Hyponatremia
  Hypochloremia
  Alkalosis
Gastrointestinal system
  Elevated serum concentration of liver enzymes
  Delayed gastric emptying
  Constipation
Endocrine system
  Diminished thyroxine level with normal thyroid-stimulating hormone level
  Elevated plasma cortisol level
  Diminished secretion of luteinizing hormone, follicle-stimulating hormone, estrogen, or testosterone
Bone
  Osteoporosis

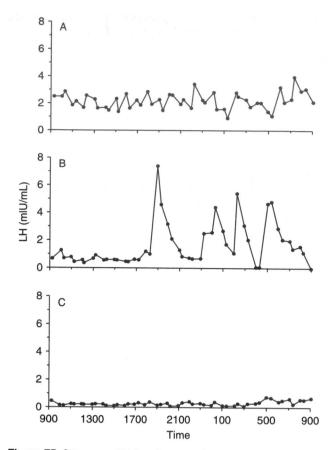

**Figure 75–4** *Patterns of 24-hour luteinizing hormone (LH) secretion of a normal adult woman (A), of a woman with anorexia nervosa showing a pattern normally seen in adolescence (B), and of a woman with anorexia nervosa showing a pattern normally seen before puberty (C).*

failure occasionally develops in individuals during overly rapid refeeding. The electrocardiogram shows sinus bradycardia and a number of nonspecific abnormalities. Arrhythmias may develop, often in association with fluid and electrolyte disturbances. It has been suggested that significant prolongation of the QT interval may be a harbinger of life-threatening arrhythmias in some individuals with anorexia nervosa, but this has not been conclusively demonstrated.

The motility of the gastrointestinal tract is diminished, leading to delayed gastric emptying and contributing to complaints of bloating and constipation. Rare cases of acute gastric dilatation or gastric rupture, which is often fatal, have been reported in individuals with anorexia nervosa who consumed large amounts of food when binge-eating.

As already noted, virtually all of the physiological abnormalities described in individuals with anorexia nervosa are also seen in other forms of starvation, and most improve or disappear as weight returns to normal. Therefore, weight restoration is essential for physiological recovery. More surprisingly, perhaps, weight restoration is believed to be essential for psychological recovery as well. Accounts of human starvation amply document the profound impact of starvation on mental health. Starving individuals lose their sense of humor, their interest in friends and family fades, and mood generally becomes depressed. They may develop peculiar behavior similar to that of patients with anorexia nervosa, such as hoarding food or concocting bizarre food combinations. If starvation disrupts psychological and behavioral functioning in normal individuals, it presumably does so as well in those with anorexia nervosa. Thus, correction of starvation is a prerequisite for the restoration of both physical and psychological health.

## Diagnosis and Differential Diagnosis

### Phenomenology

Anorexia nervosa often begins innocently. Typically, an adolescent girl or young woman who is of normal weight or, perhaps, a few pounds overweight decides to diet. This decision may be prompted by an important but not extraordinary life event, such as leaving home for camp, attending a new school, or a casual unflattering remark by a friend or family member. Initially, the dieting seems no different from that pursued by many young women, but as weight falls, the dieting intensifies. The restrictions become broader and more rigid; for example, desserts may first be eliminated, then meat, then any food that is thought to contain fat. The person becomes increasingly uncomfortable if she is seen eating and avoids meals with others. Food seems to assume a moral quality so that vegetables are viewed as "good" and anything with fat is "bad." The individual has idiosyncratic rules about how much exercise she must do, and when, where, and how she can eat.

Food avoidance and weight loss are accompanied by a deep and reassuring sense of accomplishment, and weight gain is viewed as a failure and a sign of weakness. Physical activity, such as running or aerobic exercise, often increases as the dieting and weight loss develop. Inactivity and complaints of weakness usually occur only when emaciation has

seriously impaired so that the serum albumin concentration and the prothrombin time are usually within normal limits. Serum cholesterol levels are sometimes elevated in anorexia nervosa, although the basis of this abnormality remains obscure. In some patients, self-imposed fluid restriction and excessive exercise produce dehydration and elevations of serum creatinine and blood urea nitrogen. In others, water loading may lead to hyponatremia. The status of serum electrolytes is a reflection of the individual's salt and water intake and the nature and the severity of the purging behavior. A common pattern is hypokalemia, hypochloremia, and mild alkalosis resulting from frequent and persistent self-induced vomiting.

It has become clear that individuals with anorexia nervosa have decreased bone density compared with age- and sex-matched peers and, as a result, are at increased risk for fractures. Low levels of estrogen, high levels of cortisol, and poor nutrition have been cited as risk factors for the development of reduced bone density in anorexia nervosa. Theoretically, estrogen treatment might reduce the risk of osteoporosis in women who are chronically amenorrheic because of anorexia nervosa, but controlled studies indicate that this intervention is of limited, if any, benefit.

Abnormalities of cardiac function include bradycardia and hypotension, which are rarely symptomatic. The pump function of the heart is compromised, and congestive heart

become extreme. The person becomes more serious and devotes little effort to anything but work, dieting, and exercise. She may become depressed and emotionally labile, socially withdrawn, and secretive, and she may lie about her eating and her weight. Despite the profound disturbances in her view of her weight and of her calorie needs, reality testing in other spheres is intact, and the person may continue to function well in school or at work. Symptoms usually persist for months or years until, typically at the insistence of friends or family, the person reluctantly agrees to see a physician.

In general, anorexia nervosa is not difficult to recognize. Uncertainty surrounding the diagnosis sometimes occurs in young adolescents, who may not clearly describe a drive for thinness and the fear of becoming fat. Rather, they may acknowledge only a vague concern about consuming certain foods and an intense desire to exercise. It can also be difficult to elicit the distorted view of shape and weight (criterion C) from patients who have had anorexia nervosa for many years. Such individuals may state that they realize they are too thin and may make superficial efforts to gain weight, but they do not seem particularly concerned about the physical risks or deeply committed to increasing their calorie consumption.

## Assessment

### Special Issues in Psychiatric Examination and History

In assessing individuals who may have anorexia nervosa, it is important to obtain a weight history including the individual's highest and lowest weights and the weight he or she would like to be now. For women, it is useful to know the weight at which menstruation last occurred, because it provides an indication of what weight is normal for that individual. The patient should be asked to describe a typical day's food intake and any food restrictions and dietary practices such as vegetarianism. The psychiatrist should ask whether the patient ever loses control over eating and engages in binge-eating and, if so, the amounts and types of food eaten during such episodes. The use of self-induced vomiting, laxatives, diuretics, enemas, diet pills, and syrup of ipecac to induce vomiting should also be queried.

Probably the greatest problem in the assessment of patients with anorexia nervosa is their denial of the illness and their reluctance to participate in an evaluation. A straightforward but supportive and nonconfrontational style is probably the most useful approach, but it is likely that the patient will not acknowledge significant difficulties in eating or with weight and will rationalize unusual eating or exercise habits. It is therefore helpful to obtain information from other sources such as the patient's family.

### Physical Examination and Laboratory Findings

The patient should be weighed, or a current weight should be obtained from the patient's general physician. Blood pressure, pulse, and body temperature are often below the lower limit of normal. On physical examination, lanugo, a fine, downy hair normally seen in infants, may be present on the back or the face. The extremities are frequently cold and have a slight red-purple color (acrocyanosis). Edema is rarely observed at the initial presentation but may develop transiently during the initial stages of refeeding.

The basis for laboratory abnormalities is presented in the earlier section on pathophysiology. Common findings are a mild to moderate normochromic, normocytic anemia and leukopenia, with a deficit in polymorphonuclear leukocytes leading to a relative lymphocytosis. Elevations of blood urea nitrogen and serum creatinine concentrations may occur because of dehydration, which can also artificially elevate the hemoglobin and hematocrit. A variety of electrolyte abnormalities may be observed, reflecting the state of hydration and the history of vomiting and diuretic and laxative abuse. Serum levels of liver enzymes are usually normal but may transiently increase during refeeding. Cholesterol levels may be elevated.

The electrocardiogram typically shows sinus bradycardia and, occasionally, low QRS voltage and a prolonged QT interval; a variety of arrhythmias have also been described.

### Differences in Presentation

The symptoms of anorexia nervosa are remarkably homogeneous, and differences between patients in clinical manifestations are fewer than in most psychiatric illnesses. As described before, younger patients may not express verbally the characteristic fear of fatness or the overconcern with shape and weight, and some patients with long-standing anorexia nervosa may express a desire to gain weight but be unable to make persistent changes in their behavior. It has been suggested that in other cultures, the rationale given by patients for losing weight differs from the fear of fatness characteristic of cases in North America. For example, the features of weight phobia, fear of fatness, and pursuit of thinness have been described as being absent in some patients in Hong Kong and India who, in other regards, present symptoms that closely resemble those of anorexia nervosa; reasons for food refusal given by such patients include lack of appetite and epigastric bloating (Hsu and Lee 1993).

Men have anorexia nervosa far less frequently than women. However, when the syndrome does develop in a man, it is typical. There may be an increased frequency of homosexuality among men with anorexia nervosa.

### Differential Diagnosis

Although depression, schizophrenia, and obsessive–compulsive disorder may be associated with disturbed eating and weight loss, it is rarely difficult to differentiate these disorders from anorexia nervosa. Individuals with major depression may lose significant amounts of weight but do not exhibit the relentless drive for thinness characteristic of anorexia nervosa. In schizophrenia, starvation may occur because of delusions about food, for example, that it is poisoned. Individuals with obsessive–compulsive disorder may describe irrational concerns about food and develop rituals related to meal preparation and eating but do not describe the intense fear of gaining weight and the pervasive wish to be thin that characterize anorexia nervosa.

A wide variety of medical problems cause serious weight loss in young people and may at times be confused with anorexia nervosa. Examples of such problems include gastric outlet obstruction, Crohn's disease, and brain tumors. Individuals whose weight loss is due to a general medical illness generally do not show the drive for thinness, the fear of gaining weight, and the increased physical activity characteristic of anorexia nervosa. However, the psychiatrist is well advised to consider any chronic medical illness associated with weight loss, especially when evaluating individuals with unusual clinical presentations such as late age at onset or prominent physical complaints, for example, pain and gastrointestinal cramping while eating.

## Course and Natural History

The course of anorexia nervosa is enormously variable. Some individuals have mild and brief illnesses and either never come to medical attention or are seen only briefly by their pediatrician or general medical physician. It is difficult to estimate the frequency of this phenomenon because such individuals are rarely studied.

Most of the literature on course and outcome is based on individuals who have been hospitalized for anorexia nervosa. Although such individuals presumably have a relatively severe illness and adverse outcomes, a substantial fraction, probably between one-third and one-half, make full and complete psychological and physical recoveries. On the other hand, anorexia nervosa is also associated with an impressive long-term mortality. The best data currently available suggest that 10 to 20% of patients who have been hospitalized for anorexia nervosa will, in the next 10 to 30 years, die as a result of their illness. Much of the mortality is due to severe and chronic starvation, which eventually terminates in sudden death. In addition, a significant fraction of patients commit suicide.

Between these two extremes are a large number of individuals whose lives are impaired by persistent difficulties with eating. Some are severely affected maintaining a chronic state of semistarvation, bizarre eating rituals, and social isolation; others may gain weight but struggle with bulimia nervosa and strict rules about food and eating; and still others may recover initially but then relapse into another full episode. There is a high frequency of depression among individuals who have had anorexia nervosa and a significant frequency of drug and alcohol abuse, but psychotic disorders develop only rarely. Thus, in general, individuals either recover or continue to struggle with psychological and behavioral problems that are directly related to the eating disorder. It is of note that it is rare for individuals who have had anorexia nervosa to become obese.

It is difficult to specify factors that account for the variability of outcome in anorexia nervosa. A significant body of experience suggests that the illness has a better prognosis when it begins in adolescence, but there are also suggestions that prepubertal onset may portend a difficult course. It is likely that the severity of the illness (e.g., the lowest weight reached, the number of hospitalizations) and the presence of associated symptoms, such as binge-eating and purging, also contribute to poor outcome. However, it is impossible to predict course and outcome in an individual with any certainty.

## Goals of Treatment

The first goal of treatment is to engage the patient and her or his family. For most patients with anorexia nervosa, this is challenging. Patients usually minimize their symptoms and suggest that the concerns of the family and friends, who have often been instrumental in arranging the consultation, are greatly exaggerated. It is helpful to identify a problem that the patient can acknowledge, such as weakness, irritability, difficulty concentrating, or trouble with binge-eating. The psychiatrist may then attempt to educate the patient regarding the pervasive physical and psychological effects of semistarvation and about the need for weight gain if the acknowledged problem is to be successfully addressed.

A second goal of treatment is to assess and address acute medical problems, such as fluid and electrolyte disturbances and cardiac arrhythmias. Depending on the severity of illness, this may require the involvement of a general medical physician.

The additional but most difficult and time-consuming goals are the restoration of normal body weight, the normalization of eating, and the resolution of the associated psychological disturbances. The final goal is the prevention of relapse.

## Treatment

A common major impediment to the treatment of patients with anorexia nervosa is their disagreement with the goals of treatment; many of the features of their illness are simply not viewed by patients as a problem. In addition, this may be compounded by a variety of concerns of the patient, such as basic mistrust of relationships, feelings of vulnerability and inferiority, and sensitivity to perceived coercion. Such concerns may be expressed through considerable resistance, defiance, or pseudocompliance with the psychiatrist's interventions and contribute to the power struggles that often characterize the treatment process. The psychiatrist must try to avoid colluding with the patient's attempts to minimize problems but at the same time allow the patient enough independence to maintain the alliance. Dealing with such dilemmas is challenging and requires an active approach on the part of the psychiatrist. In most instances, it is possible to preserve the alliance while nonetheless adhering to established limits and the need for change.

The initial stage of treatment should be aimed at reversing the nutritional and behavioral abnormalities (Figure 75–5). The intensity of the treatment required and the need for partial or full hospitalization should be determined by the current weight, the rapidity of weight loss, and the severity of associated medical and behavioral problems and of other symptoms such as depression. In general, patients whose weights are less than 75% of expected should be viewed as medically precarious and require intensive treatment such as hospitalization.

Most inpatient or day treatment units experienced in the care of patients with anorexia nervosa use a structured treatment approach that relies heavily on supervision of calorie intake by the staff. Patients are initially expected to consume sufficient calories to maintain weight, usually requiring 1,500 to 2,000 kcal/day in four to six meals. After the initial medical assessment has been completed and weight has stabilized, calorie intake is gradually increased to an amount necessary to gain 2 to 5 lb/week. Because the consumption of approximately 4,000 kcal beyond maintenance requirements is needed for each pound of weight gain,

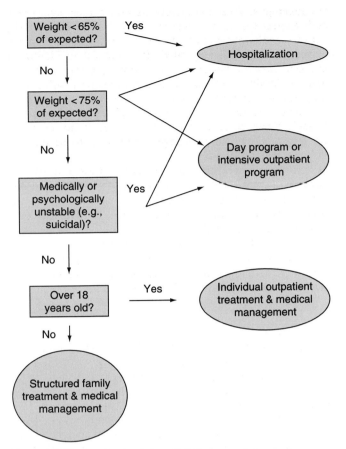

**Figure 75–5** *Algorithm for choice of initial treatment of anorexia nervosa.*

the daily calorie requirements become impressive, often in the range of 4,000 kcal/day. Some eating disorder units provide only food while others rely on nutritional supplements such as Ensure or Sustacal. During this phase of treatment it is necessary to monitor patients carefully; many will resort to throwing food away or vomiting after meals. Careful supervision is also required to obtain accurate weights; patients may consume large amounts of fluid before being weighed or hide heavy articles under their clothing.

During the weight restoration phase of treatment patients require substantial emotional support. It is probably best to address fears of weight gain with education about the dangers of semistarvation and with the reassurance that patients will not be allowed to gain "too much" weight. Most eating disorders units impose behavioral restrictions, such as limits on physical activity, during the early phase of treatment. Some units use an explicit behavior modification regimen in which weight gain is tied to increased privileges and failure to gain weight results in bed rest.

A consistent and structured treatment approach, with or without an explicit behavior modification program, is generally successful in promoting weight recovery but requires substantial energy and coordination to maintain a supportive and nonpunitive treatment environment. In most experienced treatment units, parenteral methods of nutrition, such as nasogastric feeding or intravenous hyperalimentation, are only rarely needed. Nutritional counseling

and behavioral approaches can also be effective in helping patients expand their dietary repertoire to include foods they have been frightened of consuming.

As weight increases, individual, group, and family psychotherapy can begin to address other issues in addition to the distress engendered by gaining weight (Garner and Garfinkel 1997). For example, it is typically important for patients to recognize that they have come to base much of their self-esteem on dieting and weight control and are likely to judge themselves according to harsh and unforgiving standards. Similarly, patients should be helped to see how the eating disorder has interfered with the achievement of personal goals such as education, sports, or making friends.

There is, at present, no general agreement about the most useful type of psychotherapy or the specific topics that need to be addressed. Most eating disorders programs employ a variety of psychotherapeutic interventions. A number of psychiatrists recommend the use of individual and group psychotherapy using cognitive–behavioral techniques to modify the irrational overemphasis on weight. Although most authorities see little role for traditional psychoanalytic therapy, individual and group psychodynamic therapy can address such problems as insecure attachment, separation and individuation, sexual relationships, and other interpersonal concerns. There is good evidence supporting the involvement of the family in the treatment of younger patients with anorexia nervosa. Family therapy can be helpful in addressing family members' fears about the illness; interventions typically emphasize parental cooperation, mutual support and consistency, and establishing boundaries regarding the patient's symptoms and other aspects of his or her life (Lock et al. 2000).

Despite the multiple physiological disturbances associated with anorexia nervosa, there is no clearly established role for medication (Zhu and Walsh 2002). The earliest systematic medication trials in anorexia nervosa focused on the use of neuroleptics. Theoretically, such agents might help to promote weight gain, to reduce physical activity, and to diminish the distorted thinking about shape and weight, which often reaches nearly delusional proportions. Early work in the late 1950s and 1960s using chlorpromazine led to substantial enthusiasm, but two placebo-controlled trials of the neuroleptics, sulpiride and pimozide, were unable to establish significant benefits. In recent years interest has grown in taking advantage of the impressive weight gain associated with some atypical antipsychotics; however, no controlled data supporting this intervention have yet appeared.

Four controlled studies, three of tricyclic antidepressants and one of fluoxetine, have examined the use of antidepressants in the treatment of anorexia nervosa. The benefits of the antidepressants compared to placebo were small and of uncertain clinical significance. Therefore, despite the frequency of depression among patients with anorexia nervosa, there is no good evidence supporting the use of antidepressant medication in their treatment.

One of the more interesting pharmacological interventions examined in controlled trials of anorexia nervosa is the use of cyproheptadine. Cyproheptadine is an antihistamine used in the treatment of a variety of allergic conditions that has been associated with weight gain. The weight gain is thought to be related to cyproheptadine's potency as a serotonin antagonist because animal studies suggest that decreases in hypothalamic serotonin are usually associated with increases in food consumption. Unfortunately, although controlled trials have provided some evidence of benefit, the impact of cyproheptadine in anorexia nervosa appears limited.

A large percentage of patients with anorexia nervosa remain chronically ill; 30 to 50% of patients successfully treated in the hospital require rehospitalization within 1 year of discharge. Therefore, posthospitalization out-patient treatments are recommended to prevent relapse and improve overall short- and long-term functioning. Several studies have attempted to evaluate the efficacy of various outpatient treatments for anorexia nervosa including behavioral, cognitive–behavioral, and supportive psychotherapy, as well as a variety of nutritional counseling interventions. Although most of these treatments seem to be helpful, the clearest findings to date support two interventions. For patients whose anorexia nervosa started before age 18 years and who have had the disorder for less than 3 years, family therapy is effective, and for adult patients, cognitive–behavioral therapy reduces the rate of relapse. Preliminary information suggests that fluoxetine treatment may reduce the risk of relapse among patients with anorexia nervosa who have gained weight, but additional controlled data are required to document the usefulness of this intervention.

## Refractory Patients

Some patients with anorexia nervosa refuse to accept treatment and thereby can raise difficult ethical issues. If weight is extremely low or if there are acute medical problems, it may be appropriate to consider involuntary commitment. For patients who are ill but more stable, the psychiatrist must weigh the short-term utility of involuntary treatment against the disruption of a potential alliance with the patient.

The goals of treatment may need to be modified for patients with chronic illness who have failed multiple previous attempts at inpatient and outpatient care. Treatment may be appropriately aimed at preventing further medical, psychological, and social deterioration in the hope that the anorexia nervosa may eventually improve with time.

## BULIMIA NERVOSA

### Definition

Overeating has presumably been a problem for humans for millennia. However, interest in a disorder related to anorexia nervosa but characterized behaviorally by persistent binge-eating grew dramatically in the late 1970s and early 1980s, driven by the appearance of increasing numbers of patients with the chief complaint of binge-eating. In an article published in 1979, Russell (1979) clearly delineated the syndrome of bulimia nervosa, and in 1980, bulimia was formally recognized as a disorder in the newly published *Diagnostic and Statistical Manual of Mental Disorders*, Third Edition (DSM-III). Although discussion continues about the best method of defining the syndrome, there have been no major changes in its conceptualization.

---

**DSM-IV-TR Criteria** 307.51

**Bulimia Nervosa**

A. Recurrent episodes of binge-eating. An episode of binge-eating is characterized by both of the following:

  (1) eating, in a discrete period of time (e.g., within any 2-hour period), an amount of food that is definitely larger than most people would eat during a similar period of time and under similar circumstances.

  (2) a sense of lack of control over eating during the episode (e.g., a feeling that one cannot stop eating or control what or how much one is eating).

B. Recurrent inappropriate compensatory behavior in order to prevent weight gain, such as self-induced vomiting; misuse of laxatives, diuretics, enemas, or other medications; fasting; or excessive exercise.

C. The binge-eating and inappropriate compensatory behaviors both occur, on average, at least twice a week for 3 months.

D. Self-evaluation is unduly influenced by body shape and weight.

E. The disturbance does not occur exclusively during episodes of anorexia nervosa.

*Specify* type:

**Purging type:** during the current episode of bulimia nervosa, the person has regularly engaged in self-induced vomiting or the misuse of laxatives, diuretics, or enemas.

**Nonpurging type:** during the current episode of bulimia nervosa, the person has used other inappropriate compensatory behaviors, such as fasting or excessive exercise, but has not regularly engaged in self-induced vomiting or the misuse of laxatives, diuretics, or enemas.

The salient behavioral disturbance of bulimia nervosa is the occurrence of episodes of binge-eating. During these episodes, the individual consumes an amount of food that is unusually large considering the circumstances under which it was eaten. Although this is a useful definition and conceptually reasonably clear, it can be operationally difficult to distinguish normal overeating from a small episode of binge-eating. Indeed, the available data do not suggest that there is a sharp dividing line between the size of binge-eating episodes and the size of other meals. On the other hand, while the border between normal and abnormal eating may not be a sharp one, both patients' reports and laboratory studies of eating behavior clearly indicate that, when binge-eating, patients with bulimia nervosa do indeed consume larger than normal amounts of food (Walsh et al. 1992).

Episodes of binge-eating are associated, by definition, with a sense of loss of control. Once the eating has begun, the individual feels unable to stop until an excessive amount has been consumed. This loss of control is only subjective, in that most individuals with bulimia nervosa will abruptly stop eating in the midst of a binge episode if interrupted, for example, by the unexpected arrival of a roommate.

After overeating, individuals with bulimia nervosa engage in some form of inappropriate behavior in an attempt to avoid weight gain. Most patients who present to eating disorders clinics with this syndrome report self-induced vomiting or the abuse of laxatives. Other methods include misusing diuretics, fasting for long periods, and exercising extensively after eating binges.

The DSM-IV-TR criteria require that the overeating episodes and the compensatory behaviors both occur at least twice a week for 3 months to merit a diagnosis of bulimia nervosa. This criterion, although useful in preventing the diagnostic label from being applied to individuals who only rarely have difficulty with binge-eating, is clearly an arbitrary one.

Criterion D in the DSM-IV-TR definition of bulimia nervosa requires that individuals with bulimia nervosa exhibit an overconcern with body shape and weight. That is, they tend to base much of their self-esteem on how much they weigh and how slim they look.

Finally, in the DSM-IV-TR nomenclature, the diagnosis of bulimia nervosa is not given to individuals with anorexia nervosa. Individuals with anorexia nervosa who recurrently engage in binge-eating or purging behavior should be given the diagnosis of anorexia nervosa, binge-eating/purging subtype, rather than an additional diagnosis of bulimia nervosa. This is a change from the *Diagnostic and Statistical Manual of Mental Disorders*, Third Edition, Revised (DSM-III-R) system, in which both diagnoses could be given simultaneously.

In DSM-IV-TR, a subtyping scheme was introduced for bulimia nervosa in which patients are classed as having either the purging or the nonpurging type of bulimia nervosa. This scheme was introduced for several reasons. First, those individuals who purge are at greater risk for the development of fluid and electrolyte disturbances such as hypokalemia. Second, data suggest that individuals with the nonpurging type of bulimia nervosa weigh more and have less psychiatric illness compared with those with the purging type. Finally, most of the published literature on the treatment of bulimia nervosa has been based on studies of individuals with the purging type of this disorder.

## Epidemiology

Soon after bulimia nervosa was recognized as a distinct disorder, surveys indicated that many young women reported problems with binge-eating, and it was suggested that the syndrome of bulimia nervosa was occurring in epidemic proportions. Later careful studies have found that although binge-eating is frequent, the full-blown disorder of bulimia nervosa is much less common, probably affecting 1 to 2% of young women in the US (Fairburn and Beglin 1990).

Although sufficient research data do not exist to pinpoint specific epidemiological trends in the occurrence of bulimia nervosa, research suggests that women born after 1960 have a higher risk for the illness than those born before 1960 (Kendler et al. 1991).

Evidence suggests an important role of sociocultural influences in the development of bulimia nervosa. For example, the frequency of the disorder has been reported to be increasing among immigrants to the US and UK from non-Western countries (Hsu 1990). Although the rate of the disorder appears to be lower among nonwhite and non-Western cultures, the frequency of bulimia nervosa has been reported to be increasing among these groups, especially among the higher socioeconomic classes. Surprisingly, several epidemiological and clinical studies in the US found no relationship between bulimia nervosa and social class (Kendler et al. 1991).

Among patients with bulimia nervosa who are seen at eating disorders clinics, there is an increased frequency of anxiety and mood disorders, especially major depressive disorder and dysthymic disorder, of drug and alcohol abuse, and of personality disorders. It is not certain whether this comorbidity is also observed in community samples or whether it is a characteristic of individuals who seek treatment.

## Etiology

As in the case of anorexia nervosa, the etiology of bulimia nervosa is uncertain. Several factors clearly predispose individuals to the development of bulimia nervosa, including being an adolescent girl or young adult woman. A personal or family history of obesity and of mood disturbance also appears to increase risk. Twin studies have suggested that inherited factors are related to the risk of developing bulimia nervosa, but what these factors are and how they operate are unclear.

Many of the same psychosocial factors related to the development of anorexia nervosa are also applicable to bulimia nervosa, including the influence of cultural esthetic ideals of thinness and physical fitness. Similarly, bulimia nervosa primarily affects women; the ratio of men to women is approximately 1:10. It also occurs more frequently in certain occupations (e.g., modeling) and sports (e.g., wrestling, running).

Although not proven, it seems likely that several factors serve to perpetuate the binge-eating once it has begun (Figure 75–6). First, most individuals with bulimia nervosa, because of both their concern regarding weight and their worry about the effect of the binge-eating, attempt to restrict their food intake when they are not binge-eating. The psychological and physiological restraint that is thereby entailed presumably makes additional binge-eating more likely. Second, even if mood disturbance is not present at the outset, individuals become distressed about their inability to control their eating, and the resultant lowering of self-esteem contributes to disturbances of mood and to a reduced ability to control impulses to overeat. In addition, cognitive–behavioral theories emphasize the role of rigid rules regarding food and eating, and the distorted and dysfunctional thoughts that are similar to those seen in anorexia nervosa. Interpersonal theories also implicate interpersonal stressors as a primary factor in triggering

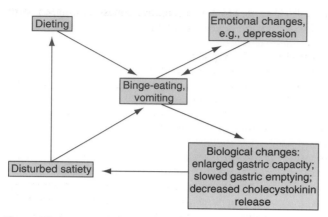

**Figure 75–6** *Diagram illustrating factors that may perpetuate bulimia nervosa.*

binge-eating. There is no evidence to suggest that a particular personality structure is characteristic of women with bulimia nervosa (Wonderlich 2002).

There are also indications that bulimia nervosa is accompanied by physiological disturbances that disrupt the development of satiety during a meal and therefore increase the likelihood of binge-eating. These disturbances include an enlarged stomach capacity, a delay in stomach emptying, and a reduction in the release of cholecystokinin, a peptide hormone secreted by the small intestine during a meal that normally plays a role in terminating eating behavior (Geracioti and Liddle 1988, Geliebter et al. 1992). All these abnormalities appear to predispose the individual to overeat and therefore to perpetuate the cycle of binge-eating.

It has been suggested that childhood sexual abuse is a specific risk factor for the development of bulimia nervosa. Scientific support for this hypothesis is weak. The best studies to date have found that compared with women without psychiatric illness, women with bulimia nervosa do indeed report increased frequencies of sexual abuse. However, the rates of abuse are similar to those found in other psychiatric disorders and occur in a minority of women with bulimia nervosa. Thus, while early abuse may predispose an individual to psychiatric problems generally, it does not appear to lead specifically to an eating disorder, and most patients with bulimia nervosa do not have histories of sexual abuse (Welch and Fairburn 1994).

## Pathophysiology

In a small fraction of individuals, bulimia nervosa is associated with the development of fluid and electrolyte abnormalities that result from the self-induced vomiting or the misuse of laxatives or diuretics. The most common electrolyte disturbances are hypokalemia, hyponatremia, and hypochloremia. Patients who lose substantial amounts of stomach acid through vomiting may become slightly alkalotic; those who abuse laxatives may become slightly acidotic.

There is an increased frequency of menstrual disturbances such as oligomenorrhea among women with bulimia nervosa. Several studies suggest that the hypothalamic–pituitary–gonadal axis is subject to the same type of disruption as is seen in anorexia nervosa but that the abnormalities are much less frequent and severe.

Patients who induce vomiting for many years may develop dental erosion, especially of the upper front teeth (Figure 75–7). The mechanism appears to be that stomach acid softens the enamel, which in time gradually disappears so that the teeth chip more easily and can become reduced in size. Some patients develop painless salivary gland enlargement, which is thought to represent hypertrophy resulting from the repeated episodes of binge-eating and vomiting. The serum level of amylase is sometimes mildly elevated in patients with bulimia nervosa because of increased amounts of salivary amylase.

Most patients with bulimia nervosa have surprisingly few gastrointestinal abnormalities. As indicated earlier, it appears that the disorder is associated with an enlarged gastric capacity and delayed gastric emptying, but these abnormalities are not so severe as to be detectable on routine clinical examination. Potentially life-threatening complications such as an esophageal tear or gastric rupture occur, but fortunately rarely.

The long-standing use of syrup of ipecac to induce vomiting can lead to absorption of some of the alkaloids and to permanent damage to nerve and muscle.

## Diagnosis and Differential Diagnosis

### Phenomenology

Bulimia nervosa typically begins after a young woman who sees herself as somewhat overweight starts a diet and, after some initial success, begins to overeat. Distressed by her lack of control and by her fear of gaining weight, she decides to compensate for the overeating by inducing vomiting or taking laxatives, methods she has heard about from friends or seen in media reports about eating disorders. After discovering that she can successfully purge, the individual may, for a time, feel pleased in that she can eat large amounts of food and not gain weight. However, the episodes of binge-eating usually increase in size and in frequency and occur after a variety of stimuli, such as transient depression or anxiety or a sense that she has begun to overeat. Patients often describe themselves as "numb" while they are binge-eating, suggesting that the eating may serve to avoid uncomfortable emotional states. Patients usually feel intensely ashamed of their "disgusting" habit

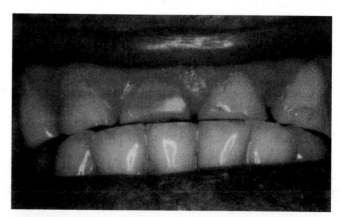

**Figure 75–7** *Dental erosion of upper front teeth of a patient with long-standing bulimia nervosa.*

and may become depressed by their lack of control over their eating.

The binge-eating tends to occur in the late afternoon or evening and almost always while the patient is alone. The typical patient presenting to eating disorders clinics has been binge-eating and inducing vomiting 5 to 10 times weekly for 3 to 10 years. Although there is substantial variation, binges tend to contain 1,000 or more calories and to consist of sweet, high-fat foods that are normally consumed as dessert, such as ice cream, cookies, and cake. Although patients complain of "carbohydrate craving," they only rarely binge-eat foods that are pure carbohydrates, such as fruits. Patients usually induce vomiting or use their characteristic compensatory behavior immediately after the binge and feel substantial relief that the calories are "gone." In reality, it appears that vomiting is the only purging method capable of disposing of a significant number of ingested calories. The weight loss associated with the misuse of laxatives and diuretics is primarily due to the loss of fluid and electrolytes, not calories.

When not binge-eating, patients with bulimia nervosa tend to restrict their calorie intake and to avoid the foods usually consumed during episodes of binge-eating. Although there is some phenomenological resemblance between binge-eating and substance abuse, there is no evidence that physiological addiction plays any role in bulimia nervosa.

## Assessment

### Special Issues in Psychiatric Examination and History

The assessment of individuals who may have bulimia nervosa is similar to that described for anorexia nervosa. The patient should be asked to describe a typical day's food intake and a typical binge, and the interviewer should assess whether the patient does indeed consume an unusually large amount of food as required by the DSM-IV definition of a binge. The interviewer should explicitly inquire about self-induced vomiting and whether syrup of ipecac is ever used to promote vomiting. The interviewer should ask about the use of laxatives, diuretics, diet pills, and enemas. A weight history should be obtained, so the interviewer can determine whether the binge-eating was preceded by obesity or by anorexia nervosa, as is often the case. Because there is substantial comorbidity, the interviewer should ascertain whether there is a history of anxiety or mood disturbance or of substance abuse.

### Physical Examination and Laboratory Findings

The patient should be weighed and the presence of dental erosion noted. Routine laboratory testing reveals an abnormality of fluid and electrolyte balance such as those described in the section on pathophysiology in about 10% of patients with bulimia nervosa.

### Differences in Presentation

Probably the greatest difference in presentation is between those individuals who purge and those who do not. Individuals with the nonpurging form of bulimia nervosa are more likely to be overweight at the time of presentation and to exhibit less general psychiatric illness compared with individuals who induce vomiting.

### Differential Diagnosis

Bulimia nervosa is not difficult to recognize if a full history is available. The binge-eating/purging type of anorexia nervosa has much in common with bulimia nervosa but is distinguished by the characteristic low body weight and, in women, amenorrhea. Some individuals with atypical forms of depression overeat when depressed; if the overeating meets the definition of a binge described previously (i.e., a large amount of food is consumed with a sense of loss of control), and if the binge-eating is followed by inappropriate compensatory behavior, occurs sufficiently frequently, and is associated with overconcern regarding body shape and weight, an additional diagnosis of bulimia nervosa may be warranted. Some individuals become nauseated and vomit when upset; this and similar problems are probably not closely related to bulimia nervosa and should be viewed as a somatoform disorder.

Many individuals who believe they have bulimia nervosa have a symptom pattern that fails to meet full diagnostic criteria because the frequency of their binge-eating is less than twice a week or because what they view as a binge does not contain an abnormally large amount of food. Individuals with these characteristics fall into the broad and heterogeneous category of atypical eating disorders. Binge-eating disorder (see section on binge-eating disorder), a category currently included in the DSM-IV appendix B for categories that need additional research, is characterized by recurrent binge-eating similar to that seen in bulimia nervosa but without the regular occurrence of inappropriate compensatory behavior.

### Course and Natural History

Over time, the symptoms of bulimia nervosa tend to improve although a substantial fraction of individuals continue to engage in binge-eating and purging (Keel et al. 1999). On the other hand, some controlled clinical trials have reported that structured forms of psychotherapy have the potential to yield substantial and sustained recovery in a significant fraction of patients who complete treatment (Fairburn et al. 1993, Pyle et al. 1990). It is not clear what factors are most predictive of good outcome, but those individuals who cease binge-eating and purging completely during treatment are least likely to relapse (Olmstead et al. 1994).

### Goals of Treatment

The goals of the treatment of bulimia nervosa are straightforward. The binge-eating and inappropriate compensatory behaviors should cease and self-esteem should become more appropriately based on factors other than shape and weight.

### Treatment

The power struggles that often complicate the treatment process in anorexia nervosa occur much less frequently in the treatment of patients with bulimia nervosa. This is largely because the critical behavioral disturbances, binge-eating and purging, are less ego-syntonic and are more distressing to these patients. Most bulimia nervosa patients

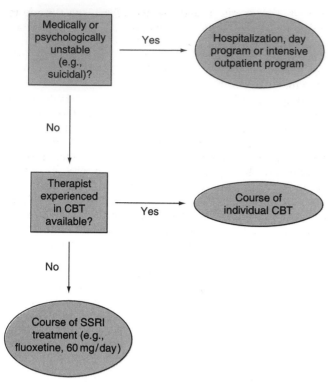

**Figure 75–8** *Algorithm for choice of initial treatment of bulimia nervosa.*

who pursue treatment agree with the primary treatment goals and wish to give up the core behavioral features of their illness.

The treatment of bulimia nervosa has received considerable attention in recent years and the efficacies of both psychotherapy and medication have been explored in numerous controlled studies (Figure 75–8). The form of psychotherapy that has been examined most intensively is cognitive–behavioral therapy, modeled on the therapy of the same type for depression (Agras 1993). Cognitive–behavioral therapy for bulimia nervosa concentrates on the distorted ideas about weight and shape, on the rigid rules regarding food consumption and the pressure to diet, and on the events that trigger episodes of binge-eating. The therapy is focused and highly structured and is usually conducted in 3 to 6 months. Approximately 25 to 50% of patients with bulimia nervosa achieve abstinence from binge-eating and purging during a course of cognitive–behavioral therapy, and in most, this improvement appears to be sustained. The most common form of cognitive–behavioral therapy is individual treatment, although it can be given in either individual or group format. The effect of cognitive–behavioral therapy is greater than that of supportive psychotherapy and of interpersonal therapy, indicating that cognitive–behavioral therapy should be the treatment of choice for bulimia nervosa.

The other commonly used mode of treatment that has been examined in bulimia nervosa is the use of antidepressant medication (Zhu and Walsh 2002). This intervention was initially prompted by the high rates of depression among patients with bulimia nervosa and has now been tested in more than a dozen double-blind, placebo-controlled studies using a wide variety of antidepressant medications. Active medication has been consistently

found to be superior to placebo, and although there have been no large "head-to-head" comparisons between different antidepressants, most antidepressants appear to possess roughly similar antibulimic potency (Figure 75–9). Fluoxetine at a dose of 60 mg/day is favored by many investigators because it has been studied in several large trials and appears to be at least as effective as, and better tolerated than, most other alternatives. It is notable that it has not been possible to link the effectiveness of antidepressant treatment for bulimia nervosa to the pretreatment level of depression. Depressed and nondepressed patients with bulimia nervosa respond equally well in terms of their eating behavior to antidepressant medication.

Although antidepressant medication is clearly superior to placebo in the treatment of bulimia nervosa, several studies suggest that a course of a single antidepressant medication is generally inferior to a course of cognitive–behavioral therapy. However, patients who fail to respond adequately to, or who relapse following a trial of psychotherapy, may still respond to antidepressant medication.

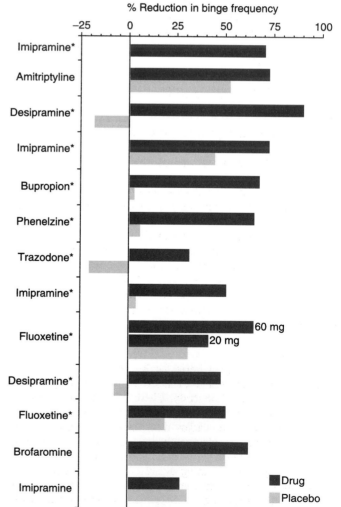

**Figure 75–9** *Results of controlled trials of antidepressants in bulimia nervosa. (*indicates a statistically significant difference between the active medication and placebo; Source: Walsh BT and Devlin MJ [1995] Eating disorders. Child Adolesc Psychiatr Clin N Am 4, 343–357.)*

## Special Features Influencing Treatment

A major factor influencing the treatment of bulimia nervosa is the presence of other significant psychiatric or medical illness. For example, it can be difficult for individuals who are currently abusing drugs or alcohol to use the treatment methods described, and many psychiatrists suggest that the substance abuse needs to be addressed before the eating disorder can be effectively treated. Other examples include the treatment of individuals with bulimia nervosa and serious personality disturbance and those with insulin-dependent diabetes mellitus who "purge" by omitting insulin doses. In treating such individuals, the psychiatrist must decide which of the multiple problems must be first addressed and may elect to tolerate a significant level of eating disorder to confront more pressing disturbances.

## Refractory Patients

Although psychotherapy and antidepressant medication are effective interventions for many patients with bulimia nervosa, some individuals have little or no response. There is no clearly established algorithm for the treatment of such refractory patients. Alternative interventions that may prove useful include other forms of psychotherapy and other medications such as opiate antagonists and the serotonin agonist fenfluramine. Hospitalization should also be considered as a way to normalize eating behavior, at least temporarily, and perhaps to initiate a more effective outpatient treatment.

## BINGE-EATING DISORDER

### History

As noted earlier, binge-eating disorder is a proposed diagnostic category related to, but quite distinct from, bulimia nervosa. Individuals with binge-eating disorder, like individuals with bulimia nervosa, repeatedly engage in episodes of binge-eating but, unlike patients with bulimia nervosa, do not regularly utilize inappropriate compensatory behaviors. The phenomenon of binge-eating without purging among the obese was clearly described by Stunkard (1959), 20 years before bulimia nervosa was recognized. Yet binge-eating disorder has been the focus of sustained attention only in the last decade. The clinical utility of the information which quickly developed following the recognition of bulimia in the DSM nomenclature was an important source of interest in binge-eating disorder.

### Definition

Suggested diagnostic criteria for binge-eating disorder are included in an appendix of DSM-IV-TR which provides criteria sets for further study. These criteria require recurrent episodes of binge-eating, which are defined just as for bulimia nervosa. The major difference from bulimia nervosa is that individuals with binge-eating disorder do not regularly use inappropriate compensatory behavior, although the precise meaning of "regularly" is not specified. Other differences from the definition of bulimia nervosa relate to the frequency of binge-eating: individuals with bulimia nervosa must binge-eat, on average, at least two times per week over the last 3 months, whereas individuals with binge-eating disorder must binge-eat at least 2 days per week over the last 6 months. A major reason for the differ-ence in the criteria is that the end of a binge episode in bulimia nervosa is usually clearly marked by the occurrence of inappropriate compensatory behavior, like purging, whereas in binge-eating disorder, the end of a binge episode may be more difficult to identify precisely. The criteria attempt to deal with this definitional difficulty by requiring the frequency of binge-eating to be measured in terms of the number of days per week on which episodes occur, and, because of the potential difficulty in distinguishing "normal" overeating from binge-eating, to require a 6 month duration, rather than 3 months for bulimia nervosa. In addition, the suggested DSM-IV-TR criteria for binge-eating disorder require that individuals report behavioral evidence of a sense of loss of control over eating, such as eating large amounts of food when not physically hungry. Finally, while there is some evidence that individuals with binge-eating disorder tend to be more concerned about body image than individuals of similar weight, the criteria for binge-eating disorder require only that there is marked distress over the binge-eating. Thus, the criteria for binge-eating disorder do not require that self-evaluation be overly influenced by concerns regarding body weight and shape, as is required for bulimia nervosa.

### Epidemiology

The epidemiology of binge-eating disorder is uncertain. Cross-sectional studies suggest that the prevalence of binge-eating disorder among adults is a few percent and that the prevalence is higher among obese individuals in the community and among obese individuals who attend weight loss clinics. Similarly, the frequency of binge-eating disorder increases with the degree of obesity. In contrast to anorexia nervosa and bulimia nervosa, individuals with binge-eating disorder are more likely to be men (the female to male ratio is roughly 1.5:1 compared to approximately 10:1 for anorexia nervosa and bulimia nervosa), from minority ethnic groups, and middle-aged (Yanovski 1993).

### Etiology

Very little is known about the etiology of binge-eating disorder. Binge-eating disorder is clearly associated with obesity, but it is uncertain to what degree the binge-eating is a contributor to, and to what degree a consequence of, the obesity.

## Diagnosis and Differential Diagnosis

### Phenomenology

In theory, binge-eating disorder should be easy to recognize on the basis of patient self-report: the individual describes the frequent consumption of large amounts of food in a discrete period of time about which he or she feels distressed and unable to control. Difficulties arise, however, because of uncertainty about what precisely constitutes a "large amount of food," especially for an obese individual, and regarding what constitutes a discrete period of time. Many individuals describe eating continuously during the day or evening, thereby consuming a large amount of food, but it is not clear whether such behavior is best viewed as binge-eating.

Individuals who meet the proposed definition of binge-eating disorder clearly have increased complaints of depression and anxiety compared to individuals of similar weight without binge-eating disorder.

## Assessment

The assessment of individuals who may have binge-eating disorder parallels that of individuals who may have bulimia nervosa. It is important to obtain a clear understanding of daily food intake and of what the individual considers a binge. As in the assessment of bulimia nervosa, the interviewer should inquire about the use of purging and other inappropriate weight control methods. Individuals who describe binge-eating disorder are likely to be obese, and it is important to obtain a history of changes in weight and of efforts to lose weight. The interviewer should also inquire about symptoms of mood disturbance and anxiety.

## Physical Examination and Laboratory Findings

The salient general medical issue is that of obesity. Individuals with binge-eating disorder who are obese should be followed by a primary care physician for assessment and treatment of the complications of obesity. There is no evidence suggesting that the behavioral disturbances characteristic of binge-eating disorder add to the physical risks of obesity. Whether the presence of binge-eating disorder affects the natural history of obesity is an intriguing but unanswered question.

## Differential Diagnosis

As noted above, the most difficult issue in the diagnostic assessment of binge-eating disorder is determining whether the eating pattern of concern to the individual meets the proposed definition of binge-eating. There are numerous varieties of unhealthy eating, such as the consumption of high fat foods, and the nosology of these patterns of eating is poorly worked out.

Some individuals with atypical depression binge-eat when depressed; if the individual meets criteria for both binge-eating disorder and an atypical depression, both diagnoses should be made.

## Course and Natural History

As the recognition of binge-eating disorder is quite recent, there is little definitive information about the natural history of this disorder. However, both controlled treatment studies and follow-up studies of community samples indicate that there is substantial fluctuation over time in the frequency and severity of the cardinal symptoms of this disorder.

## Goals of Treatment

For most individuals with binge-eating disorder, there are three related goals. One is behavioral, to cease binge eating. A second focuses on improving symptoms of mood and anxiety disturbance which frequently are associated with binge-eating disorder. The third is weight loss for individuals who are also obese.

## Treatment

Treatment approaches to binge-eating disorder are currently under active study. There is good evidence that psychological (e.g., CBT) and pharmacological (e.g., SSRI) interventions which are effective for bulimia nervosa are also useful in reducing the binge frequency of individuals with binge-eating disorder and in alleviating mood disturbance. However, it is not clear how helpful these approaches are in facilitating weight loss. Standard behavioral weight loss interventions employing caloric restriction appear useful in helping patients to control binge-eating, but the benefits of such treatment have not been compared to those of more psychologically-oriented treatments, such as CBT.

---

### Clinical Vignette 1

When Ms. A was first evaluated for admission to an inpatient eating disorders program, she had been restricting her food intake for approximately 5 years and had been amenorrheic for 4 years. At the time of her admission, this 24-year-old, single, white woman weighed 71 lb at a height of 5 feet 1.5 inches. In 12th grade, Ms. A menstruated for the first time and also developed "very large" breasts. She had a difficult first year at college, where she gained to her maximum weight of 120 lb. The following year, Ms. A transferred to a smaller college, became a vegetarian "for ethical reasons," and began to significantly restrict her food intake. She limited herself to a total of 700 to 800 cal/day, with a maximum of 200 calories per meal, and gradually lost weight in the next 5 years. Ms. A did not binge, vomit, abuse laxatives, or engage in excessive exercise. She considered herself to be "obsessed with calories" and observed a variety of rituals regarding food and food preparation (e.g., obsessively weighing her food).

Although Ms. A excelled academically, she had no close friends and had never been involved in a romantic relationship. She was quite close to her mother and sister and had always been dependent on her parents. After graduating (with honors) from college, Ms. A worked at a series of temporary jobs but was unemployed and living at home with her mother at the time of admission. She had been in outpatient psychotherapy with two different therapists during the previous 2 years. The first therapist did not address her eating disorder, and Ms. A continued to lose weight, from 90 to 80 lb. Although her second therapist confronted her about her anorexia nervosa and started her on desipramine at 20 mg/day for depressive symptoms, Ms. A continued to lose weight.

During her first 5-month hospitalization, Ms. A was treated with a multimodal program (behavioral weight gain protocol, individual and family therapy, fluoxetine at 60–80 mg for obsessive–compulsive traits and depressive symptoms) and gained to a weight of 98 lb. At discharge, she was maintaining her weight on food but remained concerned about her weight and was particularly frightened of reaching "the triple digits" (i.e., 100 lb). After leaving the hospital, Ms. A continued with outpatient psychotherapy and fluoxetine for several months. She was then seriously injured in a car accident and, during a prolonged convalescent period, discontinued treatment for her eating disorder. Ms. A remained unemployed, eventually moved in with her sister and her sister's family, and gradually lost weight.

About 3.5 years after discharge, at age 27 years, Ms. A again sought inpatient treatment. At admission, she weighed 83 lb but still felt "fat." During hospitalization, she steadily gained weight and was prescribed sertraline at 100 mg/day for feelings of low self-esteem, anxiety, and obsessional thinking. When she was discharged 5 months later, at a weight of 108 lb, she noted menstrual bleeding for the first time in more than 7 years. After leaving the hospital, Ms. A continued taking medication and began outpatient cognitive–behavioral psychotherapy. For the next year, she continued to struggle with eating and weight issues but managed to maintain her weight and successfully expand other aspects of her life by independently supporting herself with a full-time job, making new friends, and becoming involved in her first romantic relationship.

---

### Clinical Vignette 2

When Ms. B, a 20-year-old white college student, was first evaluated for treatment at an outpatient eating disorders program, she had been binge-eating and purging for approximately 5 years. Each evening, she consumed large quantities of food, vomited three or four times, and took two to six laxatives. She also occasionally used herbal diuretics but had never abused diet pills or prescription diuretics. Ms. B's weight was well within the normal range (106 lb at a height of 5 feet 2 inches). She was extremely concerned about her shape and weight, was afraid of becoming fat, and wanted to weigh no more than 100 lb ("the double digits are nice too … maybe 90 lb, but I don't think I could run at that weight").

Ms. B always binged alone in her dormitory room while watching television and flipping through magazines. A typical binge might consist of two packages of cookies, a half-gallon of ice cream, one box of cereal, one can of spaghetti, one bag of pretzels, one can of soup, one package of fishsticks, one bag of candy, and six bagels with butter, eaten during a 3- to 4-hour period. She would vomit every hour or so, each time making room for more food. Throughout the day, she would severely restrict her food intake, usually eating nothing but fruit, salad, oatmeal, diet hot chocolate, coffee, and chewing gum. She was an avid cross-country runner, totaling about 50 miles per week, but denied running to compensate for eating binges.

Ms. B was raised on the East Coast by her parents, who were college graduates, and had an older brother. She had a history of always being thin, and when she was in the sixth grade, she weighed 75 lb at a height of 4 feet 9 inches. She began binge-eating and purging at age 16 years, after her father was hospitalized for a suicide attempt. She read many books about eating disorders, because she "wanted to be anorexic," and within 2 months, she was binge-eating and purging every day. She had periodically been treated for her eating disorder, both with individual psychotherapy and with 20 mg of fluoxetine; none of these treatments was significantly helpful. She was also hospitalized for 7 weeks at age 17 years and stopped binge-eating and purging, but anorexia nervosa developed. Her weight dropped to 95 lb, which was 80% of her ideal body weight. She had not menstruated since she began binge-eating and purging, and she did not menstruate again until she was 19 years old.

Other than her father's depression, there was no family history of psychiatric illness or eating disorders. Ms. B had also had several major depressive episodes since she was 16 years old, during which she experienced depressed mood, lessened interest in her usual activities, tiredness, decreased concentration, and suicidal thoughts. She had never used drugs and drank only rarely.

Soon after she began a 4-month course of cognitive–behavioral therapy plus desipramine, 100 mg/day, Ms. B's eating disorder improved substantially. By the time she completed treatment, she was still binge-eating and vomiting occasionally, but she felt much more in control of her

bulimia. Her self-esteem was greatly improved, and she was more aware of distortions in her thoughts about her eating and body shape and weight. She was optimistic yet realistic about maintaining the gains she had achieved. Ms. B was prescribed desipramine for 3 months more, and then for the following 9 months, she was treated with fluoxetine, 30 mg/day, and met occasionally with another therapist. Ms. B continued to be much improved, but not entirely well, binge-eating and purging once or twice a month.

## Comparison of DSM-IV/ICD-10 Diagnostic Criteria

The ICD-10 Diagnostic Criteria for Research and the DSM-IV-TR criteria for anorexia nervosa differ in several ways. ICD-10 specifically requires that the weight loss be self-induced by the avoidance of "fattening foods" and that in men there be a loss of sexual interest and potency (corresponding to the amenorrhea requirement in women). Finally, in contrast to DSM-IV-TR which gives anorexia nervosa precedence over bulimia nervosa, ICD-10 excludes a diagnosis of anorexia nervosa if regular binge eating has been present.

For bulimia nervosa, the ICD-10 Diagnostic Criteria for Research and the DSM-IV-TR criteria for bulimia nervosa are similar except that ICD-10 requires a "persistent preoccupation with eating and a strong desire or sense of compulsion to eat." Furthermore, whereas the ICD-10 definition requires a self-perception of being too fat (identical to an item in anorexia nervosa), the DSM-IV-TR criteria set requires instead that "self-evaluation is unduly influenced by body shape and weight."

Both DSM-IV-TR and ICD-10 include categories unique to their systems. DSM-IV-TR has a category for "Binge-Eating Disorder" in its appendix of research categories whereas ICD-10 has categories for "Overeating associated with other psychological disturbances" and "Vomiting associated with other psychological disturbances."

## References

Agras WS (1993) Short-term psychological treatments for binge-eating. In Binge Eating: Nature, Assessment, and Treatment, Fairburn CG and Wilson GT (eds). Guilford Press, New York, p. 270.

Bedoyere MDL (1947) Catherine: Saint of Sienna. Hollis and Carter, London.

Bell RM (1985) Holy Anorexia. University of Chicago Press, Chicago.

Bruch H (1973) Eating Disorders. Obesity, Anorexia Nervosa, and the Person Within. Basic Books, New York.

Bruch H (1982) Anorexia nervosa: Therapy and theory. Am J Psychiatr 132, 1531.

Casper RC, Hedeker D, and McClough JF (1992) Personality dimensions in eating disorders and their relevance for subtyping. J Am Acad Child Adolesc Psychiatr 31, 830.

Fairburn CG and Beglin SJ (1990) Studies of the epidemiology of bulimia nervosa. Am J Psychiatr 147, 401.

Fairburn CG and Walsh BT (2002) Atypical eating disorders. In Eating Disorders and Obesity: A Comprehensive Textbook, 2nd ed., Brownell KD and Fairburn CG (eds). Guilford Press, New York, p. 171.

Fairburn CG, Jones R, Peveler RC, et al. (1993) Psychotherapy and bulimia nervosa: Longer-term effects of interpersonal psychotherapy, behavior therapy and cognitive behavior therapy. Arch Gen Psychiatr 50, 419.

Garner DM and Garfinkel PE (eds) (1997) Handbook of Psychotherapy for Anorexia Nervosa and Bulimia, 2nd ed. Guilford Press, New York.

Geliebter A, Melton P, McCray RS, et al. (1992) Gastric capacity, gastric emptying, and test-meal intake in normal and bulimic women. Am J Clin Nutr 56, 656.

Geracioti TD and Liddle RA (1988) Impaired cholecystokinin secretion in bulimia nervosa. New Engl J Med 319, 683.

Gordon RA (1990) Anorexia and Bulimia: Anatomy of a Social Epidemic. Basil Blackwell, Cambridge, MA.

Halmi KA, Eckert ED, LaDu TJ, et al. (1986) Anorexia nervosa: Treatment efficacy of cyproheptadine and amitriptyline. Arch Gen Psychiatr 43, 177.

Hsu KL (1990) Eating Disorders. Guilford Press, New York.

Hsu LK (1996) Epidemiology of the eating disorders. Psychiatr Clin N Am 19, 681.

Hsu LK and Lee S (1993) Is weight phobia always necessary for a diagnosis of anorexia nervosa? Am J Psychiatr 150, 1466.

Kaye WH (1997) Anorexia nervosa, obsessional behavior, and serotonin. Psychopharmacol Bull 33, 335.

Keel PK, Mitchell JE, Miller KB, et al. (1999) Long-term outcome of bulimia nervosa. Arch Gen Psychiatr 56, 63.

Kendler KS, Maclean C, Neale M, et al. (1991) The genetic epidemiology of bulimia nervosa. Am J Psychiatr 148, 1627.

Klump KL, Kaye W, and Strober M (2001) The evolving genetic foundations of eating disorders. Psychiatr Clin N Am 24, 215.

Lock J, le Grange D, Agras WS, et al. (2000) Treatment Manual for Anorexia Nervosa. Guilford Press, New York.

Minuchin S, Rosman BL, and Baker L (1978) Psychosomatic Families. Anorexia Nervosa in Context. Harvard University Press, Cambridge, MA.

Morton R (1689) Phthisiologica: Or a Treatise of Consumptions. London.

Olmstead MP, Kaplan AS, and Rockert W (1994) Rate and prediction of relapse in bulimia nervosa. Am J Psychiatr 151, 738.

Pyle RL, Mitchell JE, Eckert ED, et al. (1990) Maintenance treatment and 6-month outcome for bulimic patients who respond to initial treatment. Am J Psychiatr 147, 871.

Russell G (1979) Bulimia nervosa: An ominous variant of anorexia nervosa. Psychol Med 9, 429.

Seidell JC and Thjhuis MAR (2002) Obesity and quality of life. In Eating Disorders and Obesity: A Comprehensive Textbook, 2nd ed., Brownell KD and Fairburn CG (eds). Guilford Press, New York, p. 388.

Srinivasagam NM, Kaye WH, Plotnicov KH, et al. (1995) Persistent perfectionism, symmetry, and exactness after long-term recovery from anorexia nervosa. Am J Psychiatr 152, 1630.

Striegel-Moore RH, Schreiber GB, Lo A, et al. (2000) Eating disorder symptoms in a cohort of 11- to 16-year-old black and white girls: The NHLBI growth and health study. Int J Eat Disord 27, 49.

Stunkard AJ (1959) Eating patterns and obesity. Psychiatr Q 33, 284.

Van Hoeken D, Lucas AR, and Hoek HW (1998) Epidemiology. In Neurobiology in the Treatment of Eating Disorders, Hoek HW, Treasure JL, and Katzman MA (eds). John Wiley, Chichester, p. 97.

Walsh BT (2001) Eating disorders. In Harrison's Principles of Internal Medicine, 15th ed., Braunwald E, Fauci AS, Kasper DL, et al. (eds). McGraw-Hill, New York, p. 486.

Walsh BT and Devlin MJ (1995) Eating disorders. Child Adolesc Psychiatr Clin N Am 4, 343–357.

Walsh BT, Hadigan CM, Kissileff HR, et al. (1992) Bulimia nervosa: A syndrome of feast and famine. In The Biology of Feast and Famine: Relevance to Eating Disorders, Anderson GH and Kennedy SH (eds.) Academic Press, Orlando, p. 3.

Welch SL and Fairburn CG (1994) Sexual abuse and bulimia nervosa: Three integrated case control comparisons. Am J Psychiatr 151, 402.

Wonderlich SA (2002) Personality and eating disorders. In Eating Disorders and Obesity: A Comprehensive Textbook, 2nd ed., Brownell KD and Fairburn CG (eds). Guilford Press, New York, p. 204.

Yanovski SZ (1993) Binge eating disorder: Current knowledge and future directions. Obes Res 1, 306.

Zhu AJ and Walsh BT (2002) Pharmacological treatment of eating disorders. Can J Psychiatr 47, 227.

# 76  Sleep and Sleep–Wake Disorders

J. Christian Gillin
Sonia Ancoli-Israel
Milton Erman

Clinical psychiatrists and psychologists of the new millennium will need to master a general basic knowledge of sleep and chronobiology, the disorders of sleep and circadian rhythms, their clinical manifestations and differential diagnosis, and their clinical management (American Psychiatric Association 1994, Kryger et al. 2000). This chapter provides an overview of the main topics in basic and clinical sciences of sleep.

## PHENOMENOLOGY AND ORGANIZATION OF SLEEP

### Physiological Regulation of Sleep and Wakefulness

Three physiological processes regulate sleep and wakefulness (Borbely and Ackermann 1992).

**Ultradian Rhythm of Rapid Eye Movement (REM) and Non-Rapid Eye Movement (Non-REM) Sleep.** Sleep consists of two major REM and non-REM sleep, which alternate throughout the sleep period (Kryger et al. 2000). Sleep normally begins in the adult with non-REM sleep and is followed after about 70 to 90 minutes by the first REM period. Thereafter, non-REM sleep and REM sleep oscillate with a cycle length (the interval between onset of each non-REM or REM period) of about 80 to 110 minutes. This cycle of REM and non-REM sleep is an example of an ultradian rhythm, a biological rhythm with a cycle length considerably less than 24 hours (Figure 76–1).

On the basis of electroencephalographical (EEG) characteristics, non-REM sleep in humans is further divided into four stages: stage 1, a brief transitional stage between wakefulness and sleep; stage 2, which occupies the greatest amount of time during sleep; and stages 3 and 4, sometimes called delta sleep because of the characteristic high-amplitude slow EEG waves (delta waves) (Table 76–1). The amount of ocular activity per minute of REM sleep is quantified as REM density; this can be measured by either

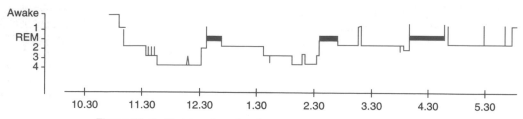

**Figure 76–1** *All-night polygraphic sleep stages in a normal young volunteer.*

visual scoring (e.g., on an analogue scale from 0 to 8 per minute) or by computer analysis. Dreaming is commonly reported and is usually vivid when subjects are awakened from REM sleep but also occurs during non-REM sleep, especially at sleep onset during stage 1 sleep.

**Circadian (24-Hour) Rhythm of Sleep and Wakefulness.** The rest–activity or sleep–wake cycle is an example of a

circadian rhythm (Table 76–2). Other examples include the hypothalamic–pituitary–adrenal axis, thyroid-stimulating hormone, and core body temperature. [Circadian rhythms can be characterized by three difference measures: (a) cycle length (tau) (e.g., the time between two peaks of the ∼24 hour temperature curve); (b) amplitude (e.g., the difference between the minimum value of the cycle (nadir) and maximum value (acrophase), for example, the difference between the lowest and highest points in the ∼24 hour temperature curve; and (c) phase position of the rhythm (e.g., the time of day when the acrophase occurred)] (Kryger et al. 2000, Moore-Ede et al. 1982).

The propensity for sleep and wakefulness varies in a circadian fashion, at least after infancy, and is modulated in part by one or more biological clocks. The suprachiasmatic nucleus (SCN) in the anterior hypothalamus plays a decisive role in the regulation of most circadian rhythms in humans and animals. The endogenous activity rhythms of the SCN are synchronized with the environment primarily by ambient light. Information regarding light reaching the retina is conveyed to the SCN directly through the retinohypothalamic tract and indirectly through the intergeniculate leaflet of the lateral geniculate body. Changes in light intensity, especially at dawn and dusk, are particularly important in synchronizing endogenous oscillators controlling rhythms of sleep–wake, cortisol, melatonin, and core body temperature with one another and with the outside world.

If humans are allowed to choose their sleep–wake cycles in the absence of time cues such as daily light–dark signals or clocks, they usually show, as most mammalian species do, a sleep–wake cycle longer than 24 hours. The self-selected rest–activity cycle is typically about 24.5 to 25 hours in length, although it may increase, for example, to 36 hours (24 hours awake and 12 hours asleep). These observations imply that neurons within the SCN have an inherent rhythmicity of approximately 24.5 to 25 hours. Subjects in a time-free environment are said to be "free-running" because endogenous processes, such as a circadian oscillator, rather than environmental cues, determine their sleep–wake, endocrine, and other rhythms.

The propensity for, character, and duration of sleep are closely related to the phase position of the underlying circadian oscillator. If the daily temperature curve is used to index the phase position of the biological clock, sleep in general and REM sleep in particular occur most commonly near the nadir of the temperature rhythm. Thus, in persons who live a conventional sleep schedule (11 PM–7 AM), REM sleep is more common in the last half of the night when core body temperature is lowest than in the first half and more likely in morning naps than in afternoon naps. Further-

| Table 76–1 | Commonly Used Terms in Human Sleep Studies |
|---|---|
| Term | Definition |
| Delta wave | Electroencephalographic pattern conventionally defined as 75 mV, 0.5 Hz or cycles per second wave; the amplitude tends to decrease with normal aging |
| Non-REM sleep | Stages 1, 2, 3, and 4 sleep |
| Total sleep time | Non-REM and REM sleep time |
| REM latency | Time from onset of sleep to onset of REM sleep; declines from about 70–100 min in the 20s to 55–70 min in the elderly, short REM latency associated with narcolepsy, depression, and a variety of clinical conditions |
| REM sleep | Rapid eye movement sleep; characterized by low-voltage, relatively fast frequency EEG, bursts of rapid eye movements, and loss of tone (atonia) in the major antigravity muscles; associated with dreaming |
| Sleep efficiency | Percentage of time in bed spent in sleep; usually above 90% in the young, falls somewhat with age |
| Sleep latency | Time from "lights out" to onset of sleep |
| Stage 1 sleep | A brief transitional state of sleep between wakefulness and sleep, characterized by low-voltage, mixed-frequency EEG, and slow eye movements; about 5% of total sleep time |
| Stage 2 sleep | Characterized by K complexes and sleep spindles (12–14 per cycle rhythms) in the EEG; usually about 45–75% of total sleep time |
| Stages 3 and 4 sleep | Sometimes referred to as delta sleep, based on amount of sleep delta waves in EEG, 20–50% of an epoch (i.e., 30 or 60 s) for stage 3, more than 50% for stage 4; amount per night declining from about 20–25% of total sleep time in the teens to nearly zero in the elderly |
| WASO | Wake time sleep onset |
| REM density | A measure of amount of ocular activity per minute of REM sleep |

| Table 76–2 | Commonly Used Terms in Chronobiology |
|---|---|
| Term | Definition |
| Acrophase | The time, at which the maximal point of a circadian rhythm occurs, i.e., maximal secretion of cortisol normally occurs at midmorning in humans. |
| Circadian rhythm | Refers to biological rhythms having a cycle length of about 24 h, derived from Latin *circa dies*, "about 1 d"; examples include the sleep–wake cycle in humans, temperature, cortisol, and psychological variation in the 24-h day; characterized by exact cycle length (tau), amplitude, and phase position. |
| Constant routine | An experimental method used to estimate amplitude and phase position of circadian temperature and neuroendocrine rhythms; the subject remains awake for about 36 h under dim light, with head elevated slightly, eating frequent equal-calorie meals, while blood samples are withdrawn unobtrusively every 20–30 min and rectal temperature is measured about once a minute. |
| Dim light melatonin onset (DLMO) | An experimental method for estimating the phase of melatonin onset; under dim light conditions starting in late afternoon, blood samples are withdrawn every 20–30 min to determine when melatonin secretion begins. |
| Nadir | Time when the minimal point of a circadian rhythm occurs. |
| Phase position | Temporal relationship between rhythms or between one rhythm and the environment; e.g., maximal daily temperature peak (acrophase) usually occurs in the late afternoon. |
| Phase-advanced rhythm | Phase position of biological rhythm occurs earlier than reference, i.e., the patient retires and arises early. |
| Phase-delayed rhythm | Phase position of biological rhythm occurs later than reference, i.e., the patient retires and arises late. |
| Phase-response curve | Graph showing the magnitude and direction of change in phase position of circadian rhythm depending upon timing of Zeitgeber with reference to the endogenous oscillator. |
| Tau | Cycle length, e.g., from one acrophase to the next of temperature. |
| Zeitgebers | Time cues, such as social activities, meals, and bright lights, that influence phase position of rhythm. |

The phase position of the circadian oscillator can also be estimated in humans by the 24-hour rhythms of cortisol or melatonin secretion. Because these rhythms can be affected by exercise, meals, light, and so forth, the conditions under which they are measured should be controlled. For example, clinical investigators may use a "constant routine" condition in which the subjects are kept awake in bed for 36 hours, under constant low-intensity light (Minors and Waterhouse 1984). An alternative is to determine the onset of melatonin secretion under dark conditions (dim light melatonin onset) (Lewy and Sack 1989). As discussed later, various strategies are under experimental development with the hope that appropriate administration of light–dark cycles, melatonin, vitamin $B_{12}$, or specific medications will "nudge" and "squash" the circadian oscillator correctly to better manage clinical disorders of sleep–wakefulness, such as jet lag, delayed sleep syndrome, and shift work problems (Lewy and Sack 1989, Czeisler et al. 1990). In addition, bright light has been shown to have antidepressant effects in patients with winter depression, some patients with major depressive disorder, and patients with premenstrual dysphoric disorder.

If animals suffer lesions of the SCN, they no longer exhibit circadian rhythms of temperature, cortisol secretion, eating, drinking, or sleep–wakefulness. Sleep and wakefulness, for example, are taken in brief bouts throughout the 24-hour day. Total sleep time, however, may increase under these circumstances. Although no selective lesion of the human SCN has been documented, a case report has been published of a 34-year-old woman who suffered damage to the anterior hypothalamus, presumably ablating the SCN, and who exhibited a polyphasic sleep–wake cycle (Cohen and Albers 1993).

**Homeostatic Regulation of Sleep–Wakefulness.** Common experience suggests that the longer one is awake, the more likely one is to fall asleep. Furthermore, sleep reverses the

more, subjects tend to awaken on the rising phase of the temperature rhythm.

Appropriate exposure to light and darkness can change the phase position of the underlying biological oscillator or, in some circumstances, the amplitude of circadian rhythms (Czeisler et al. 1989). Bright light at the beginning of the subjective evening in conjunction with dark during the subjective morning delays and resets the phase position of the temperature, cortisol, melatonin, and sleep–wake rhythms; dark in the subjective evening and bright light in the subjective morning have the opposite effect. The magnitude and direction of the changes induced by bright light or other Zeitgebers ("timegivers") at any particular time form the *phase-response curve* (Figure 76–2).

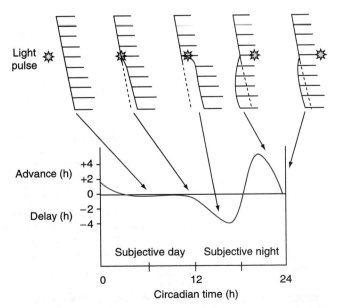

**Figure 76–2** *The phase-response curve in the hamster, demonstrating the magnitude and direction of phase-shifting properties of bright light, depending on when the light is presented with relationship to circadian time.*

sleepiness and other consequences of wakefulness. Thus, sleep can be said to perform a homeostatic function; it is a time of rest and restoration that overcomes the "ravages of wakefulness" (Daan et al. 1984). Consistent with the hypothesis, sleep deprivation usually decreases sleep latency and increases sleep efficiency and delta sleep on recovery nights.

The precise regulation of sleep and wakefulness remains an area of intense investigation and theory. Two of the current theories of sleep–wake regulation include the two-process model (Daan et al. 1984) and the opponent process model (Edgar et al. 1993). The first postulates that sleep and wakefulness are regulated by a circadian process (process C), which sets the circadian thresholds for sleep and wakefulness, and a homeostatic process (process S), in which sleep propensity builds up with wakefulness and dissipates during non-REM sleep, especially delta sleep. The opponent process model postulates that the SCN promotes alertness and that duration of wakefulness facilitates sleep.

## Normal Age-Related Changes in Sleep and Wakefulness

The newborn spends nearly 50% of total sleep time in REM sleep. Because infants may sleep up to 16 hours a day, the infant may spend 8 hours in REM sleep per day. Often to the consternation of the parents, the newborn has a polyphasic sleep–wake pattern, with short bouts of sleep and wakefulness throughout the 24-hour day, until several months of age when the child eventually sleeps through the night. Daytime napping, however, often persists until the age of 4 to 6 years. Stages 3 and 4 sleep increase in the early years. Maximal "depth" of sleep may occur during the prepubertal period, when children are often difficult to awake at night. Adolescents often still need at least 10 hours of sleep. Yet, during adolescence, stages 3 and 4 sleep decline and daytime sleepiness increases, partially in association with the normal Tanner stages of pubertal development (Carskadon et al. 1980). Teenagers are also phase delayed which means that they may not get sleepy until the early morning hours (e.g., 2–3 AM) and do not naturally wake up until the later morning hours. Early school start times and social pressures may produce mild sleep deprivation during weekdays, with some catch-up on weekends.

As adults enter middle age and old age, sleep often becomes more shallow, fragmented, and variable in duration and circadian timing compared with that of young adults. Stages 1 and 2 and wake time after sleep onset tend to increase; REM latency and stages 3 and 4 decline, probably at an earlier age in men than in women and possibly related to changes in brain structure and metabolism (Feinberg 1974, Feinberg et al. 1990). Daytime sleepiness and napping usually increase with age, often as a function of disturbed nocturnal sleep. The elderly frequently choose an "early-to-bed, early-to-rise" pattern reflecting, in part, an apparent phase advance of the circadian clock. Even when they retire at the same time that they did when they were young, they still tend to wake up early, thus sleep-depriving themselves. This can lead to daytime sleepiness and napping. Although average total sleep time actually increases slightly after age 65 years, greater numbers of

persons fall into either long-sleeping (>8 hours) or short-sleeping (<7 hours) subgroups. Psychiatrists should always consider the role of chronobiological factors when evaluating patients with sleep disorders, especially the elderly, who have more sleep–wake complaints than younger persons. The sleep–wake patterns of the early bedtimes of the elderly, short REM latency, sleep fragmentation at night, and napping during the day may reflect a phase-advance and reduced amplitude of the circadian oscillator (Duffy and Czeisler 2002, Duffy et al. 2002).

Factors that could contribute to these age-related patterns include loss of influence from Zeitgebers (light, work schedules, social demands, physical exercise) and a weaker signal from the circadian oscillator to effector systems. Indoor living conditions or loss of hearing and sight may deprive individuals of cues that synchronize the circadian system. In a significant number of totally blind persons, for example, the circadian oscillator free-runs in the normal environment, with resulting regular periods of insomnia and hypersomnia every 3 weeks as the circadian oscillator delays by about 45 minutes each 24 hours while the subject tries to maintain a normal sleep period (11PM–7AM). In a study of normally sighted elderly individuals in San Diego, California, exposure to self-selected bright light averaged 45 minutes and 90 minutes per day for healthy women and men, respectively; 30 minutes per day for patients with Alzheimer's disease living at home; and 2 minutes for chronically ill, institutionalized patients (Campbell et al. 1988, Jacobs et al. 1989). Perhaps not surprisingly, the elderly in one nursing home study never spent more than an hour in either consolidated sleep or wakefulness throughout a 24-hour period (Jacobs et al. 1989, Ancoli-Israel et al. 1989).

## Neurophysiology and Neurochemistry of Sleep

The non-REM–REM sleep cycle is regulated within the brain stem (Steriade and McCarley 1990) (Figure 76–3). The so-called pontine preparation, made by a transection at the pontomesencephalic junction in the cat, blocks input to the pons from the forebrain. The isolated brain stem generates periodic episodes of rapid eye movements and muscle atonia, the physiological signatures of REM sleep. In contrast, the forebrain of this preparation generates alternating periods of EEG slow waves and EEG arousal, suggestive of non-REM sleep and wakefulness, respectively.

Consistent with the concept that the brain stem regulates REM sleep, an Israeli soldier ceased having REM sleep after suffering a shrapnel wound to the brain stem (Lavie et al. 1984). Some antidepressant medications, notably monoamine oxidase inhibitors (MAOIs), completely eliminate REM sleep when they are taken at high clinical doses for more than 2 weeks (Landolt et al. 2001). No specific deleterious effects have been attributed to the loss of REM sleep in these patients. These observations underscore the mystery about the fundamental functions of REM sleep in particular and sleep in general.

Lesions of the locus subcoeruleus in the cat result in REM sleep without atonia, in which the animal appears to act out dreams (i.e., fighting, stalking, or playing while still in REM sleep) (Hendricks et al. 1982). A clinical analogue of REM sleep without atonia is the REM sleep

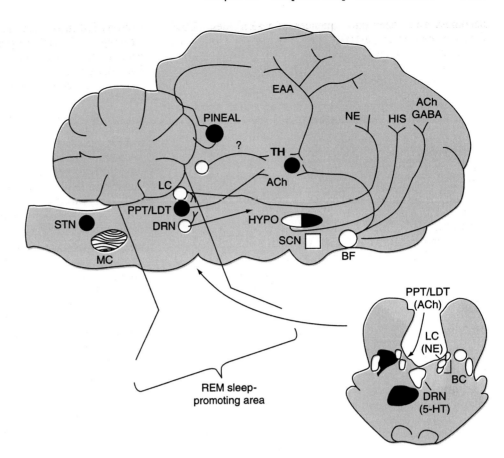

**Figure 76–3** *The neuroanatomy of sleep and wakefulness. ACh, acetylcholine; BC, brachium conjunctivum; BF, basal forebrain; DRN, dorsal raphe nucleus; EAA, excitatory amino acid; GABA, γ-aminobutyric acid; HIS, histamine; 5-HT, 5-hydroxytryptamine; HYPO, hypothalamus; LC, locus coeruleus; MC, magnocellular; NE, norepinephrine; PPT/LDT, pedunculopontine tegmental/lateral dorsal tegmental; SCN, suprachiasmatic nucleus; STN, solitary tract nucleus; TH, thalamus.*

behavior disorder (Mahowald and Schenck 1992). Patients with this disorder maintain muscle tone during REM sleep and act out the content of dreams (e.g., a man ran across his bedroom and crashed into a dresser as he dreamed that he was a linebacker in a football game).

At least five anatomical sites have been implicated in non-REM sleep: the basal forebrain area, thalamus, hypothalamus, dorsal raphe nucleus, and solitary nucleus (Steriade and McCarley 1990). Thalamocortical and corticothalamic loops play an especially important role in the generation of the EEG patterns that define wakefulness, non-REM sleep, and REM sleep (Steriade et al. 1994). Cholinergic, aminergic, histaminergic, and other projections to the thalamus determine the membrane potential of thalamocortical cells. As these cells progressively hyperpolarize, they develop bursting patterns of firing that drive assemblies of cortical cells at the frequencies of the spindle wave (12–14 Hz) and the delta wave (0.3–2.0 Hz).

As a clinical correlate of the role of thalamus in non-REM sleep, Lugaresi (1992) characterized a syndrome known as fatal familial insomnia. The earliest symptoms are an inability to sleep or to generate EEG sleep patterns. Neuropathological examination demonstrates degeneration of the anterior or anteroventral and dorsomedial thalamic nuclei. The disorder is inherited as an autosomal dominant gene, apparently the result of a mutation at codon 178 of the prion protein gene.

No specific "sleep neurotransmitter" has been identified that is responsible for the induction or maintenance of sleep, but many different types of neurochemicals (neurotransmitters, neuromodulators, neuropeptides, immune modulators) have been implicated. Adenosine is a potential sleep promoting neurotransmitter; its concentration in basal forebrain increases with prolonged wakefulness. Caffeine probably promotes alertness by blocking the adenosine $A_1$-receptor. Of particular importance to psychiatry, acetylcholine, released from neurons originating in the dorsal tegmentum, induces REM sleep and cortical activation. Serotonin and norepinephrine, on the other hand, inhibit REM sleep, possibly by inhibition of cholinergic neurons responsible for REM sleep. These physiological mechanisms may be involved in both depression and the sleep disturbances associated with depression and other neuropsychiatric disorders, such as short REM latency (see later). For example, depression may be associated with a functional serotonin deficiency. The suppression of REM sleep during treatment with antidepressants may reflect either enhanced serotoninergic or noradrenergic neurotransmission or anticholinergic effects.

In addition, considerable current research suggests that sleep and immunological processes are intimately related. Several neuroimmunomodulators, such as specific interleukins or tumor necrosis factor, may promote sleep (Kapas et al. 1993). In contrast, sleep deprivation may alter immune function, for example, reducing activity of natural killer cells (Irwin et al. 1992).

## SLEEP DISORDERS

Sleep disorders can be divided into four major categories: (1) insomnias, disorders associated with complaints of insufficient, disturbed, or nonrestorative sleep; (2) hypersomnias, disorders of excessive sleepiness; (3) disturbances of the circadian sleep–wake cycle; and (4) parasomnias, abnormal behaviors or abnormal physiological events in sleep (American Psychiatric Association 1994, Kryger et al. 2000). By definition, the *Diagnostic and Statistical Manual of Mental Disorders*, Fourth Edition (DSM-IV) limits itself to chronic disorders (at least 1 month in duration) (American Psychiatric Association 1994). On the other hand, the *International Classification of Sleep Disorders* includes sleep disorders of short-term and intermediate duration, which in fact are more common than chronic disorders (Diagnostic Classification Steering Committee Thorpy MJC 1990).

### General Approach to the Patient with a Sleep Disorder

Disorders of sleep and wakefulness are common. Insomnia complaints are reported by about one-third of adult Americans during a 1-year period; clinically significant obstructive sleep apnea may be seen in as many as 10% of working, middle-aged men; and sleepiness is an underrecognized cause of dysphoria, automobile accidents, and mismanagement of patients by sleep-deprived physicians. Nearly all physicians will hear complaints of sleep problems. Psychiatrists may be even more likely than other medical specialists to receive these complaints. Of particular importance for mental disorders, prospective epidemiological studies suggest that persistent complaints of either insomnia (Ford and Kamerow 1989, Livingston et al. 1993) or hypersomnia (Ford and Kamerow 1989) are risk factors for the later onset of depression, anxiety disorders, and substance abuse.

This chapter attempts to provide a framework for psychiatrists and other mental health specialists to use in understanding the multiple causes of the sleep disorders, their diagnostic evaluation, and their treatment. To assist the patient with a sleep complaint, the psychiatrist needs to have a diagnostic framework with which to obtain the information needed about both the patient as a person and his or her disorder. Two issues are particularly important: (i) How long has the patient had the sleep complaint? Transient insomnia and short-term insomnia, for example, usually occur in persons undergoing acute stress or other disruptions, such as admission to a hospital, jet lag, bereavement, or change in medications. Chronic sleep disorders, on the other hand, are often multidetermined and multifaceted. (ii) Does the patient suffer from any preexisting or comorbid disorders? Does another condition cause the sleep complaint, modify a sleep complaint, or affect possible treatments? In general, because common sleep disorders are frequently secondary to underlying causes, treatment should be directed at underlying medical, psychiatric, pharmacological, psychosocial, or other disorders.

A detailed history of the complaint and attendant symptoms must be obtained (Tables 76–3 and 76–4). Special attention should be given to the timing of sleep and wakefulness; qualitative and quantitative subjective measures of sleep and wakefulness; abnormal sleep-related behaviors; respiratory difficulties; medications or other substances affecting sleep, wakefulness, or arousal; expectations, concerns, attitudes about sleep, and efforts used by the patient to control symptoms; and the sleep–wake environment. The psychiatrist must be alert to the possibility that sleep complaints are somatic symptoms, which reflect individual ways of experiencing, expressing, and coping with psychosocial distress, stress, or psychiatric disorders.

Sleep disorders vary with age and gender and, possibly, with culture and social class. As mentioned previously, the circadian timing of rest–activity, sleep duration at night, and daytime napping and sleepiness vary with age and gender. In addition, parasomnias are most common in boys, Kleine–Levin syndrome in adolescent boys, delayed sleep phase syndrome in adolescents and young adults, insomnia in middle-aged and elderly women, REM sleep behavior disorder and sleep-related breathing disorders in middle-aged men, and advanced sleep phase syndrome in the elderly. Sleep–wake patterns are also influenced by cultural or geographical factors, such as the siesta and late bedtime commonly associated with tropical climates, or the winter hypersomnia and summer hyposomnia said to occur near the arctic circle. Insomnia is more common in lower

| Table 76–3 | Office Evaluation of Chronic Sleep Complaints |
|---|---|

Detailed history and review of the sleep complaint: predisposing, precipitating, and perpetuating factors

Review of difficulties falling asleep, maintaining sleep, and awakening early

Timing of sleep and wakefulness in the 24-h day

Evidence of excessive daytime sleepiness and fatigue

Bedtime routines, sleep setting, physical security, preoccupations, anxiety, beliefs about sleep and sleep loss, fears about consequences of sleep loss

Medical and neurological history and examination, routine laboratory examinations: look for obesity, short fat neck, enlarged tonsils, narrow upper oral airway, foreshortened jaw (retrognathia), and hypertension

Psychiatric history and examination

Use of prescription and nonprescription medications, alcohol, stimulants, toxins, insecticides, and other substances

Evidence of sleep-related breathing disorders: snoring, orthopnea, dyspnea, headaches, falling out of bed, nocturia

Abnormal movements or behaviors associated with sleep disorders: "jerky legs," leg movements, myoclonus, restless legs, leg cramps, cold feet, nightmares, enuresis, sleepwalking, epilepsy, bruxism, sleep paralysis, hypnagogic hallucinations, cataplexy, night sweats, and so on

Social and occupational history, marital status, living conditions, financial and security concerns, physical activity

Sleep–wake diary for 2 wk

Interview with bed partners or persons who observe patient during sleep

Tape recording of respiratory sounds during sleep to screen for sleep apnea

| | |
|---|---|
| **Table 76–4** | **Selected Disorders and Terms Used in Clinical Sleep Disorders Medicine** |

| Term | Definition |
|---|---|
| Apnea index | Number of apneic events per hour of sleep; usually is considered pathological if ≥ 5. |
| Cataplexy | Sudden, brief loss of muscle tone in the waking stage, usually triggered by emotional arousal (laughing, anger, surprise), involving either a few muscle groups (i.e., facial) or most of major antigravity muscles of the body; may be related to muscle atonia normally occurring during REM sleep; is associated with narcolepsy. |
| Hypopnea | 50% or more reduction in respiratory depth for 10 s or more during sleep. |
| Multiple Sleep Latency Test | An objective method for determining daytime sleepiness; sleep latency and REM latency are determined for four or five naps (i.e., a 20-min opportunity to sleep every 2 h between 10 AM and 6 PM); normal mean values are above 15 min. |
| Periodic limb movements in sleep index | Number of leg kicks per hour of sleep; usually is considered pathological if ≥ 5. |
| Polysomnography | Describes detailed, sleep laboratory-based, clinical evaluation of patient with sleep disorder; may include electroencephalographical measures, eye movements, muscle tone at chin and limbs, respiratory movements of chest and abdomen, oxygen saturation, electrocardiogram, nocturnal penile tumescence, esophageal pH, as indicated. |
| Respiratory disturbance index | Number of apneas and hypopneas per hour of sleep. |
| Sleep apnea | Sleep-related breathing disorder characterized by at least five episodes of apnea per hour of sleep, each longer than 10 s in duration. |

than in middle and upper socioeconomic classes, perhaps reflecting the stress of poverty, crowding and lack of privacy, poor medical care, drugs and alcohol, lack of physical security, and so forth.

One approach to the differential diagnosis of persistent sleep disorders is suggested in the algorithm in Figure 76–4. First, determine whether the sleep complaint is due to another medical, psychiatric, or substance abuse disorder. Second, consider the role of circadian rhythm disturbances and sleep disorders associated with abnormal events predominantly during sleep. Finally, evaluate in greater detail complaints of insomnia (difficulty initiating or maintaining sleep) and excessive sleepiness.

## Role of the Sleep Laboratory in Clinical Sleep Disorders

Psychiatrists can usually diagnose most sleep disorders by traditional, simple but systematic clinical methods. Referral

to a specialized sleep disorders center, however, should be considered in patients suspected of having severe intractable insomnia, persistent excessive daytime sleepiness, and sleep disorders due to a general medical condition (such as narcolepsy, REM sleep behavior disorder, sleep apnea, periodic limb movements in sleep [PLMS], or sleep-related epilepsy). Specialists in sleep disorders medicine will evaluate the patient and, if necessary, arrange for sleep laboratory or ambulatory diagnostic procedures.

One of the most important and common laboratory examinations is all-night polysomnography, which typically records the EEG activity's eye movements with the electro-oculogram, and muscle tone with the electromyogram from the chin (submental) muscles (Figure 76–5). These measures are used to determine sleep stages visually scored as 20- or 30-second epochs by a sleep technician. To evaluate sleep-related respiration and cardiovascular function, measures are made of nasal and oral air flow with a thermistor; of sounds of breathing and snoring with a small microphone near the mouth; of respiratory movements of the chest and abdominal walls; of heart rate with the electrocardiogram; and of blood-oxygen saturation with finger oximetry. To evaluate PLMS, an electromyogram from the shin (anterior tibial) muscles is obtained. Other more specialized tests include intraesophageal pressures, which increase during the upper airway resistance syndrome if respiration is impeded, nocturnal penile tumescence in the evaluation of impotence, and core body temperature (usually rectal or tympanic membrane).

Daytime sleepiness can be evaluated in the sleep laboratory with the Multiple Sleep Latency Test, which measures sleep latency during opportunities for napping during the day (see Table 76–4). In addition, subjective sleepiness can be assessed by a questionnaire, the Stanford Sleepiness Scale, in which the subject rates sleepiness on a 7-point scale at set intervals throughout the day.

Two research laboratory procedures have been developed for experimental measurement of circadian phase in humans: the constant routine method for temperature and neuroendocrine secretions, and the dim light melatonin onset method for melatonin (see Table 76–2).

According to DSM-IV-TR definitions (American Psychiatric Association 1994), primary sleep disorders are presumed to arise from endogenous abnormalities in sleep–wake-generating mechanisms, timing mechanisms, sleep hygiene, or conditioning, rather than occurring secondary to medical or psychiatric disorders. Two types of primary sleep disorders are defined: *dyssomnias* (abnormalities in the amount, quality, or timing of sleep) and *parasomnias* (abnormal behaviors associated with sleep, such as nightmares or sleepwalking). In addition, sleep disorders may be related to other mental disorders, general medical conditions, and substance abuse.

## Dyssomnias

### Primary Insomnia

According to DSM-IV-TR criteria, primary insomnia is a subjective complaint of poor, insufficient, or nonrestorative sleep lasting more than a month; associated with significant distress or impairment; and without obvious relationships to another sleep, medical, or psychiatric disorder or

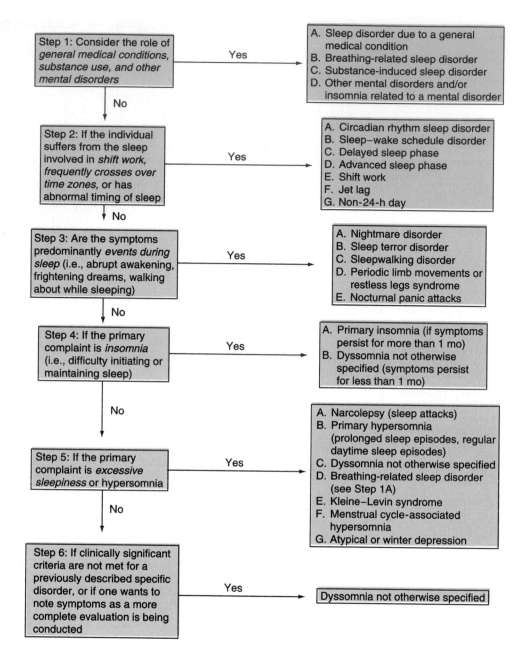

Step 1: Consider the role of *general medical conditions, substance use, and other mental disorders* → Yes →
A. Sleep disorder due to a general medical condition
B. Breathing-related sleep disorder
C. Substance-induced sleep disorder
D. Other mental disorders and/or insomnia related to a mental disorder

No ↓

Step 2: If the individual suffers from the sleep involved in *shift work, frequently crosses over time zones,* or has abnormal timing of sleep → Yes →
A. Circadian rhythm sleep disorder
B. Sleep–wake schedule disorder
C. Delayed sleep phase
D. Advanced sleep phase
E. Shift work
F. Jet lag
G. Non-24-h day

No ↓

Step 3: Are the symptoms predominantly *events during sleep* (i.e., abrupt awakening, frightening dreams, walking about while sleeping) → Yes →
A. Nightmare disorder
B. Sleep terror disorder
C. Sleepwalking disorder
D. Periodic limb movements or restless legs syndrome
E. Nocturnal panic attacks

No ↓

Step 4: If the primary complaint is *insomnia* (i.e., difficulty initiating or maintaining sleep) → Yes →
A. Primary insomnia (if symptoms persist for more than 1 mo)
B. Dyssomnia not otherwise specified (symptoms persist for less than 1 mo)

No ↓

Step 5: If the primary complaint is *excessive sleepiness* or hypersomnia → Yes →
A. Narcolepsy (sleep attacks)
B. Primary hypersomnia (prolonged sleep episodes, regular daytime sleep episodes)
C. Dyssomnia not otherwise specified
D. Breathing-related sleep disorder (see Step 1A)
E. Kleine–Levin syndrome
F. Menstrual cycle-associated hypersomnia
G. Atypical or winter depression

No ↓

Step 6: If clinically significant criteria are not met for a previously described specific disorder, or if one wants to note symptoms as a more complete evaluation is being conducted → Yes → Dyssomnia not otherwise specified

**Figure 76–4** *An algorithm for the differential diagnosis of persistent sleep disorder complaints.*

physiological effects of a substance. Primary insomnia is similar to some insomnia diagnoses in the *International Classification of Sleep Disorders*, including psychophysiological insomnia, which is often ascribed to conditioned arousal factors; sleep state misperception, in which the magnitude of the subjective complaint often exceeds that of the objective abnormality; and idiopathic insomnia, with a childhood onset and lifelong course.

The etiology of primary insomnia is unclear, but it may be dependent more on the factors that perpetuate it than on those that precipitated it.

In general surveys of the prevalence of insomnia in the population, about 1 in 3 people reported "insomnia" during the previous year, about 1 in 6 described it as "serious," and about 1 in 12 called it "chronic" (Ancoli-Israel and Roth 1999).

The rates of insomnia are higher in women than in men, in the elderly than in the young, and in the lower than in the higher socioeconomic classes. In a survey conducted by the Gallup Poll for the National Sleep Foundation (Ancoli-Israel and Roth 1999, Roth and Ancoli-Israel 1999), the most common complaint of insomniacs is waking up feeling drowsy rather than specific complaints about sleep, implying that the sleepiness insomniacs experience could be associated with some morbidity. Compared with transient insomniacs or normal control subjects, chronic insomniacs reported greater difficulty enjoying family and social relationships, greater difficulty concentrating, more problems with memory, greater frequency of falling asleep while visiting friends, and more automobile accidents due to sleepiness. Nevertheless, only about 5% of patients with chronic insomnia ever sought medical attention specifically

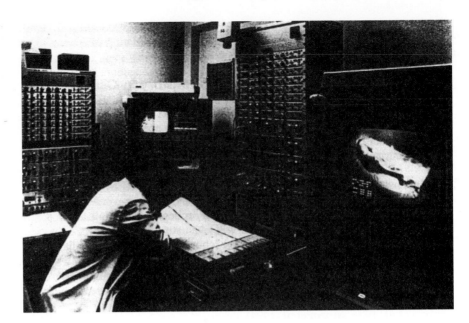

**Figure 76–5** *The polysomnographic evaluation of patients in the sleep laboratory.*

---

### DSM-IV-TR Criteria 307.42

#### Primary Insomnia

A. The predominant complaint is difficulty initiating or maintaining sleep, or nonrestorative sleep, for at least 1 month.

B. The sleep disturbance (or associated daytime fatigue) causes clinically significant distress or impairment in social, occupational, or other important areas of functioning.

C. The sleep disturbance does not occur exclusively during the course of narcolepsy, breathing-related sleep disorder, circadian rhythm sleep disorder, or a parasomnia.

D. The disturbance does not occur exclusively during the course of another mental disorder (e.g., major depressive disorder, generalized anxiety disorder, a delirium).

E. The disturbance is not due to the direct physiological effects of a substance (e.g., a drug of abuse, a medication) or a general medical condition.

---

Reprinted with permission from the Diagnostic and Statistical Manual of Mental Disorders, Fourth Edition, Text Revision. Copyright 2000 American Psychiatric Association.

---

for insomnia. Only a minority of patients have ever used prescription sleeping pills. On the other hand, most psychiatrists do not routinely inquire about difficulties with sleep and wakefulness. If these patients with chronic or serious insomnia are to be helped, psychiatrists must be proactive and ask specific questions about sleep and its disorders.

The prevalence of primary insomnia is not known. Treatment of insomnia should, insofar as possible, be directed at identifiable causes, or those factors that perpetuate the disorders, such as temperament and lifestyle, ineffective coping and defense mechanisms, inappropriate use of alcohol or other substances, maladaptive sleep–wake schedules, and excessive worry about poor sleep. The harder these individuals try to sleep, the worse it is. They keep themselves awake by their apprehensions: "If I don't get to sleep right now, I'll make a bad impression tomorrow." Cognitive–behavioral therapy (CBT) therefore is very effective, as shown by Morin and colleagues (1993). An 8-week group intervention aimed at changing maladaptive sleep habits and altering dysfunctional beliefs and attitudes about sleeplessness was effective in reducing sleep latency, waking up after sleep onset, and early morning awakening, and in increasing sleep efficiency. In a second study, Morin and colleagues (1999) found that CBT and pharmacological approaches were both effective for the short-term management of insomnia but that improvement was better sustained over time with the behavioral treatment.

### Diagnosis

Diagnosis and treatment of chronic insomnia are often challenging and difficult (Hauri 1991). Both the psychiatrist and the patient must be forbearing and realistic as they jointly explore the evolution, causes, manifestations, and ramifications of the sleep complaint. In part, the diagnosis of primary insomnia is reached by exclusion after a careful differential diagnosis of other causes. Simple answers and simple solutions are rare. Even if insomnia is initially precipitated by a single event or condition, chronic insomnia is usually maintained by various predisposing and perpetuating factors. For example, a business woman in her early thirties had insomnia during a period of intense stress in her business, but it continued long after the stress had been satisfactorily resolved. Factors that contributed to chronicity included her lifelong somewhat obsessive, anxious personality structure and after the onset of her insomnia, her gradually escalating concerns about her insomnia; these resulted in advanced sleep phase as she tried to spend more time in bed for "rest" and use of wine and sleeping pills at bedtime to sleep. If all these factors can be properly sorted out and dealt with, both the psychiatrist and the patient will be gratified.

## Treatment of Chronic Primary Insomnia

Clinical management is often multidimensional, involving psychosocial, behavioral, and pharmacological approaches. The relationship with the psychiatrist can often be important since many insomniac patients are skeptical that they can be helped overtly. They are focused on the symptom rather than the underlying causes, and are not psychologically minded. Behavioral treatments, in combination with addressing sleep hygiene, may be helpful in treating psychophysiological and other insomnias. Relaxation training (progressive relaxation, autogenic training, meditation, deep breathing) can all be effective if overtaught to become automatic. Two other behavioral therapies have been shown to be effective for insomnia: stimulus control and sleep restriction therapy (Bootzin and Nicassio 1978, Spielman et al. 1987, Morin et al. 1994).

The aim of stimulus control therapy is to break the negative associations of being in bed unable to sleep (Table 76–5). It is especially helpful for patients with sleep-onset insomnia and prolonged awakenings. Sleep restriction therapy (Table 76–6) is based on the observation that more time spent in bed leads to more fragmented sleep. Both therapies may take 3 to 4 weeks or longer to be effective.

A wide variety of sedating medications have commonly been used as sleeping pills including benzodiazepines, imidazopyridines (zolpidem), pyrazolopyrimidines (zaleplon), chloral hydrate, antihistamines (diphenhydramine, hydroxyzine, doxylamine), certain antidepressants (amitriptyline, doxepin, trimipramine, and trazodone), barbiturates, and over-the-counter medications. However, they do vary in their pharmacokinetic properties and side effects (Table 76–7). The ideal sleeping pill would shorten latency to sleep; maintain normal physiological sleep all night without blocking normal behavioral responses to the crying baby or the alarm clock; leave neither hangover nor withdrawal effects the next day; and be devoid of tolerance and side effects such as impairment of breathing, cognition, ambulation, and coordination (Gillin and Byerley 1990).

| Table 76–5 | Sleep Hygiene and Stimulus Control Rules |
|---|---|

Curtail time spent awake while in bed.
Go to bed only when sleepy.
Do not remain in bed for more than 20–30 min while awake.
Get up at the same time each day.
Avoid looking at the bedroom clock.
Avoid caffeine, alcohol, and tobacco near bedtime.
Exercise during the morning or afternoon.
Eat a light snack before bed.
Adjust sleeping environment for optimal temperature, sound, and
　darkness.
Do not worry right before and in bed. Use the bed for sleeping.
Do not nap during the day.

| Table 76–6 | Sleep Restriction Therapy |
|---|---|

Stay in bed for the amount of time you think you sleep each night,
　plus 15 min.
Get up at the same time each day.
Do not nap during the day.
When sleep efficiency is 85% (i.e., sleeping for 85% of the time in
　bed), go to bed 15 min earlier.
Repeat this process until you are sleeping for 8 h or the desired
　amount of time.
Example: if you report sleeping only 5 h a night and you normally
　get up at 6 AM, you are allowed to be in bed from 12:45 AM
　until 6 AM.

Furthermore, sleeping pills should not be habit-forming or addictive. Unfortunately, the ideal sleeping pill has not yet been found. Sleeping pills, if given in appropriate doses, are effective compared with placebo at least from a few days to a few weeks. More recent, developed sleeping pills (such as zaleplon) have demonstrated their superiority after 1 year in double-blind studies with a parallel placebo group. The question, however, is what is the lowest adequate dose for an individual patient, that is, the dose that will promote sleep with the least number of side effects.

The duration of action of these medications is important for several reasons (Table 76–8). Drugs with long half-life metabolites may have next-day hangover effects and tend to accumulate with repeated nightly administration, especially in the elderly, who metabolize and excrete the drugs more slowly than the young do. In addition, long half-life metabolites may act addictively or synergistically the next day with alcohol, with drugs with sedative side effects, or during periods of decreased alertness, such as the afternoon dip in arousal levels. Because the elderly are more sensitive to both the benefits and the side effects at a given dose than are younger patients, a dose for the elderly and debilitated patient should normally be about half of that for young and middle-aged patients.

Short half-life hypnotics usually produce less daytime sedation than long half-life drugs, but they often result in more rebound insomnia when they are discontinued (Gillin et al. 1989). Whereas nearly all hypnotics and sedatives can produce amnesia, the problem may be more common with some short half-life drugs, especially for material that is learned during the periods of peak concentrations of drugs, for example, if the subject is awakened during the middle of the night. Administration of zaleplon 4 hours or more before arising in the morning does not appear to be associated with impairment in motor performance (Vermeeren et al. 2002).

Patients should be educated about the anticipated benefits and limitations of sleeping pills, side effects, and appropriate use, and should be followed up by office visits or phone calls regularly if prescriptions are renewed. Although hypnotics are usually prescribed for relatively short periods of time (2–6 weeks at most), about 0.5 to 1% of the population uses a hypnotic nearly every night for months or years. Whether this practice is good, useless, or bad remains controversial. Treatment of these patients should focus on the lowest possible effective dose—intermittently if possible—for the treatment of insomnia.

| Table 76–7 | Clinical Characteristics of Sedative–Hypnotics | | | |
|---|---|---|---|---|
| Name | Dose (mg) | Absorption | Active Metabolite | Half-Life |
| Chlordiazepoxide (Librium) | 5–10 | Intermediate | Yes | 2–4 d |
| Diazepam (Valium) | 2–10 | Fast | Yes | 2–4 d |
| Estazolam (ProSom)* | 0.5–2.0 | Intermediate | Yes | 17 h |
| Flurazepam (Dalmane)* | 7.5–30 | Intermediate to fast | Yes | 2–4 d |
| Clorazepate (Tranxene) | 7.5–15 | Fast | Yes | 2–4 d |
| Clonazepam (Klonopin) | 0.5–1.0 | Intermediate | Yes | 2–3 d |
| Quazepam (Doral)* | 7.5–15 | Intermediate | Yes | 2–4 d |
| Oxazepam (Serax) | 10–15 | Slow | No | 8–12 h |
| Lorazepam (Ativan) | 0.5–4.0 | Intermediate | No | 10–20 h |
| Temazepam (Restoril)* | 7.5–15 | Slow | No | 10–20 h |
| Alprazolam (Xanax) | 0.25–2 | Intermediate | No | 14 h |
| Zoplicone† | 7.5–15 | Fast | Yes | 4–6.5 h |
| Triazolam (Halcion)* | 0.125–0.5 | Intermediate | No | 2–5 h |
| Zolpidem (Ambien)* | 5–10 | Fast | No | 2–5 h |
| Zaleplon (Sonata)* | 5–10 | Fast | No | 1 h |

*Marketed as a sleeping pill in the US.

†Not yet marketed in the US.

Hypnotics are relatively contraindicated in patients with sleep-disordered breathing; during pregnancy; in substance abusers, particularly alcohol abusers; and in those individuals who may need to be alert during their sleep period (e.g., physicians on call). In addition, caution should be used in prescribing hypnotics to patients who snore loudly; to patients who have renal, hepatic, or pulmonary disease; and to the elderly.

## Melatonin

Melatonin received enormous coverage in the popular press in the mid-1990s, with extravagant claims that it can prevent all ills from aging to cancer and treat everything from jet lag and insomnia to depression and acquired immunodeficiency syndrome (AIDS). The scientific reality is still far removed from most of these claims at the present time.

| Table 76–8 | Comparison of Long and Short Half-Life Hypnotics | |
|---|---|---|
| | Half-Life | |
| Measure | Short | Long |
| Sedative hangover effects | + | ++++ |
| Accumulation with consecutive nightly use | 0 | +++ |
| Tolerance | +++ | + |
| Withdrawal insomnia | +++ | + |
| Anxiolytic effects next day | 0 | +++ |
| Amnesia | +++ | ++ |
| Full benefits the first night | +++ | ++ |

*Note*: Although zaleplon is short acting, research suggests that it does not have some of the problems of other short-acting hypnotics, such as tolerance or withdrawal insomnia.

What is known is that melatonin is synthesized and released from the pineal gland under dark ambient conditions at a time that is determined by the individual's internal biological clock located within the SCN at the anterior portion of the hypothalamus. For individuals who are synchronized with the local light–dark environment, melatonin is usually secreted at night. The duration of secretion is approximately 8 to 12 hours, depending partially on age, season of the year, and lighting conditions. Bright light prevents or terminates secretion of melatonin. For these reasons, melatonin has sometimes been called the "hormone" of the night or of sleep. In addition, nocturnal melatonin secretion appears to be blunted with normal aging, with administration of beta-adrenergic blockers (propranolol, pindolol, metoprolol), and in some populations of patient (including patients with mood disorders, premenstrual depression, and panic disorder).

The functions of melatonin in humans are poorly understood, although in animals it has been implicated in seasonal behaviors, breeding, reproductive physiology, and timing of adolescence.

The limited database available suggests that melatonin may eventually have a role in the prevention and treatment of circadian and sleep disturbances. Some evidence suggests that it has intrinsic hypnotic effects. Laboratory studies suggest that people are more likely to sleep during the period of endogenous melatonin secretion than during periods of the day without melatonin secretion. Furthermore, some but not all studies suggest that melatonin (0.3–10.0 mg) may induce and maintain sleep when administered to normal subjects or, in a few studies, to individuals with insomnia, jet lag, or other circadian rhythm disturbances. In addition, it is possible that melatonin administration can shift the phase position of the underlying biological clock. The entraining effects of a dose of 0.5 mg melatonin act like a "dark pulse," that is, the phase-response curve is nearly opposite that of light. Melatonin-induced phase-advanced rhythms when administered in the late afternoon or early evening, and it delayed the circadian clock when administered in the early morning. Future research is needed to fulfill the promise that melatonin can be used to prevent or treat some forms of insomnia or other sleep disorders, especially in the elderly, or in cases associated with circadian rhythm disorders (jet lag, shift work, the non-24-hour-day syndrome, phase displacement), neurological disorders, or psychiatric disorders.

The scientific clinical database for the use of melatonin in humans is limited at this time (Brown 1995). Few well-designed clinical trials exist to establish clinical benefits or risks in specific disorders or conditions. Little is known about optimal doses, timing of melatonin administration, duration of treatment, drug interactions, or populations at risk, if any. The safety of melatonin, especially melatonin available in health food stores, is unknown. Melatonin is currently treated by the US Food and Drug Administration as a nutritional supplement rather than a medication. Therefore, purity of the product, safety, efficacy, and claims by manufacturers are not carefully regulated in the US. Physicians are advised to maintain a watchful eye at this time and to be prudently cautious about recommendations to patients and the public about the uses and benefits of melatonin.

Because the timing of melatonin secretion is regulated by the SCN, investigators and clinicians can measure plasma levels of melatonin in dim light conditions to determine the phase position of the circadian clock. A useful revision of this technique is called the dim light melatonin onset (DLMO, pronounced "dil-mo") (Lewy and Sack 1989).

Using repeated measures of DLMO over periods of weeks, Lewy and Sack (1989) demonstrated that the circadian clock was "free-running" in a significant proportion of totally blind individuals, that is, the time of day at which melatonin secretion began completely drifted around the clock in a clockwise direction about every 3 weeks. Since the patients tried to maintain a conventional bedtime (approximately 11PM–7AM), their wake–sleep cycle was in and out of synchrony with their own internal clock, creating significant difficulties in sleep and alertness at times during the month. Furthermore, Lewy and Sack found that appropriately-timed administration of melatonin synchronized the internal clock with the external light–dark cycle.

## Primary Hypersomnia

A specific diagnostic category for primary hypersomnia exists in DSM-IV-TR, defining a disorder characterized by clinically significant excessive sleepiness of at least 1 month's duration, with significant distress or impairment. The hypersomnia is not caused by another primary sleep disorder, a psychiatric disorder, a medical disorder, or a substance. Patients with primary hypersomnia usually present with complaints of long and nonrestorative nocturnal sleep, difficulty awakening ("sleep drunkenness"), and daytime sleepiness and intellectual dysfunction; do not experience the accessory symptoms of narcolepsy such as cataplexy, sleep paralysis, and hypnagogic hallucinations; and often report frequent headaches and Raynaud's phenomena.

### Differential Diagnosis

Previously called non-REM narcolepsy, this relatively rare disorder is represented by perhaps 5 to 10% of patients

---

**DSM-IV-TR Criteria** 307.44

**Primary Hypersomnia**

A. The predominant complaint is excessive sleepiness for at least 1 month (or less if recurrent) as evidenced by either prolonged sleep episodes or daytime sleep episodes that occur almost daily.

B. The excessive sleepiness causes clinically significant distress or impairment in social, occupational, or other important areas of functioning.

C. The excessive sleepiness is not better accounted for by insomnia and does not occur exclusively during the course of another sleep disorder (e.g., narcolepsy, breathing-related sleep disorder, circadian rhythm sleep disorder, or a parasomnia) and cannot be accounted for by an inadequate amount of sleep.

D. The disturbance does not occur exclusively during the course of another mental disorder.

E. The disturbance is not due to the direct physiological effects of a substance (e.g., a drug of abuse, a medication) or a general medical condition.

*Specify* if:

**Recurrent:** if there are periods of excessive sleepiness that last at least 3 days occurring several times a year for at least 2 years

Reprinted with permission from the Diagnostic and Statistical Manual of Mental Disorders, Fourth Edition, Text Revision. Copyright 2000 American Psychiatric Association.

---

presenting to sleep disorders centers for evaluation of hypersomnia. The diagnosis must be made on the basis of polysomnographic confirmation of hypersomnia; subjective complaints of excessive sleepiness are not adequate. A family history of excessive sleepiness may be present.

Although usually seen as a persistent complaint, primary hypersomnia includes recurrent forms, well defined with periods of excessive sleepiness of at least 3 days' duration occurring several times a year for at least 2 years. Among the recurrent or intermittent hypersomnia disorders are Kleine–Levin syndrome, usually seen in adolescent boys, and menstrual cycle-associated hypersomnia syndrome. In addition to hypersomnia (up to 18 hours per day), patients with Kleine–Levin syndrome often demonstrate aggressive or inappropriate sexuality, compulsive overeating, and other bizarre behaviors. The rare nature of this syndrome and its unusual behaviors may be mistaken for psychosis, malingering, or a personality disorder (Waller et al. 1984).

Another syndrome, idiopathic recurring stupor, has been described and may be confused with hypersomnia (Rothstein et al. 1992). Patients experience attacks of stupor or coma as infrequently as once or twice a year to as often as once a week. The duration of each episode varies from 2 hours to 4 days. Unlike patients with hypersomnia, these patients are in a stuporous coma-like state and cannot be easily aroused or awakened. Furthermore, unlike the EEG of hypersomnia with its sleep spindles and K complexes, the EEG during stupor is characterized by diffuse activity at 13 to 18 Hz. Because the episode can be promptly but temporarily reversed by administration of flumazenil, a benzodiazepine receptor antagonist, a search was made for an endogenous ligand for the benzodiazepine receptor in plasma and cerebrospinal fluid. The investigators discovered significantly increased levels of "endozepine 4" in blood and cerebrospinal fluid during periods of coma or stupor, suggesting that this syndrome is caused by this endogenous benzodiazepine-like compound. The syndrome occurs predominantly in men; mean age at onset is age 47 years (range, age 22–67 years). The cause is unknown.

Aside from associated medical and psychiatric disorders, the frequency and importance of hypersomnia and daytime sleepiness in otherwise healthy individuals have been increasingly recognized. Sleepiness, for example, as a result of sleep deprivation, disrupted sleep, or circadian dyssynchronization, probably plays a major role in mistakes and accidents in sleepy drivers, interns and medical staff, and industrial workers. Psychiatrists have an obligation to recognize and advise their patients about the dangers inherent in acute or chronic sleepiness.

## Treatment

Clinical management is controversial owing to the lack of controlled studies. As in narcolepsy, the stimulant compounds are the most widely used and most often successful of the treatment options available. However, some patients are intolerant of stimulants or report no significant therapeutic effects. For patients intolerant of, or insensitive to, stimulants, some success has been obtained with the use of stimulating antidepressants, both of the MAOI and the selective serotonin reuptake inhibitor (SSRI) classes. Methysergide, a serotonin receptor antagonist, may be effective in some treatment-resistant cases but must be used with caution in view of the possibility of pleural and retroperitoneal fibrosis with persistent, uninterrupted use. Careful documentation should be maintained of interruption of drug use at regular intervals and of physical examinations that find the absence of obvious side effects of any sort.

## Narcolepsy

Narcolepsy is associated with a pentad of symptoms: (1) excessive daytime sleepiness, characterized by irresistible "attacks" of sleep in inappropriate situations such as driving a car, talking to a supervisor, or social events; (2) cataplexy, which is sudden bilateral loss of muscle tone, usually lasting seconds to minutes, generally precipitated by strong emotions such as laughter, anger, or surprise; (3) poor or disturbed nocturnal sleep; (4) hypnagogic hallucinations, varied dreams at sleep onset; and (5) sleep paralysis, a brief period of paralysis associated with the transitions into, and out of, sleep.

The disorder is lifelong. The first symptom is usually excessive sleepiness, typically developing during the late teens and early twenties. The full syndrome of cataplexy and other symptoms unfolds in several years.

### DSM-IV-TR Criteria 347

**Narcolepsy**

A. Irresistible attacks of unrefreshing sleep that occur daily for at least 3 months.

B. The presence of one or both of the following:

(1) cataplexy (i.e., brief episodes of sudden bilateral loss of muscle tone, most often in association with intense emotion)

(2) recurrent intrusions of elements of REM sleep into the transition between sleep and wakefulness, as manifested by either hypnopompic or hypnagogic hallucinations or sleep paralysis at the beginning or end of sleep episodes

C. The disturbance is not due to the direct physiological effects of a substance (e.g., a drug of abuse, a medication) or another general medical condition.

Reprinted with permission from the Diagnostic and Statistical Manual of Mental Disorders, Fourth Edition, Text Revision. Copyright 2000 American Psychiatric Association.

Narcolepsy is now understood as an inherited, physiological disturbance of REM sleep regulation (Mignot et al. 1991, 1993a). It is also seen in dogs and other mammals. Genetic markers in humans (Mignot et al. 1991, 1993a) and basic neurochemical and neurophysiological studies in canine narcolepsy (Siegel et al. 1992, Mignot et al. 1993b) may clarify the basic pathophysiological process of human narcolepsy. Narcoleptic patients often enter REM sleep right after sleep onset (the "sleep-onset REM periods"), reflecting an abnormally short or even nonexistent first non-REM sleep period (Figure 76–6). Several of the core symptoms of narcolepsy can be understood as abnormal physiological representations of normal REM sleep. For example, cataplexy can be understood as an abrupt presentation during wakefulness of the paralysis normally seen in REM sleep. Cataplexy is usually triggered by an emotional stimulus. Sleep-onset REM periods may be subjectively appreciated as hypnagogic hallucinations, which may be accompanied by sleep paralysis. Dissociated REM sleep inhibition of the voluntary musculature may lead to complaints of cataplexy and sleep paralysis.

A strong association between narcolepsy and the human leukocyte antigen HLA-DR2 phenotype has been demonstrated (Honda et al. 1986, Rosenthal et al. 1991). Studies to date suggest that between 90 and 100% of Asian and white narcoleptics have the HLA-DR2 and DQwl phenotype, versus 20 to 40% of nonnarcoleptic control subjects. The frequent occurrence of this trait in "normal" populations limits the utility of this test for diagnostic purposes.

In recent years, a potential biochemical abnormality has been identified in both canine and human narcolepsy. Narcoleptic dogs appear to have a nonfunctional receptor (OX2R) for orexin (hypocretin), a peptide neurotransmitter

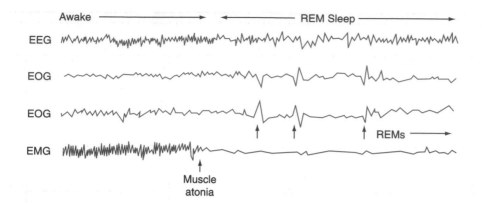

**Figure 76–6** *REM-onset sleep in a patient with narcolepsy. EEG, electroencephalogram; EOG, electrooculogram; EMG, electromyogram; REMs, rapid eye movements.*

that has also been associated with feeding and energy metabolism. "Knockout" mice, which no longer make this peptide, appear to have a narcoleptic-like syndrome. Levels of orexin/hypocretin have been reported to be low in both autopsied brains and spinal fluid in human narcoleptics.

## Diagnosis

Narcolepsy is not a rare disease; the prevalence rate of 0.03 to 0.16% approximates that of multiple sclerosis. Observers may mistake classic sleepiness in its mild form as withdrawal, poor motivation, negativism, and hostility. The hypnagogic imagery and sleep paralysis symptoms, alone and in combination, may resemble bizarre psychiatric illness. Like many medical disorders, narcolepsy presents a wide range of severity, from mild to cases so severe that employment is functionally impossible. Partial remissions and exacerbations occur. Sleep paralysis and hypnagogic imagery may be seen without cataplexy; cataplexy may present in isolation without other REM-associated phenomena. The presence of REM sleep onset at night or during daytime naps, an important sleep laboratory parameter, remains the most valid and reliable method available for diagnosing narcolepsy. Because of the seriousness of the disorder and likelihood that amphetamine or other stimulants will be used to treat the patient at some time, it is important that the diagnosis of narcolepsy be objectively verified as soon as possible. Furthermore, stimulant abusers have been known to feign symptoms of narcolepsy to obtain prescriptions.

Narcolepsy is associated with significant social and financial impairment for affected individuals and their families (Broughton and Ghanem 1976). For example, automobile accidents may result from either sleepiness or cataplexy. Most states prohibit narcoleptic patients from driving, at least as long as they are symptomatic.

## Treatment

The major goals of treatment of narcolepsy include: (a) to improve quality of life, (b) to reduce excessive daytime sleepiness (EDS), and (c) to prevent cataplectic attacks.

The major wake-promoting medications are: modafinil, amphetamine, dextraamphetamine, and methylphenidate. Modafinil is preferred on grounds of efficacy, safety, availability, and low risk of abuse and diversion. Pemoline is helpful but it carries the rare risk of hepatic toxicity, which

can be fatal. The pharmacological treatment of cataplexy, sleep paralysis, and hypnogogic hallucinations includes administration of activating SSRIs such as fluoxetine and tricyclic antidepressants such as protriptyline. Another new drug, sodium oxybate xyrem, appears to be well tolerated and beneficial for the treatment of cataplexy, daytime sleepiness, and inadvertent sleep attacks (Littner et al. 2001, US Xyrem Multicenter Study Group 2002).

## Breathing-Related Sleep Disorder

The essential feature of this disorder is sleep disruption resulting from sleep apnea or alveolar hypoventilation, leading to complaints of insomnia or, more commonly, excessive sleepiness. The disorder is not accounted for by other medical or psychiatric disorders or by medications or other substances. Breathing-related sleep disorder (BRSD) was first described in 1877, yet it was recognized as a serious problem only about 30 years ago.

## Diagnosis

The major diagnostic criterion for sleep apnea is cessation of breathing lasting at least 10 seconds and an apnea index (number of apneic events per hour of sleep) of 5 or more (Figure 76–7). Most apneic episodes are terminated by transient arousals. Hypopneas (50% decrease in respiration) may also produce arousal or hypoxia even when complete apneas do not occur. Therefore, rather than just the apnea index, a respiratory disturbance index (number of respiratory events, or number of apneas plus hypopneas per hour of sleep) is used. Whereas the criterion for the respiratory disturbance index has not been fully established, many psychiatrists use a respiratory disturbance index of 10 or greater for purposes of diagnosis. Each time respiration ceases, the individual must awaken to start breathing again. Once the person goes back to sleep, breathing stops again. This pattern continues throughout the night. Clinically, however, it is not unusual to see patients who stop breathing for 60 to 120 seconds with each event and experience hundreds of events per night. Many individuals with BRSD cannot sleep and breathe at the same time and therefore spend most of the night not breathing and not sleeping. In contrast, the central alveolar hypoventilation syndrome is not associated with either apneas or hypopneas, but impaired ventilatory control or hypoventilation results in hypoxemia. It is most common in morbid obesity.

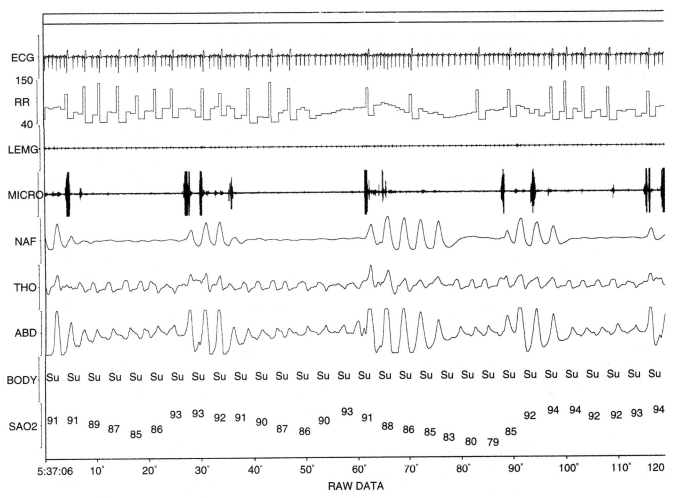

**Figure 76–7** *Mixed sleep apnea. EEG, electroencephalogram; EOG, electrooculogram; EMG, electromyogram; ECG, electrocardiogram.*

Sleep apnea is characterized by repetitive episodes of upper airway obstruction that occur during sleep, resulting

in numerous interruptions of sleep continuity, hypoxemia, hypercapnia, bradytachycardia, and pulmonary and systemic hypertension (Shepard 1992). It may be associated with snoring, morning headaches, dry mouth on awakening, excessive movements during the night, falling out of bed, enuresis, cognitive decline and personality changes, and complaints of either insomnia or, more frequently, hypersomnia and excessive daytime sleepiness (Guilleminault et al. 1973, Roehrs et al. 1985, Aldrich and Chauncey 1990). The typical patient with clinical sleep apnea is a middle-aged man who is overweight or who has anatomical conditions narrowing his upper airway.

There are three types of apnea. The first is obstructive sleep apnea, which involves the collapse of the pharyngeal airway during inspiration, with partial or complete blockage of airflow. The person still attempts to breathe, and one can observe the diaphragm moving, but the airway is blocked and therefore there is no air exchange. It can be caused by bagginess or excessive pharyngeal mucosa and a large uvula, fatty infiltration at the base of the tongue, or collapse of the pharyngeal walls. The resulting decreased air passage compromises alveolar ventilation and causes blood-oxygen desaturation and strenuous attempts at inspiration through the narrowed airway, all of which lighten and disrupt sleep. Hypercapnia, which results either from obstructive sleep apnea or from lung disease, reduces breathing without the presence of disruptive inspiratory efforts.

The second type is central sleep apnea, which results from failure of the respiratory neurons to activate the phrenic and intercostal motor neurons that mediate respiratory movements. There is no attempt to breathe, and although the airway is not collapsed, there is no respiration. This type of apnea is more commonly associated with heart disease (Olson and Strohl 1986).

The third type is mixed sleep apnea, which is a combination, generally beginning with a central component and ending with an obstructive component.

The lifetime prevalence of BRSD in adults has been estimated to be 9% in men and 4% in women (Young et al. 1993). The prevalence does increase with age, particularly in postmenopausal women. The prevalence in the elderly has been estimated to be 28% in men and 19% in women (Ancoli-Israel et al. 1991c).

During apneas and hypopneas, the blood-oxygen level often drops to precarious levels. In addition, one often sees cardiac arrhythmias and nocturnal hypertension in association with the respiratory disturbances. The cardiac arrhythmias include bradycardia during the events and tachycardia after the end of the events. It is not unusual to see premature ventricular contractions, trigeminy and bigeminy, asystole, second-degree atrioventricular block, atrial tachycardia, sinus bradycardia, and ventricular tachycardia. However, the electrocardiogram taken during the waking state might be normal. It is only during the respiratory events during sleep that the abnormalities appear.

BRSD, especially central sleep apnea, is commonly seen in patients with congestive heart failure (Findley et al. 1985). Cor pulmonale may also be a consequence of long-standing BRSD and is seen in both sleep apnea syndrome and primary hypoventilation. Patients may present with unexplained respiratory failure, polycythemia, right ventricular failure, and nocturnal hypertension. About 50% of patients with BRSD have hypertension, and about one-third of all hypertensive patients have BRSD. In the large cross-sectional study, it was found that both systolic and diastolic blood pressure (SDB) as well as the prevalence of hypertension increased significantly with increasing SDB (Nieto et al. 2000). It has also been shown that there is a dose–response association between SDB at baseline and hypertension 4 years later suggesting that SDB may be a risk factor for hypertension and consequent cardiovascular morbidity (Peppard et al. 2000).

The most common symptoms of BRSD include excessive daytime sleepiness and snoring. The excessive daytime sleepiness probably results from sleep fragmentation caused by the frequent nocturnal arousals occurring at the end of the apneas, and possibly from hypoxemia. The excessive daytime sleepiness is associated with lethargy, poor concentration, decreased motivation and performance, and inappropriate and inadvertent attacks of sleep. Sometimes the patients do not realize they have fallen asleep until they awaken.

The second complaint is loud snoring, sometimes noisy enough to be heard throughout or even outside the house. Often the wife has complained for years about the snoring and has threatened to sleep elsewhere if she has not moved out already. Bed partners describe a characteristic pattern of loud snoring interrupted by periods of silence, which are then terminated by snorting sounds. Snoring results from a partial narrowing of the airway caused by multiple factors, such as inadequate muscle tone, large tonsils and adenoids, long soft palate, flaccid tissue, acromegaly, hypothyroidism, or congenital narrowing of the oral pharynx (Fairbanks 1987). Snoring has been implicated not only in sleep apnea but also in angina pectoris, stroke, ischemic heart disease, and cerebral infarction, even in the absence of complete sleep apneas (Koskenvuo et al. 1985, Partinen and Palomaki 1985). Because the prevalence of snoring increases with age, especially in women (Kripke et al. 1990), and because snoring can have serious medical consequences, the psychiatrist must give serious attention to complaints of loud snoring. Snoring is not always a symptom of BRSD. Approximately 25% of men and 15% of women are habitual snorers.

Patients with BRSD are frequently overweight. In some patients, a weight gain of 20 to 30 lb might bring on episodes of BRSD. The same fatty tissue seen on the outside is also present on the inside, making the airway even more narrow. Because obstructive sleep apnea is always caused by the collapse of the airway, in patients of normal weight, anatomical abnormalities (such as large tonsils, long uvula) must be considered.

Other symptoms of BRSD include unexplained morning headaches, nocturnal confusion, automatic behavior, dysfunction of the autonomic nervous system, or night sweats. The severity of BRSD will depend on the severity of the cardiac arrhythmias, hypertension, excessive daytime sleepiness, respiratory disturbance index, amount of sleep fragmentation, and amount of oxygen desaturation.

Mild to moderate sleep-related breathing disturbances increase with age, even in elderly subjects without major complaints about their sleep. The frequency is higher in men than in women, at least until the age of menopause, after which the rate in women increases and may approach that of men. With use of the apnea index of 5 or more apneic episodes per hour as a cutoff criterion, prevalence rates range from 27 to 75% for older men and from 0 to 32% for older women (Ancoli-Israel 1989). In general, the severity of apnea in these older persons is mild (an average apnea index of about 13) compared with that seen in patients with clinical sleep apnea. However, older men and women with mild apnea have been reported to fall asleep at inappropriate times significantly more often than older persons without apnea. Furthermore, the frequency of sleep apnea and other BRSDs is higher in individuals with hypertension, congestive heart failure, obesity, dementia, and other medical conditions.

Increased mortality rates have been noted in excessively long sleepers (Kripke et al. 1990); therefore sleep apnea may account for some of these excess deaths (Kripke 1983). This is also consistent with evidence that excess deaths from all causes increase between 2 and 8 AM, specifically deaths related to ischemic heart disease in patients older than 65 years (Mitler et al. 1987). There have been several studies suggesting that untreated sleep apnea in the elderly may lead to shorter survival (Bliwise et al. 1988, Fleury 1992, Ancoli-Israel et al. 1996).

The clinical significance of relatively mild "subclinical" sleep apneas is not fully understood yet. Psychiatrists

| Table 76–9 | Clinical Symptoms of Breathing-Related Sleep Disorders |
|---|---|
| Daytime Symptoms | Nighttime Symptoms |
| Excessive daytime sleepiness | Loud snoring |
| Memory loss | Hypertension |
| Decreased mental function | Cardiac arrhythmias |
| Morning headache | Leg kicks |
| Automatic behavior | Confusion |
| Lethargy | Impotence |
| | Choking–gasping |

should be aware, however, that such disturbances might be associated with either insomnia or excessive daytime sleepiness. Furthermore, for some patients with sleep apnea, administration of hypnotics, alcohol, or other sedating medications is relatively contraindicated. The risk is not yet known, but reports indicate that benzodiazepines as well as alcohol may increase the severity of mild sleep apnea (Mendelson et al. 1981, Block et al. 1983). Therefore, psychiatrists should inquire about snoring, gasping, and other signs and symptoms of sleep apnea before administering a sleeping pill. If patients have excessive sleepiness or morning hangover effects while taking benzodiazepines, major tranquilizers, or other sedating medications, the psychiatrist should consider the possibility of an iatrogenic BRSD due to medications.

The diagnosis of BRSD must be differentiated from other disorders of excessive sleepiness such as narcolepsy (Table 76–9). Patients with BRSD will not have cataplexy, sleep-onset paralysis, or sleep-onset hallucination. Narcolepsy is not usually associated with loud snoring or sleep apneas. In laboratory recordings, patients with BRSD do not usually have sleep-onset REM periods either at night or in multiple naps on the Multiple Sleep Latency Test. However, one must be aware that both BRSD and narcolepsy can be found in the same patient. BRSD must also be distinguished from other hypersomnias, such as those related to major depressive disorder or circadian rhythm disturbances.

## Treatment of Sleep Apnea

Sleep apnea is sometimes alleviated by weight loss, avoidance of sedatives, use of tongue-retaining devices, and breathing air under positive pressure through a face mask (continuous positive airway pressure [CPAP]) (Guilleminault and Stoohs 1990, Aubert 1992). Oxygen breathed at night may alleviate insomnia associated with apnea that is not accompanied by impeded inspiration. Surgery may be helpful, for example, to correct enlarged tonsils, a long uvula, a short mandible, or morbid obesity. Pharyngoplasty, which tightens the pharyngeal mucosa and may also reduce the size of the uvula, or the use of a cervical collar to extend the neck, may relieve heavy snoring (Rodenstein 1992). Although tricyclic antidepressants are sometimes used in the treatment of clinical sleep apnea in young adults, they may cause considerable toxic effects in older people. The newer shorter-acting non-

benzodiazepine hypnotics seem to be safer in these patients and may be considered in those patients who snore.

## Circadian Rhythm Sleep Disorder (Sleep–Wake Schedule Disorders)

Circadian rhythm disturbances result from a mismatch between the internal or endogenous circadian sleep–wake system and the external or exogenous demands on the sleep–wake system. The individual's tendency to sleep–wakefulness does not match that of her or his social circumstances or of the light–dark cycle. Although some individuals do not find this mismatch to be a problem, for others the circadian rhythm disturbance interferes with the ability to function properly at times when alertness or sleepiness is desired or required. For those individuals, insomnia, hyper-

---

**DSM-IV-TR Criteria** 307.45

### Circadian Rhythm Sleep Disorder

A. A persistent or recurrent pattern of sleep disruption leading to excessive sleepiness or insomnia that is due to a mismatch between the sleep–wake schedule required by a person's environment and his or her circadian sleep–wake pattern.

B. The sleep disturbance causes clinically significant distress or impairment in social, occupational, or other important areas of functioning.

C. The disturbance does not occur exclusively during the course of another sleep disorder or other mental disorder.

D. The disturbance is not due to the direct physiological effects of a substance (e.g., a drug of abuse, a medication) or a general medical condition.

*Specify* type:

**Delayed sleep phase type:** a persistent pattern of late sleep onset and late awakening times, with an inability to fall asleep and awaken at a desired earlier time

**Jet lag type:** sleepiness and alertness that occur at an inappropriate time of day relative to local time, occurring after repeated travel across more than one time zone

**Shift work type:** insomnia during the major sleep period or excessive sleepiness during the major awake period associated with night shift work or frequently changing shift work

**Unspecified type**

Reprinted with permission from the Diagnostic and Statistical Manual of Mental Disorders, Fourth Edition, Text Revision. Copyright 2000 American Psychiatric Association.

somnia, sleepiness, and fatigue result in significant discomfort and impairment. The circadian rhythm disturbances include delayed sleep phase, advanced sleep phase, shift work, jet lag, and non-24-hour-day syndrome.

## Diagnosis

The diagnosis is based on a careful review of the history and circadian patterns of sleep–wakefulness, napping, alertness, and behavior. According to DSM-IV criteria, the diagnosis of circadian rhythm sleep disorder requires significant social or occupational impairment or marked distress related to the sleep disturbance. It is often useful for patients with chronic complaints to keep a sleep–wake diary covering the entire 24-hour day each day for several weeks. If possible, an ambulatory device that measures rest–activity, such as a wrist actigraph, might supplement the sleep–wake diary. Wrist actigraphs record acceleration of the wrist at frequent intervals, such as every minute, and save it for later display. Because the wrist is mostly at rest during sleep, the record of wrist rest–activity provides a fairly accurate estimate of the timing and duration of sleep–wakefulness. In addition, some commercial wrist activity devices have a built-in photometer, which provides a record of ambient light–darkness against which the rest–activity pattern can be compared.

### Delayed and Advanced Sleep Phase Disorders

Delayed sleep phase refers to a delay in the circadian rhythm in the sleep–wake cycle (Vignau et al. 1993). These individuals are generally not sleepy until several hours after "normal" bedtime (i.e., 2–3 AM). If allowed to sleep undisturbed, they will sleep for 7 or 8 hours, which means they awaken at 10 to 11 AM. People with delayed sleep phase are considered extreme "owls." They may or may not complain of sleep-onset insomnia. They usually enjoy their alertness in the evening and night and have little desire to sleep beginning at 10 PM or midnight. Their problem is trying to wake up at normal times (i.e., 6–7 AM). In essence, their rhythm is shifted to a later clock time relative to conventional rest–activity patterns.

Individuals with delayed sleep phase often choose careers that allow them to set their own schedules, such as freelance writers. Delayed sleep phase occurs commonly in late adolescence and young adulthood, such as in college students. As many of these individuals age, however, their endogenous sleep–wake rhythm advances and they eventually are able to conform themselves to a normal rest period at night.

For others, however, this phase shift of the endogenous oscillator may lead at a later age to the advanced sleep phase (Richardson 1990). In this condition, individuals become sleepy earlier in the evening (e.g., 7–8 PM). They will also sleep for 7 to 8 hours, but that means they awaken at 2 to 3 AM. These individuals are "larks," being most alert in the morning. They complain of sleep maintenance insomnia, that is, they cannot stay asleep all night long. This condition is more prevalent in the elderly than in the young.

The etiology of extreme "night owls" and "larks" is probably multifaceted but, in some cases, appears to reflect genetic factors. Jones and colleagues (1999) described a family in which extreme phase advance (bedtime about 7 PM) appeared to be consistent with an autosomal dominant trait. One member of the family was studied in a temporal isolation facility; as predicted, her endogenous sleep–wake cycle averaged less than 24 hours, clearly different from most subjects who average about 24.2 to 24.5 hours. Members of this family appear to have a mutation of one of the "clock genes" (Jones et al. 1999). In addition, Ancoli-Israel and colleagues (2001) identified a pedigree of one family with phase delay.

**Treatment.** Clinical management includes chronobiological strategies to shift the phase position of the endogenous circadian oscillator in the appropriate direction. For example, exposure to bright light in the morning advances the delayed sleep phase, that is, individuals will become sleepy earlier in the evening (Rosenthal et al. 1990). On the other hand, administration of bright light in the evening acts to delay the circadian rhythm, that is, individuals will get sleepy later in the evening. Light is usually administered in doses of 2,500 lux for a period of 2 hours per day, although the ideal intensity and duration are yet to be determined. For some individuals, spending more time outdoors in bright sunlight may be sufficient to treat the sleep phase. For example, individuals with delayed sleep phase should be encouraged to remove blinds and curtains from their windows, which would allow the sunlight to pour into their bedrooms in the morning when they should arise. In addition, gradual adjustments of the timing of the sleep–wake cycle may be used to readjust the phase position of the circadian oscillator. For example, patients with delayed phase disorder can be advised to delay the onset of sleep by 2 to 3 hours each day (i.e., from 4 to 7 to 10 AM, and so on) until the appropriate bedtime. After that, they should maintain regular sleep–wake patterns, with exposure to bright light in the morning.

### Shift Work

Shift work problems occur when the circadian sleep–wake rhythm is in conflict with the rest–activity cycle imposed by the externally determined work schedule (Akerstedt 1991). Nearly a quarter of all American employees have jobs that require them to work outside the conventional 8 AM to 5 PM schedule. Different patterns include rotating schedules and more or less permanent evening and night schedules. Rotating schedules, particularly rapidly shifting schedules, are difficult because constant readjustment of the endogenous circadian oscillator to the imposed sleep–wake cycle is necessary. In both rotating and shift work schedules, further difficulties are encountered because the worker is usually expected to readjust to a normal sleep–wake cycle on weekends and holidays. Even if the worker can adjust his or her circadian system to the work schedule, he or she is then out of synchrony with the rhythm of family and friends during off-duty hours. These individuals, therefore, are constantly sleep deprived and constantly sleepy. They endure impaired performance and increased risk of accidents, somatic complaints, and poor morale; hypnotics, stimulants, and alcohol are used excessively in relationship to unusual or shifting work schedules (Moore-Ede 1986, Akerstedt 1991, Czeisler et al. 1990). Shift work schedules may have played a role in human errors that contributed to the Three Mile Island and Chernobyl accidents and the Challenger disaster.

**Treatment.** No totally satisfactory methods currently exist for managing shift work problems. Because people vary in their ability to adjust to these schedules, self-selection or survival of the fittest may be involved for those who can find other employment or work schedules. Older individuals appear to be less flexible than younger persons in adjusting to shift work. Some experiments suggest that the principles of chronobiology may be useful in reducing the human costs of shift work. For example, because the endogenous pacemaker has a cycle length (tau) longer than 24 hours, rotating shift workers do better when their schedules move in a clockwise direction (i.e., morning to evening to night) rather than in the other direction. Appropriate exposure to bright lights and darkness may push the circadian pacemaker in the correct direction and help stabilize its phase position, especially in association with the use of dark glasses outside and blackout curtains at home to maintain darkness at the appropriate times for promotion of sleep and shifting of the circadian pacemaker (Czeisler et al. 1990). Naps may also be useful in reducing sleep loss. Modest amounts of coffee may maintain alertness early in the shift but should be avoided near the end of the shift.

### Jet Lag

Jet lag occurs when individuals travel across several time zones. Traveling east advances the sleep–wake cycle and is typically more difficult than traveling west (which delays the cycle). Jet lag may be associated with difficulty initiating or maintaining sleep or with daytime sleepiness, impaired performance, and gastrointestinal disturbance after rapid transmeridian flights (Moore-Ede 1986). Individuals older than 50 years appear to be more vulnerable to jet lag than are younger persons.

**Management.** Considerable research and theorizing are under way to better prevent and manage the problems associated with jet lag. Some efforts before departure may be useful to prevent or ameliorate these problems. For persons who plan to readjust their circadian clock to the new location, it may be possible to move the sleep–wake and light–dark schedules appropriately before departure. In addition, good sleep hygiene principles should be respected before, during, and after the trip. For example, many people are sleep deprived or in alcohol withdrawal when they step on the plane because of last-minute preparations or farewell parties. Whereas adequate fluid intake on the plane is necessary to avoid dehydration, alcohol consumption should be avoided or minimized because it causes diuresis and may disrupt sleep maintenance.

On arriving at the destination, it may be preferable to try to maintain a schedule coinciding with actual home time if the trip is going to be short. For example, the individual should try to sleep at times that correspond to the usual bedtime or with the normal midafternoon dip in alertness. If, on the other hand, the trip will be longer and it is desirable to synchronize the biological clock with local time, exposure to appropriate schedules of bright light and darkness may be helpful, at least theoretically. Unfortunately, the exact protocols have not been established in all instances yet and require further research and experimentation. In addition, some of these protocols require avoidance of bright light at certain times, necessitating wearing dark goggles, for example, when traveling.

In addition to synchronizing the clock with the new environment, sleep and rest should be promoted by good sleep hygiene principles, by avoidance of excessive caffeine and alcohol, and, possibly, by administration of short-duration hypnotics. Care should be taken, however, to avoid hangover effects or amnesia associated with hypnotics. Because individual responses to sleeping pills vary considerably from person to person, it is often helpful to develop experience with specific compounds and doses before departure.

### Non-24-Hour-Day Syndrome

The non-24-hour-day (or "hypernyctohemeral") syndrome is characterized by free-running in the natural environment, that is, the subject goes to bed and arises about 45 minutes later each day. The average duration of the sleep–wake cycle is about 24.5 to 25.0 hours. During the course of about 3 weeks, the subject's sleep–wake cycle "goes around the clock" as the timing of the sleep period gradually delays. The lengthened sleep–wake cycle of these patients in the natural environment is similar to that of normal subjects living in a time-free environment. The disorder appears to be relatively common in patients with total blindness, because they no longer perceive visual Zeitgebers. In many cases, the cause is unknown, but it is sometimes observed in individuals who are socially or linguistically isolated. Management may include bright light therapy in the morning to entrain the endogenous oscillator. Administration of vitamin $B_{12}$ may be helpful, perhaps by enhancing the effectiveness of Zeitgebers (Kamgar-Parsi et al. 1983).

The prevalence of circadian rhythm disturbances has not been established. Approximately two-thirds of shift workers have difficulty with their schedules. Circadian rhythm disturbances must be differentiated from sleep-onset insomnia due to other causes (such as pain, caffeine consumption), early morning insomnia due to depression or alcohol use, and changes in sleep patterns due to lifestyle or lifestyle changes.

## Periodic Limb Movements in Sleep

Periodic limb movements in sleep (PLMS), previously called nocturnal myoclonus, is a disorder in which repetitive, brief, and stereotyped limb movements occur during sleep, usually about every 20 to 40 seconds. Dorsiflexions of the big toe, ankle, knee, and sometimes the hip are involved (Ancoli-Israel et al. 1991b, Chesson et al. 1999) (Table 76–10 and Figure 76–8).

| Table 76–10 | Features of Periodic Limb Movements in Sleep |
|---|---|

Leg kicks every 20–40 s
Duration of 0.5–5 s
Complaints of:
   Insomnia
   Excessive sleepiness
   Restless legs
   Very cold or hot feet
   Uncomfortable sensations in legs

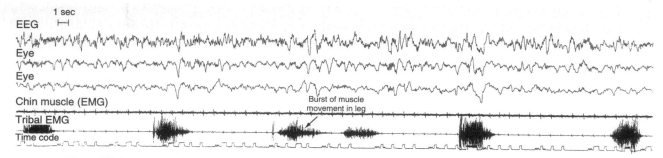

EEG

Eye

Eye

Chin muscle (EMG)

Burst of muscle movement in leg

Tribal EMG

Time code

**Figure 76–8** *Periodic limb movements in sleep. Time scale: 1 cm = 1 s. EEG, electroencephalogram; EMG, electromyogram.*

## Diagnosis

Questioning of the patient or bed partner often yields reports of restlessness, kicking, unusually cold or hot feet, disrupted and torn bedclothes, unrefreshing sleep, insomnia, or excessive daytime sleepiness. Patients may be unaware of these pathological leg movements or arousals, although their bed partners may be all too aware of the kicking, frequent movements, and restlessness (Coleman et al. 1983, Ancoli-Israel et al. 1986). If these disorders are strongly suspected, the patient should probably be referred to a sleep disorders laboratory for evaluation and an overnight polysomnogram with tibial electromyograms. These disorders are often associated with transient arousals in the EEG recording. Diagnosis is made when the periodic limb movement index (number of leg jerks per hour of sleep) is 5 or greater, accompanied by arousals. The jerks occur primarily in the legs but may also appear in less severe forms in the arms. The movements can be bilateral or unilateral and occur in stage 1 and stage 2 sleep. Patients often have reduced deep sleep because the jerks continually awaken them.

A related disturbance, restless legs syndrome, is associated with disagreeable sensations in the lower legs, feet, or thighs that occur in a recumbent or resting position and cause an almost irresistible urge to move the legs (Walters et al. 1995).

Whereas almost all patients with restless legs syndrome have PLMS, not all patients with PLMS have restless legs syndrome. Restless legs syndrome may be frequent in patients with uremia and rheumatoid arthritis or in pregnant women.

Both PLMS and restless legs syndrome usually occur in middle-aged people, but many patients report having had the same sensations as adolescents and even as children. It has been suggested that both conditions are familial, perhaps due to an autosomal dominant gene.

Individuals with PLMS are reported to sleep about an hour less per night than control subjects without PLMS (Ancoli-Israel et al. 1991b). Interestingly, the prevalence of PLMS is not higher in insomniac patients than in those without insomnia. Complaints of excessive daytime sleepiness increase in individuals with PLMS, probably consequent to the numerous sleep interruptions. The psychiatrist may find it useful to talk with a bed partner, who will often describe kicking and leg twitches during sleep in individuals with PLMS.

The myoclonic movements are not related to seizure disorder but should be distinguished from seizures. Because complaints of insomnia and daytime sleepiness are not uncommon, other insomnias, sleep apnea, and narcolepsy should be ruled out.

Prevalence of PLMS in young and middle-aged adults has not been fully established. In sleep disorders clinic populations, about 11% of those complaining of insomnia are diagnosed with PLMS. In the elderly, however, this condition is extremely common; more than 45% have at least five leg kicks per hour of sleep (Ancoli-Israel et al. 1985, 1991b).

## Treatment

Because the pathogenesis of PLMS is usually unknown, treatment is often symptomatic (Table 76–11). Some studies suggest that the movements arise subcortically from the brain or spinal cord; others suggest subclinical peripheral neuropathy. At the present time, dopaminergic agents such as levodopa (L-dopa), pergolide, or pramipexole generally provide the most effective treatment for both PLMS and restless legs syndrome (Walters et al. 1988, Chesson et al. 1999, Heninger et al. 1999, Montplaisir et al. 2000, 2002). Opiates, such as oxycodone and propoxyphene, have also been demonstrated to be effective in the treatment of PLMS and restless legs syndrome. Anticonvulsants, such as carbamazepine and gabapentin, have been shown to be effective in treatment of restless legs syndrome. Clonazepam, a benzodiazepine anticonvulsant, is effective in the treatment of PLMS and possibly for restless legs syndrome. Other benzodiazepines have also been used to treat these conditions, as they will decrease some of the awakenings but may have no effect on the number of leg movements (Chesson et al. 1999, Heninger et al. 1999).

## Parasomnias

The parasomnias are a group of disorders characterized by disturbances of either physiological processes or behavior associated with sleep, but not necessarily causing disturbances of sleep or wakefulness.

## Nightmare Disorder

The essential feature of this disorder is the repeated occurrence of frightening dreams that lead to full awakenings from sleep (Hartmann 1991, 1994). The dreams or awakenings cause the individual significant distress or dysfunction. By DSM-IV-TR definition, the disorder is excluded if the nightmare occurs in the course of another mental or medical disorder or as a direct result of a medication or substance. Many, but not all, nightmares occur during REM sleep;

| Table 76-11 | Pharmacologic Treatment Options in RLS/PLMS | | | |
| --- | --- | --- | --- | --- |
| Medication | Dosage Range | Side Effects | Advantages | Disadvantages |
| L-dopa/carbidopa | 25/100–100/400/D | Dyskinesia Nausea Hallucinations | Low cost | Breakthrough restlessness Loss of efficacy |
| Pergolide | 0.05–1 mg | Dyskinesia Nausea Rhinitis Dizziness | High rate of response | Frequent side effects |
| Pramipexole | 0.25–0.875 mg | Orthostasis Dizziness Sedation | High rate of response Good tolerance | Expense |
| Anticonvulsants | Variable | Sedation | Low cost Sleep promotion | Variable response |
| Opiates | Variable | Nausea Constipation | Low cost | Variable response Abuse potential |
| Clonazepam | 0.5–2 mg | Sedation Dizziness | Sleep promotion | Variable response Abuse potential |

## DSM-IV-TR Criteria 307.47

### Nightmare Disorder

A. Repeated awakenings from the major sleep period or naps with detailed recall of extended and extremely frightening dreams, usually involving threats to survival, security, or self-esteem. The awakenings generally occur during the second half of the sleep period.

B. On awakening from the frightening dreams, the person rapidly becomes oriented and alert (in contrast to the confusion and disorientation seen in sleep terror disorder and some forms of epilepsy).

C. The dream experience, or the sleep disturbance resulting from the awakening, causes clinically significant distress or impairment in social, occupational, or other important areas of functioning.

D. The nightmares do not occur exclusively during the course of another mental disorder (e.g., a delirium, posttraumatic stress disorder) and are not due to the direct physiological effects of a substance (e.g., a drug of abuse, a medication) or a general medical condition.

Reprinted with permission from the Diagnostic and Statistical Manual of Mental Disorders, Fourth Edition, Text Revision. Copyright 2000 American Psychiatric Association.

REM nightmares take place most often during the last half of the night when REM sleep is most common (see nightmares in posttraumatic stress disorder).

Whereas more than half of the adult population probably experiences an occasional nightmare, nightmares start more commonly in children between the ages of 3 and 6 years. The exact prevalence is unknown.

## Treatment

The disorder is usually self-limited in children but can be helped sometimes with psychotherapy, desensitization, or rehearsal instructions (Bakwin 1970). Secondary nightmares, as in posttraumatic stress disorder (PTSD), can be difficult to treat.

## Sleep Terror Disorder

This disorder is defined as repeated abrupt awakenings from sleep characterized by intense fear, panicky screams, autonomic arousal (tachycardia, rapid breathing, and sweating), absence of detailed dream recall, amnesia for the episode, and relative unresponsiveness to attempts to comfort the person (Kales et al. 1980, Gordon 1992). Because sleep terrors occur primarily during delta sleep, they usually take place during the first third of the night. These episodes may cause distress or impairment, especially for caretakers who witness the event. Sleep terrors may also be called night terrors, *pavor nocturnus*, or incubus.

The prevalence of the disorder is estimated to be about 1 to 6% in children and less than 1% in adults. In children, it usually begins between the ages of 4 and 12 years and resolves spontaneously during adolescence. It is more common in boys than in girls. It does not appear to be associated with psychiatric illness in children. In adults, it usually begins between 20 and 30 years of age, has a chronic undulating course, is equally common in men and women, and may be associated with psychiatric disorders, such as PTSD, generalized anxiety disorder, borderline personality disorder, and others. An increased frequency of enuresis and somnambulism has been reported in the first-degree relatives of patients with night terrors.

## Treatment

Nocturnal administration of benzodiazepines has been reported to be beneficial, perhaps because these drugs suppress delta sleep, the stage of sleep during which sleep terrors typically occur.

### Sleep Terror Disorder

A. Recurrent episodes of abrupt awakening from sleep, usually occurring during the first third of the major sleep episode and beginning with a panicky scream.

B. Intense fear and signs of autonomic arousal, such as tachycardia, rapid breathing, and sweating, during each episode.

C. Relative unresponsiveness to efforts of others to comfort the person during the episode.

D. No detailed dream is recalled and there is amnesia for the episode.

E. The episodes cause clinically significant distress or impairment in social, occupational, or other important areas of functioning.

F. The disturbance is not due to the direct physiological effects of a substance (e.g., a drug of abuse, a medication) or a general medical condition.

## Sleepwalking Disorder

This disorder is characterized by repeated episodes of motor behavior initiated in sleep, usually during delta sleep in the first third of the night. While sleepwalking, the patient has a blank staring face, is relatively unresponsive to others, and may be confused or disoriented initially on being aroused from the episode. Although the person may be alert after several minutes of awakening, complete amnesia for the episode is common the next day. Sleepwalking may cause considerable distress, for example, if a child cannot sleep away from home or go to camp because of it. By DSM-IV definition, pure sleepwalking is excluded if it occurs as a result of a medication or substance or is due to a medical disorder. However, sleepwalking may be an idiosyncratic reaction to specific drugs, including tranquilizers and sleeping pills (Glassman et al. 1986).

Most behaviors during sleepwalking are routine and of low-level intensity, such as sitting up, picking the sheets, or walking around the bedroom. More complicated behaviors may also occur, however, such as urinating in a closet, leaving the house, running, eating, talking, driving, or even committing murder (Luchins et al. 1978). A real danger is that the individual will be injured by going through a window or falling from a height.

Whereas about 10 to 30% of children have at least one sleepwalking episode, only about 1 to 5% have repeated episodes. The disorder most commonly begins between the ages of 4 and 8 years and usually resolves spontaneously during adolescence. Genetic factors may be involved, because sleepwalkers are reported to have a higher than expected frequency of first-degree relatives with either sleepwalking or sleep terrors (Bakwin 1970).

### Sleepwalking Disorder

A. Repeated episodes of rising from bed during sleep and walking about, usually occurring during the first third of the major sleep episode.

B. While sleepwalking, the person has a blank, staring face, is relatively unresponsive to the efforts of others to communicate with him or her, and can be awakened only with great difficulty.

C. On awakening (either from the sleepwalking episode or the next morning), the person has amnesia for the episode.

D. Within several minutes after awakening from the sleepwalking episode, there is no impairment of mental activity or behavior (although there may initially be a short period of confusion or disorientation).

E. The sleepwalking causes clinically significant distress or impairment in social, occupational, or other important areas of functioning.

F. The disturbance is not due to the direct physiological effects of a substance (e.g., a drug of abuse, a medication) or a general medical condition.

Sleepwalking may be precipitated in affected patients by gently sitting them up during sleep, by fever, or by sleep deprivation. Adult onset of sleepwalking should prompt the search for possible medical, neurological, psychiatric, pharmacological, or other underlying causes, such as nocturnal epilepsy.

### Treatment

No treatment for sleepwalking is established, but some patients respond to administration of benzodiazepines or sedating antidepressants at bedtime. The major concern should be the safety of the sleepwalker, who may injure herself or himself or someone else during an episode.

### REM Sleep Behavior Disorder

First described in 1986, this disorder, like sleepwalking, is associated with complicated behaviors during sleep such as walking, running, singing, and talking (Schenk et al. 1986). In contrast to sleepwalking, which occurs during the first third of the night during delta sleep, REM sleep behavior disorder usually occurs during the second half of the night during REM sleep. It apparently results from an intermittent loss of the muscle atonia that normally accompanies REM sleep, thus allowing the patient to act out her or his dream. Also, in contrast to sleepwalking, memory for the dream content is usually good. Furthermore, the idiopathic form typically occurs in men during the sixth or seventh decade of life. The cause or causes remain unknown. It has been reported in a variety of neurological disorders and during withdrawal from sedatives or alcohol; during treatment with tricyclic antidepressants or biperiden (Akineton); and in various neurological disorders including dementia, subarachnoid hemorrhage, and degenerative neurological disorders.

## Treatment

Nocturnal administration of clonazepam, 0.5 to 1 mg, is usually remarkably successful in controlling the symptoms of this disorder. Patients and their families should be educated about the nature of the disorder and warned to take precautions about injuring themselves or others.

## Nocturnal Panic Attacks

The typical daytime panic attack, as bizarre and frightening as it may seem to the patient experiencing it, is often fairly obvious to the assessing psychiatrist. Symptoms of anxiety, sweating, tremor, dizziness, chest pain, and palpitations occur "out of the blue" with or without specific behavioral or associational stimuli. Once it has been diagnosed, treatment options may include pharmacotherapy with one of several classes of drugs, behavioral therapy, or a combined approach.

When these symptoms occur at night, the task of the assessing psychiatrist is greatly complicated. The patient may assume that the cause is a nightmare or a night terror and may be resistant to the diagnosis of an anxiety disorder, particularly if the symptoms are absent or mild during the daytime. Patients with panic disorder often have not only disturbed subjective sleep but also panic attacks during sleep (Stein et al. 1993, Koenigsberg et al. 1994). Psychiatrists should remember that panic attacks could occur exclusively during sleep, without daytime symptoms, in some patients.

Conversely, a report of "awakening in a state of panic" may be associated with a variety of other disorders including obstructive sleep apnea, gastroesophageal reflux, nocturnal angina, orthopnea, nightmares, night terrors, and others.

## Sleep-Related Epilepsy

Some forms of epilepsy occur more commonly during sleep than during wakefulness and may be associated with parasomnia disorders. Nocturnal seizures may at times be confused with sleep terror, REM sleep behavior disorder, paroxysmal hypnogenic dystonia, or nocturnal panic attacks (Culebras 1992). They may take the form of generalized convulsions or may be partial seizures with complex symptoms. Nocturnal seizures are most common at two times: the first 2 hours of sleep, or around 4 to 6 AM. They are more common in children than in adults. The chief complaint may be only disturbed sleep, torn up bedsheets and blankets, morning drowsiness (a postictal state), and muscle aches. Some patients never realize they suffer from nocturnal epilepsy until they share a bedroom or bed with someone who observes a convulsion.

## Sleep Disturbances Related to Other Psychiatric Disorders

Subjective and objective disturbances of sleep are common features of many psychiatric disorders. General abnormal-

ities include dyssomnias (such as insomnia and hypersomnia), parasomnias (such as nightmares, night terrors, and nocturnal panic attacks), and circadian rhythm disturbances (early morning awakening). Before assuming that a significant sleep complaint invariably signals a psychiatric diagnosis, mental health specialists should go through a careful differential diagnostic procedure to rule out medical, pharmacological, or other causes. Even if the sleep complaint is primarily related to an underlying psychiatric disorder, sleep disorders in the mentally ill may be exacerbated by many other factors, such as increasing age; comorbid psychiatric, sleep, and medical diagnoses; alcohol and substance abuse; effects of psychotropic or other medications; use of caffeinated beverages, nicotine, or other substances; lifestyle; past episodes of psychiatric illness (persisting "scars"); and cognitive, conditioned, and coping characteristics such as anticipatory anxiety about sleep as bedtime nears. Some features of these sleep disorders may persist during periods of clinical remission of the psychiatric disorder and may be influenced by genetic factors. Finally, even if the sleep complaint is precipitated by a nonpsychiatric factor, psychiatric and psychosocial skills may be useful in ferreting out predisposing and perpetuating factors involved in chronic sleep complaints.

Although signs and symptoms of sleep disturbance are common in most psychiatric disorders, an additional diagnosis of insomnia or hypersomnia related to another mental disorder is made according to DSM-IV-TR criteria only when the sleep disturbance is a predominant complaint and is sufficiently severe to warrant independent clinical attention. Many of the patients with this type of sleep disorder diagnosis focus on the sleep complaints to the exclusion of other symptoms related to the primary psychiatric disorder. For example, they may seek professional help with complaints of insomnia or oversleeping when they should be at work, excessive fatigue, or desire for sleeping pills, but initially, they minimize or strongly deny signs and symptoms related to poor mood, anxiety, obsessive rumination, alcohol abuse, or a personality disorder.

## Sleep Disturbances in Psychiatric Disorders: "Chicken or Egg?"

Whether sleep disturbances "cause" psychiatric disorders can be debated. At one level, this hypothesis seems unlikely because normal subjects vary considerably in their amount and type of sleep. Occasional extreme short sleepers, "needing" and sleeping as little as an hour a day for many years, have been reported, who appeared to be psychologically and medically normal in other respects. Furthermore, prolonged partial or selective sleep deprivation in normal volunteers does not apparently precipitate major psychiatric disorders. Normal control subjects have been kept awake for as long as 11 consecutive days in experiments to test the effect of sleep deprivation. Such experiments may cause dysphoria and dysfunction but not depression or dementia. Moreover, patients with narcolepsy or depression have been deprived of REM sleep for more than a year while being treated with high doses of MAOIs; if anything, they were better because their primary mood disorder improved during the course of treatment (Landolt et al. 2001). Finally, total or partial sleep deprivation for one night has antidepressant effects in about half of depressed patients, including severely depressed melancholic, endogenous, or delusional patients (Hillman et al. 1990).

These observations neither prove nor disprove the hypothesis that sleep disturbance does not cause psychiatric disorders. After all, experimental disruption of sleep in normal control subjects is highly artificial, usually conducted in supportive environments in well-screened, self-selected, healthy subjects. Likewise, people may vary in their sleep needs, but as far as we know, everyone needs to sleep; it may just be that individuals vary in the threshold of sleep disturbance beyond which they can go before manifesting psychiatric symptoms. Most important, chronic subjective sleep disturbances may be risk factors for certain vulnerable individuals. For example, two longitudinal epidemiological studies reported that a persistent complaint of insomnia for a year was also a risk factor for the later onset of major depressive disorder, anxiety disorder, and substance abuse (Ford and Kamerow 1989, Livingston et al. 1993). One of these studies also assessed persistent hypersomnia and found that this complaint was a risk factor. In addition, a questionnaire study suggested that nonalcoholic college-age men who reported that they "need less than 6 hours of sleep to feel comfortable" had a higher frequency of alcoholic first-degree relatives and drank more than did men who slept more (Schuckit and Bernstein 1981). Thus, specific sleep characteristics may predispose to, or be a risk factor for, later development of psychiatric or substance abuse disorders. Again, the complaint of chronic insomnia or hypersomnia or normal short sleep cannot always be equated with objective sleep abnormalities, but it should at least alert the psychiatrist to the possibility that the patient deserves careful monitoring for a time.

Sleep disruption may be particularly harmful to some persons, for example, bipolar disorder patients, whether euthymic or depressed, in whom sleep deprivation may precipitate a manic episode (Wehr 1992). Mania is not uncommon with jet lag or work-related sleep deprivation in bipolar disorder patients. Behavioral and apparent personality changes with sleep deprivation are probably common but more often ignored in everyday life. The irritability of sleep-deprived children is known to most parents; and who of us has not had a "bad day" after a "bad night"? More seriously, scattered case reports exist of apparently normal control subjects who had psychiatric complications in the midst of experimental manipulations of the light–dark cycle (Rockwell et al. 1978, Wehr et al. 1993) or, possibly, in association with disruptions of the circadian system (Mendlewicz et al. 1989). Thus, the role of subjective insomnia and sleep loss in the prediction and prevention of mood disorders deserves further attention from psychiatrists and researchers.

Whereas insomnia is probably the most common sleep complaint in most psychiatric disorders, hypersomnia is not infrequently reported, especially in association with the following: bipolar mood disorder during depressed periods; major depressive disorder with atypical features (i.e., hypersomniac, hyperphagic patients with "leaden paralysis" and loss of energy); seasonal (winter) depression; stimulant abusers during withdrawal; some patients with personality disorders; and patients who are heavily sedated with anxiolytic, antipsychotic, or antidepressant medications, among other disorders (Table 76–12).

## Polysomnographic Features of Sleep in Psychiatric Disorders

Polygraph recordings have now been obtained in most psychiatric disorders, especially during episodes of illness rather than remission (Benca et al. 1992, Gillin et al. 1993). As summarized in Table 76–13, no single measure or constellation of measures has yet been found to be diagnostically pathognomonic for any specific disorder. Most diagnostic disorders are associated with insomnia, characterized by increased sleep latency and reduced total sleep, sleep efficiency, and delta sleep. Whereas short REM latency was once proposed as a biological marker for depression, studies suggest that it may also be associated with schizophrenia and some eating disorders.

More studies of sleep and sleep-related phenomenology have been conducted in *depression* than in any other disorder (Table 76–14 and Figure 76–9). Despite the

---

**Table 76–12** Selected Disorders of Apparent Hypersomnia or Excessive Daytime Sleepiness

| Disorder | Sex | Hyperphagia | Depression | Hypersomnia | Excessive Daytime Sleepiness | Seasonality | Light Therapy |
|---|---|---|---|---|---|---|---|
| Atypical depression | F > M | ++ | +++ | ++ | + | – | – |
| Seasonal affective disorder | F > M | ++ | +++ | ++ | ++ | +++ | +++ |
| Bipolar depression | F = M | ± | +++ | + | + | + | + |
| Delayed sleep phase | M > F | – | ± | – | AM | – | ++ |
| Klein–Levin syndrome | M > F | ++ | + | +++ | +++ | – | – |
| Non-24-hour-day syndrome | M = F | – | – | – | – | – | + |
| Narcolepsy | M = F | – | ± | + | +++ | – | – |
| Sleep drunkenness | M = F | – | ± | +++ | AM | – | – |
| Sleep apnea | M > F | + | ± | ++ | +++ | – | – |
| Withdrawal from stimulants | M > F | ++ | + | ++ | ++ | – | – |

**Table 76–13   Generalized Polygraphic Sleep Features of Patients with Psychiatric Disorders***

| Disorder | Total Sleep Time | Sleep Efficiency | Sleep Latency | REM Latency | Delta % | REM % | REM Density |
|---|---|---|---|---|---|---|---|
| Depression | ↓↓ | ↓↓ | ↑↑ | ↓↓ | ↓↓ | ↓↓ | ↑ |
| Alcoholism | ↓ | ↓/= | ↑ | = | ↓ | ↑ | ↑= |
| Panic disorder | ↓/= | ↓↓ | ↑↑ | = | = | = | = |
| Generalized anxiety disorder | = | = | ↑ | = | = | = | = |
| Posttraumatic stress disorder | ↓↓ | ↓↓ | = | ↑/= | = | ↓↑ | ↑/= |
| Borderline disorder | ↓/= | ↓/= | ↑/= | ↓/= | = | = | = |
| Eating disorders | ↓/= | ↓/= | = | ↓/= | = | = | ↓/= |
| Schizophrenia | ↓↓ | ↓↓ | ↑↑ | ↓↓ | ↓/= | = | ↓ |
| Insomnia | ↓↓ | ↓↓ | ↑↑ | = | ↓↓ | = | = |
| Narcolepsy | = | ↓ | ↓↓ | ↓↓ | = | = | = |

*Two arrows (↑↑ or ↓↓) signify predominance of evidence; one arrow (↑ or ↓) signifies weak evidence; equal sign (=) means no difference; ↓/= or ↑/= means mixed results.

*Source*: Data from Benca RM, Obermeyer WH, Thisted RA, et al. (1992) Sleep and psychiatric disorders: A meta-analysis. Arch Gen Psychiatr 49, 651–668; Gillin JC, Dow BM, Thompson P, et al. (1993) Sleep in depression and other psychiatric disorders. Clin Neurosci 1, 90–96; Dow BM, Kelsoe JRJ, and Gillin JC (1996) Sleep and dreams in Vietnam PTSD and depression. Biol Psychiatr 39, 42–50.

common clinical impression that early morning wakefulness is a predominant symptom in depression, most of the objective measures in recent years have implicated abnormalities occurring at sleep onset and during the first non-REM and REM periods: prolonged sleep latency; reduced stages 3 and 4 sleep; increased duration and REM density of the first REM period; and associated neuroendocrine abnormalities, including growth hormone, thyroid-stimulating

**Table 76–14   Sleep-Related Characteristics Associated with Depression**

Short REM latency (state, possibly trait)

Reduced amounts of stages 3 and 4 sleep (state and trait)

Difficulties initiating and maintaining sleep

Increased amounts of ocular movement during REM sleep (REM density), especially during the first REM period

A redistribution of REM sleep toward the beginning of sleep: increased duration of the first REM period

Low arousal thresholds to auditory stimulation

Elevated core body temperature during sleep

Blunted or reduced levels of plasma growth hormone (state and trait)

Elevated levels of plasma cortisol, increased number of pulses, and earlier onset of the morning rise in cortisol levels

Reduced levels of plasma testosterone

Blunted levels of thyroid-stimulating hormone at sleep onset

Reduced nocturnal levels of plasma melatonin

Longer but flattened periods of prolactin release

Elevated cerebral glucose metabolic rate during the first non-REM period

Faster induction of REM sleep after administration of cholinergic agonists

Antidepressant effect of total and partial sleep deprivation and, possibly, selective REM sleep deprivation

hormone, and melatonin. Furthermore, some studies have suggested that short REM latency (Giles et al. 1988) or reduced delta sleep ratio (amount of delta waves in first non-REM periods compared with second non-REM periods) (Kupfer et al. 1990) may predict relapse in depressed patients. Some of these sleep-related abnormalities appear to persist during periods of clinical remission, such as short REM latency, loss of stages 3 and 4 sleep, and blunted nocturnal growth hormone release. Genetic factors may influence some of these measures, including short REM latency. Preliminary data suggest that short REM latency may be a genetic marker for depression in first-degree relatives of patients with mood disorders (Mendlewicz et al. 1989).

Given the prevalence of sleep disturbance in depression, one puzzle is the well-established observation that sleep deprivation and some other manipulations of sleep have antidepressant effects in about half of depressed patients (Table 76–15). Total and partial sleep deprivation for one night has the best documented benefits but, unfortunately, has not gained widespread clinical utility because most patients usually wake up depressed again after napping or sleeping. One exception may be premenstrual depression: partial sleep deprivation for one night at the onset of symptoms often aborts the symptoms for that month.

Even though the polygraphic sleep findings in depression do not appear to be diagnostically specific, they remain among the best documented biological abnormalities of any psychiatric disorder at this time. One challenge is to understand their pathophysiological mechanism. Because of the shallow, fragmented sleep and response to sleep deprivation, the sleep of patients with depression has been described as "overaroused." For instance, the antidepressant response of sleep deprivation may "dampen down" an overly aroused limbic system in a subgroup of patients. Several studies have shown that responders to sleep

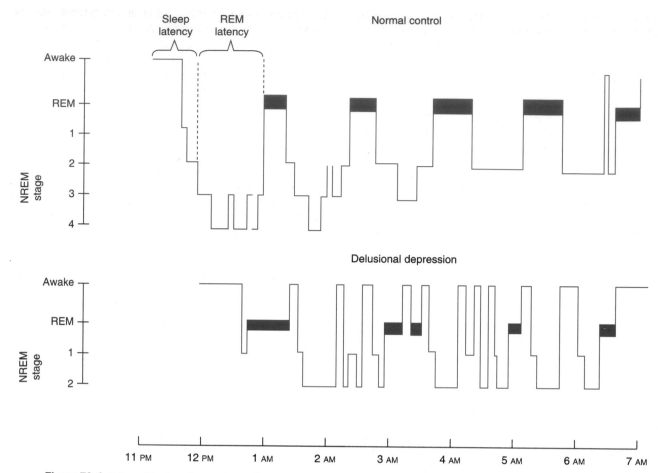

**Figure 76–9** *Polygraphic sleep characteristics of a patient with delusional depression compared with those of a normal control subject.*

deprivation differ from nonresponders at baseline assessment before sleep deprivation by having a higher level of metabolic activity in the cingulate gyrus and that this overactivity approaches normality with clinical improvement (Wu et al. 1992, Ebert et al. 1994, Gillin et al. 2001a). Consistent with the overarousal hypothesis, a preliminary

study using positron emission tomography to measure cerebral glucose metabolism suggested that depressed patients are more metabolically active during the first non-REM period of the night than are normal control subjects (Ho et al. 1996). Because cholinergic projections from brain stem and basal forebrain are involved in central physiological arousal mechanisms, it is not surprising that depressed patients are more likely than control subjects to awaken to an intravenous infusion of physostigmine (a cholinesterase inhibitor that facilitates cholinergic neurotransmission) during the first non-REM period (Berger et al. 1983). Moreover, depressed patients enter REM sleep more rapidly after administration of cholinergic agonists, whether they are given orally before bed (Berger et al. 1983) or during non-REM sleep (Gillin et al. 1991).

The sleep disturbances of *schizophrenic* patients are often similar to those of depressed patients, including short REM latency and reduced delta sleep, total sleep time, and sleep efficiency. Interestingly, while making nightly "sleep checks" on hospitalized patients, nurses are more accurate in judging sleep time in schizophrenic patients than in depressive patients, who often appear to be asleep when they are actually awake.

Although less well studied, the sleep of patients with *anxiety* disorders, such as generalized anxiety disorder, panic disorder, obsessive–compulsive disorder, acute stress disorder, and PTSD, is often disturbed (Uhde 1994). *Panic*

| Table 76–15 | Sleep Therapies for Depression | | |
|---|---|---|---|
| Sleep Manipulation | Duration | Response Rate | Comment |
| Total sleep deprivation | All night | 25–60% | Temporary benefits Well documented |
| Partial sleep deprivation | First or second half of night | 25–60% | Same Well documented |
| REM sleep deprivation | 2–3 wk | 50% | Long-term benefits Only one study |
| Advance of sleep period (i.e., 5 PM–2 AM) | 1–2 wk | 25–50% | Only a few studies |

attacks, for example, may occur occasionally during sleep itself, usually at the transition between stage 2 and delta sleep. Patients with panic disorders during sleep are also likely to experience panic attacks during wakefulness either with relaxation or after sleep deprivation.

Patients with *obsessive–compulsive* disorder frequently endure difficulties in the initiation and maintenance of sleep. They often have elaborate compulsive rituals before going to bed, for example, concerns about "germs" may necessitate long showers and fresh, clean "sterilized" pajamas and sheets each night. Polysomnographic features are sometimes similar to those described in major depressive disorder, even though the patients do not have symptoms that meet full diagnostic criteria for major depressive disorder.

Classic symptoms of *posttraumatic stress* disorder include nightmares, night terrors, and violent thrashing about during sleep. These patients are easily aroused. Combat survivors with PTSD sometimes seek a physically "secure" sleeping environment in which to sleep and wake up frequently during the night to "check the perimeter." These sleep problems in Vietnam veterans who suffer from PTSD are often complicated by chronic conditioning, alcohol and substance abuse, depression, anxiety, and significant interpersonal and social problems. Total sleep time is usually reduced with variable and inconsistent disturbances of REM sleep (Dow et al. 1996). Successful treatment of the disorder and the sleep complaints has been traditionally difficult. The nightmares of PTSD appear to occur in both non-REM and REM sleep. While SSRIs are often recommended in the treatment of PTSD, some of the activating antidepressants appear to worsen subjective complaints of sleep. Nefazodone, a sedative antidepressant, slowly improved subjective sleep quality, mood, and the number of reported nightmares during a 12-week open label study (Gillin et al. 2001b). Phenelzine and other MAOIs have also been reported to improve sleep and nightmares, but the possibility of serious drug interactions, alcoholism, and poor compliance limit their usefulness.

More recently, Raskin and colleagues have reported a significant reduction in nightmares and overall improvement in combat veterans with PTSD who were treated with prazosin, an alpha-1-adrenergic receptor antagonist (Taylor and Raskin 2002).

Changes in sleep patterns may occur in patients with eating disorders (Blois et al. 1981). Night bingeing and increased sleep after eating are commonly reported in bulimic patients, who are also reported to eat and shop for food while sleepwalking. The patient frequently does not remember these nocturnal episodes; they often become known from family or friends who have observed the behavior or from physical evidence of shopping or eating behaviors. Patients with anorexia are often hyperactive, needing little sleep. Given the degree of physical and psychic stress associated with eating disorders, it is surprising how limited are the objective sleep disturbances associated with these disorders.

## General Approaches to the Clinical Management of Sleep Disorders in Psychiatric Patients

The sleep complaint in the patient with an apparent psychiatric disorder deserves the same careful diagnostic and therapeutic attention that it does in any patient. Just because a patient is depressed does not mean that the complaint of insomnia or hypersomnia can be explained away as a symptom of depression. Too many patients with depression have been found to have a BRSD; too many patients with panic disorder to have insomnia secondary to caffeinism. Chronic sleep complaints are multidetermined and multifaceted, even in many psychiatric patients. Differential diagnosis remains the first obligation of the psychiatrist before definitive treatment, which should be aimed at the underlying cause or causes.

Nonspecific treatments, such as use of sleep hygiene principles, are often helpful for both the sleep complaints and the underlying psychiatric disorders. In particular, bipolar disorder patients and patients whose daily activities are poorly organized (like patients with chronic schizophrenia and patients with certain personality disorders) may benefit from fairly rigid sleep–wake and light–dark schedules to synchronize circadian rhythms and impose structure on their behavior. Physical exercise, meditation, relaxation methods, sleep restriction therapy, and cognitive psychotherapy may help patients manage anxiety, rumination, and conditioned psychophysiological insomnia that often cause sleeplessness at night and fatigue during the day. Partial or total sleep deprivation may be like "paradoxical intention" therapy in the treatment of major depressive disorder or premenstrual dysphoric disorder but should probably be avoided in bipolar depression.

Medications may either help or hurt. Whether the patient should have drugs with sedating or activating properties should be considered. Timing and dose are important considerations in the context of pharmacokinetic and pharmacodynamic properties of drugs. Nighttime administration of sedating drugs may improve sleep and reduce daytime oversedation. Clinically significant drug side effects such as oversedation or activation may be more likely early in treatment than later, after tolerance has developed. On the other hand, some sedating medications, even short half-life sleeping aids, may have disinhibiting effects, even late into the next day, especially in elderly and cognitively impaired individuals. Doses of sleeping pills and other medications should usually be reduced by about half in the elderly compared with the dose for a young adult.

In general, avoid polypharmacy. Sleeping pills should be prescribed reluctantly to patients who receive adequate doses of antidepressants. Although coadministration of a benzodiazepine may improve sleep during the first week of antidepressant therapy, a low dose of zolpidem, zaleplon, trazodone, or other sedating antidepressant at night in addition to the antidepressant may be less likely to produce tolerance and may have additive antidepressant benefits. Antipsychotic medications should not be administered as sleeping aids unless the patient is psychotic or otherwise unresponsive to other medications.

## Sleep Disorders in Other Medical Conditions

A sleep disorder due to a general medical condition is defined in DSM-IV-TR as a prominent disturbance in sleep severe enough to warrant independent clinical attention. Subtypes include insomnia, hypersomnia, parasomnia, and mixed types.

As a general rule, any disease or disorder that causes pain, discomfort, or a heightened state of arousal in the waking state is capable of disrupting or interfering with sleep. Examples of this phenomenon include pain syndromes of any sort, arthritic and other rheumatological disorders, prostatism and other causes of urinary frequency or urgency, chronic obstructive lung disease, and other pulmonary conditions. Many of these conditions increase in prevalence with advancing age, suggesting at least one reason that sleep disorders are more likely to be seen in senior populations. A few examples of sleep disorders due to general medical conditions follow.

## Rheumatological Disorders

Rheumatological disorders often cause disturbances of sleep depth and continuity. The pain and discomfort associated with flares of rheumatoid arthritis lead to markedly disrupted sleep, with complaints of increased pain and stiffness the following day (Hirsch et al. 1994). Similar (although somewhat less intense) complaints are seen in association with untreated (or insufficiently treated) osteoarthritis. In both disorders, normal movements associated with shifts in position and stage in sleep may trigger awakenings from which return to sleep may be difficult or impossible. Similar problems may be seen with injuries to, or inflammation of, the back or ribs, with a report of awakening with pain associated with all shifts of position while asleep.

## Fibromyalgia

Fibromyalgia is typically associated with complaints of chronic, relapsing fatigue with shallow, unrefreshing sleep and localized tenderness in different muscle groups ("trigger points") (Jennum et al. 1993). No laboratory evidence of articular, nonarticular, musculoskeletal, or metabolic disease exists. Onset usually begins in young women. Although increased amounts of alpha-wave intrusion and disruption of other sleep stages have been described in some patients with fibromyalgia, this is not a uniform finding and is probably not important in the pathophysiological process (Saskin et al. 1986, Manu et al. 1994).

## Pulmonary Conditions

Chronic obstructive pulmonary disease, asthma, cough, and other respiratory conditions are often associated with complaints of light and disturbed sleep. The basis for these complaints is physiological and transparent. In sleep, minute ventilation decreases. Variability in ventilation is also greater in REM sleep than in non-REM sleep, with decreases in hypoxic and hypercapnic ventilatory drive in REM. Thus, patients with mild chronic obstructive pulmonary disease may report awakenings every few hours in sleep (in REM), whereas patients with more severe lung disease may report repetitive arousals throughout the night and difficulty sustaining sleep for any protracted period. Nocturnal oximetry studies demonstrate the problem, and appropriate use of supplemental oxygen at night will diminish the severity of the complaint.

Cough is a good example of the impact of breathing disturbance on sleep. Because it is impossible to cough while asleep, the irritation of the lungs or oral mucosa that leads to cough necessitates an arousal of at least transient duration to recruit and coordinate the muscles needed to expel the rush of air that generates the cough. Chronic cough may be exacerbated in sleep. In addition, two occult causes for nocturnal coughing are nocturnal gastroesophageal reflux and occult obstructive sleep apnea. Sleep apnea may also lead to the presentation or exacerbation of asthmatic episodes in sleep. Administration of theophylline may be helpful (Mulloy and McNicholas 1993).

## Congestive Heart Failure and Other Cardiac Disorders

Paroxysmal nocturnal dyspnea, orthopnea, and nocturia are classic symptoms of congestive heart failure but may be associated with or confused with sleep apnea, sleep terrors, or nocturnal panic disorder (Shepard 1992). Nocturnal angina may also lead to awakenings, with the possibility of exacerbation in REM sleep (as may be the case for some types of cardiac arrhythmias).

## Gastrointestinal Conditions

Sleep disturbance is particularly associated with peptic ulcer disease and gastroesophageal reflux (Orr et al. 1983), and rectal urgency in patients with colitis or ileitis. Patients with a colostomy may find sleep disrupted as a consequence of short transit time through remaining gut.

## Cerebral Degenerative Disorders

Sleep disturbances are common in patients with Parkinson's disease, Huntington's chorea, advanced Alzheimer's disease, hereditary progressive dystonia, and other similar disorders.

## Sleep in Elderly with Dementia

The sleep of older adults with dementia is extremely disturbed, with severely fragmented sleep, often to the extent that there is not a single hour in a 24-hour day that is spent fully awake or asleep (Jacobs et al. 1989). Patients with mild to moderate dementia have extremely fragmented sleep at night, while those with severe dementia are extremely sleepy during both the day and night (Pat-Horenczyk et al. 1998). Sleep stages also change with dementia, with significantly lower amounts of stages 3, 4, and REM sleep, and significantly more awakenings, as well as more time spent awake during the night (Prinz et al. 1982a). This results in increased stage 1 sleep and decreased sleep efficiency (Bliwise 1994). It has also been shown that there is a high prevalence of sleep apnea in patients with dementia, with as many as 80% having symptoms that meet the criteria for diagnosis (Ancoli-Israel et al. 1991a, 1997, Bliwise 1996). The sleep changes and disruption seen are likely due to the neuronal degeneration found in Alzheimer's disease.

Neuronal structures damaged in patients with dementia include the basal forebrain and the reticular formation of the brain stem, the same structures implicated in sleep regulation (Prinz et al. 1982b).

The nocturnal awakenings seen in dementia patients are often accompanied by agitation, confusion, and wandering. These behaviors have been referred to as "sundowning" as it was believed that they typically occurred as the sun set. A recent study (Martin et al. 2000) challenged the idea of sundowning by showing that peak levels of agitation occur during various times of the day, but more often in the afternoon, rather than in the evening or night.

It has been suggested that agitation or sundowning may be a circadian rhythm disorder (Bliwise et al. 1993, Martin et al. 2000). These authors found an association between circadian rhythms of activity, agitation and light exposure, indicating that sleep disruption in demented individuals may be amenable to treatment using bright light exposure. Others have tested this theory by exposing patients with dementia to bright light. The results have been mixed, but in general support the theory that increased light exposure, whether during the morning or evening, will improve both sleep and behavior to some extent (Satlin et al. 1992, Mishima et al. 1994, Ancoli-Israel et al. 2002).

## Parkinson's Disease

Sleep difficulties are particularly common in patients with Parkinson's disease with over half complaining of difficulty falling asleep and almost 90% complaining of difficulty staying asleep (Factor et al. 1990). Sleep recordings confirm that these patients do in fact have a prolonged sleep latency and are awake about one-third of the night (Kales et al. 1971). The sleep disruption may be secondary to the Parkinson's disease itself or to the medication used to treat the disease. Neurochemical changes caused by the disease include reductions in serotonergic, noradrenergic, and cholinergic neurons, all of which are involved in sleep regulating mechanisms (Jellinger 1986). Dopaminergic agonists used to treat the disease affect sleep–wake patterns (Aldrich 1994). Motor activity, including tremors, muscle contractions, increased muscle tone, vocalizations, and PLMS all disrupt sleep. Respiratory disorders, most common in patients with autonomic disturbance (Apps et al. 1985), are likely to contribute to sleep fragmentation. Finally, sleep–wake schedules are easily disrupted, either due to the medications, or to circadian rhythm abnormalities such as advanced or delayed sleep phase (Aldrich 1994). Sleep disruption often increases with the progression of the disease.

Sleep hygiene education may improve sleep in patients with Parkinson's disease. For example, since patients often complain of difficulty getting to the bathroom at night, having a commode available at the bedside may be extremely helpful (Shochat et al. 2001). The spouse or bed partner might consider sleeping in a different bed since the patient's disrupted sleep may impact the sleep of the bed partner. Since the bed partner is often also the caregiver, this sleep disruption may lead to early institutionalization. In addition to behavioral treatment of sleep problems, adjusting the time and dose of the dopaminergic medications used for treating Parkinson's disease may improve the problem. Low doses in the evening may prevent insomnia but may not sufficiently control nocturnal rigidity. Higher evening doses will promote sleep by minimizing nocturnal rigidity, however, this may cause sleep-onset insomnia. Withdrawal from dopamine agonists may lead to severe akinesia, which is associated with sleep disruption (Shochat et al. 2001). Some of the intermediate-acting sedative–hypnotics, such as clonazepam or temazepam, may improve the insomnia caused by nocturnal dyskinesia (Shochat et al. 2001). The shorter-acting benzodiazepines, such as zolpidem or zaleplon, are also indicated to help stabilize the sleep–wake schedule. Sedating tricyclic antidepressants such as amitriptyline may improve both sleep-onset insomnia and some daytime parkinsonian symptoms. However,

since they can cause nocturnal delirium, they are contraindicated for cognitively impaired patients.

Dopaminergic agents taken in the evening can cause sleep-onset insomnia. Chronic use of L-dopa causes vivid dreams, nightmares, and night terrors, particularly with demented patients (Scharf et al. 1978). Therefore, for Parkinson's disease patients with dementia suffering from nocturnal hallucinations and confusion, only very small doses of L-dopa can be used, and the sleep disruption is particularly difficult to manage.

## Substance-Induced Sleep Disorder

An important aspect of the evaluation of any patient, particularly those with sleep disorders, is the review of medications and other substances (including prescription, over-the-counter and recreational drugs, as well as alcohol, stimulants, narcotics, coffee and caffeine, and nicotine) and exposure to toxins, heavy metals, and so forth (Gillin and Drummond 2000). These substances may affect sleep and wakefulness during either ingestion or withdrawal, causing most commonly insomnia, hypersomnia, or, less frequently, parasomnia or mixed types of difficulties. On the basis of DSM-IV-TR criteria, a diagnosis of substance-induced sleep disorder may be made if the disturbance of sleep is sufficiently severe to warrant independent clinical attention and is judged to result from the direct physiological effects of a substance. Substance-induced sleep disorder cannot result from mental disorder or occur during delirium. If appropriate, the context for the development of sleep symptoms may be indicated by specifying with onset during intoxication or with onset during withdrawal.

The recognition of substance-related sleep disturbances usually depends on active searching by the psychiatrist, beginning with a careful history, physical examination, laboratory and toxicological testing, and information (with permission) from former health care providers or friends and relatives. Patients may not know what prescription medications they are taking or the doses, and may forget to mention over-the-counter medications, coffee, occupational or environmental toxins, and so forth. In the case of alcohol and drugs of abuse, they may deny to themselves and others their use, or quantity, or frequency of use. Substance dependence and abuse is often associated with other psychiatric diagnoses or symptoms. When comorbidity does exist, it is important to establish, if possible, whether the sleep disturbance is primary or secondary, that is, whether the sleep disturbance is substance-induced (secondary) or whether the substance use functions as a form of "self-medication" for sleep disturbance, in which the sleep disturbance would be considered primary. Many patients with alcoholism experience secondary depression during the first few weeks of withdrawal from alcohol and exhibit short REM latency and other sleep changes similar to those reported in primary depression (Moeller et al. 1993). This secondary depression usually remits spontaneously. Likewise, about one-third of patients with unipolar depression and about three-fifths of patients with bipolar disorder, manic type, have a substance use pattern that meets diagnostic criteria for alcoholism or substance abuse at some point. Prognosis and treatment may be altered in comorbid states, depending on whether the sleep disturbance is primary or secondary. In general, treatment should be aimed at

**DSM-IV-TR Criteria**

**Substance-Induced Sleep Disorder**

A. A prominent disturbance in sleep that is sufficiently severe to warrant independent clinical attention.

B. There is evidence from the history, physical examination, or laboratory findings of either (1) or (2):

  (1) the symptoms in criterion A developed during, or within a month of, substance intoxication or withdrawal

  (2) medication use is etiologically related to the sleep disturbance

C. The disturbance is not better accounted for by a sleep disorder that is not substance induced. Evidence that the symptoms are better accounted for by a sleep disorder that is not substance induced might include the following: the symptoms precede the onset of the substance use (or medication use); the symptoms persist for a substantial period of time (e.g., about a month) after the cessation of acute withdrawal or severe intoxication, or are substantially in excess of what would be expected given the type or amount of the substance used or the duration of use; or there is other evidence that suggests the existence of an independent non-substance-induced sleep disorder (e.g., a history of recurrent non-substance-related episodes).

D. The disturbance does not occur exclusively during the course of a delirium.

E. The sleep disturbance causes clinically significant distress or impairment in social, occupational, or other important areas of functioning.

**Note:** This diagnosis should be made instead of a diagnosis of substance intoxication or substance withdrawal only when the sleep symptoms are in excess of those usually associated with the intoxication or withdrawal syndrome, and when the symptoms are sufficiently severe to warrant independent clinical attention.

*Code*

[specific substance]–induced sleep disorder: (291.8 alcohol; 292.89 amphetamine; 292.89 caffeine; 292.89 cocaine; 292.89 opioid; 292.89 sedative, hypnotic, or anxiolytic; 292.89 other [or unknown] substance)

*Specify* type:

**Insomnia type:** if the predominant sleep disturbance is insomnia

**Hypersomnia type:** if the predominant sleep disturbance is hypersomnia

**Parasomnia type:** if the predominant sleep disturbance is a parasomnia

**Mixed type:** if more than one sleep disturbance is present and none predominates

*Specify* if:

**With onset during intoxication:** if criteria are met for intoxication with the substance and the symptoms develop during the intoxication syndrome

**With onset during withdrawal:** if criteria are met for withdrawal from the substance and the symptoms develop during, or shortly after, a withdrawal syndrome

Reprinted with permission from the Diagnostic and Statistical Manual of Mental Disorders, Fourth Edition, Text Revision. Copyright 2000 American Psychiatric Association.

the primary diagnosis after management of any acute withdrawal condition that may exist.

## Alcohol

Alcohol is probably the most commonly self-administered "sleeping aid." Although it may be sedating, especially in middle-aged or elderly or sleep-deprived persons, its usefulness as a hypnotic is limited by potential disinhibiting and arousing effects, gastric irritation, falling blood-alcohol levels in the early part of the night with mild withdrawal symptoms and sleep fragmentation at the end of the night, morning headaches and hangover effects, tolerance with repeated use, and exacerbation of BRSDs such as apnea.

Virtually any type of sleep disturbance has been attributed to the effects of alcohol or alcohol withdrawal in patients with alcohol abuse or dependence. Insomnia may occur during episodes of drinking and acute and chronic withdrawal. Complaints of insomnia and objective disruption of sleep continuity and stages 3 and 4 sleep have been reported for up to several years in some abstinent patients. Hypersomnia may occur during heavy bouts of drinking, sometimes with peripheral compression neuropathies, or as "terminal hypersomnia" after delirium tremens. Circadian sleep disturbances may also occur during bouts of drinking, including periods of short polyphasic sleep–wake episodes. Parasomnias include sleepwalking and enuresis.

Because alcohol may temporarily improve the poor sleep of the chronic alcoholic individual, sleep disturbance may be a factor in relapse (Landolt and Gillin 2001). Treatment of the sleep disturbances of the chronic but abstinent alcoholic individual is difficult. Nonpharmacological approaches include sleep hygiene and sleep restriction, as well as attention to general nutrition, physical health, and psychosocial supports. Use of benzodiazepines or other hypnotics is not generally recommended because of cross-tolerance or deliberate or inadvertent overdose. In a preliminary report, Brower and colleagues (Karam-Hage and Brower 2000) reported that the sleep of abstinent alcoholic patients improved when treated with gabapentin. It has been reported that increased REM percentage and short REM latency at admission to an inpatient alcohol treatment program are risk factors for relapse in primary alcoholic patients without depression (Gillin et al. 1994).

## Nicotine

Aside from medical complications, such as coughing that may interfere with sleep, smoking has been associated with both difficulty in falling asleep and getting up in the morning (Wetter and Young 1994), suggesting that nicotine may phase delay the circadian oscillator. Furthermore, compared with nonsmokers, men who smoked reported more nightmares—women who smoked reported more daytime sleepiness. Furthermore, as blood-nicotine levels fall during the night, smokers go into relative withdrawal and start craving a cigarette. One of the best measures of nicotine dependence is how long the smoker can wait in the morning for the first smoke. Abstinence from smoking is associated with lighter and more fragmented sleep, daytime sleepiness on the Multiple Sleep Latency Test, irritability, craving, and other subjective emotional distress (Prosise et al. 1994).

## Amphetamines and Cocaine

Stimulants initially prolong sleep onset and reduce REM sleep, sleep continuity, and sleep duration, but tolerance usually develops. During acute withdrawal, hypersomnia and excessive REM sleep occur for the first week or so but may be followed by a few days of insomnia (Weddington et al. 1990, Watson et al. 1992).

## Caffeine

Like the stimulants, caffeine usually promotes arousal and delays sleep, but withdrawal may be associated with hypersomnia. It is probably the most commonly self-administered stimulant (Walsh et al. 1990), for example, the morning cup of coffee to "get going." Caffeine has some benefits as a mild stimulant to overcome sleepiness.

## Opiates

Short-term use of opiates may increase sleep and subjective sleep quality and reduce REM sleep, especially in patients who need an analgesic for relief of pain, but these drugs may also disrupt sleep. Tolerance usually develops with repeated administration. Withdrawal may be associated with hypersomnia or the "nods."

## Sedatives, Hypnotics, and Anxiolytics

Tolerance usually develops with repeated administration of the sedating effects of barbiturates, chloral hydrate, and even benzodiazepines. This is true especially with short half-life agents, with the possible exception of zaleplon. As mentioned earlier, 1 or 2 days of withdrawal insomnia may occur after a few days of administration of short half-life benzodiazepines, such as triazolam (Gillin et al. 1989), but not with the newer nonbenzodiazepine hypnotics, such as zolpidem and zaleplon.

Potential side effects associated with sedating medications during the sleep period include falls and fractures, difficulty arousing to the telephone or the crying infant, amnesia, impairment of cognitive and motor skills, drug-induced sleepwalking, and possibly, BRSDs.

## Other Substances

Many medications produce sleep disturbance, including those with central or autonomic nervous system effects, like adrenergic agonists and antagonists, dopamine agonists and antagonists, cholinergic agonists and antagonists, antihistamines, and steroids. Among the prescription drugs associated frequently with sleep disorders are the SSRIs, which have been connected with overarousal and insomnia in some patients and, more commonly, sedation in other patients (Beasley et al. 1991). Coadministration of trazodone at night has been shown, in a double-blind, placebo-controlled study, to be effective in managing fluoxetine-induced insomnia in depressed patients (Nierenberg et al. 1994). Additional sleep-related disturbances occasionally associated with the SSRIs include sleepwalking, REM sleep behavior disorder, and rapid eye movements during non-REM sleep.

---

Clinical Vignette 1

> When first seen in evaluation in 1998, Mr. SV was a 48-year-old married male. His chief complaint was of leg, arm, and occasional body jerking throughout the night, which caused awakenings and led to lightened and fragmented sleep. He also reported restlessness in his legs at sleep onset, interfering with his capacity to fall asleep. He reported that it typically took him 40 minutes to fall asleep, but that occasionally his initial sleep latency could be as long as 2 hours. He would typically awaken four to five times per night, then have difficulty falling back to sleep.
>
> He reported that symptoms had been present for about 7 years, but had become much worse in the 2 months prior to his evaluation. He questioned whether this might have resulted from a more active exercise schedule that he had undertaken in an effort to lose weight.
>
> Mr. SV reported that his sleep in recent weeks had been disrupted to the extent that he was sleeping only 4 to 5 hours per night. This reflected a significant decrease from his historic average of 7 hours of sleep per night. However, he denied any sleepiness as a consequence of his disturbed sleep, reporting an Epworth Sleepiness Scale Score of 0, consistent with no perceived hypersomnia tendencies.
>
> He reported mild snoring but denied awareness of pauses in breathing. His wife confirmed the absence of any episodes of the "breath-holding" suggestive of sleep apnea. She confirmed the presence of "restless sleep," with frequent twitches and jerks of the arms and legs, which disrupted her sleep, as well as that of her husband.
>
> Mr. SV reported a history of asthma, not requiring treatment with medication at that time. He denied any other significant health problems, specifically denying a history of anemia or of any type of kidney disease. Physical examination was normal, with a normal body mass index and neck circumference, and with a normal-appearing oral airway.
>
> The presumptive diagnosis at this time was restless legs syndrome (RLS) and periodic limb movements in sleep (PLMS). A trial of L-dopa/carbidopa was initiated at a dose of 25/100 mg, with directions to increase the dose as needed.

Clinical Vignette 1 *continued*

Three weeks later, Mr. SV reported an excellent response at the initial dose of 25/100 taken 2 hours before bedtime, with a reported sleep latency of 5 to 10 minutes, and a reduction in awakenings to two to three times per night. When he did wake up in the night, he reported that he could fall back to sleep without great difficulty.

Over the next 6 months, Mr. SV reported the need for a progressive increase in doses of L-dopa/carbidopa, to the point where he was taking 3 tablets of the 25/100 mg dose. He was beginning to experience an increase in sensations of restlessness prior to his evening dose of medication, as well as a return of movement symptoms in the early morning hours.

Rather than a further increase in medications, Mr. SV requested a trial of a different medication. He discontinued the L-dopa/carbidopa and was started on pergolide 0.05 mg, with instructions to begin with 1 tablet 2 hours before bedtime and to increase as needed and tolerated. He reported doing well at a dose of $3 \times 0.05$ mg, with sustained sleep throughout the night and no complaints of restlessness at the start of the night.

He continued to do well with this regimen for 1 year. At that time he noted a return of some symptoms of restlessness and excessive movement. The dose was raised to $4 \times 0.5$ mg, with good symptomatic relief. He has remained symptom-free at this dose, with no complaints of side effects or intolerance of the medication.

**Discussion**

Mr. SV presented with a typical RLS/PLMS history, although many patients with these complaints that have persisted over a longer period of time will also complain of daytime fatigue or sleepiness.

No sleep studies were performed. Although it would have been of interest to confirm the clinical diagnosis of RLS/PLMS with a polysomnographic study, there were no symptoms present suggestive of another disorder, such as sleep apnea, which could have caused his complaints and which could have been confirmed or excluded on the basis of polysomnography.

Had he not responded to a first or second course of pharmacologic therapy for his presumed RLS/PLMS, a sleep study could have been ordered to confirm the diagnosis.

From a historical perspective, the absence of anemia or of kidney disease were of importance to rule out treatable causes of RLS/PLMS (iron deficiency or renal failure). However, treatment for these conditions (iron replacement or dialysis) does not always lead to resolution of the RLS/PLMS complaints, particularly in early phases of treatment for iron deficiency anemia.

The history of loss of benefit from treatment with L-dopa/carbidopa is also not unusual. Patients taking this medication often experience a "breakthrough" of RLS symptoms over time, and may report that, as medication is given earlier in the evening to reduce symptoms of restlessness, symptoms begin to appear progressively earlier, frustrating efforts at effective treatment.

Clinical Vignette 2

When seen in consultation, Ms. A was a 56-year-old married woman, the wife of a physician, referred by her rheumatologist for evaluation of long-standing sleep complaints. She described her sleep complaint as follows:

"With the help of medications, I am able to sleep for 2 to 4 hours. When I wake up, I am fully awake no matter what the hour."

She stated that her sleep problems had been present for approximately 15 years. She described in great detail her severe problems with fibromyalgia, which had led to a substantial decline in functioning. She reported that she had experienced a significant degree of improvement under the care of her rheumatologist and noted that sedating antidepressants, particularly amitriptyline, had been helpful to her in controlling pain and improving her sleep. Other antidepressants that had been used singly or in combination included doxepin and nortriptyline. Cyclobenzaprine had been of some benefit but led to a complaint of mouth dryness. She had received various sedative medications in treatment of sleep complaints, including clonazepam, triazolam, temazepam, chloral hydrate, meprobamate, ethchlorvynol, and various barbiturates. In reviewing her history of hypnotic use, it became apparent that she had in fact used hypnotic medications on a nightly basis for more than 30 years. She had also used L-tryptophan in the past and had experienced a well-documented eosinophilia–myalgia syndrome.

She reported that she took her sleep medication (at time of evaluation, temazepam at 30 mg) 2 to 2.5 hours before her regular hour of retiring of 11 PM. She awakened several hours later without awareness of any specific cause and reported difficulty in returning to sleep on a nightly basis. She listened to a tape recorder on a nightly basis, using self-help and relaxation tapes and keeping the recorder running throughout the night whether she was awake or asleep.

She reported that she "rested" for an hour at a time several times a day, although she denied feeling truly sleepy at any point in the daytime, acknowledging instead symptoms of fatigue and low energy. She acknowledged that "on rare occasions," she might briefly fall asleep during these periods of daytime rest.

A Minnesota Multiphasic Personality Inventory was performed a year before evaluation and demonstrated an elevation in the depression (D) scale. No formal psychiatric treatment had been recommended or obtained.

Treatment was initiated to reduce reliance on medications, to improve sleep hygiene, and to improve nocturnal sleep continuity. Use of her tape recorder during the night was forbidden because it may have activated her, and her sleep medication was changed to zolpidem to allow more rapid onset of action and shorter duration of action. She was instructed to discontinue her periods of rest during the daytime, with the exception of a single 20-minute period of rest or sleep in the afternoon. She was told not go to bed until she felt tired in the evening and to take her sleep medication at that time. She was instructed to avoid clock watching during the night and to read something relaxing or boring in another room until she felt sleepy, at which point she could return to bed. She was asked to complete a sleep diary on a daily basis. Her initial perception was of somewhat less sleep than she had previously been obtaining, with a further decline in daytime performance. In a period of 4 weeks, her reported sleep time at night climbed to 5 hours, with improvement in perceived daytime function. After a year of further support of behavioral interventions and good sleep hygiene, she was able to taper and discontinue use of hypnotics and antidepressants, reported a substantial improvement in her fibromyalgia complaint, and had essentially complete resolution of her sleep complaints.

## Sleep Societies and Associations: Resources for Professional and Patient Information

| Name | Address | Phone | Website |
|---|---|---|---|
| American Academy of Sleep Medicine (AASM) | One Westbrook Corporate Center Suite 920 Westchester, IL 60154 | (708) 492-0930 | www.apss.org |
| Academy of Dental Sleep Medicine (ADSM) | 10592 Perry Hwy, #220 Wexford, PA 15090-9244 | (724) 935-0836 | www.dentalsleepmed.org |
| Associated Professional Sleep Societies (APSS) | One Westbrook Corporate Center Suite 920 Westchester, IL 60154 | (708) 492-0930 | www.apss.org |
| American Sleep Apnea Association (ASAA) | 1424 K St. NW, Suite 302 Washington DC 20005 | (202) 293-3650 | www.sleepapnea.org |
| Narcolepsy Network | 10921 Reed Hartman Hwy Cincinnati, OH 45242 | (513) 891-3522 | www.narcolepsynetwork.org |
| National Sleep Foundation (NSF) | 1522 K St. NW, Suite 500 Washington DC 20005 | (202) 347-3471 | www.sleepfoundation.org |
| Sleep Medicine Education and Research Foundation (SMERF) | 6301 Bandel Rd., Suite 101 Rochester, MN 55901 | (507) 287-6008 | www.aasmnet.org |
| Sleep Research Society (SRS) | One Westbrook Corporate Center Suite 920 Westchester, IL 60154 | (708) 492-0930 | www.sleepresearchsociety.org |
| Society for Light Treatment and Biological Rhythms (SLTBR) | PO Box 591687 San Francisco, CA 94159 | (415) 876-0716 | www.sltbr.org |

## Comparison of DSM-IV/ICD-10 Diagnostic Criteria

For primary insomnia, the ICD-10 Diagnostic Criteria for Research and the DSM-IV-TR criteria are almost identical except that ICD-10 requires a frequency of at least three times a week for at least a month, whereas DSM-IV-TR does not specify a required frequency. For primary hypersomnia, the ICD-10 Diagnostic Criteria for Research and the DSM-IV-TR criteria are almost identical except that ICD-10 also counts sleep drunkenness as a presenting symptom. Furthermore, ICD-10 requires that the problems occur nearly every day for at least 1 month (or recurrently for shorter periods of time).

Since narcolepsy and breathing-related sleep disorder are included in chapter VI (Diseases of the Nervous System) in ICD-10, there are no diagnostic criteria provided for these conditions.

For circadian rhythm sleep disorder, the ICD-10 Diagnostic Criteria for Research and the DSM-IV-TR criteria are almost identical except that ICD-10 specifies that the problems occur nearly every day for at least 1 month (or recurrently for shorter periods of time) (DSM-IV-TR has no specified duration). This condition is referred to in ICD-10 as "Nonorganic disorder of the sleep–wake cycle."

The ICD-10 Diagnostic Criteria for Research and the DSM-IV-TR criteria for nightmare disorder and sleepwalking disorder are essentially identical. The ICD-10 Diagnostic Criteria for Research and the DSM-IV-TR criteria sets for sleep terror disorder are almost identical except that ICD-10 explicitly limits the duration of the episode to less than 10 minutes.

## References

Akerstedt T (1991) Shift work and sleep disturbances. In Sleep and Health Risk, Peter JH, Penzel T, Podszus T, et al. (eds). Springer-Verlag, New York, pp. 265–278.

Aldrich MS (1994) Parkinsonism. In Principles and Practice of Sleep Medicine, Kryger MH, Roth T, and Dement WC (eds). WB Saunders, Philadelphia, pp. 783–789.

Aldrich MS and Chauncey JB (1990) Are morning headaches part of obstructive sleep apnea syndrome? Arch Intern Med 150, 1265–1267.

American Psychiatric Association (1994) Diagnostic and Statistical Manual of Mental Disorders. APA, Washington DC.

Ancoli-Israel S (1989) Epidemiology of sleep disorders. In Clinics in Geriatric Medicine, Roth TR and Roehrs TA (eds). WB Saunders, Philadelphia, pp. 347–362.

Ancoli-Israel S and Roth T (1999) Characteristics of insomnia in the United States: I. Results of the 1991 National Sleep Foundation Survey. Sleep 22, S347–S353.

Ancoli-Israel S, Klauber MR, Butters N, et al. (1991a) Dementia in institutionalized elderly: Relation to sleep apnea. Am Geriatr Soc 39, 258–263.

Ancoli-Israel S, Kripke DF, Klauber MR, et al. (1991b) Periodic limb movements in sleep in community-dwelling elderly. Sleep 14(6), 496–500.

Ancoli-Israel S, Kripke DF, Klauber MR, et al. (1991c) Sleep disordered breathing in community-dwelling elderly. Sleep 14(6), 486–495.

Ancoli-Israel S, Kripke DF, Klauber MR, et al. (1996) Morbidity, mortality, and sleep disordered breathing in community dwelling elderly. Sleep 19, 277–282.

Ancoli-Israel S, Kripke DF, Mason W, et al. (1985) Sleep apnea and periodic movements in an aging sample. J Gerontol 40, 419–425.

Ancoli-Israel S, Martin JL, Kripke DF, et al. (2002) Effect of light treatment on sleep and circadian rhythms in demented nursing home patients. Am Geriatr Soc 50, 282–289.

Ancoli-Israel S, Parker L, Sinaee R, et al. (1989) Sleep fragmentation in patients from a nursing home. J Gerontol 44, M18–M21.

Ancoli-Israel S, Poceta JS, Stepnowsky C, et al. (1997) Identification and treatment of sleep problems in the elderly. Sleep Med Rev 1, 3–17.

Ancoli-Israel S, Schnierow B, Kelsoe J, et al. (2001) A pedigree of one family with delayed sleep phase syndrome. Chronobiol Int 18, 831–841.

Ancoli-Israel S, Seifert AR, and Lemon M (1986) Thermal biofeedback and periodic movements in sleep: Patient's subjective reports and a case study. Biofeedback Self-Reg 11, 177–188.

Apps MCP, Sheaff PC, Ingram DA, et al. (1985) Respiration and sleep in Parkinson's disease. J Neurol Neurosurg Psychiatr 48, 1240–1245.

Aubert G (1992) Alternative therapeutic approaches in sleep apnea syndrome. Sleep 15, S69–S72.

Bakwin H (1970) Sleepwalking in twins. Lancet 2, 446–447.

Beasley CM Jr., Sayler ME, Bosomworth JC, et al. (1991) High-dose fluoxetine efficacy and activating-sedating effects in agitated and retarded depression. J Clin Psychopharmacol 11(3), 166–174.

Benca RM, Obermeyer WH, Thisted RA, et al. (1992) Sleep and psychiatric disorders: A meta-analysis. Arch Gen Psychiatr 49, 651–668.

Berger M, Lund R, Bronisch T, et al. (1983) REM latency in neurotic and endogenous depression and the cholinergic REM induction test. Psychiatr Res 10, 113–123.

Bliwise DL (1994) Sleep in dementing illness. Annu Rev Psychiatr 13, 757–777.

Bliwise DL (1996) Is sleep apnea a cause of reversible dementia in old age? J Am Geriatr Soc 44, 1407–1409.

Bliwise DL, Bliswise NG, Partinen M, et al. (1988) Sleep apnea and mortality in an aged cohort. Am J Pub Health 78(5), 544–547.

Bliwise DL, Carroll JS, Lee KA, et al. (1993) Sleep and "sundowning" in nursing home patients with dementia. Psychiatr Res 48, 277–292.

Block AJ, Dolly FR, and Slayton PC (1983) Does flurazepam ingestion affect breathing and oxygenation during sleep in patients with chronic obstructive lung disease? Am Rev Respir Dis 129, 230–233.

Blois R, Monnier M, Tissot R, et al. (1981) Effect of DSIP on diurnal and nocturnal sleep in man. In Sleep 1980, Koella WP (ed). S. Karger, Basel, pp. 301–303.

Bootzin RR and Nicassio PM (1978) Behavioral treatments for insomnia. In Progress in Behavior Modification, Hersen M, Eisler RM, and Miller PM (eds). Academic Press, New York, pp. 1–45.

Borbely AA and Ackermann P (1992) Concepts and models of sleep regulation: An overview. J Sleep Res 1, 63–79.

Broughton R and Ghanem Q (1976) The impact on compound narcolepsy in the life of the patient. In Narcolepsy, Advances in Sleep Research, Guilleminault C, Dement W, Passant P, et al. (eds). Spectrum Publications, Hollingswood, New York, pp. 201–220.

Brown GM (1995) Melatonin in psychiatric and sleep disorders. CNS Drugs 3, 209–226.

Campbell SS, Kripke DF, Gillin JC, et al. (1988) Exposure to light in healthy elderly subjects and Alzheimer's patients. Physiol Behav 42, 141–144.

Carskadon MA, Harvey K, Duke P, et al. (1980) Pubertal changes in daytime sleepiness. Sleep 2, 453–460.

Chesson AL Jr., Wise M, Davila D, et al. (1999) Practice parameters for the treatment of restless legs syndrome and periodic limb movement disorder. An American Academy of Sleep Medicine Report. Standards of Practice Committee of the American Academy of Sleep Medicine. Sleep 22, 961–968.

Cohen RA and Albers HE (1993) Disruption of human circadian and cognitive regulation following a discreet hypothalamic lesion: A case study. Neurology 41, 726–729.

Coleman R, Bliwise DL, Sajben N, et al. (1983) Epidemiology of periodic movements during sleep. In Sleep/Wake Disorders: Natural History, Epidemiology, and Long-Term Evolution, Guilleminault C and Lugaresi E (eds). Raven Press, New York, pp. 217–229.

Culebras A (1992) Neuroanatomic and neurologic correlates of sleep disturbances. Neurology 42(Suppl 6), 19–27.

Czeisler CA, Johnson MP, Duffy JF, et al. (1990) Exposure to bright light and darkness to treat physiologic maladaption to night work. New Engl J Med 322(18), 1253–1259.

Czeisler CA, Kronauer RE, Allan JS, et al. (1989) Bright light induction of strong (type 0) resetting of the human circadian pacemaker. Science 244, 1328–1332.

Daan S, Beersma DGM, and Borbely AA (1984) Timing of human sleep: Recovery process gated by a circadian pacemaker. Am J Physiol 246, R161–R183.

Diagnostic Classification Steering Committee, Thorpy MJ (Chair) (1990) International Classification of Sleep Disorders: Diagnostic and Coding Manual, Rev. American Academy of Sleep Medicine, Rochester.

Dow BM, Kelsoe JRJ, and Gillin JC (1996) Sleep and dreams in Vietnam PTSD and depression. Biol Psychiatr 39, 42–50.

Duffy J and Czeisler CA (2002) Age-related change in the relationship between circadian period, circadian phase, and diurnal preference in humans. Neurosci Lett 318, 117–120.

Duffy J, Zeitzer JM, Rimmer DW, et al. (2002) Peak of circadian melatonin rhythm occurs later within the sleep of older subjects. Am J Physiol Endocrinol Metab 282, E297–E303.

Ebert D, Feistel H, Barocka A, et al. (1994) Increased limbic blood flow and total sleep deprivation in major depression with melancholia. Psychiatr Res Neuroimag 55, 101–109.

Edgar DM, Dement WC, and Fuller CA (1993) Effect of SCN lesions on sleep in squirrel monkeys: Evidence for opponent processes in sleep-wake regulation. J Neurosci 13(3), 1065–1079.

Factor SA, McAlarney T, Sanchez-Ramos JR, et al. (1990) Sleep disorders and sleep effect in Parkinson's disease. Movt Disord 5, 280–285.

Fairbanks DNF (1987) Snoring: An overview with historical perspectives. In Snoring and Obstructive Sleep Apnea, Fairbanks DNF, Fujita S, Ikematsu T, et al. (eds). Raven Press, New York, pp. 1–18.

Feinberg I (1974) Changes in sleep cycle patterns with age. J Psychiatr Res 10, 283–306.

Feinberg I, Thode HC Jr., Chugani HT, et al. (1990) Gamma distribution model describes maturational curves for delta wave amplitude, cortical metabolic rate, and synoptic density. J Theoret Biol 142, 149–161.

Findley LJ, Zwillich CW, Ancoli-Israel S, et al. (1985) Cheyne-Stokes breathing during sleep in patients with left ventricular heart failure. South Med J 78, 11–15.

Fleury B (1992) Sleep apnea syndrome in the elderly. Sleep 16(6), S39–S41.

Ford DE and Kamerow DB (1989) Epidemiologic study of sleep disturbance and psychiatric disorders: An opportunity for prevention? JAMA 262, 1479–1484.

Giles DE, Jarrett RB, Roffwarg HP, et al. (1988) Reduced REM latency: A predictor of recurrence in depression. Neuropsychopharmacology 1, 33–39.

Gillin JC and Byerley WF (1990) The diagnosis and management of insomnia. New England Journal of Medicine 322, 239–248.

Gillin JC and Drummond SPA (2000) Medication and substance abuse. In Principles and Practice of Sleep Medicine, Kryger MH, Roth T, and Dement WC (eds). WB Saunders, Philadelphia, pp. 1176–1195.

Gillin JC, Buchsbaum M, Wu J, et al. (2001) Sleep deprivation as a model experimental antidepressant treatment: Findings from functional brain imaging. Depress Anx 14, 37–49.

Gillin JC, Dow BM, Thompson P, et al. (1993) Sleep in depression and other psychiatric disorders. Clin Neurosci 1, 90–96.

Gillin JC, Smith TL, Irwin M, et al. (1994) Increased pressure for rapid eye movement sleep at time of hospital admission predicts relapse in nondepressed patients with primary alcoholism at 3-month follow-up. Arch Gen Psychiatr 51, 189–197.

Gillin JC, Smith-Vaniz A, Schnierow B, et al. (2001b) An open-label, 12 week clinical and sleep EEG study of nefazodone in chronic combat-related posttraumatic stress disorder. J Clin Psychiatr 62, 789–796.

Gillin JC, Spinweber CL, and Johnson LC (1989) Rebound insomnia: A critical review. J Clin Psychopharmacol 9, 161–172.

Gillin JC, Sutton L, Ruiz C, et al. (1991) The cholinergic rapid eye movement induction test with arecoline in depression. Arch Gen Psychiatr 48, 264–270.

Glassman JN, Darko DF, and Gillin JC (1986) Medication-induced somnambulism in a patient with schizoaffective illness. J Clin Psychiatr 47, 523–524.

Gordon N (1992) The more unusual sleep disturbances of childhood. Brain Dev 14, 182–184.

Guilleminault C and Stoohs R (1990) Obstructive sleep apnea syndrome: Whom to treat and how to treat. In Sleep and Respiration, Issa FG, Suratt PM, and Remmers JE (eds). Wiley-Liss, New York, pp. 417–426.

Guilleminault C, Eldridge F, and Dement W (1973) Insomnia with sleep apnea: A new syndrome. Science 181, 856–858.

Hartmann E (1991) Boundaries in the Mind. Basic Books, New York.

Hartmann E (1994) Nightmares and other dreams. In Principles and Practice of Sleep Medicine, Kryger M, Roth T, and Dement W (eds). WB Saunders, Philadelphia, pp. 407–410.

Hauri PJ (1991) Case Studies in Insomnia. Plenum Medical Book Publishers, New York.

Hendricks JC, Morrison AR, and Mann GL (1982) Different behaviors during paradoxical sleep without atonia depend on pontine lesion site. Brain Res 239, 81–105.

Heninger W, Allen R, Earley C, et al. (1999) The treatment of restless legs syndrome and periodic limb movement disorder (Review). Sleep 22, 970–999.

Hillman E, Kripke DF, and Gillin JC (1990) Sleep restriction, exercise and bright lights: Alternate therapies for depression. In American Psychiatric Press Review of Psychiatry. Treatment of Refractory Affective Disorder, Tasman A, Kaufmann C, and Goldfinger S (eds). American Psychiatric Press, Washington DC, pp. 132–144.

Hirsch M, Carlander B, Verg M, et al. (1994) Objective and subjective sleep disturbances in patients with rheumatoid arthritis: A reappraisal. Arthritis Rheum 37, 41–49.

Ho AP, Gillin JC, Buchsbaum MS, et al. (1996) Brain glucose metabolism during non-rapid eye movement sleep in major depression. A positron emission tomography study. Arch Gen Psychiatr 53, 645–652.

Honda Y, Juji T, Matsuki K, et al. (1986) HLA-DR2 and Dw2 in narcolepsy and in other disorders of excessive somnolence without cataplexy. Sleep 9, 133–142.

Irwin M, Smith TL, and Gillin JC (1992) Electroencephalographic sleep and natural cytotoxicity in depressed patients and control subjects. Sleep Res 6, 128.

Jacobs D, Ancoli-Israel S, Parker L, et al. (1989) 24-hour sleep/wake patterns in a nursing home population. Psychol Aging 4(3), 352–356.

Jellinger K (1986) Pathology of parkinsonism. In Recent Developments in Parkinson's Disease, Fahn S, Marsden CD, Jenner P, et al. (eds). Raven Press, New York, pp. 33–66.

Jennum P, Drewes AM, Andreasen A, et al. (1993) Sleep and other symptoms in primary fibromyalgia and in healthy controls. J Rheumatol 20, 1756–1759.

Jones CR, Campbell SS, Zone SE, et al. (1999) Familial advanced sleep-phase syndrome: A short-period circadian rhythm variant in humans. Nat Med 5, 1062–1065.

Kales A, Ansel RD, Markham CH, et al. (1971) Sleep in patients with Parkinson's disease and normal subjects prior to and following levodopa administration. Clin Pharm Ther 12, 397–406.

Kales JD, Kales A, Soldatos CR, et al. (1980) Night terrors. Arch Gen Psychiatr 37, 1413–1417.

Kamgar-Parsi B, Wehr TA, and Gillin JC (1983) Successful treatment of human non-24-hour sleep-wake syndrome. Sleep 6, 257–264.

Kapas L, Obal F, and Krueger JM (1993) Humoral regulation of sleep. Int Rev Neurobiol 36, 131–160.

Karam-Hage M and Brower KJ (2000) Gabapentin treatment for insomnia associated with alcohol dependence (letter). Am J Psychiatr 157, 151.

Koenigsberg HW, Pollak CP, Fine J, et al. (1994) Cardiac and respiratory activity in panic disorder: Effects of sleep and sleep lactate infusions. Am J Psychiatr 151, 1148–1152.

Koskenvuo M, Kaprio J, Partinen M, et al. (1985) Snoring as a risk factor for hypertension and angina pectoris. Lancet 1(8434) 893–896.

Kripke DF (1983) Epidemiology of sleep apnea among the aged: Is sleep apnea a fatal disorder? In Sleep Wake Disorders: Natural History, Epidemiology, and Long-Term Evolution, Guilleminault C and Lugaresi E (eds). Raven Press, New York, pp. 137–142.

Kripke DF, Ancoli-Israel S, Mason WJ, et al. (1990) Sleep apnea: Association with deviant sleep durations and increased mortality. In Obstructive Sleep Apnea Syndrome, Guilleminault C and Partinen M (eds). Raven Press, New York, pp. 9–14.

Kryger MH, Roth T, and Dement WC (2000) Principles and Practice of Sleep Medicine. WB Saunders, Philadelphia.

Kupfer DJ, Frank E, McEachran AB, et al. (1990) Delta sleep ratio: A biological correlate of early recurrence in unipolar affective disorder. Arch Gen Psychiatr 47, 1100–1105.

Landolt HP and Gillin JC (2001) Sleep abnormalities during abstinence in alcohol-dependent patients. Aetiology and management. CNS Drugs 15, 413–425.

Landolt HP, Raimo EB, Schnierow BJ, et al. (2001) Sleep and sleep electroencephalogram in depressed patients treated with phenelzine. Arch Gen Psychiatr 58, 268–276.

Lavie P, Pratt H, Scharf B, et al. (1984) Localized pontine lesion: Nearly total absence of REM sleep. Neurology 34, 118–120.

Lewy AJ and Sack RL (1989) The dim light melatonin onset as a marker for circadian phase position. Chronobiol Int 6, 93–102.

Littner M, Johnson SF, McCall WV, et al. (2001) Practice parameters for the treatment of narcolepsy: An update for 2000. Sleep 24, 451–466.

Livingston G, Blizard B, and Mann A (1993) Does sleep disturbance predict depression in elderly people? Br J Gen Pract 43, 445–448.

Luchins DJ, Sherwood PM, Gillin JC, et al. (1978) Filicide during psychotropic-induced somnambulism: A case report. Am J Psychiatr 135, 1404–1405.

Lugaresi E (1992) The thalamus and insomnia. Neurology 42(Suppl 6), 28–33.

Mahowald MW and Schenck CH (1992) Dissociated states of wakefulness and sleep. Neurology 42(Suppl 6), 44–52.

Manu P, Lane TJ, Matthews DA, et al. (1994) Alpha-delta sleep in patients with a chief complaint of chronic fatigue. South Med J 87, 465–470.

Martin J, Marler M, Shochat T, et al. (2000) Circadian rhythms of agitation in institutionalized Alzheimer's disease patients. Chronobiol Int 17, 405–418.

Mendelson WB, Garnett D, and Gillin JC (1981) Single case study: Flurazepam-induced respiratory changes. J Nerv Ment Dis 169, 261–264.

Mendlewicz J, Sevy S, and de Maertelaer V (1989) REM sleep latency and morbidity risk of affective disorders in depressive illness. Neuropsychobiology 22(1), 14–17.

Mignot E, Nishino S, Hunt Sharp L, et al. (1993a) Heterozygosity at the canarc-1 locus can confer susceptibility for narcolepsy: Induction of cataplexy in heterozygous asymptomatic dogs after administration of a combination of drugs acting on monoaminergic and cholinergic systems. J Neurosci 13, 1057–1064.

Mignot E, Renaud A, Nishino S, et al. (1993b) Canine cataplexy is preferentially controlled by adrenergic mechanisms: Evidence using monoamine selective uptake inhibitors and release enhancers. Psychopharmacology (Berl) 113, 76–82.

Mignot E, Wang C, Rattazzi C, et al. (1991) Genetic linkage of autosomal recessive canine narcolepsy with a μ immunoglobulin heavy-chain switch-like segment. Proc Natl Acad Sci USA 88, 3475–3478.

Minors DS and Waterhouse JM (1984) The use of the constant routine in unmasking the endogenous component of human circadian rhythms. Chronobiol Int 1, 205–216.

Mishima K, Okawa M, Hishikawa Y, et al. (1994) Morning bright light therapy for sleep and behavior disorders in elderly patients with dementia. Acta Psychiatr Scand 89, 1–7.

Mitler MM, Hajdukovic RM, Shafor R, et al. (1987) When people die. Cause of death versus time of death. Am J Med 82, 266–274.

Moeller FG, Gillin JC, Irwin M, et al. (1993) A comparison of sleep EEGs in patients with primary major depression and major depression secondary to alcoholism. J Affect Disord 27, 39–42.

Montplaisir J, Denesle R, and Petit D (2000) Pramipexole in the treatment of restless legs syndrome: A follow-up study. Eur J Neurol 7(Suppl), 27–31.

Montplaisir J, Nicolas A, Denesle R, et al. (2002) Restless legs syndrome improved by pramipexole: A double-blind randomized trial. Neurology 52, 938–943.

Moore-Ede MC (1986) Jet lag, shift work, and maladaption. NIPS 1, 156–160.

Moore-Ede MC, Sulzman FM, and Fuller CA (1982) The Clocks That Time Us: Physiology of the Circadian Timing System. Harvard University Press, Cambridge.

Morin CM, Colecchi C, Stone J, et al. (1999) Behavioral and pharmacological therapies for late life insomnia. JAMA 281, 991–999.

Morin CM, Culbert JP, and Schwartz SM (1994) Nonpharmacological interventions for insomnia: A meta-analysis of treatment efficacy. Am J Psychiatr 151, 1172–1180.

Morin CM, Kowatch RA, Barry T, et al. (1993) Cognitive–behavior therapy for late-life insomnia. J Consult Clin Psychol 61, 137–146.

Mulloy E and McNicholas WT (1993) Theophylline improves gas exchange during rest, exercise, and sleep in severe chronic obstructive pulmonary disease. Am J Respir Crit Care Med 148, 1030–1036.

Nierenberg AA, Adler LA, Peselow E, et al. (1994) Trazodone for antidepressant-associated insomnia. Am J Psychiatr 151, 1069–1072.

Nieto FJ, Young T, Lind B, et al. (2000) Sleep-disordered breathing, sleep apnea, and hypertension in a large community-based study. JAMA 283, 1829–1836.

Olson LG and Strohl KP (1986) Pathophysiology and treatment of central sleep apnea. Chest 90, 154–155.

Orr W, Lackey C, Robinson M, et al. (1983) Acid reflux and clearance in sleep in Barrett's esophagus. Gastroenterology 84, 1265.

Partinen M and Palomaki H (1985) Snoring and cerebral infarction. Lancet 2, 1325–1326.

Pat-Horenczyk R, Klauber MR, Shochat T, et al. (1998) Hourly profiles of sleep and wakefulness in severely versus mild-moderately demented nursing home patients. Aging Clin Exp Res 10, 308–315.

Peppard P, Young T, Palta M, et al. (2000) Prospective study of the association between sleep-disordered breathing and hypertension. New Engl J Med 342, 1378–1384.

Prinz PN, Peskind E, Raskind MA, et al. (1982a) Changes in sleep and waking EEG in nondemented and demented elderly. J Am Geriatr Soc 30, 86–93.

Prinz PN, Vitaliano PP, Vitiello MV, et al. (1982b) Sleep, EEG, and mental function changes in senile dementia of the Alzheimer's type. Neurobiol Aging 3, 361–370.

Prosise GL, Bonnet MH, Berry RB, et al. (1994) Effects of abstinence from smoking on sleep and daytime sleepiness. Chest 105, 1136–1141.

Richardson GS (1990) Circadian rhythms and aging. Biol Aging 13, 275–305.

Rockwell DA, Winget CM, Rosenblatt LS, et al. (1978) Biological aspects of suicide: Circadian disorganization. J Nerv Ment Dis 166, 851–858.

Rodenstein DO (1992) Assessment of uvulopalatopharyngoplasty for the treatment of sleep apnea syndrome. Sleep 15(6), S56–S62.

Roehrs T, Conway W, Wittig R, et al. (1985) Sleep–wake complaints in patients with sleep-related respiratory disturbances. Am Rev Respir Dis 132, 520–523.

Rosenthal L, Roehrs TA, Hayashi H, et al. (1991) HLA DR2 in narcolepsy with sleep-onset REM periods but not cataplexy. Biol Psychiatr 30, 830–836.

Rosenthal NE, Joseph-Vanderpool JR, Levendosky A, et al. (1990) Phase-shifting effects of bright morning light as treatment for delayed sleep phase syndrome. Sleep 13(4), 354–361.

Roth T and Ancoli-Israel S (1999) Daytime consequences and correlates of insomnia in the United States: II. Results of the 1991 National Sleep Foundation Survey. Sleep (Suppl 2), S354–S358.

Rothstein JD, Guidotti A, Tinuper P, et al. (1992) Endogenous benzodiazepine receptor ligands in idiopathic recurring stupor. Lancet 340, 1002–1004.

Saskin P, Moldofsky H, and Lue FA (1986) Sleep and posttraumatic rheumatic pain modulation disorder (fibrositis syndrome). Psychosom Med 48, 319–323.

Satlin A, Volicer L, Ross V, et al. (1992) Bright light treatment of behavioral and sleep disturbances in patients with Alzheimer's disease. Am J Psychiatr 149, 1028–1032.

Scharf B, Moskovitz C, Lupton MD, et al. (1978) Dream phenomena induced by chronic levodopa therapy. J Neural Transm 43, 143–151.

Schenk C, Bundlie S, Ettinger M, et al. (1986) Chronic behavioral disorders of human REM sleep: A new category of parasomnia. Sleep 9, 293–308.

Schuckit MA and Bernstein LI (1981) Sleep time and drinking history: A hypothesis. Am J Psychiatr 138, 528–530.

Shepard JW Jr. (1992) Hypertension, cardiac arythmias, myocardial infarction, and stroke in relation to obstructive sleep apnea. Clin Chest Med 13(3), 437–458.

Shochat T, Loredo JS, and Ancoli-Israel S (2001) Sleep disorders in the elderly. Curr Treat Opt Neurol 3, 19–36.

Siegel JM, Nienhuis R, Fahringer HM, et al. (1992) Activity of medial mesopontine units during cataplexy and sleep-waking states in the narcoleptic dog. J Neurosci 12, 1640–1646.

Spielman AJ, Saskin P, and Thorpy MJ (1987) Treatment of chronic insomnia by restriction of time in bed. Sleep 10, 45–56.

Stein MB, Chartier M, and Walker JR (1993) Sleep in nondepressed patients with panic disorder: I. Systematic assessment of subjective sleep quality and sleep disturbance. Sleep 16, 724–726.

Steriade M and McCarley RW (1990) Brainstem Control of Wakefulness and Sleep. Plenum Press, New York.

Steriade M, Contreras D, and Amzica F (1994) Synchronized sleep oscillations and their paroxysmal developments. Trends Neurosci 17, 199–208.

Taylor F and Raskin MA (2002) The alpha-1-adrenergic antagonist prazosin improves sleep and nightmares in civilian trauma posttraumatic stress disorder. J Clin Psychopharmacol 1, 82–85.

Uhde TH (1994) The anxiety disorders. In Principles and Practise of Sleep Medicine, Kryger M, Roth T, and Dement WC (eds). WB Saunders, Philadelphia, pp. 871–898.

US Xyrem Multicenter Study Group (2002) A randomized, double-blind, placebo-controlled multicenter trial comparing the effects of three doses of orally administered sodium oxybate with placebo for the treatment of narcolepsy. Sleep 25, 42–49.

Vermeeren A, Riedel WJ, van Boxtel MP, et al. (2002) Differential residual effects of zaleplon and zopiclone on actual driving: A comparison with a low dose of alcohol. Sleep 25, 224–231.

Vignau J, Dahlitz M, Arendt J, et al. (1993) Biological rhythms and sleep disorders in man: The delayed sleep phase syndrome. In Light and Biological Rhythms in Man, Wettering L (ed). Pergamon Press, Stockholm, pp. 261–271.

Waller D, Jarriel S, Erman M, et al. (1984) Recognizing and managing the adolescent with Kleine–Levin syndrome. J Adolesc Health 5, 139–141.

Walsh JK, Muehlbach MJ, Humm TM, et al. (1990) Effect of caffeine on physiological sleep tendency and ability to sustain wakefulness at night. Psychopharmacology 101, 271–273.

Walters AS, Aldrich MS, Allen R, et al. (1995) Toward a better definition of the restless legs syndrome. Movt Disord 10, 634–642.

Walters AS, Hening WA, Kavey N, et al. (1988) A double-blind randomized crossover trial of bromocriptine and placebo in restless legs syndrome. Ann Neurol 24, 455–458.

Watson R, Bakos L, Compton P, et al. (1992) Cocaine use and withdrawal: The effect on sleep and mood. Am J Drug Alcohol Abuse 18, 21–28.

Weddington WW, Brown BS, Haertzen CA, et al. (1990) Changes in mood, craving, and sleep during short-term abstinence reported by male cocaine addicts. Arch Gen Psychiatr 47, 861–868.

Wehr TA (1992) Improvement of depression and triggering of mania by sleep deprivation. JAMA 267, 548–551.

Wehr TA, Moul DE, Barbato G, et al. (1993) Conservation of photoperiod-responsive mechanisms in humans. Am J Physiol 265, R846–R857.

Wetter DW and Young TB (1994) The relationship between cigarette smoking and sleep disturbance. Prev Med 23, 328–334.

Wu JC, Gillin JC, Buchsbaum MS, et al. (1992) Effect of sleep deprivation on brain metabolism of depressed patients. Am J Psychiatr 149, 538–543.

Young T, Palta M, Dempsey J, et al. (1993) The occurrence of sleep-disordered breathing among middle-aged adults. New Engl J Med 328, 1230–1235.

# 77 Impulse Control Disorders

Ronald M. Winchel
Daphne Simeon
Yoram Yovell

Intermittent Explosive Disorder
Kleptomania
Pyromania
Pathological Gambling
Trichotillomania

Although dissimilar in behavioral expressions, the disorders in this chapter share the feature of impulse dyscontrol. Individuals who experience such dyscontrol are overwhelmed by the urge to commit certain acts that are often apparently illogical or harmful (McElroy et al. 1992). The phrase monomanias instinctives (instinctive monomanias) was suggested more than 150 years ago (Esquirol 1838). Its meaning reflects the understanding that individuals may be driven toward particular behaviors for which there is no clear motive. The outcome of each of these behaviors is often harmful, either for the afflicted individual (trichotillomania, pathological gambling) or for others (intermittent explosive disorder, pyromania, kleptomania).

The trait of impulsivity has been the subject of increasing interest in psychiatry. New research findings seem to associate various forms of impulsive behavior with biological markers of altered serotonergic function. These include impulsive suicidal behavior, impulsive aggression, and impulsive fire-setting (Stein et al. 1993). Impulsivity is also a focus of interest in the increasing attention paid to the behavioral phenomenology of borderline personality disorder. In all these circumstances, impulsivity is conceived of as the rapid expression of unplanned behavior, occurring in response to a sudden thought. (This is seen by some as the polar opposite of obsessional behavior, in which deliberation over an act may seem never-ending.) Although the sudden and unplanned aspect of the behavior may be present in the impulse disorders (such as in intermittent explosive disorder and kleptomania), the primary connotation of the word impulsivity, as used to describe these conditions, is the irresistibility of the urge to act.

Trichotillomania, pyromania, and pathological gambling may involve episodes in which a sudden desire to commit the act of hair-pulling, fire-setting, or gambling is followed by rapid expression of the behavior. But in these conditions, the individual may spend considerable amounts of time fighting off the urge, trying not to carry out the impulse. The inability to resist the impulse is the common core of these disorders, rather than the rapid transduction of thought to action. A decision tree for the differential diagnosis of impulsive behaviors may be seen in Figure 77–1.

Other than sharing the essential feature of impulse dyscontrol, it is unclear whether the conditions in this chapter bear any relationship to each other. Emerging perspectives on the neurobiology of impulsivity suggest that impulsive behaviors, across diagnostic boundaries, may share an underlying pathophysiological diathesis. As noted earlier, markers of altered serotonergic neurotransmission have been associated with a variety of impulsive behaviors: suicidality, aggressive violence, pyromania, and conduct disorder. These observations have led to speculation that decreased serotonergic neurotransmission may result in decreased ability to control urges to act. In accord with this model, these disorders may be varying expressions of a single disturbance—or closely related disturbances—of serotonergic function. Although such markers of altered serotonergic function have been demonstrated among impulsive fire-setters and impulsive violent offenders, there is, as yet, insufficient research on these conditions to accept or dismiss this theory.

It has been noted that these conditions are embedded in similar patterns of comorbidity with other psychiatric disorders. High rates of comorbid mood disorder and anxiety disorder appear typical of these disorders. This contextual similarity, combined with the common feature of impulsivity, may further support the notion that these conditions are—at the level of core diathesis—related to each other.

Although these conditions have historically been considered uncommon, later investigations suggest that some

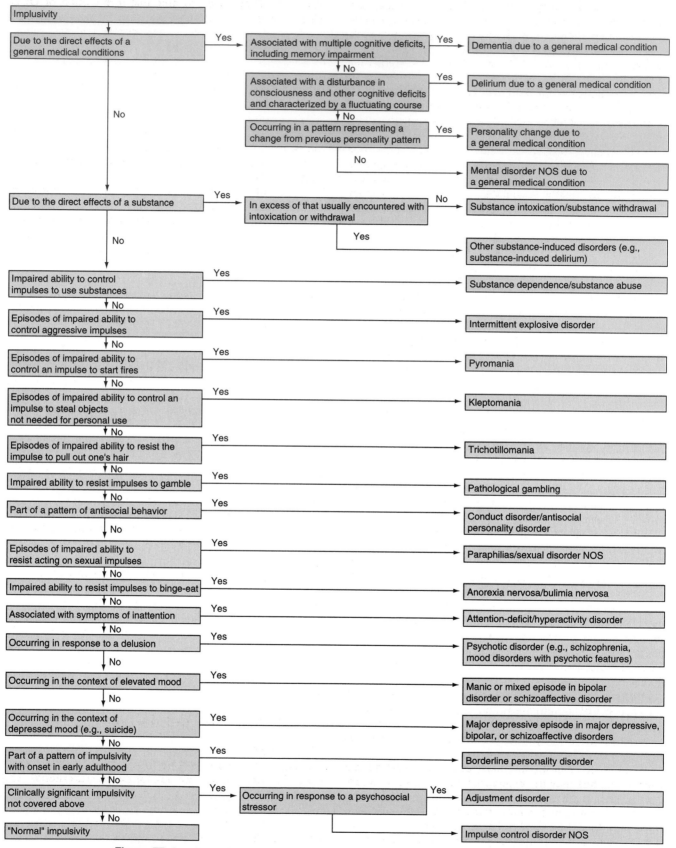

**Figure 77–1** *Differential diagnosis of impulsivity. Impulsivity is a tendency to act in a sudden, unpremeditated, and excessively spontaneous fashion. Other decision trees that should be considered are those for aggressive behavior, catatonia, delusions, depressed mood, euphoric or irritable mood, disorganized or unusual behavior, distractibility, eating behavior, self-mutilation, and suicide ideation or attempt. (NOS, not otherwise specified.)*

of them may be fairly common. Trichotillomania, for example, was once considered rare. However, surveys indicate that the lifetime prevalence of the condition may exceed 1% of the population. Pathological gambling may be present in up to 3% of the population. Extrapolation from the known incidence of comorbid conditions suggests that kleptomania may have a 0.6% incidence. It would seem reasonable to suspect that individuals with pyromania and kleptomania may seek to avoid detection and may therefore be underrepresented in research and clinical samples.

Treatment protocols for these conditions have not been well studied. Few treatment studies of these specific conditions have been performed. Attempts to treat these conditions are usually formulated by extrapolation from treatments that have been developed for other conditions.

The treatment literature for most of these conditions reflects the general development of psychiatric theory. Papers from the early decades of the 20th century are largely restricted to reports of the psychoanalytic treatment of individual cases or of small series. The aggressive quality of kleptomania, pyromania, and intermittent explosive disorder and the self-damaging nature of trichotillomania and pathological gambling have presented tempting substrates for the application of traditional analytical concepts. From this perspective, these behaviors have been seen as symptomatic expressions of unconscious conflict, often sexual in nature. Other formulations include desires for oral gratification and masochistic wishes to be caught and punished, motivated by a harsh, guilt-inducing superego. The increasing influence of object relations theory was reflected in increasing emphasis on narcissistic psychopathology and histories of disturbed early parenting. As successful behavioral interventions were developed for other conditions, case reports of behavioral treatments for these conditions emerged. Reports of hypnotic treatments are also prominent in the literature.

The contemporary medical and psychological literature reflects, not surprisingly, prevailing general interests in current research and theory. As pharmacological treatments are applied to an increasing range of symptoms, the impulse disorders in this chapter present new opportunities to widen the application of thymoleptic and anxiolytic and, more recently, (atypical) neuroleptic medication. Some are reconceptualizing the idea of mood and obsessional disorders, widening them into affective and obsessional spectrums, encompassing various impulse disorders into these domains.

As part of the ongoing dynamic of evolving theory, the very concept of impulsivity is still in ferment. Attempts to further refine the idea of impulsivity are reflected in a perspective offered by Van Ameringen and associates (1999).

In a discussion of preliminary evidence indicating that trichotillomania may be preferentially responsive to neuroleptics, they suggest that individuals with trichotillomania may have features in common with the subgroup of obsessive compulsive disorder (OCD) patients who have comorbid Tourette's syndrome (TS). These authors offer a thoughtful model, applying the idea of an "Impulsion" (Shapiro and Shapiro 1992), an action performed until a sense of "rightness" is achieved, rather than a compulsion, which is designed to reduce an anxiety brought on by an obsession. They go on to note one formulation of OCD, which divides symptoms into three types: symmetry/hoarding, pure obsessions and contamination/cleaning. The symmetry/hoarding factor—impulsion-driven behavior—was differentially related to OCD with comorbid TS (Baer 1994). They point to recent data suggesting that the OCD/TS subgroup is not as responsive to SSRI medication alone as other OCD subtypes—but responds better to SSRI/neuroleptic combinations. These observations, taken together with their report of enhanced response of trichotillomania to neuroleptics, is the basis for their argument that trichotillomania should be seen as more similar to OCD/TS than OCD, more impulsion than compulsion. The idea of anxiously seeking "rightness" is consistent with the clinical experience of many individuals with trichotillomania and is a thoughtful addition to the other attributes associated with impulsivity: anxiety reduction, irresistibility of action, and rapidity of its execution.

Trichotillomania provides an example of the convergence of current research techniques and treatment perspectives. Psychodynamic theories of motivation are rare in the current literature on trichotillomania, and ethologically based models are proposed. The absence of new dynamic formulations would seem to reflect not an abandonment of dynamic theory but an acceptance that such models are most useful in understanding individual patients rather than providing universal explanations for the symptom. Dynamic considerations may be useful in trying to understand why particular circumstances may provoke episodes of the problem behavior for a particular individual. But there is no available evidence that dynamic therapy, when employed as a sole mode of treatment, is efficacious in the treatment of trichotillomania or other conditions in this chapter.

Not all these conditions are, as yet, receiving significant attention. Trichotillomania, intermittent explosive disorder, and pathological gambling have become the focus of increasing interest. Kleptomania and pyromania, however, remain stepchildren of research. Perhaps the legal implications of these behaviors and their entanglement with similar—but not impulsively motivated—behaviors complicate the availability of sufficient cases to facilitate research.

Because of the limited body of systematically collected data, the following sections largely reflect accumulated clinical experience. Therefore, the practicing psychiatrist should be particularly careful to consider the exigencies of individual patients in applying treatment recommendations.

## Intermittent Explosive Disorder

### Definition

Patients with intermittent explosive disorder have a problem with their temper (see box for diagnostic criteria). This definition highlights the centrality of impulsive aggression in intermittent explosive disorder. Impulsive aggression, however, is not specific to intermittent explosive disorder. It is a key feature of several psychiatric disorders and nonpsychiatric conditions and may emerge during the course of yet other psychiatric disorders. Therefore, the definition of intermittent explosive disorder as formulated in the DSM-IV-TR is essentially a diagnosis of exclusion. As described

### DSM-IV-TR Criteria 312.34

**Intermittent Explosive Disorder**

A. Several discrete episodes of failure to resist aggressive impulses that result in serious assaultive acts or destruction of property.

B. The degree of aggressiveness expressed during the episodes is grossly out of proportion to any precipitating psychosocial stressors.

C. The aggressive episodes are not better accounted for by another mental disorder (e.g., antisocial personality disorder, borderline personality disorder, a psychotic disorder, a manic episode, conduct disorder, or attention-deficit/hyperactivity disorder) and are not due to the direct physiological effects of a substance (e.g., a drug of abuse, a medication) or a general medical condition (e.g., head trauma, Alzheimer's disease).

Reprinted with permission from the Diagnostic and Statistical Manual of Mental Disorders, Fourth Edition, Text Revision. Copyright 2000 American Psychiatric Association.

in criterion C, a diagnosis of intermittent explosive disorder is made only after other mental disorders that might account for episodes of aggressive behavior have been ruled out. The individual may describe the aggressive episodes as "spells" or "attacks." The symptoms appear within minutes to hours and, regardless of the duration of the episode, may remit almost as quickly. As in other impulse control disorders, the explosive behavior may be preceded by a sense of tension or arousal and is followed immediately by a sense of relief or release of tension.

Although not explicitly stated in the DSM-IV-TR definition of intermittent explosive disorder, impulsive aggressive behavior may have many motivations that are not meant to be included within this diagnosis. Intermittent explosive disorder should not be diagnosed when the purpose of the aggression is monetary gain, vengeance, self-defense, social dominance, or expressing a political statement or when it occurs as a part of gang behavior. Typically, the aggressive behavior is ego-dystonic to individuals with intermittent explosive disorder, who feel genuinely upset, remorseful, regretful, bewildered, or embarrassed about their impulsive aggressive acts.

Awareness of the existence of individuals who perform behaviors that are harmful to themselves or others in response to overpowering, irresistible, uncontrollable, or "morbid" impulses is not new to psychiatry, dating to the early 19th century. In his monograph about mental illnesses, the French psychiatrist Esquirol (1838) coined the term monomanies instinctives (instinctive monomanias) to describe a form of mental illness, which he classified as "partial insanity," that was characterized by the performance of senseless impulsive acts without motive. These acts were performed in response to "instinctive," or involuntary, irresistible impulses (Esquirol 1838). Many subsequent reports in the psychiatric literature described individuals with similar syndromes that were labeled impulsive insan-

ity, psychopathic forms of reaction, or impulse neuroses. Because the essential feature of intermittent explosive disorder is the occurrence of serious assaultive acts or destruction of property, it is a diagnosis relevant to the interface between psychiatry and the law.

## Etiology and Pathophysiology

Theories about the etiology of impulsive aggressive outbursts and intermittent explosive disorder have been part of psychiatry from its origins. Possession by spirits, humoral imbalances, and "moral weakness" were all suggested to play a role. Since the second half of the 19th century, two main lines of explanation, which are to a large extent complementary, have been developed to account for the existence of individuals with episodic impulsive aggression. One line of explanation viewed the etiology of impulsive aggression as stemming from the effects of early childhood experiences and possibly childhood trauma on the development of self-control, frustration tolerance, planning ability, and gratification delay, which are all important for self-prevention of impulsive aggressive outbursts. Early experiences with "good-enough" mothering that fosters phase-appropriate delay of gratification and the development of the potential for imitation and identification with the mother are considered important for normal development. Too much or too little frustration, as well as overgratification or undergratification, may impair the normal development of the ability to anticipate frustration and delay gratification (Khantzian and Mack 1983).

A second line of explanation, which has yielded numerous positive findings during the past 15 years, views impulsive aggression as the result of variations in brain mechanisms that mediate behavioral arousal and behavioral inhibition. A rapidly growing body of evidence has shown that impulsive aggression may be related to defects in the brain serotonergic system, which acts as an inhibitor of motor activity (Kavoussi et al. 1997, Staner and Mendlewicz 1998). Animal studies suggest that serotonergic neurons play a role in behavioral inhibition and thus provide an impetus to explore the role of serotonin in human impulsivity. Although the majority of the human studies involved patients who suffered from impulsive aggression in the context of disorders other than intermittent explosive disorder, their findings may be relevant to the behavioral dimension of impulsive aggression, of which intermittent explosive disorder is a "pure" form. Siever and colleagues (1991) and Stein and colleagues (1993) have confirmed a relationship between levels of 5-hydroxyindoleacetic acid (5-HIAA) in the CSF and impulsive or aggressive behaviors. Linnoila and coworkers (1989) who divided aggressive behaviors into impulsive and nonimpulsive forms, found that reduced CSF 5-HIAA levels were correlated with impulsive aggression only. Pharmacological challenge studies of the serotonergic system have also demonstrated that low serotonergic responsiveness (as measured by the neuroendocrine response to serotonergic agonists) correlates with scores of impulsive aggression. Studies of impulsive aggression among alcoholics have further defined a probable relationship between such behaviors and diminished serotonergic function (Virkkunen et al. 1995, Virkkunen and Linnoila 1993).

The literature on serotonin and suicide, which may be viewed as an extreme form of self-directed aggression, suggests another link between serotonin and aggression. Postmortem studies found that brain stem levels of serotonin were decreased in suicide victims, and reduced imipramine binding, which is thought to be associated with reduced presynaptic serotonergic binding sites, was found in the brains of suicide completers. Furthermore, an increase in postsynaptic 5-hydroxytryptamine (5-HT$_2$) receptors was found in the brains of suicide completers, and this finding was confirmed in subsequent studies. An increase in 5-HT$_2$ receptors, which are thought to be mostly postsynaptic, may reflect the brain's reaction to a decrease in functional serotonergic neurons, with consequent up-regulation of postsynaptic serotonin binding sites (Stanley and Mann 1988).

Another line of neurobiological evidence links impulsive aggression with dysfunction of the prefrontal cortex. Studies of neuropsychiatric patients with localized structural brain lesions have demonstrated that some bilateral lesions in the prefrontal cortex may be specifically associated with a chronic pattern of impulsive aggressive behaviors. Neurological studies suggest that the prefrontal cortical regions associated with impulsive aggression syndromes are involved in the processing of affective information and the inhibition of motor responsiveness, both of which are impaired in patients with impulsive aggression. Interictal episodes of aggression may occur among some individuals with epilepsy. In a quantitative MRI study of such episodes among individuals with temporal lobe epilepsy (TLE) (Woermann et al. 2000) three groups (24 TLE patients with aggressive behavior, 24 TLE patients without such behavior and 35 nonpatient controls) were compared. The researchers concluded that the aggressive behavior was associated with a reduction of frontal neocortical grey matter.

Further evidence linking the prefrontal cortex with the serotonergic system and impulsive aggression comes from postmortem and animal studies suggesting that the prefrontal cortex is rich in excitatory 5-HT$_2$ receptors, whose number is increased in suicide victims and correlated with aggressive social behavior in primates. Lower levels of CSF 5-HIAA were found in neurological patients who suffered frontal brain injuries than in patients with injuries in other brain regions. Furthermore, the fenfluramine challenge test, a neuroendocrine challenge to the serotonergic system, was found to increase cerebral prefrontal glucose metabolism in normal control subjects. Brain imaging studies with positron emission tomography have found selective reductions in glucose metabolism in the prefrontal and frontal cortex of patients with impulsive aggression. The regional reductions in glucose metabolism in impulsive aggressive patients were more significant during the continuous performance task, whose performance was impaired in neurological patients with frontal lesions and was found to increase frontal glucose metabolism in normal subjects (Raine et al. 1994).

Thus, biological studies implicate the serotonergic system and the prefrontal cortex in the pathogenesis of impulsive aggression. The diagnosis of intermittent explosive disorder is sometimes considered in forensic settings; the biological correlates of impulsive aggression focus attention on, but do not solve, the complicated problem of personal responsibility for impulsive violent acts that are correlated with objective biological findings.

Data from a study of visual-evoked potentials and EEGs in a large group of children and adolescents who demonstrated aggressive behavior also suggest that such behavior may be associated with altered innate characteristics of central nervous system function (Bars et al. 2001).

## Assessment and Differential Diagnosis

### Phenomenology and Variations in Presentation

Violence is underreported in Western societies. As discussed by Lion (1992) although violence is commonly encountered in clinical psychiatric practice, its diagnostic acknowledgment within psychiatry has always been problematical (McElroy et al. 1992). To a large extent, this difficulty also reflects history: Freud himself never fully developed a theory of aggression and came to consider the existence of a "primary" destructive drive only late in his life, after the death and devastation of World War I (*Beyond the Pleasure Principle*, published in 1920) (Freud 1955).

Episodes of violent behavior appear in several common psychiatric disorders such as antisocial personality disorder, borderline personality disorder, and substance use disorders and need to be distinguished from the violent episodes of patients with intermittent explosive disorder, which are apparently rare. The study of Felthous and coworkers (1991) in which 15 men with rigorously diagnosed DSM-III-R intermittent explosive disorder were identified from among a group of 443 men who complained of violence, permitted some systematic observations about the "typical violent episode" as reported by patients with intermittent explosive disorder.

In the vast majority of instances, the subjects with intermittent explosive disorder identified their spouse, lover, or girlfriend or boyfriend as a provocateur of their violent episodes. Only one was provoked by a stranger. For most, the reactions occurred immediately and without a noticeable prodromal period. Only one subject stated that the outburst occurred between 1 and 24 hours after the perceived provocation. All subjects with intermittent explosive disorder denied that they intended the outburst to occur in advance. Most subjects remained well oriented during the outbursts, although two claimed to lose track of where they were. None lost control of urine or bowel function during the episode. Subjects reported various degrees of subjective feelings of behavioral dyscontrol. Only four felt that they completely lost control. Six had good recollection of the event afterward, eight had partial recollection, and one lost memory of the event afterward. Most subjects with intermittent explosive disorder attempted to help or comfort the victim afterward.

### Assessment

#### Special Issues in the Psychiatric Examination and History

The DSM-IV-TR diagnosis of intermittent explosive disorder is essentially a diagnosis of exclusion, and the psychiatrist should evaluate and carefully rule out more common diagnoses that are associated with impulsive violence. The lifelong nonremitting history of impulsive aggression associated with antisocial personality disorder and borderline personality disorder, together with other features of antisocial behavior (in antisocial personality disorder) or impulsive behaviors in other spheres (in borderline personality disorder) may distinguish them from intermittent explosive disorder, in which baseline behavior and functioning are in marked contrast to the violent outbursts. Other features of borderline personality disorder such as unstable and intense interpersonal relationships, frantic efforts to avoid abandonment, and identity disturbance may also be elicited by a careful history. More than in most psychiatric diagnoses, collateral information from an independent historian may be extremely helpful. This is especially true in forensic settings. Of note, patients with intermittent explosive disorder are usually genuinely distressed by their impulsive aggressive outbursts and may voluntarily seek psychiatric help to control them. In contrast, patients with antisocial personality disorder do not feel true remorse for their actions and view them as a problem only insofar as they suffer their consequences, such as incarceration and fines. Although patients with borderline personality disorder, like patients with intermittent explosive disorder, are often distressed by their impulsive actions, the rapid development of intense and unstable transference toward the psychiatrist during the evaluation period of patients with borderline personality disorder may be helpful in distinguishing it from intermittent explosive disorder.

Other causes of episodic impulsive aggression are substance use disorders, in particular alcohol abuse and intoxication. When the episodic impulsive aggression is associated only with intoxication, intermittent explosive disorder is ruled out. However, as discussed earlier, intermittent explosive disorder and alcohol abuse may be related, and the diagnosis of one should lead the psychiatrist to search for the other.

Neurological conditions such as dementias, focal frontal lesions, partial complex seizures, and postconcussion syndrome after recent head trauma may all present as episodic impulsive aggression and need to be differentiated from intermittent explosive disorder. Other neurological causes of impulsive aggression include encephalitis, brain abscess, normal-pressure hydrocephalus, subarachnoid hemorrhage, and stroke. In these instances, the diagnosis would be personality change due to a general medical condition, aggressive type, and it may be made with a careful history and the characteristic physical and laboratory findings.

Individuals with intermittent explosive disorder may have comorbid mood disorders. Although the diagnosis of a manic episode excludes intermittent explosive disorder, the evidence for serotonergic abnormalities in both major depressive disorder and impulse control disorders supports the clinical observation that impulsive aggression may be increased in depressed patients, leading ultimately to completed suicide.

### Physical Examination and Laboratory Findings

The physical and laboratory findings relevant to the diagnosis of intermittent explosive disorder and the differential diagnosis of impulsive aggression may be divided into two main groups: those associated with episodic impulsive aggression but not diagnostic of a particular disorder and those that suggest the diagnosis of a psychiatric or medical disorder other than intermittent explosive disorder. No laboratory or physical findings are specific for intermittent explosive disorder.

The first group of findings that are associated with impulsive aggression across a spectrum of disorders includes soft neurological signs such as subtle impairments in hand–eye coordination and minor reflex asymmetries. These signs may be elicited by a comprehensive neurological examination and simple pencil-and-paper tests such as parts A and B of the Trail Making Test. Measures of central serotonergic function such as CSF 5-HIAA levels, the fenfluramine challenge test, and positron emission tomography of prefrontal metabolism also belong to this group. Although these measures advanced our neurobiological understanding of impulsive aggression, their utility in the diagnosis of individual cases of intermittent explosive disorder and other disorders with impulsive aggression is yet to be demonstrated.

The second group of physical and laboratory findings is useful in the diagnosis of causes of impulsive aggression other than intermittent explosive disorder. The smell of alcohol on a patient's breath or a positive alcohol reading with a Breathalyzer may help reveal alcohol intoxication. Blood and urine toxicology screens may reveal the use of other substances, and track marks on the forearms may suggest intravenous drug use. Partial complex seizures and focal brain lesions may be evaluated by use of the EEG and brain imaging. In cases without a grossly abnormal neurological examination, magnetic resonance imaging may be more useful than computed tomography of the head. Magnetic resonance imaging can reveal mesiotemporal scarring, which may be the only evidence for a latent seizure disorder, sometimes in the presence of a normal or inconclusive EEG. Diffuse slowing on the EEG is a nonspecific finding that is probably more common in, but not diagnostic of, patients with impulsive aggression. Hypoglycemia, a rare cause of impulsive aggression, may be detected by blood chemistry screens.

### Differences in Cultural Presentations

Amok is an extremely rare culture-specific syndrome of episodic aggression first described in the Malay Peninsula but later found in Africa and Papua New Guinea. Amok is an episode of sudden, unprovoked rage in which the affected individual runs around with a weapon and attempts to kill a number of people or animals. Sometimes the perpetrator, typically a man, then kills himself. If captured alive, the individual with amok claims no memory of the acts. The etiology of amok and its relation to intermittent explosive disorder are unclear.

### Differential Diagnosis

As discussed earlier, the differential diagnosis of intermittent explosive disorder covers the differential diagnosis of impulsivity and aggressive behavior in general. Aggression and impulsivity are defined as follows:

Aggression is defined as forceful physical or verbal action, which may be appropriate and self-protective or inappropriate as in hostile or destructive behavior. It may be directed against another person, against the environment, or toward the self. The psychiatric nosology of aggression is still preliminary.

Impulsivity is defined as the tendency to act in a sudden, unpremeditated, and excessively spontaneous fashion.

The diagnosis of intermittent explosive disorder should be considered only after all other disorders that are associated with impulsivity and aggression have been ruled out. Chronic impulsivity and aggression may occur as part of a cluster B personality disorder (antisocial and borderline); during the course of substance use disorders and substance intoxication; in the setting of a general medical (usually neurological) condition; and as part of disorders first diagnosed during childhood and adolescence such as conduct disorder, oppositional defiant disorder, attention-deficit/hyperactivity disorder, and mental retardation. In addition, impulsive aggression may appear during the course of a mood disorder, especially during a manic episode, which precludes the diagnosis of intermittent explosive disorder, and during the course of an agitated depressive episode. Impulsive aggression may also be an associated feature of schizophrenia, in which it may occur in response to hallucinations or delusions. Impulsive aggression may also appear in variants of OCD, which may present with concurrent impulsive and compulsive symptoms.

A special problem in the differential diagnosis of impulsive aggression, which may arise in forensic settings, is that it may represent purposeful behavior. Purposeful behavior is distinguished from intermittent explosive disorder by the presence of motivation and gain in the aggressive act, such as monetary gain, vengeance, or social dominance. Another diagnostic problem in forensic settings is malingering, in which individuals may claim to have intermittent explosive disorder to avoid legal responsibility for their acts.

Figure 77–2 presents the differential diagnosis of aggression.

Common disorders that should be excluded before intermittent explosive disorder is diagnosed and features that may be helpful in the differential diagnosis are summarized in Table 77–1.

## Epidemiology

### Prevalence and Incidence

Intermittent explosive disorder has been subjected to little systematic study. As formulated in DSM-IV-TR, intermittent explosive disorder is probably a rare disorder. The exclusionary criterion in the DSM-IV-TR definition (criterion C) reflects an ongoing debate over the boundaries of this disorder. The current definition of intermittent explosive disorder is the result of a succession of attempts by researchers to classify syndromes associated with impulsive aggression. The *Diagnostic and Statistical Manual of Mental Disorders*, First Edition (DSM-I), in 1952, did not specifically address impulsive aggression as an isolated or episodic behavior but listed an aggressive type of passive-aggressive personality that was described as "a persistent reaction to frustration with irritability, temper tantrums, and destructive behavior." A distinct diagnosis of episodic impulsive aggression was included in the second edition (DSM-II), in 1968, which introduced the diagnostic category of "explosive personality (epileptoid personality disorder)." The diagnostic term "intermittent explosive disorder" first appeared in the 1980 *Diagnostic and Statistical Manual of Mental Disorders*, Third Edition (DSM-III). The DSM-III and the revised third edition (DSM-III-R) definitions of intermittent explosive disorder required the absence of signs of generalized impulsivity or aggressiveness between episodes. Episodic behavioral disorders are quite common and exist across a continuum between ictal causes (excessive neuronal discharges) and purely motivational causes (psychogenic). Temper proneness is a relatively common clinical syndrome that is associated with a wide variety of psychiatric disorders and is usually found in patients with central nervous system dysfunction, character disorders, and psychoactive substance abuse. "Pure" intermittent explosive disorder, on the other hand, was found to be a rare clinical entity.

Intermittent explosive disorder is assumed to be more common in men than in women, and men with the disorder are more likely to be encountered in forensic settings, whereas women with the disorder are more likely to be found in psychiatric settings. This difference in presentation may reflect the reduced severity of the aggressive acts committed by women with intermittent explosive disorder. Given the rarity of pure intermittent explosive disorder, reliable information about age at onset and course is lacking. Anecdotal case reports suggest that the disorder usually appears by the second or third decade of life and persists into middle life. It may become attenuated or remit completely as the

| **Table 77–1**   Differential Diagnosis of Intermittent Explosive Disorder | |
|---|---|
| Intermittent Explosive Disorder Must Be Differentiated from Aggressive Behavior in | In Contrast to Intermittent Explosive Disorder, the Other Condition |
| Substance intoxication or withdrawal | Is due to the direct physiological effects of a substance |
| Delirium or dementia (substance induced or due to a general medical condition) | Includes characteristic symptoms (e.g., memory impairment, impaired attention)<br>Requires the presence of an etiological general medical condition or substance use |
| Personality change due to a general medical condition, aggressive type | Requires presence of an etiological general medical condition |
| Conduct disorder or antisocial personality disorder | Is characterized by more general pattern of antisocial behavior |
| Other mental disorders (schizophrenia, manic episode, oppositional defiant disorder, borderline personality disorder) | Includes the characteristic symptoms of the other mental disorder |

*Source*: First M and Frances A (eds) (1995) DSM-IV Handbook of Differential Diagnosis. American Psychiatric Press, Washington DC, p. 200.

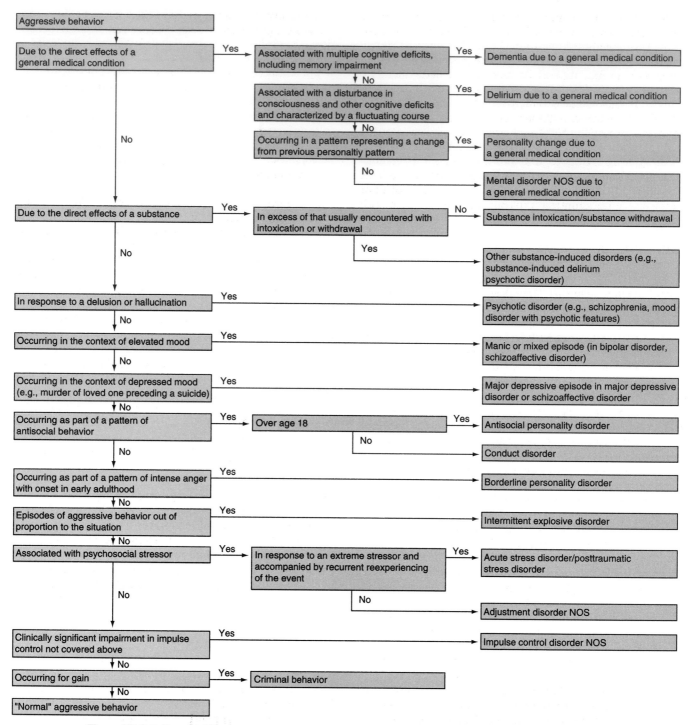

**Figure 77–2** *Differential diagnosis of aggression. The psychiatric nosology of aggression has not been well worked out and requires much additional study. This is a particularly unfortunate state of affairs because the attribution (or misattribution) of aggression to a mental disorder is a frequent focus of forensic attention and can mean the difference between a life term in prison or a promotional tour for a bestseller. Because of the inherent difficulties in making these determinations, psychiatric testimony in this regard should be interpreted with caution. Other decision trees that may be of interest include those for catatonia; delusions; euphoria or irritability; disorganized, agitated, or unusual behavior; impulsivity; hallucinations; substance use; and general medical condition.*

individual ages. However, cognitive impairment caused by Alzheimer's disease and other age-related causes of dementia may result in the reappearance of impulsive aggressive behavior. The mode of onset of intermittent explosive disorder may be abrupt and without a prodromal period.

In one of the few studies of the prevalence of DSM-III-R intermittent explosive disorder among violent men, Felthous and colleagues (1991) found that of 443 subjects who complained of violence, only 15 (3.4%) met criteria for intermittent explosive disorder. The DSM-III-R definition of intermittent explosive disorder was more restrictive than the current DSM-IV-TR diagnosis because it required the absence of signs of generalized impulsivity or aggressiveness between episodes. The mean age of the 15 subjects who met these strict diagnostic criteria was 31.1 years. By design, they were all men. Most were white, with only one black and one Hispanic subject included. Seven (47%) were married, 5 (33%) were single, and 3 (20%) were divorced. Most (8, or 53%) were employed full-time and 80% were employed either full-time or part-time. Most (10, or 67%) graduated from high school. Their estimated level of intellectual functioning ranged from intelligence quotients (IQs) of 75 to 125 with a mean of 102.5. The EEGs of 13 of the men with intermittent explosive disorder were normal; two showed excessive slowing.

## Comorbidity

In contrast to the more restrictive DSM-III and DSM-III-R criteria, the DSM-IV-TR definition of intermittent explosive disorder allows signs of generalized impulsivity or aggressiveness to be present between episodes. It also allows the psychiatrist to give an additional diagnosis of intermittent explosive disorder in the presence of another disorder if the episodes are not better accounted for by the other disorder. These changes were deemed necessary because the clinical reality is that most individuals who have intermittent episodes of aggressive behavior also have some impulsivity between episodes and often present with other past or current psychiatric disorders. There is minimal research-based data available regarding comorbidity. But the literature on the comorbidity of impulsive aggressive episodes suggests that it often occurs with three classes of disorders:

(1) Personality disorders, especially antisocial personality disorder and borderline personality disorder. By definition, antisocial personality disorder and borderline personality disorder are chronic and include impulsive aggression as an essential feature. Therefore, their diagnosis effectively excludes the diagnosis of intermittent explosive disorder (Figure 77–2).

(2) A history of substance use disorders, especially alcohol abuse. A concurrent diagnosis of substance intoxication excludes the diagnosis of intermittent explosive disorder. However, many patients with intermittent explosive disorder report past or family histories of substance abuse, and in particular alcohol abuse. In light of evidence linking personal and family history of alcohol abuse with impulsive aggression (Linnoila 1989) and the evidence (reviewed later) linking both with low central serotonergic function, this connection may be clinically relevant. Therefore, when there is evidence suggesting that alcohol abuse may be present, a systematic evaluation of intermittent explosive disorder is warranted, and vice versa.

(3) Neurological disorders, especially severe head trauma, partial complex seizures, dementias, and inborn errors of metabolism. Intermittent explosive disorder is not diagnosed if the aggressive episodes are a direct physiological consequence of a general medical condition. Such cases would be diagnosed as personality change due to a general medical condition, delirium, or dementia. However, individuals with intermittent explosive disorder often have nonspecific findings on neurological examination, such as reflex asymmetries, mild hand–eye coordination deficits, and childhood histories of head trauma with or without loss of consciousness. Their EEGs may show nonspecific changes. Such isolated findings are compatible with the diagnosis of intermittent explosive disorder and preempt the diagnosis only when they are indicative of a definitely diagnosable general medical or neurological condition. Such "soft" neurological signs may be diagnosed by a full neurological examination and neuropsychological testing.

McElroy and coworkers (McElroy et al. 1998, McElroy 1999) studied 27 individuals who had symptoms that met criteria for Intermittent explosive disorder (IED) and reported: "Twenty-five (93%) subjects had lifetime DSM-IV-TR diagnoses of mood disorders; 13 (48%), substance use disorders; 13 (48%), anxiety disorders; 6 (22%), eating disorders; and 12 (44%), an impulse-control disorder other than intermittent explosive disorder. Subjects also displayed high rates of comorbid migraine headaches. First-degree relatives displayed high rates of mood, substance use, and impulse-control disorders."

Some children with Tourette's disorder may be prone to rage attacks (Budman et al. 1998, 2000). The clinical manifestation of these rage attacks are similar to IED and may be more common among children with Tourette's who have comorbid mood disorders. On the basis of these observations, the rage attacks of these children may flow from an underlying dysregulation of brain function (Budman et al. 1998, 2000).

## Course, Natural History, and Prognosis

Little systematic study has been done on the course of intermittent explosive disorder. The onset of the disorder appears to be from late adolescence to the third decade of life, and it may be abrupt and without a prodromal period. Intermittent explosive disorder is apparently chronic and may persist well into middle life unless treated successfully. In some cases, it may decrease in severity or remit completely with old age.

## Treatment

Given the rarity of pure intermittent explosive disorder, it is not surprising that few systematic data are available on its response to treatment and that some of the recommended treatment approaches to intermittent explosive disorder are based on treatment studies of impulsivity and aggression in the setting of other mental disorders and general medical conditions. Thus, no standard regimen for the treatment of intermittent explosive disorder can be recommended at this time. Both psychological and somatic therapies have been utilized in the treatment of intermittent explosive disorder. A prerequisite for both modalities is the willingness of the individual to acknowledge some responsibility for the behavior and participate in attempts to control it.

### Psychological Treatment

Lion (1992) has described the major psychotherapeutic task of teaching individuals with intermittent explosive disorder how to recognize their own feeling states and especially the affective state of rage. Lack of awareness of their own mounting anger is presumed to lead to the buildup of intolerable rage that is then discharged suddenly and inappropriately in a temper outburst. Patients with intermittent explosive disorder are therefore taught how to first recognize and then verbalize their anger appropriately. In addition, during the course of insight-oriented psychotherapy, they are encouraged to identify and express the fantasies surrounding their rage. Group psychotherapy for temper-prone patients has also been described. The cognitve–behavioral model of psychological treatment may be usefully applied to problems with anger and rage management.

## Somatic Treatments

Several classes of medications have been used to treat intermittent explosive disorder. The same medications have also been used to treat impulsive aggression in the context of other disorders. These included beta-blockers (propranolol and metoprolol), anticonvulsants (carbamazepine and valproic acid), lithium, antidepressants (tricyclic antidepressants and serotonin reuptake inhibitors), and antianxiety agents (lorazepam, alprazolam, and buspirone). Mattes (1990) compared the effectiveness of two commonly used agents, carbamazepine and propranolol, for the treatment of rage outbursts in a heterogeneous group of patients. He found that although carbamazepine and propranolol were overall equally effective, carbamazepine was more effective in patients with intermittent explosive disorder and propranolol was more effective in patients with attention-deficit/hyperactivity disorder. A substantial body of evidence supports the use of propranolol—often in high doses—for impulsive aggression in patients with chronic psychotic disorders and mental retardation. Lithium has been shown to have anti-aggressive properties and may be used to control temper outbursts. In patients with comorbid major depressive disorder, OCD, or cluster B and C personality disorders, SSRIs may be useful. Overall, in the absence of more controlled clinical trials, the best approach may be to tailor the psychopharmacological agent to coexisting psychiatric comorbidity. In the absence of comorbid disorders, carbamazepine, titrated to antiepileptic blood levels, may be used empirically.

---

Clinical Vignette 1

Mr. A is a 42-year-old separated man who works as a bank clerk. He came to seek outpatient psychiatric treatment after an angry outburst that led to the breakdown of his second marriage: his wife issued an order of protection against him after a rage attack in which he slapped her across the face and destroyed most of the kitchen and living room furniture. His rage was triggered by his wife's decision to buy a new microwave oven without consulting him. Mr. A, who remembered the episode clearly and with remorse, said that he realized how angry he was only after he actually struck at his wife.

During the course of his evaluation, Mr. A became tearful and admitted to several similar episodes during the course of his current and previous marriages. These episodes were rare, occurring once or twice a year. They were brief and apparently unpredictable and resulted in his separation from his first wife. Except during those episodes, Mr. A was a pleasant, rather timid man who deferred to his wife in most important decisions. There was no history suggestive of

antisocial or borderline personality disorder. Mr. A, who described himself as a shy, withdrawn child, gave a history of head trauma at the age of 12, while he was ice-skating, with loss of consciousness for 10 minutes. Other than this, his medical history was normal. There were no neurological or behavioral sequelae. Mr. A also described prolonged physical abuse by his alcoholic father. Mr. A himself denied a history of substance abuse, involvement with the criminal justice system, and prior psychiatric treatment. He denied a history of manic and depressive episodes. Mr. A had few friends and was not popular at his job. Although he had never lost his temper there, he believed that his boss and coworkers could sense his "stress" while dealing with clients.

Mr. A's physical and neurological examination was notable only for mild bilateral difficulty with rapid alternating hand movements. Except for his tearfulness while describing the episode, Mr. A's Mental Status Examination was unremarkable. Results of routine laboratory blood work and computed tomography of the head were within normal limits. An EEG was notable for diffuse slowing without an epileptic focus.

Mr. A's treatment was started with carbamazepine. He also received a short course of psychotherapy that focused on recognizing his anger and venting it appropriately, on his memories of childhood physical abuse, and on his current sense of himself as a helpless person who was being controlled by his wife and boss. In addition, it was recommended that he transfer to a position that would not involve contact with clients. During a 2-year follow-up, Mr. A had no further rage episodes. He continued to have few friends but was able to maintain a long-term relationship with a woman he was planning to marry.

## Kleptomania

### Definition

Kleptomania shares with all other impulse control disorders the recurrent failure to resist impulses. Unfortunately, in the absence of epidemiological studies, little is known about

---

**DSM-IV-TR Criteria** 312.32

**Kleptomania**

A. Recurrent failure to resist impulses to steal objects that are not needed for personal use or for their monetary value.

B. Increasing sense of tension immediately before committing the theft.

C. Pleasure, gratification, or relief at the time of committing the theft.

D. The stealing is not committed to express anger or vengeance and is not in response to a delusion or a hallucination.

E. The stealing is not better accounted for by conduct disorder, a manic episode, or antisocial personality disorder.

kleptomania. Clinical case series and case reports are limited. Family, neurobiological, and genetic investigations are not available. There are no established treatments of choice. Therefore, in reading this section the reader must keep in mind that much of what is described is based on limited data or on anecdotal information.

## Etiology and Pathophysiology

The etiology of kleptomania is essentially unknown, although various models have been proposed in an effort to conceptualize the disorder. At present, the available empirical data are insufficient to substantiate any of these models.

With the exception of scant information on family history, data regarding possible familial or genetic transmission of a kleptomania diathesis are unavailable. One study found the risk for major mood disorders in first-degree relatives of probands with kleptomania to be 0.31—similar to the familial risk for probands with major depressive disorder (McElroy et al. 1991a). In the same study, 7% of first-degree relatives of patients with kleptomania had histories of OCD. These findings, combined with other lines of evidence, might suggest that kleptomania shares a common biological diathesis with mood disorders or OCD.

The affective spectrum model suggests that kleptomania and other impulse control disorders may share a common underlying biological diathesis with other disorders, such as depression, panic disorder, OCD, and bulimia nervosa (McElroy et al. 1992, 1991b, Hudson and Pope 1990). The apparent high comorbidity of kleptomania with depression and bulimia nervosa has already been noted. As early as 1911, Janet (1911) recognized the alleviation of depressive symptoms on the commission of kleptomanic acts. In some individuals, kleptomania responds to treatment with thymoleptic agents or electroconvulsive therapy. These observations are cited as support for an affective spectrum model.

Although the affective spectrum has been claimed to encompass obsessive–compulsive pathology (Hudson and Pope 1990) there exists a more specific model conceptualizing kleptomania and other impulse disorders as obsessive–compulsive spectrum disorders (McElroy et al. 1993). Several lines of evidence support this model. First, there are phenomenological similarities between the classical obsessions and compulsions of OCD and the irresistible impulses and repetitive actions characteristic of kleptomania. In addition, there appears to be a greater than chance occurrence of OCD in probands with kleptomania and in their relatives. In addition, both conditions have significant comorbidity with mood, anxiety, substance use, and eating disorders. However, OCD rituals are more clearly associated with relief of anxiety and harm avoidance, whereas kleptomanic acts seem to be associated with gratification or pleasure. In addition, OCD is associated with a clear preferential response to SSRIs as opposed to general thymoleptics. The limited treatment literature (see later) does not support a similar response pattern in kleptomania. Unfortunately, the role of the serotonergic or of any other neurotransmitter system has not been investigated in kleptomania. Interestingly, a large study found subjects with mixed anorexia and bulimia nervosa to have a higher lifetime prevalence of kleptomania than those with either anorexia or bulimia nervosa alone (Herzog et al. 1992). This could suggest a relationship between kleptomania and both the obsessive–compulsive (anorexic) and affective (bulimic) spectrum.

Alternatively, kleptomania could be conceptualized as an addictive disorder. The irresistible impulse to steal is reminiscent of the urge and the high associated with drinking or using drugs (McElroy et al. 1992). Marks (1990) has proposed a constellation of behavioral (i.e., nonchemical) addictions encompassing OCD, compulsive spending, gambling, binging, hypersexuality, and kleptomania. This model postulates certain concepts thought to be common in all these disorders, such as craving, mounting tension, "quick fixing," withdrawal, external cuing, and habituation. These components have not yet been well investigated in kleptomania.

It should be emphasized that the lack of neurobiological or prospective pharmacological treatment data for kleptomania limits any conclusions that can be drawn with regard to biological models.

In addition to the foregoing theories, numerous psychological formulations of kleptomania have been postulated over the years. A frequent theme, reported by numerous authors and reviewed by Goldman (1991) and McElroy and coworkers (1991b) is that of kleptomania as an acting-out aimed at alleviating depressive symptoms. Fishbain (1987) has carefully described the case of a woman whose kleptomanic episodes were closely related to depressive bouts and who experienced an apparent antidepressant effect from the thrill and excitement of her risk-taking behavior.

From a psychodynamic point of view, kleptomania has been viewed over the decades as a manifestation of a variety of unconscious conflicts, with sexual conflicts figuring prominently in the literature. Case reports have described conscious sexual gratification, sometimes accompanied by frank masturbation or orgasm during kleptomanic acts (Fishbain 1987, Fenichel 1945). Thus, it has been suggested, kleptomanic behavior serves to discharge a sexual drive that may have forbidden connotations similar to those of masturbation, and the stolen object itself may have unconscious symbolic or overt fetishistic significance. Although no systematic studies exist, there has long been an implication in the literature on kleptomania that those afflicted with kleptomania suffer disproportionately from a variety of sexual dysfunctions. Turnbull (1987) described six patients with a primary diagnosis of kleptomania, all of whom had dysfunctional sexual relationships with their partners, compulsive promiscuity, or anorgasmia.

Other cases of kleptomania have been understood as reflecting conflictual infantile needs and attempts at oral gratification, masochistic wishes to be caught and punished related to a harsh guilt-inducing superego or primitive aggressive strivings, penis envy or castration anxiety with the stolen object representing a penis, a defense against unwelcome passive homosexual longings, restitution of the self in the presence of narcissistic injuries, or the acquisition of transitional objects (Beldoch 1991). These various formulations are presented in more detail in Goldman's review (1991). One should probably conclude that the psychodynamics associated with kleptomania ought to be carefully tailored to the individual patient. The literature on kleptomania has frequently implicated disturbed childhoods, inadequate parenting, and significant character disturbances in kleptomanic patients. From this perspective kleptomania can be more effectively understood in the context of an individual's overall character. Unfortunately, no clinical studies exist that systematically explore Axis II psychopathology in these patients.

## Assessment and Differential Diagnosis

### Phenomenology and Presentation

At presentation, the typical patient suffering from kleptomania is a 35-year-old woman who has been stealing for about 15 years and may not mention kleptomania as the presenting complaint or in the initial history (Goldman 1991, McElroy 1991a). The patient may complain instead of anxiety, depression, lability, dysphoria, or manifestations of character pathology. There is often a history of a tumultuous childhood and poor parenting, and in addition acute stressors may be present, such as marital or sexual conflicts. The patient experiences the urge to steal as irresistible, and the thefts are commonly associated with a thrill, a high, a sense of relief, or gratification. Generally, the behavior has been hard to control and has often gone undetected by others. The kleptomania may be restricted to specific settings or types of objects, and the patient may or may not be able to describe rationales for these preferences. Quite often, the objects taken are of inherently little financial value, or have meaningless financial value relative to the income of the person who has taken the object. Additionally, the object may never actually be used. These factors often help distinguish theft from kleptomania. The theft is followed by feelings of guilt or shame and, sometimes, attempts at atonement. The frequency of stealing episodes may greatly fluctuate in concordance with the degree of depression, anxiety, or stress. There may be periods of complete abstinence. The patient may have a past history of psychiatric treatments including hospitalizations or of arrests and convictions, whose impact on future kleptomanic behavior can be variable.

### Assessment

Generally, the diagnosis of kleptomania is not a complicated one to make. However, kleptomania may frequently go undetected because the patient may not mention it spontaneously and the psychiatrist may fail to inquire about it as part of the routine history. The index of suspicion should rise in the presence of commonly associated symptoms such as chronic depression, other impulsive or compulsive behaviors, tumultuous backgrounds, or unexplained legal troubles. It could convincingly be argued that a cursory review of compulsivity and impulsivity, citing multiple examples for the patient, should be a part of any thorough and complete psychiatric evaluation. In addition, it is important to do a careful differential diagnosis and pay attention to the various exclusion criteria before diagnosing theft as kleptomania. Possible diagnoses of sociopathy, mania, or psychosis should be carefully considered. In this regard, the psychiatrist must inquire about the affective state of the patient during the episodes, the presence of delusions or hallucinations associated with the occurrence of the behavior, the motivation behind the stealing, and the fate and subsequent use of the objects.

Although the typical patient may be a 35-year-old woman, it is important to remember that men, children, and elderly persons may present with or engage in kleptomania. Interestingly, Goldman's review (1991) suggested that men may first present for evaluation 15 years later than women. Kleptomania occurs transculturally and has been described in various Western and Eastern cultures. Asian observers have also noted an overlap with eating disorders (Lee 1994). Atypical presentations should raise a greater suspicion of an organic etiology, and a medical evaluation is then indicated. Medical conditions that have been associated with kleptomania include cortical atrophy, dementia, intracranial mass lesions, encephalitis, normal-pressure hydrocephalus, benzodiazepine withdrawal, and temporal lobe epilepsy. A complete evaluation when such suspicions are present includes a physical and neurological examination, general serum chemistry and hematological panels, and an EEG with temporal leads or computed tomography of the brain (Chiswick 1976, Khan and Martin 1977, Mendez 1988, Wood and Garralda 1990, Coid 1984, McIntyre 1990).

## Epidemiology and Comorbidity

### Prevalence and Incidence

No epidemiological studies of kleptomania have been conducted, and thus its prevalence can be calculated only grossly and indirectly. In a thorough review of the existing literature, Goldman (1991) found that in a series of shoplifters, the estimate of kleptomania ranged from 0 to 24%. The frequency of kleptomania may be indirectly extrapolated from incidence rates of kleptomania in comorbid disorders with known prevalence, such as bulimia nervosa. Such speculations suggest at least a 0.6% prevalence of kleptomania in the general population (Goldman 1991). However, given that people who shoplift are often not caught, this is almost certainly an underestimate. Its presence may be further obscured because the behavior is often shameful and, consequently, treatment may not be sought. In addition, studies examining comorbidity of other disorders may neglect to inquire about kleptomania.

Despite the lack of valid epidemiological data, there is general agreement that kleptomania is more common among women than among men. In a retrospective review of 56 cases that appeared to fulfill DSM-III-R criteria for kleptomania, McElroy and colleagues (1991b) found that 77% were women. Similarly, in a prospective series of 20 patients with DSM-III-R kleptomania, 75% were women (McElroy 1991a). However, women generally seek psychiatric help more frequently than men, whereas men are more likely to become involved with the penal system. Consequently, this may not reflect true gender distribution.

### Comorbidity

Among individuals with kleptomania who present for treatment, there is a high incidence of comorbid mood, anxiety, and eating disorders, when compared with rates in the general population. In reviewing 26 case reports of kleptomania, Goldman (1991) reported mention of histories of depression in 13 patients (50%), anxiety in 8 patients (31%), and bulimia nervosa in 3 patients (12%). Similar percentages are noted by McElroy and colleagues (1991b) in the review of 56 patients with probable kleptomania: 57% with mood disorder symptoms, 34% with anxiety disorder symptoms, and 11% with bulimic symptoms. Comorbidity patterns among individuals who present for treatment may be greater than among random samples. More reliable comorbidity rates can be found in a prospective investigation of 20 individuals with kleptomania conducted by McElroy and coworkers (1991a). Lifetime DSM-III-R comorbidity rates were 40% major depressive disorder, 50% substance abuse, 40% panic disorder, 40% social phobia, 45% OCD, 30% anorexia nervosa, 60% bulimia nervosa, and 40% other impulse control disorders. Dissociative symptoms, significant character pathology, and trauma histories are commonly encountered among this group (Goldman 1991, McElroy et al. 1991b). Unfortunately, Axis I dissociative pathology and Axis II pathology have not yet been systematically investigated in these patients.

## Course
In two separate studies, the mean age at onset of kleptomania was reported to be 20 years (Goldman 1991, McElroy et al. 1991a). The subjects included individuals who had begun stealing as early as 5 to 7 years of age. The disorder appears to be chronic, lasting for decades, albeit with varying intensity. Fifteen or 16 years may elapse before treatment is sought (Goldman 1991, McElroy et al. 1991a). Onset in and beyond the fifth decade of life appears to be unusual, and in some of these cases remote histories of past kleptomania can be elicited (Goldman 1991). At peak frequency, McElroy and colleagues (1991a) found a mean of 27 episodes a month, essentially daily stealing, with one patient reporting four acts daily. The majority of patients may eventually be apprehended for stealing once or more, and a minority may even be imprisoned; more often than not these repercussions do not result in more than a temporary remission of the behavior. Individuals with kleptomania may also have extensive histories of psychiatric treatments, including hospitalization for other conditions, most commonly depression or eating disorders. Because of the unavailability of longitudinal studies, the prognosis is not known. It appears, however, that without treatment the behavior may be likely to persist for decades, sometimes with significant associated morbidity. There may be transient periods of remission.

## Treatment

### Treatment Goals
The general goal of treatment is the eradication of kleptomanic behavior. Treatment typically occurs in the outpatient setting, unless comorbid conditions such as severe depression, eating disturbances, or more dangerous impulsive behaviors dictate hospitalization. In the initial contact with the psychiatrist, as described earlier, it is important that the appropriate differential diagnoses be considered. The interview must be conducted in a respectful climate that ensures confidentiality. Patients not only may experience considerable guilt or shame for stealing but also may be

unrevealing because of the fear of legal repercussions. In the acute treatment phase, the aim is to decrease significantly or, ideally, eradicate episodes of stealing during a period of weeks to months. Concurrent conditions may compound the problem and require independently targeted treatment.

The acute treatment of kleptomania has not been, to date, systematically investigated. Recommendations are based on retrospective reviews, case reports, and small case series. Maintenance treatment for kleptomania has not been investigated either, and only anecdotal data exist for patients who have been followed up for significant periods after initial remission.

### Psychiatrist–Patient Relationship
As with any condition that may be associated with intense guilt or shame, kleptomania must be approached respectfully by the psychiatrist. Patients can be reassured and their negative feelings alleviated to some degree with proper initial psychoeducation. The treatment alliance can be strengthened by consistently maintaining a nonjudgmental and supportive stance. In addition, patients' fears regarding breaks of confidentiality and criminal repercussions must be addressed.

No treatments have been systematically shown to be effective for kleptomania. These treatment recommendations are supported by case reports and retrospective reviews only. In general, it appears that thymoleptic medications and behavioral therapy may be the most efficacious treatments for the short term, whereas long-term psychodynamic psychotherapy may be indicated and have good results for selected patients.

### Pharmacological and Somatic Treatments
Mixed results have been reported regarding the pharmacological treatment of kleptomania. In a literature review of 56 cases of kleptomania, McElroy and coworkers (1991b) noted that somatic treatments were described for eight patients. Significant improvement was reported for seven of these. Treatment included antidepressants alone, antidepressants combined with antipsychotics or stimulants, electroconvulsive therapy alone, or electroconvulsive therapy with antidepressants. The medications most commonly used to treat kleptomania are the antidepressants. In a series of 20 patients fulfilling DSM-III-R criteria for kleptomania, McElroy and colleagues (1991a) found that 18 had received antidepressants and of those 56 patients 10 had partial or complete remission of both kleptomanic urges and behavior. It has been suspected that kleptomania may respond selectively to SSRIs because of the anticompulsive and anti-impulsive properties of these compounds. Of these 18 patients, 10 were administered fluoxetine alone and only 2 had a full response and 1 had a partial response. These data are not suggestive of a high response rate to SSRIs, but dose and duration of treatment were not explicitly stated. In a report on three patients with concurrent DSM-III-R kleptomania and bulimia nervosa treated with serotonergic antidepressants, two received high-dose fluoxetine and one trazodone; all three showed significant improvement in kleptomania, independent of the course of bulimia nervosa and depression (McElroy et al. 1989). It is still unclear whether kleptomania responds

preferentially to serotonergic antidepressants, and this question awaits further study. Other agents reported to have treated kleptomania successfully include nortriptyline (McElroy et al. 1991b) and amitriptyline (Fishbain 1987). In addition, it remains unclear if the antikleptomanic effect of thymoleptics is dependent on or independent of their antidepressant effect.

A number of other medications have been employed to treat kleptomania. These include antipsychotics (McElroy et al. 1991b, Fishbain 1987), stimulants (McElroy et al. 1991b), valproic acid (McElroy et al. 1991a), carbamazepine (McElroy et al. 1991a), clonazepam (McElroy et al. 1991a) and lithium (McElroy et al. 1991a, Monopolis and Lion 1983). Lithium augmentation may be of benefit when kleptomania does not respond to an antidepressant alone (Burstein 1992). Finally, there have been some reports of successful treatment of kleptomania with electroconvulsive therapy, which may have been administered for a concurrent mood disorder (McElroy et al. 1991b).

Although little is known about maintenance pharmacological treatment for kleptomania, there is a suggestion in the literature that symptoms tend to recur with cessation of thymoleptic treatment and again remit when treatment is reinstituted (McElroy et al. 1991a, Fishbain 1987).

## Psychosocial Treatments

Formal studies of psychosocial interventions for kleptomania have not been performed. However, a number of clinical reports have supported behavioral therapy for kleptomania. The available clinical literature suggests that for most patients this may be a more efficacious approach than insight-oriented psychotherapy. Different behavioral techniques have been employed with some success, including aversive conditioning (Guidry 1969, Keutzer 1972) systematic desensitization (Marzagao 1972) covert sensitization (Gauthier and Pellerin 1982, Glover 1985) and behavior modification (Fishbain 1987, Wetzel 1966). In their review of 56 reported cases of kleptomania, McElroy and colleagues (1991a) noted that the eight patients who were treated with behavioral therapy—mostly aversive conditioning—showed significant improvement. We give here some specific examples of behavioral techniques that have been successfully employed and described. One patient was taught to hold her breath as a negative reinforcer whenever she experienced an impulse to steal (Keutzer 1972). Another patient was taught to use systematic desensitization techniques to control the mounting anxiety associated with the impulse to steal (Marzagao 1972). A patient treated by covert sensitization learned to associate images of nausea and vomiting with the desire to steal (Glover 1985). A woman who experienced sexual excitement associated with shoplifting and would masturbate at the site of the act was instructed to practice masturbation at home, while fantasizing kleptomanic acts (Fishbain 1987). There is a suggestion in the literature that these techniques remain effective over the long term (Gauthier and Pellerin 1982, Glover 1985).

Finally, it appears that the most effective behavioral treatment of all may be complete abstinence, that is, the patient should no longer visit any of the stores or settings where kleptomanic acts occur. A number of patients who never come to psychiatric attention apparently employ this technique successfully, and it may be an appropriate treatment goal if it does not result in excessive restrictions of activity and lifestyle.

The psychodynamic treatment of kleptomania centers on the exploration and working through of the underlying conflict or conflicts. In a review of 26 case reports, McElroy and associates (1991b) reported that four of five patients had a good response to psychoanalysis or related therapy. However, in another review of 20 cases (meeting DSM-III-R criteria) McElroy and coworkers (1991a) reported that of 11 patients treated with psychotherapy, none showed improvement. There are case reports in the literature of successful psychodynamic treatment of kleptomania (Schwartz 1992). Such treatment, possibly in combination with other approaches, may be indicated for patients for whom a clear conflictual basis for the behavior can be formulated, who also have the needed insight and motivation to undertake this type of treatment. In proposing such treatments, which may be long term, the psychiatrist should consider whether there are immediate risks that must be addressed, such as a high risk of legal consequences.

## Special Treatment Considerations

Little is known about treating kleptomania and therefore special treatment considerations have not been elucidated. However, it is clear that comorbid conditions, such as depression, bulimia nervosa, OCD, or substance abuse, must be addressed along with the kleptomania. In addition to the inherent suffering and morbidity of these other disorders, their course and severity could compound the kleptomanic behavior. In the rare cases of a precipitating or exacerbating organic etiology, the underlying organic cause must be treated. In addition, the treatment of particular groups such as children or the elderly should take into account special contributing life stage or situational factors. The involvement of family or others on whom the patient is dependent may be indicated.

## Refractoriness to Initial Treatment

There has not been sufficient study of the treatment of kleptomania to systematically delineate approaches to the refractory patient. However, general clinical principles can be applied. Medication trials should be maximized, predominantly employing antidepressants and mood stabilizers, alone or in combination. In addition, it is important that comorbid conditions such as depression or OCD be monitored and treated, because they complicate the course of kleptomania. For patients who have no response or a partial response to pharmacotherapy alone or who do not want medication treatment, behavioral therapy is indicated. Behavioral therapy can be used alone or in combination with medication. There are no systematic comparisons of medication, behavioral therapy, or combined treatments. Therefore, the initial treatment choice is based in the assessment of the particular circumstances of each presentation. The patient's past treatment history, comorbid diagnoses, and personal resources should be weighed in choosing a course of treatment. Finally, there may be refractory patients for whom a multiple combination approach is helpful. Fishbain (1987) described the treatment of a middle-aged woman with a long history of kleptomania, depression, and suicidality and extensive past psychiatric treatments who responded to a combination of supportive and insight-oriented therapy, medication, and behavior modification.

## Pyromania and Fire-Setting Behavior

### Definition

The primary characteristics of pyromania are recurrent, deliberate fire-setting, the experience of tension or affective arousal before the fire-setting, an attraction or fascination with fire and its contexts, and a feeling of gratification or relief associated with the setting of a fire or its aftermath.

True pyromania is present in only a small subset of fire-setters. Multiple motivations are cited as causes for fire-setting behavior. These include arson for profit, crime concealment, revenge, vandalism, and political expression. In addition, fire-setting may be associated with other psychiatric diagnoses. (See the following discussion of differential diagnosis.) But true pyromania is rare.

Fire-setting behavior may be a focus of clinical attention, even when criteria for pyromania are not present. Because the large majority of fire-setting events are not associated with true pyromania, this section also addresses fire-setting behavior in general.

### Fire-Setting as a Planned, Nonimpulsive Behavior

Prins and colleagues (1985) have suggested the following motivations for intentional arson: financial reward, to conceal another crime, for political purposes, as a means of revenge, as a symptom of other (nonpyromania) psychiatric

---

### DSM-IV-TR Criteria 312.33

**Pyromania**

A. Deliberate and purposeful fire-setting on more than one occasion.

B. Tension or affective arousal before the act.

C. Fascination with, interest in, curiosity about, or attraction to fire and its situational contexts (e.g., paraphernalia, uses, consequences).

D. Pleasure, gratification, or relief when setting fires, or when witnessing or participating in their aftermath.

E. The fire-setting is not done for monetary gain, as an expression of sociopathical ideology, to conceal criminal activity, to express anger or vengeance, to improve one's living circumstances, in response to a delusion or hallucination, or as a result of impaired judgment (e.g., in dementia, mental retardation, substance intoxication).

F. The fire-setting is not better accounted for by conduct disorder, a manic episode, or antisocial personality disorder

Reprinted with permission from the Diagnostic and Statistical Manual of Mental Disorders, Fourth Edition, Text Revision. Copyright 2000 American Psychiatric Association.

---

conditions (e.g., in response to a delusional belief), as attention-seeking behavior, as a means of deriving sexual satisfaction, and as an act of curiosity when committed by children. Revenge and anger appear to be the most common motivations for fire-setting (O'Sullivan and Kelleher 1987).

### Etiology and Pathophysiology

Because pyromania is rare, there is little reliable scientific literature available regarding individuals who fit diagnostic criteria. But because of the morbid impact that arson has on society, fire-setting behavior (which often does not fulfill criteria for pyromania) has been the focus of scientific investigation and literature.

Arson has been the subject of several investigations of altered neuroamine function. These findings include the observation that platelet monoamine oxidase is negatively correlated with fire-setting behavior of adults who had been diagnosed with attention-deficit disorder in childhood (Kuperman et al. 1988).

Investigation of the function of serotonergic neurotransmission in individuals with aggressive and violent behaviors has included studies of CSF concentrations of 5-HIAA in individuals with a history of fire-setting. 5-HIAA is the primary metabolite of serotonin, and its concentration in the CSF is a valid marker of serotonin function in the brain. Virkkunnen and colleagues (1987, 1994) demonstrated that impulsive fire-setting was associated with low CSF concentrations of 5-HIAA. This finding was consistent with other observations associating impulsive behaviors with low CSF 5-HIAA levels (such as impulsive violence and impulsive suicidal behavior). A history of suicide attempt strongly predicts recidivism of arson (68 sensitivity) (DeJong et al. 1992).

### Assessment and Differential Diagnosis

#### Presentation

The diagnosis of pyromania emphasizes the affective arousal, thrill, or tension preceding the act, as well as the feeling of tension relief or pleasure in witnessing the outcome. This is useful in distinguishing between pyromania and fire-setting elicited by other motives (i.e., financial gain, concealment of other crimes, political, arson related to other mental illness, revenge, attention seeking, erotic pleasure, part of conduct disorder).

The onset of pyromania has been reported to occur as early as age 3 years, but the condition may initially present in adulthood. Because of the legal implications of fire-setting, individuals may not admit previous events, which may result in biased perceptions of the common age at onset. Men greatly outnumber women with the disorder.

In children and adolescents, the most common elements are excitation caused by fires, enjoyment produced by fires, relief of frustration by fire-setting, and expression of anger through fire-setting (Brandford and Dimock 1986).

Fire-setting behavior may be common among more impaired psychiatric patients. In a study of 191 nongeriatric patients in a psychiatric hospital who were admitted for other reasons, 26 had some form of fire-setting behavior (including threats). Of these, 70% had actually set fires. None had a diagnosis of true pyromania (Soltys 1992).

## Assessment

### *The Psychiatric Interview*

The interviewer must bear in mind that the circumstances of arson, whatever the motive, may pose legal and criminal problems for the individual. This may provide motivation to skew the reporting of events. Individuals who may be at risk for the legal consequences of fire-setting may be motivated to represent themselves as victims of psychiatric illness, hoping that a presumed psychiatric basis of the behavior may attenuate legal penalties. Therefore, the interviewer must maintain a guarded view of the information presented.

### Differential Diagnosis

Other causes of fire-setting must be ruled out. Fire-setting behavior may be motivated by circumstances unrelated to mental disorders. Such motivations include profit, crime concealment, revenge, vandalism, and political statement or action (Geller 1987, Lowenstein 1989). Furthermore, fire-setting may be a part of ritual, cultural, or religious practices in some cultures.

Fire-setting may occur in the presence of other mental disorders. A diagnosis of fire-setting is not made when the behavior occurs as a part of conduct disorder, antisocial personality disorder, or a manic episode or if it occurs in response to a delusion or hallucination. The diagnosis is also not given if the individual suffers from impaired judgment associated with mental retardation, dementia, or substance intoxication.

## Epidemiology and Comorbidity

### Prevalence and Incidence

No data are available on the prevalence or incidence of pyromania, but it is apparently uncommon.

Although pyromania is a rare event, fire-setting behavior is common in the histories of psychiatric patients. Geller and Bertsch (1985) found that 26 of 191 nongeriatric state hospital patients had histories of some form of fire-setting behavior. Unlike pyromania, which is rare among women, fire-setting behavior was common in the histories of female patients (22%), as well as male patients (28.8%).

Among children with psychiatric conditions, fire-setting behavior is apparently quite common. Kolko and Kadzin (1988) found that among a sample of children attending an outpatient psychiatry clinic, approximately 20 had histories of fire-setting. For a sample of inpatient children, the rate was approximately 35% (Kolko and Kazdin 1988).

### Comorbidity

Limited data are available regarding individuals with pyromania. Reported data of comorbid diagnoses are generally derived from forensic samples and do not distinguish between criminally motivated fire-setters and compulsive fire-setters. Fire-setting behavior may be associated with other mental conditions. These include mental retardation, conduct disorder, alcohol and other substance use disorders, personality disorders, and schizophrenia.

Repo and coworkers (1997) examined the medical and criminal records of 282 arsonists in order to examine factors that predicted recidivism. They concluded "Alcohol dependence and antisocial personality disorder were common among recidivist offenders. This finding was especially prominent among offenders who committed violent crimes. Recidivist offenders commonly had a history of long-lasting enuresis during their childhood. They were younger at the time of their first offence, and were more often intoxicated with alcohol during the arson attempt. Psychosis was a common diagnosis among subjects who had no record of recidivist criminal offences." Puri and coauthors (1995) also examined a group of 36 forensically referred fire-setters. They found that about one-third had no other evidence of mental illness, about a quarter were female, psychoactive substance abuse was common and interpersonal relationships were often disturbed.

## Course

There are no data regarding the course of and prognosis for pyromania. However, the impulsive nature of the disorder suggests a repetitive pattern. Again, because legal consequences may occur, the individual may be motivated to represent the index episode as a unique event. Fire-setting for nonpsychiatric reasons may be more likely to be a single event.

## Treatment

### Treatment Goals

Because of the danger inherent in fire-setting behavior, the primary goal is elimination of the behavior. The treatment literature does not distinguish between pyromania and fire-setting behavior of other causes.

Much of the literature is focused on controlling fire-setting behavior in children and adolescents.

### Psychiatrist–Patient Relationship

Because of the potential legal risks for individuals who acknowledge fire-setting behavior, the psychiatrist must take particular pains to ensure an environment of empathy and confidentiality. A corollary concern involves obligations that may be incumbent on the psychiatrist. Because of the legal implications of these behaviors and the potential for harm to another individual should fire-setting recur, the psychiatrist should be careful to consider both the ethical and the legal constraints that may follow from information learned in the course of treatment.

### Pharmacotherapy

There are no reports of pharmacological treatment of pyromania. Because fire-setting may be frequently embedded in other psychiatric illness, therapeutic attention may be directed primarily to the underlying disorder. However, the dangerous nature of fire-setting requires that the behavior be controlled. Much in the same fashion that one would seek to educate impaired patients about the functional risks associated with their symptoms—and to establish boundaries of acceptable behavior—the fire-setting behavior must be directly addressed, even if it is not a core symptom of the associated disorder.

### Psychosocial Treatments

It has been estimated that up to 60% of childhood fire-setting is motivated by curiosity. Such behavior often responds to direct educational efforts. In children and adolescents, focus on interpersonal problems in the family and clarification of events preceding the behavior may help to control the behavior (Lowenstein 1989). The treatments described for fire-setting are largely behavioral or focused on intervening in family or intrapersonal stresses that may precipitate episode of fire-setting.

One technique combines overcorrection, satiation, and negative practice with corrective consequences. The child is supervised in constructing a controlled, small fire in a safe location. The fire is then extinguished by the child. Throughout the process, the parent verbally instructs the child in safety techniques.

The graphing technique has been used as the basis of several intervention programs with fire-setters. The psychiatrist and the patient agree on a goal of stopping the fire-setting behavior. The psychiatrist and the patient construct a graph that details the events, feelings, and behaviors associated with fire-setting episodes. These factors are described on a chronological line graph. The graph is utilized to help the patient see the cause-and-effect relationships between personal events, feelings, and subsequent behaviors. The specific intent is to educate patients so that they are able to identify the events that put them at risk for fire-setting. Then patients are equipped to label the feelings as a signal that may allow them to use alternative modes for discharging their feelings. This technique may help the individual curtail other maladaptive behaviors as well. Follow-up reports suggest that individuals who have successfully completed a graphing intervention may be at substantially lower risk for future fire-setting.

Relaxation training may be used (or added to graphing techniques) to assist in the development of alternative modes of dealing with the stress that may precede fire-setting.

Principles of cognitive–behavioral therapy have been recently applied to childhood fire-setting (Kolko 2001).

## Treatment of Comorbid Conditions

As noted earlier, fire-setting behavior may be associated with other mental conditions (mental retardation, conduct disorder, alcohol and other substance use disorders, personality disorders, and schizophrenia.) Usual treatment approaches for these conditions are followed. To protect the patient and others, additional precautions may be needed if the patient is at continued high risk for fire-setting in these conditions.

---

**Clinical Vignette 2**

A 34-year-old man came to a medical emergency department for the treatment of third-degree burns on his hands and face. He claimed to have been accidentally caught in a fire at a warehouse. Because of the patient's severe agitation and inability to explain the circumstances of the injury coherently, the treating surgeon asked that the patient be seen by a psychiatrist.

On meeting the psychiatrist the patient became even more severely agitated. He began to complain of the pain caused by his burns and was reluctant to speak with the psychiatrist. The patient insisted that he was in substantial pain and that he had no need to speak with "some shrink."

Because the patient was going to be admitted for medical monitoring, the psychiatrist withdrew, planning to visit the patient again the next day in his hospital room. The next day the young man was more amenable to an interview. At this time he seemed sad and, although anxious, less visibly agitated than he was on the preceding day. He no longer questioned the psychiatrist's purpose in visiting him and participated in a brief discussion about his burns, the pain they caused, and the misfortune he suffered, having been caught in a fire. The psychiatrist again decided to withdraw after this brief conversation. Despite the passive cooperation the patient offered, the psychiatrist was still impressed with how guarded he seemed about the question of the events that led up to the fire. The psychiatrist concluded that the patient seemed to want to avoid discussing the details and decided that several visits might be necessary to engage the patient sufficiently to obtain an adequate history.

On the following day the patient seemed relieved when the psychiatrist entered the room. He said that he had something to tell the psychiatrist. He then proceeded to describe a history of fascination with fire since age 16 years. He had set a couple of small fires in wastebaskets at that age and found himself drawn to trade magazines that specialized in fire control equipment. He would often walk by the local firehouse and tried to follow the fire crews when they responded to a fire alarm. For a number of years he was aware of a growing urge to set fires. He worried about this compulsion and managed to avoid acting on it.

In the past 3 years his forbearance began to erode. In that period he had set several fires in isolated parts of the city. He was careful to do so in areas where he knew few people might be caught in the fire. He tried to arrange circumstances in which the fire would be quickly discovered. Indeed, he reported one of the fires himself—both because he was fearful of the harm that might occur and because he had a great urge to see the firefighters arrive and battle the flames. In a recent fire a firefighter had been mildly injured. At that point he realized the dangers of his compulsion. Several days ago he went out to set another fire. He did not realize how quickly the fire would progress and he was injured. After telling the psychiatrist this story he expressed great relief that he finally had shared his shame with someone. He also expressed the hope that it would be understood that he suffered from a compulsion and asked the psychiatrist if there might be some way to reduce or erase the need to set fires. He realized he faced criminal prosecution but felt relieved that his behavior had been interrupted before another person was seriously hurt.

## Pathological Gambling

### Definition

Gambling as a behavior is common. Current estimates suggest that approximately 80% of the adult population in the US gamble. The amount of money wagered legally in the US grew from $17 billion in 1974 to $210 billion in 1988, an increase of more than 1,200%, making gambling the fastest growing industry in America (Lesieur and Rosenthal 1991). DSM-IV-TR, like DSM-III-R before it, covertly recognized the ubiquity of gambling behavior and the desire to gamble by the careful wording of criterion A for pathological gambling: "Persistent and recurrent maladaptive gambling behavior as indicated by five (or more) of the following." This definition of pathological gambling differs from some

**Pathological Gambling**

A. Persistent and recurrent maladaptive gambling behavior as indicated by five (or more) of the following:

   (1) is preoccupied with gambling (e.g., preoccupied with reliving past gambling experiences, handicapping or planning the next venture, or thinking of ways to get money with which to gamble)

   (2) needs to gamble with increasing amounts of money in order to achieve the desired excitement

   (3) has repeated unsuccessful efforts to control, cut back, or stop gambling

   (4) is restless or irritable when attempting to cut down or stop gambling

   (5) gambles as a way of escaping from problems or of relieving a dysphoric mood (e.g., feelings of helplessness, guilt, anxiety, depression)

   (6) after losing money gambling, often returns another day to get even ("chasing" one's losses)

   (7) lies to family members, therapist, or others to conceal the extent of involvement with gambling

   (8) has committed illegal acts such as forgery, fraud, theft, or embezzlement to finance gambling

   (9) has jeopardized or lost a significant relationship, job, or educational or career opportunity because of gambling

   (10) relies on others to provide money to relieve a desperate financial situation caused by gambling

B. The gambling behavior is not better accounted for by a manic episode.

other definitions of impulse control disorders not elsewhere classified, which are worded as "Failure to resist an impulse to." This difference implies that neither gambling behavior nor failure to resist an impulse to engage in it is viewed as pathological in and of itself. Rather, the maladaptive nature of the gambling behavior is the essential feature of pathological gambling and defines it as a disorder.

## Etiology and Pathophysiology

Pathological gambling has been included in DSM-III, DSM-III-R, and DSM-IV as a disorder of impulse con-

trol. Pathological gambling can also be viewed as an addictive disorder (Murray 1993), an affective spectrum disorder (McElroy et al. 1992) and an obsessive–compulsive spectrum disorder (Hollander et al. 1992) DSM-IV-TR maintains a close relationship between pathological gambling and addictive disorders in that several of the diagnostic criteria for pathological gambling were intentionally made to resemble criteria for substance dependence (Table 77–2).

The parallels between pathological gambling and addictive disorders are manifold. Pathological gambling has been viewed as the "pure" addiction, because it involves several aspects of addictive behavior without the use of a chemical substance. The parallels between substance dependence, in particular alcohol dependence, and pathological gambling have led to the successful adoption of the self-help group model of Alcoholics Anonymous to Gamblers Anonymous. Patterns of comorbidity also suggest a possible link between pathological gambling and addictions, in particular alcoholism. In addition to the comorbidity of pathological gambling and substance use disorders, family studies have demonstrated a familial clustering of alcoholism and pathological gambling. Ramirez and colleagues (1983) found that 50% of their patients with pathological gambling had a parent with alcoholism; other studies have also found high rates of a family history of substance dependence in patients with pathological gambling. There is also a greater prevalence of pathological gambling in parents of patients with pathological gambling.

The links between pathological gambling and affective disorders are also supported by family studies that demonstrate high rates of affective disorders in first-degree relatives of patients with pathological gambling (McElroy et al. 1992), as well as by high rates of comorbidity of pathological gambling and affective disorders. In addition, as noted by many authors and incorporated in the DSM-IV-TR criteria for pathological gambling, many patients with pathological gambling gamble as a way of relieving dysphoric moods (criterion A5), and cessation of gambling may be associated with depressive episodes in the majority of recovering gamblers (Linden 1986).

The links between pathological gambling and obsessive spectrum disorders are less clear. Although a popular name for pathological gambling is compulsive gambling, the vast majority of patients with pathological gambling do not experience the urge to gamble as ego-dystonic until late in the course of their illness, after they have suffered some of its consequences. The rates of comorbidity of pathological gambling and OCD and obsessive–compulsive personality disorder are not nearly as high as the rates of comorbidity of pathological gambling and affective and addictive disorders. Nevertheless, pathological gambling shares several characteristics with compulsions: it is repetitive, often has ritualized aspects, and is meant to relieve or reduce distress. Moreover, sporadic reports on the effectiveness of SSRIs in the treatment of pathological gambling suggest a possible link to obsessive spectrum disorders (Hollander et al. 1992).

**Neurotransmitter Function in Pathological Gambling.** The association between altered function of the serotonin

| Table 77-2 | Comparison of DSM-IV-TR Criteria for Pathological Gambling and Substance Dependence |
|---|---|

| Pathological Gambling | Substance Dependence |
|---|---|
| A. Persistent and recurrent maladaptive gambling behavior as indicated by at least five (or more) of the following: | A maladaptive pattern of substance use, leading to clinically significant impairment or distress, as manifested by three (or more) of the following: |
|    A1. Is preoccupied with gambling (e.g., preoccupied with reliving past gambling experiences, handicapping or planning the next venture, or thinking of ways to get money with which to gamble) | 5. A great deal of time is spent in activities necessary to obtain the substance or recover from its effects |
|    A2. Needs to gamble with increasing amounts of money to achieve the desired excitement | 1 (tolerance) (a). A need for markedly increased amounts of the substance to achieve intoxication or desired effect or (b). markedly diminished effect with continued use of the same amount of substance |
|    A3. Has repeated unsuccessful efforts to control, cut back, or stop gambling | 4. There is a persistent desire or unsuccessful attempts to cut down or control substance use |
|    A4. Is restless or irritable when attempting to cut down or stop gambling | 2 (withdrawal) (a). The characteristic withdrawal syndrome for the substance |
|    A5. Gambles as a way of escaping from problems or relieving a dysphoric mood | |
|    A6. After losing money gambling, often returns another day to get even ("chasing" one's losses) | 2 (withdrawal) (b). The same substance is taken to relieve or avoid withdrawal symptoms |
| | 3. The substance is often taken in larger amounts or over a longer period than was intended |
|    A7. Lies to family members, therapist, or others to conceal the extent of involvement with gambling | |
|    A8. Has committed illegal activities such as forgery, fraud, theft, or embezzlement to finance gambling | |
|    A9. Has jeopardized or lost a significant relationship, job, or educational opportunity because of gambling | 6. Important social, occupational, or recreational activities are given up or reduced because of substance use |
|    A10. Relies on others to provide money to relieve a desperate financial situation caused by gambling | |
| B. The gambling behavior is not better accounted for by a manic episode | |
| | 7. The substance use is continued despite knowledge of having a persistent or recurrent physical or psychological problem that is likely to have been caused or exacerbated by the substance |

*Source*: Adapted from American Psychiatric Association (2000) Diagnostic and Statistical Manual of Mental Disorders, 4th ed., Text Rev. APA, Washington DC.

neurotransmitter system and impulsive behaviors has focused attention on a potential role for serotonin function in the neurophysiology of pathological gambling. Several studies have provided data supporting such a link. These findings include: blunted prolactin response after intravenous administration of the serotonin reuptake inhibitor, clomipramine (Moreno et al. 1991), increased prolactin response after the administration of a serotonin agonist, m-CPP (DeCaria et al. 1996), low platelet MAO-B activity (a correlate central nervous system concentrations of the serotonin metabolite 5-HIAA) (Blanco et al. 1996, Carrasco et al. 1994). However, direct measure of cerebrospinal fluid 5-HIAA in pathological gamblers has yielded mixed results (Roy et al. 1988, Bergh et al. 1997, Ibanez et al. 2002). Preliminary data supports potential utility of serotonin reuptake inhibitor medications in the treatment of pathological gambling (Hollander et al. 1998, 2000, Ibanez et al. 2002). A potential role for noradrenergic function has been explored as well. In preliminary support for such a role, pathological gamblers have been shown to have higher urinary and cerebrospinal fluid concentrations of noradrenaline and metabolites (Roy et al. 1988, Bergh et al. 1997). In addition, increased growth hormone secretion, a measure of noradrenergic reactivity, has been found in response to oral administration of clonidine, an alpha-2-adrenergic agonist (Ibanez et al. 2002).

Because of the "addictive" aspects of pathological gambling—and the role that dopaminergic function plays in chemical addictions—attention has ben directed at dopamine function among pathological gamblers. Two available studies have yielded contradictory data (Roy et al. 1988, Bergh et al. 1997).

**Genetic Contribution.** The incidence of pathological gambling among first degree family members of pathological gamblers appears to be approximately 20% (Ibanez et al. 2002). Inherited factors may explain 62% of variance in the diagnosis (Eisen et al. 1998) and some of these genetic factors may also contribute to the risk for conduct disorder, antisocial personality disorder, and alcohol abuse (Eisen et al. 2001). At this time, early molecular genetics studies of pathological gamblers point to possible associated polymorphisms in genes that code for both serotonergic and dopaminergic factors (Ibanez et al. 2002).

**Psychodynamic Considerations.** Psychoanalytic theories of gambling were the first systematic attempts to account for pathological gambling. Erotization of the fear, tension, and aggression involved in gambling behavior, as well as themes of grandiosity and exhibitionism, were explored by several authors during the first quarter of the 20th century. Freud (1961) in his influential essay on Dostoyevsky, suggested that the pathological gambler actually gambled to lose, not to win, and traced the roots of the disorder to the ambivalence felt by the young man toward his father. The father, the object of his love, is not only loved but also hated, and this results in unconscious guilt. The gambler then loses to punish himself, in what Freud labeled "moral masochism." Freud also spoke of "feminine masochism" in which losing is a way of gaining love from the father, who will somehow reward the loser for loyalty. To lose is to suffer, and for the feminine masochist, suffering equals love. Interestingly, in the later spirit of DSM-IV-TR, Freud also conceptualized pathological gambling as an addiction and included it in a triad with alcoholism and drug dependence. He saw all three as manifestations of that primary addiction, masturbation, or at least masturbatory fantasies. Like most researchers after him, Freud focused only on male gamblers.

Bergler, a psychoanalyst who actually treated many patients with pathological gambling, expanded on Freud's idea that the pathological gambler gambles to lose (Lesieur and Rosenthal 1991). He traced the roots of this desire to lose to the rebellion of gamblers against the authority of their parents and against the parents' intrusive introduction of the reality principle into their lives. The rebellion causes guilt, and the guilt creates the need for self-punishment. Bergler thought that the gambler's characteristic aggression is actually pseudoaggression, a craving for defeat and rejection. He saw the gambler as one who perpetuates an adversarial relationship with the world. The dealer in the casino, the gambler's opponents at the card table, the stock exchange, and the roulette wheel are all unconsciously identified with the refusing mother or the rejecting father. Overall, psychoanalytic approaches to pathological gambling (Lesieur and Rosenthal 1991) generally conceptualized it as either a compulsive neurosis (Freud, Bergler, Rosenthal) or an impulse disorder (Fenichel). Fenichel focused on the gambler's entitlement and intense need to "get the stuff," an oral fixation. Several published case reports documented the successful treatment of pathological gambling by psychoanalysis.

Learning theories of pathological gambling focus on the learned and conditioned aspects of gambling and use the quantifiable nature of the behavior to test specific hypotheses. One hypothesis was that patients with pathological gambling crave the excitement and tension associated with their gambling, as evidenced by the fact that they are much more likely to place last-second wagers than are low-frequency gamblers, to prolong their excitement. Higher wagers placed by patients with pathological gambling also produce greater excitement, and greater amounts of money are required to achieve the same "buzz" over time, an observation incorporated in the diagnostic criteria for pathological gambling (criterion A2).

## Assessment and Differential Diagnosis

It is not difficult to diagnose pathological gambling once one has the facts. It is much more of a challenge to elicit the facts, because the vast majority of patients with pathological gambling view their gambling behavior and gambling impulses as ego-syntonic and may often lie about the extent of their gambling (criterion A7). Patients with pathological gambling may first seek medical or psychological attention because of comorbid disorders. Given the high prevalence of addictive disorders in pathological gambling and the increased prevalence of pathological gambling in those with alcoholism and other substance abuse, an investigation of gambling patterns and their consequences is warranted for any patient who presents with a substance abuse problem. Likewise, the high rates of comorbidity with mood disorders suggest the utility of investigating gambling patterns of patients presenting with an affective episode.

The spouses and significant others of patients with pathological gambling deserve special attention. Individuals with pathological gambling usually feel entitled to their behavior and often rely on their families to bail them out (criterion A10). As a consequence, it is often the spouse of the patient with pathological gambling who first realizes the need for treatment and who bears the consequences of the disorder. Lorenz (1981) conducted a survey of 103 wives of pathological gamblers who attended Gam-Anon meetings (for family members of patients with pathological gambling). She found that most spouses had to borrow money and were harassed or threatened by bill collectors. Most spouses physically assaulted the gambler, verbally abused their children, and experienced murderous or destructive impulses toward the gambler. Although the gamblers themselves appeared less violent than the general population norms, their spouses were more violent, possibly because of desperation and anger. Eleven percent of the spouses of patients with pathological gambling admitted to having attempted suicide, and this result was replicated in a later study. These findings have two main implications for the assessment of pathological gambling: first, the spouse may be a valuable and motivated informant who should be questioned about the patient's behavior, and second, spouses should be specifically asked about the effects of the patient's illness on their own well-being and functioning and about suicidal ideation and attempts and the control of their own impulsivity.

An important and understudied area is the clinical presentation of pathological gambling in women. Women constitute a third of all patients with pathological gambling in epidemiological studies. However, they are extremely underrepresented in treatment populations, and most psychoanalytic theories of pathological gambling ignore them completely. Part of this bias may be due to the fact that gambling carries a greater social stigma for women, that women gamblers are more likely to live and to gamble alone, and that treatment programs for pathological gambling in the US were first pioneered in Veterans Hospitals. Compared with men with pathological gambling, women with pathological gambling are more likely to be depressed and to gamble as an escape rather than because of a craving for action and excitement. Pathological gambling begins at a later age in female than in male gamblers, often after adult roles have been established. Big winning is usually less important than the need to impress. Women typically play less competitive forms of gambling in which luck is more important than skill, and they play alone. Their progression into the disorder is often more rapid, and the time between the onset of the disorder and the time they present for treatment is usually much shorter than for men (3 years compared with 20 years). The shorter duration makes for a better prognosis in treatment, but, unfortunately, few of the women with pathological gambling ever come to treatment.

The choice of gambling activities is dictated by local availability and cultural norms. Horseracing, cockfights, roulette, slot machines, casino card games, state-sponsored lotteries, and the stock market may all be used by the pathological gambler. Likewise, the extent of gambling considered normal varies across cultures. DSM-IV-TR approaches this issue by concentrating on the consequences of gambling rather than on its frequency and type.

The differential diagnosis of pathological gambling is relatively simple (Table 77–3). Pathological gambling should be differentiated from professional gambling, social gambling, and a manic episode. Social gambling, engaged in by the vast majority of adult Americans, typically occurs with friends or colleagues, lasts for a specified time, and is limited by predetermined acceptable losses. Professional gambling is practiced by highly skilled and disciplined individuals and involves carefully limited risks. Many individuals with pathological gambling may feel that they are actually professional gamblers. Chasing behavior and unplanned losses distinguish the pathological gamblers. Patients in a manic episode may exhibit a loss of judgment and excessive gambling resulting in financial disasters. A diagnosis of pathological gambling should be given only if a history of maladaptive gambling behavior exists at times other than during a manic episode. Problems with gambling may also occur in individuals with antisocial personality disorder. If criteria are met for both disorders, both can be diagnosed.

| Table 77–3 | Differential Diagnosis of Pathological Gambling |
| --- | --- |
| **Pathological Gambling Must Be Differentiated From** | **In Contrast to Pathological Gambling, the Other Condition** |
| Professional gambling | Is characterized by discipline and limited risk taking<br>Is intended to be a source of income |
| Social gambling | Usually occurs among friends<br>Is characterized by limited time spent on gambling and limited risk taking |
| Manic episode | Involves episodes of characteristic symptoms (e.g., flight of ideas)<br>Is characterized by symptoms that persist at times when individual is not gambling |

*Source*: First M and Frances A (eds) (1995) DSM-IV Handbook of Differential Diagnosis. American Psychiatric Press, Washington DC, pp. 196–197.

## Epidemiology and Comorbidity

### Prevalence and Incidence
Pathological gambling is considered to be the most common of the impulse control disorders not elsewhere classified. The number of people whose gambling behavior meets criteria for pathological gambling in the US is estimated to be between 2 million and 6 million (Volberg 1988). The prevalence of pathological gambling in several communities in the US has been assessed. Surveys conducted between 1986 and 1990 in Maryland, Massachusetts, New York, New Jersey, and California estimated the prevalence of "probable pathological gamblers" among the adult population to be between 1.2 and 2.3%. These states have a broad range of legal wagering opportunities and a heterogeneous population. Similar surveys in Minnesota and Iowa, states with limited legal wagering opportunities and more homogeneous populations, yielded prevalence rates of 0.9 and 0.1%, respectively (Rosenthal 1992). It thus appears that availability of gambling opportunities as well as demographic makeup may influence the prevalence of pathological gambling. A 1998 study of national prevalence, using DSM-IV-TR criteria, determined that the prevalence of pathological gambling was 1.2% (1.7% for men and 0.8% for women). In addition to these individuals who fulfilled DSM-IV-TR criteria, the researchers classified an addition 1.5% as "problem gamblers." The combined total of "pathological gamblers" and "problem gamblers" is 5.5 million adult Americans (Gerstein et al. 1999). During the past 20 years, many states have turned to lotteries as a way of increasing their revenues without increasing taxes. At this time, some form of gambling is legal in 47 of the 50 states, as well as in more than 90 countries worldwide. From 1975 to 1999 revenues from legal gambling in the US has risen from $3 to 58 billion (Volberg 2002). (Given the dramatic increase in the amounts of money wagered in legal gambling activities during the past 20 years, the prevalence and incidence of pathological gambling are expected to increase.)

It is estimated that women make up to one-third of all Americans with pathological gambling. Nevertheless, they are underrepresented in Gamblers Anonymous, in which only 2 to 4% of the members are women. This pattern is echoed in England and Australia, where women make up 7 and 10% of Gamblers Anonymous members, respectively. The reason for this discrepancy was postulated to be the greater social stigma attached to pathological gambling in women and the characteristic pattern of solitary gambling in women. Nonwhites and those with less than a high school education are more highly represented among pathological gamblers than in the general population. The demographic makeup of patients in treatment for pathological gambling differs substantially from the demographics of all patients with pathological gambling. Jewish persons are overrepresented in treatment settings and in Gamblers Anonymous, whereas women, minorities, and those younger than age 30 years are underrepresented in Gamblers Anonymous and in treatment (Lesieur and Rosenthal 1991).

### Comorbidity
Overall, patients with pathological gambling have high rates of comorbidity with several other psychiatric disorders and conditions. Individuals presenting for clinical treatment of pathological gambling apparently have impressive rates

of comorbidity. Ibanez and coworkers (2001) reported 62.3% of one group seeking treatment had a comorbid psychiatric disorder. The most frequent diagnosis they found were personality disorders (42%), alcohol abuse or dependence (33.3%), and adjustment disorders (17.4%).

**Mood Disorders.** There is evidence for extensive comorbidity of pathological gambling with major depressive disorder and with bipolar disorder. In several surveys, between 70 and 80% of all patients with pathological gambling also had mood symptoms that met criteria for a major depressive episode, a manic episode, or a hypomanic episode at some point in their life. More than 50% had recurrent major depressive episodes (Lesieur and Rosenthal 1991). A complicating factor is that recovering pathological gamblers may experience depressive episodes after cessation of gambling. In addition, some patients with pathological gambling may gamble to relieve feelings of depression (criterion A5). Despite criterion B for pathological gambling, which essentially precludes the diagnosis of pathological gambling if the behavior occurs exclusively during the course of a manic episode, many patients have a disturbance that meets criteria for both disorders because they gamble both during and between manic and hypomanic episodes. Between 32 and 46% of patients with pathological gambling were reported also to have mood symptoms that meet criteria for bipolar disorder, bipolar II disorder, or cyclothymic disorder (McElroy et al. 1992).

**Suicide.** Although data is not yet conclusive, a meaningful association between problem gambling and suicidal behavior and/or ideation appears to exist. Phillips and coworkers (1997) conclude that "Las Vegas, the premier US gambling setting, displays the highest levels of suicide in the nation, both for residents of Las Vegas and for visitors to that setting. In general, visitors to and residents of major gaming communities experience significantly elevated suicide levels. In Atlantic City, abnormally high suicide levels for visitors and residents appeared only after gambling casinos were opened. The findings do not seem to result merely because gaming settings attract suicidal individuals." In other reports, between 12 and 24% of patients with pathological gambling in various settings have had a history of at least one suicide attempt. In one study, 80% of patients with pathological gambling had a history of either suicide attempts or suicidal ideation (Lesieur and Rosenthal 1991).

**Substance Abuse and Dependence.** Studies of prevalence of comorbid substance use disorders yield widely varying results; from 9.9% for alcohol and other substance dependence (Gerstein et al. 1999) to 44% for alcohol dependence and 40% for illicit drug dependence (Bland et al. 1993, Cunningham-Williams et al. 1998). Using a structured instrument, between 5 and 25% of substance-abusing patients in several settings were found to meet criteria for pathological gambling and an additional 10 to 15% were considered to have "gambling problems" (Lesieur and Rosenthal 1991). Among individuals with pathological gambling, individuals with higher socioeconomic status (SES) are more likely to have concurrent problems with alcohol abuse then are gamblers with lower SES (Welte et al. 2001).

**Other Disorders.** Again, current data are inconclusive, but OCD, panic disorder, generalized anxiety disorder, and eating disorders have all been reported present in higher rates in patients with pathological gambling than in the general population. The reported prevalence of OCD among pathological gamblers ranges from 0.9% (Cunningham-Williams et al. 1998) to 16% (Bland et al. 1993). Narcissistic and antisocial personality disorders are believed to be overrepresented in patients with pathological gambling, and pathological narcissism is assumed by some psychoanalysts to underlie the entitlement displayed by many patients with pathological gambling. In addition, retrospective studies suggest that many patients with pathological gambling may have had symptoms that met criteria for attention-deficit/hyperactivity disorder as children (McElroy et al. 1992). In addition to psychiatric disorders, patients with pathological gambling may manifest greater prevalences of stress-related medical conditions, like peptic ulcer disease, hypertension, and migraine.

## Course

Pathological gambling usually begins in adolescence in men and later in life in women. The onset is usually insidious, although some individuals may be "hooked" by their first bet. There may be years of social gambling with minimal or no impairment followed by an abrupt onset of pathological gambling that may be precipitated by greater exposure to gambling or by a psychosocial stressor. The gambling pattern may be regular or episodic, and the course of the disorder tends to be chronic. Over time, there is usually a progression in the frequency of gambling, the amounts wagered, and the preoccupation with gambling and with obtaining money with which to gamble. The urge to gamble and gambling activity generally increase during periods of stress or depression, as an attempted escape or relief (criterion A5). Rosenthal (1992) described four typical phases in the course of a typical male patient with pathological gambling: winning, losing, desperation, and hopelessness (Linnoila et al. 1989).

### Typical Phases

**Winning.** Many male gamblers become involved with gambling because they are good at it and receive recognition for their early successes. Women with pathological gambling are less likely to have a winning phase. Traits that foster a winning phase and are typical of male patients with pathological gambling are competitiveness, high energy, ability with numbers, and interest in the strategy of games. The early winnings lead to a state in which a large proportion of the gambler's self-esteem derives from gambling, with accompanying fantasies of winning and spectacular success.

**Losing.** A string of bad luck or a feeling that losing is intolerable may be the precipitant of chasing behavior; previous gambling strategies are abandoned as the gambler attempts to win back everything all at once. The gambler experiences a state of urgency, and bets become more frequent and heavy. Debts accumulate, and only the most essential are paid. Covering up and lying about gambling become more frequent. As this is discovered, relationships with family members deteriorate. Losing gamblers use their own and their family's money, go through savings, take out loans, and finally exhaust all legitimate sources. Eventually, they cannot borrow any more, and faced with threats from creditors or loss of a job or marriage, they go to their family and finally confess. This results in the "bailout": debts are paid in return for a promise to stop or cut down gambling. Any remission, if achieved at all, is short-lived. After the bailout there is an upsurge of omnipotence; the gambler believes that it is possible to get away with anything, bets more heavily, and loses control altogether.

**Desperation.** This stage is reached when the gambler begins to do things that would previously be inconceivable: writing bad checks, stealing from an employer, or other illegal activities. Done once, these behaviors are much more likely to be repeated. The behavior is rationalized as a short-term loan with an intention to pay it back as soon as the winning streak arrives. The gambler feels just one step away from winning and solving all the problems. Attention is increasingly taken up with illegal loans and various scams to make money. The gambler becomes irritable and quick tempered. When reminded of responsibilities or put in touch with guilt feelings, the gambler responds with anger and projective blame. Appetite and sleep deteriorate and life holds little pleasure. A common fantasy at this stage is of starting life over with a new name and identity, the ultimate "clean slate."

**Hopelessness.** For some gamblers, there is a fourth stage in which they suddenly realize that they can never get even, but they no longer care. This is often a revelation, and the precise moment when it occurred is often remembered. From this point on, just playing is all that matters. Gamblers often acknowledge knowing in advance that they will lose and play sloppily so that they lose even if they have the right horse or a winning hand. They seek action or excitement for its own sake and gamble to the point of exhaustion.

Few gamblers seek help in the winning phase. Most seek help only during the later phases and only after a friend, family member, or employer has intervened. Two-thirds of the gamblers have committed illegal activities by then, and the risk of suicide increases as the gambler progresses through the phases of the illness.

## Prognosis

Without treatment, the prognosis of pathological gambling is poor. It tends to run a chronic course with increasing morbidity and comorbidity, gradual disruption of family and work roles and relationships, depletion of financial reserves, entanglement with criminals and the criminal justice system, and, often, suicide attempts. In the hands of an experienced psychiatrist, it is an "extremely treatable disorder" with a favorable prognosis (Rosenthal 1992). The difference between a poor and a good prognosis depends on treatment, and treatment depends on a diagnosis. As noted earlier, the diagnosis of pathological gambling is often missed in clinical settings because mental health professionals do not think to ask about it. Because most patients with pathological gambling do not see themselves as having a disorder and many of them do not even consider themselves as having a problem with gambling, collateral information from a family member may be extremely helpful.

## Treatment

### Overall Goals of Treatment

The goals of treatment of an individual with pathological gambling are the achievement of abstinence from gambling,

rehabilitation of the damaged family and work roles and relationships, treatment of comorbid disorders, and relapse prevention. This approach echoes the goals of treatment of an individual with substance dependence. There are many similarities and several important differences between the treatment of pathological gambling and the treatment of substance dependence. For most patients without severe acute psychiatric comorbidity, such as major depressive disorder with suicidal ideation or alcohol dependence with a history of delirium tremens, treatment may be given on an outpatient basis. Inpatient treatment in specialized programs may be considered if the gambler is unable to stop gambling, lacks significant family or peer support, or is suicidal, acutely depressed, multiply addicted, or contemplating some dangerous activity.

No standard treatment of pathological gambling has emerged. Despite many reports of behavioral and cognitive interventions for pathological gambling, there are minimal data available from well-designed or clearly detailed treatment studies (Petry 2002). Pharmacologic treatments (described further below) offer promise, but research-guided approaches are still insufficient to offer a standardized approach. Therefore, general approaches, based in clinical experience and available resources (such as Gamblers Anonymous or other support groups) should be considered.

The treatment of pathological gambling may consist of participation in Gamblers Anonymous, individual therapy, family therapy, treatment of comorbid disorders, and medication treatment. As is the case for substance dependence, the gambler needs to be abstinent to be accessible to any or all of these treatment modalities. For many gamblers, participation in Gamblers Anonymous is sufficient, and it is an essential part of most treatment plans. Gamblers Anonymous is a 12-step group built on the same principles as Alcoholics Anonymous. It utilizes empathic confrontation by peers who struggle with the same impulses and a group approach. Gam-Anon is a peer support group for family members of patients with pathological gambling. Extensive data are lacking, but overall Gamblers Anonymous appears somewhat less effective than Alcoholics Anonymous in achieving and maintaining abstinence.

Individual therapy is often useful as an adjunct to Gamblers Anonymous. Rosenthal (1992) stressed that to maintain abstinence and use Gamblers Anonymous successfully, many gamblers need to understand why they gamble. Therapy involves confronting and teasing out the vicissitudes of the patient's sense of omnipotence and dealing with the various self-deceptions, the defensive aspects of the patient's lying, boundary issues, and problems involving magical thinking and reality. Relapse prevention involves knowledge and avoidance of specific triggers. In addition to psychodynamic therapy, behavioral treatment of pathological gambling has been proposed, with imagined desensitization achieving better rates of remission than aversive conditioning.

The greatest differences between the treatment of pathological gambling and other addictions are in the area of family therapy. Because relapse may be difficult to detect (there is no substance to be smelled on the patient's breath, no dilated or constricted pupils, no slurred speech or staggered gait) and because of a long history of exploitative behavior by the patient, the spouse and other family members tend to be more suspicious of, and angry at, the patient with pathological gambling compared with families of alcoholic patients. Frequent family sessions are often essential to offer the gambler an opportunity to make amends, learn communication skills, and deal with preexisting intimacy problems. In addition, the spouse and other family members have often acquired their own psychiatric illnesses during the course of the patient's pathological gambling and need individualized treatment to recover.

## Medication

Although research reports of the pharmacological treatment of pathological gambling have begun to emerge, there are still, as yet, insufficient data to come to any conclusions about the utility of medication. The effectiveness of selective serotonin reuptake inhibitors has been examined in a limited number of double-blind trials, but do show promise. The opiate antagonist, naltrexone, has also shown preliminary evidence of efficacy. Doses at the higher end of the usual treatment range should be considered with both these classes of agents. The use of mood stabilizers (lithium and carbamazepine) has been the subject of a limited number of reports. At this time, no clear guidelines for pharmacologic treatment have emerged (Grant and Kim 2002, Haller and Hinterhuber 1994, Hollander et al. 2000, Kim and Grant 2001, Kim et al. 2001).

---

Clinical Vignette 3

Mr. Z is a 44-year-old automobile mechanic who is married and has two adolescent children. He was referred for inpatient treatment from the emergency department of his local hospital after an overdose of a full bottle of over-the-counter sleeping pills taken as a suicide attempt. He took the pills in the setting of a major depressive episode without psychotic features. This was his first psychiatric contact. During his initial evaluation, Mr. Z admitted to several past depressive episodes for which he did not seek treatment and which resolved spontaneously. He also admitted to a history of alcohol abuse and stated that his drinking may have escalated recently. His family history was significant for a father with alcohol dependence and a mother with bipolar disorder. Mr. Z was treated as an inpatient with fluoxetine and improved rapidly, with full resolution of his suicidal ideation and other depressive symptoms.

Two days before his planned discharge from the hospital, a family meeting was held. During the meeting, his treatment team was surprised when his wife announced that she refused to let Mr. Z return home before "the other problem" was taken care of. At this point, a parallel history was taken and revealed that Mr. Z has had a problem with "excessive gambling" for the last 25 years. His wife meant that Mr. Z gambled with money that he did not have and went on gambling sprees that ended only when he lost all the money available to him and exhausted his current abilities to borrow money. During such episodes he had lost the family home, was caught stealing spare parts from his job and was fired, and borrowed several thousand dollars from his in-laws and his sister, which he was unable to repay. More recently he became involved with loan sharks, who were now threatening him physically. His suicide attempt followed a threat to hurt him and his family if his debts were not paid.

Mr. Z began to gamble when he was 16 years old and stated that "there is nothing else like it." He frequented off-track-betting establishments and considered himself an expert in horseracing. His only social acquaintances were other gamblers, and he found other recreational activities dull and unsatisfying. When he was confronted with this history, Mr. Z felt that his wife was "being hysterical." He admitted that he loved to gamble but described himself as a professional gambler and cited several occasions on which he won significant amounts of money. He was not interested in any kind of treatment but agreed to attend Gamblers Anonymous if his extended family would help him out of his current financial problems.

During the course of a 2-year follow-up, Mr. Z continued to gamble and lose money. He stopped going to meetings. He was fired from his job again, discontinued his medication, became depressed, and started drinking. At that time, he came to treatment with his wife, who was attending Gam-Anon and began seeing a psychiatrist for the treatment of her own mild depression. Mr. Z agreed to an arrangement in which his wife would have complete power of attorney over his financial affairs. His participation in Gamblers Anonymous and Alcoholics Anonymous became a prerequisite for his continued living at home. He was again given fluoxetine and began a course of individual psychotherapy with biweekly family sessions. For the first time in his adult life, Mr. Z was able to abstain from gambling for a period of 3 months.

## Trichotillomania

### Definition

The essential feature of trichotillomania is the recurrent failure to resist impulses to pull out one's own hair. Resulting hair loss may range in severity from mild (hair loss may be negligible) to severe (complete baldness and

---

**DSM-IV-TR Criteria** 312.39

**Trichotillomania**

A. Recurrent pulling out of one's hair resulting in noticeable hair loss.

B. An increasing sense of tension immediately before pulling out the hair or when attempting to resist the behavior.

C. Pleasure, gratification, or relief when pulling out the hair.

D. The disturbance is not better accounted for by another mental disorder and is not due to a general medical condition (e.g., a dermatological condition).

E. The disturbance causes clinically significant distress or impairment in social, occupational, or other important areas of functioning.

Reprinted with permission from the Diagnostic and Statistical Manual of Mental Disorders, Fourth Edition, Text Revision. Copyright 2000 American Psychiatric Association.

involving multiple sites on the scalp or body). Individuals with this condition do not want to engage in the behavior, but attempts to resist the urge result in great tension. Thus, hair-pulling is motivated by a desire to reduce this dysphoric state. In some cases, the hair-pulling results in a pleasurable sensation, in addition to the relief of tension. Tension may precede the act or may occur when attempting to stop. Distress over the symptom and the resultant hair loss may be severe.

## Etiology and Pathophysiology

The etiology of trichotillomania is unknown. The phenomenological similarities between trichotillomania and OCD have prompted speculations that the pathophysiology of the two conditions may be related. The apparent association between altered serotonergic function and OCD has guided attention toward the possible role of serotonergic function in the underlying cause of trichotillomania. Thus, interest has been spurred in examining serotonergic function in patients with trichotillomania. As yet, however, only limited laboratory investigations have emerged.

Ninan and coworkers (1992) obtained CSF from eight individuals with trichotillomania and measured concentrations of the primary serotonin metabolite 5-HIAA. Baseline concentrations of 5-HIAA did not differ from those of control subjects, nor was there a relationship between the baseline 5-HIAA concentration and the severity of trichotillomania symptoms. However, seven of these patients were then treated with SSRIs (fluoxetine and clomipramine). The researchers found a negative correlation between baseline CSF 5-HIAA concentration and the degree of improvement after treatment. This observation does not, however, directly support a conclusion that altered serotonin function is etiologically related to trichotillomania.

Swedo and associates (1991) used positron emission tomography to measure regional brain glucose in three groups: patients with trichotillomania, patients with OCD, and normal control subjects. Like the patients with OCD, those with trichotillomania had altered patterns of glucose utilization compared with normal control subjects. However, the regional patterns of altered glucose utilization were not the same in the trichotillomania and OCD groups.

A morphometric MRI study compared volumes of brain structures in 10 female subjects with trichotillomania versus 10 normal controls. Left putamen volume was found to be significantly smaller in trichotillomania subjects as compared with normal matched controls (O'Sullivan et al. 1997).

Performance on particular neuropsychological tests may offer an additional basis for defining the underlying neuropathological process in individuals with trichotillomania. In addition, because impaired performance on such tests may indicate altered function in particular brain regions, they may help localize brain regions in which altered function may be associated with trichotillomania.

On the basis of such tests, Rettew and colleagues (1991) have suggested that patients with trichotillomania may have deficits in spatial processing. Patterns of deficits on such tests may provide further support for a relationship between trichotillomania and other psychiatric conditions. Rettew and coworkers found similarities between subjects with trichotillomania and subjects with OCD.

Keuthen and colleagues (1996) also speculated that individuals with trichotillomania would demonstrate alterations in neuropsychological function similar to individuals with OCD, who have been shown to have impairments in executive, visual–spatial and nonverbal memory function. In a study of 20 subjects with trichotillomania and 20 matched healthy-controls, they demonstrated the presence of impaired performance on two of these three parameters (nonverbal memory and executive function). These results were interpreted as supporting the presumed relationship between trichotillomania and OCD.

However, Stanley and colleagues (1997), in their study of 21 trichotillomania subjects (compared with 17 healthy controls) did not find evidence of deficits in visual–spatial ability, motor function, or executive function. But, differences were found on measures of divided attention, leading to the suggestion that trichotillomania might be more properly conceptualized as an affective or anxiety-based disorder, and that any demonstrated similarities with OCD may be related to their shared overlap with anxiety/affective disorders.

Additional support for a possible relationship between trichotillomania and OCD may come from family history studies. In a preliminary investigation of psychiatric diagnoses among first-degree relatives of probands with trichotillomania, Lenane and associates (1992) found increased frequencies (compared with normal control subjects) of OCD, as well as mood and anxiety disorders. Bienvenue and Colleagues (2000) examined 300 first-degree relatives of 343 patients with OCD, and found increased rates of "grooming" conditions (e.g., nail-biting, skin-picking, trichotillomania), and other impulse control disorders (e.g., kleptomania, pathological gambling, pyromania).

In summary, few data are available to support any particular model of the etiological pathophysiology of trichotillomania. Early studies point to some alteration of brain activity. Inconsistent support has been found in these early explorations for a relationship with OCD.

## Assessment and Differential Diagnosis

### Presentation

Typically, the person complaining of unwanted hair-pulling is a young adult or the parent of a child who has been seen pulling out hair (Winchel 1992). Hair-pulling tends to occur in small bursts that may last minutes to hours. Such episodes may occur once or many times each day. Hairs are pulled out individually and may be pulled out rapidly and indiscriminately. Often, however, the hand of the individual may roam the afflicted area of scalp or body, searching for a shaft of hair that may feel particularly coarse or thick. Satisfaction with having pulled out a complete hair (shaft and root) is frequently expressed. Occasionally the experience of hair-pulling is described as quite pleasurable. Some individuals experience an itch-like sensation in the scalp that is eased by the act of pulling. The person may then toss away the hair shaft or inspect it. A substantial number of people then chew or consume (trichophagia) the hair. Hair-pulling is most commonly limited to the eyebrows and eyelashes. The scalp is the next most frequently afflicted site. However, hairs in any location of the body may be the focus of hair-pulling urges, including facial, axillary, chest, pubic, and even perineal hairs.

Anxiety is almost always associated with the act of hair-pulling. Such anxiety may occur in advance of the hair-pulling behavior. A state of tension may occur spontaneously—driving the person to pull out hair in an attempt to reduce dysphoric feelings. Varying lengths of time must pass before the tension abates. Consequently, the amount of hair that may be extracted in an episode varies from episode to episode and from person to person. Frequently, hair-pulling begins automatically and without conscious awareness. In such circumstances, individuals discover themselves pulling out hairs after some have already been pulled out. In these situations, dysphoric tension is associated with the attempt to stop the behavior.

Circumstances that seem to predispose to episodes of hair-pulling include both states of stress and, paradoxically, moments of particular relaxation. Frequently hair-pulling occurs when at-risk individuals are engaged in a relaxing activity that promotes distraction and ease (e.g., watching television, reading, talking on the phone).

It is common for hair-pullers to report that the behavior does not occur in the presence of other people. A frequent exception may be that many pull hair in the presence of members of the nuclear family.

Some individuals have urges to pull hairs from other people and may sometimes try to find opportunities to do so surreptitiously (such as initiating bouts of play fighting). There have been reports of affected individuals pulling hairs from pets, dolls, and other fibrous materials, such as sweaters or carpets (Tabatabai 1981).

The distress that usually accompanies trichotillomania varies in severity. Concerns tend to focus on the social and vocational consequences of the behavior. Themes of worry include fear of exposure, a feeling that "something is wrong with me," anxiety about intimate relationships, and sometimes inability to pursue a vocation. Because certain kinds of work, such as reading and writing at a desk, seem to precipitate episodes of hair-pulling, some afflicted individuals make career choices based on the avoidance of desk work. Leisure activities that may involve a risk of exposure (ranging from gymnastics class to sexual intimacy) may be avoided.

Patterns of hair-pulling behavior among children are less well described. Usually, the parent observes a child pulling out hair and may note patches of hair loss. Children may sometimes be unaware of the behavior or may, at times, deny it. Childhood trichotillomania has been reported to be frequently associated with thumb-sucking or nail-biting (Friman 1987). It has been suggested that trichotillomania with onset in early childhood may occur frequently with spontaneous remissions. Consequently, some have recommended that trichotillomania in early childhood may be considered a benign habit with a self-limited course. However, many individuals who present with chronic trichotillomania in adulthood report onset in early childhood (Reeve et al. 1992).

## Assessment

In general, the diagnosis of trichotillomania is not complicated. The essential symptom—recurrently pulling out hair in response to unwanted urges—is easily described by the patient. When the patient acknowledges the hair-pulling behavior and areas of patchy hair loss are evident, the diagnosis is not usually in doubt. Problems in diagnosis may arise when the diagnosis is suspected but the patient denies it. Such denial may occur in younger individuals and some adults. When the problem is suspected but denied by the patient, a skin biopsy from the affected area (see later) may aid in making the diagnosis.

### The Psychiatric Interview

The psychiatrist should carefully inquire into the nature of the distress and concerns that may be present in a person with this problem. Although the cosmetic impact may appear slight, distress may be severe. Concerns about disclosure, anticipation of social rejection, and concerns about limitations in career choices are frequent and may result in chronic dysphoria. The psychiatrist should be aware of the embarrassment that may accompany inspection of the hair loss, particularly when located in regions of the body that are not usually accessible in the course of a standard psychiatric examination. Because of the apparent frequency of comorbid mood disorders (past or current), the interviewer should pay special attention to the presence of these features.

### Physical Examination and Laboratory Findings

Areas of hair loss can be marked by complete alopecia or can appear diffusely thinned or "ratty." Altered scalp appearance can range from small areas of thinned hair to complete baldness. For unclear reasons, several patterns of scalp loss are typical. Frequently, coin-sized areas of alopecia are noted at the vertex or at temporal or occipital regions. Among more severely afflicted people a peculiar pattern, so-called tonsure trichotillomania, may appear: a completely bald head except for a narrow, circular fringe circumscribing the outer boundary of the scalp, producing a look reminiscent of medieval friars.

Despite the hair loss, most individuals with this condition have no overtly unusual appearance on cursory inspection. If the hair loss is not covered by clothing or accessories, artful combing of hair or use of eyeliner and false eyelashes may easily hide it. The ease with which the condition may often be hidden may explain the general underappreciation of its apparent frequency and potential associated distress.

### Associated Laboratory Findings

Histological findings are considered characteristic and may aid diagnosis when it is suspected despite denial by the individual. Biopsy samples from involved areas may have the following features. Short and broken hairs are present. The surface of the scalp usually shows no evidence of excoriation. On histological examination, normal and damaged follicles are found in the same area, as well as an increased number of catagen (i.e., nongrowing) hairs. Inflammation is usually minimal or absent. Some hair follicles may show signs of trauma (wrinkling of the outer root sheath). Involved follicles may be empty or contain a deeply pigmented keratinous material. The absence of inflammation distinguishes trichotillomania-induced alopecia from alopecia areata, the principal condition in the differential diagnosis (Mehregan 1970, Muller 1990).

## Specific Age-, Culture-, and Gender-Related Features

Secondary avoidance of intimate relationships, which occurs among some individuals with trichotillomania, may be exacerbated for women in cultures in which physical appearance is weighted differently for men and women. Avoidance of sports activities, in which disguised hair loss can be revealed, may also have gender-related effects in cultures in which athletic participation has different social meanings for men and women. Although culture-based expectations regarding appearance may make hair loss a greater burden for women, women may have a greater opportunity to hide hair loss through the use of wigs, hats, and scarves.

Reliable data regarding sex ratio in the general population are not yet available. It has long been suggested that women greatly outnumber men. But, as noted earlier, surveys of college students suggest that the true ratio may be near parity. Although the apparent preponderance of women presenting for treatment may reflect the true sex ratio, it may alternatively reflect self-selection for presentation for treatment. Self-selection may reflect gender-related, culturally based attitudes regarding appearance, as well as an acceptance of normative hair loss among men. Because such gender-related distinctions may not be made by parents who are concerned about hair-pulling habits in their children, the apparent equal presentation of male and female children may more accurately reflect the true sex ratio.

For many women hair-pulling may worsen during the premenstrual phase (Keuthen et al. 1997).

## Differential Diagnosis

Among individuals presenting with alopecia who complain of hair-pulling urges, the diagnosis is not usually in doubt. When patients deny hair-pulling, other (dermatological) causes of alopecia should be considered. These include alopecia areata, male pattern hair loss, chronic discoid lupus erythematosus, lichen planopilaris, folliculitis decalvans, pseudopelade, and alopecia mucinosa.

Trichotillomania is not diagnosed when hair-pulling occurs in response to a delusion or hallucination.

Many people twist and play with their hair. This may be exacerbated in states of heightened anxiety but does not qualify for a diagnosis of trichotillomania.

Some individuals may present with features of trichotillomania but hair damage may be so slight as to be virtu- ally undetectable, even under close examination. In such conditions the disorder should be diagnosed only if it results in significant distress to the individual.

Trichotillomania may have a short, self-limited course among children and may be considered a temporary habit. Therefore, among children the diagnosis should be reserved for situations in which the behavior has persisted during several months.

## Epidemiology and Comorbidity

### Prevalence and Incidence

Trichotillomania was long thought to be an uncommon condition, often accompanied by other psychiatric conditions. Although definitive studies of frequency rates in the general population are still lacking, three surveys of college-age samples support the emerging view that trichotillomania is quite common. In two of these samples, totaling approximately 3000 undergraduate students, a lifetime incidence of self-identified trichotillomania (reaching full symptom criteria as described in DSM-III-R) was present in about 1% of the respondents. Some features of the condition—but not meeting full criteria—were identified in an additional 1 to 2% (Rothbaum et al. 1993, Christenson et al. 1991a).

These may be underestimates of the lifetime incidence of the disorder. Had these studies applied DSM-IV-TR criteria, which have become slightly less restrictive than DSM-III-R criteria, the rates might be higher. In addition, because onset may occur later in life than the mean ages of individuals in these groups, the true lifetime incidence would probably be higher. Moreover, these samples consist of a selected population—largely first-year college students—and may not reflect the general population. Nonetheless, these studies indicate that the condition is likely to be far more common than previously assumed. But definitive, controlled studies of the prevalence of the condition have not yet been performed.

### Comorbidity

Individuals with trichotillomania have increased risk for mood disorders (major depressive disorder, dysthymic disorder) and anxiety symptoms (Table 77–4). The frequency of specific anxiety disorders (such as generalized anxiety disorder and panic disorders as well as OCD) may be increased as well. Although it has been suggested that trichotillomania in childhood or adolescence is associated

| Table 77–4 | Lifetime Comorbidity and Trichotillomania | | | | | |
|---|---|---|---|---|---|---|
| Reference | No Axis I | Anxiety Disorder | Mood Disorder | PSUD* | OCD | Eating Disorder |
| Christenson et al. (1991a) (n = 60) | 18% | 57% | 65% | 22% | 15% | 20% |
| Winchel et al. (1992) (n = 20) | 45% | 5% | 45% | 15% | 5% | 0% |
| Swedo et al. (1989) (n = 14) | ? | 43% | 57% | 29% | † | 0% |

*PSUD, Psychoactive substance use disorder.

†Patients with OCD were excluded from this sample, as were patients with psychosis.

with schizophrenia or severe disruptions of the family system, no systematically collected data support such conclusions.

## Course

The age at onset typically ranges from early childhood to young adulthood. Peak ages at presentation may be bimodal, with an earlier peak about age 5 to 8 years among children in whom it has a self-limited course, whereas among patients who present to clinicians in adulthood the mean age at onset is approximately 13 years (Rothbaum et al. 1993, Winchel 1992, Swedo et al. 1989). Initial onset after young adulthood is apparently uncommon. There have been reports of onset as early as 14 months of age and as late as 61 years.

Trichotillomania may be one of the earliest occurring conditions in psychiatry. Some parents insist that their child began pulling hair before 1 year of age. When trichotillomania begins before age 6 years it tends to be a milder condition. It often responds to simple interventions and may be self-limited, with a duration of several weeks to several months, even if not treated. It often occurs in association with thumb-sucking. In some cases it remits spontaneously when therapeutic attention is directed at concurrent, severe thumb-sucking (Watson and Allen 1993). It has been suggested that trichotillomania in childhood may be associated with severe intrapsychic or familial psychiatric conditions. But there is no reliable evidence that supports such a conclusion. Indeed, some have suggested that because it may be common and frequently self-limiting, it should be considered a normal behavior among young children.

Some individuals have continuous symptoms for decades. For others, the disorder may come and go for weeks, months, or years at a time. Sites of hair-pulling may vary over time. Circumscribed periods of hair-pulling (weeks to months) followed by complete remission are reported among children.

Progression of the condition appears to be unpredictable. Waxing and waning of the severity of hair-pulling and number of hair-pulling sites occur in most individuals. It is not known which factors may predict a protracted and unremitting course.

## Prognosis

Because of the unavailability of longitudinal studies of trichotillomania, generalizations about prognosis cannot be made. Patients who present in research clinics typically have histories of many years (up to decades) of hair-pulling. Presentation after age 40 years appears to be far less common than in the previous three decades of life, suggesting that the condition may eventually remit spontaneously, even when untreated. It is likely that the persistent cases seen in research environments reflect the more severe end of the spectrum. As noted earlier, trichotillomania in children may often be a time-limited phenomenon.

## Treatment

### Treatment Goals

Treatment of trichotillomania typically occurs in an outpatient setting. Eradication of hair-pulling behavior is the general focus of treatment. Distress, avoidant behaviors, and cosmetic impairment are secondary to the hair-pulling behavior and would be likely to remit if the hair-pulling behavior is controlled. However, if sufficient control of hair-pulling cannot be attained, treatment goals should emphasize these associated problems as well. Even if hair-pulling persists, therapeutic interventions may be targeted at reducing secondary avoidance and diminishing distress.

Treatment may be considered in three phases:

**Initial Contact.** The diagnosis is made and the patient and psychiatrist agree on a strategy that may incorporate both pharmacological and psychological interventions. If distress is severe, supportive interventions should be immediately considered in anticipation of incomplete treatment response or of a delay of weeks to months before interventions may be beneficial.

**Acute Treatment.** Even when treatment of hair-pulling behavior is optimally successful, there may be a delay of several weeks to months before adequate control is attained. Therefore, the acute treatment phase may be prolonged.

**Maintenance.** It is not known how long patients must maintain active treatment interventions to prevent relapse. It should be anticipated that a substantial number of patients require ongoing treatment for an extended time. Pharmacological treatments may need to be maintained for open-ended periods. Behavioral or hypnotic intervention may require periodic "booster shots" to support continuation of benefits.

### Psychiatrist–Patient Relationship

It is important to bear in mind the particular nature of embarrassment that often accompanies this condition. Several factors contribute to feelings of shame for many people with trichotillomania. When hair-pulling has had its onset in childhood or adolescence, there is often a history of the hair-pulling being treated as a family secret. Patients have been frequently castigated by parents or spouses for lack of self-control. In addition, there may be a feeling that the problem is largely cosmetic, causing some individuals to fear they do not have the "right" to utilize health resources for its treatment. This may also be manifest as fears of having their problem minimized or of being derided for seeking help. It is helpful for the psychiatrist to share with patients an understanding that the problem pervades their daily life and may result in meaningful distress and functional inhibition.

A variety of treatment approaches have been advocated for trichotillomania. However, there have, as yet, been few controlled studies of the efficacy of any treatment approach. A number of investigations of the use of antidepressants with specific inhibition of serotonin reuptake (i.e., fluoxetine and clomipramine) have yielded mixed results (Rothbaum et al. 1993, Winchel et al. 1992, Swedo et al. 1989 Stein et al. 1997 Jaspers 1996). A multimodal approach, simultaneously utilizing several complementary treatment options, may turn out to be the most effective approach for most patients.

While a number of treatment options can be currently offered to individuals with trichotillomania, the durability of long-term outcomes is unclear. Keuthen and colleagues (1998, 2001) followed a group of hair-pullers who had "naturalistic" treatment in the community. Treatments were pharmacologic, behavioral or both. Among those who had benefits, improvements were often lost over time, and persistent treatment and ongoing treatment was common over the course of several years.

## Stress Management

Before embarking on a course of treatment, the psychiatrist and the patient should first consider the course and severity of the individual's condition. Because early remission may occur in cases of recent onset, mild trichotillomania of short duration does not necessarily require immediate intervention. In particular, if the hair-pulling first occurred during a period of stress, the behavior may spontaneously diminish as the stressful circumstances abate. In such circumstances, therapeutic attention may best be directed toward examining and seeking to diminish the basis for stress. Teaching alternative stress reduction methods may be useful in reducing recent-onset trichotillomania. However, when individuals with trichotillomania present to the psychiatrist, it is often likely to have been a persistent condition and may have been present for many years or decades. Among such patients, stress reduction may also be useful in reducing trichotillomania but complete remission is less likely.

## Pharmacotherapy

A variety of medications have been used in the treatment of trichotillomania. In 1989, initial reports appeared demonstrating the apparent benefits of fluoxetine and clomipramine. Clomipramine was found to be superior to desipramine (Swedo et al. 1989). Fluoxetine was reported beneficial in open treatment (Winchel et al. 1992). Although reports for more than 60 patients have subsequently added support for the use of these medications, the two double-blind studies in which fluoxetine has been compared with placebo did not demonstrate any improvement compared to placebo (Christenson et al. 1991b, Streichenwein and Thornby 1995). Fluvoxamine (Stanley et al. 1997b), citalopram (Stein et al. 1997), and venlafaxine (Ninan et al. 1998) have been reported to be efficacious in open trials. Although further controlled studies of SSRIs are needed, the use of such medications would be a prudent first step if a pharmacological approach has been agreed upon.

Initial evidence of improvement is usually first reported by the patient as greater awareness of the inclination to pull hair. This is usually followed by an ability to abort hair-pulling episodes more quickly than in the past. The ability to resist the urge follows. In cases with a good outcome, the inclination to pull diminishes and may eventually disappear. Patients who pull from several sites may find that the rate of improvement varies from site to site.

There have been conflicting reports of early relapse of symptoms in some patients treated with clomipramine or fluoxetine. Although good maintenance of benefit has been reported for some patients 6 months and longer after the initiation of treatment, early relapse after several weeks to months has been reported as well. Keuthen and coworkers (2001) have provided long-term data on maintenance of response over time. Following a group of individuals who had varying forms of treatment (pharmacologic and psy-

chological) for several years after an index evaluation, the authors concluded that initial improvement was common, but over time there was an increase in symptom scores and self-esteem scores worsened in the group over time. This problem remains to be further evaluated in long-term treatment studies. If early relapse does turn out to be common, it would distinguish trichotillomania from depression and OCD, in which, once established, medication benefits are often well maintained as long as medication is continued. Optimal duration of treatment for well-treated individuals is also still unknown. In accordance with standards developed for the treatment of other conditions, it would be reasonable to continue medication for at least 6 months before tapering. Reinitiation of treatment may be necessary.

## Other Medications

Christenson and coworkers (1991c) have reported successful treatment with lithium. This observation awaits replication.

Because trichotillomania is often accompanied by other manifestations of anxiety—and for many individuals is exacerbated by stressful conditions—attempts at treatment with anxiolytic agents may be useful. There are no published reports of such treatments.

Adjunctive treatment with pimozide, a neuroleptic agent, has been advocated for some patients who are refractory to other medications (Stein and Hollander 1992). The potential benefits of neuroleptics has been reported now by several authors (Potenza et al. 1998, Gabriel 2001, Gupta and Gupta 2000, Epperson et al. 1999). Most of these reports describe individuals for whom SSRIs provided insufficient benefits. The addition of atypical neuroleptics much improved their outcomes. The greater margin of safety and tolerability associated with atypical neuroleptics have made this a more viable treatment option.

Van Ameringen and colleagues (1999) described the use of haloperidol in nine patients with trichotillomania. Six had previously failed treatment with SSRIs. Eight of nine patients responded to the haloperidol. The possible superiority of neuroleptics prompted these authors to speculate that trichotillomania may be similar to Tourette's syndrome (TS), which responds preferentially to neuroleptics.

## Psychosocial Treatments

**Behavioral Treatment.** Various behavioral techniques have been tried (Diefenbach et al. 2000). The most successful technique, habit reversal, is based on designing competitive behaviors that should inhibit the behavior of hair-pulling (Azrin and Nunn 1977, Azrin et al. 1980, Rosenbaum and Ayllon 1981). For example, if hair-pulling requires raising the arm to the scalp and contracting the muscles of the hand to grasp a hair, the behaviorist may design a behavioral program in which the patient is taught to lower the arm and extend the muscles of the hand. As with behavioral techniques in general, these interventions are most successful when the patient is strongly motivated and compliant. In addition, the treating psychiatrist should be experienced in the use of such techniques. If necessary, a referral should be made to such an experienced individual.

Modified behavioral approaches have been described for children and adolescents (Vitulano et al. 1992, Rapp et al. 1998).

**Cognitive Behavioral Therapy (CBT).** CBT has been developed for, and applied to, individuals with trichotillomania. At this time, the potential for the efficacy of this treatment approach appears good. Ninan and colleagues (2000) compared CBT to clomipramine in the treatment of trichotillomania. The authors reported that CBT had a dramatic effect in reducing symptoms of trichotillomania and was significantly more effective than clomipramine ($P = 0.016$) or placebo ($P = 0.026$). Clomipramine resulted in symptom reduction greater than that with placebo, but the difference fell short of statistical significance. Placebo response was minimal.

**Hypnotherapy.** There are no formal studies of the use of hypnosis for trichotillomania, but there are many published reports of beneficial treatment (Barabasz 1987, Cohen et al. 1999, Fabbri and Dy 1974, Kohen 1996, Rowen 1981, Zalsman et al. 2001). Benefits may be variable. Some patients may have dramatic improvement. For some who improve, the benefits may be short-lived. As with behavioral interventions, the benefits of this approach are sometimes dependent on a highly motivated patient who can regularly carry out self-hypnotic measures as instructed by the psychiatrist. Some patients who have obtained partial benefits from either hypnosis or medication do well when both treatments are combined. Successful use of hypnotherapy for children with trichotillomania has also been reported (Cohen et al. 1999).

**Dynamic Psychotherapy.** Many psychoanalytically oriented descriptions of individuals with trichotillomania have been published. These reports generally describe the psychodynamic formulations of individual cases and should not be the basis for generalizations about most individuals with trichotillomania. Although patients with trichotillomania may benefit from exploration and attempts to reduce intrapsychic conflict, the literature does not provide persuasive evidence of the efficacy of this approach in reducing hair-pulling.

**Self-help and Other Groups.** Self-help groups for patients with trichotillomania have appeared. Some are based in the structure of other 12-step programs. Some patients appear to experience meaningful reduction in hair-pulling symptoms after beginning participation in such a group. Although the efficacy of such groups in reducing symptoms remains to be established, most patients with trichotillomania can benefit from meeting other individuals with similar symptoms. Because of the lack of general awareness of trichotillomania, these individuals frequently believe that they are "oddball" individuals with a behavior that is unique. Many have experienced parental condemnation for the behavior and have been frequently castigated for a "habit" that may be viewed by others as under their voluntary control. The experience of meeting others with the condition is extremely supportive for such individuals and may help to reduce the attendant stress while supporting self-esteem. Where programs specifically oriented toward trichotillomania may not be generally available, these individuals may benefit from groups oriented toward OCD.

## Treatment of Comorbid Conditions

Depression, dysthymic disorder, and anxiety symptoms occur frequently in patients with trichotillomania. Successful treatment of depression may not be associated with reduction in trichotillomania. If depression or dysthymic disorder is present and independently provides an indication for medication, one of the antidepressants discussed earlier should be chosen. If fluoxetine is used, the psychiatrist should be aware that a dose that is sufficient for reduction of the depressive symptoms may not be sufficient for reduction of trichotillomania. If panic disorder is present, either medication may still be used, but fluoxetine may initially exacerbate panic attacks in such patients and initiation of treatment at low doses (2.5–5 mg/day) should be considered. With slow titration upward, the patient should generally be able to tolerate usual doses with concomitant amelioration of the panic disorder. Combined treatment with anxiolytics may be useful for some and may contribute to the reduction in symptoms of trichotillomania. Other conditions that may be present, such as OCD or eating disorders, may require special attention. Although fluoxetine may be useful for patients with eating disorders, medication treatment alone is unlikely to be adequate and the usual multimodal approaches for the treatment of bulimia nervosa or anorexia are appropriate. OCD may respond to treatment directed at trichotillomania, but adjunctive behavioral treatment of symptoms of OCD may be desirable.

## Demographical Features

When trichotillomania presents in early childhood, as discussed earlier, the condition may be likely to be inherently self-limited. Often, all that may be necessary is to draw the child's attention to the behavior in some systematic way and to clarify for the child that the behavior is undesirable. Such methods include daily application of a nonmedicinal ointment to the affected region and reminding the child that the purpose is elimination of the hair-pulling habit. Some suggest that the child be given the responsibility of applying the ointment with parental supervision. Others suggest that parents should monitor the child as much as possible and respond with reminders that the hair should not be pulled and rewards with verbal encouragement for ceasing to pull hair. There have been no systematic studies of the benefits of such interventions, but dermatologists who specialize in the treatment of children have noted that hair-pulling behavior may frequently disappear within a few weeks of initiating such an approach. In circumstances in which childhood trichotillomania is more persistent, the parent and psychiatrist are faced with a dilemma. More elaborate behavioral interventions, such as habit reversal, should be tried. This, however, may be difficult with a child. Rosenbaum and Ayllon (1981) have described a modified version of habit reversal that may be employed with children. Hypnosis has been also used in the treatment of habit disorders in children. Medication should be cautiously considered in the treatment of childhood trichotillomania. Although medication may be useful, the absence of data supporting the benefits of such treatments in children indicates a conservative approach. If medication is considered, the use of medication in the treatment of childhood OCD should serve as a guideline.

Should the psychiatrist be presented with trichotillomania in a person of advanced age, special attention should be paid to usual concerns regarding the use of these medications in the elderly. Lower doses of medication should be considered because of potential altered pharmacokinetics in older persons. Medications with anticholinergic side effects (such as clomipramine) may present greater hazards for the older person. Sedative-hypnotic anxiolytics should be used sparingly because of greater vulnerability to cognitive side effects and the increased risk of falling.

Women of childbearing potential (perhaps the majority of individuals who may present for treatment) should be advised regarding the potential risks of these medications to a developing fetus. If the patient is pregnant or considering pregnancy, behavioral treatments may be favored.

The psychiatrist should be sensitive to the interaction between cultural values and trichotillomania. Women of certain cultures may be more prone to distress if trichotillomania is perceived as a hindrance to achieving valued goals, such as marriage. It should also be noted that in some communities, wigs and other hair accessories are generally acceptable and may present a comfortable means of diminishing the cosmetic impact of hair loss. In other communities, such accoutrements may themselves draw undesired attention.

## Refractory Response or Nonresponse to Initial Treatment

Because research in the treatment of trichotillomania is still limited, it is not possible to recommend an initial best treatment for all patients. However, the decision is often determined by available resources. Support groups may not be easily found in many areas. Hypnotherapy and behavioral therapy may be more easily available, but psychiatrists with these skills may not be experienced in the specific techniques used in this condition. Pharmacological interventions may be more readily available. Wherever possible, simultaneous multimodal interventions should be considered. Pharmacological, behavioral, and hypnotic interventions, which may each be only partially useful, may be synergistic when used in combination.

If therapy with a single medication is not successful, the psychiatrist may consider augmenting one agent with another. Augmentation strategies in the treatment of trichotillomania have not been studied. General principles of augmentation used in the treatment of depression or OCD may be considered. There may be particular benefit in combining anxiolytic agents (such as buspirone or clonazepam) with an SSRI antidepressant. As noted above, the advent of atypical neuroleptics may offer a new and possibly efficacious treatment option. Despite the increasing safety of these medications, caution should be used in the introduction of a neuroleptic for the treatment of a persistent condition.

---

Clinical Vignette 4

Mr. G, a 32-year-old podiatrist, began pulling out hairs in his second year of college. He had always been a generally anxious person and thought of it as a nervous habit. Never particularly concerned about his appearance and noting the familial disposition to male pattern hair loss, he felt resigned to eventual baldness and thought little about it. He noted that his hair-pulling tended to be worse in a variety of circumstances: before examinations, after a breakup with a girlfriend, while studying, and while watching television. He thought the last circumstance surprising. The others seemed to be situations of understandable stress, but television relaxed him. Indeed, at those times he was hardly aware of it until he would find his hands roaming searchingly through his scalp and would then find a small pile of hairs beside him on the sofa. Occasionally an acquaintance would comment—with varying degrees of tact—on the ratty appearance of his hair, particularly above the left temple. Nevertheless, he was still not too concerned. He did note a progression of the habit until he was pulling from virtually every spot on his body where hair grew, including his perineum.

Despite Mr. G's relative lack of concern, his new wife was not so resigned to the habit. She could not deny the mild revulsion she felt when she saw the range of locations from which he pulled hair. (In the beginning of their courtship, she was aware of only the thinned scalp.) She insisted that he go to a psychiatrist.

Mr. G's new psychiatrist tried a variety of interventions. Noting Mr. G's general anxiety, the psychiatrist instructed him in relaxation techniques, while exploring with him the sources of stress in his life. This was not too helpful. They then embarked on a course of medication trials, including three different SSRIs. There was encouraging improvement at first, but a partial relapse occurred and the benefits were limited. The psychiatrist then heard about a local therapist who led a group therapy for people with trichotillomania and also practiced hypnotic techniques for the problem. With some hesitancy, Mr. G joined the group. He was initially uncomfortable, being the only man in the group, and he did not identify with many of the concerns expressed by the women. But he settled in, became an active participant, and was surprised to find that his hair-pulling diminished further. He found that he was pulling from fewer sites and was able to abort hair-pulling episodes more quickly. Fortified by the partial successes and encouraged by the other group members, he went to a behavioral psychologist, who used a technique called habit reversal to supply him with a repertoire of skills he could employ to control urges to pull his hair. Finally, with this multimodal approach (medication, hypnosis, and group and behavioral therapy) his hair-pulling virtually disappeared. He had occasional relapses when under significant stress, but by and large he was relieved of his symptom. He and his wife thought the substantial efforts he had made to rid himself of the problem were worthwhile.

## Comparison of DSM-IV/ICD-10 Diagnostic Criteria

The ICD-10 Diagnostic Criteria for Research do not include diagnostic criteria for intermittent explosive disorder. It is included in ICD-10 as an "other habit and Impulse Control Disorder."

The ICD-10 Diagnostic Criteria for Research and the DSM-IV-TR criteria for kleptomania, pyromania, and trichotillomania are essentially equivalent.

Finally, the ICD-10 Diagnostic Criteria for Research for pathological gambling are monothetic (i.e., A plus B plus C plus D are required) whereas the DSM-IV-TR criteria set is polythetic (i.e., 5 out of 10 required) with different items. Furthermore, the ICD-10 criteria specify "two or more episodes of gambling over a period of at least 1 year," whereas DSM-IV-TR does not specify a duration.

## References

American Psychiatric Association (2000) Diagnostic and Statistical Manual of Mental Disorders, 4th ed., Text Rev. APA, Washington DC.

Azrin NA and Nunn R (1977) Habit Control in a Day. Simon & Schuster, New York.

Azrin NS, Nunn RG, and Frantz SE (1980) Treatment of hair-pulling (trichotillomania): A comparitive study of habit reversal and negative practice training. J Behav Ther Exp Psychiatr 11, 13–20.

Baer L (1994) Factor analysis of symptom subtypes of obsessive–compulsive disorder and their relation to personality and tic disorders. J Clin Psychiatr 55, 18–23.

Barabasz M (1987) Trichotillomania: A new treatment. Int J Clin Exp Hypn 35, 146–154.

Bars DR, Heyrend FL, Simpson CD, et al. (2001) Use of visual evoked-potential studies and EEG data to classify aggressive, explosive behavior of youths. Psychiatr Serv 52, 81–86.

Beldoch M (1991) Stolen objects as transitional objects. Am J Psychiatr 148, 1754.

Bergh C, Eklund T, Sodersten P, et al. (1997) Altered dopamine function in pathological gambling. Psychol Med 27, 473–475.

Bienvenu OJ, Samuels JF, Riddle MA, et al. (2000) The relationship of obsessive–compulsive disorder to possible spectrum disorders: Results from a family study. Biol Psychiatr 48, 287–293.

Blanco C, Orensanz-Munoz L, Blanco-Jerez C, et al. (1996) Pathological gambling and platelet MAO activity: A psychobiological study. Am J Psychiatr 153, 119–121.

Bland RC, Newman SC, Orn H, et al. (1993) Epidemiology of pathological gambling in Edmonton. Can J Psychiatr 38, 108–112.

Brandford J and Dimock J (1986) A comparative study of adolescents and adults who wilfully set fires. Psychiatr J Univ Ottawa 11, 228–234.

Budman CL, Bruun RD, Park KS, et al. (1998) Rage attacks in children and adolescents with Tourette's disorder: A pilot study. J Clin Psychiatr 59, 576–580.

Budman CL, Bruun RD, Park KS, et al. (2000) Explosive outbursts in children with Tourette's disorder. J Am Acad Child Adolesc Psychiatr 39, 1270–1276.

Burstein A (1992) Fluoxetine-lithium treatment for kleptomania. J Clin Psychiatr 53, 28–129.

Carrasco JL, Saiz-Ruiz J, Hollander E, et al. (1994) Low platelet monoamine oxidase activity in pathological gambling. Acta Psychiatr Scand 90, 427–431.

Chiswick D (1976) Shoplifting, depression and an unusual intracranial lesion (a case report). Med Sci Law 16, 266–268.

Christenson GA, Mackenzie TB, and Mitchell JE (1991a) Characteristics of 60 adult chronic hair pullers. Am J Psychiatr 148, 365–370.

Christenson GA, Mackenzie TB, Mitchell JE, et al. (1991b) A placebo-controlled, double-blind crossover study of fluoxetine in trichotillomania. Am J Psychiatr 148, 1566–1571.

Christenson GA, Popkin MK, Mackenzie TB, et al. (1991c) Lithium treatment of chronic hair-pulling. J Clin Psychiatr 52, 116–120.

Cohen HA, Barzilai A, and Lahat E (1999) Hypnotherapy: An effective treatment modality for trichotillomania. Acta Paediatr 88, 407–410.

Coid J (1984) Relief of diazepam-withdrawal syndrome by shoplifting. Br J Psychiatr 145, 552–554.

Cunningham-Williams RM, Cottler LB, Compton WM, et al. (1998) Taking chances: Problem gamblers and mental health disorders—results from the St. Louis Epidemiologic Catchment Area Study. Am J Pub Health 88, 1093–1096.

DeCaria CM, Hollander E, Grossman R, et al. (1996) Diagnosis, neurobiology, and treatment of pathological gambling. J Clin Psychiatr 57, 80–83; discussion 83–84.

DeJong J, Virkkunen M, and Linnoila M (1992) Factors associated with recidivism in a criminal population. J Nerv Ment Dis 180, 543–550.

Diefenbach GJ, Reitman D, and Williamson DA (2000) Trichotillomania: A challenge to research and practice. Clin Psychol Rev 20, 289–309.

Eisen SA, Lin N, Lyons MJ, et al. (1998) Familial influences on gambling behaviour: An analysis of 3359 twin pairs. Addiction 93, 1375–1384.

Eisen SA, Slutske WS, Lyons MJ, et al. (2001) The genetics of pathological gambling. Semin Clin Neuropsychiatr 6, 195–204.

Epperson CN, Fasula D, Wasylink S, et al. (1999) Risperidone addition in serotonin reuptake inhibitor-resistant trichotillomania: Three cases. J Child Adolesc Psychopharmacol 9, 43–49.

Esquirol E (1838) Des Maladies Mentales. Bailliere, Paris.

Fabbri R Jr. and Dy AJ (1974) Hypnotic treatment of trichotillomania: Two cases. Int J Clin Exp Hypn 22, 210–215.

Felthous AR, Bryant SG, Wingerter CB, et al. (1991) The diagnosis of intermittent explosive disorder in violent men. Bull Am Acad Psychiatr Law 19, 71–79.

Fenichel O (1945) The Psychoanalytic Theory of Neurosis. WW Norton, New York.

First M and Frances A (eds) (1995) DSM-IV Handbook of Differential Diagnosis. American Psychiatric Press, Washington DC, pp. 196–197.

Fishbain DA (1987) Kleptomania as risk-taking behavior in response to depression. Am J Psychother 41, 598–603.

Freud S (1955) Beyond the pleasure principle. In The Standard Edition of the Complete Psychological Works of Sigmund Freud, Vol. 18, Strachey J (ed). Hogarth Press, London, pp. 7–64. (Originally published in 1920)

Freud S (1961) Dostoevsky and parricide. In The Standard Edition of the Complete Psychological Works of Sigmund Freud, Vol. 21, Strachey J (ed). Hogarth Press, London.

Friman PC and Hove G (1987) Apparent covariation between child habit disorders: Effects of successful treatment for thumb-sucking on untargeted chronic hair-pulling. J Appl Behav Anal 20, 421–425.

Gabriel A (2001) A case of resistant trichotillomania treated with risperidone-augmented fluvoxamine. Can J Psychiatr 46, 285–286.

Gauthier J and Pellerin D (1982) Management of compulsive shoplifting through covert sensitization. J Behav Ther Exp Psychiatr 13, 73–75.

Geller JL (1987) Firesetting in the adult psychiatric population. Hosp Comm Psychiatr 38, 501–506.

Geller JL and Bertsch G (1985) Fire-setting behavior in the histories of a state hospital population. Am J Psychiatr 142, 464–468.

Gerstein DR, Volberg RA, Harwood R, et al. (1999) Gambling Impact and Behavior Study: Report to the National Gambling Impact Study Commission. National Opinion Research Center at the University of Chicago, Chicago, IL.

Glover JH (1985) A case of kleptomania treated by covert sensitization. Br J Clin Psychol 24, 213–214.

Goldman MJ (1991) Kleptomania: Making sense of the nonsensical. Am J Psychiatr 148, 986–996.

Grant JE and Kim SW (2002) Pharmacotherapy of pathological gambling. Psychiatr Ann 32, 186–191.

Guidry LS (1969) Use of a covert punishing contingency in compulsive stealing. J Behav Ther Exp Psychiatr 6, 169.

Gupta MA and Gupta AK (2000) Olanzapine is effective in the management of some self-induced dermatoses: Three case reports. Cutis 66, 143–146.

Haller R and Hinterhuber H (1994) Treatment of pathological gambling with carbamazepine. Pharmacopsychiatry 27, 129.

Herzog DB, Keller MB, Sacks NR, et al. (1992) Psychiatric comorbidity in treatment-seeking anorexics and bulimics. J Am Acad Child Adolesc Psychiatr 31, 810–818.

Hollander E, DeCaria CM, Finkell JN, et al. (2000) A randomized double-blind fluvoxamine/placebo crossover trial in pathologic gambling. Biol Psychiatr 47, 813–817.

Hollander E, DeCaria CM, Mari E, et al. (1998) Short-term single-blind fluvoxamine treatment of pathological gambling. Am J Psychiatr 155, 1781–1783.

Hollander E, Frenkel M, Decaria C, et al. (1992) Treatment of pathological gambling with clomipramine. Am J Psychiatr 149, 710–711.

Hudson JI and Pope HG (1990) Affective spectrum disorder: Does antidepressant response identify a family of disorders with a common pathophysiology? Am J Psychiatr 147, 552–564.

Ibanez A, Blanco C, and Saiz-Ruiz J (2002) Neurobiology and genetics of pathological gambling. Psychiatr Ann 32, 181–185.

Ibanez A, Blanco C, Donahue E, et al. (2001) Psychiatric comorbidity in pathological gamblers seeking treatment. Am J Psychiatr 158, 1733–1735.

Janet P (1911) La Kleptomanie et al. depression mentale. J Psychol Norm Pathol 8, 97–103.

Jaspers JP (1996) The diagnosis and psychopharmacological treatment of trichotillomania: A review. Pharmacopsychiatry 29, 115–120.

Kavoussi R, Armstead P, and Coccaro E (1997) The neurobiology of impulsive aggression. Psychiatr Clin N Am 20, 395–403.

Keuthen NJ, Fraim C, Deckersbach T, et al. (2001) Longitudinal follow-up of naturalistic treatment outcome in patients with trichotillomania. J Clin Psychiatr 62, 101–107.

Keuthen NJ, O'Sullivan RL, Goodchild P, et al. (1998) Retrospective review of treatment outcome for 63 patients with trichotillomania. Am J Psychiatr 155, 560–561.

Keuthen NJ, O'Sullivan RL, Hayday CF, et al. (1997) The relationship of menstrual cycle and pregnancy to compulsive hair-pulling. Psychother Psychosom 66, 33–37.

Keuthen NJ, Savage CR, O'Sullivan RL, et al. (1996) Neuropsychological functioning in trichotillomania. Biol Psychiatr 39, 747–749.

Keutzer CS (1972) Kleptomania: A direct approach to treatment. Br J Med Psychol 45, 159–163.

Khan K and Martin IC (1977) Kleptomania as a presenting feature of cortical atrophy. Acta Psychiatr Scand 56, 168–172.

Khantzian EJ and Mack JE (1983) Self-preservation and the care of the self. Ego instincts reconsidered. Psychoanal Stud Child 38, 209–232.

Kim SW and Grant JE (2001) The psychopharmacology of pathological gambling. Semin Clin Neuropsychiatr 6, 184–194.

Kim SW, Grant JE, Adson DE, et al. (2001) Double-blind naltrexone and placebo comparison study in the treatment of pathological gambling. Biol Psychiatr 49, 914–921.

Kohen DP (1996) Hypnotherapeutic management of pediatric and adolescent trichotillomania. J Dev Behav Pediatr 17, 328–334.

Kolko DJ (2001) Efficacy of cognitive–behavioral treatment and fire safety education for children who set fires: Initial and follow-up outcomes. J Child Psychiatr 42, 359–369.

Kolko DJ and Kazdin AE (1988) Parent–child correspondence in identification of firesetting among child psychiatric patients. J Child Psychol Psychiatr 29, 175–184.

Kuperman S, Kramer J, and Loney J (1988) Enzyme activity and behavior in hyperactive children grown up. Biol Psychiatr 24, 375–383.

Lee S (1994) The heterogeneity of stealing behaviors in Chinese patients with anorexia nervosa in Hong Kong. J Nerv Ment Dis 182, 304–307.

Lenane MC, Swedo SE, Rapoport JL, et al. (1992) Rates of obsessive–compulsive disorder in first degree relatives of patients with trichotillomania: A research note. J Child Psychol Psychiatr 33, 925–933.

Lesieur HR and Rosenthal RJ (1991) Pathological gambling: A review of the literature. J Gambling Stud 7, 5–39.

Linden RD, Pope HG Jr., and Jonas JM (1986) Pathological gambling and major affective disorder: Preliminary findings. J Clin Psychiatr 47, 201–203.

Linnoila M, De Jong J, and Virkkunen M (1989) Family history of alcoholism in violent offenders and impulsive fire setters. Arch Gen Psychiatr 46, 613–616.

Lion JR (1992) The intermittent explosive disorder. Psychiatr Ann 2, 64–66.

Lorenz V (1981) Differences found among Catholic, Protestant, and Jewish families of pathological gamblers. In Fifth National Conference on Gambling and Risk Taking, Lake Tahoe, CA.

Lowenstein LF (1989) The etiology, diagnosis and treatment of the fire-setting behaviour of children. Child Psychiatr Hum Dev 19, 186–194.

Marks I (1990) Behavioural (nonchemical) addictions. Br J Addict 85, 1389–1394.

Marzagao LR (1972) Systemic desensitization treatment of kleptomania. J Behav Ther Exp Psychiatr 3, 327–328.

Mattes JA (1990) Comparative effectiveness of carbamazepine and propranolol for rage outbursts. J Neuropsychiatr Clin Neurosci 2, 159–164.

McElroy SL (1999) Recognition and treatment of DSM-IV intermittent explosive disorder. J Clin Psychiatr 60, 12–16.

McElroy SL, Hudson JI, Phillips KA, et al. (1993) Clinical and theoretical implications of a possible link between obsessive–compulsive and impulse control disorders. Depression 1, 121–132.

McElroy SL, Hudson JI, Pope HG, et al. (1991a) Kleptomania: Clinical characteristics and associated psychopathology. Psychol Med 21, 93–108.

McElroy SL, Hudson JI, Pope HG Jr., et al. (1992) The DSM-III-R impulse control disorders not elsewhere classified: Clinical characteristics and relationship to other psychiatric disorders. Am J Psychiatr 149, 318–327.

McElroy SL, Keck PE Jr., Pope HG Jr., et al. (1989) Pharmacological treatment of kleptomania and bulimia nervosa. J Clin Psychopharmacol 9, 358–360.

McElroy SL, Pope HG Jr., Hudson JI, et al. (1991b) Kleptomania: A report of 20 cases. Am J Psychiatr 148, 652–657.

McElroy SL, Soutullo CA, Beckman DA, et al. (1998) DSM-IV intermittent explosive disorder: A report of 27 cases. J Clin Psychiatr 59, 203–210; quiz 211.

McIntyre AW and Emsley RA (1990) Shoplifting associated with normal-pressure hydrocephalus: Report of a case. J Geriatr Psychiatr Neurol 3, 229–230.

Mehregan AH (1970) Trichotillomania. A clinicopathologic study. Arch Dermatol 102, 129–133.

Mendez MF (1988) Pathological stealing in dementia. J Am Geriatr Soc 36, 825–826.

Monopolis S and Lion JR (1983) Problems in the diagnosis of intermittent explosive disorder. Am J Psychiatr 140, 1200–1202.

Moreno I, Saiz-Ruiz J, and Lopez-Ibor JJ (1991) Serotonin and gambling dependence. Hum Psychopharmacol Clin Exp 6, 9–12.

Muller SA (1990) Trichotillomania: A histopathologic study in sixty-six patients. J Am Acad Dermatol 23, 56–62.

Murray JB (1993) Review of research on pathological gambling. Psychol Rep 72, 791–810.

Ninan PT, Knight B, Kirk L, et al. (1998) A controlled trial of venlafaxine in trichotillomania: Interim phase I results. Psychopharmacol Bull 34, 221–224.

Ninan PT, Rothbaum BO, Marsteller FA, et al. (2000) A placebo-controlled trial of cognitive–behavioral therapy and clomipramine in trichotillomania. J Clin Psychiatr 61, 47–50.

Ninan PT, Rothbaum BO, Stipetic M, et al. (1992) CSF 5-HIAA as a predictor of treatment response in trichotillomania. Psychopharmacol Bull 28, 451–455.

O'Sullivan GH and Kelleher MJ (1987) A study of fire-setters in the southwest of Ireland. Br J Psychiatr 151, 818–823.

O'Sullivan RL, Rauch SL, Breiter HC, et al. (1997) Reduced basal ganglia volumes in trichotillomania measured via morphometric magnetic resonance imaging. Biol Psychiatr 42, 39–45.

Petry NM (2002) Psychosocial treatments for pathologiocal gambling: Current status and future directions. Psychiatr Ann 32, 192–196.

Phillips DP, Welty WR, and Smith MM (1997) Elevated suicide levels associated with legalized gambling. Suicide Life-Threat Behav 27, 373–378.

Potenza MN, Wasylink S, Epperson CN, et al. (1998) Olanzapine augmentation of fluoxetine in the treatment of trichotillomania. Am J Psychiatr 155, 1299–3000.

Prins H, Tennent G, and Trick K (1985) Motives for arson (fire raising). Med Sci Law 25, 275–278.

Puri BK, Baxter R, and Cordess CC (1995) Characteristics of fire-setters. A study and proposed multiaxial psychiatric classification. Br J Psychiatr 166, 393–396.

Raine A, Buchsbaum MS, Stanley J, et al. (1994) Selective reductions in prefrontal glucose metabolism in murderers. Biol Psychiatr 36, 365–373.

Ramirez LF, McCormick RA, Russo AM, et al. (1983) Patterns of substance abuse in pathological gamblers undergoing treatment. Addict Behav 8, 425–428.

Rapp JT, Miltenberger RG, Long ES, et al. (1998) Simplified habit reversal treatment for chronic hair-pulling in three adolescents: A clinical replication with direct observation. J Appl Behav Anal 31, 299–302.

Reeve EA, Bernstein GA, and Christenson GA (1992) Clinical characteristics and psychiatric comorbidity in children with trichotillomania. J Am Acad Child Adolesc Psychiatr 31, 132–138.

Repo E, Virkkunen M, Rawlings R, et al. (1997) Criminal and psychiatric histories of Finnish arsonists. Acta Psychiatr Scand 95, 318–323.

Rettew DC, Cheslow DL, Rapoport JL, et al. (1991) Neuropsychological test performance in trichotillomania: A further link with obsessive–compulsive disorder. J Anx Disord 5, 225–235.

Rosenbaum MS and Ayllon T (1981) The habit-reversal technique in treating trichotillomania. Behav Ther 12, 473–481.

Rosenthal RJ (1992) Pathological gambling. Psychiatr Ann 22, 72–78.

Rothbaum BO, Shaw L, Morris R, et al. (1993) Prevalence of trichotillomania in a college freshman population. J Clin Psychiatr 54, 72–73.

Rowen R (1981) Hypnotic age regression in the treatment of a self-destructive habit: Trichotillomania. Am J Clin Hypn 23, 195–197.

Roy A, Adinoff B, Roehrich L, et al. (1988) Pathological gambling. A psychobiological study. Arch Gen Psychiatr 45, 369–373.

Schwartz HJ (1992) Psychoanalytic psychotherapy for a woman with diagnoses of kleptomania and bulimia. Hosp Comm Psychiatr 43, 109–110.

Shapiro AK and Shapiro E (1992) Evaluation of the reported association of obsessive–compulsive symptoms or disorder with Tourette's disorder. Compr Psychiatr 33, 152–165.

Siever LJ, Kahn RS, Lawlor BA, et al. (1991) Critical issues in defining the role of serotonin in psychiatric disorders. Pharmacol Rev 43, 509–525.

Soltys SM (1992) Pyromania and firesetting behaviors. Psychiatr Ann 22, 79–83.

Staner L and Mendlewicz J (1998) Heredity and role of serotonin in aggressive impulsive behavior. Encephale 24, 355–364.

Stanley M and Mann JJ (1988) Biological factors associated with suicide. In Review of Psychiatry, Vol. 7, Frances AJ and Hales RE (eds). American Psychiatric Press, Washington DC.

Stanley MA, Breckenridge JK, Swann AC, et al. (1997a) Fluvoxamine treatment of trichotillomania. J Clin Psychopharmacol 17, 278–283.

Stanley MA, Hannay HJ, and Breckenridge JK (1997b) The neuropsychology of trichotillomania. J Anx Disord 11, 473–488.

Stein DJ and Hollander E (1992) Low-dose pimozide augmentation of serotonin reuptake blockers in the treatment of trichotillomania. J Clin Psychiatr 53, 123–126.

Stein DJ, Bouwer C, and Maud CM (1997) Use of the selective serotonin reuptake inhibitor citalopram in treatment of trichotillomania. Eur Arch Psychiatr Clin Neurosci 247, 234–236.

Stein DJ, Hollander E, and Liebowitz MR (1993) Neurobiology of impulsivity and the impulse control disorders. J Neuropsychiatr Clin Neurosci 5, 9–17.

Streichenwein SM and Thornby JI (1995) A long-term, double-blind, placebo-controlled crossover trial of the efficacy of fluoxetine for trichotillomania. Am J Psychiatr 152, 1192–1196.

Swedo SE, Leonard HL, Rapoport JL, et al. (1989) A double-blind comparison of clomipramine and desipramine in the treatment of trichotillomania (hair-pulling). N Engl J Med 321, 497–501.

Swedo SE, Rapoport JL, Leonard HL, et al. (1991) Regional cerebral glucose metabolism of women with trichotillomania. Arch Gen Psychiatr 48, 828–833.

Tabatabai SE and Salari-Lak M (1981) Alopecia in dolls! Cutis 28, 206.

Turnbull JM (1987) Sexual relationships of patients with kleptomania. South Med J 80, 995–998.

Van Ameringen M, Mancini C, Oakman JM, et al. (1999) The potential role of haloperidol in the treatment of trichotillomania. J Affect Disord 56, 219–226.

Virkkunen M and Linnoila M (1993) Brain serotonin, type II alcoholism and impulsive violence. J Stud Alcohol (Suppl 11), 163–169.

Virkkunen M, Goldman D, Nielsen DA, et al. (1995) Low brain serotonin turnover rate (low CSF 5-HIAA) and impulsive violence. J Psychiatr Neurosci 20, 271–275.

Virkkunen M, Nuutila A, Goodwin FK, et al. (1987) CSF monoamine metabolites in male arsonists. Arch Gen Psychiatr 3, 241–247.

Virkkunen M, Rawlings R, Tokola R, et al. (1994) CSF biochemistries, glucose metabolism, and diurnal activity rhythms in alcoholic, violent offenders, fire setters, and healthy volunteers. Arch Gen Psychiatr 51, 20–27.

Vitulano LA, King RA, Scahill L, et al. (1992) Behavioral treatment of children and adolescents with trichotillomania. J Am Acad Child Adolesc Psychiatr 31, 139–146.

Volberg RA (2002) The epidemiology of pathological gambling. Psychiatr Ann 32, 171–178.

Volberg RA and Steadman HJ (1988) Refining prevalence estimates of pathological gambling. Am J Psychiatr 145, 502–505.

Watson TS and Allen KD (1993) Elimination of thumb-sucking as a treatment for severe trichotillomania. J Am Acad Child Adolesc Psychiatr 32, 830–834.

Welte J, Barnes G, Wieczorek W, et al. (2001) Alcohol and gambling pathology among US adults: Prevalence, demographic patterns and comorbidity. J Stud Alcohol 62, 706–712.

Wetzel R (1966) Use of behavior techniques in a case of compulsive stealing. J Consult Psychol 5, 367–374.

Winchel RM (1992) Trichotillomania: Presentation and treatment. Psychiatr Ann 22, 8–89.

Winchel RM, Jones JS, Stanley B, et al. (1992) Clinical characteristics of trichotillomania and its response to fluoxetine. J Clin Psychiatr 53, 304–308.

Woermann FG, van Elst LT, Koepp MJ, et al. (2000) Reduction of frontal neocortical grey matter associated with affective aggression in patients with temporal lobe epilepsy: An objective voxel by voxel analysis of automatically segmented MRI. J Neurol Neurosurg Psychiatr 68, 162–169.

Wood A and Garralda ME (1990) Kleptomania in a 13-year-old boy. A sequel of a "lethargic" encephalitic/depressive process? Br J Psychiatr 157, 770–772.

Zalsman G, Hermesh H, and Sever J (2001) Hypnotherapy in adolescents with trichotillomania: Three cases. Am J Clin Hypn 44, 63–68.

# 78 Adjustment Disorders

James J. Strain
Jeffrey H. Newcorn

Adjustment Disorders
Adjustment Disorder Subtypes

## Definition

The *Diagnostic and Statistical Manual of Mental Disorders*, Fourth Edition, Text Revision (DSM-IV-TR) states that the essential feature of adjustment disorder (AD) is the development of clinically significant emotional or behavioral symptoms in response to an identifiable psychosocial stressor (American Psychiatric Association 2000). The symptoms must develop within 3 months after the onset of the stressor (criterion A). The clinical significance of the reaction is indicated either by marked distress that is in excess of what would be expected given the nature of the stressor or by significant impairment in social or occupational (academic) functioning (criterion B). This disorder should not be used if the emotional and cognitive disturbances meet the criteria for *another* specific Axis I disorder (e.g., a specific anxiety or mood disorder) or are merely an exacerbation of a preexisting Axis I or Axis II disorder (criterion C). AD may be diagnosed if other Axis I or II disorders are present, but do not account for the pattern of symptoms that have occurred in response to the stressor. The diagnosis of AD does not apply when the symptoms represent bereavement (criterion D). By definition, AD must resolve within 6 months of the termination of the stressor or its consequences (criterion E). However, the symptoms may persist for a prolonged period (i.e., longer than 6 months) if they occur in response to a chronic stressor (e.g., a chronic, disabling general medical condition) or to a stressor that has enduring consequences (e.g., the financial and emotional difficulties resulting from a divorce) (American Psychiatric Association 2000).

Although the above definition provides a certain structure for identifying and describing AD, there is still uncertainty as to when the impairment in functioning or the severity of the psychiatric symptoms that develop in response to a stressor are sufficient to warrant a diagnosis of AD. The DSM-IV-TR describes the boundary issues between conditions that may be a focus of clinical attention (V codes), *subthreshold* disorders (NOS disorders), and the specific mental disorders (American Psychiatric Association 2000). A compelling literature documents that there is much "physical" in mental disorders and much "mental" in physical disorders (p. xxx). No definition adequately specifies precise boundaries for the concept of a "mental disorder."

"The concept...lacks a consistent operational definition that covers all situations....Whatever its original cause, it must currently be considered a manifestation of a behavioral, psychological, or biological dysfunction in the individual" (p. xxxi). The issue of defining boundaries is especially problematic in the subthreshold diagnoses, for example, the AD, in which there are no symptom checklists, algorithms, or guidelines for the "quantification of attributes" (p. xxxii).

AD is a subthreshold diagnosis, which has undergone a major evolution since the original Diagnostic and Statistical Manual of the American Psychiatric Association 1952.

The symptoms of AD are defined in terms of their being a maladaptive response to a psychosocial stressor. There are, in fact, no specific symptoms of AD; any combination of behavioral or emotional symptoms that occur in association with a stressor may qualify. The nature of the symptomatology is described by a variety of possible "subtypes" (Appendix 1). Mezzich and colleagues (1981) and Strain (1981) observed that many of the subtypes of AD were infrequently used (e.g., "with mixed emotional features"), whereas "with physical complaints," a DSM-III-R category had insufficient time to be observed (American Psychiatric Association 1987). Both were deleted in DSM-IV.

The lack of specific symptoms or quantifiable criteria of the AD permits the labeling of early or temporary mental states when the clinical picture does not meet full evidence for a more specific mental disorder, but the morbid state is more than expected in a normal reaction and treatment or intervention may be indicated. AD are an essential "linchpin" in the psychiatric–taxonomic spectrum-hierarchy: (1) disorders with specific diagnostic criteria; (2) disorders not otherwise specified (NOS); (3) adjustment disorders; (4) other conditions that may be a focus of clinical attention (V codes) (American Psychiatric Association 2000); and (5) normal fluctuations of mental states. Demoralization has been suggested as another V-code category and should be distinguished from AD and other pathological conditions (Slavney 1999). Understandably, the AD are a diagnostic group with a significant evolution since 1952 (Table 78–1). As the diagnosis of AD has evolved, the recognition of other stress-related disorders, for example, posttraumatic stress disorder (PTSD) has occurred. A new acute stress disorder diagnosis—those stress reactions that follow a disaster or cataclysmic personal event (e.g., acute stress disorder) (Spiegel 1994)—was introduced into DSM-IV.

---

### DSM-IV-TR Criteria 309.xx

**Adjustment Disorders**

A. The development of emotional or behavioral symptoms in response to an identifiable stressor(s) occurring within 3 months of the onset of the stressor(s).

B. These symptoms or behaviors are clinically significant as evidenced by either of the following:

   (1) marked distress that is in excess of what would be expected from exposure to the stressor

   (2) significant impairment in social or occupational (academic) functioning

C. The stress-related disturbance does not meet the criteria for another specific Axis I disorder and is not merely an exacerbation of a preexisting Axis I or Axis II disorder.

D. The symptoms do not represent bereavement.

E. Once the stressor (or its consequences) has terminated, the symptoms do not persist for more than an additional 6 months.

*Specify* if:
**Acute**: if the disturbance lasts less than 6 months

**Chronic**: if the disturbance lasts for 6 months or longer

Adjustment disorders are coded based on the subtype, which is selected according to the predominant symptoms. The specific stressor(s) can be specified on Axis IV.

**309.0**   **With depressed mood**

**309.24**   **With anxiety**

**309.28**   **With mixed anxiety and depressed mood**

**309.3**   **With disturbance of conduct**

**309.4**   **With mixed disturbance of emotions and conduct**

**309.9**   **Unspecified**

---

**Table 78–1**   **Diagnostic Categories of Adjustment Disorders**

**DSM-I (1952) Transient Situational Personality Disorder**

Gross stress reactions
Adult situational reaction
Adjustment reaction of infancy
Adjustment reaction of childhood
Adjustment reaction of adolescence
Adjustment reaction of late life
Other transient situational personality disturbance

**DSM-II (1968) Transient Situational Disturbance**

Adjustment reaction of infancy
Adjustment reaction of childhood
Adjustment reaction of adolescence
Adjustment reaction of adult life
Adjustment reaction of late life

**DSM-III (1980) Adjustment Disorder**

Adjustment disorder with depressed mood
Adjustment disorder with anxious mood
Adjustment disorder with mixed emotional features
Adjustment disorder with disturbance of conduct
Adjustment disorder with mixed disturbance of emotions and conduct
Adjustment disorder with work (or academic) inhibition
Adjustment disorder with withdrawal
Adjustment disorder with atypical features

**DSM-III-R (1987) Adjustment Disorder**

Adjustment disorder with depressed mood
Adjustment disorder with anxious mood
Adjustment disorder with mixed emotional features
Adjustment disorder with disturbance of conduct
Adjustment disorder with mixed disturbance of emotions and conduct
Adjustment disorder with work (or academic) inhibition
Adjustment disorder with withdrawal
Adjustment disorder with physical complaints
Adjustment disorder not otherwise specified (NOS)

**DSM-IV (1994) Adjustment Disorder**

Adjustment disorder with depressed mood
Adjustment disorder with anxiety
Adjustment disorder with mixed anxiety and depressed mood
Adjustment disorder with disturbance of conduct
Adjustment disorder with mixed disturbance of emotions and conduct
Adjustment disorder unspecified

**Acute:** This specifier can be used to indicate persistence of symptoms for less than 6 mo.

**Chronic:** This specifier can be used to indicate persistence of symptoms for 6 mo or longer. By definition, symptoms cannot persist for more than 6 mo after the termination of the stressor or its consequences. The chronic specifier therefore applies when the duration of the disturbance is longer than 6 mo in response to a chronic stressor or a stressor that has enduring consequences.

---

Disorders that do not fulfill the criteria for a specific mental disorder may be accorded a lesser interest by mental health care workers, research institutes, and third-party payers, even though they present with serious (or incipient) symptoms that require intervention or treatment. Given this concept, the AD are formulated as a means of classifying psychiatric morbidity that is clinically significant; when the symptom profile is as yet insufficient to meet the more specifically operationalized criteria for another mental disorder; when the symptoms, disturbance of mood, and vocational or interpersonal dysfunction are in excess of a normal reaction to the stressors in question; and for which treatment is indicated. For example, a diagnosis of AD is not given when the clinical picture is a psychosocial problem (V code) requiring clinical attention, such as noncompliance, phase of life problem, bereavement, or occupational (academic) problem. Their etiological and dynamic attributes make the AD a fascinating group of disorders that serve as a fulcrum between normality and more specific mental disorders (Figure 78–1).

Attention to less severe mental symptoms (and psychiatric morbidity) may forestall the evolution to more serious disorders and allow remediation before relationships, work, and functioning are so impaired that they are disrupted or permanently sundered. Yet, in the gray area in which early diagnosis may have enormous value with modest therapeutic investment, guidelines are the most tenuous. It is the professionals at the "front door"—primary care physicians, triage personnel, emergency department staff, walk-in clinic staff—who need assistance in making this difficult call: Is there sufficient psychiatric morbidity to warrant mental health intervention?

Problems with the use of the AD diagnosis in clinical practice were highlighted in a survey of child and adolescent psychiatrists. Of those who responded, 55% indicated that they used AD to avoid the stigmatization of patients (in this case children and youth). More of those who favored the use of this category were psychodynamically oriented, not formally trained in the DSM-III-R, and not inclined to use NOS categories (Setterberg et al. 1991, American Psychiatric Association 1987). More than half of these psychiatrists did not consider the temporal onset criterion or the

exclusionary criteria in applying this diagnosis. The survey results suggested that some psychiatrists, in part to protect their patients from the feared adversities of major psychiatric nomenclature, use the AD diagnosis excessively and incorrectly.

Because AD is a nonpejorative psychiatric condition (Kovacs et al. 1993), it may also have been overdiagnosed in youths (Kovacs et al. 1994). Andreasen and Wasek (1980) observed that 25% of a sample of adolescents with AD had attempted suicide and that 17% probably "would have met DSM-III criteria for major depressive disorder" because they had the required symptoms. Kovacs and colleagues (1993) stated, "Suicide attempts among clinically referred youths occur mostly in the context of specific psychiatric disorders, including major depressive and dysthymic disorders, and rarely in the context of AD, further suggesting that AD may have been incorrectly diagnosed in some cases." Reports that 5 to 12% of young inpatients with psychiatric disorders have been assigned a diagnosis of AD also raise the possibility of mislabeling (Andreasen and Wasek 1980, Faulstich et al. 1986). Nevertheless, in psychological autopsy studies of adolescent suicide completers, approximately 20% do not meet the criteria for any single psychiatric diagnosis, although they present with significant functional impairment and life-threatening behavior.

The problem of how to diagnose individuals with suicidal behavior who do *not* meet criteria for a specific mental disorder has received considerable recent attention. De Leo and colleagues (1986a, 1986b) reported on the association of AD and suicidality. Runeson and colleagues (1996) observed from psychological autopsy methods that there was a very short median interval between first suicidal communication and suicide in AD (less than 1 month) compared to major depressive disorder (3 months), borderline personality disorder (30 months), or schizophrenia (47 months).

Recent life events, which would constitute an acute stress, were commonly found to correlate with suicidal behavior in a group that included those with AD (Isometsa et al. 1996). Spalletta and colleagues (1996) observed that assessment of suicidal behavior to be an important tool in differentiating major depressive disorder, dysthymic disorder, and AD. Furthermore, AD patients were observed to be among the most common recipients of a deliberate self-harm (DSH) diagnosis, with the majority involving self-poisoning (Vlachos et al. 1994). Thus, DSH with all its variants, e.g., reckless driving, is more common in AD patients (Vlachos et al. 1994), whereas the percentage of completed suicidal behavior per se was found to be higher in depressed patients (Spalletta et al. 1996). Of note, biological findings in suicidal patients with AD suggest characteristic patterns of monoamine oxidase (MAO) and noradrenaline turnover (Tripodianakis et al. 2000). Clearly, what is regarded, as a subthreshold diagnosis—AD—does not necessarily imply the presence of subthreshold symptomatology.

## Epidemiology

AD has principally been studied in clinical samples. Epidemiological data in adults are not available. The AD diagnosis was not included in the Epidemiologic Catchment Area Study conducted in five disparate sites throughout the US, and there are only a few studies in children and adolescents.

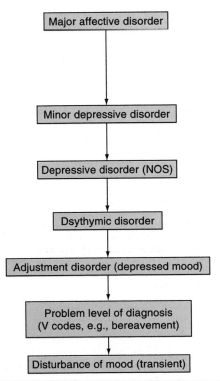

**Figure 78–1** *Descending order of depressive states, from most serious to least depressed mood, as a state of being for an occurrence of the moment.*

Andreasen and Wasek (1980) reported that 5% of an inpatient and outpatient sample were labeled AD. Fabrega and coworkers (1987) observed that 2.3% of a sample of patients presenting to a walk-in diagnostic and evaluation center clinic met criteria for AD with no other Axis I or Axis II diagnoses. When patients with other Axis I diagnoses (Axis I comorbidities) were also included, 20% had the diagnosis of AD. Of a sample of more than 11,000 patients (all ages) 10% were found to have AD (Table 78–2), making it the second largest diagnostic category (Fabrega et al. 1986, 1987, Mezzich et al. 1989). In the Pittsburgh sample studied, 16% of the children and adolescents younger than 18 years were diagnosed with AD (Fabrega et al. 1986). In adults, women predominated over men by approximately 2:1. The sex ratio was more equal in children and adolescents, although there was still a slight excess of female patients.

Prevalence estimates of AD in other clinical populations have been characterized by considerable variability (see Table 78–2). In general hospital inpatient and psychiatric consultation populations, AD was diagnosed in 21.5 and 11.5%, respectively (Popkin et al. 1988, Snyder and Strain 1990). Strain and coworkers (1998b) examined the consultation–liaison data from seven university teaching hospitals in the US, Canada, and Australia. The sites had all used a common clinical database to examine 1,039 consecutive referrals. AD was diagnosed in 125 patients (12.0%); as the sole diagnosis in 81 (7.8%); and comorbidly with other Axis I and II diagnoses in 44 (4.2%) (Strain et al. 1998a). It had been considered as a "rule-out" diagnosis in an additional 110 (10.6%). AD with depressed mood, anxious mood, or mixed emotions were the most common sub-categories used. AD was diagnosed comorbidly most frequently with personality disorder and organic mental disorder. Sixty-seven (6.4%) were assigned a V code diagnosis only. Patients with AD compared to other diagnostic categories were referred significantly more often for problems of anxiety, coping, and depression; had less past psychiatric illness; and were rated as functioning better—all consistent with the construct of AD as a maladaptation to a psychosocial stressor. Interventions employed for this general hospital inpatient cohort were similar to those for other Axis I and II diagnoses, in particular, the prescription of antidepressant medications. Patients with AD required a similar amount of clinical time and resident supervision.

Oxman and coworkers (1994) observed that 50.7% of elderly patients (aged 55+ years) receiving elective surgery for coronary artery disease developed AD related to the stress of surgery. Thirty percent had symptomatic and functional impairment 6 months following surgery. It is reported that 27% of elderly patients examined 5 to 9 days following a cerebral vascular accident had symptoms that fulfilled the criteria for AD (Kellermann et al. 1999). Spiegel (1996) observed that half of all cancer patients have a psychiatric disorder, usually an AD with depression. Since patients treated for their mental states had longer survival time, treatment of depression in cancer patients should be considered integral to their medical treatment. AD is a frequently made diagnosis in patients with head and neck surgery (16.8%) (Kugaya et al. 2000), patients with HIV dementia (73%) (Pozzi et al. 1999), cancer patients from a multicenter survey of consultation–liaison psychiatry in oncology (27%) (Grassi et al. 2000), dermatology patients (29% of the 9% who had psychiatric diagnosis) (Pulimood et al. 1996), and suicide attempters (22%) examined in an emergency room (Schnyder and Valach 1997). Other studies include diagnosis of AD in more than 60% of inpatients being treated for severe burns (Perez-Jimenez et al. 1994), 20% of patients in early stages of multiple sclerosis (Sullivan et al. 1995), and 40% of poststroke patients (Shima et al. 1994).

In a study of emergency department visits, it was reported that 13% of adults and 42% of adolescents were diagnosed with AD (Hillard et al. 1987). Among adolescents in that study, AD was twice as common as any other diagnosis, including substance abuse. Faulstich and coworkers (1986) reported the prevalence of DSM-III conduct disorder and AD for adolescent psychiatric inpatients. Mezzich and coworkers (1981) and Fabrega and coworkers (1987) evaluated walk-in clinic patients (mainly adults) for the current presence of 64 symptoms in three diagnostic cohorts: (1) specific diagnoses, (2) AD, and (3) "not ill." Vegetative,

| Table 78–2 | Prevalence of Adjustment Disorder | | | |
|---|---|---|---|---|
| Study | Sample Type | Sample Size | Assessment Method | Prevalence |
| Bird et al. (1988) | Epidemiological, general population | Probability estimate of 2,036 households | Structured rating scales; clinical interview | 7.6% (CGAS* < Ld70) 4.2% (CGAS < Ld60) |
| Weiner and Del Gaudio (1976) | Epidemiological, clinical services | 1,344 | Clinical diagnosis | 27% of all cases |
| Mezzich et al. (1989) | Clinical screening evaluation (all services) | 11,282 | Semistructured assessment instrument | 10% (all ages) 16% (< Ld18 yr) |
| Faulstich et al. (1986) | Clinical (adolescent inpatient) | 392 | Chart review, clinical diagnosis | 12.5% |
| Hillard et al. (1987) | Clinical (emergency room department) | 100 adolescents 100 adults (random) | Chart review, clinical diagnosis | 42% of adolescents 13% of adults |
| Doan and Petti (1989) | Clinical (partial hospital) | 796 | Chart review, clinical diagnosis | 7% |
| Jacobson et al. (1980) | Clinical (four outpatient pediatric clinics) | 20,000 pediatric patients | Clinical diagnosis | 25–65% of cases with psychiatric diagnosis |

*CGAS, Children's Global Assessment Scale.

substance use or abuse, and characterological symptoms were greatest in specific diagnoses, intermediate with the AD, and least in the "not ill." The symptoms of mood and affect, general appearance, behavior, disturbance in speech and thought pattern, and cognitive functioning had a similar distribution (specific diagnosis > AD > "not ill"). The patients with AD were significantly different from the "not ill" group with regard to more "depressed mood" and "low self-esteem" ($P < 0.0001$). The patients with AD and the "not ill" group had minimal disturbance of thought content and perception. Twenty-nine percent of the patients with AD versus 9.0% of the "not ill" patients had a positive response on the suicide indicators. The three cohorts did not differ on the kinds or amounts of general medical conditions.

Andreasen and Wasek (1980) using a chart review, reported that more inpatient adolescents experienced acting-out and behavioral symptoms than adults who were observed to have significant depressive symptoms (87.2 and 63.8%, respectively). Anxiety symptoms were frequent at all ages. They also observed that in their AD cohorts, 21.6% of the adolescents and 11.8% of the adults' fathers had problems with alcohol.

There are two published epidemiological studies in populations of children and adolescents that included AD. One, conducted in Puerto Rico, employed a two-stage screening process using standardized rating scales as well as structured and unstructured clinical interviews (Bird et al. 1988, Bird et al. 1989). The prevalence rate of AD was determined to be 7.6% if an upper limit of 70 on the Children's Global Assessment Scale (CGAS) is applied (Shaffer et al. 1983). However, if an upper limit of 60 is imposed (corresponding to "moderate" impairment on the CGAS), the prevalence of AD dropped to 4.2%. This indicates that up to 40% of AD diagnosed patients have only mild impairment, more than for any other diagnosis. A recent study conducted in a very large birth registry in Finland found that AD with mixed disturbance of emotions and conduct was the most frequent AD diagnosis, and occurred in 3.4% of the population at the time of the assessment (Almqvist et al. 1999). Other studies conducted in pediatric patients who presented with psychiatric disturbance from four different clinics indicated rates of AD across the clinics ranging from 25 to 65% (Jacobson et al. 1980). The prevalence of AD in children and adolescents may be somewhat higher than it is in adults, but varies considerably according to the population studied.

The relationship between family functioning and AD was evaluated by administering the Family Assessment Devise (FAD) to families who had a member with one of seven mental disorders: schizophrenia, bipolar disorder, major depression, anxiety disorder, eating disorder, substance abuse, and adjustment disorder (Friedmann et al. 1997). Regardless of which specific psychiatric diagnosis was present in the family member, having a family member in an acute phase of any of these psychiatric disorders—even a subthreshold diagnosis such as AD, was a risk factor for poor family functioning. AD in a family member was a significant family stressor.

## Etiology

By definition, the ADs are stress-related phenomena in which a psychosocial stressor results in the development of maladaptive states and psychiatric symptoms. The condition is presumed to be time limited, that is, a transitory reaction; symptoms recede when the stressor is removed or a new state of adaptation is defined. There are also other stress-related disorders in DSM-IV-TR, such as PTSD and acute stress disorder those stress reactions that follow a disaster or cataclysmic personal event (American Psychiatric Association 2000). These stress disorders are among the few conditions in DSM-IV-TR, along with substance-induced disorders and mental disorders due to a general medical condition, with a *known cause* and for which the etiological agent is *essential* to establishing the diagnosis. For the most part, the DSM-IV-TR is relatively atheoretical with regard to etiology and is instead phenomenologically driven in its definitions of disorders (Feighner et al. 1972). However, the DSM-IV-TR stress-induced disorders, including the AD, require the diagnostician to impute etiological significance to a life event—a stressor—and relate its effect in clinical terms to the patient, his/her symptoms, and his/her behavior.

That the relationship between stress and the occurrence of a psychiatric disorder is both complex and uncertain has caused many to question the theoretical basis of AD (Rutter 1981, Weiner and Del Gaudio 1976, Holmes and Rahe 1967). The linear model of stress–disease interaction, which serves as the model for AD has been questioned (Woolsten 1988, Paykel et al. 1971). The linear model presupposes that a direct and clearly identifiable pathological reaction may follow a stressful event, a scenario that no doubt occurs in some individuals with AD but may not accurately characterize others. For example, there may be multiple stressors, insidious or chronic, as opposed to discrete events. Furthermore, relatively minor precipitating events may generate a disturbance in an individual who has previously been sensitized to stress.

Several authors have criticized the stressor criterion in AD because stressors are difficult to specify and measure, and their clinical implications and impact are uncertain (Fabrega and Mezzich 1987). Questions pertain to whether patients with AD are unusually sensitive to psychosocial events not likely to cause disturbance in others. Are there individuals who have been exposed to high levels of stress, the severity or accumulation of which would probably produce negative consequences in most people?

Diverse variables and modifiers are involved in the presentation of AD after exposure to a stress. Cohen (1981) argued that acute stresses are different from chronic ones in both psychological and physiological terms; that the meaning of the stress is affected by "modifiers"—ego strengths, support systems, prior mastery—and that one must differentiate manifest and latent meaning of the stressors (e.g., loss of a job may be a relief or a catastrophe). An objectively overwhelming stress could have little impact on one individual, whereas another individual could regard a minor one as cataclysmic. A recent minor stress superimposed on a previous underlying (major) stress (which had no observable effect on its own) may have a significant impact, not operating independently but by its additive effect—the concatenation of events (Hamburg, personal communication).

Proper use of the AD diagnosis also requires a careful understanding of the timing of the stressor and the subsequent emotional or behavioral symptoms; by definition, this must occur within 3 months of the stressor. Until DSM-IV-TR, a time limit was also imposed regarding how long after the occurrence of the stressor this diagnosis could be employed. Before DSM-IV-TR, AD was a "transitory" diagnosis that, by definition, could not exceed 6 months; after 6 months, the diagnosis had to be changed to another psychiatric disorder. However, there are limited data with regard to the timing of symptoms following the occurrence of the stressor. Depue and Monroe (1986) and Rahe (1990) stated that the model of a single stressor impinging on an undisturbed individual to cause symptoms at a single point in time is insufficient to account for the many presentations of stress and illness in the clinical situation. Holmes and Rahe (1967) assigned relative values to specific stressors. Other life events scales have also been shown to be inconsistent in their ability to link stress and illness (Paykel et al. 1971, Dohrenwend et al. 1978, Tennant 1983). Depue and Monroe (1986) and Skodol and colleagues (1990) identified significant methodological problems in evaluating the quality, quantity, and timing of both stressors and symptoms. It was difficult to establish interrater reliability with regard to these three entities of a stressor. With regard to another attempt to assess and document stress in a multiaxial diagnostic schema, Axis IV of DSM-III, and DSM-III-R, was designed to allow the psychiatrist to quantify the stress as a diagnostic attribute of psychiatric disorders. Unfortunately, this measure was confounded by low reliability, which made its use a problem (Spitzer and Forman 1979, Zimmerman 1987, Rey et al. 1988). As a result, the DSM-IV-TR Axis IV is now a qualitative list of psychosocial–circumstantial problems.

Andreasen and Wasek (1980) described the differences between the types of stressors found in adolescents and those of adults; respectively, 59 and 35% of the precipitants had been present for a year or more, and 9 and 39% for 3 months or less. Fabrega and colleagues (1987) reported that their group of patients with AD described stressors compared with the other cohorts: "specific diagnoses" and "not ill." There was a significant difference in the amount of stressors reported relevant to the clinical request for evaluation; the group with AD, compared with the "specific diagnoses" and "not ill" patients, were overrepresented in the "higher stress" categories. Popkin and associates (1988) reported that in their general hospital inpatient consultation cohort, 68.6% of the patients were judged to have their medical illness as the primary psychosocial stressor. Snyder and Strain (1990) observed that the assessment of stressors on Axis IV was significantly more severe ($P = 0.0001$) for inpatient psychiatric consultation patients with AD compared with patients with other diagnostic disorders.

Despite these findings suggesting a correlation between the acknowledgment of stress and the assignment of an AD diagnosis, stress is *not* universally related to the development of psychiatric illness, and this has implications for understanding the meaning of stressors in AD. Specific types of stressful events and individual patterns of stress response appear to be preferentially related to the development of psychiatric symptoms in vulnerable individuals.

## Diagnosis and Differential Diagnosis

Each of the diagnostic constructs required for the diagnosis of AD is difficult to assess and measure: (1) the stressor, (2) the maladaptive reaction to the stressor, and (3) the time and relationship between the stressor and the psychological response. None of these three components has been operationalized for a diagnostic decision tree, which consequently plagues the AD diagnosis with limited reliability.

In contrast to other DSM-IV-TR disorders, the diagnostic criteria for AD include no clear and specific symptoms (or checklist) that collectively compose a psychiatric (medical) syndrome or disorder.

First, with regard to the maladaptive reaction, it is unclear how this concept can or should be operationalized. The social, vocational, and relationship dysfunctions, which are unspecified qualitatively or quantitatively, do not lend themselves to reliable or to valid assessment. The elements of culture (i.e., the expectable reactions within a specific cultural environment), differences in gender responses, developmental level differences, and differences in the "meaning" of events and reactions to them by a specific individual further confound it.

The concepts of "average expectable environment" (e.g., the expectation of adequate food in a household in an industrial society) and "patient's explanatory belief model" are examples of an attempt to weigh cultural and subjective differences in the assessment of an individual's mental state and reaction (Hartman 1986, Klineman 1980). Such individual cultural–social considerations often require an understanding on the part of the psychiatrist and thereby often render the assessment of whether a reaction is excessive or maladaptive a judgment call.

Mixed anxiety–depressive disorder is another subthreshold diagnosis that is included as an unofficial category in the appendix of research criteria needing further study in DSM-IV-TR. This research category is similar to AD with mixed anxiety and depression that does not meet criteria for a specific mood or anxiety disorder, thus making it difficult to draw a boundary between the two disorders except that there is less emphasis on a stressor as a precipitating cause. Furthermore, using the DSM-III-R definition of AD which limited the duration to 6 months, the main difference between the two diagnoses was the chronicity of the mixed anxiety–depressive disorder, as was noted in the mixed anxiety–depression field trial (Zinbarg et al. 1994). Now, with the change in criterion C for AD allowing for chronic forms of AD, the problem of differentiating the two subthreshold diagnoses remains difficult. This uncertainty is further complicated by the question of treatment. Is this an anxiety accompanied by depression that should be treated with anxiolytics, such as benzodiazepines or is this a depression accompanied by anxiety that should be treated with an antidepressant, such as a selective serotonin reuptake inhibitor (SSRI)?

The criterion and predictive validity of the diagnosis of AD in 92 children who had new onset insulin-dependent diabetes mellitus were examined. DSM-III criteria were employed plus requiring four clinically significant signs or symptoms, and the time frame extended to 6 months (instead of the 3 months specified in the definition) after the diagnosis of diabetes. Thirty-three percent of the cohort developed AD (mean 29 days after the medical diagnosis) and the average episode length was 3 months with a recovery rate of 100%. The five-year cumulative probability of a new psychiatric disorder was 0.48 in comparison to 0.16 for the non-AD subjects. The findings support the criterion validity of the AD diagnosis using the criterion of predicting the future development of psychiatric disorder.

## Maladaptation

Although the diagnosis of AD requires evidence of maladaption, it is notable that no specific requirement for functional impairment has been included (e.g., there is no requirement for a certain decrement in the Global Assessment of Functioning Scale score in order to make the diagnosis). Fabrega and colleagues (1986) stated that both subjective symptoms and decrement in social function can be considered maladaptive and that the severity of either of these is subject to great individual variation. However, they could not conclude that the level of severity of psychiatric illness observed correlates with impaired functioning in three areas: occupational status, family, or other individuals.

The psychiatrist needs to examine the patient's behavior to see whether it is beyond what is expected in a particular situation, and for that patient. In order to do this, the psychiatrist needs to take into account the patient's cultural beliefs and practices, his or her developmental age, and the transient nature of the behavior. If the behavior lasts a few moments or is an impulsive outburst, it would not qualify for a maladaptive response to justify the diagnosis of AD. The behavior in question should be maladaptive for that patient, in his/her culture, and sufficiently persistent to qualify for the maladaptation attribute of the AD diagnosis.

## Stresses

No criteria or guidelines are offered in DSM-IV-TR to quantify the degree of stress required for the diagnosis of AD or assess its effect or meaning for a particular individual at a given time. Many of the statements regarding the problem of assessing maladaptation described above apply equally well to the assessment of stressors (Woolston 1988, Zilberg et al. 1982, Perris 1984). Mezzich and coworkers (1981) attempted to classify and quantify the psychosocial stressors in 13 domains (i.e., health, bereavement, love and marriage, parental, family stressors for children and adolescents, other familial relationships, work, school, financial, legal, housing, and miscellaneous). The measurement of the severity of the stressor and its temporal and causal relationship to demonstrable symptoms are often uncertain.

According to DSM-IV-TR, even if a specific and presumably causal stressor is identified, if enough symptoms develop so that diagnostic criteria are met for a specific disorder, then that diagnosis should be made instead of a diagnosis of AD (American Psychiatric Association 1980, 1987, 2000). Therefore, the presence of stressors does not automatically signify a diagnosis of AD, and conversely, a diagnosis of a specific disorder (e.g., major depressive or anxiety disorder) does not imply the absence of concomitant or concurrent stressful events (Setterberg et al. 1991).

The modifications introduced in DSM-IV-TR, which differentiate between acute and chronic forms of AD, solved the problem of a 6-month limitation in DSM-III-R's criteria. This change was validated by Despland and colleagues (1995), who observed that 16% of patients with AD required treatment for longer than 1 year, with the mean length exceeding the prior limitation of 6 months.

## Assessment of the Subtypes of Adjustment Disorder, Comorbidity, and Diagnostic Boundaries

The diagnostic criteria for AD define the contextual and temporal characteristics of a subthreshold response to a psychosocial stressor; the specific quality and nature of the resultant psychological morbidity have been used as a means of subtyping.

DSM-IV-TR identifies six AD subtypes; two of the subtypes define discrete disturbances of mood (e.g., depressed, anxious); two describe mixed clinical presentations (e.g., mixed emotional features, mixed disturbance of emotions and conduct); one specifies disturbance of conduct; and the final subtype, unspecified, is a residual category.

Significant occurrence of comorbidity has been reported in studies of AD using structured diagnostic instruments. In a cohort of children, adolescents, and adults, approximately 70% of AD patients had at least one additional Axis I diagnosis (Fabrega et al. 1987). In the study of correlates of depressive disorders in children, 45% of those with AD with depressed mood had another disorder (Kovacs et al. 1984). However, comorbidity in AD was less than in dysthymic disorder or major depressive disorder, suggesting a "purer" or more encapsulated disturbance in AD.

Several studies reported an association of suicidal behavior in adolescents and young adults with AD. One study found that 56% of those hospitalized for suicidal behavior in an urban hospital setting met the DSM-II criteria for transient situational disturbance (an earlier diagnostic label for what came to be called AD) (Minnaar et al. 1980). A retrospective review of 325 consecutive hospital admissions for deliberate self-poisoning revealed that 58% of all cases met criteria for AD with depressed mood, the majority of whom were female patients aged 15 to 24 years (McGrath 1989). In a Scandinavian sample of 58 consecutive suicide victims aged 15 to 29 years, 14% were classified as AD with depressed mood (Runeson 1989); in a US population, 9% of suicide victims aged 10 to 29 years were reported to have AD (Fowler et al. 1986). These studies underscore the seriousness of AD in a subset of individuals and suggest that although the diagnosis may be subthreshold, its morbidity can be serious and at times even fatal.

The issue of boundaries between the specific mood and anxiety disorders, depressive disorder or anxiety disorder NOS, and the AD remains problematic. The specific mood and anxiety disorders are often associated with and, even precipitated by stress. Therefore, it is not always possible to say one group of diagnoses is accompanied by stress (the AD) and another (e.g., major depressive disorder) is not. Stress may accompany many of the psychiatric diagnoses, but it is not an essential component to make certain diagnoses (e.g., major depressive disorder).

More research is needed to carefully demarcate the boundaries or the meaning of these boundaries among the problem-level, subthreshold, and threshold disorders, in particular with regard to the role of stressors as etiological precipitants, concomitants, or factors essentially unrelated to the occurrence of a particular psychiatric diagnosis. Furthermore, serial and ongoing observation of the clinical course is required to ascertain whether the AD is a transitory remitting event, the prodromal state of a more serious and developing disorder, or an intermittent chronic state of a low-level mood disorder. There is considerable evidence indicating that major depressive disorder is a highly recurrent, often chronic condition that is frequently associated with low-grade symptoms prior to, and between, major episodes (Keller et al. 1995). Thus, the differential diagnoses of depressed mood must be linked to ongoing assessment, not cross-sectional evaluation, which is so often the case; it is essential to maintain a longitudinal view of the subthreshold disorders to know their place in an individual's affective history. Keller and coworkers (1995) described the need for a longitudinal taxonomy, a "course-based classification system."

Boundary issues with subthreshold (i.e., so-called "minor") disorders of mood and anxiety were studied in the DSM-IV Field Trial for mixed anxiety and depression. Zinbarg and colleagues (1994) and Liebowitz (1993) reported that subsyndromal disorders were common and could be differentiated from other anxiety disorders. The "subdefinitional threshold" cases were often recurrent or chronic (of more than 6 months' duration) and thereby, according to DSM-III-R criteria used in the field trial, would not have been labeled AD. However, in DSM-IV-TR, AD can now also have a chronic form that persists longer than 6 months, so that the duration boundary becomes less clear between the subthreshold disorders, anxiety or depressive disorder NOS, and AD. Angst and Ernst (1993) argued that most diagnostic subgroups of depression are artificial and not diagnostic entities, but subtypes of the same spectrum disorder.

These data suggest that AD could be placed in an innovative category of "stress response syndromes," or for that matter, in several diverse locations within the DSM classification (Strain et al. 1993). However, the literature does not offer data to support such alternative groupings. In the extreme, AD could be eliminated altogether, with the advantage of maintaining the atheoretical approach of the DSM. This solution, however, does not seem beneficial in view of the findings that demonstrate AD to be a valid diagnosis (Kovacs et al. 1994, 1995).

Construct validity was also observed in a retrospective data study comparing outpatients with single episode major depressive disorder, recurrent major depressive disorder, dysthymic disorder, depressive disorder NOS, and AD with depressed mood with or without mixed anxiety (Jones et al. 1999). The Medical Outcomes Study 36-item Short Form Health Status Survey (SF-36) was completed before and 6 months after treatment. The diagnostic categories were significantly different at baseline, but did not differ with regard to outcome at follow-up. Females were significantly more likely to be diagnosed with major depressive disorder or dysthymic disorder than with AD. Females were also more likely to score lower on the Mental Component Summary scales of the SF-36 scales at admission. AD patients scored higher on all SF-36 scales, as did the other diagnostic groups at baseline and again at follow-up. There was no significant difference among diagnostic groups with regard to treatment outcome. The authors concluded that the results support the construct validity of the AD diagnostic category (Jones et al. 1999).

In reviewing the diagnosis of AD for DSM-IV, one issue emerges as fundamental. The effect of the imprecision of this diagnosis on reliability and validity, because of the lack of behavioral or operational criteria, must be determined. One study (Aoki et al. 1995), however, found three psychological tests, Zung's Self-Rating Anxiety Scale (Zung 1971), Zung's Self-Rating Depression Scale (Zung 1965), and Profile of Mood States (McNair et al. 1971), to be useful tools for AD diagnosis among physical rehabilitation patients. Although Aoki and colleagues (1995) succeeded in reliably differentiating patients with AD from healthy patients, they did not distinguish them from patients with major depression or PTSD.

## Course and Natural History

Andreasen and Hoenk (1982) demonstrated at a 5-year follow-up that there were important differences in adolescents and adults with regard to prognosis. It would be important to extend this long-term observation to cohorts of the elderly and the "old elderly" (those older than 75 years). Although the prognosis was favorable and most adult patients with AD were symptom free at 5 years (71% were completely well, 8% had an intervening problem, and 21% had a major depressive disorder or alcoholism), adolescents had a far different outcome. At a 5-year follow-up, 43% had a major psychiatric disorder (e.g., schizophrenia, schizoaffective disorder, major depressive disorder, substance abuse disorder, and personality disorder); 13% had an intervening psychiatric illness; and 44% had no psychiatric diagnosis (Andreasen and Hoenk 1982). In adolescents, behavioral symptoms and the chronicity of the morbidity were the major predictors for psychopathological disorders at the 5-year follow-up. This was not so with the adults in the study, and raises the question of whether these adolescents were diagnosed as having AD as part of a prodrome of another more serious disorder.

Kovacs and associates (1994) reported a much different set of findings. The authors report that children who were older at the time of onset of AD recovered faster, and there was a trend for subjects with the depressed mood subtype to recover faster than subjects with other symptoms. The researchers concluded that among young, school-aged, clinic-based patients, AD has clinical information value, and is associated with a favorable short-term prognosis, but is often associated with comorbid psychiatric disorders which complicates assessment. When effects of comorbidity were controlled for, there was no compelling evidence for a negative long-term prognosis during a follow-up period of 7 to 8 years specifically attributable to the earlier AD (Andreasen and Hoenk 1982).

Thus, even if AD is properly diagnosed, the negative prognosis that has been reported could be attributable to comorbid disorders such as depressive, anxiety, or conduct disorders that were not recognized (Andreasen and Hoenk 1982). Kovacs and colleagues (1994) furthermore reported that comorbid psychiatric disorders had no discernible effect on the speed of recovery from AD. Among both patients with AD and the control subjects, similar rates of dysfunction were detected during the follow-up, probably attributable to the specific psychiatric conditions that were present initially.

Snyder and Strain (1989) observed that in the acute care inpatient hospital setting, many of the psychiatric consultation patients initially thought to have an AD did not maintain that diagnosis at the time of discharge. These same authors also observed that many patients initially diagnosed as having major depressive disorder were reclassified to AD at discharge. It remains to be seen if either the major depressive disorder or the AD diagnosis is significantly altered at a 6-week follow-up and, in particular, when the patient has left the hospital. This evolution of psychiatric morbidity within the acute care general medical setting cautions the psychiatrist to go slowly with treatment until there is a level of certainty to justify an intervention, in particular with a chemotherapeutic modality.

Attempting to diagnose disorders in an early state or before there is a full-blown syndrome or disorder often means that a patient will qualify for the AD criteria or the subsyndromal condition. Just as it is difficult to know when a patient has crossed the diagnostic line (threshold) from normal to disturbed behavior, it is difficult to know how quickly the symptoms will remit with a remission of the stressor, which for the general medical–surgical inpatient include (1) acute hospitalization, (2) uncertain medical diagnosis, (3) pain, (4) medications, (5) separation, and (6) lack of ability to function or contain emotions. The AD must be looked at as a *transitory state* for most patients, in that it may subside, respond with treatment, evolve to another diagnosis, or be maintained as the stressor continues.

Furthermore, Monroe and associates (1992) pointed out that "stress does not credit a more favorable treatment course for patients with recurrent depression." For these patients, stress occurring before treatment entry suggests the likelihood of a poorer early treatment response and a longer time to attain relief. Psychiatrists working with recurrent depression should not expect more rapid recovery from patients reporting these types of stress and should not become discouraged if treatment progress is slower or more erratic than usual. The severity of the stressor should be studied as well as its recurrence and its meaning to the patient, all in conjunction with treatment outcome in those with AD.

## Treatment

There are no reported randomized controlled trials regarding the psychological, social, or pharmacological treatment of AD (Adams and Gelder 1994, Chalmers et al. 1992, Conte and Karasu 1992). In lieu of any substantive randomized controlled trials to guide treatment, the choice of intervention remains a clinical decision. The Institute of Medicine has developed *Guidelines for Clinical Practice: From Development to Use* (Field and Lohr 1992). A critical attribute of a guideline is the *strength of the evidence*. "Practice guidelines should be accompanied by descriptions of the strength of the evidence and the expert judgment behind them. [They] should be accompanied by estimates of the health and cost outcomes expected from the interventions in question, compared with alternative practice" (Field and Lohr 1992, p. 8). Therefore, with no evidence from randomized controlled trials, the treatment recommendations for

the AD remain based on consensus rather than evidence. However, there has not been an official consensus conference on the optimal way to treat this disorder. Recommendations of clinical experts may differ from the results of meta-analyses of randomized controlled trials (Antman et al. 1992).

There are two approaches to treatment. One is based on the understanding that this disorder emanates from a psychological reaction to a stressor. The stressor needs to be identified, described, and shared with the patient; plans must be made to mitigate it, if possible. The abnormal response may be attenuated if the stressor can be eliminated or reduced. Popkin and coworkers (1990) have shown that in the medically ill, the most common stressor is the medical illness itself; and the AD may remit when the medical illness improves or a new level of adaptation is reached. The other approach to treatment is to provide intervention for the symptomatic presentation, despite the fact that it does not reach threshold level for a specific disorder, on the premise that it is associated with impairment and that treatments that are effective for more pronounced presentations of similar pathology are likely to be effective. This may include psychotherapy, pharmacotherapy, or a combination of the two (Schatzberg 1990).

## Psychotherapy

Psychotherapeutic intervention in AD is intended to reduce the effects of the stressor, enhance coping to the stressor that cannot be reduced or removed, and establish a mental state and support system to maximize adaptation. Psychotherapy can involve any one of several approaches: cognitive–behavioral treatment, interpersonal therapy, psychodynamic efforts, or counseling.

The first goal of these psychotherapies is to analyze the nature of the stressors affecting the patient to see whether they may be avoided or minimized (e.g., assuming excessive responsibility out of keeping with realistic goals; putting oneself at risk, such as dietary indiscretions for a type I diabetic). It is necessary to clarify and interpret the meaning of the stressor for the patient. For example, an amputation of the leg may have devastated a patient's feelings about himself or herself, especially if the individual was a runner. It is necessary to clarify that the patient still has enormous residual capacity; that he or she can engage in much meaningful work, does not have to loose valued relationships, and can still be sexually active; and that it does not necessarily mean that further body parts will be lost. (However, it will also involve redirecting the physical activity to another pastime.) Otherwise, the patient's pernicious fantasies ("all is lost") may take over in response to the stressor (i.e., amputation), make the patient dysfunctional (at work, sex), and precipitate a painful dysphoria or anxiety reaction.

Some stressors may elicit an overreaction (e.g., the patient's attempted suicide or homicide after the abandonment by a lover). In such instances of overreaction with feelings, emotions, or behaviors, the therapist would help the patient put his or her feelings and rage into words rather than into destructive actions and gain some perspective. The role of verbalization and the joining of affects and conflicts cannot be overestimated in an attempt to reduce the pressure of the stressor and enhance coping. Drugs and alcohol are to be discouraged.

Psychotherapy, medical crisis counseling, crisis intervention, family therapy, group treatment, cognitive–behavioral treatment, and interpersonal therapy all encourage the patient to express affects, fears, anxiety, rage, helplessness, and hopelessness to the stressors imposed (Pollin and Holland 1992). They also assist the patient to reassess reality in the service of adaptation. Following the example given above, the loss of a leg is not the loss of one's life. But it is a major loss. Sifneos (1989) believed that patients with AD could profit most from brief psychotherapy. The psychotherapy should attempt to reframe the meaning of the stress, find ways to minimize it, and diminish the psychological deficit due to its occurrence. The treatment should expose the concerns and conflicts that the patient is experiencing; help the patient gain perspective on the adversity; and encourage the patient to establish relationships and to attend support groups or self-help groups for assistance in the management of the stressor and the self.

Wise (1988), drawing from his experience in military psychiatry, emphasized the variables of **b**revity, **i**mmediacy, **c**entrality, **e**xpectance, **p**roximity, and **s**implicity (BICEPS principles). The treatment structure encompasses a simple straightforward approach dealing with the immediate situation at hand which is troubling the patient. The treatment approach is brief, usually no more than 72 hours (True and Benway 1992).

In another sample, interpersonal psychotherapy was applied to depressed outpatients with human immunodeficiency virus, (HIV), infection and found to be useful (Markowitz et al. 1992). Some of the attributes of interpersonal psychotherapy are psychoeducation regarding the sick role; using a here-and-now framework; formulation of the problems from an interpersonal perspective; exploration of options for changing dysfunctional behavior patterns; and identification of focused interpersonal problem areas. Lazarus (1992) described a seven-pronged approach in the treatment of minor depression. The therapy includes assertiveness training, enjoyable events, coping, imagery, time projection, cognitive disputation, role-playing, desensitization, family therapy, and biological prophylaxis.

Support groups have been demonstrated to help patients adjust and enhance their coping mechanisms, and they may prolong life as well. Spiegel and coworkers (1989) showed that women with stage IV breast cancer lived longer after ongoing group therapy than those with standard cancer care. However, these findings on group psychological intervention and mortality have not been confirmed in at least two replication trials reported to date (Goodwin et al. 2001, Cunningham et al. 1998).

## Pharmacotherapy

Stewart and colleagues (1992) emphasized the need to consider psychopharmacological interventions as well as psychotherapy for the treatment of minor depression, and this recommendation might be extrapolated to other subthreshold disorders. This group recommends antidepressant therapy if there is no benefit from 3 months of psychotherapy or other supportive measures. Although psychotherapy is the first choice treatment, psychotherapy combined with benzodiazepines may be helpful, especially for patients with severe life stress(es) and a significant anxious component (Uhlenhuth et al. 1995, Shaner 2000). Tricyclic antidepres-

sants or buspirone were recommended in place of benzodiazepines for patients with current or past heavy alcohol use because of the greater risk of dependence in these patients (Uhlenhuth et al. 1995).

Psychotropic medication has been used in the medically ill, in the terminally ill, and in patients who have been refractory to verbal therapies. Rosenberg and associates (1991) described in the medically ill with depressive disorders (the type of depression was unspecified) that 16 of 29 patients (55%) improved within 2 days of treatment with the maximal dose of amphetamine derivatives. The presence of delirium was associated with a decreased response. Whether methylphenidate is similarly useful in AD with depressed mood remains to be examined. Reynolds (1992), reviewing randomized controlled trials, concluded that bereavement-related syndromal depression also appears to respond to antidepressant medication. The medication chosen should reflect the nature of the predominant mood that accompanies the AD (e.g., benzodiazepines for AD with anxious mood; antidepressants for AD with depressed mood). For example, Schatzberg (1990) recommended that the therapist consider both psychotherapy and pharmacotherapy in the AD with anxious mood and that the psychiatrist prescribe anxiolytics as part of the treatment. The degree to which pharmacotherapy is used for AD has remained elusive. Olfson and colleagues (1998) report an increase in the use of antidepressants among less severely ill patients, including those with AD. However, Kaplan and coworkers (1994) suggest that those with less severe conditions are overall less likely to receive psychopharmacologic treatment.

Other authors have begun to examine the effect of homeopathic treatments. From a 25-week multicenter randomized placebo-controlled double-blind trial, a special extract from kava-kava was reported to be effective in AD with anxiety and without the adverse side effect profile associated with tricyclics and benzodiazepines (Volz and Kieser 1997). Tianeptine, alprazolam, and mianserin were found to be equally effective in symptom improvement in patients with AD and anxious mood (Ansseau et al. 1996). In a random double-blind study trazodone was more effective than clorazepate in cancer patients for the relief of anxious and depressed symptoms (Razavi et al. 1999). Similar findings were observed in HIV positive patients with AD (DeWit et al. 1999).

## Refractory Patients and Nonresponse to Initial Treatment

Those patients who do not respond to counseling or the various modes of psychotherapy that have been outlined and to a trial of antidepressant or anxiolytic medications should be regarded as treatment nonresponders. It is essential to reevaluate the patient to ensure that the diagnostic impression has not altered and, in particular, that the patient has not developed a major mental disorder, which would require a more aggressive treatment, often biological. The psychiatrist must also consider that an Axis II disorder might be interfering with the patient's resolution of the AD. Finally, if the stressor continues and cannot be removed (e.g., the continuation of a seriously impairing chronic illness), additional support and management strategies need to be employed to assist the patient in optimally adapting to the stressor that she or he is confronting (e.g., experiencing the progression of HIV infection).

DSM-IV allows the use of the diagnosis of AD even after 6 months, and then it is described as AD, chronic. With such a contingency (e.g., AD lasting a few years), it is necessary to ensure that the patient is not experiencing dysthymic disorder or an unremitting depressive disorder. However, these diagnoses have a symptom profile that should distinguish them from the AD.

## Conclusion

Appropriate and timely treatment is essential for patients with AD so that their symptoms do not worsen; do not further impair their important relationships; and do not compromise their capacity to work, study, or be active in their interpersonal pursuits. Treatment must attempt to forestall further erosion of the patient's capacity to function that could ultimately have grave and untoward consequences. Maladaptation may so impede the patient that irreversible losses in important sectors of his or her life occur. Although this diagnosis lacks rigorous specificity, its treatment is no less challenging or less important. AD's lack of a designated symptom profile results in this diagnosis having insufficient specificity. However, it is this lack of specificity, which permits the psychiatrist to have a "diagnosis" to use when the patient is presenting with early, vague, nonconcrete symptomatology, which should be noted, identified, and followed. This is similar to the situation with early fever, or fever of unknown origin, which, by the way, may never go on to a specific medical diagnosis, but be at discharge simply diagnosed as a "fever of unknown origin." Unspecified chest pain is another example where the patient may never have a specific diagnosis even over time. Spitzer has described the ADs as a "wild card" in the psychiatric lexicon, that allows a place for an uncertain, early, not completely developed diagnosis to be housed until it disappears, develops into a full blown category, persists in a subsyndromal state, or disappears. As said above, this is not uncommon with physical or mental subsyndromal states.

DSM-III-R has been described as "medical illness and age unfair" (i.e., it does not sufficiently take into account the issues of age and/or medical illness) (L. George, personal communication, Strain 1981). DSM-IV-TR has tried to take this into account with considerable effort placed on those psychological interface disorders that border between physical and mental phenomena, for example, the somatoform disorders, AD, dissociation, and so on. However, in addition to enhancing reliability and validity, the psychiatric taxonomy needs to consider the impact of developmental epochs (e.g., children and youth, adults, young elderly, and "old" elderly) and medical illness on symptomatology. With regard to the latter issue, Endicott (1984) has described replacing vegetative with ideational symptoms when evaluating depressed patients with medical illness. Rapp and Vrana (1989) confirmed Endicott's proposed changes in the diagnostic criteria for depression in medically ill elderly persons and observed maintenance of specificity and sensitivity, respectively, when substituting ideational for vegetative symptoms. Recent studies found AD patients to be significantly younger compared with patients who have a major psychiatric diagnosis (Despland

et al. 1995, Mok and Walter 1995). Zarb's (1996) study suggests that cognitively impaired elderly, when evaluated using individual items of the Geriatric Depression Scale exhibited AD rather than major depressive disorder. In addition, Despland and colleagues (1995) reported that the patients' group with AD with depressive or mixed symptoms included more women, thus exhibiting a sex ratio resembling that for major depressive disorder or dysthymic disorder. Therefore, future editions of DSM may be able to take into account the differences encountered in symptom profiles for gender, various developmental epochs, and medical and psychiatric comorbidity. Finally, longitudinal observations would describe the outcome of AD over time. Their resolution, evolution to another diagnosis, their response to a variety of treatments would augment our understanding and approach to this important subthreshold diagnosis.

---

### Clinical Vignette 1

A 35-year-old married woman, mother of three children, was desperate when she learned she had cancer and would need mastectomy followed by chemotherapy and radiation. She was convinced that she would not recover, that her body would be forever distorted and ugly, that her husband would no longer find her attractive, and that her children would be ashamed of her baldness and the fact that she had cancer. She wondered whether anyone would ever want to touch her again. Because her mother and sister had also experienced breast cancer, the patient felt she was fated to an empty future. Despite several sessions dealing with her feelings, the patient's dysphoria remained profound. It was decided to add antidepressant medication (fluoxetine, 20 mg/day) to her psychotherapy to decrease the patient's continuing unpleasant symptoms. Two weeks later, the patient reported that she was feeling less despondent and less concerned about the future and that she had a desire to start resuming her former activities with her family. As the patient came to terms with the overwhelming stressor and, assisted with antidepressant agents, her depressed mood improved, more adequate coping strategies to handle her serious medical illness were mobilized.

Although it is uncommon to use psychotropic medication for the majority of the adjustment disorders, this clinical vignette illustrates the effective use of antidepressant therapy in a patient who was not responding to counseling and psychotherapy; she never had symptoms that met the DSM-IV criteria for a major depressive disorder. It has been found that the addition of a psychotropic medication in adjustment disorder, on the basis of the mood disturbance, may assist those patients who continue to experience disordered mood and adjustment to the stressor despite treatment with verbal therapies. The antidepressant medications have also been found helpful in the terminally ill who exhibit adjustment disorder with depressed mood and who have not responded to counseling alone.

---

### Clinical Vignette 2

Mr. L, a 48-year-old laborer, had his right leg amputated below the knee as a result of vascular and neurological damage secondary to diabetes mellitus. He manifested both anxious and depressed moods, became difficult in his relationship with his wife, and refused to take care of himself even in those areas that he could despite his recent surgery. Mr. L complained that he could not function in his wheelchair without assistance, despite upper body capacity to both transfer and propel the chair on his own. Previous to the surgery, he had been independent and turned away assistance, maintaining that he could do it on his own. Despite his distress, he did not evidence the criteria for a major or minor depression (e.g., difficulties in eating, sleeping, guilt, hopelessness, or suicidal ideation). The stressor of his recent surgery had resulted in his maladaptation to his illness and his performance at home and in a depressed and anxious mood.

Mr. L illustrates the occurrence of an adjustment disorder in response to the stressor of chronic illness and the loss of a body part essential to his usual occupational pursuit. Although bereavement is reserved for those patients who have lost a loved one, the loss of a body part or a body function constitutes a major stressor that can precipitate an adjustment disorder. The patient's "giving in" and "giving up" were unlike his customary extreme independence and resulted in a maladaptation to the stressor, out of all keeping with the physical limitations imposed by the surgery. It was also out of keeping with his family and cultural ideals that they kept going the "best they could" and maintained responsibilities and self-care even if it meant discomfort and extra effort.

Clinical Vignette 3

A 38-year-old woman who had lost her sister 5 days before in the attack on the World Trade Center was convinced that she was responsible for the sister's death in that she did not stop by and have coffee with her that morning, thereby delaying her arrival at work which would have preserved her life. She was having difficulty sleeping, her diabetes was out of control, she found herself crying, unable to function at work, and having difficulty coping with her three children. She was anxious, depressed and felt guilty that she was the only one who could have saved the sister, if she had not avoided her usual routine, which usually resulted in making the sister about 30 minutes late for her employment. The 30 minutes would have made the difference in arriving too late to enter the burning building. This patient did not have a posttraumatic stress response because it had not been 30 days since the stressor. She did not qualify for an acute stress disorder as she did not have derealization, depersonalization, or amnesia (i.e., at least 3 out of 5 symptoms are required). Could the patient be labeled as in bereavement? The patient has significant maladaptation to a major stressor characterized by a depressed and anxious mood. The degree of the patient's belief that she was responsible for the sister's death, and the degree of her nonfunctional capacity at work or to perform at home, does not support that bereavement would be a preferred diagnosis. Medications were prescribed to assist her with sleep and to reduce the daytime anxiety. What was the most appropriate diagnosis in the early days of this disaster, if the patient did not achieve the criteria for an acute stress response? It would seem that appropriate follow-up may highlight the trajectory of symptom

development and whether the person goes on to develop other diagnoses or into a remission toward normalcy. Medications were temporarily prescribed to assist with the intense sleep and anxiety disturbances.

## Comparison of DSM-IV/ICD-10 Diagnostic Criteria

In contrast to DSM-IV-TR (which requires the onset of symptoms within 3 months of the stressor), the ICD-10 Diagnostic Criteria for Research specify an onset within 1 month. Furthermore, ICD-10 excludes stressors of "unusual or catastrophic type." In contrast, DSM-IV-TR allows extreme stressors so long as the criteria are not met for posttraumatic or acute stress disorder. ICD-10 also provides for several different subtypes, including "brief depressive reaction" (depressive state lasting 1 month or less), "prolonged depressive reaction" (depressive state lasting up to 2 years).

## Acknowledgment
This work was funded by the Malcomb Gibbs Foundation, Inc., New York.

## References

Adams C and Gelder M (1994) The case for establishing a register of randomized controlled trials of mental health care. Br J Psychiatr 164, 433–436.

Almquist F, Puura K, Kumpulainen K, et al. (1999) Psychiatric disorders in 8–9-year-old children based on a diagnostic interview with the parents. Eur Child Adolesc Psychiatr 8(Suppl 4), 17–28.

American Psychiatric Association (1980) Diagnostic and Statistical Manual of Mental Disorders, 3rd ed. APA, Washington DC.

American Psychiatric Association (1987) Diagnostic and Statistical Manual of Mental Disorders, 3rd ed., Rev. APA Washington DC.

American Psychiatric Association (2000) Diagnostic and Statistical Manual of Mental Disorders, 4th ed., Text Rev. APA, Washington DC.

Andreasen NC and Hoenk PR (1982) The predictive value of adjustment disorders: A follow-up study. Am J Psychiatr 139, 589.

Andreasen NC and Wasek P (1980) Adjustment disorders in adolescents and adults. Arch Gen Psychiatr 37, 1166–1170.

Angst J and Ernst C (1993) Current concepts of the classification of affective disorders. Int Clin Psychopharmacol 8, 211–215.

Ansseau M, Bataille M, Briole G, et al. (1996) Controlled comparison of tianeptin, alprazolam and mianserin in the treatment of adjustment disorders with anxiety and depression. Hum Psychopharmacol Clin Exp 11, 293–298.

Antman EM, Lau J, Kupelnick B, et al. (1992) A comparison of results of meta-analyses of randomized control trials and recommendations of clinical experts. JAMA 268, 240–248.

Aoki T, Hosaka T, and Ishida A (1995) Psychiatric evaluation of physical rehabilitation patients. Gen Hosp Psychiatr 17, 440–443.

Bird HR, Canino G, Rubio-Stipec M, et al. (1988) Estimates of the prevalence of childhood maladjustment in a community survey in Puerto Rico. Arch Gen Psychiatr 45, 1120–1126.

Bird HR, Gould MS, Yager T, et al. (1989) Risk factors for maladjustment in Puerto Rican children. J Am Acad Child Adolesc Psychiatr 28, 847–850.

Chalmers I, Dickersin K, and Chalmers TC (1992) Getting to grips with Archie Cochrane's agenda. BMJ 305, 786–788.

Cohen F (1981) Stress and bodily illness. Psychiatr Clin N Am 4, 269–286.

Conte HR and Karasu TB (1992) A review of treatment studies of minor depression: 1980–1991. Am J Psychother 46, 58–74.

Cunningham AJ, Edmonds CV, Jenkins GP, et al. (1998) A random-ized controlled trial of the effects of group psychological therapy on survival in women with metastatic breast cancer. Psycho-Oncology 7, 508–517.

De Leo D, Pellegrini C, and Serraiotto L (1986a) Adjustment disorders and suicidality. Psychol Rep 59, 355–358.

De Leo D, Pellegrini C, Serraiotto L, et al. (1986b) Assessment of severity of suicide attempts: A trial with the dexamethasone suppression test and two rating scales. Psychopathology 19, 186–191.

Depue RA and Monroe SM (1986) Conceptualization and measurement of human disorder in life stress research: The problem of chronic disturbance. Psychol Bull 99, 36–51.

Despland JN, Monod L, and Ferrero F (1995) Clinical relevance of AD in DSM-III-R and DSM-IV. Comp Psychiatr 36, 456–460.

DeWit S, Cremers L, Hirsch D, et al. (1999) Efficacy of trazodone versus clorazepate in the treatment of HIV-positive subjects with adjustment disorder: A pilot study. J Int Med Res 27, 223–232.

Doan RJ and Petti TA (1989) Clinical and demographic characteristics of child and adolescent partial hospital patients. J Am Acad Child Adolesc Psychiatr 28(1) (Jan), 66–69.

Dohrenwend BS, Krasnoff L, Askenasy AR, et al. (1978) Exemplification of a method for scaling life events: The PERI Life Event Scale. J Health Soc Behav 19, 205–229.

Endicott J (1984) Measurement of depression in patients with cancer. Cancer 53, 2243–2249.

Fabrega H Jr. and Mezzich J (1987) Adjustment disorder and psychiatric practice: Cultural and historical aspects. Psychiatry 50, 31–49.

Fabrega H Jr, Mezzich J, Mezzich AC, et al. (1986) Descriptive validity of DSM-I. II. Depressions. J Nerv Ment Dis 174, 573–584.

Fabrega H Jr., Mezzich JE, Mezzich AC, et al. (1987) Adjustment disorder as a marginal or transitional illness category in DSM-III. Arch Gen Psychiatr 44, 567–572.

Faulstich ME, Moore JR, Carey MP, et al. (1986) Prevalence of DSM-III conduct and adjustment disorders for adolescent psychiatric inpatients. Adolescence 21, 333–337.

Feighner JP, Robins E, Guze SB, et al. (1972) Diagnostic criteria for use in psychiatric research. Arch Gen Psychiatr 26, 57–63.

Field M and Lohr KN (1992) Guidelines for Clinical Practice. From Development to Use. National Academy Press, Washington DC.

Fowler RC, Rich CL, and Young D (1986) San Diego suicide study II. Substance abuse in young cases. Arch Gen Psychiatr 43, 962–965.

Friedmann MS, McDermut WH, Solomon DA, et al. (1997) Family functioning and mental illness: A comparison of psychiatric and nonclinical families. Fam Process 36, 357–367.

Goodwin PJ, Leszcz M, Ennis M, et al. (2001) The effect of group psychosocial support on survival in metastatic breast cancer. N Engl J Med 345, 1719–1726.

Grassi L, Gritti P, Rigatelli M, et al. (2000) Psychosocial problems secondary to cancer: An Italian multicenter survey of consultation-liaison psychiatry in oncology. Italian Consultation Liaison Group. Eur J Cancer 36, 579–585.

Hartmann H (1986) Ego Psychology and the Problem of Adaptation. International Universities Press, New York, pp. 23, 35, 46.

Hillard JR, Slomowitz M, and Levi LS (1987) A retrospective study of adolescents' visits to a general hospital psychiatric emergency service. Am J Psychiatr 144, 432.

Holmes TH and Rahe RH (1967) The Social Readjustment Rating Scale. J Psychosom Res 11, 213–218.

Isometsa E, Heikkinen M, Henriksson M, et al. (1996) Suicide in non-major depressions. J Affect Disord 36, 117–127.

Jacobson AM, Goldberg ID, Burns BJ, et al. (1980) Diagnosed mental disorder in children and use of health services in four organized health care settings. Am J Psychiatr 137, 559–565.

Jones R, Yates WR, Williams S, et al. (1999) Outcome for adjustment disorder with depressed mood: Comparison with other mood disorders. J Affect Disord 55, 55–61.

Kaplan SL, Simms RM, and Busner J (1994) Prescribing practices of out-patient child psychiatrists. J Am Acad Child Adolesc Psychiatr 33, 35–44.

Keller M, Klein DN, Hirschfeld RMA, et al. (1995) Results of the DSM-IV mood disorders field trial. Am J Psychiatr 152, 843–849.

Kellermann M, Fekete I, Gesztelyi R, et al. (1994) Screening for depressive symptoms in acute phase of a stroke. Gen Hosp Psychiatr 21, 116–121.

Klineman A (1980) Patients and Healers in the Context of Culture: An Exploration of the Borderland between Anthropology, Medicine and Psychiatry. University of California Press, Berkeley, CA.

Kovacs M, Feinberg TL, Crouse-Novak MA, et al. (1984) Depressive disorders in childhood. I. A longitudinal prospective study of character-istics and recovery. Arch Gen Psychiatr 41, 643–649.

Kovacs M, Gatsonis C, Pollock M, et al. (1994) A controlled prospective study of DSM-III adjustment disorder in childhood. Arch Gen Psychiatr 51, 535–541.

Kovacs M, Goldston D, and Gatsonis C (1993) Suicidal behaviors and childhood-onset depressive disorders: A longitudinal investigation. J Am Acad Child Adolesc Psychiatr 32, 8–20.

Kovacs M, Ho V, and Pollock MH (1995) Criterion and predictive validity of the diagnosis of adjustment disorder: A prospective study of youths with new-onset insulin-dependent diabetes mellitus. Am J Psychiatr 152, 523–528.

Kugaya A, Akechi T, Okuyama T, et al. (2000) Prevalence, predictive factors, and screening for psychological distress in patients with newly diagnosed head and neck cancers. Cancer 88, 2817–2823.

Lazarus AA (1992) The multimodal approach to the treatment of minor depression. Am J Psychother 46, 50–57.

Liebowitz MR (1993) Mixed anxiety and depression: Should it be included in DSM-IV? J Clin Psychiatr 54(Suppl), 4–7; discussion 17–20.

Markowitz JC, Klerman GL, and Perry SW (1992) Interpersonal psychotherapy of depressed HIV-positive outpatients. Hosp Comm Psychiatr 43, 885–890.

McGrath J (1989) A survey of deliberate self-poisoning. Med J Austral 150, 317–318.

McNair DM, Lorr M, and Doppelman LF (eds) (1971) Manual for the Profile of Mood States. Educational and Industrial Testing Service, San Diego, CA.

Mezzich JE, Dow JT, Rich CL, et al. (1981) Developing an efficient clinical information system for a comprehensive psychiatric institute. II. Initial evaluation form. Behav Res Methods Instr 13, 464–478.

Mezzich JE, Fabrega H Jr, Coffman GA, et al. (1989) DSM-III disorders in a large sample of psychiatric patients: Frequency and specificity of diagnoses. Am J Psychiatr 146, 212–219.

Minnaar GK, Schlebusch L, and Levin A (1980) A current study of parasuicide in Durban. S Afr Med J 57, 204–207.

Mok H and Walter C (1995) Brief psychiatric hospitalization: Preliminary experience with an urban sort-stay unit. Can J Psychiatr 40, 415–417.

Monroe SM, Kupfer DJ, and Frank E (1992) Life stress and treatment course of recurrent depression. I. Response during index episode. J Consult Clin Psychol 60, 718–724.

Olfson MM, Pincus HA, Zito JM, et al. (1998) Antidepressant prescribing practices of outpatient psychiatrists. Arch Gen Psychiatr 55, 310–316.

Oxman TE, Barrett JE, Freeman DH, et al. (1994) Frequency and correlates of adjustment disorder relates to cardiac surgery in older patients. Psychosomatics 35, 557–568.

Paykel ES, Prusoff BA, and Uhlenhuth EH (1971) Scaling of life events. Arch Gen Psychiatr 25, 340–347.

Perez-Jimenez JP, Gomez-Bajo GJ, LopezCatillo JJ, et al. (1994) Psychiatric consultation and posttraumatic stress disorder in burned patients. Burns 20, 532–536.

Perris H, von Knorring L, Oreland L, et al. (1984) Life events and biological vulnerability: A study of life events and platelet MAO activity in depressed patients. Psychiatr Res 12, 111–120.

Pollin IS and Holland J (1992) A model for counseling the medically ill: The Linda Pollin Foundation approach. Gen Hosp Psychiatr 14(Suppl 6), 15–25.

Popkin MK, Callies AL, and Colon EA (1988) The treatment and outcome of adjustment disorders in medically ill inpatients. National Institute of Mental Health Conference, Pittsburgh, PA.

Popkin MK, Callies AL, Colon EA, et al. (1990) Adjustment disorders in medically ill patients referred for consultation in a university hospital. Psychosomatics 31, 410–414.

Pozzi G, Del Borgo C, Del Forna A, et al. (1999) Psychological discomfort and mental illness in patients with AIDS: Implications for home care. STDS 13, 555–564.

Pulimood S, Rajagopalan B, Rajagopalan M, et al. (1996) Psychiatric morbidity among dermatology inpatients. Nat Med J India 9, 208–210.

Rahe RH (1990) Psychosocial stressors and adjustment disorder: Van Gogh's life chart illustrates stress and disease. J Clin Psychiatr 51(Suppl), 13–24.

Rapp SR and Vrana S (1989) Substituting nonsomatic for somatic symptoms in the diagnosis of depression in elderly male medical patients. Am J Psychiatr 146, 1197–1200.

Razavi D, Kormoss N, Collard A, et al. (1999) Comparative study of the efficacy and safety of trazodone versus clorazepate in the treatment of adjustment disorders in cancer patients: A pilot study. J Int Med Res 27, 264–272.

Rey JM, Stewart GW, Plapp JM, et al. (1988) DSM-III Axis IV revisited. Am J Psychiatr 145, 286–292.

Reynolds CF (1992) Treatment of depression in special populations. J Clin Psychiatr 53(Suppl), 45–53.

Rosenberg PB, Ahmed I, and Hurwitz S (1991) Methylphenidate in depressed medically ill patients. J Clin Psychiatr 52, 263–267.

Runeson B (1989) Mental disorder in youth suicide: DSM-III-R Axes I and II. Acta Psychiatr Scand 79, 490–497.

Runeson BS, Beskow J, and Waern M (1996) The suicidal process in suicides among young people. Acta Psychiatr Scand 93, 35–42.

Rutter M (1981) Stress, coping and development: Some issues and some questions. J Child Psychol Psychiatr 22, 323–356.

Schatzberg AF (1990) Anxiety and adjustment disorder: A treatment approach. J Clin Psychiatr 51(Suppl), 20–24.

Schnyder U and Valach L (1997) Suicide attempters in a psychiatric emergency room population. Gen Hosp Psychiatr 19, 119–129.

Setterberg SR, Ernst M, Rao U, et al. (1991) Child psychiatrists' views of DSM-III-R: Survey of usage and opinions. J Am Acad Child Adolesc Psychiatr 30, 652–658.

Shaffer D, Gould MS, Brasic J, et al. (1983) A Children's Global Assessment Scale (CGAS). Arch Gen Psychiatr 40, 1228–1231.

Shaner R (2000) Benzodiazepines in psychiatric emergency settings. Psychiatr Ann 30, 268–289.

Shima S, Kitagawa Y, Kitamura T, et al. (1994) Poststroke depression. Gen Hosp Psychiatr 16, 286–289.

Sifneos PE (1989) Brief dynamic and crisis therapy. In Comprehensive Textbook of Psychiatry, Vol. 2, 5th ed., Kaplan HI and Sadock BJ (eds). Williams & Wilkins, Baltimore, pp. 1562–1567.

Skodol AE, Dohrenwend BP, Line BG, et al. (1990) The nature of stress: Problems of measurement. In Stressors and the Adjustment Disorder, Noshpitz JD and Coddington RD (eds). John Wiley, New York, pp. 3–22.

Slavney PR (1999) Diagnosing demoralization in consultation psychiatry. Psychosomatics 40, 325–329.

Snyder S and Strain JJ (1989) Differentiation of major depression and adjustment disorder with depressed mood in the medical setting. Gen Hosp Psychiatr 12, 159–165.

Snyder S and Strain JJ (1990) Diagnostic instability in psychiatric consultations. Hosp Comm Psychiatr 41, 10–13.

Spalletta G, Troisi A, Saracco M, et al. (1996) Symptom profile: Axis II comorbidity and suicidal behaviour in young males with DSM-III-R depressive illnesses. J Affect Disord 39, 141–148.

Spiegel D (1994) DSM-IV Options Book. American Psychiatric Association, Washington DC.

Spiegel D (1996) Cancer and depression. Br J Psychiatr 168(Suppl 30), 109–116.

Spiegel D, Bloom JR, Kraemer HC, et al. (1989) Effect of psychosocial treatment on survival in breast cancer. Lancet 1, 888–891.

Spitzer RL and Forman JBW (1979) DSM-III field trials. II. Initial experience with the multiaxial system. Am J Psychiatr 136, 818–820.

Stewart JW, Quitkin FM, and Klein DF (1992) The pharmacotherapy of minor depression. Am J Psychother 46, 23–36.

Strain JJ (1981) Diagnostic considerations in the medical setting. Psychiatr Clin N Am 4, 287–300.

Strain JJ, Newcorn J, Wolf D, et al. (1993) Considering changes in adjustment disorder. Hosp Comm Psychiatr 44, 13–15.

Strain JJ, Newcorn JH, Mezzich JE, et al. (1998a) Adjustment disorder: The MacArthur reanalysis. In DSM-IV Sourcebook, Vol. 4. American Psychiatric Association, Washington DC, pp. 403–424.

Strain JJ, Smith GC, Hammer JS, et al. (1998b) Adjustment disorder: A multisite study of its utilization and interventions in the consultation-liaison psychiatry. Gen Hosp Psychiatr 20, 139–149.

Sullivan MJ, Winshenker B, and Mikail S (1995) Screening for major depression in the early stages of multiple sclerosis. Can J Neurol Sci 22, 228–231.

Tennant C (1983) Life events and psychological morbidity: The evidence from prospective studies [editorial]. Psychol Med 13, 483–486.

Tripodianakis J, Markianos M, Sarantidis D, et al. (2000) Neurochemical variables in subjects with adjustment disorder after suicide attempts. Eur Psychiatr 15, 190–195.

True PK and Benway MW (1992) Treatment of stress reaction prior to combat using the "BICEPS" model. Mil Med 157, 380–381.

Uhlenhuth EH, Balter MB, Ban TA, et al. (1995) International study of expert judgment on therapeutic use of benzodiazepines and other psychotherapeutic medications. III. Clinical features affecting experts' therapeutic recommendations in anxiety disorders. Psychopharmacol Bull 31, 289–296.

Vlachos IO, Bouras N, Watson JP, et al. (1994) Deliberate self-harm referrals. Eur J Psychiatr 8, 25–28.

Volz HP and Kieser M (1997) Kava-kava extract WS 1490 versus placebo in anxiety disorders: A randomized placebo-controlled 25-week out-patient trial. Pharmacopsychiatry 30, 1–5.

Weiner IB and Del Gaudio AC (1976) Psychopathology in adolescence: An epidemiological study. Arch Gen Psychiatr 33, 187–193.

Wise MG (1988) Adjustment disorders and impulse control disorders not otherwise classified. In Textbook of Psychiatry, Talbot JA, Hales R, and Yodofsky SC (eds). American Psychiatric Press, Washington DC, pp. 605–620.

Woolston JL (1988) Theoretical considerations of the adjustment disorders. J Am Acad Child Adolesc Psychiatr 27, 280.

Zarb J (1996) Correlates of depression in cognitively impaired hospitalized elderly referred for neuropsychological assessment. J Clin Exp Neuropsychol 18, 713–723.

Zilberg NJ, Weiss DS, and Horowitz MJ (1982) Impact of Event Scale: A cross-validation study and some empirical evidence supporting a conceptual model of stress response syndromes. J Consult Clin Psychol 50, 407–414.

Zimmerman M, Pfohl B, Coryell W, et al. (1987) The prognostic validity of DSM-III Axis IV in depressed inpatients. Am J Psychiatr 144, 102–106.

Zinbarg RE, Barlow DH, Liebowitz M, et al. (1994) The DSM-IV field trial for mixed anxiety-depression. Am J Psychiatr 151, 1153–1162.

Zung W (1965) A self-rating depression scale. Arch Gen Psychiatr 12, 63–70.

Zung W (1971) A rating instrument for anxiety disorders. Psychosomatics 12, 371–379.

# 79    Personality Disorders

Thomas A. Widiger
Stephanie Mullins

Personality Disorder
Paranoid Personality Disorder
Schizoid Personality Disorder
Schizotypal Personality Disorder
Antisocial Personality Disorder
Borderline Personality Disorder
Histrionic Personality Disorder
Narcissistic Personality Disorder
Avoidant Personality Disorder
Dependent Personality Disorder
Obsessive–Compulsive Personality Disorder
Passive–Agressive Personality Disorder
Depressive Personality Disorder

Personality traits have long been the focus of considerable research. Their heritability, cross-situational consistency, temporal stability, functional relevance to work, well-being, marital stability, and even physical health have been well established across many studies (Pervin and John 1999, Hogans et al. 1997). Everybody has a personality, or a characteristic manner of thinking, feeling, behaving, and relating to others. Some persons are typically introverted and withdrawn, others are more extraverted and outgoing. Some persons are invariably conscientious and efficient, whereas other persons might be consistently undependable and negligent. Some persons are characteristically anxious and apprehensive, whereas others are typically relaxed and unconcerned. These personality traits are often felt to be integral to each person's sense of self, as they involve what persons value, what they do, and their innate tendencies and preferences.

It is "when personality traits are inflexible and maladaptive and cause significant functional impairment or subjective distress [that] they constitute Personality Disorders" (American Psychiatric Association 2000, p. 686). The *Diagnostic and Statistical Manual of Mental Disorders*, Fourth Edition, Text Revision (DSM-IV-TR) (American Psychiatric Association 2000) provides the diagnostic criteria for 10 personality disorders. Two additional diagnoses are placed within an appendix to DSM-IV for criteria sets provided for further study (passive–aggressive and depressive).

This chapter begins with a discussion of the definition, etiology, assessment, epidemiology, course, and treatment of personality disorders in general, followed by a discussion of these issues for the 12 individual personality disorders.

## Personality Disorder

### Definition

A personality disorder is defined in DSM-IV-TR as "an enduring pattern of inner experience and behavior that deviates markedly from the expectations of the individual's culture, is pervasive and inflexible, has an onset in adolescence or early adulthood, is stable over time, and leads to distress or impairment" (American Psychiatric Association 2000, p. 686). The DSM-IV-TR general diagnostic criteria for a personality disorder are provided below.

Personality disorder is the only class of mental disorders in DSM-IV-TR for which an explicit definition and criterion set are provided. A general definition and criterion set can be useful to psychiatrists because the most common personality disorder diagnosis in clinical practice is often the diagnosis "not otherwise specified" (NOS) (Clark et al. 1995). Psychiatrists provide the NOS diagnosis when they determine that a personality disorder is present but the symptomatology fails to meet the criterion set for one of the 10 specific personality disorders. A general definition of

## DSM-IV-TR Criteria

### General Diagnostic Criteria for Personality Disorder

A. An enduring pattern of inner experience and behavior that deviates markedly from the expectations of the individual's culture. This pattern is manifested in two (or more) of the following areas:

   1. cognition (i.e., ways of perceiving and interpreting self, other people, and events)

   2. affectivity (i.e., the range, intensity, lability, and appropriateness of emotional response)

   3. interpersonal functioning

   4. impulse control

B. The enduring pattern is inflexible and pervasive across a broad range of personal and social situations.

C. The enduring pattern leads to clinically significant distress or impairment in social, occupational, or other important areas of functioning.

D. The pattern is stable and of long duration and its onset can be traced back at least to adolescence or early adulthood.

E. The enduring pattern is not better accounted for as a manifestation or consequence of another mental disorder.

F. The enduring pattern is not due to the direct physiological effects of a substance (e.g., a drug of abuse, a medication) or a general medical condition (e.g., head trauma).

Reprinted with permission from the Diagnostic and Statistical Manual of Mental Disorders, Fourth Edition, Text Revision. Copyright 2000 American Psychiatric Association.

what is meant by a personality disorder is therefore helpful when determining whether the NOS diagnosis should in fact be provided. Points worth emphasizing with respect to the general criterion set are presented in the following discussion of the assessment, differential diagnosis, epidemiology, and course of personality disorders.

### Etiology and Pathophysiology

A primary purpose of a diagnosis is to lead to scientific knowledge concerning the etiology for a patient's condition and the identification of a specific pathology for which a particular treatment (e.g., medication) would ameliorate the condition (Frances et al. 1995). However, many of the mental disorders in DSM-IV-TR, including the personality disorders, may not in fact have single etiologies or even specific pathologies. The DSM-IV-TR personality disorders might be, for the most part, constellations of maladaptive personality traits that are the result of multiple genetic dis-

positions interacting with a variety of detrimental environmental experiences (Clark and Watson 1999, Widiger and Sankis 2000). The DSM-IV-TR personality disorder diagnoses do provide the clinician with a substantial amount of important information concerning the etiology and pathology for a patient's particular personality syndrome, but there are likely to be alternative pathways to the development of maladaptive personality traits and alternative neurophysiological, cognitive–behavioral, interpersonal, and psychodynamic models for their pathology (Livesley 2001).

### Assessment and Differential Diagnosis

One of the innovations of DSM-III was the provision of a multiaxial system for clinical diagnosis (American Psychiatric Association 1980, Spitzer et al. 1980). However, prior to DSM-III psychiatrists rarely diagnosed a personality disorder when a patient's symptoms met the diagnostic criteria for an anxiety, mood, or other mental disorder. In an extensive, widely cited, and historically influential study of psychiatric diagnosis, Ward and colleagues (1962, p. 202) concluded that psychiatric diagnoses were excessively unreliable and that the greatest basis of disagreement was determining "whether the neurotic symptomatology or the characterological pathology is more extensive or basic". They criticized the assumption that a clinician must choose between a "neurotic condition" and a personality disorder when both in fact appeared to be present. A personality disorder will predate the onset of most other mental disorders and its presence is likely to have a considerable impact on the treatment of these other disorders (Dolan-Sewell et al. 2001, Millon et al. 1996). DSM-III, therefore, moved the personality disorders to a separate axis so that psychiatrists could diagnose both conditions "rather than being forced to arbitrarily and unreliably make a choice between them" (Frances 1980, p. 1050). The multiaxial system does appear to have been successful in encouraging psychiatrists to no longer make arbitrary distinctions between personality disorders and other mental disorders (Loranger 1990). Ironically, however, the placement of the personality disorders on a separate axis may have also contributed to the development of false assumptions and misleading expectations concerning the distinctions between personality disorders and other mental disorders with respect to etiology, pathology, or treatment (Livesley 1998).

The second most frequently cited cause for unreliable clinical diagnosis identified by Ward and colleagues (1962) was the absence of specific, explicit diagnostic criteria. Another innovation of DSM-III (American Psychiatric Association 1980, Spitzer et al. 1980) was the provision of specific and explicit diagnostic criterion sets that have facilitated the obtainment of more reliable clinical diagnosis. This innovation, however, has been problematic for the personality disorders as it is difficult to provide a brief list of specific diagnostic criteria for the broad and complex behavior patterns that constitute a personality disorder. The only personality disorder to be diagnosed reliably in general clinical practice has been antisocial and the validity of this diagnosis has been questioned precisely because of its emphasis on overt and behaviorally specific acts of criminality, irresponsibility, and delinquency (Hare et al. 1991, Widiger and Corbitt 1995).

There are assessment instruments, however, that will help psychiatrists obtain more reliable and valid personality disorder diagnoses. Semistructured interviews will obtain reliable diagnoses of personality disorders and are therefore the preferred method for the assessment of personality disorders in clinical research (Kaye and Shea 2000, Widiger and Coker 2002, Zimmerman 1994). Semistructured interviews provide a researched set of required and recommended interview queries and observations to assess each of the personality disorder diagnostic criteria. Psychiatrists can find the administration of a semistructured interview to be constraining (Westen 1997) but a major strength of semistructured interviews is their assurance through an explicit structure that each relevant diagnostic criterion has in fact been systematically assessed. Idiosyncratic and subjective interviewing techniques are much more likely to result in gender- and culturally-biased assessments relative to unstructured clinical interviews (Garb 1997, Widiger 1998). The manuals that accompany a semistructured interview also provide useful information for understanding the rationale of each diagnostic criterion, for interpreting vague or inconsistent symptomatology, and for resolving diagnostic ambiguities. There are currently five semistructured interviews for the assessment of the DSM-IV-TR (American Psychiatric Association 2000) personality disorder diagnostic criteria: (1) Diagnostic Interview for Personality Disorders (Zanarini et al. 1995); (2) International Personality Disorder Examination (Loranger 1999); (3) Personality Disorder Interview-IV (Widiger et al. 1995); (4) Structured Clinical Interview for DSM-IV-TR Axis II Personality Disorders (First et al. 1997); and (5) Structured Interview for DSM-IV-TR Personality Disorders (Pfohl et al. 1997). The particular advantages and disadvantages of each particular interview have been discussed extensively (Clark and Harrison 2001, Kaye and Shea 2000, Widiger and Coker 2002, Zimmerman 1994).

The administration of an entire personality disorder semistructured interview can take 2 hours, an amount of time that is impractical for routine clinical practice. However, this time can be reduced substantially by first administering a self-report questionnaire that screens for the presence of the DSM-IV-TR personality disorders (Widiger and Coker 2002). A psychiatrist can then confine the interview to the few personality disorders that the self-report inventory suggested would be present. Self-report inventories are useful in ensuring that all of the personality disorders were systematically considered and in alerting the clinician to the presence of maladaptive personality traits that might otherwise have been missed. There are a number of alternative self-report inventories that can be used and the advantages and disadvantages of each of them have been discussed extensively (Clark and Harrison 2001, Kaye and Shea 2000, Millon et al. 1996, Widiger and Coker 2002).

Gender and cultural biases are one potential source of inaccurate personality disorder diagnosis that are worth noting in particular (Alarcon 1996, Garb 1997, Widiger 1998). One of the general diagnostic criteria for personality disorder is that the personality trait must deviate markedly from the expectations of a person's culture (see DSM-IV-TR general diagnostic criteria for personality disorders). The purpose of this cultural deviation requirement is to compel clinicians to consider the cultural background of the patient. A behavior pattern that appears to be aberrant from the perspective of one's own culture (e.g., submissiveness or emotionality) could be quite normative and adaptive within another culture. The cultural expectations or norms of the psychiatrist might not be relevant or applicable to a patient from a different cultural background. However, one should not infer from this requirement that a personality disorder is primarily or simply a deviation from a cultural norm. Deviation from the expectations of one's culture is not necessarily maladaptive, nor is conformity to one's culture necessarily healthy. Many of the personality disorders may even represent (in part) extreme or excessive variants of behavior patterns that are valued or encouraged within a particular culture. For example, it is usually adaptive to be confident but not to be arrogant, to be agreeable but not to be submissive, or to be conscientious but not to be perfectionistic. Gender and cultural biases of particular relevance to individual personality disorders will be discussed further in the chapter.

## Epidemiology and Comorbidity

Virtually all patients must have had a characteristic manner of thinking, feeling, behaving, and relating to others prior to the onset of an Axis I disorder that could have an important impact on the course and treatment of the respective mental disorder (Harkness and Lilienfeld 1997) and many of these persons would be diagnosed with a DSM-IV-TR personality disorder (Dolan-Sewell et al. 2001, Mattia and Zimmerman 2001). Estimates of the prevalence of personality disorder within clinical settings is typically above 50% (Mattia and Zimmerman 2001). As many as 60% of inpatients within some clinical settings would be diagnosed with borderline personality disorder (American Psychiatric Association 2000, Gunderson 2001) and as many as 50% of inmates within a correctional setting could be diagnosed with antisocial personality disorder (Widiger and Corbitt 1995). Although the comorbid presence of a personality disorder is likely to have an important impact on the course and treatment of an Axis I disorder (Dolan-Sewell et al. 2001) the prevalence of personality disorder is generally underestimated in clinical practice due in part to the failure to provide systematic or comprehensive assessments of personality disorder symptomatology and perhaps as well to the lack of funding for the treatment of personality disorders (Zimmerman and Mattia, 1999).

Approximately 10 to 15% of the general population would be diagnosed with one of the 10 DSM-IV-TR personality disorders, excluding PDNOS (Mattia and Zimmerman 2001, Torgersen et al. 2001). Table 79–1 provides prevalence data reported by the best available studies to date for estimating the prevalence of individual personality disorders within a community population. All of these studies have important limitations, though, that qualify their results. For example, many of the studies sampled persons who would probably have less personality disorder pathology than a randomly selected sample (e.g., some studies have sampled persons without any history of Axis I psychopathology) and the studies have used either the DSM-III (American Psychiatric Association 1980) or DSM-III-R (American Psychiatric Association 1987) criterion sets rather than DSM-IV-TR (American Psychiatric Association 2000). Nevertheless, the prevalence estimates are

| Table 79–1 | Epidemiology of Personality Disorders | | | | | | | | | | | | | | |
|---|---|---|---|---|---|---|---|---|---|---|---|---|---|---|---|
| | Sample | N | Int | DSM | PRN | SZD | STP | ATS | BDL | HST | NCS | AVD | DPD | OCP | PAG |
| Black et al. (1993) | R-HN | 127 | SIDP | III | 1.6 | 0.0 | 3.9 | 0.0 | 5.5 | 3.9 | 0.0 | 3.2 | 2.4 | 7.9 | 12.6 |
| Black et al. (1993) | R-OCD | 120 | SIDP | III | 1.7 | 0.0 | 2.5 | 0.8 | 0.8 | 2.5 | 0.0 | 0.8 | 0.8 | 10.8 | 8.3 |
| Coryell et al. (1989) | R-HN | 185 | SIDP | III | 0.5 | 1.6 | 2.2 | 1.6 | 1.1 | 1.6 | 0.0 | 1.6 | 0.5 | 3.2 | 2.2 |
| Drake et al. (1988) | Men(47) | 369 | Clinical | III | 1.1 | 4.1 | 2.4 | 0.8 | 0.5 | 3.8 | 3.5 | 1.6 | 10.3 | 0.5 | 7.8 |
| Klein et al. (1995) | R-DP | 258 | PDE | III-R | 1.7 | 0.9 | 0.0 | 2.2 | 1.7 | 1.7 | 3.9 | 5.2 | 0.4 | 2.6 | 1.7 |
| Lenzenweger et al. (1997) | Stdts | 1646 | PDE | III-R | 0.4 | 0.4 | 0.0 | 0.8 | 0.0 | 1.9 | 1.2 | 0.4 | 0.4 | 0.0 | 0.0 |
| Maier et al. (1992) | Comm | 452 | SCID-II | III-R | 1.8 | 0.4 | 0.7 | 0.2 | 1.1 | 1.3 | 0.0 | 1.1 | 1.5 | 2.2 | 1.8 |
| Moldin et al. (1994) | HN | 302 | PDE | III-R | 0.0 | 0.0 | 0.7 | 2.6 | 2.0 | 0.3 | 0.0 | 0.7 | 1.0 | 0.7 | 1.7 |
| Samuels et al. (1994) | Comm | 762 | Clinical | III | 0.0 | 0.0 | 0.1 | 1.5 | 0.4 | 2.1 | 0.0 | 0.0 | 0.1 | 1.7 | 0.1 |
| Torgersen et al. (2001) | Comm | 2053 | SIDP-R | III-R | 2.4 | 1.7 | 0.6 | 0.7 | 0.7 | 2.0 | 0.8 | 5.0 | 1.5 | 2.0 | 1.7 |
| Median | | | | | 1.4 | 0.4 | 0.7 | 0.8 | 1.0 | 2.0 | 0.0 | 1.4 | 0.9 | 2.1 | 1.7 |
| DSM-IV estimates | | | | | .5-2.5 | uncm | 3.0 | 2.0 | 2.0 | 2-3 | <1 | .5-1 | — | 1.0 | |

*Note*: N, number of persons in study; Int, interview that was used; DSM=Edition of Diagnostic and Statistical Manual that was used (DSM-III or DSM-III-R); PRN, paranoid; SZD, schizoid; STP, schizotypal; ATS, antisocial; BDL, borderline; HST, histrionic; NCS, narcissistic; AVD, avoidant; DPD, dependent; OCP, obsessive–compulsive; PAG, passive–aggressive; R-HN, relatives of hyper-normal (persons without history of mental disorder); R-OCD, relatives of persons with obsessive–compulsive anxiety disorder; Men(47), males of approximate age of 47 years; R-DP, relatives of persons with depression; Stdts, students; Comm, community; SIDP, Structured Interview for Personality Disorder (Pfohl B, Blum N, and Zimmerman M [1997] Structured Interview for DSM-IV-TR Personality Disorder. American Psychiatric Press, Washington DC.); SCID-II, Structured Clinical Interview for DSM personality disorder (First M, Gibbon M, Spitzer RL, et al. [1997] User's Guide for the Structured Clinical Interview for DSM-IV Axis II Personality Disorders. American Psychiatric Press, Washington DC.); Clinical, unstructured or unspecified semistructured interview; PDE, Personality Disorder Examination; uncm, uncommon.

generally close to those provided in DSM-IV-TR. Prevalence rates for individual personality disorders will be discussed later in this chapter.

There is also considerable personality disorder diagnostic co-occurrence (Bornstein 1998, Lilienfeld et al. 1994, Oldham et al. 1992, Widiger and Trull 1998). Patients who meet the DSM-IV diagnostic criteria for one personality disorder are likely to meet the diagnostic criteria for another. Table 79–2 provides the co-occurrence among the DSM-III-R (American Psychiatric Association 1987) personality disorder diagnoses that were obtained for the development of DSM-IV (Widiger and Trull 1998). DSM-IV instructs psychiatrists that all diagnoses should be recorded because it can be important to consider (for example) the presence of antisocial traits in someone with a borderline personality disorder or the presence of paranoid traits in someone with a dependent personality disorder. However, the extent of diagnostic co-occurrence is at times so extensive that most researchers prefer a more dimensional description of personality (Cloninger 2000, Livesley 1998, Oldham and Skodol 2000, Widiger 2000). Diagnostic categories provide clear, vivid descriptions of discrete personality types but the personality structure of actual patients might be more accurately described by a constellation of maladaptive personality traits.

Alternative dimensional models of personality disorder are being developed. One such model, based on a theory of temperament and character, consists of seven dimensions. Cloninger (2000) proposes that there are four temperaments (reward dependence, harm avoidance, novelty seeking, and persistence), each governed by a particular neurotransmitter system, and three character dimensions

| Table 79–2 | DSM-III-R Personality Disorder Diagnostic Co-Occurrence Aggregated Across Six Research Sites | | | | | | | | | | |
|---|---|---|---|---|---|---|---|---|---|---|---|
| | PRN | SZD | SZT | ATS | BDL | HST | NCS | AVD | DPD | OCP | PAG |
| Paranoid (PRN) | — | 8 | 19 | 15 | 41 | 28 | 26 | 44 | 23 | 21 | 30 |
| Schizoid (SZD) | 38 | — | 39 | 8 | 22 | 8 | 22 | 55 | 11 | 20 | 9 |
| Schizotypal (SZT) | 43 | 32 | — | 19 | 44 | 17 | 26 | 68 | 34 | 19 | 18 |
| Antisocial (ATS) | 30 | 8 | 15 | — | 59 | 39 | 40 | 25 | 19 | 9 | 29 |
| Borderline (BDL) | 31 | 6 | 16 | 23 | — | 30 | 19 | 39 | 36 | 12 | 21 |
| Histrionic (HST) | 29 | 2 | 7 | 17 | 41 | — | 40 | 21 | 28 | 13 | 25 |
| Narcissistic (NCS) | 41 | 12 | 18 | 25 | 38 | 60 | — | 32 | 24 | 21 | 38 |
| Avoidant (AVD) | 33 | 15 | 22 | 11 | 39 | 16 | 15 | — | 43 | 16 | 19 |
| Dependent (DPD) | 26 | 3 | 16 | 16 | 48 | 24 | 14 | 57 | — | 15 | 22 |
| Obs–Compulsive (OCP) | 31 | 10 | 11 | 4 | 25 | 21 | 19 | 37 | 27 | — | 23 |
| Pass–Aggressive (PAG) | 39 | 6 | 12 | 25 | 44 | 36 | 39 | 41 | 34 | 23 | — |

Sites used DSM-III-R criterion sets. Data obtained for purposes of informing the development of the DSM-IV-TR personality disorder diagnostic criteria.

*Source*: Widiger TA and Trull TJ (1998) Performance characteristics of the DSM-III-R personality disorder criteria sets. In DSM-IV Sourcebook, Vol. 4, Widiger TA, Frances AJ, Pincus HA, et al. (eds). American Psychiatric Association, Washington DC.

(self-directedness, cooperativeness, and self-transcendence). The presence of a personality disorder is said to be determined primarily by the four temperaments and the particular form or manner of the personality disorder by the three character dimensions.

Another approach has been to apply the predominant model of general personality functioning to the study of personality disorders. Five broad domains of personality functioning have been identified empirically through the study of the languages of a number of different cultures (Hogan et al. 1997, Pervin and John 1999). Language can be understood as a sedimentary deposit of the observations of persons over the thousands of years of the language's development and transformation. The most important domains of personality functioning would be those with the greatest number of terms to describe and differentiate their various manifestations and nuances, and the structure of personality will be evident by the empirical relationship among the trait terms. Such lexical analyses of languages have typically identified five fundamental dimensions of personality: neuroticism (or negative affectivity) versus emotional stability, introversion versus extraversion, conscientiousness versus undependability, antagonism versus agreeableness, and closedness versus openness to experience (Costa and McCrae 1992). Each of these five broad domains can be differentiated further in terms of underlying facets. For example, the facets of antagonism versus agreeableness include suspiciousness versus trusting gullibility, tough-mindedness versus tender-mindedness, confidence and arrogance versus modesty and meekness, exploitation versus altruism and sacrifice, oppositionalism and aggression versus compliance, and deception and manipulation versus straightforwardness and honesty (Costa and McCrae 1992). Each of the DSM-IV-TR personality disorders can be understood as maladaptive variants of these personality traits that are evident in all persons to varying degrees (Widiger et al. 2002).

Table 79–3 provides a description of the DSM-IV-TR personality disorders in terms of this five factor model. For example, the schizoid personality disorder may represent an extreme variant of introversion, avoidant may represent extreme neuroticism and introversion, and antisocial personality disorder an extreme variant of antagonism and undependability. Advantages of understanding personality disorders in terms of this dimensional model are the provision of more specific descriptions of individual patients (including adaptive as well as maladaptive personality functioning) and the avoidance of arbitrary categorical distinctions. An additional factor is the ability to bring to bear on an understanding of personality disorders the extensive amount of research on the heritability, temperament, development, and course of general personality functioning (Costa and Widiger 2002).

## Course

Personality disorders must be evident since adolescence or young adulthood and have been relatively chronic and stable throughout adult life (see DSM-IV-TR criteria for personality disorders). The World Health Organization's (WHO) *International Classification of Diseases*, 10th Revision (ICD-10, World Health Organization 1992) does recognize the existence of personality change secondary to catastrophic experiences and to brain injury or disease, but only the latter is included within DSM-IV-TR (American Psychiatric Association 2000). A 75-year-old man can be diagnosed with a DSM-IV-TR dependent personality disorder but the symptoms must have been present throughout the duration of his adulthood (e.g., since the age of 18 years) unless the dependent behavior was a direct, explicit expression of a neurochemical disease or lesion.

The requirement that a personality disorder be evident since late adolescence and be relatively chronic thereafter has been a traditional means with which to distinguish a personality disorder from an Axis I disorder (Millon et al. 1996, Spitzer et al. 1980). Mood, anxiety, psychotic, sexual, and other mental disorders have traditionally been conceptualized as conditions that arise at some point during a person's life and that are relatively limited or circumscribed in their expression and duration. Personality disorders, in contrast, are conditions that are evident as early as late adolescence (and in some instances prior to that time), are evident in everyday functioning, and are stable throughout adulthood. However, the consistency of this distinction across disorders in the classification has been decreasing with each edition of the DSM, as early-onset and chronic variants of Axis I disorders are being added to the diagnostic manual (e.g., early-onset dysthymia and generalized social phobia). Some researchers have in fact suggested abandoning the concept of personality disorders and replacing them with early-onset and chronic variants of existing Axis I disorders. For example, avoidant personality disorder could become generalized social phobia, obsessive–compulsive personality disorder could become an early-onset variant of obsessive–compulsive anxiety disorder, and borderline personality disorder could become an early-onset and chronic mood dyscontrol. A precedent for this revision of the diagnostic manual is that ICD-10 currently does not include a diagnosis of schizotypal personality disorder, including instead a diagnosis of schizotypal disorder that is an early-onset and chronic variant of schizophrenia (World Health Organization 1992).

## Treatment

One of the mistaken assumptions or expectations of Axis II is that personality disorders are untreatable. In fact, maladaptive personality traits are often the focus of clinical treatment (Beck and Freeman 1990, Benjamin 1993, Gabbard 2000, Gunderson and Gabbard 2000, Millon et al. 1996, Markovitz 2001, Paris 1998, Stone 1993). Personality disorders are among the more difficult of mental disorders to treat as they involve entrenched behavior patterns, some of which will be integral to a patient's self-image (Millon et al. 1996, Stone 1993). Nevertheless, there is compelling empirical support to indicate that meaningful responsivity to psychosocial and pharmacologic treatment does occur (Markovitz 2001, Perry et al. 1999, Sanislow and McGlashan 1998). Treatment of a personality disorder is unlikely to result in the development of a fully healthy or ideal personality structure, but clinically and socially meaningful change to personality structure and functioning does occur. In fact, given the considerable social, occupational, medical, and other costs that are engendered by such personality disorders as the antisocial and borderline, even marginal reductions in symptomatology can represent

| Table 79–3 | DSM-IV-TR Personality Disorders from the Perspective of the Five-Factor Model of General Personality Functioning |

|  | PRN | SZD | SZT | ATS | BDL | HST | NCS | AVD | DPD | OCP |
|---|---|---|---|---|---|---|---|---|---|---|
| **Neuroticism** |  |  |  |  |  |  |  |  |  |  |
| Anxiousness |  |  | High |  | High |  |  | High | High |  |
| Angry hostility | High |  |  | High | High |  | High |  |  |  |
| Depressiveness |  |  |  |  | High | High |  | High |  |  |
| Self-consciousness |  |  | High |  |  | High | High | High | High |  |
| Impulsivity |  |  |  |  | High |  |  |  |  |  |
| Vulnerability |  |  |  |  | High |  |  | High | High |  |
| **Extraversion** |  |  |  |  |  |  |  |  |  |  |
| Warmth |  | Low | Low |  |  | High |  |  | High |  |
| Gregariousness |  | Low | Low |  |  | High |  | Low |  |  |
| Assertiveness |  |  |  |  |  |  |  | Low | Low | High |
| Activity |  |  |  |  |  |  |  |  |  |  |
| Excitement-seeking |  |  |  | High |  | High |  | Low |  |  |
| Positive emotionality |  | Low | Low |  |  | High |  |  |  |  |
| **Openness** |  |  |  |  |  |  |  |  |  |  |
| Fantasy |  |  | High |  |  | High | High |  |  |  |
| Aesthetics |  |  |  |  |  |  |  |  |  |  |
| Feelings |  | Low |  |  |  | High |  |  |  |  |
| Actions |  |  | High |  |  |  |  |  |  |  |
| Ideas |  |  | High |  |  |  |  |  |  |  |
| Values |  |  |  |  |  |  |  |  |  | Low |
| **Agreeableness** |  |  |  |  |  |  |  |  |  |  |
| Trust | Low |  | Low |  | Low | High |  |  | High |  |
| Straightforwardness | Low |  |  | Low |  |  |  |  |  |  |
| Altruism |  |  |  | Low |  |  | Low |  | High |  |
| Compliance | Low |  |  | Low | Low |  |  |  | High | Low |
| Modesty |  |  |  |  |  |  | Low |  | High |  |
| Tender-mindedness |  |  |  | Low |  |  | Low |  |  |  |
| **Conscientiousness** |  |  |  |  |  |  |  |  |  |  |
| Competence |  |  |  |  | Low |  |  |  |  | High |
| Order |  |  |  |  |  |  |  |  |  | High |
| Dutifulness |  |  |  | Low |  |  |  |  |  | High |
| Achievement-striving |  |  |  |  |  |  | High |  |  | High |
| Self-discipline |  |  |  | Low |  |  |  |  |  |  |
| Deliberation |  |  |  | Low |  |  |  |  |  |  |

quite significant and meaningful public health care, social and clinical benefits (Linehan 1993, 2000).

DSM-IV-TR includes 10 individual personality disorder diagnoses that are organized into three clusters: (a) paranoid, schizoid, and schizotypal (placed within an odd–eccentric cluster); (b) antisocial, borderline, histrionic, and narcissistic (dramatic–emotional–erratic cluster); and (c) avoidant, dependent, and obsessive–compulsive (anxious–fearful cluster) (American Psychiatric Association 2000). Each of these personality disorders, along with the two that are included in the appendix to DSM-IV-TR for disorders needing further study (i.e., passive–aggressive and depressive), will be discussed in turn.

## Paranoid Personality Disorder

### Definition

Paranoid personality disorder (PPD) involves a pervasive and continuous distrust and suspiciousness of the motives of others (American Psychiatric Association 2000) but the disorder is more than just suspiciousness. Persons with this disorder are also hypersensitive to criticism, they respond with anger to threats to their autonomy, they incessantly seek out confirmations of their suspicions, and they tend to be quite rigid in their beliefs and perceptions of others (Millon et al. 1996, Widiger et al. 1995). The presence of PPD is indicated by four or more of the seven diagnostic criteria presented in the DSM-IV criteria for PPD.

### Etiology and Pathology

Research has indicated a genetic contribution to the development of suspiciousness and mistrust (Jang et al. 1998, Nigg and Goldsmith 1994, Plomin and Caspi 1999). There is some support for a genetic relationship of PPD with schizophrenia but these findings have not always been replicated and the findings may have been due to the overlap of PPD with the schizotypal personality disorder (Siever 1992). There is only limited support for a genetic relationship with delusional disorder, persecutory type (Nigg and Goldsmith 1994).

**Paranoid Personality Disorder**

A. A pervasive distrust and suspiciousness of others such that their motives are interpreted as malevolent, beginning by early adulthood, and present in a variety of contexts, as indicated by four (or more) of the following:

(1) suspects, without sufficient basis, that others are exploiting, harming, or deceiving him or her

(2) is preoccupied with unjustified doubts about the loyalty or trustworthiness of friends or associates

(3) is reluctant to confide in others because of unwarranted fear that the information will be used maliciously against him or her

(4) reads hidden demeaning or threatening meanings into benign remarks or events

(5) persistently bears grudges, i.e. is unforgiving of insults, injuries, or slights

(6) perceives attacks on his or her character or reputation that are not apparent to others and is quick to react angrily or to counterattack

(7) has recurrent suspicions, without justification, regarding fidelity of spouse or sexual partner

B. Does not occur exclusively during the course of schizophrenia, a mood disorder with psychotic features, or another psychotic disorder, and is not due to the direct physiological effects of a general medical condition.

**Note:** if criteria are met prior to the onset of schizophrenia, add "premorbid," e.g., paranoid personality disorder (premorbid).

There are no systematic studies on possible psychosocial contributions to the development of PPD. There is some support for the contribution of excessive parental criticism and rejection but there has not yet been adequate prospective longitudinal studies (Miller et al. 2001). Paranoid belief systems could develop through parental modeling, a history of discriminatory exploitation or abandonment, or the projection of anger, resentment, and bitterness onto a group that is external to, and distinct from, oneself. Mistrust and suspicion is often evident in members of minority groups, immigrants, refugees, and other groups for whom such distrust can be a realistic and appropriate response to the social environment. It is conceivable that a comparably sustained experience through childhood and adolescence could contribute to the development of excessive paranoid beliefs that are eventually applied inflexibly and inappropriately to a wide variety of persons, but it can be very difficult to determine what is excessive or unrealistic suspicion and mistrust within a member of an oppressed minority (Alarcon and Foulks 1997). Paranoid suspiciousness could in fact be more closely associated with prejudicial attitudes, wherein a particular minority group in society becomes the inappropriate target of one's anger, blame, and resentment.

There has been little consideration given to the neurophysiological concomitants of nonpsychotic paranoid personality traits. More attention has been given to cognitive, interpersonal, and object-relational models of pathology. Paranoid beliefs do appear to have a self-perpetuating tendency resulting from the narrow and limited focus on signs and evidence for malicious intentions (Beck and Freeman 1990). The pathology of PPD, from this perspective, is inherent to the irrationality of the person's belief systems and is sustained by the biased information processing. There may also be an underlying motivation or need to perceive threats in others and to externalize blame that help to sustain the accusations and distortions (Gabbard 2000, Millon et al. 1996).

**Differential Diagnosis**

PPD paranoid ideation is inconsistent with reality and is resistant to contrary evidence but the ideation is not psychotic, absurd, inconceivable, or bizarre. PPD also lacks other features of psychotic and delusional disorders (e.g., hallucinations) and is evident since early adulthood, whereas a psychotic disorder becomes evident later within a person's life or remits after a much briefer period of time. Persons with PPD can develop psychotic disorders but to diagnose PPD in such cases the paranoid personality traits must be evident prior to and persist after the psychotic episode. If PPD precedes the onset of schizophrenia, then it should be noted that it is premorbid to the schizophrenia (American Psychiatric Association 2000). However, it may not be meaningful to diagnose a person with both PPD and schizophrenia, as the premorbid paranoid traits may in some cases have simply represented a prodromal phase of the schizophrenic pathology.

**Epidemiology and Comorbidity**

Trust versus mistrust is a fundamental personality trait along which all persons vary (Pervin and John 1999). Thirteen percent of the adult male population and 6% of the adult female population may be characteristically mistrustful of others (Costa and McCrae 1992). However, only 0.5 to 2.5% of the population are likely to meet the DSM-IV-TR diagnostic criteria for a PPD (see DSM-IV-TR Criteria for PPD). It is suggested in DSM-IV-TR that approximately 10 to 30% of persons within inpatient settings and 2 to 10% within outpatient settings have this disorder (American Psychiatric Association 2000) but the lower end of these rates may represent the more accurate estimate. It does appear that more males than females have the disorder (Corbitt and Widiger 1995).

Paranoid personality traits are evident in other personality disorders. Persons with avoidant personality disorder are socially withdrawn and apprehensive of others; borderline, antisocial, and narcissistic persons may be impatient, irritable, and antagonistic; and schizotypal persons may display paranoid ideation. The diagnosis of PPD often co-occurs with these other personality disorder diagnoses (see Table 79–2). Persons with PPD are prone to develop a variety of Axis I disorders, including substance-related, obsessive–compulsive anxiety, agoraphobia, and depressive disorders (American Psychiatric Association 2000).

## Course

Premorbid traits of PPD may be evident prior to adolescence in the form of social isolation, hypersensitivity, hypervigilance, social anxiety, peculiar thoughts, angry hostility, and idiosyncratic fantasies (American Psychiatric Association 2000). As children, they may appear odd and peculiar to their peers and they may not have achieved to their capacity in school. Their adjustment as adults is particularly poor with respect to interpersonal relationships. They may become socially isolated or fanatic members of groups that encourage or at least accept their paranoid ideation. They might maintain a steady employment but are difficult coworkers, as they tend to be rigid, controlling, critical, blaming, and prejudicial. They are likely to become involved in lengthy, acrimonious, and litigious disputes that are difficult, if not impossible, to resolve (Millon et al. 1996, Stone 1993).

## Treatment

Persons with PPD rarely seek treatment for their feelings of suspiciousness and distrust. They experience these traits as simply accurate perceptions of a malevolent and dangerous world (i.e., ego-syntonic). They may not consider the paranoid attributions to be at all problematic, disruptive, or maladaptive. They are not delusional but they also fail to be reflective, insightful, or self-critical. They may recognize only that they have difficulty controlling their anger and getting along with others. They might be in treatment for an anxiety, mood, or substance-related disorder or for various marital, familial, occupational, or social (or legal) conflicts that are secondary to their personality disorder but they also externalize the responsibility for their problems and have substantial difficulty recognizing their own contribution to their internal dysphoria and external conflicts. They consider their problems to be due to what others are doing to them, not to how they perceive, react, or relate to others.

The presence of paranoid personality traits complicate the treatment of an Axis I disorder or a relationship problem (Dolan-Sewell et al. 2001). Trust is central to the development of an adequate therapeutic alliance, yet it is precisely the absence of trust that is central to this disorder (Gabbard 2000, Stone 1993). It can be tempting to be less than forthright and open in the treatment of excessively suspicious persons because they distort, exaggerate, or escalate minor errors, misunderstandings, or inconsistent statements. However, therapists find that they weave an increasingly tangled web as they walk gingerly around the truth. Also, persons with PPD seize upon any kernel of deception to confirm their suspicion that the therapist is not to be trusted. It is preferable to be especially forthright and precise with paranoid patients. Details that are inconsequential and of no interest to most patients can be important to provide to persons with PPD so that they are ensured that nothing is being withheld or hidden from them.

Clinicians agree on several general principles in the treatment of paranoid personality traits (Beck and Freeman 1990, Gabbard 2000, Millon et al. 1996, Stone 1993). It is usually pointless and often harmful to rapport or to confront (or argue with) the paranoid beliefs. Such efforts may only alienate the patient and confirm his or her suspicions. The therapist should maintain a sincere and consistent respect for their autonomy and for their right to make their own decisions. However, one should not attempt to ingratiate oneself by being overly acquiescent and compliant. This can appear to be obviously patronizing, insincere, or manipulative. The goal is to develop, in a nonthreatening way, more self-reflection and self-awareness (e.g., recognition of the contribution of the paranoid traits and behaviors to the difficulties they are experiencing within their lives). A useful approach can be to communicate a sincere and respectful willingness to explore the implications, logic, and reality of the suspicions (Beck and Freeman 1990). Whenever one appears to be endangering rapport by moving too quickly, one should retreat to a more neutral and accepting position.

One must also be careful to avoid defensive reactions to the inevitable accusations. Any one of the conflicts they have had with others can develop within the therapeutic relationship (Benjamin 1993, Gabbard 2000) and persons with PPD have a tendency to be contentious, rigid, accusatory, suspicious, and litigious that can tax the empathy and patience of the therapist. One must attempt to maintain an empathic concern for their feelings of betrayal, and reassure them in an understanding, forthright manner that is neither patronizing nor disrespectful. Termination of treatment may at times be necessary if continuation would only result in further acrimony.

The suspicions, accusations, and acrimony often makes the person with PPD a poor candidate for group therapies. There is the potential to learn much about themselves within a group, but it is usually very difficult for them to develop the feelings of trust, respect, and security that are necessary for successful group therapy. Their propensity to make unfair hostile accusations alienate them from other group members, and they may quickly become a scapegoat for difficulties and conflicts that develop within the group.

There have been a variety of studies on the pharmacologic treatment of psychotic paranoid ideation and of schizotypal PD (which often includes paranoid personality traits) but little to no research on the pharmacologic responsivity of the nonpsychotic suspiciousness and ego-syntonic paranoid ideation of PPD (Markovitz 2001, Perry et al. 1999). Persons with PPD may also perceive the use of a medication to represent an effort to simply suppress or control their accusations and suspicions rather than to respectfully consider and address them. However, they may be receptive and responsive to the benefits of a medication to help control feelings of anxiousness or depression that are secondary to their personality disorder.

## Schizoid Personality Disorder

### Definition

The schizoid personality disorder (SZPD) is a pervasive pattern of social detachment and restricted emotional expression. Introversion (versus extraversion) is one of the

**Schizoid Personality Disorder**

A. A pervasive pattern of detachment from social relationships and a restricted range of expression of emotions in interpersonal settings, beginning by early adulthood and present in a variety of contexts, as indicated by four (or more) of the following:

(1) neither desires nor enjoys close relationships, including being part of a family

(2) almost always chooses solitary activities

(3) has little, if any, interest in having sexual experiences with another person

(4) takes pleasure in few, if any, activities

(5) lacks close friends or confidants other than first-degree relatives

(6) appears indifferent to the praise or criticism of others

(7) emotional coldness, detachment, or flattened affectivity

B. Does not occur exclusively during the course of schizophrenia, a mood disorder with psychotic features, another psychotic disorder, or a pervasive developmental disorder, and is not due to the direct physiological effects of a general medical condition.

**Note:** if criteria are met prior to the onset of schizophrenia, add "premorbid," e.g., schizoid personality disorder (premorbid).

fundamental dimensions of general personality functioning (Pervin and John 1999). Facets of introversion include low warmth (e.g., cold, detached, impersonal), low gregariousness (socially isolated, withdrawn), and low positive emotions (reserved, constricted or flat affect, anhedonic), which define well the central symptoms of SZPD (Widiger et al. 2002; see Table 79–3). The presence of SZPD is indicated by four or more of the seven diagnostic criteria presented in the DSM-IV criteria for SZPD.

## Etiology and Pathology

A fundamental distinction for schizophrenic symptomatology is between positive and negative symptoms. Positive symptoms include hallucinations, delusions, inappropriate affect, and loose associations; negative symptoms include flattened affect, alogia, anhedonia, and avolition. SZPD has been conceptualized as representing subthreshold negative symptoms, comparable to the subthreshold positive symptoms (cognitive–perceptual aberrations) that

predominate schizotypal personality disorder (STPD). However, a genetic link of SZPD to schizophrenia that cannot be accounted for by comorbid STPD symptomatology has not been well established (Miller et al. 2001). Research has supported heritability for the personality dimension of introversion–extraversion (Jang et al. 1998, Jang and Vernon 2001, Plomin and Caspi 1999) and for the association of SZPD with introversion (Costa and Widiger 2002). The central pathology of SZPD does appear to be anhedonic deficits, or an excessively low ability to experience positive affect (Kalus et al. 1993, Rothbart and Ahardi 1994). Psychosocial models for the etiology of SZPD are lacking. It is possible that a sustained history of isolation during infancy and childhood, with an encouragement and modeling by parental figures of interpersonal withdrawal, indifference, and detachment could contribute to the development of schizoid personality traits (Bernstein and Travaglini 1999).

## Differential Diagnosis

SZPD can be confused with the schizotypal and avoidant personality disorders as both involve social isolation and withdrawal (Kalus et al. 1993, Widiger et al. 1995). Schizotypal personality disorder, however, also includes an intense social anxiety and cognitive–perceptual aberrations. The major distinction with avoidant personality disorder is the absence of an intense desire for intimate social relationships. Avoidant persons will also exhibit substantial insecurity and inhibition, whereas the schizoid person is largely indifferent toward the reactions or opinions of others (Widiger et al. 1995).

The presence of premorbid schizoid traits can have prognostic significance for the course and treatment of schizophrenia (Siever 1992) but, more importantly, it might not be meaningful to suggest that a person has a schizoid personality disorder that is independent of or unrelated to a comorbid schizophrenia. The negative, prodromal, and residual symptoms of schizophrenia resemble closely the features of SZPD. Once a person develops schizophrenia, a diagnosis of SZPD can become rather pointless as all of the schizoid symptoms can then be understood as (prodromal or residual) symptoms of schizophrenia.

## Epidemiology and Comorbidity

Approximately half of the general population will exhibit an introversion within the normal range of functioning. However, only a small minority of the population would be diagnosed with a schizoid personality disorder (Mattia and Zimmerman 2001). Estimates of the prevalence of SZPD within the general population have been less than 1% (see Table 79–1) and SZPD is among the least frequently diagnosed personality disorders within clinical settings. Many of the persons who were diagnosed with SZPD prior to DSM-III are probably now diagnosed with either the avoidant or the schizotypal personality disorders (Widiger et al. 1988) and prototypic (pure) cases of SZPD are likely to be quite rare within the population.

## Course

Persons with SZPD are socially isolated and withdrawn as children. They may not have been accepted well by their peers, and may have even borne the brunt of some ostracism (American Psychiatric Association 2000). As adults, they have few friendships. The friendships that do occur are likely to be initiated by their peers or colleagues. They have few sexual relationships and may never marry. Relationships fail to the extent to which the other person desires or needs emotional support, warmth, and intimacy. Persons with SZPD may do well and even excel within an occupation, as long as substantial social interaction is not required. They prefer to work in isolation. They may eventually find employment and a relationship that is relatively comfortable, but they could also drift from one job to another and remain isolated throughout much of their life. If they do eventually become a parent, they have considerable difficulty providing warmth and emotional support, and they may appear neglectful, detached, and disinterested.

## Treatment

Prototypic cases of SZPD rarely present for treatment, whether it is for their schizoid traits or a concomitant Axis I disorder. They feel little need for treatment, as their isolation is often ego-syntonic. Their social isolation is of more concern to their relatives, colleagues, or friends than to themselves. Their disinterest in and withdrawal from intimate or intense interpersonal contact is also a substantial barrier to treatment. They at times appear depressed but one must be careful not to confuse their anhedonic detachment, withdrawal, and flat affect with symptoms of depression.

If persons with SZPD are seen for treatment for a concomitant Axis I disorder (e.g., a sexual arousal disorder or a substance dependence) it is advisable to work within the confines and limitations of the schizoid personality traits (Beck and Freeman 1990, Stone 1993). Charismatic, engaging, emotional, or intimate therapists can be very uncomfortable, foreign, and even threatening to persons with SZPD. A more business-like approach can be more successful (Beck and Freeman 1990).

It is also important not to presume that persons with SZPD are simply inhibited, shy, or insecure. Such persons are more appropriately diagnosed with the avoidant personality disorder. Persons with SZPD are perhaps best treated with a supportive psychotherapy that emphasizes education and feedback concerning interpersonal skills and communication (Stone 1993). One may not be able to increase the desire for social involvements but one can increase the ability to relate to, communicate with, and get along with others. Persons with SZPD may not want to develop intimate relationships but they will often want to interact and relate more effectively and comfortably with others. The use of role playing and videotaped interactions can at times be useful in this respect. Persons with SZPD can have tremendous difficulty understanding how they are perceived by others or how their behavior is unresponsive to and perceived as rejecting by others.

Group therapy is often useful as a setting in which the patient can gradually develop self-disclosure, experience the interest of others, and practice social interactions with immediate and supportive feedback (Beck and Freeman 1990, Gabbard 2000). However, persons with SZPD are prone to being rejected by a group due to their detachment, flat affect, and indifference to the feelings of others. If the group is patient and accepting, they can benefit from the experience.

There have been many studies on the pharmacologic treatment of the schizotypal PD but no comparable studies on SZPD (Markovitz 2001, Perry et al. 1999). The schizotypal and schizoid PDs share many features, but the responsivity of the schizotypal PD to pharmacotherapy will usually reflect schizotypal social anxiety and cognitive–perceptual aberrations that are not seen in prototypic, pure cases of SZPD.

## Schizotypal Personality Disorder

### Definition

Schizotypal PD (STPD) is a pervasive pattern of interpersonal deficits, cognitive and perceptual aberrations, and eccentricities of behavior (American Psychiatric Association 2000). The interpersonal deficits are characterized in large part by an acute discomfort with and reduced capacity for close relationships. The symptomatology of STPD has been differentiated further into components of positive (cognitive, perceptual aberrations) and negative (social aversion and withdrawal) symptoms comparable to the distinctions made for schizophrenia (Squires-Wheeler et al. 1997). The presence of STPD is indicated by five or more of the nine diagnostic criteria listed in the DSM-IV criteria for STPD.

### Etiology and Pathology

There is substantial empirical support for a genetic association of STPD with schizophrenia (Jang and Vernon 2001, Nigg and Goldsmith 1994, Siever 1992) which is not surprising given that the diagnostic criteria were obtained from the observations of biological relatives of persons with schizophrenia. Research has indicated further that the positive and negative symptoms may even have a distinct genetic relationship with the comparable symptoms of schizophrenia (Fanous et al. 2001). This suggests that the influence of familial etiological factors determining the expression of these symptom dimensions reaches across the boundary of psychotic illness to phenomena currently classified under the rubric of personality (Fanous et al. 2001, p. 672).

A predominant model for the psychopathology of STPD is deficits or defects in the attention and selection processes that organize a person's cognitive–perceptual evaluation of and relatedness to his or her environment (Raine et al. 1995). These defects may lead to discomfort within social situations, misperceptions and suspicions, and to a coping strategy of social isolation. Correlates of central nervous system dysfunction seen in persons with schizophrenia have been observed in laboratory tests of persons with STPD, including performance on tests of visual and auditory attention (e.g., backward masking and sensory gating tests) and smooth pursuit eye movement (Raine et al. 1997, Roitman et al. 1997). This dysfunction may be the result of dysregulation along dopaminergic pathways, which could be serving to modulate the expression of an underlying schizotypal genotype (Raine et al. 1995).

### Differential Diagnosis

Avoidant personality disorder and STPD share the features of social anxiety and introversion, but the social anxiety of STPD does not diminish with familiarity, whereas the

**DSM-IV-TR Criteria** 301.22

**Schizotypal Personality Disorder**

A. A pervasive pattern of social and interpersonal deficits marked by acute discomfort with, and reduced capacity for, close relationships as well as by cognitive or perceptual distortions and eccentricities of behavior, beginning by early adulthood, and present in a variety of contexts, as indicated by five (or more) of the following:

  (1) ideas of reference (excluding delusions of reference)

  (2) odd beliefs or magical thinking that influences behavior and is inconsistent with subcultural norms (e.g., superstitiousness, belief in clairvoyance, telepathy, or "sixth sense"; in children and adolescents, bizarre fantasies or preoccupations)

  (3) unusual perceptual experiences, including bodily illusions

  (4) odd thinking and speech (e.g., vague, circumstantial, metaphorical, overelaborate, or stereotyped)

  (5) suspiciousness or paranoid ideation

  (6) inappropriate or constricted affect

  (7) behavior or appearance that is odd, eccentric, or peculiar

  (8) lacks close friends or confidants other than first-degree relatives

  (9) excessive social anxiety that does not diminish with familiarity and tends to be associated with paranoid fears rather than negative judgments about self

B. Does not occur exclusively during the course of schizophrenia, a mood disorder with psychotic features, another psychotic disorder, or a pervasive developmental disorder.

**Note:** if criteria are met prior to the onset of schizophrenia, add "premorbid," e.g., schizotypal personality disorder (premorbid).

Reprinted with permission from the Diagnostic and Statistical Manual of Mental Disorders, Fourth Edition, Text Revision. Copyright 2000 American Psychiatric Association.

anxiety of avoidant PD (AVPD) is concerned primarily with the initiation of a relationship (Widiger et al. 1995). STPD is also a more severe disorder that includes a variety of cognitive and perceptual aberrations that are not seen in persons with AVPD.

An initial concern of many clinicians when confronted with a person with STPD is whether the more appropriate diagnosis is schizophrenia. Persons with STPD closely resemble persons within the prodromal or residual phases of schizophrenia. This differentiation is determined largely by the absence of a deterioration in functioning. It is indicated in DSM-IV that one should note that STPD is "premorbid" if the schizotypal symptoms were present prior to the onset of schizophrenia (American Psychiatric Association 2000). Premorbid schizotypal traits will have prognostic significance for the course and treatment of schizophrenia and such traits should then be noted (Siever 1992). However, as discussed for SZPD, in most of these cases the schizotypal PD symptoms could then be readily understood as prodromal symptoms of schizophrenia.

**Epidemiology and Comorbidity**

STPD may occur in as much as 3% of the general population although most studies with semistructured interviews have suggested a somewhat lower percent (see Table 79–1). STPD might occur somewhat more often in males (Corbitt and Widiger 1995, Raine et al. 1995). STPD co-occurs most often with the schizoid, borderline, avoidant, and paranoid personality disorders (see Table 79–2). Common Axis I disorders are major depressive disorder, brief psychotic disorder, and generalized social phobia (Miller et al. 2001).

**Course**

STPD is classified within the same diagnostic grouping as schizophrenia in ICD-10 (World Health Organization 1992) because of its close relationship in phenomenology, etiology, and pathology (Raine et al. 1995). However, it is classified as a personality disorder in DSM-IV-TR (American Psychiatric Association 2000) because its course and phenomenology are more consistent with a disorder of personality (i.e., early onset, evident in everyday functioning, characteristic of long-term functioning, and egosyntonic). Persons with STPD are likely to be rather isolated in childhood. They may have appeared peculiar and odd to their peers, and may have been teased or ostracized. Achievement in school is usually impaired, and they may have been heavily involved in esoteric fantasies and peculiar interests, particularly those that do not involve peers. As adults, they may drift toward esoteric–fringe groups that support their magical thinking and aberrant beliefs. These activities can provide structure for some persons with STPD, but they can also contribute to a further loosening and deterioration if there is an encouragement of aberrant experiences. Only a small proportion of persons with STPD develop schizophrenia (Raine et al. 1995). The symptomatology of STPD does not appear to remit with age (Siever 1992). The course appears to be relatively stable, with some proportion of schizotypal persons remaining marginally employed, withdrawn, and transient throughout their lives.

**Treatment**

Persons with STPD may seek treatment for their feelings of anxiousness, perceptual disturbances, or depression. Treatment of persons with STPD should be cognitive, behavioral, supportive, and/or pharmacologic, as they will often find the intimacy and emotionality of reflective, exploratory psychotherapy to be too stressful and they have the potential for psychotic decompensation.

Persons with STPD will often fail to consider their social isolation and aberrant cognitions and perceptions to be particularly problematic or maladaptive. They may consider themselves to be simply eccentric, creative, or nonconformist. Rapport can be difficult to develop as increasing familiarity and intimacy may only increase their level of discomfort and anxiety (Siever 1992). They are unlikely to be responsive to informality or playful humor. The sessions should be well-structured to avoid loose and tangential ideation.

Practical advice is usually helpful and often necessary (Beck and Freeman 1990). The therapist should serve as the patient's counselor, guide, or "auxiliary ego" to more adaptive decisions with respect to everyday problems (e.g., finding an apartment, interviewing for a job, and personal appearance). Persons with STPD should also receive social skills training directed at their awkward and odd behavior, mannerisms, dress, and speech. Specific, concrete discussions on what to expect and do in various social situations (e.g., formal meetings, casual encounters, and dates) should be provided. The rate of progress will tend to be slow, and it is helpful if there remains a continuity in the therapeutic relationship (Stone 1993).

Most of the systematic empirical research on the treatment of STPD has been confined to pharmacologic interventions. Low doses of neuroleptic medications (e.g., thiothixene) have shown some effectiveness in the treatment of schizotypal symptoms, particularly the perceptual aberrations and social anxiousness (Markovitz 2001, Siever 1992). Group therapy has also been recommended for persons with STPD but only when the group is highly structured and supportive (Millon et al. 1996). The emotional intensity and intimacy of unstructured groups will usually be too stressful. Schizotypal patients with predominant paranoid symptoms may even have difficulty in highly structured groups.

---

Clinical Vignette 1

LK was a 34-year-old male. He was referred to the Day Hospital Treatment Program by his parents. He had been living with them since his graduation from high school, with no apparent prospects of leaving home. They did not object to his staying at home, but they were now approaching retirement and they were worried that he might not be able to support himself. He was unemployed, had no close friends, and spent much of his time in his room with a computer.

LK was first diagnosed with schizotypal personality disorder at the age 26 years. The diagnosis was influential in his obtainment of disability income. He had been unemployed since the age of 19 years. His career goal was to become a successful fortune-teller. He had no history of psychotic episodes, although he had at times become intensely involved in fringe belief systems. The only time he had left home for any significant period was to participate on a quest for a close encounter with an alien in the deserts of Arizona. No concrete, physical encounters occurred but he did claim to have experienced a variety of signs of alien communication. He was also an active student of "numerology," or the study of the symbolic and spiritual significance of numbers. He described himself as "a 3-8-4."

He did not complain of any clinical symptoms other than chronic feelings of anxiousness, which at times escalated to the point that he felt unable to leave the house. He was also rather odd in his appearance. For example, he would often wear thick red flannel shirts in the summer with lime green pants, and then switch to red pants and a green flannel shirt the next week. He cut his own hair, creating an erratic, peculiar appearance. He described a history of fleeting, superficial relationships. He would at times feel lonely but stated that he found most people to be "discomforting."

His treatment consisted of group therapy, supportive psychotherapy, and a (low dosage) neuroleptic. He found the group therapy to be helpful in providing feedback regarding his appearance and mannerisms, such as staring intently at persons and then exclaiming "what, what, what?!" when eye contact was made or drifting off into tangential topics during conversations. The supportive psychotherapy focused on improving his social judgment and awareness, including grooming, hygiene, and dress. Therapy also included discussions of his experiences, misperceptions, and difficulties with persons within the group and elsewhere. He was also referred to the Occupational Activities Program for counseling and guidance regarding employment. He eventually obtained a trainee position within a wholesale computer dealership. He found the job to be quite satisfying, as it allowed him to work with computers and required little contact with others.

## Antisocial Personality Disorder

### Definition

Antisocial PD (ASPD) is a pervasive pattern of disregard for and violation of the rights of others (American Psychiatric Association 2000). Persons with ASPD will also be irresponsible and exploitative in their sexual relationships, and irresponsible as employees and parents. They may display a lack of empathy, an inflated or arrogant self-appraisal, a callous, cynical, and contemptuous response to the suffering of others, and a glib, superficial charm (Hare et al. 1991). This disorder has also been referred to as psychopathy (Hare et al. 1991), sociopathy, or dissocial (World Health Organization 1992) personality disorder. The presence of ASPD is indicated by the occurrence of a conduct disorder prior to age 15 years and by three of the seven adult diagnostic criteria presented in DSM-IV Criteria for ASPD.

### Etiology and Pathology

There is considerable support from twin, family, and adoption studies for a genetic contribution to the etiology of the criminal, delinquent tendencies of persons with ASPD (Nigg and Goldsmith 1994, Stoff et al. 1997). The genetic disposition may be somewhat stronger in ASPD females due perhaps to a greater social pressure on females against aggressive, exploitative, and criminal behavior (Hare et al. 1991). What is inherited by persons with ASPD, however, is unclear; it could be impulsivity, antagonistic callousness, or abnormally low anxiousness.

A predominant theory for the etiology of ASPD is that it results from abnormally low levels of behavioral inhibition and high levels of behavioral activation systems that

## DSM-IV-TR Criteria 301.7

### Antisocial Personality Disorder

A. There is a pervasive pattern of disregard for and violation of the rights of others (occurring since age 15 years), as indicated by three (or more) of the following:

 (1) failure to conform to social norms with respect to lawful behaviors as indicated by repeatedly performing acts that are grounds for arrest

 (2) deceitfulness, as indicated by repeated lying, use of aliases, or conning others for personal profit or pleasure

 (3) impulsivity or failure to plan ahead

 (4) irritability and aggressiveness, as indicated by repeated physical fights or assaults

 (5) reckless disregard for safety of self or others

 (6) consistent irresponsibility, as indicated by repeated failure to sustain consistent work behavior or honor financial obligations

 (7) lack of remorse, as indicated by being indifferent to or rationalizing having hurt, mistreated, or stolen from another

B. The individual is at least age 18 years.

C. Evidence of conduct disorder with onset before age 15 years.

D. The occurrence of antisocial behavior is not exclusively during the course of schizophrenia or a manic episode.

Reprinted with permission from the Diagnostic and Statistical Manual of Mental Disorders, Fourth Edition, Text Revision. Copyright 2000 American Psychiatric Association.

are important for normal, adaptive functioning (Fowles 2001, Widiger and Lynam 1998). The behavioral inhibition system (BIS) is responsible for inhibiting behavior in response to punishment and acts in opposition to the behavioral activation system (BAS) that activates behavior in response to reward. The BIS has input into the reticular activating system providing experiences of anxiety or arousal. The clinical symptoms of ASPD might be manifestations of a weak or deficient BIS in combination with a normal or strong BAS that reduce normal sensitivity and anxiety in response to threatening and stressful situations. Activities that the average person would find stimulating, antisocial persons would find dull, impelling them to engage in risky, reckless, prohibited, and impulsive activities. Low arousal would also help minimize feelings of anxiety, guilt, or remorse and help resist aversive conditioning. Studies have indicated an electrodermal response hyporeactivity in psychopathic persons (Fowles 2001, Stoff et al. 1997). This hyporeactivity may be particularly associated with a deficit in anticipatory anxiety and worrying, while not impairing

the alarm reactions of flight versus fight. Abnormally low levels of behavioral inhibition may be mediated by the septohippocampal system (and the neurotransmitter serotonin). Deficiencies in response modulation (difficulties suspending a dominant set in response to negative feedback) are apparent in animals with septohippocampal dysfunction (Newman and Wallace 1993).

There are also substantial data to support the contribution of family, peer, and other environmental factors (Stoff et al. 1997). No single environmental factor appears to be specific to its development. Modeling by parental figures and peers, excessively harsh, lenient, or erratic discipline, and a tough, harsh environment in which feelings of empathy and warmth are discouraged (if not punished) and tough-mindedness, aggressiveness, and exploitation are encouraged (if not rewarded) have all been associated with the development of ASPD (Sutker and Allain 2001). For example, ASPD in some cases could be the result of an interaction of early experiences of physical or sexual abuse, exposure to aggressive parental models, and erratic discipline that develop a view of the world as a hostile environment, which is further affirmed over time through selective attention on cues for antagonism, encouragement and modeling of aggression by peers, and the immediate benefits that result from aggressive, exploitative behavior (Dodge et al. 1990). Persons with ASPD may have had their feelings of anxiety, guilt, and remorse extinguished through progressive and cumulative experiences of harsh aggression, violence, abuse, and exploitation.

The development of adequate guilt, conscience, and shame may also require a degree of distress-proneness (anxiousness or neuroticism) and attentional self-regulation (constraint). Normal levels of neuroticism will promote the internalization of a conscience (the introjection of the family's moral values) by associating distress and anxiety with wrongdoing, and the temperament of self-regulation will help modulate impulses into a socially acceptable manner (Clark et al. 2000, Fowles and Kochanska 2000, Kochanska and Murray 2000, Rothbart and Ahadi 1994), Studies have indicated that high levels of arousal at age 15 years serve as a protective factor against criminal activities at age 30 years in persons at high risk for becoming criminals (Raine et al. 1995, 1998). Additional factors may also help to avoid the development of ASPD, such as high intelligence which may contribute to the availability of alternative life paths, while other factors may exacerbate or escalate its development, such as drug or alcohol dependence (Sher and Trull 1994). In sum, ASPD appears to be the result of a constellation of factors, including genetic predisposition, experiences within the family, and sociological factors, coupled with the absence of preventive factors (Stoff et al. 1997, Sutker and Allain 2001).

### Assessment and Differential Diagnosis

All of the DSM-IV-TR assessment instruments described earlier include the assessment of ASPD. However, an instrument that is focused on the assessment of ASPD is the Psychopathy Checklist—Revised (PCL-R, Hare 1991). The PCL-R is commonly used within forensic and prison settings and is particularly well suited for the assessment of this disorder within settings that are heavily populated by persons with a criminal history (Kaye and Shea 2000,

Widiger and Coker 2002). The PCL-R includes the assessment of psychopathic traits that are relatively more specific to ASPD within prison settings, such as lack of empathy, glib charm, and arrogance (Widiger et al. 1996). However, as suggested by its title, it is perhaps better described as a checklist than as a semistructured interview. Many of its items are scored primarily (if not solely) on the basis of a person's legal, criminal record rather than on the basis of interview questions. The availability of a detailed criminal history within prison settings has contributed to the PCL-R's excellent interrater reliability and predictive validity, but an application of the PCL-R within most other clinical settings will need to rely more heavily on PCL-R interview questions, the administration and scoring of which will be unclear for some PCL-R items (Lilienfeld 1994, Widiger and Coker 2002).

ASPD will at times be difficult to differentiate from a substance dependence disorder in young adults because many persons with ASPD develop a substance-related disorder and many persons with a substance dependence engage in antisocial acts. The requirement that the ASPD features be evident prior to the age of 15 years will usually assure the onset of ASPD prior to the onset of a substance-related disorder. If both are evident prior to the age of 15 years, then it is likely that both disorders are in fact present and both diagnoses should then be made. ASPD and substance dependence will often interact, exacerbating and escalating each other's development (Myers et al. 1998, Sher and Trull 1994, Stoff et al. 1997, Sutker and Allain 2001).

Antisocial acts will also be evident in the histrionic and borderline personality disorders, as persons with these disorders will display impulsivity, sensation-seeking, self-centeredness, manipulativeness, and a low frustration tolerance. Females with antisocial PD are often misdiagnosed with histrionic personality disorder (Widiger 1998). Prototypic cases of ASPD might be distinguished from other personality disorders by the presence of the childhood history of conduct disorder and the cold, calculated exploitation, abuse, and aggression (Millon et al. 1996, Widiger et al. 1995). Persons with narcissistic personality disorder are also characterized by a lack of empathy and may often exploit and use others. In fact, many of the traits of narcissistic personality disorder are evident in psychopathy, including a lack of empathy, glib and superficial charm, and arrogant self-appraisal (Widiger et al. 1996).

## Epidemiology and Comorbidity

The National Institute of Mental Health Epidemiologic Catchment Area (ECA) study indicated that approximately 3% of males and 1% of females have ASPD (Robins et al. 1991). This rate has been replicated in subsequent studies, but it has also been suggested that the ECA finding may have underestimated the prevalence in males due to the failure to consider the full range of ASPD features. Other estimates have been as high as 6% in males (Kessler et al. 1994, Robins et al. 1991). The rate of ASPD within prison and forensic settings has been estimated at 50% (Hare et al. 1991, Robins et al. 1991) but the ASPD criteria may exaggerate the rate within such settings due to the emphasis given to overt acts of criminality, delinquency, and irresponsibility that are common to the persons within these settings (Sutker and Allain 2001, Widiger et al. 1996). More specific criteria for psychopathy provide a more conservative estimate of 20 to 30% of male prisoners with ASPD (Hare et al. 1991).

ASPD is much more common in males than in females (Corbitt and Widiger 1995, Robins et al. 1991). A sociobiological explanation for the differential sex prevalence is the presence of a genetic advantage for social irresponsibility, infidelity, superficial charm, and deceit in males that contributes to a higher likelihood of developing features of ASPD (Stoff et al. 1997, Sutker and Allain 2001). It has also been suggested that ASPD and histrionic personality disorder share a biogenetic disposition (perhaps towards impulsivity or sensation-seeking) that is mediated by gender-specific biogenetic and sociological factors toward respective gender variants (Hamburger et al. 1996, Lilienfeld and Hess 2001).

Persons with ASPD are at a high risk for developing substance-related and impulse dyscontrol disorders (Stoff et al. 1997, Sutker and Allain 2001). They are also likely to display borderline, narcissistic, and paranoid personality traits (see Table 79–2). Females with ASPD will also display histrionic personality traits (Hamburger et al. 1996, Widiger 1998).

## Course

ASPD is evident in childhood in the form of a conduct disorder (Lynam 1996). Evidence of a conduct disorder prior to the age of 15 years is in fact required for a DSM-IV ASPD diagnosis (American Psychiatric Association 2000). The continuation into adulthood is particularly likely to occur if multiple delinquent behaviors are evident prior to the age of 10 years (Lynam 1996, Moffitt 1993, Moffit et al. 1996). As adults, persons with ASPD are unlikely to maintain steady employment and they may even become impoverished, homeless, or spend years within penal institutions (Robins et al. 1991). However, some persons with ASPD characterized by high rather than low levels of conscientiousness may express their psychopathic tendencies within a socially acceptable or at least legitimate profession (Hare 1991, Widiger and Lynam 1998). They may in fact be quite successful as long as their tendency to bend or violate the norms or rules of their profession and exploit, deceive, and manipulate others, contribute to a career advancement. Their success, however, may at some point unravel when their psychopathic behaviors become problematic or evident to others. The same pattern may also occur within sexual and marital relationships. They may at first appear to be charming, engaging, and sincere, but most relationships will end due to a lack of empathy, responsibility, and fidelity.

There does tend to be a gradual remission of antisocial behaviors, particularly overt criminal acts, as the person ages (Stoff et al. 1997, Sutker and Allain 2001). Persons with ASPD, however, are more likely than the general population to have died prematurely by violent means (e.g., accidents or homicides) and to engage in quite dangerous, high-risk behavior (Stoff et al. 1997).

## Treatment

The presence of ASPD is important to recognize in the treatment of any Axis I disorder, as their tendency to be manipulative, dishonest, exploitative, aggressive, and irresponsible will often disrupt and sabotage treatment. It is also very easy to be seduced by psychopathic charm. Persons with ASPD can be seductive in their engaging friendliness, expressions of remorse, avowed commitment to change, and apparent response to or even fascination with the success, skills, and talents of the therapist, none of which will be sincere or reliable.

The extent to which ASPD is untreatable has at times been overstated and exaggerated (Salekin 2002). Nevertheless, ASPD is the most difficult personality disorder to treat (Gunderson and Gabbard 2000, Stone 1993, Stoff et al. 1997). Persons with ASPD will often lack a motivation or commitment to change. They might see only the advantages of their antisocial traits and not the costs (e.g., risks of arrest and failure to sustain lasting or meaningful relationships). They are prone to manipulate, abuse, or exploit their fellow patients and the staff (Gabbard 2000). The immediate motivation for treatment is often provided by an external source, such as a court order or the demands of an employer or relative. Motivation may last only as long as an external pressure remains.

The most effective treatment is likely to be prevention through an identification and intervention early in childhood (Lynam 1996, Stoff et al. 1997). In adulthood, the most effective treatment may at times be simply some form of sustained incarceration (e.g., imprisonment), as many antisocial behaviors do tend to dissipate (or burnout) with time (Robins et al. 1991, Sutker and Allain 2001). The tendency to rationalize irresponsibility, minimize the consequences of acts, and manipulate others needs to be confronted on a daily and immediate basis. Community residential or wilderness programs that provide a firm structure, close supervision, and intense confrontation by peers have been recommended (Gabbard 2000) The involvement of family members in the treatment has been shown to be helpful, but there are also data to suggest that interventions with little professional input are less successful and are times counterproductive (Salekin 2002).

There is some research to suggest that the ability to form a therapeutic alliance is an important indicator of treatment success. Factors to consider are the demographic similarity of the therapist and patient, the quality of the patient's past relationships, and the therapist's positive regard for the patient (Stoff et al. 1997, Sutker and Allain 2001). Many psychiatrists may also experience strong feelings of animosity and distaste for antisocial persons who have a history of abusive and exploitative acts (Gunderson and Gabbard 2000). Rational, utilitarian approaches that help the person consider the long-term consequences of behavior can be helpful (Beck and Freeman 1990, Salekin 2002). This approach does not attempt to develop a sense of conscience, guilt, or even regret for past actions, but focuses instead on the material value and future advantages to be gained by a more prosocial behavior pattern. There are data to suggest the use of pharmacotherapy in the treatment of impulsive aggression but it is unclear whether these findings would generalize to the full spectrum of ASPD psychopathology (Markovitz 2001).

Clinical Vignette 2

MF was a 24-year-old male born in Miami, Florida. His biological mother died when he was 3 years old as the result of a stray bullet during a drug-related dispute. It was unclear whether his mother was herself involved in this dispute. He was taken from his biological father at the age of 6 years because of a history of neglect and physical abuse. He then lived in a series of foster homes until the age of 10 years when he was adopted by Mr. and Mrs. F.

Mr. and Mrs. F adopted M because they felt too old to raise a child from birth and wished to "give back to society what they had received." They were quite wealthy and wanted to provide a chance in life for a child from a disadvantaged background. However, they had difficulty from the beginning controlling M. He was first referred to treatment at the age of 13 years for setting fire to the school. He was diagnosed with a conduct disorder but was described by his therapist as being tearful, remorseful, and ashamed. Treatment was said to be successful.

At the age of 16 years he was remanded to treatment by a juvenile court for assaulting a police officer who had caught him trying to break into a neighbor's home. Mr. and Mrs. F acknowledged at his court hearing that he had a history of criminal behavior. Since his arrival within their home he had pawned expensive articles from home and repeatedly vandalized the house. His parents, however, felt that he simply needed more patience, understanding, and love. They noted that after each "incident" he was always very remorseful. They characterized his various aggressive and criminal acts as "occasional setbacks" or "falling off the wagon."

Treatment at this time revealed an apparent history of sexual abuse by an older male sibling within one of the foster homes. MF tearfully recounted lurid episodes of sexual victimization and attributed his difficulty controlling his behavior to the abuse he had received from this sibling and his father. Treatment was terminated after 1.5 years of outpatient therapy with no apparent recurrence of criminal or aggressive acts.

MF, however, was again referred to treatment at the age of 24 years when he was arrested for attempting to sexually abuse a neighbor's child. He presented as an intelligent, cultured young man who was ashamed, mortified, and distraught over his "inability" to control his sexual urges. He was diagnosed with pedophilia and referred to both individual and group treatment within a sexual offender's program. He discussed within his therapies of being sexually abused not only by a foster brother but also by his father.

However, his involvement within the program was questioned when he was discovered at night within the treatment center. He explained that he was simply trying to find his wallet that he left there after one of the group sessions. However, he had no explanation for how he had managed to enter the locked building. He claimed that the entry and office doors had not been locked. Members of his group spoke passionately on his behalf to be allowed to remain within the program. The staff was also painfully ambivalent. On the one hand, he was indeed the result of an abusive and neglectful history; on the other hand, he had committed a serious violation of the treatment program. The decision, however, became easier when it was discovered that he was sexually involved with a member of the staff, another program violation. He had stolen the keys from her. His motivation for treatment was also diminished substantially by the withdrawal of the sexual abuse charges by the neighbor's child and parents. MF's parents had apparently interceded on his behalf. The parents, however, continued to insist that he receive some form of treatment. He was then transferred to a summer residential program. After he left the sexual offenders program, group members acknowledged having been intimidated and threatened. Staff and patients concluded that he was in the building in order to obtain copies of the patients' confidential files.

The new treatment program was more actively confrontational and less tolerant. He eventually acknowledged that his past claims of being sexually abused were fraudulent. He had been physically abused by his biological father but he had not been sexually abused by him or anyone else. It was also discovered that he had gambled and lost a substantial amount of his parents' money, and had avoided a series of possible arrests by soliciting and obtaining the support of his parents and sympathetic victims.

MF proved to be very difficult to treat. It was never clear when he was being honestly remorseful and insightful, or simply saying what he believed the staff wanted to hear. His level of intelligence, verbal skills, and engaging charm were very compelling. He was indeed troubled by his past neglect and abuse. He would at times be able to acknowledge the bitterness, anger, and hurt from the past, yet he would then use whatever sympathy or empathy this history elicited to attempt to manipulate the staff. When confronted with this disingenuous manipulation he would then confess, express regret and remorse, and attempt a new ploy. None of the staff felt that they were able to develop a really meaningful relationship. He completed the summer program but the staff was pessimistic regarding his future.

## Borderline Personality Disorder

### Definition

Borderline personality disorder (BPD) is a pervasive pattern of impulsivity and instability in interpersonal relationships and self-image (American Psychiatric Association 2000). A broad domain of general personality functioning is neuroticism (or emotional instability; Pervin and John 1999), characterized by facets of angry hostility, anxiousness, depressiveness, impulsivity, and vulnerability; BPD is essentially the most extreme and highly maladaptive variant of emotional instability (Widiger et al. 2002). This disorder is indicated by the presence of five or more of the nine diagnostic criteria presented in the DSM-IV-TR criteria for BPD.

### Etiology and Pathology

There are studies to indicate that BPD may breed true but most research has suggested an association with mood and impulse dyscontrol disorders (Silk 2000, Torgersen 2000). There is also consistent empirical support for a childhood history of physical and/or sexual abuse, as well as parental conflict, loss, and neglect (Johnson et al. 1999, Zanarini 2000). It appears that past traumatic events are important in many if not most cases of BPD, contributing to the overlap and association with posttraumatic stress and dissociative disorders (Brodsky et al. 1995, Gunderson 2001,

**DSM-IV-TR Criteria** 301.83

### Borderline Personality Disorder

A. A pervasive pattern of instability of interpersonal relationships, self-image, and affects, and marked impulsivity beginning by early adulthood and present in a variety of contexts, as indicated by five (or more) of the following:

   (1) frantic efforts to avoid real or imagined abandonment. **Note:** do not include suicidal or self-mutilating behavior covered in criterion 5

   (2) a pattern of unstable and intense interpersonal relationships characterized by alternating between extremes of idealization and devaluation

   (3) identity disturbance: markedly and persistently unstable self-image or sense of self

   (4) impulsivity in at least two areas that are potentially self-damaging (e.g., spending, sex, substance abuse, reckless driving, binge eating). **Note:** do not include suicidal or self-mutilating behavior covered in criterion 5

   (5) recurrent suicidal behavior, gestures, or threats, or self-mutilating behavior

   (6) affective instability due to a marked reactivity of mood (e.g., intense episodic dysphoria, irritability, or anxiety usually lasting a few hours and only rarely more than a few days)

   (7) chronic feelings of emptiness

   (8) inappropriate, intense anger or difficulty controlling anger (e.g., frequent displays of temper, constant anger, recurrent physical fights)

   (9) transient, stress-related paranoid ideation or severe dissociative symptoms

Hefferman and Cloitre 2000) but the nature and age at which these events have occurred will vary. BPD may involve the interaction of a genetic disposition towards dyscontrol of mood and impulses (i.e., emotionally unstable temperament), with a cumulative and evolving series of intensely pathogenic relationships (Gunderson 2001, Morey and Zanarini 2000).

There are numerous theories regarding the pathogenic mechanisms of BPD, most concern issues regarding abandonment, separation, and/or exploitative abuse, which is one of the reasons that frantic efforts to avoid abandonment is the first item in the DSM-IV-TR diagnostic criterion set (Gunderson et al. 1991, Zanarini et al. 1997). Persons with BPD have quite intense, disturbed, and/or abusive relationships with the significant persons of their past, including their parents (Gunderson 2001), contributing to the development of malevolent perceptions and expectations of others (Ornduff 2000). These expectations, along with an impairment in the ability to regulate affect and impulses (Linehan 1993), may contribute to the perpetuation of intense, angry, and unstable relationships. Neurochemical dysregulation is evident in persons with BPD but it is unclear whether this dysregulation is a result, cause, or correlate of prior interpersonal traumas (Gunderson 2001, Silk 2000).

## Assessment and Differential Diagnosis

All of the DSM-IV assessment instruments described earlier include the assessment of BPD. However, an instrument that is focused on the assessment of BPD is the Diagnostic Interview for Borderlines-Revised (DIB-R; Zanarini et al. 1989). The DIB-R provides a more thorough assessment of components of BPD (e.g., impulsivity, affective dysregulation, and cognitive–perceptual aberrations) than is provided by more general DSM-IV-TR personality disorder semi-structured interviews, but psychiatrists might find it impractical to devote up to 2 hours to assess one particular personality disorder, especially when it is likely that other maladaptive personality traits not covered by the DIB-R are also likely to be present (Kaye and Shea 2000, Widiger and Coker 2002, Zanarini et al. 1998b).

Most persons with BPD develop mood disorders (Links et al. 1998) and it is at times difficult to differentiate BPD from a mood disorder if the assessment is confined to the current symptomatology (Gunderson 2001, Widiger and Coker 2002). A diagnosis of BPD requires that the borderline symptomatology be evident since adolescence, which should differentiate BPD from a mood disorder in all cases other than a chronic mood disorder. If there is a chronic mood disorder, then the additional features of transient, stress-related paranoid ideation, dissociative experiences, impulsivity, and anger dyscontrol that are evident in BPD should be emphasized in the diagnosis (Gunderson 2001, Widiger et al. 1995).

## Epidemiology and Comorbidity

Approximately 1 to 2% of the general population would meet the DSM-IV criteria for BPD (see Table 79–1). BPD is the most prevalent personality disorder within maximum clinical settings. Approximately 15% of all inpatients (51% of inpatients with a personality disorder) and 8% of all outpatients (27% of outpatients with a personality disorder) have a borderline personality disorder. Approximately 75% of persons with BPD will be female (Corbitt and Widiger 1995, Gunderson 2001). Persons with BPD meet DSM-IV-TR criteria for at least one Axis I disorder. The range of potential Axis I comorbid psychopathology includes mood (major depressive disorder), anxiety (posttraumatic stress disorder), eating (bulimia nervosa), substance (alcohol dependence), dissociative (dissociative identity disorder), and psychotic (brief psychotic) disorders (Gunderson 2001, Links et al. 1998, Zanarini et al. 1998a). Persons with BPD also meet DSM-IV-TR criteria for at least one other personality disorder, particularly histrionic, dependent, antisocial, schizotypal, or passive–aggressive (see Table 79–2 Links et al. 1998, Zanarini et al. 1998b). Researchers and

clinicians have at times responded to this extensive co-occurrence by imposing a diagnostic hierarchy whereby other disorders are not diagnosed in the presence of BPD because BPD is generally the most severely dysfunctional disorder (Gunderson et al. 2000). A potential limitation of this approach is that it resolves the complexity of personality by largely ignoring it. This approach may fail to recognize the presence of maladaptive personality traits that could be important for understanding a patient's dysfunctions and for developing an optimal treatment plan (Zimmerman and Mattia 1999).

## Course

As children, persons with BPD are likely to have been emotionally unstable, impulsive, and angry or hostile. Their chaotic impulsivity and intense affectivity may contribute to involvement within rebellious groups as a child or adolescent, along with a variety of Axis I disorders, including eating, substance use, and mood disorders. BPD is often diagnosed in children and adolescents but considerable caution should be used when doing so as some of the symptoms of BPD (e.g., identity disturbance and unstable relationships) could be confused with a normal adolescent rebellion or identity crisis (Ad-Dab'bagh and Greenfield 2001, Gunderson 2001). As adults, persons with BPD may require numerous hospitalizations due to their affect and impulse dyscontrol, psychotic-like and dissociative symptomatology, and risk of suicide (Gunderson 2001, Zanarini et al. 1998a). Minor problems quickly become crises as the intensity of affect and impulsivity result in disastrous decisions. They are at a high risk for developing depressive, substance-related, bulimic, and posttraumatic stress disorders. The potential for suicide increases with a comorbid mood and substance-related disorder. Approximately 3 to 10% commit suicide by the age of 30 years (Gunderson 2001). Relationships tend to be very unstable and explosive, and employment history is poor (Daley et al. 2000, Stone 2001). Affectivity and impulsivity, however, may begin to diminish as the person reaches the age of 30 years, or earlier if the person becomes involved with a supportive and patient sexual partner (Stone 2001). Some, however, may obtain stability by abandoning the effort to obtain a relationship, opting instead for a lonelier but less volatile life. The mellowing of the symptomatology, however, can be easily disrupted by the occurrence of a severe stressor (e.g., divorce by or death of a significant other) that results in a brief psychotic, dissociative, or mood disorder episode.

## Treatment

Persons with BPD often develop intense, dependent, hostile, unstable, and manipulative relationships with their therapists as they do with their peers. At one time they might be very compliant, responsive, and even idealizing, but later angry, accusatory, and devaluing. Their tendency to be manipulatively as well as impulsively self-destructive is often very stressful and difficult to treat (Stone 2000).

Persons with BPD are often highly motivated for treatment. Psychotherapeutic approaches tend to be both supportive and exploratory (Gabbard 2001, Gunderson 2001, Stone 1993, 2000). Therapists should provide a safe, secure environment in which anger can be expressed and actively addressed without destroying the therapeutic relationship.

The historical roots of current bitterness, anger, and depression within past familial relationships should eventually be explored, but immediate, current issues and conflicts must also be explicitly addressed. Suicidal behavior should be confronted and contained, by hospitalization when necessary. Patients with BPD can be very difficult to treat because the focus of the patient's love and wrath will often be shifted toward the therapist, and the treatment may itself become the patient's latest unstable, intense relationship. Immediate and ongoing consultation with colleagues is often necessary, as it is not unusual for therapists to be unaware of the extent to which they are developing or expressing feelings of anger, attraction, annoyance, or intolerance toward their borderline patient.

A particular form of cognitive–behavioral therapy, dialectical behavior therapy, has been shown empirically to be effective in the treatment of BPD (Linehan 1993, 2000). Part of the strategy entails keeping patients focused initially on the priorities of reducing suicidal threats and gestures, behaviors that can disrupt or resist treatment, and behaviors that effect the immediate quality of life (e.g., bulimia, substance abuse, or unemployment). Once these goals are achieved, the focus can then shift to a mastery of new coping skills, management of reactions to stress, and other individualized goals. Individual therapy is augmented by skills-training groups that may be highly structured (e.g., comparable to a classroom format). Patients are taught skills for coping with identity diffusion, tolerating distress, improving interpersonal relationships, controlling emotions, and resolving interpersonal crises. Patients are given homework assignments to practice these skills that are further addressed and reinforced within individual sessions. Negative affect is also addressed through a mindful meditation that contributes to an acceptance and tolerance of past abusive experiences and current stress. The dialectical component of the therapy is that "the dialectical therapist helps the patient achieve synthesis of oppositions, rather than focusing on verifying either side of an oppositional argument" (Linehan 1993, p. 204). An illustrative list of dialectical strategies is presented in Table 79–4.

DBT, however, also includes more general principles of treatment that are important to emphasize in all forms of therapy for BPD (Linehan 1993, Stone 1993, 2000), some of which are presented in Table 79–5. For example, exasperated therapists may unjustly experience and even accuse borderline patients of being unmotivated or unwilling to work. It is important to appreciate that they do want to improve and are doing the best that they can. One should not make the therapy personal, but instead identify the sources of the inhibition or interference to their motivation to change. One should take seriously their complaints that their lives are indeed unbearable but not absolve them of their responsibility to solve their own problems. They are unlikely to change simply through a passive reception of insight, nurturance, support, and medication. They will need to actively work on changing their lives. Therapists will often be tempted to rescue their patients, particularly when they are within a crisis. However, it is precisely at such times that there will be the best opportunity to develop and learn new coping strategies. Failures can occur, and it is a failure of the therapy that should be conscientiously and effectively addressed by the therapist. Finally, therapists need to honestly recognize their own limitations. All therapists have their own flaws and limits and patients with BPD invariably strain and overwhelm these limits. Therapists need to be open and receptive to outside support, advice, and criticism.

Pharmacologic treatment of patients with BPD is varied, as it depends primarily on the predominant Axis I symptomatology (Markovitz 2001, Soloff 2000). Persons with BPD can display a wide variety of Axis I symptoms, including anxiety, depression, hallucinations, delusions, and dissociations. It is important in their pharmacologic treatment not to be unduly influenced by transient symptoms or by symptoms that are readily addressed through exploratory or supportive techniques. On the other hand, it is equally important to be flexible in the use of medications and not to be unduly resistant to their use. Relying solely upon one's own psychotherapeutic skills can be unnecessary and even irresponsible.

| Table 79–4 | Dialectical Behavior Therapy Strategies |
|---|---|

Alternate between acceptance and change strategies.
Balance nurturing with demands for self-help
Balance persistence and stability with flexibility
Balance capabilities with limitations and deficits
Move with speed, keeping the patient slightly off balance
Take positions wholeheartedly
Look for what is not included in patient's own points of view
Provide developmental descriptions of change
Question intransigence of boundary conditions of the problem
Highlight importance of interrelationships in identity
Advocate a middle path
Highlight paradoxical contradictions in patient's own behavior, in the therapeutic process, and in life in general
Speak in metaphors and tell parables and stories
Play the devil's advocate
Extend the seriousness or implications of patient's statements
Add intuitive knowing to emotional experience and logical analysis
Turn problems into assets
Allow natural changes in therapy
Assess the patient, therapist, and process dialectically

*Source*: Linehan MM (1993) Cognitive–Behavioral Treatment of Borderline Personality Disorder. Guilford Press, New York, p. 206.

| Table 79–5 | Basic Propositions of BPD Treatment from DBT |
|---|---|

1. Patients are doing the best they can.
2. Patients want to improve.
3. Patients need to do better, try harder, and be more motivated to change.
4. Patients may not have caused all of their own problems, but they have to solve them anyway.
5. The lives of suicidal, borderline individuals are unbearable as they are currently being lived.
6. Patients must learn new behaviors in all relevant contexts.
7. Patients cannot fail in therapy.
8. Therapists treating borderline patients need support.

*Source*: Linehan MM (1993) Cognitive–Behavioral Treatment of Borderline Personality Disorder. Guilford Press, New York, pp. 106–108.

---

**Clinical Vignette 3**

SC was a 36-year-old female. She was referred to a Day Hospital Borderline Personality Disorders Treatment Program after her fourth hospitalization for depression and suicidality. SC had not known her father. She was raised by her mother who had a polysubstance dependence. Her relationship with her mother was described as negligent and distant. She had two brothers. The oldest brother abused her sexually for 3 years since she was 13 years old. The abuse ended when he was drafted into the army. She denied any feelings of anger or bitterness towards him, and in fact described substantial feelings of fondness and affection. He died while serving in Vietnam.

She obtained good to excellent grades in school but had a history of indiscriminant sexual behavior, substance abuse, and bulimia (her common method for purging was to attempt to swallow a belt, thereby inducing vomiting). Her first treatment was at the age of 19 years. She became significantly depressed when she discovered that her fiance was sexually involved with her best friend. Her hospitalization was precipitated by the ingestion of a lethal amount of drugs. Subsequent to this hospitalization she began to mutilate herself by scratching or cutting her arms with broken plates, dinner knives, or metal. The self-mutilation was usually precipitated by episodes of severe loneliness and feelings of emptiness.

She had a very active social life and a large network of friends. However, her relationships were very unstable. She could be quite supportive, engaging, and personable, but would overreact to common conflicts, disagreements, and difficulties. She would feel intensely hurt, depressed, angry, or enraged, and would hope that her friends would relieve her pain through some gesture. However, they would typically feel frustrated, annoyed, or overwhelmed by the intensity of her affect and her reactions.

Her sexual relationships were even more problematic. She would quickly develop intense feelings of attraction, involvement, and dependency. However, she would soon experience her lovers as disappointing and neglectful, which at times had more than a kernel of truth. Many were neglectful, unempathic, or abusive, but all of them found the intensity of the inevitable conflicts and her anger to be intolerable.

She was also questioning her sexual orientation. She had never been sexually involved with a woman, but she did have fantasies of an involvement with various women that she had known. It was conceivable that she might find a relationship with a woman to be more stable and satisfying, but it was likely that as much conflict would occur with women as had occurred with men.

She attended the Day Hospital BPD Program for 2 years. Treatment included group therapy, individual psychotherapy (using both cognitive–behavioral and insight), and antidepressant medication. The cognitive–behavioral treatment focused on daily management of problems, exploring alternative perceptions of and means for addressing conflicts with others and gradually developing more effective coping strategies. The irrationality of her reactions became more apparent to her as their source within her past relationships were better understood. Treatment was successful in ending her reliance on self-mutilation and in decreasing the intensity of her interpersonal conflicts. She continued to have unstable relationships, but she was much more successful in acknowledging and resolving conflicts in ways that were more realistic and appropriate.

## Histrionic Personality Disorder

### Definition

Histrionic personality disorder (HPD) is a pervasive pattern of excessive emotionality and attention-seeking (American Psychiatric Association 2000). Histrionic persons tend to be emotionally manipulative and intolerant of delayed gratification (American Psychiatric Association 1980, 1987, Bornstein 1999). HPD is indicated by the presence of five or more of the eight diagnostic criteria presented in DSM-IV criteria for HPD.

### Etiology and Pathology

There is little research on the etiology of HPD. There is a suggestion that HPD may share a genetic disposition toward impulsivity or sensation-seeking with the antisocial personality disorder (Hamburger et al. 1996, Lilienfeld and Hess 2001). It has also been suggested that HPD is (in part) a severe, maladaptive variant of the personality dimensions of

---

**DSM-IV-TR Criteria** 301.50

**Histrionic Personality Disorder**

A pervasive pattern of excessive emotionality and attention seeking, beginning by early adulthood and present in a variety of contexts, as indicated by five (or more) of the following:

(1) is uncomfortable in situations in which he or she is not the center of attention

(2) interaction with others is often characterized by inappropriate sexually seductive or provocative behavior

(3) displays rapidly shifting and shallow expression of emotions

(4) consistently uses physical appearance to draw attention to self

(5) has a style of speech that is excessively impressionistic and lacking in detail

(6) shows self-dramatization, theatricality, and exaggerated expression of emotion

(7) is suggestible, i.e. easily influenced by others or circumstances

(8) considers relationships to be more intimate than they actually are

extraversion and neuroticism (Widiger et al. 2002). Extraversion includes the facets of excitement seeking, gregariousness, and positive emotionality, and neuroticism includes the facets of angry hostility, self-consciousness, and vulnerability (Costa and McCrae 1992) that are all characteristic of persons with HPD (Trull et al. 1998) and there is considerable empirical support for the heritability of these personality dimensions (Jang et al. 1998, Jang and Vernon 2001, Nigg and Goldsmith 1994, Plomin and Caspi 1999).

Environmental and social–cultural factors, however, may also play a significant role in the development of HPD (Bornstein 1999). Kernberg (1991a), for example, speculates that the fathers of females with HPD combine early sexual seductiveness with subsequent authoritarian puritanical attitudes, while the mother tends to be domineering, controlling, and intrusive. Such a history may indeed occur in some cases of HPD but there is unlikely to be a specific, common pattern to all cases. The tendency of a family to emphasize, value, or reinforce attention-seeking in a person with a genetic disposition toward emotionality may represent a more general pathway toward HPD (Cooper and Ronningstam 1992).

Affective instability is an important feature of HPD, which may be associated with a hyperresponsiveness of the noradrenergic system. This instability in the catecholamine functioning may contribute to a pronounced emotional reactivity to rejection and loss (Markovitz 2001). However, the attention-seeking of HPD can be as important to the disorder as the emotionality. The purpose of the exaggerated emotionality is often to evoke the attention and maintain the interest of others (Bornstein 1999, Gunderson and Gabbard 2000, Stone 1993). Persons with HPD are intensely insecure regarding the extent to which others appreciate, desire, or want their company. They need to be the center of attention to reassure themselves that they are valued, desired, attractive, or wanted.

## Assessment and Differential Diagnosis

HPD involves to some extent maladaptive variants of stereotypically feminine traits (Sprock et al. 1990). The DSM-IV-TR diagnostic criteria for HPD are sufficiently severe that a normal woman would not meet these criteria, but studies have indicated that clinicians will at times diagnose HPD in females who in fact have antisocial traits (Widiger 1998). Both of these disorders can involve impulsivity, sensation-seeking, low frustration tolerance, and manipulativeness, and the presence of a female gender may at times contribute to a false presumption of HPD. It is therefore important to adhere closely to the DSM-IV-TR diagnostic criteria when confronted with histrionic and antisocial symptoms in female patients.

Persons with HPD will often have borderline, dependent, or narcissistic personality traits (see Table 79–2). Prototypic cases of HPD can be distinguished from other personality disorders (Widiger et al. 1995, 2002). For example, the prototypic narcissistic person ultimately desires admiration whereas the histrionic person desires whatever attention, interest, or concern can be obtained. As a result, the histrionic person will at times seek attention through melodramatic helplessness and emotional outbursts that could be experienced as denigrating and humili-

ating to the narcissistic person. However, most cases will not be prototypic and the most accurate description of a patient's constellation of maladaptive personality traits will be the provision of multiple diagnoses (Oldham et al. 1992, Oldham and Skodol 2000).

## Epidemiology and Comorbidity

Approximately 1 to 3% of the general population may be diagnosed with HPD (see Table 79–1; Mattia and Zimmerman 2001, Torgersen 2001). A controversial issue is its differential sex prevalence (Bornstein 1999, Sprock et al. 1990, Widiger 1998). It is stated in DSM-IV-TR that the sex ratio for HPD is "not significantly different than the sex ratio of females within the respective clinical setting" (American Psychiatric Association 2000, p. 712). However, this should not be interpreted as indicating that the prevalence is the same for males and females. It has typically been found that at least two-thirds of persons with HPD are female, although there have been a few exceptions (Corbitt and Widiger 1995). Whether or not the rate will be significantly higher than the rate of women within a particular clinical setting depends upon many factors that are independent of the differential sex prevalence for HPD (Widiger 1998).

## Course

Little is known about the premorbid behavior pattern of persons with HPD (Bornstein 1999). During adolescence they are likely to be flamboyant, flirtatious, and attention-seeking. As adults, persons with HPD readily form new relationships but have difficulty sustaining them. They may fall in love quite quickly, but just as rapidly become attracted to another person. They are unlikely to be reliable or responsible. Relationships with persons of the same sexual orientation are often be strained due to their competitive sexual flirtatiousness. Employment history is likely to be erratic, and may be complicated by the tendency to become romantically or sexually involved with colleagues, by their affective instability, and by their suggestibility. Persons with HPD may become devoted converts to faddish belief systems. They have a tendency to make impulsive decisions that will have a dramatic (or melodramatic) effect on their lives. The severity of the symptomatology may diminish somewhat as the person ages.

## Treatment

Persons with HPD readily develop rapport but it is often superficial and unreliable. Therapists may also fail to appreciate the extent of influence they can have on the highly suggestible HPD patient (Bornstein 1999, Horowitz 1997). Persons with HPD can readily become converts to whatever the therapist may suggest or encourage. The transformation to the theoretical model or belief system of the psychiatrist is unlikely to be sustained.

A key task in treating the patient with HPD is countering their global and diffuse cognitive style by insisting on attending to structure and detail within sessions and to the practical, immediate problems encountered in daily life (Beck and Freeman 1990, Gunderson and Gabbard 2000, Horowitz 1997, Stone 1993). It is also important to explore within treatment the historical source for their needs for attention and involvement. Persons with HPD are prone to superficial and transient insights but they will benefit from a carefully reasoned and documented exploration of their current and past relationships.

Many clinicians recommend the use of group therapy for persons with HPD (Beck and Freeman 1990, Gabbard 2000, Millon et al. 1996). It is quite easy for them to become involved within a group, which may then be very useful in helping them recognize and explore their attention-seeking, suggestibility, and manipulation, as well as develop alternative ways to develop more meaningful and sustained relationships. However, it is also important to closely monitor their involvements within the group, as they are prone to dominate and control sessions and they may escalate their attention-seeking to the point of suicidal gestures. The intense affectivity of persons with HPD may also be responsive to antidepressant treatment, particularly those patients with substantial mood reactivity, hypersomnia, and rejection sensitivity (Markovitz 2001).

## Narcissistic Personality Disorder

### Definition

Narcissistic PD (NPD) is a pervasive pattern of grandiosity, need for admiration, and lack of empathy (American Psychiatric Association 2000). Persons with NPD can be very vulnerable to threats to their self-esteem. They may react defensively with rage, disdain, or indifference but are in fact struggling with feelings of shock, humiliation, and shame. NPD is indicated by the presence of five or more of the nine diagnostic criteria presented in the DSM-IV-TR Criteria for NPD.

### Etiology and Pathology

There are no data on the heritability of the narcissistic PD (Jang and Vernon 2001, Nigg and Goldsmith 1994), although there are data on the heritability of arrogance, modesty, and conceit (Jang et al. 1998, Plomin and Caspi 1999). The etiological theories have been primarily sociological, psychodynamic, and interpersonal. For example, it has been suggested that current Western society has become overly self-centered with the decreasing importance of familial bonds, traditional social, religious, and political values or ideals, and rising materialism (Cooper and Ronningstam 1992, Millon et al. 1996).

Narcissism may also develop through unempathic, neglectful, and/or devaluing parental figures (Kernberg 1991b). The child may develop the belief that a sense of worth, value, or meaning is contingent upon accomplishment or achievement. Kohut (1977) has suggested that the parents failed to adequately mirror an infant's natural need for idealization. Benjamin (1993) and Millon and colleagues (1996) suggest that narcissistic persons received excessive idealization by parental figures, which they incorporated into their self-image. The irrationality of this idealization, or its being coupled with inconsistent indications of an actual disinterest and devaluation, may contribute to the eventual difficulties and conflicts surrounding self-image.

Conflicts and deficits with respect to self-esteem have been shown empirically to be central to the pathology of NPD (Raskin et al. 1991, Rhodewalt et al. 1998). Narcissistic persons must continually seek and obtain signs and

**DSM-IV-TR Criteria** 301.81

**Narcissistic Personality Disorder**

A pervasive pattern of grandiosity (in fantasy or behavior), need for admiration, and lack of empathy, beginning by early adulthood and present in a variety of contexts, as indicated by five (or more) of the following:

(1) has a grandiose sense of self-importance (e.g. exaggerates achievements and talents, expects to be recognized as superior without commensurate achievements)

(2) is preoccupied with fantasies of unlimited success, power, brilliance, beauty, or ideal love

(3) believes that he or she is "special" and unique and can only be understood by, or should associate with, other special or high-status people (or institutions)

(4) requires excessive admiration

(5) has a sense of entitlement, i.e. unreasonable expectations of especially favorable treatment or automatic compliance with his or her expectations

(6) is interpersonally exploitative, i.e., takes advantage of others to achieve his or her own ends

(7) lacks empathy: is unwilling to recognize or identify with the feelings and needs of others

(8) is often envious of others or believes that others are envious of him or her

(9) shows arrogant, haughty behaviors or attitudes

Reprinted with permission from the Diagnostic and Statistical Manual of Mental Disorders, Fourth Edition, Text Revision. Copyright 2000 American Psychiatric Association.

symbols of recognition to compensate for feelings of inadequacy (Cooper and Ronningstam 1992, Stone 1993, Gabbard 2000). They are not persons who feel valued for their own sake. Value is contingent upon a success, accomplishment, or status. Their feelings of insecurity may be masked by a disdainful indifference towards rebuke and by overt expressions of arrogance, conceit, and even grandiosity. However, the psychopathology is still evident in such cases by the excessive reliance and importance that is continually placed upon status and recognition. Some narcissistic persons may in fact envy those who are truly indifferent to success and who can enjoy a modest, simple, and unassuming life.

### Assessment and Differential Diagnosis

All of the semistructured interviews and self-report inventories described earlier include scales for the assessment of NPD. There is also a semistructured interview devoted to the assessment of narcissism (Diagnostic Interview for Narcissism [DIN]; Gunderson et al. 1990), the research with which was highly influential in the development of the DSM-IV-TR diagnostic criteria (Gunderson et al. 1991). There are also a number of self-report inventories devoted to the assessment of narcissistic personality traits, including the Narcissistic Personality Inventory (NPI) that has been used in a number of informative personality and social–psychological studies of narcissism (Rhodewalt and Morf 1995). The DIN and NPI have the useful feature of subscales for the assessment of various components of narcissism (e.g., NPI scales for superiority, vanity, leadership, authority, entitlement, exploitativeness, and exhibitionism).

Individuals with narcissistic PD may often appear relatively high functioning. Exaggerated self-confidence may in fact contribute to success in a variety of professions and narcissistic traits will at times be seen in highly successful persons (Kernberg 1991b, Ronninstam and Gunderson 1990, Widiger et al. 1995). A diagnosis of NPD requires the additional presence of interpersonal exploitation, lack of empathy, a sense of entitlement, and other symptoms beyond simply arrogance and grandiosity.

Both narcissistic and antisocial persons may exploit, deceive, and manipulate others for personal gain, and both may demonstrate a lack of empathy or remorse. As indicated above, many of the traits of narcissism, such as arrogance and glib charm, are seen in psychopathic persons (Hare et al. 1991, Widiger et al. 1996). Prototypic cases can be distinguished, as the motivation for the narcissistic person will be for recognition, status, and other signs of success, whereas the prototypic antisocial person would be motivated more for material gain or for the subjugation of others (Widiger et al. 1995). Antisocial persons will also display an impulsivity, recklessness, and lax irresponsibility that may not be seen in narcissistic persons.

### Epidemiology and Comorbidity

Approximately 18% of males and 6% of females may be characterized as being excessively immodest (i.e., arrogant or conceited; Costa and McCrae 1992) but only a small percent of these persons would be diagnosed with NPD. In fact, the median prevalence rate obtained across 10 community data collections was zero (see Table 79–1). The absence of any cases within community studies, however, may reflect inadequacies within the diagnostic criteria or limitations of semistructured interview assessments of narcissism (Hilsenroth et al. 1996, Westen 1997). NPD is observed within clinical settings (approximately 2 to 20% of patients) although it is also among the least frequently diagnosed personality disorders (American Psychiatric Association 2000, Gunderson et al. 1991). Persons with NPD are considered to be prone to mood disorders, as well as anorexia and substance-related disorders, especially cocaine (American Psychiatric Association 2000, Cooper and Ronninstam 1992). Persons with NPD are likely to have comorbid antisocial (psychopathic), histrionic, paranoid, and borderline personality traits (see Table 79–2).

### Course

Little is known about the premorbid behavior pattern of NPD, other than through retrospective reports of persons diagnosed when adults (Cooper and Ronningstam 1992, Kernberg 1991b, Kohut 1977, Mattia and Zimmerman

2001). As adolescents, persons with NPD are likely to be self-centered, assertive, gregarious, dominant, and perhaps arrogant. They may have achieved well in school or within some other activity. As adults, many persons with NPD will have experienced high levels of achievement (Ronningstam and Gunderson 1990). However, their relationships with colleagues, peers, and staff will eventually become strained as their exploitative use of others and self-centered egotism become evident. Success may also be impaired by their difficulty in acknowledging or resolving criticism, deficits, and setbacks. Interpersonal and sexual relationships are usually easy for them to develop but difficult to sustain due to their low empathy, self-centeredness, and need for admiration. Persons who are deferential and obsequious, or who share a mutual need for status and recognition, may help sustain a relationship. As parents, persons with NPD may attempt to live through their children, valuing them as long as they are a source of pride. Their personal sense of adjustment may be fine for as long as they continue to experience or anticipate success. Some may not recognize the maladaptivity of their narcissism until middle age, when the emphasis given to achievement and status may begin to wane.

### Treatment

Persons with narcissistic personality traits seek treatment for feelings of depression, substance-related disorders, and occupational or relational problems that are secondary to their narcissism. Their self-centeredness and lack of empathy are particularly problematic within marital, occupational, and other social relationships, and they usually lack an appreciation of the contribution of their conflicts regarding self-esteem, status, and recognition (Gunderson and Gabbard 2000, Stone 1993). It is difficult for them even to admit that they have a psychological problem or that they need help, as this admission is itself an injury to their self-esteem. In addition, one of the characteristics of NPD is the belief that they can only be understood by persons of a comparably high social status or recognition. They may be unable to accept advice or insight from persons they consider less intelligent, talented, or insightful than themselves, which may eventually effectively eliminate most other persons.

When they are involved in treatment, persons with NPD will often require some indication that their therapist is among the best or at least worth their time. They are prone to idealizing their therapists (to affirm that he or she is indeed of sufficient status or quality) or to devalue them (to affirm that they are of greater intelligence, capacity, or quality than their therapist, to reject the insights that they have failed to identify, and to indicate that they warrant or deserve an even better therapist). How best to respond is often unclear. It may at times be preferable to simply accept the praise or criticism, particularly when exploration will likely be unsuccessful, whereas at other times it is preferable to confront and discuss the motivation for the devaluation (or the idealization).

Psychodynamic approaches to the treatment of NPD vary in the extent to which emphasis is given to an interpretation of underlying anger and bitterness, or to the provision of empathy and a reflection (or mirroring) of a positive regard and self-esteem (Cooper and Ronningstam

1992, Kernberg 1991b, Kohut 1977, Gabbard 2000). It does appear to be important to identify the current extent and historical source of the conflicts and sensitivities regarding self-esteem. Active confrontation may at times be useful, particularly when the therapeutic alliance is strong, but at other times the vulnerability of the patient may require a more unconditional support (Stone 1993). Cognitive–behavior approaches to NPD emphasize increasing awareness of the impact of narcissistic behaviors and statements on interpersonal relationships (Beck and Freeman 1990). The idealization and devaluation can be responsive to role playing and rational introspection, an intellectual approach that may itself be valued by some persons with NPD. However, therapists must be careful not to become embroiled within intellectual conflicts (or competitions). This approach may not work well with the narcissistic person who is motivated to defeat or humiliate the therapist (Kernberg 1991b).

Group therapy can be useful for increasing awareness of the grandiosity, lack of empathy, and devaluation of others. However, these traits not only interfere with the narcissistic person's ability to sustain membership within groups (and within individual therapy), they may also become quite harmful and destructive to the rapport of the entire group. There is no accepted pharmacologic approach to the treatment of narcissism (Markovitz 2001).

---

**Clinical Vignette 4**

RP was a well-regarded clinician with a good publication record and a successful private practice. However, one of his patients filed a complaint with the state board after their sexual relationship ended. He offered in his defense that his behavior was simply the result of marital stress. His license to practice was suspended indefinitely. One of the terms of his probation was to complete successfully 2 years of psychotherapy. RP agreed that treatment would be beneficial but questioned whether any clinician within his local community was sufficiently qualified, as he considered himself to be among the leading clinicians within this community.

Treatment was problematic from the very beginning. RP felt that their discussions should be quid pro quo: if he was going to reveal aspects of himself then the therapist should do likewise. When confronted with the understanding that he was the one in treatment, RP argued that the therapist must be having "narcissistic conflicts" if he is unwilling to accept the insight and guidance that he could offer. Some of the difficulty within the treatment was attributable to the situation (i.e., it would probably be difficult for most therapists to be mandated to receive therapy from a colleague) but as treatment progressed it became apparent that he had similar conflicts with other persons in his life.

RP's wife was threatening divorce in part because of a history of extramarital affairs. RP did not deny the existence of these affairs but argued that his wife was exaggerating their importance: the other women meant little to him, why should they be of concern to her? He said that he did not keep his affairs secret from her prior to marriage (at least those that he was unable to keep secret), and therefore she knew from the beginning that extramarital affairs would occur. In addition, he felt that his affairs were only petty philandering and that his wife should tolerate them because she was "frankly lucky" to have him for a husband. He was good looking, wealthy, and professionally successful, and felt that if he had been more patient he might have found someone better than her.

RP was popular with women, at least at the beginning of relationships. He was charming, engaging, and verbally facile. However, he acknowledged during the course of therapy that some women eventually became unhappy, dissatisfied, and at times even angry with him. It is quite possible that his perception of his past relationships even understated the extent of the dissatisfaction. He attributed their dissatisfaction to "unrealistic and neurotic expectations." He stated that women would flirt with him because he is an "attractive catch" and that he was only fulfilling their fantasies by letting them become involved with him. He would soon lose interest though in the women with whom he became involved, and he acknowledged that it was not always easy to extricate himself from a relationship without any cost to himself.

He evidenced only a marginal insight into the potential harm he had caused the patient with whom he had the sexual relationship. He argued that the proscription against sexual involvements should not have been enforced in this instance because he had been very careful in determining that their relationship was not the intended target of the ethical guidelines: she was herself a "competent" professional who had "freely" entered the relationship and, in any case, no complaint would have been filed if he had been willing to continue the relationship. She was a well-known public figure. She testified to the state board that he repeatedly suggested to her that she accompany him on his business trips, and it was her impression that he wanted to show her off as a "trophy" to his colleagues. She stated that she ended the relationship when she discovered from her colleagues that he was bragging to others about their relationship and revealing details of their sexual activities.

Treatment was terminated by RP after 6 months of treatment upon reading the biannual report by his therapist to the state board regarding his progress. RP felt that he had been making substantial progress that was not being adequately appreciated by his therapist. He noted, for example, that his wife was no longer seeking a divorce and that his ex-patient was engaged to be married. He did indicate that he was dissatisfied with treatment, and felt that progress would be improved by "a more experienced and respected" clinician. He attributed the therapist's negative evaluation of his progress to professional jealousy.

## Avoidant Personality Disorder

### Definition

Avoidant personality disorder (AVPD) is a pervasive pattern of timidity, inhibition, inadequacy, and social hypersensitivity (American Psychiatric Association 2000). Persons with AVPD may have a strong desire to develop close, personal relationships but feel too insecure to approach others or to express their feelings. AVPD is indicated by the presence of four or more of the seven diagnostic criteria presented in the DSM criteria for AVPD.

### Etiology and Pathology

AVPD appears to be an extreme variant of the fundamental personality traits of introversion and neuroticism (Widiger

## DSM-IV-TR Criteria 301.82

### Avoidant Personality Disorder

A pervasive pattern of social inhibition, feelings of inadequacy, and hypersensitivity to negative evaluation, beginning by early adulthood and present in a variety of contexts, as indicated by four (or more) of the following:

(1) avoids occupational activities that involve significant interpersonal contact, because of fears of criticism, disapproval, or rejection

(2) is unwilling to get involved with people unless certain of being liked

(3) shows restraint within intimate relationships because of the fear of being shamed or ridiculed

(4) is preoccupied with thoughts of being criticized or rejected in social situations

(5) is inhibited in new interpersonal situations because of feelings of inadequacy

(6) views self as socially inept, personally unappealing, or inferior to others

(7) is unusually reluctant to take personal risks or to engage in any new activities because they may prove embarrassing

Reprinted with permission from the Diagnostic and Statistical Manual of Mental Disorders, Fourth Edition, Text Revision. Copyright 2000 American Psychiatric Association.

et al. 2002). Introversion includes such facets as passivity, social withdrawal, and inhibition, while neuroticism includes self-consciousness, vulnerability, and anxiousness (Costa and McCrae 1992). The personality dimensions of neuroticism and introversion have substantial heritability, as do the more specific traits of social anxiousness, shyness, and inhibition (Jang et al. 1998, Jang and Vernon 2001, Nigg and Goldsmith 1994, Plomin and Caspi 1999).

In childhood, neuroticism appears as a distress-prone or inhibited temperament (Rothbart and Ahadi 1994). Shyness, timidity, and interpersonal insecurity might be exacerbated further in childhood through overprotection and excessive cautiousness (Schmidt et al. 2001). Parental behavior coupled with a distress-prone temperament has been shown to result in social inhibition and timidity (Burgess et al. 2001, Rothbart and Ahadi 1994). Most children and adolescents will have many experiences of interpersonal embarrassment, rejection, or humiliation, but these will be particularly devastating to the person who is already lacking in self-confidence or is temperamentally passive, inhibited, or introverted.

AVPD may involve elevated peripheral sympathetic activity and adrenocortical responsiveness, resulting in excessive autonomic arousal, fearfulness, and inhibition (Siever and Davis 1991). Just as ASPD may involve deficits in the functioning of a behavioral inhibition system, AVPD may involve excessive functioning of this same system

(Depue and Lenzenweger 2001). The pathology of AVPD, however, may also be more psychological than neurochemical, with the timidity, shyness, and insecurity being a natural result of a cumulative history of denigrating, embarrassing, and devaluing experiences (Schmidt et al. 2001). Underlying AVPD may be excessive self-consciousness, feelings of inadequacy or inferiority, and irrational cognitive schemas that perpetuate introverted, avoidant behavior (Beck and Freeman 1990, Clark 2001, Dreessen et al. 1999).

### Differential Diagnosis

The most difficult differential diagnosis for AVPD is with generalized social phobia (Tillfors et al. 2001, van Velzen et al. 2000, Widiger 2001). Both involve an avoidance of social situations, social anxiety, and timidity, and both may be evident since late childhood or adolescence. Many persons with AVPD in fact seek treatment for a social phobia. To the extent that the behavior pattern pervades the person's everyday functioning and has been evident since childhood, the diagnosis of a personality disorder would be more descriptive. There are arguments to subsume all cases of AVPD into the diagnosis of generalized social phobia (as was done for schizoid disorder of childhood in DSM-IV-TR) but there is considerable empirical support for the existence of the personality dimensions of introversion and neuroticism and for an understanding of AVPD as a maladaptive variant of these personality traits (Costa and Widiger 2002, Trull et al. 1998, Widiger 2001).

Many persons with AVPD may also meet the criteria for dependent personality disorder (DPD). This might at first glance seem unusual, given that AVPD involves social withdrawal whereas DPD involves excessive social attachment. However, once a person with AVPD is able to obtain a relationship, he or she will often cling to this relationship in a dependent manner. Both disorders include feelings of inadequacy, needs for reassurance, and hypersensitivity to criticism and neglect (i.e. abnormally high levels of anxiousness, self-consciousness, and vulnerability). A distinction between AVPD and DPD is best made when the person is seeking a relationship (Widiger et al. 1995). Avoidant persons tend to be very shy, inhibited, and timid (and are therefore slow to get involved with someone) whereas dependent persons urgently seek another relationship as soon as one ends (i.e., avoidant persons are high in introversion whereas dependent persons are high in extraversion). Avoidant persons may also be reluctant to express their feelings whereas dependent persons can drive others away by continuous expressions of neediness. The differentiation of AVPD from the schizoid, paranoid, and schizotypal personality disorders was discussed in previous sections.

### Epidemiology and Comorbidity

Timidity, shyness, and social insecurity are not uncommon problems (Crozier and Alden 2001) and AVPD is one of the more prevalent personality disorders within clinical settings, occurring in 5 to 25% of all patients (American Psychiatric Association 2000, Mattia and Zimmerman 2001). However, AVPD may be diagnosed in only 1 to 2% of the general population (see Table 79–1). It appears to occur equally among males and females, with some studies reporting more males and others reporting more females (Corbitt and Widiger 1995). Persons with AVPD are likely to have symptoms that meet the DSM-IV criteria for a generalized social phobia, and others may have a mood disorder.

## Course

Persons with AVPD are shy, timid, and anxious as children (Bernstein and Travaglini 1999). Many are diagnosed with a social phobia during childhood. Adolescence is a particularly difficult developmental period due to the importance at this time of attractiveness, dating, and popularity. Occupational success may not be significantly impaired, as long as there is little demand for public performance. Persons with AVPD may in fact find considerable gratification and esteem through a job or career that they are unable to find within their relationships. The job may serve as a distraction from intense feelings of loneliness. Their avoidance of social situations will impair their ability to develop adequate social skills, and this will then further handicap any eventual efforts to develop relationships. As parents, they may be very responsible, empathic, and affectionate, but may unwittingly impart feelings of social anxiousness and awkwardness. Severity of the AVPD symptomatology diminishes as the person becomes older.

## Treatment

Persons with AVPD seek treatment for their avoidant personality traits, although many initially seek treatment for symptoms of anxiety, particularly social phobia (generalized subtype). It is important in such cases to recognize that the shyness is not due simply to a dysregulation or dyscontrol of anxiousness. There is instead a more pervasive and fundamental psychopathology, involving feelings of interpersonal insecurity, low self-esteem, and inadequacy (Millon et al. 1996, Stone 1993, Widiger 2001).

Social skills training, systematic desensitization, and a graded hierarchy of *in vivo* exposure to feared social situations have been shown to be useful in the treatment of AVPD (Beck and Freeman 1990, Clark 2001, Millon et al. 1996). However, it is also important to discuss the underlying fears and insecurities regarding attractiveness, desirability, rejection, or intimacy (Stone 1993, Gabbard 2000, Gunderson and Gabbard 2000). Persons with AVPD are at times reluctant to discuss such feelings, as they may feel embarrassed, they may fear being ridiculed, or they may not want to "waste the time" of the therapist with such "foolish" insecurities. They may prefer a less revealing or involved form of treatment. It is important to be understanding, patient, and accepting, and to proceed at a pace that is comfortable for the patient. Insecurities and fears can at times be addressed through cognitive techniques as the irrationality is usually readily apparent (Beck and Freeman 1990, Clark 2001). It remains useful though to identify the historical source of their development as this understanding will help the patient appreciate the irrationality or irrelevance of their expectations and perceptions for their current relationships.

Persons with AVPD often find group therapies to be helpful. Exploratory and supportive groups can provide them with an understanding environment in which to discuss their social insecurities, to explore and practice more assertive behaviors, and to develop an increased self-confidence to approach others and to develop relationships outside of the group. Focused and specialized social skills training groups would be preferable to unstructured groups that might be predominated by much more assertive and extraverted members.

Many persons with AVPD will respond to anxiolytic medications, and at times to antidepressants, particularly such monoamine oxidase inhibitors as phenelzine (Markovitz 2001). Normal and abnormal feelings of anxiousness can be suppressed or diminished through pharmacologic interventions (Widiger 2001). This approach may in fact be necessary to overcome initial feelings of intense social anxiety that are markedly disruptive to current functioning (e.g., inability to give required presentations at work or to talk to new acquaintances). However, it is also important to monitor closely a reliance on medications. Persons with AVPD could be prone to rely excessively on substances to control their feelings of anxiousness, whereas their more general feelings of insecurity and inadequacy would require a more comprehensive treatment.

---

Clinical Vignette 4

LW was a 26-year-old female. She was first seen in treatment at the age of 19 years when she entered an anxiety disorders treatment program. She was a music major (specializing in the flute) at a prominent university. However, she suffered from substantial feelings of anxiety to the point that she was unable to perform in front of an audience. She was diagnosed with a generalized social phobia when it was discovered that she was anxious within a wide variety of other social situations. She was generally timid, insecure, shy, and introverted. She was treated with phenelzine, and found substantial improvement within a few weeks in her more severe feelings of anxiety. She was able to complete the music program and graduated with honors.

However, she subsequently sought outpatient therapy at the age of 23 years for feelings of depression. She complained of substantial feelings of inadequacy, worthlessness, and helplessness. She was currently married to a man who was sexually abusive and emotionally detached. She had in fact been involved in a series of disappointing and often exploitative relationships. She described herself as being undesirable, yet she was in fact bright, attractive, responsible, and affectionate. Her past boyfriends had been either socially inadequate or domineering males who failed to provide her with much emotional support or meaningful involvement. Her current husband was attractive to her primarily because she perceived him as successful, strong, and protective. However, he was also continually critical, derogatory, and often required her to perform sexual acts that she found humiliating.

Her employment history was equally disappointing. She would rarely apply for any quality employment because she assumed that she would be rejected. When she did find employment, she would quit within just a few weeks because of feelings of tension and anxiety. Her feelings of anxiety were not confined to performing in front of others. She described a terror over the thought of disappointing any employer. She was in fact very capable, responsible, and even talented, but she was certain that she would eventually be shown to be inadequate and incompetent.

She described her mother as having been continually anxious and nervous, with a history of depression in her biological relatives. She described her father as being alcoholic, derogatory, and hostile. A typical example of his emotional abuse consisted of him interrogating at dinner each sibling in turn regarding their behavior (or failures) that day. Those that met with his disapproval were sent from the table. She performed very well in school because she was intensely afraid of his anger if she did less than excellent. She was cognitively aware that his criticisms were usually inappropriate and always excessive, but she could not help feeling fearful and hurt. He was her father and how he felt about her meant a great deal to her. In fact, she had largely incorporated his attitude to her as her own attitude toward herself.

She was treated with an antidepressant, group therapy for interpersonal assertiveness, and 3 years of outpatient psychotherapy that focused on her self-image. The therapist emphasized the irrationality and maladaptivity of her statements regarding her self-image, and their development within her relationships and within her family. In treatment, she gradually developed increasing feelings of self-confidence and assertion. Medication was terminated at the end of 6 months. By the end of the group and individual psychotherapy she had obtained employment within a department store and had been promoted to floor manager. She divorced her husband during treatment. She continued to suffer from feelings of anxiousness when dating, but the relationships were now more satisfying, meaningful, and promising.

## Dependent Personality Disorder

### Definition

Dependent personality disorder (DPD) involves a pervasive and excessive need to be taken care of that leads to submissiveness, clinging, and fears of separation (American Psychiatric Association 2000, Bornstein 1999, Pincus and Wilson 2001). Persons with DPD will also have low self-esteem, and will often be self-critical and self-denigrating. DPD is indicated by the presence of five or more of the eight diagnostic criteria presented in DSM-IV-TR Criteria for DPD.

### Etiology and Pathology

Central to the etiology and pathology of DPD is an insecure interpersonal attachment (Bornstein 1999, Pincus and Wilson 2001, Stone 1993). Insecure attachment and helplessness may be generated through a parent–child relationship, perhaps by a clinging parent or a continued infantilization during a time in which individuation and separation normally occurs (Gabbard 2000, Thompson and Zuroff 1998). However, DPD may also represent an interaction of an anxious–inhibited temperament with inconsistent or overprotective parenting (Bornstein 1999, O'Neill and Kendler 1998, Rothbart and Ahadi 1994). Dependent persons may turn to a parental figure to provide a reassurance, security, and confidence that they are unable to generate for themselves. They may eventually believe that their self-worth is contingent upon the worth or importance they have to another person (Beck and Freeman 1990).

## DSM-IV-TR Criteria 301.6

**Dependent Personality Disorder**

A pervasive and excessive need to be taken care of that leads to submissive and clinging behavior and fears of separation, beginning by early adulthood and present in a variety of contexts, as indicated by five (or more) of the following:

(1) has difficulty making everyday decisions without an excessive amount of advice and reassurance from others.

(2) needs others to assume responsiblity for most major areas of his or her life.

(3) has difficulty expressing disagreement with others because of fear of loss of support or approval (**Note:** Do not include realistic fears of retribution).

(4) has difficulty initiating projects or doing things on his or her own (because of a lack of self-confidence in judgment or abilities rather than to a lack of motivation or energy).

(5) goes to excessive lengths to obtain nurturance and support from others, to the point of volunteering to do things that are unpleasant.

(6) feels uncomfortable or helpless when alone, because of exaggerated fears of being unable to care for himself or herself.

(7) urgently seeks another relationship as a source of care and support when a close relationship ends.

(8) is unrealistically preoccupied with fears of being left to take care of himself or herself

### Differential Diagnosis

Excessive dependency will often be seen in persons who have developed debilitating mental and general medical disorders such as agoraphobia, schizophrenia, mental retardation, severe injuries, and dementia. However, a diagnosis of DPD requires the presence of the dependent traits since late childhood or adolescence (American Psychiatric Association 2000). One can diagnose the presence of a personality disorder at any age during a person's lifetime, but if, for example, a DPD diagnosis is given to a person at the age of 75 years, this presumes that the dependent behavior was evident since the age of approximately 18 years (i.e., predates the onset of a comorbid mental or physical disorder).

Deference, politeness, and passivity will also vary substantially across cultural groups. It is important not to confuse differences in personality that are due to different cultural norms with the presence of a personality disorder (Alarcon 1996, Alarcon and Foulks 1997, Bornstein 1999). The diagnosis of DPD requires that the dependent behavior be maladaptive, resulting in clinically significant functional impairment or distress.

Many persons with DPD will also meet the criteria for histrionic and borderline personality disorders (see Table 79–2). Persons with DPD and HPD may both display strong needs for reassurance, attention, and approval. However, persons with DPD tend to be more self-effacing, docile, and altruistic, whereas persons with HPD tend to be more flamboyant, assertive, and self-centered and persons with BPD will tend to be much more dysfunctional and emotionally dysregulated (Bornstein 1999, Widiger et al. 1995).

## Epidemiology and Comorbidity

DPD is among the most prevalent of the personality disorders (American Psychiatric Association 2000), occurring in 5 to 30% of patients and 2 to 4% of the general community (Mattia and Zimmerman 2001). A controversial issue is its differential sex prevalence (Bornstein 1999, Widiger 1998). DPD is diagnosed more frequently in females but there is some concern that there might be a failure to recognize adequately the extent of dependent personality traits within males (Bornstein 1999, Corbitt and Widiger 1995). Many studies have indicated that dependent personality traits provide a vulnerability to the development of depression in response to interpersonal loss (Hammen et al. 1995, Robins et al. 1995, Widiger et al. 1999).

## Course

Persons with DPD are likely to have been excessively submissive as children and adolescents, and some may have had a chronic physical illness or a separation anxiety disorder during childhood (American Psychiatric Association 2000). Persons with DPD fear intensely a loss of concern, care, and support from others, particularly the person with whom they have an emotional attachment (Bornstein 1999, Stone 1993). They are unable to be by themselves, as their sense of self-worth, value, or meaning is obtained by or through the presence of a relationship. They have few other sources of self-esteem. Along with the need for emotional support, are perpetual doubts and insecurities regarding the current source of support. Persons with DPD constantly require reassurance and reaffirmation that any particular relationship will continue, because they anticipate or fear that at some point they may again be alone (Overholser 1996). Because of their intense fear of being alone they may become quickly attached to persons who are unreliable, unempathic, and even exploitative or abusive. More desirable or reliable partners are at times driven away by their excessive clinging and continued demands for reassurance. Occupational functioning is impaired to the extent that independent responsibility and initiative are required. Persons with DPD are prone to mood disorders, particularly major depressive disorder and dysthymic disorder, and to anxiety disorders, particularly agoraphobia, social phobia, and perhaps panic disorder. However, the severity of the symptomatology tends to decrease with age, particularly if the person has obtained a reliable, dependable, and empathic partner.

## Treatment

Persons with DPD are often in treatment for one or more Axis I disorders, particularly a mood (depressive) or an anxiety disorder. They tend to be very agreeable, compliant, and grateful patients, at times to excess. An important issue in the treatment of persons with DPD is not letting the relationship with the therapist become an end in itself (Stone 1993). Many persons with DPD find the therapeutic relationship to satisfy their need for support, concern, and involvement. The therapist can be perceived as a nurturing, caring, and dependable partner who is always available for as long as the patient desires. Successful treatment can in fact be feared because it suggests the termination of the relationship, an outcome that is at times avoided at all costs. As a result, they be may be excessively compliant, submissive, agreeable, and cooperative in order to be the patient that the therapist would want to retain. Therapists need to be careful not to unwittingly encourage or exploit this submissiveness, nor to commit the opposite error of rejecting and abandoning them to be rid of their needy and clinging dependency. Such responses are common in the interpersonal (marital and sexual) history of persons with DPD, and are at times experienced as well within therapeutic relationships. Persons with DPD tend to have unrealistic expectations regarding their therapist. They may attempt to have the therapist take control of their lives, and may make unrealistic requests or demands for their therapist's time, involvement, and availability.

Exploration of the breadth and source of the need for care and support is often an important component of treatment (Gunderson and Gabbard 2000). Persons with DPD often have a history of exploitative, rejecting, and perhaps even abusive relationships that have contributed to their current feelings of insecurity and inadequacy (Bornstein 1999). Cognitive–behavioral techniques are useful in addressing the feelings of inadequacy, incompetence, and helplessness (Beck and Freeman 1990). Social skills, problem-solving, and assertiveness training also makes important contributions.

Persons with DPD may also benefit from group therapy. A supportive group is useful in diffusing the feelings of dependency onto a variety of persons, in providing feedback regarding their manner of relating to others, and in providing practice and role models for more assertive and autonomous interpersonal functioning. There is no known pharmacologic treatment for DPD (Markovitz 2001).

---

Clinical Vignette 5

LC was a 21-year-old college sophomore who unexpectedly returned home in the middle of the first semester, proclaiming that she could no longer suffer the anxiety and depression she felt at college. Neither she nor her parents felt that they had a clear understanding of what was making her feel so distraught. She was doing fine in her classes and was actively involved in a number of college organizations. Her mother called her academic advisor at college for advice and LC was referred to a clinician for consultation and treatment.

LC indicated at the initial session that she had been intensely ambivalent about attending college, and had in fact delayed enrollment for 2 years in the hope that she could convince her parents that she would not have to leave home. She indicated that she felt overwhelmingly frightened and tearful away from home. She had been calling her parents three to five times each week, seeking their advice and reassurance but also simply to maintain regular contact. LC's level of anxiety decreased substantially when she returned home but quickly emerged at the thought of leaving home again.

LC's parents were concerned that she was returning home to be close to a boy that she had once dated. LC, however, denied this motivation, indicating that she had long abandoned any hope of a future in that particular relationship. LC was a popular young woman, generally considered to be quite amicable, modest, friendly, warm, attractive, bright, and engaging. However, she acknowledged that she often felt very insecure in her relationships, requiring reassurances from her girlfriends and boyfriends that she was not a burden to them as she in fact grew increasingly burdensome in part from her need for their reassurance. She indicated that she had often fallen in love but had repeatedly felt crushed and devastated when the object of her love failed to become as attached. She said that one boyfriend broke up with her explicitly because he experienced her as being too "needy" and "clinging." She admitted that this was "not far from the truth" but had pleaded to him that she would no longer be so needy if only he would not leave her.

LC described her relationship with parents, particularly her mother, as being very close, supportive, and dependable. LC's childhood history, however, included many examples of failures to develop an independent self-confidence. For example, she felt unable to attend a summer camp attended by her best friends because of fears of separation from her parents; she did attend the following summer but taxed the patience of the camp counselors with her demands for attention and support. Her parents verbally encouraged her to develop greater independence and self-confidence but they also would repeatedly give in to her requests for protection and support. LC's mother in fact often appeared to be somewhat reluctant to let LC separate from her.

LC was seen in twice-weekly individual psychotherapy. Pharmacotherapy was provided for her anxious and depressive symptoms but was discontinued after 2 months due to complaints of side effects. Cognitive therapy focused on her self-denigrating beliefs of helplessness, behavioral therapy included a gradual shaping of independence from her parents, and insight therapy explored the relationship of her self-image with her relationships with her parents. Treatment was successful in developing sufficient independence and self-esteem for LC to feel comfortable and confident enough to return the following year to college. She successfully completed college although abandoned aspirations to pursue a social work career after she married and had children of her own.

## Obsessive–Compulsive Personality Disorder

### Definition

Obsessive–compulsive PD (OCPD) includes a preoccupation with orderliness, perfectionism, and mental and interpersonal control (American Psychiatric Association 2000). OCPD is indicated by the presence of four or more of the eight diagnostic criteria presented in DSM criteria for OCPD.

**DSM-IV-TR Criteria** 301.4

### Obsessive–Compulsive Personality Disorder

A pervasive pattern of preoccupation with orderliness, perfectionism, and mental and interpersonal control at the expense of flexibility, openness, and efficiency, beginning by early adulthood and present in a variety of contexts, as indicated by four (or more) of the following:

(1) is preoccupied with details, rules, lists, order, organization, or schedules to the extent that the major point of the activity is lost

(2) shows perfectionism that interferes with task completion (e.g., is unable to complete a project because his or her own overly strict standards are not met)

(3) excessive devotion to work and productivity to the exclusion of leisure activities and friendships (not accounted for by obvious economic necessity)

(4) is overconscientious, scrupulous, and inflexible about matters of morality, ethics, or values (not accounted for by cultural or religious identification)

(5) is unable to discard worn-out or worthless objects even when they have no sentimental value

(6) is reluctant to delegate tasks or to work with others unless they submit to exactly his or her way of doing things

(7) adopts a miserly spending style toward both self and others; money is viewed as something to be hoarded for future catastrophes

(8) shows rigidity and stubbornness

### Etiology and Pathology

A variety of studies have indicated heritability for the trait of obsessionality (Nigg and Goldsmith 1994). OCPD may also relate to the adult personality trait of conscientiousness–constraint (Costa and McCrae 1992, Widiger et al. 2002) and the childhood temperament of attentional self-regulation, both of which have demonstrated substantial heritability (Jang and Vernon 2001, Plomin and Caspi 1999, Rothbart and Ahadi 1994).

Early psychoanalytic theories regarding OCPD concerned issues of unconscious guilt or shame (Gunderson and Gabbard 2000). A variety of underlying conflicts have since been proposed, including a need to maintain an illusion of infallibility to defend against feelings of insecurity, an identification with authoritarian parents, or an excessive, rigid control of feelings and impulses (Gabbard 2000, Oldham and Frosch 1991, Stone 1993). Any one or more of these conflicts might be relevant for a particular person with OCPD but there is quite limited empirical support for these particular models of etiology and pathology. OCPD includes personality traits that are highly valued within most cultures (e.g., conscientiousness) and some instances of OCPD may reflect exaggerated or excessive responses to the expectations of or pressures by parental figures.

## Differential Diagnosis

Devotion to work and productivity will vary substantially across cultural groups. One should be careful not to confuse normal cultural variation in conscientiousness with the presence of this personality disorder. A diagnosis of OCPD requires that the devotion to work be maladaptive or to the exclusion of leisure activities and friendships (American Psychiatric Association 2000).

OCPD resembles to some extent the obsessive–compulsive anxiety disorder (OCAD). However, many persons with OCPD fail to develop OCAD, and vice versa (Pfohl and Blum 1991). OCAD involves intrusive obsessions or circumscribed and repetitively performed rituals whose purpose is to reduce or control feelings of anxiety (American Psychiatric Association 2000). OCPD, in contrast, involves rigid, inhibited, and authoritarian behavior patterns that are more ego-syntonic. If both behavior patterns are present, both diagnoses should be given as these disorders are sufficiently distinct that it is likely that in such cases two different disorders are in fact present (Widiger et al. 1995).

OCPD may at times resemble narcissistic PD, as both disorders can involve assertiveness, domination, achievement, and a professed perfectionism. However, the emphasis in OCPD will be on work for its own sake whereas narcissistic persons will work only to achieve status and recognition (Widiger et al. 1995). Persons with OCPD will also be troubled by doubts, worries, and self-criticism, whereas the narcissistic person will tend to be overly self-assured.

## Epidemiology and Comorbidity

Conscientiousness is one of the fundamental dimensions of personality (Hogan et al. 1997, Pervin and John 1999), characterized by the tendency to emphasize duty, order, deliberation, discipline, competence, and achievement (Costa and McCrae 1992). Persons who are excessively organized, ordered, deliberate, dutiful, and disciplined would be characterized as having OCPD (Widiger et al. 2002). Only 1 to 2% of the general community may meet the diagnostic criteria for the disorder (see Table 79–1) but this could be an underestimation (Oldham and Frosch 1991). Up to 10% of the population has been estimated to be maladaptively stubborn, 4% excessively devoted to work, and 8% excessively perfectionistic (Nestadt et al. 1991). OCPD is one of the less frequently diagnosed personality disorders within inpatient settings, occurring in approximately 3 to 10% of patients (American Psychiatric Association 2000) but its prevalence may be much higher within private practice settings. This disorder does appear to occur more often in males than in females but exceptions to this finding have been reported (Corbitt and Widiger 1995).

## Course

As children, some persons with OCPD may have appeared to be relatively well-behaved, responsible, and conscientious. However, they may have also been overly serious, rigid, and constrained (Rothbart and Ahadi 1994). As adults, many will obtain good to excellent success within a job or career. They can be excellent workers to the point of excess, sacrificing their social and leisure activities, marriage, and family for their job (Oldham and Frosch 1991, Stone 1993). Relationships with spouse and children are likely to be strained due to their tendency to be detached and uninvolved, yet authoritarian and domineering with respect to decisions. A spouse may complain of a lack of affection, tenderness, and warmth. Relationships with colleagues at work may be equally strained by the excessive perfectionism, domination, indecision, worrying, and anger. Jobs that require flexibility, openness, creativity, or diplomacy may be particularly difficult. Persons with OCPD may be prone to various anxiety and physical disorders that are secondary to their worrying, indecision, and stress. Those with concomitant traits of angry hostility and competitiveness may be prone to cardiovascular disorders. Mood disorders may not develop until the person recognizes the sacrifices that have been made by their devotion to work and productivity, which may at times not occur until middle-age. However, most will experience early employment or career difficulties or even failures that may result in depression.

## Treatment

Persons with OCPD may fail to seek treatment for the OCPD symptomatology. They may seek treatment instead for disorders and problems that are secondary to their OCPD traits, including anxiety disorders, health problems (e.g., cardiovascular disorders), and problems within various relationships (e.g., marital, familial, and occupational). Treatment will be complicated by their inability to appreciate the contribution of their personality to these problems and disorders (Gunderson and Gabbard 2000, Oldham and Frosch 1991, Stone 1993). It is not unusual for persons with OCPD to perceive themselves as being simply conscientious, dutiful, moral, and responsible, rather than perfectionistic, stubborn, rigid, domineering, and unavailable. Their understanding is complicated further by the contribution of their traits to various achievements and successes (e.g., career advancement) and to the control of negative affect (e.g., ability to control feelings of dysphoria during a crisis). The OCPD traits are not invariably or always maladaptive, and persons with this disorder may not appreciate the disorder's cost to their physical health, psychological well-being, and personal relationships.

Cognitive–behavioral techniques that address the irrationality of excessive conscientiousness, moralism, perfectionism, devotion to work, and stubborness can be effective in the treatment of OCPD (Beck and Freeman 1990). Persons with OCPD may in fact appreciate the rational approach to treatment provided by cognitive–behavioral therapy. A common difficulty though is the tendency to drift into lengthy and unproductive ruminations and intellectualized speculations (Beck and Freeman 1990, Gunderson and Gabbard 2000, Stone 1993). Therapeutic techniques that emphasize the acknowledgment, recognition, and acceptance of feelings will therefore be useful (Gabbard 2000). Gestalt techniques that focus upon and confront feeling states will often feel threatening to persons with OCPD but precisely for this reason they can also be quite revealing and useful. Persons with OCPD will attempt to control therapeutic sessions, and techniques that encourage uncontrolled, freely expressed associations to explore historical motivations for control, perfectionism, and workaholism are often helpful.

Persons with OCPD can be problematic in groups. They will tend to be domineering, constricted, and judgmental. There is no accepted pharmacologic treatment for OCPD (Markovitz 2001). Some persons with OCPD will benefit from anxiolytic or antidepressant medications, but this will typically reflect the presence of associated features or comorbid disorders. The core traits of OCPD might not be affected by pharmacologic interventions.

## Personality Disorder Not Otherwise Specified

As indicated earlier, DSM-IV includes a diagnostic category, personality disorder not otherwise specified (PDNOS), for persons with a personality disorder who do not meet the diagnostic criteria for any one of the ten officially recognized diagnoses. PDNOS has in fact been the singly most commonly used personality disorder diagnosis in almost every study in which it has been considered (Clark et al. 1995, Widiger and Coker 2002). It would not, of course, be possible to discuss the etiology, pathology, course, or treatment of the PDNOS disorder as the diagnosis refers to a wide variety of personality types. However, one usage of PDNOS is for the two personality disorders presented in the appendix to DSM-IV for criterion sets provided for further study, the passive–aggressive and the depressive (American Psychiatric Association 2000).

## Passive–Aggressive (Negativistic) Personality Disorder

### Definition

Passive–aggressive personality disorder (PAPD) is a pervasive pattern of negativistic attitudes and passive resistance to authority, demands, responsibilities, or obligations (American Psychiatric Association 2000). PAPD would be diagnosed by the presence of four or more of the seven criteria presented in DSM-IV-TR criteria for PAPD.

PAPD was an officially recognized diagnosis in DSM-III-R (American Psychiatric Association 1987). It is in the appendix of DSM-IV because there has been little research to support its validity. There was concern that the DSM-III-R diagnosis described a situational reaction rather than a pervasive and chronic personality disorder, and the criteria were revised substantially for DSM-IV-TR to describe a more general and pervasive negativism (Gunderson 1998, Widiger et al. 1995). Compelling objections were raised in response to the decision to downgrade the recognition of this longstanding diagnosis (Wetzler and Morey 1999) and the new criteria may eventually prove to have more validity and clinical utility than the DSM-III-R version (McCann 1988, Millon 1993) but this additional research needs to be conducted in order for the diagnosis to be given an official recognition.

---

### DSM-IV-TR Criteria

**Passive–Aggressive Personality Disorder**

A. A pervasive pattern of negativistic attitudes and passive resistance to demands for adequate performance, beginning by early adulthood and present in a variety of contexts, as indicated by four (or more) of the following:

(1) passively resists fulfilling routine social and occupational tasks

(2) complains of being misunderstood and unappreciated by others

(3) is sullen and argumentative

(4) unreasonably criticizes and scorns authority

(5) expresses envy and resentment toward those apparently more fortunate

(6) voices exaggerated and persistent complaints of personal misfortune

(7) alternates between hostile defiance and contrition

B. Does not occur exclusively during major depressive episodes and is not better accounted for by dysthymic disorder.

Reprinted with permission from the Diagnostic and Statistical Manual of Mental Disorders, Fourth Edition, Text Revision. Copyright 2000 American Psychiatric Association.

### Etiology and Pathology

Central to the psychopathology of PAPD appears to be bitter resentment (Millon et al. 1996). Passive–aggressive persons have a hostile, angry, and bitter attitude towards the world. There are no data on its heritability or psychosocial etiology. It has been suggested that passive–aggressive behavior is due in part to conflicts concerning dependency and resentment, or a history of mistreatment and neglect (McCann 1988). One might find a history of being exploited, neglected, mistreated, or abused by persons upon whom the person with PAPD relied. Negativistic traits may also be modeled by parental figures.

### Assessment and Differential Diagnosis

Most of the DSM-IV semistructured interviews include items for the assessment of PAPD (First et al. 1997, Pfohl et al. 1997, Widiger et al. 1995, Zanarini et al. 1995). It is particularly important when assessing for PAPD to recognize that passive–aggressive behavior might be confined to settings in which persons have lost freedom, responsibility, or decision-making authority that was previously available to them and overt expressions of assertiveness or opposition are being discouraged. For example, it would not be surprising to observe passive–aggressive behavior within the military, prison, or some inpatient hospitals. It is important in such settings to verify that the negativistic behavior was evident earlier and is currently evident within other situations.

## Epidemiology and Comorbidity

Approximately 1 to 2% of the community will meet the DSM-III-R criteria for PAPD (see Table 79–1). Up to 5% of patients were being diagnosed with PAPD earlier (McCann 1988, Millon 1993, Wetzler and Morey 1999). The rate was higher when semistructured interviews were used but still low compared to most other personality disorders. The prevalence rate with the DSM-IV criteria are likely to be higher, given the expansion of the disorder from simply a passive resistance to demands for adequate performance to a more general negativism (Millon 1993). An approximately equal prevalence of males and females have traits that met the criteria for the disorder based upon the DSM-III and DSM-III-R criteria (Corbitt and Widiger 1995). However, the broader formulation of negativism resembles closely the general trait of oppositionalism (characterized by the tendency to be complaining, discontented, grumbling, whining, and argumentative) which does appear to occur more often in males than in females (Costa and McCrae 1992).

## Course

Many persons with PAPD may have met the criteria for an oppositional defiant disorder during childhood, which is also characterized by the tendency to be irritable, complaining, oppositional, argumentative, and negativistic (American Psychiatric Association 1980). As adults, impairment is likely to be most evident with respect to employment. Persons with PAPD are irresponsible, lax, and negligent employees, as well as resistant, oppositional, and even hostile. Resolution of interpersonal conflicts is difficult due to the tendency of the passive–aggressive person to blame others. They are argumentative, sullen, and critical of their peers and friends, who may not tolerate their antagonism.

## Treatment

Persons with PAPD rarely enter treatment to make effective changes to their personality or behavior. They are more likely to seek treatment for Axis I disorders (e.g., depression, anxiety, or somatoform disorder), or for marital, family, or occupational problems. The initiation of treatment is often at the insistence of a spouse, relative, or employer (Gabbard 2000, Stone 1993). They can be very difficult patients to treat due to their tendency to be blaming, argumentative, pessimistic, and passively resistant (Millon et al. 1996). It is important for the therapist to remain supportive and empathic; carefully and benignly offering observations, suggestions, and reflections on the patient's tendency to be their own worst enemy. Cognitive treatment can be useful to directly address the false perceptions, assumptions, and attributions (Beck and Freeman 1990) as long as the therapist is not drawn into unproductive disagreements and arguments. It is common for therapists to become frustrated, impatient, and defensive in response to the negativism, criticism, and complaints. Periodic consultation with colleagues are advisable. Group therapy is often helpful once the patient has developed a commitment to the group, as the various members can provide consistent and confirmatory feedback regarding the negativistic and passive–aggressive behavior. There is no known pharmacologic treatment for PAPD (Markovitz 2001).

## Depressive Personality Disorder

### Definition

Depressive personality disorder (DPPD) is a pervasive pattern of depressive cognitions and behaviors that have been evident since adolescence and characteristic of everyday functioning (American Psychiatric Association 2000). These are persons who characteristically display a gloominess, cheerlessness, pessimism, brooding, rumination, and dejection. DPPD would be diagnosed by the presence of five or more of the seven criteria presented in the DSM criteria for DPPD.

DPPD was proposed for inclusion in DSM-III and DSM-III-R but there were concerns that it may not be adequately distinguished from the mood disorder of dysthymia (Klein 1999, Phillips et al. 1995, 1998, Ryder and Bagby 1999, Widiger 1999). However, a field trial by the DSM-IV Mood Disorders Work Group indicated that many persons do meet diagnostic criteria for DPPD rather than early-onset dysthymia (Phillips et al. 1995, Widiger 1999). In addition, many persons diagnosed with early-onset dysthymia may not be adequately described as having a disorder that is confined to the regulation or control of their mood (Klein 1999, Phillips et al. 1998). However, the DSM-IV diagnostic criteria for DPPD lack sufficient empirical support to warrant full recognition (Gunderson 1998).

### Etiology and Pathology

DPPD may represent a characterologic variant of mood disorder, in the same manner that STPD is perhaps a char-

---

**DSM-IV-TR Criteria**

**Depressive Personality Disorder**

A. A pervasive pattern of depressive cognitions and behaviors beginning by early adulthood and present in a variety of contexts, as indicated by five (or more) of the following:

   (1) usual mood is dominated by dejection, gloominess, cheerlessness, joylessness, unhappiness

   (2) self-concept centers around beliefs of inadequacy, worthlessness, and low self-esteem

   (3) is critical, blaming, and derogatory toward self

   (4) is brooding and given to worry

   (5) is negativistic, critical, and judgmental toward others

   (6) is pessimistic

   (7) is prone to feeling guilty or remorseful

B. Does not occur exclusively during major depressive episodes and is not better accounted for by dysthymic disorder.

Reprinted with permission from the Diagnostic and Statistical Manual of Mental Disorders, Fourth Edition, Text Revision. Copyright 2000 American Psychiatric Association.

acterologic variant of schizophrenia. Support for this hypothesis is provided by recent family history and biogenetic studies (Klein 1999). Trait depression is also a facet of the personality trait of neuroticism or negative affectivity, which has demonstrated substantial heritability within the general population (Jang et al. 1998, Jang and Vernon 2001, Pervin and John 1993). A characteristically low self-esteem, self-criticism, pessimism, brooding, and guilt may also result from continued, sustained criticism, derogation, and discouragement by a significant parental figure that is accepted and incorporated by the child (Stone 1993).

## Assessment and Differential Diagnosis

Most of the DSM-IV-TR semistructured interviews include items for the assessment of DPPD (First et al. 1997, Pfohl et al. 1997, Widiger et al. 1995, Zanarini et al. 1995) and there is also available a semistructured interview that is devoted to its assessment, the Diagnostic Interview for Depressive Personality (Gunderson et al. 1994).

DPPD overlaps substantially with early-onset dysthymia. Early-onset dysthymia was in fact conceptualized previously as depressive personality or a characterologic depression prior to DSM-III-R (Keller 1989) and the alternative criteria for dysthymia that were placed in the appendix to DSM-IV-TR were developed in part on research on DPPD (Phillips et al. 1995, Widiger 1999). It is in fact noted in DSM-IV that there may not be a meaningful distinction between these diagnoses (American Psychiatric Association 2000). Some may prefer to use the diagnosi of early-onset dysthymia, but a dysregulation in mood may not adequately explain why some persons are characterized by chronic attitudes of pessimism, negativism, hopelessness, and dejection.

## Epidemiology and Comorbidity

There are not yet published data on the prevalence of DPPD within the general population. DPPD is likely to be comorbid with early onset dysthymia, although not all cases of DPPD will meet the DSM-IV-TR criteria for dysthymia (Klein 1999, Phillips et al. 1995). Many of the persons who meet the DSM-IV-TR criteria for DPPD will also likely meet the DSM-IV-TR criteria for PAPD and BPD.

## Course

As children, persons with DPPD are pessimistic, gloomy, passive, and withdrawn. Performance in school is often inadequate to poor. This behavior pattern continues essentially unchanged into and through adulthood. Some, however, may eventually become good workers, exhibiting tremendous discipline and devotion to their work (Phillips et al. 1995). Relationships with peers and sexual partners, however, are invariably problematic. They are gloomy and irritable company, and have difficulty finding pleasure, joy, or satisfaction in leisure activities (Millon et al. 1996). They may also be quite withdrawn and lonely, but lack an apparent motivation or energy to seek or maintain relationships.

## Treatment

Many persons with DPD are referred or seek treatment for a depressive mood disorder. It is important in such cases to recognize the extent to which the depressed mood reflects their fundamental view of themselves and the world. Their pessimism involves more than simply a dysregulation of mood. Cognitive–behavioral techniques have demonstrated efficacy in the treatment of depressive personality traits (Beck and Freeman 1990). The depressive individual's pessimistic view of themselves and their future should be systematically challenged. Explorations of the faulty reasoning, arbitrary inferences, selective perceptions, and misattributions can be influential in overcoming the pessimistic, gloomy, critical, and negativistic attitudes. Audio- or video-taped role playing is useful in helping the person recognize the occurrence and pervasiveness of the depressive cognitions, and in generating, developing, and rehearsing more realistic and accurate reasoning. However, exploration of the source for and historical development of self-defeating behaviors may also be helpful, not only to undermine their credibility and validity within current relationships and situations but also to address any motivation for their perpetuation (Stone 1993). Persons with DPPD will also be responsive to antidepressant pharmacotherapy, particularly tricyclic antidepressants (Klein 1999, Markovitz 2001, Widiger 1999).

## Comparison of DSM-IV/ICD-10 Diagnostic Criteria

The items sets for paranoid, schizoid, schizotypal, antisocial, histrionic, avoidant, dependent, and obsessive–compulsive personality disorders in the ICD-10 Diagnostic Criteria for Research and the DSM-IV-TR criteria differ but define essentially the same condition. Furthermore, ICD-10 does not consider schizotypal to be a personality disorder and instead includes this condition in the section containing schizophrenia and other psychotic disorders. ICD-10 also refers to several of the DSM-IV-TR disorders by different names: antisocial is called "dissocial," borderline is called "emotionally unstable personality disorder, borderline type," and obsessive–compulsive is called "anankastic."

ICD-10 includes an "emotionally unstable personality disorder" with two subtypes: impulsive type and borderline type; criteria are provided for each subtype but not for emotionally unstable personality disorder. Neither of these subtypes by themselves correspond to the DSM-IV-TR borderline personality disorder, which includes some items from each of these subtypes. Narcissistic personality disorder in DSM-IV-TR is not included in ICD-10 as a specific personality disorder, although the DSM-IV-TR criteria set is included in Annex I of ICD-10 (i.e., "provisional criteria for selected disorders").

## References

Ad-Dab'bagh Y and Greenfield B (2001) Multiple complex developmental disorder: The "multiple and complex" evolution of the "childhood borderline syndrome" construct. J Am Acad Child Adolesc Psychiatr 40, 954–964.

Alarcon RD (1996) Personality disorders and culture in DSM-IV: A critique. J Pers Disord 10, 260–270.

Alarcon RD and Foulks EF (1997) Cultural factors and personality disorders: A review of the literature. In DSM-IV Sourcebook, Vol. 3, Widiger TA, Frances AJ, Pincus HA, et al. (eds). American Psychiatric Association, Washington DC, pp. 975–982.

American Psychiatric Association (1980) Diagnostic and Statistical Manual of Mental Disorders, 3rd ed. APA, Washington DC.

American Psychiatric Association (1987) Diagnostic and Statistical Manual of Mental Disorders, 3rd ed., Rev. APA, Washington DC.

American Psychiatric Association (2000) Diagnostic and Statistical Manual of Mental Disorders, 4th ed., Text Rev. APA, Washington DC.

Beck AT and Freeman A (1990) Cognitive Therapy of Personality Disorders. Guilford Press, New York.

Benjamin LS (1993) Interpersonal Diagnosis and Treatment of Personality Disorders. Guilford Press, New York.

Bernstein DP and Travaglini L (1999) Schizoid and avoidant personality disorders. In Oxford Textbook of Psychopathology, Millon T, Blaney PH, and Davis RD (eds). Oxford University Press, New York, pp. 523–534.

Black DW, Noyes R, Pfohl B, et al. (1993) Personality disorder in obsessive–compulsive volunteers, well comparison subjects, and their first degree relatives. Am J Psychiatr 150, 1226–1232.

Bornstein RF (1998) Reconceptualizing personality disorder diagnosis in the DSM-V: The discriminant validity challenge. Clin Psychol: Sci Pract 5, 333–343.

Bornstein RF (1999) Dependent and histrionic personality disorders. In Oxford Textbook of Psychopathology, Millon T, Blaney PH, and Davis RD (eds). Oxford University Press, New York, pp. 535–554.

Brodsky BS, Cloitre M, and Dulit RA (1995) Relationship of dissociation to self-mutilation and childhood abuse in borderline personality disorder. Am J Psychiatr 152, 1788–1792.

Burgess KB, Rubin KH, Chea CSL, et al. (2001) Behavioral inhibition, social withdrawal, and parenting. In International Handbook of Social Anxiety, Crozier WR and Alden LE (eds). John Wiley, New York, pp. 137–158.

Clark DM (2001) A cognitive perspective on social phobia. In International Handbook of Social Anxiety, Crozier WR and Alden LE (eds). John Wiley, New York, pp. 405–430.

Clark LA and Harrison JA (2001) Assessment instruments. In Handbook of Personality Disorders, Livesley WJ (ed). Guilford Press, New York, pp. 277–306.

Clark LA and Watson D (1999) Personality, disorder, and personality disorder: Toward a more rational conceptualization. J Pers Disord 13, 142–151.

Clark LA, Kochanska G, and Ready R (2000) Mothers' personality and its interaction with child temperament as predicting parenting behavior. J Pers Soc Psychol 79, 274–285.

Clark LA, Watson D, and Reynolds S (1995) Diagnosis and classification of psychopathology: Challenges to the current system and future directions. Annu Rev Psychol 46, 121–153.

Cloninger CR (2000) A practical way to diagnosis personality disorders: A proposal. J Pers Disord 14, 99–108.

Cooper AM and Ronningstam E (1992) Narcissistic personality disorder. In Review of Psychiatry, Vol. 11, Tasman A and Riba MB (eds). American Psychiatric Press, Washington DC, pp. 80–97.

Corbitt EM and Widiger TA (1995) Sex differences among the personality disorders. An exploration of the data. Clin Psychol: Sci Pract 2, 225–238.

Coryell WH and Zimmerman M (1989) Personality disorder in the families of depressed, schizophrenic, and never-ill probands. Am J Psychiatr 146, 496–502.

Costa PT and McCrae RR (1992) Revised NEO Personality Inventory (NEO PI-R) and NEO Five-Factor Inventory (NEO-FFI) Professional Manual. Psychological Assessment Resources, Odessa, FL.

Costa PT and Widiger TA (eds) (2002) Personality Disorders and the Five Factor Model of Personality, 2nd ed. American Psychological Association, Washington DC.

Crozier WR and Alden LE (eds) (2001) International Handbook of Social Anxiety. Concepts, Research, and Interventions Relating to the Self and Shyness. John Wiley, New York.

Daley SE, Burge D, and Hammen C (2000) Borderline personality disorder symptoms as predictors of 4-year romantic relationship dysfunction in young women: Addressing issues of specificity. J Abnorm Psychol 109, 451–460.

Depue RA and Lenzenweger MF (2001) A neurobehavioral dimensional model. In Handbook of Personality Disorders, Livesley WJ (ed). Guilford Press, New York, pp. 136–176.

Dodge KA, Bates JE, and Pettit GS (1990) Mechanisms in the cycle of violence. Science 250, 1678–1683.

Dolan-Sewell RG, Krueger RF, and Shea MT (2001) Co-occurrence with syndrome disorders. In Handbook of Personality Disorders, Livesley WJ (ed). Guilford Press, New York, pp. 84–104.

Drake RE, Adler DA, and Vaillant GE (1988) Antecedents of personality disorders in a community sample of men. J Pers Disord 2, 60–68.

Dreessen L, Arntz A, Hendriks T, et al. (1999) Avoidant personality disorder and implicit schema-congruent information processing bias: A pilot study with a pragmatic inference task. Behav Res Ther 37, 619–632.

Fanous A, Gardner C, Walsh D, et al. (2001) Relationship between positive and negative symptoms of schizophrenia and schizotypal symptoms in nonpsychotic relatives. Arch Gen Psychiatr 58, 669–673.

First M, Gibbon M, Spitzer RL, et al. (1997) User's Guide for the Structured Clinical Interview for DSM-IV Axis II Personality Disorders. American Psychiatric Press, Washington DC.

Fowles DC (2001) Biological variables in psychopathology: A psychobiological perspective. In Comprehensive Handbook of Psychopathology, 3rd ed., Adams HE and Sutker PB (eds). Kluwer Academic/Plenum Publishers, New York, pp. 85–104.

Fowles DC and Kochanska G (2000) Temperament as a moderator of pathways to conscience in children: The contribution of electrodermal activity. Psychophysiology 37, 788–795.

Frances AJ (1980) The DSM-III personality disorders section: A commentary. Am J Psychiatr 137, 1050–1054.

Frances AJ, First MB, and Pincus HA (1995) DSM-IV Guidebook. American Psychiatric Press, Washington DC.

Gabbard GO (2000) Psychodynamic Psychiatry in Clinical Practice, 3rd ed. American Psychiatric Press, Washington DC.

Gabbard GO (2001) Psychodynamic psychotherapy of borderline personality disorder: A contemporary approach. Bull Menn Clin 65, 41–57.

Garb HN (1997) Race bias, social class bias, and gender bias in clinical judgment. Clin Psychol: Sci and Pract 4, 99–120.

Gunderson JG (1998) DSM-IV personality disorders: Final overview. In DSM-IV Sourcebook, Vol. 4, Widiger TA, Frances AJ, Pincus HA, et al. (eds). American Psychiatric Association, Washington DC, pp. 1123–1140.

Gunderson JG (2001) Borderline Personality Disorder: A Clinical Guide. American Psychiatric Press, Washington DC.

Gunderson JG and Gabbard GO (2000) Psychotherapy for Personality Disorders. American Psychiatric Press, Washington DC.

Gunderson JG, Phillips KA, Triebwasser JT, et al. (1994) The diagnostic interview for depressive personality. Am J Psychiatr 151, 1300–1304.

Gunderson JG, Ronningstam E, and Bodkin A (1990) The diagnostic interview for narcissistic patients. Arch Gen Psychiatr 47, 676–680.

Gunderson JG, Ronningstam E, and Smith LE (1991) Narcissistic personality disorder: A review of data on DSM-III-R descriptions. J Pers Disord 5, 167–177.

Gunderson JG, Shea MT, Skodol AE, et al. (2000) The Collaborative Longitudinal Personality Disorders Study. I. Development, aims, design, and sample characteristics. J Pers Disord 14, 300–315.

Gunderson JG, Zanarini MC, and Kisiel CL (1991) Borderline personality disorder: A review of data on DSM-III-R descriptions. J Pers Disord 5, 340–352.

Hamburger ME, Lilienfield SO, and Hogben M (1996) Psychopathy, gender, and gender roles: Implications for antisocial and histrionic personality disorder. J Pers Disord 10, 41–55.

Hammen CL, Burge D, Daley SE, et al. (1995) Interpersonal attachment cognitions and predictions of symptomatic responses to interpersonal stress. J Abnorm Psychol 104, 436–443.

Hare RD (1991) The Hare Psychopathy Checklist-Revised Manual. Multi-Healthy Systems, North Tonawanda, New York.

Hare RD, Hart SD, and Harpur TJ (1991) Psychopathy and the DSM-IV criteria for antisocial personality disorder. J Abnorm Psychol 100, 391–398.

Harkness AR and Lilienfeld SO (1997) Individual differences science for treatment planning: Personality traits. Psychol Assess 9, 349–360.

Heffernan K and Cloitre M (2000) A comparison of posttraumatic stress disorder with and without borderline personality disorder among women with a history of childhood sexual abuse: Etiological and clinical characteristics. J Nerv Ment Dis 188, 589–595.

Hilsenroth MJ, Handler L, and Blais MA (1996) Assessment of narcissistic personality disorder: A multi-method review. Clin Psychol Rev 16, 655–683.

Hogan R, Johnson J, and Briggs S (eds) (1997) Handbook of Personality Psychology. Academic Press, New York.

Horowitz MJ (1997) Psychotherapy for histrionic personality disorder. J Psychother Pract Res 6, 93–104.

Jang KL, McCrae RR, Angleitner A, et al. (1998) Heritability of facet-level traits in a cross-cultural twin sample: Support for a hierarchical model of personality. J Pers Soc Psychol 74, 1556–1565.

Jang KL and Vernon PA (2001) Genetics. In Handbook of Personality Disorders, Livesley WJ (ed). Guilford Press, New York, pp. 177–195.

Johnson JG, Cohen P, Brown J, et al. (1999) Childhood maltreatment increases risk for personality disorders during early adulthood. Am J Psychiatr 56, 600–606.

Kalus O, Bernstein DP, and Siever LJ (1993) Schizoid personality disorder: A review of current status and implications for DSM-IV. J Pers Disord 7, 43–52.

Kaye AL and Shea MT (2000) Personality disorders, personality traits, and defense mechanisms. In Handbook of Psychiatric Measures, Pincus HA, Rush AJ, First MB, et al. (eds). American Psychiatric Association, Washington DC, pp. 713–749.

Keller M (1989) Current concepts in affective disorders. J Clin Psychiatr 50, 157–162.

Kernberg OF (1991a) Hysterical and histrionic personality disorders. In Psychiatry, Vol. 1, Ch. 19, Michels R (ed). JB Lippincott, Philadelphia, PA, pp. 1–11.

Kernberg OF (1991b) Narcissistic personality disorder. In Psychiatry, Vol. 1, Ch. 18, Michels R (ed). JB Lippincott, Philadelphia, PA, pp. 1–12.

Kessler K, McGonagle K, Zhao S, et al. (1994) Lifetime and 12 month prevalence of DSM-III-R Psychiatric Disorders in the United States. Arch Gen Psychiatr 51, 8–19.

Klein DN (1999) Commentary on Ryder and Bagby's "Diagnostic Validity of Depressive Personality Disorder: Theoretical and Conceptual Issues". J Pers Disord 13, 118–127.

Klein DN, Riso LP, Donaldson SK, et al. (1995) Family study of early-onset dysthymia: Mood and personality disorders in relatives of outpatients with dysthymia and episodic major depressive and normal controls. Arch Gen Psychiatr 52, 487–496.

Kochanska G and Murray KT (2000) Mother–child responsive orientation and conscience development: From toddler to early school age. Child Dev 71, 417–431.

Kohut H (1977) The Restoration of the Self. International Universities Press, New York.

Lenzenweger MF, Loranger AW, Korfine L, et al. (1997) Detecting personality disorders in a nonclinical population. Arch Gen Psychiatr 54, 345–351.

Lilienfeld SO (1994) Conceptual problems in the assessment of psychopathy. Clin Psychol Rev 14, 17–38.

Lilienfeld SO and Hess TH (2001) Psychopathic personality traits and somatization: Sex differences and the mediating role of negative emotionality. J Psychopathol Behav Assess 23, 11–24.

Lilienfeld SO, Waldman ID, and Israel AC (1994) A critical examination of the use of the term "comorbidity" in psychopathology research. Clin Psychol: Sci Pract 1, 71–83.

Linehan MM (1993) Cognitive–Behavioral Treatment of Borderline Personality Disorder. Guilford Press, New York.

Linehan MM (2000) The empirical basis of dialectical behavior therapy: Development of new treatments vs. evaluation of existing treatments. Clin Psychol: Sci Pract 7, 113–119.

Links PS, Heslegrave R, and van Reekum R (1998) Prospective follow-up study of borderline personality disorder: Prognosis, prediction of outcome, and Axis II comorbidity. Can J Psychiatr 43, 265–270.

Livesley WJ (1998) Suggestions for a framework for an empirically based classification of personality disorder. Can J Psychiatr 43, 137–147.

Livesley WJ (ed) (2001) Handbook of Personality Disorders. Guilford Press, New York.

Loranger AW (1990) The impact of DSM-III on diagnostic practice in a university hospital. Arch Gen Psychiatr 47, 672–675.

Loranger AW (1999) International Personality Disorder Examination (IPDE). Psychological Assessment Resources, Odessa, Florida.

Lynam DR (1996) The early identification of chronic offenders: Who is the fledgling psychopath? Psychol Bull 120, 209–234.

Maier W, Lichtermann D, Klinger T, et al. (1992) Prevalences of personality disorders (DSM-III-R) in the community. J Pers Disord 6, 187–196.

Markovitz P (2001) Pharmacotherapy. In Handbook of Personality Disorders, Livesley WJ (ed). Guilford Press, New York, pp. 475–493.

Mattia JI and Zimmerman M (2001) Epidemiology. In Handbook of Personality Disorders, Livesley WJ (ed). Guilford Press, New York, pp. 107–123.

McCann J (1988) Passive–aggressive personality: A review. J Pers Dis 2, 170–179.

Miller MB, Useda JD, Trull TJ, et al. (2001) Paranoid, schizoid, and schizotypal personality disorders. In Comprehensive Handbook of Psychopathology, 3rd ed., Adams HE and Sutker PB (eds). Kluwer Academic/Plenum Publishers, New York, pp. 535–558.

Millon T (1993) Negativistic (passive–aggressive) personality disorder. J Pers Disord 7, 78–85.

Millon T, Davis RD, Millon CM, et al. (1996) Disorders of Personality. DSM-IV and Beyond. John Wiley, New York.

Moldin SO, Rice JP, Erlenmeyer-Kimling L et al. (1994) Latent structure of DSM-III-R Axis II psychopathology in a normal sample. J Abnorm Psychol 103, 259–266.

Moffitt TE (1993) Adolescence limited and life-course persistent antisocial behavior: A developmental taxonomy. Psychol Rev 100, 674–701.

Moffitt TE, Caspi A, Dickson N, et al. (1996) Childhood-onset versus adolescent onset antisocial conduct problems in males: Natural history from ages 3 to 18 years. Dev Psychopathol 8, 399–424.

Morey LC and Zanarini MC (2000) Borderline personality: Traits and disorder. J Abnorm Psychol 109, 733–737.

Myers MG, Stewart DG, and Brown SA (1998) Progression from conduct disorder to antisocial personality disorder following treatment for adolescent substance abuse. Am J Psychiatr 155, 479–485.

Nestadt G, Romanoski AJ, Brown CH, et al. (1991) DSM-III compulsive personality disorder: An epidemiological survey. Psychol Med 21, 461–471.

Newman JP and Wallace JF (1993) Psychopathy and cognition. In Psychopathology and Cognition, Kendall PC and Dobson KS (eds). Academic Press, New York, pp. 293–349.

Nigg JT and Goldsmith HH (1994) Genetics of personality disorders: Perspectives from personality and psychopathology research. Psychol Bull 115, 346–380.

Oldham JM and Frosch WA (1991) Compulsive personality disorder. In Psychiatry, Vol. 1, Ch. 22, Michels R (ed). JB Lippincott, Philadelphia, PA, pp. 1–8.

Oldham JM and Skodol AE (2000) Charting the future of Axis II. J Pers Disord 14, 17–29.

Oldham JM, Skodol AE, Kellman HD, et al. (1992) Diagnosis of DSM-III-R personality disorders by two semistructured interviews: Patterns of comorbidity. Am J Psychiatr 149, 213–220.

O'Neill FA and Kendler KS (1998) Longitudinal study of interpersonal dependency in female twins. Br J Psychiatr 172, 154–158.

Ornduff SR (2000) Childhood maltreatment and malevolence: Quantitative research findings. Clin Psychol Rev 20, 991–1018.

Overholser JC (1996) The dependent personality and interpersonal problems. J Nerv Ment Dis 184, 8–16.

Paris J (1998) Working with Traits: Psychotherapy of Personality Disorders. Jason Aronson, Northvale, New Jersey.

Perry JC, Banon E, and Ianni F (1999) Effectiveness of psychotherapy for personality disorders. Am J Psychiatr 156, 1312–1321.

Pervin LA and John OP (eds) (1999) Handbook of Personality. Theory and Research, 2nd ed. Guilford Press, New York.

Pfohl B and Blum N (1991) Obsessive–compulsive personality disorder: A review of available data and recommendations for DSM-IV. J Pers Disord 5, 363–375.

Pfohl B, Blum N, and Zimmerman M (1997) Structured Interview for DSM-IV Personality Disorder. American Psychiatric Press, Washington DC.

Phillips KA, Gunderson JG, Triebwasser J, et al. (1998) Reliability and validity of depressive personality disorder. Am J Psychiatr 155, 1044–1048.

Phillips KA, Hirschfeld RMA, Shea MT, et al. (1995) Depressive personality disorder. In The DSM-IV Personality Disorders, Livesley WJ (ed). Guilford Press, New York, pp. 287–302.

Pincus AL and Wilson KR (2001) Interpersonal variability in dependent personality. J Pers 69, 223–252.

Plomin R and Caspi A (1999) Behavioral genetics and personality. In Handbook of Personality, 2nd ed., Pervin L and John O (eds). Guilford Press, New York, pp. 251–276.

Raine A, Benishay D, Lencz T, et al. (1997) Abnormal orienting in schizotypal personality disorder. Schizophr Bull 23, 75–82.

Raine A, Lencz T, and Mednick SA (eds) (1995) Schizotypal Personality. Cambridge University Press, New York.

Raine A, Reynolds C, Venables PH, et al. (1998) Fearlessness, stimulus-seeking, and large body size at age 3 as early predispositions to childhood aggression at age 11 years. Arch Gen Psychiatr 55, 745–751.

Raine A, Venables PH, and Williams M (1995) High autonomic arousal and electrodermal orienting at age 15 years as protective factors against criminal behavior at age 29 years. Am J Psychiatr 152, 1595–1600.

Raskin R, Novacek J, and Hogan R (1991) Narcissistic self-esteem management. J Pers Soc Psychol 60, 911–918.

Rhodewalt F and Morf CC (1995) Self and interpersonal correlates of the narcissistic personality inventory: A review and new findings. J Res Pers 29, 1–23.

Rhodewalt F, Madrian JC, and Cheney S (1998) Narcissism, self-knowledge, organization, and emotional reactivity: The effect of daily experience on self-esteem and affect. Pers Soc Psychol Bull 24, 75–87.

Robins CJ, Hayes AH, Block P, et al. (1995) Interpersonal and achievement concerns and the depressive vulnerability and symptom specificity hypothesis: A prospective study. Cogn Ther Res 19, 1–20.

Robins LN, Tipp J, and Przybeck T (1991) Antisocial personality. In Psychiatric Disorders in America, Robins LN and Regier DA (eds). The Free Press, New York, pp. 258–290.

Roitman SE, Cornblatt BA, Bergman A, et al. (1997) Attentional functioning in schizotypal personality disorder. Am J Psychiatr 154, 655–660.

Ronningstam E and Gunderson JG (1990) Identifying criteria for narcissistic personality disorder. Am J Psychiatr 147, 918–922.

Rothbart MK and Ahadi SA (1994) Temperament and the development of personality. J Abnor Psychol 103, 55–66.

Ryder AG and Bagby RM (1999) Diagnostic viability of depressive personality disorder: Theoretical and conceptual issues. J Pers Disord 13, 99–117.

Salekin RT (2002) Psychopathy and therapeutic pessimism. Clinical lore or clinical reality? Clin Psychol Rev 22, 79–112.

Samuels JF, Nestadt G, Romanoski AJ, et al. (1994) DSM-III personality disorders in the community. Am J Psychiatr 151, 1055–1062.

Sanislow CA and McGlashan TH (1998) Treatment outcome of personality disorders. Can J Psychiatr 43, 237–250.

Schmidt LA, Polak CP, and Spooner AL (2001) Biological and environmental contributions to childhood shyness: A diathesis-stress model. In International Handbook of Social Anxiety, Crozier WR and Alden LE (eds). John Wiley, New York, pp. 29–52.

Sher KJ and Trull TJ (1994) Personality and disinhibitory psychopathology: Alcoholism and antisocial personality disorder. J Abnorm Psychol 103, 92–102.

Siever LJ (1992) Schizophrenia spectrum disorders. In Review of Psychiatry, Vol. XI, Tasman A and Riba MB (eds). American Psychiatric Press, Washington DC, pp. 25–42.

Siever LJ and Davis KL (1991) A psychobiological perspective on the personality disorders. Am J Psychiatr 148, 1647–1658.

Silk KR (2000) Borderline personality disorder. Overview of biologic factors. Psychiatr Clin N Am 23, 61–75.

Soloff PH (2000) Psychopharmacology of borderline personality disorder. Psychiatr Clin N Am 23, 169–192.

Spitzer RL, Williams JBW, and Skodol AE (1980) DSM-III: The major achievements and an overview. Am J Psychiatr 137, 151–164.

Sprock J, Blashfield RK, and Smith B (1990) Gender weighting of DSM-III-R personality disorder criteria. Am J Psychiatr 147, 586–590.

Squires-Wheeler E, Friedman D, Amminger GP, et al. (1997) Negative and positive dimensions of schizotypal personality disorder. J Pers Disord 11, 285–300.

Stoff DM, Breiling J, and Maser JD (eds) (1997) Handbook of Antisocial Behavior. John Wiley, New York.

Stone MH (1993) Abnormalities of Personality. Within and Beyond the Realm of Treatment. WW Norton, New York.

Stone MH (2000) Clinical guidelines for psychotherapy with borderline personality disorder. Psychiatr Clin N Am 23, 193–210.

Stone MH (2001) Natural history and long-term outcome. In Handbook of Personality Disorders, Livesley WJ (ed). Guilford Press, New York, pp. 259–273.

Sutker PB and Allain AN (2001) Antisocial personality disorder. In Comprehensive Handbook of Psychopathology, 3rd ed., Sutker PB and Adams HE (eds). Kluwer Academic/Plenum Publishers, New York, pp. 445–490.

Thompson S and Zuroff DC (1998) Dependent and self-critical mothers' responses to adolescent autonomy and competence. Pers Indiv Diff 24, 311–324.

Tillfors M, Furmark T, Ekselius L, et al. (2001) Social phobia and avoidant personality disorder as related to parental history of social anxiety: A general population study. Behav Res Ther 39, 289–298.

Torgersen S (2000) Genetics of patients with borderline personality disorder. Psychiatr Clin N Am 23, 1–9.

Torgersen S, Kringlen E, and Cramer V (2001) The prevalence of personality disorders in a community sample. Arch Gen Psychiatr 58, 590–596.

Trull TJ, Widiger TA, Useda JD, et al. (1998) A structured interview for the assessment of the five-factor model of personality. Psychol Assess 10, 229–240.

van Velzen CJ, Emmelkamp PM, and Scholing A (2000) Generalized social phobia versus avoidant personality disorder: Differences in psychopathology, personality traits, and social and occupational functioning. J Anx Disord 14, 395–411.

Ward CH, Beck AT, Mendelson M, et al. (1962) The psychiatric nomenclature. Reasons for diagnostic disagreement. Arch Gen Psychiatr 7, 198–205.

Westen D (1997) Divergences between clinical and research methods for assessing personality disorders: Implications for research and the evolution of Axis II. Am J Psychiatr 154, 895–903.

Wetzler S and Morey LC (1999) Passive–aggressive personality disorder: The demise of a syndrome. Psychiatry 62, 49–59.

Widiger TA (1998) Sex biases in the diagnosis of personality disorders. J Pers Disord 12, 95–118.

Widiger TA (1999) Depressive personality traits and dysthymia: A commentary on Ryder and Bagby. J Pers Disord 13, 135–141.

Widiger TA (2000) Personality disorders in the 21st century. J Pers Disord 14, 3–16.

Widiger TA (2001) Social anxiety, social phobia, and avoidant personality disorder. In International Handbook of Social Anxiety, Crozier WR and Alden L (eds). John Wiley, New York, pp. 335–356.

Widiger TA and Coker LA (2002) Assessing personality disorders. In Clinical Personality Assessment: Practical Approaches, 2nd ed., Butcher JN (ed). Oxford University Press, New York, pp. 407–434.

Widiger TA and Corbitt EM (1995) Antisocial personality disorder in DSM-IV. In The DSM-IV Personality Disorders, Livesley WJ (ed). Guilford Press, New York, pp. 103–126.

Widiger TA and Lynam DR (1998) Psychopathy from the perspective of the five-factor model of personality. In Psychopathy: Antisocial, Criminal, and Violent Behaviors, Millon T, Simonsen E, Birket-Smith M, et al. (eds). Guilford Press, New York, pp. 171–187.

Widiger TA and Sankis L (2000) Adult psychopathology: Issues and controversies. Annu Rev Psychol 51, 377–404.

Widiger TA and Trull TJ (1998) Performance characteristics of the DSM-III-R personality disorder criteria sets. In DSM-IV Sourcebook, Vol. 4, Widiger TA, Frances AJ, Pincus HA, et al. (eds). American Psychiatric Association, Washington DC, pp. 357–373.

Widiger TA, Cadoret R, Hare R, et al. (1996) DSM-IV antisocial personality disorder field trial. J Abnorm Psychol 105, 3–16.

Widiger TA, Frances AJ, Spitzer RL et al. (1988) The DSM-III-R personality disorders: An overview. Am J Psychiatr 145, 786–795.

Widiger TA, Mangine S, Corbitt EM, et al. (1995) The Personality Disorder Interview—IV: A Semistructured Interview for the Diagnosis of Personality Disorders. Psychological Assessment Resources, Odessa, Florida.

Widiger TA, Trull TJ, Clarkin JF, et al. (2002) A description of the DSM-IV personality disorders with the five-factor model of personality. In Personality Disorders and the Five-Factor Model of Personality, 2nd ed., Costa PT and Widiger TA (eds). American Psychological Association, Washington DC, pp. 89–99.

Widiger TA, Verheul R, and van den Brink W (1999) Personality and psychopathology. In Handbook of Personality, 2nd ed., Pervin L and John O (eds). Guilford Press, New York, pp. 347–366.

World Health Organization (1992) The ICD-10 Classification of Mental and Behavioural Disorders. Clinical Descriptions and Diagnostic Guidelines. World Health Organization, Geneva.

Zanarini MC (2000) Childhood experiences associated with the development of borderline personality disorder. Psychiatr Clin N Am 23, 89–101.

Zanarini MC, Frankenburg FR, Dubo ED, et al. (1998a) Axis I comorbidity of borderline personality disorder. Am J Psychiatr 155, 1733–1739.

Zanarini MC, Frankenburg FR, Dubo ED, et al. (1998b) Axis II comorbidity of borderline personality disorder. Compre Psychiatr 39.

Zanarini MC, Frankenburg FR, Sickel AE, et al. (1995) Diagnostic Interview for DSM-IV Personality Disorders (DIPD-IV). McLean Hospital, Boston, MA.

Zanarini MC, Gunderson JG, Frankenburg FR, et al. (1989) The Revised Diagnostic Interview for Borderlines: Discriminating BPD from other Axis II disorders. J Pers Disord 3, 10–18.

Zanarini MC, Williams AA, Lewis RE, et al. (1997) Reported childhood experiences associated with the development of borderline personality disorder. Am J Psychiatr 154, 1101–1106.

Zimmerman M (1994) Diagnosing personality disorders. A review of issues and research methods. Arch Gen Psychiatr 51, 225–245.

Zimmerman M and Mattia JI (1999) Differences between clinical and research practices in diagnosing borderline personality disorder. Am J Psychiatr 156, 1570–1574.

# 80 Psychological Factors Affecting Medical Condition

James L. Levenson

Psychological Factors Affecting Physical Condition
Psychological Factors Affecting Medical Condition

## Definition

This diagnostic category recognizes the variety of ways in which specific psychological or behavioral factors can adversely affect medical illnesses. Such factors may contribute to the initiation or the exacerbation of the illness, interfere with treatment and rehabilitation, or contribute to morbidity and mortality. Psychological factors may themselves constitute risks for medical diseases, or they may magnify the effects of nonpsychological risk factors. The effects may be mediated directly at a pathophysiological level (e.g., psychological stress inducing myocardial ischemia) or through the patient's behavior (e.g., noncompliance).

The criteria in the *Diagnostic and Statistical Manual of Mental Disorders*, Third Edition, Revised (DSM-III-R) for this diagnosis were brief and emphasized the temporal relationship of psychological factors to the initiation or exacerbation of the medical condition (DSM-III-R, B). The criteria in the *Diagnostic and Statistical Manual of Mental Disorders*, Fourth Edition (DSM-IV) were expanded in two ways. The overall category was expanded to include situations in which psychological factors interfered with medical treatment, posed health risks, or caused stress-related pathophysiological changes. This diagnosis was also structured in DSM-IV so that both the psychological factor and the general medical condition are to be specified. The psychological factor can be an Axis I or Axis II mental disorder (e.g., major depressive disorder aggravating coronary artery disease), a psychological symptom (e.g., anxiety exacerbating asthma), a personality trait or coping style (e.g., type A behavior contributing to the development of coronary artery disease), maladaptive health behaviors (e.g., unsafe sex in a person with human immunodeficiency virus [HIV] infection), a stress-related physiological response (e.g., tension headache), or other unspecified psychological factors. The medical condition is noted on Axis III. The expansion and elaboration of diagnostic criteria in DSM-IV were based on an extensive review of the literature by a DSM-IV work group organized by organ system and medical specialty categories. Their work has been published and is a source of more detail for the interested reader (Stoudemire et al. 1996, Stoudemire 1995).

The subject of psychological factors affecting medical condition (PFAMC) has become the focus of intense research because of the illumination it may provide of basic disease mechanisms (e.g., psychoneuroimmunology) and because of the deep interest in improving both the outcomes and the efficiency of health care delivery. In epidemiological studies, several psychiatric disorders increase the likelihood of mortality (Bruce et al. 1994), especially depression, bipolar disorder, schizophrenia, and alcohol abuse or dependence. Psychiatric disorders or symptoms in patients with medical illness may increase their use of health care services, particularly the length of costly hospital stays. (Levenson et al. 1990b, Saravay and Lavin 1994, Strain et al. 1994,

---

### DSM-III-R Criteria 316

**Psychological Factors Affecting Physical Condition**

A. Psychologically meaningful environmental stimuli are temporally related to the initiation or exacerbation of a specific physical condition or disorder (recorded on Axis III).

B. The physical condition involves either demonstrable organic pathology (e.g., rheumatoid arthritis) or a known pathophysiological process (e.g., migraine headache).

C. The condition does not meet the criteria for a somatoform disorder.

**Psychological Factors Affecting Medical Condition**

A. A general medical condition (coded on Axis III) is present.

B. Psychological factors adversely affect the general medical condition in one of the following ways:

    (1) the factors have influenced the course of the general medical condition as shown by a close temporal association between the psychological factors and the development or exacerbation of, or delayed recovery from, the general medical condition

    (2) the factors interfere with the treatment of the general medical condition

    (3) the factors constitute additional health risks for the individual

    (4) stress-related physiological responses precipitate or exacerbate symptoms of the general medical condition

*Choose* name based on the nature of the psychological factors (if more than one factor is present, indicate the most prominent):

**Mental disorder affecting... [indicate the general medical condition]** (e.g., an Axis I disorder such as major depressive disorder delaying recovery from a myocardial infarction)

**Psychological symptoms affecting... [indicate the general medical condition]** (e.g., depressive symptoms delaying recovery from surgery; anxiety exacerbating asthma)

**Personality traits or coping style affecting... [indicate the general medical condition]** (e.g., pathological denial of the need for surgery in a patient with cancer; hostile, pressured behavior contributing to cardiovascular disease)

**Maladaptive health behaviors affecting... [indicate the general medical condition]** (e.g., overeating; lack of exercise; unsafe sex)

**Stress-related physiological response affecting... [indicate the general medical condition]** (e.g., stress-related exacerbations of ulcer, hypertension, arrhythmia, or tension headache)

**Other or unspecified psychological factors affecting... [indicate the general medical condition]** (e.g., interpersonal, cultural, or religious factors)

Reprinted with permission from the Diagnostic and Statistical Manual of Mental Disorders, Fourth Edition, Text Revision. Copyright 2000 American Psychiatric Association.

Deykin et al. 2001). Interest has been further increased by intervention trials aimed at psychological factors or disorders that have demonstrated improvements in medical outcomes and in quality of life in patients with serious medical disorders.

It should be evident that this diagnosis is not really a discrete diagnostic category but rather a label for the interactive effects of psyche on soma. Mind–body interactions have long been a focus of interest, both in health and in disease. Psychiatric illness and medical disease frequently coexist. Psychiatrists and investigators of past eras were misled by this frequent comorbidity into premature conclusions that the psychological factors were preeminent in the causation of the medical disorders, and these were designated psychosomatic (Alexander 1950). A more modern approach has been to recognize that all medical illnesses are potentially affected by many different factors in the biological, psychological, and social realms. The earlier designation of certain disorders as psychosomatic (e.g., peptic ulcer disease) overvalued the contribution of psychological factors to those disorders and undervalued their contribution to other medical disorders (e.g., cancer). Furthermore, whereas labeling medical illnesses as psychosomatic drew attention to the importance of mind–body interactions, it unfortunately and falsely implied to many patients and physicians that the illness was basically psychogenic, that the symptoms were not "real," and that the illness was somehow the patient's fault.

The diagnosis of PFAMC focuses attention on one causal direction in the interactions between psyche and soma, that is, the effects of psychological factors on the medical condition (Figure 80–1). This represents a heuristic simplification, highlighting a particular process for further exploration, understanding, and intervention. In most patients, there are effects in the other direction as well (i.e., the effects of general medical illness on psychological function). Furthermore, both mind and body interact with social and environmental factors both dramatic (e.g., poverty, racism, war) and more subtle (e.g., employment status, neighborhood) (Roux et al. 2001), that affect the incidence and outcome of medical illness. Diagnosing PFAMC may help psychiatrist and patient address an important dimension of care, but the other "arrows" of Figure 80–1 often warrant attention too.

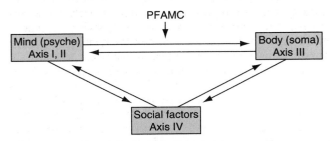

**Figure 80–1** *Psychological factors affecting medical condition (PFAMC): Interaction between psyche and soma. Social factors warrant attention as well.*

## Etiology and Pathophysiology

How do psychological factors affect medical illnesses? Physicians have long recognized that psychological factors seem to affect medical illnesses, and research elucidating the intervening causal mechanisms is now rapidly growing. From their clinical experience, physicians recognize many ways in which psychological factors affect the onset, progression, and outcome of their patients' illnesses. First, psychological factors may promote other known risks for medical illness. Smoking is a risk factor for heart disease, cancer, and pulmonary and many other diseases, and individuals with schizophrenia or depression are much more likely to smoke than the general population. A wide variety of psychiatric illnesses are associated with an increased likelihood of abuse of other substances. Depression and schizophrenia also are associated with a sedentary lifestyle. Patients with affective disorders often have chronic pain and chronically tend to overuse analgesics. Individuals with schizophrenia, bipolar disorder, and some personality disorders are more likely to engage in unsafe sex, which in turn increases the risk of sexually transmitted diseases, including HIV infection and hepatitis B. Depression, eating disorders, and other emotional and behavioral factors affect the pattern and content of diet.

In addition to promoting known risk factors for medical illness, psychological factors also have an impact on the course of illness by influencing how patients respond to their symptoms, including whether and how they seek care. For example, the defense mechanism of denial may lead an individual to ignore anginal chest pain, attribute it to indigestion, delay seeking medical attention, or minimize the pain when describing it to a physician. This tends to result in treatment delay after the acute onset of coronary symptoms, with consequently greater morbidity and mortality. Anxiety is also a common cause of avoidance or delay of health care; phobic fears of needles, sight of blood, surgery, and other health care phobias are common (Noyes et al. 2000). Patients may also neglect their symptoms and fail to promptly seek medical care because of depression, psychosis, or personality traits (e.g., procrastination).

Psychological factors also affect the course of illness through their effects on the physician–patient relationship, since they influence both patients' health behaviors and physicians' diagnostic and treatment decisions. A substantial proportion of the excess mortality experienced by individuals with mental disorders is explained by their receiving poorer quality medical care (Druss et al. 2001a). One explanation for the poorer quality and outcomes of medical care in patients with both serious medical and mental illnesses is the lack of integration between their medical and mental health care (Druss et al. 2001b). Psychological factors can also reduce a patient's compliance with diagnostic recommendations, treatment, and lifestyle change, and can interfere with rehabilitation through impairment of motivation, understanding, optimism, or tolerance. A recent meta-analysis found that patients with depression are three times as likely to be noncompliant with medical treatment than patients without (DiMatteo et al. 2000). In addition, many of the effects of psychological factors on medical illness appear to be mediated through a wide array of social factors, including social support, job strain, disadvantaged socioeconomic and educational status, and marital stress.

There is an increasing body of scientific evidence that psychological factors, in addition to their impact on classic (nonpsychological) risk factors, patient behaviors, and the physician–patient interaction, have direct effects on pathophysiological processes. For example, stress has been experimentally shown to cause myocardial ischemia in patients with coronary disease. Stress and depression are associated with a wide range of immunological effects (Irwin 1999, Yang and Glaser 2000). Many psychiatric disorders (especially mood disorders) are associated with disruptions in homeostasis including sleep architecture, other circadian rhythms, and endocrine secretion and feedback. For example, depression causes increased bone remodeling and decreased bone density (Herran et al. 2000). That such effects occur is well established, but the magnitude of their clinical significance in medical disease is often unclear, and full explanatory causal linkages have for the most part not been demonstrated yet. Nevertheless, investigators have learned a great deal about changes in autonomic, hematologic, endocrine, immunologic, and sensory function, as well as gene expression that bring us closer to understanding how psychological factors may affect medical illness. These issues of pathophysiology are discussed later in this chapter for each organ system or specialty category.

## Assessment and Diagnosis

The diagnosis of PFAMC differs from most other psychiatric diagnoses in its focus on the interaction between the mental and medical realms. As noted, the criteria require more than that the patient have both a medical illness and contemporaneous psychological factors, because their coexistence does not always include significant interactions between them. To make the diagnosis of PFAMC, either the factors must have influenced the course of the medical condition, interfered with its treatment, contributed to health risks, or physiologically aggravated the medical condition.

Let us consider each of these four ways of making the diagnosis of PFAMC in more detail. The psychological factor's influence on the course of a general medical condition can be inferred from a close temporal relationship between the factor and the development or exacerbation of the medical condition (or delayed recovery). For example, a 45-year-old male executive reports symptoms sounding like typical angina, but occurring only on weekends. Further questioning reveals that he is depressed over deterioration in his marriage. During the week he works late and has limited contact with his family but he spends the weekend at home. The symptoms began after he and his wife started arguing every weekend. The temporal link between onset and recurrence of angina and marital arguments supports a diagnosis of PFAMC.

PFAMC can also be diagnosed when the psychological factor interferes with treatment including not seeking medical care, not following up, nonadherence to prescribed drugs or other treatment, or maladaptive modifications in treatment made by the patient or family. The executive with angina rejected his physician's recommendations for further assessment and treatment. He said, "I do get upset at home but I feel just fine at the office, so there couldn't be anything really wrong with me." The patient is able to acknowledge marital discord, but the defense of denial clouds his perception of his physical health and blocks appropriate medical care. This is another form of PFAMC.

PFAMC can also be diagnosed when the psychological factor contributes to health risks, exemplified by the executive increasing his smoking and drinking despite his physician's warnings. ("Its the only way I can cope with my wife.") Finally, PFAMC is an appropriate diagnosis when there are stress-related physiological responses precipitating or exacerbating symptoms of the medical condition. The same man observes that angina is most likely to occur after marital arguments during which he becomes irate, yells, slams doors, and throws things.

When a patient's medical illness is faring worse than expected and not responding well to standard treatment, physicians should and often do consider whether a psychological factor may be responsible for the poorer than expected outcome. This is a far from trivial task. To ignore the possibility of PFAMC may miss the crucial barrier to the patient's recovery. On the other hand, premature or facile attribution to psychological factors may lead the physician to overlook medical or social explanations for "treatment-resistant disease" and unfairly blame the patient, with resultant further deterioration in health outcomes and the physician–patient relationship.

To illustrate, a common clinical problem is the brittle diabetic adolescent with labile blood glucose levels and frequent episodes of ketoacidosis and hypoglycemia, despite vigorous attempts by the physician to improve diabetic management and glucose control. The considerable difficulty in controlling such patients' diabetes is often attributed to adolescents' dislike of lifestyle restrictions, their tendency to act out and rebel against authority figures, their denial of vulnerability, their ambivalence about their need for nurturance, and their wish to be "normal." There are many adolescent (and some adult) diabetic patients for whom these psychological issues do play an important role in undermining diabetes management through noncompliance regarding medication, diet, visits to the physician, substance use, and activity limitations. However, psychological factors do not always account for brittleness and are sometimes incorrectly suspected. It has been demonstrated that much of the difficulty in achieving stable glucose control in adolescent diabetics is the result of the dramatically labile patterns of hormone secretion (cortisol, growth hormone) typical of adolescence, independent of psychological status.

PFAMC has descriptive names for subcategories described as follows:

## Mental Disorder Affecting a General Medical Condition

If the patient has a mental disorder meeting criteria for an Axis I or Axis II diagnosis, the diagnostic name is mental disorder affecting medical condition, with the particular medical condition specified. In addition to coding PFAMC, the specific mental disorder is also coded on Axis I or Axis II. Examples include major depressive disorder that reduces energy and compliance in a hemodialysis patient; panic disorder that makes an asthmatic patient hypersensitive to

dyspnea; and schizophrenia in a patient with recurrent ventricular tachycardia who refuses placement of an automatic implantable defibrillator because he fears it will control his mind.

## Psychological Symptoms Affecting a General Medical Condition

Patients who have psychological symptoms that do not meet the threshold for an Axis I diagnosis may still experience important effects on their medical illness, and the diagnosis would be psychological symptoms affecting a medical condition. Examples include anxiety that aggravates irritable bowel syndrome; depressed mood that hinders recovery from hip replacement surgery; and anger that interferes with rehabilitation after spinal cord injury.

## Personality Traits or Coping Style Affecting a General Medical Condition

This may include personality traits or coping styles that do not meet criteria for an Axis II disorder and other patterns of response considered to be maladaptive because they may pose a risk for particular medical illnesses. An example is the competitive hostility component of the type A behavior pattern, and its impact on coronary artery disease. Maladaptive personality traits or coping styles are particularly likely to interfere with the physician–patient relationship as well as the patient's relationships with other caregivers.

## Maladaptive Health Behaviors Affecting a General Medical Condition

Many maladaptive health behaviors have significant effects on the course and treatment of many medical conditions. Examples include sedentary lifestyle, smoking, abuse of alcohol or other substances, and unsafe sexual practices. If the maladaptive behaviors can be better accounted for by an Axis I or Axis II disorder, the first subcategory (mental disorder affecting a medical condition) should be used instead.

## Stress-Related Physiological Response Affecting a General Medical Condition

Examples of stress-related physiological responses affecting a medical condition include the precipitation by psychological stress of angina, cardiac arrhythmia, migraine, or attack of colitis in medically vulnerable individuals. In such cases, stress is not the cause of the illness or symptoms; the patient has a medical condition that etiologically accounts for the symptoms (e.g., coronary artery disease, migraine, or ulcerative colitis), and the stressor instead represents a precipitating or aggravating factor.

## Other or Unspecified Psychological Factors Affecting a General Medical Condition

There are other psychological phenomena that may not fit within one of these subcategories. An interpersonal example is marital dysfunction. A cultural example is the extreme discomfort women from some cultures may experience being alone with a male physician, even while they are fully dressed. A religious example is a Jehovah's Witness who ambivalently refuses blood transfusion. These fall under the residual category of other or unspecified psychological factors affecting a medical condition.

## Differential Diagnosis

As noted before, the close temporal association between psychiatric symptoms and a medical condition does not always reflect PFAMC. If the two are considered merely coincidental, then separate psychiatric and medical diagnoses should be made. In some cases of coincident psychiatric and medical illness, the mental symptoms are actually the result of the medical condition (i.e., the causality is in a direction opposite from that of PFAMC). When a medical condition is judged to be pathophysiologically causing the mental disorder (e.g., hypothyroidism causing depression), the correct diagnosis is the appropriate mental disorder due to a general medical condition (e.g., mood disorder due to hypothyroidism, with depressive features). In PFAMC, the psychological or behavioral factors are judged to precipitate or aggravate the medical condition.

Substance use disorders may adversely affect many medical conditions, and this can be described through PFAMC. However, in some patients, all of the psychiatric and medical symptoms are direct consequences of substance abuse, and it is usually parsimonious to use just the substance use disorder diagnosis. For example, a patient with delirium tremens after alcohol withdrawal would receive a diagnosis of alcohol withdrawal delirium, not PFAMC, but a patient with alcohol dependence who repeatedly missed hemodialysis treatments because of intoxication would receive diagnoses of alcohol dependence and PFAMC (mental disorder affecting end stage renal disease).

Patients with somatoform disorders (e.g., somatization disorder, hypochondriasis) present with physical complaints which may mimic a medical illness, but the somatic symptoms are actually accounted for by the psychiatric disorder. In principle, it might seem that somatoform disorders are easily distinguished from PFAMC, because PFAMC requires the presence of a diagnosable medical condition. The distinction in practice is sometimes difficult because the patient may have both a somatoform disorder and one or more medical disorders. For example, a patient with seizures regularly precipitated by emotional stress might have true epilepsy aggravated by stress (PFAMC), pseudoseizures (conversion disorder), or both.

## Epidemiology and Comorbidity

Because this diagnosis describes a variety of possible interactions between the full range of psychiatric disorders (as well as symptoms and behaviors) on the one hand and the complete range of medical diseases on the other, it is impossible to estimate overall rates of prevalence or incidence. We can start, however, by noting how frequently medical and psychiatric disorders coexist. Psychiatric problems are common in medical patients, although the measured frequency varies, depending on the criteria and method of measurement used. A reasonable estimate is that 25 to 30% of medical outpatients and 40 to 50% of general medical inpatients have diagnosable psychiatric disorders (Table 80–1). Most common in medical outpatients are depression, anxiety, and substance abuse; medical inpatients most often have cognitive impairment (delirium, dementia), depression, and substance abuse. Depression, both as a diagnosis and as a symptom has been better studied in the medically ill than any other psychiatric syndrome. Major depressive disorder occurs in 18 to 25% of patients

| Table 80–1 | Prevalence of Selected Psychiatric Disorders | | |
|---|---|---|---|
| Disorder | Community | Primary Care Patients | Medical Inpatients |
| All psychiatric disorders | 15–20% | 25–30% | 40–50% |
| Depression | | | |
| Depressive symptoms | 10–15% | 10–30% | 20–35% |
| Major depressive disorder | 2–4% | 5–10% | 5–25% |
| Anxiety | | | |
| Anxiety symptoms | 10–20% | 12–20% | 20–30% |
| Panic disorder | 1–2% | 2–15% | — |
| Cognitive disorders | | | |
| | 1% | — | 15–20% |
| | 5–10% | — | 30–50% |
| | (>65 yr) | | (>65 yr) |

*Source*: Levenson JL (1994) Common psychological reactions to medical illness and treatment. In Clinical Psychiatry for Medical Students, 2nd ed., Stoudemire A (ed). JB Lippincott, Philadelphia, pp. 580B–609.

with serious coronary disease, in 25% of those with cancer, and at three times the normal rate in diabetic patients. Individuals presenting with symptoms of chronic fatigue have a 50 to 75% lifetime prevalence of major depression (Wessely et al. 1998).

Nonpsychiatric physicians underdiagnose and undertreat psychiatric disorders in the medically ill. Medical disorders are also common in patients seen for mental health treatment, and mental health specialists often underrecognize the presence and significance of coexisting medical disorders. Regardless of whether the patient has come seeking medical care or mental health care, medical and psychiatric problems are often both present. Such coincidence by itself is not sufficient for the diagnosis of PFAMC. In some cases, the illnesses may coexist with little effect on each other; in other cases, the effects of the medical illness on the psychiatric condition may be more important. The diagnosis of PFAMC in DSM-IV is reserved for patients in whom psychological factors adversely affect a medical condition in a specifiable way.

## Course

Given the wide range of psychiatric disorders and psychological factors that may affect medical illness and the large number of different medical disorders that may be influenced, there are no general rules about the course of the PFAMC interaction. Psychological factors may have minor or major effects at a particular point or throughout the course of a medical illness. We do know in general that patients with medical disorders who also have significant psychological symptoms have poorer outcomes and higher medical care costs than those patients with the same medical disorders but without psychological distress. A number of studies now document that psychological or psychiatric problems (particularly cognitive disorder, depression, and anxiety) in general medical inpatients are associated with significant increases in length of hospital stay (Levenson et al. 1990b, Saravay and Lavin 1994, Stevens et al. 1998). Psychosocial interventions have been able to improve outcomes in medical illness, sometimes with an attendant savings in health care costs (Strain et al. 1994, Smith 1994, Katon and Gonzales 1994).

The impact of psychological factors on the course and natural history of medical disorders is discussed further in this chapter in the context of specific diseases.

## Treatment

Management of psychological factors affecting the patient's medical condition should be tailored both to the particular psychological factor of relevance and to the medical outcome of concern. Some general guidelines, however, can be helpful. The physician, whether in primary care or a specialty, should not ignore apparent psychiatric illness. Unfortunately, this occurs all too often because of discomfort, stigma, lack of training, or disinterest. Referring the patient to a mental health specialist for evaluation is certainly better than ignoring the psychological problem but should not be regarded as "disposing" of it, because the physician must still attend to its potential impact on the patient's medical illness. Similarly, psychiatrists and other mental health practitioners should not ignore coincident medical disease and should not assume that referral to a nonpsychiatric physician absolves them of all responsibility for the patient's medical problem.

## Mental Disorder Affecting a Medical Condition

If the patient has a treatable Axis I disorder, treatment for it should be provided. Whereas this is obviously justified on the basis of providing relief from the Axis I disorder, psychiatric treatment is further supported by the myriad ways in which the psychiatric disorder may currently or in future adversely affect the medical illness. The same psychopharmacological and psychotherapeutic treatments used for Axis I mental disorders are normally appropriate when an affected medical condition is also present. However, even well-established psychiatric treatments supported by randomized controlled trials have seldom been validated in the medically ill, who are typically excluded from the controlled trials. Thus, psychiatric treatments may not always be directly generalizable to, and often must be modified for, the medically ill.

When prescribing psychiatric medications for patients with significant medical comorbidity, the psychiatrist should keep in mind potential adverse effects on impaired organ systems (e.g., anticholinergic exacerbation of postoperative ileus; tricyclic antidepressant causing completion of heart block), changes in pharmacokinetics (absorption, protein binding, metabolism, and excretion), and drug–drug interactions. Psychotherapy may also require modification in patients with comorbid medical illness, including greater flexibility regarding the length and frequency of appointments, and deviations from standard therapeutic abstinence and neutrality. Psychotherapists treating patients with PFAMC should usually be much more active in communicating with other health care professionals caring for the patient (with the patient's consent) than is usually the case in psychotherapy.

If the patient has an Axis II personality disorder or other prominent personality or coping style, the psychiatrist should modify the patient's treatment accordingly, which is usually more easily accomplished than trying to change the patient's personality. For example, patients who tend to be paranoid or mistrustful should receive more careful explanations, particularly before invasive or anxiety-provoking procedures. With narcissistic patients, the psychiatrist should avoid relating in ways that may seem excessively paternalistic or authoritarian to the patient. With some dependent patients, it may be advisable to be more directive, without overdoing it and fostering excessive dependency.

## Psychological Symptoms Affecting a General Medical Condition

In some instances, psychiatric symptoms not meeting the threshold for an Axis I diagnosis will respond positively to the same treatments used for the analogous Axis I psychiatric disorder, with appropriate modifications as noted before. There is not a great amount of treatment research on subsyndromal psychiatric symptoms, and even less in patients with comorbid medical illness, so this area of practice remains less evidence-based. Some psychiatric symptoms affecting a medical condition may be amenable to stress management and other behavioral techniques as well as appropriate reassurance.

Any intervention directed by the psychiatrist at a particular patient's psychological symptoms or behavior should be grounded in exploratory discussion with the patient. Interventions without such grounding tend to seem at best superficial and artificial and at worst are entirely off the mark. For example, if the psychiatrist wrongly presumes to know why a particular patient seems anxious without asking, the patient is likely to feel misunderstood. Facile, nonspecific reassurance can undermine the physician–patient relationship because the patient is likely to feel that the psychiatrist is out of touch with and not really interested in the patient's experience. It is especially important with depressed patients that psychiatrists avoid premature or unrealistic reassurance or an overly cheerful attitude; this tends to alienate depressed patients, who feel that their psychiatrist is insensitive and either does not understand or does not want to hear about their sadness. Physicians *should* provide specific and realistic reassurance, emphasize on a constructive treatment plan, and mobilize the patient's support system.

## Personality Traits or Coping Style Affecting a General Medical Condition

As with Axis II disorders affecting a medical condition, psychiatrists should be aware of the personality style's effects on the physician–patient relationship and modify management to better fit the patient. For example, with type A "time urgent" patients, psychiatrists may need to be more sensitive to issues of appointment scheduling and waiting times. Group therapy interventions can enhance active coping with serious medical illnesses like cancer, heart disease, and renal failure but to date have usually been designed to be broadly generalizable rather than targeted to one particular trait or style (with the exception of type A behavior).

Another general guideline is not to attack or interfere with a patient's defensive style unless the defense is having an adverse impact on the medical illness or its management. Psychiatrists are particularly tempted to intervene when the defense is dramatic, breaks with reality, or makes the psychiatrist uncomfortable.

For example, denial is a defense mechanism that reduces anxiety and conflict by blocking conscious awareness of thoughts, feelings, or facts that an individual cannot face. Denial is common in the medically ill but varies in its timing, strength, and adaptive value. Some patients are aware of what is wrong with them but consciously suppress this knowledge by avoiding thinking about or discussing it. Others cope with the threat of being overwhelmed by their illness by unconsciously repressing it and thereby remain unaware of their illness. Marked denial, in which the patient emphatically refuses to accept the existence or significance of obvious symptoms and signs of the disease, may be seen by the psychiatrist as an indication that the patient is "crazy" because the patient seems impervious to rational persuasion. In the absence of signs of another major psychiatric disorder (e.g., paranoid delusions), such denial is not often a sign of psychosis but rather represents a defense against overwhelming fear.

The adaptive value of denial may vary, depending on the nature or stage of illness. When a patient's denial does not preclude cooperation with treatment, the psychiatrist should leave it alone. The psychiatrist does have an ethical and professional obligation to ensure that the patient has been informed about the illness and treatment. After that, if the patient accepts treatment but persists with an irrationally optimistic outlook, the psychiatrist should respect the patient's need to use denial to cope. For some, the denial is fragile, and the psychiatrist must decide whether the defense should be supported and strengthened, or if the patient had better give up the denial to discuss fears directly and receive reassurance from the psychiatrist. The psychiatrist should not support denial by giving the patient false information, but rather encourage hope and optimism. When denial is extreme, patients may refuse vital treatment or threaten to leave against medical advice. Here, the psychiatrist must try to help reduce denial but not by directly assaulting the patient's defenses. Because such desperate denial of reality usually reflects intense underlying anxiety, trying to scare the patient into cooperation will intensify denial and the impulse to flight. A better strategy for the psychiatrist is to avoid directly challenging the patient's claims while simultaneously reinforcing concern for the patient and maximizing the patient's sense of control.

## Maladaptive Health Behavior Affecting a General Medical Condition

This is an area of research with many promising approaches. To achieve smoking cessation, bupropion, nicotine replacement, behavioral therapies, and other pharmacological strategies all warrant consideration. Behavioral strategies are also useful in promoting better dietary practices, sleep hygiene, safe sex, and exercise. For some patients, change can be achieved efficiently through support groups, whereas others change more effectively through a one-to-one relationship with a health care professional.

## Stress-Related Physiological Response Affecting a Medical Condition

Biofeedback, relaxation techniques, hypnosis, and other stress management interventions have been helpful in reducing stress-induced exacerbations of medical illness including cardiac, gastrointestinal, headache, and other symptoms. Pharmacological interventions have also been useful (e.g., the widespread practice of prescribing benzodiazepines during acute myocardial infarction to prevent stress-induced increase in myocardial work).

## Psychological Factors in Specific Medical Disorders

In the remainder of this chapter, the effects of psychological factors on selected medical disorders are reviewed. The primary focus is on those effects for which there is reasonable evidence from controlled studies. Space considerations preclude inclusion of all valuable studies and all medical disorders.

Most of the early research suffers from serious methodological flaws, including use of small biased samples, limited or no statistical analysis, poor (if any) controls, and retrospective designs subject to recall and other biases (Levenson et al. 1990a). This early work generated excitement and interest in psychosomatic medicine but also produced ideas that in retrospect were intellectually appealing but erroneous and simplistic regarding the special designation of certain diseases as psychosomatic.

Later research has shown improvements in methodology, but problems in design and interpretation continue. Several studies that seem to show significant effects of psychological factors on medical disease are inconclusive because of nonequivalence in groups at baseline either in medical disease severity or in treatments received (many studies do not even monitor this possibility). Some studies fail to attend to important potential confounding factors such as smoking or diet. A number of studies measure too many psychological variables and then overly emphasize the few "discovered" positive associations in the published results. Failure to standardize measures of initial psychological factors and measures of medical outcome has also been frequent. Despite these and other critiques, a large and growing body of disease-specific research is illuminating the full range of PFAMC.

## Psychological Factors in Oncology

Many health professionals and lay people believe that psychological factors play a major role in cancer onset and progression. The media have promoted popular ideas of overcoming cancer through "mind over body." Enthusiasm for these optimistic theories and practices should be tempered by the recognition that scientific evidence clarifying the relationship between psychological factors and cancer lags far behind. Nevertheless, there is an exciting frontier of exploration of immune and endocrine mechanisms that may provide a pathophysiological basis for some PFAMC in cancer (Spiegel and Sephton 2001). In this section, aspects of PFAMC in oncology that have received support in the research literature are reviewed.

## Mental Disorders and Psychological Symptoms Affecting Cancer

The most active area of study has been the linking of affective states, particularly depression (as a symptom or as a disorder), with the onset and course of cancer. An early large epidemiological study of more than 2,000 employees of Western Electric reported that depressive symptoms were associated with a higher than normal frequency of cancer and twice as high a risk for death from cancer (Shekelle et al. 1981, Persky et al. 1987). Later epidemiological studies, however, have generally not found such associations (Vogt et al. 1994, Gallo et al. 2000). A meta-analysis of studies relating depression to later cancer development found a small statistically significant but clinically insignificant association (McGee et al. 1994). The interpretation of epidemiologic studies is complex with many methodological problems, discussed in detail elsewhere (Levenson and McDonald 2002).

Besides epidemiologic studies, other research has focused on the impact of affective states on outcome in cancer patients. Emotional distress may predict lower survival with lung cancer (Faller et al. 1999), as may anger in metastatic melanoma patients (Butow et al. 1999). Other studies have found positive, negative, or mixed associations between depression and mortality in cancer patients (Garssen and Goodkin 1999, Watson et al. 1999). Besides survival, depression in cancer patients may result in poorer pain control (Glover et al. 1995), poorer compliance (Ayres et al. 1994), and less desire for life-sustaining therapy (Lee and Ganzini 1992).

Bereavement has also been considered a possible risk factor. Whereas most studies have not supported this (Helsing and Szklo 1981), interest has been kindled by the finding that bereavement is associated with a decrement in immune function (Schleifer et al. 1983). Bereavement may result in reduction in natural killer-cell activity and changes in the ratios of T-cell subpopulations (Irwin et al. 1987), but the clinical significance of such findings remains uncertain. A meta-analysis of 46 studies found only a modest association between separation and loss experiences and development of breast cancer (McKenna et al. 1999). Bereavement (death of a son) after, but not before, diagnosis of cancer was associated with accelerated demise (Levav et al. 2000). However, neither cancer onset nor progression have been clearly shown to be influenced by bereavement.

## Personality Traits or Coping Style Affecting Cancer

A large body of literature has described cancer patients' degree of emotional expressiveness and its purported effect on prognosis. Descriptive case reports began appearing in the 1950s, noting shorter survival in patients with depressed, resigning characteristics compared with patients who were able to express more negative emotions such as anger. Using a variety of conceptualizations of the "expressive" versus "repressive" dichotomy, in an assortment of cancer types, several investigators have found reduced cancer risks in the more expressive subjects (Temoshok et al. 1985, Kune GA et al. 1991). Other clinical studies, again with varying definitions and study populations, have not supported an influence of this personality style

(Cassileth et al. 1985, Buddeberg et al. 1991). Epidemiological studies have not supported a relationship between emotional suppression and cancer occurrence or mortality (Shekelle et al. 1981, Ragland et al. 1987).

Breast cancer patients who demonstrated a "fighting spirit" or who used denial, were found to have a higher survival rate than those with stoic acceptance or expressed hopelessness and helplessness (Greer et al. 1979). Fighting spirit also was associated with longer survival after bone marrow transplantation for leukemia (Tschushke et al. 2001), but other outcome studies in cancer have found no association (Watson et al. 1999).

## Other Psychological Factors in Cancer

An enormous literature documents the adverse effects of maladaptive health behaviors as risk factors for the development of various cancers, especially smoking but also excessive alcohol use, unsafe sex, and dietary practices. Relatively less research has examined the effects of interpersonal variables on cancer, but there is some evidence that the quality of relationships may affect cancer onset and its course (Graves et al. 1991, Waxler-Morrison et al. 1991). Social relations and social support and their effects on cancer patients (as with other diseases) are complex phenomena and may vary with cancer site and extent of disease (Helgeson and Cohen 1996).

A number of human studies have shown an increased frequency of stressful life events preceding the onset of cervical, pancreatic, gastric, lung, colorectal, and breast cancer (Kune S et al. 1991, Geyer 1991). Some research has tentatively linked life stressors with cancer recurrence or progression, although not unequivocally (Ramirez et al. 1989). Many other studies have failed to find any association between preceding stressful life events and cancer onset, relapse, or progression (Giraldi et al. 1997, Maunsell et al. 2001). Recent studies have suggested that occupational stress might increase the risk of lung cancer (Jahn et al. 1995, Lynge and Anderson 1997) and colorectal cancer (Courtney et al. 1993).

## Psychosocial Intervention and Cancer Outcome

A number of studies have shown improvement in the quality of life in cancer patients receiving group therapy including improved mood and vigor, decreased pain, and better adjustment (Trijsburg et al. 1992, Anderson 1992, Fawzy et al. 1993, Spiegel et al. 1981, Goodwin et al. 2001). The possibility that cancer patients receiving psychotherapy might have increased survival time as well as improved quality of life has generated intense study, (Spiegel et al. 1989, Cunningham et al. 1998, Gellert et al. 1993, Goodwin et al. 2001) with more evidence showing improvement in pain control and mood than for increased survival.

# Psychological Factors in Cardiology

## Coronary Disease

One of the most studied examples of PFAMC is the type A behavior pattern and its relationship to coronary artery disease. Type A is a complex set of traits including impatience, hostility, intense achievement drive, and time urgency, among others. Strong epidemiological evidence appeared that type A behavior pattern was a risk factor for the development of coronary artery disease (Haynes et al. 1980, Rosenman et al. 1975). A possible mechanism is through premature atherosclerosis (Sparagon et al. 2001). However, the relationship between type A behavior pattern and coronary disease has come under serious question. Later epidemiological studies have not strongly supported type A behavior pattern as a coronary risk factor, and most angiographic studies have failed to find an association between type A behavior and the extent of coronary artery disease (Dimsdale 1988). The possibility that type A behavior pattern is nevertheless an important risk factor should be kept in mind, considering that the evidence for other risk factors (e.g., exercise or cholesterol) has often been ambiguous (Haynes and Matthews 1988). Whereas global type A behavior ratings are probably not reliable predictors of coronary artery disease outcome, the component behavior of hostility may be (Dembroski et al. 1989), although here too there are serious doubts (Marata et al. 1993, Myrtek 2001). A number of relatively small, short-term studies have demonstrated that type A behavior can be targeted for structured treatment and can possibly be modified (Levenkron and Moore 1988). Only one large randomized study has been reported, in which men were assigned after myocardial infarction to receive cardiac group counseling with or without type A counseling. The coronary artery disease recurrence rate was 7.2% in the group that received type A behavior counseling and 13% in the control subjects, with no difference in mortality (Friedman et al. 1986).

Although it has received less media attention than type A, the evidence that depression is a risk factor affecting both the onset and course of coronary artery disease is stronger than that for type A (Musselman et al. 1998, Glassman and Shapiro 1998). The weighting of depression as an independent risk factor in coronary artery disease has had to adjust for its interrelationships with other risk factors, especially smoking. Depression in coronary artery disease is associated with increased morbidity and mortality, which cannot be accounted for by other variables including severity of cardiac disease (Frasure-Smith et al. 1993, Ladwig et al. 1991, Ahern et al. 1990). Frasure-Smith and coworkers (1993) reported a fourfold increase in mortality 6 months after myocardial infarction in patients with major depression compared to those without depression. In a large epidemiologic study, major depression tripled the relative risk of cardiac mortality in those without heart disease, and quadrupled it in those who did have heart disease (Penninx et al. 2001). Depression is also associated with an increased risk for serious arrhythmia. The severity of depressive symptoms has more impact on disability than does the number of stenosed coronary arteries (Sullivan et al. 1997). Depression also reduces the return to work in patients with coronary artery disease (Ladwig et al. 1991).

While the mechanisms by which depression increases morbidity and mortality in coronary artery disease has not been firmly established, evidence is mounting regarding depression's adverse effects on heart rate variability (Carney et al. 2001), autonomic imbalance and arrhythmia (Carney et al. 1993, Roose et al. 1991), and platelet activation (Musselman et al. 2000, Markovitz et al.

2000). In coronary artery disease, depression also reduces functional capacity (Wells et al. 1989), amplifies somatic symptoms (especially pain) (Light et al. 1991), and reduces motivation and compliance with medication, lifestyle change, and cardiac rehabilitation (Ziegelstein et al. 2000, Carney et al. 1995). Multicenter intervention studies are currently under way to determine whether treatment of depression in coronary artery disease can improve medical as well as quality of life outcomes.

One specific mechanism by which psychological factors can affect coronary artery disease (CAD) has been demonstrated experimentally. Silent myocardial ischemia (ischemic changes on the electrocardiogram without symptoms of angina) can be precipitated by acute mental stress (Rozanski et al. 1988). Those who experience it are twice as likely to have major cardiac events compared to those who do not (Jiang et al. 1996). Silent ischemia may be partly a consequence of cognitive or defensive traits such as denial, hyposensitivity to somatic sensation, or systematic misperception of angina (Barsky et al. 1990). Psychological stress also changes the balance between procoagulation and fibrinolysis (von Kanel et al. 2001). Psychological factors may also affect outcome in CAD via differences in health care received. After myocardial infarction, patients with mental disorders are less likely to undergo cardiac catheterization and coronary revascularization than those without mental disorder (Druss et al. 2000).

Although the diagnosis and treatment of anxiety in patients with cardiac symptoms have received much attention, there has been less examination of anxiety as a risk factor affecting CAD. Increases in myocardial infarction and/or sudden death have been documented in epidemiologic studies of populations undergoing missile attacks, earthquakes, and other disasters (Leor et al. 1996, Krantz et al. 2000). A cohort study of 34,000 initially healthy men showed that phobic anxiety predicted deaths from CAD, although not nonfatal myocardial infarctions (MI) (Kawachi et al. 1994). Anxiety following MI may lead to more frequent readmission for unstable angina and more MI recurrences (Frasure-Smith et al. 1995), as well as higher mortality (Moser and Dracup 1996). Anxiety's adverse effects on CAD outcome may occur via effects on heart rate variability, QT prolongation, or other autonomically-mediated phenomena, like the stress-induced silent ischemia described above (Januzzi et al. 2000).

Denial is another common and significant psychological factor in patients with coronary disease. Denial may prevent individuals from acknowledging acute cardiac symptoms and promptly seeking medical care. The length of delay between the onset of symptoms of a myocardial infarction and hospitalization is a powerful predictor of morbidity and mortality, so denial at the onset of symptoms has an adverse impact on acute coronary disease. In contrast, denial *during* hospitalization may have adaptive value, perhaps even reducing morbidity and mortality (Levenson et al. 1989, Levine et al. 1990).

There are other psychological factors deserving of study. Women with severe marital stress have triple the risk of recurrent coronary events than those without marital stress (Orth-Gomer et al. 2000). Many studies have also examined maladaptive health behaviors as risk factors in coronary disease, with the effects of smoking better established than those of sedentary lifestyle, obesity, or specific diet. The effects of psychopathology and of smoking on heart disease are easily confounded, as persons with psychiatric disorders are overall twice as likely to smoke as others, with the increased risk found with all the major anxiety, mood, and psychotic disorders (Lasser et al. 2000).

## Arrhythmias

There is evidence that psychological stressors can also play an important role in precipitating serious ventricular arrhythmias (Ahern et al. 1990, Carney et al. 1993, Follick et al. 1988). Sudden cardiac death after psychological distress has been reported anecdotally for a long time but is difficult to study scientifically. A systematic review of published cases of ventricular fibrillation in patients without known cardiac disease could identify preceding psychological distress in 22% (Viskin and Belhassen 1990). A recent review of 96 published studies investigating psychosocial risk factors for arrhythmia found that 92% were positive (Hemingway et al. 2001). Whether type A personality traits predict sudden cardiac death after myocardial infarction remains controversial (Ahern et al. 1990).

## Congestive Heart Failure

Depression is especially common in patients with congestive heart failure (Koenig 1998, Jiang et al. 2001). In patients hospitalized for congestive heart failure, major depression is independently associated with increased mortality and readmission 3 and 12 months later (Jiang et al. 2001).

## Hypertension

The stress-related physiological response subcategory of PFAMC is particularly relevant to hypertension. There are some data suggesting that blood pressure reactivity to stress is a risk factor for the development of hypertension (Pickering and Gerin 1988) and may influence progression of disease as well (Shapiro 1988). Many studies have examined relationships between personality, coping style, blood pressure reactivity, and hypertension, but conflicting results and methodological limitations have precluded any consensus conclusions (Friedman et al. 2001). Findings regarding the effects of stress, anger, hostility, or anxiety on blood pressure in normotensive individuals are not necessarily relevant to clinical hypertension. A high level of anxiety at baseline evaluation independently predicted twice the risk for development of hypertension in middle-aged men but not in women in one study, (Markovitz et al. 1993) but in another study by the same investigators, anxiety did predict hypertension in women (Markovitz et al. 1991). Some epidemiologic studies have found depression and/or anxiety symptoms predictive of later development of hypertension even after controlling for confounding factors (Davidson et al. 2000, Jonas et al. 1997). Several measures of occupational stress appear to be independent risk factors for hypertension in the general population (Schnell and Pieper 1990, Levenstein et al. 2001). Some of the apparent association between psychological distress and hypertension is chiefly attributable to health risk behaviors (obesity, smoking, alcohol, and sedentary lifestyle) (Levenstein et al. 2001).

Studies of psychological treatments for hypertension (mainly biofeedback and relaxation techniques) have demonstrated the possibility of modest but clinically significant sustained reduction in blood pressure but less effectively than with drug therapy (De-Ping Lee et al. 1988). The major limiting factor in using behavioral treatments for hypertension is compliance, because the treatments must be self-administered indefinitely. Behavioral therapies may be helpful as an adjunctive treatment in patients receiving antihypertensive drugs; psychological treatment should seldom be given as the sole treatment for hypertension.

## Psychological Factors in Endocrinology

### Diabetes Mellitus

Despite some of the early psychosomatic literature, there is no unique diabetic personality, but physicians who take care of diabetic patients attest to a close interrelationship between psychological factors and glucose control. There is conflicting evidence whether psychological factors directly affect the onset of diabetes (Helz and Templeton 1990, Mooy et al. 2000, Wales 1995). That psychological stress can adversely affect glucose control in diabetics seems expectable because the hormones of the stress response are part of the counterregulatory response to insulin. A number of studies have shown that glycemic control is poorer in those diabetic patients who have more perceived stress (Halford et al. 1990, Garay-Sevilla et al. 2000, Lloyd et al. 1999, Herpetz et al. 2000). As assessed by hemoglobin A1c, metabolic control was poorer in depressed children (Lernmark et al. 1999), and in adult depressed type 1 but not type 2 diabetics (de Groot et al. 1999, Van Tilburg et al. 2001). A recent meta-analysis of 24 studies concluded that depression consistently is associated with a small-to-moderate increase in hyperglycemia in both type 1 and type 2 diabetes (Lustman et al. 2000). Depression is associated with more diabetic complications (Lloyd et al. 1992, de Groot et al. 2001). Most such research has been retrospective or cross-sectional, leaving it unclear which came first—poor metabolic control and complications or the psychological factor—and what is the relationship between them.

When psychiatric illness antedates and adversely affects the course of diabetes, it may be mediated by noncompliance (diet, medication, activity, visits to the physician, self-care) (Ciechanowski et al. 2000, Van Tiburg et al. 2001) or by neurohumoral mechanisms. The adverse effects in diabetic control cannot all be attributed to noncompliance. Psychological stress administered under laboratory conditions can impair glucose control in both insulindependent (Halford et al. 1990, Gonder-Frederick et al. 1990) and noninsulin-dependent diabetes (Goetsch et al. 1993). In insulin-dependent diabetes, this effect appears to be mediated by mental stress-induced insulin resistance (Moberg et al. 1994).

Randomized controlled trials have demonstrated improvements in glucose control in diabetics receiving psychological interventions (Delamater et al. 2001, Lustman et al. 1998). Antidepressants are effective in the treatment of depression in diabetics, but can cause increases or decreases in blood glucose by themselves. Deterioration in glucose control in schizophrenic diabetics may be due to some of the newer antipsychotic drugs, but diabetes was a major problem for schizophrenics before their advent, presumably because of obesity (a side effect of almost every antipsychotic), unhealthy diet, and poorer health care (Dixon et al. 2000). Optimal management of diabetes requires a degree of organization very difficult for most patients with schizophrenia.

### Thyroid Disease

It is well established that too little or too much thyroid hormone can result in disturbances in mood and activity. In the other direction, the effects of emotion and stress on thyroid function, although long a focus of interest, are less well established. Parry's original report in 1825 described a woman who had hypothyroidism 4 months after she accidentally fell down stairs in a wheelchair. A number of classic studies reported a relationship between antecedent traumatic stress and the onset of thyrotoxicosis, particularly as part of Graves' disease. However, these studies were retrospective, uncontrolled, and too methodologically flawed by current standards to support the validity of such a link. More recent studies have supported stressful life events as a risk factor for Graves' disease (Radosavljevic et al. 1996, Sonino et al. 1993, Yoshiuchi et al. 1998a). Psychological stress may also be a result of less optimal control of hyperthyroidism (Yoshiuchi et al. 1998b).

Whereas there has been little well-substantiated evidence of the impact of psychological factors on thyroid disease, alterations in thyroid function or its hypothalamic–pituitary control have been demonstrated in relation to affective disorders, schizophrenia, and posttraumatic stress disorder (Mason et al. 1994, 1989). Depression has been most studied, revealing a variety of thyroid abnormalities, most frequently a relative increase in thyroxine without changes in the activated (triiodothyronine) and inactive (reverse triiodothyronine) forms and a blunting of the thyroid-stimulating hormone response to thyrotropin-releasing hormone (Goodwin and Jamison 1990). There is no agreement regarding the relationship between these endocrine changes and depressive pathophysiological processes, and it remains unknown whether depression modifies endocrine measures in clinical thyroid disease.

### Psychological Factors in Pulmonary Disease

Although asthma was once regarded as a classic psychosomatic disorder, it is currently viewed as a primary respiratory disease with varying immunological and autonomic pathophysiological changes. Many physicians still believe that psychological factors play an important role in the precipitation and aggravation of asthma, particularly anxiety. One must remember, however, that respiratory distress itself causes a wide array of anxiety symptoms (panic attacks, generalized and anticipatory anxiety, phobic avoidance), and most of the drugs used to treat asthma have anxiety as a potential side effect. Brittle asthmatic patients, like brittle diabetic patients, are more likely to have current or past psychiatric disorder (particularly anxiety disorders) than are other asthmatic individuals, but which came first is not established (Garden and Ayres 1993). There is no typical personality type susceptible to development of asthma. Studies have shown that anxiety and depression are associated in asthmatic patients with more respiratory symptom complaints but no differences in objective measures of respiratory function (Janson et al. 1994, Rietveld et al. 1999). However, psychological factors and psychosocial problems in hospitalized asthmatics were a more powerful predictor of which ones required intubation than any other examined variable (e.g., smoking, infection, prior hospitalization, etc.) (Le Son and Gershwin 1996). Psychological morbidity is associated with high levels of denial and delays in seeking medical care, which may be life-threatening in severe asthma (Campbell et al. 1995, Miles et al. 1997), as well as less medication adherence and consequently poorer control of asthma (Cluley and Cochrane 2001). Not surprisingly then psychopathology in severe asthmatics is associated with increased health care utilization including hospitalizations, and outpatient and emergency room visits, independent of asthma severity (Ten Brinke et al. 2001).

Similar problems exist in interpreting relationships between anxiety or depression and other chronic obstructive pulmonary diseases (COPD) (chronic bronchitis, emphysema). Depression and anxiety are common in COPD (Yohannes et al. 2000, Aydin and Ulusahin 2001, Withers et al. 1999), though this partly reflects their increased prevalence in past or current smokers. As in asthma, psychological distress in COPD amplifies dyspnea without usually causing changes in objective pulmonary functions. Depression and anxiety do lead to lower exercise tolerance (Withers et al. 1999), noncompliance with treatment (Bosley et al. 1996), and increased disability in COPD (Aydin and Ulusahin 2001). Anxious COPD patients can improve their exercise tolerance through cognitive–behavioral therapy and pulmonary rehabilitation (Withers et al. 1999, Eiser et al. 1997). Smoking is a well-established maladaptive health behavior causing and exacerbating chronic obstructive pulmonary disease, and its elimination is the most beneficial intervention available.

### Psychological Factors in Rheumatoid Arthritis

Rheumatoid arthritis (RA) was also once thought to be a psychosomatic disorder, but studies in the modern era have provided little or no support for this belief. There is no particular personality type susceptible to development of RA. Earlier research suggesting that stressful events play a role in the development or onset of RA has not been supported by more recent studies (Carette et al. 2000, Leymarie et al. 1997). Psychological factors and disease manifestations account for comparable proportions of disability in RA (Escalante and del Rincon 1999). Psychological morbidity in RA results in more pain, poorer quality of life, more joint surgery, lower compliance, and increased use of health care resources (Newman and Mulligan 2000, Wolfe 1999, Kroll et al. 1999).

Depression has been the most frequently studied psychological disturbance in RA; depression is very common, as in other chronic medical conditions (Creed 1990, Soderlin et al. 2000). Depression appears to adversely affect outcome in rheumatoid arthritis, aggravating chronic pain, increasing health care use, and increasing social isolation (Creed 1990, Young 1992). Randomized controlled trials of antidepressants in depressed RA patients demonstrate improvements in pain, morning stiffness, and disability in addition to depression (Bird and Broggini 2000, Ash et al. 1999).

There is a consensus among investigators that passive, avoidant, emotion-laden coping strategies (e.g., wish-fulfilling fantasy, self-blame) are associated with poorer adjustment to illness in RA compared with active, problem-focused coping (e.g., information seeking, cognitive restructuring) (Young 1992, Covic et al. 2000). Rheumatoid arthritis patients with high helplessness are more likely to receive psychotropic, analgesic, and anti-inflammatory drugs and to be less adherent with treatment than those with low helplessness (Stein et al. 1988). Patients with RA may be more vulnerable to stress-induced increases in immune and endocrine function (Hirano et al. 2001). A randomized controlled trial of cognitive–behavioral therapy as an adjunct to standard treatment in recently diagnosed patients with rheumatoid arthritis showed it efficacious in reducing both psychological and physical morbidity (Sharpe et al. 2001).

## Psychological Factors in Neurology

Depression is frequent after stroke, particularly in the acute phase during hospitalization and the first few weeks after stroke (Astrom et al. 1993). The presence of depression is associated with poorer outcome, including higher later mortality (Robinson and Price 1982, Robinson et al. 1986, House et al. 2001), and functional status is improved with treatment of depression after stroke (Lipsey et al. 1984). A negative attitude after stroke (i.e., feeling there is nothing one can do to help oneself) is associated with decreased survival (Lewis et al. 2001). Research has focused on depression as a complication of stroke but there is also evidence that depression and other psychological factors constitute risks for stroke, consistent with widespread lay and folk beliefs regarding stress and stroke. There is preliminary evidence that anger and hostility may pose a risk for carotid atherosclerosis just as it may for coronary disease (Matsumoto et al. 1993). In a longitudinal prospective epidemiological study, depression appeared to significantly predict greater stroke frequency, but the finding disappeared when other significant predictors were taken into consideration (e.g., age, sex, smoking, hypertension, diabetes) (Colantonio et al. 1992). More recent studies have found depressive symptoms increase the risk of stroke in older adults (Simons et al. 1998, Everson et al. 1998, Ostir et al. 2001). As with many other major medical illnesses, stroke patients with extensive social support have better functional outcomes than those who do not (Colantonio et al. 1993).

Depression is common in Parkinson's disease, may antedate the development of motor symptoms, and is associated with cognitive dysfunction (Tandberg et al. 1997, Errea and Ara 1999). Physicians observe that depression and other psychological factors interact to affect the course and outcome of Parkinson's disease, but there has been little formal study of such relationships (Ellgring et al. 1993). Depression is also common and erodes quality of life in multiple sclerosis (MS) (Fruewald et al. 2001) and in epilepsy (Barry et al. 2000). The study of depression as an independent risk factor affecting the onset or course of neurological diseases is challenging because depression may also be consequence of the disease, a psychological reaction to the illness, or a complication of pharmacother-apy (Zorzon et al. 2001). In MS depression may increase and its treatment decrease production of proinflammatory cytokines (Mohr et al. 2001). Depression is especially difficult to study in MS because of its uncertain relationship to the MS-fatigue syndrome (Bakshi et al. 2000).

Patients with chronic migraine headaches have often been described as having a "typical" personality characterized as conscientious, perfectionistic, ambitious, rigid, tense, and resentful, but controlled studies have not supported any consistent conclusion. Specific personality traits in migraine appear more likely to be a consequence rather than a cause of suffering from recurrent headaches (Stronks et al. 1999). Migraine and depression are highly comorbid (Lipton et al. 2000). A community-based survey found more personality disturbance and 2.5 times more psychological distress in migraine sufferers than in matched control subjects, but there was no relationship between headache frequency and the severity of psychological distress or personality abnormality (Brandt et al. 1990). Thus, the relationship between psychological factors and migraine remains to be worked out.

## Psychological Factors in End-Stage Renal Disease

Studies of the influence of psychological factors upon the course of end-stage renal disease (ESRD) have nearly all focused on depression or noncompliance. There has been essentially no investigation of psychological factors in chronic renal failure before end stage.

Depression has been shown in at least one study to be a better predictor of (shorter) survival than age or pathophysiological variables in dialysis patients (Burton et al. 1986). Other studies have reached similar conclusions (Shulman et al. 1989), although negative results have also appeared (Devins et al. 1990, Kutner et al. 1994). Depression is associated with smoking, alcoholism, and other forms of substance abuse that are highly prevalent in ESRD patients (Hegde et al. 2000). More recent studies have done a better job of controlling for ESRD severity and other potential confounds, and still find that depression predicts higher mortality (Kimmel et al. 2000).

Other outcome studies have focused on the impact of noncompliance in ESRD (Manley and Sweeney 1986). Compliance is a complex, multidimensional array of behaviors, and its relationship with health outcomes in dialysis patients is difficult to study. Thus, whereas effects of noncompliance on dialysis patients' outcomes are well recognized by physicians, they have not been adequately characterized empirically. Nevertheless, the widespread belief among physicians and nurses that noncompliance results in worse outcomes including higher mortality in ESRD is supported by a large multicenter study (Leggat et al. 1998). The chronic overuse of nonsteroidal anti-inflammatory agents and analgesics is a maladaptive health behavior recognized as a fairly common contributing cause of chronic renal insufficiency (Fored et al. 2001). One psychosocial intervention outcome study in ESRD found that patients who participated in a support group lived longer than nonparticipants even after multiple psychosocial and psychological variables were controlled, but this was a naturalistic nonrandomized study (Friend et al. 1986).

## Psychological Factors in Gastroenterology

### Inflammatory Bowel Disease

Ulcerative colitis is another disorder that was described in the early literature as a psychosomatic disease, but no specific psychogenic factor contributing to the development of ulcerative colitis or Crohn's disease has ever been substantiated. As with other chronic medical diseases, patients with more psychological distress tend to be those with more severe physical disease and poorer functional capacity, but the causal relationships are not clear (Addolorato et al. 1997, Sewitch et al. 2001). Psychological stress does appear to aggravate both symptom complaints and mucosal disease activity in ulcerative colitis (Levenstein et al. 1994). Disability and distress in patients with inflammatory bowel disease are increased by the presence of a concurrent psychiatric disorder (Walker et al. 1996). In fact, depression is a better predictor of subjective impairment in inflammatory bowel disease than is inflammatory activity (Cuntz et al. 1999). Psychotherapy has the potential to improve outcomes in inflammatory bowel disease, as suggested by controlled trials (Payne and Blanchard 1995, Jantschek et al. 1998).

### Peptic Ulcer Disease

The direct effects of emotion on gastric secretion were first demonstrated in 1833 by William Beaumont, who made observations through a Canadian lumberjack's gastric fistula resulting from an injury. Early psychosomatic investigators studied the role of specific psychological risk factors for duodenal ulcer. In a classical empirical study, Weiner and colleagues (1957) successfully predicted which men in a large cohort of Army draftees would have duodenal ulcers by combining psychological criteria with the biological criterion of high baseline pepsinogen secretion. Since then, the central role of the bacterium *Helicobacter pylori* (*H. pylori*) in the etiology of peptic ulcer disease (PUD) has been clearly established. Many physicians have consequently discarded the longstanding belief that stress causes PUD, and concluded that PUD is an infectious disease, except when attributable to nonsteroidal anti-inflammatory drugs (NSAIDS). Nevertheless, psychological factors appear to be a significant part of the explanation for why only a fraction of those colonized by *H. pylori* or taking NSAIDS develop ulcers. Psychological stress is an independent risk factor for the development (Armstrong et al. 1994) and recurrence of duodenal ulcer (Levenstein et al. 1995a). The frequency of peptic ulcer increases following catastrophic stressful events, including bombardment, earthquake, economic crisis, or being a prisoner of war or "boat people" refugee (Levenstein 2000). Overall, psychosocial factors contribute between 30 and 65% of peptic ulcers (Levenstein 2000), and are most likely to be present in patients with duodenal ulcers who do not have conventional medical risk factors (*H. pylori*, NSAIDS) (Levenstein et al. 1995b). Occupational stress, family conflicts, depression, maladjustment and hostility also are prospectively associated with PUD (Levenstein et al. 1997).

Psychological factors appear to influence PUD through both health risk behaviors (smoking, alcohol abuse, overuse of NSAIDS, poor diet, poor sleep) and psychophysiologic mechanisms (pepsinogen and acid secretion, altered blood flow, impairment of mucosal defenses, and slowing of healing related to the action of cortisol) (Levenstein 2000).

### Irritable Bowel Syndrome

Irritable bowel syndrome (IBS) is a heterogeneous condition with a high frequency of comorbid anxiety especially panic attacks, depression, and somatization. Whereas patients with IBS are psychologically more distressed than normal subjects, they do not have a common profile of psychological symptoms or personality traits (Walker et al. 1990). Patients with IBS are more likely to have a history of childhood sexual abuse than are those with other gastrointestinal disorders in studies of patients seeking care at tertiary referral centers (Walker et al. 1993). In fact, almost all psychological characteristics and psychopathology thought to be more common in IBS are differentially increased only in those who seek medical care for their symptoms (Herschbach et al. 1999).

Both IBS patients and their physicians observe that their gastrointestinal symptoms seem aggravated by stress, but there is no clear evidence that stress causes a different gastrointestinal smooth muscle response than in control subjects (Camilleri and Neri 1989). Instead, psychological factors' effects on IBS appear predominantly on perception of pain and other somatic symptoms, and on health care seeking behaviors. After an acute episode of infectious gastroenteritis, individuals with more life stress, and who were more hypochondriacal, were the ones most likely to go on to develop IBS, without any differences in intestinal physiology (Gwee et al. 1999).

## Psychological Factors in Dermatology

Dermatologists routinely observe the effect of psychological factors, especially anxiety, in the aggravation of a wide variety of dermatological conditions. There are few systematic studies, and perhaps the most important relationships are not uniquely related to particular dermatological disorders. Both anxiety and depression appear to worsen pruritus (itching). So-called neurotic excoriation complicates many dermatological disorders and is aggravated by anxiety, depression, and other behavioral factors (Gupta et al. 1996). That so many skin diseases appear to be precipitated or exacerbated by psychological stress also suggests a nonspecific impairment of cutaneous function. There is now evidence in both animals and humans that stress negatively affects skin's function as a permeability barrier (Garg et al. 2001).

Dermatologists clinically observe important relationships between psychological factors and urticaria, angioedema, atopic dermatitis, hyperhidrosis, acne, and psoriasis, (Arnold 2000) but controlled studies are lacking. Excessive sun exposure is a maladaptive health behavior contributing to skin cancer and various other dermatological conditions.

## Psychological Factors Affecting Infectious Diseases

HIV infection is the most destructive example of unsafe sexual practices, as a maladaptive health behavior, contributing to development and transmission of an infectious medical condition. Once contracted, HIV infection appeared to be a likely candidate for important effects of psychological factors, because of the work demonstrating changes in normal immune function after stress, bereavement, and depression. The effects of stress and depression on disease progression, immune function, and mortality in HIV infection have been an active field of investigation, with varying conclusions (Burack et al. 1993, Leserman et al. 1999, Evans et al. 1997, Psychd et al. 2000). There is less doubt that anxiety worsens symptoms and functioning in HIV patients (Sewell et al. 2000). No research has demonstrated that depression predicts the onset of somatic symptoms in HIV infection, acquired immunodeficiency syndrome, or death (Lyketsos et al. 1993). Psychological factors in HIV infection remain an area of active research.

Psychological factors influence other infectious diseases as well, including the common cold (Takkouche et al. 2001), pneumonia (Mehr et al. 2001), genital herpes (Levenson et al. 1987), and recurrent urinary tract infections (Hunt and Waller 1992). A number of studies have convincingly shown that psychological stress suppresses the secondary (but not primary) antibody response to immunization (Cohen et al. 2001).

## Psychological Factors in Obstetrics

While much more attention has been paid to postpartum depression, antepartum depression also adversely affects pregnancy outcome (Tony et al. 2001). Both antepartum anxiety and depression have been associated with growth retardation and premature birth, resulting in lower birth weights, but potential confounding factors have often not been adequately controlled for. Whether depression and other psychological dysfunction cause poorer obstetric outcomes through poor nutrition, substance abuse (including tobacco), poor adherence or no prenatal care, and/or physiological (hormonal, vascular) effects require further investigation.

## Psychological Factors in Infertility

Psychological factors are likely to affect fertility because frequency and timing of sexual intercourse are important determinants of fertility. Nonconsummation, avoidance of intercourse, vaginismus, and psychogenic amenorrhea are attributable to psychological origins. Psychogenic causes do not account for most male impotence but may play a secondary role in many cases (Tay et al. 1996).

Whereas some prospective data support psychological factors influencing fertility in the general population (Stoleru et al. 1993, 1996), psychological factors appear less potent in predicting pregnancy outcome in couples receiving treatment for infertility (Schover et al. 1994). In general, measures of stress, but not of psychopathology, have been associated with infertility (Griel 1997). This is a particularly complex subject for study because it involves potential psychological factors in both members of the couple and interactions between them as well as their effects on sexual behavior and fertility (Carr et al. 1990, Stoleru et al. 1996). Most psychological distress seen in infertile couples is a result of, rather than a cause of, infertility.

Clinical Vignette 1

Ms. A, a 46-year-old married attorney was referred for psychiatric evaluation by her gastroenterologist who follows her for long-standing irritable bowel syndrome. She has had irritable bowel syndrome since the age of 20 years, with complaints of intermittent constipation, diarrhea, crampy abdominal pain, and bloating. She feels that these symptoms have gradually worsened, particularly in the last month. She describes a highly pressured job and a stressful marriage. She has specifically noticed a precipitous increase in intestinal symptoms immediately after arguments with her husband and when facing deadlines at work. Three months ago, she developed depressed mood, early morning awakening, anorexia, fatigue, crying spells, impaired concentration, irritability, and preoccupation with thoughts of ill health. Her family physician diagnosed major depression and prescribed amitriptyline, which was discontinued after it caused worsening of her constipation. Her psychiatrist then tried fluoxetine (discontinued because of diarrhea) and trazodone (too sedating). She then responded well to nortriptyline with disappearance of the symptoms of depression and improvement in her irritable bowel syndrome. However, severe irritable bowel syndrome symptoms continued to follow the frequent marital arguments. The psychiatrist asked the patient to invite her husband to join one of their sessions so that marital issues could be further explored. He did so, resulting in the discovery that her husband was himself significantly depressed. He was referred to another psychiatrist for treatment, the marital discord abated, and her irritable bowel syndrome symptoms returned to a manageable level.

In this clinical vignette, the patient had features of both mental disorder (major depression) affecting a general medical condition and stress-related physiological response affecting a general medical condition. Treatment included individual psychotherapy and antidepressant medication as well as marital assessment and intervention. Pharmacotherapy required modification because of gastrointestinal sensitivity to side effects.

Clinical Vignette 2

Mr. B is a 60-year-old married judge with coronary artery disease. He was referred for psychiatric evaluation by his cardiologist because he declined coronary artery bypass surgery despite strong and repeated recommendations for surgery by the cardiologist. The cardiologist perceived that the patient's resistance to surgery was not due to lack of information or understanding.

Mr. B had no acute psychiatric symptoms, although he had several lifelong phobias including fear of cats, fear of being buried alive, and claustrophobia (recent episodes in the hospital elevator and during magnetic resonance imaging). His only previous psychiatric contact was some marital therapy 20 years earlier. His coronary artery disease was severe, with two myocardial infarctions and recurrent malignant arrhythmias. He continued to have recurrent angina despite maximal medical management; his pain occurred mainly at night as "a predictable consequence of pushing too hard at work" (he typically worked 12-hour days). He had also had a stroke 3 months ago, from which he had made a complete recovery with no sequelae. Twenty years earlier, he had surgery for a renal stone that was complicated postoperatively with five pulmonary emboli. He said that he has had "eight near-death experiences" amidst his various illnesses.

Mr. B was eager to discuss his reluctance to have coronary bypass surgery. He had not decided against the surgery but had been unable to reach a decision. He brought to the

**Clinical Vignette 2** *continued*

appointment with the psychiatrist a two-page list of arguments for and against surgery and other variables that could influence the decision and outcome. He was aware that he was approaching the question of surgery with the same style of carefully balanced consideration of all sides of an issue that he prided himself on in his occupation as a judge. He worked longer days than his colleagues because he believed it took more time to make fair, proper, and legally correct decisions. His analysis of the pros and cons of surgery, as well as intervening factors affecting and affected by the decision, appeared to the psychiatrist to be well informed, accurate, flexible, and appropriate. There was no evidence of rigidity in his thinking, premature closure, or distorted perceptions. Whereas the thought processes were logical, they had not enabled him to reach a decision, despite extensive discussions with the cardiologist over a period of months. He was aware that this was another decision in his life that was taking much longer than average, but he thought it could not be resolved any other way.

This case represents an example of personality trait or coping style affecting a general medical condition. His obsessional style was largely adaptive in his chosen occupation, although it reduced his efficiency. Now confronted with a major health care decision, and mindful of major complications he had suffered after surgery in the past, the need to weigh all sides of an issue had paralyzed his decision-making. The presence of phobias in his history raised the possibility of these too affecting his decision-making, but he denied feeling fearful of the surgery, anesthesia, intubation, and the like. The anxiety he was experiencing was entirely focused around making the right decision.

## Comparison of DSM-IV/ICD-10 Diagnostic Criteria

Although the corresponding ICD-10 category ("Psychological and behavioural factors associated with disorders or diseases classified elsewhere") does not have specified diagnostic criteria, it is defined in essentially the same way as DSM-IV-TR.

## References

Addolorato G, Capristo E, Stefanini GF, et al. (1997) Inflammatory bowel disease: A study of the association between anxiety and depression, physical morbidity, and nutritional status. Scand J Gastroenterol 32, 1013–1021.

Ahern DK, Gorkin L, Anderson JL, et al. (1990) Biobehavioral variables and mortality or cardiac arrest in the Cardiac Arrhythmia Pilot Study (CAPS). Am J Cardiol 66, 59–62.

Alexander F (1950) Psychomatic Medicine. WW Norton, New York.

Andersen BL (1992) Psychological interventions for cancer patients to enhance the quality of life. J Consult Clin Psychol 60, 552–568.

Armstrong D, Arnold R, Classen M, et al. (1994) RUDER—a prospective, two-year, multicenter study of risk factors for duodenal ulcer relapse during maintenance therapy with ranitidine. RUDER Study Group. Digest Dis Sci 39, 1425–1433.

Arnold LM (2000) Dermatology. In Psychiatric Care of the Medical Patient, 2nd ed., Stoudemire A, Fogel BS, and Greenberg DB (eds). Oxford University Press, New York, pp. 821–834.

Ash G, Dickens CM, Creed FH, et al. (1999) The effects of dothiepin on subjects with rheumatoid arthritis and depression. Rheumatology 38, 959–967.

Astrom M, Adolfsson R, and Asplund K (1993) Major depression in stroke patients. A 3-year longitudinal study. Stroke 24, 976–982.

Aydin IO and Ulusahin A (2001) Depression, anxiety comorbidity, and disability in tuberculosis and chronic obstructive pulmonary disease patients: Applicability of GHQ-12. Gen Hosp Psychiatr 23, 77–83.

Ayres A, Hoon PW, Franzoni JB, et al. (1994) Influence of mood and adjustment to cancer on compliance with chemotherapy among breast cancer patients. J Psychosom Res 38, 393–402.

Bakshi R, Shaikh ZA, Miletich RS, et al. (2000) Fatigue in multiple sclerosis and its relationship to depression and neurologic disability. Mult Scler 6, 181–185.

Barry JJ, Huynh N, and Lembke A (2000) Depression in individuals with epilepsy. Curr Treat Opt Neurol 2, 571–585.

Barsky AJ, Hochstrasser B, Coles NA, et al. (1990) Silent myocardial ischemia. Is the person or the event silent? JAMA 264, 1132–1135.

Bird H and Broggini M (2000) Paroxetine versus amitriptyline for treatment of depression associated with rheumatoid arthritis: A randomized, double-blind, parallel group study. J Rheumatol 27, 2791–2797.

Bosley CM, Corden ZM, Rees PJ, et al. (1996) Psychological factors associated with the use of home nebulized therapy for COPD. Eur Res J 9, 2346–2350.

Brandt J, Celentano D, Stewart W, et al. (1990) Personality and emotional disorder in a community sample of migraine headache sufferers. Am J Psychiatr 147, 303–308.

Bruce ML, Leaf PJ, Rozal GPM, et al. (1994) Psychiatric status and 9-year mortality data in the New Haven Epidemiological Catchment Area Study. Am J Psychiatr 151, 716–721.

Buddeberg C, Wolf C, Sieber M, et al. (1991) Coping strategies and course of disease of breast cancer patients. Results of a 3-year longitudinal study. Psychother Psychosom 55, 151–157.

Burack JH, Barrett DC, Stall RD, et al. (1993) Depressive symptoms and CD4 lymphocyte decline among HIV-infected men. JAMA 270, 2568–2573.

Burton HJ, Kline SA, Lindsay RM, et al. (1986) The relationship of depression to survival in chronic renal failure. Psychosom Med 48, 251–258.

Butow PN, Coates AS, and Dunn SM (1999) Psychosocial predictors of survival in metastatic melanoma. J Clin Oncol 17, 2256.

Camilleri M and Neri M (1989) Motility disorders and stress. Digest Dis Sci 34, 1777–1786.

Campbell DA, Yellowlees PM, McLennan G, et al. (1995) Psychiatric and medical features of near fatal asthma. Thorax 50, 254–259.

Carette S, Surtees PG, Wainwright NW, et al. (2000) The role of life events and childhood experiences in the development of rheumatoid arthritis. J Rheumatol 27, 2123–2130.

Carney RM, Blumenthal JA, Stein PK, et al. (2001) Depression, heart rate variability, and acute myocardial infarction. Circulation 104, 2024–2028.

Carney RM, Freedland KE, Eisen SA, et al. (1995) Major depression and medication adherence in elderly patients with coronary artery disease. Health Psychol 14, 88–90.

Carney RM, Freedland KE, Rich MW, et al. (1993) Ventricular tachycardia and psychiatric depression in patients with coronary artery disease. Am J Med 95, 23–28.

Carr EK, Friedman T, Lannon B, et al. (1990) The study of psychological factors in couples receiving artificial insemination by donor: A discussion of methodological difficulties. J Adv Nurs 15, 906–910.

Cassileth BR, Lusk EJ, Miller DS, et al. (1985) Psychological correlates of survival in advanced malignant disease? New Engl J Med 312, 1551–1555.

Ciechanowski PS, Katon WJ, and Russo JE (2000) Depression and diabetes: Impact of depressive symptoms on adherence, function, and costs. Arch Intern Med 160, 3278–3285.

Cluley S and Cochrane GM (2001) Psychological disorder in asthma is associated with poor control and poor adherences to inhaled steroids. Respir Med 95, 37–39.

Cohen S, Miller GE, and Rabin BS (2001) Psychological stress and antibody response to immunization: A critical review of the human literature. Psychosom Med 63, 7–18.

Colantonio A, Kasi SV, and Ostfeld AM (1992) Depressive symptoms and other psychosocial factors as predictors of stroke in the elderly. Am J Epidemiol 136, 884–894.

Colantonio A, Kasi SV, and Ostfeld AM (1993) Psychosocial predictors of stroke outcomes in an elderly population. J Gerontol 48, S261–S268.

Courtney JG, Longnecker MP, Theorell T, et al. (1993) Stressful life events and the risk of colorectal cancer. Epidemiology 4, 407–414.

Covic T, Adamson B, and Hough M (2000) The impact of passive coping on rheumatoid arthritis pain. Rheumatology 39, 1027–1030.

Creed F (1990) Psychological disorders in rheumatoid arthritis: A growing consensus? Ann Rheum Dis 49, 808–812.

Cunningham AJ, Edmonds CV, Jenkins GP, et al. (1998) A randomized controlled trial of the effects of group psychological therapy on survival in women with metastatic breast cancer. Psychooncology 7, 508–517.

Cuntz U, Welt J, Ruppert E, et al. (1999) Determination of subjective burden from chronic inflammatory bowel disease and its psychosocial consequences. Results from a study of 200 patients. Psychother Psychosom Med Psychol 49, 494–500.

Davidson K, Jonas BS, Dixon KE, et al. (2000) Do depression symptoms predict early hypertension incidence in young adults in the CARDIA study? Coronary Artery Risk Development in Young Adult. Arch Intern Med 160, 1495–1500.

de Groot M, Anderson R, Freedland KE, et al. (2001) Association of depression and diabetes complications: A meta-analysis. Psychosom Med 63, 619–630.

de Groot M, Jacobson AM, Samson JA, et al. (1999) Glycemic control and major depression in patients with type 1 and type 2 diabetes mellitus. J Psychosom Res 46, 425–435.

Delamater AM, Jacobson AM, Anderson B, et al. (2001) Psychosocial therapies in diabetes: Report of the Psychosocial Therapies Working Group. Diabet Care 24, 1286–1292.

Dembroski TM, MacDougall JM, Cista PT Jr, et al. (1989) Components of hostility as predictors of sudden death and myocardial infarction in the Multiple Risk Factor Intervention Trial. Psychosom Med 51, 514–522.

De-Ping Lee D, DeQuattro V, Allen J, et al. (1988) Behavioral vs. beta-blocker therapy in patients with primary hypertension: Effects on blood pressure, left ventricular function and mass, and the pressor surge of social stress anger. Am Heart J 116, 637–644.

Devins GM, Mann J, Mandin H, et al. (1990) Psychosocial predictors of survival in end-stage renal disease. J Nerv Ment Dis 178, 127–133.

Deykin EY, Keane TM, Kaloupek D, et al. (2001) Posttraumatic stress disorder and the use of health services. Psychosom Med 63, 835–841.

DiMatteo MR, Lepper HS, and Croghan TW (2000) Depression is a risk factor for noncompliance with medical treatment: Meta-analysis of the effects of anxiety and depression on patient adherence. Arch Intern Med 160, 2101–2107.

Dimsdale JE (1988) A perspective on type A behavior and coronary disease. New Engl J Med 318, 110–112.

Dixon L, Weiden P, Delahanty J, et al. (2000) Prevalence and correlates of diabetes in national schizophrenia samples. Schizophr Bull 26, 903–912.

Druss BG, Bradford WD, Rosenheck RA, et al. (2001a) Quality of medical care and excess mortality in older patients with mental disorders. Arch Gen Psychiatr 58, 565–572.

Druss BG, Rohrbaugh RM, Levinson CM, et al. (2001b) Integrated medical care for patients with serious psychiatric illness. Arch Gen Psychiatr 58, 861–868.

Eiser N, West C, Evans S, et al. (1997) Effects of psychotherapy in moderately severe COPD: A pilot's study. Eur Res J 10, 1581–1584.

Ellgring H, Seiler S, Perleth B, et al. (1993) Psychosocial aspects of Parkinson's disease. Neurology 43, S41–S44.

Errea JM and Ara JR (1999) Depression and Parkinson disease. Rev Neurol 28, 694–698.

Escalante A and del Rincon I (1999) How much disability in rheumatoid arthritis is explained by rheumatoid arthritis? Arthritis Rheum 42, 1712–1721.

Evans DL, Leserman J, Perkins DO, et al. (1997) Severe life stress as a predictor of early disease progression in HIV infection. Am J Psychiatr 154, 630–634.

Everson SA, Roberts RE, Goldberg DR, et al. (1998) Depressive symptoms and increased risk of stroke mortality over a 29-year period. Arch Intern Med 158, 1133–1138.

Faller H, Bulzebruck H, Drungs P, et al. (1999) Coping, distress, and survival among patients with lung cancer. Arch Gen Psychiatr 56, 756–762.

Fawzy FI, Fawzy NW, Ryan OS, et al. (1993) Malignant melanoma. Effects of an early structured psychiatric intervention, coping, and affective state on recurrences and survival 6 years later. Arch Gen Psychiatr 60, 681–689.

Follick MJ, Gorkin L, Capone RJ, et al. (1988) Psychological distress as a predictor of ventricular arrhythmias in a postmyocardial infarction population. Am Heart J 116, 32–36.

Fored CM, Ejerblad E, Lindblad P, et al. (2001) Acetaminophen, aspirin, and chronic renal failure. New Engl J Med 345, 1801–1808.

Frasure-Smith N, Lesperance F, and Talajic M (1993) Depression following myocardial infarction: Impact on 6-month survival. JAMA 270, 1819–1825.

Frasure-Smith N, Lesperance F, and Talajic M (1995) The impact of negative emotions on prognosis following myocardial infarction: Is it more than depression? Health Psychol 14, 388–398.

Friedman R, Schwartz JE, Schnall PL, et al. (2001) Psychological variables in hypertension: Relationship to casual or ambulatory blood pressure in men. Psychosom Med 63, 19–31.

Friedman M, Thoresen CE, Gill JJ, et al. (1986) Alteration of type A behavior and its effect on cardiac recurrences in postmyocardial infarction patients: Summary results of the Recurrent Coronary Prevention Project. Am Heart J 112, 653–665.

Friend R, Singletary Y, Mendell N, et al. (1986) Group participation and survival among patients with end-stage renal disease. Am J Pub Health 76, 670–672.

Fruewald S, Loeffler-Stastka H, Eher R, et al. (2001) Depression and quality of life in multiple sclerosis. Acta Neurol Scand 104, 257–261.

Gallo JJ, Armenian HK, Ford DE, et al. (2000) Major depression and cancer: The 13-year follow-up of the Baltimore epidemiologic catchment area sample (United States). Cancer Causes Control 11, 751–758.

Garay-Sevilla ME, Malacara JM, Gonzalez-Contreras E, et al. (2000) Perceived psychological stress in diabetes mellitus type 2. Rev Invest Clin 52, 241–245.

Garden GM and Ayres JG (1993) Psychiatric and social aspects of brittle asthma. Thorax 48, 501–505.

Garg A, Chren MM, Sands LP, et al. (2001) Psychological stress perturbs epidermal permeability barrier homeostasis: Implications for the pathogenesis of stress-associated skin disorders. Arch Dermatol 137, 53–59.

Garssen B and Goodkin K (1999) On the role of immunological factors as mediators between psychosocial factors and cancer progression. Psychiatr Res 85, 51–61.

Gellert GA, Maxwell RM, and Siegel BS (1993) Survival of breast cancer patients receiving adjunctive psychosocial support therapy: A 10-year follow-up study. J Clin Oncol 11, 66–69.

Geyer S (1991) Life events prior to manifestation of breast cancer: A limited prospective study covering eight years before diagnosis. J Psychosom Res 35, 355–363.

Giraldi T, Rodani MG, Cartei G, et al. (1997) Psychosocial factors and breast cancer: A 6-year Italian follow-up study. Psychother Psychosom 66, 229–236.

Glassman AH and Shapiro PA (1998) Depression and the course of coronary artery disease. Am J Psychiatr 155, 4–11.

Glover J, Dibble SL, Dood MJ, et al. (1995) Mood states of oncology outpatients: Does pain make a difference? J Pain Sympt Manag 10, 120–128.

Goetsch VL, VanDorsten B, Pbert LA, et al. (1993) Acute effects of laboratory stress on blood glucose in noninsulin-dependent diabetes. Psychosom Med 55, 492–496.

Gonder-Frederick LA, Carter WR, Cox DJ, et al. (1990) Environmental stress and blood glucose change in IDDM. Health Psychol 9, 503–515.

Goodwin FK and Jamison KR (1990) Manic-Depressive Illness. Oxford University Press, New York, pp. 454–455.

Goodwin PJ, Leszcz M, Ennis M, et al. (2001) The effect of group psychological support on survival in metastatic breast cancer. N Engl J Med 345, 1719–1726.

Graves PJ, Thomas CB, and Mead LA (1991) Familial and psychological predictors of cancer. Cancer Detect Prev 15, 59–64.

Greer S, Morris T, and Pettingale KW (1979) Psychological response to breast cancer: Effect on outcome. Lancet 2, 785–787.

Greil AL (1997) Infertility and psychological distress: A critical review of the literature. Soc Sci Med 45, 1679–1704.

Gupta MA, Gupta AK, and Shork NJ (1996) Psychological factors affecting self-excoriative behavior in women with mild-to-moderate facial acne vulgaris. Psychosomatics 37, 127–130.

Gwee KA, Leong YL, Graham C, et al. (1999) The role of psychological and biological factors in postinfective gut dysfunction. Gut 44, 400–406.

Halford WK, Cuddily S, and Mortimer RH (1990) Psychological stress and blood glucose regulation in type 1 diabetic patients. Health Psychol 9, 516–528.

Haynes SG and Matthews DA (1988) Review and methodologic critique of recent studies on type A behavior and cardiovascular disease. Ann Behav Med 10, 47–59.

Haynes SG, Feinleib M, and Kannel WB (1980) The relationship of psychosocial factors to coronary heart disease in the Framingham Study: III. Eight-year incidence of coronary heart disease. Am J Epidemiol 111, 37–58.

Hegde A, Veis JH, Seidman A, et al. (2000) High prevalence of alcoholism in dialysis patients. Am J Kidney Dis 35, 1039–1043.

Helgeson VS and Cohen S (1996) Social support and adjustment to cancer: Reconciling descriptive, correlational, and intervention research. Health Psychol 15, 135–148.

Helsing KJ and Szklo M (1981) Mortality after bereavement. Am J Epidemiol 114, 41–52.

Helz JW and Templeton B (1990) Evidence of the role of psychosocial factors in diabetes mellitus: A review. Am J Psychiatr 147, 1275–1282.

Hemingway H, Malik M, and Marmot M (2001) Social and psychosocial influences on sudden cardiac death, ventricular arrhythmia and cardiac autonomic function. Eur Heart J 22, 1082–1101.

Herpertz S, Johann B, Lichtblau K, et al. (2000) Patients with diabetes mellitus: Psychosocial stress and the use of psychosocial support: A multicenter study. Med Klin 95, 369–377.

Herran A, Amado JA, Garcia-Unzueta MT, et al. (2000) Increased bone remodeling in first-episode major depressive disorder. Psychosom Med 62, 779–782.

Herschbach P, Henrich G, and von Rad M (1999) Psychological factors in functional gastrointestinal disorders: Characteristics of the disorder or of the illness behavior? Psychosom Med 61, 148–153.

Hirano D, Nagashima M, Ogawa R, et al. (2001) Serum levels of interleukin 6 and stress related substances indicate mental stress condition in patients with rheumatoid arthritis. J Rheumatol 28, 490–495.

House A, Knapp P, Bamford J, et al. (2001) Mortality at 12 and 24 months after stroke may be associated with depressive symptoms at 1 month. Stroke 32, 696–701.

Hunt JC and Waller G (1992) Psychological factors in recurrent uncomplicated urinary tract infection. Br J Urol 69, 460–464.

Irwin M (1999) Immune correlates of depression. Adv Exp Med Biol 46, 1–24.

Irwin M, Daniels M, and Weiner H (1987) Immune and neuroendocrine changes during bereavement. Psychiatr Clin N Am 10, 449–465.

Jahn I, Becker U, Jockel KH, et al. (1995) Occupational life course and lung cancer risk in men. Findings from a socio-epidemiological analysis of job-changing histories in a case–control study. Soc Sci Med 40, 961–975.

Janson C, Bjornnson E, Hetta J, et al. (1994) Anxiety and depression in relation to respiratory symptoms and asthma. Am J Res Crit Care Med 149, 930–934.

Jantschek G, Zeitz M, Pritsch M, et al. (1998) Effect of psychotherapy on the course of Crohn's disease. Result of the German prospective multicenter psychotherapy treatment study of Crohn's disease. German study group on psychosocial intervention in Crohn's disease. Scand J Gastroenterol 33, 1289–1296.

Januzzi JL, Stern TA, Pasternak RC, et al. (2000) The influence of anxiety and depression on outcomes of patients with coronary artery disease. Arch Intern Med 160, 1913–1921.

Jiang W, Alexander J, Christopher E, et al. (2001) Relationship of depression to increased risk of mortality and rehospitalization in patients with congestive heart failure. Arch Intern Med 161, 1849–1856.

Jiang W, Babyak M, Krantz DS, et al. (1996) Mental stress—induced myocardial ischemia and cardiac events. JAMA 275, 1651–1656.

Jonas BS, Franks P, and Ingram DD (1997) Are symptoms of anxiety and depression risk factors for hypertension? Longitudinal evidence from the National Health and Nutrition Examination Survey I Epidemiologic Follow-up Study. Arch Fam Med 6, 43–49.

Katon W and Gonzales J (1994) A review of randomized trials of psychiatric consultation-liaison studies in primary care. Psychosomatics 35, 268–278.

Kawachi I, Colditz GA, Acherio A, et al. (1994) Prospective study of phobic anxiety and risk of coronary heart disease in men. Circulation 89, 1992–1997.

Kimmel PL, Peterson RA, Weihs KL, et al. (2000) Multiple measurements of depression predict mortality in a longitudinal study of chronic hemodialysis outpatients. Kidney Int 57, 2093–2098.

Koenig HG (1998) Depression in hospitalized older patients with heart failure. Gen Hosp Psychiatr 20, 29–43.

Krantz DS, Sheps DS, Carney RM, et al. (2000) Effects of mental stress in patients with coronary artery disease. Evidence and clinical implications. JAMA 283, 1800–1802.

Kroll T, Barlow JH, and Shaw K (1999) Treatment adherence in juvenile rheumatoid arthritis—a review. Scand J Rheumatol 28, 10–18.

Kune GA, Kune S, Watson LF, et al. (1991) Personality as a risk factor in large bowel cancer: Data from the Melborune Colorectal Cancer Study. Psychol Med 21, 29–41.

Kune S, Kune GA, Watson LF, et al. (1991) Recent life change and large bowel cancer. Data from the Melbourne Colorectal Cancer Study. J Clin Epidemiol 44, 57–68.

Kutner NG, Lin LS, Fielding B, et al. (1994) Continued survival of older hemodialysis patients: Investigation of psychosocial predictors. Am J Kidney Dis 24, 42–49.

Ladwig KH, Kieser M, Konig J, et al. (1991) Affective disorders and survival after acute myocardial infarction: Results from the post-infarction late potential study. Eur Heart J 12, 959–964.

Lasser K, Boyd JW, Woolhandler S, et al. (2000) Smoking and mental illness: A population-based prevalence study. JAMA 284, 2606–2610.

Lee MA and Ganzini L (1992) Depression in the elderly: Effect on patient attitudes toward life-sustaining therapy. J Am Geriat Soc 40, 983–988.

Leggat JE Jr, Orzol SM, Hulbert-Shearin TE, et al. (1998) Noncompliance in hemodialysis: Predictors and survival analysis. Am J Kidney Dis 32, 139–145.

Leor J, Poole WK, and Kloner RA (1996) Sudden cardiac death triggered by an earthquake. New Engl J Med 334, 413–419.

Lernmark B, Persson B, Fisher L, et al. (1999) Symptoms of depression are important to psychological adaptation and metabolic control in children with diabetes mellitus. Diabet Med 16, 14–22.

Leserman J, Jackson ED, Petitto JM, et al. (1999) Progression to AIDS: The effects of stress, depressive symptoms, and social support. Psychosom Med 61, 397–406.

Le Son S and Gershwin ME (1996) Risk factors for asthmatic patients requiring intubation. III. Observations in young adults. J Asthma 33, 27–35.

Levav I, Kohn R, Iscovich J, et al. (2000) Cancer incidence and survival following bereavement. Am J Pub Health 90, 1601–1607.

Levenkron JC and Moore LG (1988) The type A behavior pattern: Issues for intervention research. Ann Behav Med 10, 78–83.

Levenson JL (1994) Common psychological reactions to medical illness and treatment. In Clinical Psychiatry for Medical Students, 2nd ed., Stoudemire A (ed). JB Lippincott, Philadelphia, pp. 580B–609.

Levenson JL, Colenda C, Larson DB, et al. (1990a) Methodology in consultation-liaison research: A classification of biases. Psychosomatics 31, 367–376.

Levenson JL, Hamer RM, Myers T, et al. (1987) Psychological factors predict symptoms of severe recurrent genital herpes infection. J Psychosom Res 31, 153–159.

Levenson JL, Hamer RM, and Rossiter LF (1990b) Relation of psychopathology in general medical inpatients to use and cost of services. Am J Psychiatr 147, 1498–1503.

Levenson JL and McDonald K (2002) The role of psychological factors in cancer onset and progression. A critical appraisal. In The Psychoimmunology of Human Cancer, Lewis CE, O'Sullivan C, and Barraclough (eds). Oxford University Press, Oxford, UK.

Levenson JL, Mishra A, Hamer RM, et al. (1989) Denial and medical outcome in unstable angina. Psychosom Med 51, 27–35.

Levenstein S (2000) The very model of a modern etiology: A biopsychosocial view of peptic ulcer. Psychosom Med 62, 176–185.

Levenstein S, Kaplan GA, and Smith M (1995a) Sociodemographic characteristics, life stressors, and peptic ulcer: A prospective study. J Clin Gastroenterol 21, 185–192.

Levenstein S, Kaplan GA, and Smith MW (1997) Psychological predictors of peptic ulcer incidence in the Alameda County Study. J Clin Gastroenterol 24, 140–146.

Levenstein S, Prantera C, Varvo V, et al. (1994) Psychological stress and distress activity in ulcerative colitis: A multidimensional cross-sectional study. Am J Gastroenterol 89, 1219–1225.

Levenstein S, Prantera C, Varvo V, et al. (1995b) Patterns of biologic and psychologic risk factors in duodenal ulcer patients. J Clin Gastroenterol 21, 110–117.

Levenstein S, Smith MW, and Kaplan GA (2001) Psychosocial predictors of hypertension in men and women. Arch Intern Med 161, 1341–1346.

Levine J, Warrenburg S, Kerns R, et al. (1990) The role of denial in recovery from coronary heart disease. Psychosom Med 49, 109–117.

Lewis SC, Dennis MS, O'Rourke SJ, et al. (2001) Negative attitudes among short-term stroke survivors predict worse long-term survival. Stroke 32, 1640–1645.

Leymarie F, Jolly D, Sanderman R, et al. (1997) Life events and disability in rheumatoid arthritis: A European cohort. Br J Rheumatol 36, 116–112.

Light KC, Herbst MC, Bragdon EE, et al. (1991) Depression and type A behavior pattern in patients with coronary artery disease: Relationships to painful versus silent myocardial ischemia and beta-endorphin responses during exercise. Psychosom Med 53, 669–683.

Lipsey JR, Robinson RG, Pearlson GD, et al. (1984) Nortriptyline treatment of poststroke depression: A double-blind study. Lancet 11, 297–300.

Lipton RB, Hamelsky SW, Kolodner KB, et al. (2000) Migraine, quality of life, and depression: A population-based case–control study. Neurology 55, 629–635.

Lloyd CE, Dyer PH, Lancashire RJ, et al. (1999) Associated between stress and glycemic control in adults with type 1 (insulin-dependent) diabetes. Diabet Care 22, 1278–1283.

Lloyd CE, Matthews KA, Wing RR, et al. (1992) Psychosocial factors and complications of IDDM. The Pittsburgh Epidemiology of Diabetes Complications Study VIII. Diabet Care 15, 166–172.

Lustman PJ, Anderson RJ, Freedland KE, et al. (2000) Depression and poor glycemic control: A meta-analytic review of the literature. Diabet Care 23, 934–942.

Lustman PJ, Griffith LS, Freedland KE, et al. (1998) Cognitive–behavior therapy for depression in type 2 diabetes mellitus. A randomized, controlled trial. Ann Intern Med 129, 613–621.

Lyketsos CG, Hoover DR, Guccione M, et al. (1993) Depressive symptoms as predictors of medical outcome in HIV infection. JAMA 270, 2563–2567.

Lynge E and Andersen O (1997) Unemployment and cancer in Denmark, 1970–1975 and 1986–1990. IARC Sci Publ 138, 353–359.

Manley M and Sweeney J (1986) Assessment of compliance in hemodialysis adaptation. J Psychosom Res 30, 153–161.

Marata T, Hamburgen ME, Jennings CA, et al. (1993) Keeping hostility in perspective. Coronary heart disease and the hostility scale on the Minnesota Multiphasic Personality Inventory. Mayo Clin Proc 68, 109–114.

Markovitz JH, Matthews KA, Kannel WB, et al. (1993) Psychological predictors of hypertension in the Framingham Study. Is there tension in hypertension? JAMA 270, 2439–2443.

Markovitz JH, Matthews KA, Wing RR, et al. (1991) Psychological biological, and health behavior predictors of blood pressure changes in middle-aged women. J Hypertens 7, 399–406.

Markovitz JH, Shuster JL, Chitwood WS, et al. (2000) Platelet activation in depression and effects of sertraline treatment: An open-label study. Am J Psychiatr 157, 1006–1008.

Mason J, Southwick S, Yehuda R, et al. (1994) Elevation of serum free triiodothyronine, total triiodothyronine, thyroxine-binding globulin, and total thyroxine levels in combat-related posttraumatic stress disorder. Arch Gen Psychiatr 51, 625–641.

Mason JW, Kennedy JL, Kosten TR, et al. (1989) Serum thyroxine levels in schizophrenic and affective disorder diagnostic subgroups. J Nerv Ment Dis 177, 351–358.

Matsumoto Y, Uyama O, Shimizu S, et al. (1993) Do anger and aggression affect carotid atherosclerosis? Stroke 24, 983–986.

Maunsell E, Brisson J, Mondor M, et al. (2001) Stressful life events and survival after breast cancer. Psychosom Med 63, 306 315.

McGee R, Williams S, and Elwood M (1994) Depression and the development of cancer: A meta-analysis. Soc Sci Med 38, 187–192.

McKenna MC, Zevon MA, Corn B, et al. (1999) Psychosocial factors and the development of breast cancer: A meta-analysis. Health Psychol 18, 520–531.

Mehr DR, Binder EF, Kruse RL, et al. (2001) Predicting mortality in nursing home residents with lower respiratory tract infection. JAMA 286, 2427–2436.

Miles JF, Garden GM, Tunnicliffe WS, et al. (1997) Psychological morbidity and coping skills in patients with brittle and nonbrittle asthma: A case–control study. Clin Exp Allergy 27, 1151–1519.

Moberg E, Kollind M, Lins PE, et al. (1994) Acute mental stress impairs insulin sensitivity in IDDM patients. Diabetologia 37, 247–251.

Mohr DC, Goodkin DE, Islar J, et al. (2001) Treatment of depression is associated with suppression of nonspecific and antigen-specific T (H) 1 responses in multiple sclerosis. Arch Neurol 58, 1081–1086.

Mooy JM, deVries H, Gootenhuis PA, et al. (2000) Major stressful life events in relation to prevalence of undetected type 2 diabetes: The Hoorn Study. Diabet Care 23, 197–201.

Moser DK and Dracup K (1996) Is anxiety early after myocardial infarction associated with subsequent ischemic and arrhythmic events? Psychosom Med 58, 395–401.

Musselman DL, Evans DL, and Nemeroff CB (1998) The relationship of depression to Cardiovascular disease: Epidemiology, biology, and treatment. Arch Gen Psychiatr 55, 580–592.

Musselman DL, Marzec UM, Manatunga A, et al. (2000) Platelet reactivity in depressed patients treated with paroxetine: Preliminary findings. Arch Gen Psychiatr 57, 875–882.

Myrtek M (2001) Meta-analyses of prospective studies on coronary heart disease, type A personality, and hostility. Int J Cardiol 79, 245–251.

Newman S and Mulligan K (2000) The psychology of rheumatic diseases. Baillieres Best Pract Res Clin Rheumatol 14, 773–786.

Noyes R Jr, Hartz AJ, Doebbeling CC, et al. (2000) Illness fears in the general population. Psychosom Med 62, 318–325.

Orth-Gomer K, Wamala SP, Horsten M, et al. (2000) Marital stress worsens prognosis in women with coronary heart disease: The Stockholm Female Coronary Risk Study. JAMA 284, 3008–3014.

Ostir GV, Markides KS, Peek MK, et al. (2001) The association between emotional well-being and the incidence of stroke in older adults. Psychosom Med 63, 210–215.

Payne A and Blanchard EB (1995) A controlled comparison of cognitive therapy and self-help support groups in the treatment of irritable bowel syndrome. J Consult Clin Psychol 63, 779–786.

Penninx BW, Beekman AT, Honig A, et al. (2001) Depression and cardiac mortality: Results from community-based longitudinal study. Arch Gen Psychiatr 58, 221–227.

Persky VW, Kempthorne-Rawson J, and Shekelle RB (1987) Personality and risk of cancer: 20-year follow-up of the Western Electric Study. Psychosom Med 49, 435–449.

Pickering TG and Gerin W (1988) Ambulatory blood pressure monitoring and cardiovascular reactivity for the evaluation of the role of psychosocial factors and prognosis in hypertensive patients. Am Heart J 116, 665–672.

Psychd ST, Troop M, Burgess AP, et al. (2000) The relationship of psychological variables and disease progression among long-term HIV infected men. Int J STD AIDS 11, 734–742.

Radosavljevic VR, Jankovic SM, and Marinkovic JM (1996) Stressful life events in the pathogenesis of Graves' disease. Eur J Endocrinol 134, 699–701.

Ragland DR, Brand RJ, and Fox BH (1987) Type A behavior and cancer mortality in the Western Collaborative Group Study [abstract]. Psychosom Med 49, 209.

Ramirez AJ, Craig TK, Watson JP, et al. (1989) Stress and relapse of breast cancer. BMJ 298, 291–293.

Rietveld S, van Beest I, and Everaerd W (1999) Stress-induced breathlessness in asthma. Psychol Med 29, 1359–1366.

Robinson RG, Bolla-Wilson K, Kaplan E, et al. (1986) Depression influences intellectual impairment in stroke patients. Br J Psychiatr 148, 541–547.

Robinson RG and Price TR (1982) Poststroke depressive disorders: A follow-up of 103 patients. Stroke 13, 635–641.

Roose SP, Dalack GW, and Woodring S (1991) Death, depression, and heart disease. J Clin Psychiatr 52, 34–39.

Rosenman RH, Brand RJ, Jenkins CD, et al. (1975) Coronary heart disease in the Western Collaborative Group Study: Final follow-up experience of eight and one-half years. JAMA 233, 872–877.

Roux AVD, Merkin SS, Arnett D, et al. (2001) Neighborhood of residence and incidence of coronary heart disease. New Engl J Med 345, 99–106.

Rozanski A, Bairey CN, Krantz DS, et al. (1988) Mental stress and the induction of silent myocardial ischemia in patients with coronary artery disease. New Engl J Med 318, 1005–1012.

Saravay M and Lavin M (1994) Psychiatric comorbidity and length of stay in the general hospital: A critical review of outcome studies. Psychosomatics 35, 233–252.

Schleifer SJ, Keller SE, Camerino M, et al. (1983) Suppression of lymphocyte stimulation following bereavement. JAMA 250, 374–377.

Schnell PL and Pieper C (1990) The relationship between "job strain," workplace diastolic blood pressure, and left ventricular mass index. Results of a case–control study. JAMA 263, 1929–1935.

Schover LR, Greenhalgh LF, Richards SI, et al. (1994) Psychological screening and the success of donor insemination. Hum Reprod 9, 176–178.

Sewell MC, Goggin KJ, Rabkin JG, et al. (2000) Anxiety syndromes and symptoms among men with AIDS: A longitudinal controlled study. Psychosomatics 41, 294–300.

Sewitch MJ, Abrahamowicz M, Bitton A, et al. (2001) Psychological distress, social support, and disease activity in patients with inflammatory bowel disease. Am J Gastroenterol 96, 1470–1479.

Shapiro PA (1988) Psychological factors in hypertension: An overview. Heart J 116, 632–637.

Sharpe K, Sensky T, Timberlake N, et al. (2001) A blind, randomized, controlled trial of cognitive–behavioral intervention for patients with recent onset rheumatoid arthritis: Preventing psychological and physical morbidity. Pain 89, 275–283.

Shekelle RB, Raynor WJ, Ostfeld AM, et al. (1981) Psychological depression and 17-year risk of death from cancer. Psychosom Med 43, 117–125.

Shulman R, Price JD, and Spinelli J (1989) Biopsychosocial aspects of long-term survival on end-stage renal failure therapy. Psychol Med 19, 945–954.

Simons LA, McCallum J, Friedlander Y, et al. (1998) Risk factors for ischemic stroke: Dubbo Study of the elderly. Stroke 29, 1341–1346.

Smith G (1994) The course of somatization and its effects on utilization of health care resources. Psychosomatics 35, 263–267.

Soderlin MK, Hakala M, and Nieminen P (2000) Anxiety and depression in a community-based rheumatoid arthritis population. Scand J Rheumatol 29, 177–183.

Sonino N, Girelli ME, Boscaro M, et al. (1993) Life events in the pathogenesis of Graves' disease. A controlled study. Acta Endocrinol 128, 293–296.

Sparagon B, Friedman M, Breall WS, et al. (2001) Type A behavior and coronary atherosclerosis. Atherosclerosis 156, 145–149.

Spigel D and Sephton SE (2001) Psychoneuroimmune and endocrine pathways in cancer: Effects of stress and support. Semin Clin Neuropsychiatr 6, 252–265.

Spiegel D, Bloom JR, and Yalom ID (1981) Group support for patients with metastatic cancer: A randomized prospective outcome study. Arch Gen Psychiatr 38, 527–533.

Spiegel P, Bloom JR, Kraemer HC, et al. (1989) Effects of psychosocial treatment on survival of patients with metastatic breast cancer. Lancet 2, 888–891.

Stein MJ, Wallston KA, Nicassio PM, et al. (1988) Correlates of a clinical classification schema for the Arthritis Helplessness Subscale. Arthritis Rheum 31, 876–881.

Stevens LE, de Moore GM, and Simpson JM (1998) Delirium in hospital: Does it increase length of stay? Aust N Z J Psychiatr 32, 805–808.

Stoleru S, Teglas JP, Fermanian J, et al. (1993) Psychological factors in the etiology of infertility: A prospective cohort study. Hum Reprod 8, 1039–1046.

Stoleru S, Teglas JP, Spira A, et al. (1996) Psychological characteristics of infertile patients: Discriminating etiological factors from reactive changes. J Psychosom Obstet Gynaecol 17, 103–118.

Stoudemire A (ed) (1995) Psychological Factors Affecting Medical Conditions. American Psychiatric Press, Washington DC.

Stoudemire A, Beardsley G, Folks DG, et al. (1996) Psychological factors affecting physical condition (PFAPC). In DSM-IV Sourcebook, Vol. 2, Widiger TA, Frances AJ, Pincus HA, et al. (eds). American Psychiatric Association, Washington DC, pp. 1051–1078.

Strain JJ, Hammer JS, and Fulop G (1994) APM Task Force on psychosocial interventions in the general hospital inpatient setting: A review of cost-offset studies. Psychosomatics 35, 253–262.

Stronks DL, Tulen JH, Pepplinkhuizen L, et al. (1999) Personality traits and psychological reactions to mental stress of female migraine patients. Cephalagia 19, 566–574.

Sullivan MD, La Croix AZ, Baum C et al. (1997) Functional status in coronary artery disease: A one-year prospective study of the role of anxiety and depression. Am J Med 103, 348–356.

Takkouche B, Regueira C, and Gestal-Otero JJ (2001) A cohort study of stress and the common cold. Epidemiology 12, 345–349.

Tandberg E, Larsen JP, Aarsland D, et al. (1997) Risk factors for depression in Parkinson disease. Arch Neurol 54, 625–630.

Tay HP, Juma S, and Joseph AC (1996) Psychogenic impotence in spinal cord injury patients. Arch Phys Med Rehabil 77, 391–393.

Temoshok L, Heller BW, Sageviel RW, et al. (1985) The relationship of psychological factors of prognostic indicators in cutaneous malignant melanoma. J Psychosom Res 29, 138–153.

Ten Brinke A, Ouwerkerk ME, Zwinderman AH, et al. (2001) Psychopathology in patients with severe asthma is associated with increased health care utilization. Am J Respir Crit Care Med 163, 1093–1096.

Tony KH, Chung MD, Franzcog TK, et al. (2001) Antepartum depressive symptomatology is associated with adverse obstetric and neonatal outcomes. Psychosom Med 63, 830–834.

Trijsburg RW, van Knippenberg FC, and Rijpma SE (1992) Effects of psychological treatment on cancer patients: A critical review. Psychosom Med 54, 489–517.

Tschuschke V, Hertenstein B, Arnold R, et al. (2001) Associations between coping and survival time of adult leukemia patients receiving allogeneic bone marrow transplantation: Results of a prospective study. J Psychosom Res 50, 277–285.

Van Tilburg MA, McCaskill CC, Lane JD, et al. (2001) Depressed mood is a factor in glycemic control in type 1 diabetes. Psychosom Med 63, 551–555.

Viskin S and Belhassen B (1990) Idiopathic ventricular fibrillation. Am Heart J 120, 661–671.

Vogt T, Pope C, Mullooly J, et al. (1994) Mental health status as a predictor of morbidity and mortality: A 15-year follow-up of members of a health maintenance organization. Am J Pub Health 84, 227–231.

von Kanel R, Mills PJ, Fainman C, et al. (2001) Effects of psychological stress and psychiatric disorders on blood coagulation and fibrinolysis: A biobehavioral pathway to coronary artery disease? Psychosom Med, 63, 531–544.

Wales JK (1995) Does psychological distress cause diabetes? Diabet Med 12, 109–112.

Walker EA, Gelfand MD, Gelfand AN, et al. (1996) The relationship of current psychiatric disorder to functional disability and distress in patients with inflammatory bowel disease. Gen Hosp Psychiatr 18, 220–229.

Walker EA, Katon WJ, Roy-Byrne RP, et al. (1993) Histories of sexual victimization in patients with irritable bowel syndrome or inflammatory bowel disease. Am J Psychiatr 150, 1502–1506.

Walker EA, Roy-Byrne RP, and Katon WJ (1990) Irritable bowel syndrome and psychiatric illness. Am J Psychiatr 174, 565–572.

Watson M, Haviland JS, Greer S, et al. (1999) Influence of psychological response on survival in breast cancer: A population-based cohort study. Lancet 354, 1331–1336.

Waxler-Morrison N, Hislop TG, Mears B, et al. (1991) Effects of social relationships on survival for women with breast cancer: A prospective study. Soc Sci Med 33, 177–183.

Weiner H, Thaler M, Reiser MF, et al. (1957) Etiology of duodenal ulcer. I. Relation of specific psychological characteristics to rate of gastric secretion (serum pepsinogen). Psychosom Med 19, 1–10.

Wells KB, Stewart A, Mays RD, et al. (1989) The functioning and well-being of depressed patients. Results from the Medical Outcomes Study. JAMA 262, 914–919.

Wessely S, Hotoph M, and Sharpe M (1998) Oxford University Press, Oxford, UK.

Withers NJ, Rudkin ST, and White RJ (1999) Anxiety and depression in severe chronic obstructive pulmonary disease: The effects of pulmonary rehabilitation. J Cardiopulm Rehabil 19, 362–365.

Wolfe F (1999) Psychological distress and rheumatic disease. Scand J Rheumatol 28, 131–136.

Yang EV and Glaser R (2000) Stress-induced immunomodulation: Impact on immune defenses against infectious disease. Biomed Pharmacother 54, 245–250.

Yohannes AM, Baldwin RC, and Connolly MJ (2000) Depression and anxiety in elderly outpatients with chronic obstructive pulmonary disease: Prevalence and validation of the BASDEC screening questionnaire. Int J Geriatr Psychiatr 15, 1090–1096.

Yoshiuchi K, Kumano H, Nomura S, et al. (1998a) Stressful life events and smoking were associated with Graves' disease in women, but not in men. Psychsom Med 60, 182–185.

Yoshiuchi K, Kumano H, Nomura S, et al. (1998b) Psychological factors influencing the short-term outcome of antithyroid drug therapy in Graves' disease. Psychosom Med 60, 592–596.

Young L (1992) Psychological factors in rheumatoid arthritis. J Consult Clin Psychol 60, 619–627.

Ziegelstein RC, Fauerbach JA, Stevens SS, et al. (2000) Patients with depression are less likely to follow recommendations to reduce cardiac risk during recovery from a myocardial infarction. Arch Intern Med 160, 1818–1823.

Zorzon M, de Masi R, Nasuelli D, et al. (2001) Depression and anxiety in multiple sclerosis. A clinical and MRI study in 95 subjects. J Neurol 248, 416–421.

# 81    Medication-Induced Movement Disorders

Dilip V. Jeste
Christian R. Dolder

Neuroleptic-Induced Acute Dystonia
Neuroleptic-Induced Parkinsonism
Neuroleptic-Induced Acute Akathisia
Neuroleptic-Induced Tardive Dyskinesia
Neuroleptic Malignant Syndrome
Medication-Induced Postural Tremor

## Introduction

Modern medical practice presents physicians with choices of numerous medications to treat various ailments. Most medications have some side effects, and psychotropic medications are no exception. With the discovery of the antipsychotic effect of chlorpromazine in the early 1950s, psychiatry moved into the modern age of psychopharmacology, and there have been a number of advances since then. Along with these advances has come the awareness that many of these medications can produce disturbing side effects.

Perhaps the most uncomfortable side effects from psychotropic medications (especially antipsychotics or neuroleptics) are the acute and chronic movement disorders. Any psychiatrist in clinical practice has witnessed the intense distress that medication-induced movement disorders may bring to patients. Perhaps most disturbing is that unlike other medications, antipsychotics can produce "tardive" or late-occurring movement disorders that may be persistent or even irreversible. Patients in whom movement disorders develop may have more than subjective distress; they may suffer psychosocial embarrassment that makes them avoid being seen in public, and they may even suffer occupational impairment in severe cases. The responsibility this places on the prescribing psychiatrist is significant. Careful and reasoned thought must go into the analysis of whether the benefit of treatment with a medication exceeds the risk to the patient. This includes adequately explaining and obtaining informed consent from patients.

When a psychiatrist prescribes a medication that has the potential to induce a movement disorder, the physician–patient relationship becomes particularly important. Patients who require these medications are sometimes not amenable to trusting relationships (i.e., the paranoid patient). Working with a patient who has a psychotic illness requires that the psychiatrist establish a therapeutic bond with the patient.

## Historical Background

The presence of so-called extrapyramidal motor reactions to drugs was first described in the 1940s with reserpine. It was, however, in the early 1950s that attention was first focused on the motor effects of the antipsychotic drugs. In 1952, Delay and Deniker (1968) noticed extrapyramidal signs (EPS) after treatment with the antipsychotic medication chlorpromazine. Many of these EPS appeared similar to Parkinson's disease (PD), and some investigators proposed that the presence of EPS equated with the onset of antipsychotic benefit (Haase 1961).

Approximately 5 years after chlorpromazine was observed to be effective for psychotic disorders, Schonecker (1957) noted the onset of orobuccal dyskinesias after prolonged exposure to chlorpromazine. This condition lasted nearly 3 months after the medication was stopped. This was in marked contrast to the parkinsonism-like EPS that had been previously described to reverse on discontinuation of antipsychotics. Similar reports soon followed in France, England, Denmark, and the US (Lohr and Jeste 1988a). The term *tardive dyskinesia* (TD) was first used in 1964 by Faurbye and coworkers (1964) to describe this condition. The number of reports grew rapidly in a period of years, and many of the cases were reported to be irreversible.

## Classification

There are different types of movement disorders that may result from treatment with psychotropic (especially neuroleptic) medications. They can generally be divided into those that occur acutely or subacutely and those that occur late in treatment (tardive). For the purpose of this discussion, we group the movement disorders into the

| Table 81–1 | Time of Emergence of Neuroleptic-Induced Movement Disorders |
|---|---|
| Condition | Highest Risk of Emergence |
| Acute dystonia | Days 0–7 |
| Neuroleptic malignant syndrome | Days 0–7 (continues at lesser degree until end of first mo) |
| Akathisia | Days 7–14 (continues at lesser degree until 2.5 mo) |
| Parkinsonism | Days 14–30 (continues at lesser degree until 2.5 mo) |
| Tardive dyskinesia | Month 3* → onward (risk increases with increasing time on neuroleptic) |

*In patients older than 60 yr, month 1 → onward.

relatively acute neuroleptic-induced disorders (acute dystonia, parkinsonism, and akathisia), neuroleptic-induced TD, and neuroleptic malignant syndrome (NMS). We also devote a section to the discussion of medication-induced postural tremor that predominantly focuses on lithium-induced tremor. This covers the major diagnostic groupings contained within the *Diagnostic and Statistical Manual of Mental Disorders*, Fourth Edition, Text Revision (DSM-IV-TR) under the general title medication-induced movement disorders.

A time line for the emergence of the neuroleptic-induced movement disorders is provided in Table 81–1.

## Informed Consent and Medicolegal Issues

In general, the more a patient is able to understand the nature of his or her illness and the reason that a particular medication is being prescribed, the more likely he or she is to be adherent. When the psychiatrist does not devote adequate time to informing and instructing the patient, the result may be poor trust, poor communication, and possible legal difficulties for everyone involved. Unless declared incompetent by a court of law, a patient is considered to be legally competent to consent to or refuse psychotropic medications. The only exception to this rule is when an emergency situation exists and a patient must be medicated to prevent harm to self or others. The psychiatrist must provide information to the patient or the patient's decision-maker about the nature and purpose of the medication, its risks and benefits, alternatives to the proposed treatment, and prognosis without treatment (Wettstein 1988). Obtaining a written informed consent is one way of documenting the consent process. Another way is noting in the chart a summary of the discussion with a patient (or caregiver) about the consent to neuroleptic treatment.

Although the antipsychotics can produce unpleasant side effects, a patient who has been prepared openly and honestly for their possibility is more likely to view the side effects as evidence of the psychiatrist's excellent fund of knowledge rather than as a terrible surprise thrust on him or her by a dishonest or ignorant physician. On a final note, it may not be assumed that a patient already receiving antipsychotics prescribed by another physician has received an adequate informed consent. The process must begin anew with the new treating physician.

A new twist in the legal issues surrounding antipsychotic agents is the lower incidence of EPS and TD with atypical agents. The question of what is standard of care and how this relates to patients' prescribed conventional antipsychotics who are at a higher risk of developing a movement disorder such as TD presents interesting legal issues (Slovenko 2000).

In general, the literature continues to expand with trials demonstrating reduced incidence of new onset neuroleptic-induced movement disorders with atypical antipsychotics and at least partial improvement of existing movement disorders caused by conventional antipsychotics. While atypical antipsychotics are not without a risk of movement disorders, the improved motor side effect profile of the atypical agents provides a compelling argument for the use of atypical antipsychotics when initiating therapy, especially in susceptible populations such as the elderly. Switching to an atypical agent should be considered for those patients maintained on a conventional agent who develop or have a high risk of movement disorders.

## ACUTE NEUROLEPTIC-INDUCED MOVEMENT DISORDERS

A summary of the treatment of these disorders is provided in Table 81–2.

## Neuroleptic-Induced Acute Dystonia

### Definition
This long-lasting contraction or spasm of musculature develops in conjunction with the use of antipsychotic medication.

### Etiology and Pathophysiology
The pathophysiological mechanism of neuroleptic-induced acute dystonia is presently unknown. Because no consistent pathological abnormality has been located in the brain, dystonia was often regarded in the past as a disorder of psychogenic origin. There is currently no evidence to support psychological factors as being the source of dystonia.

In neuroleptic-induced dystonia, the finding that anticholinergic medication reverses the dystonia consistently may suggest that a hypercholinergic state is a correlate of dystonia (Rupniak et al. 1986, Burke et al. 1985). There is some suggestion of a correlation with changing blood–brain levels of antipsychotic medication (Miller and Jankovic 1992). It is also possible that dystonia is related to the changing ratio of dopamine $D_2$ to $D_1$ receptors that accompany the normal aging process (Wong et al. 1984).

Abnormalities in dopamine–acetylcholine balance have been suggested as a possible mechanism because cholinergic antagonists and dopaminergic agonists seem to improve the dystonia in many patients, in contrast to dopaminergic antagonists, which seem to exacerbate or even cause dystonia (Burke et al. 1985, Stahl and Berger 1982, Lang 1985, Fahn 1983). In contrast, other investigators have proposed that dopaminergic excess may be the responsible factor (Marsden and Jenner 1980).

### Epidemiology and Comorbidity
Acute dystonia is generally less common than most other extrapyramidal side effects of antipsychotics. Its frequency

| Table 81-2 | Treatment of Acute Neuroleptic-Induced Movement Disorders | | |
| --- | --- | --- | --- |
| Condition | First Choice | Second Choice | Third Choice |
| Acute dystonia | Anticholinergic medication, e.g., 2 mg benztropine PO, IM, IV 50 mg diphenhydramine PO, IM, IV | Benzodiazepine, e.g., lorazepam 1 mg IM, IV | — |
| Parkinsonism | Decrease neuroleptic to lowest effective dose; Consider change to lower potency neuroleptic | Anticholinergic, e.g., benztropine at 2 mg/d | Consider high-dose anticholinergic; Consider discontinuation of neuroleptic; Consider experimental treatment |
| Akathisia | | | |
| with high-potency neuroleptic | β-blocker, e.g., propranolol 10–30 mg t.i.d. | Anticholinergic, e.g., 2 mg/d benztropine | Benzodiazepine, e.g., lorazepam, e.g., 1 mg t.i.d. |
| with low-potency neuroleptic | β-blocker | Benzodiazepine | Anticholinergic |
| with other extrapyramidal signs | Anticholinergic | Anticholinergic plus β-blocker | Anticholinergic plus benzodiazepine |

*Source*: Data from Arana GW and Rosenbaum JF (2000) Handbook of Psychiatric Drug Therapy, 4th ed. Lippincott, Williams & Wilkins, Philadelphia, pp. 6–52.

has been reported to range from 2 to 12% of patients taking conventional antipsychotic medication (Lohr and Jeste 1988a). For patients who receive high doses of high-potency conventional agents, however, the frequency may be as high as 50% (Ayd 1961, Swett 1975). Incidence of acute dystonia can probably be reduced to approximately 2% if low-dose treatment strategies are employed (Rupniak et al. 1986). Furthermore, acute dystonia is considerably less likely to occur with atypical antipsychotic medications (i.e., less than

5% of individuals) (American Psychiatric Association 2000). For example, dystonic reactions occurred in less than 5% of patients in a study of ziprasidone (Tandon et al. 1997) and 1% in a dose comparison study with quetiapine (King et al. 1998).

Large doses of high-potency conventional antipsychotics appear to be the most consistent risk factor reported for acute dystonia (Rupniak et al. 1986). Other factors that also seem to predispose to dystonia are young age and male sex.

### DSM-IV-TR Criteria 333.7

**Neuroleptic-Induced Acute Dystonia**

A. One (or more) of the following signs or symptoms has developed in association with the use of neuroleptic medication:

(1) abnormal positioning of the head and neck in relation to the body (e.g., retrocollis, torticollis)

(2) spasms of the jaw muscles (trismus, gaping, grimacing)

(3) impaired swallowing (dysphagia), speaking, or breathing (laryngeal–pharyngeal spasm, dysphonia)

(4) thickened or slurred speech due to hypertonic or enlarged tongue (dysarthria, macroglossia) tongue protrusion or tongue dysfunction

(5) eyes deviated up, down, or sideward (oculogyric crisis)

(6) abnormal positioning of the distal limbs or trunk

B. The signs or symptoms in criterion A developed within 7 days of starting or rapidly raising the dose of neuroleptic medication, or of reducing a medication used to treat (or prevent) acute extrapyramidal symptoms (e.g., anticholinergic agents).

C. The symptoms in criterion A are not better accounted for by a mental disorder (e.g., catatonic symptoms in schizophrenia). Evidence that the symptoms are better accounted for by a mental disorder might include the following: the symptoms precede the exposure to neuroleptic medication or are not compatible with the pattern of pharmacological intervention (e.g., no improvement after neuroleptic lowering or anticholinergic administration).

D. The symptoms in criterion A are not due to a nonneuroleptic substance or to a neurological or other general medical condition. Evidence that the symptoms are due to a general medical condition might include the following: the symptoms precede the exposure to the neuroleptic medication, unexplained focal neurological signs are present, or the symptoms progress in the absence of change in medication.

Reprinted with permission from the Diagnostic and Statistical Manual of Mental Disorders, Fourth Edition, Text Revision. Copyright 2000 American Psychiatric Association.

A prior dystonic reaction is a good predictor of a repeated episode when the same antipsychotic at the same dose is reapplied (Keepers and Casey 1986).

## Assessment and Differential Diagnosis

Neuroleptic-induced dystonia (sometimes referred to as a dystonic reaction) usually begins 12 to 36 hours after a new antipsychotic is started or the dosage of a preexisting one is increased. It is unusual to see a dystonia after 2 weeks of antipsychotic treatment, and probably 90% of all neuroleptic-induced dystonias occur within the first 5 days of antipsychotic treatment (Ayd 1961). Patients may report a sense of tongue "thickness" or difficulty in swallowing in the 3 to 6 hours preceding the acute dystonia (Arana and Rosenbaum 2000).

Acute dystonia presents as a sustained, painful muscle spasm that produces twisting, squeezing, and pulling movements of the muscle groups involved. The most common muscle groups affected are the eyes, jaw, tongue, and neck, but any muscle group in the body can be involved. On occasion, the larynx or pharynx may be involved, and this can result in rapid respiratory compromise (American Psychiatric Association 2000).

Neuroleptic-induced acute dystonias are dramatic and usually easy to diagnose. There are, however, a number of other conditions that can present similarly and need to be ruled out. Spontaneously occurring focal or segmental dystonias may persist for days to weeks independent of medication. Neurological conditions such as temporal lobe seizures, infections, trauma, or tumors can produce symptoms similar to the neuroleptic-induced acute dystonia. A number of medications, while generally less common than antipsychotics, can cause dystonias (e.g., anticonvulsant medications and selective serotonin reuptake inhibitors) (American Psychiatric Association 2000).

Neuroleptic malignant syndrome (NMS) can produce muscle contractions that look similar to acute dystonia but can be distinguished by generalized "lead pipe" type of rigidity, fever, fluctuating consciousness, and unstable vital signs. Catatonia associated with an affective or psychotic disorder can be difficult to distinguish from dystonia clinically but does not respond to the administration of anticholinergic or antihistaminic medication. Furthermore, patients with catatonia are typically not concerned about their stiffness, whereas the patient with dystonia are likely to be extremely distressed (American Psychiatric Association 2000).

On occasion, an acute dystonic reaction may resemble tardive dyskinesia (TD). This is easily clarified by administering anticholinergic medications, which rapidly clear dystonia and do not affect (or may worsen) TD. Making a differential diagnosis between an acute dystonia and tardive dystonia can be difficult. Tardive dystonia (similar to TD) is a diagnosis made late in the course of antipsychotic treatment and is generally a chronic condition compared with acute dystonia, which occurs early in the course of medication treatment and typically responds rapidly to pharmacological intervention.

## Course

A neuroleptic-induced acute dystonia typically subsides spontaneously within hours after onset. However, treatment should be started as soon as the dystonia is diagnosed because the experience is "intensely" distressing to the patient.

## Treatment

The standard approach to treatment is the immediate administration of an anticholinergic or antihistaminic agent. In most cases, this medication may be administered orally, intramuscularly, or intravenously. The first dose of medication should be the equivalent of 2 mg of benztropine or 50 mg of diphenhydramine. This should be repeated if the first dose does not produce a robust response within 30 minutes (Lohr and Jeste 1988a). This standard approach is usually successful in resolving the dystonia.

In the unusual refractory case, intramuscular or intravenous anticholinergic or antihistaminic drugs should be used at more frequent dosing intervals, and consideration should be given to adding an intramuscular injection of lorazepam for additional sedation (Arana and Rosenbaum 2000). Since even the milder dystonias respond much more quickly to intramuscular or intravenous medication, it may therefore be worth avoiding the use of oral medication in treating dystonia. Oral medication takes much longer to work and is likely to result in unnecessarily prolonged distress of the patient.

In cases of laryngeal or pharyngeal dystonias with airway compromise, repeated dosing of medication should occur at shorter intervals until resolution is achieved. Arana and Rosenbaum (2000) recommended that the patient receive 4 mg of intravenous benztropine within 10 minutes followed by 1 to 2 mg of intravenous lorazepam. If airway compromise continues for any appreciable amount of time, emergent support from an anesthesiologist should be obtained and the patient should receive general anesthesia with airway protection. Fortunately, the need for such measures is rare.

After a dystonia, a patient should be maintained with oral anticholinergic or antihistaminic medication for at least 48 hours. If there is a history of previous dystonias, the medication should be continued for 2 weeks. Consideration should be given to decreasing the previous dose of the antipsychotic or possibly switching to a low-potency neuroleptic or atypical agent if the patient has been prescribed a conventional antipsychotic. The use of prophylactic anticholinergic medication will be discussed later.

## Neuroleptic-Induced Parkinsonism

### Definition

Neuroleptic-induced parkinsonism (NIP) is defined as parkinsonian signs or symptoms (tremor, muscle rigidity, or akinesia) that develop in association with the use of an antipsychotic medication.

### Etiology and Pathophysiology

NIP is presumed to result from blockade of postsynaptic dopamine ($D_2$) receptors in the corpus striatum causing a pathological state functionally resembling the loss of dopaminergic cells in the striatum in idiopathic Parkinson's disease (PD). However, it is not clear whether nigrostriatal dopamine loss is adequate to explain the clinical symptoms seen in NIP or PD (Lohr and Jeste 1988a). It is possible that

**Neuroleptic-Induced Parkinsonism**

A. One (or more) of the following signs or symptoms has developed in association with the use of neuroleptic medication:

   (1) parkinsonian tremor (i.e., a coarse, rhythmic, resting tremor with a frequency between 3 and 6 cycles per second, affecting the limbs, head, mouth, or tongue)

   (2) parkinsonian muscular rigidity (i.e., cogwheel rigidity or continuous "lead-pipe" rigidity)

   (3) akinesia (i.e., a decrease in spontaneous facial expressions, gestures, speech, or body movements)

B. The symptoms in criterion A developed within a few weeks of starting or raising the dose of a neuroleptic medication, or of reducing a medication used to treat (or prevent) acute extrapyramidal symptoms (e.g., anticholinergic agents).

C. The symptoms in criterion A are not better accounted for by a mental disorder (e.g., catatonic or negative symptoms in schizophrenia, psychomotor retardation in a major depressive episode). Evidence that the symptoms are better accounted for by a mental disorder might include the following: the symptoms precede the exposure to neuroleptic medication or are not compatible with the pattern of pharmacological intervention (e.g., no improvement after lowering the neuroleptic dose or administering anticholinergic medication).

D. The symptoms in criterion A are not due to a nonneuroleptic substance or to a neurological or other general medical condition (e.g., Parkinson's disease, Wilson's disease). Evidence that the symptoms are due to a general medical condition might include the following: the symptoms precede the exposure to neuroleptic medication, unexplained focal neurological signs are present, or the symptoms progress despite a stable medication regimen.

other neurochemical abnormalities may coexist with dopaminergic depletion to produce the syndrome. Abnormalities in norepinephrine and serotonin have also been reported to be involved in the mechanism (Hornykiewicz 1982, Mitchell et al. 1985, Langston and Irwin 1986).

Positron emission tomography (PET) and other technologies have been utilized to examine the relationship between $D_2$ receptor blockade in the basal ganglia with antipsychotic efficacy and NIP. Clinically effective doses of conventional antipsychotics have been shown to block 70 to 90% of $D_2$ receptors in the basal ganglia. Of note are findings that with conventional agents at least 60% occupancy is needed for satisfactory antipsychotic response but that NIP tends to occur with 80% or greater occupancy of the $D_2$ receptors (Glazer 2000, Farde et al. 1992, Kapur et al. 1998). With regard to atypical agents, the lower $D_2$ receptor blockade at recommended dosages with some agents and the serotonergic blockade seen with these medications are believed to lead to the reduced risk of NIP. Similar to conventional antipsychotics, higher doses of some atypical agents also appear to be related to an increase in NIP, as greater $D_2$ receptor blockade has been reported (Glazer 2000).

## Epidemiology and Comorbidity

The reported frequency of NIP varies 5 to 90%, depending on the study reviewed (Lohr and Jeste 1988a). This wide variation is due to different definitions of parkinsonism in different studies as well as the inclusion of mild bradykinesia as a sign of NIP in some investigations. The usual incidence of "clinically significant" NIP with conventional antipsychotics is 10 to 15% (Miller and Jankovic 1992). When, however, high-potency conventional agents are used without anticholinergic drugs and signs of rigidity are carefully assessed, one is likely to find that the majority of patients have some NIP. Rates of parkinsonism induced by atypical antipsychotics are considerably lower (American Psychiatric Association 2000). The incidence of NIP in older psychiatric patients is considerably greater. A study of newly medicated older patients on low doses of conventional antipsychotics found 32% of patients met criteria for NIP (Caligiuri et al. 1999). In an investigation of extrapyramidal side effects in patients with Alzheimer disease treated with very low dose conventional antipsychotics, 67% of patients met criteria for NIP at some time during the 9-month follow-up period (Caligiuri et al. 1998).

A number of patient-related and medication-related risk factors have been proposed. A history of prior episodes of NIP, older age, and concomitant dementia or delirium are thought to predispose to NIP (American Psychiatric Association 2000). Neuroleptic potency and preexisting extrapyramidal symptoms may also increase the risk of NIP (Sweet et al. 1994, Caligiuri and Lohr 1997, Chakos et al. 1992).

Rapid increases in antipsychotic dosage, administration of higher absolute doses of antipsychotics, and absence of concurrent anticholinergic medication represent other risk factors for NIP initiation (American Psychiatric Association 2000). Highly anticholinergic antipsychotics (i.e., chlorpromazine and thioridazine) are less likely to cause NIP than less anticholinergic agents (i.e., haloperidol and fluphenazine).

## Assessment and Differential Diagnosis

NIP symptoms may develop quickly after the initiation of an antipsychotic or insidiously during the course of treatment. It most typically develops 2 to 4 weeks after antipsychotic initiation. The three cardinal symptoms of NIP are tremor, muscle rigidity, and akinesia.

Parkinsonian tremor is a steady, rhythmical, oscillatory motion generally at an alternating rhythm of 3 to 6 Hz. The most affected body area tends to be the upper extremities, but the tremor may spread to the head, neck, jaw, face, tongue, legs, and trunk. The tremor is typically suppressed during action and increases during times of anxiety, stress, or fatigue (American Psychiatric Association 2000).

Parkinsonian muscle rigidity appears clinically as a firmness and spasm of muscles at rest that may affect all skeletal muscles or be confined to just a few specific muscle groups. It can appear as a continuous lead pipe-type rigidity that resists movement or a cogwheel-type rigidity that presents a "ratchet-like" resistance when a muscle is moved around a joint. Cogwheeling may represent an extremely high frequency (8–12 Hz) "action" tremor that is physiologically imposed on the rigidity (Lance and McLeod 1981). The psychiatrist may diagnose cogwheel rigidity by placing his or her hand over the joint that is being passively moved. Generalized muscle pain, body aches, and discoordination are features associated with NIP rigidity (American Psychiatric Association 2000).

Parkinsonian akinesia is seen clinically as decreased spontaneous motor activity and a global slowness in the initiation and execution of movements. It can be associated with drooling, bent over neck, stooped shoulders, and masked facial expression (the so-called masked facies) (American Psychiatric Association 2000).

Parkinsonism occurs in numerous medical and neurological conditions and can be caused by many medications or substances. Idiopathic PD can be difficult to distinguish from NIP and we refer the reader to Hausner (1983) for methods of attempting to make a differential diagnosis between the two conditions.

The tremor of NIP must be distinguished from tremor caused by other conditions. In general, nonparkinsonian tremors are finer, faster, and worse on intention. Tremor associated with substance withdrawal typically presents with associated hyperreflexia and increased autonomic signs. Cerebellar disease-induced tremor may present with associated nystagmus, ataxia, or scanning speech. Strokes and other central nervous system lesions usually have associated focal neurological symptoms. NMS can often present with akinesia and lead pipe-type rigidity but also has other associated findings, such as fever, elevated creatine kinase, and fluctuating consciousness (American Psychiatric Association 2000).

Tremor in neuroleptic-induced TD does not typically have the steady rhythm associated with NIP. In the past, it has been hypothesized that NIP and TD would not be likely to coexist in the same patient. If true, this would provide another means of making a differential diagnosis between the two conditions. A review and a study by Caligiuri and colleagues (1991) do not support this hypothesis, however, and it appears that TD and NIP frequently coexist in the same patient.

A number of primary psychiatric illnesses may mimic symptoms of NIP and may be difficult to separate. These include major depressive disorder, catatonic-type schizophrenia, mood disorder with catatonic features, schizophrenia with a predominance of negative features, delirium, dementia, anxiety disorders, and certain conversion disorders (American Psychiatric Association 2000). It may be particularly easy to confuse negative symptoms of schizophrenia and depression with the akinesia and rigidity of NIP. Catatonia and NIP may also be difficult to differentiate, and there is evidence that the two conditions are related to each other (Lohr et al. 1987b). Often, the diagnosis of NIP should be made provisionally and clarified by a dosage reduction of antipsychotic or trial of anticholinergic medication (American Psychiatric Association 2000).

## Course

NIP symptoms usually continue unchanged or diminish slowly in 2 to 3 months after onset. The signs and symptoms typically improve with a dose reduction, discontinuation of antipsychotic medication, or switch to an atypical antipsychotic in patients previously receiving a conventional antipsychotic. Improvement is also seen with the addition of antiparkinsonian agents.

## Treatment

Many milder cases of NIP do not require treatment because they are not bothersome to the patient. A switch to an atypical agent should be strongly considered if troublesome NIP develops while on a conventional antipsychotic. Large randomized controlled trials have demonstrated reductions in parkinsonian symptoms in patients treated with atypical antipsychotics (Arvanitis et al. 1997, Beasley et al. 1997, Chouinard et al. 1993, Simpson and Lindenmayer 1997, Kane et al. 1988a). If symptoms become troublesome, the initial step should be to decrease the dose of antipsychotic to the lowest effective dose for the patient. The next step is to add a low dosage of an anticholinergic medication. The equivalent of 2 mg/day of benztropine generally represents a reasonable starting point. Periodic attempts should be made to wean the patient from the anticholinergic agent. As many as 90% of patients do not require anticholinergic medication at the end of 3 months (Coleman and Hays 1975, Johnson 1978). Anticholinergic medication should always be tapered slowly to avoid the rapid redevelopment of parkinsonian symptoms as well as the possibility of uncomfortable cholinergic rebound symptoms.

Refractory cases of NIP do occur and may require more aggressive management. Increasing the dose of the anticholinergic medication is a good starting point because some patients may require up to the equivalent of 20 mg/day of benztropine to achieve relief from NIP. If such high doses are to be employed, they should be used for the shortest possible time, and rigorous attention should be paid to the possibility of untoward anticholinergic effects (i.e., delirium, urinary retention, fecal impaction). Consideration may be given to starting a dopamine-releasing agent, such as amantadine or perhaps even levodopa. A major concern with this treatment approach is the possibility of exacerbating the psychosis for which the antipsychotic medication was prescribed in the first place. Trials of dopaminergic agents are therefore best attempted in an inpatient setting or with careful outpatient observation and assessment. A number of experimental treatment strategies have been proposed for the treatment of the refractory cases including vitamin E, calcium supplementation, electroconvulsive therapy, and L-deprenyl (Osser 1992).

Another treatment approach for the refractory case is to lower the dose of the antipsychotic medication or even discontinue it until the NIP resolves, then resume the antipsychotic (preferably a different one) at a lower dose. This treatment strategy may also need to be carried out in an inpatient setting to monitor early emergence of psychotic symptoms.

## Neuroleptic-Induced Acute Akathisia

### Definition
Neuroleptic-induced acute akathisia is defined as a subjective feeling of restlessness and an intensely unpleasant need to move occurring secondary to antipsychotic treatment.

### Etiology and Pathophysiology
The pathophysiological mechanism of akathisia remains unknown. A number of theories have been offered by investigators. Early theories about the etiology of akathisia proposed that it represented a subjective response to the presence of the rigidity and akinesia of NIP (Tarsy 1992). Akathisia has also been suggested to be a primary sensory disturbance in which motor disturbance occurs as a direct response to the sensory disturbance (Sovner and Dimascio 1978). In contrast, others have proposed that akathisia simply represents another EPS because it frequently occurs with other EPS and is often reversed by anticholinergic medications.

Marsden and Jenner (1980) suggested that dopamine blockade in the mesocortical system may account for the hyperactive symptoms of akathisia. Mesocortical dopaminergic neurons that innervate the prefrontal cortex seem to be resistant to depolarization induced by long-term antipsychotic treatment, suggesting a possible explanation for why akathisia often does not improve with time (Lohr and Jeste 1988a).

The possibility that excessive noradrenergic activity plays a role in the pathogenesis of akathisia is supported by the efficacy of beta-adrenergic blockers in improving some cases of akathisia. Additionally, opioid mechanisms have been proposed to contribute to akathisia on the basis of reported therapeutic effects of opioid drugs (Walters et al. 1986). The lower likelihood of akathisia with atypical antipsychotics and reports of selective serotonin reuptake inhibitors causing akathisia have implicated serotonin as having a possible role in akathisia, however this is still under investigation (Miller and Fleischhacker 2000).

### Epidemiology and Comorbidity
Akathisia is a common side effect of antipsychotic treatment. It is estimated to occur in 20 to 75% of all patients treated with conventional agents. The wide discrepancy in reported prevalence may result from a lack of consistency in the definition of akathisia, different prescribing practices, different study designs, and differences in population demographics (American Psychiatric Association 2000). While atypical antipsychotics are less likely to cause akathisia compared to typical agents (Arvanitis et al. 1997, Tollefson et al. 1997), prevalence rates have varied (Miller and Fleischhacker 2000). Clozapine-induced akathisia has ranged from 0 to 39% (Safferman et al. 1993, Kurz et al. 1998, Cohen et al. 1991) and a point prevalence of 13% was reported for risperidone (Miller et al. 1998). Akathisia is thought by many psychiatrists to be a leading cause of nonadherence.

---

**DSM-IV-TR Criteria** 333.99

**Neuroleptic-Induced Acute Akathisia**

A. The development of subjective complaints of restlessness after exposure to a neuroleptic medication.

B. At least one of the following is observed:

   (1) fidgety movements or swinging of the legs

   (2) rocking from foot to foot while standing

   (3) pacing to relieve restlessness

   (4) inability to sit or stand for at least several minutes

C. The onset of the symptoms in criteria A and B occurs within 4 weeks of initiating or increasing the dose of the neuroleptic, or of reducing medication used to treat (or prevent) acute extrapyramidal symptoms (e.g., anticholinergic agents).

D. The symptoms in criterion A are not better accounted for by a mental disorder (e.g., schizophrenia, substance withdrawal, agitation from a major depressive or manic episode, hyperactivity in attention-deficit/hyperactivity disorder). Evidence that symptoms may be better accounted for by a mental disorder might include the following: the onset of symptoms preceding the exposure to the neuroleptics, the absence of increasing restlessness with increasing neuroleptic doses, and the absence of relief with pharmacological interventions (e.g., no improvement after decreasing the neuroleptic dose or treatment with medication intended to treat the akathisia).

E. The symptoms in criterion A are not due to a nonneuroleptic substance or to a neurological or other general medical condition. Evidence that symptoms are due to a general medical condition might include the onset of the symptoms preceding the exposure to neuroleptics or the progression of symptoms in the absence of a change in medication.

Reprinted with permission from the Diagnostic and Statistical Manual of Mental Disorders, Fourth Edition, Text Revision. Copyright 2000 American Psychiatric Association.

---

Higher doses of high-potency conventional antipsychotics appear to be most frequently associated with the appearance of akathisia (American Psychiatric Association 2000). Previous episodes of neuroleptic-induced akathisia increase the risk for future episodes if antipsychotics are restarted.

### Assessment and Differential Diagnosis
Akathisia tends to occur within the first 4 weeks of initiating or increasing the dose of antipsychotic medication. It can

develop rapidly after the initiation or the dose increase of an antipsychotic. Patients with akathisia tend to have subjective complaints of "inner restlessness," most often in the legs. It may be difficult for the patients to describe their feelings. They feel that they must move, and this manifests as fidgeting, frequent changes in posture, crossing and uncrossing of the legs, rocking while sitting, and shuffling when walking (American Psychiatric Association 2000).

Akathisia is often associated with severe dysphoria, anxiety, and irritability. When the akathisia is particularly severe, aggression or suicide attempts may be a possible result, although this is controversial. Akathisia in a psychotic patient can easily be mistaken for worsening of psychotic features, resulting in an increase in antipsychotic dose and an exacerbation of the akathisia.

The strange subjective discomfort associated with akathisia is the feature that seems to be most useful in making a differential diagnosis between neuroleptic-induced akathisia and other neuroleptic-induced movement disorders. TD is often associated with a lack of sensory perception of having a movement disorder. This contrasts with akathisia in which patients tend to be acutely aware of their distress. When patients with TD are uncomfortable, it is usually a result of social factors such as embarrassment and functional factors such as frustration over not being able to perform certain tasks. Another differentiating factor is that TD usually involves the face, mouth, and upper extremities, whereas akathisia more commonly involves the lower extremities.

The rhythmical appearance of akathisia may sometimes suggest a tremorous condition. Thus, the tremor of NIP and idiopathic PD may be mistaken for akathisia, especially if the feet and legs are involved. Iron deficiency anemia can also present with symptoms phenomenologically similar to neuroleptic-induced akathisia. A number of other medications but particularly selective serotonin reuptake inhibitor antidepressant medications may produce akathisia clinically identical to that produced by antipsychotics (American Psychiatric Association 2000).

It is critical to differentiate akathisia from other psychiatric disorders presenting with agitation, such as depressive episodes, manic episodes, anxiety disorders, schizophrenia, dementia, delirium, substance intoxication or withdrawal, and attention-deficit/hyperactivity disorder. The reason for the importance of this differentiation is that mistaking akathisia for a primary psychiatric disorder can result in an intervention that would be the exact opposite of what is appropriate (i.e., increasing the dose of an antipsychotic instead of decreasing it because akathisia is mistaken for worsening psychosis) (American Psychiatric Association 2000).

### Course
Neuroleptic-induced akathisia typically lasts as long as antipsychotic treatment is continued but may have variable intensity in time (American Psychiatric Association 2000). Treatment of akathisia may or may not alter the course of the akathisia.

### Treatment
Akathisia may be difficult to treat effectively. The best initial approach is to try and reduce the chance of developing akathisia by minimizing the dosage of antipsychotic medication. The use of atypical antipsychotics should be considered as a result of their lower risk of akathisia (Sachdev et al. 1995). If using conventional antipsychotics, a switch to a low-potency agent such as thioridazine or chlorpromazine may prove helpful because these antipsychotics seem to have somewhat lower propensity to cause akathisia than high-potency conventional antipsychotics. After these initial steps, consideration should be given to initiation of an anti-akathisic drug regimen. A number of agents have been reported to be effective, including beta-adrenergic blockers, anticholinergic drugs, benzodiazepines, and clonidine (American Psychiatric Association 2000).

When choosing an agent to treat akathisia, a beta-blocker such as propranolol should generally be considered first-line as its efficacy has been proven and it has been shown to be superior to other possible treatments such as benztropine and lorazepam (Adler et al. 1986, 1987, 1993a). In terms of antiakathisic effects, the beta-blocker chosen should be lipophilic so as to cross the blood–brain barrier and should also have activity at the beta-2 receptor (Miller and Fleischhacker 2000). Benzodiazepines such as clonazepam and lorazepam have been shown to be efficacious in the treatment of akathisia and are also a reasonable therapeutic option, especially when considering the interplay between anxiety and akathisia, however, their side effects and abuse potential should be considered. Anticholinergic agents such as benztropine may also be tried, but less evidence exists to supports their use. A limited number of studies have also shown possible roles for clonidine and amantadine in the treatment of akathisia (Miller and Fleischhacker 2000). Agents with serotonin receptor blocking activity (i.e., ritanserine, mianserin) have also been reported to be of benefit in akathisia (Bersani et al. 1990, Poyurovsky et al. 1999).

## PROPHYLACTIC ANTICHOLINERGIC MEDICATION?

One issue that remains controversial among researchers and psychiatrists is whether preventive anticholinergic medication should be given to patients who are starting antipsychotics. Arguments against this practice include the risk of anticholinergic side effects such as dry mouth, blurry vision, constipation, and urinary retention. Further, anticholinergic medication is associated with cognitive side effects, such as memory impairment, confusion, and delirium (Simpson 1970, McClelland et al. 1974, Dimascio and Demergian 1970, Raleigh 1977, Syndulko et al. 1981). The relationship between anticholinergic medications and TD is not definitive (Kiloh et al. 1973, Jeste and Caligiuri 1993).

Arguments in favor of initiating prophylactic anticholinergic therapy point to the decrease in the frequency of EPS (including dystonias, akathisia, and akinesia) when anticholinergic drugs are prescribed prophylactically (Stern and Anderson 1979, Winslow et al. 1986). Furthermore, medication nonadherence and decompensation may relate to inadequately treated NIP, especially akathisia and akinesia (Rifkin et al. 1975, 1978, Van Putten 1975, Van Putten et al. 1974). With the introduction and increased use of atypical antipsychotics, the risk of EPS and TD has decreased, thus reducing the need for prophylactic anticholinergic medication for many patients prescribed atypical agents.

Although this complicated issue remains unresolved, some basic guidelines can be proposed. When psychosis is severe and unmanageable and adherence with medications needs to be rigorously enforced, antipsychotic and anticholinergic medication may be administered concurrently, with the anticholinergic medication tapered slowly within the next few weeks. When the psychosis is milder and antipsychotic medication may be gradually increased, it may be best to avoid anticholinergic medications until such time as they become clinically necessary. In patients with any degree of cognitive impairment (especially the elderly or demented patient with agitation or psychosis), it is best to aim for the administration of less anticholinergic medication. In younger patients, especially young men (who have a high frequency of dystonia), it may be preferable to use anticholinergic medication prophylactically because it may prevent an uncomfortable dystonic reaction and can generally be used with relative impunity of serious side effects. In general, long-term prophylactic use of anticholinergic medication is not recommended (Ungvari et al. 1999) nor its use in the elderly (Mamo et al. 1999).

## NEUROLEPTIC-INDUCED TARDIVE DYSKINESIA

### Definition
Neuroleptic-induced tardive dyskinesia (TD) is a syndrome consisting of abnormal, involuntary movements caused by long-term treatment with antipsychotic medication. The movements are typically choreoathetoid in nature and principally involve the mouth, face, limbs, and trunk. TD, by definition, occurs late in the course of drug treatment.

### Etiology and Pathophysiology
Historically, striatal dopamine receptor supersensitivity had been proposed to be responsible for TD. It now seems more likely that a number of separate neurotransmitter systems are involved in the pathogenesis of TD. There may be different subtypes of TD, each perhaps involving a unique profile of neurochemical imbalance (Jeste and Wyatt 1982).

Neuroleptic-induced striatal pathological change represents another possibility for explaining mechanisms of TD (Jeste et al. 1992). Lohr and Jeste (1988b) suggested that long-term antipsychotic use may produce "toxic free radicals" that damage neurons and result in persistent TD.

### Epidemiology and Comorbidity
The reported prevalence of TD has been somewhat variable as a result of differences in populations of patients and in the methods used (Jeste and Wyatt 1981). Yassa and Jeste (1992) reviewed 76 studies of the prevalence of TD published from 1960 to 1990. In a total population of approximately 40,000 patients, the overall prevalence of TD was 24.2%, although it was much higher (about 50%) in studies of elderly patients treated with antipsychotics.

There have been relatively few studies of the incidence of TD. Kane and coworkers (1988b) prospectively studied more than 850 patients (mean age 29 years) and found the incidence of TD after cumulative exposure to conventional antipsychotics to be 5% after 1 year, 18.5% after 4 years,

**DSM-IV-TR Criteria** 333.82

**Neuroleptic-Induced Tardive Dyskinesia**

A. Involuntary movements of the tongue, jaw, trunk, or extremities have developed in association with the use of neuroleptic medication.

B. The involuntary movements are present over a period of at least 4 weeks and occur in any of the following patterns:

(1) choreiform movements (i.e., rapid, jerky, nonrepetitive)

(2) athetoid movements (i.e., slow, sinuous, continual)

(3) rhythmic movements (i.e., stereotypies)

C. The signs or symptoms in criteria A and B develop during exposure to a neuroleptic medication or within 4 weeks of withdrawal from an oral (or within 8 weeks of withdrawal from a depot) neuroleptic medication.

D. There has been exposure to neuroleptic medication for at least 3 months (1 month if age 60 years or older).

E. The symptoms are not due to a neurological or general medical condition (e.g., Huntington's disease, Sydenham's chorea, spontaneous dyskinesia, hyperthyroidism, Wilson's disease), ill-fitting dentures, or exposure to other medications that cause acute reversible dyskinesia (e.g., L-dopa, bromocriptine). Evidence that the symptoms are due to one of these etiologies might include the following: the symptoms precede the exposure to the neuroleptic medication or unexplained focal neurological signs are present.

F. The symptoms are not better accounted for by a neuroleptic-induced acute movement disorder (e.g., neuroleptic-induced acute dystonia, neuroleptic-induced acute akathisia).

Reprinted with permission from the Diagnostic and Statistical Manual of Mental Disorders, Fourth Edition, Text Revision. Copyright 2000 American Psychiatric Association.

and 40% after 8 years. Incidence in older populations has been found to be much higher. Saltz and colleagues (1991) reported an incidence of 31% after 43 weeks of conventional antipsychotic treatment in a population of elderly patients. Jeste and colleagues (1995, 1999c) evaluated 439 psychiatric patients with a mean age of 65 years and found that 28.8% of the sample met criteria for TD during the first 12 months of study treatment; 50.1% had TD by the end of 24 months, and 63.1% by the end of 36 months. The risk of severe TD has also been reported to be higher in older patients (Caligiuri et al. 1997).

Evidence supporting a reduced risk of TD with atypical antipsychotics is beginning to emerge. The lower risk of EPS with atypical agents has led to the widespread conclusion that these agents will also have reduced TD risk. The low risk of tardive dyskinesia in clozapine-treated individuals has been well established (Kane et al. 1993). In addition, a lower incidence of TD has been reported in patients treated with risperidone (Jeste et al. 1999a, 1999b, Chouinard et al. 1993) and olanzapine (Tollefson et al. 1997). More long-term prospective studies are needed with the atypical agents.

Aging consistently appears to be the most important risk factor for the development of TD. Prevalence and severity of TD seem to increase with age (Smith and Baldessarini 1980). The reasons for this increased risk of TD with aging are not known but may be related to the propensity of the nigrostriatal system to degenerate with age as well as pharmacokinetic and pharmacodynamic factors (Jeste and Caligiuri 1993).

Gender (female) was thought to be a risk factor for TD. A meta-analysis of the published reports demonstrated a greater prevalence of TD in women (26.6%) compared with that in men (21.6%) (Yassa and Jeste 1992). Interestingly, studies of incidence of TD in older patients failed to confirm the reported propensity of women to have TD at a higher rate than men (Saltz et al. 1991, Jeste et al. 1995). A possible relationship between gender and age of onset of schizophrenia to severity of dyskinesia has been reported as women with late-onset schizophrenia (LOS) and men with early-onset schizophrenia (EOS) had more severe dyskinesia that men with LOS and women with EOS (Lindamer et al. 2001).

Mood disorders (especially unipolar depression) have been reported to be risk factors for TD in a number of publications, although findings have been mixed (Kane et al. 1988b, Saltz et al. 1991, Casey 1988, Casey and Keepers 1988, Jeste et al. 1995).

There are conflicting reports regarding ethnicity as a risk factor for TD. In a study of 491 chronic psychiatric patients, no significant differences in TD prevalence were found among blacks, whites, and Hispanics (Sramek et al. 1991). Higher incidence rate of TD in African-Americans than in whites, however, was reported by Morgenstern and Glazer (1993) and, to a smaller extent, by Lacro and Jeste (1997). There is some evidence that Asian patients may have the lowest prevalence rate of TD.

People with diabetes mellitus may be at a higher risk for development of TD (Ganzini et al. 1991, Woerner et al. 1993). Sewell and Jeste (1992a) proposed that diabetes mellitus might be a risk factor for TD in patients treated with metoclopramide.

The presence of dementia or delirium may or may not be a risk factor for TD. Yassa and associates (1984) determined central nervous system damage predisposed to TD, but two prospective TD studies of older patients found organic diagnosis not to be associated with TD susceptibility (Saltz et al. 1991, Jeste et al. 1995).

Patients who experience an acute neuroleptic-induced movement disorder (especially parkinsonism or akathisia) are likely to be at a greater risk for development of TD if antipsychotic treatment is continued (Kane et al. 1992).

Total exposure to typical antipsychotic agents has been correlated with TD risk (Casey 1997) and within elderly populations, cumulative amount of typical antipsychotics has also been associated with TD risk, especially with high-potency conventional agents (Jeste et al. 1995).

The observation that anticholinergic drugs exacerbate some symptoms of TD does not appear to indicate that the drugs promote the onset of the disorder (Gardos and Cole 1983).

## Assessment and Differential Diagnosis

TD may develop at any age and typically has an insidious onset. It may develop during exposure to antipsychotic medication or within 4 weeks of withdrawal from an oral antipsychotic (or within 8 weeks of withdrawal from a depot neuroleptic). There must be a history of at least 3 months of antipsychotic use (or 1 month in the elderly) before TD may be diagnosed (American Psychiatric Association 2000).

The most common features of TD are involuntary movements of the tongue, face, and neck muscles. Less common are movements in the upper and lower extremities as well as in the trunk (Brandon et al. 1971, Edwards 1970, Guy et al. 1986). Most rare of all are involuntary movements of the muscle groups involved with breathing and swallowing. The earliest symptoms typically involve buccolingual–masticatory movements. The movements of TD are choreiform (rapid, jerky), athetoid (slow, sinuous), or rhythmical (stereotypical) (American Psychiatric Association 2000).

Severe choreoathetoid dyskinesia differs from the milder forms, mainly in the frequency and amplitude of the abnormal movements (Gardos and Cole 1992). Some cases of severe dyskinesia consist of generalized choreoathetosis of the face, trunk, and all four limbs (Gardos et al. 1987, Mann et al. 1983, Casey and Rabins 1978). TD may be accompanied by dystonias (Tarsy et al. 1977, Nasrallah et al. 1980, McLean and Casey 1978), parkinsonism, (Brandon et al. 1971, Bitton and Melamed 1984) and akathisia (Brandon et al. 1971, Chouinard and Bradwein 1982).

TD is worsened by stimulants, short-term withdrawal of antipsychotic medication, anticholinergic medication, emotional arousal, stress, and voluntary movements of other parts of the body. It is improved by relaxation, voluntary movements of the involved parts of the body, sleep, and increased dose of antipsychotics.

The differential diagnosis of TD is extensive. The major task for the psychiatrist is to rule out other causes of dyskinesia. It may be useful for the psychiatrist to keep in mind three questions for the facilitation of the differential diagnosis: (1) Does the patient have dyskinesia? (2) Does another disorder fully explain the cause of the dyskinesia? (3) If the dyskinesia is related to antipsychotic use, is it TD? (Jeste and Wyatt 1982).

A number of nondyskinetic movement disorders are part of the differential diagnosis of TD. Tremor can be confused with TD, including the tremor of neuroleptic-induced parkinsonism, rabbit syndrome, Wilson's disease, and cerebellar disease. Further, fine tremors of the fingers and hands are produced by anxiety states, alcoholism, hyperthyroidism, and drugs. Acute dystonias, myoclonus, tics, mannerisms, compulsions, and akathisia must be differentiated from TD. The differentiation is made on the basis of the clinical assessment. For further details, the reader is referred to Jeste and Wyatt (1982).

Once it has been established that the patient suffers from a dyskinesia, the main cause must be determined. In children and young adults, a number of conditions may cause dyskinesia besides antipsychotic treatment. The use of drugs, especially amphetamines and antihistamines, are associated with dyskinesia. Sydenham's chorea can produce choreiform movements. Conversion disorder and malingering are conditions that can present with apparently involuntary movements. Hyperthyroidism and hypoparathyroidism are two endocrinological conditions that can produce dyskinesias similar to TD. Huntington's disease is a condition that can be difficult to distinguish clinically from TD, but certain characteristics may aid in the diagnosis, including (1) a family history of Huntington's disease, (2) the presence of dementia, (3) a slowly progressive downhill course, and (4) atrophy of the caudate nucleus on computed tomography scan.

In the middle-aged or elderly patient, denture or dental problems may commonly mimic TD. Lesions of the basal ganglia may result in dyskinesias. The use of antiparkinsonian medications such as levodopa, amantadine, and bromocriptine can cause dyskinetic movements. The presence of spontaneous dyskinesias must also be ruled out.

When it has been established that antipsychotics are responsible for the dyskinesia, it does not follow that the dyskinesia is necessarily TD. Acute dyskinesia occurring early in antipsychotic treatment is common and responds well to antihistaminic or anticholinergic medications. Withdrawal–emergent dyskinesia also occurs in a variable proportion of patients. This phenomenon refers to the appearance or worsening of dyskinetic movements on reduction or discontinuation of antipsychotic medication. Withdrawal–emergent dyskinesia is phenomenologically similar to TD and often has the full range of involuntary choreiform and athetoid movements. A typical case may begin within a few days after a sudden decrease in dosage and worsen as the antipsychotic is withdrawn. This phase is followed by rapid improvement in a period of weeks to months. A history of antipsychotic exposure and remission of dyskinetic symptoms within 3 months of antipsychotic withdrawal are suggestive of the diagnosis of withdrawal–emergent dyskinesia (Gerhard 1992).

Finally, tardive Tourette's disorder must be differentiated from TD. A number of cases of tardive Tourette's disorder have been reported as a result of treatment with antipsychotics, emerging during treatment or after cessation of treatment (Jeste and Wyatt 1982, Klawans et al. 1978, DeVaugh-Geiss 1980, Stahl 1980, Seeman et al. 1981, Muller and Aminoff 1982, Munetz et al. 1985). Tardive Tourette's disorder presents with symptoms similar to those of idiopathic Tourette's disorder. Motor tics are usually compulsive organized stereotypies that may, in certain cases, be difficult to distinguish from the choreoathetoid movements of TD. Typically, vocal tics (including barks, grunts, coughs, and yelps) represent part of tardive Tourette's disorder but not TD. Tardive Tourette's disorder seems to show a pharmacological response similar to that of TD, leading to the assumption that the syndrome may be a type of the more commonly seen TD. Thus, tardive Tou-

rette's disorder may be masked by an increase in antipsychotics and exacerbated by withdrawal (Jeste et al. 1986).

## Course

One-third of the TD patients experience remission within 3 months of discontinuation of antipsychotic medication, and approximately half have remission within 12 to 18 months of antipsychotic discontinuation (American Psychiatric Association 2000). Elderly patients are reported to have lower rates of remission, especially if antipsychotics are continued. When TD patients must be maintained with antipsychotics, TD seems to be stable in 50%, worsen in 25%, and improve in the rest.

Time may be the most important factor in outcome of TD. In studies that have followed up patients for longer than 5 years, TD seems to improve in half of patients with or without antipsychotic treatment. Furthermore, TD may improve as slowly as it develops and may exist on a spectrum between resolution and persistence (Kane et al. 1992).

Severe TD may lead to numerous physical complications and psychosocial problems. Dental and denture problems are common sequelae of severe oral dyskinesia (Yassa and Jones 1985), as are ulcerations of the tongue, cheeks, and lips. Hyperkinetic dysarthria has been described by Maxwell and coworkers (1970) and Portnoy (1979). Swallowing disorders represent another complication (Massengil and Nashold 1952). Respiratory disturbances, although fairly rare, have been reported by a number of investigators (Casey and Rabins 1978, Ayd 1979, Jackson et al. 1980, Weiner et al. 1978). These disturbances are usually manifested by shortness of breath at rest, irregularities in respiration, and various grunts, snorts, and gasps. Respiratory alkalosis may be seen on laboratory tests. Gastrointestinal complications of severe TD may involve vomiting and dysphagia secondary to disruption of the normal activity of the esophagus (Yassa and Jones 1985); weight loss may result from such a disturbance.

Subjective distress is a common accompaniment of severe dyskinesia. Suicidal ideation may result from distress over the dyskinesia, and there have been reports of some successful suicides. General impairment of functioning may be related to the severity of the dyskinetic disorder. Social embarrassment as a result of TD may represent a reason that some patients with TD tend to be reluctant to leave their homes. Even mild dyskinesia may lead to anxiety, guilt, shame, and anger. These symptoms can lead to severe depressive episodes (Yassa and Jones 1985).

## Treatment

Despite intense effort, there is as yet no consistently reliable therapy for TD. As a result, the psychiatrist must focus primary efforts toward prevention of the disorder. The use of atypical antipsychotics are recommended due to their probable lower risk of TD. Antipsychotic use should be minimized in all patients. Patients with nonpsychotic mood or other disorders who need antipsychotics should receive the minimal necessary amounts of antipsychotic treatment and should have the medication tapered and then stopped once the clinical need is no longer present. In general, there must be enough clinical evidence to show that the benefits outweigh the potential risks of TD development (Arana and Rosenbaum 2000). Antipsychotics should be used with particular caution in elderly patients because of their high risk for development of TD (Figure 81–1).

Gradual taper of the antipsychotic medication may be attempted as long as the risk/benefit ratio of antipsychotic maintenance versus withdrawal does not preclude such a strategy. Gilbert and colleagues (1995) suggested that a slow taper of medication to the lowest effective dose is probably the preferred strategy for the treatment of chronic schizophrenia in a large number of stable patients.

Paradoxically, antipsychotics themselves represent the most effective short-term treatment for TD. An increase in dosage of a conventional agent usually (approximately 66% of patients) results in a clinically significant but temporary reduction in TD symptoms (Jeste et al. 1988). The most

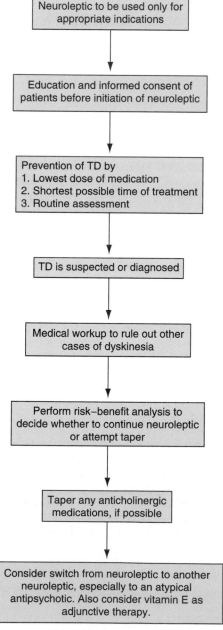

**Figure 81–1** *Management of tardive dyskinesia (TD).*

exciting development in the treatment of TD has been the use of the atypical antipsychotics. Clozapine has been shown to be effective in reducing TD in patients with existing TD (Simpson et al. 1978, Lieberman et al. 1991, Kane et al. 1993, Small et al. 1987), however, side effects such as agranulocytosis and clozapine's affinity for anticholinergic side effects limits its use. Additional studies have noted a beneficial effect of other atypical agents (i.e., risperidone and olanzapine) on preexisting TD (Littrell et al. 1998, Street et al. 2000, Jeste et al. 1997). The reduced risk of TD with all atypical agents (when used at appropriate doses) supports their use as preventive measures and as therapeutic options for those who develop TD on a conventional antipsychotic.

A number of experimental studies have attempted to treat TD with alternative strategies. Jeste and colleagues (1988) reviewed these treatments and noted that they had varying degrees of success but were inconsistent. One treatment that has demonstrated some efficacy has been the use of vitamin E alpha-tocopherol). Lohr and Jeste (1988b) have proposed that antipsychotic treatment results in the production of free radicals that damage the neuronal components. An antioxidant such as vitamin E would therefore, theoretically, result in improvement in the symptoms of TD. Vitamin E is a possible agent for the treatment and prophylaxis of TD (Gupta et al. 1999, Gardos 1999). A number of studies of varying design have shown benefit of vitamin E in TD (Lohr et al. 1987a, Elkashef et al. 1990, Egan et al. 1992, Adler et al. 1993b, Shriqui et al. 1992, Adler et al. 1998, Sajjad 1998); however, a recent double-blind, placebo-controlled multicenter trial failed to show a difference between vitamin E and placebo after 1 year of treatment (Adler et al. 1999). Although the results are far from conclusive, vitamin E remains a reasonably safe treatment modality for a patient with recently diagnosed TD. Doses are usually in the range of 1,200 to 1,600 mg/day. Other agents have been investigated such as calcium channel blockers (i.e., diltiazem, verapamil, nifedipine), and clonazepam, but more studies are warranted (Gupta et al. 1999).

Psychiatrists must regularly assess for the presence and progression of TD and present the patient (or the patient's guardian, when appropriate) with information about the risks of treatment; they may also give written information sheets, assess understanding by the patient or guardian, and accurately record evidence of the informed consent in the patient's record (Wettstein 1988).

## NEUROLEPTIC MALIGNANT SYNDROME

### Definition
Neuroleptic Malignant Syndrome (NMS) is a potentially fatal reaction to antipsychotic medications that is characterized clinically by muscle rigidity, fever, autonomic instability, and changes in level of consciousness.

### Etiology and Pathophysiology
The pathophysiological mechanism of NMS remains unclear. The hypothesis of most interest is that of reduced dopaminergic activity secondary to neuroleptic-induced dopamine blockade. This reduced dopamine activity in different parts of the brain (hypothalamus, nigrostriatal

**DSM-IV-TR Criteria** 333.92

**Neuroleptic Malignant Syndrome**

A. The development of severe muscle rigidity and elevated temperature associated with the use of neuroleptic medication.

B. Two (or more) of the following:

  (1) diaphoresis

  (2) dysphagia

  (3) tremor

  (4) incontinence

  (5) changes in level of consciousness ranging from confusion to coma

  (6) mutism

  (7) tachycardia

  (8) elevated or labile blood pressure

  (9) leukocytosis

  (10) laboratory evidence of muscle injury (e.g., elevated CPK [creatine kinase])

C. The symptoms in criteria A and B are not due to another substance (e.g., phencyclidine) or a neurological or other general medical condition (e.g., viral encephalitis).

D. The symptoms in criteria A and B are not better accounted for by a mental disorder (e.g., mood disorder with catatonic features).

Reprinted with permission from the Diagnostic and Statistical Manual of Mental Disorders, Fourth Edition, Text Revision. Copyright 2000 American Psychiatric Association.

system, and corticolimbic tracts) may serve to explain the various clinical features of NMS. Dopamine reduction in the hypothalamus may cause fever and autonomic instability; in the nigrostriatal system, dopamine reduction may lead to the rigidity; and the reduction in corticolimbic dopamine activity may explain the altered consciousness (Sewell and Jeste 1992b). This hypothesis is based on the fact that antipsychotics are dopamine-blocking agents, whereas certain dopamine agonists are reported to help resolve NMS.

The dopaminergic blocking theory does not, however, explain why NMS may develop at a given time and in a given patient. There are probably other genetic (possibly a predisposition similar to that seen in malignant hyperthermia) (Sewell and Jeste 1992b), constitutional, environmental, and pharmacological factors that interact to produce the syndrome. A number of investigators have proposed that other neurotransmitter abnormalities may be responsible for the syndrome, including serotonergic hyperfunction in the hypothalamus (Yamawaki et al. 1986), excessive catecholamine secretion (Addonizio et al. 1987), and gamma-aminobutyric acid deficiency (Addonizio et al. 1987).

**Epidemiology and Comorbidity**

The exact frequency of NMS is unknown. A number of retrospective and prospective studies have found 0.02 to 3.2% of patients treated with antipsychotics to be affected with NMS. Several factors probably account for this large variability in frequency, including differences in study methods and diagnostic criteria for NMS (Sewell and Jeste 1992b, Adityanjee et al. 1999).

A number of retrospective studies have attempted to isolate possible risk factors for the development of NMS. A prior episode of NMS appears to predispose to future episodes of NMS. Rosebush and colleagues (1989) found that the longer the time elapsed after an episode of NMS, the lower the risk of a recurrence of NMS.

Any preexisting medical problems, especially those associated with agitation or dehydration, may increase the likelihood of NMS development when antipsychotics are used. Patients with a neurological condition as well as patients with presumed psychosis due to human immunodeficiency virus infection may be at higher risk for development of NMS (Shalev et al. 1989, Harris et al. 1991). A number of potential risk factors related to antipsychotic treatment have been identified. Higher doses of antipsychotic, rapid increases in dosage (especially "rapid neuroleptization") (Keck et al. 1989a), and intramuscular injections of high-potency conventional agents (e.g., haloperidol and fluphenazine) (Deng et al. 1990) have been reported to be risk factors for NMS. A combination of lithium with an antipsychotic has been proposed as a possible risk factor for NMS development, but results from different investigators have been contradictory (Sewell and Jeste 1992b). NMS can occur (but rarely) in patients prescribed atypical antipsychotics and a review of atypical-induced NMS concluded that symptoms appear similar to NMS induced by conventional antipsychotics (Hasan and Buckley 1998).

NMS is more frequently reported in men than in women and is more frequently seen in a younger population. A previous diagnosis of a mood disorder may place patients at a higher risk for NMS (Pearlman 1986, Addonizio et al. 1987). Warm, humid climates may also predispose to the disorder (American Psychiatric Association 2000).

**Assessment and Differential Diagnosis**

NMS usually presents in the first month of antipsychotic treatment but may develop at any time. Two-thirds of the cases manifest within the first week of treatment (American Psychiatric Association 2000). One study found that NMS occurred as soon as 45 minutes and as late as 65 days after initiation of treatment (Shalev and Munitz 1986).

The two key diagnostic features for the disorder are severe muscle rigidity (classically referred to as lead pipe rigidity) and elevated temperature. A number of other features are also seen (see DSM-IV-TR criteria). For the psychiatrist, the most suggestive features are fluctuating consciousness (from confusion to coma), labile vital signs (tachycardia, unstable or elevated blood pressure), laboratory evidence of muscle injury (elevation of creatine kinase), and leukocytosis. Other features include diaphoresis, dysphagia, tremor, incontinence, and mutism (American Psychiatric Association 2000). The DSM-IV-TR criteria are broader than earlier criteria proposed by Pope and co-workers (1986) and revised by Keck and colleagues (1989b). The Pope criteria require the following three items for a definite diagnosis: (1) oral temperature of at least 38°C in the absence of another known cause; (2) at least two extrapyramidal side effects from the following list: lead pipe-type muscle rigidity, cogwheeling, sialorrhea, oculogyric crisis, retrocollis, opisthotonos, trismus, dysphagia, choreiform movements, dyskinetic movements, festinating gait, and flexor–extensor posturing; and (3) autonomic dysfunction characterized by two or more of the following: hypertension, tachycardia, tachypnea, prominent diaphoresis, and incontinence.

The differential diagnosis of NMS can be difficult (Table 81–3). The most important point is that the psychiatrist must start by suspecting NMS and then carefully rule out other possible organic problems. Because medical illness is a likely predisposing factor, it is important to consider that NMS may be present even if a definitive organic disease is found to explain the NMS-like symptoms. Sewell

and Jeste (1991) retrospectively examined the records of 34 hospitalized patients with suspected NMS and found that 24 seemed to have had NMS and 10 had acute medical problems. Hence, it is critical to consider the diagnosis of NMS as well as to rule out other acute illnesses when a patient receiving antipsychotics becomes medically ill.

Numerous general medical and neurological conditions can present with symptoms that may resemble NMS. Examples include central nervous system infection, status epilepticus, subcortical brain lesions, porphyria, and tetanus (American Psychiatric Association 2000). The presence of significantly elevated temperature and severe muscle rigidity makes the diagnosis of NMS more likely.

The syndrome of lethal catatonia (seen in patients with uncontrolled manic excitement or catatonic schizophrenia) can mimic NMS (with increased temperature, autonomic irregularities, and elevated creatine kinase), and the differential diagnosis can be difficult. It is obviously important to determine whether the patient is indeed being treated with an antipsychotic. Although NMS may clinically look like catatonia, NMS does not typically have alternating periods of catatonic excitement and catatonic mutism. A past history of catatonic episodes is also important in making the differential diagnosis. One report suggested that lorazepam was useful in alleviating the symptoms of catatonia (Salam and Kilzieh 1988). Lorazepam has not been shown to be useful in treatment of NMS. Therefore, it is possible that a brief lorazepam trial could provide a useful and relatively easy method of distinguishing between these two conditions. The problem, of course, is that not all cases of catatonia respond to lorazepam.

Heat stroke may also look like NMS but typically differs in that it presents with hypotension, dry skin, and

**Table 81-3  Differential Diagnosis of Neuroleptic Malignant Syndrome**

| Feature | Lethal Catatonia | Heat Stroke | Malignant Hyperthermia | Serotonin Syndrome | Neuroleptic Malignant Syndrome |
|---|---|---|---|---|---|
| Previous psychiatric illness | Yes | No | No | Yes | Yes |
| Onset of symptoms | + Prodromal psychotic symptoms | − Prodromal symptoms; development in several hours | − Prodromal symptoms; development after anesthesia | − Prodromal symptoms; development days to months after serotoninergic medication | − Prodromal symptoms; development hours to months after neuroleptic |
| Preceding anesthesia with muscle cell-depolarizing agents | No | No | Yes | No | No |
| Preceding neuroleptics | Maybe | Maybe | Maybe | Maybe | Yes |
| Preceding serotoninergic agents | Maybe | Maybe | Maybe | Yes | Maybe |
| Autonomic dysfunction | Maybe | No | No | No | Yes |
| Episodes: stupor mixed with episodes of excitement | Yes | No | No | No | Maybe |
| Diaphoresis | Maybe | No | Maybe | Maybe | Yes |
| Rigidity | Fluctuating | No | Yes | Yes | Yes |

*Source*: Modified from Sewell DD and Jeste DV (1991) Distinguishing neuroleptic malignant syndrome (NMS) from NMS-like acute medical illnesses: A study of 34 cases. J Neuropsychiatr Clin Neurosci 4, 265–269.

limb flaccidity (American Psychiatric Association 2000). Malignant hyperthermia can also have a similar presentation but generally occurs within the context of a patient's receiving halogenated anesthetic agents or succinylcholine. This condition typically begins immediately after administration of the anesthetic agent and only in genetically susceptible individuals (American Psychiatric Association 2000).

Medications can cause a number of conditions that may present as syndromes similar to NMS. Allergic drug reactions may produce fever and autonomic instability but not rigidity (Pelonero et al. 1998). Serotonin syndrome (Sternbach 1991), with common clinical characteristics including fever, resting tremor, rigidity, myoclonus, and generalized seizures should also be considered. A medication history can usually help distinguish between the two syndromes, but patients receiving antipsychotics may also be treated with selective serotonin reuptake inhibitors, thus making the clinical picture more confusing. Lithium intoxication and anticholinergic delirium can both resemble NMS, as can intoxication with amphetamines, cocaine, and phencyclidine as well as rapid termination of antiparkinsonian medication.

## Course

The course of NMS is variable. Some cases may progress to fatality, whereas others may follow a mild self-limited course. Once the syndrome is recognized and the antipsychotic medication is discontinued, the syndrome usually resolves between 2 weeks and 1 month (American Psychiatric Association 2000).

Mortality rate is reported to be 4 to 25% (Sewell and Jeste 1992b). The most common medical complications leading to morbidity and mortality are respiratory failure and renal failure. Shalev and coworkers (1989) reported that myoglobinemia and renal failure are the best predictors of mortality in NMS; the presence of either condition imparted a 50% mortality risk. In general, complications are a result of physiologic consequences of severe rigidity and immobilization such as deep vein thrombosis, pulmonary embolism, dehydration, and an increased risk for rhabdomyolysis (Pelonero et al. 1998).

## Treatment

The most critical step in treatment (Table 81–4) is to recognize the clinical features of the syndrome and rapidly discontinue the antipsychotic. The importance of this initial step mandates that psychiatrists who use antipsychotics in their practice be cognizant of the early clinical features and recognize that the syndrome can occur at any time during the course of treatment. Once the antipsychotic has been stopped, supportive care remains the core of treatment (Arana and Rosenbaum 2000) and often must be carried out in the context of a medical intensive care unit. Each supportive intervention should be targeted to a specific symptom. Examples of interventions include cooling blankets for fever, cardiac monitoring for arrhythmias, parenteral hydration for dehydration, and monitoring for urine output and renal function. Dialysis may also be considered for acute renal failure.

Some specific treatments for NMS have been proposed, but their beneficial effect is unclear. The muscle relaxant dantrolene is thought by some investigators to be

| Table 81–4 | Treatment of Neuroleptic Malignant Syndrome |
|---|---|
| Step 1 | Assess medication regimen<br>• Stop dopamine antagonists<br>• Restart any recently stopped dopamine agonists |
| Step 2 | Supportive care<br>• Monitor vital signs<br>• Administer intravenous fluids<br>• Provide cooling blankets<br>• Administer antipyretics<br>• Consider dialysis for acute renal failure |
| Step 3 | No improvement within 24–28 h<br>• Administer oral bromocriptine 5 mg PO t.i.d. to be increased daily by 5 mg increments until positive response<br>• Continue bromocriptine for 10 d, then withdraw in period of 1 wk<br>• Monitor for relapse |
| Step 4 | If patient cannot tolerate bromocriptine or cannot take oral medications<br>• Administer intravenous dantrolene 1–3 mg/kg/body weight q.i.d.<br>• Gradually increase dose until positive response |
| Step 5 | Consider adding bromocriptine to dantrolene |
| Step 6 | Consider discontinuing all medications and giving supportive care only |
| Step 7 | Consider electroconvulsive therapy after 3–4 d, if no improvement |

*Source*: Modified from Sewell DD and Jeste DV (1991) Distinguishing neuroleptic malignant syndrome (NMS) from NMS-like acute medical illnesses: A study of 34 cases. J Neuropsychiatr Clin Neurosci 4, 265–269.

helpful in decreasing rigidity, hyperthermia, and tachycardia. Dosing of 1 to 3 mg/kg/day orally or intravenously in four divided doses is currently advocated (Arana and Rosenbaum 2000). The dopamine agonist bromocriptine may also provide some relief of the symptoms, especially for muscle rigidity. Dosing is usually in the range of 5 to 10 mg orally three times a day (Arana and Rosenbaum 2000). The two medications can be administered together. Gelenberg (1992), however, pointed out that a study by Rosebush and coworkers (1991) not only has cast doubt on the benefit of the use of these agents in the treatment of NMS but may also point to the possibility that these agents actually retard the course of improvement of NMS. In the Rosebush study, 8 of 20 patients with presumed NMS received dantrolene, bromocriptine, or both along with supportive care, and 12 of 20 received supportive care only. There was a suggestion that the resolution of the NMS episodes took longer in the patients treated with the additional medications. The treatments in the investigation were not randomized or controlled.

Electroconvulsive therapy is another treatment option in NMS presumably because it increases dopamine turnover in the brain (Pearlman 1986). Electroconvulsive therapy is particularly indicated when there is difficulty in distinguishing between NMS and lethal catatonia and when there seems to be a significant risk of recurrence of NMS on restarting neuroleptics (Addonizio et al. 1987). Some psychiatrists report rapid and dramatic success in use of electroconvulsive therapy for NMS.

At present, the appropriate course is to begin with antipsychotic discontinuation and supportive care and to consider antidote therapy only if improvement in symptoms is not seen within the first few days (Gelenberg 1992). Caroff and colleagues suggested that treatment of NMS should be individualized for each patient based on clinical signs and symptoms. For example, supportive care may be sufficient in mild and early cases of NMS. Trials of bromocriptine, dantrolene, or amantadine are suggested for patients with moderate symptoms. Anticholinergics can be used in managing afebrile patients with neuroleptic-induced parkinsonian symptoms and benzodiazepines may be useful for agitation in NMS. ECT is recommended in situations where lethal catatonia is suspected, when NMS symptoms are treatment refractory, and in patients who remain psychotic in the immediate post-NMS period (Caroff and Mann 1998).

A particular difficulty for the psychotic patient who has NMS is that rechallenge with antipsychotics may cause NMS to recur. Successful rechallenge seems to be positively related to the length of time elapsed after resolution of NMS (Rosebush et al. 1989). There is some evidence to suggest that clozapine may have relatively little propensity to induce NMS. There are some case reports indicating that clozapine may have caused NMS but only in conjunction with other medications (carbamazepine in one case and lithium carbonate in another) (Pope et al. 1986, Muller et al. 1988). Clozapine, therefore, may represent one option for the patient who has experienced NMS with a conventional agent. It is likely but not yet known definitively that atypical antipsychotics will prove to have a lower frequency of NMS. In general, it is recommended to switch to an agent in a different chemical class and with a lower $D_2$ affinity compared to the causal agent (Pelonero et al. 1998).

## MEDICATION-INDUCED POSTURAL TREMOR

### Definition

This category refers to fine postural action tremor that develops as a result of a medication. Medications that have been reported to cause such an effect are lithium, beta-adrenergic agonist medications, stimulants, dopaminergic medications, anticonvulsant medications, antipsychotics, antidepressant medications, and methylxanthines (e.g., caffeine) (American Psychiatric Association 2000). The psychotropic medication most typically associated with such tremor is lithium, and most of the available information on medication-induced tremor relates to that caused by lithium.

### Etiology and Pathophysiology

Normal muscle contractions are accompanied by tremor as a result of contractions of muscle fiber recruitment. This tremor is typically low in amplitude and is referred to as a physiological tremor. When these contractions are maintained, the amplitude of the tremor increases and it becomes visible. This is referred to as an enhanced physiological tremor (Young 1992). A number of medications, including lithium and bronchodilators, produce an enhanced physiological tremor. The pathophysiological mechanism of these tremors is not well understood but seems to relate to adrenergic changes (probably mediated in the locus coeruleus) in the mechanical properties of the skeletal muscle (Young 1992). The response of these tremors to beta-adrenergic

---

> **DSM-IV-TR Criteria** 333.1
>
> **Medication-Induced Postural Tremor**
>
> A. A fine postural tremor that has developed in association with the use of a medication (e.g., lithium, antidepressant medication, valproic acid).
>
> B. The tremor (i.e., a regular, rhythmic oscillation of the limbs, head, mouth, or tongue) has a frequency between 8 and 12 cycles per second.
>
> C. The symptoms are not due to a preexisting nonpharmacologically induced tremor. Evidence that the symptoms are due to a preexisting tremor might include the following: the tremor was present prior to the introduction of the medication, the tremor does not correlate with serum levels of the medication, and the tremor persists after discontinuation of the medication.
>
> D. The symptoms are not better accounted for by neuroleptic-induced parkinsonism.

Reprinted with permission from the Diagnostic and Statistical Manual of Mental Disorders, Fourth Edition, Text Revision. Copyright 2000 American Psychiatric Association.

---

blocking agents and their exacerbation as a result of beta-adrenergic agonists seem to lend support to the notion of adrenergic mediation.

### Epidemiology and Comorbidity

Estimates of the frequency of lithium-induced tremor vary widely across the literature and range between 4 and 65% (Goodwin and Jamison 1990). Lifetime incidence of tremor is estimated to be 25 to 50% of patients starting lithium therapy (Price and Heninger 1994).

A number of possible risk factors have been proposed to predispose a person to development of a lithium-induced tremor. These include older age, greater serum lithium levels, concomitant use of antidepressant or antipsychotic medication, greater caffeine intake, history of tremor, alcohol dependence, and anxiety (American Psychiatric Association 2000).

### Assessment and Differential Diagnosis

Lithium-induced tremor may appear as soon as treatment is initiated. As the lithium level increases, the tremor becomes more severe and coarse and may have associated muscle twitching or fasciculations (American Psychiatric Association 2000). Complaints about the tremor are typically greatest at the beginning of therapy. There is disagreement as to whether the tremor typically remains stable or improves with time on lithium.

The lithium-induced tremor is reasonably easy to diagnose. It is a rhythmical action tremor. It is most commonly seen in the hands or fingers but can occasionally be seen in the head, mouth, or tongue (American Psychiatric Association 2000). The frequency of the tremor is typically 8 to 12 Hz and is similar in appearance to an essential tremor

(Arana and Rosenbaum 2000). It may usually be seen by asking the patient to hold the affected body part in a stable position. The tremor is made worse by anxiety, stress, fatigue, hypoglycemia, thyrotoxicosis, pheochromocytoma, hypothermia, alcohol withdrawal, performance of voluntary movements, and concomitant administration of cyclic antidepressant medications (Arana and Rosenbaum 2000, American Psychiatric Association 2000).

The most difficult differential diagnosis involves distinguishing a lithium-induced tremor from a tremor that was preexisting. To be classified as a medication-induced tremor, it must have a temporal relationship to the medication, it must relate to the serum level of the medication, and it must not persist after the medication is discontinued. A similar postural tremor is essential tremor, and differentiation between the two is nearly impossible clinically without the medication history.

Any of the factors listed that may exacerbate a medication-induced tremor can also cause a similar tremor in the absence of the medication. Medication-induced tremor may resemble NIP. NIP, however, is generally worse at rest, is lower in frequency, and has other associated features of parkinsonism (American Psychiatric Association 2000).

## Course

The literature suggests that there is some risk that tremor may be embarrassing for certain patients and could impair activities that require delicate movements (Arana and Rosenbaum 2000). The actual percentage of patients who are bothered by their tremor is unknown. There do not appear to be any long-term sequelae as a result of having a medication-induced postural tremor. A sudden worsening of tremor may be indicative of the beginning of lithium intoxication.

## Treatment

Most treatment options have been described for treatment of lithium-induced tremor. Typically the tremor is benign, is not bothersome to the patient, and requires no specific intervention. Some cases, however, require treatment because of the patient's concern about the side effect. Preliminary measures include possibly reducing the lithium dose (if clinically feasible), changing the lithium dose to one-time evening administration, or changing the lithium preparation. Caffeine intake should be reduced or eliminated, and anxiety should be pharmacologically or behaviorally treated.

Beta-blockers represent the best-studied method for gaining pharmacological control of the tremor if the preliminary measures are ineffective. Arana and Rosenbaum (2000) recommended starting propranolol on an as-needed basis. They suggested 10 to 20 mg a half-hour before the activity in which the tremor must not be present. If a patient requires chronic relief from the tremor, propranolol should be initiated at 10 to 20 mg b.i.d and increased until adequate dose for suppression of the tremor is attained. Propranolol may decrease glomerular filtration rate and may result in a reduction in renal lithium clearance. This suggests that patients who require long-term beta-blocker suppression for tremor need to have lithium levels checked more regularly even when they are taking a stable dose of lithium.

There is little information in the literature as to the possible treatment of tremor induced by medications other than lithium and further investigations are needed to elucidate this syndrome.

---

**Clinical Vignette 1 • Treatment of Tardive Dyskinesia**

Mr. A, a 67-year-old single man, was diagnosed with paranoid schizophrenia at the age of 23 while in the Army. Between the ages of 23 and 38 years, Mr. A received no medication, was able to hold a job as a security guard, and his symptoms did not interfere substantially with his daily functioning.

At 38 years of age, Mr. A began having visual hallucinations of snakes, and his paranoid delusions became more severe. He was treated with a conventional antipsychotic and was seen regularly by a psychiatrist. He functioned well for the next 10 years (able to hold a job, live independently) while continuing to take an antipsychotic and see his psychiatrist.

At ages 50 and 56 years, Mr. A was hospitalized once each time for 2 weeks for exacerbation of psychotic symptoms. During the second hospitalization, he was switched to a high potency conventional antipsychotic. At age 61 years, Mr. A's psychiatrist attempted to taper the dose of his neuroleptic. This attempt was unsuccessful as a result of a psychotic decompensation.

At the age of 66 years, Mr. A's neuroleptic was discontinued and olanzapine (maintenance dose 10 mg daily) was initiated because of the development of abnormal involuntary mouth and tongue movements associated with TD. He experienced some worsening of his mouth and tongue movements on withdrawal of the conventional antipsychotic. The TD symptoms improved moderately after 3 months. One year after discontinuing the neuroleptic, and beginning olanzapine, Mr. A's TD remains significantly reduced.

---

**Clinical Vignette 2 • Confusion Between Neuroleptic-Induced Akathisia and Psychotic Agitation**

Ms. B, a 77-year-old widow, lived in a nursing home. As a result of severe degenerative arthritis and neuropathic pain due to type 2 diabetes, she was confined mainly to her bed and a wheelchair. She had a past psychiatric history significant for Alzheimer-type dementia diagnosed at age 74. Ms. B was started on haloperidol 1 mg b.i.d. 6 weeks ago due to frequent, bothersome delusions regarding her roommate and health care personnel.

Two weeks ago, Ms. B's roommate complained that Ms. B was increasingly agitated, restless, and boisterous throughout the day while in bed. Believing that her behavioral disturbance was inadequately controlled, Ms. B's physician increased her haloperidol to 2 mg b.i.d. A few days later, Ms. B was noted to be increasingly agitated and restless. Subjective discomfort was noted upon further interviews with the patient. Since the haloperidol-induced akathisia worsened by increased dosages of haloperidol, Ms. B was started on low-dose risperidone and haloperidol was stopped over the course of 1 week. Ms. B is currently receiving risperidone 0.5 mg b.i.d. without any symptoms of akathisia and noted reductions in her delusions.

## Acknowledgment

The authors would like to recognize David Naimark for his outstanding contribution to the previous edition of this chapter.

## Comparison of DSM-IV/ICD-10 Diagnostic Criteria

Some of these categories are included in Chapter VI of ICD-10 (Diseases of the Nervous System) but no diagnostic criteria or definitions are provided.

## References

Addonizio G, Susman VL, and Roth SD (1987) Neuroleptic malignant syndrome: Review and analysis of 115 cases. Biol Psychiatr 22, 1004–1020.

Adityanjee, Aderibigbe YA, and Mathews T (1999) Epidemiology of neuroleptic malignant syndrome. Clin Neuropharmacol 22, 151–158.

Adler L, Angrist B, Peselow E, et al. (1986) A controlled assessment of propranolol in the treatment of neuroleptic-induced akathisia. Br J Psychiatr 149, 42–45.

Adler LA, Reiter S, Angrist B, et al. (1987) Pindolol and propranolol in neuroleptic-induced akathisia. Am J Psychiatr 144, 1241–1242.

Adler LA, Peselow E, Rosenthal M, et al. (1993a) A controlled comparison of the effects of propranolol, benztropine, and placebo on akathisia: An interim analysis. Psychopharmacol Bull 29, 283–286.

Adler LA, Peselow E, Rotrosen J, et al. (1993b) Vitamin E treatment of tardive dyskinesia. Am J Psychiatr 150, 1405–1407.

Adler LA, Edson R, Lavori P, et al. (1998) Long-term treatment effects of vitamin E for tardive dyskinesia. Biol Psychiatr 43, 868–872.

Adler LA, Rotrosen J, Edson R, et al. (1999) Vitamin E treatment for tardive dyskinesia. Arch Gen Psychiatr 56, 836–841.

American Psychiatric Association (2000) Diagnostic and Statistical Manual of Mental Disorders, 4th ed., Text Rev. APA, Washington DC.

Arana GW and Rosenbaum JF (2000) Handbook of Psychiatric Drug Therapy, 4th ed. Lippincott, Williams & Wilkins, Philadelphia.

Arvanitis LA, Miller BG, and the Seroquel Trial 13 Study Group (1997) Multiple fixed doses of "seroquel" (quetiapine) in patients with acute exacerbation of schizophrenia: A comparison with halopericol and placebo. Biol Psychiatr 42, 233–246.

Ayd FJ (1961) A survey of drug-induced extrapyramidal reactions. J Am Med Assoc 175, 1054–1060.

Ayd FJ (1979) Respiratory dyskinesias in patients with neuroleptic-induced extrapyramidal reaction. Int Drug Ther News 14, 1–4.

Beasley CM, Hamilton SH, Crawford AM, et al. (1997) Olanzapine versus haloperidol: Acute phase results of the international double-blind olanzapine trial. Eur J Neuropsychopharmacol 7, 125–137.

Bersani G, Grispini A, Marini S, et al. (1990) 5-HT$_2$ antagonist ritanserin in neuroleptic-induced parkinsonism: A double-blind comparison with orphenadrine and placebo. Clin Neuropharmacol 13, 500–506.

Bitton V and Melamed E (1984) Coexistence of severe parkinsonism and tardive dyskinesia as side effects of neuroleptic therapy. J Clin Psychiatr 45, 28–30.

Brandon S, McClelland HA, and Protheroe C (1971) A study of facial dyskinesia, in a mental hospital population. Br J Psychiatr 118, 171–184.

Burke RE, Reches A, Traub MM, et al. (1985) Tetrabenazine induces acute dystonic reactions. Ann Neurol 17, 200–202.

Caligiuri MP and Lohr JB (1997) Instrumental motor predictors of neuroleptic-induced parkinsonism in newly medicated schizophrenia patients. J Neuropsychiatr Clin Neurosci 9, 562–567.

Caligiuri MP, Lohr JB, Bracha HS, et al. (1991) Clinical and instrumental assessment of neuroleptic-induced parkinsonism in patients with tardive dyskinesia. Biol Psychiatr 29, 139–148.

Caligiuri MP, Lacro JP, Rockwell E, et al. (1997) Incidence and risk factors for severe tardive dyskinesia in older patients. Br J Psychiatr 171, 148–153.

Caligiuri MP, Rockwell E, and Jeste DV (1998) Extrapyramidal side effects in patients with Alzheimer's disease treated with low-dose neuroleptic medication. Am J Geriatr Psychiatr 6, 75–82.

Caligiuri MP, Lacro JP, and Jeste DV (1999) Incidence and predictors of drug-induced parkinsonism in older psychiatric patients treated with very low doses of neuroleptics. J Clin Psychopharmacol 19, 322–328.

Caroff SN and Mann SC (1998) Specific treatment of the neuroleptics malignant syndrome. Biol Psychiatr 44, 378–381.

Casey DE (1988) Affective disorders and tardive dyskinesia. L'Encephale 14, 221–226.

Casey DE (1997) Will the new antipsychotics bring hope of reducing the risk of developing extrapyramidal syndromes and tardive dyskinesia? Int Clin Psychopharmacol 12, S19–S27.

Casey DE and Keepers GA (1988) Neuroleptic side effects: Acute extrapyramidal syndromes and tardive dyskinesia. In Psychopharmacology: Current Trends, Casey DE and Christensen AV (eds). Springer-Verlag, Berlin, pp. 74–93.

Casey DE and Rabins P (1978) Tardive dyskinesia as a life-threatening illness. Am J Psychiatr 135, 486–488.

Chakos MH, Mayerhoff DI, Loebel AD, et al. (1992) Incidence and correlates of extrapyramidal symptoms in first episode of schizophrenia. Psychopharmacol Bull 28, 81–86.

Chouinard G and Bradwein J (1982) Reversible and irreversible tardive dyskinesia: A case report. Am J Psychiatr 139, 360–362.

Chouinard G, Jones B, Remington G, et al. (1993) A Canadian multicenter placebo-controlled study of fixed doses of risperidone and haloperidol in the treatment of chronic schizophrenic patients. J Clin Psychopharmacol 13, 25–40.

Cohen BM, Keck PE, Satlin A, et al. (1991) Prevalence and severity of akathisia in patients on clozapine. Biol Psychiatr 29, 1215–1219.

Coleman JH and Hays PE (1975) Drug-induced extrapyramidal effects—a review. Dis Nerv Syst 36, 591–593.

Delay J and Deniker P (1968) Drug-induced extrapyramidal syndromes. In Diseases of the Basal Ganglia, Vinken PJ and Bruyn GW (eds). North-Holland, Amsterdam, pp. 248–266.

Deng MZ, Chen GQ, and Phillips MR (1990) Neuroleptic malignant syndrome in 12 of 9,792 Chinese inpatients exposed to neuroleptics: A prospective study. Am J Psychiatr 147, 1149–1155.

DeVaugh-Geiss J (1980) Tardive Tourette syndrome. Neurology 30, 562–563.

Dimascio A and Demergian E (1970) Antiparkinson drug overuse. Psychosomatics 11, 596–601.

Edwards H (1970) The significance of brain damage in persistant oral dyskinesia. Br J Psychiatr 116, 271–275.

Egan MF, Hyde TM, Albers GW, et al. (1992) Treatment of tardive dyskinesia with vitamin E. Am J Psychiatr 149, 773–777.

Elkashef AM, Ruskin PE, Bacher N, et al. (1990) Vitamin E in the treatment of tardive dyskinesia. Am J Psychiatr 147, 505–506.

Fahn S (1983) High dosage anticholinergic therapy in dystonia. Neurology 33, 1255–1261.

Farde L, Nordstrom AL, and Wiesel FA (1992) Positron emission tomographic analysis of central D$_1$ and D$_2$ dopamine receptor occupancy in patients treated with classical neuroleptics and clozapine: Relation to extrapyramidal side effects. Arch Gen Psychiatr 49, 538–544.

Faurbye A, Rasch PJ, Petersen PB, et al. (1964) Neurological symptoms in pharmacotherapy of psychoses. Acta Psychiatr Scand 40, 10–27.

Ganzini L, Heintz RT, Hoffman WF, et al. (1991) The prevalence of tardive dyskinesia in neuroleptic-treated diabetics: A controlled study. Arch Gen Psychiatr 48, 259–263.

Gardos G (1999) Managing antipsychotic-induced tardive dyskinesia. Drug Safety 20, 187–193.

Gardos G and Cole JO (1983) Tardive dyskinesia and anticholinergic drugs. Am J Psychiatr 140, 200–202.

Gardos G and Cole JO (1992) Severe tardive dyskinesia. In Movement Disorders in Neurology and Neuropsychiatry, Joseph AB and Young RR (eds). Blackwell Scientific, Boston, pp. 40–45.

Gardos G, Cole JO, Schniebolk S, et al. (1987) Comparison of severe and mild tardive dyskinesia: Implications for etiology. J Clin Psychiatr 48, 359–362.

Gelenberg AJ (1992) The best treatment for NMS. Biol Ther Psychiatr 15, 13 and 16.

Gerhard AL (1992) Withdrawal dyskinesia. In Movement Disorders in Neurology and Neuropsychiatry, Joseph AB and Young RR (eds). Blackwell Scientific, Boston, pp. 81–82.

Gilbert PL, Harris MJ, McAdams LA, et al. (1995) Neuroleptic withdrawal in schizophrenic patients. Arch Gen Psychiatr 52, 173–188.

Glazer WM (2000) Extrapyramidal side effects, tardive dyskinesia, and the concept of atypicality. J Clin Psychiatr 61, 16–21.

Goodwin FK and Jamison KR (1990) Manic–Depressive Illness, 1st ed. Oxford University Press, New York.

Gupta S, Mosnik D, Black DW, et al. (1999) Tardive dyskinesia: Review of treatments past, present, and future. Ann Clin Psychiatr 11, 257–266.

Guy W, Ban TA, and Wilson WH (1986) The prevalence of abnormal involuntary movements among chronic schizophrenics. Int Clin Psychopharmacol 1, 134–144.

Haase HJ (1961) Extrapyramidal system and neuroleptics: A "conditio sine qua non." In Systéme Extra-Pyramidal et Neuroleptiques (Extrapyramidal System and Neuroleptics), Bordeleau LM (ed). Editions Psychiatriques, Montreal, pp. 329–353.

Harris MJ, Jeste DV, Gleghorn A, et al. (1991) New-onset psychosis in HIV-infected patients. J Clin Psychiatr 52, 352–376.

Hasan S and Buckley P (1998) Novel antipsychotics and the neuroleptics malignant syndrome: A review and critique. Am J Psychiatr 155, 1113–1116.

Hausner RS (1983) Neuroleptic-induced parkinsonism and Parkinson's disease: Differential diagnosis and treatment. J Clin Psychiatr 44, 13–16.

Hornykiewicz O (1982) Brain neurotransmitter changes in Parkinson's disease. In Movement Disorders, Marsden CD and Fahn S (eds). Butterworth Scientific, London, pp. 41–58.

Jackson IV, Volavka J, James B, et al. (1980) The respiratory components of tardive dyskinesia. Biol Psychiatr 15, 485–487.

Jeste DV and Caligiuri MP (1993) Tardive dyskinesia. Schizophr Bull 19, 303–315.

Jeste DV and Wyatt RJ (1981) Changing epidemiology of tardive dyskinesia—an overview. Am J Psychiatr 138, 297–309.

Jeste DV and Wyatt RJ (1982) Understanding and Treating Tardive Dyskinesia. Guilford Press, New York.

Jeste DV, Wisniewski A, and Wyatt RJ (1986) Neuroleptic-associated "Tardive" syndromes. In Schizophrenia: The Psychiatric Clinics of North America, Vol. 9:1, Roy A (ed). Plenum Press, New York, pp. 183–192.

Jeste DV, Lohr JB, Clark K, et al. (1988) Pharmacological treatment of tardive dyskinesia in the 1980s. J Clin Psychopharmacol 8, 38S–48S.

Jeste DV, Lohr JB, and Manley M (1992) Study of neuropathologic changes in the striatum following 4, 8 and 12 months of treatment with fluphenazine in rats. Psychopharmacology 106, 154–160.

Jeste DV, Caligiuri MP, Paulsen JS, et al. (1995) Risk of tardive dyskinesia in older patients: A prospective longitudinal study of 266 patients. Arch Gen Psychiatr 52, 756–765.

Jeste DV, Klausner M, Brecher M, et al. (1997) A clinical evaluation of risperidone in the treatment of schizophrenia: A 10-week, open-label, multicenter trial involving 945 patients. Psychopharmacology 131, 239–247.

Jeste DV, Lacro JP, Bailey A, et al. (1999a) Lower incidence of tardive dyskinesia with risperidone compared with haloperidol in older patients. J Am Geriatr Soc 47, 716–719.

Jeste DV, Lacro JP, Palmer BW, et al. (1999b) Incidence of tardive dyskinesia in early stages of low-dose treatment with typical neuroleptics in older patients. Am J Psychiatr 156, 309–311.

Jeste DV, Rockwell E, Harris MJ, et al. (1999c) Conventional versus newer antipsychotics in elderly patients. Am J Geriatr Psychiatr 7, 70–76.

Johnson DAW (1978) Prevalence and treatment of drug-induced extrapyramidal symptoms. Br J Psychiatr 132, 27–30.

Kane JM, Honigfeld G, Singer J, et al. (1988a) Clozapine for the treatment resistant schizophrenic: A double-blind comparison with chlorpromazine. Arch Gen Psychiatr 45, 789–796.

Kane JM, Woerner M, and Lieberman J (1988b) Tardive dyskinesia: Prevalence, incidence, and risk factors. J Clin Psychopharmacol 8(4), 52S–56S.

Kane JM, Jeste DV, Barnes TRE, et al. (1992) Tardive Dyskinesia: A Task Force Report of the American Psychiatric Association. American Psychiatric Association, Washington DC.

Kane JM, Woerner MG, Pollack S, et al. (1993) Does clozapine cause tardive dyskinesia? J Clin Psychiatr 54, 327–330.

Kapur S, Zipursky RB, Remington G, et al. (1998) 5-HT$_2$ and D$_2$ receptor occupancy of olanzapine in schizophrenia: A PET investigation. Am J Psychiatr 155, 921–928.

Keck PE, Pope HG, and Cohen BM (1989a) Risk factors for neuroleptic malignant syndrome: A case-control study. Arch Gen Psychiatr 46, 914–918.

Keck PE, Sebastianelli J, Pope HG, et al. (1989b) Frequency and presentation of neuroleptic malignant syndrome in a state psychiatric hospital. J Clin Psychiatr 50, 352–355.

Keepers GA and Casey DE (1986) Prediction of neuroleptic-induced dystonia. J Clin Psychopharmacol 7, 342–344.

Kiloh LG, Smith JS, and Williams SE (1973) Antiparkinson drugs as causal agents in tardive dyskinesia. Med J Austral 2, 591–593.

King DJ, Link CG, and Kowalcyk B (1998) A comparison of b.i.d. and t.i.d. dose regimens of quetiapine (Seroquel) in the treatment of schizophrenia. Psychopharmacology 137, 139–146.

Klawans HL, Falk DK, Nausieda PA, et al. (1978) Gille de la Tourette's syndrome after long-term chlorpromazine therapy. Neurology 28, 1064–1068.

Kurz M, Hummer M, Kemmler G, et al. (1998) Long-term pharmacokinetics of clozapine. Br J Psychiatr 173, 341–344.

Lacro JP and Jeste DV (1997) The role of ethnicity in the development of tardive dyskinesia. In Neuroleptic-Induced Movement Disorders, Yassa R, Nair NVP, and Jeste DV (eds). Cambridge University Press, New York, pp. 298–310.

Lance JW and McLeod JG (1981) A Physiological Approach to Clinical Neurology, 3rd ed. Butterworth, London.

Lang AE (1985) Dopamine agonists in the treatment of dystonia. Clin Neuropharmacol 8, 38–57.

Langston JW and Irwin I (1986) MPTP: Current concepts and controversies. Clin Neuropharmacol 9, 485–507.

Lieberman JA, Saltz BL, Johns CA, et al. (1991) The effects of clozapine on tardive dyskinesia. Br J Psychiatr 158, 503–510.

Lindamer LA, Lohr JB, Caligiuri MP, et al. (2001) Relationship of gender and age of onset of schizophrenia to severity of dyskinesia. J Neuropsychiatr Clin Neurosci 13, 399–402.

Littrell KH, Johnson CG, Littrell S, et al. (1998) Marked reduction of tardive dyskinesia with olanzapine. Arch Gen Psychiatr 55, 279–280.

Lohr JB and Jeste DV (1988a) Neuroleptic-induced movement disorders: Acute and subacute disorders. In Psychiatry, Rev. ed., Michels R, Cavenar JO Jr., Brodie NKH, et al. (eds). JB Lippincott, Philadelphia, pp. 1–19.

Lohr JB and Jeste DV (1988b) Neuroleptic-induced movement disorders: Tardive dyskinesia and other tardive syndromes. In Psychiatry, Rev. ed., Michels R, Cavenar JO Jr., Brodie NKH, et al. (eds). JB Lippincott, Philadelphia, pp. 1–17.

Lohr JB, Cadet JL, Lohr MA, et al. (1987a) Alpha-tocopherol in tardive dyskinesia (letter). Lancet 1, 913–914.

Lohr JB, Lohr MA, Wasli E, et al. (1987b) Self-perception of tardive dyskinesia and neuroleptic-induced parkinsonism: A study of clinical correlates. Psychopharmacol Bull 23, 211–214.

Mamo DC, Sweet RA, and Keshavan MS (1999) Managing antipsychotic-induced parkinsonism. Drug Safety 20, 252–275.

Mann SC, Greenstein RA, and Eilers R (1983) Early onset of severe dyskinesia following lithium-haloperidol treatment. Am J Psychiatr 140, 1385–1386.

Marsden CD and Jenner P (1980) The pathophysiology of extra-pyramidal side-effects of neuroleptic drugs. Psychol Med 10, 55–72.

Massengil R Jr. and Nashold B (1952) A swallowing disorder denoted in tardive dyskinesia patients. Acta Oto-Laryngol 68, 457–458.

Maxwell S, Massengil R, and Nashold B (1970) Tardive dyskinesia. J Speech Hear Disord 35, 33–36.

McClelland HA, Blessed G, and Bhata S (1974) Abrupt withdrawal of antiparkinsonian drugs in schizophrenic patients. Br J Psychiatr 124, 151–159.

McLean P and Casey D (1978) Tardive dyskinesia in an adolescent. Am J Psychiatr 8, 952–971.

Miller CH and Fleischhacker WW (2000) Managing antipsychotic-induced acute and chronic akathisia. Drug Safety 22, 73–81.

Miller CH, Mohr F, Umbricht D, et al. (1998) The prevalence of acute extrapyramidal signs and symptoms in patients treated with clozapine, risperidone, and conventional antipsychotics. J Clin Psychiatr 59, 52–75.

Miller LG and Jankovic J (1992) Drug-induced movement disorders: An overview. In Movement Disorders in Neurology and Neuropsychiatry, Joseph AB and Young RR (eds). Blackwell Scientific, Boston, p. 7.

Mitchell IJ, Cross AJ, and Sambrook MA (1985) Sites of the neurotoxic action of 1-methyl-4-phenyl-1,2,3,6-tetrahydropyridine in the macaque monkey include the ventral tegmental area and the locus ceruleus. Neurosci Lett 61, 195–200.

Morgenstern H and Glazer WM (1993) Identifying risk factors for tardive dyskinesia among long-term outpatients maintained with neuroleptic medications: Results of the Yale tardive dyskinesia study. Arch Gen Psychiatr 50, 723–733.

Muller J and Aminoff MJ (1982) Tourette-like syndrome after long-term neuroleptic drug treatment. Br J Psychiatr 141, 191–193.

Muller T, Becker T, and Fritze J (1988) Neuroleptic malignant syndrome after clozapine plus carbamazepine. Lancet 2, 1500.

Munetz MR, Slawsky RC, and Neil JF (1985) Tardive Tourette's syndrome treated with clonidine and mesoridazine. Psychosomatics 26, 254–257.

Nasrallah HA, Pappas NJ, and Crowe RR (1980) Oculogyric dystonia in tardive dyskinesia. Am J Psychiatr 137, 850–851.

Osser DN (1992) Neuroleptic-induced pseudoparkinsonism. In Movement Disorders in Neurology and Neuropsychiatry, Joseph AB and Young RR (eds). Blackwell Scientific, Boston, pp. 73–74.

Pearlman CA (1986) Neuroleptic malignant syndrome: A review of the literature. J Clin Psychopharmacol 6, 257–273.

Pelonero AL, Levenson JL, and Pandurangi AK (1998) Neuroleptic malignant syndrome: A review. Psychiatr Serv 49, 1163–1172.

Pope HG, Keck PE, and McElroy SL (1986) Frequency and presentation of neuroleptic malignant syndrome in a large psychiatric hospital. Am J Psychiatr 143, 1227–1233.

Portnoy RA (1979) Hyperkinetic dysarthria as an early indicator of impending tardive dyskinesia. J Speech Hear Disord 44, 214–219.

Poyurovsky M, Shardorodsky M, Fuchs C, et al. (1999) Treatment of neuroleptic-induced akathisia with the 5-HT$_2$ antagonist mianserin. Double-blind, placebo-controlled study. Br J Psychiatr 174, 238–242.

Price LH and Heninger GR (1994) Lithium in the treatment of mood disorders. Neurology 34, 1348–1353.

Raleigh FR Jr. (1977) Reducing unnecessary antiparkinsonian medication in antipsychotic therapy. J Am Pharmaceut Assoc 17, 101–105.

Rifkin A, Quitkin F, and Klein DF (1975) Akinesia: A poorly recognized drug-induced extrapyramidal behavioral disorder. Arch Gen Psychiatr 32, 672–674.

Rifkin A, Quitkin F, and Kane J (1978) Are prophylactic antiparkinson drugs necessary? Arch Gen Psychiatr 35, 483–489.

Rosebush PI, Stewart TD, and Gelenberg AJ (1989) Twenty neuroleptic rechallenges after neuroleptic malignant syndrome in 15 patients. J Clin Psychiatr 50, 295–298.

Rosebush PI, Stewart T, and Mazurek MF (1991) The treatment of neuroleptic malignant syndrome: Are dantrolene and bromocriptine useful adjuncts to supportive care? Br J Psychiatr 159, 709–712.

Rupniak NMJ, Jenner P, and Marsden CD (1986) Acute dystonia induced by neuroleptic drugs. Psychopharmacology 88, 403–419.

Sachdev P, Kruk J, Kneebone M, et al. (1995) Clozapine-induced neuroleptic malignant syndrome: Review and report of new cases. J Clin Psychopharmacol 15, 365–371.

Safferman AZ, Lieberman JA, Pollack S, et al. (1993) Akathisia and clozapine treatment. J Clin Psychopharmacol 13, 286–287.

Sajjad SH (1998) Vitamin E in the treatment of tardive dyskinesia: A preliminary study over 7 months at different doses. Int Clin Psychopharmacol 13, 147–155.

Salam SA and Kilzieh N (1988) Lorazepam treatment of psychogenic catatonia: An update. J Clin Psychiatr 49, 16–21.

Saltz BL, Woerner MG, Kane JM, et al. (1991) Prospective study of tardive dyskinesia incidence in the elderly. J Am Med Assoc 266, 2402–2406.

Schonecker M (1957) Ein eigentumliches syndrom im oralen Bereich bei Megaphen Applikation. Nervenarzt 28, 35.

Seeman MJ, Patel J, and Pyke J (1981) Tardive dyskinesia with Tourette-like syndrome. J Clin Psychiatr 42, 357–358.

Sewell DD and Jeste DV (1991) Distinguishing neuroleptic malignant syndrome (NMS) from NMS-like acute medical illnesses: A study of 34 cases. J Neuropsychiatr Clin Neurosci 4, 265–269.

Sewell DD and Jeste DV (1992a) Metoclopramide-associated tardive dyskinesia: An analysis of 67 cases. Arch Fam Med 1, 271–278.

Sewell DD and Jeste DV (1992b) Neuroleptic malignant syndrome: Clinical presentation, pathophysiology, and treatment. In Medical Psychiatric Practice, Stoudemire A and Fogel BS (eds). American Psychiatric Press, Washington DC, pp. 425–452.

Shalev A and Munitz H (1986) The neuroleptic malignant syndrome: Agent and host interaction. Acta Psychiatr Scand 73, 337–347.

Shalev A, Hermesh H, and Munitz H (1989) Mortality from neuroleptic malignant syndrome. J Clin Psychiatr 50, 18–25.

Shriqui CL, Bradwejn J, Annable L, et al. (1992) Vitamin E in the treatment of tardive dyskinesia: A double-blind placebo-controlled study. Am J Psychiatr 149, 391–393.

Simpson GM (1970) Long-acting antipsychotic agents and extrapyramidal side effects. Dis Nerv Syst 31, 12–14.

Simpson GM and Lindenmayer JP (1997) Extrapyramidal symptoms in patients treated with risperidone. J Clin Psychopharmacol 17, 194–201.

Simpson GM, Lee JM, and Shrivastava RK (1978) Clozapine in tardive dyskinesia. Psychopharmacology 56, 75–80.

Slovenko R (2000) Update on legal issues associated with tardive dyskinesia. J Clin Psychiatr 61, 45–57.

Small JG, Milstein V, Marhenke JD, et al. (1987) Treatment outcome with clozapine in tardive dyskinesia, neuroleptic sensitivity, and treatment-resistant psychosis. J Clin Psychiatr 48, 263–267.

Smith JM and Baldessarini RJ (1980) Changes in prevalence, severity, and recovery in tardive dyskinesia with age. Arch Gen Psychiatr 37, 1368–1373.

Sovner R and Dimascio A (1978) Extrapyramidal syndromes and other neurological side effects of psychotropic drugs. In Extrapyramidal Syndromes and Other Neurological Side Effects of Psychotropic Drugs, Lipton MA, Dimascio A, and Killam KF (eds). Raven Press, New York, pp. 1021–1032.

Sramek J, Roy S, Ahrens T, et al. (1991) Prevalence of tardive dyskinesia among three ethnic groups of chronic psychiatric patients. Hosp Comm Psychiatr 42, 590–592.

Stahl SM (1980) Tardive Tourette syndrome in an autistic patient after long-term neuroleptic administration. Am J Psychiatr 137, 1267.

Stahl SM and Berger PA (1982) Bromocriptine, physostigmine, and neurotransmitter mechanisms in the dystonias. Neurology 32, 889–892.

Stern TA and Anderson WH (1979) Benztropine prophylaxis of dystonic reactions. Psychopharmacol 61, 261–262.

Sternbach H (1991) The serotonin syndrome. Am J Psychiatr 148, 705–713.

Street JS, Tollefson GD, Tohen M, et al. (2000) Olanzapine for psychotic conditions in the elderly. Psychiatr Ann 30, 191–196.

Sweet RA, Pollock BG, Rosen J, et al. (1994) Early detection of neuroleptic-induced parkinsonism in elderly patients with dementia. J Geriatr Psychiatr Neurology 7, 251–253.

Swett C Jr. (1975) Drug-induced dystonia. Am J Psychiatr 132, 532–534.

Syndulko K, Gilden ER, and Hansch EC (1981) Decreased verbal memory associated with anticholinergic treatment in Parkinson's disease patients. Int J Neurosci 14, 61–66.

Tandon R, Harrigan E, and Zorn SH (1997) Ziprasidone: A novel antipsychotic with unique pharmacology and therapeutic potential. J Serotonin Res 4, 159–177.

Tarsy D (1992) Akathisia. In Movement Disorders in Neurology and Neuropsychiatry, Joseph AB and Young RR (eds). Blackwell Scientific, Boston, pp. 88–99.

Tarsy D, Granacher R, and Bralower M (1977) Tardive dyskinesia in young adults. Am J Psychiatr 134, 1032–1034.

Tollefson GD, Beasley CM, Tran PV, et al. (1997) Olanzapine versus haloperidol in the treatment of schizophrenia and schizoaffective and schizophreniform disorders: Results of an international collaborative trial. Am J Psychiatr 154, 457–465.

Ungvari GS, Chiu HF, Lam LC, et al. (1999) Gradual withdrawal of long-term anticholinergic antiparkinson medication in Chinese patients with chronic schizophrenia. J Clin Psychopharmacol 19, 141–148.

Van Putten T (1975) The many faces of akathisia. Compr Psychiatr 16, 43–47.

Van Putten T, Mutalipassi LR, and Malkin MD (1974) Phenothiazine-induced decompensation. Arch Gen Psychiatr 30, 102–105.

Walters A, Hening W, Chokroverty S, et al. (1986) Opioid responsiveness in patients with neuroleptic-induced akathisia. Movt Disord 1, 119–127.

Weiner WJ, Goetz CG, Nausieda PA, et al. (1978) Respiratory dyskinesias: Extrapyramidal dysfunction and dyspnea. Ann Intern Med 88, 327–331.

Wettstein RM (1988) Psychiatry and the law. In Textbook of Psychiatry, Talbot JA, Hales RE, and Yudofsky SC (eds). American Psychiatric Press, Washington DC, pp. 1078–1079.

Winslow RS, Stillner V, and Coons DJ (1986) Prevention of acute dystonic reactions in patients beginning high-potency neuroleptics. Am J Psychiatr 143, 706–710.

Woerner MG, Saltz BL, Kane JM, et al. (1993) Diabetes and development of tardive dyskinesia. Am J Psychiatr 150, 966–968.

Wong DF, Wagner HN Jr., Dannals RF, et al. (1984) Effects of age on dopamine and serotonin receptors measured by positron emission tomography in the living human brain. Science 226, 1393–1396.

Yamawaki S, Yanagawa K, and Morio M (1986) Possible central effect of dantrolene sodium in neuroleptic malignant syndrome. J Clin Psychopharmacol 6, 378–379.

Yassa R and Jeste DV (1992) Gender differences in tardive dyskinesia: A critical review of the literature. Schizophr Bull 18(4), 701–715.

Yassa R and Jones BD (1985) Complications of tardive dyskinesia: A review. Psychosomatics 26, 305–313.

Yassa R, Nair V, and Schwartz G (1984) Tardive dyskinesia: A two-year follow-up study. Psychosomatics, 25, 852–855.

Young RR (1992) Tremor: An overview. In Movement Disorders in Neurology and Neuropsychiatry, Joseph AB and Young RR (eds). Blackwell Scientific, Boston, pp. 565–566.

# 82 Relational Problems

Martha C. Tompson
David J. Miklowitz
John F. Clarkin

Relational Problem Related to a Mental
    Disorder or General Medical Condition
Parent–Child Relational Problem
Partner Relational Problem
Sibling Relational Problem
Relational Problem Not Otherwise Specified

## Introduction

A relational problem is a situation in which two or more emotionally attached individuals (i.e., family members, romantic partners) engage in communication or behavior patterns that are destructive or unsatisfying, or both, to one or more of the individuals. Relational problems deserve clinical attention because, once initiated, they tend to be perpetuating and chronic, and are frequently contemporaneous with or are followed by other serious problems, such as individual symptoms in the most vulnerable members of the family (e.g., depression) or social unit dissolution (e.g., divorce). They may be diagnosed either in the presence or absence of individual disorders given in the *Diagnostic and Statistical Manual of Mental Disorders* (DSM).

The strength and direction of causality between the individual and the relational problem are empirically undetermined. Few empirical investigations of the relational problems that are "precursors" to individual pathology have been conducted. Most of the existing research selects disturbed family units in which one member has an existing disorder (e.g., schizophrenia, depression) and examines the communication difficulties that accompany the disorder. Thus, cause-and-effect relations between individual disorders and relational difficulties have not been experimentally specified.

There is also the issue of generalization: Do those who manifest relational problems with a spouse or other family member manifest these same problems with others and in other contexts? Only a beginning literature exists on this issue. However, preliminary data suggest that some individuals manifest severe communication difficulties with their spouses or other family members but not with persons outside the family.

## Definition

Relational problems are placed in the fourth edition of the DSM (DSM-IV-TR) section on other conditions that may be a focus of clinical attention. Five specific relational problems are described:

1. **Relational problem related to a mental disorder or general medical condition:** a pattern of impaired family interaction in the presence of a mental disorder or medical condition in a family member.
2. **Parent–child relational problem:** a pattern of family interaction between parent and child that shows signs of impairment, such as faulty communication, overprotection, or inadequate discipline. The family interaction is associated with clinically significant impairment or symptoms in an individual or in family functioning, or both.
3. **Partner relational problem:** a pattern of interaction between spouses or partners characterized by negative and distorted communication or noncommunication, which is associated with clinically significant impairment in one or both partners.
4. **Sibling relational problem:** a pattern of interaction between siblings that is associated with clinically significant impairment in individual or family functioning.
5. **Relational problem not otherwise specified:** relational problems not listed here, such as extra-family relational problems or difficulties with others, such as coworkers.

*Source*: American Psychiatric Association (1994) Diagnostic and Statistical Manual of Mental Disorders, 4th ed. APA, Washington DC.

## Constructs and Manifestations of Relational Problems

The empirical data substantiate the existence of relational difficulties that can be reliably assessed and have clinical significance (Clarkin and Miklowitz 1994). The data are sparse in reference to each DSM disorder and coexisting family relational difficulties, with the exceptions of depression and schizophrenia.

In our examination of the construct of relational problems, we emphasize those constructs that have shown reliable assessment in research and that have been found to (1) distinguish distressed from nondistressed couples or families, or (2) to identify couples or families in which one or more members manifest significant individual pathologic conditions. Some constructs with theoretical importance were found to lack one or both of these criteria and were not included in this review.

Four major constructs (Table 82–1) have been investigated that describe nodal areas of relational difficulty in the family and marital environment: structure, communication, expression of affect, and problem solving. Relational difficulties in other environments (e.g., work) have not been described in the clinical literature.

It is interesting to compare the constructs investigated in the couples and family contexts. The areas of affective communication and conflict resolution are almost identical in conceptualization, behavioral criteria, and importance in the spouse–spouse and parent–child communication domains. However, three other rather sharply defined constructs in the parent–child literature are not fully represented in the spouse–spouse literature: communication deviance (CD), emotional overinvolvement, and coercive process. In the cognitive realm, the CD construct (unclear, amorphous, or fragmented communication) has been investigated primarily among schizophrenic patients and their parents; comparable work has not been done with couples. The more general construct of communication has been explored with marital couples, with no theoretical link to thought disorder and schizophrenia.

Coercive processes—the shaping of the behavior of parents by negative behavior on the part of the child—is similar to negative escalation in couples. Although not yet investigated in couples, it is quite conceivable that one

spouse could effectively utilize a coercive process with the other spouse. Overinvolvement, which has been explored in the parent–child literature may have a related domain in the marital literature—specifically, structure. Indeed, the overinvolvement construct has been seen as most relevant with children and parents and has little predictive utility in adult couple samples (Vaughn and Leff 1976a, Butzlaff and Hooley 1998, Hooley et al. 1986). However, it seems that the concept of structure, with the issues of leadership, dominance and submission, and distribution of functions, is an area that needs further exploration in reference to both couples and the entire family.

The Global Assessment of Relational Functioning Scale included in DSM-IV-TR for rating relational units utilizes the constructs that we have found in the empirical literature. The scale anchor points refer to structure ("agreed-on patterns or routines exist that help meet the usual needs of each family/couple member"), affect expression ("a range of feeling is expressed"; "despair and cynicism are pervasive"), communication ("communication is frequently inhibited"), and problem solving and conflict resolution ("decision making is usually competent"; "decision making is tyrannical or quite ineffective"; "unresolved conflicts often interfere with daily routines"). Descriptions and a review of the relevant research on each of these constructs—structure, communication, affect expression, and problem solving—will be reviewed below, both for couples and for families.

## Structure

For a marriage or family to function as a unit requires leadership and distribution of functions. Leadership, dominance, and power distribution can all have a profound effect on the quality of interaction satisfaction and on adequate functioning of both couples and families, both in ordinary and in stressful circumstances.

### Couples

Dominance as measured by verbal frequency has not distinguished functional and dysfunctional families (Jacob 1975). When one spouse is depressed, the power distribution is not always as theoretically hypothesized (i.e., depressed spouse submissive to dominance of the nondepressed partner). Contrary to expectation, Hooper and colleagues (1977) found that depressed patients produced substantial control-oriented communication with their spouses during an acute depressed episode. In a hospitalized sample, Merikangas and coworkers (1979) found that during early therapy sessions, the patient was strongly influenced by the behavior of his or her spouse; however, by the last session, there was a more equal balance of power. In contrast, introversion and interpersonal dependency may reflect enduring abnormalities in the functioning of individuals with remitted depression (Barnett and Gotlib 1988).

### Families

Some parent–offspring relationships are marked by unclear boundaries and overdependence, often inhibiting the offspring's ability to separate, individuate, or recover from illness (Minuchin 1974). With respect to psychiatric and sometimes medical disorders, it is not unusual to see a pairing of an overprotective, overinvolved parent with a

| Table 82–1 | Empirically Derived Family Relational Constructs |
|---|---|
| Structure | Leadership and distribution of functions |
| Overinvolvement | Unclear boundaries; overdependence |
| Communication | Amount and clarity of information exchange |
| Communication deviance | Unclear, amorphous, fragmented, and/or unintelligible communication |
| Coercion | Behavior control by use of aversive communication |
| Expression of affect | Implicit or explicit verbalization of affective tone |
| Problem solving | Definition of problems, consideration of alternative lines of action, agreement to use optimal line of action |
| Conflict and its resolution | Process of resolving differences of opinion |

highly disabled, passive, withdrawn offspring. Because ill offspring in these families often elicit such responses, an overinvolved relationship is best thought of as a dyadic attribute rather than a problem generated by a parent. Overinvolvement is often difficult to define or assess in parents of school-age or adolescent children (Asarnow et al. 1987). However, among studies of youth, those focusing on separation anxiety, and school refusal in particular, describe parental overinvolvement and protectiveness as complicating features (Kearney and Silverman 1995).

A number of inadequately designed studies in the 1950s and 1960s indicated that overprotectiveness characterized the parents of patients with schizophrenia (Tietze 1949, Reichard and Tillman 1950, Clardy 1951, Wahl 1954, 1956, Lidz et al. 1964, Gerard and Siegel 1950, Mark 1953, Freeman and Grayson 1955, Kohn and Clausen 1956, Lane and Singer 1957, Horowitz and Lovell 1960, Lu 1961, Garmezy et al. 1961, McGhie 1950, 1961, McKeown 1950, Alanen 1958, 1966). The term *expressed emotion* (EE) is used to refer to critical comments, hostility, and/or overinvolvement as expressed by a family member toward another family member with a mental disorder. Studies suggest that overinvolvement is a risk factor for later episodes of psychosis among patients diagnosed with schizophrenia, independent of the level of criticism demonstrated by the family (Brown et al. 1972, Vaughn and Leff 1976a, Vaughn et al. 1984, Leff and Vaughn 1985).

Subsequent EE studies and studies of family interaction have delineated other characteristics of overinvolved relationships in families of patients with schizophrenia. In terms of premorbid social adjustment, patients with schizophrenia in emotionally overinvolved families are more likely than those in normally involved families to have had poor premorbid social adjustment and a high level of residual symptoms after acute episodes (Miklowitz et al. 1983). Overinvolvement is reasonably common among families of patients with chronic schizophrenia (Miklowitz et al. 1986) but is infrequently observed among parents of recent-onset patients with schizophrenia (Neuchterlein et al. 1986). Emotionally overinvolved parents of patients with schizophrenia are more likely than normally involved parents to use an excessive number of intrusive, "mind-reading" statements in direct family interaction (Miklowitz et al. 1984). They are also characterized by high levels of CD (Miklowitz et al. 1986).

Several other studies suggest that parental overinvolvement combined with low levels of caring are retrospectively reported by patients with neurotic depression (Parker 1979, 1983) and borderline personality disorder (Zweig-Frank and Paris 1991). Interestingly, parental overinvolvement was associated with a better course of illness in one sample of individuals with borderline personality disorder (Hooley and Hoffman 1999), suggesting that its impact varies across different forms of psychiatric disorder.

## Communication of Information

Verbal communication between two or more individuals involves the various aspects of information exchange, including the amount and clarity of the information and the reception of the information by another. This broad concept of communication implies the willingness to convey information, the accuracy and clarity of the information, and the accurate decoding of the information by the other.

## Couples

The amount and quality of verbal communication have differentiated distressed and nondistressed couples, and treatment leads to an improvement in communication (Ely et al. 1973). Measures of communication quality taken early in marriage are predictive of marital satisfaction 4 years later (Rogge and Bradbury 1999). In the area of information exchange, there are more inaccuracies in the communication of distressed couples than in that of nondistressed couples owing to encoding (sending clear messages) rather than decoding (understanding partner's messages) errors. Distressed husbands were distinguished by more encoding and decoding errors than nondistressed husbands (Noller 1981, 1984). Although both distressed and nondistressed couples are relatively inaccurate observers of their own interactional behavior, distressed couples are comparatively less reliable (Elwood and Jacobson 1982, 1988).

In addition to the overt verbal communication, various cognitive constructs are thought to be intimately related to the nature and quality of communication. Five areas of cognitive phenomena are hypothesized to play important roles in marital communication and maladjustment: selective attention, attributions, expectancies, assumptions, and standards (Baucom et al. 1989, Robinson and Price 1980). Not all of these areas have been equally investigated.

Distressed spouses focus on negative behavior; positive interactions often are ignored (Fincham and O'Leary 1983). Distressed spouses tend to attribute their partner's undesired communication behavior as global and stable (Camper et al. 1988, Holtzworth-Munroe and Jacobson 1985), and the partner is blamed for her or his negative behavior, which is seen as intentional, global, stable, and originating from internal factors. In contrast, nondistressed individuals give each other credit for positive behavior and overlook or exonerate their spouses for negative behavior (Jacobson et al. 1985, Fincham et al. 2000). While the evolution or developmental history of these cognitive sets has not been clearly delineated, current evidence suggests that negative attributions for partner behavior may predict marital satisfaction over time.

The relationship between these attributions and marital satisfaction may be mediated by spouses' efficacy expectations for the relationship (Markman 1981). Data on premarital communication patterns and later marital conflict also suggest that certain forms of premarital communication (as opposed to specific content areas) predict a growing negative cognitive set held by partners toward each other (Buehlman et al. 1992). Indeed, among both newlywed couples and couples with young children, spouses' cognitions about the relationship were highly predictive of divorce or stability over time (Carrere et al. 2000, Epstein and Eidelson 1981). In the area of distorted assumptions that can affect marital behavior, it has been found that distressed spouses make the assumption that their partners cannot change the relationship and that overt disagreement is destructive (Jordan and McCormick 1987). Likewise, unrealistic assumptions and standards about relationships are predictive of general marital distress (Patterson 1982, Patterson et al. 1991). In the area of expectations, Pretzer and colleagues (1991) found that spouses' low efficacy expectations regarding their ability to solve their marital problems were associated with marital distress and depression.

## Families

Many of the same disordered processes (e.g., expression of hostility or excessive criticism, poor information exchange, lack of conflict resolution) in the spousal communication literature are presumed to disrupt healthy family functioning. Unlike in the marital literature, however, the independent variable in family studies is often the presence or absence of a psychopathologic condition in an offspring or parent rather than high or low levels of marital distress. This section reviews disordered processes within families that have empirical validity in distinguishing disordered from nondisordered states, including coercive family processes and communication deviance.

## *Coercive Communication Processes*

When two individuals within a family (i.e., a parent and child) are controlling each others' behavior via aversive stimuli or responses that are perceived by these individuals or by others in the family as unpleasant, a "coercive entrapment" has developed (Patterson 1982). The key ingredient to such entrapment is negative reinforcement. In this model, children first learn to perform mild, relatively innocuous aversive behaviors (e.g., whining, teasing, running back and forth, negativism) as a way of terminating aversive behaviors that have been issued from a parent (e.g., scolding, issuing negative commands). The result is that the parent eventually withdraws his/her demands in order to terminate the child's aversive behavior. For the child, her or his aversive behavior has terminated the original aversive parental behavior (e.g., scolding). For the parent, her or his acquiescence has terminated the child's aversive behavior (e.g., whining). In this manner, the parent's attempts to discipline the child often have the effect of reinforcing the child's coercive behaviors and subsequent aggression (Patterson 1982, Patterson et al. 1991).

The coercive behaviors on the part of the child may escalate as this family interactional pattern continues, from minor coercive behaviors (e.g., whining) to more intense (if less frequent) coercive behaviors (e.g., hitting, temper tantrums, stealing). Indeed, coercive exchanges can be thought of as a series of "rounds" that escalate in severity and increase the probability that one or more family members (the child or the parent) will react aggressively (Robinson and Jacobson 1987).

A number of studies provide validation for the association between highly coercive family relationships and antisocial/aggressive behavior (Burgess and Conger 1978, Kopfstein 1972, Lobitz and Johnson 1975, Patterson 1976, 1980, 1982, Patterson and Cobb 1971, Patterson et al. 1991, Robinson and Jacobson 1987, Snyder 1977, Wahler and Dumas 1987) and substance abuse (Hops et al. 2000) in offspring. For example, members of families containing children who are socially aggressive or who steal engage in higher rates of aversive behavior than do members of families containing normal children (Patterson 1982, Patterson et al. 1991). Mothers of children with conduct problems have been found to be more likely to initiate and continue unpleasant, aversive interchanges with the index child than mothers of normal children (Lobitz and Johnson 1975, Patterson 1982, Patterson and Cobb 1971). In addition, children with behavior problems are more likely to continue coercive interchanges with their mothers than are control children (Patterson 1982). Perhaps as a consequence, coercive relationships are frequently associated with depression in one or more family members (Patterson 1980). It is not clear, however, whether coercive processes simply reflect the parents' response to the child's aggressive behavior or whether these processes play a direct role in causing aggression in the child.

## *Communication Deviance*

Wynne and Singer (1963a, 1963b) observed that the transactional processes of families of concurrently hospitalized patients with schizophrenia were often unclear, amorphous, fragmented, or unintelligible. In their research, these high levels of CD discriminated parents of children with schizophrenia from parents of children with borderline personality, neurotic, antisocial, or autistic disorders and from parents of normal children (Singer and Wynne 1963, 1965a, 1965b). The authors believed that CD was present before, and was etiologically associated with, the appearance of schizophrenia in genetically prone offspring. Direct evidence for this view derives from one high-risk study demonstrating that high levels of CD among parents of disturbed but nonpsychotic adolescents predicted the onset of disorders within the schizophrenia spectrum (i.e., schizophrenic or schizotypal, schizoid, paranoid, or borderline personality disorders) among these adolescents who had follow-up into adulthood (Goldstein 1987). However, CD may covary with the severity of the offspring's diagnosis rather than the presence of a specific diagnosis. Indeed, high CD is characteristic of the parents of bipolar, as well as schizophrenic, offspring (Miklowitz et al. 1991) and may increase with severity of offspring psychopathology (i.e., from normal to neurotic to borderline to psychotic) (Wynne et al. 1977).

Although CD appears to be correlated with a diagnosis of schizophrenia, a number of mechanisms may explain this association (Miklowitz and Tompson in press). Two in particular have garnered empirical support. First, CD in parents may be internalized by the child and lead to the development of difficulties in processing information and perceiving reality. Thus, CD contributes to the development of vulnerability to schizophrenia. This view receives modest support from the diagnostic discrimination studies and high-risk study cited above. More recently, Wahlberg and colleagues (1997) demonstrated that individuals with high genetic risk (having a schizophrenic biological parent) who were exposed to high CD adoptive parents were at particularly high risk for developing thought disorder. Second, CD may reflect an indirect expression of the genetic vulnerability to schizophrenia in parents of affected offspring. One study suggested that parents of schizophrenic patients who show high levels of the perceptual–cognitive forms of CD also show dysfunction on information-processing tasks (Wagener et al. 1986). Two other studies demonstrated cross-generational correlations between CD in parents and the degree of attentional and information-processing dysfunction in their diagnosed schizophrenic offspring (Nuechterlein et al. 1989, Asarnow et al. 1988). However, levels of CD are not correlated with the presence or absence of DSM-III-R (American Psychiatric Association 1987) diagnoses in parents (current or past) (Goldstein et al. 1990).

In summary, studies suggest that high levels of CD are a correlate of severe psychiatric conditions and may influence the development, and possibly the course, of these conditions. It is premature to refer to CD as an etiological agent in schizophrenia or other disorders.

## Expression of Affect

All messages have cognitive and emotional content and overtones, but it is conceivable that family units could be relatively proficient in one area while deficient and disturbed in the other. Negatively toned communication can consist of intensely personal, "character-assassinating" remarks (e.g., "You are an incompetent person") or, alternatively, an excessive number of specifically delineated criticisms of a person's behavior (e.g., "You never try hard in school"). It is also common to observe "negatively escalating cycles," which become increasingly pejorative and personal as they continue. Often, these cycles are accompanied by negative, defensive, nonverbal behavior that also escalates (Hahlweg et al. 1989, Simoneau et al. 1998).

### Couples

When spousal communication is extremely negative or pejorative, the marriage is likely to be at high risk and symptoms may develop in one or both mates. Because the direct and indirect expressions of affects such as anger, hostility, and resentment seem central to both poor problem-solving behavior and low marital satisfaction, we isolate affect from cognition for conceptual clarity and emphasis.

Depressed and distressed spouses are more likely to express dysphoric affect than are nondepressed and nondistressed spouses (Hautzinger et al. 1982, Kowalik and Gotlib 1987). In addition, distressed spouses exchange more negative affect than do nondistressed spouses (Schaap 1984). As the EE literature indicates, a subgroup of spouses of depressed patients demonstrate critical remarks and nonacceptance of the mate, which are associated with a poor prognosis for the depressed partner (Hooley et al. 1986).

Distressed couples, compared with nondistressed couples, are more *affectively reactive* to ongoing negative and positive stimuli (Jacobson et al. 1980, 1982). There is a greater likelihood that distressed spouses, compared with nondistressed spouses, will react negatively to displeasing behavior by the other spouse (Jacobson et al. 1980). This type of behavior predicted marital dissatisfaction in at least one longitudinal study (Markman 1981).

A *circular interactional pattern* has been described in the literature on depression and marriage. This pattern resembles the coercive processes of families of aggressive children described above. In this marital pattern, negative communication and a lack of positive support and responsiveness on the depressed spouse's part elicit hostility and withdrawal from the nondepressed partner, which in turn elicits more depression and more calls for reassurance by the depressed individual (Baucom and Epstein 1990, Birchler et al. 1975, Hinchcliffe et al. 1978, Klerman et al. 1984). Spouses of depressed mates rated as high in EE showed interactions characterized by negative and critical remarks, frequent disagreement with the depressed spouse, and nonacceptance of what the mate has said to them. In turn, depressed mates showed low frequencies of self-disclosure and high levels of neutral nonverbal behavior (Hooley 1986).

Depressed couples, compared with control subjects, are characterized by negative affect after interactions and negative appraisals of the other spouse's behavior (Gotlib and Whiffen 1989). Couples with a depressed partner exhibit negative and asymmetrical communication, with frequent expression of dysphoric and uncomfortable feelings (Hautzinger et al. 1982). In general, depressed couples tend to be characterized by negative affect (Kowalik and Gotlib 1987).

### Families

As in couples, families may be able to communicate clearly but may deliver messages that are highly critical, pejorative, hostile, or vilifying. Although some degree of this type of communication is to be expected in every family, an excessive number or duration of negatively toned interactions may become associated with disturbance in one or more family members. Although it is not unusual for one family member to be the primary source of hostile emotional communication and another the primary target, it is also common for other family members to "aid and abet" these types of interchanges.

Throughout childhood, the emotional quality of parent–child interaction impacts development and adjustment. Negatively toned parental feedback may lead to the internalization of a more negative self-concept and set the stage for future difficulties (Harter 1999). In addition, parental expression of affect in parent–child interactions may be strongly linked to children's social development and acceptance by peers over time. Expressions of positive affect among mothers predict greater acceptance by the child's peers, whereas expressions of negative affect among fathers predict poorer acceptance by peers (Isley 1996).

There is now evidence from more than 35 studies to suggest that excessive criticism, hostility, or emotional overinvolvement (high EE), or a combination of these from parents, as measured by the individually administered Camberwell Family Interview (Vaughn and Leff 1976b), are prospectively associated with the course of numerous psychiatric difficulties (Butzlaff and Hooley 1998), including schizophrenia (Miklowitz 1994, Kavanagh 1992, Parker and Hadzi-Pavlovic 1990), bipolar affective disorder (Miklowitz et al. 1988), nonpsychotic depression (Hooley et al. 1986, Vaughn and Leff 1976a), alcoholism (Fichter et al. 1997, O'Farrell et al. 1998), and obesity (Fischmann-Havstad and Marston 1984). High family EE is also predictive of poorer outcome among individuals undergoing behavioral treatments for obsessive–compulsive disorders, agoraphobia (Chambless and Steketee 1999), and posttraumatic stress disorder (Tarrier et al. 1999).

A separate domain of inquiry has concerned negatively toned family interactions. In a 15-year prospective study of nonpsychotic, disturbed adolescents (Goldstein 1987), affective negativity in parent to adolescent interactions (i.e., criticism, guilt induction, intrusiveness) was independently predictive (along with the family's level of CD) of the severity of outcomes observed in these adolescents at 15-year follow-up. Two other studies (Doane et al. 1985, Miklowitz et al. 1988) using similar procedures and construct definitions found that the level of affective negativity during interactions between parents and their schizophrenic or bipolar offspring, measured after the patient's hospital discharge, was associated with the risk of the patient's relapse at a 9-month follow-up. Finally, Doane and co-workers (1986) in a controlled family treatment study found that family treatment was effective in delaying new episodes of schizophrenia if it was successful in reducing the number of critical comments and intrusive, "mind-reading" statements observed among parents during pretreatment family interaction assessments. Thus, there is strong evidence for the prognostic validity of negative affective communication or attitudes within families containing a patient with a severe psychiatric illness.

## Problem Solving

Problem solving is a general construct relating to the manner in which two or more people define conflict issues, consider alternative lines of action, and proceed to the most optimal action as demanded by a problem situation (Falloon et al. 1984). The impact of negative life events within a relational unit may be impacted by the strategies they use for approaching and solving problems (Cohan and Bradbury 1997). It is common for families seeking treatment to be unable to solve major family problems—this is often the very reason that they seek treatment. However, when families do not have the skills for solving problems in general, such as the ability to define a problem or generate possible solutions, they may become "stuck" in ways that prevent the growth or individuation of one or more members.

### Couples

Distressed couples manifest more negative communication and fewer positive communication behaviors when solving problems, as rated by observational coding systems (Birchler et al. 1975, Gottman 1979, Gottman et al. 1977, Revenstorf et al. 1984, Schaap 1984). Problem-solving behavior is less frequent (Biglan et al. 1985), more negative (Vincent et al. 1975), and often results in ineffective solutions in distressed couples (Winemiller and Mitchell 1994). Problem escalation (i.e., problem solving by spouse 1, followed by negativity by spouse 2, followed by negativity by spouse 1) is also more characteristic of distressed couples (Revenstorf et al. 1984). Furthermore, negative reciprocity, involving mutual fault finding, cross-complaining (Gottman 1994), and the communication of global and negative attributions, is also greater among distressed than nondistressed couples (Billings 1979, Gottman et al. 1976a, 1976b, Margolin and Wampold 1981, Rausch et al. 1974, Revenstorf et al. 1984). Positive reciprocity is more characteristic of nondistressed couples (Revenstorf et al. 1984), but not in all samples (Margolin and Wampold 1981). Poor problem-solving ability has been associated with depression among spouses (Basco et al. 1992) and this association is over and above the effects of marital discord and depression alone (Christian et al. 1994).

Conflict resolution is a specific subset of problem-solving behaviors (i.e., resolving differences of opinion between two or more people). Whereas all couples display conflict, it is especially chains of disagreement that characterize distressed couples (Gottman et al. 1977, Margolin and Wampold 1981, Hahlweg et al. 1984a, 1984b). The reciprocity of negative rather than positive behavior distinguishes distressed from nondistressed couples (Revenstorf et al. 1984, Schaap 1984).

Christensen and Shenk (1991) used a self-report instrument to investigate the role of constructive communication, avoidance of communication, and demand–withdrawal communication (in which demands by one partner are consistently met with withdrawal by the other partner). Distressed couples in this study (clinic-referred couples and divorcing couples) had less mutual constructive communication, more avoidance of communication, and more demand–withdrawal communication than did nondistressed couples.

From a longitudinal perspective, predictors of short-term and long-term marital satisfaction appear to be different (Gottman and Krokoff 1989). Although disagreement and angry exchanges relate to dissatisfaction in the short run, they may not be harmful across time. In contrast, longitudinal marital deterioration is best predicted by defensiveness, whining, stubbornness, and withdrawal from interaction. Stonewalling, in which one partner adamantly refuses to discuss a problem, is particularly associated with divorce (Gottman 1994). Interestingly, in a large longitudinal study of marriage and economic stress, Conger and colleagues (1999) found that effective problem solving among couples reduced the impact of marital conflict on perceived marital satisfaction. Thus, when couples are able to generate and implement effective problem solutions, disagreement per se does not lead to unhappiness with the relationship.

### Families

When a family is deficient in solving problems, the tension level in the household is likely to increase and conflict between members tends to escalate. In such a family climate, children do not learn to recognize the steps necessary to solve interpersonal problems and may develop psychiatric problems or their social or academic competence may suffer (Blechman 1990).

In general, a strong relation has been found in the literature between the way parents solve socialization problems of their children and the cognitive abilities of these children (Baumrind 1975, Bee et al. 1982, Bradley and Cadwell 1980, Gottfried and Gottfried 1983, Hess and Shipman 1965). For example, in a study of school-age children, Blechman and McEnroe (1985) found that those families that built the tallest towers in a cooperative task were those with the most academically and socially competent children.

Compared to nonclinic families, families seeking help at a mental health clinic demonstrated less problem solving (Krinsley and Bry 1991) and more disagreement (Whittaker and Bry 1991) in problem-solving discussions. Poor family problem solving has been noted in the families of youth with depression (Sheeber and Sorenson 1998). Forehand and associates (1990) found that during direct interaction between mothers and these adolescents, mothers' problem-solving scores (i.e., ability to define a problem clearly and propose alternative solutions) and positive communication scores (i.e., acknowledgments, openness to others' opinions) were higher when these mothers were from intact rather than divorced families. In addition, conflict initiation occurred more frequently among divorced than married mothers. Perhaps most significantly, these parenting skills predicted adolescent functioning in the domains of cognitive and social competence. Similarly, Goodman and colleagues (1999) found that frequent, negative conflict between parents was associated with poorer social problem-solving skills among youth.

Finally, findings from intervention studies indicate that problem-solving skills are amenable to intervention and that improvements in family problem solving are associated with decreases in conflict and enhanced family functioning. Falloon and coworkers (1984) found that communication-oriented and problem-solving-oriented family treatment (behavioral family management) was far more effective in delaying episodes of psychosis among recently hospitalized schizophrenic patients than was individual treatment of similar duration. In a reanalysis of Falloon and colleagues' data, Doane and coworkers (1986) found a marked increase, during the period from baseline to 3-month follow-up, in the number of spontaneously occurring problem-solving statements among families in family treatment. Little or no change in the frequency of these statements occurred among families in which patients received individual treatment. Furthermore, increases in problem-solving ability were most notable when a decrease in emotional negativity among parents as measured by number of critical and intrusive statements was also observed. Thus, an improved ability by the family to address problems in a structured manner may reduce its need to "ventilate."

Barkley and colleagues (2001) compared problem-solving communication training (PSCT) alone to a combination of PSCT and behavior management training (BMT) among families of youth with attention-deficit/hyperactivity disorder and oppositional defiant disorder. Both treatments used behavioral techniques to enhance problem-management skills. While the two treatments did not differ in outcomes, they both produced positive change in observed and self-reported measures of parent–child conflict. Thus, teaching problem-solving skills to parents and adolescents may address family conflicts associated with disruptive behavior disorders.

## Diagnosis of Relational Disorders

Although research on structure, expression of affect, communication, and problem solving in couples and families has lead to a greater understanding of the difficulties that can afflict these relational units, specific relational problems have only been recently included as a diagnostic entity in the DSM (see DSM-III-R, DSM-IV-TR) and clear diagnostic criteria have yet to be developed. Current textual descriptions of these conditions refer to impairment in the "pattern of interaction" in these relational units (American Psychiatric Association 2000, p. 736), reflecting the broad range of specific difficulties subsumed under these diagnostic entities.

## Phenomenology

Five specific relational problems are noted in DSM-IV (see the definition section earlier in the chapter). Family relational problems and partner relational problems are delineated below. These difficulties may also afflict relational units in the presence of a mental disorder or medical condition. The phenomenology of sibling relational problems and relational problems with other individuals have not been well explored.

### Partner Relational Problems

Clinical experience and the research descriptions suggest that marital (and couples) relational problems manifest in the following ways:

1. Couple does not clarify mutual requests, provide information, or accurately describe problems.
2. Spouse or spouses verbalize underlying attributions, assumptions, and expectations that are negative (e.g., spouse is globally negatively intentioned) or exaggerated (e.g., couples should never fight).
3. Affective communication is characterized by negative affect (e.g., anger, hostility, jealousy), critical remarks, disagreement with spouse, and nonacceptance of what the mate has communicated.
4. There is a low frequency of self-disclosure of thoughts, feelings, and wishes.
5. Couple demonstrates inadequate problem solving characterized by poor problem definition, lack of task focus, mutual criticism and complaint, and negative escalation.
6. Couple displays sequences of negative communication characterized by criticism, disagreement, negative listening, and refusal to agree.
7. Couple avoids conflict by withdrawal, lack of discussion, and subsequent nonresolution.

**Associated Features.** Associated features of marital communication difficulties or disorders include poor marital satisfaction, psychiatric disorder in one or both spouses, threatened and contemplated separation and divorce, or concentration and job performance difficulties.

### Family Relational Problems

Family relational problems manifest as the following:

1. Family is unable to communicate clearly, cannot communicate closure, or cannot share a focus of attention (CD).
2. Family communication is characterized by unidirectional hostility or frequent criticism or by bidirectional, negatively escalating cycles of pejorative or critical comments.
3. Parent–offspring relationships are characterized by overprotectiveness, overconcern, unnecessarily self-sacrificing behaviors, intrusiveness, or overdependence (emotional overinvolvement).
4. Parent–offspring interchanges are marked by negatively reinforcing coercive cycles that tend to perpetuate antisocial or aggressive behavior in one or more family members.
5. A broad array of family problems cannot be solved because of the family's inability to agree to try to solve,

define, generate, or evaluate solutions to, or implement solutions to, existing problems.

**Associated Features.** The associated features of parent–child communication difficulties or disorders include adolescent acting out and disruptive behavior, major psychiatric disorders in one or more family members (i.e., schizophrenia, affective disorder), poor parental morale, and parenting dissatisfaction.

## Assessment of Relational Disorders

### Overall Relationship Functioning

The Global Assessment of Relational Functioning Scale (GARF) (Group for Advancement of Psychiatry 1996) included in DSM-IV-TR is a 1 to 100 scale of overall relationship functioning, akin to the Global Assessment Scale for individuals. Recent studies have indicated that the GARF is reliable in clinical settings (Dausch et al. 1996, Rosen et al. 1997, Hilsenroth et al. 2000, Mottarella et al. 2001) and that changes in GARF scores are positively associated with both client and therapist-reported change in treatment and with treatment satisfaction (Ross and Doherty 2001).

### Structure

Family structure can be measured with self-report instruments as control subscales on both the Family Assessment Measure (Skinner et al. 1983) and the Family Environment Scale (Moos and Moos 1981) and as an organizational subscale on the latter. In interaction research, it has been recommended (Markman and Notarius 1987) that dominance be measured in terms of procedures that assess the consequences of behavior (e.g., influence of dominant member on decision making) rather than on who speaks first and/or for the greatest proportion of the time.

Parental overinvolvement has been defined in various ways in the psychiatric literature (Parker 1982), but the criteria used within the EE coding system (Leff and Vaughn 1985) are the best operationalized: a tendency to be overprotective of, overly concerned about, overly controlling of, or domineering toward an offspring; to engage in numerous self-sacrificing behaviors in the name of good parenting (e.g., the parent denies himself or herself social relationships to satisfy the needs of the offspring); to engage in intrusive, boundary-crossing, or mind-reading interactions with the offspring; and to react to minor events affecting the offspring with exaggerated emotional responses and to overdramatize these incidents. In return, the offspring may react with overt struggles for independence or autonomy or, in contrast, passivity, withdrawal, and overdependency. Parker and coworkers' (1979) well-validated Parental Bonding Instrument provides a working definition of overprotection: parental overcontrol, intrusion, and excessive contact, and preventing the child from acting independently (Parker 1983).

### Communication

Communication is measured in family and marital questionnaires—for example, with a communication subscale of the Family Assessment Measure (FAM-III) (Skinner et al. 1983); the Dyadic Adjustment Scale (Spanier 1976) with a dyadic cohesion subscale; and the Primary Communication Inventory (Navran 1967) with its verbal communication subscale.

Ratings of interpersonal behavior involving self-disclosure, positive solution, negative solution, justification, direct expression, criticism, critique, positive communication, and negative communication can be seen as relating to the general category of communication skills (Markman and Notarius 1987). As an example, Kategoriensystem für Partnerschaftliche Interaktion (KPI) (Hahlweg et al. 1984a) codes, such as self-disclosure ("I'm too angry to listen to you at the moment"), positive solutions ("I'll sweep the floor if you play with the kids"), problem description ("We've got a problem with the kids"), and disagreement ("That's not true"), provide evidence of communication skills. The brief Communication Patterns Questionnaire (Heavey et al. 1996) has shown strong associations with both marital satisfaction and the constructiveness of spousal behavior during video-taped problem-solving discussions.

Recently, measures have been developed to evaluate partner's cognitions that have been associated with communication difficulties. The Relationship Attribution Measure (Fincham and Bradbury 1992) assesses the manner in which partners assign responsibility for their spouses' behavior. The Marital Attitudes Survey (Pretzer et al. 1991) assesses spouses' attributions regarding their partners' attitudes and behaviors in the relationship and expectancies about the possibility of relationship change.

Communication deviance consists of two primary components: disorders of linguistic–verbal reasoning (i.e., unfinished phrases, unintelligibility, odd word usage) and perceptual–cognitive disturbances (i.e., inability to integrate multiple pieces of information into a coherent message; inability to perceive and describe an object or concept accurately). The majority of studies of CD have relied on transcripts of projective test (i.e., the Rorschach Inkblot Test or Thematic Apperception Test) responses from parents as the primary data source for coding CD. One study (Velligan et al. 1990) found a correspondence between levels of parental CD as measured in a projective and an interactional context, although not all forms of CD were measurable in both contexts.

Measurement of coercive processes usually requires that the observer watch the family interact directly, because these processes often occur on a behavior-exchange rather than a verbal-exchange level. In this way, coercive processes are to be distinguished from affectively negative verbal exchanges.

Perhaps the best-known system for coding coercive processes is the Family Interaction Coding System (Patterson 1982, Patterson et al. 1969). It is a home observation system in which positive, neutral, and negative behaviors on the part of all family members are coded sequentially by live observers, in contiguous 6-second time blocks. Interrater reliabilities for the system have been consistently high across studies (Robinson and Jacobson 1987).

### Expression of Affect

Family and marital questionnaires address affect in terms of expressiveness, a subscale of the Family Environment Scale (Moos and Moos 1981); affective communication, a subscale of the Marital Satisfaction Inventory (Snyder 1979, 1981); affectional expression, a subscale of the Dyadic Adjustment Scale (Spanier 1976); and the affective expression and involvement subscales of the Family Assessment Measure (Skinner et al. 1983). Studies using self-report instruments have also yielded interesting results (Hooley and Teasdale 1989, Kreisman et al. 1979, Haas et al. 1988).

For interaction research, it has been recommended that affect be coded by observing the affective content of both verbalizations and nonverbal behavior (Markman and Notarius 1987). Negatively toned family communication has been measured primarily via structured interviews of individual family members (e.g., the Camberwell Family Interview for rating EE) or observation and coding of family interactions (e.g., the affective style coding system or the KPI).

## Problem Solving

On self-report instruments, the Marital Satisfaction Inventory (Snyder 1979) has a problem-solving communication subscale. In addition, problem-solving behavior is often sampled directly, both as it spontaneously occurs in free-flowing discussion and in the context of solving assigned tasks, such as card sorting (Oliveri and Reiss 1981) or the revealed differences technique (Strodbeck 1951) and its modifications (Ferreira 1963).

Conflict is measured on the dyadic consensus subscale of the Dyadic Adjustment Scale (Spanier 1976) and on the conflict subscale of the Family Environment Scale (Moos and Moos 1981). It is measured in terms of disagreement about finances, sexual dissatisfaction, and conflict over child-rearing on the Marital Satisfaction Inventory (Snyder 1979); the Conflict Tactics Scales (Straus 1979) obtain self-report on strategies used to resolve conflicts in families, including reasoning, verbal aggression, and violence.

Interactional ratings of conflict are similar in content. Interactional ratings of agreement, disagreement, sequences of positive and negative communication, such as on the KPI, are all under the umbrella of conflict. Conflict has also been operationalized in interactional speech samples as speech interruptions, simultaneous speech, agreement/disagreement ratios (Jacob 1975, Riskin and Faunce 1970) and failure to reach agreement (Farina 1960).

In the family literature, measurement of problem-solving skills has typically involved an unstructured or semistructured task, such as a family problem-solving discussion (Strodbeck 1954) or a tower-building game (Goldberg and Maccoby 1965). Criterion variables generated by these tasks have included tabulations of problem-solving enhancement statements during interaction (Doane et al. 1986), the number of tower blocks the family puts together (Blechman and McEnroe 1985), or the family's self-rated satisfaction with the problem-solving task (Blechman and McEnroe 1985). In other studies (Reiss et al. 1986), problem solving may be measured by such attributes as the level of coordination shown by family members in solving a given problem (e.g., recognizing patterns in an array of symbols) or the family's openness to new information from each other or its ability to change solutions to accommodate new data ("delayed closure").

## Epidemiology of Relational Disorders

The raw frequency of relational disorders (broadly defined) in the general population is unknown. No epidemiological studies have been done, in part because of the absence of accepted diagnostic criteria for these disorders. There are rather vague "proxies" of relational disorders that are useful in making estimations of their prevalence, such as the approximate frequencies of divorce in the general populus (40–50% of all couples) or of marital violence (12–33% of couples) (Sagrestano et al. 1999, Straus and Gelles 1986, US Bureau of the Census 1992). Factors such as divorce or violence, however, are best thought of as relational events rather than relational disorders. A single incident of marital violence does not necessarily signal the presence of a family relational disorder (in the absence of confirmatory information), nor is a diagnosable relational disorder in a spousal couple necessarily associated with divorce. Thus, the prevalence of specific types of relational disorders, as described in this chapter, is difficult to estimate.

A further difficulty in making these estimations in the normal population is that certain of the constructs conveyed, such as expressed emotion (EE) as based on the Camberwell Family Interview (Vaughn and Leff 1976b), assume the presence of a psychiatric disorder in an index family member. Also, the goal of EE and other family psychopathological studies has been to examine family attribute–outcome relationships on a within-group basis in psychiatric disorders rather than to making comparisons between families of psychiatric patients and nonpsychiatric control subjects. Thus, data are lacking on the frequencies of high-EE attitudes or other family attributes in normal control groups.

Estimating the normal prevalence of EE is aided by the availability of the Five-Minute Speech Sample EE coding system (Magana et al. 1986), which simply requires that the parent talk for 5 minutes, uninterrupted, about the relationship with an index offspring (ill or well). This coding system yields an EE rating that has a close but not perfect correspondence (72–89.7%) (Magana et al. 1986, Moore and Kuipers 1999) with EE ratings based on the Camberwell Family Interview, the traditional measure of EE (Vaughn and Leff 1976b). Stubbe and associates (1993), in a population-based study of inner-city preadolescents, found that 22% of parents of children with no psychiatric disorders met the Five-Minute Speech Sample coding criteria for high EE, in contrast with 40% of parents of children having one or more psychiatric disorders.

A number of the studies of CD have examined rates of speech deviance in the normal population, but most have selected normal comparison groups to match with samples of patients with schizophrenia and, thus, do not reflect a random cross-section of the population. Given this limitation, high levels of CD (defined in various ways) appear to occur in about 16% (range 0–39%) of the parents of normal persons, compared with about 63% (range 19–76%) of the parents of patients with schizophrenia (Miklowitz 1994, Miklowitz and Stackman 1992). The significant variability in rates across samples probably reflects differences in methods of assessing CD as well as sampling variabilities.

The paucity of studies on the frequency of family relational disorders points to the need to develop strict operational criteria for these disorders and to conduct epidemiological studies using random sampling techniques, much as is done for individual disorders. The availability of epidemiological data would allow us to determine not only the need for treatment of specific relational disorders, but also their comorbidity with individual or other relational disorders, their associated features, and the social conditions under which they are most likely to arise.

## Treatment

### Specific Goals of Treatment

The primary goal of treatment is to bring the relational unit to a more satisfying, organized, and less conflictual level of functioning. The mediating goals of treatment are focused on improvement in the specific areas of functioning of the relational unit (i.e., structure, communication, affect expression, problem solving). In relational units where one member is suffering from a mental disorder or medical condition (e.g., schizophrenia, depression, childhood disruptive behavior disorder), additional goals include the reduction of individual symptoms and improvements in psychosocial functioning.

### Treatment Format

Relational problems are best observed and treated directly in a family format in which the conflicted family members are present with the therapist. However, there may be certain situations in which relational problems are more conducive to change within an individual treatment format. For example, relational problems related to an individual with a mental disorder (e.g., a 25-year-old son with schizophrenia, in conflict with his mother and father) may in some cases best be approached by individual sessions with the affected person. Further, when one adult in a family unit is depressed, individual interpersonal or cognitive psychotherapies may be used and focused on conflict resolution.

### Treatment Strategies and Techniques

The specific techniques available to family therapists can be divided into five categories: psychoeducational, cognitive–behavioral, structural, strategic–systemic, and insight-oriented. Psychoeducational approaches are most helpful when there is a family member with a specific medical or psychiatric disorder, and the family can utilize information on how to manage the disorder with the least tension and stress on the patient (Clarkin 1989). Cognitive–behavioral techniques are useful in improving communication and problem-solving skills and the positive interactive behaviors in marital-family units. Structural and strategic–systemic approaches are most useful in rearranging the repetitive interactions in a family that constitute the boundaries and alliances in the social system.

In practice, there are many common elements and much eclectic usage of strategies and techniques across the various schools of family intervention. Family therapy shares many of the common treatment elements with other forms of psychotherapy. All psychosocial treatments require the development and maintenance of a good patient–therapist relationship, or therapeutic alliance. There is an assumption that most patients experience

some degree of corrective emotional experience, or reliving of significant life experiences in the presence of an empathic therapist who demonstrates new ways of relating. In this context, the patient (or patients) is able to identify with the therapist and utilize the behaviors discussed and modeled. In all forms of psychotherapy, there is a certain degree of transmission of new information. The learning can be about methods of behavior, ways of thinking, or increased awareness of complex emotions. Most therapies involve some shaping of people's behavior through implicit and explicit rewards for behavior considered appropriate, and discouragement of behaviors considered harmful. This shaping can occur through advice, suggestion, persuasion, role playing, and practice.

### Standard Approach to Treatment

There is increasing evidence for the efficacy of family and marital interventions in the treatment of a broad range of relational problems and psychopathology, and extensive reviews of this literature can be found elsewhere (Pinsof and Wynne 1995). However, several specific questions about treatment efficacy can be asked here in reference to the previous review of relational difficulties:

1. Do the specific relational difficulties (i.e., structure, communication, affect, and problem solving) respond to intervention?
2. Do the individual disorders associated with relational problems (e.g., schizophrenia, affective disorders, adolescent delinquent behavior) show improvements in illness course when the relational problems are at least part of the focus of intervention?

### Empirical Investigations of the Efficacy of Family or Marital Treatment

**Partner Relational Difficulties.** Difficulties between romantic partners, including marital distress and relationship conflict, are most often addressed using couples-based interventions. A number of treatment models have been articulated and investigated, including "emotionally-focused marital therapy" (Johnson 1999), "insight-oriented marital therapy" (Snyder and Wills 1989), and "integrative couples therapy" (Lawrence et al. 1999). Recent meta-analysis examining findings from 15 couples intervention studies found that, when compared to no treatment, couples therapy resulted in significant positive changes in partners' behavior and evaluations of the relationship (Dunn and Schwebel 1995). The most well-researched therapy is behavioral marital therapy (BMT) (Alexander et al. 1994, Christensen et al. 1995), in which partners are coached on methods for increasing positive interactions and decreasing aversive ones, improving communication, and enhancing problem solving. Although BMT has received extensive empirical support and testing, longitudinal follow-up studies conducted by Jacobson (1984) and colleagues (Jacobson et al. 1987) indicate that almost half of couples engaged in these interventions fail to make clinically meaningful improvement and many fail to maintain gains achieved within these interventions. Modifications of the BMT approach have included a greater emphasis on facilitating "acceptance" of one's partner (Lawrence et al.

1999). In a small clinical trial (Jacobson et al. 2000), this modified approach yielded more substantial increases in marital satisfaction than did traditional BMT.

**Parent–Child Difficulties.** Difficulties between parents and their offspring can take the form of child and adolescent behavioral problems; child abuse and neglect; and difficulties, deficits, or excesses in parenting. An outstanding investigation of the effectiveness of treating these kinds of difficulties was conducted by Kazdin and colleagues (1992), who randomly assigned children (aged 7–13 years) with a variety of conduct disorders and problems to a manualized problem-solving skills training or parent-management training, or a combination of the two. Problem-solving skills training used cognitive–behavioral strategies to assist the child in negotiating interpersonal situations. The parents were brought in on the sessions to assist the therapist and to foster problem-solving steps in the home. In parent-management training, the parent was seen individually to improve child-rearing practices and to use contingencies to support prosocial behavior by the child. Although both treatments resulted in improved child functioning and increased social competence, the combination treatment resulted in more marked changes in child and parent functioning and placed a larger proportion of children within the range of nonclinical levels of functioning. This and other studies (Sayger et al. 1988, Singer et al. 1989) suggest that family therapy has promise in reducing specific problematical child behaviors with behavioral techniques and that the parents have a better personal adjustment after learning parenting skills.

**Nonspecific Parent–Adolescent Conflicts and Adolescent Behavioral Problems and Delinquency.** Numerous studies have been completed in this area. The most well-researched intervention for serious behavior problems in youth is the aforementioned parent-management training. This intervention has shown efficacy in the treatment of a wide range of serious behavior problems in youth, including conduct problems and delinquency, oppositionality, and aggressive behavior (Kazdin 1997, Mabe et al. 2001). Henggeler and associates (1992) developed multisystemic therapy and applied it to the treatment of juvenile offenders with records of serious crime. Multisystemic therapy had a duration of 3 months and employed intervention strategies similar to those in family and behavioral therapy (i.e., individualized treatment plans sometimes involving home visits in addition to therapy meetings). Compared with "treatment as usual" (incarceration or probation), multisystemic therapy led to greater reductions in both incarceration and criminal behavior for boys in the treatment condition.

**Substance Abuse.** More research is needed with patients and families suffering from alcohol and substance abuse, a major problem area in our society. The existing family studies show some promise for the use of family therapy (Friedman 1989, Liddle 1999, Stanton and Todd 1979, 1982) but it may be most effective with specific subgroups, possibly with younger abusers still at home and where family assets are substantial. The poor response to any treatment of the cocaine abuser (Kang et al. 1991) is disappointing. It is unclear whether cocaine abusing patients can

benefit from verbal therapies regardless of the format (i.e., individual, family, or group).

**Eating Disorders.** The early theoretical and clinical work of Salvador Minuchin, one of the leaders of the family movement, focused on eating disorders. Recent research lends increasing empirical support to the role of family-based treatments in a comprehensive strategy for addressing eating disorders. Russell and collaborators (1987) randomly assigned patients (57 with anorexia nervosa and 23 with bulimia nervosa) to either family therapy or individual supportive treatment after an inpatient treatment intended to bring the patient to normal weight. The goal of treatment was to help the family support the patient's recovery from eating disorder. After 1 year of treatment, the patients were reassessed for body weight and menstrual functioning. Treatment effects were still apparent at a 5-year follow-up (Eisler et al. 1997). The results are relevant to differential treatment planning, as those patients whose eating disorder was not chronic and had begun before the age of 19 years were more effectively treated with family therapy.

Comparing conjoint family therapy to a separated family therapy (in which parents and the adolescent were seen in separate sessions), Eisler and colleagues (2000) found separated family treatment to be associated with significant reductions in parental EE and greater symptom improvement. Robin and colleagues (1999) compared Behavior Family Systemic Treatment to individual treatment for anorexia nervosa. While improvements were apparent in both treatments, symptom improvement was greater in the family intervention. Group family treatments have also been shown to facilitate recovery from anorexia nervosa (Geist et al. 2000).

**Schizophrenia.** Family treatments for patients with schizophrenia and their families have been found to have strong beneficial effects. There are at least eight studies of family interventions of longer-term (i.e., 9 months or more) duration (Barrowclough and Tarrier 1990, Falloon et al. 1985, 1987, Falloon and Pederson 1985, Hogarty et al. 1986, 1991, Leff et al. 1982, 1985, 1989, Randolph et al. 1994, Tarrier et al. 1988, 1989, 1994, Xiong et al. 1994).

Illustrative is the treatment approach articulated by Anderson and colleagues (Anderson et al. 1986, Hogarty et al. 1986), which is broad based and extensive, including survival skills workshops for the families, reentry of the patient into the family, enhancing work and social adjustment of the patient, problem solving, and maintenance of therapeutic gains. Results of randomized studies (Hogarty et al. 1986, 1991) show the superiority (in terms of relapse rates and social adjustment of patients) of family therapy to individual social skills training or a no-therapy, medication-only control group during a 2-year follow-up.

Both the number and the quality of family therapy studies are impressive. The family treatments have been manualized, and the existing outcome literature suggests that family therapy is a useful and effective part of the overall treatment of these seriously disturbed individuals (Bellack and Mueser 1993, Goldstein and Miklowitz 1995, Penn and Mueser 1996). Recent studies suggest that multiple family group interventions may be more cost-effective than those focused on individual family units (McFarlane 1995). It may be that a focus on the individual family is appropriate early in the course of illness, whereas later on, a multiple family group format may be optimal (Tompson et al. 1996).

Questions remain as to the most important focus of family intervention (e.g., lowering EE versus increasing family coping); which families (at what point in the illness of the patient) are most likely to respond positively to family intervention?

**Mood Disorders.** Most of the studies of family intervention in families where one member is suffering from a mood disorder have been done in the marital treatment format, reflecting the age at onset of affective disorders (Beach and O'Leary 1992, Jacobson et al. 1991). There are a few studies involving families. Data from the Cornell Medical Center study of inpatient family intervention with patients with bipolar or major depressive disorders (Clarkin et al. 1990) suggest that inpatient family intervention may be fruitful for some subgroups. These patients and their families were randomly assigned to psychoeducational inpatient treatment with or without family intervention. At both 6- and 18-month follow-up times, patients who received family intervention showed better outcome than those without it. These treatment effects were limited, however, to the female bipolar patients. In contrast, those patients with unipolar depression did better without family intervention.

Clarkin and colleagues (1998) randomly assigned 33 married bipolar I patients to a psychoeducational marital therapy with medication or to a standard medication treatment. Although the marital treatment did not have differential effects on relapse rates, it was associated with gradually improving Global Assessment Scale scores over 11 months of treatment. Patients in marital treatment also were more consistent with their use of medication than those in standard medical treatment.

Two recent clinical trials examined a family-focused treatment for bipolar I patients (Miklowitz and Goldstein 1997) following hospitalization for mania or depression. Family-focused treatment, delivered along with mood stabilizing medication and consisting of education, communication skills training, and problem-solving skills training, was found to reduce risk of both relapse and hospitalization when compared to treatments consisting of crisis intervention and medication (Miklowitz et al. 2000) or individual therapy and medication (Rea et al. in press).

**Summary.** The research suggests that family treatment is effective with schizophrenia, affective disorders, adolescent and child acting-out difficulties, and eating disorders (Pinsof and Wynne 1995). In terms of strategies and techniques used in the family and marital treatment formats, there is substantial evidence for the effectiveness of cognitive–behavioral and psychoeducational techniques, with few data on the other approaches. Future studies should compare the efficacy of (and estimate the relative treatment effect sizes attributable to) family therapy versus competing therapies (i.e., individual or group therapies). Future research should also determine the optimal format in which to administer family treatment (i.e., home-based versus clinic-based; individual families versus multifamily educational groups).

## Medical Comorbidity

Relational problems can co-occur with virtually any general medical condition. In most cases, it can be convincingly argued that a medical condition in one member (e.g., cancer) can promulgate relational problems between this member and other members or between two other members of the family (e.g., a husband and wife who develop marital problems stemming from disagreements as to how to treat their daughter's juvenile-onset diabetes). In some cases, the relational problems may have prognostic value for the course of the medical condition and thus may become a focus of ancillary treatment.

Numerous attempts have been made to link the family constructs listed earlier (i.e., structure, communication, expression of affect, and problem solving) to the concurrent severity or future outcome of various medical conditions. For example, Koenigsberg and coworkers (1993) examined levels of spousal EE in relation to glucose control in diabetic patients. The number of critical comments made by the spouse during a modified Camberwell Family Interview significantly predicted glycosylated hemoglobin levels (a measure of glucose control) in the patient, the latter having been measured for the 2- to 3-month period before the interview. Levels of emotional overinvolvement among spouses were not predictive.

Vitaliano and colleagues (1989) reported that spouses of Alzheimer's disease patients (with early-to-middle-stage dementia) infrequently (22%) exhibited high-EE attitudes on the Five-Minute Speech Sample (a measure that may underestimate the prevalence of high-EE attitudes relative to the Camberwell Family Interview). When spouses had high EE, they reported more depression, feelings of being burdened, anger turned inward, and problems in anger control than those who had low EE. However, it was also the case that patients paired with high-EE spouses were rated by interviewers as having higher levels of functional impairment than those paired with low-EE spouses. During a prospective follow-up, the Alzheimer's disease patients with high-EE spouses showed more externalizing behavioral problems (i.e., paranoia, violence, wandering) than those with low-EE spouses, despite the absence of differences over the follow-up in levels of cognitive decline (Vitaliano et al. 1993).

There is evidence that medical conditions often covary with communication disturbances in marital couples. For example, Hudgens (1979) found that 18 of 24 couples in which one member had chronic pain had communication disturbances. However, extensive communication between spouses where one has chronic pain also carries certain disadvantages. For example, in one study, higher levels of agreement between pain patients and their spouses in their evaluations of the severity and impact of the pain problem predicted poorer outcome for the pain disorder (Swanson and Murata 1980, Roy 1988). Chronic pain in one family member requires changes in the structure or hierarchical organization of the family, such that the well spouse must become the primary wage earner or take over a considerable proportion of the family's decision making (Rowat and Knafl 1985). Perhaps in couples where spouses strongly agreed, they had made an accommodation to the chronic pain, and there was reduced motivation to address this condition.

There is evidence that enhanced family problem-solving may be a protective factor in the course of certain medical conditions. Using a pattern-recognition procedure, Reiss and associates (1986) examined the problem-solving interactions of families in which one member had end-stage renal disease requiring long-term hemodialysis. High family scores on "delayed closure" during a problem-solving task indicated that a family was "environmentally sensitive," open to new information in choosing solutions, and willing to introduce new solutions when new information was available. The authors found these high scores predicted fewer medical complications in the affected family member during a 9-month follow-up period.

While family-based interventions for medical conditions have not been sufficiently investigated, there is some evidence of their utility, particularly for the treatment of chronic childhood diseases (Campbell and Patterson 1995) where families are faced with numerous challenges in promoting health and adjusting to often-complex medical regimens. Family-based psychoeducational interventions in the treatment of sickle cell disease (Kaslow et al. 2000) have resulted in greater disease knowledge among participating families when compared to treatment as usual. In a clinical trial, behavior family systems therapy with adolescents with insulin-dependent diabetes mellitus resulted in lower diabetes-specific family conflict and improvements in the parent–child relationship when compared to treatment as usual and to an educational support group (Wysocki et al. 2000).

It is clear that chronic and progressive medical illness co-occurs with a host of relational difficulties that may in some cases bode poorly for the outcome of the medical condition. In most instances, these relational disturbances seem to arise in reaction to the medical condition and are not apparently causally related to the disorder itself. Family or marital intervention in medical conditions may, however, reduce the tension in the household and the level of burden and psychosocial stress experienced by the caretaking family member(s), which could in turn provide a more protective environment for the ill family member.

The following case description illustrates one manifestation of relational problem. The case is conceptualized with regard to the relational constructs reviewed above, including structure, communication, expression of affect, and problem solving. A typical treatment strategy is then briefly presented.

---

**Clinical Vignette**

Mr. A, a 26-year-old man employed as an air conditioning mechanic, was referred by a local marital therapist with the recommendation of individual therapy for anxiety and adjustment disorder. He arrived 10 minutes early for his session and entered the therapist's office with an air of anxiety and deference to the therapist's authority. He immediately leaped into his personal story, almost before the therapist could sit down. He and his wife of some 15 months had just had their first child, a son, born 3 weeks ago. In addition, the couple had moved to the suburban

area only 6 months ago, and the move had taken them from a city apartment near the wife's parents to a suburban single-family house located near his parents. The problem, according to Mr. A, was his wife's overattachment to her parents and her related dislike of his parents, which spilled over into resentment toward him. This disturbance had led Mr. A to be distracted and less efficient at work. His boss, who had paternal concern toward him, noticed his upset and suggested that he seek counseling. Mr. A had gone to a marital therapist, who told him he could do nothing because the wife refused to attend marital sessions. Mr. A indicated that his wife would not see the present therapist either. The therapist asked Mr. A to talk to his wife about the current therapy and ask her if the therapist, in the effort to help Mr. A, could telephone her. The wife agreed to a telephone call and, subsequent to the call, was willing to come to the therapist's office for an individual session.

She arrived for her appointment, accompanied by Mr. A, who was holding their 4-week-old son, who appeared well clothed and content. The wife's story was consistent with that of her husband's but quite different in emphasis and focus. She indicated that her husband's loyalty and involvement with his parents, especially his mother, had come to a head with the birth of their son. The mother-in-law had "invaded" her hospital room the day after the son's birth and insisted that Ms. A come directly from the hospital after discharge to her house with the newborn child and stay with her. Although Ms. A had difficulty opposing her mother-in-law, she stated that she was going to their own home and that her own mother would be with them for a couple of days. After receiving that message, the mother-in-law instantly became quiet and abrupt. Indeed, Ms. A felt that from that time on, Mr. A, influenced by the mother, had also become aloof and abrupt with her.

**Diagnostic Evaluation**

Currently, Mr. A exhibits the following diagnoses using the multiaxial system:

| | |
|---|---|
| Axis I | 309.24 Adjustment Disorder with Anxiety |
| | V61.10 Partner Relational Problem |
| Axis II | 799.9 Diagnosis Deferred |
| Axis III | None |
| Axis IV | Recent move to new neighborhood; birth of child |
| Axis V | GAF = 60 |

Mr. A's symptoms of anxiety and agitation in the last few months were clearly related temporally to the difficulties with his wife and their families of origin and possibly exacerbated by the birth of his son. Currently, the patterns of interaction within the relationship are impaired and the relational unit has become increasingly distressed and dysfunctional. In addition to Mr. A's distress, Ms. A has been isolated and experienced depressed mood after the birth of her child. Thus, the most efficient approach to the individual difficulties lies in an evaluation of the family situation.

Mr. A clearly has a partner relational problem. In terms of the family relational constructs enunciated in this chapter, the situation can be described as follows. In terms of family structure, there are diffuse and nonfunctional boundaries between the young couple and the families of origin. Mr. A and Ms. A are both heavily involved with their families of origin, possibly to the neglect of their marital relationship. In particular, Mr. A's pattern of communication with his mother and related lack of intimacy with his wife is quite disturbing to Ms. A. In terms of communication, interactions between husband and wife are characterized by periods of silence and then bursts of verbal exchange characterized by suspicion and accusation, especially about their families of origin. Both parties feel aggrieved and each feels victimized by the other's parents.

In terms of expression of affect, the interactions between the two are characterized by negative emotions of anger, sadness, and mutual withdrawal. Very little positive affect is expressed. In terms of problem solving, few attempts are made to resolve the difficulties, and daily issues become not occasions for normal problem resolution but rather, opportunities for mutual recrimination. For example, Mr. A recently decided that he did not have the time to drop off their annual tax return to the accountant, so he took the returns in an unsealed envelope to his mother to deliver. The wife was enraged at this manner of delivering their private financial accounts and once again accused him of being too close to his parents. This "lack" of problem-solving ability is "situation specific," however, as both husband and wife can effectively problem-solve in other settings (e.g., work).

**Treatment**

Treatment began with further individual meetings with both spouses. These meetings focused on understanding the history of the relationship, the nature of interactions and expectations within each of their families of origin, and exploration of their individual goals. Conjoint sessions with husband and wife then focused on their relationship. The tasks of therapy can be understood in terms of the previously discussed constructs. First, in terms of structure, the partners needed to develop clearer boundaries within and around the relationship. The therapist repeatedly pointed out how both partners had brought with them, from their families of origin, certain expectations for family relationships. As these expectations became clearer to both partners, the therapy shifted to helping the partners examine their relationship and develop clearer boundaries between the husband/wife subsystem and their respective parents. Second, in terms of communication, listening skills were practiced by each, as the other partner explained his/her expectations and hopes in the relationship. The partners were taught specific communication skills, including giving and receiving positive and negative feedback and making requests for behavior change. Homework assignments between sessions were used to practice and generalize these skills.

In terms of affect expression, improvements in communicating led to decreases in negative exchanges. In addition, partners were encouraged to review the positive aspects in each which had initially brought them into the relationship, and, through homework, to practice noticing and commenting on positive aspects of each other's behavior. Finally, problem-solving skills were taught and practiced in and out of sessions. As the couple tried to establish clearer boundaries within and around the relationship, numerous opportunities arose to practice solving problems related to their families of origin.

# References

Alanen YO (1958) The mothers of schizophrenic patients. Acta Psychiatr Scand 124 (Suppl), 1–361.

Alanen YO (1966) The family in the pathogenesis of schizophrenic and neurotic disorders. Acta Psychiatr Scand 190 (Suppl), 1–654.

Alexander JF, Holtzworth-Munroe A, and Jameson PB (1994) The process and outcome of marital and family therapy: Research review and evaluation. In Handbook of Psychotherapy and Behavior Change, 4th ed., Bergin AE and Garfield SL (eds). John Wiley, New York, pp. 595–630.

American Psychiatric Association (1987) Diagnostic and Statistical Manual of Mental Disorders, 3rd ed., Rev. APA, Washington DC.

American Psychiatric Association (1994) Diagnostic and Statistical Manual of Mental Disorders, 4th ed. APA, Washington DC.

American Psychiatric Association (2000) Diagnostic and Statistical Manual of Mental Disorders, 4th ed., Text Rev. APA, Washington DC.

Anderson CM, Reiss DJ, and Hogarty GE (1986) Schizophrenia and the Family. Guilford Press, New York.

Asarnow JR, Ben-Meir SL, and Goldstein MJ (1987) Family factors in childhood depressive and schizophrenia-spectrum disorders: A preliminary report. In Understanding Major Mental Disorder: The Contribution of Family Interaction Research, Hahlweg K and Goldstein MJ (eds). Family Process Press, New York, pp. 123–138.

Asarnow JR, Goldstein MJ, and Ben-Meir S (1988) Parental communication deviance in childhood onset schizophrenia spectrum and depressive disorders. J Child Psychol Psychiatr 29, 825–838.

Barkley RA, Edward G, Laneri M, et al. (2001) The efficacy of problem-solving communication training alone, behavior management training alone and their combination for parent-adolescent conflict in teenagers with ADHD and ODD. J Consult Clin Psychol 69, 926–941.

Barnett PA and Gotlib IH (1988) Psychosocial functioning and depression: Distinguishing among antecedents, concomitants, and consequences. Psychol Bull 104, 97–126.

Barrowclough C and Tarrier N (1990) Social functioning in schizophrenic patients: The effects of expressed emotion and family intervention. Soc Psychiatr Psychiatr Epidemiol 25, 125–130.

Basco MR, Prager KJ, Pita JM, et al. (1992) Communication and intimacy in the marriages of depressed patients. J Fam Psychol 6, 184–194.

Baucom DH and Epstein N (1990) Cognitive–Behavioral Marital Therapy. Brunner/Mazel, New York.

Baucom DH, Epstein N, Sayers S, et al. (1989) The role of cognitions in marital relationships: Definitional, methodological, and conceptual issues. J Consult Clin Psychol 57, 31–38.

Baumrind D (1975) The contributions of the family to the development of competence in children. Schizophr Bull 14, 12–37.

Beach ARS and O'Leary KD (1992) Treating depression in the context of marital discord: Outcome and predictors of response for marital therapy vs. cognitive therapy. Behav Ther 23, 507–528.

Bee HL, Barnard KE, Eyres SJ, et al. (1982) Predictions of IQ and language skill from perinatal status, child performance, family characteristics, and mother–infant interaction. Child Dev 53, 1134–1156.

Bellack AS and Mueser KT (1993) Psychosocial treatment for schizophrenia. Schizophr Bull 19(2), 317–336.

Biglan A, Hops H, Sherman L, et al. (1985) Problem-solving interactions of depressed women and their husbands. Behav Ther 16, 431–451.

Billings A (1979) Conflict resolution in distressed and nondistressed married couples. J Consult Clin Psychol 47, 368–376.

Birchler G, Weiss R, and Vincent J (1975) Multimethod analysis of social reinforcement exchange between maritally distressed and nondistressed spouses and partners. J Pers Soc Psychol 31, 349–360.

Blechman EA (1990) Effective communication: Enabling multi-problem families to change. In Advances in Family Research, Vol. 2, Cowan P and Hetherington ME (eds). Lawrence Erlbaum, New Jersey.

Blechman EA and McEnroe MJ (1985) Effective family problem solving. Child Dev 56, 429–437.

Bradley RH and Caldwell BM (1980) The relation of home environment, cognitive competence, and IQ among males and females. Child Dev 51, 1140–1148.

Brown GW, Birley JLT, and Wing JK (1972) Influence of family life on the course of schizophrenic disorders: A replication. Br J Psychiatr 121, 241–258.

Buehlman KT, Gottman JM, and Katz LF (1992) How a couple views their past predicts their future: Predicting divorce from an oral history interview. J Fam Psychol 5, 295–318.

Burgess RL and Conger RD (1978) Family interaction in abusive, neglectful, and normal families. Child Dev 49, 1163–1173.

Butzlaff RL and Hooley JM (1998) Expressed emotion and psychiatric relapse. Arch Gen Psychiatr 55, 547–552.

Campbell TL and Patterson JM (1995) The effectiveness of family interventions in the treatment of physical illness. J Marital Fam Ther 21, 545–583.

Camper PM, Jacobson NS, Holtzworth-Munroe A, et al. (1988) Causal attributions for interactional behaviors in married couples. Cogn Ther Res 12, 195–209.

Carrere S, Buehlman KT, and Gottman JM (2000) Predicting marital stability and divorce in newlywed couples. J Fam Psychol 14, 42–58.

Chambless DL and Steketee G (1999) Expressed emotion and behavior therapy outcome: A prospective study with obsessive–compulsive and agoraphobic outpatients. J Consult Clin Psychol 67, 658–665.

Christensen A and Shenk JL (1991) Communication, conflict, and psychological distance in nondistressed, clinic, and divorcing couples. J Consult Clin Psychol 59, 458–463.

Christensen A, Jacobson NS, and Babcock JC (1995) Integrative behavioral couple therapy. In Clinical Handbook of Couple Therapy, Jacobson NS and Gurman AS (eds). Guilford Press, New York, pp. 31–64.

Christian JL, O'Leary DK, and Vivian D (1994) Depressive symptomatology in maritally discordant women and men: The role of individual and relationship variables. J Fam Psychol 8, 32–42.

Clardy ERA (1951) A study of the development and course of schizophrenic children. Psychiatr Q 25, 81–90.

Clarkin JF (1989) Family education. In A Clinical Guide for the Treatment of Schizophrenia, Bellack A (ed). Plenum Press, New York, pp. 187–205.

Clarkin JF and Miklowitz DJ (1994) Marital and family communication difficulties: A review for DSM-IV. In DSM-IV Sourcebook, Widiger TA, Frances AJ, Pincus HA, et al. (eds). American Psychiatric Press, Washington DC, pp. 631–672.

Clarkin JF, Carpenter D, Hull J, et al. (1998) Effects of psychoeducational intervention for married patients with bipolar disorder and their spouses. Psychiatr Serv 49, 531–533.

Clarkin JF, Glick ID, Haas GL, et al. (1990) A randomized clinical trial of inpatient family intervention v. results for affective disorders. J Affect Disord 18, 17–28.

Cohan CL and Bradbury TN (1997) Negative life events, marital interaction, and the longitudinal course of newlywed marriage. J Pers Soc Psychol 73, 114–128.

Conger RD, Rueter MA, and Elder GH (1999) Couple resilience to economic pressure. J Pers Soc Psychol 76, 54–71.

Dausch BM, Miklowitz DJ, and Richards JA (1996) Global Assessment of Relational Functioning Scale (GARF): II. Reliability and validity in a sample of families of bipolar patients. Fam Process 35, 175–189.

Doane JA, Falloon IRH, Goldstein MJ, et al. (1985) Parental affective style and the treatment of schizophrenia: Predicting course of illness and social functioning. Arch Gen Psychiatr 42, 34–42.

Doane JA, Goldstein MJ, Miklowitz DJ, et al. (1986) The impact of individual and family treatment on the affective climate of families of schizophrenics. Br J Psychiatr 148, 279–287.

Dunn RL and Schwebel AI (1995) Meta-analytic review of marital therapy outcome research. J Fam Psychol 9(1), 58–68.

Eisler I, Dare C, Hodes M, et al. (2000) Family therapy for adolescent anorexia nervosa: The results of a controlled comparison of two family interventions. J Child Psychol Psychiatr Allied Disc 41, 727–736.

Eisler I, Dare C, Russell GFM, et al. (1997) Family and individual therapy in anorexia nervosa: A 5-year follow-up. Arch Gen Psychiatr 54, 1025–1030.

Elwood RW and Jacobson NS (1982) Spouse agreement in reporting their behavioral interactions: A clinical replication. J Consult Clin Psychol 50, 783–784.

Elwood RW and Jacobson NS (1988) The effects of observational training on spouse agreement about events in their relationship. Behav Res Ther 26, 159–167.

Ely AL, Guerney BG, and Stover L (1973) Efficacy of the training phase of conjugal therapy. Psychother Theor Res Pract 10, 201–207.

Epstein NB and Eidelson RJ (1981) Unrealistic beliefs of clinical couples: Their relationship to expectations, goals, and satisfaction. Am J Fam Ther 9, 13–22.

Falloon IRH and Pederson J (1985) Family management in the prevention of morbidity of schizophrenia: The adjustment of the family unit. Br J Psychiatr 147, 156–163.

Falloon IRH, Boyd JL, and McGill CW (1984) Family Care of Schizophrenia. Guilford Press, New York.

Falloon IRH, Boyd JL, McGill CW, et al. (1985) Family management in the prevention of morbidity of schizophrenia: Clinical outcome of a two-year longitudinal study. Arch Gen Psychiatr 42, 887–896.

Falloon IRH, McGill C, Boyd J, et al. (1987) Family management in the prevention of morbidity of schizophrenia: Social outcome of a two-year longitudinal study. Psychol Med 17, 59–66.

Farina A (1960) Patterns of role dominance and conflict in parents of schizophrenic patients. J Abnorm Soc Psychol 61, 31–38.

Ferreira AJ (1963) Decision-making in normal and pathological families. Arch Gen Psychiatr 13(8), 68–73.

Fichter MM, Glynn SM, Weyerer S, et al. (1997) Family climate and expressed emotion in the course of alcoholism. Fam Process 36, 202–221.

Fincham FD and Bradbury TN (1992) Assessing attributions in marriage: The relationship attribution measure. J Pers Soc Psychol 62, 457–468.

Fincham FD and O'Leary KD (1983) Causal inferences for spouse behavior in maritally distressed and nondistressed couples. J Soc Clin Psychol 1, 42–57.

Fincham FD, Harold GT, and Gano-Phillips S (2000) The longitudinal association between attributions and marital satisfaction: Direction of effects and role of efficacy expectations. J Fam Psychol 14(2), 267–285.

Fischmann-Havstad L and Marston AR (1984) Weight loss maintenance as an aspect of family emotion and process. Br J Clin Psychol 23, 265–271.

Forehand R, McCombs TA, Wierson M, et al. (1990) Role of maternal functioning and parenting skills in adolescent functioning following parental divorce. J Abnorm Psychol 99, 278–283.

Freeman RV and Grayson HM (1955) Maternal attitudes in schizophrenia. J Abnorm Soc Psychol 50, 45–52.

Friedman AS (1989) Family therapy v. parent groups: Effects on adolescent drug abusers. Am J Fam Ther 17, 335–347.

Garmezy N, Clarke AR, and Stockner C (1961) Child rearing attitudes of mothers and fathers as reported by schizophrenics and normal patients. J Abnorm Soc Psychol 63, 176–182.

Geist R, Heinmaa M, Stephen D, et al. (2000) Comparison of family therapy and family group psychoeducation in adolescents with anorexia nervosa. Can J Psychiatr 45, 173–178.

Gerard DL and Siegel J (1950) The family background of schizophrenia. Psychiatr Q 24, 47–73.

Goldberg MH and Maccoby EE (1965) Children's acquisition of skill in performing a group task under two conditions of group formation. J Pers Soc Psychol 2, 898–902.

Goldstein MJ (1987) Family interaction patterns that antedate the onset of schizophrenia and related disorders: A further analysis of data from a longitudinal prospective study. In Understanding Major Mental Disorder: The Contribution of Family Interaction Research, Hahlweg K and Goldstein M (eds). Family Process Press, New York, pp. 11–32.

Goldstein MJ and Miklowitz DJ (1995) The effectiveness of psychoeducational family therapy in the treatment of schizophrenic disorders. J Marital Fam Ther 21, 361–376.

Goldstein MJ, Talovic SA, and Nuechterlein KH (1990) Family interaction v. individual psychopathology: Do they indicate the same processes in the families of schizophrenics? Presented at the Third International Schizophrenia Symposium, Transactional Processes in Onset and Course of Schizophrenic Disorders, Bern, Switzerland.

Goodman SH, Barfoot B, Frye AA, et al. (1999) Dimensions of marital conflict and children's social problem-solving skills. J Fam Psychol 13, 33–45.

Gotlib IH and Whiffen VE (1989) Depression and marital functioning: An examination of specificity and gender differences. J Abnorm Psychol 98, 23–30.

Gottfried AW and Gottfried AE (1983) Home environment and mental development in young children of middle-class families. In Home Environment and Early Mental Development: Longitudinal Research, Gottfried AW (ed). Academic Press, New York.

Gottman JM (1979) Marital Interaction: Empirical Investigation. Academic Press, New York.

Gottman JM (1994) What Predicts Divorce? The Relationship Between Marital Processes and Marital Outcomes. Lawrence Erlbaum, Hillsdale, NJ.

Gottman J and Krokoff LJ (1989) Marital interaction and satisfaction: A longitudinal view. J Consult Clin Psychol 57, 47–52.

Gottman J, Markman H, and Notarius C (1977) The topography of marital conflict: A sequential analysis of verbal and nonverbal behavior. J Marriage Fam 39, 461–477.

Gottman J, Notarius C, Gonso J, et al. (1976a) A Couple's Guide to Communication. Research Press, Champaign, Il.

Gottman J, Notarius C, Markman H, et al. (1976b) Behavior exchange theory and marital decision making. J Pers Soc Psychol 34, 14–23.

Group for the Advancement of Psychiatry, Committee on the Family (1996) Global assessment of relational functioning scale (GARF): I. Background and rationale. Fam Process 35, 155–172.

Haas GL, Glick ID, Clarkin JF, et al. (1988) Inpatient family intervention: A randomized clinical trial. II. Results at hospital discharge. Arch Gen Psychiatr 45, 217–224.

Hahlweg K, Goldstein MJ, Nuechterlein KH, et al. (1989) Expressed emotion and patient-relative interaction in families of recent-onset schizophrenics. J Consult Clin Psychol 57, 11–18.

Hahlweg K, Reisner L, Kohli G, et al. (1984a) Development and validity of a new system to analyze interpersonal communication (KPI). In Marital Interaction: Analysis and Modification, Hahlweg K and Jacobson NS (eds). Guilford Press, New York.

Hahlweg K, Revenstorf D, and Schindler L (1984b) Effects of behavioral marital therapy on couples' communication and problem-solving skills. J Consult Clin Psychol 52, 553–566.

Harter S (1999) The construction of the self: A developmental perspective. Guilford Press, New York.

Hautzinger M, Linden M, and Hoffman N (1982) Distressed couples with and without a depressed partner: An analysis of their verbal interaction. J Behav Ther Exp Psychiatr 13, 307–314.

Heavey CL, Larson BM, Sumtobel DC, et al. (1996) The Communication Patterns Questionnaire: The reliability and validity of a constructive communication measure. J Marriage Fam 58, 796–800.

Henggeler SW, Melton GB, and Smith LA (1992) Family perseveration using multisystemic therapy: An effective alternative to incarcerating serious juvenile offenders. J Consult Clin Psychol 60, 953–961.

Hess RD and Shipman VC (1965) Early experience and the socialization of cognitive modes in children. Child Dev 36, 869–886.

Hilsenroth MJ, Ackerman SJ, Blagys MD, et al. (2000) Reliability and validity of DSM-IV Axis V. Am J Psychiatr 157, 1858–1863.

Hinchcliffe M, Hooper D, Roberts FJ, et al. (1978) The melancholy marriage: An inquiry into the interaction of depression. IV. Disruptions. Br J Med Psychol 51, 15–24.

Hogarty GE, Anderson CM, Reiss DJ, et al. (1986) Family psychoeducation, social skills training, and maintenance chemotherapy in the aftercare treatment of schizophrenia. I. One-year effects of a controlled study on relapse and expressed emotion. Arch Gen Psychiatr 43, 633–642.

Hogarty GE, Anderson CM, Reiss DJ, et al. (1991) Family psychoeducation, social skills training, and maintenance chemotherapy in the aftercare treatment of schizophrenia. II. Two-year effects of a controlled study on relapse and adjustment. Arch Gen Psychiatr 48, 340–347.

Holtzworth-Munroe A and Jacobson NS (1985) Causal attributions of married couples: When do they search for causes? What do they conclude when they do? J Pers Soc Psychol 48, 1398–1412.

Hooley JM (1986) Expressed emotion and depression: Interactions between patients and high versus low EE spouses. J Abnorm Psychol 95, 237–246.

Hooley JM and Hoffman PD (1999) Expressed emotion and clinical outcome in borderline personality disorder. Am J Psychiatr 156, 1557–1562.

Hooley JM and Teasdale JD (1989) Predictors of relapse in unipolar depressives: Expressed emotion, marital distress, and perceived criticism. J Abnorm Psychol 98, 229–235.

Hooley JM, Orley J, and Teasdale JD (1986) Levels of expressed emotion and relapse in depressed patients. Br J Psychiatr 148, 642–647.

Hooper D, Roberts FJ, Hinchcliffe MK, et al. (1977) The melancholy marriage: An inquiry into the interaction of depression. I. Introduction. Br J Med Psychol 50, 113–124.

Hops H, Andrews JA, Duncan SC, et al. (2000) Adolescent drug use development: A social interactional and contextual perspective. In Handbook of Developmental Psychopathology, 2nd ed., Sameroff AJ, Lewis M, and Miller SM (eds). Kluwer Academic/Plenum Publishers, New York, pp. 589–605.

Horowitz FD and Lovell LL (1960) Attitudes of mothers of female schizophrenics. Child Dev 31, 299–305.

Hudgens AJ (1979) Family-oriented treatment of chronic pain. J Marriage Fam Ther 5, 67–78.

Isley S, O'Neil R, and Parke RD (1996) The relation of parental affect and control behaviors to children's classroom acceptance: A concurrent and predictive analysis. Early Educ Dev 7, 7–23.

Jacob T (1975) Family interaction in disturbed and normal families: A methodological and substantive review. Psychol Bull 82, 33–65.

Jacobson NS (1984) A component analysis of behavioral marital therapy: The relative effectiveness of behavior exchange and communication/problem-solving training. J Consult Clin Psychol 52, 295–305.

Jacobson NS, Christensen A, Prince SE, et al. (2000) Integrative behavioral couple therapy: An acceptance-based, promising new treatment for couple discord. J Consult Clin Psychol 68(2), 351–355.

Jacobson NS, Dobson K, Fruzzetti AE, et al. (1991) Marital therapy as a treatment for depression. J Consult Clin Psychol 59, 547–557.

Jacobson NS, Follette WC, and McDonald DW (1982) Reactivity to positive and negative behavior in distressed and nondistressed married couples. J Consult Clin Psychol 50, 706–714.

Jacobson NS, McDonald DW, Follette WC, et al. (1985) Attributional processes in distressed and nondistressed married couples. Cogn Ther Res 9, 35–50.

Jacobson NS, Schmaling KB, and Holtzworth-Munroe A (1987) Component analysis of behavioral marital therapy: 2-year follow-up and prediction of relapse. J Marital Fam Ther 13(2), 187–195.

Jacobson NS, Waldron H, and Moore D (1980) Toward a behavioral profile of marital distress. J Consult Clin Psychol 48, 696–703.

Johnson SM (1999) Emotionally focused couple therapy: Straight from the heart. In Short-Term Couple Therapy, Donovan J (ed). Guilford Press, New York, pp. 13–42.

Jordan TJ and McCormick NB (1987) The role of sex beliefs in intimate relationships. Presented at the Annual Meeting of the American Association of Sex Educators, Counselors, and Therapists, New York.

Kang SY, Kleinman PH, Woody GE, et al. (1991) Outcomes for cocaine abusers after once-a-week psychosocial therapy. Am J Psychiatr 148, 630–635.

Kaslow NJ, Collins MH, Rashid FL, et al. (2000) The efficacy of a pilot family psychoeducational intervention for pediatric sickle cell disease (SCD). Fam Sys Health 18, 381–404.

Kavanagh D (1992) Recent developments in expressed emotion and schizophrenia. Br J Psychiatr 160, 601–620.

Kazdin AE (1997) Parent management training: Evidence, outcomes, and issues. J Am Acad Child Adolesc Psychiatr 36, 1349–1356.

Kazdin AE, Siegel TC, and Bass D (1992) Cognitive problem-solving skills training and parent management training in the treatment of antisocial behavior in children. J Consult Clin Psychol 60, 733–747.

Kearney CA and Silverman WK (1995) Family environment of youngsters with school refusal behavior: A synopsis with implications for assessment and treatment. Am J Fam Ther 23, 59–72.

Klerman GL, Weissman MM, Rounsaville BJ, et al. (1984) Interpersonal Psychotherapy of Depression. Basic Books, New York.

Koenigsberg HW, Klausner E, Pelino D, et al. (1993) Expressed emotion and glucose control in insulin-dependent diabetes mellitus. Am J Psychiatr 150, 1114–1115.

Kohn M and Clausen JA (1956) Parental authority behavior and schizophrenia. Am J Orthopsychiatr 26, 297–313.

Kopfstein D (1972) Effects of accelerating and decelerating consequences on the social behavior of trainable retarded children. Child Dev 43, 800–809.

Kowalik D and Gotlib H (1987) Depression and marital interaction: Concordance between intent and perception of communications. J Abnorm Psychol 96, 127–134.

Kreisman DE, Simmens SJ, and Joy VD (1979) Rejecting the patient: Preliminary validation of a self-report scale. Schizophr Bull 5, 220–222.

Krinsley KE and Bry BH (1991) Sequential analysis of adolescent, mother, and father behaviors in distressed and nondistressed families. Child Fam Behav Ther 13, 45–62.

Lane RC and Singer JL (1957) Familial attitudes in paranoid schizophrenics and normals from two socioeconomic classes. J Abnorm Soc Psychol 59, 328–329.

Lawrence E, Eldridge K, Christensen A, et al. (1999) Integrative couple therapy: The dyadic relationship of acceptance and change. In Short-Term Couple Therapy, Donovan J (ed). Guilford Press, New York, pp. 226–261.

Leff J and Vaughn C (1985) Expressed Emotion in Families. Guilford Press, New York.

Leff J, Berkowitz R, Sitavit N, et al. (1989) A trial of family therapy versus a relatives' group for schizophrenia. Br J Psychiatr 154, 58–66.

Leff J, Kuipers L, Berkowitz R, et al. (1982) A controlled trial of social intervention in the families of schizophrenic patients. Br J Psychiatr 141, 121–134.

Leff J, Kuipers L, Berkowitz R, et al. (1985) A controlled trial of social intervention in the families of schizophrenic patients: Two-year follow-up. Br J Psychiatr 146, 594–600.

Liddle HA (1999) Theory development in a family-based therapy for adolescent drug abuse. J Clin Child Psychol 28, 521–532.

Lidz T, Cornelison AR, Singer MT, et al. (1964) The mothers of schizophrenic patients. In Schizophrenia and the Family, Lidz T, Fleck S, and Cornelison AR (eds). International Universities Press, New York.

Lobitz WC and Johnson SM (1975) Parental manipulation of the behavior of normal and deviant children. Child Dev 46, 719–726.

Lu Y-C (1961) Mother–child role relations in schizophrenia. Psychiatry 24, 133–142.

Mabe PA, Turner MK, and Josephson AM (2001) Parent management training. Child Adolesc Psychiatr Clin N Am 10, 451–464.

Magana AB, Goldstein MJ, Karno M, et al. (1986) A brief method for assessing expressed emotion in relatives of psychiatric patients. Psychiatr Res 17, 203–212.

Margolin G and Wampold BE (1981) Sequential analysis of conflict and accord in distressed and nondistressed marital partners. J Consult Clin Psychol 49, 554–567.

Mark JC (1953) The attitudes of the mothers of male schizophrenics towards child behavior. J Abnorm Soc Psychol 48, 185–189.

Markman HJ (1981) The prediction of marital distress: A five-year follow-up. J Consult Clin Psychol 49, 760–762.

Markman HJ and Notarius CI (1987) Coding marital and family interaction: Current status. In Family Interaction and Psychopathology, Jacob T (ed). Plenum Press, New York, pp. 329–390.

McFarlane WR, Link B, Dushay R, et al. (1995) Psychoeducational multiple family groups: Four-year relapse outcome in schizophrenia. Fam Process 34(2), 127–144.

McGhie A (1950) A comparative study of the mother–child relationship in schizophrenia. Br J Med Psychol 34, 195–208.

McGhie A (1961) A comparative study of the mother–child relationship in schizophrenia. II. Psychological testing. Br J Med Psychol 34, 209–221.

McKeown JE (1950) The behavior of parents of schizophrenic, neurotic, and normal children. Am J Soc 56, 75–179.

Merikangas KR, Ranelli CJ, and Kupfer DJ (1979) Marital interaction in hospitalized depressed patients. J Nerv Ment Dis 167, 689–695.

Miklowitz D and Tompson MC (in press) Family variables and interventions in schizophrenia, Ch. 17. In Textbook of Marital and Family Therapy, Sholevar P (ed). APPI, Washington DC.

Miklowitz D, Velligan D, Goldstein M, et al. (1991) Communication deviance in families of schizophrenic and manic patients. J Abnorm Psychol 100, 163–173.

Miklowitz DJ (1994) Family risk indicators in schizophrenia. Schizophr Bull 20, 137–149.

Miklowitz DJ and Goldstein MJ (1997) Bipolar Disorder: A Family Focused Treatment Approach. Guilford Press, New York.

Miklowitz DJ, Goldstein MJ, and Falloon IRH (1983) Premorbid and symptomatic characteristics of schizophrenics from families with high and low levels of expressed emotion. J Abnorm Psychol 92, 359–367.

Miklowitz DJ, Goldstein MJ, Falloon IRH, et al. (1984) Interactional correlates of expressed emotion in the families of schizophrenics. Br J Psychiatr 144, 482–487.

Miklowitz DJ, Goldstein MJ, Nuechterlein KH, et al. (1988) Family factors and the course of bipolar affective disorder. Arch Gen Psychiatr 45, 225–231.

Miklowitz DJ, Simoneau TL, George EL, et al. (2000) Family-focused treatment of bipolar disorder: One-year effects of a psychoeducational program in conjunction with pharmacotherapy. Biol Psychiatr 48, 582–592.

Miklowitz DJ and Stackman D (1992) Communication deviance in families of schizophrenic and other psychiatric patients: Current state of the construct. In Progress in Experimental Personality and Psychopathology Research, Vol. 15, Walker EF, Dworkin RH, and Cornblatt BA (eds). Springer-Verlag, New York, pp. 1–46.

Miklowitz DJ, Strachan AM, Goldstein JA, et al. (1986) Expressed emotion and communication deviance in the families of schizophrenics. J Abnorm Psychol 95, 60–66.

Minuchin S (1974) Families and Family Therapy. Harvard University Press, Cambridge.

Moore E and Kuipers E (1999) The measurement of expressed emotion in relationships between staff and service users: The use of short speech samples. Br J Clin Psychol 38, 345–356.

Moos R and Moos BS (1981) Family Environment Scale: Manual. Consulting Psychologists Press, Palo Alto, CA.

Mottarella KE, Philpot CL, and Fritzsche BA (2001) Don't take out this appendix! Generalizability of the global assessment of relational functioning scale. Am J Fam Ther 29, 271–278.

Navran L (1967) Communication and adjustment in marriage. Fam Process 6, 173–184.

Neuchterlein KH, Snyder KS, Dawson ME, et al. (1986) Expressed emotion, fixed dose fluphenazine decanoate maintenance, and relapse in recent-onset schizophrenia. Psychopharmacol Bull 22, 633–639.

Noller P (1981) Gender and marital adjustment level differences in decoding messages from spouses and strangers. J Pers Soc Psychol 41, 272–278.

Noller P (1984) Nonverbal Communication and Marital Interaction. Pergamon Press, New York.

Nuechterlein KH, Goldstein MJ, Ventura J, et al. (1989) Patient-environment relationships in schizophrenia: Information processing, communication deviance, autonomic arousal, and stressful life events. Br J Psychiatr 155(5), 84–89.

O'Farrell TJ, Hooley J, Fals-Stewart W, et al. (1998) Expressed emotion and relapse in alcoholic patients. J Consult Clin Psychol 66, 744–752.

Oliveri ME and Reiss D (1981) A theory-based empirical classification of family problem-solving behavior. Fam Process 20, 409–418.

Parker G (1979) Parental characteristics in relation to depressive disorders. Br J Psychiatr 134, 138–147.

Parker G (1982) Re-searching the schizophrenogenic mother. J Nerv Ment Dis 170, 452–462.

Parker G (1983) Parental Overprotection: A Risk Factor in Psychosocial Development. Grune & Stratton, New York.

Parker G and Hadzi-Pavlovic D (1990) Expressed emotion as a predictor of schizophrenia relapse: An analysis of aggregated data. Psychol Med 20, 961–965.

Parker G, Tupling H, and Brown LB (1979) A parental bonding instrument. Br J Med Psychol 52, 1–10.

Patterson GR (1976) The aggressive child: Victim and architect of a coercive system. In Behavior Modification and Families, Vol. 1, Theory and Research, Mash EJ, Hamerlynck LA, and Handy LC (eds). Brunner/Mazel, New York, pp. 267–316.

Patterson GR (1980) Mothers: The unacknowledged victims. Monogr Soc Res Child Dev 45, 5.

Patterson GR (1982) A Social Learning Approach to Family Intervention. III. Coercive Family Process. Castalia, Eugene, OR.

Patterson GR and Cobb JA (1971) A dyadic analysis of "aggressive" behaviors. In Minnesota Symposia on Child Psychology, Vol. 5, Hill JP (ed). University of Minnesota Press, Minneapolis, pp. 72–129.

Patterson GR, Capaldi D, and Bank L (1991) An early starter model for predicting delinquency. In The Development and Treatment of Childhood Aggression, Pepler DJ and Rubin KH (eds.) Lawrence Erlbaum, Hillsdale, NJ, pp. 139–168.

Patterson GR, Ray RS, and Shaw D (1969) Manual for the Coding of Family Interactions. Available from ASIS National Auxiliary Publications Service under document no. 01234.

Penn DL and Mueser KT (1996) Research update on the psychosocial treatment of schizophrenia. Am J Psychiatr 153, 607–617.

Pinsof WM and Wynne LC (1995) The efficacy of marital and family therapy: An empirical overview, conclusions, and recommendations. J Marital Fam Ther 21, 585–613.

Pretzer J, Epstein N, and Fleming B (1991) Marital attitude survey: A measure of dysfunctional attributions and expectancies. J Cogn Psychother 5, 131–114.

Randolph ET, Eth S, Glynn S, et al. (1994) Behavioural family management in schizophrenia: Outcome of a clinic-based intervention. Br J Psychiatr 64, 501–506.

Rausch HL, Barry WA, Hertel RK, et al. (1974) Communication, Conflict and Marriage. Jossey-Bass, San Francisco.

Rea MM, Tompson MC, Miklowitz DJ, et al. (in press) Family-focused treatment vs. individual treatment for bipolar disorder: Results of a randomized clinical trial. J Consult Clin Psychol.

Reichard S and Tillman C (1950) Patterns of parent–child relationships in schizophrenia. Psychiatry 13, 247–257.

Reiss D, Gonzalez S, and Kramer N (1986) Family process, chronic illness, and death. Arch Gen Psychiatr 43, 795–804.

Revenstorf D, Hahlweg K, Schindler L, et al. (1984) Interactional analysis of marital conflict. In Marital Interaction: Analysis and Modification, Hahlweg K and Jacobson NS (eds). Guilford Press, New York, pp. 159–181.

Riskin J and Faunce E (1970) Family Interaction Scales I. Theoretical framework and method. Arch Gen Psychiatr 22, 504–512.

Robin AL, Siegel PT, and Moye AW (1999) A controlled comparison of family versus individual therapy for adolescents with anorexia nervosa. J Am Acad Child Adolesc Psychiatr 38, 1482–1489.

Robinson EA and Jacobson NS (1987) Social learning theory and family psychopathology: A kantian model in behaviorism? In Family Interaction and Psychopathology, Jacob T (ed). Plenum Press, New York, pp. 117–162.

Robinson EA and Price MG (1980) Pleasurable behavior in marital interaction: An observational study. J Consult Clin Psychol 48, 117–118.

Rogge RM and Bradbury TN (1999) Recent advances in the prediction of marital outcomes. In Preventive Approaches in Couples Therapy, Berger T and Hannah MT (eds). Brunner/Mazel, Philadelphia, pp. 331–360.

Rosen KH, McCollum EE, Middleton K, et al. (1997) Interrater reliability and validity of the global assessment of relational functioning (GARF) scale in a clinical setting: A preliminary study. Am J Fam Ther 25, 357–360.

Ross NM and Doherty WJ (2001) Validity of the global assessment of relational functioning (GARF) when used by community-based therapists. Am J Am Ther 29, 239–253.

Rowat KM and Knafl KA (1985) Living with chronic pain: The spouse's perspective. Pain 23, 259–271.

Roy R (1988) Impact of chronic pain on marital partners: Systems perspective. In Proceedings of the Fifth World Congress on Pain, Dauber R, Gebhart GF, and Bond MR (eds). Elsevier Science, New York, pp. 286–297.

Russell GFM, Szmukler GI, Dare C, et al. (1987) An evaluation of family therapy in anorexia nervosa and bulimia nervosa. Arch Gen Psychiatr 44, 1047–1056.

Sagrestano LM, Heavey CL, and Christensen A (1999) Perceived power and physical violence in marital conflict. J Soc Issues 55(1), 65–79.

Sayger TV, Horne AM, Walker JM, et al. (1988) Social learning family therapy with aggressive children: Treatment outcome and maintenance. J Fam Psychol 1, 261–285.

Schaap C (1984) A comparison of the interaction of distressed and nondistressed married couples in a laboratory situation: Literature survey, methodological issues, and an empirical investigation. In Marital Interaction: Analysis and Modification, Hahlweg K and Jacobson NS (eds). Guilford Press, New York, pp. 133–158.

Sheeber L and Sorensen E (1998) Family relationships of depressed adolescents: A multimethod assessment. J Clin Child Psychol 27, 268–277.

Simoneau TL, Miklowitz DJ, and Saleem R (1998) Expressed emotion and interactional patterns in the families of bipolar patients. J Abnorm Psychol 107, 497–507.

Singer GH, Irvin LK, Irvine B, et al. (1989) Evaluation of community-based support services for families of persons with developmental disabilities. J Assoc Pers Severe Handicaps 14, 312–323.

Singer M and Wynne L (1963) Differentiating characteristics of parents of childhood schizophrenics, childhood neurotics, and young adult schizophrenics. Am J Psychiatr 120, 234–243.

Singer M and Wynne L (1965a) Thought disorder and family relations of schizophrenics. III. Methodology using projective techniques. Arch Gen Psychiatr 12, 187–200.

Singer M and Wynne L ( 1965b) Thought disorder and family relations of schizophrenics. IV. Results and implications. Arch Gen Psychiatr 12, 201–212.

Skinner HA, Steinhauer PD, and Santa-Barbara F (1983) The family assessment measure. Can J Comm Ment Health 2, 91–105.

Snyder DK (1979) Multidimensional assessment of marital satisfaction. J Marriage Fam 41, 813–823.

Snyder DK (1981) Marital Satisfaction Inventory (MSI) Manual. Western Psychological Services, Los Angeles.

Snyder DK and Wills RM (1989) Behavioral versus insight-oriented marital therapy: Effects on individual and interspousal functioning. J Consult Clin Psychol 57, 39–46.

Snyder JJ (1977) Reinforcement analysis of interaction in problem and nonproblem families. J Abnorm Psychol 86, 528–535.

Spanier GB (1976) Measuring dyadic adjustment: New scales for assessing the quality of marriage and similar dyads. J Marriage Fam 38, 15–30.

Stanton MD and Todd TC (1979) Structural family therapy with drug addicts. In The Family Therapy of Drug and Alcohol Abuse, Kaufman E and Kaufman P (eds). Gardner Press, New York, pp. 55–69.

Stanton MD and Todd TC (1982) The Family Therapy of Drug Abuse and Addiction. Guilford Press, New York.

Straus MA (1979) Measuring intrafamily conflict and violence: The conflict tactics (CT) scales. J Marriage Fam 41, 75–88.

Straus MA and Gelles RJ (1986) Social change and change in family violence from 1975–1985 as revealed by two national surveys. J Marriage Fam 48, 465–479.

Strodbeck FL (1951) Husband–wife interaction over revealed differences. Am Sociol Rev 16, 468–473.

Strodbeck FL (1954) The family as a three-person group. Am Sociol Rev 19, 23–29.

Stubbe DE, Zahner GEP, Goldstein MJ, et al. (1993) The diagnostic specificity of a brief measure of expressed emotion in a community sample of children and families. J Child Psychol Psychiatr Allied Disc 34, 139–154.

Swanson DW and Murata T (1980) The family's view of chronic pain. Pain 8, 163–166.

Tarrier N, Barrowclough C, Porcedov K, et al. (1994) The Salford Family Intervention Project: Relapse rates of schizophrenia at five and eight years. Br J Psychiatr 165, 829–832.

Tarrier N, Barrowclough C, Vaughn C, et al. (1988) The community management of schizophrenia: A controlled trial of behavioural intervention with families to reduce relapse. Br J Psychiatr 153, 532–542.

Tarrier N, Barrowclough C, Vaughn C, et al. (1989) Community management of schizophrenia. A two-year follow-up of a behavioural intervention with families. Br J Psychiatr 154, 625–628.

Tarrier N, Sommerville C, and Pilgrim H (1999) Relatives expressed emotion (EE) and PTSD treatment outcome. Psychol Med 29, 801–811.

Tietze T (1949) A study of mothers of schizophrenic patients. Psychiatry 12, 55–65.

Tompson MC, Goldstein MJ, and Rea MM (1996) Psychoeducational family intervention: Individual differences in response to treatment. In Advanced Prelapse Education: Compliance and Relapse in Practice: Papers Presented at a Lundbeck Symposium, Kane JM and van den Bosch RJ (eds). Lundbeck Publications, Denmark, pp. 21–28.

US Bureau of the Census (1992) Current Population Reports, P23–180. How We Are Changing; The Demographic State of The Nation. US Government Printing Office, Washington DC.

Vaughn CE and Leff JP (1976a) The influence of family and social factors on the course of psychiatric illness. Br J Psychiatr 129, 125–137.

Vaughn CE and Leff JP (1976b) The measurement of expressed emotion in the families of psychiatric patients. Br J Soc Psychol 15, 157–165.

Vaughn CE, Snyder KS, Jones S, et al. (1984) Family factors in schizophrenic relapse: Replication in California of British research on expressed emotion. Arch Gen Psychiatr 41, 1169–1177.

Velligan DI, Goldstein MJ, Nuechterlein KH, et al. (1990) Can communication deviance be measured in a family problem-solving interaction? Fam Process 29, 213–226.

Vincent JP, Weiss RL, and Birchler GR (1975) A behavioral analysis of problem solving in distressed and nondistressed married and stranger dyads. Behav Ther 6, 475–487.

Vitaliano PP, Becker J, Russo J, et al. (1989) Expressed emotion in spouse caregivers of patients with Alzheimer's disease. J Appl Soc Sci 13, 215–250.

Vitaliano PP, Young H, Russo J, et al. (1993) Does expressed emotion in spouses predict subsequent problems among care recipients with Alzheimer's disease? J Gerontol 48, 202–209.

Wagener DK, Hogarty GE, Goldstein MJ, et al. (1986) Information processing and communication deviance in schizophrenic patients and their mothers. Psychiatr Res 18, 365–377.

Wahl CW (1954) Some antecedent factors in the family histories of 392 schizophrenics. Am J Psychiatr 110, 668–676.

Wahl CW (1956) Some antecedent factors in the family histories of 568 male schizophrenics of the US Navy. Am J Psychiatr 113, 201–210.

Wahlberg KE, Wynne L, Oja H, et al. (1997) Gene-environment interaction in vulnerability to schizophrenia: Findings from the Finnish Family Study of Schizophrenia. Am J Psychiatr 154(3) 355–362.

Wahler RG and Dumas JE (1987) Family factors in childhood psychology: Toward a coercion-neglect model. In Family Interaction and Psychopathology, Jacob T (ed). Plenum Press, New York, pp. 581–627.

Whittaker S and Bry BH (1991) Overt and covert parental conflict and adolescent problems: Observed marital interaction in clinic and nonclinic families. Adolescence 26, 865–876.

Winemiller DR and Mitchell ME (1994) Development of a coding system for marital problem solving efficacy. Behav Res Ther 32, 159–164.

Wynne LC and Singer M (1963a) Thought disorder and family relations of schizophrenics. II. A classification of forms of thinking. Arch Gen Psychiatr 9, 199–206.

Wynne LC and Singer MT (1963b) Thought disorder and family relations of schizophrenics. I. A research strategy. Arch Gen Psychiatr 9, 191–198.

Wynne L, Singer M, Bartko J, et al. (1977) Schizophrenics and their families: Recent research on parental communication. In Developments in Psychiatric Research, Tanner JM (ed). Hodder & Stoughton, London, pp. 254–286.

Wysocki T, Harris MA, Greco P, et al. (2000) Randomized, controlled trial behavior therapy for families of adolescents with insulin-dependent diabetes mellitus. J Pediatr Psychol 25, 23–33.

Xiong W, Phillips MR, Hu X, et al. (1994) Family-based intervention for schizophrenic patients in China: A randomised controlled trial. Br J Psychiatr 165, 239–247.

Zweig-Frank H and Paris J (1991) Parents' emotional neglect and overprotection according to recollections of patients with borderline personality disorder. Am J Psychiatr 148, 648–651.

SECTION

# VI

Michele Pato, Section Editor

# *Therapeutics*

# 83 Individual Psychoanalytic Psychotherapy

Jerald Kay
Rena L. Kay

Psychoanalytic theory provides the modern clinician with a comprehensive system for the understanding of personality development, the meaningfulness of human conflict and emotional pain, and the mutative factors within the doctor–patient relationship. Psychoanalysis is a general psychology, a developmental theory, and a specific treatment. Since its inception, psychoanalytic theory has undergone numerous and substantial revisions. Its history and the movements that contributed to its evolution are described in Chapter 27. With respect to psychoanalysis as a treatment approach, its history has been punctuated by persistent attempts both to simplify psychoanalytic technique and to shorten its duration of treatment. The synonymous terms psychoanalytic psychotherapy, psychoanalytically oriented psychotherapy, psychodynamic psychotherapy, and expressive psychotherapy have come to represent the most coherent of these attempts.

For many years after World War II there was intense controversy among psychoanalysts about the merit of psychoanalytic psychotherapy because it was considered to be a diluted form of psychoanalysis with poorly defined techniques and goals. Today, for a number of reasons, this issue seems to be less important. First, and most recently, managed care, with its emphasis on cost containment and fiscal accountability, has attributed greater importance to episodic care through briefer psychotherapeutic interventions. Second, compared with 15 years ago, psychoanalysis as a treatment option is no longer equitably reimbursed by third-party payers. As a result, many analysts devote more of their professional time to psychoanalytic psychotherapy than psychoanalysis. Third, with only a few notable exceptions, psychoanalysis has all but moved out of psychiatry departments in academic health centers, and most residency training curricula now focus much more on the basic and practical applications of psychoanalytic theory and technique and not on more traditional psychoanalytic metapsychology. Moreover, during the last 35 years, many new, brief, psychoanalytically informed psychotherapies have been developed. These include, but are not limited to, the methods of Malan (1976), Mann (1973), Sifneos (1979), Davanloo (1978), Horowitz and colleagues (1984), Luborsky (1984), and Strupp (Strupp et al. 1984). Manual-driven psychotherapies with demonstrated treatment efficacy, such as interpersonal psychotherapy and some forms of cognitive–behavioral psychotherapy, also incorporate many traditional psychoanalytic notions about the physician–patient relationship and the role of interpretation. Last, psychoanalytic theory has remained relatively dynamic and has integrated and consolidated the advances from object relations theory, self psychology, interpersonal theory, and the renewed interest in the study of psychic trauma. This has permitted, in the case of severe personality disorders and serious developmental trauma, the psychodynamic treatment of a broader range of psychological problems than was previously considered possible through classical psychoanalysis.

## What Is Psychotherapy?

It is customary to define psychotherapy in a broad fashion as being composed of three distinct components: a healing agent, a sufferer, and a healing or therapeutic relationship (Frank and Frank 1991). Strupp (1986) specified that psychotherapy is the systematic use of a human relationship for therapeutic purposes of alleviating emotional distress by effecting enduring changes in a patient's thinking, feelings, and behavior. The mutual engagement of the patient and the psychotherapist, both cognitively and emotionally, is the foundation for effective psychotherapeutic work.

Whereas there are many different types of psychotherapy (Figure 83–1), the core task of the psychoanalytic psychotherapist is to make contact with and comprehend, as thoroughly as possible, the patient's subjective inner world to engage in an analytical (i.e., interpretive) conversation about it (Ornstein and Kay 1990). This core task implies that all psychoanalytic psychotherapies may be further defined in terms of three operations: accepting, understanding, and explaining (Ornstein and Ornstein 1985) (Table 83–1). First, and more specifically, the therapist must engage with the patient by accepting the subjective experience of the patient's emotional pain and conflict. This is achieved through the establishment of a therapeutic dialogue based on an empathic, nonjudgmental rapport. Second, within the process of listening to, and feeling with, the patient, the therapist will begin to develop an understanding of the intricacies of the patient's plight. Much of what the therapist observes may at first remain outside of the patient's conscious aware-

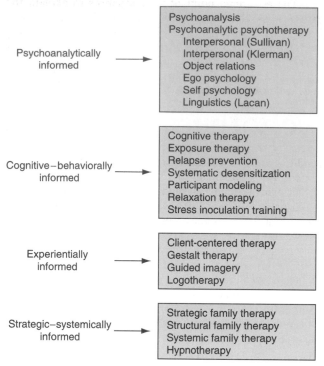

**Figure 83–1** *Some types of psychotherapy.*

ness, manifested in the form of reenactments and reliving of earlier experiences within the therapy, rather than in deliberate, conscious, descriptive communication. Last, by the sharing of this beginning understanding with the patient through a simultaneously empathic and interpretive mode, both arrive at a deeper appreciation for the genesis of, and the reasons for, the patient's symptoms. The shared relationship in which understanding is gained is no less instrumental in achieving change than are the insights and modified perceptions that may result from the psychotherapeutic experience.

## Expressive–Supportive Continuum

Traditionally, to the degree that psychoanalytic psychotherapy has focused on the recovery of repressed psychological material, it has been called "expressive" and has been distinguished from the supportive psychotherapies, which have concentrated on the shoring up of certain defense mechanisms. Supportive psychotherapy has been the traditional treatment approach for more disturbed patients, for example, those with debilitating thought and personality disorders. Supportive treatment has also been helpful to

| Table 83–1 | Essential Operations of Psychoanalytic Psychotherapy |
|---|---|
| Accepting | The therapist affirms the patient's past and present subjective experience |
| Understanding | The therapist appreciates both the conscious and the unconscious contributions to the patient's emotional problems |
| Explaining | The therapist expresses, through interpretations, his or her understanding to the patient |

*Source*: Adapted from Ornstein PH and Ornstein A (1985) Clinical understanding and explaining: The empathic vantage point. In Progress in Self Psychology, Vol. 1, Goldberg A (ed). Guilford Press, New York, pp. 43–61.

patients who are not necessarily suffering from serious underlying impairments but whose symptoms are reactive to immediate identifiable precipitants, such as loss, illness, or other major life change. Expressive psychotherapy, on the other hand, has been concerned with the uncovering of unconscious beliefs, wishes, needs, and memories through the analysis of defense mechanisms and has been indicated for the treatment of neuroses and related conditions, as well as traumatic disorders and less dysfunctional personality disorders.

Such a clear-cut distinction is now viewed as arbitrary and scientifically unsound. Indeed, all effective psychoanalytic psychotherapies, including psychoanalysis, use supportive measures. Moreover, effective supportive psychotherapy is frequently psychoanalytically informed, and no systematic studies have demonstrated that the behavioral change and symptom relief from supportive treatment are inferior to, or less enduring than, those gained from expressive therapies (Wallerstein 1986).

It is more appropriate, therefore, to conceptualize psychoanalytic psychotherapy as being on a continuum of expressive to supportive (Luborsky 1984, Gabbard 1994). This implies that any given treatment might employ more or less expressive and supportive interventions, depending on what is transpiring within the psychotherapeutic process. An important skill of the psychoanalytic psychotherapist is then the ability to employ the appropriate balance of both expressive and supportive interventions as dictated by the needs of the patient. Finally, the conceptualization of an expressive–supportive continuum also facilitates the establishment of therapeutic goals, interventional plans, and indications for individual psychoanalytic psychotherapy (Gabbard 1994) (Table 83–2).

The following clinical vignette illustrates the combination of expressive and supportive measures.

### Clinical Vignette 1

Ms. S entered twice-weekly psychotherapy because of the discouraging lack of career advancement. It became abundantly clear to the therapist that each time the patient was acknowledged by her peers for her outstanding contributions to her law firm, she became profoundly depressed and the quality of her work deteriorated. The therapist shared this observation with Ms. S, who became anxious and frightened. The patient worried that perhaps her reaction to the therapist's words indicated she was "sicker" than she thought. The therapist reassured the patient that she was not "going crazy," and stated that it was important to understand the meaningfulness of the response to the intervention as had been the case with all issues in the psychotherapy.

## Theory of Psychoanalytic Psychotherapy

### Basic Concepts

Because psychoanalytic psychotherapy is derived from psychoanalysis, it is necessary to appreciate the fundamental contributions. Five different but complementary views of mental phenomena constitute the metapsychology or theoretical edifice of psychoanalysis. Whereas none of the five constructs is comprehensive or sufficient to explain all of human behavior, each one has contributed a significant

| Table 83–2 | Comparative Interventions | |
|---|---|---|
| **Expressive** | ←Continuum→ | **Supportive** |
| Confrontation | | Suggestion |
| Clarification | | Reassurance |
| Interpretation | | Advice giving |
| Interpretation of transference | | Praise |
| | | Environmental intervention and manipulation |

component to the current theory and technique underlying psychoanalytic psychotherapy. Freudian or classical psychoanalysis is, above all, a psychology based on conflict in which human beings are constantly defending against strong, unconscious, biologically based, intrapsychic needs and desires. The five metapsychological viewpoints attempt to explain this psychology (Table 83–3).

The topographical point of view states that there are varying levels of mental awareness. Feelings and thoughts may be unconscious, preconscious, or conscious. Repression, about which there is recent neuroscientific support (Anderson and Green 2001), is the most basic of defense mechanisms that keep conflicted feelings and thoughts inaccessible, thereby preventing emotional discomfort.

The dynamic point of view postulates that mental processes are both fluid and the result of opposing forces. This point of view supports the concepts of both conflict and defense. Defense refers to that universal unconscious process whereby patients struggle against the conscious awareness of anxiety-provoking mental content, such as memories, needs, wishes, or fears. There is neurobiological evidence for the existence of signal anxiety which functions as an alerting or warning system to prompt defense mechanisms (Wong 1999). Resistance refers to defenses as they appear in the therapy when the patient unconsciously protects himself or herself against the anticipated pain of such awareness and therefore, to some degree, against progress in treatment.

The structural point of view is based on a tripartite model of the mind consisting of ego, superego, and id. Each of these theoretical concepts is associated with certain functions. The id is considered the repository of irrational and illogical infantile wishes and impulses; the superego, narrowly defined, represents moral and ethical prohibitions; and the ego is that executive portion of the mind that mediates between the id and superego by allowing a person to establish a stable balance between early powerful feelings and impulses and the demands of socialization. The ego mediates, therefore, between the demands of the unconscious and those of external reality. The ego is conceptualized as containing not only the defense mechanisms but the experiencing and observing functions of the mind as well.

| Table 83–3 | Five Psychoanalytic Viewpoints and Associated Constructs |
|---|---|
| Topographical | Conscious, preconscious, unconscious |
| Dynamic | Conflict and resistance |
| Structural | Ego, id, and superego |
| Economic | Psychological investment in ideas and affects |
| Genetic | Past lives in the present, repetition–compulsion |

The economic point of view attempts to explain the nature of psychic energy as it relates to the expression of feelings and ideas and is helpful in understanding defense mechanisms, those unconscious processes that ward off anxiety and other painful affects. As will be explicated, appreciating the role of defense mechanisms is critical both to understanding why patients behave in specific ways and to appreciating the concept of transference.

The genetic point of view, the fifth perspective, addresses the centrality of those childhood experiences, especially traumas, that may account for strong feelings, conflicts, and symptoms later in life. This view is best expressed by the statement that the past lives in the present. It also provides an explanation as to why certain dysfunctional or self-defeating behaviors are repeated throughout life in an attempt to master earlier psychological problems. It is responsible for the unique transference perceptions and reenactments each patient experiences in relation to persons in her or his present life, including the therapist within the process of psychoanalytic psychotherapy.

The theoretical concepts that derived from these five points of viewing mental activity constitute, more or less, the assumptions behind all psychoanalytic psychotherapy. These include, most importantly, the role of the unconscious; the centrality of transference; the characterological defense mechanisms; and the resistance to self-awareness and thereby to progress in the therapeutic setting. Of secondary importance, but nevertheless closely related to the unconscious, is the concept of psychic determinism, namely, that people behave in specific ways for specific reasons. No experience or memory, according to psychoanalysis, is ever lost but resides in the unconscious, which continues to influence current and future ways of experiencing feelings, thoughts, and behaviors. Advances in cognitive neuroscience have supported the notion that many significant experiences throughout life remain outside of awareness.

## Transference and Resistance, Countertransference and Counterresistance

Transference and resistance constitute the two most distinctive features of psychoanalytic psychotherapies. Transference is defined as those perceptions of, and responses to, a person in the here and now that more appropriately reflect past feelings about, or responses to, important people earlier in one's life, especially parents and siblings. Whereas transference experiences are ubiquitous in everyday life as well as in psychotherapy, the development of a transference neurosis, or the recreation of a sustained, intensely affective, conflictual relationship to the person of the psychoanalyst, is more likely to occur within the analytical setting. It is promoted by characteristics of that therapeutic interaction (e.g., use of couch, frequent sessions, therapeutic regression, abstinent position of the analyst) and is more likely to be the focus of interpretation in psychoanalysis. However, supportive measures traditionally characteristic of other forms of treatment also have an important role in psychoanalysis. Psychoanalytic psychotherapy stresses the importance of transference within the treatment relationship, but it differs from psychoanalysis in that it does not, to the same degree, promote the depth and intensity of the transference.

Transference is demonstrated by the two patients in this brief clinical vignette.

---

A patient comments at the end of the first session that the therapist reminds her of her beloved sister who is bright and generous, and whose style of home decorating is beautiful and warm. The patient was apprehensive about beginning psychotherapy but feels more hopeful and comfortable now that she has met the therapist and seen her office.

Another patient finds the office of this same therapist "sterile, not warm or homey and intentionally unrevealing" of who the therapist is as a person. The patient interprets this "professional decor" as an indication that she should not hope for warmth or emotional involvement from the therapist.

Countertransference is variously defined as (1) the analyst's or psychotherapist's transference reactions to the patient; (2) his or her reactions to the patient's transferences; and (3) any reactions, feelings, and attitudes of the analyst or therapist toward the patient, regardless of their source. Such responses to the patient were once viewed as deviations from the ideal of a consistently bland and comfortable experiencing of the patient by the analyst or therapist. Countertransference reactions were also conceptualized as impediments to progress within the treatment, that is, as interferences in the therapist's ability to understand the patient. They are currently more broadly understood as manifestations of the requisite engagement by the therapist or analyst in the emotional process of treatment. Moreover, these reactions are a rich source of understanding of the patient's experience as it touches the therapist affectively. Although countertransference feelings are at times uncomfortable for the therapist and a challenge to monitor and process, they are understood as a reflection of the glue of the relationship without which no real connection or significant change can occur.

The following clinical vignette illustrates a countertransference reaction in response to intense feelings of helplessness.

---

Dr. J was treating a 30-year-old depressed cardiac transplant patient in brief psychotherapy. The onset of the patient's depression coincided with clinical evidence that his new heart was being rejected. The patient's course deteriorated rapidly, and he was hospitalized. Dr. J continued to see the patient as he awaited the highly unlikely possibility of a new donor. After each of the sessions, Dr. J noted that he was exceptionally tired. On the way to his session with the patient that occurred on Christmas Eve, Dr. J stopped at the nursing station and prepared a plate of Christmas cookies for the patient, something he had never done for a patient regardless of the treatment setting.

Resistance is broadly defined as the conscious or, more often, unconscious force within the patient opposing the emergence of unconscious material. Resistance must be understood not as something the patient does to the therapist, but rather as the patient's attempt to protect herself or himself by avoiding the anticipated emotional discom-

| Table 83–4 | Some Common Defense Mechanisms* |
|---|---|
| Repression | Relegation of threatening wishes, needs, or impulses into unawareness |
| Projection | Attribution of conflicted thoughts or feelings to another or to a group of people |
| Denial | Refusal to appreciate information about oneself or others |
| Identification | Patterning of oneself after another |
| Projective identification | Attribution of unacceptable personality characteristics onto another followed by identification with that other |
| Regression | A partial return to earlier levels of adaptation to avoid conflict |
| Splitting | Experiencing of others as being all good or all bad, i.e., idealization or devaluation |
| Reaction formation | Transformation of an unwanted thought or feeling into its opposite |
| Isolation | Divorcing a feeling from its unpleasant idea |
| Rationalization | Using seemingly logical explanations to make untenable feelings or thoughts more acceptable |
| Displacement | Redirection of unpleasant feelings or thoughts onto another object |
| Dissociation | Splitting off of thought or feeling from its original source |
| Conversion | Transformation of unacceptable wishes or thoughts into body sensations |
| Sublimation | A mature mechanism whereby unacceptable thoughts and feelings are channeled into socially acceptable ones |

*All defense mechanisms are involuntary and unconscious.

fort that accompanies the emergence of conflictual, dangerous, or painful experiences, feelings, thoughts, memories, needs, and desires. Resistance occurs through the use of unconscious mental operations called defense mechanisms, for which there is substantial research support (Vaillant 1992, Horowitz et al. 1995) (Table 83–4). The recognition, clarification, and interpretation of resistance constitute important activities of the psychoanalyst and the psychoanalytic psychotherapist, both of whom must first appreciate how a patient is warding off anxiety before understanding why he or she is so compelled.

An example of resistance is illustrated in the following encounter.

---

Ms. C entered psychotherapy because of anxiety and depression. Later in the treatment, evidence emerged that many of the patient's symptoms were related to her significant sexual conflicts and inhibitions. The therapist noted that each time the subject of her sexual activities was approached, Ms. C became confused and anxious and was unable to remember what had been discussed from one session to the next. This pattern of response was involuntary and left the patient frustrated and pessimistic about the ultimate success of therapy.

Counterresistance refers to those psychological processes within the therapist that impede therapeutic progress. These are reactions to some aspect of the treatment experience that unconsciously create anxiety in the therapist. Such occurrences become accessible first to conscious awareness and then to self-study or self-analytical work often in the form of a mistake or a symptom experienced in a therapy session. As an example, the therapist might forget the patient's appointment time or feel sleepy or bored during a therapy session. Countertransference feelings may also be manifested in dreams or fantasies about the patient. Analysis of such symptoms of countertransference not only can facilitate progress in a stalled treatment but may lead to significant growth in self-understanding by the therapist, as well as improved understanding of the patient.

## Basic Technique

As noted, the analysis of transference by the repeated interpretation of resistance is the primary activity of the psychoanalyst and an important one for the psychoanalytic psychotherapist. To promote the patient's examination of the phenomena of transference and resistance, both the analyst and the therapist are guided by principles that establish a confidential, safe, and predictable environment geared toward maximizing the patient's introspection and focus on the therapeutic relationship. The patient is encouraged to free associate, that is, to notice and report as well as she or he can whatever comes into conscious awareness. In the case of psychoanalysis, the depth of the therapeutic process is enhanced by the patient's lying down with the analyst out of the patient's visual range, with a modest level of verbal activity by the analyst, and by meeting frequently, usually four or five times weekly for 45 to 50 minutes for a number of years (American Psychiatric Association 1985) (Tables 83–5 and 83–6).

Therapeutic neutrality and abstinence are related concepts. Both foster the unfolding and deepening of the transference, as well as the opportunity for its interpretation.

**Table 83–5  Characteristics of Psychoanalysis**

| Goals | Personality reorganization<br>Resolution of childhood conflicts |
|---|---|
| Patient's characteristics | Psychoneuroses and mild to moderate personality disorders<br>Psychological mindedness<br>Introspectiveness<br>Can experience and learn from intense affects or conflicts without acting them out<br>Reasonable object relationships<br>High motivation<br>Can tolerate frustration and therapeutic regression |
| Techniques | Use of couch<br>Four or five sessions weekly<br>Free association<br>Neutrality<br>Abstinence<br>Analysis of defenses<br>Analysis of transference<br>Dream interpretation<br>Genetic reconstruction<br>Less frequent use of medication |
| Length of treatment | 3–6 yr or longer |

**Table 83–6  Characteristics of Psychoanalytic Psychotherapy**

| Goals | Partial personality reorganization<br>Appreciation of conflicts and related defense mechanisms<br>Partial reconstruction of the past<br>Symptom relief<br>Improved interpersonal relationships |
|---|---|
| Patient's characteristics | Includes all criteria for psychoanalysis<br>Moderate to severe personality disorders (e.g., borderline)<br>Some affective disorders with and without medication (e.g., major depression, dysthymia) |
| Techniques | Active therapeutic stance<br>Face to face (sitting up)<br>One to three sessions weekly<br>Limited free association<br>Active focus on current life issues<br>Limited transference analysis<br>Some supportive techniques<br>Liberal use of medication<br>Clarification and interpretation |
| Length of treatment | Months to years (may or may not be shorter than psychoanalysis) |

The analyst and psychoanalytic psychotherapist assume a neutral position vis-à-vis the patient's psychological material by neither advocating for the patient's wishes and needs nor prohibiting against these. Essentially, from the structural point of view, the analyst and therapist side with neither the id nor the superego. That is, the patient is encouraged in the therapeutic relationship to develop the capacity for self-observation, a function of the ego, to the best of his or her ability. Neutrality does not mean nonresponsiveness. It is nonjudgmental nondirectiveness, a principle emphasized by psychoanalysts in reaction to the prevalence of suggestion, including posthypnotic suggestions, in the practices of the earliest psychiatrists.

Abstinence refers to the position assumed by the analyst and psychoanalytic psychotherapist of recognizing and accepting the patient's wishes and emotional needs, particularly as they emanate from transference distortions, while abstaining from direct gratification of those needs through action. Abstinence is a principle that guards against the therapist's gratification at the patient's expense. For example, in psychoanalysis, as the treatment experience deepens into a more consolidated transference neurosis, there will be a strong tendency by the patient to experience the analyst as *the* important person in the patient's life around whom the characteristic conflictual issues are manifested. Although it is technically proper to speak of the development of a transference neurosis only in psychoanalysis, many patients in psychoanalytic psychotherapy also develop strong transferences within their treatment experiences. By maintaining a neutral and abstinent position with respect to the patient's needs and wishes, the analyst and psychotherapist create a safe atmosphere for the experiencing and expression of even highly charged affects, the safety required for the patient's motivation for continued therapeutic work. Although there is a persistent caricature of the psychoanalyst, and to a lesser degree of the psychoanalytic psychotherapist, as working in a withholding and aloof fashion, the concepts of optimal frustration and optimal gratification imply that there is a position held by the psychiatrist that is neither sterile nor overstimulating and that promotes the establishment of a meaningful therapeutic relationship.

The rule of free association dictates that the patient's primary obligation within the psychoanalytic situation is that of verbalizing to the best of her or his ability whatever comes into awareness, including thoughts, feelings, physical sensations, memories, dreams, fears, wishes, fantasies, and perceptions of the analyst. This rule is relevant to psychoanalytic psychotherapy as well. Whereas at first glance this requirement appears to be unscientific, in fact, the psychiatrist and patient quickly come to appreciate that no thought or feeling is random or irrelevant but rather that all mental content is relevant to the patient's emotional problems. Indeed, much productive therapeutic work is focused on those instances when the patient is not able to speak what is on his or her mind. As an example, a patient suddenly stops talking after enthusiastically reporting the recent achievements of her son. In response to the therapist's asking what is making it difficult to continue, the patient at first states that her mind is blank and then apologizes for "bragging." Further exploration reveals the fear of the therapist's jealousy and resentment of her child's possibly outperforming the therapist's children.

Dream interpretation has been a significant feature of psychoanalysis since the turn of the century. Many psychoanalytic psychotherapists also use this technique, although recently there may be less emphasis on this. Freud placed great emphasis on the interpretation of dreams not only because it was pivotal in his self-analysis but because he discovered that such a technique provided insights into the working of the unconscious. In a similar fashion, slips of the tongue, jokes, puns, and some types of forgetfulness are attended to carefully by the therapist because they are non-sleep activities that also provide insight into the patient's unconscious mental processes. Good technique does not necessarily include pointing out to the patient these events each time they occur, for they may often be a source of intense embarrassment. Rather, the slips are noted as helpful data in assessing the patient's inner thoughts.

All of these techniques are embedded in a unique manner of listening to the patient's verbalizations within the context of the treatment situation. In particular, two related but specific components initially attributed to the analyst's listening process are worthy of note. First, the concept of the analyst's evenly hovering or evenly suspended attention implies that listening to the patient requires of the analyst that he or she be nonjudgmental and give equal attention to every topic and detail that the patient provides. It also embraces the notion that the effective therapist is one who can remain open to her or his own thoughts and feelings as they are evoked while listening to the patient. Such internal responses often supply important insights into the patient's concerns. Second, empathic listening is of equal importance to both parties. Empathy permits the patient to feel understood, as well as provides the therapist with a method to achieve vicarious introspection. Indeed, one of the major contributions of self psychology has been the identification of empathic listening and interpretation (the immersion by the therapist into the subjectivity of the patient's experience) as basic to the methodology of psychoanalysis and psychoanalytic psychotherapy (Kohut 1978, 1971). Interferences to successful empathic listening are often the product of countertransference reactions, which should be suspected whenever, for example, the therapist experiences irritation, strong erotic feelings, or inattention during a treatment session.

## How Does Psychoanalytic Psychotherapy Work?

Classical psychoanalysis has held that patients are helped by the acquisition of insight into their intrapsychic conflicts. More specifically, conflict is resolved through precise and accurate transference interpretations, which eventually permit the patient to experience the analyst with fewer distortions from childhood experiences. From a structural point of view, the outcome of this interpretive process is a strengthening of the ego and often a softening of the superego. From a different vantage point, it could be said that psychoanalysis helps by permitting the patient to become increasingly conscious of troublesome feelings, conflicts, and wishes that heretofore had remained out of awareness and that produced unhappiness by promoting repetitive self-defeating behaviors.

Whereas insight has always been valued as a goal of psychoanalysis, insight by itself is insufficient. The process whereby insight is acquired is a lengthy and arduous one that is inextricably linked with the recall of painful affects, memories, and traumatic experiences. For treatment to be effective, there must be then both cognitive and affective experiences for the patient. Neither a purely intellectual nor a purely cathartic experience is likely to result in relief or behavioral change. The support provided by the treatment relationship, which includes commitment, respect, reliability, honesty, and care, is a powerful factor in the curative process. It is this atmosphere that makes bearable the emotional pain that accompanies the healing of the wounds first experienced in isolation, so often inflicted by the first objects of the patient's love, need, and trust. All of these considerations are central to psychoanalytic psychotherapy as well.

The concept of "working through" is helpful in appreciating the lengthy and complex psychoanalytic and psychotherapeutic processes. Working through is that stage or aspect of treatment characterized by repeated identification of reenactment and reliving of earlier experiences through confrontation, clarification, and interpretation of resistance and transference that ultimately promotes the patient's self-awareness. In effect, the working through process frees the patient from the position of being at the mercy of unconscious conflicts and fears that have compromised interpersonal relationships and achievement. This is accomplished not only through the analysis of the transference but also of current interpersonal relationships outside of the analysis or psychotherapy. Ultimately, a thorough understanding of the transference and of current relationships permits the patient to appreciate their relationship to important early experiences and ultimately to ameliorate the influence of the past on the present.

## Therapeutic Alliance

The "curative" process as first conceptualized in psychoanalysis rested on the analyst's strict interpretation of intrapsychic conflicts as manifested within the transference neurosis. Accurate transference interpretations ultimately permitted the patient to appreciate the limiting or self-defeating distortions in her or his current life that more appropriately resided in early childhood perceptions. Currently, psychoanalysis places greater importance on the role of the *therapeutic* or *working* alliance than was previously emphasized (Zetzel 1956, Greenson 1967). Both of these terms relate to the real component, as distinguished from the transference component, of the therapist–patient relationship. The real component is composed of the patient's conscious, rational, and nonconflictual feelings toward the therapist that permit a collaborative relationship and that provide the motivation for working toward symptom relief.

A great deal of research in the outcome of psychoanalytic psychotherapy has focused on the importance of the therapeutic alliance (Docherty 1985). Increasing appreciation for the role of supportive factors, such as the rapport between the patient and therapist that constitutes the therapeutic relationship, has balanced the earlier and more narrowly defined position that attributed therapeutic success exclusively to insight resulting from the analyst's specific interpretive activity. The clinical consequences of this appreciation of the helpfulness of nonspecific factors have been the psychoanalytic psychotherapist's paying much greater attention to the initial phases of engaging the patient in psychotherapy and a greater respect for those positive and negative factors that the therapist brings to the working relationship. More specifically, earlier psychoanalysis was more likely to understand the patient's responses and attitudes toward the analyst as products exclusively of transference distortions. Currently, psychoanalysis and psychoanalytic psychotherapy hold that the psychiatrist's personality and interventional technique have equal influence on the therapeutic process. In essence, the contemporary view is more dyadic, and places greater importance on the contributions of the therapist (both the conscious and the unconscious), as well as of the patient with respect to progress and impasse in the psychotherapeutic process.

## Drives

Freud's psychoanalytic model of the mind continually changed throughout his career. His first conceptualization was based on an id psychology, which directed the analyst to attend to the patient's hidden sexual and aggressive drives in the form of wishes, needs, and impulses. His second model, ego psychology, focused more on bringing to the patient's awareness both repressed and disavowed mental content and the role of the unconscious defense mechanisms of the ego as it mediated conflict. Early psychoanalysis then focused on the analysis of drives; later psychoanalysis emphasized drives and their defenses. Analysis based on the later model had limitations as well, especially when the patient did not have a typical symptom neurosis but rather had more characterological problems. It is fair to say that today many psychoanalysts and psychoanalytic psychotherapists attribute less importance to the concept of drives.

## Interpersonal and Object Relationships

One significant clinical and theoretical revision that attempted to transcend the limitations of ego psychology was object relations theory. Some object relationists

retained drive theory (Jacobson 1964, Kernberg 1975, Mahler et al. 1975) whereas others did not (Sullivan 1953, Guntrip 1971). All, however, gave greater credence to the role of internalized object relations both in normal development and in psychiatric illness. Integrating "good and bad objects" was considered the goal of normal development, whereas psychiatric illness resulted when these objects remained separate or "split."

Others (Kohut 1978, Sullivan 1953) thought that object relations theory did not effectively close the gap between theory and practice, especially with respect to the treatment of severe personality disorders. Self psychology deleted drives as central organizing principles and raised the development of self-esteem to a supraordinate theoretical and clinical position. Although the contributions of self psychology have been debated for the last 30 years, much of self psychology has now become a part of modern psychoanalysis and psychoanalytic psychotherapy. This is especially true regarding the importance of empathy in treatment, as well as the appreciation of the so-called self-object transference configurations: the idealizing transference, twinship transference, and the mirror transference.

In summary, contemporary psychoanalysis and psychoanalytic psychotherapy still emphasize elucidation of the unconscious, especially within the transference, and still use interpretation as the primary clinical intervention but recognize more fully the important role of the mutual emotional engagement of therapist and patient and the curative role of this relationship in addition to other supportive factors. They adhere to a much broader perspective on human development and psychiatric disorders. Psychological problems can result not only from early intrapsychic conflict but also from developmental deficits or failures as well as from psychological trauma (Table 83–7).

| Table 83–7 | Indications for Psychoanalysis |
| --- | --- |

Psychoanalysis is the treatment of choice for repetitive, long-standing, maladaptive problems involving personality or character and chronic, repetitive behavioral, affective, or mental disturbances or symptoms that do not respond to cheaper or quicker forms of treatment. In general, it is used for all the character disorders or personality disorders, except antisocial and schizotypal disorders, as well as numerous symptom disorders.

The chronic symptoms must reflect both
1. Intrapsychic conflict
2. Developmental arrest or inhibition

As well, the psychiatrist must expect that
3. The patient's symptoms are likely to continue unless analysis is undertaken
4. Treatments that are less intensive than analysis would likely result in excessive personal or social cost for the patient or just provide temporary relief of acute symptoms related to a current stress, without dealing with underlying issues, hence predisposing the patient to difficulties in future.

Finally, the patient must be able to use psychoanalysis. In general, this rules out the psychotic disorders and a number, but not all, of the borderline disorders.

*Source*: American Psychiatric Association (1985) Peer Review Manual, 3rd ed. APA, Washington DC.

The following clinical vignette is a segment of process from the third year of a 4.5-year psychotherapy conducted by a woman therapist illustrating

- Free association
- Working alliance (threats to and the reestablishment of)
- Transference perceptions and reactions based on experiences both with mother and with father
- Defense and resistance, including denial, projection, reaction formation, and acting out
- Failure of defenses, manifested by symptoms of anxiety, depression, and somatization
- Use of confrontation, clarification, and interpretation of wishes and impulses, defenses and resistances
- Dream interpretation
- Genetic reconstruction
- Role of neutrality and abstinence in maintaining the safety requisite to the patient's experiencing and expressing highly charged, previously unconscious wishes and fears
- Development of insight, accompanied by a decrease in symptoms

---

### Clinical Vignette 5

Ms. J began treatment at age 35 years because of anxiety, work inhibitions, and a tendency to "martyr" herself. She also wanted help with her highly ambivalent relationships with her husband of 15 years and with her married lover of 8 of those years. Ms. J had been subjected to chronic verbal, physical, and sexual abuse by her alcoholic father throughout her childhood. Her mother, depressed and overburdened with many children, was hurtful primarily in her collusive blindness to the father's predations.

Two months before the therapist's planned summer vacation, the patient terminated her sexual involvement with her lover. She became increasingly ambivalent about this decision as the interruption approached. She imagined that her therapist (1) valued men more than women and felt that a man's wishes should always be gratified; (2) found her needs burdensome and preferred that she turn to her lover for the attention she wanted; and (3) was going on vacation to punish her for refusing sex with her lover (projection). Together, the patient and therapist understood these feelings and ideas (transference) as aspects of the patient's re-experiencing, within the treatment, the relationship with the mother of her childhood who had left her to the father, fostering the incest.

Moreover, the patient felt that the therapist was possessive of her attention and did *not* want her to resume the affair. The patient experienced the therapist as withholding attention from her during the vacation, preferring to be with others as her father had sometimes preferred to be with the mother or siblings. The patient recognized that her own angry jealousy of the therapist's family and the wish for retaliation against the therapist played a role in her renewed interest in the extramarital involvement.

During the first psychotherapy session after the vacation, Ms. J reported that as soon as the therapist had left town, she had lost interest in understanding her feelings before acting on them and had resumed her sexual affair (acting out). She soon stopped the sexual involvement when she experienced an insight: she had been hoping unconsciously that by discontinuing the extramarital affair, she would please her therapist and make her cancel the vacation (insight). She

spoke next about having been given a raise at work, which made her depressed and guilty and fearful of the therapist's competitive anger. Ms. J then reported a dream in which she made sure that her lover's wife got more loaves of bread than she. The dream was understood (dream interpretation) as representing both an attempt to undo the sexual betrayal and a protection against the danger of outdoing the therapist with the new "dough" (reaction formation and denial). The extra income from the raise also ensured funding of the psychotherapy. This fact made the therapist wonder (silently) whether the patient's depression in response to learning about the raise implied that she was ambivalent about continuing the therapy, fearful of what might lie ahead (resistance).

The next session began with the patient's reporting that she had felt hurt, inappropriately she thought, when her husband did not want her to touch him. She linked this reaction to her fear of the therapist's rejection because of her sexual behavior during the vacation. She also talked about having "needs that you are unwilling to meet" (neutrality and abstinence). Whereas she had felt last month that the affair was a harmless way of having needs met that were "not being met elsewhere" (displacement), she now stated ambiguously that by "not choosing between the relationships" she was "putting a ceiling on things." The therapist better understood the resistance function of the sexual acting out: it had discharged unconscious sexual impulses in relation to the therapist that were threatening both because of fears of disapproval and of gratification of those wishes through action. That is, the patient was afraid that the therapist would respond sexually as had the father in childhood. Putting a ceiling on things seemed to be the patient's attempt to keep things safe, to keep the therapist under control. Testing this hypothesis, the therapist asked, "Might the affair be putting a ceiling on things here with me as well?" The patient stated that it would be dangerous to want or ask more of the therapist because of the risk of rejection and punishment; also, although getting attention from her lover was "illegitimate, it was less wrong than getting it from you would be. Part of it's sexual," she said, and went on to discuss the role her lover played as mentor and advisor.

Confronting that which was being resisted, the therapist asked, "What about the sexual part?" The patient talked about the "infantile part," wanting to be rocked and held by the therapist, and went on to label her physical needs and desires as "excessive, bad, something that should be repressed." In an attempt to interpret both impulse and defense, the therapist used the somewhat ambiguous action word from the patient's statement at the start of the hour, saying, "It's uncomfortable when you're aware of wanting me to touch you." The patient acknowledged that because the psychotherapeutic relationship did not include physical contact, she turned to the sexual affair to have those needs met (displacement). Interpreting the defense, the therapist said, "When you find it threatening to want me to meet that need sexually, you find it safer to return to your lover." "Yes. It protects both of us. I see it as a threat to the relationship. It might ruin things." The therapist interpreted more specifically the patient's fear of her own desires: "I think that you're feeling that the desire might ruin things not only because I might disapprove, but also because you're afraid there will be some actual behavior that would ruin things." The patient agreed. "That's right. I think I'm afraid the desire would lead to behavior. When I was a child, other ways weren't found to deal with things. I think the desire makes me afraid you'll become my father" (transference and genetic reconstruction).

The next day the patient reported that during the latter part of this hour she had been experiencing back pain (an example of somatization as a failure of defenses), a symptom that throughout the psychotherapy accompanied memories of past sexual abuse. The pain, anxiety, and depression she had been feeling the day before had dissipated after the hour (insight accompanied by decrease in symptoms).

## How Does Psychoanalytic Psychotherapy Differ from Psychoanalysis?

The answer to this question has occupied many researchers and psychiatrists throughout the last 50 years. Efforts have been made continually not only to elucidate the differences between the two treatments but, more important, to define the underlying principles of psychoanalytic psychotherapy. Whereas some prefer definitions of psychoanalysis and psychotherapy as distinct separate entities, it is more useful to many psychiatrists to conceptualize psychoanalysis and psychoanalytic psychotherapy as residing on a therapeutic continuum. As discussed, there is much in the conduct of psychoanalytic psychotherapy that has been borrowed from psychoanalysis. Free association, clarification, and interpretation in psychoanalytic psychotherapy are such examples. The centrality of transference is another, although early psychiatrists and researchers advocated that transferences were to be recognized and acknowledged in psychoanalytic psychotherapy and "managed" rather than interpreted so that patients were not subject to the intense therapeutic regressions characteristic of psychoanalysis. Today, such a distinction regarding the approach to transference in psychoanalytic psychotherapy is less rigid.

On the other hand, certain supportive and more directive techniques, such as greater activity of the therapist through focusing the patient on specific current problems and relationships, reassuring and affirming the patient, and the giving of advice, are used much more in psychoanalytic psychotherapy than in psychoanalysis. Therefore, the adherence to the therapist's neutrality is less strict, and as a result, there is often but not always less frustration for the patient in psychoanalytic psychotherapy. The length of treatment may not distinguish the two approaches, but the frequency of sessions (four or five per week) and the use of the couch, however, are characteristic of psychoanalysis (see Table 83–5).

Overall, it is fair to say that psychoanalytic psychotherapy

- Places greater emphasis on the here and now in terms of the patient's current interpersonal relationships and experiences outside of the therapy; whereas in psychoanalysis, there is greater emphasis on the experiences within the analysis and the relationship between analyst and analysand
- Incorporates, more than does psychoanalysis, various other techniques from other dynamic and behavioral psychotherapies
- Emphasizes the usefulness of focusing on current (dynamic) problems and less on genetic issues
- Establishes more modest goals of treatment

The last point is particularly important in that it facilitated the development of brief dynamic psychotherapies which address focal problems generally in up to 20 sessions.

## Tasks of the Psychoanalytic Psychotherapist

What are the challenges of the psychotherapist in performing psychoanalytic psychotherapy? First, the therapist must ensure that the patient can feel both emotionally and physically safe within the therapeutic relationship. This is accomplished by acknowledging the goals of the treatment and defining the role of the therapist and through establishing professional boundaries. Boundaries refer to those constant and highly predictable components of the treatment situation that constitute the framework of the working relationship. For example, agreeing to meet with the patient for a specified amount of time, in a professional office, and for an established fee are some of the elements of the professional framework. Boundaries also have ethical dimensions best summarized as the absolute adherence by the therapist to the rule of never taking advantage of the patient: through sexual behavior; for personal, financial, or emotional gain; or by exploiting the patient's need and love for the therapist in any fashion (e.g., by using the therapy sessions to discuss the therapist's own problems). The concepts of neutrality, abstinence, and confidentiality further define the role of the therapist.

A critical task of the psychoanalytic psychotherapist is to detect when a breach in either role or boundary has occurred and to restore the patient's security through clarifying and interpreting the meaningfulness of such a breach. As an example, a patient and a therapist were suddenly interrupted in their session by hospital maintenance personnel who obtained entry into the office through the use of a master key. After dismissing the workers, the therapist observed that the patient became uncharacteristically silent. The therapist acknowledged the unanticipated disruption and its impact on the patient, and requested that the patient share what he was thinking during and after the intrusion. The patient told of the effects of a childhood incident in which his bathroom privacy was violated by a distant family member.

The explication of a boundary violation is but one specific example of the technique of interpretation. Successful interpretation is based on a number of prerequisite skills. These include the capacity to empathize with the patient's plight, the ability to recognize the meaning of one's own fantasies about, and responses to, a patient (countertransference), the ability to maintain the patient's verbal flow through the use of open-ended or focused questions, and the capacity to tolerate a relatively high level of ambiguity within the therapeutic relationship. One important professional characteristic of the skilled psychotherapist is patience. Psychotherapy is often arduous, and the capacity to "stay in the chair" with the patient is critical.

The identification of repeated patterns of behavior both within the therapy and in the patient's outside life is a fundamental technique in making sense of the patient's emotional life. This, of course, involves the appreciation of transference and the art of knowing how and when to share this recognition with the patient. Interpretation relies on both appropriate timing and dosage. That is, the psychoanalytic psychotherapist must appreciate when the patient can best integrate the therapist's observations and must respect the patient's defenses, taking care not to overwhelm the patient by insisting that she or he confront more than is tolerable. A poor interpretation is exemplified by this next clinical vignette.

A patient talks about how unimportant therapy is in his life compared with other things, stating that he never thinks about the treatment or the therapist between appointments. The therapist notes that the patient always arrives early for his sessions and has come even when ill, evidence that he has formed an attachment and does need the therapist despite what he asserts. The patient then cancels all appointments for the next month.

Psychoanalytic psychotherapy requires the successful engagement of the patient and the establishment of a therapeutic or working alliance. The alliance can be threatened by a number of phenomena including, but not limited to, the following:

- The therapist's countertransferences or other limitations in his or her capacity to tolerate the emotions stirred by the patient, resulting in empathic failures and mistakes
- The emergence of intense feelings and needs within the patient, for example, when an accurate well-timed intervention evokes feelings in relation to the therapist of appreciation and love accompanied by feelings of vulnerability, erotic desire, or inferiority which the patient wants to flee
- The patient's being reminded of the existence of others in the therapist's life, such as other patients or family (e.g., during interruptions due to the therapist's vacations), triggering painful and embarrassing feelings of jealousy and possessiveness

The therapist's ability to appreciate and respectfully to acknowledge to the patient the impact of these temporal events is critical to the progress of treatment.

From another vantage point, the therapist must also be able to "pass the test" (Weiss 1993). That is, in addition to transference reactions, patients may turn the passive into active by replicating within the therapeutic relationship the original conflictual, disappointing, or traumatic parental experience but reversing the roles. Essentially, the patient does to the psychotherapist what was initially done to her or him. For example, a patient whose parents seemed never to have time to listen has the habit of ending the session 2 minutes early to avoid feeling interrupted and rejected. Such behavior is an adaptive, largely unconscious, interpersonal strategy whose objective is to assess the level of safety within the therapeutic dyad and ultimately to master a psychological problem. If the psychotherapist can pass the test, that is, responds differently from the patient's early negative childhood expectations or pathogenic beliefs, the patient feels more secure and can allow deepening of the therapeutic process. The following clinical vignette illustrates this concept of passing the test, a central component of control–mastery theory (Weiss 1995).

Dr. S was placed on academic leave by his university because he was unable to get to his classes on time. He grew up in a family dominated by a cold, intimidating, and frequently abusive father. In the second session to which he was 10 minutes late, he shared an early memory of keeping his father waiting in the car each Sunday immediately before church. He acknowledged that only on Sunday mornings would his father not beat him for his tardiness. The patient came late to each of the four successive meetings, after which time the therapist interpreted that by being late, the patient was attempting to determine whether the therapist would treat him in the same fashion as did his abusive father. By not becoming enraged or disappointed with the patient, as was frequently the case with the patient's father, the therapist passed the test. The patient experienced greater security in the therapeutic relationship, and his tardiness to sessions ceased.

All of the psychotherapist's skills and techniques must be embedded in a consistent and coherent theoretical viewpoint that provides the therapist with a framework to understand the etiology and meaning of a patient's symptoms and dysfunctional behaviors both in the past and in the present in each of the phases of psychotherapy (Table 83–8). This includes an organized method for understanding the therapist's unconscious and conscious responses to the patient as well. It requires that the therapist listen to the patient's communications in a manner that is markedly different from other forms of social discourse. So-called "process communication" speaks to the therapist on multiple levels and through displacement, through passing remarks and jokes, through shifts in topics, and through metaphors and symbols. To assist in understanding complicated process communication, psychiatrists often ask themselves, Why is the patient telling me this now? What might the patient be trying to say about his or her uncomfortable feelings? Is something being said about the therapeutic relationship? To illustrate, a patient begins the session by being angry about a bill he received for a medical procedure that had not alleviated his physical symptoms. Its high cost and ineffectiveness seem to reflect the physician's uncaring attitude and willingness to make money at the patient's expense. The therapist asks whether the patient recently

| Table 83–8 | Phases of Psychoanalytic Psychotherapy |
|---|---|
| Beginning phase | Patient is educated about roles of both parties<br>Therapeutic alliance is formed → symptomatic relief from nonspecific relationship factors |
| Middle phase | Usually the longest phase of therapy<br>Reexperiencing of patient's conflicts within dyad<br>Interpretation of conscious and previously unconscious material → new insightfulness about current, past, and sometimes previously forgotten experiences |
| Termination phase | Begins with agreed-on end of treatment<br>Anxiety evoked by impending loss of therapist<br>Initial symptoms may recur<br>Integration and consolidation of therapeutic gains<br>Therapist is viewed with less distortion |

received his bill for the psychotherapy and could his concerns about the physician apply to his psychotherapy relationship as well.

As noted, psychoanalytic psychotherapy differs from psychoanalysis in the weight given to the use of supportive measures and in the establishment of more circumscribed goals. Both the psychoanalytic psychotherapist and the psychoanalyst must be skillful in supporting the patient at times of emotional disequilibrium but they may differ in the degree and manner in which support is provided to the patient. Psychoanalysis has always striven for an extensive transformation of the patient's characterological problems and a thorough analysis of the patient's transference neurosis. The psychoanalytic psychotherapist must be skillful in setting more limited goals with a patient regarding the reconstruction of the patient's past. The objective of this type of treatment is to improve the patient's quality of life largely through enhancing interpersonal relationships by promoting greater insight into perceptual distortion and intrapsychic and interpersonal conflict. Psychoanalytic psychotherapy accomplishes this objective by focusing much more on the patient's current predicaments as manifested in both life activities and relationship with the therapist. Compared with psychoanalysis, it is often, but not always, less concerned with the analysis of transference and the complete discovery of the underlying genetic precursors of the patient's current psychological problems.

## Indications for Psychoanalytic Psychotherapy

Although current psychotherapy research attempts to ascertain what specific disorder in what type of patient is most effectively treated by what specific psychotherapeutic approach, studies have not as yet provided the answers to these questions. At this time, it is possible only to speak in generalities based on case reports and limited studies. Conditions and disorders for which psychoanalytic psychotherapy appears to be indicated include personality disorders (except antisocial personality disorder); posttraumatic stress disorders; symptom neuroses or neurotic conflicts; adjustment disorders; paraphilias; and *some* mood, anxiety, somatoform, sexual and gender identity, eating, substance abuse, and dissociative disorders (Table 83–9). In addition, psychoanalytic psychotherapy is often employed in treating patients who present with relational problems and those problems that are the result of abuse or neglect. It may also be useful to patients with certain impulse disorders and to patients whose psychological problems are affecting or are the result of their primary medical illnesses. In short, psychoanalytic psychotherapy, often in combination with medication, is an appropriate intervention in a broad range of disorders, conditions, and psychiatric illnesses (Karasu 1989, Gabbard 1995).

With increasing frequency, patients who are suitable for psychoanalysis are treated in psychoanalytic psychotherapy because of extrinsic demands such as financial resources, time limitations, and job and family conflicts. The characteristics of the patient assumed to be correlated with positive outcome in psychoanalytic psychotherapy include introspectiveness (psychological mindedness); ability to establish and maintain human relationships, even "unhealthy" ones; vocational stability; high degree of

| Table 83–9 | Putative Indications for Psychoanalytic Psychotherapy |
|---|---|

Neuroses
Personality disorders (except antisocial personality disorder)
Posttraumatic stress disorders
Adjustment disorders
Paraphilias*
Mood disorders*
Anxiety disorders*
Somatoform disorders*
Sexual and gender identity disorders*
Eating disorders*
Substance abuse disorders*
Dissociative disorders*
Relational problems
Impulse control disorders*
Psychological problems affecting medical illnesses

*Not indicated for all disorders in these categories.

motivation; absence of formal thought disorder; and psychological resources sufficient to withstand the frustration of the treatment and its characteristic therapeutic regression and accompanying strong affects.

## Contraindications to Psychoanalytic Psychotherapy

Although it is no longer the case, psychoanalytic psychotherapy had been traditionally reserved for patients who could not tolerate the inherent frustration and therapeutic regression of psychoanalysis. More often than not, the issue of analyzability (roughly comparable to treatability) was framed in terms of the assessment of the patient's ego strengths. If a patient was thought to have insufficient psychological resources to withstand the rigors of a psychoanalysis, especially a patient with severe personality disorders and significant thought disorders, psychoanalytic psychotherapy might be prescribed. Similarly, if the patient was considered to be poorly motivated or had some cognitive deficit that might prevent the integration of interpretations, she or he was urged toward a treatment with more supportive elements. For the most part, contraindications to any psychoanalytic psychotherapy that is heavily weighted toward the expressive end of the therapeutic continuum are as follows (Table 83–10):

- Poor impulse control
- Significant cognitive deficits
- Severely dysfunctional interpersonal relationships
- Little ability to tolerate frustration, anxiety, and depression
- Significant lack of introspective capacity

## Supportive Psychoanalytic Psychotherapy

Although only recently systematized, this form of psychotherapy provides psychological stabilization to the patient through the vehicle of a consistent and predictable caring therapist–patient relationship (Werman 1984, Rockland 1989, Novalis et al. 1993, Hellerstein et al. 1994, Misch 2000). The provision of emotional support to patients with psychiatric disorders can be traced to the 18th century

| Table 83–10 | Contraindications to Expressive Psychoanalytic Psychotherapy |
|---|---|

Major ego deficits
Poor motivation
Significant cognitive deficits
Inability to obtain symptom relief through understanding
Inability to verbalize affects
Lack of psychological mindedness
Minimal impulse control
No social support network
Low frustration tolerance
Inability to form therapeutic alliance

moral treatment movement advocated by Pinel and others. Supportive psychotherapy attempts to shore up the patient's defenses and enhance his or her ability to cope with the trials of illness or psychological deficits and the challenges they impose on the patient's daily activities (Table 83–11). Not unexpectedly, it also strives to prevent decompensation and regression. As such, psychoanalytic supportive psychotherapy employs a psychodynamic understanding of the patient's difficulties but does not emphasize interpretation of the patient's internal world. Rather, supportive psychotherapy focuses on assisting the patient to address interpersonal and environmental challenges in the here and now.

Despite its noninterpretive emphasis, supportive psychotherapy can have substantial impact in the lives of patients with significant ego deficits and those with major mental illness. These patients may include those with high levels of aggressivity, poor impulse control, overreliance on action rather than verbal expression of emotions, compromised reality testing, and limited psychological mindedness. It is also highly effective with higher functioning patients who have experienced recent psychic trauma (e.g., through natural disasters, illness, physical or sexual assault, and unexpected devastating losses).

Supportive psychotherapy techniques consist predominantly of empathically listening to the patient's feelings and experiences; giving advice and reassurance; offering suggestion and helpful coping techniques; and for some patients with severe and chronic maladaptations, gently revealing their misperceptions and how they interfere in daily functioning. Although often unexpressed, the patient's identification with the therapist's values, ideals, and approaches to problems is exceptionally therapeutic. Environmental interventions through helping agencies and the patient's significant others are also effective supportive techniques. Although nonspecific to some degree, these interventions are nevertheless based on a comprehensive understanding of the patient's strengths and weaknesses, and are frequently instrumental in curbing self-destructive and self-defeating behaviors. Transference is appreciated but the therapist rarely interprets it in supportive psychoanalytic psychotherapy, choosing rather to foster a positive working relationship through other means (Pinsker et al. 1992).

Although frequently disparaged, effective supportive psychoanalytic psychotherapy is often more challenging to provide than some forms of expressive psychotherapy. Appreciating the psychological forces that are impinging on a marginally functioning patient whose communicative abilities are suboptimal requires a sophisticated clinical approach. Moreover, in supportive psychotherapy, the therapist must assist the patient to modulate intense affective states that are often frightening to the patient and to those in his or her environment. Needless to say, such affects can be directed at the therapist as well. The establishment with the patient of the requisite safe and caring relationship, which may be frequently disrupted by both internal and external forces, is often a significant clinical challenge.

Supportive psychotherapy can produce significant and lasting behavioral change through the reinforcement of health-promoting behaviors; increased capacity for self-

| Table 83–11 | Characteristics of Supportive Psychoanalytic Psychotherapy | |
|---|---|---|
| Goals | Maintain current level of psychological functioning | |
| | Restore premorbid adaptation, if possible | |
| | Enhance coping mechanisms | |
| | Strengthen defense mechanisms unless they are maladaptive | |
| | Support reality testing | |
| | Relieve symptoms | |
| | Decrease mental distress | |
| Patient's characteristics | Severe character disorders | |
| |   Chronic ego deficits | |
| |   Thought disorders | |
| |   Limited psychological mindedness | |
| |   Limited motivation | |
| |   Poor interpersonal relationships | |
| |   Poor impulse control | |
| |   Low frustration tolerance | |
| |   Regression proneness | |
| |   Some potential for therapeutic alliance | |
| |   Extreme passivity | |
| |   Inability to verbalize affects | |
| | Those in crisis situations (catastrophic loss, acute psychic trauma, medical illness) | |
| |   Psychologically healthy | |
| |   Effective social network | |
| |   High premorbid adaptation | |
| |   Flexible defenses | |
| Techniques | Predictability and consistency of therapist | |
| | Conversational style | |
| | Confrontation, clarification, education | |
| | Problem-solving focus | |
| | Provide encouragement, advice, praise, reassurance | |
| | Environmental intervention | |
| | Strengthen reality testing | |
| | Shore up defense mechanisms | |
| | Discourage regression | |
| | Infrequent genetic reconstruction | |
| | Infrequent transference analysis | |
| | Less therapeutic neutrality | |
| | Frequent use of medication | |
| Length of treatment | Usually once weekly or less | |
| | Duration of sessions flexible | |
| | Varies from brief therapy for those reactive disorders in individuals who do not need or are not motivated for further help to lifelong treatment of patients with some chronic disorders | |

reflection; anxiety reduction; and development of new defenses such as intellectualization that enable the patient to acquire a cognitive, anxiety-reducing conceptualization of her or his difficulties.

## Gender Issues in Psychotherapy

Does the gender of the psychotherapist have any effect on the psychotherapeutic relationship and treatment outcome? Are certain psychological problems best treated by therapists whose gender is different from that of the patient? Do different phenomena appear in the treatment of those patients whose therapists are of the same gender? Is the duration of treatment affected by the therapist's gender? Does gender have any influence on the choice of therapist by a patient? These are important questions that have been debated in psychotherapy and psychoanalytic literature for more than 50 years.

The influence of the therapist's gender on the treatment relationship was first raised by Freud (1931) who suggested that women analysts might have the ability to promote a greater variety of transferences than their male counterparts. Shortly thereafter, Thompson (1939) articulated what has become of the traditional psychoanalytic psychotherapeutic position regarding the gender of the therapist, namely, that the therapist's personality is much more critical to the treatment outcome than is his or her gender. A classic study of sex role stereotypical beliefs held by psychotherapists (psychiatrists, social workers, and psychologists) demonstrated that psychological health was defined in terms of normative development for men, whereas for women alone, dimensions such as emotional lability, submissiveness, and dependency were denoted as healthy (Broverman et al. 1970). Although the existence of some influence on the therapy of such attitudes is intuitively compelling, studies examining actual behavior of the therapist rather than beliefs and attitudes do not conclusively demonstrate that gender stereotyping of the therapist has direct effects on the treatment process, length of treatment, or outcome (Schwartz and Abromowitz 1975, Abromowitz et al. 1976, Blasé 1979, Orlinsky and Howard 1976). Women psychotherapists, however, do have an advantage over their male counterparts in terms of satisfaction for both female and male patients (Kirshner et al. 1978).

Although the literature regarding the advantages and disadvantages of gender matching of patients and therapists consists largely of anecdotal and negative reports (Zlotnick et al. 1998), it is nevertheless evocative. A number of common themes have emerged, including that

- The gender of the therapist may be more critical in supportive treatments that rely on identification with the therapist (Cavenar and Werman 1983)
- The therapist's gender may be less important in psychoanalysis than in face-to-face psychoanalytic psychotherapies, because in the latter, the transference can be less intense (Mogul 1982)
- Beginning women therapists have less difficulty with empathy but more difficulty with authority issues than do their male counterparts (Kaplan 1979)

The wish for a woman to be treated by a female psychotherapist, an increasingly common event, may be related to a number of different issues. For example, the woman may wish to rectify an unfulfilling experience with her own mother; seek permission from another woman to be assertive and accomplished; anticipate feeling understood more readily by another woman than by a man; or feel greater physical safety in the therapeutic relationship with another woman, particularly if she has experienced past sexual abuse or has been the victim of sexual misconduct by a previous male therapist.

Similarly, a woman might choose a male therapist if she is fearful of becoming dependent on another woman (Nadelson and Notman 1991). A female psychotherapist could also be valued in the early portion of therapy but then subsequently be devalued as the female patient begins to experience the therapist competitively (Notman et al. 1978) or as other more hostile transferences unfold.

Male patients can have comparable conscious and unconscious reasons for selecting a psychotherapist by gender. For instance, men who are frightened of male competition or intense homosexual concerns might gravitate toward female psychotherapists. Men who have been unsuccessful in establishing meaningful relationships with women might select a female therapist in the hope that she could teach him how to be successful with women. The same might be true for a male patient suffering from sexual dysfunction who yearns for the secret of what sexually pleases women. Conversely, a man fearful of strong women, a man hungry for a strong male figure with whom he can identify, or a man seeking to avoid dependent or strong heterosexual feelings in the treatment relationship might prefer a male therapist.

In short, although there is only one controlled study and it showed no difference regarding the influence of the therapist's gender on the therapeutic process (Zlotnick et al. 1996), there is much to consider about the influence of actual gender and gender-related beliefs of both patient and therapist on the emergence of transference and countertransference. However, the best psychoanalytic psychotherapies will include ample opportunities for the working through of the patient's issues related to important figures of both genders.

## Ethnocultural Issues in Psychotherapy

Culture refers to meanings, values, and behavioral norms that are learned and transmitted in the dominant society and within its social groups. Culture powerfully influences cognitions, feeling, and "self" concept, as well as the diagnostic process and treatment decisions. Ethnicity, a related concept, refers to social groupings which distinguish themselves from other groups based on ideas of shared descent and aspirations, as well as to behavioral norms and forms of personal identity associated with such groups (Mezzich et al. 1993).

The *Diagnostic and Statistical Manual of Mental Disorders*, Fourth Edition (DSM-IV) advocates a cultural formulation that augments the multiaxial diagnostic assessment of culturally diverse patients (American Psychiatric Association 1994). The cultural formulation is derived from the traditional biopsychosocial case formulation, and it emphasizes how culture may influence the expression of symptoms, the patient's conceptualization of illness, the treatment, and the treating relationship (Mezzich et al. 1993). The guideline for cultural formulation that served

| Table 83-12 | Guideline for Cultural Formulation |
| --- | --- |

The following guidelines for cultural formulation are meant to supplement the multiaxial diagnostic assessment and to address difficulties that may be encountered in applying DSM-IV criteria in a multicultural environment. The cultural formulation provides a systematic review of the individual's cultural background, the role of the cultural context in the expression and evaluation of symptoms and dysfunction, and the effect cultural differences may have on the relationship between the individual and the clinician.

It is important that the clinician take into account the individual's ethnic and cultural context in the evaluation of each of the DSM-IV axes. In addition, the cultural formulation suggested below provides an opportunity to describe systematically the individual's cultural and social reference group and ways in which cultural context is relevant to clinical care. The clinician should provide a narrative summary of each of the following areas:

| Area | Summary |
| --- | --- |
| Cultural identity of the individual | The clinician should specify the individual's cultural reference groups. Attend particularly to language abilities, use, and preferences (including multilingualism). For immigrants and ethnic minorities, note separately the degree of involvement with both the culture of origin and the host or majority culture. |
| Cultural explanations of the individual's illness | Identify (1) the predominant idioms of distress through which symptoms are communicated (e.g., "nerves," possessing spirits, somatic complaints, inexplicable misfortune); (2) the meaning and perceived severity of the individual's symptoms in relation to norms of the cultural reference group; (3) any local illness category used by the individual's family and community to identify the condition; (4) the perceived causes or explanatory models that the individual and the reference group employ to explain the illness; and (5) current preferences and past experience with professional and popular sources of care. |
| Cultural factors related to psychosocial environment and functioning | Note culturally relevant interpretations of social stressors, available social supports, and levels of functioning and disability. Special attention should be given to stresses in the local social environment and to the role of religion and kin networks in providing emotional, instrumental, and informational support. |
| Cultural elements of the relationship between the individual and the clinician | Indicate differences in culture and social status between the individual and the clinician and problems that these differences may cause in diagnosis and treatment (e.g., difficulty in communicating in the individual's first language, in eliciting symptoms or understanding their cultural significance, in negotiating an appropriate relationship or level of intimacy, in determining whether a behavior is normative or pathological). |
| Overall cultural assessment for diagnosis and care | The formulation should conclude with a discussion of how these cultural considerations specifically influence comprehensive diagnosis and care. |

*Source*: Mezzich JE, Kleinman A, Fabrega J, et al. (eds) (1993) Revised Cultural Proposals for DSM-IV (Technical Report). NIMH Cultural and Diagnosis Group, Pittsburgh, PA.

as the template for the DSM-IV-TR outline is presented in Table 83–12.

In the establishment of a therapeutic alliance, the patient's cultural difference from the therapist may add another level of complexity to the therapeutic process. For example, in engaging a Japanese patient, the psychotherapist must be cognizant of the patient's need for formality because an informal style may lead to embarrassment for the patient (Marsella 1989). In the treatment of some Asian patients, there may be an inherent cultural expectation that the therapist teach the patient how to correct her or his behavior (Blue and Gonzalez 1992). The ability to trust the psychotherapist is a fundamental task of any psychotherapy. Establishing trust with an African-American patient, for example, may be more complicated for a white psychotherapist if the patient's experiences with the dominant culture or white physicians have been disappointing or demeaning. An African-American psychotherapist might have to encounter early in the treatment overt or covert prejudice from a white patient. A Native American patient may have great distrust for a white therapist who represents a dominant culture. In some circumstances, a patient from a different culture might be obsequious in an attempt to please the psychotherapist.

Comas-Diaz and Jacobsen (1991, 2001) have introduced the concept of ethnocultural allodynia to describe an intense sensitivity and response to relatively innocuous or neutral stimuli emanating from previous culturally based painful experiences. They describe how sociocultural and ethnic emotional injuries can have profound impact on self-cohesiveness and object relationships. As is the case in Herman's concept of complex posttraumatic stress disorder (PTSD) (Herman 1992), alterations in self-perception and perception of others, affective lability, interpersonal relationships, world view, and hope can accompany traumatic ethnocultural experiences which, when present, require attention within the treatment relationship (Comas-Diaz and Jacobsen 2001).

Countertransference reactions, too, may be influenced by the patient's culture. For example, novice psychotherapists often become so intrigued by the culturally diverse patient that they behave as if they were clinical anthropologists and neglect the patient's emotional pain by focusing exclusively on the patient's culture (Comas-Diaz and Jacobsen 1991). For other therapists, the struggle with impulses to right historical or sociological wrongs may be expressed in persistent rescue feelings. Under certain circumstances, when culturally diverse therapists treat patients from their own culture, they may distance themselves from their patients or may overidentify with them.

Given the increasing multiculturalism of many cities in the US, how should the psychoanalytic psychotherapist treat patients from cultures other than his or her own? Whereas therapists are obligated to be culturally informed, Foulks and colleagues (1995) have argued against the promotion of culturally specific psychotherapies. Although acknowledging that some cross-cultural psychiatrists believe expressive–supportive psychotherapy to be an ethnotherapy appropriate only to the citizens of the Western world, they emphasized the overwhelming problems in establishing separate therapies and clinics devoted to patients from a multitude of specific cultures. Also, they stated that the principles of psychotherapy elucidated in this chapter—accepting, understanding, and explaining—are appropriate for the culturally diverse patient.

## Is Psychoanalytic Psychotherapy Effective?

The short answer to this question is yes. The longer answer would require an extensive chapter on the history of psychotherapy research (Talley et al. 1994, Wallerstein 1995). The effectiveness of psychotherapies was first challenged by the argument that responses to psychotherapeutic treatment were no greater than those achieved through spontaneous remission (Eysenck 1952). Many studies have criticized this finding, the latest of which was based on a reevaluation of Eysenck's (McNeilly and Howard 1991) original data, which demonstrated that approximately 15 sessions of psychotherapy can accomplish the same result as a spontaneous remission that takes 2 years. Meta-analytical studies of psychotherapy have demonstrated unequivocally that psychotherapy is effective (Luborsky et al. 1975, Smith et al. 1980, Lambert et al. 1986). The study by Smith and coworkers (1980), for example, demonstrated that 80% of those patients treated in psychotherapy fared better on outcome measures than those who received no treatment. Psychological growth achieved through psychotherapy is also enduring (Husby 1985).

The helpfulness of psychotherapy for those patients suffering from significant medical illness has been documented. Spiegel and colleagues (1989) demonstrated that breast cancer patients enrolled in expressive–supportive group psychotherapy lived an average of 18 months longer than control subjects who were not treated with group therapy. The most recent study of the effect of group psychotherapy on survival of patients with metastatic breast cancer however failed to replicate prolonged survival but did note that women receiving supportive–expressive psychotherapy had significant mood improvement and pain perception particularly in those subjects who were initially more distressed (Goodwin et al. 2001). Similarly, patients with lymphoma, leukemia, and malignant melanoma fared better with their illnesses when treated with supportive individual and group interventions (Richardson et al. 1990, Fawzy et al. 1993). Expressive–supportive psychotherapy is also effective in opioid-dependent patients attending community methadone maintenance programs and is superior to counseling (Woody et al. 1995).

Other cost-offset studies have repeatedly demonstrated the helpfulness of psychotherapy in reducing general health care services by as much as one-third (Mumford et al. 1984, Krupnick and Pincus 1992, Olfson and Pincus 1994). These include reduction in hospital stays for surgical and cardiac patients (Mumford et al. 1982) and decreased treatment costs for those with respiratory illnesses, diabetes, and hypertension (Schlesinger et al. 1983). Brief psychotherapy has also been shown to be effective in general medical clinics, where those patients with significant medical and psychiatric problems improve substantially more than those treated by primary care physicians alone (Meyer et al. 1981).

Whereas earlier meta-analyses addressed psychoanalytic, cognitive, and behavioral therapies as an aggregate, Luborsky and coworkers (1993) have demonstrated that psychoanalytic psychotherapy is as effective as cognitive, behavioral, experiential, and group therapies and hypnotherapy. For this meta-analysis, rigorous inclusion criteria were established including, but not limited to, adequate sample size with random assignment, suitable length and frequency of sessions, sound outcome measures, adherence by therapists to treatment manuals, and comparable skill levels among therapists.

Milrod and colleagues (2001) have demonstrated the usefulness of their manualized brief psychodynamic psychotherapy in the treatment of panic disorder. In this open trial, 21 patients on no medication received twice-weekly therapy for 24 sessions. Sixteen of the 17 subjects who completed treatment experienced remission of panic and agoraphobic symptoms. Eighty-one percent of patients had a comorbid disorder and those with depression also improved dramatically. In addition, improvements in quality of life were significant and were sustained at 6-month follow-up.

A study of brief psychodynamic psychotherapy in patients with panic disorder combined with medication demonstrated that combined treatment was superior to medication alone (Wilborg and Dahl 1996). In this comparative study, subjects were treated with either clomipramine or 15 sessions of dynamic psychotherapy with clomipramine. After discontinuation of medication at 9 months, the relapse rate for those treated with medication alone was significantly higher. Those treated with combined treatment functioned at higher levels which was attributed to the gains made in psychotherapy.

A randomized controlled study of psychoanalytic psychotherapy and medication versus standard psychiatric care (which included no psychotherapy) in the treatment of 44 patients with borderline personality disorder demonstrated the effectiveness of psychoanalytic psychotherapy (Bateman and Fonagy 2001). At 18-month follow-up, those who had received psychotherapy in the context of a partial hospital program of a year-and-a-half, not only maintained their improvement in functioning but also demonstrated increased gains in a number of significant domains while receiving ongoing twice-weekly psychoanalytic group psychotherapy. These gains included fewer suicide attempts, less self-mutilating behavior, a lower number and shorter duration of inpatient admissions, and less use of other psychiatric services. There was also continued symptomatic improvement in anxiety, depression, and general symptom distress, as well as gains in interpersonal relationships and social adjustment.

Swiss researchers (Burnand et al. 2002) conducted a randomized controlled trial of combined psychodynamic psychotherapy and clomipramine in the outpatient treatment of major depression. Seventy-four patients with major depression received either 10 sessions of psychodynamic psychotherapy with medication or medication and supportive psychotherapy. Those in the former group were treated by nurses who received 6 months of training, followed a manualized protocol, and were supervised weekly by an experienced psychoanalyst. While both treatment groups demonstrated significant improvement, medication plus dynamic psychotherapy was associated with both better work and higher global functioning. Moreover, in the psychodynamic psychotherapy treatment group there were fewer treatment failures and posttreatment hospitalizations which resulted in cost savings (direct and indirect costs) of $2,311 per patient. For those patients who were employed at the onset of the study, savings amounted to $3,394 in indirect costs.

At this time, however, the therapist is left with few data supporting the superiority of one type of psychotherapy over another for a given condition or disorder (Smith et al. 1980). This dilemma must be tempered by the recognition of the enormous complexity of psychotherapy research. The important research questions with respect to brief psychoanalytic psychotherapy have been summarized by Barber (1994) and are relevant to all psychoanalytic psychotherapies (Table 83–13).

The majority of studies examining psychoanalysis and psychoanalytic psychotherapy have been outcome studies rather than comparative. Although many early outcome studies of psychoanalysis were methodologically unsound (Wallerstein 1995), a number of these that examined both outcome and therapeutic process were sophisticated (Bachrach et al. 1991). In general, process studies have attempted to examine important variables, such as how interpretation and therapeutic alliance are related to outcome and how transference, central conflict, and internalization are measured in a reliable and valid manner (Barber 1994). The Menninger Psychotherapy Research Project, for example, attempted to answer not only outcome (what changes accrued from treatment) but also how such changes were brought about in those patients receiving psychoanalysis, psychoanalytic psychotherapy, and supportive psychoanalytic psychotherapy (Wallerstein 1986). The Psychotherapy Research Project's most significant findings centered on the unanticipated effectiveness of supportive psychoanalytic psychotherapy in the treatment of patients

with significant psychiatric illness. In short, across all three forms of psychoanalytic psychotherapy, changes emanating from supportive interventions were substantial and in no way inferior to the more expressive interventions of psychoanalysis that were aimed at structural change.

## Long-Term Versus Brief Psychotherapies

Despite the massive economic forces impinging on the current practice of long-term psychoanalytic psychotherapies, both brief and extended expressive and supportive treatments are required in the psychiatrist's therapeutic armamentarium. Whereas the research on brief psychoanalytic psychotherapies has been impressive, patients successfully treated by these techniques have generally met inclusion criteria that place them in the less dysfunctional range of psychiatric illness; that is, they tend to have less severe character disorder. Moreover, more than 80% of patients entering psychoanalysis have previously been unsuccessful in less intensive forms of treatment (Doidge et al. 1994). Up to 25% of all depressed patients do not tolerate medications or they respond poorly to them (American Psychiatric Association 1993), and of course there are always patients who will not agree to take antidepressants. Even the National Institute of Mental Health Collaborative Study of Depression, which assessed cognitive–behavioral therapy and interpersonal psychotherapy and tricyclic antidepressant medication, demonstrated the exceptional efficacy of psychotherapy. Shea and colleagues (1992) have argued that 16 weeks of treatment appears to be insufficient for many patients to achieve a full recovery. The need for maintenance psychotherapy in treating unipolar depression has been substantiated (Frank et al. 1990). A significant study of the relationship between the number of sessions and patient improvement in psychotherapy has shown that by eight sessions and 26 sessions of weekly psychotherapy, 50 and 75% of patients, respectively, improve (Howard et al. 1986). When chronic distress and characterological symptoms are examined however, 74 to 89% of patients with chronic distress and only 60% of patients with character problems improve after a year of treatment (Kopta et al. 1992). In short, patients with more complex conditions often require longer treatment.

## Disconnection Between Psychotherapy Practice and Research

There is a persistent tension in the psychotherapy research literature relating to the perception that therapists do not integrate the findings from psychotherapy research and that psychotherapy researchers fail to study the relevant clinical issues (Stiles 1992). From the therapist's point of view, most psychotherapy research lacks a therapeutic context and fails to answer basic questions such as: How is a treatment altered when the patient has unusual characteristics? What intervention should the therapist use if the prescribed treatment is failing? How should therapeutic change be assessed? The tension between therapists and researchers has been made all the more strident because of pressures placed on both parties to prove cost-effectiveness for all psychotherapeutic interventions. Unfortunately, nationally funded research in psychotherapy has not been a priority, and when such research is funded, more often than not, it must embrace a clinical trials methodology, which may or may not be able to ask the relevant clinical questions.

| Table 83–13 | Research Challenges for Psychoanalytic Psychotherapy |
|---|---|

Determining efficacy for specific disorders

Developing treatment guidelines for interpersonal problems and personality disorders

Developing reliable and valid self-report measures for core conflicts

Measuring potential cost-offset of different therapies

Determining efficacy of short-term vs. long-term psychotherapies

Matching patients to treatment on basis of personality, functional level, or developmental stage

Examining whether and how experienced therapists can be trained in short-term psychoanalytic treatments

Learning the limits of brief therapy and conditions or symptoms for which longer-term psychotherapy should be recommended

*Source*: Barber JP (1994) Efficacy of short-term dynamic psychotherapy: Past, present, and future. J Psychother Pract Res 3, 108–121.

What can be done about bridging the chasm between psychotherapy practice and research? Talley and colleagues (1994) have advocated five practices likely to be helpful in creating a rapprochement between researchers and therapists. First, case studies should no longer be disparaged, for they have the ability to be scientifically rigorous by testing specific hypotheses. Second, wherever possible, researchers should endeavor to include clinical vignettes in their published work and emphasize the clinical applicability of specific findings. Third, studies must be conducted that determine what type of psychotherapy research is helpful to therapists. Fourth, the accessibility of psychotherapy research findings to therapists should be studied with respect to knowledge of new findings as well as understandability. Last, training programs must assist students to integrate new research findings, as well as train a new generation of researchers to ask the clinically significant questions.

## Towards a Neurobiology of Psychotherapy

Exciting new research in psychiatry, brain imaging, cognitive neuroscience, genetics, and molecular biology has provided striking insights into how psychotherapy actually changes both brain structure and function (Liggan and Kay 1999, Gabbard 2000, Lehrer and Kay 2002). Learning and memory are associated with alterations in central nervous system (CNS) neuronal plasticity including increased synaptic strength and number of synapses. Neurogenesis, or the creation of new brain cells, occurs daily in the human hippocampus (Eriksson et al. 1998), the central location for the formation of new explicit memories. Not only does memory consolidation lead to persistent modifications in synaptic plasticity, but psychotherapy, a form of learning, also produces changes in the permanent storage of information acquired throughout an individual's life and pro-

vides new resources to address important psychobiological relationships between affect, attachment, and memory which is of fundamental importance in psychiatric disorders. Rapidly accruing knowledge about the different types of memory and the role of the amygdala now support the influence of memories that reside outside of the awareness of our patients (LeDoux 1996). Implicit memories formed in infancy and childhood persistently affect the manner in which patients experience themselves and their worlds as manifested, for example, in transference reactions within and outside of the therapeutic relationship.

Research beginning in the last decade has demonstrated that psychotherapy affects cerebral metabolic rates. One study has provided preliminary evidence that psychoanalytic psychotherapy alters serotonin metabolism in borderline personality disorder and depression (Viinamaki et al. 1998). Comparative imaging studies testing psychotherapy versus medication have shown normalizing changes in regional cerebral blood flow (rCBF) and neurotransmitter metabolism in patients with obsessive–compulsive disorder (OCD) and major depression (Baxter et al. 1992, Brody et al. 2001, Martin et al. 2001). Other studies have shown restoration of sleep architecture and thyroid hormone levels after psychotherapeutic treatment of patients with major depression (Thase et al. 1998, Joffe et al. 1996) (Table 83–14).

Psychotherapy may have profound impact on neuroimmunology. As noted, providing psychotherapy to patients who have metastatic breast cancer or malignant melanoma can reduce morbidity and perhaps mortality (Spiegel et al. 1989, Fawzy et al. 1993). Elucidating the role of the hypothalamic–pituitary–adrenal system (HPA axis) has also clarified the impact of stress on learning, memory, and lifelong psychological adaptation during important periods of attachment in mammals (Suomi 1991, Rosenblum and Andrews 1994, Kaufman et al. 2000). Many studies have demonstrated enduring elevated levels

| Table 83–14 | Neurobiological Studies of Psychotherapy | | | |
|---|---|---|---|---|
| Investigators | Treatment | Disorder | *N* | Findings |
| Baxter et al. (1992) (PET) | Fluoxetine vs. exposure/response prevention therapy | OCD | 9 patients 9 patients | < activity in the head of the right caudate nucleus in responders with both psychotherapy (6/9) + pharmacotherapy (7/9) |
| Joffe et al. (1996) | CBT | Major depression | 30 patients | Increased $T_4$ in all 17 responders Decreased $T_4$ in nonresponders |
| Schwartz et al. (1996) (PET) | Exposure/response prevention therapy | OCD | 9 new patients 9 patients from previous study | < caudate activity (R>L) in responders |
| Thase et al. (1998) (EEG) | CBT | Major depression | 78 patients | Psychotherapy + pharmacotherapy restored normal sleep architecture |
| Viinamaki et al. (1998) (SPECT) | Psychodynamic psychotherapy vs. no treatment | Borderline PD + depression | 2 patients (10 controls) | > 5-HT metabolism PFC + thalamus |
| Brody et al. (2001) (PET) | IPT vs. paroxetine | Major depression | 24 patients | Normalization of PFC, AC + temporal lobe with both treatments |
| Martin et al. (2001) (SPECT) | IPT vs. venlafaxine | Major depression | 28 patients | Increase (r) CBF to basal ganglia in both treatments. Increase (r) CBF in limbic system for IPT only |

CBT, cognitive–behavioral therapy;  IPT, interpersonal psychotherapy;  PFC, prefrontal cortex;  AC, anterior cingulate.

of cortisol, adrenocorticotrophic hormone (ACTH), and corticotrophin-releasing factor (CRF) following episodes of maternal separation. Even with appropriate substitute nurturing, animals respond to stress in a more intense fashion throughout their lives. Early experiences therefore can have profound impact on future psychosocial and neurobiological development as has been demonstrated in reduced hippocampal volumes of children who have experienced abuse and maltreatment (Bremner et al. 1997).

Last, genetic and epidemiological studies have clarified the role of experiences on gene expression and vulnerability to psychiatric illness. Kendler's large study of groups of female twins, both at low and high risk for major depression, eloquently demonstrated that the meaning and valence of a stressor have great influence on illness onset (Kendler et al. 1995). The probability for depression for low-risk twins and high-risk twins who experienced a recent death, assault, or marital problems increased from 0.5 to 6.2% and 1.1 to 14.6% respectively, over a 17-month period. Similarly, by studying large numbers of teenagers from variously configured families, Reiss demonstrated that the inherited psychological and temperamental characteristics of children can evoke very different types of relatedness from their parents (Reiss et al. 1995). Compared to their siblings, teenagers who had highly conflictual relationships with their parents, for example, a negative way of relating accounted for nearly two-thirds of variance in antisocial behavior and more than one-third the variance in depressive symptomatology. The experience of a nonshared family environment expressed by the differential treatment of adolescents has significant explanatory power as to why some are at greater risk for mental illness.

The study of psychotherapy from a neurobiological perspective is likely to provide greater understanding of how words in the context of therapeutic relationships can heal. It may be that there are similar mechanisms and anatomical regions that are involved in the successful treatment of psychiatric illness with psychotherapy and pharmacotherapy as monotherapies, as well as in the combined treatment situation (Sacheim 2001). It is also likely to yield a greater understanding of pathogenesis and delineate helpful interventions to decrease genetic vulnerability to emotional disorders.

## Conclusion

The practice of psychoanalytic psychotherapy by psychiatrists is currently under scrutiny. Nevertheless, the majority of all encounters with patients in American psychiatry involve some form of psychotherapy, and many of these interventions are based on the principles of psychoanalytic psychotherapy.

At this time, the theory and technique of psychoanalytic psychotherapy provide the most comprehensive orientation to the continuum of expressive–supportive psychotherapy. Psychoanalytic psychotherapy is a potent intervention and, as such, holds great promise when it is used in a sophisticated fashion for appropriate patients with appropriate psychiatric problems. Like medication, psychoanalytic psychotherapy has specific indications, contraindications, and undoubtedly, potentially negative effects. As an effective therapeutic intervention, it requires that the therapist be highly skilled in assessing the inner experience of those who come for help. It also requires extensive training and education in techniques of this treatment modality. As well, the therapist must acquire significant self-knowledge, sophistication, and dedication in working so intensively with human pain.

## References

Abromowitz S, Roback H, Schwartz J, et al. (1976) Sex bias in psychotherapy: A failure to confirm. Am J Psychiatr 133, 706–709.

American Psychiatric Association (1985) Peer Review Manual, 3rd ed. APA, Washington DC.

American Psychiatric Association (1993) Practice guideline for major depressive disorder in adults. Am J Psychiatr 150(Suppl), 1–26.

American Psychiatric Association (1994) Diagnostic and Statistical Manual of Mental Disorders, 4th ed. APA, Washington DC, pp. 843–844.

Anderson MC and Green C (2001) Suppressing unwanted memories by executive control. Nature 410, 366–369.

Bachrach HM, Galatzer-Levi R, Skolnikoff A, et al. (1991) On the efficacy of psychoanalysis. J Am Psychoanal Assoc 39, 871–916.

Barber JP (1994) Efficacy of short-term dynamic psychotherapy: Past, present, and future. J Psychother Pract Res 3, 108–121.

Bateman A and Fonagy P (2001) Treatment of borderline personality disorder with psychoanalytically oriented partial hospitalization program: An 18-month follow-up. Am J Psychiatr 158, 36–42.

Baxter LR, Schwartz JM, Bergman KS, et al. (1992) Caudate glucose metabolic rate changes with both drug and behavior therapy for OCD. Arch Gen Psychiatr 49, 681–689.

Blasé J (1979) A study on the effects of sex of the client and sex of the therapist on client's satisfaction with psychotherapy. Diss Abstr Int 49, 6107–6107B.

Blue HC and Gonzalez CA (1992) The meaning of ethnocultural difference: Its impact on and use in the psychotherapeutic process. New Dir Ment Health Serv 55, 73–84.

Bremner JD, Randall P, Vermetten E, et al. (1997) Magnetic resonance imaging based measurement of hippocampal volume in posttraumatic stress disorder related to childhood physical and sexual abuse: A preliminary report. Biol Psychiatr 41, 23–31.

Brody AL, Saxena S, Stoessel P, et al. (2001) Regional brain metabolism changes in patients with major depression treated with either paroxetine or interpersonal therapy. Arch Gen Psychiatr 58, 631–640.

Broverman I, Broverman D, Clarkson F, et al. (1970) Sex role stereotypes and clinical judgements of mental health. J Consult Clin Psychol 32, 1–7.

Burnand Y, Andreoli A, Kolatte E, et al. (2002) Psychodynamic psychotherapy and clomipramine in the treatment of major depression. Psychiatr Serv 53, 585–590.

Cavenar JO and Werman DS (1983) The sex of the psychotherapist. Am J Psychiatr 140, 85–87.

Comas-Diaz L and Jacobsen FM (1991) Ethnocultural transference and countertransference in the therapeutic dyad. Am J Orthopsychiatr 61, 392–402.

Comas-Diaz L and Jacobsen FM (2001) Ethnocultural allodynia. J Psychother Pract Res 10, 246–252.

Davanloo H (1978) Short-Term Dynamic Psychotherapy. Jason Aronson, New York.

Docherty JP (section ed) (1985) Therapeutic alliance and treatment outcome. In Psychiatry Update. American Psychiatric Association Annual Review, Vol. 4, Hales RE and Francis AJ (eds). American Psychiatric Press, Washington DC, pp. 525–633.

Doidge N, Simon B, Gillies LA, et al. (1994) Characteristics of psychoanalytic patients under a nationalized health plan: DSM-III-R diagnoses, previous treatment and childhood traumata. Am J Psychiatr 151, 586–590.

Eriksson PS, Perfilieva E, Bjork-Eriksson T, et al. (1998) Neurogenesis in the adult hippocampus. Nat Med 11, 1313–1317.

Eysenck HJ (1952) The effects of psychotherapy: An evaluation. Consult Psychol 16, 319–324.

Fawzy FI, Fawzy NW, Hyun CS, et al. (1993) Malignant melanoma. Effects of an early structured psychiatric intervention, coping, and affective state on recurrence and survival 6 years later. Arch Gen Psychiatr 50, 681–689.

Foulks EF, Bland IJ, and Shervington D (1995) Psychotherapy across cultures. In American Psychiatric Press Review of Psychiatry, Vol. 14,

Oldham JM and Riba MB (eds). American Psychiatric Press, Washington DC, pp. 511–528.

Frank E, Kupfer D, Perel JM, et al. (1990) Three-year outcomes for maintenance therapies in recurrent depression. Arch Gen Psychiatr 46, 1093–1099.

Frank JD and Frank JB (1991) Persuasion and Healing: A Comparative Study of Psychotherapy, 3rd ed. Johns Hopkins University Press, Baltimore.

Freud S (1961) Female sexuality. In The Standard Edition of the Complete Psychological Works of Sigmund Freud, Vol. 21, Strachey J (trans-ed). Hogarth Press, London, pp. 223–243. (Originally published in 1931)

Gabbard GO (1994) Psychodynamic Psychiatry in Clinical Practice, DSM-IV ed. American Psychiatric Press, Washington DC.

Gabbard GO (ed in chief) (1995) Treatments of Psychiatric Disorders, 2nd ed. American Psychiatric Press, Washington DC.

Gabbard GO (2000) A neurobiologically informed perspective on psychotherapy. Br J Psychiatr 177, 117–122.

Goodwin PJ, Leszcz M, Ennis M, et al. (2001) The effect of group psychosocial support on survival in metastatic breast cancer. NEJM 345, 1719–1726.

Greenson RR (1967) The Technique and Practice of Psychoanalysis. International Universities Press, New York.

Guntrip JS (1971) Psychoanalytic Theory, Therapy, and the Self. Basic Books, New York.

Hellerstein DJ, Pinsker H, Rosenthal RN, et al. (1994) Supportive Therapy as the Treatment Model of Choice. J Psychother Pract Res 3, 300–306.

Herman JL (1992) Trauma and Recovery. Basic Books, New York.

Horowitz MJ, Marmar C, Krupnick J, et al. (1984) Personality Styles and Brief Psychotherapy. Basic Books, New York.

Horowitz MJ, Milbrath C, and Stinson CH (1995) Signs of defensive control locate conflicted topics in discourse. Arch Gen Psychiatr 52, 1040–1047.

Howard KI, Kopta SM, Krause MS, et al. (1986) The dose-effect relationship in psychotherapy. Am Psychol 41, 159–164.

Husby R (1985) Short-term dynamic psychotherapy IV: Comparison or recorded changes in 33 neurotic patients 2 and 5 years after end of treatment. Psychother Psychosom 43, 23–27.

Jacobson E (1964) The Self and the Object World. International Universities Press, New York.

Joffe R, Segal Z, and Singer W (1996) Change in thyroid hormone levels following response to cognitive therapy for major depression. Am J Psychiatr 153, 411–413.

Kaplan A (1979) Toward an analysis of sex-role issues in the therapeutic relationship. Psychiatry 42, 112–120.

Karasu TB (ed) (1989) Treatment of Psychiatric Disorders. American Psychiatric Association, Washington DC.

Kaufman J, Plotsky P, Nemeroff C, et al. (2000) Effects of adverse experiences on brain structure and function: Clinical implications. Biol Psychiatr 48, 778–790.

Kendler KS, Kessler RC, Neale MC, et al. (1995) Stressful life events, genetic liability, and onset of major depression in women. Am J Psychiatr 152, 833–842.

Kernberg OF (1975) Borderline Conditions and Pathological Narcissism. Jason Aronson, New York.

Kirshner LA, Hauser ST, and Genack A (1978) Effects of gender on short-term therapy. Psychotherapy 15, 158–167.

Kohut H (1971) The Analysis of the Self. International Universities Press, New York.

Kohut H (1978) Introspection, empathy and psychoanalysis. In The Search for the Self, Ornstein P (ed). International Universities Press, New York, pp. 205–232.

Kopta SM, Howard KI, Lowery JL, et al. (1992) The psychotherapy dosage model and clinical significance: Estimating how much is enough for psychological symptoms. Paper presented at the Society for Psychotherapy (June), Berkley, CA.

Krupnick JL and Pincus HA (1992) The cost-effectiveness of psychotherapy: A plan for research. Am J Psychiatr 149, 1295–1305.

Lambert MJ, Shapiro DA, and Bergin AE (1986) The effectiveness of psychotherapy. In Handbook of Psychotherapy and Behavior Change, 3rd ed., Garfield SL and Bergin AE (eds). John Wiley, New York, pp. 157–211.

LeDoux J (1996) The Emotional Brain: The Mysterious Underpinnings of Emotional Life. Touchstone Books, New York.

Lehrer DS and Kay J (2002) The neurobiology of psychotherapy. In The Encyclopedia of Psychotherapy, Hersen M and Sledge W (eds). Academic Press, New York, pp. 207–221.

Liggan DY and Kay J (1999) Some neurobiological aspects of psychotherapy. J Psychother Pract Res 8, 103–114.

Luborsky L (1984) Principles of Psychoanalytic Psychotherapy: A Manual for Supportive–Expressive (SE) Treatment. Basic Books, New York.

Luborsky L, Diguer L, Luborsky E, et al. (1993) The efficacy of psychodynamic psychotherapy: Is it true that "everyone has won and all must have prizes"? In Psychodynamic Treatment Research: A Handbook for Clinical Practice, Miller NE, Luborsky L, Barber JP, et al. (eds). Basic Books, New York, pp. 447–514.

Luborsky L, Singer B, and Luborsky L (1975) Comparative studies of psychotherapies: Is it true that "everyone has won and all must have prizes"? Arch Gen Psychiatr 32, 995–1008.

Mahler MS, Pine F, and Bergman A (1975) The Psychological Birth of the Human Infant: Symbiosis and Individuation. Basic Books, New York.

Malan DH (1976) The Frontier of Brief Psychotherapy. Plenum Press, New York.

Mann J (1973) Time-Limited Psychotherapy. Harvard University Press, Cambridge, MA.

Marsella AJ (1989) Ethnocultural issues in the assessment of psychopathology. In Measuring Mental Illness: Psychometric Assessment for Clinicians, Wetler S (ed). American Psychiatric Press, Washington DC, pp. 231–256.

Martin SD, Martin E, Rai SS, et al. (2001) Brain blood flow changes in depressed patients treated with venlafaxine or interpersonal interpersonal psychotherapy. Arch Gen Psychiatr 58, 641–648.

McNeilly CL and Howard KI (1991) The effects of psychotherapy: A reevaluation based on dosage. Psychother Res 1, 74–78.

Meyer E, Derogatis LR, Miller MJ, et al. (1981) Addition of time-limited psychotherapy to medical treatment in a general medical clinic: Results at one-year follow-up. J Nerv Ment Dis 169, 780–790.

Mezzich JE, Kleinman A, Fabrega J, et al. (eds) (1993) Revised Cultural Proposals for DSM-IV (Technical Report). NIMH Cultural and Diagnosis Group, Pittsburgh, PA.

Milrod B, Busch F, Leon AC, et al. (2001) A pilot open trial of brief psychodynamic psychotherapy for panic disorder. J Psychother Pract Res 10, 239–245.

Misch DA (2000) Basic Strategies of Dynamic Supportive Psychotherapy. J Psychother Pract Res 9, 173–189.

Mogul KM (1982) Overview: The sex of the therapist. Am J Psychiatr 139, 1–11.

Mumford E, Schlesinger HJ, and Glass GV (1982) The effects of psychological intervention on recovery from surgery and heart attacks: An analysis of the literature. Am J Pub Health 72, 141–152.

Mumford E, Schlesinger HJ, Glass GV, et al. (1984) A new look at evidence about reduced cost of medical utilization following mental health treatment. Am J Psychiatr 141, 1145–1158.

Nadelson CC and Notman MT (1991) The impact of the new psychology of men and women on psychotherapy. In American Psychiatric Press Review of Psychiatry, Vol. 10, Tasman A and Goldfinger SM (eds). American Psychiatric Press, Washington DC, pp. 608–626.

Notman MT, Nadelson CC, and Bennett M (1978) Achievement conflict in women: Psychotherapeutic considerations. Psychother Psychosom 29, 203–213.

Novalis PN, Rojcewicz SJ, and Peele R (1993) Clinical Manual of Supportive Psychotherapy. American Psychiatric Press, Washington DC.

Olfson M and Pincus HA (1994) Outpatient psychotherapy in the United States, I: Volume, costs, and user characteristics. Am J Psychiatr 151, 1281–1288.

Orlinsky D and Howard K (1976) The effects of sex of therapist on the therapeutic experiences of women. Psychotherapy 13, 82–88.

Ornstein PH and Kay J (1990) Development of psychoanalytic self psychology: A historical-conceptual overview. In American Psychiatric Press Review of Psychiatry, Vol. 9, Tasman A, Goldfinger SM, and Kaufmann CA (eds). American Psychiatric Press, Washington DC, pp. 303–322.

Ornstein PH and Ornstein A (1985) Clinical understanding and explaining: The empathic vantage point. In Progress in Self Psychology, Vol. 1, Goldberg A (ed). Guilford Press, New York, pp. 43–61.

Pinsker H, Rosenthal R, and McCullough L (1992) Dynamic supportive psychotherapy. In Handbook of Short-term Dynamic Psychotherapy, Crits-Christoph P and Barber JP (eds). Basic Books, New York, pp. 220–247.

Reiss D, Hetherington EM, and Plomin R (1995) Genetics questions for environmental studies: Differential parenting and psychopathology in adolescence. Arch Gen Psychiatr 52, 925–936.

Richardson JL, Shelton DR, Krailo M, et al. (1990) The effect of compliance with treatment on survival among patients with hematologic malignancies. J Clin Oncol 8, 356–364.

Rockland LH (1989) Supportive Therapy: A Psychodynamic Approach. Basic Books, New York.

Rosenblum LA and Andrews MW (1994) Influences of environmental demand on maternal behavior and infant development. Acta Paediatr Suppl 397, 57–63.

Sacheim HA (2001) Functional brain circuits in major depression and remission. Arch Gen Psychiatr 58, 649–650.

Schlesinger HJ, Mumford E, Glass GV, et al. (1983) Mental health treatment and medical care utilization in a fee-for-service system: Outpatient mental health treatment following the onset of a chronic disease. Am J Pub Health 73, 423–429.

Schwartz J and Abromowitz S (1975) Value-related effects in psychiatric judgement. Arch Gen Psychiatr 32, 1525–1529.

Schwartz JM, Stoessal PW, Baxter LR, et al. (1996) Systematic changes in cerebral glucose metabolism rate after successful behavior modification treatment of obsessive–complusie disorder. Arch Gen Psychiatr 53, 109–113.

Shea T, Elkin I, Imber S, et al. (1992) Course of depressive symptoms over follow-up: Findings from the National Institute of Mental Health Treatment of Depression Collaborative Research Program. Arch Gen Psychiatr 49, 782–787.

Sifneos P (1979) Short-Term Dynamic Psychotherapy. Plenum Press, New York.

Smith ML, Glass GV, and Miller TI (1980) The Benefits of Psychotherapy. The Johns Hopkins University Press, Baltimore.

Spiegel D, Bloom JR, Kraemer HC, et al. (1989) Effect of psychosocial treatment on survival of patients with metastatic breast cancer. Lancet 2, 888–891.

Stiles WB (1992) Producers and consumers of psychotherapy research ideas. J Psychother Pract Res 1, 305–307.

Strupp HH (1986) The nonspecific hypothesis of therapeutic effectiveness: A current assessment. Am J Orthopsychiatr 56, 513–552.

Strupp HH and Binder JL (1984) Psychotherapy in a New Key: A Guide to Time-Limited Dynamic Psychotherapy. Basic Books, New York.

Sullivan HS (1953) The Interpersonal Theory of Psychiatry. WW Norton, New York.

Suomi S (1991) Early stress and adult emotional reactivity in rhesus monkeys. In Childhood Environmental and Adult Disease: Symposium No. 156, CIBA Foundation Symposium Staff (ed). John Wiley, Chichester, pp. 171–188.

Talley PF, Strupp HH, and Butler SF (eds) (1994) Psychotherapy Research and Practice: Bridging the Gap. Basic Books, New York.

Thase ME, Fasiczka AL, Berman SR, et al. (1998) Electroencephalographic sleep profiles before and after. Arch Gen Psychiatr 55, 138–144.

Thompson C (1939) Notes on the psychoanalytic significance of the choice of analyst. Psychiatr 1, 205–206.

Vaillant GE (1992) Ego Mechanisms of Defense: A Guide for Clinicians and Researchers. American Psychiatric Press, Washington DC.

Viinamaki J, Kuikka J, Tiilonen J, et al. (1998) Change in monamine transporter density relation to clinical recovery: A case-controlled study. Nordic J Psychiatr 52, 39–44.

Wallerstein RS (1986) Forty-two Lives in Treatment: A Study of Psychoanalysis and Psychotherapy. Guilford Press, New York.

Wallerstein RS (1995) Research in psychodynamic psychotherapy. In Psychodynamic Concepts in General Psychiatry, Schwartz HJ, Bleiberg E, and Weissman SH (eds). American Psychiatric Press, Washington DC, pp. 431–456.

Weiss J (1993) How Psychotherapy Works: Process and Technique. Guilford Press, New York.

Weiss J (1995) Clinical applications of control-mastery theory. Curr Opin Psychiatr 8, 154–156.

Werman DS (1984) The Practice of Supportive Psychotherapy. Brunner/Mazel, New York.

Wilborg IM and Dahl AA (1996) Does brief psychodynamic psychotherapy reduce the relapse rate of panic disorder? Arch Gen Psychiatr 53, 689–694.

Wong PS (1999) Anxiety, signal anxiety, and unconscious anticipation: Neuroscientific evidence for unconscious signal function in human. Am J Psychoanal 47, 817–841.

Woody GE, McLellan AT, Luborsky L, et al. (1995) Psychotherapy in community methadone programs: A validation study. Am J Psychiatr 152, 1302–1308.

Zetzel ER (1956) Current concepts of transference. Int J Psychoanal 37, 369–378.

Zlotnick C, Elkin I, and Shea T (1998) Does the gender of a patient or the gender of a therapist affect treatment of patients with major depression? J Consul Clin Psychol 66, 655–659.

Zlotnick C, Shea T, Pilkonis P, et al. (1996) Gender, type of treatment, dysfunctional attitudes, social support, life events, and depressive symptoms over naturalistic follow-up. Am J Psychiatr 153, 10–17.

# CHAPTER
# 84  Group Psychotherapy

Walter N. Stone

Human beings live in a social world in which their ability to gain self-esteem and self-definition significantly follows from their success in personal relationships. Psychotherapy in a group setting provides a social arena in which members can learn about their assets and deficits through interactions with peers (fellow members) and authority (the therapist). Members also have opportunities to experiment with newly learned behaviors in the protected atmosphere of the group in preparation for using them in their external world.

A broad spectrum of theoretical approaches informs therapists about which aspects of group behaviors they should attend to. Some focus on individuals as seen through the psychoanalytic lens of transference and resistance; others stress interpersonal transactions in which distortions arising from childhood are played out within the group and are subject to feedback, while others focus on properties of the group as a whole, which emphasize group dynamics and systems theories as the central organizing concepts. Learning principles are contained in almost all of these orientations and are the central emphases in cognitive–behavioral approaches. Successful integration of these approaches has not been accomplished. Therapists may maintain a central theoretical orientation and pragmatically adapt elements from other orientations to address particular problems as they emerge in the treatment process.

The concepts in this chapter primarily address working with adults in an outpatient setting in the psychodynamic tradition. Individuals' internal psychopathologies emerge in the microcosm of the group. They are expressed in interpersonal transactions, which are influenced by the dynamics of the therapeutic system.

## History
Joseph Pratt, an internist, is generally credited as the founder of modern group psychotherapy, treating tuberculosis patients in organized classes (Pratt 1969). Most early contributors to the group therapy field were schooled in psychoanalytic concepts which they modified for the group setting. Jacob Moreno emphasized action and spontaneity in founding a psychodramatic approach to treatment. S.R. Slavson, a self-taught psychotherapist, expanded his initial interest in children's groups to adults and was a central figure in the founding of the American Group Psychotherapy Association in 1942.

Group therapy received a stimulus during World War II when many therapists were initially exposed to group work during their military experience. Theoreticians in England (Bion, Bridger, Ezriel, Foulkes, Rickman, and Sutherland) and in the US (Horwitz, Glatzer, Lieberman, Scheidlinger, Schwartz, Whitaker, Wolf, and Yalom) applied psychoanalytic or interpersonal (Sullivan) concepts to a rapidly expanding interest in group treatment.

Interest in group processes, stimulated by the work of Kurt Lewin, led to the educational experiments in group dynamics at Bethel, Maine. The social upheavals of the 1960s resulted in a burgeoning of sensitivity training experiences (T-groups) and a variety of personal growth groups. The emergence of transactional analysis, gestalt therapy, bioenergetics, existential models for group therapy, and many additional innovative variations have enriched the group therapy field.

Activity groups for children began in 1930 and later developed into verbal groups for both children and adolescents. Groups for special populations have gained popularity and are used in schools to address issues such as parental divorce, substance abuse, and acquired immunodeficiency syndrome (AIDS) prevention. Short-term models are also widely applied to special adult issues, such as bereavement and a host of medical and social situations. Time-limited psychoeducational groups, with an emphasis on imparting information and sharing experiences, provide additional therapeutic opportunities.

The self-help movement, which traces its origins to the efforts of Alexander Low and Recovery Inc. in the 1930s, and the emergence of Alcoholics Anonymous and the 12-step model, which is also applied to other addictions, have increased the awareness of the therapeutic potential of collective interaction in the recovery and maintenance of individual emotional well-being.

The future will continue to see the use of a broad spectrum of group modalities and a variety of different models as the entire psychotherapeutic field endeavors to find a balance between efficiency and effectiveness. For an excellent review of 9 decades of group psychotherapy see Scheidlinger (1994).

## Group Development and Group Dynamics
The basic science informing group treatment is group development and dynamics. Understanding of these concepts provides a foundation for the therapist's integration of individual, interpersonal, and intrapsychic dynamics with those of group membership (Table 84–1).

| Table 84–1 | Stages of Group Development | |
| --- | --- | --- |
| Stage | Theme | Dynamics |
| Orientation (forming) | Engagement | Dependency<br>Safety<br>Norms |
| Differentiation (storming) | Power | Testing<br>Competition<br>Autonomy |
| Maturation (performing) | Work | Affect tolerance<br>Leadership<br>Self-reflection |
| Termination (departing) | Separation | Loss<br>Hope |

## Group Development

The seminal work of Bennis and Shepard (1956) produced a spate of studies demonstrating that groups have a natural developmental sequence. Groups must accomplish certain tasks as they move from a collection of individuals to a functioning and working organization. In this discussion, the focus is on developmental sequences in groups conducted along psychodynamic principles.

### Initial (Engagement, Orientation) Phase

Individuals entering a psychotherapy group are faced with two major tasks: they have to decide how they will use the treatment to accomplish their goals, and simultaneously they have to determine the limits of emotional safety. Members turn to the therapist in hope of gaining information on how to proceed. They anticipate that the leader, a person they already know and who fulfills a traditional role, will provide guidance and smooth the way in getting to know the strangers in the room. In the main, these "dependency" strivings are frustrated. Members tentatively reveal themselves to others. Gradually, unwritten and primarily unconscious rules (norms) develop, which help contain anxiety and set standards for acceptable behavior. Therapists help shape behavior by providing information on how to proceed and by clarifying (interpreting) underlying anxieties. Common themes and concerns may be highlighted, which serve to diminish members' sense of isolation and enhance cohesion.

### Reactive (Power, Differentiation) Phase

Many groups move into this phase by rebelliously rejecting their leader. This may be followed by a relatively short-lived sense of well-being and harmony. However, norms are often experienced as restrictive, and members may begin to feel as though they are controlled by the group (group tyranny). In response, they assert individuality and demonstrate their own power. Struggles between members emerge, and angry exchanges are not uncommon. Usual norms against expression of intense intragroup affects are tested and modified in accordance with members' personal capacities. Some members may threaten to quit, or they remain silent during this phase as they grapple with their ability to tolerate conflict. The therapist assists in helping members understand and tolerate responses to intense feelings and differences.

### Mature (Working) Phase

In this phase, groups have developed considerable cohesion. Members can tolerate differences, and they can contain anxiety and allow conflicts to emerge without having to interrupt exchanges. They have learned to provide and receive feedback from others without undue defensiveness. A considerable portion of the group transactions is focused on the here and now, and exchanges are appreciated as containing both, reactions to the present and vestiges from prior relationships (transferences). Members attempt to understand one another at both surface and in-depth levels. The therapist no longer is the sole expert, and members are valued for their emotional and cognitive uniqueness. Therapists continue to help patients understand their in-group reactions and assist in broadening their perspectives to include the sources (genetic) of their feelings and their manifestations in their outside world.

### Termination Phase

Ending treatment is the final stage. It is filled with mixed feelings: those of success and looking to the future and those surrounding separations (Schermer and Klein 1996). Often there is a regression as anxieties over departing are addressed. This provides an additional opportunity to explore the problems that emerge. Members respond with pleasure at seeing someone "graduate," but they also experience loss of a valued contributor to the work and envy over a colleague's achievement. A successful termination also offers hope for those who remain. The therapist monitors the dynamic forces and enables members to say their farewells within a context of therapeutic accomplishments and continuing psychological work. In the process, remaining members experience and integrate their responses to the departure.

### Summary

Groups do not uniformly traverse these developmental phases, and they undergo shifts to earlier stages under stress, such as vacations or change in membership. A considerable amount of therapeutic work takes place at each developmental level. For instance, a group of individuals experiencing problems with basic trust may spend a good deal of time in an initial stage, where these feelings may be explored. Patients who need to address competitive feelings may alternate between the reactive and the working phases. Understanding group development provides a framework for therapists to appreciate the forces that have an impact on members' feelings and behavior.

## Group Dynamics

Group dynamics refer to norms and cultures that are unique to each group. They are influenced by group size, members' race, gender, age, and the social environment. Group dynamics are also a product of members' personalities, the leader's functioning, and their subsequent interactions. The dynamics emerge as members go about their tasks of determining how they will achieve their goals and maintain personal safety. Norms are rules defining what is acceptable, that is, how people express themselves, what one can do or say. Illustrative of norms are the pressures of using "politically correct" (PC) expressions. There are sanctions, both conscious and unconscious, against violating norms. In part, norms are initially defined in the therapeutic agreement (discussed later) as presented by the therapist, but they are modified as a result of group development.

The concept of role is intimately linked with group therapy. Roles are essential functions that help the group achieve its goals and support members' emotional tasks. Four general roles can be defined for groups (MacKenzie 1997): structural, sociable, divergent, and cautionary roles. The structural or leadership role helps the group address its work. The therapist is the primary occupant of this role, but members also function in keeping the group on task, organizing the experience and maintaining a perspective of the group process. The social or emotional role helps contain feelings and assists in managing social relationships among the members and with the leader. Some individuals relieve group tensions by changing the topic, making a joke, smoothing ruffled feelings, or by encouraging others to express their less acceptable and/or painful feelings. The divergent role is filled by persons who seem oppositional, who "don't go along with the crowd," or seem to fight authority. They are likely to become a container for unacceptable thoughts or emotions. Such individuals are vulnerable to becoming scapegoated, a process in which inadmissible feelings are seen (or placed) in one person and thereby kept out of awareness in the others. The cautionary or silent role may be played by a member who seldom speaks or keeps his thoughts and feelings hidden. These persons often are a threat to the others because they keep secrets or avoid painful affects. When a group is ready to take action, members often attempt to "recruit" the silent person into their ranks; this process is most frequently seen when there is preparation for fight-or-flight (see discussion of Bion below). Roles may be filled by one or several persons. They are essential for group functioning, and, theoretically, each member has the psychological potential to fill varying roles.

## Theories of Group Therapy

The theoretical spectrum informing the practice of group therapy is broad. Within psychodynamics, some emphasize drive theory, object relations, or self psychology. Other therapists favor interpersonal theory and cognitive–behavioral approaches. Transactional analysis, originating from the work of Berne (1966), and Gestalt therapy (Perls et al. 1951) emphasize interpersonal transactions arising from more traditional psychodynamic theory.

Group theoreticians are generally categorized along a continuum of group as a whole, interpersonal, and intrapsychic. Moreover, therapists using object relations, self psychology, or psychodynamic theories integrate their theoretical preferences along this continuum (Kibel 1992, Harwood and Pines 1998, Rutan and Stone 2001). There are few purists, and varying degrees of integration is the norm (Table 84–2).

A common thread in many of these theories is that individuals in their interaction and discourse within the group will exhibit their difficulties in relationships, which in turn provides a window into their internal world. In short, the group becomes a microcosm of their external world (Slater 1966).

## Group-as-a-Whole Approaches

These theories emphasize whole-group processes as the primary therapeutic vehicle. They subscribe to notions that

| Table 84–2 | Group Theories | |
|---|---|---|
| Theory | Authors | Key Phrases |
| Group-as-a-whole | Bion | Basic assumption, Work group |
| | Whitaker and Lieberman | Group focal conflict |
| | Ezriel | Required, Avoided, Calamitous relationship |
| | Foulkes | Group analysis, Group matrix, Figure/ground |
| | Horwitz | Integrative, Inductive |
| Interpersonal | Yalom | Cohesion, Therapeutic factors, Feedback |
| | Gustafson and Cooper | Unconscious planning |
| Intrapsychic | Slavson | Limited regression, Transference |
| | Wolff and Schwartz | Standard analytic, Alternate sessions |
| | Durkin | Group-as-preoedipal mother, Transference neurosis |
| | Glatzer | |
| General system | Durkin | Exchange across boundaries |
| | Agazarian | Subgrouping |
| | Ettin | Social and cultural values and attitudes |
| | Hopper | Social unconscious |

members are influenced by the group dynamics and that one or more persons may speak for the entire group, including those who are silent.

Bion (1960), working within a Kleinian object relations model, conceptualized groups as having two levels: work and basic assumptions. Work groups operate on a reality principle and are goal directed. Basic assumptions groups function *as if* the group were meeting to satisfy members' emotional needs. Bion identified three basic assumptions that suffuse the work group: dependency, fight-or-flight, and pairing. Therapists working in this model focus on members' relationship to the leader, particularly as expressed through basic assumptions.

Tripartite conflict models, in which an impulse, a wish, or an object need was met with a counterreaction or a fear leading to a compromise, were applied to group therapy by Whitaker and Lieberman (1964) (group focal conflict with the three elements: the disturbing motive, reactive motive, and solution) and Ezriel (1973) (psychoanalytic group therapy with the three elements: required, calamitous, and avoided relationships). Foulkes (1961) formulated group analysis, in which communication and relations among members formed a group matrix. The conductor's (therapist's) attention shifts between group and individual, with one representing the figure and the other the ground in the gestalt of the group interaction.

Horwitz (1977) proposed that individuals' contributions to the central theme be addressed before making group-as-a-whole interventions. This inductive approach attends to individuals' needs for attention and strengthens the therapeutic alliance before intervening at a whole-group level, which links members and strengthens cohesion.

## Interpersonal Approaches

On the basis of Sullivanian principles, Yalom (1995) emphasized the centrality of transactions in the here and now of the group as the primary, but not exclusive, therapeutic force for change. His formulation of "therapeutic factors" brought into sharp focus the importance of cohesion (which is a dynamic concept that implies that the group is attractive, "safe," and that members have a commitment to the group goals and ideals). Yalom pays particular attention to members' capacity to give and receive feedback. He asserts that maladaptive interpersonal transactions are the consequence of parataxic distortions (having some similarity to transference responses, i.e., arising from childhood experiences) that can be therapeutically altered by authentic human interaction, that is, feedback and consensual validation.

The contributions of Gustafson and Cooper (1979), based on the work of Weiss and Sampson subsequently published as a monograph (1986), posited that individuals enter groups with unconscious and conscious plans to determine if they will be traumatized in the group as they had been in the (developmental) past. They present "tests" to determine if they will be attacked or to learn new ways of problem solving.

## Intrapsychic Approaches

Intrapsychic theories are primarily application of dyadic theory into the group setting. The emphasis is on unconscious processes with the group providing opportunities for patients to regress to a level of internal conflict or developmental arrest. These theories explore individual transferences, resistances, and developmental arrests as the primary therapeutic focus. Peers may be experienced as siblings or as displacement objects from parental figures (Slavson 1950, Wolf and Schwartz 1962). Groups may either dilute or intensify transferences to the leader (Horwitz 1994), which enables "stuck" patients to resolve impasses occurring in dyadic treatment. Regression is limited, and the presence of others creates a balance between the external and the internal worlds (Durkin 1964). Integration of an intrapsychic framework with that of the group as a whole is contained in descriptions of members' transferences to the group as a preoedipal maternal experience (Glatzer 1953, Scheidlinger 1974).

## General Systems Approaches

General systems theory is based on open systems theory (von Bertalanffy 1966). Emphasis is placed on the boundaries separating the group from the external world and members or subgroups from one another (Durkin 1981). Emphasis on boundaries as worthy of therapeutic concern is evident in the group agreement. Agazarian (1997) elaborated systems concepts into a model of group treatment that focused on subgroups as the primary site of therapeutic attention. She asserted that by focusing on subgroups, which contain individual differences and similarities, members are more prepared to address intrapsychic defenses and resistances.

Greater attention has been paid to participants' cultural background and the impact of such forces on conscious and unconscious values and attitudes (Ettin 1994). Similarly, events in the culture and "politically correct attitudes" may constrain or stimulate members and are transported into the consultation room often outside of awareness as a social unconscious (Hopper 1996).

## Therapeutic Factors

As in all dynamic therapies, specific and nonspecific elements contribute to therapeutic change. Nonspecific factors are embedded in the relationships that are established through a consistent, accepting, nonjudgmental, and supportive environment. Groups provide a corrective emotional experience in which patients experience others responding to them differently than those in their past. Members share their stories (catharsis) and feel less isolated when others have shared similar stories (universalization); they have opportunities to be helpful to others through both cognitive understanding and emotional linking (imparting information, providing feedback, and altruism). They also see others improve, which conveys hope. These elements contribute to the sense of collaboration and a willingness to adopt norms (i.e., discuss feelings about the interactions in the meeting) that further members' sense of efficacy and belonging. Taken together, these nonspecific elements add to group cohesion, which has been likened to the therapeutic alliance in dyadic treatment. They contribute to an experience of support and acceptance, which may be sufficient therapeutic gain for a number of patients.

Additional nonspecific elements that contribute to change are opportunities for imitative learning. Patients observe and imitate others' successful interactions. Members may model and practice new ways of interacting in the protected setting of the group and thereby disaffirm prior beliefs that their behaviors will elicit noxious responses.

Each theoretical school emphasizes its own specific contributions to therapeutic change. Yalom (1995), in the interpersonal tradition, places giving and receiving feedback about behaviors in the here and now as central therapeutic factors. Other psychodynamic theorists emphasized resolution of transferences, resistances, or unblocking developmental arrests. The group is conceptualized as re-creating the family of origin where enactments of previous experiences with parents or siblings will emerge. Those transferences will be subject to modification through interpretations. The group is often conceived of as a microcosm (Slater 1966) in which members emotionally display their unresolved conflicts or developmental needs. These then become available for modification through the relational experiences and interpretation.

Within the psychodynamic tradition, change mechanisms of confrontation, clarification, and interpretation promote imitation and identification optimally leading to internalization and change in psychic organization (Rutan and Stone 2001). Members and therapist contribute to these processes, albeit in an unequal manner. Indeed, an asset of group treatment is that participants learn to appreciate less than conscious motivations in themselves and in others and develop a capacity to empathize with others in the immediacy of the group setting. Moreover, they can experiment with novel ways of behaving. Individuals successfully completing group treatment cite the help of member-to-member interactions; those who fail are more likely to focus on therapists' shortcomings (Dies 1983).

## Beginning a Group

### Group Organization

Forming a psychotherapy group is a complex task, and attention to organizational details will anticipate some of the potential hazards and smooth the path. Composition, size, fees, place, duration, and time of meetings are elements that require decisions in advance of recruiting and preparing potential members.

The size of dynamically-oriented groups ranges from 6 to 10 members. Groups at the upper size range generally meet for lengthier periods to provide sufficient "airtime" for each person. Smaller groups (four members or less) may be threatened by fears of dissolution (Fulkerson et al. 1981). The duration of meetings is set for 75 to 120 minutes, the norm being 90 minutes. Most groups meet once weekly. Attention must be paid to the group space. An optimal room will comfortably seat 8 to 10 persons with unobstructed views of one another. Seats do not have to be identical. Both the position and the type of seat members choose may assume considerable emotional significance. Access to the room needs consideration. Is there time for members to gather in the group room before the meeting, or is a waiting room necessary? In private settings, meetings are occasionally held in a waiting room, and therapists must ensure that others do not intrude on that space.

The therapist should make advance decisions for the meeting time. Most outpatient adult groups meet in the evening, when there are greater opportunities to gather sufficient members. It is best to remain firm and not attempt to adjust time or day if one or two likely prospects are unable to make a particular schedule. The time can then be used to interview candidates. This procedure clarifies one essential selection criterion—can the patient attend at the established time?

Most therapists prefer to establish a uniform group fee. The charges are generally in the range that is manageable for most persons. There are obvious limitations to such a policy, as managed care often stipulates charges, and "balance billing" is not permissible. Policies about charges for missed appointments should be decided in advance. Whatever the ultimate arrangements, as set in the agreement (discussed later), therapists have the task of helping patients be responsible for their fees. In clinic settings, this may mean cooperating with administrative procedures. Groups that openly address fees, in either private or clinic settings, are rated by their therapists as more cohesive than those that avoid such discussions (Englander 1989).

Careful thought must be given to optimal group composition (Table 84–3).

Patients chosen for groups that will explore intrapsychic elements should have a capacity for self-reflection and empathy with others. If possible, members with different personality styles should be selected to provide a spectrum of interactive patterns. Other long-term groups may

| Table 84–3 | Selection of Patients | |
| --- | --- | --- |
| Type of Group | Positive Attributes | Negative Attributes |
| Dynamic | Ego strength | Crisis situation |
| | Motivation for change | Active substance abuse-related disorder |
| | Capacity for insight | Sociopathy |
| | History of satisfying relationship | Cognitive disorder or mental retardation |
| Supportive | Diminished ego strength | Acute psychosis |
| | Limited reflective capacity | Disabling cognitive disorders |
| | Motivation for support | Substance abuse |
| | Most relationships problematical | |
| Specialized focus | Common characteristic | Psychosis |
| | Focus on single problem | Motivation for personality change |

be established with supportive goals and include patients with significant ego deficits. (Groups for the chronically mentally ill are discussed separately later.) Groups designed with a specialized format (e.g., women survivors of sexual abuse, male perpetrators, or individuals with eating disorders) generally are more focused on a symptom or a specific behavior and in such cases balanced membership is of lesser importance.

Using gender as an illustration, groups can be started with unequal numbers of men or women, but open places should be used to equalize membership. A single man or woman tends to become stereotyped, and, if possible, at least two members of each sex should be included to reduce initial feelings of isolation and to promote identifications. Age ranges might be limited in groups composed of late teenagers, young adults, or elderly persons; however, in groups whose members have attained their late twenties, the range may be quite broad. Each individual is distinct and represents a singleton. The task is not to exclude differences but to create a group where the differences are not so great that an emotional link cannot be achieved.

### Recruiting, Selecting, and Preparing Patients

Few applicants requesting psychotherapy consider group treatment. Thus, gathering 6 to 10 individuals together may not be a simple task. The optimal place to recruit patients is from the therapist's own individual practice. These are individuals who have a relationship with the therapist and are in an optimal position to collaborate in a decision to join a group. Colleagues also become helpful referral sources, but in many instances they may be unfamiliar with indications for group therapy. The therapist will then need to provide them with the necessary information. In clinic settings, special attention should be paid to persons responsible for screening of new admissions. They are in a critical position to recommend group therapy when it is appropriate.

Patients are more likely to agree to enter a group if the rationale is explained to them in some detail. Thus, the therapist needs to be clear about the relationship between group goals and patient goals (to be discussed below). The therapist also needs to be familiar with the patient's history, coping style, symptoms, and personality configurations. In obtaining a patient's developmental history, the therapist can specifically search for the person's interaction in group settings, such as school, church, recreation, and family. Discussion of the person's typical reactions to group situations helps engage the patient in examining his or her roles in interpersonal situations. The screening and preparatory interviews have five major tasks (Rutan and Stone 2001):

1. Establish a preliminary alliance between patient and therapist.
2. Define the patients' therapeutic goals.
3. Provide information about the nature of group treatment.
4. Explore the patients' anticipatory anxiety.
5. Discuss the group agreement and gain the patient's acceptance.

Sufficient time should be allowed to accomplish these tasks. In most instances, several individual interviews are necessary. During the interview process, patients engage with the therapist who serves as an important anchor as they enter into the anxiety-laden experience of revealing themselves to strangers. It is not unusual for some persons, after an initial meeting, to decide not to enter a group. Inevitably some individuals drop out shortly after they join, which interferes with group formation. Careful screening helps patients anticipate the tasks of entering a group. Such preparation will decrease, but not eliminate premature termination which may range from 20 to 50% of members in newly formed groups.

In traditional psychodynamic group treatment the clinician begins with a goal of establishing a group in which there is free-flowing interaction and discussion that will provide an arena in which members may experience and learn about problematic aspects of themselves and their relationships with others. For the individual, treatment goals may be formulated in both interpersonal and intrapsychic terms, which can then be explained within the broader group goals. It may be worthwhile to indicate that for many persons the group, alone, may be optimal treatment; others may benefit from combined individual and group treatment (these formats will be discussed below).

An example of setting goals might be a patient who wishes to address his difficulty in sustaining closeness. This person may establish a goal of intensely examining his feeling states in the context of differing interactions in order to determine which interactions stimulate or diminish wishes for intimacy. Previously unrecognized issues often emerge during treatment leading to new goals. The person may choose to remain in the group in order to explore the previously unrecognized issues.

Prospective members often have questions about the group format. They should be informed about the physical arrangements (place, time, day), that groups are characteristically composed of strangers, both men and women will be present, and that one of their initial goals will be in learning about themselves in the process of meeting strangers. This structuring helps assuage some anxiety by defining an initial task.

Individuals vary in their capacity to attend to their fears about entering a group. Therapists should be alert to indicators of anxiety and work to bring such feelings to the surface. Role-playing or showing a videotape of a group has been used to impart information or address pretreatment anxieties, but most concerns can be uncovered by careful exploration of a patient's prior experiences in entering novel group situations. Inquiry into a patient's recent dreams, either in anticipation of preparatory sessions or between screening interviews, will expose less conscious aspects of their anxieties. After these explorations, some individuals choose to delay entry and work on understanding their feelings more thoroughly before joining.

Therapists often are discouraged or frustrated by the difficulties they encounter in gathering sufficient members to begin treatment. Consultation may be useful in providing support and may expose countertransference responses to some prospects or uncover resistance to assuming the leadership tasks. An illustration of a countertransference might be of an applicant who was rejected for group treatment because the therapist experienced the person as similar to an important and noxious figure from his past—that is, mother, father, or difficult supervisor.

## The Group Agreement

The agreement represents the framework in which treatment will proceed. It promotes a structure that defines boundaries between the group and the environment, among the members and with the therapist. Although members accept the agreement, they also break it. Such disruptions are valuable windows into understanding a person's inner world. The therapist must distinguish between acts that are disruptive to the group and those that carry more benign communications (Nitsun 1996).

Rutan and Stone (2001) list the elements of the agreement as shown in Table 84–4.

The initial element in the agreement addresses patients' ability to attend all sessions. Those who have responsibilities that interfere with attendance should not be admitted into the group (e.g., executives whose conflicts make them unavailable once every third or fourth week). Similarly, persons who have time conflicts and would consistently

| Table 84–4 | The Group Agreement |
| --- | --- |

Attend all meetings, be on time, and remain throughout the session

Actively work toward treatment goals, remain until they have been achieved, and discuss plans to stop treatment

Observe one's inner reactions to interactions in the group and comment on them

Use the group for therapeutic and not social purposes

Put feelings into words and not action

Be responsible for fees

Understand the therapist's role

Protect the confidentiality of the meetings and the anonymity of members

come late or leave early should delay entry until their schedule can be adapted to that of the group.

In establishing goals, the patient and therapist enter into a conscious agreement to work toward specified change. However, unconscious elements contributing to a patient's behaviors are likely to emerge in the therapeutic process that may point to additional goals worthy of pursuit. Instructions regarding termination are an additional part of this agreement element. Patients generally have little idea how to stop treatment, and leaders can indicate that sufficient time to take leave of the group is an important part of the therapy. Plans to leave should be discussed and then a date for departure established that allows sufficient time to say goodbye.

The succeeding three elements in the agreement address patient behaviors within the group. Patients slowly learn that one of the major benefits of therapy follows from addressing feelings and reactions to one another and to the therapist. Consistent attainment of this goal suggests that the group is functioning at a mature level. Physical contact and verbal abuse are prohibited. Patients unable to contain these behaviors may be asked to leave the session temporarily. Although physical touching or hugging may seem soothing and reassuring to some individuals, for others it is a threat to their personal boundaries. Those behaviors are open to analysis.

Members will have contact with one another outside the sessions. Contact may be limited to brief encounters immediately before or after the meeting, or it may include plans to eat together after a session. On occasion, patients develop social relationships with one another. The therapeutic aim is to create an environment in which these contacts can be discussed and their meaning addressed. Rarely do these extra-group meetings lead to sexual liaisons, which may be destructive to treatment. With patients understanding that continuing such liaisons will interfere with their remaining in the group, most will discontinue their sexual relationships. The greatest danger to the group exists in silence surrounding outside contacts.

Patients and therapists alike have difficulty in processing paperwork in the era of managed care. Members may be asked to file insurance forms and to be responsible for their fees and copayments. If payments are not made within the agreed time frame, the failure should be openly raised within the group. The leader must overcome a natural resistance to discussing money in a "public" forum. Yet money often assumes major importance in patients' lives, with linkages to self-esteem, shame, competition, and power. The therapist "swims upstream" when she or he introduces problems with fees in the group but failure to do so excludes important aspects of patients' inner experiences.

Therapists even the playing field by including a description of their own role to this basic agreement. They may indicate that they will try to help members understand themselves and others. Instructions regarding their own absences, or how members should notify the group when they will be absent, are additional elements that are often added to the agreement.

The element of confidentiality is left to last in presenting the agreement to emphasize its importance. No guarantee can be made about member confidentiality, but stressing the significance of maintaining others' anonymity if material from the group is discussed is easily understood and does not interfere with members' freedom to process their treatment experience with persons outside the group.

Considerable ambiguities exist within the agreement that enable a group to develop its own interpretations and norms. The underlying principle, however, is to create a structure within which the therapeutic work can proceed. The agreement is presented to prospective members before joining and should be repeated at the time of the initial group session when new members are added, and subsequently woven through the treatment process.

## Therapist's Role

The group leader assumes a major, but not the sole, responsibility for the treatment. The therapist's special role is established in part by the agreement. Within that framework, clinicians begin to shape the group to provide participants a way of using their experience to learn about themselves. Assuming that patients' optimal learning begins with a focus on transactions within the group, psychodynamically-oriented therapists try to find ways of helping members examine resistances and defenses against such engagement. In contrast, clinicians using a more strictly interpersonal (Yalom 1995) or a system-centered orientation (Agazarian 1997) may actively instruct members to address one another directly in the here and now of the meeting. The goals of the different approaches are similar—to use the intragroup processes to promote personal change. Therapists with an intersubjective view examine their own contributions to the construction of the group dialogue (Harwood 1998).

The therapist's focus, however, is not exclusively on in-group processes. Rutan and Stone (2001) list six foci for the therapist's attention (Table 84–5):

The major but not exclusive focus promoting change is members learning from the here and now of treatment. Groups develop a rhythm in which members might address outside events as a warm-up to exploring in-group interactions, or they might focus on current feelings and then expand on those experiences in respect to their outside lives, now, in the past, or in the future. Integration of a person's experiences across an extended period enhances feelings of continuity and stability of the self.

In a similar fashion, to-and-fro movement takes place in the therapist's focus from group as a whole to interpersonal to individual. Whole-group processes seldom completely disappear. Clinicians may choose to address an individual, subgroup, or the entire group, recognizing that whatever intervention is made, all levels will be affected. Group-as-a-whole or subgroup interventions may be helpful in linking individuals but are never completely accurate for each person. They tend to address earlier developmental levels than do more interpersonal or intrapsychic interventions

| Table 84–5 | Therapist's Focus |
|---|---|
| Past ——————(here and now)——————future |
| In group ——————————out of group |
| Group as a whole——(subgroup)—(interpersonal)——individual |
| Affect ——————————cognition |
| Process ——————————content |
| Understanding——————corrective emotional experience |

(Kernberg 1975). Horwitz (1977), addressing the failure to establish a therapeutic alliance with singular attention to whole group processes, proposed that a group theme be identified and elaboration of individual experiences be undertaken before making a whole-group interpretation.

The therapist monitors the ebb and flow of affects which reflect the group developmental stage. Members' capacity to tolerate intense feelings is enhanced as trust and cohesion increase. The dialectical tension between affect and cognition is seen in members' roles as they attempt to contain dysphoric states and sustain emotional contacts with one another. Patients may find ways of managing intense feelings through scapegoating or externalizing. These are group-wide processes and should be addressed as such. Some individuals require cognitive understanding before risking immersion into feelings, whereas others search for affective connections before integrating their experience cognitively.

The therapeutic process is fueled by members' searching for new solutions to their developmental arrests and conflicts. In general, members communicate feelings about their in-group experience through associations (not always conscious) to events in their outside world. As such, the associations can be understood as metaphoric communication that informs the treatment process. After a successful interpretation or clarification, associations to external or historical events may represent integration of those experiences into members' psychic structure.

Considerable individual change takes place via the group relationship without overt cognitive integration. The sense of sharing, of being understood, of having needs met, of being responded to in an empathic (corrective) manner may stabilize a shaky psychic structure, and, some patients, to their therapist's surprise, may successfully terminate treatment without having achieved understanding (Stone 1985). These are the powerful forces for change, labeled "corrective emotional" experiences. Patients also strive for cognitive integration of their thoughts and feelings, and, through experiencing and then understanding the here-and-now, external, and developmental incidents, they consolidate their learning. Patients are then more prepared to transfer their learning from therapy to situations in their outside world (Ezriel 1973).

## Initiating Treatment

Beginning a group is suffused with anxiety for all involved. Even the therapist is not immune to apprehensive feelings, such as "Will anyone come? Will the members get along? Will they learn to work together? Will affects get out of control?" Patients are subject to similar feelings, and they face the dual tasks of figuring out how to meet strangers and how to use the group to achieve their therapeutic goals.

The therapist provides the initial structure, which can be accomplished by reviewing the agreement and asking individuals to introduce themselves. A simple statement that members can continue in any way they wish usually suffices to continue the process. On occasion, patients will question the therapist about aspects of the treatment. Whether the therapist chooses to answer some questions directly or to explore anxieties underlying questions is a matter of style. However, extended silence is often counterproductive, particularly in initial meetings.

**Clinical Vignette 1**

In the opening minutes of a new group's first session, a member asked the therapist how he would like to be addressed—as "doctor" or by his first name? He did not reply. Subsequent associations included several references to rudeness, followed by emergence of angry and destructive themes, quite uncharacteristic of a new group. The members appeared to have reacted to the therapist's nonresponse as a narcissistic injury that led to displaced rage.

As patients orient themselves to the relatively unstructured situation, they utilize coping mechanisms, which may have been derived from childhood (regressive solutions). They search for answers from the therapist as an authority and a person with whom they have had prior contact (dependency themes), or they cautiously test to determine what they can reveal about themselves to strangers (safety themes). Stories may be told about other novel experiences or of travels which symbolically represent the therapeutic journey. Personal roles will emerge that fulfill collective needs.

The following is a fictive illustration of a group opening: After the therapist's introduction, a member may tell about the history of his or her "illness," which may be a harbinger of an emotional leader role. A second person may respond by telling about a recently encountered dangerous situation, a potential cautionary role. A third person may inquire how this discussion fits with what the members are trying to do, a potential task role. Finally, someone may protest that this is a waste of time, a divergent, potential scapegoat role. Although each person may be speaking as an individual, each comment most likely represents internal aspects of each member that is expressed through another's voice.

In the opening phase, people attempt to orient themselves and determine what can be discussed safely. They are often uncertain about what they have to offer others, and commonly share a (false) belief that only the leader has the skills to be helpful. Providing suggestions or antidotes to others' problems is typical early behavior. This almost invariably fails, and making suggestions may be understood as members' efforts to be helpful or as a demonstration of their own ineffectiveness, which contains a covert plea for the therapist to help them. Another common early process, by no means consciously planned, is for individuals to take turns in telling their story as a way of structuring the treatment and avoiding competitive conflicts. Sometimes a single individual's problems become the primary group focus, suggesting that others may not feel safe in exposing their own difficulties until they determine the fate of the person who has been the center of attention.

Therapists help members make linkages so that no individual feels isolated. They draw themes from associations that help members appreciate commonalities despite external differences. Processes of universalization, linking, acceptance, altruism, and feeling that one can be helpful to another (i.e., by observing a behavior or identifying a feeling) are emphasized. A beginning effort is made to focus members' attention on their in-group experiences. However, premature exploration of anger or rage can disrupt a sense of safety and cohesion in early formative phases. These feelings, which may emerge among members, are often displaced reactions to disappointments with the clinician and may be redirected to their primary source. For example, a member who arrives late may be the recipient of anger in his or her own right, but covert anger may be present regarding the therapist's inability to control behavior and maintain a level of internal comfort.

In early sessions the group may seem unstable. Some members may become dissatisfied and terminate treatment, sometimes without notice. Early terminations vary from 20 to 50% of the membership, and therapists must examine the impact of these events on the remaining group, as well as find replacements (Roback and Smith 1987, Stone and Rutan, 1984). Too many dropouts lead to demoralization among the members, a feeling that requires immediate attention.

Despite the stress, the majority of members derive benefit from this treatment phase by sharing problems, and experiencing diminished isolation and shame about psychological problems. Not surprisingly, many individuals report feeling better and, as a consequence of their membership, they may experience a disappearance of somatic or emotional symptoms (Tschuschke and Anbeh 2000).

## Treatment Course

Members' level of self and ego development influence the course of the group as a therapeutic agent. Persons suffering from archaic conflicts of trust or psychic safety, as expressed in a variety of personality disorders (the difficult patient), may require an extended period of therapy exploring these issues. Transferences to the group, leader, or peers emerge that reflect these developmental levels. For instance, the group may be experienced in an archaic maternal image as warm and protective or hostile and destructive (Scheidlinger 1974). The therapist may be cast in a similar light or splits may occur in which the therapist is experienced as the bad parent and the group as the good parent (Kauff 1991). Interactions may be conceptualized in the paradigm of self psychology, with the therapist experienced as an idealized self-object (Stone 1992). Patients with these limited goals may not be readily identified in preparatory interviews.

For some individuals, achieving a treatment alliance in which others are experienced as separate and unique may be a sufficient treatment goal (Masterson 1978). Stabilizing the self, as a result of feeling understood or accepted, may be sufficient for some patients, who may terminate treatment, often to the surprise of the therapist (Ornstein and Ornstein 1977).

For those desiring greater self-understanding, treatment continues as power struggles take place. Patients learn to address their in-group transactions and are able to sustain examination of those relationships despite anxiety. Use of tension-deflecting mechanisms diminishes (e.g., scapegoating, invoking humor, or externalizing), and, if they occur, a member may take the lead in redirecting the conversation. Members develop a useful memory of the group history and can make linkages between current interactions and those in past meetings as part of the working-through process. They remember details that the therapist may have forgotten and in the process reinforce their own

sense of self by becoming more empathic with each other, more independent from the leader, and contributing to group work. Triangular themes emerge, and patients examine competitive strivings and their envy, jealousy, guilt, and shame (Gibbard and Hartman 1973, Alonso and Rutan 1988).

Termination is an emotionally important treatment phase. The therapist may be aware of patients' change and begin to wonder about ending treatment before a member will directly address leaving. Until a person successfully terminates treatment, groups do not reach their full potential. There is generally resistance to fully facing the feelings associated with saying goodbye. Some individuals abruptly announce that they are leaving in the following one or two sessions. Even though the therapist may be in agreement that termination is appropriate, for a person who has been a member for a significant period, this is too brief a time frame. Some therapists build into their initial agreement a clause that asks a member to remain for a specified number of sessions after her or his decision to leave. Optimally, members will discuss their thoughts about terminating over the course of a number of sessions and make a final decision. Then a future date should be set.

Not infrequently, deciding on the date is followed by a denial of the termination, and all members respond as if such a significant decision had not been reached. However, often earlier patterns of interacting emerge (regression) that enable the departing person to gain additional self-knowledge (Kauff 1977). Other members also become embroiled in feelings of saying goodbye, and they often tend to become critical or search for defects in the departing member that would contraindicate termination. Feelings of envy about the departure or shame that they have not achieved similar success fuel these affects. Under these circumstances, the therapist must carefully assess the situation and as a result may need to "protect" the person's decision to leave. Affect contagion may spread to the leader and interfere with judgment during this emotion-packed period. Moreover, therapists may experience countertransferences in the face of losing a member who may have served as a significant process facilitator. In most instances, the patient's final session is filled with considerable sadness as well as pleasure at the departure.

## Special Treatment Considerations

### Dreams

Patients may have dreams that they present to the group. Some dreams include members, whereas others may be of collective situations in which emotionally important aspects of group transactions regarding individuals or the therapist are prominent. These latter dreams may be presented initially without the dreamer's awareness that a connection exists to the group experience. The therapist's posture in relation to dreams has an impact on the members. When presenting the agreement, many therapists comment that if a person has dreams, they may be related to experiences in the group, and it would be useful to discuss them. If the therapist helps the presenter and others examine dreams, and in the process previously unexpressed emotions within the group are exposed, members will find it valuable to report their dreams.

The dreamer should be provided an initial opportunity to examine the dream. The therapist may inquire if others have responses and, after their associations are made, may ask about feelings or unexplored dream elements. An important clue to the meaning of the dream may be in the interactions that immediately precede the dreamer's report or in the associations following inquiry of the dreamer and other members. Complete analysis of dreams is infrequent. Dream work may help surface many unexpressed conscious feelings, expose unconscious conflicts, and facilitate more direct interaction.

---

**Clinical Vignette 2**

In a session in which members had been discussing feelings of attraction to one another and consequent jealousies, Ms. K reported the following dream: Ms. L (a member) was in the corner of the room watching some little children. The therapist was having a heart attack, and she (Ms. K) ran out into the hall trying to find someone to help.

Ms. K said that she had been angry with the therapist, and that is why she dreamed about his having a heart attack. A member wondered what kind of help Ms. K was seeking in the dream, leading to a discussion of cardiac resuscitation, which became elaborated into ideas of mouth-to-mouth resuscitation, and then exposed sexual feelings. Ms. L's position in the dream, her interest in playing with the children, isolated her from the competition. Prior and present competitive and romantic feelings among the members and toward the therapist emerged and were more sharply focused in the ensuing discussion. The concrete expression "heart attack" had a clear double meaning of both wishing ill on the therapist for not reciprocating Ms. K's romantic feelings and simultaneously exposing those feelings more directly.

---

## Scapegoating

Group psychotherapy has been called a hall of mirrors (Foulkes 1961) where aspects of oneself are seen reflected in others. Scapegoating is the process in which individuals, by "observing" characteristics in another that are unacceptable in themselves, try to deny their feelings and place them in the "offending" person. This process, involving projective identification, is universal and frequently activated during treatment. It is by no means entirely conscious but patients often have an initial awareness that they are attempting to rid themselves of unacceptable feelings or behaviors.

Scapegoating may lead to the "scapegoat's" extrusion from the group. It depletes the group, in the sense that specific emotional responses are not available for examination. Many affects may serve as the stimulus to evoke scapegoating, such as anger, envy, or romantic feelings. Scapegoating becomes virulent because of affect contagion (Freud 1955), in which feelings become greatly magnified in the communication process and adds a destructiveness to scapegoating.

The therapist's task of protecting the scapegoat is primarily accomplished through assisting members in "taking back" feelings that they are attributing to the scapegoat. A simple illustration is members' anger with an individual who habitually arrives late. That person might be accused of wanting to avoid the group. Analysis of the members' vitriol may reveal that they are also avoiding other intense group feelings. Such an analysis enables the scapegoat to become linked with the others rather than have an isolating experience.

## Nonverbal Communication

Patients communicate powerful feelings nonverbally. Discrepancy between verbal and nonverbal messages is confusing, but frequently the latter element is received as the "truth." Patients may tell sad stories and laugh, or they may relate a success in a dreary manner. Members may pull their chairs outside the group circle, sit close to or opposite the therapist, shift position in their chair, or not look at one another during emotionally laden interchanges. White knuckles, crimson blushing, or a black dress are additional colorful communications.

Patients learn to address these meaningful communications as they become comfortable examining in-group behaviors. However, many times the person may be unaware of sending nonverbal messages, and confrontations can be experienced as intrusive and threatening. Stereotyping certain behaviors as carrying predetermined meanings is a common error, and patients learn, sometimes through painful experience, that the sender may have highly personal meanings attached to the behavior. Exploration of nonverbal behaviors often is a powerful entry into the recipient's and the sender's current and past feelings.

## Difficult Patients

A number of individuals appear to be good group candidates, but they prove to benefit little from participation or they seem to obstruct the treatment process. These individuals, generically labeled "difficult patients," can be conceptualized as having significant relational problems that interact with a particular group culture (Roth et al. 1990, Stone and Gustafson 1982). Although such individuals are often diagnosed as having borderline or narcissistic personality disorder, not all such patients can readily be given those specific diagnoses. Nitsun's (1996) felicitous expression, "the anti-group," characterizes these individuals as having the potential to disrupt the entire therapeutic endeavor.

The difficult patient should be seen in context. Some groups can accept individuals who seldom speak, whereas others see such a person as seriously harming cohesion and, therefore, as "difficult." Difficult patients fill roles and are frequently labeled "monopolizer," "help-rejecting complainer," or "the silent one." The role embodies both the individual personality and a group function. Evidence for this assertion is found when the difficult individual is removed and another rises to fill his or her place, which suggests that, in part, the role was necessary to deal with members' anxieties.

A more careful examination of the processes involved in the emergence of a difficult patient may expose that such individuals are covertly coconstructed by others in the group (Gans and Alonso 1998). Interactions among members and the therapist tend to evoke and/or exaggerate particular character tendencies of members who often have underlying issues of forming intimate relationships. The therapeutic challenge is to deconstruct the processes so all can see their contributions to the difficult individual. This is similar to scapegoating described previously.

Nevertheless, some patients persist in behaviors that do not change and that become destructive to the treatment process. They evoke responses in others, including the therapist, that interfere with a sense of safety and limit members' willingness to expose their inner thoughts and feelings. Many difficult patients seem unable to process their interactions cognitively but remain enmeshed in emotional exchange. Others may interrupt emotional exchange with intellectual dissertations.

Not infrequently, these individuals prematurely terminate treatment, leaving those remaining with feelings of relief, frustration, and anger. Other difficult patients remain in the group, and at times the therapist is faced with making a decision that favors the group over an individual. The patient is informed that she or he is not benefiting from the treatment modality and is asked to leave. Such a decision should be reached only after the therapist has completed a thorough self-scrutiny and has sought consultation to explore countertransference contributions to the impasse.

## Alternative Treatment Formats

### Cotherapy

In some settings, groups are conducted by cotherapists. This format provides opportunities for clinicians to learn from one another, share leadership responsibilities, more readily recruit members, and provide continuity in the absence of one leader. Cotherapy uniquely offers therapists chances to directly observe another clinician's work and to learn about countertransferences. The model is utilized for training neophyte group therapists who can be paired with a more experienced therapist. For patients, this model is thought to offer a recreation of the family, as therapists are cast in parental roles, whether or not the therapists are of the same or different gender.

The conduct of cotherapy is not without special problems (Lang and Halperin 1989). Cotherapists need to attend to their relationship because they are susceptible to a variety of transference responses to one another, most commonly competitive and narcissistic strivings. They will need to predetermine under what circumstances they might address their inevitable disagreements directly in the session.

It is inadvisable to use the cotherapy format unless both therapists are committed to spending time between sessions reviewing the therapeutic process and their emotional responses to the members and to one another. Patients, in their reactions (transference or realistic), will assign roles to therapists and may split them into good and bad. These are not comfortable configurations and considerable effort is required by the leaders to examine their contributions to the role assignment. Consultation may be advisable when therapists seem to reach an impasse in resolving conflicts or the group seems stuck.

An unresolved problem involves determining patient fees for cotherapy sessions. Some therapists set a fee that remains the same with one or both therapists present. Some cotherapists charge individually for the sessions in which they are present. This method is compatible with insurance company policies of paying only for services provided. The set fee has the advantage of charging for the treatment, but often therapists will earn less for their time than if they work singly. Patients will certainly wonder about having identical charges in the presence of one or both therapists. The therapist should be prepared to explain the policy but also to examine transferences. It is important to recall that money is a difficult topic in our culture and often evokes countertransferences.

### Concurrent Therapy

The practice of combining individual and group psychotherapy has gained considerable acceptance. Patients may be seen either by the same (combined) or by a second (conjoint) therapist. Each modality potentially complements the other. In dyadic settings, therapists can focus in greater detail and explore developmental (transference) contributors to group transactions. Subsequently, patients can observe their group interactional patterns that have been addressed in the dyadic setting.

In the combined model, therapists have opportunities to observe individuals in both settings. Most therapists draw a firm boundary between the two modalities—that is, they will not introduce information into the group that was learned elsewhere; the patient is encouraged to assume that responsibility (Lipsius 1991).

In the concurrent model, the majority of therapists obtain the patient's consent to communicate about the treatments. For some, the absence of consent rules out this treatment format. Therapists, by exchanging information, can alert one another to the emerging transferences. The format may stimulate splitting, in which a patient may denigrate one treatment and idealize the other. Through consultation with one another, therapists can sort out precipitants for those behaviors and diminish the potential for countertransference responses.

Not uncommonly, some members may be treated in concurrent formats, whereas others are not. The dynamics stimulate direct questions or allusions to specialness, favoritism, and degree of illness that require exploration. (Persons in concurrent treatment may be viewed as sicker by others.) The patient may be the one to mention her or his individual sessions (at least initially), and the timing of such references often carry considerable meaning that can be examined therapeutically.

Fees for patients in combined or concurrent therapy require discussion, particularly for individuals whose treatment is covered by insurance. Insurance companies limit payments, whether by amount of payments or number of sessions, and fees for the two modalities generally differ significantly. If treatment will extend beyond the limits—a likely situation—the patient should decide, in advance if possible, where he/she will pay out of pocket and where insurance will be filed.

### Pharmacotherapy and Group Therapy

The inclusion of patients receiving pharmacotherapy in dynamic psychotherapy groups is common practice. Eighty-three percent of surveyed psychiatrists included patients requiring medication in group therapy, which was not significantly greater than the percentage of psychologists

(70%) or social workers (60%) (Stone et al 1991). Mood disorder patients (dysthymia, unipolar and bipolar disorders) were most frequently included, followed by those with personality or anxiety disorders. Medicated schizophrenic patients represented less than 1% of the total and were least likely to be in group therapy.

Clearly, inclusion of medicated individuals broadens the population available for treatment. Medications are often seen as helping patients utilize the dynamic treatment focus more effectively. A common dynamic process is exposure of attitudes derogating medicated members and a "we–they" split, which may result in medicated patients becoming scapegoated as "too ill." Focusing on medication may become a group resistance (Rodenhauser and Stone 1993).

Arguments against combining medication with group therapy include therapists' attitudes about the "purity" of change. Some clinicians believe medication interferes with patients feeling ownership over themselves. Nonmedical therapists may be adverse to introducing such patients to group therapy because of problems in collaboration with physicians who are unfamiliar with the group model or do not choose to provide such services.

Combining medications with psychotherapy has become widespread. The evidence for modification, if not cure, of major debilitating symptoms is substantial, and yet patients will be left with emotional responses and unexplored meaning of their illness. Moreover, discontinuation of medication is highly correlated with recurrence of symptoms. In my opinion, clinicians' and patients' objections to the combined treatment approach can be sensitively addressed, and inclusion of patients receiving medications in groups offers opportunities to effectively treat a wider patient population.

## Time-Limited Groups

As pressure mounts to conduct therapy in briefer periods, interest in time-limited groups has increased (MacKenzie 1997). The number of sessions may range from 12 to 30. Many insurance companies limit coverage to 20 sessions, and thus a 16-session model allows for preparatory interviews and, if necessary, one or two sessions after termination of the group.

Time-limited goals are established by the therapist. Groups may be organized along specific symptom constellations, such as bereavement, sexual abuse, bulimia, or anorexia nervosa, or they may explore a personality sector with the expectation that the individual will continue to utilize the learning after termination.

Selection of patients for time-limited groups is of central importance. Therapists may opt to organize groups with ability to work with interpretations or one that is primarily supportive. Members should be assessed for their degree of psychological mindedness, that is, are they able to reflect on themselves and their interactions, and on their ability to find a focus, not necessarily of recent origin. Difficulties should be formulated in interpersonal terms to facilitate the exploration of the problems in the group setting (e.g., a delayed grief reaction).

In most circumstances, once treatment begins additional members are not accepted. The agreement is similar to that of longer-term groups with the exception that the number of sessions is limited. Using this format, the therapist needs to be more active in defining the focus for the members. In the context of group development, interventions are made that focus on the interpersonal aspects of the particular dynamic stage. These groups can be particularly useful in addressing issues of engagement, trust, unfulfilled hopes, separation, and loss. The combination of time pressure, maintaining focus on interpersonal processes, and providing encouragement to apply learning in the external world has produced a treatment format that may be as effective as individual treatment (Budman et al. 1988).

## Chronically Mentally Ill

This special population of patients requires modification of traditional dynamic approaches (Kanas 1996, Stone 1996, Schermer and Pines 1999). The population is broader than individuals with major psychiatric disorders (schizophrenia or bipolar disorders) and includes some disabling anxiety or personality disorders. Indeed, chronicity is determined primarily by duration and disability rather than by diagnosis. In some instances, groups are organized homogeneously for patients with schizophrenia or bipolar disorder (Cerbone et al. 1992). These groups often emphasize the importance of continuing with medication and include important educational components. They may have greater structure and focus on particular topics, such as managing hallucinations, paranoid thinking, or social relations (Stone 1996).

More typically, groups are structured to include a spectrum of patients within a relatively small range of disability. Patients are prone to attend erratically, and a flexible format that accepts this propensity may serve these individuals well (Stone 1996). The sessions are usually shorter, 45 to 60 minutes, and the group census may range from 12 to 16 persons. In the flexible format, core and peripheral subgroups develop and, over extended periods, groups develop a sense of continuity and cohesion.

Treatment goals should be concordant with patients' strengths and are generally formulated to help in adaptation to everyday problems, improving social relations, and managing feelings. The agreement is modified, and patients may be encouraged to socialize outside of the meetings. Therapists attempt to help patients manage their isolation and sense of shame over their illness.

Countertransferences require particular attention in part due to the difficulty patients have in linking to their therapists, which may leave the clinician expecting more than the patients can deliver. Moreover, in the current climate, particularly for major mental illness, medications are valorized, and therapy is depreciated, a state of affairs that affects the therapist (Della Badia 1999).

## Treatment Failures

Treatment failures may be examined from an individual or group perspective. Failures may be further classified by individuals who fail to benefit and those who are harmed by the treatment.

Individuals who terminate treatment abruptly are generally considered failures. The early dropout rate is substantial (Roback and Smith 1987) and can probably never be reduced to zero. Some patients terminate treatment prematurely because they have been poorly prepared for psychotherapy and find themselves overwhelmed by the intensity of interactions. Others may have wished for supportive treatment and find themselves in an atmosphere that is supportive but also confrontational. Occasional patients may be placed in a group that functions at a level below that of their own development and they drop out. Some patients express themselves in a fashion that invites rejection. Patients may be familiar with being extruded from social situations and enter a group to find a new way of managing old solutions but in the process repeat old patterns. These persons have often filled roles labeled monopolizer, help-rejecting complainer, or isolate. Some patients initially reveal themselves extensively, then feel overexposed and terminate treatment abruptly. They may be injured by their treatment. Similarly, an individual who becomes enmeshed in a scapegoat role from which he or she cannot be extricated may be injured by the experience.

Therapists have become more willing to include more difficult patients who represent a risk of not benefiting from treatment. They may remain for extended periods, participating in their stereotypical patterns, without any evidence of change. Certain patients continually violate group boundaries, and their behavior seems impossible to change after examination of collective and individual factors. Extragroup socializing (which might include sexual liaisons), inability to refrain from attacking others, and schedules that preclude regular attendance are examples of situations that suggest that continued treatment might be harmful. At times, an open discussion with such a person might lead to a mutual decision to discontinue the treatment format.

Therapy impasses and failures must also be examined from the perspective of the functional state of the group. Groups enmeshed in an intense resistance or a negative transference to the therapist might act in a fashion to reject certain personality types. This creates the potential for members to feel that they too are failures. Ambitious therapists who have overestimated members' psychological strengths may push for interaction or demand insights beyond that of the members' capabilities, resulting in a flurry of terminations or a whole-group failure (Stone et al. 1980).

Therapists who find themselves experiencing extended periods of boredom, frustration, or anger may be reflecting group-wide affects (via projective identification). The members may be attempting to communicate through this channel their experiences of being stuck or that the therapy is ineffective. Therapist's affect can be very useful in identifying misunderstandings or errors. The clinician's emotional state may be used then in finding ways to address the misunderstanding and prevent a treatment failure (Stone 2001). For clinicians experiencing recurrent treatment failures or dropouts, consultation is in order.

## Research

Research in treatment outcome in group therapy is considerably more complicated than dyadic treatment. Group treatment adds a large number of elements that must be taken into account. Some of these elements are the type of group (psychoeducation, counseling, or dynamic psychotherapy), duration of treatment, experience of the therapist (trainee or seasoned), age (children, adolescents, adults), functional level (chronically mentally ill or

"typical" outpatient), and the more complex question of patient–therapist fit.

Several large meta-analyses of the effectiveness of treatment have been conducted. Toseland and Siporin (1986) reviewed 32 well-controlled experimental studies and reported that in 24 (75%) no significant differences in effectiveness were found between individual and group treatments and that in the other eight (25%), group treatment was more effective. Tillitski (1990) conducted a meta-analysis of nine studies that compared group, individual, and control conditions. Group and individual therapies yielded similar outcomes, and the average effect size indicated that 80% of the treated patients were improved in comparison with the control group.

A study of patients randomized either to time-limited individual therapy or group therapy was reported by Budman and colleagues (1988). On multiple measures, patients in both treatments showed similar improvement and maintained these changes at a 1-year follow-up. However, the authors carefully reported that almost nine times (26 versus 3) the number of patients withdrew from the study after they were informed that they had been assigned to group treatment (i.e., they had time conflicts, job changes). Moreover, patients' subjective responses indicated a strong preference for individual treatment. A well-controlled study of patients suitable for psychoanalytically oriented therapy failed to identify characteristics that would predict outcome (de Carufel and Piper 1988).

Reviews of the status of research in group psychotherapy (Dies 1993, Piper 1993) have proposed that greater attention needs to be paid to the problems of characteristics and preparation of patients and the question of group composition. The fit of patients in a particular group may well be instrumental to outcome. Patients' coping styles may differentially interact with the type of therapy (cognitive, focused expressive, and supportive) and affect outcome (Beutler et al. 1991). Several studies linking outcome with group cohesion are beset with problems of definition and operational measures and have not yielded significant findings. A valuable addition to the group research literature focuses on the variety of measurement systems used to assess change (Beck and Lewis 2000). The editors provided a transcript of a group session to researchers who were to apply their model of measuring change. The publication illustrates the strengths and weaknesses of process analyses.

In a report of a randomized clinical trial, Piper and colleagues (2001) investigated two patients' personal characteristics (quality of object relations [QOR] and psychological mindedness [PM]) with either interpretive or supportive forms of time-limited short-term group therapy for patients with "complicated grief." Patients in both therapies improved, though those with high PM did better. For grief symptoms an interaction was found with high QOR doing better in interpretive therapy and low QOR doing better in supportive treatment.

The general finding that group therapy is as effective as individual treatment has substantial research support. The complexity of conducting this research has limited continuing efforts to define more precisely many of the elements contributing to that success. A somewhat worrisome tendency is for clinics under pressures from funding agencies to substitute consumer satisfaction in place of other evaluative measures. As the study of Budman and coworkers (1988) illustrated, there may be a dissociation between improvement and satisfaction, particularly in short-term groups.

## Training

Therapists with a background in dyadic treatment do not find the shift to conducting groups simple. Adequate training is necessary to ensure that the therapist and patients alike have a satisfactory experience (Alonso 1993).

The components of training include: (1) didactic presentations; (2) opportunities to observe groups conducted by experienced therapists; (3) participation as a member in an experiential group or as a patient in a therapy group; (4) coleadership of a group with an experienced clinician; and (5) solo leadership of a group (Day 1993, Alonso 1993). Supervision is essential to assist therapists in achieving increasingly sophisticated understanding of group dynamics and process, intervention options, transferences, and countertransferences. An important additional element of training in groups is exploration of ethical issues, including confidentiality, dealing with sexual contacts (between patients and those involving the therapist), dangerousness, and informed consent (Lakin 1991).

Therapists are subjected to many powerful emotional forces evoked by the group setting, and they often try to translate individual approaches to the multiperson setting, where dynamic forces have a different impact. Increased awareness of these forces is gained through participating in a group. The American Group Psychotherapy Association offers brief group experiences at their annual conference and regional societies, or independent psychotherapy training centers may provide additional opportunities to participate as a member.

The most important element in training is supervision. Beginning supervision is most often provided individually. However, many therapists continue supervision well beyond learning the basics, and they often participate in small-group supervision of their therapy endeavors. This format provides support and an opportunity for the therapist again to reexperience group dynamics in action. Often unconscious aspects of the therapist's behavior (countertransferences) emerge in the supervisory group in a manner that can be utilized to gain greater understanding of the therapeutic process.

Many graduate-level training programs (psychiatry, psychology, social work, and nursing) provide only a modicum of training in group dynamics and therapy, and clinicians turn to other training settings, which may include a 2-year program combining the elements described earlier.

## The Future

While, historically, group psychotherapy was sometimes misrepresented as a less expensive, watered-down treatment, work by many has helped establish it as an effective, cost efficient, and rigorous therapeutic modality applicable to a wide variety of patient problems. It provides a more direct experience for patients working with peers, as well as with those in "authority." The individual's difficulties with people is not limited to the experience of a particular individual therapist but emerges in the relational context of a number of individuals, thereby broadening the entire treatment context. In this era of emphasis on cost containment and efforts to provide rapid, brief therapies, groups can provide for some a positive time-limited treatment and for others an extended opportunity to address and alter significant intrapsychic and interpersonal difficulties.

Effective group treatment, like any other therapeutic modality, depends on opportunities for training and ongoing exchange among colleagues to enhance skills and provide the best possible treatment experience for group members.

## References

Agazarian YM (1997) Systems-Centered Therapy for Groups. Guilford Press, New York.

Alonso A (1993) Training for group psychotherapy. In Group Therapy in Clinical Practice, Alonso A and Swiller HI (eds). American Psychiatric Press, Washington DC, pp. 521–532.

Alonso A and Rutan JS (1988) The experience of shame and the restoration of self-respect in group psychotherapy. Int J Group Psychother 38, 1–14.

Beck AP and Lewis CM (2000) The Process of Group Psychotherapy: Systems for Analyzing Change. American Psychological Association, Washington DC.

Bennis WG and Shepard HA (1956) A theory of group development. Hum Rel 9, 415–437.

Berne E (1966) Games People Play. Grove Press, New York.

Beutler LE, Engle D, and Mohr D (1991) Predictors of differential response to cognitive, experiential and self-directed psychotherapeutic procedures. J Consult Clin Psychol 59, 333–340.

Bion W (1960) Experiences in Groups. Basic Books, New York.

Budman SH, Bennett MJ, and Wisnecki MJ (1988) Comparative outcome of time-limited individual and group psychotherapy. Int J Group Psychother 38, 63–86.

Cerbone MJA, May JA, and Cuthbertson BA (1992) Group therapy as an adjunct to medication in the management of bipolar affective disorder. Group 16, 174–187.

Day M (1993) Training and Supervision in Group Psychotherapy. In Group Therapy in Clinical Practice, Alonso A and Swiller HI (eds). American Psychiatric Press, Washington DC, pp. 656–667.

de Carufel FL and Piper WE (1988) Group psychotherapy or individual psychotherapy: Patient characteristics as predictive factors. Int J Group Psychother 38, 169–188.

Della Badia E (1999) Supervision of group psychotherapy with chronic psychotic patients. In Group Psychotherapy of the Psychoses: Concepts, Interventions and Contexts, Schermer VL and Pines M (eds). Jessica Kingsley, London, pp. 301–323.

Dies RR (1983) Clinical implications of research on leadership in short-term group psychotherapy. In Advances in Group Psychotherapy: Integrating Research and Practice, Dies RR and MacKenzie KR (eds). International Universities Press, New York, pp. 27–78.

Dies RR (1993) Research on group psychotherapy: Overview and clinical applications. In Group Therapy in Clinical Practice, Alonso A and Swiller HI (eds). American Psychiatric Press, Washington DC, pp. 473–518.

Durkin HE (1964) The Group in Depth. International Universities Press, New York.

Durkin JE (ed) (1981) Living Groups. Brunner/Mazel, New York.

Englander T (1989) The facilitating environment: Cohesion and the contract in group psychotherapy (Thesis). The Fielding Institute, Santa Barbara, CA.

Ettin MF (1994) Links between group process and social, political and cultural issues. In Comprehensive Group Psychotherapy, 3rd ed., Kaplan HI and Sadock BJ (eds). Williams & Wilkins, Baltimore, pp. 699–716.

Ezriel H (1973) Psychoanalytic group therapy. In Group Therapy: 1973 An Overview, Wolberg LR and Schwartz E (eds). Intercontinental Medical Book, Stratton, New York, pp. 183–210.

Foulkes SH (1961) Group process and the individual in the therapeutic group. Br J Med Psychol 34, 23–31.

Freud S (1955) Group psychology and the analysis of the ego. In The Standard Edition of the Complete Psychological Works of Sigmund Freud, Vol. 18, Strachey J (trans-ed). Hogarth Press, London, pp. 69–143. (Originally published in 1921)

Fulkerson CCF, Hawkins DM, and Alden AR (1981) Psychotherapy groups of insufficient size. Int J Group Psychother 31, 73–81.

Gans JS and Alonso A (1998) Difficult patients: Their construction in group therapy. Int J Group Psychother 48, 311–326.

Gibbard GS and Hartman JS (1973) The oedipal paradigm in group development: A clinical and empirical study. Small Group Behav 4, 305–354.

Glatzer HT (1953) Handling transference resistance in group therapy. Psychoanal Rev 40, 36–43.

Gustafson JP and Cooper L (1979) Unconscious planning in small groups. Hum Rel 32, 1039–1064.

Harwood INH (1998) Advances in group psychotherapy and self psychology: An intersubjective approach. In Self Experiences in Group: Intersubjective and Self Psychological Pathways to Human Understanding, Harwood INH and Pines M (eds). Jessica Kingsley, London, pp. 30–46.

Harwood INH and Pines M (eds) (1998) Self Experiences in Group: Intersubjective and Self Psychological Pathways to Human Understanding. Jessica Kingsley, London.

Hopper E (1996) The social unconscious in clinical work. Group 20, 7–42.

Horwitz L (1977) A group-centered approach to group psychotherapy. Int J Group Psychother 27, 423–440.

Horwitz L (1994) Depth of transference in groups. Int J Group Psychother 44, 271–290.

Kanas N (1996) Group Therapy for Schizophrenic Patients. American Psychiatric Press, Washington DC.

Kauff PF (1977) The termination process: Its relationship to the separation–individuation phase of development. Int J Group Psychother 27, 13–18.

Kauff PF (1991) The unique contributions of analytic group therapy to the treatment of preoedipal character pathology. In Psychoanalytic Group Theory and Therapy: Essays in Honor of Saul Scheidlinger, Tuttman S (ed). International Universities Press, Madison, CT, pp. 175–190.

Kernberg OF (1975) A systems approach to priority setting of interventions in groups. Int J Group Psychother 25, 251–275.

Kibel HD (1992) The clinical application of object relations theory. In Handbook of Contemporary Group Psychotherapy, Klein RH, Bernard HS, and Singer DL (eds). International Universities Press, Madison, CT, pp. 141–176.

Lakin M (1991) Coping with Ethical Dilemmas in Psychotherapy. Pergamon Press, Elmsford, NY.

Lang E and Halperin DA (1989) Coleadership in groups: Marriage a la mode? In Group Psychodynamics: New Paradigms and New Perspectives, Halperin DA (ed). Year Book Medical Publishers, Chicago, pp. 76–86.

Lipsius SH (1991) Combined individual and group psychotherapy: Guidelines at the interface. Int J Group Psychother 41, 313–337.

MacKenzie KR (1997) Time-Managed Group Psychotherapy: Effective Clinical Applications. American Psychiatric Press, New York.

Masterson JF (1978) The borderline adult: Therapeutic alliance and transference. Am J Psychiatr 135, 437–441.

Nitsun M (1996) The Anti-Group: Destructive Forces in the Group and Their Creative Potential. Routledge, London.

Ornstein PH and Ornstein A (1977) On continuing evolution of psychoanalytic psychotherapy: Reflections upon recent trends and some predictions for the future. Annu Psychoanal 5, 329–370.

Perls F, Hefferline R, and Goodman P (1951) Gestalt Therapy. Julian, New York.

Piper WE (1993) Group psychotherapy research. In Comprehensive Group Psychotherapy, 3rd ed., Kaplan HI and Sadock BJ (eds). Williams & Wilkins, Baltimore, pp. 673–682.

Piper WE, McCallum M, Joyce AS, et al. (2001) Patient personality and time-limited group psychotherapy for complicated grief. Int J Group Psychother 51, 525–552.

Pratt JH (1969) The home sanatorium treatment of consumption. In Group Therapy Today, Ruitenbeek H (ed). Atherton Press, New York, pp. 9–14. (Originally published in 1906)

Rice CA (1996) Premature termination of group therapy: A clinical perspective. Int J Group Psychother 46, 5–23.

Roback HB and Smith M (1987) Patient attrition in dynamically oriented treatment groups. Am J Psychiatr 144, 426–431.

Rodenhauser P and Stone WN (1993) Combining psychopharmacotherapy and group psychotherapy: Problems and advantages. Int J Group Psychother 43, 11–28.

Roth BE, Stone WN, and Kibel HD (eds) (1990) The Difficult Patient in Group. International Universities Press, Madison, CT.

Rutan JS and Stone WN (2001) Psychodynamic Group Psychotherapy, 3rd ed. Guilford Press, New York.

Scheidlinger S (1974) On the concept of the mother-group. Int J Group Psychother 24, 417–428.

Scheidlinger S (1994) An overview of nine decades of group psychotherapy. Hosp Comm Psychiatr 45, 217–225.

Schermer VL and Klein RH (1996) Termination in group psychotherapy from the perspectives of contemporary object relations theory and self psychology. Int J Group Psychother 46, 99–115.

Schermer VL and Pines M (eds) (1999) Group Psychotherapy of the Psychoses: Concepts, Interventions and Contexts. Jessica Kingsley, London.

Slater P (1966) Microcosm: Structural, Psychological and Religious Evolution in Groups. John Wiley, New York.

Slavson SR (1950) Analytic Group Psychotherapy. Columbia University Press, New York.

Stone WN (1985) The curative fantasy in group psychotherapy. Group 9, 3–14.

Stone WN (1992) The place of self psychology in group psychotherapy: A status report. Int J Group Psychother 42, 335–350.

Stone WN (1996) Group Psychotherapy for People with Chronic Mental Illness. Guilford Press, New York.

Stone WN (2001) The role of the therapist's affect in the detection of empathic failures, misunderstandings, and injury. Group 25, 13–14.

Stone WN and Gustafson JP (1982) Technique in group psychotherapy of narcissistic and borderline patients. Int J Group Psychother 32, 29–47.

Stone WN, Blase M, and Bozzuto J (1980) Late dropouts from group psychotherapy. Am J Psychother 34, 401–412.

Stone WN and Rutan JS (1984) Duration of treatment in group psychotherapy. Int J Group Psychother 34, 101–117.

Stone WN, Rodenhauser P, and Markert RJ (1991) Combining group psychotherapy and pharmacotherapy: A Survey. Int J Group Psychother 34, 401–412.

Tillitski CJ (1990) A meta-analysis of estimated effect sizes for group versus individual versus control treatments. Int J Group Psychother 40, 215–224.

Toseland RW and Siporin M (1986) When to recommend group treatment: A review of the clinical and the research literature. Int J Group Psychother 36, 171–201.

Tschuschke V and Anbeh T (2000) Early treatment effects of long-term outpatient group therapies — First preliminary results. Group Anal 33, 397–411.

von Bertalanffy L (1966) General system theory and psychiatry. In American Handbook of Psychiatry, Arieti S (ed). Basic Books, New York, pp. 705–721.

Weiss J, Sampson H, and the Mount Zion Psychotherapy Research Group (1986) The Psychoanalytic Process: Theory, Clinical Observations and Empirical Research. Guilford Press, New York.

Whitaker DS and Lieberman MA (1964) Psychotherapy Through the Group Process. Atherton Press, New York.

Wolf A and Schwartz EK (1962) Psychoanalysis in Groups. Grune & Stratton, New York.

Yalom ID (1995) The Theory and Practice of Group Psychotherapy, 4th ed. Basic Books, New York.

# 85 Time-Limited Psychotherapy

Holly A. Swartz
John C. Markowitz

## Introduction

The dominant model of psychotherapy during most of the 20th century was open-ended, long-term, and psychodynamic. At the beginning of the 21st century, driven by growing economic pressures, shorter psychotherapies moved to the forefront of clinical practice. Unfortunately, although many therapists are mandated to administer psychotherapy over a limited number of health care visits, few have training in specific, evidence-based, brief psychotherapies. As a result, most "short" psychotherapies administered in clinical practice are nonspecific, truncated versions of open-ended psychotherapy. By contrast, time-limited psychotherapy as discussed in this chapter refers to treatments of specified duration and structure that are designed for delivery over a relatively short time-period.

In an earlier edition of this textbook, the chapter on time-limited psychotherapy (TLP) focused on the historical progression of psychodynamic psychotherapy from psychoanalysis to the more circumscribed treatments of Malan, Sifneos, Davanloo, and so on. Over the past decades, the field has evolved considerably: brief, psychodynamic psychotherapy, what we shall call the "first generation" of TLP, has largely been supplanted by more formally time-limited, empirically tested psychotherapies such as interpersonal psychotherapy, cognitive–behavioral therapy, and behavior therapy. The first generation of brief treatments was relatively long by today's standards and rarely empirically tested. By contrast, the "second generation" treatments were developed and designed for use in clinical research trials that compared psychotherapy to pharmacotherapy or other psychotherapies. Reflecting these changes, the chapter now focuses primarily on empirically supported TLPs, although we still draw from the first generation psychotherapies to illustrate specific points and will summarize, for historical purposes, the approaches used by major practitioners of brief psychodynamic psychotherapy.

Increasing numbers of TLPs have been evaluated in clinical trials and have demonstrated efficacy for the treatment of specific disorders. In the face of this growing body of research, the Accreditation Council of Graduate Medical Education (ACGME), the organization responsible for oversight of psychiatric residency training programs in the US, now requires graduating residents to demonstrate "competence" in TLP. In addition, many seasoned therapists, pressured by the constraints of their patients' mental health benefits, express interest in acquiring expertise in TLP.

In this chapter, we offer an overview of the field of TLP. Given the explosive growth in the field of brief psychotherapy research, it is impossible to review all extant, empirically supported, TLPs. Instead, we focus on concepts common to second generation TLPs, practical strategies associated with brief treatments, and problems typical to this modality. To illustrate these principles, we use examples from several evidence-based treatments, with a focus on interpersonal psychotherapy—as it is not covered elsewhere in this text—as a paradigm of TLP.

## What Is Time-Limited Psychotherapy?

Time-limited psychotherapy refers to a psychosocial intervention, usually an individual psychotherapy, of relatively brief duration. Many of the defining features of TLPs follow from the fact that these treatments are intensive or compressed. Over a short period of time, the therapist identifies necessarily circumscribed treatment goals, working actively to maintain the treatment focus and preserve the treatment structure. Thus, TLPs are characterized by (1) specified treatment duration or time limit, (2) narrow treatment focus, (3) rapid and succinct case formulation, (4) structured treatment format, and (5) active therapist role. We elaborate these principles below.

Despite these similarities, TLPs comprise a heterogeneous array of treatments used to treat a plethora of conditions over quite variable time periods. "Brief" treatments can last anywhere from a single session to a year, and the therapeutic techniques deployed may range from transference interpretation (in brief psychodynamic psychotherapy) to a fear hierarchy (in behavioral therapy). Although brief therapies are not indicated for the management of long-standing character disorders or chronic and persistent mental illness such as schizophrenia or bipolar disorder, TLPs have been used to treat conditions as diverse as oedipal conflicts and mood, anxiety, and eating disorders.

Given that (a) not all TLPs are the same and (b) experience in delivering one treatment does not confer expertise in all TLP modalities, it would be overwhelming to attempt mastery of TLPs in general. Thus, a reasoned approach to acquiring "competence" in brief interventions might include acquainting oneself with the general principles of TLP, learning the techniques and strategies associated with one evidence-based therapy, and then obtaining clinical training (including expert supervision that involves review of audiorecorded or videotaped sessions) in the selected TLP modality. Although standards for "competence" vary across TLP modalities (in some cases, they are not defined at all), true competence is typically obtained after completion of a course in a specific psychotherapy followed by several carefully supervised cases (Markowitz 2001). This chapter will facilitate the first step in this process: familiarity with the concepts common to most evidence-based TLPs.

## Historical Background

Time-limited psychotherapy has its roots—like most psychotherapies—in the work of Freud and other early psychoanalysts. Sandor Ferenczi and Otto Rank, two of Freud's contemporaries, first articulated theoretical models for briefer psychodynamic treatments. In the early 1900s, Ferenczi, experimenting with a technique called "active therapy" (Ferenczi 1950), anticipated the more active stance required of the TLP therapist (in contrast to the neutral stance of the traditional psychoanalyst). Otto Rank, however, was the earliest theorist to focus on the primacy of time limitation per se. He formulated a 9-month treatment which, in recapitulating duration of gestation, sought to undo the "trauma of birth" (Rank 1952). Central to Rank's work was the idea that treatment must have a time limit imposed from the start. He then used the feelings that emerged around termination to process the seminal issues of separation and individuation.

Interest in briefer psychodynamic psychotherapies increased in the years following World War II. In the 1950s and 1960s, Balint and his colleagues at the Tavistock Clinic and Cassel Hospital in England formed the Focal Therapy Workshop. This group's intent was to develop a short-term psychotherapy with limited aims for use as an alternative to psychoanalysis (Balint et al. 1972). Balint's innovation lay in explicitly drawing attention to the primacy of "focus" in time-limited treatments. He called his technique "focal psychotherapy," and his student, David Malan, continued to elaborate this work after Balint's death in 1970. Malan believes that the selection of a clear focus appropriate to the patient constitutes the most important aspect of shorter treatments. Using the transference as a therapeutic tool, Malan's therapy explores triangular links among the transference relationship, a current problematic relationship, and past problematic relationships (usually with a parent), as well as links among anxiety, defenses, and underlying impulses, to bring about insight and therapeutic change. He believes that transference interpretations are the most meaningful because of their current emotional valence (Malan 1975). The importance of selecting a clear and relevant treatment focus, a concept emphasized by Balint and Malan, remains a central principle of most (if not all) TLPs.

Working at the Boston University School of Medicine in the 1960s, James Mann attempted to solve the problem of lengthy waiting lists in the University Mental Health Clinic by developing a TLP (Mann 1973). Although he writes eloquently about the philosophical and existential import of time, the impetus for his novel treatment approach was pragmatic; he needed to service an expanding cadre of patients with a fixed number of personnel. Thus Mann's treatment has, as its primary concern, a specific limitation of time. Patients receive 12 hours of therapy, which can be divided in any way that makes sense for the patient. In practice, most patients are treated for a 50-minute hour weekly for 12 weeks, although other permutations are permissible. The date of the last session is set during the initial session, allowing the treatment to have a clear beginning, middle, and end. Mann writes, "The most significant dynamic element in the treatment agreement lies in the exact prescription of time" (Mann 1973, p. 30). This general concept is central to many of the TLPs that follow.

Peter Sifneos, another pioneer in the evolution of brief psychodynamic psychotherapy, developed short-term anxiety-provoking psychotherapy (STAPP) while working at Massachusetts General Hospital in Boston in the 1960s and 1970s. He describes STAPP as a time-limited approach to resolving well-defined oedipal conflicts (Sifneos 1979). The therapy is prescribed as weekly 45-minute sessions for up to 20 weeks. The precise duration of treatment is *not* specified at the outset—although both therapist and patient agree ahead of time that the treatment will be "brief." In delineating the nature of an acceptable treatment focus, Sifneos specifically chooses an oedipal or triangular problem area: "This implies that problems must have developed between the patient and his parents in early childhood and are being repeated in his current interpersonal relations. These problems have to do with a competition with a parent of the same sex for the love and affection of the parent, or a parent surrogate, of the opposite sex" (Sifneos 1979, p. xi). STAPP uses "anxiety-provoking" techniques, which he distinguishes from the "anxiety-suppressing" techniques of supportive psychotherapy. Sifneos believes that a high level of anxiety must be maintained in order to sustain the patient's motivation for improvement. The therapist is encouraged to actively confront the patient's defenses in an effort to uncover the underlying impulse or drive. This strategy differs from the traditional analytic approach in which defenses are interpreted first.

Habib Davanloo, working at Montreal General Hospital, developed a short-term treatment, short-term dynamic psychotherapy (STDP), that was originally intended for patients with serious problems such as severe phobias and obsessive–compulsive symptoms in addition to patients with triangular oedipal problems (Davanloo 1978). Treatment can last anywhere from 1 to 40 sessions, but typically takes about 20 sessions. As in STAPP, a termination date is not set at the beginning of treatment but both therapist and patient know that the duration will be brief. The initial diagnostic interview, known as "Trial Therapy," can last anywhere from 45 minutes to 3 hours, depending on the degree of the resistance the therapist encounters. This initial evaluation establishes a focus of treatment through a process known as "unlocking the unconscious." Davanloo identifies a central dynamic issue, rapidly identifies and clarifies the patient's defenses, pressurizes the patient to acknowledge the defenses, directly challenges the defenses, clarifies and challenges the transference resistance, and eventually expects an exhaustion of the resistance. There follows an intrapsychic crisis, a period of consolidation, and a new understanding of the central dynamic issue. This forms the focus for the remaining treatment sessions. At the heart of STDP is Davanloo's "gentle but relentless" confrontation of defenses. Davanloo facilitates the rapid formation of a positive therapeutic alliance which allows the patient to tolerate a rather invasive, insistent process of clarification and interpretation. Davanloo recommends modifying these techniques for very fragile patients.

## Overview of Interpersonal Psychotherapy

Throughout the chapter, we use examples from interpersonal psychotherapy (IPT) to illustrate many of the general principles of TLP. In order to acquaint the reader with IPT, we offer a brief overview of this modality, introducing IPT-specific concepts such as the interpersonal inventory, the four interpersonal problem areas, and the interpersonal formulation. The reader is referred to the treatment manual (Weissman et al. 2000) for a more thorough discussion of IPT.

IPT was developed in the 1970s by Klerman and Weissman as a 16-session psychotherapy for outpatients with nonpsychotic depression (Klerman et al. 1984). IPT grew out of the interpersonal theories of Harry Stack Sullivan and Adolf Meyer as well as several empirical studies demonstrating the bidirectional link between interpersonal stresses and onset of depression. Although IPT was initially intended as a research tool that could be used reliably to deliver a standardized treatment in clinical trials, its research success has sparked demand for its clinical dissemination. In its original form IPT is an acute treatment for depression. It can be used alone or in combination with medication to treat the patient's depressive symptoms and the interpersonal problems that contribute to or are affected by the depression. IPT makes no inference about causality, simply linking the depressive symptoms to a patient's particular interpersonal issues. Regardless of which came first, IPT assumes, based on empirical evidence, that one can achieve improvement in mood by addressing interpersonal problems.

IPT uses a medical model of psychiatric illness. The therapist explains to the patient that he or she has "major depression" which is a medical illness, like diabetes or heart disease, and instills the hopeful and empirically validated idea that IPT is a good treatment for this specific disorder. Using Parsons's concept of the "sick role" (Parsons 1951), the patient is assigned the responsibility to work toward better health in exchange for being relieved of unmanageable social obligations. The patient is also educated about the relationship between depression and interpersonal problems, and, in collaboration with the therapist, selects an "interpersonal problem area" (see later) as the focus of treatment.

In the process of assessing the patient, the IPT therapist conducts the "interpersonal inventory." The interpersonal inventory consists of a review of all important past and present relationships as they relate to the current depressive episode. The therapist asks about the patient's life circumstances and requests a description of the important people in his or her life. In addition to outlining the "cast of characters" in the patient's life, the therapist probes the quality of those relationships, asking the patient to describe satisfying and unsatisfying aspects, unmet expectations with others, and aspects of relationships that the patient would like to change. The interpersonal inventory helps the therapist establish the "interpersonal problem area."

One of four interpersonal problem areas—grief, role dispute, role transition, or interpersonal deficits—serves as the explicitly agreed upon focus of treatment. It typically consists of issues such as the incompletely mourned loss of a loved one (i.e., complicated bereavement), conflict with a spouse or an employer (i.e., role dispute), an important life event (i.e., role transition), or, in the absence of one of these acute precipitants, long-standing, impoverished interpersonal relationships (i.e., interpersonal deficits). The therapist offers the patient an "interpersonal formulation": having emphasized that depression is a medical disorder with a constellation of psychological and physical symptoms, the therapist links the patient's current interpersonal problem to the depression and offers IPT as a powerful treatment for both the depression and the interpersonal problems. In the ensuing weeks (total of 16 weekly sessions), the therapist uses a variety of techniques outlined in the manual to help the patient work through these "real life" problems.

## General Principles of Time-Limited Psychotherapy

The hallmark of TLP is its specified treatment duration. Because of this compression, TLPs share attributes that both link them to one another and distinguish them from long-term treatment modalities. These general principles are summarized in Table 85–1.

### Time Limit

The time limit distinguishes TLPs from open-ended psychotherapies such as psychoanalysis (Brenner 1974). Most TLPs last 12 to 20 sessions, although they may range from 1 to 40 sessions (Koss and Shiang 1994). There is great variability in time requirements among the brief treatments. The first generation of TLPs was defined in relation to psychoanalysis—that is, they were time-limited in the sense that they were *not* open-ended. Their treatment duration is more flexible than the TLPs that followed. The second generation of TLPs tends to have more formal time constraints, usually specifying an exact number of sessions from the outset. For patients who have responded acutely, some TLPs provide monthly continuation and maintenance sessions to promote a full recovery and prevent relapse (Frank 1991). Table 85–2 groups psychotherapies commonly administered in a time-limited format by treatment approach and lists representative examples of strategies and typical treatment durations.

TLPs differ from truncated long-term treatments that are interrupted by attrition, noncompliance, or the pressures of managed care organizations. The duration of these latter therapies may coincide with that of a TLP, but they do not constitute fully formed brief treatments. TLPs

| Table 85–1 | General Principles of Time-Limited Versus Open-Ended Psychotherapies | |
|---|---|---|
| Principle | Time-Limited Psychotherapy | Open-Ended Psychotherapy |
| Duration of treatment | Specified time frame, 1–40 sessions | Duration not specified; may last several years |
| Scope of treatment | Well-defined treatment focus; circumscribed goals | Flexible treatment goals, varying over time, often not well defined |
| Treatment goals | Remission of specific symptoms or intrapsychic conflict | Character change, improved functioning, or ongoing support |
| Case formulation | Rapid; succinct; drives treatment goals; often explicitly stated to patient | Strives for depth of understanding; subject to ongoing revision and reassessment as treatment unfolds |
| Characteristics of suitable patients* | Acute illness; good premorbid functioning; limited resources; focused problem area | Chronic illnesses; poor premorbid functioning; extensive resources; multiple targets of change |
| Treatment structure | Defined stages of treatment; clearly specified termination phase; often specified in a manual | Flexible structure; no specified end point; treatment stages vary widely; not codified as a manual |
| Therapeutic stance | Active; direct suggestion may be permitted; functions to maintain treatment focus | Less directive; neutral |

Adapted from Frances A, Clarkin J, and Perry S (1984) Differential Therapeutics in Psychiatry: The Art and Science of Treatment Selection. Brunner/Mazel, New York.

| Table 85–2 | Major Models of Time-Limited Psychotherapy | |
|---|---|---|
| Psychotherapy Type/Major Theorists | Techniques | Typical Time Duration |
| Interpersonal psychotherapy (IPT)<br>□ Klerman<br>□ Weissman | • *Medical model* of illness.<br>• Life events affect mood, and vice versa.<br>• Link symptoms to one of four *interpersonal problem areas*.<br>• Work through an affectively meaningful problem area using role-play, communication analysis, and direct suggestion.<br>• Focus on the *here and now*, outside rather than inside the office. | 12–16 wk |
| Cognitive–behavioral therapy (CBT)<br>□ Beck<br>□ Rush<br>□ Barlow | • Identify distorted thoughts that lead to maladaptive feelings and behaviors.<br>• Homework assignments to recognize, test, and challenge underlying *automatic negative thoughts* or maladaptive behaviors.<br>• *Relaxation techniques* to manage anxiety.<br>• Encourage *rational*, scientific, collaboration between patient and therapist. | 12–16 wk |
| Behavior therapy (BT)<br>□ Foa<br>□ Mynors-Wallis | • Based on principles of operant conditioning, social learning theory.<br>• Gradual *exposure* to anxiety-producing stimuli.<br>• Self-monitoring, graded task assignment. | 8–12 wk |
| Brief psychodynamic psychotherapy<br>□ Balint<br>□ Davanloo<br>□ Luborsky<br>□ Malan<br>□ Mann<br>□ Sifneos<br>□ Strupp | • Identify problematic relationship themes that are resolved through *transference interpretations*.<br>• Offer *support* through the formal aspects of treatment such as regular appointments and collaboration.<br>• Select central issue that has current relevance and past antecedent.<br>• *Transference interpretations and clarification* to develop insight and resolve conflict.<br>• *Confront defenses*—despite emergence of anxiety—to uncover underlying impulse.<br>• Explore past *conflicts*, ego *defenses*, and *resistances*. | 12–20 sessions |
| Motivational interviewing<br>□ Miller<br>□ Rollnick | • Patient-centered, directive method for *enhancing motivation* to change.<br>• Encourage articulation and resolution of *ambivalence*.<br>• Diminish resistance and strengthen patient's *commitment to change*. | 2–4 sessions |
| Psychodynamic–interpersonal<br>□ Hobson<br>□ Shapiro | • Less emphasis on interpretation than most psychodynamic treatments.<br>• Greater emphasis on patient–therapist relationship than in IPT.<br>• Help patient learn new ways of relating to therapist and, by extension, others.<br>• Enhance interpersonal skills. | 3–8 sessions |

have distinctly defined beginnings, middles, and ends—regardless of their absolute duration. Knowledge from the outset that therapy has a defined end-point indeed may constitute a key active ingredient of time-limited therapy. It suggests that relief may be near at hand. Marmor speculates that this approach "counters the patient's impulse to see himself as helpless, inadequate, and in need of dependent support" (Marmor 1979, p. 153). Our experience with IPT as a treatment for depression in individuals who are HIV-seropositive suggests that these individuals, despite shortened life spans, use the brevity of treatment as an impetus to effect radical, rapid changes in their lives (Swartz and Markowitz 1998). The time limit, in a variety of ways, seems to provide an important motivation to speed the patient toward health.

A meta-analysis of many psychotherapy studies (none of them TLPs) found that most (75%) patients achieve symptom relief within 26 sessions of an open-ended treatment (Howard et al. 1986). Most treatments included in this meta-analysis were naturalistic (e.g., not controlled) studies of patients suffering from very heterogeneous symptoms (diagnoses are not specified). This finding suggests that many patients may respond quickly, even if psychotherapy is open-ended. Although no studies have compared prospectively response rates of TLPs to open-ended treatments, we predict that treatment response would be more rapid for patients receiving time-limited interventions because of explicit expectations that therapy will conclude within a specified time frame.

TLPs are generally dosed with a frequency of once a week, although this varies as well. Mann, for example, limits psychotherapy to 12 treatment hours, but distributes it according to the needs of the patient. He may, for instance, prescribe 12 weekly 1-hour sessions, 24 weekly half-hour sessions, or six twice-weekly hour-long sessions (Mann 1974). Investigators at the University of Sheffield experimented with a "two-plus-one" strategy in which patients with subsyndromal depressive symptoms were seen for two sessions separated by a week and then a review session 3 months later. Interestingly, this dosing strategy seemed efficacious, regardless of whether the content of the intervention was cognitive–behavioral or psychodynamic-interpersonal (Barkham et al. 1999). The same group of investigators also demonstrated no long-term advantage of 16 sessions of cognitive–behavioral therapy (CBT) for depression over eight sessions of CBT. By contrast, subjects who received eight sessions of psychodynamic–interpersonal therapy (PI) had worse outcomes than those receiving 16 sessions of PI, 8 sessions of CBT, or 16 sessions of CBT (Shapiro et al. 1995). In a randomized, controlled study of patients suffering from panic disorder ($N$=43), investigators from the University of Oxford found no differences in outcomes between a full course of cognitive therapy (12 hour-long sessions) and brief cognitive therapy (five hour-long sessions plus self-study materials administered over 11 weeks) (Clark et al. 1999).

Unfortunately, dose-finding studies are expensive. As there is no psychotherapeutic equivalent of the pharmaceutical industry which finances dose-ranging studies on all of its promising compounds, limited resources are available to conduct dose-ranging studies of psychotherapy. Therefore, the optimal duration and dosage of TLP, although empirical questions, remain largely unanswered to date. In practice, treatment duration is often defined by convention, the exigencies of a research protocol or managed care organization, or even the inclinations of the therapist.

## IPT: Duration of Treatment

IPT was originally designed as a 16-week intervention so that it could be administered over the same period as an acute course of pharmacotherapy, allowing an assessment of the relative efficacy of the two interventions (DiMascio et al. 1979). IPT is also administered as a 14-session intervention (Markowitz unpublished data), a 12-session intervention (Mufson et al. 1999, O'Hara et al. 2000), and an 8-session intervention (Swartz et al. 2002), but there are no data comparing the relative benefits of varying doses of acute IPT. Investigators at the University of Pittsburgh recently completed a study comparing weekly, bimonthly, and monthly doses of maintenance IPT; however, these results are not yet published (Frank E personal communication, January 2002).

## Treatment Focus

An important characteristic of TLP is careful definition of treatment goals, which are usually agreed upon by the patient and therapist, and often specified at the beginning of treatment. Because therapy is brief, the scope of the treatment is circumscribed and focused. Unlike psychoanalysis and long-term psychodynamic psychotherapy, TLPs do not attempt sweeping changes in character. Rather, treatments target a specific diagnosis, set of symptoms, or a narrow aspect of character. Typical and appropriate treatment goals for TLPs include remission of depressive symptoms, reduction in frequency of binge-eating, and resolution of a specific interpersonal conflict.

Again, it is useful to distinguish between psychodynamically oriented TLPs and evidence-based TLPs. Time-limited psychodynamic psychotherapies focus on unresolved unconscious conflicts while evidence-based TLPs, employing a more heterogeneous array of techniques, focus on addressing DSM-IV symptoms. By definition, evidence-based treatments have been proved to work in controlled clinical trials, whereas psychodynamic TLPs rely on the time-honored (but not necessarily scientifically tested) principles of psychoanalysis. Time-limited psychodynamic psychotherapies retain the somewhat nebulous goal, "facilitating of health-seeking behaviors and mitigating obstacles to normal growth" (Ursano and Hales 1986, p. 1511). In practice, most "brief" psychodynamic treatments (empirically validated or otherwise) are longer than the second generation of TLPs, permitting correspondingly less focused treatment goals. For instance, Sifneos includes in his selection criteria "the ability of the patient to have a circumscribed chief complaint" (Sifneos 1979, p. xi). He urges therapists to concentrate on an unresolved oedipal conflict, such as an ambivalent relationship with a partner that stems from difficulties moving through the oedipal phase of development (Sifneos 1978).

By contrast, second generation TLPs define treatment goals by diagnostic criteria, in much the manner of pharmacotherapies. IPT focuses on two discrete goals: remission of depressive symptoms and resolution of an interpersonal problem area (Weissman et al. 2000). Cognitive–behavioral therapy for panic disorder focuses on reduction in frequency of panic attacks and relief of general anxiety symptoms (Barlow 1997). Motivational interviewing, a brief intervention designed to facilitate behavior change, is often administered for the sole purpose of helping patients reduce or eliminate their alcohol consumption (Miller and Rollnick 1991). Thus, although the treatments vary in their focus, in all cases their treatment goals are narrow and usually specified from the outset.

## Case Formulation

Treatment focus is closely allied with the broader concept of case formulation. According to Eells, psychotherapy case formulation is "a hypothesis about the causes, precipitants, and maintaining influences of a person's psychological, interpersonal, and behavioral problems. . . .It should serve as a blueprint, guiding treatment" (Eells 1997, pp. 1–2). In the process of evaluating a patient and beginning a course of psychotherapy, the therapist evaluates the patient's psychological and social difficulties, using this material to generate hypotheses about the patient's difficulties. This anamnesis is then synthesized into a rational explanation for the patient's problems and linked to treatment goals. In TLP, because time is short, the process of generating a case formulation is also compressed. The therapist must identify the most important components of the patient's narrative, balancing the urge to learn more about the patient's life circumstances with the time constraints of the TLP. Thus, the TLP therapist typically conducts an overview of the patient's psychosocial circumstances and then selects a few "hot" topics—relevant both to the current complaint and the nature of the therapy—to consider in greater depth. This approach allows the therapist to develop an informed, timely case formulation. The ability to rapidly develop and deliver such a formulation is for many therapists among the more difficult but also most valuable aspects of learning a TLP.

## IPT: Case Formulation

Case formulation in IPT builds on two core IPT concepts: (1) depression is a treatable illness and (2) events in one's psychosocial environment affect one's mood, and vice versa. The IPT therapist defines depression as a medical illness that, like asthma, is both treatable and affected by the patient's circumstances. The therapist notes that, in a biologically vulnerable individual, when painful events occur, mood worsens and depression may result. Conversely, depressed mood compromises one's ability to handle one's social role, generally leading to negative events. IPT therapists use the connections among mood, environment, and social role to help patients understand their depressions within an interpersonal context, and to teach them to handle their social role and environment so as to both solve their interpersonal problems and relieve their depressive syndrome.

The therapist's formulation includes a diagnosis of depression as a medical illness, the provision of reassurance and hope, the assignment of the sick role and, most importantly, the identification of one (or at most two) interpersonal problem areas that become the agenda for the remainder of the treatment. The therapist directly states

this case formulation to the patient and elicits his or her agreement with the proposed strategy before moving ahead with the next phase of treatment. Thus, in IPT, case formulation constitutes an important treatment tool that links the patient's mood symptoms to life events and introduces a specific interpersonal problem area as the focus of treatment for the ensuing sessions (Markowitz and Swartz 1997). See Clinical Vignette 1 for an example of an IPT case formulation.

---

**Clinical Vignette 1**

Ms. A is a 38-year-old divorced mother of three children, working as a clerk at a local hospital. Her depression began a year before treatment, around the time that her 18-year-old daughter became pregnant, dropped out of school, and moved out of the house to live with her boyfriend. Ms. A's 21-year-old son had moved out of the house several years previously, but often came to stay with her because of problems resulting from substance abuse. Her 13-year-old son was beginning to get into trouble at school and had been previously diagnosed with attention-deficit/hyperactivity disorder. By contrast, her 18-year-old daughter, Gloria, was the "good child." She had always excelled in school, never used drugs, and was close to her mother. Because Ms. A had also dropped out of high school because of a pregnancy, she had always hoped her daughter would not repeat her mistakes. She was devastated when her daughter's life took this unexpected turn. Her family practitioner suggested she see a therapist when Ms. A expressed reluctance to take antidepressant medication. At the time of her evaluation for treatment, her 17-item Hamilton Depression Rating Scale score was 25 (significantly elevated), and she easily met DSM-IV criteria for major depression, single episode. After conducting a psychiatric interview and diagnosing a major depressive episode, the therapist and patient discussed treatment options. Ms. A declined pharmacotherapy but was open to a trial of CBT or IPT, both empirically supported, time-limited psychotherapies for depression. After a review of Ms. A's interpersonal relationships and recent life events, the therapist suggested that IPT might be preferable to CBT because it would help Ms. A with both her depression and numerous interpersonal stressors. Ms. A agreed, and the therapist offered her the following IPT case formulation.

*You have been depressed for the past year, and depression is a medical illness, just like diabetes or asthma. As we discussed, it's not your fault, not something to blame yourself for, but we do need to treat it. Your job over the next several weeks will be to be a patient with the medical illness called major depression. You should focus on your treatment and not worry too much if you don't yet feel like your usual self. The good news is that depression is very treatable—feeling hopeless is just one of its symptoms—and I expect that you'll be feeling much better in a matter of a few weeks. There are a number of proven ways to treat depression. One way is with interpersonal psychotherapy, which is a brief antidepressant treatment that focuses on the connection between your mood disorder and what's going on in your life. Understanding that connection and using that understanding should allow you to choose the best options to deal with your situation, and help you feel better.*

Clinical Vignette 1 *continued*

*From what you've told me, I think your depression has something to do with your worries about your daughter. You had always hoped that she would go to college and put off having children so that she would not live with the same kind of regrets that you have. It sounds like you and Gloria have different ideas about how she should run her life and how your relationship should be, now that she has a baby and lives on her own. You want to help her with the baby but also help her "make something of her life." She wants you to help her with babysitting but does not want any of your advice about what to do with her life. It's hard for you to communicate with her right now, and you are very worried that she will continue to make "bad" decisions. We call this a role dispute. If you're willing, and this makes sense to you, what I'd suggest is that we spend the next 12 weeks working on this dispute with Gloria. IPT has been carefully tested in research studies and shown to be effective in treating the kind of depression you have. So we have a good chance of doing two things in the next 12 weeks: helping you solve your role dispute and, at the same time, getting you out of this horrible episode of depression.*

The brevity of treatment leaves little room for error in formulating the IPT case—or any TLP case, for that matter. The therapist must use the initial treatment sessions to aggressively pursue all potential areas and to determine the treatment focus prior to embarking on the middle phase of treatment. It is unlikely that a diligent therapist will discover, midway through treatment, that he or she has seriously misjudged the salience of a chosen problem area. If a covert and imposing problem area should arise in the middle phase, however, the therapist would have to renegotiate the treatment contract to address it.

## Structured Treatment

Although all interventions, by default, have beginnings, middles, and ends, these phases of therapy may be difficult to discern in a treatment whose termination may occur 7 to 10 years hence. For instance, the midpoint of psychoanalysis is apparent to neither patient nor therapist until after treatment has concluded. By contrast, in TLP, the structure of the intervention is clearly delineated and referenced throughout the treatment period. The therapist will often call the patient's attention to important landmarks in the treatment: "Today we've reached the halfway point" or "We only have three sessions left." In manualized treatments, each of these time intervals has specified tasks or strategies. For instance, in IPT, the initial phase can last up to three sessions. During that time, the therapist has specific tasks (viz., obtain a psychiatric history and interpersonal inventory, offer a case formulation). Similarly, the middle and end phases of treatment have a specified duration and associated tasks.

In support of the treatment structure, TLP requires the therapists to make formal or informal "treatment contracts" in which the patient and therapist explicitly or implicitly agree to goals, duration, and other parameters of treatment. The therapist may discuss with the patient the exact number of sessions planned, rules for missed sessions or rescheduled sessions, fees, and so on. Although some aspects of treatment contracts are common to all psychotherapies, TLPs tend to specify more elements in the contract from the outset, including expected treatment responses (e.g., "At the end of 16 weeks, your mood will likely be much better") and specific requirements of the patient (e.g., homework assignments in Prolonged Exposure and CBT). Patients often find the transparent structure of TLPs reassuring, removing some of the unnecessary mystery (and perhaps stigma) historically associated with psychotherapy.

The structures of all evidence-based TLPs and some psychodynamically oriented TLPs are delineated in treatment manuals (Beck et al. 1979, Luborsky 1984, Mann 1974, McCullough 2000, Miller and Rollnick 1991, Milrod et al. 1997, Sifneos 1979, Weissman et al. 2000). Manuals generally include an overview of the theoretical underpinnings of treatment, case material, and a step-by-step "how to" outline of the treatment itself. Some treatments and their manuals detail very specific instructions for each session, much like a recipe in a cookbook. Other manuals outline treatment structure in broader strokes, identifying some concrete tasks as well as more general treatment principles.

In routine practice settings, manuals get mixed reviews (Addis and Krasnow 2000). Some therapists find the structure manuals helpful in guiding treatment. Manuals provide goals and fallback interventions that may keep therapists from getting demoralized in frustrating circumstances, and thus improve outcome. Other therapists worry that manuals may take the "art" out of psychotherapy and reduce rapport with patients. Some therapists (especially new therapists) may adhere too rigidly to the manuals, which could create difficulties with the nonspecific treatment tasks of forming an alliance and empathic listening. On balance, however, evidence-based treatments can only be practiced by adhering to specified techniques, and current data suggest that patients who receive evidence-based TLPs designed to address specific disorders fare better than those receiving generic supportive treatments (Markowitz et al. 1998).

Most second generation TLPs call for serial assessments of symptoms. In research protocols, therapists rely on rater-administered instruments such as the Hamilton Rating Scale for Depression (Hamilton 1960) to evaluate symptoms over time. In clinical practice (and in clinical trials), it is often more practical to administer a self-report measure such as the Beck Depression Inventory (Beck and Steer 1993) or the Beck Anxiety Inventory (Beck and Steer 1990). Regardless of the instrument chosen, it is important to build into the weekly therapy session time to complete and review a standardized symptom measure and track change over time. Serial symptom assessment provides the patient with additional psychoeducation (i.e., symptom recognition) and a reliable means of tracking improvement (or lack thereof).

## Active Therapist

In order to maintain the treatment focus, the therapist must be active in TLP. He or she must move the treatment process forward under the pressure of an inexorably ticking clock. This demands constant attention to the treatment focus and redirection of the patient if the focus falters. The therapist gently keeps the patient on task, shaping the treatment rather than simply following the patient's lead. Many brief treatments encourage the therapist to make direct suggestions when the patient is unable to solve a problem by him/her. In CBT, for example, the therapist assigns homework exercises and readings (Beck et al. 1979). In IPT, without assigning specific weekly homework, the therapist helps the patient identify a current interpersonal problem that is amenable to change during the treatment interval. A challenge in TLP is to balance strict adherence to the treatment focus with an empathic stance that supports the treatment alliance. Although it is important to attend to the agreed upon problem area in IPT, it is also important that the patient feel "heard" and that the therapist allows time in the session for the patient to express his or her feelings unimpeded.

## Common Factors of Psychotherapy

An overview of the extant literature, including all psychotherapeutic modalities and a wide variety of research techniques, suggests that nonspecific, "common factors" of psychotherapy significantly mediate psychotherapy treatment outcomes (Lambert 1998). These principles seem to hold for time-limited treatments as well as long-term psychotherapies.

Researchers and theorists alike have expended great effort delineating the nature of these effects. Frank identified six therapeutic factors common to all forms of psychotherapy: (1) "An intense, emotionally charged, confiding relationship"; (2) "A rationale, or myth, which includes an explanation of the cause of the patient's distress"; (3) "Provision of new information concerning the nature and sources of the patient's problems and possible alternative ways of dealing with them"; (4) "Strengthening the patient's expectations of help"; (5) "Provision of success experiences"; and (6) "Facilitation of emotional arousal". (Frank 1971, pp. 355–357). Marmor's list includes such concepts as identification with the therapist, therapeutic alliance, and "working through" (Marmor 1979, p. 153). Available data on the effects of these general psychotherapeutic factors are limited, although many points seem reasonable on the basis of common sense. For instance, in a short period of time, a positive therapeutic alliance is likely to hasten treatment response; facilitation of affect is likely to make treatment feel meaningful and thereby increase the patient's commitment to the process; and instilling hope is unlikely to cause harm.

Studies suggest that treatment outcomes are highly correlated with therapeutic alliance (Blatt et al. 2000, Krupnick et al. 1996, Marmar et al. 1989), a parameter that captures many of the common factors described above. Interestingly, this aspect of treatment seems to correlate with pharmacotherapy—as well as psychotherapy—outcomes (Krupnick et al. 1996, Weiss et al. 1997), suggesting that the common factors have clinical importance in all therapeutic interventions, including TLPs.

The "common factors" may be considered the bedrock of psychotherapy, the foundation on which specific interventions of particular therapies may be built. Without a therapeutic alliance, therapists might have the most sophisticated and powerful tools in the world, but fail to deliver them to a dysphoric patient. Novice therapists who read TLP manuals may marvel at the unique characteristics of a particular therapy and ignore the common factors supporting them, yet do so at their peril. Yet, even though the common factors are shared and important, some studies have shown differences in treatment outcome between TLPs.

## Practical Issues in Time-Limited Therapy

### Patient Selection

Which patients are appropriate for time-limited approaches? Are there patient characteristics that predict a better response to psychotherapy over medication, or one psychotherapy over another? Are there genetic factors that predict a better response to one class of medication over another? Should we consider patient preferences when recommending treatments? These important questions are much discussed throughout the field of psychiatry. Frances and colleagues (1984) laid out important issues in differential therapeutics, concerned that "therapists tend to recommend preferentially the treatment they have to offer rather than to consider systematically each of the alternative possibilities"; they advised a more rigorous approach to clinical judgment.

At one end of the spectrum, researchers are beginning to identify biologic markers that may predict differential treatment response. Thase and colleagues (1997) demonstrated that patients with recurrent major depression who had markedly abnormal EEG sleep profiles were less likely to respond to psychotherapy alone. Since in clinical practice, obtaining sleep studies is difficult, we often rely on less specific markers to guide treatment recommendations. Frances and colleagues (1984) identified patients with chronic illnesses, poor premorbid functioning, extensive resources, and multiple targets of change as good candidates for longer treatments, and patients with acute illnesses, good premorbid functioning, limited resources, and focused problem areas as good candidates for shorter treatments, such as TLPs.

Because of their limited focus, TLPs are ideally suited to patients with acute symptomatology and relatively favorable baseline functioning. Resource availability may also influence decisions to use a time-limited or open-ended approach. Most evidence-based treatments are designed for and have been tested in samples of patients who meet DSM-IV criteria for Axis I disorders (predominantly mood and anxiety disorders, as well as specific behavioral problems such as substance abuse or eating disorders). Thus, it is important to conduct a thorough diagnostic interview, identify target diagnoses and symptoms, and select a TLP that has been empirically validated for that population. It would be inappropriate to treat a patient with a primary diagnosis of a specific phobia with IPT, as IPT has not been tested in this population; a behavioral approach would be preferable. A patient suffering from major depression, however, might reasonably be treated with either CBT or IPT.

How do we make informed TLP recommendations for individual patients among several efficacious treatment options? Relatively few clinical trials have been conducted comparing multiple active treatments, largely because such trials are laborious and expensive. Moreover, it is difficult to show differences between competing active treatments without very large sample sizes. Nevertheless, data from clinical trials provide some clues about patient and therapeutic characteristics that might predict differential responses to TLPs. IPT, CBT, behavior, and cognitive therapies have clearly demonstrated efficacy for the treatment of major depression (Thase 2001). A *post hoc* analysis of data from the Treatment of Depression Collaborative Research Program (TDCRP), a large (*N*=250) randomized, controlled study comparing IPT, CBT, imipramine, and placebo plus clinical management for the treatment of major depression, suggested that patients with low social dysfunction (i.e., good interpersonal skills) responded better to IPT, whereas patients with low cognitive dysfunction responded better to CBT. The data further suggest that severely depressed patients responded better to imipramine and to IPT (Sotsky et al. 1991). Thus, a severely depressed patient with good interpersonal skills might ideally receive IPT, whereas a cognitively intact but interpersonally deficient, less severely depressed individual might fare better with CBT. We speculate that severely depressed individuals with both cognitive dysfunction and marked social deficits might benefit most from medication administered in the context of a supportive therapeutic relationship, but might not be able to fully avail themselves of either CBT or IPT. The same study showed that medication worked faster than did the psychotherapies.

The indications for brief psychodynamic treatments are more ambiguous patient variables—such as the capacity to sustain a focus in treatment, motivation for insight, and good outside relationships (Malan 1976)—rather than DSM-IV diagnoses. Some brief dynamic treatments (such as Luborsky's supportive–expressive psychotherapy) are intended for "a broad range of problems from mild situational maladjustments to borderline psychotic" (Luborsky 1984, p. 56). Because these parameters have not been operationalized for routine clinical practice, it is difficult to intuit which patients may be appropriate for some psychodynamic TLPs. Furthermore, many of the studies/reports of first generation TLPs included predominantly healthier patients who are easier to treat, regardless of treatment modality. An exception to this is the recent manualized psychodynamic treatment by Milrod and colleagues (1997, 2000) for DSM-IV panic disorder, a "second generation" treatment, which has shown promising results in an open study.

Patient preferences may also drive treatment decisions. Some patients may voice a preference for psychotherapy over medication, or endorse a model of understanding their symptoms based on cognitive distortions. Patients will sometimes prefer a therapist of the same (or, occasionally different) gender. Studies, however, have not demonstrated effects of therapist matching for gender (Zlotnick et al. 1998).

How do we select treatments for patients who suffer from more than one psychiatric disorder? Epidemiologic studies indicate that the majority of individuals with a lifetime history of any psychiatric illness meet diagnostic criteria for more than one psychiatric disorder (Kessler et al. 1994). Patients with comorbid Axis I disorders display more recurrent and severe psychopathology (Andrade et al. 1994, Coryell et al. 1992, Grunhaus et al. 1988, 1994), poorer

psychosocial functioning (Grunhaus et al. 1988, Hollifield et al. 1997), and poorer response to both psychotherapeutic and pharmacologic treatments (Coryell et al. 1992, Frank et al. 2000b, Grunhaus et al. 1988). Data are limited on the efficacy of TLPs in comorbid populations. From a clinical standpoint, it makes sense to identify a primary diagnosis and direct treatment towards those symptoms first. If a patient fails to respond or experiences a partial response, the clinician can then augment or switch treatments.

## Engagement

The closely allied concepts of engagement and treatment alliance respectively refer to the patient's commitment to the treatment enterprise and the relationship between therapist and patient. Positive treatment alliance typically correlates with better treatment adherence and engagement. Given the brevity of treatment, one challenge of TLP is to establish rapidly a relationship with the patient in order to facilitate engagement in treatment. Maintaining this alliance throughout treatment is also important because nonattendance, while disruptive to any psychotherapy, is particularly costly in a time-limited treatment.

### IPT: Therapeutic Relationship

While many of the so-called "common" factors of psychotherapy function to facilitate this process, in IPT the therapist's stance is specifically intended to create a positive relationship with a depressed patient. The IPT therapist maintains a warm, encouraging stance that counters the depressed patient's pessimism with an equal and opposite optimistic realism. In psychodynamic terms, the IPT therapist cultivates a positive transference. He or she handles negative transference as illness-derived, treatment-interfering behaviors: for instance, tardiness or lack of participation would be defined as sequelae of depression. The therapist might intervene by saying, "It's hard to feel enthusiastic about therapy when your depression makes it hard to enjoy anything." In addition, the therapist might address it on a practical level, saying, "We only have five sessions left. We need all the remaining time to get to the bottom of your problem with your wife and to treat your depression." These strategies both promote the therapeutic alliance and enhance treatment engagement.

## Maintaining the Focus

As previously discussed, it is imperative that the TLP therapist identify clear treatment goals and maintain focus during the brief treatment period. It can be challenging to keep the patient on task and manage material that emerges in sessions unrelated to the primary treatment goal. To address this important issue, the therapist must clarify from the outset the goals and potential limitations of treatment.

### IPT: Treatment Focus

In IPT, treatment goals are specifically stated during the initial phase of treatment. The IPT therapist might say, "The goal of this treatment is to help you with this depression and your unresolved feelings about your mother's death last year. At the end of 16 weeks, we can discuss whether you need additional treatment for your bulimia, but let's first see how you feel when the depression has lifted." It is important that the patient explicitly agree to the stated treatment goals. In the case described above, the patient would need to agree to defer treatment for a possible eating disorder, focusing on her depression and grief for the immediate future.

In IPT, a clear treatment contract helps the patient and therapist remain focused. For instance, if the patient brings up feelings of dissatisfaction in the workplace during a therapy designed to address problematic relationships with a spouse (role dispute), the therapist may first briefly explore whether these complaints relate to the treatment focus. Thus, if demands from the spouse lead the patient to accept an unsatisfactory job, or if a dispute at work parallels that at home, the therapist can refocus the comments in light of the ongoing marital dispute. However, if there is no obvious connection to the main treatment focus, the therapist might gently redirect the patient by saying, "Although your work concerns are important too, at the beginning of therapy we agreed that we should spend these few months working through your problems with your spouse. I wonder how that has been going."

In TLP, time is the therapist's ally. Time can be used as leverage if the therapy falters. The therapist can remind the patient of time constraints should the patient digress, urging the patient to stay on task lest the clock run out before the work is done. In general, it is helpful to intermittently remind the patient of the time-frame (e.g., "we have six sessions left") to enhance motivation. The more fragile (severely depressed) the patient, the more important it is to balance the pressure to make changes with empathic support, reassurance, and the selection of graded activation strategies that do not overwhelm the patient (Linehan 1993).

## Termination

As the end of treatment nears, the therapist reiterates the date and time of the final session, actively eliciting responses to the end of treatment if the patient does not spontaneously offer them. Termination provides an opportunity to review treatment gains (which are often impressive), support the patient's sense of competence and independence, grieve the end of treatment, and identify unaddressed problems. The termination phase is more crucial and more complicated in psychodynamic psychotherapies because of their emphasis on the importance of the therapeutic relationship.

### IPT: Termination

In IPT, termination is handled as a graduation or role transition. In the termination phase of IPT (typically the last two to three sessions), the therapist helps the patient express expectable sad feelings (which are distinguished from recrudescent depressive affect) about the end of treatment, but underscores patient progress in having treated the depressive episode and problems at work, love relationships, and so on. While concerns about the patient's ability to manage without the therapist's help are inevitable, the therapist counters with examples of the patient's hard therapeutic work outside of the office. The therapist commends the patient's "real world" victories, reminding the patient that IPT has helped him or her to develop new skills that he or she will continue to use after treatment ends. Termination promotes patient independence while grieving the loss of the treatment relationship. The therapist and patient also review the symptoms of depression and identify "warning signs" which might lead the patient to a reevaluation in the future.

In the event of partial response or nonresponse, the therapist suggests alternative treatments and makes appropriate referrals for follow-up. If the therapist judges that additional treatment is warranted for management of persistent symptoms, it is critically important that the therapist blames the therapy rather than the patient for failing to bring about a full remission. The therapist can gently point out that all of our treatments for depression are imperfect and that we cannot yet predict which treatments will work for any individual patient. The therapist confidently reassures the patient that there are other options (i.e., medication, CBT), helping the patient select follow-up treatment that fits his or her needs. Another reasonable strategy (though not backed by any empirical data) would be to extend the treatment duration of IPT by a fixed number of sessions (e.g., six or eight additional sessions). This option would probably be best for a patient who has had at least a partial response to IPT and may need a few extra sessions to complete therapeutic work that is already underway. In keeping with the spirit of IPT, it would be important to explain this rationale to the patient explicitly and to set a second termination point to help maintain the focus of treatment. See later the section on nonresponse and partial response for a fuller discussion of treatment options for patients who are not well at the end of 16 sessions.

When the patient experiences a remission of symptoms by the end of 16 sessions, it may be tempting to refer the patient for additional psychotherapy such as marital treatment or an insight-oriented psychotherapy to address residual interpersonal issues or longstanding personality problems. However, it may be preferable to encourage a treatment-free period of 3 to 6 months to help clarify and consolidate treatment gains, particularly if the patient has presented with a first episode of relatively acute illness. Greater symptom chronicity and number of episodes suggest the need for continuation and maintenance treatment.

## Therapist Training

TLPs are optimally conducted by relatively skilled and experienced therapists. Because of time constraints, the therapist must assess the patient rapidly, formulate the case succinctly, and identify an appropriate treatment focus. In TLPs, therapists necessarily have to do more and faster, than in therapies of more desultory framework. In addition, with manualized treatments, there is the risk that beginners will adhere too mechanically to the manual and lose touch with the patient's affect. On the other hand, inexperienced therapists may find that the framework of a TLP is more easily mastered than the less specified strategies of an open-ended treatment. Beginning psychotherapists may find the structure these treatments provide reassuring and instructive. Therefore, in some training programs, residents are introduced to outpatient psychotherapy by learning one of the TLPs.

Few studies in the literature examine what constitutes adequate experience for a therapist practicing TLP. Curiously, Sifneos' clinical observations suggested that "the less experienced [therapists] were better therapists and more often obtained successful results than did their more experienced counterparts" but offer a "possible explanation" noting that "younger supervisees...lack...certain preconceived ideas about psychotherapy in contrast to the older ones" (Sifneos 1978 pp. 492–493). Sifneos insisted on a relatively healthy "patient" population, which may account for the relative "success" of these inexperienced clinicians. By contrast, in a naturalistic study of depressed patients treated with CBT, Burns and Nolen-Hoeksema (1997) found that patients of beginning therapists showed significantly less improvement in depressive symptoms than did the patients of therapists with 4 or more years of clinical experience. An exhaustive review of the literature concludes that, in general, "increased levels of systematic training on the part of the therapist enhance patient outcome, lower rates of attrition, and decrease recidivism" (Koss and Shiang 1994 p. 676). It seems likely that with sicker patients, skilled therapists will have more success than novices.

Most modalities require that experienced practitioners undertake additional specialized training to learn the specific time-limited technique (Markowitz 2001). Although the data on training are scarce, a clinician wishing to practice a time-limited treatment should seek additional education at a site offering programs in the specific modality of interest. In addition to reviewing the manual, training typically consists of completing several videotaped, training cases in supervision with an expert. Some institutions (such as Beck's Center for Cognitive Therapy in Philadelphia) offer courses in time-limited treatments. In the US, training for IPT practitioners is currently conducted primarily in research centers; however, useful updates on international training opportunities can be found on the website of the International Society for Interpersonal Psychotherapists (ipt@list.medicine.uiowa.edu). We encourage new practitioners of TLP to treat patients with psychotherapy alone, avoiding the concomitant prescribing of medication. From a training perspective, this offers the clinician an opportunity to gain confidence in their clinical skills and see first hand the effects of the psychotherapy.

## Common Problems in Time-Limited Psychotherapy

### Nonresponse and Partial Response
There are no clear guidelines to determine the optimal next step for patients who fail to respond or do not respond fully to an initial course of psychotherapy. In the case of nonresponse to a given treatment, which may be defined as failure to achieve at least a 25% decrease in baseline symptoms over a 6- to 8-week time period (Nierenberg and DeCecco 2001), the usual approach would be to stop the unhelpful therapy and consider alternatives. Patients who show no benefit from a TLP should be evaluated for the typical sources of treatment failure such as misdiagnosis, the presence of a comorbid psychiatric disorder, or comorbid general medical conditions (Kornstein and Schneider 2001), and referred for appropriate treatment. If the TLP psychotherapist is also a physician, it would be reasonable at this point to initiate pharmacotherapy. If the clinician decides that it is in the best interest of the patient to abandon a course of TLP, it is important that the therapist help the patient understand that the "fault" lies with the TLP rather than the patient. The therapist should be certain to offer the patient support during the transition to an alternate treatment, instilling hope that the new treatment will offer relief and making sure that continuity of care is preserved.

Partial response to a treatment has been defined as "somewhere below response and above nonresponse" (Nierenberg and DeCecco 2001). Clinically, this translates into a patient who feels somewhat better than when he or she started off, but continues to experience some symptoms or functional impairment. As for partial response to pharmacotherapy, clinicians have the option of augmenting the current treatment or switching to a different treatment (Thase and Rush 1995). Options would include adding a medication to psychotherapy, stopping psychotherapy and treating a patient with medication alone, or switching from one kind of psychotherapy to another.

In most cases of partial response to a TLP, clinicians choose to add medication as their first strategy. Unless the therapist suspects that psychotherapy may have worsened the patient's condition, continuing psychotherapy usually makes sense. The preexisting therapeutic relationship can provide a supportive holding environment for the patient while medication is initiated that may help the patient tolerate initial medication side effects and the delayed onset of action associated with antidepressant medication. Among depressed patients who fail to respond to an initial course of pharmacotherapy, response rates to a second antidepressant hover around 50% (Marangell 2001). By contrast, in a sample of depressed women, the addition of an SSRI to IPT among those who failed to respond to IPT alone brought about remission in almost 80% of subjects (Frank et al. 2000a). Thus, depressed patients who do not remit with psychotherapy alone may be excellent candidates for combination treatment with psychotherapy and medication.

If a patient refuses medications or prefers a trial of a different psychotherapy, it may be reasonable to change TLP modalities or consider an open-ended treatment. Issues to consider include whether it makes sense to switch therapists, the qualifications of the therapist to administer multiple types of psychotherapy, and the availability of alternate treatments in the patient's geographic area. Whereas psychopharmacologists can easily change prescriptions and proceed with a consistent therapeutic approach, a psychotherapist who suddenly begins acting differently may confuse an already uncomfortable patient. In one study, patients suffering from bipolar disorder who were changed from one psychotherapy to another (administered by the same therapist) had a greater risk of recurrence than patients who continued to receive the same form of psychotherapy (Frank et al. 1999). Thus, changing from one TLP to another should be undertaken with caution. Finally, patients who have had a partial response to a TLP may require a few extra sessions of the same therapy to consolidate further treatment gains.

### IPT: Handling Nonresponse to Treatment
In IPT, we make every effort to blame the treatment rather than the patient when symptoms persist beyond termination. Depressed patients are inclined to blame themselves,

so it is important for therapists to maintain their objective stance, pointing out treatment successes (there are usually some) and underscoring the fact that not all patients respond to any single treatment. Patients with histories of chronic or recurrent depression who respond to an acute course of IPT are generally considered candidates for continuation and/or maintenance of IPT sessions (usually administered at a reduced frequency) to help achieve a full remission and prevent relapse and/or recurrence (Frank 1991, Markowitz 1998).

## Mid-Treatment Crises

During the course of any psychotherapy, unanticipated crises may occur in the patient's life, temporarily derailing treatment. For instance, if the patient suddenly developed new, life-threatening symptoms such as active suicidal ideation or frank psychosis, the case formulation would be abandoned in order to attend to patient safety. Alternately, if the patient experienced an unexpected life crisis mid-treatment (i.e., the death of an important person, significant changes in socioeconomic status, etc.), it would be reasonable to reevaluate the treatment focus in order to attend to the patient's pressing needs.

Regardless of treatment modality, patient safety supersedes the treatment paradigm. In TLP, it is desirable to address the crisis as quickly as possible in order to return to the treatment focus and complete the treatment within the specified time frame. If the therapist can address the crisis rapidly and resume the prior focus, it may be possible to regain the original treatment trajectory. If multiple sessions are required to address crisis, the therapist must ask, "Is this TLP salvageable?" and "Can we meet our treatment goals within the remaining allotted time?" If not, the therapist should consider altering the treatment focus or abandoning the current treatment approach entirely. As we have emphasized throughout, changes in treatment approach should be handled carefully, reassuring the patient that they are not to blame and providing support as the patient shifts to a new intervention.

## Enduring Effects of Brief Therapies?

Do the effects of TLPs continue beyond the acute treatment phase? What are the roles of continuation and maintenance treatment? Which patients can be managed with an acute course of psychotherapy alone? These questions are important because many psychiatric disorders are recurrent, and studies suggest that many patients continue to experience functional impairments, even after acute symptoms remit (Keller et al. 2000). Thus, in circumstances of high risk of relapse or recurrence, it may be preferable to follow the successful acute treatment of an illness with some form of maintenance treatment.

Frank and Kupfer (1990) at the University of Pittsburgh demonstrated that patients with recurrent major depression treated acutely with IPT plus imipramine have an 80% chance of experiencing a recurrence over a 3-year period in the absence of ongoing maintenance treatment. In this study, monthly IPT sessions prevented recurrence in about 30% of subjects and imipramine (with or without IPT) prevented recurrence in 80% of subjects. This study did not address whether maintenance treatment is indicated for patients who respond to psychotherapy alone in the acute phase, since all patients initially received combined IPT and pharmacotherapy.

Other studies have suggested that the effects of TLPs persist at follow-up. Barkham and colleagues (1999) found that patients treated for subsyndromal depressive symptoms with CBT had significantly fewer depressive symptoms at 1-year follow-up than those treated acutely with PI. Follow-up data from the TDCRP suggest that among patients who responded acutely to either IPT, CBT, or imipramine, only about 20% remained completely well throughout the 18-month follow-up period (Shea et al. 1992). Subsequent analyses demonstrated that, at 18 months, patients treated acutely with IPT or CBT reported greater ability to establish and maintain interpersonal relationships and to identify symptoms of depression than those treated with imipramine (Blatt et al. 2000). Evans and colleagues (1992) found that CBT had enduring effects beyond the acute treatment phase but that antidepressant medication (when stopped after 3 months) did not. Other studies have also suggested that, unlike medication, the effects of psychotherapy may continue even after treatment is stopped (Blackburn et al. 1986, Simons et al. 1986).

## Contraindication to Time-Limited Psychotherapy

For all psychoactive treatments it is important to consider instances in which a specific therapy is *not* indicated for a disorder or kind of patient. Unfortunately, thus far there are no well-designed empirical studies of a psychotherapy's potential "toxicities"—although there is speculation about the kinds of individuals who would be predicted to respond poorly to time-limited treatments.

In the brief psychodynamic psychotherapy literature, time-limited treatments are generally not recommended for those individuals who might have difficulty in quickly forming a therapeutic alliance or might develop severe difficulties in the face of termination (Marmor 1979). In practice, this usually translates into a reluctance to treat borderline, suicidal, substance abusing, or psychotic patients with brief psychotherapy (Davanloo 1980, Mann 1974, Sifneos 1979). Also excluded are "acting out," cognitively impaired, very dependent, or "unrestrainably" anxious patients (Koss and Shiang 1994).

Although Sifneos (1979) and Mann (1974) consider severe psychopathology a contraindication to their brief psychodynamic psychotherapies, other time-limited treatments specifically target serious mental disorders. IPT and CBT, for example, were developed for the treatment of major depression; these and other brief psychotherapies have been used to treat a spectrum of significant pathologies including bulimia (Fairburn 1998), alcohol dependence (Miller et al. 1998), panic disorder (Barlow 1997, Milrod et al. 2000), and posttraumatic stress disorder (Foa et al. 1991).

Patients suffering from personality disorders have often been excluded from trials of time-limited psychotherapies, thus we know little about the effects of these treatments on Axis II pathology. Markowitz and colleagues (1998) reported that HIV-positive patients with depressive symptoms who had comorbid personality disorders had slightly higher depression scores, both at baseline and at the end of 16 weeks of treatment with TLPs, than did comparable patients without personality disorders, but the extent of symptomatic improvement was equivalent between the groups. Data from the TDCRP suggest that patients suffering from both major depression and a personality disorder experience greater residual depressive symptomatology than patients with MDD alone, although there were no differences in mean depression scores between the groups at termination (Shea et al. 1990). Similarly, an open study of CBT for the treatment of a range of mood disorders found that patients with comorbid personality disorders had more severe depressive symptoms at intake and more residual depressive symptoms at the end of treatment (Kuyken et al. 2001). Although it is unlikely that a personality disorder will remit following a course of brief psychotherapy, we also know that it is often difficult to accurately diagnose personality disorders in the presence of an Axis I disorder (Hirschfeld et al. 1983). Hence *seeing* Axis II pathology should rarely be an exclusion in the presence of an appropriate Axis I target disorder. Furthermore, the structure and brevity of time-limited treatments may help the therapist to manage or circumvent some of the treatment-interfering behaviors characteristic of cluster B personality disorders. Thus, it may be reasonable to treat patients with moderate character pathology for an Axis I disorder with a TLP and then refer them for a different kind of psychotherapy once the acute symptoms have remitted.

## Empirical Data

Because these treatments are relatively short, it is easier (though by no means easy) to conduct psychotherapy outcome studies with TLPs than with longer-term psychotherapies. The past decade has witnessed the publication of relatively large numbers of TLP studies. Because of these studies, we have more confidence that TLPs work, at least for particular indications, than other forms of psychotherapy. In Table 85–3, we summarize findings from empirical studies of TLPs as treatments for mood disorders. In Table 85–4 we summarize population-specific indications for selected TLPs.

## IPT Studies

IPT has been tested in several large, randomized clinical trials evaluating its efficacy for the treatment of depression. The landmark study in this area, conducted by Elkin and colleagues (1989), was the NIMH TDCRP. In clinical trials conducted at three different sites, over 200 outpatients meeting DSM-III criteria for depression were randomly assigned to one of four treatment cells: IPT, CBT, imipramine plus clinical management (CM), or placebo plus CM.

| Table 85–3 | Summary of Empirical Evidence Supporting Efficacy of TLPs for Mood Disorders (Randomized Trials Only) | | | |
|---|---|---|---|---|
| Diagnosis | N | Study Design | Results | Reference |
| Major depressive disorder | 81 | 16 wk of IPT, amitriptyline (AMI), IPT plus AMI, or nonscheduled control | IPT plus AMI > IPT = AMI > control | DiMascio et al. (1979) |
| Major depressive disorder in the elderly | 91 | 16–20 wk of behavioral (BT), cognitive (CT), or brief psychodynamic (BPT) therapy or wait-list control (WLC) | BT = CT = BPT > WLC | Thompson et al. (1987) |
| Major depressive disorder | 250 | 16 wk of IPT, CBT, imipramine (IMI) or Placebo (PLA) plus clinical management (CM) | IMI > IPT > CBT > PLA plus CM (differences were nonsignificant) | Elkin et al. (1989) |
| Recurrent major depressive disorder | 128 | 3 yr of maintenance treatment: monthly maintenance IPT (IPT-M), IMI plus IPT-M, IPT-M plus PLA, CM plus PLA, IMI plus CM | IMI plus IPT-M = IMI plus CM > IPT-M = IPT-M plus PLA > CM plus PLA | Frank et al. (1990) |
| Major depressive disorder | 107 | 12 wk of CT, IMI, or CT plus IMI | CT plus IMI > IMI = CT (differences were nonsignificant) | Hollon et al. (1992) |
| Depressive symptoms in HIV-positive individuals | 101 | 16 wk of IPT, CBT, IMI plus supportive therapy (SP), or SP alone | IMI plus SP = IPT > CBT = SP alone (differences were nonsignificant) | Markowitz et al. (1998) |
| Recurrent major depressive disorder in the elderly | 180 | 3 yr of maintenance treatment: Nortriptyline (NTP), IPT-M, IPT-M plus NTP, IPT-M plus PLA, or CM plus PLA | NTP plus IPT-M > NTP > IPT-M plus PLA > CM plus PLA | Reynolds et al. (1999) |
| Major depressive disorder in adolescents | 48 | 12 wk of IPT or CM | IPT > CM | Mufson et al. (1999) |
| Severe, refractory, nonpsychotic illness | 110 | 8 wk of psychodynamic interpersonal therapy (PI) or usual care (UC) | PI > UC | Guthrie et al. (1999) |
| Postpartum depression | 120 | 12 wk of IPT or WLC | IPT > WLC | O'Hara et al. (2000) |
| Chronic depression | 681 | 12 wk of nefazodone (NFZ), cognitive–behavioral analysis system of psychotherapy (CBASP), or NFZ plus CBASP | NFZ plus CBASP > NFZ = CBASP | Keller et al. (2000) |

| Table 85-4 | Time-Limited Therapies with Demonstrated Efficacy for Specific Disorders | |
|---|---|---|
| Disorder | Psychotherapy | Efficacy |
| Major depression, acute | IPT | 1* |
| | CBT | 1 |
| | PI | 2 |
| Major depression, recurrent | Maintenance IPT | 1 |
| Major depression in the elderly | Cognitive therapy | 2 |
| | Behavior therapy | 2 |
| | Horowitz's stress-response psychotherapy | 2 |
| Depressive symptoms in HIV seropositive men | IPT | 2 |
| Chronic depression | Cognitive–behavioral analysis system of psychotherapy | 1 |
| Dysthymia | CBT | 2 |
| | IPT | 2 |
| Opiate addiction | Luborsky's SE plus drug counseling | 2 |
| | CBT plus drug counseling | 2 |
| Alcohol addiction | CBT | 1 |
| | Motivational enhancement therapy | 1 |
| | Twelve-step facilitation | 1 |
| Bulimia | CBT | 1 |
| | IPT | 2 |
| PTSD | Prolonged exposure | 2 |
| Panic Disorder | CBT | 1 |
| | Panic-focused psychodynamic therapy | 2 |

*, tentative classification; 1, rigorously proven; 2, promising results.

Independent raters assessed patient progress with standardized rating instruments. Although all four groups showed improvement, nonstatistically significant differences existed among the cells: imipramine was slightly better than IPT which was considerably better than CBT which, in turn, was somewhat better than placebo plus CM. A secondary analysis of the data suggested that imipramine and IPT were more effective for the more severely depressed patients than were placebo plus CM and CBT (Sotsky et al. 1991).

Markowitz and colleagues (1998) conducted a study (N = 101) comparing IPT, CBT, supportive psychotherapy (SP), and imipramine plus SP for the treatment of HIV-seropositive individuals who were depressed. Subjects were mostly male (85%), gay or bisexual (80%), and white (58%). Although all groups improved, subjects who received IPT alone or imipramine plus SP had significantly greater improvement in depressive symptoms than those receiving CBT or SP alone. The authors speculate that some of the properties of IPT such as encouragement to make life changes and recognition of the connection between mood and real life events may be inherently more helpful to HIV-positive patients with depressive symptoms—who face a surfeit of such life events—than the cognitive restructuring and refocusing techniques employed in CBT. Limitations of the above study include constricted patient demographics (i.e., primarily homosexual, relatively well-educated men), failure of some subjects to meet strict DSM criteria for a current mood disorder, and relatively small numbers of subjects per cell.

Frank and colleagues (1990) at the University of Pittsburgh examined the role of maintenance therapies in the treatment of recurrent depression. One hundred and twenty-five patients with multiply recurrent major depression were randomly assigned to one of five treatment cells: a monthly maintenance form of IPT (IPT-M) alone, IPT-M plus imipramine, IPT-M plus placebo, medication clinic plus placebo, or medication clinic plus imipramine. Imipramine was given in high doses throughout the 3-year trial, whereas IPT was given at its lowest dose (monthly sessions). Both imipramine and IPT-M yielded significantly longer survival times (i.e., relapse prevention) than did placebo. High dose imipramine performed better than "low dose" IPT, and additional IPT-M conferred no additional benefit to treatment with imipramine alone.

Predating these large studies, a smaller controlled trial, the New Haven–Boston study, comparing IPT with amitriptyline (DiMascio et al. 1979), provided initial evidence for IPT's superiority to placebo for the treatment of depression. Subsequent randomized controlled trials have demonstrated that IPT is an efficacious treatment for postpartum depression (O'Hara et al. 2000), depression in primary care settings (Schulberg et al. 1996), and as maintenance strategy for late-life depression (Reynolds et al. 1999). Open studies suggest that IPT may also be efficacious for the treatment of antenatal depression (Spinelli 1997) and depressed adolescents (Mufson et al. 1999). On the other hand, IPT was not better than control conditions in two studies of patients with substance abuse (Carroll et al. 1991, Rounsaville et al. 1983).

## Cognitive Therapy, Behavior Therapy, and CBT Studies

Numerous studies have used cognitive and/or behavioral therapies to treat depression (Thase 2001). A few studies stand out, however, as examples of sophisticated work employing "clean" research methodologies. In addition to the large TDCRP study of Elkin and colleagues (1989) discussed earlier, Thompson and colleagues (1987), Hollon and colleagues (1992), and Evans and colleagues (1992) have done excellent work demonstrating the efficacy of cognitive and/or behavioral therapy for depression.

Thompson and colleagues (1987) randomly assigned 91 depressed geriatric patients to one of four treatment cells: cognitive therapy (CT), behavior therapy (BT), Horowitz's psychodynamically oriented stress-response psychotherapy (Horowitz et al. 1984), and a waitlist. All three active treatments produced greater improvement at 16 to 20 weeks than waitlist, with no significant differences among them. There was a nonsignificant trend showing the highest response rates in the behavioral group followed by the psychodynamic group and then by the cognitive group.

Hollon and colleagues (1992) randomly assigned over 100 depressed outpatients to either imipramine plus clinical management, CT alone, or CT plus imipramine. Twenty CBT sessions were administered over 12 weeks. Despite high attrition (64 of 107 patients completed the study), all three treatments showed efficacy, with a nonsignificant trend suggesting that the combined treatment did better than either treatment alone. As discussed previously, follow-up data suggested that the effects of CBT were more enduring than the effects of an acute course of imipramine, albeit medication was stopped after a brief 3-month course (Evans et al. 1992).

In one of the more provocative studies in the TLP literature, Fairburn and colleagues (1995) randomly assigned patients suffering from bulimia nervosa ($N = 89$) to 18 sessions of CBT, BT, or IPT. Investigators had originally included IPT in this study as an "inactive" control condition, but at long-term follow-up (mean 5.8 years), there were no differences between IPT and CBT in the number of patients who remained remitted. A follow-up, multicenter comparison of CBT to IPT for the treatment of bulimia ($N = 220$) found that patients assigned to CBT remitted faster than those assigned to IPT but also found no significant differences between treatments at 12-month follow-up (Agras et al. 2000).

A large, multicenter study ($N = 681$) randomly assigned subjects diagnosed with chronic depression to 12 weeks of nefazodone ($N = 226$), cognitive–behavioral analysis system of psychotherapy (CBASP) ($N = 228$), or their combination ($N = 227$). In intent-to-treat analyses, significantly more subjects assigned to nefazodone plus CBASP responded to treatment (73%) than those assigned to either nefazodone (48%) or CBASP (48%) alone (for both, $p < 0.001$). The mean scores on the 24-item version of the Ham-D posttreatment (week 12) were 14.7 ($\pm 0.70$), 15.1 ($\pm 0.69$), and 9.7 ($\pm 0.65$) for the nefazodone, CBASP, and combination treatment groups, respectively. These relatively high posttreatment scores suggest that many patients experienced clinically significant residual symptoms after treatment (Keller et al. 2000).

Prolonged exposure (PE) is a treatment for PTSD that uses techniques such as imaginal exposure to help patients emotionally reprocess a traumatic event (Foa and Rothbaum 1998). Stress inoculation training (SIT) uses the techniques of relaxation, breathing retraining, and thought stopping to manage anxiety and intrusive thoughts. Foa and colleagues (1991) randomly assigned 45 rape victims with PTSD to nine biweekly sessions of PE, SIT, supportive counseling, or to a waitlist control. All subjects improved on measures of anxiety, depression, and PTSD symptoms, although SIT produced greater improvement in PTSD symptoms than supportive counseling or waitlist immediately posttreatment. At 3-month follow-up, however, there was a trend for subjects assigned to PE to show further improvement in PTSD scores relative to posttreatment. They hypothesized that while SIT resulted in immediate reductions in anxiety symptoms, PE produced a more enduring change through emotional processing of the traumatic event (Foa et al. 1991). In a follow-up study, 96 victims of an assault who suffered from PTSD were randomly assigned to PE, SIT, combination PE plus SIT, or a waitlist control. All active treatments were superior to waitlist but were not different from each other at posttreatment and follow-up. In intent-to-treat analyses, PE had larger effect on PTSD severity, depression, and anxiety than the other active treatments (Foa et al. 1999).

Cognitive and behavioral therapies have also demonstrated efficacy for the treatment of other disorders, in particular, anxiety spectrum disorders, eating disorders, sexual disorders, and substance abuse. For a fuller discussion of these issues, see Chapter 86 in this book.

## Brief Psychodynamic Psychotherapy Studies

These first generation treatments, extensively reviewed in an earlier version of this chapter (Swartz and Markowitz 1997), have not been subjected to the same kind of rigorous studies as the second generation TLPs, with one notable exception. Luborsky and colleagues at the University of Pennsylvania developed and tested a psychodynamic psychotherapy—supportive–expressive therapy (SE) that can be used in an open-ended or time-limited format (Luborsky 1984). Luborsky credits Sifneos and Malan as significant influences in the evolution of his technique.

Most of the Penn Psychotherapy Project's research has been directed toward process variables (i.e., identifying treatment variables that affect the process of psychotherapy). Woody, however, used SE in a controlled outcome trial looking at the treatment of opiate addicts (Woody et al. 1983). One hundred and ten opiate addicts in a methadone maintenance program were randomly assigned to one of three clinical conditions: drug counseling alone (a treatment that addresses external coping skills); drug counseling plus CBT; or drug counseling plus SE. The two psychotherapies were administered for 6 months. Outcome measures included standardized ratings of mood, function, and addiction behaviors. The SE and CBT groups showed statistically significant improvement compared to the control group in social function (e.g., number of days worked) and psychiatric symptoms (e.g., ratings on the Beck Depression Inventory, Symptom Check List 90, and Maudsley Personality Inventory). There were no statistically significant differences in efficacy on any measure between the two psychotherapy groups. A reanalysis of the data showed no differences among the three groups on any measures of illicit or prescribed drug use (Woody et al. 1990). Crits-Christoph and colleagues (1999) randomly assigned 487 subjects with cocaine dependence to 6 months of treatment: individual drug counseling plus group drug counseling (GDC), cognitive therapy (CT) plus GDC, SE plus GDC, or GDC alone. Subjects assigned to individual drug counseling plus GDC showed greater improvement on a variety of measures, including addiction behaviors, than subjects assigned to CT plus GDC, SE plus GDC, or GDC alone. Typical of studies treating substance abusers, attrition was very high in this study (only 28% of subjects enrolled completed the study). In contrast to the earlier study of opioid addiction, it seems that there are no advantages to adding CT or SE to drug counseling for the treatment of cocaine addiction.

## Motivational Interviewing Studies

Motivational interviewing (MI) has been used primarily as a treatment for maladaptive behaviors such as substance abuse or smoking. A meta-analysis found motivational interviewing to be among the best-supported interventions for alcohol problems (Miller et al. 1998). For instance, Brown and Miller (1993) showed that subjects ($N = 28$) entering a residential alcohol program who participated in a single session of MI exhibited lower alcohol consumption at 3 months than subjects who did not participate in an MI session. Project Matching Alcoholism Treatments to Client Heterogeneity (MATCH), a large ($N = 1,726$), randomized study, compared three manualized treatments for alcohol abuse: 12 sessions of CBT, a four-session psychotherapy based on MI principles called motivational enhancement therapy (MET), and a 12-session twelve-step facilitation (TSF) treatment administered over 12 weeks. There were no differences in outcomes among groups on measures of percent days abstinent or drinks per drinking day, with all treatments leading to significant reductions in these behaviors (Kadden 1996, Project MATCH Research Group 1997). MET was the least expensive treatment of the three (Cisler et al. 1998).

## Psychodynamic–Interpersonal Psychotherapy Studies

Investigators from the UK have published several reports on the efficacy and effectiveness of psychodynamic–interpersonal (PI) psychotherapy for the treatment of various psychiatric disorders. This treatment is based on both psychodynamic and interpersonal principles (Hobson 1985), but can be distinguished from both psychodynamic psychotherapy and IPT (Guthrie et al. 1998). As in IPT, PI focuses on the connection between mood and interpersonal relationships but uses transference and metaphor as tools for resolving interpersonal difficulties. In contrast to traditional psychodynamic psychotherapies, there is relatively *less* emphasis on the interpretation of the transference;

however, in contrast to IPT, transference feelings are examined. Guthrie and colleagues (1999) recruited a sample of patients with severe, refractory, nonpsychotic, psychiatric illness, defined as failing to improve following at least 6 months of usual psychiatric care. Subjects ($N = 110$) were randomly assigned to eight weekly sessions of PI or continued usual care from a mental health provider. At 6-month follow-up, subjects assigned to PI experienced significantly greater improvement than controls on measures of global illness severity, depressive symptoms, and social functioning. The same team of investigators conducted a separate study of a four-session version of PI to treat patients who had attempted to kill themselves by overdose or toxic ingestion. One hundred and nineteen subjects were randomly assigned to either brief PI ($N = 58$) or treatment as usual ($N = 61$). At 6-month follow-up, those assigned to PI were significantly less likely to have made another suicide attempt and had significantly lower scores on an instrument assessing suicidal ideation (Guthrie et al. 2001). These studies are remarkable for both their strong research designs (internal validity) and generalizability to routine practice settings (external validity).

In earlier studies, depressed subjects ($N = 117$) were randomly assigned to 8 or 16 sessions of CBT or PI. On most acute outcome measures, CBT and PI were equally effective, irrespective of duration of treatment. (Shapiro et al. 1994). Among subjects who completed a mailed assessment 1 year after completing treatment ($N = 104$), those who had received only eight sessions of PI had a greater chance of relapse than those assigned to 16 sessions of PI or 8 or 16 sessions of CBT (Shapiro et al. 1995). Although data from the acute phase of the study suggested that the more severely depressed patients assigned to 16 sessions of CBT fared better than those assigned to eight sessions, at 1-year follow-up, there were no measurable benefits of 16 sessions of CBT over eight sessions.

## Conclusion

In 1975, Luborsky asked the question, "Is it true that 'everyone has won and all must have prizes'?" (Luborsky and Singer 1975). In other words, are all psychotherapies equally efficacious for all conditions and all patients all of the time? In the ensuing decades, through more systematic studies of TLPs, we have begun to establish the efficacy of specific psychotherapies for specific disorders. Moving beyond the first generation TLPs that used psychodynamic principles to treat mildly ill patients with heterogeneous diagnoses, the second generation of TLPs are characterized by written manuals that specify treatment interventions for defined disorders and populations. Research questions have become more pointed and evidence has begun to accumulate documenting the efficacy of specific treatments for specific conditions.

In the process of focusing the lens, however, we may have lost sight of the big picture. As Guthrie (2000) points out, although patients in real world settings experience chronic symptoms and multiple disorders, psychotherapy researchers have typically excluded these patients from outcome studies. Since the first version of this chapter was published in 1997, there have been great strides in the field of TLP research. The next challenge will be to develop strategies to disseminate these evidence-based (*efficacy* proven) TLPs into general clinical settings and to conduct new (*effectiveness*) psychotherapy studies of their relevance in general psychiatric populations.

It seems likely, however, that the supremacy of psychoanalysis has ended and that TLPs are here to stay. Their indications are not universal, but they do address many of the syndromes with which patients present for treatment. Future empirical work may focus on further defining psychotherapy duration, with the dual goals of establishing the fewest number of sessions that can be used to treat a given problem and identifying those patients for whom longer courses of therapy are indicated.

## Acknowledgment

The authors would like to thank Danielle Novick for her assistance in the preparation of the chapter.

Preparation of this chapter was supported, in part, by a grant from the National Institute of Mental Health, MH-64519 (H.A.S.).

## References

Addis ME and Krasnow AD (2000) A national survey of practicing psychologists' attitudes toward psychotherapy treatment manuals. J Consult Clin Psychol 68(2), 331–339.

Agras WS, Walsh T, Fairburn CG, et al. (2000) A multicenter comparison of cognitive–behavioral therapy and interpersonal psychotherapy for bulimia nervosa. Arch Gen Psychiatr 57(5), 459–466.

Andrade L, Eaton WW, and Chilcoat H (1994) Lifetime comorbidity of panic attacks and major depression in a population-based study. Symptom profiles. Br J Psychiatr 165(3), 363–369.

Balint M, Ornstein PH, and Balint E (1972) Focal Psychotherapy. Tavistock, Wiltshire, England.

Barkham M, Shapiro DA, Hardy GE, et al. (1999) Psychotherapy in two-plus-one sessions: Outcomes of a randomized controlled trial of cognitive–behavioral and psychodynamic–interpersonal therapy for subsyndromal depression. J Consult Clin Psychol 67(2), 201–211.

Barlow DH (1997) Cognitive–behavioral therapy for panic disorder: Current status. J Clin Psychiatr 58(Suppl 2), 32–36; discussion 36–37.

Beck AT and Steer RA (1990) Manual for the revised Beck Anxiety Inventory. Psychological Corporation, San Antonio, TX.

Beck AT and Steer RA (1993) Manual for the Beck Depression Inventory. Psychological Corporation, San Antonio, TX.

Beck AT, Rush AJ, Shaw BF, et al. (1979) Cognitive therapy of depression. Guilford Press, New York.

Blackburn IM, Eunson KM, and Bishop S (1986) A two-year naturalistic follow-up of depressed patients treated with cognitive therapy, pharmacotherapy and a combination of both. J Affect Disord 10(1), 67–75.

Blatt SJ, Zuroff DC, Bondi CM, et al. (2000) Short- and long-term effects of medication and psychotherapy in the brief treatment of depression: Further analyses of data from the NIMH TDCRP. Psychother Res 10(2), 215–234.

Brenner C (1974) An Elementary Textbook of Psychoanalysis, revised and expanded edition. Anchor Press/Doubleday, New York.

Brown JM and Miller WR (1993) Impact of motivational interviewing on participation and outcome in residential alcoholism treatment. Psychol Addict Behav 7(4), 211–218.

Burns DD and Nolen-Hoeksema S (1992) Therapeutic empathy and recovery from depression in cognitive–behavioral therapy: A structural equation model. J Consult Clin Psychol 60(3), 441–449.

Carroll KM, Rounsaville BJ, and Gawin FH (1991) A comparative trial of psychotherapies for ambulatory cocaine abusers: Relapse prevention and interpersonal psychotherapy. Am J Drug Alcohol Abuse 17(3), 229–247.

Cisler R, Holder HD, Longabaugh R, et al. (1998) Actual and estimated replication costs for alcohol treatment modalities: Case study from Project MATCH. J Stud Alcohol 59(5), 503–512.

Clark DM, Salkovskis PM, Hackmann A, et al. (1999) Brief cognitive therapy for panic disorder: A randomized controlled trial. J Consult Clin Psychol 67(4), 583–589.

Coryell W, Endicott J, and Winokur G (1992) Anxiety syndromes as epiphenomena of primary major depression: Outcome and familial psychopathology. Am J Psychiatr 149(1), 100–107.

Crits-Christoph P, Siqueland L, Blaine J, et al. (1999) Psychosocial treatments for cocaine dependence: National Institute on Drug Abuse Collaborative Cocaine Treatment Study. Arch Gen Psychiatr 56(5), 493–502.

Davanloo H (ed) (1978) Basic Principles and Techniques in Short-Term Dynamic Psychotherapy. Spectrum, New York.

Davanloo H (ed) (1980) Short-Term Dynamic Psychotherapy. Jason Aronson, Northvale, NJ.

DiMascio A, Weissman MM, Prusoff BA, et al. (1979) Differential symptom reduction by drugs and psychotherapy in acute depression. Arch Gen Psychiatr 36(13), 1450–1456.

Eells TD (ed) (1997) Handbook of Psychotherapy Case Formulation. Guilford Press, New York.

Elkin I, Shea MT, Watkins JT, et al. (1989) National Institute of Mental Health Treatment of Depression Collaborative Research Program: General effectiveness of treatments. Arch Gen Psychiatr 46(11), 971–982.

Evans MD, Hollon SD, DeRubeis RJ, et al. (1992) Differential relapse following cognitive therapy and pharmacotherapy for depression. Arch Gen Psychiatr 49(10), 802–808.

Fairburn CG (1998) Interpersonal psychotherapy for bulimia nervosa. In (ed) Interpersonal Psychotherapy. Review of Psychiatry Series, JC Markowitz American Psychiatric Press, Washington DC, pp. 99–128.

Fairburn CG, Norman PA, Welch SL, et al. (1995) A prospective study of outcome in bulimia nervosa and the long-term effects of three psychological treatments. Arch Gen Psychiatr 52(4), 304–312.

Ferenczi S (1950) The further development of an active therapy in psychoanalysis (1920). In Further Contributions to the Theory and Technique of Psychoanalysis, S Ferenczi (ed). The Hogarth Press, London.

Foa EB and Rothbaum BO (1998) Treating the trauma of rape: Cognitive–behavioral therapy for PTSD. Guilford Press, New York.

Foa EB, Dancu CV, Hembree EA, et al. (1999) A comparison of exposure therapy, stress inoculation training, and their combination for reducing posttraumatic stress disorder in female assault victims. J Consult Clin Psychol 67(2), 194–200.

Foa EB, Rothbaum BO, Riggs DS, et al. (1991) Treatment of posttraumatic stress disorder in rape victims: A comparison between cognitive–behavioral procedures and counseling. J Consult Clin Psychol 59(5), 715–723.

Frances A, Clarkin J, and Perry S (1984) Differential Therapeutics in Psychiatry: The Art and Science of Treatment Selection. Brunner/Mazel, New York, pp. xviii, 147.

Frank E (1991) Interpersonal psychotherapy as a maintenance treatment for patients with recurrent depression. Psychotherapy 28(2), 259–266.

Frank E, Grochocinski VJ, Spanier CA, et al. (2000a) Interpersonal psychotherapy and antidepressant medication: Evaluation of a sequential treatment strategy in women with recurrent major depression. J Clin Psychiatr 61(1), 51–57.

Frank E, Kupfer DJ, Perel JM, et al. (1990) Three-year outcomes for maintenance therapies in recurrent depression. Arch Gen Psychiatr 47(12), 1093–1099.

Frank E, Shear MK, Rucci P, et al. (2000b) Influence of panic–agorophobic spectrum symptoms on treatment response in patients with recurrent major depression. Am J Psychiatr 157(7), 1101–1107.

Frank E, Swartz HA, Mallinger AG, et al. (1999) Adjunctive psychotherapy for bipolar disorder: Effects of changing treatment modality. J Abnorm Psychol 108(4), 579–587.

Frank J (1971) Therapeutic factors in psychotherapy. Am J Psychother 25, 350–361.

Grunhaus L, Harel Y, Krugler T, et al. (1988) Major depressive disorder and panic disorder. Effects of comorbidity on treatment outcome with antidepressant medications. Clin Neuropharmacol 11(5), 454–461.

Grunhaus L, Pande AC, Brown MB, et al. (1994) Clinical characteristics of patients with concurrent major depressive disorder and panic disorder. Am J Psychiatr 151(4), 541–546.

Guthrie E (2000) Psychotherapy for patients with complex disorders and chronic symptoms. The need for a new research paradigm. Br J Psychiatr 177, 131–137.

Guthrie E, Kapur N, Mackway-Jones K, et al. (2001) Randomized controlled trial of brief psychological intervention after deliberate self poisoning. BMJ 323(7305), 135–138.

Guthrie E, Moorey J, Barker H, et al. (1998) Brief psychodynamic–interpersonal therapy for patients with severe psychiatric illness which is unrepsonsive to treatment. Br J Psychother 15(2), 155–166.

Guthrie E, Moorey J, Margison F, et al. (1999) Cost-effectiveness of brief psychodynamic–interpersonal therapy in high utilizers of psychiatric services. Arch Gen Psychiatr 57(6), 519–526.

Hamilton M (1960) A rating scale for depression. J Neurol Neurosurg Psychiatr 25, 56–62.

Hirschfeld RM, Klerman GL, Clayton PJ, et al. (1983) Assessing personality: Effects of the depressive state on trait measurement. Am J Psychiatr 140(6), 695–699.

Hobson RF (1985) Forms of Feeling. Tavistock, London.

Hollifield M, Katon W, Skipper B, et al. (1997) Panic disorder and quality of life: Variables predictive of functional impairment. Am J Psychiatr 154(6), 766–772.

Hollon SD, DeRubeis RJ, Evans MD, et al. (1992) Cognitive therapy and pharmacotherapy for depression. Singly and in combination. Arch Gen Psychiatr 49(10), 774–781.

Horowitz MJ, Marmar C, Weiss DS, et al. (1984) Brief psychotherapy of bereavement reactions. The relationship of process to outcome. Arch Gen Psychiatr 41(5), 438–448.

Howard KI, Kopta SM, Krause MS, et al. (1986) The dose–effect relationship in psychotherapy. Am Psychol 41(2), 159–164.

Kadden RM (1996) Project MATCH: Treatment main effects and matching results. Alcohol Clin Exp Res 20(Suppl 8), 196A–197A.

Keller MB, McCullough JP, Klein DN, et al. (2000) A comparison of nefazodone, the cognitive–behavioral analysis system of psychotherapy, and their combination for the treatment of chronic depression. New Engl J Med 342(20), 1462–1470.

Kessler RC, McGonagle KA, Zhao S, et al. (1994) Lifetime and 12-month prevalence of DSM-III-R psychiatric disorders in the United States: Results from the National Comorbidity Study. Arch Gen Psychiatr 51(1), 8–19.

Klerman GL, Weissman MM, Rounsaville BJ, et al. (1984) Interpersonal Psychotherapy of Depression. Basic Books, New York.

Kornstein SG and Schneider RK (2001) Clinical features of treatment-resistant depression. J Clin Psychiatr 62(Suppl 16), 18–25.

Koss MP and Shiang J (1994) Research on brief psychotherapy. In Handbook of Psychotherapy and Behavior Change, Bergin AE and Garfield SL (eds). John Wiley, New York, pp. 664–700.

Krupnick JL, Sotsky SM, Simmens S, et al. (1996) The role of the therapeutic alliance in psychotherapy and pharmacotherapy outcome: Findings in the National Institute of Mental Health Treatment of Depression Collaborative Research Program. J Consult Clin Psychol 64(3), 532–539.

Kuyken W, Kurzer N, DeRubeis RJ, et al. (2001) Response to cognitive therapy in depression: The role of maladaptive beliefs and personality disorders. J Consult Clin Psychol 69(3), 560–566.

Lambert MJ (1998) What are the implications of psychotherapy research for clinical practice and training. Nord J Psychiatr 52(Suppl 41), 38–49.

Linehan MM (1993) Cognitive–Behavioral Treatment of Borderline Personality Disorder. Guilford Press, New York.

Luborsky L (1984) Principles of Psychoanalytic Psychotherapy: A Manual for Supportive–Expressive Treatment. Basic Books, New York.

Luborsky L and Singer B (1975) Comparative studies of psychotherapies. Is it true that "everyone has won and all must have prizes"? Arch Gen Psychiatr 32(8), 995–1008.

Malan DH (1975) A Study of Brief Psychotherapy. Plenum Press, New York.

Malan DH (1976) The Frontier of Brief Psychotherapy. Plenum Medical Books, New York.

Mann J (1973) Time-Limited Psychotherapy. Harvard University Press, Cambridge, Mass.

Mann J (1974) Time-Limited Psychotherapy. Harvard University Press, Cambridge, Mass.

Marangell LB (2001) Switching antidepressants for treatment-resistant major depression. J Clin Psychiatr 62(Suppl 18) 12–17.

Markowitz JC (1998) Interpersonal Psychotherapy for Dysthymic Disorder. American Psychiatric Press, Washington DC.

Markowitz JC (2001) Learning new psychotherapies. In Treatment of Depression: Bridging the 21st Century, MM Weissman (ed). American Psychiatric Press, Washington DC, pp. 281–300.

Markowitz JC and Swartz HA (1997) Case formulation in interpersonal psychotherapy of depression. In Handbook of psychotherapy case formulation, Eells TD (ed). Guilford Press, New York, pp. 192–222.

Markowitz JC, Kocsis JH, Fishman B, et al. (1998) Treatment of depressive symptoms in human immunodeficiency virus-positive patients. Arch Gen Psychiatr 55(5), 452–457.

Marmar CR, Gaston L, Gallagher D, et al. (1989) Alliance and outcome in late-life depression. J Nerv Ment Dis 177(8), 464–472.

Marmor J (1979) Short-term dynamic psychotherapy. Am J Psychiatr 136, 149–155.

McCullough JP Jr. (2000) Treatment for Chronic Depression: Cognitive Behavioral Analysis System of Psychotherapy (CBASP). Guilford Press, New York.

Miller WR and Rollnick S (1991) Motivational Interviewing: Preparing People to Change Addictive Behavior. Guilford Press, New York.

Miller WR, Andrews NR, and Wilbourne P (1998) A wealth of alternatives: Effective treatments for alcohol problems. In Treating Addictive Behaviors, 2nd ed., Miller WR and Heather N (eds). Plenum Press, New York, pp. 203–216.

Milrod B, Busch F, Cooper A, et al. (1997) A Manual for Panic-Focused Psychodynamic Psychotherapy. American Psychiatric Press, Washington DC.

Milrod B, Busch F, Leon AC, et al. (2000) Open trial of psychodynamic psychotherapy for panic disorder: A pilot study. Am J Psychiatr 157(11), 1878–1880.

Mufson L, Weissman MM, Moreau D, et al. (1999) Efficacy of interpersonal psychotherapy for depressed adolescents. Arch Gen Psychiatr 57(6), 573–579.

Nierenberg AA and DeCecco LM (2001) Definitions of antidepressant treatment response, remission, nonresponse, partial response, and other relevant outcomes: A focus on treatment-resistant depression. J Clin Psychiatr 62(Suppl 16), 5–9.

O'Hara MW, Stuart S, Gorman LL, et al. (2000) Efficacy of interpersonal psychotherapy for postpartum depression. Arch Gen Psychiatr 57(11), 1039–1045.

Parsons T (1951) Illness and the role of the physician: A sociological perspective. Am J Orthopsychiatr 21, 452–460.

Project MATCH Research Group (1997) Matching alcoholism treatments to client heterogeneity: Project MATCH posttreatment drinking outcomes [see comments]. J Stud Alcohol 58(1), 7–29.

Rank O (1952) The Trauma of Birth (1924) Robert Brunner, New York.

Reynolds CF III, Frank E, and Perel JM (1999) Nortriptyline and interpersonal psychotherapy as maintenance therapies for recurrent major depression: A randomized controlled trial in patients older than 59 years. J Am Med Assoc 281(1), 39–45.

Rounsaville BJ, Glazer W, and Wilber CH (1983) Short-term interpersonal psychotherapy in methadone-maintained opiate addicts. Arch Gen Psychiatr 40(6), 629–636.

Schulberg HC, Block MR, and Madonia MJ (1996) Treating major depression in primary care practice: Eight-month clinical outcomes. Arch Gen Psychiatr 53(10), 913–919.

Shapiro DA, Barkham M, and Rees A (1994) Effects of treatment duration and severity of depression on the effectiveness of cognitive–behavioral and psychodynamic–interpersonal psychotherapy [see comments]. J Consult Clin Psychol 62(3), 522–534.

Shapiro DA, Rees A, Barkham M, et al. (1995) Effects of treatment duration and severity of depression on the maintenance of gains after cognitive–behavioral and psychodynamic–interpersonal psychotherapy [see comments]. J Consult Clin Psychol 63(3), 378–387.

Shea MT, Elkin I, Imber SD, et al. (1992) Course of depressive symptoms over follow-up. Findings from the National Institute of Mental Health Treatment of Depression Collaborative Research Program. Arch Gen Psychiatr 49(10), 782–787.

Shea MT, Pilkonis PA, Beckham E, et al. (1990) Personality disorders and treatment outcome in the NIMH Treatment of Depression Collaborative Research Program. Am J Psychiatr 147(6), 711–718.

Sifneos PE (1978) The teaching and supervising of STAPP. In Basic Principles and Techniques in Short-Term Dynamic Psychotherapy, Davanloo H (ed). Spectrum, New York, pp. 491–499.

Sifneos PE (1979) Short-Term Dynamic Psychotherapy: Evaluation and Technique. Plenum Press, New York.

Simons AD, Murphy GE, Levine JL, et al. (1986) Cognitive therapy and pharmacotherapy for depression. Sustained improvement over one year. Arch Gen Psychiatr 43(1), 43–48.

Sotsky SM, Glass DR, Shea MT, et al. (1991) Patient predictors of response to psychotherapy and pharmacotherapy: Findings in the NIMH Treatment of Depression Collaborative Research Program. Am J Psychiatr 148(8), 997–1008.

Spinelli MG (1997) Interpersonal psychotherapy for depressed antepartum women: A pilot study. Am J Psychiatr 154(7), 1028–1030.

Swartz HA and Markowitz JC (1997) Time-limited psychotherapy. In Psychiatry, Vol. 2, Tasman A, Kay J, and Lieberman JA (eds). WB Saunders, Philadelphia, pp. 1405–1417.

Swartz HA and Markowitz JC (1998) Interpersonal psychotherapy for the treatment of depression in HIV-positive men and women. In Interpersonal Psychotherapy. Review of Psychiatry Series, Markowitz JC (ed). American Psychiatric Press, Washington DC, pp. 129–155.

Swartz HA, Frank E, Shear MK, et al. (2002) Pilot study of brief interpersonal psychotherapy. Poster presented at the Second Annual Research Day, Western Psychiatric Institute and Clinic, Pittsburgh, PA.

Thase ME (2001) Depression-focused psychotherapies. In Treatment of Psychiatric Disorders, 3rd ed., Gabbard GO (ed). American Psychiatric Press, Washington DC, pp. 1181–1227.

Thase ME and Rush AJ (1995) Treatment-resistant depression. In Psychopharmacology: The Fourth Generation of Progress, Bloom FE and Kupfer DJ (eds). Raven Press, New York.

Thase ME, Buysse DJ, Frank E, et al. (1997) Which depressed patients will respond to interpersonal psychotherapy? The role of abnormal EEG sleep profiles. Am J Psychiatr 154(4), 502–509.

Thompson LW, Gallagher D, and Breckenridge JS (1987) Comparative effectiveness of psychotherapies for depressed elders. J Consult Clin Psychol 55(3), 385–390.

Ursano RJ and Hales RE (1986) A review of brief individual psychotherapies. Am J Psychiatr 143(12), 1507–1517.

Weiss M, Gaston L, Propst A, et al. (1997) The role of the alliance in the pharmacologic treatment of depression. J Clin Psychiatr 58(5), 196–204.

Weissman MM, Markowitz JC, and Klerman GL (2000) Comprehensive Guide to Interpersonal Psychotherapy. Basic Books, New York.

Woody G, Luborsky L, McLellan AT, et al. (1990) Corrections and revised analyses for psychotherapy in methadone maintenance patients. Arch Gen Psychiatr 47(8), 788–789.

Woody GE, Luborsky L, McLellan AT, et al. (1983) Psychotherapy for opiate addicts. Does it help? Arch Gen Psychiatr 40(6), 639–645.

Zlotnick C, Elkin I, and Shea MT (1998) Does the gender of a patient or the gender of a therapist affect the treatment of patients with major depression? J Consult Clin Psychol 66(4), 655–659.

# 86 Cognitive and Behavioral Therapies

Edward S. Friedman
Michael E. Thase
Jesse H. Wright

The cognitive and behavioral therapies have evolved over the past 40 years as an alternative to more traditional non-directive and insight-oriented modes of psychotherapy (Beck 1991, Wolpe 1982, Kazdin 1982, Robins and Hays 1993). The family of cognitive and behavioral therapies includes a diverse group of interventions. Nevertheless, the treatments share several pragmatic and theoretical assumptions. First, these therapies emphasize a psychoeducational orientation, by which patients learn about the nature of their difficulties and the rationale for use of particular treatment strategies. Second, the cognitive and behavioral therapies typically employ homework and self-help assignments to provide patients the opportunity to practice therapeutic methods to enhance generalization outside of the therapy hour. Third, objective assessment of psychiatric illness is considered an integral part of treatment, and selection of therapeutic strategies derives logically from such assessments. Fourth, the therapeutic methods used are generally structured, are directive, and require a high level of therapist activity. As such, the cognitive and behavioral therapies tend to be easier than other approaches to describe in treatment manuals. Fifth, for most disorders, the cognitive and behavioral therapies are time-limited interventions. Sixth, and perhaps most important, these therapies are built on empirical evidence that validates the theoretical orientation and guides the choice of therapeutic techniques. Specifically, learning theories (i.e., classical, operant, and observational models of learning) and the principles of cognitive psychology are relied on heavily in constructing cognitive–behavioral treatment models.

## Cognitive Model

The basic theories of the cognitive model are rooted in a long tradition of viewing cognitions as primary determinants of emotion and behavior. Cognitive therapy concepts have been traced as far as the writings of the Greek Stoic philosophers (Beck 1976, Ellis 1989, Dobson and Block 1988) and have been linked to a number of other influences, including the phenomenological school of philosophy, Albert Ellis' rational emotive therapy, and the contributions of Adler and other neo-Freudians (Wright and Beck 1994). However, the greatest impetus for the development of cognitively oriented therapy has been the work of Aaron T. Beck (1963, 1964, 1967, 1976, 1991, 1993). For an excellent review of the historical bases of cognitive therapy, see Dobson and Block (1988) and Clark, Beck, and Alford (1999). Clark and coworkers (1999) also provide an excellent review of the philosophical and theoretical assumptions of the cognitive theory of depression.

At the time Beck began to formulate his theories, the predominant treatment approach was psychoanalytically oriented therapy. Freud conceived of depression as resulting from anger turned inward (Freud 1950). However, when Beck attempted to study depression from this perspective, he noted stereotypical patterns of pessimistic and self-critical thinking, and distorted information processing were essential characteristics of depression (Beck 1963). This early work led to development of a cognitive model of depression (Beck 1964), the description of specific treatment interventions, and a substantial research effort to study cognitive functioning and treatment outcome in a variety of disorders. (Beck 1976, Wright and Beck 1994, Beck et al. 1979, Beck and Rush 2000).

Along the way, contributions from cognitive psychologists, behavioral therapists, and other clinical practitioners have been incorporated into the cognitive model (Meichenbaum 1977, Nelson and Craighead 1977, Hollan and Kendall 1980, Lewinsohn et al. 1982, Clark 1986, Dobson and Shaw 1986, Barlow and Cerny 1988, Wright and Thase 1992). The description of cognitive theories given here is based largely on Beck's concepts. This model of therapy tends to give somewhat more emphasis to cognitive than behavioral factors in treatment interventions, but both are considered to be integral parts of the model (Figure 86–1).

Depending on the case formulation and the phase of therapy, attention may be directed primarily at cognitive or behavioral aspects of the disorder. In most cases, a combination of cognitive and behavioral techniques is used. For this reason, we use the term cognitive–behavioral therapy (CBT) throughout the chapter unless referring to a specific form of behavioral treatment.

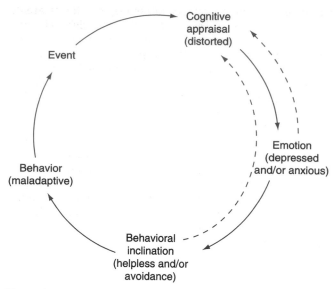

**Figure 86–1** *A working model for cognitive–behavioral therapy. (Source: Wright JH [1988] Cognitive therapy of depression. In The American Psychiatric Press Review of Psychiatry, Vol. 7, Frances AJ and Hales RE [eds]. American Psychiatric Press, Washington DC, pp. 554–590.)*

Figure 86–2 displays a simplified model for understanding the relationships between environmental events, cognitions, emotion, and behavior (Wright and Beck 1994, Wright 1988, Thase and Beck 1993). This model is based on the theoretical assumption that environmental stimuli trigger cognitive processes and the ensuing cognitions give the event personal meaning and elicit subsequent physiological and affective arousal. These emotions, in turn, have a potent reciprocal effect on cognitive content and information processing, such that cascades of dysfunctional thoughts and emotions can occur. The individual's behavioral responses to stimuli and thoughts are viewed as both a product and a cause of maladaptive cognitions. Thus, treatment interventions may be targeted at any or all components of the model.

Of course, many other factors are involved in psychiatric disorders, including genetic predisposition, state-

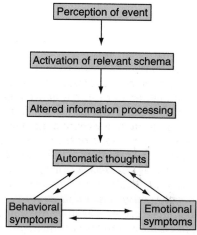

**Figure 86–2** *Cognitive model of information processing.*

dependent neurobiological changes, and various interpersonal variables. These influences are also included in the case conceptualization in CBT. Wright and Thase (1992) have outlined an expanded cognitive–biological model that can be used for synthesizing cognitive and neurobiological factors in a combined therapy approach. Contemporary psychiatric research is striving to understand how best to combine and/or sequence CBT and pharmacotherapy, and relate CBT technique to new understandings in cognitive neuroscience. Nevertheless, the working model in Figure 86–2 can be used as a practical template to guide the therapist's case formulation and interventions.

## Automatic Thoughts and Schemas

Dysfunctional information processing is apparent in many psychiatric disorders at two major levels of cognition–automatic thoughts and schemas (Beck 1976, Dobson and Shaw 1986, Teasdale 1983, Segal 1988, Alfrod and Correia 1994). Automatic thoughts are cognitions that stream rapidly through an individual's mind, whether spontaneously or in response to some prompt or stimulus. Automatic thoughts may be triggered by affective arousal (i.e., anger, anxiety, or sadness), or conversely, affective shifts are generally accompanied by automatic negative thoughts (Teasdale 1983). Their automatic nature refers to their speed of entry into awareness and their implicit believability. In this way, automatic thoughts have emotional validity (Thase and Beck 1993). For most people, before therapy, automatic thoughts are usually not examined carefully for validity. In fact, many people susceptible to anxiety or depression are likely to use an affectively focused logic referred to as emotional reasoning (i.e., "I *feel* that this is correct, therefore it is correct"). Although we all experience automatic thoughts, in depression, anxiety, and other psychiatric disorders the thoughts are distinguished by their greater intensity and frequency (LeFebvre 1981).

Beck (1967) coined the term *cognitive triad* to describe the content of automatic negative thoughts. Typically, automatic negative thoughts may be grouped by themes pertaining to self, world (i.e., significant others or people in general), and future. As described subsequently, the themes revealed in one's characteristic automatic negative thoughts may be used to infer deeper levels of cognition: beliefs, rules, and schemas. Patients can be taught to examine their beliefs and their operational rules. Although patients are not fully aware of their schemas, these cognitions are usually accessible through the questioning techniques used in CBT (Wright and Beck 1994).

Beck and coworkers (Beck et al. 1979, Beck and Emery 1985, Wright and Beck 1983) have noted that stereotypic errors in logic (termed cognitive errors or cognitive distortions) also shape the content of automatic thoughts. Examples of these processes include personalization, magnification and minimization, all-or-nothing thinking, jumping to conclusions, and ignoring the evidence or selective abstraction. Definitions of a number of common cognitive errors are included in Table 86–1. Cognitive errors help to translate between the "surface" level of cognition (revealed in automatic negative thoughts) and deeper cognitive structures such as basic assumptions, rules, and schemas (Thase and Beck 1993, Segal 1988, Young and Lindermann 1992). It has been proposed that such appar-

| Table 86–1 | Common Patterns of Irrational Thinking in Anxiety and Depression |
|---|---|
| Cognitive Error | Definition |
| Overgeneralization | Evidence is drawn from one experience or a small set of experiences that reach an unwarranted conclusion with far-reaching implications. |
| Catastrophic thinking | An extreme example of overgeneralization, in which the impact of a clearly negative event or experience is amplified to extreme proportions, e.g, "If I have a panic attack, I will lose *all* control and go crazy (or die)." |
| Maximizing and minimizing | The tendency to exaggerate negative experiences and minimize positive experiences in one's activities and interpersonal relationships. |
| All-or-none (black or white, absolutistic) thinking | An unnecessary division of complex or continuous outcomes into polarized extremes, e.g., "Either I am a success at this, or I am a total failure." |
| Jumping to conclusions | Use of pessimism or earlier experiences of failure to prematurely or inappropriately predict failure in a new situation; also known as fortune-telling. |
| Personalization | Interpretation of an event, situation, or behavior as salient or personally indicative of a negative aspect of self. |
| Selective negative focus—"ignoring the evidence" or "mental filter" | Undesirable or negative events, memories, or implications are focused on at the expense of recalling or identifying other, more neutral or positive information; in fact, positive information may be ignored *or* disqualified as irrelevant, atypical, or trivial. |

*Source*: Adapted from Beck AT, Rush AJ, Shaw BF, et al. (1979) Cognitive Therapy of Depression. Guilford Press, New York.

ently illogical thinking during times of heightened emotion may have had evolutionary value (Thase and Beck 1993). Specifically, cognitive distortions during periods of affective arousal tend to narrow one's focus of attention, simplify information processing, and intensify behavioral responses. Thus, the individual may be primed to respond decisively to the crisis at hand. This is consistent with recent findings that elucidate the neurocircuitry of brain fear pathways (distinct affective and cognitive pathways). LeDoux has shown that activation of the fear pathway causes a sequential activation of affective (limbic-amygdala branch) and cognitive (hippocampal-cortical branch) pathways. However, the affective pathway is shorter allowing activation milliseconds before the cognitive pathway. This primes the system with a sequenced affective/cognitive response to fearful environmental stimuli (LeDoux 1988).

Schemas represent the sum of one's beliefs and attitudes. They are the basic assumptions or unspoken rules that act as templates for screening and decoding information from the environment (Segal 1988, Wright and Beck 1983, Young and Lindermann 1992). Psychological well-being may be understood in part by development of a set of schemas that yield realistic appraisals of self in relation to

world (e.g., "I'm reasonably attractive, but looks aren't everything," "I can be loved under the right circumstances," or "I must work harder to compensate for an average intellect"). Although unspoken, schemas may be inferred from one's beliefs and attitudes. In the cognitive model, dysfunctional attitudes are the structural "bridge" between pathological schemas and automatic negative thoughts. Schemas pertaining to safety, vulnerability to threat, self-evaluation, one's lovability, and one's competence or self-efficacy contain the ground rules for personal behavior that are particularly relevant to the understanding of disorders such as anxiety, depression, or characterological disturbances. (Segal 1988, Young and Lindermann 1992, Blackburn et al. 1986, Beck et al. 1990). A number of schemas relevant to psychiatric illness are listed in Table 86–2. Bowlby (1985) has noted that most psychopathologically relevant schemas are developed early in life, when the individual is relatively powerless and dependent on caregivers.

The cognitive model of psychiatric illness emphasizes the concept of stress-diathesis (Thase and Beck 1993, Metalsky et al. 1987). From this perspective, a schema such as "I must be loved to have worth," might remain latent until activated by a relevant life stressor (i.e., a romantic breakup). Thus, being "dumped" by a romantic partner may trigger marked emotional response in a person with a "matching" schematic vulnerability but only a normal amount of sadness in someone with a healthier schema (e.g., "I am a worthwhile person that people can love") (Hammen et al. 1989). Some schemas may be influenced by neurobiological factors. In panic disorder, exquisite sensitivity to neurobiological signals, such as the evolutionarily ancient "suffocation alarm," may simultaneously trigger noradrenergic arousal and fearful cognitions (Klein 1993). This combination may underpin the schema "I am weak and unable to cope with distress." In recurrent depression, neurobiological changes may exaggerate stress responsivity, undermine the individual's hardiness in the face of adversity, and dampen hedonic capacity (Wright and Thase 1992). As a result, the individual may develop the dysfunctional attitude "I am powerless to change my destiny."

Underlying schemas may be buttressed by either maladaptive or adaptive attitudes (e.g., "No matter how hard I try, I'm bound to fail" versus "I'm a survivor; if I just hang in there things will be okay"), but many of these cognitive structures have mixed features (Wright and Beck 1994). Schemas such as "If I'm not perfect, I'm a failure" may lead to driven obsessional behavior, rigid attitudes and beliefs, and frequent bouts of dysphoric or irritable moods. However, basic perfectionistic beliefs such as these can also result in high levels of performance and success.

The concept of attributional style (Hammen et al. 1989) describes an alternative view of cognitive vulnerability. Derived from human studies of the learned helplessness paradigm (Seligman 1975), attributional style refers to the characteristic way that people explain the causality, controllability, and impact of events. People susceptible to depression are more likely to have an attributional style in which negative events are perceived to be personally controllable (i.e., internality), far-reaching (i.e., globality), and enduring (i.e., stability) (Peterson et al. 1985, Abramson

| Table 86–2 | Proposed Maladaptive Schemas |
|---|---|

**Autonomy**

| | |
|---|---|
| Dependence | The belief that one is unable to function with the constant support of others |
| Subjugation/lack of individuation | The voluntary or involuntary sacrifice of one's own needs to satisfy others' needs |
| Vulnerability to harm or illness | The fear that disaster (i.e., natural, criminal, medical, or financial) is about to strike at any time |
| Fear of losing self/control | The fear that one will involuntarily lose control of one's own impulses, behavior, emotions, mind, and so on |

**Connectedness**

| | |
|---|---|
| Emotional deprivation | The expectation that one's needs for nurturance, empathy, or affect will never be adequately met by others |
| Abandonment/loss | The fear that one will imminently lose significant others or be emotionally isolated forever |
| Mistrust | The expectation that others will hurt, abuse, cheat, lie, or manipulate you |
| Social isolation/ alienation | The belief that one is isolated from the rest of the world, is different from other people, or does not belong to any group or community |

**Worthiness**

| | |
|---|---|
| Defectiveness/ unlovability | The assumption that one is inwardly defective or that, if the flaw is exposed, one is fundamentally unlovable |
| Social undesirability | The belief that one is outwardly undesirable to others (e.g., ugly, sexually undesirable, low in status, dull, or boring) |
| Incompetence/failure | The assumption that one cannot perform competently in areas of achievement, daily responsibilities, or decision-making |
| Guilt/punishment | The conclusion that one is morally bad or irresponsible and deserving of criticism or punishment |
| Shame/ embarrassment | Recurrent feelings of shame or self-consciousness experienced because one believes that one's inadequacies (as reflected in the preceding maladaption schemas of worthiness) are totally unacceptable to others |

**Limits and Standards**

| | |
|---|---|
| Unrelenting standards | The relentless striving to meet extremely high expectation of oneself, at all costs (i.e., at the expense of happiness, pleasure, health, or satisfactory relationships) |
| Entitlement | Insistence that one should be able to do, say, or have whatever one wants immediately |

*Source*: Thase ME and Beck AT (1992) An overview of cognitive therapy. In Cognitive Therapy with Inpatients: Developing a Cognitive Milieu, Wright JH, Thase ME, Beck AT et al. (eds). Guilford Press, New York, p. 9; adapted from Young (1999) Cognitive Therapy for Personality Disorders: A Schema-Focused Approach. Professional Resource Exchange, Sarasota, FL.

et al. 1989, Sweeney et al. 1986). There is an obvious parallel between the depressogenic attributional style of Abramson and colleagues (1978) and Beck's cognitive triad.

In general, studies of people suffering from depression and anxiety have confirmed that pathological information processing is an important part of these disorders. Negative automatic thoughts and cognitive errors have been found to be more common in depressed patients than in control subjects (Dobson and Shaw 1986, Blackburn et al. 1986b, LeFebvre 1981, Watkins and Rush 1983). Similarly, automatic thoughts concerning uncontrollability, threat, or danger have been documented in patients with high levels of anxiety (Kendall and Hollon 1989, Ingram and Kendall 1987). In clinical studies, depressed subjects also demonstrated elevated levels of dysfunctional attitudes, (Blackburn et al. 1986b, Simons et al. 1984, DeRubeis et al. 1990), distorted attributions to life events, (Abramson et al. 1978, Peterson et al. 1985, Sweeney et al. 1986, Zautra et al. 1985, Deutscher and Cimbolic 1990), and negatively biased responses to feedback (DeMonbreun and Craighead 1977, Rizley 1978, Wenzloff and Grozier 1988). Anxious individuals have been found to have an unrealistic view of the danger or threat in situations (Mathews and MacLeod 1987, Fitzgerald and Phillips 1991), an attentional bias toward threatening stimuli (Mathews and MacLeod 1987), and an enhanced memory for anxiety-provoking situations (Ingram and Kendall 1987, Cloitre and Liebowitz 1991).

Taken together, the results of these studies suggest that disturbances in information processing are essential features of depression and anxiety. Theoretical assumptions and treatment strategies for CBT of many other conditions, including the eating disorders, substance abuse, personality disturbances, and psychoses, have been articulated. The reader is referred to publications on these topics for descriptions of how the cognitive model can be adapted for treatment of a wide variety of psychiatric disorders (Beck et al. 1990, Linehan et al. 1993, Freeman et al. 1989, Sensky and Wright 1993, Beck et al. 1993, Wright et al. 1993, Kingdon and Turkington 1995, Wilkes et al. 1994, Beck and Emery 1985). Specific applications of cognitive and behavioral treatment strategies are described later in the chapter.

## Behavioral Model

The learning theories underpinning the behavioral therapies date to the work of Pavlov (Pavlov and Gantt 1928) and Skinner (1938). Voluminous laboratory research on learning in animals subsequently established certain lawful relationships in the acquisition and maintenance of behavior (Hull 1943, Mowrer 1947, Spence 1956). Moreover, demonstrations that abnormal or "neurotic" behaviors in animals could be either induced by repeated pairings of a noxious stimulus with a neutral one (i.e., classical conditioning) or shaped by controlling reinforcement schedules (i.e., operant conditioning) suggested that these approaches were relevant to psychiatric illness as well (Watson and Rayner 1920, Masserman 1943, Skinner 1948, Wolpe 1952, Lindsley 1956).

By the late 1950s, there was considerable dissatisfaction with the medical and psychoanalytic models of psychopathological processes and treatment, particularly from within academic clinical psychology (Kazdin 1982). Such ferment was underpinned by the low levels of diagnostic reliability, even for well-established illnesses such as schizophrenia (Kanfer and Saslow 1965, Mischel 1968), as well as by the lack of evidence supporting the effectiveness of psychodynamic psychotherapy (Eysenck 1952, Zubin 1953). Moreover, the revolution that has become modern psychopharmacology was still in its infancy; no alternative paradigm at the time had adequate scientific currency. The behavioral therapy movement was thus born, emphasizing the use of scientific principles of investigation with a focus on learned and measurable behaviors (Kazdin 1982, Beck et al. 1990). Further demonstrations of the utility of operant conditioning (i.e., behavior modification experiments in institutionalized, chronically mentally ill patients by use of contingent reinforcement or extinction [Ayllon and Azrin 1968, Ullmann and Krasner 1965]) and counterconditioning treatment of anxiety disorders (such as systematic desensitization [Marks and Gelder 1965, Paul 1966]) triggered a surge of enthusiasm for these more objective treatment methods. By the late 1970s, behavioral therapy had become the most academically influential model of treatment outside of the medical setting (Kazdin 1982, Beck and Emery 1985).

The behavioral model is based on the relatively straightforward chain of events and responses illustrated in Figure 86–3. Through the years, considerable effort and debate have concerned whether stimulus–response and response–reinforcement relationships could be invoked to account for the complexity of human behavior (Kazdin 1982, Staats 1964). In its maturity, behavioral therapy has broadened beyond an exclusive focus on observable behaviors (i.e., radical behaviorism) and now incorporates cognitive processes and other individual variables that affect one's preparedness to learn (Bandura 1977b, Goldfried and Davison 1994). For example, in observational learning, the stimulus–response contingency relationship is established vicariously, by watching, reading about, or imagining the event in question. Reinforcement does not have to take place explicitly; it may occur vicariously, or it may simply be imagined. Other factors, such as the individual's past history, inherent talents, or skillfulness of his or her pertinent response repertoire, help account for the wealth of interindividual variability in stimulus–response relationships. Bandura's cognitive–behavioral formulation of self-efficacy is one example of a "mental" construct that has abiding behavioral implications. This modifiable attitude or belief (roughly akin to self-confidence) influences persistence, willingness to try new things, optimism, and capacity to endure setbacks (Bandura 1977a).

One of the most important enduring experimental models of depression (learned helplessness) is the direct descendant of studies of animal learning (Seligman 1975, Maier and Seligman 1976, Miller and Seligman 1975). Learned helplessness is a state of behavioral passivity and apparent apathy induced by repeated exposure to noxious, yet inescapable, stimuli. The learned helplessness paradigm is based on a modification of escape or avoidance condi-

tioning. A wide variety of species, ranging from goldfish to humans, can readily learn to avoid or escape from a setting when given advance notice (i.e., a light or tone) of an impending noxious event (i.e., a painful shock) (Maier and Seligman 1976). However, when escape is impossible (e.g., a dog is harnessed, or the walls of the experimental box are too high to be scaled), the animal learns to "lie still and take it." During such "helplessness training," the animal's affect and behavior shift progressively from a state of apprehensive arousal (anxiety, perhaps?) to one that may be analogous to depression. After repeated pairings, the animal will become unable or unwilling to escape from the stimulus when unharnessed. The parallels to human experiences are obvious, although it is not known if the animal cognates helpless thoughts ("It won't work...why bother to try...I'm better off just to be still") (Oakes and Curtis 1982). Nevertheless, neurochemical and pharmacological studies underscore the phenomenological similarities between learned helplessness and depression (Weiss and Simson 1985, Willner 1991). Further, "helpless" dogs can be retrained to escape with techniques much like those use in behavioral therapy (Klein and Seligman 1976).

## Cognitive and Behavioral Treatment Strategies

The cognitive and behavioral therapies are well known for their use of specific treatment techniques. Commonly used CBT procedures are directly linked to the theoretical constructs and empirical research of this school of therapy. Although techniques are given somewhat more emphasis in CBT than in other forms of psychotherapy, there is still considerable room for therapists to be creative and flexible in developing a treatment plan. In fact, novice therapists sometimes focus too much on applying techniques at the expense of nurturing the therapeutic alliance and case formulation. Development of a productive therapeutic relationship and an individualized case conceptualization should always take precedence over the implementation of specific cognitive or behavioral techniques. A number of the more important CBT strategies are described briefly here. More detailed accounts of CBT interventions can be found elsewhere (Beck et al. 1979, Beck 1995, Barlow and Cerny 1988, Freeman et al. 1989, Persons 1989).

## Collaborative Empiricism

The therapeutic relationship is as important in CBT as in any of the other effective psychotherapies. However, interchanges between therapist and patient often differ from those observed in supportive or dynamically oriented treatment. One difference is that the therapist is responsible for managing the pace of the session and uses an agenda to help make each session as efficient as possible. Cognitive–behavioral therapists strive for a therapeutic relationship that emphasizes: (1) a high degree of collaboration and (2) a scientific attitude toward testing the validity or usefulness of particular cognitions and behavior. This therapeutic stance is referred to as collaborative empiricism. The empirical nature of the relationship reflects that therapist and patient work together as an investigative team to develop hypotheses about cognitive or behavioral patterns, examine data, and explore alternative ways of thinking or behaving. At first, therapists usually spend more time teaching and

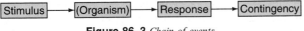

Stimulus → (Organism) → Response → Contingency

**Figure 86–3** *Chain of events.*

explaining in CBT than in other forms of therapy, yet in the course of therapy, patients are actively engaged to become increasingly involved in the work of treatment.

Critics of CBT sometimes suggest that the patient–therapist relationship is compromised by the therapist's attempt to replace negative thoughts with positive ones. One jaded senior colleague referred to CBT as a "feel-good therapy," and another stated that CBT's unspoken strategy was to teach people to lie to themselves. CBT *is* a cautiously optimistic therapy, but effective therapists do not use a "Polyanna" approach to treatment. The data demonstrating CBT's efficacy, discussed below, is the basis for our prognostic optimism. The collaborative empirical stance requires that the therapist and patient work together to make an *honest* appraisal of the validity of cognitions as well as of the adaptive or maladaptive nature of beliefs and behaviors. If a negative assessment proves to be accurate (e.g., the patient actually has made serious mistakes, the individual's spouse is highly likely to leave, or the patient has engaged in a repetitive self-defeating behavior pattern), then the therapist and patient need to work together in a problem-solving mode to develop a plan to cope with the problems at hand or practice more adaptive strategies for use in the future.

Wright and Beck (1994), and others (Clark et al. 1999), have recommended several strategies for enhancing collaborative empiricism. These include: (1) adjusting the therapist's level of activity to match the patients' symptom severity or the phase of treatment; (2) encouraging use of self-help procedures; (3) attending to the "nonspecific" variables important in all therapeutic relationships (e.g., empathy, respect, equanimity, kindness, and good listening skills); (4) promoting frequent two-way feedback; (5) devising coping strategies to help deal with real losses or implementing a plan of action to address maladaptive behavior; (6) recognizing transference phenomena; (7) customizing therapeutic interventions; and (8) using humor judiciously. It is also important to recognize and account for the wide variety of individual differences in cultural backgrounds, social attitudes, and expectations that each patient brings to the therapy encounter (Wright and Davis 1994).

## Psychoeducation

Most forms of CBT integrate explicit psychoeducational procedures as a core element of the treatment process. Psychoeducational procedures are typically blended into treatment sessions in a manner that de-emphasizes formal teaching. There is a concerted effort to teach the patient *why* it is important to challenge automatic thoughts, identify cognitive errors, and practice implementing a more rational thinking style. Behavioral interventions are also preceded by psychoeducation to convey the background for principles such as extinction, reinforcement, self-monitoring, exposure, and response prevention.

There are a number of ways in which therapists employ psychoeducation in CBT. Perhaps the most important is the demonstration of basic concepts, which usually begins in the first therapy session (Beck et al. 1979, Thase and Wright 1991). If patients can see the relevance of cognitive–behavioral principles for situations that are personally significant, they are more likely to grasp and implement therapy concepts. On occasion, therapists may give "mini-lectures" (Epstein et al. 1988), but an interactive and guided method of instruction usually predominates (Beck et al. 1979, Overholser 1993a, 1993b, 1993c).

In the early phases of treatment, special attention is paid to socializing the patient to CBT. The basic cognitive–behavioral model is demonstrated, and expectations for both patient and therapist are conveyed. Some of the frequently used psychoeducational procedures in CBT include brief, impromptu explanations (often written on a chalkboard or a pad of paper to increase the chances of comprehension and retention) and reading assignments, such as *Coping with Depression* (Beck and Greenberg 1974), *Feeling Good* (Burns 1980), *Mind Over Mood* (Greenberger and Padesky 1995), or *Getting Your Life Back* (Wright and Basco 2001). Psychoeducational initiatives typically become more complex as therapy proceeds. For example, detailed explanations and repeated exercises may be needed before the patient fully grasps abstract concepts such as attributional style or schemas. As therapy progresses, homework assignments continue to explicitly reinforce material covered during therapy sessions.

As in other forms of learning, individual differences in homework compliance may influence the progress of therapy. For example, some evidence suggests that homework compliance is correlated with treatment outcome (Whisman 1993, Burns and Spangler 2000). We have found that homework compliance is influenced partly by the therapist's consistency, enthusiasm, and ability to integrate the assignments into the treatment plan.

Because psychoeducation can be time consuming and is a routine part of therapy, several investigators have developed computer programs that provide education on cognitive therapy, encourage homework completion, and actively involve patients in self-help exercises. One of the earliest programs, developed by Selmi and coworkers (1990, 1991), was found to be efficacious in the treatment of depression. Although this software relies completely on written text for conveying information and is not available for clinical use, it demonstrated the potential benefits of computer tools for CBT. More recently, Wright and coworkers (Wright and Wright 1997, Wright et al. 2001) have introduced a multimedia form of computer-assisted CBT ("Good Days Ahead") that uses full screen video and vivid graphics to engage users in the learning process. Research with this program has demonstrated strong effects on learning, high levels of acceptance by patients, and evidence for efficacy in the treatment of depression (Wright et al. 2001, 2002b). Some investigators (Shaw et al. 1999, Kenwright et al. 2001) have been using a text-based computer program ("Fear Fighter") in Great Britain for treating anxiety disorders with exposure therapy. Significant increases in treatment efficiency have been reported when the computer program is used to provide psychoeducation and involve patients in exposure protocols (Kenwright et al. 2001). The use of computers as treatment adjuncts has been reviewed by Locke and Rezza (1996) and Wright and Wright (1997). Computer-assisted treatment is still in the early stages of development, but there appears to be considerable potential for using these new technologies to augment the process of psychotherapy.

## Modifying Automatic Thoughts

The first step in changing automatic thoughts is to help the patient recognize when she or he is having them. The therapist is often able to illustrate the presence of automatic negative thoughts during the initial session by gently calling attention to a change in the patient's mood. Such "mood shifts" can be excellent learning experiences that give personally relevant illustrations of the linkage between cognitions and feelings. Use of a mood shift to identify automatic thoughts is illustrated in the following interchange.

> *Therapist: I noticed a moment ago that your mood appeared to change. All of a sudden, you looked very sad. Do you mind if we talk about what was going through your mind?*
>
> *Patient: No... but I'm not really sure what you mean... I guess I just felt that this therapy might be too hard to handle.*
>
> *Therapist: I'd like to make a distinction between what you thought and what you felt. It looked like you were sad. Am I right? (patient nods) And, at about that time, you had the thought that this therapy might be too difficult? (patient nods) This could be an example of what we call a negative automatic thought. Let's spend a few minutes to see if it is one, and if so, what it might mean.*

One common misconception of CBT is that its practitioners disregard the role of affect or feelings in the etiology and treatment of psychiatric disorders. Actually, one of the principal components of CBT is the stimulation and modulation of emotion (see Figure 86–1). In fact, Beck referred to emotion as "the royal road to cognition" (Beck 1991). In contrast to experiential therapies, variations in emotion are used in CBT to establish links with cognition and identify errors in information processing. Getting in touch with feelings is thus not a goal in CBT but only a means by which therapy helps patients to gain greater control over the processes that influence their moods and behaviors.

## Socratic Questioning

The most frequently used technique to uncover and modify automatic negative thoughts is Socratic questioning (or guided discovery) (Beck et al. 1979, Overholser 1993a, 1993b, 1993c). Socratic questioning teaches the use of rationality and inductive reasoning to challenge whether what is thought or felt is actually true. The therapist models the use of Socratic questioning and encourages the patient to start raising questions about the validity of his or her thinking. There are few formal guidelines for Socratic questioning (Overholser 1993a). Rather, therapists learn to use their experience and ingenuity to frame good questions that engage the patient in a process aimed at recognizing and modifying a biased or distorted cognitive style. Typical questions include: What ran through your mind at that time? What is the evidence that your impression is accurate? Could there be any alternative explanations? If this were true, what would be the worst thing that would happen? When guided discovery methods are not sufficient to draw out automatic thoughts, the therapist may turn to several alternative ways of eliciting dysfunctional cognitions, as described in the following.

## Imagery Techniques and Role-Playing

Imagery techniques and role-playing are used when direct questioning does not fully reveal important underlying cognitions. When imagery is used, the therapist sets the scene by asking the patient to visualize the situation that caused distress. Although some patients can readily imagine themselves in a previous scene, many need prompts or imagery induction to encourage their active participation in the exercise. Several types of questions can be used to help frame the scene. These include inquiries about: (1) the physical details of the setting, (2) occurrences immediately before the interaction, and (3) descriptions of the other people in the scene (Wright and Beck 1994). In role-playing exercises, the therapist and patient act out an interpersonal vignette to uncover automatic thoughts or to try out a revised pattern of thinking. This technique is used less frequently than imagery by most cognitive–behavioral therapists and may be reserved for situations in which transference distortions are unlikely (Wright and Beck 1994).

## Thought Recording

Thought recording is one of the most useful procedures for identifying and changing automatic thoughts. This technique is first presented in relatively simple two- or three-column versions in the early stages of therapy. When the two-column procedure is used, patients are instructed to write down events in one column and thoughts in the other. Alternatively, they can record events, thoughts, and emotions in the three columns. The purpose of this exercise is to encourage patients to begin to use self-monitoring to increase awareness of their thought patterns. Next, the strength of the emotion and the believability of the automatic negative thoughts are rated on a scale of 0 to 100. In subsequent sessions, a more complex five-column thought record, the Daily Record of Dysfunctional Thoughts (DRDT) is introduced (Figure 86–4). The fourth column of the DRDT encourages the patient to develop rational alternatives that rebut the automatic negative thoughts; the fifth column is used for a reevaluation of the mood and cognitive ratings. Work on identifying cognitive errors can also be included in this form of thought recording.

## Examining the Evidence

The examining the evidence procedure is a collaborative exercise used to test the validity of automatic negative thoughts. Cognitions are set forth as hypotheses rather than established facts. The patient is encouraged to write down evidence that either supports or refutes the automatic thought using a two-column form (i.e., pros and cons). For example, examining the evidence for the automatic thought "everyone always looks down on me" might reveal data in support of both sides of the question. It is likely that the patient will recall many times when he or she felt looked down on, treated disrespectfully, or criticized unfairly. On the other hand, it would be virtually impossible that he or she has *always* been seen in this way by others. Specific evidence of good job performance, positive relationships with relatives and friends, and successes in school or recreational activities may then be used to help counterbalance the

| Date | Event | Automatic thoughts | Emotions | Rational thoughts | Outcome |
|---|---|---|---|---|---|
| | a. Describe actual event preceding unpleasant emotion or<br>b. Stream of thoughts, daydream, or memories preceding unpleasant emotion. | a. Write automatic thought(s) that led to emotion(s).<br>b. Rate of belief in automatic thought(s), 0–100%. | a. Specify sad, anxious, angry, tense, and so on.<br>b. Rate degree of emotion, 0–100. | a. Identify cognitive errors.<br>b. Write rational response to automatic thought(s).<br>c. Rate belief in rational response, 0–100%. | a. Specify and rate subsequent emotion(s), 0–100. |
| 1/30/95 | My boss asks for a progress report. | I'm in big trouble. (85)<br>I can't handle this job. (90)<br>I've messed everything up. (95) | Anxious (95)<br>Sad (80) | Magnification, ignoring the evidence, overgeneralization.<br><br>I'm slightly behind schedule, but I can catch up. (95)<br>I've had a good track record with this job. (100)<br>I'm doing O.K. in some other areas of my life. (95) | Anxious (40)<br>Sad (20) |
| | My son comes home late from a party. | Nobody listens to me. (90)<br>He doesn't care. (75)<br>What's the use of trying? (80) | Angry (75)<br>Sad (85) | All or none thinking, ignoring the evidence, personalizing.<br><br>My son pays attention a fair amount of the time, but he doesn't always do what I want. (90)<br>There's plenty of evidence that he cares about me. (100)<br>We need to improve how we communicate. (95)<br>I need to tell him that I'm angry. (100) | Angry (30)<br>Sad (25) |

**Figure 86–4** *Daily record of dysfunctional thoughts.*

patient's negatively biased overgeneralized automatic thought. More ambiguous examples may also be revealed in which the evidence does not clearly point in one direction or the evidence is not clear. In these situations, the therapist may suggest homework to collect additional information. Cognitive errors such as magnification, personalization, and all-or-nothing thinking are frequently revealed in these situations.

Next, the therapist helps to guide revision of the automatic negative thought in light of the evidence (e.g., "I *often* feel inferior to others, even when there's no good evidence that they feel that way" or "I have had a number of difficulties with my teachers and employers, but not all relationships have been bad"). The process thus moves from the patient's general and globally negative interpretations to more specific, factually based statements.

When an honest appraisal uncovers evidence in support of negative cognitions, the therapist may choose to focus on the patient's attributions of causality or internality. The patient who posits a negative attribution for poor work evaluation (e.g., "My performance was poor because I don't have what it takes") can usually be aided to consider a more neutral attribution (e.g., "My performance was poor because I was underprepared . . . my depression also prevented more energetic preparation"). The treatment plan may also be revised to develop better methods of coping in similar situations or to work on ways of remediating skill deficits. Sometimes, particular difficulties cannot be changed (e.g., physical handicaps, markedly unattractive physical looks, or severe financial limitations). A trainee once remarked to one of us, "I'm not sure that CBT is the right treatment for my patient. He really *is* ugly and dumb, and as far as I can tell, no one has ever loved him!" Before turning supervisory attention to the patient's problems, the therapist-in-training was engaged in a guided discovery exercise to clarify *his* assumptions and beliefs about the essential importance of physical beauty, intelligence, and romantic love. Subsequently, the patient was able to address these issues successfully in therapy as well.

## Generating Alternatives

If automatic thoughts prove to be largely dysfunctional, the patient is encouraged to generate alternatives that are more accurate or factual. Many of the techniques discussed earlier can be used to help generate alternatives to automatic thoughts. Socratic questioning is used in therapy sessions to help the patient start to think more creatively. Also, psychoeducational procedures may be employed to teach brainstorming techniques. For example, the patient may be taught to use "expert testimony" or the opinions of someone who knows her or him well (i.e., a sibling, spouse, or best friend) to help develop more rational alternatives.

Thought records are often used to record alternatives to automatic thoughts. We often encourage patients to collect their thought records in notebook form for ongoing use. Figure 86–4 illustrates the use of rational alternatives during CBT for a depressed patient.

Many patients with depression, anxiety, and related conditions have relatively rigid cognitive styles that perpetuate dysfunctional thought and behavior patterns. These individuals frequently experience "second-order" automatic negative thoughts, that is, negative thoughts that are triggered by rational alternatives ("that's a cop-out...quit making excuses"). These thoughts about thoughts tend to undermine the credibility of the rational responses and may dampen the patient's enthusiasm for using the procedure. The therapist may notice a particular facial expression or a change in the patient's posture that suggests the existence of second-order thoughts. In such cases, more active therapeutic assistance may be needed. For example, the therapist may need to act as a teacher or coach in the area of adaptive cognitive functioning, rapidly rebutting automatic thoughts as they arise. Coping cards, which are index cards with helpful reminders on the use of CBT methods (in this case, rational responses to repetitive automatic negative thoughts), may be written during sessions and carried by the patient in his or her pocket, wallet, or purse for later use.

## Cognitive–Behavioral Rehearsal

Cognitive–behavioral rehearsal is a treatment strategy that is particularly useful for preparing patients to put their experiences in CBT to work in real-life circumstances. After automatic thoughts have been elicited and modified through procedures described before, the therapist guides the patient in a series of rehearsal exercises to try out alternative cognitions in a variety of situations. By using imagery and role-playing scenarios to practice generating more adaptive cognitions, the patient may become aware of problems that could interfere with implementation of the new style of thinking. Further practice and targeted homework assignments may then be needed before alternative cognitions can be fully used. For example, the effects of cognitive–behavioral rehearsal may be extended to real situations by assigning homework to test use of the modified automatic thoughts.

## Modifying Schemas

The emphasis in the early phases of therapy is usually on behavioral activation, identifying and changing automatic thoughts, and the reduction of symptoms. However, as the patient gains knowledge of cognitive–behavioral principles and acute symptoms begin to subside, the focus of the treatment sessions usually shifts toward work on the schema level. Because schemas serve as underlying templates for making sense of new information, they play a major role in the modulation of more superficial cognitions (automatic thoughts), regulation of affect, self-esteem, and control of the behavioral repertoire. Thus, schema modification is an important component of cognitively oriented therapies.

With Axis I disorders such as major depressive disorder and panic disorder, schema revision efforts are directed at correcting dysfunctional attitudes that may predispose the patient to symptomatic recurrences. After several months of productive therapy, schema modification may be placed in the context of reducing future vulnerability. CBT of personality disorders typically requires that a major portion of therapy be devoted to modifying schemas and related patterns of behavioral dysfunction (Beck et al. 1990). When schematic work cannot be fully addressed in time-limited therapy, the model of ongoing change may be introduced. Thus, the patient may begin to change her or his "life course" by development of a long-term self-help plan. Jarrett and colleagues (2001) have proposed continuation and maintenance phases of CBT treatment of depression, and they argue for focusing on schema change in these phases of treatment if it is not accomplished in the acute phase of treatment.

Many of the techniques used to test and modify automatic thoughts are also used to identify and revise schemas. Psychoeducational interventions are usually required as a first step. Most patients are not aware of their "guiding principles," so the therapist may need to begin by introducing and illustrating this concept. It is often useful to use synonyms for the term schema (such as basic assumptions or core beliefs) and to demonstrate how schemas are linked to automatic negative thoughts using material from the patient's own experience (Wright and Beck 1994). Socratic questioning is the core procedure used for schema modification (Beck et al. 1979, Overholser 1993c).

The downward arrow technique (Figure 86–5) is a particularly powerful way to move from surface cognitions to deeper cognitive structures (Thase and Beck 1993). This technique describes asking the patient a question such as: "If this automatic thought were true, what would it mean about you as a person?" Another useful approach is to examine patterns of automatic thoughts from thought records to sort out common themes. The therapist may suggest a thematic collation based on her or his knowledge of the patient's automatic negative thoughts. In some situations, it may be helpful to have patients review a description of common pathological schemas to recognize some of their core beliefs (see Table 86–2). On occasion, it may be useful to have the patient write a brief autobiography to help elucidate the historical antecedents of the schema. Computerized learning programs can also be employed to help patients uncover their schemas (Wright et al. 1995, 2002a).

Because schemas are so strongly held (in essence, they have helped define reality and mold behavior for years), they may require intensive work in a number of therapy sessions to undergo significant change. Sometimes long-term continuation and maintenance CBT is required to accomplish schematic restructuring. Therapists can select from a number of CBT techniques, including examining the evidence, listing advantages and disadvantages, generating alternatives, cognitive response prevention, and cognitive–behavioral rehearsal, as they attempt to modify schemas (Wright and Beck 1994). Examining the evidence, generating alternatives, and cognitive–behavioral rehearsal were described earlier as methods of changing automatic thoughts.

## Cognitive Response Prevention

In cognitive response prevention, the patient agrees to complete a homework assignment in which she or he must

| Patient | Therapist |
|---|---|
| "I think the date went poorly (*chuckles with gallows humor*). . . I'm so depressed!" | |
| ↓ | "Is it true that the date went poorly? Could this be an example of how negative thinking is involved with feeling depressed?" |
| "No—It's true. He didn't mention another date and hasn't called me since." | |
| ↓ | "Okay . . . that sounds convincing enough. So, if the date went badly, what's that really say about you?" |
| "Stuff like this happens to me a lot!" | |
| ↓ | "And, if that's true?" |
| "There is something seriously wrong with me." (*There is a visible shift in affect.*) | |
| ↓ | "Such as . . . " |
| "I must be a reject . . . a social basket case . . . I'm so pathetic!" (*tearful*) | |
| ↓ | "And, if that's true, which we still have to test out, what does that say about your world and future?" |
| "It says that no one will ever love me . . . I'll be lonely forever . . . an old maid . . . " (*more tears*) | |
| ↓ | "I can see from your tears that these thoughts really hit you where it hurts. I've written down some of the more dramatic and hurtful statements. Do you feel up to taking a look at them and testing their accuracy?" |

**Figure 86–5** *The downward arrow technique.*

behave in a way that is inconsistent with the pathological schema. For example, a person with perfectionistic attitudes may be engaged in an assignment in which she or he must perform in a "so-so" manner. This is intended to activate the schema which is triggering automatic negative thoughts (e.g., "They'll think I'm a sloth" or "I'll never be trusted with an important assignment again"). By not responding to the perfectionistic demands dictated by the schema, the individual thus has the opportunity to cope with the automatic negative thoughts consequent to this "rule violation."

## Listing Advantages and Disadvantages

The listing advantages and disadvantages procedure is particularly useful when a schema appears to have both adaptive and maladaptive features. Schemas that have damaging effects are often maintained because they also have a positive side. For example, the schema "I must be perfect to be accepted" can have significant benefits (e.g., hard work and attention to detail often lead to success in work or school). Nevertheless, because perfection is seldom possible, the individual may remain vulnerable to setbacks. Other schemas, such as "I'm a complete loser," may not seem to have any advantages at first glance. However, even such a markedly negative basic assumption can have certain behavioral reinforcers associated with it. For example, a person who believes that he or she is a loser may avoid making commitments, withdraw from challenging assignments, or refuse to exert a sustained effort to solve a difficult problem. This strategy may thus protect the person from painful setbacks. The advantages and disadvantages analysis provides the patient and therapist with essential information for planning modifications. Revised schemas are most likely to be used when they take into account both the maladaptive and the adaptive features of the old basic assumption.

In general, it is recommended that patients keep a list of the schemas as they have been identified. The schema list helps to focus the patient's attention on the overarching nature of these maladaptive principles. Because schemas often become manifest only during periods of increased stress or symptom expression, they may appear to fade in significance as the patient begins to improve. For example, behavioral treatment programs that neither endorse nor aim to modify schemas are generally as effective as CBT in the short run. However, there may be a false security engendered by symptom relief. The cognitive model posits that the individual will remain vulnerable to the depressogenic impact of "matching" life events unless schema revision is accomplished (Thase and Beck 1993).

## Behavioral Techniques

In CBT, behavioral methods are usually integrated with cognitive restructuring in a comprehensive treatment plan. Behavioral strategies may be given a greater emphasis earlier in therapy with more severely symptomatic patients such as those with intense depression, bipolar symptoms, or schizophrenia (Beck et al. 1979, Thase and Wright 1991, Kingdon and Turkingdon 1995, Basco and Rush 1996, Scott and Wright 1997). Some cognitive–behavior therapists may rely primarily on behavioral interventions for conditions such as obsessive–compulsive disorder (OCD) or simple phobias. Commonly used behavioral strategies are described here in alphabetical order.

## Activity Scheduling, Graded Tasks, and Mastery–Pleasure Exercises

Depressed people may spend excessive amounts of time alone or have tangible reductions of pleasurable activity. One of the earliest behavioral formulations of depression viewed the disorder as an "extinction state" resulting from the loss of reinforcers (Ferster 1973). Neurobiological changes accompanying prolonged stress may also dampen hedonic capacity, which in turn reduces the salience of reinforcers (Weiss and Simson 1985, Willner 1991). Thus, the learned helplessness paradigm brings together behavioral and neurobiological domains. Depressed operant (i.e., goal-directed) behavior may elicit negative cognitions as well (Teasdale 1983). For example, depressed people often procrastinate against performing potentially "overwhelming" chores or tasks. Procrastination, in turn, elicits guilty thoughts and self-criticisms. Moreover, the depressive cognitive state increases the likelihood that individuals will minimize the positive value of the activities they are able to complete. As a result, it may also be said that depressed people suffer from a deficit of self-reinforcement (Rehm 1977).

One key to the behavioral approach for treatment of depression is the interruption of the downward spiral linking mood, inactivity, and negative cognition (Beck et al. 1979, Lewinsohn et al. 1982) (Figure 86–6). Completing an activity schedule is often the first behavioral homework assignment used in CBT (Beck and Greenberg 1974). Depressed patients are asked to begin to keep a daily log that is used to chart the relationship between their moods and their activities (Figure 86–7).

The nature of the activities is examined, and deficits in activities that might elicit pleasure or feelings of competence are identified. Next, assignments are made to engage in discrete pleasurable activities (or, in the case of an anhedo-nic individual, activities that were rewarding before becoming depressed). If needed, a "menu" of reinforcers can be generated by having the patient fill out a Pleasant Events Schedule (Lewinsohn et al. 1982). Following operant principles, activities that have been "high-grade" reinforcers in the past are scheduled during times of low moods or decreased activity. Next, subjective ratings of mastery or competence and pleasure are added to the activity schedule by use of a simple scale (i.e., 0–5), to avoid the tendency of dichotomous thinking. In this way, achieving a small degree of pleasure or mastery during a scheduled activity may be framed as an accomplishment, particularly early in the course of therapy.

The activity schedule may also be used to begin to tackle overdue chores or other dreaded activities. The graded task approach is based on the premise that in a depressed state, many normal activities are indeed too demanding for depressed patients to complete according to their usual standards or with their characteristic efficiency. Thus, the task is broken down into units or components. The first homework assignment is typically to identify and complete a minimally acceptable initial step. For example, a depressed businessman had concealed from his family that he was 6 months behind in paying their income taxes. When he tried to tackle the project, he thought, "I'm too tired to do it now.... I can't concentrate on this stuff.... I'll get more depressed if I try and fail." These cognitions were so discouraging that he invariably postponed working on the taxes. As a result, he felt some relief immediately (a reinforcer for procrastination). However, within minutes he was plagued by automatic negative thoughts about the implications of putting off such an important task yet again. He also had shameful thoughts about what his family or friends would think about him when his secret was discovered. In this case, the man

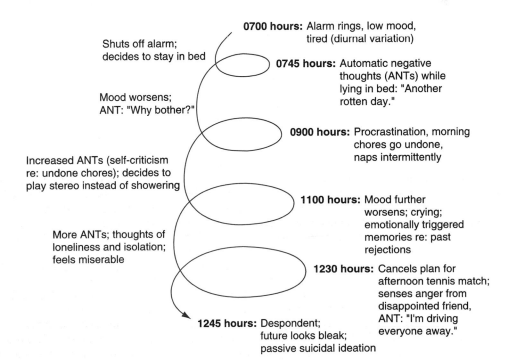

**Figure 86–6** *The downward spiral: interaction of affect, behavior, and cognition in severe depression. ANTs, Automatic negative thoughts.*

Shuts off alarm; decides to stay in bed

Mood worsens; ANT: "Why bother?"

Increased ANTs (self-criticism re: undone chores); decides to play stereo instead of showering

More ANTs; thoughts of loneliness and isolation; feels miserable

**0700 hours:** Alarm rings, low mood, tired (diurnal variation)

**0745 hours:** Automatic negative thoughts (ANTs) while lying in bed: "Another rotten day."

**0900 hours:** Procrastination, morning chores go undone, naps intermittently

**1100 hours:** Mood further worsens; crying; emotionally triggered memories re: past rejections

**1230 hours:** Cancels plan for afternoon tennis match; senses anger from disappointed friend, ANT: "I'm driving everyone away."

**1245 hours:** Despondent; future looks bleak; passive suicidal ideation

**Note:** Grade activities **M** for mastery and **P** for pleasure

| | | Monday | Tuesday | Wednesday | Thursday | Friday | Saturday | Sunday |
|---|---|---|---|---|---|---|---|---|
| AM | 6:00<br>6:30 | | | | | | | |
| | 7:00<br>7:30 | | | | | | | |
| | 8:00<br>8:30 | | | | | | | |
| | 9:00<br>9:30 | | | | | | | |
| | 10:00<br>10:30 | | | | | | | |
| | 11:00<br>11:30 | | | | | | | |
| PM | 12:00<br>12:30 | | | | | | | |
| | 1:00<br>1:30 | | | | | | | |
| | 2:00<br>2:30 | | | | | | | |
| | 3:00<br>3:30 | | | | | | | |
| | 4:00<br>4:30 | | | | | | | |
| | 5:00<br>5:30 | | | | | | | |

Mastery, accomplished, achieved something
Pleasure, fun, amusement, enjoyment

Scale: 0–5; 0, none, 5, most

**Figure 86–7** *Weekly activity schedule.*

estimated that the task would require at least 10 hours *if he were well.* He also estimated that he had only about 50% of his normal energy and ability to concentrate. Therefore, 20 hours of work was planned in small blocks spaced out for the next 20 days. The first assignment was for the man to spend only 15 minutes organizing the forms necessary to do the overdue income taxes. Self-instruction and visual imagery may be used to help initiate action, and self-reinforcement after completion of each step helps to maintain therapeutic momentum.

## Breathing Control

An important component of CBT for anxiety disorders involves teaching the patient breathing exercises that may be used to counteract hyperventilation and/or reduce tension (Clark et al. 1985). Slow, deep breathing can have a calming effect not unlike progressive muscle relaxation (Bernstein and Borkovec 1973). These exercises also help to distract the patient from autonomic cues. After initial instruction and practice, the breathing skills are then applied in progressively more anxiety-provoking situations.

A note of caution is in order when teaching patients breathing control exercises. We have seen many patients who have misunderstood instructions and who have developed a pattern of deep overbreathing in response to stress. Instead of helping reduce anxiety, their breathing

changes may increase the chances of hyperventilation. Thus, we typically recommend that patients be taught about the pace and form of normal breathing patterns. Next clinicians can model normal, calm breathing as compared to overbreathing during an anxiety attack. The second hand of a watch can be used to time breaths so that they can be slowed to a normal rate. Positive, calming images can also be used to reduce anxiety during the breathing exercises. Finally, we suggest that patients practice breathing exercises regularly to gain mastery of this anxiety management technique.

## Contingency Contracting and Behavior Exchange

These strategies use the principles of operant conditioning (Skinner 1938) to modify the probability of occurrence of either undesired or desired behaviors. An excellent introduction to these methods is presented by Malott and colleagues (1993). One key to applied behavioral analysis is control over the contingencies or reinforcers. Another important factor is that the terms of the contract are negotiated and should be specific and relatively straightforward. The positive contingency or reinforcer should be desirable and available shortly after the terms of the contract have been met. A paycheck is a good example of a contingency contract. Another common strategy is to chain, or pair, a high-frequency behavior (e.g., reading, watching television, or listening to music) to a low-frequency one (e.g., doing paperwork, doing housework, spending time with the children). Contingencies should generally start out relatively "rich" (e.g., 1 hour of video game time after 15 minutes of paperwork) and may be progressively "thinned" in time (Malott et al. 1993). Punishments or "response cost" contingencies are less widely used because of their negative affective responses (Azrin and Holz 1966).

Behavior exchange contracts are used with couples or families. For example, a distressed couple may voice dissatisfaction about two distinctly different behavioral tendencies, as illustrated.

> **Partner 1**: *You never help me out around the house.*
> **Partner 2**: *That's not true, I'm always pitching in. My problem is that on the weekends you never want to go out and have fun.*
> **Partner 1**: *That's partly true... but if I wasn't so sick and tired of being stuck with all the housework, maybe I'd feel more like going out.*

Rather than join the debate to ascertain which partner is right about what, the therapist suggests a contract to objectify the communication and increase the likelihood of mutually rewarding experiences. The contingencies used in the contract represent an exchange of desired behaviors. In the example, partner 1 desires assistance with specific household tasks (e.g., wash the dishes, fold the laundry). A desired frequency is also determined (e.g., nightly). For partner 2, a weekend outing is specified, and a mutually acceptable activity is chosen. The contract is written and signed by both parties and the therapist. Consequences for nonadherence may also need to be formulated.

Behavioral contracts may be particularly useful for assisting patients with medication adherence. For example, the therapist may help the patient identify barriers to taking medication as prescribed and then work out behavioral solutions which are written in contract form. Behavioral methods may include pairing medication taking with routine activities such as brushing teeth or meals, reminder systems, and reinforcement from significant others. We recommend explicit discussion of adherence problems and mutual agreement on a plan for taking medications when patients have difficulty in following the pharmacotherapy plan.

## Desensitization and Relaxation Training

Systematic desensitization (Wolpe 1958) was one of the first behavioral strategies to gain wide acceptance. Systematic desensitization relies on exposure through a progressive hierarchy of fear-inducing situations. This procedure may use pairing of progressive deep muscle relaxation and visualization of the target behavior to decondition fearful responses. Systematic desensitization is useful for treatment of simple phobias, social phobia, panic attacks, and generalized anxiety (Wolpe 1982). Some evidence suggests that the active ingredient of systematic desensitization is exposure to the feared situation, first in imagination and later in reality, rather than an actual counterconditioning through the relaxation response (Kazdin and Wilcoxin 1976). Progressive deep muscle relaxation is also useful as a self-directed coping strategy and for treatment of sleep-onset insomnia (Goldfried and Davison 1994, Bernstein and Borkovec 1973).

## Exposure and Flooding

The purpose of these strategies is to speed extinction of conditioned fear or anxiety responses. Behavioral theory dictates that fearfulness is reinforced by avoidance and escape behaviors (Rachman et al. 1986). Because the basis of the fear or phobia is irrational, the optimal strategy is to increase exposure to the feared activity without aversive consequences. In obsessive–compulsive disorder, the ritualistic behavior (e.g., hand washing or checking) is presumed to be reinforced by the relief of the anxiety associated with the compulsion (e.g., hand washing temporarily relieves the fear of contamination) (Rachman et al. 1986). In exposure, there are at least three means of fear reduction: autonomic habituation, recognition that the fear is irrational, and explicit enhancement of morale or self-efficacy that accompanies mastering the previously dreaded activity.

In graded or progressive exposure, a hierarchy is established, ranging from least to most anxiety-provoking situations. The individual is taught one or more ways to cope with anxiety (e.g., relaxation or self-instruction), and with the help of the therapist, the items on the hierarchy are worked through, one item at a time. Mastery is predicated on maintaining a sufficient duration of exposure for the fear to extinguish or dissipate. In some cases, imagery (exposure *in vitro*) is used before moving to exposure to the actual feared stimulus. Exposure may also be enhanced by guided support (i.e., the therapist's presence during the session) or by use of coping cognitions for the duration of the exposure exercise.

Flooding, which relies on the same principles, dispatches with the hierarchical approach. The individual is exposed to the maximal level of anxiety as quickly as possible. The rationale for this accelerated approach is that it may hasten autonomic habituation. To be effective, flooding needs to be accompanied by response prevention. In response prevention treatment of OCD, the individual agrees not to perform the compulsion despite strong urges to do so. Because obsessions are more private than compulsions, there can be less certainty that the individual has fully participated in response prevention exercises (Stern 1978).

Simple phobias may be rapidly treated by an accelerated form of exposure referred to as participant modeling or contact desensitization. The therapist serves as a supportive coach or guide and assists the patient through a progressively more demanding level of exposure to the feared situation. In most cases, lifelong fears of air travel, tunnels, heights, matches, dogs, water, or insects can be fully treated in a few hours of guided exposure.

## Social Skills Training

Satisfactory interpersonal relationships require a complex set of skills, including reciprocity, respect for another's opinion, appropriate modulation of self-disclosure, the tempered ability to yield on some occasions and to set limits at other times, the natural use of social reinforcers, and the capacity to express anger and resolve conflicts in a constructive manner (Lewinsohn et al. 1982; Hersen et al.

1984). Many people with psychiatric disorders suffer from either a state-dependent deterioration of these social skills or lifelong deficits of such skills. Once established, social skills deficits can increase the likelihood of experiencing stressful life events as well as "turn off" family members and other sources of social support that may help to buffer people against stressors (Coyne et al. 1987).

Problems as diverse as underassertiveness, temper "attacks," excessive self-disclosure, monopolistic conversational style, underreinforcement of significant others, and splitting (i.e., playing one against another) are amenable to social skills training. The methods employed include modeling (i.e., the therapist demonstrates a more effective alternative approach), role-playing and role reversal, behavior rehearsal, and specific practice assignments. Often, the interpersonal anxiety and lack of self-confidence that go hand in hand with social skills deficits lessen in response to successful mastery of targeted assignments.

## Thought Stopping and Distraction

Automatic negative thoughts and repetitive, intrusive ruminations are sometimes too intense to address with purely cognitive interventions. The technique of thought stopping capitalizes on the individual's ability to use a selectively narrowed attentional focus to suppress the intrusive cognitions. For example, a ruminative individual may be asked to visualize a large red "stop" sign, including its octagonal shape and white lettering. The command "Stop!" is paired with the image. The image and command are then used to interrupt a "run" of ruminations. At first, the technique is practiced in sessions at times when automatic thoughts or ruminations are mild. After initial success, the technique is next applied to more intensely disturbing cognitions. For individuals who find visualization difficult or ineffective, a rubber band may be worn on the wrist as a distractor. In a manner similar to that described before, the command "Stop!" is paired with a brisk snap of the rubber band.

Anxious patients may benefit from use of other distraction techniques to cope with panicky thoughts or increased sensitivity to interoceptive cues. Specifically, patients susceptible to panic often have a heightened awareness of otherwise normal physiological cues (e.g., heart rate, dryness in the throat, tightness in the chest, or increased peristalsis). In turn, such sensitivity triggers automatic negative thoughts about the imagined impending calamity. Distractions such as counting backward, praying, or imagining a calming scene may be applied to direct attention away from the internal stimuli. Distraction techniques thus help the individual exert some control over the symptoms, permitting greater exposure and a growing sense of self-efficacy.

## Formulation of Treatment

## Indications for Treatment

The cognitive and behavioral therapies are indicated as primary treatments for adults suffering from several non-psychotic, nonorganic Axis I disorders in the *Diagnostic and Statistical Manual of Mental Disorders*, Fourth Edition (DSM-IV). These include major depressive disorder, dys-

thymic disorder, panic disorder, social phobia, OCD, post-traumatic stress disorder (PTSD), generalized anxiety disorder, and bulimia nervosa (Wright et al. 2002b). Cognitive and behavioral therapies are also useful as adjunctive treatments for patients with bipolar disorder (Basco and Rush 1996, Basco and Thase 1998, Lam et al. 2000) and schizophrenia (Mueser 1998, Kingdon and Turkington 1995, Senky et al. 2000). Although not extensively studied, cognitive and behavioral therapies incorporating coping skills training and relapse prevention strategies may also improve the outcome of individuals with substance abuse disorders (Wright et al. 2002b).

Cognitive and behavioral therapies, like most other types of treatment, have not been studied widely in patients with Axis II disorders. However, the CBT approach to problem specification and explicit training in coping skills may be well suited for treatment of individuals willing to work on changing these habitual, ingrained patterns of thinking and behavior (Beck et al. 1990). Specific cognitive–behavioral formulations have been developed for each of the personality disorders, and modifications of CBT methods have been described for working with patients with Axis II problems. (Beck et al. 1990) Linehan's model of CBT (dialectical behavior therapy) has been shown to be efficacious in reducing parasuicidal behavior in patients with borderline personality disorder (Linehan et al. 1991, 1993).

## Selection of This Modality

Perhaps the greatest "rate-limiting step" in selection of CBT is having access to a well-trained therapist. However, there are a growing number of training programs in CBT, and centers for CBT are available in many cities throughout the world. CBT is now a required element in the education of psychiatry residents and is the major orientation of many psychology graduate programs. The Academy of Cognitive Therapy (www.academyofct.org) certifies therapists in this approach.

Selection of CBT for an individual patient should be based on the appropriateness of CBT for the treatment situation. Relevant questions include: Is the patient psychotic? If so, are there specific target behaviors and has psychopharmacological treatment been optimized? Does the patient suffer from a disorder known to be responsive to CBT? Within groups of patients with potentially treatable disorders, other indicators of responsivity include chronicity, severity, and comorbidity (Whisman 1993, Thase et al. 1993). A good general rule is that patients with acute, mild to moderately severe, mood and anxiety disorders are the best candidates for treatment with CBT alone (Thase 1995). Patients with more chronic, severe, or complicated illnesses may be better candidates for combined treatment strategies than for CBT alone (Wright and Thase 1992, Thase and Howland 1994, Friedman 1997). McCullough (2000) has developed a variant of CBT for chronic depression that has shown much promise alone and combined with antidepressant medication.

An outpatient trial of acute phase CBT typically ranges from 10 to 20 weekly treatment sessions (Wright and Beck 1983, Beck et al. 1979, Barlow and Cerny 1988, Persons 1989). However, shorter courses of treatment have been shown to be efficacious in some situations. Deterioration or noncompliance of the patient may warrant early termination of a treatment trial, and for certain chronic conditions such as borderline personality disorder and bipolar disorder, longer courses of therapy may be indicated (Beck et al. 1990, Linehan 1993, Basco and Rush 1996). Jarrett and coworkers (Jarrett and Kraft 1997, Jarrett et al. 2001) have conceptualized treatment across the acute, continuation, and maintenance phases of the depressive disorder. We will discuss these phases of treatment in greater detail below. During treatment of major depressive disorder and panic disorder, a majority of patients who will benefit from CBT will show a significant reduction in symptoms within 6 to 8 weeks of starting therapy (Ilardi and Craighead 1994). Moreover, those who show a late response to CBT (i.e., between weeks 12 and 16) may be at high risk for subsequent relapse (Thase et al. 1992).

## Issues of Gender, Race, and Ethnicity

The cognitive and behavioral therapies appear equally effective for men and women and people of various races (Dobson 1989, Thase et al. 1994a). As with other forms of psychotherapy, a productive CBT working alliance is based on mutual respect for individual differences (Wright and Davis 1994). For some persons with gender, racial, or ethnically related issues, it may be useful to select therapists with special skills or experiences (e.g., therapists specializing in gay and lesbian issues or posttraumatic stress syndromes due to rape or incest). It has been recommended that cognitive–behavioral therapists receive special training and supervision in methods of responding to gender, race, and ethnicity variations (Wright and Davis 1994).

## Preparation of the Patient

The cognitive and behavioral therapies explicitly incorporate strategies to increase involvement and preparedness of the patient for therapy. Patients are typically encouraged to read relevant written materials describing the theory and strategies of the therapy; for common disorders, such as major depressive disorder and panic disorder, self-help manuals for patients are now available (Burns 1990, Greenberger and Padesky 1995, Wright and Basco 2001). It is likely that multimedia programs will have an increasing role in therapy preparation (Locke and Rezza 1996, Wright and Wright 1997, Wright et al. 2002a). Regardless of the mode of application, patients beginning CBT need to become acculturated to the following: (1) they will be active participants in trying out new strategies; (2) they will be expected to do homework; (3) the outcome of therapy will be measured and strategies will be altered if they are not helping; (4) therapy will be focused on symptoms and social functioning and generally will be time limited in nature; and (5) the chances of success after treatment termination can be gauged by the patients' incorporation of the therapy into their day-to-day life.

## Phases of Treatment

Most cognitive and behavioral therapies may be viewed as using a three-stage process. The initial phase includes the processes of clinical assessment, case formulation, establishment of a therapeutic relationship, socialization of the patient to therapy, psychoeducation, and introduction to treatment procedures. The middle stage involves the sequential application and mastery of cognitive and behavioral treatment strategies. The second stage ends when the patient has obtained the desired symptomatic outcome. The final phase of therapy is characterized by preparation for termination. The frequency of sessions is reduced, and there is a steady transfer of the responsibility for the continued use of therapeutic strategies from the therapist to the patient. The third stage of treatment also focuses on relapse prevention. Strategies used at this point include anticipation of reaction to future stressors or high-risk situations, identification of prodromal symptoms, rehearsal of self-help procedures, and establishment of guidelines for return to treatment (Otto et al. 1993, Thase 1993). The failure to achieve a remission of depressive symptoms after 16 to 20 weeks of treatment may indicate a need for continuation phase treatment to achieve these goals and maintenance phase treatment for relapse prevention. Incomplete symptomatic remission after 20 weeks of CBT may also indicate the need for adding pharmacotherapy to the treatment plan as we discuss in greater detail below.

## Intensity of Treatment

Outpatient CBT is normally conducted once or twice a week. In selected cases, three-times-weekly or even daily sessions may be useful, but the cost-effectiveness of such a labor-intensive approach is uncertain. One of the authors (J.H.Wright), who often uses CBT in combination with pharmacotherapy and computer-assisted treatment, has found that he can reduce sessions for ambulatory patients to every other week or to a shortened time frame (i.e., 20–25-minute sessions) when a good therapeutic relationship has been established and the patient has started to make significant progress.

When patients are seen in a day treatment hospital or inpatient setting, sessions are typically provided on a daily or every-other-day basis. Many programs blend individual and group therapies (Wright et al. 1993). In our experience, more frequent sessions help to offset symptom severity and demoralization in severely ill patients (Thase and Wright 1991). The cost-effectiveness of more and less intensive cognitive–behavioral strategies has not been systematically studied. Nevertheless, we believe that therapists should adjust the frequency and intensity of treatment in concert with the needs of patients as well as the therapy resources that are available.

## Duration of Treatment

In most cases, treatment is conducted in a period of 3 to 6 months. For those who begin therapy as inpatients, a similar period of aftercare is strongly recommended (Thase 1993). Unsuccessful therapy (e.g., failure to effect significant symptomatic improvement) should generally not continue past 12 to 16 weeks for outpatients. Therapy should not be terminated until patients have achieved symptomatic remission. Ideally, at least two or three sessions are planned on an every-other-week basis in preparation for termination.

## Outcome Assessment

Cognitive and behavioral therapies are, in part, distinguished by their integrated use of objective assessment methods. For depression and the anxiety disorders, a number of well-established rating scales are available. Therapist-administered scales include the Hamilton Anxiety Rating Scale (Hamilton 1959) and the Hamilton Depression Rating Scale (Hamilton 1960) as well as the Yale-Brown Obsessive–Compulsive Scale (Goodman et al. 1989). Self-report assessments of symptoms include the Beck Depression Inventory (Beck et al. 1961), the Beck Anxiety Inventory (Beck et al. 1988), the Fear Survey Schedule (Wolpe and Lang 1964), the Fear Questionnaire, (Marks and Matthews 1979), and the Hopkins Symptom Checklist (Derogatis et al. 1974). These scales are typically administered before treatment and repeated periodically (e.g., weekly or monthly) to monitor progress. The Dysfunctional Attitudes Scale, the Attributional Style Questionnaire, and the Automatic Thoughts Questionnaire may be used to evaluate distorted cognitions (Dobson and Shaw 1986). As suggested earlier, high residual levels of cognitive symptoms most likely convey an increased risk for relapse after termination of treatment (Thase et al. 1992, Simons et al. 1986). Similarly, high scores on the Hopelessness Scale (Beck et al. 1974) have been associated with a high risk for subsequent suicidal behavior (Beck et al. 1985b).

## Augmentation of Therapy

One of the major methods of augmenting a cognitive and behavioral therapy is to add an appropriate form of pharmacotherapy. For example, a depressed or agoraphobic person who has not benefited much from 8 weeks or more of CBT alone should probably be considered for pharmacotherapy. In such cases, the neurobiological substrate of the illness may be too severely disturbed to be responsive to the CBT without concomitant pharmacotherapy (Wright and Thase 1992, Jindal et al. 2002). In clinical practice, psychiatrists who are trained in CBT often combine cognitive therapy and pharmacotherapy from the beginning of treatment unless the patient expresses a strong desire to receive only a single form of therapy.

There are no contraindications to combining CBT and pharmacotherapy (Hollon et al. 1991, Wright and Thase 1992). In fact, these modalities are highly compatible in theory and practice. As noted earlier, pharmacological stabilization is a prerequisite for CBT for some Axis I disorders (e.g., psychotic depressions, schizophrenia, and bipolar disorder). When these treatments are used in combination, the treatment team should have a well-defined division of labor, open lines of communication, and an explicit sense of collaboration. Treatment of patients with severe, refractory, or incapacitating mood and anxiety disorders may represent the best use of combined therapies (Thase and Howland 1994, Bowers 1990, Otto et al. 1994, Scott 1992, Whisman et al. 1991). Other strategies used to enhance CBT include increasing the frequency of visits, switching emphasis (i.e., from cognitive to behavioral or vice versa), or involving the spouse or significant others in the therapy (Beach et al. 1994, Emmelkamp and Gerlsma 1994). The last strategy has been shown to be particularly useful in cases of depression associated with marital discord (Jacobson et al. 1991, Beach and O'Leary 1992). Computer augmentation is a new addition to the tools available for CBT (Selmi et al. 1991, Wright and Wright 1997, Kenwright et al. 2001, Wright et al. 2002a). Greater availability of personal computers with multimedia capability and increased pressure to reduce the cost of treatment may make this form of therapy augmentation a more common practice in clinical settings.

## Continuation and Maintenance Phase CBT

When Beck and associates (1979) described CBT in the late 1970s, depression researchers were primarily concerned with the issue of response to treatment—is psychotherapy or pharmacotherapy effective in reducing the symptoms of the disorder over a given period of time (generally 4–10 weeks for efficacy studies of the tricyclic antidepressants, 6–12 weeks for efficacy studies of selective serotonin reuptake inhibitors [SSRIs], and 12–20 weeks for studies of psychotherapies)? This phase of treatment has come to be called the "acute phase." Because some patients do not completely achieve a remission of symptoms (their return to premorbid well state) and because many patients experience depression as a recurring illness, there is a need for longer-term treatment methods for major depression (Kupfer et al. 1986). Furthermore, incomplete remission of depression leads to recurrence, and this conveys many adverse economic, interpersonal, and medical consequences (Thase 1992).

Over the past 18 years, studies conducted by Thase and coworkers at the University of Pittsburgh have identified and replicated correlates of relapse (return of symptoms during continuation phase treatment) and recurrence (return of symptoms after 1 year of remission of the illness) following the termination of acute-phase CT (A-CT). Failure to achieve a complete remission of the index episode by the sixth week of A-CT is associated with a three- to fivefold increase in the subsequent risk of relapse or recurrence. Thase and coworkers have found that between 50 to 60% of A-CT responders meet this criteria for risk and Jarrett's group has demonstrated that an 8-month course of continuation-CBT (C-CT) essentially neutralizes this higher risk of relapse. C-CT focuses on the vulnerabilities for recurrent depression in three domains: biologic (genetics, biology, familial, and developmental), psychosocial (personality, interpersonal, and social), and cognitive (Jarrett et al. 2001). By identifying and modifying risks and vulnerabilities and learning more effective ways of managing mood symptoms, C-CT helps prevent relapse and recurrence.

Fava and associates (1994) has developed another interesting approach to reduce the risk of relapse, the sequencing of treatment depending upon the degree of response following acute therapy. They found that a 12-session course of CBT focusing on healthy lifestyle changes significantly reduced depressive symptoms (Fava et al. 1994), increased the likelihood of successfully withdrawing from antidepressants (Fava et al. 1996, 1998a), and decreased the risk of subsequent relapse after withdrawing antidepressant medications (Fava et al. 1998b). Other studies (Blackburn and Moore 1997, Paykel et al. 1999) support the strategy of using a short course of focused CBT to offset the risks of relapse and recurrence of major depression.

## Efficacy of CBT

The cognitive and behavioral therapies are, as a class, the best studied type of psychotherapy. Numerous research studies have demonstrated the efficacy for a variety of Axis I disorders.

## Mood Disorders

Most of the evidence for the effectiveness of Beck's model of CBT for mood disorders is derived from studies of outpatients with major depressive disorder (nonbipolar, nonpsychotic subtype). There is no doubt that CBT is an effective treatment of major depression compared with a waiting list control condition (Thase 1995, Dobson 1989, Depression Guideline Panel 1993). Dating to an initial study by Rush and associates (1977), one major research focus has been to establish the efficacy of CBT vis-á-vis antidepressant pharmacotherapy. At this time, eight controlled trials contrasting CBT and tricyclic antidepressants have been completed (McCullough 2000), as have a legion of studies using other designs and other comparison groups (Thase 1995, Jarrett and Rush 1994). Several meta-analytical reviews have been published (Dobson 1989, Depression Guideline Panel 1993). Results of these studies indicate that CBT is generally comparable in efficacy (in 12–16 weeks) to tricyclic antidepressant pharmacotherapy (Watkins et al. 1993).

Thase and coworkers (2000) have recently published a report of a retrospective comparison of consecutive cohorts treated with CBT or supportive counseling and pill-placebo. The findings of this analysis suggest that CBT has greater therapeutic effects than this competently administered control condition, the ideal comparator for pharmacology efficacy studies.

The results of the National Institute of Mental Health's Treatment of Depression Collaborative Research Program (TDCRP) (Elkin et al. 1989), a large, controlled three-site clinical trial, initially appeared to be inconsistent with these findings. The study reported that CBT was as effective as the tricyclic antidepressant imipramine in the full sample, but neither CBT or imipramine was significantly more effective than the control condition, supportive clinical management, and pill-placebo. Furthermore, in the more severely ill patients or in patients with greater functional impairment, CBT appeared to be less effective than imipramine. Moreover, the study results suggested that CBT was slightly, although not statistically, less effective than interpersonal psychotherapy, especially when recovery (stable symptomatic remission lasting greater than 8 consecutive weeks) was the outcome measure examined. However, when this same cohort was observed over the course of 18 months of follow-up (Shea et al. 1992), it was determined that there was no significant difference among any of the treatments with respect to the number of patients that recovered and remained well. When the follow-up outcome of the CBT patients was reviewed, the authors found that CBT patients had the lowest rates of receiving some kind of treatment during the follow-up period and CBT patients had the lowest rates of relapse after 18 months. This led the authors to be encouraged about the prophylactic value of CBT.

Ablon and Jones (2002) also question the validity of the results of the psychotherapy findings of the TDCRP. The authors used actual transcripts of the interpersonal therapy (IPT) and CBT sessions and rated CBT and IPT sessions with respect to therapy process, therapy technique, and intervention styles. They report that both the IPT and CBT sessions adhered most strongly to the ideal prototype of CBT. In addition, adherence to the CBT prototype yielded more positive correlations with outcome measures across both types of treatment.

The acute-phase treatment findings of the TDCRP have raised questions about the suitability of CBT as a treatment of severe depression (American Psychiatric Association 2000). Alternatively, the adequacy of CBT provided in the TDCRP trial has been challenged by some who believe CBT therapists may need a longer period of training than that required to become proficient at interpersonal psychotherapy (Thase 1994). Nevertheless, in other groups' hands, CBT is fully the equal of pharmacotherapy (Blackburn et al. 1981, Murphy et al. 1984, Hollon et al. 1992). CBT has also been demonstrated to be effective for inpatients with severe and chronic depression (DeJong et al. 1986). An intensive CBT protocol has been demonstrated to be an effective treatment of 60 to 70% of unmedicated depressed inpatients suffering from nonpsychotic major depression (Thase et al. 1991, 1993).

Furthermore, in a large multisite randomized clinical trial of a difficult cohort of severe and chronically depressed patients, McCullough's CBT-based treatment, the Cognitive–Behavioral Analysis System for Psychotherapy (Keller et al. 2000, McCullough 2000), has shown equal efficacy to the serotonin–norepinephrine reuptake inhibitor, nefazodone, each being effective in 55% of cases, but the combination of the two treatments produced an impressive response rate of 85% at the end of 12 weeks of treatment. Thus, a version of CBT modified to specifically address the problems of severe and chronic depression has shown efficacy. Also see Thase and coworkers (1994b).

Interestingly, group CBT strategies for treatment of depression have been found to be nearly as effective as individual treatment in both direct comparisons (Ross and Scott 1985) and composite meta-analytical comparisons (Depression Guideline Panel 1993, DeRubeis and Crits-Christoph 1998). These studies, which have not yet dramatically affected practice habits, suggest that a significant savings in cost-effectiveness might be gained by more regular use of group treatments. One study (Ravindran et al. 1999) in dysthymic patients compared the efficacy of sertraline and group CBT, alone or in combination. These authors found the group CBT to be less effective than sertraline in alleviating clinical symptoms. However, CBT augmented the effects of sertraline with respect to some functional changes, and in a subgroup of patients it attenuated the functional impairments characteristic of dysthymia.

Marital CBT also appears to be as effective as individual CBT in treatment of depression associated with marital discord (Jacobson et al. 1991, Beach and O'Leary 1992). When effective, this marital therapy also typically produces concomitant improvement in dyadic adjustment, whereas effects of individual CBT are primarily limited to symptom variables (Jacobson et al. 1991, Beach and O'Leary 1992). Because marital discord plays a major role in the pathogenesis of many depressive episodes, greater use of couples treatment strategies may be indicated (Beach et al. 1994, Baucom et al. 1990) and such strategies have been described (Baucom and Epstein 1990).

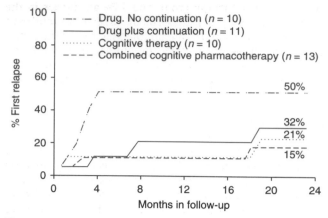

**Figure 86–8** *Risk of relapse after cognitive therapy and pharmacotherapy, singly or in combination. (Source: Evans MD, Hollon SD, DeRubeis RJ, et al. [1992] Differential relapse following cognitive therapy and pharmacotherapy for depression. Arch Gen Psychiatr 49, 802–808. Copyright 1992 American Medical Association.)*

Some evidence suggests that CBT reduces the risk for relapse after termination of treatment (vis-á-vis patients withdrawn from antidepressants) (Simons et al. 1986, Evans et al. 1992, Blackburn et al. 1986a). In the study by Evans and colleagues (1992), CBT responders had the same degree of prophylaxis against relapse at more that 1 year of follow-up as did antidepressant responders treated with continuation phase pharmacotherapy (Figure 86–8). The risk for relapse after CBT may be particularly low for patients who achieve a complete remission before ending treatment (Thase et al. 1992). The use of CBT for relapse prevention by Fava's group (1994) has been discussed.

Other models of cognitive and behavioral therapy have also been studied in randomized clinical trials of major depressive disorder, and they have generally matched or exceeded the results of the antidepressant condition (McLean and Hakstian 1979, Wilson 1982, Hersen et al. 1984). In two studies, the combination of behavioral therapy and antidepressants resulted in significantly more rapid improvement (Wilson 1982, Roth et al. 1982). Behavioral strategies emphasizing self-control skills, problem-solving skills, and increased pleasant activities have also been consistently found to be superior to waiting list control conditions, although these approaches have not yet been subjected to trials against antidepressants or other active treatments (Thase 1995, Depression Guideline Panel 1993).

## Anxiety Disorders

Controlled studies have established the efficacy of cognitive and behavioral therapies for generalized anxiety disorder, obsessive–compulsive disorder, simple phobia, social phobia, panic disorder, and agoraphobia (Wolpe 1982, Clum et al. 1993, Beck and Zebb 1994, Chambless and Gillis 1993, Durham and Allan 1993, Butler et al. 1991, Barlow et al. 2000). CBT has also been shown in a randomized clinical trial to be an effective treatment for anxiety disorders in older adults at the end of therapy and over 12 months of follow-up. These authors included patients with a wide range of anxiety disorders to allow generalization of their findings to a greater "real-world" population (Barrowclough et al. 2001).

For *simple phobias*, cognitive and behavioral treatments emphasizing progressive (graded) exposure, systematic desensitization, relaxation training, and homework assignments are so well established that they should be considered the psychotherapeutic treatment of first choice (Wolpe 1982, Rachman and Wilson 1980, Chambless and Gillis 1993).

*Obsessive–compulsive disorder*, often refractory to traditional psychosocial treatments, is also amenable to cognitive–behavioral interventions; response rates of 50 to 70% are typically reported (Emmelkamp and Beens 1991, Foa et al. 1992, Stekette 1994). Behavioral strategies generally take precedence over cognitive interventions, with the paired strategies of exposure and response prevention proving particularly useful (Emmelkamp and Beens 1991, Foa et al. 1992, Salkovskis and Westbrook 1989). Although comparative studies are fewer, therapies emphasizing exposure and response prevention have been found to be comparable to antiobsessional agents such as clomipramine in patients with behavioral compulsions (Foa et al. 1992, Marks et al. 1988). Interestingly, in a small study by Baxter and colleagues (1992), behavioral treatment of obsessive–compulsive disorder produced a change in glucose metabolism in the caudate nucleus (a putative neurobiological marker of obsessive–compulsive disorder) comparable to that observed in patients treated with pharmacotherapy. It remains to be seen whether pharmacological and cognitive–behavioral strategies can be used fruitfully in combination or in sequence (Marks et al. 1980, Turner et al. 1980).

*Generalized anxiety disorder* and *social phobia* are common and protean conditions, often presenting with much depressive and Axis II comorbidity. CBT emphasizing relaxation training, cognitive coping skills, social skills training, and graded exposure to feared situations has generally been shown to be superior to waiting list or nonspecific therapy control conditions. (Blowers et al. 1987, Borkovec et al. 1987, Borkovec and Mathews 1988, Butler et al. 1991, Durham et al. 1994, Heimberg 1990). An average of 60 to 80% of patients treated in clinical trials have responded to cognitive and behavioral methods (Gelernter et al. 1991, Power et al. 1990). In a controlled trial of patients with generalized anxiety disorder comparing CBT to behavioral therapy (BT) and a waiting list control group, results show a clear advantage for CBT over BT. There was a consistent pattern of change favoring CBT in measures of anxiety, depression, and cognition. A randomized, controlled trial in older adults with generalized anxiety disorder of CBT versus a nondirective supportive psychotherapy found no significant differences between the treatments although both reduced worry, anxiety, and depression (Stanley et al. 1997). Further comparative research is needed, especially with respect to long-term outcomes.

The comparative efficacy of cognitive and behavioral treatments and pharmacotherapy for *panic disorder* and *agoraphobia* is currently a topic of intensive investigation. (Clark et al. 1994, Clum et al. 1993, Beck and Zebb 1994, Margraf et al. 1993, National Institutes of Health 1991). These treatments teach patients to disregard or deemphasize internal cues linked to sensitivity to anxiety while mastering behavioral self-control strategies such as breathing exercises and deep muscle relaxation. Cognitive strategies are also used in these models to decrease exaggerated thinking patterns (e.g., catastrophization) and reduce worrying.

In general, between 70 and 90% of patients treated with CBT become panic free within 2 to 4 months of beginning therapy (Clum et al. 1993, Chambless and Gillis 1993, National Institutes of Health 1991). The specific models of CBT introduced by Beck and Emery (1985), Clark (1986), and Barlow and Cerny (1988) were shown to be superior to waiting list or nonspecific control conditions (Margraf et al. 1993, Barlow et al. 1989, Beck et al. 1992). In a study using an across-subjects design, CBT was found to be significantly superior to information-based therapy in reducing panic attacks in patients with panic disorder and secondary depression (Laberge et al. 1993). Meta-analyses (Beck et al. 1985a, Chambless and Gillis 1993) suggest comparability of CBT and pharmacotherapy (i.e., tricyclic antidepressants or potent benzodiazepines) during acute phase therapy. In one trial, the SSRI fluvoxamine was superior to CBT (Black et al. 1993). However, in other studies, similar advantages favored CBT (Margraf et al. 1993, Klosko et al. 1990, Marks et al. 1993).

Even if it is comparably effective, the cost-efficiency of pharmacological treatment may be reduced (relative to CBT) by high rates of relapse after discontinuation of pharmacotherapy (DuPont et al. 1992, Noyes et al. 1991, Pollack et al. 1993). Evidence collected to date suggests that there may be fewer relapses after cessation of CBT compared with relapse rates after medication discontinuation (Otto et al. 1993). This prophylactic effect may be related to significant changes in neurophysiological sensitivity (Beck and Zebb 1994). For example, Shear and colleagues (1991) found that successful CBT resulted in a significant reduction in patients' sensitivity to sodium lactate, a biological probe that reliably induces panic attacks in a significant number of patients susceptible to panic.

As with treatment of depression, CBT has shown value when it is used sequentially to reduce the risk of relapse after withdrawal of pharmacotherapy (Otto et al. 1993, Spiegel et al. 1994). To date, evidence does not indicate that the combination of CBT and pharmacotherapy yields a strongly synergistic effect (Clum et al. 1993, Marks et al. 1993, Hegel et al. 1994, Mavissakalian and Michelson 1986, Gelder 1998).

There is also interest in the application of CBT to PTSD. A recent review of controlled outcome studies indicated that CBT is the psychological treatment of choice and that is more effective than eye movement desensitivization and reprocessing (Bryant and Friedman 2001).

## Eating Disorders

Many research studies have demonstrated the efficacy of CBT for bulimia nervosa (Agras et al. 1992, 1994, 2000, Fairburn et al. 1991, 1992, 1993, 1995, Garner 1992, Goldbloom et al. 1997, Walsh et al. 1997). Reviews of controlled studies of CT have found strong evidence for the efficacy of CBT (Wilson 1999, Ricca et al. 2000). Combined cognitive and behavioral therapy has been shown to be superior to a behavior therapy–alone approach to bulimia (Thackwray et al. 1993). At the 6-month follow-up assessment after treatment, 69% of the subjects who received CBT reported no binge eating and purging as compared to 38% abstinence

in the behavior therapy group and 15% abstinence in the attention placebo group. Reviews of research on combined CBT and pharmacotherapy for bulimia have found that CBT has an additive effect to antidepressant therapy (Wilson 1999, Ricca et al. 2000). But, there appears to be no advantage to adding medication to CBT for bulimia nervosa.

## Other Disorders

Although CBT is not as well established as a primary treatment for other disorders, promising preliminary data are available in studies of borderline personality disorder (Lineham et al. 1991, 1993, Salkovskis et al. 1990). Cognitive and behavioral therapies have also been studied in substance abuse disorders and tend to be more effective than standard counseling approaches only with patients with concomitant psychiatric illness (Woody et al. 1984, Carroll et al. 1994, Higgins et al. 1994). The directive methods employed by cognitive–behavioral therapists may help to lessen the resistance characteristic of more sociopathic substance-abusing patients, who may have limited ability to make use of reflective and insight-oriented strategies (Kadden et al. 1989).

For the psychotic Axis I disorders, including schizophrenia and bipolar disorder, the cognitive and behavioral therapies have been shown to be useful adjunctive treatments for patients stabilized with appropriate psychotropic agents (Perris 1989). The first trials of CBT for psychosis were uncontrolled but suggested that this treatment approach could be used effectively for hallucinations, delusions, and other symptoms of schizophrenia (Fowler and Morley 1989, Chadwick and Birchwood 1994, Kingdon and Turkington 1991). Subsequently, several randomized controlled trials have found that CBT can add to the effect of medication (Hogarty et al. 1986, Drury et al. 1996a, 1996b, Kuipers et al. 1997, Tarrier et al. 1993, Sensky et al. 2000).

For example, Drury and coworkers (1996a, 1996b) observed that positive symptoms improved more in hospitalized patients who received CBT than those patients receiving nonspecific and supportive treatment. This research group also observed reduced time required for recovery in those treated with CBT. Sensky and coworkers (2000) studied 90 patients with schizophrenia who had persistent, drug resistant symptoms. In this study both forms of psychotherapy (CBT and an equal amount of time in "befriending") were effective at the end of active treatment. However, 9 months after treatment subjects who received CBT had significantly lower ratings on measures of positive and negative symptoms.

There are two randomized control trials of CBT in patients with bipolar disorder. The first studied whether CBT improved lithium compliance at 6 and 12 months after treatment as compared to a control group. The results indicated no difference in lithium compliance on the self-reports, informant-reports, or serum lithium levels, but the physician (who was not blind to which group the patient belonged) reported more compliance on the part of the patient exposed to CBT (Cochran 1984). The second randomized controlled trial of CBT in patients with bipolar disorder examined the efficacy of CBT to prevent relapse in patients also taking mood stabilizer medications. The authors modified CBT by (1) a psychoeducational component that modeled bipolar illness as a stress-diathesis illness; (2) adaptive CBT skills to cope with producers (identifying the onset of symptoms of bipolar disorder characteristic of the patient's illness pattern); (3) promoting the importance of circadian regularity by emphasizing the importance of routine and sleep; and (4) dealing with the long-term vulnerabilities and difficulties of the illness. Therapy consisted of 12 to 20 sessions and lasted 6 months and outcomes were measured at 6- and 12-month points. The CBT group had significantly fewer bipolar episodes, higher social functioning, better coping strategies for bipolar problems, evidence of less fluctuation in symptoms of mania and depression, less hopelessness, better medication compliance, and they used significantly less neurologic medication (Lam et al. 2000).

## Conclusion

The cognitive and behavior therapies are based on well-articulated theories that have a strong empirical basis. These therapies emphasize objective assessments and use of directive interventions aimed at reducing symptomatic distress, enhancing interpersonal skills, and improving social and vocational functioning. Cognitive interventions are focused primarily on identifying and modifying distorted thoughts and pathological schemas. Behavioral techniques to increase exposure, increase activity, enhance social skills, and improve anxiety management are useful modalities, and can complement or amplify the effects of cognitive strategies. Similarly, the cognitive perspective can add depth to behavioral models for therapy by teaching patients how to recognize and modify their attitudinal vulnerabilities.

The cognitive and behavioral therapies are the best-studied psychological treatments of major depressive, panic, generalized anxiety, and obsessive–compulsive disorders. Overall, there is good evidence for the effectiveness of these interventions within these indications. Cognitive and behavioral therapies are being adapted for adjunctive use with pharmacotherapy for treatment of bipolar disorder and schizophrenia. There are no contraindications for use in combination with pharmacotherapy. The cognitive and behavioral therapies have become one of the standard psychosocial treatment approaches for mental disorders.

## References

Ablon JS and Jones EE (2002) Validity of controlled clinical trials of psychotherapy: Findings from the NIMH treatment of depression collaborative research program. Am J Psychiatr 159(5), 775–783.

Abramson LY, Metalsky GI, and Alloy LB (1989) Hopelessness depression: A theory-based subtype of depression. Psychol Rev 96, 358–372.

Abramson LY, Seligman MEP, and Teasdale J (1978) Learned helplessness in humans: Critique and reformulation. J Abnorm Psychol 87, 49–74.

Agras WS, Rossiter EM, Arnow B, et al. (1992) Pharmacologic and cognitive–behavioral treatment for bulimia nervosa: A controlled comparison. Am J Psychiatr 149, 82–87.

Agras WS, Telch CF, Arnow B, et al. (1994) Weight loss, cognitive–behavioral, and desipramine treatments in binge eating disorder: An additive design. Behav Ther 25, 225–238.

Agras WS, Walsh BT, Fairburn CG, et al. (2000) A multicenter comparison of cognitive–behavioral therapy and interpersonal psychotherapy for bulimia nervosa. Arch Gen Psychiatr 57(5), 459–466.

Alfrod BA and Correia CJ (1994) Cognitive therapy of schizophrenia: Theory and empirical status. Behav Ther 25, 17–33.

American Psychiatric Association (2000) Practice guideline for major depressive disorder in adults. Am J Psychiatr 157(Suppl), 1–45.

Ayllon T and Azrin NH (1968) The Token Economy: A Motivational System for Therapy and Rehabilitation. Appleton-Century-Crofts, New York.

Azrin NH and Holz WC (1966) Punishment. In Operant Behavior: Areas of Research and Application, Honig WK (ed). Appleton-Century-Crofts, New York, pp. 12–32.

Bandura A (1977a) Self-efficacy: Toward a unifying theory of behavioral change. Psychol Rev 84, 191–215.

Bandura A (1977b) Social Learning Theory. Prentice-Hall, Englewood Cliffs, NJ.

Barlow DH and Cerny JA (1988) Psychological Treatment of Panic. Treatment Manual for Practitioners. Guilford Press, New York.

Barlow DH, Craske MG, Cerny JA, et al. (1989) Behavioral treatment of panic disorder. Behav Ther 20, 261–282.

Barlow DH, Gorman JM, Shear MK, et al. (2000) Cognitive–behavioral therapy, imipramine, or their combination for panic disorder: A randomized controlled trial. JAMA 283(19), 2529–2536.

Barrowclough C, King P, Colville J, et al. (2001) A randomized trial of the effectiveness of cognitive–behavioral therapy and supportive counseling for anxiety symptoms in older adults. J Consult Clin Psychol 69(Suppl), 756–762.

Basco RM and Rush AJ (1996) Cognitive–Behavior Therapy for Bipolar Disorder. Guilford Press, New York.

Basco RM and Thase ME (1998) Cognitive–behavioral treatment of bipolar disorder. In International Handbook of Cognitive and Behavioral Treatments for Psychological Disorders, Caballo VE (ed). Elsevier Science, Oxford, pp. 521–550.

Baucom D and Epstein N (1990) Cognitive–Behavioral Marital Therapy. Brunner/Mazel, New York.

Baucom D, Sayers S, and Scher T (1990) Supplemental behavioral marital therapy with cognitive restructuring and emotional expressiveness training: An outcome investigation. J Consult Clin Psychol 58, 636–645.

Baxter LR, Schwartz JM, Bergman KS, et al. (1992) Caudate glucose metabolic rate changes with both drug and behavior therapy for obsessive–compulsive disorder. Arch Gen Psychiatr 49, 681–689.

Beach SRH and O'Leary KD (1992) Treating depression in the context of marital discord: Outcome and predictors of response of marital therapy versus cognitive therapy. Behav Ther 23, 507–528.

Beach SRH, Whisman MS, and O'Leary KD (1994) Marital therapy for depression: Theoretical foundation, current status, and future directions. Behav Ther 25, 345–371.

Beck AT (1963) Thinking and depression. Arch Gen Psychiatr 9, 324–333.

Beck AT (1964) Thinking and depression, 2: Theory and therapy. Arch Gen Psychiatr 10, 561–571.

Beck AT (1967) Depression: Clinical, Experimental, and Theoretical Aspects. Harper & Row, New York.

Beck AT (1976) Cognitive Therapy and the Emotional Disorders. International Universities Press, New York.

Beck AT (1991) Cognitive therapy: A 30-year retrospective. Am Psychol 46, 368–375.

Beck AT (1993) Cognitive therapy: Past, present, and future. J Consult Clin Psychol 61, 194–198.

Beck AT and Emery G (1985) Anxiety Disorders and Phobias: A Cognitive Perspective. Basic Books, New York.

Beck AT and Greenberg RL (1974) Coping with Depression [booklet]. Institute for Rational Living, New York.

Beck AT and Rush AJ (2000) Cognitive therapy. In Comprehensive Textbook of Psychiatry, Vol. 7, Kaplan HI and Saddock BJ (eds). Williams & Wilkins, Baltimore.

Beck AT, Emery G, and Greenberg RL (1985a) Anxiety Disorders and Phobias: A Cognitive Perspective. Basic Books, New York.

Beck AT, Epstein N, Brown G, et al. (1988) An inventory for measuring clinical anxiety: Psychometric properties. J Consult Clin Psychol 56, 893–897.

Beck AT, Freeman A, and Associates (1990) Cognitive Therapy of Personality Disorders. Guilford Press, New York.

Beck AT, Rush AJ, Shaw BF, et al. (1979) Cognitive Therapy of Depression. Guilford Press, New York.

Beck AT, Sokol L, Clark DA, et al. (1992) A crossover study of focused cognitive therapy for panic disorder. Am J Psychiatr 149, 778–783.

Beck AT, Steer RA, Kovacs M, et al. (1985b) Hopelessness and eventual suicide: A ten-year prospective study of patients hospitalized with suicidal ideation. Am J Psychiatr 142, 559–563.

Beck AT, Ward CH, Mendelson M, et al. (1961) An inventory for measuring depression. Arch Gen Psychiatr 4, 561–571.

Beck AT, Weissman A, Lester D, et al. (1974) The measurement of pessimism: The hopelessness scale. J Consult Clin Psychol 42, 861–865.

Beck AT, Wright FD, Newman CF, et al. (1993) Cognitive Therapy of Substance Abuse. Guilford Press, New York.

Beck JS (1995) Cognitive Therapy: Basics and Beyond. Guilford Press, New York.

Beck JS and Zebb BJ (1994) Behavioral assessment and treatment of panic disorder: Current status, future directions. Behav Ther 25, 581–611.

Bernstein DA and Borkovec TD (1973) Progressive Relaxation Training. Research Press, Champaign, IL.

Black DW, Wesner R, Bowers W, et al. (1993) A comparison of fluvoxamine, cognitive therapy, and placebo in the treatment of panic disorder. Arch Gen Psychiatr 50, 44–50.

Blackburn IM and Moore RG (1997) Controlled acute and follow-up trial of cognitive therapy and pharmacotherapy in out-patients with recurrent depression. Br J Psychiatr 171, 328–334.

Blackburn IM, Bishop S, Glen AIM, et al. (1981) The efficacy of cognitive therapy in depression. A treatment trial using cognitive therapy and pharmacotherapy, each alone and in combination. Br J Psychiatr 139, 181–189.

Blackburn IM, Eunson KM, and Bishop S (1986a) A two-year naturalistic follow-up of depressed patients treated with cognitive therapy, pharmacotherapy and a combination of both. J Affect Disord 10, 67–75.

Blackburn IM, Jones S, and Lewin RJP (1986b) Cognitive style in depression. Br J Clin Psychol 25, 241–251.

Blowers C, Cobb J, and Mathews A (1987) Generalized anxiety: A controlled treatment study. Behav Res Ther 25, 493–502.

Borkovec TD and Mathews AM (1988) Treatment of nonphobic anxiety disorders: A comparison of nondirective, cognitive, and coping desensitization therapy. J Consult Clin Psychol 56, 877–884.

Borkovec TD, Mathews AM, Chambers A, et al. (1987) The effects of relaxation training with cognitive or nondirective therapy and the role of relaxation-induced anxiety in the treatment of generalized anxiety. J Consult Clin Psychol 55, 883–888.

Bowers WA (1990) Treatment of depressed inpatients. Cognitive therapy plus medication, relaxation plus medication, and medication alone. Br J Psychiatr 156, 73–78.

Bowlby J (1985) The role of childhood experience in cognitive disturbance. In Cognition and Psychotherapy, Mahoney MJ and Freeman A (eds). Plenum Press, New York, pp. 181–200.

Bryant R and Friedman M (2001) Medication and nonmedication treatments of posttraumatic stress disorder. Curr Opin Psychiatr 14(2), 119–123.

Burns DD (1980) Feeling Good. William Morrow, New York.

Burns DD (1990) The Feeling Good Handbook. Penguin Books, New York.

Burns DD and Spangler DL (2000) Does psychotherapy homework lead to improvements in depression in cognitive-behavioral therapy or does improvement lead to increased homework compliance? J Consult Clin Psychol 68(1), 46–56.

Butler G, Fennell M, Robson P, et al. (1991) Comparison of behavior therapy and cognitive behavior therapy in the treatment of generalized anxiety disorder. J Consult Clin Psychol 59, 167–175.

Carroll KM, Rounsaville BJ, Gordon LT, et al. (1994) Psychotherapy and pharmacotherapy for ambulatory cocaine abusers. Arch Gen Psychiatr 51, 177–187.

Chadwick P and Birchwood M (1994) The omnipotence of voices: A cognitive approach to auditory hallucinations. Br J Psychiatr 164, 190–201.

Chambless DL and Gillis MM (1993) Cognitive therapy of anxiety disorders. J Consult Clin Psychol 62, 248–260.

Clark D (1986) A cognitive approach to panic. Behav Res Ther 24, 461–470.

Clark DA, Beck AT, and Alford BA (1999) Scientific Foundations of Cognitive Theory and Therapy of Depression. John Wiley, New York, pp. 36–76.

Clark DM, Salkovskis PM, and Chalkley AJ (1985) Respiratory control as a treatment for panic attacks. J Behav Ther Exp Psychiatr 16, 23–30.

Clark DM, Salkovskis PM, Hackmann A, et al. (1994) A comparison of cognitive therapy, applied relaxation, and imipramine in the treatment of panic disorder. Br J Psychiatr 164, 759–769.

Cloitre M and Liebowitz MR (1991) Memory bias in panic disorder: An investigation of the cognitive avoidance hypothesis. Cogn Ther Res 15, 371–386.

Clum GA, Clum GA, and Surls R (1993) A meta-analysis of treatments of panic disorder. J Consult Clin Psychol 61, 317–326.

Cochran SD (1984) Preventing medical noncompliance in the outpatient treatment of bipolar affective disorders. J Consult Clin Psychol 52, 873–878.

Coyne JC, Kessler RC, Tal M, et al. (1987) Living with a depressed person. J Consult Clin Psychol 55, 347–352.

DeJong R, Treiber R, and Henrich G (1986) Effectiveness of two psychological treatments for inpatients with severe and chronic depressions. Cogn Ther Res 10, 645–663.

DeMonbreun BG and Craighead WE (1977) Distortion of perception and recall of positive and neutral feedback in depression. Cogn Ther Res 1, 311–329.

Depression Guideline Panel (1993) Depression in Primary Care, Vol. 2, Treatment of Major Depression. Clinical Practice Guideline, No. 5, US Department of Health and Human Services, Agency for Health Care Policy and Research, publication 93–0551, Rockville, MD.

Derogatis L, Lipman R, and Rickels K (1974) The Hopkins Symptom Checklist (HSCL): A self-report symptom inventory. Behav Sci 19, 1–16.

DeRubeis RJ and Crits-Christoph P (1998) Empirically supported individual and group psychological treatments for adult mental disorder. J Consult Clin Psychol 66(1), 37–52.

DeRubeis RJ, Evans MD, Hollon SD, et al. (1990) How does cognitive therapy work? Cognitive change and symptom change in cognitive therapy and pharmacotherapy for depression. J Consult Clin Psychol 58, 862–869.

Deutscher S and Cimbolic P (1990) Cognitive processes and their relationship to endogenous and reactive components of depression. J Nerv Ment Dis 178, 351–359.

Dobson KS (1989) A meta-analysis of the efficacy of cognitive therapy for depression. J Consult Clin Psychol 57, 414–419.

Dobson KS and Block L (1988) Historical and philosophical bases of the cognitive–behavioral therapies. In Handbook of Cognitive Behavioral Therapies, Dobson KS (ed). Guilford Press, New York, pp. 3–38.

Dobson KS and Shaw BF (1986) Cognitive assessment with major depressive disorders. Cogn Ther Res 10, 13–29.

Drury V, Birchwood M, Cochrane R, et al. (1996a) Cognitive therapy and recovery from acute psychosis: A controlled trial I: Impact on psychotic symptoms. Br J Psychiatr 169, 593–601.

Drury V, Birchwood M, Cochrane R, et al. (1996b) Cognitive therapy and recovery from acute psychosis: A controlled trial II: Impact on recovery time. Br J Psychiatr 169, 602–607.

DuPont RL, Swinson RP, Ballenger JC, et al. (1992) Discontinuation of alprazolam after long-term treatment of panic-related disorders. J Clin Psychopharmacol 12, 352–354.

Durham RC and Allan T (1993) Psychological treatment of generalized anxiety disorder. A review of the clinical significance of results in outcome studies since 1980. Br J Psychiatr 163, 19–26.

Durham RC, Murphy T, Allan T, et al. (1994) Cognitive therapy, analytic psychotherapy and anxiety management training for generalized anxiety disorder. Br J Psychiatr 165, 315–323.

Elkin I, Shea MT, Watkins JT, et al. (1989) National Institute of Mental Health Treatment of Depression Collaborative Research Program. General effectiveness of treatments. Arch Gen Psychiatr 46, 971–982.

Ellis A (1989) The history of cognition in psychotherapy. In Comprehensive Handbook of Cognitive Therapy, Freeman A, Simon KM, Beutler LE, et al. (eds). Plenum Press, New York, pp. 5–19.

Emmelkamp PMG and Beens H (1991) Cognitive therapy with obsessive-compulsive disorder: A comparative evaluation. Behav Res Ther 29, 293–300.

Emmelkamp PMG and Gerlsma C (1994) Marital functioning and the anxiety disorders. Behav Ther 25, 407–429.

Epstein N, Schlesinger SE, and Dryden W (1988) Cognitive–Behavioral Therapy with Families. Brunner/Mazel, New York.

Evans MD, Hollon SD, DeRubeis RJ, et al. (1992) Differential relapse following cognitive therapy and pharmacotherapy for depression. Arch Gen Psychiatr 49, 802–808.

Eysenck HJ (1952) The effects of psychotherapy: An evaluation. J Consult Clin Psychol 16, 319–324.

Fairburn CG, Agras WS, and Wilson GT (1992) The research on treatment of bulimia nervosa: Practical and theoretical implications. In

The Biology of Feast and Famine: Relevence to Eating Disorders, Anderson GH and Kennedy SH (eds). Academic Press, San Diego, pp. 318–340.

Fairburn CG, Jones R, Peveler RC, et al. (1991) Three psychological treatments for bulimia nervosa. Arch Gen Psychiatr 48, 463–469.

Fairburn CG, Jones R, Peveler RC, et al. (1993) Psychotherapy and bulimia nervosa. Arch Gen Psychiatr 50, 419–428.

Fairburn CG, Norman PA, Welch SL, et al. (1995) A prospective study of outcome in bulimia nervosa and the long-term effects of three psychological treatments. Arch Gen Psychiatr 52, 304–312.

Fava GA, Grandi G, Zielezny M, et al. (1994) Cognitive–behavioral treatment of residual symptoms in primary major depressive disorder. Am J Psychiatr 151(9), 1295–1299.

Fava GA, Grandi G, Zielezny M, et al. (1996) Four-year outcome for cognitive behavioral treatment of residual symptoms in major depression. Am J Psychiatr 153(7), 945–947.

Fava GA, Rafanelli C, Grandi S, et al. (1998a) Prevention of recurrent depression with cognitive–behavioral therapy. Arch Gen Psychiatr 55, 816–820.

Fava GA, Rafanelli C, Grandi S, et al. (1998b) Six-year outcome for cognitive–behavioral treatment of residual symptoms in major depression. Am J Psychiatr 155(10), 1443–1445.

Ferster CB (1973) A functional analysis of depression. Am Psychol 28, 857–870.

Fitzgerald TE and Phillips W (1991) Attentional bias and agoraphobic avoidance: The role of cognitive style. J Anx Disord 5, 333–341.

Foa EB, Kozak MJ, Steketee GS, et al. (1992) Treatment of depressive and obsessive–compulsive symptoms in OCD by imipramine and behaviour therapy. Br J Clin Psychol 31, 279–292.

Fowler D and Morley S (1989) The cognitive–behavioral treatment of hallucinations and delusions: A preliminary study. Behav Psychother 17, 262–282.

Freeman A, Simon KM, Beutler LE, et al. (eds) (1989) Comprehensive Handbook of Cognitive Therapy. Plenum Press, New York.

Freud S (1950) Mourning and melancholia. In Collected Papers, Vol. 4. Hogarth Press and the Institute of Psychoanalysis, London, pp. 152–172. (Originally published in 1917)

Friedman ES (1997) Combined therapy for depression. J Pract Psychiatr Behav Health 3(4), 211–222.

Garner DM (1992) Psychotherapy for eating disorders. Curr Opin Psychiatr 5, 391–395.

Gelder MG (1998) Combined pharmacotherapy and cognitive–behavioral therapy in the treatment of panic disorder. J Clin Psychopharmacol 18(Suppl), 2S–5S.

Gelernter CS, Uhde TW, Cimbolic P, et al. (1991) Cognitive–behavioral and pharmacological treatments of social phobia. Arch Gen Psychiatr 48, 938–945.

Goldbloom DS, Olmsted M, Davis R, et al. (1997) A randomized controlled trial of fluoxetine and cognitive–behavioral therapy for bulimia nervosa: Short-term outcome. Behav Res Ther 35(9), 803–811.

Goldfried MR and Davison GC (1994) Clinical Behavior Therapy, Expanded Version. John Wiley, New York.

Goodman WK, Price LH, Rasmussen SA, et al. (1989) The Yale-Brown Obsessive–Compulsive Scale. II. Validity. Arch Gen Psychiatr 46, 1012–1016.

Greenberger D and Padesky CA (1995) Mind Over Mood: A Cognitive Therapy Treatment Manual for Clients. Guilford Press, New York.

Hamilton M (1959) The assessment of anxiety states by rating. Br J Med Psychol 32, 50–55.

Hamilton M (1960) A rating scale for depression. J Neurol Neurosur Psychiatr 23, 56–62.

Hammen C, Ellicott A, Gitlin M, et al. (1989) Sociotropy/autonomy and vulnerability to specific life events in patients with unipolar depression and bipolar disorders. J Abnorm Psychol 98, 154–160.

Hegel MT, Ravaris CL, and Ahles TA (1994) Combined cognitive–behavioral and time-limited alprazolam treatment of panic disorder. Behav Ther 25, 183–195.

Heimberg RG, Dodge CS, Hope DA, et al. (1990) Cognitive–behavioral group treatment for social phobia: Comparison with a credible placebo-control. Cogn Ther Res 14, 1–23.

Hersen M, Bellack AS, Himmelhoch JM, et al. (1984) Effects of social skill training, amitriptyline, and psychotherapy in unipolar depressed women. Behav Ther 15, 21–40.

Higgins ST, Budney AJ, Bickel WK, et al. (1994) Incentives improve outcome in outpatient behavioral treatment of cocaine dependence. Arch Gen Psychiatr 51, 568–576.

Hogarty G, Anderson CM, Reiss DJ, et al. (1986) Environmental personal indicators in the course of schizophrenia research group. Family psychoeducation, social skills training and maintenance chemotherapy in the aftercare of schizophrenia: 1. One year effects of a controlled study on relapse and expressed emotion. Arch Gen Psychiatr 43, 633–642.

Hollan SD and Kendall PC (1980) Cognitive self-statements in depression: Development of an automatic thought questionnaire. Cogn Ther Res 4, 383–395.

Hollon SD, DeRubeis RJ, Evans MD, et al. (1992) Cognitive therapy and pharmacotherapy for depression: Singly and in combination. Arch Gen Psychiatr 49, 774–781.

Hollon SD, Shelton RC, and Loosen P (1991) Cognitive therapy and pharmacotherapy for depression. J Consult Clin Psychol 59, 88–99.

Hull CL (1943) Principles of Behavior. Appleton-Century-Crofts, New York.

Ilardi SS and Craighead WE (1994) The role of nonspecific factors in cognitive–behavior therapy for depression. Clin Psychol Sci Pract 1, 138–156.

Ingram RE and Kendall PC (1987) The cognitive side of anxiety. Cogn Ther Res 11, 523–536.

Jacobson NS, Dobson K, Fruzzetti AE, et al. (1991) Marital therapy as a treatment for depression. J Consult Clin Psychol 59, 547–557.

Jarrett RB and Kraft D (1997) Prophylactic cognitive therapy for major depressive disorder. In Session: Psychotherapy in Practice, 3(3), 65–79.

Jarrett RB and Rush AJ (1994) Short-term psychotherapy of depressive disorders: Current status and future directions. Psychiatry 57, 115–132.

Jarrett RB, Kraft D, Doyle J, et al. (2001) Preventing recurrent depression using cognitive therapy with and without a continuation phase: A randomized clinical trial. Arch Gen Psychiatr 58, 381–388.

Jindal R, Thase ME, Fasiczka AL, et al. (2002) Electroencephalographic sleep profiles in single-episode and recurrent unipolar forms of major depression: II. Comparison during remission. Biol Psychiatr 51(3), 230–236.

Kadden RM, Conney NL, Getter H, et al. (1989) Matching alcoholics to coping skills or interactional therapies: Pretreatment results. J Consult Clin Psychol 57, 698–704.

Kanfer FH and Saslow G (1965) Behavioral analysis: An alternative to diagnostic classification. Arch Gen Psychiatr 12, 529–538.

Kazdin AE (1982) History of behavior modification. In International Handbook of Behavior Modification and Therapy, Bellack AS, Hersen M, and Kazdin AE (eds). Plenum Press, New York, pp. 3–32.

Kazdin AE and Wilcoxin LA (1976) Systematic desensitization and nonspecific treatment effects: A methodological consideration. Psychol Bull 83, 729–758.

Keller MB, McCullough JP, Klein DN, et al. (2000) A comparison of nefazodone. The cognitive–behavioral-analysis system for psychotherapy, and their combination for the treatment of chronic depression. New Engl J Med 342, 1462–1470.

Kendall PC and Hollon SD (1989) Anxious self-talk: Development of the Anxious Self-Statements Questionnaire (ASSQ). Cogn Ther Res 13, 81–93.

Kenwright M, Liness S, and Marks IM (2001) Reducing demands on clinicians by offering computer-aided self-help for phobia/panic: A feasibility study. Br J Psychiatr 179, 456–459.

Kingdon DG and Turkington D (1991) The use of cognitive–behavior therapy with a normalizing rationale in schizophrenia. J Nerv Ment Dis 179, 207–211.

Kingdon DG and Turkington D (1995) Cognitive–Behavioral Therapy of Schizophrenia. Guilford Press, New York.

Klein DC and Seligman MEP (1976) Reversal of performance deficits in learned helplessness and depression. J Abnorm Psychol 85, 11–26.

Klein DF (1993) False suffocation alarms, spontaneous panics, and related conditions: An integrative hypothesis. Arch Gen Psychiatr 50, 306–317.

Klosko JS, Barlow DH, Tassinari RB, et al. (1990) Comparison of alprazolam and behavior therapy in the treatment of panic disorder. J Consult Clin Psychol 58, 77–84.

Kuipers E, Garety P, and Fowler D (1997) London-East Anglia randomized controlled trial of cognitive–behavioral therapy for psychosis I: Effects of the treatment phase. Br J Psychiatr 171(10), 319–327.

Kupfer DJ, Frank E, Perel JM, et al. (1986) Five-year outcome for maintenance therapies in recurrent depression. Arch Gen Psychiatr 43, 43–50.

Laberge B, Gouthier JG, Cote G, et al. (1993) Cognitive–behavioral therapy of panic disorder with secondary depression: A preliminary investigation. J Consult Clin Psychol 61(6), 1028–1037.

Lam DL, Bright J, Jones S, et al. (2000) Cognitive therapy for bipolar illness—A pilot study of relapse prevention. Cogn Ther Res 24(5), 503–520.

LeDoux J (1988) Fear and the brain: Where have we been, and where are we going. Biol Psychiatr 44, 1229–1238.

LeFebvre MF (1981) Cognitive distortion and cognitive errors in depressed psychiatric and low back pain patients. J Consult Clin Psychol 49, 517–525.

Lewinsohn PM, Sullivan JM, and Grosscup SJ (1982) Behavioral therapy: Clinical applications. In Short-Term Psychotherapies for Depression, Rush AJ (ed). Guilford Press, New York, pp. 50–87.

Lindsley OR (1956) Operant conditioning methods applied to research in chronic schizophrenia. Psychiatr Res Rep 5, 118–139.

Linehan MM, Armstrong HE, Suarez A, et al. (1991) Cognitive–behavioral treatment of chronically parasuicidal borderline patients. Arch Gen Psychiatr 48, 1060–1064.

Linehan MM, Heard HL, and Armstrong HE (1993) Naturalistic follow-up of a behavioral treatment for chronically parasuicidal borderline patients. Arch Gen Psychiatr 50, 971–974.

Locke SE and Rezza MEH (1996) Computer-based education in mental health. MD Comput 13, 10–45.

Maier SF and Seligman MEP (1976) Learned helplessness: Theory and evidence. J Exp Psychol 105, 3–46.

Malott RW, Whaley DL, and Mallott ME (1993) Elementary Principles of Behavior. Prentice-Hall, Englewood Cliffs, NJ.

Margraf J, Barlow DH, Clark DM, et al. (1993) Psychological treatment of panic: Work in progress on outcome, active ingredients, and follow-up. Behav Res Ther 31, 1–8.

Marks IM and Gelder MG (1965) A controlled retrospective study of behaviour therapy in phobic patients. Br J Psychiatr 111, 561–573.

Marks IM and Matthews AM (1979) Brief standard self-rating for phobic patients. Behav Res Ther 17, 263–267.

Marks IM, Lelliott P, Basoglu M, et al. (1988) Clomipramine, self exposure and therapist-aided exposure for obsessive–compulsive rituals. Br J Psychiatr 152, 522–534.

Marks IM, Stern RS, Mawson D, et al. (1980) Clomipramine and exposure for obsessive–compulsive rituals. Br J Psychiatr 136, 1–25.

Marks IM, Swinson RP, Basoglu M, et al. (1993) Alprazolam and exposure alone and combined in panic disorder with agoraphobia: A controlled study in London and Toronto. Br J Psychiatr 162, 776–787.

Masserman JH (1943) Behavior and Neurosis. University of Chicago Press, Chicago.

Mathews A and MacLeod C (1987) An information-processing approach to anxiety. J Cogn Psychother 1, 105–115.

Mavissakalian M and Michelson L (1986) Agoraphobia: Relative and combined effectiveness of therapist-assisted in-vivo exposure and imipramine. J Consult Clin Psychol 47, 117–122.

McCullough JP (2000) Treatment for Chronic Depression: Cognitive–Behavioral Analysis System of Psychotherapy. Guilford Press, New York.

McLean PD and Hakstian AR (1979) Clinical depression: Comparative efficacy of outpatient treatments. J Consult Clin Psychol 47, 818–836.

Meichenbaum DB (1977) Cognitive–Behavior Modification: An Integrative Approach. Plenum Press, New York.

Metalsky GI, Halberstadt LJ, and Albramson LY (1987) Vulnerability to depressive mood reactions: Toward a more powerful test of the diathesis-stress and causal mediation components of the reformulated theory of depression. J Pers Soc Psychol 52, 386–393.

Miller WR and Seligman MEP (1975) Depression and learned helplessness in man. J Abnorm Psychol 84, 228–238.

Mischel W (1968) Personality and Assessment. John Wiley, New York.

Mowrer OH (1947) On the dual nature of learning—a re-interpretation of 'conditioning' and 'problem-solving.' Harv Educ Rev 16, 102–140.

Mueser KT (1998) Cognitive–behavioral treatment of schizophrenia. In International Handbook of Cognitive and Behavioral Treatments for Psychological Disorders, Caballo VE (ed). Elsevier Science, Oxford, pp. 551–570.

Murphy GE, Simons AD, Wetzel RD, et al. (1984) Cognitive therapy and pharmacotherapy: Singly and together in the treatment of depression. Arch Gen Psychiatr 41, 33–41.

National Institutes of Health (1991) Treatment of panic disorder. NIH Consens Statement 9(2), 25–27.

Nelson RE and Craighead WE (1977) Selective recall of positive and negative feedback, self-control behaviors and depression. J Abnorm Psychol 86, 379–388.

Noyes R, Garvey MJ, Cook B, et al. (1991) Controlled discontinuation of benzodiazepine treatment for patients with panic disorder. Am J Psychiatr 148, 517–523.

Oakes WF and Curtis N (1982) Learned helplessness: Not dependent upon cognitions, attributions, or other such phenomenal experiences. J Pers 50, 387–408.

Otto MW, Gould RA, and Pollack MH (1994) Cognitive–behavioral treatment of panic disorder: Considerations for the treatment of patients over the long term. Psychiatr Ann 24, 307–315.

Otto MW, Pollack MH, Sachs GS, et al. (1993) Discontinuation of benzodiazepine treatment: Efficacy of cognitive–behavioral therapy for patients with panic disorder. Am J Psychiatr 150(10), 1485–1490.

Overholser JC (1993a) Elements of the Socratic method: I. Systematic questioning. Psychotherapy 30, 67–74.

Overholser JC (1993b) Elements of the Socratic method: II. Inductive reasoning. Psychotherapy 30, 75–85.

Overholser JC (1993c) Elements of the Socratic method: III. Universal definitions. 31, 286–293.

Paul GL (1966) Insight Versus Desensitization in Psychotherapy: An Experiment in Anxiety Reduction. Stanford University Press, Stanford, CA.

Pavlov IP and Gantt WH (trans) (1928) Lectures on Conditioned Reflexes. International Publishers, New York.

Paykel ES, Scott J, Teesdale JD, et al. (1999) Prevention of relapse in residual depression by cognitive therapy. 56, 829–837.

Perris C (1989) Cognitive Therapy with Schizophrenic Patients. Guilford Press, New York.

Persons JB (1989) Cognitive Therapy in Practice: A Case Formulation Approach. WW Norton, New York.

Peterson C, Villanova P, and Raps CS (1985) Depression and attributions: Factors responsible for inconsistent results in the published literature. J Abnorm Psychol 94, 165–168.

Pollack MH, Otto MW, Tesar GE, et al. (1993) Long-term outcome after acute treatment with clonazepam and alprazolam for panic disorder. J Clin Psychopharmacol 13, 257–263.

Power KG, Simpson RJ, Swanson V, et al. (1990) A controlled comparison of cognitive–behavior therapy, diazepam, and placebo, alone, and in combination, for the treatment of generalized anxiety disorder. J Anx Disord 4, 267–292.

Rachman SJ and Wilson GT (1980) The Effects of Psychological Therapy. Pergamon Press, New York.

Rachman SJ, Craske MG, Tallman K, et al. (1986) Does escape behavior strengthen agoraphobic avoidance? A replication. Behav Res Ther 26, 41–52.

Ravindran AV, Anisman H, Merali Z, et al. (1999) Treatment of primary dysthymia with group cognitive therapy and pharmacotherapy: Clinical symptoms and functional impairment. Am J Psychiatr 156(10), 1608–1617.

Rehm LP (1977) A self-control model of depression. Behav Ther 8, 787–804.

Ricca V, Mannucci E, Zucchi T, et al. (2000) Cognitive–behavioral therapy for bulimia nervosa and binge eating disorder: A review. Psychother Psychosom 69, 287–295.

Rizley R (1978) Depression and distortion in the attribution of causality. J Abnorm Psychol 87, 32–48.

Robins CJ and Hayes AM (1993) An appraisal of cognitive therapy. J Consult Clin Psychol 61, 205–214.

Ross M and Scott M (1985) An evaluation of the effectiveness of individual and group cognitive therapy in the treatment of depressed patients in an inner city health center. J Roy Coll Gen Pract 35, 239–242.

Roth D, Bielski R, Jones M, et al. (1982) A comparison of self-control therapy and antidepressant medication in the treatment of depression. Behav Ther 13, 133–144.

Rush AJ, Beck AT, Kovacs M, et al. (1977) Comparative efficacy of cognitive therapy and pharmacotherapy in the treatment of depressed outpatients. Cogn Ther Res 1, 17–37.

Salkovskis PM and Westbrook D (1989) Behavior therapy and obsessional ruminations: Can failure be turned into success? Behav Res Ther 27, 149–160.

Salkovskis PM, Atha C, and Storer D (1990) Cognitive–behavioral problem solving in the treatment of patients who repeatedly attempt suicide. A controlled trial. Br J Psychiatr 157, 871–876.

Scott J (1992) Chronic depression: Can cognitive therapy succeed when other treatments fail? Behav Psychother 20, 25–36.

Scott J and Wright JH (1997) Cognitive therapy for chronic and severe mental disorders. In American Psychiatric Press Review of Psychiatry, Vol. 16, Dickstein LJ, Riba MB, and Oldham JM (eds). American Psychiatric Press, Washington DC, pp. 1135–1170.

Segal ZV (1988) Appraisal of the self-schema construct in cognitive models of depression. Psychol Bull 103, 147–162.

Seligman MEP (1975) Helplessness: On Depression, Development, and Death. WH Freeman, San Francisco.

Selmi PM, Klein MH, Greist JH, et al. (1990) Computer-administered cognitive–behavioral therapy for depression. Am J Psychiatr 147, 51–56.

Selmi PM, Klein MH, Greist JH, et al. (1991) Computer-administered therapy for depression. MD Comput 8, 98–102.

Sensky T and Wright JH (1993) Cognitive therapy with medical patients. In The Cognitive Milieu: Inpatient Applications to Cognitive Therapy, Wright JH, Thase ME, Ludgate J, et al. (eds). Guilford Press, New York, pp. 219–246.

Sensky T, Turkington D, Kingdon D, et al. (2000) A randomized controlled trial of cognitive–behavioral therapy for persistent symptoms in schizophrenia resistant to medication. Arch Gen Psychiatr 57(2), 176–172.

Shaw SC, Marks IM, and Toole S (1999) Lessons from pilot tests of computer self-help for agoraphobia, claustrophobia, and panic. MD Comput 16(4), 44–48.

Shea MT, Elkin I, Imber SD, et al. (1992) Course of depressive symptoms over follow-up: Findings from the National Institute of Mental Health Treatment of Depression Collaborative Research Program. Arch Gen Psychiatr 49, 782–787.

Shear MK, Fyer AJ, Ball G, et al. (1991) Vulnerability to sodium lactate in panic disorder patients given cognitive–behavioral therapy. Am J Psychiatr 148, 795–797.

Simons AD, Garfield SL, and Murphy CE (1984) The process of change in cognitive therapy and pharmacotherapy for depression. Arch Gen Psychiatr 41, 45–51.

Simons AD, Murphy GE, and Levine JL (1986) Cognitive therapy and pharmacotherapy of depression: Sustained improvement over one year. Arch Gen Psychiatr 43, 43–48.

Skinner BF (1938) The Behavior of Organisms. Appleton-Century-Crofts, New York.

Skinner BF (1948) 'Superstition' in the pigeon. J Exp Psychol 38, 168–170.

Spence KW (1956) Behavior Theory and Conditioning. Yale University Press, New Haven.

Spiegel DA, Bruce TJ, Gregg SF, et al. (1994) Does cognitive–behavior therapy assist slow-taper alprazolam discontinuation in panic disorder?. Am J Psychiatr 151, 876–881.

Staats AW (1964) Human Learning: Studies Extending Conditioning Principles to Complex Behavior. Holt, Rinehart & Winston, New York.

Stanley MA, Beck JG, and Glosso DJ (1997) Treatment of generalized anxiety in older adults: A preliminary comparison of cognitive–behavioral and supportive approaches. Behav Ther 27, 285–296.

Stekette G (1994) Behavioral assessment and treatment planning with obsessive–compulsive disorder: A review emphasizing clinical application. Behav Ther 25, 613–633.

Stern RS (1978) Obsessive thoughts: The problem of therapy. Br J Psychiatr 133, 200–205.

Sweeney PD, Anderson K, and Bailey S (1986) Attributional style in depression: A meta-analysis review. J Pers Soc Psychol 50, 974–991.

Tarrier N, Beckett R, Harwoods S, et al. (1993) A trial of two cognitive–behavioral methods of treating drug-resistant residual psychotic symptoms in schizophrenic patients: I: Outcome. Br J Psychiatr 162, 524–532.

Teasdale JD (1983) Negative thinking in depression: Cause, effect, or reciprocal relationship? Adv Behav Res Ther 5, 3–25.

Thackwray DE, Smith MC, Bodfish JW, et al. (1993) A comparison of behavioral and cognitive–behavioral interventions for bulimia nervosa. J Consult Clin Psychol 61, 639–645.

Thase ME (1992) Long-term treatments of recurrent depressive disorders. J Clin Psychiatr 53(Suppl 9), 32–44.

Thase ME (1993) Transition and aftercare. In Cognitive Therapy with Inpatients, Wright JH, Thase ME, Beck AT, et al. (eds). Guilford Press, New York, pp. 414–435.

Thase ME (1994) After the fall: Cognitive–behavior therapy of depression in the "postcollaborative" era. Behav Ther 17, 48–52.

Thase ME (1995) Reeducative psychotherapy. In Treatments of Psychiatric Disorders: The DSM-IV Edition, Gabbard GO (ed). American Psychiatric Press, Washington DC.

Thase ME and Beck AT (1992) An overview of cognitive therapy. In Cognitive Therapy with Inpatients: Developing a Cognitive Milieu, Wright JH, Thase ME, Beck AT et al. (eds). Guilford Press, New York, p. 9.

Thase ME and Beck AT (1993) Cognitive therapy: An overview. In The Cognitive Milieu: Inpatient Applications to Cognitive Therapy, Wright JH, Thase ME, Ludgate J, et al. (eds). Guilford Press, New York.

Thase ME and Howland R (1994) Refractory depression: Relevance of psychosocial factors and therapies. Psychiatr Ann 24, 232–240.

Thase ME and Wright JH (1991) Cognitive–behavior therapy manual for depressed inpatients: A treatment protocol outline. Behav Ther 22, 579–595.

Thase ME, Bowler K, and Harden T (1991) Cognitive–behavior therapy of endogenous depression: Part 2: Preliminary findings in 16 unmedicated inpatients. Behav Ther 22, 469–477.

Thase ME, Friedman ES, Berman S, et al. (2000) Is cognitive behavior therapy just a 'nonspecific' intervention for depression? A retrospective comparison of consecutive cohorts treated with cognitive–behavior therapy or supportive counseling and pill placebo. J Affect Disord 57, 63–71.

Thase ME, Reynolds CF III, Frank E, et al. (1994a) Do depressed men and women respond similarly to cognitive–behavior therapy? Am J Psychiatr 151, 500–505.

Thase ME, Reynolds CF III, Frank E, et al. (1994b) Response to cognitive–behavior therapy in chronic depression. J Psychother Pract Res 3, 204–214.

Thase ME, Simons AD, and Reynolds CF III (1993) Psychobiological correlates of poor response to cognitive–behavior therapy: Potential indications for antidepressant pharmacotherapy. Psychopharmacol Bull 29, 293–301.

Thase ME, Simons AD, McGeary J, et al. (1992) Relapse after cognitive–behavior therapy of depression: Potential implications for longer courses of treatment? Am J Psychiatr 149, 1046–1052.

Turner SM, Hersen M, Bellack AS, et al. (1980) Behavioral and pharmacological treatment of obsessive–compulsive disorders. J Nerv Ment Dis 168, 651–657.

Ullmann LP and Krasner L (eds) (1965) Case Studies in Behavior Modification. Holt, Rinehart & Winston, New York.

Walsh BT, Wilson GT, Loeb KL, et al. (1997) Medication and psychotherapy in the treatment of bulimia nervosa. Am J Psychiatr 154(4), 523–531.

Watkins J, Leber W, Imber S, et al. (1993) Temporal course of change in depression. J Consult Clin Psychol 61, 858–864.

Watkins JT and Rush AJ (1983) Cognitive response test. Cogn Ther Res 7, 425–436.

Watson JB and Rayner R (1920) Conditioned emotional reactions. J Exp Psychol 3, 1–14.

Weiss JM and Simson PG (1985) Neurochemical mechanisms underlying stress-induced depression. In Stress and Coping, Field TM, McCabe PM, and Schneiderman N (eds). Lawrence Erlbaum, Hillsdale, NJ, pp. 93–113.

Wenzloff RM and Grozier SA (1988) Depression and the magnification of failure. J Abnorm Psychol 97, 90–93.

Whisman MA, Miller IW, Norman WH, et al. (1991) Cognitive therapy with depressed inpatients: Specific effects on dysfunctional cognitions. J Consult Clin Psychol 59, 282–288.

Whisman MS (1993) Mediators and moderators of change in cognitive therapy of depression. Psychol Bull 114, 248–265.

Wilkes TCR, Belsher G, Rush AJ, et al. (1994) Cognitive Therapy for Depressed Adolescents. Guilford Press, New York.

Willner P (1991) Animal models as simulations of depression. Trends Pharmacol Sci 12, 131–136.

Wilson GT (1999) Cognitive–behavior therapy for eating disorders: Progress and problems. Behav Res Ther 37, S79–S95.

Wilson PH (1982) Combined pharmacological and behavioral treatment of depression. Behav Res Ther 29, 173–184.

Wolpe J (1952) Experimental neuroses as learned behavior. Br J Psychol 43, 243–268.

Wolpe J (1958) Psychotherapy by Reciprocal Inhibition. Stanford University Press, Stanford, CA.

Wolpe J (1982) The Practice of Behavior Therapy. Pergamon Press, New York.

Wolpe J and Lang PJ (1964) A fear survey schedule for use in behavior therapy. Behav Res Ther 2, 27–30.

Woody GE, McLellan AT, and Luborsky L (1984) Psychiatric severity as a predictor of benefits from psychotherapy. Am J Psychiatr 141, 1171–1177.

Wright JH (1988) Cognitive therapy of depression. In The American Psychiatric Press Review of Psychiatry, Vol. 7, Frances AJ and Hales RE (eds). American Psychiatric Press, Washington DC, pp. 554–590.

Wright JH and Basco MR (2001) Getting Your Life Back: The Complete Guide to Depression. The Free Press, New York.

Wright JH and Beck AT (1983) Cognitive therapy of depression: Theory and practice. Hosp Comm Psychiatr 34, 1119–1127.

Wright JH and Beck AT (1994) Cognitive therapy. In American Psychiatric Press Textbook of Psychiatry, Vol. 13, Hales RE, Yudofsky SC, and Talbott JA (eds). American Psychiatric Press, Washington DC, pp. 1083–1114.

Wright JH and Davis D (1994) The therapeutic relationship in cognitive–behavioral therapy: Patient perceptions and therapist responses. Cogn Behav Pract 1, 25–45.

Wright JH and Thase ME (1992) Cognitive and biological therapies: A synthesis. Psychiatr Ann 22, 451–458.

Wright JH and Wright AS (1997) Computer-assisted psychotherapy. J Psychother Prac Res 315–329.

Wright JH, Salmon P, Wright AS, et al. (1995) Cognitive Therapy: A Multimedia Learning Program. MindStreet Multimedia, Louisville, KY.

Wright JH, Thase ME, Beck AT, et al. (1993) Cognitive Therapy With Inpatients: Developing a Cognitive Milieu. Guilford Press, New York.

Wright JH, Wright AS, and Beck AT (2002a) Good Days Ahead: The Multimedia Program for Cognitive Therapy. Mindstreet, Louisville, KY.

Wright JH, Wright AS, Basco MR, et al. (2001) Controlled trial of computer-assisted cognitive therapy for depression. Poster presentation, World Congress of Cognitive Therapy (July), Vancouver, Canada.

Wright JH, Wright AS, Salmon P, et al. (2002b) Development and initial testing of a multimedia program for computer-assisted cognitive therapy. Am J Psychother 56(1), 76–86.

Young JE (1999) Cognitive Therapy for Personality Disorders: A Schema-Focused Approach. Professional Resource Exchange, Sarasota, FL.

Young JE and Lindermann MD (1992) An integrative schema-focused model for personality disorders. J Cogn Psychother 6, 11–23.

Zautra JH, Guenther RT, and Chartier GM (1985) Attributions for real and hypothetical events: Their relation to self-esteem and depression. J Abnorm Psychol 94, 530–540.

Zubin J (1953) Evaluation of therapeutic outcome in mental disorders. J Nerv Ment Dis 117, 95–111.

# 87

# Family Therapy

James L. Griffith
Lois Slovik

## Introduction

Family therapy is psychotherapy that directly involves family members in addition to the identified patient, and/or explicitly attends to the interactions among family members (Pinsof and Wynne 1995). Family therapy thus engages relational and communicational processes of families and social networks as a primary context for solving clinical problems or treating psychiatric disorders, even though one family member may be the sole bearer of distress or symptoms. By educating family members or altering family patterns of relating or communicating, such clinical problems as depression, anxiety, marital conflict, or disruptive childhood behavior can be resolved or attenuated.

Although social workers met therapeutically with families as early as the late 1880s, family therapy as known today emerged in the 1940s (Broderick and Schrader 1981). The sudden reuniting of families at the conclusion of World War II precipitated marital discord, divorce, delinquency, and emotional breakdowns, leading to requests for professional help (Goldenberg and Goldenberg 1980). The subsequent failure of psychoanalysis to find therapeutic breakthroughs for such problems as schizophrenia and juvenile delinquency shifted attention away from the interior emotional life of individuals to their family relationships as a potential point of intervention. During the late 1940s and 1950s isolated pockets of family therapy practitioners proliferated across the US. Each group brought its unique perspective to the observation of families, and from each a distinct "school" of family therapy developed (Slovik and Griffith 1992).

Over the ensuing decades, these different clinical approaches to family therapy began coalescing into clinical traditions defined by their core theoretical assumptions and methods, supported to varying extents by research. Each of the major family therapy traditions has contributed to the repertoire of mental health professionals, its unique framework for understanding clinical problems, and an associated set of interventions. Some approaches have insisted that whole families be involved in most sessions, while others have worked focally with individuals or subunits of families. The different family therapy traditions can be usefully contrasted by comparing how each structures perceptual, cognitive, and executive processes when clinicians work with families—from each of these perspectives:

- What does a therapist look for?
- What does a therapist think about?
- What does a therapist do?

When multiple traditions or schools of psychotherapy are considered, the question naturally arises: which works best? There has been ample clinical evidence that each tradition "works," somewhat better than others for particular problems, or with particular families, or in the hands of particular therapists, or at different phases of recovery from illness (Pinsof and Wynne 1995). The evolution of mental health services, however, has led not to a dominance of any one of the family therapy traditions, but to comprehensive family-centered programs that now draw broadly from multiple traditions. These family-centered programs for preventing or treating psychiatric disorders have been validated to a substantial extent in empirical research studies, as discussed below. Different family therapy traditions are themselves best regarded as different sets of ideas and interventions to be valued as potential tools within comprehensive, multimodality treatment programs.

In the following paragraph we will illustrate the range of perspectives and interventions available in the different traditions by examining, in turn, how psychodynamic, structural, strategic, cognitive–behavioral, and postmodern family therapy traditions each might approach an identical clinical problem. The problem is explained in Clinical Vignette 1.

---

**Clinical Vignette 1**

Bill and Roberta requested therapy due to the fights they were having over parenting their two stepchildren. Roberta's 11-year-old son, David, with significant problems from attention-deficit disorder with hyperactivity, lived with them. Bill's 10-year-old son, whom he coparented with his former wife, lived with them every other weekend and one night each week. The arguments were so severe that they threatened the marriage.

---

## Psychodynamic Family Therapy

Psychodynamic psychotherapy helps family members solve relational problems by understanding better how emotional processes influence the perceptions, feelings, and actions of those involved. The early psychoanalysts noted that intrapsychic processes of an individual powerfully shape his or her interactions with other people, and most so in emotionally intimate relationships of couples and families. Extending the concepts and language of psychoanalysis to family behavior was a logical next step for those who began meeting with parents and children, couples, and whole families. In particular, object relations theory provided a bridge from the individual intrapsychic processes to the interpersonal processes of families (Scharff and Scharff 1987, Framo 1991, Slipp 1991).

The era of ascendancy for psychoanalytic thinking coincided with development of general systems theory and cybernetics as conceptual models for understanding, controlling, and predicting the behavior of complex physical and biological systems. Psychodynamic family therapists adopted such systems concepts as boundaries and levels of hierarchy, and such cybernetics concepts as negative feedback and homeostasis. Such systems described complex family interactions, while preserving the psychological language of psychoanalysis in describing such motivational processes as projective identification.

**What to Think About.** In order to understand how one family member acts in relation to other family members, psychodynamic family therapy concentrates upon motivations, conflicts, defenses, and relationships from the past that currently influence the present. Family interactions are explained in terms of internal processes within individual family members. Therapeutic change is sought through family members gaining conscious insight into previously unconscious processes that have been generating problems in family relationships.

**What to Look For.** Psychodynamic family therapy grounds its work in historical information. Extensive individual and family histories are elicited in order to understand family members' experiential models of the world. These experiential models govern how meanings are attributed to such family patterns as rules for how people should respond and models for being a man or a woman, husband or wife, or mother or father. These models have developed out of each family member's personal history, the family's history and mythology, and their cultural history. Some of the diagnostic patterns upon which psychodynamic family therapists focus when assessing families include the following:

- *Projective Identification.* Projective identification is an ego defense to which psychodynamic family therapists have attributed a crucial role in conflictual family relationships. In projective identification, one family member (a parent or couple partner) relates to another family member (a particular child or the other couple partner) as if he or she embodied a projected part of self. The projecting family member then interacts with, or relates to, the projected part of self as if that part were an internalized part of himself or herself. The projecting family member unconsciously prompts the other to conform to the way in which he or she is being perceived, evoking in the other the associated feelings and behaviors as if they were authentic. When viewed from the outside by the therapist, it appears as if the two are in collusion with one another in order to sustain these mutual, projected perceptions. Projection of disavowed elements of the self, whether positive or negative, has the effect of charging the relationship with

emotion that has been transposed from an intrapsychic sphere into an interpersonal one. Acted out interpersonally, it serves to decrease psychic anxiety at the expense of an increase in tension and impasse in the relationship.

- *Unresolved Grief.* When a family member, or the family as a whole, has not fully grieved losses, the family can become developmentally frozen. While so preoccupied with the past, it can be difficult to focus enough time and energy on current problems.

- *Clarity of Ego Boundaries and Capacity for Intimacy/ Separateness.* Conflicted family relationships can represent an alternative method for stabilizing emotional distance when the involved family members lack the emotional maturity to regulate closeness and distance in more differentiated ways. This has been a common model for understanding couples who chronically fight yet never separate.

**What to Do.** Psychodynamic family therapists employ the fundamental tools of psychodynamic psychotherapy (opening emotional expression, clarifying communications, encouraging family members to speak from the "I" position, and interpretation of unconscious conflicts) to resolve projective processes, cut-off relationships, and difficulties in modulating closeness and distance in family relationships. Psychodramatic techniques, such as doubling and role reversal, can play useful roles in implementing these interventions (Blatner 1994). Therapeutic rituals are particularly useful in facilitating grief over losses and in facilitating developmental transitions, such as a young adult leaving home or a couple moving into retirement years (Imber-Black and Roberts 1992).

Psychodynamic family therapists commonly utilize family genograms when taking a family history. A genogram can provide a map of family life over time in a visual form that can help family members grasp interactional patterns, particularly when the patterns extend across the generations (McGoldrick and Gerson 1985). A psychodynamic family therapy with Roberta and Bill might begin as given in Clinical Vignette 2.

---

Clinical Vignette 2

The therapist asked to meet with Roberta and Bill as parents before meeting with 11-year-old David. Utilizing a genogram she elicited a history, not only of their current nuclear family but also for Roberta's and Bill's parents' and grandparents' generations. She learned that Roberta had been ashamed of her family of origin. She characterized her mother as "a slut who stayed out all night." Eventually, Roberta's mother was diagnosed with bipolar disorder, but it was poorly controlled with multiple hospitalizations. Roberta was the oldest of six children, all from different fathers. Roberta stated, "Nobody raised me, but I raised my brothers and sisters." At age 12 years, a new stepfather entered the family but was verbally and emotionally abusive towards her. Consequently, "stepfathers" have had a negative connotation in Roberta's mind. Out of her childhood experiences, Roberta came to believe that "I'm okay so long as I can be on my own, because I can't trust or depend on anybody."

Bill, on the other hand, was the second oldest child in a strict, rigid family. Both parents were emotionally and physically abusive, his father more than his mother. At one

Clinical Vignette 2 *continued*

point Bill tried to stop his father from beating his older brother and was himself badly beaten. Although angry and afraid of his father's violence, Bill also blamed his brother's out-of-control behavior for provoking his father. At 16, Bill pinned his father to the wall and said, "If you hit me, I'll kill you." His father never hit him again. Bill's mother was also abusive. Once she kept hitting him across the face, and he responded by telling her, "I hope you like it" and let her hit him until she finally stopped.

The therapist used the genogram session as an opportunity for Roberta and Bill to hear the stories from each others' childhoods that so charged with emotion their discussions about disciplining David, that arguing always had ensued. The therapist actively interpreted to them how Roberta's aversive experiences with a stepfather put her on guard with Bill and made her more protective of David whenever Bill tried to discipline him. In contrast, Bill's experiences with his brother and parents, people he described as "having out-of-control behavior," led him to overreact to David's attention-deficit/hyperactivity disorder (ADHD). Each of them, operating out of their own well-meaning logic, was making the problem worse. The therapist then used psychodramatic techniques and had them create and then practice ways in which they could work as a team in disciplining David.

## Structural Family Therapy

Structural family therapy considers problems involving a particular family member to be inextricably linked to the organizational context of the entire family. It solves problems by changing the family's organizational context. Structural family therapy thus emphasizes an understanding of a family in terms of the family rules and roles that shape its members' actions.

Family structure is the internal organization of the family that dictates how, when, and to whom family members relate while carrying out the various functions of the family (Aponte and VanDeusen 1981, Colapinto 1991). Some important elements of family structure for clinical work are boundaries, hierarchy, alliances, and coalitions:

- *Boundaries*. Rules defining who participates and how, in particular moments of family-life. For example, a boundary around the parental couple means that the children are included in discussions of certain topics but not in others;
- *Hierarchy*. Relative influence of each family member upon the outcome of an activity. For example, all family members may have opinions about spending money, but the parents as a couple typically have the final say;
- *Alliances*. Family members joining together to support another family member. For example, older children may join the well-parent in organizing to parent younger children if the other parent were to become seriously ill;
- *Coalitions*. Family members joining together in opposition to another family member. For example, a grandchild and grandmother might quietly ally together for the child to stay up late at night against the mother's wishes when the child is at grandmother's house.

The family structure should provide cohesive and flexible responses to life-stresses so that important family functions—parenting, providing income, marital intimacy, recreation, and other activities—can be carried out successfully, and family members can grow and mature in their individual lives.

**What to Look For.** A structural family therapist observes closely the flow of family structures as family members talk about and interact together around the presenting problem of the therapy. The therapist wishes to witness how sequences of family behaviors are enacted during interactions in the sessions, particularly the occurrence of a symptom as it is embedded within different configurations of organized family interactions. The therapist observes how boundaries, hierarchy, alliances, and coalitions are associated with the presenting symptom, as well as any repetitive-behavioral sequences (verbal or nonverbal) that involve symptomatic behavior.

**What to Think About.** The structural family therapist considers the problem to be sustained by the current family structure and its community ecosystem. Important questions to answer in assessing these relationships include:

- To what elements of family structure—boundaries, hierarchy, alliances, coalitions—do occurrences of the presenting problem appear linked?
- What family functions are blocked by the problem? If not for the problem, what would be happening that is not happening now?
- For whom is the problem a concern? Who is most affected? Who would need to change for the symptom to disappear?

**What to Do.** Structural family therapists ameliorate symptoms by shifting family structure. Boundaries can be strengthened or weakened by behavioral assignments that exclude a particular family member from certain moments of family life (e.g., an assignment for parents to leave children with a baby sitter to go on a date alone) or include a particular family member where that person had been absent (e.g., involving both parents in collaborative disciplining of a misbehaving child when the father had been only peripherally involved). Alliances are encouraged when they support the individual development of family members and strengthen the family as a whole. Secret coalitions, particularly when they cross generational boundaries, are targeted for therapeutic disruption as when one parent covertly supports a child's oppositional behavior with the other parent. A structural family therapy with Roberta and Bill might include the following as given in Clinical Vignette 3.

Clinical Vignette 3

Before Roberta's marriage to Bill, Roberta and David had lived together as a unit for years, which had fostered an intense bond between them. In order to shift successfully to the structure of a stepfamily, Roberta needed to let a relationship build between David and Bill, and that between her and David to loosen. She also needed to build a relationship with Bill's son.

In their spousal relationship, both Bill and Roberta needed to enhance their sexual intimacy. They needed to develop a style of working together as a parental team. Bill, in addition, needed to limit appropriately his involvement with his ex-wife. Both boys needed to have time to create a relationship with each other.

In planning a strategy to counter fights around disciplining the two boys, the therapist began by viewing Roberta and David as an enmeshed-couple. That is, Roberta would "know" what David felt when Bill attempted to discipline him, so she stood up for David "to protect him." Although she saw herself as a protective parent, she was not allowing Bill and David to work things out for themselves. Moreover, David learned how to provoke Bill in order to prompt his mother to side with him.

The therapist gave Bill and Roberta an assignment to go out to dinner in a quiet, comfortable restaurant and to make a list of David's positive qualities and actions that they felt good about. They were then told to make a list of those behaviors, which they felt were destructive, and what they thought should be done about them. The therapist then met with Bill and Roberta alone and discussed their lists. As the therapist had anticipated, a fight ensued about David's behavior in the subsequent family meeting with David present. Through this spontaneous enactment, the therapist helped the family rechoreograph the sequence of interactions. In a new pattern, the couple would first establish decisions together, then would support each other in avoiding David's moves to side his mother against Bill.

## Strategic Family Therapy

Strategic therapy is built upon the premise that a therapist is responsible for planning a strategy that solves successfully the family's presenting problem. The therapist sets clear goals that intervene by changing relational and communicational processes in the family (Madanes 1981, Stanton 1981). Strategic therapy was designed as a counterpoint to psychodynamic psychotherapy by emphasizing "how" people can behave differently in order to solve problems, rather than "why" they behave as they do. Its development was heavily informed by Ericksonian hypnotherapy and application of cybernetics principles to human systems (Madanes 1981). Its impetus also came from the discovery of the one-way mirror, permitting detailed tracking of repetitive family processes that triggered symptoms. Strategic therapy planned interventions that would disrupt such behavioral sequences, whether by direct behavioral prescriptions or by indirect paradoxical interventions.

**What to Think About.** The focus of strategic therapy is upon problem solving. Problems are viewed as persistent efforts by one or more family members to apply a solution that makes sense but is inadequate for the problem at hand, such that "the solution becomes the problem." Commonsense understandings often lead people to pursue unsuccessful strategies even though it ought to be apparent that the problem is not resolving. For example, people intuitively attempt to cheer up a person who is depressed, even though cheering up (a solution) usually makes the depression (the problem) worse.

Strategic therapists commonly view clinical problems as emerging out of difficult life-cycle transitions, both predictable ones (e.g., marriage, birth of a child, separating/individuating of an adolescent) and unpredictable ones (e.g., loss of job, sudden illness, a death in the family) that necessitate shifting to new patterns of perceiving and acting.

At such times when innovative problem-solving is needed, people nevertheless persist with once successful strategies that are now outdated.

**What to Look For.** Strategic therapists are most interested in the here-and-now context of the problem, rather than in its history. They seek to learn what each involved person believes about the problem and how these beliefs are acted upon in efforts to generate a solution. Questions are asked about who, what, when, where, and how people are involved, in order to ascertain how moves are sequenced in the family game.

**What to Do.** The central aim of a strategic therapist is to motivate family members to try novel solutions, rather than repeating what has been tried in the past. Psychoeducation, direct behavioral assignments, and paradoxical or defiance-based directives are the cornerstones of strategic therapy. In-session interventions and out-of-session homework are used. Strategic therapists have become best known for their paradoxical directives. Paradoxical directives include:

- *Reframing or Relabeling the Symptom.* By changing the context of actions constituting the symptom, the meaning of the event is reframed. For example, a husband's emotional distancing could be reframed as "his way of getting his wife to notice him."
- *Prescribing the Symptom or Behavioral Sequence.* By using a rationale that is plausible in its logic, a therapist can encourage family members to engage in the very behavior that needs to be eliminated. For example, a wife whose husband is emotionally distancing might be told to continue to pursue her husband because "this lets him know that he is the center of her life and that there is nothing else about her life that she finds valuable or interesting." She might be instructed to continue in her behavior for his sake, even though it may give her friends a distorted idea about her. When the reframe "fits," yet the new meaning feels distasteful, the rebound against the directive can paradoxically propel therapeutic change.
- *Restraining the System.* The therapist can attempt to discourage or even deny the possibility of change. For example, a therapist may tell couple-partners to "go slow" or may emphasize dangers of improvement. Family members may then react against the therapist's conservative outlook by pressing forward to change.
- *Positioning.* The therapist attempts to shift a problematic "position" (usually an assertion that the patient is making about self, the problem, or a partner) by accepting but exaggerating that position. This intervention is used when the partner's position is thought to be maintained by its complementary, reciprocal response from the other partner. For example, when one partner takes an optimistic stance and the other a pessimistic one, a therapist may suggest the pessimistic spouse to worry even more so that the optimistic spouse can feel more secure and even more happily optimistic. Here, too, if a new explanation has a plausible logic, but frames the behavior in a manner that renders it aversive, the behavior will change. A strategic therapist might have tracked the characteristic pattern of arguments between Bill and Roberta as given in Clinical Vignette 4.

When Roberta felt unheard, she yelled louder. As her voice became louder, Bill became more emotionally distant and coldly rational. As the fight escalated, Roberta first threw an object at Bill, then asked him to leave, then threatened divorce. The strategic therapist considered each of these behaviors to be efforts at a solution that likely had worked successfully in past conflicts, but now, was amplifying the problem.

The therapist noted that each time the couple "made up" each reported having "the greatest sex." She referred to their pattern as an "accordion dance" and told them that should they persist in it, they would in time reach a point of no-return. She then modified its rules by suggesting that Bill ask Roberta to leave the room to cool off when she appeared to be losing control. If Roberta refused to leave, then Bill would say that he needed to take a walk to clear his head.

Alternatively, the therapist might have suggested to Roberta that "if you don't want to be heard, then you should continue to scream louder … but if you do want Bill to hear you, then you should do an 'EF Hutton,' that is, to whisper instead of yell."

## Cognitive–Behavioral Family Therapy

Cognitive–behavioral family therapy applies principles of learning theory to help family members solve problems by modifying cognitive distortions and repetitive problem-inducing interactions, and by learning new knowledge and skills. Cognitive–behavioral family therapy relies heavily upon family psychoeducation and a teaching/coaching stance of the therapist.

Behavioral family therapy emerged from behavioral modification programs for young children with such problems as bedtime tantrums, nocturnal enuresis, and aggressive behavior (Falloon 1991, Arias 1992). It is based upon the influence family members hold by offering positive and negative reinforcements to other family members. Parents and spouses are trained to eliminate reinforcement contingencies for undesirable behaviors.

Cognitive interventions engage family members as coinvestigators who study the ecology of family problems and symptoms and discern how thoughts, feelings, and behaviors interplay. A therapist assists family members in identifying when such cognitive distortions as catastrophic thinking, overgeneralization, or misattributions lead to conflicts in relationships (Epstein et al. 1988, Freeman et al. 1989) (see Clinical Vignette 5).

**What to Look For.** Families presenting problems for therapy often have

- difficulties in recognizing deviant behavior
- lack of clearly-defined family rules
- problems in emotional communication among family members, usually a paucity of expression of positive feelings coupled with an excess of negative expressions
- relational conflict associated with either a paucity of relational skills or interpretive errors based on faulty assumptions or cognitive distortions.

**What to Think About.** A cognitive–behavioral family therapist considers each member of the family to be doing his or her best to cope with the behavioral contingencies perceived at that point in time, given the practical and emotional restraints experienced. Family members need to acquire knowledge about cognitive and behavioral principles, to gain skills needed to reinforce desired behaviors, to eliminate reinforcement of undesired behaviors, to modify faulty assumptions and interpretations of others' actions, and to learn skills for communicating clearly and effectively.

**What to Do**

- *Psychoeducation.* Educational modules about the presenting problem are taught when family members appear to lack a significant understanding of issues, ranging from such general topics as developmental milestones of children and principles of learning theory, to specific information about a particular psychiatric disorder (Falloon 1991)
- *Communication Training.* Empathic listening, expressing positive feelings, and speaking negative communications more respectfully are taught as skills (Falloon 1991)
- *Problem-Solving Training.* Family members practice consistent, structured approaches for resolving conflicts (Falloon 1991)
- *Operant-Conditioning Strategies.* Behavior shaping and time-out procedures are taught to increase desirable behaviors among children (Falloon 1991)
- *Contingency Contracting.* Coercive, blaming patterns of family behavior are replaced by contracts that specify what behaviors involved family members each to agree to perform (Falloon 1991)
- *Thought Diaries.* Out-of-session, assignments are made to track habitual patterns of thoughts, feelings, and behaviors in generating symptoms (Freeman et al. 1989).

Addressing David's attention-deficit disorder was an important aspect of the therapy, and Bill and Roberta began reading materials about the disorder. In sessions, they were taught to make distinctions in David's behavior according to Green's (2000) concept of three baskets: In Basket A steps relevant to safety that must be taken regardless whether the child becomes agitated in response; in Basket B are new skills to be taught and practiced, pacing the teaching according to the child's capacity to respond; in Basket C are the child's behaviors that should be ignored. During the family sessions the therapist worked on problem-solving techniques and empathic listening, helping family members to notice and comment on positive feelings and to speak negative feelings respectfully.

## The Postmodern Family Therapies

The postmodern family therapies as a group include narrative, solution-focused, collaborative language systems, and feminist family therapies (Andersen 1987, 1997, de Shazer 1985, Epston 1989, Epston and White 1992, Freedman and Combs 1995, Griffith and Griffith 1994, Madsen 1999,

O'Hanlon and Weiner-Davis 1989, Penn 2001, Tomm 1987, Weiner-Davis 1992, Weingarten 1995, White 1989, 1995 2000). Innovations introduced by postmodern therapies have opened new ways for families to solve problems by valuing and learning from their own experiences, histories, traditions, values, and identities, instead of seeking answers from mental health experts. These alternative therapies developed out of critical inquiries into ways that academic traditions, scientific programs, and professional communities have often emphasized practices that sustained their own power and economic well-being, rather than practices that prioritize the interests of families. The postmodern therapies have sought to empower families by helping them to develop reflective processes for exercising choice, to build supportive communities with other families, and to clarify undesirable ways in which cultural influences have limited appreciation and utilization of the family's own practical wisdom. In these ways, the postmodern family therapies have rendered family therapy more usable for those whose lives vary from the stereotypic American two-parent, middle-class, nuclear families, traditionally the largest consumers of private-practice family therapy.

The postmodern therapies have made contributions that have broadly influenced the clinical practice of family therapy through:

- the art of crafting interview questions for fostering reflection and creative problem-solving;
- clinical methods that help patients and families to identify and use skills, competencies, and resources from their everyday lived-experiences;
- clinical methods that counter adverse influences of culture in generating and maintaining problems that families face.

The hallmark of the postmodern family therapies has been the empowerment of families to honor and to utilize their own lived-experience in solving problems. Narrative therapy has sought to ground therapy in significant narratives of human experience and their influences, rather than the constructs of psychological theories. Stories guiding the lives of individuals are commonly related to broader cultural narratives that organize social practices of gender, race, ethnicity, political power, religion, and social class. Narrative therapy has worked to give a particularly privileged status to the stories of local cultures—those from the daily lives of patients and their families and those providing a sense of identity as "who we are as a people."

Solution-focused therapists have examined how people construct solutions to problems in daily life. Their clinical methods have helped people to learn from those occasions when the problem is "not" occurring and to learn from those "exceptions" when the problem might have been expected to occur but did not. By studying occasions when the problem didn't happen, behavioral assignments could be constructed that would amplify the frequency and intensity of these "solution sequences."

**What to Think About.** Each person makes sense out of his or her life experiences by attributing meaning to them. This meaning is shaped by a canon of personal narratives as they are told and retold to self and to others. Among the most important of these narratives are those of identity about who one is as a person and as a family. There are certain dominant narratives in a person's life that, more than others, organize one's perceptions, cognitions, and actions. How a family member views oneself and the other family members is shaped by the limits of the language—the metaphors, stories, and beliefs—he or she employs.

Impasses occur in family relationships, and problems emerge when:

- one or more family members lack either the needed emotional vocabulary or the needed narrative skills to make one's personal experience understandable to others;
- the available narratives preclude ways of relating other than conflictual ones;
- specific words hold very different meanings for different family members due to different personal narratives connected to the language (e.g., "loyalty," "trust," "safety");
- family members have become positioned relationally such that they cannot hear, tell, and/or expand their stories in conversation, i.e., they have become confused by or habituated to the conflict such that they have stopped listening.

Therapy provides a context where narratives that limit and constrain relationships can be identified. The power of constraining narratives can be attenuated through careful interviewing that renders visible the specific historical, cultural, or political contexts from which they emerged and the hidden interpretive assumptions upon which they rest. Alternatively, more useful narratives often lie unnoticed within forgotten experiences the partners have had with one another, but are now outside their recollection.

### What to Look For
- Listen for the exact words and precise manner in which people use language. The focus of therapy is the language itself and the limits of its possibilities, not what this language is interpreted to mean.
- Metaphors, phrases, and prominent or repetitive words in the family members' specific uses of language are noted as "doors to be knocked upon" by asking specific questions about stories of lived-experience that have given them meaning.
- "Unique outcomes" or "exceptions" when problems might have been expected to occur, but did not.

**What to Do.** Narrative approach to therapy consists of two phases:

- First Phases: A first priority is creation of a therapeutic relationship within which important first-person narratives can be safely told, heard, and changed. In particular, the therapist carefully watches for nonverbal signs that the dialogue is opening up or closing down, such as family members' breathing, posture, and flow and tone of speech. Creating a relationship and a conversation favorable for the telling of important personal stories is the priority, not gathering data.

- Second Phase: As important first-person narratives relevant to the problem are told, the therapist asks carefully designed questions that facilitate:
  a. retrieval of other forgotten, or unnoticed, narratives that might enhance solving the problem of the therapy, in contrast to the dominant narrative;
  b. cocreation of an alternative narrative to a form that holds more possibilities for resolving the problem of the therapy;
- The therapist utilizes such questions as circular, reflexive, unique outcome, or relative influence questions (Tomm 1987, White 1989)
- A solution-focused therapist may assign couple-partners the task of studying segments of time when the problem is "not" occurring, looking for "exceptions..." Examples of solution-focused questions include:
  a. "Between now and the next time we meet, I would like you to observe—so that you can describe to us next time—what happens between both of you that you do value, would NOT want to change, and would like to see continue to happen in the future."
  b. The Miracle Question (de Shazer 1985)—"Suppose that one night, while you were asleep, there was a miracle and this problem was solved. How would you know? What would be different? How would your partner know without your even saying a word about it?" [The therapist then negotiates with the partner(s) what part of this new reality the partner(s) would be willing to implement the next day, as if the miracle had occurred.]
  c. (Weiner-Davis 1992) "If the problems between you and your partner got resolved all of a sudden, what would you do with the time and energy you have been spending on fixing or worrying about the marriage? Describe what you would do instead."
  d. (Weiner-Davis 1992) "What might be one or two small things that you can do this week that will take you one step closer to your goal?"
  e. (Weiner-Davis 1992) "What, if anything, might present a challenge to your taking these steps this week, and how will you meet the challenge?"

Family interviewing methods associated with the postmodern therapies are illustrated in Clinical Vignette 6:

---
Clinical Vignette 6

Roberta repeatedly referred to her anger as a "flash flood." Noting her selection of this metaphor, the therapist asks what important stories of her life experience gave special meaning to "flash flood." She described growing up in the Southwest where in the middle of an arid summer, a thunderstorm could trigger a flash flood that suddenly and without warning swept away everything in its path. Later during a couple's session with Bill present, the therapist asked Roberta: "Were there times when, to your surprise, you felt the thunder and lightening of your emotion, but instead of overflowing the river ran smoothly?" Roberta responded with an account of a time when she suddenly felt angry with Bill, but had "used words instead of action" and

said, "I am mad." The therapist then asked more detailed questions about what each of them noticed, thought, felt, and enacted on this occasion that had been different. She then said to Roberta, "Between now and the next time that we meet, I would like you to observe those times when your emotions begin to churn but you are able to ride the rough waters to a successful conclusion." She then instructed Bill to notice those times when he would have expected Roberta to "blow up," but she didn't ... and to notice what happened and how each of them felt at the time. In subsequent sessions a new plan for engaging in conflict was constructed out of their observations and reflections on this "unique outcome."

## Family Psychoeducation Therapies

The earliest approaches to family therapy were built upon individual psychotherapy and simply extended to the family their ideas about diagnosing and treating psychopathology, referring to "family pathology" instead of psychopathology. Early versions of psychodynamic, structural, strategic, and cognitive–behavioral family therapies each assessed underlying family pathology and engaged families in corrective treatments. By the 1990s, however, family therapies were shifting to more collaborative therapeutic relationships in which families were regarded as allies, rather than sources of pathology, with education, rather than treatment, as the central focus.

This shift brought a sea change in how family therapy began to be practiced. Instead of diagnostic scrutiny, clinicians became preoccupied with learning to convey respect to families, to protect them from stigma, and to learn from their real life experiences coping with illness. A focus on "looking at" families diagnostically in order "to intervene" in the family system, was gradually eclipsed by a commitment to "looking with" families as they coped with illness in order "to collaborate" with them in countering effects of illness on the family.

Family therapy for schizophrenia best illustrates this evolution from pathology-focused family therapy to collaborative family-centered treatment. Early family therapists had hoped that a family approach would open new venues for treating schizophrenia where both psychoanalysis and the then available psychopharmacology had faltered. Murray Bowen, for example, hospitalized entire families for extended periods of time at the National Institutes of Mental Health in order to observe reciprocal relationships between exacerbations of psychosis and family processes (Hoffman 1985). The Bateson project in Palo Alto made famous the double-bind theory of schizophrenia; concluding from analyses of audiotaped family conversations that psychosis was a coherent response to communications with conflicting directives between the explicit verbal message and the implicit nonverbal one (Sluzki and Vernon 1971). Jay Haley, a Bateson research team member, tailored family interventions around a Hamlet-like assumption that psychotic behavior represented a move by the psychotic family member to wield power through force of illness (Haley 1976, 1980). The Milan team extended the Bateson model by viewing psychosis as a compromise solution to a dilemma in the family system and designed counter tactics to neutralize the moves of the family members in this family game (Selvini-Palazzoli et al. 1978).

These family therapy models that located the genesis of schizophrenia in family relationships and communications never gained strong support from empirical research. Moreover, family advocates were alienated by the implicit pathologizing of families with psychotic members. By the 1980s, some family therapists working with these disorders were proposing that family therapy could be more effectively applied by engaging families as partners in treatment, instead as sources of psychopathology. These efforts were characterized by a fresh set of assumptions (Dixon and Lehman 1995):

- Severe psychiatric disorders, such as schizophrenia and bipolar disorder, are regarded as illnesses.
- The family environment does not cause the disorder but can influence its course and severity.
- Support is provided to families who are enlisted as partners and collaborators in treatment.
- Family interventions are only one component in a treatment program that includes routine drug treatment and outpatient clinical management.

These new clinical approaches mixed psychoeducation, behavioral problem-solving training, family support, and crisis management in interventions with either individual families or groups of families.

As a research contribution, the construct of expressed emotion (EE) played a significant role in the evolution of family psychoeducation (Leff and Vaughn 1985). During a structured interview, families were given an EE rating based on observations of critical comments, hostility, and overinvolvement. Over 2 decades an enormous body of research suggested that patients living with families characterized by high levels of EE were more vulnerable to relapse (Anderson et al. 1986). Interventions were then designed that relied heavily upon family psychoeducation in order to enable high EE families to change to a low EE status.

Development of family psychoeducation interventions was also propelled by the self-help family education movement that emerged after the Reagan assassination attempt by a man with schizophrenia. Families mobilized by the National Alliance Against Mental Illnesses and related advocacy organizations demanded information that would help families cope with severe mental illnesses. Family psychoeducation approaches emerged that sought to "put the illness in its place" (Gonzalez et al. 1989) by helping families acquire the knowledge, skills, and resources needed to minimize the loss of time, money, and energy from a chronic medical or psychiatric disorder. These approaches avoided promising a cure. Rather, treatment was considered successful when family members accepted the presence of the illness but refused for it to organize the life of the family. Unlike the early family therapies that rejected psychiatric treatments, family psychoeducation approaches made maximal use of psychotropic medications to control disruptive symptoms and openly embraced interventions drawn from other individual, family, or social network therapies.

Family psychoeducation for schizophrenia was honed into a systematic therapeutic approach by well-conducted empirical research programs during the 1970s and 1980s

and validated by empirical research studies (Goldstein et al. 1978, Leff et al. 1982, Hogarty et al. 1986). For example, the University of Pittsburgh Schizophrenia Research Project, by using intramuscular depot antipsychotic medications, determined that the benchmark relapse rate for psychosis in schizophrenia was 40 to 50% over a 2-year period, even with optimal adherence to medication treatment, and that rates were still higher among patients with multiple past relapses (Hogarty et al. 1986). They designed a family psychoeducation program in which family alliance-building and education about the illness began before hospital discharge. Groups of families were gathered for a "survival skills workshop" consisting of discussions about schizophrenia diagnosis, etiology, use of antipsychotic medication, and the needs of patients and family members when there is a psychotic member. They made practical suggestions for adjusting performance expectations, diminishing high expressed emotion, simplifying family communications, normalizing family routines, and making best use of professionals. Subsequent family meetings after discharge then addressed both adherence to antipsychotic medications and family psychosocial processes in a phased plan covering the first-year "re-entry phase," social and occupational rehabilitation, and latter stages of treatment. Family meetings focused particularly upon elements of schizophrenia for which therapeutic responses by family members would be often counterintuitive—the need to soften criticism and lessen expectations for high performance because of vulnerability to emotional overstimulation and confusion from negative symptoms of schizophrenia (apathy, isolation, amotivation) are considered to be symptoms of the illness rather than laziness or a flawed character.

The subsequent treatment outcomes were impressive: The first-year relapse rate dropped from the expected 50%, with antipsychotic medications alone, to 19% when family psychoeducation was added, and to 0% when medications, family psychoeducation, and social skills training for the patient were combined.

The effectiveness of family psychoeducation was shown to be further amplified when applied to family groups, rather than to individual families in isolation. Single-family therapies often involve only two or three people, while a multifamily group commonly involves 10 or more people. Multifamily groups thus expand the patient's and family's social network (McFarlane 2002). Their usefulness has been demonstrated not only for psychiatric, but also for nonpsychiatric disabling medical conditions (Gonzalez et al. 1989, Steinglass 1998).

For schizophrenia, William McFarlane and colleagues designed a multifamily group therapy that has shown particularly robust therapeutic effects in empirical studies (McFarlane 2002, McFarlane et al. 1995, 1996). A group of families meets regularly to work towards creating home and social environments in which affects would be relatively warm, communications clear and simple, change kept to a minimum, the impact of life events cushioned, and graduated expectations set at a level consistent with the patient's state of symptoms. In an initial workshop, patients do not join other family members during the initial orientation and educational sessions but do join them for later illness management sessions. Each multifamily group meets biweekly, led by two cotherapists and including patients. An individual patient's or family's problem is addressed by the entire multifamily group in a structured, problem-solving process guided by the clinician. These family meetings focus upon management issues for different symptoms and families' uncertainties about how best to promote recovery and rehabilitation. After the second year, the ongoing groups typically evolve into natural social networks for mutual support in enhancing rehabilitation and quality of life.

McFarlane's multifamily group treatment, which included family psychoeducation and maintenance antipsychotic medications, reduced risk of relapse for an extended period of time and did so more effectively than family psychoeducation with individual families. Elements that appeared to be tied to its outcome effectiveness included:

• Creation of social contacts and support
• Problem-solving with others bearing the burden of the same disorder
• Countering stigma
• Cross-parenting of adolescents
• Normalizing family communications
• Intervening effectively during crises.

In a cost-saving estimate, the multifamily psychoeducational groups achieved a 1:16.50 ratio, saving $16.50 for every dollar spent on mental health services.

Family-focused psychoeducational interventions have been developed for other psychiatric disorders. Family-focused treatment for bipolar disorder, for example, integrates family psychoeducation, communication training, and problem-solving into a 20-session therapy extending over most of a year. This intervention in a controlled study has been shown to delay relapse of bipolar disorder (Miklowitz and Goldstein 1997, Miklowitz et al. 2000).

## Family Resilience Therapies

While family psychoeducation approaches have focused on roles that families can play in reducing frequency of illness relapse or buffering its severity, family resilience interventions extend this strategy to identify salutary family processes that not only buffer severity of illness, but prevent its onset for those at risk. Key processes can be identified that enable couples and families facing disruptive crises or persistent stresses to strengthen relationships, regain functioning, and further the growth of its individual members (Walsh 1998, Wolin and Wolin 1993). For example, twin studies of schizophrenia have identified some families who seemed capable of reducing the risk of illness onset for genetically at-risk adopted children. In addition, some children exposed to horrific childhood experiences with alcoholism, mentally-ill parents, physical abuse, sexual abuse, or emotional deprivation, nevertheless have grown up to be psychologically healthy and hardy adults. Michael Rutter's (1985, 1987) research found that even combinations of severe risk factors were predictive of mental illness for no more than half the affected children.

Family resilience refers to coping and adaptational processes in the family as a functional unit (Walsh 1998; Wolin and Wolin 1993). From this perspective, a stressor affects at-risk children only to the extent that they disrupt crucial family processes that otherwise would neutralize or buffer

the stressor (Patterson 1983). Family resilience rests upon several systemic principles (Walsh 1998, p. 24):

• The hardiness of individuals is best understood and fostered in the context of the family and larger social world, as a mutual interaction of individual, family, and environmental processes.
• Crisis events and persistent stresses affect the entire family, posing risks not only for individual dysfunction but for relational conflict and family breakdown.
• Family processes mediate the impact of stress on all members and their relationships, with protective processes fostering resilience by buffering stress and promoting recovery, and maladaptive responses heightening vulnerability and risks for individual and relationship distress.
• All families have the potential for resilience, which can be maximized by encouraging their best efforts and strengthening key processes.

Innovative research programs during the 1980s and 1990s sought to identify family factors contributing to the resilience of at-risk children and to design interventions that could help families better protect vulnerable children. These family resilience programs regarded resilience not to be embedded within the character of the person, but immanent within the communicational and relational systems of the person's family and social networks.

The family resilience program best validated by empirical research has been the family-based program of William Beardslee and colleagues at Boston Children's Hospital to reduce risk of onset of depression for children reared by a parent with a major depressive disorder. Epidemiological studies have established that children growing up in a home with a depressed parent have a 50% likelihood of developing a depressive disorder during adolescence and a four- to sixfold greater likelihood of receiving a psychiatric diagnosis in adulthood, particularly a depression diagnosis, than children growing up in a home with neither parent depressed (Beardslee 1998, Beardslee et al. 1999). Beardslee's group studied children who ultimately showed no signs of adult life depression, despite growing up with a depressed parent, in order to identify individual and family processes that could attenuate this risk. Factors conferring protection upon children at risk for depression were identified as:

• Becoming activists and doers
• Becoming heavily involved in school and extra-curricular activities
• Developing deep commitments to and involvement in interpersonal relationships
• Seeking self-understanding as a way to deal with a parent's depression
• Expressing articulate understanding of the parent's illness and problems ensuing from it
• Refusing to feel blame or guilt for the parent's illness.

Beardslee and colleagues designed a family-based cognitive–behavioral intervention that attempted to educate families about depression, using either a clinician's visit or group lecture as format. The intervention sought to enhance understanding of depression in all family members and to promote resilience in children at risk. Its steps consisted of an initial assessment of all family members. A program of psychoeducational material about affective disorders not only taught facts but linked the educational material to that family's life experiences. Family members were counseled to counter children's feelings of guilt and blame. Children were encouraged to develop relationships, both within and outside the family. Parents were encouraged to facilitate their children's independent functioning in school and outside home (Beardslee 1998). This clinician-facilitated format was conducted over four to eight sessions, initially alone with parents then individually with the children, ending with a whole family session and a wrap-up session. Follow-up studies have validated sustained reduction in family risk-factors for depression 3 years after intervention including an improved understanding of the parent's illness by the child; better communication between parents and children about the illness; and enhanced attunement of parents to their child's experience; and higher adaptive functioning by the child. Children who began showing symptoms of depression were identified early in the course and treated (Beardslee et al. 1999). Two notable processes that appeared correlated with effectiveness of the intervention were:

1. Active linking of life experiences of the family to information presented, rather than simply delivering factual information;
2. Giving the child an active voice in family discussions about the illness.

With programs such as Beardslee's, family resilience programs have moved past treatment of acute illness and relapse prevention, to primary prevention of the disorder itself. Such programs identify risk factors and protective factors for onset of illness; relate these factors to family organization, communications, and knowledge of the disorder; and design family interventions that enhance family understanding, attenuate risk factors, and amplify protective factors (see Table 87–1).

| **Table 87–1** | **Resilience Factors That Protect Children At Risk for Depression Due to Living with a Depressed Parent** |
|---|---|

- Becoming activists and doers
- Becoming heavily involved in school and extracurricular activities
- Developing deep commitments to and involvement in interpersonal relationships
- Seeking self-understanding as a way to deal with a parent's depression
- Expressing articulate understandings of the parent's illness and problems ensuing from it
- Refusing to feel blame or guilt for the parent's illness
- Learning to link life experiences in the family to factual information about depressive disorders
- Acquiring an active voice in family discussions about the illness

*Source:* Beardslee WR (1998) Prevention and the clinical encounter. Am J Orthopsychiatr 69(4), 521–533; Beardslee W, Versage EM, Salt P, et al. (1999) The development and evaluation of two preventive intervention strategies for children of depressed parents. In Rochester Symposium on Developmental Psychopathology, Vol. 9, Development Approaches to Prevention and Intervention, Cicchetti D and Toth SL (eds). University of Rochester Press, Rochester, New York.

## Family-Centered Approaches in International Mental Health

The extent to which North America values differentiation by individuals has arguably made it a less favorable climate for family-focused approaches than other cultures of the world. High divorce rates, fluid urban lifestyles, and frequent geographic relocations, all served to weaken the bonds of both nuclear and extended families during the latter half of the 20th century. Although couples therapy is firmly established in the American mental health system, family therapy has remained marginal.

People worldwide, however, both in their local cultures and in American immigrant groups are far more based within their families. In many world cultures, a person is more a family member than an individual, psychologically as well as in commitments of time and personal resources. Consequently family-centered therapies are often more fitting for non-Western cultures than the individual psychotherapies developed in North America and Western Europe (Weine et al. 2002). Moreover, family-centered approaches hold an advantage in resource utilization in many countries where there are few mental health professionals and little funding of mental health programs for large, poor populations (Baron 2002, Baron et al. 2002). Treating non-Western patients as individuals outside their family and community contexts has been described as the most common cross-cultural error among psychotherapists (Elsass 1997, p. 118).

Family therapy can serve as a medium in which Western psychological methods and local culture can meet on more equal footing than in individual psychotherapies. Rebuilding family and social networks after migration is vital to successful adaptation in a new land (Sluzki 1992, 1998). Culturally-sensitive family therapy focuses upon the problems of a family in transition between old and new cultures. It rests upon negotiation and collaboration and the capacity of a therapist to hold multiple perspectives simultaneously, moving back and forth between the family culture "insider" view and the "outsider" Western psychiatric view of a clinical problem. Such family therapy utilizes family meetings to create a context in which family predicaments can be presented through the narratives of everyday family life, while interweaving clinical methods for working with and making sense of these stories in their cultural contexts (DiNicola 1997).

Family-centered community mental health services has emerged as an organizing principle for mental health recovery programs in refugee communities and post-war settings following the campaigns of genocide, ethnic violence, and civil warfare of last quarter of the 20th century (Barron 2002, Barron et al. 2002, Weine et al. 2003). The Kosovar Family Professional Educational Collaborative (KFPEC) is an example of a successful family-centered approach towards community mental health services in Kosovo, a country with many mental health needs but few available funds or trained mental health professionals (Griffith 2002, Griffith et al. 2001, Weine et al. 2003). The KFPEC incorporated the strengths of family psychoeducation and family resilience-building programs discussed above, in a collaboration with Kosovar mental health professionals to train Kosovar clinicians in family therapy skills and to organize mental health services around the strengths and needs of Kosovar families.

Kosovo, a Kentucky-size country of 2 million, was left after the 1999 war with only 5 psychiatrists, 2 psychologists, no psychiatric social workers or nurses, and no hospital for the chronically mentally-ill. In recognition of the extended family as the core unit of Kosovar society, the KFPEC was established to link the University of Prishtina School of Medicine with American university and professional organizations (Griffith et al. 2001, Griffith 2002). The KFPEC has supported development of a family-focused community mental health system by training clinicians and developing services fitted to the strengths, skills, and traditions of Kosovar families. The following vignette illustrates the application of this family resilience approach with a traditional Kosovar family who were coping with the loss of five family members from the violence of the war:

---

**Clinical Vignette 7**

The T family suffered the murder of five family members during an attack upon their rural village during the war and ethnic violence of 1999. Soldiers ordered the women into the street and the men into the barnyard. As the women listened to the gunshots, the grandfather, two adult sons, and two grandsons, 8- and 10-year old, were each executed. A surviving son who had been working in Germany returned to the village to care for his mother, his sister with schizophrenia, two widowed daughters-in-law, and nine fatherless nephews and nieces.

A University of Prishtina team of psychiatrist, psychologist, and psychiatry resident conducted eight home visits to the T family, spread over several months. They supported the grandmother in her new position as head of the family, an unprecedented female role within traditional Albanian culture. They administered acute, in-home treatment for the daughter with schizophrenia whose psychosis had been exacerbated by the violence. Family sessions with adults and children provided a context for the shared expression of sorrow, grieving, and open communication. They encouraged reorganization of the family around the needs of the nine children. Team members visited the graves together with the family members and met with the family during Ramadan, when it was expected that their grief would be most intense.

Follow-up interviews conducted periodically for 2 years after the in-home family therapy found that the family had successfully reorganized with the grandmother heading the household, and the other adults sharing roles as needed to parent the children and provide support for the family. The children were excelling academically and socially in school. The daughter's psychosis was in remission, and the other family members appeared free of clinical symptoms.

---

The T family was engaged as the primary unit of therapy by the University of Prishtina clinicians. They met with T family members in their family home, drawing upon family and cultural traditions, and helping them adapt where flexibility and innovation were needed. Kosovar families particularly in villages and rural areas, are distinguished by a well-defined hierarchy of authority and clearly specified roles for each family member, determined largely by age and gender. Loyalty among family members is intense. Decisions about work, marriage, and the handling of money are all made in the context of what is best for the family as a whole. Amplifying these family strengths in recovery from trauma was an approach that can be contrasted with one more commonly employed in North America, in which individuals are screened for posttraumatic symptoms and then treated in professional offices.

## Summary

Family therapy has evolved from a treatment modality that searched family relationships for the causes of mental illness to a framework for engaging the strengths and competencies of families in solving clinical problems and treating psychiatric disorders. The various clinical traditions of family that matured during the 1960s and 1970s remain rich sources of ideas and interventions that can be integrated into multimodality programs alongside family psychoeducation, individual psychotherapy, and psychopharmacology. Such family-centered approaches as multifamily psychoeducation groups are sufficiently supported by empirical research to be regarded as evidenced-based practices. Family-centered models for primary prevention of major psychiatric disorders and family-centered community mental health programs for immigrant, refugee, and international populations represent the developing frontiers of family therapy.

## Appendix I

### Psychodynamic Family Therapy
**What to Look For**
- Projective identification
- Unresolved grief
- Clarity of ego boundaries and capacity for intimacy/separateness

**What to Think About**
- Internal processes within individual family members shape family interactions.
- Family members' motivations, conflicts, defenses, and relationships from the past, currently influence present relationships.
- Therapeutic change occurs through family members gaining conscious insight into previously unconscious processes generating problems in family relationships.

**What to Do**
- Opening emotional expression in family relationships
- Clarifying communications
- Encouraging family members to speak from the "I" position
- Interpretation of unconscious conflicts to resolve projective processes, cut-off relationships, and difficulties in modulating closeness and distance in family relationships
- Psychodramatic techniques, such as doubling and role reversal
- Therapeutic rituals to facilitate developmental transitions and grief over losses
- Family genograms

### Structural Family Therapy
**What to Look For**
Contrasting the particular family structure with that "normal" to the culture and developmental stage in terms of:

- Organization (structure)
- Rules (sequences of action)
- Roles that shape family members' actions
- Boundaries
- Hierarchy of power
- Alliances
- Coalitions
- Verbal and nonverbal behavioral sequences.

**What to Think About**

Presenting problem results from a family structure out of alignment with the culture and the developmental stage of the family.

**What to Do**

- Actively shift the family structure
- In-session enactments
- Out-of-session homework assignments

## Strategic Family Therapy

**What to Look For**

- Here-and-now context of the problem
- Who, what, when, where, and how people are involved in trying to solve the problem

**What to Think About**

- "The solution to the problem is the problem."
- Difficult life-cycle transitions give birth to clinical problems when people persist in old coping strategies but relational and communication processes need to change to meet new life contexts.

**What to Do**

- Psychoeducation
- Direct behavioral assignments to adopt new problem-solving strategies
- Defiance-based, paradoxical interventions

## Cognitive–Behavioral Family Therapy

**What to Look For**

- Family member difficulties in recognizing deviant behavior
- Lack of clearly-defined family rules
- Problems in emotional communication among family members, usually a paucity of expression of positive feelings coupled with an excess of negative expressions
- Relational conflict due to a paucity of relational skills
- Relational conflict due to interpretive errors based on faulty assumptions or cognitive distortions

**What to Think About**

- Each member of the family is assumed to be doing his or her best to cope with the behavioral contingencies perceived at that point in time, given the practical and emotional restraints experienced.
- Family members need to learn cognitive and behavioral principles of learning.
- Family members need to gain skills needed:
  1. To reinforce desired behaviors;
  2. To eliminate reinforcement of undesired behaviors;
  3. To modify faulty assumptions and interpretations about other family member's actions;

4. To learn skills for communicating clearly and effectively.

**What to Do**

- Conduct psychoeducation about the presenting problem.
- Conduct skill training in empathic listening expressing positive feelings, and speaking negative communications respectfully.
- Conduct training in problem-solving and conflict-resolution skills.
- Teach operant conditioning strategies for behavior shaping with children.
- Teach principles for contingency contracting to replace coercive and blaming behaviors with contracts specifying what each family members agrees to perform.
- Teach family members to utilize behavioral observation and thought diaries in out-of-session assignments to track patterns of thoughts, feelings, and behaviors that generate symptoms.

## Postmodern Family Therapies

**What to Look For**

- Listen for exact usage of language expressed as metaphors, stories, and beliefs
- Listen for first-person narratives from family members' lived-experiences that imbue with meaning such abstractions as "love," "trust," and other important language of relationships
- Note exceptions, or unique outcomes, when problems might have occurred but surprisingly did not
- Note what is happening at times when problems are absent

**What to Think About**

- The limits of a person's language constitutes the limits of his or her experiential world.
- Narratives, or stories, are the basic units of human experience.
- A canon of personal narratives shapes the meaning each family attributes to his or her experience.
- Narratives of identity, about who one is as a family member, and who we are as a family, strongly influence family interactions.
- Family conflicts emerge:
  1. When lack of narrative skills makes their experiences unintelligible to others;
  2. When the available narratives preclude ways of relating other than conflictual ones;
  3. When specific words or expressions hold very different meanings for different family members due to the personal narratives with which they are associated;
  4. When family members become positioned relationally such that they cannot hear, tell, and/or expand their stories in conversation.

**What to Do**

- Focus on creating a dialogue in which important personal narratives can be safely expressed, heard, and reflected upon by family members.
- Ask questions that elicit forgotten, or unnoticed, narratives of family life that open better possibilities for solving problems than the current narratives that have dominated the family dialogue.

- Engage family members in an inquiry of:
  1. What is happening in family interactions when problems are being solved successfully and symptoms are not occurring.
  2. Skills, practical knowledge, competencies, and resources of the family that can be brought to bear upon the problem.

## References

Andersen T (1987) The reflecting team: Dialogue and meta-dialogue in clinical work. Fam Process 26, 415–428.

Anderson CM, Reiss DJ, and Hogarty GE (1986) Schizophrenia and the Family: A Practitioner's Guide to Psychoeducation and Management. Guilford Press, New York.

Anderson H (1997) Conversation, Language, and Possibilities. Basic Books, New York.

Aponte JH and VanDeusen JM (1981) Structural family therapy. In The Handbook of Family Therapy, Gurman A and Kniskern D (eds). Brunner/Mazel, New York, pp. 310–360.

Arias I (1992) Behavioral marital therapy. In Handbook of Clinical Behavior Therapy, Turner SM, Calhoun KS, and Adams HE (eds). John Wiley, New York, pp. 437–455.

Baron N (2002) Community-based psychosocial and mental health services for southern Sudanese refugees in long-term exile in Uganda. In Trauma, War and Violence: Public Mental Health in a Socio-Cultural Context, de Jong JTVM (ed). Kluwer Academic/Plenum Publishing, New York.

Baron N, Jensen SB, and de Jong JTVM (2002) Mental health of refugees and internally displaced people. In Guidelines for Psychosocial Policy and Practice in Social and Humanitarian Crises: Report to the United Nations, Fairbanks J, Friedman M, de Jong J, et al. (eds). United Nations, New York.

Beardslee W, Versage EM, Salt P, et al. (1999) The development and evaluation of two preventive intervention strategies for children of depressed parents. In Rochester Symposium on Developmental Psychopathology, Vol. 9, Development Approaches to Prevention and Intervention, Cicchetti D and Toth SL (eds). University of Rochester Press, Rochester, New York, pp. 111–151.

Beardslee WR (1998) Prevention and the clinical encounter. Am J Orthopsychiatr 69(4), 521–533.

Beardslee WR, Swatling S, Hoke L, et al. (1998) From cognitive information to shared meaning: Healing principles in prevention intervention. Psychiatry 61, 112–129.

Blatner A (1994) Psychodramatic methods in family therapy. In Family Play Therapy, Schaefer CE and Carey LJ (eds). Jason Aronson, Northvale, NJ.

Broderick C and Schrader S (1981) The history of professional marriage and family therapy. In The Handbook of Family Therapy, Gurman A and Kniskern D (eds). Brunner/Mazel, New York, pp. 5–35.

Colapinto J (1991) Structural family therapy. In The Handbook of Family Therapy, Vol. 2, Gurman A and Kniskern D (eds). Brunner/Mazel, New York, pp. 417–443.

de Shazer S (1985) Keys to Solution in Brief Therapy. WW Norton, New York.

DiNicola V (1997) A Stranger in the Family: Culture, Families, and Therapy. WW Norton, New York.

Dixon LB and Lehman AF (1995) Family interventions for schizophrenia Schizophr Bull 21, 631–643.

Elsass P (1997) Treating Victims of Torture and Violence: Theoretical, Cross-Cultural and Clinical Implications. New York University Press, New York, p. 118.

Epstein N, Schlesinger SE, and Dryden W (eds) (1988) Cognitive–Behavioral Therapy With Families. Brunner/Mazel, New York.

Epston D (1989) Collected Papers. Dulwich Centre Publications, Adelaide, South Australia.

Epston D and White M (eds) (1992) Experience, Contradiction, Narrative, and Imagination. Dulwich Centre Publications, Adelaide, South Australia.

Falloon IRH (1991) Behavioral family therapy. In The Handbook of Family Therapy, Vol. 2, Gurman A and Kniskern DP (eds). Brunner/Mazel, New York, pp. 65–95.

Framo JL (1991) Family of Origin Consultations: An Intergenerational Approach. Brunner/Mazel, New York.

Freeman A, Simon K, Beutler L, et al. (eds) (1989) Comprehensive Handbook of Cognitive Therapy. Plenum Press, New York.

Freedman J and Combs G (1995) Narrative Therapy: The Social Construction of Preferred Realities. WW Norton, New York.

Goldenberg I and Goldenberg H (eds) (1980) Family Therapy: An Overview. Brooks/Cole, Monterey, CA.

Goldstein MJ, Rodnick EH, Evans JR, et al. (1978) Drug and family therapy in the aftercare of schizophrenia. Arch Gen Psychiatr 43, 633–642.

Gonzalez S, Steinglass P, and Reiss D (1989) Putting the illness in its place: Discussion groups for families with chronic medical illnesses. Fam Process 28, 69–87.

Green RW (2000) The Explosive Child: A New Approach for Understanding and Parenting Easily Frustrated, Chronically Inflexible Children. Harper Collins, New York.

Griffith JL (2002) Living with threat and uncertainty: What the Kosovars tell us. Fam Process 41, 24–27.

Griffith JL and Griffith ME (1994) The Body Speaks: Therapeutic Dialogues for Mind/Body Problems. Basic Books, New York.

Griffith JL, Blyta A, Ukshini S, et al. (2001) Promoting family resistance to effects of culturecide: The Kosovar Family Professional Educational Collaborative. Presented at the 154th Annual Meeting of the American Psychiatric Association (May 21), Philadelphia, PA.

Haley J (1976) Problem-Solving Therapy. Jossey-Bass, San Francisco.

Haley J (1980) Leaving Home. McGraw-Hill, New York.

Hoffman L (1985) Foundations of Family Therapy. Basic Books, New York.

Hogarty GE, Anderson CM, Reiss DJ, et al. (1986) Family education, social skills training, and maintenance chemotherapy in the aftercare of schizophrenia. Arch Gen Psychiatr 43, 633–642.

Imber-Black E and Roberts J (1992) Rituals for Our Times: Celebrating, Healing, and Changing Our Lives and Our Relationships. Harper-Perennial, New York.

Leff J and Vaughn CE (1985) Expressed Emotion in Families. Guilford Press, New York.

Leff J, Kuipers L, Berkowitz R, et al. (1982) A controlled trail of social intervention in the families of schizophrenia patients. Br J Psychiatr 141, 121–134.

Madanes C (1981) Strategic Family Therapy. Jossey-Bass, Washington.

Madsen W (1999) Collaborative Therapy with Multi-Stressed Families: From Old Problems to New Futures. Guilford Press, New York.

McFarlane WR (2002) Multifamily Groups in the Treatment of Severe Psychiatric Disorders. Guilford Press, New York.

McFarlanen WR, Dushay RA, Stasny P, et al. (1996) A comparison of two levels of family-aided assertive community treatment. Psychiatr Serv 47, 744–750.

McFarlane WR, Link B, Dushar B, et al. (1995) Psychoeducational multiple family groups: Four-year relapse outcome in schizophrenia. Fam Process 34, 127–144.

McGoldrick M and Gerson R (1985) Genograms in Family Assessment. WW Norton, New York.

Miklowitz DJ and Goldstein MJ (1997) Bipolar Disorder: A Family-Focused Treatment Approach. Guilford Press, New York.

Miklowitz DJ, Simoneau TL, George EL, et al. (2000) Family-focused treatment of bipolar disorder: One year effects of a psychoeducational program in conjunction with pharmacotherapy. Biol Psychiatr 48, 582–592.

O' Hanlon W and Wiener-Davis M (1989) In Search of Solutions: Creating a Context for Change. WW Norton, New York.

Patterson G (1983) Stress: A change agent for family processes. In Stress, Coping, and Development in Children, Garmezy N and Rutter M (eds). McGraw-Hill, New York.

Penn P (2001) Chronic illness: Trauma, language, and writing: Breaking the silence. Fam Process 40, 33–52.

Pinsof WM and Wynne LC (1995) The efficacy of marital and family therapy: An empirical overview, conclusions, and recommendations. J Marital Fam Ther 21, 585–613.

Rutter M (1985) Resilience in the face of adversity: Protective factors and resistance to psychiatric disorder. Br J Psychiatr 147, 598–611.

Rutter M (1987) Psychosocial resilience and protective mechanisms. Am J Orthopsychiatr 57, 316–331.

Scharff DE and Scharff JS (1987) Object Relations Family Therapy. Jason Aronson, Northvale, NJ.

Selvini-Palazzoli M, Boscolo L, Cecchin G, et al. (1978) Paradox and Counterparadox. Jason Aronson, New York.

Slipp S (1991) The Technique and Practice of Object Relations Family Therapy. Jason Aronson, Northvale, NJ.

Slovik LS and Griffith JL (1992) The current face of family therapy. In Psychotherapy for the 1990's, Rutan JS (ed). Guilford Press, New York.

Sluzki CE (1992) Disruption and reconstruction of networks following migration/relocation. Fam Syst Med 10, 359–363.

Sluzki CE (1998) Migration and the disruption of the social network. In Re-Visioning Family Therapy: Race, Culture, and Gender in Clinical Practice, McGoldrick M (ed). Guilford Press, New York, pp. 360–369.

Sluzki CE and Vernon E (1971) The double blind as a universal pathogenic situation. Fam Process 10, 397–417.

Stanton MD (1981) Strategic approaches to family therapy. In The Handbook of Family Therapy, Gurman A and Kniskern D (eds). Brunner/Mazel, New York, pp. 361–402.

Steinglass P (1998) Multiple family discussion groups for patients with chronic medical illness. Fam Syst Health 16, 55–70.

Tomm K (1987) Interventive interviewing: Part II. Reflexive questioning as a means to enable self-healing. Fam Process 26, 167–183.

Walsh F (1998) Strengthening Family Resilience. Guilford Press, New York.

Weine SM, Feetham S, Kulauzovic Y, et al. (2003) Family Interventions in a Services Research Framework with Refugee Communities. In From Clinic to Community: Ecological Approaches to Refugee Mental Health, Miller K and Rasco L (eds). Lawrence Erlbaum, New York. (in press)

Weiner-Davis M (1992) Divorce Busting. Simon & Schuster, New York.

Weingarten K (1995) Radical listening: Challenging cultural beliefs for and about mothers. J Feminist Fam Ther 7, 7–22.

White M (1989) Selected Papers. Dulwich Centre Publications, Adelaide, South Australia.

White M (1995) Re-Authoring Lives: Interviews and Essays. Dulwich Centre Publications, Adelaide, South Australia.

White M (2000) Reflections on Narrative Practices: Essays and Interviews. Dulwich Centre Publications, Adelaide, South Australia.

Wolin S and Wolin S (1993) The Resilient Self: How the Survivors of Troubled Families Rise Above Adversity. Villard Books, New York.

# 88 Couples Therapy

Eva Ritvo

Ira D. Glick

With 50% of all marriages ending in divorce, it is no wonder that there exists a large need and demand for couples therapy. Relationship distress is a common presenting complaint in most psychotherapy practices as some periods of dysfunction are inevitable in any long-term relationship. The tremendous complexities involved in meeting intimacy, social, financial, and parenting needs mean that all couples will clash over some aspects of life. It is common for marriages to undergo periodic stages of crisis and reorganization. Problems occur when couples lose faith in the marriage or lose a sense of respect and warmth for each other. Partners who have had poor role models, who have had a childhood of loss or violence, or who are poorly suited to each other by style or inclination may have increasing difficulty as time goes by.

There can be no single model to describe a functional couple just as no single therapeutic treatment modality can be universally applied. The task of the therapist is to understand the needs of a particular couple at the time they come for treatment and help them function as effectively as possible in the many domains that couples must navigate. Integrative treatment approaches are often the most effective. Not all marriages or relations can or should be held together and at times it becomes the role of the therapist to facilitate a separation in as constructive a manner as possible.

> Visions of permanent togetherness are delusions. People die; people break up; people end up alone. Yet humans will always push the fantasy of couplehood to the limit. That's why people call each other to express eternal love 2 seconds before they burn up. Coupling is a primal human urge. People team up because they need other people to watch their backs. We look out for each other. People stay hooked together despite scheduled or unplanned events, separation, death. Whatever happens, bonding with someone is the best—sometimes, the only—defense we have against life's contingencies and randomness. (Matthew Klam, *The New York Times Magazine*, October 14, 2001, p. 74)

The above quotation succinctly captures the rapidly changing nature of (and fantasies about) joining another as a couple on the "walk through life." For the student and clinician, the point is, that a couples therapist must determine what a couple wants, what the problems are in achieving it, and how to fix it.

Accordingly, in this chapter we provide a capsule summary of several models (including our own for couples therapy, i.e., an integrated model), ways of evaluating couples, formulating a broad-based diagnosis, setting goals, and formulating a treatment plan. Detailed basic strategies and techniques of couples treatment including how to treat comorbid sexual problems, medical and/or psychiatric problems, and special issues related to gay or lesbian couples are also included. This chapter closes with the essential issues related to, results of, and indications for, couples therapy. Heuristically, this chapter is based (in part) on the preceding chapter covering "family therapy"—building on that, rather than repeating it. It is also distilled from our text '*Marital and Family Therapy*' (Glick et al. 2000). There too, the authors provide the systems-oriented theoretical foundation in conjunction with new neuroscience and treatment outcome data to compliment the basics presented here.

## What Is "Couples Therapy?"

Marital or couples therapy can be defined as a format of intervention involving both members of a dyad in which the focus of intervention is the problematic interactional patterns of the couple. In this chapter, we will use marital and couples therapy interchangeably as the majority of the issues are the same. The focus of couples therapy is on the dyad and its intimate emotional and sexual aspects.

Couples therapy is distinguished by the peer relationship of the participants, the ever-present question of commitment, and a need to carefully attend to gender issues. In general, even behaviorally focused couples therapy must attend particularly to the feeling level with the goals being positive feeling between the partners and more reasonable behavior.

It is important to understand that when considering different types of psychotherapy—individual, group, and family therapy—"couples therapy" is considered as a subtype of "family therapy." Further, we should make explicit the obvious—a couple is an example of a "family" (broadly defined).

Currently, there are various models and strategies for treating couples. Each may emphasize different assumptions and types of interventions. Some therapists prefer to operate with one strategy in most cases, whereas others intermix these strategies, depending on the presenting problem and the phase of treatment. At times, the type of strategy used is made explicit by the therapist, whereas in other instances it remains covert; irrespective of whether a therapist specializes in one or another approach or is eclectic, some hypotheses will be formed about the nature of the couple's difficulty and the preferable approach to adopt.

Some therapists emphasize reconstruction of past events, whereas others choose to deal only with current behavior as manifested during the therapy session. Some therapists favor verbal exploration and interpretation, whereas others are more in favor of utilizing an action or experiential mode of treatment, either in the session itself or by requiring new behavior outside the interview. Some therapists think in terms of problems and symptoms and attempt to decode or understand possible symbolic meanings of symptomatology, whereas other therapists focus on the potentials for growth and differentiation that are not being fulfilled. Some therapists utilize one or a very limited number of methods in dealing with a whole range of "problems," but others are more eclectic and attempt to tailor the treatment techniques to what they consider the specific requirements of the situation.

Therapists may choose one school or another based on their training or their personality. For example, a very organized and directive person would probably prefer cognitive–behavioral methods, while a person who prefers long-term emotional intensity over problem solving might gravitate to experiential models. Individuals and families as well may prefer some ways of working over others. This chapter encourages the integration of a variety of techniques depending on the particular problem and personalities of the couple as well as the skill-set of the therapist. It also encourages the therapist to look beyond the problem at hand, that is, the presenting complaint, to issues of power, intimacy, and personal growth. Our approach is to emphasize models that have (at least some) empirical data.

With the therapeutic focus on one person, the emphasis is often on the individual's perceptions, reactions, and feelings, and also on the equality of status between the individual and the therapist; when two people are the operative system, attention is directed to interactions and relationships. Therapists who think in terms of a unit of three people look at coalitions, structures, and hierarchies of status and power. The number of people actually involved in the interviews may not be as important as how many people are involved in the therapist's way of thinking about the problem.

### Marriage in its Historical Context

The marital relationship in all societies is a peculiar combination of the most idiosyncratic and intimate and the most culturally patterned of relationships. Each society varies in its emphasis on the external aspects of the marriage (as a mechanism for the transfer of property and privilege, and management of paternity) and the intimate aspects (the friendship, love, and sexual issues, binding the couple). In general, the more Westernized the culture, the more free marital choice and issues of love and intimacy

become paramount. However, there are still strong cultural sanctions to marry within one's race or class.

Westernized, current marriage practices are characterized by freedom to choose a spouse, equality in terms of marriage vows (though not in terms of situation), emancipation from relatives, and an increased emphasis on intimacy. Marriage of all family relationships is most distinguished by the peculiar set of power differentials dictated by gender. In an emotional sense, at the level of intimacy and connection, the couple are equal partners. The issue of power inequality in relationships bound by love is complex (Goldner et al. 1990). Reasons include man's greater power in the culture, his greater physical strength, and the fact that marital choice usually involves women marrying men who are older and more financially successful. Marriage is also distinguished among family relationships by its voluntary nature; while you can never truly be an "ex-parent" or an "ex-child," it is possible to be an ex-spouse, to choose to truly sever the relationship. This lends the relationship a particular complexity which is central to treatment.

## Couples Function and Dysfunction

### Couples Development

Dym (1993) has described how couples relationships evolve over time. Members of couples are influenced by past and present relationships and tend to form ties that have a distinct character that emerges through regular cycles of conflict and resolution. Dym draws attention to broad, normative changes in couples, characterizing these developmental shifts as periods of expansion, contraction, and resolution. For example, in the early expansive years of a committed romantic relationship, the lives of two are in a sense woven into one. Some refer to this period of optimism, promise, and fusion as moving from "I" to "We."

In the next years of the relationship, Dym describes a predictable stage of contraction and a feeling of betrayal, in which members of the couple reconnect with a need for an "I." This desire can be marked by experiences of doubts, fears, and insecurities, and many couples retreat from their established routines. Partners may find themselves feeling "out of synch" with their own personal ambitions, describe themselves as feeling trapped or lonely, and may believe they are progressing at different tempos from each other. Stormy times may ensue with bitter conflict and blame. During the resolution stage couples may resort to compromise, negotiation, or even a more radical restructuring of their relationship in an effort to make room for both the individual and the relationship. In considering this dialectical movement from expansion to contraction to resolution, this cycle repeats several times over the course of the relationship. Dym notes that many couples have what he calls a "home base" where they tend to reside, in terms of the sense of "We," "I," or "working on it." A home base is the point of the cycle of expansion and contraction where the couples find themselves most often.

### Sexual Functioning of Couples

Schnarch (1997) contends that for many married people the magnetic force that drew them together eventually weakens to the point where sexuality and eroticism play a minor role in their lives. Sometimes, specific problems in sexual functioning affect the couple's relationship. Although the DSM-IV (American Psychiatric Association 1994) and most of the early sex therapists make a dichotomous distinction between sexual function and dysfunction, sexuality is probably best thought of as a set of experiences on a continuum of satisfaction. It is possible, for example, to have a sexual life in which there is, physiologically, sexual arousal and orgasm, but the experience feels passionless and boring, while the same "functioning" couple could have more passionate and exciting sex after therapy. It is possible to have an erotic sexual experience even if there is technical "dysfunction" as in the case of the male partner being unable to achieve erection because of physical illness, but the couple uses other methods of sexual expression. It is possible to have a good sexual experience even if there are serious arguments between the couple around issues of frequency or type of sexual practice.

It has been estimated that 50% of American marriages have some sexual problems. These can be divided into "difficulties" (such as inability to agree on frequency) which are clearly dyadic issues; and dysfunction which are specific problems with desire, arousal, and orgasm, as listed in the DSM-IV (American Psychiatric Association 1994). Dysfunctions may be organic or psychological at base, and may be lifelong or acquired, generalized or situational. They may be deeply embedded in relational power or intimacy struggles, or may be the only problem in an otherwise well-functioning relationship. While most family therapists believe that there is no uninvolved partner when one member of a couple presents with sexual dysfunction, that is different from saying that the relationship itself is the cause of the dysfunction. The job of the therapist is to ascertain as best as possible the etiology of the problem and to choose the most effective therapy, whether medical, individual, or relational. It is also within the therapist's purview to inquire about whether the couple would like to improve a technically functional but not very satisfying sexual relationship, in the same way that the therapist can offer methods or directions to increase intimacy in a couple that wishes personal growth.

### Diagnosis/Systems Issues

Sexual dysfunction or dissatisfaction is seldom caused by a psychiatric disorder (although depression and anxiety may often decrease sexual desire). It is commonly caused by ignorance of sexual anatomy and physiology, negative attitudes and self-defeating behavior, anger, power or intimacy issues with the partners, or medical/physiological problems. Medication side effects are a particularly common cause of sexual dysfunction in patients who are receiving selective serotonin reuptake inhibitors (SSRIs). Male erection problems are proving increasingly amenable to medical forms of treatment. It is also important to remember that people vary enormously in the importance they place on sex or eroticism in their lives. For example, in *The Social Organization of Sexuality: Sexual Practices in the US* (Laumann and Michael 1994), about a third of the people surveyed have sex at least twice a week, about a third a few times a month, and the rest, sex with a partner a few times a year or not at all. In general, when sex is not part of a marriage over a long period of time, the relationship has less vitality and life. However, even well-functioning marriages may have periods in which sexuality is much less part of their lives (such as after the birth of a first child, or during a family or health crisis). Different people have vastly different tolerance for such periods.

### Some Parameters of Sexual Function

Healthy sexual functioning can be thought of as resulting from relatively nonconflicted and self-confident attitudes about sex and the belief that the partner is pleased by one's performance. In this type of situation, a reinforcing positive cycle can be activated.

However, when either partner has doubts about his or her sexual abilities or the ability to please the other, his or her sexual performance may suffer. This self-absorption and anxiety will characteristically produce a decrease in sexual performance and enjoyment and can lead to impotency and orgasmic difficulties. Couple and individual difficulties of various sorts might then follow. A vicious cycle may be activated, with worries being increased, leading to increasingly poor sexual performance.

Because sex is a way of each person being vulnerable to the other, it is difficult to have sex when one is angry or not in a mood to be close (although some people can block out other feelings and keep the sexual area more separate). In addition, people who feel abused, mistreated, or ignored in a relationship are less likely to want to please the other. For some who feel that they have no voice in the relationship, lack of desire is sometimes the only way they feel able to manifest displeasure.

Couples who continue in marital or individual treatment for long periods of time can resolve some of their marital problems but can still suffer from specific sexual difficulties in their marriage. It is also true that specific sexual problems may be dramatically reversed after relatively brief periods of sex therapy, even though such problems may have proven intractable following long periods of more customary psychotherapy. However, sexual functioning which is suffering because the partners do not want to be close is not likely to respond to sex therapy unless other issues are also addressed.

Usually, when a marital couple has a generally satisfactory relationship, any minor sexual problems may be only temporary. Resolution of sexual problems, however, will not inevitably produce positive effects in other facets of a relationship as well.

Marital and sexual problems interact in various ways:

1. The sexual dysfunction produces or contributes to secondary marital discord. Specific strategies focused on the sexual dysfunctions would usually be considered the treatment of choice in these situations, especially if the same sexual dysfunction occurred in the person's other relationships.
2. The sexual dysfunction is secondary to marital discord. In such situations, general strategies of marital treatment might be considered the treatment of choice. If the marital relationship is not too severely disrupted, a trial of sex therapy might be attempted because a relatively rapid relief of symptoms could produce beneficial effects on the couple's interest in pursuing other marital issues.
3. Marital discord co-occurs with sexual problems. This situation would probably not be amenable to sex

therapy because of the partners' hostility to each other. Marital therapy would usually be attempted first, with later attention given to sexual dysfunction.

4. Sexual dysfunction occurs without marital discord. This case might be found in instances where one partner's medical illness has affected his or her sexual functioning, forcing the couple to learn new ways to manage the change. Another example might be when one partner has a history of sexual abuse or a sexual assault that creates anxiety related to the sexual experience. While individual therapy can be helpful in both of these cases, couples therapy can be especially useful in creating a safe place to address painful feelings and anxious expectations, and to provide education and guidance for couples undergoing these transitions.

## Secrets and Confidentiality

Unless a therapist sees both parties together at all times, he/she will eventually face a situation in which family secrets are disclosed in individual sessions. Since secrets are a common source of dysfunction, discovering and dealing with them is a frequent occurrence. As Imber-Black (1993) says, "secrets, decisions about secrecy and openness, and the management of information are woven into the fabric of our society. The paradoxes of what is to be kept secret and what is to be shared and with whom are all around us and are embedded in each encounter between family and therapist."

The therapist needs to make a distinction between *secrecy* and *privacy*. Privacy is usually considered to mean information held by one person that they would prefer not to share but that does not directly affect their relationship with others. It usually implies a zone of comfort free from intrusion. Secrets are usually considered to be feelings or information that would directly affect a relationship. They are most often connected to fear, anxiety, and shame, and are often shared—that is, some people in the system know, whereas some do not. There is also a gray area in which different people have different ideas about whether the information is important or not. (Does a spouse consider an extramarital affair that ended 10 years ago private or secret?)

Secrets define hierarchy and relationships, leaving the unaware mystified and out of alliance. Some are about the past such as an affair many years ago, and some about the present such as an ongoing affair, or an impending bankruptcy. The majority of toxic secrets are in some way related to sex (including abortions and illegitimate birth), money, or betrayal.

In general, the best rule of thumb is that a secret should be disclosed if it is seriously affecting connections between people, posing danger to a family member (sexual abuse), or shaping family coalitions and alliances. In general, keeping secrets is such a serious barrier that it is better to disclose them, even if painful—because otherwise the sense of mystification and isolation in the unaware is very strong. (This seems to be true in many areas affecting children that were formerly always kept secret, such as adoption, out-of-wedlock birth, and artificial insemination.) Such issues are however very dependent on situation. For example, if a husband is bisexual or homosexual and does not tell his wife but engages in unprotected (or even protected) intercourse with men, the wife is in serious danger and needs to know. Since the husband's sexuality is definitely the wife's concern, not telling her this secret is a serious threat to the relationship.

The therapist must carefully consider the timing and type of disclosure. Premature disclosure, before the therapist has an alliance with the family, can cause the family to leave therapy with no place to deal with potentially explosive material. This is particularly true when there has been a history of violence or abuse. It is generally believed that if a family member refuses to disclose a secret so serious that therapy will be derailed, the therapist may terminate therapy but should not disclose the secret himself or herself. An exception is in cases of potential violence to another, especially in child abuse or threats to murder, where the therapist is required to report to the authorities and the potential victim, so the secret will have to be disclosed. The confusion many therapists feel—faced with the requirement for reporting and knowing this may end their relationship with the family—is difficult to manage, and these cases must be discussed with a supervisor or mentor. Issues around disclosure also arise in cases where one partner is HIV positive and has not disclosed. Legally, the therapist is not obliged to do so—ethically it is extraordinarily hard not to. The patient should be strongly urged to share this important information.

In the following section, guidelines for assessing and treating couples are offered. Although these guidelines do not sufficiently cover all couples' problems and situations, they do represent a generic set of ideas that therapists may apply to the specifics of many marital issues.

## Evaluation of the Couple

The evaluation of a couple involves obtaining data on the current point in the marital and/or family life cycle, why the couple approaches for assistance at a particular time, and each partner's view of the marital or relationship problem (Table 88–1). Often the couple's therapist will hold

| Table 88–1 | Outline for Family Evaluation |
|---|---|

I. Current phase of family life cycle and identifying data

II. Explicit interview data:
   A. What is the current family problem?
   B. Why does the family come for treatment at the present time?
   C. What is the background of the family problem?
   D. What is the history of past treatment attempts or other attempts at problem solving in the family?
   E. What are the family's goals and expectations of the treatment? What are their motivations and resistances?

III. Formulating the family problem areas:
   A. Rating important dimensions of family functioning:
     1. Communication
     2. Problem solving
     3. Roles and coalitions
     4. Affective responsiveness and involvement
     5. Behavior control
     6. Operative family beliefs
   B. Family classification and "diagnosis"

IV. Planning the therapeutic approach and establishing the treatment contract

one individual session with each partner after the first or second conjoint session. This gives each partner an opportunity to divulge information that might otherwise not be obtainable. Issues of confidentiality need to be carefully addressed.

In formulating the marital difficulties, the evaluator will want to consider the couple's communication, problem solving, roles, affective expression and involvement, and behavioral expression, especially in sexual and aggressive areas. The clinician will also want to evaluate gender roles, cultural and racial issues, and power inequities resulting from gender, class, age, or financial status. It is critical to ask about alcohol, health and reproductive issues, and violence (Table 88–2).

Even if the partners do not mention their children as a problem, it is wise to spend some time developing a sense of how the children are doing, is there a favored child or problem with any of them, and whether the children are being pulled into marital conflicts. At times children can be the source of a couple's conflict and at other times they may function as the glue that keeps the relationship together. If a large part of the couple's difficulty centers around issues with the children, family therapy may be the preferred treatment modality (see Chapter 87).

The clinician must always ascertain whether there is a concomitant psychiatric condition, especially on Axis I (see later). If one exists, the impact of the condition on each member of the couple must be explored.

Other areas deserving special attention include each spouse's commitment to the marital union and the couple's sexual life. Assessment is complicated when one spouse is keeping commitment doubts or extramarital sex a secret. Conjoint and individual sessions with each partner may be needed. When infidelity or serious commitment questions arise, the therapist and couple must address whether or not the couple should stay together.

## Genograms for Evaluation

A helpful device when evaluating a couple is the use of a genogram. The therapist can collect and organize historical data through the use of a genogram, the three-generational family tree depicting the family's patterns regarding either specific problems or general family functioning. The genogram technique suggests possible connections between present family events and the prior experiences that family members have shared (e.g., regarding the management of serious illnesses, losses, and other critical transitions), thereby placing the presenting problem in a historical context (Shorter 1977, McGoldrick and Gerson 1985). Constructing a genogram early on in treatment can provide a wealth of data that frequently offers clues about pressures, expectations, and hopes regarding the marriage. This pictorial way of gathering a history allows each member of the couple to learn about beliefs or themes that characterize his/her family background. An example of a genogram can be seen in Figure 88–1.

## Assessment of Concomitant Psychiatric Illness

Having a spouse with a serious Axis I disorder, such as anxiety disorder, mood disorder, or substance abuse puts

| Table 88-2 | Guidelines for Interviewing Couples—The Process |
| --- | --- |

- Can you tell me about yourself? As individuals? As a couple? (Joining, forming an alliance with each member and the couple, creating a safe place)
- What brings you here? How do you understand the problem? What feelings does it elicit for each of you? (Developing an interactional problem focus)
- How does the problematic pattern actually work? Can you show me how it works? (Observing by staging an "enactment")
- How did this pattern originate? How did you create it? (Placing the problem in context of their relationship, family of origin, and their own individual development)
- How have you maintained this pattern? What have you done to keep it going? (Placing the pattern or problem under their joint control)
- Tell me about what you believe should be happening. (Myths, stories, ideas, expectations about love, sexuality, marriage, and closeness)
- In what other ways is the pattern currently reinforced? What do your family and friends believe is the problem? (How do jobs, extended family members, and friends contribute to the pattern's resilience?)
- Is this pattern always occurring or are there exceptions? (How pervasive is it, is it chronic, or related to a life transition?)
- What have you done to try to change the pattern? (Trying to avoid redundancy by inquiring about solution behavior)
- Have your efforts to change the pattern made things better or worse? (Looking at the problem as "attempted solutions")
- What has been the influence of this problem in your lives? (Again looking for the "influence" of the problem over their lives)
- How motivated are you to change the pattern now? (Assessing individual and couples motivation)
- What would happen if you succeeded in changing the pattern? (Anticipating possible consequences of change, both positive and negative)
- What patterns of relating have you created that you want to keep? (Identifying and honoring assets and resources)
- Are you ready to make a change? How about trying something different? (Preparing the couple for exploring new patterns of interaction)

The therapist is then free to track themes (always keeping an interactional focus), invent tasks and experiments designed to provide new experiences for the couple, and to evaluate the changes that occur or do not occur as a result of the couple's efforts to change their patterns of interaction.

realistic strain on the marital relationship. The marital interaction prior to, during, and following the onset of the symptoms in the spouse is influenced by numerous factors and is quite variant across dyads. It is incorrect to assume that in all cases the interaction between the spouses brought on, or caused, or even helped trigger the mental disorder and symptoms in the other. Whatever the symptoms in one spouse, the relationship of symptoms to the marital interaction is on a continuum and can take any one of the following forms:

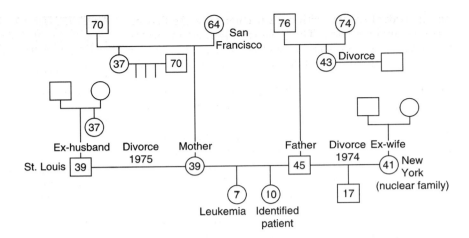

**Figure 88–1** *Example of a genogram.*

1. The marital interaction neither causes the symptoms nor stresses the psychologically vulnerable spouse.
2. The marital interaction does not stress the vulnerable individual but following onset of symptoms the marital interaction declines and becomes dysfunctional, thus causing more distress.
3. The marital interaction acts as a stressor that contributes to the onset of symptoms in a vulnerable spouse.
4. The symptoms can be explained totally as under the control and function of the interactional patterns between the spouses.

The therapist meeting a new couple therefore can entertain a range of different ideas that may help illuminate and explain their distressing circumstances. The Axis I condition can be a useful focus and often is what brings the couple in for help.

## Evaluation of Sexual Disorders

A careful evaluation of the couple's total interactions needs to be done by the therapist as well as a physical assessment when dysfunction is present. When it appears that the basic marriage is a sound one, but that the couple suffers from specific sexual difficulties (which may also lead to various secondary marital consequences), the primary focus might be sex therapy per se. In many cases, however, specific sex therapy cannot be carried out until the relationship between the two partners has been improved in other respects; indeed, the sexual problems may clearly be an outgrowth of the marital difficulties. When marital problems are taken care of, the sexual problems may readily be resolved. It may be difficult to disentangle marital from sexual problems or to decide which came first. The priorities for therapy may not always be clear.

The DSM-IV (American Psychiatric Association 1994) recognizes the following as dysfunctions:

- Sexual desire disorders: hypoactive sexual desire disorder (HSDD), sexual aversion disorder
- Sexual arousal disorders: female sexual arousal disorder, male erectile disorder
- Orgasmic disorders: female orgasmic disorder, male orgasmic disorder, premature ejaculation

- Sexual pain disorders: dyspareunia (not due to a general medical condition), vaginismus (not due to a general medical condition), vaginismus (due to a general medical condition). They are coded separately if they are due to a general medical condition or are substance induced.

Many people have more than one dysfunction (e.g., HSDD plus orgasmic disorder) and frequently each member of a couple will have a dysfunction, for example, premature ejaculation in the man with hypoactive desire in the woman. It is important to understand the sequencing of the onset of the dysfunctions to understand how they influence each other. As we have said, many sexual problems are not dysfunctions but are relationally based dissatisfactions.

Specific techniques are available which have been devised for eliciting a sexual history and for evaluating sexual functioning. The marital therapist should become familiar with these ideas and obtain experience in their utilization. A systemic assessment of sexual difficulties includes, at the minimum, the following details as listed in Table 88–3.

In addition, in couples where there is any possibility that the problems may have an organic component, it is crucial to insist on a medical workup. This is particularly key for men, for whom small physiological changes in potency may produce anxiety that exacerbates the problem.

The taking of an intimate sexual history of husband and wife should, of course, be conducted with the couple without children present. The process of taking a sexual history should be handled with care and regard for each person's level of comfort.

What type of language should be used when discussing sexual topics? Obviously, one should not use terms that would be offensive or uncomfortable for either the therapist or the couple. At the same time, care must be taken to avoid using bland generalities which fail to elicit specific sexual information. Frankness is encouraged, and when there is vagueness, the therapist needs to follow up with more specific questions.

The therapist should use simple language or use the simplest technical sexual term that the patient is comfortable with. Some patients will misunderstand technical terms. For others, the use of the vernacular by the therapist

| Table 88-3 | Assessment of Sexual Problems |
|---|---|

1. Definition of the problem
   (a) How does the couple describe the problem? What are their theories about its etiology? How do they generally relate to their sexuality, as reflected in their language, attitudes toward sexuality, comfort level, and their permission system?
   (b) How is the problem a problem for them? What is the function of the problem in their relationship system? Is the relationship problem the central problem? Why now?
2. Relationship history
   (a) Current partner
   (b) Previous relationship history
   (c) Psychosexual history, including information about early childhood experiences, nature of sexual encounters prior to the relationship, sexual orientation, and feelings about masculinity and femininity.
   (d) Description of current sexual functioning, focusing on conditions for satisfactory sex, positive behaviors, specific technique, etc. Who initiates sex, who leads, or do both? How does their sexual pattern of intimacy and control reflect on or compensate for other aspects of their relationship?
3. Developmental life-cycle issues (births, deaths, transitions)
4. Medical history, focusing on current physical status, medications, and present medical care, especially endocrine, vascular, metabolic.
5. Goals (patients' and therapist's viewpoints): The task is to examine whether goals are realistic and what previous attempted solutions have yielded.

may be inappropriate. The problem faced in the choice of language is itself an indication of our general cultural discomfort with sexuality. The therapist's own use of a particular sexual vocabulary can be a model to help the marital partners feel comfortable in communicating with each other more openly.

Taking a sexual history of lesbian and gay couples may be particularly difficult for a heterosexual therapist, either because of discomfort with homosexuality or lack of knowledge of homosexual norms and mores. In addition, the couple may have a wider or different set of sexual practices than the therapist is used to (of course, this may be true with heterosexual couples as well). Therapists have the options of educating themselves about homosexual sexuality, either by reading books available in mainstream bookstores about gay and lesbian life, and/or asking the couple about their own and other common practices. If the therapist is very anxious in this situation, he/she must decide when the therapy is not proving effective and if he/she should refer to another therapist. Gay and lesbian couples may present with any of the dysfunctions or dissatisfactions of heterosexual couples.

## Indications for Couples Therapy

The process of choosing a type of therapy is complex and research is just beginning to develop guidelines for such decisions. The therapist must most often base his or her judgment on clinical intuition, general clinical opinion, and the wishes and judgments of the people involved.

## Marital Versus Individual Therapy

One of the most common questions for clinicians who are proficient in both therapies is regarding the decision about type and timing of therapy. The basic theoretical premise of couple/family therapy is that many problems are purely relational, that individual symptoms in one person can be viewed as interpersonal in terms of etiology or problem maintenance, and that they can be changed by altering the system. The basic principle of individual therapy is that problems or symptoms develop because of the biochemistry or dynamics of the individual, and that change occurs in the individual (either behaviorally or because of cognitive understanding of the problems) in the presence of an intense and exclusive relationship with the therapist. In truth, for many people, both forms of therapy may be useful or necessary. Self-knowledge does not always help the person understand the complex family system and how one's behavior affects and is affected by family members. In addition, family therapy does not allow for intense exploration of psychodynamic issues. Individual therapy also does not allow the clinician to see how the problems of other family members may also be affecting the system. For example, a woman who requested individual treatment for depression was found on family evaluation to have a husband who had an untreated bipolar condition, that is, had symptoms of mania. Much of her depression was due to his behavior in manic or hypomanic states, and one of the key factors in treating her depression was treating his symptoms and having him acknowledge the truth of her concerns about him. On the other hand, for many people symptoms occur regardless of the different systems around them over time.

Since people tend to pick partners at similar stages of differentiation, it is not unusual for people with psychological difficulties to have spouses with similar or complementary but equally severe problems. In addition to the need to evaluate the partner, it must be recognized that such couples create problems maintaining systems that need to be addressed directly. Children in such families often suffer either from genetically based similar illnesses (such as depression) or symptoms as a result of dealing with parental problems. These are often best treated with family therapy, but this does not rule out special time just for the child. For many people, both types of therapy are helpful, allowing for increased pleasure with the partner and also a context for personal and private growth.

The choice of timing of therapy is always of interest. If the person is highly symptomatic and has a problem which is usually amenable to medications, it is often helpful to begin medication and family therapy first, in order to reduce the symptoms and educate the family, as well as to eliminate family sources of stress.

In general, one tries to deal with the most acute problems first. If it is possible in terms of timing and finances, it is easily possible to do individual and couples therapy at the same time. It is often recommended that the therapies be done by different therapists, however, in this strategy it is imperative that the therapists remain in contact to avoid splitting or conflicting treatment. Others, including therapists on occasion, have treated both the couple and one member of the couple individually, although this can present some additional challenges to the therapist to remain neutral and unbiased. The therapist's criteria depend more on the characteristics of the couple and how they function than on the particular diagnosis or problem area. The bias of the couple or individual must also be taken into account.

## Individual, Couple, or Sex Therapy for Sexual Problems

This distinction was clearer 10 years ago when sex therapy was primarily focused on a specific and highly detailed behavioral protocol. Sex therapy in the last few years has moved in the direction of further understanding of the physiologic causes of sex dysfunction on one hand, and cognitive–behavioral issues on the other. It is clear at this point that, in general, sexual problems do not disappear with couple therapy unless specific attention is paid to the nature and quality of the sexual problems. Usually, it is most effective to deal with severe couple conflict before beginning to deal with sexual issues directly (Table 88–4). Sex therapy includes education, a focus on the intimacy and power aspects of sex, and often homework assignments that in some way deal with sexual anxiety and expansion of sexual options. Individual therapy is indicated if the problems are clearly related to the partner's history (sexual abuse, hatred of women), have occurred in multiple relationships, and are not amenable to being worked on in the couple. Individual therapy is the most inefficient way of dealing with most couple centered sexual problems. It is also important to consider the possible role of organic problems in any dysfunction.

Recent research has demonstrated that no one school of therapy is definitively superior to another (Shadish et al. 1995). In general the trend in the last few years has been toward a more integrative approach, drawing from a variety of models and allowing for a more fluid type of work (Lebow 1997). Integrative models are likely to combine some form of here and now work (cognitive or behavioral) with some type of historical understanding of the patterns that led to the current problem.

## Contraindications for Couples Therapy

Couples therapy is not indicated for every couple in distress. In fact, at times, it may even be contraindicated. If one member is keeping an important secret, an attempt to

work with them as a pair may fail and the therapist often has to take a strong stand and refuse to treat the couple, as in the case of an HIV positive male who refused to share this information with his wife. At times, one member of a couple may be too ill to benefit from couples therapy. This may be the case when one partner has a bipolar disorder or schizophrenia and is acutely psychotic.

Other couples feel more comfortable when each partner has his or her own therapist. At times it can be more effective to have each member in individual therapy with good coordination between the two therapists. Finally, cases may arise where seeing a couple together may put one member of the couple in physical danger. When one member has a history of violence toward the partner, the therapist must often see each party alone to ensure the safety of a partner. Discussing areas of conflict together may risk increasing the violent behavior of one partner.

Sex therapy may be contraindicated in the same situations as above. In addition, many couples do not feel comfortable in a therapy exclusively focusing on sex. These couples may make more progress if the sex therapy is carefully included in the overall treatment of the couple. When referring to a sex therapist, it is particularly important to be familiar with the skill and credentials of the therapist.

## Treatment

We believe that for most people the strongest predictor of overall life satisfaction is the quality of the person's central relationship. In addition, "a good and stable relationship buffers against the genetic vulnerability to both medical and psychiatric disorder." Thus, helping a couple achieve a more satisfying relationship can have widespread and profound influence on their life and lives of those with whom they interact.

The treatment of each couple is unique and may require a combination of couples therapy, individual therapy, group therapy (particularly self-help groups such as Alcoholics Anonymous) family therapy, and medication management. By using an integrative approach with each couple, the therapist maximizes the chances for success. Identifying goals of treatment will help determine which modalities will be most effective and in what order they need to be applied. Goals most likely attained by employing couples therapy include the following: specification of the interactional problem, recognition of mutual contributions to the problems, clarification of marital boundaries, clarification and specification of each spouse's needs and desires in the relationship, increased communication skills, decreased coercion and blame, and increased differentiation and resolution of marital transference distortions. Final goals of the marital intervention may involve resolution of presenting problems, reduction of symptoms, increased intimacy, increased role flexibility, balance of power, clear communication, resolution of conflictual interaction, and improved relations with children and families of origin.

The treatment of couples is often conceived of as a relatively brief therapy (though it need not be), usually meeting once weekly, with a focus on the marital interaction. The major indication for marital intervention is the presence of marital conflict but other indications include symptomatic behaviors that impact both parties such as

| **Table 88–4** | **Criteria for Sex and Marital Therapy** |
|---|---|
| Sex Therapy | Marital Therapy |
| The marital problem is clearly focused on sexual dysfunction | Sexuality not an issue, or it is one of many issues in marital dysfunction. |
| Enabling Factors | |
| Willingness and ability to carry out the sexual functioning tasks that would be assigned by therapist. | Anger and resistance too intense to carry out extra-session tasks around sexual functioning. |
| Strong attachment to marital partner; both partners interested in reversing the sexual dysfunction. | Couple not committed to each other; there are covert and/or overt behaviors to dissolve the marriage. |

depression, anxiety disorders, substance abuse, and illness in a child, marital partner, or other family member.

## Strategies and Techniques of Intervention

Couples therapy utilizes strategies for imparting new information, opening up new and expanded individual and marital experiences, psychodynamic strategies for individual and interactional insight, communication and problem-solving strategies, and strategies for restructuring the repetitive interactions between the spouses or partners.

As the divisive spirit of the era of the earlier schools of psychotherapy recedes and pluralism and clinical pragmatism grows, clinicians attempt to integrate the various strategies into a coherent treatment approach that can be adapted to the individual case. The authors advocate an integrative marital therapy model that utilizes psychodynamic, behavioral, and structural-strategic strategies of intervention (see later).

Data suggests that the diagnosis and symptom picture of one spouse and characteristics of the other spouse stand in complex relationship to the issues in the marital interaction and should, therefore, influence the planning of intervention, that is, the goals. For example, if one spouse has a nonendogenous, unipolar depression with no clear precipitating stressful life events, the marital interaction could be a chronic stressor and contributor to the condition. Marital therapy in this situation could well be a preferred mode of intervention. On the other hand, if the spouse is suffering from a bipolar illness, manic episode, and the marital interaction has been good prior to the episode, psychoeducational intervention with the couple may be in order with little or no attention to the ongoing marital interaction.

Sometimes, couples present with chronic histories of unresolved and unrelenting conflict. Other couples are in a state of transition, perhaps moving from the initial expansion stage of their marriage to the inevitable crisis related to the reevaluation of the contraction stage. In either case, clarifying the couples' process and their reoccurring patterns of behavior represents the starting place for couples therapy.

The focus should be primarily on the interpersonal distortions between husband and wife, and not on the couple–therapist transference. However, negative transference distortions toward the therapist must be addressed quickly and overtly.

There are three strategies in this focused, active treatment of marital discord:

1. The therapist interrupts collusive processes between the spouses. The interaction may involve either spouse failing to perceive positive or negative aspects of the other that are clear to an outsider (e.g., cruelty or alternately generosity) or when either spouse behaves in a way aimed at protecting the other from experiences that are inconsistent with the spouse's self-perception, (e.g., husband working part time views himself as breadwinner, whereas wife works full time and manages checkbook to shield husband from reality of their income and finances).
2. The therapist links individual experience, including past experience and inner thoughts, to the marital relationships.
3. The therapist creates and allocates tasks that are constructed to (a) encourage the spouses to differentiate between the impact of the other's behavior versus (the other's) intent, (b) to bring into awareness the concrete behavior of the partner that contradicts (anachronistic) past perceptions of that partner, and (c) to encourage each spouse to acknowledge his/her own behavior changes that are incompatible with the maladaptive ways each sees himself/herself and is seen by the marital partner. These tasks also help reconstruct the couple's narrative to make it more positive.

The last (c) is most important. In fact, in the initial stage of marital treatment the authors ask that each partner focus on what they want to change in themselves, not how they want the other spouse to be different.

In this integrative model, the focus is on three related domains: the functional relationships between the antecedents and consequences of discrete interactional sequences; the recurrent patterns of interaction including their implicit rules; and each spouse's individual schemata for intimate relationships. In the initial stage, alliances must be developed between the therapist and each marital partner, with the therapist offering empathy, warmth, and understanding. The therapist must also ally with the couple as a whole and learn their shared language as well as their different problem-solving styles and attitudes.

Behavioral techniques, including giving between-session homework, in-session tasks, communication skills, and problem-solving training, can facilitate the process of helping marital partners reintegrate denied aspects of themselves and of each other. However, the focus is not on behavioral change alone, as overt behavior is seen as reflecting the interlocking feelings and perceptions of each spouse. Ideally, the process of treatment should be one where each partner can consider what they want to change in themselves as opposed to how they want the other spouse to be different; safely explores new beliefs, feelings, and behaviors; and experiments with new patterns of interaction that are unfamiliar and even anxiety-provoking.

## Treatment of Sexual Dysfunction

Treatment of psychosexual disorders, in the form developed by Masters and Johnson (1966), consisted of a thorough assessment of the partners and their relationship, education about sexual functioning, and a series of behavioral exercises. The model was based on three fundamental postulates: (a) a parallel sequence of physiological and subjective arousal in both genders, (b) the primacy of psychogenic factors, particularly learning deficits and performance anxiety, and (c) the amenability of most sexual disorders to a brief, problem-focused treatment approach—that is, sensate focus. These sensate focus exercises were designed predominantly for behavioral desensitization, but also functioned to teach the partners about their own and the other's sexual desires, and also served to elicit relationship problems. In these exercises, the couple pleasures each other, alternating in the role of giver and receiver, first in nongenital areas, then genitally, and then with intercourse. In the traditional form, intercourse is prohibited during the early stages to remove performance anxiety. There are also specific exercises for each of the sexual dysfunctions.

Different authors developed different exercises and ways of approaching them. For a complete description of these exercises, we recommend Kaplan (1995), LoPiccolo and Stock (1996), and Zilbergeld (1992). This method works best when there is ignorance, shame, or specific dysfunction such as premature ejaculation. These exercises are difficult to complete if the couple feels angry or unloving toward each other.

Many of the patients who saw Masters and Johnson in the 1970s had issues related to sexual ignorance and inexperience. Two decades later, the increase in premarital sex and the proliferation of easily available articles and books on sexuality and information on the Internet have decreased the number of these couples, and allowed some couples with sexual dysfunction to work on their issues at home. Recent studies of couples requesting sex therapy have shown a higher proportion having concomitant, complicated marital problems. Recent writers in the field, notably Schnarch (1997), have focused on cognitive/emotional issues in sexuality, and especially on the meanings attached to a particular act, and the level of intimacy involved. Having learned a great deal about the more mechanical and organic issues related to arousal and orgasm, it is important to rethink other aspects of sex, such as eroticism, passion, mystery and dominance/submission which make the act itself meaningful. This is particularly true in areas of sexual boredom or situational lack of desire. These therapists do not use rigidly staged exercises, but focus on the couple's relatedness during sex; they may, however, suggest specific homework to help a couple focus on a particular aspect of their sexuality.

Although not mentioned in the DSM-IV, the issue of sexual compulsions or addictions may be seen in couples. In these cases, one partner's unceasing compulsion to think about, view (print or on-line), talk about, and/or have sex may be very wearing to the other partner or to oneself. A key component of this problem is that such persons may become extremely anxious if sex is denied. They may present with multiple affairs or with constant demands on the partners. However, most people who have affairs do not have a sexual compulsion.

Treatment for these disorders is still controversial. Some therapists use a 12-step addiction model along with group therapy; some treat it as a compulsion with individual therapy and medication (particularly with SSRIs such as fluoxetine). Couples therapy is still a critical component part of treatment—to educate the couple, and if multiple affairs have taken place, to discuss the viability of the marriage.

In recent years, emphasis has shifted to the role of biomedical and organic factors in the etiology of sexual dysfunction, along with the growing use of medical and surgical treatment interventions. Particular focus has been given to their role on vascular disorders and neuroendocrine problems, as well as the tendency for many medications to effect sexual functioning. It is critical for the patient to have a thorough physical workup. For a good review on the interaction of medication and sexuality, see Abramowicz (1992).

A variety of medical approaches to the treatment of erectile disorders in men have been developed in recent years. These include, but are not limited to, surgical prostheses or penile implants (seldom used in the last few years),

intracorporal injection of vasoactive drugs such as papavarine, constriction rings and vacuum pump devices, and urethral suppositories. In 1998, oral medications for the treatment of impotence were introduced (sildenafil, Viagra). Because our understanding and treatment of impotence is developing so rapidly, it is important to stay current on new research in the field. Surgical treatments are available for the correction of arterial insufficiency or venous leakage problems. These methods may be more or less acceptable both to the man and his partner. The partner's response to the changes is often a key element in their success. There has been some success in treating premature ejaculation with SSRIs and clomipramine; however, since these may also decrease sexual desire, caution and careful monitoring are indicated (Abramowicz 1992). Wellbutrin is sometimes helpful in preventing loss of sexual desire in patients treated with SSRIs.

In women, most medical interventions have been for dyspareunia. Female dyspareunia due to the decreased lubrication of aging can be treated with topical estrogen cream or lubricant jelly. Even when an organic cause is found and treated, the conditioned anxiety and lack of arousal associated with sex usually require an additional course of couples therapy with a sexual focus. Hormone treatment for lack of desire has not proven effective (Rosen and Lieblum 1995).

**Clinical Vignette 1**

Mrs. L had problems with anger during adolescence, generally due to feeling neglected by her busy parents. During adolescence, she had a period of intense sexual activity which was related to looking for affection through sexuality. She reported that she had no sexual problems during this time. Through twice-a-week individual psychotherapy in her twenties she worked through these problems, married Mr. L, and had a child. Mr. L was a kind but rather distant man who soon after the marriage made a series of career moves that kept him extremely busy. For the first 2 years there were no sexual problems. Then, marital problems developed, and Mrs. L's desire decreased. Mr. L became more sexually demanding. Frequency and enjoyment of sex for both partners was markedly decreased. Mrs. L refused to have sex, saying that she was too upset. When they had sex occasionally, however, both were orgasmic.

Mr. and Mrs. L had both been raised in traditional backgrounds, and had been taught that sex should not be discussed. Although both had previous sexual experiences, they were unable to talk about their sexual problems. Mrs. L began fantasizing about other men. Although fantasies of other partners are not unusual, Mrs. L's fantasies only occurred when she was particularly angry with her husband. While at one time individual psychotherapy for Mrs. L might have been the treatment of choice, the therapist decided to use both marital therapy and sex therapy. Marital therapy helped open communication between the couple. It was discovered that Mrs. L was feeling very abandoned by her extremely hard working husband and feeling that she was being ignored as she had been in her childhood. In addition, she was angry at her husband for not helping with child-rearing responsibilities. Her fantasies

Clinical Vignette 1 *continued*

about other men, which seemed to be a way of wishing for the affection she craved earlier in her life, were upsetting her and making her wonder if she loved her husband. Mr. L's inability to challenge her and insist on her connecting with him emotionally before demanding sex was experienced as further withdrawal from her.

Using psychodynamic techniques, the couple was encouraged to deal more directly with their differences and with the disappointments underlying their anger. Issues related to each partner's family of origin were brought up. Roles were restructured and Mr. L took over more of the child-rearing responsibilities. As the marital relationship improved, their sexual problems decreased. Using the cognitive–behavioral model, the couple was given a series of sensate focus exercises in which they were asked to focus on giving and receiving pleasure. They were encouraged to share their feelings and fantasies, to talk to each other about their sexual wishes, and to pay attention to the connection between them while being sexual (the experiential model). They also discussed deepening their nonsexual physical connection, that is, "constructing" a new reality for themselves as a couple.

This case demonstrates the use of combining different models and strategies to change behaviors which are complex in origin.

## Homosexuality or Bisexuality

The authors believe that couples therapists should be adequately educated in the area of human sexual orientation and sexual identity. These terms in themselves are confusing. *Sexual orientation* is another way of indicating an individual's tendency to be attracted to one or both sexes. Sexual orientation, like most psychological phenomenon, is not an absolute or mutually exclusive trait. One may be sexually attracted to the opposite sex, the same sex, or both. Sexual orientation falls along a continuum, with completely homosexual and completely heterosexual preferences falling at the extreme ends, and many gradations in between. Sexual orientation may also change over time. Some persons change from heterosexual to homosexual or the reverse in their thirties, forties, or fifties. Some remain bisexual during their adult lives.

Observations of human sexual behavior, affectional attachments, erotic fantasies, arousal, and erotic preference have suggested that sexual orientation and identity are not static. In fact, both may fluctuate over a person's lifetime. Sometimes changes in sexuality are "just phases"; sometimes they become the predominant disposition of sexual relation. Regardless, deviation from heterosexuality in western society is frequently accompanied by rejection, not only by one's immediate family, but also by one's peers and, in some cases, society in general. Accusations of discrimination and violence, "gay bashing," have been a constant news story in metropolitan headlines. Bisexuals have the added nonacceptance by gay and lesbian friends or associates who may accuse them of "fence-sitting," of "sleeping with the enemy," or of being deviant because they are unable to choose whether to be hetero- or homosexual. For the therapist, the issue should be centered on understanding and listening to other's experiences, even if they are quite different than our own.

Many persons who are bisexual or whose homosexuality is admitted consciously later in life may spend some years in heterosexual marriages. Many such people are able to function well heterosexually, changing their sexual focus when they realize that "something is missing" or that their level of desire and love is greater for their own sex. Some have low levels of sexual desire in the marriage and develop affairs. Because there may be a great deal of love and affection between the marital partners, the discovery that one member is homosexual is very painful. The desire to remain in the marriage may be strong on one or both sides. Although sex therapy can improve sexual functioning, there is no treatment which has proven effective in decreasing homosexual desires and fantasies. The couple must decide how to handle the situation—that is, whether to divorce, remain in the relationship and allow for alternative sexual behaviors, or whether the homosexual person can remain monogamous in the marriage and give up expressing the other parts of themselves. Therapy can help the couple clarify these alternatives and make decisions. Experience shows that even with the most loving spouses the most common final event is divorce.

## Sexual Problems After Medical Illness

Adults treated for cancer, diabetes, heart disease, prostatitis, HIV, and chemical dependency may face extraordinary sexual challenges due to the underlying disorder, their treatment, or the illness' effect on the couple's relationship. Two separate kinds of problems can occur. In one, the illness specifically affects sexual functioning. For example, surgery for prostate cancer may produce erectile dysfunction. This is now generally treated medically with alprostadil or similar medication in various forms; in few cases penile prosthesis may be necessary. Close communication with the urologist is necessary. The therapist should also help partners expand their repertoire of nonintercourse sexual behaviors. In the second type of situation, sex is still possible but the couple is anxious that having sex will injure one person. The classic example here is sex following myocardial infarction (Cobb and Schaffer 1975). There is no evidence that sex with a known partner in familiar surroundings is problematic for the heart. The very few heart attacks related to sex are most likely to involve affair partners and heavy intake of food or alcohol. The couple should be advised to resume sex as soon as any reasonable exercise is permissible.

Erectile dysfunction may be the predictable side effect of certain antihypertensive medications. Narcotics such as heroin, barbiturates, and alcohol have a similar effect. Obviously, addictive drugs should be stopped or efforts made to change necessary medications. Many of the newer antidepressants, especially SSRIs, can decrease sexual desire and delay orgasm. In general, the treatment of choice is to lower the dose or change antidepressants, although adjunctive pharmacologic therapy is sometimes helpful in reducing these side effects. Serious illness of any kind, plus treatment for certain illness like cancer, may leave the person with no sexual interest. In this case, the couple may have to live with it, and the therapist's task is to help the couple decide the best way to handle it within the marital relationship.

Similarly, surgery, chemotherapy, or radiation for cervical, ovarian, and prostate cancer can reduce desire and performance. HIV and AIDS should alter a couple's approach to sex, and safe sexual practices must be recommended.

## Treatment of Axis I Disorders

With increasing evidence of the multiple causes (including genetic, neurochemical, familial, and environmental) of many psychiatric syndromes, attention must be paid to both individual diagnoses and family interactions. In the last 20 years as diagnostic categories have become clearer, our treatment approaches have also become clearer. Many DSM-IV-TR diagnoses are now treated with pharmacotherapy at some point in the course of the illness. For example, antipsychotic medications are used to treat the positive symptoms of schizophrenia while antidepressants are usually indicated when an individual is diagnosed with a major depression. In most instances, treatment is also indicated for the problems of a couple and interactions accompanying these conditions. Couples therapy has been shown to be effective in providing psychoeducation and enhancing compliance with medication and psychosocial interventions when one member is suffering from any DSM-IV-TR diagnosed conditions including, but not limited to, schizophrenia, depression, bipolar disorder, anxiety disorders, dementia, substance abuse, and some Axis II conditions. Disorders diagnosed in infancy, childhood, and adolescence such as pervasive developmental disorders, attention deficit disorder, conduct disorders, mood and anxiety disorders, and eating disorders most often require family therapy as part of the overall treatment program.

Some of the problems may be related to the etiology of the individual illness, some may be secondary to it, others may adversely affect the course of the illness, and still others may not be connected at all. For example, if panic disorder with agoraphobia has developed in a spouse early in the marriage, the therapist's attention must be directed not only to treating the illness but also to the nature of the marital interaction, including its possible role in exacerbating or ameliorating the illness. In addition, if a major psychiatric diagnosis occurs in one spouse, attention must be paid to the partner's ability to cope with the illness. A child may respond to his or her mother's severe depressive illness by becoming a caretaker for a younger sibling, risking his or her own development, or the child may begin acting out. Moreover, the treatment of a child with a DSM-IV diagnosis will be greatly assisted by the couple's recognition of the problem and adherence to the treatment program.

## Effectiveness and Efficacy of Couples Therapy

There are two major sources for reviews of efficacy of couples therapy. Shadish and coworkers (1995) summarized 163 randomized studies, 62 marital, and 101 family therapy. Pinsof and Wynne (1995) in a commentary have summarized the data. These studies point to the following general conclusions:

1. Family treatment is more effective than no treatment. This conclusion is manifest in studies that contrast family and marital treatment to no-treatment control groups. Roughly 67% of marital cases and 70% of family

cases improve. The outcome may be slightly better if the identified patient is a child or an adolescent than if he or she is an adult. These findings were statistically significant. No one therapy method was demonstrated clearly to be better than another.

2. The deterioration rate (i.e., the percentage of patients who become worse or experience negative effects of therapy) is estimated at about 10%—lower than for individual therapy. Pinsof and Wynne (1995) believe the rate is lower than 5 to 10% and describe family therapy as not harmful.

3. In several areas evidence indicates that family treatment is the preferred intervention strategy. In other areas family therapy and individual therapy were tied—often in situations in which the identified patient had a significant Axis I problem (Shadish et al. 1995). These treatments of choice are of great importance for practitioners and students.

## Couple Distress or Problems

The data over 3 decades suggest that couples therapy is superior to individual therapy for marital conflict situations (Pinsof and Wynne 1995). The strongest effects are for increasing marital satisfaction and reducing conflict. (It should be pointed out that these are not synonymous—some people who have high marital conflict still report high marital satisfaction, and some couples have low conflict because the marriages are "dead.") Not surprisingly, couples who are less distressed show more improvement. Some of these effects wash out over time, as is common in chronic conditions.

## Sexual Difficulties

Twenty-five years of experience in treating sexual difficulties with some combination of sex and couples therapy has shown the combination to be consistently superior to individual therapy in the treatment of sexual dysfunction. Although Masters and Johnson's (1970) original success rates have not been repeated in later studies, 60 to 95% of sexual dysfunctions can be treated, depending on the type of sexual problem. Recent advances in sex therapy have seen a movement from mostly behavioral to more integrative treatment models with more attention to cognitive and systemic factors, and increasing focus on organic causes and medical treatment for male dysfunction, especially erectile dysfunction (Rosen and Lieblum 1995).

## Mood Disorder in Women Who Have Couple or Marital Problems

Prince and Jacobson's review (1995) suggests that medication plus marital therapy is better than individual therapy alone. In these cases, individual therapy does little to moderate the "toxic" marital problems that increase the depression. Drugs alone are also ineffective for this type of problem. Most therapy for depression has been done on depressed women so we have little information on working with depressed married men. However, some men are deeply troubled by the experience of talking about problems, preferring to work on them in private. Many depressed men have wives who are very angry, which might increase their depression if discussed in therapy. Parenthetically, there is some evidence that women with other Axis I conditions respond better to couples therapy than men with other Axis I conditions (Haas et al. 1990).

What happens if the outcome of marital treatment is separation or divorce? One might automatically assume that such an outcome is deleterious and that marital and family therapy should be designed to hold the families together. On reflection, experience seems to indicate otherwise. Marital therapy allows the partners to examine whether or not it is to their advantage to stay together, and it gives them permission to separate if that is what they need to do.

---

**Clinical Vignette 2**

In the A family the couple were in their thirties. He was a dentist, she a housewife who had previously been a teacher. She came from a family in which her father had been a chronic "run-around," and she married her husband because he appeared to be reliable and stable. He came from a family in which the mother was dull and masochistic, and he married his wife because she seemed exciting and interesting.

The couple came to therapy after 5 years of marriage when it was "discovered that the husband was having extramarital affairs" (he had left around several notes from his girlfriends). Exploration of the situation revealed that, soon after marriage, Mrs. A had become slowly and imperceptibly disillusioned with her husband when she found that he was very insecure about himself, was very unreliable, and characteristically "lied and cheated." Dr. A perceived after several years that his wife was not as exciting as he had thought and would not fulfill the role he had envisioned for her—that is, being the "slave" to a professional husband.

The therapy allowed the couple to examine some of the original premises on which they had gotten together and they found them faulty. The process of therapy, and not the therapist's values, gave them the necessary permission to separate.

---

## Dropouts

The dropout rate in the early stage of couple or family therapy is relatively high. In one study, about 30% of all the families or couples referred for family treatment failed to appear for the first session (defected) and another 30% terminated in the first three sessions, leaving about 40% who continued (Shapiro and Budman 1973). The main reason families gave for termination was a lack of activity on the part of the therapist, whereas defectors in general had a "change of heart," and denied that a problem existed. The issue usually is that no matter how bad a situation was, it was preferable to what might happen if a couple changed their behaviors. The motivation of the husband appeared to play a crucial role—the more motivated he was, the more likely the family was to continue treatment. The idea that a dropout is "denying a problem" may or may not be true. Because the process of entering therapy is frightening for many people and because the therapist must meet the needs of several people, it is unsurprising that the process of engagement is rocky.

## Ethical Issues in Couples Therapy

The fundamental ethical dilemmas inherent in psychotherapy: confidentiality, limits of control, duty to warn/reporting of abuse, and therapist–patient boundaries become more complex when the treatment involves more than one person. The couple's therapist has an ethical responsibility to everyone in the family. In some cases, individual needs and system needs may be in conflict. For example, a husband may wish to conceal a brief episode of unprotected sex with another woman, while his wife is better protected, for health reasons as well as psychological reasons, if she knows about it. A wife's wish to be divorced from a psychiatrically ill and demanding husband may conflict with his need for her care. Such clinical situations provide a set of ethical dilemmas for the therapist. The therapist must be clear that his/her job in most cases (such as impending divorce) is to help the partners sort out their values, obligations, and options rather than making a decision for them. In some cases, however (such as the reporting of child abuse), the ethical decision must be the therapist's. And in some cases the therapist faces difficult gray areas which must be decided on a case-by-case basis. The therapist also has certain unalterable ethical obligations such as not engaging in "dual relationships" (see later) with patients or exploiting them for their own benefit.

While the operative concept is "first do no harm," the issues of how one defines harm, and who will or will not be harmed by a certain action, are complex and difficult questions, especially when treating a couple or family.

## The Conflicting Interests of Family Members

It is not unusual for the interests of each member of the couple to conflict at some point. Boszormenyi-Nagy and Spark (1973) years ago emphasized the contractual obligations and accountability between persons in the multigenerations of a family. Relational ethics are concerned with the balance of equitable fairness between people. To gauge the balance of fairness in the here-and-now, and across time and generations, each member must consider both his/her own interests and the interests of each of their partner. The basic issue is one of equitability, that is, everyone is entitled to have his or her welfare and interests considered in a way that is fair to the related interests of other family members.

There may be times when it is difficult to decide whether a therapeutic action or suggestion may be helpful for one individual, but not helpful or even temporarily harmful to the other individual. In their concern for the healthy functioning of the system as a whole, therapists may inadvertently ignore what is best for one individual. An ethical issue is how the decision is made. Should it be the therapist's concern alone or should it be shared with the couple? How much information should they be given on the pros and cons of modalities? The authors' bias is to negotiate and give the couple all the relevant information so that they can make the most informed decision possible (for further discussion, see also Hare-Mustin et al. 1979, Hare-Mustin 1980).

## Boundaries

The issue of boundaries and dual relationships is a critical one in all forms of psychotherapy. Because couples therapy involves more than one patient in the consulting room, there is less likelihood of inappropriate sexual contact between therapist and patient. However, there have been cases in which a therapist, working with a couple, began an affair with one of the spouses, either during couple's therapy or after the couple separated. The American Association of Marital and Family Therapy (AAMFT) Code of Ethics (1998) has a very sensible code of ethics making clear the inappropriateness of this kind of behavior.

Other confusing issues may arise because the issues that couples face are the same as issues therapists face in their own lives, making it very likely that at some point countertransference issues may become ethical ones. For example, seeing a couple going through a separation at the same time one is going through the early stages of one's own divorce is an extremely difficult thing to do, and the likelihood of remaining neutral to both parties is not great. While it is obviously impossible for a therapist to stop treating patients while going through a divorce, he or she could certainly choose not to accept a new patient whose situation is very similar to their own or who reminds them of their departing spouse. Issues of "confidentiality" and "boundaries" are issues mentioned in the AAMFT Code of Ethics (1998). Three of these have special relevance to couples therapists:

(1) Marriage and family therapists are aware of their influential position with respect to clients, and they avoid exploiting the trust and dependency of such persons. Therapists, therefore, make every effort to avoid dual relationships with clients that could impair professional judgment or increase the risk of exploitation. When a dual relationship cannot be avoided, therapists take appropriate professional precautions to ensure judgment is not impaired and no exploitation occurs. Examples of such dual relationships include, but are not limited to business or close personal relationships with clients. Sexual intimacy with clients is prohibited. Sexual intimacy with former clients for 2 years following the termination of therapy is prohibited.
(2) Marriage and family therapists respect the right of clients to make decisions and help them understand the consequences of these decisions. Therapists clearly advise a client that a decision on marital status is the responsibility of the client.
(3) Marriage and family therapists have unique confidentiality concerns because the client in a therapeutic relationship may be more than one person. Therapists respect and guard confidences of each individual client.

## Financial Issues

Who pays the bill is relatively simple in individual treatment with adult patients, but is not necessarily so in couples therapy. The ethical issues of who pays the bill become especially tense in marital treatment of spouses in conflict. For example, if both spouses have insurance coverage from their respective employers, the question arises as to whose insurance should be used? This becomes most delicate when the spouses have conflicting views of the matter for any number of reasons, for example, "I don't

want my secretary seeing the insurance forms," "using my insurance makes me the patient," and so on. As with many concrete issues of conflict, the family therapist should approach the matter with a sense of fairness. The symbolic meanings of who pays should be thoroughly explored. When both partners have separate income and separate financial arrangements, they should each pay half the bill. Other financial questions involve sudden changes of fortune. If a woman married to a well-to-do man divorces her and her income drops severely and suddenly, should the therapist be willing to continue treatment even if the husband refuses to pay? For many therapists and many clients, money is the most taboo subject, even more than sex. It is the therapist's job to clarify their own understanding and feelings about money so they can support discussions with patients.

## Conclusion

Couples and sex therapy are important forms of psychotherapy. There is little question that developing the skills needed to successfully work with couples presenting with a wide range of difficulties requires an understanding of how normal couples' relationships change over time, how problems emerge and are maintained, and how focused marital treatment can alleviate distress and dysfunction. The rewards, however, are great when therapists can assist couples in recognizing and shifting the patterns that inhibit their abilities to live rich, intimate lives together.

This chapter provides the basics of evaluation and treatment of the most common types of couples. It also succinctly details the kinds of results a therapist might expect and discusses not only when to prescribe couples therapy, but also the practical issues in carrying it out to successful completion.

As mentioned in the introduction to this chapter, long-term relationships that are mutually supportive with a high level of intimacy are rare. As societies around the world (including our own) continue to evolve, unexpected events create havoc even for very stable families. What couples ask of their psychiatrists is the basic knowledge and skills, artfully applied to their joint relationships, to improve the quality of their lives.

## References

Abramowicz ME (1992) Drugs that cause sexual dysfunction: An update. Med Lett 34, 95–111.
American Association of Marital and Family Therapy (1998) Code of Ethics.
American Psychiatric Association (1994) Diagnostic and Statistical Manual of Mental Disorders, 4th ed. APA, Washington DC.
Borzormenyi-Nagy I and Spark G (1973) Invisible Loyalties: Reciprocity in Intergenerational Family Therapy. Harper & Row, New York.
Cobb LA and Schaffer WE (1975) Letter to the editor. N Engl J Med 293, 1100.
Dym B (1993) Couples: Exploring and Understanding the Cycles of Intimate Relationships. HarperCollins, Boston, MA.
Glick ID, Berman E, Clarkin JK, et al. (2000) Marital and Family Therapy, 4th ed. American Psychiatric Press, Washington DC.
Goldner V, Penn P, Sheinberg M, et al (1990) Love and violence: Gender paradoxes in volatile attachments. Fam Process 29, 343–364.
Haas GL, Glick ID, Clarkin JF, et al. (1990) Gender and schizophrenia outcome: A clinical trial of an inpatient family intervention. Schizophr Bull 16, 277–292.
Hare-Mustin R (1980) Family therapy may be dangerous to your health. Prof Psychol 11, 935–938.

Hare-Mustin R, Marecek J, Caplan K, et al. (1979) Rights of clients, responsibilities of therapists. Am Psychol 34, 3–16.

Imber-Black E (1993) Secrets in Families and Family Therapy. WW Norton, New York.

Kaplan HS (1995) The Sexual Desire Disorders: Dysfunctional Regulation of Sexual Motivation, Ch. 18. Brunner/Mazel, New York.

Laumann E and Michael E (1994) The Social Organization of Sexuality: Sexual Practices in the US. University of Chicago Press, Chicago, IL.

Lebow J (1997) The integrative revolution in couple and family therapy. Fam Process 36, 1–19.

LoPiccolo J and Stock W (1996) Treatment of sexual dysfunction. J Consult Clin Psychol 54, 158–167.

Masters W and Johnson V (1966) Human Sexual Response. Little, Brown, Boston, MA.

Masters W and Johnson V (1970) Human Sexual Inadequacy. Little, Brown, Boston, MA.

McGoldrick M and Gerson R (1985) Genograms in Family Assessment. WW Norton, New York.

Pinsof WM and Wynne LC (1995) The efficacy of marital and family therapy: An empirical review, conclusions and recommendations. J Marital Fam Ther 21, 585–613.

Prince SE and Jacobson NS (1995) A review and evaluation of marital and family therapies for affective disorders. J Marital Fam Ther 21, 401.

Rosen R and Lieblum S (1995) Treatment of sexual disorders in the 1990s: An integrated approach. J Consult Clin Psychol 63, 877–890.

Schnarch D (1997) Passionate Marriage. WW Norton, New York.

Shadish WR, Ragsdale K, Glaser RR, et al. (1995) The efficacy and effectiveness of marital and family therapy: A perspective from meta-analysis. J Marital Fam Ther 21, 345–361.

Shapiro R and Budman S (1973) Defection, termination and continuation in family and individual therapy. Fam Process 12, 55–67.

Shorter E (1977) The Making of the Modern Family. Basic Books, New York.

Zilbergeld B (1992) The New Male Sexuality. Bantam, New York.

# 89   Hypnosis

José R. Maldonado
David Spiegel

Hypnosis is a natural state of attentive, focused concentration. As such, most individuals are able to experience trance-like states at different times in their daily lives. An example is the alteration of awareness experienced by some persons as they concentrate intently on a movie or a play while disconnecting from awareness of the surrounding environment. Depending on the degree of natural ability to enter a trance state (hypnotic capacity or hypnotizability), a given subject will require more or less help to enter and use his or her hypnotic capacity. That is, highly hypnotizable individuals enter trance states with ease, on many occasions even without being fully aware of it. Individuals with low hypnotizability require more direction or help from the therapist who facilitates the trance experience. High hypnotic capacity may actually become a liability to patients who are unaware of their hypnotic capacity or of their unconscious use of this mechanism, as is the case of individuals suffering from a dissociative disorder. Even when we do not intend to use hypnosis formally, we must remember that the ability to enter a trance state is widely and naturally distributed throughout the normal population. Thus, some of our patients may be experiencing trance states even without our planning.

## Historical Background

The phenomenon of "trance experiences" has been described throughout history. In ancient Greece, trance-like states were used as a vehicle for treatment of mental or physical illness by allowing or facilitating contact with gods or spirits deemed causative of human malaise. Official reports of the use of hypnosis in the modern world date to the 18th century (Table 89–1). Friedrich (Franz) Anton Mesmer (1734–1815) is considered the father of hypnosis. He described the use of "mesmeric passes" (manipulations) by which he believed he was able to influence the "magnetic fluid" throughout his patients' bodies. Despite the fact that his work was discredited by a panel of French experts appointed by King Louis XVI (1784), it represented the first formal method of psychological treatment, or psychotherapy (Ellenberger 1970). The Royal Commission did acknowledge that the phenomenon of suggestion, the influence of one individual on another, was at the root of social order as well as personal change. Now we know that suggestibility not only is one of the main components of the hypnotic experience but also is ever present in any form of therapeutic interaction between physicians of any specialty and their patients.

In the late 18th century, José Custodi Di Faria (1756–1819) proposed the theory of expectancy and receptivity as the clue for hypnotic success. He also moved away from the mesmeric passes to the use of verbal suggestions. During the 19th century, interest in hypnosis persisted in America through the writings of William James (1902), Boris Sidis (1905), and Morton Prince (1906), who founded the *Journal of Abnormal Psychology*. They were fascinated by the extreme symptoms observed in patients with such dissociative symptoms as conversion reactions and multiple personality disorder.

The use of hypnosis has not been limited to the field of psychiatry. In fact, we owe the name hypnosis to the British surgeon James Braid (1785–1860), who initially coined the name *neurohypnology* or nervous sleep (Braid 1843), which was later shortened to the current term, hypnosis. The earliest reported use of hypnoanesthesia is attributed to the French surgeon Jules Cloquet, who in 1829 used it while performing a mastectomy (Fourmestraux 1934). In 1836, the first use of hypnosis as an anesthetic in the US was reported in Boston (West 1836). John Elliotson (1843) is credited with the introduction of hypnosis as a form of anesthesia in Great Britain. The British surgeon James Esdaile (1846) reported excellent surgical success rates (up to 85%) using hypnosis as the only form of anesthesia while practicing in India. Throughout the years, the routine use of hypnosis as a form of anesthesia has declined, probably because of the uniformity of results obtained by chemical agents. Nevertheless, the use of hypnosis in medicine has been extended to the treatment of other medical symptoms, including chronic pain and procedural anxiety.

In France, the noted neurologist Jean Martin Charcot (1825–1893) reported cases of patients suffering from pseudo-neurological disorders that responded to the use of suggestion (1890). Later he found that these "hysterical symptoms" could be both induced and removed by hypnosis. Following the steps of his predecessor, Pierre Janet (1859–1947) built a theory of the unconscious involving compartmentalization of memory (1920). This differed from Freud's model in being horizontal rather than vertical and archeological. According to Janet's dissociative model, information kept out of awareness was relatively untransformed, but it could be accessed directly by use of

| Table 89–1 | History of Hypnosis |
|---|---|
| 1734–1815 | Friedrich (Franz) Anton Mesmer, the father of modern hypnosis; "magnetic fluid theory." |
| 1751–1825 | Marquis Armand De Puygseur described the forerunner steps of the "cathartic cure" or spontaneous talk in a somnambulistic state. |
| 1756–1819 | José Custodio Di Faria proposed the theory of expectancy and receptivity as the clue for hypnotic success; moved from "mesmeric passes" to verbal inductions. |
| 1785–1860 | James Braid initially called it neurohypnology or nervous sleep, later shortened to hypnosis; introduced the principle of monoideism as hypnotic induction. |
| 1791–1860 | John Elliotson, professor of surgery at the University College in London, is attributed with the introduction of hypnosis as anesthetic in England. |
| 1808–1859 | James Esdaile performed surgery using hypnosis as the only form of anesthesia. |
| 1823–1904 | Auguste-Ambroise Liebault stressed the role of "suggestibility" in hypnosis; combined Braid's eye fixation procedure with Di Faria's verbal suggestions. |
| 1825–1893 | Jean Marie Charcot discovered that many hysterical symptoms could be both induced and removed by hypnosis; erroneously identified hypnosis as a disease of the central nervous system and stated that only sick (hysterical) people could be hypnotized. |
| 1829–1838 | Hypnosis as anesthesia in the Western Hemisphere.<br>    1829, France: Jules Cloquet—mastectomy<br>    1836, Boston: Hypnosis used as anesthetic for dental surgery<br>    1838, England: John Elliotson—orthopedic surgery |
| 1837–1919 | Hippolyte Bernheim hypothesized that the causes of hypnotic induction were psychological and not organic; described suggestion as the main factor underlying hypnosis. |
| 1842–1925 | Josef Breuer suggested that hysteria was the result of repressed memories and emotions. Along with his colleague, Freud, he discovered that these symptoms could be removed by asking the patient to talk about these memories and emotions. This made Breuer move from attempting to remove the symptoms by direct hypnotic removal to uncovering of the original traumatic memories under hypnotic trance, by either age regression or hypnotic reenactment. This became the precursor to the cathartic method. |
| 1854–1919 | Morton Prince used hypnosis on the treatment of multiple personality disorders and conversion disorder; founded the *Journal of Abnormal Psychology.* |
| 1856–1939 | Sigmund Freud became interested in hypnosis after watching Breuer at work. In 1885, he went to study with Charcot (Paris) and later with Bernheim and Liebault (Nancy). He believed, at first, that hypnosis gave access to the unconscious and therefore could be used in the treatment of neurotic symptoms. It was not until 1889 that Freud used the cathartic method with his patients. He described the treatment of his patients with this method and detailed their progress in "Studies in hysteria" (1895). As he developed his psychoanalytic theories, he used hypnosis less frequently. Soon after the publication of the hypnosis-based "Studies in hysteria," he abandoned its use as a treatment modality in favor of his psychoanalytic method. |
| 1859–1947 | Pierre Janet proposed that "while under hypnosis the conscious mind is gradually suppressed, which allows the unconscious mind to take over." |
| 1947 | Kardiner and Spiegel described the usefulness of hypnosis in the treatment of traumatic neurosis or shell shock syndrome during World War II. |
| 1949 | The Society for Clinical and Experimental Hypnosis was founded. |
| 1957 | Milton Erickson founded the American Society of Clinical Hypnosis. |
| 1959 | Weitzenhoffer and Hilgard published the Stanford Hypnotic Susceptibility Scale for research purposes. |
| 1960 | Hypnosis is officially recognized as a legitimate therapeutic tool in both medicine and psychiatry by the American Medical Association and the American Psychiatric Association. |
| 1975 | Hilgard and Hilgard published the first hypnotizability scale designed for clinical settings, the Stanford Hypnotic Clinical Scale. |
| 1978 | Spiegel and Spiegel introduced the Hypnotic Induction Profile specifically designed to assess hypnotic capacity and clinical applications. |

techniques such as hypnosis. Janet used the ability of highly hypnotizable individuals as evidence of experimentally induced psychiatric illness. Hippolyte Bernheim and Herter (1964) took a contrary (and ultimately correct) view that hypnotic phenomena were essentially normal rather than evidence of disease, a viewpoint developed further by Freud's early collaborator Joseph Breuer. Breuer suggested that hysteria was the result of an uncontrolled hypnotic-like state driven by repressed memories and emotions. Later, Breuer and Freud (1955) discovered that these symptoms could be alleviated by asking the patient to talk about these memories and emotions. Thus they began the use of hypnotic age regression or hypnotic reenactment (the "ca-

thartic method") to treat hysterical symptoms. This led to the development of their theory linking unconscious determinants to conscious symptoms. They believed that "hypnoid-like" states constituted the building blocks of hysterical symptoms. This became one of the first recognitions that hypnotic processes are indeed normal and yet could often be mobilized in the service of resolving an unconscious conflict. Later, as he developed his psychoanalytic theories, Freud (1958) abandoned hypnosis in favor of free association, viewing it as a manipulation of transference phenomena.

During the early part of the 20th century hypnosis was rarely used in the clinical setting. Interest in its utility revived during World War II. At the time, army psychiatrists described its usefulness in treating so-called shell shock or traumatic neurosis (Kardiner and Spiegel 1947). In the 1950s, an era of serious laboratory investigation of the phenomenon began with the development of several hypnotizability scales, such as the Stanford Hypnotic Susceptibility Scales (Hilgard 1965, Weitzenhoffer 1962, Weitzenhoffer and Hilgard 1959). This was followed by the development of several shorter hypnotizability scales in the 1970s, which were designed for use in clinical settings (Stanford Hypnotic Clinical Scale [Hilgard and Hilgard 1975], Hypnotic Induction Profile [Spiegel and Spiegel 1978]).

In 1960, the American Medical Association and the American Psychiatric Association (APA) officially recognized hypnosis as a legitimate therapeutic tool. Two professional hypnosis societies emerged at the national level, each publishing a journal. The Society for Clinical and Experimental Hypnosis emphasizes research in the field of experimental hypnosis, and the American Society for Clinical Hypnosis focuses more on the clinical applications of hypnosis. Hypnosis is currently part of the curriculum in many medical schools and psychiatric residency programs. The American Psychological Association has devoted a division (Division 30) to its study. At present, the uses of hypnosis in clinical and investigational areas continue to grow, as does research on the neuropsychological mechanisms involved in the hypnotic process.

## Definition

Hypnosis is a psychophysiological state of attentive, receptive concentration, with a relative suspension of peripheral awareness. Hypnotic phenomena occur spontaneously, and the alteration of consciousness that hypnotized individuals experience has a variety of therapeutic applications. The hypnotic experience may be understood as involving three main factors (Table 89–2).

## Absorption

By absorption we refer to the tendency to engage in self-altering and highly focused attention with complete immersion in a central experience at the expense of contextual orientation (Hilgard 1970b, Tellegen 1981, Tellegen and Atkinson 1974). As one becomes deeply involved in a central focus of consciousness, one tends to ignore more peripheral perceptions, thoughts, memories, or motor activities. Hypnotized individuals can become so intensely absorbed in their trance experience that they often choose to ignore the environmental context and other peripheral events. This intense exclusion of information that is considered by the subject to be peripheral to the trance state allows the phenomenon known as *trance logic*.

Trance logic implies a thinking pattern that does not obey the rules of "normal" logical processes. For example, it may be suggested that the individual sustain a conversation with a person who is not present in the room. A highly hypnotizable subject may hallucinate the experience without "thinking twice" about the absurdity of talking to an empty chair. An extreme form of pathological absorption is seen in cases of traumatic flashbacks. In these instances, patients become so absorbed in the experience triggered by an environmental cue that they act as though they were reliving the whole experience, despite the impossibility of it.

There is abundant scientific evidence that demonstrates a correlation between hypnotizability and a spontaneous tendency for people to undergo absorbing or self-altering experiences (Tellegen and Atkinson 1974). If this is true, we can assume that individuals who tend to get deeply caught up in external or internal experiences, such as watching a movie or imagining something, are highly hypnotizable. This is because individuals with hypnotic ability may use it spontaneously, not simply when formally instructed to do so. This tendency of highly hypnotizable individuals to enter spontaneous hypnotic states may be a liability to them and has important interpersonal and clinical implications.

## Dissociation

By dissociation we imply the ability to separate mental processes so they seem to occur independently from each other. The process of dissociation is complementary to absorption. Thus, there is nonpathological and pathological dissociation. During hypnosis, the intense absorption characteristic of the hypnotic state permits keeping out of conscious awareness many routine experiences that would ordinarily be conscious by the process of nonpathological dissociation. When working properly in our daily lives it allows us to carry out several complex tasks simultaneously (e.g., knitting while conversing or watching television).

On the other hand, pathological dissociation may arise as a result of severe trauma or abuse (Maldonado and Spiegel 1994). Even complex emotional states, motor functions, or sensory experiences may be dissociated. Dissociated perception of the internal or external world results in depersonalization or derealization. Restricted access to memory results in cases of dissociative amnesia or dissociative fugue. Motor dysfunction elicited by dissociated phenomena may include cases of conversion disorder, such as conversion paralysis or psychogenic paresthesias. As described by Charcot (1890), most of these phenomena can be both induced and reversed with the structured use of hypnosis.

| Table 89–2 | Components of the Hypnotic Process |
|---|---|
| Component | Explanation |
| Absorption | Refers to the tendency to engage in self-altering and highly focused attention with complete immersion in a central experience at the expense of contextual orientation and more peripheral perceptions, thoughts, memories, or motor activities. |
| Dissociation | Permits keeping out of conscious awareness many routine experiences that ordinarily would be conscious. Dissociated material may be temporarily and reversibly unavailable to consciousness, but it continues to influence conscious and unconscious experiences and behavior. |
| Suggestibility | Involves heightened responsiveness to social cues. It allows subjects to suspend the usual conscious curiosity that makes us question the reason for our actions, making subjects more prone to accept suggestions given no matter how irrational. |

Dissociated memories may be temporarily and reversibly unavailable to consciousness, but they continue to influence conscious (or other unconscious) experiences and behavior (Hilgard 1977, Kilhstrom 1984). Out of sight does not mean out of mind. Many of the symptoms experienced by patients suffering from posttraumatic stress disorder (PTSD – DSM-IV-TR) can be explained by the influence exerted by memories unavailable to consciousness. This is the case when a sensory stimulus trigger a flashback in a trauma survivor. The process of absorption complements that of dissociation; the state of intense focal attention (absorption) facilitates putting information outside of conscious awareness (dissociation).

## Suggestibility

Suggestibility implies the ability to influence someone's beliefs or behaviors by suggestion. Owing to the intense absorption experienced during trance, hypnotized individuals have a heightened responsiveness to social cues, including suggestions given by the therapist. This enhanced suggestibility allows hypnotized subjects to accept instructions relatively easily. Hypnotized individuals are not deprived of their will, but they do have a tendency to accept instructions in an uncritical way when under trance. This quality of the hypnotic process allows subjects to suspend the usual conscious curiosity that makes us question the reason for our actions. Because of this, hypnotized individuals are more likely to accept suggestions or directions, no matter how irrational they might be. Subjects under hypnosis are less likely to distinguish an instruction coming from an outside source (i.e., from the therapist) from those coming themselves (a phenomenon known as hypnotic source amnesia). This allows highly suggestible individuals to act on another person's ideas as though they were their own. This aspect of hypnosis may be used by conscientious therapists to bypass the patient's defenses and mobilize the patient's strengths. On the other hand, a hypnotized patient is less likely to correct a therapist's mistakes and may be confused by hypnotic instructions that are vague or misguided.

## Hypnosis: What It Is and What It Is Not

Several principles provide guidance for the use of hypnosis in medicine and psychiatry. We attempt to clarify some of the myths and misconceptions about hypnosis by establishing what hypnosis is and what it is not (Table 89–3).

**Hypnotizability is a stable and measurable trait.** Not everyone is hypnotizable. Hypnotizability, or hypnotic capacity varies throughout the population. Just as some people have more or less ability to play a musical instrument or no ability at all, there is considerable variation in individuals' ability to undergo and use hypnosis, and these differences are stable over time (Hilgard 1965, Hilgard and Hilgard 1975, Spiegel and Spiegel 1978). Hypnotizability is as consistent as intelligence for a 30-year interval in adulthood (Piccione et al. 1989). Hypnotizability is highest in late childhood and declines gradually throughout adulthood. Recognizing this fact is helpful in demystifying hypnosis and reducing anxiety on the part of both the physician inducing hypnosis and the patient. About 75% of the population has some usable hypnotic capacity; of these, about

| Table 89–3 | What Is Hypnosis? |
| --- | --- |

**What It Is**

Hypnosis is a form of focused concentration.
Hypnotizability is a stable and measurable trait.
Hypnosis is something you do with, rather than to, a subject or patient.
All hypnosis is self-hypnosis.

**What It Is Not**

Hypnosis is not sleep.
There are no apparent sex differences in hypnotizability.
Hypnotizability is not a sign of weak-mindedness.
Hypnosis is not intrinsically dangerous.
Hypnosis is not therapy.
There is nothing you can do with hypnosis that you cannot do without it.

10% are highly hypnotizable. This means that about one of four adults has no usable hypnotic capacity (Spiegel and Spiegel 1978). It is advantageous to determine this early and encourage those with the ability to use it; other treatment modalities are offered to those who are not hypnotizable.

**Hypnosis is something you do *with*, not something you do *to*, a subject or patient.** A therapist inducing hypnosis is in the position of the Socratic teacher, helping students discover what they already know. A useful metaphor to share with subjects is that of a coach. A correctly performed hypnotic induction allows the patient and physician to assess and explore the patient's hypnotic capacity or lack of it, just as a trainer assesses the athlete's natural capacities and then attempts to maximize them. This approach tends to minimize power struggles between the physician and the patient. For example, there is less chance of misinterpreting a patient's inability to experience a hypnotic trance as resistance.

**All hypnosis is self-hypnosis.** The therapist helps the patient use his or her own hypnotic capacity to undergo a trance state. Helping patients to understand the degree of control they have over their mental processes is a good way to foster mastery and control. By doing this, patients may be able to comprehend the extent to which the unconscious use of their hypnotic abilities may create or contribute to their psychiatric symptoms, as in the case of dissociative disorders (Bliss 1980, 1984, Spiegel 1974, Spiegel and Fink 1979). Similarly, hypnosis may help patients understand how certain physical symptoms may have unconscious etiological factors, as in the case of conversion phenomena (i.e., psychogenic blindness, pseudoseizures) or psychosomatic conditions (i.e., asthma, headache) (Maldonado and Spiegel 2000).

**There are no apparent sex differences in hypnotizability.** Men and women are equally hypnotizable (Hilgard 1965, Stern et al. 1979).

**Hypnosis is not sleep.** The most prevalent misunderstanding derives from the name itself. Unfortunately, in the late 1800s, James Braid coined the word neurohypnology to describe what he considered to be a special kind of sleep. Later, this was shortened to its current name, derived from the Greek root *hypnos*, which means "sleep." The hypnotized individual is not asleep but rather awake and alert. To an outside observer, hypnotized individuals may appear asleep owing to their apparent lack of responsiveness to the environment. This is due to their intense absorption and concentration on their internal experience, rather than due to their lack of will.

**Hypnotizability is not a sign of weak-mindedness.** Charcot described the ability to undergo a hypnotic trance as a sign of a defective central nervous system. Today, we know that on the contrary, a hypnotic trance requires an intact capacity for focused concentration. If anything, high hypnotizability is associated with the absence of serious psychotic and neurological disorders (Lavoie and Sabourin 1980, Pettinati 1982, Spiegel et al. 1982).

**Hypnosis is not intrinsically dangerous.** For the most part, it is a benign process. The same cognitive flexibility that allows patients to enter the trance facilitates their exit from it with clear structure and support from the therapist. The dangers of hypnosis lay not in the process itself but in how it is used. There are few contraindications for the use of hypnosis. An occasional paranoid schizophrenic patient may incorporate an attempt at inducing hypnosis into a delusional system. A severely depressed individual may interpret a failure to benefit from hypnosis as further evidence of little self-worth. These problems can be avoided in part by use of hypnotizability testing at the beginning of the intervention. The most serious problem involves possible effects of hypnosis on memory. This is discussed at length under the section "Forensic Applications of Hypnosis," later in the chapter.

**Hypnosis is not therapy.** Entry into a hypnotic state does not have any therapeutic effects of its own, although many find it pleasant and relaxing. Therapeutic change comes not from the state itself but from what happens during it. In this regard, hypnosis is not a treatment itself but rather a facilitator of a variety of treatment strategies. The state of intense concentration elicited in hypnosis can facilitate attention to a variety of strategies that enhance control over somatic function, reduce pain, allow the recovery and restructuring of memories, elicit the reproduction and control of conversion symptoms or fugue episodes, and provide control of dissociated states.

**There is nothing you can do with hypnosis that you cannot do without it.** As an adjunct to therapy, hypnosis may help speed the process by which information can be accessed and processed because of its ability to heighten concentration and focus attention; however, it is not a treatment in and of itself.

## Hypnotizability Scales

Most of the hypnotizability scales developed in the early part of the 20th century were designed for use in research settings, most notably the Stanford Hypnotic Susceptibility Scale of Weitzenhoffer and Hilgard (Hilgard 1965, Weitzenhoffer and Hilgard 1959, 1962). Research scales are very accurate, but lengthy, making their frequent use impractical in the clinical setting. More recently, hypnotizability scales have been developed for clinical use (Hypnotic Induction Profile [Spiegel and Spiegel 1978], Stanford Hypnotic Clinical Scale [Hilgard and Hilgard 1975]). These scales are briefer (about 5–10 minutes for the Hypnotic Induction Profile and 20 minutes for the Stanford Hypnotic Clinical Scale, compared with 1 hour for the research scales) and are designed for comfortable use even with patients who have severe psychiatric disturbances (Spiegel and Spiegel 1978, Spiegel et al. 1982, 1988). They are well accepted by patients and help to bypass anxiety by shifting the focus of the interaction from one in which the therapist tries to make the patient have a hypnotic experience to one in which the therapist assesses the patient's response to a set of instructions, like any other medical or psychological test (Spiegel and Spiegel 1978). The therapist focuses on evaluating the patient's ability to enter the state rather than on getting the person into the state. They all involve a structured hypnotic induction and an assessment of the subject's response to a variety of instructions, such as alterations in the sense of control over body movements, physical sensations, orientation to time and space, and perception. Furthermore, such a standardized testing induction permits an important deduction regarding the hypnotic capacity of the subject. The restricted range of input from the therapist maximizes the information provided by variations in subjects' responses. After the results of the testing are discussed with the subject, both can proceed knowledgeably, choosing to use hypnosis or other techniques in the service of an agreed on treatment goal.

The use of this kind of objective measurement has several clinical advantages and therapeutic implications (Table 89–4):

It takes the pressure off both the therapist and the patient. Hypnotizability testing helps to clarify the hypnotic interaction. The therapist objectively assesses the patient's natural ability to use her or his hypnotic capacity, if any, rather than pushing the patient to respond in a certain manner. By objectively determining the patient's ability, there is no pressure on the therapist to see whether he or she can hypnotize the patient. Likewise, it reduces the sense of pressure on the patient to either comply or resist. The test setting creates an atmosphere of scientific exploration that encourages rather than coerces involvement.

**Table 89–4    Benefits of the Use of Hypnotizability Measures**

It objectively assesses the patient's natural ability to use his or her hypnotic capacity.

It relieves performance pressure on both therapist and patient.

It provides objective data about the patient's ability to respond to treatment employing hypnosis.

It provides the therapist with scientific data to make rational treatment choices.

It provides helpful information about the subject's interpersonal style and possible psychiatric illness.

It helps predict the patient's likely response to psychotherapeutic treatment.

Hypnotizability testing provides objective data about the patient's ability to respond to treatment via hypnosis. If the patient is a highly hypnotizable individual, she or he can be rationally encouraged to proceed with the use of hypnosis. Nonhypnotizable individuals can be offered an alternative approach that is likely to be more efficacious, such as relaxation techniques, biofeedback, or medication.

Objective standardized tests of hypnotic capacity used across a large population provide the therapist with scientific data to make rational inferences about the patient's expected response. Patients' relative ability, or inability, to restructure their inner experience by hypnosis will provide helpful information to the therapist about the subject's interpersonal style and/or level of psychiatric disturbance.

The intense concentration and increased receptivity characteristic of the trance phenomenon will make us predict that the capacity to experience hypnosis correlates with responsiveness to psychological treatment. Indeed, research has found a high correlation between high hypnotizability scores and a number of selected clinical problems, such as pain (Hilgard and Hilgard 1975), cigarette smoking (Spiegel and Spiegel 1978, Spiegel et al. unpublished data), and asthma (Collison 1975). High hypnotizability scores have also been correlated with the increased likelihood of responding to treatments that do not explicitly employ hypnosis, such as acupuncture (Katz et al. 1974, Lu and Lu 1999).

## Hypnosis Induction Profile

The Hypnotic Induction Profile (Figure 89–1) is a useful clinical screening test for hypnotic capacity. It consists of a number of the simple instructions that allow the measurement of patients' natural ability to tap into and use their hypnotic capacity. It begins with a simple and quick induction, counting from 1 to 3, accompanied by the eye roll. This involves instructed upward gaze and lowering of the eyelids (Figure 89–2). The dissociation between upward gaze and lowering of the eyelid can be scored (Figure 89–3), providing the therapist with an initial prediction of the subject's hypnotic capacity. The eye roll is then followed by a series of instructions to briefly influence the subject's behavior during and shortly after the test (posthypnotic suggestions). The Hypnotic Induction Profile allows the therapist to rate the subject on five items (Table 89–5) assessing cognitive and behavioral aspects of the single continuous but brief hypnotic experience elicited during the test. These are: (1) ability to experience a sense of dissociation of the left hand from the rest of the body; (2) hand levitation, or floating of the hand back up in the air after being pulled down; (3) sense of involuntariness or unconscious compliance while elevating the hand; (4) response to the cutoff signal ending the hypnotic experience; and (5) sensory alteration in the hand or elsewhere in the body.

Scores on the Hypnotic Induction Profile are significantly but moderately correlated with those on the Stanford scales (Orne et al. 1979) and provide useful discrimination among different psychiatric disorders, as described in the following section.

| Table 89–5 | Items Tested by the Hypnotic Induction Profile |
|---|---|
| | Body dissociation |
| | Hand levitation |
| | Level of unconscious compliance |
| | Response to posthypnotic suggestion |
| | Sensory alteration |

## Hypnotizability in Psychiatric Disorders

Charcot described a relationship between conversion phenomena and hypnotizability. He later incorrectly attributed both phenomena to a pathological process afflicting the central nervous system. Charcot believed that only sick or hysterical people could be hypnotized. Others, including Bernheim, Janet, and Breuer, refuted the idea. They attributed the symptoms of conversion to unconscious mechanisms and viewing hypnosis as a tool useful in both the elicitation and removal of such states. Research in hypnosis has lately been directed at understanding the relationship between hypnotizability and psychiatric illness.

It is true that some psychiatric disorders are associated with high hypnotizability scores (Table 89–6). Such is the case in patients with PTSD (DSM-IV-TR) (Kluft 1993, Putnam 1992, Spiegel 1992, Spiegel et al. 1988, Stuntman and Bliss 1985). Several studies have shown significantly higher hypnotizability among individuals with PTSD than among similar individuals without PTSD (Stuntman and Bliss 1985) or in comparison to psychiatric patients with other disorders (Spiegel et al. 1988). Those with dissociative disorders (DSM-IV-TR) such as fugue, amnesia, or dissociative identity disorder (DTD) (multiple personality disorder) also tend to be highly hypnotizable (Allen and Smith 1993, Bliss 1986, Braun and Sachs 1985, Carlson and Putnam 1989, Coons and Milstein 1986, Frischholz 1985, Maldonado and Spiegel 2002a, Frischholz et al. 1992, Kluft 1985a, 1993, Spiegel 1984, Spiegel et al. 1989b). Most patients with DID report histories of severe physical and sexual abuse in childhood (Braun and Sachs 1985, Kluft

| Table 89–6 | Psychiatric Disorders Associated with High Hypnotizability |
|---|---|
| | Victims of overwhelming trauma |
| |    Adjustment disorders |
| |    Acute stress disorder |
| |    PTSD |
| | Dissociative disorders |
| |    Fugue states |
| |    Dissociative amnesia |
| |    Dissociative identity disorder |
| | Anxiety disorders |
| |    Phobias |
| |    Performance anxiety |
| | Bulimia nervosa |
| | Borderline personality disorder |
| | Conversion disorder |

Hypnotic Induction Profile score sheet

Name _____    Date _____

Sequence ☐ Initial _____ Previous _____    When _____

Item    Position of subject ☐ Standing _____ Supine _____ Chair _____ Chair-stool _____

A    *Up-gaze*                                                    *0 – 1 – 2 – 3 – 4*

B                                        Roll:    0 – 1 – 2 – 3 – 4

C                                        Squint:    0 – 1 – 2 – 3 – 4

D    Eye-roll sign (roll and squint)              0 – 1 – 2 – 3 – 4

E    *Arm (R-L) levitation instruction*              *0 – 1 – 2 – 3 – 4*

F    *Tingle*                        0 –                – 1 – 2

G_____    Dissociation                0 –                – 1 – 2

H_____    Levitation          ⎧ No reinforcement ⎫                    3 – 4
           (postinduction)     ⎪ 1st      "       ⎪                    2 – 3
                               ⎨ 2nd      "       ⎬              1 – 2    Smile _____
                               ⎪ 3rd      "       ⎪              1 –
                               ⎩ 4th      "       ⎭        0 –    Surprise _____

I _____    Control differential          0 –                – 1 – 2

J _____    Cut-off                0 –                – 1 – 2

K_____    *Amnesia to cut-off*          0 –                – 1 – 2
           *or no-test* _____

L_____    Floating sensation          0 –                – 1 – 2

Summary scores

_____ Induction score    Profile score    0 – 1 – 2 – 3 – 4 – 5

_____ Soft            _____ Zero            _____ Intact

_____ Minutes    _____ Decrement    _____ Special zero    _____ Special intact

**Figure 89–1** *Hypnotic Induction Profile score sheet. (Source: Spiegel H and Spiegel D [1978] Trance and Treatment: Clinical Uses of Hypnosis. Basic Books, New York, p. 40. Reprinted 1987 American Psychiatric Press, Washington DC.)*

1985b, Maldonado and Spiegel 1995, 2002a, Spiegel 1984). It is thought that these patients enhanced their natural ability to dissociate by separating themselves from painful physical experiences over time. Later, the same defenses are unconsciously mobilized during periods of extreme anxiety or stress. The same temporary dissociation that allowed the victim to tolerate overwhelming fear and pain earlier in life becomes an ongoing part of the personality structure. This tendency to compartmentalize memories and experiences by the processes of repression and dissociation allows the victim of PTSD to split into multiple dissociated selves. Some of them suffered the pain and humiliation, others took on themselves the function of protecting the patient from the experience of further injury.

The literature on posttraumatic and dissociative disorders reveals a close relationship between trauma, dissociation, and hypnotizability. The data on DID (DSM-IV-TR) highlights that most patients with DID are highly hypnotizable (Frischholz 1985, Maldonado and Spiegel 2002a) (see also Chapter 73 in this textbook). It also stresses the fact that many of these patients have a history of severe neglect, physical and/or sexual abuse during childhood (Kluft 1985a, Maldonado and Spiegel 2002a, 2002b, Maldonado et al. 2000, Spiegel 1984, Stuntman and Bliss 1985). Together

Eye-roll sign for hypnotizability

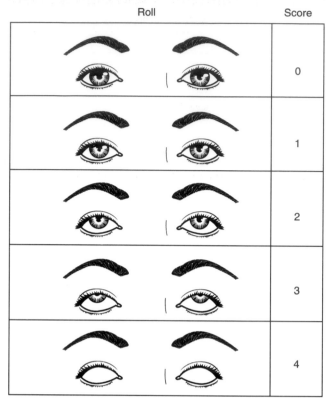

**Figure 89–2** *Eye-roll sign for hypnotizability. (Source: Spiegel H and Spiegel D [1978] Trance and Treatment: Clinical Uses of Hypnosis. Basic Books, New York, p. 52. Reprinted 1987 American Psychiatric Press, Washington DC.)*

these observations have led to the recognition that the capacity to dissociate—that is, to separate psychological material from the physical experience—is mobilized during and after extreme trauma, such as rape or assault (Bremner and Brett 1997, Bryant et al. 2001, Butler et al. 1996, Eriksson and Lundin 1996, Kluft 1984, Koopman et al. 1995, Putnam 1985, Spiegel 1984, 1986, 1988, 1990, Spiegel et al. 1988, Stuntman and Bliss 1985, van der Kolk and van der Hart 1989, Wood and Sexton 1997).

Years ago, a syndrome resembling histrionic personality disorder was described (DSM-IV-TR) but in this particular group, the capacity for hypnotic dissociation was deemed to be central. It was labeled the "Grade 5" syndrome (Spiegel 1974). These patients are described to be highly hypnotiz-

Eye-roll measurement

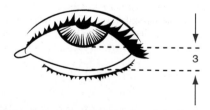

**Figure 89–3** *Eye-roll measurement. (Source: Spiegel H and Spiegel D [1978] Trance and Treatment: Clinical Uses of Hypnosis. Basic Books, New York, p. 53. Reprinted 1987 American Psychiatric Press, Washington DC.)*

able, to repeatedly establish naive and dependent relationships, and to express their distress in dramatic ways. They are slow in becoming aware of their internal cues, requiring much external reassurance. They tend to develop superficial but intense affiliations with new ideas and people that tend not to last over time. Because of their tendency to become overly dependent, they require a therapeutic environment that is highly structured. The goal of therapy with these patients is to help them recognize their tendency to repeatedly seek relationships in which they make themselves vulnerable owing to their tendency to relinquish control.

As in the case of dissociative disorders, several studies described an increased hypnotic capacity in patients suffering from anxiety disorders, especially phobias (Bodden 1991, Frankel and Orne 1976, Gerschman et al. 1987, Menzies and Clarke 1993, Rodolfa et al. 1990, Smith 1990). Some explain this increased hypnotizability as being secondary to a heightened dissociative response triggered by phobic symptoms. The symptoms of phobia or anxiety may represent a state of absorption in the fearful situation, with subsequent suspension of critical judgment. This is not true for all anxiety disorders. Other researchers failed to replicate this finding (Frischholz et al. 1982). At least one other study showed that patients suffering from generalized anxiety disorder (DSM-IV-TR) obtained markedly lower hypnotizability scores than normal subjects (Spiegel et al. 1982).

Impulse–control behaviors characteristic of eating disorders (Covino et al. 1994, Evans and Staats 1989, Kranhold et al. 1992) and personality disorders (Baker 1983, Copeland 1986, Murray-Jobsis 1991, Pettinati et al. 1990), especially borderline personality disorder, may represent a state of dissociation associated with higher hypnotizability scores. Indeed, Pettinati and colleagues (1990) administered both the Stanford Hypnotic Susceptibility Scale (Form C) and the Hypnotic Induction Profile to patients with eating disorders. They observed higher hypnotizability in bulimic patients compared with restrictors (e.g., anorexia nervosa). Many bulimic subjects reported being in a trance-like state when they engaged in compulsive binging and purging behavior. Likewise, many patients suffering from self-destructive behavior described dissociative or trance-like states surrounding periods of self-mutilation. This is not uncommon among individuals with DID. The literature suggests that some patients with this disorder also meet criteria for borderline personality disorder (DSM-IV-TR). These individuals also indulge in self-cutting and other kinds of body injury. This subgroup may have higher hypnotizability scores than individuals with other personality disorders.

Patients with psychosis, suffering from delusions, loosening of associations, and hallucinations, might be expected to do poorly in tests requiring attention and concentration. Hypnosis represents a state of heightened concentration and focused attention. If these two premises are true, we could predict that severely psychotic patients would not be hypnotizable. Indeed, Copeland and Kitching (1937) made the observation that some previously diagnosed psychotic patients who proved to be hypnotizable had been, in fact, misdiagnosed. Somewhat lower scores have been obtained on the Hypnotic Induction Profile (Pettinati 1982, Pettinati et al. 1990, Spiegel et al. 1982), and a restricted range of scores and the absence of high hypnotizability scores have been found in studies employing the Stanford Hypnotic Susceptibility Scale among schizophrenic subjects (Lavoie and Elie 1985, Lavoie and Sabourin 1980, Pettinati 1982, Pettinati et al. 1990, Weitzenhoffer and Hilgard 1959, 1962). Even though hallucinatory activity can be artificially produced in hypnotic states, psychotic patients, especially those with schizophrenia, have shown impairment in their ability to sustain a high level of attention, which interferes with hypnotic concentration. Patients suffering from a major affective disorder have been found to score between normal subjects and schizophrenic patients in hypnotizability (Spiegel et al. 1982). These findings were independent of psychoactive medication use (Spiegel 1980a).

Thus, several psychiatric syndromes (schizophrenia, generalized anxiety disorder, and to a lesser extent major affective disorder) (DSM-IV-TR) have been associated with generally lower hypnotic responsiveness. It may be that the primary illness process impairs the use of a patient's natural capacity for hypnotic concentration. Because of this, hypnotizability testing can sometimes be used to clarify diagnoses. As always, the presence or absence of hypnotic capacity should be interpreted within the context of the presentation, medical and psychiatric histories, and genetic background. In the case of an acute psychosis in which there is no familial background, the presentation is later in life than normal, there is a past history of physical or sexual abuse, and the patient has a high hypnotizability score, a diagnosis of hysterical psychosis or a dissociative disorder should be strongly considered when the possibility of schizophrenia is evaluated (Spiegel and Fink 1979, Steingard and Frankel 1985).

## Applications of Hypnosis

### General Considerations
Because of the intrinsic qualities of the hypnotic state, it can be an effective adjunct to the treatment of a variety of symptoms and problems, both in psychiatry and in medicine in general. The first criterion to consider is the patient's level of hypnotizability. Once it has been determined that the patient has usable hypnotic capacity (defined by high scores in hypnotizability scales), a discussion about the nature of the hypnotic process follows. It is important at this point to dispel any myths and correct misconceptions the patient may have about the process. This includes the cooperative nature of the hypnotic process, rather than the "tell me what to do" most patients expect. Finally, the therapist must decide whether the problem presented by the patient is amenable to hypnotic intervention or whether other steps should be taken instead.

We have divided the discussion of the applications of hypnosis into five areas: general psychiatry, general medicine, psychosomatic disorders, habit control, and forensic psychiatry (Table 89–7).

### Application in Psychiatric Disorders
The use of hypnosis in the context of conventional psychotherapy can facilitate the therapeutic process in a number of ways. For example, hypnotherapeutic techniques may be used to enhance the patient's sense of self, restructure traumatic and phobic experiences, or access to repressed memories that have not emerged with use of other techniques.

| Table 89–7 | Applications of Hypnosis |
|---|---|

**General Psychiatry**

Anxiety disorders
  Phobias
  PTSD
Dissociative disorders
  Dissociative amnesia
  Dissociative identity disorder
Sleep disorders
  Insomnia

**General Medicine**

Anxiety associated with medical and surgical procedures
Pain control
Psychosomatic disorders
  Bronchial asthma
  Warts and other skin conditions
  Gastrointestinal disturbances (irritable bowel syndrome, peptic ulcer disease)
  Cardiovascular diseases
Adjuvant to chemotherapy
Emesis (chemotherapy, hyperemesis gravidarum)

**Habit Control**

Smoking cessation
Weight control

**Forensic Psychiatry**

Memory enhancement

This is true not only of painfully repressed memories but also of situations in which both the patient and the therapist have worked on resistance issues and feel that some additional leverage is necessary. In conventional psychotherapy, the transference is observed and analyzed; in hypnosis, the transference is used as part of the therapeutic process.

Conventional psychoanalytic psychotherapy involves observation and analysis of the meaning of the transference reaction that arises during therapeutic interactions. On the other hand, when hypnosis is used, transference is not avoided or bypassed but may be amplified. All the usual therapeutic rules and processes of psychotherapy apply when hypnosis is used in the psychotherapy context, which may intensify or accelerate the therapeutic process (see Clinical Vignette 1).

**Clinical Vignette 1**

A young woman sought consultation with me (JRM) because of a phobia about crossing bridges that had begun 5 years earlier. The patient, a psychiatric nurse, was psychologically minded and despite having seen several therapists for her problem had not been able to resolve it using psychotherapy. The problem was now a major issue in her life because she had just bought a car and was angry that her problem impeded her "new freedom."

She reported that her phobia initially occurred when she was driving in her sister's car down a long bridge in one of the coastal eastern states. As she was midway across the bridge, she looked around, noticing that her sister, her sister's boyfriend, and a cousin were all asleep. She reported becoming slowly anxious. Then, all of a sudden, she became extremely frightened. She slammed on the car brakes and stopped the car in the middle of the bridge. Since then, she has not been able to drive across a bridge again. She proceeded to describe her multiple attempts to do so in the preceding few months.

She agreed to try hypnosis and proved to be an excellent candidate. Her Hypnotic Induction Profile score was 9 out of a possible maximum of 10. After induction of a hypnotic state, age regression was used to return her to the first known episode of panic. It was suggested that she would become both physically and mentally relaxed, then allow her unconscious mind to take her to the first time she ever felt this way. The patient spontaneously curled up in the chair; she began to sob and then scream, "Please, mommy, don't leave me."

After the abreaction was over, she spontaneously exited her hypnotic state, and we proceeded to examine and reframe the experience. She reported that under trance, she was able to remember how when she was 7 years of age her mother came home with a box full of plastic bags and began to pack the belongings of each of her children. The mother then put the children and the bags in her car and drove out of town, over the bridge, and into a neighboring state where many of her relatives lived. The patient ended up staying with her grandmother while her siblings lived with two different aunts. She had completely forgotten these facts even though she had always been fully aware that she had been raised by her grandmother.

Still, the question of timing remained. Why did it begin 5 years ago and not before? She closed her eyes and easily entered a hypnotic state. This time she was able to review the events surrounding the initial episode of phobia. She remembered how before initiating her trip down the East Coast, she had arrived home one day and found a message from her long disappeared mother. In it, her mother said that she was going to visit the East Coast and that she intended to visit her and her sisters. The patient contacted her sisters, but their conversation was limited. "Did she also call you?" "Yes," replied her sister; that was all. She had completely avoided talking or thinking about what was going to happen shortly after her trip. As she was driving over the bridge, noticing that everyone was asleep, her mind began to wander. Fear about what was to happen came to mind. She wished that there was a way by which she could avoid the encounter. Suddenly, she froze. The car stopped and she was unable to continue. She just could not cross the bridge. Once again, she spontaneously exited the trance state and began to provide her own appropriate explanation about what might have happened. She saw this long bridge as a kind of umbilical cord that would reunite her with her mother. Then conflict arose accompanied by feelings of ambivalence, then fear. The only way to avoid the situation was not getting there, and because she was in control of the car, her only way out was to panic, to freeze, and to stop.

After a debriefing session and reframing of her past and how to reinterpret the original trauma as well as the phobia, she expressed feeling confident about her skills as a survivor. She was able to move from being in the position of the indefensible victim (the 7-year-old child) or the handicapped adult and talked about the new challenge that lay ahead. She politely agreed to a plan to test her ability to drive across a bridge. For the third and final time in this session, she entered (now on her own) a hypnotic state and saw herself being able to drive through the bridge. She agreed to return in 2 weeks, after stating that she planned to test herself the following weekend.

Two weeks after the initial contact, the patient returned. She proceeded to recount the events of the three trips she had made by the second session, each of increasing difficulty. To this day, 11 years later, the patient has not had any further episodes of phobia associated with bridges and has an amicable but distant relationship with her mother.

Because of the intense emotions that are characteristic of the hypnotic retrieval (which facilitates expression of inner fantasies), intense feelings and deep personal experiences may be elicited. Some patients may find that the hypnotic state facilitates a sense of infantile dependency in which the therapist becomes the transferential object. The quality of this transference reaction will be based on the patient's early object relations, just as in any other therapeutic relationship. Indeed, the transference reaction may develop so fast that the inexperienced therapist may not have the opportunity to recognize it or may do so too late. The difference here is the intensity of the feelings developed as a result of the strong emotions that arise during trance. As in the case of victims of abuse, the therapist may use the transference relationship under hypnosis to foster the patient's ability to help herself or himself.

An example of this is the use of self-mothering techniques in which, for example, patients are able to go beyond the anger toward a parent or perpetrator and become able to provide for themselves the nurturing and protection that they needed but never had. The therapist may also use the influence he or she has over the patient to suggest alternative ways to deal with problems. Sometimes a patient recovers a memory under hypnosis but then forgets it once the trance state has ended. The therapist who is aware of this may lead the patient to the goal, always respecting the principle that the patient will remember when she or he is ready to remember.

Finally, we do not use the term hypnotherapist, because there are no hypnotherapists. Instead, there are therapists who use hypnosis within the context of the therapeutic practice to achieve a specific therapeutic result. The difficult aspect of doing hypnosis is not the induction of the hypnosis trance, but what happens once the patient is under trance. Remember that all hypnosis is self-hypnosis. Thus, there are two factors which will predict the success of the hypnosis intervention: the patients' hypnotizability and the therapeutic skills of the therapist.

## Anxiety Disorders

Anxiety disorders are among the most widely prevalent psychiatric disturbances. They afflict as much as 15% of the population (Myers et al. 1984). Anxiety can be seen as a state of hyperarousal experienced by both emotional and somatic discomfort. Patients describe their experience in physical terms, such as palpitations, gastrointestinal discomfort, chest pain, sweating, and motor restlessness. Among anxiety disorders most responsive to hypnotic intervention are generalized anxiety disorder, panic disorder, phobias, and posttraumatic anxiety disorders (these will be discussed in the section that follows).

Generalized anxiety disorder (GAD) can be seen as a chronic state of anxiety that usually inhibits psychological comfort and social functioning. GAD involves excessive anxiety, occurring more days than not and lasting over a 6 month period. The anxiety is more like a "free floating" worry or fear about a number of events or activities, and is commonly associated with multiple symptoms, including restlessness, muscle tension, fatigue, insomnia, difficulty in concentrating, and irritability. In contrast, panic attacks are sudden and intense states associated with extreme anxiety, physical and emotional distress, and usually occurs in a very discrete period of time. The disorder is usually associated with irrational avoidance behavior and anticipatory anxiety. In between are discrete episodes of fear associated with specific stimuli or phobias. Phobic reactions involve marked, excessive fear cued by the presence or anticipation of an object or specific situation. Invariably, the exposure to the stimulus provokes an immediate and extreme anxiety response. Hypnosis can be helpful as an adjunctive tool for treating anxiety disorders because of its ability to help patients control their somatic response to anxiety-provoking stimuli. This enables patients to attend to the stimuli long enough to alter their point of view about them and achieve a sense of mastery over them.

Most of the strategies in the treatment of anxiety disorders employing hypnosis combine instructed physical relaxation with a restructuring of cognition, using imagery coupled with physical relaxation. As in the treatment of anxiety disorders by systematic desensitization (Marks et al. 1968) or progressive relaxation, patients are instructed to maintain a physical sense of relaxation (e.g., floating) while picturing the feared situation or stimulus. It is important that the relaxation instruction use an image that connotes reduced somatic tension, such as floating or lightness, rather than being a direct instruction to relax. The more cognitive term "relax" may actually induce more anxiety, whereas affiliation with a somatic metaphor usually produces some reduction in tension. Unlike systematic desensitization, hypnosis produces a physically relaxed state that can be rapidly achieved with a quick induction. Also different from systematic desensitization, the coupling of relaxation to a fearful stimulus does not require the development or working through of a hierarchy.

A typical self-hypnosis induction can be rapid. For example, a patient can be told:

> Now just get as comfortable as you can. There are many ways to enter a state of self-hypnosis. One simple but useful method is to count to yourself from 1 to 3. On 1, do one thing: look up. On 2, do two things: slowly close your eyes and take a deep breath. On 3, do three things: let your eyes relax but keep them closed, let your breath out, and let your body float. Then let one hand or the other float up into the air like a buoyant balloon. This is your signal to yourself and to me that you are ready to concentrate.

Initially, the use of hypnosis in the session can help in demonstrating to patients that they have a greater degree of control over somatic responsiveness than they had imagined. It is often useful to begin by teaching patients to create a place in their mind's eye where they feel safe and secure. On occasion, it helps the subjects to learn how to project their image onto an imaginary screen. Later, they can learn to manipulate the screen by making it either bigger or smaller, having the screen nearer or farther away, as needed:

> Just allow your body to float, as if you were floating in a bath, a lake, or a hot tub. Enjoy this sense of floating lightness. Now, picture in your mind's eye an imaginary screen. It might be a movie screen, a television screen, or a piece of clear blue sky. First picture a pleasant scene, somewhere you enjoy being.

Allow the patient to experience this state for a minute or two, then inquire about the experience:

> With your eyes closed and remaining in this state of concentration, describe how your body is feeling right now. What image are you picturing?

After receiving the answers, add:

> Notice how you can use your store of memories and fantasies to help yourself and your body feel better.

After they have learned to manipulate the screen and their physical sensations, patients may be ready to do therapy work. They may, for example, learn to re-create the physical state of relaxation while projecting the fearful situation onto the screen. This, then, becomes a useful procedure by which to control and obtain mastery over anxiety-producing situations by dissociating the somatic reaction from the psychological response to the feared stimulus. Initially, the patient is asked to re-create the physical feeling of relaxation. Then, the patient projects onto the screen images associated with the feared situation, only this time the somatic reactions associated with anxiety do not develop. On occasion, it helps for patients to foresee likely physical sensations or situations associated with a fearful experience to master them. For example, in the case of plane phobia, the patient can learn to couple the real sensation of floating in the air with the hypnotic experience: "Learn to float with the plane."

Patients may also use the trance state as a means of facing their concerns more directly. As in the preceding cases, they may make use of the screen technique. They can achieve this by placing an image of an upcoming performance or fearful situation on one side of the screen, testing out various strategies for mastering the situation on the other side.

Other approaches using hypnosis have included instructing patients in a trance to imagine that they are literally somewhere else, away from the fearful stimulus, thus separating themselves from the anxiety-producing experience (Erickson and Haley 1967). Positive reinforcement or "ego-strengthening" techniques have also been used; for example, hypnotic instructions are given to patients suggesting that their capacity to master the situation and their response to it will improve (Crasilneck and Hall 1985). There is little reason to use uncovering techniques seeking to link anxiety to some early traumatic experience in cases of phobia or generalized anxiety disorders. This is different in cases of PTSD (DSM-IV-TR), however, in which more work may be needed to confront and place into context the traumatic experience.

Certainly, in some cases, understanding the cause of the feared situation may help resolve the conflict. One of the techniques used to facilitate the recovery of traumatic memories associated with fearful situations is the affect bridge technique (Watkins 1987).

## Posttraumatic Stress Disorder

The use of hypnosis for treatment of traumatic experiences was initially described by Breuer and Freud (1955). At the time, they observed that an abreaction is accompanied by a release of psychic tension and, on occasion, relief of physical symptoms. That was the premise behind the use of the cathartic method. The idea was that some intense affect associated with the traumatic event needed to be released, and that simply repeating the event with its associated emotion in the trance state would suffice to resolve the symptoms. That was particularly true in cases of hysterical conversion.

It did not take long for Freud to realize that conscious, cognitive work must be done on the recovered material for it to be successfully worked through (Freud 1946, 1958). For psychotherapy to be effective, the patient must cognitively recollect the traumatic events with an enhanced sense of control over the memories of the experience; abreaction alone is not enough. The idea is not to reexperience the trauma, patients do that on their own every time they experience a traumatic flashback. In fact, there is actually a risk of further retraumatization in the continuous reliving of traumatic experience without adequate restructuring (Spiegel and Spiegel 1978). The cognitive restructuring technique takes the form of a symbolic restructuring of the traumatic experiences under hypnosis and the use of a grief work model (Spiegel 1981). As adapted for the treatment of PTSD (DSM-IV-TR), hypnosis can be used to provide controlled access to the dissociated or repressed memories of the traumatic experience and then to help patients restructure their memories of the events (Maldonado and Spiegel 1994, 1995).

Trauma constitutes a sudden discontinuity in both physical and mental experiences. The effect of the traumatic experience forces the victim to reorganize mental and psychophysiological processes to buffer the immediate impact of the trauma. This process is meant to be an adaptive mechanism to maintain psychological control during a time of enormous stress. Unfortunately, a number of trauma victims go on to suffer acute or chronic symptoms, such as dissociation, intrusive thoughts, anxiety, withdrawal, and hyperarousal, leading to a diagnosis of acute stress disorder or PTSD.

Multiple authors have described how victims use dissociation to cope with a traumatic event as it is occurring (Spiegel 1986, 1988, 1990, Spiegel et al. 1988, van der Kolk and van der Hart 1989). Others have suggested that major stress and trauma are common antecedents of dissociative phenomena, including some of the symptoms observed in PTSD victims (Cardeña and Spiegel 1993, Classen et al. 1993, Coons et al. 1989, Keane and Wolfe 1990, Maldonado and Spiegel 2002a, Maldonado et al. 2000, McFarlane 1986, 1988, Solomon et al. 1989, Spiegel et al. 1985, Spiegel 1986, 1990, Wilkinson 1983, van der Kolk and van der Hart 1989).

There may be a relationship during childhood between stress, such as early trauma, and high hypnotizability. In support of this idea are reports of high hypnotizability in children who were victims of severe punishment during childhood (Nash and Lynn 1986, Spiegel and Cardeña 1991). It is possible that the impact of the stress suffered encouraged them to use their self-hypnotic abilities more effectively (Kluft 1984, 1992, Spiegel et al. 1982).

The major categories of symptoms in PTSD are similar to the components of the hypnotic process (American Psychiatric Association 1994, Maldonado and Spiegel 2002a). Hypnotic absorption is similar to the intrusive reliving of traumatic events experienced by these patients. When in a flashback, trauma victims become so absorbed in the memories of the traumatic event, they lose touch with their present surroundings and even forget that the events took place in the past. Likewise, highly hypnotizable individuals may become so intensely absorbed in the trance experience that they can reenact a previous life event (during hypnotic age regression) as if they were reliving it. A hypnotized patient may dissociate a body part to the extent of not recognizing it as part of his or her body. Similarly, PTSD patients may dissociate feelings to the extent of experiencing the so-called psychic numbing. This allows them to disconnect current affects from their everyday experience in an attempt to avoid emotions triggering memories associated with the trauma. Finally, suggestibility is comparable to hyperarousal. The heightened sensitivity to environmental cues observed in those patients suffering from PTSD is similar to that experienced by a hypnotized individual who responds to suggestions of coldness by shivering.

Because many patients suffering from PTSD are highly hypnotizable, and because of the resemblance between the symptoms of PTSD and the hypnotic phenomena, it makes sense to use hypnosis in its treatment. If patients suffering from PTSD are unknowingly using their own hypnotic capacities (Kluft 1991, 1992, Maldonado and Spiegel 2002a, Spiegel 1986, 1989, Spiegel et al. 1988), it is therapeutically useful to teach them how to enter, access, and control their trance potential. Hypnosis may be invaluable as a tool to access previously dissociated traumatic material.

We do not refer here to uncontrolled abreaction. The purpose is not simply to help the patient remember the trauma, because in a way, every time a patient goes through a flashback, an uncontrolled abreaction is experienced. An abreaction that is not conducted within the context of cognitive restructuring and before new defenses are in place can lead to the further retraumatization of the patient (Kluft 1992, Spiegel 1981). At the end of the following section (Dissociative Disorders), we summarize a comprehensive approach to the use of hypnosis in the treatment of psychiatric syndromes associated with severe trauma.

## Dissociative Disorders

Hypnosis is one of the most helpful tools in the treatment of patients suffering from dissociative disorders (Maldonado and Spiegel 2002a, Maldonado et al. 2000). As a rule, these patients experience their symptoms (i.e., fugue states, dissociated identities, and blackouts) as occurring unexpectedly and beyond their control. Because these patients are unknowingly using their hypnotic capacities, it makes sense to teach them how to turn their weakness into a strength (Maldonado and Spiegel 1995). Hypnosis can be used formally both as a diagnostic tool and for therapeutic purposes. The hypnotic state can be seen as a controlled form of dissociation (Nemiah 1985). Hypnosis is useful in the treatment of these patients, first in determining whether they have a dissociative disorder, and second in providing rapid access to these dissociated states. When used by the therapist in the context of treatment, it can demonstrate to patients the amount of control they have over this state, which they normally experience as "automatic and unpredictable." This not only serves to teach patients how to control dissociation but also allows them to establish a process of communication that will eventually lead to a reduction in spontaneous dissociative symptoms. Therapists must remember that many of these patients have suffered physical, emotional, or sexual abuse. It is imperative that we recognize and take account of the impact of whatever trauma occurred and help patients work through their reactions to it, as in the case of PTSD. Recognizing and teaching patients with dissociative disorders how to master their capacity to dissociate are among the most important psychotherapeutic tasks in the course of their treatment (Maldonado and Spiegel 2002a, Maldonado et al. 2000).

Studies have demonstrated a high frequency of dissociative-like defenses in victims of early childhood abuse, and it is possible that exposure to traumatic events may be one of the natural paths toward developing high hypnotizability. Indeed, studies have shown a positive correlation between severity of punishment during childhood and hypnotizability (Hilgard 1970a, Nash and Lynn 1986). It is possible that the impact of the stress suffered by the victims of childhood abuse allows a more effective use of hypnotic traits naturally found in children. Whether these children do so consciously or not, the frequent use of their hypnotic capacity in an attempt to "avoid" repeated exposure to abuse, may prevent its extinction later in life (Morgan and Hilgard 1973). The unconscious "practicing" of this trance-like trait may account in part for the high level of hypnotizability seen in adults who were once victims of abuse (Kluft 1985b, 1990, Maldonado and Spiegel 1994, 1995, Spiegel et al. 1982).

We can make use of hypnotic techniques as a way to help patients access repressed and dissociated memories. Teaching patients to use self-hypnosis allows them to obtain a sense of control over their symptoms and eventually their lives. The repression or dissociation of traumatic events and the realities that surround them may serve a defensive purpose of avoiding painful affect associated with the memories. The memories are there, either transformed or interspersed with fantasy. Our approach to the treatment of these victims is directed at helping them acknowledge the extent of the emotional pain caused by the trauma. Then, through therapy, we can assist in the development of mature and adequate coping mechanisms that will allow the patient to place the experience into proper perspective. The goal is to allow the patient to come to terms with the trauma and to redefine herself or himself in view of the past, but with a firm hold on the realities of the present.

Dissociation as a defense serves a dual purpose. It represents an effort to preserve some form of control, safety, and identity when faced with overwhelming stress. At the same time, victims use it in an attempt to separate themselves from the full impact of the trauma. Unfortu-nately, these individuals may ward off memories of the trauma so well that they may act as if it is not happening and later as if it never happened. Some individuals can so effectively repress traumatic memories that they become unable to consciously work through them. As a consequence, they are unable to put the facts surrounding the events associated with the trauma into perspective, but slowly, the dissociated feelings and memories leak into consciousness. This creates some of the classic symptoms associated with PTSD and DID, such as flashbacks or intrusive thoughts.

The advantage of using hypnosis comes from the facilitation of the recovery of affect or memories, the ability to dissociate memories from cognition, and the speed with which the process is achieved. Finally, because of the relationship between a history of childhood abuse and trance, these patients are usually highly hypnotizable (Chu and Dill 1990, Hilgard 1984, Nash and Lynn 1986, Putman 1993, Spiegel 1988, 1990, Spiegel et al. 1988).

Many former victims of childhood abuse may unknowingly use their hypnotic capacities to keep out of awareness the content of traumatic memories, and in effect create different degrees of psychiatric illness (Sanders and Giola 1991, Spiegel 1984, 1986, 1989, Spiegel et al. 1988, Terr 1991). Teaching these patients self-hypnosis is a way of turning a weakness into a strong tool for self-mastery and control. The controlled use of hypnosis, then, becomes a way to systematically access previously dissociated material.

A hypnotic-like state may be spontaneously elicited during traumatic experiences. The principle of state-dependent memory teaches us that we store memories along with their associated affect (Bower 1981). If this is indeed true, the experience of a situation with similar affective charge may facilitate the retrieval of the initial memory. While working with hypnosis in the context of psychotherapy, we may elicit memories of a traumatic experience, resulting in the reactivation of the formerly repressed painful affect. The transition into the hypnotic trance can facilitate access to memories related to a dissociated state, as might have happened at the time of the trauma.

### The Condensed Hypnotic Approach

The use of hypnosis in the treatment of PTSD and dissociative disorders can be conceptualized as having two major goals, which can be achieved by the use of six different techniques (Maldonado and Spiegel 1994, 1995, 2002b, Spiegel 1992) (Table 89–8). The goals are to bring into *consciousness* previously repressed memories and to develop a sense of *congruence* between memories associated with the traumatic experience and current self-images. By making conscious previously repressed memories, the patient has the opportunity to understand, accept, and restructure them. These goals are achieved by working through six treatment stages: confrontation, condensation, confession, consolation, concentration, and control.

First the patient must *confront* the trauma. The therapist helps the patient recognize and understand the factors involved in the development of the symptoms for which help is now being sought. Hypnosis is then used to help the patient *condense* the traumatic memories. The hypnotic experience can be used to define a particularly frightening

| Table 89–8 | Condensed Hypnotic Approach |
|---|---|
| **Goals** | |
| To bring into consciousness previously repressed memories | |
| To develop a sense of congruence between the traumatic memories and the self | |
| **Treatment Stages** | |
| Confrontation | |
| Condensation | |
| Confession | |
| Consolation | |
| Concentration | |
| Control | |

memory during the revision of the patient's history, which summarizes or condenses the main conflicts. The focused concentration achieved during the hypnotic state not only can facilitates recall of traumatic material but also helps place boundaries around it. After memories are recovered, we can help patients restructure them and even "become aware of things you did at the moment of trauma to survive." Once memories are recovered, patients usually need to *confess* feelings and experiences of which they are profoundly ashamed. These are usually things that they may have told no one else before; in fact, they have been running from them all their lives. At this time, the therapist must convey a sense of "being present" for the patient while remaining as neutral as possible. This is followed by the stage of *consolation*. Here, the therapist needs to be emotionally available to the patient. This stage must be carried on with caution and in a most professional manner. Therapists should be aware that the body and emotional boundaries of these patients may have been violated in the past. Then comes the stage of *concentration*. This component of the trance experience allows patients to have access or "turn on" the traumatic memories during the psychotherapeutic session and then "shut them off" once the work has been done. During the final stage, the patient comes to define herself or himself as being in *control* again.

The underlying principle to remember is that the most damaging effect of overwhelming trauma is that it renders its victims defenseless. Because of the lack of physical and emotional control, patients activate dissociative defenses in an attempt to master their experiences. By using self-hypnosis, the therapist can model and teach the patient to regain control over her or his memories. Patients must be encouraged to remember as much as they feel is safe to remember at a given time. The goal is that patients learn how to think about traumatic experiences, rather than negating their existence. The use of self-hypnosis teaches patients that they are in control of their experiences. Patients must dispel the magical beliefs that therapists "can take away the memories." Rather, by modeling this sense of trust in their therapists, patients learn to trust themselves. They relearn trust in their own feelings and perceptions.

The challenge in treating victims of abuse is to achieve a new sense of unity within the patient after the initial fragmentation caused by the traumatic experience. Over-

whelming trauma tends to cause sudden and radical discontinuities in consciousness, which leaves the victims with a polarized view of themselves involving, on one hand the old self (before the trauma) and, on the other, the helpless, defenseless, and traumatized victim. Our goal is to find ways to integrate these two aspects of the self. Here, the patient's task is to acknowledge and place into perspective painful life events, thereby making them acceptable to conscious awareness.

One of the advantages of the use of hypnosis is that the affect elicited can be so powerful that most patients do not need to remember every single event of abuse or trauma. In fact, through the use of hypnosis, the therapist may help the patient consolidate the memories in a constructive way, thus facilitating recovery. After a condensation of the traumatic experiences, patients become ready to accept the victimized self. Instead of continuing the self-blame and shame because of what happened to them, they can learn to acknowledge and even thank themselves for what they did to survive. This restructuring allows them to shift their perception of self, changing their self-image from that of a victim to that of a survivor.

**Therapeutic Precautions.** Therapeutic precautions are shown in Table 89–9. The strength of transference during the psychotherapy of trauma victims is enormous. The use of hypnosis does not prevent development of a transference reaction; it may actually facilitate its emergence earlier than in regular therapy owing to the intensity with which the material is expressed and memories are recovered (Maldonado and Spiegel 1994, 1995, 2002b).

Reliving the traumatic experience along with the patient may allow a special feeling of "being there with them" at the moment of trauma. This allows the therapist to provide guidance, support, protection, and comfort as the patient goes through the difficult path of reprocessing traumatic memories. On the other hand, this kind of *traumatic transference* between the therapist and the victim of sexual assault is different in the sense that the feelings transferred are related not so much to early object relationships but to the abuser or circumstances that are associated with the trauma (Spiegel 1992). Instead of seeing this expressed anger at the therapist as a form of negative transference reaction, we should explore the possibility that this may be a healthy attempt for the patient to experience anger toward the perpetrator. As therapists, we should not minimize or shut off these feelings. This will only confirm the patient's former perception that there was something wrong with him or her for having these feelings, which will probably activate further use of primitive defenses, including dissociation or acting out.

| Table 89–9 | Therapeutic Precautions |
|---|---|
| Traumatic transference | |
| Confabulation | |
| Concreting | |
| Contamination of memories | |
| False memories | |
| Possible compromise of patient's ability to testify in court | |
| Electronic recording of all contacts with patient | |

A more serious complication of the use of hypnosis with trauma victims is the possible creation of *false memories*. Hypnosis, with its heightened sense of concentration, allows the patient to focus intensely on a given time or place, enhancing memory recall. The principle of state-dependent memory also makes it plausible that the mere entrance into this trance state can facilitate retrieval of memories associated with a similar state of mind that may have occurred during the trauma and subsequent flashbacks. However, not every memory recovered with the use of hypnosis is necessarily true. Hypnosis can facilitate improved recall of true as well as confabulated material (Dywan and Bowers 1983). Suggestibility is increased in hypnosis, and information can be implanted or imagined and reported as verdict (Laurence and Perry 1983, McConkey 1992). Because of this, therapists are warned about "believing" everything a patient is able to recall. Just as we use therapeutic judgment to analyze and interpret our patients' (nontraumatic) childhood memories, fantasies, and dreams, so should we treat hypnotically recovered material with caution.

To this date, no evidence proves that the patient's confrontation with alleged perpetrators of childhood abuse or pursuit of legal retribution toward the perpetrator provides any therapeutic benefit. As therapists, we cannot be certain of which memories are real, which are completely confabulated, and which are a combination of both. Because of this, we should not encourage our patients to take legal actions. If, on the other hand, our patients insist in pursuing this avenue, it is our duty to warn them of our concerns but to be supportive of whatever final decision they make. Certainly we will do a service to our patients if we inform them of all the legal ramifications that the use of hypnosis, or any other form of memory enhancement, may have for their defense, including their ability to testify in court or to use the material recovered by such techniques.

## Applications in General Medicine

### Medical Procedures

Because hypnosis can be used to produce a state of relaxation and to reduce anxiety, it has proved to be valuable as an adjuvant to medical procedures. Once patients have been trained in the use of self-hypnosis, they can use it both in preparation for a hospital visit and while in the clinic or hospital. Once in that state, they can imagine themselves being somewhere they enjoy and feel safe, thereby dissociating their mental experience from the physical (and possibly painful or unpleasant) aspects of the procedure (see Clinical Vignette 2). It can also be used as a way of mastering the anxiety associated with potentially threatening procedures, either diagnostic such as computed tomography (Cadranel et al. 1994, Chandler 1996, Covino and Frankel 1993, Ellis and Spanos 1994, Hilgard and LeBaron 1982, Kessler and Dane 1996, Lambert 1996, Lang et al. 1996, Mize 1996, Rape and Bush 1994), bone marrow aspirations (Liossi and Hatira 1999), needle injections (Bell et al. 1983), phlebotomy (Dash 1981, Morse and Cohen 1983, Nugent et al. 1984), needle biopsy (Adams and Stenn 1992), lumbar punctures (Kellerman et al. 1983), or therapeutic interventions, such as chemotherapy (Covino and Frankel 1993, Faymonville et al. 1995, Genuis 1995, Hilgard and LeBaron 1982, Jacknow et al. 1994, Renouf 1998, Zeltzer et al. 1984), external beam radiation therapy (Steggles 1999), and dental procedures (Hammarstrand et al. 1995, Lu 1994, Moore et al. 1996, Peretz 1996, Robb and Crothers 1996, Rustvold 1994, Shaw and Niven 1996, Shaw and Welbury 1996, Wilks 1994).

---

### Clinical Vignette 2

A 43-year-old woman who suffered several episodes of convulsions refused to undergo magnetic resonance imaging (MRI) testing because of feelings of claustrophobia. On two previous occasions she agreed to try, but even after several milligrams of diazepam, she was unable to relax sufficiently to lie comfortably during the procedure. Finally, she accepted a referral to psychiatric consultation. In my office (JRM.), she proved to be highly hypnotizable (a score of 9 of 10 on the Hypnotic Induction Profile). During hypnosis, we explored the associations between the scanner and her anxiety. Images of a coffin came to mind. These were then followed by memories of her father lying in the funeral home—he had died of a massive stroke. We then proceeded to explore her anxiety as it related to fears of what the test might show, including the possibility of a malformed blood vessel or other pathological change affecting her brain, as had happened to her father. Once this was discussed, she felt that it "was better to know than to avoid." She was trained in self-hypnosis. After inducing a relaxed state, she was instructed, "Create in your mind's eye a place where you can feel safe and comfortable, knowing that sounds and people in the room will not disturb you." We also "practiced" going to the scanner room by having her imagine that she was both the patient in the room and the technician operating the machine. In this fashion, she felt more "in control" of the situation.

The next day, I met her at the scanner room. Once she was on the imaging table, the patient followed the procedure we practiced. When the test began, I left the room with the agreement that the technician would let her know when the test was over. She imagined herself walking through a forest and crossing a river. As she walked to the riverbank, instead of floating, she sank slowly as she followed the contours of the river. Once on the bottom, she held on to some algae. When she exhaled her breath, it formed a gigantic bubble or cocoon that allowed her to breathe underwater and be safe. As the magnets in the magnetic resonance imager shifted in position, she imagined that this was the clanking sound of motorboat engines on the surface. She remained in this state for approximately 2 hours while tests were performed with and without contrast material. She tolerated the procedure well and easily came out of the trance state when the signal was given.

---

### Pain Control

Pain is always a psychosomatic phenomenon, combining somatic with subjective distress. It never exists in a vacuum and always represents a combination of tissue injury and the emotional reaction to it. James Esdaile (1846), a Scottish surgeon working in India, described 80% surgical anesthesia for amputations with use of hypnosis. He also reported a lower mortality rate (5%) with his procedures than the mortality rates in Great Britain (40%), probably because of the high risks of anesthesia or the difficulty of performing surgery without anesthesia at that time. Unfortunately, he later withdrew his findings after being severely censured by his colleagues.

Despite the organic factors causing pain, it is clear that psychological factors are major variables in the intensity of the pain experience. More than 100 years after Esdaile, at the Massachusetts General Hospital, Beecher (1956) demonstrated that the intensity of pain was directly associated with its meaning. For example, to the extent that pain represented threat and the possibility of future disability, it was more intense than it was among a group of combat soldiers to whom the pain of injury meant that they were likely to get out of combat alive.

Hypnosis can facilitate an alteration in the subjective experience of pain (Brose and Spiegel 1992). Several techniques can be used to achieve this goal. Most techniques involve the production of physical relaxation coupled with visual or somatic imagery that provides a substitute focus of attention for the painful sensation.

The use of hypnosis as an adjunct to anesthesia has been described in patients undergoing angioplasty (Westein and Au 1991), plastic surgery (Faymonville et al. 1995), thyroidectomies (Meurisse et al. 1996), orthopedic surgery (Mauer et al. 1999), surgical neck dissection and exploration (Meurisse et al. 1999), management of burn injuries (Patterson et al. 1997, Ohrbach et al. 1998), limb fracture reduction (Iserson 1999), chronic tension-type headaches (Gysin 1999, Spinhoven and ter Kuile 2000), and migraine headache (Matthews and Flatt 1999). It has also been described as effective in the management of pain (Benhaiem et al. 2001, Crawford et al. 1998, Freeman et al. 2000, Anonymous 1996, Montgomery et al. 2000, Moskowitz 1996, Sandrini et al. 2000).

The specific technique employed may depend on the degree of hypnotic ability of the subject. For example, patients can be taught to develop a comfortable floating sensation on the affected body part. Highly hypnotizable individuals may simply imagine an injection of procaine hydrochloride (Novocain) in the affected area, producing a sense of tingling numbness similar to that experienced in previous dental work. Other patients may prefer to move the pain to another part of their body or to dissociate the affected part from the rest of the body. As an extreme form of hypnotically induced, controlled dissociation, some patients may imagine themselves floating above their body, creating distance between themselves and the painful sensation or experience.

For some more moderately hypnotizable patients, it may be easier to focus on a change in temperature, either warmth or coolness. A sensation of warmth could be elicited while patients imagine they are floating in a warm bath or applying a heating pad to a given area of the body. A cooling sensation can be elicited by imagining that the afflicted extremity is immersed in an ice-cold mountain stream or in a bucket of ice chips. Temperature metaphors are especially effective. This may be related to the fact that pain and temperature fibers run together in the lateral spinothalamic tract.

The images or metaphors used for pain control employ certain general principles. First, the hypnotically controlled image may serve to "filter the hurt out of the pain." Patients also learn to transform the pain experience. They acknowledge that it exists (the pain), but there is a distinction between the signal itself and the discomfort the signal causes.

The hypnotic experience that patients create and control helps them transform the signal into one that is less uncomfortable. Patients expand their perception from an experience in which the pain either is there or is not, to a third option—the pain is there but transformed by the presence of such competing sensations as tingling, numbness, warmth, or coolness.

Finally, patients are taught not to fight the pain. Fighting pain only enhances it by focusing attention on the pain, enhancing related anxiety and depression, and increasing physical tension that can literally put traction on painful parts of the body and increase the pain signals generated peripherally.

For patients undergoing painful procedures, such as bone marrow aspirations, the main focus is on the hypnotic imagery rather than on relaxation. This works especially well with children because they are so highly hypnotizable and easily absorbed in images (Hilgard and Hilgard 1975, Zeltzer and Le Baron 1982). Patients may be guided through the experience while the procedure is performed, or a given scenario may be suggested, and the patient later undergoes the experience hypnotically while the procedure is under way. This enables patients to restructure their experience of what is going on and dissociate themselves psychologically from pain and fear of the procedure.

Even though the precise mechanism for hypnotic analgesia is not known, it is suspected to have components of two complementary mechanisms: physical relaxation and attention control. Patients in pain tend to splint the painful area instinctively, which in turn increases muscle tension around the painful area, often resulting in increased pain. Therefore, creating a state of hypnotically induced relaxation may easily decrease their experience or perception of pain.

This can be more easily achieved by creating images that facilitate a relaxing response, such as a warm bath, floating on an air mattress in a pool, or just floating out in space. Second, and probably more important, because hypnosis involves an intensification and narrowing of the focus of attention, it allows patients to pay selective attention to the action or ideas contained in the metaphor or images, therefore placing pain at the periphery of their awareness. It thus diminishes the amount of attention they pay to painful stimuli. A third possible mechanism affecting the pain experience may be related to the psychological meaning of the pain itself (Clinical Vignette 3). Some patients have been in pain so long that pain has become an intrinsic part of their existence.

---

Clinical Vignette 3

A 62-year-old woman was referred to me (JRM) with hopes that hypnosis would help alleviate her experience of chronic pain associated with cancer. A formal test of hypnotizability demonstrated that she was in the highly hypnotizable range. Under hypnosis, she was instructed that all the pain would "go away," or at least she would be able to block it, but as soon as she exited the trance state, the pain returned. Because of the curious dynamics of this phenomenon, I decided to explore the meaning pain had for her. She told me how her oncologist had warned her that she would be in pain as long as she is alive. It became clear that she associated pain with being alive and that she would be "pain free" only on the day she died.

After I explored this and discussed it with the patient, she decided that it was "not fair that after suffering so much, I still have to deal with the pain." She gave herself permission to live without pain and to enjoy as many of her remaining days as she could. She ended her trance experience and discussed it. Shortly afterward, she left the office, inadvertently leaving her cane behind. A few hours later, I called her home to let her know she had forgotten her cane in my office. To which she replied, "You can keep it as a souvenir."

Hypnotic analgesia cannot be explained by simple social compliance alone—merely enacting a role and telling the therapist what he or she wants to hear. Rather, there is evidence that it involves neurophysiological changes in information processing. Studies of the effects of hypnosis on cortical event-related potentials indicate that highly hypnotizable individuals diminish the P100 and P300 components of their event-related response to a somatosensory stimulus by focusing on a hallucinated image that blocks their perception of the stimulus (Spiegel et al. 1989a).

A number of studies have tested the idea that endogenous opiates are involved in hypnotic analgesia. With one partial exception (Frid and Singer 1979), studies with both volunteers (Goldstein and Hilgard 1975) and patients in chronic pain (Spiegel and Albert 1983) have shown that hypnotic analgesia is not blocked and reversed by a substantial dose of naloxone given in double-blind, crossover fashion. Therefore, the cortical attention deployment mechanism is at the moment the most plausible explanation for hypnotic reduction of pain.

Regardless of the underlying mechanism, there is no doubt about the efficacy of hypnotic analgesia. Hypnosis has been shown to be superior to an attentional control condition for analgesia among children undergoing painful procedures (Zeltzer and LeBaron 1982). Furthermore, in a randomized prospective study, a combination of hypnosis and group psychotherapy was shown to result in a 50% reduction in pain among patients with metastatic breast cancer (Spiegel and Bloom 1983). This was accompanied by a significant reduction in mood disturbance (Spiegel et al. 1981a).

Studies have also shown the superiority of hypnotic analgesia to the level of analgesia provided by either placebo (McGlashan et al. 1969) or acupuncture (Knox and Shum 1977). Katz and colleagues (1974) have shown a correlation between hypnotizability and responsiveness to acupuncture, proving that hypnotic mechanisms of pain control may be mobilized by other treatment techniques. Nevertheless, the explicit use of hypnosis with hypnotizable patients has proved to be the most powerful means of controlling pain. Hilgard and Hilgard (1975) estimated a 0.5 correlation between hypnotizability and treatment responsiveness for pain control. It is believed that the ability of highly hypnotizable patients to focus their attention on and alter their response to perception while at the same time producing a physical state of relaxation gives them an unusual ability to restructure their experience of pain,

which in turn allows them to develop a sense of mastery over it.

## Insomnia

As we discussed earlier, hypnosis is a state of increased concentration and awareness. From this point of view, the hypnotic state is far from sleep, although both are restful altered mental states with reduced awareness of the peripheral environment. So, it might seem paradoxical to use hypnosis to help people fall asleep. Nevertheless, hypnosis can be helpful for inducing a state of physical relaxation that is at least compatible with sleep. As in the treatment of anxiety, a relaxing trance state may diminish the sympathetic arousal usually associated with anxious preoccupation and could facilitate entering into a restful sleep. Patients can be instructed to enter a state of self-hypnosis, then to induce a sense of floating and physical relaxation. Once this is achieved, they may use one of many different mechanisms to put worries or thoughts on hold "for tonight," knowing that they can always deal with them tomorrow. For example, the patients can project these thoughts onto an imaginary screen. Then they can become a kind of "traffic director" for their thoughts, dealing with them on the screen, thereby dissociating them from the physical response to them while remaining in a quiet and relaxed state (Spiegel and Spiegel 1978).

Another useful method is to have patients imagine themselves lying restfully in a comfortable and safe place while they see themselves placing the disturbing thoughts "onto the clouds, watching the breeze slowly carry them away," or they can even imagine their worries to be like "leaves floating on the surface of a river, flowing with the current," rather than holding on to any particular thought. Such approaches can be helpful in conjunction with standard sleep hygiene practices, which include keeping the bedroom as a place to sleep, avoiding working and other anxiety-arousing activities in bed, and avoiding looking at the clock when awakened. It is also important to distinguish routine insomnia due to situational reactions and anxiety from the more severe forms that are associated with major depression, an anxiety disorder, or a sleep disorder such as sleep apnea syndrome (DSM-IV-TR).

## Psychosomatic Disorders

Most patients with high hypnotizability also have an unusual capacity for psychological control of somatic function. This is especially evidenced in psychosomatic disorders as well as in cases of conversion reactions. It is possible that somehow these individuals have turned their capacity for somatic control against themselves, producing rather than controlling symptoms. If this is true, then it makes sense that hypnosis could be used in the treatment of these symptoms. For example, Andreychuk and Skriver (1975) found that high hypnotizability was a good predictor of both pretreatment symptom severity and treatment response for migraine headache patients. That is, more highly hypnotizable individuals complained of more severe migraine symptoms before treatment but responded better to intervention.

Hypnosis is useful in both the diagnosis and the treatment of psychosomatic illness. By using hypnosis with these patients, the therapist may assist in diagnosing the symptoms as psychosomatic. Under hypnosis, many of the symptoms may improve or be completely reversed. It is important not to "force a cure" in any patient, but rather to allow patients to improve at a pace that feels comfortable, or to give up the symptom when ready. This allows patients not only to feel in control of the treatment and recovery process but also to slowly get back their sense of control over their body. Some patients obtain insight into what is happening to their bodies owing to the ability to explore the meaning and cause of the symptoms hypnotically.

In most instances, it is better if hypnosis is used as an adjuvant to any other medical treatment, including physical rehabilitation or any other treatment modality typically used in the treatment of the "real illness." Most such problems involve a combination of somatic and psychological symptoms. Using a rehabilitation model avoids the trap of humiliating the patient who improves with the inference that the problem was "all in the mind."

Patients suffering from psychosomatic diseases are indeed suffering from a true organic process. This is the case in the disorders classically included under the rubric of psychosomatic, such as asthma (Aronoff et al. 1975, Clarke 1970, Collison 1975, Ewer and Stewart 1986, Kohen 1986, Gluzman and Zisel'son 1989, Hackman et al. 2000, Inoue et al. 1995, Kelly and Zeller 1969, Kohen 1987, Kohen and Wynne 1997, Luparello et al. 1968, Maher-Loughnan 1970, McFadden et al. 1969, Moorefield 1971, Morrison 1988, Mun 1969, Smith et al. 1970), cystic fibrosis and chronic dyspnea (Anbar 2000, 2001), peptic ulcer disease (Colgan et al. 1988), Francis and Houghton 1996, Klein and Spiegel 1989), irritable bowel syndrome (Barabasz and Spiegel 1989, Francis and Houghton 1996, Houghton et al. 1996, Snape 1994, Vidakovic-Vukic 1999, Whorwell et al. 1984, 1987), warts, (Arone di Bertolino 1983, Ewin 1992, Johnson and Barber 1978, Spanos et al. 1988, 1990, Steele and Irwin, 1988), and psoriasis (Kantor 1990, Tausk and Whitmore 1999, Winchell and Watts 1988). If these processes go untreated, serious body damage may occur. The goal of hypnosis then includes allowing patients to see the effects of their affect and emotional stress on their body, sometimes by demonstrating, under hypnosis, their ability to recreate the condition for which they now seek help. Afterward, they are helped to retrain their minds to control their response to the somatic symptoms.

Hypnosis can be invaluable in the treatment of a number of psychosomatic conditions. In particular, disorders affecting the gastrointestinal system are among those conditions in which studies demonstrated a dramatic response. In cases of ulcerative colitis and regional enteritis, patients have found it helpful to imagine in trance something soothing in their gut. This gives them a sense of control over a symptom that causes them to feel especially helpless, thereby diminishing the cycle of reactive anxiety. Whorwell and colleagues (1984, 1987) demonstrated that 15 patients with irritable bowel syndrome who were treated with hypnosis reported significant improvement in pain, abdominal distention, and diarrhea as well as emotional well-being, compared with a randomly assigned control group. Follow-up of these patients showed continued remission of the symptoms.

In studies related to peptic ulcer disease, Klein and Spiegel (1989) observed significant hypnotic control of gastric acid secretion among highly hypnotizable subjects. They were initially instructed (under hypnosis) to consume an imaginary meal. This was accompanied by a rise in basal acid output of 89%. This was followed by another study in which subjects were instructed to use hypnosis to experience deep relaxation. These patients experienced a significant drop of 39% in basal acid output. In a third trial, subjects were given an injection of pentagastrin to stimulate maximal parietal cell output. Even with this chemical stimulus, there was a significant 11% reduction in peak acid output when hypnosis was used. An independent study by Colgan and colleagues (1988) randomly assigned a group of patients with peptic ulcer disease to either hypnosis or no treatment (control) after an initial treatment with ranitidine. They reported that 100% of the patients in the control group relapsed, compared with only 53% of those in the hypnosis group.

Hypnosis has been found effective in reducing the gastrointestinal side effects of chemotherapy, especially conditioned nausea and vomiting (Redd et al. 1982). Useful techniques include imagining being elsewhere than the hospital and clinic with smells and sights that trigger associations with the effects of the chemotherapy infusion. It is often useful to instruct patients to imagine that they are at a favorite vacation spot or comfortable at home. One woman absorbed herself in an imaginary project of redecorating a large castle on the Rhine. There are hypnotic means of dissociating the emetic stimulus from the response. Zeltzer and associates (1984) reported significant reduction in chemotherapy-induced nausea and vomiting among patients trained in self-hypnosis compared with control subjects.

Several studies have proved the efficacy of hypnosis in the treatment of other psychosomatic conditions, including warts (Ewin 1992, Spanos et al. 1988, 1990), bronchial asthma (Aronoff et al. 1975, Ewer and Stewart 1986, Kohen et al. 1984, Morrison 1988), and cardiovascular problems such as angina pectoris (Greenleaf et al. 1992, Weinstein and Au 1991).

These examples further emphasize that high hypnotizability is a two-edged sword. It may positively or adversely affect a given physiological parameter, depending on the mental content during the hypnotic state. Unfortunately, many patients unconsciously use it to their detriment. The goal of treatment then is to train them how to master their hypnotic capacity and use it to normalize and regulate body functions.

## Applications of Hypnosis in Habit Control

### Smoking Cessation
A number of studies demonstrate the efficacy of hypnosis as a tool to facilitate control of smoking. These studies show success rates in cigarette abstinence after treatment with hypnosis ranging from 13 to 64%. In these studies, abstinence is defined as no smoking during a follow-up time of at least 6 months (Schwartz 1987). Spiegel (1970) developed a single-session approach for smoking cessation that is widely used (Schwartz 1987). His results have been replicated and shown to produce outcomes of 20 to 35%

long-term complete abstinence (Barabasz et al. 1986, Berkowitz et al. 1979, Covino and Bottari 2001, Frank et al. 1986, Spiegel 1970, Spiegel and Spiegel 1978). Others have reported abstinence rates as high as 64% at 6 months (Crasilneck and Hall 1985, Holroyd 1980, 1991, Hyman et al. 1986, Schwartz 1987, Spiegel 1970, Williams and Hall 1988). These numbers are better than the rates of unassisted quitting (Gritz and Bloom 1987). Studies have also shown that higher hypnotizability predicts better outcome (Barabasz et al. 1986, Spiegel and Spiegel 1978, Spiegel et al., unpublished data).

There are several mechanisms by which hypnosis may contribute to success in smoking cessation. The ritualistic process of the hypnotic exercise may provide a kind of substitute physical relaxation for the "breathing exercise" that accompanies the act of smoking; the positive affirmations in self-hypnosis provide positive reinforcement for behavior change and promote positive self-image; its use enhances self-observation and self-monitoring; and finally it can facilitate cognitive restructuring of the smoking habit.

The single-session method developed by Spiegel (1970) emphasizes teaching patients self-hypnosis rather than having multiple sessions with a therapist. It uses a strategy that is intrinsically self-reinforcing and meaningful to the patient. It can be practiced whenever the urge to smoke comes on the patient. This method of cognitive restructuring involves emphasizing that the act of smoking is destructive specifically to the patient's body and thereby limits what the patient can do with his or her life by shortening the life span and deteriorating the quality of life. Hypnosis is used to emphasize the patient's commitment to protect the body from the poison in cigarettes. This approach gives the patient the ability to examine priorities and to balance the urge to smoke against the urge to protect his or her body from damage. Smokers are instructed to focus on what they are *for*—protecting their bodies—rather than what they are *against*—smoking. This reduces the amount of attention they pay to smoking or its absence and provides immediate internal reinforcement for attending to care of the body (Spiegel and Spiegel 1978).

In summary, there is no evidence that treatments employing hypnosis are more effective than other interventions for smoking. Nevertheless, they may be more efficient because they enable patients to employ a self-administered treatment strategy (self-hypnosis) to reinforce a more adaptive cognitive restructuring while providing patients with an exercise in physical relaxation.

## Weight Control

Seldom will the use of hypnosis alone be sufficient for the treatment of weight problems. It is usually employed as an adjunct to a comprehensive dietary and exercise control program for weight reduction and management. Similar to the use of self-hypnosis in the control of smoking, the purpose in dietary control is to restructure the patient's experience with overeating. Patients are asked to examine their excess food intake and to pay attention to the damaging effects to their body. This then translates into an exercise about learning to eat with respect for one's body. Once again, the emphasis is on what the patient is *for*, rather than being *against* food.

An important component of such an approach consists of teaching the patient to use self-hypnosis training to control the urge to overeat. This is better accomplished by preparing a list of food items that constitute eating with respect and then comparing an urge for a particular food item with the list. If the desired food is on the list, the patient is encouraged to eat it like a gourmet, focusing intently on all aspects of the eating experience and enjoying it. If the food is not on the list, the patient is asked to recognize the desire rather than fight the urge. Then the patient is encouraged to use self-hypnosis to compare this urge with her or his overall commitment to protect and treat her or his body with respect and therefore to eat with respect. This involves dissociating the urge to eat from the need to act on that urge. By using this method, patients can see their desire to eat not as an occasion to feel deprived but rather as one in which they are enhancing their mastery over the urge by choosing to protect their body. Patients are also instructed to pay more attention to their somatic signals of hunger and satiety; to eat when they are hungry, but stop eating as soon as they are full.

Unfortunately, long-term outcome studies on the usefulness of hypnosis for weight control are lacking. Clinical experience suggests that those within 20% of their ideal body weight may obtain some benefit from such restructuring techniques with self-hypnosis, combined with a regimen of a balanced diet and exercise. Anderson (1985) described that high hypnotizability is correlated with weight reduction. Barabasz and Spiegel (1989) performed a study comparing the usefulness of hypnosis with a self-management group for weight reduction. All members in the study were highly motivated. The control group was exposed to an active self-management treatment program resulting in adequate weight reduction. On the other hand, the hypnosis subjects were given suggestions emphasizing their desire to protect and care for their bodies rather than to fight the desire for certain foods, along with a behavioral intervention. The results showed significant effects for the hypnosis plus behavioral intervention group (mean weight loss, 6.4 kg) as contrasted with the group using behavioral intervention only (mean weight loss, 1.3 kg). One of the most important aspects of the study was the significant relationship between weight loss and hypnotizability. The study demonstrated a significant correlation between hypnotizability scores and weight loss.

Other studies employing hypnosis for weight loss have proven effective (Stradling et al. 1998). This has also been the case when hypnosis has been added to other cognitive–behavioral treatments for weight reduction (Anderson 1985, Kirsch et al. 1995, Kirsch 1996).

## Applications in Forensic Psychiatry

The most serious problem involves possible effects of hypnosis on memory. There is evidence that hypnosis can distort memory in two ways: through *confabulation*, the creation of pseudomemories that are reported as real, or through *concreting*, an unwarranted increase in the confidence with which hypnotized individuals report their memories, either true or false (McConkey 1992, Orne et al. 1985, Spiegel and Spiegel 1986, Spiegel and Vermutten 1994). Hypnosis can facilitate the recall of dissociated memories, especially when recall is hampered by the strong affect associated with trauma (Kardiner and Spiegel 1947, Spiegel 1984, 1992). However, the research literature indicates that the most clearly reproducible problem is the production of confident errors, exaggerating the true value of memories unearthed in hypnosis.

This is especially a problem when the memories involve witnessing a crime and civil or criminal action in court is a possibility. Most states prohibit the use of hypnotically induced testimony, but some prescribe witnesses who have been hypnotized regarding the content of their potential testimony (Spiegel and Scheflin 1994). If the possibility exists that a patient may be required to testify, it is wise to discuss the use of hypnosis with the patient and (with the patient's permission) the patient's attorney or the district attorney and obtain written agreement regarding its use. If the patient is likely to be called to testify, the therapist should obtain electronic recording of all contact with the patient (preferably on videotape) so the court can examine for possible suggestive influences. Full guidelines for use of hypnosis in the forensic setting include careful debriefing of the subject before hypnosis is employed, the use of non-leading questions, complete videotaping of all contact with the patient, and careful debriefing afterward (Spiegel and Spiegel 1986).

The controversies surrounding so-called false memory syndrome have reignited questions regarding the validity of the material recovered by the use of hypnosis. One of the most common applications of hypnosis in the court and legal settings had been refreshing recollection of witnesses and victims of crimes. Even though the current controversy focuses on the dangers of hypnotically induced confabulation or excessive confidence in memories (Diamond 1980), there have been some positive results. A well-known example is the case involving the driver of a hijacked school bus in Chowchilla, California (*People v. Schoenfeld* 1980). Under hypnosis, the bus driver was able to recall the license plate number of the car driven by the kidnappers. This information, not consciously available to him before hypnotic intervention, led to the arrest and conviction of the criminals.

Because hypnosis involves a suspension of critical judgment, and therefore a state of heightened suggestibility or responsivity to social cues, it is important that the interview be conducted with a minimum of inserted information. To minimize the risk of contaminating subjects' memories, it is important to use open-ended questions, such as, "What happens next?" rather than, "How did he sexually abuse you?"

Information retrieved with the aide of hypnosis may simply be the result of an additional recall trial (Erdelyi and Kleinbard 1978), it may be new and true (Dywan and Bowers 1983), or it may be a confabulation (Laurence and Perry 1983). It may indeed be a combination of all three (Orne et al. 1985). As a result, courts have long been unwilling to admit the testimony of a person hypnotized while testifying and have also begun to exclude testimony of witnesses who have previously been hypnotized about the event in question. Even when a subject is acting in good faith, hypnosis can amplify both truth and falsehood. A good guideline is that hypnosis increases the recovery of memories, both true and confabulated. Spiegel (1980b) described what he called the "honest liar," a hypnotized witness who in his or her desire to please the hypnotist or simply as a result of being in the suggestible state of hypnosis makes up material and believes the newly created story to be real. This poses obvious dangers for the legal system. A witness who produces "confident errors" (McConkey 1992) may mislead a jury looking for signs of discomfort or insecurity in their evaluation of the veracity of testimony. This has been termed *concreting* (Diamond 1980, Orne 1979).

On the other hand, people do dissociate during trauma, often failing to recall events despite being conscious at the time (Cardeña and Spiegel 1993, Spiegel and Cardeña 1991). There is evidence that such memory gaps may persist for years or even decades after such traumatic events as physical or sexual abuse (Williams 1994).

Therapists treating victims of sexual abuse must be aware that the use of hypnosis may compromise the ability of a witness to testify in court. Indeed, several states (Arizona (*State ex rel Collins v. Superior Court* 1982), California (*People v. Guerra* 1984, *People v. Shirley* 1982), New Jersey (*People v. Hurd* 1980), and New York (*People v. Hughes* 1983) restrict the testimony of victims or witnesses who have used hypnosis to refresh their recollection. The reason for the courts' objection to the use of hypnosis is a combination of real and exaggerated dangers of hypnosis.

After much legal battling, some courts now allow witnesses to testify after the use of hypnosis provided that certain guidelines are followed (California Legislature 1985). These relate primarily to the training and independence of the professional doing the hypnotic interrogation and the electronic recording of the entire process (Spiegel and Spiegel 1986).

To address this controversial issue, the Council on Scientific Affairs of the American Medical Association convened a panel of experts to examine the research evidence relevant to this problem. The report issued by the panel concluded that the existing evidence indicates that the use of hypnosis tends to increase the productivity of witnesses, resulting in new memories, some of which are true and some of which are incorrect (Orne et al. 1985). Furthermore, some studies showed an increase in the confidence assigned by hypnotized subjects to their memories despite the fact that their percentage of correct responses had not improved. The panel noted that the analogy between the laboratory setting in which most of the studies were done and the real-life situation in the courtroom must be drawn with great caution and that situations in which extreme emotional and physical trauma had occurred differ markedly. The panel recommended that careful guidelines similar to the ones adopted by the state of California be followed when hypnosis is used in the forensic setting (Table 89–10).

As a rule, it is advisable to caution attorneys and witnesses that the use of hypnosis might open the possibility of challenge to the credibility or even the admissibility of a witness. The kind of situation in which hypnosis is most likely to be worth the risk is one in which there is a traumatic amnesia for the events of a crime or in which all other avenues of exploration have been exhausted. Hypnosis is by no means a truth serum, and the courts must weigh the effects of any hypnotic procedure on a witness.

| Table 89–10 | Hypnosis and Forensic Psychiatry |
|---|---|

If you consider the use of hypnosis in a trial case, certain guidelines need to be observed:

- Caution attorneys and witnesses that the use of hypnosis might open the possibility of challenge to the credibility or even the admissibility of a witness.
- Carefully document memory before hypnosis of the witness.
- Use an expert psychiatrist or psychologist as a hypnosis consultant.
- Electronically record all interaction preceding, during, and after hypnosis sessions. Document and record all contact with the victim.
- Conduct the interview in a neutral tone. Guide the victim through the experience but avoid using leading or suggestive questions. Avoid introducing information during the interrogation.

Because it is almost impossible not to add some degree of contamination to the procedure, we recommend that at least the following steps be undertaken. First (with the patient's permission), consult with the victim's attorney. If an investigation is in progress or court proceedings are likely, you may also want to contact the district attorney's office or the police. Second, make a video (preferably) or audio recording of all contact with the victim. Make certain that you can clearly hear the voice of the victim and your own voice or that of anyone else participating in the process. Third, conduct the interview in a neutral tone. Guide the victim through the experience but avoid using leading or suggestive questions. It is imperative to avoid introducing information during the interrogation. This is best achieved by asking open-ended, neutral questions based on the information already provided by the victim. For example, ask questions such as "Now what is happening?" rather than "Did he knock you down?" or "Who raped you? Was it your father?"

The medico–legal aspects of the use of hypnosis in psychiatric practice have already been discussed at length elsewhere (Maldonado and Spiegel 2002a, 2002b).

## Treatment Outcome Studies in Hypnosis

Most outcome studies have resulted in two main conclusions related to the therapeutic uses of hypnosis. First, there is no doubt that hypnosis is effective. Second, the degree of hypnotizability is predictive of treatment response (Spiegel et al. 1981b). A study of 178 patients treated with a single session of self-hypnosis for flying phobia indicated that 52% were either improved or cured at a 7-year follow-up. Hypnotizable patients did significantly better than nonhypnotizable patients. Several studies have shown hypnosis for the treatment of smoking to produce outcomes of 20 to 35% abstinence at 6 months of follow-up (Barabasz et al. 1986, Berkowitz et al. 1979, Frank et al. 1986, Spiegel 1970, Spiegel and Spiegel 1978). Kohen (1986) reported dramatic and sustained improvement in the management of asthma in children 2 years after training in self-hypnosis. Studies have described a success rate for employing hypnosis in the treatment of warts ranging from 27 (Johnson and Barber 1978) to 55% (Bloch 1927). Even more remarkable is Ewin's (1992) observation regarding the use of hypnosis in the treatment of warts: "I use the term *cure* because there is not a single case report in the literature of recurrence after healing with hypnosis." Ewin reported an 80% cure rate in his study. In general, it has been observed that hypnosis is particularly useful and yields better results when it is specifically requested by the patient (Glick 1970, Lazarus 1973).

## Neurophysiological Correlates of Hypnosis

Since the earliest days of hypnosis, scientists have been trying to understand its neurophysiological underpinnings. Mesmer initially explained the mechanism of action of his technique as the manipulation of the body's energies, or magnetic fluid. One of the most memorable debates occurred between Charcot (1890), who described hypnosis as a disease of the nervous system and argued that normal people could not be hypnotized, and Bernheim (1964), who challenged Charcot's ideas of hypnotizability as a disease and rather described it as a trait exhibited to different degrees by normal individuals.

Since those early times, many research efforts have attempted to correlate the hypnotic experience with actual physiological or cerebral physiology changes. To date, a "seat of hypnosis" has not been found in the brain. Nevertheless, there is ample clinical and research experience indicating that the hypnotic process affects both electrical and metabolic processes in the brain. Similarly, as we have observed in clinical experience, hypnotic activity is capable of causing various physiological changes. Some of these have been simulated under laboratory conditions.

The ability of highly hypnotizable individuals to control peripheral skin temperature and blood flow has been replicated in several well-controlled experiments (Grabowska 1971, Kistler et al. 1999, Zimbardo et al. 1970). Conn and Mott (1984) demonstrated plethysmographic measure changes caused by hypnotically mediated rapid vasodilation after direct suggestion in cases of Raynaud's disease treated with hypnosis. Fox and coworkers (1999) were able to demonstrate the effects of hypnosis in clinically significant immunological functioning. They use hypnosis to treat patients suffering from frequently recurrent genital herpes simplex virus (rgHSV). Following hypnosis intervention, they recorded a significant overall reduction in the number of reported episodes of rgHSV, accompanied by a corresponding increase in the numbers of CD3 and CD8 lymphocytes, significant rises in natural killer (NK) cell counts, HSV specific lymphokine activated killer (LAK) activity, and reduced levels of anxiety when compared to nonimprovers.

Gemignani and coworkers (2000) studied the physiological and electroencephalographic (EEG) responses of highly hypnotizable volunteers suffering from simple phobia. Under hypnotic suggestion, subjects exposed to aversive stimuli experienced significant increases in heart rate (HR) and respiratory rate (RR) with a shift of the sympatho–vagal indexes towards a sympathetic predominance. These subjects also experienced a significant increase in the EEG gamma band with a left fronto-central prevalence.

Finally, Williamson and colleagues (2001) using healthy, highly hypnotizable volunteers demonstrated dramatic changes in ratings of perceived exertion (RPE) when asked to imagine themselves in an uphill bicycle grade. They found significant increases in RPE, HR, mean blood pressure (BP), regional cerebral blood flow (rCBF) in the right insular cortex and right thalamic activation. Conversely, when subjects were asked to imagine themselves on a perceived downhill grade they observed decrements in both the ratings of perceived exertion RPE and rCBF in the left insular cortex and anterior cingulate cortex, but it did not alter exercise HR or BP responses.

## Neurotransmitters

Hypnotizability has been found to be significantly correlated with cerebrospinal fluid levels of homovanillic acid, a metabolite of dopamine (Spiegel and King 1992) (Table 89–11). This provides evidence for the involvement of the frontal cortex in the hypnotic process because levels of homovanillic acid in the cerebrospinal fluid primarily reflect activity in the frontal cortex and basal ganglia, which are rich in dopaminergic synapses. Sjoberg and Hollister (1965) suggested that the administration of dopaminergic agents such as amphetamine may enhance hypnotizability. It has been postulated that the automaticity observed in hypnotic motor behavior could represent an activation of the basal ganglia, which is involved in both implicit memory (Mishkin and Murray 1994, Schacter 1987) and routine motor activity.

## Brain Electrical Activity

Even though it was initially described as a form of nervous sleep, today we know that hypnosis and sleep share no common characteristics. The brain electrical pattern of a hypnotized subject actually resembles that of a fully awake and attentive individual more than the pattern of a person who is asleep (see Table 89–11). Power spectral analysis of brain electrical activity has provided some limited understanding into the physiological mechanism of the hypnotic state.

Various researchers (Edmonston and Grotevant 1975, Morgan et al. 1974) have reported an increased alpha activity among highly hypnotizable individuals. This difference is present whether or not the subjects were in trance. They also found an alpha laterality difference favoring the left hemisphere among highly hypnotizable individuals. This difference suggested that hypnosis might preferentially in-

volve the right cerebral hemisphere, because alpha is the noise the brain makes when resting but alert, so relatively less alpha on the right suggests more activity. These findings are supported by observations that highly hypnotizable individuals tend to be left-lookers, preferring to activate their right hemisphere (Bakan 1969, Gur and Rehyer 1973). Finally, Meszaros and Szabo (1999) demonstrated that in highly susceptible subjects the right parieto-temporal region shows more electric power than the left one while the low susceptibles have left side predominance or equilibrated power in all derivations.

More recent studies have questioned the right hemispheric dominance theory of the hypnotic process. Edmonston and coworkers (1990) obtained bilateral EEG measures on highly hypnotizable subjects while performing hemisphere-specific tasks during hypnosis and no-hypnosis control conditions. These studies suggest a lack of task appropriate activity during hypnosis, indicating that data analysis techniques were the source of potential misinterpretations of previously obtained data.

Jasiukaitis and colleagues (1997) raised new questions regarding the old theory of right cerebral hemisphere dominance of brain activity during hypnosis. They conducted a review of the literature and included in their analysis data from electrodermal responding, visual event-related potentials (VERPs), and Stroop interference. Their analysis suggests, instead, that although hemispheric activation on hypnotic challenge may depend in large part on the kind of task the challenge might involve, several general aspects of hypnosis might be more appropriately seen as left-hemisphere rather than right-hemisphere brain functions, including concentrated attentional focus and the role of language in the establishment of hypnotic reality.

There may also be frontal versus posterior topographical differences among high and low hypnotizable individuals. In fact, more recent studies of power spectral analysis suggest that theta power, especially in the frontal region, best differentiates highly hypnotizable from poorly hypnotizable individuals (Sabourin et al. 1990). Similarly, Graffin and coworkers (1995) found greater theta power in the more frontal areas of the cortex for highly hypnotizable subjects. During the actual hypnotic induction, theta power increased markedly for both groups in the more posterior areas of the cortex, whereas alpha activity increased across all sites. In the period just preceding and following the hypnotic induction, poorly hypnotizable subjects displayed an increase in theta activity, whereas highly hypnotizable subjects displayed a decrease. Taken together, these findings suggest that anterior/posterior cortical differences may be more important than hemispheric laterality for understanding the hypnotic processes.

Event-related potentials (ERP) have been used to study the effects of hypnotic hallucination on brain electrical activity. These studies are based on the premise that hypnotically induced changes in perception should be reflected in alterations in ERP amplitude. The results of early studies showed varying and contradictory effects. Halliday and Mason (1964) and Amadeo and Yanovski (1975) found no effect of hypnotic hallucinations on the EEG, but studies by Clynes and associates (1964) and Wilson (1968) did. These studies were limited because of small sample sizes, nonquantitative analysis of EEGs,

| Table 89–11 | Neurophysiology of Hypnosis |
| --- | --- |

| Neurotransmitters |
| --- |
| High correlation between cerebrospinal fluid levels of homovanillic acid and hypnotizability. |

| Brain Electrical Activity |
| --- |
| Alpha laterality difference favoring the left hemisphere among highly hypnotizable individuals. |
| Theta power, especially in the right frontal region, best differentiates highly hypnotizable individuals from subjects with low hypnotizability. |
| Highly hypnotizable subjects experiencing a hypnotic hallucination revealed significant reductions in P300 amplitude of event-related potentials. |

limited use of hypnotizability testing, and use of subjects with comorbid neurological or psychiatric disorders.

On the other hand, new evidence suggests that highly hypnotizable subjects experiencing a hypnotic hallucination may alter their perception of an external stimulus with corresponding amplitude changes in the response evoked to an external stimulus (Clynes et al. 1964, Wilson 1968). Spiegel and colleagues (1985) found that highly hypnotizable subjects who experience a visual hallucination obstructing their view of a monitor showed significant reductions in P300 amplitude throughout the scalp and of N200 in the occipital region. This alteration occurred only in highly hypnotizable subjects in which a hallucination was suggested. It was not seen in any other hypnotic condition, and it was not evident among a group of subjects with low hypnotizability attempting to experience the same perceptual alteration.

Jasiukaitis and colleagues (unpublished data) replicated the results of Spiegel and coworkers (1985) with visual hypnotic obstruction but included an additional condition in which highly hypnotizable subjects were instructed to simply ignore half of their visual field (selective inattention) outside of the hypnotic trance. Both hypnotic obstruction and selective inattention reduced P100 and P300 peaks of visual evoked potential (Figure 89–4). However, the P200 peak differentiated hypnotic from nonhypnotic conditions. Hypnotic obstruction decreased P200, whereas selective inattention actually increased it. These results suggest that subjects performing positive hypnotic hallucination employ, to a degree, elements of inattention along with processes unique to hypnosis. Later, in new visual-ERP research, Jasiukaitis and colleagues (1996) implicated the left cerebral hemisphere in hypnotic perceptual alteration. He demonstrated a greater reduction of occipital P200 amplitude during hypnotic obstructive hallucination when visual stimuli were presented to the right visual field than

when they were presented to the left visual field, which demonstrates a stronger hypnotic effect of imagery in the left than the right occipital cortex.

The effect of auditory hallucination has been studied with similar results. Sigalowitz and colleagues (1991) found P300 differences among highly hypnotizable individuals hallucinating a reduction or increase in tones; subjects with low hypnotizability did not show such a change. The amplitude reduction did not reach statistical significance, but the increase during positive hallucination did. Crawford and colleagues (1996) studied the effect of hypnotic susceptibility levels on auditory event-related potentials (AERPs) and found that high hypnotizable individuals appeared to divert greater attentional processing to the tasks at hand and were also slower to respond to not-to-be-attended stimuli. These findings confirmed the hypothesis that hypnotic susceptibility is associated with efficient attentional processing such that highs can more effectively partition attention towards relevant stimuli and away from irrelevant stimuli than can low hypnotizables. Lamas and Valle-Inclan (1998) found that there were increases in reaction times and P300 latencies as a function of noise and spatial stimulus–response incompatibility (Simon effect), and that hypnotic suggestions decreased the response times for all types of trials nonsignificantly indicating a specific effect of hypnotic suggestions in the processing of hallucinated stimuli, which is consistent with the hallucinatory experience reported by the subjects.

A study by Barabasz and colleagues (1999) examined the effects of positive obstructive and negative obliterating instructions on simultaneous visual and auditory ERPs— P300 signals. Subjects were selected on the basis of high and low hypnotizability and were requested to perform identical tasks during waking and alert hypnotic conditions. The study found that highly hypnotizable subjects showed greater ERP amplitudes while experiencing negative

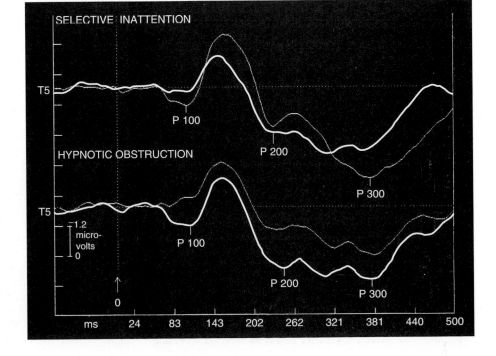

**Figure 89–4** *Grand mean (N = 22) visual evoked potentials to right visual field stimuli at electrode T₅. (Top) Dark waveform is the visual evoked potential while the visual field is attended. Light waveform is the visual evoked potential while the right visual field is ignored. (Bottom) Dark waveform is the visual evoked potential while the right visual field is not obstructed during hypnosis. Light waveform is the visual evoked potential while the right visual field is obstructed by positive hypnotic hallucination. Note that from 140 to 320 ms after the stimulus, hypnotic obstruction and selective inattention appear to exert opposite effects on the visual evoked potential.*

hallucinations and lower ERP amplitudes while experiencing positive obstructive hallucinations, in contrast with low hypnotizables and their own waking imagination-only conditions. These results constitute a rather robust physiological marker of hypnosis, an alteration in consciousness that correspond to participants' subjective experiences of perceptual alteration.

Hypnotically induced hallucinated experiences in other sensory modalities have yielded similar results. Similar to the use of hypnosis for pain control, hypnotic suggestions given to filter somatosensory (electrical) stimulation applied to peripheral nerves affect event-related potential amplitude. Suggestions of a tingling, cool, numbing sensation were given with the idea that it would filter out any other sensations in the area. This approach produced a significant reduction in P300 amplitude and also in P100 amplitude, suggesting earlier filtering of the somatosensory signal in the hypnotic hallucination condition. The interpretation of these data suggests that these subjects responded cortically as though the stimulus were less intense. When suggestions to increase attention to the stimuli were given, a significant increase in P100 but not in P300 amplitude were observed. This is further evidence that highly hypnotizable subjects were capable of producing bidirectional changes in ERP amplitude to sensory stimuli, depending on the cognitive task employed during hypnosis (Spiegel et al. 1989a). Subjects with low hypnotizability or volunteers trying to simulate these conditions were not able to reproduce these findings. De Pascalis and Carboni (1997) studied somatosensory target selection in women and found that highly hypnotizable subjects demonstrated significant suppression of P3 peak amplitude to target stimuli in the left frontal and posterior scalp sites during hypnotic obstructive hallucination as compared to a normal attention condition. The researchers concluded that hypnotically induced obstructive hallucination to somatosensory stimuli involve alterations in neural and autonomic responses which are consistent with a trait conception of hypnotizability. Crawford and colleagues (1998) studied the somatosensory responses under hypnotic analgesia of moderate to highly hypnotizable adults with chronic low back pain. They found that hypnotic analgesia led to highly significant mean reductions in perceived sensory pain and distress suggesting that this was an active process that required inhibitory effort, dissociated from conscious awareness, where the anterior frontal cortex participates in a topographically specific inhibitory feedback circuit that cooperates in the allocation of thalamocortical activities.

In a related topic, the somatosensory event-related potential (SERP) literature (Naatanen and Michie 1979) demonstrated the presence of a clearly defined response to SERP's selective attention, evidenced by a negative deflection 140 milliseconds after the stimulus was administered, known as the N140. This negative deflection is consistently seen as a response to selective attention to somatic stimulation (Allison 1982, Michie 1984, Naatanen and Michie 1979). While postulating that somatic conversion disorders may represent a form of selective attention (Maldonado 1996, 2001) Maldonado and Jasiukaitis (1996) set out to study a group of patients presenting with lateralized (i.e., unilateral) deficits using SERPs. If indeed these patients are constantly monitoring the affected body part or side, they should show an enhanced N140 on the affected side. This proved to be the case. They found that subjects exhibited a "normal N140" on the unaffected side (as expected in all "normal controls"), but an *enhanced* N140 on the affected side (Maldonado et al. 2000, Maldonado and Spiegel 2001). Even more remarkably, when the researchers provided suggestions for time regression (e.g., 2 weeks prior to the onset of symptoms) subjects experienced complete normalization of the SERP's response, showing only the "classic" N140 bilaterally (Figure 89–5).

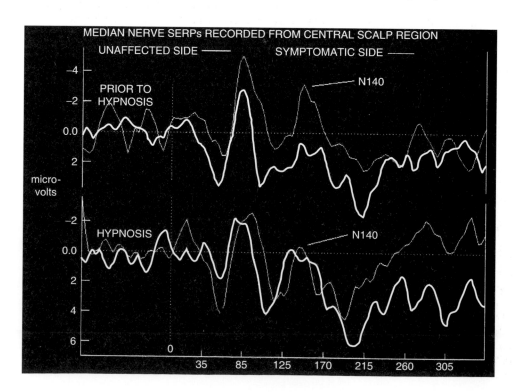

**Figure 89–5** *Somatosensory evoked potentials (SERPs) of a patient diagnosed with a lateralized conversion paralysis affecting the right side of the body. (Top) Baseline recording. The dark waveform represents the patient's response to electrical stimulation of the nonaffected side; the light waveform represents response to stimulation of the affected side. The affected side exhibits a larger N140 peak than the nonaffected side. (Bottom) Recording obtained during hypnosis. Suggestions were given for symptom resolution. The patient appeared clinically to have no neurological deficits. As above, dark and light waveforms represent nonaffected and affected sides, respectively. Under hypnosis, along with a resolution of symptoms observed, the N140 peaks for both sides are now equal.*

At the end of the trial, the SERP's tracing returned to the previous pattern; that is a classic N140 on the unaffected side and an enhanced N140 in the affected side. These findings suggest the possibility of an unconscious, auto-hypnotic model used by patients suffering from conversion disorder in order to create their symptoms.

## Brain Imaging

Despite the relatively limited research on hypnosis using newer brain imaging techniques such as positron emission tomography (PET), single photon emission computed tomography (SPECT), and magnetic resonance imaging (MRI) new data is slowly emerging. Ulich and associates (1987), using PET, have demonstrated a global increase in cerebral perfusion during hypnosis. There was no change observed during the use of autogenic training in normal subjects. Work using PET of the brain has led to the discovery that attentional processes can be subdivided into a series of components with different neuroanatomical localizations (Posner and Peterson 1990). The posterior attentional system involves orienting, with activation of the posterior or pre-striate cortex. Focusing of attention is associated with activity in the anterior cingulate gyrus. Arousal involves activity in the right frontal cortex. We have defined hypnosis as a state of focal attention and heightened concentration. Indeed, most studies demonstrate a significant correlation between hypnosis and alteration in amplitude of ERPs in similar regions of the brain.

These findings relate primarily to alterations involving the P300, with maximal changes over the frontal and central cortex. This suggests that during hypnosis, there is specific activation of the anterior attentional systems involving focusing (anterior cingulate) and arousal (frontal, especially on the right). Therefore, these imaging techniques may prove useful in identifying subsystems within the brain devoted to specific types of perceptual and cognitive processing in the hypnotic process.

In the last few years new studies shed further light into the neurophysiology of hypnotic phenomena. Rainville and coworkers (1997) demonstrated that hypnotic reduction of the perceived unpleasantness of a stimulus was associated with significant changes in pain-evoked activity within anterior cingulate but not somatosensory cortex in PET studies. PET scans were also used by Szechtman and colleagues (1998) to measure rCBF of highly hypnotizable subjects asked to produce vivid auditory hallucinations. They found that subjects capable of producing the hallucinations had increased rCBF in the right anterior cingulate gyrus. Of interest, the "externality" and "clarity" of the hallucinations were highly correlated with blood flow in this region.

Rainville and colleagues (1999) investigated the effects of hypnosis and suggestions to alter pain perception on the PET measured rCBF and the EEG measures of brain electrical activity, in highly hypnotizable subjects under different experimental conditions. Pain was induced by immersion of a hand in either water at room temperature or painfully hot water. The findings suggest that hypnosis was accompanied by significant increases in both occipital rCBF and delta EEG activity, which were highly correlated with each other ($r = 0.70$, $P < 0.0001$). Peak increases in rCBF were also observed in the caudal part of the right

anterior cingulate sulcus and bilaterally in the inferior frontal gyri. Hypnosis-related decreases in rCBF were found in the right inferior parietal lobule, the left precuneus, and the posterior cingulate gyrus. Hypnosis-with-suggestions produced additional widespread increases in rCBF in the frontal cortices predominantly on the left side. Moreover, the medial and lateral posterior parietal cortices showed suggestion-related increases overlapping partly with regions of hypnosis-related decreases. Results support a state theory of hypnosis in which occipital increases in rCBF and delta activity reflect the alteration of consciousness associated with decreased arousal and possible facilitation of visual imagery. Frontal increases in rCBF associated with suggestions for altered perception might reflect the verbal mediation of the suggestions, working memory, and top–down processes involved in the reinterpretation of the perceptual experience.

Hypnotic alteration of perception involves changes in primary sensory association cortex as demonstrated by Kosslyn and colleagues (2000). They obtained PET scans using $^{15}$O-CO$_2$ of highly hypnotizable subjects asked to see a colored pattern in color in a number of visual stimuli, included gray and white stimulus. Under hypnosis, both the left and right hemisphere color areas were activated when they were asked to perceive color, whether they were actually shown the color or the gray-scale stimulus; moreover, these brain regions had decreased activation when subjects were told to see the gray scale, whether they were actually shown the color or gray scale stimulus. Similarly Faymonville and coworkers (2000) used PET scans to identify the brain areas in which hypnosis modulates cerebral responses to noxious stimuli. They compared brain images of subjects in a hypnotic resting state with mental imagery and a hypnotic state with stimulation (warm nonnoxious versus hot noxious stimuli applied to right thenar eminence). Statistical parametric mapping demonstrated that noxious stimulation caused an increase in rCBF in the thalamic nuclei, anterior cingulate, and insular cortices. The hypnotic state induced a significant activation of a right-sided extra-striate area and the anterior cingulate cortex. The interaction analysis showed that the activity in the anterior (mid-) cingulate cortex was related to pain perception and unpleasantness differently in the hypnotic state than in control situations. Results also showed that hypnosis decreased both pain sensation and the unpleasantness of noxious stimuli and suggest that hypnotic modulation of pain is mediated by the anterior cingulate cortex.

Thus, the observed changes in subjective experience achieved while in a hypnotic state are reflected by changes in brain function similar to those that occur in perception. These findings suggest that hypnotic alteration of perception is more than mere compliance with suggestion, but rather it involves alteration in sensory experience.

## Conclusion

Hypnosis is a natural state of mind. As a trait, it can be measured and mastered. Even though it occurs naturally, not everybody has the same hypnotic capacity. It involves the ability to concentrate intensely, the capacity to receive new information, and the flexibility to change behavior. The capacity to experience hypnosis constitutes a therapeutic resource in the patient that can be mobilized by formal hypnosis during the therapy session and self-hypnosis exercises afterward. Strategies such as cognitive restructuring under hypnosis can help patients alter their perspective on their symptoms by experiencing symptom resolution as an occasion to enhance their sense of mastery. Many therapeutic approaches using hypnosis involve changing the patient's perspective on the relationship between the psychological and the physical state, dissociating mental from physical stress and suffering (i.e., pain), adopting a stance of protectiveness toward the body rather than fighting destructive urges (i.e., quality of life versus smoking), or learning to see sudden discontinuities in consciousness (i.e., flashbacks and episodes of dissociation) as understandable and controllable hypnotic phenomena.

Training patients in the use of self-hypnosis can facilitate the therapeutic process. This use of hypnosis can communicate the therapist's desire to enhance the patient's mastery and independence. Thus, patients can learn to use their hypnotic capacity rather than be used by it. This newly developed ability can be understood as an exercise in self-control rather than submission to the will of the therapist. It can be used to enhance control of somatic processes, reactions to anxiety-provoking stimuli, and impulsive behavior.

## References

Adams PC and Stenn PG (1992) Liver biopsy under hypnosis. J Clin Gastroenterol 15(2) (Sept), 122–124.

Allen JG and Smith WH (1993) Diagnosing dissociative disorders. Bull Menn Clin 57, 328–343.

Allison T (1982) Scalp and cortical recordings of initial somatosensory cortex to median nerve stimulation in man. In Evoked Potentials: Annals of the New York Academy of Sciences, Vol. 388, Bodis-Wollner I (ed). The New York Academy of Sciences, New York.

Amadeo M and Yanovski A (1975) Evoked potentials and selective attention in subjects capable of hypnotic analgesia. Int J Clin Exp Hypn 23, 200–210.

American Psychiatric Association (1994) Diagnostic and Statistical Manual of Mental Disorders, 4th ed. APA, Washington DC.

Anbar RD (2000) Self-hypnosis for patients with cystic fibrosis. Pediatr Pulmonol 30(6), 461–465.

Anbar RD (2001) Self-hypnosis for management of chronic dyspnea in pediatric patients. Pediatrics 107(2), E21.

Anderson MS (1985) Hypnotizability as a factor in the treatment of obesity. Int J Clin Exp Hypn 33, 150–159.

Andreychuk T and Skriver C (1975) Hypnosis and biofeedback in the treatment of migraine headache. Int J Clin Exp Hypn 23, 172–183.

Anonymous (1996) Integration of behavioral and relaxation approaches into the treatment of chronic pain and insomnia. NIH Technology Assessment Panel. JAMA 276(4), 313–318.

Arone di Bertolino R (1983) Hypnosis in dermatology. Minerva Med 74(51–52), 2969–2973.

Aronoff GM, Aronoff S, and Peck LW (1975) Hypnotherapy in the treatment of bronchial asthma. Ann Allergy 42, 356–362.

Bakan P (1969) Hypnotizability, laterality of eye movements and functional brain asymmetry. Percept Mot Skills 28, 927–932.

Baker EL (1983) The use of hypnotic dreaming in the treatment of the borderline patient: Some thoughts on resistance and transitional phenomena. Int J Clin Exp Hypn 31, 19–27.

Barabasz A, Baer L, Sheehan DV, et al. (1986) A three-year follow-up of hypnosis and restricted environmental stimulation therapy for smoking. Int J Clin Exp Hypn 34, 169–181.

Barabasz A, Barabasz M, Jensen S, et al. (1999) Cortical event-related potentials show the structure of hypnotic suggestions is crucial. Int J Clin Exp Hypn 47(1), 5–22.

Barabasz M and Spiegel D (1989) Hypnotizability and weight loss in obese subjects. Int J Eat Disord 8, 335–341.

Beecher HK (1956) Relationship of significance of wound to pain experienced. JAMA 161, 1609–1616.

Bell DS, Christian ST, and Clements RS Jr. (1983) Acuphobia in a long-standing insulin-dependent diabetic patient cured by hypnosis. Diabet Care 6(6), 622.

Benhaiem JM, Attal N, Chauvin M, et al. (2001) Local and remote effects of hypnotic suggestions of analgesia. Pain 89(2–3), 167–173.

Berkowitz B, Ross-Townsend A, and Kohberger R (1979) Hypnotic treatment of smoking: The single-treatment method revisited. Am J Psychiatr 136, 83–85.

Bernheim H and Herter CA (trans) (1964) Hypnosis and Suggestion in Psychotherapy: A Treatise on the Nature of Hypnotism. University Books, New Hyde Park, NY. (Originally published in 1889)

Bliss EL (1980) Multiple personalities: A report of 14 cases with implications for schizophrenia and hysteria. Arch Gen Psychiatr 37, 1388–1397.

Bliss EL (1984) Hysteria and hypnosis. J Nerv Ment Dis 172, 203–206.

Bliss EL (1986) Multiple Personality Allied Disorders and Hypnosis. Oxford University, New York.

Bloch B (1927) Über die Heilung de Warzen durch Suggestion. Klin Wochenschr 6, 2271–2275.

Bodden JL (1991) Accessing state-bound memories in the treatment of phobias: Two case studies. Am J Clin Hypn 34, 24–28.

Bower GH (1981) Mood and memory. Am Psychol 36, 129–148.

Braid J (1843) Neurohypnology, or the Rationale of Nervous Sleep Considered in Relation with Animal Magnetism, Illustrated by Numerous Cases of Its Successful Application in the Relief and Cure of Disease. John Churchill, London.

Braun BG and Sachs RG (1985) The development of multiple personality disorder: Predisposing, precipitating, and perpetuating factors. In Childhood Antecedents of Multiple Personality, Kluft RP (ed). American Psychiatric Press, Washington DC, pp. 37–64.

Bremner JD and Brett E (1997) Trauma-related dissociative states and long-term psychopathology in posttraumatic stress disorder. J Traum Stress 10, 37–49.

Breuer J and Freud S (1955) Studies on hysteria. In The Standard Edition of the Complete Psychological Works of Sigmund Freud, Vol. 2, Strachey J (trans-ed). Hogarth Press, London, pp. 1–309.

Brose WG and Spiegel D (1992) Neuropsychiatric aspects of pain management. In The American Psychiatric Press Textbook of Neuropsychiatry, 2nd ed., Yudofsky SC and Hales RE (eds). American Psychiatric Press, Washington DC, pp. 245–275.

Bryant RA, Guthrie RM, and Moulds ML (2001) Hypnotizability in acute stress disorder. Am J Psychiatr 158(4), 600–604.

Butler LD, Duran RE, Jasiukaitis P, et al. (1996) Hypnotizability and traumatic experience: A diathesis-stress model of dissociative symptomatology. Am J Psychiatr 153(Suppl 7), 42–63.

Cadranel JF, Benhamou Y, Zylberberg P, et al. (1994) Hypnotic relaxation: A new sedative tool for colonoscopy? J Clin Gastroenterol 18, 127–129.

California Legislature: AB 2669 Chapter 7 (1985) Hypnosis of Witnesses, added to Chapter 7, Division 6 of the Evidence Code, Enacted January 1.

Cardeña E and Spiegel D (1993) Dissociative reactions to the Bay Area earthquake. Am J Psychiatr 150, 474–478.

Carlson EB and Putnam FW (1989) Integrating research on dissociation and hypnotizability: Are there two pathways to hypnotizability? Dissociation 2, 32–38.

Chandler T (1996) Techniques for optimizing MRI relaxation and visualization. Admin Radiol J 15, 16–18.

Charcot JM (1890) Oeuvres Completes de JM Charcot, Tome IX. Lecrosnier et Babe, Paris.

Chu DA and Dill DL (1990) Dissociative symptoms in relation to childhood physical and sexual abuse. Am J Psychiatr 147, 887–892.

Clarke PS (1970) Effects of emotion and cough on airways obstruction in asthma. Med J Austral 1(11), 535–537.

Classen C, Koopman C, and Spiegel D (1993) Trauma and dissociation. Bull Menn Clin 2, 179–194.

Clynes M, Kohn M, and Lifshitz K (1964) Dynamics and spatial behavior of light-evoked potentials, their modification under hypnosis, and on-line correlation in relation to rhythmic components. Ann NY Acad Sci 112, 468–509.

Colgan SM, Faragher EB, and Whorwell PJ (1988) Controlled trial of hypnotherapy in relapse prevention of duodenal ulceration. Lancet 1, 1299–1300.

Collison DR (1975) Which asthmatic patients should be treated by hypnotherapy? Med J 1, 776–781.

Conn L and Mott T Jr. (1984) Plethysmographic demonstration of rapid vasodilation by direct suggestion: A case of Raynaud's disease treated by hypnosis. Am J Clin Hypn 26(3), 166–170.

Coons PM and Milstein V (1986) Psychosexual disturbances in multiple personality: Characteristics, etiology, and treatment. J Clin Psychiatr 47, 106–110.

Coons PM, Bowman ES, and Pellow TA (1989) Posttraumatic aspects of the treatment of victims of sexual abuse and incest. Psychiatr Clin N Am 12, 325–337.

Copeland DR (1986) The application of object relations theory to the hypnotherapy of developmental arrests: The borderline patient. Int J Clin Exp Hypn 34, 157–168.

Copeland MD and Kitching EH (1937) Hypnosis in mental hospital practice. J Ment Sci 83, 316–329.

Covino NA and Bottari M (2001) Hypnosis, behavioral theory, and smoking cessation. J Dent Educ 65(4), 340–347.

Covino NA and Frankel FH (1993) Hypnosis and relaxation in the medically ill. Psychother Psychosom 60, 75–90.

Covino NA, Jimerson DC, Wolfe BE, et al. (1994) Hypnotizability, dissociation, and bulimia nervosa. J Abnorm Psychol 103, 455–459.

Crasilneck HD and Hall JA (1985) Clinical Hypnosis: Principles and Applications, 2nd ed. Grune & Stratton, New York.

Crawford HJ, Corby JC, and Kopell BS (1996) Auditory event-related potentials while ignoring tone stimuli: Attentional differences reflected in stimulus intensity and latency responses in low and highly hypnotizable persons. Int J Neurosci 85(1–2), 57–69.

Crawford HJ, Knebel T, Kaplan L, et al. (1998) Hypnotic analgesia: 1. Somatosensory event-related potential changes to noxious stimuli and 2. Transfer learning to reduce chronic low back pain. Int J Clin Exp Hypn 46(1), 92–132.

Dash J (1981) Rapid hypno-behavioral treatment of a needle phobia in a 5-year-old cardiac patient. J Pediatr Psychol 6(1) (Mar), 37–42.

De Pascalis V and Carboni G (1997) P300 event-related-potential amplitudes and evoked cardiac responses during hypnotic alteration of somatosensory perception. Int J Neurosci 92(3–4), 187–207.

Diamond BL (1980) Inherent problems in the use of pretrial hypnosis on a prospective witness. Calif Law Rev 68, 313–349.

Dywan S and Bowers KS (1983) The use of hypnosis to enhance recall. Science 222, 184–185.

Edmonston WE Jr. and Grotevant WR (1975) Hypnosis and alpha density. Am J Clin Hypn 17(4), 221–232.

Edmonston WE Jr. and Moscovitz HC (1990) Hypnosis and lateralized brain functions. Int J Clin Exp Hypn 38(1), 70–84.

Ellenberger H (1970) The Discovery of the Unconscious. Basic Books, New York.

Elliotson J (1843) Numerous Cases of Surgical Operations Without Pain in the Mesmeric State. Lea & Blanchard, Philadelphia.

Ellis JA and Spanos NP (1994) Cognitive–behavioral interventions for children's distress during bone marrow aspirations and lumbar punctures: A critical review. J Pain Sympt Manag 9, 96–108.

Erdelyi MH and Kleinbard J (1978) Has Ebbinghaus decayed with time? The growth of recall (hypermnesia) over days. J Exp Psychol Hum Learn Mem 4, 275–289.

Erickson MH and Haley J (eds) (1967) Advanced Techniques of Hypnosis and Therapy. Selected Papers of Milton H. Erickson, M.D. Grune & Stratton, New York.

Eriksson NG and Lundin T (1996) Early traumatic stress reactions among Swedish survivors of the Estonia disaster. Br J Psychiatr 169, 713–716.

Esdaile J (1846) Mesmerism in India and Its Practical Applications in Surgery and Medicine. Longmans, Brown, Green & Longmans, London.

Esdaile J (1957) Hypnosis in Medicine and Surgery. Julian Press, New York. (Originally published in 1846)

Evans FJ and Staats JM (1989) Suggested posthypnotic amnesia in four diagnostic groups of hospitalized psychiatric patients. Am J Clin Hypn 32, 27–35.

Ewer TC and Stewart DE (1986) Improvement in bronchial hyper-responsiveness in patients with moderate asthma after treatment with a hypnotic technique: A randomized controlled trial. Br Med J Clin Res 293, 1129–1132.

Ewin DM (1992) Hypnotherapy for warts (verruca vulgaris): 41 consecutive cases with 33 cures. Am J Clin Hypn 35, 1–10.

Faymonville ME, Fissette J, Mambourg PH, et al. (1995) Hypnosis as adjunct therapy in conscious sedation for plastic surgery. Reg Anesth 20, 145–151.

Faymonville ME, Laureys S, Degueldre C, et al. (2000) Neural mechanisms of antinociceptive effects of hypnosis. Anesthesiology 92(5), 1257–1267.

Fourmestraux I (1934) Histoire de la Chirurgie Française (1790–1920). Masson, Paris.

Fox PA, Henderson DC, Barton SE, et al. (1999) Immunological markers of frequently recurrent genital herpes simplex virus and their response to hypnotherapy: A pilot study. Int J STD AIDS 10(11), 730–734.

Francis CY and Houghton LA (1996) Use of hypnotherapy in gastro-intestinal disorders. Eur J Gastroenterol Hepatol 8, 525–529.

Frank RG, Umlauf RL, Wonderlich SA, et al. (1986) Hypnosis and behavioral treatment in a worksite smoking cessation program. Addict Behav 11, 59–62.

Frankel FH and Orne MT (1976) Hypnotizability and phobic behavior. Arch Gen Psychiatr 33, 1259–1261.

Freeman R, Barabasz A, Barabasz M, et al. (2000) Hypnosis and distraction differ in their effects on cold pressor pain. Am J Clin Hypn 43(2), 137–148.

Freud A (1946) The Ego and Mechanisms of Defense. International Universities Press, New York.

Freud S (1958) Remembering, repeating, and working-through (further recommendations on the technique of psycho-analysis II). In The Standard Edition of the Complete Psychological Works of Sigmund Freud, Vol. 12, Strachey J (trans-ed). Hogarth Press, London, pp. 145–156. (Originally published in 1914)

Frid M and Singer G (1979) Hypnotic analgesia in conditions of stress is partially reversed by naloxone. Psychopharmacology (Berl) 61, 211–215.

Frischholz EJ (1985) The relationship among dissociation, hypnosis, and child abuse in the development of multiple personality disorder. In Childhood Antecedents of Multiple Personality Disorder, Kluft RP (ed). American Psychiatric Press, Washington DC, pp. 99–126.

Frischholz EJ, Lipman LS, Braun BG, et al. (1992) Psychopathology, hypnotizability, and dissociation. Am J Psychiatr 149, 1521–1525.

Frischholz EJ, Spiegel D, Spiegel H, et al. (1982) Differential hypnotic responsivity of smokers, phobics, and chronic pain control patients: A failure to confirm. J Abnorm Psychol 91, 269–272.

Gemignani A, Santarcangelo E, Sebastiani L, et al. (2000) Changes in autonomic and EEG patterns induced by hypnotic imagination of aversive stimuli in man. Brain Res Bull 53(1), 105–111.

Genuis ML (1995) The use of hypnosis in helping cancer patients control anxiety, pain, and emesis: A review of recent empirical studies. Am J Clin Hypn 37, 316–325.

Gerschman J, Burrows GD, and Reade P (1987) Hypnotizability and dental phobic disorders. Int J Psychosom 34, 42–47.

Glick BS (1970) Conditioning therapy with phobic patients. Success and failure. Am J Psychother 24, 92–101.

Gluzman SA and Zisel'son AD (1989) Psychotherapy of bronchial asthma in children. Pediatriia 5, 107–108.

Goldstein E and Hilgard E (1975) Failure of opiate antagonist naloxone to modify hypnotic analgesia. Proc Natl Acad Sci USA 71, 1041–1043.

Grabowska MJ (1971) The effect of hypnosis and hypnotic suggestions on the blood flow in the extremities. Pol Med J 10, 1044–1051.

Graffin NF, Ray WJ, and Lundy R (1995) EEG concomitants of hypnosis and hypnotic susceptibility. J Abnorm Psychol 104, 123–131.

Greenleaf M, Fisher S, Miaskowski C, et al. (1992) Hypnotizability and recovery from cardiac surgery. Am J Clin Hypn 35, 119–128.

Gritz E and Bloom J (1987) Psychosocial sequelae of cancer in longterm survivors and their families. Presented at the Western Regional Conference of American Cancer Society (Jan), Los Angeles, CA.

Gur RE and Rehyer J (1973) Relationship between style of hypnotic induction and direction of lateral eye movements. J Abnorm Psychol 82, 499–505.

Gysin T (1999) Clinical hypnotherapy/self-hypnosis for unspecified, chronic and episodic headache without migraine and other defined headaches in children and adolescents. Forschende Komplementarmedizin 1(Suppl 6), 44–46.

Hackman RM, Stern JS, and Gershwin ME (2000) Hypnosis and asthma: A critical review. J Asthma 37(1), 1–15.

Halliday AM and Mason AA (1964) Cortical evoked potentials during hypnotic anaesthesia. Electroencephalogr Clin Neurophysiol 16, 312–314.

Hammarstrand G, Berggren U, and Hakeberg M (1995) Psychophysiological therapy v. hypnotherapy in the treatment of patients with dental phobia. Eur J Oral Sci 103, 399–404.

Hilgard ER (1965) Hypnotic Susceptibility. Harcourt, Brace & World, New York.

Hilgard ER (1970a) Toward a neo-dissociation theory: Multiple controls in human functioning. Persp Biol Med 17, 301–316.

Hilgard JR (1970b) Personality and Hypnosis: A Study of Imaginative Involvement. University of Chicago Press, Chicago.

Hilgard ER (1977) Divided Consciousness: Multiple Controls in Human Thought and Action. John Wiley, New York.

Hilgard ER (1984) The hidden observer and multiple personality. Int J Clin Exp Hypn 32, 248–253.

Hilgard ER and Hilgard JR (1975) Hypnosis in the Relief of Pain. William Kaufmann, Los Altos, CA.

Hilgard JR and LeBaron S (1982) Relief of anxiety and pain in children and adolescents with cancer: Quantitative measures and clinical observations. Int J Clin Exp Hypn 30, 417–442.

Holroyd J (1980) Hypnosis treatment for smoking: An evaluative review. Int J Clin Exp Hypn 28, 341–357.

Holroyd J (1991) The uncertain relationship between hypnotizability and smoking treatment outcome. Int J Clin Exp Hypn 39, 93–102.

Houghton LA, Heyman DJ, and Whorwell PJ (1996) Symptomatology, quality of life and economic features of irritable bowel syndrome—the effect of hypnotherapy. Aliment Pharmacol Ther 10, 91–95.

Hyman GJ, Stanley RO, Burrows GD, et al. (1986) Treatment effectiveness of hypnosis and behavior therapy in smoking cessation: A methodological refinement. Addict Behav 11, 355–365.

Inoue H, Kobayashi H, and Chiba T (1995) Classification for bronchial asthma from the viewpoint of autonomic nerve function and airway hyperreactivity (in Japanese). Nippon Kyobu Shikkan Gakkai Zasshi 33(Suppl), 104–105.

Iserson KV (1999) Hypnosis for pediatric fracture reduction. J Emerg Med 17(1) (Jan–Feb), 53–56.

Jacknow DS, Tschann JM, Link MP, et al. (1994) Hypnosis in the prevention of chemotherapy-related nausea and vomiting in children: A prospective study. J Dev Behav Pediatr 15, 258–264.

James W (1902) Varieties of Religious Experiences. Random House, New York.

Janet P (1920) The Major Symptoms of Hysteria. Macmillan, New York.

Jasiukaitis P, Nouriani B, and Spiegel D (1996) Left hemisphere superiority for event-related potential effects of hypnotic obstruction. Neuropsychologia 34(7), 661–668.

Jasiukaitis P, Nouriani B, Hugdahl K, et al. (1997) Relateralizing hypnosis: Or, have we been barking up the wrong hemisphere? Int J Clin Exp Hypn 45(2), 158–177.

Johnson RFQ and Barber TX (1978) Hypnosis, suggestions and warts: An experimental investigation implicating the importance of "believed-in efficacy." Am J Clin Hypn 20, 165–174.

Kantor SD (1990) Stress and psoriasis. Cutis 46(4), 321–322.

Kardiner A and Spiegel H (1947) War Stress and Neurotic Illness. Paul Hoeber, New York.

Katz RL, Kao CY, Spiegel H, et al. (1974) Pain, acupuncture, and hypnosis. Adv Neurol 4, 819–825.

Keane TM and Wolfe J (1990) Comorbidity in posttraumatic stress disorder: An analysis of community and clinical studies. J Appl Soc Psychol 20, 1776–1788.

Kellerman J, Zeltzer L, Ellenberg L, et al. (1983) Adolescents with cancer. Hypnosis for the reduction of the acute pain and anxiety associated with medical procedures. Adolesc Health Care 4(2) (June), 85–90.

Kelly E and Zeller B (1969) Asthma and the psychiatrist. J Psychosom Res 13(4), 377–395.

Kessler R and Dane JR (1996) Psychological and hypnotic preparation for anesthesia and surgery: An individual differences perspective. Int J Clin Exp Hypn 44, 189–207.

Kilhstrom JF (1984) Conscious, subconscious, unconscious: A cognitive perspective. In The Unconscious Reconsidered, Bowers KS and Meichenbaum D (eds). John Wiley, New York, pp. 149–211.

Kirsch I (1996) Hypnotic enhancement of cognitive–behavioral weight loss treatments—another meta-reanalysis. J Consult Clin Psychol 64, 517–519.

Kirsch I, Montgomery G, and Sapirstein G (1995) Hypnosis as an adjunct to cognitive–behavioral psychotherapy: A meta-analysis. J Consult Clin Psychol 63, 214–220.

Kistler A, Mariauzouls C, Wyler F, et al. (1999) Autonomic responses to suggestions for cold and warmth in hypnosis. Forschende Komplementarmedizin 6(1), 10–14.

Klein KB and Spiegel D (1989) Modulation of gastric acid secretion by hypnosis. Gastroenterology 96, 1383–1387.

Kluft RP (1984) Treatment of multiple personality disorder. Psychiatr Clin N Am 7, 9–29.

Kluft RP (ed) (1985a) Childhood antecedents of multiple personality. In Clinical Insights. American Psychiatric Press, Washington DC.

Kluft RP (ed) (1985b) Childhood multiple personality disorder: Predictors, clinical findings, and treatment results. In Childhood Antecedents of Multiple Personality Disorder. American Psychiatric Press, Washington DC, pp. 167–196.

Kluft RP (ed) (1990) Incest-Related Syndromes of Adult Psychopathology. American Psychiatric Press, Washington DC.

Kluft RP (1991) Clinical presentations of multiple personality disorder. Psychiatr Clin N Am 14, 605–629.

Kluft RP (1992) The use of hypnosis with dissociative disorders. Psychiatr Med 10, 31–46.

Kluft RP (1993) Multiple personality disorder. In Dissociative Disorders: A Clinical Review, Spiegel D (ed). Sidran Press, Lutherville, MD.

Knox VJ and Shum K (1977) Reduction of cold-processor pain with acupuncture analgesia in high- and low-hypnotic subjects. J Abnorm Psychol 86, 639–643.

Kohen DP (1986) Application of relaxation/mental imagery (self-hypnosis) to the management of asthma: Report of behavioral outcomes of a two year, prospective controlled study. Am J Clin Hypn 34, 283–294.

Kohen DP (1987) A biobehavioral approach to managing childhood asthma. Child Today 16(2), 6–10.

Kohen DP and Wynne E (1997) Applying hypnosis in a preschool family asthma education program: Uses of storytelling, imagery, and relaxation. Am J Clin Hypn 39, 169–181.

Kohen DP, Olness KN, Colwell SO, et al. (1984) The use of relaxation-mental imagery (self-hypnosis) in the management of 505 pediatric behavioral encounters. J Dev Behav Pediatr 5, 21–25.

Koopman C, Classen C, Cardeña E, et al. (1995) When disaster strikes, acute stress disorder may follow. J Traum Stress 8, 29–46.

Kosslyn SM, Thompson WL, Costantini-Ferrando MF, et al. (2000) Hypnotic visual illusion alters color processing in the brain. Am J Psychiatr 157(8), 1279–1284.

Kranhold C, Baumann U, and Fichter M (1992) Hypnotizability in bulimic patients and controls. A pilot study. Eur Arch Psychiatr Clin Neurosci 242(2–3), 72–76.

Lamas JR and Valle-Inclan F (1998) Effects of a negative visual hypnotic hallucination on ERP's and reaction times. Int J Psychophysiol 29(1), 77–82.

Lambert SA (1996) The effects of hypnosis/guided imagery on the postoperative course of children. J Dev Behav Pediatr 17, 307–310.

Lang EV, Joyce JS, Spiegel D, et al. (1996) Self-hypnotic relaxation during interventional radiological procedures: Effects on pain perception and intravenous drug use. Int J Clin Exp Hypn 44, 106–119.

Laurence JR and Perry C (1983) Hypnotically created memory among highly hypnotizable subjects. Science 222, 523–524.

Lavoie G and Elie R (1985) The clinical relevance of hypnotizability in psychosis: With reference to thinking processes and sample variances. In Modern Trends in Hypnosis, Waxman D, Misra P, Gibson M, et al. (eds). Plenum Press, New York, pp. 41–66.

Lavoie G and Sabourin M (1980) Hypnosis and schizophrenia: A review of experimental and clinical studies. In Handbook of Hypnosis and Psychosomatic Medicine, Burrows GD and Dennerstein L (eds). Elsevier/North-Holland, Amsterdam, pp. 377–420.

Lazarus AA (1973) "Hypnosis" as a facilitator in behavior therapy. Int J Clin Exp Hypn 21, 25–31.

Liossi C and Hatira P (1999) Clinical hypnosis versus cognitive behavioral training for pain management with pediatric cancer patients undergoing bone marrow aspirations. Int J Clin Exp Hypn 47(2), 104–116.

Lu DP (1994) The use of hypnosis for smooth sedation induction and reduction of postoperative violent emergencies from anesthesia in pediatric dental patients. ASDC J Dent Child 61, 182–185.

Lu DP and Lu GP (1999) Clinical management of needle-phobia patients requiring acupuncture therapy. Acupunc Electro-Therap Res 24(3–4), 189–201.

Luparello T, Lyons HA, Bleecker ER, et al. (1968) Influences of suggestion on airway reactivity in asthmatic subjects. Psychosom Med 30(6), 819–825.

Maher-Loughan GP (1970) Hypnosis and autohypnosis for the treatment of asthma. Int J Clin Exp Hypn 18, 1–14.

Maldonado JR (1996) Physiological correlates of conversion disorders. Paper presented at the 149th Annual Meeting of the American Psychiatric Association (May) New York.

Maldonado JR (2001) Reviews in Psychiatry: Conversion disorder. Paper presented at the 154th annual meeting of the American Psychiatric Association (May) New Orleans, LA.

Maldonado JR and Jasiukaitis P (1996) Psychological and physiological factors in the production of conversion disorder. Paper presented at the annual meeting of the Society for Clinical and Experimental Hypnosis, Tampa, FL.

Maldonado JR and Spiegel D (1994) Treatment of posttraumatic stress disorder. In Dissociation: Clinical, Theoretical and Research Perspectives, Lynn SJ and Rhue J (eds). Guilford Press, New York, pp. 215–241.

Maldonado JR and Spiegel D (1995) Using hypnosis. In Treating Women Molested in Childhood, Classen C (ed). Jossey-Bass, San Francisco, pp. 163–186.

Maldonado JR and Spiegel D (2000) Conversion disorder. In Review of Psychiatry, Vol. 20, Somatoform and Factitious Disorders, Phillips KA (ed). American Psychiatric Press, Washington DC, pp. 95–128.

Maldonado JR and Spiegel D (2002a) Dissociative disorders. In Textbook of Psychiatry, 4th ed., Talbot J and Yudosky S (eds). American Psychiatric Press, Washington DC.

Maldonado JR and Spiegel D (2002b) Hypnosis. In Textbook of Psychiatry, 4th ed., Talbot J and Yudosky S (eds). American Psychiatric Press, Washington DC.

Maldonado JR, Butler L, and Spiegel D (2000) Treatment of dissociative disorders. In A Guide to Treatments That Work, 2nd ed., Nathan PE and Gorman JM (eds). Oxford University Press, New York, pp. 463–496.

Marks IM, Gelder MG, and Edwards G (1968) Hypnosis and desensitization for phobias: A controlled prospective trial. Br J Psychiatr 114, 1263–1274.

Matthews M and Flatt S (1999) The efficacy of hypnotherapy in the treatment of migraine. Nurs Std 14(7), 33–36.

Mauer MH, Burnett KF, Ouellette EA, et al. (1999) Medical hypnosis and orthopedic hand surgery: Pain perception, postoperative recovery, and therapeutic comfort. Int J Clin Exp Hypn 47(2), 144–161.

McConkey KM (1992) The effects of hypnotic procedures on remembering. In Contemporary Hypnosis Research, Fromm E and Nash MR (eds). Guilford Press, New York, pp. 405–426.

McFadden ER Jr., Luparello T, Lyons HA, et al. (1969) The mechanism of action of suggestion in the induction of acute asthma attacks. Psychosom Med 31(2), 134–143.

McFarlane AC (1986) Posttraumatic morbidity of a disaster: A study of cases presenting for psychiatric treatment. J Nerv Ment Dis 174, 4–13.

McFarlane AC (1988) The longitudinal course of posttraumatic morbidity: The range of outcomes and their predictors. J Nerv Ment Dis 176, 30–39.

McGlashan TD, Evans FJ, and Orne MT (1969) The nature of hypnotic analgesia and the placebo response to experimental pain. Psychosom Med 31, 227–246.

Menzies RG and Clarke JC (1993) The etiology of fear of heights and its relationship to severity and individual response patterns. Behav Res Ther 31, 355–365.

Meszaros I and Szabo C (1999) Correlation of EEG asymmetry and hypnotic susceptibility. Acta Physiol Hung 86(3–4), 259–263.

Meurisse M, Faymonville ME, Joris J, et al. (1996) Endocrine surgery by hypnosis. From fiction to daily clinical application. Ann Endocrinol 57(6), 494–501.

Meurisse M, Hamoir E, Defechereux T, et al. (1999) Bilateral neck exploration under hypnosedation: A new standard of care in primary hyperparathyroidism? Ann Surg 229(3), 401–408.

Michie P (1984) Selective attention effects on somatosensory event-related potentials. In Brain and Information: Event-Related Potentials, Karrer R, Cohen J, and Tueting P (eds). (Ann NY Acad Sci 425). The New York Academy of Sciences, NY.

Mishkin M and Murray EA (1994) Stimulus recognition. Curr Opin Neurobiol 4, 200–206.

Mize WL (1996) Clinical training in self-regulation and practical pediatric hypnosis: What pediatricians want pediatricians to know. J Dev Behav Pediatr 17, 317–322.

Montgomery GH, DuHamel KN, and Redd WH (2000) A meta-analysis of hypnotically induced analgesia: How effective is hypnosis? Int J Clin Exp Hypn 48(2), 138–153.

Moore R, Abrahamsen R, and Brodsgaard I (1996) Hypnosis compared with group therapy and individual desensitization for dental anxiety. Eur J Oral Sci 104, 612–618.

Moorefield CW (1971) The use of hypnosis and behavior therapy in asthma. Am J Clin Hypn 13(3), 162–168.

Morgan AH and Hilgard ER (1973) Age differences in susceptibility to hypnosis. Int J Clin Exp Hypn 21, 78–85.

Morgan AH, MacDonald H, and Hilgard ER (1974) EEG alpha: Lateral asymmetry related to task and hypnotizability. Psychophysiology 11, 275–282.

Morrison JB (1988) Chronic asthma and improvement with relaxation induced by hypnotherapy. J R Acad Med 81, 701–704.

Morse DR and Cohen BB (1983) Desensitization using meditation-hypnosis to control "needle" phobia in two dental patients. Anesth Prog 30(3) (May–June), 83–85.

Moskowitz L (1996) Psychological management of postsurgical pain and patient adherence. Hand Clin 12(1), 129–137.

Mun CT (1969) The value of hypnotherapy as an adjunct in the treatment of bronchial asthma. Sing Med J 10(3), 182–186.

Murray-Jobsis J (1991) An exploratory study of hypnotic capacity of schizophrenic and borderline patients in a clinical setting. Am J Clin Hypn 33, 150–160.

Myers JK, Weissman MM, Tischler GL, et al. (1984) Six-month prevalence of psychiatric disorders in three communities 1980 to 1982. Arch Gen Psychiatr 41, 959–967.

Naatanen R and Michie PT (1979) Early selective attention effects on the evoked potential. A critical review and interpretation. Biol Psychol 8, 81–136.

Nash MR and Lynn SJ (1986) Child abuse and hypnotic ability. Imagin Cogn Pers 5, 211–218.

Nemiah JC (1985) Dissociative disorders. In Comprehensive Textbook of Psychiatry, 4th ed., Kaplan H and Sadock B (eds). Williams & Wilkins, Baltimore, pp. 942–957.

Nugent WR, Carden NA, and Montgomery DJ (1984) Utilizing the creative unconscious in the treatment of hypodermic phobias and sleep disturbance. Am J Clin Hypn 26(3) (Jan), 201–205.

Ohrbach R, Patterson DR, Carrougher G, et al. (1998) Hypnosis after an adverse response to opioids in an ICU burn patient. Clin J Pain 14(2), 167–175.

Orne MT (1979) The use and misuse of hypnosis in court. Int J Clin Exp Hypn 27, 311–341.

Orne MT, Axelrad AD, Diamond BL, et al. (1985) Scientific status of refreshing recollection by the use of hypnosis. JAMA 253, 1918–1923.

Orne MT, Hilgard ER, Spiegel H, et al. (1979) The relation between the Hypnotic Induction Profile and the Stanford Hypnotic Susceptibility Scales, Forms A and C. Int J Clin Exp Hypn 27, 85–102.

Patterson DR, Adcock RJ, and Bombardier CH (1997) Factors predicting hypnotic analgesia in clinical burn pain. Int J Clin Exp Hypn 45(4), 377–395.

People v. Guerra (1984) 37 Cal. App. 3d 385, 208 Cal. Rptr. 162,690 P.2d Orange County Supreme Court, CA.

People v. Hughes (1983) 59 NY2d 523, 466 NYS2d 255, 543 NE2d, 484.

People v. Hurd (1980) NJ.

People v. Schoenfeld (1980) 168 Cal Rptr 762, 111 CA3d 671.

People v. Shirley (1982) 31 Cal 3d 18, 641 P2d 775, modified 918a (1982).

Peretz B (1996) Relaxation and hypnosis in pediatric dental patients. J Clin Pediatr Dent 20, 205–207.

Pettinati HM (1982) Measuring hypnotizability in psychotic patients. Int J Clin Exp Hypn 30, 404–416.

Pettinati HM, Kogan LG, Evans FJ, et al. (1990) Hypnotizability of psychiatric inpatients according to two different scales. Am J Psychiatr 147, 69–75.

Piccione C, Hilgard ER, and Zimbardo PG (1989) On the degree of stability of measured hypnotizability over a 25-year period. J Pers Soc Psychol 56, 289–295.

Posner MI and Peterson SE (1990) The attention system of the human brain. Annu Rev Neurosci 13, 25–42.

Prince M (1906) The Dissociation of a Personality. Longmans-Green, New York.

Putnam FW (1985) Dissociation as a response to extreme trauma. In Childhood Antecedents of Multiple Personality Disorder, Kluft RP (ed). American Psychiatric Press, Washington DC, pp. 65–97.

Putnam FW (1992) Using hypnosis for therapeutic abreactions. Psychiatr Med 10, 51–65.

Putman FW (1993) Dissociative disorders in children: Behavioral profiles and problems. Child Abuse Negl 17, 39–45.

Rainville P, Duncan GH, Price DD, et al. (1997) Pain affect encoded in human anterior cingulate but not somatosensory cortex. Science 277, 968–971.

Rainville P, Hofbauer RK, Paus T, et al. (1999) Cerebral mechanisms of hypnotic induction and suggestion. J Cogn Neurosci 11(1), 110–125.

Rape RN and Bush JP (1994) Psychological preparation for pediatric oncology patients undergoing painful procedures: A methodological critique of the research. Child Health Care 23, 51–67.

Redd WH, Andresen GV, and Minagawa RY (1982) Hypnotic control of anticipatory emesis in patients receiving cancer chemotherapy. J Consult Clin Psychol 50, 14–19.

Renouf D (1998) Hypnotically induced control of nausea: A preliminary report. J Psychosom Res 45(3), 295–296.

Robb ND and Crothers AJ (1996) Sedation in dentistry, part 2: Management of the gagging patient. Dent Update 23, 182–186.

Rodolfa ER, Kraft W, and Reilley RR (1990) Etiology and treatment of dental anxiety and phobia. Am J Clin Hypn 33, 22–28.

Rustvold SR (1994) Hypnotherapy for treatment of dental phobia in children. Gen Dent 42, 346–348.

Sabourin ME, Cutcomb SD, Crawford HJ, et al. (1990) EEG correlates of hypnotic susceptibility and hypnotic trance: Spectral analysis and coherence. Int J Psychophysiol 10, 125–142.

Sanders B and Giolas MH (1991) Dissociation and childhood trauma in psychologically disturbed adolescents. Am J Psychiatr 148, 50–54.

Sandrini G, Milanov I, Malaguti S, et al. (2000) Effects of hypnosis on diffuse noxious inhibitory controls. Physiol Behav 69(3), 295–300.

Schacter DL (1987) Implicit memory: History and current status. J Exp Psychol Learn Mem Cogn 13, 501–518.

Schwartz JL (1987) Smoking Cessation Methods: United States and Canada 1978–85. Division of Cancer Prevention and Control Publication NIH 87-2940, National Cancer Institute, Washington DC.

Shaw AJ and Niven N (1996) Theoretical concepts and practical applications of hypnosis in the treatment of children and adolescents with dental fear and anxiety. Br Dent J 180, 11–16.

Shaw AJ and Welbury RR (1996) The use of hypnosis in a sedation clinic for dental extractions in children: Report of 20 cases. ASDC J Dent Child 63, 418–420.

Sidis B and Goodhart SP (1905) Multiple Personality. Appleton-Century-Crofts.

Sigalowitz SJ, Dywan J, and Ismailos L (1991) Electrocortical evidence that hypnotically-induced hallucinations are experienced. Presented at the Society for Clinical and Experimental Hypnosis Meeting as part of a symposium entitled Dissociations in Conscious Experience: Electrophysical and Behavioural Evidence, October (9–13), New Orleans, LA.

Sjoberg BM and Hollister LE (1965) The effects of psychotomimetic drugs on primary suggestibility. Psychopharmacologia 8, 251–262.

Smith MM, Colebatch HJ, and Clarke PS (1970) Increase and decrease in pulmonary resistance with hypnotic suggestion in asthma. Am Rev Respir Dis 102(2), 236–242.

Smith WH (1990) Hypnosis in the treatment of anxiety. Bull Menn Clin 54, 209–216.

Snape WJ Jr. (1994) Current concepts in the management of the irritable bowel syndrome. Rev Gastroenterol Mex 59(2), 127–132.

Solomon Z, Mikulincer M, and Benbenishty R (1989) Combat stress reaction: Clinical manifestations and correlates. Mil Psychol 1, 35–47.

Spanos NP, Stenstrom RJ, and Johnston JC (1988) Hypnosis, placebo and suggestion in the treatment of warts. Psychosom Med 50, 245–260.

Spanos NP, Williams V, and Gwynn MI (1990) Effects of hypnotic, placebo, and salicylic acid treatments on warts regression. Psychosom Med 52, 109–114.

Spiegel D (1980a) Hypnotizability and psychoactive medication. Am J Clin Hypn 22, 217–222.

Spiegel D (1981) Vietnam grief work using hypnosis. Am J Clin Hypn 24, 33–40.

Spiegel D (1984) Multiple personality as a posttraumatic stress disorder. Psychiatr Clin N Am 7, 101–110.

Spiegel D (1986) Dissociating damage. Am J Clin Hypn 29, 123–131.

Spiegel D (1988) Dissociation and hypnosis in posttraumatic stress disorder. J Traum Stress 1, 17–33.

Spiegel D (1989) Hypnosis in the treatment of victims of sexual abuse. Psychiatr Clin N Am 12, 295–305.

Spiegel D (1990) Hypnosis, dissociation and trauma: Hidden and overt observers. In Repression and Dissociation, Singer JL (ed). University of Chicago Press, Chicago, pp. 121–142.

Spiegel D (1992) The use of hypnosis in the treatment of PTSD. Psychiatr Med 10, 21–30.

Spiegel D and Albert L (1983) Naloxone fails to reverse hypnotic alleviation of chronic pain. Psychopharmacology (Berl) 81, 140–143.

Spiegel D and Bloom JR (1983) Group therapy and hypnosis reduce metastatic breast carcinoma pain. Psychosom Med 45, 333–339.

Spiegel D and Cardeña E (1991) Disintegrated experience: The dissociative disorders revisited. J Abnorm Psychol 100, 366–378.

Spiegel D and Fink R (1979) Hysterical psychosis and hypnotizability. Am J Psychiatr 136, 777–781.

Spiegel D and King R (1992) Hypnotizability and CSF HVA levels among psychiatric patients. Biol Psychiatr 31, 95–98.

Spiegel D and Scheflin AW (1994) Dissociated or fabricated? Psychiatric aspects of repressed memory in criminal and civil cases. Int J Clin Exp Hypn 42, 411–432.

Spiegel D and Spiegel H (1986) Forensic uses of hypnosis. In Handbook of Forensic Psychology, Weiner IB and Hess AK (eds). John Wiley, New York, pp. 490–507.

Spiegel D and Vermutten E (1994) Physiological correlates of hypnosis and dissociation. In Dissociation: Culture, Mind and Body, Spiegel D (ed). American Psychiatric Press, Washington DC, pp. 185–209.

Spiegel D, Bierre P, and Rootenberg J (1989a) Hypnotic alteration of somatosensory perception. Am J Psychiatr 146, 749–754.

Spiegel D, Bloom JR, and Yalom ID (1981a) Group support for patients with metastatic cancer: A randomized prospective outcome study. Arch Gen Psychiatr 38, 527–533.

Spiegel D, Cutcomb S, Ren C, et al. (1985) Hypnotic hallucination alters evoked potentials. J Abnorm Psychol 94, 249–255.

Spiegel D, Detrick D, and Frischholz EJ (1982) Hypnotizability and psychopathology. Am J Psychiatr 139, 431–437.

Spiegel D, Frischholz EJ, Lipman LS, et al. (1989b) Dissociation, hypnotizability and trauma. Presented at the annual meeting of the American Psychiatric Association, San Francisco, CA.

Spiegel D, Frischholz EJ, Maruffi B, et al. (1981b) Hypnotic responsivity and the treatment of flying phobia. Am J Clin Hypn 23, 239–247.

Spiegel D, Hunt T, and Dondershine H (1988) Dissociation and hypnotizability in posttraumatic stress disorder. Am J Psychiatr 145, 301–305.

Spiegel H (1970) Termination of smoking by a single treatment. Arch Environ Health 20, 736–742.

Spiegel H (1974) The Grade 5 Syndrome. The highly hypnotizable person. Int J Clin Exp Hypn 22, 303–319.

Spiegel H (1980b) Hypnosis and evidence: Help or hindrance? Ann NY Acad Sci 347, 73–85.

Spiegel H and Spiegel D (1978) Trance and Treatment: Clinical Uses of Hypnosis. Basic Books, New York. (Reprinted 1987 American Psychiatric Press, Washington DC)

Spinhoven P and ter Kuile MM (2000) Treatment outcome expectancies and hypnotic susceptibility as moderators of pain reduction in patients with chronic tension-type headache. Int J Clin Exp Hypn 48(3), 290–305.

State ex rel Collins v. Superior Court (1982) 132 Ariz 180, 644 P2d 1266. Supplemental opinion filed May 4, 1982.

Steele K and Irwin WG (1988) Treatment options for cutaneous warts in family practice. Fam Pract 5(4), 314–319.

Steggles S (1999) The use of cognitive–behavioral treatment including hypnosis for claustrophobia in cancer patients. Am J Clin Hypn 41(4), 319–326.

Steingard S and Frankel FH (1985) Dissociation and psychotic symptoms. Am J Psychiatr 142, 953–955.

Stern DL, Spiegel H, and Nee JCM (1979) The Hypnotic Induction Profile: Normative observations, reliability, and validity. Am J Clin Hypn 21, 109–132.

Stradling J, Roberts D, Wilson A, et al. (1998) Controlled trial of hypnotherapy for weight loss in patients with obstructive sleep apnoea. Int J Obes Rel Metab Disord 22(3), 278–281.

Stuntman RK and Bliss EL (1985) Posttraumatic stress disorder, hypnotizability and imagery. Am J Psychiatr 142, 741–743.

Szechtman H, Woody E, Bowers KS, et al. (1998) Where the imaginal appears real: A positron emission tomography study of auditory hallucinations. Proc Natl Acad Sci 95, 1956–1960.

Tausk F and Whitmore SE (1999) A pilot study of hypnosis in the treatment of patients with psoriasis. Psychother Psychosom 68(4), 221–225.

Tellegen A (1981) Practicing the two disciplines for relaxation and enlightenment: Comment on "Role of the Feedback Signal in Electromyograph Biofeedback: The Relevance of Attention," by Qualls and Sheegan. J Exp Psychol Gen 110, 217–226.

Tellegen A and Atkinson G (1974) Openness to absorbing and self-altering experiences ("absorption"), a trait related to hypnotic susceptibility. J Abnorm Psychol 83, 268–277.

Terr LC (1991) Childhood traumas: An outline and overview. Am J Psychiatr 148, 10–20.

Ulich P, Meyer HJ, Biehl B, et al. (1987) Cerebral blood flow in autogenic training and hypnosis. Neurosurg Rev 10, 305–307.

van der Kolk BA and van der Hart O (1989) Pierre Janet and the breakdown of adaptation in psychological trauma. Am J Psychiatr 146, 1530–1540.

Vidakovic-Vukic M (1999) Hypnotherapy in the treatment of irritable bowel syndrome: Methods and results in Amsterdam. Scand J Gastroenterol 230(Suppl), 49–51.

Watkins JG (1987) Hypnotherapeutic Technique: The Practice of Clinical Hypnosis. Irvington Publishers, New York.

Weinstein EJ and Au PK (1991) Use of hypnosis before and during angioplasty. Am J Clin Hypn 34, 29–37.

Weitzenhoffer AM and Hilgard ER (1959) Stanford Hypnotic Susceptibility Scale, Forms A & B. Consulting Psychologists Press, Palo Alto, CA.

Weitzenhoffer AM and Hilgard ER (1962) Stanford Hypnotic Susceptibility Scale, Form C. Consulting Psychologists Press, Palo Alto, CA.

West BH (1836) Experiments in animal magnetism. Boston Med Surg J 14, 349–351.

Whorwell PJ, Prior A, and Colgan SM (1987) Hypnotherapy in severe irritable bowel syndrome: Further experience. Gut 28, 423–425.

Whorwell PJ, Prior A, and Faragher EB (1984) Controlled trial of hypnotherapy in the treatment of severe refractory irritable-bowel syndrome. Lancet 1, 1232–1234.

Wilkinson CB (1983) Aftermath of a disaster: The collapse of the Hyatt Regency Hotel skywalks. Am J Psychiatr 140, 1134–1139.

Wilks CG (1994) The use of hypnosis in the management of gagging and intolerance to dentures (letter). Br Dent J 176, 332.

Williams JM and Hall DW (1988) Use of single session hypnosis for smoking cessation. Addict Behav 13, 205–208.

Williams LM (1994) Recall of childhood trauma: A prospective study of women's memories of childhood sexual abuse. J Consult Clin Psychol 62, 1167–1176.

Williamson JW, McColl R, Mathews D, et al. (2001) Hypnotic manipulation of effort sense during dynamic exercise: Cardiovascular responses and brain activation. J Appl Physiol 90(4), 1392–1399.

Wilson NJ (1968) Neurophysiologic alterations with hypnosis. Dis Nerv Syst 29, 618–620.

Winchell SA and Watts RA (1988) Relaxation therapies in the treatment of psoriasis and possible pathophysiologic mechanisms. J Am Acad Dermatol 18(1, Pt 1), 101–104.

Wood DP and Sexton JL (1997) Self-hypnosis training and captivity survival. Am J Clin Hypn 39, 201–211.

Zeltzer L and LeBaron S (1982) Hypnosis and nonhypnotic techniques for reduction of pain and anxiety during painful procedures in children and adolescents with cancer. J Pediatr 101, 1032–1035.

Zeltzer L, LeBaron S, and Zeltzer PM (1984) The effectiveness of behavioral intervention for reduction of nausea and vomiting in children and adolescents receiving chemotherapy. J Clin Oncol 2, 683–690.

Zimbardo PG, Maslach C, and Marshall G (1970) Hypnosis and the Psychology of Cognitive and Behavioral Control. Department of Psychology, Stanford University, Stanford, CA.

# 90 Behavioral Medicine

Mark A. Slater
Andrew Steptoe
Anne L. Weickgenant
Joel E. Dimsdale

## Overview

Founded in the 1970s, behavioral medicine is a relatively new subspecialty that emerged out of curious roots. Foremost among these was the realization that many medical problems have their genesis, and perhaps cure, in behavioral actions. In the previous edition of this text, we observed that behavioral medicine was frequently an object of mystery to physicians and allied health professionals. Although some confusion persists, behavioral medicine has become more recognized and accepted as a part of mainstream medicine than was the case just 5 years ago. Perhaps one of the clearest examples of the mainstreaming of behavioral medicine is the *Healthy People 2010* initiative of the US Department of Health and Human Services (2000). This initiative is explicitly biobehavioral in perspective, formulating health as the interplay of behavior and biology interacting with the social and physical environment. The goals of this initiative are to increase both the quality and years of healthy life, and to eliminate health disparities. The approach to achieving these goals recognizes the importance of behavioral factors and focuses on leading health indicators that impact health and well-being (i.e., physical activity, overweight and obesity, tobacco use, substance abuse, responsible sexual behavior, mental health, injury and violence, environmental quality, immunization, and access to health care). This integrative approach to the determinants of health is central to behavioral medicine.

The second founding attribute of behavioral medicine is a conviction that behavior is a crucial subject matter in its own right in medicine and that underlying motivations and personality structure, although interesting, may not be crucial in determining change in health. Thus, the focus on behavior alone reflects one pole in the familiar and doctrinaire struggles between psychodynamic and behaviorist intellectual traditions.

Perhaps a third characteristic of behavioral medicine is its opportunism. We use this term advisedly and without any pejorative connotations. Psychosomatic medicine flourished as a research discipline to study the physiological and psychological underpinnings of many diseases. As a clinical subspecialty, it provided psychotherapy for patients determined to have "psychosomatic illnesses" but focused par-

ticularly on a limited subset of illnesses (the so-called "holy seven"). General psychiatry and even consultation–liaison psychiatry also left certain important clinical areas uncovered. None of these movements in psychiatry was oriented toward improving patients' compliance or modifying their many risk-enhancing behaviors. Similarly, psychiatry did not seem to offer special programs other than supportive psychotherapy for specialized groups of patients with diverse medical problems, such as chronic pain or anticipatory nausea associated with chemotherapy.

Despite the extraordinarily successful growth in consultation psychiatry, such services were oriented primarily toward inpatient settings. Little was being done in outpatient settings to address the intersection of psychiatry and medicine. Thus, a fourth characteristic of behavioral medicine is its interdisciplinary focus on outpatient settings. As the economics of medicine have shifted from inpatient settings and specialty consultation to managed care, outpatient treatment, and health maintenance, new opportunities for the emerging field of behavioral medicine have arisen, and behavioral medicine concepts have become more integrated into mainstream care.

Finally, behavioral medicine straddles medicine, psychiatry, psychology, and public health. It tends to focus not just on the patient but also larger health policy matters such as social class, race and ethnicity, risk screening, and communication of medical information to diverse populations.

Before the specific accomplishments, limitations, and developments of behavioral medicine are discussed, it may be useful to review clinical vignettes concerning how the same patient might be approached by two related professionals: the consultation–liaison psychiatrist and the behavioral psychologist. We are indebted to Aaron Lazare (1973) for his articulate discussion of "hidden conceptual models" in psychiatry. Presenting the same case from different theoretical vantage points, he demonstrated the remarkably diverse ways we try to make sense of patients' histories and that treatment can be inappropriate and ineffective when it is based on a limited assessment of the patient. It is our thesis that both of these clinical approaches (consultation–liaison and behavioral psychology) are extremely valuable, but when complex medical problems are confronted, the greatest value comes from an integration of these traditions that includes the synthesis of diverse sources of medical information and perspectives. This integration provides a new interdisciplinary conceptualization and treatment approach known as behavioral medicine.

---

**Clinical Vignette 1 • The Consultation–Liaison Approach**

Mr. H, a 51-year-old man undergoing dialysis for end-stage renal disease, was referred because of noncompliance with the numerous dietary restrictions required for dialysis. The psychiatrist noted that his wife had died 2 years earlier, and he still had difficulties adjusting to her loss. His 25-year-old daughter tried to cheer him up by eating with him, but he seemed sad all the time. He did not sleep well, ate irregularly and carelessly, and blamed himself for not having been more demonstrative to his wife while she was alive. As further history was obtained, the psychiatrist eventually diagnosed Mr. H with a major depressive disorder and prescribed an antidepressant and short-term psychotherapy oriented toward enhancing his adjustment to bereavement. The patient's mood lifted but he was still noncompliant with diet and died of hyperkalemia after a 3-day weekend marked by consumption of high-potassium foods.

---

**Clinical Vignette 2 • The Behavioral Psychology Approach**

Mr. H, a 51-year-old man undergoing dialysis for end-stage renal disease, was referred because of noncompliance with the numerous dietary restrictions required for dialysis. The therapist noted that he was unable to remember the complex dietary limitations or medication requirements. With carefully designed education, individually tailored reminder notes on the refrigerator, and the use of an alarm clock to cue eating, the therapist attempted to engineer the task to be less daunting. In addition, the therapist encouraged the patient's married daughter to congratulate (i.e., reinforce) him whenever he ordered appropriate foods while they dined together at restaurants. The patient seemed to be doing better with his diet until the anniversary of his wife's death, when he binged on a high-potassium diet, developed a cardiac arrhythmia, and died.

---

Both therapists may have considered their interventions successful until the final denouement. Each diagnosed carefully and arranged for astutely monitored interventions. Each failed. The reader may complain that these are overdramatized and oversimplified cases. We agree. We have seen many such cases, however, and their message is clear: unless practitioners have a clear understanding of the broader behavioral medicine ramifications of their cases, they will be at risk for providing inadequate care. These two clinicians failed by not addressing both behavior (and behavioral change) and psychopathology in the conceptualization of the case or in the treatment advised.

## What Is Behavioral Medicine?

Behavioral medicine is an interdisciplinary field concerned with the development and integration of behavioral and biomedical science, knowledge, and techniques relevant to health and illness and the application of this knowledge and these techniques to prevention, diagnosis, treatment, and rehabilitation (Schwartz and Weiss 1978). This classic definition of the field emphasizes several essential aspects of behavioral medicine that are highlighted and expanded in Table 90–1. Among these, five primary factors deserve further comment in characterizing the unique nature of behavioral medicine approaches to health care.

First, behavioral medicine is inherently and absolutely interdisciplinary. Traditional (Western) medical care divided problems and patients by disciplinary boundaries and encouraged independent treatment approaches. Contemporary care, often characterized as multidisciplinary, is organized as a summation of component disciplines. True interdisciplinary care involves an integration and melding of the component disciplinary approaches, such that the original component distinctions are no longer important and a new complex approach is created that is more than the sum of its parts.

Second, behavioral medicine is staunchly entrenched in the scientific method and is founded in empirical data. An emphasis on scientific research and empirical support for theories and interventions has been a hallmark of the field. The field has always emphasized the development of knowledge at least as much as the application of knowledge and

| Table 90–1 | Characteristics of Behavioral Medicine | |
|---|---|---|
| Interdisciplinary | A primary characteristic of the field | |
| | Emphasis on interaction and integration within and across disciplines to develop a coherent, comprehensive conceptualization of health problems and solutions | |
| Field | Not simply a therapeutic technique or group of techniques or a subspecialization of another discipline | |
| | A field of study and application dedicated to the development of information, knowledge, and technologies | |
| | Empirically grounded and based on a scientific approach to health care | |
| | Distinct from alternative medicine, which is based on a mistrust of the scientific method | |
| Integration of behavioral and biomedical sciences | Two primary sources: behavioral and biomedical sciences | |
| | Emphasis on the integration of findings and approaches from these fields into a coherent single entity | |
| Medical health | In contrast to most traditional psychiatry, medical problems primarily addressed rather than psychiatric or behavioral problems and disorders | |
| Health and illness | Not solely an approach to remediation of illness; provides an approach to illness prevention and health maintenance and enhancement | |
| | Recognizes that health and illness represent arbitrary points on continua of well-being | |
| All aspects of health care | Not limited to assessment or intervention, acute or chronic illness, or particular illness categories | |
| | A general approach to health care, health service delivery, medical research, and public health | |

technology to care of patients. In this way, behavioral medicine is different from "alternative medicine" approaches, which are based on a fundamental mistrust of science and a disregard for scientific (Western) method.

A third characteristic of behavioral medicine is one of the clearest distinctions between it and conventional psychiatry and psychology. Emphasis is placed on a medical disorder rather than on a psychiatric or behavioral problem. The behavioral medicine specialist addresses foremost that which is held to be the principal problem of the patient, a medical disease, while understanding that secondary psychiatric symptoms are common with health problems and must also be treated to ensure optimal health.

Fourth, behavioral medicine has a primary focus on the integration of behavioral and biomedical sciences to solve problems related to health and illness. Behavioral medicine assumes equally strong understanding of and familiarity with biomedical and behavioral sciences (Epstein 1992). It is the integration of these disciplines that truly distinguishes the field from other areas of medicine. With this approach, behavioral medicine is applicable (potentially) at any point along the health–illness continuum.

Thus, a fifth characteristic of behavioral medicine is that it is not limited to particular diseases, disorders, or syndromes; nor is it limited to particular activities (e.g., epidemiology, assessment, intervention) or techniques (e.g., biofeedback, education, medication). Behavioral medicine is a general approach to health care, health service delivery, medical research, and public health.

Returning to the clinical vignette; a behavioral medicine physician evaluating and treating Mr. H would require scientific knowledge of the biological, psychological, and social aspects of renal problems and their treatment (e.g., dialysis). The physician would need to be thoroughly familiar with the appropriate diagnostic techniques and treatments for such a condition along with possible side effects. In addition, behavioral approaches specifically tailored to this disease process (e.g., behavioral contracting, self-monitoring, behavioral reminders, tailoring medical regimen, cognitive restructuring, principles of reinforcement) and personal and social aspects of Mr. H's present life circumstance (death of spouse; daughter as primary caretaker) and health problem (depression and shame associated with his medical problem) would be evaluated and addressed as part of Mr. H's total treatment package.

The behavioral medicine approach cuts across health care disciplines in an attempt to fully address the complex array of *biopsychosocial* factors in any particular disease presentation. With regard to discipline, the behavioral medicine practitioner could be a primary care physician, internal medicine specialist, psychiatrist, psychologist, or nurse; more likely, an interdisciplinary team of experts that represents all of these, and perhaps additional, disciplines.

## History and Development of the Field

The recognition that behavioral factors influence health and illness dates from Hippocrates. Intellectual and clinical interest in behavioral factors in health and health care, however, has waxed and waned through the years. Four major factors came together in the late 1960s and early 1970s to renew such interest and motivate the establishment of behavioral medicine.

Morbidity and mortality patterns were changing, as were health care programs. Infectious diseases, the primary killers of the previous generation, were treated and prevented with unparalleled success. Now the major health problems in terms of morbidity, mortality, and disability were chronic illnesses with undeniable lifestyle and behavioral correlates (e.g., heart disease, cancer, diabetes, chronic pain syndromes). These disorders did not appear to fit readily into the traditional infectious disease model, which had been so successful with the major illnesses of the past. Moreover, with improved health, demystification of medicine, and the knowledge that many chronic illnesses have predisposing lifestyle factors, patients became more interested in what they could do to influence their health (self-management). This recognition culminated with the US government publication of *Healthy People 2000* (US Department of Health and Human Services 1991), which articulated the major health goals for the millennium. The report indicated that the major health issues for the nation have behavioral and lifestyle components and called for prevention and intervention programs that address these issues.

Consultation–liaison psychiatry focused on delivery of pragmatic (often crisis-based) care to medical–surgical inpatients but offered relatively little in the way of preventive services, health promotion, or outpatient services. Psychosomatic medicine, moving away from its roots in psychoanalysis, became increasingly oriented toward research (both physiological and epidemiological) concerning mind–body or biopsychosocial relationships. Behavioral approaches had demonstrated success in several areas of mental health (Masters et al. 1987). In part because clear operational goals are implicit in any behavioral intervention, the data from such techniques were measurable and the efficacy was impressive. For the first time, data were available that demonstrated reliable change elicited by behavioral technologies. An interest developed at this time for broadening the application of behavioral technologies.

Developments in the area of psychophysiology combined with behavior theory to create biofeedback. The pioneering work of Neil Miller (DiCara and Miller 1968, Miller 1978) demonstrating operant control of autonomic responses in animals and humans had a profound influence in fostering the field's development. Biofeedback demonstrated possible mechanisms by which behavior change can affect physiological mechanisms of disease.

The combination of these factors provided the foundation for this new field, and by the mid-1970s behavioral medicine emerged. In the last 25 years, the field has grown, developed subspecializations, and begun to face challenges, just as psychosomatic medicine and biofeedback did previously. It is apparent that the field has thrived and made significant contributions to many areas of medicine. Still, significant questions remain. Can the field live up to its promise? Has it promised more than it can deliver? Should the field remain distinct or be subsumed into a larger rubric?

The concepts of stress and coping have been a major underpinning of the field of behavioral medicine, because these concepts have commonly been seen as linking the mind and the body. Whereas traditional psychiatry has been interested in stress as a cause or effect of many mental disorders, behavioral medicine has emphasized stress as it relates to medical illness and health behaviors. Behavioral medicine has posed questions such as: does exposure to stress put individuals at risk for the development of health problems? If so, are certain ways of reacting to and handling life stress more adaptive than others? Are there effective treatments or can we teach coping skills to persons exposed to a variety of stressful conditions, such as those in our daily environment and those associated with chronic physical and mental illness?

## Relationship of Health Behaviors to Illness and Wellness

For the three leading causes of death in the US—heart disease, cancer, and stroke—factors that are causally related include tobacco, diet, lack of exercise, and alcohol, each the result of behavioral choices (McGinnis and Foege 1993, US Department of Health and Human Services 2000). Cigarette smoking is a proven risk factor for heart disease, malignant neoplasms, and stroke (Lichtenstein and Glasgow 1992). Sedentary lifestyle has been implicated as a risk factor for many major medical diseases including coronary heart disease and diabetes (US Department of Health and Human Services 1996). Poor dietary habits and obesity are associated with diabetes, hypertension, and coronary artery disease (Wolf and Coditz 1998). Excessive consumption of alcohol is associated with gastrointestinal problems, liver disease, dementia, and fatal traffic accidents (Harwood et al. 1998).

The personal cost of these behavior-related illnesses is immense (e.g., 390,000 Americans die each year as a result of smoking [US Department of Health and Human Services 1991]), and the cost to treat these personal lifestyle choices is staggering (Table 90–2). Although the data in Table 90–2 are now 10 years old, they provide a useful context for the magnitude of the problem. More recent data suggest that the burden of preventable, chronic, and behaviorally linked illness persists unabated. For example, behavioral factors play a major role in each of the top 10 causes of death (see Table 90–3). These 10 leading causes of death account for approximately 80% of all deaths. In terms of costs, data from the 2000 Healthcare Cost and Utilization Project demonstrates the enormity of the burden of providing care for these diseases (see Table 90–4). Statistics such as these have fueled the growth and focus of behavioral medicine as a field, as well as national efforts such as *Healthy People 2010* and political pressures on health care reform. It is becoming clear that health attitudes and resultant behaviors may have various effects on physiological characteristics of individuals—sometimes assisting their general well-being, but often posing serious adverse consequences to them.

## Physical Activity

Mounting research provides ever more compelling evidence of the merits of an active lifestyle (Center for Disease Control 1993, US Department of Health and Human Services 1996). Exercise can have marked benefits on cardiovascular and

| Table 90–2 | Costs in 1990 of Treatment for "Preventable" Conditions | | |
|---|---|---|---|
| Condition | Overall Magnitude | Intervention* | Cost per Patient† |
| Heart disease | 7 million with CAD‡<br>500,000 deaths/yr<br>284,000 bypasses/yr | Coronary bypass surgery | $30,000 |
| Cancer | 1 million new/yr<br>510,000 deaths/yr | Lung cancer treatment<br>Cervical cancer treatment | $29,000<br>$28,000 |
| Stroke | 600,000 strokes/yr | Hemiplegia treatment and rehabilitation | $22,000 |
| Injuries | 2.3 million hospitalizations/yr<br>142,500 deaths/yr<br>177,000 with spinal cord injuries in US | Quadriplegia treatment and rehabilitation<br>Hip fractures and rehabilitation<br>Severe head injury treatment and rehabilitation | $570,000 (lifetime)<br><br>$40,000<br>$310,000 |
| HIV injuries | 1–1.5 million infected<br>118,000 AIDS‡ cases (as of 1/90) | AIDS treatment | $75,000 |
| Alcoholism | 18.5 million abuse alcohol<br>105,000 alcohol-related deaths/yr | Liver transplant | $250,000 |
| Drug abuse | Regular users: 1–3 million<br>375,000 drug-exposed babies | Treatment of drug-affected babies | $63,000 (5 yr) |
| Low-birth-weight baby | 260,000 born/yr<br>23,000 deaths/yr | Neonatal intensive care | $10,000 |
| Inadequate immunization | 20–30% lack basic immunization series | Congenital rubella syndrome treatment | $345,000 (lifetime) |

*Examples (other interventions may apply).

†Representative first-year costs, except as noted. Does not include nonmedical costs, such as loss of productivity to society.

‡CAD, coronary artery disease; HIV, human immunodeficiency virus infection; AIDS, acquired immunodeficiency syndrome.

*Source*: US Department of Health and Human Services (1991) National Health Promotion and Disease Prevention Objectives, Full Report with Commentary, Healthy People 2000. US Government Printing Office, (PHS) 91-S0212, Washington DC.

| Table 90-3 | Top Ten Causes of Death | |
|---|---|---|
| | | **Percentage of Deaths** |
| Heart disease | | 31.4 |
| Malignant neoplasms | | 23.3 |
| Stroke | | 6.9 |
| Chronic obstructive pulmonary disease | | 4.7 |
| Unintentional injury and adverse effects | | 4.1 |
| Pneumonia or influenza | | 3.7 |
| Diabetes | | 2.7 |
| Suicide | | 1.3 |
| Kidney disease | | 1.1 |
| Chronic liver disease | | 1.1 |

respiratory fitness, body composition (i.e., body mass, fat content), muscle strength, endurance, and flexibility (Dubbert 1992). In addition, physical activity is associated with (1) reduced risk for osteoporosis or bone loss in postmenopausal women using weight-bearing exercise, (2) increased strength from resistance weight training in geriatric populations, (3) psychological health and effective treatment of some emotional disorders (e.g., anxiety, depression, and addictive behaviors), (4) prevention and treatment of obesity, (5) significant improvement in chronic pain conditions (arthritis and low back pain), (6) increased longevity, and (7) improvements in quality of life. Yet, only an estimated 15% of American adults regularly engage in moderate physical exercise, and 40% engage in no leisure physical activity at all (Center for Disease Control 1992).

The physiological mechanism linking health improvement with activity is unknown, but some suggestions include (1) strengthening of the heart muscle, increasing its size, and improving its functioning; (2) increase of high-density lipoprotein cholesterol; (3) reduction of triglycerides; (4) decreased likelihood for development of hypertension and reduction of diastolic blood pressure; (5) reduction of blood glucose levels, increasing insulin receptors and the effectiveness of insulin; (6) promotion of skeletal muscle size and weight, increased burning of calories, and increased resting metabolic rate; and (7) reduction of the stickiness of fibrins that leads to blood clots (Haskell et al. 1992).

Data contradict previous beliefs that exercise should be at least 20 continuous minutes of vigorous activity, three or four times per week, to have significant health benefits and fitness improvement (Dubbert 1992, American College of Sports Medicine 1991). Although frequent vigorous activity may be required for cardiovascular fitness, newer data support instead the value of regular moderate activity

(DeBusk et al. 1990, Leon et al. 1993). Studies have also shown that the greatest increment in fitness occurred in individuals going from a sedentary status to briskly walking 30 to 60 minutes each day. In summary, physical activity is now thought to be an independent determinant of health and well-being and is a leading target of treatment in behavioral medicine interventions (Dubbert 1992).

## Dietary Risk Factors

The influence of diet on health has changed considerably through the years as common nutritional-deficiency diseases such as rickets and scurvy have become rare in the US. Although dietary habits still contribute significantly to ill health, the primary cause tends to no longer be a deficiency of nutrients, but rather an oversupply. Whereas animals have a strong evolutionary defense against undernutrition, some researchers have suggested that they have a weak response to the effects of overnutrition (Blundell and Lawton 1993). Thus, modern society brings in its wake many health problems not commonly experienced previously during times of food scarcity. In the top 10 causes of death, dietary fats are associated with increased risk of coronary heart disease, some cancers, stroke, diabetes, and atherosclerosis (US Department of Health and Human Services 1991, 2000). In addition, increases in dietary fiber can mitigate important health problems, such as diabetes, cardiovascular disease, and cancer; excessive sodium use increases the likelihood of hypertension for some individuals; and supplemental calcium not only can decrease blood pressure but also helps maintain bone density.

Data on the ill effects of obesity suggest that increases in body mass index (weight in kilograms divided by the square of the height in meters) are strongly associated with increases in morbidity and mortality. Excess visceral adipose tissue is associated with metabolic disorders, such as diabetes, hypercholesterolemia, hypertriglyceridemia, and hypertension (Stunkard and Wadden 1993). Similar to the data showing health benefits from less exercise, data from newer studies suggest greater health benefit from small weight losses. A 10% loss of body weight, for instance, has been found to normalize blood pressures in obese hypertensive patients (Brownell and Wadden 1992) and to reduce blood glucose levels and blood lipid and lipoprotein levels (Brownell and Rodin 1994).

## Smoking

Addiction to nicotine may be the most serious medical problem in the US. Tobacco use causes more deaths than alcohol, firearms, motor vehicles, and illegal drugs combined (McGinnis and Foege 1993). On the basis of a review of the literature from 1977 to 1993, cigarette smoking was

| Table 90-4 | Healthcare Cost and Utilization Project Cost Data | | |
|---|---|---|---|
| | **US Hospital Discharges in 2000** | **Percentage of Discharges** | **Aggregate Charges($)** |
| Coronary atherosclerosis | 1,360,507 | 3.7 | 30,753,753,045 |
| Acute myocardial infarction | 768,495 | 2.1 | 20,643,624,141 |
| Congestive heart failure | 1,025,295 | 2.8 | 14,676,657,106 |
| Acute cerebrovascular disease | 580,054 | 1.6 | 10,800,301,598 |

found to cause 30% of all cancer deaths, 21% of deaths from heart disease, and 19% of all deaths combined (McGinnis and Foege 1993). It is thought that 20% of low-weight births, 8% of preterm deliveries, and 5% of all perinatal deaths could be prevented by eliminating smoking during pregnancy (US Department of Health and Human Services 1990). Furthermore, evidence accumulated in the last 10 years implicates environmental tobacco smoke as a risk factor for nonsmokers (Lichtenstein and Glasgow 1992). Despite intensive programs, low cessation rates have remained a perplexing problem. Hence, structured interventions of late have attempted to incorporate methods that individuals have used on their own to quit. These programs are aimed at targeting the specific "stage" of quitting in which the individual is operating (Prochaska et al. 1993) (Table 90–5).

## Screening Behavior and Risk Appraisal

Screening and risk assessment are becoming increasingly important in clinical medicine, and behavioral medicine is focusing more on the complexity of the problems attendant with such assessment. Screening involves the systematic application of a test to identify individuals at sufficient risk of a specific disease to benefit from further investigation or direct preventive action, among people who have not sought medical action on account of symptoms (Wald 1994). The aim of most screening is to detect disease at an early stage or in a predisease stage. Risk appraisal involves providing people with risk information on which to base medical and lifestyle decisions. Of course, screening has been with us for many years in forms such as chest X rays and amniocentesis, while appraisal of risks such as cigarette smoking are very familiar. However, two factors have led to recent growth in the area.

The first is the increased sophistication with which biological pathways related to disease are being identified. For example, cardiovascular risk assessment has advanced beyond the measurement of blood pressure and total cholesterol; now such screening can extend to consideration of apolipoproteins, hemostatic factors, and inflammatory markers in the risk profile. Similarly, there are many

screening indications in cancer. Premalignant polyps (adenomas) are early markers for colorectal cancer, prostate-specific antigen for prostate cancer, and human papillomavirus seropositivity is a marker for cervical cancer.

The second factor leading to increased focus on screening is the explosion of genetic sophistication, which has led to the identification of specific genotypes for several common disorders such as breast cancer, colon cancer, and early onset Alzheimer's disease. This new knowledge has led to the development of genetic screening, aimed at identifying genetic susceptibility to disease in individuals or their offspring. Genetic counseling, in which people are advised about disease risk usually on the basis of family history, has also been expanding.

This growth of medical screening and risk appraisal raises important issues in behavioral medicine. Individuals who previously regarded themselves as healthy may be identified as being ill or at high risk for illness. The World Health Organization has argued that screening is only justified if there is evidence for an effective treatment, together with reason to believe that early treatment will result in better outcome. Unfortunately, screening tests are often developed more rapidly than treatments, so clinical conditions may be identified without any treatment or preventive action being available. Early identification can have undesirable consequences, such as the lowering of parental and school expectations in children, difficulties with employment and insurance in adults, and the need to make difficult decisions about preventive surgery which may have unpleasant side effects or uncertain benefits.

There is concern that medical and genetic screening may have adverse emotional effects. Some screening procedures involve a period of distress and uncertainty, even for individuals who prove to have negative results, because test findings may not be instantly available. Fortunately, while transient distress is common, few studies have as yet identified long-term adverse emotional effects of screening (Wardle and Pope 1992). Nevertheless, screening requires careful attention to the psychological experience of participants as well as to clinical outcomes, and counseling programs may be required for emotionally vulnerable individuals. The need for counseling in conjunction with screening has been recognized for many years in relation to HIV and Huntington's disease, but now with the profusion of screening indications, this knowledge is increasingly relevant to larger numbers of patients.

Another important behavioral aspect of screening concerns participation rates. Screening and risk appraisal programs are useful in reducing disease in the population only if used widely. But while participation is generally good in research studies, screening and clinical practice often reach fewer than 50% of the target population, even when services are free. Several factors are relevant, including lack of motivation, inconvenience, and fear and denial concerning the outcome. Social cognition models of human action such as a health belief model and the theory of planned behavior have proved useful in helping to understand screening participation. Thus, it has been found that individuals who take advantage of screening programs perceive themselves as more susceptible to the disease, believe that screening will be beneficial, and are knowledgeable about the condition and report high self-efficacy, while screening

| Table 90–5 | Stages of Readiness to Quit Smoking |
|---|---|
| Stage | Description |
| Precontemplation | Smoker is not seriously considering quitting. Smoker is not amenable to smoking cessation program. |
| Contemplation | Smoker is seriously thinking about stopping in the next 6 mo. |
| Preparation | Smoker has firmly decided to quit within the next 6 mo. |
| Action | Ranges from 0 to 6 mo after smoker has made overt attempts to stop. This period has been the focus of traditional cessation programs. |
| Maintenance | This period is 6 mo after behavior change of quitting smoking. One continues to maintain action until eventual termination of the problem. |

is less common in those who describe major practical, financial, or emotional barriers to taking part.

Screening is likely to become increasingly central to behavioral medicine over the next few years. Already, screening clinics are being seen as valuable sites for health behavior change and preventive advice, since people attending them may be sensitive to general health issues and therefore responsive to advice. Genetic screening may also interact with health behavior change programs. For example, there is evidence that particular genetic polymorphisms may increase the risk, among smokers, of coronary heart disease and lung cancer; information of this type may enhance motivation for smoking cessation. However, screening results can have complex effects on health behavior that are not yet well understood. Negative results may lead to a false sense of security, while positive results can be greeted with fatalism rather than providing an added impetus for taking preventive action.

## Personality Factors

Personality factors have long been thought to predispose an individual to illness. Probably the best known personality risk factor is the type A behavior pattern, a term first coined in the 1950s (Friedman and Rosenman 1959), and its association with coronary artery disease. The original definition described type A behavior as an action–emotion complex that individuals use to confront their environment and challenges. This hard-driving behavior pattern included aggression; competitiveness; impatience; and specific behaviors, such as muscle tension, alertness, rapid and emphatic vocal style, accelerated pace of activities, emotional responses of irritability or covert hostility, and above-average anger (Rosenman 1993). Early studies found approximately two times the frequency of coronary artery disease compared with that of non-type A persons, five times the frequency of having a second myocardial infarction, and two times the chance of having a fatal heart attack (Rosenman et al. 1975).

However, the validity of the original concept of type A behavior pattern and its relationship to heart disease have been challenged as newer studies have failed to replicate earlier findings (Rosenman et al. 1975, Dimsdale 1988, Ragland and Brand 1988). The concept of type A behavior pattern itself has undergone further refinement. Initially described as unrelated to formal psychiatric syndromes or marked psychiatric illness, type A behavior pattern nonetheless has been associated with certain maladaptive personality features. Type A behavior pattern has been related to a covert anxiety that is associated with insecurity and fear of failure (Suls and Wan 1989), and it has also been associated with maladaptive coping and particular risk behaviors (Rosenman 1993). Current conceptualizations of type A behavior pattern have focused on hostility, suspiciousness, and cynicism as the critical factors that increase risk (Goldstein and Niaura 1992) and on poor health behaviors (e.g., smoking and alcohol abuse; high-fat, high-cholesterol diet; and sedentary lifestyle) (Lichtenstein and Glasgow 1992). Thus, the notion of a type A behavior pattern now encompasses a broader array of risk behaviors—health habits, personality, and coping style—all of which combine and interact to create a greater risk for cardiac health problems (Williams 1987).

## Stress, Coping, and Illness

The most common psychosocial variable associated with illness onset has to do with the ever-elusive concept of stress, one of the most controversial and pervasive notions in health care today. Poor management of stress has been associated with an increased occurrence of heart disease, coronary artery disease, poor diabetes control, chronic pain conditions, and significant emotional distress (Kaplan et al. 1993).

The experience of stress has been defined vaguely as the process of adapting to challenge (Friedman and DiMatteo 1989). This challenge involves a transaction between the person and the situation (Lazarus and Folkman 1984). Although stress and illness relationships have become recognized as "fact" and everyone "knows" that stress is related to disease, objective evidence for a causal relationship (how stress actually translates into frequency, severity, or duration of illness) has been controversial and not impressive, at best. Nevertheless, data thus far collected are promising and demonstrate that stress is complex, with many interacting factors that feed back on each other to produce change in health.

Stressors have been associated with numerous pathological changes in biochemical and immunological activities. Research on the relationship of stress and the likelihood of becoming ill has clearly pointed out that exposure to stress alone is almost never a sufficient explanation for illness in ordinary human experience, just as genetics alone does not cause mental illness. Characteristics of the stressor presumed to mediate its impact include its magnitude, duration, novelty, and predictability and the temporal sequence of events. Relevant person factors include biological vulnerabilities, response thresholds, age at exposure, personality style (e.g., self-efficacy, optimism, and sense of coherence), and coping styles (i.e., habitual patterns of response). In addition, the person's appraisal of the stressful situations (i.e., the degree of threat, perception of control, previous experience, and what coping resources or options are available) has been found to be critical in determining psychological and physiological reactions to stress. Individuals who appraise situations as more threatening, important, and uncontrollable report more physical symptoms and emotional distress (Affleck et al. 1987). Table 90–6 summarizes the multiple stress factors influencing health outcome. On the basis of the empirical evidence, coping skills training programs teach patients the importance of particular coping strategies in enhancing health (Chesney et al. 1995).

One way in which stress might lead to illness is by altering nervous, immune, or endocrine systems, creating modifications in heart rate, blood pressure, hypothalamic and pituitary activity, and other physiological processes. Physiological reactivity (particularly sympathetic nervous system reactivity) in response to stressful events has been proposed as a factor contributing to the progression of cardiovascular disease through increased plasma catecholamine levels, which may facilitate plaque accumulation or damage endothelial cells in blood vessels (Clarkson et al. 1986). Sympathetic and parasympathetic balance in response to stress may also lead to occurrence of fatal arrhythmias (Coumel and Leenhardt 1991). Moreover, research in psychoneuroimmunology has demonstrated that stressors may lead to

| Table 90–6 | Stress Factors Determining Health Outcome | | |
|---|---|---|---|
| Person–Environment | Stressor | Appraisal | Coping |
| Biology | Type | Threat | Information and support seeking |
| Age exposure | Magnitude | Importance | Positive reappraisal |
| Personality | Duration | Challenge | Concrete action |
| Demographics | Novelty | Control | Minimizing, denial, fantasy |
| Social resources | Predictability | Experience | Accepting the situation |
| Environmental system | Temporal sequence | Coping resources | Seeking negative or alternative reinforcers |
| | | | Venting negative emotions |

the suppression of immune functioning (Ader and Cohen 1975). Situations that repeatedly tax the individual's ability to adapt (crowding, maternal separation, isolation, torture, and so forth) have been linked to increased frequency of hypertension, heart disease, and ulcers and decreased resistance to virus and tumor cells (Weiner 1977).

A second way in which stress may lead to illness is by fostering activities that increase the likelihood of disease or injury. For instance, by managing life's difficulties with heavy use of tobacco and alcohol or drugs, using poor dietary habits, and leading a sedentary lifestyle, one increases the chances of morbidity and mortality.

A third way in which stress and maladaptive coping may lead to illness is by psychological and social influences that consistently lead a person to minimize the significance of various symptoms or to fail to comply with treatment regimens. Lack of information, minimizing or denying important medical assessments and treatment, and failure to take prophylactic health measures may delay medical care and lead to illness or even fatality. For instance, when individuals do not know the utility of prostate, cholesterol, or breast cancer screening, they may neglect to seek medical evaluations crucial to preventing major illness. When a person delays seeking medical attention at the time of experiencing symptoms of cancer or a heart attack, chances of survival are lower.

These factors may operate simultaneously in patients to produce multiple risks for illness. The temperamentally aggressive person who in time becomes insecure and socially aloof, avoids self-disclosure, and passively copes with life's frustrations and micro-aggressions by smoking cigarettes and drinking excessively, provides such an example. Habitual cynicism, hostility, and anger may (1) produce chronic physiological overarousal, (2) increase the likelihood of poor health habits (such as less physical activity, less self-care, and more frequent episodes of drinking and driving), and (3) discourage social supports that facilitate access to medical care and buffer the deleterious effects of stress—all of which may tax the cardiovascular, neuroendocrine, and immune systems.

In summary, a multifactorial model of health and illness includes the consideration not only of individuals but also of their biology, psychological functioning, and environment. In addition, the nature of the stressor itself and the many potential mediating factors in the stress exposure must be considered. All of these factors feed back on each other. Hence, the notion of stress as it relates to illness is best described by an extremely complex interaction of biopsychosocial issues.

## The Population Perspective: Sociodemographic Factors

The origins of behavioral medicine as a discipline lie in individual biobehavioral processes and the impact of emotions and behavior on health outcomes. Another major strand has been added to this interdisciplinary field via behavioral and psychosocial epidemiology. It has been known for centuries that the experience of illness depends on the social environment as well as individual behavior and biology. People living in poverty, migrants, and ethnic minorities have suffered a greater disease burden and more premature mortality since records began. In the 19th and early 20th century, much of this excess was caused by material deprivation, undernutrition, unsanitary living conditions and exposure to infectious organisms. But despite the general improvements in living conditions and the conquering of much infectious disease in the 20th century, social inequalities in morbidity and mortality have persisted. There are socioeconomic gradients in many of the leading causes of death, including coronary heart disease, stroke, respiratory diseases and many cancers, chronic conditions such as arthritis and ulcers, and in suicide and mental illness. Behavioral medicine researchers have been very involved in tracing these pathways in the hopes of influencing public policy. After all, the "etiology" of so much of the premature mortality is "behavioral" or "societal" in nature.

Figure 90–1, modified from the work of Professor Sir Michael Marmot, schematically diagrams the putative pathways by which socioeconomic factors act. Note that these pathways involve some of the major themes of behavioral medicine, in particular health behavior and stress–related psychophysiological mechanisms. Marmot notes that social structures influence risk of disease through experiences in adult working and nonworking life, building on the substrate of early life and genetic factors. These chronic experiences determine patterns of health behavior and disturbances in stress-related autonomic, neuroendocrine, and immunological function, leading to emotional and biological risk factor profiles that are prejudicial for health. For example, people in lower socioeconomic status categories (as defined by occupation, income, and educational background) tend to have jobs over which they have little control; they have relatively little influence over decision making, the pace of work, or how their work is carried out. Low job control in turn leads to heightened blood pressure and disturbances in the diurnal rhythm of the output of the hypothalamic–pituitary–adrenocortical axis. Monotonous, uncontrollable work may also increase depressive symptoms, and be associated with deleterious health habits such

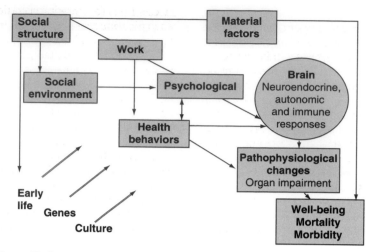

**Figure 90–1** *Potential behavioral medicine pathways linking social position and ill health. (Source: Modified from Stansfeld SA and Marmot MG [2002] Introduction. In Stress and the Heart, Stansfeld SA and Marmot MG [eds]. BMJ Books, London, pp. 1–4.)*

as lack of physical exercise (Stansfeld et al. 1999). Thus behavioral medicine operates within a population framework and touches on issues of culture and social organization as well as on individual health outcomes (Adler et al. 1999).

## Behavioral Medicine Techniques: Clinical Applications

Although behavioral medicine shares many applications and techniques with traditional medical and behavioral approaches to health care, several aspects are unique and characteristic of the field. Five specific clinical activities have been synonymous with behavioral medicine across several areas of application and clinical populations.

## Biobehavioral Assessment

Biobehavioral assessment involves the coordinated and integrated evaluation of biomedical and behavioral factors in the health status and quality of life of the patient. Careful behavioral analysis is a hallmark of this approach with a detailed specification of the frequency, amplitude, duration, quality, and correlates of key health behaviors. Behavioral analysis emphasizes a systematic search for functional (contingent) relationships of the cues in the environment (discriminative stimuli), "signs, symptoms, or problems" (behavioral responses), and consequences of the behaviors (reinforcers). The frequent clinical observation that chronic pain patients in the presence of the floor nurse (discriminative stimulus) increase their rates and intensity of pain complaints and behaviors (behavioral responses), resulting in greater likelihood of narcotics administration (positive reinforcement), exemplifies these contingent relationships. Direct observation of the patient's behavior in problem settings is preferred to self-reports of symptoms and analysis of internal (mental) "causes."

## Behavior Management

Behavior management is the use of learning principles (particularly operant and classical conditioning) to encourage and direct health behavior change. This approach emphasizes a functional analysis and contingency management to assist patients in making desired behavior change to achieve health goals. A functional analysis is a case conceptualization, similar to the case of the pain patient with an escalating narcotic intake described before, that emphasizes empirical contingent (predictable) relationships between the person's behavior and the environment. Contingency management is the systematic manipulation of the probabilistic relationships (contingencies) between the terms of the functional analysis (i.e., discriminative stimuli, behavioral responses, and reinforcing stimuli). An example of this strategy is to schedule narcotics administration at regular intervals (time contingent) rather than as needed (pain behavior contingent), which removes the contingency between pain behaviors and narcotic reinforcement, thereby decreasing (after perhaps an initial extinction burst) the probability (and strength) of the behavioral response (pain complaints and behaviors). Again, these clinical techniques have been direct outgrowths of basic psychological laboratory research.

## Cognitive–Educational Approaches

Cognitive–educational approaches have been based primarily on the health belief model (Rosenstock 1966, Janz and Becker 1984). The health belief model emphasizes the role of the individual's beliefs about health and the meaning of symptoms, including beliefs about the likely effects of behavior change on health outcomes and beliefs about the ability to make worthwhile behavior change. This model asserts that such beliefs and anticipated costs and benefits of health behaviors, whether accurate or not, are critical determinants of health choices that have direct effects on clinical outcomes. Clinical approaches from this perspective emphasize education and cognitive change as key factors for improving health. The social and educational psychology literatures provide extensive information about variables (e.g., credibility, perceived similarity) that enhance persuasion and provide the empirical foundation for efforts toward cognitive change. These health education-based approaches have played a particularly significant role in community and public health interventions.

## Self-control Theory

Self-control theory has been a primary conceptual underpinning of behavioral medicine. Behavioral medicine approaches are based on the notion that systems within and across individuals self-regulate on the basis of feedback from the environment. Thus, patients are encouraged to be active participants in their care, to take responsibility for their health, and to attend to appropriate feedback to assist them in self-management of health and illness. Care providers in this model provide specialized technical services and consultation to patients to assist their self-regulation.

## Stress Management and Biofeedback

Stress management and biofeedback are related techniques that teach patients (1) self-regulation of arousal, (2) predictability and control of cognitive and overt responses to stressors, and (3) awareness and control of psychophysiological relationships. Biofeedback is the application of physiological monitoring for the express purpose of facilitating the patient's learning to modulate physiological responses directly. This technology was a direct outgrowth of operant psychophysiological research and has been applied to many clinical problems. Biofeedback is often combined with perception-modification techniques (e.g., relaxation training, distraction, mental visualization, and suggestion) to provide pain and symptom control.

## Examples of the Application of Behavioral Medicine Techniques

Behavioral medicine interventions target dietary risk factors, such as helping individuals reduce saturated fat and cholesterol to lower serum cholesterol levels, reduce calories to control weight, reduce sugar intake to lower triglyceride levels and control weight, reduce sodium while increasing potassium and calcium to control blood pressure, and reduce alcohol to lower blood pressure as well as prevent detrimental effects on organ tissue. Behavioral medicine programs have offered education in nutrition and instruction in behavior modification to alter food choices, cooking methods, shopping habits, and attention to prevention of relapse to realistically change dietary habits in the long run. These programs have shown considerable promise.

Most behavioral programs aimed at smoking cessation now include a variety of methods. Self-control procedures are always included, such as self-monitoring (e.g., identification of triggers to anticipate, modify, or avoid), stimulus control (e.g., training in cognitive and behavioral strategies to reduce cravings and avoidance of smoking-related activities (such as parties or bars), and development of substitute behaviors (e.g., chewing gum, using toothpicks, drinking water, exercising, engaging in hobbies) for smoking (Fiore et al. 1992). Relaxation training, stress management, and contingency contracts may also be implemented (Lichtenstein 1982). The core assumption in behavioral smoking interventions and relapse prevention is that participants who learn, practice, and use behavioral and cognitive coping skills for managing cravings and smoking triggers will be more successful at quitting. The use of nicotine replacement has been examined as both a sole treatment and an adjunctive treatment to behavioral programs. A comprehensive review of the research literature found that success rates for smoking cessation were significantly higher when nicotine replacement was incorporated into a comprehensive behavioral treatment package (Fiore et al. 1992).

Behavioral medicine programs for chronic pain management have also been effective and employ a broad range of the techniques described above (Atkinson and Slater 1992, Slater and Good 1991, Slater and Kodiath 1991, Fordyce 1976, Turk et al. 1983, Morley et al. 1999, Haddock et al. 1997, Holroyd and Penzien 1990). Central to the behavioral approach to pain management is an analysis of behavior patterns related to pain and daily functioning. Patients are taught self-monitoring and contingency management skills, as well as, in many cases, relaxation and coping skills. Medication use is brought under systematic control and functional capacity is gradually increased with self-monitoring, contingency management, and self-control techniques. Attendant psychiatric disorders such as depression are treated, and psychosocial issues such as family discord are addressed. Patients are encouraged to assume greater responsibility for self-management with guidance from their physicians. Similar approaches have also provided successful models for case management of other chronic illnesses such as congestive heart failure (Riegel et al. 2002).

## Treatment for Stress-Related Illness

Stress responses are complex reaction patterns with physiological, cognitive, behavioral, and social components. As a result, prevention and treatment of stress-related illness have concentrated on several important dimensions. The characteristic approach of behavioral medicine is to help individuals be more competent in managing their behaviors and emotions in reaction to taxing aspects of their environment or their medical illness. Self-management and effective command of one's health and environment depend on possessing the necessary cognitive and behavioral skills and being able to employ those skills. Goals for treatment do not entail eliminating stress (or the medical problem) but aim toward helping the patient to learn the skills to function adequately despite stressful situations.

Individuals who rely more on active coping efforts to manage problems generally tend to adapt better to life stressors and experience fewer physiological and psychiatric symptoms than those who cope by avoiding (Manne and Zautra 1990, Parker et al. 1988). Active efforts to seek information and support and to problem solve have been related to better adjustment in a variety of populations, including medical patients with diverse disorders, family caregivers, and healthy adults. Furthermore, research has shown that persistent avoidance or passive coping, such as denying, fantasizing, minimizing, accepting the situation, and venting negative emotions, is maladaptive and an important risk factor associated with many medical illnesses as well as emotional distress.

One of the key areas of focus has been on arousal-reducing techniques (Jacobson 1938), such as biofeedback, relaxation training, diaphragmatic breathing, meditation, self-hypnosis, and the use of exercise to reduce or counter stress (Table 90–7). The rationale for these stress management techniques assumes that an increased level of physiological arousal is manifested by a combination of increased

| Table 90–7 | Behavioral Arousal Control Methods |
|---|---|
| Progressive muscle relaxation | Systematic tensing and relaxing of major skeletal muscles |
| Diaphragmatic breathing | Repeated deep abdominal breathing |
| Autogenic training | Self-statements of rhythmical breathing, limb heaviness, and warmth |
| Guided imagery | Use of imagination and fantasy to visualize relaxing images |
| Hypnosis | Focused attention with suggestion for specific responses |
| Meditation | Repetitious inward attention with no specific suggestions |
| Biofeedback | Providing physiological information to facilitate self-regulation |
| Exercise | Physical activity, particularly aerobic activity |
| Cognitive therapy | Analysis and modification of thoughts contributing to arousal |
| Coping skills training | Analysis and modification of inefficacious responses to stress |

muscle tension and increased sympathetic nervous system activity. In addition, specific training in reducing thoughts that increase arousal and learning more adaptive behaviors in response to a variety of stressful situations are emphasized in behavioral medicine's integrated multicomponent approach to managing stress-related illness.

## Biofeedback

Biofeedback as a tool for the treatment of tension dates to the early 1970s and has been used to provide information on physiological changes that were once thought involuntary (Miller 1969). With repeated training, patients can produce and detect physiological changes to bring under control many aspects of autonomic arousal (e.g., blood pressure, heart rate, musculoskeletal tension, and peripheral vascular blood flow).

The effects of biofeedback are often produced by the person's attempts at relaxation or mental imagery. Treatment of a range of problems, such as anxiety, headaches, temporomandibular joint difficulties, and a variety of chronic pain problems, has been useful with the techniques of biofeedback. However, for the most part, it is fair to say that biofeedback has not shown to be any more effective in reducing arousal and helping with these illnesses than the following stress management strategies.

## Relaxation Training

The oldest arousal-reducing or stress management techniques for a variety of medical problems, especially cardiovascular reactivity, are the various forms of relaxation training: (1) progressive muscle relaxation, the systematic tensing and relaxing of major muscle groups; (2) autogenic training, specific self-instructions to relax; (3) various forms of meditation, including the "relaxation response" (Benson 1976); and (4) diaphragmatic breathing. These nonpharmacological treatments for stress-related disorders have been a major landmark in the field; a large body of evidence has accumulated showing diminished stress-related symptoms. The various techniques allow an individual a way of

countering arousal in anticipation, moderating its intensity, inhibiting it, or assisting in recovery from stressful encounters.

Tension is associated with physiological changes that may or may not be noticeable (e.g., heart rate, blood pressure, and respiratory rates). Regular practice of progressive muscle relaxation teaches individuals to gradually relax skeletal muscles and quiet the autonomic nervous system. Individuals are taught to become more familiar with the effects of stress on musculoskeletal tension and to counteract these reactions by acquainting themselves with the sensations of both tight and relaxed musculature throughout the whole body. Training begins with the tensing and relaxing of multiple muscle groups, and individuals are eventually asked to achieve relaxation by merely recalling the sensations associated with the release of tension. Successful training aids the individual in greater awareness of muscle tension and its physiological effects and provides an ability to reduce arousal in an efficient manner. Emphasis is placed on transferring the relaxation effects to real-life situations (also called applied relaxation)—the physician's office, work site, traffic jams, or everyday interactions with others.

## Exercise

Whereas a formidable body of evidence has accumulated underscoring the long-term benefits of exercise, the specific stress-reducing effects have been more anecdotal than empirical. Evidence indicates that aerobic exercise tends to lower blood pressure across a wide variety of hypertensive individuals—from mildly to moderately hypertensive patients, in adolescent to geriatric populations, and even in those with advanced end-organ damage such as renal dialysis patients. Persons who are aerobically fit are better able to meet a physical demand with less sympathetic activation than their less fit counterparts. Fit individuals secrete less catecholamine, have reduced heart rates, and have lower peripheral vasoconstriction at the same exercise workload (Clausen 1977). Moreover, review of the literature suggests that exercise may be effective in reducing the risk for development of essential hypertension (Siegel and Blumenthal 1991).

## Cognitive Therapy

Another focus of stress management techniques has been on the specific thoughts that decrease arousal and reduce the effects of stress. The area that has shown the greatest promise has been cognitive therapy (Beck 1976, Burns 1980). To decrease persistent negative emotions and help patients adapt to events for which they have little or no control, individuals are taught cognitive strategies, such as restructuring irrational beliefs and replacing distorted, unrealistic, negative, or worry thoughts with rational, optimistic, and "wait and see" beliefs.

Aside from unusual catastrophic events (e.g., prisoner of war, rape, victimization by terrorists), stress is often a perception or an attribution by the patient. Moreover, thoughts about a situation always precede arousal (whether the individual is aware of the thought or not). Therefore, individuals are taught to identify events that increase emotional distress or arousal, analyze specific aspects of the event that are upsetting, and learn whether they are overreacting or distorting events unnecessarily. When events are determined to be realistically difficult, then learning more positive ways to think about the situation may decrease negative reactions to such stressors.

## Skills Training

Behavioral coping skills training teaches a variety of skills: problem-solving strategies, time management skills, assertiveness training, and use of social supports. Assertiveness training, a cognitive–behavioral technique used to alter significant components of the stress response, involves learning to stand up for one's personal and reasonable rights and to express appropriate thoughts, feelings, and beliefs in a direct, honest, and appropriate way (Lange and Jakubowski 1971). Assertiveness training emphasizes responding to the environment in a healthier fashion and feeling more confident and capable. Aggressive, nonassertive, and assertive behaviors are clearly distinguished as reflected by eye contact, body posture, physical contact, gestures, facial expressions, verbal tone, verbal content, and thoughts. Nonassertive behavior typically entails inhibition of action and denial of feelings so that such individuals often do not get what they want. Persons who act aggressively may get what they desire but at the expense of others. Assertiveness, on the other hand, does not necessarily entail a positive outcome, but individuals who use such an approach express themselves honestly and stand up for what they want while respecting the wishes of others.

A particular variant of assertiveness training has been designed to alter excessively angry or aggressive responses and includes education concerning the function of anger, triggers to hostility (persons and situations), and appraisal of events leading to angry feelings. Emphasis is placed on the harmful physiological aspects of anger, and individuals are taught the difference between healthy and constructive expressions of anger and those that are indirect or hurtful. Alberti and Emmons (1995) summarized coping strategies used to manage anger (Table 90–8).

## Social Support

An extensive literature has reviewed the protective effects of social support as a mediator of stress and an important resource for those suffering from chronic disease (Goldberger and Breznitz 1993). The construct of social support has been defined as the product of any activity that enhances an individual's sense of mastery through sharing tasks, giving material and cognitive assistance, and providing emotional comfort (Hobfoll and Vaux 1993). Three types of social supports have been distinguished: (1) support network resources, the available social relationships that objectively may be called on for help in times of need and that offer stable attachment to a social group; (2) supportive behavior, an exchange of resources between at least two individuals intended to enhance the well-being of the person receiving the support; and (3) subjective appraisal of support, the assessment of the person's supportive behaviors within the relationship (Hobfoll and Vaux 1993). Access to positive social supports appears to beneficially influence a variety of health problems, including cardiovascular morbidity and mortality, cancer, arthritis, renal disease, childhood leukemia, stroke, and diabetes (Taylor and Aspinwall 1993).

| Table 90–8 | Effective Techniques for Coping with Anger |
| --- | --- |

Keep an anger diary.

Write a self-management contract, including an affirmation to yourself.

Learn alternative behaviors.

Learn to tune out provocation.

Develop early warning systems.

Know your own "buttons."

Know your body feelings.

Count to 10, delay your response.

Read about dealing with anger—especially in history and great literature and ancient philosophy.

Learn to express anger assertively.

Focus on the task on hand and your goals.

Exaggerate your feelings to a ridiculous extreme—then laugh at yourself.

Talk yourself out of angry feelings.

Look for humor in the situation.

Develop a rational belief system—overcome irrational beliefs, such as "The world should be fair."

Develop a relaxation response.

Develop cool, friendly ways of responding to potential angry situations or hostility in others.

Learn stress inoculation techniques.

*Source*: Alberti RE and Emmons ML (1995) Your Perfect Right: A Guide to Assertive Living, 7th ed. Impact Publishers, San Luis Obispo, CA. Copyright 1995 Robert E. Alberti and Michael L. Emmons. Reproduced for John Wiley & Sons by permission of Impact Publishers, Inc., P.O. Box 1094, San Luis Obispo, CA 93406. Further reproduction prohibited.

As with stress, social support has a complex effect on well-being. Social supports may function by changing the individual's assessment of the stressful event or may prevent damaging behavioral or physiological responses to stress. Social supports may reduce the distress of managing a chronic illness and have been associated with greater adherence to medical regimens and use of health services (Wallston et al. 1983). Moreover, it is believed that social support may be most influential when it is used under highly stressful conditions.

When stress increases, people are more likely to seek more social support. In a review of the social support literature, Hobfoll and Vaux (1993, pp. 695–696) summarized the role of social support and stress by stating that social support may prevent the occurrence of stressors, inoculate against them, facilitate accurate appraisal of an ambiguous encounter, facilitate reappraisal as an encounter unfolds, act directly to meet the demand, suggest coping options, and sustain efficacy or facilitate recovery of emotional equilibrium through either emotional support or diversion. Whereas empirical work is only starting to demonstrate these proposed relationships, social support is overall considered a valuable resource. Patients are taught the importance of social supports for maintaining health, how to elicit and retain support, and how to identify support that is appropriate to the demands of relevant stressors.

## Pain Management: An Example of Adaptation and Progress in Behavioral Medicine

Pain management has been a significant emphasis of behavioral medicine since its earliest days. Pain control is also one of the areas of greatest success and documented efficacy. The development of pain management approaches in behavioral medicine parallels the development of the field in general and the historical, political, and socioeconomic factors of the times.

## Phase I: Mental Control of Pain Sensations

Initial efforts to conceptualize chronic pain syndromes emphasized psychiatric concepts that influence pain reports (e.g., somatization, hypochondriasis, hysteria, secondary gain) (Pilowsky 1978, Freud and Breuer 1974). Psychotherapeutic approaches were then employed to resolve conflicts and redirect attention. Most notable was the use of mental techniques like hypnosis to redirect attention and modify perception directly at a cognitive level (Hilgard 1978). Considerable success was attained, particularly with painful procedures, acute pain, and relatively circumscribed pain syndromes. Dissatisfaction grew out of inconsistency of results, lack of generalization to chronic pain, and inattention to dysfunction and disability.

## Phase II: Biofeedback to Regulate Painful Processes

Biofeedback approaches offered an integrated psychophysiological (mind–body) approach to pain. Biofeedback developed out of the need to address disease process and dysfunction. Moreover, biofeedback was congruent with the basic notion of self-regulation that permeates the field and arose from successful laboratory research demonstrating reliable visceral learning phenomena (Miller 1969). Biofeedback approaches enjoyed considerable success when disease processes were well understood, although the mechanism of action is still under considerable debate (Gaupp et al. 1994). Dissatisfaction grew out of limited applications, lack of generalization, and limited attention to disability.

## Phase III: Behavioral Rehabilitation to Restore Function

The marriage of operant psychology and rehabilitation medicine brought the next wave of influence on behavioral medicine pain management (Fordyce 1976). This approach indirectly addressed pain by directly modifying pain behaviors, functional capacities, and use of health care technologies. For example, patients were taught to gradually increase their exercise tolerance while staff and families systematically reinforced attempts at healthy functional behavior and did not reinforce "pain behaviors" (e.g., guarding, bracing, limping, grimacing, complaints of pain). Greater emphasis was placed on reducing impairment and disability associated with pain than on alleviation of the subjective experience of pain. For the first time, rigorous outcome data were available supporting behavioral approaches to reducing pain, distress, and disability. Dissatisfaction grew out of limited acceptability to patients, lack of generalization, and limited attention to pain.

## Phase IV: Comprehensive Integrated Biomedical and Behavioral Technologies

Before the 1980s, pain management approaches were primarily singular. Practitioners adopted one of the aforementioned approaches or gradually converted and retrained as

the prevailing modes developed. Moreover, behavioral care was not well integrated with biomedical approaches. The 1980s saw the development of the multidisciplinary pain center, providing a conscious attempt to integrate the preceding three behavioral approaches with each other and with biomedical technologies (Loeser and Egan 1989). Patients were typically treated in highly structured inpatient settings to control their environments and were exposed to mental techniques, biofeedback, operant conditioning, cognitive therapy, physical rehabilitation, occupational therapy, vocational counseling, analgesic management, and innovative neurosurgical pain control technologies. With such comprehensive approaches, it was difficult to determine which elements were primarily responsible for observed effects. Dissatisfaction grew out of limited access, limited generalizability of findings and techniques, and high costs of treatment.

## Phase V: Health Services Delivery Accountability Models

The 1990s brought a renewed emphasis on accountability. Clinical outcomes were weighed against costs of treatment in ever more sophisticated ways. Most multidisciplinary inpatient pain centers have closed or are in financial trouble at this time. The emphasis in care has centered on cost containment, and comprehensive inpatient programs have found it difficult to justify sufficient incremental benefits over more focused outpatient programs. Current research focuses on distilling the findings from comprehensive treatment packages, determining essential treatment components, evaluating patient–treatment matching, and exploring more efficient delivery systems. Prevention of chronicity and disability management have taken center stage in the new millennium.

## Conclusion

In this chapter, we have tried to describe some of the historical and ideological underpinnings of behavioral medicine. The field has made impressive strides in a short time by offering unique behavioral interventions in diverse medical settings. What is the future of this approach?

Paradoxically, the interdisciplinary focus, which is responsible for much of its progress, also entails some problems. Behavioral medicine programs are rarely found in their own "departments" and instead are typically housed in departments of psychiatry, psychology, or family medicine. In such settings, the behavioral medicine practitioner or academic may be relatively isolated as a lone voice for the behavioral medicine perspective. More recently some free-standing departments and programs in behavioral medicine have been developed at several notable institutions such as Harvard and the University of California, San Francisco, and behavioral medicine has become a part of many medical school curricula. Professional societies such as the Society of Behavioral Medicine and the American Psychosomatic Society provide academic and clinical leadership through their journals and annual conferences. It remains to be determined what setting is best for long-term flourishing of behavioral medicine programs.

Issues of health care cost are predominant in the current climate. Behavioral medicine clinical activities are effective but are under increasing scrutiny as to their cost-effectiveness. The prevention programs are relatively inexpensive. Many of the clinical interventions, although relatively low-technology in nature, are costly in terms of personnel time and costly indeed in terms of the time and effort required of patients. Thus, it is unlikely that behavioral medicine programs will grow for treatment of conditions such as hypertension, for which numerous effective medications are available. On the other hand, behavioral medicine interventions not only are effective but are frequently unchallenged by any other interventions for diverse problems such as smoking cessation, pain management, and anticipatory nausea.

Curiously, behavioral medicine may be threatened most by its own success. With greater acceptance of the critical role of behavior in health through major initiatives such as *Healthy People 2010* (US Department of Health and Human Services 2000) and the foundation of the Office of Behavioral and Social Sciences Research within the National Institutes of Health in 1995, many are eager to jump on the bandwagon. It is striking to note that 8 of the 10 leading health indicators in *Healthy People 2010* are either behaviors (physical activity, tobacco use, substance abuse, responsible sexual behavior, injury, and violence) or else have substantial behavioral determinants (overweight and obesity, immunization, access to health care). It is gratifying to note that behavioral and psychosocial processes are beginning to be recognized as fundamental to comprehensive understanding of disease etiology and promotion of health and well-being (Singer and Ryff 2001), but it is concerning to see the highly variable quality of efforts attempting to establish credibility through association with behavioral medicine. The rising popularity of alternative medicine further contributes to this trend. As with other areas of medicine and psychiatry, attention to quality of care issues will be paramount for behavioral medicine in the next decade (Kohn et al. 2000, Institute of Medicine Committee 2001). Indeed, the renewed emphasis on patient safety, diffusion of innovation, and improved outcomes for patients with chronic illnesses provides new opportunities for the field. As efficacy and effectiveness are established, issues related to diffusion of innovations will become central. The current emphasis on integrating behavioral medicine with primary care highlights both the successes and limitations of the transition from a subspecialty focus to broader application.

As for so many approaches in psychiatry, behavioral medicine enthusiasts have a tendency toward grandiosity and all-inclusiveness. We have certainly learned from the experience of psychoanalysis and community psychiatry that there is peril in promising too much. There is certainly no shame in accumulating data regarding the efficacy of specific treatments for specific health problems. Indeed, this cautious methodical approach to intervention is one of the prime characteristics of the field. In many instances, behavioral medicine interventions are a vital component of care for patients, either in conjunction with other interventions such as consultation psychiatry or standing alone as in smoking cessation programs. Behavioral medicine requires a disciplined integration of many components—from the individual patient's body, to the society he or she lives in, to the environment with which he or she interacts. In the future, it is conceivable that a behavioral medicine approach will be the first choice of treatment in certain conditions—a choice based on efficacy, overall cost containment, and maximal wellness achieved for the patient.

## References

Ader R and Cohen N (1975) Behaviorally conditioned immunosuppression. Psychosom Med 37, 333–340.

Adler NE, Marmot M, McEwen BS, et al. (eds) (1999) Socioeconomic status and health in industrial nations: Social, psychological and biological pathways. Ann NY Acad Sci 896, 1–500.

Affleck G, Tennen H, Pfeiffer C, et al. (1987) Appraisal of control and predictability in adapting to chronic disease. J Pers 53, 273–279.

Alberti RE and Emmons ML (1995) Your Perfect Right: A Guide to Assertive Living, 7th ed. Impact Publishers, San Luis Obispo, CA.

American College of Sports Medicine (1991) Guidelines for Exercise Testing and Prescription, 4th ed. Lea and Febiger, Philadelphia.

Atkinson JH and Slater MA (1992) Behavioral medicine approaches to chronic back pain. In Rothman and Simeone's The Spine, 3rd ed., Herkowitz H, Bell G, Wiesel S, et al. (eds). WB Saunders, Philadelphia, pp. 1961–1982.

Beck AT (1976) Cognitive Therapy and the Emotional Disorders. International Universities Press, New York.

Benson H (1976) The Relaxation Response. Avon, New York.

Blundell JE and Lawton CL (1993) Pharmacological aspects of appetite. In Obesity: Theory and Therapy, 2nd ed., Stunkard AJ and Wadden TA (eds). Raven Press, New York, pp. 63–96.

Brownell KD and Rodin J (1994) The dieting maelstrom: Is it possible and advisable to lose weight? Am Psychol 49, 781–791.

Brownell KD and Wadden TA (1992) Etiology and treatment of obesity: Understanding a serious, prevalent, and refractory disorder. J Consult Clin Psychol 60, 505–517.

Burns DD (1980) Feeling Good: The New Mood Therapy. Avon, New York.

Center for Disease Control (1992) Prevalence of Sedentary Leisure-Time Behavior Among Adults in the United States. Health E-Stats. Atlanta, GA: CDC. NCHS. 1999.

Center for Disease Control (1993) Physical activity and the prevention of coronary heart disease. Morbid Mortal Week Rev 42, 669–672.

Chesney MA, Lurie P, and Coates TJ (1995) Strategies of addressing the social and behavioral challenges of prophylactic HIV vaccine trials. J AIDS Hum Retro 9, 30–35.

Clarkson TB, Manuck SB, and Kaplan JR (1986) Potential role of cardiovascular reactivity in atherogenesis. In Handbook of Stress, Reactivity, and Cardiovascular Disease, Matthews KA, Weiss SM, Detre T, et al. (eds). John Wiley, New York, pp. 35–47.

Clausen JP (1977) Effect of physical training on cardiovascular adjustments to exercise in men. Physiol Rev 57, 779–816.

Coumel P and Leenhardt A (1991) Mental activity, adrenergic modulation, and cardiac arrhythmias in patients with heart disease. Circulation 83(Suppl 2), 58–70.

DeBusk RF, Stenestrand U, Sheenan M, et al. (1990) Training effects of long versus short bouts of exercise in healthy subjects. Am J Cardiol 65, 1010–1013.

DiCara LV and Miller NE (1968) Instrumental learning of vasomotor responses by rats: Learning to respond differently in two ears. Science 159, 1485–1486.

Dimsdale J (1988) Perspective on type A and coronary disease. New Engl J Med 318, 110–112.

Dubbert P (1992) Exercise in behavioral medicine. J Consult Clin Psychol 60, 613–618.

Epstein LH (1992) The role of behavior therapy in behavioral medicine. J Consult Clin Psychol 60, 493–498.

Fiore MC, Jorenby DE, Baker TB, et al. (1992) Tobacco dependence and the nicotine patch: Clinical guidelines for effective use. JAMA 268, 2687–2694.

Fordyce WE (1976) Behavioral Methods for Chronic Pain and Illness. Mosby, St. Louis.

Freud S and Breuer J (1974) Studies on Hysteria. Pelican, London.

Friedman HS and DiMatteo MR (1989) Health Psychology. Prentice-Hall, Englewood Cliffs, NJ.

Friedman M and Rosenman RH (1959) Association of specific overt behavior pattern with blood and cardiovascular findings. JAMA 169, 1286–1296.

Gaupp LA, Flinn DE, and Weddige RL (1994) Adjunctive treatment techniques. In Handbook of Pain Management, 2nd ed., Tollison CD, Satterthwaite JR, and Tollison JW (eds). Williams & Williams Baltimore, pp. 108–135.

Goldberger L and Breznitz S (eds) (1993) Handbook of Stress: Theoretical and Clinical Aspects, 2nd ed. Free Press, New York.

Goldstein MG and Niaura R (1992) Psychological factors affecting physical condition: Cardiovascular disease literature review. Part 1. Psychosomatics 33, 134–145.

Haddock CK, Rowan AB, Wilson PG, et al. (1997) Home-based behavioral treatments for chronic benign headache: A meta-analysis of controlled trials. Cephalalgia 17, 113–118.

Harwood H, Fountain D, and Livermore G (1998) The Economic Costs of Alcohol and Drug Abuse in the United States, 1992. HHS, NIH, NIH Pub. No. 98-4327, Rockville, MD.

Haskell WL, Leon AS, Casperson CJ, et al. (1992) Cardiovascular benefits and assessment of physical activity and fitness in adults. Med Sci Sports Exer 24, S201–S220.

HCUPnet, Healthcare Cost and Utilization Project. Agency for Healthcare Research and Quality, Rockville, MD. http://www.ahrq.gov/data/hcup/hcupnet.htm

Hilgard ER (1978) Hypnosis and pain. In The Psychology of Pain, Sternbach RA (ed). Raven Press, New York, pp. 219–240.

Hobfoll SE and Vaux A (1993) Social support: Social resources and social context. In Handbook of Stress: Theoretical and Clinical Aspects, 2nd ed., Goldberger L and Breznitz S (eds). Free Press, New York, pp. 685–705.

Holroyd KA and Penzien DB (1990) Pharmacological versus non-pharmacological prophylaxis of recurrent migraine headache: A meta-analytic review of clinical trials. Pain 42, 1–13.

Institute of Medicine Committee on Quality of Health Care in America (2001) Crossing the Quality Chasm: A New Health System for the 21st Century. National Academy Press, Washington DC.

Jacobson E (1938) Progressive Relaxation. University of Chicago Press, Chicago.

Janz NK and Becker MH (1984) The health beliefs model: A decade later. Health Educ Q 11, 1–47.

Kaplan RM, Sallis JF, and Patterson TL (1993) Health and Human Behavior. McGraw-Hill, New York.

Kohn LT, Corrigan JM, and Donaldson MS (eds) (2000) To Err is Human: Building a Safer Health System. Committee on Quality of Health Care in America. Institute of Medicine. National Academy Press, Washington DC.

Lange AJ and Jakubowski P (1971) Responsible Assertive Behavior: Cognitive/Behavioral Procedures for Trainers. Research Press, Champaign, IL.

Lazare A (1973) Hidden conceptual models in clinical psychiatry. New Engl J Med 288, 345–351.

Lazarus RS and Folkman S (1984) Stress, Appraisal, and Coping. Springer-Verlag, New York.

Leon AS, Connett J, Jacobs DR, et al. (1993) Leisure-time physical activity levels and risk of coronary heart disease and death. JAMA 258, 2388–2395.

Lichtenstein E (1982) The smoking problem: A behavioral perspective. J Consult Clin Psychol 50, 804–819.

Lichtenstein E and Glasgow RE (1992) Smoking cessation: What have we learned over the past decade? J Consult Clin Psychol 60, 518–527.

Loeser JD and Egan KJ (1989) Managing the Chronic Pain Patient: Theory and Practice at the University of Washington Multidisciplinary Pain Center. Raven Press, New York.

Manne SL and Zautra AJ (1990) Couples coping with chronic illness: Women with rheumatoid arthritis and their healthy husbands. J Behav Med 13, 327–342.

Masters JC, Burish TG, Holland SD, et al. (1987) Behavior Therapy: Techniques and Empirical Findings. Harcourt Brace Jovanovich, San Diego, CA.

McGinnis JM and Foege WH (1993) Actual causes of death in the United States. JAMA 270, 2207–2212.

Miller NE (1969) Learning of visceral and glandular responses. Science 163, 434–445.

Miller NE (1978) Biofeedback and visceral learning. Annu Rev Psychol 29, 373–404.

Morley S, Eccleston C, and Williams A (1999) Systematic review and meta-analysis of randomized controlled trials of cognitive behaviour therapy and behaviour therapy for chronic pain in adults, excluding headache. Pain 80, 1–13.

Parker JC, McCrae C, Smarr K, et al. (1988) Coping strategies in rheumatoid arthritis. J Rheumatol 15, 1376–1383.

Pilowsky I (1978) Psychodynamic aspects of the pain experience. In The Psychology of Pain, Sternbach RA (ed). Raven Press, New York, pp. 203–217.

Prochaska JO, DiClemente CC, Velicer WF, et al. (1993) Standardized, individualized, interactive, and personalized self-help programs for smoking cessation. Health Psychol 12, 399–405.

Ragland DR and Brand RJ (1988) Type A behavior and mortality from coronary heart disease. New Engl J Med 318, 65–69.

Riegel B, Carlson B, Kopp Z, et al. (2002) Under A: Effect of a standardized nurse case-management telephone intervention on resource use in patients with chronic heart failure. Arch Intern Med 162, 705–712.

Rosenman RH (1993) Relationships of the type A behavior pattern with coronary heart disease. In Handbook of Stress, 2nd ed., Goldberger L and Breznitz S (eds). Free Press, New York, pp. 449–476.

Rosenman RH, Brand RJ, Jenkins CD, et al. (1975) Coronary heart disease in the Western Collaborative Group Study: Final follow-up experience of 8 years. JAMA 233, 872–877.

Rosenstock IM (1966) National study of health beliefs. J Health Hum Behav 7, 248–254.

Schwartz GE and Weiss SM (1978) Yale conference on behavioral medicine: A proposed definition and statement of goals. J Behav Med 1, 3–12.

Siegel WC and Blumenthal JA (1991) The role of exercise in the prevention and treatment of hypertension. Ann Behav Med 13, 23–30.

Singer BH and Ryff CD (eds) (2001) New Horizons in Health: An Integrative Approach. Committee on Future Directions for Behavioral and Social Sciences Research at the National Institutes of Health. National Academy Press, Washington DC.

Slater MA and Good AB (1991) Behavioral management of chronic pain. Holis Nurs Pract 6, 66–75.

Slater MA and Kodiath M (1991) Comprehensive management of the chronic pain patient: A case study. Holis Nurs Pract 6, 1–8.

Stansfeld SA and Marmot MG (2002) Introduction. In Stress and the Heart, Stansfeld SA and Marmot MG (eds). BMJ Books, London, pp. 1–4.

Stansfeld SA, Fuhrer R, Shipley MJ, et al. (1999) Work characteristics predict psychiatric disorder: Prospective results from the Whitehall II Study. Occup Environ Med 56, 302–307.

Stunkard AJ and Wadden TA (eds) (1993) Obesity: Theory and Therapy, 2nd ed. Raven Press, New York.

Suls J and Wan CK (1989) Effects of sensory and procedural information on coping with stressful medical procedures and pain: A meta-analysis. J Consult Clin Psychol 3, 372–379.

Taylor SE and Aspinwall LG (1993) Coping with chronic illness. In Handbook of Stress: Theoretical and Clinical Aspects, 2nd ed., Goldberger L and Breznitz S (eds). Free Press, New York, pp. 511–531.

Turk DC, Meichenbaum D, and Genest M (1983) Pain and behavioral medicine: A cognitive–behavioral approach. Guilford Press, New York.

US Department of Health and Human Services (1990) The Health Benefits of Smoking Cessation: A Report of the Surgeon General. US Government Printing Office, CDC 90-8416, Washington DC.

US Department of Health and Human Services (1991) National Health Promotion and Disease Prevention Objectives, Full Report with Commentary, Healthy People 2000. US Government Printing Office, (PHS) 91-S0212, Washington DC.

US Department of Health and Human Services (1996) Physical Activity and Health: A Report of the Surgeon General. CDC, National Center for Chronic Disease Prevention and Health Promotion (NCCDPHP), Atlanta, GA.

US Department of Health and Human Services (2000) With Understanding and Improving Health and Objectives for Improving Health, Vol. 1 and 2, Healthy People 2010, 2nd ed. Government Printing Office, Washington DC.

Wald NJ (1994) Guidance on terminology. J Med Screen 1, 76.

Wallston BS, Alagna SW, DeVellis BM, et al. (1983) Social support and physical health. Health Psychol 2, 367–391.

Wardle J and Pope R (1992) The psychological costs of screening for cancer. J Psychosom Res 36, 609–624.

Weiner H (1977) Psychobiology and Human Disease. Elsevier, New York.

Williams RB Jr. (1987) Psychological factors in coronary artery disease: Epidemiological evidence. Circulation 76(1), 117–123.

Wolf AM and Coditz GA (1998) Current estimates of the economic cost of obesity in the United States. Obes Res 6, 97–106.

# 91 Psychosocial Rehabilitation

Alan S. Bellack

Evidence accumulated over the last several decades has led to a general consensus that schizophrenia is a brain disease or set of related diseases caused by genetic and/or prenatal and perinatal insult (Weinberger 1987, Roberts 1991). Replicated data point to problems in neural structure (e.g., enlarged cerebral ventricles, hippocampus), neurotransmitter systems (including dopamine, serotonin, acetylcholine, and glutamate, among others), neural circuitry (e.g., especially including circuits mediated by frontal cortex), and cerebral blood flow and metabolism (especially in dorsolateral prefrontal cortex, cingulate gyrus) (Thaker and Carpenter 2001, Selemon 2001).

While the definitive neurobiological substrate of the illness remains to be determined, it is clear that treatment for schizophrenia must be based on effective biological/medical intervention. Conversely, no extant medical treatment is sufficient. Twenty percent or more of patients are not responsive to antipsychotic medication, and the majority although responsive, are residually symptomatic. In addition, many patients are substantially noncompliant. Even among those who are judged to be responsive and compliant, only a small proportion achieve adequate outcomes, including a return to premorbid levels of function. Schizophrenia is a multiply handicapping disorder marked by poor social role performance, chronic unemployment (or under-employment), excess medical morbidity and mortality, shortened life expectancy (including a markedly elevated risk for suicide), high levels of substance abuse, and increased risk for criminal victimization. Antipsychotic medications are demonstrably effective in reducing positive symptoms and have a modest effect on negative symptoms (especially on secondary negative symptoms), but they have limited impact on cognitive impairment and psychosocial functioning (Sharma and Harvey 2000). Even the new generation drugs are insufficient to restore premorbid levels of functioning, produce normative role performance, or substantially improve quality of life for most patients.

Moreover, it seems highly unlikely that medication alone can be sufficient until and unless discoveries emanating from genetics and genomics lead to different and more effective compounds for pharmacotherapy. Accumulating evidence indicates that schizophrenia is a neurodevelopmental disorder in which many patients demonstrate subtle attentional, cognitive, and neuromotor abnormalities in early childhood, long before the onset of overt psychotic illness, in keeping with "neurodevelopmental" models of the illness (Cornblatt and Keilp 1994, Walker et al. 1994, Weinberger 1995). Perhaps the most remarkable investigation demonstrating this was performed by Jones and colleagues (1994) who followed up subjects originally studied as part of the Medical Research Council National Survey of Health and Development, a study of all births in England, Scotland, and Wales during 1 week in 1946. These children were assessed at multiple time points with measures of developmental milestones, educational achievement, and social-behavioral assessments. Of the 4,746 English subjects, 30 developed schizophrenia by the age of 43, with cases identified and diagnosed on the basis of multiple medical record sources and direct interview data when subjects were aged 36. These subjects demonstrated delayed achievement of motor and speech milestones in infancy, lower estimated IQ scores by middle childhood, and increased social anxiety by early adolescence in comparison to the 4,716 controls. These data suggest that adult schizophrenia is preceded by multiple manifestations of subtle developmental compromise across neurological, intellectual, and social domains.

The developmental consequences of the illness are magnified with the first psychotic episode in late adolescence or young adulthood. People with schizophrenia become progressively more removed from their peer group, fail to achieve (or sustain) adult milestones such as marriage, higher education, and employment, and often become socially isolated. These functional, psychosocial consequences become more severe and entrenched as illness duration increases, and result in multiple treatment needs that are superimposed on the neurobiological aspects of illness. While innovative new medications could potentially ameliorate (or compensate for) some of the consequences of anomalous neural development, it is unlikely that any pharmacological approach could restore normal brain function. Furthermore, no medication could undo the lifelong consequences of impaired learning, failure to master adult developmental tasks, and social withdrawal. These impairments mandate a multifaceted approach to treatment that includes an array of psychosocial strategies, of which rehabilitation plays a key role (Bellack 1989). This conclusion is supported by a series of consensus treatment guidelines developed in the latter half of the 1990s (American Psychiatric Association 1997, Canadian Psychiatric Association 1998, Lehman and Steinwachs 1998, McEvoy et al. 1999).

In the following sections critical issues involved in effective use of rehabilitation and other psychosocial interventions are discussed and brief reviews of the most promising approaches are provided. The term *rehabilitation* is not precisely defined in our field. It is generally used to imply a subcategory of psychosocial treatment in which there is an emphasis on teaching/training, rather than discussion, and the focus is primarily on behaviors and functioning, rather than on intrapsychic processes (thinking and feeling). Reference is made later to *psychosocial intervention* when the issues have generality to the broader domain of psychological treatment.

## Issues in the Design of Psychosocial Interventions

The potential benefits of psychosocial treatment are often not achieved in the community due to poor understanding of the special needs and liabilities of schizophrenia patients. Five factors need to be taken into account when implementing psychosocial interventions and evaluating the results: (1) timing and duration of treatment; (2) individual differences in treatment needs; (3) the role of the patient in treatment; (4) the limitations imposed by impairments in information processing; and (5) the need to base interventions on a compensatory model.

## Timing and Duration of Treatment

The APA *Practice Guidelines for the Treatment of Patients with Schizophrenia* (American Psychiatric Association 1997, p. 1) makes a number of important points that are germane to rehabilitation programming, not the least of which pertains to the need for multimodal, long-term care: "Schizophrenia is a chronic condition that frequently has devastating effects on many aspects of the patient's life and carries a high risk of suicide and other life-threatening conditions. The care of most patients involves multiple efforts to reduce the frequency and severity of episodes and to reduce the overall morbidity and mortality of the disorder. Many patients require comprehensive and continuous care over the course of their lives with no limits as to duration of treatment." This guideline is widely reflected in case management and pharmacotherapy but has not been adequately addressed in rehabilitation programs.

Most research on psychosocial interventions has focused on time-limited strategies, typically in the range of 3 to 6 months (e.g., see sections on social skills training and cognitive rehabilitation, later in the chapter). This treatment duration is generally guided more by the pragmatics of grant design than by an analysis of patient needs. Nevertheless, such brief treatments have been found to be helpful for achieving specific goals, such as teaching patients how to discuss medication side effects with a physician, how to engage in safe sex, and how to communicate more effectively with family members. Research indicates that gains from such brief, focused treatments can be maintained over time (Bellack et al. 1984, Eckman et al. 1992). However, given the pervasive neurodevelopmental and psychosocial effects of the illness, these brief interventions are unlikely to produce broad-based improvement in overall functioning, or enduring changes in vulnerability to symptom exacerbations and relapse. Brief and highly focused rehabilitation programs designed to accomplish specific goals (e.g., to teach patients how to negotiate with health care providers or to go grocery shopping) can be quite effective. However, most patients will require intermittent booster treatment even for such circumscribed skills training programs, while others will need continuing support (e.g., prompting to perform activities of daily living) throughout their lives.

Unfortunately, the literature does not give much guidance in how to predict individual patient needs or systematically plan how long the course of rehabilitation treatment should be. Many community agencies have responded to this uncertainty by permanently enrolling patients in day treatment. However, few patients can, or do, actively participate in such endless treatment programs. They may come to the treatment center, especially if directed to do so by family members or residential managers, but that does not mean that they are actively participating or learning new skills. Our own experience, while not supported by data, strongly supports the use of time limited training curricula that address current needs and goals. The patient may repeat a curriculum (e.g., begin a new 3–6-month period in social skills training) if she/he desires but this should be a mutual choice between patient and program that reflects continuing motivation and need, not a reflection of diagnosis or economics (e.g., agencies cannot bill unless the patient receives some intervention). This latter point relates to another issue addressed in the APA guidelines: timing of treatment. The guidelines contend that the illness transpires in three phases: (1) *Acute*, during which the primary aim is to reduce acute symptoms; (2) *Stabilization*, during which aims are to minimize likelihood of relapse, further reduce symptoms, and enhance adaptation in the community; and (3) *Stable*, during which aims are to maintain or improve level of functioning and quality of life, while continuing to monitor. Rehabilitation is generally not applicable during acute stages of illness. With hospital stays often limited to a few days to 1 week there is little opportunity to conduct a systematic rehabilitation program, and acutely ill patients generally are unable to effectively participate in cognitive–behavioral interventions during this period.

The role for psychosocial treatment increases as the patient becomes more stable and shifts from support and stress reduction to specific rehabilitation strategies such as social skills training and cognitive rehabilitation. This three stage model and associated treatment emphasis has good face validity. However, both the model and assumptions about shifting goals of psychosocial treatment are based more on anecdotal evidence and clinical assumptions than on empirical data. In the concluding section on research needs, the guidelines aptly indicate that, "More precision is needed in specifying types of patients appropriate for specific treatment approaches at particular phases of the illness" (American Psychiatric Association 1997, p. 96).

## Individual Differences in Treatment Needs

Schizophrenia is a heterogeneous disorder, with wide variability in symptom presentation, severity, course, and treatment response. Indeed, the term *schizophrenias* may be more applicable. This heterogeneity has been interpreted as reflecting either multiple etiologies or multiple disease entities (Tsuang et al. 1990, Carpenter et al. 1993). It also undoubtedly reflects the idiosyncratic impact of each patient's environment and experiences throughout life, which influence both how the illness manifests itself and individual differences unrelated to the core illness (e.g., comorbid vulnerability to depression or substance abuse). For example, Mueser and colleagues (1991a) found that 50% of schizophrenia patients had persistent deficits in social skill over a 1-year period, while 11% did not differ from nonpatient controls, and the remainder showed variable performance. Thus, the common assumption that patients with schizophrenia have deficits in their social skill is true for many but not all patients.

Similar evidence of heterogeneity exists in regard to neuropsychological deficits. Schizophrenia patients, as a group, perform very poorly on the Wisconsin Card Sorting Test (WCST) (Heaton 1981), a measure of prefrontal cortical functioning and performance deficits are associated with hypoactivation of the dorsolateral prefrontal cortex (Berman et al. 1986, Weinberger et al. 1986). Yet, as many as 20% of patients may perform within normal levels on the WCST, and poor-performing patients appear to have a broader pattern of neuropsychological deficits than those who can perform at normative levels (Braff et al. 1991, Goldstein et al. 1996). Stratta and colleagues (1997) suggest that there are important differences in how different patients perform the task, as well as in how well they do. They subdivided patients into good- and poor-performing groups on the basis of categories correct at baseline, and then requested them to enunciate their selection strategy on readministration. The good-baseline performers improved significantly with this technique, while the poor performers got worse. The additional task demand apparently further disrupted their already impaired ability to solve the task. There is also considerable variability in the extent to which patients can be taught to improve their performance (Goldberg et al. 1987, Bellack et al. 1990) and in the extent to which performance improvements generalize to other tasks (Bellack et al. 2001).

In a creative study of patient heterogeneity that has considerable implications for rehabilitation, (Bellack et al. 1999) groups of schizophrenia patients with good and poor vocational outcomes on a battery of neuropsychological tests and brain morphology were compared with the help of MRI. Robust differences between the two groups in both domains were found. Poor vocational outcome patients performed more poorly on measures of processing speed and social judgment, and they showed evidence of reduced cortical asymmetries. These results have two implications for a consideration of rehabilitation in schizophrenia. First, the data suggest that good outcome patients have certain strengths and basic competencies that may compensate for liabilities. It is important to be able to identify patients who appear to have these competencies but who are not currently functioning well in order to provide special clinical attention, as their treatment needs should be different than the needs of patients who lack these strengths. Second, the fact that poor outcome is associated with greater abnormality of brain morphology is not surprising; previous reports

have documented relationships between poor outcome and ventricular size (Pearlson et al. 1984, Vita et al. 1991, van Os et al. 1995). It is also not a cause for therapeutic nihilism. It appears likely that such patients may require very different services to achieve maximal independence than patients who have much more intact cognitive performance. However, it will not be possible to develop such services in an effective manner until we have achieved a clearer understanding of the determinants of disability in schizophrenia.

In addition to the variability between patients, significant changes occur within patients over time that have a bearing on their treatment needs. Young patients need special help in dealing with the fact that they have a serious illness which may interfere with their personal goals and their ability to achieve independence, a problem which may contribute to their high vulnerability to suicide and substance abuse (Test et al. 1989, Caldwell and Gottesman 1990). Older patients may adjust to the difficulties of the illness through withdrawal or positive coping strategies (Wing 1987, Strauss 1989), but they face unique problems of their own. For example, as parents grow older they are generally less able to continue caring for an offspring with schizophrenia, necessitating a shift in care taking responsibility to either siblings (Horwitz et al. 1992) or the mental health system. A survey of the needs of schizophrenia patients in regular contact with their families indicated that concern over what happens when a parent dies was ranked fourth highest out of 45 topics (parents ranked this concern fifth) (Mueser et al. 1992).

Taken together, these data underscore that treatment planning must be individualized. While this might seem like a given, many outpatient treatment systems are designed with a *one-size-fits-all* model, in which most patients are assigned to a standard set of group treatments paired with case management. This is a strategy that maximizes dropouts and minimizes effectiveness. This is a population that is difficult to treat effectively under the best of circumstances. Positive outcomes are likely only if both the content of treatment and the format of treatment are tailored to the individual patient's needs and learning capacities.

## The Role of the Patient
The combination of psychosis, thought disorganization, and negative symptoms (especially anergia, apathy, and anhedonia) often lead to the false assumption that patients are not capable of being active participants in their own treatment. Indeed, many patients seem unmotivated and are noncompliant, but such seeming disinterest and passivity should not be interpreted as accurate reflections of the person's goals and desires or as immutable traits. Negative symptoms are not always stable, and they may be secondary to demoralization, psychotic symptoms, medication side effects, and other factors that vary over time (Carpenter et al. 1988, McGlashan and Fenton 1992). Paul and Lentz (1977) have shown that even extremely withdrawn, chronic schizophrenia patients can be motivated by a systematic incentive program. Similarly, desire to change and inclination to do the work required for treatment also vary over time in the same way that motivation to lose weight or quit smoking varies in nonpatient populations.

As cogently argued by Strauss (1989), schizophrenia patients have an active "will." Much of their behavior is goal directed and reflects an attempt to cope with the illness as best they can. Consequently, it is essential to view the patient as a potentially active partner and involve him or her in goal setting and treatment planning. Too often, treatments are imposed on patients by the treatment team and family members, with little consideration of the patient's own desires. It should not be surprising in such circumstances if the patient fails to adhere to treatment recommendations, increasing the risk of relapse and creating tensions in relationships with family members and treatment providers. To be sure, engaging the patient to establish treatment goals can be a long, arduous process, but failure to do so courts the larger risk of undermining the very purpose of the intervention.

Assessing engagement and "motivation" is not a straightforward process as illustrated by data from a clinical trial we are conducting to evaluate a new treatment program for substance abuse in schizophrenia. All patients were volunteers who signed informed consent documents confirming their desire to participate in treatment for their substance use, yet participation after signing consent has varied dramatically. Some 30% of volunteers never begin treatment. Initial results from those who do begin suggest a bimodal distribution of participation and outcome; about half of the patients come regularly and do very well and half drop out or participate intermittently and do poorly. It appears as if we can make very good predictions of outcome with the pretreatment score on the University of Rhode Island Change Assessment (URICA), a self-report measure of motivation to reduce substance abuse. If these preliminary results are maintained, we could potentially determine when to enroll patients, or triage highly motivated patients to active treatment and poorly motivated (but cooperative) patients to a motivation enhancement intervention. This approach warrants investigation for other interventions as well.

## Impairments in Information Processing

It is now well established that impaired information processing represents one of the most significant areas of dysfunction in schizophrenia. The illness is marked by neuropsychological deficits in multiple domains, including verbal memory, working memory, attention, speed of processing, abstract reasoning, and sensorimotor integration (Braff 1991, Green and Nuechterlein 1999). These deficits are highly related to social functioning and role performance in the community, as well as to performance in skills training programs (Green 1996, Green et al. 2000). For example, Mueser and colleagues (1991b) found that poor memory had a deleterious effect on learning in social skills training, while pretreatment symptomatology was unrelated to social skill acquisition. Kern and colleagues (1992) also found that memory impairment as well as poor sustained attention (on the Continuous Performance Test) was associated with decreased learning in social skills training.

A related issue concerns the impact of neurocognitive deficits on the generalization of treatment effects. A basic assumption of all psychotherapies is that skills acquired in treatment sessions must be transferred or generalized to the patient's natural environment. Yet, such generalization is contingent upon cognitive processes that are often disrupted in schizophrenia, especially "executive functions" mediated by the dorsolateral prefrontal cortex (Weinberger 1987). Several analog studies suggest that generalization is limited at best, even when explicitly programmed (Bellack et al. 1996, 2000).

Unfortunately, clinical rehabilitation programs have lagged behind the experimental literature in this arena and neurocognitive deficits have not been addressed in a systematic manner. To be sure, most sophisticated rehabilitation programs do adjust the rate at which information is presented and the amount of detail or nuance provided. Allowance is also generally made for the need for repetition and regular review. However, these adjustments do not necessarily compensate for deficits in working memory and higher level executive processes. For example, there are impairments in the ability to perceive the continuity of experience over time and to plan behavior accordingly: that is, to see how past experiences relate to current circumstances, or how what is currently being discussed can be applied in the future (Hemsley 1996). This problem would interfere with the ability to utilize newly acquired skills at appropriate times, to pursue goals in a systematic manner, or to use past experience to solve the problem. While there are strong data to document that rehabilitation programs are effective in teaching new behavior (Smith et al. 1996), the literature does not document that newly acquired skills are applied in the community. Even in cases where interventions result in better clinical outcomes, the data do not support the face valid assumption that changes are due to what has been taught. This point was amply illustrated in the Treatment Strategies in Schizophrenia Project, in which family treatment was associated with reduced relapse rates despite an absence of any change in communication patterns, the purported mechanism of change (Bellack et al. 2000). Determination of the mechanisms that mediate behavior change in the community is perhaps the greatest challenge facing the field over the next decade if we are to develop more effective treatments.

## Adoption of a Compensatory Model

As indicated above, schizophrenia is a multiply handicapping disorder. It impacts on the ability to perform activities of daily living (ADLs) and the ability to fulfill social roles, including worker, homemaker, student, parent, and spouse; it increases the risk of substance abuse and disease, including HIV; and it interferes with performance of appropriate health care behaviors, including compliance with both medical and psychiatric treatment. A large proportion of patients also have residual psychotic symptoms and periodic exacerbations and they experience high levels of depression and anxiety. Overall, they suffer from poor quality of life. In light of this panoply of impairments, no single treatment is likely to have a sufficiently broad-based impact. This circumstance stands in marked contrast to less severe disorders such as unipolar depression and anxiety disorders in which a single intervention may be expected to produce substantial amelioration of the condition. Nevertheless, psychosocial treatments for schizophrenia have often been held to this same standard leading to the faulty conclusion that they are not effective.

A rehabilitation model, the primary focus of this chapter, is more appropriate than the standard treatment model as: (1) it implies a narrower focus on specific skills and behaviors, and (2) it aims to improve functioning in specific areas, rather than eliminating or curing an entire condition. As indicated above, cognitive impairment is a central feature of the disorder, evident in childhood and progressing sharply with the onset of psychotic illness. It is reasonable to speculate that the impairments observed in ill adult patients are at least of two types: (1) those present from early in development; and (2) those that are related to clinical psychotic illness. The existence of such early, developmentally based impairments suggest that the concept of "premorbid" functioning in schizophrenia may no longer be tenable; rather, there is a prepsychotic period during which there is subtle evidence of the "morbid" process. Thus, the challenge confronting attempts at cognitive enhancement may not be restoration of function, but instead may be the development of critical competencies and strategies for coping with deficits.

Consistent with this hypothesis, a compensatory approach to treatment may be more appropriate than the restorative or reparative approach characteristic of most treatment programs. For example, rehabilitation for people with visual impairments involves teaching them to rely more on other senses, to use special appliances such as Braille keyboards, to use aides such as canes and guide dogs, and to systematically arrange their environment to minimize the need for sight. Success is achieved by improving independence, role functioning, and quality of life, not by restoring vision. Comparable rehabilitation programming is provided for stroke patients, individuals with paralysis, and amputees. Of note, these activist, goal oriented approaches are inconsistent with either the short-term up-and-out philosophy or the lifelong day care approach often seen in public mental health centers. Patients receive ongoing support, but the support is oriented to skill development and solving problems in daily living, not restoration of premorbid functioning. Conversely, effective rehabilitation is neither infantalizing nor paternalistic; it is supportive, but it is also task and goal oriented.

### Clinical Vignette

Susan R was a single white woman first diagnosed with schizophrenia when she was 24. She had been working as a clerk in a small store and living with her parents when she first became ill. She had had few friends and dated infrequently. She was 32 when she began to participate in our rehabilitation program. She was living in a group home and had been unable to work since her first psychotic episode. She was described by her case manager as a passive, shy woman who was frequently taken advantage of by other residents in the group home and the day treatment program she attended. She was referred to us because of concerns that: (1) she needed to be more assertive with other patients who were borrowing her money and personal items, and (2) that she had expressed an interest in getting a job but was so quiet that she was unable to get past interviews.

Susan was well-maintained on medication, she did not have significant negative symptoms, and she did not manifest behavioral problems that would prevent her from working. Based on the case manager's report and a review of Susan's medical record we focused our attention on social skills. She was appropriately groomed and did not present herself as a "patient" (e.g., no inappropriate mannerisms, no intrusions of psychotic or tangential thoughts, able to track conversation and provide appropriate responses to questions). However, she had a *deer in the headlights* quality. She seemed quite ill at ease; she scarcely made eye contact, looking mostly at the floor; her arms were wrapped round herself and she seemed to be physically tense; her shoulders were hunched and her head tilted toward the floor; she spoke haltingly in a very soft voice, such that the interviewer frequently had to ask her to repeat what she had said and to speak more loudly. When asked about her case manager's concerns about lending things to peers she indicated she didn't always want to give away her money and things, but that she was afraid people would get angry with her if she refused. She expressed the desire to return to work as a clerk, especially if the job did not involve much pressure. She reported that she always felt nervous during job interviews even when she thought she could do the work.

In response to our evaluation and Susan's expressed desire to be more assertive and to be able to get a job, we contracted with her to participate in a social skills training group for 3 months. The group included six other patients and met twice per week for 60 to 90 minutes. Susan's program consisted of three inter related curriculum units: (1) assertiveness training to teach her how to be more effective in refusing unreasonable requests from peers; (2) job interview skills; and (3) sexual assertion skills. The unit on sex was based on our concern that Susan was vulnerable to unwanted sexual advances, and addressed refusal skills (how to say "no") and safe sex skills (how to get a partner to use a condom). Skills training for all three units consisted primarily of role-play rehearsals. A theme was defined for each sessions (e.g., telling a friend you cannot lend them money) and each patient was prompted to identify a specific situation which had recently occurred or might occur in the near future. Patients then took turns engaging in repeated role plays in which the therapist portrayed someone in the patient's environment. In Susan's case, she identified other patients who frequently asked her for things and she rehearsed saying no to typical requests. Training Susan in job interview skills was coordinated with efforts by her case manager to arrange for interviews, as training is invariably more effective when it has near-term relevance and the new skills can be practiced in the real world. Training in safe sex skills proved to be very relevant as Susan admitted that she was being pressured to have sex by other patients.

Susan responded well to treatment. She was able to secure a part time job as a clerk within a few months of training, and had maintained the job when we followed up some 6 months later. Her case manager reported that she was better able to refuse requests for money, although it was arranged for staff to bank her paychecks and keep a minimal amount of cash on hand just to be safe. The case manager also reported that Susan had a boyfriend, another patient attending the day treatment center. While there is no assurance that Susan was practicing safe sex skills, she had not become pregnant, there was no evidence of an STD, and the boyfriend was known to be taking condoms from the bowl at the reception desk.

Cognitive adaptation training (CAT) is a creative compensatory approach developed by Velligan and colleagues (2000). Case managers provide patients with home-based, compensatory environmental strategies to help structure the patient's living environment which maximizes the likelihood that she/he can complete requisite activities of daily living. Examples include posting reminders about appointments on the exit door from the apartment, listing items of clothing to be worn on the closet door, and placing medications in a location that makes it maximally likely that the patient will see it and be reminded to take it. Prompts and other environmental aides are individually tailored to the patients' level of apathy, disinhibition, and executive dysfunction. CAT can be administered in a time limited fashion, but may be a lifelong service for severely impaired patients. Velligan and colleagues found 9-months of CAT to be superior to an attention placebo and standard outpatient care on positive symptoms, negative symptoms, motivation, community functioning, global functioning, and incidence of rehospitalization. This is an excellent model for compensatory interventions, and warrants further study (Table 91–1).

## Rehabilitation Strategies

The following sections will briefly describe and evaluate the two types of rehabilitation programs that have had the greatest clinical and heuristic impact on the field in the 1990s, social skills training and cognitive rehabilitation, and promising directions in vocational rehabilitation.

## Social Skills Training

Social dysfunction is a defining characteristic of schizophrenia that is semi-independent of other domains of the illness (Strauss et al. 1974, Lenzenwerger et al. 1991). Social functioning is also predictive of the course and outcome of the illness (McGlashan 1986, Johnstone et al. 1990). The most useful perspective for understanding social functioning and social dysfunction in the illness has been the "social skills model" (Meier and Hope 1998, Morrison and Bellack 1984). Social skills are specific response capabilities necessary for effective performance. They include verbal response skills (e.g., the ability to start a conversation or to say "No" when needed), paralinguistic skills (e.g., use of appropriate voice volume and intonation), and nonverbal skills (e.g., appropriate use of gaze, hand gestures, and facial expressions). These skills tend to be stable over time and make a unique contribution to the performance of social roles and quality of life (Bellack et al. 1990, Mueser et al. 1991a). Increasing social competence and improving social role functioning has been a major focus of rehabilitation efforts for the past 25 years, and a well-developed technology for teaching social skills has been developed and empirically tested: social skills training (SST) (Bellack et al. 1997, Liberman 1995) (see Table 91–1).

The basic technology for training social skills was developed in the 1970s and has not changed substantially in the intervening years. It is a highly structured educational procedure that is generally conducted in small groups. Complex social repertoires such as making friends and

**Table 91–1** Examples of Promising Rehabilitation Strategies

| Strategy | Representative Source | Brief Description |
|---|---|---|
| Social skills training | Bellack et al. (1997) | A small group intervention for teaching patients social skills. Social behaviors are broken down into component units (e.g., making eye contact). Patients receive instruction on how to perform the units, and then rehearse effective social behaviors in simulated social encounters, analogous to learning motor skills. |
| | In Vivo Amplified Social Skills Training (Liberman et al. 2001) | A program designed to foster generalization to the community by combining social skills training with intensive case management. |
| Cognitive rehabilitation | Integrated Psychological Therapy (Brenner et al. 1990) | A small group approach that attempts to reduce cognitive impairment that interferes with social functioning. Program involves a series of stages beginning with basic cognitive processing and ending with social skills training. |
| | Neuropsychological Educational Approach to Remediation (Medalia and Revheim 1999) | A training program that employs commercially produced educational software that is selected to be of high intrinsic interest to patients. Patients select from a variety of software programs that involve diverse neurocognitive capacities and work at their own pace. |
| | Cognitive Remediation Therapy (Wykes et al. 1999) | A one-on-one training program that focuses on executive functioning and higher level cognitive capacities using paper and pencil tasks and neurocognitive tests. Emphasis is placed on teaching response strategies (e.g., problem solving) in a graduated fashion that minimizes errors and frustration. |
| Vocational rehabilitation | Integrated Placement and Support Model (Drake et al. 1999) | An innovative approach that employs a train and place model, rather than the traditional train and place approach. Patients work with a case manager who helps them find a real job in the community, and then provides ongoing support at the workplace to help the person succeed. |
| Cognitive adaptation training | Velligan et al. (2000) | Based on the assumption that many patients cannot monitor and manage their own behavior in the community, a clinician goes to the person's home to help structure the environment in ways that minimize demands on limited cognitive capacity. Techniques include: (1) organizing drawers and closets so person automatically selects appropriate clothing items; (2) placing signs and other prompts in highly visible places in the apartment (e.g., bathroom mirror) to remind patient to perform ADLs (activities of daily life); (3) to take medicine, etc. |

dating are broken down into steps or component elements such as maintaining eye contact and asking questions. Patients are first taught to perform the elements and then gradually learn to smoothly combine them. Each session has a specific focus such as how to initiate conversations with strangers and how to refuse an unreasonable request. Trainers are more like teachers than traditional therapists. They first give patients simple instructions about how the behavior is to be performed, then they model appropriate behavior in a simulated conversation, and then they engage patients in role playing of simulated social encounters as a vehicle for practicing new skills. The therapists provide social reinforcement after each role played response and shape improved performance.

A large number of single case studies and small group designs have demonstrated the efficacy of SST for teaching a wide range of skills, including conversational skill, assertiveness, and medication management (Benton and Schroeder 1990, Halford and Hayes 1991). Over the past decade, six larger group studies have been conducted (Brown and Munford 1983, Spencer et al. 1983, Bellack et al. 1984, Liberman et al. 1986, Hogarty et al. 1986, Eckman ct al. 1992). The findings have been consistent with the smaller trials and indicate that effects of SST are maintained for at least 6 to 12 months.

Four of the six studies examined the effects of SST on symptoms, relapse, and social adjustment, with mixed results. Bellack and colleagues (1984) compared 3 months of group SST in a day hospital with day hospital treatment alone. At the 6-month follow-up, patients who received SST were less symptomatic and had better social adjustment, but there were no differences in relapse at the 1-year follow-up. Liberman and colleagues (1986) compared 2 months of intensive SST with "holistic health" treatment for long-term residents of a state hospital awaiting discharge. At the 2-year follow-up, the SST patients were better on several symptom measures and social adjustment, but relapse rates did not differ significantly. Eckman and colleagues (1992) and Marder and colleagues (1993) compared 1 year of intensive group SST with a supportive group. At the 2-year follow-up, patients who had received SST had better social adjustment, although their relapse rates did not differ from the control group.

In the only well-controlled study to examine individual SST, Hogarty and colleagues (1986, 1991) compared SST, family psychoeducation, SST plus family psychoeducation, and medication only. All patients were living with, or in contact with, high expressed emotion (EE) family members. SST, alone and in combination with family therapy, was associated with reduced relapse rates throughout the first 21 months of the study. By the 24th month, however, the effect of SST was no longer significant due to several relapses in the last 3 months for this group. The effect of SST on social functioning was not effectively assessed in this study, so it is unclear as to how well SST was administered. SST was also not specifically designed to help patients interact with their high EE relatives, an important factor in relapse.

Several trends emerge from these studies. SST is clearly effective in increasing the use of specific behaviors (e.g., gaze, asking questions, voice volume) and improving functioning in the specific domains that are the primary focus of the treatment (e.g., conversational skill, ability to perform on a job interview). However, it is unclear whether other more diffuse dimensions of social functioning are affected, or the extent to which learning in the clinic translates into improved role functioning in the community. The effects of SST on relapse rate and symptoms appear to be negligible, although this is not surprising given the narrow focus of the intervention. Several recent reviews of empirically supported treatments rated SST as no more than "promising," a somewhat disappointing evaluation after 25 years of study (DeRubeis and Crits-Christoph 1998, Scott and Dixon 1995). SST is clearly an effective teaching technology that is well-received by both patients and clinicians. Nevertheless, it may well be that no time-limited, compartmentalized, office-based treatment can have broad-based effects. As discussed earlier in this chapter, it may be necessary to employ longer-term treatments that extend into the community and that are integrated with an array of intervention strategies.

Liberman and colleagues (2001) have approached the problem of generalization with an innovative approach referred to as *in vivo* amplified skills training (IVAST). It combines standard skills training with intensive case management, based on the assertive community treatment (ACT) model (Stein and Test 1985). Office-based SST is supplemented and extended by a case manager who helps guide and reinforce appropriate behaviors in the community such as by helping a patient make a doctor's appointment or learn how to use public transportation. IVAST requires careful assessment of individual skills and needs and the extent to which the living environment is concordant with the patient's capacity to succeed. The case manager/trainer helps develop skills and/or shape the environment as needed, rather than putting the onus for success on the patient. IVAST has not yet been evaluated empirically but it is a creative approach that warrants careful study.

## Cognitive Rehabilitation

Recognition of the importance of neurocognitive deficits has stimulated increasing interest in the prospects for cognitive remediation. It is difficult to trace the history of interest in this approach, but it certainly goes back at least as far as the early 1970s (Meichenbaum and Cameron 1973, Platt and Spivack 1972a, 1972b). However, these somewhat anomalous studies were not replicated and interest in cognitive training languished. Two reports in the late 1980s rekindled interest in the possibility of cognitive rehabilitation. Hans Brenner and his colleagues (1990) developed a multistage approach, integrated psychological therapy (IPT), that attempted to marry cognitive training with higher level social skills training. Results have not been particularly robust but the work has had tremendous heuristic value.

The second study that had a significant impact was influential for very different reasons. Goldberg and colleagues (1987) reported that patients with schizophrenia were unable to benefit from explicit instructions and practice on the WCST. Coupled with data demonstrating diminished blood flow while responding to the WCST, these data implied that schizophrenia was marked by an unmodifiable abnormality of the dorsolateral prefrontal cortex. The NIH (National Institutes of Health) work stimulated a series of mostly successful demonstrations that WCST performance deficits, albeit widespread, are neither endemic to the illness nor immutable. To examine the malleability of WCST performance, it was demonstrated that performance on the WCST could be improved by reinforcement and specific instructions (Bellack et al. 1990). Other laboratories have been able to produce comparable effects using this training strategy (Nisbet et al. 1996, Vollema et al. 1995) and slightly different variations, with improvements lasting from several weeks (Kern et al. 1992, Metz et al. 1994) to 1 month (Young and Freyslinger 1995).

Several studies have employed cognitive remediation strategies to improve performance on other measures of information processing as well. For example, Benedict and colleagues (1994) employed a computer-based training program that had been developed to enhance attention in brain-injured patients. Performance improved on the training tasks, but there was no associated improvement on Asarnow and Nuechterlein's span of apprehension test or degraded stimulus for continuous performance test. Wexler and colleagues (1997) provided subjects with extensive practice on a motor dexterity task and either a visual reading task or a dot spatial memory task. Improved performance was gradually shaped over 10 weeks. A majority of subjects reached normative levels on the reading and dot tasks, and most showed improvement on the dexterity task as well. These results are consistent with other studies demonstrating that modest improvements can be observed on a variety of tasks using practice, shaping, and errorless learning (Silverstein et al. 2001).

The studies described above were not designed to produce clinically significant change. However, a recent review of the literature identified 15 studies in which the duration and intensity of training was (putatively) sufficient to produce a clinical impact, and which include: (1) a control group for comparison, and (2) measures of change that were independent of tasks used in training (Twamley et al. 2002). It is difficult to compare these studies due to significant differences in training approach, duration, and focus (e.g., attention, memory, executive processing), but overall, the data are promising, with most studies generating small to medium effect sizes. The reader is referred to Twamley and colleagues (2002) and Wykes and van der Gaag (2001) for reviews of this literature.

Several programs warrant comment either because they have been widely discussed or because they are particularly innovative. Brenner (Brenner et al. 1990, 1994), and Spaulding (Spaulding et al. 1997, 1999) evaluated the effects of IPT, a small group treatment program which first targets problems in basic cognitive capacities (e.g., concept formation, memory) followed by training in problem solving and social skill. The program has lead to improvements on several of the neuropsychological tasks targeted in training, akin to the practice effects reported in several of the analog studies referred to above. However, there has not been evidence of widespread improvements in cognitive functioning, or generalization to higher level domains (e.g., social skill).

Wykes and colleagues (1999) developed an intervention called *cognitive remediation therapy*, that focuses on executive functioning (e.g., cognitive flexibility, working memory, and planning). The approach employs a sophisticated training model that is based on principles of errorless learning, targeted reinforcement, and guided practice on cognitive tasks. Training media consist of a variety of paper and pencil games and neurocognitive tests. A preliminary trial yielded improvement on several neuropsychological measures and modest retention of training effects over a 6-month follow-up interval. A limitation of this program is that it employs a highly tailored individual treatment model and demands high levels of therapist skill to slowly shape patient behavior. However, the focus on executive functioning seems much more likely to lead to transferable effects than narrowly focused programs designed to strengthen working memory or attention.

An alternative approach to cognitive rehabilitation capitalizes on the ease of standardization and flexibility provided by computer software. Wexler and colleagues (1997) and Bell and colleagues (2001) reported positive results for similar programs that provide self-directed practice on basic attention, memory, and reasoning tasks (e.g., visual tracking, pyramids). These programs are limited in that patients find the tasks repetitive and boring, and they do not receive training per se. Patients may become more skilled on the specific tasks but they do not necessarily learn effective strategies that normalize dysfunctional neural circuitry or foster generalization to other situations.

Medalia (Medalia and Revheim 1999, Medalia et al. 2000) developed an innovative program called neuropsychological educational approach to remediation (NEAR) that employs commercially available educational software. These tasks are intrinsically interesting to subjects and have built-in feedback mechanisms to guide performance. The intervention is administered in an open classroom format in which patients attend, on an *ad lib* basis, select tasks they are interested in working on each day and move at their own pace. Medalia emphasizes self-guided practice, rather than structured training, in order to foster "intrinsic motivation" for learning and to allow patients to enhance their preferred problem-solving styles. This is an appealing approach, but reliance on self-guided practice seems unlikely to lead to learning. Neuroimaging data suggest that patients use inefficient neurocognitive operations and are unable to utilize appropriate (i.e., normal) neural circuits to perform cognitive tasks (Frith 1995, Weinberger et al. 1992). Consequently, practice without training may improve performance on the specific task practiced but it is not likely to normalize functioning or lead to transferable gains.

Judging the potential for cognitive rehabilitation based on existing trials (analog or clinical) is difficult due to the risk of Type II error (e.g., incorrectly concluding that it is ineffective). It may be safe to conclude that a particular strategy is not effective, but one cannot extrapolate from any single trial or group of trials to the broader domain. For example, a particular technique that fails to produce an effect in 10 training sessions might be effective after 50. Ten sessions of practice on computerized memory tasks may not be sufficient to produce a generalizable increase in processing capacity but meaningful changes may beg apparent after 100 sessions. Alternatively, an innovative program based on a different conceptual model could produce results that the simpler practice/rehearsal strategies currently in vogue do not. In summary, existing approaches are promising but none have yet demonstrated the ability to produce clinically meaningful change in neurocognitive capacity or shown that training has a significant impact on community functioning (see Table 91–1).

## Vocational Rehabilitation

The ability to perform productive work, earn money, and achieve a degree of independence is generally regarded as a major factor in self-esteem, quality of life, and relationships with significant others. Yet it is a domain that is particularly difficult for schizophrenia patients. Rates of competitive employment for persons with schizophrenia are generally less than 25%, and participation in sheltered employment is not much better (Lehman 1995). There have been numerous hypotheses to explain the poor employment performance of schizophrenia patients, many of which place the onus on symptomatology, especially the sequelae of negative symptoms. Conversely, evidence suggests that employment history, work adjustment, and ability to get along or function socially with others are better predictors of employment (Anthony and Jansen 1984). Social skill and ability to get along with others appear to be critical factors in both securing work (Charisiou et al. 1989) and maintaining employment (Chadsey-Rusch 1992, Cook et al. 1994, Lehman 1995).

There are many forms of vocational programs available in the community, including sheltered workshops, job clubs, transitional employment, the Boston University model, and programs of job support. With the exception of programs involving job support, there is little evidence that these types of vocational interventions often result in sustained competitive employment among patients with severe mental illness (Lehman 1995). Such programs, however, appear to provide many patients with structured opportunities for socialization and meaningful daily activity. Such limited goals may be appropriate for certain patients. However, for patients who are interested in competitive employment, it is clear that traditional approaches to psychiatric rehabilitation have proven to be disappointingly ineffective. In part, this lack of efficacy may be attributed to the severe cognitive disability that is common among patients with schizophrenia. Further, the negative financial incentives that have traditionally been built into the SSI (Supplemental Security Income) and SSDI (Social Security Disability Income) systems may have played an important role in patients choosing long-term involvement with rehabilitation programs rather than actual competitive employment. Thus, there are both illness and system of care factors that may contribute to the limited efficacy of traditional rehabilitation approaches. Even allowing for these factors, it is clear that improvement of vocational functioning among patients with severe mental illness remains a critical goal for psychosocial intervention.

Recent evidence from several well-controlled studies suggests that the integrated placement and support (IPS) model of vocational rehabilitation may provide a distinct advantage in increasing rates of competitive employment among patients with severe mental illness (Drake et al. 1999, Lehman et al. 2002). The IPS model emphasizes the integration of vocational and mental health services by having an employment specialist becoming a member of the multidisciplinary clinical management team. The employment specialist helps patients search for real jobs in the community, rather than for placement in sheltered workshops or training programs. After employment is secured, the specialist provides follow-along support in a time-unlimited manner, including intervening with the employer if necessary. A manual has been developed to ensure fidelity of implementation of the approach. There have now been several independent reports of superior efficacy of the IPS model for initiating employment. However, job retention is a major problem. For example, Lehman and colleagues (2002) reported that while 42% of subjects randomized to an IPS condition achieved competitive employment during a 2-year treatment period compared to 11% in a control condition, monthly employment rates averaged only 15 to 20%, and there were no between-group differences in length of employment, hourly wages, or hours worked. Clearly, job retention is a critical problem that requires different strategies than job finding. Given the high priority placed on employment by patients, family members, and the community, improved employment services should be a major focus of research efforts in the future (see Table 91–1).

## Summary and Conclusion

This chapter has provided an overview of issues involved in providing effective rehabilitation programming for people with schizophrenia. Interest in psychosocial treatment, including rehabilitation has waxed and waned over the last several decades, but there is now widespread agreement that it plays a critical role in comprehensive care for people with schizophrenia. The illness is the result of a failure in normal neurodevelopment, with subtle manifestations evident long before the first exacerbation. There appears to be a lifelong disruption of normal socialization coupled with enduring neurocognitive impairments that make it unlikely that medication alone can be sufficient to produce adequate quality of life. That being said, several factors were discussed that must be addressed if psychosocial treatments are to be effective, including: (1) timing and duration of treatment; (2) individual differences in treatment needs; (3) the role of the patient in treatment; (4) the limitations imposed by impairments in information processing; and (5) the need to base interventions on a compensatory model.

Three rehabilitation strategies that have received considerable attention were then reviewed: social skills training (SST), cognitive rehabilitation, and vocational rehabilitation. SST is an effective teaching/training strategy but it is not clear that the intervention can produce meaningful changes in community performance unless it is embedded in a comprehensive, community oriented intervention program. The potential for cognitive rehabilitation is less clear. Several approaches seem to be based on an overly simplistic model of neurocognitive functioning and rely primarily on a naive "exercise" model that attempts to alter brain function by repeated practice. This may be overly optimistic about the potential for neurocognitive repair or restoration of function. Newer strategies that focus on improving higher level integrative processes may prove to be more effective, especially those that employ computerized educational software that clients find inherently engaging. Traditional vocational training that emphasizes sheltered workshops and job training have not been highly effective. The integrated placement and support model is an innovative new approach that helps place clients in competitive employment and provides ongoing support in the real workplace. Initial results are very promising, although durability of effects and job retention remain highly problematic.

As evidenced by these three approaches, the scientific literature is moving away from long-term, unfocused day treatment approaches to targeted intervention strategies designed to deal with specific problems. This approach, which is much more likely to produce useful outcomes has not yet had adequate penetration of community services. Further research is required to match interventions with patients to determine when specific interventions should be provided, and to build in sufficient booster or follow-up procedures to maximize the chances for enduring change in the community. It is by now very apparent that neither a *one-size-fits-all* nor a time-limited, up-and-out approach works with this population.

## Acknowledgment

Preparation of this manuscript was supported by the Mental Illness Research, Education, and Clinical Center at the VA Capitol Health Care Network, and by NIH grants DAO9406 and DA11753 from NIDA.

## References

American Psychiatric Association (1997) Practice Guideline for the Treatment of Patients with Schizophrenia. APA, Washington DC.

Anthony WA and Jansen MA (1984) Predicting the vocational capacity of the chronically mentally ill. Am Psychol 39, 537–544.

Bell M, Bryson G, Tamasine G, et al. (2001) Neurocognitive enhancement therapy with work: Effects on neuropsychological test performance. Arch Gen Psychiatr 58, 763–768.

Bellack AS (1989) A comprehensive model for the treatment of schizophrenia. In A Clinical Guide for the Treatment of Schizophrenia, Bellack AS (ed). Plenum Press, New York, pp. 1–22.

Bellack AS, Blanchard JJ, Murphy P, et al. (1996) Generalization effects of training on the Wisconsin Card Sorting Test for schizophrenia patients. Schizophr Res 19, 189–194.

Bellack AS, Gold JM, and Buchanan RW (1999) Cognitive rehabilitation for schizophrenia: Problems, prospects, and strategies. Schizophr Bull 25, 257–274.

Bellack AS, Haas GL, Schooler NR, et al. (2000) The effects of behavioral family treatment on family communication and patient outcomes in schizophrenia. Br J Psychiatr 177, 434–439.

Bellack AS, Morrison RL, Wixted JT, et al. (1990) An analysis of social competence in schizophrenia. Br J Psychiatr 156, 809–818.

Bellack AS, Mueser KT, Gingerich S, et al. (1997) Social Skills Training for Schizophrenia: A Step-By-Step Guide. Guilford Press, New York, NY.

Bellack AS, Mueser KT, Morrison RL, et al. (1990) Remediation of cognitive deficits in schizophrenia. Am J Psychiatr 147, 1650–1655.

Bellack AS, Turner SM, Hersen M, et al. (1984) An examination of the efficacy of social skills training for chronic schizophrenic patients. Hosp Comm Psychiatr 35, 1023–1028.

Bellack AS, Weinhardt LS, Gold JM, et al. (2001) Generalization of training effects in schizophrenia. Schizophr Res 48, 255–262.

Benedict RHB, Harris AE, Markow T, et al. (1994) Effects of attention training on information processing in schizophrenia. Schizophr Bull 20, 537–546.

Benton MK and Schroeder HE (1990) Social skills training with schizophrenics: A meta-analytic evaluation. J Consult Clin Psychol 58, 741–747.

Berman KF, Zec RF, and Weinberger DR (1986) Physiologic dysfunction of dorsolateral prefrontal cortex in schizophrenia II. Role of neuroleptic treatment, attention, and mental effort. Arch Gen Psychiatr 43, 126–135.

Braff DL (1991) Information processing and attentional abnormalities in the schizophrenia disorders. In Cognitive Bases of Mental Disorders, Magaro PA (ed). Sage Publications, Newbury Park, CA, pp. 262–307.

Braff DL, Heaton R, Kuck J, et al. (1991) The generalized pattern of neuropsychological deficits in outpatients with chronic schizophrenia with heterogeneous Wisconsin Card Sorting Test results. Arch Gen Psychiatr 48, 891–898.

Brenner HD, Kraemer S, Hermanutz M, et al. (1990) Cognitive treatment in schizophrenia. In Schizophrenia: Models and Interventions, Straube E and Hahlweg K (eds). Springer-Verlag, New York, pp. 161–191.

Brenner HD, Roder V, Hodel B, et al. (1994) Integrated Psychological Therapy for Schizophrenic Patients (IPT). Hogrefe & Huber, Goettingen, Germany.

Brown MA and Munford AM (1983) Life skills training for chronic schizophrenics. J Nerv Ment Dis 17, 466–470.

Caldwell CB and Gottesman II (1990) Schizophrenics kill themselves too: A review of risk factors for suicide. Schizophr Bull 16, 571–589.

Canadian Psychiatric Association (1998) Canadian clinical practice guidelines for the treatment of schizophrenia. Can J Psychiatr 43, 25–39.

Carpenter WT, Buchanan RW, Kirkpatrick B, et al. (1993) Strong inference, theory testing, and the neuroanatomy of schizophrenia. Arch Gen Psychiatr 50, 825–831.

Carpenter WT, Heinrichs DW, and Wagman AMI (1988) Deficit and nondeficit forms of schizophrenia: The concept. Am J Psychiatr 145, 578–583.

Chadsey-Rusch J (1992) Toward defining and measuring social skills in employment settings. Am J Ment Retard 96, 405–418.

Charisiou, J, Jackson HJ, Boyle GJ, et al. (1989) Which employment interview skills best predict the employability of schizophrenic patients? Psychol Rep 64, 683–699.

Cook JA, Razzano LA, Straiton DM, et al. (1994) Cultivation and maintenance of relationships with employers of people with psychiatric disabilities. Psychol Rehabil J 17, 103–116.

Cornblatt BA and Keilp JG (1994) Impaired attention, genetics, and the pathophysiology of schizophrenia. Schizophr Bull 20, 31–46.

DeRubeis RJ and Crits-Christoph P (1998) Empirically supported individual and group psychological treatments for adult mental disorders. J Consult Clin Psychol 16, 37–52.

Drake RE, McHugo GJ, Bebout RR, et al. (1999) A randomized clinical trial of supported employment for inner-city patients with severe mental disorders. Arch Gen Psychiatr 56, 627–633.

Eckman TA, Wirshing WC, Marder SR, et al. (1992) Technology for training schizophrenics in illness self-management: A controlled trial. Am J Psychiatr 149, 1549–1555.

Frith C (1995) Functional imaging and cognitive abnormalities (review). Lancet 346, 615–620.

Goldberg TE, Weinberger DR, Berman KF, et al. (1987) Further evidence for dementia of the prefrontal type in schizophrenia? Arch Gen Psychiatr 44, 1008–1014.

Goldstein G, Beers SR, and Shemansky WJ (1996) Neuropsychological differences between schizophrenic patients with heterogeneous Wisconsin Card Sorting Test performance. Schizophr Res 21, 13–18.

Green MF (1996) What are the functional consequences of neurocognitive deficits in schizophrenia? Am J Psychiatr 153, 321–330.

Green MF and Nuechterlein KH (1999) Should schizophrenia be treated as a neurocognitive disorder? Schizophr Bull 25, 309–318.

Green MF, Kern RS, Braff DL, et al. (2000) Neurocognitive deficits and functional outcome in schizophrenia: Are we measuring the "right stuff"? Schizophr Bull 26, 119–136.

Halford WK and Hayes R (1991) Psychological rehabilitation of chronic schizophrenic patients: Recent findings on social skills training and family psychoeducation. Clin Psychol Rev 11, 23–44.

Heaton RK (1981) Wisconsin Card Sorting Test Manual. Psychological Assessment Resources, Odessa, FL.

Hemsley DR (1996) Schizophrenia: A cognitive model and its implications for psychological intervention. Behav Modif 20, 139–169.

Hogarty GE, Anderson CM, Reiss DJ, et al. (1986) Family psychoeducation, social skills training, and maintenance chemotherapy in the aftercare treatment of schizophrenia, I. One-year effects of a controlled study on relapse and expressed emotion. Arch Gen Psychiatr 43, 633–642.

Hogarty GE, Anderson CM, Reiss DJ, et al. (1991) Family psychoeducation, social skills training, and maintenance chemotherapy in the aftercare treatment of schizophrenia, II. Two-year effects of a controlled study on relapse and adjustment. Arch Gen Psychiatr 48, 340–347.

Horwitz AV, Tessler RC, Fisher GA, et al. (1992) The role of adult siblings in providing social support to the severely mentally ill? J Marriage Fam 54, 233–241.

Johnstone EC, Macmillan JF, Frith CD, et al. (1990) Further investigation of the predictors of outcome following first schizophrenic episodes. Br J Psychiatr 157, 182–189.

Jones P, Rodgers B, Murray R, et al. (1994) Child development risk factors for adult schizophrenia in the British 1946 birth cohort. Lancet 344, 1398–1402.

Kern RS, Green MF, and Satz P (1992) Neuropsychological predictors of skills training for chronic psychiatric patients. Psychiatr Res 43, 223–230.

Lehman A (1995) Vocational rehabilitation in schizophrenia. Schizophr Bull 21, 645–656.

Lehman AF and Steinwachs DM (1998) Translating research into practice: The schizophrenia patient outcomes research team (PORT) treatment recommendations. Schizophr Bull 24, 1–10.

Lehman AF, Goldberg R, Dixon LB, et al. (2002) Improving employment outcomes for persons with severe mental illnesses. Arch Gen Psychiatr 59, 165–172.

Lenzenwenger MF, Dworkin RH, and Wethington E (1991) Examining the underlying structure of schizophrenic phenomenology: Evidence for a three-process model. Schizophr Bull 17, 515–524.

Liberman RP (1995) Social and Independent Living Skills: The Community Re-entry Program. Liberman, Los Angeles.

Liberman RP, Blair KE, Glynn SM, et al. (2001) Generalization of skills training to the natural environment. In The Treatment of Schizophrenia: Status and Emerging Trend, Brenner HD, Boker W, and Genner R (eds). Hogrefe & Huber, Seattle, WA, pp. 104–120.

Liberman RP, Mueser KT, and Wallace CJ (1986) Social skills training for schizophrenic individuals at risk for relapse. Am J Psychiatr 143, 523–526.

Marder SR, Wirshing WC, Eckman T, et al. (1993) Psychosocial and pharmacological strategies for maintenance therapy: Effects on two-year outcome. Schizophr Res 9, 260.

McEvoy JP, Scheifler PL, and Frances A (1999) Treatment of schizophrenia. J Clin Psychiatr 60(Suppl 11).

McGlashan TH (1986) The prediction of outcome in chronic schizophrenia, IV. The Chestnut Lodge follow-up study. Arch Gen Psychiatr 43, 167–175.

McGlashan TH and Fenton WS (1992) The positive-negative distinction in schizophrenia: Review of natural history validators. Arch Gen Psychiatr 49, 63–72.

Medalia A and Revheim N (1999) Computer assisted learning in psychiatric rehabilitation. Psychiatr Rehabil Skills 3(1), 77–98.

Medalia A, Revheim N, and Casey M (2000) Remediation of memory disorders in schizophrenia. Psychol Med 30, 1451–1459.

Meichenbaum DH and Cameron R (1973) Training schizophrenics to talk to themselves: A means of developing attentional controls. Behav Ther 4, 515–534.

Meier VJ and Hope DA (1998) Assessment of social skills. In Behavioral Assessment, 4th ed., Bellack AS and Hersen M (eds). Allyn & Bacon, Needham Heights, MA, pp. 232–255.

Metz JT, Johnson MD, Pliskin NH, et al. (1994) Maintenance of training effects on the Wisconsin Card Sorting Test by patients with schizophrenia or affective disorders. Am J Psychiatr 151, 120–122.

Morrison RL and Bellack AS (1984) Social skills training. In Schizophrenia: Treatment, Management, and Rehabilitation, Bellack AS (ed). Grune & Stratton, Orlando, FL, pp. 247–279.

Mueser KT, Bellack AS, Douglas MS, et al. (1991a) Prevalence and stability of social skill deficits in schizophrenia. Schizophr Res 5, 167–176.

Mueser KT, Bellack AS, Douglas MS, et al. (1991b) Prediction of social skill acquisition in schizophrenic and major affective disorder patients from memory and symptomatology. Psychiatr Res 37, 281–296.

Mueser KT, Bellack AS, Wade JH, et al. (1992) An assessment of the educational needs of chronic psychiatric patients and their relatives. Br J Psychiatr 160, 674–680.

Nisbet H, Siegert R, Hunt M, et al. (1996) Improving Wisconsin card-sorting performance. Br J Clin Psychol 35, 631–633.

Paul GL and Lentz RJ (1977) Psychosocial Treatment of Chronic Mental Patients: Milieu Versus Social-Learning Programs. Harvard University Press, Cambridge, MA.

Pearlson GD, Garbacz DJ, Breakey WR, et al. (1984) Lateral ventricular enlargement associated with persistent unemployment and negative symptoms in both schizophrenia and bipolar disorder. Psychiatr Res 12, 1–9.

Platt JJ and Spivack G (1972a) Problem-solving thinking of psychiatric patients. J Consult Clin Psychol 39, 148–151.

Platt JJ and Spivack G (1972b) Social competence and effective problem-solving thinking in psychiatric patients. J Clin Psychol 28, 3–5.

Roberts GW (1991) Schizophrenia: A neuropathological perspective. Br J Psychiatr 158, 8–17.

Scott JE and Dixon LB (1995) Psychological interventions for schizophrenia. Schizophr Bull 21, 621–630.

Selemon LD (2001) Regionally diverse cortical pathology in schizophrenia: Clues to the etiology of the disease. Schizophr Bull 27, 349–377.

Sharma T and Harvey PD (2000) Cognitive enhancement as a treatment strategy in schizophrenia. In Cognition in Schizophrenia: Impairments, Importance, and Treatment Strategies, Sharma T and Harvey PD (eds). Oxford University Press, Oxford, England, pp. 286–302.

Silverstein SM, Menditto AA, and Stuve P (2001) Shaping attention span: An operant conditioning procedure to improve neurocognition and functioning in schizophrenia. Schizophr Bull 27, 247–257.

Smith TE, Bellack AS, and Liberman RP (1996) Social skills training for schizophrenia: Review and future directions. Clin Psychol Rev 16, 599–617.

Spaulding W, Reed D, Elting D, et al. (1997) Cognitive changes in the course of rehabilitation. In Towards a Comprehensive Therapy for Schizophrenia, Brenner HD, Boker W, and Genner R (eds). Hogrefe & Huber, Seattle, WA, pp. 106–117.

Spaulding WD, Reed D, Sullivan M, et al. (1999) Effects of cognitive treatment in psychiatric rehabilitation. Schizophr Bull 25, 657–676.

Spencer PG, Gillespie CR, and Ekisa EG (1983) A controlled comparison of the effects of social skills training and remedial drama on the conversational skills of chronic schizophrenic inpatients. Br J Psychiatr 143, 165–172.

Stein LI and Test MA (eds) (1985) The Training in Community Living Model: A Decade of Experience (New directions for Mental Health Services, No. 26). Jossey-Bass, San Francisco.

Stratta P, Mancini F, Mattei P, et al. (1997) Remediation of Wisconsin card sorting test performance in schizophrenia. Psychopathology 30, 59–66.

Strauss JS (1989) Subjective experiences of schizophrenia: Toward a new dynamic psychiatry II. Schizophr Bull 15, 179–187.

Strauss JS, Carpenter WT Jr., and Bartko JJ (1974) The diagnosis and understanding of schizophrenia. Part III. Speculations on the processes that underlie schizophrenic symptoms and signs. Schizophr Bull 11, 61–69.

Test MA, Wallisch LS, Allness DJ, et al. (1989) Substance use in young adults with schizophrenic disorders. Schizophr Bull 15, 465–476.

Thaker GK and Carpenter WT (2001) Advances in schizophrenia. Nat Med 7, 667–671.

Tsuang MT, Lyons MJ, and Faraone SV (1990) Heterogeneity of schizophrenia: Conceptual models and analytic strategies. Br J Psychiatr 156, 17–26.

Twamley EW, Jeste DV, and Bellack AS (2002) A review of cognitive training in schizophrenia. (Manuscript submitted for publication)

van Os J, Fahy TA, Jones P, et al. (1995) Increased intracerebral cerebrospinal fluid spaces predict unemployment and negative symptoms in psychotic illness: A prospective study. Br J Psychiatr 166, 750–758.

Velligan DI, Bow-Thomas CC, Huntzinger C, et al. (2000) Randomized controlled trial of the use of compensatory strategies to enhance adaptive functioning in outpatients with schizophrenia. Am J Psychiatr 157, 1317–1323.

Vita A, Dieci M, Giobbio GM, et al. (1991) CT scan abnormalities and outcome of chronic schizophrenia. Am J Psychiatr 148, 1577–1579.

Vollema MG, Geutsen GJ, and van Voorst AJP (1995) Durable improvements in Wisconsin Card Sorting Test performance in schizophrenic patients. Schizophr Res 16, 209–215.

Walker EF, Savoie T, and Davis D (1994) Neuromotor precursors of schizophrenia. Schizophr Bull 20, 441–451.

Weinberger DR (1987) Implications of normal brain development for the pathogenesis of schizophrenia. Arch Gen Psychiatr 44, 660–669.

Weinberger DR (1995) Neurodevelopmental perspectives on schizophrenia. In Psychopharmacology: The Fourth Generation of Progress, Bloom FE and Kupfer DJ (eds). Raven Press, New York, pp. 1171–1183.

Weinberger DR, Berman KF, Suddath R, et al. (1992) Evidence of dysfunction of a prefrontal-limbic network in schizophrenia: A magnetic resonance imaging and regional cerebral blood flow study of discordant monozygotic twins. Am J Psychiatr 149, 890–897.

Weinberger DR, Berman KF, and Zec RF (1986) Physiologic dysfunction of dorsolateral prefrontal cortex in schizophrenia I. Regional cerebral blood flow evidence. Arch Gen Psychiatr 43, 114–124.

Wexler BE, Hawkins KA, Rounsaville B, et al. (1997) Normal neurocognitive performance after extended practice in patients with schizophrenia. Schizophr Res 26, 173–180.

Wing JK (1987) Psychosocial factors affecting the long-term course of schizophrenia. In Psychosocial Treatment of Schizophrenia, Strauss JS, Boker W, and Brenner HD (eds). Hans Huber, Toronto, Canada, pp. 13–29.

Wykes T and van der Gaag M (2001) Is it time to develop a new cognitive therapy for psychosis—cognitive remediation therapy (CRT)? Clin Psychol Rev 21, 227–1256.

Wykes T, Reeder C, Corner J, et al. (1999) The effects of neurocognitive remediation on executive processing in patients with schizophrenia. Schizophr Bull 25, 291–307.

Wykes T, Reeder C, Williams C, et al. (in press) Are the effects of cognitive remediation therapy (CRT) durable? Results from an exploratory trial. Schizophr Res.

Young DA and Freyslinger MG (1995) Scaffolded instruction and the remediation of Wisconsin Card Sorting Test deficits in chronic schizophrenia. Schizophr Res 16, 199–207.

# 92 Electroconvulsive Therapy

Matthew V. Rudorfer
Michael E. Henry
Harold A. Sackeim

Although major depression can often be treated successfully, there is a great need for progress in developing treatments that can achieve and maintain recovery for patients with depressive disorders that do not respond readily to currently available treatments.

*Glass 2001*

The profound advances in pharmacotherapy for mental disorders described in previous chapters are widely assumed to correlate with the demise of the older physical or somatic treatments. Indeed, both within and outside the field many assume that electroconvulsive therapy (ECT), as insulin shock treatment and crude forms of psychosurgery, has been confined to the dustbin of psychiatric history. In fact, following 6.5 decades of uneven use, modern ECT has found a narrow but crucial niche among contemporary treatments in psychiatry (US Department of Health and Human Services 1999, American Psychiatric Association 2001). A large body of controlled data supports the efficacy and safety of ECT in the treatment of major depression and other severe psychiatric disorders (American Psychiatric Association 2001).

## History and Utilization

### History

In contrast to the serendipitous discovery of most biological treatments of mental disorders, the introduction of induced generalized seizures for therapeutic purposes was based on a theoretical construct: the belief in a biological antagonism between schizophrenia and epilepsy. This hypothesis was later rejected. Nonetheless, the demonstration by Ladislas Meduna of the successful reversal of a 4-year catatonic stupor by a series of generalized convulsions induced by intramuscular camphor in oil led to research efforts that permanently altered the attitudes and approaches to treatment of the severely mentally ill. Using the more reliable convulsant agent, pentylenetetrazol (Metrazol), Meduna went on to treat more than 100 patients with schizophrenia

during the mid-1930s, reporting a 50% response rate in those ill for less than 10 years (Fink 1984).

As word spread of the efficacy of convulsive therapy in dementia praecox, investigators sought to overcome its limitations, including difficulty in consistently inducing the desired generalized seizures. Having demonstrated the safety of electrically induced seizures in animals, in 1938 Ugo Cerletti and Lucio Bini applied this technique in the treatment of a delusional, incoherent man found wandering the streets of Rome. The patient showed improvement after a single treatment, recovered after a series of 11—proclaiming his enthusiasm about the new treatment at discharge—and was well and working at 1-year follow-up (Pallanti 1999). Thus "electro convulsive therapy," or ECT was born, along with the general principle, still debated today, that the "active ingredient" of convulsive therapy is the generalized seizure, and its means of production is unimportant (Cerletti 1956). Primed by a widely reported 1937 conference in Switzerland on convulsive and insulin coma therapies, clinicians around the world hastened to apply the new ECT to their schizophrenic patients.

The initial 2 decades of ECT use brought a continual stream of refinements in the treatment, as well as abuses, which continue to blemish its reputation and public image. Although an influential 1947 report by the Group for the Advancement of Psychiatry decried what many in the then predominant psychodynamic community felt to be overuse of ECT at the expense of more desirable psychotherapy, by then a wave of unprecedented therapeutic optimism was fueled by ECT, as its efficacy was demonstrated in the mood disorders and its adverse effects reduced by modifications in treatment technique. In the ensuing years, the introduction of general anesthesia, oxygenation, and muscle relaxing agents; and refinements in electrode placement, the seizure-inducing electrical waveform, and the informed consent process have helped to improve the benefit–risk ratio of convulsive therapy over the past half century (see Table 92–1).

Just as the more modern era of modified ECT was beginning, however, it was overtaken in many settings by the psychopharmacology revolution in the 1950s (Fink 1984, Rudorfer and Goodwin 1993). The introduction of effective medications that were easier to use and less expen-

| Table 92–1 | Central Events in the History of Electroconvulsive Therapy |
|---|---|
| 1500s | The 16th century Swiss physician, Paracelsus, uses camphor by mouth to produce seizures to treat psychiatric conditions. |
| 1764 | Leopold von Auenbrugger treats "mania vivorum" with camphor every 2 h, producing seizures. |
| 1785 | Oliver reports in the *London Medical Journal* the therapeutic use of seizure induction to treat a case of mania, using camphor by mouth. |
| 1934 | Von Meduna introduces the modern use of convulsive therapy, unaware of the previous history. On January 23, 1934, Von Meduna begins treatment of a patient with schizophrenia who had been in catatonic stupor for 4 yr, using intramuscular injection of camphor in oil. He soon replaced this technique with intravenous infusion of pentylenetetrazol. |
| 1937 | The Swiss psychiatrist, Müller, organizes an international meeting on convulsive therapy in Münsingen. Meeting proceedings are published in the *American Journal of Psychiatry*, and use of convulsive therapy spreads worldwide. |
| 1938 | The Italian psychiatrist and neurophysiologist, Cerletti and Bini, introduce the use of electricity as a means of seizure induction. A mute, catatonic patient is first treated with ECT in mid-April 1938. The patient begins to talk after the first treatment. |
| 1939 | Lothar Kalinowsky, who observed the second treatment administered by Cerletti and Bini, introduces ECT in England. |
| 1940 | ECT is introduced to the US. Within a few weeks, two facilities in New York City and one in Cincinnati conduct the first treatments. Through the 1940s and 1950s use of ECT becomes widespread, and its particular efficacy in mood disorders is noted. |
| 1940 | The psychiatrist, A.E. Bennett, pioneers the extraction of curare from *Chondodendron tomentosum*. Curare is originally developed to serve as a muscle relaxant in ECT. |
| 1951 | Fatalities resulting from the use of synthetic forms of curare lead to the introduction of succinylcholine, which becomes the standard agent used for muscle relaxation. The routine use of general anesthesia ensues. |
| 1958 | The British psychiatrist, Lancaster, publishes the first controlled study of the use of unilateral ECT. From the outset, it is evident that cognitive side effects were lessened with unilateral relative to bilateral electrode placement. The controversy concerning the equivalency in efficacy continues to the present. |
| 1960 | The Swedish psychiatrist, Ottosson, reports a classic study demonstrating that interference with the seizure discharge by administration of an anticonvulsant medication reduces the efficacy of ECT. The view that the seizure activity provides the necessary and sufficient conditions for treatment efficacy is supported. |
| 1962 | Greenblatt in the US, and later, in 1965, the Medical Research Council in Great Britain, report large-scale, randomized clinical trials of the efficacy of ECT and medications in the treatment of depression. Antidepressant response rates are substantially higher with ECT than with pharmacotherapy. |
| 1965 | May and Tuma compare the use of neuroleptics, ECT, psychotherapy, and milieu treatment for "middle prognosis" schizophrenia. Neuroleptic medication shows superior short-term efficacy, although ECT is more effective than the other interventions on long-term follow-up. |
| 1975 | The popular movie, *One Flew Over the Cuckoo's Nest*, is released, portraying ECT as a form of punishment and behavioral control. In this era, use of pharmacological treatment increases and use of ECT in public sector facilities decreases markedly. |
| 1976 | The American psychiatrist, Blatchley, develops a constant current, brief pulse ECT device. This form of treatment ultimately replaces constant voltage, sine wave stimulation due to a substantial advantage with respect to cognitive side effects. |
| 1978 | The American Psychiatric Association releases its first Task Force Report on ECT. New standards are introduced regarding consent, and use of unilateral electrode placement is encouraged. |
| 1984 | A set of six double-blind, randomized trials, conducted in England in the late 1970s and early 1980s, compares the efficacy of ECT with administration of anesthesia alone. ECT is shown to be more effective than sham treatment in major depression. |
| 1985 | The National Institutes of Health/National Institute of Mental Health Consensus Conference on ECT confirms its role for special populations and calls for additional research and national standards of care. |
| 1987 | Sackeim and colleagues at Columbia University report that the combination of low dosage and right unilateral electrode placement is ineffective. By demonstrating that generalized seizures can be produced that lack efficacy, the long-standing view that the seizure provides the necessary and sufficient conditions for ECT response is contradicted. |
| 1988 | Following 50 yr of empirical use of ECT in the treatment of acute mania, Small and associates at Indiana University publish the first random-assignment controlled clinical trial. ECT and lithium are shown to be equally effective. This finding is soon replicated in medication-resistant manic patients in New York in a prospective trial that has to be aborted after several staff members are assaulted by the medication-free subjects. |
| 1990 | The American Psychiatric Association releases its second Task Force Report on ECT. Detailed recommendations for treatment delivery, education, and training are provided. |
| 1993 | A study reported in the *New England Journal of Medicine* provides the first demonstration that electrical dosage can influence the efficacy, speed of response, and cognitive side effects of ECT. An accompanying editorial offers evidence to the field of the contemporary role of ECT as "a modern medical procedure." |
| 1995 | Publication of the autobiographical book, *Undercurrents* by psychologist Martha Manning presents to a broad audience a compelling account of the life-saving potential of ECT by an initially reluctant recipient. |
| 2000 | Independent research groups confirm and extend the dose–response relationship in right unilateral ECT, demonstrating an equivalent clinical response between high-dose unilateral and bilateral ECT, but with a decided cognitive advantage to right unilateral electrode placement. Previous recommendation of unilateral stimulation at 150% above seizure threshold is found to be inadequate. |
| 2001 | The American Psychiatric Association publishes another ECT Task Force Report, this one constituting the 2nd edition of its highly successful ECT guidelines for practice, education, and training. Additional emphasis is placed on informed consent and avoiding narrow interpretations of potential ECT responders; position on combined medications plus ECT is softened. |
| 2001 | *Journal of the American Medical Association* publishes the largest modern trial of post-ECT continuation pharmacotherapy, demonstrating superiority of combined treatment with a tricyclic antidepressant (nortriptyline) plus lithium compared to nortriptyline alone or placebo in preventing relapse during the 6 mo following a successful course of ECT. An accompanying editorial (quoted at the beginning of this chapter) welcomes ECT to the medical mainstream. |
| 2002 | Ongoing research includes a multisite controlled trial of continuation ECT vs. optimal pharmacotherapy in relapse prevention, and further development of potentially alternative somatic treatments, including rTMS, magnetic stimulation therapy, and VNS. |

sive than ECT led to the curtailment of convulsive therapy in many public institutions. This development was also driven by political factors, which, aided by outdated and, at times distorted media presentations, cast convulsive therapy as an oppressive, dangerous tool of the psychiatric establishment. The net effect was that during the 1960s and 1970s many training programs in psychiatry stopped the teaching of ECT and the treatment appeared to be dying.

The subsequent reemergence of ECT and its role today as a valued member of the treatment armamentarium can be accounted for by several factors. First, critical limitations of psychopharmacology and other treatment approaches have been recognized, including a significant rate of treatment resistance in the major psychiatric disorders and medication toxicities. Second, a series of critical reexaminations of ECT by professional organizations around the world, including Britain (Pippard and Ellam 1981, Royal College of Psychiatrists 1995), Scandinavia (Heshe and Roeder 1976, Frederiksen and d'Elia 1979), Canada (Clark 1985), and, in the US, a National Institutes of Health (NIH)/National Institute of Mental Health (NIMH) consensus conference (1985), three sets of recommendations by American Psychiatric Association (APA) Task Forces (1978, 1990, 2001), and the first-ever Surgeon General's report on mental health (US Department of Health and Human Services 1999), have supported the important role of convulsive therapy in modern medicine (Potter and Rudorfer 1993). Finally, coincident with advances in the clinical science of ECT and with the personal testimonies to the benefits of convulsive therapy by a number of public and private figures (Manning 1995, Hartmann 2002), media accounts of this treatment have become notably more balanced over the past decade.

## Utilization

Throughout its long history, the actual usage of ECT has been determined not only by the results of clinical trials and experience, but by the status of alternative treatments, cost, rates of institutionalization, diagnostic shifts, and, more than any other extant psychiatric treatment, public and professional attitudes about the procedure. A consistent feature of the utilization of ECT over the past several decades has been its unevenness—regionally (Hermann et al. 1995, Olfson et al. 1998) and even locally (Westphal et al. 1997, Glen and Scott 2000, Prudic et al. 2001). Current use of ECT is influenced most by treatment setting, demographic features of patients (including psychiatric and medical diagnoses, age, and ethnicity), and, in several instances, local legal restrictions. In addition, there remain wide variations in the rate of utilization or recommendation of ECT within the mental health professions, on both sides of the Atlantic (Glen and Scott 2000, Prudic et al. 2001). Hermann and associates (1998) have described some of the characteristics of the relatively few (<8%) American psychiatrists who perform ECT, including a greater likelihood of being a male international medical graduate not having performed residency during the ECT "training deficit" in the 1970s, and practicing in private care settings in the southeast or mid-Atlantic sections of the country. Despite the low rate of ECT utilization in Texas, state hospital psychiatrists there profess a favorable attitude toward the use of

ECT in generally accepted circumstances (Finch et al. 1990).

## Rates of ECT Use

Several surveys in this country and abroad between the 1970s and early 1990s documented the extent of ECT use over time. Representative psychiatric inpatient data collected by NIMH demonstrated a 46% decline in ECT use in the American hospitals between 1975 and 1980 (Thompson and Blaine 1987) totaling only 2.4% of psychiatric admissions in 1980. However, ECT use during the 1980s remained constant or actually increased, reaching 36,558 US inpatients in 1986 (Thompson et al. 1994), some 5,000 more individuals than had been counted at the start of the decade. Among Medicare beneficiaries, the number of patients treated with ECT continued to rise into the next decade, from 12,000 in 1987 to 15,560 in 1992 (Rosenbach et al. 1997); during that 5-year period, the rate of ECT use increased from 4.2 to 5.1 individuals for every 10,000 Medicare beneficiaries. More recently, a large-scale national survey of representative acute-care hospital records sponsored by the US government yielded a wealth of information on more than 2,000 inpatients who received ECT in 1993, representing 9.4% of sampled individuals discharged with a diagnosis of recurrent major depression (Olfson et al. 1998). By the mid-1990s, legislative restrictions on the use of ECT in some states, for example, Texas, were associated with relatively low rates of use of this modality (Finch et al. 1990).

## ECT Setting

Even more striking was the shift in the type of institutional setting where ECT is used. In contrast to its origins in the public mental health sector, in the US ECT now is primarily a treatment offered in private general and psychiatric hospitals (Thompson and Blaine 1987, Kramer 1990, Thompson et al. 1994, Olfson et al. 1998). Approximately 10% of admissions to academic and private psychiatric facilities receive ECT (Asnis et al. 1978, Fink 1992). In contrast, relatively few public institutions provide ECT (Asnis et al. 1978, Kramer 1990, Malsch et al. 1991, Fink 1992, Rosenbach et al. 1997, Olfson et al. 1998, Reid et al. 1998, Sylvester et al. 2000). For example, in a recent survey, only 164 of the more than 10,000 inpatients, that is <2%, in the New York state hospital system received ECT over a 2-year period. Data from other countries conform in general to the American experience, including a reduced use of ECT in the 1970s in countries like Great Britain (Lambourn and Gill 1978) followed by an increase in usage the next decade, as shown in Denmark (Stromgren 1991). In England, where most ECT is performed in National Health System hospitals, the decline in the prescription of convulsive therapy continued throughout the 1980s, but in an uneven fashion, such that Pippard (1992) found 12-fold differences in ECT use across health districts. Similarly, 22-fold differences in ECT use were seen among hospitals in the Republic of Ireland, where more ECT is performed per capita than in England (Latey and Fahy 1985). Across the entire UK, current estimates of ECT use are approximately 150 per 100,000 population annually.

It should be noted that most of the large surveys of ECT use to date have not accounted for the outpatient administration of convulsive therapy (Thompson et al. 1994, Fink et al. 1996), a growing but still less-common practice with considerable cost-effectiveness potential (Komrad 1988, Rosenbach et al. 1997, Prudic et al. 2001). Indeed, the cost implications for ECT in general constitute the proverbial two-edged sword. On the one hand, a course of ECT per se, even without the additional charge for hospitalization, costs thousands of dollars, putting it out of reach for many poorly insured patients (Olfson et al. 1998). On the other hand, the appropriate use of ECT may save money over the long haul, especially if its timely application prevents weeks or months of fruitless medication trials and hospitalization (Markowitz et al. 1987). Thus, among patients hospitalized for recurrent depression in the early 1990s, those who received ECT beginning in the first 5 days in hospital, compared to those whose ECT started later in their hospital stay, experienced (controlling for several demographic and other variables) a hospital stay that was on average 6 days shorter and nearly $6,000 less expensive (Olfson et al. 1998). The savings in time and money were even greater for the subgroup of inpatients with psychotic depression. However, it must be borne in mind that even with prompt institution of ECT, these patients' total hospital charges were more than $5,000 greater than those of similar inpatients who did not receive ECT at all (Olfson et al. 1998). Similarly, the use of ECT in very old (at least 75 years) depressed patients (Manly et al. 2000) and in patients with Parkinson's disease (Moellentine et al. 1998) has been associated with increased hospitalization length of stay, compared to similar cohorts treated pharmacologically.

## Demographic Factors

Patient characteristics associated with the use of ECT were identified in several large surveys (Thompson and Blaine 1987, Thompson et al. 1994, Olfson et al. 1998). These include the following:

### Gender

As depression is diagnosed more commonly in women than in men, it is not surprising that most individuals who receive ECT are female. For example, 71% of ECT recipients in 1986 were women, a figure that was virtually unchanged in the 1993 nationwide survey (Olfson et al. 1998), a British survey of ECT in geriatric patients (Gormley et al. 1998), and a contemporary review of ECT use in a Pennsylvania state hospital (Sylvester et al. 2000). Olfson and associates (1998) did find that a slightly greater proportion of women with a diagnosis of recurrent depression were treated with ECT compared to their male counterparts (10.1 versus 8.0%). Consistent with that finding, men did not share in the increase in ECT use among Medicare beneficiaries in the 1987 to 1992 survey (Rosenbach et al. 1997).

### Age

More than one-third of ECT patients in 1986 were at least 65 years old, a fourfold greater representation than among the psychiatric inpatient population. Among adult inpatients with recurrent depression in 1993, the rate of ECT use approximately doubled with every 15-year age increment, rising from 10.6% of patients between age 50 and 64 years to 21.2% of those older than 65 years (Olfson et al. 1998). Similar results were obtained in Norway, where 22% of 239

patients consecutively admitted to a geriatric psychiatry unit received ECT (Kujala et al. 2002). A retrospective survey of ECT use at 59 of the New York City metropolitan area facilities in 1996 found that >50% of ECT recipients were older than age 60 years (Prudic et al. 2001). Similar findings have been reported in other surveys in the US (Westphal et al. 1997, Reid et al. 1998, Sylvester et al. 2000) and abroad (Jorm and Henderson 1989, Glen and Scott 2000) consistent with the well-recognized advantages of ECT in the elderly, such as safety in the face of concomitant medical illness (NIH/NIMH 1985, Sackeim 1993, American Psychiatric Association 2001). However, the increased utilization of ECT seen in the Medicare population in the late 1980s to early 1990s was actually driven by individuals younger than age 65 years (Rosenbach et al. 1997).

While ECT can be safely and effectively administered to children and adolescents, such use remains rare (Duffett et al. 1999), for example only 0.17% of inpatients younger than age 18 years with recurrent major depression received ECT in 1993 (Olfson et al. 1998). None of the ECT patients in the 1996 New York City area survey were younger than age 13 years, and few were between age 13 and 18 years (Prudic et al. 2001). Only 20 patients younger than age 19 years received ECT for mood disorder over a decade, according to a Paris survey of five centers, three of which specialized in adolescent psychiatry (Taieb et al. 2001). Prospectively collected data for the city of Edinburgh, Scotland, during the 1990s documented an extremely low annual rate of ECT use in young people of 0.5 patients per 100,000 total population (or 2.5 patients per 100,000 population < age 18 years; no one younger than age 17 years actually received this treatment) (Scott and Glen 2000). During the same time period, ECT was administered to Edinburgh adults between age 18 and 64 years at a rate of 26.3 patients per 100,000 population. In some US locales the administration of ECT to young people is restricted by law; for example, between 1974 and 1993, legislation in the states of California, Tennessee, Colorado, and Texas prohibited the use of ECT in anyone younger than a cutoff age that ranged from 12 to 18 years (Reid et al. 1998, Taieb et al. 2001).

### Race/Ethnicity

In the US, ECT is predominantly used for the treatment of the white individuals. For example, in 1986 the African-American patients (23% of the total inpatient sample) were grossly under represented among ECT subjects (1.5%) (Thompson et al. 1994). Seven years later the black and Hispanic inpatients with recurrent major depression remained less likely than their white counterparts to receive ECT (Olfson et al. 1998). During that time span, the increased use of ECT among Medicare recipients did not include a proportionate number of minority individuals (Rosenbach et al. 1997).

## Indications for ECT

### General Considerations

In contrast to its origins as a treatment of schizophrenia, ECT today is generally utilized more frequently in patients with depression (NIH/NIMH 1985, Thompson et al. 1994, Olfson et al. 1998, US Department of Health and Human Services 1999, American Psychiatric Association 2001).

Mania and schizophrenia account for most of the remainder of convulsive therapy use, across the life span (Rey and Walter 1997, Van Gerpen et al. 1999, Kramer 1999). The decision about when to use ECT is based on signs and symptoms of severe mental disorders that cut across diagnostic lines (Fink 1994). These have been most clearly spelled out by the American Psychiatric Association Task Force (now Committee) on ECT (American Psychiatric Association 1990, 2001), which identified "primary" and "secondary" use of convulsive therapy. Primary indications are those for which ECT may appropriately be used as a first-line treatment. These include situations where the patient's medical or psychiatric condition requires rapid clinical response, where the risk of alternative treatments is excessive, or where, based on past history, response to ECT or nonresponse to medications is anticipated. In line with these findings, Prudic and associates (2001) reported that the New York area clinicians cited as the immediate indication for ECT previous successful use of the treatment almost 30% of the time and psychiatric urgency in nearly 20% of patients. If these conditions are not met, medication or other alternative treatment is recommended first, with ECT reserved for cases of nonresponse to adequate trial(s), unacceptable adverse effects of the alternative treatment, or deterioration of the patient's condition, increasing the urgency of the need for response (American Psychiatric Association 2001). These general principles in turn require individualized interpretation in the presence of specific psychiatric and medical disorders. Even where ECT is not used as treatment of first choice, its introduction sooner in the decision tree rather than being reserved as a "last resort" may spare the patient multiple unsuccessful medication trials, thereby avoiding months of suffering and possibly reducing the likelihood of treatment resistance (Potter and Rudorfer 1993, American Psychiatric Association 2001, Glass 2001). Modern diagnostic and clinical considerations in the recommendation of ECT are summarized in Table 92–2.

Contemporary use of ECT overwhelmingly conforms to evidence-based indications. Hermann and associates (1999) surveyed nearly 1,000 ECT recipients in one New England health plan and found 86.5% to conform to evidence-based indications, with most of the remainder suffering from disorders with substantial depressive components; no indiscriminant use of ECT was identified.

## Depression

More than 30,000 individuals hospitalized with mood disorders in the US in 1986 (about 1 in 20 with those diagnoses) received ECT, accounting for 84% of the use of this treatment (Thompson et al. 1994). Of these, the vast majority suffered from severe major depression. Similar data were obtained in the more recent survey of the New York City area facilities (Prudic et al. 2001). It is well established that major depression is a heterogeneous disorder, encompassing mildly ill, functioning outpatients, as well as profoundly disturbed, dysfunctional, or often psychotic inpatients. Along this spectrum, ECT appears higher in the treatment hierarchy for the more severe presenting depression, usually defined by the presence of neurovegetative signs, psychosis, or suicidality (Abrams 1982, American Psychiatric Association 2000, 2001). Contemporary use of ECT reflects this severity spectrum, with rates of inpatient ECT administra-

| Table 92–2 | Indications for Electroconvulsive Therapy |
|---|---|

### I. Diagnostic Considerations

A. Major depression: unipolar, especially primary *psychotic* (but other subtypes may respond); bipolar
B. Mania
C. Schizophrenia: acute
D. Schizoaffective disorder
E. Neurologic disorders: Parkinson's disease
                              catatonia
                              neuroleptic malignant syndrome

### II. Clinical Considerations

A. Need for rapid response on medical or psychiatric grounds (e.g. suicidality, inanition)
B. History of treatment-resistance or excessive risk of alternative treatments
C. Severity of illness
D. History of previous positive response to ECT
E. Patient preference
F. Informed consent required

tion falling from 9.4% in patients with recurrent major depression to 3.2% of those with a single episode of major depression and only 0.5% of patients with a discharge diagnosis of dysthymia (Olfson et al. 1998).

This severity of depression also partly determines whether alternative treatments will be attempted prior to a trial of convulsive therapy. While there are no absolute rules, severely melancholic or psychotic patients are often appropriate candidates for ECT as treatment of first choice, whereas more moderately ill individuals might not be considered for ECT until adequate medication trials have failed. In the presence of primary, melancholic depression, a case can be made that a single adequate unsuccessful trial of appropriate antidepressant medication is a sufficient prerequisite for ECT (Potter and Rudorfer 1993). On the other hand, a patient with mood shifts secondary to a personality disorder may not be a candidate for ECT even after multiple medication failures (Kramer 1982).

## Clinical Trials

The evidence supporting the efficacy of ECT in depression is overwhelming. Three main types of data have appeared, to a large part sequentially, over the past half century: uncontrolled case series in the early years, followed in the 1950s and 1960s by controlled comparisons of ECT and psychotropic medications, and finally, in the 1970s and 1980s, the use of sham ECT-treated patient samples to control for the nonspecific effects of the procedure and its associated anesthesia and other medications. Janicak and associates (1985) conducted a meta-analysis of ECT comparison studies in depression. Their results were clear-cut: ECT was found to have superior efficacy to all comparison groups, being 41% more effective than placebo, 32% more effective than sham ECT, 20% more effective than generally adequate doses of tricyclic antidepressants (TCAs), and 45% better than monoamine oxidase inhibitors (MAOIs). Although this sweeping conclusion has been challenged (Rifkin 1988), due to the shortcomings of some studies by today's methodological standards, the extraordinary efficacy of ECT is now well accepted (NIH/NIMH 1985, Potter and Rudorfer 1993), with no controlled study ever showing any other treatment to have superior efficacy to ECT in the treatment of depression.

Controlled comparisons of ECT with the modern generation of antidepressants are sparse, in large part due to the difficulty in recruiting patients for such a random assignment study. A notable exception is a German clinical trial that entailed randomization of 39 patients with major depression resistant to at least two previous medication trials to either a course of brief-pulse right unilateral ECT or a trial of the standard selective serotonin reuptake inhibitor (SSRI), paroxetine (Folkerts et al. 1997). The ECT group (mean of 7.2 treatments) showed superiority to the paroxetine subjects (mean daily dose of 44 mg), both in magnitude of clinical improvement (71 versus 28% response rate) and speed of antidepressant effect (Folkerts et al. 1997). As a useful, if uncontrolled reference point, the recent New York survey of ECT practice in the community (Prudic et al. 2001) found an acute clinical benefit for >84% of patients, the vast majority of whom were suffering from depression. Although published reports describe a 63% ECT response rate in depressed children and adolescents, there have been no controlled trials in this population (Rey and Walter 1997).

## Predictors of Response

The literature describes an overall response rate to ECT of 75 to 85% in depression (Crowe 1984, O'Connor et al. 2001). Efforts to delineate subtypes of depression particularly responsive to ECT have yielded inconsistent results. ECT is most likely to be helpful in an acute episode of severe depression of relatively brief duration (Rich et al. 1984). Combined data from two simulated ECT-controlled trials (Brandon et al. 1984, Buchan et al. 1992) identified the presence of delusions and psychomotor retardation as predictive of preferential response. A later open British study (Hickie et al. 1990) replicated the finding of psychomotor retardation as a positive predictor.

Psychotic depression, increasingly recognized as a distinct subtype of mood disorder that responds poorly to antidepressants alone, has emerged as a powerful indication for ECT (Potter et al. 1991, Petrides et al. 2001). In this subgroup, ECT is at least as effective as a combination trial of antidepressant and antipsychotic medications. On balance, the evidence supports the early use of ECT in psychotic depression, particularly in lieu of prolonged, complicated medication trials that may be poorly tolerated in the elderly (Khan et al. 1987, Potter et al. 1991, Sackeim 1993). Indeed, in one modern study in three academic medical centers, only 4% of psychotically depressed patients referred for ECT had received adequate pharmacotherapy trials (Mulsant et al. 1997). By the 1990s, these findings were incorporated into routine clinical practice, as evidenced by the relatively high rates of ECT used with patients hospitalized with major depression with psychotic features, both recurrent (11.8%) and single episode (5.5%) (Olfson et al. 1998). Nearly half of the geriatric patients receiving ECT at three UK hospitals in the mid-1990s exhibited psychotic features associated with unipolar or bipolar depression (Gormley et al. 1998), twice the rate seen in a smaller US retrospective survey of very old

patients (Casey and Davis 1996). The most definitive contemporary data comparing ECT effectiveness in psychotic versus nonpsychotic depression emerge from the acute treatment phase of an ongoing NIMH-supported four-site Consortium for Research in ECT (CORE) trial of continuation treatments (Petrides et al. 2001). Among 253 patients with unipolar major depression who underwent an acute course of bilateral ECT were 77 individuals, of similar age and gender distribution to the group as a whole, with psychotic features. More than a third of the old–old patients in this group had psychotic features, compared to less than a quarter of those aged 45 years and younger (O'Connor et al. 2001). The remission rate among treatment completers was significantly greater for the psychotic patients (95%) than the still impressively high 83% remission rate for the nonpsychotic completers; there was no difference in the number of treatments between the groups. Time to remission was also shorter in the psychotically depressed patients (Petrides et al. 2001).

Data from the acute phase of another NIMH-supported three-site trial (Sackeim et al. 2001) have shown a history of antidepressant medication resistance to predict nonresponse to a subsequent course of ECT (Prudic et al. 1996). The predictive power of medication resistance applied only to heterocyclic antidepressants, not SSRIs or MAOIs. It is also relevant that the 100 patients analyzed for this relationship were all nonpsychotic; psychotically depressed patients typically fail to respond to antidepressant medication alone, yet, as noted, consistently demonstrate high response rates to ECT (Petrides et al. 2001). Recent advances in optimizing right unilateral ECT, to be reviewed later, may help overcome the reported resistance to convulsive therapy (Prudic et al. 1996).

In general, beyond psychosis, individual clinical features, even melancholia, the predictor of long-standing conventional wisdom (Rush and Weissenburger 1994), and psychomotor retardation (Sobin et al. 1996) have not proven to be reliable indicators of response to ECT in modern studies (Zimmerman et al. 1986, American Psychiatric Association 2001). Indeed, recent data have shown ECT effectiveness even in so-called "atypical depression" (McClintock et al. 2002). While bipolar (discussed later) and unipolar depressions are equally responsive to ECT (Zorumski et al. 1986a, Zornberg and Pope, 1993, American Psychiatric Association 2002), response may be less likely with secondary than primary depression, in both adults (Kramer 1982, Zorumski et al. 1986b, Zimmerman et al. 1986a)—including the elderly (Zorumski et al. 1988)—and adolescents (Schneekloth et al. 1993). This may be especially true when depression is secondary to another psychiatric disorder, rather than to a medical illness (Winokur et al. 1988, Zorumski et al. 1988). A family history of nonaffective psychiatric disorder, specifically alcohol dependence or sociopathy, may also lessen responsivity to ECT among primary depressives (Coryell and Zimmerman 1984).

Suicidal ideation is of special relevance in evaluating the potential role of ECT in the treatment of an individual with major depression. While commonly regarded as an indication for the prescription of ECT, suicidal ideation has not been shown by itself to predict responsivity (Tanney 1986, Prudic and Sackeim 1999). While historically, the introduction of ECT was regarded as associated with a reduction in completed suicides, careful review of the literature (Prudic and Sackeim 1999) revealed considerable methodological limitations in most relevant surveys; a more accurate interpretation of the data may be that ECT is associated with a reduction in mortality from all causes, not necessarily specifically suicide. Indeed, retrospective reports continue to appear claiming a failure of ECT to prevent suicide, based on similar rates of utilization of the treatment in depressed patients who did or did not go on to commit suicide (Sharma 1999).

However, recent data have indicated a significant acute antisuicidality effect of ECT. Prudic and Sackeim (1999) found a significant reduction in the suicide item score on the Hamilton depression rating scale following a course of ECT, both in responders ($N = 72$) and, to a lesser but still significant extent, in nonresponders ($N = 76$). Similar results are being observed in the acute phase of the ongoing CORE trial. Among the first 235 patients rated as suicidal at baseline, two-thirds had a suicidality item rating of zero after three bilateral ECT treatments, and 90% were free of suicidal ideation after completion of seven treatments (Kellner et al. 2002). As with its general antidepressant effect, this apparent antisuicidal action of ECT should be regarded as acute and not long-term without the introduction of appropriate continuation and maintenance treatment, as will be discussed further.

Biological measures have proven unhelpful as predictors of ECT response, including the initially promising dexamethasone suppression test (DST) (Coryell and Zimmerman 1984, Scott 1989, Devanand et al. 1991). Similarly, although the pretreatment blunting of the thyroid-stimulating hormone (TSH) response to thyrotrophin-releasing hormone (TRH) challenge has been reported to return to normal following successful ECT (Kirkegaard and Faber 1986, 1998), the state versus trait nature of this challenge paradigm remains under investigation, making its clinical application at this time premature (Golden and Potter 1986). While assurance of an adequate seizure induction at each treatment session is necessary for a successful outcome (Sackeim et al. 1993, Abrams 2000), efforts at constructing a "dose–response" relationship based on total seizure duration over an ECT course, likewise have proven disappointing (Zorumski et al. 1986a). A number of physiological responses to ECT, including release of posterior pituitary peptides (Scott 1989, Scott et al. 1991) and changes in sensitivity to the barbiturate anesthesia (Barry et al. 1991) remain under investigation as possible predictors of outcome. Others, such as the typical rise in seizure threshold over a course of ECT (Scott 1989, Sackeim et al. 1993), have proven unrelated to clinical response (Scott et al. 2000).

Finally, a previous history of antidepressant medication failure is emerging as a potent predictor of ECT nonresponse and early relapse (Prudic et al. 1990, Sackeim et al. 1990a, 1990b). This concept challenges decades of generally retrospective case series claiming considerable (often >70%) success rates with ECT in pharmacotherapy-resistant depressed patients (Avery and Lubrano 1979, Paul et al. 1981, Magni et al. 1988). These earlier findings have been questioned based on methodological limitations of these uncontrolled treatment trials, most notably inadequacies in the definition of treatment response and resistance

(Prudic et al. 1990). In one prospective trial of bilateral ECT administered to 53 patients with major depression (Prudic et al. 1990, Sackeim et al. 1990a), only a 50% clinical response rate was obtained in the 24 patients who previously had failed to respond to adequate pharmacotherapy. In contrast, 86% of patients lacking a history of medication resistance responded to ECT. A range of clinical factors potentially might account for these results and requires further prospective study. Nonetheless, in community surveys, medication resistance is the cited precipitating factor leading to a course of ECT in about two-thirds of cases (Prudic et al. 2000).

## Bipolar Disorder

ECT is an extremely effective and rapidly acting treatment for both acute mania and bipolar depression (American Psychiatric Association 2002). However, it is infrequently used for mania, because of the availability of pharmacological strategies (Goodwin and Jamison 1990). Nonetheless, ECT has been repeatedly endorsed as an accepted second- or third-line treatment of acute manic episodes, particularly in cases of medication resistance, in patients of all ages (NIH/NIMH 1985, Goodwin and Jamison 1990, Mukherjee et al. 1994, Van Gerpen et al. 1999, American Psychiatric Association 2002). Although 20 to 30% of bipolar patients are refractory to lithium and other medications, mania accounts for only approximately 3% of ECT use in this country. Under certain circumstances, such as manic delirium, ECT can be life-saving (Fink 2002), a reminder that prior to the development of somatic treatments, mania had a mortality rate of at least 10%. Thus, in medical emergencies associated with mania, ECT should be regarded as a treatment of first choice (American Psychiatric Association 2002). The same is true for medical conditions accompanying acute mania (including pregnancy, discussed later) that contraindicate or render intolerable the use of psychotropic medications.

### Clinical Trials

The methodological problems that hamper research in ECT generally (Rudorfer 1994, Potter 1994) are starkly illustrated in the case of mania. The imperatives of securing informed consent and withdrawing confounding psychotropic drugs are difficult to reconcile with the clinical realities of dealing with a severely ill, often irritable and aggressive, patient population. Indeed, hospital staff were injured and hospitalized in one prospective trial (Mukherjee 1989). Another pilot study that sought to avoid use of neuroleptics in manic patients scheduled for an ECT versus lithium trial (Small et al. 1988) was aborted when all four subjects dropped out within 10 days. Adjunctive antipsychotic medications had to be permitted to allow the study to go forward.

Half a century's worth of uncontrolled case series on the use of ECT in mania has only recently been supplemented by a trio of prospective clinical trials (totaling 69 patients) and several large and small retrospective chart reviews (Mukherjee et al. 1994). In a comprehensive review of the literature, Mukherjee and associates (1994) tabulated a total of nearly 600 manic patients, of whom 80% showed marked clinical improvement or remission following convulsive therapy. Most compelling were two controlled retrospective studies from the 1970s and early 1980s (McCabe 1976, McCabe and Norris 1977, Thomas and Reddy 1982), a large but uncontrolled naturalistic survey (Black et al. 1987), and the three controlled prospective trials (Small et al. 1988, Mukherjee 1989, Sikdar et al. 1994).

Related record reviews at the University of Iowa demonstrated the superiority of ECT in acute mania over no active treatment (in historical controls from the 1930s) (McCabe 1976) or chlorpromazine (McCabe and Norris 1977). In the latter study, all 10 of 28 chlorpromazine-treated patients who failed to improve subsequently responded to ECT, joining the 18 of 28 initial ECT responders. A later retrospective study (Thomas and Reddy 1982) found very high (100% in the case of ECT), and not significantly different, antimanic response rate to convulsive therapy, lithium, or chlorpromazine. Naturalistic surveys have found higher response rates when ECT was used as a first-line treatment of mania (100%) (Mukherjee and Debsikdar 1992) than when it was reserved for medication-resistant manic patients (Alexander et al. 1988, Stromgren 1988). Black and colleagues (1986, 1987) found a 78% response rate to ECT, superior to the approximately 60% response rate with lithium. In contrast to recent experience with depressed patients discussed above, subsequent ECT in manic lithium nonresponders yielded an impressive response rate of 69%.

The first prospective and randomized comparison of ECT and lithium was obtained in 34 manic inpatients (Small et al. 1988). ECT resulted in greater improvement during the 8-week trial than lithium. However, at the end of the acute treatment period, the two groups did not differ in clinical improvement, and went on to similar rates of relapse and recurrence during a subsequent 2-year trial of lithium maintenance. As noted, the primary confound in the Indiana study (Small et al. 1988) was the use of concurrent neuroleptic medication. Different methodology was applied in the other American prospective trial of ECT in mania, where patients were preselected for nonresponse to lithium or a neuroleptic in the index episode (Mukherjee 1989, Mukherjee et al. 1994). In this New York study, amobarbital, but no antipsychotics, was permitted as prn medication. Either unilateral or bilateral ECT was associated with clinical improvement in most (59%) of 22 patients, compared to no responders among five patients assigned to an intensive lithium plus haloperidol combination. The efficacy of ECT in acute mania was also demonstrated in the only non-US prospective trial (Sikdar et al. 1994), in which bilateral ECT was compared to sham ECT. Both groups received concurrent chlorpromazine 600 mg/day, but no patients received lithium. Twelve of 15 patients who received real ECT, compared to only one manic patient treated with sham ECT, showed complete recovery, with improvement in all manic symptoms. Follow-up neuroleptic requirements were accordingly lower in the real ECT group. Looking at another way, the addition of ECT to the antipsychotic medication regimen cut the duration of the index manic episode in half (Sikdar et al. 1994).

## Predictors of Response

There is little information on which manic patients benefit most from ECT or on optimal ECT treatment in mania. The Indiana group (Small et al. 1986, Milstein et al. 1987)

suggested that bilateral electrode placement was superior to unilateral ECT in treating manic symptoms. However, the naturalistic Iowa study (Black et al. 1987) and the prospective New York trial (Mukherjee 1989) failed to find significant differences in the response rates of manic patients treated with bilateral, unilateral, or mixed electrode placements. In terms of clinical features associated with response, Small and associates (1988) found baseline depression rating most highly related to 8-week outcome. Extreme manic behavior and mixed symptoms of mania and depression were also associated with a superior response to ECT over lithium. However, in contrast to the situation in psychotic depression, discussed earlier, the presence or absence of psychosis has not been found to affect the high response rate of mania to ECT (Black et al. 1987). Schnur and colleagues (1992) reported that response to ECT was reduced among manic patients with prominent symptoms of anger, irritability, and aggression, consistent with findings regarding lithium.

Bipolar depression responds as well as unipolar depression to ECT, in both adult and geriatric patients (Gormley et al. 1998, American Psychiatric Association 2002). In the early years of psychopharmacology, several controlled trials in bipolar depression found ECT superior to first-generation antidepressant (MAO inhibitor or tricyclic) medications (American Psychiatric Association 2002). Hypomania or mania is a risk of using ECT for depression in bipolar patients, but this is not different from the experience with any antidepressant treatment in this disorder (Gormley et al. 1998, American Psychiatric Association 2001, American Psychiatric Association 2002). A number of small trials over the years have described a beneficial role of maintenance ECT for some patients with bipolar disorder, an approach endorsed by the American Psychiatric Association (2002) for those patients who fail to respond or cannot tolerate maintenance medication. In one recent study by Gagné and colleagues (2000), discussed in detail later, the 12 depressed patients with bipolar disorder had long-term outcomes with maintenance medications, alone or in combination with maintenance ECT, that were similar to those of the 46 unipolar depressed patients studied.

While Small and colleagues (1988) identified mixed mood states as predictors of ECT response in bipolar disorder, little systematic research has addressed that issue in the intervening decade and a half. A chart review by Devanand and associates (2000) confirmed the responsiveness of mixed bipolar disorder to ECT, but these patients seemed more difficult to treat, tending toward longer hospital stays and more ECT sessions, compared to matched samples of pure bipolar depressed and manic inpatients; however, multiple potentially confounding variables, including presence of psychosis, ECT treatment parameters, and concurrent medications were not controlled. A prospective but also uncontrolled Italian study was more encouraging about the role of ECT in medication-resistant mixed mood states. Ciapparelli and colleagues (2001) found a higher response rate (56 versus 26%) and a greater reduction in suicidality in consecutive ECT patients with mixed mania ($N = 41$) compared with those with bipolar depression ($N = 23$). While additional definitive controlled trials are required, the existing database strongly supports a role for ECT in the treatment of all phases of bipolar disorder in the face of clinical urgency or refractoriness or excessive risk associated with psychotropic medications (American Psychiatric Association 2001, 2002).

## Schizophrenia

Among the changes undergone by convulsive therapy over its 60-year history, few are as striking as those associated with its use in chronic psychotic illness. ECT has evolved from a treatment of first choice for 1930s dementia praecox to often a treatment of last resort for DSM-IV schizophrenia. Advances in diagnostic assessment and classification, shifting some of the former overabundance of would-be schizophrenics to more appropriate, often mood disorder categories, partly accounted for this change. Perhaps more critical were the general factors noted earlier, that is the psychopharmacology revolution, deinstitutionalization, disappointment with ECT effects in chronically psychotic patients, and the limited availability of ECT in public care settings. More recently, the development of clozapine and other atypical antipsychotic medications provides another treatment option for the refractory patient with schizophrenia, further rendering ECT more likely to be unnecessary. Thus, throughout the 1980s the use of ECT for schizophrenia fell in this country, representing 16.5% of inpatient ECT in 1980, but only 6.5% of the increased 1986 pool of ECT recipients (Thompson et al. 1994). In another modern survey, only 1% of hospitalized schizophrenic patients received ECT (Thompson et al. 1994). However, the efficacy of ECT for depressive symptoms associated with psychotic illness is reflected in recent nationwide data showing the use of convulsive therapy in almost 12% of patients with recurrent major depression comorbid with schizophrenia (Olfson et al. 1998), a utilization rate higher than that seen in uncomplicated recurrent depressive disorder.

### Clinical Trials

Much of the early literature on ECT in schizophrenia is methodologically unacceptable by modern standards. Diagnoses were assigned by clinical judgment, treatment and assessment paradigms were rarely standardized, and control groups often were absent (Ridell 1963, Salzman 1980, Kreuger and Sackeim 1995). From Meduna's time on, however, it was observed that ECT efficacy in schizophrenia appeared inversely related to length of illness, such that the more acutely ill patients responded best. Some evidence for the need for a large number of treatments (20 treatments were common), sometimes given intensely, also emerged in the early work. However, until the 1960s, little controlled data supported the efficacy of ECT in true "Schneiderian" chronic schizophrenia (Turek and Hanlon 1977). Controlled studies in the 1960s and 1970s positioned ECT between the more-effective neuroleptics and the less-useful milieu or psychotherapy (May 1968, Greenblatt 1977). May and associates (1976), in a conclusion that still stands, observed that pharmacotherapy is generally superior to ECT alone in chronic schizophrenia, but that convulsive therapy may be helpful in some patients who fail to respond to medication. Long-term follow-up 2 to 5 years after acute treatment showed no significant differences between neuroleptic and ECT groups, but on a variety of quality-of-life and symptom measures the outcome in chronic schizophrenia was "grim" (May et al. 1981). The potential value of ECT in combination with antipsychotic medications also began to be appreciated once appropriate studies were performed (Krueger and Sackeim 1995).

These preliminary observations have been solidified over the past 2 decades in a new generation of controlled studies of ECT in schizophrenia (Crowe 1984). Small (1985) reviewed the prospective trials conducted between 1953 and 1985, including five studies of real versus sham ECT and six trials comparing ECT with neuroleptics. She concluded that ECT alone is effective over the short-term in acutely ill schizophrenic patients, but that the majority of "middle prognosis" patients fared better on medication. In such individuals, ECT should be reserved for cases of drug resistance or intolerance.

The latest update of the Cochrane Review of the still inadequate research data (Tharyan and Adams 2002), based on 24 controlled trials in schizophrenia, found a higher rate of improvement with active versus sham ECT or placebo. Other advantages of ECT over inactive control conditions included trends toward increased likelihood of hospital discharge and fewer relapses on short-term follow-up. Another eight randomized clinical trials, however, favored antipsychotic medications over ECT, although, as noted, the addition of continuation ECT to antipsychotic drugs was superior to medications alone (Tharyan and Adams 2002). The potential value of ECT for acute and maintenance treatment in older patients with medication-resistant schizophrenic spectrum disorders—mainly schizoaffective disorder—also has been described in open case series (Kramer 1999).

Additionally, three studies were noted to support a more rapid and complete short-term response to the combination of ECT and neuroleptics than to medication alone. Subsequently, the apparent potentiation of antipsychotic drugs by ECT in medication-refractory schizophrenic patients has been reported in additional clinical samples (Friedel 1986, Gujavarty et al. 1987, Sajatovic and Meltzer 1993), but the presence of affective symptoms and relatively short duration of illness in some patients again raised the question of diagnostic heterogeneity (Christison et al. 1991, Meltzer 1992). A limited controlled database finds continuation treatment in schizophrenia with combined ECT and antipsychotic medications superior to either modality alone (Tharyan and Adams 2002).

With the development of clozapine and other atypical antipsychotic drugs, ECT has been pushed further back in the treatment algorithm for medication-resistant schizophrenia. Case reports and series, often with positive outcomes (Frankenburg et al. 1993, Hirose et al. 2001) are now appearing on the next logical step: clozapine or other atypical antipsychotics combined with ECT. The mechanisms of action of combined ECT–antipsychotic drug treatment remain undefined (Kellner et al. 1991, Klapheke 1993).

The net effect of this body of not particularly well-controlled data is that the American Psychiatric Association Task Force on ECT (American Psychiatric Association 2001) and the Canadian Psychiatric Association (Enns and Reiss 1992) identified a role for ECT as a second-line treatment for selected patients with schizophrenia, particularly when associated with a brief duration of illness and/or affective symptoms. Both groups found chronic schizophrenia to respond no better to real ECT than to sham treatment. Accenting these views is the speculation by Wyatt (1991) that the long-term presence of psychosis per se may be biologically "toxic" to the brain—in addition to the clear debilitating psychological and social costs of chronic mental illness—suggesting that no treatment option, including ECT, be overlooked in the service of inducing a prompt remission in newly ill, "first-break" patients (Sakar et al. 1994, Fink and Sackeim 1996). Indeed, a substantial proportion of such patients prove on follow-up to be suffering from a mood disorder, for which ECT would be expected to help, but which might be worsened by a neuroleptic (Van Valkenburg and Clayton 1985). Additionally, should ECT enable the delay or reduction in life-time exposure to neuroleptic drugs, the risk of tardive dyskinesia or other adverse effects of medications might be decreased. Reports of even occasional response to ECT in the more chronically ill schizophrenic individual indicate that convulsive therapy should not be abandoned altogether in this poor-prognosis patient population (Van Valkenburg and Clayton 1985, Hertzman 1992, Fink and Sackeim 1996, Tang and Ungvari 2001b).

## Predictors of Response

Despite the considerable variability in methodology across the studies over the past 50 years, several trends have emerged regarding ECT use in schizophrenia. It has been consistently found that the schizophrenic patients most likely to respond to ECT are those with good prognosis signs: mood disturbances, short duration of illness, predominance of positive rather than negative symptoms, and over-excitement (Fink and Sackeim 1996). The potential responsiveness of acute psychotic symptoms in schizophrenia to ECT is more emphatically stated in the 2001 revision of the American Psychiatric Association Task Force Report compared to the previous edition, based on research conducted and compiled in the intervening decade (Fink and Sackeim 1996). Diagnostic subtypes of schizophrenia associated with a positive response to ECT include acute, schizophreniform, schizoaffective, catatonic, and paranoid (Milstein et al. 1990, Rudorfer and Harris in press). Two prospective studies addressing the issue of predictors of outcome in schizophrenic and schizoaffective patients treated with ECT and concurrent neuroleptics found positive treatment response to be associated with recent onset of illness, shorter duration of current episode, dearth of premorbid schizoid personality traits, the presence of perplexity, mood-congruent delusions or hallucinations, and a lesser family history of schizophrenia (Dodwell and Goldberg 1989, Chanpattana and Chakrabhand 2001). Successful ECT in schizophrenia may require a greater number of treatments than is typical in the treatment of mood disorders. No evidence has emerged favoring either bilateral or unilateral electrode placement in the treatment of schizophrenia (Small 1985). A recent report from Hong Kong notes that the benefits of ECT in chronic schizophrenia may extend beyond symptomatic change (Tang and Ungvari 2001b). Although only modest improvement in positive and negative symptoms was observed in six long-term hospitalized patients completing at least eight ECT treatments, four of these individuals experienced clinically significant enhancement of occupational and social functioning (Tang and Ungvari 2001b). This enabled patients with schizophrenia to benefit

further from rehabilitative psychosocial interventions. These factors of social and occupational functioning are probably important in determining subjective feelings of improvement following ECT for all chronically ill patients (Rohland 2000), and are especially important as data emerge showing that even where ECT (plus neuroleptics) benefits positive symptoms of schizophrenia, negative symptoms are not improved (Chanpattana and Chakrabhand 2001); the impact of newer atypical antipsychotics on these effects awaits further study.

## Other Axis I Disorders

As reiterated in the recent Surgeon General's report on mental health (US Department of Health and Human Services 1999), ECT has no demonstrated efficacy in dysthymia, substance abuse, or anxiety disorder. Nonetheless, ECT may play a role when the severity of a secondary major depression is severe and/or treatment refractory (Olfson et al. 1998, American Psychiatric Association 2001). In such circumstances, ECT can be expected to improve the comorbid mood component, leaving the underlying primary disorder untreated; in some circumstances, removal of the burden of overlying depression may indirectly benefit the underlying disorder. A case in point is obsessive–compulsive disorder (OCD). Despite half a century of literature describing the use of ECT in this anxiety disorder, there is no convincing evidence for the efficacy of convulsive therapy in combating the core symptoms of OCD. Rather, what efficacy has been described can more parsimoniously be traced to a therapeutic action of ECT against the comorbid depression that commonly accompanies OCD (Rudorfer 2000). On the other hand, in the face of a potentially ECT-responsive major depressive episode, the presence of a nonmood Axis I disorder, even substance abuse, should not constitute a contraindication to the use of convulsive therapy (Olfson et al. 1998, American Psychiatric Association 2001).

## Axis II Disorders

There are no evidence-based biological treatments for DSM-IV Axis II personality disorders, including ECT. Given the high incidence of comorbid, often treatment-refractory depression that accompanies Axis II pathology, ECT has been used in personality disordered patients, with inconsistent—but generally negative—reports of success, for many years. Most of the literature has focused on what today falls under DSM-IV cluster B personality disorders, especially borderline personality disorder (BPD). In the absence of controlled clinical trials, the perceived clinical wisdom has been along the lines of one recent Canadian retrospective survey (Sareen et al. 2000), which found that compared to ECT candidates with major depression and no Axis II diagnosis, those with comorbid personality disorders had a poorer acute response to ECT and a higher rate of depressive relapse during 1-year follow-up after completion of the treatment course. Even in that methodologically challenged chart review, most patients with comorbid depression and personality disorder did respond acutely to ECT, and more than a quarter of that cohort successfully completed 1-year follow-up without relapse into depression (Sareen et al. 2000).

Even in prospective trials with standardized diagnostic criteria, totaling some 75 patients with major depression plus personality disorder, the role of ECT is not well defined. This is true of all treatment studies with personality disorder patients, who commonly endorse symptoms on depression rating scales that may reflect Axis II rather than I pathology, confounding the measurement of antidepressant treatment response. In a comprehensive review of the literature, DeBattista and Mueller (2001) summed up current understanding of this dilemma by observing that "the depressed, borderline patient appears to have two distinct disorders, one which is responsive to ECT and the other which is not." Definitive, randomized studies are necessary to determine whether the mixed and often disappointing effects of ECT in patients with comorbid Axis I and II disorders reflect a reduced efficacy of the intervention or is consistent with the treatment-resistant nature of depression in these individuals. However, based on present knowledge, in an individual case, the presence of a major depressive episode that is clearly separate and distinct from the underlying personality disorder should determine the appropriateness and likelihood of response to ECT (DeBattista and Mueller 2001).

## Neurologic Disorders

Only 1% of patients admitted with a primary diagnosis other than a mood disorder or schizophrenia are treated with ECT in this country (Thompson et al. 1994). Nonetheless, individuals with neurologic or other medical problems often suffer from primary or secondary mood or motor disorders that are ECT-responsive.

## Catatonia

From the inception of convulsive therapy, its efficacy in the syndrome of catatonia, which is dominated by motor signs, has been consistent and often dramatic (Fink and Sackeim 1996). Nearly always successful in this situation, ECT typically induces remission in catatonia in less than a week with only two to four closely spaced, for example daily, treatments (Fink 2002). The use of ECT in this behavioral disorder marked by extremes in activity has been extremely selective, due in large part to the confluence of mostly practical factors. Thus, until recent years the official classification system relegated catatonia exclusively to a subtype of schizophrenia which, according to prevailing wisdom, was not a primary indication for ECT. Moreover, immobile and unresponsive catatonic patients as a rule are unable to give informed consent, and ECT is not typically available in general medical settings, complicating the use of a nonpharmacological somatic treatment (Fink 2002). In recent years, as catatonia has been identified as a component of mood disorders, especially mania (Taylor and Abrams 1977) and "depressive stupor," as well as systemic medical disorders, such as lupus, DSM-IV-TR has broadened its classification beyond schizophrenia.

The case report literature describes the generally prompt and complete response to ECT of catatonic syndromes associated with both primary psychiatric (Pataki et al. 1992, Fink and Sackeim 1996) and systemic disorders (Fricchione et al. 1990). ECT may justifiably be described as life-saving where catatonia leads to inanition and in the often fatal, malignant form of catatonia (Mann et al. 1990b, Philbrick and Rummans 1994). However, controlled trials are lacking and, in the absence of sham ECT comparisons, questions have been raised as to the potential efficacy of the

barbiturate anesthesia per se without seizure induction in the catatonic syndrome (Rosebush et al. 1992). A review of the literature over the past 3 decades, however, found all three uncontrolled trials of ECT in catatonia to be efficacious (Hermann et al. 1999); 40 of 43 catatonic patients described in published case reports also responded to ECT. Three quarters of 24 children and adolescents with catatonia associated with mood disorders, schizophrenia, or physical illness are described in an uncontrolled literature as showing marked improvement with ECT (Rey and Walter 1997).

Over the past decade, benzodiazepines have emerged as the pharmacological treatment of choice for catatonia (Rosebush et al. 1992, Ungavari et al. 1994). However, in medication-unresponsive patients, prolonged drug trials with continuing clinical deterioration should be avoided in favor of a course of ECT (Ungavari et al. 1994). Reflecting current understanding of the syndrome and its treatment, Fricchione (1989) recommended that "given the significant morbidity and mortality associated with catatonia, ECT should be considered if an expeditious 48- to 72-hour benzodiazepine trial is unsuccessful." As a practical point, given the now-common initial use of benzodiazepines in this condition, the catatonic patient may come to ECT with an initially elevated seizure threshold, and treatment parameters should be adjusted accordingly (Fink 2002).

## Neuroleptic Malignant Syndrome

This clinical syndrome of fever, muscle rigidity with elevated serum creatine phosphokinase, autonomic instability, and mental status changes occurring in patients treated with neuroleptics, may be a form of malignant catatonia (Philbrick and Rummans 1994). Thus, ECT would be expected to be useful. Nevertheless, in the absence of controlled trials, the efficacy of ECT in this syndrome was questioned as recently as the mid-1980s (Levenson 1985).

A subsequent comprehensive review (Davis et al. 1991) refuted this uncertainty and established ECT as a safe and effective treatment of neuroleptic malignant syndrome (NMS). Tabulating 665 detailed cases of NMS, Davis and colleagues (1991) identified 48 who had received ECT, 29 of them during the acute phase of the syndrome. The mortality rate for the ECT-treated patients (10.3%) was comparable to that (9.7%) with accepted dopaminergic pharmacotherapy (bromocriptine, amantadine, levodopa, dantrolene) and half that associated with supportive care alone (21%). Critically, failure to respond or death in ECT-treated patients was associated with continued use of high-potency neuroleptics. Careful physiological monitoring of patients undergoing ECT in the face of ongoing NMS is essential (Hughes 1986, Devanand et al. 1987). Although formal controlled trials will probably never be feasible, the use of ECT is indicated in NMS patients unresponsive to supportive care or use of one of the dopaminergic or benzodiazepine medication options (Lazarus 1986, Fink 2000). Moreover, ECT may be a feasible alternative treatment for the underlying mental disorder in the NMS patient for whom continuation or reintroduction of an antipsychotic is inadvisable (Pelonero et al. 1998).

A theoretical concern was raised regarding the use of ECT in NMS: that exposure to succinylcholine as an ECT premedication might precipitate malignant hyperthermia—possibly related pathophysiologically to NMS—in these vulnerable individuals. This fear has not been borne out (Addonizio and Susman 1987, Davis et al. 1991).

Although the incidence of NMS can be expected to drop with the decreasing use of conventional neuroleptics in favor of atypical antipsychotics, ECT retains a place in the treatment algorithm for delirium of any cause, including metabolic, infectious, and toxic brain and systemic disorders, particularly where ongoing symptoms interfere with the necessary correction of an underlying systemic etiology (Fink 2000).

## Parkinson's Disease

A great deal of interest currently attends the use of ECT for this disabling, progressive neurodegenerative disease. Kellner and Bernstein (1993) compiled 22 reports from the literature between 1959 and 1991, totaling 77 Parkinson's disease patients, who had received ECT, most often for a concomitant mood disorder. Most showed a positive response of both motor signs (often improving first) and mood disturbance, but occasional patients showed a dissociation, whereby one or the other syndrome improved with no change in the other (Young et al. 1985). Tallying the literature through 1998, Hermann and associates (1999) described antidepressant efficacy in patients with Parkinson's disease in both published controlled trials (one of which was randomized), in three of the four uncontrolled trials, and in 24 of 30 case reports. In the largest case series, investigators at the Mayo Clinic (Moellentine et al. 1998) retrospectively compared 25 patients with Parkinson's disease with an equal number of neurologically healthy psychiatric patients, all of whom received ECT, typically for major depression and generally utilizing unilateral electrode placement. Ratings of depression and anxiety, by nonblind raters, fell significantly in both groups; 14 of the 25 Parkinson's disease patients also demonstrated improvement in motor function at hospital discharge, although further follow-up was not available (Moellentine et al. 1998).

The presence of psychosis may predict lack of an antidepressant effect in patients with Parkinson's disease (Price and McAllister 1989). Clinical response of parkinsonian signs to ECT in general occurs early in the treatment course but often is transient, lasting for hours to months. Right unilateral electrode placement has been reported effective, for example in the Mayo Clinic series (Moellentine et al. 1998), with a switch to bilateral electrode placement recommended if early response to ECT is not observed (Rasmussen and Abrams 1991).

Most of the work in Parkinson's disease uncomplicated by psychiatric illness has been performed in Sweden and consisted of two parts. In an open case series of nine patients, five responded to bilateral ECT with significant reductions in rigidity and bradykinesia ("off time"), lasting from 1 to 10 months (Balldin et al. 1981). A later double-blind trial by Andersen and colleagues (1987) found bilateral or unilateral ECT effective in all nine patients receiving active convulsive therapy, with improvement in motor signs continuing for 2 to 6 weeks. In contrast, neither patient assigned to sham ECT responded. Similar positive findings have been reported for refractory Parkinson's disease patients openly treated with ECT in the US (Douyon et al. 1989, Zervas and Fink 1991). Older patients have done especially well on ECT for parkinsonian signs

(Balldin et al. 1981, Andersen et al. 1987, Douyon et al. 1989).

Taking the treatment paradigm the next step, two reports (Zervas and Fink 1991, Wengel et al. 1998) have described the use of maintenance ECT in nondepressed Parkinson's disease patients, an intervention that has been recommended, given the frequent finding of relapse within weeks of completion of ECT in these individuals (Rasmussen and Abrams 1991, Kellner and Bernstein 1993, Kellner et al. 1994). Positive results were seen in five of six patients completing maintenance ECT, typically every 3 to 4 weeks, up to 12 months (Zervas and Fink 1991, Wengel et al. 1998). Motor improvement was most evident in reductions in off time, with little effect on other parkinsonian signs, such as tremor (Wengel et al. 1998).

In general, the baseline cognitive impairment commonly associated with Parkinson's disease is not worsened by ECT and may actually improve (Moellentine et al. 1998, Wengel et al. 1998). The effects of ECT on dopamine systems are consistent with its antiparkinsonian properties (Rudorfer et al. in press), and may also account for its toxicity in this clinical context. Moellentine and others (1998) reported transient interictal delirium in 13 (of 25) Parkinson's disease patients during a course of ECT, 10 of whom were on levodopa at the time of ECT initiation. Indeed, the commonly observed dyskinesias or delirium late in the course of ECT in these patients responds to reductions in dose of levodopa and carbidopa (Douyon et al. 1989, Rasmussen and Abrams 1991, Oh et al. 1992, Kellner and Bernstein 1993, Kellner et al. 1994), perhaps reflecting the increased dopamine receptor sensitivity (Balldin et al. 1982, Rudorfer et al. 1992) or number (Fochtmann et al. 1989) that accompanies a course of ECT.

## Other Neurologic Illness

The remaining neurological indications for ECT can be considered to fall into two major categories: (1) those for which, as with any medical illness (see later), ECT is considered for treatment of a secondary depression when benefit–risk analysis favors ECT over antidepressant medications and (2) those for which ECT may play a special role by virtue of its unique actions compared to alternative treatment options.

In the first category are such conditions as poststroke depression (Murray et al. 1986, Currier et al. 1992) and mood disturbance in the context of brain trauma, tumor, or dementia (Hsiao et al. 1987, Liang et al. 1988, Kohler and Burock 2001). Medication may be difficult to tolerate by these neurologically ill patients, tilting the potential benefit–risk ratio in favor of ECT (Price and McAllister 1989). The case report literature is encouraging in that ECT can successfully treat a secondary depression in, for example, patients with primary dementia (Liang et al. 1988, Mulsant et al. 1991) or poststroke (Currier et al. 1992), while the underlying cognitive and neurological deficits are most often unaffected. Although the outcomes are not presented, the 1993 national survey of ECT use in the community (Olfson et al. 1998) found that one in six patients with recurrent major depression with underlying dementia was treated with ECT, making dementia the most common comorbidity associated with depression among ECT recipients.

Despite a high rate of mental disorders in people with mental retardation, there are no controlled trials of ECT in these individuals. In a comprehensive review of the field, Dutch investigators (Van Waarde et al. 2001) culled published reports of 44 mentally retarded patients, most of whom suffered from psychotic depression, who had received ECT. With an 84% response rate and no unusual adverse effects reported, Van Waarde and associates (2001) concluded that the apparent underuse of ECT in patients with mental retardation and severe mental disorders results more from diagnostic, legal, and ethical challenges in this population rather than an inherent lessened efficacy or increased risk.

Potential contraindications to ECT are very few and rarely are absolute (American Psychiatric Association 2001). Although ECT generally should not be performed in the presence of raised intracranial pressure, it has been given safely even in the face of brain tumors and other mass lesions (Hsiao et al. 1987, Fried and Mann 1988, Abrams 1991, 1992, Kohler and Burock 2001) with special steps taken to protect against the ECT-associated hemodynamic changes; intracranial pressure may be reduced with the use of oral or parenteral steroids (Beale et al. 1997). Postsurgical patients may require individualized ECT electrode placement to avoid skull defects (Lisanby et al. 2001a). Patients with Down syndrome require careful pre-ECT assessment for atlantoaxial instability, found in 1 to 2% of these individuals, which would render neck hyperextension during ventilation contraindicated (Van Waarde et al. 2001). However, although structural brain abnormalities are not induced or worsened by ECT (Currier et al. 1992, Devanand et al. 1994) their presence at pretreatment may increase the likelihood of ECT-associated transient cognitive deficits or interictal delirium (Botteron et al. 1991). In younger neurologically impaired patients, the literature describes 15 individuals with multiple sclerosis who received ECT for treatment of depression (Mattingly et al. 1992); the high rate of antidepressant response (80%) must be tempered by a disproportionate (20%) incidence of delirium or other neurologic deficit these patients developed during the course of treatment. On the other hand, despite the neurotropic properties of the human immunodeficiency virus (HIV), nondemented depressed patients with HIV seropositivity or acquired immune deficiency syndrome (AIDS) have responded to ECT without cognitive decline (Schaerf et al. 1989). Similarly, ECT has been used successfully, without reported cognitive deterioration, in individuals suffering from depression or delirium following closed head injury (Kant et al. 1999).

The second group of neurologic indications for ECT, of which Parkinson's disease is the prototype, include intractable epilepsy or status epilepticus (Price and McAllister 1989, Kellner and Bernstein 1993, Lisanby et al. 2001a). In this condition, should anticonvulsant medications prove insufficient to adequately control seizures, a trial of ECT would seek to take advantage of its anticonvulsant properties (Sackeim et al. 1983, 1987a). Achievement of an adequate seizure during ECT in such circumstances may require tapering of what is often a complex anticonvulsant medication regimen and/or use of a benzodiazepine antagonist to temporarily reduce seizure threshold at the time of treatment (Lisanby et al. 2001a).

Maintenance ECT or anticonvulsant medication would be required to sustain these otherwise-transient effects beyond the acute ECT trial. Although case reports have been published for decades (Caplan 1946, Sackeim et al. 1983, Regenold et al. 1998, Lisanby et al. 2001); no controlled ECT studies have been conducted for this potential indication.

## Other Considerations in the Use of ECT

It can be appreciated that while accurate psychiatric diagnosis is essential to prioritize treatment options, it is far from the only consideration for the clinician weighing the advantages and potential problems of prescribing ECT (American Psychiatric Association 2001). Two often-related variables are the patient's state of physical health and age. A disproportionate number of individuals receiving ECT in this country are elderly, many of whom are physically compromised. Fortunately, advances in the understanding and practice of ECT, according to Abrams (1991), "now enable its routine and successful application in a population of patients previously believed to be too old or too physically ill to undergo the stress of induced convulsions."

### Advanced Age

More vulnerable than younger individuals to both the symptoms of depression, particularly psychosis, decreased nutritional intake, and suicidal ideation, and the adverse effects of antidepressant medications, the elderly represent a growing segment of the patient base for ECT (Benbow 1989, Blazer 1989, Sackeim 1993, Olfson et al. 1998). A substantial proportion of geriatric depressed patients referred for ECT suffer from significant concurrent medical illness, which often preclude adequate trials of pharmacotherapy (Tew et al. 1999). Indeed, interpretation of case–control studies of geriatric depression treatment is fraught with difficulty, as elderly patients able to successfully undergo medication trials often have less severe physical illness than those undergoing ECT (Kroessler and Fogel 1993). With the introduction of SSRIs and other newer and potentially less toxic medications, that factor may be changing. However, the benefit–risk ratio, influenced by speed of response, tolerability, and adherence factors, still often favors ECT over pharmacotherapy in the older person with severe depression.

Even with a dearth of controlled studies, the efficacy of ECT in geriatric depression is well established (Sackeim 1993) and is often perceived as even superior to that in younger age groups (Benbow 1989). In addition to the usual clinical criteria for recommending ECT, as discussed earlier, some have suggested that anxiety or agitation, commonly regarded as a negative prognostic sign in younger individuals, may be predictive of a good response to ECT in the older depressed patients (Salzman 1982, Benbow 1989). More than 1,000 elderly depressed patients (some with dementia) were treated with ECT in 14 mostly retrospective reports published in the 1980s (Mulsant et al. 1991). Most patients responded to treatment, with significant medical complications noted in 6% and confusion or delirium in 11%. Similar findings emerged in one of the few prospective, albeit naturalistic, studies of ECT in 40 patients with late-life depression (Mulsant et al. 1991).

Systematic retrospective surveys on both sides of the Atlantic have focused on those at greatest physical risk from all invasive procedures: the "old–old," commonly defined as individuals over age 75 years. In 22 courses of mostly bilateral, brief pulse ECT, investigators at Louisville (Casey and Davis 1996) found a very high (86.3%) response rate. Although the adverse effect rate of 22.7% was notable, only two patients experienced cardiovascular complications, and most adverse effects, including one case of prolonged confusion, were transient and did not interfere with completion of the ECT course. No pretreatment patient characteristics or treatment parameters were associated with adverse effects of ECT in this sample (Casey and Davis 1996). Similarly impressive efficacy (85% moderate or marked response) was observed in 93 courses of ECT administered to patients over age 75 years at three British and Irish hospitals in the last decade (Gormley et al. 1998). The observed 10% rate of complications consisted mainly of confusion and hypomania, which resolved within two weeks following completion of ECT; one case each of hypertension and headache was also transient. It is noteworthy that in addition to the use of brief pulse (albeit mainly bilateral) stimulation, in accord with usual British and European practice this study utilized a twice-weekly ECT schedule, rather than the usual American three times per week approach (Gormley et al. 1998). Employing a matched control group treated only with medication, Manly and associates (2000) demonstrated better antidepressant outcome, with fewer cardiovascular and gastrointestinal adverse effects, in old–old inpatients treated with ECT. The convulsive therapy patients, however, had significantly longer hospital stays.

These retrospective findings have been confirmed and extended by recent prospective data emerging from the acute phase of a pair of NIMH-sponsored continuation treatment studies. In a three-site trial, old–old patients actually showed greater antidepressant efficacy to ECT (67%) than the 54% response rate seen in adults up to age 59 years (Tew et al. 1999). The greatest ECT response (73%) occurred, however, in an intermediate "young–old" cohort aged 60 to 74 years, despite the fact that they as well as the old–old group aged 75 years and above presented for treatment with a greater burden of physical illness and global cognitive impairment than did the younger adults (Tew et al. 1999). The four-site CORE trial described above (Petrides et al. 2001, O'Connor et al. 2001) similarly found a higher rate of remission and response in geriatric patients, without a significant difference between "old–old" and "young–old" patients. Following a brief-pulse bilateral acute ECT course in CORE, those patients under age 45 years had a 75% remission rate (57% if all the dropouts are counted as nonresponders), compared to 93% of the middle age group (age 46–64 years; 86% including dropouts) and 90% for those over age 65 years (80% for complete group). Similar findings were seen for the less stringent outcome of response, obtained for the complete sample in 68% for the young adults, 91% for the middle group, and 90% for the old–old. Considering age as a continuous variable, there was a highly significant positive correlation between age and degree of change in the Hamilton depression score with ECT. Beyond the effect of age per se, in this study the geriatric patients also exhibited a higher incidence of psychotic features (Petrides et al. 2001), an older age of

onset of depression, and a lower number of previous episodes than the younger age groups, which may have contributed to the superior ECT response in older individuals (O'Connor et al. 2001).

Two general points should be made about the use of ECT in the elderly: (1) the physiological changes associated with ECT—cardiovascular (elevated blood pressure, arrhythmias), cognitive (confusion, memory loss), risk of traumatic injury to bones and teeth—that are benign and easily tolerated in young and middle-aged patients are prominent sources of potential ECT-associated morbidity in geriatric patients and (2) the safety of ECT is appreciably enhanced if the foregoing effects on the older body, whether healthy or diseased, are anticipated and controlled. For example, Casey and Davis (1996) noted that a "rigorous falls prevention protocol" helped protect their elderly ECT patients from a potentially dangerous complication seen in earlier studies.

## Younger Age

The very limited use of ECT in children and adolescents at present has been noted above. Only a generation ago, it was not unusual for the American textbooks of child psychiatry to omit any mention of convulsive therapy. As with adults, early use of ECT in young patients focused on childhood schizophrenia, which is no longer considered an appropriate primary indication for this intervention. Rather, modern practice guidelines direct that the use of ECT in children and adolescents with schizophrenia "be reserved for those cases where several trials of medication therapy (including a trial of clozapine) have failed. ECT may also be considered for catatonic states" (American Academy of Child and Adolescent Psychiatry 2001). When intractable psychotic illnesses in adolescents, including schizophrenia and schizoaffective disorder, are in fact treated with ECT, clinical response typically is less complete than that seen in mood disorders (Cohen et al. 2000a). The limited use of modern ECT in young people is generally reserved for cases of depression or mania complicated by medication resistance or the need for an urgent clinical response. However, even today, the literature in this area consists of case reports and series, with no controlled trials (Baldwin and Oxlad 1996, Cohen et al. 2000b, Rabheru 2001). Nonetheless, where ECT is utilized in younger patients, its efficacy and safety appear comparable to those in adults (Rey and Walter 1997, Cohen et al. 2000b), although additional controlled research is needed (Rabheru 2001).

In using ECT with children and adolescents, attention must be paid to the lower seizure threshold in young people, with appropriately low initial stimulus parameters and careful dose titration during an ECT course (American Psychiatric Association 2001). Although young patients may be at greater risk for prolonged seizures, other adverse effects are no more likely, aided by the more common lack of comorbid physical illness in younger patients (Rey and Walter 1997).

## Physical Health

Recent national survey data across all age groups found the presence of physical illness comorbid with recurrent major depression to be associated with a >25% higher utilization rate of ECT compared with uncomplicated depressive disorder alone (Olfson et al. 1998). As the common occurrence of underdiagnosis and undertreatment of depression associated with serious medical illnesses, such as cancer, is increasingly recognized and rectified, the demonstrated efficacy and safety of ECT in such clinical circumstances should not be overlooked (Beale et al. 1997). Preliminary data suggesting improvement in chronic pain and associated affective symptoms suggest areas for further research (Bloomstein et al. 1996). Thus, careful pretreatment evaluation of the patient's medical and neurological status, as well as review of concurrent medications and their potential impact on ECT are crucial (Salzman 1982, Rasmussen and Zorumski 1993).

A special physical health challenge to the treatment of mental disorders is presented by pregnancy. According to clinical lore, the efficacy and safety of ECT in this circumstance were discovered accidentally in the early 1940s when, following successful treatment, a patient's "abdominal mass" was determined to be a fetus. More systematic, if uncontrolled, experience over the ensuing decades, totaling >300 published cases (Miller 1994)—combined with the introduction of effective, but potentially teratogenic psychotropic medications—has confirmed this initial favorable impression. When used with appropriate care and modifications, ECT is relatively safe and effective during all trimesters of pregnancy and in the postpartum period (Miller 1994, American Psychiatric Association 2001, Rabheru 2001). These are times of high risk for mood disorders, certainly detrimental to the well-being of the pregnant patient and her baby, yet the very circumstance in which many women and their physicians wish to avoid medications which could be harmful to the developing fetus. Hence, the niche for non-pharmacological somatic interventions, particularly ECT, has persisted throughout the last half century of medication development, especially for severe depression or mania during pregnancy (American Psychiatric Association 2002). Advantages of ECT that operate in favor of persons with medical illness are especially pertinent for the pregnant woman: the times of highest risk are the times of treatment sessions, at which close monitoring of the patient and the fetus can take place, with the obstetrician in attendance, and brief and transient exposure to anesthesia and ECT premedications that cross the placenta. Fewer than 10% of published cases of ECT in pregnancy have described adverse effects, the majority of these described as benign and self-limited (Miller 1994, Bhatia et al. 1999). Guidelines for the administration of ECT in the pregnant patient, incorporating measures such as intravenous hydration, avoidance of hyperventilation and nonessential anticholinergic medication, measures against gastric reflux, proper positioning of the patient during treatment, and uterine and fetal cardiac monitoring, have been developed and incorporated into modern practice (Miller 1994, Walker and Swartz 1994, American Psychiatric Association 2001).

Appropriate precautions and monitoring during and following ECT can minimize complications and permit safe and effective convulsive therapy even in the medically compromised patient of any age (Rasmussen et al. 2002a).

## Pretreatment Evaluation

Once the decision has been made to proceed with a course of ECT, specific steps are taken by the treatment team to maximize the benefits and minimize the risks. In some instances these procedures are part of the initial workup, and the results may influence treatment decisions, as when certain psychiatric or physical disorders are ruled in or out.

The psychiatrist will want to make liberal use of appropriate consultants, especially representing the fields of anesthesiology and, when indicated, internal medicine (often cardiology) or obstetrics. However, the careful and complete history and physical examination will often abrogate the need for unnecessary tests in the interest of "defensive medicine." Given the current regulatory climate, the physician needs to be aware of local requirements regarding the need for second opinions or other pretreatment procedures in certain circumstances, or to arrange for guardianship or court proceedings where the patient's capacity to consent to ECT is in question, to assure that the initiation of treatment is not unduly delayed.

### Psychiatric Considerations

The pre-ECT evaluation is a good time to confirm psychiatric diagnosis, including Axis II and III, which often must be given short shrift in the course of the admission process. In many settings, a specific ECT consultation may be helpful in evaluating the patient for a potentially ECT-responsive disorder and weighing the various treatment options (Klapheke 1997). Input from nursing and other professional staff that have been working with the patient should be factored in. Should the indications for ECT remain present, baseline assessments of mental status including evaluation of suicidality, orientation, and memory will help monitor changes in both therapeutic and adverse effects over the course of treatment. The history and effects of previous treatment with ECT should be obtained. Also, this time, decisions must be made regarding ongoing psychotropic medications particularly those increasing the risk of toxicity in combination with ECT, for example lithium, and those affecting seizure threshold, such as benzodiazepines and anticonvulsants—and steps instituted to adjust, taper, or discontinue these medications, when appropriate.

### Other Medical Considerations

History and physical examination should focus on the cardiovascular and neurological systems, the areas of greatest risk. The consulting internist, anesthesiologist, or other physician should advise the treatment team regarding cardiovascular risk of ECT and the need for any modifications in treatment technique, such as medications to moderate hemodynamic changes (Dolinski and Zvara 1997). The safety of possible treatment adjuncts, such as intravenous caffeine, should also be addressed where baseline cardiovascular function is compromised. Appropriate pretreatment optimization and monitoring of medical conditions that may be affected by ECT, such as diabetes, should be arranged at this time.

In the uncomplicated situation, the routine laboratory workup for ECT is that indicated for any procedure involving general anesthesia: complete blood count, serum electrolyte levels, and electrocardiogram (ECG) (American Psychiatric Association 2001, Chaturvedi et al. 2001). Chest X-ray is often obtained as well. The need for further pretreatment workup, such as serum chemistries, urinalysis, HIV antibody titers, and medication blood concentrations, is determined on an individual basis (Lafferty et al. 2001). Given a normal neurologic and fundoscopic examination, computerized tomography (CT) or magnetic resonance imaging (MRI) of the brain is not indicated. Lumbosacral spine films, historically routine prior to institution of muscle relaxation in the ECT premedication protocol, have become optional for many patients. This remains appropriate for older patients with a history of or at risk for osteoporosis, and for any patient with a history of bone trauma. A formal anesthesiology consultation should result in an assignment of the degree of anesthesia risk and recommendations for any necessary modification in the ECT protocol (Folk et al. 2000). A personal or family history of anesthesia complications may call for assessment of the hydrolyzing capacity of plasma pseudocholinesterase to determine the safety of succinylcholine. The condition of dentition should be routinely assessed to avoid the treatment-associated risk of aspiration or fracture of loose teeth or bridgework. Especially in elderly patients, a formal dental examination may be helpful to assure proper protection of the teeth during ECT.

## Informed Consent

Among the unique features of ECT compared with other standard psychiatric treatments is the requirement for written informed consent by the patient or legal guardian or other substitute. Guidelines regarding the content of a standard informed consent form for ECT have been published (American Psychiatric Association 2001). Supplemental information regarding ECT for patients and their families in a variety of media is also available and its distribution is encouraged (Fink 1999, American Psychiatric Association 2001). Informed consent entails the patient being provided the rationale for the recommendation for ECT, along with information regarding the potential benefits and risks of available alternative treatments, including no treatment. The consent form encompasses information regarding the series of treatment sessions that constitute a course of ECT, with the explicit understanding that consent may be withdrawn and treatments terminated at any point, at the patient's discretion. A separate consent form is necessary for continuation or maintenance ECT following completion of the (acute phase treatment) course (see further). In some locales specific procedures for obtaining consent for ECT are regulated by the state, a recent example being legislation passed in Vermont in 2000. As with all medical procedures, special challenges attend the informed consent process for children and adolescents. In addition to seeking the parents' or guardians' consent, and, if possible, the patient's assent, current professional (and, in some locales, regulatory) standards call for consultation with an independent colleague prior to initiating ECT in a young person (American Psychiatric Association 2001, Taieb et al. 2001). Reviewing the current knowledge of the potential benefits and risks of convulsive therapy for adolescents with severe mental disorders, child psychiatrists in France have warned that "the consequence of overprotection is that the adolescent may remain untreated because of unrealistic fears regarding ECT" and conclude that "there is no ethical reason to ban the use of ECT in adolescents" (Cohen et al. 2000a).

The NIH/NIMH Consensus Development Conference on ECT (1985) emphasized that informed consent is a process that continues throughout the treatment course. Given the transient cognitive impairments common in depression and during an ECT course, it is particularly necessary to maintain a dialogue with the patient as treatment progresses to assure that all of the patient's questions and concerns are addressed, even if repetitive discourse ensues. With appropriate modification of the presentation of information, including use of nonverbal demonstration of the procedure, even patients with mental retardation often can make informed decisions about consent for ECT (Van Waarde et al. 2001).

Most candidates for ECT are voluntarily admitted inpatients. Questions about the capacity of the patient to make treatment decisions or the refusal of the dangerously ill patient (e.g. catatonic, malnourished, continually suicidal) to agree to ECT that is medically indicated constitute legal issues, for which judicial intervention should be sought promptly; this appears to be more common in public rather than private settings. Despite local variations in relevant laws and regulations, many ECT practitioners can cite instances of court ordered ECT in carefully selected cases where the potentially life-saving necessity of ECT had been clearly demonstrated to a judge. At the same time, good communication with the patient's family or friends is imperative in dealing with the complex dynamics involved in considering an intervention over the patient's objections (Boronow et al. 1997).

## Initiation of Treatment

Once informed consent has been obtained, the initiation of treatment involves several decisions. These include selection of ECT device, electrode placement, dose of electricity, choice of premedications, and frequency of treatment.

Several different types of devices for administering ECT have been used. They differ in two major respects: the waveform of the stimulus delivered, and whether they deliver constant current, constant voltage, or constant energy (Stephens et al. 1991, Abrams 1982). The waveforms available for delivering stimuli in the US include sine wave and brief pulse (Abrams 1997b, 2000). The older sine wave devices have the disadvantage of requiring more energy, thereby producing greater cognitive side effects than the more recently developed, and now standard, brief pulse devices (Weiner et al. 1986, Stephens et al. 1991, Abrams 1997b, Sackeim et al. 1994).

The other respect in which ECT devices differ is whether constant current, constant voltage, or constant energy is delivered. With constant current devices, the current is set and the device dynamically adjusts the voltage to maintain that current. In devices where the voltage is kept constant, an increase in resistance results in a decrease in the current delivered, which may lead to induction of subtherapeutic seizures. Lastly, with constant energy machines the amount of energy delivered is kept fixed. Increased resistance, such as poor skin contact, will also decrease the amount of current delivered and possibly result in a subtherapeutic or missed seizure (Sackeim et al. 1994). Research is now underway regarding the possible role of various components of the electrical stimulus waveform, for example, pulse width in determining the therapeutic and adverse effects of brief pulse ECT.

In choosing electrode placement there are two important factors to consider: antidepressant efficacy and cognitive side effects. The choices of electrode placement can be divided into unilateral placement over the nondominant (generally right) hemisphere and bilateral electrode placement (Figure 92–1), traditionally bifrontotemporal. The advantage of unilateral placement is that there is less memory loss and confusion than with bilateral electrode placement (Horne et al. 1985, Weiner et al. 1986, Abrams 1982). The disadvantage of unilateral ECT is that it appears to be less effective when the dose of electricity given is close to seizure threshold (Sackeim et al. 1993), and the seizure

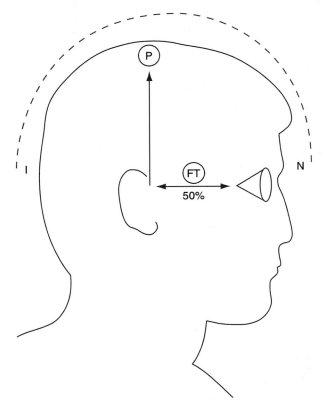

**Figure 92–1** *Positioning of stimulus electrodes with bilateral and right unilateral ECT. For the standard bifrontotemporal (bilateral) placement, the electrodes are placed in position FT (frontotemporal). The midpoint of the line connecting the external canthus and the tragus is determined on both sides of the head. The center of the electrode is positioned 1 inch above this point. In the US, stimulus electrodes are typically 2 inches in diameter, so the bottom of the electrode is adjacent to this point. For the commonly used d'Elia placement with right unilateral ECT, one electrode is in the FT position on the right side. The other electrode (P) is over parietal cortex and is positioned by determining the intersection between the line connecting the left and right tragus and the inion (I) and nasion (N). The center of this electrode is 1 inch below this intersection. (Source: American Psychiatric Association [2001] The Practice of Electroconvulsive Therapy: Recommendations for Treatment, Training and Privileging—A Task Force Report, 2nd ed. American Psychiatric Press, Washington DC.)*

*As potential but still experimental alternatives to traditional bifrontotemporal electrode placement, novel bifrontal and asymmetric placements are undergoing investigation as to whether they confer cognitive advantages by reducing electrical stimulation in left temporal areas while retaining therapeutic efficacy (Bailine et al. 2000). The bifrontal placement of Lawson and coworkers (1990) positions the center of each electrode approximately 5 cm above the lateral angle (external canthus) of each orbit, about 14 to 16 cm apart. The asymmetric (anterior bilateral) placement of Swartz (1994) positions the left-sided electrode above the left eye, with the lateral edge bordering the bony ridge between the forehead and the temple. The right-sided electrode is placed in an identical position to that used for the right-sided electrode in the traditional bifrontotemporal placement.*

threshold can vary more than 40-fold from individual to individual (Sackeim et al. 1987a, 1991). With bilateral placement, seizure threshold is less of a concern, and the degree and speed of response appears greater with (high dose) bilateral than unilateral ECT (Nobler et al. 1997, Sackeim et al. 2000b). Although bifrontotemporal placement has been more widely used, a limited number of studies suggest that bifrontal electrode placement may offer comparable treatment efficacy with fewer cognitive side effects (Weiner 1994). NIMH-supported research currently underway seeks to compare the efficacy and cognitive safety of standard bilateral (bifrontotemporal) electrode placement with high-dose right unilateral ECT and with bifrontal electrode placement. In short, electrode placement should be individualized based on the relative benefits and risks for a given patient (Abrams 1997b, 2000, Farah and McCall 1993). Individuals who are unresponsive to several adequately dosed unilateral treatments may benefit from a switch to bilateral electrode placement.

The initial dose of electricity should therefore be chosen to deliver a moderately suprathreshold stimulus. A dose that excessively exceeds the seizure threshold is likely to cause unnecessary memory difficulties and confusion (Abrams 1992, Sackeim et al. 1993). One method used to individualize the starting dose of electricity is to determine the initial seizure threshold using a titration method such as that described by Sackeim and colleagues (1987b) and then choose settings for unilateral ECT which are sufficiently above those required to elicit an adequate seizure. Previous recommendations for unilateral ECT dosing at 150% above initial seizure threshold have been revised upwards in light of recent data showing a continued dose–response relationship for unilateral ECT up to 5- to 12-times above seizure threshold (Sackeim et al. 2000b, McCall et al. 2000). Sackeim and associates (2000b) demonstrated an equivalent clinical response to bilateral and high-dose (500% above seizure threshold) right unilateral ECT, but with more severe and persistent retrograde and anterograde memory disturbance associated with bilateral electrode placement. For most patients, a reasonable balance between efficacy and cognitive toxicity can be achieved with right unilateral ECT beginning with a stimulus intensity 250% above seizure threshold. It must be kept in mind that the seizure threshold rises during a course of ECT (Sackeim et al. 1987a) and a dose that was adequately suprathreshold at the start of treatment may be inadequate by the end of the course. Stimulus parameters should be reevaluated if the patient does not continue to improve throughout the course of ECT.

A contemporary survey of ECT practices (Farah and McCall 1993) revealed that several methods for determining initial parameters are used in clinical practice. Some of them include adjusting dosage on the basis of age and sex, to compensate for the effects of these parameters on seizure threshold; others utilize a fixed set of parameters for individuals which does not take into account the range in variation of seizure threshold (Farah and McCall 1993, Abrams 2000). The main conceptual point is that dose of electricity relative to seizure threshold is an important variable (especially with unilateral electrode placement) and that optimum clinical results are most likely to be obtained when the stimulus intensity is significantly higher than seizure threshold (Sackeim et al. 1993, Weiner 1994).

From the start of the treatment procedure (see Table 92–3) EKG, heart rate, and blood pressure are monitored and oxygen saturation is measured via pulse oximetry. Pure oxygen by mask is typically administered after the induction of anesthesia and until the return of spontaneous respiration. Depending upon the preference of the treatment team, patients may or may not be premedicated with an anticholinergic agent. Atropine and glycopyrrolate are the agents most commonly used (Abrams 1997). The rationale for using these premedications is twofold. First, they reduce the bradycardia observed immediately after the delivery of the stimulus, and second, they dry secretions during anesthesia (Sommer et al. 1989). The decrease in heart rate initially observed during seizure induction is the result of increased vagal tone which occurs immediately after the stimulus (Elliot et al. 1982).

The patient is rendered unconscious with a short-acting general anesthetic. Methohexital 0.75 to 1.0 mg/kg given intravenously is the agent most commonly used (Folk et al. 2000). Other agents in use include thiopental, propofol, etomidate, and ketamine. The usual, but in this context undesired, elevation of seizure threshold associated with the use of barbiturate anesthetics such as methohexital or thiopental has fueled the search for alternative anesthetic agents (Swartz 1993, Weiner 1994). Thiopental may also be associated with an increased risk of postictal cardiac arrhythmias. Propofol attenuates the hypertension and tachycardia during the seizure (Elliot et al. 1982) but also decreases seizure duration (Boey and Lai 1990, Villalonga et al. 1993) with uncertainty regarding possible decreased efficacy of ECT (Swartz 1993, Nishihara and Saito 2002). In animal studies, ketamine lengthened seizure duration relative to animals administered ECS without anesthesia, but in human use may cause patients to hallucinate in the postoperative period (Lunn et al. 1981). Etomidate compares favorably with the barbiturates and may be a useful alternative for ECT anesthesia (Kovac and Pardo 1992); while repeated dosing of etomidate may suppress adrenal function, this is unlikely to be clinically significant when given for brief periods as in ECT (Kovac and Pardo 1992).

Once the patient is unconscious, a muscle relaxant is administered. Intravenous succinylcholine 0.5 to 1.0 mg/kg is almost always used for this purpose. The goal of the muscle relaxant is to dampen the tonic–clonic movements from the seizure and reduce the risk of musculoskeletal injury (Elliot et al. 1982, Lippmann et al. 1993, Weiner 1994). The *cuff technique* (Fink and Johnson 1982) may be applied to an ankle or forearm, preventing localized circulation of the muscle relaxant, thereby facilitating monitoring of the motor seizure duration. The degree of relaxation is somewhat dependent upon the preference of the practitioner; however, when there is a history of skeletal disease the paralysis should be nearly complete. The fasciculations induced by succinylcholine can cause myalgias which can be prevented by administration of a small dose of the nondepolarizing agent, curare, prior to dosing with the succinylcholine. When curare is used in this manner it is necessary to increase the succinylcholine dosage by approximately 25% to achieve the same level of muscle relaxation as previously.

When the patient is unconscious and relaxed, the stimulus is delivered, using the desired electrode placement. Initially, the jaw will clench as a result of direct electrical stimulation. The heart rate will slow and the patient will generally have tonic contraction of the extremities (Elliot et al. 1982). This initial period, which lasts anywhere from 2 to 5 seconds, is usually followed by a marked increase in blood pressure and heart rate (McCall 1993). This is secondary to a centrally mediated catecholamine surge (Elliot et al. 1982, Swartz 1993). The extremities change to tonic–clonic contractions, the intensity of which depends on the degree to which they have been modified by the muscle relaxant.

Excessive increases in heart rate and blood pressure can be reduced by a number of prophylactic agents (Elliot et al. 1982, Lippmann et al. 1993, McCall 1993, Weiner 1994). Esmolol is an ultrashort-acting beta-blocker with a half-life of approximately 9 minutes. Because of its receptor selectivity, it is usually more effective for controlling heart rate than blood pressure. However, it is often sufficient to keep the cardiovascular response within an acceptable range. Labetalol is another beta-blocker which is frequently used as an alternative to esmolol. Doses of esmolol in excess of 200 mg and labetalol doses > 20 mg may decrease seizure duration (McCall 1993). When the beta-blockers are sufficient to control the increase in heart rate, but not blood pressure, a calcium channel blocker such as nifedipine may be used (Abrams 1991). Alternatively, nitroglycerin, which is more specific for blood pressure, may be helpful. Caution must be taken when using these agents to avoid excessively decreasing blood pressure and heart rate, particularly in the context of subconvulsive stimulation (Decina et al. 1984); as noted earlier, anticholinergic premedication may be helpful in this regard.

During the treatment, seizure duration should be monitored via a one- or two-channel electroencephalogram (EEG), an integral component of modern ECT devices (Stephens et al. 1991). Combining motor movement timing with EEG monitoring yields the most reliable seizure duration determinations in the clinical setting (Lippmann et al. 1993). Although dose of electricity relative to seizure threshold is the important variable, in general, an adequate seizure is usually between 20 seconds and 2 minutes in duration. Seizures lasting over 3 minutes are considered prolonged. Should this occur the practitioner may attempt to terminate the seizure with an intravenous benzodiazepine. Diazepam given intravenously enters the brain within seconds and can terminate status epilepticus within 1 minute (Bauer and Elger 1994, Fink 1994b). Peak heart rate during ECT has been proposed as an index of seizure quality (Swartz 2000).

Although many practitioners continue to seek a minimum "therapeutic" seizure duration, for example 25 seconds, a growing body of evidence points to a more complex neurophysiological mediation of ECT response (Nobler et al. 1993, Krystal et al. 1993, Weiner 1994, Delva et al. 2000). Once the seizure terminates, the patient is continuously supported and monitored until breathing spontaneously and responsive to voice commands, with return of muscle strength. The patient's vital signs are monitored every 15 minutes until stable.

This process is repeated for an average of 6 to 12 sessions in the treatment of depression. In the US, ECT is usually performed three times per week, while in the UK and Europe twice-a-week schedule is more common. The available data suggest that the twice-a-week schedule produces an equivalent therapeutic response with fewer treatments, but the speed of clinical improvement is slower than the three times per week schedule (Lerer et al. 1995, Shapira et al. 2000). On the other hand, the more rapid therapeutic response to thrice weekly ECT is accompanied by greater cognitive adverse effects than those associated with the slower rate of treatments (Lerer et al. 1995, Shapira et al. 2000).

A small percentage of ECT practitioners utilize a treatment schedule known as *multiple monitored ECT*, or just *multiple ECT* (MECT), as today EEG and EKG monitoring capability is integral to all modern ECT devices. In this paradigm, multiple seizures are elicited per anesthesia session, resulting in a course of fewer sessions (but similar or increased number of seizures) than in standard ECT. In the recent New York area survey, only 15% of responding centers reported some use of MECT (Prudic et al. 2001). Although the intent of MECT was to speed clinical response, this potential advantage appears to be overshadowed by an increase in cognitive and cardiovascular adverse effects (Weiner 1994). Most of the literature on MECT is anecdotal and uncontrolled. Indeed, the seven published comparative studies on this approach include only a single randomized controlled trial (Roemer et al. 1990). In that study, depressed patients were randomly assigned to standard or "double-seizure" bilateral ECT. Although a more rapid reduction in depression scores occurred in the MECT group, by the end of the treatment course depression ratings in the two treatment groups were not significantly different. However, even though cognitive effects were rated only on the basis of chart notes, clinically significant confusion was reported for 10 of the 16 MECT patients, but only 2 of 13 patients receiving standard ECT (Roemer et al. 1990). While other retrospective studies and case reports are rife with methodological limitations, and in spite of the risk of observer bias, the literature is replete with unexpected and severe adverse effects associated with MECT, including instances of myocardial infarction and prolonged seizures and confusional states. Research on MECT appears to have ended. Weighing the knowledge of the potential benefits and risks of MECT, most professional societies now recommend against its use for the treatment of mental disorders (NIH/NIMH Consensus Conference (1985), American Psychiatric Association (2001)). Although the database is anecdotal, under limited, urgent conditions there may remain a role for MECT (up to two seizures per session) in the treatment of NMS or intractable seizures (American Psychiatric Association 2001).

Regardless of the treatment schedule, the rate of response will vary for each patient. Often, the patient's vegetative symptoms will respond before the patient feels subjectively improved. In the US, ECT devices are approved for marketing by the FDA as a Class III (most restricted medical device, having been "grandfathered" in based on their use prior to the 1976 medical device regulatory system). A proposed reclassification of ECT devices to the less restricted Class II category has been stalled since 1990, with opponents of ECT arguing against less restrictive regulation and many clinicians concerned about draft language limited the acceptable indication for ECT as major depression with melancholia. Indeed, some practitioners

---

**Clinical Vignette**

Mr. A, a 47-year-old married Asian engineer, presented with a 7-month history of depressed mood. The patient reported that he began to feel depressed after he made a "lateral move" at work to another department. In particular, his new job required that he do significantly more conflict resolution and he felt that his performance was below par. In addition, Mr. A's second child had just started college and he was very concerned about finances. At the time of presentation, the patient reported that his depressed mood was 7 on a scale of 1 to 10. Accompanying this low mood, he described middle insomnia nightly, anhedonia, decreased energy and concentration, diminished appetite with a 10 lb weight loss in the preceding 3 weeks, and passive suicidal ideation. There was no past psychiatric history prior to 7 months earlier, and no history of substance abuse or physical illness. Family history was positive for a poststroke depressive episode in father.

Treatment to date of the presenting episode consisted of three successive medication trials, each lasting 6 to 8 weeks: fluoxetine 20 mg/day, venlafaxine 300 mg/day, and bupropion 300 mg/day (added to ongoing venlafaxine). At presentation, Mr. A was taking bupropion 200 mg qAM and 100 mg qPM. ECT was recommended.

After a discussion of the potential advantages and drawbacks of ECT compared with other treatment options, Mr. A consented to a course of ECT. He expressed concern about possible memory problems related to ECT and the detrimental effect this would have on his work, and was relieved to hear that high-dose unilateral ECT has been shown to be effective with a low risk of cognitive dysfunction.

On the first treatment, a right unilateral d'Elia electrode placement was used. Seizure threshold was titrated to 40 mC after anesthesia was induced with methohexital 80 mg, and premedication with succinylcholine 60 mg and glycopyrrolate 0.2 mg. The stimulus parameters were increased to 192 mC for the next seven treatments, during which a remission of Mr. A's depressive symptoms were achieved. Subsequently, the patient was started on nortriptyline and achieved a steady-state therapeutic plasma level of 78 µg/mL. One month after completion of ECT, Mr. A returned to work and remained in his job. However, 2 months after the last ECT treatment, he relapsed back into depression. Olanzapine was added to his medication regimen for some ruminative thoughts. With worsening of depression, Mr. A then was given two additional ECT treatments within a week on an outpatient basis, with notable improvement. At that point, ECT was continued on a tapering schedule, reaching one treatment session monthly. Mr. A remains in remission, with no adverse effects, on monthly maintenance ECT.

---

have argued in favor of regulatory change to permit the marketing of more powerful ECT devices, such as those used internationally, capable of delivering an electrical stimulus greater than the present US limit under 600 millicoulombs (Abrams 2000). An estimated 5 to 10% of patients are unable to experience an adequate seizure with one popular current device (Krystal et al. 2000a, Sackeim et al. 2000b), although this figure can be reduced somewhat with the use of a narrower electrical pulse width and longer stimulus duration, as provided on the newest devices.

A typical example of the use of ECT in modern psychiatric practice is illustrated in the above clinical vignette.

## Adverse Effects

The potential adverse effects from ECT range from mild complications such as myalgias, to serious events such as fractured bones, to catastrophes such as death. In the era that predated anesthesia for this procedure, serious complications occurred in up to 40% of cases. At present, the risk of serious complication is about 1 in 1,000 patients. The risk of death is about 1 in 10,000 patients, which approximates the risk of general anesthesia for a minor surgical procedure (NIH/NIMH 1985) and is actually lower than the spontaneous death rate in the community (Abrams 1997a). The most detailed modern account of ECT-associated mortality is derived from the database in Texas, where all deaths occurring within 14 days of ECT must be reported to state authorities (Shiwach et al. 2001). In the first 5 years since the law's inception in 1993, only one death (of 30 reported), from laryngospasm on the day of treatment, could be clearly associated with the anesthestic procedure. A conservative interpretation of the death reports yielded a mortality rate of two to ten deaths per 100,000 treatments, confirming ECT's status as one of the safest procedures for which general anesthesia is employed (Shiwach et al. 2001). Of note, the two most common fatal occurrences in this naturalistic series, cardiac events and suicide, in no cases were established as caused by ECT.

Nonetheless, cardiac complications are the most frequent medical side effects associated with ECT. The arrhythmias range in severity from the common and benign sinus tachycardia to life threatening or fatal ventricular arrhythmias. The initial parasympathetically-mediated bradycardia during ECT—blocked by atropine or glycopyrrolate premedication—has been associated with clinically insignificant transient asystole in many patients (Burd and Kettle 1998) and at times has led to discontinuation of the treatment (Tang and Ungvari 2001a). However, ECT is not associated with persistent EKG changes or myocardial damage (Dec et al. 1985). The most common cardiovascular effect frequently observed is hypertension, occurring in 6% of one sample of geriatric ECT patients (Kujala et al. 2002). Related to the medically high-risk nature of many candidates for ECT, during most of its history convulsive therapy was frequently complicated by major cardiovascular morbidity in the medically ill (Gerring and Shields 1982) and the most common cause of death during ECT is from cardiac complications. Today, with careful pretreatment evaluation and consultation and the judicious use of prophylactic and therapeutic medications, including beta-blockers and calcium channel blockers, many arrhythmias, dangerous elevations of blood pressure, and other cardiovascular complications may be avoided, even in the medically high-risk patients (Zielinski et al. 1993, Rice et al. 1994, Roose et al. 1994). Indeed, 8 of the 10 cardiac deaths in the Texas series occurred between 2 days and 2 weeks after ECT, with none during treatment (Shiwach et al. 2001). Furthermore, depression per se is now recognized as an important risk factor for coronary heart disease as well as suicide (Rugulies 2002). Data regarding the effect of ECT on some cardiac parameters,

| Table 92–3 | Typical Electroconvulsive Therapy Schedule of Events |
|---|---|
| 12:00 AM | Patient begins NPO. |
| 7:45 AM | Patient is escorted to the ECT suite. |
| 7:50 AM | Nurse ascertains that patient has voided, has remained NPO, has dentures and jewelry removed, has clean and dry hair, and orders for ECT are completed properly. |
| 7:55 AM | Psychiatrist and anesthesiologist review medical chart and determine any change in medical or mental status or medications. |
| 8:00 AM | An intravenous line is placed; EKG, EEG, blood pressure, and oximetry monitoring are instituted; stimulus parameters are selected on the ECT device. |
| 8:02 AM | Sites of the ECT electrodes are prepared to reduce impedance. |
| 8:05 AM | Anticholinergic premedication with glycopyrrolate or atropine is given; other adjunctive medications are administered as needed. |
| 8:07 AM | Short-acting barbiturate anesthetic (e.g., methohexital or thiopental) is administered through IV; positive pressure respiratory support is instituted. |
| 8:08 AM | Loss of consciousness is ascertained (eyelash reflex); blood pressure cuff is inflated over a lower or upper extremity to block distribution of the muscle relaxant (succinylcholine), which is then administered through IV. |
| 8:09 AM | Fasciculations are noted in the cuffed extremity; a nerve stimulator may be used to ensure adequate muscle relaxation. |
| 8:10 AM | Electrodes are positioned, and integrity of the electrical circuit is checked; bite block or mouth guard is put in place; electrical stimulus is applied. |
| 8:11 AM | Seizure activity is monitored and duration timed for both motor and EEG manifestations; cardiac status is closely monitored; respiratory support is provided until patient is breathing spontaneously. |
| 8:12 AM | Vital signs are monitored frequently until return to baseline level. |
| 8:20 AM | When the patient is breathing spontaneously, is responsive to commands, and vital signs are stable, the patient is transferred by stretcher to a recovery room. |
| 8:25 AM | Patient is assessed for recovery of orientation; with continued stability of vital signs, the patient is discharged from recovery when reoriented and able to ambulate without assistance, usually 30–60 min following the treatment. |

for example vagally-mediated heart rate variability, which may be reduced in depression and pose a risk factor to heart disease, are still contradictory (Schultz et al. 1997, Nahshoni et al. 2001). While minor side effects, for example headache, are common in young people given ECT, cardiovascular complications are rare (Rey and Walter 1997).

Confusion and memory loss are also commonly occurring side effects. These adverse effects are the major factor limiting the use of ECT. Transient confusion occurs universally as a postictal event. Memory disturbance also occurs quite frequently (Calev 1994). In one typical naturalistic series of ECT-treated geriatric patients, impaired memory was the most common adverse effect (14%), followed by a 6% incidence of clinically significant confusion (Kujala et al.

2002). The extent and persistence of the confusion and memory impairment are highly variable—affecting between 0 and 100% of patients across 59 New York facilities (Prudic et al. 2001)—and sensitive to technical factors in ECT, such as electrode placement (Weiner et al. 1986, Sackeim et al. 1993) electrical dosage (Sackeim et al. 1993) stimulus wave form (Weiner et al. 1986) and frequency of treatments (Lerer et al. 1995). In general, during the acute course of ECT, both retrograde and anterograde memory are impaired to some degree (NIH/NIMH 1985, Calev 1994). Retrograde amnesia is generally felt to be more problematic, and until recently, conventional wisdom held that autobiographical memory was specifically disrupted by ECT. However, Lisanby and associates (2000) have demonstrated that in fact, following completion of a course of ECT, memory of impersonal events was more impaired; retrograde amnesia was seen only in patients treated with bilateral, not right unilateral electrode placement, and was not affected by electrical dosage or clinical response. A neurophysiological dissociation between the cognitive and therapeutic effects of ECT has been demonstrated (Sackeim et al. 2000a). Some patients can be shown to experience nonverbal memory impairment with right unilateral ECT, although it is not common for this to interfere with functioning. Learning ability is impaired by depression, but not ECT (Vakil et al. 2000); implicit memory, for example perceptual priming, is also unaffected by ECT. After the treatments end, the memory difficulties gradually resolve over the ensuing weeks to months (Lisanby et al. 2000). Some patients may have permanent spottiness in memory for events that occurred in the weeks to months before, during, and following the ECT course. Rarely, patients have complained of persistent memory difficulties severe enough to interfere with social and/or occupational functioning (NIH/NIMH 1985). However, the infrequency with which this occurs, and certain technical factors such as the lack of nondepressed pretreatment memory and other neuropsychiatric measures, (Coffey 1994) has made it difficult to study these individuals systematically. Subjective impressions of post-ECT memory deficits appear to correlate more closely with clinical outcome and mood state than with objective cognitive measures (Prudic et al. 2000). Although evidence to date points to only a transient and tolerable degree of cognitive impairment with continuation and maintenance ECT (Datto et al. 2001) as these treatment strategies continue to play an increasing role in the long-term treatment of mood disorders, more definitive research on their effects on memory will help guide clinicians. Several decades of appropriately controlled animal and human studies, supplemented in recent years by modern brain scanning techniques (Coffey 1994, Ende et al. 2000) and biochemical analysis of cerebrospinal fluid (CSF) constituents (Zachrisson et al. 2000) have demonstrated that ECT does not cause brain damage (Lippmann et al. 1985, Devanand et al. 1994).

Few formal studies of ECT effects on cognitive functioning in children and adolescents have been conducted in the past 50 years. The limited database in young people—generally with pastgeneration ECT methodology—shows transient confusion and decrements in visuomotor and intellectual performance in some patients, with no lasting deficits (Rey and Walter 1997). Preliminary long-term follow-up data, collected an average of 3.5 years after ECT in a small group of adolescents, found no difference in cognitive testing of these patients compared to controls, even in those individuals who had experienced acute memory problems after treatment (Cohen et al. 2000b).

Moreover, despite continuing negative perceptions of ECT among segments of the public—including many depressed patients lacking personal experience with the treatment (Pettinati et al. 1994)—adults and adolescents whose depression has been treated with ECT report favorable attitudes toward convulsive therapy (Freeman and Kendell 1980, Calev et al. 1991, Pettinati et al. 1994, Manning 1995, Taieb et al. 2001, Hartmann 2002). The majority of surveyed parents of adolescent recipients of ECT would support a physician's recommendation for additional ECT for their child in the future (Walter et al. 1999, Taieb et al. 2001). Patients' positive feelings regarding ECT—comparing it favorably with visits to the dentist (Freeman and Kendell 1980)—are present with both bilateral (Calev et al. 1991) and unilateral (Pettinati et al. 1994) electrode placement and are maintained at 6-month follow-up after completion of the treatment course (Calev et al. 1991, Pettinati et al. 1994).

## ECT–Drug Combinations and Interactions

As most patients referred for ECT already are taking psychotropic medications, many ECT–drug interactions result from the inadvertent or intentional continuation of preexisting medication regimens with the initiation of convulsive therapy. Community surveys indicate that fewer than half of patients have discontinued all previous psychotropic medications at the time of ECT (Prudic et al. 2000). Although the controlled database is sparse, substantial anecdotal and case series document possible changes in the efficacy or safety of ECT in the face of concurrent drug treatment of psychiatric or comorbid medical illness (Kellner et al. 1991, Fink 1994). In the face of a dearth of controlled data, expert opinion on the potential advantages and drawbacks of combining psychotropic medications with ECT is mixed and evolving. In the 11 years between the last two editions of the American Psychiatric Association Task Force Report, the 1990 recommendation that antidepressants be discontinued prior to starting ECT is undergoing reconsideration (American Psychiatric Association 2001), based on limited data suggesting possible augmentation of ECT's therapeutic effects with concomitant antidepressants (Royal College of Psychiatrists 1995). The heterocyclic antidepressants are generally thought of as promoting seizures, although they have also demonstrated anticonvulsant effects as well. The cardiovascular effects of the heterocyclics have been an area of concern when they are combined with ECT. However, on the whole there is little evidence that the two treatment modalities pose an excessive cardiac risk (Fink 1994). The only published controlled trial of the past decade on the subject was a Danish study comparing the TCA, imipramine, with the SSRI, paroxetine and placebo in combination with ECT in inpatients with severe major depression (Lauritzen et al. 1996); only patients free of EKG abnormalities were permitted to receive imipramine. Acute antidepressant response in the

ECT + imipramine group was superior to that in the other two groups, although paroxetine proved a more effective continuation treatment after completion of ECT (see further). Bernardo and colleagues (2000) have also specifically demonstrated the cardiovascular safety of combining tertiary amine tricyclics with ECT in physically healthy individuals. While more definitive research is underway, the American Psychiatric Association Task Force recommends that, particularly for patients with a history of treatment resistance, "concurrent treatment with an antidepressant medication and ECT should be considered" (American Psychiatric Association 2001).

The limited data on the newer antidepressants suggest that bupropion and the SSRIs beyond paroxetine also may be safely combined with ECT. Despite early concerns of prolonged seizures, the initial studies and most case reports combining fluoxetine with ECT have not found a significant effect on seizure duration (Fink 1994), at least one case of therapeutic lengthening of previously inadequate ECT seizure duration with the addition of concurrent fluoxetine has been described. Double-blind, single-dose administration of the SSRIs fluoxetine or citalopram shortly prior to ECT does not cause adverse effects or change in seizure duration compared to placebo (Papakostas et al. 2000). Initial case reports with bupropion suggest that it may lengthen seizure duration, perhaps related to its dopaminergic action, and caution is recommended, particularly when high doses of bupropion are continued during ECT (Rudorfer et al. 1991, American Psychiatric Association 2001). In one recent case, a single prolonged seizure was reported following the first ECT stimulation of a patient taking therapeutic doses of bupropion, lithium, and venlafaxine (Conway and Nelson 2001); while the exact cause cannot be determined with certainty, venlafaxine alone has been safely combined with ECT (Bernardo et al. 2000).

Although today primarily of historic interest, there remain patients who still take a member of the original class of antidepressants, the MAOIs. For many years, it was standard to recommend that clinicians avoid combining MAOIs with general anesthesia, due to reports of hyper- or hypotension or other serious adverse effects. Although the data are limited, however, several studies have successfully combined ECT with an MAOI without significant adverse effects. Thus, in most cases there is no need for a long washout period after MAOI discontinuation prior to introduction of ECT. However, no increase in efficacy was found with the combination (Kellner et al. 1991). Data are sparse with the newer, selective MAOIs, for example selegiline, but there are no reports of dangerous interactions with ECT (American Psychiatric Association 2001).

The combination of lithium and ECT has been a subject of debate (Rudorfer et al. 1987). There have been several case reports indicating that the combination of the two increases the risk of delirium or prolonged seizures (Rudorfer and Linnoila 1987) but this is not a universal finding (Jha et al. 1996). Conventional clinical practice is to discontinue lithium prior to ECT (American Psychiatric Association 2001, NIH/NIMH 1985) unless a specific indication for the combination shifts the benefit–risk ratio of combination treatment for a given patient (Rudorfer et al. 1987). For instance, patients receiving maintenance ECT who require ongoing lithium for mood stabilization may have one or two doses of medication withheld prior to each ECT session (American Psychiatric Association 2001).

Although not generally used for mood stabilization or antidepressant effect, the calcium channel blocker, nicardipine, was incidentally found to be associated with lower Hamilton depression rating scores when given throughout a course of ECT to nonpsychotically depressed patients in a placebo-controlled trial (Dubovsky et al. 2001); no differences in seizure length or adverse effects between the two groups were noted.

In contrast to lithium, the combination of neuroleptics or atypical antipsychotics and ECT has been reported to be safe and possibly to increase the efficacy of ECT in psychotic patients (Chanpattana and Chakrabhand 2001).

Benzodiazepines and antiepileptic drugs increase the seizure threshold and may decrease the efficacy of ECT (Pettinati et al. 1990, Jha and Stein 1996). Over the past dozen years, conventional practice has been to discontinue benzodiazepines or decrease them to the lowest possible dose prior to the start of ECT, unless there is a clinical contraindication (American Psychiatric Association 2001). If they cannot be discontinued, the bilateral electrode placement may be preferred because with that technique the dose of electricity relative to seizure threshold appears to be less important to a successful therapeutic outcome (Pettinati et al. 1990, Sackeim et al. 1993, Jha and Stein 1996). In some instances, however, it may prove necessary or desirable to continue benzodiazepines in the ECT patient, either to treat an underlying anxiety disorder or to calm fears related to the treatment situation. Low doses of the short-acting benzodiazepine lorazepam have been found in prospective research to lack significant effect on seizure threshold, although lorazepam dose did correlate with decreased EEG-monitored seizure duration during ECT (Boylan et al. 2000). Thus, where clinically necessary, modest daily doses of lorazepam or similarly short half-life benzodiazepine may be continued without interfering with ECT, provided dosing is withheld for 8 hours prior to each treatment (American Psychiatric Association 2001); administration of a benzodiazepine antagonist, such as flumazenil, has been considered for the benzodiazepine-dependent patient, but is not routine at this point. Similarly, usual doses of pre-ECT barbiturate anesthesia are unlikely to impact seizure threshold (Boylan et al. 2000). However, since it is typically difficult to gauge seizure "adequacy" beyond duration, it is considered prudent to discontinue anticonvulsants being used as mood stabilizers prior to instituting a course of ECT, or to withhold one or two doses before each maintenance ECT session (American Psychiatric Association 2001).

Conversely, medications that lower the seizure threshold (such as theophylline) and/or prolong seizure duration (such as caffeine) may, in excess, contribute to ECT toxicity, for example status epilepticus. Carefully titrated, however, such agents may be useful therapeutically in augmenting the actions of ECT, particularly during a course when seizure threshold has risen (Sackeim et al. 1987a,b) and seizure duration has shortened (Sackeim et al. 1987b, Young et al. 1991, Calev et al. 1993, Nobler and Sackeim 1993, Fink 1994a).

Medications to combat the acute cardiovascular effects of ECT, when necessary, have been discussed earlier. Efforts at pharmacological prevention or treatment of ECT-associated cognitive adverse effects have to date been disappointing (Krueger et al. 1992, Dubovsky et al. 2001). The revised American Psychiatric Association (2000) Practice Guidelines on the treatment of major depression identify the potential efficacy and safety implications of combinations of ECT and psychotropic medications as one of the most pressing areas for further research in convulsive therapy.

## Continuation and Maintenance Treatment

Among the unique features of ECT is the time-limited nature of its use in the treatment of acute episodes of illness. Following completion of an acute treatment course, ECT is generally terminated abruptly, coincident both with clinical response and, in many cases, impending inpatient discharge. It is now clearly established that left untreated after completion of ECT, at least half of patients will relapse, most within 6 months (American Psychiatric Association 2001, Sackeim et al. 2001a). A questionnaire survey in New York, without independent documentation, reported what may have been an optimistic relapse rate in the year after ECT of only about 20% (Prudic et al. 2001). Naturalistic follow-up of adolescents after ECT has shown a relapse rate of about 40% after 1 year (Cohen et al. 2000a). Risk factors for post-ECT relapse include the change in ECT patient samples over the past generation to a more medication-refractory population (Sackeim 1994) certain clinical features of the presenting illness including the presence of psychotic features (Meyers et al. 2001) or underlying dysthymia ("double depression"), and biological factors, most notably persistent cortisol hypersecretion and dexamethasone nonsuppression (Bourgon and Kellner 2000). Most contemporary authors adhere to the distinction between *continuation* treatment, over 6 months or so, to prevent relapse into the index episode, and *maintenance* treatment beyond that point, with the goal of avoiding recurrence, that is a new episode of illness. Nearly all published data on continuation and maintenance treatment have dealt with ECT administered for the treatment of depression.

## Continuation Pharmacotherapy

No longer novel, the use of continuation pharmacotherapy following completion of a course of ECT is now routine, occurring with >80% of patients in community surveys (Prudic et al. 2001). The strategy of introducing or continuing antidepressant medication following a course of ECT was endorsed by British controlled studies in the 1960s that showed a significant drop in 6-month relapse rate from 50% on placebo to 20% with continuation tricyclic or MAOI treatment (Seager and Bird 1962, Imlah et al. 1965, Kay et al. 1970). A decade later, two studies evaluated post-ECT pharmacotherapy in unipolar depressed patients. In one retrospective review lacking a placebo group, tricyclic or lithium therapy was found effective during 6 months' maintenance (Perry and Tsuang 1979). Another small trial (Coppen et al. 1981) used a placebo control and failed to find benefit from maintenance lithium until after the first 6 months post-ECT. However, subsequent naturalistic stud-

ies, both retrospective and prospective, documented a high relapse rate of 50 to 75% during the first 6 months following successful ECT despite clinician's choice continuation pharmacotherapy (Karlinsky and Shulman 1984, Currier et al. 1992) with the highest rate seen in patients who had received ECT for psychotic depression (Spiker et al. 1985, Aronson et al. 1987). Longer follow-up revealed continued occurrence of relapse in one prospective trial (Malcolm et al. 1991) such that nearly 75% of patients were rehospitalized within 2 years of the original ECT course.

Sackeim and colleagues (1990a, 1993) closely monitored two overlapping samples of ECT responders ($N = 58$ and 70). At least 50% of each group relapsed, most within 4 to 6 months post-ECT, despite (uncontrolled) continuation pharmacotherapy. Relapse was a function of the adequacy of the unsuccessful pharmacotherapy that had preceded the ECT trial, occurring in patients who had failed an adequate medication trial at a rate (64%) twice that of those who had not received a full antidepressant medication trial before ECT (Sackeim et al. 1990a). This effect was independent of the polarity of depressive illness or the presence of psychosis in the index episode. These results suggested that clinicians would best be advised to use for continuation purposes a class of antidepressant medication or combination treatment that is different from that which failed before ECT (Sackeim 1994). Fewer than half of patients on maintenance antidepressant medication (plus mood stabilizer or neuroleptic where clinically indicated) relapsed during 2-year follow-up post-ECT in another American retrospective study (Gagné et al. 2000); however, patients with the strongest history of previous medication nonresponse at that center were offered continuation and maintenance ECT in addition to medication (see later).

The stage was thus set for a definitive prospective trial to address these issues regarding optimal post-ECT pharmacotherapy for relapse prevention. With NIMH support, the first-ever placebo-controlled maintenance medication trial in the US for this indication was undertaken at three sites throughout most of the 1990s (Sackeim et al. 2001a). Following the achievement of remission from unipolar depression with an open course of bilateral or unilateral ECT, 84 medication-free patients were randomized to one of three treatment groups, stratified by history of medication resistance and psychotic symptoms. In addition to placebo, active double-blind treatment arms were the tricyclic antidepressant, nortriptyline (no longer a first-line treatment by the 1990s), alone or combined with lithium; tricyclic and lithium levels were used to assure therapeutic dosing throughout the trial. As expected, most (84%) patients receiving placebo after ECT relapsed during the 24-week trial, consistent with previous uncontrolled studies. Monotherapy with nortriptyline was somewhat more effective (60% relapse), but only reached trend significance. A statistically significant benefit over placebo was seen for combined lithium (at low therapeutic levels) and nortriptyline, which was associated with a 39.1% relapse rate during the trial. Eight of the 9 patients who relapsed while taking combined nortriptyline plus lithium did so during the first 5 weeks of the trial, while relapses in the placebo and nortriptyline-only groups continued throughout the 6 months of study. Across the treatment conditions, highest relapse rates were observed in patients with the highest post-ECT depression rating scores, those with a history of medication resistance, and in women. This study thus established without question the necessity of post-ECT continuation treatment, while refuting suggestions from earlier trials that tricyclic monotherapy was adequate for relapse prevention in the modern era. Combined nortriptyline and lithium, while superior to placebo or to the tricyclic alone, nonetheless prevented relapse in only 6 of every 10 patients.

Combined antipsychotic and antidepressant medications, the pharmacotherapy option of choice in the acute treatment of psychotic depression, are also used frequently as continuation treatment after completion of an ECT course in such individuals (Gagné et al. 2000). In a prospective 26-week trial assessing the value of such a combination in preventing relapse, Meyers and associates (2001) randomized older (nearly all > 60 years of age) patients whose delusional depression had responded to ECT to one of two active treatment groups: either a tricyclic antidepressant alone (nortriptyline, the same as used by Sackeim et al. 2001a) or nortriptyline plus a conventional high-potency neuroleptic, perphenazine. One quarter of the 28 evaluable patients had relapsed at the 6 months follow-up. Contrary to expectation, combination pharmacotherapy was not superior to antidepressant monotherapy, and, in fact, was associated with a nonsignificantly greater frequency of relapse. Furthermore, the combined-medication group experienced more adverse effects, including falls (even though the nortriptyline dose was adjusted downward in the group to account for pharmacokinetic interactions with perphenazine) and typical neuroleptic-associated side effects, including extrapyramidal symptoms and even tardive dyskinesia, despite the relatively brief neuroleptic exposure (Meyers et al. 2001).

Additional research is necessary to develop even more effective strategies to prevent relapse after completion of ECT. Such approaches could include the use of newer antidepressants and/or mood stabilizers, or atypical antipsychotics, and the introduction of medication (other than lithium) during an ECT course to reduce the latency of pharmacotherapy response once ECT is completed (Sackeim et al. 2001). One trial that did utilize antidepressants concurrently with ECT led to an initial favorable foray into the use of an SSRI post-ECT, with paroxetine more effective than imipramine at preventing relapse in geriatric patients (prevalence of psychotic depression not stated); at 6-month follow-up, relapse rates were 10% for paroxetine, 30% for imipramine, and 65% for placebo (Lauritzen et al. 1996). In that trial, only patients without cardiac disease received the tricyclic. On the other hand, introduction of fluoxetine after completion of successful ECT was associated with a 28% relapse rate over 3 months in a small Israeli study (Grunhaus et al. 2001); the addition of double-blind melatonin to the continuation regimen did not affect the outcome.

## Continuation/Maintenance ECT

Given both the logic of continuing the same treatment that achieved acute improvement to prevent relapse or recurrence and the historical reality that ECT achieved widespread use more than a decade prior to the introduction of effective psychotropic medications, it is not surprising that much of the literature on the use of follow-up ECT

after completion of an acute course is decades old (Monroe 1991).

However, the chief concern in the earlier eras was the issue of avoiding new episodes of illness. The newer concept of continuation treatment after a successful series of ECT treatments has led to modern case series in patients with a known history of relapse on medications. Decina and associates (1987) offered a detailed protocol of outpatient continuation ECT at progressively longer intervals over several months. This was adapted in one prospective series (Clarke et al. 1989) which avoided a prime confounding factor in most continuation ECT studies, that of concomitant medication (Gagné et al. 2000). In that 5-month series of 27 depressed patients, the rehospitalization rate was 8% in patients who completed an outpatient ECT trial versus 47% in those who did not, a significant difference (Clarke et al. 1989).

In another contemporary series (Petrides et al. 1994) a third of 21 patients with mood disorder treated with continuation ECT required rehospitalization within 1 year of response to a full course of inpatient ECT. Of particular interest were the results in patients with delusional depression, a disorder previously associated with a 95% 1-year relapse rate during post-ECT pharmacological treatment at the same institution (Aronson et al. 1987). In contrast, with the introduction of continuation ECT, the comparable relapse rate in psychotic depressives fell to 42% (Petrides et al. 1994). Marked drops in rate of rehospitalization during extended follow-up periods of 18 months (Thornton et al. 1990) to 4 years (Schwarz et al. 1995) are reported following maintenance ECT in patients with recurrent depression. One of the longest follow-up periods ever monitored for maintenance ECT (mean of > 5 years) was reported by Gagné and associates (2000) in a retrospective, case-controlled study, though only one of 29 patients was medication free, and a number of the others were on multiple medications throughout the course of maintenance. Compared to a matched group of pharmacotherapy-only post-ECT continuation treatment patients, the combination maintenance ECT + medication patients had higher cumulative survival rates at 2 and 5 years (93 and 73% for ECT versus 52 and 18% for medication), as well as a longer mean survival time (6.9 versus 2.7 years) (Gagné et al. 2000).

By the mid-1980s, ECT practitioners in one survey (Kramer 1987) reported treating a median of three patients per year with some form of continuation or maintenance ECT. As the use of ECT in outpatient settings increases, in all likelihood so will the application of continuation ECT, now up to one in six patients in the New York City area (Grunhaus et al. 1990, Jaffe et al. 1990, Stephens et al. 1993, Sackeim 1994, Prudic et al. 2001, Fox 2001). Although the optimal methodology for this extension of the traditional ECT course—including electrode placement, frequency, and duration of treatment—is yet to be determined (Scott et al. 1991) it has become the subject of the ongoing NIMH-supported four-site CORE trial (O'Connor et al. 2001). Following an acute course of generally successful bilateral ECT (see earlier), patients in the CORE trial are being randomized for the next 6 months to either a weekly to monthly maintenance ECT trial or to an active control pharmacotherapy condition, consisting of the most effective post-ECT medication regimen (combined nortriptyline plus lithium) identified by Sackeim et al. (2001a). Moreover, additional data are required on the risk of cognitive and other adverse effects of continuation and maintenance ECT, and the best means of minimizing untoward effects of this potentially valuable intervention (Fox 2001). In the meantime, there is general agreement that new written informed consent, beyond that obtained for the acute series of treatments, must be secured for continuation/maintenance ECT. In the event of prolonged maintenance ECT, the American Psychiatric Association (2001) Task Force recommends that the informed consent process be repeated every 6 months.

## Theories of Mechanisms of Therapeutic Action

### General Considerations

Despite the early recognition of the essential role of generalized seizure activity in producing the therapeutic effects of convulsive therapy, the exact mechanisms of action of ECT have remained elusive. There are several reasons for this. First, mechanistic research in ECT is difficult to perform, (Rudorfer 1994, Potter 1994) given the myriad of possible confounding variables, including diagnostic heterogeneity, concomitant medications, treatment parameters and severity of patient illness. Study of the acute treatment process, in particular, entails the challenge of accounting for the many physiological changes induced by general anesthesia, muscle relaxation, the evoked seizure, and the subsequent postictal state. Moreover, many of the tools required to investigate human brain function did not exist during most of the life span of ECT. It has proven easier to find changes in various physiological and biochemical processes associated with convulsive therapy than to prove a casual relation with efficacy (Nutt et al. 1989). Ironically, the very high response rate to ECT in some clinical studies removed the opportunity to correlate any biological findings with treatment outcomes (Krahn et al. 2000). Animal studies are proving helpful in understanding the mechanisms of ECT's therapeutic and adverse effects (Fochtmann 1994), but interpretations of preclinical electroconvulsive shock (ECS) are of necessity limited by the species differences between animals, generally rodents, and human patients, as well as the lack of adequate illness models in most such investigations. In one promising line of investigation, ECS shared with antidepressant drugs an ability to restore responsivity to reward that was lost in a chronic mild stress model of depression in rats and mice; interestingly, the response to ECS took only 1 week, versus 3 to 5 weeks for medications, paralleling clinical results in human patients (Willner 1997). In the following text, we review the primary areas of hypothesized mechanisms of ECT's therapeutic action—the neuropsychological, neurophysiological, endocrine, and biochemical—with an emphasis on areas of promising investigation.

### Neuropsychological Theories

Early theories related the efficacy of ECT to the harsh physical and psychological conditions of 1940s-era treatment. Psychodynamic interpretations focused on themes of punishment, fear, and pain. Neuropsychological deficits, including confusion and amnesia, which are secondary to the unmodified seizure and accompanying hypoxia, were also invoked as therapeutic correlates. These notions were casualties of the advances in ECT technique, described in detail later. Thus, the introduction of general anesthesia, muscle relaxation, and oxygenation eliminated many of the more traumatic and fearful aspects of treatment. The use of sham ECT procedures in double-blind clinical trials controlled for nonspecific psychological aspects of the treatment, and removed them from consideration as the agents of therapeutic change. Finally, the placement of stimulating electrodes over one cerebral hemisphere (unilateral ECT) clearly demonstrated the independence of therapeutic actions from cognitive adverse effects, as many patients show complete therapeutic response to unilateral ECT with little demonstrable loss of memory (Horne et al. 1985). Thus, theories ascribing the efficacy of ECT to neuropsychological deficits are no longer regarded as credible.

### Neurophysiological/Structural Theories

ECT results in a change in brain physiology, including transiently increased permeability of the blood–brain barrier. Recent work has centered on ECT-associated modification of brain electrical activity and regional cerebral blood flow. It has long been recognized that seizure threshold rises throughout a course of ECT (Sackeim et al. 1987a). Support for this phenomenon as a therapeutic mechanism is provided by its correlation with clinical response in both depression (Sackeim et al. 1987b) and mania (Mukherjee 1989) and by the latency of its appearance. This is consistent with preclinical studies in which chronic ECS, but not a single session, produces an anticonvulsant effect (Post et al. 1986). Other preclinical data have demonstrated production of a small anticonvulsant protein with opiate-like properties in the CSF of animals following repeated ECS (Isaac and Swanger 1983, Tortella and Long 1985) as well as GABAergic effects of ECS (Fochtmann 1994). The antimanic and mood-stabilizing clinical efficacy of anticonvulsant drugs, clearly established over the past 20 years, gives new currency to an anticonvulsant mechanism of ECT's therapeutic action, particularly in mood disorders (Post 1990). A related issue is the occurrence of postictal EEG suppression after each ECT session, which appears to correlate with clinical improvement (Nobler et al. 1993). Further investigation of the implications of ECT-associated EEG changes is underway (Krystal et al. 1993, 1998). For example, Krystal and associates (2000b) have developed an ictal EEG model capable of retrospectively distinguishing therapeutically effective versus ineffective seizures during ECT, although the potential clinical utility of this approach is unclear, pending further investigation (Nobler et al. 2000). While some EEG measures, such as intensity of prefrontal seizure intensity during treatment, seem to relate to clinical efficacy of ECT, others, including degree of bilateral generalization of seizure expression, do not (Luber et al. 2000).

Although cerebral blood flow (CBF) is often reduced in untreated depression (Sackeim and Prohovnik 1993) particularly in frontal regions, the effects of ECT on this measure have been inconsistent to date (Milo et al. 2001). Nobler and coworkers (2000) found successful ECT results in further generalized and regional (primarily frontal) CBF decreases, both in depression and mania. The extent of CBF decline was correlated with degree of clinical improvement, with the CBF changes localized to the side of electrode placement with unilateral ECT (Nobler et al. 1994). Other investigators have reported increased CBF in several brain regions in ECT responders (Bonne et al. 1996). Seeking to resolve this issue, Milo and associates (2001) compared rCBF in 15 patients before and after ECT, as well as 11 healthy volunteers. In the five patients showing excellent clinical response to ECT, following treatment there was both an increase in the initially reduced perfusion in frontal regions and a decrease in blood flow in several hyperperfused areas. While demographic differences between patients and controls confounded interpretation of these findings, they were consistent with a return toward normal rCBF associated with response to ECT (Milo et al. 2001).

Similarly, there are still inconclusive data pointing to a reduction in regional brain glucose utilization following ECS or ECT (Ackermann et al. 1986, Yatham et al. 2000, Nobler et al. 2001). Although still preliminary, positron emission tomography (PET) studies in small patient samples have shown variable decreases in glucose metabolism after ECT, particularly in frontal, prefrontal, and parietal cortexes (Yatham et al. 2000, Nobler et al. 2001, Henry et al. 2001). In at least one trial, changes in frontal glucose metabolism correlated with decrements in depression ratings with ECT (Henry et al. 2001). Moreover, relative increases in glucose metabolism in brain regions with dopaminergic innervation may relate to putative effects of ECT on this catecholamine neurotransmitter (see further) (Henry et al. 2001). Other brain imaging studies have addressed possible toxicity of ECT. For example, the lack of a decrease in the hippocampal $N$-acetylaspartate signal after ECT suggests that any ECT-associated memory impairment is not due to cell death in this brain structure (Ende et al. 2000).

## Neurotransmitter/Biochemical Theories

Discerning the therapeutic "signal" from the "noise" created by the plethora of biochemical changes that accompany ECT is daunting (Nutt et al. 1989, Glue et al. 1990, Rudorfer 1994). Advances in methodology in both animal and human studies have been applied to this task in recent years, yielding a number of provisional clues to the mechanisms of action of ECT. This area has been comprehensively reviewed (Lerer and Shapira 1986, Lerer 1987, Fochtmann 1994, Mann and Kapur 1994, Mann 1998). Several areas of ongoing study are of particular clinical relevance.

Both the similarities and differences between the biochemical effects of ECT and those of antidepressant medications are instructive (Rudorfer et al. 1988). Thus, ECS in a rat model produces the familiar beta-receptor down regulation (Kellar et al. 1981a) associated with antidepressant medications, with a time course that roughly coincides with the clinical effects of ECT in patients. The down regulation is complete in about a week, sustained during ongoing treatment, reverses about a week after withdrawal of ECS, but remains unchanged with sufficiently intensive maintenance ECS (Francis and Fochtmann 1993). Pre- and postsynaptic alpha-2-receptors are also down regulated by chronic ECS (Heal et al. 1991, Fochtmann 1994). For

instance, a clonidine pharmacologic probe has been used to demonstrate a time-dependent alpha-2-receptor down regulation in rat brain following repeated, but not single, ECS; this receptor effect was sustained with a maintenance ECS schedule (Andrade and Sudha 2000). However, translation of these noradrenergic findings to the clinical situation remains suggestive but unproven. Plasma norepinephrine (NE) is increased about threefold acutely at each ECT session (Cooper et al. 1985, Khan et al. 1985, Mann et al. 1990a, Weinger et al. 1991). However, by the completion of an ECT course, there is little change in plasma NE or CSF and urinary noradrenergic measures (Rudorfer et al. 1988, Rudorfer et al. in press) in contrast to the effects of antidepressant medications. An increase in plasma biopterin after successful ECT has been suggested as the driving force behind accompanying increases in synthesis of amino acids, especially tyrosine, driving catecholaminergic function (Hoekstra et al. 2001).

The effects of ECT on the serotonergic system are also unclear. Preclinical data have long suggested enhanced responsivity of serotonin-mediated behaviors after repeated ECS, and increased density of 5-hydronytryptamine (5-HT$_2$) receptors. This is opposite to the 5-HT$_2$ receptor down regulation obtained with antidepressant medications (Kellar et al. 1981b, Fochtmann 1994). More recent data suggest that there is no alteration in presynaptic functioning of serotonergic neurons with chronic ECS (Blier and Bouchard 1992). In humans, although a course of ECT leads to increased CSF levels of the primary metabolite of serotonin in most patients (Rudorfer et al. 1991, Mann and Kapur 1994, Rudorfer et al. in press) which is opposite to the effect of chronic antidepressants, no consistent change in response to a serotonergic agonist challenge (Manji et al. 1992) or in platelet imipramine binding sites (Langer et al. 1986, Wägner et al. 1987) accompanies a series of treatments. Furthermore, in contrast to the transient reemergence of depressive symptoms to a tryptophan depletion challenge in patients successfully treated with serotonergic antidepressant medications, no such effect was observed in a small group of newly responsive ECT patients, suggesting that maintenance of ECT-induced improvement did not depend on the availability of presynaptic serotonin (Cassidy et al. 1997). Dutch investigators have also reported that initially low plasma tryptophan levels rose in responders to ECT (Hoekstra et al. 2001).

More robust is a significant dopaminergic effect of ECS and ECT. This is reflected preclinically in acute elevation in brain content of dopamine with each ECS (Glue et al. 1990, Zis et al. 1991) increased D$_1$ receptors in regions of rat brain (Fochtmann et al. 1989) and enhanced dopamine-mediated behaviors (Fochtmann 1994). Although dopamine measures are little affected by most antidepressant treatments, repeated ECT is associated with a significant elevation in CSF concentrations of homovanillic acid (HVA), the main metabolite of dopamine (Rudorfer et al. in press). In delusionally depressed geriatric patients, there was a trend for successful treatment with ECT, but not with psychotropic drugs, to be associated with an increase in initially diminished levels of dopamine beta-hydroxylase, which catalyzes the conversion of dopamine to norepinephrine (Meyers et al. 1999). There may be a strong clinical correlation to these findings, as dopaminergic mechanisms have been invoked as part of the pathophysiology of a number of the leading indications for ECT, including delusional depression, mania, and Parkinson's disease. Thus, region-specific increases in dopaminergic activity following ECT could be tied to a variety of therapeutic actions (Glue et al. 1990, Rudorfer et al. in press).

Additional preclinical findings of potential clinical relevance are represented by increased opioid and gamma-aminobutyric acid (GABA) activity, correlating with the anticonvulsant effect of ECT (Tortella et al. 1989, Nakajima et al. 1989, Ferraro et al. 1990) and enhanced cholinergic activity, which may relate to the cognitive adverse effects of convulsive therapy (Lerer 1984, Fochtmann 1994). Continuing advances in research methodology, for example PET scans utilizing ligands for specific receptor subtypes, (Rudorfer 1994) may help define further the specific biochemical mechanisms of therapeutic action among these many possibilities.

## Neuromodulator/Endocrine Theories

Although the endocrine effects of ECT are legion, most of the observed changes can be accounted for by the nonspecific effects of stress or the seizure per se and are not associated with the therapeutic effects of ECT. Most studied is the acute treatment situation. Within minutes of the ECT seizure, there are increases in plasma levels of prolactin, adrenocorticotropic hormone (ACTH), cortisol, oxytocin, vasopressin, beta-endorphin, and, less consistently, growth hormone (Whalley et al. 1982, Apëria et al. 1984, Abrams and Swartz 1985, Linnoila et al. 1984, Devanand et al. 1989, Papakostas et al. 1990, Kronfol et al. 1991, Weinger et al. 1991, Young et al. 1991, Bernardo et al. 1993).

Among these hormones, prolactin has been studied most intensively, being released acutely with each session of ECT and peaking at 15 to 30 minutes postseizure (Whalley et al. 1982, Apëria et al. 1985, Papakostas et al. 1990, Swartz 2000). This effect is greater with bilateral than with unilateral ECT in some studies (Papakostas et al. 1984) but not others (Kronfol et al. 1991). Attempting to definitively resolve this issue, McCall and associates (1996) controlled for stimulus intensity relative to seizure threshold and did, in fact, confirm the greater increase in prolactin levels with bilateral electrode placement. The absolute levels and pattern of response to prolactin after a session of ECT are not influenced by a single dose of the SSRI, citalopram (Papakostas et al. 2000). During a series of ECT, the acute prolactin response often attenuates over the course (Deakin et al. 1983, Apëria et al. 1985, Abrams and Swartz 1985, Swartz 1985). A number of studies have sought to characterize the kinetics of the prolactin response to ECT (McGuire et al. 1989, Swartz 2000) and to control for some of the myriad of confounding variables influencing this stress-sensitive hormone, which is under multiple neurotransmitter control (Swartz et al. 1988). Despite the heuristic appeal of suggestions that increased postsynaptic dopamine activity developing during a course of ECT might be responsible for inhibition of the prolactin surge late in the treatment series (Apëria et al. 1985, Abrams and Swartz 1985), the data related to both the mechanisms of the prolactin response to ECT and its correlation with treatment outcome remain inconclusive (Abrams and Swartz 1985, Deakin et al. 1983, Swartz et al. 1988, McGuire et al. 1989).

A more promising area of endocrine inquiry into ECT mechanisms may be the thyroid axis. Most investigators have reported an increase in TSH acutely following ECT, with a peak at 30 minutes (Apëria et al. 1985, Papakostas et al. 1990). Reduction in TSH output at the last treatment compared to the first correlates with the expected decline in seizure length during a course of ECT, but not with clinical outcome (Scott 1989). On a preclinical level, rat brain concentrations of thyrotropin-releasing hormone (TRH), a behaviorally active peptide, is increased after ECS (Kubek et al. 1989). A single study found no alteration in CSF concentrations of TRH in depressed patients following a course of ECT (Kirkegaard and Faber 1998, Kirkegaard et al. 1979). Independent of these hypothalamic/pituitary findings, peripheral levels of free T4 (which are normal to high at depressed baseline) decline by 10 to 20%, while remaining within or entering the normal range, during a course of ECT (Kirkegaard and Faber 1986, 1998, Scott et al. 1990). Joffe and Sokolov (1994) have noted that T4 may affect brain function and, thus, the reduction in circulating T4 levels with ECT may be as important to ECT's antidepressant action as changes higher up the thyroid axis. Of clinical significance is a recent study by Stern and associates (1993) who suggest that the addition of triiodothyronine (T3) to ECT enhances the antidepressant response, while also reducing cognitive adverse effects.

The acute increase in oxytocin-associated neurophysine during ECT is worth noting as, unlike many other transient endocrine effects, in some studies its magnitude has correlated with clinical response (Scott et al. 1986, 1991). This hormonal change reflects the intensity of the ECT stimulation of relevant parts of the brain necessary for a therapeutic effect (Riddle et al. 1993). On the other hand, the pattern of increase of beta-endorphin at each treatment is inconsistent (Young et al. 1991) with a long-term decrease in CSF levels of this polypeptide late in the course of ECT (Nemeroff et al. 1991). Similarly, corticotrophin-releasing hormone (CRH) concentrations in CSF are unchanged (Rudorfer et al. 1991) or decline significantly (Nemeroff et al. 1991) after completion of at least most of the course of ECT. In contrast, CSF somatostatin, which has been reported to decrease in untreated depression, increases significantly over a course of ECT (Nemeroff et al. 1991, Mathé et al. 1996). CSF levels of other peptides, including endothelin, neurokinin A, and neuropeptide Y also rise after completion of a course of ECT (Mathé et al. 1996), but the dearth of clinical nonresponders in that study did not permit determination of relations with outcome. Similar findings have been reported in parallel ECS studies in rat brains, but may have been confounded by the effects of the seizure activity per se (Mathé et al. 1996). In a human treatment study, the additional confounding factors of mood change and resulting normalization of circadian rhythms complicate interpretation of a decrease in daily (mainly daytime) excretion of the main urinary metabolite of melatonin after successful ECT (Krahn et al. 2000).

Sprouting of the mossy fiber pathway in hippocampus of animals with repeated ECS and increased hippocampal choline signal in humans after ECT are prompting study of neurotrophic factors in the pathophysiology of depression and the mechanisms of action of ECT and antidepressant drugs (Ende et al. 2000).

## Treatment Failure

Given the still widespread view of ECT as a treatment of last resort, it is not surprising that failure to respond to ECT is often regarded as synonymous with "hopeless case." In fact, most patients have other, if less attractive, treatment alternatives available at the time ECT is initially selected, a fact which can be called upon in the event that ECT is not successful.

The total population of patients who are considered ECT treatment failures can be divided into three categories: true nonresponders; relative nonresponders for whom ECT can yet be made to work; and individuals for whom, upon closer inspection and examination, ECT was not the right treatment choice. Thus, the first approach to the ECT-resistant patient is to assure that an appropriately intensive trial of convulsive therapy has been attempted. Then reassessment, removal of any obstacles to treatment responsivity, and, in most cases, entry into a treatment-resistant depression algorithm are indicated.

## Adequacy of ECT Trial

A course of 8 to 12 bilateral ECT treatments should be completed before any patient is declared ECT resistant. Patients who fail to respond to several treatments with unilateral electrode placement should be switched to bilateral ECT and offered an opportunity to respond to a full trial of that modality (Delva et al. 2001). The treatment history of the ECT-refractory patient should be reviewed to ensure that seizures were generalized and of adequate duration, and that in the case of unilateral electrode placement, stimulus intensity was sufficiently above seizure threshold. Some patients who are still resistant may respond to an unusually intensive ECT trial. For instance, 79% of the medication-resistant patients who had failed to respond to a standard course of ECT in the Prudic and coworkers' study (1990) improved during a second trial of bilateral ECT at high electrical intensity (Sackeim 1994). Some resistant patients may require additional ECT sessions in order to respond (Sackeim et al. 1990b). Adjunctive treatment, for example intravenous caffeine to prolong induced seizures of inadequate duration, may be considered, although the popularity of this approach has waned in recent years in the absence of definitive evidence of its value in the refractory patient. As noted, despite their frequent empirical use controlled studies of other ECT-medication (e.g. antidepressant) combinations are only now underway (Sackeim 1994).

## Reevaluation

Even in carefully selected patients, lack of response to a course of ECT may occur in 10 to 30% of individuals (NIH/NIMH 1985). Nonetheless, this degree of refractoriness should trigger a reassessment of the patient, with confirmation of the original diagnosis. The additional information learned during a hospitalization may enable a more accurate assessment of the chronicity of illness, presence of medical disease, degree of mood congruence of symptoms, vegetative functioning, mood reactivity, Axis II pathology, alcohol or other substance abuse, and outstanding psychosocial issues than was available on admission. Such data may both help explain the lack of response to ECT and open avenues to further evaluation or treatment efforts.

## Alternative Pharmacotherapy Options

Despite the prior history of medication nonresponse in most ECT candidates, the majority of ECT nonresponders will go on to successful treatment with single or combination drug treatment (Sackeim 1994). A careful review of past pharmacotherapy efforts is essential to avoid repeating previous failures and to identify promising untried approaches. While in many cases this will entail antidepressant potentiation strategies, for example with lithium, or creative combinations, for example a tricyclic antidepressant plus an MAOI or SSRI or neuroleptic, often an opportunity for monotherapy will be identified (Sackeim et al. 1990). For instance, it is increasingly common that patients are referred for ECT from the community following two or three unsuccessful trials of SSRIs or other newer antidepressants (Sackeim 1994). Should ECT fail in such individuals, a trial of a tricyclic antidepressant or MAOI alone, then potentiated with lithium if necessary, generally is indicated.

This approach was deemed successful in an Israeli report (Shapira et al. 1988) of 12 ECT nonresponders, most with a prior history of tricyclic nonresponse. All 12 went on to respond to tricyclic treatment (all but two with clomipramine) following the unsuccessful ECT trial, including three potentiated with lithium and one with lithium plus haloperidol combined with clomipramine (Shapira et al. 1988). Sackeim and associates (1990) likewise were able to effect clinical response in a mostly antidepressant, as well as ECT-resistant sample of 19 research patients. Aside from two patients who were rediagnosed and treated accordingly, all but three patients showed response to either an additional course of high-dose bilateral ECT ($N = 8$) or pharmacotherapy with a variety of antidepressants alone ($N = 2$) or combined with lithium ($N = 1$) or a neuroleptic ($N = 3$). Other investigators, however, report less success with pharmacotherapy in ECT nonresponders (Zimmerman et al. 1990). In sum, experience to date suggests that with careful attention to diagnosis and assurance of adequacy of both ECT and pharmacotherapy, the cumulative response rate of ECT-resistant patients can be well worth the effort. As in many of the topics discussed in this chapter, further controlled research is necessary (Rudorfer and Lebowitz 1999).

## Novel Somatic Treatments

Coincident with the considerable advances in clinical research aimed at optimizing the use of ECT, the past decade has also witnessed renewed interest in the development of new somatic, nonpharmacologic interventions for mental disorders, particularly depression. Ongoing research supports the antidepressant efficacy of repetitive transcranial magnetic stimulation (rTMS) (Holtzheimer et al. 2001) and possibly, vagus nerve stimulation (Sackeim et al. 2001b). These and other related interventions under study stimulate the brain in manners less direct but more focused than does ECT. Should additional research establish an acceptable benefit–risk ratio for these or related new somatic interventions, they may enter treatment algorithms as options for ECT nonresponders or even as alternatives to ECT. The potential role of new somatic therapies with respect to ECT is specifically under study in the case of rTMS. In contrast to the application of an electrical stimulus to the scalp, as in

ECT, a more precisely localized electrical current can be produced within the brain by pulsing a magnetic wave (generated through a coil on the head), which passes undistorted through the skull. A train of TMS pulses, delivered to the left prefrontal cortex repeatedly but at a subconvulsive rate up to 20 minutes/day to an awake and alert patient, has demonstrated antidepressant efficacy in several small open and sham-controlled trials. To date, antidepressant effects have been relatively modest, and few patients have been medication free or followed systematically beyond a 1- or 2-week rTMS treatment trial. Encouraging further research is the apparent safety of this noninvasive procedure, which does not require anesthesia and has rarely been associated with adverse effects beyond mild headache noise-related discomfort. Although controlled trials to date have been small and not entirely consistent, recently five meta-analyses have confirmed the superior antidepressant efficacy of several weeks' treatment with high-frequency TMS over the left prefrontal area compared to a sham condition. For example, based on a review of 23 such published trials, Burt and colleagues (2002) calculated a combined effect size for rTMS of 0.67 (largest in TMS versus ECT rather than sham procedure studies), consistent with a moderate to large antidepressant effect for rTMS. The threshold for TMS clinical efficacy appears to be 2 weeks of treatment.

Of particular interest are several prospective studies where depressed patients for whom ECT is clinically indicated have been randomized to treatment with either ECT or rTMS. In a mixed inpatient/outpatient sample of 40 subjects with major depression who continued existing medication regimens, Grunhaus and coworkers (2000) found ECT (initially unilateral, switched to bilateral in nonresponders) to be superior to rTMS (up to 4 weeks) in patients with psychotic depression, but the two treatments were similarly effective in nondelusional depression. After replicating this finding in a larger sample, this Israeli group followed 41 patients who had responded to either ECT or rTMS while they received continuation clinician's choice of open-label pharmacotherapy (antidepressants, in several patients combined with an antipsychotic or mood stabilizer). During 6-month follow-up, the relapse rate was low (20%) and did not differ in the two treatment groups (Dannon et al. 2002), suggesting that the clinical gains from rTMS could be sustained with continuation treatment in a manner similar to ECT.

Similar results have been reported by other investigators, including Janicak and coworkers (2002), who randomly assigned depressed patients to either bilateral ECT or 2 to 4 weeks of rTMS; efforts were made to minimize concomitant medications. Using rigorous response criteria, 22 completers showed statistically equivalent response rates to ECT (56%) or rTMS (46%) (Janicak et al. 2002). Pridmore (2000) also found similar antidepressant effects for standard bilateral ECT or a combination of ECT (one treatment per week) and rTMS (4 treatment sessions per week).

If rTMS can achieve the desired efficacy in a given patient, it possesses several intrinsic advantages over ECT, including reduced stigma, elimination of the need for anesthesia, and apparent absence of cognitive toxicity. In the best-case scenario, these desirable properties could translate into increased adherence and cost savings compared to ECT. As the field achieves growing consensus on appropriate treatment parameters for rTMS and true double-blind sham control conditions, it is expected that further research will more definitively determine the relative efficacy and adverse effects of ECT and TMS.

While rTMS is designed as a nonconvulsive intervention, some investigators have begun to explore the possibility of using magnetic stimulation as an alternative to ECT to deliberately induce seizures, which presumably may be therapeutic. This line of research is being most actively pursued in nonhuman primates, and its feasibility in humans has been demonstrated (Lisanby et al. 2001b). Although magnetic seizure therapy, like ECT, requires general anesthesia, if future research demonstrates an ability to more finely control the dosing and localization of the resulting seizure activity, this new intervention could offer advantages over ECT, both in therapeutic action and diminished unwanted cognitive effects.

A different aspect of ECT action is being investigated as a nonconvulsive alternative intervention. Burst suppression therapy (BST) uses repeated administrations of certain general anesthetics—without any brain stimulation—to mimic the transient postictal EEG quiescence that typically follows ECT. While the presumed absence of cognitive adverse effects is appealing, the evidence supporting clinically meaningful antidepressant efficacy of BST is mixed, and definitive trials are still being planned.

Much as anticonvulsant drugs were carried over from neurology to psychiatry for mood stabilization, vagus nerve stimulation (VNS) is an effective treatment of refractory seizure disorders that is showing promise as an antidepressant intervention. Approved by the US Food and Drug Administration in 1997 for selected cases of epilepsy, VNS was first reported to be associated with improved mood in neurology patients and more recently has shown partial efficacy in refractory mood disorders. The afferent connections of the left vagus nerve with locus coeruleus, dorsal raphe, and limbic structures have been implicated in the putative antidepressant effect of this intervention.

An initial surgical procedure is required for implantation of a small pacemaker-like stimulus generator beneath the clavicle, with an attached lead wrapped around the left vagus nerve in the neck. The generator can be programmed to automatically deliver a fixed duration of vagus nerve stimulation, for example 30 seconds of stimulation every 5 minutes. Many patients notice physical concomitants of vagal stimulation, such as coughing or hoarseness (Sackeim et al. 2001b). While this may defeat the masking of no-stimulation programming as a control condition in research studies, the intervention otherwise appears well tolerated. In the event of disturbing adverse effects, a magnet held over the stimulus generator will abort a stimulation. Safety experience thus far with seizure disorder patients has been satisfactory; stimulation of the left vagus nerve has no cardiac effects.

In a published industry-sponsored pilot study (Rush et al. 2000), 30 neurologically healthy patients with nonpsychotic treatment-resistant depression underwent VNS while maintained on stable medication regimens. Device implantation was followed by an initial 2-week no-stimulation recovery period. Then 10 weeks of active VNS was associated with a 50% or greater drop in Hamilton depression scores in 40% of patients. However, only 17% of patients demonstrated full remission, as reflected in a posttreatment Hamilton depression score < 10 (Rush et al. 2000). With expansion of the trial to include an additional 29 completers, the overall response rate fell to 30.5%, with complete remission in 15.3% (Sackeim et al. 2001b). Those patients with the strongest histories of treatment resistance were least likely to respond to VNS, suggesting that VNS would not be a feasible alternative for the ECT nonresponder. A subsequent industry-sponsored multisite pivotal trial of VNS in major depression was not successful in showing superior efficacy of real versus sham VNS. However, most patients who did respond in the acute trials maintained their improvement, and others converted to responder or remitter status, during a 1- and 2-year naturalistic follow-up (Marangell et al. 2002). Further research is necessary to define those patients for whom an invasive intervention such as VNS is likely to be appropriate and beneficial.

In conclusion, ECT retains a limited but important role in the treatment of selected patients with severe mood and other mental disorders. While efforts to continue to minimize the adverse effects, particularly cognitive, of ECT while retaining its effectiveness, other research is underway at developing additional or alternative nonpharmacologic somatic interventions for depression and other mental illnesses (Rasmussen et al. 2002b). Optimal treatment for a given individual continues to require the determination of the benefit–risk ratio for each particular person and situation.

## References

Abrams R (1982) Clinical prediction of ECT response in depressed patients. Psychopharmacol Bull 18, 48–50.

Abrams R (1991) Electroconvulsive therapy in the medically compromised patient. Psychiatr Clin N Am 14, 871–885.

Abrams R (1997a) Electroconvulsive Therapy, 3rd ed. Oxford University Press, New York.

Abrams R (1997b) The mortality rate with ECT. Convuls Ther 13, 125–127.

Abrams R (2000) Electroconvulsive therapy requires higher dosage levels: Food and Drug Administration action is required. Arch Gen Psychiatr 57, 445–446.

Abrams R and Swartz CM (1985) Electroconvulsive therapy and prolactin release: Relation to treatment response in melancholia. Convuls Ther 1, 38–42.

Ackermann RF, Engel J Jr., and Baxter L (1986) Positron emission tomography and autoradiographic studies of glucose utilization following electroconvulsive seizures in humans and rats. Ann NY Acad Sci 462, 263–269.

Addonizio G and Susman VL (1987) ECT as a treatment alternative for patients with symptoms of neuroleptic malignant syndrome. J Clin Psychiatr 48, 102–105.

Alexander RC, Salomon M, Pioggia MI, et al. (1988) Convulsive therapy in the treatment of mania: McLean Hospital. Convuls Ther 4, 115–125.

American Academy of Child and Adolescent Psychiatry (2001) Practice parameter for the assessment and treatment of children and adolescents with schizophrenia. J Am Acad Child Adolesc Psychiatr 40(Suppl 7), 4S–23S.

American Psychiatric Association (1990) The Practice of ECT: Recommendations for Treatment, Training and Privileging. American Psychiatric Press, Washington DC.

American Psychiatric Association (2000) Practice Guideline for the Treatment of Patients With Major Depressive, 2nd ed., American Psychiatric Publishing, Washington DC.

American Psychiatric Association (2001) The Practice of Electroconvulsive Therapy: Recommendations for Treatment, Training and Privileging—A Task Force Report, 2nd ed. American Psychiatric Press, Washington DC.

American Psychiatric Association (2002) Practice guideline for the treatment of patients with bipolar disorder (revision). Am J Psychiatr 159(Suppl 4), 1–50.

American Psychiatric Association Task Force on ECT (1978) Electro-Convulsive Therapy, Task Force Report #14. APA, Washington DC.

Andersen K, Balldin J, Gottfries CG, et al. (1987) A double-blind evaluation of electroconvulsive therapy in Parkinson's disease with "on-off" phenomena. Acta Neurol Scand 76, 191–199.

Andrade C and Sudha S (2000) Electroconvulsive therapy and the alpha-2 noradrenergic receptor: Implications of treatment schedule effects. J ECT 16, 268–278.

Apëria B, Bergman H, Engelbrektson K, et al. (1985) Effects of electroconvulsive therapy on neuropsychological function and circulating levels of ACTH, cortisol, prolactin, and TSH in patients with major depressive illness. Acta Psychiatr Scand 72, 536–541.

Apëria B, Thorën M, Zettergren M, et al. (1984) Plasma pattern of adrenocorticotropin and cortisol during electroconvulsive therapy in patients with major depressive illness. Acta Psychiatr Scand 70, 361–369.

Aronson TA, Shukla S, and Hoff A (1987) Continuation therapy after ECT for delusional depression: A naturalistic study of prophylactic treatments and relapse. Convuls Ther 3, 251–259.

Asnis GM, Fink M, and Saferstein S (1978) ECT in metropolitan New York hospitals: A survey of practice, 1975–1976. Am J Psychiatr 135, 479–482.

Avery D and Lubrano A (1979) Depression treated with imipramine and ECT: The DeCarolis study reconsidered. Am J Psychiatr 136, 559–562.

Bailine SH, Rifkin A, Kayne E, et al. (2000) Comparison of bifrontal and bitemporal ECT for major depression. Am J Psychiatr 157, 121–123.

Baldwin S and Oxlad M (1996) Multiple case sampling of ECT administration with 217 minors: Review and meta-analysis. J Ment Health 5, 451–463.

Balldin J, Granërus AK, Lindstedt G, et al. (1981) Predictors for improvement after electroconvulsive therapy in parkinsonian patients with on-off symptoms. J Neural Transm 52, 199–211.

Balldin J, Granërus AK, Lindstedt G, et al. (1982) Neuroendocrine evidence for increased responsiveness of dopamine receptors in humans following electroconvulsive therapy. Psychopharmacology 76, 371–376.

Barry S, Rowan MJ, Mulhall J, et al. (1991) Change in barbiturate anaesthetic sensitivity as a prognostic indicator of electroconvulsive therapy outcome. Acta Psychiatr Scand 83, 251–255.

Bauer J and Elger CE (1994) Management of status epilepticus in adults. CNS Drugs 1, 26–44.

Beale MD, Kellner CH, and Parsons PJ (1997) ECT for the treatment of mood disorders in cancer patients. Convuls Ther 13, 222–226.

Benbow SM (1989) The role of electroconvulsive therapy in the treatment of depressive illness in old age. Br J Psychiatr 155, 147–152.

Bernardo M, Gaya J, Escobar R, et al. (1993) Hypophyseal response to ECT: A higher and faster vasopressin peak. Biol Psychiatr 33, 670–672.

Bernardo M, Navarro V, Salvá J, et al. (2000) Seizure activity and safety in combined treatment with venlafaxine and ECT: A pilot study. J ECT 16, 38–42.

Bhatia SC, Baldwin SA, and Bhatia SK (1999) Electroconvulsive therapy during the third trimester of pregnancy. J ECT 15, 270–274.

Black DW, Winokur G, and Nasrallah A (1986) ECT in unipolar and bipolar disorders: A naturalistic evaluation of 460 patients. Convuls Ther 2, 231–237.

Black DW, Winokur G, and Nasrallah A (1987) Treatment of mania: A naturalistic study of electroconvulsive therapy versus lithium in 438 patients. J Clin Psychiatr 48, 132–139.

Blazer D (1989) Depression in the elderly. N Engl J Med 320, 164–166.

Blier P and Bouchard C (1992) Effect of repeated electroconvulsive shocks on serotonergic neurons. Eur J Pharmacol 211, 365–373.

Bloomstein JR, Rummans TA, Maruta T, et al. (1996) The use of electroconvulsive therapy in pain patients. Psychosomatics 37, 374–379.

Boey WK and Lai FO (1990) Comparison of propofol and thiopentone as anaesthetic agents for electroconvulsive therapy. Anaesthesia 45, 623–628.

Bonne O, Krausz Y, Shapira B, et al. (1996) Increased cerebral blood flow in depressed patients responding to electroconvulsive therapy. J Nucl Med 37, 1075–1080.

Boronow J, Stoline A, and Sharfstein SS (1997) Refusal of ECT by a patient with recurrent depression, psychosis, and catatonia. Am J Psychiatr 154, 1285–1291.

Botteron K, Figiel GS, and Zorumski CF (1991) Electroconvulsive therapy in patients with late-onset psychoses and structural brain changes. J Geriatr Psychiatr Neurol 4, 44–47.

Bourgon LN and Kellner CH (2000) Relapse of depression after ECT: A review. J ECT 16, 19–31.

Boylan LS, Haskett RF, Mulsant BH, et al. (2000) Determinants of seizure threshold in ECT: Benzodiazepine use, anesthetic dosage, and other factors. J ECT 16, 3–18.

Brandon S, Cowley P, McDonald C, et al. (1984) Electroconvulsive therapy: Results in depressive illness from the Leicestershire trial. Br Med J 288, 22–25.

Buchan H, Johnstone E, McPherson K, et al. (1992) Who benefits from electroconvulsive therapy? Combined results of the Leicester and Northwick Park trials. Br J Psychiatr 160, 355–359.

Burd J and Kettle P (1998) Incidence of asystole in electroconvulsive therapy in elderly patients. Am J Geriatr Psychiatr 6, 203–211.

Burt T, Lisanby SH, and Sackeim HA (2002) Neuropsychiatric applications of transcranial magnetic stimulation: A meta analysis. Neuropsychopharmacology 5, 73–103.

Calev A (1994) Neuropsychology and ECT: Past and future research trends. Psychopharmacol Bull 30, 461–469.

Calev A, Fink M, Petrides G, et al. (1993) Caffeine pretreatment enhances clinical efficacy and reduces cognitive effects of electroconvulsive therapy. Convuls Ther 9, 95–100.

Calev A, Kochav-lev E, Tubi N, et al. (1991) Change in attitude toward electroconvulsive therapy: Effects of treatment, time since treatment, and severity of depression. Convuls Ther 7, 184–189.

Caplan G (1946) Electrical convulsive therapy in the treatment of epilepsy. J Ment Sci 92, 784–794.

Casey DA and Davis MH (1996) Electroconvulsive therapy in the very old. Gen Hosp Psychiatr 18, 436–439.

Cassidy F, Murry E, Weiner RD, et al. (1997) Lack of relapse with tryptophan depletion following successful treatment with ECT. Am J Psychiatr 154, 1151–1152.

Cerletti U (1956) Electroshock therapy. In The Great Physiodynamic Therapies in Psychiatry, Marti-Ibanez F, Sackler AM, and Sackler RR. Hoeber Harper, New York, pp. 91–120.

Chanpattana W and Chakrabhand MLS (2001) Combined ECT and neuroleptic therapy in treatment-refractory schizophrenia: Prediction of outcome. Psychiatr Res 105, 107–115.

Chaturvedi S, Chadda RK, Rusia U, et al. (2001) Effect of electroconvulsive therapy on hematological parameters. Psychiatr Res 104, 265–268.

Christison GW, Kirch DG, and Wyatt RJ (1991) When symptoms persist: Choosing among alternative somatic treatments for schizophrenia. Schizophr Bull 17, 217–245.

Ciapparelli A, Dell'Osso L, Tundo A, et al. (2001) Electroconvulsive therapy in medication-nonresponsive patients with mixed mania and bipolar depression. J Clin Psychiatr 62, 552–555.

Clark CJ (1985) Report of the Electro-Convulsive Therapy Review Committee. Ontario Ministry of Health, Toronto.

Clarke TB, Coffey CE, Hoffman GW, et al. (1989) Continuation therapy for depression using outpatient electroconvulsive therapy. Convuls Ther 5, 330–337.

Coffey CE (1994) The role of structural brain imaging in ECT. Psychopharmacol Bull 30, 477–483.

Cohen D, Flament M, Taieb O, et al. (2000a) Electroconvulsive therapy in adolescence. Eur Child Adolesc Psychiatr 9, 1–6.

Cohen D, Taieb O, Flament M, et al. (2000b) Absence of cognitive impairment as long-term follow-up in adolescents treated with ECT for severe mood disorder. Am J Psychiatr 157, 460–462.

Conway CR and Nelson LA (2001) The combined use of bupropion, lithium, and venlafaxine during ECT: A case of prolonged seizure activity. J ECT 17, 216–218.

Cooper SJ, Kelly JG, and King DJ (1985) Adrenergic receptors in depression: Effects of electroconvulsive therapy. Br J Psychiatr 147, 23–29.

Coppen A, Abou-Saleh MT, Milln P, et al. (1981) Lithium continuation therapy following electroconvulsive therapy. Br J Psychiatr 139, 284–287.

Coryell W and Zimmerman M (1984) Outcome following ECT for primary unipolar depression: A test of newly proposed response predictors. Am J Psychiatr 141, 862–867.

Crowe RR (1984) Current concepts. Electroconvulsive therapy—A current perspective. N Engl J Med 311, 163–167.

Currier MB, Murray GB, and Welch CC (1992) Electroconvulsive therapy for post-stroke depressed geriatric patients. J Neuropsychiatr Clin Neurosci 4, 140–144.

Dannon PN, Dolberg OT, Schreiber S, et al. (2002) Three and six-month outcome following courses of either ECT or rTMS in a population of severely depressed individuals – Preliminary report. Biol Psychiatr 51, 687–690.

Datto CJ, Levy S, Miller DS, et al. (2001) Impact of maintenance ECT on concentration and memory. J ECT 17, 170–174.

Davis JM, Janicak PG, Sakkas P, et al. (1991) Electroconvulsive therapy in the treatment of the neuroleptic malignant syndrome. Convuls Ther 7, 111–120.

Deakin JF, Ferrier IN, Crow TJ, et al. (1983) Effects of ECT on pituitary hormone release: Relationship to seizure, clinical variables and outcome. Br J Psychiatr 143, 618–624.

DeBattista C and Mueller K (2001) Is electroconvulsive therapy effective for the depressed patient with comorbid borderline personality disorder? J ECT 17, 91–98.

Dec GW Jr., Stern TA, and Welch C (1985) The effects of electroconvulsive therapy on serial electrocardiograms and serum cardiac enzyme values: A prospective study of depressed hospitalized patients. JAMA 253, 2525–2529.

Decina P, Guthrie EB, Sackeim HA, et al. (1987) Continuation ECT in the management of relapses of major affective episodes. Acta Psychiatr Scand 75, 559–562.

Decina P, Malitz S, Sackeim HA, et al. (1984) Cardiac arrest during ECT modified by beta-adrenergic blockade. Am J Psychiatr 141, 298–300.

Delva NJ, Brunet D, Hawken ER, et al. (2000) Electrical dose and seizure threshold: Relations to clinical outcome and cognitive effects in bifrontal, bitemporal, and right unilateral ECT. J ECT 16, 361–369.

Delva NJ, Brunet DG, Hawken ER, et al. (2001) Characteristics of responders and nonresponders to brief-pulse right unilateral ECT in a controlled clinical trial. J ECT 17, 118–123.

Devanand DP, Bowers MBJ, Hoffman FJJ, et al. (1989) Acute and subacute effects of ECT on plasma HVA, MHPG, and prolactin. Biol Psychiatr 26, 408–412.

Devanand DP, Dwork AJ, Hutchinson ER, et al. (1994) Does ECT alter brain structure? Am J Psychiatr 151, 957–970.

Devanand DP, Polanco P, Cruz R, et al. (2000) The efficacy of ECT in mixed affective states. J ECT 16, 32–37.

Devanand DP, Sackeim HA, and Finck AD (1987) Modified ECT using succinylcholine after remission of neuroleptic malignant syndrome. Convuls Ther 3, 284–290.

Devanand DP, Sackeim HA, Lo ES, et al. (1991) Serial dexamethasone suppression tests and plasma dexamethasone levels: Effects of clinical response to electroconvulsive therapy in major depression. Arch Gen Psychiatr 48, 525–533.

Dodwell D and Goldberg D (1989) A study of factors associated with response to electroconvulsive therapy in patients with schizophrenic symptoms. Br J Psychiatr 154, 635–639.

Dolinski SY and Zvara DA (1997) Anesthetic considerations of cardiovascular risk during electroconvulsive therapy. Convuls Ther 13, 157–164.

Douyon R, Serby M, Klutchko B, et al. (1989) ECT and Parkinson's disease revisited: A "naturalistic" study. Am J Psychiatr 146, 1451–1455.

Dubovsky SL, Buzan R, Marshall T, et al. (2001) Nicardipine improves the antidepressant action of ECT but does not improve cognition. J ECT 17, 3–10.

Duffett R, Hill P, and Lelliott P (1999) Use of electroconvulsive therapy in young people. Br J Psychiatr 175, 228–230.

Elliot DL, Linz DH, and Kane JA (1982) Electroconvulsive therapy: Pretreatment medical evaluation. Arch Intern Med 142, 979–981.

Ende G, Braus DF, Walter S, et al. (2000) The hippocampus in patients treated with eletroconvulsive therapy: A proton magnetic resonance spectroscopic imaging study. Arch Gen Psychiatr 57, 937–943.

Enns MW and Reiss JP (1992) Electroconvulsive therapy. Can J Psychiatr 37, 671–686.

Farah A and McCall WV (1993) Electroconvulsive therapy stimulus dosing: A survey of contemporary practices. Convuls Ther 9, 90–94.

Ferraro TN, Golden GT, and Hare TA (1990) Repeated electroconvulsive shock selectively alters gamma-aminobutyric acid levels in the rat brain: Effect of electrode placement. Convuls Ther 6, 199–208.

Finch JM, Sobin PB, Carmody TJ, et al. (1990) A survey of psychiatrists' attitudes toward electroconvulsive therapy. Psychiatr Serv 50, 264–265.

Fink M (1984) Meduna and the origins of convulsive therapy. Am J Psychiatr 141, 1034–1041.

Fink M (1992) ECT and public mental health services. Convuls Ther 8, 87–91.

Fink M (1994a) Combining electroconvulsive therapy and drugs: A review of safety and efficacy. CNS Drugs 1, 370–376.

Fink M (1994b) Diazepam or lorazepam for prolonged seizures? Convuls Ther 10, 236.

Fink M (1994c) Indications for the use of ECT. Psychopharmacol Bull 30, 269–275.

Fink M (1999) Electroshock: Restoring the Mind. Oxford University Press, New York.

Fink M (2002) Catatonia and ECT: Meduna's biological antagonism hypothesis reconsidered. World J Biol Psychiatr 3, 105–108.

Fink M and Johnson L (1982) Monitoring the duration of electroconvulsive therapy seizures: 'Cuff' and EEG methods compared. Arch Gen Psychiatr 39, 1189–1191.

Fink M and Sackeim HA (1996) Convulsive therapy in schizophrenia? Schizophr Bull 22, 27–39.

Fink M, Abrams R, Bailine S, et al. (1996) Ambulatory electroconvulsive therapy: Report of a task force of the Association for Convulsive Therapy. Convuls Ther 12, 42–55.

Fochtmann LJ (1994) Animal studies of electroconvulsive therapy: Foundations for future research. Psychopharmacol Bull 30, 321–444.

Fochtmann LJ, Cruciani R, Aiso M, et al. (1989) Chronic electroconvulsive shock increases D-1 receptor binding in rat substantia nigra. Eur J Pharmacol 167, 305–306.

Folk JW, Kellner CH, Beale MD, et al. (2000) Anesthesia for electroconvulsive therapy: A review. J ECT 16, 157–170.

Folkerts HW, Michael N, Tolle R, et al. (1997) Electroconvulsive therapy vs. paroxetine in treatment-resistant depression—a randomized study. Acta Psychiatr Scand 96, 334–342.

Fox HA (2001) Extended continuation and maintenance ECT for long-lasting episodes of major depression. J ECT 17, 60–64.

Francis A and Fochtmann L (1993) Sustained downregulation of cortical adrenergic receptor density with maintenance electroconvulsive stimulation. Convuls Ther 9, 185–191.

Frankenburg FR, Suppes T, and McLean PE (1993) Combined clozapine and electroconvulsive therapy. Convuls Ther 9, 176–180.

Frederiksen SO and d'Elia G (1979) Electroconvulsive therapy in Sweden. Br J Psychiatr 134, 283–287.

Freeman CP and Kendell RE (1980) ECT: I. Patients' experiences and attitudes. Br J Psychiatr 137, 8–16.

Fricchione G (1989) Catatonia: A new indication for benzodiazepines? Biol Psychiatr 26, 761–765.

Fricchione GL, Kaufman LD, Gruber BL, et al. (1990) Electroconvulsive therapy and cyclophosphamide in combination for severe neuropsychiatric lupus with catatonia. Am J Med 88, 442–443.

Fried D and Mann JJ (1988) Electroconvulsive treatment of a patient with known intracranial tumor. Biol Psychiatr 23, 176–180.

Friedel RO (1986) The combined use of neuroleptics and ECT in drug resistant schizophrenic patients. Psychopharmacol Bull 22, 928–930.

Gagné GG Jr., Furman MJ, Carpenter LL, et al. (2000) Efficacy of continuation ECT and antidepressant drugs compared to long-term antidepressants alone in depressed patients. Am J Psychiatr 157, 1960–1965.

Gerring JP and Shields HM (1982) The identification and management of patients with a high risk for cardiac arrhythmias during modified ECT. J Clin Psychiatr 43, 140–143.

Glass RM (2001) Electroconvulsive therapy: Time to bring it out of the shadows (editorial). JAMA 285, 1346–1348.

Glen T and Scott AIF (2000) Variation in rates of electroconvulsive therapy use among consultant terms in Edinburgh (1993–1996). J Affect Disord 58, 75–78.

Glue P, Costello MJ, Pert A, et al. (1990) Regional neurotransmitter responses after acute and chronic electroconvulsive shock. Psychopharmacology 100, 60–65.

Golden RN and Potter WZ (1986) Neurochemical and neuroendocrine dysregulation in affective disorders. Psychiatr Clin N Am 9, 313–327.

Goodwin FK and Jamison KR (1990) Manic–Depressive Illness. Oxford University Press, New York.

Gormley N, Cullen C, Walters L, et al. (1998) The safety and efficacy of electroconvulsive therapy in patients over age 75. Int J Geriatr Psychiatr 13, 871–874.

Greenblatt M (1977) Efficacy of ECT in affective and schizophrenic illness. Am J Psychiatr 134, 1001–1005.

Grunhaus L, Dannon PN, Schreiber S, et al. (2000) Repetitive transcranial magnetic stimulation is as effective as electroconvulsive therapy in the treatment of nondelusional major depressive disorder: An open study. Biol Psychiatr 47, 314–324.

Grunhaus L, Hirschman S, Dolberg OT, et al. (2001) Coadministration of melatonin and fluoxetine does not improve the 3-month outcome following ECT. J ECT 17, 124–128.

Grunhaus L, Pande AC, and Haskett RF (1990) Full and abbreviated courses of maintenance electroconvulsive therapy. Convuls Ther 6, 130–138.

Gujavarty K, Greenberg LB, and Fink M (1987) Electroconvulsive therapy and neuroleptic medication in therapy-resistant positive-symptom psychosis. Convuls Ther 3, 185–195.

Hartmann CE (2002) Personal Accounts—Life as death: Hope regained with ECT. Psychiatr Serv 53, 413–414.

Heal DJ, Prow MR, and Buckett WR (1991) Determination of the role of noradrenergic and 5-hydroxytryptaminergic neurones in postsynaptic alpha-2-adrenoceptor desensitization by desipramine and ECS. Br J Pharmacol 103, 1865–1870.

Henry ME, Schmidt ME, Matochik JA, et al. (2001) The effects of ECT on brain glucose: A pilot FDG PET study. J ECT 17, 33–40.

Hermann RC, Dorwart RA, Hoover CW, et al. (1995) Variation in ECT use in the United States. Am J Psychiatr 152, 869–875.

Hermann RC, Ettner SL, Dorwart RA, et al. (1998) Characteristics of psychiatrists who perform ECT. Am J Psychiatr 155, 889–894.

Hermann RC, Ettner SL, Dorwart RA, et al. (1999) Diagnoses of patients treated with ECT: A comparison of evidence-based standards with reported use. Psychiatr Serv 50, 1059–1065.

Hertzman M (1992) ECT and neuroleptics as primary treatment for schizophrenia. Biol Psychiatr 31, 217–220.

Heshe J and Roeder E (1976) Electroconvulsive therapy in Denmark. Br J Psychiatr 128, 241–245.

Hickie I, Parsonage B, and Parker G (1990) Prediction of response to electroconvulsive therapy: Preliminary validation of a sign-based typology of depression. Br J Psychiatr 157, 65–71.

Hirose S, Ashby CR Jr., and Mills MJ (2001) Effectiveness of ECT combined with risperidone against aggression in schizophrenia. J ECT 17, 22–26.

Hoekstra R, van den Broek WW, Fekkes D, et al. (2001) Effect of electroconvulsive therapy on biopterin and large neutral amino acids in severe, medication-resistant depression. Psychiatr Res 103, 115–123.

Holtzheimer PE, Russo J, and Avery DH (2001) A meta-analysis of repetitive transcranial magnetic stimulation in the treatment of depression. Psychopharmacol Bull 35, 149–169.

Horne RL, Pettinati HM, Sugerman AA, et al. (1985) Comparing bilateral to unilateral electroconvulsive therapy in a randomized study with EEG monitoring. Arch Gen Psychiatr 42, 1087–1092.

Hsiao JK, Messenheimer JA, and Evans DL (1987) ECT and neurological disorders. Convuls Ther 3, 121–136.

Hughes JR (1986) ECT during and after the neuroleptic malignant syndrome: Case report. J Clin Psychiatr 47, 42–43.

Imlah NW, Ryan E, and Harrington JA (1965) The influence of antidepressant drugs on the response to electroconvulsive therapy and on subsequent relapse rates. Neuropsychopharmacology 4, 438–442.

Isaac L and Swanger J (1983) Alteration of electroconvulsive threshold by cerebrospinal fluid from cats tolerant to electroconvulsive shock. Life Sci 33, 2301–2304.

Jaffe R, Dubin W, Shoyer B, et al. (1990) Outpatient electroconvulsive therapy: Efficacy and safety. Convuls Ther 6, 231–238.

Janicak PG, Davis JM, Gibbons RD, et al. (1985) Efficacy of ECT: A meta-analysis. Am J Psychiatr 142, 297–302.

Janicak PG, Dowd SM, Martis B, et al. (2002) Repetitive transcranial magnetic stimulation versus electroconvulsive therapy for major depression: Preliminary results of a randomized trial. Biol Psychiatr 51, 659–667.

Jha AK and Stein GS (1996) Decreased efficacy of combined benzodiazepines and unilateral ECT in treatment of depression. Acta Psychiatr Scand 94, 101–104.

Jha AK, Stein GS, and Fenwick P (1996) Negative interaction between lithium and electroconvulsive therapy—A case-control study. Br J Psychiatr 168, 241–243.

Joffe RT and Sokolov STH (1994) The thyroid and electroconvulsive treatment. Psychopharmacol Bull 30, 485–488.

Jorm AF and Henderson AS (1989) Use of private psychiatric services in Australia: An analysis of Medicare data. Austral N Z J Psychiatr 23, 461–468.

Kant R, Coffey CE, and Bogyi AM (1999) Safety and efficacy of ECT in patients with head injury: A case series. J Neuropsychiatr Clin Neurosci 11, 32–37.

Karlinsky H and Shulman KI (1984) The clinical use of electroconvulsive therapy in old age. J Am Geriatr Soc 32, 183–186.

Kay DW, Fahy T, and Garside RF (1970) A 7-month double-blind trial of amitriptyline and diazepam in ECT-treated depressed patients. Br J Psychiatr 117, 667–671.

Kellar KJ, Cascio CS, Bergstrom DA, et al. (1981a) Electroconvulsive shock and reserpine: Effects on beta-adrenergic receptors in rat brain. J Neurochem 37, 830–836.

Kellar KJ, Cascio CS, Butler JA, et al. (1981b) Differential effects of electroconvulsive shock and antidepressant drugs on serotonin-2 receptors in rat brain. Eur J Pharmacol 69, 515–518.

Kellner CH and Bernstein HJ (1993) ECT as a treatment for neurologic illness. In The Clinical Science of Electroconvulsive Therapy, Coffey CE (ed). American Psychiatric Press, Washington, DC, pp. 183–210.

Kellner CH, Beale MD, Prichett JT, et al. (1994) Electroconvulsive therapy and Parkinson's disease: The case for further study. Psychopharmacol Bull 30, 495–500.

Kellner CH, Knapp R, Petrides G, et al. (2002) Bilateral ECT rapidly relieves suicidality: Findings from phase I of the CORE ECT study. Poster presentation at 42nd annual NCDEU meeting, June 11. Boca Raton, FL.

Kellner CH, Nixon DW, and Bernstein HJ (1991) ECT—drug interactions: A review. Psychopharmacol Bull 27, 595–609.

Khan A, Cohen S, Stowell M, et al. (1987) Treatment options in severe psychotic depression. Convuls Ther 3, 93–99.

Khan A, Nies A, Johnson G, et al. (1985) Plasma catecholamines and ECT. Biol Psychiatr 20, 799–804.

Kirkegaard C and Faber J (1986) Influence of free thyroid hormone levels on the TSH response to TRH in endogenous depression. Psychoneuroendocrinology 11, 491–497.

Kirkegaard C and Faber J (1998) The role of thyroid hormones in depression. Eur J Endocrinol 138, 1–9.

Kirkegaard C, Faber J, Hummer L, et al. (1979) Increased levels of TRH in cerebrospinal fluid from patients with endogenous depression. Psychoneuroendocrinology 4, 227–235.

Klapheke MM (1993) Combining ECT and antipsychotic agents: Benefits and risks. Convuls Ther 9, 241–255.

Klapheke MM (1997) Electroconvulsive therapy consultation: An update. Convuls Ther 13, 227–241.

Kohler CG and Burock M (2001) ECT for psychotic depression associated with a brain tumor. Am J Psychiatr 158, 2089

Komrad MS (1988) Electroconvulsive therapy. I. Indications. Md Med J 37, 167.

Kovac AL and Pardo M (1992) A comparison between etomidate and methohexital for anesthesia in ECT. Convuls Ther 8, 118–125.

Krahn LE, Gleber E, Rummans TA, et al. (2000) The effects of electroconvulsive therapy on melatonin. J ECT 16, 391–398.

Kramer BA (1982) Poor response to electroconvulsive therapy in patients with a combined diagnosis of major depression and borderline personality disorder. Lancet 2, 1048.

Kramer BA (1987) Maintenance ECT: A survey of practice, 1986. Convuls Ther 3, 260–268.

Kramer BA (1990) ECT use in the public sector: California. Psychiatr Q 61, 97–103.

Kramer BA (1999) ECT in elderly patients with schizophrenia. Am J Geriatr Psychiatr 7, 171–174.

Kroessler D and Fogel BS (1993) Electroconvulsive therapy for major depression in the oldest old: Effects of medical comorbidity on post-treatment survival. Am J Geriatr Psychiatr 1, 30–37.

Kronfol Z, Hamdan-Allen G, Goel K, et al. (1991) Effects of single and repeated electroconvulsive therapy sessions on plasma ACTH, prolactin, growth hormone and cortisol concentrations. Psychoneuroendocrinology 16, 345–352.

Krueger RB and Sackeim HA (1995) Electroconvulsive therapy and schizophrenia. In Schizophrenia, Hirsch S and Weinberger D (eds). Blackwell, Oxford, UK.

Krueger RB, Sackeim HA, and Gamzu ER (1992) Pharmacological treatment of the cognitive side effects of ECT: A review. Psychopharmacol Bull 28, 409–424.

Krystal AD, Coffey CE, Weiner RD, et al. (1998) Changes in seizure threshold over the course of electroconvulsive therapy affect therapeutic response and are detected by ictal EEG ratings. J Neuropsychiatr Clin Neurosci 10, 178–186.

Krystal AD, Dean MD, Weiner RD, et al. (2000a) ECT stimulus intensity: Are present ECT devices too limited? Am J Psychiatr 157, 963–967.

Krystal AD, Weiner RD, Lindahl V, et al. (2000b) The development and retrospective testing of an electroencephalographic seizure quality-based stimulus dosing paradigm with ECT. J ECT 16, 338–349.

Krystal AD, Weiner RD, McCall WV, et al. (1993) The effects of ECT stimulus dose and electrode placement on the ictal electroencephalogram: An intraindividual crossover study. Biol Psychiatr 34, 759–767.

Kubek MJ, Low WC, Sattin A, et al. (1989) Role of TRH in seizure modulation. Ann NY Acad Sci 553, 286–303.

Kujala L, Rosenvinge B, and Bekkelund SI (2002) Clinical outcome and adverse effects of electroconvulsive therapy in elderly psychiatric patients. J Geriatr Psychiatr Neurol 15, 73–76.

Lafferty JE, North CS, Spitznagel E, et al. (2001) Laboratory screening prior to ECT. J ECT 17, 158–165.

Lambourn J and Gill D (1978) A controlled comparison of simulated and real ECT. Br J Psychiatr 133, 514–519.

Langer SZ, Sechter D, Loo H, et al. (1986) Electroconvulsive shock therapy and maximum binding of platelet tritiated imipramine binding in depression. Arch Gen Psychiatr 43, 949–952.

Latey R and Fahy T (1985) Electroconvulsive therapy in the Republic of Ireland 1982: A summary of findings. Br J Psychiatr 147, 438–439.

Lauritzen L, Odgaard K, Clemmesen L, et al. (1996) Relapse prevention by means of paroxetine in ECT-treated patients with major depression: A comparison with imipramine and placebo in medium-term continuation therapy. Acta Psychiatr Scand 94, 241–251.

Lawson JS, Inglis J, Delva NJ, et al. (1990) Electrode placement in ECT: Cognitive Effects. Psychol Med 20, 335–344.

Lazarus A (1986) Therapy of neuroleptic malignant syndrome. Psychiatr Dev 4, 19–30.

Lerer B (1984) Electroconvulsive shock and neurotransmitter receptors: Implications for mechanism of action and adverse effects of electroconvulsive therapy. Biol Psychiatr 19, 361–383.

Lerer B (1987) Neurochemical and other neurobiological consequences of ECT: Implications for the pathogenesis and treatment of affective disorders. In Psychopharmacology: The Third Generation of Progress, Meltzer HY (ed). Raven Press, New York, pp. 577–588.

Lerer B and Shapira B (1986) Neurochemical mechanisms of mood stabilization: Focus on electroconvulsive therapy. Ann NY Acad Sci 462, 366–375.

Lerer B, Shapira B, Calev A, et al. (1995) Antidepressant and cognitive effects of twice- versus three-times-weekly ECT. Am J Psychiatr 152, 564–570.

Levenson JL (1985) The neuroleptic malignant syndrome. Am J Psychiatr 142, 1137–1145.

Liang RA, Lam RW, and Ancill RJ (1988) ECT in the treatment of mixed depression and dementia. Br J Psychiatr 152, 281–284.

Linnoila M, Litovitz G, Scheinin M, et al. (1984) Effects of electroconvulsive treatment on monoamine metabolites, growth hormone, and prolactin in plasma. Biol Psychiatr 19, 79–84.

Lippmann S, Haas S, and Quast G (1993) Procedural complications of electroconvulsive therapy: Assessment and recommendations. South Med J 86, 1110–1114.

Lippmann S, Manshadi M, Wehry M, et al. (1985) 1, 250 electroconvulsive treatments without evidence of brain injury. Br J Psychiatr 147, 203–204.

Lisanby SH and Sackeim HA (2001) New developments in convulsive therapy for major depression. Epilepsy Behav 2, S68–S73.

Lisanby SH, Bazil CW, Resor SR, et al. (2001a) ECT in the treatment of status epilepticus. J ECT 17, 210–215.

Lisanby SH, Luber B, Finck AD, et al. (2001b) Deliberate seizure induction with repetitive transcranial magnetic stimulation in nonhuman primates. Arch Gen Psychiatr 58, 199–200.

Lisanby SH, Maddox JH, Prudic J, et al. (2000) The effects of electroconvulsive therapy on memory of autobiographical and public events. Arch Gen Psychiatr 57, 581–590.

Luber B, Nobler MS, Moeller JR, et al. (2000) Quantitative EEG during seizures induced by electroconvulsive therapy: Relations to treatment modality and clinical features. II. Topographic analyses. J ECT 16, 229–243.

Lunn RJ, Savageau MM, Beatty WW, et al. (1981) Anesthetics and electroconvulsive therapy seizure duration: Implications for therapy from a rat model. Biol Psychiatr 16, 1163–1175.

Magni G, Fisman M, and Helmes E (1988) Clinical correlates of ECT-resistant depression in the elderly. J Clin Psychiatr 49, 405–407.

Malcolm K, Dean J, Rowlands P, et al. (1991) Antidepressant drug treatment in relation to the use of ECT. J Psychopharm 5, 255–258.

Malsch E, Ho L, Booth MJ, et al. (1991) Survey of anesthetic coverage of electroconvulsive therapy in the state of Pennsylvania, 1988. Convuls Ther 7, 262–274.

Manji HK, Hsiao JK, Risby ED, et al. (1992) Failure of blunted prolactin response to IV clomipramine to normalize following successful ECT. J Psychopharmacol 6, 501–508.

Manly DT, Oakley SP Jr., and Bloch RM (2000) Electroconvulsive therapy in old–old patients. Am J Geriatr Psychiatr 8, 232–236.

Mann JJ (1998) Neurobiological correlates of the antidepressant action of electroconvulsive therapy. J ECT 14, 172–180.

Mann JJ and Kapur S (1994) Elucidation of biochemical basis of the antidepressant action of electroconvulsive therapy by human studies. Psychopharmacol Bull 30, 445–454.

Mann JJ, Manevitz AZ, Chen JS, et al. (1990a) Acute effects of single and repeated electroconvulsive therapy on plasma catecholamines and blood pressure in major depressive disorder. Psychiatr Res 34, 127–137.

Mann SC, Caroff SN, Bleier HR, et al. (1990b) Electroconvulsive therapy of the lethal catatonia syndrome. Convuls Ther 6, 239–247.

Manning M (1995) Undercurrents: A Life Beneath the Surface. Harper, San Francisco.

Marangell LB, Rush AJ, George MS, et al. (2002) Vagus nerve stimulation (VNS) for major depressive episodes: One year outcomes. Biol Psychiatr 51, 280–287.

Markowitz J, Brown R, Sweeney J, et al. (1987) Reduced length and cost of hospital stay for major depression in patients treated with ECT. Am J Psychiatr 144, 1025–1029.

Mathé AA, Rudorfer MV, Stenfors C, et al. (1996) Effects of electroconvulsive treatment on somatostatin, neuropeptide Y, endothelin and neurokinin A concentrations in cerebrospinal fluid of depressed patients. Depression 3, 250.

Mattingly G, Baker K, Zorumski CF, et al. (1992) Multiple sclerosis and ECT: Possible value of gadolinium-enhanced magnetic resonance scans for identifying high-risk patients. J Neuropsychiatr Clin Neurosci 4, 145–151.

May PR (1968) Treatment of Schizophrenia: A Comparative Study of Five Treatment Methods. Science House, New York.

May PR, Tuma AH, Dixon WJ, et al. (1981) Schizophrenia: A follow-up study of the results of five forms of treatment. Arch Gen Psychiatr 38, 776–784.

May PR, Tuma AH, Yale C, et al. (1976) Schizophrenia—A follow-up study of results of treatment. Arch Gen Psychiatr 33, 481–486.

McCabe M (1976) ECT in the treatment of mania: A controlled study. Am J Psychiatr 133, 688–691.

McCabe M and Norris B (1977) ECT versus chlorpromazine in mania. Biol Psychiatr 12, 245–254.

McCall WV (1993) Antihypertensive medications and ECT. Convuls Ther 9, 317–325.

McCall WV, Reboussin DM, Weiner RD, et al. (2000) Titrated moderately suprathreshold vs fixed high-dose right unilateral electroconvulsive therapy: Acute antidepressant and cognitive effects. Arch Gen Psychiatr 57, 438–444.

McCall WV, Weiner RD, Carroll BJ, et al. (1996) Serum prolactin, electrode placement, and the convulsive threshold during ECT. Convuls Ther 12, 81–85.

McClintock SM, Husain MM, Claassen C, et al. (2002) Atypical depression and electroconvulsive therapy: A preliminary report. Poster presentation at 42nd annual NCDEU meeting, June 11. Boca Raton, FL.

McGuire RJ, Scott AI, Bennie J, et al. (1989) Reliability of the application of a kinetic model of hormone release: Prolactin and oestrogen-stimulated neurophysin after electroconvulsive therapy. Convuls Ther 5, 131–139.

Meltzer HY (1992) Treatment of the neuroleptic-nonresponsive schizophrenic patient. Schizophr Bull 18, 515–542.

Meyers BS, Alexopoulos GS, Kakuma T, et al. (1999) Decreased dopamine beta-hydroxylase activity in unipolar geriatric delusional depression. Biol Psychiatr 45, 448–452.

Meyers BS, Klimstra SA, Gabriele M, et al. (2001) Continuation treatment of delusional depression in older adults. Am J Geriatr Psychiatr 9, 415–422.

Miller J (1994) Use of electroconvulsive therapy during pregnancy. Hosp Comm Psychiatr 45, 444–450.

Milo TJ, Kaufman GE, Barnes WE, et al. (2001) Changes in regional cerebral blood flow after electroconvulsive therapy for depression. J ECT 17, 15–21.

Milstein V, Small JG, Klapper MH, et al. (1987) Uni- versus bilateral ECT in the treatment of mania. Convuls Ther 3, 1–9.

Milstein V, Small JG, Miller MJ, et al. (1990) Mechanisms of action of ECT: Schizophrenia and schizoaffective disorder. Biol Psychiatr 27, 1282–1292.

Moellentine C, Rummans T, Ahlskog JE, et al. (1998) Effectiveness of ECT in patients with parkinsonism. J Neuropsychiatr Clin Neurosci 10, 187–193.

Monroe R (1991) Maintenance electroconvulsive therapy. Psychiatr Clin N Am 14, 947–960.

Mukherjee S (1989) Mechanisms of the antimanic effect of electroconvulsive therapy. Convuls Ther 5, 227–243.

Mukherjee S and Debsikdar V (1992) Unmodified electroconvulsive therapy of acute mania: A retrospective naturalistic study. Convuls Ther 8, 5–11.

Mukherjee S, Sackeim HA, and Schnur DB (1994) Electroconvulsive therapy of acute manic episodes: A review of 50 years' experience. Am J Psychiatr 151, 169–176.

Mulsant BH, Haskett RF, Prudic J, et al. (1997) Low use of neuroleptic drugs in the treatment of psychotic major depression. Am J Psychiatr 154, 559–561.

Mulsant BH, Rosen J, Thornton JE, et al. (1991) A prospective naturalistic study of electroconvulsive therapy in late-life depression. J Geriatr Psychiatr Neurol 4, 3–13.

Murray GB, Shea V, and Conn DK (1986) Electroconvulsive therapy for poststroke depression. J Clin Psychiatr 47, 258–260.

Nahshoni E, Aizenberg D, Sigler M, et al. (2001) Heart rate variability in elderly patients before and after electroconvulsive therapy. Am J Geriatr Psychiatr 9, 255–260.

Nakajima T, Daval JL, Gleiter CH, et al. (1989) C-fos mRNA expression following electrical-induced seizure and acute nociceptive stress in mouse brain. Epilepsy Res 4, 156–159.

National Institutes of Health/NIMH consensus conference (1985) Electroconvulsive therapy. JAMA 254, 2103–2108.

Nemeroff CB, Bissette G, Akil H, et al. (1991) Neuropeptide concentrations in the cerebrospinal fluid of depressed patients treated with electroconvulsive therapy: Corticotrophin-releasing factor, beta-endorphin and somatostatin. Br J Psychiatr 158, 59–63.

Nishihara F and Saito S (2002) Pre-ictal bispectral index has a positive correlation with seizureduration during electroconvulsive therapy. Anesth Analg 94, 1249–1252

Nobler MS and Sackeim HA (1993) Augmentation strategies in electroconvulsive therapy. Convuls Ther 9, 331–351.

Nobler MS, Luber B, Moeller JR, et al. (2000) Quantitative EEG during seizures induced by electroconvulsive therapy: Relations to treatment modality and clinical features. I. Global analyses. J ECT 16, 211–228.

Nobler MS, Oquendo MA, Kegeles LS, et al. (2001) Decreased regional brain metabolism after ECT. Am J Psychiatr 158, 305–308.

Nobler MS, Sackeim HA, Moeller JR, et al. (1997) Quantifying the speed of symptomatic improvement with electroconvulsive therapy: Comparison of alternative statistical methods. Convuls Ther 13, 208–221.

Nobler MS, Sackeim HA, Prohovnik I, et al. (1994) Regional cerebral blood flow in mood disorders, III. Treatment and clinical response. Arch Gen Psychiatr 51, 884–897.

Nobler MS, Sackeim HA, Solomou M, et al. (1993) EEG manifestations during ECT: Effects of electrode placement and stimulus intensity. Biol Psychiatr 34, 321–330.

Nutt DJ, Gleiter CH, and Glue P (1989) Neuropharmacological aspects of ECT: In search of the primary mechanism of action. Convuls Ther 5, 250–260.

O'Connor MK, Knapp R, Husain M, et al. (2001) The influence of age on the response of major depression to electroconvulsive therapy: A C.O.R.E. Report. Am J Geriatr Psychiatr 9, 382–390.

Oh JJ, Rummans TA, O'Connor MK, et al. (1992) Cognitive impairment after ECT in patients with Parkinson's disease and psychiatric illness. Am J Psychiatr 149, 271.

Olfson M, Marcus S, Sackeim HA, et al. (1998) Use of ECT for the inpatient treatment of recurrent major depression. Am J Psychiatr 155, 22–29.

Pallanti S (1999) Images in Psychiatry: Ugo Cerletti. Am J Psychiatr 156, 630.

Papakostas Y, Markianos M, Papadimitriou G, et al. (1990) Thyrotropin and prolactin secretion during ECT: Implications for the mechanism of ECT action. Convuls Ther 6, 214–220.

Papakostas YG, Markianos M, Zervas IM, et al. (2000) Administration of citalopram before ECT: Seizure duration and hormone responses. J ECT 16, 356–360.

Papakostas Y, Stefanis C, Sinouri A, et al. (1984) Increases in prolactin levels following bilateral and unilateral ECT. Am J Psychiatr 141, 1623–1624.

Pataki J, Zervas IM, and Jandorf L (1992) Catatonia in a university inpatient service (1985–1990). Convuls Ther 8, 163–173.

Paul SM, Extein I, Calil HM, et al. (1981) Use of ECT with treatment-resistant depressed patients at the National Institute of Mental Health. Am J Psychiatr 138, 486–489.

Pelonero AL, Levenson JL, and Pandurangi AK (1998) Neuroleptic malignant syndrome: A review. Psychiatr Serv 49, 1163–1172.

Perry P and Tsuang MT (1979) Treatment of unipolar depression following electroconvulsive therapy: Relapse rate comparisons between lithium and tricyclics therapies following ECT. J Affect Disord 1, 123–129.

Petrides G, Dhossche D, Fink M, et al. (1994) Continuation ECT: Relapse prevention in affective disorders. Convuls Ther 10, 189–194.

Petrides G, Find M, Husain MM, et al. (2001) ECT remission rates in psychotic versus nonpsychotic depressed patients: A report from CORE. J ECT 17, 244–253.

Pettinati HM, Stephens SM, Willis KM, et al. (1990) Evidence for less improvement in depression in patients taking benzodiazepines during unilateral ECT. Am J Psychiatr 147, 1029–1035.

Pettinati HM, Tamburello TA, Ruetsch CR, et al. (1994) Patient attitudes toward electroconvulsive therapy. Psychopharmacol Bull 30, 471–476.

Philbrick KL and Rummans TA (1994) Malignant catatonia. J Neuropsychiatr Clin Neurosci 6, 1–13.

Pippard J (1992) Audit of electroconvulsive treatment in two National Health Service regions. Br J Psychiatr 160, 621–637.

Pippard J and Ellam L (1981) Electroconvulsive Treatment in Great Britain, 1980. Gaskell, London.

Post RM (1990) ECT: The anticonvulsant connection. Neuropsychopharmacology 3, 89–92.

Post RM, Putnam F, Uhde TW, et al. (1986) Electroconvulsive therapy as an anticonvulsant: Implications for its mechanism of action in affective illness. Ann NY Acad Sci 462, 376–388.

Potter WZ (1994) ECT methodologic issues. Psychopharmacol Bull 30, 455–460.

Potter WZ and Rudorfer MV (1993) Electroconvulsive therapy—A modern medical procedure. N Engl J Med 328, 882–883.

Potter WZ, Rudorfer MV, and Manji H (1991) The pharmacologic treatment of depression. N Engl J Med 325, 633–642.

Price TR and McAllister TW (1989) Safety and efficacy of ECT in depressed patients with dementia: A review of clinical experience. Convuls Ther 5, 61–74.

Pridmore S (2000) Substitution of rapid transcranial magnetic stimulation treatments for electroconvulsive therapy treatments in a course of electroconvulsive therapy. Depress Anx 12, 118–123.

Prudic J and Sackeim HA (1999) Electroconvulsive therapy and suicide risk. J Clin Psychiatr 60(Suppl 2), 104–110.

Prudic J, Haskett RF, Mulsant B, et al. (1996) Resistance to antidepressant medications and short-term clinical response to ECT. Am J Psychiatr 153, 985–992.

Prudic J, Olfson M, and Sackeim HA (2001) Electro-convulsive therapy practices in the community. Psychol Med 31, 929–934.

Prudic J, Peyser S, and Sackeim HA (2000) Subjective memory complaints: A review of patient self-assessment of memory after electroconvulsive therapy. J ECT 16, 121–132.

Prudic J, Sackeim H, and Devanand D (1990) Medication resistance and clinical response to electroconvulsive therapy. Psychiatr Res 31, 287–296.

Rabheru K (2001) The use of electroconvulsive therapy in special patient populations. Can J Psychiatr 46, 710–719.

Rasmussen K and Abrams R (1991) Treatment of Parkinson's disease with electroconvulsive therapy. Psychiatr Clin N Am 14, 925–933.

Rasmussen KG and Zorumski CF (1993) Electroconvulsive therapy in patients taking theophylline. J Clin Psychiatr 54, 427–431.

Rasmussen KG, Rummans TA, and Richardson JW (2002a) Electroconvulsive therapy in the medically ill. Psychiatr Clin N Am 25, 177–193.

Rasmussen KG, Sampson SM, and Rummans TA (2002b) Electroconvulsive therapy and newer modalities for the treatment of medication-refractory mental illness. Mayo Clin Proc 77, 552–556.

Regenold WT, Weintraub D, and Taller A (1998) Electroconvulsive therapy for epilepsy and major depression. Am J Geriatr Psychiatr 6, 180–183.

Reid WH, Keller L, Leatherman M, et al. (1998) ECT in Texas: 19 months of mandatory reporting. J Clin Psychiatr 59, 8–13.

Rey JM and Walter G (1997) Half a century of ECT use in young people. Am J Psychiatr 154, 595–602.

Rice EH, Sombrotto LB, Markowitz JC, et al. (1994) Cardiovascular morbidity in high-risk patients during ECT. Am J Psychiatr 151, 1637–1641.

Rich CL, Spiker DG, Jewell SW, et al. (1984) The efficiency of ECT: I. Response rate in depressive episodes. Psychiatr Res 11, 167–176.

Riddle WJ, Scott AI, Bennie J, et al. (1993) Current intensity and oxytocin release after electroconvulsive therapy. Biol Psychiatr 33, 839–841.

Ridell SA (1963) The therapeutic efficacy of ECT. Arch Gen Psychiatr 8, 42–52.

Rifkin A (1988) ECT versus tricyclic antidepressants in depression: A review of the evidence. J Clin Psychiatr 49, 3–7.

Roemer RA, Dubin WR, Jaffe R, et al. (1990) An efficacy study of single-versus double-seizure induction with ECT in major depression. J Clin Psychiatr 51, 473–478.

Rohland BM (2000) Self-report of improvement following hospitalization for electroconvulsive therapy: Relationship to functional status and service use. Admin Policy Ment Health 28, 193–203.

Roose SP, Glassman AH, Attia E, et al. (1994) Comparative efficacy of selective serotonin reuptake inhibitors and tricyclics in the treatment of melancholia. Am J Psychiatr 151, 1735–1739.

Rosebush PI, Hildebrand AM, and Mazurek MF (1992) The treatment of catatonia: Benzodiazepines or ECT? Am J Psychiatr 149, 1279–1280.

Rosenbach ML, Hermann RC, and Dorwart RA (1997) Use of electroconvulsive therapy in the Medicare population between 1987 and 1992. Psychiatr Serv 48, 1537–1542.

Royal College of Psychiatrists (1995) The ECT Handbook: The Second Report of The Royal College of Psychiatrists' Special Committee on ECT. London, England.

Rudorfer MV (1994) New directions for ECT research: Overview. Psychopharmacol Bull 30, 261–264.

Rudorfer MV (2000) Electroconvulsive therapy in treatment-refractory obsessive–compulsive disorder. In Obsessive–Compulsive Disorder: Contemporary Issues in Treatment, Goodman WK, Rudorfer MV, and Maser JD (eds). Lawrence Erlbaum Associates, Mahwah, New Jersey, pp. 431–455.

Rudorfer MV and Goodwin FK (1993) Introduction. In The Clinical Science of Electroconvulsive Therapy, Coffey CE (ed). American Psychiatric Press, Washington DC, pp. xvii–xxi.

Rudorfer MV and Harris HW (in press) Schizoaffective disorder: Past, present, and future. Schizophr Bull.

Rudorfer MV and Lebowitz BD (1999) Progress in ECT research (letter to editor). Am J Psychiatr 156, 975.

Rudorfer MV and Linnoila M (1987) Electroconvulsive therapy. In Lithium Therapy Monographs, Vol. 1: Lithium Combination Treatment, Johnson FN (ed). Karger, Basel, Switzerland, pp. 164–178.

Rudorfer MV, Linnoila M, and Potter WZ (1987) Combined lithium and electroconvulsive therapy: Pharmacokinetic and pharmacodynamic interactions. Convuls Ther 3, 40–45.

Rudorfer MV, Manji HK, and Potter WZ (1991) Bupropion, ECT, and dopaminergic overdrive (letter to editor). Am J Psychiatr 148, 1101–1102.

Rudorfer MV, Manji HK, and Potter WZ (1992) ECT and delirium in Parkinson's disease. Am J Psychiatr 149, 1758–1759.

Rudorfer MV, Manji HK, Osman OT, et al. (in press) The biochemical effects of electroconvulsive therapy in depressed patients: Changes in cerebrospinal fluid monoamine metabolite concentrations. J ECT.

Rudorfer MV, Risby ED, Hsiao JK, et al. (1988) Disparate biochemical actions of electroconvulsive therapy and antidepressant drugs. Convuls Ther 4, 133–140.

Rudorfer MV, Risby ED, Osman OT, et al. (1991) Hypothalamic-pituitary-adrenal axis and monoamine transmitter activity in depression: A pilot study of central and peripheral effects of electroconvulsive therapy. Biol Psychiatr 29, 253–264.

Rugulies R (2002) Depression as a predictor for coronary heart disease: A review and meta-analysis. Am J Prev Med 23, 51–61.

Rush AJ and Weissenburger JE (1994) Melancholic symptom features and DSM-IV. Am J Psychiatr 151, 489–498.

Rush AJ, George MS, Sackeim HA, et al. (2000) Vagus nerve stimulation (VNS) for treatment-resistant depressions: A multicenter study. Biol Psychiatr 47, 276–286.

Sackeim HA (1993) The use of electroconvulsive therapy in late life depression. In Diagnosis and Treatment of Depression in Late Life, Schneider LS, Reynolds III CF, Lebowitz BD, et al. (eds). American Psychiatric Press, Washington DC, pp. 259–277.

Sackeim HA (1994) Continuation therapy following ECT: Directions for future research. Psychopharmacol Bull 30, 501–521.

Sackeim HA and Prohovnik I (1993) Brain imaging studies in depressive disorders. In Biology of Depressive Disorders, Mann JJ and Kupfer D (eds). Plenum Press, New York, pp. 205–258.

Sackeim HA, Decina P, Portnoy S, et al. (1987b) Studies of dosage, seizure threshold, and seizure duration in ECT. Biol Psychiatr 22, 249–268.

Sackeim HA, Decina P, Prohovnik I, et al. (1987a) Seizure threshold in electroconvulsive therapy: Effects of sex, age, electrode placement, and number of treatments. Arch Gen Psychiatr 44, 355–360.

Sackeim HA, Decina P, Prohovnik I, et al. (1983) Anticonvulsant and antidepressant properties of electroconvulsive therapy: A proposed mechanism of action. Biol Psychiatr 18, 1301–1310.

Sackeim HA, Devanand DP, and Prudic J (1991) Stimulus intensity, seizure threshold, and seizure duration: Impact on the efficacy and safety of electroconvulsive therapy. Psychiatr Clin N Am 14, 803–843.

Sackeim HA, Haskett RF, Mulsant BH, et al. (2001a) Continuation pharmacotherapy in the prevention of relapse following electroconvulsive therapy: A randomized controlled trial. JAMA 285, 1299–1307

Sackeim HA, Long J, Luber B, et al. (1994) Physical properties and quantification of the ECT stimulus: I. Basic principles. Convuls Ther 10, 93–123.

Sackeim HA, Luber B, Moeller JR, et al. (2000a) Electrophysiological correlates of the adverse cognitive effects of electroconvulsive therapy. J ECT 16, 110–120.

Sackeim HA, Prudic J, Devanand DP, et al. (1993) Effects of stimulus intensity and electrode placement on the efficacy and cognitive effects of electroconvulsive therapy. N Engl J Med 328, 839–846.

Sackeim HA, Prudic J, Devanand DP, et al. (1990a) The impact of medication resistance and continuation pharmacotherapy on relapse following response to electroconvulsive therapy in major depression. J Clin Psychopharmacol 10, 96–104.

Sackeim HA, Prudic J, and Devanand DP (1990b) Treatment of medication-resistant depression with electroconvulsive therapy. In Annual Review of Psychiatry, Vol. 9. Tasman A, Goldfinger SM, and Kaufmann CA (eds). American Psychiatric Press, Washington DC, pp. 91–115.

Sackeim HA, Prudic J, Devanand DP, et al. (2000b) A prospective, randomized, double-blind comparison of bilateral and right unilateral electroconvulsive therapy at different stimulus intensities. Arch Gen Psychiatr 57, 425–434.

Sackeim HA, Rush AJ, George MS, et al. (2001b) Vagus nerve stimulations (VNS) for treatment-resistant depression: Efficacy, side effects, and predictors of outcome. Neuropsychopharmacology 25, 713–728.

Sajatovic M and Meltzer HY (1993) The effect of short-term electroconvulsive treatment plus neuroleptics in treatment-resistant schizophrenia and schizoaffective disorder. Convuls Ther 9, 167–175.

Sakar P, Andrade C, Kapur B, et al. (1994) An exploratory evaluation of ECT in haloperidol-treated DSM-III-R schizophreniform disorder. Convuls Ther 10, 271–278.

Salzman C (1980) The use of ECT in the treatment of schizophrenia. Am J Psychiatr 137, 1032–1041.

Salzman C (1982) Electroconvulsive therapy in the elderly patient. Psychiatr Clin N Am 5, 191–197.

Sareen J, Enns MW, and Guertin JE (2000) The impact of clinically diagnosed personality disorders on acute and one-year outcomes of electroconvulsive therapy. J ECT 16, 43–51.

Schaerf FW, Miller RR, Lipsey JR, et al. (1989) ECT for major depression in four patients infected with human immunodeficiency virus. Am J Psychiatr 146, 782–784.

Schneekloth TD, Rummans TA, and Logan KM (1993) Electroconvulsive therapy in adolescents. Convuls Ther 9, 158–166.

Schnur DB, Mukherjee S, Sackeim HA, et al. (1992) Symptomatic predictors of ECT response in medication-nonresponsive manic patients. J Clin Psychiatr 53, 63–66.

Schultz SK, Anderson EA, and van de Borne P (1997) Heart rate variability before and after treatment with electroconvulsive therapy. J Affect Disord 44, 13–20.

Schwarz T, Loewenstein J, and Isenberg KE (1995) Maintenance ECT: Indications and outcome. Convuls Ther 11, 14–23.

Scott AI (1989) Which depressed patients will respond to electroconvulsive therapy? The search for biological predictors of recovery. Br J Psychiatr 154, 8–17.

Scott AI, Milner JB, Shering PA, et al. (1990) Fall in free thyroxine after ECT: Real effect or an artefact of assay? Biol Psychiatr 27, 784–786.

Scott AI, Phil M, and Boddy H (2000) The effect of repeated bilateral electroconvulsive therapy on seizure threshold. J ECT 16, 244–251.

Scott AI, Shering PA, Legros JJ, et al. (1991) Improvement in depressive illness is not associated with altered release of neurophysins over a course of ECT. Psychiatr Res 36, 65–73.

Scott AI, Walley LJ, Bennie J, et al. (1986) Oestrogen-stimulated neurophysin and outcome after electroconvulsive therapy. Lancet 1, 1411–1414.

Scott AI, Weeks DJ, and McDonald CF (1991) Continuation electroconvulsive therapy: Preliminary guidelines and an illustrative case report. Br J Psychiatr 159, 867–870.

Seager CP and Bird RL (1962) Imipramine with electrical treatment in depression: A controlled trial. J Ment Sci 108, 704–707.

Shapira B, Kindleer S, and Lerer B (1988) Medication outcome in ECT-resistant depression. Convuls Ther 4, 192–198.

Shapira B, Tubi N, and Lerer B (2000) Balancing speed of response of ECT in major depression and adverse cognitive effects: Role of treatment schedule. J ECT 16, 97–109.

Sharma V (1999) Retrospective controlled study of inpatient ECT: Does it prevent suicide? J Affect Disord 56, 183–187.

Shiwach RS, Reid WH, and Carmody TJ (2001) An analysis of reported deaths following electroconvulsive therapy in Texas, 1993–1998. Psychiatr Serv 52, 1095–1097.

Sikdar S, Kulhara P, Avasthi A, et al. (1994) Combined chlorpromazine and electroconvulsive therapy in mania. Br J Psychiatr 164, 806–810.

Small JG (1985) Efficacy of electroconvulsive therapy in schizophrenia, mania, and other disorders. I. Schizophrenia. Convuls Ther 1, 263–270.

Small JG, Klapper MH, Kellams JJ, et al. (1988) Electroconvulsive treatment compared with lithium in the management of manic states. Arch Gen Psychiatr 45, 727–732.

Small JG, Milstein V, Klapper MH, et al. (1986) Electroconvulsive therapy in the treatment of manic episodes. In Electroconvulsive Therapy—Clinical and Basic Research Issues, Malitz S and Sackeim HA (eds). New York Academy of Sciences, New York, pp. 37–49.

Sobin C, Prudic J, Devanand DP, et al. (1996) Who responds to electroconvulsive therapy? A comparison of effective and ineffective forms of treatment. Br J Psychiatr 169, 322–328.

Sommer BR, Satlin A, Friedman L, et al. (1989) Glycopyrrolate versus atropine in post-ECT amnesia in the elderly. J Geriatr Psychiatr Neurol 2, 18–21.

Spiker DG, Stein J, and Rich CL (1985) Delusional depression and electroconvulsive therapy: One year later. Convuls Ther 1, 167–172.

Stephens SM, Greenberg RM, and Pettinati HM (1991) Choosing an electroconvulsive therapy device. Psychiatr Clin N Am 14, 989–1006.

Stephens SM, Pettinati HM, Greenberg RM, et al. (1993) Continuation and maintenance therapy with outpatient ECT. In The Clinical Science of Electroconvulsive Therapy, Coffey CE (ed). American Psychiatric Press, Washington DC, pp. 143–164.

Stern RA, Steketee MC, Durr AL, et al. (1993) Combined use of thyroid hormone and ECT. Convuls Ther 9, 285–292.

Stromgren LS (1988) Electroconvulsive therapy in Aarhus, Denmark, in 1984: Its application in nondepressive disorders. Convuls Ther 4, 306–313.

Stromgren LS (1991) Electroconvulsive therapy in the Nordic countries, 1977–1987. Acta Psychiatr Scand 84, 428–434.

Swartz CM (1985) Characterization of the total amount of prolactin released by electroconvulsive therapy. Convuls Ther 1, 252–257.

Swartz CM (1993) Anesthesia for ECT. Convuls Ther 9, 301–316.

Swartz CM (1994) Asymmetric bilateral right frontotemporal left frontal stimulus electrode placement for electroconvulsive therapy. Neuropsychobiology 29, 174–178.

Swartz CM (2000) Physiological response to ECT stimulus dose. Psychiatr Res 97, 229–235.

Swartz CM, Abrams R, and Drews V (1988) Serotinin and electroconvulsive shock-induced prolactin release. Convuls Ther 4, 141–145.

Sylvester AP, Mulsant BH, Chengappa KN, et al. (2000) Use of electroconvulsive therapy in a state hospital: A 10-year review. J Clin Psychiatr 61, 534–539.

Taieb O, Flament MF, Corcos M, et al. (2001) Electroconvulsive therapy in adolescents with mood disorder: Patients' and parents' attitudes. Psychiatr Res 104, 183–190.

Tang WK and Ungvari GS (2001a) Asystole during electroconvulsive therapy: A case report. Austral N Z J Psychiatr 35, 382–385.

Tang WK and Ungvari GS (2001b) Electroconvulsive therapy in rehabilitation: The Hong Kong experience. Psychiatr Serv 52, 303–306.

Tanney BL (1986) Electroconvulsive therapy and suicide. Suicide Life Threat Behav 16, 198–222.

Taylor MA and Abrams R (1977) Catatonia: Prevalence and importance in the manic phase of manic–depressive illness. Arch Gen Psychiatr 34, 1223–1225.

Tew JD Jr., Mulsant BH, Haskett RF, et al. (1999) Acute efficacy of ECT in the treatment of major depression in the old–old. Am J Psychiatr 156, 1865–1870.

Tharyan P and Adams CE (2002) Electroconvulsive therapy for schizophrenia. Cochrane Database Syst Rev 2, CD000076.

Thomas J and Reddy B (1982) The treatment of mania: A retrospective evaluation of the effects of ECT, chlorpromazine, and lithium. J Affect Disord 4, 85–92.

Thompson JW and Blaine JD (1987) Use of ECT in the United States in 1975 and 1980. Am J Psychiatr 144, 557–562.

Thompson JW, Weiner RD, and Myers CP (1994) Use of ECT in the United States in 1975, 1980, and 1986. Am J Psychiatr 151, 1657–1661.

Thornton JE, Mulsant BH, Dealy R, et al. (1990) A retrospective study of maintenance electroconvulsive therapy in a university-based psychiatric practice. Convuls Ther 6, 121–129.

Tortella FC and Long JB (1985) Endogenous anticonvulsant substance in rat cerebrospinal fluid after a generalized seizure. Science 228, 1106–1108.

Tortella FC, Long JB, Hong J, et al. (1989) Modulation of endogenous opioid systems by electroconvulsive shock. Convuls Ther 5, 261–273.

Turek IS and Hanlon TE (1977) The effectiveness and safety of electroconvulsive therapy (ECT). J Nerv Ment Dis 164, 419–431.

Ungavari GS, Leung CM, Wong MK, et al. (1994) Benzodiazepines in the treatment of catatonic syndrome. Acta Psychiatr Scand 89, 285–288.

US Department of Health and Human Services (1999) Mental Health: A Report of the Surgeon General. US Department of Health and Human Services, Substance Abuse and Mental Health Services Administration/ Center for Mental Health Services, National Institutes of Health/ National Institute of Mental Health, Rockville, MD.

Vakil E, Grunhaus L, Nagar I, et al. (2000) The effect of electroconvulsive therapy (ECT) on implicit memory: Skill learning and perceptual priming in patients with major depression. Neuropsychologia 38, 1405–1414.

Van Gerpen MW, Johnson JE, and Winstead DK (1999) Mania in the geriatric patient population. Am J Geriatr Psychiatr 7, 188–202.

Van Valkenburg C and Clayton PJ (1985) Electroconvulsive therapy and schizophrenia. Biol Psychiatr 20, 699–700.

Van Waarde JA, Stolker JJ, and van der Mast RC (2001) ECT in mental retardation: A review. J ECT 17, 236–243.

Villalonga A, Bernardo M, Gomar C, et al. (1993) Cardiovascular response and anesthetic recovery in electroconvulsive therapy with propofol or thiopental. Convuls Ther 9, 108–111.

Wägner A, Aberg-Wistedt A, Asberg M, et al. (1987) Effects of antidepressant treatments on platelet tritiated imipramine binding in major depressive disorder. Arch Gen Psychiatr 44, 870–877.

Walker R and Swartz CM (1994) Electroconvulsive therapy during high-risk pregnancy. Gen Hosp Psychiatr 16, 348–353.

Walter G, Koster K, and Rey JM (1999) Views about treatment among parents of adolescents who received electroconvulsive therapy. Psychiatr Serv 50, 701–702.

Weiner RD (1994) Treatment optimization with ECT. Psychopharmacol Bull 30, 313–320.

Weiner RD, Rogers HJ, Davidson JR, et al. (1986) Effects of stimulus parameters on cognitive side effects. Ann NY Acad Sci 462, 315–325.

Weinger MB, Partridge BL, Hauger R, et al. (1991) Prevention of the cardiovascular and neuroendocrine response to electroconvulsive therapy: I. Effectiveness of pretreatment regimens on hemodynamics. Anesth Analg 73, 556–562.

Wengel SP, Burke W, Pfeiffer RF, et al. (1998) Maintenance electroconvulsive therapy for intractable Parkinson's disease. Am J Geriatr Psychiatr 6, 263–269.

Westphal JR, Horswell R, Kumar S, et al. (1997) Quantifying utilization and practice variation of electroconvulsive therapy. Convuls Ther 13, 242–252.

Whalley LJ, Rosie R, Dick H, et al. (1982) Immediate increases in plasma prolactin and neurophysin but not other hormones after electroconvulsive therapy. Lancet 2, 1064–1068.

Willner P (1997) Validity, reliability, and utility of the chronic mild stress model of depression: A 10-year review and evaluation. Psychopharmacology 134, 319–329.

Winokur G, Black DW, and Nasrallah A (1988) Depressions secondary to other psychiatric disorders and medical illnesses. Am J Psychiatr 145, 233–237.

Wyatt RJ (1991) Neuroleptics and the natural course of schizophrenia. Schizophr Bull 17, 325–351.

Yatham LN, Clark CC, and Zis AP (2000) A preliminary study of the effects of electroconvulsive therapy on regional brain glucose metabolism in patients with major depression. J ECT 16, 171–176.

Young EA, Grunhaus L, Haskett RF, et al. (1991) Heterogeneity in the beta-endorphin immunoreactivity response to electroconvulsive therapy. Arch Gen Psychiatr 48, 534–539.

Young RC, Alexopoulos GS, and Shamoian CA (1985) Dissociation of motor response from mood and cognition in a parkinsonian patient treated with ECT. Biol Psychiatr 20, 566–569.

Zachrisson OGG, Balldin J, Ekman R, et al. (2000) No evident neuronal damage after electroconvulsive therapy. Psychiatr Res 96, 157–165.

Zervas IM and Fink M (1991) ECT for refractory Parkinson's disease. Convuls Ther 7, 222–223.

Zielinski RJ, Roose SP, Devanand DP, et al. (1993) Cardiovascular complications of ECT in depressed patients with cardiac disease. Am J Psychiatr 150, 904–909.

Zimmerman M, Coryell W, Pfohl B, et al. (1986a) ECT response in depressed patients with and without a DSM-III personality disorder. Am J Psychiatr 143, 1030–1032.

Zimmerman M, Coryell W, Pfohl B, et al. (1990) What happens when ECT does not work? A prospective follow-up study of ECT failures. Ann Clin Psychiatr 2, 47–51.

Zimmerman M, Coryell W, Stangl D, et al. (1986b) An American validation study of the Newcastle scale. III. Course during index hospitalization and six-month prospective follow-up. Acta Psychiatr Scand 73, 412–415.

Zis AP, Nomikos GG, Damsma G, et al. (1991) In vivo neurochemical effects of electroconvulsive shock studied by microdialysis in the rat striatum. Psychopharmacology 103, 343–350.

Zornberg GL and Pope HJ (1993) Treatment of depression in bipolar disorder: New directions for research. J Clin Psychopharmacol 13, 397–408.

Zorumski CF, Burke WJ, Rutherford JL, et al. (1986a) ECT: Clinical variables, seizure duration, and outcome. Convuls Ther 2, 109–119.

Zorumski CF, Rubin EH, and Burke WJ (1988) Electroconvulsive therapy for the elderly: A review. Hosp Comm Psychiatr 39, 643–647.

Zorumski CF, Rutherford JL, and Burke WJ (1986b) ECT in primary and secondary depression. J Clin Psychiatr 47, 298–300.

CHAPTER

# 93 Neurosurgery for Treatment-Refractory Psychiatric Disorders: Obsessive–Compulsive Disorder and Major Depressive Disorder

Brian Martis
Rees Cosgrove
Michael Jenike

## Introduction

The history of palliative neurosurgical treatments of refractory psychiatric disorders has not been without controversy (Feldman and Goodrich 2001). Though Burckhardt is credited with the first report of intentional brain lesioning to alter behavior in 1891 (Feldman and Goodrich 2001), Egaz Moniz and Almeida Lima of Portugal introduced prefrontal leucotomy for intractable psychotic illness in 1936 and coined the term *psychosurgery* (Moniz 1937). From the 1930s to the 1950s thousands of prefrontal leukotomy/lobotomy procedures were performed with the foremost proponents in the US being Freeman and Watts (1942). Severe overcrowding of institutionalized chronic psychiatric patients and the unavailability of effective treatments (prior to 1954) were important factors that contributed to the enthusiastic use of surgery. The early surgical procedures often consisted of poorly conceived and crudely executed prefrontal white matter lesions and were associated with many adverse effects on motivation, personality, and neurological functioning. Nevertheless, many patients in the prepsychopharmacologic era improved after surgery but the overall experience has understandably sensitized both the professional and lay communities. This memory lives on in the form of severe restrictions and even bans on the use of these procedures in some countries.

A few neurosurgical procedures have however stood the test of time and are utilized for patients with treatment-refractory obsessive–compulsive disorder (OCD) and major depressive disorder (MDD). Stereotactic neurosurgical procedures were introduced in 1954 in an attempt to optimize outcomes and reduce the morbidity of earlier interventions. Over the next 3 decades, a more cautious application of neurosurgical procedures evolved aided by advances in both psychiatry and neurosurgery. This evolution resulted in the development of four procedures (cingulotomy, capsulotomy, subcaudate tractotomy, and limbic leukotomy) that continue to be performed at various centers today. Significant progress in the diagnosis and treatment of psychiatric disorders continues, and the availability of precision neurosurgical techniques and sophisticated clinical and neuroimaging assessment strategies promises better data to help guide researchers and clinicians in the refinement of these palliative strategies. Indeed, over the past decade, more sophisticated prospective studies in psychiatric neurosurgery are being reported in an ongoing attempt to provide relief in a scientific and ethical manner (Baer et al. 1995, Poynton et al. 1995, Dougherty et al. 2002).

Despite these recent developments, the paucity of carefully controlled prospective studies of neurosurgical intervention for refractory psychiatric illness compels us to constantly review the risk/benefit ratio of such treatments. This chapter discusses psychiatric aspects of palliative neurosurgical procedures for treatment-refractory psychiatric disease, specifically treatment-refractory OCD and treatment-refractory MDD.

## Characteristics of Patients Undergoing Neurosurgery for Treatment-Refractory OCD and MDD

Though selection criteria have not been standardized across centers, a review of most reported studies from several countries suggests that only OCD or MDD patients who have not responded to a variety of exhaustive treatments are considered for palliative neurosurgery. Treatments include multiple adequate medication trials, an adequate trial of behavioral treatment/psychotherapy, and electroconvulsive therapy (ECT) for MDD—patients are severely disabled for several years despite these efforts (Table 93–1). In addition to the essential informed consent of the patient, a panel of specialists, usually constituted at the institutional level, carefully reviews all aspects of the patient's condition before making a consensus decision on surgery. In England, Wales, Belgium as well as in the state of Victoria in Australia, a clinical assessment and informed consent from the patient has to be accompanied by approval of an independent panel appointed by the Mental Health Act Commission (Malhi and Bartlett 2000).

Severe, chronic OCD and MDD referrals commonly present with comorbidities including depression, obsessive–compulsive "psychosis," substance abuse, history of harmful behavior, and personality disorders. The decision to offer surgery must be evaluated on a case-by-case basis, carefully considering the benefits and risks of intervention, alongside those of nonintervention. Tables 93–1 and 93–2 contain guidelines for indications and relative contraindications for these procedures evolved in the context of 25 years of experience with the stereotactic cingulotomy procedure for intractable psychiatric disorder at one center.[1] At this center, the Cingulotomy Assessment Committee

| Table 93–2 | Suggested Guidelines: RELATIVE Contraindications to Neurosurgical Intervention |
|---|---|

1. Age younger than 18 yr or older than 65 yr.
2. The patient has another current or lifetime Axis I diagnosis (e.g., organic brain syndrome, delusional disorder, somatization or current or recent substance abuse) that substantially complicates diagnosis, treatment, or the patient's ability to comply with treatment or a chronically unstable clinical course (e.g., history of multiple impulsive suicidal attempts).
3. A complicating current DSM-IV Axis II diagnosis from cluster A (e.g., paranoid personality disorder) or B (e.g., borderline, antisocial, or histrionic personality disorder). A current cluster C personality disorder (e.g., avoidant or obsessive–compulsive personality disorder) is generally not a contraindication.
4. The patient has a current Axis III diagnosis with brain pathology, such as moderate or marked cerebral atrophy, stroke, or tumor or has undergone previous neurosurgical procedures that have a high likelihood of producing unacceptable complications.

(CAC), a multidisciplinary team (consisting of psychiatrists, neurologists, neurosurgeons, psychologists, and experienced clinic staff), meets on a monthly basis to review referrals for cingulotomy and repeat procedures, as well as to discuss follow-up, quality control issues, and outcomes.

## Interventions

Currently, only a few specialized centers in the world conduct neurosurgical procedures for treatment-refractory OCD and treatment-refractory MDD. These procedures have evolved at particular centers more by convention and experience than by controlled research studies and direct comparison of the various procedures. The modern neurosurgical procedures include (1) cingulotomy, (2) anterior capsulotomy, (3) subcaudate tractotomy, and (4) limbic leukotomy. All four procedures involve magnetic resonance (MR) imaging guided stereotactic lesions placed bilaterally in the various target regions, after which they are named.

### Cingulotomy

Initially reported as an open procedure in the 1950s (Whitty et al. 1952), anterior cingulotomy has been performed stereotactically since the 1960s for intractable anxiety and mood disorders. This procedure has since evolved into the neurosurgical intervention of choice for the past 25 years in North America for treatment-refractory pain, major depression, and OCD (Ballantine et al. 1987, Jenike 1998).

Earlier stereotactic cingulotomy was performed using indirect targeting with ventriculography. Currently, cingulotomy is an MR imaging guided stereotactic procedure. Briefly, a preoperative MR image is taken while the patient wears an MR compatible stereotactic frame for localization and demarcation of targets in the rostral anterior cingulum (Broadmann's Area 24 and 32). Then, in the operating room, under local anesthesia and intravenous sedation, electrodes with a 10 mm exposed tip are introduced via bilateral burr holes, using a stereotactic frame to the predetermined cingulate targets approximately 7 mm from the midline and

| Table 93–1 | Suggested Guidelines: Indications for Neurosurgical Intervention for IOCD (Intractable Obsessive–Compulsive Disorder) |
|---|---|

1. Patient fulfills the diagnostic criteria for OCD/MDD (SCID derived DSM-IV OR comparable such as ICD-10).
2. The duration of illness exceeds 5 yr.
3. The disorder is severe (while not necessarily reflective of overall disability, OCD patients usually have YBOCS scores of ≥20) and is causing substantial distress.
4. The disorder is causing substantial reduction in the patient's psychosocial functioning (e.g., Global Assessment of Functioning (GAF) of 40 and below).
5. Current treatment options* tried systematically for at least 5 yr either have been without appreciable effect on the symptoms or must be discontinued owing to intolerable side effects.
6. The prognosis, without neurosurgical intervention, is considered poor.
7. The patient gives informed consent.
8. The patient agrees to participate in the preoperative evaluation and postoperative rehabilitation programs respectively.
9. The patients' local referring physician is willing to acknowledge responsibility for the postoperative long-term management of the patient.

*OCD: Adequate trials (at least 12 weeks at the maximally tolerated dose) of all serotoninergic agents (clomipramine, paroxetine, fluoxetine, fluvoxamine, sertraline), and possibly a serotoninergic–noradrenergic agent (venlafaxine) and MAO-I as well; as augmentation of at least one of these drugs for 1 month: lithium, clonazepam, buspirone or other experimental agents; all patients must have had an adequate trial of behavioral therapy (at least 20 hours of "real" exposure and response prevention therapy).

[1] Massachusetts General Hospital (MGH): OCD Clinic and Cingulotomy Program, Boston, MA, USA.

20 mm posterior to the tip of the frontal horn. Radiofrequency thermolesions are then created by heating the electrode tips to 80 to 85° for 90 seconds. This results in a 1 cm lesion in the cingulate bundles. Usually one or more lesions are made bilaterally in the rostral anterior cingulate cortex (Figure 93–1).

Multiple studies (discussed later) have reported modest benefit at a high benefit/adverse effects ratio (Jenike et al. 1991, Baer et al. 1995, Dougherty et al. 2002) making cingulotomy a useful palliative procedure with a relatively benign risk profile. Second and even third repeat cingulotomies in psychiatric subjects are not uncommon.

## Anterior Capsulotomy

Two surgical techniques for creating lesions in the anterior limb of the internal capsule (Ant. IC), the radiofrequency thermolesion and the radiosurgical or "gamma" capsulotomy, were developed in Sweden (Figure 93–2). The primary indications for these procedures over the past 3 decades have been OCD and treatment-refractory "anxiety." More recently, these procedures are being done in US centers as well. In the stereotactic radiofrequency thermolesion procedure developed by Lars Leksell (Bingley et al. 1977, Burzaco 1981, Mindus 1991), the operation is performed under local anesthesia and light sedation. After determining the coordinates of the target in the Ant. IC with MRI, small bilateral burr holes are made just behind the coronary suture. Monopolar electrodes with a 5 mm exposed tip are inserted into the target area stereotactically. Thermolesions are then produced by heating the uninsulated tip of the electrode for 75 seconds to approximately 75°, creating a lesion approximately 15 to 18 mm long and 4 mm wide. Patients do not report any subjective sensations during lesion induction. Immediate postoperative confusion and urinary incontinence are common. A transient mild

decrease in initiative and mental drive may be noted during the first 2 to 3 postoperative months. Most patients are reported to gain weight postoperatively (less than 11 pounds) (Meyerson and Mindus 1988; based on 68 patients who underwent the procedure between 1970 and 1985).

In the radiosurgical technique (gamma capsulotomy), also developed by Leksell and colleagues, bilateral lesions are produced by cross firing approximately 200 narrow beams of cobalt 60 gamma irradiation from a stereotactic gamma unit. While an individual beam exerts negligible biological effects, the combined effect of multiple beams converging on a single point of locus produces a radiosurgical lesion. Using a standardized dose of 140 to 160 gray and a 4 mm collimator, the typical lesions measure approximately 15 to 20 mm high × 8 mm wide. There is however considerable variability in lesion size due to individual radiobiological differences. The advantage of this procedure is that it can be performed noninvasively and on an outpatient basis. While experience with the gamma capsulotomy technique is less extensive than that of the radiofrequency thermolesion, comparable results have been reported (Meyerson and Mindus 1988, Mindus et al. 1987). No case of radiation-induced malignancy has been reported in the 2 decades during which the procedure has been in use.

## Subcaudate Tractotomy

The original subcaudate tractotomy procedure was developed by Geoffrey Knight in London in the 1960s and has been used for the ensuing 3 decades primarily for the palliative treatment of refractory mood disorder (Strom-Olsen and Carlisle 1971, Göktepe et al. 1975, Hodgkiss et al. 1995). In the original procedure, lesions were created by yttrium (Y-90) beta radiation (half-life 60

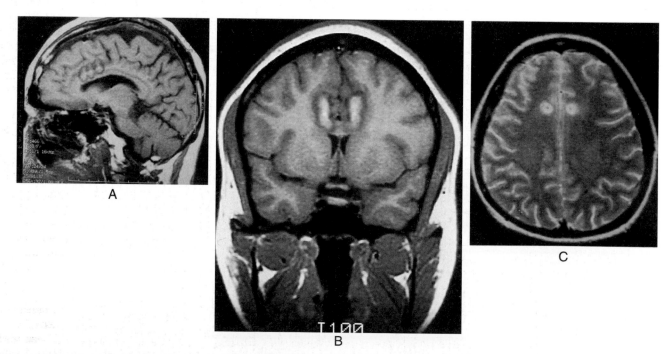

A

B

C

**Figure 93–1** Anterior cingulotomy. (A) *Acute sagittal MRI demonstrating three contiguous cingulotomy lesions;* (B) *Acute coronal view;* (C) *Chronic axial MRI demonstrating single cingulotomy lesion.*

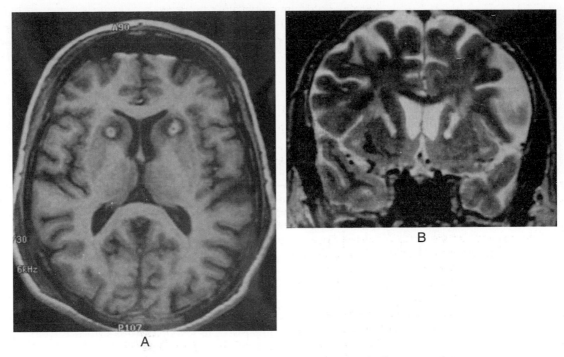

**Figure 93–2** *Anterior capsulotomy* (A) *Acute axial view;* (B) *Chronic coronal view.*

hours) 7 mm × 1 mm seeds, stereotactically implanted via low frontal burr holes bilaterally in the white matter, beneath and just anterior to the caudate head. Early postoperative confusion that seemed to correlate with radiologically verified transient edema was reported as a possible side effect (Malizia 1991). More recently, Y-90 rods have been replaced by stereotactically directed

radiofrequency electrocoagulation lesions (Figure 93–3) (Malhi and Bartlett 1998).

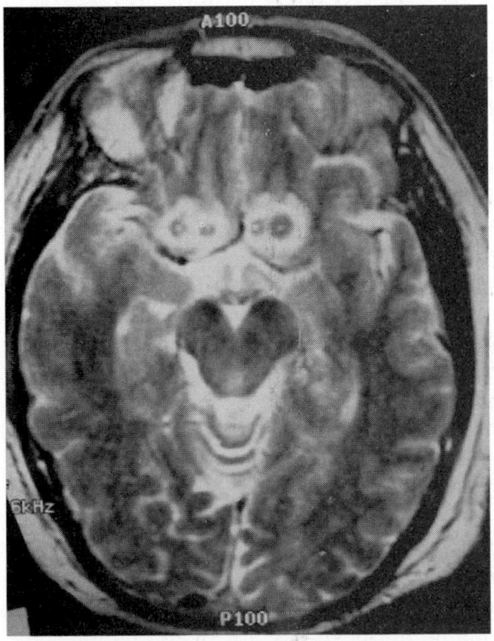

## Limbic Leukotomy

Developed by Kelly and colleagues (1973) in the UK, this procedure involves creation of lesions bilaterally in the subcaudate area and the cingulum bundle simultaneously (Figure 93–4). The theory was that two lesions affecting the limbic and paralimbic connections might be more effective than either single lesion. Twenty-six of 40 patients (65%) in their initially reported cohort were operated on for treatment-refractory OCD or anxiety (Kelly et al. 1973).

In the original procedure, after preparation with local or general anesthesia, bilateral burr holes were made 9.5 cm posterior to the nasion and 15 mm from the midline, and targets were localized by ventriculograms and intraoperative stimulation (to elicit autonomic responses) in the subcaudate area. Usually 8 to 12 lesions (cingulate and lower medial quadrant of frontal lobe, bilaterally), each approximately 6 to 10 mm in diameter, were then produced by means of radiofrequency-induced heated electrodes. Side effects reported included transient postoperative confusion and headache. Currently this procedure is done via MR guided stereotactic placement of lesions in the cingulum and subcaudate area.

## Neuroanatomic Basis for Obsessive–Compulsive Symptoms: Understanding the Effects of Neurosurgical Interventions in Treatment-Refractory OCD

Although a number of hypotheses exist, much remains unclear about the exact mechanism by which certain

**Figure 93–3** *Subcaudate tractotomy. Acute axial view.*

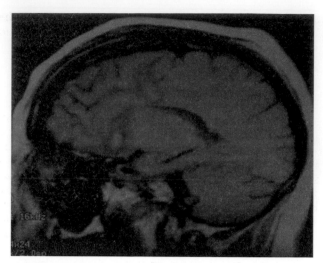

**Figure 93–4** *Limbic leukotomy. Acute sagittal combined cingulotomy and subcaudate lesions.*

neurosurgical procedures improve symptoms in some patients. Important questions to consider include: Why does interrupting certain neural pathways affect OCD and mood symptoms? What is the specificity of response to specific lesions? How can we use our accumulated neurosurgical experience, along with current neurobiological understanding, to better understand brain function in these disorders? While there are more questions than answers, we will examine some of these issues using OCD as an example.

Findings from clinical neuropsychiatry, neuroimaging, and neurosurgery, and advances in understanding the functional neuroanatomy of frontal–striatal circuits lend evidence that specific neurobiological deficits may underlie the OCD syndrome. The familial nature of OCD and the phenomenological and genetic overlap with Tourette syndrome in some patients; the association of obsessive and compulsive symptoms with neuroautoimmune syndromes like Sydenham's chorea; the association of OCD with specific brain lesions in the frontal, temporal, and cingulate areas (Berthier et al. 1996); indirect evidence of the involvement of serotonin, dopamine, and other neurotransmitters in OCD; the benefit of neurosurgical procedures in treatment-refractory OCD; and evidence from several positron emission tomography (PET) studies provide these clues.

From a neuroanatomic perspective, accumulating evidence suggests involvement of the basal ganglia in the OCD syndrome. Several neurological syndromes such as Sydenham's chorea and Tourette syndrome (TS) known to affect the basal ganglia have been associated with OC symptoms (Cummings and Frankel 1985, LaPlane et al. 1989, Weilburg et al. 1989). These observations have received further support from several recent lines of research. A subgroup of OCD patients with tics/TS or history of tics has been described: patients are usually younger, male, with obsessions and compulsions related to symmetry, religion, and aggression, and have tics (Leonard et al. 1992). In some patients with OCD (with or without tic disorders), low doses of dopaminergic antagonists (used in the treatment of tics/TS) may enhance treatment response rather than a serotoninergic agent alone (McDougle et al. 1994, 2000).

Several studies have reported a familial overlap between OCD and TS (Pauls et al. 1995). The other line of evidence involves the observation of an association between infections with group-A beta-hemolytic streptococci (GABHS) and the dramatic onset or exacerbation of neuropsychiatric symptoms including those of OCD and tics (Swedo et al. 1989). This has led to the hypotheses that OCD and TS may be different phenotypic manifestations of similar basal ganglia pathology (Baxter et al. 1990). The proposed research model suggesting a relationship between neuropsychiatric symptoms and poststreptococcal, immune mediated adverse effects on the basal ganglia, may offer clues about etiology in at least some of these patients.

Research has also implicated the orbitomedial region of the frontal lobe in OCD. The involvement of the frontal lobe in disease is associated with characteristic syndromes (depending on the region involved). Some of these features, such as decreased response inhibition, inflexibility, and difficulty getting a gestalt accompanied by excessive attention to irrelevant details, are reminiscent of the OC syndrome. While overt frontal lobe deficits have not been impressive in OCD, there is evidence from neuropsychological and structural imaging studies of OCD for subtle frontal lobe dysfunction (Savage et al. 2000, Garber et al. 1989).

PET studies have provided perhaps the most compelling evidence for implicating orbitofrontal cortex and basal ganglia dysfunction in OCD. Resting state PET [18]F-fluorodeoxyglucose studies in children and adults have consistently reported significant elevation of absolute glucose metabolic rates for the whole cerebral hemispheres and orbital gyri (OG), and somewhat less consistently for the caudate nucleus and the thalamus in OCD patients (Baxter et al. 1987, 1988, Nordahl et al. 1989, Swedo et al. 1989). Symptom provocation studies have shown increased metabolism in the OG, caudate, and thalamus among other areas (Rauch et al. 1994, Breiter et al. 1996). Treatment studies (pre–post) using various modalities such as clomipramine (Swedo et al. 1992), selective serotonin reuptake inhibitors (SSRIs) (Baxter et al. 1992, Saxena et al. 1999), and behavioral therapy (BT) (Schwartz et al. 1996) have demonstrated reduction in metabolism in corresponding areas with successful symptom attenuation. In some studies increased pretreatment local metabolic rates in the OG predicted a poorer response to fluoxetine while decreased OG metabolism predicted better response to BT (Baxter et al. 1992). These findings have been mostly replicated (Schwartz et al. 1996, Saxena et al. 2002), suggesting that these regions are involved in the symptomatic state, and may be directly or indirectly relevant to the pathophysiology of the disorder.

These findings along with a recent better understanding of basal ganglia function have prompted several authors to develop a neuroanatomical model of dysfunction in OCD. This model is based on dysfunctional activity in the frontal–striatal–pallidal–thalamic–frontal loops in the brain (Baxter et al. 1990, Insel 1992, Modell et al. 1989, Rapoport et al. 1981). Neuroanatomical evidence supports the existence of functional circuits linking cortical, striatal, and thalamic nuclei in a series of topographically defined segregated loops (Alexander et al. 1986, 1990). The basal ganglia have been described to separately influence at least five different pathways, including the orbitofrontal–mediodorsal thalamic circuit, of primary interest in OCD. This loop has two components, direct (stimulatory) and indirect (inhibitory), that modulate frontal-thalamic transmission via opposing influences on this circuit. Hypothetically, in patients with OCD, dysfunction in the modulatory activity of these complementary loops on frontal-thalamic transmission results in an overactive frontal-thalamic circuit associated with obsessive and anxiety symptoms. Subsequent activation of limbic pathways would cause increasing anxiety and discomfort. Compulsions are hypothesized to be ritualized activities in a compensatory yet dysfunctional attempt to recruit the striatum to regulate frontal-thalamic overactivity. Thus in theory, lesions placed in these circuits might serve to either interrupt aberrant overactivity or reroute compensatory strategies more efficiently.

It appears that differing interpretations of a similar notion—that the separation of cognitive elements (ascribed to frontal cortex) from the affective elements (limbic functions) was somehow desirable in both OCD and depression—have given rise to differing targets and procedures. It has been suggested that there may be two particularly salient components in the neuroanatomy of OCD: the obsessive–compulsive component and the associated anxiety component (mediated through the limbic circuit which includes the cingulum bundle, the target of cingulotomy) (Martuza et al. 1990, Kelly 1980). Thus in cingulotomy, the cingulum bundle that connects parts of the frontal cortex to the subcortical limbic structures is severed. Similarly anterior capsulotomy disconnects the frontal-thalamic projections (including the implicated frontal–striatal–pallidal–thalamic–frontal loop) and in subcaudate tractotomy, the orbitomedial–subcortical connections are interrupted.

Currently, due to lack of specific data, one can only speculate that disruption of different pathways are achieving changes by direct or compensatory effects on the frontal–striatal–thalamic pathways so as to normalize activity leading to symptom attenuation. In humans, it has been shown that lesions in one region of the brain induce degeneration in distal regions that are part of the anatomically (and by extension, functionally) connected circuit; for example, extensive degeneration in the ventral portion of the internal capsule following *substantia innominata* lesions in subcaudate tractotomy (Corsellis and Jack 1973). This degeneration can be traced back to the dorsomedial nucleus of the thalamus, which has extensive interconnections with various parts of the limbic system (Nauta 1986). More recently Rauch and colleagues (2000) reported atrophy in the caudate body and tail in subjects who had undergone one or more cingulotomies approximately 6 months after surgery. While these few studies currently do not afford broader conclusions in OCD, they demonstrate the functional connectivity of the relevant cortical and subcortical brain regions.

Additionally, preliminary evidence suggests that OCD and MDD patients do not improve immediately after surgery but that several weeks to months are required for positive clinical effects to be fully manifested. Thus, it is likely that secondary nerve degeneration or metabolic alter-

ations in brain areas, other than the region where the lesions are actually made, are involved in the therapeutic effect.

## Methodological Problems in Evaluating Retrospective Neurosurgical Reports

Most published reports of neurosurgery for treatment-refractory OCD and MDD are retrospective and usually involve a relatively small number of patients at a single center with varying assessment strategies and outcome parameters. Compounding this issue is the variability the surgical techniques used, differing entry criteria, the irregular use of validated clinical outcome rating scales, the paucity of blinded ratings, and the inability to perform an appropriate "control" procedure (i.e., a sham procedure) due to obvious ethical reasons. Most early studies have determined outcome using simple outcome scales such as the Pippard Scale, a neurosurgical outcome scale modified for OCD patients (Pippard 1955). This creates obvious difficulties in comprehensively assessing efficacy in a complex chronic disorder such as OCD. Additionally, introduction of newer, more effective treatments may result in fewer number of referrals and a decrease in "good outcome" patients (Malhi and Bartlett 2000, Jenike et al. 1991). This complicates meaningful comparison of older and newer studies.

Hopefully future studies will strive to use modern outcome measurements that are reasonably comparable over centers. An important advance is the emergence of the ability to stringently test some procedures (like gamma knife capsulotomy as well as deep brain stimulation and vagal nerve stimulation) which lend themselves to an ethically justifiable and scientifically acceptable control procedure (discussed later). On this cautionary note we review existing data.

## Neurosurgery for Treatment-Refractory OCD and Treatment-Refractory MDD: Outcome Studies

### Cingulotomy

Ballantine reviewed the long-term results of cingulotomy performed on 198 patients with a variety of chronic intractable psychiatric disorders at the Massachusetts General Hospital (MGH) between 1962 and 1985. Using subjective outcomes rating scales, the authors found that 62% of patients with treatment-resistant depression and 56% of those with treatment-refractory OCD had worthwhile improvement (long-term follow-up of 8.6 years) (Ballantine et al. 1987).

Jenike and colleagues (1991) conducted a more rigorous retrospective evaluation of the 33 patients who underwent one or more cingulotomies for treatment-refractory OCD at the MGH during that same time period (mean illness duration before first surgery: $17.9 \pm 11.3$ years; mean age at first cingulotomy: $37.3 \pm 11.3$ years). Using conservative criteria including the Yale-Brown Obsessive–Compulsive Scale (YBOCS) change (retrospective presurgical report minus current report) they reported that at least 25 to 30% of the patients "benefited substantially from the intervention." The most serious side effects in this cohort included well-controlled seizures in three patients (9%).

Four patients (12%) were reported to have committed suicide at the follow-up evaluation and one patient with pre-existing heart disease died of a myocardial infarction 6 weeks after surgery.

The same group subsequently reported findings from a prospective study of 18 treatment-refractory OCD patients (mean onset age: 14.7 years; mean age at cingulotomy: 34.9 years) assessed before and at a mean follow-up of 26.8 months after bilateral anterior cingulotomy (Baer et al. 1995). These patients were evaluated carefully with comprehensive diagnostic and outcome measures for efficacy and safety. Five patients (28%) met conservative criteria (> 35% improvement in YBOCS score) for treatment responders, and three others (17%) were possible responders. The group as a whole improved significantly in mean functional status, and few serious adverse events were found.

Spangler and colleagues (1996) reported a retrospective analysis of 34 patients (mean age 37 years; range 16–71 years) who underwent MR guided stereotactic cingulotomies for treatment-refractory affective disorder and OCD (between May 1991 and February 1995). Of the 15 treatment-refractory OCD patients using clinical global improvement scales completed by the referring/treating psychiatrist, 54% were classified responders and possible responders (27% each), while 46% were classified as nonresponders. The corresponding numbers for the treatment-refractory depressive disorder group (n=15) were: responders 53%, possible responders 20%, and nonresponders 27%. Side effects included seven patients (22%) with transient postoperative urinary retention and two patients (with prior history of seizure activity) with isolated seizure episodes. The authors noted that of the 14 patients who were considered nonresponders after one cingulotomy, 36% were responders after multiple cingulotomies and 36% possible responders. Some patients with only limited response to surgery report that treatment modalities that were ineffective before surgery seemed to give them at least some symptom relief postoperatively (Jenike et al. 1991, Dougherty et al. 2002). This important information requires further study but offers some hope to the patient who has had a poor response to the initial surgical procedure. It also underscores the need for continued pharmacological and behavioral therapy.

Dougherty and colleagues (2002) conducted an open prospective study where 44 treatment-refractory OCD patients were evaluated carefully before and at various intervals after a single or multiple stereotactic cingulotomies (mean age at time of operation 34.4 years; SD 11.8; range 16–69 years). Patients received comprehensive modern rating scales and the criteria for response were stringent for responders: 35% improvement on YBOCS and CGI less than or equal to 2 (moderately to much better on obsessions, depression, and anxiety, and the patient does not attribute improvement to a treatment other than cingulotomy). At mean follow-up of 32 months following one or more cingulotomies, 14 (32%) met criteria for treatment response and six (14%) for partial response. Nine patients (20%) reported at least one transient side effect and two patients (5%) reported enduring sequelae (including one who developed seizure disorder that has required ongoing anticonvulsant treatment). The main limitation of this study was the absence of a control group, which the authors appropriately acknowledge.

## Anterior Capsulotomy

Bingley and colleagues (1977) reported on 35 patients (mean age 40 years; mean illness duration 17 years) who had undergone stereotactic anterior internal capsulotomy. Using subjective outcomes rating scales, 71% of 35 patients were reported to be either "free of symptoms" or "much improved" (some residual symptoms but considerably alleviated) after a mean follow-up period of 35 months. Of note, 20 (of 24 preoperatively completely disabled) subjects were reported to have regained partial or full work capacity postsurgically. Postoperative transient confusion was described in many patients and two patients suffered from transient hemiparesis due to subcortical hemorrhages. There were no seizures reported in this cohort.

The same group (Meyerson and Mindus 1988) reported on an additional 30 OCD subjects who underwent anterior internal capsulotomy and reported a 70% good outcome response rate (duration of illness 5–30 years, mean 15 years, followed up for 1–9 years, mean 4 years). One patient (out of 68) developed seizures postoperatively and another had transient target area hematoma requiring drainage. The authors reported that no significant long-term cognitive or personality deficits were observed in this cohort.

Lippitz and colleagues (1999) prospectively monitored psychiatric and brain MR imaging data (mean follow-up: 9.6 years; range 2.4–20.3 years) of 29 OCD patients (mean age 40.5 years; range 25.5–66.2 years) who underwent thermocapsulotomy (n=19) and gamma knife capsulotomy (n=10). The authors reported a significant correlation between an MR defined right sided anterior capsular common lesional area and good response (defined as 50–100% reduction in target symptom score) postoperatively in responders in both groups. These results await replication in a larger number of patients.

Rasmussen and colleagues (Hollander et al. 2002) recently presented encouraging preliminary findings in treatment-refractory OCD patients undergoing initial double lesion (versus single lesion) gamma knife capsulotomy (38–50% patients were "clinically improved" versus none in the single shot group). A larger controlled trial is awaited.

## Subcaudate Tractotomy

Subcaudate tractotomy has been used extensively for intractable MDD and a few reports concerning this procedure in treatment-refractory OCD exist. Earlier reports reported a 50% good outcome rate for a small number of OCD subjects (Strom-Olsen and Carlisle 1971, Göktepe et al. 1975). Low rates of postoperative epilepsy and of adverse behaviors such as overeating, volubility, and extravagance were reported by the authors.

Bridges and colleagues (1973) compared 24 patients with treatment-refractory OCD (mean onset age: 25.4 years; mean time to first surgery: 11.5 years; mean interview age: 42.4 ± 13) to 24 matched controls of depression OCD (mean onset age: 30.5 years; mean time to first surgery: 11.3 years; mean interview age: 46.5 ± 12.8), both of whom had undergone (at least 3 years prior) stereotactic subcaudate tractotomies (SST) as described by Knight (1969). At this stage of follow-up they reported that 16 (67%) of the OCD patients were determined to fall into categories I and II (symptom free or much improved) compared to the depressive patients where 17 (71%) were assigned to these categories. Only two (8%) patients in each diagnostic group reported no improvement at the 3-year follow-up and none were considered to have worsened. In the improved OCD group, the number of hospital admissions fell from a mean of seven per year to one per year. Of note in this study, OCD patients with a poor response to subcaudate tractotomy were found to have an earlier age at onset of disease (mean = 22 years) compared with those who did well (mean = 28.8 years).

Göktepe and colleagues (1975) reported a 2.5- to 4.5-year follow-up study on 208 patients who underwent SST; 134 patients were fully assessed, 25 were dead, and partial data existed for 49 patients. Out of the fully assessed patients, 53/78 (68%) patients with depression were reported to have a good outcome (categories I and II on the Pippard Scale), while the corresponding number for patients with OCD was 9/18 (50%). A striking reduction in inpatient hospitalizations and need for ECT was noted in patients who fell into this category. Adverse events included postoperative epilepsy (3/134; 2.2%), reports of undesirable social behaviors (9/134; 6.7%), and one death related to the operative procedure. There were three suicides reported over this period, the rest of the 25 deaths being attributed to various causes.

Hodgkiss and colleagues (1995) reported on a 12-month follow-up study of 286 patients who underwent SST between 1979 and 1991 (249 were completely evaluated including 74 who were evaluated by an independent rater); 63/183 (34%) MDD patients and 5/15 (33%) of OCD patients were classified as good outcome (I and II). There were six deaths during this period though none was attributed to neurosurgery or suicide. The authors noted that most deaths involved patients over 70 and cautioned the use of this procedure for the elderly.

Poynton and colleagues (1995) from the same group reported a more rigorously conducted prospective SST study in 23 patients followed up at 2 weeks, 6 months, and 1 year postsurgery. Patient characteristics were as follows: mean age 49.0 (range 21–74 SD 12.9); mean age at onset of psychiatric disorder: 33.9 (range 15–69 SD 15.4); mean number of drug treatments preop: 3.4 (range 0–6 SD 2.6); mean number of total ECT preop: 29 (range 0–98 SD 24); mean number of total suicide attempts preop: 2.17 (range 0–20 SD 4.2). Patients were assessed with standardized scales, underwent tests of general cognition and frontal lobe functions, and independent global assessment at 1 year (22/23). There was a significant reduction in the total Hamilton score at 6 months and global assessment revealed 13/22 (59%) to be in the good outcome category (I and II).

## Limbic Leukotomy

Kelly and colleagues (1973) conducted a prospective 6-week postoperative follow-up study of 40 patients (mean symptom duration 11 years) who underwent limbic leukotomy (between 1970 and 1972); 2/5 (40%) MDD patients and 7/17 (41%) OCD patients were categorized as good outcome (Pippard I and II ). Side effects included transient confusion, lethargy, and transient incontinence.

Mitchell-Heggs and colleagues (1976) in an extension of this report described 66 patients (mean symptoms: 11 years, range 3–27 years) followed up for a mean of 16 months (9–37 months). This study involved an independent rater

and side effects were reported to be low. There were no seizures reported (all patients were on seizure prophylaxis for 6 months), 18/27 (66%) OCD patients fell into categories I and II, while the corresponding number for MDD was 5/9 (55%). Montoya and colleagues (2002) reported a retrospective chart review of 21 refractory patients (15 with OCD and 6 with MDD) who underwent one or more stereotactic procedures that culminated in a limbic leukotomy (mean follow-up 26 months). In the OCD group, using conservative YBOCS (>35% improvement) criteria, 36% were considered responders at the follow-up period, though based on physician CGI and CGPS (available in 12/15) the percentage was 50. Adverse effects reported were: incontinence in three (14%), seizures in one (5%), short-term memory (STM) disorder (1%), and headache (5%).

## Results of Comparative Reviews

With the usual methodological caveats mentioned above, a few authors have compiled reviews on outcome of various procedures for treatment-refractory OCD. Herner (1961) reviewed nine studies ($n=116$) where treatment-refractory OCD subjects underwent frontal stereotactic thermolesions. A meta-analysis revealed that 89 (55%) patients were reported to be markedly improved. Three patients were considered to have worsened after (but not necessarily due to) limbic leukotomy, one was worse after subcaudate tractotomy, and three, included in an early series from 1961, were worse after capsulotomy.

Chiocca and Martuza (1990) reviewed 10 studies ($n=210$) involving all four current procedures to investigate comparative efficacy. After acknowledging the inherent limitations of such a comparison, the authors concluded that the percentages of patients who improved with each of these four procedures were roughly the same. This latter conclusion may be disputed, however, because the number of outcome categories was not identical (e.g., A, B, and C for limbic leukotomy; A and B only for capsulotomy).

Waziri (1990) reviewed 12 studies ($n=253$) of patients undergoing stereotactic interventions for treatment-refractory OCD and noted that 38% of patients were reported to be symptom free, 29% markedly improved, 10% unchanged, and 3% worse or dead on follow-up (including one suicide). An overall figure for satisfactory response to surgery of 67% was found in these 253 OCD patients.

The methodological issues discussed earlier and the lack of rigorous, controlled, and/or head to head comparison studies prevent comment on which of these procedures is superior. This is further complicated by the heterogeneous profile of OCD patients. At present, there is little evidence to suggest the clear superiority of one procedure over another. More research addressing these issues is desirable.

## Predictors of Outcome

Most investigators reporting outcome studies concerning various procedures have naturally attempted to identify predictors of outcome, though these have been elusive. Bridges and colleagues (1973) reported that OCD subjects who were considered responders in their study had an older age of onset (mean 28.5 years) versus nonresponders (mean 22 years). In a prospective cingulotomy study, using comprehensive assessment strategies, Baer and colleagues (1995) reported that the presence of symmetry obsessions, ordering and hoarding compulsions were predictive of lower YBOCS score at final follow-up (partial correlations). More recently, Rauch and colleagues (2001) utilizing a retrospective design, reported that higher preoperative metabolic rates in a single right posterior cingulate locus (determined by FDG-PET) was associated with better post-cingulotomy outcome in II OCD patients. The advantages of predicting response in such invasive palliative procedures are obvious and need further study.

## Risks of Neurosurgical Intervention

### Surgical Risks

Surgical risks include acute and subacute complications like hemorrhage, postoperative infections and seizures, as well as more serious enduring side effects such as focal neurological deficits, cognitive or personality change, and weight gain.

In an earlier retrospective report, Ballantine and colleagues (1987) reported no deaths in their series of 696 cingulotomies performed over a 25-year period in patients with various psychiatric disorders. The incidence of hemiplegia has been estimated to be 0.3% after cingulotomy (Ballantine et al. 1987). The risk of postoperative epilepsy after these interventions has been estimated to be less than 1% (Jenike et al. 1991, Ballantine et al. 1987) and these cases were usually easily controlled with antiseizure medications. Dougherty and colleagues (2002) in their long-term follow-up of 44 patients after one or more cingulotomies, noted the following surgical complications: urinary disturbances ($n=3$; 7%), seizure disorder ($n=1$; 2%), and postoperative hydrocephalus ($n=1$; 2%). In most patients, these adverse effects resolved over a few days to a year post-surgery, though in two patients (5%) they were enduring.

Weight gain has been reported after capsulotomy (Bingley et al. 1977, Meyerson and Mindus 1988) but the specificity of weight gain to this procedure is unclear. Overall the risk of neurosurgery for severe OCD compares favorably with that of stereotactic operations for nonpsychiatric illnesses; in one study of 243 consecutive stereotactic interventions for various neurological illnesses, 15 complications were noted, including one death (Blaauw and Braakman 1988).

### Neuropsychiatric Risks

#### Cognitive/Intellectual Domain

With regard to cingulotomy, an independent study of a cohort of patients was performed for the US government by the Department of Psychology at the Massachusetts Institute of Technology. The authors reported that they found no evidence of lasting neurological, intellectual, personality, or behavioral deficits after surgery (Corkin et al. 1979, Corkin 1980). In fact, a comparison of preoperative and postoperative scores revealed modest gains in the Wechsler IQ ratings. The only apparent irreversible decrement identified by these investigators was a decrease in performance on the Taylor Complex Figure Test in patients older than age 40 years. Several authors, using varying assessment strategies and batteries pre- and postoperatively, have reported the relative lack of serious adverse cognitive effects following cingulotomy (Corkin et al. 1979, Corkin 1980), subcaudate tractotomy (Bartlett and Bridges 1977, Göktepe et al. 1975), limbic leukotomy (Mitchell-Heggs et al. 1976, Kelly 1980), and capsulotomy (Herner 1961, Bingley et al. 1977, Vasko and Kullberg 1979). Nevertheless, the need to include carefully thought out (based on the procedure involved) neurocognitive assessments before and at regular intervals after the surgery/surgeries cannot be overstated. Long-term studies are desirable for the existing procedures to better inform patients and clinicians of the risks as well to help rehabilitative efforts.

#### Affective/Social and Personality Domains

As these neurosurgical procedures may be expected to influence, directly or indirectly, frontal lobe and other functions comprising one's "personality," it is important that this is an integral part of the pre- and postoperative assessment. Important domains that need to be addressed are executive functions, impulsivity/aggressiveness, social propriety, and mood changes. Ideally this would involve input from both the patient as well as the family and treating clinician. In general, anecdotal evidence from most reported studies concerning the different procedures suggest a remarkable freedom from significant adverse personality changes. On the contrary, the few studies that have directly addressed this issue report an improvement in negative personality traits at follow-up.

One of the better researched instruments is the Karolinska Scales of Personality (KSP), developed by Schalling and coworkers (1987). The KSP contains subscales measuring traits related to frontal lobe function as well as those reflecting anxiety proneness. In capsulotomy studies reported from Sweden, the KSP was administered to 24 consecutive patients 1 year and 8 years after radiofrequency capsulotomy. Small changes in mean scores towards normalization were apparent on all 15 KSP subscales at the 1-year follow-up and significant improvement was reported in anxiety proneness at the 8-year follow-up (Mindus et al. 1999).

One would expect that the more precise modern procedures should further reduce this risk. In fact most recent studies report a low incidence of adverse behaviors postsurgery. However, this remains a potential risk and conclusions based on observations made on groups of patients may not preclude negative adverse effects in an individual patient.

#### Suicide

While suicide is not considered a known complication of neurosurgical procedures in nonpsychiatric patients undergoing these procedures, the possibility of contributing directly or indirectly to this process in psychiatric patients is theoretically present. However, it is important to note that severe major depression is associated with high lifetime suicide rates (approximately 3–8%) (Nierenberg et al. 2001). Thus, of the suicides reported in psychiatric neurosurgical cohorts, it is difficult to ascertain whether these are a result of existing psychopathology or whether the surgery contributed in some way to this process.

For example, Jenike and colleagues (1991) found that 4 of 33 patients who had undergone cingulotomy for OCD had died by suicide at follow-up that averaged 13 years. Chart reviews revealed that each of these suicide completers had been noted to suffer from extensive comorbid disease (especially severe depression) with prominent suicidal ruminations at initial evaluation for cingulotomy. On the contrary, none of the OCD patients without baseline suicidality became suicidal after the operation. In the large ($n=44$) prospective long-term follow-up study following one or more cingulotomies, Dougherty and colleagues (2002) reported one suicide (2%) in a patient having severe depression with chronic suicidal ideation and a past history of a suicide attempt. Thus, in most published studies, the suicide rate has been low and these patients have been noted to have had significant presurgical suicidality. This highlights the need to carefully assess for and monitor suicidality in this severely ill population.

Patients with a poor response to surgery may be at increased risk for suicide (Jenike et al. 1991). Preventative strategies therefore include careful assessment of suicidality at baseline and follow-ups, assessment of family and clinician support networks, clear explanations of the scope of the procedure as well as the long response latency (usually a year for cingulotomy), education that presurgical nonresponders sometimes respond to treatment postsurgery, and the need for secondary or tertiary lesions in case of cingulotomy in some patients to achieve response.

### Risk of Nonintervention

The World Health Organization (WHO) lists OCD and depression among the top 10 causes of medical disability worldwide along with ischemic heart disease, stroke, and schizophrenia. Untreated OCD and MDD are associated with considerable morbidity and comorbidity and resultant suffering for not only patients but also their families and the community at large. Approximately 6 to 14% of OCD patients unfortunately suffer a progressively downhill course, resulting in severe disability, and personal and economic loss. An estimated 3 to 8% of people with severe MDD commit suicide during their lifetime. Thus, the physician of a patient with truly treatment-refractory OCD and/or MDD has the challenging task of helping the patient and family weigh the risks/benefits of neurosurgical intervention against the considerable risk of nonintervention while making their decision.

## Recent Advances

### Neurosurgical Advances and Imaging Strategies

The routine use of MR guided stereotactically placed neurosurgical lesions and the increasing availability of the gamma knife offer more precise procedures with objectively quantifiable lesions. High resolution structural MRI studies are being used to track volumetric changes local and distal to the lesions (Rauch et al. 2000) and PET studies are providing information about blood flow and regional metabolism that may serve as predictors of response (Rauch et al. 2001). Recordings in implicated brain structures such as the cingulum (similar to intracortical recordings and microdialysis in the temporal lobe in surgical epilepsy patients) may provide useful additional information. Strategies such as magnetic resonance spectroscopy (MRS) and newer methods such as diffusion tensor imaging (DT-MRI) can provide information about regional neurochemistry and white matter tract integrity, respectively. They offer the exciting possibility of collecting valuable neurobiological data, which may aid in monitoring changes as well as predicting response.

### Newer Strategies

Recently, several new experimental strategies have emerged and are being investigated in refractory OCD and MDD. These are invasive modalities currently being offered only in the context of research studies and thus have not been proven or approved for treatment. We include them in this discussion for the sake of completion.

### Deep Brain Stimulation

Deep brain stimulation (DBS) involves stimulation of target regions via stereotactically placed electrodes that can be programmed to deliver low voltage electrical stimulation to modulate transmission of specific brain pathways. While DBS of different regions has been experimentally investigated for treatment-refractory pain syndromes, movement disorders, and seizure disorders, only DBS for treatment-refractory Parkinson's disease or essential tremor is currently FDA approved in the US. Recently following a preliminary report of deep brain stimulation in the anterior limb of the internal capsule in four patients with treatment-refractory OCD (Nuttin et al. 1999), a few specialized centers in the world (including the US) are conducting ongoing controlled studies of DBS in treatment-refractory OCD patients. Nuttin and colleagues described four patients with treatment-refractory OCD who underwent DBS with bilateral stereotactically implanted quadripolar electrodes in the anterior limb of the internal capsule (instead of anterior capsulotomy) and reported "beneficial effects" in three of the four patients. It is important to note that this remains an experimental procedure at this stage for treatment-refractory OCD. Nevertheless these developments offer the exciting possibility of reversible "lesions" as well as ethically justifiable sham procedures (controls can be implanted but the stimulation not turned on or at lower voltage undetectable by the patient who can subsequently receive the benefit of the treatment) (Greenberg, personal communication).

### Vagal Nerve Stimulation

Vagal nerve stimulation is currently used as an FDA approved treatment strategy for some patients with drug-resistant, partial-onset epilepsy due to its seizure attenuating effects. Mood improvement in epilepsy patients treated with VNS, in addition to its known effects on brain neurotransmitter systems, prompted an investigation of its effects for treatment-refractory depression. Recently Sackeim and colleagues (2001) reported that a 12-week open-label multicenter study conducted in the US on 60 treatment-refractory MDD patients (2-week single-blind recovery period after implantation followed by 10 weeks of VNS) resulted in a 30% response rate (50% reduction in $HDRS_{28}$ scores). Low to moderate treatment resistance (those with less than seven adequate trials of antidepressants) was significantly associated with better outcome. Voice alteration/hoarseness was reported to be the most common side effect (33/60; 55%). Following completion of this acute study, 30 adults received an additional 9 months of VNS (where changes in stimulus parameters and medications were permitted). The remission rate (Hamilton Depression Rating Scale$_{28}$ < 10) was reported to have significantly improved (17 [5/30] – 29% [8/28]; $p = 0.045$) along with significant improvement in function (Marangell et al. 2002). The promising results of this open

| **Table 93–3** | **Suggested Guidelines for Neurosurgical Intervention in Neurosurgery for Intractable Psychiatric Illness** |
|---|---|

1. Center and expertise

Center/s with stereotactic neurosurgical expertise and integrated multidisciplinary expertise in the evaluation, neurosurgical treatment, and management of patients with intractable psychiatric disorders.

2. Patient selection

Suggested guidelines for patient selection presented in Tables 93–1 and 93–2. A clinical psychiatrist with OCD expertise evaluates patients and orders a presurgical workup (below).

3. Profiles

Workup should be carefully thought out and relevant to the specific procedures as well as to enhance comparability. Information should be collected from multiple sources (patient, family, psychiatrist, etc.).

   Psychiatric:

      Preferably a structured clinical interview (e.g., SCID-CV* for DSM-IV). Reliable and valid scales (inventories and clinician administered) of mood, obsessions and compulsions, and anxiety (e.g., BDI[†], HDRS[‡]; YBOCS[§]).

   Neuropsychological

      Batteries of both general cognition as well as specific to lesion: (e.g., general intellectual functioning, executive functions, memory, personality assessment)

   Neuromedical

      General surgical risk workup.

      Specific neurological issues: neurological examination, pre-lesion MRI (for lesion demarcation), documentation of past neurological problems, especially seizures.

4. Raters and schedule

Assessors and raters should be blinded to the extent possible.

5. Documentation of neurosurgical effects

Documentation of lesion site, size, and extent. Pre- and poststructural and functional scans would be highly desirable.

6. Postsurgical follow-up

Should involve administration of selected profiles mentioned above at various intervals (e.g., 1 wk postsurgery, 3, 6, 9, and 12 mo and longer when possible.

Enhancing comparability of data

- Centers should attempt to use universally accepted/equivalent patient selection criteria, psychiatric instruments, neuropsychological batteries, and objective quantification and monitoring of lesions.
- Establishment of a database to remove inherent bias of only publishing positive studies.
- Consortium of centers investigating different procedures.

*First MB, Spitzer RL, Gibbon M, et al. (1996) Structured Clinical Interview for DSM-IV Axis I Disorders, Clinical Version (SCID-IV). American Psychiatric Press, Washington DC.

†Beck AT, Steer RA, and Brown GK (1996) Manual for Beck Depression Inventory-II. Psychological Corporation, San Antonio, TX.

‡Hamilton M (1986) The Hamilton Rating Scale for depression. In Assessment of Depression, Sartorius N and Ban TA (eds). Springer-Verlag, Berlin.

§Goodman WK, Price LH, Rasmussen SA, et al. (1989) The Yale-Brown Obsessive–Compulsive Scale. I. Development, use, and reliability. Arch Gen Psychiatr 46(11) (Nov), 1006–1011.

trial await replication. Like DBS, VNS is an invasive experimental procedure for refractory MDD and must be conducted only in centers that have the personnel and expertise.

## Conclusion

A small but significant number of psychiatric patients remain refractory to state-of-the-art treatments and are severely disabled. Based on the existing data, palliative neurosurgery continues to be an option for these patients. The impressive advances in psychiatry as well as stereotactic and radioneurosurgery and neuroimaging have resulted in promising outcomes with a better benefit/risk ratio, suggesting that these options should be further pursued. Improvement of study design as well as improved communication between interested specialized centers is desirable to further advance the field. See Table 93–3 for suggested guidelines. Meanwhile newer, less invasive strategies, such as the gamma knife as well as potentially reversible manipulation of the CNS such as DBS and VNS have emerged and could potentially change the nature of this field. Till we have data from more sophisticated controlled studies, it is highly recommended that these procedures be done only in centers that have the necessary expertise, personnel, and resources to undertake and follow through with such procedures.

### Clinical Vignette

JS, a 44-year-old, single, Caucasian male, living on a disability income in a semi-independent living facility, was referred for neurosurgical evaluation by his treating psychiatrist. He was first diagnosed to have OCD when he was a 20-year-old sophomore in college and has suffered a progressively deteriorating course despite treatment, leading to his being unable to work as well as care for himself adequately, over the past 10 years. He had failed adequate trials of treatments including fluoxetine, sertraline, and clomipramine as well as multiple courses of exposure and response prevention, including long-term intensive residential treatments. His most disabling symptoms have been his fear of contamination and related washing and checking compulsions. He spends most of his day locked in his room engaged in repeatedly washing and showering and often has to be supervised by his family (who live close by) to feed and groom himself. This has taken a significant toll on his family who have to constantly monitor his progress. John has also suffered from several depressive episodes, is chronically dysthymic, and has attempted suicide in the past due to feeling hopeless about his situation.

At the specialized center, a psychiatrist with experience in presurgical evaluations evaluated John. He also underwent neuropsychological and psychosocial evaluations and a medical fitness examination. His case was then discussed by a panel of experts at the institutional level to review his eligibility for anterior cingulotomy. After informed consent from John and his family, he underwent a magnetic resonance guided, stereotactic, bilateral anterior cingulotomy. The immediate postsurgical period was notable for some transient confusion and urinary incontinence. After recovery, John was referred back to his psychiatrist and his medications were continued. At the 3-month follow-up, John did not report any change in his symptoms. At the 6-month and 1-year follow-ups, however, John and his family reported that the frequency of "getting stuck" in his washroom had observably reduced. He still reported contamination obsessions but with less frequency and severity. When they did occur, he was able to "unstick" himself with less difficulty. His mood and self-care was better and he had begun to socialize more. He was considering participating in a day program at the facility. His psychiatrist corroborated these reports.

## Acknowledgment

We thank Ms. Christen Ebens for her generous help in the preparation of this manuscript.

## References

Alexander GE, Crutcher MD, and DeLong MR (1990) Basal ganglia-thalamocortical circuits: Parallel substrates for motor, oculomotor, "prefrontal" and "limbic" functions. Prog Brain Res 85, 119–146.

Alexander GE, DeLong MR, and Strick PL (1986) Parallel organization of functionally segregated circuits linking basal ganglia and cortex. Annu Rev Neurosci 9, 357–381.

Baer L, Rauch SL, Ballantine HT Jr., et al. (1995) Cingulotomy for treatment refractory obsessive–compulsive disorder: Prospective long-term follow-up of 18 patients. Arch Gen Psychiatr 52, 384–392.

Ballantine HT Jr., Bouckoms AJ, Thomas EK, et al. (1987) Treatment of psychiatric illness by stereotactic cingulotomy. Biol Psychiatr 22, 807–819.

Bartlett JR and Bridges PK (1977) The extended subcaudate tractotomy lesion. In Neurosurgical Treatment in Psychiatry, Pain and Epilepsy, Sweet W, Obrador S, and Martin-Rodriguez JG (eds). University Park Press, Baltimore, p. 387.

Baxter LR, Phelps ME, Mazziotta JC, et al. (1987) Local cerebral glucose metabolic rates in obsessive–compulsive disorder. A comparison with rates in unipolar depression and in normal controls. Arch Gen Psychiatr 4, 211–218.

Baxter LR, Schwartz JM, Bergman KS, et al. (1992) Caudate glucose metabolic rate changes with both drug and behavior therapy for OCD. Arch Gen Psychiatr 49, 681–689.

Baxter LR, Schwartz JM, Guze BH, et al. (1990) Neuroimaging in obsessive–compulsive disorder: Seeking the mediating neuroanatomy. In Obsessive–Compulsive Disorders: Theory and Management, 2nd ed., Jenike MA, Baer L, and Minichiello WE (eds). Year Book Medical Publishers, Chicago, pp. 167–188.

Baxter LR, Schwartz JM, Mazziotta JC, et al. (1988) Cerebral glucose metabolic rates in nondepressed patients with obsessive–compulsive disorder. Am J Psychiatr 145, 1560–1563.

Beck AT, Steer RA, and Brown GK (1996) Manual for Beck Depression Inventory-II. Psychological Corporation, San Antonio, TX.

Berthier ML, Kulisevsky J, Gironell A, et al. (1996) Obsessive–compulsive disorder associated with brain lesions: Clinical phenomenology, cognitive function, and anatomic correlates. Neurology 47(2) (Aug), 353–361.

Bingley T, Leksell L, Meyerson BA, et al. (1977) Long term results of stereotactic capsulotomy in chronic obsessive–compulsive neurosis. In Neurosurgical Treatment in Psychiatry, Pain and Epilepsy, Sweet W, Obrador S, and Martin-Rodriguez JG (eds). University Park Press, Baltimore, p. 287.

Blaauw G and Braakman R (1988) Pitfalls in diagnostic stereotactic brain surgery. Acta Neurosurg 42(Suppl), 161.

Breiter HC, Rauch SL, Kwong KK, et al. (1996) Functional magnetic resonance imaging of symptom provocation in obsessive–compulsive disorder. Arch Gen Psychiatr 53(7) (July), 595–606.

Bridges PK, Goktepe EO, and Maratos J (1973) A comparative review of patients with obsessional neurosis and with depression treated by psychosurgery. Br J Psychiatr 123(577) (Dec), 663–674.

Burzaco J (1981) Stereotactic surgery in the treatment of obsessive–compulsive neurosis. In Biological Psychiatry, Perris C, Struwe G, and Jansson B (eds). Elsevier/North Holland Biomedical Press, Amsterdam, p. 1103.

Chiocca EA and Martuza RL (1990) Neurosurgical therapy of obsessive–compulsive disorder. In Obsessive–Compulsive Disorders: Theory and Management, Jenike MA, Baer L, and Minichiello WE (eds). Year Book Medical Publishers, Chicago, p. 283.

Corkin S (1980) A prospective study of cingulotomy. In The Psychosurgery Debate, Valenstein ES (ed). WH Freeman, San Francisco, p. 264.

Corkin S, Twitchell TE, and Sullivan EV (1979) Safety and efficacy of cingulotomy for pain and psychiatric disorder. In Modern Concepts in Psychiatric Surgery, Hitchcock ER, Ballantine HT, and Myerson BA (eds). Elsevier/North Holland, New York, pp. 253–272.

Corsellis J and Jack AB (1973) Neuropathological observations on yttrium implants and on undercutting in the orbito-frontal areas of the brain. In Surgical Approaches in Psychiatry, Laitinen LV and Livingston KE (eds). University Park Press, Baltimore, p. 90.

Cummings JL and Frankel M (1985) Gilles de la Tourette syndrome and the neurological basis of obsessions and compulsions. Biol Psychiatr 20, 1117–1126.

Dougherty DD, Baer L, Cosgrove GR, et al. (2002) Prospective long-term follow-up of 44 patients who received cingulotomy for treatment-refractory obsessive–compulsive disorder. Am J Psychiatr 159(2) (Feb), 269–275.

Feldman RP and Goodrich JT (2001) Psychosurgery: A historical overview. Neurosurgery 48(3) (Mar), 647–657; discussion 657–659.

First MB, Spitzer RL, Gibbon M, et al (1996) Structured Clinical Interview for DSM-IV Axis I Disorders, Clinical Version (SCID-IV). American Psychiatric Press, Washington DC.

Freeman W and Watts JW (1942) Psychosurgery: Intelligence, Emotion, and Social Behavior Following Prefrontal Lobotomy for Mental Disorders. Charles C Thomas, Springfield, IL.

Garber HJ, Ananth JV, Chiu LC, et al. (1989) Nuclear magnetic resonance study of obsessive–compulsive disorder. Am J Psychiatr 146(8) (Aug), 1001–1005.

Göktepe EO, Young LB, and Bridges PK (1975) A further review of the results of stereotactic subcaudate tractotomy. Br J Psychiatr 126, 270.

Goodman WK, Price LH, Rasmussen SA, et al. (1989) The Yale-Brown Obsessive–Compulsive Scale. I. Development, use, and reliability. Arch Gen Psychiatr 46(11) (Nov), 1006–1011.

Hamilton M (1986) The Hamilton Rating Scale for depression. In Assessment of Depression, Sartorius N and Ban TA (eds). Springer-Verlag, Berlin.

Herner T (1961) Treatment of mental disorders with frontal stereotactic thermo-lesions. A follow-up of 116 cases. Acta Psychiatr Scand 36(Suppl) 158, 1–140.

Hodgkiss AD, Malizia AL, Bartlett JR, et al. (1995) Outcome after the psychosurgical operation of stereotactic subcaudate tractotomy, 1979–1991. J Neuropsychiatr Clin Neurosci 7(2) (Spring), 230–234.

Hollander E, Bienstock CA, Koran LM, et al. (2002) Refractory obsessive–compulsive disorder: State-of-the-art treatment. J Clin Psychiatr 63(Suppl 6), 20–29.

Insel TR (1992) Toward a neuroanatomy of obsessive–compulsive disorder. Arch Gen Psychiatr 49(9) (Sept), 739–744.

Jenike MA (1998) Neurosurgical treatment of obsessive–compulsive disorder. Br J Psychiatr 35(Suppl), 79–90.

Jenike MA, Baer L, Ballantine HT, et al. (1991) Cingulotomy for refractory obsessive–compulsive disorder. A long-term follow-up of 33 patients. Arch Gen Psychiatr 48, 548–555.

Kelly D (1980) Anxiety and Emotions. Physiological Basis and Treatment. Charles C Thomas, Springfield, IL.

Kelly D, Richardson A, Mitchell-Heggs N, et al. (1973) Stereotactic limbic leucotomy: A preliminary report on forty patients. Br J Psychiatr 123(573) (Aug), 141–148.

Knight G (1969) Stereotactic surgery for the relief of suicidal and severe depression and intractable psychoneurosis. Postgrad Med J 45, 1–13.

LaPlane E, Levasseur M, Pillon B, et al. (1989) Obsessions–compulsions and other behavioral changes with bilateral basal ganglia lesions: A neuropsychological, magnetic resonance imaging, and positron tomography study. Brain 112, 699–725.

Leonard HL, Lenane MC, Swedo SE, et al. (1992) Tics and Tourette's disorder: A 2- to 7-year follow-up of 54 obsessive–compulsive children. Am J Psychiatr 149(9), 1244–1251.

Lippitz BE, Mindus P, Meyerson BA, et al. (1999) Lesion topography and outcome after thermocapsulotomy or gamma knife capsulotomy for obsessive–compulsive disorder: Relevance of the right hemisphere. Neurosurgery 44(3) (May), 452–458; discussion 458–460.

Malhi GS and Bartlett JR (1998) A new lesion for the psychosurgical operation of stereotactic subcaudate tractotomy (SST). Br J Neurosurg 12(4) (Aug), 335–339.

Malhi GS and Bartlett JR (2000) Depression: A role for neurosurgery? Br J Neurosurg 14(5) (Oct), 415–422.

Malizia A (1991) Indications for psychosurgery. Biol Psychiatr (Suppl 11S), Abstract S-13-12-02.

Marangell LB, Rush AJ, George MS, et al. (2002) Vagus nerve stimulation (VNS) for major depressive episodes: One year outcomes. Biol Psychiatr 51(4) (Feb 15), 280–287.

Martuza RL, Chiocca EA, Jenike MA, et al. (1990) Stereotactic radiofrequency thermal cingulotomy for obsessive–compulsive disorder. J Neuropsychiatr Clin Neurosci 2, 331–336.

McDougle CJ, Epperson CN, Pelton GH, et al. (2000) A double-blind, placebo-controlled study of risperidone addition in serotonin reuptake inhibitor-refractory obsessive–compulsive disorder. Arch Gen Psychiatr 57(8), 794–801.

McDougle CJ, Goodman WK, Leckman JF, et al. (1994) Haloperidol addition in fluvoxamine-refractory obsessive–compulsive disorder:

A double-blind, placebo-controlled study in patients with and without tics. Arch Gen Psychiatr 51(4), 302–308.

Meyerson BA and Mindus P (1988) Capsulotomy as treatment of anxiety disorders. In Modern Stereotactic Neurosurgery, Lunsford LD (ed). Martinus Nijhoff, Boston, p. 353.

Mindus P (1991) Capsulotomy in anxiety disorders. A multidisciplinary study. Thesis. Karolinska Institute, Stockholm.

Mindus P, Bergström K, Levander SE, et al. (1987) Magnetic resonance images related to clinical outcome after psychosurgical intervention in severe anxiety disorder. J Neurol Neurosurg Psychiatr 50, 1288.

Mindus P, Edman G, and Andreewitch S (1999) A prospective, long-term study of personality traits in patients with intractable obsessional illness treated by capsulotomy. Acta Psychiatr Scand 99(1) (Jan), 40–50.

Mitchell-Heggs N, Kelly D, and Richardson A (1976) Stereotactic limbic leucotomy—a follow-up at 16 months. Br J Psychiatr 128, 226–240.

Modell JG, Mountz JM, Curtis GC, et al. (1989) Neurophysiologic dysfunction in basal ganglia/limbic striatal and thalamocortical circuits as a pathogenetic mechanism of obsessive–compulsive disorder. J Neuropsychiatr 1, 27–36.

Moniz E (1937) Prefrontal leucotomy in the treatment of mental disorders. Am J Psychiatr 93, 1379.

Montoya A, Weiss AP, Price BH, et al. (2002) Magnetic resonance imaging-guided stereotactic limbic leukotomy for treatment of intractable psychiatric disease. Neurosurgery 50(5) (May), 1043–1049.

Nauta WJH (1986) Circuitous connections linking cerebral cortex, limbic system, and corpus striatum. In The Limbic System. Functional Organization and Clinical Disorders, Doane BK and Livingston KE (eds). Raven Press, New York, p. 43.

Nierenberg AA, Gray SM, and Grandin LD (2001) Mood disorders and suicide. J Clin Psychiatr 62(Suppl 25), 27–30.

Nordahl TE, Benkelfat C, Semple WE, et al. (1989) Cerebral glucose metabolic rates in obsessive–compulsive disorder. Neuropsychopharmacology 2, 23–28.

Nuttin B, Cosyns P, Demeulemeester H, et al. (1999) Electrical stimulation in anterior limbs of internal capsules in patients with obsessive–compulsive disorder. Lancet 354(9189) (Oct 30), 1526.

Pauls DL, Alsobrook JP, Goodman W, et al. (1995) A family study of obsessive–compulsive disorder. Am J Psychiatr 152(1), 76–84.

Pippard J (1955) Rostral leucotomy: A report on 240 cases personally followed up after one and one-half to five years. J Met Sci 101, 756.

Poynton AM, Kartsounis LD, and Bridges PK (1995) A prospective clinical study of stereotactic subcaudate tractotomy. Psycho Med 25(4) (July), 763–770.

Rapoport J, Elkins R, Langer DH, et al. (1981) Childhood obsessive–compulsive disorder. Am J Psychiatr 138, 12.

Rauch SL, Dougherty DD, Cosgrove GR, et al. (2001) Cerebral metabolic correlates as potential predictors of response to anterior cingulotomy for obsessive–compulsive disorder. Biol Psychiatr 50(9) (Nov 1), 659–667.

Rauch SL, Jenike MA, Alpert NM, et al. (1994) Regional cerebral blood flow measured during symptom provocation in obsessive–compulsive disorder using oxygen 15-labeled carbon dioxide and positron emission tomography. Arch Gen Psychiatr 51(1), 62–70.

Rauch SL, Kim H, Makris N, et al. (2000) Volume reduction in the caudate nucleus following stereotactic placement of lesions in the anterior cingulate cortex in humans: A morphometric magnetic resonance imaging study. J Neurosurg 93(6) (Dec), 1019–1025.

Sackeim HA, Rush AJ, George MS, et al. (2001) Vagus nerve stimulation (VNS) for treatment-resistant depression: Efficacy, side effects, and predictors of outcome. Neuropsychopharmacology 25(5) (Nov), 713–728.

Savage CR, Deckersbach T, Wilhelm S, et al. (2000) Strategic processing and episodic memory impairment in obsessive–compulsive disorder. Neuropsychology 14(1) (Jan), 141–151.

Saxena S, Brody AL, Ho ML, et al. (2002) Differential cerebral metabolic changes with paroxetine treatment of obsessive–compulsive disorder vs. major depression. Arch Gen Psychiatr 59(3) (Mar), 250–261.

Saxena S, Brody AL, Maidment KM, et al. (1999) Localized orbitofrontal and sub-cortical metabolic changes and predictors of response to paroxetine treatment in obsessive–compulsive disorder. Neuropsychopharmacology 21(6) (Dec), 683–693.

Schalling D, Åsberg M, Edman G, et al. (1987) Markers of vulnerability to psychopathy: Temperament traits associated with platelet MAO activity. Acta Psychiatr Scand 16, 172.

Schwartz JM, Stoessel PW, Baxter LR Jr., et al. (1996) Systematic changes in cerebral glucose metabolic rate after successful behavior modification treatment of obsessive–compulsive disorder. Arch Gen Psychiatry 53(2) (Feb), 109–113.

Spangler WJ, Cosgrove GR, Ballantine HT Jr., et al. (1996) Magnetic resonance image-guided stereotactic cingulotomy for intractable psychiatric disease. Neurosurgery 38(6) (June), 1071–1076; discussion 1076–1078.

Strom-Olsen R and Carlisle S (1971) Bi-frontal stereotactic tractotomy: A follow-up study of its effects on 210 patients. Br J Psychiatr 118, 141–154.

Swedo SE, Pietrini P, Leonard HL, et al. (1992) Cerebral glucose metabolism in childhood-onset obsessive–compulsive disorder. Revisualization during pharmacotherapy. Arch Gen Psychiatr 49(9) (Sep), 690–694.

Swedo SE, Rapoport JL, Chelsea DL, et al. (1989) High prevalence of obsessive–compulsive symptoms in patients with Sydenham's chorea. Am J Psychiatr 146(2) (Feb), 246–249.

Vasko T and Kullberg G (1979) Results of psychological testing of cognitive functions in patients undergoing stereotactic psychiatric surgery. In Modern Concepts in Psychiatric Surgery, Hitchcock ER, Ballantine HT Jr., and Meyerson BA (eds). Elsevier/North Holland Biomedical Press, Amsterdam, p. 303.

Waziri R (1990) Psychosurgery for anxiety and obsessive–compulsive disorders. In Handbook of Anxiety. Treatment of Anxiety, Noyes R Jr., Roth M, and Burrows GD (eds). Elsevier Science, Amsterdam.

Weilburg JB, Mesulam MM, Weintraub S, et al. (1989) Focal striatal abnormalities in a patient with obsessive–compulsive disorder. Arch Neurol 46, 233–235.

Whitty CWM, Duffield JE, Tow PM, et al. (1952) Anterior cingulectomy in the treatment of mental disease. Lancet 1, 475–481.

# 94  Psychopharmacology: Ethnic and Cultural Perspectives

Keh-Ming Lin
Michael W. Smith
Margaret T. Lin

The advent of the modern era of psychopharmacology in the last half century represents one of the most significant milestones in the history of psychiatry. This relatively young field has not only provided a myriad of interventions that are increasingly safe and efficacious, but has also invigorated research to enrich our understanding of the function of the brain, both in normal and abnormal states (Bloom et al. 1995). As more effective medications enable a greater number of severely disturbed patients to move from confined settings to community living, the field of psychopharmacology has furthermore, contributed toward the development of psychosocial rehabilitation programs and the reshaping of the mental health care delivery system.

The power of these modern day wonder drugs is demonstrated by the fact that, within a few years of their discovery, they were introduced into practically all geographic areas in the world, and quickly became the mainstay for treatment of the mentally ill in all societies (Lin et al. 1993). Similarly, along with the rapid diversification of populations in the US and other industrialized countries, it has now become clear that the effectiveness and specificity of different classes of psychotropics seem to transcend cultural and ethnic boundaries (Lin et al. 1993, Lin and Cheung 1999). It appears that, in general, psychiatric medications are widely accepted and are regarded as useful and helpful by patients and their families, irrespective of their cultural backgrounds.

Without disputing the universally important role that psychopharmacotherapy plays across different cultures, accumulated practice experiences in divergent cultural and ethnic settings have also revealed numerous reports of cross-cultural/cross-ethnic variations in psychotropic responses (Lin and Poland 1995). Until most recently, practically all psychiatric medications have been developed and tested in North America and Western Europe, involving predominantly "young white males." Consequently, scientifically based information regarding the extent of cultural and ethnic influences has been incomplete and scattered (Lin and Cheung 1999). However, both theoretical considerations and data derived from divergent fields have made it increasingly clear that cultural and ethnic factors, similar to age and gender, deserve much more careful consideration than previously thought necessary (Jensvold et al. 1996).

## Dispelling the "Color Blind" Approach

Substantial individual variation in drug responses, at times up to 100-fold in terms of optimal dosing, is the rule rather than the exception. Although the current understanding of such remarkable variability remains incomplete, it is clear that the interplay between genetics and environmental factors plays a pivotal role in pharmacotherapeutic responses, particularly in the context of an individual's ethnic origin, lifestyle, and other socio-demographic variables. Clinicians and researchers have tended to ignore such variables for several reasons: (1) There has been a profound tendency in our field to equate biology with universality, and to regard response variations to biomedical interventions as "noise," (2) There is a history of recurrent racist misinterpretation, distortion, and/or outright fabrication of scientific data, making the discussion of biological diversity an anxiety-ridden topic for many different ethnic groups, (3) When taken out of the context of the often equally substantial, or greater, individual variability that exists in any population groups, findings of ethnic differences run the risk of being interpreted simplistically and stereotypically. Because of these and other reasons, ethnic variations in pharmacological responses have often been regarded with suspicion, and are not taken seriously (Lin and Cheung 1999).

However, as shown in Figure 94–1, virtually all factors affecting pharmacological responses are significantly influenced by culture and ethnicity. Furthermore, patterns of genetic polymorphism, often with substantial ethnic variation, exist in a large number of genes encoding drug metabolizing enzymes as well as receptors and transporters believed to be targets of pharmaceutical agents. The expression of these genes is often significantly modified by a large

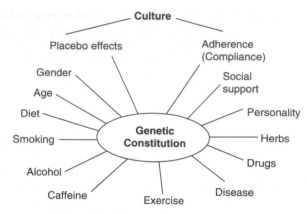

**Figure 94–1** *Factors affecting drug response.*

number of environmental factors, including diet and exposure to various substances (e.g., tobacco). Of even greater importance, the success of any therapy, including pharmacotherapy, depends on the participation of the patient and as such, depends significantly on the quality of interaction between the clinician and the patient. The importance of culture in this regard is paramount.

## The Cultural Context of Psychopharmacotherapy

Perhaps one of the biggest problems in contemporary medical healing practice is its tendency to focus, often exclusively, on technological, biomedical interventions (Kleinman 1988). This tendency frequently obscures the fact that treatment almost always takes place in the context of interactions among individuals. In these interactions, all participants bring their own knowledge, predispositions, values, priorities, modes of thinking, and belief systems into play. Further, perhaps reflecting the bias of the Western culture, these interactions are traditionally discussed in terms of the dyadic relationship between the clinician and the patient (Marsella et al. 1985). However, both members of the dyad act in concert. No matter how isolated a patient may be, she or he almost always makes decisions within the context of real or imagined input from other people. Similarly, as members of professional groups, clinicians are profoundly influenced by the opinions of their peers and the prevailing ideologies of the field. Moreover, as medical care in most societies becomes increasingly organized, institutional control and influences over the practice of physicians become progressively more prominent. The pharmaceutical industry represents a powerful source of influence on clinicians' prescription behaviors as well as researchers' focus and priorities. Thus, while most pharmacotherapeutic decisions may be technical and straightforward in appearance, on closer look they are always imbedded in the rich sociocultural milieus that both the patient and the clinician bring into the transaction (Smith et al. 1993).

Despite their apparent significance, these contextual issues have rarely received adequate attention from both clinicians and researchers. Often they are regarded as "noise" or even "nuisance." Consequently, there has been a dearth of information regarding the nature and determi-

nants of related issues, such as adherence and the "expectation effect" (including the placebo effect). Even less is known on how sociocultural factors impact these processes. While much awaits further clarification, the extant literature in aggregate does support the suggestion that social and cultural forces play a major role in determining the expectations and behaviors of both clinicians and patients. These in turn affect the process and outcome of the treatment.

## Clinicians' Attitudes

A large body of literature indicates that patients' cultural/ethnic backgrounds significantly determine the way clinicians conceptualize and label their problems, which in turn dictate the choices for therapeutic intervention (Mezzich et al. 1995). Using case vignettes that are identical except for ethnic group identification, a number of studies demonstrated that cases identical in every other aspect were nevertheless given significantly more severe diagnoses if the patients were identified as being of ethnic minority origin (Gaw 1993, Lopez 1989). Paralleling such a tendency, African-American psychiatric patients are more likely to have been given a diagnosis of schizophrenia as compared to their Caucasian counterparts (Littlewood 1992, Lopez 1989). Interestingly, in studies where patients were reassessed with the use of structured interviews, such differences largely disappeared, suggesting that such a differential diagnostic pattern is largely determined by variables related to clinicians' biases rather than to the patients' clinical conditions (Adebimpe 1981, Marquez et al. 1985, Mukherjee et al. 1983, Roukema et al. 1984). It is likely that similar biases led to the pervasive use of higher doses of neuroleptics in treating African-American patients, irrespective of diagnosis. Similarly, studies have shown that African-American patients were more likely than their Caucasian counterparts to be treated with depot neuroleptics, presumably due to a general perception of their problem with nonadherence (Strickland et al. 1991, Price et al. 1985).

The potential consequence of these diagnostic and treatment biases may be far from innocuous. Several large scaled studies have documented that the rate of tardive dyskinesia is significantly higher in African-Americans (Swartz et al. 1997, Sramek et al. 1991, Morgenstern and Glazer 1993). Although other reasons for this heightened risk for tardive dyskinesia among African-Americans have not been ruled out, it is very likely that their increased exposure to neuroleptics accounts for at least part of such a risk.

## Adherence

The magnitude of the problem with nonadherence to psychotropic medications has commonly been estimated in the range of 20–90% (Becker and Maiman 1980, Becker 1985, Chen 1991, Sackett and Haynes 1976). Although factors such as insight and motivation may render treatment adherence particularly challenging for psychiatric patients, the problem is far from unique for mental health. In fact, similar high rates of nonadherence have been reported with the treatment of a large number of chronic medical conditions requiring long-term pharmacotherapy (Sackett and Haynes 1976). Most studies exploring correlates of nonadherence have focused on patient and treatment variables, and have shown that a large number of factors significantly predict problems with adherence. These include the sociodemographics of the patient, the financial burden of the treatment, and the side effect profile of the medications (Manne 1998, Fenton et al. 1997). The health belief model has served as the theoretical framework for a large number of seminal research endeavors, which in aggregate demonstrate that the beliefs held by patients and those significant in their lives to a large extent determine their participation in and response to treatment decisions (Hughes et al. 1997). The model has also been proven useful in guiding the development of intervention strategies that effectively enhance treatment adherence (Becker 1985, Haynes et al. 1987). In comparison, little empirical data are available on the influence of factors related to clinician(s) involved in the treatment transaction, the institution(s) where such transactions take place, as well as the nature and quality of the interactions between the clinician(s) and the patient (and those close to him or her).

Following the logic of the health belief model, one would expect adherence to be an even larger problem in cross-cultural clinical situations. This has been substantiated by a number of clinical observations and reports of the service utilization of particular ethnic minority groups (Sue et al. 1991). Compared to Caucasians, ethnic minority patients are often found to enter treatment at a significantly delayed stage, and they also are more likely to drop out of psychiatric treatment prematurely. Programs aiming at bridging cultural gaps have been shown to significantly improve treatment retention and outcome (Acosta et al. 1982).

Findings from two studies underscore the importance of cultural factors in determining medication adherence: Kinzie and colleagues (1987) reported that 61% of their depressed medicated refugee patients showed no tricyclic antidepressants (TCA) in their blood, and that another 24% of them revealed only very low TCA serum levels, even though all of them were treated with adequate TCA dosage. When questioned, these patients admitted to nonadherence for a variety of reasons. Education emphasizing the importance of long-term medication and the maintenance of appropriate blood levels resulted in significant improvement in adherence in some, but not all refugee groups. Similarly, a study in South Africa (Gillis et al. 1987) followed 406 patients belonging to three ethnic groups (whites, blacks, and Asian Indians) for a 2-year period after discharge from a psychiatric hospital. They found that the nonadherence rate for oral phenothiazines was approximately two-thirds for black patients, one half for Asian-Indian patients, and one quarter for white patients. The authors noted that the understanding of the treatment protocols by the relatives of the black and Asian-Indian families was particularly poor, with the possibility of culture and communication being significant factors contributing to the results; but one must also consider the impact of structural barriers such as cost and availability of transportation, as well as discrimination. Perhaps for analogous reasons, blacks in the US are reportedly less compliant (D'Mello et al. 1989, Marcolin et al. 1991) and consequently more likely to be placed on injectable antipsychotics (Price et al. 1985).

Adverse effects of psychotropics are often substantial. Various drug-induced symptoms, including not only the classical extrapyramidal and anticholinergic side effects, but also problems such as paradoxical agitation and weight gain, have been found to significantly contribute towards nonadherence and treatment termination. Some of the most dramatic and disabling untoward effects of these therapeutic agents undoubtedly would be regarded with alarm by patients irrespective of their ethnic/cultural backgrounds (Glazer and Ereshefsky 1996). However, depending on their beliefs and expectations, many other drug effects could be interpreted either as negative or positive. For example, in a study of Hong Kong Chinese bipolar patients treated with lithium, Lee and colleagues (1992) found that, unlike Western patients, the Chinese rarely complained of "missing the highs," and "loss of creativity," and actually regarded polydipsia, polyuria, and weight gain as part of the therapeutic effect of the medicine. In contrast, lethargy, drowsiness, and poor memory represented serious concerns for many of these patients, and were prominent in their complaints, even though objectively they were not likely to be due to the medications they were taking, since they occurred at similar rates among matched controls. Such findings highlight the importance of culturally based beliefs and expectations in determining how physical and psychological experiences associated with drug treatment and recovery are attributed.

The Explanatory Model (EM) approach, as originally proposed by Kleinman (1978), may be a particularly effective way for the systematic assessment of such beliefs and expectations. By methodically eliciting the patient's perspectives on the symptoms that are most salient and worrisome to them (patterns of distress), their attributions (perceived causes), their help-seeking experiences and preference, as well as their perception on stigma, discrepancy between the patients' and the professionals' EMs could be systematically identified and bridged (Weiss 1997). Elements of the EM are included in Appendix I of the DSM-IV manual as part of the Outline for Cultural Formulation (American Psychiatric Association 1994). It is likely that the routine use of tools such as this one will enable clinicians to more effectively enhance adherence, without which no therapeutic interventions can exert their effects.

## Expectation ("Placebo") Effects

Although placebo control is an essential ingredient of modern clinical trials, the nature and determinants of the so-called "placebo" effect remain largely elusive and unexplored (Kleinman 1988, White et al. 1985). Researchers generally recognize that such effects are typically substantial and, in fact, often account for a larger proportion of the improvement than that attributable to the "specific" effect of the therapeutic agent being tested (Swartzman and Burkell 1998, Shepherd 1993). Despite the potency of the "placebo," it has rarely been the focus of attention to researchers. Consequently, much ambiguity currently exists in regard to this important phenomenon, and there is no consensus regarding which term to use when referring to such effects. The most commonly used term, "placebo," carries a negative connotation, and is easily misunderstood as implying deception as well as ineffectiveness. The term "nonspecific effect" could be similarly misleading, since much of the therapeutic effects elicited by "inert" agents might well be mediated through specific biological mechanisms (Weiner and Weiner 1996).

The concept of "expectations effect," commonly used in the field of psychotherapy research, may represent a broader, and at the same time, less controversial notion for such a phenomenon (Kirsch 1990, Tinsley et al. 1988). This term reflects the importance and power of expectation and beliefs on treatment effects in determining patients' response to any therapy, whether psychosocial or pharmacological. Expectations regarding the safety and effectiveness of any therapeutic interventions, in turn, are shaped by patients' sociocultural backgrounds as well as individual "idiosyncratic" experiences (e.g., past experiences of side effects). Since patients' beliefs regarding medical treatments are often shaped by their cultural backgrounds, it stands to reason that patients' expectation regarding the therapeutic effect of the offered treatment would be largely affected by their cultural construct of the illness.

Despite rapid modernization, traditional medical theories and practices remain deeply rooted and influential in determining individuals' health beliefs and behaviors in many societies (Wolffers 1989, Okpaku 1998, Wig 1989, Rappaport 1977). For example, most traditional medical systems emphasize the importance of maintaining a dynamic balance between "coldness" and "hotness" (Castro et al. 1994) or between "Yin" and "Yang" in the case of the Chinese system (Lin 1981). These principles provide guidance for assessment as well as for formulating treatment approaches. For patients who subscribe to such beliefs, a perceived mismatch between the therapeutic agents and the afflictions may significantly lower the expectation effect. For example, red-colored pills might be regarded as capable of enhancing the "hot" element, and might be regarded as less effective in the treatment of conditions perceived as a result of excessive "hotness" (e.g., fever, anxiety state, or mania). Interestingly, Buckalew and Coffield (1982) reported findings from a well-controlled study showing significant ethnic differences in response to placebo pills with different colors. In this study, white capsules were seen as analgesics by Caucasian subjects but as stimulants by their African-American counterparts. In contrast, black capsules were seen as stimulants by Caucasians and as analgesics by African-Americans.

## The Concomitant Use of Alternative/ Indigenous Treatment and Healing Methods

As mentioned above, the worldwide ascendancy of modern "cosmopolitan" ("Western") medicine has not replaced the traditional or "indigenous" medical and healing systems (Frank 1974, Engebretson and Wardell 1993, Lin et al. 1990, Moerman 1979). Instead, "alternative" traditions (e.g., Chinese medicine and Ayurvedic medicine) seemed to have responded well to challenges and have continued to evolve and thrive (Landy 1977, Leslie 1976). Multiple medical and healing traditions and treatment modalities coexist in all societies, and patients often utilize these services simultaneously or sequentially, frequently without informing their physicians. This phenomenon has long been observed in "non-Western" countries (Kleinman 1988) as well as ethnic minority populations in the US (Chan and Chang 1976, Sankury 1983, Vermeer and

Farrel 1985, Westermeyer 1989) although its significance in Western societies has not been adequately appreciated until recent years. When Eisenberg and colleagues (1993) first reported that middle class Americans (predominantly Caucasians) utilized more "alternative" medical than "orthodox" medical services, their findings came as a surprise to most health professionals. In the ensuing years, it appears that, both in North America and Western Europe, the popularity of several "alternative" medical and healing methods, including many imported from non-Western traditions, has increased exponentially (Eisenberg 1998, Wetzel et al. 1998). Thus, problems with drug–drug interactions that could potentially arise from such a practice are no longer limited to particular ethnic groups, and constitute an important consideration for clinicians prescribing medications.

Contrary to general perceptions, alternative treatments are not always mild or "benign," and are capable of inducing severe toxic effects. Indeed, various herbs utilized by traditional practitioners and healers are biologically active (it has been estimated that approximately 40% of our "modern" pharmacotherapeutic agents originated from natural sources [Balick and Cox 1996]). Although much remains unclear, herbal preparations do exert significant impact on various biological systems, including those crucial for the functioning of the central nervous system (Cott 1997, Duke 1995). For example, many herbal preparations possess potent anticholinergic properties (Smith and Smith 1999), and may cause atropine psychosis, particularly when used concomitantly with psychotropics with similar side effect profiles. Numerous herbs have distinctive stimulant or sedative properties, and may either potentiate or attenuate the intended effects of medications prescribed by mental health clinicians (Amadi et al. 1991, Lewis et al. 1991). Since most patients do not regard herbs as medicines and typically fail to inform their physicians of such uses unless specifically inquired, toxicities or treatment failures due to "herb–drug interactions" are likely widespread and unsuspected.

As will be further elaborated later, a limited number of enzymes are involved in the biotransformation of all drugs, including psychotropics. Although the activity of these enzymes are crucial for determining the pharmacokinetics and hence the fate and disposition of modern drugs, their primary substrates are not the medications prescribed by physicians, but are xenobiotics (natural substances) existing in the environment (Gonzalez and Nebert 1990). Many herbs are thus natural substrates for these "drug metabolizing enzymes." Further, through inhibition and/ or induction, xenobiotics, including a large number of herbs (Liu 1991), exert powerful influences on the expression of these enzymes, which then determine the rate of metabolism of the prescription medications.

Herbal preparations may modulate the effect of modern therapeutic agents, including psychotropics, not only at the pharmacodynamic level (the effect of the drugs on the organism), but also at the pharmacokinetic level. Pharmacokinetic herb–drug interactions occur when the coadministration of an herbal remedy results in the alteration of the absorption, distribution, metabolism, or excretion of the prescribed drug. For example, tetracycline's antibiotic efficacy is diminished when taken concurrently with the herb, cassia cinnamon (D'Arcy 1991). In this example, tetracycline is absorbed by the cassia bark in the herbal remedy, thereby decreasing its bioavailability. Additionally, tannins contained in tea have been shown to bind psychotropic medications, preventing their gastrointestinal absorption and subsequent entrance into the blood stream and central nervous system (D'Arcy 1991, 1993). Herbal medications can also impact the metabolism of a number of different medications, including psychotropics. For example, a number of case studies have cited a decrease in effectiveness of medications such as cyclosporine (Ruschitzka et al. 2000), oral contraceptives (Fugh-Berman 2000), the anticoagulants phenprocomon (Maurer et al. 1999), and warfarin (Yue et al. 2000), and the HIV antiviral agent, indinavir (Piscitelli et al. 2000), when taken in combination with St. John's Wort (Ernst 1999). The proposed mechanism for these herb–drug interactions is induction of CYP enzymes and/or the p-glycoprotein drug transport system (PGP) involved in their metabolism by St. John's Wort (Fugh-Berman 2000). In contrast to the inductive effects of St. John's Wort, significant inhibition of CYP3A4 and resultant toxicity of medications that are substrates of this enzyme have been noted with grape fruit juice (Ameer and Weintraub 1997, Benton et al. 1996). The results of these studies suggest that grapefruit juice–drug interactions may be due to compounds such as flavonoids which are also found in fruits, vegetables, and many commonly used herbals (Fukuda et al. 1997, Ha et al. 1995).

## Biological Diversity and Its Consequence in Psychotropic Responses

The central importance of biodiversity in maintaining and ensuring the survival of any species and promoting its adaptation to the local environment is a fundamental principle that unfortunately has not been adequately appreciated (Hughes et al. 1997, Marwick 1995). Possibly because of this under-appreciation of the extent and significance of biological diversity in the past, recent findings of the widespread existence of genetic polymorphisms have appeared surprising to many researchers. Emerging data now convinc-

| Table 94–1 | Genetically Variable Enzymes of Drug Metabolism |
|---|---|
| *Alcohol dehydrogenase (ADH) | Dopamine β-hydroxylase |
| *Aldehyde dehydrogenase (ALDH) | Dihydropyrimidine dehydrogenase |
| Butyryl cholinersterase | *Glucuronyl transferase (UDPGT) |
| Catalase | *Glutathione-S-transferase (class mu) |
| *Catechol-*O*-methyltransferase (COMT) | Monoamine oxidase |
| CYP1A2 | *N-Acetyl transferase (NAT2) |
| *CYP2A6 | *Phenol sulfotransferase |
| *CYP2C19 | *Serum paroxanase/ arylesterase |
| CYP2D6 | Superoxide dismutase |
| *CYP2E1 | *Thiol methyltransferase |
| *CYP3A4 | *Thiopurine methyltransferase |

*Indicates polymorphic variation.

Adapted from Kalow W (1992) Pharmacogenetics of Drug Metabolism. Pergamon Press, New York; Lin KM and Poland RE (1995) Ethnicity, Culture, and Psychopharmacology in Psychopharmacology: The Fourth Generation of Progress, Bloom FE and Kupfer DI (eds). Raven Press, New York.

ingly demonstrate that for the majority of the genes, polymorphism is the rule rather than the exception. Furthermore, the frequency and distribution of alleles responsible for such polymorphisms often vary substantially across ethnic groups, effectively requiring that ethnicity always be considered in genetic studies (National Institute of Mental Health 1997). These phenomena have long been known in blood and human lymphocyte antigen (HLA) typing (Polednak 1989). In recent years, it has become increasingly clear that equally extensive polymorphisms exist in genes governing key aspects of how drugs are metabolized (see Table 94–1) as well as how they affect the target organs. These processes, commonly called pharmacokinetics and pharmacodynamics, are depicted in Figure 94–2 (Greenblatt 1993). Together, these

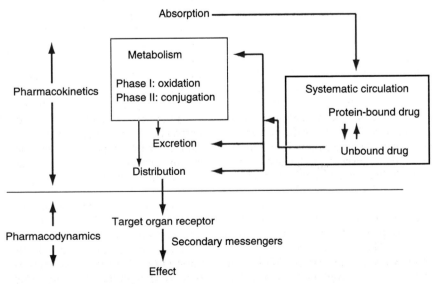

**Figure 94–2** *Pharmacokinetics and pharmacodynamics.*

genetic factors may explain to a large extent the often extensive inter-individual cross-ethnic variations in drug responses (Kalow 1992, Lin et al. 1993). Some of the relevant findings in these regards will be highlighted in the following section.

## Genetic Polymorphism of Genes Encoding "Drug-Metabolizing Enzymes"

As shown in Figure 94–2, of the four factors (absorption, distribution, metabolism, and excretion) that together determine the fate and disposition of most drugs, variability in the process of metabolism is most substantial and usually is the reason for inter-individual and cross-ethnic variation in drug responses (Lin and Poland 1995). Most drugs are metabolized via two phases: Phase I, commonly mediated by one or more of the cytochrome P-450 enzymes (CYPs), leads to the oxidation of the substrate; Phase II involves conjugation, and is usually mediated by one of the transferases. There is clear evidence of inter-individual and cross-ethnic variations in the activity of enzymes in both phases, the genetic basis of which has been increasingly elucidated in recent years (Kalow 1992, Weber 1997). Since far more information is currently available in regard to the CYPs than the Phase II enzymes, and since the CYPs appear to control the rate-limiting steps in the metabolism of most psychotropics, the following discussion will focus mainly on these enzymes.

Table 94–2 includes a list of major CYPs that are responsible for the Phase I metabolism of commonly used psychotropics as well as selected substances that are psychoactive and are commonly used by psychiatric patients. With very few exceptions (e.g., lithium does not require biotransformation; lorazepam and oxazepam are directly conjugated without first going through oxidation), the pharmacokinetics of practically all psychotropics are dependent on one or more of the CYPs, whose activity significantly influences the tissue concentrations, dose requirement and side effect profiles of their substrates.

Functionally significant genetic polymorphisms exist in most of the CYPs (Lin and Poland 1995), leading to extremely large variations in the activity of these enzymes in any given population (Table 94–2). CYP2D6 represents the most dramatic example, with more than 20 mutations that inactivate, impair, or accelerate its function (Daly et al. 1996). Significantly, most of these mutant alleles are to a large extent ethnically specific. For example, CYP2D6*4, which leads to the production of defective proteins, is found in approximately 25% of Caucasians, but is rarely identified in other ethnic groups. This mutation is mainly responsible for the poor metabolizers (PM) in Caucasians (5–9%), who are extremely sensitive to drugs metabolized by CYP2D6. Instead of CYP2D6*4, extremely high frequencies of CYP2D6*17 (Leathart et al. 1998, Masimirembwa and Hasler 1997) and CYP2D6*10 (Wang et al. 1993, Dahl et al. 1995, Roh et al. 1996) were found among those of African and Asian origins, respectively. Both of these alleles are associated with lower enzyme activities and slower metabolism of CYP2D6 substrates (Figure 94–3), and may be in part responsible for previous findings of slower pharmacokinetic profiles and lower therapeutic dose ranges observed in Asians in regard to both classes of psychotropics, and in African-Americans in regard to tricyclic antidepressants (Lin and Poland 1995). Interestingly, our recent study showed that Mexican-Americans had very low rates of any of these "impairing" mutations. Correspondingly, they also showed significantly faster overall CYP2D6 activity.

CYP2D6 also is unique in that the gene often is duplicated or multiplied (up to 13 copies). Those possessing these duplicated or multiple genes have proportionally more enzymes and faster enzyme activity, and are termed "ultra-rapid" metabolizers (UMs). This is found in 1% of Swedish, 5% in Spaniards (white Americans are in between these two figures), 19% in Arabs, and 29% in Ethiopians. UM patients are likely to fail to respond to usual doses of medications biotransformed by CYP2D6, since they typically will fail to achieve therapeutic levels unless treated with extremely high doses of the same drugs. There have been reports of UM patients being regarded as nonadherent because they did not show any evidence of drug effect while given seemingly adequate doses of medications (Akullu et al. 1996).

CYP2C19 represents another dramatic example for the existence of both cross-ethnic and inter-individual variations in drug metabolism. This enzyme is involved in the metabolism of commonly used psychotropics such as diazepam and tertiary tricyclic antidepressants, as well as one of the new antidepressants, citalopram. Using S-mephenytoin as the probe, earlier studies demonstrated that up to 20% of East Asians (Chinese, Japanese, and Koreans) are PM, which is true only in 3–5% of Caucasians. After the gene for the enzyme had been identified and sequenced, it became clear that such enzyme deficiency is caused by two unique mutations (CYP2C19*2 and CYP2C19*3). While *2 can be found in all ethnic groups, *3 appears to be specific to those with Eastern Asian origins. The presence of *3, together with a higher rate of *2, are responsible for the higher rate of PM among Asians, as well as their often increased sensitivity in the clinical setting to drugs such as diazepam (de Morais et al. 1994, Goldstein et al. 1997).

Genetic polymorphism also exists in CYP2C9, CYP2E1, CYP3A4 as well as the majority of other drug metabolizing enzymes (see Tables 94–1 and 94–2). It is interesting to note that, almost without exception, wherever genetic polymorphism is identified, the allele frequency of the mutations typically show substantial ethnic variations (Stephens et al. 1994, Gill et al. 1999, Kidd et al. 1999).

## Factors Affecting the Expression of Drug-Metabolizing Enzymes

In addition to genetic endowment, a large number of nongenetic factors also significantly influence the expression of the genes. These factors are both external and internal. External factors include nutrients, various plant products, pharmaceutical agents, and other chemicals. Internal factors include steroid hormones and other endogenous substances (Anderson et al. 1987, Bolt 1994). These substances either inhibit or induce the activity of the enzyme, and thus affect the metabolism of drugs that are dependent on a particular enzyme. Such shifts in the enzyme status could at times lead to serious clinical consequence. The following are selected examples that have caught the field's attention in recent years: (1) A number of the newer antidepressants, including fluoxetine and paroxetine, two of the most widely used selective serotonin reuptake inhibitors (SSRIs), are potent

| Table 94-2 | Major Human Cytochrome P-450 Enzymes and Their Psychotropic Substrates | |
|---|---|---|
| | Substrates | Genetic Polymorphisms |
| CYP1A2 | ANTIDEPRESSANTS: amitriptyline, clomipramine, imipramine, fluvoxamine<br>NEUROLEPTICS: haloperidol, phenothiazines, thiothixine, clozapine, olanzapine<br>OTHERS: tacrine, caffeine, theophylline, acetominophen, phenacetin | No report of polymorphism until 1999; the significance of the following findings remain unclear (Nakajima 1999)<br>*1C: reduced activity; 23% in Japanese<br><br>*1F: higher inducibility; 32% in Caucasians |
| CYP2C19 | BENZODIAZEPINES: diazepam<br><br>ANTIDEPRESSANTS: imipramine, amitriptyline, clomipramine, citalopram<br>OTHERS: propranolol, hexobarbital, mephobarbital, proguanil, omeprazole, S-mephenytoin | *2: no activity; 23–39% in Asians; 13% in Caucasians; 25% in African-Americans<br>*3: no activity; 6–10% in Asians; 0% in others<br><br>*6 *7 and *8 contain mutations that result in the poor metabolizer phenotype in Caucasians (Ibeanu 1998, 1999) |
| CYP2D6 | ANTIDEPRESSANTS: amitriptyline, clomipramine, imipramine, desipramine, nortriptyline, trimipramine, N-desmethyl-clomipramine, fluoxetine, norfluoxetine, paroxetine, venlafaxine, seltraline<br>NEUROLEPTICS: chlorpromazine, thioridazine, perphenazine, haloperidol, reduced haloperidol, risperidone, clozapine, sertindole<br>OTHERS: codeine, opiate, propranolol, dextromethorphan | *2: accounts for 60% of intermediate metabolizers in Caucasians (Raimundo 2000).<br><br>*3: no activity; 1% in Caucasians (Shimada 2001)<br>*4: no activity; 25% in Caucasians; 0–10% in others<br><br>*5: no activity; 2–10% in all groups<br><br>*10: reduced activity; 47–70% in Asians, 5% in others (Mendoza 2001)<br>*17: reduced activity; 25–40% in blacks, 0% in others (Wan 2001)<br>*2XN: increased activity; 19–29% in Arabs and Ethiopians; 5% in others |
| CYP3A4 | ANTIDEPRESSANTS: mirtazepine, nefazadone, sertraline<br><br>NEUROLEPTICS: thioridazine, haloperidol, clozapine, quetiapine, risperidone, sertindole, ziprasidone<br>MOOD STABILIZERS: carbamazepine, gabapentin, lamotrigine<br><br>BENZODIAZEPINES: alprazolam, clonazepam, diazepam, midazolam, triazolam, zolpidem<br>CALCIUM CHANNEL BLOCKERS: diltiazem, nifedipine, nimodipine, verapamil<br>STEROIDS: androgens, estrogens, cortisol<br>OTHERS: erthyromycin, terfenadine, cyclosporine, dapsone, ketaconazole, lovastatin, lidocaine, alfentanil, amiodarone, astemiazole, codeine, sildenafil | Several single nucleotide polymorphisms have been identified with racial variability in their frequency. However, functional significance of these polymorphisms have not been clearly elucidated (Dai et al. 2001)<br><br>Recent reports of the functional significance of a variant with mutation in the regulatory region (*1B) has been suggested. The prevalence of *1B is 10% in Caucasians, and unknown in other ethnic groups.<br><br>There are preliminary reports of two other promising alleles (*2 and *3), but details of these mutations are not yet available.<br><br>*4, *5, *6 have been suggested to possibly decrease 3A4 activity in Chinese subjects but the incidences of these mutations are rare and their prevalence in other ethnic groups is unknown (Hsieh 2001) |

Other important human CYPs include CYP2A6, CYP2B6, CYP2C8, CYP2C9, and CYP2E1. CYP2A6 is involved in the metabolism of nicotine and cotinine, CYP2C9 is responsible for the biotransformation of drugs including phenytoin and warfarin, CYP2E1 metabolizes acetaminophen, theophylline as well as alcohol and is associated with the production of free radicals.

inhibitors of CYP2D6, capable of converting an extensive metabolizer into a poor metabolizer. Thus, when these drugs are prescribed for a patient who is already been taking a CYP2D6 substrate (e.g., tricyclic antidepressants or neuroleptics), the concentration of the latter could be pushed unexpected into the toxic range (Aranow et al. 1989, Bergstrom et al. 1992, Brosen 1995), (2) Smoking has long been known to significantly reduce the serum concentration of psychotropics, and it is likely that many patients suffer from relapse soon after discharge from the hospital because they resume smoking (Guengerich et al. 1994). This effect is now known to be due to the induction of CYP1A2 by

constituents of tobacco (DeVane 1994), (3) Many drugs and natural substances significantly inhibit the activity of CYP3A4, altering its ability to metabolize drugs that are dependent on this enzyme for their biotransformation. A widely known example is the grape fruit juice (Oesterheld and Kallepalli 1997, Fuhr et al. 1993), which is capable of increasing the blood level of antiviral drugs as well as psychotropics such as nefazodone and alprazolam by several folds, if taken concurrently. In addition, reports of lethality caused by the combination of ketoconazole and terfenadine has led to the withdrawal of the latter from the market (Jurima-Romet et al. 1994), (4) A large body of

Serum Haloperidol (ng)

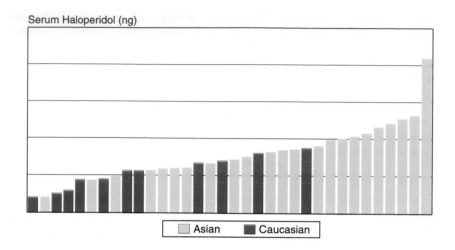

Asian  Caucasian

**Figure 94–3** *Variability of haloperidol concentrations in normal volunteers after the administration of haloperidol (0.5 mg, IM). The graph shows: (1) substantial interindividual variability within each of the ethnic groups; (2) dramatic differences in the pharmacokinetics of haloperidol between the two ethnic groups; and (3) overlap of the pharmacokinetics between the two groups. (Source: Lin KM, Poland RE, Lan JK, et al. [1988] Haloperidol and prolactin concentrations in Asians and Cancasians. J Clin Psychopharmacol 8, 195–201.)*

literature indicates that macronutrients (i.e., high protein versus high carbohydrate diet) also significantly influence the activity of cytochrome P-450 enzymes. High protein diet accelerates the metabolism of drugs such as antipyrine and theophylline, and high carbohydrate diet appears to have the opposite effect (Branch et al. 1978, Fraser et al. 1979, Anderson and Kappas 1991).

These examples demonstrate the importance of environmental factors in substantially modifying the activity of these drug-metabolizing enzymes. Patients from different ethnic/cultural backgrounds live divergent lifestyles, and are likely to be exposed to unique substances that may have strong effects on the expression and activity of drug metabolizing enzymes. Thus, what we currently know about environmental influences on drug metabolism may represent only the tip of the iceberg. This may be especially true in regard to ethnic minority and other non-Western populations. For example, studies have shown that Asian Indians and Africans were significantly slower in metabolizing substrates of CYP1A2, such as theophylline, antipyrine, and clomipramine. However, after they immigrated to Europe and adapted to the new dietary habits, their metabolic profiles for these drugs became indistinguishable from the "native" Westerner's (Allen et al. 1977).

As discussed earlier, herbal medicines are routinely and extensively used by people worldwide. Since patients typically are not aware of the potential of herb–drug interactions, they often combine the use of herbs and "Western medicines." When severe toxic effects subsequently emerge, they usually blame them on drugs prescribed by clinicians, rather than on herbal preparations obtained over-the-counter, or from traditional/alternative practitioners (Smith et al. 1993). Since thousands of herbs are widely in use, and the indication and popularity of these herbs vary greatly across cultural traditions, the potential for interactions between herbs and modern pharmaceutical agents is endless and largely unexplored (Smith and Smith 1999).

### Genetic Polymorphism of Genes Encoding Receptors, Transporters, or Other Therapeutic Targets

Monoamines, including dopamine (DA), serotonin (5-HT), and norepinephrine (NE), have been the focus of intensive

research attention in the past several decades. In addition to being implicated in the pathogenesis of psychiatric disorders including schizophrenia and major depression, they have also been regarded as the putative targets of psychotropics (Schatzberg and Schildkraut 1995, Barker and Blakely 1995). Confirming the importance of the 5-HT system in affective and other psychiatric disorders, a number of SSRIs have been developed and are now widely in use for a wide range of clinical conditions. At the same time, although the far more diffuse receptor binding profiles of the "atypical neuroleptics" call into question the primacy of the "dopamine hypothesis" in schizophrenia research, the function of the dopaminergic system remains important in understanding the schizophrenic process and its pharmacological management (Bloom and Kupfer 1995).

Along with the cloning and sequencing of the genes encoding the receptors and transporters that mediate and regulate the function of these important neurotransmitters, it has become apparent that, contrary to earlier predictions (Kalow 1990), these genes are almost without exception highly polymorphic, and the pattern of these polymorphisms vary significantly across ethnicity (Gelenter et al. 1997, Goldman et al. 1996, Hodge 1994, Dean et al. 1994, Chang et al. 1996). For example, the frequency of the TaqI A RFLP polymorphism of the dopamine $D_2$ receptor (DRD2), one of the most extensively investigated brain receptors, ranges from 5 to 18% in Caucasians to approximately 36% in African-Americans and 37 to 42% in Asians (Blum et al. 1995). Earlier studies suggesting the existence of an association between this allele and alcoholism have been criticized because ethnicity as a potential confounding variable was not taken into consideration. Similarly, dramatic ethnic variations exist in the pattern of genetic polymorphism of many other receptor and transporter genes. These include other DRD2 mutations (Taq1 B, 311Ser/Cys and exon 8 A/G substitution), other dopamine receptors such as DRD4 and DRD3 (Parsian et al. 1999, Sander et al. 1995, Sullivan et al. 1998), the dopamine transporter gene (DAT1; locus symbol SLC6A3) (Vandenbergh et al. 1992), the serotonin transporter gene (5-HTT), and a number of serotonin receptors (5-HT$_{2A}$-1438 A/G and 5-HT$_{2A}$-102 T/C) (Greenberg et al. 1998, Smeraldi et al. 1998, Michaelovsky et al. 1999).

These polymorphisms are likely to have functional significance and hence might be associated with the risk for psychopathology as well as the response to treatment regimens. For example, recent studies show that the basal transcriptional activity of the serotonin transporter gene (5-HTT) is significantly higher in those possessing a long variant in the promoter region of this gene, which results in differential 5-HTT expression and 5-HT cellular uptake (Greenberg et al. 1998). The clinical significance of these findings was recently demonstrated in a study of the effect of SSRIs in treating psychotic depression (Smeraldi et al. 1998). In this study, patients who were either homozygote or hctcrozygotc long variant (5-*IITTLPR l/l* and *l/s*) responded significantly better than those who were homozygote short variant (*s/s*). Similarly, DRD2 TaqI A restriction fragment length polymorphism (RFLP), located in the 3' flanking region of the DRD2 gene, has been shown in brain imaging (Hietala et al. 1994) and postmortem (Noble et al. 1991) studies to affect $D_2$ receptor density in different parts of the brain, and thus might affect the receptor's response to neuroleptics, in addition to its possible association with the risk for alcoholism. It is, however, at present unclear if such associations might be true across ethnic groups, and if ethnic differences in the polymorphisms might result in ethnic variations in the pharmacodynamics of drugs whose effects are mediated by these receptors/transporters.

## Genetic Polymorphism of Other Genes Affecting Pharmacological Responses

The synthesis and catabolism of the catecholamines are controlled by a number of enzymes including tryptophan hydroxylase, tyrosine hydroxylase, catechol-*O*-methyl-transferase (COMT), and the monoamine oxidases (MAO). Tryptophan hydroxylase controls the rate limiting step for the production of 5-HT from tryptophan (Smeraldi et al. 1998), and tyrosine hydroxylase plays a central role in the production of DA and NE. On the catabolic side, MAO mediates the oxidation and deamination of 5-HT into 5-hydroxyindole-3-acetic acid (5-HIAA) and other metabolites, and both MAO and COMT are responsible for the metabolism of the catecholamines (DA and NE). Interestingly, all of these enzymes are highly polymorphic (Jonsson et al. 1997). For example, COMT activity has long been known to have a trimodal distribution (McLeod et al. 1994, Li et al. 1997). Recent studies demonstrate that the reduction of its activity is caused by a single nucleotide mutation whose allele frequency is approximately 26% in African-Americans, 18% in Asians, and 50% in Caucasians. Higher COMT activity is correlated with the ratio between 3-O-methyldopa and levodopa, which in turn predicts the occurrence of side effects of levodopa in treating Parkinsonism. Reflecting this, a higher percentage of Asians have been found to be poor responders to levodopa (Rivera-Calimlim and Reilly 1984). It is at present unclear whether, and to what extent, such inter-individual and cross-ethnic variations in the polymorphism of these enzymes might influence the pharmacodynamics of psychotropics used in the clinical settings.

Although much less understood, it is commonly agreed that the signal transduction cascade is also of tremendous importance in mediating the effect of psychotropics. Components of this cascade include G-proteins, ion channels, "secondary messengers," and protein kinases (Manji et al. 1995). Inter-individual and cross-ethnic variations in the genes coding these proteins are likely to exist, and may also be responsible for the individual variability in drug response as observed clinically.

## Summary and Future Research Directions

This brief survey serves to highlight the significance as well as the complexity of issues surrounding the influence of cultural and ethnic forces on psychotropic responses. Taken together, the literature reviewed above clearly demonstrates the importance of these factors in psychopharmacotherapy. At the same time, it is equally important that any findings regarding ethnic variations in pharmacological responses not be interpreted stereotypically. In this regard, it is useful to keep in mind that almost all ethnic and cultural contrasts are superimposed on usually very substantial inter-individual variations in all human groups. This is true not only in regard to biological traits such as the ones reviewed above, but equally so (or even more so) with regard to "cultural" and psychosocial variables. Stereotypic interpretations of cultural and ethnic differences in either psychological or biological characteristics are not only misleading but also potentially divisive and dangerous.

Further, in interpreting biological diversity, both within and across populations, it is important to keep in mind that biological systems are dynamic rather than static, and the expression of genetic predisposition is constantly modified by environmental exposure. This is most clearly demonstrated in the case of the induction and inhibition of the drug metabolizing enzymes, which could radically alter an individual's metabolic profile, such that a genetically "extensive metabolizer" might appear to possess nonfunctioning gene(s). Although it is reasonable to believe that social and psychological events would similarly exert powerful influences on the functioning of relevant genes, such influences are likely to be far more subtle and complex, and have remained largely unexplored.

In addition to culture and ethnicity, other key sociodemographic variables, such as age and gender, have also been known to significantly influence the pharmacokinetics and pharmacodynamics of psychotropics and other pharmaceutical agents (Jensvold et al. 1996). For example, the activity of most P-450 enzymes shows significant decline in older individuals (Kinirons and Crome 1997, Tanaka, 1998), who are also likely to suffer from progressive loss of neuron cells as well as receptors targeted by psychotropics (Salzman 1984). Both of these changes render the elderly more sensitive to the effects of medications in general. Similarly, steroid hormones including sex hormones have been demonstrated to be substrates of some of the P-450 enzymes, and have the capacity to alter the activity of these enzymes through competitive inhibition and/or other mechanisms. They have also been known to exert powerful influences on some of the brain receptors that might directly or indirectly affect the pharmacodynamics of psychotropics (Jensvold et al. 1996). It is at present unclear to what extent such age and gender effects interact with the effect of ethnicity, and whether such interactions are "synergistic" or "additive." Studies examining such interactions might be of utmost clinical importance, since they might help identify groups with heightened possibility of "unusual" dose response and side effect profiles.

Progress in the research on P-450 enzymes and other drug metabolizing enzymes in the past 3 decades has led to the development of a number of laboratory procedures that could be used for determining the activity of these enzymes as well as polymorphisms of the genes encoding these enzymes. These procedures have been found to be predictive of the pharmacokinetics and side effect profiles of a number of psychotropics. In addition, emergent data suggest that some of the polymorphisms of genes encoding neurotransmitter transporters and/or receptors might also predict treatment outcome. Thus, it appears that technology may be in place for researchers to systematically test the utility of these procedures in the clinical settings. It is likely that progress in this direction will eventually lead to the development of a panel of genotyping and/or phenotyping procedures that could be used by clinicians to guide their decisions in terms of the choice of antidepressants, the starting dosage, strategies for titration, as well as the prediction of likely side effects. Such a panel will not only enhance the treatment response rate, but also reduce the duration for dose titration, minimize the development of untoward effects, and thus ensure better treatment compliance. Thus, it should also result in treatment strategies that are not only more effective but also more cost-effective than "traditional" titration methods. With the development of high throughput of gene array technologies (Hacia et al. 1998), such as the matrix-assisted laser desorption ionization time-of-flight mass spectroscopy (TOLFI MS) (Ross et al. 1998), thousands of samples could be processed on a daily basis, so that the turnaround time for test results could be short enough to be useful for clinicians ordering such tests. Together, these exciting new developments should help make psychopharmacotherapy increasingly more rational, evidence based, and effective.

The progress in pharmacogenetics might also stimulate research on "nonbiological" issues such as cultural influences on adherence and other factors that determine patients' perception and help-seeking behavior, which in turn contribute toward their sense of satisfaction and their being able to maximally benefit from psychotropic treatment. With such an integrative approach, we would be best able to define elements for optimal pharmacotherapeutic practices that would take both cultural and biological diversity into consideration and tailor treatment to individual characteristics rather than relying on global guidelines.

---

Clinical Vignette

A 32-year-old Vietnamese female with no prior psychiatric history and unclear family history of mental problems presented with complaints of chronic fatigue and hearing voices telling her to kill herself. She was born in Vietnam and immigrated with her parents to the US from Vietnam when she was 22 years old. She attended school till the fifth grade in Vietnam and has had no formal education in the US. She worked on the family farm in Vietnam, and once moved to the US, began working at a family friend's donut shop as a cashier. Family reported that she has always been a shy person and has always preferred to be alone. For the last few months, family began to notice her hoarding little pieces of trash papers which she claimed to be evidence that the communists have followed them to the US. She was also noticed by others to be more isolative and would sometimes mumble to herself. One week prior to her presentation to the community mental health clinic, she became tearful while watching TV with her family and began talking about her body being controlled by the government through electric transmissions in the air. She became agitated when family tried to calm her down and threatened to kill herself. In the psychiatrist office, patient was observed to be responding to internal stimuli. She admitted to hearing voices telling her to kill herself. She also complained of fatigue, headaches, neck and eye pains.

After the initial history and physical, the psychiatrist started her on Risperdal, titrated over 1 month to 4 mg and Paxil, titrated over the same period of time to 20 mg/day. Six weeks after the initial evaluation, patient was noted to be very restless, pacing back and forth in the office and extremely agitated. Her Risperdal was lowered to 2 mg and in the subsequent weeks her symptoms of restlessness resolved as well as her complaints of auditory hallucinations. Two months later, although patient appeared to be doing better, she continued to complain of chronic fatigue. Upon further questioning, she admitted to the psychiatrist that Paxil 20 mg/day was helpful for sleep; however, she had discontinued taking it because of concerns that she may become "addicted to sleeping pills."

## References

Acosta FX, Yamamoto J, and Evans LA (1982) Effective Psychotherapy for Low-Income and Minority Patients. Plenum Press, New York.

Adebimpe VR (1981) Overview: White norms and psychiatric diagnosis of Black patients. Am J Psychiatr 138, 279–285.

Akullu E, Persson I, Bertilsson L, et al. (1996) Frequent distribution of ultrarapid metabolizers of debrisoquine in an Ethiopian population carrying duplicated and multiduplicated functional CYP2D6 alleles. J Pharmacol Exp Ther 278, 441–446.

Allen JG, Rack P, and Vaddadi K (1977) Differences in the effects of clomipramine on English and Asian volunteers: Preliminary report on a pilot study. Postgrad Med J 53, 79–86.

Amadi E, Offiah N, and Akah P (1991) Neuropychopharmacologic properties of a Schumanniophyton problematicum root extract. J Ethnopharmacol 33, 73–77.

Ameer B and Weintraub RA (1997) Drug interactions with grapefruit juice. Clin Pharmacokinet 33, 103–121.

American Psychiatric Association (1994) Diagnostic and Statistical Manual of Mental Disorders, 4th ed. APA, Washington, DC.

Anderson KE, Rosner W, Khan MS, et al. (1987) Diet-hormone interactions: Protein/carbohydrate ratio alters reciprocally the plasma levels of testosterone and cortisol and their respective binding globulins in man. Life Sci 40, 1761–1768.

Anderson KE and Kappas A (1991) Dietary regulation of cytochrome P450. Annu Rev Nutr 11, 141–167.

Aranow RB, Hudson JI, Pope HG, et al. (1989) Elevated antidepressant plasma levels after addition of fluoxetine. Am J Psychiatr 146, 911–913.

Balick MJ and Cox PA (1996) Plants, People, and Culture: The Science of Ethnobotany. Scientific American Library, New York.

Becker MH (1985) Patient adherence to prescribed therapies. Med Care 23, 539–555.

Becker M and Maiman L (1980) Strategies for enhancing patient compliance. J Comm Health 6, 113–135.

Benton RE, Honig PK, Zamani K, et al. (1996) Grapefruit juice alters terfenadine pharmacokinetics, resulting in prolongation of repolarization on the electrocardiogram. Clin Pharmacol Ther 59, 383–388.

Bergstrom RF, Peyton AL, and Lemberger L (1992) Quantification and mechanism of the fluoxetine and tricyclic antidepressant interaction. Clin Pharmacol Ther 51, 239–248.

Bloom FE, Kupfer D, Bunney B, et al. (1995) Psychopharmacology: The Fourth Generation of Progress. An official publication of the American College of Neuropsychopharmacology. Raven Press, New York.

Blum K, Sheridan PJ, Wood RC, et al. (1995) Dopamine D$_2$ receptor gene variants: Association and linkage studies in impulsive–addictive–compulsive behaviour. Pharmacogenetics 5, 121–141.

Bolt HM (1994) Interactions between clinically used drugs and oral contraceptives. Environ Health Persp 102(Suppl 9), 35–38.

Branch RA, Salih SY, and Homeida M (1978) Racial differences in drug metabolizing ability: A study with antipyrine in the Sudan. Clin Pharmacol Ther 24, 283–286.

Brosen K (1995) Drug interactions and the cytochrome P450 system. Clin Pharmacokinet 29, 20–25.

Buckalew LW and Coffield K (1982) Drug expectations associated with perceptual characteristics: Ethnic factors. Percept Motor Skills 55, 915–918.

Castro, FG, Furth P, and Karlow H (1994) The health beliefs of Mexican, Mexican-American and Anglo-American women. Hispanic J Behav Sci 6, 365–383.

Chan CW and Chang JK (1976) The role of Chinese medicine in New York City's Chinatown. Am J Chin Med 4, 31–45, 129–146.

Chang FM, Kidd JR, Livak KJ, et al. (1996) The world-wide distribution of allele frequencies at the human dopamine D$_4$ receptor locus. Hum Genet 98, 91–101.

Chen A (1991) Noncompliance in community psychiatry: A review of clinical interventions. Hosp Comm Psychiatr 42, 282–287.

Cott JM (1997) In vitro receptor binding and enzyme inhibition by hypericum perforatum extract. Pharmacopsychiatry 30, 108–112.

Dai D, Tang J, Rose R, et al. (2001) Identification of variants of CYP3A4 and characterization of their abilities to metabolize testosterone and chlorpyrifos. J Pharmacol Exp Ther 299(3), 825–831.

D'Arcy PF (1991) Adverse reactions and interactions with herbal medicines. Part 1. Adverse reactions. Adverse Drug React Toxicol Rev 10, 189–208.

D'Arcy PF (1993) Adverse reactions and interactions with herbal medicines. Part 2. Drug interactions. Adverse Drug React Toxicol Rev 12, 147–162.

D'Mello DA, McNeil JA, and Harris W (1989) Multi-ethnic variance in psychiatric diagnosis and neuroleptic dosage. APA 142nd Annual Meeting in San Francisco (May 6–11), CA.

Dahl ML, Yue QY, Roh HK, et al. (1995) Genetic analysis of the CYP2D locus in relation to debrisoquine hydroxylation capacity in Korean, Japanese and Chinese subjects. Pharmacogenetics 5, 159–164.

Daly AK, Brockmoller J, Broly F, et al. (1996) Nomenclature for human CYP2D6 alleles. Pharmacogenetics 6, 193–201.

de Morais SM, Wilkinson GR, Blaisdell J, et al. (1994) The major genetic defect responsible for the polymorphism of S-mephenytoin metabolism in humans. J Biol Chem 269, 15419–15422.

Dean M, Stephens JC, Winkler C, et al. (1994) Polymorphic admixture typing in human ethnic populations. Am J Hum Genet 55, 788–808.

DeVane CL (1994) Pharmacogenetics and drug metabolism of newer antidepressant agents. J Clin Psychiatr 55(Suppl), 38–45.

Duke JA (1995) Commentary—novel psychotherapeutic drugs: A role for ethnobotany. Psychopharmacol Bull 31, 177–184.

Eisenberg DM, Davis RB, Ettner SL, et al. (1998) Trends in alternative medicine use in the United States, 1990–1997: Results of a follow-up national survey. JAMA 280, 1569–1575.

Eisenberg DM, Kessler RC, Foster C, et al. (1993) Unconventional medicine in the United States: Prevalence, cost, and patterns of use. N Engl J Med 328, 246–252.

Engebretson J and Wardell D (1993) A contemporary view of alternative healing modalities. Nurse Pract 18, 51–55.

Ernst E (1999) Second thoughts about safety of St. John's wort. Lancet 354, 2014–2016.

Fenton WS, Blyler CR, and Heinssen RK (1997) Determinants of medication compliance in schizophrenia: Empirical and clinical findings. Schizophr Bull 23, 637–651.

Frank JD (1974) Persuasion and Healing: A Comparative Study of Psychotherapy. Schocken Books, New York.

Fraser HS, Mucklow JC, Bulpitt CJ, et al. (1979) Environmental factors affecting antipyrine metabolism in London factory and office workers. Br J Clin Pharmacol 7, 237–243.

Fugh-Berman A (2000) Herb–drug interactions. Lancet 355, 134–138.

Fuhr U, Klittich K, and Staib AH (1993) Inhibitory effect of grapefruit juice and its bitter principal, naringenin, on CYP1A2 dependent metabolism of caffeine in man. Br J Clin Pharmacol 35, 431–436.

Fukuda K, Ohta T, and Yamazoe Y (1997) Grapefruit component interacting with rat and human P450 CYP3A: Possible involvement of non-flavonoid components in drug interaction. Biol Pharm Bull 20, 560–565.

Gaw A (1993) Culture, Ethnicity, and Mental Illness. American Psychiatric Press, Washington DC.

Gelenter J, Kranzler H, Cubells JF, et al. (1997) Serotonin transporter protein (SLC6A4) allele and haplotype frequencies and linkage disequilibria in African- and European-American and Japanese populations in alcohol-dependent subjects. Hum Genet 101, 243–246.

Gill HJ, Tijia JF, Kitteringham NR, et al. (1999) The effect of genetic polymorphisms in CYP2C9 on suphamethoxazole N-hydroxylation. Pharmacogenetics 9, 43–53.

Gillis L, Trollip D, Jakoet A, et al. (1987) Non-compliance with psychotropic medication. S Afr Med J 72, 602–606.

Glazer WM and Ereshefsky L (1996) A pharmacoeconomic model of outpatient antipsychotic therapy in "revolving door" schizophrenic patients. J Clin Psychiatr 57, 337–345.

Goldman D, Lappalainen J, and Ozaki N (1996) Direct analysis of candidate genes in impulsive behaviors. Ceiba Found Sump 194, 139–152.

Goldstein JA, Faletto MB, Romkes-Sparks M, et al. (1994) Evidence that CPY2C19 is the major (S)-mephenytoin 4″-hydroxylase in humans. Biochemistry 33, 1743–1752.

Goldstein JA, Ishizaki T, Chiba K, et al. (1997) Frequencies of the defective CYP2C19 alleles responsible for the mephenytoin poor metabolizer phenotype in various Oriental, Caucasian, Saudi Arabian and American black populations. Pharmacogenetics 7, 59–64.

Gonzalez FJ and Nebert DW (1990) Evolution of the P450 gene superfamily: Animal-plant 'warfare', molecular drive and human genetic differences in drug oxidation. Trends Genet 6, 182–186.

Greenberg BD, McMahon FJ, and Murphy DL (1998) Serotonin transporter candidate gene studies in affective disorders and personality: Promises and potential pitfalls. Guest Editorial. Mol Psychiatr 3, 186–189.

Greenblatt DJ (1993) Basic phamacokinetic principles and their application to psychotropic drugs. J Clin Psychiatr 54, 8–13.

Guengerich FP, Shimada T, Yun CH, et al. (1994) Interactions of ingested food, beverage, and tobacco components involving human cytochrome P4501A2, 2A6, 2E1, and 3A4 enzymes. Environ Health Persp 102(Suppl 9), 49–53.

Ha HR, Chen J, Leuenberger PM, et al. (1995) In vitro inhibition of midazolam and quinidine metabolism by flavonoids. Eur J Clin Pharmacol 48, 367–371.

Hacia JG, Brody LC, and Collins FS (1998) Applications of DNA chips for genomic analysis. Mol Psychiatr 3, 483–492.

Haynes R, Wang E, and da Mota Gomez M (1987) A critical review of interventions to improve compliance with prescribed medications. Patient Educ Couns 10, 155–166.

Herrera J, Lawson W, and Sramek J (1999) Cross Cultural Psychiatry. John Wiley, New York, pp. 3–5, 45–52.

Hietala J, West C, Syvalahti E, et al. (1994) Striatal D$_2$ dopamine receptor binding characteristics in vivo in patients with alcohol dependence. Psychopharmacology 116, 285–290.

Hodge SE (1994) What association analysis can and cannot tell us about the genetics of complex disease. Am J Med Genet 54, 318–323.

Hsieh KP, Lin YY, Cheng CL, et al. (2001) Novel mutations of CYP3A4 in Chinese. Drug Metab Dispos 29(3), 268–273.

Hughes JB, Daily GC, and Ehrlich PR (1997) Population diversity: Its extent and extinction. Science 278, 689–692.

Ibeanu GC, Blaisdell J, Ferguson RJ, et al. (1999) A novel transversion in the intron 5 donor splice junction of CYP2C19 and a sequence polymorphism in exon 3 contribute to the poor metabolizer phenotype for the anticonvulsant drug S-mephenytoin. J Pharmacol Exp Ther 290(2), 635–640.

Ibeanu GC, Goldstein JA, Meyer U, et al. (1998) Identification of new human CYP2C19 alleles (CYP2C19&6 and CYP2C19*2B) in a Caucasian poor metabolizer of mephenytoin. J Pharmacol Exp Ther 286(3), 1490–1495.

Jensvold MF, Halbreich U, and Hamilton JA (1996) Psychopharmacology and Women: Sex, Gender, and Hormones. American Psychiatric Press, Washington DC, pp. 121–136.

Jonsson EG, Goldman D, Spurlock G, et al. (1997) Tryptophan hydroxylase and catechol-O-methyltransferase gene polymorphisms: Relationships to monoamine metabolite concentrations in CSF of healthy volunteers. Eur Arch Psychiatr Clin Neurosci 247, 297–302.

Jurima-Romet M, Crawford K, Cyr T, et al. (1994) Terfenadine metabolism in human liver: In vitro inhibition by macrolide antibiotics and azole antifungals. Drug Metab Dispos 22, 849–857.

Kalow W (1990) Pharmacogenetics: Past and future. Life Sci 47, 1385–1397.

Kalow W (1992) Pharmacogenetics of Drug Metabolism. Pergamon Press, New York.

Kidd RS, Straughn AB, Meyer MC, et al. (1999) Pharmacokinetics of chlorpheniramine, phenytoin, glipizide and nifedipine in an individual homozygous for the CYP2C9*3 allele. Pharmacogenetics 9, 71–80.

Kinirons MT and Crome P (1997) Clinical pharmacokinetic considerations in the elderly: An update. Clin Pharmacokinet 33, 302–312.

Kinzie JD, Leung P, Boehnlein J, et al. (1987) Tricyclic antidepressant plasma levels in Indochinese refugees: Clinical implication. J Nerv Ment Disord 175, 480–485.

Kirsch I (1990) Changing Expectations: A Key to Effective Psychotherapy. Brooks/Cole, Pacific Grove, CA.

Kleinman A, Eisenberg L, and Good BJ (1978) Culture, illness, and care: Clinical lessons from anthropologic and cross-cultural research. Annu Intern Med 88(2), 251–258.

Kleinman A (1988) Rethinking Psychiatry. Free Press, New York.

Landy D (1977) Culture, Disease, and Healing. Macmillan, New York.

Leathart JB, London SJ, Steward A, et al. (1998) CYP2D6 phenotype-genotype relationships in African-Americans and Caucasians in Los Angeles. Pharmacogenetics 8, 529–541.

Lee S, Wing YK, and Wong KC (1992) Knowledge and compliance towards lithium therapy among Chinese psychiatric patients in Hong Kong. Aust NZ J Psychiatr 26, 444–449.

Leslie C (1976) Asian Medical Systems: A Comparative Study. University of California Press, Berkeley, CA.

Lewis W, Kennelly E, and Bass G (1991) Ritualistic use of the holly ilex guayusa by Amazonian Jivaro Indians. J Ethnopharmacol 33, 25–30.

Li T, Vallada H, Curtis D, et al. (1997) Catechol-O-methyltransferase Val158Met polymorphism: Frequency analysis in Han Chinese subjects and allelic association of the low activity allele with bipolar affective disorder. Pharmacogenetics 7, 349–353.

Lin KM (1981) Traditional Chinese medical beliefs and their relevance for mental illness and psychiatry. In Normal and Abnormal Behavior in Chinese Culture, Kleinman S and Lin TY (eds). Dordrecht, Boston, Reidel, Hingham, MA.

Lin KM and Cheung F (1999) Mental health issues for Asian-Americans. Psychiatr Serv 50, 774–780.

Lin KM and Poland RE (1995) Ethnicity, Culture, and Psychopharmacology in Psychopharmacology: The Fourth Generation of Progress, Bloom FE and Kupfer DI (eds). Raven Press, New York.

Lin KM, Demonteverde L, and Nuccio I (1990) Religion, healing and mental health among Filipino-Americans. Int J Mental Health 19, 40–44.

Lin KM, Poland RE, Lan JK, et al. (1988) Haloperidol and prolactin concentrations in Asians and Cancasians. J Clin Psychopharmacol 8, 195–201.

Lin KM, Poland RE, and Nakasaki G (1993) Psychopharmacology and Psychobiology of Ethnicity. American Psychiatric Press, Washington DC.

Lin KM, Poland RE, and Nakasaki G (1993) Psychopharmacology. American Psychiatric Press, Washington DC.

Littlewood R (1992) Psychiatric diagnosis and racial bias: Empirical and interpretative approaches. Soc Sci Med 34, 141–149.

Liu G (1991) Effects of some compounds isolated from Chinese medicinal herbs on hepatic microsomal cytochrome P-450 and their potential biological consequences. Drug Metab Rev 23, 439–465.

Lopez SR (1989) Patient variable biases in clinical judgment: Conceptual overview and methodological considerations. Psychol Bull 106, 184–203.

Manji HK, Potter WZ, Lenox RH, et al. (1995) Signal transduction pathways: Molecular targets for lithium's actions. Arch Gen Psychiatr 52, 531–543.

Manne SL (1998) Treatment adherence and compliance. In Handbook of Pediatric Psychology and Psychiatric, Vol. 2: Disease, Injury, and Illness. Allyn & Bacon, Boston, MA.

Marquez C, Taintor Z, and Schwartz MA (1985) Diagnosis of manic depressive illness in Blacks. Compr Psychiatr 26, 337–341.

Marsella AJ, DeVos G, and Hsu FLK (1985) Culture and Self: Asian and Western Perspectives. Tavistock, New York.

Marwick C (1995) Scientists stress biodiversity–human health links. JAMA 273, 1246.

Masimirembwa CM and Hasler JA (1997) Genetic polymorphism of drug metabolising enzymes in African populations: Implications for the use of neuroleptics and antidepressants. Brain Res Bull 44, 561–571.

Maurer A, Johne A, and Bauer S (1999) Interaction of St. John's wort extract with phenprocoumon. Eur J Clin Pharmacol 55(A22).

Mendoza, R, Wan YJY, Poland RE, et al. (2001) CYP2D6 polymorphism in a Mexican American population. Clin Pharmacol Therap 70(6), 552–560.

McLeod HL, Fang L, Luo X, et al. (1994) Ethnic differences in erythrocyte catechol-O-methyltransferase activity in black and white Americans. J Pharmacol Exp Ther 270, 26–29.

Mezzich JE, Kleinman A, Fabrega H, et al. (1995) Culture and Psychiatric Diagnosis. American Psychiatric Press, Washington DC.

Michaelovsky E, Frisch A, Rockah R, et al. (1999) A novel allele in the promoter region of the human serotonin transporter gene. Mol Psychiatr 4, 97–99.

Moerman D (1979) Anthropology of symbolic healing. Cur Anthropol 20, 59–80.

Morgenstern H and Glazer WM (1993) Identifying risk factors for tardive dyskinesia among long-term outpatients maintained with neuroleptic medications. Arch Gen Psychiatr 50, 723–733.

Mukherjee S, Shukla S, Woodle J, et al. (1983) Misdiagnosis of schizophrenia in bipolar patients: A multiethnic comparison. Am J Psychiatr 140, 1571–1574.

National Institute of Mental Health (1997) Genetics and Mental Disorders: Report of the National Institute of Health's Genetics Workgroup. www.nimh.nih.gov/research/genetics.htm.

Nakajima M, Yodoi T, Mizutani M, et al. (1999) Genetic polymorphism in the 5'-flanking region of human CYP1A2 gene: Effect on the CYP1A2 inducibility in humans. J Biochem (Tokyo) 125(4), 803–808.

Noble EP, Blum K, Ritchie T, et al. (1991) Allelic association of the $D_2$ dopamine receptor gene with receptor-binding characteristics in alcoholism. Arch Gen Psychiatr 48, 648–654.

Oesterheld J and Kallepalli BR (1997) Grapefruit juice and clomipramine: Shifting metabolic ratios. J Clin Psychopharmacol 17, 62–63.

Okpaku SO (1998) Clinical Methods in Transcultural Psychiatry. American Psychiatric Press, Washington, DC.

Parsian A, Chakraverty S, Fisher L, et al. (1999) No association between polymorphisms in the human dopamine $D_3$ and $D_4$ receptors genes and alcoholism. Am J Med Genet 74, 281–285.

Pi E, Gutierrez M, and Gray G (1993) Tardive Dyskinesia: Cross-cultural Perspectives in Psychopharmacology and Psychobiology of Ethnicity, Lin KM, Poland R, and Nakasaki G (eds). American Psychiatric Press, Washington, DC, pp. 153–167.

Pi E, Gutierrez M, and Gray G (1993) Cross-cultural studies in tardive dyskinesia. Am J Psychiatr 150, 991.

Piscitelli SC, Burstein AH, Chaitt D, et al. (2000) Indinavir concentrations and St. John's Wort [letter]. Lancet 355, 547–548.

Polednak A (1989) Racial and Ethnic Differences in Disease. Oxford University Press, New York.

Price N, Glazer WM, and Morgenstern H (1985) Race and the use of fluphenazine decanoate. Am J Psychiatr 142, 1491–1492.

Raimundo S, Fischer J, Eischelbaum M, et al. (2000) Elucidation of the genetic basis of the common 'intermediate metabolizer' phenotype for drug oxidation by CYP2D6. Pharmacogenetics 10(7), 577–581.

Rappaport H (1977) The tenacity of folk psychotherapy: A functional interpretation. Soc Psychiatr 12(3), 127–132.

Rivera-Calimlim L and Reilly DK (1984) Difference in erythrocyte catechol-O-methyltransferase activity between Orientals and Caucasians: Difference in levodopa tolerance. Clin Pharmacol Ther 35, 804–809.

Roh HK, Dahl ML, Johansson I, et al. (1996) Debrisoquine and S-mephenytoin hydroxylation phenotypes and genotypes in a Korean population. Pharmacogenetics. 6, 441–447.

Ross P, Hall L, Smirnov I, et al. (1998) High level multiplex genotyping by MALDI-TOF mass spectrometry. Nat Biotechnol 16, 1347–1351.

Roukema R, Fadem BH, James B, et al. (1984) Bipolar disorder in a low socioeconomic population: Difficulties in diagnosis. J Nerv Ment Dis 72, 76–79.

Ruschitzka F, Meier PJ, Turina M, et al. (2000) Acute heart transplant rejection due to Saint John's Wort [letter]. Lancet 355, 548–549.

Sackett D and Haynes R (1976) Compliance with Therapeutic Regimens. Johns Hopkins University Press, Baltimore.

Salzman C (1984) Clinical Geriatric Psychopharmacology. McGraw-Hill, New York.

Sander T, Harms H, Podschus J, et al. (1995) Dopamine $D_1$, $D_2$ and $D_3$ receptor genes in alcohol dependence. Psychiatr Genet 5, 171–176.

Sankury T (1983) Lead poisoning from Mexican folk remedies—California (letter). JAMA 250, 3149.

Shepherd M (1993) The placebo: From specificity to the nonspecific and back. Psychol Med 23, 569–578.

Shimada T, Tsumura F, Yamazaki H, et al. (2001) Characterization of (+/−)-bufuralol hydroxylation activities in liver microsomes of Japanese and Caucasian subjects genotyped for CYP2D6. Pharmacogenetics 1(2), 143–156.

Smeraldi E, Zanardi R, Benedetti F, et al. (1998) Polymorphism within the promoter of the serotonin transporter gene and antidepressant efficacy of fluvoxamine. Mol Psychiatr 3, 508–511.

Smith M, Lin KM, and Mendoza R (1993) "Non-Biological" Issues affecting psychopharmacotherapy: Cultural Considerations in Psycho-Pharmacology and Psychobiology of Ethnicity, Lin KM, Poland R, and Nakasaki G. (eds). American Psychiatric Press, Washington, DC. 37–58.

Smith M and Smith J (1999) Herbal toxicity. Ess Psychopharmacol 19, 363–378.

Sramek J, Roy S, Ahrens T, et al. (1991) Prevalence of tardive dyskinesia among three ethnic groups of chronic psychiatric patients. Hosp Comm Psychiatr 42, 590–592.

Stephens EA, Taylor JA, Yang CH, et al. (1994) Ethnic variation in the CYP2E1 gene: Polymorphism analysis of 695 African-Americans, European-Americans and Taiwanese. Pharmacogenetics 4, 185–192.

Strickland TL, Ranganath V, Lin KM, et al. (1991) Psychopharmacologic considerations in the treatment of black American populations. Psychopharmacol Bull 27, 441–448.

Sue S, Fujino DC, Hu LT, et al. (1991) Community mental health services for ethnic minority the cultural responsiveness hypothesis. J Consult Clin Psychol 59, 533–540.

Sullivan G, Wells KB, Morgenstern H, et al. (1995) Identifying modifiable risk factors for rehospitalization: A case-control study of seriously mentally ill persons in Mississippi. Am J Psychiatr 152(12), 1749–1756.

Sullivan PF, Fifield WJ, Kennedy MA, et al. (1998) No association between novelty seeking and the type 4 dopamine receptor gene (DRD4) in two New Zealand samples. Am J Psychiatr 155, 98–101.

Swartz R, Burgoyne K, Smith M, et al. (1997) Tardive dyskinesia and ethnicity: Review of the literature. Ann Clin Psychiatr 9, 53–59.

Swartzman LC and Burkell J (1998) Expectations and the placebo effect in clinical drug trials: Why we should not turn a blind eye to unblinding, and other cautionary notes. Clin Pharmacol Ther 64, 1–7.

Tanaka E (1998) In vivo age-related changes in hepatic drug-oxidizing capacity in humans. J Clin Pharm Ther 23, 247–255.

Tinsley H, Bowman S, and Ray S (1988) Manipulation of expectancies about counselling and psychotherapy: Review and analysis of expectancy manipulation strategies and results. J Couns Psychol 35(1), 99–108.

Vandenbergh DJ, Persico AM, Hawkins AL, et al. (1992) Human dopamine transporter gene (DAT1) maps to chromosome 5p15.3 and displays a VNTR. Genomics 14, 1104–1106.

Vermeer D and Farrell R (1985) Nigerian geophagical clay: A traditional antidiarrheal pharmaceutical. Science 227, 634–636.

Wan YJY, Poland RE, Han G, et al. (2001) Analysis of the CYP2D6 gene polymorphism and enzyme activity in African-Americans in Southern California. Pharmacogenetics 11, 489–499.

Wang SL, Huang JD, Lai MD, et al. (1993) Molecular basis of genetic variation in debrisoquin hydroxylation in Chinese subjects: Polymorphism in RFLP and DNA sequence of CYP2D6. Clin Pharmacol Ther 53, 410–418.

Weber WW (1997) Pharmacogenetics. Oxford University Press, New York.

Weiner M and Weiner GJ (1996) The kinetics and dynamics of responses to placebo. Clin Pharmacol Ther 60, 247–254.

Weiss M (1997) Explanatory Model Interview Catalogue (EMIC): Framework for comparative study of illness. Transcult Psychiatr 34, 235–263.

Westermeyer J (1989) Psychiatric Care of Migrants: A Clinical Guide. American Psychiatric Press, Washington DC.

Wetzel MS, Eisenberg DM, and Kaptchuk TJ (1998) Courses involving complementary and alternative medicine at US medical schools. JAMA 280, 784–787.

White L, Tursky B, and Schwartz GE (1985) Placebo: Theory, Research, and Mechanisms. The Guilford Press, New York.

Wig NN (1989) Indian concepts of mental health and their impact on care of the mentally ill. Int J Ment Health 18(3), 71–80.

Wolffers I (1989) Traditional practitioners' behavioral adaptations to changing patients' demands in Sri Lanka. Soc Sci Med 29(9), 1111–1119.

Yue QY, Bergquist C, and Gerden B (2000) Safety of St. John's Wort (Hypericum perforatum). Lancet 355, 576–577.

# 95 Antipsychotic Drugs

Seiya Miyamoto
Jeffrey A. Lieberman
W. Wolfgang Fleischhacker
Anri Aoba
Stephen R. Marder

## Introduction

Information about antipsychotic drugs and theoretical developments in the treatment of psychosis is rapidly expanding, and more agents with antipsychotic efficacy are being developed. The advent of newer second-generation antipsychotics in the wake of clozapine represents the first significant advances in the pharmacologic treatment of schizophrenia and related psychotic disorders, and many clinicians in the US are prescribing these second-generation antipsychotics as the first-choice agent for acute and maintenance therapy for these illnesses (Buckley 2001, McEvoy et al. 1999).

There is growing evidence that most of the new medications can offer advantages over conventional neuroleptics such as improvement in negative symptoms, cognitive impairment, fewer extrapyramidal symptoms, and less tardive dyskinesia. Treatment successes have contributed to the increased use of newer antipsychotic agents and have also allowed psychiatrists to expand clinical expectations. In addition, these second-generation drugs are being used increasingly for various conditions beyond schizophrenia as happened with the conventional antipsychotics (Glick et al. 2001). This chapter reviews history, pharmacology, indications, efficacy, and side effects of antipsychotic drugs on the basis of the currently available evidence, and discusses how newer antipsychotic medications have revolutionized the management of the symptoms and improved the quality of life of patients with psychosis, and their broadening utilization to other disorders.

## History of Antipsychotic Drug Development

The era of antipsychotic pharmacotherapy began with the discovery of the antipsychotic properties and introduction of chlorpromazine in the early 1950s by Delay and Deniker (1952). Since then, a number of neuroleptics were developed based on the hypothesis that schizophrenia reflected a disorder of hyperdopaminergic activity, with the dopamine $D_2$ receptor most strongly associated with antipsychotic response (Seeman 1992). In many patients with schizophrenia, the widely used typical antipsychotic drugs (phenothiazines, butyrophenones, and thioxanthenes), which are also referred to as conventional, standard, classical, traditional, or typical antipsychotic drugs, are effective in the treatment of the positive symptoms of schizophrenia, and also in preventing psychotic relapse (Kane 1989). Almost a half century of experience, however, has revealed their substantial limitations in the use. As many as 25 to 60% of patients treated with conventional antipsychotics remain symptomatic and are labeled either treatment-refractory, or partially responsive (Miyamoto et al. 2000). Moreover, these drugs at best only modestly improve negative symptoms of the deficit syndrome and a range of cognitive impairments, which may be fundamental to the disease (Meltzer 1999a). Further, first-generation antipsychotics cause a variety of troublesome side effects both acutely (e.g., extrapyramidal side effects [EPS]) and with long-term exposure (e.g., tardive dyskinesia [TD]) (Fleischhacker 1995, Campbell et al. 1999). Such side effects may reduce compliance, which in turn leads to relapse and rehospitalization, and thus they represent a major drawback of first-generation drugs.

For a number of years, there was a widely held view that any compound that was an effective antipsychotic agent must also induce EPS. The availability of clozapine and other newer second-generation antipsychotic agents have, however, disproved this concept. The development of second-generation antipsychotic drugs was aimed at increasing the ratio between doses that produce therapeutic effects and those that produce side effects, as well as improving efficacy (e.g., against a broader spectrum of psychopathological symptoms and the treatment-resistant aspects of the disorder) (Lieberman 1996). Although there is currently no standardized definition of the term "atypical," in its broadest sense it is used to refer to drugs that have at least equal antipsychotic efficacy compared to conventional drugs, without producing the same degree of EPS or prolactin elevation (Kinon and Lieberman 1996, Lieberman 1996). A more restrictive definition would require that atypical drugs also have superior antipsychotic efficacy (i.e., they are effective in treatment-resistant schizophrenic patients, and against negative symptoms and/or cognitive deficits) (Remington and Chong 1999).

The agents like thioridazine were first suggested to have atypical characteristics, but it now is generally accepted that clozapine, first synthesized in 1958, is the prototypical "atypical" antipsychotic (Meyer and Simpson 1997). Clozapine underwent extensive clinical testing in the 1970s, but its development was halted in the US, and limited in other countries, because of a relatively high incidence of a potential fatal side effect, agranulocytosis. Nonetheless, its superior outcomes ultimately led to further development and eventual reintroduction beginning in 1990 (Lieberman et al. 1989). The renaissance of clozapine was based on several advantages: it appears to be superior to conventional drugs (e.g., chlorpromazine and haloperidol) in treatment-resistant schizophrenia (Kane et al. 1988); it can ameliorate some of the negative as well as positive symptoms of schizophrenia (Lieberman 1993); it can reduce relapse; it may improve certain cognitive impairments (Buchanan et al. 1994a, Meyer-Lindenberg et al. 1997); it may alleviate mood symptoms associated with schizophrenia and reduce the likelihood of suicidal behavior; it has very low liability for EPS and TD; and it does not induce sustained hyperprolactinemia (Lieberman et al. 1989, Remington and Chong 1999).

The reintroduction of clozapine represented a breakthrough in the treatment of schizophrenia. In recent years, concerted research and development efforts have been made to produce a second generation of "atypical" antipsychotic drugs (Table 95–1), with the therapeutic advantages of clozapine, without the associated risk of blood dyscrasias (Duncan et al. 1999b). In early 2002, iloperidone was in late phase III trials in the US. Sertindole, amisulpiride, and zotepine are not marketed in the US. Amisulpiride and zotepine are widely used in Europe and other countries. Sertindole has just been relaunched in Europe solely for the purpose of using it in clinical trials. The others are all approved by the US Food and Drug Administration (FDA). Ongoing clinical evaluation of the new "second-generation" antipsychotic drugs will eventually allow comprehensive assessment of their clinical efficacy and safety.

## Mechanism of Action of Antipsychotic Agents

### Receptor Blockade

The classical dopamine hypothesis of schizophrenia postulates a hyperactivity of dopaminergic transmission at the dopamine $D_2$ receptor (Snyder et al. 1974, Seeman et al. 1976). The hypothesis remains the preeminent neurochemical theory (Seeman and Kapur 2000, Abi-Dargham et al.

2000), despite several limitations (Duncan et al. 1999a). The notion was initially supported by a tight correlation between the therapeutic doses of conventional antipsychotic drugs and their binding affinity for the $D_2$ receptor (Creese et al. 1976, Seeman et al. 1976, Seeman 1987, Miyamoto et al. 2001b).

Recent positron emission tomography (PET) and single photon emission computed tomography (SPECT) studies have further elucidated the importance of dopamine receptor occupancy as a predictor of antipsychotic response and adverse effects (Remington and Kapur 1999). Prospective studies have demonstrated that antipsychotic effects require a striatal $D_2$ receptor occupancy of 65 to 70% (Farde et al. 1992, Kapur et al. 1996, 2000, Nordstrom et al. 1993), and $D_2$ occupancy greater than 80% significantly increases the risk of EPS (Farde et al. 1992). Thus, a threshold between 65 and 80% $D_2$ occupancy appears to represent the optimal therapeutic range to minimize the risk of EPS for first-generation antipsychotic drugs (Remington and Kapur 1999, Nyberg and Farde 2000, Kapur et al. 2000a). It should be noted, however, that despite adequate $D_2$ occupancy, many patients do not respond to medication (Nordstrom et al. 1993). Nevertheless, the results to date support the hypothesis that some degree of $D_2$ antagonism is still required to achieve antipsychotic effects (Lieberman et al. 1998). Moreover, results of studies with second-generation drugs, such as olanzapine indicate that $D_2$ occupancy levels above 80% are not invariably associated with the occurrence of EPS, thus casting some doubt over the generalizability of the $D_2$ occupancy model with regard to second-generation antipsychotics (Lieberman et al. 1998).

PET studies showing that therapeutic doses of risperidone and olanzapine produce greater than 70% occupancy of $D_2$ receptors suggest that $D_2$ receptor antagonism could be a predominant mechanism of action of these second-generation drugs (Kapur et al. 1998, 1999). Clozapine and quetiapine, however, do not exhibit high levels of $D_2$ receptor occupancy (less than 70%) at therapeutically effective dose (Farde et al. 1992, Nordstrom et al. 1995, Kapur et al. 1999, 2000b), suggesting that $D_2$ receptor antagonism alone cannot explain the greater therapeutic efficacy of clozapine (Duncan et al. 1999b). The low occupancy of striatal $D_2$ receptors by clozapine and quetiapine could account for its low EPS liability (Nordstrom et al. 1995, Seeman and Tallerico 1998, Kapur et al. 2000b, Nyberg and Farde 2000).

Clozapine, risperidone, olanzapine, and ziprasidone occupy more than 80% of cortical $5\text{-HT}_{2A}$ receptors in the therapeutic dose range in humans (Farde et al. 1992, 1995, Kapur et al. 1998, 1999, Nordstrom et al. 1995, Fischman et al. 1996). Although $5\text{-HT}_{2A}$ receptor antagonism is likely to be associated with the low EPS liability of risperidone and olanzapine, the role of this molecular action in the superior therapeutic responses to clozapine is unclear (Duncan et al. 1999b). Moreover, at this point it is unclear what clinical effects $5\text{-HT}_{2A}$ antagonism confers, in addition to mitigating the adverse effect of striatal $D_2$ antagonism, and propensity to cause EPS (Lieberman et al. 1998). The apparent lack of efficacy of monotherapy with the selective $5\text{-HT}_{2A}$ receptor antagonists M-100907 indicates that $5\text{-HT}_{2A}$ antagonism alone cannot explain the efficacy of second-generation antipsychotic drugs. Further studies examining combination therapy with $D_2$ antagonist and

| Table 95–1 | List of Second-Generation Antipsychotics | |
|---|---|---|
| Drug | Pharmaceutical Company | Trade Name |
| Clozapine | Sandoz, Novartis | Clozaril (Leponex) |
| Risperidone | Janssen | Risperdal |
| Olanzapine | Eli Lilly | Zyprexa |
| Quetiapine | Zeneca, AstraZeneca | Seroquel |
| Ziprasidone | Pfizer | Geodon (Zeldox) |
| Sertindole | Lundbeck | Serdolect |
| Amisulpride | Lorex, Sanofi | Solian |
| Zotepine | Orion, Fujisawa | Zoleptil (Lodopin) |
| Aripiprazole | Otsuka, Bristol-Myers Squibb | Abilify |
| Iloperidone | Hoechst, Novartis | Zomaril |

M-100907 are necessary to evaluate the potential role of $5\text{-HT}_{2A}$ antagonism in the mechanism of action of second-generation antipsychotic drugs.

Recently, aripiprazole, a partial dopamine agonist with some affinity for $5\text{-HT}_{2A}$ and $5\text{-HT}_{1A}$, has been introduced, which may act through a novel mechanism of action, has proved effective. This raises further questions about the requisite pharmacodynamic actions at $D_2$ receptors for therapeutic effects and whether 5-HT actions have an integral role.

## Depolarization Inactivation

Although antipsychotic drugs can achieve a high level of $D_2$ receptor occupancy in humans within hours after acute oral administration (Farde et al. 1992, Nordstrom et al. 1993, Kapur et al. 1999), antipsychotics must be administered to schizophrenics for several weeks before their clinical effects can be fully produced (Johnstone et al. 1978). The slowly developing onset of therapeutic efficacy cannot be explained only by $D_2$ receptor blockade induced by antipsychotics.

Acute administration of first-generation antipsychotic agents (e.g., haloperidol and chlorpromazine) induces an increase in dopamine neuron firing in both the *substantia nigra pars compacta* (A9, which projects primarily to the striatum) and the ventral tegmental area (A10, which projects primarily to the limbic cortical regions) in rats (Bunney and Grace 1978, Chiodo and Bunney 1983). Repeated treatment with first-generation antipsychotics for 3 weeks or more, however, resulted in a decrease in the number of spontaneously active dopamine neurons in both A9 and A10 regions (Bunney and Grace 1978, Chiodo and Bunney 1983, White and Wang 1983). After chronic treatment, the dopamine neurons were not in a hyperpolarized, inactive state, but were instead tonically depolarized to such an extent that their spike-generating mechanism was inactive. The neuroleptic-induced inhibition of spontaneous cell firing was termed "depolarization inactivation" or "depolarization block" (Grace 1992). The depolarization inactivation hypothesis is supported in part by studies demonstrating that systematic administration of a dopamine agonist apomorphine, which hyperpolarizes dopamine cells in control animals, can reverse the effects of chronic treatment with antipsychotics by causing previously nonfiring dopamine cells to become active (Grace and Bunney 1986, Grace 1992).

In contrast to the first-generation antipsychotics, chronic treatment with second-generation antipsychotic drugs, including clozapine, olanzapine, quetiapine, and iloperidone, resulted in the depolarization inactivation of A10 neurons, but not A9 dopamine cells (Chiodo and Bunney 1983, Stockton and Rasmussen 1996, White and Wang 1983, Goldstein et al. 1993, Hesselink 2000). It is suggested that the inability of these drugs to decrease A9 dopamine neuronal activity may contribute to their lower incidence of EPS, thought to be a key factor in second-generation antipsychotic profile, and that the inactivation of mesolimbic (A10) dopamine areas may be involved in the delayed onset of therapeutic effects during treatment (Chiodo and Bunney 1983, Stockton and Rasmussen 1996, White and Wang 1983).

## Receptor Cycling and Internalization

For neurotransmitter receptors, receptor mobility or receptor trafficking to distinct locations within the cell, plays important roles not only in biosynthesis of the receptor, but also in the transmembrane and intracellular signaling process (Hollenberg 1991). The binding of an agonist to the receptor, which is randomly distributed on the membrane, triggers a number of mobile receptor reactions. The initial microclustering of the receptor is followed by aggregation into patches at sites of internalization (frequently, but not necessarily always, coated pit regions). After internalization, the receptor aggregate, localized to an endosomal organelle, can (1) migrate to a variety of intracellular locales (intracellular redistribution), (2) be degraded, or (3) recycle back to the cell surface (Hollenberg 1991, Kallal and Benovic 2000).

Using micrography, Willins and colleagues (1999) have discovered that clozapine, olanzapine, and risperidone, but not drugs which have no affinity for the $5\text{-HT}_{2A}$ receptor, induced a rapid internalization of the $5\text{-HT}_{2A}$ receptor from the cell surface in fibroblasts *in vitro*. Furthermore, treatment with clozapine or olanzapine, but not haloperidol, induced a loss of $5\text{-HT}_{2A}$ receptor-like immunoreactivity ($5\text{-HT}_{2A}$-LI) on apical dendrite of pyramidal neurons, and dramatically increased intracellular $5\text{-HT}_{2A}$-LI within the soma in the medial prefrontal cortex. These results suggest that several second-generation antipsychotics with high $5\text{-HT}_{2A}$ receptor affinities can induce a subcellular redistribution of $5\text{-HT}_{2A}$ receptors through a direct action at $5\text{-HT}_{2A}$ receptors both *in vivo* and *in vitro*, and that these drugs may share a common ability to induce $5\text{-HT}_{2A}$ receptor internalization (Willins et al. 1999). However, the precise mechanism and therapeutic significance of antipsychotics-induced internalization of $5\text{-HT}_{2A}$ receptors remain unknown.

## Effects on Intracellular Signal Transduction

It has been suggested that the slow onset of the action of antipsychotic drugs is associated with long-lasting adaptive modifications in neural functioning that implicate changes in intracellular signal transduction, and ultimately, in gene expression of target neurons (Rogue and Malviya 1994). The currently available antipsychotic drugs have affinity for a number of receptors, such as dopamine, serotonin, muscarinic, cholinergic, adrenergic, and histamine receptors (Table 95–2). Most of these receptors belong to the G-protein-coupled receptor superfamily (Neer 1995). Signaling to the nucleus through receptors involves different second messenger systems (Figure 95–1). Activation of G-protein-coupled receptors by agonists stimulates specific heterotrimeric G-proteins, whose subunits can then regulate multiple downstream effectors such as adenylate cyclase, phospholipases, and various ion channels (Neer 1995). In the phosphatidylinositol (PI)-signaling pathway, protein kinase C (PKC) and phospholipase C (PLC) play important roles in mediating receptor-induced cellular responsiveness (Majewski and Iannazzo 1998). Recent evidence indicates that the regulation of phosphorylation mediated by specific PKC and PLC isozymes may represent an intracellular target of both first- and second-generation antipsychotics, and modulation of the expression of specific PKC and PLC isozymes by these drugs may cause changes in various physiological functions, which in turn may be of relevance to their antipsychotic effects (Dwivedi and Pandey 1999).

There has been a surge of interest in immediate early gene (IEG) induction in response to antipsychotics adminis-

**Table 95–2  Relative Neurotransmitter Receptor Affinities for Antipsychotics at Therapeutic Doses**

| Receptor | Clozapine | Risperidone | Olanzapine | Quetiapine | Ziprasidone | Sertindole | Amisulpride | Zotepine | Aripiprazole | Iloperidone | Haloperidol |
|---|---|---|---|---|---|---|---|---|---|---|---|
| D$_1$ | + | + | ++ | − | + | ++ | − | + | + | + | + |
| D$_2$ | ++ | ++++ | +++ | + | +++ | ++++ | ++++ | ++ | ++++ | +++ | ++++ |
| D$_3$ | ++ | ++ | + | − | ++ | ++ | ++ | ++ | ++ | ++ | +++ |
| D$_4$ | ++ | − | ++ | − | +++ | + | − | ++ | + | ++ | +++ |
| 5-HT$_{1A}$ | − | − | − | | +++ | | | | + | | − |
| 5-HT$_{1D}$ | − | + | − | | +++ | | | | | | |
| 5-HT$_{2A}$ | +++ | ++++ | +++ | + | ++++ | ++++ | − | +++ | + | +++ | + |
| 5-HT$_{2C}$ | ++ | ++ | ++ | − | + | ++ | | ++ | | ++ | − |
| 5-HT$_6$ | ++ | − | ++ | − | ++ | | | ++ | | | |
| 5-HT$_7$ | +++ | +++ | − | − | ++ | | | ++ | ++ | +++ | +++ |
| α$_1$ | +++ | +++ | ++ | +++ | ++ | ++ | − | ++ | | +++ | +++ |
| α$_2$ | + | ++ | + | + | − | + | − | ++ | | + | − |
| H$_1$ | +++ | − | +++ | ++ | − | + | − | ++ | | + | − |
| m$_1$ | ++++ | − | +++ | ++ | − | − | − | + | | | − |
| DA Transporter | ++ | | ++ | | ++ | | | | | − | |
| NA Transporter | + | | ++ | | ++ | | | ++ | | − | |
| 5-HT Transporter | | | | | ++ | | | | | | |

−, minimal to none; +, low; ++, moderate; +++, high; ++++, marked

Adapted and modified with permission from Blin O (1999) A comparative review of new antipsychotics. Can J Psychiatr 44, 235–244; Burns MJ (2001) The pharmacology and toxicology of atypical antipsychotic agents. J Clin Toxicol 39, 1–14.

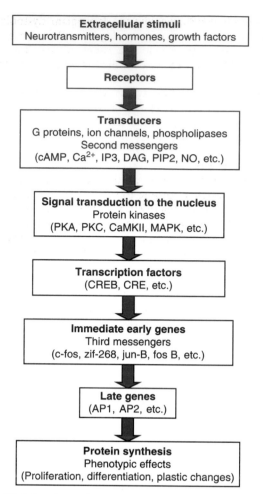

**Figure 95–1** *Signaling pathways for neurotransmitter control of gene expression.*

tration as a method for analyzing the anatomical sites and mechanisms by which they act (Rogue and Vincendon 1997). Acute treatment with conventional antipsychotics (e.g., haloperidol and fluphenazine) increases the expression of IEG *c-fos* mRNA or its protein product Fos in the dorsolateral striatum, as well as the shell of nucleus accumbens in rats (Dragunow et al. 1990, Robertson and Fibiger 1992, Merchant and Dorsa 1993, Semba et al. 1996, Leveque et al. 2000). Neuroleptic-induced expression of Fos in the nucleus accumbens has been postulated to relate to the antipsychotic activity of both conventional and second-generation drugs (Deutch et al. 1992, Robertson et al. 1994). The ability of second-generation antipsychotics to induce Fos expression in the medial prefrontal cortex could be related to their therapeutic efficacy for negative symptoms of schizophrenia (Robertson and Fibiger 1992, 1996, Ohashi et al. 2000). The Fos expression in the dorsolateral striatum has been proposed to be predictive of a liability to induce EPS (Robertson and Fibiger 1992, Robertson et al. 1994, Leveque et al. 2000). For example, clozapine and sertindole can induce Fos expression in the prefrontal cortex as well as the nucleus accumbens, and no change in the dorsolateral striatum (Fink-Jensen and Kristensen 1994, Ananth et al. 2001, Waddington and Casey 2000). Risperidone induces Fos expression in the nucleus accumbens, but unlike clozapine, it modestly induces Fos in

the dorsolateral striatum in the absence of induction in the prefrontal cortex (Wan et al. 1995, Waddington and Casey 2000). Olanzapine shares the action of clozapine to increase Fos expression in the prefrontal cortex as well as the nucleus accumbens, but unlike clozapine, olanzapine induces Fos expression in the dorsolateral striatum at high doses (10 mg/kg) in rats (Robertson and Fibiger 1996, Bymaster et al. 1999).

The *N*-methyl-D-aspartate receptor (NMDA-R) antagonist MK-801 can attenuate *c-fos* and Fos increase produced by antipsychotics in the nucleus accumbens and striatum, suggesting the involvement of the NMDA-R in the regulation of IEG expression induced by antipsychotics (Dragunow et al. 1990, Ziolkowska and Hollt 1993, Leveque et al. 2000). Konradi and colleagues have suggested the intracellular pathway involved in the *c-fos* expression induced by haloperidol: (i) acute haloperidol administration can activate the NMDA-R via cyclic AMP-protein kinase A-mediated phosphorylation of the NR1 subtype of the NMDA-R (Leveque et al. 2000); (ii) the NMDA-R may activate a signal transduction pathway that translocates to the nucleus and causes phosphorylation of the transcription factor, cyclic AMP response element binding protein (CREB) (Konradi and Heckers 1995, Rajadhyaksha et al. 1998); and (iii) phosphorylation of CREB leads to an increase in mRNA synthesis of the *c-fos* genes in the striatum (Rajadhyaksha et al. 1999, Leveque et al. 2000).

It should be noted, however, that long-term treatment with haloperidol or clozapine can reduce the acute response of Fos induction in most brain regions, except the lateral septum for haloperidol and except the nucleus accumbens for clozapine (Sebens et al. 1995). Thus, it is suggested that in most brain areas, high Fos-protein levels are not necessary to maintain antipsychotic activity or side effects, and the persisting effect of clozapine in the nucleus accumbens may be of significance to its superior clinical efficacy.

## Neuroplasticity
A number of studies have demonstrated that certain antipsychotic drugs can produce structural changes in the brain (Harrison 1999). For example, striatal enlargement after chronic treatment with conventional antipsychotics, but not second-generation drugs, has been reported by several investigators in both schizophrenic patients (Keshavan et al. 1994, Chakos et al. 1994, 1995, Doraiswamy et al. 1995, Gur et al. 1998, Corson et al. 1999) and rats (Chakos et al. 1998). Although the underlying pharmacological and cellular mechanisms are poorly understood, these changes appear to be indicative of antipsychotic-induced neuroplastic effects in the striatum (Harrison 1999).

The studies of Meshul and colleagues have shown that chronic treatment of rats with haloperidol, but not with clozapine, can increase the number of asymmetrical synapses associated with a perforated postsynaptic density in the striatum (Meshul et al. 1992a, 1992b, Meshul and Tan 1994). Perforated postsynaptic densities demonstrate a sign of a newly formed or forming synapse (Geinisman et al. 1989). Thus, the higher proportion of synapses with perforated postsynaptic densities induced by haloperidol may reflect increased synaptic formation or turnover (Harrison 1999).

It has been shown that chronic haloperidol administration induces an increase in dopamine $D_2$ receptor density and $D_{2L}$ receptor mRNA in the striatum (Buckland et al. 1993, Rogue et al. 1991, Inoue et al. 1997). $D_2$-like receptors are coupled to different intracellular transduction pathways, each of which could be involved in the control of synaptic and neuronal plasticity-associated gene expression (Rogue and Malviya 1994, Eastwood et al. 1997). In fact, the expression of several synaptic protein genes is upregulated by chronic haloperidol treatment in the striatum (Eastwood et al. 1994, 1997, Kroesen et al. 1995). More recently, it has been reported that haloperidol, but not clozapine, acutely increased the IEG, arc (activity-regulated cytoskeleton-associated gene) mRNA levels (Nakahara et al. 2000). Arc is selectively localized in neural dendrites and thought to play a significant role in activity-dependent synaptic plasticity (Kodama et al. 1998, Steward et al. 1998). Riva and colleagues (1999) also found that acute or chronic administration of clozapine increased basic fibroblast growth factor (FGF-2) levels in the striatum, suggesting neuroprotective activity of clozapine. Thus, available data suggest that antipsychotic drugs may induce long-term neuroplastic changes that lead to morphological and/or functional alterations in the striatum, probably in a different way between conventional and second-generation drugs. However, it is unclear whether the neuroplastic changes relate primarily to the therapeutic action of antipsychotic drugs, or more likely to their propensity to produce side effects (e.g., EPS and TD).

## Molecular Basis of "Typicality" and "Atypicality"

Recent research in molecular pharmacology has led to new insight into the mechanisms of action of antipsychotic drugs. Although all antipsychotics block dopamine $D_2$ receptors, the looseness of attachment of the agent to dopamine $D_2$ receptors seems to differentiate "typical" and "atypical" antipsychotics (Kapur and Seeman 2001). Kapur and colleagues have recently proposed that a low affinity and fast dissociation from the $D_2$ receptor (not high affinity at multiple receptors), may be the key to "atypicality" (Kapur and Seeman 2001, Kapur and Remington 2001). In animal models, Robertson and colleagues (1994) proposed that if the number of Fos-positive cells in the core of nucleus accumbens is greater than those in the striatum, the drug should be considered "atypical." In addition, as we mentioned in this section, the antipsychotics-induced depolarization inactivation of A10 neurons, internalization of 5-$HT_{2A}$ receptors, or neuroplastic effects in the striatum may differentiate "typicality" and "atypicality." With knowledge of the molecular action of antipsychotic drugs, more precise definitions of "atypicality" could be proposed and evaluated.

## Pharmacology of Antipsychotic Agents

### First-Generation Antipsychotic Agents

The first-generation antipsychotic agents are equally effective in the treatment of psychotic symptoms of schizophrenia, while they vary in potency, their pharmacological properties, and their propensity to induce side effects (Davis et al. 1980, American Psychiatric Association 2000). The effect that is common to all first-generation antipsychotics is a high affinity for dopamine $D_2$ receptors (Marder and Van Putten 1995). In addition, all of the first-generation agents produce EPS, including parkinsonism, dystonia, akathisia, and TD, to a varying degree and increase serum prolactin concentration in the usual clinical dose range (Meltzer 1985). These are described in greater detail in the section "Adverse Effects."

The first-generation agents are usually classified into three groups: phenothiazines, butyrophenones (e.g., haloperidol), and others (e.g., thiothixene, molindone, and loxapine), based on their structure.

### Phenothiazines

The phenothiazine antipsychotics are usually categorized into three classes according to substitutions at position 10 (Marder and Van Putten 1995). The aliphatic class (e.g., chlorpromazine) consists of agents that have relatively low potency at $D_2$ receptors compared with other first-generation antipsychotics, more antimuscarinic activity, more sympathetic and parasympathetic activity, and more sedation. The piperidine class (e.g., thioridazine) has a similar clinical profile to the aliphatic class, with somewhat reduced affinity for $D_2$ sites. The piperazine class (e.g., fluphenazine) has fewer antimuscarinic and autonomic effects, but greater potency at $D_2$ sites, and thus can produce more EPS.

### Butyrophenones

The butyrophenone antipsychotics, represented by haloperidol, tend to be potent $D_2$ antagonists and have minimal anticholinergic and autonomic effects (Marder and Van Putten 1995). PET studies demonstrate that low doses of haloperidol (2–5 mg/day) would be expected to induce 60 to 80% dopamine $D_2$ receptor occupancy (Kapur et al. 1996, 1997). While theoretically this dosage should be enough for optimal clinical efficacy correlated to an optimal $D_2$ receptor antagonism, dosages 5 to 20 times as high are prescribed in current clinical practice (Stip 2000) (see section "Dose of Antipsychotic Agent").

## Second-Generation and Novel Antipsychotic Agents

The pharmacological properties that confer the unique therapeutic properties of second-generation antipsychotic drugs are poorly understood despite intensive research efforts by the pharmaceutical industry and the psychopharmacology research community. Since clozapine is the prototype "atypical" drug, defining the role of the individual complex actions of this drug, that are responsible for its unique therapeutic profile, is necessary for rational design of new and improved second-generation (clozapine-like) antipsychotics (Miyamoto et al. 2002a). In this chapter, second-generation antipsychotics refer to clozapine, risperidone, olanzapine, quetiapine, ziprasidone, sertindole, amisulpride, zotepine, aripiprazole, and iloperidone.

### Clozapine

A distinguishing feature of clozapine in comparison to conventional antipsychotics is the relatively high affinity of clozapine for 5-$HT_{2A}$ receptors, and lower affinity for $D_2$ receptors (Lieberman 1993, Duncan et al. 1999b). Meltzer and colleagues (1989) provided evidence that combined 5-$HT_{2A}$/$D_2$ antagonistic actions, with greater relative potency at the 5-$HT_{2A}$ receptor, may be critical to "atypicality," in terms of enhanced efficacy and reduced EPS liability.

Clozapine has modest affinity for some dopamine receptors ($D_4$, as well as $D_2$ and $D_1$), but also considerably high antagonist affinity for $H_1$ histaminergic, muscarinic, and alpha-adrenergic receptors (Bymaster et al. 1996) (Table 95–2).

## Risperidone

Risperidone emulated the relative $5\text{-HT}_{2A}/D_2$ affinities of clozapine, but has substantially higher affinity for both receptors than clozapine (Table 95–2). A PET study indicated risperidone to occupy 75 to 80% of striatal $D_2$ receptors at 6 mg/day, while occupying 78 to 88% of cortical $5\text{-HT}_2$ receptors in schizophrenic patients (Farde et al. 1995). The reduced EPS side effects associated with low-dose risperidone treatment (4–6 mg/day), even at high levels of $D_2$ receptor occupancy, may be due to the $5\text{-HT}_{2A}$ antagonistic properties of the drug (Meltzer et al. 1989, Gerlach 1991). However, at higher doses, risperidone produces EPS (Marder and Meibach 1994), indicating that $5\text{-HT}_{2A}$ receptor antagonism alone cannot completely eliminate EPS associated with high $D_2$ receptor blockade. Risperidone, like clozapine, has relatively high affinity for alpha-1- and alpha-2-adrenergic receptors (Table 95–2), but the potential therapeutic significance of the adrenergic receptor blocking properties of clozapine and risperidone is uncertain.

## Olanzapine

Olanzapine is closely related in chemical structure to clozapine, and the two drugs have many common receptor binding characteristics (Miyamoto et al. 2001a). Primary considerations in selection of olanzapine for development were the drug's relatively potent antagonistic effects at both $D_2$ and $5\text{-HT}_{2A}$ receptors (Bymaster et al. 1996, 1997). Olanzapine is more potent at $5\text{-HT}_{2A}$ than $D_2$ receptors (Table 95–2), similar to clozapine and risperidone. In addition, receptor-binding characteristics of olanzapine in regard to other dopaminergic, serotonergic, cholinergic, and adrenergic receptor subtypes are similar to clozapine, but there are also some notable distinctions between the two drugs. For example, clozapine has substantially higher affinity for $5\text{-HT}_{1A}$ and $5\text{-HT}_7$ receptors in comparison to olanzapine (Table 95–2). A PET study showed a striatal $D_2$ receptor occupancy of 71 to 80% in the usual clinical dose range of olanzapine (10–20 mg/day), while doses of 30 mg/day and higher are associated with more than 80% $D_2$ occupancy in schizophrenic patients (Kapur et al. 1998).

## Quetiapine

Quetiapine is another drug with greater relative affinity for $5\text{-HT}_{2A}$ than for $D_2$ receptors, but also some affinity for alpha-1-adrenergic and $H_1$ receptors (Markowitz et al. 1999) (Table 95–2). PET studies indicate quetiapine to occupy 22 to 68% of striatal $D_2$ receptors at therapeutic doses, while occupying 48 to 70% of cortical $5\text{-HT}_2$ receptors in schizophrenic patients (Gefvert et al. 1998). Interestingly, quetiapine produces transiently high striatal $D_2$ occupancy in schizophrenic patients, but the effect lasts for only the first few hours (Kapur et al. 2000b). Thus, the $D_2$-occupying properties of quetiapine, as with clozapine, appear to be prominent only for a short duration (Seeman and Kapur 2000). This suggests that transient occupancy of $D_2$ receptors may be sufficient to produce therapeutic antipsychotic effects.

## Ziprasidone

Ziprasidone has potent $5\text{-HT}_{2A}$ and $D_2$ affinities, and like clozapine, it exhibits $5\text{-HT}_{1A}$ agonist properties that could potentially act as protective effects on the development of EPS (Ferris 2000, Sprouse et al. 1999). Ziprasidone also has significant affinity for $5\text{-HT}_{1D}$ and $5\text{-HT}_{2C}$, as well as $H_1$ and alpha-1-adrenergic receptors (Arnt and Skarsfeldt, 1998) (Table 95–2). Ziprasidone inhibits the reuptake of NA and 5-HT (Waddington and Casey 2000). Ziprasidone exhibits high levels of $D_2$ occupancy at doses of 20 to 40 mg (Bench et al. 1993, 1996) that are much lower than the therapeutically effective dose (120–160 mg/day) (Keck et al. 1998, Goff et al. 1998). Thus, pharmacological properties other than $D_2$ receptor antagonism may account for the clinical efficacy of ziprasidone.

## Sertindole

Sertindole is an indole derivative with high affinity antagonism for $5\text{-HT}_{2A}$, $5\text{-HT}_{2C}$, alpha-1-adrenergic, and $D_2$-like receptors (Schotte et al. 1996) (Table 95–2). In conventional preclinical models, the profile of sertindole is one that would predict antipsychotic efficacy with reduced EPS liability (Arnt and Skarsfeldt 1998). In schizophrenic patients, SPECT studies found that sertindole shares the action of risperidone to occupy a high percentage both of striatal $D_2$-like receptors and of cortical $5\text{-HT}_{2A}$ receptors (Bigliani et al. 2000, Travis et al. 1997, Pilowsky et al. 1997, Kasper et al. 1998). Electrophysiologically, sertindole also exhibited dose-dependent marked limbic selectivity (Daniel and Copeland 2001).

## Amisulpride

Amisulpride, a substituted benzamide analogue of sulpiride, is a selective antagonist of $D_2$ and $D_3$ receptors with little affinity for $D_1$-like or nondopaminergic receptors (Waddington and Casey 2000) (Table 95–2). Animal studies suggest that low doses of the drug preferentially block presynaptic $D_2$-like autoreceptors, and thus lead to an increase in dopaminergic neurotransmission, while higher doses reduce certain postsynaptic $D_2$ receptor-mediated behaviors to predict antipsychotic efficacy, but with little or no production of catalepsy to predict low EPS liability (Perrault et al. 1997, Waddington and Casey 2000). PET studies in schizophrenia demonstrate lower doses of amisulpride (50–100 mg) to occupy 4 to 26% of striatal $D_2$-like receptors, while higher doses (200–800 mg) occupy 38 to 76% thereof (Martinot et al. 1996).

## Zotepine

Zotepine is a dibenzothiepine analogue of clozapine with high affinity for $5\text{-HT}_{2A}$, $5\text{-HT}_{2C}$, $5\text{-HT}_6$, $5\text{-HT}_7$, alpha-1-adrenergic, and $H_1$ receptors (Needham et al. 1996) (Table 95–2). It has modest affinity for $D_2$, $D_3$, $D_4$, and $D_1$ receptors. It is also a potent NA reuptake inhibitor (Blin 1999). Preclinical studies suggest that low-dose zotepine increases dopaminergic neurotransmission while, at higher doses, it acts as a dopaminergic antagonist (Blin 1999). There are as yet no studies on zotepine in human subjects using PET (Waddington and Casey 2000). In schizophrenic patients, SPECT studies indicate zotepine to occupy 68 to 78% of striatal $D_2$-like receptors at conventional clinical doses (Barnas et al. 2001).

## Aripiprazole

Aripiprazole (OPC-14597) is a partial dopamine agonist with a high affinity for $D_2$ and $D_3$ receptors, but no appreciable affinity for $D_1$ receptors (Kikuchi et al. 1995, Lawler et al. 1999, Semba et al. 1995). It has modest affinity for 5-$HT_{2A}$, 5-$HT_6$, and 5-$HT_7$ receptors, where it acts as a full antagonist, and for the 5-$HT_{1A}$ receptor where it acts as a partial agonist (Lawler et al. 1999) (Table 95–2). Aripiprazole decreased striatal dopamine release (Semba et al. 1995), and inhibited the activity of dopamine neurons when applied locally to the ventral tegmental area in rats (Momiyama et al. 1996). Animal behavioral studies showed that aripiprazole exhibited weak cataleptogenic effects compared to haloperidol and chlorpromazine despite the fact it has almost identical $D_2$ receptor antagonistic activity (Kikuchi et al. 1995). The potency of aripiprazole to up-regulate striatal $D_2$ receptors in response to chronic treatment was much smaller than that of haloperidol, suggesting lower potential for EPS, including TD (Inoue et al. 1997). It has been proposed that aripiprazole induces "functionally selective" activation of $D_2$ receptors coupled to diverse G-proteins (and hence different functions), thereby explaining its unique clinical effects (Lawler et al. 1999). Based on available data, it would appear that aripiprazole is the first compound with partial $D_2$ agonist properties to be a clinically effective antipsychotic agent (Kane et al. 2002).

## Iloperidone

Iloperidone is a piperidin-1-ylbenzisoxazole derivative, and does not have the tricyclic structure of other second-generation antipsychotics such as olanzapine, clozapine, and quetiapine (Hesselink 2000). Iloperidone has greater affinity for 5-$HT_{2A}$ and alpha-1-adrenergic receptors, and moderate affinity for $D_2$, $D_3$, and 5-$HT_6$ receptors (Szewczak et al. 1995, Kalkman et al. 2001) (Table 95–2). It induced a depolarization blockade of the A10 mesolimbic dopaminergic neurons, but not the A9 nigrostriatal neurons, similar to clozapine and olanzapine (Hesselink 2000). In conventional preclinical models, the profile of iloperidone would predict antipsychotic efficacy with reduced EPS liability (Hesselink 2000).

## Antipsychotic Medications for Different Indications

Antipsychotic agents are effective for treating nearly every medical and psychiatric condition where psychotic symptom or aggression is the predominant feature. The development of second-generation antipsychotics has been a major clinical advance for the treatment of schizophrenia. At present, these second-generation drugs are being used for schizophrenia as the first-line treatment, and are being used increasingly for various conditions beyond schizophrenia as happened with the first-generation antipsychotics (Marder 1997, Glick et al. 2001). The low incidence of EPS and TD associated with second-generation agents is highly beneficial in several neuropsychiatric conditions. A summary of various indications for second-generation antipsychotics is shown in Table 95–3. Some uses have gained general acceptance, whereas others depend on moderate or preliminary evidence.

## Schizophrenia and Schizoaffective Disorder

Nearly all acute episodes of schizophrenia and schizoaffective disorder, including first episode psychosis and recurrence in chronic schizophrenia, should be treated with antipsychotic medications (American Psychiatric Association 2000). The psychiatrist should evaluate the patient's mental status and physical condition before establishing a baseline for the administration of antipsychotic medications.

Once the patient is diagnosed, pharmacotherapy should be applied as early in this phase as possible (Marder 1996, Lieberman and Fenton 2000). Renewed attention has focused on treatment response of first episode schizophre-

| Table 95–3 | Indications for Second-Generation Antipsychotic Use Other than Schizophrenia | | |
|---|---|---|---|
| **Strong Evidence** | **Moderate Evidence** | **Preliminary Evidence** | |
| **Risperidone** | | | |
| Dementia | Bipolar disorder, Stuttering | Pediatric psychoses | |
| Pervasive developmental disorders | Conduct disorder, Tourette's disorder | | |
| **Olanzapine** | | | |
| Bipolar disorder | Dementia | Borderline personality disorder | |
| | Substance-induced psychosis | Depression, Pediatric psychoses | |
| | | Childhood schizophrenia | |
| **Quetiapine** | | | |
| Bipolar disorder | Dementia | Borderline personality disorder | |
| L-dopa-induced psychosis | | Substance-induced psychosis | |
| | | Depression, Pediatric psychoses | |
| **Clozapine** | | | |
| L-dopa-induced psychosis | Pediatric psychoses | | |
| | Prophylaxis of treatment resistant bipolar disorder | | |
| **Ziprasidone** | | Bipolar disorder | |
| | | Tourette's disorder | |
| **Zotepine** | | Psychotic depression | |
| **Amisulpride** | | | |

nia because of the widely-held belief that early intervention with antipsychotic agents after the onset of psychosis may favorably alter the following course of the illness (Wyatt 1991, 1995, Lieberman 1996). This notion, which often invokes the "toxic psychosis hypothesis" as a mechanism (Lieberman et al. 1996, Lieberman 1999a), is largely based on several studies (Loebel et al. 1992, Scully et al. 1997, Waddington et al. 1995, Wyatt et al. 1997, McGorry et al. 1996). Lieberman (1999a) has hypothesized that a limited neurodegenerative process may be involved in the pathophysiology of schizophrenia, and that the pathologic process may be reflected by the psychotic symptoms and most active in the early stages of the illness. In addition, the duration and number of periods of active psychosis during the first episode, prior to receiving antipsychotics, appear to be a significant predictor of the time to treatment response, relapse, and long-term outcome (Huber et al. 1980, May et al. 1981, Crow et al. 1986, Lieberman et al. 1990, Wyatt 1991, Loebel et al. 1992). Specifically, the treatment response and outcome are diminished with longer duration of psychosis before treatment is initiated (McGlashan 1996, Lieberman et al. 1997). These findings have important consequences for the development of early detection and intervention strategies for acute episodes (McGlashan 1996, Gaebel and Marder 1996, Lieberman 1999a).

Other naturalistic studies, however, have found no significant association between the duration of prior or untreated psychosis and clinical outcome (Craig et al. 2000, Ho et al. 2000, Robinson et al. 1999). Larsen and colleagues (2001) have recently reviewed the literature on early intervention programmes in schizophrenia. They conclude that the existence of a causal relationship between longer duration of untreated psychosis and poorer outcome is not yet perfectly established. Thus, prospective controlled trials are necessary to determine whether early intervention with specific antipsychotics improves the early course of the illness in first episode patients (Lieberman and Fenton 2000).

Theoretically, it would be reasonable to withhold antipsychotic agents from patients who will recover without them or those who will not improve with them (Marder 1997). In fact, several studies have suggested that some schizophrenic patients may remit without medication or with a placebo effect (Kane et al. 1982, Crow et al. 1986, National Institute of Mental Health—Psychopharmacology Service Center Collaborative Study Group 1964, Kane 1999). However, this is a very small number and the literature is not particularly helpful in supplying reliable predictors of drug response (Marder 1997). Moreover, in the practical treatment setting of acute schizophrenia, it is impossible to identify reliably patients who will recover spontaneously unless they are first tried without medication (Hirsch and Barnes 1995). In addition, the initial treatment without medication appears to be impractical, since a delay in the treatment of acute exacerbations may be associated with poorer clinical outcomes as mentioned above (May et al. 1976, Wyatt 1995), and rapid treatment and discharge are often required in day-to-day clinical practice situations (Hirsch and Barnes 1995).

It has been postulated that patients with schizophrenia might be better treated in the long term by offering them a period off medication when they were feeling well and only reinstitutional treatment if they experienced early signs of relapse. This so-called "targeted" or "intermittent" strategy would allegedly reduce the long-term risks and subjective discomfort associated with adverse effects of medication (Carpenter et al. 1987, Hirsch and Barnes 1995). This strategy has been tested in a number of controlled studies (Gaebel 1995, Kane 1999), all of which reported that relapse rates with intermittent treatment were approximately twice as high as those with continuous treatment with the possible exception of first episode patients (Gaebel et al. 2002). Therefore, continuous medications may be preferable for most patients with schizophrenia, even if they are symptom free (Marder 1997).

## Major Depression with Psychotic Features

Clear psychotic symptoms, such as delusions or hallucinations, are observed in approximately 25% of patients with major depressive disorder (Rothschild 1996). These symptoms often respond poorly to antidepressants when they are administered alone, and usually require the use of adjunctive antipsychotic agents (Marder 1997). Conventional antipsychotic drugs are likely to expose patients to the development of TD and EPS, which may occur more frequently in patients with affective disorders than in those with schizophrenia (Casey 1999). Thus, second-generation antipsychotics may have a more beneficial effect for this patient population. A few case reports and chart review studies have suggested that clozapine may be useful in the treatment of psychotic depression (Rothschild 1996), with one study suggesting that it may be more effective for bipolar psychotic depression than for unipolar psychotic depression (Banov et al. 1994). Hillert and colleagues (1992) first found evidence that risperidone might reduce psychotic and affective symptoms in patients with major depression with psychotic features. In a retrospective chart review, Rothschild and colleagues (1999) found that olanzapine, either alone or in combination with antidepressants, was efficacious in patients with major depression with psychotic features. However, no controlled studies of second-generation antipsychotics in the treatment of major depression with psychotic features have been published.

There is clinical evidence that some of the second-generation antipsychotics may have antidepressant effects in addition to their antipsychotic properties, and thus may improve depressive symptoms in schizophrenia (Tollefson et al. 1999, Buckley 2001). Although depressive symptoms have traditionally been treated with antidepressants, a number of case reports and open trials have shown risperidone and olanzapine to be efficacious as monotherapy or adjunctive treatment for the treatment of depression without psychotic features (Jacobsen 1995, Ostroff and Nelson 1999) (for review, see Buckley 2001). In a recent 8-week double-blind study of 28 patients with treatment-resistant depression without psychotic features, olanzapine combined with fluoxetine produced significantly greater improvement compared to either monotherapy (Shelton et al. 2001).

## Mania

In almost 50% of manic episodes, clear psychotic symptoms, such as delusions or hallucinations, are observed (Goodwin and Jamison 1990). Antipsychotic medications can effectively treat the symptoms of acute mania, particularly in patients, who present with prominent agitation, in advance of the onset of action of lithium or mood stabilizers (Marder

1997, Buckley 2001). Over the past few years, second-generation antipsychotics have gained increasing favor over the conventional neuroleptics for the treatment of bipolar disorder because of their fewer EPS, a presumably lower risk of TD, and antimanic or mood stabilizing effects (Thase and Sachs 2000). Currently, second-generation antipsychotics are being used as second-choice treatments for bipolar disorder and/or adjunctive therapy with lithium, carbamazepine, or sodium valproate (Ghaemi 2000). Evidence from three double-blind studies supports the efficacy of olanzapine in the short-term treatment of acute mania (Berk et al. 1999, Tohen et al. 1999, 2000). It is noteworthy that olanzapine is the first antipsychotic approved by the USFDA in 2000 for short-term treatment of acute manic episodes associated with bipolar disorder. One controlled comparison study supports the effectiveness of risperidone in acute bipolar mania (Segal et al. 1998). One double-blind monotherapy trial has preliminarily found that ziprasidone is superior to placebo for treating acute mania (Giller et al. 2001). There are currently no double-blind, controlled monotherapy studies of clozapine or quetiapine in the treatment of acute bipolar mania, but clozapine has been shown to be helpful in the management of treatment-refractory bipolar disorder (Ciapparelli et al. 2000, Green et al. 2000).

## Tourette's Disorder

Tourettes's disorder is a neurobehavioral disorder characterized clinically by motor and vocal tics (Jimenez-Jimenez and Garcia-Ruiz 2001). Tics are usually present in childhood and may persist throughout life. The pathophysiology of the illness is not well known. When the tics interfere with the functioning of the patient, an antipsychotic medication can be effective in reducing the severity of both motor and vocal tics (Marder 1997). Although haloperidol and pimozide have been the most commonly used agents for the disease, second-generation antipsychotics are considered as promising agents for the control of tics, because of their better adverse event profiles. Several open trials and case studies have demonstrated that risperidone and olanzapine may be a good anti-tic agent in youth with Tourettes's disorder (Jimenez-Jimenez and Garcia-Ruiz 2001, Toren et al. 1998). In a small, randomized, controlled trial, ziprasidone (5–40 mg/day) appears to be effective and well tolerated in the treatment of Tourettes's syndrome (Sallee et al. 2000).

## Borderline Personality Disorder

Antipsychotic agents are occasionally used in the treatment of borderline personality disorder (BPD). They may be useful as adjunctive therapy to reduce anxiety, tension, and suicidality (Schulz et al. 1999). A number of studies indicate that these individuals improve when they receive low doses of a conventional antipsychotic agent such as thiothixene or haloperidol (Marder 1997). Several case reports and open-labeled studies have shown that risperidone (Khouzam and Donnelly 1997, Szigethy and Schulz 1997), olanzapine (Hough 2001, Schulz et al. 1999), or clozapine (Benedetti et al. 1998, Chengappa et al. 1999) may be beneficial for BPD. In a recent double-blind, placebo-controlled study of olanzapine in 28 female patients suffering from BPD, olanzapine was effective for core areas of borderline psychopathology such as affect, cognition, impulsivity, and interpersonal relationships (Zanarini and Frankenburg 2001). As yet, there are no published studies examining the efficacy of quetiapine or ziprasidone in the management of patients with BPD (Buckley 2001).

## Substance-Related Disorders

A variety of substances, including amphetamines, cocaine, alcohol, and phencyclidine, can cause schizophrenia-like symptoms that occur while the patient is intoxicated or during drug withdrawal (Marder 1997). While clinical trials have not yet established the efficacy of the second-generation antipsychotics for substance use disorders, several case reports and open-labeled studies offer suggestions of the effectiveness of new agents in these off-label uses (Misra and Kofoed 1997, Smelson et al. 1997). One open trial has shown that olanzapine may be beneficial for treatment-refractory schizophrenic patients with a history of substance abuse who have a greater tendency for EPS and TD (Conley et al. 1998). McEvoy and colleagues (1999) have demonstrated that patients with treatment-refractory schizophrenia who smoke have a better therapeutic response to clozapine and they smoke less after switching from a first-generation antipsychotic to clozapine.

## Behavioral Disturbances in the Elderly

Dementia, whether due to Alzheimer's disease or other causes, is frequently associated with behavioral disturbance, agitation, and psychotic phenomena (e.g., persecutory delusions, hallucinations) (Stoppe et al. 1999). The management of behavioral disturbance and psychosis in the elderly is complicated by age-related decline in drug metabolism, vulnerability to drug–drug interactions, high incidence of concomitant physical illnesses, and heightened sensitivity to EPS and TD (Marder 1997, Buckley 2001). Usually, lower dosages are more necessary for the elderly than for younger patients. Although evidence from a number of double-blind studies supports the efficacy of traditional antipsychotics for treating agitated elderly patients, the use of older agents is limited by EPS, TD, anticholinergic adverse effects, sedation, and orthostatic hypotension, which may result in falls and fractures. Available data for the use of newer antipsychotics demonstrates lower rates of these adverse effects (Stoppe et al. 1999). Two placebo-controlled studies demonstrate the effectiveness of low-dose risperidone (1 mg/day) in the treatment of behavioral symptoms, particularly agitation, in elderly patients with dementia (De Deyn et al. 1999, Katz et al. 1999). In a placebo-controlled trial of olanzapine, low-dose olanzapine (5 and 10 mg/day) was superior to placebo and well tolerated in treating agitation/aggression and psychosis in patients with Alzheimer's disease (Street et al. 2000). Thus far, there are no controlled studies evaluating clozapine or quetiapine in the treatment of behavioral disturbance and psychosis in the elderly. However, in an open-label trial of quetiapine (25–800 mg/day; mean dose = 100 mg/day) in 151 elderly patients with psychotic disorders, quetiapine was well tolerated and demonstrated significant improvement in the 18-item Brief Psychiatric Rating Scale (BPRS) total score and the Clinical Global Impressions (CGI) scale severity score (McManus et al. 1999).

## Other Organic Syndromes

Patients with Parkinson's disease (PD) are sometimes accompanied with psychotic symptoms. First-generation neuroleptics were effectively used to alleviate psychotic symptoms in these patients, but the worsening of motor dysfunction was intolerable (Buckley 2001). Second-generation antipsychotics can offer a true benefit to this patient population (Friedman and Factor 2000). Open-label trials involving over 400 patients and two multicenter, double-blind, placebo-controlled studies demonstrated that low doses of clozapine are effective in treating psychosis without worsening motor features of PD (The Parkinson Study Group 1999). Limited data provide conflicting information on both risperidone and olanzapine (Friedman and Factor 2000). A number of open-labeled trials and case series suggest that quetiapine may be a preferred treatment in patients with PD (Juncos 1999, Parsa and Bastani 1998, Targum and Abbott 2000, Weiner et al. 2000, Menza et al. 1999).

Patients with Huntington's disease (HD) can also benefit from antipsychotic medications (Marder 1997). As with PD, the use of conventional agents worsens chorea movement disturbance (Buckley 2001). Several case reports and open-labeled studies suggest that risperidone (Dallocchio et al. 1999, Madhusoodanan et al. 1998, Madhusoodanan and Brenner 1998) and olanzapine (Dipple 1999, Squitieri et al. 2001) may be effective in the treatment of motor disability and psychiatric symptoms in HD. In a double-blind randomized trial comparing clozapine with placebo, clozapine demonstrated little beneficial effect in patients with HD, although individual patients may tolerate doses high enough to reduce chorea (van Vugt et al. 1997). As yet, there are no reports evaluating quetiapine or ziprasidone in HD (Buckley 2001).

## Childhood Schizophrenia

Children with schizophrenia may need neuroleptics for a long term. The value of first-generation antipsychotics in this population is diminished by various side effects, particularly dysphoria, cognitive impairment, parkinsonism, akathisia, and dyskinesia (Toren et al. 1998). Second-generation antipsychotics may be beneficial and tolerable in children and adolescents with schizophrenia who are especially susceptible to the adverse effects of conventional antipsychotic medication (Fleischhacker 2002). For example, one double-blind controlled trial, comparing the efficacy and adverse effects of clozapine and haloperidol in treatment-refractory childhood-onset schizophrenia, demonstrated that clozapine has striking superiority for positive and negative symptoms (Kumra et al. 1996). At present, no controlled trials have been published on the use of risperidone, olanzapine, quetiapine, or ziprasidone for the pediatric population with schizophrenia, thus definitive evidence is lacking. A number of open clinical trials and case reports of these new agents, however, indicate a possible effectiveness, though pediatric patients seem to have a greater propensity than adults for side effects, particularly EPS, weight gain, and dysphoria, but also prolactin increase and white blood count aberrations (Kumra et al. 1998, Toren et al. 1998, Wudarsky et al. 1999, McConville et al. 2000).

## Other Indications in Children and Adolescents

Patients with pervasive developmental disorders may demonstrate periods of hyperactivity, screaming, and agitation with combativeness (Marder 1997). Although there are no controlled trials available regarding the effectiveness of treatment with second-generation antipsychotic drugs, a number of case reports and open clinical trials with clozapine, risperidone, or olanzapine showed an improvement in behavioral symptoms (Toren et al. 1998, Potenza et al. 1999). Second-generation antipsychotics, such as risperidone, have also shown to be helpful in the management of autism, conduct disorder (Findling et al. 2000), and behavioral disturbances in children with borderline intellectual functioning (Van Bellinghen and De Troch 2001).

## Effects of Antipsychotic Agents on Symptoms of Schizophrenia

### Positive Symptoms

Antipsychotic agents have a specific effect on positive symptoms of schizophrenia including hallucinations, delusions, and thought disorder (Hirsch and Barnes 1995). First-generation antipsychotic drugs (e.g., chlorpromazine and haloperidol) are effective for alleviating positive symptoms and in preventing their recurrence in many schizophrenic patients (Miyamoto et al. 2000, 2002a). Approximately 30% of patients with acutely exacerbated psychotic symptoms, however, have little or no response to conventional antipsychotics, and up to 50% of patients have only a partial response to medication (Kane 1989, Fleischhacker 1995). At this time, the only groups of patients in which the first-generation antipsychotics are clearly preferable are those for whom there is a clear indication for short- or long-acting injectable preparations, or who have a history of excellent response to an older agent with minimal side effects (Sharif 1998, Schulz and McGorry 2000).

Although the proportion of patients who improve and the magnitude of therapeutic effects vary greatly, second-generation antipsychotics appear to be at least as effective for psychotic symptoms as conventional drugs (Markowitz et al. 1999, Remington and Kapur 2000). There have been a number of double-blind studies comparing the efficacy and tolerability of second-generation antipsychotic drugs with first-generation agents in chronic schizophrenic patients with acute exacerbations.

Nine double-blind clinical trials have demonstrated that clozapine is at least as effective as conventional antipsychotics for positive symptoms in acutely psychotic patients with schizophrenia (Buchanan 1995, Buchanan and McKenna 2000). Four double-blind trials of risperidone have reported that the antipsychotic effect size favors risperidone over first-generation antipsychotics in patients with acute exacerbations of schizophrenia (Borison et al. 1992, Hoyberg et al. 1993, Huttunen et al. 1995, Blin et al. 1996). At selected doses, risperidone is as effective as haloperidol in treating positive symptoms (Marder and Meibach 1994, Borison et al. 1992, Claus et al. 1992), and faster in onset of action (Borison et al. 1992, Chouinard et al. 1993, Claus et al. 1992).

The efficacy of olanzapine in comparison to haloperidol was evaluated in two large double-blind clinical trials in acutely exacerbated patients with chronic schizophrenia. In the North American clinical trials of 335 patients, the high dose ranges of olanzapine (12.5–17.5 mg/day) was superior to haloperidol (10–20 mg/day) for overall symptomatology, as measured by the Brief Psychiatric Rating Scale (BPRS) total score (Beasley et al. 1996b). However, in an international clinical trial of 431 patients, response to three dosage ranges of olanzapine (5, 10, or 15 ± 2.5 mg/day) did not significantly differ from haloperidol (15 ± 5 mg/day), as measured by the BPRS, the Positive and Negative Syndrome Scale (PANSS), and the Clinical Global Impression (CGI) score (Beasley et al. 1997). In an international trial comparing olanzapine (5–20 mg/day) with haloperidol (5–20 mg/day) over 6 weeks in 1,996 patients with schizophrenia, schizophreniform disorder, or schizoaffective disorder, olanzapine demonstrated significantly greater overall efficacy than haloperidol in the BPRS total score, and CGI severity score (Tollefson et al. 1997b). Duggan and colleagues (2000) reviewed the data from nine published and unpublished studies of olanzapine versus first-generation antipsychotics, and found that olanzapine has advantages in positive symptoms in short-term studies.

Two double-blind studies compared the efficacy of quetiapine to a first-generation antipsychotic in patients with an acute exacerbation of chronic schizophrenia. In a 6-week, double-blind, placebo-controlled multicenter trial in 361 patients, quetiapine was comparable to haloperidol (12 mg/day) in reducing positive symptoms at doses ranging from 150 to 750 mg/day (Arvanitis et al. 1997). Results of a double-blind quetiapine (mean dose, 407 mg/day) versus chlorpromazine (mean dose, 384 mg/day) trial among 201 patients also demonstrated similar efficacy in the treatment of positive symptoms (Peuskens and Link 1997).

There has been only one study published comparing ziprasidone to a first-generation antipsychotic. Goff and colleagues (1998) found that ziprasidone (160 mg/day) was comparable to haloperidol (15 mg/day) in alleviating overall psychopathology and positive symptoms in 90 patients with an acute exacerbation of schizophrenia or schizoaffective disorder. In a 6-week, double-blind trial of 302 acutely ill patients, ziprasidone (80 and 160 mg/day) was more effective than placebo in improving the PANSS total, BPRS total, BPRS core items, and CGI-S (Daniel et al. 1999).

A double-blind, placebo-controlled clinical trial has demonstrated that sertindole (12, 20, or 24 mg/day) is as effective as haloperidol (4, 8, or 16 mg/day) in treating positive symptoms in 497 hospitalized schizophrenics (Zimbroff et al. 1997). Two double-blind clinical trials have demonstrated that amisulpride (400–800 mg/day) is at least as effective as haloperidol (16–20 mg/day) for positive symptoms in patients with acute exacerbations of schizophrenia (Moller et al. 1997, Puech et al. 1998). In a meta-analysis of 11 randomized controlled trials of acutely ill patients with schizophrenia on amisulpride, Leucht and colleagues (2002) concluded that amisulpride was superior to conventional antipsychotics in reducing global schizophrenic symptoms (measured with the BPRS).

The efficacy of zotepine in comparison to first-generation antipsychotics was evaluated in two large 8-week, double-blind clinical trials in acutely exacerbated patients with schizophrenia. A comparison of zotepine (150–300 mg/day) versus haloperidol (6–20 mg/day) demonstrated equivalent efficacy in reducing positive symptoms (Petit et al. 1996). A comparison of zotepine (150 or 300 mg/day) versus chlorpromazine (300 or 600 mg/day) and pla-

cebo demonstrated greater efficacy for zotepine against both in improving mean BPRS scores (Cooper et al. 2000).

Tran and colleagues (1997) carried out the first randomized, double-blind head-to-head study comparing olanzapine (10–20 mg/day; mean dose 17.2 mg/day) with risperidone (4–12 mg/day; mean dose 7.2 mg/day) in the treatment of 339 patients with schizophrenia and other psychotic disorders over 28 weeks. They demonstrated that olanzapine was as effective as risperidone in treating positive symptoms (Tran et al. 1997). Olanzapine induced less EPS than risperidone and showed advantages over risperidone in an analysis of response rates. This study has, however, received several criticisms including the relatively high dosages of risperidone used and the statistical methods (Lieberman 2001). Conley and Mahmoud (2001) compared risperidone (2–6 mg/day; mean modal dose 4.8 mg/day) with olanzapine (5–20 mg/day; mean modal dose 12.4 mg/day) in a randomized, double-blind treatment trial of 377 patients with schizophrenia or schizoaffective disorder over 8 weeks. The study found significantly greater efficacy of risperidone than olanzapine in reducing positive symptoms at week 8 (subjects who completed the study), but not at end-point (all subjects, including dropouts) (Conley and Mahmoud 2001).

Within a short period of time, clozapine, risperidone, olanzapine, quetiapine, and ziprasidone have become the drugs of choice over conventional antipsychotic drugs in the treatment of schizophrenia and schizoaffective disorder (Buckley 2001). There is, however, still considerable debate with regard to the clinical superiority of second-generation over conventional antipsychotics. Geddes and colleagues (2000) carried out a systematic overview and meta-analyses of 52 randomized trials comparing second-generation antipsychotics (clozapine, olanzapine, risperidone, quetiapine, sertindole, and amisulpride) with conventional drugs (haloperidol or chlorpromazine). There was no difference in efficacy between first- and second-generation antipsychotics, if only trials that used 12 mg or less of haloperidol were considered. For example, the advantages of second-generation antipsychotics in terms of efficacy and dropout rates were not seen if haloperidol is used at doses of 12 mg/day or less, although atypicals still caused fewer EPS (Geddes et al. 2000). There is, therefore, a growing need to consider the comparator dose of drugs in order to evaluate the relative efficacy and tolerability of first- and second-generation antipsychotics (Miyamoto and colleagues 2002b). In contrast to the report by Geddes and colleagues (2000), Leucht and colleagues (1999) have also performed a meta-analysis and have come to the conclusion that second-generation antipsychotics have efficacy and tolerability advantages over traditional neuroleptics. Volavka and colleagues examined the comparative effects of clozapine, olanzapine, risperidone, and haloperidol in 160 treatment refractory patients with schizophrenia in a fourteen week randomized double-blind trial. They found that all three atypical drugs produced statistically significant reductions in PANSS ratings of symptoms from baseline while haloperidol did not. However, only clozapine and olanzapine were statistically superior to haloperidol. The World Psychiatric Association (Sartorius et al. 2002) and the National Institute of Clinical Excellence (NICE 2000 Web Page) both conclude that second-generation antipsychotics should be among the options for first-line treatment of schizophrenia patients, especially when dealing with first breaks of the illness.

## Negative Symptoms

Negative symptoms can be divided into three components that are usually difficult to distinguish: (1) primary or deficit-enduring negative symptoms, (2) primary nonenduring negative symptoms, and (3) secondary negative symptoms that may be associated with positive symptoms, EPS, depression, and environmental deprivation (Buchanan and Gold 1996, Collaborative Working Group on Clinical Trial Evaluations 1998a). Studies of the early course of illness have shown that about 70% of schizophrenics develop primary negative symptoms, such as affective blunting, emotional withdrawal, poverty of speech, anhedonia, and apathy, before the onset of positive symptoms (Hafner et al. 1992). Negative symptoms may represent core features of the illness, and may be associated with poor outcome and prolonged hospitalization for patients (Buchanan and Gold 1996).

Conventional antipsychotics are generally less effective against negative than positive symptoms of schizophrenia (Miyamoto et al. 2002a). Thus, the efficacy of second-generation antipsychotics on negative symptoms compared with that of first-generation drugs has received much attention. In double-blind studies, risperidone at selected doses, was significantly superior to haloperidol or perphenazine for the management of negative symptoms of schizophrenia (Hoyberg et al. 1993, Marder and Meibach 1994, Marder et al. 1997). Olanzapine was also significantly better than haloperidol for the treatment of negative symptoms in a post hoc analysis of the two pivotal efficacy trials (Beasley et al. 1996b, Tollefson et al. 1997b). Quetiapine was superior to placebo in reducing negative symptoms, but it was not significantly better than haloperidol or chlorpromazine (Borison et al. 1996, Small et al. 1997, Arvanitis et al. 1997, Peuskens and Link 1997). The results of long-term efficacy trials of ziprasidone have not been published, but preliminary data suggest that ziprasidone may be more effective than placebo and haloperidol in improving negative symptoms (Keck et al. 2001). Amisulpride is the only second-generation antipsychotic that has been studied in independent placebo-controlled clinical trials with regard to its efficacy against primary or prevailingly negative symptoms in schizophrenia patients (Leucht et al. 2002). All studies have found a profound positive effect (Boyer et al. 1995, Paillere-Martinot et al. 1995, Loo et al. 1997, Danion et al. 1999). Zotepine has also been evaluated in this group of patients, the evidence being less compelling but still encouraging (Muller-Spahn et al. 1991, Barnas et al. 1992). In a recent prospective double-blind, randomized study, Volavka and colleagues (2002) compared the effects of clozapine, olanzapine, risperidone, and haloperidol, for 14 weeks in 157 chronic inpatients with a history of suboptimal response to treatment. These second-generation agents demonstrated significantly greater efficacy than haloperidol in reducing negative symptoms, and clozapine was the most effective (Volavka et al. 2002).

Although second-generation antipsychotics have been shown to be more effective than conventional agents in treating negative symptoms, there is a continuing debate as to whether these effects are related to a reduction in EPS, or to a direct effect on primary negative symptoms (Marder and Meibach 1994, Kane et al. 2001, Remington and Kapur

2000, Carpenter et al. 1995, Conley et al. 1994, Meltzer 1995). Moreover, the effect sizes of improvement on negative symptoms for second-generation agents are usually moderate to small in comparison with placebo or conventional agents (Marder et al. 1997, Goff and Evins 1998, Leucht et al. 1999). Path analyses, however, have suggested that both risperidone and olanzapine exert direct effects on (primary) negative symptoms independent of differences in psychotic, depressive, or extrapyramidal symptoms (Moller 1993, Tollefson and Sanger 1997). A collaborative working group concluded that second-generation drugs are superior in terms of the "totality" of negative symptoms, but their impact on specific components is still under investigation (Collaborative Working Group on Clinical Trial Evaluations 1998a).

Few data are available from controlled trials to guide treatment of negative symptoms that persist despite optimal treatment with second-generation antipsychotics (Goff and Evins 1998). Augmentation strategies are commonly employed by psychiatrists to treat residual negative symptoms of chronic schizophrenia, but evidence supporting this practice is derived mostly from an older literature describing combinations of augmenting agents added to first-generation antipsychotics (Miyamoto et al. 2002a).

## Cognitive Symptoms

Cognitive impairment appears to be an integral characteristic of schizophrenia and may be evident in up to 60% of patients (Tollefson 1996, Sharma 2000). Measurable deficits are prominent in tasks involving attention, verbal fluency, memory, and executive function (Tollefson 1996, Collaborative Working Group on Clinical Trial Evaluations 1998b). A wide range of cognitive deficits are usually present at the time of the first psychotic episode (Mohamed et al. 1999), and remain relatively stable or only slowly progressive during the course of the illness, independent of psychotic symptoms (Aleman et al. 1999, Gold et al. 1999, Harvey et al. 1999). Cognitive deficits are particularly prominent in patients meeting criteria for the deficit syndrome (Buchanan et al. 1994b) and in patients with TD (Waddington et al. 1990). Cognitive impairments are more strongly related to social and vocational functioning than psychotic symptoms, and may influence the quality of life of patients (Green 1996, Harvey et al. 1998). Thus, targeting cognitive impairments appears to be a major focus of the treatment of schizophrenia.

Conventional neuroleptics produce small and inconsistent effects on cognitive functioning (Spohn and Strauss 1989, Meltzer et al. 1996, Collaborative Working Group on Clinical Trial Evaluations 1998b). Some studies of schizophrenia report worsening, improvement, or no change in cognitive function with first-generation neuroleptic treatment (Meltzer et al. 1996). For example, they improved sustained attention, whereas motor control (finger tapping) declined, and memory and executive functioning were minimally affected (Asarnow et al. 1988, King 1990). These discrepancies may be due, in part, to differences in patient populations, specific tests used, and response of psychopathology to antipsychotics (Meltzer et al. 1996). Cognitive impairment may be worsened by adjunctive anticholinergic medications or other antiparkinsonian agents, which are frequently required to treat EPS caused by first-generation agents (Tollefson 1996).

Studies of the effect of second-generation antipsychotics on cognition have been limited, and the findings have been inconsistent (Keefe et al. 1999, Meltzer and McGurk 1999, Worrel et al. 2000) (Table 95–4). It is at present unclear whether this effect is dependent or independent of psychotic symptoms (Buckley 2001). Improvement in global cognitive functioning with second-generation antipsychotics may be secondary to less EPS liability and greater efficacy in the treatment of negative symptoms.

Treatment with clozapine in patients with schizophrenia has been reported to show either no effect (Goldberg et al. 1993), or improvements in a wide range of cognitive functions, including verbal fluency, attention, and reaction time (Buchanan et al. 1994a, Meyer-Lindenberg et al. 1997, Keefe et al. 1999, Meltzer and McGurk 1999). In general, clozapine, risperidone, and olanzapine have demonstrated superior efficacy compared to first-generation antipsychotics on tests of verbal fluency, digit–symbol substitution, fine motor function, and executive function (Green et al. 1997, Keefe et al. 1999, Meltzer and McGurk 1999). Measures of learning and memory were least affected by second-generation agents (Keefe et al. 1999). Because these tests all measure performance during a timed trial, enhanced performance with second-generation drugs could result, in part, from reduced parkinsonian side effects (Keefe et al. 1999). Although methodological issues such as small sample sizes, lack of control groups, no baseline measurements, or short drug trial periods, limit comparisons between second-generation agents, preliminary evidence suggests that risperidone may be more effective for visual and working memory than clozapine (Meltzer and McGurk 1999).

In a recent double-blind trial in the treatment of cognitive impairment in early phase schizophrenia, risperidone (mean dose, 6 mg/day) and olanzapine (mean dose, 11 mg/day) produced significantly greater improvement in verbal fluency compared to haloperidol (mean dose, 10 mg/day), and olanzapine was superior to both haloperidol and risperidone in effects on motor skills, nonverbal fluency, and immediate recall (Purdon et al. 2000). This finding is, however, complicated by the high incidence of anticholinergic administration prior to the final cognitive assessment, and other problems in methodology (Harvey and Keef 2001, Weiss et al. 2002). Two small double-blind clinical studies

have demonstrated that quetiapine relative to haloperidol has a positive impact on important domains of cognitive performance, including executive function, attention, verbal reasoning, fluency skills, immediate recall, and verbal memory (Purdon et al. 2001, Velligan et al. 2002). A small double-blind, randomized trial has suggested that zoptepine may be more effective than clozapine in improving cognitive impairment (Meyer-Lindenberg et al. 1997). As in efficacy studies for negative symptoms, dose equivalency is an important factor in trials comparing cognitive effects of second-generation drugs, particularly since excessive dosing can impair performance on time-sensitive tasks and can increase anticholinergic exposure.

## Phases of Schizophrenia

## Mood Symptoms and Suicidal Behavior

Depressive symptoms frequently occur in the context of psychotic symptoms or intercurrently between psychotic episodes (Siris 2001). Antidepressant medication used adjunctively to antipsychotic drugs is generally indicated and effective (Siris 2001). Atypical antidepressants have been reported to have selective benefits against mood symptoms in schizophrenia, both manic and depressive (Sartorius et al. 2002).

Suicidal behavior presents a particular problem in patients with schizophrenia. Recently the FDA approved clozapine for use in suicidal patients with schizophrenia on the basis of results in the InterSePT study. This study found that clozapine treatment produced a lower rate of suicidal behavior than the comparison treatment olanzapine in patients with active or histories of suicidal behavior (Meltzer et al. 2003).

## Treatment of Different Phases of Schizophrenia

## Treatment During the Acute Phase

## Route of Administration
In clinical situations, antipsychotic medications can be administered in oral forms, including oral tablets, oral liquid

| Table 95–4 | Clinical Profile of Second-Generation Antipsychotic Drug Efficacy | | | | | | | | |
|---|---|---|---|---|---|---|---|---|---|
| Drug | Clozapine | Risperidone | Olanzapine | Quetiapine | Ziprasidone | Sertindole | Amisulpride | Aripiprazole | Iloperidone |
| **Clinical effect** | | | | | | | | | |
| Psychotic symptoms | +++ | +++ | +++ | ++ | ++ | +++ | +++ | +++ | +++ |
| Negative symptoms | + | + | + | + | + | ++ | ++ | ++ | ++ |
| Cognitive symptoms | ++ | ++ | ++ | + | ? | ? | ? | ++ | ? |
| Mood symptoms | +++ | ++ | +++ | ++ | ++ | ++ | ++ | ++ | ? |
| Refractory symptoms | +++ | +++ | +++ | ++ | ? | ? | ++ | ? | ? |

+ to +++, weakly to strongly active; ?, questionable to unknown activity.

*Source*: Adapted with permission and modified from Dawkins K, Lieberman JA, Lebowitz BD, et al. (1999) Antipsychotics: Past and future. National Institute of Mental Health Division of Services and Intervention Research Workshop (July 14, 1998). Schizophr Bull 25, 395–404.

concentrates, and orally dissolving formulations, as short-acting intramuscular preparations, or as long-acting depot preparations (American Psychiatric Association 2000). In most cases, patients who are cooperative prefer oral administration to parenteral medications (Marder 1997). Oral antipsychotic medications tend to be rapidly and well absorbed from the gastrointestinal tract, and reach a peak plasma concentration in 1 to 10 hours (Burns 2001). The long average half-life (12–24 hours) and active metabolites of most oral antipsychotic drugs allow for once- to twice-daily dosing (Marder 1997, Burns 2001). Among the second-generation agents, quetiapine and ziprasidone have relatively shorter half-lives (Table 95–5), and should be administered in divided doses (Markowitz et al. 1999). A single or twice-daily dose of an oral preparation will result in steady-state blood levels in 2 to 5 days (Dahl 1990). Oral medications have the disadvantage of being less dependable than parenteral administration (Marder 1997). Occasionally, there are patients who appear to accept oral medication but do not swallow it, so-called "cheeking or spitting" (Allen 2000). In addition, concurrent medications (i.e., antacids), hepatic disease, or slow absorption may increase the half-life of an antipsychotic agent, and the time required to attain steady-state concentrations (Marder 1997, Baldessarini 1996).

Short-acting intramuscular (IM) medications are particularly useful in the management of acute pathologic excitement and agitation (Buckley 1999). The main indication for the use of a short-acting parenteral form in the acute situation is to treat severely disturbed patients who cannot be verbally redirected, who may be violent, and who may have to be medicated over objection (Sharif 1998). Short-acting IM preparations can reach a peak concentration 30 to 60 minutes after the medication is administered (Dahl 1990). In addition, parenteral administration bypasses first-pass metabolism in the liver and gut, resulting in greater bioavailability (Marder 1997). A single IM injection of a high potency conventional drug such as haloperidol or fluphenazine can result in rapid calming without an excess of sedation. This calming effect on agitation may be different from the true antipsychotic effect of these medications, which may require several days or weeks (American Psychiatric Association 2000), as has been shown by Möller and colleagues (1982) who have demonstrated that the advantages of an intravenous administration of haloperidol is only apparent in the first few days of treatment. For younger patients, high doses of high-potency drugs can, however, lead to dystonia, which may increase the patient's agitation (Marder 1996).

Among second-generation antipsychotics, a short-acting IM parenteral form of olanzapine is currently licensed in some countries, and ziprasidone is available in many European countries (Potkin and Cooper 2000, Breier et al. 2000). Two double-blind clinical trials have demonstrated that ziprasidone (10 or 20 mg) IM is well tolerated and substantially reduces the symptoms of acute agitation in patients with psychotic disorders (Daniel et al. 2001, Lesem et al. 2001). In a randomized, open-label trial, ziprasidone IM appears to be at least as effective as haloperidol IM in reducing the symptoms of acute agitation associated with psychosis (Swift et al. 1999). Furthermore, ziprasidone IM may be rapidly effective with significantly less liability for EPS than haloperidol (Swift et al. 1999, Potkin and Cooper 2000, Lesem et al. 2001). In a recent large double-blind study, olanzapine (10 mg) IM rapidly and effectively produced a sustained and safe alleviation of acute agitation in patients with schizophrenia (Wright et al. 2001).

Several first-generation antipsychotic drugs (e.g., haloperidol or fluphenazine) are available in long-acting depot formulations. Long-acting depot medications are seldom prescribed for acute psychotic episodes, since they take months to reach a stable steady state and are eliminated very slowly (Marder et al. 1989). They are, however, especially advantageous in patients with suspected compliance problems, those with a history of severe relapses upon medication discontinuation, and patients with active substance abuse, who are more likely to be noncompliant with oral medications (Sharif 1998, Kane et al. 1998). In general, they make compliance monitoring much easier, as patients who

| Table 95–5 | Recommended Dosages for Second-Generation Antipsychotic Agents | | | | |
|---|---|---|---|---|---|
| | Half-life (hr) | Starting Dose | Average Dose Range (mg/day) | | Average Maintenance Dose (mg/day) | Routes of Administration |
| | (Mean) | (Total mg/day) | First Episode | Recurrent Episode | | |
| **Clozapine** | 10–105 (16) | 25–50 | 150–300 | 400–600 | 400 | Oral |
| **Risperidone** | 3–24 (15) | 1–2 | 2–4 | 4–6 | 4–6 | Oral, depot |
| **Olanzapine** | 20–70 (30) | 5–10 | 10–20 | 15–30 | 10–20 | Oral, IM |
| **Quetiapine** | 4–10 (7) | 50–100 | 300–400 | 500–800 | 400–500 | Oral |
| **Ziprasidone** | 4–10 | 40–80 | 80–120 | 120–200 | 120–160 | Oral, IM |
| **Zotepine** | 12–30 (15) | 50–100 | 75–150 | 150–450 | 75–300 | Oral |
| **Amisulpride** | (12) | 50–100 | 50–300 | 400–800 | 400–800 | Oral |
| **Aripiprazole** | (75–96) | 10–15 | 10–30 | 15–30 | 15–30 | Oral |

*Source*: Adapted with permission and modified from McEvoy JP, Scheifler PL, and Frances A (1999) The expert consensus guideline series: Treatment of schizophrenia 1999. J Clin Psychiatr 60, 1–80; Burns MJ (2001) The pharmacology and toxicology of atypical antipsychotic agents. J Clin Toxicol 39, 1–14; Worrel JA, Marken PA, Beckman SE, et al. (2000) Atypical antipsychotic agents: A critical review. Am J Health Syst Pharm 57, 238–255.

are noncompliant will easily be recognized, when not showing up for their depot-injection. This type of medication is therefore thought to be especially helpful in the maintenance phase. In fact, they have lowered relapse rates by an average of 15% compared to oral neuroleptics in six double-blind, randomized trials (Glazer and Kane 1992). As of August 2002, a long-acting depot formulation of risperidone is licensed in several European countries.

There is a short-acting depot of clopenthixol, a neuroleptic of the thioxanthenes group, which is said to be especially helpful in the treatment of manic or acutely agitated schizophrenic patients. However, recommendations on the use of zuclopenthixol acetate, the cis(Z)-isomer of clopenthixol, in emergency psychiatry should be viewed with caution because of lack of evidence from well-conducted randomized controlled trials (Coutinho et al. 2000, Fenton et al. 2001).

## Selection of an Antipsychotic Agent

Selection of an agent in emergency settings for the management of the gross agitation, excitement, and violent behavior associated with psychosis might be based on clinical symptoms, differences in efficacy or side effects of candidate drugs, or, more pragmatically, the formulation of a drug as it affects route of administration, onset, and duration (Hirsch and Barnes 1995, Allen 2000). Most agitated patients will assent to oral medication and, in a survey of 51 psychiatric emergency services, the medical doctors estimated that only 10% of emergency patients require injectable medications (Currier 2000). Practice and legal requirements concerning injectable medications differ substantially across the globe. The US Health Care Finance Administration's (HCFA) regulations regarding so-called "chemical restraint" call for it to be a last resort, which would suggest that oral medication should be offered whenever it is possible to speak with the patient (Allen 2000). Intramuscular treatments, however, remain necessary for some agitated or aggressive patients who refuse oral medications of any kind (Allen et al. 2001). In these situations, many clinicians avoid high doses on antipsychotic medications in favor of a combination of an antipsychotic and a benzodiazepine (Miyamoto et al. 2002b).

**First-Generation Antipsychotics.** The use of high doses of first-generation antipsychotics during the first days of treatment ("rapid neuroleptization") should be avoided because of lack of efficacy and risk of side effects (Hirsch and Barnes 1995, American Psychiatric Association 2000). The use of intravenous (IV) first-generation antipsychotics may be associated with rapid onset (Möller et al. 1982), yet IV care is available in a small minority of psychiatric settings, because of the risk of cardiac arrythmias and other autonomic complications (Hirsch and Barnes 1995, Allen 2000). Prior to the development of second-generation antipsychotics, many clinicians favored IM preparations of high-potency first-generation antipsychotics because of the perceived benefits of reliable drug delivery (Hillard 1998). They were generally viewed as much safer than low-potency first-generation antipsychotics and barbiturates (Allen 2000). The onset of action of IM administration is generally slower than that of IV. However, droperidol IM is absorbed so rapidly that there is little difference between IM and IV administration (Cressman et al. 1973). In a randomized, double-blind, pro-

spective study in 68 violent or agitated patients, Thomas and colleagues (1992) found IM droperidol (5 mg) to have a faster onset of efficacy for agitation than haloperidol (5 mg), but the two agents were equivalent at 1 hour.

**Second-Generation Antipsychotics.** First-line treatments for behavioral emergencies have changed significantly with the advent of second-generation antipsychotics. By 1999, the newer second-generation agents were recommended as first-line treatment for schizophrenia by the medication experts in the US in most clinical situations, including in an acute episode (McEvoy et al. 1999, APA 2000, Sartorius et al. 2002). The experts consider risperidone and olanzapine the first-line choices for emergency medication among the oral atypical drugs (Allen et al. 2001).

The use of oral second-generation antipsychotics and benzodiazepines in combination appears to be the most common medication strategy in psychiatric emergency settings (Currier 2000, Allen et al. 2001). It would be best to avoid combining antipsychotics in favor of sequential trials of monotherapy with different antipsychotics (Feifel 2000). It is possible to safely escalate the dose of second-generation antipsychotics more rapidly than is usual in outpatient settings to achieve target doses typically utilized for the treatment of schizophrenia (Feifel 2000, Karagianis et al. 2001). Once behavioral control is achieved, benzodiazepines should be discontinued and the patient should be maintained on the atypical antipsychotics alone (Sharif 1998).

One of the major advantages of second-generation antipsychotics is a lower rate of the worrisome side effects, such as akathisia, that may worsen agitation. The anti-aggressive characteristics of clozapine are well established in chronically psychotic patients (Glazer and Dickson 1998, Buckley 1999), yet clozapine initiation is contraindicated at sedative doses in the psychiatric emergency service, because of its serious potential side effects, including seizures and agranulocytosis (Currier 2000). Czobor and colleagues (1995), in a subanalysis of the US multicenter comparative trial between risperidone and haloperidol, noted a greater selective effect of risperidone (2–16 mg/day) on hostility than haloperidol (20 mg/day) in 139 patients with schizophrenia. Moreover, risperidone (5–15 mg/day) has been shown to be more effective than perphenazine (16–48 mg/day) in controlling hostility associated with psychosis in a double-blind study in 107 chronic schizophrenic patients with acute exacerbations (Hoyberg et al. 1993). In a subanalysis conducted on the results of a large, international, randomized, double-blind trial, Kinon and colleagues (2001b) demonstrated that olanzapine (5–20 mg/day) is superior to haloperidol (5–20 mg/day) in reducing agitation and positive symptoms in 1,996 patients in the acute phase of schizophrenia. Quetiapine was preliminarily found to be superior to haloperidol (12.5 mg/day) in reducing agitation at a dose of 600 mg/day in two 6-week, double-blind, randomized studies (Goldstein 1998, Hellewell et al. 1998). For patients who are intolerant of the side effects that can occur in greater frequency with the second generation drugs including weight gain and alterations in glucose and lipid metabolism, ziprasidone and aripiprazole may be specifically indicated as they do not produce these effects to any significant degree.

A final concern is the patient who appears to accept oral medication but does not swallow it, so-called "cheeking or spitting" (Allen 2000). Currier and Simpson (2001) have recently found that the combination of oral risperidone liquid concentrate (2 mg) and oral lorazepam (2 mg) was equivalent in efficacy to IM haloperidol (5 mg) and IM lorazepam (2 mg) in agitated psychotic patients who accept oral medications. Kinon and colleagues (2001a) preliminarily reported a prospective open-label study, assessing the efficacy and safety of the orally disintegrating tablet formation of olanzapine that dissolves shortly after contact with saliva, for up to 6 weeks in 85 acutely ill, noncompliant schizophrenic patients (Kinon et al. 2001a). Orally disintegrating olanzapine (10–20 mg/day), demonstrated significant efficacy in improving overall psychopathology and reducing noncompliant attitudes and behaviors. The unique oral formulation of olanzapine was well tolerated (Kinon et al. 2001a).

Psychiatrists can now select between the available formulations of several second-generation antipsychotics when treating agitated patients with schizophrenia. Because the usefulness of these drugs in acute emergency situations has been largely unexplored, and there has been less clinical experience with them compared with conventional agents, clinicians must determine how to use the new agents most effectively and safely (Miyamoto et al. 2002b). When interpreting studies that include hostile patients, one always has to keep in mind that, as patients that enter clinical trials need to sign informed consent, patients in such studies are likely to represent a selected minority.

## Dose of Antipsychotic Agent

**Rapid Neuroleptization.** Rapid neuroleptization has been proposed as a strategy for providing rapid and effective control of excitement and agitation in acute psychotic patients (Donlon et al. 1979). This practice involves the use of high doses of high-potency conventional antipsychotics, usually haloperidol, administered intramuscularly over brief intervals of time within a 24-hour period, until the patient demonstrates obvious sedation or side effects (Polak and Laycob 1971, Donlon et al. 1979). A number of well-controlled, double-blind studies comparing high-dose strategies with standard dosage regimens revealed no significant superiority for high dosage in either degree or rapidity of response in acute psychotic patients (Neborsky et al. 1981, Escobar et al. 1983, Coffman et al. 1987). Moreover, higher doses of antipsychotics produced a significantly higher incidence of EPS (Neborsky et al. 1981, Escobar et al. 1983, Coffman et al. 1987). Thus, the rapid neuroleptization technique has largely been discontinued as a therapeutic strategy.

**Effective Doses of First-Generation Antipsychotics.** The goal of pharmacotherapy is to maximize efficacy and minimize adverse effects with the lowest effective dose (Janicak and Davis 1996). The neuroleptic threshold hypothesis, first considered by Haase (1961), and subsequently revised by McEvoy and colleagues (1991), states that fine motor side effects as opposed to classic EPS signal the minimum effective dose for many acutely psychotic patients (Haase 1961, McEvoy et al. 1991, Janicak and Davis 1996). Determining the optimal dose of first-generation antipsychotics for an acute schizophrenic episode, however, has been an elusive goal, with the possible exception of chlorpromazine or haloperidol (Hirsch and Barnes 1995, Janicak and Davis 1996).

Patients are likely to demonstrate an optimal therapeutic response at 300 to 1,000 mg/day of chlorpromazine equivalents (Baldessarini et al. 1988, American Psychiatric Association 2000). Raising the dose above this range is unlikely to lead to more rapid response or greater improvement, and lower doses may be insufficient for many acutely psychotic patients (Baldessarini et al. 1988, Marder 1996, Gaebel and Marder 1996). A number of dosage comparison studies have failed to support the routine use of higher doses of first-generation antipsychotics (Levinson et al. 1990, Van Putten et al. 1990, McEvoy et al. 1991, Volavka et al. 1992, Janicak et al. 1993). When groups of patients are assigned to higher doses, such as more than 2,000 mg chlorpromazine or 40 mg haloperidol, the rate and amount of improvement are no greater than for those assigned to more moderate doses (Marder 1996). Moreover, these higher doses are frequently associated with neurological side effects, particularly akathisia and akinesia, that can cause discomfort and worsen the outcome of treatment (Van Putten et al. 1990, Levinson et al. 1990, Gaebel and Marder 1996).

Recent data from imaging studies have provided some new guidance for antipsychotic dosing strategies in acute schizophrenia. For example, the findings from PET studies demonstrate that low doses (e.g., 2 mg) of haloperidol induce high levels of striatal $D_2$ receptor occupancy (53–74%) with substantial clinical improvement (Kapur et al. 1996). The data may support the efficacy of lower doses of conventional drugs, particularly for first-episode schizophrenic patients (Kapur et al. 2000a).

**Effective Doses of Second-Generation Antipsychotics.** The dosage recommendations for second-generation antipsychotic drugs are summarized in Table 94–5. Although clinical trial data show that second-generation antipsychotics are efficacious and cause fewer EPS than the conventional agents, optimal dosing constitutes a critical issue in their effective use. For example, when risperidone was first released, a final dose of 6 mg/day was recommended on the basis of data from large fixed-dose trials, particularly the North American trials (Chouinard et al. 1993, Marder and Meibach 1994), which demonstrated that 6 mg/day was associated with the greatest improvement and similar EPS to placebo. However, Kasper (1998) reviewed clinical trials and market research with risperidone and concluded that the most effective dose with minimal side effects is 4 to 6 mg/day (Kasper 1998). Brain imaging studies have provided a scientific rationale in support of the clinical observations relating to those of lower doses of risperidone. For example, a PET study by Nyberg and colleagues (1999) demonstrated that mean $D_2$ occupancy in 8 first-episode or drug-free schizophrenic patients who received 6 mg/day of risperidone was 82%, which is probably higher than necessary for achieving optimal clinical effects without EPS. After dose reduction to 3 mg/day, mean $D_2$ occupancy was 72%, suggesting that 3 to 4 mg/day may be an optimal dose (Nyberg et al. 1999). On the basis of naturalistic trials, clinical audit, phase 4 trials, PET data, and 5 years of practical experience, Williams (2001) has suggested that the currently recommended target dose with respect to efficacy and tolerability of risperidone is 4 mg/day for most schizophrenic patients.

The recommended starting dosage of olanzapine is 5 to 10 mg/day (Bhana et al. 2001). The effective dosage of olanzapine in clinical trials may be between 10 and 20 mg/day for most schizophrenic patients (Beasley et al. 1996b, 1997, Tollefson et al. 1997b, Tran et al. 1997, Sacristan et al. 2000, Nemeroff 1997). These data, however, do not indicate whether higher doses of olanzapine are more efficacious. Kapur and colleagues (1998) demonstrated in PET studies that striatal $D_2$ occupancy in schizophrenic patients treated with olanzapine varied from 71 to 80% in the dose range of 10 to 20 mg/day. At doses above 20 mg/day, which led to higher than 80% $D_2$ occupancy, EPS and prolactin elevation were observed in the patients (Kapur et al. 1998).

Dosing recommendations for clozapine vary two- to threefold between the US and Europe (Fleischhacker et al. 1994). This may be due to the fact that in the US clozapine use is restricted to patients with clear-cut severe treatment resistance, while European psychiatrists use the drug a little more liberally. Quetiapine has shown superiority over placebo for the treatment of positive symptoms at dosage of more than 150 mg/day, and for negative symptoms at a dosage of 300 mg/day (Arvanitis et al. 1997). Clinical trials have shown that 150 to 300 mg/day of zotepine may be as effective as first-generation antipsychotics in improving positive and negative symptoms of schizophrenia (Muller-Spahn et al. 1991, Barnas et al. 1992, Petit et al. 1996, Cooper et al. 2000). Sertindole in the dose range of 12 to 24 mg/day may reduce positive symptoms, whereas only 20 mg/day of sertindole was more effective than placebo in reducing negative signs (Zimbroff et al. 1997). Lower doses of amisulpride (50–300 mg/day) has a beneficial effect on negative symptoms (Boyer et al. 1995, Paillere-Martinot et al. 1995, Loo et al. 1997, Speller et al. 1997, Danion et al. 1999). At higher doses (400–800 mg/day), amisulpride is highly effective in controlling positive symptoms (Moller et al. 1997, Puech et al. 1998).

## Treatment Resistance

Patients with schizophrenia may manifest poor response to treatment because of intolerance to medication, poor compliance, inappropriate dosing, as well as true resistance of their illness to antipsychotic medications (Conley and Kelly 2001). It has been consistently reported that approximately 10 to 15% of patients with first-episode schizophrenia are resistant to drug treatment (Lieberman et al. 1993), and between 30 to 60% of patients become only partially responsive or completely unresponsive to treatment during the course of the illness (Davis and Casper 1977, Essock et al. 1996b, Lieberman 1999b). Before a patient is considered treatment-resistant, an optimized medication and treatment trial should be employed (Conley and Kelly 2001). The definition of treatment resistance remains controversial in spite of its importance (Peuskens 1999). The most accepted criteria for defining treatment resistance in schizophrenia were initially utilized by Kane and collaborators (1988) in the Multicenter Clozapine Trial (MCT). These criteria appeared to be quite strict to try to obtain a true population of resistant patients (Conley and Kelly 2001). Thus, in recent clinical trials, the modified criteria have been used to define treatment resistance (Table 95–6), which may be helpful in standardizing treatment and clinical trials (Kinon et al. 1993, Shalev et al. 1993, Conley and Kelly 2001). Although most definitions of treatment resistance focus on the persistence of positive symptoms, there is growing awareness of the problems of persistent negative symptoms and cognitive impair-

| Table 95–6 | Proposed Guidelines for Determining Treatment Resistance in Schizophrenia |
|---|---|

1. Drug-refractory condition
   At least two prior drug trials of 4- to 6-weeks duration at 400 to 600 mg of chlorpromazine (or equivalent) with no clinical improvement
2. Persistence of illness
   >5 years with no period of good social or occupational functioning
3. Persistent psychotic symptoms
   BPRS total score > 45 (on 18 item scale) and item score >4 (moderate) on at least two of four positive symptom items

BPRS, Brief Psychiatric Rating Scale.

*Source*: Adapted with permission from Conley RR and Kelly DL (2001) Management of treatment resistance in schizophrenia. Biol Psychiatr 50, 898–911.

ments, which may have an important impact on level of functioning, psychosocial integration, and quality of life (Conley and Kelly 2001, Peuskens 1999).

As noted previously, only clozapine has consistently demonstrated efficacy for psychotic symptoms in well-defined treatment refractory patients; the mechanism responsible for this therapeutic advantage remains uncertain (Kane et al. 1988, Fleischhacker 1999, Conley and Kelly 2001). In the study by Kane and associates, comparing clozapine with chlorpromazine in 268 patients prospectively established to be treatment resistant, 30% in the clozapine group met criteria for response at 6 weeks compared to 7% treated with chlorpromazine (Kane et al. 1988). Chakos and associates (2001), in a review and meta-analysis of seven controlled trials comparing clozapine to a first-generation antipsychotic in treatment-resistant schizophrenia, found that clozapine is superior to first-generation antipsychotics in terms of overall psychopathology, EPS, and compliance rate. Thus, clozapine remains the "gold standard" for treatment of this patient population. The evidence is strongest in support of clozapine monotherapy as an intervention for treatment-resistant patients; serum levels of 350 µg/mL or greater have been associated with maximal likelihood of response (Miller 1996).

Since the approval of clozapine, attention has shifted to a greater focus on the use of other second-generation antipsychotics for managing treatment resistance in schizophrenia, but the relative efficacy of other second-generation antipsychotics is less clear. There is one well-controlled, double-blind trial comparing risperidone with haloperidol (Wirshing et al. 1999). In 67 patients with treatment-refractory schizophrenia, risperidone (6 mg/day) significantly improved total BPRS scores compared to haloperidol (15 mg/day) at 4 weeks, but response did not differ between groups at 8 weeks (Wirshing et al. 1999). The differential efficacy of risperidone was not as large as what is typically seen with clozapine. Three controlled trials have found comparable efficacy for risperidone and clozapine (Bondolfi et al. 1998, Klieser et al. 1995, Breier et al. 1999). However, in one 4-week trial, the 59 participants were not screened for treatment resistance at baseline and, despite equivalence in outcomes between groups using a last observation carried forward (LOCF) analysis, 25% of the risperidone group dropped out due to lack of efficacy compared to only 5% in the clozapine group (Klieser et al. 1995). In addition, a recent large double-blind comparative study of risperidone and clozapine found clozapine to have superior efficacy over risperidone (Azorin et al. 2001).

In a 6-week trial designed to mirror the landmark Clozapine Collaborative Trial (Kane et al. 1988), only 7% of patients prospectively determined to be treatment-resistant to haloperidol responded to olanzapine (25 mg/day), a response rate that did not differ from chlorpromazine (1,200 mg/day) (Conley et al. 1998). Conley and colleagues (1999) reported that treatment-resistant patients who failed to respond to olanzapine responded to a subsequent trial of clozapine at about the rate that would have been expected in any other treatment-resistant group. In addition, open trials in which patients have been switched from clozapine to olanzapine or risperidone have reported a high incidence of clinical deterioration, casting doubt upon claims for therapeutic equivalence between clozapine and the second-generation agents, at least at the doses tested (Henderson and Goff 1996, Still et al. 1996). However, Tollefson and collaborators (2001) have recently reported that both olanzapine (15–25 mg/day) and clozapine (200–600 mg/day) were similarly effective in reducing overall psychotic symptoms in treatment-resistant patients clinically eligible for treatment with clozapine. Some preliminary reports suggest that higher doses of olanzapine may be more effective (Dursun et al. 1999, Reich 1999); however, dosage issues of olanzapine have not yet been adequately addressed in more controlled conditions (Conley and Kelly 2001). There are also several reports of beneficial effects of quetiapine in treatment-resistant patients with schizophrenia (Fabre et al. 1995, Szigethy et al. 1998, Brooks 2001), but no controlled studies of quetiapine in strictly treatment-resistant patients have been published (Emsley et al. 2000).

Given the risk of agranulocytosis, the burden of side effects, and the requirement of white blood cell monitoring, the second-generation agents (risperidone, olanzapine, quetiapine, and ziprasidone) should be tried before proceeding to clozapine in almost all patients (Conley and Kelly 2001, Miyamoto et al. 2002a). Many clinicians express the impression that certain patients do respond preferentially to a single agent of this class. Sequential controlled trials of the newer agents in treatment-resistant patients will be necessary to fully examine this issue.

## Treatment During the Resolving Phase

During the resolving phase, the goals of treatment are to minimize stress on the patient, to facilitate the patient's return to community life, and to establish a long-term maintenance plan (Marder 1999, American Psychiatric Association 2000). If a particular antipsychotic medication has improved the acute symptoms, it should be continued at the same dose for the next 6 months, before a lower maintenance dose is considered for continued treatment (American Psychiatric Association 2000). Rapid dose reduction or discontinuation of the medications during the resolving phase may result in relatively rapid relapse (American Psychiatric Association 2000). If the psychiatrist has decided to switch the therapy to a long-acting depot antipsychotic agent, this can often be accompanied during this phase. This may also be a reasonable time to educate the patient and family regarding the course and outcome of schizophrenia, as well

as factors that influence the outcome such as drug compliance (Marder 1997, American Psychiatric Association 2000). Patients should be helped to begin formulating a rehabilitation plan through realistic goal setting (Marder 1997).

## Treatment During the Stable Phase (Maintenance Treatment)

The goals of treatment during the stable or maintenance phase are to maintain symptom remission, to prevent psychotic relapse, to implement a plan for rehabilitation, and to improve the patient's quality of life (Marder 1999, American Psychiatric Association 2000). In a review of 24 double-blind studies of maintenance treatment with conventional antipsychotics, Davis noted that approximately 70% of patients who were switched to a placebo had relapses during the subsequent year, whereas only about 30% of patients receiving an antipsychotic agent suffered a relapse (Davis 1975, Gilbert et al. 1995). Even those patients who have been successfully maintained in the community for 2 to 3 years on antipsychotic drugs will have a relapse rate of 66% by a year after their treatment is discontinued (Hogarty et al. 1976, Johnson et al. 1983). In addition, double-blind studies indicate that 40 to 60% of first-episode patients with schizophrenia will relapse within a year if their medications are discontinued (Kane et al. 1982, Crow et al. 1986). These results indicate that antipsychotic medications are effective in preventing relapse in most stabilized patients (Marder 1999). Current guidelines recommend that first-episode patients should be treated for 1 to 2 years; however, 75% of patients will have relapses after their treatment is discontinued (Kissling 1991, Davis et al. 1994, Lehman and Steinwachs 1998, American Psychiatric Association 2000). Patients who have had multiple episodes should receive at least 5 years of maintenance therapy (Kissling 1991, Davis et al. 1994, American Psychiatric Association 2000). Patients with severe or dangerous episodes should probably be treated indefinitely (American Psychiatric Association 2000).

For conventional antipsychotics, the risk of long-term side effects such as the development of TD inspired a search for strategies to reduce patients' exposure to these agents, and strategies for preventing relapse during the maintenance phase has focused on finding dosages that minimize drug adverse effects and provide adequate protection against psychotic relapse (Marder 1999). Maintenance studies of the dose–response relationship found that lowering the dose prescribed for acute treatment by about 80% may be relatively safe for maintenance, although relapse rates are excessively high when doses are reduced to about 10% of an acute dose (Marder et al. 1987, Hogarty et al. 1988, Kane et al. 1983). The international consensus conference recommended a gradual reduction in antipsychotic dose of approximately 20% every 6 months until a minimal maintenance dose is reached (Kissling 1991). A minimal maintenance dose was considered to be as low as 2.5 mg/day of oral fluphenazine or haloperidol, 50 mg of haloperidol decanoate every 4 weeks, or 5 mg of fluphenazine decanoate every 2 weeks (Kissling 1991). The use of the lower effective dose of maintenance antipsychotic agents may be associated with milder side effects and better compliance (Marder 1999, American Psychiatric Association 2000). As noted previously, a targeted or intermittent therapy has not been found more effective than continuous administration of maintenance medication and is associated with risks of symptom exacerbation, relapse, and rehospitalization (Gaebel 1995, Kane 1999, Carpenter et al. 1990, Herz et al. 1991, Jolley et al. 1990, Gaebel et al. 1993, Schooler et al. 1997).

Newer second-generation antipsychotics may have important advantages for treatment during the stable phase of schizophrenia, since they are associated with fewer discomforting side effects, and with their effectiveness in negative and cognitive symptoms (Marder 1999). In a randomized trial of clozapine in 227 patients with schizophrenia, Essock and colleagues (1996a) compared patients who were assigned to clozapine with patients who were maintained on their usual antipsychotics for 2 years. Those patients treated with clozapine showed significantly greater reductions in side effects, disruptiveness, and hospitalizations, but not lower overall symptoms or improved quality of life (Essock et al. 1996a). However, clozapine-treated patients had a higher likelihood of remaining in the community after discharge (Essock et al. 1996a), suggesting that clozapine may be associated with a reduced risk of relapse compared with conventional agents (Marder 1999).

Recently, Csernansky and colleagues (2002) conducted a long-term, double-blind, prospective study in outpatients with schizophrenia and schizoaffective disorder to compare risperidone and haloperidol for preventing relapse. They found that the patients treated with risperidone (mean dose 4.9 mg/day) had a lower risk of relapse (34 versus 60%, $P < 0.001$) analyzed by the Kaplan–Meier estimates, as well as greater reductions in the mean severity of psychotic symptoms and EPS, than the patients treated with haloperidol (mean dose, 11.7 mg/day).

The efficacy of olanzapine in preventing relapse was evaluated in the double-blind extensions of acute studies. In North American trials, therapeutic doses of olanzapine (5–20 mg/day) were found to be significantly more effective than placebo or low-dose olanzapine (1 mg/day) in maintenance treatment (Dellva et al. 1997). Olanzapine (5–20 mg/day) was also significantly superior to haloperidol (5–20 mg/day) in long-term maintenance of response in double-blind extension phases (Tran et al. 1998) of 3 randomized, controlled comparative trials (Beasley et al. 1996b, 1997, Tollefson et al. 1997b). The estimated 1-year risk of relapse was 19.7% with olanzapine and 28% with haloperidol (Tran et al. 1998). In a double-blind, comparative trial, quality of life tended to be improved to a greater extent with olanzapine than haloperidol (Hamilton et al. 1998). Furthermore, a significantly greater proportion of the olanzapine (10–20 mg/day)-treated responders than of the risperidone (4–12 mg/day)-treated responders maintained their improvement in the extended follow-up after 28 weeks of therapy (Tran et al. 1997). It is not clear whether the lower relapse rates of olanzapine are due to increased prophylactic efficacy or better treatment compliance due to better tolerability (Miyamoto et al. 2001a).

In a 26-week, double-blind study comparing zotepine (150 mg or 300 mg/day) versus placebo in 121 schizophrenic patients with a history of relapse on their previous treatment, the estimated 26-week risk of recurrence was six times lower for zotepine than placebo (8.7% versus 52.8%) (Cooper et al. 2000). Daniel and colleagues (1998) conducted a long-term, double-blind, prospective study in 282 outpatients with schizophrenia to compare sertindole (24 mg/day) and halo-

peridol (10 mg/day) for long-term efficacy and safety. Time to treatment failure was statistically indistinguishable between the sertindole and haloperidol-treated patients. However, sertindole-treated patients remained free of hospitalization for psychotic decompensation and remained medically compliant significantly longer than did haloperidol-treated patients. Furthermore, there were significantly fewer reports of EPS in sertindole-treated patients.

There is hope that long-term trials with second-generation antipsychotic drugs will demonstrate their greater efficacy, as measured by reduced rates of relapse, more global symptom remission, and improved social reintegration, accompanied by a significantly decreased risk of TD. Additional information, from trials not sponsored by the pharmaceutical industry, however, appears to be necessary to inform physicians and policy makers regarding an appropriate role of newer agents. A multicenter, National Institute of Mental Health-funded double-blind trial (Clinical Antipsychotic Trials of Intervention Effectiveness-Schizophrenia Trial: CATIE) is now underway to determine the long-term (over a 24-month period) efficacy, effectiveness, and tolerability of the newer second-generation antipsychotics (clozapine, risperidone, olanzapine, quetiapine, and ziprasidone) relative to each other and to a first-generation antipsychotic agent (perphenazine). In addition, the European Foundation for Research in Schizophrenia is conducting the European First Episode Schizophrenia Treatment Study (EUFEST) in which risperidone, olanzapine, quetiapine, and amisulpride are compared to a low dose of haloperidol (2–4 mg/day) and to each other in patients with a first episode of schizophrenia.

## Use of Plasma Levels of Antipsychotic Drugs

The use of plasma levels as a guide for dosing or determining lack of response to an antipsychotic medication is relatively common in clinical settings, yet it remains controversial (Marder 1997). There is a wide interindividual difference in blood levels in patients on the same dose of an antipsychotic drug, and a narrow dose range between therapeutic efficacy and increasing risk of adverse effects (Van Putten et al. 1991, Kane and Marder 1993, Marder 1997). Although plasma levels among first-generation antipsychotics have been established for several compounds, there is at best a moderate correlation between these levels and clinical effects (Kane and Marder 1993).

It may be useful to monitor the plasma level of an antipsychotic medication under certain circumstances (Fleischhacker 2001). For example, before deciding that the agent is ineffective despite an adequate trial at a sufficient dose, it is important to determine whether it may be due to alterations in the pharmacokinetics of the drug or nonadherence to medications (Van Putten et al. 1991, Conley and Kelly 2001). A low plasma level (e.g., less than 5 µg/mL of haloperidol) may require raising the dose or addressing compliance issues. A higher plasma level (e.g., greater than 15 µg/mL of haloperidol) may require lowering the dose because medication side effects may be overshadowing therapeutic effects (Marder 1997). Other instances when plasma level monitoring may be useful is when decreasing the dose of drug during maintenance therapy, since too low plasma levels may indicate an increased risk of relapse (Marder 1997).

Some researchers have suggested monitoring the plasma level of clozapine as a guide to dose titration, with the goal to achieve levels between 200 and 400 μg/mL (typically associated with a dose of 300–400 mg/day) (American Psychiatric Association 2000). For example, Miller and colleagues reported that plasma clozapine concentrations greater than 350 μg/mL are associated with maximal likelihood of response in treatment-resistant schizophrenia (Miller et al. 1994, Miller 1996). On the other hand, VanderZwaag and colleagues (1996) have submitted that a number of patients also respond to considerably lower concentrations of the drug. Whether plasma levels of clozapine correlate with therapeutic efficacy or side effects, however, remains uncertain (American Psychiatric Association 2000).

## Drug Interactions and Antipsychotic Agents

Most antipsychotics are metabolized by hepatic microsomal oxidases (cytochrome P450 system). The major isoenzyme systems involved are CYP1A2, CYP2C19, CYP2D6, and CYP3A4 (Ereshefsky 1996). Induction or inhibition of these enzymes by other drugs may occasionally produce clinically important drug interactions (Burns 2001). Table 95–7 summarizes clinically significant pharmacokinetic drug interactions involving second-generation antipsychotic drugs. Selective serotonin uptake inhibitors, particularly fluoxetine and paroxetine, can increase plasma concentrations of antipsychotic medications by inhibiting hepatic enzymes and decreasing the clearance of antipsychotics, possibly leading to toxicity (Preskorn 1993, Burns 2001). Conventional antipsychotic drug clearance can be decreased by 50% with concurrent administration of certain heterocyclic antidepressants, beta-blockers, some antibiotic/antifungal agents, and cimetidine (Ereshefsky 1996). Clozapine toxicity has occurred following coadministration with the CYP1A2 inhibitors cimetidine, erythromycin, and fluvoxamine (Ereshefsky 1996, Burns 2001). Inhibitors of

CYP3A4, such as erythromycin, fluoxetine, nefazadone, and protease inhibitors, may produce quetiapine and ziprasidone toxicity or prolong recovery from poisoning by these drugs (Nudelman et al. 1998, Burns 2001).

In contrast, other drugs, particularly carbamazepine, phenobarbital, and phenytoin, can reduce plasma concentrations of antipsychotic drugs by increasing the metabolism of the antipsychotic agent. For example, carbamazepine, commonly combined with antipsychotic medications, can reduce the plasma concentration of haloperidol by 50% (Jann et al. 1985). Anticonvulsants, however, may not have a significant effect on the metabolic clearance of olanzapine or risperidone (Ereshefsky 1996). Cigarette smoking has been shown to induce CYP1A2 and increases drug clearance for many antipsychotic drugs, including clozapine and olanzapine (Ereshefsky 1996). Inhaled smoke can decrease the plasma concentrations of high potency first-generation antipsychotics by up to 20 to 100% (Ereshefsky 1996). The clearance rate of clozapine and olanzapine are similarly increased by 20 to 50% (Ereshefsky 1996, Haring et al. 1990).

There are other common interactions that will concern clinicians. Antacids can decrease the absorption of the antipsychotic agent from the gut. Antipsychotic medications can antagonize the effects of dopamine agonists or levodopa when these drugs are used to treat parkinsonism. Antipsychotic agents may also enhance the effects of central nervous system depressants such as analgesics, anxiolytics, and hypnotics. If patients require preanesthetic medication or general anesthetics, the doses of these drugs may need to be reduced (Marder 1997).

## Antipsychotic Medications and Pregnancy

Most antipsychotic agents readily cross the placenta and are secreted in breast milk to some degree (Trixler and Tenyi 1997). There is little data to demonstrate whether prenatal

| Table 95–7 | Pharmacokinetic Drug Interactions Involving Second-Generation Antipsychotic Agents | |
|---|---|---|
| Drug and Cytochrome P-450 Isoenzyme(s) | Inhibitors | Inducers |
| **Clozapine** | | |
| 1A2 | Fluoroquinolones, fluvoxamine | Smoking, PAHs[a] |
| 3A4 | Erythromycin, ketoconazole, ritonavir, sertraline,[b] cimetidine | Carbamazepine, phenytoin |
| 2D6 | Ritonavir, quinidine, risperidone,[b] fluoxetine,[b] sertraline[b] | None |
| **Risperidone** | | |
| 2D6 | Paroxetine, fluoxetine | None |
| **Olanzapine** | | |
| 1A2 | Fluvoxamine | Smoking, PAHs, carbamazepine |
| 2D6 | None | Phenytoin |
| **Quetiapine** | | |
| 3A4 | Ketoconazole, erythromycin | Rifampin, carbamazepine, phenytoin |
| **Ziprasidone** | | |
| 3A4 | None | None |
| **Aripiprazole** | None | None |
| 3A4 | | |
| 2D6 | | |

[a]PAHs, polycyclic aromatic hydrocarbons.

[b]Case reports of mild to moderate elevations in serum concentration.

Adapted and modified with permission from Worrel JA, Marken PA, Beckman SE, et al. (2000) Atypical antipsychotic agents: A critical review. Am J Health Syst Pharm 57, 238–255.

exposure to antipsychotic agents is linked to spontaneous abortion, congenital malformations, carcinogenesis, intrauterine growth retardation, or behavioral teratogenicity (Trixler and Tenyi 1997). It has, however, been suggested that fetal exposure over the course of pregnancy may affect development of the dopamine system (Altshuler et al. 1996). Physicians must consider the benefits of controlling psychotic symptoms during pregnancy versus the possible risks to the mother and the fetus of withdrawing treatment and the risks to the fetus of continuing treatment (Trixler and Tenyi 1997). Thus far, second-generation antipsychotics have not been shown to be teratogenic in animal studies or in preliminary human reports (Goldstein et al. 2000, Stoner et al. 1997, Trixler and Tenyi 1997). However, if possible, use of antipsychotic medication should be avoided, at least during the first trimester, especially between weeks 6 and 10, unless the patient's psychosis places the mother and/or her fetus at significant risk (Trixler and Tenyi 1997, American Psychiatric Association 2000). Antipsychotic medications may be relatively safe during the second and third trimesters of pregnancy. If a first-generation antipsychotic agent is used, high-potency agents appear to be preferable for first-line management, because they have a lower propensity to cause orthostasis (Trixler and Tenyi 1997). Low doses should be given, administration of antipsychotic medication should be as brief as possible, and the medication should be discontinued 5 to 10 days before delivery to minimize the chances of the newborn experiencing EPS (Trixler and Tenyi 1997, American Psychiatric Association 2000). This notion, however, has been reevaluated (Altshuler et al. 1996), since discontinuation of medication before delivery may put the mother at risk for decompensation (Trixler and Tenyi 1997). Anticholinergic agents should also be avoided during pregnancy, especially for the first trimester (American Psychiatric Association 2000). Since antipsychotics are also secreted into breast milk, the infants should not be breast-fed if the mother resumes taking antipsychotic medication postpartum.

## Adverse Effects

### Acute Extrapyramidal Side Effects (Dystonia, Parkinsonism, Akathisia)

Antipsychotic-induced EPS occur both acutely and after chronic treatment. All antipsychotic medications are capable of producing EPS. In general, first-generation antipsychotics are more likely to cause EPS than second-generation antipsychotics when the drugs are used at usual therapeutic doses. Among second-generation drugs, clozapine and quetiapine have been shown to carry minimal to no risk for EPS within the therapeutic dosage range (Kane et al. 1988, Small et al. 1997, Dev and Raniwalla 2000). Risperidone can produce dose-related EPS ($\geq 6$ mg/day) (Chouinard 1995, Csernansky and Okamoto 2000). With the exception of akathisia (Tran et al. 1997), the incidence of EPS with olanzapine and ziprasidone is not significantly different from that with placebo (Tollefson et al. 1997a, Ferris 2000) (Table 95–8). The relative liability of the individual second-generation agents to produce EPS will become apparent only when they have been directly compared with each other in prospective clinical trials.

Commonly occurring acute EPS include akathisia, dystonia, and parkinsonism, with each having a characteristic time of onset. This group of acute EPS develops relatively soon after the initiation of antipsychotic medications and remits soon after the drugs are discontinued. These movement disorders are dose-dependent and reversible (Casey 1995). It has been estimated that 60% of patients who receive conventional antipsychotic medications acutely develop some form of EPS (American Psychiatric Association 2000). The increasing use of second-generation antipsychotics is believed to have substantially reduced the problem of EPS.

Dystonias tend to be sudden in onset, the most dramatic form of acute EPS, and extremely distressing to patients. They present as sustained muscle contraction with contorting, twisting, or abnormal postures affecting mainly the musculature of the head and neck but sometimes the trunk and lower extremities (Marder 1997). Dystonic reactions usually occur within the first few days of therapy (American Psychiatric Association 2000). Laryngeal dystonias are the most serious, and are potentially fatal. Risk factors for acute dystonias include a history of prior dystonias, young age, male gender, use of high-potency neuroleptic agents such as haloperidol or fluphenazine, high dose of medication, and parenteral administration (American Psychiatric Association 2000).

Medication-induced parkinsonism is characterized by the symptoms of idiopathic parkinsonism, including rigidity, tremor, akinesia, and bradykinesia (American Psychiatric Association 2000). It occurs in approximately 30% of patients who receive long-term treatment with conventional antipsychotics (Marder 1997), and up to 90% of cases occur within the first 10 weeks of treatment (American Psychiatric Association 1994). Medication-induced parkinsonism occurs more commonly with high-potency antipsychotics, especially when concomitant anticholinergic medications are not administered (Marder 1997). Other risk factors include older age, higher dose, a history of parkinsonism, and underlying damage in the basal ganglia (Marder 1997).

Patients with akinesia or bradykinesia appear to suffer from slow movement, apathy, with unspontaneous speech, and difficulty in initiating usual activities (American Psychiatric Association 2000, Marder 1997). These symptoms need to be distinguished from negative symptoms of schizophrenia, depressive symptoms, and catatonia (American Psychiatric Association 2000).

Akathisia, the most common EPS of conventional antipsychotics agents, is characterized by both the subjective and objective somatic restlessness. Patients with akathisia may usually experience an inner tension, discomfort, irritation, anxiety, or irresistible urge to move various parts of their bodies (American Psychiatric Association 2000). Akathisia appears objectively as psychomotor agitation, such as continuous pacing, rocking from foot to foot, or the inability to sit still (American Psychiatric Association 2000). Akathisia is typically witnessed in a few hours to days after medication administration (Casey 1993). This side effect can be seen in up to 20 to 25% of patients treated with conventional agents (Braude et al. 1983). Akathisia is frequently cited as a reason for poor drug compliance, since it is often extremely distressing to patients. It can also result in dysphoria and aggressive or suicidal behavior (Barnes and McPhillips 1998, American Psychiatric Association 2000).

The treatment of acute EPS depends on the specific side effect (Casey 1993). Dystonia can be quickly and success-

| Table 95-8 | Side-Effect Profile of Second-Generation Antipsychotic Drugs | | | | | | | | | |
|---|---|---|---|---|---|---|---|---|---|---|
| Drug | Conventional Agents | Clozapine | Risperidone | Olanzapine | Quetiapine | Ziprasidone | Sertindole | Amisulpride | Aripiprazole | Iloperidone |
| **Side effect** | | | | | | | | | | |
| EPS[a] | +++ | 0 | ++ | + | 0 | + | 0 | ++ | + | + |
| TD | +++ | 0 | ++ | + | 0 | + | 0 to + | + | + | + |
| NMS | ++ | + | + | + | ? | + | + | + | ? | ? |
| Prolactin elevation | +++ | 0 | +++ | 0 to + | 0 | 0 to + | 0 to + | ++ | 0 | 0 to + |
| Weight gain | + to ++ | +++ | + | +++ | + | 0 | + | + | 0 | ? |
| Prolonged QT[a] | + to +++ | 0 | + | 0 | + | ++ | +++ | + | 0 | 0 |
| Hypotension[a] | + to ++ | +++ | + | ++ | ++ | + | + | 0 | + | + |
| Sinus tachycardia[a] | + to +++ | +++ | + | ++ | ++ | + | + | 0 | 0 | + |
| Anticholinergic effects[a] | + to +++ | +++ | 0 | ++ | + | 0 | 0 | 0 | 0 | 0 |
| Hepatic transaminitis | + to ++ | ++ | + | ++ | + | + | + | + | 0 | + |
| Agranulo-cytosis | 0 to + | ++ | 0 | 0 | 0 | 0 | 0 | 0 | 0 | 0 |
| Sedation | + to +++ | +++ | + | ++ | +++ | + | + | + | + | + |
| Seizures[a] | 0 to + | +++ | 0 | 0 to + | 0 to + | 0 to + | 0 to + | 0 to + | 0 to + | 0 to + |

EPS, extrapyramidal side effects; TD, tardive dyskinesia; NMS, neuroleptic malignant syndrome.

+ to +++, active to strongly active; 0, minimal to none; ?, questionable to unknown activity.

[a]Dose dependent.

Adapted and modified with permission from Dawkins K, Lieberman JA, Lebowitz BD, et al. (1999) Antipsychotics: Past and future. National Institute of Mental Health Division of Services and Intervention Research Workshop (July 14, 1998). Schizophr Bull 25, 395–404; Burns MJ (2001) The pharmacology and toxicology of atypical antipsychotic agents. J Clin Toxicol 39, 1–14.

fully treated with an intramuscular injection of an anti-cholinergic (i.e., benztropine) or an antihistaminic (i.e., diphenhydramine) agent. Dystonias can usually be prevented, either by pretreatment with antiparkinsonian medications or by limiting the neuroleptic dosage prescribed (Lavin and Rifkin 1991, Winslow et al. 1986). Dystonic reactions occur in about 40% of patients who are treated with high-potency drugs without prophylactic antiparkinsonian medications. However, these anticholinergic antiparkinsonian drugs also have side effects, including dry mouth, constipation, urinary retention, blurry vision, and cognitive impairment (Gelenberg et al. 1989, Marder 1997).

The initial treatment of parkinsonian side effects is lowering the dose of antipsychotic. If an adequate response is not achieved, adding an anticholinergic, an antihistaminic drug, or amantadine (a weak dopamine agonist), may be efficacious (American Psychiatric Association 2000). If symptoms persist, switching to an second-generation antipsychotic or a low-potency conventional antipsychotic should be considered.

Akathisia is less responsive to treatment than are other acute EPS (American Psychiatric Association 2000). The first step of the treatment of akathisia is lowering the antipsychotic dose. The next step is individual trials of beta-adrenergic blockers (i.e., propranolol), antiparkinsonian agents, and benzodiazepines (i.e., lorazepam and clonazepam) (Casey 1993, American Psychiatric Association 2000, Fleischhacker 2001, Miller and Fleischhacker 2000).

## Tardive Dyskinesia and Other Tardive Syndromes

TD is a repetitive, involuntary, hyperkinetic movement disorder caused by sustained exposure to antipsychotic medication. TD is characterized by choreiform movements, tics and grimaces of the orofacial muscles, and dyskinesia of distal limbs, often the paraspinal muscles, and occasionally the diaphragm (Glazer 2000). Younger patients with TD tend to exhibit slower athetoid movements of the trunk, extremities, and neck (Marder 1997). In addition to the more frequently observed orofacial and choreoathetoid signs of TD, tardive dystonias (sustained abnormal postures or positions) and tardive akathisia (persistent subjective and/or objective signs of restlessness) have been described (Casey 1999). The abnormal movements of TD are usually increased with emotional arousal and are absent when the individual is asleep (Marder 1997). According to the diagnostic criteria proposed by Schooler and Kane (1982), the movements should be present for at least 4 weeks, and exposure to antipsychotic drugs should have totaled at least 3 months. The onset of the abnormal movements should occur either while the patient is receiving an antipsychotic agent or within a few weeks of discontinuing the offending agent.

Prevalence surveys indicate that mild forms of TD occur in approximately 20% of patients who receive chronic treatment with conventional antipsychotic medication (Kane and Lieberman 1992, Casey 1995). A major prospective research demonstrates that the cumulative incidence of TD is 5% in the first year, 10% the second year, 15% the third year, and 19% the fourth year in a patient who receives a typical neuroleptic (Kane et al. 1986). Prevalence rates of TD may exceed 50% in high-risk groups, such as the elderly (Casey 1995). The reported prevalence of tardive dystonia is around 1.5 to 4% (Barnes and McPhillips 1998). Nearly every patient who receives antipsychotic medication has one or more identifiable risk factors for TD. Among the most significant predictors of TD are older age, female gender, presence of EPS, diabetes mellitus, affective disorders, and certain parameters of neuroleptic exposure such as dose and duration of therapy (Casey 1999).

All first-generation antipsychotic agents are associated with a risk of TD (Marder 1997). Studies of newer antipsychotics suggest that TD liability is much lower with the second-generation agents, and clozapine is associated with a substantially lower risk for development of TD than other antipsychotic medications (Kane et al. 1988, Casey 1999). In a double-blind, random assignment study of 1,714 patients, Beasley and colleagues (1999) found a 0.52% long-term risk of TD with olanzapine treatment, as compared to a 7.45% risk with haloperidol. Another published double-blind randomized study showed a significantly lower risk of TD in olanzapine-treated patients (1%) than haloperidol-treated schizophrenic patients (4.6%) (Tollefson et al. 1997a). Among a sample of geriatric patients, Jeste and colleagues (1999) reported a lower incidence of TD in patients treated with risperidone than in those treated with haloperidol at least over a 9-month period. The rate of TD with risperidone has been reported to be low (0.6%) for doses currently used (2–8 mg/day) (Chouinard 1995, Csernansky and Okamoto 2000). The incidence of TD with quetiapine is preliminarily reportedly low or virtually nonexistent, although this remains to be demonstrated prospectively (Dev and Raniwalla 2000). The risk of TD with ziprasidone is not known. Although some studies suggest that higher doses of antipsychotic drugs are a risk factor for TD, this has not been a consistent finding (Marder 1997).

For most patients, TD dose not appear to be progressive or irreversible (Gardos et al. 1994). The onset of TD often tends to be insidious with a fluctuating course (American Psychiatric Association 1992). With time, TD will either stabilize or improve even if the antipsychotic medication is continued, although there are reports of TD worsening during continued drug therapy (American Psychiatric Association 1992, Gardos et al. 1994). After discontinuation of antipsychotic medication, a significant proportion of patients with TD will have remission of symptoms, especially if the TD is of recent onset or the patient is young (Glazer et al. 1984). Unfortunately, withdrawal of antipsychotic agents is seldom an option for patients with serious psychosis (Marder 1997).

The American Psychiatric Association Task Force on TD (1992) issued a report in which a number of recommendations were made for preventing and managing TD. These include (1) establishing objective evidence that antipsychotic medications are effective for an individual; (2) using the lowest effective dose of antipsychotic drugs; (3) prescribing cautiously for children, elderly patients, and patients with mood disorders; (4) examining patients on a regular basis for evidence of TD; (5) considering alternatives to antipsychotic drugs, obtaining informed consent, and also considering a reduction in dosage when TD is diagnosed; and (6) considering a number of options if the TD worsens, including dis-

continuing the antipsychotic medication, switching to a different drug, or considering a trial of clozapine.

Although a large number of agents have been studied for their therapeutic effects on TD, there is no definitive drug treatment for it (American Psychiatric Association 2000). Second-generation antipsychotics, in particular clozapine, have been used in clinical practice to treat TD, but there have been no adequately controlled trials to date support this practice. Casey (1999), however, suggested that second-generation antipsychotics should be used as first-line treatment for patients who have TD or are at risk for TD. Guidelines for treating TD recommend using second-generation agents for mild TD symptoms, and clozapine or a newer agent for more severe symptoms (McEvoy et al. 1999).

## Neuroleptic Malignant Syndrome

Neuroleptic malignant syndrome (NMS), another type of acute EPS, is characterized by the triad of rigidity, hyperthermia (101–104°F), and autonomic instability in association with the use of an antipsychotic medication (American Psychiatric Association 1994). NMS is often associated with elevation of creatine kinase (greater than 300 U/mL), leukocytosis (greater than 15,000 mm$^3$), and change in level of consciousness (American Psychiatric Association 2000). NMS can be of sudden and unpredictable onset, usually occurring early in the course of antipsychotic treatment, and can be fatal in 5 to 20% of untreated cases (American Psychiatric Association 2000).

The incidence of NMS varies from 0.02 to 3.23%, reflecting differences in criteria (Caroff and Mann 1993). Prevalence rates are unknown, but are estimated to vary from 1 to 2% of patients treated with antipsychotic medication (American Psychiatric Association 2000). The relative risk of second-generation antipsychotics for NMS is likely to be lower, but conclusive data is not yet available (Burns 2001). NMS has been reported with clozapine, risperidone, olanzapine, and quetiapine (Burns 2001). Proposed risk factors include prior episode of NMS, younger age, male gender, physical illness, dehydration, use of high-potency antipsychotics, rapid dose titration, use of parenteral (IM) preparations, and preexisting neurological disability (Caroff and Mann 1993, American Psychiatric Association 2000).

If NMS is suspected, the offending antipsychotic agent should be discontinued and supportive and symptomatic treatment started (Marder 1997). Both dantrolene and dopamine agonists such as bromocriptine have also been used in the treatment of NMS (American Psychiatric Association 2000). These agents, however, have not shown greater efficacy compared to supportive treatment (Caroff and Mann 1993, Levenson 1985).

The usual course of treatment is between 5 and 10 days. Long acting depot preparations will prolong recovery time. After several weeks of recovery, treatment may be cautiously resumed with a different antipsychotic medication with gradually increased doses (American Psychiatric Association 2000).

## Endocrine and Sexual Effects

All standard antipsychotic drugs elevate serum prolactin levels by blocking the tonic inhibitory actions of dopamine on lactotrophic cells in the pituitary (Marder 1997). Among second-generation antipsychotics, risperidone and amisulpride can produce dose-dependent hyperprolactinemia to a greater extent than first-generation antipsychotics (Grunder et al. 1999, Yasui-Furukori et al. 2002), whereas clozapine, olanzapine, and quetiapine do not cause a sustained elevation of prolactin above normal levels (Lieberman 1993, Small et al. 1997, Worrel et al. 2000, Small 2001, Turrone et al. 2002). Aripiprazole being a partial DA agonist produces no elevation of prolactin and even suppresses prolactin levels slightly (Lieberman, in press). Although some patients treated with traditional antipsychotics acquire tolerance to this elevation after several weeks (Meltzer 1985), most have chronic elevations. Hyperprolactinemia in women can lead to menstrual disturbances, including anovulatory cycles and infertility, menses with abnormal luteal phases, or frank amenorrhea and hypoestrogenemia (Marder 1997). Women have also reported decreased libido and anorgasmia, and increased long-term risk of osteoporosis (Petty 1999). Antipsychotic-induced gynecomastia has been reported in 3% of women and 6% of men (Petty 1999). The resultant hyperprolactinemia can also lead to galactorrhea in 2.7% of men and 10 to 50% of women (Windgassen et al. 1996). The major effects of hyperprolactinemia in men are loss of libido, impotence, hypospermatogenesis, and erectile or ejaculatory disturbances (Petty 1999). Although amisulpride and risperidone cause significant elevations of prolactin levels, a number of studies have found only a small incidence of sexual dysfunctions in patients treated with these drugs (Kleinberg et al. 1999). This may be due to the fact that these reports have relied on spontaneous reporting of sexual side effects. In a drug monitoring study, in which side effects profiles of haloperidol and clozapine were investigated, Hummer and colleagues (1999) found a significantly higher frequency of sexual disturbances. Using a side effect rating scale, these authors showed that the prevalence of these adverse events was high during the first weeks of the study. They remitted spontaneously despite continuous treatment in the majority of patients.

## Metabolic Effects

Various degrees of weight gain have been recognized as a common problem with conventional antipsychotic medications. Weight gain is an important issue in the management of patients, because this adverse effect may be associated with noncompliance and certain medical illnesses, such as diabetes mellitus, cardiovascular disease, certain cancers, and osteoarthritis (Lader 1999, Sussman 2001, Kurzthaler and Fleischhacker 2001).

Differences have been discovered among second-generation antipsychotics with respect to their ability to induce weight gain (Table 95–8). A recent meta-analysis, which estimates the weight change after 10 weeks of treatment at a standard dose, demonstrated that mean increases were 4.45 kg for clozapine, 4.15 kg for olanzapine, 2.10 kg for risperidone, and 0.04 kg for ziprasidone (Allison et al. 1999). The long-term risk of weight gain with quetiapine appears to be less than that with olanzapine and clozapine (Dawkins et al. 1999, Brecher et al. 2000), minimal short-term weight gain (2.16 kg over 10 weeks) has been reported with quetiapine (Sussman 2001). Ziprasidone has been associated with minimal weight gain, which could distinguish it among other second-generation antipsychotics (Hummer and Fleischhacker 2000). Similarly, aripiprazole appears to

cause little or no weight gain (Lieberman, in press). During long-term treatment, clozapine and olanzapine have the largest effects on weight gain; risperidone produces intermediate weight gain; quetiapine and ziprasidone produce the least weight gain (Sussman 2001). It does not appear to be dose-dependent and tends to plateau between 6 and 12 months after initiation of treatment (Allison et al. 1999, Haupt and Newcomer 2001). Eder and colleagues (2001) have found that this weight gain is mainly due to an increase in body fat. The mechanism by which weight gain occurs during treatment with antipsychotics is poorly understood, but the broader receptor affinities of the agents and their antagonism of histamine $H_1$ and serotonin 5-$HT_{2C}$ receptors have been implicated (McIntyre et al. 2001a). There is currently no standard approach to the management of weight gain induced by antipsychotic medication. Patient education prior to initiating treatment should be provided, and regular exercise should be encouraged in all patients receiving antipsychotic medication. Switching to other second-generation antipsychotics with fewer propensities for producing weight gain may be the most efficient way to deal with antipsychotic-induced weight gain.

Abnormalities in peripheral glucose regulation and diabetes mellitus (DM) occur more commonly in schizophrenic patients compared with the general population (Mukherjee et al. 1996, Dixon et al. 2000). There is growing concern with metabolic disturbances associated with antipsychotic use, including hyperglycemia, hyperlipidemia, exacerbation of existing type 1 and 2 DM, new-onset type 2 DM, and diabetic ketoacidosis (Henderson et al. 2000, Haupt and Newcomer 2001, Meyer 2001). A number of case reports have implicated both clozapine and olanzapine in the emergence of noninsulin-dependent (type 2) DM and diabetic ketoacidosis (Wirshing et al. 1998, Haupt and Newcomer 2001, Henderson 2001). There are fewer reports describing an association between DM and quetiapine or risperidone, but these drugs do appear to have this side effect potential albeit to a lesser degree. In contrast there are no reports for ziprasidone and aripiprazole which suggests they may have less or no metabolic side affect liability (Haupt and Newcomer 2001, Lieberman, in press). The limited reporting for ziprasidone may be related to the relatively limited use of the agent at the present time. Although no clear mechanism of action of the second-generation agents has been established, significant weight gain or antagonism of specific serotonin receptor subtypes may contribute to the development of these abnormalities (Wirshing et al. 1998). Physicians employing second-generation agents should routinely monitor weight, fasting blood glucose, and lipid profiles (McIntyre et al. 2001b).

## Cardiovascular Effects

Orthostatic hypotension is usually seen with low-potency conventional antipsychotic agents (e.g., chlorpromazine or thioridazine) and clozapine through alpha-l-adrenergic antagonism (Marder 1997). It is most likely to occur during the first few days after initiation of treatment, or when increasing the dose of medications. Most patients develop tolerance to it in the following 4 to 6 weeks (Young et al. 1998). Elderly patients are particularly vulnerable to this side effect and it may predispose them to falls and increase the incidence of serious injuries or fractures (American Psychiatric Association 2000). A gradual upward titration of dosage may help to reduce the risk of hypotension (Cutler and Sramek 2000). Patients should be advised to change posture slowly.

Tachycardia may occur as a result of the anticholinergic effects of antipsychotic medications on vagal inhibition, or secondary to orthostatic hypotension (American Psychiatric Association 2000). Clozapine produces the most pronounced tachycardia; approximately 25% of patients will have a sinus tachycardia with an increase of about 10 to 15 beats per minute (Lieberman 1998). While quetiapine has virtually no cholinergic activity, tachycardia is a possible side effect, perhaps secondary to its adrenergic effects on blood pressure (Barnes and McPhillips 1999). Most patients will develop tolerance to this side effect over time. If tachycardia is sustained or becomes symptomatic, an electrocardiogram (ECG) should be obtained. Low doses of a peripherally acting beta-blocker such as atenolol can be useful to treat medication-induced tachycardia without hypotension (Young et al. 1998, Lieberman et al. 1989, Lieberman 1998).

ECG changes are observed with many antipsychotic agents (Buckley and Sanders 2000, Glassman and Bigger 2001). Chlorpromazine may cause prolongation of the QT and PR intervals, ST depression, and T-wave flattening or inversion, and thioridazine may cause QT and T-wave changes (Marder 1997). These effects rarely cause clinically relevant symptoms within therapeutic dose ranges. In a postmarketing study, QTc prolongation (>456 ms) was present in 11 and 7% of patients taking therapeutic doses of risperidone and clozapine, respectively (Burns 2001). Therapeutic doses of sertindole and ziprasidone can also prolong the QT interval (Burns 2001). This has led to a temporary suspension of the marketing authorization of sertindole in the European Union. It has now become available again, but solely for the treatment of patients with schizophrenia in clinical trials. Ziprasidone, which has also been shown to prolong the QTc-interval more than other second-generation drugs (with the exception of sertindole), but less so than thioridazine, has very specific recommendations in the package insert as to the types of patients it should not be used in. Needless to say, antipsychotics that lead to QTc-prolongation must not be combined with other, also nonpsychotropic, drugs that have similar effects. The effect of many but not all antipsychotic drugs on the QT interval appears to be dose related (Reilly et al. 2000). Several antipsychotic drugs have infrequently been associated with malignant arrhythmias such as *torsade de pointes* (Janicak et al. 1997). To date, *torsade de pointes* has not been reported following therapeutic doses or overdose with second-generation antipsychotics (Burns 2001).

Sudden unexplained deaths have been rarely reported with therapeutic doses of antipsychotic drugs, and such deaths could result from cardiac arrhythmias in the absence of another explanation (Burns 2001). There is, however, currently no evidence that antipsychotic drugs are associated with an increased prevalence of sudden deaths due to cardiac events (Marder 1997), although a number of case reports and case series concerning death following cardiomyopathy, potentially induced by clozapine are a matter of concern (Buckley and Sanders 2000).

## Gastrointestinal Effects
The anticholinergic effects of antipsychotic medications can induce dry mouth and constipation as well as tachycardia,

urinary retention, and blurring of vision (American Psychiatric Association 2000). These adverse effects are relatively commonly encountered with low-potency first-generation antipsychotics and may be dose related (Marder 1997). Patients with severe dry mouth should be advised to rinse their mouths frequently, use sugarless gum or drops, and have regular dental care (Janicak et al. 1997). Severe constipation can usually be treated with stool softeners or laxatives. In cases of more serious gastrointestinal adverse events, such as paralytic ileus, which has been reported following treatment with haloperidol, medication must be discontinued immediately and relevant medical or surgical interventions may become necessary. Anticholinergic manifestations are common with poisoning from clozapine and olanzapine (Burns 2001).

## Hepatic Effects
Asymptomatic mild, transient, and reversible elevations of liver enzyme levels occur infrequently with both first- and second-generation antipsychotic drugs (Casey 1997, Barnes and McPhillips 1999, Hummer et al. 1997). These abnormalities are idiosyncratic and seldom a serious concern (Marder 1997). They usually occur during the first 3 months of treatment (Burns 2001). With first-generation antipsychotic agents, especially phenothiazines, obstructive or cholestatic jaundice occurs infrequently. Approximately 0.1 to 0.5% of patients treated with chlorpromazine develop cholestatic jaundice, usually within the first month of treatment (Janicak et al. 1997). Rarely, symptomatic hepatotoxicity (cholestatic or hepatitic) may be associated with second-generation antipsychotics (Burns 2001). In these cases, the offending medication should be discontinued (American Psychiatric Association 2000). Recovery occurs in up to 75% of patients within 2 months and 90% recover within 1 year (Janicak et al. 1997). Patients taking antipsychotics who have nausea, fever, abdominal pain, and rash should have their liver function evaluated to exclude hepatotoxicity. Since antipsychotic-induced jaundice is infrequent, other etiologies should be ruled out before the cause is judged to be antipsychotic treatment (American Psychiatric Association 2000).

## Hematological Effects
Antipsychotic medications may cause blood dyscrasias, including neutropenia, leukopenia, leukocytosis, thrombopenia, and agranulocytosis. Leukopenia, usually transient, commonly occurs early in treatment, and resolves spontaneously. Chlorpromazine has been associated with benign leukopenia, which occurs in up to 10% of patients (American Psychiatric Association 2000, Kane and Lieberman 1992). This phenomenon is even more common following clozapine administration (Hummer et al. 1994).

Agranulocytosis (granulocyte count less than 500/mm$^3$) is a fatal side effect of antipsychotic drugs. Approximately 0.32% of patients receiving chlorpromazine, and 1% treated with clozapine will experience agranulocytosis (American Psychiatric Association 2000, Lieberman et al. 1989). Early reports of this risk led to clozapine's withdrawal in many countries and severe restrictions of its use in others (Amsler et al. 1977, Idanpaan-Heikkila et al. 1977, Jungi et al. 1977). It carries a mortality rate of approximately 3% (Lieberman et al. 1989). The risk of agranulocytosis is greatest early in treatment, usually within the first 8 to 12 weeks of treatment (Novartis Pharmaceuticals 2000). It tends to occur slightly more often in women, the elderly, and young patients (less than 21 years old). Agranulocytosis from clozapine is usually reversible if the drug is withdrawn immediately (Lieberman et al. 1988). Olanzapine is not associated with severe agranulocytosis (Beasley et al. 1996a, 1996b, Dossenbach et al. 2000). Despite these encouraging studies, there are a number of case studies reporting agranulocytosis during treatment with olanzapine (and quetiapine) in patients who had suffered this adverse event during previous clozapine exposure (Ruhe et al. 2001, Tolosa-Vilella et al. 2002).

Before initiating treatment with clozapine, patients in the US must be registered in a program that ensures that they receive weekly monitoring of their white blood cell (WBC) count during the first 6 months of treatment (Marder 1997). Clozapine is prescribed on a weekly basis unless the WBC count is less than $3,500/mm^3$ or if there is a substantial drop in the WBC count (Marder 1997). If the WBC count is 3,000 to $3,500/mm^3$ and the absolute neutrophil count (ANC) is greater than $1,500/mm^3$, patients should be monitored twice weekly. If the WBC count is 2,000 to $3,000/mm^3$ or the ANC count is 1,000 to $1,500/mm^3$, clozapine treatment should be discontinued and patients should be monitored daily. If the WBC count falls below $2,000/mm^3$ or the ANC is less than $1,000/mm^3$, clozapine should be discontinued and bone marrow aspiration should be considered (American Psychiatric Association 2000). If this occurs, the patient should be given immediate intensive treatment and considered protective isolation. Current guidelines require weekly monitoring for 1 month after the termination of clozapine treatment (American Psychiatric Association 2000). Guidelines on the use of clozapine vary between different countries.

## Other Side Effects

Sedation is the single most common side effect among low-potency conventional antipsychotics, as well as clozapine, zoteapine, and quetiapine (American Psychiatric Association 2000, Young et al. 1998). Although sedation is often beneficial at the beginning of treatment to calm down an anxious or aggressive patient, it usually impairs functioning during long-term treatment (Hummer and Fleischhacker 2000). Most patients usually develop tolerance over time, or it may be possible to minimize sedation by dose reduction or by shifting most of the medication to night to reduce daytime sleepiness (Hummer and Fleischhacker 2000).

Antipsychotic medications can lower the seizure threshold to some degree (Kane and Lieberman 1992). Seizure is more common with low-potency first-generation antipsychotics and clozapine (American Psychiatric Association 2000). Clozapine is associated with dose-related increase in seizures. For example, Devinsky and colleagues (1991) reported that doses of clozapine below 300 mg/day have a seizure rate of about 1%, doses between 300 and 600 mg/day have a seizure rate of 2.7%, and doses above 600 mg/day have a rate of 4.4%. Strategies to reduce the risk for seizures include slower dose titration, a lower dose, and the addition of an anticonvulsant agent (i.e., valproic acid) (Hummer and Fleischhacker 2000).

## Future Directions in Antipsychotic Drug Treatment

The development and investigation of second-generation antipsychotics has advanced our understanding of schizo-

phrenia. Undoubtedly, these advances will help set the stage for further gains. However, second-generation agents are not a panacea for the treatment of psychotic disorders (Remington and Chong 1999, Miyamoto et al. 2000); they are not effective in all patients and against all symptom dimensions and clearly there is a need for the development of new agents with novel pharmocologic mechanisms (Table 95–4). With respect to cognitive symptoms, cognitive effects of the antipsychotics are now targets of treatment and are becoming considered as part of the efficacy of the drug; additional study of these impairments is required to refine both theory and clinical practice in the treatment of schizophrenia (Collaborative Working Group on Clinical Trial Evaluations 1998b, Keefe et al. 1999). Even with success with clozapine in treatment-resistant schizophrenia, a substantial number of patients remain refractory to treatment such that further advances in pharmacotherapy are needed. In addition, it is clear that for many patients the atypical drugs are unable to fully reverse already-established impairment in cognition, negative symptoms, and social disability (Meltzer 1999b). Thus, the possible use of these agents in the prodromal period of schizophrenia or high risk individuals, before the emergence of psychosis, is an important issue in need of research and clarification (Meltzer 1999b). As the pharmacological profiles of the second-generation antipsychotics differ substantially between each other, there is also a likelihood that these drugs may differ from each other with respect to their efficacy against different target symptoms or syndromes and concerning safety and tolerability. As more and more direct comparisons of these antipsychotics become available, evidence-based differential indications will follow suit.

Finally, the second-generation antipsychotics cost considerably more than the conventional they may replace. Existing evidence does not adequately address long-term effectiveness and cost issues. The effects of second-generation agents on long-term outcome, relapse prevention, social and vocational functioning, suicide prevention, quality of life, and family and caregiver burden have just begun to be explored.

## Conclusion

The second-generation and novel antipsychotics have substantially changed our view of the opportunities for treating psychosis. There is now strong evidence that atypical antipsychotics are at least as effective as conventional agents in reducing positive symptoms in schizophrenia, and that second-generation antipsychotics are associated with lower risk of EPS than older agents (Leucht et al. 1999, NICE 2000 Web Page, Sartorius et al. 2002). This evidence is, however, predominantly based on short-term efficacy studies. Moreover, second-generation antipsychotics have their own limitations and different side effect profiles as described in this chapter. A comprehensive understanding of the long-term nature and extent of any clinical advantages of second-generation antipsychotics over conventional agents remains to be explored. There is, however, a hope that second-generation antipsychotics may improve the breadth and depth of clinical response and overall patient outcomes. Thus far, we do not yet have the ultimate ideal antipsychotic drug, but the growing number of potentially novel compounds based on a variety of pharmacological strategies are now moving through preclinical and clinical testing. The search for new antipsychotic drugs and their use in clinical practice could lead to more effective treatments for psychosis in the future. Clearly, the use of pharmacological treatment in patients suffering from schizophrenia needs to be supplemented by psychosocial measures, as outlined in Chapters 86, 91, and 105.

---

### Clinical Vignette

Ms. A is a 54-year-old single woman who has the DSM-IV diagnoses of schizophrenia, chronic undifferentiated type. She had a history of psychotic episode beginning at around age 23 years. She repeated psychotic episodes until she was admitted to hospital approximately 15 years ago. She has been hospitalized continuously since that time, as her disorder has remained resistant to a variety of conventional antipsychotic medications. For the last 3 years, symptoms of auditory hallucinations and persecutory delusions were partially controlled with haloperidol 18 mg/day, chlorpromazine 25 mg/day, and levomepromazine 150 mg/day, but she suffered from persistent negative symptoms, cognitive impairment, and persistent adverse effects, including tremor, excess salivation, tardive dystonia, constipation, and orthostatic hypotension. Therefore, she seemed to be an ideal candidate to switch to a second-generation antipsychotic. She was started on olanzapine (10 mg orally every night) with the plan to discontinue the first-generation antipsychotics after several weeks. After 2 weeks, the dose of olanzapine was increased to 15 mg/day, and after 4 weeks to 20 mg/day. The EPS disappeared 8 weeks later, and she went on to have a dramatic response to olanzapine in terms of psychotic symptoms and negative symptoms. She reported an overall improved condition, and denied any problems with adverse effects. During this time, Ms. A was less withdrawn, less socially isolated, and more interested in ward activities; her grooming improved, and she was better able to handle her family visits. Over a period of several subsequent months, she continued to be treated with olanzapine with a significant improvement in mental status, and without adverse effects. This is a typical case whose clinical status and quality of life have improved significantly after switching from first-generation antipsychotics to a second-generation agent.

## Acknowledgment

The authors would like to acknowledge with appreciation the support of Janssen Pharmaceutical K.K. (Japan) for preparing this manuscript.

## References

Abi-Dargham A, Rodenhiser J, Printz D, et al. (2000) Increased baseline occupancy of $D_2$ receptors by dopamine in schizophrenia. Proc Natl Acad Sci USA 97, 8104–8109.

Aleman A, Hijman R, de Haan EH, et al. (1999) Memory impairment in schizophrenia: A meta-analysis. Am J Psychiatr 156, 1358–1366.

Allen MH (2000) Managing the agitated psychotic patient: A reappraisal of the evidence. J Clin Psychiatry 61(Suppl 14), 11–20.

Allen MH, Currier GW, Hughes DH, et al. (2001) The expert consensus guideline series. Treatment of behavioral emergencies. Postgrad Med (Spec No) 1–88.

Allison DB, Mentore JL, Heo M, et al. (1999) Antipsychotic-induced weight gain: A comprehensive research synthesis. Am J Psychiatr 156, 1686–1696.

Altshuler LL, Cohen L, Szuba MP, et al. (1996) Pharmacologic management of psychiatric illness during pregnancy: Dilemmas and guidelines. Am J Psychiatr 153, 592–606.

American Psychiatric Association (1994) Diagnostic and Statistical Manual of Mental Disorders, 4th ed. APA, Washington DC.

American Psychiatric Association (2000) Practice guideline for the treatment of patients with schizophrenia. In Practice Guidelines for the Treatment of Psychiatric Disorders, Anonymous. APA, Washington DC, pp. 299–412.

American Psychiatric Association Task Force on TD (1992) Tardive Dyskinesia: A Task Force Report of the American Psychiatric Association. APA, Washington DC.

Amsler HA, Teerenhovi L, Barth E, et al. (1977) Agranulocytosis in patients treated with clozapine. A study of the Finnish epidemic. Acta Psychiatr Scand 56, 241–248.

Ananth J, Burgoyne KS, Gadasalli R, et al. (2001) How do the atypical antipsychotics work? J Psychiatr Neurosci 26, 385–394.

Arnt J and Skarsfeldt T (1998) Do novel antipsychotics have similar pharmacological characteristics? A review of the evidence. Neuropsychopharmacology 18, 63–101.

Arvanitis LA, Miller BG, and The Seroquel Trial 13 Study Group (1997) Multiple fixed doses of "Seroquel" (quetiapine) in patients with acute exacerbation of schizophrenia: A comparison with haloperidol and placebo. Biol Psychiatr 42, 233–246.

Asarnow RF, Marder SR, Mintz J, et al. (1988) Differential effect of low and conventional doses of fluphenazine on schizophrenic outpatients with good or poor information-processing abilities. Arch Gen Psychiatr 45, 822–826.

Azorin JM, Spiegel R, Remington G, et al. (2001) A double-blind comparative study of clozapine and risperidone in the management of severe chronic schizophrenia. Am J Psychiatr 158, 1305–1313.

Baldessarini RJ (1996) Drugs and the treatment of psychiatric disorders: Psychosis and anxiety. In Goodman & Gilman's The Pharmacological Basis of Therapeutics, 9th ed., Hardman JG, Limbird LE, Molinoff PB, et al. (eds). McGraw-Hill, New York, pp. 399–420.

Baldessarini RJ, Cohen BM, and Teicher MH (1988) Significance of neuroleptic dose and plasma level in the pharmacological treatment of psychoses. Arch Gen Psychiatr 45, 79–91.

Banov MD, Zarate CA Jr., Tohen M, et al. (1994) Clozapine therapy in refractory affective disorders: Polarity predicts response in long-term follow-up. J Clin Psychiatry 55, 295–300.

Barnas C, Quiner S, Tauscher J, et al. (2001) In vivo (123)I IBZM SPECT imaging of striatal dopamine 2 receptor occupancy in schizophrenic patients. Psychopharmacology (Berl) 157, 236–242.

Barnes TR and McPhillips MA (1998) Novel antipsychotics, extrapyramidal side effects and tardive dyskinesia. Int Clin Psychopharmacol 13(Suppl 3), S49–S57.

Barnes TRE and McPhillips MA (1999) Critical analysis and comparison of the side-effect and safety profiles of the new antipsychotics. Br J Psychiatr 174(Suppl 38), 34–43.

Beasley CM, Dellva MA, Tamura RN, et al. (1999) Randomized double-blind comparison of the incidence of tardive dyskinesia in patients with schizophrenia during long-term treatment with olanzapine or haloperidol. Br J Psychiatr 174, 23–30.

Beasley CMJ, Hamilton SH, Crawford AM, et al. (1997) Olanzapine versus haloperidol: Acute phase results of the international double-blind olanzapine trial. Eur Neuropsychopharmacol 7, 125–137.

Beasley CMJ, Sanger T, Satterlee W, et al. (1996a) Olanzapine versus placebo: Results of a double-blind, fixed-dose olanzapine trial. Psychopharmacology (Berl) 124, 159–167.

Beasley CMJ, Tollefson G, Tran P, et al. (1996b) Olanzapine versus placebo and haloperidol: Acute phase results of the North American double-blind olanzapine trial. Neuropsychopharmacology 14, 111–123.

Bench CJ, Lammertsma AA, Dolan RJ, et al. (1993) Dose dependent occupancy of central dopamine $D_2$ receptors by the novel neuroleptic CP-88,059-01: A study using positron emission tomography and 11C-raclopride. Psychopharmacology (Berl) 112, 308–314.

Bench CJ, Lammertsma AA, Grasby PM, et al. (1996) The time course of binding to striatal dopamine $D_2$ receptors by the neuroleptic ziprasidone (CP-88,059-01) determined by positron emission tomography. Psychopharmacology (Berl) 124, 141–147.

Benedetti F, Sforzini L, Colombo C, et al. (1998) Low-dose clozapine in acute and continuation treatment of severe borderline personality disorder. J Clin Psychiatry 59, 103–107.

Berk M, Ichim L, and Brook S (1999) Olanzapine compared to lithium in mania: A double-blind randomized controlled trial. Int Clin Psychopharmacol 14, 339–343.

Bhana N, Foster RH, Olney R, et al. (2001) Olanzapine: An updated review of its use in the management of schizophrenia. Drugs 61, 111–161.

Bigliani V, Mulligan RS, Acton PD, et al. (2000) Striatal and temporal cortical D2/D3 receptor occupancy by olanzapine and sertindole in vivo: A [123I]epidepride single photon emission tomography (SPET) study. Psychopharmacology (Berl) 150, 132–140.

Blin O (1999) A comparative review of new antipsychotics. Can J Psychiatr 44, 235–244.

Blin O, Azorin JM, and Bouhours P (1996) Antipsychotic and anxiolytic properties of risperidone, haloperidol, and methotrimeprazine in schizophrenic patients. J Clin Psychopharmacol 16, 38–44.

Bondolfi G, Dufour H, Patris M, et al. (1998) Risperidone versus clozapine in treatment-resistant chronic schizophrenia: A randomized double-blind study. The Risperidone Study Group. Am J Psychiatr 155, 499–504.

Borison RL, Arvanitis LA, and Miller BG (1996) ICI 204,636 an atypical antipsychotic: Efficacy and safety in a multicenter, placebo-controlled trial in patients with schizophrenia. US SEROQUEL Study Group. J Clin Psychopharmacol 16, 158–169.

Borison RL, Pathiraja AP, Diamond BI, et al. (1992) Risperidone: Clinical safety and efficacy in schizophrenia. Psychopharmacol Bull 28, 213–218.

Braude WM, Barnes TR, and Gore SM (1983) Clinical characteristics of akathisia: A systematic investigation of acute psychiatric inpatient admissions. Br J Psychiatr 143, 139–150.

Brecher M, Rak IW, Melvin K, et al. (2000) The long-term effect of quetiapine (seroquel) monotherapy on weight in patients with schizophrenia. Int J Psychiatr Clin Pract 4, 287–291.

Breier A and Hamilton SH (1999) Comparative efficacy of olanzapine and haloperidol for patients with treatment-resistant schizophrenia. Biol Psychiatr 45, 403–411.

Breier A, Wright P, Birkett M, et al. (2000) A double-blind dose response study comparing intramuscular olanzapine, haloperidol, and placebo in acutely agitated schizophrenic patients. In ACNP 39th Annual Meeting Abstract, Anonymous. American college of Neuropsychopharmocology, Puerto Rico, p. 348.

Breier AF, Malhotra AK, Su TP, et al. (1999) Clozapine and risperidone in chronic schizophrenia: Effects on symptoms, Parkinsonian side effects, and neuroendocrine response. Am J Psychiatr 156, 294–298.

Brooks JO (2001) Successful outcome using quetiapine in a case of treatment-resistant schizophrenia with assaultive behavior. Schizophr Res 50, 133–134.

Buchanan R and McKenna P (2000) Clozapine: Clinical use and experience. In Schizophrenia and Mood Disorders: The New Drug Therapies in Clinical Practice, Buckley PF and Waddington JL (eds). Butterworth-Heinemann, Woburn, MA, pp. 21–31.

Buchanan RW (1995) Clozapine: Efficacy and safety. Schizophr Bull 21, 579–591.

Buchanan RW and Gold JM (1996) Negative symptoms: Diagnosis, treatment and prognosis. Int Clin Psychopharmacol 11 (Suppl 2), 3–11.

Buchanan RW, Holstein C, and Breier A (1994a) The comparative efficacy and long-term effect of clozapine treatment on neuropsychological test performance. Biol Psychiatr 36, 717–725.

Buchanan RW, Strauss ME, Kirkpatrick B, et al. (1994b) Neuropsychological impairments in deficit vs. nondeficit forms of schizophrenia. Arch Gen Psychiatr 51, 804–811.

Buckland PR, O'Donovan MC, and McGuffin P (1993) Both splicing variants of the dopamine D2 receptor mRNA are up-regulated by antipsychotic drugs. Neurosci Lett 150, 25–28.

Buckley PF (1999) The role of typical and atypical antipsychotic medications in the management of agitation and aggression. J Clin Psychiatr 60(Suppl 10), 52–60.

Buckley PF (2001) Broad therapeutic uses of atypical antipsychotic medications. Biol Psychiatr 50, 912–924.

Buckley NA and Sanders P (2000) Cardiovascular adverse effects of antipsychotic drugs. Drug Saf 23, 215–228.

Bunney BS and Grace AA (1978) Acute and chronic haloperidol treatment: Comparison of effects on nigral dopaminergic cell activity. Life Sci 23, 1715–1728.

Burns MJ (2001) The pharmacology and toxicology of atypical antipsychotic agents. J Clin Toxicol 39, 1–14.

Bymaster F, Perry KW, Nelson DL, et al. (1999) Olanzapine: A basic science update. Br J Psychiatr 174, 36–40.

Bymaster FP, Calligaro DO, Falcone JF, et al. (1996) Radioreceptor binding profile of the atypical antipsychotic olanzapine. Neuropsychopharmacology 14, 87–96.

Bymaster FP, Rasmussen K, Calligaro DO, et al. (1997) In vitro and in vivo biochemistry of olanzapine: A novel, atypical antipsychotic drug. J Clin Psychiatr 58(Suppl 10), 28–36.

Campbell M, Young PI, Bateman DN, et al. (1999) The use of atypical antipsychotics in the management of schizophrenia. Br J Clin Pharmacol 47, 13–22.

Caroff SN and Mann SC (1993) Neuroleptic malignant syndrome. Med Clin N Am 77, 185–202.

Carpenter WT Jr., Conley RR, Buchanan RW, et al. (1995) Patient response and resource management: Another view of clozapine treatment of schizophrenia. Am J Psychiatr 152, 827–832.

Carpenter WT Jr., Hanlon TE, Heinrichs DW, et al. (1990) Continuous versus targeted medication in schizophrenic outpatients: Outcome results. Am J Psychiatr 147, 1138–1148.

Carpenter WT Jr., Heinrichs DW, and Hanlon TE (1987) A comparative trial of pharmacologic strategies in schizophrenia. Am J Psychiatr 144, 1466–1470.

Casey DE (1993) Neuroleptic-induced acute extrapyramidal syndromes and tardive dyskinesia. Psychiatr Clin N Am 16, 589–610.

Casey DE (1995) Neuroleptic-induced extrapyramidal syndromes and tardive dyskinesia. In Schizophrenia, Hirsch SR and Weinberger DR (eds). Blackwell, Oxford, UK, pp. 546–565.

Casey DE (1997) The relationship of pharmacology to side effects. J Clin Psychiatr 58(Suppl 10), 55–62.

Casey DE (1999) Tardive dyskinesia and atypical antipsychotic drugs. Schizophr Res 35(Suppl), S61–S66.

Chakos M, Lieberman J, Hoffman E, et al. (2001) Effectiveness of second-generation antipsychotics in patients with treatment-resistant schizophrenia: A review and meta-analysis of randomized trials. Am J Psychiatr 158, 518–526.

Chakos MH, Lieberman JA, Alvir J, et al. (1995) Caudate nuclei volumes in schizophrenic patients treated with typical antipsychotics or clozapine. Lancet 345, 456–457.

Chakos MH, Lieberman JA, Bilder RM, et al. (1994) Increase in caudate nuclei volumes of first-episode schizophrenic patients taking antipsychotic drugs. Am J Psychiatr 151, 1430–1436.

Chakos MH, Shirakawa O, Lieberman J, et al. (1998) Striatal enlargement in rats chronically treated with neuroleptic. Biol Psychiatr 44, 675–684.

Chengappa KN, Ebeling T, Kang JS, et al. (1999) Clozapine reduces severe self-mutilation and aggression in psychotic patients with borderline personality disorder. J Clin Psychiatr 60, 477–484.

Chiodo LA and Bunney BS (1983) Typical and atypical neuroleptics: Differential effects of chronic administration on the activity of A9 and A10 midbrain dopaminergic neurons. J Neurosci 3, 1607–1619.

Chouinard G (1995) Effects of risperidone in tardive dyskinesia: An analysis of the Canadian multicenter risperidone study. J Clin Psychopharmacol 15, 36S–44S.

Chouinard G, Jones B, Remington G, et al. (1993) A Canadian multicenter placebo-controlled study of fixed doses of risperidone and haloperidol in the treatment of chronic schizophrenic patients. J Clin Psychopharmacol 13, 25–40.

Ciapparelli A, Dell'Osso L, Pini S, et al. (2000) Clozapine for treatment-refractory schizophrenia, schizoaffective disorder, and psychotic bipolar disorder: A 24-month naturalistic study. J Clin Psychiatr 61, 329–334.

Claus A, Bollen J, De Cuyper H, et al. (1992) Risperidone versus haloperidol in the treatment of chronic schizophrenic inpatients: A multicentre double-blind comparative study. Acta Psychiatr Scand 85, 295–305.

Coffman JA, Nasrallah HA, Lyskowski J, et al. (1987) Clinical effectiveness of oral and parenteral rapid neuroleptization. J Clin Psychiatr 48, 20–24.

Collaborative Working Group on Clinical Trial Evaluations (1998a) Assessing the effects of atypical antipsychotics on negative symptoms. J Clin Psychiatr 59(Suppl 12), 28–34.

Collaborative Working Group on Clinical Trial Evaluations (1998b) Evaluating the effects of antipsychotics on cognition in schizophrenia. J Clin Psychiatr 59(Suppl 12), 35–40.

Conley R, Gounaris C, and Tamminga C (1994) Clozapine response varies in deficit versus nondeficit schizophrenic subjects. Biol Psychiatr 35, 746–747.

Conley RR and Kelly DL (2001) Management of treatment resistance in schizophrenia. Biol Psychiatr 50, 898–911.

Conley RR and Mahmoud R (2001) A randomized double-blind study of risperidone and olanzapine in the treatment of schizophrenia or schizoaffective disorder. Am J Psychiatr 158, 765–774.

Conley RR, Tamminga CA, Bartko JJ, et al. (1998) Olanzapine compared with chlorpromazine in treatment-resistant schizophrenia. Am J Psychiatr 155, 914–920.

Conley RR, Tamminga CA, Kelly DL, et al. (1999) Treatment-resistant schizophrenic patients respond to clozapine after olanzapine nonresponse. Biol Psychiatr 46, 73–77.

Corson PW, Nopoulos P, Miller DD, et al. (1999) Change in basal ganglia volume over 2 years in patients with schizophrenia: Typical versus atypical neuroleptics. Am J Psychiatr 156, 1200–1204.

Craig TJ, Bromet EJ, Fennig S, et al. (2000) Is there an association between duration of untreated psychosis and 24-month clinical outcome in a first-admission series? Am J Psychiatr 157, 60–66.

Creese I, Burt DR, and Snyder SH (1976) Dopamine receptor binding predicts clinical and pharmacological potencies of antischizophrenic drugs. Science 192, 480–483.

Cressman WA, Plostnieks J, and Johnson PC (1973) Absorption, metabolism and excretion of droperidol by human subjects following intramuscular and intravenous administration. Anesthesiology 38, 363–369.

Crow TJ, MacMillan JF, Johnson AL, et al. (1986) A randomized controlled trial of prophylactic neuroleptic treatment. Br J Psychiatr 148, 120–127.

Csernansky J and Okamoto A (2000) Risperidone vs. haloperidol for prevention of relapse in schizophrenia and schizoaffective disorders. A long-term double-blind comparison. In The 10th Biennial Winter Workshop on Schizophrenia, Anonymous. Davos, Switzerland.

Csernansky JG, Mahmoud R, and Brenner R (2002) A comparison of risperidone and haloperidol for the prevention of relapse in patients with schizophrenia. New Engl J Med 346, 16–22.

Currier GW (2000) Atypical antipsychotic medications in the psychiatric emergency service. J Clin Psychiatr 61(Suppl 14), 21–26.

Cutler NR and Sramek J (2000) Atypical antipsychotics and QT prolongation: A class effect. Curr Opin CPNS Invest Drugs 2, 52–57.

Dahl SG (1990) Pharmacokinetics of antipsychotic drugs in man. Acta Psychiatr Scand 358(Suppl), 37–40.

Dallocchio C, Buffa C, Tinelli C, et al. (1999) Effectiveness of risperidone in Huntington chorea patients. J Clin Psychopharmacol 19, 101–103.

Daniel DG and Copeland LF (2001) Second generation antipsychotics in the treatment of schizophrenia: Sertindole. In Current Issues in the Psychopharmacology of Schizophrenia, Breier A, Tran PV, Herrera JM, et al. (eds). Lippincott Williams & Wilkins Healthcare, Philadelphia, pp. 262–276.

Daniel DG, Zimbroff DL, Potkin SG, et al. (1999) Ziprasidone 80 mg/day and 160 mg/day in the acute exacerbation of schizophrenia and schizoaffective disorder: A 6-week placebo-controlled trial. Neuropsychopharmacology 20, 491–505.

Davis JM (1975) Overview: Maintenance therapy in psychiatry: I. Schizophrenia. Am J Psychiatr 132, 1237–1245.

Davis JM and Casper R (1977) Antipsychotic drugs: Clinical pharmacology and therapeutic use. Drugs 14, 260–282.

Davis JM, Matalon L, Watanabe MD, et al. (1994) Depot antipsychotic drugs. Place in therapy. Drugs 47, 741–773.

Davis JM, Schaffer CB, Killian GA, et al. (1980) Important issues in the drug treatment of schizophrenia. Schizophr Bull 6, 70–87.

Dawkins K, Lieberman JA, Lebowitz BD, et al. (1999) Antipsychotics: Past and future. National Institute of Mental Health Division of Services and Intervention Research Workshop (July 14, 1998). Schizophr Bull 25, 395–404.

De Deyn PP, Rabheru K, Rasmussen A, et al. (1999) A randomized trial of risperidone, placebo, and haloperidol for behavioral symptoms of dementia. Neurology 53, 946–955.

Delay J and Deniker P (1952) Le traitement des psychoses par une méthode neurolytique dérivée de l' libérothérapie. Comptes Rendus du Congr Alien Neurol 50, 503–513.

Dellva MA, Tran P, Tollefson GD, et al. (1997) Standard olanzapine versus placebo and ineffective-dose olanzapine in the maintenance treatment of schizophrenia. Psychiatr Serv 48, 1571–1577.

Deutch AY, Lee MC, and Iadarola MJ (1992) Regionally specific effects of atypical antipsychotic drugs on striatal Fos expression: The nucleus accumbens shell as a locus of antipsychotic action. Mol Cell Neurosci 3, 332–341.

Dev V and Raniwalla J (2000) Quetiapine: A review of its safety in the management of schizophrenia. Drug Safety 23, 295–307.

Devinsky O, Honigfeld G, and Patin J (1991) Clozapine-related seizures. Neurology 41, 369–371.

Dipple HC (1999) The use of olanzapine for movement disorder in Huntington's disease: A first case report. J Neurol Neurosurg Psychiatr 67, 123–124.

Dixon L, Weiden P, Delahanty J, et al. (2000) Prevalence and correlates of diabetes in national schizophrenia samples. Schizophr Bull 26, 903–912.

Donlon PT, Hopkin J, and Tupin JP (1979) Overview: Efficacy and safety of the rapid neuroleptization method with injectable haloperidol. Am J Psychiatr 136, 273–278.

Doraiswamy PM, Tupler LA, and Krishnan KR (1995) Neuroleptic treatment and caudate plasticity. Lancet 345, 734–735.

Dossenbach MRK, Beuzen JN, Avnon M, et al. (2000) The effectiveness of olanzapine in treatment-refractory schizophrenia when patients are nonresponsive to or unable to tolerate clozapine. Clin Ther 22, 1021–1034.

Dragunow M, Robertson GS, Faull RL, et al. (1990) D₂ dopamine receptor antagonists induce Fos and related proteins in rat striatal neurons. Neuroscience 37, 287–294.

Duggan L, Fenton M, Dardennes RM, et al. (2000) Olanzapine for schizophrenia. Coch Database Syst Rev CD001359.

Duncan GE, Sheitman BB, and Lieberman JA (1999a) An integrated view of pathophysiological models of schizophrenia. Brain Res Rev 29, 250–264.

Duncan GE, Zorn S, and Lieberman JA (1999b) Mechanisms of typical and atypical antipsychotic drug action in relation to dopamine and NMDA receptor hypofunction hypotheses of schizophrenia. Mol Psychiatr 4, 418–428.

Dursun SM, Gardner DM, Bird DC, et al. (1999) Olanzapine for patients with treatment-resistant schizophrenia: A naturalistic case series outcome study. Can J Psychiatr 44, 701–704.

Dwivedi Y and Pandey GN (1999) Effects of treatment with haloperidol, chlorpromazine, and clozapine on protein kinase C (PKC) and phosphoinositide-specific phospholipase C (PI-PLC) activity and on mRNA and protein expression of PKC and PLC isozymes in rat brain. J Pharmacol Exper Therapeut 291, 688–704.

Eastwood SL, Burnet PW, and Harrison PJ (1994) Striatal synaptophysin expression and haloperidol-induced synaptic plasticity. Neuroreport 5, 677–680.

Eastwood SL, Heffernan J, and Harrison PJ (1997) Chronic haloperidol treatment differentially affects the expression of synaptic and neuronal plasticity-associated genes. Mol Psychiatr 2, 322–329.

Eder U, Mangweth B, Ebenbichler C, et al. (2001) Association of olanzapine-induced weight gain with an increase in body fat. Am J Psychiatr 158, 1719–1722.

Emsley RA, Raniwalla J, Bailey PJ, et al. (2000) A comparison of the effects of quetiapine ("seroquel") and haloperidol in schizophrenic patients with a history of and a demonstrated, partial response to conventional antipsychotic treatment. PRIZE Study Group. Int Clin Psychopharmacol 15, 121–131.

Ereshefsky L (1996) Pharmacokinetics and drug interactions: Update for new antipsychotics. J Clin Psychiatr 57(Suppl 11), 12–25.

Escobar JI, Barron A, and Kiriakos R (1983) A controlled study of neuroleptization with fluphenazine hydrochloride injections. J Clin Psychopharmacol 3, 359–362.

Essock SM, Hargreaves WA, Covell NH, et al. (1996a) Clozapine's effectiveness for patients in state hospitals: Results from a randomized trial. Psychopharmacol Bull 32, 683–697.

Essock SM, Hargreaves WA, Dohm FA, et al. (1996b) Clozapine eligibility among state hospital patients. Schizophr Bull 22, 15–25.

Fabre LF Jr., Arvanitis L, Pultz J, et al. (1995) ICI 204, 636, a novel, atypical antipsychotic: Early indication of safety and efficacy in patients with chronic and subchronic schizophrenia. Clin Ther 17, 366–378.

Farde L, Nordstrom AL, Wiesel FA, et al. (1992) Positron emission tomographic analysis of central D₁ and D₂ dopamine receptor occupancy in patients treated with classical neuroleptics and clozapine. Relation to extrapyramidal side effects. Arch Gen Psychiatr 49, 538–544.

Farde L, Nyberg S, Oxenstierna G, et al. (1995) Positron emission tomography studies on D₂ and 5-HT₂ receptor binding in risperidone-treated schizophrenic patients. J Clin Psychopharmacol 15, 19S–23S.

Feifel D (2000) Rationale and guidelines for the inpatient treatment of acute psychosis. J Clin Psychiatr 61(Suppl 14), 27–32.

Ferris P (2000) Ziprasidone. Curr Opin CPNS Invest Drugs 2, 58–70.

Fink-Jensen A and Kristensen P (1994) Effects of typical and atypical neuroleptics on Fos protein expression in the rat forebrain. Neurosci Lett 182, 115–118.

Fischman AJ, Bonab AA, Babich JW, et al. (1996) Positron emission tomographic analysis of central 5-hydroxytryptamine2 receptor occupancy in healthy volunteers treated with the novel antipsychotic agent, ziprasidone. J Pharmacol Exper Therapeut 279, 939–947.

Fleischhacker WW (1995) New drugs for the treatment of schizophrenic patients. Acta Psychiatr Scand 388(Suppl), 24–30.

Fleischhacker WW (1999) Clozapine: A comparison with other novel antipsychotics. J Clin Psychiatr 60, 30–34.

Fleischhacker WW (2001) Drug treatment of patients with schizophrenia. In Contemporary Psychiatry, Vol. 3, Henn F, Sartorius N, Helmchen H, et al. (eds). Springer-Verlag, Berlin, Heidelberg; New York, pp. 139–158.

Friedman JH and Factor SA (2000) Atypical antipsychotics in the treatment of drug-induced psychosis in Parkinson's disease. Mov Disord 15, 201–211.

Gaebel W (1995) Is intermittent, early intervention medication an alternative for neuroleptic maintenance treatment? Int Clin Psychopharmacol 9(Suppl 5), 11–16.

Gaebel W and Marder S (1996) Conclusions and treatment recommendations for the acute episode in schizophrenia. Int Clin Psychopharmacol 11(Suppl 2), 93–100.

Gaebel W, Frick U, Kopcke W, et al. (1993) Early neuroleptic intervention in schizophrenia: Are prodromal symptoms valid predictors of relapse? Br J Psychiatr 21(Suppl), 8–12.

Gaebel W, Janner M, Frommann N, et al. (2002) First vs multiple episode schizophrenia: Two-year outcome of intermittent and maintenance medication strategies. Schizophr Res 53, 145–159.

Gardos G, Casey DE, Cole JO, et al. (1994) Ten-year outcome of tardive dyskinesia. Am J Psychiatr 151, 836–841.

Geddes J, Freemantle N, Harrison P, et al. (2000) Atypical antipsychotics in the treatment of schizophrenia: Systematic overview and meta-regression analysis. BMJ 321, 1371–1376.

Gefvert O, Bergstrom M, Langstrom B, et al. (1998) Time course of central nervous dopamine-$D_2$ and 5-$HT_2$ receptor blockade and plasma drug concentrations after discontinuation of quetiapine (Seroquel) in patients with schizophrenia. Psychopharmacology (Berl) 135, 119–126.

Geinisman Y, Morrell F, and de Toledo-Morrell L (1989) Perforated synapses on double-headed dendritic spines: A possible structural substrate of synaptic plasticity. Brain Res 480, 326–329.

Gelenberg AJ, Van Putten T, Lavori PW, et al. (1989) Anticholinergic effects on memory: Benztropine versus amantadine. J Clin Psychopharmacol 9, 180–185.

Gerlach J (1991) New antipsychotics: Classification, efficacy, and adverse effects. Schizophr Bull 17, 289–309.

Ghaemi SN (2000) New treatments for bipolar disorder: The role of atypical neuroleptic agents. J Clin Psychiatr 61(Suppl 14), 33–42.

Gilbert PL, Harris MJ, McAdams LA, et al. (1995) Neuroleptic withdrawal in schizophrenic patients. A review of the literature. Arch Gen Psychiatr 52, 173–188.

Giller ER, Mandel F, and Keck PE (2001) Ziprasidone in the acute treatment of mania: A double-blind, placebo controlled, randomized trial. Schizophr Res 49, 229.

Glassman AH and Bigger JT Jr. (2001) Antipsychotic drugs: Prolonged QTc interval, torsade de pointes, and sudden death. Am J Psychiatr 158, 1774–1782.

Glazer WM (2000) Expected incidence of tardive dyskinesia associated with atypical antipsychotics. J Clin Psychiatr 61(Suppl 4), 21–26.

Glazer WM and Dickson RA (1998) Clozapine reduces violence and persistent aggression in schizophrenia. J Clin Psychiatr 59(Suppl 3), 8–14.

Glazer WM and Kane JM (1992) Depot neuroleptic therapy: An underutilized treatment option. J Clin Psychiatr 53, 426–433.

Glazer WM, Moore DC, Schooler NR, et al. (1984) Tardive dyskinesia: A discontinuation study. Arch Gen Psychiatr 41, 623–627.

Glick ID, Murray SR, Vasudevan P, et al. (2001) Treatment with atypical antipsychotics: New indications and new populations. J Psychiatr Res 35, 187–191.

Goff DC and Evins AE (1998) Negative symptoms in schizophrenia: Neurobiological models and treatment response. Harv Rev Psychiatr 6, 59–77.

Goff DC, Posever T, Herz L, et al. (1998) An exploratory haloperidol-controlled dose-finding study of ziprasidone in hospitalized patients with schizophrenia or schizoaffective disorder. J Clin Psychopharmacol 18, 296–304.

Gold S, Arndt S, Nopoulos P, et al. (1999) Longitudinal study of cognitive function in first-episode and recent-onset schizophrenia. Am J Psychiatr 156, 1342–1348.

Goldberg TE, Greenberg RD, Griffin SJ, et al. (1993) The effect of clozapine on cognition and psychiatric symptoms in patients with schizophrenia. Br J Psychiatr 162, 43–48.

Goldstein DJ, Corbin LA, and Fung MC (2000) Olanzapine-exposed pregnancies and lactation: Early experience. J Clin Psychopharmacol 20, 399–403.

Goldstein JM (1998) "Seroquel" (quetiapine fumarate) reduces hostility and aggression in patients with acute schizophrenia. Presented at the 151st annual meeting of the American Psychiatric Association. Anonymous. Toronto, Canada,

Goldstein JM, Litwin LC, Sutton EB, et al. (1993) Seroquel: Electrophysiological profile of a potential atypical antipsychotic. Psychopharmacology (Berl) 112, 293–298.

Goodwin FK and Jamison KR (1990) Manic–Depressive Illness. Oxford University Press, New York.

Grace AA (1992) The depolarization block hypothesis of neuroleptic action: Implications for the etiology and treatment of schizophrenia. J Neural Transm 36(Suppl), 91–131.

Grace AA and Bunney BS (1986) Induction of depolarization block in midbrain dopamine neurons by repeated administration of haloperidol: Analysis using in vivo intracellular recording. J Pharmacol Exp Therap 238, 1092–1100.

Green AI, Tohen M, Patel JK, et al. (2000) Clozapine in the treatment of refractory psychotic mania. Am J Psychiatr 157, 982–986.

Green MF (1996) What are the functional consequences of neurocognitive deficits in schizophrenia? Am J Psychiatr 153, 321–330.

Green MF, Marshall BDJ, Wirshing WC, et al. (1997) Does risperidone improve verbal working memory in treatment-resistant schizophrenia? Am J Psychiatr 154, 799–804.

Gur RE, Maany V, Mozley PD, et al. (1998) Subcortical MRI volumes in neuroleptic-naive and treated patients with schizophrenia. Am J Psychiatr 155, 1711–1717.

Haase HJ (1961) Extrapyramidal modification of fine movements: A "conditio sine qua non" of the fundamental therapeutic action of neuroleptic drugs. In Systeme Extrapyramidal et Neuroleptique, Bordeleau JM (ed). Editions Psychiatriques, Montreal, pp. 329–353.

Hafner H, Riecher-Rossler A, Maurer K, et al. (1992) First onset and early symptomatology of schizophrenia. A chapter of epidemiological and neurobiological research into age and sex differences. Eur Arch Psychiatr Clin Neurosci 242, 109–118.

Hamilton SH, Revicki DA, Genduso LA, et al. (1998) Olanzapine versus placebo and haloperidol: Quality of life and efficacy results of the North American double-blind trial. Neuropsychopharmacology 18, 41–49.

Haring C, Fleischhacker WW, Schett P, et al. (1990) Influence of patient-related variables on clozapine plasma levels. Am J Psychiatr 147, 1471–1475.

Harrison PJ (1999) The neuropathological effects of antipsychotic drugs. Schizophr Res 40, 87–99.

Harvey PD and Keefe RS (2001) Studies of cognitive change in patients with schizophrenia following novel antipsychotic treatment. Am J Psychiatr 158, 176–184.

Harvey PD, Howanitz E, Parrella M, et al. (1998) Symptoms, cognitive functioning, and adaptive skills in geriatric patients with lifelong schizophrenia: A comparison across treatment sites. Am J Psychiatr 155, 1080–1086.

Harvey PD, Silverman JM, Mohs RC, et al. (1999) Cognitive decline in late-life schizophrenia: A longitudinal study of geriatric chronically hospitalized patients. Biol Psychiatr 45, 32–40.

Haupt DW and Newcomer JW (2001) Hyperglycemia and antipsychotic medications. J Clin Psychiatr 62(Suppl 27), 15–26.

Hellewell JSE, Cameron-Hands D, and Cantillon M (1998) Seroquel: Evidence for efficacy in the treatment of hostility and aggression. Schizophr Res 29, 154–155.

Henderson DC (2001) Clinical experience with insulin resistance, diabetic ketoacidosis, and type 2 diabetes mellitus in patients treated with atypical antipsychotic agents. J Clin Psychiatr 62(Suppl 27), 10–14.

Henderson DC and Goff DC (1996) Risperidone as an adjunct to clozapine therapy in chronic schizophrenics. J Clin Psychiatr 57, 395–397.

Henderson DC, Cagliero E, Gray C, et al. (2000) Clozapine, diabetes mellitus, weight gain, and lipid abnormalities: A five-year naturalistic study. Am J Psychiatr 157, 975–981.

Herz MI, Glazer WM, Mostert MA, et al. (1991) Intermittent vs maintenance medication in schizophrenia. Two-year results. Arch Gen Psychiatr 48, 333–339.

Hesselink JMK (2000) Iloperidone. Curr Opin CPNS Invest Drugs 2, 71–78.

Hillard JR (1998) Emergency treatment of acute psychosis. J Clin Psychiatr 59(Suppl 1), 57–60.

Hillert A, Maier W, Wetzel H, et al. (1992) Risperidone in the treatment of disorders with a combined psychotic and depressive syndrome—a functional approach. Pharmacopsychiatry 25, 213–217.

Hirsch SR and Barnes TRE (1995) The clinical treatment of schizophrenia with antipsychotic medication. In Schizophrenia, Hirsch SR and Weinberger DR (eds). Blackwell Science, Oxford, pp. 443–468.

Ho BC, Andreasen NC, Flaum M, et al. (2000) Untreated initial psychosis: Its relation to quality of life and symptom remission in first-episode schizophrenia. Am J Psychiatr 157, 808–815.

Hogarty GE, McEvoy JP, Munetz M, et al. (1988) Dose of fluphenazine, familial expressed emotion, and outcome in schizophrenia. Results of a two-year controlled study. Arch Gen Psychiatr 45, 797–805.

Hogarty GE, Ulrich RF, Mussare F, et al. (1976) Drug discontinuation among long term, successfully maintained schizophrenic outpatients. Dis Nerv Syst 37, 494–500.

Hollenberg MD (1991) Structure-activity relationships for transmembrane signaling: The receptor's turn. FASEB J 5, 178–186.

Hough DW (2001) Low-dose olanzapine for self-mutilation behavior in patients with borderline personality disorder. J Clin Psychiatr 62, 296–297.

Hoyberg OJ, Fensbo C, Remvig J, et al. (1993) Risperidone versus perphenazine in the treatment of chronic schizophrenic patients with acute exacerbations. Acta Psychiatr Scand 88, 395–402.

Huber G, Gross G, Schuttler R, et al. (1980) Longitudinal studies of schizophrenic patients. Schizophr Bull 6, 592–605.

Hummer M and Fleischhacker WW (2000) Nonmotor side effects of novel antipsychotics. Curr Opin CPNS Invest Drugs 2, 45–51.

Hummer M, Kurz M, Barnas C, et al. (1994) Clozapine-induced transient white blood count disorders. J Clin Psychiatr 55, 429–432.

Hummer M, Kurz M, Kurzthaler I, et al. (1997) Hepatotoxicity of clozapine. J Clin Psychopharmacol 17, 314–317.

Huttunen MO, Piepponen T, Rantanen H, et al. (1995) Risperidone versus zuclopenthixol in the treatment of acute schizophrenic episodes: A double-blind parallel-group trial. Acta Psychiatr Scand 91, 271–277.

Idanpaan-Heikkila J, Alhava E, Olkinuora M, et al. (1977) Agranulocytosis during treatment with clozapine. Eur J Clin Pharmacol 11, 193–198.

Inoue A, Miki S, Seto M, et al. (1997) Aripiprazole, a novel antipsychotic drug, inhibits quinpirole-evoked GTPase activity but does not up-regulate dopamine $D_2$ receptor following repeated treatment in the rat striatum. Eur J Pharmacol 321, 105–111.

Jacobsen FM (1995) Risperidone in the treatment of affective illness and obsessive–compulsive disorder. J Clin Psychiatr 56, 423–429.

Janicak PG and Davis JM (1996) Antipsychotic dosing strategies in acute schizophrenia. Int Clin Psychopharmacol 11(Suppl 2), 35–40.

Janicak PG, Davis JM, Preskorn SH, et al. (1993) Principles and Practice of Psychopharmacology. Williams & Wilkins, Baltimore, MD.

Janicak PG, Davis JM, Preskorn SH, et al. (1997) Principles and Practice of Psychopharmacology, 2nd ed. Williams & Wilkins, Baltimore, MD.

Jann MW, Ereshefsky L, Saklad SR, et al. (1985) Effects of carbamazepine on plasma haloperidol levels. J Clin Psychopharmacol 5, 106–109.

Jeste DV, Lacro JP, Bailey A, et al. (1999) Lower incidence of tardive dyskinesia with risperidone compared with haloperidol in older patients. J Am Geriatr Soc 47, 716–719.

Jimenez-Jimenez FJ and Garcia-Ruiz PJ (2001) Pharmacological options for the treatment of Tourette's disorder. Drugs 61, 2207–2220.

Johnstone EC, Crow TJ, Frith CD, et al. (1978) Mechanism of the antipsychotic effect in the treatment of acute schizophrenia. Lancet 1, 848–851.

Jolley AG, Hirsch SR, Morrison E, et al. (1990) Trial of brief intermittent neuroleptic prophylaxis for selected schizophrenic outpatients: Clinical and social outcome at two years. BMJ 301, 837–842.

Juncos JL (1999) Management of psychotic aspects of Parkinson's disease. J Clin Psychiatr 60(Suppl 8), 42–53.

Jungi WF, Fischer J, Senn HJ, et al. (1977) Frequent cases of agranulocytosis due to clozapin (leponex) in eastern Switzerland. Schweiz Med Wochenschr 107, 1861–1864.

Kalkman HO, Subramanian N, and Hoyer D (2001) Extended radioligand binding profile of iloperidone: A broad spectrum dopamine/serotonin/norepinephrine receptor antagonist for the management of psychotic disorders. Neuropsychopharmacology 25, 904–914.

Kallal L and Benovic JL (2000) Using green fluorescent proteins to study G-protein-coupled receptor localization and trafficking. Trends Pharmacol Sci 21, 175–180.

Kane J, Honigfeld G, Singer J, et al. (1988) Clozapine for the treatment-resistant schizophrenic. A double-blind comparison with chlorpromazine. Arch Gen Psychiatr 45, 789–796.

Kane JM (1989) The current status of neuroleptic therapy. J Clin Psychiatr 50, 322–328.

Kane JM (1999) Management strategies for the treatment of schizophrenia. J Clin Psychiatr 60, 13–17.

Kane JM and Lieberman JA (1992) Adverse Effects of Psychotropic Drugs. Guilford Press, New York.

Kane JM and Marder SR (1993) Psychopharmacologic treatment of schizophrenia. Schizophr Bull 19, 287–302.

Kane JM, Gunduz H, and Malhortra AK (2001) Second generation antipsychotics in the treatment of schizophrenia: Clozapine. In Current Issues in the Psychopharmacology of Schizophrenia, Breier A, Tran PV, Herrera JM, et al. (eds). Lippincott Williams & Wilkins Healthcare, Philadelphia, pp. 209–223.

Kane JM, Rifkin A, Quitkin F, et al. (1982) Fluphenazine vs placebo in patients with remitted, acute first-episode schizophrenia. Arch Gen Psychiatr 39, 70–73.

Kane JM, Rifkin A, Woerner M, et al. (1983) Low-dose neuroleptic treatment of outpatient schizophrenics. I. Preliminary results for relapse rates. Arch Gen Psychiatr 40, 893–896.

Kane JM, Woerner M, Borenstein M, et al. (1986) Integrating incidence and prevalence of tardive dyskinesia. Psychopharmacol Bull 22, 254–258.

Kane JM, Carson WH, Sana AR, et al. (2002) Efficacy and safety of aripiprazole and haloperidol versus placebo in patients with schizophrenia and schizoaffective disorder. J Clin Psychiatr 63, 763–771.

Kapur S and Remington G (2001) Dopamine $D_2$ receptors and their role in atypical antipsychotic action: Still necessary and may even be sufficient. Biol Psychiatr 50, 873–883.

Kapur S and Seeman P (2001) Does fast dissociation from the dopamine $D_2$ receptor explain the action of atypical antipsychotics? A new hypothesis. Am J Psychiatr 158, 360–369.

Kapur S, Remington G, Jones C, et al. (1996) High levels of dopamine $D_2$ receptor occupancy with low-dose haloperidol treatment. A PET study. Am J Psychiatr 153, 948–950.

Kapur S, Zipursky R, Jones C, et al. (2000a) Relationship between dopamine $D_2$ occupancy, clinical response, and side effects: A double-blind PET study of first-episode schizophrenia. Am J Psychiatr 157, 514–520.

Kapur S, Zipursky R, Jones C, et al. (2000b) A positron emission tomography study of quetiapine in schizophrenia: A preliminary finding of an antipsychotic effect with only transiently high dopamine $D_2$ receptor occupancy. Arch Gen Psychiatr 57, 553–559.

Kapur S, Zipursky R, Roy P, et al. (1997) The relationship between $D_2$ receptor occupancy and plasma levels on low dose oral haloperidol: A PET study. Psychopharmacology (Berl) 131, 148–152.

Kapur S, Zipursky RB, Remington G, et al. (1998) 5-HT$_2$ and $D_2$ receptor occupancy of olanzapine in schizophrenia: A PET investigation. Am J Psychiatr 155, 921–928.

Kapur S, Zipursky RB, and Remington G (1999) Clinical and theoretical implications of 5-HT$_2$ and $D_2$ receptor occupancy of clozapine, risperidone, and olanzapine in schizophrenia. Am J Psychiatr 156, 286–293.

Karagianis JL, Dawe IC, Thakur A, et al. (2001) Rapid tranquilization with olanzapine in acute psychosis: A case series. J Clin Psychiatr 62(Suppl 2), 12–16.

Kasper S (1998) Risperidone and olanzapine: Optimal dosing for efficacy and tolerability in patients with schizophrenia. Int Clin Psychopharmacol 13, 253–262.

Kasper S, Tauscher J, Kufferle B, et al. (1998) Sertindole and dopamine $D_2$ receptor occupancy in comparison to risperidone, clozapine, and haloperidol—a 123I-IBZM SPECT study. Psychopharmacology (Berl) 136, 367–373.

Katz IR, Jeste DV, Mintzer JE, et al. (1999) Comparison of risperidone and placebo for psychosis and behavioral disturbances associated with dementia: A randomized, double-blind trial. Risperidone Study Group. J Clin Psychiatr 60, 107–115.

Keck PE Jr. McElroy SL, and Arnold LM (2001) Ziprasidone: A new atypical antipsychotic. Expert Opin Pharmacother 2, 1033–1042.

Keck PJ, Buffenstein A, Ferguson J, et al. (1998) Ziprasidone 40 and 120 mg/day in the acute exacerbation of schizophrenia and schizoaffective disorder: A 4-week placebo-controlled trial. Psychopharmacology (Berl) 140, 173–184.

Keefe RSE, Silva SG, Perkins DO, et al. (1999) The effects of atypical antipsychotic drugs on neurocognitive impairment in schizophrenia: A review and meta-analysis. Schizophr Bull 25, 201–222.

Keshavan MS, Bagwell WW, Haas GL, et al. (1994) Changes in caudate volume with neuroleptic treatment. Lancet 344, 1434.

Khouzam HR and Donnelly NJ (1997) Remission of self-mutilation in a patient with borderline personality during risperidone therapy. J Nerv Ment Dis 185, 348–349.

Kikuchi T, Tottori K, Uwahodo Y, et al. (1995) 7-(4-[4-(2,3-Dichlorophenyl)-1-piperazinyl]butyloxy)-3,4-dihydro-2(1H)-quinolinone (OPC-14597), a new putative antipsychotic drug with both presynaptic dopamine autoreceptor agonistic activity and postsynaptic $D_2$ receptor antagonistic activity. J Pharmacol Exp Therap 274, 329–336.

King DJ (1990) The effect of neuroleptics on cognitive and psychomotor function. Br J Psychiatr 157, 799–811.

Kinon BJ and Lieberman JA (1996) Mechanisms of action of atypical antipsychotic drugs: A critical analysis. Psychopharmacology (Berl) 124, 2–34.

Kinon BJ, Kane JM, Chakos M, et al. (1993) Possible predictors of neuroleptic-resistant schizophrenic relapse: Influence of negative symptoms and acute extrapyramidal side effects. Psychopharmacol Bull 29, 365–369.

Kinon BJ, Milton DR, and Hill AL (2001a) Efficacy of olanzapine orally-disintegrating tablet in the treatment of acutely ill noncompliant schizophrenic patients. Biol Psychiatr 49, 171S.

Kinon BJ, Roychowdhury SM, Milton DR, et al. (2001b) Effective resolution with olanzapine of acute presentation of behavioral agitation and positive psychotic symptoms in schizophrenia. J Clin Psychiatr 62(Suppl 2), 17–21.

Kissling W (1991) Guidelines for Neuroleptic Relapse Prevention in Schizophrenia. Springer-Verlag, Berlin.

Klieser E, Lehmann E, Kinzler E, et al. (1995) Randomized, double-blind, controlled trial of risperidone versus clozapine in patients with chronic schizophrenia. J Clin Psychopharmacol 15, S45–S51.

Kodama M, Akiyama K, Ujike H, et al. (1998) A robust increase in expression of arc gene, an effector immediate early gene, in the rat brain after acute and chronic methamphetamine administration. Brain Res 796, 273–283.

Konradi C and Heckers S (1995) Haloperidol-induced Fos expression in striatum is dependent upon transcription factor cyclic AMP response element binding protein. Neuroscience 65, 1051–1061.

Kroesen S, Marksteiner J, Mahata SK, et al. (1995) Effects of haloperidol, clozapine, and citalopram on messenger RNA levels of chromogranins A and B and secretogranin II in various regions of rat brain. Neuroscience 69, 881–891.

Kumra S, Frazier JA, Jacobsen LK, et al. (1996) Childhood-onset schizophrenia. A double-blind clozapine-haloperidol comparison. Arch Gen Psychiatr 53, 1090–1097.

Kumra S, Jacobsen LK, Lenane M, et al. (1998) Childhood-onset schizophrenia: An open-label study of olanzapine in adolescents. J Am Acad Child Adolesc Psychiatr 37, 377–385.

Kurzthaler I and Fleischhacker WW (2001) The clinical implications of weight gain in schizophrenia. J Clin Psychiatr 62(Suppl 7), 32–37.

Lader M (1999) Some adverse effects of antipsychotics: Prevention and treatment. J Clin Psychiatr 60, 18–21.

Lavin MR and Rifkin A (1991) Prophylactic antiparkinson drug use: I. Initial prophylaxis and prevention of extrapyramidal side effects. J Clin Pharmacol 31, 763–768.

Lawler CP, Prioleau C, Lewis MM, et al. (1999) Interactions of the novel antipsychotic aripiprazole (OPC-14597) with dopamine and serotonin receptor subtypes. Neuropsychopharmacology 20, 612–627.

Lesem MD, Zajecka JM, Swift RH, et al. (2001) Intramuscular ziprasidone, 2 mg versus 10 mg, in the short-term management of agitated psychotic patients. J Clin Psychiatr 62, 12–18.

Leucht S, Pitschel-Walz G, Abraham D, et al. (1999) Efficacy and extrapyramidal side effects of the new antipsychotics olanzapine, quetiapine, risperidone, and sertindole compared to conventional antipsychotics and placebo. A meta-analysis of randomized controlled trials. Schizophr Res 35, 51–68.

Levenson JL (1985) Neuroleptic malignant syndrome. Am J Psychiatr 142, 1137–1145.

Leveque JC, Macias W, Rajadhyaksha A, et al. (2000) Intracellular modulation of NMDA receptor function by antipsychotic drugs. J Neurosci 20, 4011–4020.

Levinson DF, Simpson GM, Singh H, et al. (1990) Fluphenazine dose, clinical response, and extrapyramidal symptoms during acute treatment. Arch Gen Psychiatr 47, 761–768.

Lieberman J, Jody D, Geisler S, et al. (1993) Time course and biologic correlates of treatment response in first-episode schizophrenia. Arch Gen Psychiatr 50, 369–376.

Lieberman JA (1993) Understanding the mechanism of action of atypical antipsychotic drugs: A review of compounds in use and development. Br J Psychiatr 163, 7–18.

Lieberman JA (1996) Atypical antipsychotic drugs as a first-line treatment of schizophrenia: A rationale and hypothesis. J Clin Psychiatr 57(Suppl 11), 68–71.

Lieberman JA (1998) Maximizing clozapine therapy: Managing side effects. J Clin Psychiatr 59(Suppl 3), 38–43.

Lieberman JA (1999a) Is schizophrenia a neurodegenerative disorder? A clinical and pathophysiological perspective. Biol Psychiatr 46, 729–739.

Lieberman JA (1999b) Pathophysiologic mechanisms in the pathogenesis and clinical course of schizophrenia. J Clin Psychiatr 60(Suppl 12), 9–12.

Lieberman JA (2001) Hypothesis and hypothesis testing in the clinical trial. J Clin Psychiatr 62(Suppl 9), 5–8.

Lieberman JA (press) Aripiprazole in Textbook of Psychopharmacology, Eds. Nemeroff C and Schatzberg A. APPI, Washington, DC.

Lieberman JA and Fenton WS (2000) Delayed detection of psychosis: Causes, consequences, and effect on public health. Am J Psychiatr 157, 1727–1730.

Lieberman JA, Johns CA, Kane JM, et al. (1988) Clozapine-induced agranulocytosis: Noncross-reactivity with other psychotropic drugs. J Clin Psychiatr 49, 271–277.

Lieberman JA, Kane JM, and Johns CA (1989) Clozapine: Guidelines for clinical management. J Clin Psychiatr 50, 329–338.

Lieberman JA, Kinon BJ, and Loebel AD (1990) Dopaminergic mechanisms in idiopathic and drug-induced psychoses. Schizophr Bull 16, 97–109.

Lieberman JA, Koreen A, Chakos M, et al. (1996) Factors influencing treatment response and outcome of first-episode schizophrenia implications for understanding the pathophysiology of schizophrenia. J Clin Psychiatr 57, 5–9.

Lieberman JA, Mailman RB, Duncan G, et al. (1998) Serotonergic basis of antipsychotic drug effects in schizophrenia. Biol Psychiatr 44, 1099–1117.

Lieberman JA, Sheitman BB, and Kinon BJ (1997) Neurochemical sensitization in the pathophysiology of schizophrenia deficits and dysfunction in neuronal regulation and plasticity. Neuropsychopharmacology 17, 205–229.

Loebel AD, Lieberman JA, Alvir JMJ, et al. (1992) Duration of psychosis and outcome in first-episode schizophrenia. Am J Psychiatr 149, 1183–1188.

Madhusoodanan S and Brenner R (1998) Use of risperidone in psychosis associated with Huntington's disease. Am J Geriatr Psychiatr 6, 347–349.

Madhusoodanan S, Brenner R, Moise D, et al. (1998) Psychiatric and neuropsychological abnormalities in Huntington's disease: A case study. Ann Clin Psychiatr 10, 117–120.

Majewski H and Iannazzo L (1998) Protein kinase C: A physiological mediator of enhanced transmitter output. Prog Neurobiol 55, 463–475.

Marder SR (1996) Pharmacological treatment strategies in acute schizophrenia. Int Clin Psychopharmacol 11(Suppl 2), 29–34.

Marder SR (1997) Antipsychotic drugs. In Psychiatry, Tasman A, Kay J, and Lieberman JA (eds). WB Saunders, Philadelphia, pp. 1569–1585.

Marder SR (1999) Antipsychotic drugs and relapse prevention. Schizophr Res 35, S87–S92.

Marder SR and Meibach RC (1994) Risperidone in the treatment of schizophrenia. Am J Psychiatr 151, 825–835.

Marder SR and Van Putten T (1995) Antipsychotic medications. In The American Psychiatric Press Textbook of Psychopharmacology, Schatzberg AF and Nemeroff CB (eds). American Psychiatric Press, Washington DC, pp. 247–261.

Marder SR, Davis JM, and Chouinard G (1997) The effects of risperidone on the five dimensions of schizophrenia derived by factor analysis: Combined results of the North American trials. J Clin Psychiatr 58, 538–546.

Marder SR, Hubbard JW, Van Putten T, et al. (1989) Pharmacokinetics of long-acting injectable neuroleptic drugs: Clinical implications. Psychopharmacology (Berl) 98, 433–439.

Marder SR, Van Putten T, Mintz J, et al. (1987) Low- and conventional-dose maintenance therapy with fluphenazine decanoate. Two-year outcome. Arch Gen Psychiatr 44, 518–521.

Markowitz JS, Brown CS, and Moore TR (1999) Atypical antipsychotics Part I: Pharmacology, pharmacokinetics, and efficacy. Ann Pharmacother 33, 73–85.

Martinot JL, Paillere-Martinot ML, Poirier MF, et al. (1996) In vivo characteristics of dopamine $D_2$ receptor occupancy by amisulpride in schizophrenia. Psychopharmacology (Berl) 124, 154–158.

Mauri MC, Bravin S, Bitetto A, et al. (1996) A risk-benefit assessment of sulpiride in the treatment of schizophrenia. Drug Safety 14, 288–298.

May PR, Tuma AH, and Dixon WJ (1981) Schizophrenia—a follow-up study of the results of five forms of treatment. Arch Gen Psychiatr 38, 776–784.

May PR, Tuma AH, Yale C, et al. (1976) Schizophrenia—a follow-up study of results of treatment. Arch Gen Psychiatr 33, 481–486.

McConville BJ, Arvanitis LA, Thyrum PT, et al. (2000) Pharmacokinetics, tolerability, and clinical effectiveness of quetiapine fumarate: An open-label trial in adolescents with psychotic disorders. J Clin Psychiatr 61, 252–260.

McEvoy JP, Hogarty GE, and Steingard S (1991) Optimal dose of neuroleptic in acute schizophrenia. A controlled study of the neuroleptic threshold and higher haloperidol dose. Arch Gen Psychiatr 48, 739–745.

McEvoy JP, Scheifler PL, and Frances A (1999) The expert consensus guideline series: Treatment of schizophrenia 1999. J Clin Psychiatr 60, 1–80.

McGlashan TH (1996) Early detection and intervention in schizophrenia: Research. Schizophr Bull 22, 327–345.

McIntyre RS, Mancini DA, and Basile VS (2001a) Mechanisms of antipsychotic-induced weight gain. J Clin Psychiatr 62(Suppl 23), 23–29.

McIntyre RS, McCann SM, and Kennedy SH (2001b) Antipsychotic metabolic effects: Weight gain, diabetes mellitus, and lipid abnormalities. Can J Psychiatr 46, 273–281.

Meltzer HY (1985) Long-term effects of neuroleptic drugs on the neuroendocrine system. Adv Biochem Psychopharmacol 40, 59–68.

Meltzer HY (1995) Clozapine: Is another view valid? Am J Psychiatr 152, 821–825.

Meltzer HY (1999a) Outcome in schizophrenia: Beyond symptom reduction. J Clin Psychiatr 60(Suppl 3), 3–7.

Meltzer HY (1999b) Treatment of schizophrenia and spectrum disorders: Pharmacotherapy, psychosocial treatments, and neurotransmitter interactions. Biol Psychiatr 46, 1321–1327.

Meltzer HY and McGurk SR (1999) The effects of clozapine, risperidone, and olanzapine on cognitive function in schizophrenia. Schizophr Bull 25, 233–255.

Meltzer HY, Matsubara S, and Lee JC (1989) Classification of typical and atypical antipsychotic drugs on the basis of dopamine $D_1$, $D_2$ and Serotonin2 pKi values. J Pharmacol Exp Therap 251, 238–246.

Meltzer HY, Thompson PA, Lee MA, et al. (1996) Neuropsychologic deficits in schizophrenia: Relation to social function and effect of antipsychotic drug treatment. Neuropsychopharmacology 14, 27S–33S.

Meltzer HY, Alphs L, Green AI (2003) Clozapine Treatment for Suicidality in Schizophrenia: International Suicide Prevention Trial (InterSePT). Arch Gen Psychiatr 60(1), 82–91.

Menza MM, Palermo B, and Mark M (1999) Quetiapine as an alternative to clozapine in the treatment of dopamimetic psychosis in patients with Parkinson's disease. Ann Clin Psychiatr 11, 141–144.

Merchant KM and Dorsa DM (1993) Differential induction of neurotensin and c-fos gene expression by typical versus atypical antipsychotics. Proc Natl Acad Sci USA 90, 3447–3451.

Meshul CK and Tan SE (1994) Haloperidol-induced morphological alterations are associated with changes in calcium/calmodulin kinase II activity and glutamate immunoreactivity. Synapse 18, 205–217.

Meshul CK, Janowsky A, Casey DE, et al. (1992a) Coadministration of haloperidol and SCH-23390 prevents the increase in "perforated" synapses due to either drug alone. Neuropsychopharmacology 7, 285–293.

Meshul CK, Janowsky A, Casey DE, et al. (1992b) Effect of haloperidol and clozapine on the density of "perforated" synapses in caudate, nucleus accumbens, and medial prefrontal cortex. Psychopharmacology (Berl) 106, 45–52.

Meyer JM (2001) Effects of atypical antipsychotics on weight and serum lipid levels. J Clin Psychiatr 62(Suppl 27), 27–34.

Meyer JM and Simpson GM (1997) From chlorpromazine to olanzapine: A brief history of antipsychotics. Psychiatr Serv 48, 1137–1139.

Meyer-Lindenberg A, Gruppe H, Bauer U, et al. (1997) Improvement of cognitive function in schizophrenic patients receiving clozapine or zotepine: Results from a double-blind study. Pharmacopsychiatry 30, 35–42.

Miller CH and Fleischhacker WW (2000) Managing antipsychotic-induced acute and chronic akathisia. Drug Safety 22, 73–81.

Miller DD (1996) The clinical use of clozapine plasma concentrations in the management of treatment-refractory schizophrenia. Ann Clin Psychiatr 8, 99–109.

Miller DD, Fleming F, Holman TL, et al. (1994) Plasma clozapine concentrations as a predictor of clinical response: A follow-up study. J Clin Psychiatr 55(Suppl B), 117–121.

Misra L and Kofoed L (1997) Risperidone treatment of methamphetamine psychosis. Am J Psychiatr 154, 1170.

Miyamoto S, Duncan GE, Goff DC, et al. (2002a) Therapeutics of schizophrenia. In Neuropsychopharmacology: The Fifth Generation of Progress, Davis KL, Charney D, Coyle JT, et al. (eds). Lippincott Williams & Wilkins, Philadelphia, pp. 775–807.

Miyamoto S, Duncan GE, and Lieberman JA (2001a) Second-generation antipsychotics in the treatment of schizophrenia: Olanzapine. In Current Issues in the Psychopharmacology of Schizophrenia, Breier A, Tran PV, Herrera JM, et al. (eds). Lippincott Williams & Wilkins Healthcare, Philadelphia, pp. 224–242.

Miyamoto S, Duncan GE, Mailman RB, et al. (2000) Developing novel antipsychotic drugs: Strategies and goals. Curr Opin CPNS Invest Drugs 2, 25–39.

Miyamoto S, Mailman RB, Lieberman JA, et al. (2001b) Blunted brain metabolic response to ketamine in mice lacking $D_{1A}$ dopamine receptors. Brain Res 894, 167–180.

Miyamoto S, Stroup TS, Duncan GE, et al. (2002b) Acute pharmacologic treatment of schizophrenia. In Schizophrenia, 2nd ed., Hirsch SR and Weinberger DR (eds). Blackwell Science, London.

Mohamed S, Paulsen JS, O'Leary D, et al. (1999) Generalized cognitive deficits in schizophrenia: A study of first-episode patients. Arch Gen Psychiatr 56, 749–754.

Möller HJ (1993) Neuroleptic treatment of negative symptoms in schizophrenic patients. Efficacy problems and methodological difficulties. Eur Neuropsychopharmacol 3, 1–11.

Möller HJ, Kissling W, Lang C, et al. (1982) Efficacy and side effects of haloperidol in psychotic patients: Oral versus intravenous administration. Am J Psychiatr 139, 1571–1575.

Momiyama T, Amano T, Todo N, et al. (1996) Inhibition by a putative antipsychotic quinolinone derivative (OPC-14597) of dopaminergic neurons in the ventral tegmental area. Eur J Pharmacol 310, 1–8.

Mukherjee S, Decina P, Bocola V, et al. (1996) Diabetes mellitus in schizophrenic patients. Compr Psychiatr 37, 68–73.

Nakahara T, Kuroki T, Hashimoto K, et al. (2000) Effect of atypical antipsychotics on phencyclidine-induced expression of arc in rat brain. Neuroreport 11, 551–555.

National Institute of Mental Health-Psychopharmacology Service Center Collaborative Study Group (1964) Phenothiazine treatment in acute schizophrenia. Arch Gen Psychiatr 10, 246–261.

Neborsky R, Janowsky D, Munson E, et al. (1981) Rapid treatment of acute psychotic symptoms with high- and low-dose haloperidol. Behavioral considerations. Arch Gen Psychiatr 38, 195–199.

Needham PL, Atkinson J, Skill MJ, et al. (1996) Zotepine: Preclinical tests predict antipsychotic efficacy and an atypical profile. Psychopharmacol Bull 32, 123–128.

Neer EJ (1995) Heterotrimeric G proteins: Organizers of transmembrane signals. Cell 80, 249–257.

Nemeroff CB (1997) Dosing the antipsychotic medication olanzapine. J Clin Psychiatr 58(Suppl 10), 45–49.

Nordstrom AL, Farde L, Nyberg S, et al. (1995) $D_1$, $D_2$, and 5-$HT_2$ receptor occupancy in relation to clozapine serum concentration: A PET study of schizophrenic patients. Am J Psychiatr 152, 1444–1449.

Nordstrom AL, Farde L, Wiesel FA, et al. (1993) Central $D_2$–dopamine receptor occupancy in relation to antipsychotic drug effects: A double-blind PET study of schizophrenic patients. Biol Psychiatr 33, 227–235.

Novartis Pharmaceuticals (2000) Product Information: Clozaril (Clozapine). In Physicians' Desk Reference, 54th ed. Anonymous Medical Economics Company, Montvale, NJ, pp. 2008–2012.

Nudelman E, Vinuela LM, and Cohen CI (1998) Safety in overdose of quetiapine: A case report. J Clin Psychiatr 59, 433.

Nyberg S and Farde L (2000) Non-equipotent doses partly explain differences among antipsychotics—implications of PET studies. Psychopharmacology (Berl) 148, 22–23.

Nyberg S, Eriksson B, Oxenstierna G, et al. (1999) Suggested minimal effective dose of risperidone based on PET-measured $D_2$ and 5-$HT_{2A}$ receptor occupancy in schizophrenic patients. Am J Psychiatr 156, 869–875.

Ohashi K, Hamamura T, Lee Y, et al. (2000) Clozapine- and olanzapine-induced Fos expression in the rat medial prefrontal cortex is mediated by beta-adrenoceptors. Neuropsychopharmacology 23, 162–169.

Ostroff RB and Nelson JC (1999) Risperidone augmentation of selective serotonin reuptake inhibitors in major depression. J Clin Psychiatr 60, 256–259.

Parsa MA and Bastani B (1998) Quetiapine (Seroquel) in the treatment of psychosis in patients with Parkinson's disease. J Neuropsychiatr Clin Neurosci 10, 216–219.

Perrault G, Depoortere R, Morel E, et al. (1997) Psychopharmacological profile of amisulpride: An antipsychotic drug with presynaptic $D_2/D_3$ dopamine receptor antagonist activity and limbic selectivity. J Pharmacol Exp Therap 280, 73–82.

Petty RG (1999) Prolactin and antipsychotic medications: Mechanism of action. Schizophr Res 35(Suppl), S67–S73.

Peuskens J (1999) The evolving definition of treatment resistance. J Clin Psychiatr 60(Suppl 12), 4–8.

Peuskens J and Link CG (1997) A comparison of quetiapine and chlorpromazine in the treatment of schizophrenia. Acta Psychiatr Scand 96, 265–273.

Pilowsky LS, O'Connell P, Davies N, et al. (1997) In vivo effects on striatal dopamine $D_2$ receptor binding by the novel atypical antipsychotic drug sertindole—a 123I IBZM single photon emission tomography (SPET) study. Psychopharmacology (Berl) 130, 152–158.

Polak P and Laycob L (1971) Rapid tranquilization. Am J Psychiatr 128, 640–643.

Potkin S and Cooper S (2000) Ziprasidone and zotepine: Clinical use and experience. In Schizophrenia and Mood Disorders: The New Drug Therapies in Clinical Practice, Buckley PF and Waddington JL (eds). Butterworth-Heinemann, Woburn, MA, pp. 49–58.

Preskorn SH (1993) Pharmacokinetics of antidepressants: Why and how they are relevant to treatment. J Clin Psychiatr 54(Suppl), 14–34.

Purdon SE, Jones BD, Stip E, et al. (2000) Neuropsychological change in early phase schizophrenia during 12 months of treatment with olanzapine, risperidone, or haloperidol. The Canadian Collaborative Group for research in schizophrenia. Arch Gen Psychiatr 57, 249–258.

Rajadhyaksha A, Barczak A, Macias W, et al. (1999) L-Type Ca(2+) channels are essential for glutamate-mediated CREB phosphorylation and c-fos gene expression in striatal neurons. J Neurosci 19, 6348–6359.

Rajadhyaksha A, Leveque J, Macias W, et al. (1998) Molecular components of striatal plasticity: The various routes of cyclic AMP pathways. Dev Neurosci 20, 204–215.

Reich J (1999) Use of high-dose olanzapine in refractory psychosis. Am J Psychiatr 156, 661.

Reilly JG, Ayis SA, Ferrier IN, et al. (2000) QTc-interval abnormalities and psychotropic drug therapy in psychiatric patients. Lancet 355, 1048–1052.

Remington G and Chong SA (1999) Conventional versus novel antipsychotics: Changing concepts and clinical implications. J Psychiatr Neurosci 24, 431–441.

Remington G and Kapur S (1999) $D_2$ and 5-$HT_2$ receptor effects of antipsychotics: Bridging basic and clinical findings using PET. J Clin Psychiatr 60(Suppl 10), 15–19.

Remington G and Kapur S (2000) Atypical antipsychotics: Are some more atypical than others? Psychopharmacology (Berl) 148, 3–15.

Riva MA, Molteni R, Tascedda F, et al. (1999) Selective modulation of fibroblast growth factor-2 expression in the rat brain by the atypical antipsychotic clozapine. Neuropharmacology 38, 1075–1082.

Robertson GS and Fibiger HC (1992) Neuroleptics increase c-fos expression in the forebrain: Contrasting effects of haloperidol and clozapine. Neuroscience 46, 315–328.

Robertson GS and Fibiger HC (1996) Effects of olanzapine on regional c-fos expression in rat forebrain. Neuropsychopharmacology 14, 105–110.

Robertson GS, Matsumura H, and Fibiger HC (1994) Induction patterns of neuroleptic-induced Fos-like immunoreactivity as predictors of atypical antipsychotic activity. J Pharmacol Exp Therap 271, 1058–1066.

Robinson DG, Woerner MG, Alvir JM, et al. (1999) Predictors of treatment response from a first episode of schizophrenia or schizoaffective disorder. Am J Psychiatr 156, 544–549.

Rogue P and Malviya AN (1994) Regulation of signalling pathways to the nucleus by dopaminergic receptors. Cell Signal 6, 725–733.

Rogue P and Vincendon G (1997) Modulation of signal-regulated transcription factors by antipsychotics. Eur Neuropsychopharmacol 7, S109–S110.

Rogue P, Hanauer A, Zwiller J, et al. (1991) Up-regulation of dopamine $D_2$ receptor mRNA in rat striatum by chronic neuroleptic treatment. Eur J Pharmacol 207, 165–168.

Rothschild AJ (1996) Management of psychotic, treatment-resistant depression. Psychiatr Clin N Am 19, 237–252.

Rothschild AJ, Bates KS, Boehringer KL, et al. (1999) Olanzapine response in psychotic depression. J Clin Psychiatr 60, 116–118.

Sacristan JA, Gomez JC, Montejo AL, et al. (2000) Doses of olanzapine, risperidone, and haloperidol used in clinical practice: Results of a prospective pharmacoepidemiologic study. EFESO Study Group. Estudio Farmacoepidemiologico en la Esquizofrenia con Olanzapina. Clin Therap 22, 583–599.

Sallee FR, Kurlan R, Goetz CG, et al. (2000) Ziprasidone treatment of children and adolescents with Tourette's syndrome: A pilot study. J Am Acad Child Adolesc Psychiatr 39, 292–299.

Sartorius N, Fleischhacker WW, Gjerris A, et al. (2002) The usefulness and use of Second-Generation Antipsychotic Medications. Current Opinion in Psychiatry 15(Suppl 1).

Schooler NR and Kane JM (1982) Research diagnoses for tardive dyskinesia. Arch of Gen Psychiatr 39, 486–487.

Schooler NR, Keith SJ, Severe JB, et al. (1997) Relapse and rehospitalization during maintenance treatment of schizophrenia. The effects of dose reduction and family treatment. Arch Gen Psychiatr 54, 453–463.

Schotte A, Janssen PFM, Gommeren W, et al. (1996) Risperidone compared with new and reference antipsychotic drugs: In vitro and in vivo receptor binding. Psychopharmacology (Berl) 124, 57–73.

Schulz C and McGorry P (2000) Traditional antipsychotic medications: Contemporary clinical use. In Schizophrenia and Mood Disorders: The New Drug Therapies in Clinical Practice, Buckley PF and Waddington JL (eds). Butterworth-Heinemann, Woburn, pp. 14–20.

Schulz SC, Camlin KL, Berry SA, et al. (1999) Olanzapine safety and efficacy in patients with borderline personality disorder and comorbid dysthymia. Biol Psychiatr 46, 1429–1435.

Scully PJ, Coakley G, Kinsella A, et al. (1997) Psychopathology, executive (frontal) and general cognitive impairment in relation to duration of initially untreated versus subsequently treated psychosis in chronic schizophrenia. Psychol Med 27, 1303–1310.

Sebens JB, Koch T, Ter Horst GJ, et al. (1995) Differential Fos-protein induction in rat forebrain regions after acute and long-term haloperidol and clozapine treatment. Eur J Pharmacol 273, 175–182.

Seeman P (1987) Dopamine receptors and the dopamine hypothesis of schizophrenia. Synapse 1, 133–152.

Seeman P (1992) Dopamine receptor sequences. Therapeutic levels of neuroleptics occupy $D_2$ receptors, clozapine occupies $D_4$. Neuropsychopharmacology 7, 261–284.

Seeman P and Kapur S (2000) Schizophrenia: More dopamine, more $D_2$ receptors. Proc Nat Acad Sci USA 97, 7673–7675.

Seeman P and Tallerico T (1998) Antipsychotic drugs which elicit little or no parkinsonism bind more loosely than dopamine to brain $D_2$ receptors, yet occupy high levels of these receptors. Mol Psychiatr 3, 123–134.

Seeman P, Lee T, Chau-Wong M, et al. (1976) Antipsychotic drug doses and neuroleptic/dopamine receptors. Nature 261, 717–719.

Segal J, Berk M, and Brook S (1998) Risperidone compared with both lithium and haloperidol in mania: A double-blind randomized controlled trial. Clin Neuropharmacol 21, 176–180.

Semba J, Sakai M, Miyoshi R, et al. (1996) Differential expression of c-fos mRNA in rat prefrontal cortex, striatum, N. accumbens and lateral septum after typical and atypical antipsychotics: An in situ hybridization study. Neurochem Int 29, 435–442.

Semba J, Watanabe A, Kito S, et al. (1995) Behavioural and neurochemical effects of OPC-14597, a novel antipsychotic drug, on dopaminergic mechanisms in rat brain. Neuropharmacology 34, 785–791.

Shalev A, Hermesh H, Rothberg J, et al. (1993) Poor neuroleptic response in acutely exacerbated schizophrenic patients. Acta Psychiatr Scand 87, 86–91.

Sharif ZA (1998) Common treatment goals of antipsychotics: Acute treatment. J Clin Psychiatr 59(Suppl 19), 5–8.

Sharma T (2000) Effects of antipsychotic agents on cognitive function in schizophrenia. Curr Opin CPNS Invest Drugs 2, 40–44.

Shelton RC, Tollefson GD, Tohen M, et al. (2001) A novel augmentation strategy for treating resistant major depression. Am J Psychiatr 158, 131–134.

Siris SG (2001) Depression and Schizophrenia: Perspective in the era of 'Atypical' antipsychotic agents. Am J Psychiatr 157(9), 1379–1389.

Small JG (2001) Second generation antipsychotics in the treatment of schizophrenia: Quetiapine. In Current Issues in the Psychopharmacology of Schizophrenia, Breier A, Tran PV, Herrera JM, et al. (eds). Lippincott Williams & Wilkins, Philadelphia, pp. 252–261.

Small JG, Hirsch SR, Arvanitis LA, et al. (1997) Quetiapine in patients with schizophrenia. A high- and low-dose double-blind comparison with placebo. Seroquel Study Group. Arch Gen Psychiatr 54, 549–557.

Smelson DA, Roy A, and Roy M (1997) Risperidone and neuropsychological test performance in cocaine-withdrawn patients. Can J Psychiatr 42, 431.

Snyder SH, Banerjee SP, Yamamura HI, et al. (1974) Drugs, neurotransmitters, and schizophrenia. Science 184, 1243–1253.

Spohn HE and Strauss ME (1989) Relation of neuroleptic and anticholinergic medication to cognitive functions in schizophrenia. J Abnorm Psychol 98, 367–380.

Sprouse JS, Reynolds LS, Braselton JP, et al. (1999) Comparison of the novel antipsychotic ziprasidone with clozapine and olanzapine: Inhibition of dorsal raphe cell firing and the role of 5-$HT_{1A}$ receptor activation. Neuropsychopharmacology 21, 622–631.

Squitieri F, Cannella M, Piorcellini A, et al. (2001) Short-term effects of olanzapine in Huntington disease. Neuropsychiatr Neuropsychol Behav Neurol 14, 69–72.

Stahl SM (1999) Selecting an atypical antipsychotic by combining clinical experience with guidelines from clinical trials. J Clin Psychiatr 60, 31–41.

Steward O, Wallace CS, Lyford GL, et al. (1998) Synaptic activation causes the mRNA for the IEG Arc to localize selectively near activated postsynaptic sites on dendrites. Neuron 21, 741–751.

Still DJ, Dorson PG, Crismon ML, et al. (1996) Effects of switching inpatients with treatment-resistant schizophrenia from clozapine to risperidone. Psychiatr Serv 47, 1382–1384.

Stip E (2000) Novel antipsychotics: Issues and controversies. Typicality of atypical antipsychotics. J Psychiatr Neurosci 25, 137–153.

Stockton ME and Rasmussen K (1996) Electrophysiological effects of olanzapine, a novel atypical antipsychotic, on A9 and A10 dopamine neurons. Neuropsychopharmacology 14, 97–105.

Stoner SC, Sommi RW Jr., Marken PA, et al. (1997) Clozapine use in two full-term pregnancies. J Clin Psychiatr 58, 364–365.

Stoppe G, Brandt CA, and Staedt JH (1999) Behavioural problems associated with dementia: The role of newer antipsychotics. Drugs Aging 14, 41–54.

Street JS, Clark WS, Gannon KS, et al. (2000) Olanzapine treatment of psychotic and behavioral symptoms in patients with Alzheimer disease in nursing care facilities: A double-blind, randomized, placebo-controlled trial. The HGEU Study Group. Arch Gen Psychiatr 57, 968–976.

Sussman N (2001) Review of atypical antipsychotics and weight gain. J Clin Psychiatr 62(Suppl 23), 5–12.

Swift RH, Harrigan EP, and Van Kammen DP (1999) A comparison of intramuscular ziprasidone with intra-muscular haloperidol. Schizophr Res 36, 298.

Szewczak MR, Corbett R, Rush DK, et al. (1995) The pharmacological profile of iloperidone, a novel atypical antipsychotic agent. J Pharmacol Exp Ther 274, 1404–1413.

Szigethy E, Brent S, and Findling RL (1998) Quetiapine for refractory schizophrenia. J Am Acad Child Adolesc Psychiatr 37, 1127–1128.

Szigethy EM and Schulz SC (1997) Risperidone in comorbid borderline personality disorder and dysthymia. J Clin Psychopharmacol 17, 326–327.

Targum SD and Abbott JL (2000) Efficacy of quetiapine in Parkinson's patients with psychosis. J Clin Psychopharmacol 20, 54–60.

Thase ME and Sachs GS (2000) Bipolar depression: Pharmacotherapy and related therapeutic strategies. Biol Psychiatr 48, 558–572.

The Parkinson Study Group (1999) Low-dose clozapine for the treatment of drug-induced psychosis in Parkinson's disease. New Engl J Med 340, 757–763.

Thomas H Jr., Schwartz E, and Petrilli R (1992) Droperidol versus haloperidol for chemical restraint of agitated and combative patients. Ann Emerg Med 21, 407–413.

Tohen M, Jacobs TG, Grundy SL, et al. (2000) Efficacy of olanzapine in acute bipolar mania: A double-blind, placebo-controlled study. The Olanzipine HGGW Study Group. Arch Gen Psychiatr 57, 841–849.

Tohen M, Sanger TM, McElroy SL, et al. (1999) Olanzapine versus placebo in the treatment of acute mania. Olanzapine HGEH Study Group. Am J Psychiatr 156, 702–709.

Tollefson GD (1996) Cognitive function in schizophrenic patients. J Clin Psychiatr 57(Suppl 11), 31–39.

Tollefson GD and Sanger TM (1997) Negative symptoms: A path analytic approach to a double-blind, placebo- and haloperidol-controlled clinical trial with olanzapine. Am J Psychiatr 154, 466–474.

Tollefson GD, Andersen SW, and Tran PV (1999) The course of depressive symptoms in predicting relapse in schizophrenia: A double-blind, randomized comparison of olanzapine and risperidone. Biol Psychiatr 46, 365–373.

Tollefson GD, Beasley CMJ, Tamura RN, et al. (1997a) Blind, controlled, long-term study of the comparative incidence of treatment-emergent tardive dyskinesia with olanzapine or haloperidol. Am J Psychiatr 154, 1248–1254.

Tollefson GD, Beasley CMJ, Tran PV, et al. (1997b) Olanzapine versus haloperidol in the treatment of schizophrenia and schizoaffective and schizophreniform disorders: Results of an international collaborative trial. Am J Psychiatr 154, 457–465.

Tollefson GD, Birkett MA, Kiesler GM, et al. (2001) Double-blind comparison of olanzapine versus clozapine in schizophrenic patients clinically eligible for treatment with clozapine. Biol Psychiatr 49, 52–63.

Toren P, Laor N, and Weizman A (1998) Use of atypical neuroleptics in child and adolescent psychiatry. J Clin Psychiatr 59, 644–656.

Tran PV, Dellva MA, Tollefson GD, et al. (1998) Oral olanzapine versus oral haloperidol in the maintenance treatment of schizophrenia and related psychoses. Br J Psychiatr 172, 499–505.

Tran PV, Hamilton SH, Kuntz AJ, et al. (1997) Double-blind comparison of olanzapine versus risperidone in the treatment of schizophrenia and other psychotic disorders. J Clin Psychopharmacol 17, 407–418.

Travis MJ, Busatto GF, Pilowsky LS, et al. (1997) Serotonin: 5-HT$_{2A}$ receptor occupancy in vivo and response to the new antipsychotics olanzapine and sertindole. Br J Psychiatr 171, 290–291.

Trixler M and Tenyi T (1997) Antipsychotic use in pregnancy. What are the best treatment options? Drug Safety 16, 403–410.

Turrone P, Kapur S, Seeman MV, et al. (2002) Elevation of prolactin levels by atypical antipsychotics. Am J Psychiatr 159, 133–135.

Van Putten T, Marder SR, and Mintz J (1990) A controlled dose comparison of haloperidol in newly admitted schizophrenic patients. Arch Gen Psychiatr 47, 754–758.

Van Putten T, Marder SR, Wirshing WC, et al. (1991) Neuroleptic plasma levels. Schizophr Bull. 17, 197–216.

van Vugt JP, Siesling S, Vergeer M, et al. (1997) Clozapine versus placebo in Huntington's disease: A double-blind randomised comparative study. J Neurol Neurosurg Psychiatr 63, 35–39.

Vander Zwaag C, McGee M, McEvoy JP, et al. (1996) Response of patients with treatment-refractory schizophrenia to clozapine within three serum level ranges. Am J Psychiatr 153, 1579–1584.

Volavka J, Cooper T, Czobor P, et al. (1992) Haloperidol blood levels and clinical effects. Arch Gen Psychiatr 49, 354–361.

Volavka J, Czobor P, Sheitman B, et al. (2002) Clozapine, olanzapine, risperidone, and haloperidol in the treatment of patients with chronic schizophrenia and schizoaffective disorder. Am J Psychiatr 159, 255–262.

Waddington J and Casey D (2000) Comparative pharmacology of classical and novel (second-generation) antipsychotics. In Schizophrenia and Mood Disorders: The New Drug Therapies in Clinical Practice, Buckley PF and Waddington JL (eds). Butterworth-Heinemann, Woburn, pp. 3–13.

Waddington JL, Youssef HA, and Kinsella A (1990) Cognitive dysfunction in schizophrenia followed up over 5 years, and its longitudinal relationship to the emergence of tardive dyskinesia. Psychol Med 20, 835–842.

Waddington JL, Youssef HA, and Kinsella A (1995) Sequential cross-sectional and 10-year prospective study of severe negative symptoms in relation to duration of initially untreated psychosis in chronic Schizophrenia. Psychol Med 25, 849–857.

Wan W, Ennulat DJ, and Cohen BM (1995) Acute administration of typical and atypical antipsychotic drugs induces distinctive patterns of Fos expression in the rat forebrain. Brain Res 688, 95–104.

Weiner WJ, Minagar A, and Shulman LM (2000) Quetiapine for l-dopa-induced psychosis in PD. Neurology 54, 1538.

Weiss E, Kemmler G, and Fleischhacker WW (2002) Improvement of cognitive dysfunction after treatment with second-generation antipsychotics. Arch Gen Psychiatr 59, 572–573.

White FJ and Wang RY (1983) Differential effects of classical and atypical antipsychotic drugs on A9 and A10 dopamine neurons. Science 221, 1054–1057.

Williams R (2001) Optimal dosing with risperidone: Updated recommendations. J Clin Psychiatr 62, 282–289.

Willins DL, Berry SA, Alsayegh L, et al. (1999) Clozapine and other 5-hydroxytryptamine-2A receptor antagonists alter the subcellular distribution of 5-hydroxytryptamine-2A receptors in vitro and in vivo. Neuroscience 91, 599–606.

Windgassen K, Wesselmann U, and Schulze MH (1996) Galactorrhea and hyperprolactinemia in schizophrenic patients on neuroleptics: Frequency and etiology. Neuropsychobiology 33, 142–146.

Winslow RS, Stillner V, Coons DJ, et al. (1986) Prevention of acute dystonic reactions in patients beginning high-potency neuroleptics. Am J Psychiatr 143, 706–710.

Wirshing DA, Marshall BDJ, Green MF, et al. (1999) Risperidone in treatment-refractory schizophrenia. Am J Psychiatr 156, 1374–1379.

Wirshing DA, Spellberg BJ, Erhart SM, et al. (1998) Novel antipsychotics and new onset diabetes. Biol Psychiatr 44, 778–783.

Worrel JA, Marken PA, Beckman SE, et al. (2000) Atypical antipsychotic agents: A critical review. Am J Health Syst Pharm 57, 238–255.

Wright P, Birkett M, David SR, et al. (2001) Double-blind, placebo-controlled comparison of intramuscular olanzapine and intramuscular haloperidol in the treatment of acute agitation in schizophrenia. Am J Psychiatr 158, 1149–1151.

Wudarsky M, Nicolson R, Hamburger SD, et al. (1999) Elevated prolactin in pediatric patients on typical and atypical antipsychotics. J Child Adolesc Psychopharmacol 9, 239–245.

Wyatt RJ (1991) Neuroleptics and the natural course of schizophrenia. Schizophr Bull 17, 325–351.

Wyatt RJ (1995) Early intervention for schizophrenia—Can the course of the illness be altered? Biol Psychiatr 38, 1–3.

Wyatt RJ, Green MF, and Tuma AH (1997) Long-term morbidity associated with delayed treatment of first admission schizophrenic patients: A reanalysis of the Camarillo State Hospital data. Psychol Med 27, 261–268.

Young CR, Bowers MB Jr., and Mazure CM (1998) Management of the adverse effects of clozapine. Schizophr Bull 24, 381–390.

Zanarini MC and Frankenburg FR (2001) Olanzapine treatment of female borderline personality disorder patients: A double-blind, placebo-controlled pilot study. J Clin Psychiatr 62, 849–854.

Ziolkowska B and Hollt V (1993) The NMDA receptor antagonist MK-801 markedly reduces the induction of c-fos gene by haloperidol in the mouse striatum. Neurosci Lett 156, 39–42.

## Further Reading

Barnas C, Stuppack CH, Miller C, et al. (1992) Zotepine in the treatment of schizophrenic patients with prevailingly negative symptoms. A double-blind trial vs. haloperidol. Int Clin Psychopharmacol 7, 23–27.

Boyer P, Lecrubier Y, Puech AJ, et al. (1995) Treatment of negative symptoms in schizophrenia with amisulpride. Br J Psychiatr 166, 68–72.

Conley RR, Kelly DL, and Gale EA (1998a) Olanzapine response in treatment-refractory schizophrenic patients with a history of substance abuse. Schizophr Res 33, 95–101.

Cooper SJ, Butler A, Tweed J, et al. (2000a) Zotepine in the prevention of recurrence: A randomized, double-blind, placebo-controlled study for chronic schizophrenia. Psychopharmacology (Berl) 150, 237–243.

Cooper SJ, Tweed J, Raniwalla J, et al. (2000b) A placebo-controlled comparison of zotepine versus chlorpromazine in patients with acute exacerbation of schizophrenia. Acta Psychiatr Scand 101, 218–225.

Coutinho E, Fenton M, Adams C, et al. (2000) Zuclopenthixol acetate in psychiatric emergencies: Looking for evidence from clinical trials. Schizophr Res 33, 111–118.

Currier GW and Simpson GM (2001) Risperidone liquid concentrate and oral lorazepam versus intramuscular haloperidol and intramuscular lorazepam for treatment of psychotic agitation. J Clin Psychiatr 62, 153–157.

Czobor P, Volavka J, and Meibach RC (1995) Effect of risperidone on hostility in schizophrenia. J Clin Psychopharmacol 15, 243–249.

Daniel DG, Potkin SG, Reeves KR, et al. (2001) Intramuscular (IM) ziprasidone 20 mg is effective in reducing acute agitation associated with psychosis: A double-blind, randomized trial. Psychopharmacology (Berl) 155, 128–134.

Daniel DG, Wozniak P, Mack RJ, et al. (1998) Long-term efficacy and safety comparison of sertindole and haloperidol in the treatment of schizophrenia. Psychopharmacol Bull 34, 61–69.

Danion JM, Rein W, and Fleurot O (1999) Improvement of schizophrenic patients with primary negative symptoms treated with amisulpride. Amisulpride Study Group. Am J Psychiatr 156, 610–616.

Fenton M, Coutinho ES, and Campbell C (2001) Zuclopenthixol acetate in the treatment of acute schizophrenia and similar serious mental illnesses. Cochrane Database Syst Rev CD000525

Findling RL, McNamara NK, Branicky LA, et al. (2000) A double-blind pilot study of risperidone in the treatment of conduct disorder. J Am Acad Child Adolesc Psychiatry 39, 509–516.

Fleischhacker WW (2002) The first episode of schizophrenia: A challenge for treatment. Eur Psychiatr 17, 371–375.

Fleischhacker WW, Hummer M, Kurz M, et al. (1994) Clozapine dose in the United States and Europe: Implications for therapeutic and adverse effects. J Clin Psychiatr 55(Suppl B), 78–81.

Grunder G, Wetzel H, Schlosser R, et al. (1999) Neuroendocrine response to antipsychotics: Effects of drug type and gender. Biol Psychiatr 45, 89–97.

Hummer M, Kemmler G, Kurz M, et al. (1999) Sexual disturbances during clozapine and haloperidol treatment for schizophrenia. Am J Psychiatr 156, 631–633.

Kane JM, Aguglia E, Altamura AC, et al. (1998) Guidelines for depot antipsychotic treatment in schizophrenia. European Neuropsychopharmacology Consensus Conference in Siena, Italy. Eur Neuropsychopharmacol 8, 55–66.

Kleinberg DL, Davis JM, de Coster R, et al. (1999) Prolactin levels and adverse events in patients treated with risperidone. J Clin Psychopharmacol 19, 57–61.

Larsen TK, Friis S, Haahr U, et al. (2001) Early detection and intervention in first-episode schizophrenia: A critical review. Acta Psychiatr Scand 103, 323–334.

Lehman AF and Steinwachs DM (1998) Translating research into practice: The Schizophrenia Patient Outcomes Research Team (PORT) treatment recommendations. Schizophr Bull 24, 1–10.

Leucht S, Pitschel-Walz G, Engel RR, et al. (2002) Amisulpride, an unusual "atypical" antipsychotic: A meta-analysis of randomized controlled trials. Am J Psychiatr 159, 180–190.

Loo H, Poirier-Littre MF, Theron M, et al. (1997) Amisulpride versus placebo in the medium-term treatment of the negative symptoms of schizophrenia. Br J Psychiatr 170, 18–22.

McGorry PD, Edwards J, Mihalopoulos C, et al. (1996) EPPIC: An evolving system of early detection and optimal management. Schizophr Bull 22, 305–326.

McManus DQ, Arvanitis LA, and Kowalcyk BB (1999) Quetiapine, a novel antipsychotic: Experience in elderly patients with psychotic disorders. Seroquel Trial 48 Study Group. J Clin Psychiatr 60, 292–298.

Meltzer HY and Okayli G (1995) Reduction of suicidality during clozapine treatment of neuroleptic-resistant schizophrenia: Impact on risk–benefit assessment. Am J Psychiatr 152, 183–190.

Möller HJ, Boyer P, Fleurot O, et al. (1997) Improvement of acute exacerbations of schizophrenia with amisulpride: A comparison with haloperidol. PROD-ASLP Study Group. Psychopharmacology (Berl) 132, 396–401.

Muller-Spahn F, Dieterle D, and Ackenheil M (1991) [Clinical effectiveness of zotepine in treatment of negative schizophrenic symptoms. Results of an open and a double-blind controlled trial]. Fortschr Neurol Psychiatr 59(Suppl 1), 30–35.

Paillere-Martinot ML, Lecrubier Y, Martinot JL, et al. (1995) Improvement of some schizophrenic deficit symptoms with low doses of amisulpride. Am J Psychiatr 152, 130–134.

Petit M, Raniwalla J, Tweed J, et al. (1996) A comparison of an atypical and typical antipsychotic, zotepine versus haloperidol in patients with acute exacerbation of schizophrenia: A parallel-group double-blind trial. Psychopharmacol Bull 32, 81–87.

Potenza MN, Holmes JP, Kanes SJ, et al. (1999) Olanzapine treatment of children, adolescents, and adults with pervasive developmental disorders: An open-label pilot study. J Clin Psychopharmacol 19, 37–44.

Puech A, Fleurot O, and Rein W (1998) Amisulpride, and atypical antipsychotic, in the treatment of acute episodes of schizophrenia: A dose-ranging study vs. haloperidol. The Amisulpride Study Group. Acta Psychiatr Scand 98, 65–72.

Purdon SE, Malla A, Labelle A, et al. (2001) Neuropsychological change in patients with schizophrenia after treatment with quetiapine or haloperidol. J Psychiatr Neurosci 26, 137–149.

Sartorius N, Fleischhacker WW, Gjerris A, et al. (2002) The usefulness and use of second-generation antipsychotic medications. Curr Opin Psychiatr 15(Suppl 1).

Speller JC, Barnes TR, Curson DA, et al. (1997) One-year, low-dose neuroleptic study of in-patients with chronic schizophrenia characterized by persistent negative symptoms. Amisulpride v. haloperidol. Br J Psychiatr 171, 564–568.

Tolosa-Vilella C, Ruiz-Ripoll A, Mari-Alfonso B, et al. (2002) Olanzapine-induced agranulocytosis: A case report and review of the literature. Prog Neuropsychopharmacol Biol Psychiatr 26, 411–414.

Van Bellinghen M and De Troch C (2001) Risperidone in the treatment of behavioral disturbances in children and adolescents with borderline intellectual functioning: A double-blind, placebo-controlled pilot trial. J Child Adolesc Psychopharmacol 11, 5–13.

Velligan DI, Newcomer J, Pultz J, et al. (2002) Does cognitive function improve with quetiapine in comparison to haloperidol? Schizophr Res 53, 239–248.

Yasui-Furukori N, Kondo T, Suzuki A, et al. (2002) Comparison of prolactin concentrations between haloperidol and risperidone treatments in the same female patients with schizophrenia. Psychopharmacology (Berl) 162, 63–66.

Zimbroff DL, Kane JM, Tamminga CA, et al. (1997) Controlled, dose-response study of sertindole and haloperidol in the treatment of schizophrenia. Sertindole Study Group. Am J Psychiatr 154, 782–791.

# 96     Mood Stabilizers

Scott E. Moseman
Marlene P. Freeman
John Misiaszek
Alan J. Gelenberg

Although the nosological construct of manic–depressive illness was the product of Emil Kraepelin, history and literature suggest that its ravages date to antiquity (Jamison 1993). Effective treatments, on the other hand, are relatively new. Although the modern use of lithium as an antimanic agent was described by Cade (1949), it did not win approval by the US Food and Drug Administration until 1970. In a review commissioned by the National Institute of Mental Health for the US Congress, treatments for bipolar disorder demonstrated a higher degree of efficacy in controlled, clinical trials than did treatments for any other major psychiatric disorder (Gelenberg and Hopkins 1993). At the same time, however, existing medications yield less than complete symptomatic relief for many patients with bipolar disorder. Whether the drugs are not completely efficacious or patients are unable to tolerate them, mood symptoms persist, leading to suffering, dysfunction, and too commonly, loss of life. Also, students of health care delivery point to the difference between efficacy and effectiveness. Even the most efficacious agent remains ineffective sitting on a pharmacy or medicine cabinet shelf. A patient must get into the health care system, be properly diagnosed, have appropriate medication prescribed, be educated about the disorder and the medicine, and be observed and monitored appropriately for the agent to be effective.

This chapter tries to help close the gap between efficacy and effectiveness by summarizing what is known at the beginning of the 21st century about treatments for bipolar disorder. We discuss treatments for the several acute phases of the disorder—mania, depression, and mixed mania—and then describe maintenance therapy.

## Acute Mania

### General Management Considerations

Before treatment is initiated (Table 96–1), it is important to determine whether a patient is suffering from primary mania, indicative of bipolar disorder; or secondary mania, resulting from an organic dysfunction. Primary mania seldom occurs for the first time after age 40 years, but many organic factors—stroke, neoplasms, epilepsy, infec-

tions (e.g., acquired immunodeficiency syndrome), metabolic and endocrine disturbances, and substance abuse—can precipitate secondary mania. Late onset of mania should prompt a thorough physical and neurological examination, including routine laboratory and neuropsychological testing, electroencephalography, and computed tomography or magnetic resonance imaging of the head. It is also important to differentiate bipolar disorder from other psychiatric disorders. An acute manic episode could be a brief reactive psychosis, a drug-precipitated reaction, or the beginning of schizophrenic illness. Sometimes schizophrenia-related disorders can be differentiated by a personal or family history, but it may be necessary to follow the course of the illness for a time before a diagnosis can be made. While charting the illness, the psychiatrist should have regular contact with the patient; gather psychosocial, medical, and neurological data; and be available between visits in case symptoms occur.

For further details on the accurate diagnosis of acute mania and bipolar disorder please refer to Chapter 64.

A primary management consideration in acute mania is whether to hospitalize the patient (Table 96–2). As in other disorders, this typically hinges on the concern for a patient's safety outside of a secure setting. Can the patient adequately care for himself or herself, including taking prescribed medications in a safe manner? Is the patient a risk to self or others? Even if not actively suicidal or homicidal, manic patients often put themselves or others at risk through driving carelessly, taking health risks, or behaving in a provocative manner that might trigger violence. Also, manic patients can swing rapidly into depression and become acutely suicidal. Patients with mania sometimes present a clinical dilemma when a psychiatrist believes that the patient should be hospitalized but the patient refuses. In most venues, involuntary hospitalization is legal only if the patient presents an imminent and clear threat to life. Behaviors that can bankrupt or destroy a family, ruin a career, or disrupt a patient's social standing do not qualify. Although patients with hypomania may have impaired judgment, they usually do not require hospitalization. They can often be induced to comply with treatment and managed successfully as outpatients.

| Table 96–1 | Treatments for Acute Mania | |
|---|---|---|
| Treatment | Advantages | Disadvantages |
| Lithium | Efficacy: 70–80% | Side effects, low therapeutic index |
| Typical antipsychotics | Rapid onset of action | Not as effective as lithium in stabilizing mood |
| Olanzapine | Comparable to lithium | Side effects |
| Anxiolytics | Good as adjunctive sedatives, wide margin of safety | Probably not specifically antimanic |
| Valproate | Comparable to lithium | Side effects |
| Carbamazepine | Possibly comparable to lithium | Side effects |
| Other drugs (e.g., verapamil) | Not adequately studied | |
| Electroconvulsive therapy | Efficacy:~80%, safe for patients unable to take medication | More difficult to administer |

The best environment for a patient with hypomania or mania is one that is secure, predictable, unstressful, and quiet. Sleeplessness may be a trigger for mania, and conversely, sleep is essential for restoration of normal mood and thinking. It goes without saying that patients must be kept safe—from their own behavior, from the behavior of others (which their behavior may trigger), and from the hazards of medication.

The goal of treatment should be to suppress completely all symptoms of mania and return the patient to his or her mental status *quo ante*. Mood, thinking, and behavior should normalize. The patient should act and feel like herself or himself. For economic or social reasons, it is sometimes necessary to discharge a patient before total remission of symptoms has occurred. In such cases it is imperative that a patient continues to take medication as prescribed and is protected from a recrudescence of manic symptoms or a rapid slide into acute depression.

## Pharmacotherapy

The mechanism of action of antimanic drugs is more poorly understood than that of antidepressant drugs. Whereas the monoamine systems are generally believed to be involved in antidepressant responses, it is not as clear what neural systems are involved in the mechanism of antimanic drugs. That few significant changes in neurotransmitter levels have been measured suggests that the site of action may be at the receptor, intracellular level, or second-messenger systems.

## Lithium

For many patients with hypomania, lithium by itself can induce a total remission. For patients with full-blown mania, however, an adjunctive antipsychotic or antianxiety agent may be required to treat intolerable psychosis or excitement.

| Table 96–2 | When to Hospitalize an Acutely Manic Patient |
|---|---|

The patient is not safe outside a secure setting.
The patient cannot adequately care for himself or herself.
The patient cannot take prescribed medications in a safe manner.
The patient is a risk to himself or herself or others.

In four early placebo-controlled studies of lithium for acute mania, the overall response rate in 116 patients was 78% (Goodwin and Jamison 1990). There have been five small controlled trials that have shown lithium to be more effective than antipsychotic agents, which were the primary treatment for acute mania in the US before lithium became available (Johnson et al. 1968, 1971, Spring et al. 1970, Platman 1970, Takahashi et al. 1975, Shopsin et al. 1975). A meta-analysis of four of these studies found that an average of 89% of lithium-treated patients showed improvement, compared with 54% of patients taking neuroleptics (Janicak et al. 1993).

Although extensive research has uncovered much about lithium's diverse cellular actions, which of these actions are responsible for its mood-stabilizing properties has not been determined. One theory is that lithium alters neuronal function through substitution for or competition with other ions (Ward et al. 1994, Price and Heninger 1994). The lithium ion shares properties with sodium, potassium, magnesium, and calcium ions and may affect their distribution and kinetics. However, irregularities in these systems do not appear to be specific to bipolar disorder.

Lithium's mechanism of action may be related to its effects on the neurotransmitters serotonin, dopamine, norepinephrine, and acetylcholine (Ward et al. 1994). For example, lithium's antimanic properties may derive from its prevention of dopamine receptor supersensitivity, and its antidepressant effects may be a result of its enhancement of serotonin activity. Lithium also enhances acetylcholine function and has variable effects on norepinephrine.

Research, however, has focused on lithium's effects on second-messenger and signal transduction systems (Manji et al. 1995a). The behavioral and physiological manifestations of depression and mania are probably mediated by a network of interconnected neurotransmitter pathways, rather than by any single neurotransmitter system. Lithium regulates signal transduction in the brain by affecting the intracellular signal generated by multiple neurotransmitter systems. These systems, therefore, represent attractive targets for lithium's therapeutic efficacy.

One intracellular, second-messenger-generating system that may be involved in mood regulation involves phosphoinositide metabolism (Pollack et al. 1994, Baraban 1994). In this system, the plasma membrane-located lipid phosphatidylinositol 4,5-bisphosphate is hydrolyzed to postsynaptic second messengers that contribute to chronic cell stimulation by altering electrical activity in the neuron. Inositol formed during this process is recycled by the enzyme inositol monophosphatase. Central nervous system cells have limited access to plasma sources of inositol and depend on its synthesis for the transduction of neuronal signals. Lithium, in therapeutic concentrations, blocks the activity of inositol monophosphatase, inhibiting the hydrolysis of intermediate inositol phosphates into inositol, which is necessary for the resynthesis of phosphatidylinositol 4,5-bisphosphate. As a result, phosphatidylinositol 4,5-bisphosphate levels are depleted, and the lipid is no longer able to stimulate the formation of adequate quantities of the second messengers or alter electrical activity. Lithium's blockade of inositol monophosphatase becomes more effective as the substrate concentration increases, and hyperactive inositol phospholipid turnover may be associated with bipolar disorder. However, lithium's therapeutic actions occur only after long-term treatment, and they remain in effect for a while after the drug has been discontinued; therefore, they cannot be attributed only to inositol depletion.

The cyclic adenosine monophosphate (cAMP)-generating system is also significantly affected by lithium (Manji et al. 1995b). At therapeutic concentrations, lithium inhibits the accumulation of cAMP by various neurotransmitters and hormones. Lithium decreases neurotransmitter-coupled adenylate cyclase activity and cAMP formation, resulting in decreased sensitivity of adenylate cyclase receptors and decreased neuronal activity. Lithium also decreases (1) adrenoceptor stimulation of adenylate cyclase and (2) adrenoceptor function, both of which have been proposed as mechanisms of antidepressant action. These effects on the cAMP-generating system cause the physiological symptoms of polyuria and subclinical hypothyroidism, but whether they have any central nervous system manifestations is still unclear.

Because lithium has been demonstrated to affect both phosphoinositide turnover and adenylate cyclase activity, mechanisms shared by these two major second-messenger-generating systems are being studied. One of these mechanisms involves the signal-transducing guanine nucleotide-binding (G) proteins (Manji et al. 1995a). The G proteins coordinate receptor–effector activity, play widespread critical roles in the regulation of neuronal function, and maintain the functional balance between neurotransmitter systems. Studies have observed reduced receptor-G protein coupling with long-term lithium administration. G proteins may be the targets of lithium actions and possibly the molecular sites underlying the pathophysiological mechanism of bipolar disorder.

That the prophylactic action of lithium in stabilizing the mood cycling of bipolar disorder takes a few weeks to occur suggests that lithium causes alterations at the genomic level. The actions of lithium on gene expression may be mediated by protein kinase C, a calcium-activated, phospholipid-dependent enzyme that is highly enriched in the brain. Protein kinase C plays a major role in regulating presynaptic and postsynaptic aspects of neurotransmission and alters various molecules in the cell nucleus that regulate gene expression. Short-term lithium treatment activates protein kinase C, whereas prolonged administration decreases protein kinase C-mediated responses, including neurotransmitter release.

Lithium is rapidly and completely absorbed after oral administration. It is not protein bound and does not undergo metabolism. Peak plasma levels are achieved within 1.5 to 2 hours for standard preparations or 4 to 4.5 hours for slow-release forms. Lithium's plasma half-life is 17 to 36 hours. Ninety-five percent of the drug is excreted by the kidneys, with excretion proportionate to plasma concentrations. Because lithium is filtered through the proximal tubules, factors that decrease glomerular filtration rates will decrease lithium clearance. Sodium also is filtered through the proximal tubules, so a decrease in plasma sodium can increase lithium reabsorption and lead to increased plasma lithium levels. Conversely, an increase in plasma lithium levels can cause an increase in sodium excretion, depleting plasma sodium.

Tests that should be done before lithium is started include a complete blood count, electrocardiography, electrolyte determinations, and renal and thyroid panels (Table 96–3). Lithium dosage may be based on a plasma concentration sampled 12 hours after the last dose, or the drug may be gradually titrated to a dose that is tolerated and within the range usually considered "therapeutic." As with any drug, approximately five half-lives must elapse for steady state to be achieved. For an average adult, this takes about 5 days for lithium (longer in the elderly or in patients with impaired renal function). To treat acute mania, plasma concentrations should typically be greater than 0.8 mEq/L, but to avoid toxicity, the level should not usually exceed 1.5 mEq/L. It is important to know what other medications a patient may be taking, because many drugs interact with lithium and can lead to increased or decreased lithium levels and possibly adverse effects (Table 96–4).

To reach therapeutic levels rapidly in healthy younger patients with normal renal and cardiac function, the psychiatrist may prescribe 300 mg of lithium carbonate four times daily from the outset, sampling the first plasma level after 5 days (or sooner should toxic signs become apparent).

| Table 96–3 | Pretreatment Tests |
|---|---|
| Before starting any medication | Comprehensive medical history<br>Physical examination including weight<br>Pregnancy test, if applicable |
| Lithium | Complete blood count<br>Electrocardiogram<br>Electrolytes<br>Renal panel (blood urea nitrogen, creatinine, and routine urinalysis)<br>Thyroid panel plus thyroid-stimulating hormone |
| Valproate | Liver function test<br>Blood and platelet counts |
| Olanzapine | Blood glucose<br>Blood lipids |
| Carbamazepine | Blood and platelet counts<br>Urinalysis<br>Liver function test<br>Kidney function test |

| Table 96–4 | Drug Interactions with Lithium |
|---|---|

### Increase Levels of Lithium

Angiotensin-converting enzyme
Alprazolam (Xanax)
Amiloride (Midamor)
Antipsychotic agents?
Ethacrynic acid (Edecrin)
Fluoxetine (Prozac)
Ibuprofen (Motrin)
Indapamide (Lozol)
Indomethacin (Indocin)
Mefenamic acid (Ponstel)
Naproxen (Naprosyn)
Phenylbutazone (Butazolidin and others)
Some antibiotics
Spironolactone (Aldactazide, Aldactone, and others)
Sulindac (Clinoril)
Thiazide diuretics
Triamterene (Dyazide and Dyrenium)
Zomepirac (Zomax)

### Decrease Levels of Lithium

Caffeine
Carbonic anhydrase inhibitors
Laxatives
Osmotic diuretics
Theobromine diuretic (Athemol)
Theophylline (Tedral and others)

### Increase Adverse Reactions

Antithyroid effects: carbamazepine (Tegretol), iodine
Cardiovascular toxicity: hydroxyzine (Atarax, Vistaril, and others)
Confusion: electroconvulsive therapy
Extrapyramidal symptoms: neuroleptics
Hypertension: methyldopa (Aldomet and others)
Neurotoxicity: diltiazem (Cardizem), verapamil (Calan and others), clozapine (Clozaril)
Seizures: fluvoxamine (Luvox)
Somnambulism: antipsychotic agents
Toxic symptoms with normal blood levels: methyldopa (Aldomet and others)

Thereafter, the dose should be adjusted to achieve a 12-hour plasma concentration between 0.8 and 1.3 mEq/L at steady state.

In a patient with mild hypomanic symptoms, by contrast, it may be wiser to begin with a lower lithium dose, such as 300 mg b.i.d., taking longer to achieve therapeutic levels but, at the same time, minimizing side effects that could trouble the patient and hamper cooperation. Once steady state has been achieved at therapeutic concentrations and the patient is clinically stable, lithium can be administered to most patients in a once-daily dose, usually at bedtime. Not only is this schedule easier to remember, but it tends to decrease such common side effects as tremor and polyuria.

The most common acute adverse effects from lithium are nausea, vomiting, diarrhea, postural tremor, polydipsia, and polyuria (Table 96–5). If troublesome, these can usually be mitigated by a slower dosage increase. Other medications may be helpful for side effects that persist despite dosage adjustment (e.g., propranolol, 20–160 mg/day, for tremor; diuretics, such as thiazide or loop, for polydipsia or polyuria). Gastrointestinal problems may be alleviated by taking lithium with food or switching to a different preparation. More severe symptoms and signs, including confusion and ataxia, may herald toxic plasma levels and should prompt an immediate blood assay and, if necessary, temporary discontinuation or dosage reduction.

Many skin reactions have been described in association with lithium therapy, including atopic dermatitis, acne, psoriasis, and hair loss. These can usually be treated by standard dermatological means but occasionally are severe enough to force the discontinuation of therapy. Electrocardiographic effects of lithium are also usually benign and tolerable. Rarely, however, an effect such as slowing of the sinus node can lead to severe bradycardia and syncope. If continued lithium therapy is a high priority, use of a pacemaker to provide cardiac stability could be considered.

If adverse effects make lithium intolerable, the psychiatrist may need to discontinue it and try an alternative. If lithium is insufficiently effective, a new antimanic drug may be added. At times, three or more agents may be necessary to suppress mania.

| Table 96–5 | Adverse Effects of Lithium |
|---|---|

| Adverse Effect | Treatment |
|---|---|
| Weight gain | Avoid caloric beverages, watch diet, increase physical activity |
| Nausea, vomiting, diarrhea | Take lithium with food, switch to different preparation, increase dosage more slowly, check blood level to ensure against toxic levels, reduce dose* |
| Postural tremor | Administer β-blockers (if not contraindicated), increase dosage more slowly, decrease lithium level* |
| Polydipsia, polyuria | Administer diuretics, lower dosage,* take dose once a day at bedtime, decrease dietary protein |
| Confusion, ataxia | Immediately assay blood; if toxic, temporarily discontinue lithium or reduce dosage* |
| Skin reactions | Apply standard dermatological treatments, possibly discontinue lithium |
| Bradycardia, syncope | Check electrocardiogram, consider a pacemaker, possibly discontinue lithium |
| Central nervous system effects: mental dullness, memory and concentration difficulties, headache, fatigue, muscle weakness | Lower dosage,* possibly discontinue lithium |

*May decrease protection versus relapse and recurrence.

Mr. M is a 20-year-old single black male who was brought into the emergency room by his college roommate, who reported that Mr. M has been "out of control" for about 5 days. Mr. M is noticeably hyperkinetic, speaks very rapidly, and admits to racing thoughts which "have to be rapid in order to prepare himself for the President of the US who has chosen him for a secret mission." He is very tangential and states he has been doing "great" with 1 to 3 hours of sleep a night. He describes his mood as "outstanding." In talking to family and friends, they state that he never has had an episode like this in the past, although he had a depressive episode in his teens. They add that his father carries a diagnosis of bipolar disorder and has done well on lithium. All the patient's labs are within normal limits and he has neither known medical, alcohol, nor drug problems.

Mr. M presents with a euphoric mania, and would likely be a good candidate for lithium therapy. As is commonly the case, he presented with a depressive episode as an adolescent and now presents in his early twenties with his first "full-blown" manic episode. He has a positive family history in that his father suffers from a bipolar disorder that has been well controlled with lithium. In the hospital setting, Mr. M's behavioral and sleep difficulties can be ameliorated with benzodiazepines and antipsychotic medication. These adjunctive medications are usually tapered and discontinued before or soon after discharge while lithium prophylaxis is maintained.

## Antipsychotic Agents

The chemistry and pharmacology of antipsychotic drugs are presented in detail in Chapter 95, and their adverse effects and precautions are the same in the treatment of acute mania as they are for acute schizophrenia (see Chapter 62). In double-blind controlled trials, investigators have found chlorpromazine, haloperidol, pimozide, thioridazine, and thiothixene to be effective in the treatment of acute mania but, in general, not as effective as lithium (Johnson et al. 1968, 1971, Spring et al. 1970, Platman 1970, Takahashi et al. 1975, Shopsin et al. 1975, Prien et al. 1972, Post et al. 1980, Cookson et al. 1981). However, although lithium has been found to be better in stabilizing mood and ideation, first-generation antipsychotics have been found to be superior in controlling hyperactivity (Johnson et al. 1968, 1971, Shopsin et al. 1975, Johnstone et al. 1988) and to have a more rapid onset of action (Johnson et al. 1968, 1971, Shopsin et al. 1975, Prien et al. 1972, Post et al. 1980, 1987, Garfinkel et al. 1980). On the basis of these findings, combined treatment with an antipsychotic and lithium is often used (Chou 1991), but several studies have found little to no advantage in using this combination, rather than an antipsychotic alone, in the first few weeks of treatment (Johnstone et al. 1988, Garfinkel et al. 1980, Biederman et al. 1979).

Although in the 1970s it was commonplace to use ultrahigh doses of neuroleptics in attempts to suppress psychotic symptoms (sometimes in excess of 100 mg of haloperidol daily), this is seldom necessary and may be counterproductive; it can increase the risk of acute cardiovascular complications, seizures, acute dystonia, and possibly the neuroleptic malignant syndrome. For most acutely manic patients, 5 to 15 mg of haloperidol daily should suffice, augmented by a benzodiazepine to increase sedation. In emergent situations, intramuscular administration of the neuroleptic can achieve higher blood levels more rapidly than oral preparations.

As in the treatment of schizophrenia, newer ("atypical") antipsychotics are coming to replace the first generation. Emerging data suggest that clozapine may have particular benefit for acutely manic and psychotic patients. In a retrospective review at McLean Hospital, McElroy and coworkers (1991) found that 12 (86%) of 14 bipolar patients with psychotic features who were treatment resistant or intolerant of other agents showed moderate or marked improvement with clozapine after 6 weeks or more of treatment. Suppes and colleagues (1992) reported that in seven of these patients with dysphoric mania, the effects of clozapine persisted for 3 to 5 years, with no rehospitalizations for six patients who continued clozapine treatment.

Although clozapine is free from most of the extrapyramidal side effects (EPS) associated with typical neuroleptics and may not cause tardive movement disorders, it does carry the risk of serious toxic reactions, including agranulocytosis, seizures, and cardiorespiratory complications. It should be used for bipolar patients only after other options have failed. Many experienced clinicians believe clozapine is superior to traditional neuroleptics in the treatment of bipolar disorder, but definitive, controlled data are lacking.

Olanzapine has structural and pharmacologic similarities to clozapine but is generally less toxic. It shares with clozapine a low incidence of EPS and of hyperprolactinemia, as compared to typical agents. In 2000, olanzapine received approval from the US Food and Drug Administration for acute mania, joining lithium and valproate for this indication.

Two large, multicenter, double-blind, placebo-controlled studies have found olanzapine superior to placebo in the treatment of acute mania (Tohen et al. 1999, 2000). In the first 3 weeks in duration, 139 patients were randomly assigned to either olanzapine (10 mg/day) or placebo. With a response criterion of a 50% decrease in the Young Mania Rating Scale, there was a 48.6% response rate with olanzapine, compared to a 24.2% response in the placebo group, with separation from placebo occurring in week 3. In the second study, which lasted 4 weeks, 115 patients were randomly assigned to either olanzapine (5–20 mg/day) or placebo. Clinical response was achieved by 65% taking olanzapine versus 43% in the placebo group, with separation occurring at week 1 (most likely due to higher doses of olanzapine than in the previous study). In other randomized controlled trials, olanzapine has shown comparable efficacy to both lithium (Berck et al. 1999), and valproate (Tohen et al. 2002, Zajeckya et al. 2000). There is no apparent difference in treatment response to olanzapine in mania between psychotic versus nonpsychotic patients.

Ensuring compliance with treatment, and controlling agitation are important in treating mania. Currently there are no rapid-acting intramuscular formulations of FDA-approved agents for bipolar mania. However, intramuscular olanzapine is being studied. In a recent double-blind, randomized study of 201 agitated patients with mania, intramuscular olanzapine showed significantly greater reduction in agitation than intramuscular lorazepam or placebo, both at 2 hours and at 24 hours (Meehan et al. 2001).

Olanzapine, a thienobenzodiazepine (2-methyl-4-[4-methyl-1-piperazinyl]-10H-thieno<2,3-b><1,5>benzodiazepine), has a pharmacologic profile resembling clozapine (Moore et al. 1993). Like clozapine, it has a low likelihood of causing EPS or raising prolactin and greater efficacy in treating the secondary negative symptoms of schizophrenia (Casey 1989, Meltzer 1992, Beasley et al. 1996). Olanzapine has a high affinity for a variety of monoamine receptors and binds potently to $5\text{-HT}_{2A}$ and $D_2$ receptors. Its binding to $5\text{-HT}_2$ is three-times stronger than to $D_2$ (Moore et al. 1993). Its mechanism of action in treating mania is unknown but might be independent of its antipsychotic activity.

Olanzapine is rapidly absorbed after oral administration and reaches peak concentrations in approximately 6 hours. Food does not affect the rate or extent of olanzapine's absorption. It is highly protein bound (93%) and has a mean half-life of 30 hours, taking approximately a week to reach steady-state levels.

Olanzapine is metabolized by direct glucuronidation and cytochrome P450-mediated oxidation through the 1A2 and 2D6 pathways (2D6 appears to be a minor metabolic pathway). Because of olanzapine's use of the 1A2 pathway, agents such as omeprazole and rifampine, which induce 1A2, could decrease olazapine levels, while inhibitors of 1A2, such as fluvoxamine, could potentially increase them. Smokers excrete olanzapine at a rate about 40% higher than nonsmokers.

Although olanzapine is only approved for acute mania, it is frequently continued after hospital discharge. Therefore, before starting olanzapine a thorough medical exam, including weight, blood glucose, and blood lipid levels, should be obtained.

Typical starting doses of olanzapine range between 10 to 15 mg/day, with responses typically taking 1 to 3 weeks in acute mania. Unlike lithium and valproate, blood levels measurements are not needed. Once daily dosing is sufficient.

Adverse effects during the short-term use of olanzapine include constipation, weight gain, akathisia, dry mouth, tremor, increased appetite, orthostatic hypotension, and tachycardia. The most common side effect is somnolence, which is why olanzapine is usually given in one q.h.s. dose. In clinical trials, there was a 0.9% incidence of seizures, and although there were confounding factors, olanzapine should be used cautiously in patients with known seizure disorders or lowered seizure thresholds. Because of alamine aminotransferase elevations in some patients, it is also advised to use olanzapine cautiously in patients with known or suspected hepatic impairment.

Risperidone and other atypical antipsychotics also may have mood stabilizing properties. Segal and colleagues (1998) conducted a randomized, controlled trial of 45 patients taking either risperidone (6 mg/day), lithium (800–1200 mg/day), or haloperidol (10 mg/day) in the acute manic phase of bipolar illness. The study showed comparable and significant decreases in mania for all three agents. Risperidone as an adjunct to lithium or valproate may be superior to either mood stabilizer alone in acute manic episodes (Sachs and Ghaemi 2000). Data are limited on ziprasidone and quetiapine as treatments for mania.

Trials of other atypical and novel antipsychotics in mania are also being conducted but have not yet led to regulatory approval.

## Anxiolytic Agents

The pharmacology, adverse effects, and precautions associated with anxiolytic drugs are covered in Chapter 98. Among current anxiolytic agents, benzodiazepines are usually selected as adjuncts to treat acute mania because of their safety and efficacy. Although some have claimed specific antimanic efficacy for clonazepam or other benzodiazepines (Edwards et al. 1991, Chouinard 1987), most psychiatrists are more impressed with their benefits as adjunctive sedatives than with more specific antimanic activity. Because it yields predictable blood levels when administered intramuscularly, lorazepam is often the benzodiazepine selected for this indication. Benzodiazepines have a wide margin of safety and can be safely administered in even very high doses, suppressing potentially dangerous excitement and allowing patients much needed sleep. When used together with an antipsychotic agent, benzodiazepines counteract the antipsychotic agent's tendency to provoke extrapyramidal reactions and seizures. For lorazepam, 1 to 2 mg can be administered by mouth or intramuscularly as frequently as hourly.

## Valproate

After rigorous clinical investigation (Bowden et al. 1994), the anticonvulsant valproate (in the form divalproex sodium [Depakote], see later) has been approved in the US for the treatment of the acute mania of bipolar disorder. At least 16 uncontrolled and 6 controlled studies have shown valproate to be effective in treating acute mania. In the first double-blind, placebo-controlled trial, 17 patients randomized to receive valproate demonstrated a median improvement of 54% in manic symptoms versus 5% for 19 placebo-treated patients ($P = 0.003$) (Pope et al. 1991). In a double-blind, random-assignment, parallel-group study comparing valproate with lithium in manic patients, 9 of 14 valproate-treated patients and 12 of 13 lithium-treated patients responded favorably after 3 weeks of treatment (Freeman et al. 1992). In the first randomized, double-blind, parallel-group, placebo-controlled study of valproate in acute mania, 179 inpatients were randomly assigned to receive divalproex sodium, lithium, or placebo for 21 days in a 2:1:2 ratio (Bowden et al. 1994). At least 50% improvement from baseline to final analysis was seen in approximately half of the divalproex- and the lithium-treated patients, compared with one quarter of the patients who took placebo ($P < 0.025$).

Valproate's mechanism of action in treating mania is unknown but may be related to an increase in levels of gamma-aminobutyric acid, an inhibitory neurotransmitter (USP DI 1995). Valproate may be responsible for decreasing the metabolism of gamma-aminobutyric acid or its reuptake in brain tissues. An alternative theory is that valproate mimics or enhances gamma-aminobutyric acid's inhibitory action on postsynaptic receptor sites. Valproate's effects on membrane activity are not completely understood but may be related to changes in potassium conduction.

Valproate is available in the US as valproic acid or divalproex sodium, a compound containing equal parts valproic acid and sodium valproate. Divalproex is better tolerated than valproic acid, has been studied more extensively, and is more commonly used. All valproate preparations are rapidly absorbed after oral administration, reaching peak plasma levels within 2 to 4 hours of ingestion. Food may delay absorption but does not affect bioavailability. Valproate is rapidly distributed and highly bound (90%) to plasma proteins. Its half-life ranges from 9 to 16 hours, depending on whether it is taken alone or with other medications, and it takes 1 to 4 days to attain steady state.

Valproate is metabolized by the hepatic cytochrome P450 2D6 system. Unlike carbamazepine, it does not induce its own metabolism or hepatic metabolism in general, but it does appear to inhibit the degradation of other drugs metabolized in the liver (McElroy et al. 1989). Valproate inhibits drug oxidation and may increase serum levels of concomitantly administered drugs that are oxidatively metabolized, such as phenobarbital, phenytoin, and tricyclic antidepressants. Coadministration of carbamazepine, or other microsomal enzyme-inducing drugs, will decrease plasma levels of valproate, and drugs that inhibit the P450 system, such as selective serotonin reuptake inhibitors, can increase them. The coadministration of other highly protein bound drugs, such as aspirin, can increase free valproate blood levels and precipitate toxic effects.

Experts usually rank lithium as the treatment of choice for a patient with classic mania, but divalproex is an acceptable first-line alternative. It may be used singly in patients who cannot tolerate lithium. For patients who do not respond to lithium, there are no secure data on whether divalproex should be added as an adjunct or substituted, but many psychiatrists would choose the former in a patient who appears to respond at least partially to lithium and the latter in patients for whom lithium seems to afford no benefit. Increasingly, psychiatrists are turning to divalproex first for manic patients with organic brain impairment, rapid cycling, mixed or dysphoric mania, or comorbid substance abuse (Bowden et al. 1994, Calabrese et al. 1993a).

Before initiating divalproex, the psychiatrist should obtain a comprehensive medical history and insure that a physical examination has been performed, with particular attention to suggestions of liver disease or bleeding abnormalities (see Table 96–3). Baseline liver and hematological functions are measured before treatment, every 1 to 4 weeks for the first 6 months, and then every 3 to 6 months. Evidence of hemorrhage, bruising, or a disorder of hemostasis–coagulation suggests a reduction of dosage or withdrawal of therapy. The drug should be discontinued immediately in the presence of significant hepatic dysfunction.

A typical starting dose for healthy adults is 750 mg/day in divided doses. The dose can then be adjusted to achieve a 12-hour serum valproate concentration between 50 and 125 µg/mL. The time of dosing is determined by possible side effects, and if tolerated, once-a-day dosing can be employed. As with lithium, the antimanic response to valproate typically occurs after 1 to 2 weeks.

A faster response may be achieved by oral loading. In a prospective, rater-blind study, Keck and colleagues (1993) gave 19 acutely manic patients 20 mg/kg/day of divalproex sodium for 5 days. In the 15 patients who completed the study, serum concentrations greater than 50 mg/L were reached by day 2, and 10 patients had a significant decrease in manic symptoms by the end of the study. This treatment was well tolerated with few side effects.

Adverse effects that appear early in the course of therapy, are usually mild and transient, and tend to resolve in time. Gastrointestinal upset is probably the most common complaint in patients taking valproate and tends to be less of a problem with the enteric-coated divalproex sodium preparation. The administration of a histamine H2 antagonist such as famotidine (Pepcid) or cimetidine (Tagamet) may alleviate persistent gastrointestinal problems (Stoll et al. 1991). Other common complaints include tremor, sedation, increased appetite and weight, and alopecia. Weight gain is even more of a problem when other drugs are administered that also promote weight gain, such as lithium, antipsychotic, and other antiepileptics. Less common are ataxia, rashes, and hematological dysfunction, such as thrombocytopenia and platelet dysfunction. Platelet count usually recovers with a dosage decrease, but the occurrence of thrombocytopenia or leukopenia may necessitate the discontinuation of valproate. Serum hepatic transaminase elevations are common, dose related, and usually self-limiting and benign. Fatal hepatotoxicity is extremely rare, is usually restricted to young children, and usually develops within the first 6 months of valproate therapy. Other serious problems include pancreatitis and teratogenesis (McElroy et al. 1989). There is also a concern that polycystic ovary syndrome, possibly associated with weight gain, may be a risk for young women who take valproate. If at any point during administration the side effects of valproate become intolerable, the psychiatrist may need to discontinue it and try one of the other treatments described in this section as an alternative. If valproate is tolerated but not totally effective, the psychiatrist might use one of the other treatments as an adjunct.

---

**Clinical Vignette 2**

Mr. R is a 36-year-old married white male who presents for his third hospitalization for mania. He is accompanied by his wife who states that he has not slept the last 3 to 4 nights due to the fact he is "building his own coffin." On examination, the patient is agitated, hyperverbal, pacing, and continually repeating that "my day has come." The patient admits to needing only "a couple" hours of sleep a night, and adding that his "thoughts are moving in every direction, but mostly down." He expresses concurrent feelings of sadness, and vague suicidal ideation. Mr. R was previously prescribed lithium during his first hospitalization which "didn't work." During his second hospitalization, he did not tolerate a carbamazepine trial secondary to "vision problems and dizziness." A review of the record from a prior admission reveals that the patient has a history of dysphoric mania and alcohol abuse. He has no known medical problems at this time.

Mr. R presents with dysphoric mania, and has failed 2 previous drug treatments. Due to the dysphoric nature of his manic presentation and his history of alcohol and drug abuse, he would likely benefit from valproate pharmacotherapy. This could efficiently be initiated in the hospital by prescribing a loading dose of 20 mg/kg with the addition of benzodiazepines or antipsychotics to control behavior and induce sleep. Because of the resistant nature of his illness, the addition of another agent such as olanzapine could enhance mood stability.

## Carbamazepine

Double-blind studies suggest that carbamazepine is effective in the treatment of acute mania, but the methods used in many of these studies have been criticized. The results of many carbamazepine trials are confounded by the coadministration of neuroleptics or lithium. Four studies that did not use concomitant medications have been published. One compared carbamazepine with lithium in 28 patients and found no significant differences in antimanic effects between the two drugs but more consistent improvement among the lithium-treated subjects (Lerer et al. 1987). In a similar study, one-third of both the lithium-treated and carbamazepine-treated patients responded favorably (Small et al. 1991). In two studies comparing carbamazepine with chlorpromazine in a total of 87 subjects, an average of 69% of carbamazepine-treated patients showed improvement compared with 67% of the chlorpromazine-treated patients (Grossi et al. 1984, Okuma et al. 1979). In both studies, the onset of improvement was more rapid with carbamazepine.

In light of the less well-substantiated evidence for the efficacy of carbamazepine, we place this anticonvulsant fourth in the antimania algorithm—behind lithium, valproate, and olanzapine. The decision to move on to carbamazepine—and whether to use it alone or in addition to lithium, valproate, or olanzapine—hinges on the same treatment considerations listed earlier. If a patient has been treated with one or more of these agents in a previous manic episode, that experience may guide treatment of a current episode.

As with other antimanic drugs, the mechanism by which carbamazepine treats mania remains unknown. Its antimanic properties may be related to its anticonvulsant or antineuralgic effects, or to its effects on any one of a number of neurotransmitter or second-messenger systems. Carbamazepine increases acetylcholine in the striatum, decreases dopamine turnover, decreases the release of norepinephrine and cerebrospinal norepinephrine, decreases the activity of adenylate and guanylate cyclase, and decreases gamma-aminobutyric acid turnover; any or all of these actions could be relevant to its effects in mania.

Carbamazepine's absorption and metabolism are variable. Peak plasma levels occur within 4 to 6 hours after ingestion of the solid dosage form. Bioavailability is estimated at 85% but may be less when the drug is taken with meals. Eighty percent of plasma carbamazepine is protein bound, and its half-life ranges from 5 to 26 hours (after 3–4 weeks of treatment). Carbamazepine's active metabolite, 10,11-epoxide, has a half-life of about 6 hours.

Carbamazepine is metabolized by the hepatic cytochrome P450 2D6 system. It causes an induction of the cytochrome P450 enzymes, often resulting in an increased rate of its own metabolism over several weeks, as well as that of other drugs metabolized by the P450 system (Table 96–6). Because of enzyme induction, the dose of carbamazepine often must be raised after 2 to 4 months of treatment. Steady state may be attained within 4 to 5 days, but when clearance increases as a result of autoinduction, steady state may not be achieved for 3 to 4 weeks. Concomitant administration of drugs that inhibit P450 (see Table 96–6) will increase plasma levels of carbamazepine. Conversely, drugs that induce P450 enzymes—such as pheno-

| Table 96–6 | Drug Interactions with Carbamazepine |
|---|---|

**Increase Levels of Carbamazepine**

Cimetidine (Tagamet)
Diltiazem
Erythromycin
Fluoxetine (Prozac)
Fluvoxamine (Luvox)
Isoniazid (and others)
Propoxyphene (Darvon and others)
Valproate
Verapamil

**Decrease Levels of Carbamazepine**

Phenobarbital
Primidone
Phenytoin (Dilantin and others)

**Carbamazepine Decreases Levels of**

Antipsychotics
Benzodiazepines (except clonazepam)
Corticosteroids
Hormonal contraceptives
Lamotrigine
Thyroid hormone
Tricyclic antidepressants

**Others**

Lithium + carbamazepine may increase neurotoxic effects

barbital, phenytoin, or primidone—can decrease carbamazepine levels. Before carbamazepine is started, baseline blood and platelet counts, urinalysis, and liver and kidney function tests are in order (see Table 96–3). Although earlier guidelines called for routine monitoring of some or all of these indices, and some psychiatrists still obtain blood counts once or twice during the first few months of treatment and when plasma concentrations are sampled, a more general consensus at present is to instruct patients and family members to contact the psychiatrist immediately if petechiae, pallor, weakness, fever, or infection occur, at which time the psychiatrist should order relevant tests.

Used as a monotherapy, the typical starting dose for carbamazepine is 200 to 400 mg/day in three or four divided doses, increased to 800 to 1000 mg/day by the end of the first week. If clinical improvement is insufficient by the end of the second week, and the patient has not had intolerable side effects to the drug, increases to as high as 1600 mg/day may be considered. Although there are no good studies of the correlation between blood level and clinical response, a common target range for mania is 4 to 15 ng/mL. If carbamazepine is combined with lithium or neuroleptics, lower doses and blood levels of carbamazepine often are used. If valproate and carbamazepine are administered simultaneously, blood levels of each should be monitored carefully because of complex interactions between the two agents.

When the dose of carbamazepine is built up rapidly, side effects are more likely. The most common effects in the first couple of weeks are drowsiness, dizziness, ataxia,

| Table 96–7 | Adverse Effects of Carbamazepine |
|---|---|

**Common** (diminish in time or with temporary reduction in dose)
  Drowsiness
  Dizziness
  Ataxia
  Diplopia
  Nausea
  Blurred vision
  Fatigue
**Less common**
  Gastrointestinal upset
  Hyponatremia
  Skin reactions (if severe, may require discontinuation of
    carbamazepine)
**Rare**
  Transient leukopenia (carbamazepine may be continued unless
    infection develops)
**Very rare**
  Aplastic anemia
  Agranulocytosis

diplopia, nausea, blurred vision, and fatigue (Table 96–7). These tend to diminish in time or to respond to a temporary reduction in dose. Less common reactions include gastrointestinal upset, hyponatremia, and a variety of skin reactions, some of which are severe enough to require discontinuation of carbamazepine. About 10% of patients experience transient leukopenia, but unless infection develops, carbamazepine may be continued. More serious hematopoietic reactions, including aplastic anemia and agranulocytosis, are rare.

Recently oxcarbazepine, the 10-keto analogue of carbamazepine, has become available as an alternative to carbamazepine for the treatment of seizure disorders. Oxcarbazepine has less protein binding at 40%, and therefore less possibility for drug–drug interactions with highly protein bound drugs. Two small studies have shown some benefit in mania, but larger placebo-controlled studies are needed (Emrich et al. 1985, Muller and Stoll 1984).

## Other Drug Treatments

Several other drugs show promise for acute mania. The calcium-channel blocker verapamil came to the attention of psychiatric researchers in the 1980s and early 1990s. Two double-blind, crossover trials suggested that verapamil has utility in the treatment of mania (Giannini et al. 1984, Dubovsky et al. 1986). This was supported by two larger double-blind controlled trials (Höschl and Kozen 1989, Garza-Treviño et al. 1992). However, two more recent randomized, controlled trials failed to find efficacy for verapamil in acute mania (Walton et al. 1996, Janicak et al. 1998). Recent research points to a question of gender specificity. Wisner and colleagues (2002) performed an open-label trial of verapamil in 37 women, some of whom were pregnant, with the diagnosis of bipolar disorder. Twenty-seven women were being treated for episodes of acute mania or depression. In this group 100% of those treated for acute mania, and 39% of those treated for depression responded. Other calcium-channel blockers, such as nimodipine and nifedipine, may have antimanic properties as well, as suggested by anecdotal reports and small, open trials (Brunet et al. 1990, De Beaurepaire 1992).

Since carbamazepine and valproate are efficacious for acute mania, new antiepileptic medications are often tested for mania. Lamotrigine, which appears useful in maintenance, bipolar depression and rapid-cycling, has not shown efficacy in acute mania, with the exception of one recent double-blind trial (Berk 1999, Anand et al. 1999, Bowden et al. 2000a). Topirimate has shown some benefit in the treatment of acute mania as monotherapy, and as an adjunctive medication (Chengappa et al. 2001, Calabrese et al. 2001b, Gurnze et al. 2001). There is a suggestion of efficacy for zonisamide, but only in one small open trial (Knaba et al. 1994). Although there were suggestions that gabapentin has some antimanic properties in open studies (Ghaemi et al. 1998, Erfurth et al. 1998), in the only placebo-controlled study to date by Pande and colleagues (2000) it showed no efficacy. In a small open study, tiagabine showed no efficacy in eight patients (Gurnze et al. 1999).

The following drugs also have been investigated in acute mania: galanthaminehydrobromide (Snorrason and Stefansson 1991), RS 86 (Van Berkestijn et al. 1990), clonidine, acetazolamide, primidone, mephobarbital, lecithin, L-tryptophan, remoxipride, levothyroxine (Van Berkestijn et al. 1990), methysergide, cinanserin, reserpine, propranolol, amphetamine, methylphenidate, apomorphine, piribedil, physostigmine, and diltiazem. Although clonidine and L-tryptophan have shown efficacy in a few double-blind trials, and the rest have suggestive positive results in open trials or case series, none has been sufficiently tested to determine its efficacy for this indication.

## Nonpharmacotherapy: Electroconvulsive Therapy

The specifics about electroconvulsive therapy (ECT), safety data, and precautions concerning administration are covered in Chapter 92. When an acutely manic patient is unresponsive to or intolerant of medication, or if medication presents other risks (e.g., during pregnancy), ECT should be seriously considered and may be lifesaving. Although there are no coherent theories about why ECT is effective in acute mania, it has been used for more than half a century, and there are widespread clinical impressions of its safety and efficacy.

In 50-year retrospective of ECT for mania, Mukherjee and colleagues (1994) reported that ECT was associated with remission or marked clinical improvement in 78% of manic patients in early studies, 85% of patients in six retrospective studies reported since 1976, and 77% of patients in two prospective studies. In total, ECT has been associated with remission or marked clinical improvement in 470 (80%) of 589 manic patients reported in the literature.

There is a belief that ECT works faster than pharmacological treatment, making it a preferred treatment for patients who are homicidal, psychotic, or severely suicidal. However, there is little experimental evidence to support this belief. In a double-blind trial by Small and coworkers (1988), of 34 hospitalized manic patients, ECT was found to be superior to lithium during the first 8 weeks of treatment, especially for severely manic patients and those with mixed states. After 8 weeks, however, there were no significant differences between the lithium- and ECT-treated patients on ratings of manic and depressive symptoms or in the frequency of relapses, recurrences, or rehospitalizations.

## Acute Depression

### General Management Considerations

As is the case with unipolar depression, more women than men may experience bipolar depression (Angst 1978). When a patient first presents with a depressive episode, it is important to determine whether depressive symptoms result from a nonpsychiatric condition, such as primary degenerative dementia, multi-infarct dementia, amphetamine or sympathomimetic intoxication or withdrawal, or organic mood disorder (e.g., reserpine-induced depression) (Janicak et al. 1993). Once these conditions have been ruled out, the psychiatrist should determine whether the patient has a unipolar or bipolar disorder. Bipolar depression is usually indistinguishable from other forms of major depression, except that the episodes are typically shorter and more frequent. Other clues that the disorder may be bipolar include onset at a young age, a positive family history for bipolar disorder (particularly in first-degree relatives), and the occurrence of a hypomanic phase before the onset of the depressive episode.

For the most part, the treatment of a bipolar patient during an acute episode of depression is similar to that of a nonbipolar patient. The same concerns about protecting the patient from suicide and maintaining physical health and safety apply, and for the most part, the same antidepressants or ECT will be useful (Table 96–8). These antidepressants are covered in Chapter 97. Because of fears about speeding up cycling and/or precipitating mania in patients with bipolar disorder, most doctors avoid prescribing tricyclics in bipolar depression. The short section that follows addresses issues unique to treatment of bipolar depression.

### Pharmacotherapy

There is a widespread clinical impression that administering some antidepressants to bipolar patients can trigger switches into mania. Some experts also believe that antidepressants speed up mood cycles, although this point is more controversial. Because of both concerns, psychiatrists are often cautious about prescribing an antidepressant at the first sign of depression in a bipolar patient. If symptoms are mild and short-lived, many clinicians choose watchful waiting, while maintaining close contact to detect clinical deterioration

Current guidelines by the American Psychiatric Association list lithium, as well as the anticonvulsant lamotrigine

as first-line monotherapy for acute bipolar depression (Hirschfeld et al. 2002). This is a result of recent research that suggests that lamotrigine may be an effective treatment for bipolar depression, while carrying a low risk of triggering a switch into mania. Calabrese and colleagues (1999) randomized 195 patients with Bipolar I disorder during a major depressive episode to 7 weeks of treatment with either placebo or lamotrigine, 50 mg or 200 mg. There were significantly more responders (at least a 50% decrease in scores on the Ham-D 17 or Montgomery and Åsberg Depression Rating Scale (MADRS) and a Clinical Global Impression (CGI-I) score of 1–2) in the 200 mg/day lamotrogine group compared to placebo. For patients taking 50 mg/day, there was a significant difference only in the MADRS scores. There were significant differences in MADRS, CGI-S and CGI-I scores in the 200 mg/day lamotrogine group from beginning to endpoint, and a trend in the Ham-D. There was no significant treatment-emergent mania in either lamotrigine group versus placebo (5.4% versus 4.6%).

Lamotrigine is a third-generation anticonvulsant that blocks voltage-sensitive sodium channels, which inhibits release of the presynaptic excitatory amino acids aspartate and glutamate. It also blocks high-voltage activated N- and P-type calcium channels and weakly inhibits serotonin reuptake. Its mechanism of action in bipolar disorder is unknown.

Lamotrigine is completely absorbed after oral administration, with a bioavailability of 98%, which is not affected by food. Peak plasma concentrations occur between 1.4 and 4.8 hours after administration. Lamotrigine is approximately 55% protein bound, making clinical interactions with other protein-bound drugs unlikely. Its half-life is 14 to 49 hours, with steady-state levels reached in 3 to 10 days.

Lamotrigine is metabolized predominately by glucuronic acid conjugation in the liver, with the conjugate and the remaining 10% of the unmetabolized drug excreted in the urine. Clearance is markedly increased with the administration of other drugs that induce hepatic enzymes—including phenytoin, carbamazepine, and phenobarbital (Table 96–9). Adding lamotrigine to carbamazapine can decrease steady-state concentrations of lamotrigine by approximately 40%. Adding lamotrigine to valproate, however, can decrease steady-state levels of valproate by approximately 25%, while the steady-state levels of lamotrigine increases approximately twofold. In this case, the starting dose of lamotrigine should be lowered, and the titration made slowly.

The only contraindication to lamotrigine use is hypersensitivity to the drug, though there is a box warning about dermatologic events, particularly rashes. These rashes, that

| Table 96–8 | Treatments for Acute Depression | |
| --- | --- | --- |
| Treatment | Advantages | Disadvantages |
| Antidepressants | Efficacious | Possibly trigger switch into mania |
| Lamotrigine | Efficacious, possibly no switch into mania | Risk of side effects |
| Mood stabilizers | Enhance effectiveness of antidepressants, possibly protect against switch into mania | Not specifically antidepressant |
| ECT | Efficacious, safe for patients unable to take medication | More difficult to administer, possible cognitive side effects |

| Table 96–9 | Effects of Combining Lamotrigine with Other Anticonvulsants |
|---|---|

**Effects of Anticonvulsants on Lamotrigine Levels**

Carbamazepine decreases levels 40%
Oxcarbazepine decreases levels 30%
Phenobarbital decreases levels 40%
Phenytoin decreases levels 50%
Valproate increases levels 100%

occurred in approximately 10% of patients, generally occur after 2 to 8 weeks and are usually macular, papular, or erythematous in nature. Of those who develop a rash, one in 1,000 adults can precede to a Stephens–Johnson type syndrome. Because it is impossible to distinguish which rashes will develop into this serious condition, it is advised to discontinue the medication at any sign of drug-induced rash. Otherwise the most frequently encountered side effects include dizziness, ataxia, somnolence, headache, blurred vision, nausea, vomiting, and diplopia.

To reduce the risk of rash and other side effects lamotrigine should be started at low doses and titrated slowly, especially if combined with valproate therapy. Patients are commonly started on 25 to 50 mg p.o.q.d. doses for 2 weeks, with doses increased by 25 to 50 mg every 1 to 2 weeks until maintenance levels between 100 to 250 mg/day are reached. Maximum doses are lower with valproate at about 100 to 150 mg/day. Initial labs for those undergoing lamotrigine therapy should include liver function tests, renal function tests, a pregnancy test if applicable, and a complete medical workup.

Probably all available antidepressant drugs are effective in alleviating the symptoms of depression in a bipolar patient, and in fact a recent 1-year retrospective chart review by Altshuler and colleagues (2001) suggests that antidepressant discontinuation may increase the risk of depressive relapse in bipolar patients. SSRI antidepressants with clinical data supporting their use in bipolar depression include fluoxetine (Cohen et al. 1989), paroxetine (Young et al. 2001), and citalopram (Kupfer et al. 2001). In the paroxetine and citalopram studies, antidepressant medications were added to traditional mood stabilizers. Some data suggest that tranylcypromine and bupropion may be effective in bipolar depression and less likely than tricyclic antidepressants to trigger switches into mania (Himmelhoch et al. 1976, Sachs et al. 1994). Should at any point in antidepressant treatment of bipolar depression a triggered switch into mania occurs the antidepressant medication should be discontinued immediately (Himmelhoch et al. 1991).

When a patient is known to have bipolar disorder, administration of an antidepressant to reverse an acute depression is almost always used together with one of the mood-stabilizing agents, usually lithium, valproate, carbamazepine (or a combination)—or possibly one of the newer putative agents. Most bipolar patients will be taking these drugs in maintenance therapy. Moreover, mood stabilizers may enhance the effectiveness of the antidepressant and might protect against the possibility of a switch into mania.

**Clinical Vignette 3**

Mrs. L is a 46-year-old married Hispanic female with a history of one prior manic episode which required a short hospitalization in her early twenties. She presents to the outpatient clinic with a history of resistant depression. Mrs. L was treated with lithium therapy in the past but "didn't like" the blood monitoring and continued to experience depressive episodes despite treatment. Trials of several antidepressant medications, including SSRIs and buproprion, initially improved her mood but also facilitated the onset of hypomanic symptoms and problems with sleep.

Mrs. L is a good candidate for treatment with lamotrigine. Depression is the primary expression of her bipolar disorder and treatment with lamotrigine is less likely to induce manic symptoms than is treatment with antidepressant medications. The initial recommended dose is 25 to 50 mg p.o.q.d. dose for 2 weeks. The dose can be increased by 25 to 50 mg every 1 to 2 weeks until a maintenance level between 100 to 250 mg/day is reached. The patient should be closely monitored for any appearance of a rash. Should a rash occur, lamotrigine should be discontinued immediately as it is impossible to ascertain which rashes progress to the Stephens–Johnson type syndrome.

The adverse effects, pharmacology, and interactions of antidepressants are covered in Chapter 97.

## Nonpharmacotherapy: Electroconvulsive Therapy

ECT is a useful alternative to antidepressants, particularly when a patient appears not to be responding quickly or is intolerant of the medication. Early studies that claimed that ECT works faster than medication in depressed patients are now considered to be methodologically flawed. However, two later studies found a more rapid decrease in depressive symptoms with ECT than is usually observed with medications. In a total of 72 patients with major depression, approximately six ECT treatments administered in a period of about 2 weeks led to a decrease in mean Hamilton Depression Rating Scale scores from between 24 and 30 to below 10 (Abrams et al. 1991, Pettinati 1994). The authors attributed the efficacy of treatment to the use of high suprathreshold dosages. Sackeim and colleagues (1993) found that higher dosage results in more rapid improvement in both bipolar and unipolar depressed patients. There are indications that bilateral electrode placement is superior to unilateral placement (Abrams et al. 1991, Sackeim et al. 1993), but there may be an increased risk of severe cognitive side effects with bilateral ECT at ultrahigh dosages.

## Mixed States

The coexistence of manic and depressive symptoms, the so-called mixed state, is associated with poorer treatment response and prognosis than acute mania or depression (Himmelhoch et al. 1976, Keller et al. 1986, Dilsaver et al. 1993). The optimal treatment of the mixed state has not been rigorously studied, so these recommendations must be considered tentative (Table 96–10).

| Table 96–10 | Treatments for Mixed Episodes |
| --- | --- |
| General | Lithium, valproate, carbamazepine, lamotrigine (alone or in combination) |
| For severe excitement or psychosis | Antipsychotics |
| For depressive symptoms | Antidepressants, lamotrigine |
| Alternative to medication | ECT |

Almost always, these patients will be taking lithium, valproate, carbamazepine, another "mood stabilizer," or a combination. There are some suggestions that valproate may be superior to lithium alone in this condition (Freeman et al. 1992, Calabrese et al. 1993b), but this hypothesis has not been sufficiently tested. When excitement is severe or psychosis is present, antipsychotic agents may be indicated; preliminary evidence suggests that clozapine (and perhaps other atypical neuroleptics) might be particularly helpful. Antidepressants appear to treat persistent depressive symptoms. As in acute mania and acute depression, ECT can be considered an alternative to medications.

Dilsaver and colleagues (1993) found that 12 (57.1%) of 21 patients with mixed mania failed to respond to lithium, carbamazepine, valproate, and antipsychotic agents compared with 2 (11.1%) of 18 patients with pure mania. Seven of the 12 patients recovered after ECT. Four others recovered after bupropion was added to their regimens (Brown et al. 1994).

## Maintenance Therapy

### General Management Considerations

As in all psychiatric disorders, maintenance therapy of bipolar disorder is a treatment carried out for a long period, with a goal of decreasing the probability, frequency, or severity of future episodes. Because bipolar disorder is by its nature a recurrent condition, some would argue that as soon as it is definitively diagnosed (e.g., after a single manic episode not attributable to a medical or neurological cause), maintenance therapy is indicated (Table 96–11). More conservative psychiatrists advocate waiting until the frequency and severity of a patient's disorder become apparent, hoping to avoid long-term exposure to medication that may not be required. The counter to this concern is evidence suggesting that recurrent episodes in themselves may worsen treatment response and long-term outcome (Gelenberg et al. 1989).

Nowhere is the potential gap between efficacy and effectiveness more apparent than in maintenance treatment. When a patient feels well, there is little motivation to take medicine. People simply forget, and taking a "pill" is a reminder that one has an illness. Besides, medications have unwanted effects, some (like weight gain) especially troublesome in the long term. Physicians confront these problems on a daily basis with common disorders such as hypertension. It is also a major problem in treating bipolar disorder.

The most brilliant pharmacotherapy is useless in the absence of a sound physician–patient relationship with necessary education about the illness and its treatment. As we discuss in a later section on nonbiological maintenance treatments, a number of psychological interventions that are designed to amplify and advance the effectiveness of long-term medication treatments have been proposed and are being studied. Psychoeducation and other efforts to enhance compliance are common, along with techniques to stabilize patients' lives and decrease stresses.

## Pharmacological Treatments

### Lithium

For bipolar maintenance, lithium has the longest and largest database of clinical experience and by far the greatest number of patients studied in rigorous clinical trials. In a meta-analysis of all placebo-controlled studies of lithium to prevent relapse in a total of 739 bipolar patients, Janicak and colleagues (1993) found that 37.3% of lithium-treated patients relapsed compared with 79.3% of patients receiving placebo. Lithium is the only agent with the US

| Table 96–11 | Maintenance Treatment | | |
| --- | --- | --- | --- |
| Treatment | Advantages | Disadvantages |
| Lithium | Most efficacious | Side effects, low therapeutic index |
| Valproate | Possibly comparable to lithium | Side effects, not adequately studied |
| Olanzapine | Possibly comparable to lithium, no blood monitoring | Side effects, not adequately studied |
| Lamotrigine | Possibly comparable to lithium, especially for treating and preventing depressive episodes | Side effects, not adequately studied |
| Carbamazepine | Possibly comparable to lithium | Side effects, not adequately studied |
| Typical antipsychotics | Not adequately studied | Tardive movement disorders |
| Antidepressants | Comparable to lithium for preventing depressive episodes | Not as efficacious as lithium for preventing manic episodes |
| ECT | For refractory mood disorders | Not adequately studied |
| Psychotherapy | As adjunct, increases medication compliance, overall functioning | Not efficacious alone |

Food and Drug Administration's imprimatur for relapse prevention.

There are few absolute contraindications to lithium maintenance therapy. Of course, a previous adverse experience or lack of responsiveness argue against its use, but given the ready availability of blood level monitoring, even patients with impaired renal function or metabolic conditions can safely take lithium. We discuss the use of lithium in the face of various medical conditions when we cover adverse effects (see later).

Most patients starting lithium maintenance are already taking lithium after an acute episode. They should have had baseline medical tests, including assessment of thyroid function (thyroid panel plus thyroid-stimulating hormone) and renal function (blood urea nitrogen, creatinine, and routine urinalysis), a complete blood count, electrolyte determinations, an electrocardiogram, and a physical examination (see Table 96–3). A medical history should also have been obtained that included questions about past medical and family history of renal, thyroid, cardiac, and central nervous system disorders; other drugs a patient may be taking (including prescription, over-the-counter, and illicit); the use of such common substances as caffeine, nicotine, and alcohol; and special diets or diet supplements. It should also be ascertained whether the patient has a dermatological disorder or is (or may become) pregnant.

If a patient who is to start lithium maintenance therapy is not already taking lithium, it is gentlest to begin with a low dose and gradually build the daily dosage to achieve therapeutic serum concentrations. It is safe to start this slowly because the patient is by definition already in remission (that is to say, clinically stable). A physically healthy, average-size adult may be started with 300 mg of lithium carbonate twice daily. An elderly, ill, or slightly built individual can begin with as little as 150 mg twice daily (150-mg lithium capsules are available, and for even finer dose adjustments, a liquid preparation—lithium citrate—may be used). Because it takes about 5 days to achieve a steady state (longer in the elderly and those with renal impairment), blood should be drawn at approximately that interval (12 hours after the last dose) for a lithium-level assay. The dose should be adjusted until a therapeutic level has been achieved.

What is the optimal blood lithium range to protect bipolar patients against recurrent episodes? The largest, prospective, double-blind study on this question found that levels between 0.8 and 1.0 mEq/L afforded threefold greater protection against recurrent episodes than a range of 0.4 to 0.6 mEq/L[64]. Furthermore, patients in the higher range were less likely to experience subsyndromal symptoms (hypomania or minor depression) and, if such symptoms did appear, were less likely to go on to a full episode (Keller et al. 1992). However, higher blood levels were associated with more side effects and the risk of noncompliance. Sometimes education and reassurance are sufficient to keep patients at higher levels. Often contraactive therapy can help alleviate some troublesome side effects (see later). Side effects may diminish with a decrease in lithium level, but both psychiatrist and patient should be aware that this may decrease the level of protection against mood swings.

Even though an aggregated sample of bipolar patients may show fewer episodes when maintained at a higher lithium level, there probably are many individuals with this disorder who benefit from lower levels. The clinical challenge is to afford patients the greatest comfort and freedom from side effects without subjecting them to the considerable hazards of recurrent episodes. There have been no systematic studies of the lithium level–clinical response relationship in elderly patients, but because older people are more sensitive to side effects, most psychiatrists maintain their elderly bipolar patients at lower plasma lithium concentrations. (For that matter, as a patient ages, it usually takes less of a dose of lithium to achieve the same plasma level.)

Once a patient has been stabilized clinically, is taking a constant lithium dose, and has a stable serum lithium level, the blood concentration need be checked only on an occasional basis (we prefer every 3 months), usually at a follow-up visit. In addition to periodic monitoring of serum lithium levels, we like to assay the thyroid-stimulating hormone and creatinine concentrations every 6 months and, for men older than 40 years and women older than 50 years, obtain an electrocardiogram annually. During this phase of stability, a once-daily lithium regimen, usually at bedtime, tends to improve compliance and decrease side effects and is tolerable to most patients. If lithium needs to be discontinued there seems to be a lower risk of recurrence after gradual rather than rapid discontinuation of lithium (Faedda et al. 1993).

Lithium can cause a broad array of side effects (see Table 96–5). Decreased thyroid function may occur in 5% of patients and is the reason for periodic monitoring of the thyroid. (Rarely, hyperthyroidism occurs.) The psychiatrist should keep an index of suspicion for symptoms and signs that might suggest hypothyroidism and, if they occur, order an immediate thyroid panel. Hypothyroidism does not preclude continued lithium treatment but rather demands the use of thyroid hormone replacement therapy. For that matter, an elevated thyroid-stimulating hormone concentration, even in the face of normal thyroxine serum levels, often justifies the use of exogenous thyroid supplements.

Through the dysregulation of calcium metabolism, lithium may cause hypercalcemia and hyperparathyroidism, which in turn may lead to osteopenia, osteoporosis, bone resorption, and hypermagnesemia (Kingsbury and Salzman 1993). Weakness and fatigue associated with elevations of calcium may be mistaken for depression. Discontinuation of lithium should resolve these conditions.

Despite earlier fears that long-term lithium would lead to widespread renal failure, this appears to occur rarely if at all (Walker 1993). Still, it is wise to monitor renal glomerular function periodically, which is why we recommend serum creatinine assays. If creatinine level begins to rise in time, or if lithium levels rise despite a constant dosage, consultation with a nephrologist may be in order. Patients with diminished renal glomerular function or even those receiving dialysis can still be treated with lithium, but its half-life will be prolonged, and this must be accounted for in the dosage amount and interdose interval. Of course, in these cases, more intensive monitoring of serum lithium levels is called for.

Diminished renal concentrating capacity is a common side effect of lithium therapy and results in polyuria and secondary polydipsia. Patients should be encouraged to keep up with their thirst and not allow themselves to become dehydrated (which could lead to lithium intoxication). When polyuria is troublesome for a patient, one of several strategies may prove helpful. The once-daily lithium regimen we mentioned earlier often diminishes the daily urine output. A decreased daily protein intake (consistent with nutritional needs) can also be useful. Diuretics may paradoxically decrease urine volume, but because some (such as thiazides) can also raise the serum lithium concentration, it must be carefully monitored and the dose adjusted downward appropriately. Potassium levels should also be monitored; potassium supplementation may be necessary.

Lithium commonly causes a benign and reversible increase in blood neutrophils. It also produces several changes in the electrocardiogram, most commonly T wave flattening or inversion. More rarely it interferes with atrioventricular conduction or slows the sinus node. A wide range of common cutaneous reactions to lithium are listed in the lithium section under acute mania.

Gastrointestinal upset is common early in the course of therapy and later may herald a marked increase in the plasma lithium concentration. For some patients, changes in the type of lithium preparation can be helpful, whereas others may need a reduction in dose or a more gradual dose escalation.

Central nervous system effects of lithium that are more frequent at the beginning of treatment include mental dullness, memory and concentration difficulties, headache, fatigue, and muscle weakness. A number of patients develop a fine, rapid tremor while taking lithium. This is an action or postural type of tremor, more exaggerated while holding a sustained position (such as the hands outstretched). Most probably it represents an exaggeration of a physiological tremor (idiopathic, essential, senile, or familial). Tremor tends to increase with increasing plasma levels, with anxiety, or with the use of stimulants. Propranolol, 20 to 160 mg/day, can be a helpful antidote (Gelenberg and Jefferson 1994).

Weight gain is another common adverse effect troublesome in long-term treatment. Its mechanism is unknown. Patients should avoid caloric beverages, restrict food calories, and increase physical activity. Patients taking lithium are often also taking other drugs, such as antipsychotics and antiepileptics, which also can promote weight gain. Other occasional side effects of lithium are edema and a metallic taste in the mouth.

Lithium has a narrow therapeutic index: an increase in the plasma concentration to 2.0 mEq/L and above, particularly if prolonged, can cause central nervous system impairment, renal shutdown, coma, permanent brain injury, and death. To avoid this, patients and their families need to be instructed carefully on a number of matters related to lithium levels (Table 96–12). They should be alerted to early signs of intoxication—such as increased tremor, confusion, and ataxia—and directed that if these symptoms appear, the patient should immediately stop taking further lithium and report for a blood level determination and clinical evaluation. Patients and their families should be instructed to check with the psychiatrist about gastrointestinal symptoms (which can be caused by high lithium levels or, if

| Table 96–12 | Lithium Intoxication |
| --- | --- |
| Patients Should | When These Symptoms Occur |
| Call psychiatrist | Gastrointestinal symptoms |
| Stop lithium and see psychiatrist | Increased tremor, confusion, ataxia |

Patients should report any other medications they are considering taking (prescribed or over-the-counter) and be wary of diet changes (especially decreased sodium intake).

caused by an intercurrent infection, can change electrolyte and water balance sufficient to cause lithium intoxication). They should be alerted to the effects of diet changes (particularly decreased sodium intake) on lithium levels and to report to the psychiatrist any medications another physician wants to prescribe or over-the-counter medications they are contemplating (which may interact with lithium). Management of lithium intoxication may require hemodialysis and medical intensive care to maintain fluid and electrolyte balance, prevent further absorption of the drug, and maximize the rate of elimination. Concomitant use of other medications may increase levels of lithium and lead to lithium intoxication. See Table 96–4 for a list of drugs that interact with lithium.

**Managing "Breakthrough" Symptoms.** For some patients, lithium maintenance therapy is 100% successful in preventing future mood episodes. For many, lithium is helpful, but symptoms occasionally reemerge. As in all aspects of long-term therapy, a close working alliance among the patient, the family members, and the psychiatrist is an important base on which to build clinical strategies.

The first question is whether a symptom, such as a minor mood dip or insomnia, is the start of a prodrome or merely a transient event. Close telephone contact, often several times in a day, or a brief visit can be helpful. Sleep loss in particular is troublesome, because there is evidence that it can trigger a manic episode. Hypomanic symptoms are more likely to be indicative of an incipient, full-blown manic episode than are mild, depressive symptoms to predict a major recurrence of depression (Keller et al. 1992). Sometimes an incipient prodrome can be nipped in the bud. For example, use of a benzodiazepine hypnotic or specific counseling to patients and families about sleep hygiene and work and travel schedules may allow a restorative night's sleep and prevent a mood episode. Similarly, selective use of a benzodiazepine, such as lorazepam or clonazepam, may help a patient through a stressful period and prevent a full-blown episode.

Sometimes symptoms and stress are secondary to a decreased lithium level, whether it is due to poor compliance, dietary changes, or other factors. Whenever symptoms become manifest in a patient maintained with lithium, therefore, one of the first things a psychiatrist should do is order a blood level assay. If the level is low, an obvious intervention is to assess factors that led to the level change and attempt to return the patient to a therapeutic concentration.

If psychotic symptoms appear, an antipsychotic drug is indicated. Subsequent treatment should follow that described under acute mania. Similarly, a full-blown episode of depression may require the use of an antidepressant, along the lines outlined in the section on acute depression.

## Valproate

Rapid-continuous cycling, mixed states or dysphoric mania, alcohol or drug abuse, noncompliance with treatment, a cycle pattern of depression–mania–euthymia, personality disturbance, a history of poor interepisode functioning, a poor social support system, and three or more prior episodes predict a poor response to lithium prophylaxis (Table 96–13) (Prien and Potter 1990). Valproate or carbamazepine may be beneficial for many of these patients or, conceivably, one of the less-studied antiepileptics, like oxcarbazepine, topiramate, or others. In a retrospective survey, patients who responded to maintenance anticonvulsant therapy after failing to respond to standard psychotropic medication regimens, such as lithium, experienced abnormal sensory phenomena similar to those observed in epileptic patients (Hayes and Goldsmith 1991). Patients who were stable with standard medications did not experience this phenomenon. In the heterogeneous syndrome we call bipolar disorder, there may be patients with covert epileptoid discharges, who benefit specifically from antiseizure medications.

Several open trials report moderate to good results with the combination of valproate and lithium or valproate alone (Calabrese and Delucchi 1990, McElroy et al. 1992), and there has been one report of sustained prophylactic response in three patients with the combination of valproate and carbamazepine (Keck et al. 1992b).

The only published randomized, double-blinded, placebo-controlled maintenance study with valproate was conducted by Bowden and colleagues (2000b) in a 12-month trial, which compared valproate, lithium, and placebo in 372 outpatients with Bipolar I disorder. In the primary outcome measure there was no statistical difference among the three groups in time to recurrence of any mood episode. In secondary analysis, valproate was statistically superior to placebo in rates of discontinuation for either a recurrent mood episode or depressive episode. Valproate was also superior to lithium in longer duration of successful prophylaxis and in Global Assessment Scale scores. This study highlights the difficulty of studying the diverse patient group classified with this condition and points out the need for more maintenance studies.

When valproate is used for maintenance therapy, it is best to start with a low dose, such as 250 to 500 mg daily, building the dose gradually to maintain a plasma level between 50 and 125 µg/mL. Unlike carbamazepine, valproate does not induce its own metabolism, so it should not be necessary to increase the dose a few weeks after the initiation of treatment.

As noted in the section on acute mania, valproate is generally well tolerated, and most of its side effects tend to wane in time. Increased appetite with weight gain is likely to be a problem for some patients during long-term therapy and can be aggravated by concomitant administration of other medications with the same side effect (e.g., lithium, antipsychotic drugs, and some antidepressants). An essential-type tremor is a common neurological adverse reaction to valproate. If valproate is administered together with lithium, which can produce the same type of tremor, this may be more of a problem. Valproate can be teratogenic and should be avoided during pregnancy.

Some patients have alopecia, thinning, or changes in hair texture while taking valproate. Because lithium can also affect skin and hair, there is the potential for an additive problem.

Hepatotoxicity and pancreatitis were discussed in the section on acute mania. The American Medical Association's (1993) Drug Evaluations Subscription recommends tests of liver synthetic function, such as one-stage prothrombin time and fibrinogen levels, rather than enzyme measurements. A conservative schedule is to test these functions before therapy, monthly during the first 6 months, and then every 6 months (Table 96–14). Valproate can be teratogenic and should be avoided during pregnancy. Valproate increases the plasma concentrations of phenobarbital, lamotrigine, and carbamazepine, decreases those of phenytoin and ethosuximide, and may augment the sedative action of diazepam. Carbamazepine, phenobarbital, primidone, and phenytoin all decrease plasma levels of valproate, and salicylates can increase them.

If lithium has been partially although incompletely successful as a maintenance treatment for bipolar disorder, the psychiatrist may wish to add valproate to a lithium maintenance regimen. If lithium has been unsuccessful or poorly tolerated, valproate can be substituted. There are some suggestions that valproate is more likely to be successful in patients with organic brain dysfunction, dysphoric mania or mixed states, or rapid cycling (Freeman et al. 1992, Calabrese et al. 1993b). Breakthrough episodes or flurries of minor symptoms during valproate maintenance treatment should be handled in the same way as they are during lithium treatment.

| Table 96–13 | Predictors of Poor Response to Lithium Prophylaxis |
|---|---|
| Rapid or continuous cycling | |
| Mixed states or dysphoric mania | |
| Alcohol or drug abuse | |
| Noncompliance with treatment | |
| Cycle pattern of depression–mania–euthymia | |
| Personality disturbance | |
| History of poor interepisode functioning | |
| Poor social support system | |
| Three or more prior episodes | |

| Table 96–14 | Schedule of Tests of Liver Function During Valproate Therapy |
|---|---|
| Before therapy | |
| Monthly during the first 6 mo | |
| Every 6 mo after the first 6 mo | |

## Carbamazepine

Six double-blind controlled studies of carbamazepine in the maintenance treatment of bipolar disorder have been reported. In the only placebo-controlled trial, 60% of patients showed marked or moderate response to carbamazepine compared with only 22% of patients receiving placebo (Okuma et al. 1981). Four studies that compared carbamazepine with lithium found that carbamazepine-treated patients had rates of improvement either equivalent to or greater than those of patients taking lithium (Keck et al. 1992a). However, all of these studies used neuroleptics, hypnotics, or antidepressants for breakthrough episodes, and not all subjects had bipolar disorder.

One double-blind trial of carbamazepine and lithium, however, studied only bipolar patients and used concomitant medication only for nighttime sedation in one patient. Coxhead and associates (1992) randomly assigned 31 patients on stable lithium treatment to either switch to carbamazepine or continue with lithium. The relapse rate after 1 year was similar, but nearly all the carbamazepine relapses occurred in the first month of treatment, possibly as a result of lithium discontinuation.

As noted earlier, baseline blood and platelet counts, urinalysis, and liver and kidney function tests should be performed before treatment is initiated with carbamazepine (see Table 96-3). Frequent blood monitoring, previously recommended, is generally considered unnecessary after the first few months of therapy. Instead, patients and their families should be instructed to contact the psychiatrist immediately if petechiae, pallor, weakness, fever, or infection occurs. Carbamazepine can be teratogenic and should be avoided during pregnancy.

As with lithium and valproate, we recommend starting carbamazepine at a low dose, 100 mg/day, with increments of 100 mg/day every 4 to 5 days. Dosing is usually two to four times daily. Although a correlation between blood level and clinical response has yet to be established, most psychiatrists are guided by the antiepilepsy range: usually 4 to 15 µg/mL. When carbamazepine is used to control seizures, concentrations as high as 17 µg/mL are only rarely required and do not necessarily produce unacceptable side effects or toxic effects. Most patients taking carbamazepine for bipolar disorder are maintained with doses between 400 and 1800 mg/day. Because of enzyme induction, it is often necessary to increase the dose after 2 to 3 weeks of treatment to maintain the same blood level.

Most of carbamazepine's adverse effects have been described in the section on acute mania (see Table 96-7). Carbamazepine has an antidiuretic hormone-like effect, which may help counteract the opposite effect (which produces polyuria) of lithium when the two drugs are used together. By itself, carbamazepine can cause hyponatremia. Gradual buildup of carbamazepine levels and smaller, more frequent dosing can help to minimize side effects, particularly in patients concomitantly taking other drugs, such as lithium (Table 96-15).

Carbamazepine can slow atrioventricular cardiac conduction and should be avoided in patients who have heart block and administered cautiously in conjunction with other drugs that can also increase heart block, such as

| Table 96-15 | Carbamazepine Side Effects Contrasted with Lithium | | | |
|---|---|---|---|---|
| Side Effect | Carbamazepine (%) | Lithium (%) | Comments | |
| Dizziness or ataxia | 19 | <1 | Transient, associated with rapid increase in carbamazepine dose | |
| Skin problems | | | | |
|   Acne | | 1 | Essentially absent for carbamazepine | |
|   Rash | 13 | <1 | | |
|   Psoriasis | | 1 | Not uncommon in lithium-treated patients who have previously had psoriasis or have a family history of it | |
| Gastrointestinal problems | | | | |
|   Nausea | 10 | 4 | Gastrointestinal symptoms generally transient | |
|   Diarrhea | <1 | 9 | | |
| Drowsiness, sedation | 10 | 12 | Transient and dose related | |
| Visual problems | | | | |
|   Blurred vision | | 0–14 | | |
|   Diplopia | 8 | | Transient and dose related for lithium | |
| Slurred speech | 4 | | Transient and dose related for lithium | |
| Tremor | 3 | 27 | | |
| Paresthesia | 3 | | Transient and dose related | |
| Confusion | 2 | | Memory problems reported by 28% of lithium-treated patients | |
| Excessive thirst | | 36 | | |
| Excessive weight gain | | 19 | | |
| Polyuria | <1 | 30 | | |

*Source*: Goodwin FK and Jamison K (1990) Manic–Depressive Illness. Oxford University Press, New York p. 683.

tricyclic antidepressants and beta-blockers (see Table 96–6 for drug interactions involving carbamazepine).

When used in maintenance therapy for bipolar disorder, carbamazepine may be combined with lithium, valproate, and/or other putative mood stabilizers. In theory and in clinical practice, combinations of agents may help patients with this condition maintain mood stability over time, albeit at the price of adverse effects, often including weight gain. However, there is little science to underpin these practices. It has been suggested that carbamazepine, like valproate, is more likely to be effective in rapidly cycling patients or patients with other features predicting poor response to lithium (Post et al. 1987). Breakthrough episodes or flurries of minor symptoms during carbamazepine maintenance treatment should be handled the same way as they are during lithium treatment.

## Antipsychotics

Prescription surveys have shown that many bipolar patients are maintained routinely and for long periods on multiple-medication regimens (Sachs 1989). The drugs most commonly used in addition to lithium are the antipsychotics. Sernyak and Woods (1993) reviewed the long-term use of typical antipsychotic drugs in bipolar patients. In six studies of tardive dyskinesia, 90 to 100% of patients had used antipsychotics at some time, and 40 to 72% were taking an antipsychotic at the time of the study. In a study of long-term lithium use, 76% of bipolar patients had used antipsychotics before lithium therapy, and 30% were taking antipsychotics during lithium maintenance (Vestergaard and Schou 1988). Sernyak and colleagues (1994) found that 30 (75%) of 40 acutely manic inpatients who received neuroleptics during their hospitalization had received neuroleptics before they were hospitalized; 6 months after discharge, 38 (95%) were continuing to take them. Despite the popularity of using antipsychotics for the maintenance treatment of bipolar patients, there is little published evidence for their efficacy. In addition, the long-term use of typical antipsychotic drugs carries at least a 20 to 30% risk of tardive movement disorders—probably even higher among patients with mood disorders. In the six studies reviewed by Sernyak and Woods (1993), the point prevalence of tardive dyskinesia ranged from 19 to 41%. Clozapine, however, in an open trial by Suppes and colleagues (1999) has shown maintenance mood stabilization properties as an add-on treatment for patients with treatment resistant illness.

Over recent years, the new generation of antipsychotics have become agents of first-choice in schizophrenia, and they are being used more and more for patients with bipolar disorder. Olanzapine was approved for acute mania by the US Food and Drug Administration in 2000. As we write this, there is little proof of maintenance efficacy for olanzapine, though after acute hospitalizations, it is commonly left in a patient's drug regimen. Sanger and colleagues (2001) conducted a 49-week open-label extension trial using patients from an acute mania study. This study did demonstrate stability in mania and depression scales on a mean modal dose of 13.9 mg/day. During treatment 88.3% did not experience significant manic symptoms as indicated by maintaining a Young Mania Rating Scale (YMRS) of less than 12. The most common side effects were somnolence,

depression, and weight gain. As most bipolar maintenance studies, this one was plagued by a low completion rate, 39.8%. Also, 32% of patients were receiving adjunctive lithium and 33% adjunctive fluoxetine.

In maintenance therapy, it is unnecessary to monitor olanzapine blood levels. However, careful attention must be paid to patient weight and blood lipid and glucose levels. Weight gain on olanzapine has varied between 5 and 6.64 kg (Kinon et al. 2001, Melkersson et al. 2000, Osser et al. 1999, Sanger et al. 2001) and plateaus in under a year (Kinon et al. 2001). This weight gain is significant in some patients, and necessitates the need to review diet and exercise programs with patients who might benefit from the long-term use of olanzapine. It is also of note that the combination of olanzapine with agents such as lithium and valproate can lead to an even greater increase in weight. In the study by Osser and colleagues (1999) which showed a weight gain of 5.4 kg, there was a mean increase of triglycerides of 60 mg/dL, correlated with weight changes. Several case studies also show olanzapine induced hyperglycemia (Gatta et al. 1999, Ober et al. 1999, Fertig et al. 1998, Lindenmayer and Patel 1999, Von Hayek et al. 1999, Goldstein et al. 1999), with the study by Melkersson and colleagues (2000) concluding that olanzapine treatment was associated with elevated insulin and leptin levels, as well as insulin resistance. Because cardiovascular risk increases with hyperglycemia below levels necessary for the diagnosis of diabetes (Khaw et al 2001), it is important to monitor blood glucose levels in olanzapine treated patients.

Proposed antidotes to olanzapine-induced weight gain include diet and exercise, cognitive–behavioral therapy, dopamine agonists, and histamine-2 receptor antagonists (Table 96–16) (Gelenberg 2001). Topiramate, which does not promote weight gain, may promote weight loss, and might have mood-stabilizing properties, also could be an adjunct.

## Lamotrigine

Lamotrigine has been compared to placebo and lithium in two controlled maintenance studies. In the first, 326 patients with bipolar I disorder were treated after a recent manic or hypomanic episode with open-label lamotrigine (Bowden et al. 2000a). Those who stabilized were then randomized to lamotrigine, lithium, or placebo. In the study lamotrigine was significantly superior to placebo in survival in time to intervention for a mood episode, and in time to a depressive episode. In the second study, 966 patients with Bipolar I disorder were treated after a recent depressive episode (Calabrese et al. 2001a). During this trial, lamotrigine showed superiority in time to a mood

| Table 96–16 | Proposed Antidotes to Olanzapine-Induced Weight Gain |
|---|---|

Diet and exercise
Cognitive–behavioral therapy
Dopamine agonists (e.g., amantadine)
Histamine-2-receptor antagonists (e.g., cimetidine and nizatidine)

episode, as well as time to a depressive episode, but only lithium was superior to placebo on time to a manic episode.

## Other Drugs

Antidepressants are another frequently used group of drugs. The tricyclic antidepressant imipramine is less effective than lithium in preventing manic episodes but equally effective in preventing depressive episodes (Vestergaard and Schou 1988). Combining lithium and imipramine has no advantages over lithium alone (Johnstone et al. 1990, Prien et al. 1984, Quitkin et al. 1981). Tricyclic antidepressants may speed up mood cycling and possibly trigger episodes of mania.

Benzodiazepines, such as clonazepam and lorazepam, are often used for sleep and sedation in bipolar patients, and their efficacy in replacing antipsychotics in long-term treatment has been studied. Eight of 20 patients in a retrospective review were rated much or very much improved after clonazepam had been added to a regimen of lithium and other medications (Sachs et al. 1990a). In six patients who had previously required adjunctive antipsychotics, clonazepam successfully replaced the antipsychotic. Preliminary results from an open prospective study of 12 bipolar patients found no significant clinical or statistical evidence of worsening illness in patients who had been maintained with lithium and antipsychotics when they were switched to lithium and clonazepam (Sachs et al. 1990b).

On the basis of the association of long-term lithium therapy with decreased thyroid function (Souza et al. 1991, Kramlinger and Post 1990), and preliminary evidence suggesting that hypothyroidism may lead to rapid cycling. Bauer and Whybrow (1990a) studied the effects of adding levothyroxine to stable medication regimens in an open trial of 11 treatment-refractory, rapid-cycling bipolar patients (Bauer and Whybrow 1990b). Ten of the 11 patients showed a significant decrease in depressive symptoms. Manic symptoms also decreased significantly in five of the seven patients who had baseline manic symptoms. When placebo was substituted for levothyroxine in four patients under single- or double-blind conditions, three relapsed into depression or cycling.

Kusalic (1992) evaluated thyroid function in 10 rapid-cycling bipolar patients who had previously responded to lithium treatment, 10 control subjects, and 173 other lithium-treated bipolar patients. On the basis of thyrotropin-releasing hormone tests, 60% of the rapid cyclers had hypothyroidism, compared with none of the matched control subjects and 15.4% of the other patients. The six hypothyroid rapid cyclers were treated with thyroxine in addition to lithium, and the mean number of affective episodes per year decreased from 9.7 to 2.2.

Peselow and coworkers (1994) conducted a 5-year study of the prophylactic value of combination therapy versus lithium alone in bipolar patients. Patients who had experienced a manic relapse with lithium therapy were given adjunctive treatment with either a neuroleptic, carbamazepine, or a benzodiazepine (Figure 96–1). The carbamazepine-treated patients had the highest rate of remaining well after 5 years (46.2%), and the lowest rates of total relapses (30.8%) and depressive relapses (7.7%), but also the highest dropout rate (23.1%). Neuroleptics prevented manic relapses better than the other two treatments (6.3%). Patients who had experienced a depressive episode while receiving lithium alone had a tricyclic antidepressant, monoamine oxidase inhibitor, or fluoxetine added to their lithium regimens (Figure 96–2). Patients treated with monoamine oxidase inhibitors had the highest rate of remaining well after 5 years (46.2%). Fluoxetine had the lowest relapse rate (14.3%) but also the highest dropout rate (28.6%). The average probability of remaining free of an affective episode for a patient treated only with lithium was 83% after 1 year, 52% after 3 years, and 37% after 5 years.

Anecdotal reports and an open prospective study suggest that some bipolar patients may experience sustained therapeutic benefit from treatment with the barbiturate anticonvulsant primidone (Hayes 1993). Other drugs that have been proposed for the maintenance treatment of bipolar disorder include calcium channel blockers, beta-blockers, triiodothyronine, L-tryptophan, tyrosine, methylene blue, clonidine, and reserpine (Prien and Potter 1990). It is important for the psychiatrist to demonstrate that such

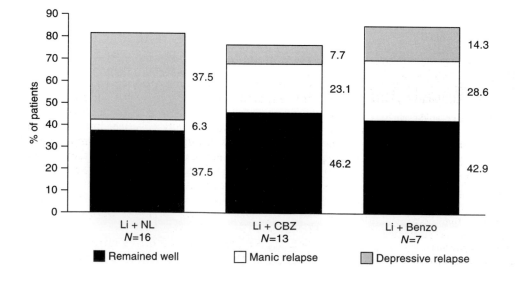

**Figure 96–1** *Five-year course of combination treatment for patients who relapsed with manic episode while receiving lithium alone. Li, Lithium; NL, neuroleptic; CBZ, carbamazepine; Benzo, benzodiazepine. (Source: Peselow ED, Fieve RR, Difiglia C, et al. [1994] Lithium prophylaxis of bipolar illness: The value of combination treatment. Br J Psychiatr 164, 208–214.)*

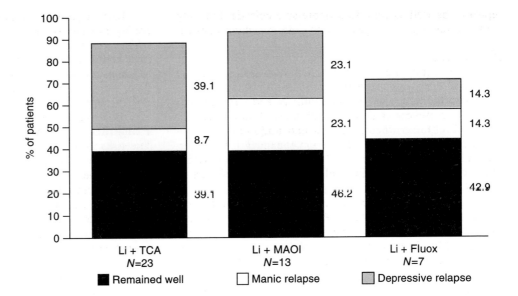

**Figure 96–2** *Five-year course of combination treatment for patients who relapsed with depressive episode while receiving lithium alone. Li, Lithium; TCA, tricyclic antidepressant; MAOI, monoamine oxidase inhibitor; Fluox, fluoxetine. (Source: Peselow ED, Fieve RR, Difiglia C, et al. [1994] Lithium prophylaxis of bipolar illness: The value of combination treatment. Br J Psychiatr 164, 208–214.)*

adjunctive medication is essential to the patient's clinical stability, because each presents its own risks.

## Rapid Cycling

Patients with rapid-cycling bipolar disorder—defined as four or more affective episodes in 1 year, with or without an intervening period of euthymia—tend to be less responsive to lithium treatment (Dunner and Fieve 1974). Whether rapid cycling is a natural progression of the illness or a separate disorder has yet to be determined. The onset of rapid cycling has been associated with antidepressant drugs (especially tricyclic antidepressants) and hypothyroidism (Wehr and Goodwin 1987, Roy-Byrne et al. 1984). Some people also experience ultrarapid cycling, switching between moods in a period of days or even hours. Various therapeutic approaches have been investigated for treating patients with rapid-cycling bipolar disorder (Table 96–17).

In one placebo-controlled study of rapid-cycling bipolar disorder, Calabrese and colleagues (2000) examined the efficacy of lamotrigine in 324 rapid-cycling bipolar I and bipolar II patients in either a manic, hypomanic, mixed or depressed phases of the illness. In a preliminary open-label

| Table 96–17 | Treatments for Rapid-Cycling Bipolar Disorder |
|---|---|
| Lithium | Less effective in rapid-cycling patients |
| Carbamazepine | Better response when combined with lithium than either drug alone |
| Lamotrigine | Possibly effective alone in some population groups |
| Valproate | Possibly effective alone or combined with lithium |
| Clozapine | Possibly effective in treatment-resistant patients |

phase, all subjects took lamotrigine, 100 to 300 mg/day, depending on tolerability, while other medications were tapered off. The 182 "responders" were then randomized to either placebo or lamotrigine monotherapy for 26 weeks. By the primary efficacy measures of time to additional pharmacotherapy for a mood episode or emerging mood symptoms, there were no significant differences between the groups. Lamotrigine did, however, show a significant overall improved survival and a trend in GAS (Global Assessment Scale) and CGI-I among bipolar II patients. Frye and colleagues (2000) compared the efficacy of lamotrigine and gabapentin versus placebo in 31 (mostly rapid cycling) patients with assorted mood disorders refractory to either lithium, valproate or carbamazepine. Mean daily doses of the medications were 274 mg for lamotrigine and 3,987 mg for gabapentin, in this double-blind randomized, crossover series of three 6-week monotherapy evaluations. During lamotrigine treatment, 52% of patients were "much" or "very much" improved versus 26% during gabapentin and 23% with placebo.

Results from one open trial and several retrospective reviews of carbamazepine in the treatment of rapid-cycling bipolar disorder have been mixed, but they suggest that lithium plus carbamazepine is more effective than either drug alone. In the open trial, two patients responded completely to carbamazepine alone, two responded to carbamazepine plus lithium, and five experienced no therapeutic benefit from carbamazepine (Joyce 1988). One retrospective review found both lithium alone and lithium plus carbamazepine to be safe and clinically effective, but the combination of the drugs brought more rapid improvement (di Costanzo and Schifano 1991). In another review, rapid-cycling patients did poorly with lithium, but 39% of them responded to the combination of lithium and carbamazepine (McKeon et al. 1992). The third review found that rapid cyclers responded poorly to both lithium and carbamazepine (Okuma 1993).

Single case reports, retrospective reviews, and prospective open-label studies have reported some degree of success using valproate, alone or combined with lithium, for the maintenance treatment of rapid-cycling patients (Sovner 1991, Sharma and Persad 1992). McElroy and coworkers (1988) conducted a retrospective review of six rapid-cycling patients treated with valproate. All had responded poorly to lithium and neuroleptics; five had also responded poorly to carbamazepine, and one was unable to tolerate it. All patients showed a moderate or marked response when valproate was added to their psychotropic regimens. Sharma and colleagues (1993) conducted an open study of valproate and lithium in nine rapid-cycling patients. Subjects had failed to respond or responded only partially to previous treatment with various agents, including a combination of carbamazepine and lithium. All but one patient showed marked or moderate improvement with valproate and lithium treatment, and the combination therapy was well tolerated.

In a prospective, naturalistic, open, ongoing trial, Calabrese and colleagues (1993a) studied 58 bipolar patients taking valproate in addition to another drug and 43 patients receiving valproate monotherapy. These 60 women and 41 men were resistant to or could not tolerate lithium monotherapy, carbamazepine monotherapy, or lithium–carbamazepine combination therapy before the study. After an average of 17 months, the investigators found that valproate protected 77% of patients against manic episodes and 38% against depressive episodes.

Jacobsen (1993) found that 11 (69%) of 16 patients with rapid-cycling Bipolar II disorder experienced sustained partial or complete stabilization of mood cycling with lower doses of valproate than currently recommended: 125 to 500 mg/day corresponding to a mean serum valproate level of 32.5 µg/mL.

Clozapine has been reported to be effective in five cases of rapid-cycling bipolar disorder in which the patients were resistant to conventional treatments (McElroy et al. 1991, Calabrese et al. 1991, Privitera et al. 1993). There are also suggestions that sleep deprivation may help alleviate depressive episodes in rapid-cycling patients, but it also may precipitate mania (Benjamin and Zohar 1992). Rapid cycling tends to be more prevalent in women, who make up 70 to 92% of the population (Dunner et al. 1977, Kukopulos et al. 1980, Cowdry et al. 1983, Wehr et al. 1988). Premenstrual syndrome has been related to major depressive disorder (Parry 1989), and Price and DiMarzio (1986) assessed the possible relationship between premenstrual syndrome and rapid-cycling bipolar disorder. These investigators found that 15 (60%) of 25 rapid-cycling female patients had severe premenstrual syndrome symptoms as opposed to 5 (20%) of 25 control subjects. In addition, bipolar patients with severe premenstrual syndrome had more affective episodes in 1 year than those with moderate or mild premenstrual syndrome symptoms.

There is no one standard protocol for the treatment of a rapidly cycling bipolar patient that can be derived from the scientific literature. First, the psychiatrist should obtain a careful history, searching for possible provocative factors. Particular attention should be paid to a precipitating effect of antidepressants and the presence of endocrinopathies, other medications, seasonal factors, psychosocial stressors, and so on. If there is no specific provocation that can be removed or remedied, attempts to stabilize the patient pharmacologically (in conjunction with psychosocial approaches) may be derived from the preceding literature review. Lithium alone may be tried but is often unsuccessful. Lithium may play a role, however, in conjunction with the anticonvulsants valproate, lamotrigine and carbamazepine. Atypical antipsychotics may be helpful. As always, ECT remains a backup option.

## Pregnancy and Lactation

The risks and benefits of treatment with mood stabilizers must be carefully assessed in the context of pregnancy and breastfeeding. All mood stabilizers are potentially teratogenic (Llewellyn et al. 1998). Reanalyses of data suggest lithium exposure during pregnancy is less harmful than previously believed. In an analysis of published studies of lithium exposure, the association between lithium use during pregnancy and fetal cardiac defects appears weaker than was assumed in the 1970s (Cohen et al. 1994). Ebstein's anomaly, a defect characterized by a malformation of the tricuspid valve, was previously considered a relatively high risk of lithium use in pregnancy (Weinstein and Goldfield 1975). Exposure to lithium in the first trimester results in 0.05 to 0.1% prevalence of Ebstein's anomaly, with a relative risk of 10 to 20% compared to population in general (Cohen and Rosenbaum 1998). By comparison, this risk is substantially lower than the risk of neural tube defects with anticonvulsants used for mood stabilization. Up to 5% prevalence of neural tube defects or other neurological problems are reported with use of anticonvulsant mood stabilizers during first trimester (Llewellyn et al. 1998).

When a patient takes lithium or anticonvulsant mood stabilizers during all or part of the first trimester, fetal development should be monitored closely. High-resolution ultrasound examination should be performed at 16 to 18 weeks' gestation and serum and amniotic fluid alpha-fetoprotein levels measured. In addition, the patient should have access to reproductive risk counseling. Serum levels should be monitored because lithium dose may need to be adjusted during pregnancy owing to changes in renal clearance and increased hepatic metabolism induced by maternal hormones.

Lithium is considered a first-line alternative for the treatment of bipolar disorder during pregnancy. However, often women chose to discontinue psychotropic medications before or during pregnancy. Viguera and colleagues (2000) demonstrated that postpartum women with bipolar disorder who had discontinued lithium during pregnancy were more likely to experience a relapse after lithium discontinuation compared to controls matched for time after lithium discontinuation. Therefore though it is recommended to continue lithium in the postpartum period, the American Academy of Pediatrics has determined that lithium use is contraindicated during breastfeeding. As reviewed by Chaudron and Jefferson (2000), lithium is passed on to a breastfeeding infant and is found in breastmilk and infant serum. Recent reviews of the literature reveal reports of 13 infants exposed to lithium in breastmilk; four experienced no adverse effects; clinical status not reported for eight; and one infant who was exposed both in utero and breastfeeding had serious adverse reactions, including cyanosis, heart murmur, and hypotonia (Burt et al. 2001, Tunnessen and Hertz 1972).

It is important to take into consideration the welfare of both the developing fetus and the mother in treating pregnant women with bipolar disorder, therefore verapamil and omega-3 fatty acids may also offer a relatively safe alternative during pregnancy. Wisner and colleagues (2002) included pregnant women in their open-label trial of verapamil for the treatment of bipolar disorder. The use of verapamil for hypertension, arrhythmias, and migraine headaches has been studied prospectively in pregnancy, and no risks of major malformations have been observed with its use compared with a control group (Magee et al. 1996). Two cases have been published in which low levels of exposure to the drug by breastfeeding infants of mothers treated with verapamil were confirmed by low infant sera levels (Andersen 1983), and the American Academy of Pediatrics (1994) has deemed verapamil compatible with breastfeeding. Also, in one double-blind study, omega-3 fatty acids were demonstrated to be efficacious in prevention of mood episodes in patients with bipolar disorder (Stoll et al. 1999). If their efficacy can be established, omega-3 fatty acids could be an ideal treatment for use in pregnancy and lactation, as they are already established as safe in pregnancy and are necessary for the baby's brain and retinal development (Olsen et al. 1992).

## Nonpharmacological Approaches

### Electroconvulsive Therapy
Although the evidence that prophylactic ECT is beneficial in bipolar disorder is limited to anecdotal reports and the results from one open clinical trial (Stevenson and Geoghegan 1951), some psychiatrists use this approach (Husain et al. 1993, Abrams 1990, Kellner et al. 1990). Systematic, controlled studies are needed to fully assess this form of maintenance therapy, but in some patients who do not respond satisfactorily to medications, it could be considered a late treatment option for preventing or attenuating future episodes.

### Psychotherapy
Probably 25 to 50% of bipolar patients fail to comply with medication regimens (Prien and Potter 1990). Psychosocial intervention, as an adjunct to pharmacotherapy, may increase medication compliance, reduce the frequency and length of hospitalization, and increase family and social functioning for patients with bipolar disorder.

In a small pilot study, 24 bipolar patients and their families were tested for family functioning and then observed for 5 years (Miller et al. 1991). Patients in families with high levels of dysfunction had more than twice the rate of rehospitalizations as those in families with low levels of dysfunction. In a follow-up study by the same investigators, 14 bipolar patients and their families were randomly assigned to receive standard treatment (pharmacotherapy and clinical management) or standard treatment and family therapy (Miller et al. 1991). During the 18-week treatment phase, 56% of the patients in the family treatment group met criteria for a full recovery compared with 20% of the patients in the standard treatment group. At 2-year follow-up, patients receiving standard treatment had been rehospitalized twice as often as the patients who had received family therapy.

Another study comparing family intervention with standard treatment found that significantly fewer patients who had been in family therapy were rehospitalized at 18 months of follow-up compared with those who had received only standard treatment (Glick et al. 1985). The patients in family therapy also functioned better in work and social roles. Of nine patients who received behavioral family management in addition to pharmacological treatment in another study, only one relapsed in the 9-month posthospitalization treatment period compared with 14 of 23 patients who did not receive family therapy (Miklowitz and Goldstein 1990).

Couples, group, and individual therapies have also demonstrated benefit in small studies. Twelve lithium-treated bipolar patients who underwent couples therapy four times a week had no rehospitalizations and no marital failures at follow-up (Davenport et al. 1977). In contrast, 18 of 53 patients who received only medication management had been rehospitalized, 15 had suffered marital failures, and 3 had committed suicide. Another study found that 15 bipolar patients with long histories of noncompliance with lithium therapy had a markedly reduced rate of relapse during and after a group therapy program integrated with lithium treatment (Shakir et al. 1979).

In a study of individual therapy, 26 bipolar patients maintained with lithium were randomly assigned to cognitive intervention or standard clinical care (Cochran 1984). Cognitive intervention produced slightly better compliance at the end of treatment, and at 6-month follow-up, therapy patients were significantly less likely to have major adherence problems, discontinue lithium against medical advice, have episodes brought on by not taking lithium, or be hospitalized.

In a study by Frank and colleagues (2000), they have investigated interpersonal and social rhythm therapy as an adjunct to prophylactic medication treatment. Primary foci included learning better coping strategies in order to regulate their daily lives, interpersonal problems, and medication compliance. It specifically looked at modulating biological and psychosocial factors in order to avoid circadian vulnerabilities, improve functioning, and better manage bipolar disorder symptoms.

## Conclusion
Whether or not a bipolar patient is engaged in formal psychotherapy, several elements are essential in the relationship between patient and psychiatrist. As in all physician–patient encounters, the relationship must be based on mutual respect, built during a period of work together. Of course, psychiatrists treating patients with bipolar disorder should be knowledgeable about the disease, its many manifestations, and the nuances of treatment.

Particularly early in the course of their illness, bipolar patients, like patients with many medical diseases, try to deny this unwanted presence in their lives. Working with a patient to accept a chronic disease is similar to assisting someone in the grieving process. Life is not as they had wished or imagined. Psychiatrists are powerless to alter the presence of disease but can assure the patient that they will be there for the long haul, offering concern, caring, and expertise.

Enlisting the patient and family members (or significant others) in a knowledgeable working alliance is also essential. Patients and their loved ones should learn to recognize prodromal signs of relapse and know what to do when they appear. They should similarly become knowledgeable about the medicines and their untoward effects, interactions, and prohibitions. Patients and family members can also learn what kind of daily routine will be most helpful for the patient during the long-term management of bipolar disorder. Sleep loss, for example, appears to be disruptive. Thus, it is best to avoid travel, work schedules, and other events that involve disruptions in sleep schedules. Spontaneous sleeplessness should be treated as a prodrome and addressed quickly and vigorously with the psychiatrist. Patients and people close to them can learn to deal better with role frictions and interpersonal stresses. "Letting it all hang out" and confrontational approaches do not tend to be optimal for patients with this condition. Drugs and alcohol are an ever-present hazard, and patients must be urged to view them as such.

In many ways, the relationship between the psychiatrist and patient with bipolar disorder is similar to all long-term relationships. If it is based on mutual trust and respect, it deepens and becomes richer through the years. Even as the feelings of elation begin to spiral, the patient with long-standing trust in his or her psychiatrist may come to trust the physician's recommendation for medication, time out, or hospitalization. Some patients with bipolar disorder are severely impaired and respond poorly to treatment—perhaps because of genetic factors, or possibly because of comorbidities, such as substance abuse. Fortunately, many can be among the most gratifying to treat. With available therapies and "a little bit of luck" many can lead productive and satisfying lives.

## References

Abrams R (1990) ECT as prophylactic treatment for bipolar disorder. Am J Psychiatr 147, 373–374.

Abrams R, Swartz CM, and Vedak C (1991) Antidepressant effects of high-dose right unilateral electroconvulsive therapy. Arch Gen Psychiatr 48, 746–748.

Altshuler L, Kiriakos L, Calcagno J, et al. (2001) The impact of antidepressant discontinuation versus antidepressant continuation on a 1-year risk for relapse of bipolar depression: A retrospective chart review. J Clin Psychiatr 62, 612–616.

American Academy of Pediatrics (1994) The transfer of drugs and other chemicals into human milk. Pediatrics 93, 137–150.

American Medical Association (1993) Drug Evaluations Subscription, Vol. 1. American Medical Association, Chicago.

Anand A, Oren DA, Berman A, et al. (1999) Lamotrigine treatment of lithium failure outpatient mania: A double-blind placebo-controlled trial. Presented at the Third International Conference on Bipolar Disorder, Pittsburgh, PA.

Andersen HJ (1983) Excretion of verapamil in human milk. Eur J Clin Pharmacol 25, 279–280.

Angst J (1978) The course of affective disorder. II. Typology of bipolar manic depressive illness. Arch Psychiatr Nervenkr 226, 65–73.

Baraban JM (1994) Toward a crystal-clear view of lithium's site of action. Proc Natl Acad Sci USA 91, 5738–5739.

Bauer MS and Whybrow PC (1990a) Rapid cycling bipolar affective disorder. I. Association with grade I hypothyroidism. Arch Gen Psychiatr 47, 427–432.

Bauer MS and Whybrow PC (1990b) Rapid cycling bipolar affective disorder. II. Treatment of refractory rapid cycling with high-dose levothyroxine: A preliminary study. Arch Gen Psychiatr 47, 435–440.

Beasley CM, Satterlee TSW, Tollefson G, et al. (1996) Olanzapine versus placebo: Results of a double-blind, fixed-dose olanzapine trial. Psychopharmacology 124, 159–167.

Benjamin J and Zohar J (1992) Sleep deprivation in rapid-cycling bipolar affective disorder: Case report. Eur Neuropsychopharmacol 2, 463–465.

Berck M, Ichim L, and Brook S (1999) Olanzapine compared with lithium in mania: A double-blind, randomized, controlled trial. Int Clin Psychopharmacol 14, 339–343.

Berk M (1999) Lamotrigine and the treatment of mania in bipolar disorder. Eur Neuropsychopharmacol 9(Suppl 4), S119–S123.

Biederman J, Lerner Y, and Belmaker RH (1979) Combination of lithium carbonate and haloperidol in schizo-affective disorder. Arch Gen Psychiatr 36, 327–333.

Bowden C, Calabrese JR, Asher J, et al. (2000a) Spectrum of efficacy of lamotrigine in bipolar disorder: Overview of double-blind placebo-controlled studies. Presented at the American College of Neuropsychopharmacolgy, 39th Annual Meeting, San Juan, Puerto Rico.

Bowden C, Calabrese JR, DeVeaugh-Geiss J, et al. (2001) Lamotrigine demonstrates long-term evidence for mood stabilization in bipolar I depression. Presented at the American College of Neuropsychopharmacolgy, 40th Annual Meeting, Waikaloa, Hawaii.

Bowden CL, Brugger AM, Swann AC, et al. (1994) Efficacy of divalproex versus lithium and placebo in the treatment of mania. JAMA 271, 918–924.

Bowden CL, Calabrese JR, McElroy SL, et al. (2000b) A randomized, placebo-controlled 12-month trial of divalproex and lithium in treatment of outpatients with bipolar I disorder. Arch Gen Psychiatr 57, 481–492.

Brown ES, Dilsaver SC, Shoaib AM, et al. (1994) Depressive mania: Response of residual depression to bupropion. Biol Psychiatr 35, 493–494.

Brunet G, Cerlich B, Robert P, et al. (1990) Open trial of a calcium antagonist, nimodipine, in acute mania. Clin Neuropharmacol 13, 224–228.

Burt VK, Suri R, Altshuler L, et al. (2001) The use of psychotropic medications during breast-feeding. Am J Psychiatr 158, 1001–1009.

Cade JFJ (1949) Lithium salts in the treatment of psychotic excitement. Med J Austral 11, 349–352.

Calabrese JR and Delucchi GA (1990) Spectrum of efficacy of valproate in 55 patients with rapid-cycling bipolar disorder. Am J Psychiatr 147, 431–434.

Calabrese JR, Bowden C, DeVeaugh-Geiss J, et al. (2001a) Lamotrigine demonstrates long term mood stabilization in recently manic patients. Presented at the American Psychiatric Association Annual Meeting, New Orleans, Louisiana.

Calabrese JR, Bowden CL, Sachs GS, et al. (1999) A double-blind placebo-controlled study of lamotrigine monotherapy in outpatients with bipolar I depression. Lamictal 602 study group. J Clin Psychiatr 60, 79–88.

Calabrese JR, Keck PE Jr., McElroy Sl, et al. (2001b) A pilot study of topiramate as monotherapy in the treatment of acute mania. J Clin Psychopharmacol 21, 340–342.

Calabrese JR, Meltzer HY, and Markovitz PJ (1991) Clozapine prophylaxis in rapid cycling bipolar disorder. J Clin Psychopharmacol 11, 396–397.

Calabrese JR, Rapport DJ, Kimmel SE, et al. (1993a) Rapid cycling bipolar disorder and its treatment with valproate. Can J Psychiatr 38(Suppl 2), S57–S61.

Calabrese JR, Suppes T, Bowden CL, et al. (2000) A double-blind, placebo-controlled, prophylaxis study of lamotrigine in rapid-cycling disorder. Lamictal 614 study group. J Clin Psychiatr 61, 841–850.

Calabrese JR, Woyshville MJ, Kimmel SE, et al. (1993b) Mixed states and bipolar rapid cycling and their treatment with divalproex sodium. Psychiatr Ann 23, 70–78.

Casey DE (1989) Clozapine: Neuroleptic-induced EPS and tardive dyskinesia. Psychopharmacology 99, S47–S53.

Chaudron LH and Jefferson JW (2000) Mood stabilizers during breastfeeding: A review. Found 11 cases of lithium use in breastfeeding infants. J Clin Psychiatr 61, 79–90.

Chengappa KNR, Gershon S, and Levine J (2001) The evolving role of topiramate among other mood stabilizers in the management of bipolar disorder. Bipolar Disord 3, 215–232.

Chou JCY (1991) Recent advances in treatment of acute mania. J Clin Psychopharmacol 11, 3–21.

Chouinard G (1987) Clonazepam in acute and maintenance treatment of bipolar affective disorder. J Clin Psychiatr 48(Suppl 10), S29–S36.

Cochran SD (1984) Preventing medical noncompliance in the outpatient treatment of bipolar affective disorders. J Consult Clin Psychol 52, 873–878.

Cohen JB, Collins G, Ashbrook E, et al. (1989) A comparison of fluoxetine, imipramine and placebo in patients with bipolar depressive disorder. Int Clin Psychopharmacol 4, 313–322.

Cohen LS and Rosenbaum JF (1998) Psychotropic use during pregnancy: Weighing the risks. J Clin Psychiatr 59, 18–28.

Cohen LS, Friedman JM, Jefferson JW, et al. (1994) A reevaluation of risk of in utero exposure to lithium. JAMA 271, 146–150.

Cookson J, Silverstone T, and Wells B (1981) Double-blind comparative clinical trial of pimozide and chlorpromazine in mania. Acta Psychiatr Scand 64, 381–397.

Cowdry RW, Wehr TA, Zis AP, et al. (1983) Thyroid abnormalities associated with rapid cycling bipolar illness. Arch Gen Psychiatr 40, 414–420.

Coxhead N, Silverstone T, and Cookson J (1992) Carbamazepine versus lithium in the prophylaxis of bipolar affective disorder. Acta Psychiatr Scand 85, 114–118.

Davenport YB, Ebert MH, Adland ML, et al. (1977) Couples group therapy as an adjunct to lithium maintenance of the manic patient. Am J Orthopsychiatr 47, 495–502.

De Beaurepaire R (1992) Treatment of neuroleptic-resistant mania and schizoaffective disorders. Am J Psychiatr 149, 1614–1615.

di Costanzo E and Schifano F (1991) Lithium alone or in combination with carbamazepine for the treatment of rapid-cycling bipolar affective disorder. Acta Psychiatr Scand 83, 456–459.

Dilsaver SC, Swann AC, Shoaib AM, et al. (1993) Depressive mania associated with nonresponse to antimanic agents. Am J Psychiatr 150, 1548–1551.

Dubovsky SL, Franks RD, Allen S, et al. (1986) Calcium antagonists in mania: A double-blind study of verapamil. Psychiatr Res 18, 309–320.

Dunner DL and Fieve RR (1974) Clinical factors in lithium carbonate prophylaxis failure. Arch Gen Psychiatr 30, 229–233.

Dunner DL, Patrick V, and Fieve R (1977) Rapid cycling manic depressive patients. Compr Psychiatr 18, 561–566.

Edwards R, Stephenson U, and Flewett T(1991) Clonazepam in acute mania: A double blind trial. Austral N Z J Psychiatr 25, 238–242.

Emrich HM, Dose M, and Von Zerssen D (1985) The use of sodium valproate, carbamazepine and oxcarbazepine in patients with affective disorder. J Affect Disord 8, 243–250.

Erfurth A, Kammerer C, Grunze H, et al. (1998) An open label study of gabapentin in the treatment of acute mania. J Psychiatr Res 32, 261–264.

Faedda GL, Tondo L, Baldessarini RJ, et al. (1993) Outcome after rapid versus gradual discontinuation of lithium treatment in bipolar disorders. Arch Gen Psychiatr 50, 448–455.

Fertig MK, Brooks VG, Shelton PS, et al. (1998) Hyperglycemia associated with olanzapine. J Clin Psychiatr 59, 687–689.

Frank E, Swartz HA, and Kupfer DJ (2000) Interpersonal and social rhythm therapy: Managing the chaos of bipolar disorder. Soc Biol Psychiatr 48, 593–604.

Freeman TW, Clothier JL, Pazzaglia P, et al. (1992) A double-blind comparison of valproate and lithium in the treatment of acute mania. Am J Psychiatr 149, 108–111.

Frye MA, Ketter TA, Kimbrell TA, et al. (2000) A placebo-controlled study of lamotrigine and gabapentin monotherapy in refractory mood disorders. J Clin Psychopharmacol 20, 607–614.

Garfinkel PE, Stancer HC, and Persad E (1980) A comparison of haloperidol, lithium carbonate, and their combination in the treatment of mania. J Affect Disord 2, 270–288.

Garza-Treviño ES, Overall JE, and Hollister LE (1992) Verapamil versus lithium in acute mania. Am J Psychiatr 149, 121–122.

Gatta B, Rigalleau V, and GinH (1999) Diabetic ketoacidosis with olanzapine treatment. Diabet Care 22, 1002–1003.

Gelenberg AJ (2001) Approaches to olanzapine-induced weight gain. Biol Ther Psychiatr 24(11), 41–42.

Gelenberg AJ and Hopkins HS (1993) Report on efficacy of treatments for bipolar disorder. Psychopharmacol Bull 29, 447–456.

Gelenberg AJ and Jefferson JW (1994) Lithium tremor. J Clin Psychiatr 56, 283–287.

Gelenberg AJ, Kane JM, Keller MB, et al. (1989) Comparison of standard and low serum levels of lithium for maintenance treatment of bipolar disorder. N Engl J Med 321, 1489–1493.

Ghaemi SN, Katzow JJ, Desai SP, et al. (1998) Gabapentin treatment of mood disorders: A preliminary study. J Clin Psychiatr 59, 426.

Giannini AJ, Houser WL Jr., Loiselle RH, et al. (1984) Antimanic effects of verapamil. Am J Psychiatr 141, 1602–1603.

Glick ID, Clarkin JF, Spencer JH, et al. (1985) A controlled evaluation of inpatient family intervention: Preliminary results of the six-month follow-up. Arch Gen Psychiatr 42, 882–886.

Goldstein LE, Sporn J, Brown S, et al. (1999) New-onset diabetes mellitus and diabetic ketoacidosis associated with olanzapine treatment. Psychosomatics 40, 438–443.

Goodwin FK and Jamison K (1990) Manic–Depressive Illness. Oxford University Press, New York.

Grossi E, Sacchetti E, Vita A, et al. (1984) Carbamazepine versus chlorpromazine in mania: A double-blind trial. In Anticonvulsants in Affective Disorders, Emrich HM, Okuma T, and Muller AA (eds). Excerpta Medica, Amsterdam, pp. 177–187.

Grunze H, Erfurth A, Marcuse A, et al. (1999) Tiagabine appears not to be efficacious in the treatment of acute mania. J Clin Psychiatr 60, 759–762.

Grunze HC, Normann C, Langosch J, et al. (2001) Antimanic efficacy of topiramate in 11 patients in an open clinical trial with and of off–on design. J Clin Psychiatr 62, 464–468.

Hayes SG (1993) Barbiturate anticonvulsants in refractory affective disorders. Ann Clin Psychiatr 5, 35–44.

Hayes SG and Goldsmith BK (1991) Psychosensory symptomatology in anticonvulsant-responsive psychiatric illness. Ann Clin Psychiatr 3, 27–35.

Himmelhoch JM, Mulla D, Neil JF, et al. (1976) Incidence and significance of mixed affective states in a bipolar population. Arch Gen Psychiatr 33, 1062–1066.

Himmelhoch JM, Thase ME, Mallinger AG, et al. (1991) Tranylcypromine versus imipramine in anergic bipolar depression. Am J Psychiatr 148, 910–916.

Hirschfeld RMA, Bowden CL, Gitlin MJ, et al. (2002) Practice guideline for the treatment of patients with bipolar disorder (Revision). 159(4), 1–50.

Höschl C and Kozen J (1989) Verapamil in affective disorders: A controlled, double-blind study. Biol Psychiatr 25, 128–140.

Husain MM, Meyer DE, Muttakin MH, et al. (1993) Maintenance ECT for treatment of recurrent mania. Am J Psychiatr 150, 985.

Jacobsen FM (1993) Low-dose valproate: A new treatment for cyclothymia, mild rapid cycling disorders, and premenstrual syndrome. J Clin Psychiatr 54, 229–234.

Jamison KR (1993) Touched with Fire. Manic–Depressive Illness and the Artistic Temperament. Free Press, New York.

Janicak PG, Davis JM, Preskorn SH, et al. (1993) Principles and Practice of Psychopharmacotherapy. Williams & Wilkins, Baltimore.

Janicak PG, Sharma RP, Pandey G, et al. (1998) Verapamil for the treatment of acute mania: A double-blind, placebo-controlled trial. Am J Psychiatr 155, 972–973.

Johnson G, Gershon S, and Hekimian LJ (1968) Controlled evaluation of lithium and chlorpromazine in the treatment of manic states: An interim report. Compr Psychiatr 9, 563–573.

Johnson G, Gershon S, Burdock EI, et al. (1971) Comparative effects of lithium and chlorpromazine in the treatment of acute manic states. Br J Psychiatr 119, 267–276.

Johnstone EC, Crow TJ, Frith CD, et al. (1988) The Northwick Park "functional" psychosis study: Diagnosis and treatment response. Lancet 2, 119–125.

Johnstone EC, Owens DGC, Lambert MT, et al. (1990) Combination tricyclic antidepressant and lithium maintenance medication in unipolar and bipolar depressed patients. J Affect Disord 20, 225–233.

Joyce PR (1988) Carbamazepine in rapid cycling bipolar affective disorder. Int Clin Psychopharmacol 3, 123–129.

Keck PE Jr., McElroy SL, and Nemeroff CB (1992a) Anticonvulsants in the treatment of bipolar disorder. J Neuropsychiatr Clin Neurosci 4, 395–405.

Keck PE, McElroy SL, Vuckovic A, et al. (1992b) Combined valproate and carbamazepine treatment of bipolar disorder. J Neuropsychiatr Clin Neurosci 4, 319–322.

Keck PE Jr., McElroy SL, Tugrul KC, et al. (1993) Valproate oral loading in the treatment of acute mania. J Clin Psychiatr 54, 305–308.

Keller MB, Lavori PW, Coryell W, et al. (1986) Differential outcome of pure manic, mixed/cycling, and pure depressive episodes in patients with bipolar illness. JAMA 255, 3138–3142.

Keller MB, Lavori PW, Kane JM, et al. (1992) Subsyndromal symptoms in bipolar disorder: A comparison of standard and low serum levels of lithium. Arch Gen Psychiatr 49, 371–376.

Kellner C, Batterson JR, and Monroe R (1990) ECT as an alternative to lithium for preventive treatment of bipolar disorder. Am J Psychiatr 147, 953.

Khaw, KT, Wareham N, Luben R, et al. (2001) Glycated haemoglobin, diabetes, and mortality in men in Norfolk cohort of European Prospective Investigation of Cancer and Nutrition (EPIC-Norfolk). BMJ, 322, 15.

Kingsbury SJ and Salzman C (1993) Lithium's role in hyperparathyroidism and hypercalcemia. Hosp Comm Psychiatry 44, 1047–1048.

Kinon BJ, Basson BR, Gilmore JA, et al. (2001) Long-term olanzapine treatment: Weight change and weight related health factors in schizophrenia. J Clin Psychiatr 62, 92–100.

Knaba S, Yagi G, Kamijima K, et al. (1994) The first open study of zonisamide, a novel anticonvulsant, shows efficacy in mania. Prog Neuropsychopharmacol Biol Psychiatr 18, 707–715.

Kramlinger KG and Post RM (1990) Addition of lithium carbonate to carbamazepine: Hematological and thyroid effects. Am J Psychiatr 147, 615–620.

Kukopulos A, Reginaldi P, Laddomada P, et al. (1980) Course of the manic depressive cycle and changes caused by treatments. Pharmacopsychiatr Neuro Psychopharmacol 13, 156–167.

Kupfer DJ, Chengappa KNR, Gelenberg AJ, et al. (2001) Citalopram as adjunctive therapy in bipolar depression. J Clin Psychiatr 62, 12.

Kusalic M (1992) Grade II and grade III hypothyroidism in rapid-cycling bipolar patients. Biol Psychiatr 25, 177–181.

Lerer B, Moore N, Meyendorff E, et al. (1987) Carbamazepine versus lithium in mania: A double-blind study. J Clin Psychiatr 48, 89–93.

Lindenmayer JP and Patel R (1999) Olanzapine-induced ketoacidosis with diabetes mellitus. Am J Psychiatr 156, 1471.

Llewellyn A, Stowe ZN, and Strader JR (1998) The use of lithium and management of women with bipolar disorder during pregnancy and lactation. J Clin Psychiatr 59, 57–64.

Magee LA, Schick B, Donnenfeld AE, et al. (1996) The safety of calcium channel blockers in human pregnancy: A prospective multicenter study. Am J Obstet Gynecol 174, 823–828.

Manji HK, Chen G, Shimon H, et al. (1995a) Guanine nucleotide-binding proteins in bipolar affective disorder: Effects of long-term lithium treatment. Arch Gen Psychiatr 52, 135–144.

Manji HK, Potter WZ, and Lenox RH (1995b) Signal transduction pathways: Molecular targets for lithium's actions. Arch Gen Psychiatr 52, 531–543.

McElroy SL, Dessain EC, Pope HG Jr., et al. (1991) Clozapine in the treatment of psychotic mood disorders, schizoaffective disorder, and schizophrenia. J Clin Psychiatr 52, 411–414.

McElroy SL, Keck PE, Pope HG, et al. (1988) Valproate in the treatment of rapid-cycling bipolar disorder. J Clin Psychopharmacol 8, 275–279.

McElroy SL, Keck PE, Pope HG, et al. (1989) Valproate in psychiatric disorders: Literature review and clinical guidelines. J Clin Psychiatr 50(Suppl 3), S23–S29.

McElroy SL, Keck PE Jr., Pope HG Jr., et al. (1992) Valproate in the treatment of bipolar disorders: Literature review and clinical guidelines. J Clin Psychopharmacol 12(Suppl 1), S42–S52.

McKeon P, Manley P, and Swanwick G (1992) Manic–depressive illness. II. Treatment outcome and bipolar disorder subtypes. Ir J Psychol Med 9, 9–12.

Meehan M, Zhang F, David S, et al. (2001) A double-blind, randomized comparison of the efficacy and safety of intramuscular injections of olanzapine, lorazepam, or placebo in treating acutely agitated patients diagnosed with bipolar mania. J Clin Psychopharmacol 21, 389–397.

Melkersson KI, Hulting AL, and Brismar KE (2000) Elevated levels of insulin, leptin, and blood lipids in olanzapine-treated patients with schizophrenia or related psychoses. J Clin Psychiatr 61, 742–749.

Meltzer HY (1992) The Mechanism of Action of Clozapine in Relation to its Clinical Advantages. Raven Press, New York, pp. 1–13.

Miklowitz DJ and Goldstein MJ (1990) Behavioral family treatment for patients with bipolar affective disorder. Behav Modif 4, 457–489.

Miller IW, Keitner GI, Epstein NB, et al. (1991) Families of bipolar patients: Dysfunction, course of illness, and pilot treatment study. Presented at the Meeting of the Association for the Advancement of Behavior Therapy, New York, NY.

Moore NA, Calligaro DC, Wong DT, et al. (1993) The pharmacology of olanzapine and other new antipsychotic agents. Curr Opin Invest Drugs 2, 281–293.

Mukherjee S, Sackeim HA, and Schnur DB (1994) Electroconvulsive therapy of acute manic episodes: A review of 50 years' experience. Am J Psychiatr 151, 169–176.

Muller AA and Stoll KD (1984) Carbamazepine and oxcarbazepine in the treatment of manic syndromes: Studies in Germany. In Anticonvulsants in Affective Disorders, Emrich HM, Okuma T, and Muller AA (eds). Excepta Medica, Amsterdam, The Netherlands, pp. 139–147.

Ober SK, Hudak R, and Rusterholtz A (1999) Hyperglycemia and olanzapine. Am J Psychiatr 156, 970.

Okuma T (1993) Effects of carbamazepine and lithium on affective disorders. Neuropsychobiology 2, 138–145.

Okuma T, Inanaga K, Otsuki S, et al. (1979) Comparison of the antimanic efficacy of carbamazepine and chlorpromazine: A double-blind controlled study. Psychopharmacology (Berl) 66, 211–217.

Okuma T, Inanaga K, Otsuki S, et al. (1981) A preliminary double-blind study of the efficacy of carbamazepine in prophylaxis of manic–depressive illness. Psychopharmacology (Berl) 73, 95–96.

Olsen SF, Sorensen JD, Secher NJ, et al. (1992) Randomised controlled trial of effect of fish oil supplementation on pregnancy duration. Lancet 339, 1003–1004.

Osser DN, Najarian DM, and Dufresne RL (1999) Olanzapine increases weight and serum triglyceride levels. J Clin Psychiatr 60, 767–770.

Pande AC, Crockatt JG, Janney CA, et al. (2000) Gabapentin in bipolar disorder: A placebo controlled trial of adjunctive therapy. Bipolar Disord 2(3), 249–255.

Parry BL (1989) Reproductive factors affecting the course of affective illness in women. Psychiatr Clin N Am 12, 207–220.

Peselow ED, Fieve RR, Difiglia C, et al. (1994) Lithium prophylaxis of bipolar illness: The value of combination treatment. Br J Psychiatr 164, 208–214.

Pettinati HM (1994) Speed of ECT? Convuls Ther 10, 69–72.

Platman SR (1970) A comparison of lithium carbonate and chlorpromazine in mania. Am J Psychiatr 127, 351–353.

Pollack SJ, Atack JR, Knowles MR, et al. (1994) Mechanism of inositol monophosphatase, the putative target of lithium therapy. Proc Natl Acad Sci USA 91, 5766–5770.

Pope HG, McElroy SL, Keck PE, et al. (1991) Valproate in the treatment of acute mania: A placebo-controlled study. Arch Gen Psychiatr 48, 62–68.

Post RM, Jimerson DC, Bunney WE, et al. (1980) Dopamine and mania: Behavioral and biochemical effects of the dopamine receptor blocker pimozide. Psychopharmacology (Berl) 67, 297–305.

Post RM, Uhde TW, Roy-Byrne PP, et al. (1987) Correlates of antimanic response to carbamazepine. Psychiatr Res 21, 71–83.

Price LH and Heninger GR (1994) Lithium in the treatment of mood disorders. N Engl J Med 331, 591–598.

Price WA and DiMarzio L (1986) Premenstrual tension syndrome in rapid-cycling bipolar affective disorder. J Clin Psychiatr 47, 415–417.

Prien RF and Potter WZ (1990) NIMH workshop report on treatment of bipolar disorder. Psychopharmacol Bull 26, 409–427.

Prien RF, Caffey EM, and Klett CJ (1972) Comparison of lithium carbonate and chlorpromazine in the treatment of mania. Arch Gen Psychiatr 26, 146–153.

Prien RF, Kupfer DJ, Mansky PA, et al. (1984) Drug therapy in the prevention of recurrences in unipolar and bipolar affective disorders. Arch Gen Psychiatr 41, 1096–1104.

Privitera MR, Lamberti JS, and Maharaj K (1993) Clozapine in a bipolar depressed patient. Am J Psychiatr 150, 986.

Quitkin FM, Kane J, Rifkin A, et al. (1981) Prophylactic lithium carbonate with and without imipramine for bipolar I patients: A double-blind study. Arch Gen Psychiatr 38, 902–907.

Roy-Byrne PP, Joffe RT, Uhde TW, et al. (1984) Approaches to the evaluation and treatment of rapid-cycling affective illness. Br J Psychiatr 145, 543–550.

Sachs GS (1989) Adjuncts and alternatives to lithium therapy for bipolar affective disorder. J Clin Psychiatr 50(Suppl 12), S31–S39.

Sachs GS and Ghaemi SN (2000) Efficacy and tolerability of risperidone versus placebo in combination with lithium or valproate in acute mania. Eur Neuropsychopharmacol 10(Suppl 3), S240.

Sachs GS, Lafer B, Stoll AL, et al. (1994) A double-blind trial of buproprion versus desipramine for bipolar depression. J Clin Psychiatr 55, 391–393.

Sachs GS, Rosenbaum JF, and Jones L (1990a) Adjunctive clonazepam for maintenance treatment of bipolar affective disorder. J Clin Psychopharmacol 10, 42–47.

Sachs GS, Weilburg JB, and Rosenbaum JF (1990b) Clonazepam versus neuroleptics as adjuncts to lithium maintenance. Psychopharmacol Bull 26, 137–143.

Sackeim HA, Prudic J, Devanand DP, et al. (1993) Effects of stimulus intensity and electrode placement on the efficacy and cognitive effects of electroconvulsive therapy. N Engl J Med 328, 839–846.

Sanger TM, Grundy SL, Gibson PJ, et al. (2001) Long-term olanzapine therapy in the treatment of bipolar I disorder: An open-label continuation phase study. J Clin Psychiatr 62, 273–281.

Segal J, Berk M, and Brook S (1998) Risperidone compared with both lithium and haloperidol in mania: A double-blind, randomized, controlled trial. Clin Neuropharmacol 21, 176–180.

Sernyak MJ and Woods SW (1993) Chronic neuroleptic use in manic–depressive illness. Psychopharmacol Bull 29, 375–381.

Sernyak MJ, Griffin RA, Johnson RM, et al. (1994) Neuroleptic exposure following inpatient treatment of acute mania with lithium and neuroleptic. Am J Psychiatr 151, 133–135.

Shakir SA, Volkmar FR, Bacon S, et al. (1979) Group psychotherapy as an adjunct to lithium maintenance. Am J Psychiatr 136, 455–456.

Sharma V and Persad E (1992) Augmentation of valproate with lithium in a case of rapid cycling affective disorder. Can J Psychiatr 37, 584–585.

Sharma V, Persad E, Mazmanian D, et al. (1993) Treatment of rapid cycling bipolar disorder with combination therapy of valproate and lithium. Can J Psychiatr 38, 137–139.

Shopsin B, Gershon S, Thompson H, et al. (1975) Psychoactive drugs in mania: A controlled comparison of lithium carbonate, chlorpromazine, and haloperidol. Arch Gen Psychiatr 32, 34–42.

Small JG, Klapper MH, Kellams JJ, et al. (1988) Electroconvulsive treatment compared with lithium in the management of manic states. Arch Gen Psychiatr 45, 727–732.

Small JG, Klapper MH, Milstein V, et al. (1991) Carbamazepine compared with lithium in the treatment of mania. Arch Gen Psychiatr 48, 915–921.

Snorrason E and Stefansson JG (1991) Galanthamine hydrobromide in mania. Lancet 337, 557.

Souza FGM, Mander AJ, Foggo M, et al. (1991) The effects of lithium discontinuation and the non-effect of oral inositol upon thyroid hormones and cortisol in patients with bipolar affective disorder. J Affect Disord 22, 165–170.

Sovner R (1991) Divalproex-responsive rapid cycling bipolar disorder in a patient with Down's syndrome: Implications for the Down's syndrome–mania hypothesis. J Ment Def Res 35, 171–173.

Spring G, Schweid D, and Gray L (1970) A double-blind comparison of lithium and chlorpromazine in the treatment of manic states. Am J Psychiatr 126, 1306–1310.

Stevenson GH and Geoghegan JJ (1951) Prophylactic electroshock: A 5-year study. Am J Psychiatr 107, 743–748.

Stoll AL, Severus WE, Freeman MP, et al. (1999) Omega-3 fatty acids in bipolar disorder: A double-blind placebo-controlled trial. Arch Gen Psychiatr 56, 407–412.

Stoll AL, Vuckovic A, and McElroy SL (1991) Histamine 2-receptor antagonists for the treatment of valproate-induced gastrointestinal distress. Ann Clin Psychiatr 3, 301–304.

Suppes T, McElroy SL, Gilbert J, et al. (1992) Clozapine in the treatment of dysphoric mania. Biol Psychiatr 32, 270–280.

Suppes T, Webb A, Paul B, et al. (1999) Clinical outcome in a randomized 1-year trial of cloazpine versus treatment and usual for patients with treatment-resistant illness and a history of mania. Am J Psychiatr 156, 1164–1169.

Takahashi R, Sakuma A, and Itoh K (1975) Comparison of efficacy of lithium carbonate and chlorpromazine in mania. Arch Gen Psychiatr 32, 1310–1318.

Tohen M, Baker RW, Altshuler LA, et al. (2002) Olanzapine versus divalproex for the treatment of acute mania. Am J Psychiatr.

Tohen M, Jacobs TG, Grundy SL, et al. (2000) Efficacy of olanzapine in acute bipolar mania: A double-blind, placebo-controlled study. Arch Gen Psychiatr 57, 841–849.

Tohen M, Sanger TM, McElroy SL, et al. (1999) Olanzapine versus placebo in the treatment of acute mania. Am J Psychiatr 156(5), 702–709.

Tunnessen WW and Hertz CG (1972) Toxic effects of lithium in newborn infants: A commentary. J Pediatr 81, 804–807.

USP DI (1995) Drug Information for the Health Care Professional, Vol. 1. United States Pharmacopeial Convention, Rockville, MD, p. 2749.

Van Berkestijn H, van der Meulen LMH, Flentge F, et al. (1990) RS 86 in manic disorder. Biol Psychiatr 27, 109–112.

Vestergaard P and Schou M (1988) Prospective studies on a lithium cohort. Acta Psychiatr Scand 78, 421–426.

Viguera AC, Nonacs R, Cohen LS, et al. (2000) Risk of recurrence of bipolar disorder in pregnant and nonpregnant women after discontinuing lithium maintenance. Am J Psychiatr 157, 179–184.

Von Hayek DV, Huttl V, Reiss J, et al. (1999) Hyperglycemia and ketoacidosis under olanzapine. Nervenarzt 70, 836–837.

Walker RG (1993) Lithium nephrotoxicity. Kidney Int 44(Suppl 42), 93–98.

Walton SA, Berk M, and Brook S (1996) Superiority of lithium over verapamil in mania: A randomized controlled, single-blind trial. J Clin Psychiatr 57, 543–546.

Ward ME, Musa MN, and Bailey L (1994) Clinical pharmacokinetics of lithium. J Clin Pharmacol 34, 280–285.

Wehr TA and Goodwin FK (1987) Can antidepressants cause mania and worsen the course of affective illness? Am J Psychiatr 144, 1403–1411.

Wehr TA, Sack DA, Rosenthal NE, et al. (1988) Rapid cycling affective disorder: Contributing factors and treatment responses of 51 patients. Am J Psychiatr 145, 179–184.

Weinstein MR and Goldfield MD (1975) Cardiovascular malformations with lithium use during pregnancy. Am J Psychiatr 132, 529–531.

Wisner, KL, Peindl KS, Perel JM, et al. (2002) Verapamil treatment for women with bipolar disorder. Biol Psychiatr.

Young LT, Joffe RT, Robb JC, et al. (2000) Double-blind comparsions of addition of second mood stabilizer versus an antidepressant to an initial mood stabilizer for treatment of patients with bipolar depression. Am J Psychiatr 157, 124–126.

Zajeckya J, Weisler R, Sachs GS, et al. (2000) Divalproex sodium versus olanzapine for the treatment of mania in bipolar disorder. American College of Neuropsychopharmacology, 39th Annual Meeting, San Juan, Puerto Rico.

# 97 Antidepressants

Robert J. Boland
Martin B. Keller

This chapter reviews current knowledge about antidepressant medications. Both theoretical and clinical data are considered and an attempt is made to focus on more recent developments in this field. The use of antidepressants in the treatment of depression remains the best-understood use of these medications, and this is the focus of the chapter. However, there is a growing list of other indications for antidepressants, and these are discussed appropriately.

## Theoretical Basis for Treatment

The discovery of antidepressants did more than provide a revolutionary therapy for depression; it changed the way we view mood disorders and, by analogy, the mind itself. It permanently transformed the appraisal of our ability to influence areas of existence previously thought unreachable through physical manipulation.

## The Development of Antidepressants

There are a number of good reviews of the history of antidepressants. A paper by Pletscher (1991) provided many of the data for this discussion.

The first antidepressant was the monoamine oxidase inhibitor (MAOI), iproniazid. It was soon followed by the tricyclic antidepressant (TCA), imipramine. Although both were developed in the early 1950s, they represented different paths of discovery: iproniazid was the result of clinical and laboratory collaboration, whereas imipramine's introduction was largely based on clinical observation. Imipramine's mechanism of action was clarified only later.

Iproniazid was synthesized from isoniazid in an attempt to improve the chemotherapy of tuberculosis. Three unexpected actions of the drug—monoamine oxidase inhibition, reversal of reserpine-induced sedation, and psychostimulation—resulted in its introduction as the first modern antidepressant. Serious side effects, particularly hypertensive crises and hepatic necrosis prevented universal acceptance of the drug.

Imipramine was synthesized from chlorpromazine. Unlike its parent, imipramine proved ineffective as an antipsychotic, and research on it was almost abandoned. Clinical investigators, however, observed that imipramine had a beneficial effect on depression. Equally important, it did not show the serious side effects associated with iproniazid. Imipramine eventually became widely accepted as a safe and effective antidepressant.

## Mechanisms of Actions

Investigations into the biochemistry of depression have taken their lead from antidepressants. All known antidepressants affect monoamine neurotransmission, and this is believed to be their mechanism of action. As imipramine, iproniazid, and related antidepressants shared an ability to augment the monoamine norepinephrine, the early neurochemical theories of depression focused on this neurotransmitter. Later, newer agents were introduced that seemed to exert their primary effect on another monoamine, serotonin. Research into these two neurotransmitters evolved into the monoamine hypothesis of depression.

### The Monoamine Hypothesis of Depression

The monoamine theory of depression suggests, in its simplest form, that depression relates to abnormal levels of monoamines: neurotransmitters thought important in the regulation of mood. Antidepressants themselves provide the strongest evidence supporting the role of monoamines in mood, as all known antidepressants affect the levels of monoamines in the brain. Other evidence for the monoamine hypothesis included the observation that reserpine (which depletes norepinephrine and serotonin) frequently causes depression.

Originally, norepinephrine was the monoamine thought to be most involved with mood, as most of the early antidepressants primarily affected this transmitter. Newer drugs had more of an effect on serotonin; as a result, this too became a focus of theories on depression. Serotonin may have a direct effect on mood, and may also interact in a regulatory way on norepinephrine. It has been shown repeatedly that tryptophan depletion (the precursor for serotonin) can render antidepressants ineffective. This is true regardless of whether the antidepressant is thought to primarily affect noradrenergic systems, thus supporting the regulatory function of serotonin (Reilly et al. 1997). TCAs also block reuptake of dopamine, and several antidepressants seem to act primarily on the dopamine system, including bupropion and nomifensine. Dopamine may interact with norepinephrine, perhaps through augmentation of alpha-1-receptors.

Several observations argue against the adequacy of the monoamine theory of depression. For example, investigators have been unable to consistently demonstrate decreased monoamine levels in depressed patients. Furthermore, there is a time lag between reuptake inhibition, and clinical response, on the order of several weeks. This effect is independent of the half-life or other pharmacokinetics of the particular drug. This latency is difficult to reconcile with simple monoamine theories, as central nervous system (CNS) monoamine levels can be altered within hours of the introduction of a drug.

## Receptors

Looking for a more complex correlate of antidepressant action, investigators focused on transmitter–receptor interactions. Vetulani and Sulser (1975) described beta-adrenoreceptor downregulation in response to antidepressant administration. This receptor effect was demonstrated in animal experiments, and observed with all antidepressants. Downregulation of the beta-receptor involves not only the noradrenergic system, but requires an intact serotonin system as well. Downregulation also shows a time lag, making it a better model of antidepressant action. When investigators administer antidepressants to animals for a significant period of time, they consistently find both reductions in the number of beta-adrenoreceptor recognition sites and a downregulation of beta-adrenoreceptor functioning. Increased monoamine availability affects not only beta-receptor downregulation, but also upregulation of the alpha-receptor, an autoreceptor that regulates neurotransmission (Ackenheil 1990). Of the serotonin receptors, 5-hydroxytryptamine type 1A (5-HT$_{1A}$) appears most related to the therapeutic effects of antidepressants, and this receptor influences norepinephrine, dopamine, acetylcholine, neuropeptides, other serotonin receptors, and probably beta-receptor downregulation.

The most compelling argument for depression-associated receptor changes would be a direct demonstration of such an association in humans. The recent availability of selective ligands for specific receptors has begun to lend support to such hypothetical associations. A number of serotonin receptor subtypes have been shown to have a reduction in sensitivity in response to selective serotonin reuptake inhibitor (SSRI) administration, including 5-HT$_{1A}$ (Cowen et al. 1994) and 5-HT$_{1D}$ (Whale et al. 2001). In both cases, these receptor changes were seen most markedly in patients with melancholic depression.

## Intracellular Systems

Current theories of depression are looking within the neuron. Second-messenger systems offer a final common pathway for the variety of transmitter and receptor effects. That is, despite the myriad of ways in which receptor and transmitters can be affected, the end result is the overall effect on intracellular mechanisms. Most of the monoamine receptors are linked to G-protein. The activation of the receptor by a neurotransmitter brings about a functional change in the G-protein, which is then able to bind to GTP, which can, in turn, affect intracellular concentrations of such second messengers as adenyl cyclase. Though the details are complicated, the relevance to antidepressants is simple: a variety of extracellular effects are transduced to a limited number of intracellular responses. This may explain how a variety of different chemicals, with different potential actions, can have the same antidepressant effect.

The role of G-protein may also explain some of the inherent limitations in antidepressant response. Alteration in G-protein synthesis and activity takes several weeks, which is consistent with the latency in effect of antidepressants.

Though G-protein may be crucial in understanding the overall antidepressant effect of drugs, it probably is not directly related to an antidepressant's mechanism of action. That is, the action of most antidepressants seems to be extracellular, and there is no evidence to suggest that any available antidepressants have a direct effect on the G-protein. Other medications, such as the lithium ion, may directly influence GTP binding, and this may explain lithium's efficacy as an adjunctive medication.

The relationship between neurotransmitter activity and the mechanism of antidepressant action is depicted in Figure 97–1.

## Antidepressants: Taxonomy and Relation to Mechanism of Action

There are several ways in which antidepressants are grouped. One is historically, in which antidepressants are roughly divided by the period in which they were introduced (e.g., such terms as "first-generation" antidepressants). Another is by chemical structure (e.g., "tricyclic antidepressants"). Alternatively, they are classified by their presumed mechanism of action ("selective serotonin reuptake inhibitors"). In practice, a combination of these is used: thus, some TCAs, which primarily act through serotonin reuptake inhibition (e.g., clomipramine), are usually included with other TCAs rather than as a serotonin reuptake inhibitor, even though they could rightly claim membership in either category.

### First-Generation Antidepressants

These are, historically, the first antidepressants, and were discovered primarily through serendipity. They include the monoamine antidepressants and the TCAs.

**Monoamine Antidepressants (MAOIs).** Historically, these are the first antidepressants discovered. However, owing largely to their side effects, and dietary restrictions, they have rarely enjoyed popular use. They are all characterized by their unique mechanism: they inhibit the action of monoamine oxidase (MAO), the primary catabolic enzyme for the monoamines. The end result is an overall increase in available monoamines.

**Tricyclic Antidepressants (TCAs).** These medications all have a structural similarity in common. They are subdivided by the number of amine groups they possess, and are usually referred to as either "tertiary" or "secondary" TCAs. Several are related by metabolism, thus the tertiary amines—amitriptyline and imipramine—are metabolized to the secondary amines—nortriptyline and desipramine—respectively. They all act through reuptake inhibition, and are generally selective for the norepinephrine transporter; several, however, have equal or greater affinity for the serotonin transporter. Normally, excess monoamine is taken up through monoamine transporters into the neuron, where it can be stored, or, more often, catabolized by intracellular MAO. Reuptake inhibitors prevent this through inhibition of the transporter; the excess neurotransmitter remains in the synaptic space where it can bind with receptors. That this is the mechanism of

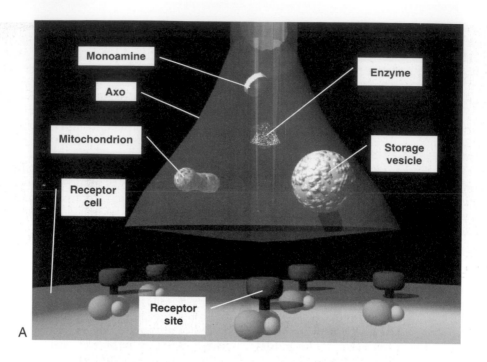

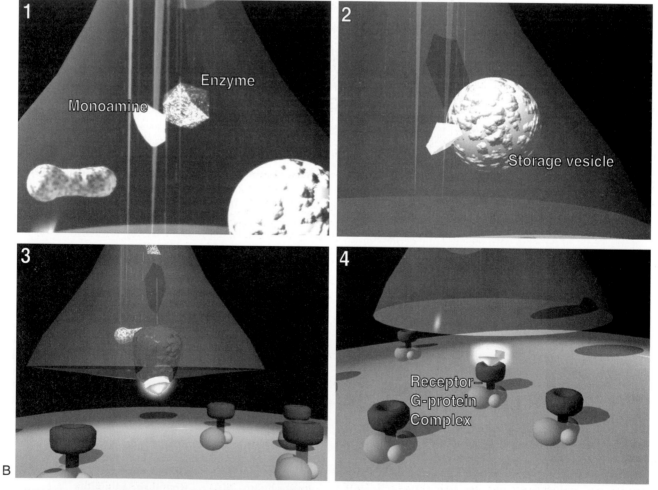

*Continues*

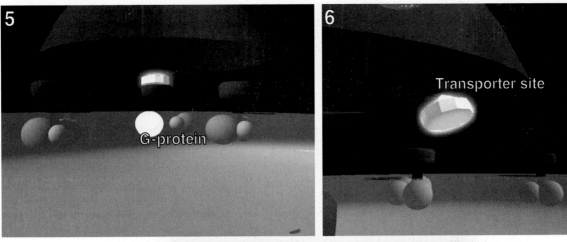

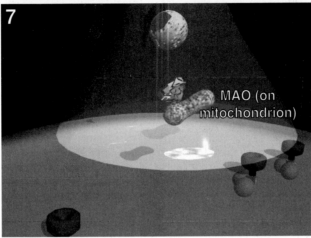

C

**Figure 97–1(A) and (B)** *The "life-cycle" of a monoamine neurotransmitter and potential sites for pharmacological intervention.*
*This presents a schematic of monoamine activity. An overview of the neuronal axon–receptor relationship is shown in the overview 1(A), with several key structures pointed out, including the axon and receptor cell, whose membranes are rendered here as transparent to illustrate key intracellular components.*
*The monoamines—norepinephrine, serotonin, and dopamine—are synthesized within the neuron (1); from dietary amino acids, and then stored within vesicles (2). This vesicle can then bind with the axonal membrane, releasing its contents into the synapse (3).*
*Upon binding to a receptor complex (4); a resultant cascade of reactions is possible. In general, the binding process causes a destabilization of the subunits comprising the receptor–G-protein complex (5). G-protein, now activated, can then regulate a number of second-messenger systems, such as adenylate cyclase and phospholipase C. The potential results can involve alterations at various levels of neuronal function: from physical structure and membrane permeability to direct regulation of genetic transcription. In this way, it is possible for the many brief and simultaneous inputs to be transduced into coherent and lasting influences on neuronal function. Neurotransmitters can even regulate their own production through binding to presynaptic autoreceptors.*
*Once the reaction is complete, the receptor–G-protein complex restabilizes, and the monoamine is released from the receptor site. The neurotransmitter can then be metabolized in the extracellular space or, more commonly, taken back in the axon through a transporter site (6). Monoamines undergoing such reuptake can be again stored within vesicles, or be deaminated by intracellular monoamine oxidase (MAO) residing on the wall of mitochondria (7).*
*Virtually all of these steps can be influenced pharmacologically. For example, enzymatic synthesis can be inhibited by such agents as alpha-methyltyrosine which inhibits tyrosine hydroxylase (1). Reserpine and tetrabenazine can inhibit uptake into the storage vesicles (2), and amphetamines increase the release of norepinephrine from synaptic vesicles (3). A number of drugs can inhibit receptor sites, such as phentolamine and phenoxybenzamine which act at alpha-receptors (4), and most antipsychotics medication, which block dopamine. The lithium ion may act directly on G-protein and second-messenger systems (5).*
*Most antidepressants appear to act either by inhibiting MAO (e.g., the monoamine oxidase inhibitors [MAOIs] which can inhibit step 7), or by preventing the reuptake on one, or more, monoamines—the TCAs and SSRIs, venlafaxine and bupropion (6). Several of the newer generation antidepressants may have a direct effect on the receptor site (4).*

action of these and many other antidepressants is reinforced by the fact that correlations have been demonstrated between transporter inhibition and clinical improvement in depressive symptoms (Hrdina et al. 1997). The TCAs were the drugs of choice for depression through the 1980s. Though very effective, their somewhat non-selective actions, acting on cholinergic, presynaptic adrenergic receptors, for example, resulted in a number of side effects.

## Second-Generation Antidepressants
These medications were developed using knowledge gained from the first-generation antidepressants. An effort was made to produce medications that were more selective for

certain actions. The primary benefit of such selectivity was a decrease in unintended side effects.

**Selective Serotonin Receptor Inhibitors (SSRIs).** The SSRIs were first introduced in the late 1980s, and within a few years eclipsed the TCAs as the drugs of choice for depression. As the name suggests, they all act through inhibition of the serotonin transporter. Though very similar, they have some subtle differences, mainly in terms of their half-life, their potency for reuptake inhibition, and their affinity for some other receptors.

These medications are not only the most popular antidepressants, but also some of the most popular drugs of any type. The US sales data demonstrate that the SSRIs remain one of the most lucrative of drugs. In 2001, for example, the producer of sertraline reported global sales of over $2 billion from the product.

**Selective Norepinephrine Reuptake Inhibitors (NRIs).** Like the SSRIs, medications in this class share a similar mechanism with the SSRIs, but act on the norepinephrine transporter and have little affinity for the serotonin transporter. Reboxetine (currently available in Europe, and expected to be available soon in the US) is an example of such a medication.

**Other Second-Generation Agents.** Sometimes referred to as "atypical antidepressants" several were introduced during the same period as the SSRIs. These include bupropion, which seems to exert primarily a dopaminergic effect, and trazodone, which was structurally related to the TCAs but has a primary serotonergic mechanism. Nomifensine, which is not commercially available after international reports of severe hemolytic anemias were reported, would be in a class similar to bupropion.

### Third-Generation Antidepressant

The next generation of antidepressants involved various attempts to expand the potential of second-generation compounds. One important feature of this group is that many of them have multiple actions. In some cases, this involves actions on multiple neurotransmitters. In other cases, it involves multiple mechanisms of action. Though, in a way this may seem a return to the broader acting first-generation compounds, the attempt with these drugs is to maximize the presumed "clinically relevant" effects of the drugs, while minimizing the less important (and potentially adverse) actions.

**Serotonin–Norepinephrine Reuptake Inhibitors (SNRIs).** Medications in this class share a common mechanism with the SSRIs, but differ in that they have equal affinity for the norepinephrine and serotonin transporter. Currently, the only medication of this type available in the US is venlafaxine. Other medications (available in other countries), such as milnacipran, have similar mechanisms of action. Though, like several of the TCAs, venlafaxine has multiple receptor effects, it is relatively free of the anticholinergic and antihistaminic side effects that are common with the TCAs.

**Mixed Serotonin Antagonist/Reuptake Inhibitors.** These agents have multiple mechanisms of action, all of which appear to be of clinical importance. Nefazodone is an example of such an agent, with both serotonin (as well as norepinephrine) transporter inhibition as well as antagonism of 5-HT$_{2A}$ and alpha-1-receptors. Trazodone may be similar; however, its effects are somewhat less specific, and as a result, it resembles the TCAs in some respects.

**Mixed Serotonin/Noradrenaline Antagonists.** Currently, the only agent in this class is mirtazapine. This agent is unique in that it appears to work primarily through receptor blockade, specifically through blockade of the alpha-2-autoreceptors on presynaptic noradrenergic neurons, which enhances noradrenergic output. They may exert a similar effect toward autoreceptors on serotonin neurons. Antagonism of 5-HT$_2$ and 5-HT$_3$ receptors may also concentrate the effect of serotonin on 5-HT$_{1A}$ receptors.

The antidepressants available in the US (as of the first quarter of 2002), their class, and relative costs are listed in Table 97–1.

## The Basis for Determining Efficacy

### Clinical Trials
As with any drug, the gold standard for proving efficacy is a double-blinded placebo-controlled trial. There have been many such studies for antidepressants. As a whole, these studies lend strong support for the efficacy of antidepressants.

There have been some limitations in these data. Some have questioned the effectiveness of the blinding techniques, and it has been demonstrated that subjects in some supposedly blinded studies can accurately guess whether they are on a drug or a placebo. Such potential bias could inflate the perceived efficacy of these drugs (Moncrieff et al. 1998). A somewhat opposing dilemma is the high placebo response in many intervention studies on depression, requiring large samples before a significant effect can be found. These biases, though important, have occasionally been exploited with the purpose of discrediting data proving the efficacy of antidepressants. However, there are very many carefully performed studies investigating antidepressants, and the sheer enormity of these adds considerable weight to the contention that these drugs are very effective in the treatment of major depressive disorder.

### First-Generation Antidepressants
Since the first reports of the efficacy of amitriptyline (Kuhn 1958) and iproniazid (Kline 1958), numerous controlled trials have demonstrated the efficacy of first-generation antidepressants. A potential antidepressant is compared to either a placebo or a gold standard antidepressant, usually imipramine. Davis and Glassman (1989) reviewed the double-blind controlled studies comparing tricyclic antidepressants with placebo or imipramine. They concluded that all tricyclic antidepressants are superior to placebo, and at least equal to imipramine, in the treatment of depression. Overall, the first-generation agents have been found to be comparable with each other (Klerman and Cole 1965), though there has been some suggestion, admittedly controversial, that the MAOIs are not as effective as the TCAs in severe "typical" depression (Thase et al. 1995), but that they may have a preferential action in patients with "atypical" depression (Quitkin et al. 1990).

| Table 97–1 | Antidepressants Available in the US | | | | | |

| | Class | Name | Brand Name(s) | Generic | How Supplied | Price Index: (Dollar Cost of Average Dose/d)* |
|---|---|---|---|---|---|---|
| First generation | TCAs | Amitriptyline | Elavil, Etrafon, others | Y | Tablets (mg): 10, 25, 50, 75, 100, 150 Oral solution: 10 mg/5mL IM: 10 mg/mL | 0.3 |
| | | Imipramine | Tofranil | Y | Tablets (mg): 10, 25, 50 | 0.6 |
| | | Nortriptyline | Pamelor, Aventyl | Y | Oral solution: 10 mg/5 mL Tablets (mg): 10, 25, 50, 75 | 0.4 |
| | | Desipramine | Norpramine, others | Y | Tablets (mg): 10, 25, 50, 75, 100, 150 | 0.7 |
| | | Amoxapine | Asendin | Y | Tablets (mg): 25, 50, 100, 150 | 1.2 |
| | | Doxepin | Sinequan, Adapin, others | Y | Oral solution: 10 mg/mL Tablets (mg): 10, 25, 50, 75, 100, 150 | 0.3 |
| | | Protriptyline | Vivactil, Triptil | N | Tablets (mg): 5, 10 | 3 |
| | | Trimipramine | Surmontil, Rhotrimine | N | Tablets (mg): 25, 50, 100 | 2.8 |
| | | Clomipramine | Anafranil | Y | Tablets (mg): 25, 50, 75 | 1.3 |
| | | Maprotiline | Ludiomil | Y | Tablets (mg): 25, 50, 75 | 1 |
| | MAOIs | Isocarboxazid | Marplan | N | Tablets: 10 mg | 2.8 |
| | | Phenelzine | Nardil | N | Tablets: 15 mg | 1.6 |
| | | Tranylcy- promine | Parnate | N | Tablets: 10 mg | 2 |
| Second generation | SSRIs | Fluoxetine | Prozac, Sarafem | Y | Oral solution: 20 mg/5mL Tablets (mg): 10, 20, 40 Extended release: 90 mg ("Prozac Weekly") | 1.5 |
| | | Sertraline | Zoloft | N | Oral solution: 20 mg/mL Tablets (mg): 25, 50, 100 | 2.2 |
| | | Paroxetine | Paxil | N | Oral solution: 10 mg/5mL Tablets (mg): 10, 20, 30, 40 | 2.5 |
| | | Fluvoxamine | Luvox | Y | Tablets (mg): 25, 50, 100 | 2 |
| | | Citalopram | Celexa | N | Oral solution: 10 mg/5 mL Tablets (mg): 10, 20, 40 | 2.1 |
| | | Escitalopram hexapro | | N | Tablets (mg): 10,20 | 2.1 |
| | Atypical | Bupropion | Wellbutrin, Zyban | N | Tablets (mg): 75, 100 Sustained release (mg): 100, 150 | 3 |
| | | Trazodone | Desyrel | Y | Tablets (mg): 50, 100, 150 | 0.5 |

*Continues*

| Table 97-1 | Antidepressants Available in the US *Continued* | | | | | |
|---|---|---|---|---|---|---|
| | Class | Name | Brand Name(s) | Generic | How Supplied | Price Index: (Dollar Cost of Average Dose/d)* |
| Third generation | SNRI | Venlafaxine | Effexor | N | Tablets (mg): 25, 37.5, 50, 75, 100 Extended release (mg): 37.5, 75, 150 | 2.5 |
| | Mixed serotonin antagonist/ reuptake inhibitors | Nefazodone | Serzone | N | Tablets (mg): 50, 100, 150, 200, 250 | 2.8 |
| | Mixed serotonin/ noradrenaline antagonists | Mirtazapine | Remeron | N | Tablets (mg): 15, 30, 45 Dissolvable tablets (mg): 15, 30, 45 | 2.4 |

*The price index is a rough calculation, assuming an average recommended dose for the treatment of major depression, and assuming that the most efficient dosing regimen, and least expensive tablet choice is prescribed. When available, generic prices are used. Prices were derived from a sampling several widely used Internet-based US pharmaceutical suppliers current as of the first quarter of 2002. Thus, in many cases, these numbers are an underestimate of the actual costs to patients.

## Second-Generation Antidepressants

Fluoxetine has been compared to both placebo and tricyclic antidepressants in numerous clinical trials. It has been available in the US since 1988, and has been used by over 40 million patients to date. Sertraline has been available in the US since 1992 and has grown to become the most prescribed antidepressant in the US. Paroxetine has been studied in over 4,000 patients in numerous clinical trials, which use placebo and TCA controls (Boyer and Feighner 1992). Citalopram and fluvoxamine, both introduced later, have similar data attesting to their efficacy in depression. Escitalopram is the S-enantiomer of the SSRI citalopram. Pharmacologic studies indicate that this form is predominantly responsible for the 5-HT reuptake by racemic citalopram. The bulk of evidence suggests that these SSRI medications are superior to placebo and equal to TCAs in the treatment of depression.

The majority of drug trials involving serotonin reuptake inhibitors have been in outpatient populations. However, there are a small but growing number of studies of SSRIs in the severely depressed (Hirschfeld 1999). Comparisons based on these studies are difficult to make, as they involve various definitions of "severe" and "recovery." Despite these limitations, comparative studies generally suggest that the SSRIs have an efficacy equal to older antidepressants in the treatment of severe depression.

Bupropion was also superior to placebo in several trials. Of interest is the suggestion that bupropion may have superior efficacy in patients who were nonresponsive to TCAs (Preskorn and Burke 1992, Stern et al. 1983). Trazodone is reported to be as effective as TCAs in a variety of double-blind comparisons (Brotman et al. 1987). Despite these numerous studies, there remains a clinical impression that trazodone is inferior to other antidepressants (Preskorn and Burke 1992). This impression may result from improper dosing of trazodone, as it is one of the few antidepressants to require divided doses. It may also be that treatment emergent side effects occur at the dosage required for therapeutic efficacy, thereby rendering trazodone of less value.

## Third-Generation Antidepressants

In six unpublished trials, with a total of 770 patients, venlafaxine was significantly superior to placebo in treating patients with major depression (Montgomery 1993). There is some evidence to suggest that it has a more rapid onset of action at high doses (doses ranged from 75 to 375 mg/day in these trials) in these trials (FDA 1993). This contention has not been supported by direct comparisons of venlafaxine with SSRIs. Some pooled comparative data does support this, and this is discussed later.

Nefazodone has been comparable to imipramine and superior to placebo in controlled trials (Rickels et al. 1995, D'Amico et al. 1990). Similarly, mirtazapine has been found to be effective in clinical trials (de Boer 1996, Sitsen and Zivkov 1995).

## Comparative Trials

The question remains whether one antidepressant is any more efficacious than another. In studies employing various comparisons, antidepressants of different classes are generally found to be equal in efficacy. There are some caveats to this statement. As already noted, placebo-response rates in many studies of depression are quite high, and it will be difficult to show a statistically significant effect. Large sample sizes are needed: assuming that any difference between two antidepressants is likely to be small (perhaps 5–10%), a study would require thousands of subjects before it could detect this difference in efficacy. Some of these limitations can be addressed by meta-analyses, which pool the results from different studies to increase the sample size. However, the use of meta-analysis has inherent limitations and a potential for bias, and cannot replace well-done controlled studies.

Most studies comparing antidepressants have not found significant differences in efficacy between agents. In general, studies comparing TCAs and SSRIs have shown equal efficacy, and meta-analyses of these studies have generally confirmed these findings (Anderson 2000,

Workman and Short 1993). However, there have been some trends in this data, with TCAs showing, perhaps, greater efficacy in patients with severe depression (Perry 1996).

Meta-analyses lend some support to the contention that drugs with multiple actions have a greater efficacy than those that are more highly selective. There is some suggestion that the antidepressants that are selective for norepinephrine and serotinin may be more effective than the SSRIs alone. Similarly, in one pooled analysis of eight double-blind studies comparing venlafaxine with SSRIs (all of which individually showed no difference between the drugs), Thase and colleagues (2001) did report a significant difference in remission rates between venlafaxine, which began at 2 weeks. Similarly, mirtazapine has not shown improved efficacy in comparative studies, but in a pooling of data from such studies, showed a more rapid onset of action (Anderson 2001). Nefazodone has been compared both with TCAs (van Moffaert et al. 1994) and with SSRIs (Baldwin et al. 1996), and generally has shown comparable efficacy, though high dosing (over 300 mg/day) is often required for equal efficacy. As these are single studies and not meta-analyses, the fact that they show no improved efficacy should not be surprising.

Though these meta-analyses are compelling, the fact that improved efficacy has yet to be demonstrated by the "gold standard" of a placebo-controlled study likely explains why the third generation of antidepressants does not yet enjoy a reputation for improved efficacy. And, even if some of the newer drugs do show improved efficacy, the proposed reason for this—multiplicity of action—may not be correct. In fact, at least one meta-analysis investigating this hypothesis, in which multiple action drugs were compared with selective drugs, did not find a difference between the two (Freemantle et al. 2000). As such, our treatment recommendations, as outlined in the summary, make the assumption that the efficacy of antidepressants is approximately equal for all agents.

## Summary

Numerous controlled studies support the efficacy of the antidepressants for the treatment of depression. Serotonin reuptake inhibitors, initially thought to be less efficacious in severe depression, now appear to be equally efficacious to the more classic antidepressants. In the near future, we can expect variations on the two primary themes: selectivity versus multiplicity. As antidepressants become even more selective for specific transmitter and receptor subtypes, there is the hope for more focused effects with less side effects. However, of these two goals, this research strategy seems more likely improve the side effect profile of antidepressants rather than dramatically improve efficacy. Modest improvements in efficacy may be possible; more dramatic ones will likely have to wait for truly unique agents to be developed.

## Development of New Antidepressants

### Animal Trials

The development of a new drug is generally divided into three phases: phase I is an initial screening for a desired activity; phase II is a more elaborate determination of desired activity and pharmacokinetics; and phase III is a definitive judgment of the drug's pharmacology. Of particular interest is the phase I, or initial screening of a drug. In the past, such a screening was largely a matter of serendipity. More analytic methods have largely supplanted this. Such methods can take two approaches: a behavioral approach, or a mechanistic approach. In a behavioral approach, investigators attempt to develop an animal model of a particular pathological condition. In a mechanistic approach, the investigator targets particular actions of a potential drug—actions that are presumed to be the basis of a therapeutic effect.

### Behavioral Models

Traditionally, investigators rely on animal models that attempt to reproduce psychiatric pathology. Three examples of such tests are the separation syndrome in rhesus monkeys (McKinney 1988), learned helplessness models (Seligman and Maier 1967), and the behavioral despair or "forced swimming" test (Porsolt et al. 1979). Most behavioral tests are complicated and expensive to perform. The behavioral despair test is probably the most practical of these tests. In this test, an investigator places a mouse or rat in a confined space filled with water. Usually, the immersed animal will first attempt to escape, and then become immobile: "behavioral despair" refers to the assumption that the animal has given up hope of escaping. On subsequent immersions, the animal becomes immobile more quickly. Most antidepressants, regardless of class, delay this effect, and the ability of a new agent to delay immobility in animals is a good predictor of antidepressant action in humans. There is even a correlation between the potency of an agent in this test and its clinical potency as an antidepressant: this feature is not demonstrable in any other animal model of depression (Willner 1990). The mechanism of this response has been shown to be mediated by both pre- and postsynaptic serotonergic 5-HT$_1$ receptors (Redrobe et al. 1996); however, the behavioral despair is not necessarily limited to these receptors alone.

### Mechanistic Models

The most common mechanistic tests evaluate antagonism of reserpine—a feature of all tricyclic antidepressants and many newer agents. Several experiments evaluate different examples of reserpine antagonism. The ability to block reserpine-induced hypothermia depends on an agent's proficiency at increasing postsynaptic norepinephrine or potentiating beta-adrenergic receptors. Antagonism of reserpine-induced ptosis is dependent on alpha-noradrenergic or serotonergic activity, and antagonism of reserpine-induced akinesia appears to be dopamine-dependent. In combination, these three tests can differentiate between a variety of monoamine-dependent effects. Other methods include antagonism of oxotremorine (related to anticholinergic activity), the high-dose apomorphine test (specific for norepinephrine reuptake), and the yohimbine test. The ability to potentiate yohimbine lethality, an alpha-2-agonist, appears to be highly specific for antidepressants.

Thus, a variety of psychopharmacological tools may be of use in screening potential antidepressants. They are generally simple to perform and relatively inexpensive, particularly when compared with clinical trials. They may also be more reliable than standard neurochemical screening in predicting the antidepressant action of an agent (Bourin 1990).

## Limitations of Behavioral and Mechanistic Models

An ideal model of depression should be able to meet the same criteria as any model of human disease. It should reproduce the symptoms and the etiology of the disease, show common biological mechanisms, and show reversal of symptoms by proven therapeutic agents (Delina-Stula 1989, McKinney and Bunney 1969). Neither the behavioral model nor the mechanistic model of depression meets all these criteria. The behavioral model suffers from inherent limitations in attempting to simulate a complex human behavior in an animal. Usually, one attempts to simulate a certain aspect of depressive behavior in an animal. Such a "target symptom" may not be a true extrapolation of human depression. Though recent attempts to selectively breed for "depressed" mice (Vaugeois and Costentin 1998) (using a predilection towards helplessness behaviors as a target symptoms) might improve the situation, the behavioral models continue to suffer from significant limitations. Behavioral models can also be cumbersome and expensive. Mechanistic models are simple and inexpensive, but suffer from limited specificity (e.g., aspirin, with no antidepressant action, can antagonize reserpine-induced hypothermia) and a reliance on available theories about the critical ingredient of antidepressants. For this reason, the mechanistic model is less likely than the behavioral model to reveal truly novel antidepressants. Used together, the two models can complement each other.

## The Formulation of Treatment

## Indications

### Acute Major Depression

All antidepressants are indicated for the treatment of acute major depressive episodes. The major depressive disorder is, most likely, a variety of neuropsychological disorders that have in common their negative effects on mood, thought and vegetative symptoms. There is much room for variation, with phenomenology ranging from individuals who are anxious and irritable to those who are anergic and melancholic. The heterogeneity of the diagnosis is recognized in the *Diagnostic and Statistical Manual of Mental Disorders* (DSM), of which the DSM-IV-Text Revision (DSM-IV-TR) (American Psychiatric Association 2000a) is the most recent edition. DSM-IV-TR lists nine possible symptoms. Of these, either depressed mood or loss of interest is required for the diagnosis, with at least four other symptoms present during a 2-week period. Though there have been some attempts to match different types of depression with different medications, there is no convincing evidence to suggest that there is a preferential efficacy between specific presentations of depression and certain medications (for an interesting review of this subject, and a partial rebuttal of our statement, see van Praag 2001).

### Prevention of Relapse and Recurrence

Beyond the acute period, there is also evidence for the use of antidepressants in the prevention of relapse and recurrence.

However, the further one gets from the initial episode, the sparser the data. Most of the commonly used antidepressants have at least one placebo-controlled study justifying their use in relapse prevention. However, few studies go beyond a year of treatment, and there is a need for more data on the use of antidepressant in long-term prevention of disease recurrence. The available data will be discussed later in this chapter.

### Other Depressive Disorders

There are a number of more minor forms of depression, many of which may also respond to antidepressant medication. Best studied of these is dysthymic disorder. Previously thought to be unresponsive to somatic therapy, a growing literature attests to the responsiveness of this chronic, minor depressive disorder to a variety of medications, including TCAs (Kocsis et al. 1985, Stewart et al. 1993) and serotonin reuptake inhibitors (Hellerstein et al. 1993, Thase et al. 1996, Ravindran et al. 1994, Vanelle 1997). As with major depression, there is no definitive data to suggest that any one agent is more efficacious than the other. The bulk of data suggests, instead, that any available agent used for major depression is likely to be effective for these other disorders.

Other minor depressive disorders include minor depression and recurrent brief depression. Though rigorous data is largely lacking in the treatment of these disorders, they seem to show an at least modest response to antidepressant medications.

### Other Uses for Antidepressants

Although the bulk of this chapter will describe the use of antidepressants in the treatment of major depression, they are also used to treat a number of other conditions (Orsulak and Waller 1989, Brotman 1993). Some uses have gained general acceptance while other uses rely on moderate or preliminary evidence. A summary of various indications is presented in Table 97–2.

### First-Generation Antidepressants

**Tricyclic Antidepressants.** There is strong evidence for the use of antidepressants in the treatment of several anxiety disorders of which, panic disorder (PD) and obsessive–compulsive disorder (OCD) are the best studied. The efficacy of antidepressants in treating these phenomena probably relates both to their downregulation of noradrenergic function and their enhancement of serotonin (Kaplan 1992). This is consistent with current theories of noradrenergic and serotonergic dysregulation with PD (Montgomery et al. 1991). Most studies suggest that the doses required to treat PD are similar to those in treating depression, with doses of at least 150 mg/day of imipramine (Klein 1984, Ballenger 1991). A few studies suggest that lower doses can be used.

The TCA clomipramine is a first-line treatment for OCD, owing to its relative selectivity for the serotonin reuptake inhibition. TCAs, either alone or in combination with cognitive therapy, can also decrease the binging and purging of bulimic patients (Mitchell et al. 1990).

TCAs are used in a number of childhood disorders as well. Perhaps the most successful use has been in the treatment of enuresis, for which imipramine is the most

| Table 97–2 | Various Uses of Antidepressants |
|---|---|

### Major Depression

Acute depression
Prevention of relapse
Other depressive syndrome
  Bipolar depression
  Atypical depression
  Dysthymia

### Other Uses

**Tricyclic Antidepressants**

Strong evidence
  Panic disorder (most)
  Obsessive–compulsive disorder (clomipramine)
  Bulimia (imipramine, desipramine)
  Enuresis (imipramine)
Moderate evidence
  Separation anxiety
  Attention-deficit/hyperactivity disorder
  Phobias
  Generalized anxiety disorder
  Anorexia nervosa
  Body dysmorphic disorder
  Migraine (amitriptyline)
  Other headaches
  Diabetic neuropathy, other pain syndromes (amitriptyline, doxepin).
  Sleep apnea (protriptyline)
  Cocaine abuse (desipramine)
  Tinnitus
Evidence for but rarely used for these disorders
  Peptic ulcer disease
  Arrhythmias

**Monoamine Oxidase Inhibitors**

Strong evidence
  Panic disorder
  Bulimia
Moderate evidence
  Other anxiety disorders
  Anorexia nervosa
  Body dysmorphic disorder

**Atypical Agents**

Trazodone
  Insomnia
  Dementia with agitation
  Minor sedative/hypnotic withdrawal
Bupropion
  Attention-deficit/hyperactivity disorder

**Serotonin Reuptake Inhibitors**

Strong evidence
  Obsessive–compulsive disorder (high dose fluoxetine, sertraline)
  Bulimia (fluoxetine)
Moderate evidence
  Panic disorder
  Obesity (high-dose fluoxetine)
  Substance abuse
  Impulsivity, anger associated with personality disorders
  Pain syndromes
Preliminary evidence
  Obsessive jealousy
  Body dysmorphic disorder

| Table 97–2 | Various Uses of Antidepressants *Continued* |
|---|---|

**Serotonin Reuptake Inhibitors** *Continued*

Preliminary evidence *Continued*
  Hypochondriasis
  Behavioral abnormalities associated with autism and mental retardation
  Anger attacks associated with depression
  Depersonalization disorder
  Social phobia
  Attention-deficit/hyperactivity disorder (as an adjunct)
  Chronic enuresis
  Paraphilic sexual disorders
  Nonparaphilic sexual disorders

frequently employed. It appears that this agent's effectiveness in enuresis is not related to its anticholinergic properties, but rather to some direct effect on the bladder muscles (Rapaport et al. 1980). Antidepressants have also been used for childhood onset psychiatric disorders such as separation anxiety or school phobia and attention-deficit/hyperactivity disorder (Ambrosini et al. 1993, Simeon 1989).

Moderate evidence exists for the use of TCAs in the treatment of additional disorders. Other anxiety disorders, such as phobias, have been treated with TCAs (Potts and Davidson 1992). In one controlled trial investigating generalized anxiety disorder (GAD), diazepam was most effective in the first 2 weeks of treatment. Imipramine and trazodone, however, were more effective in treating the disorder beyond the fourth week (Rickels et al. 1993). Anorexia nervosa may be at least partially responsive to TCA medications (Orsulak and Waller 1989). Body dysmorphic disorder can be responsive to TCAs (Phillips 1991), particularly those selective for serotonin.

Antidepressants may also be useful in a number of medical disorders. Amitriptyline is used in the treatment of headaches, particularly those due to migraine and cluster headaches (Hamilton and Halbreich 1993, Saper 1989). They have been used in a variety of other pain syndromes as well. The best-studied pain syndrome is probably diabetic neuropathy. Amitriptyline and doxepin may be more useful for diabetic neuropathy than the serotonin reuptake inhibitors (Max et al. 1992). The TCAs are probably also useful in facial pain, fibrositis, and arthritis (Krishnan and France 1989); however, they appear to be less useful for lower back pain and cancer pain (Magni 1991). Although reports vary, there is evidence to suggest that doses as low as one half the antidepressant dose are effective for pain management.

TCAs such as protriptyline may be helpful in the treatment of sleep apnea (Lilie and Lahmeyer 1991, Kaplan 1992). Desipramine has been used in the treatment of cocaine craving (Cowley 1992, Gawin and Kleber 1984). One controlled trial has demonstrated the utility of nortriptyline in treating tinnitus (Sullivan et al. 1993).

There are also several uncommon, but potential uses of TCAs. As many of these antidepressants are potent histamine blockers (particularly doxepin and amitriptyline) they could treat peptic ulcer disease (Orsulak and Waller

1989). Similarly, their quinidine-like effect makes them plausible antiarrhythmic agents (Roose and Dalack 1992). In either case, antidepressant medications are rarely used for these disorders.

**Monoamine Oxidase Inhibitors.** MAOIs have been used for the treatment of PD. They have also been reported successful in the treatment of bulimia, although the many dietary restrictions have made doctors reluctant to prescribe these agents. Moderate evidence also exists for the use of these agents in treating other anxiety disorders, anorexia nervosa, and body dysmorphic disorder (Liebowitz et al. 1990).

## Second-Generation Antidepressants

**Serotonin Reuptake Inhibitors.** There is strong evidence for this group's effectiveness in the treatment of OCD (Kasper et al. 1992). Although the recommended starting dose in OCD is the same as that for depression, higher doses, for example 60 to 80 mg for fluoxetine, may be required for adequate response (Jenike et al. 1989, Fountaine and Chouinard 1986). SSRIs are also commonly used in the treatment of bulimia nervosa (Walsh 1991, Goldbloom and Olmstead 1993). As with OCDs, there appears to be a dose–response effect, with larger doses often required (Fluoxetine Bulimia Nervose Collaborative Study Group 1992).

SSRIs are commonly used for other anxiety disorders as well, and there is good evidence for their efficacy in treating PD (Page 2002). Patients prone to panic attacks are begun at low doses (e.g., 5 mg of fluoxetine), and increased slowly to an effective dose to minimize potential side effects. Some studies also suggest that PD patients can be maintained with these lower doses with an effective response (Louie et al. 1993), although this is not a consistent finding. Other anxiety disorders for which they have shown utility include GAD, social phobia (Kosieradzki 2001, van Amerigen et al. 1993), posttraumatic stress disorder (PTSD) (Davidson et al. 2002), and depersonalization disorder (Fichtner et al. 1992).

Serotonin reuptake inhibitors are also used in a number of more complex behavioral disorders, such as obesity, substance abuse, and personality disorders (Kasper et al. 1992). Fluoxetine, in higher doses, does appear to be useful for the treatment of certain forms of obesity (Craighead and Agras 1991), and sertraline has been effective in a placebo-controlled trial of treatment for binge-eating disorder (McElroy et al. 2000). They may play a role in the treatment of substance abuse as well (Cornelius et al. 1993, Pettinati et al. 2001), that the effects are rarely robust. Serotonin reuptake inhibitors have been used to alleviate certain aggressive behaviors, such as impulsivity and uncontrolled anger, both in adults (usually with personality disorders) (Fava et al. 1993), children (Armenteros and Lewis 2002), and in the demented elderly (although the data here is not always supportive of this practice; see Sutor et al. 2001).

Given the safety of the serotonin reuptake inhibitors, they have been tried in a miscellany of disorders. Growing collections of open trials and case studies lend some support to this sometimes liberal application of psychopharmacology. Some of these applications were originally tried because the disorders appeared similar to OCD, such as obsessive jealousy (Stein et al. 1994), body dysmorphic disorder (Phillips et al. 1998), pathological gambling (Hollander et al. 2000), Tourette's syndrome (Wehr and Namerow 2001), and hypochondriasis (Viswanathan and Paradis 1991). They have also been used for the repetitive-type abnormalities associated with autism (Cook et al. 1992, Strauss et al. 2002) and mental retardation (Ricketts et al. 1993). Other uses in children include treatment for attention-deficit/hyperactivity disorder (as an adjunct to methylphenidate; Gammon and Brown 1993) and chronic enuresis (Mesaros 1993, Horrigan and Barnhill 2000).

Both paraphiliac (Stein et al. 1992), and nonparaphiliac sexual disorders (Power-Smith 1994) have been treated successfully with serotonin reuptake inhibitors. This seems understandable, as the first disorder also resembles both obsessional and impulsive disorders, and the latter resembles anxiety disorders. In the treatment of the paraphiliac disorders, the mechanism of action was thought to relate to a decrease in compulsive behaviors; thus the serotonergic drugs have been presumed to be more effective for these disorders than other antidepressants. However this presumption is not supported by a controlled trial, which found desipramine (primarily a noradrenergic agent) and clomipramine to be equally effective in the treatment of paraphilias (Kruesi et al. 1992).

The serotonin reuptake inhibitors are also used to treat pain syndromes. They appear to be less effective than the TCAs, at least in the treatment of diabetic neuropathies. They have also been used for a variety of other physical symptoms, including headaches (Tomkins et al. 2001), dizziness (Staab et al. 2002), restless leg syndrome (Dimmitt and Riley 2000), menopausal symptoms (Loprinzi et al. 2002), stuttering (Costa and Kroll 2000), and acne (Moussavian 2001), as well as the general category of vague and unexplained medical symptoms (O'Malley et al. 1999).

**Atypical Agents.** Trazodone, given its relative safety, is frequently used in the elderly, particularly as a sedative. Trazodone can cause or worsen orthostatic hypotension, particularly in the elderly, and blood pressure should be monitored when this agent is used in this group. It has been used in the demented elderly as well, and case reports and open label trials attest to its potential usefulness in treating behavioral disorders associated with dementia (Pasion and Kirby 1993, Lebert et al. 1994). Its sedative effect has also made trazodone useful in weaning patients from benzodiazepines and other sedative drugs (Ansseau and De Roeck 1993). Bupropion has been used successfully in the treatment of attention-deficit/hyperactivity disorder, both in children (Casat et al. 1989) and in adults (Wender and Reimherr 1990). Bupropion may, however, exacerbate tics in attention-deficit patients with concomitant Tourette's syndrome (Spencer et al. 1993).

## Third-Generation Antidepressants

Venlafaxine has shown efficacy in a number of anxiety disorders, including GAD (Davidson et al. 1999) and social phobia (Kelsey 1995). Nefazodone has shown efficacy in treating anxiety; however, this has generally been shown in studies of anxiety associated with major depression (Fountaine et al. 1994). Similarly, mirtazapine has shown itself to be effective in treating anxiety symptoms in general (Fawcett and Barkin 1998, Sitsen and Moors 1994), though the experience with specific anxiety disorders is more limited (Koran et al. 2001).

## Summary

All the antidepressants appear to treat more than depressive disorders. Particularly consistent has been data showing their utility for anxiety disorder, and they have begun to supplant the sedative/hypnotics for these disorders. Many other psychiatric and medical disorders have all been successfully treated with these agents. Some investigators have suggested that the usefulness of antidepressants in these various disorders suggests a common etiology, perhaps a spectrum of depression-related disorders. There is some evidence to support this assertion, such as the similar neurotransmitters that appear to be involved in these disorders. It is also compelling that many of these psychiatric and physical disorders have similar gender and inheritance patterns. Just as the use of antidepressants has affected our theoretical understanding of depression, so have they begun to influence theories about these other disorders.

## Selection of an Antidepressant

The decision whether to treat depressive symptoms with pharmacotherapy requires an assessment of both the need for intervention and the likelihood that treatment will be successful. Assessing the need for intervention involves longitudinal and cross-sectional factors. Assessing the likelihood that treatment will be successful is somewhat more difficult, but may rely on clinical, demographical, and biological factors.

## Assessing the Need for Intervention

This involves assessing the likely result if pharmacological treatment is not given. It is essential in making a useful risk–benefit assessment.

**Longitudinal Factors.** The physician should consider the course and duration of previous episodes of depression. Such episodes can predict the potential severity of the current episode, the likely time to recovery, and the probability of a subsequent recurrence. The physician should also consider the likely complications of depression for the individual patient, which may include substance abuse and suicide.

**Cross-Sectional Factors.** The physician should consider the severity of symptoms and the degree of functional impairment. Suicidal ideation is of particular concern and needs rapid and intensive treatment. Such treatment often includes hospitalization. Even with less pressing symptoms, but significant occupational or social impairment, the risk–benefit ratio generally still favors a trial of antidepressants, particularly now that safer and more easily tolerated agents are available.

## Assessing the Likelihood of Success

The ability to predict the likely response to pharmacotherapy would be invaluable for planning a treatment strategy. Such an assessment is difficult. Both clinical and biological factors have been studied in the search for more reliable predictors of response.

**Clinical Factors.** A number of symptoms have been suggested as predictors of good and poor response. In the past, depressive illness was distinguished by whether it was "endogenous" or "exogenous." Endogenous depression was thought to have a primary biological etiology, whereas exogenous depression implied a reactive response to environmental stressors. It was assumed that endogenous depression would respond better to somatic therapy and exogenous to psychosocial interventions. This distinction proved excessively simplistic. The categories did not have adequate construct validity. Usually, the attribution of cause was assigned retrospectively, and it was subject to various interpretations. As a result, these subgroups did not adequately predict treatment response.

A refinement of such categories has been the concept of "melancholic depression." This subtype contains many of the criteria thought to describe the endogenous type of depression, but it does not imply any specific etiology. This category defines a group that is most likely to respond to somatic therapy. Individuals in this subgroup tend to have a positive family history for depression and a 2:1 female–male ratio.

Another subtype, "atypical depression," describes a group of patients who differ from the melancholic type, primarily with neurovegetative symptoms: they have hypersomnia, hyperphagia, and psychomotor agitation and are more likely to be anxious or irritable. Earlier studies suggested a preferential response to certain classes of antidepressants, with MAOIs often suggested as the drug of choice (Preskorn and Burke 1992). However, more recent studies have not supported a differential effect on depression among different classes of antidepressants (McGrath et al. 2000).

Additional possible predictors of poor response include personality features (such as neurotic, hypochondriacal, and hysterical traits), multiple prior episodes, delusions, and psychomotor agitation (Kocsis 1990).

**Biological Factors**
**Neuroendocrine.** Many investigators have explored the potential usefulness of the dexamethasone suppression test (DST) in predicting antidepressant response. Unfortunately, results are mixed. Some studies show a positive correlation between nonsuppression on the DST and treatment response, others a negative correlation, and still others no correlation at all. Thus, the DST does not appear to differentiate responders from nonresponders adequately.

Other potential neuroendocrine markers, less well studied than the DST, include the thyrotropin-releasing hormone stimulation test, growth hormone response to insulin-induced hypoglycemia, and plasma cortisol levels. As with the DST, there is insufficient evidence to warrant the clinical use of any of these measures to predict treatment response (Balon 1989).

**Metabolites.** The principal metabolite of brain norepinephrine is 3-methoxy-4-hydroxyphenylglycol. Attempts to correlate levels of this metabolite with treatment response have been equivocal. The same has generally been true for other metabolites, including 5-hydroxyindo-lacetic acid and homovanillic acid. These studies are further thwarted by the fact that spinal fluid levels of these metabolites—the level usually obtained in studies—may not correlate well to brain neurotransmitter concentrations (Gjerris 1988).

### Physiological Measures

**Blood Pressure.** Several authors have correlated pretreatment orthostatic hypotension with good response to antidepressants (Jarvik et al. 1983, Davidson and Turnbull 1986), particularly in geriatric patients. Such dysregulation of blood pressure may relate to alpha-adrenergic receptor abnormalities. The simplicity and cost-effectiveness of such a test make it attractive as a screen for treatment response. However, a subsequent controlled study of these correlations in an elderly sample was not confirmatory (Diehl et al. 1993).

**Sleep.** A number of sleep electroencephalography changes have been suggested as predictors of response, particularly shortened rapid eye movement (REM) latency and increases in (REM) latency on initiation of treatment. Results of such studies are mixed. Also promising are the reports that short-term improvement in mood after sleep deprivation may predict positive antidepressant response.

**Neurophysiological Measures.** The availability of such instruments as magnetic resonance imaging (MRI), positron emission tomography (PET), or single-photon emission computed tomography (SPECT) makes possible the non-invasive investigation of drug–receptor observations. Appropriate radioligands for most of the antidepressants and receptors are available. This makes possible more direct measures of antidepressant effect, with the possibility of better predictors of treatment response. Already, PET techniques have documented receptor effects of antidepressants, such as a decrease in receptor densities following treatment with antidepressants (Yatham et al. 1999). Furthermore, the degree of receptor change has been shown to differ with different types of antidepressants (Meyer et al. 1999). Of most interest are possible correlations between neurophysiological changes and clinical response, and some such correlations have been reported. For example, one study reported a correlation between decreased prefrontal activity and antidepressant response (Cook and Leuchter 2001). These changes were observed as early as 48 hours after the initiation of treatment. Though research in this area is just beginning, it is growing rapidly and will surely be key to the future of clinical psychopharmacology.

**Drug Challenges.** Short-term responses to dextroamphetamine and methylphenidate have been studied as predictors of antidepressant response. Again, results are mixed; however, there is evidence that such challenges may predict a subgroup of depressed patients who suffer from amine metabolism disturbances (Balon 1989). Clonidine challenges have been used as measures of noradrenergic dysfunction, and there is some evidence to suggest that depressed patients who show a blunted response to clonidine challenge may preferentially respond to noradrenergic agents (Correa et al. 2001).

### Summary

No one test stands out as a definitive predictor of treatment response. This probably reflects both fundamental problems in our conception of depression, and methodological problems in the studies. Currently, the best predictors of antidepressant response remain clinical and demographical.

## Selection of a Particular Agent

Although, as noted earlier, the various antidepressants seem to have equal efficacy in the treatment of depression, a given patient may respond preferentially to one, or a class of agents. Again, cross-sectional and longitudinal factors should be taken into account.

### Longitudinal Factors

Longitudinal factors include a history of response to a particular agent, a family history of good response, a history of prior side effects (particularly if they resulted in drug discontinuation), and a history of symptoms that could suggest mania (or more minor variants of manic episodes). TCAs are less desirable for patients with prior manic episodes, as they may precipitate manic episodes. Though less well understood, MAOIs may produce the same effect (Keller et al. 1986).

### Cross-Sectional Factors

Cross-sectional factors would include data from the physical examination and laboratory work-up, which might suggest susceptibilities to certain antidepressant agents or contraindications based on physical illness. For instance, an examination that revealed prostatic hypertrophy, or an electrocardiogram that showed a conduction abnormality should influence the physician against a TCA. A seizure disorder would be a relative contraindication against using bupropion. Aspects of the psychiatric examination are useful as well. Suicidal ideation might suggest the use of a second- or third-generation antidepressants, because of their lower lethality (Montgomery 1992). In the presence of severe suicidal ideation, electroconvulsive therapy may be preferable. As previously noted, the presence of manic symptoms, indicative of a mixed bipolar illness, argues for treatment with lithium or anticonvulsants over standard antidepressants.

Anxiety has been often used as a predictive symptom. Specifically, there is often a belief that patients with anxiety symptoms do better with more sedating antidepressants. Though an early sedating effect may increase adherence in patients with prominent anxiety, there is no evidence that more sedating agents are more effective in patients with comorbid depression and anxiety. In fact the opposite is true, and a number of studies have demonstrated the equal efficacy of more and less sedating agents (Simon et al. 1998).

The presence of psychotic symptoms requires combined treatment with antidepressants and antipsychotics, as either agent alone is less effective for these symptoms. An alternative is to use electroconvulsive therapy.

An issue often neglected is that of cost. Older agents, which are available in generic form, are 10 to 100 times less expensive than newer agents. Although older agents tend to have more side effects, cost can also influence compliance. In 2001, fluoxetine became the first SSRI to be available in the US in generic form. The initial approval for generic production was given to only one company, and the result had only a moderate effect on the price of the drug. As of January 2002, however, over 15 pharmaceutical companies have received FDA approval to produce this drug, and as multiple versions become available the effect on price will certainly be more dramatic. Table 97–1 lists the relative costs of antidepressants, as of the first quarter of 2002.

## Pharmacokinetic Concerns

**First-Generation Antidepressants.** The pharmacokinetics of TCAs is complex. This complexity is reflected in the diversity of half-lives reported, which vary roughly from 10 to 40 hours. TCAs are primarily absorbed in the small intestine. They are usually well absorbed, and reach peak plasma levels 2 to 6 hours after oral administration. Absorption can be affected by changes in gut motility. The drugs are extensively metabolized in the liver on first pass through the portal system. They are lipophilic, have a large volume of distribution, and are highly protein-bound (85–95%). TCAs are metabolized in the liver by hepatic microsomal enzymes, by demethylation, oxidation, or hydroxylation. They are generally metabolized to active metabolites, and are excreted by the kidneys. There is a large range of elimination half-lives among the antidepressants.

MAOIs are also well absorbed from the gastrointestinal tract. Their metabolism, although quite efficient (they have a half-life of 1 to 2 hours) is not well understood. The short half-life of these compounds is not entirely relevant however, as they bind irreversibly with MAO. Thus, the activity of these drugs depends less on pharmacokinetics, and more on the synthesis of new MAO to restore normal enzyme activity. This synthesis requires approximately 2 weeks.

**Second-Generation Antidepressants.** All of the available serotonin reuptake inhibitors are well absorbed, and not generally affected by food administration. Sertraline is an exception to this rule, and its blood level may be increased by food. All serotonin reuptake inhibitors have large volumes of distribution and they are extensively protein-bound. They are metabolized by hepatic microsomal enzymes and are potent inhibitors of these enzymes (a fact which will be discussed later in greater detail).

The only serotonin reuptake inhibitor with an active metabolite is fluoxetine, whose metabolite norfluoxetine has a half-life of 7 to 15 days. Thus, it may take several months to achieve steady state with fluoxetine. This is considerably longer than citalopram, which has a half-life of about 1.5 days, or sertraline and paroxetine, which have half-lives of about a day.

As previously discussed, there is no correlation between half-life and time to onset. Drugs with shorter half-lives have an advantage in cases where rapid elimination is desired (for example, in the case of an allergic reaction). Drugs with a longer half-life may also have advantages: fluoxetine, for example, has been successfully given in a once-weekly dosing during the continuation phase of treatment (Burke et al. 2000), and a once-weekly formulation of this drug is currently available. All serotonin reuptake inhibitors are eliminated in the urine as inactive metabolites. Both fluoxetine and paroxetine are capable of inhibit-

ing their own clearance at clinically relevant doses. As such, they have nonlinear pharmacokinetics: changes in dose can produce proportionately large plasma levels.

As with most of the other antidepressants, bupropion undergoes extensive first pass metabolism in the liver. Although the parent compound has a half-life of 10 to 12 hours, it has three metabolites that appear to be active. One, threohydrobupropion, has a half-life of 35 hours and is relatively free in plasma (it is only 50% protein-bound). There is considerable individual variability in the levels of bupropion and its metabolites. Trazodone has a half-life that is relatively short, having a range of 3 to 9 hours. Given this, and its apparent lack of active metabolites, the plasma levels of trazodone can be quite variable during a day. For this reason, the medication requires divided dosing.

**Third-Generation Antidepressants.** Venlafaxine has a short half-life (4 hours); however, it is available in an extended release formulation that allows once-daily dosing. It appears to have a dual effect, in which at lower doses it primarily acts on the serotonin transporter, and clinically significant norepinephrine reuptake inhibition is not seen until higher doses are used (150 mg/day and above).

Nefazodone has relatively low bioavailability, and a short half-life (2–8 hours), and thus it is usually given in twice-daily doses. Mirtazapine has a half-life of 13 to 34 hours.

The relative half-lives of available antidepressants are depicted in Figure 97–2.

## Gender, Ethnic, and Racial Issues

### Gender

Women may have slower gastrointestinal absorption than men, as they have less gastric acid and slower gastric emptying. A woman's volume of distribution differs as well, given her increased ratio of adipose tissue to lean body mass. Water retention associated with the menstrual cycle may also affect the volume of distribution.

Few clinical studies specifically look at the pharmacokinetics of antidepressants in women. Existing studies show conflicting results: some studies suggest that at similar doses women will have increased plasma levels, while other studies do not show such a difference. In some of the studies, the patients used oral contraceptives, which can alter the hepatic metabolism of TCAs, and this may explain the discrepancy between studies.

There may be pharmacodynamic differences as well. Possible gender differences in responses to antidepressants have been suggested for decades (Raskin 1974), but rarely examined in detail. More recently, Kornstein and colleagues (2000) reanalyzed data from a study comparing imipramine and sertraline for chronic depression. They found that women responded better to sertraline than to imipramine whereas men had the opposite pattern of response. Women also had a longer time to response. Of interest was the fact that this effect was only seen in pre-menopausal women; postmenopausal women had similar rates of response to both medications.

### Race and Ethnicity

As with gender, there are insufficient studies available on the effects of race and ethnicity on differential dosing,

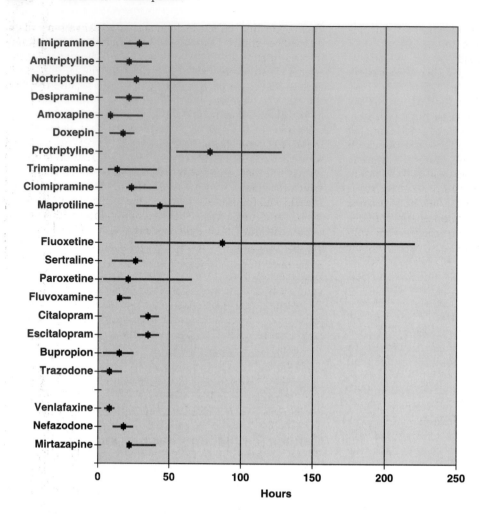

**Figure 97–2** *Approximate mean (black square) and range (colored line) of various antidepressant half-lives.*

pharmacology and treatment response. One study, comparing the use of imipramine in the Columbian and North American patients found a higher rate of response in the Columbian group. Little can be deduced from this finding, as the doses of medication in each group were not comparable (Escobar and Tuason 1980). One study reported higher nortriptyline levels in African-American patients as compared with whites; however, the plasma concentrations were not properly corrected for weight (Rifkin et al. 1978). Some studies have suggested that Hispanic patients may have an increased sensitivity to antidepressants; however, there are conflicting data on this subject (Bond 1991). Although Asians may require lower dosing with antipsychotics, this has not been demonstrated with antidepressants. Some data suggest that Asians are slower to metabolize nortriptyline than other groups. Such a hypothesis is indirectly supported by the fact that Asian countries tend to use lower doses of imipramine and amitriptyline than do western countries (Yamashita and Asano 1979).

African-Americans may be more likely than those of European descent to be slow metabolizers of antidepressant, owing to possible genetic differences in metabolic enzyme expression (Kalow 1991). A growing number of studies suggest that African-Americans will have higher plasma levels per dose of antidepressant (Strickland et al. 1997). This has been primarily demonstrated with TCAs, and data with SSRIs is lacking.

Clearly these issues need to be explored further. However, the greatest concern regarding race and ethnicity is suggested in a study by Sirey and colleagues (1999) of prescribing practices in Westchester County (New York) mental health clinics, which found that minorities were less likely than nonminorities to be offered antidepressant treatment, independent of diagnosis.

## Preparation of the Patient

### Side Effects of Antidepressants

**General Concerns.** Good preparation and reassurance are essential. Side effects—even relatively benign ones—are a major cause of treatment nonadherence. Drop-out rates ranging from 7 to 44% have been reported in various studies of TCAs, and from 7 to 23% in studies of serotonin reuptake inhibitors (Cookson 1993). Proper education and reassurance about side effects can help reduce this rate. It should help reassure the patient that many of the side effects diminish with time, or with an adjustment of dose. It may also help frame side effects in a positive light, as they represent concrete evidence that the medication is exerting its effect on the body.

The best approach may be to consider both frequency and clinical importance. That is, one should discuss those side effects that are likely to occur, as well as considering the rare but potential dangerous or irreversible side effects that should be discussed. A number of common, uncommon, and hypothetical side effects are discussed here.

The importance of discussing side effects as soon as possible is made particularly crucial given the wide variety of other sources of information at patients' disposal. Many pharmacies now include printed information to accompany medication, and these forms often include a comprehensive list of side effects. Other printed material, including the Physicians' Desk Reference (2001) and various books on medications are available and a popular offering in many bookstores and libraries. Perhaps the greatest innovation has been the explosion of electronic information that is available on the Internet. Mental health sites have become an extremely popular source of information for patients. The information on Internet sites may range from very reputable and informative, to anecdotal, to clearly hostile and misrepresentative. It should be the role of the physician to give such information context, and, if indicated, to correct misinformation.

**Specific Side Effects.** It is useful to divide side effects into "predictable" and idiosyncratic effects. Predictable side effects result from known pharmacological actions of the drug. Idiosyncratic side effects are not well understood. A number of authors have written important, and very complete reviews of medication-related side effects (e.g., Cookson 1993, Nierenberg 1992, Mir and Taylor 1997, Richelson 2001); what is intended in the following paragraphs and figures is a brief summary that incorporates data from those works.

## Predictable Side Effects

These side effects are the result of the action of the agent at various neurotransmitters and enzyme sites. The major neurotransmitters affected by antidepressants are as follows:

**Muscarinic Acetylcholine Receptors.** Blockade of this receptor produces a variety of peripheral and central effects.

Gastrointestinal effects include decreased salivation and decreased peristalsis. Decreased salivation is the most common of these effects and can cause drying of the mucous membranes. Such drying can exacerbate gum disease and dental caries. Decreased peristalsis can cause constipation and, in the extreme, paralytic ileus. Contraction of the bladder wall is inhibited, causing urinary hesitancy and even urinary retention. In the case of TCAs, concomitant sympathomimetic effects that cause constriction of the bladder neck and urethra worsen this effect on urination. Inhibition of the parasympathetically mediated accommodation reflex, in which the ciliary body muscles normally contract to thicken the lens and focus near objects on the retina, results in blurry vision and mydriasis. Such accommodation paresis can occur without other anticholinergic side effects. A more serious ocular effect is the precipitation of acute narrow-angle glaucoma, through pupillary dilatation. The iatrogenic precipitation of narrow-angle glaucoma through antidepressant use is quite rare. Anticholinergic cardiac effects include decreased vagal tone that can cause tachycardia. Central nervous effects include impaired memory and cognition. In severe cases, such cognitive impairment can reach the point of a delirium. Central anticholinergic effects can also worsen existing tardive dyskinesia.

These effects are usually dose-related, and are worse in people with preexisting defects. For example, the cardiac effects are of most concern in those with preexisting cardiac defects, and urinary blockade generally occurs only in the presence of prostatic hypertrophy. These side effects are also more common in patients taking other anticholinergic medications, which is a common feature of many over-the-counter preparations.

The relative affinities of antidepressants for blocking muscarinic receptors are compared in Figure 97–3. As MAOIs have little direct effect on receptors, and their side effects relate to enzymatic inhibition, they are not included in this section, or on the accompanying graphs.

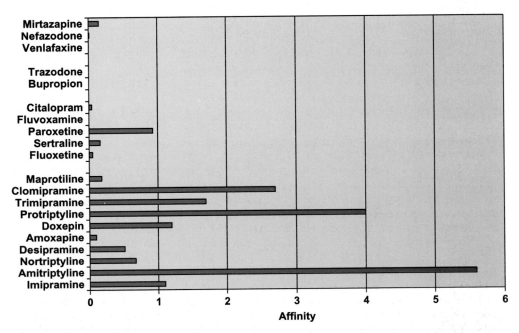

**Figure 97–3** *Relative affinities of antidepressants for blocking muscarinic receptors.*

Affinity = $10^{-7} \times 1/K_d$    ($K_d$ = dissociation constant)

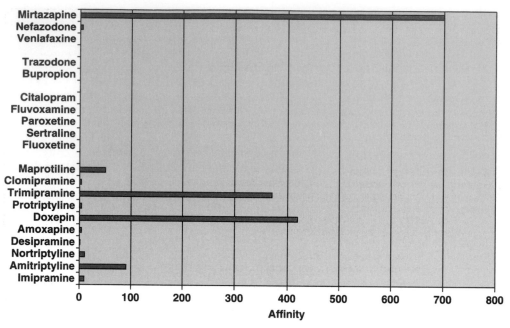

**Figure 97–4** *Relative affinities of antidepressants for blocking histaminic receptors.*

Affinity = $10^{-7} \times 1/K_d$   ($K_d$ = dissociation constant)

**Histamine.** Blockade of the histamine $H_1$-receptor is typically associated with sedation. Histamine blockade may also cause orthostatic hypotension and weight gain. It can impair psychomotor coordination and cause falls in the elderly. Cognitive impairment can occur as well. $H_2$-receptor blockade causes decreased gastric acid production. This is the mechanism of many antiulcer medications. The relative affinities of antidepressants for blocking histaminic receptors are compared in Figure 97–4.

**Norepinephrine.** Synaptic increases in norepinephrine, through either inhibition of norepinephrine reuptake or decrease in MAO degradation, cause sympathomimetic effects.

Increases in norepinephrine can cause anxiety, tremors, diaphoresis, and tachycardia. This tachycardia can potentiate anticholinergic cardiac effects. As noted, sympathomimetic effects on the bladder neck and urethra can potentiate the anticholinergic inhibition of normal urinary function. The relative potencies of antidepressants for blocking the reuptake of norepinephrine are compared in Figure 97–5.

**Receptor Blockade.** Blockade of alpha-1-receptors occurs as a chronic effect through both downregulation and desensitization of the beta- and alpha-2-receptors. Blockade of the noradrenergic alpha-1-receptor is responsible for postural hypotension. In the elderly or medically ill, this postural

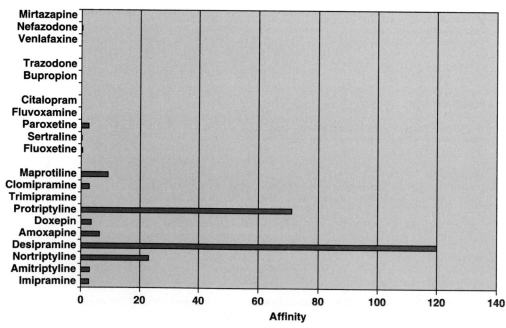

**Figure 97–5** *Relative potencies of antidepressants for blocking the reuptake of norepinephrine.*

Affinity = $10^{-7} \times 1/K_d$   ($K_d$ = dissociation constant)

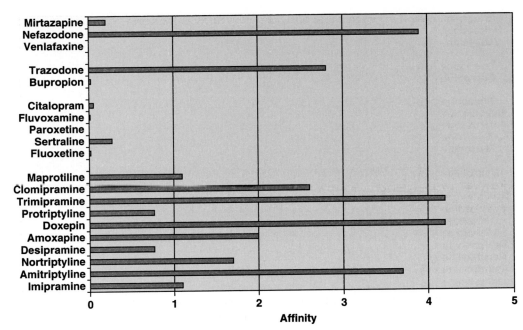

**Figure 97–6** *Relative affinities of antidepressants for blocking $\alpha_1$-adrenoceptors.*

Affinity = $10^{-7} \times 1/K_d$   ($K_d$ = dissociation constant)

hypotension can be significant, and lead to dizziness or falls. It may also be responsible for ejaculatory delay or impotence. Other potential effects include reflex tachycardia and memory dysfunction. The relative affinities of antidepressants for blocking alpha-1-adrenoceptors are compared in Figure 97–6.

**Serotonin.** Potentiation of serotonin can cause anorexia, nausea, vomiting, diarrhea, "jitteriness," and anxiety. Akathisia, a syndrome of motor restlessness usually associated with antipsychotics, may result from either the general effect of serotonin potentiation or the direct effects on the basal gan-

glia. The latter hypothesis is supported by the fact that the serotonin reuptake inhibitors—fluoxetine (Steur 1993), sertraline (Shihabuddin and Rapport 1994), and paroxetine (Choo 1993)—have all been reported to cause or exacerbate extrapyramidal reactions. Sedation, which has been reported with all serotonin reuptake inhibitors, appears to be a primary serotonin effect (Cookson 1993). Insomnia, however, is more common at higher doses, particularly with fluoxetine. A number of sexual side effects have been attributed to serotonin reuptake blockade, including anorgasmia, ejaculatory difficulties, and even spontaneous orgasms associated with yawning (Modell 1989). The relative potencies of anti-

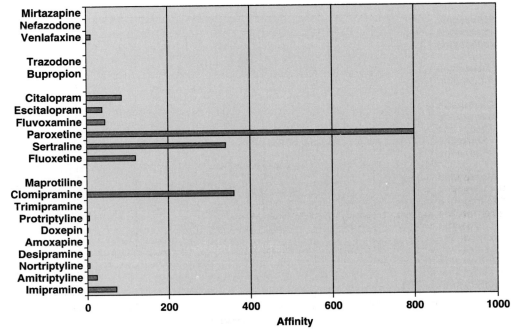

**Figure 97–7** *Relative potencies of antidepressants for blocking the reuptake of serotonin.*

Affinity = $10^{-7} \times 1/K_d$   ($K_d$ = dissociation constant)

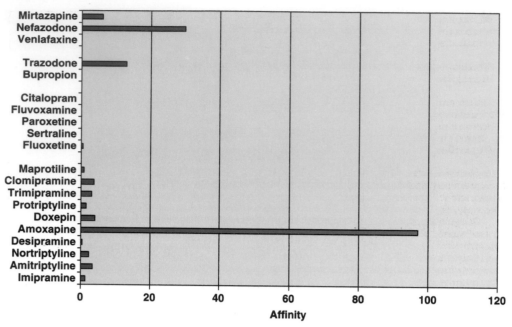

Affinity = $10^{-7} \times 1/K_d$  ($K_d$ = dissociation constant)

**Figure 97–8** *Relative affinities of antidepressants for blocking 5-HT$_{2A}$-receptors.*

depressants for blocking the reuptake of serotonin are compared in Figure 97–7.

**Receptor Antagonism.** Blockade of the 5-HT$_2$-receptors may result in hypotension and ejaculatory disturbances. Antagonism of serotonin receptors may also be responsible for weight gain and carbohydrate craving. Potency for blockade of this receptor (specifically of the 5-HT$_{2A}$-receptor) is compared in Figure 97–8.

**Dopamine.** Increases in dopamine resulting from reuptake blockade can have an antiparkinsonian effect. It can also cause psychomotor activation and aggravation of psychosis. The relative potencies of antidepressants for blocking the reuptake of dopamine are compared in Figure 97–9.

**Receptor Antagonism.** The blockade of dopamine receptors can result in extrapyramidal symptoms. These symptoms include cogwheel-type rigidity, tremor, dyskinesia, masked facies, and acute dystonia. Prolonged dopamine blockade appears to be responsible for tardive dyskinesia. Dopamine receptor blockade has also been associated with

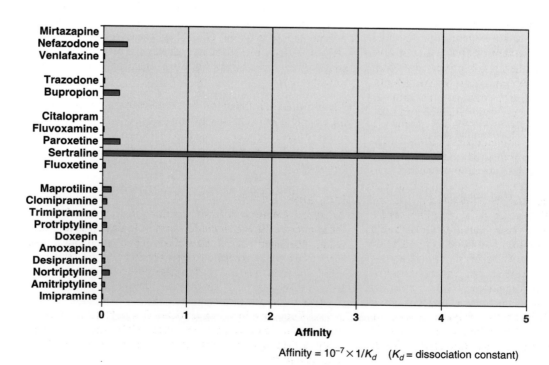

Affinity = $10^{-7} \times 1/K_d$  ($K_d$ = dissociation constant)

**Figure 97–9** *Relative potencies of antidepressants for blocking the reuptake of dopamine.*

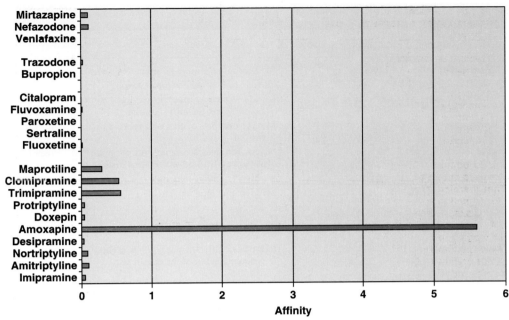

**Figure 97–10** *Relative affinities of antidepressants for blocking dopamine receptors.*

$$\text{Affinity} = 10^{-7} \times 1/K_d \quad (K_d = \text{dissociation constant})$$

endocrine changes and sexual dysfunction. The relative affinities of antidepressants for blocking dopamine receptors are compared in Figure 97–10.

**Monoamine Oxidase.** MAO is the main enzyme responsible for the metabolism of monoamines. There are two main types of MAOs, identified as types A and B. Type A is selective for serotonin and norepinephrine, and accounts for 80% of the MAO in the brain. Type B selectively deaminates phenylethylamine. Both forms oxidize dopamine and tyramine.

**Dietary Restrictions.** The dietary restrictions required when using MAOIs represent the major limitation to widespread use of these effective antidepressants. Nonselective inhibition of MAO prevents the normal hepatic metabolism of tyramine containing foods or sympathomimetic agents. The increased level of tyramine in the circulation stimulates the release of norepinephrine from sympathetic terminals. This sudden increase in norepinephrine is the basis for the "tyramine–cheese" reaction, so named because cheese is the most common source of the tyramine that causes this reaction. In fact, other pressor amines, such as levodopa, can also cause the reaction, but tyramine—a natural product of food fermentation and bacterial decarboxylation—is the most common in foods. The result of a tyramine–cheese reaction can be a hypertensive crisis. Thus, patients should be well educated as to the foods that must be avoided while using MAOIs. In the past, there has been a tendency towards conservative dietary restrictions, often based on single case reports or indirect analogies. More research and experience have suggested that not all the foods commonly restricted are equally likely to precipitate a reaction (McCabe and Tsuang 1982). Better compliance is likely if a more reasonable diet is prescribed (as suggested in Table 97–3).

Despite the best of preparation, some patients may err and suffer a hypertensive crisis. This is often experienced as a severe, pulsating, occipital headache that then generalizes. It may be alleviated with 10 mg of nifedipine, either oral or sublingual (Golwyn and Sevlie 1993).

MAOIs can cause an increase in standing systolic blood pressure, absent of tyramine containing foods or sympathomimetics. Generally, this effect is not clinically significant; however, serious unprovoked hypertensive episodes have been reported (Lavin et al. 1993), and blood pressure should be monitored for 1 to 2 hours after beginning or increasing an MAOI. Hypotension is also a reported effect of MAO, but the mechanism is not known. MAO inhibition can also cause sedation or overstimulation. Once again, the mechanism of this is not well understood.

**Membrane Stabilizing Activity.** TCAs have effects on cardiac conduction that are independent of anticholinergic or noradrenergic effects. Destabilization of the cardiac membrane can cause dysrhythmia and asystole, particularly in overdose.

## Idiopathic Effects

**Allergic Reactions.** Allergic reactions can occur with any of these agents. Effects include dermatological (rashes, urticaria, photosensitivity, Stevens-Johnson syndrome) and hematological (agranulocytosis) sensitivities. Several case reports have described a photosensitivity reaction apparently caused by desipramine that results in a blue–gray pigmentation (Narurkar et al. 1993, Steele and Ashby 1993). Fluoxetine has been associated with bleeding, inflammation (Gunzberger and Martinez 1992), and, most seriously, a fatal systemic vasculitis. It should be stopped if a rash develops.

| Table 97-3 | Suggested Diet for Patients Taking Monoamine Oxidase Inhibitors (MAOIs) | |
| --- | --- | --- |
| **Proposed Restrictions** | **Analysis** | **Can Use** |
| Most cheese and cheese products | M: accounts for most tyramine reactions | Cream, cottage, or ricotta cheese |
| Sour cream, yogurt | P: except in excess if stored too long | |
| Fermented meats (sausage, salami, pepperoni) | M: dry fermented sausage (summer sausage) has the most tyramine | Hard sausage has not been associated with hypertensive crises |
| Aged meats | M: many reports of crises for meats stored for only 2–3 d | Fresh meats |
| Liver | M: chicken liver has significant tyramine; avoid pate and other prepared dishes | Fresh beef liver |
| Smoked or pickled herring, caviar | M: high tyramine content | Fresh fish |
| Broad bean pods (Italian green beans, fava beans) | M: high levodopa content | Other fresh vegetables |
| Avocado | P: avoid if overripe; no reported reactions | |
| Sauerkraut | M | |
| Bananas | P: especially if overripe; peel has highest tyramine (eaten in the only reported case) | Other fresh fruits |
| Raisins, figs | I: based on one case report | |
| Chocolate | I: few reported cases | |
| Yeast extract (brewer's yeast, "Marmite," some packaged soups) | M | Yeast breads |
| Soy sauce | P: few case reports may be Chinese restaurant syndrome | |
| Meat tenderizers | I | |
| Chianti wine | M: most valid of alcohol restrictions | Other wines (moderate amounts) |
| Vermouth | M: may be similar to Chianti in tyramine | |
| Beers and ales | P: small amounts allowed; one ration to Irish whiskey | Other alcoholic drinks (moderate amounts) |
| Other beverages: coffee, tea, caffeinated sodas | I: a nonspecific recommendation (no reports link caffeine to reactions) | |

M, must be avoided; P, probably acceptable in moderate amounts; I, insufficient evidence to justify any restriction.

In most cases of allergic reactions, the primary treatment is to stop the agent. In one report, granulocyte colony stimulating factor was used successfully to treat severe chlomipramine-associated agranulocytosis (Hunt and Resnick 1993).

**Liver Effects.** Abnormal liver function tests have been associated with a number of antidepressants, which can be independent of dose. The risk for such effects may be worsened by chronic alcohol or anticonvulsant use.

Though sudden liver effects are possible for most antidepressants, some seem to have a heightened risk. For example, nefazodone has been reported to have a rare but notable risk of hepatic failure (Aranda-Michel et al. 1999). The manufacturer estimates that the risk of liver failure resulting in death or transplant is 1 in 250,000 to 300,000 patient-years of nefazodone treatment (Schwetz 2002). This can occur suddenly, and in individuals with previously normal liver functioning. As the rate of progressive liver damage, when it does occur, is not known, it is not yet clear whether the use of liver function tests during treatment would lessen the risk, and, if so, how often they should be performed.

**Seizures.** A preexisting seizure disorder increases an antidepressant's likelihood of precipitating a seizure. Other

predisposing factors include a family history of a seizure; an abnormal pretreatment electroencephalogram; brain damage; previous electroconvulsive treatment; abuse or withdrawal from sedatives; alcohol, or cocaine; and concurrent use of CNS-activating medications (Rosenstein et al. 1993). Seizures may be more likely to occur early in treatment, or after a large escalation in dose.

The risk of seizure with TCAs is usually reported as 0.1%. This incidence applies to outpatients, without predisposing factors for seizures, who receive low to moderate doses of medications. In higher doses the risk is probably 1.1% (Rosenstein et al. 1993); in unselected populations the risk may be as high as 2 to 2.5% (Davidson 1989). Serotonin reuptake inhibitors appear to have a lower incidence of seizures. Bupropion has a high rate of seizures in patients with a preexisting seizure history, and in patients with bulimia. In patients without these predisposing factors, the risk appears to be about 0.4%; thus, it may have a two- to fourfold risk of seizures compared with other antidepressants. Bupropion's effect on the seizure threshold has never been directly compared with other antidepressants.

**Precipitation of Mania.** Antidepressants have been associated with the precipitation of mania, and rapid cycling bipolar disorder. This appears to be most common in patients with a preexisting history of mania and in unipolar depression the rate of antidepressant-induced mania is very low (< 1%). The problem has been most frequently reported in TCAs, but has been seen in SSRIs as well (Cookson 1993). A similar problem has been found with newer agents, including nefazodone (Jeffries and al-Jeshi 1995) and venlafaxine (Shulman et al. 2001), though the data for this is more limited. Bupropion may have a lower incidence of mania (Shopsin 1983). Some research points to a particular polymorphism of the serotonin transporter as predisposing to this side effect (Mundo et al. 2001).

**Sexual Dysfunction.** A variety of sexual side effects can be caused by antidepressants, and they can affect all aspects of sexual response. Thus, antidepressants can decrease libido, increase impotence and anorgasmia, and cause delayed or retrograde ejaculation (Segraves 1992). In a study of 60 outpatients on various antidepressants, 43% experienced some type of sexual dysfunction (Balon et al. 1993). This high incidence of sexual dysfunction had no clear relation to any particular antidepressant or diagnosis.

SSRIs have a high incidence of delayed orgasm or anorgasmia. In several studies, fluoxetine adversely affected ejaculation or orgasm, with a rate ranging from 8 to 13%. All SSRIs can have similar adverse effects, but the incidence may differ with the agent. Paroxetine appears to cause the most ejaculatory delay and delayed orgasm. For example, in one direct comparison, citalopram was found to cause less delayed orgasm and ejaculation than did paroxetine (Waldinger et al. 2001a). Similarly, fluvoxamine has less effect on orgasm when compared with paroxetine, with fluoxetine and sertraline having a more intermediate effect (Waldinger et al. 1998).

Though these side effects may in part be receptor-mediated, at least some degree seems to be iatrogenic and not dose-related. As such, sexual side effects can occur at even low therapeutic doses, and dose reduction may not be possible. A change of agent may be the only alternative. Bupropion appears to have the lowest incidence of sexual side effects among the antidepressants, often not differing from placebo in studies of sexual functioning (Labbate et al. 2001). In one open study, patients using fluoxetine who experienced orgasmic dysfunction were switched to bupropion and were able to maintain an antidepressant response with less sexual side effects (Walker et al. 1993). Similarly, nefazodone has been shown to have little effect on ejaculation or orgasm (Waldinger et al. 2001b).

Trazodone has been associated with penile priapism; the risk is around 1 in 6,000 to 8,000 men. Although rare, it is notable that a third of these cases required surgical intervention, and some resulted in permanent impairment. Clitoral priapism has been reported as well (Pescatori et al. 1993). The actual cause of these sexual dysfunctions is not clear, although some of these effects may relate to dose related-anticholinergic, presynaptic alpha-2-adrenergic, or serotonergic effects.

Occasionally antidepressants can enhance sexual function. This is usually due to the alleviation of depression; however, there have been case reports of improved libido or potency after initiation of an antidepressant, which occurred independent of any antidepressant effect (Smith and Levitte 1993).

**Miscellaneous.** Fine tremors have been noticed with both TCAs and serotonin reuptake inhibitors. Although the mechanism is not clear, serotonin reuptake inhibition may be involved. Excessive sweating has been associated with both fluoxetine and paroxetine. The syndrome of inappropriate secretion of antidiuretic hormone has been seen with fluoxetine, as well as with a number of other antidepressants. Fluoxetine has also been associated with alopecia, generally—but not always—at doses above 20 mg/day (Ogilvie 1993) and there have been case reports of hair loss with sertraline as well (Bourgeois 1996). Although antidepressants are often used to treat headaches, they have on occasion been reported as causing both migraine and nonmigraine headaches (Larson 1993). These reports should be tempered by the fact that headaches are a frequent nonspecific complaint both in depressed and normal individuals, and the relationship may not always be causal (Reidenberg and Lowenthal 1968).

All serotonergic antidepressants can cause sedation; however, the Committee on Safety of Medicines in the UK has received reports of paroxetine causing a semi-stuporous state (Lewis et al. 1993).

One should always be alert to the possibility of rare, undiscovered allergic reactions. For example, the subsequent discovery of serious hepatic and hematological effects caused the withdrawal of nomifensine well after the drug's approval.

## Drug–Drug Interactions

Drugs can affect other drugs in a variety of ways. These can be divided into pharmacodynamic and pharmacokinetic interactions. Pharmacodynamic reactions involve the propensity of one drug to affect the ability of another drug to bind to its target receptor. An example of this may be found with the TCAs, which may compete with other drugs for binding sites.

Pharmacokinetic interactions involve the ability of one drug to influence the pharmacokinetics (absorption, distribution, rate of metabolism, and elimination half-life) of another drug. One way in which this can happen is through binding. Many of the antidepressants are protein-bound. If another drug is introduced that has an affinity for the same binding site, the result may be the displacement of a drug and a subsequent increase in the free drug concentration. This effect may be counteracted by a compensatory increased elimination of the now freed drug, thus the overall effect of protein binding may be hard to predict.

The most common drug–drug interaction with antidepressants is their influence on the metabolism of other drugs. Antidepressants are metabolized through catabolic enzymes located in a variety of places, but primarily in the smooth endoplasmic reticulum of hepatocytes: the cytochrome P450 (CYP) enzymes. Many other drugs are also metabolized through similar pathways: it is estimated that about half of all drugs prescribed depend on CYP for their metabolism (Bertz and Granneman 1997). Indeed, CYP is a ubiquitous enzyme, present not only in humans, but also in all animals, plants, bacteria, and fungi. There are a number of CYP enzymes, and multiple alleles for each. These are catalogued and updated by the Human Cytochrome Committee, whose web page can be found at (http://www.imm. ki.se/CYPalleles/).

Of these enzymes, most drugs are metabolized by the enzymes CYP3A4 (50%) and CYP2D6 (20%). Other clinically important CYP enzymes include CYP2C9, and CYP2C19 and CYP1A2, that latter which is found in the brain and may affect CNS distribution of antidepressant (a number of good "primers" exist on the chemistry and role of CYP, and the reader is referred to a review by Richelson [1997] for further study). A list of the enzymes and some drugs commonly affected by them is found in Table 97–4.

CYP2D6 is probably the best studied of these enzymes. It can have multiple mutations, due to an autosomal recessive trait known as "debrisoquine polymorphism" (debrisoquine is an antihypertensive, in the same chemical class as guanethidine, and its metabolism by this pathway is well understood). Thus, a person can be phenotypically an "extensive-," "intermediate-," or "poor-" metabolizer (Meier et al. 1983). These phenotypes account for much of the pharmacokinetic variability among individuals taking the numerous drugs oxidized by this pathway. Poor metabolizers can have unusually long half-lives for these drugs and a higher risk of toxicity (Tollefson 1993). The poor metabolizer phenotype occurs in about 5 to 10% of those of European heritage, and may be higher in other ethnic population, such as African-Americans. Extensive

metabolizers, on the other hand, can have great difficulty in achieving therapeutic levels with standard doses (Eichelbaum and Gross 1990).

## First-Generation Antidepressants

**Tricyclic Antidepressants.** As with any combination therapy, the side effects described previously can be additive with other similar drugs. Most problematical are the anticholinergic effects of the TCAs. Such cholinergic—particularly muscarinic—blockade is a property shared by many other medications, including numerous over-the-counter preparations. The general sedative properties of these medications can also augment any soporific. The slowing of cardiac conduction can also potentiate other medications that produce similar effects, such as type IA antiarrhythmics and anticholinergic medications. Adrenergic receptor blockade can worsen the orthostatic hypotension caused by other medications, including vasodilators and low-potency antipsychotic medications.

**Pharmacokinetic Effects.** Absorption of TCAs can be inhibited by cholestyramine, which therefore must be given at different time intervals than the antidepressants. TCA levels can be raised by substances that inhibit enzyme activity, and lowered by substances that induce it. Specific substances reported to increase TCA levels include fluoxetine, antipsychotic medications, methylphenidate, and cimetidine. In a controlled trial, methylphenidate was combined with desipramine to treat attention deficits and depression in children. The combination therapy had a higher incidence of electrocardiogram changes (particularly higher ventricular rates) and somatic side effects (nausea, dry mouth, and tremor) (Pataki et al. 1993). Enzyme "inducers" that can lower tricyclic agent levels include phenobarbital and carbamazepine. The nicotine from cigarettes can also induce enzyme activity.

Guanethidine is contraindicated with TCAs, as it relies on neuronal reuptake for its antihypertensive effect. Clonidine, a presynaptic alpha-2-receptor noradrenergic agonist, is also contraindicated, as it works in an antithetical fashion to tricyclic medications.

**Monoamine Oxidase Inhibitors.** As with the dietary proscriptions, any medication that increases tyramine can precipitate a hypertensive crisis. Such medications include numerous over-the-counter preparations for coughs, colds, and allergies. The same rule applies to sympathomimetic drugs (such as epinephrine and amphetamines) and dopaminergic drugs (such as anti-Parkinsonian medications).

The combination of MAOIs and narcotics—particularly meperidine—may cause a fatal interaction. The reaction can vary from symptoms of agitation and hyperpyrexia to cardiovascular collapse, coma, and death. The mechanism of this reaction is poorly understood, but it may result from central serotonin dysregulation. A similar reaction has also been reported when propoxyphene, diphenoxylate hydrochloride, and atropine are used with MAOIs.

The combination of an MAOI with a potentiator of serotonin (such as a serotonin reuptake inhibitor) can cause the serotonin syndrome (described later in the chapter).

| Table 97–4 | Cytochrome P-450 Isoenzymes and Common Medications Inhibiting Them | |
|---|---|---|
| | Inhibitors | Inducers |
| **1A2** | Cimetidine, fluoroquinolones, fluvoxamine, ticlopidine | Tobacco |
| **2C19** | Fluoxetine, fluvoxamine, ketoconazole, lansoprazole, omeprazole, ticlopidine | |
| **2C9** | Amiodarone, fluconazole, isoniazid, ticlopidine | Rifampin, secobarbital |
| **2D6** | Amiodarone, chlorpheniramine, cimetidine, clomipramine, fluoxetine, haloperidol, methadone, mibefradil, paroxetine, quinidine, ritonavir, | |
| **3A4,5,7** | HIV protease inhibitors: (indinavirn, elfinavir, ritonavir, saquinavir, amiodarone, but not azithromycin) cimetidine, clarithromycin, erythromycin, fluoxetine, fluvoxamine, grapefruit juice, itraconazole, ketoconazole, mibefradil, nefazodone, troleandomycin | Carbamazepine, phenobarbital, phenytoin, rifabutin, rifampin, St. John's wort, troglitazone |

Similar to the dietary restrictions, some of the drug restrictions associated with MAOIs are based on few actual data. Best established are the restrictions against the combination of MAOIs with amines, meperidine, dextromethorphan, hypoglycemic agents, L-dopa, reserpine, tetrabenazine, and tryptophan. TCAs are frequently included on this list as causing a "central excitory syndrome" in combination with MAOIs, although the two have been combined safely. Blackwell (1991) published a comprehensive review of MAOI drug interactions.

## Second-Generation Antidepressants

**Serotonin Reuptake Inhibitors.** Serotonin reuptake inhibitors are potent inhibitors of the CYP2D6 pathway, and the drug–drug interactions that can result from this have been the subject of a number of books and articles. As such, an in-depth discussion is not possible in this chapter, and some concerns will be briefly discussed. The reader is also referred to our earlier discussion of CYP-related drug interactions and to Table 97–4.

Serotonin reuptake inhibitors can slow the metabolism of any drug that is also metabolized by that pathway. Such drugs include TCAs, carbamazepine, phenothiazines, butyrophenones, opiates, diazepam, alprazolam, verapamil, diltiazem, cimetidine, and bupropion. Paroxetine appears to be the most potent inhibitor of this metabolic pathway, with fluoxetine also showing high potency. Sertraline is a somewhat less potent inhibitor.

These pharmacokinetic interactions are best managed with dosage adjustment. Fluoxetine, for example, can be safely used with tricyclic medications if TCA blood levels and, possibly, electrocardiograms are monitored (Leonard 1993). Although it binds more weakly to the CYP2D6, sertraline has also been reported to raise the level of TCAs significantly (Lydiard et al. 1993). In the case of bupropion, this relative increase in the blood level can increase the risk for seizures.

Particular caution should be used when a patient using multiple medications starts a serotonin reuptake inhibitor, as the interactions with other drugs can cause dangerous increases in levels. For example, in the cardiac patient, levels of warfarin should be monitored as fluoxetine has been reported to raise these levels (Woolfrey et al. 1993). Several case reports exist of increased antiarrhythmic levels after introduction of fluoxetine, which resulted in potential serious bradyarrhythmias.

Fluoxetine has also been reported to raise lithium levels. The mechanism for this is not clear, as lithium is primarily excreted through the kidneys.

**The Serotonin Syndrome.** Of particular concern is the serotonin syndrome. This syndrome occurs when a serotonin reuptake inhibitor is combined with another drug that can potentiate serotonin, such as MAOIs, pentazocine, and L-tryptophan. It has also been reported with the adjunctive use of less obvious serotonergic drugs, such as lithium (Muly et al. 1993) and carbamazepine (Dursun et al. 1993). This creates a toxic effect with symptoms of abdominal pain, diarrhea, diaphoresis, hyperpyrexia, tachycardia, hypertension, myoclonus, irritability, agitation, epileptic seizures, and delirium. In its severest form, it can result in coma, cardiovascular shock, and death. For this reason, a

clearance period is required before switching between a serotonin reuptake inhibitor and an MAOI. Switching from fluoxetine to an MAOI is particularly difficult, given fluoxetine's long clearance time—about 6 weeks. Clearance is considerably more rapid for sertraline or paroxetine, and a 2-week "wash-out" period is advised when changing from one of these agents to an MAOI. Occasionally, case reports have suggested that some patients tolerate a quicker switch; however, a full waiting period remains the most prudent course, as several deaths have occurred after an MAOI was begun too soon after fluoxetine was discontinued (Beasley et al. 1993).

**Other Second-Generation Antidepressants.** Few reports exist of interactions with other drugs and trazodone, although trazodone may increase levels of digoxin, phenytoin, and possibly warfarin. Bupropion causes few drug–drug interactions. The main interactions reported have occurred when bupropion is combined with another dopaminergic agent. For example, when bupropion was used with L-dopa, the combination caused excitement, restlessness, nausea, vomiting, and tremor (Goetz et al. 1984).

## Third-Generation Antidepressants

Venlafaxine does not substantially inhibit the CYP enzyme, and is not highly protein-bound, thus it tends to have few clinically significant drug–drug interactions. Nefazodone is highly protein-bound, and has several active metabolites. It is also a strong inhibitor of CYP3A4, and affects other drugs also metabolized by that pathway; however, it has little affinity for the CYP2D6 enzyme. Mirtazapine is highly protein-bound as well, but appears to only weakly affect the cytochrome enzymes.

## Initiation of Treatment

### Choosing a Drug

On average, all antidepressants are equally effective. Although an individual patient may preferentially respond to a certain antidepressant, it is difficult to predict this in advance. Without a personal or family history of such a response, side effects are the most influential factors in choosing an agent. Side effects may be particularly relevant in the following groups of patients.

### Cardiovascular Patients

**Tricyclic Antidepressants.** There is a high rate of depression in patients who have had a myocardial infarction and the presence of depression adversely affects the prognosis of cardiac disease. Indeed, there is a large literature on the relationship between depression and cardiac morbidity (Roose and Dalack 1992). It is important to appreciate this point, as a premorbid cardiac condition can cause concern, which may delay the treatment of the depressed cardiac patient. Though some concerns may be justified, they must also be weighed against the potential morbidity from undertreatment of depression in the cardiac patient.

The major cardiovascular side effect of TCAs is orthostatic hypotension. This can be clinically significant in both the hypertensive patient and the elderly patient. TCAs can more than double the risk of hip fractures in these patients (Ray et al. 1987). Some of the tricyclic medications may have a lower risk of orthostatic hypotension, notably nortriptyline and doxepin. The evidence for nortriptyline causing little or no hypotension is convincing; for doxepin it is weaker (Roose and Dalack 1992).

TCAs do not show a negative inotropic effect and do not seem to worsen congestive heart failure. Patients with congestive heart failure may, however, be at a higher risk for orthostatic hypotension. Again, nortriptyline is the safest TCA in this case.

TCAs slow conduction at the bundle of His. Their effect is analogous to type 1A antiarrhythmic agents such as quinidine and procainamide. In therapeutic doses they can slow cardiac conduction and in overdose they can cause atrioventricular blockade. These effects are of most concern in patients with preexisting cardiac conduction defects. The majority of research in this area has been done by Roose and Glassman (1989). They believe that the group at greatest risk for conduction defects from TCAs has either a bundle branch block (right or left), or a significant intraventricular conduction defect (QRS interval > 0.11 seconds). There is no evidence that any one tricyclic medication is safer than another.

Certain findings may further limit the role of tricyclic medications in heart disease. A large multicenter study found that type 1A antiarrhythmics can increase the risk of mortality among patients with ventricular arrhythmias. Data also suggest that antiarrhythmic drugs cause increased mortality in atrial fibrillation as well (Glassman et al. 1993). As a result, Glassman and coworkers (1993) recommend caution when using TCAs in all patients with ischemic heart disease, particularly patients with ventricular arrhythmias that follow a myocardial infarction.

**Serotonin Reuptake Inhibitors.** The serotonin reuptake inhibitors differ from the TCAs in that they do not prolong the PR or heart wave (QRS) interval. Thus, they probably lack any of the proarrhythmic and antiarrhythmic activities associated with TCAs. They do not cause orthostatic hypotension.

Most studies that exist suggest that SSRIs should be safe in patients with heart disease. Open studies of SSRIs have generally supported this (Roose et al. 1998). Both fluoxetine (Roose et al. 1994) and paroxetine (Nelson et al. 1999) have been compared to nortriptyline in depressed patients with ischemic heart disease. In the first case, fluoxetine had a poorer rate of response than did nortriptyline; this study was done in severe melancholic psychiatric inpatients. The paroxetine study, using moderately depressed outpatients, found similar response to the TCA with fewer cardiovascular side effects.

**Other Agents.** Trazodone has less proarrhythmic effect than the TCAs. However, there have been reports of trazodone-related ventricular ectopy and complete heart block (Martyn et al. 1993). In patients with preexisting heart disease, bupropion does not appear to cause the cardiac side effects attributed to TCAs (Roose et al. 1991).

## Elderly Patients

**Pharmacokinetic Concerns.** Two pharmacokinetic changes are of great importance in aging patients: decreased efficiency of the hepatic microoxidase system and a decreased muscle–fat ratio. Decreased efficiency of hepatic microoxi-

dases results in the slower metabolism of antidepressants and other drugs. Normal increases in body fat and a loss of muscle mass result in an alteration of the volume of distribution for a substance. Thus, lipophilic drugs—including all antidepressants—are more widely distributed in the elderly body.

Both the resulting slower metabolism and the increased volume of distribution increase the half-lives of the various antidepressants. The elderly, therefore, are likely to have a greater incidence of side effects. One dramatic example of this is the cohort study that showed a significantly greater risk for automobile accidents (relative risk of 2.2) among elderly drivers who take antidepressants (Ray et al. 1992).

The half-lives and steady state concentrations of the serotonin reuptake inhibitors are only minimally affected by age. Paroxetine may be an exception to this, and it may have an increased half-life in the elderly (Leonard 1993).

**Pharmacodynamic Concerns.** Numerous changes in the densities and sensitivities of various receptors have been reported; the clinical significance of most of these changes is not well understood. The assumption that elderly patients require lower blood levels of antidepressant medication is not correct. Although pharmacokinetic concerns may require lowering of the medication dose, plasma levels are comparable to those in young adults.

**Efficacy.** A number of antidepressants have been studied in the elderly. The consensus is that antidepressants are just as useful in the elderly as in younger adults. Most studies have been done in elderly patients who would be considered "young–old", and the patient studies are generally in good health. In some cases, the definition of "elderly" in the studies is extended to as young as 55 years of age. As such, the elderly patients used in efficacy studies may not be representative of elderly population.

Of the studies in the medically healthy elderly, there is support for the efficacy of virtually all antidepressant agents. Most TCAs (Salzman et al. 1993) and all serotonin reuptake inhibitors (Altamura et al. 1989, Guillibert et al. 1989, Cohn et al. 1990, Dunner et al. 1992) have been studied in this population. Unfortunately, existing studies that directly compare TCAs with serotonin reuptake inhibitors in the elderly tend to use low doses of the TCA and do not use placebo controls. Few studies have looked at longer-term results, although a few studies have documented the usefulness of TCAs for the continuation (Reynolds 1992) and maintenance phases (Old Age Depression Interest Group 1993) of treatment.

Few studies have looked at antidepressants in the frail elderly. One controlled trial demonstrated the superiority of nortriptyline to placebo in very old and frail elderly patients (Katz et al. 1990); however, a significant percentage of the patients studied could not tolerate nortriptyline's side effects.

It appears that antidepressants are as effective in the elderly as in the young, although the elderly may have more difficulty tolerating these medications.

## Medically Ill Patients

**General Concerns.** Few studies are available on the pharmacological treatment of depression in medically ill patients, and even less on medically ill elderly patients. At least one attempt at studying this population was discontinued because of the difficulty in recruiting such unstable patients. Although it has been suggested that depression in the setting of medical disease (or "secondary" depression) is less responsive to antidepressants than "primary" depression (Reynolds 1992), this may reflect methodological difficulties in diagnosing depression in a physically ill population. Until this is better understood, it seems ill-advised to withhold treatment for depression because of comorbid medical illness. In initiating such treatment, the physician should understand the effects of various illnesses on pharmacokinetics and the potential side effects that may result.

**Renal Impairment.** The interaction between renal impairment and TCAs is variable, with some studies reporting increased levels of TCAs in renally impaired patients and others reporting little change (Hale 1993). Fluoxetine's and sertraline's blood levels are relatively unaffected by renal impairment (Leonard 1993, Hale 1993). Dosage adjustment, therefore, does not seem necessary for these agents. In a single dose study on paroxetine, plasma levels did increase with marked renal impairment, but there was large variability in the effect (Doyle et al. 1989). This is curious, because little paroxetine is excreted unchanged in the urine. The manufacturer of paroxetine recommends dosage adjustment in the presence of renal impairment; until the excretion of this compound is better understood this appears prudent.

**Hepatic Impairment.** Most antidepressants can cause liver abnormalities. For the TCAs, these abnormalities can range from benign aberrations in biochemical tests to potentially fatal complications, such as hepatitis and cholestasis. Most of the more severe effects are unpredictable and dose-independent. As always, the potential morbidity of a depressive relapse—a likely event if effective antidepressant therapy is prematurely discontinued—must be weighed against the risk of precipitating such effects. Also to be considered is the effect of hepatic disease on the medication. Liver disease can increase the levels of TCAs, and blood levels should be monitored.

The pharmacokinetics of bupropion appears only minimally affected by alcoholic liver disease (Devane et al. 1990). There have been several reports of hepatic injury associated with trazodone, and one of trazodone-induced chronic active hepatitis in a patient with remote exposure to hepatitis B (Beck et al. 1993).

The literature suggests that the serotonin reuptake inhibitors are safe in patients with hepatic impairment, but, given their extensive liver metabolism, lower doses are required. Usually, a one half dose reduction in patients with cirrhosis is adequate.

Given its association with hepatic injury, nefazodone is not recommended for patients with hepatic disease.

**Epilepsy.** As discussed previously, the TCAs lower the seizure threshold. However, there is a high incidence of depression among epileptic patients, with estimates ranging from 19 to 31% (Hale 1993). Serotonin reuptake inhibitors appear to have a lower risk of causing seizures in patients with preexisting disorders; however, cases of seizures have been reported in which SSRIs appeared to lower the seizure threshold (Stimmel and Dopheide 1996). In at least one case report involving fluoxetine, the adverse effect appeared to be dose-dependent (Oke et al. 2001). Bupropion, which may cause more seizures than other antidepressants, is most likely to do so in patients with a previous history of seizures. As such, bupropion is contraindicated in patients with seizure disorders. Also germane to epileptic patients are the possible interactions with anticonvulsants. One study found that the serotonin reuptake inhibitor, fluvoxamine, increased carbamazepine levels to a toxic range. Other studies have not found this effect for fluvoxamine, fluoxetine, or paroxetine (Hale 1993).

**Endocrine Disorders.** Patients who have an endocrine disorder predisposing them to depression (e.g., hypothyroidism or diabetic hypoglycemia) should first undergo medical stabilization of the disorder before attempting antidepressant treatment. Of interest is data that suggests that fluoxetine may improve peripheral and hepatic insulin action in noninsulin-dependent diabetic patients (Cheer and Goa 2001).

**Iatrogenic Depression.** A wide number of medications can cause depression, and it is most likely impossible to prepare a complete list of all the medications that might induce depression in an individual patient. Many antihypertensive drugs, sedatives, steroids, antiulcer agents, digitalis-like drugs, and antiparkinsonian drugs have been reported to precipitate depression. The most obvious first step is to first try to remove the offending agent. However, at times a crucial drug has no practical substitute. In such cases, there are individual reports of antidepressants helping medication-induced depression (Levenson and Fallon 1993).

## Child and Adolescent Patients

Next to stimulants, antidepressants are the most common psychotropic medications prescribed in children (Zito et al. 2000) and adolescents (Jensen et al. 1999) and the trend to use these medications in that group is on an increase; this may relate to a decrease in a previous reluctance to use somatotherapy in children (Keller et al. 1991). It should be added, however, that the US Food and Drug Administration (FDA) has not specifically approved any antidepressant for use in children or adolescents.

In addition to depression, antidepressants are used in a number of nonaffective disorders in children and adolescents, including enuresis, attention-deficit/hyperactivity disorder, OCD, and bulimia nervosa. They are used to mitigate behaviors that are not part of a disease, for example, in suicidal adolescents who do not have a concomitant depressive disorder (American Academy of Child and Adolescent Psychiatry 2001); however, there is little empirical evidence that suggests that they can lower suicide risk (Zametkin et al. 2001). Similarly, they are used to dampen other impulsive behaviors. Though the data is growing, there continues to be a need for more controlled studies of the pharmacology of antidepressants in younger age groups. This is particularly true for the SSRIs, which are generally considered the first-line agents for children and adolescents with depression (American Academy of Child and Adolescent Psychiatry 1998).

**Dosage Concerns.** Children should generally be treated with levels of medication comparable to those used in adults, with the doses adjusted for body weight. As children have large livers (relative to body weight), they tend to be efficient metabolizers of substances, and may even need higher doses of medications (relative to body weight) than do adults.

For the SSRIs, initial dosing should be at the lowest available dose—for example, 5 to 10 mg of fluoxetine—however, many children and adolescents require dosing strategies that are similar to those for adults (Leonard et al. 1997). A number of the SSRIs have a liquid formulation, enabling very low doses. Not only do low doses minimize side effects, but also children may be more likely than adults to respond to doses of serotonin reuptake inhibitors in the low–normal range (Sylvester and Kruesi 1994). For the TCAs, the usual starting dose is 0.5 mg/kg in 2 or 3 divided doses for 2 or 3 nights. It is then increased by 0.05 mg/kg every 3 to 5 nights. The target dose can range from 0.5 to 2.5 mg/kg/day, depending on response to the drug (Janicak et al. 1993). Enuresis is generally treated only with nighttime doses, and it usually requires doses in the lower range. Attention-deficit/hyperactivity disorder and depression may require higher target doses: up to 3 mg/kg for attention-deficit/hyperactivity disorder, and as high as 5 mg/kg for childhood depression (Coffey 1986). The dose should not exceed 5 mg/kg/day. Blood level monitoring can aid proper dosing.

**Adverse Effects.** Well after the introduction of SSRIs, TCAs remained the most popular antidepressants used in children. However, there have been concerns regarding the safety of these medications. Several case studies have documented adverse cardiac affects in children treated with TCAs. Most alarming have been the reports of sudden death in children treated with desipramine (Riddle et al. 1993). In each case, desipramine was the antidepressant used, and in two of the cases, death occurred after strenuous activity. Whether desipramine was the causal agent is not known, and proposed mechanisms remain speculative. Desipramine is one of the most specific agents for norepinephrine, and can increase cardiac sympathetic tone, which in turn can predispose vulnerable individuals to arrhythmias. The Work Group on Research of the American Academy of Child and Adolescent Psychiatry (1990) conducted an extensive review of the available literature and concluded that there is minimal or no increased risk of "sudden death" in children with desipramine. It is probably wise, however, to perform an adequate cardiac work-up before starting an antidepressant in a child.

Given these issues concerning cardiotoxicity, the serotonin reuptake inhibitors have become more popular for the treatment of children and adolescents. Most of the newer agents have evidence for safety and efficacy in children, including fluoxetine (Emslie et al. 1997) and paroxetine (Keller et al. 2001). Others of the SSRIs have data for their usefulness in anxiety disorders, such as fluvoxamine (in OCD) (Riddle et al. 2001) and sertraline (which has open label data for social anxiety disorder and OCD) (Compton et al. 2001). Bupropion has been found safe and effective in children as well, although it may exacerbate tics in Tourette's disorder. Other antidepressants, including most of the first-generation antidepressants, lack any positive efficacy studies in children or adolescents.

## Pregnant and Postpartum Patients

As with many of the subjects here, the use of antidepressants in pregnant and nursing women could, and has, filled books, and some of the data are briefly reviewed here.

Of the commonly used antidepressants, none show compelling evidence of teratogenicity. Nonetheless, as is true for most medications, it is usually best to discontinue antidepressants if a patient becomes pregnant. Of the antidepressants used during pregnancy, the lengthiest experience is with the TCAs (March et al. 2001). However, the SSRIs have become more commonly used, for reasons of tolerability. Among the SSRIs, the greatest experience is with fluoxetine (Pastuszak et al. 1993). The SSRIs most likely all share a low teratogenicity (Kulin et al. 1998). There is less experience with bupropion, mirtazapine, and venlafaxine and these are not usually considered first-line drugs during pregnancy, although venlafaxine has presented data from a multicenter prospective controlled trial supporting its safety in pregnancy (Einarson et al. 2001). For all the antidepressants, including these last, one must consider a risk–benefit decision, measuring the risk of possible pregnancy-related side effects against the morbidity of a prolonged untreated depressive episode during pregnancy (Wisner et al. 2000).

Animal studies of the effect of imipramine on fetuses reveal some subtle neurobehavioral effects. These effects include delayed reflex development and decreased exploratory responses. There are too few studies of behavioral toxicity. However, one study, comparing several antidepressants, reported no differences in development when compared with sibling controls (Nulman et al. 1997). This study was with TCAs and fluoxetine; no studies with newer agents exist.

**Nursing Mothers.** All antidepressants are secreted in breast milk. The levels of these agents are difficult to predict, and their effect on the developing fetus is not known (Cohen et al. 1991). There are no systematic investigations of this issue, and what data exists is in the form of case reports and small case series (Burt et al. 2001). At least one report has documented symptoms of colic in a breast-fed infant whose mother was taking fluoxetine (Lester et al. 1993). The symptoms remitted when fluoxetine was discontinued. More serious effects have not been documented, but, given the level of uncertainty, nursing should be deferred if antidepressant treatment is required.

## Suicidal Patients

Much concern was generated by a report of six cases documenting the emergence of sudden, violent suicidal ideation with the administration of fluoxetine (Teicher et al. 1990) and sertraline (Balon 1993). Previous reports of a theoretical relationship between serotonin and violence combined with this single uncontrolled series resulted in a wild speculation—particularly among the popular media and "antipsychiatry" groups—that fluoxetine was a "suicide pill."

Subsequent meta-analysis of both world (Mann and Kapur 1991) and US (Kapur et al. 1992) and a more recent study using prospective data (Leon et al. 1999) showed no unique relationship between fluoxetine (or any antidepressant) and these behaviors. However, as with any rare event, one cannot totally discount the possibility that antidepressants may "trigger" suicidal ideation, either through a direct neurochemical effect (e.g., through an acute decrease in serotonergic transmission) or through nonspecific side effects of the drug (e.g., the induction of akathisia). If such a phenomenon exists, it is very uncommon, and probably not specific to any one antidepressant.

These concerns must be balanced over the well-proven and much greater risk of suicidal ideation and attempts when depression is not treated. Given this, and the propensity of suicidal patients to choose medication overdose as the method of suicide, the wide safety margin of the second- and third-generation antidepressants makes them preferable to first-generation agents when suicide is a concern. Bupropion has generally not been fatal in overdose, although about a third of such cases experience a seizure.

Along with concerns about toxicity, there is evidence that suggests that the serotonin reuptake inhibitors may be more effective than other antidepressants in treating depressed patients with suicidal ideation (Sachetti et al. 1991).

## Starting Doses

### First-Generation Antidepressants

**Tricyclic Antidepressants.** TCAs are usually begun at a relatively low dose. For the majority of TCAs, including imipramine, amitriptyline, desipramine, maprotiline, and doxepin, the initial starting dose is in the range of 50 to 75 mg/day. Notable exceptions include nortriptyline and protriptyline, which are more potent agents. In the case of nortriptyline, the usual starting dose is 25 to 50 mg/day, and for protriptyline, 10 to 15 mg/day (Schatzberg and Cole 1991). The lower doses are preferred in patients who are elderly. In the frail elderly, further dose reductions may be needed (about one half or less of the usual starting dose).

Once a medication is initiated, it is gradually increased to a therapeutic level. A number of strategies have been suggested for this increase. Most TCAs can be increased to 150 mg/day by the second week, and then to a range of 300 mg/day by the third or fourth week. This can be achieved through small daily increase of 25 mg or weekly increase of 75 mg. Younger patients will tolerate larger and more rapid increases, whereas the elderly benefit from smaller (25 mg/day) and less frequent (every other day) increases with a lower target dose (150 mg/day).

Protriptyline is increased by 5 to 10 mg/week to a target dose of 60 mg/day. For nortriptyline, increases of 50 mg/week are usually tolerated in the young, with the elderly requiring smaller increases (25 mg/week). Of particular interest is nortriptyline's therapeutic window: doses above and below a certain range appear to be less effective. The effective range is approximately 50 to 150 mg/day. Some authors suggest a lower range (for example, from 30 to 100 mg (Brotman et al. 1987); however, plasma blood monitoring (described later in this chapter) is a more accurate indicator of the proper level.

**Monoamine Oxidase Inhibitors.** Phenelzine is usually begun at a dose of 30 mg/day. It is increased by 15 mg after 3 days, then weekly to a target range of 45 to 90 mg/day. Tranylcypromine is started at 20 mg/day. It is increased by 10 mg after 3 days, with additional daily increases of 10 mg after 1 week, to a target range of 30 to 60 mg/day. Isocarboxazid is usually begun at 20 mg/day. It is titrated in a manner similar to tranylcypromine to a target of 30 mg/day. Schatzberg and Cole (1991) suggested that most patients require doses in the higher range, and that some may require doses above the normally recommended limits (e.g., phenelzine at 120 mg/day, tranylcypromine at 110 to 130 mg/day, and isocarboxazid at 50 mg/day).

### Second-Generation Antidepressants

**Serotonin Reuptake Inhibitors.** Although dosing strategies are less well understood with these agents, the wisest choice is to start a patient at the lowest effective dose and increase as indicated by clinical response. Reasonable doses are 20 mg/day for fluoxetine, 50 mg/day for sertraline, 20 mg/day for paroxetine and citalopram. For children, adolescents, the elderly, and patients who find medications generally difficult to tolerate, 50% reductions in these doses are reasonable starting doses.

A number of studies have shown increasing response with increasing doses of SSRIs (Leonard 1993), but the dropout rate due to side effects also increases with increasing dose. Fluoxetine, paroxetine, and citalopram should be started at a dose of 10 or 20 mg for 3 weeks (20 mg for a normal healthy adult, 10 mg for patients who are young, elderly, or particularly sensitive to medications), after which they can be increased in 10 or 20 mg increments to a dose of 40 mg/day if there is no response. A maximum dose of 60 mg/day of fluoxetine is recommended for the treatment of depression. A similar strategy can be used for sertraline, which can be begun at 25 to 50 mg, and increased in 25 to 50 mg increments to a target dose of 50 to 150 mg. Other disorders, particularly OCD and bulimia nervosa, may require 80 mg/day or more for maximal effect. The issue of dosage for SSRIs remains complicated, as some studies have suggested that fluoxetine may not have a linear dose–response curve; some patients may respond better to lower doses of the medication, such as 10 mg/day (Leonard 1993). Other studies have documented responses to fluoxetine at incredible doses and blood levels (320 mg/day and over 2,000 ng/mL, respectively) without adverse effects (Stoll et al. 1991).

As with tricyclic medications, there is a significant delay between initiation of medication and response, and there is no reason to believe that increasing the dose hastens response.

**Other Second-Generation Antidepressants.** Trazodone is generally dosed in a manner similar to TCAs, with starting doses of 50 to 75 mg/day, and target ranges of 150 to 300 mg/day, with doses not exceeding 400 mg/day in outpatients and 600 mg/day in inpatients. Unlike many of the TCAs, trazodone's short half-life requires divided doses, usually twice daily.

Bupropion, like trazodone, requires divided doses. It is available in a short acting form that requires three times a day dosing, or a longer acting form that allows twice-daily dosing. It should be begun at 100 mg b.i.d., and increased to a target of 300 mg/day after a few days. The recommended dose of the medication is 300 mg/day; however, patients not responding to that dose can be increased to 450 mg/day. Patients should be instructed to avoid taking more than 150 mg in a single dose. In the elderly, a usual starting dose is 75 mg/day of the shorter acting preparation. This is then increased to 75 mg b.i.d.

### Third-Generation Antidepressants

**Venlafaxine.** Originally available in a short acting form that required twice-daily dosing, it is currently available in a slow release preparation that enables once-daily dosing. Venlafaxine is usually begun at a dose of 37.5 mg and is increased within half to 1 week to a dose of 75 mg. If further increases are needed, it can be titrated at a rate of 75 mg every 4 days or more. Though a maximum dose of 225 mg per day is recommended by the manufacturer, doses as much as 300 to 450 mg/day have been employed to good effect in some patients.

**Mirtazapine.** Adults should be started on a dose of 15 mg/day. It is usually given as a before bedtime dose. The dosage generally needs to be increased in 15-mg intervals every half to 1 week to a target dose. The effective dose is usually between 15 and 45 mg/day; however, higher doses, such as 60 mg have been useful in some patients.

**Nefazodone.** Nefazodone is given in twice-daily doses. Patients can be started at a dose of 100 mg b.i.d. and increased at a rate of 100 to 200 mg a week. The recommended effective dose is 300 to 600 mg/day. Some clinical experience suggests that once-daily doses (given at night) are acceptable for some patients (Marathe et al. 1996).

### Therapeutic Drug Monitoring

Although blood levels are available for many antidepressants, those for imipramine, desipramine, and nortriptyline have been best established. Imipramine and desipramine appear to have a curvilinear dose–response curve with an optimal range of 150 to 300 ng/mL. Nortriptyline appears to have a therapeutic window in the range of 50 to 150 ng/mL (Preskorn et al. 1993). These blood levels are nominal, as some patients do respond above or below these ranges, and blood level monitoring should not be a substitute for clinical observation.

Drug levels have not been well established for the MAOIs and the serotonin reuptake inhibitors. For the latter compounds, as noted, there are numerous speculations about possible dose–response curves, including linear and "therapeutic window" models. Despite this, no model adequately explains the curiously flat dose–response relationship of these medications. If the therapeutic effect of the drug is indeed the inhibition of neuronal serotonin reuptake, plasma level studies suggest that these drugs are usually given in doses that well exceed saturation of this effect. The recommended starting dose of sertraline is closest to this hypothetical optimal level. Until this relationship is better understood, there is no reason to monitor blood levels of these medications, except to investigate possible toxicity, gauge adherence, or to establish clearance of the drug in preparation for an MAOI.

### Phases of Treatment

Treatment can be divided into several phases. At each phase, the goals of treatment and the potential pitfalls differ. These phases are illustrated in Figure 97–11 and described below.

### Early, or Preresponse, Period

Patients should initially be followed weekly to judge their response to treatment. The goal at this point is to manage the side effects of the various medications. Given realistic time and economic constraints, such contacts may at times be by telephone. However, it remains crucial that a patient feels that he can communicate freely with his doctor regarding any side effects or other concerns about the medication. This is of great importance as such side effects are a primary reason for treatment nonadherence, and patients may be more inclined at this early phase to simply discontinue medication rather than to first discuss it with their physician.

It can be difficult to persuade a depressed patient to remain on medication. Perhaps the greatest intervention at the disposal of the physician is reassurance. It is inevitable that patients will experience some side effects from their medications. Patients are able to tolerate this better when properly prepared. The patients may tolerate these side effects better when they are framed in a positive light—as a sign that the drug is present in their system.

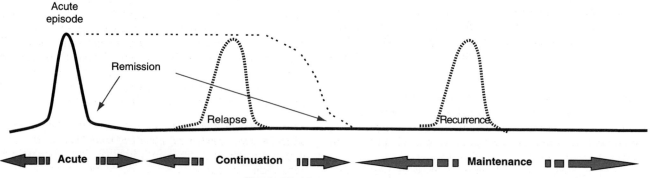

**Figure 97–11** *Phases of treatment.*

The side effects can become intolerable, and reassurance may be inadequate. There are several strategies for mitigating side effects that can be considered. Many side effects are decreased or eliminated through dose reductions or changes in the dosing regimen. SSRIs, through scored capsules or liquid preparations, can be begun at one half or one-fourth their normal starting dose in patients who are particularly sensitive to side effects. The TCAs, although often given in a single-daily dose, could be divided across the day to minimize dose-related side effects. Taking medications with food may decrease nausea. Although most physicians are aware that sedating medications should be taken in the evening, and activating ones in the morning, the patient may need these strategies reinforced. Flexibility is required as well; for example, a significant percentage of patients taking serotonin reuptake inhibitors experience sedation rather than insomnia, and this would warrant a change to evening dosing. However, the practice of starting the "less activating" SSRIs (such as paroxetine and citalopram) in the evening *a priori* seems unjustified as they still cause significant insomnia.

Failing these approaches, adjunctive agents may be employed to minimize the side effects. Anxiolytics can be added to treat the arousal and insomniac effects of the serotonin reuptake inhibitors. Although these adjunctive agents can be continued for the duration of treatment, discontinuation should be attempted after several weeks of treatment because many of the side effects may be limited to the early phase of treatment. The dry mouth caused by TCAs (and some newer agents) can be treated with saliva substitutes, although more mundane salivary stimulants such as sugar-free hard candy may be just as effective. Over-the-counter bulk-forming laxatives can treat the constipation caused by some agents (particularly TCAs but also seen with some newer agents). The cholinergic agonist bethanechol has been used to treat anticholinergic side effects, particularly urinary hesitancy and blurred vision. The usual adult dosage is 10 to 50 mg t.i.d. or q.i.d. Pilocarpine eye drops have been used to treat the blurred vision as well.

Intolerable side effects may warrant a change in medication. If side effects are the only reason for medication change, it is reasonable to choose a medication in the same class as the first, but with a different side effect profile. Anecdotal evidence suggests that patients can have variable reactions to different serotonin reuptake inhibitors despite their apparent similarity. For example, a patient who experiences significant anorgasmia with one SSRI may find little or no side effects with an equipotent dose of an alternative SSRI. The reasons for such an idiosyncratic response are not clear, but do encourage the physician to try and stay within a single class of drug if the initial response has been favorable.

## Response, or Acute Treatment, Period

This period overlaps with the initial phase of treatment and continues until response is achieved. This period usually lasts from 2 to 4 months. The goal during this phase is to control the present symptoms of depression.

It is important to differentiate between partial and complete response. Complete response implies total recovery from all symptoms of depression, whereas a partial response is usually defined as a reduction in symptoms.

The time to response varies with the patient. Few patients show a significant response before 2 weeks. The usual range for response is 3 to 4 weeks; however, it can take 6 weeks or longer. For patients who complete a satisfactory treatment regimen, the response rate for antidepressants is about 60 to 70% (American Psychiatric Association 2000b), although some of these responses will be partial. Response rates may be as high as 80% with antidepressants when an adequate dose is given for an adequate time.

There is little benefit in making treatment changes before 3 weeks (except to mitigate side effects). Changes in treatment strategy should be considered after the physician is satisfied that the patient has been treated with an adequate dosage of the antidepressant for an adequate time. In the case of TCAs, this can be confirmed with blood levels. In the case of serotonin reuptake inhibitors and MAOIs, there are fewer data available to confirm an adequate dose. For the patient showing inadequate response, these medications are increased to the limit of side effect tolerance.

In patients showing an inadequate response after a reasonable time, the physician must decide whether to continue with the same medication and augment with an additional agent, or to switch medications altogether. This decision depends on an assessment of whether the patient has shown any response to the current strategy. Partial responders may be more likely to benefit from treatment augmentations, whereas patients who show no response or worsen during treatment warrant a new agent.

### Antidepressant Augmentation

Typical augmentation strategies (Table 97–5) include the addition of lithium carbonate, thyroid hormone, or a stimulant.

**Lithium Augmentation.** Response rates as high as 65% have been reported when lithium augmentation is used. Lithium has been used successfully with most antidepressants, including TCAs, serotonin reuptake inhibitors (Dinan 1993) and bupropion (Apter and Woolfolk 1991). The blood level of lithium necessary for adjunctive use has not been well established. It is probably best to start at a low dose (300 mg b.i.d) and to increase to a therapeutic blood level (0.8 to 1.2 mEq/L) if there is no response. The trial may take 3 to 6 weeks for augmenting effect.

**Thyroid Augmentation.** For thyroid hormone supplementation, the starting dose is 25 μg/day of triiodothyronine, which can be increased to 50 μg/day in a week if there is no response (American Psychiatric Association 2000b). The trial should continue for at least 3 weeks. In the past, reported response rates for thyroid augmentation were lower than those for lithium augmentation (25%); there is little data directly comparing the two agents.

**Stimulant Augmentation.** Among the stimulants, methylphenidate and dextroamphetamine have been used for antidepressant augmentation, but there are few systematic data regarding the proper dose or length of treatment for this potential use.

| Table 97–5 | Augmentation Strategies | | | |
|---|---|---|---|---|
| Agent | Dosing Strategy | Length of Trial | Reported Response Rate | Comments |
| Lithium carbonate | Start at 300 mg b.i.d., increase to therapeutic blood level (0.8–1.2 mEq/L) | 3–6 wk | As high as 65% | Best documented strategy; has been combined with most agents |
| Triiodothyronine | Start at 25 µg/d, may increase to 50 µg/d | At least 3 wk | At 2.5% | Equal to lithium in one placebo controlled trial |
| Stimulants (methylphenidate dextroamphetamine) | † | † | † | Few systematic data |
| Combined antidepressant therapy | May need lower doses than usual (due to enzyme inhibition) † | † | † | Mainly open trials; controlled studies in progress |
| Psychotherapy | N/A | Varies by therapy | Varies by therapy | Good data for both cognitive–behavioral therapy and interpersonal therapy |

†Inadequate data.

**Combined Antidepressant Therapy.** Open trials have supported the use of combined therapy of a TCA and a serotonin reuptake inhibitor in patients for whom either class alone has failed (Seth et al. 1992). When antidepressants are combined, it is important to remember that the serotonin reuptake inhibitors can potentiate TCA levels, and this should be monitored carefully. MAOIs have also been used in combination with TCAs, although this should be monitored closely given the risk of potential toxic interactions (American Psychiatric Association 2000b). Given the risk of a serotonin syndrome, MAOIs should not be combined with serotonin reuptake inhibitors.

**Nonpharmacological Approaches.** A number of nonpharmacological augmentations should be mentioned as well, particularly the concomitant use of psychotherapy. The combination of psychotherapy and medication may offer benefits that either therapy alone cannot offer, including additional efficacy as well as prevention of relapse (Evans et al. 1992). This has been shown to some degree, for both cognitive–behavioral therapy (Hollon et al. 1992) and interpersonal therapy (Frank et al. 1990). Perhaps most compelling was a recent multicenter study comparing antidepressant medication (nefazodone) and a structured psychotherapy, which combined both cognitive–behavioral and interpersonal principles, in the treatment of patients with chronic depression (Keller et al. 2000). It was found that the combined medication–psychotherapy group had a dramatically better remission rate (85 versus 55% in the medication only group). It is notable that, in this study, the psychotherapy given was quite intensive—16 to 20 sessions were given over a 12-week period, with the sessions being as frequent as biweekly in the first 6 weeks.

### Changing to a New Agent

For the patient who shows no response or whose condition deteriorates during therapy, the physician should initiate a new trial of an alternative single agent. There remains some debate as to what type of agent should be used next. Some studies have suggested that patients who do not respond to one SSRI may respond to another (Thase et al. 1997). However, the most convincing study continues to support the more commonly held belief that it is best to switch to an agent of a different class, and approximately 50% of patients unresponsive to a first trial respond to an antidepressant of a different class (Phillips and Nierenberg 1994, Thase et al. 2002).

When the switch involves an MAOI, sufficient time must be given for medication clearance. Although seldom used, MAOIs may be very effective in patients not responsive to other classes of antidepressants (McGrath et al. 1993). Generally, 10 to 14 days for either medication is required for clearance of TCAs and MAOIs. Fluoxetine requires a much longer period—6 weeks—whereas sertraline and paroxetine require about 2 weeks when switching to an MAOI.

### Continuation Period

This period usually lasts 5 to 8 months after the end of the acute treatment period. The goal at this phase is the prevention of relapse. There is a high risk of relapse if treatment is discontinued after the acute treatment phase. The National Institutes of Health Consensus Development Conference on the Mood Disorders (1985) reported a cumulative relapse rate of 15% after 6 months and 22% after 12 months. Keller and colleagues (1982) found that the two best predictors of relapse were a high number of previous depressive episodes (greater than three predicted relapses) and underlying dysthymic disorder.

Once a patient has responded to a medication, the medication should be continued for a minimum of 4 to 6 months, beginning from the point of initial response. The World Health Organization (1989) recommended 6 months as a minimum period for continuation of treatment after the acute phase, and the American Psychiatric Association (2000b) recommended a minimum of 16 to 20 weeks of treatment following the full remission of symptoms. This period should be lengthened for the patient with a history of longer depressive episodes.

Surprisingly, few studies exist that directly look at the efficacy of antidepressants for continuation therapy. However, there exists at least one placebo-controlled study for each of the SSRIs (Montgomery et al. 1988, 1993, Montgomery and Dunbar 1993, Doogan and Caillard 1992), nefazodone (Feiger et al. 1999), and mirtazapine (Montgomery et al. 1998).

In the past, it was suggested that, on achievement of euthymia, doses could be reduced. However, it is more likely that levels similar to those needed at the acute stage of treatment will be required throughout the continuation period.

## Discontinuance of Treatment

After the continuation period, somatic therapy is usually discontinued in the patient with a single episode of major depression. Before discontinuing, however, it is important to remember that depression is often a lifelong disease with a chronic course. One should always weigh the benefits of discontinuance against the risks of recurrent depression.

In the past, a distinction between exogenous and endogenous depression was used to predict the risk of recurrence. Inferences about etiology, however, are not an accurate predictor of recurrence. More useful information are the age of onset during the initial episode and the number of episodes. Patients with a single episode of acute depression, who have an onset before age 50 years, are the best candidates for discontinuance (Greden 1993).

## Tapering and Withdrawal

For the TCAs, the usual strategy is to taper the medications at a rate of 25 to 50 mg/day every 2 to 3 days. Too rapid a discontinuation may produce symptoms of cholinergic "rebound" or supersensitivity. Such a rebound includes severe gastrointestinal symptoms (nausea, vomiting, and cramping), other signs of autonomic hyperactivity (diaphoresis, anxiety, agitation, headaches), and insomnia (often with vivid nightmares). In severe cases, a full delirium may result. Cholinergic rebound may occur as early as 48 hours or as late as 2 weeks after discontinuation. These symptoms may account for some cases of presumed early relapse from antidepressant discontinuation.

MAOIs may also have a withdrawal syndrome, including symptoms of psychosis, on abrupt withdrawal; however, this syndrome is rarer than that seen with TCAs.

Fluoxetine has a long half-life, and abrupt discontinuation should be permissible. Sertraline, citalopram, and paroxetine, with shorter half-lives of around a day, may require a 7- to 10-day taper. With the shorter-acting agents, a withdrawal syndrome including symptoms of fatigue, insomnia, abdominal distress, and influenza-like symptoms have been reported when they are too abruptly discontinued. The same may be true for venlafaxine.

Some investigators question current tapering schedules, which are based on pharmacokinetic rather than pharmacodynamic (i.e., receptor) effects. Given an antidepressant's long-term effects, they suggest that receptors will "need" more time to readjust to a new medication-free environment. Greden (1993), for instance, recommended a one-fourth reduction in dose every third month for tricyclic medication. For fluoxetine, he recommended slowly increasing the dosing interval: from daily to every other day for 3 months, then every third day for 3 months. After 3 months of dosing every 3 days, he recommended switching to a liquid form to permit 25% dose reductions each quarter year. Obviously, such a strategy would dramatically increase the taper period from several weeks to approximately a year. It will be interesting to see whether studies support the contention that extended tapers are more likely to prevent recurrence.

On discontinuance, the goal is to enable early intervention should symptoms recur. A first episode of depression has a high risk of recurrence, and the risk of recurrence is even higher in patients who show only partial response to medication. The patient should be educated to recognize symptoms of depression. The patient's own history suggests which symptoms were prodromal to the patient's full depressive episode.

## Maintenance Period

The goal of the maintenance period is to prevent the recurrence of depression. There are a number of reasons to consider long-term prophylactic therapy for depression rather than medication withdrawal. Depression is a lifelong disease, with recurrence being the norm rather than the exception (Keller et al. 1992). As the number of acute episodes increases, the risk of future episodes increases as well, and the interval between episodes shortens. Each subsequent episode carries a higher morbidity and disability. Although better understood in bipolar disorder, there is a fear that treatment response may decrease with an increasing number of depressive episodes (Greden 1993).

A number of factors can influence the decision of when it is appropriate to maintain long-term prophylaxis for depression. The seriousness of previous episodes, the severity of impairment caused by such episodes, the degree of response to previous treatments, and the ability of the patient to tolerate the drug all play a role. Central in the decision process is the concept of recurrent depression: that some patients are more likely than others to have a recurrence of the disease. Three previous episodes of depression make recurrent depression likely. The best predictors of the likelihood of recurrence appear to be older age of onset and number of episodes. Greden (1993) proposed that long-term maintenance is the treatment of choice for the following groups of patients: (1) those who were 50 years old or more at the time of the first depressive episode, (2) those who were 40 years old or more at first episode and have had at least one subsequent recurrence, and (3) anyone who has had more than three episodes.

The recommended length of maintenance treatment needs further clarification as well. Recommended lengths of time vary from 5 years of treatment to indefinite continuation. There are only a handful of studies on maintenance antidepressant treatment. One study (Prien et al. 1984) compared patients successfully treated for acute major depression, who were when randomized to a medication or placebo group for 2 years. The imipramine groups (with and without lithium) had the longest time until a recurrence, with the lithium group having an intermediate time until recovery. A second study (Kupfer et al. 1992), the longest of any such study, compared medication (imipramine) with and without psychotherapy to placebo, for 3 years, with an continuation of 2 years for a subset of the group for a total of up to 5 years. This study provided strong evidence for the efficacy of antidepressant medication: by the end of 3 years, most of the placebo group had relapsed, whereas a substantial portion of those patients on imipramine (about 80%) remained well. In the 2-year extension of the study, those patients who had remained well were randomized to imipramine or placebo, and, again, most of the patients on placebo had a recurrence of depression, whereas the majority of those on medication did not.

These two studies were in patients with recurrent depression. Another indication for maintenance treatment is for patients with chronic depression. Again, few studies have looked at this population for a sufficient time, but what studies exist does support the efficacy of antidepressants in this population. One such study compared sertraline with placebo for maintenance treatment of depression (Keller et al. 1998), and found that the placebo group was four times more likely to have a recurrence than the medication group.

Regarding choice of an agent, there are no rigorous studies comparing different antidepressants during the maintenance period. It is usually assumed that the same agent used in the acute and continuation period will also be the preferred one in the maintenance period.

## Summary

Despite limitations in data, it is reasonable to believe that most agents used for the acute treatment of depression are also effective for long-term treatment of depression.

Equally important in preventing recurrence of depression is the problem of maintaining adherence to medication long after the acute episode has resolved. Proper education and support will help with compliance. Toleration of side effects is important and evidence suggests that patients are more likely to comply with the agents that have more favorable side effect profiles. The serotonin reuptake inhibitors are generally the best tolerated antidepressants.

Although lower doses for prophylaxis have been recommended, there are few data to support this contention. Even though lower doses may increase compliance, full doses should be used until new information indicates otherwise.

## Outcome Assessment

As with all pharmacotherapy, results are simplest to judge when the original treatment is focused on clear goals. At the time of initiating pharmacotherapy for depression, the physician should document what particular symptoms justify a diagnosis of depression. The outcome of treatment can then be judged against these symptoms. It is not unusual, particularly in the case of partial response that a patient will report still feeling "depressed" and yet show observable symptom improvement.

Although clinical judgment remains the mainstay of treatment assessment, this judgment can be reinforced with a number of well-validated scales. These scales can be either interviewer-rated or self-rated scales. Some scales are more

(or less) reliable in certain groups, such as the aged, or the medically ill.

**Clinician-Rated Scales.** Perhaps the most widely used scale is the Hamilton Depression Rating Scale (HAM-D) (Hamilton 1960), a clinician-rated scale that requires some training to be performed properly. The Montgomery–Asberg Depression Rating Scale (MADRS) (Montgomery and Asberg 1979) has good interrater reliability and high validity for severity. It shows high sensitivity to change, which would be useful in monitoring the progress of treatment, and it appears useful in patients with comorbid somatic illnesses.

**Self-Rated Scales.** Self-rated scales can be easier to use and less time intensive—a patient can be filling them out while waiting for an appointment; however, they are generally less reliable than clinician-rated scales. Self-rated scales include the Beck Depression Inventory (BDI) (Beck 1978) and the Zung Depression Scale (Zung 1965). These scales, which test for a number of somatic symptoms of depression, may be less reliable in medically ill or elderly populations. The Geriatric Depression Scale (GDS) (Yesavage et al. 1983), a self-report questionnaire, is specifically intended for initial screening in the elderly. Such scales have largely been avoided in clinical practice because of added time and relative impracticality of such scales. However, the wider acceptance of computer-assisted devices, particularly palm held personal assistant devices could make such scales much simpler and practical.

## Treatment Failure

Failure to respond to treatment is most often due to inadequate treatment rather than "true" nonresponse. Inadequate treatment can be due to an inadequate length of treatment or an inadequate dose. These can result from the physician's error (either improper dosing strategies or impatience in waiting an appropriate amount of time) or the patient's error (through misunderstanding or nonadherence).

Patients will often not acknowledge nonadherence as they fear rejection from treatment, and they certainly are unlikely to admit to it if their physician does not ask them. The best remedy for nonadherence is prevention, through proper education of the patient about likely side effects that might otherwise unnerve the patient. A flexible approach is also necessary. Gentle reassurance and encouragement can be helpful; however, dogmatic insistence on adherence to a prescription leaves the patient with no choice except to hide nonadherence, or look elsewhere for treatment.

Thus, "true" nonresponse can be defined as the lack of response to an adequate dose for an adequate time. In the case of such failure, a number of issues should be examined.

**Diagnostic Issues.** The physician should reconsider the patient's diagnosis. A number of medical conditions can cause some depressive symptoms without actually causing depression. In such cases, the symptoms are unlikely to abate with treatment of the primary disorder. Similarly, a number of other psychiatric disorders have symptoms that overlap with depression, including the anxiety disorders and personality disorders. Fortunately, many of these other diagnoses may respond to antidepressants; however, this is not always the case, and therapy targeted at the alternative disorder may be preferable.

**Psychotic Depression.** The physician should also consider whether the patient has a type of depression that would predict a poor response. Psychotic depression is an example of a condition less likely to respond to antidepressants alone. It is not clear whether psychotic depression represents a qualitatively different disorder, requiring different treatment, or whether it is a more severe form of major depression. Evaluation of this question is confounded by the fact that most psychotically depressed patients are more severely depressed than nonpsychotic depressed patients. A study that matched psychotic and nonpsychotic depressed patients for severity depression showed poor response in both groups compared with moderately depressed patients, suggesting that it is the severity of disease which accounts for the poorer response of these patients (Kocsis 1990) despite adequate treatment.

Psychotic depression is usually treated with either combination pharmacotherapy (an antidepressant and an antipsychotic) or electroconvulsive therapy (Rothschild et al. 1993).

**Strategies for Treatment-Resistant Patients.** Many strategies have been suggested for treatment-resistant patients. Electroconvulsive therapy offers a safe, effective alternative somatic therapy for depression. A prior good response to electroconvulsive therapy, a need for rapid response as with life-threatening depressive symptoms (food refusal, suicide attempts) or a medical contraindication to antidepressants warrants early consideration of this treatment. It should be considered for any patient with major depression who has not responded to antidepressant medication. A number of other somatic therapies show promising preliminary results, including transcranial magnetic stimulation and vagal nerve stimulation, and these may offer additional alternatives for treatment resistant patients. For a fuller discussion of these options, see chapter 92.

Adjuvant and combination therapy, including psychotherapy, strategies that have been discussed earlier, offers additional strategies for treating the resistant patient. For a fuller discussion of these strategies, see chapter 63.

## Summary

There remain a number of important limitations regarding the pharmacotherapy of depression. Some of these limitations can be addressed by continued progress on current research. Other limitations await truly novel research into the mechanism of depression.

## Recommendations for the Use of Antidepressants

Allowing for the many limitations, we can generalize from available data to make the following recommendations:

1. All patients with acute major depression should be considered reasonable candidates for pharmacotherapy.
2. There is adequate evidence to make the same recommendation for other forms of depression. This is particularly true for dysthymia, and may be true for other minor forms of depression as well.
3. There is good evidence for the use of antidepressants for nonmood disorders as well, particularly the anxiety disorders.
4. There remains no strong evidence from choosing one medication over another, and treatment recommendations should be made on the basis of tolerability and, if appropriate, cost.
5. Extended treatment should be recommended both for patients with chronic depression and recurrent depression.
6. Maintenance treatment should consist of the same dose of antidepressant as used to achieve acute phase remission.
7. The exact length of maintenance treatment is not known. The decision for indefinite treatment should be a risks–benefit decision, made with the informed consent of the patient, who is entitled to be informed of the limitations in our knowledge.

## Unanswered Questions, Direction for Future Research

When considering the treatment of depression, the most critical unanswered question on treating depression is that of the optimal length of treatment for depression. As discussed above, most treatment guidelines recommend a length of at least 4 to 6 months. However, a significant number of relapses still occur after this period. Whether longer periods would decrease the rates of relapses remains an open question.

It continues to be a problem that, although much data suggests that there are some important differences in the different agents we use for depression, we continue to generalize across different treatments. There is a growing data on comparative efficacy; however, most of this is in the acute period of depression. We do not know whether different agents, or different classes of agents may be more likely to prevent relapses.

The issue of long-term maintenance treatment remains an important, and understudied area. The further one goes from acute treatment, the less data we have. Currently, long-term treatment is recommended for patients with recurrent depression. However, there is limited data to justify how we decide who qualifies for long-term treatment, and how long maintenance treatment should continue. Likewise, dosing strategies in the maintenance period need further study, particularly with newer agents.

Other questions remain unanswered as well. Many patients and some clinicians believe that antidepressants tend to "wear off" in their effect over a period of time (some suggest 9 to 18 months). No data exists to support this belief, but little data exists to refute it. The role of nonpharmacological treatments, and how they interact and can aid pharmacotherapy, need to be studied as well, particularly in light of some recent evidence as to the powerful additive power of psychotherapy and pharmacotherapy in combination.

Most vexing is the limitation of the current agents, which seems to be generally consistent regardless of pharmacodynamics or mechanisms of action. Though we continue to introduce new antidepressants, it remains a frustrating fact that the newest antidepressant in our modern armamentarium has basically the same efficacy and delayed onset found in the first antidepressants from half a century ago. Though it is possible that these limitations represent something inherent in major depression itself, it seems likely that the commonality in effect represents the fact that, though mechanisms of action differ, the overall effects of these drugs are similar. Though small differences might be found individually between these agents, they are modest at best. It is likely that any major improvement in either the timing of treatment or the efficacy awaits a newer class of agents that will act in a truly novel way.

Some promising areas of research into novel treatments include research into substance P antagonists and corticotropin-releasing hormone antagonists. Substance P, originally investigated for its potential role in pain transmission, has shown potential efficacy both in animal models of depression and in clinical human trials. In the latter case, the substance P antagonist MK-869 showed comparable efficacy to paroxetine in a trial of patients with major depressive disorder and moderate anxiety (Kramer et al. 1998). Most significant, the drug did not appear to interact with monoamine systems in a way typical of standard antidepressants, suggesting a novel mechanism of action. This is supported by basic research that suggests a role for substance P receptors in modulating stress within the CNS, a role that may be related to, but independent of monoamine pathways. Similarly, investigators have looked at the role of endocrine hormones in affecting depression; a reasonable inquiry given the long appreciated finding of hypothalamic–pituitary–adrenal axis dysfunction in patients who are depressed. Strategies at decreasing the hypercortisolemia in such have led to investigations with a variety of cortisol-lowering agents, including ketoconazole (Ravaris et al. 1988), metyrapone, and aminoglutethimide (Brown et al. 2001), which have all had preliminary success in depressed patients, but have been limited by side effects. A preliminary open study of the corticotropin-releasing hormone r-1 antagonist r-121919 showed promise as well, but the drug has been withdrawn because of potential liver toxicity (Zobel et al. 2000). Glucocorticoid antagonists can mitigate the effects of hypercortisolemia, and the agent RU486 (Murphy et al. 1993) has also shown promising preliminary results.

Whether these particular drugs will become part of psychiatry's clinical armamentarium is too early to say. However, the promise of new and different approaches to treating depression is exciting. Until the present, research into antidepressants has informed research in depression. In the future, the reverse will have to be true: in order to develop better antidepressants, we will have to better understand the pathophysiology of depression. With the new investigatory tools available, such discoveries seem right around the corner.

---

**Clinical Vignette 1**

Ms. W was a 34-year-old married woman who began having depressive symptoms approximately 8 months before presented to a psychiatrist. Initially, she began to notice intense fatigue, weakness, and dizziness, to the point where she was spending a good deal of time in bed. Her

primary care doctor tested her for a variety of possible medical disorders, with no abnormalities found. When he suggested an emotional disorder, she initially was reluctant; feeling convinced that her symptoms had to be medical in nature. As further months saw only worsening symptoms, she eventually agreed to psychiatric consultation.

At the time of her first psychiatric evaluation, her main complaint was of insomnia. She described herself as being constantly "on edge" during the day, often exhausted by the end of it, falling asleep briefly in the early evening, but then waking up around 3 AM, and being unable to fall back asleep. On further discussion, she admitted feeling "miserable" all the time, frequently broke into tears "for no reason." She had no interest in activities, and took no pleasure in anything. She also felt extremely guilty, particularly in her inability to be a mother to her 2-year-old child or a wife to her husband. In the latter case, she reported that her husband was perplexed by her emotions, but was very kind towards her, despite the fact that she frequently took out the bulk of her angry outbursts on him. In the context of her guilt she had fleeting thoughts that her family would be better off without her, and her fantasies ranged from leaving her husband to suicide.

The diagnosis of depression was again suggested to the patient. She again had difficulty believing this diagnosis, as she saw her physical symptoms as primary. She felt that if she could only "get a decent night's sleep" she wouldn't be so tired, and perhaps would feel better. Antidepressant medication was discussed at that time, but she declined a trial. The agreement was made to continue meeting and discussing this further. In the interim, she approached her family doctor, and received medication for sleep (temazepam).

After 2 weeks of continued misery, despite relatively good sleep, she again met with her psychiatrist. Now desperate, she reluctantly agreed to an antidepressant trial. Various options were discussed with her, and she was clearly very fearful of any medication for which anxiety might be a potential side effect. Eventually she and her psychiatrist agreed on paroxetine (though the psychiatrist noted that this drug could also cause anxiety, the patient had seen a television commercial that had convinced her that this medication would be preferable for anxiety). She was prescribed 20 mg/day, taking in the morning.

After 2 days, she called her psychiatrist, saying that the drug was making her mouth dry, and was making her feel tired during most of the day. She worried that this drug was going to turn her "into a zombie" and wondered whether she should stop it. She was encouraged to continue the medication, and her psychiatrist suggested that she should switch to evening dosing to decrease the apparent daytime sedation. She did so, but called again several days later, saying that she felt that the drug was making it hard for her to wake up in the morning. Again she suggested giving up, but was encouraged instead to halve the dose.

When she next met with her psychiatrist, she had been on the drug for 2 weeks. At that time, the side effects seemed to have partially abated. She was discouraged all the same, as her symptoms were largely unchanged. She questioned whether this was the proper drug, and indeed whether she had been diagnosed properly. Various approaches were employed, both during visits and by phone over the next few weeks, including continued education regarding the likely course of treatment, empathy for her frustration over what seemed a painstakingly slow trial, and a somewhat paternal reassurance that the psychiatrist had treated many patients like her, and that her impressions were not unusual or cause for further worry. Frequent reinforcement of these approaches was sufficient to convince the patient to continue the medication trial.

Over the next 2 weeks, the patient felt that there might have been some small improvement. She was somewhat less anxious during the days, and when asked, she admitted that she was crying less. She remained disappointed; however, her most troubling symptoms (the fatigue, weakness, and insomnia) remained, and she still reported her mood as being depressed (a word she was now more comfortably using). Her psychiatrist continued attempting to supply her with the enthusiasm she lacked, explaining that this response at 4 weeks of treatment was a very positive sign. She agreed to a dose increase of 20 mg/day.

The patient then gradually improved over the next few weeks, and within 12 weeks of beginning treatment she could declare herself to be at her baseline. In some ways, she felt that she might even be "improved" from her baseline, saying that she was more assertive with friends and relatives than she was used to being, and would seem euphoric at times. She had more energy than she was used to, and she wondered at times if she was becoming "manic," having heard that this could happen with antidepressants. On further questioning, however, her symptoms suggested nothing more than euthymia.

Soon after she improved, she began to suggest discontinuing medication. She admitted that she felt ashamed that she was taking psychiatric medication, and feared that her friends or relatives might discover what she was doing. The high risk of relapse at this early period was explained to her, and reasons for continuing medication during the asymptomatic period were reviewed with her. Though she agreed to continue, several weeks later she guiltily admitted that she instead discontinued her medication for 3 days, only to restart after feeling what she interpreted to be a relapse. The psychiatrist admitted that time course of her "relapse" combined with her description of the symptoms as "flu-like" made a withdrawal syndrome more likely than a relapse; however, this event was enough to convince her to remain on the medications for the full-time course.

Some symptoms remained during this period. Although she was largely euthymic, she admitted to continuing dissatisfaction with areas of her life, and she often reported a general sense of a lack of purpose or direction in her life. Similar dissatisfaction was reported when she discussed her marriage, though she now had great satisfaction in her role as a mother. Though psychotherapy had been suggested since the beginning of treatment, she had been even more opposed to it than she was toward medication. Now, she tentatively agreed to meet with a therapist to discuss some of these issues.

As the months passed, the patient's initial dislike for medication changed into more of an ambivalence. Though the patient still voiced wishes to be off medication, she also admitted that she was becoming apprehensive about discontinuing it. After 9 months of medication treatment, she met with her psychiatrist to discuss future options. Though she continued to feel that her episode of depression was her first, she wasn't as sure whether she had been entirely well prior to her acute episode. She noted some longstanding, though less dramatic feelings of pessimism and sadness prior to taking antidepressants. She had never considered these feeling to be abnormal until encountering

their absence. Despite these concerns, she chose to discontinue her antidepressants, a decision that seemed reasonable to her psychiatrist as well. She again felt some symptoms of withdrawal as the medication was lowered and discontinued; however, these improved over the course of a week.

Four weeks after her discontinuation, she remained well and hopeful that she would not need medication. However, by 2 months she was beginning to notice some returning symptoms. Though she did not experience the dramatic anxiety, dysphoria, and neurovegetative symptoms that first brought her into treatment, she began to feel increasingly "moody," irritable, and apathetic. Her husband noticed this as well, and though he originally had been skeptical of her need for antidepressants, he now began questioning her decision to discontinue them. After one particularly angry incident, in which she began inappropriately yelling at her child, she called her psychiatrist, asking to be put back on her medication. This was done, and she again responded after about 4 weeks of treatment.

In discussions with her psychiatrist now, she became despondent, wondering whether this meant that she would have to remain on medication for the rest of her life. It was admitted that this might be a possibility, particularly as many of her symptoms during the current episode seemed similar to her reported "usual state" prior to treatment. However, there remained the possibility that the patient had been discontinued too early from medication, and that the current symptoms represented a late relapse of the original episode. It was agreed to continue medication for a minimum of 6 months before again entertaining the idea of a discontinuation.

Though somewhat more resigned to this second period of pharmacotherapy, Ms. W became more critical of the particular medication she was taking. Initially fearful that people would discover she was on medication, she eventually was surprised to find that several of her family and friends were also taking antidepressants. The subsequent exchange of anecdotes left her curious as to whether she was on the best agent. She began to wonder whether some of the weight gain she had experienced (perhaps 5 pounds over the last year) was due to the paroxetine. An even greater complaint became apparent after a discussion between the psychiatrist and the patient's therapist, in which the therapist felt that Ms. W was minimizing her sexual problems, and that this might be an important influence on her frequent requests for the discontinuation of medication. Previously, Ms. W had rarely voiced any sexual side effects to her psychiatrist, and when asked would relate any such problems to her ongoing marital tensions. At this time, a more detailed sexual discussion led to the admission that Ms. W had been largely anorgasmic for the entire time that she had been on the paroxetine. Though she said that she preferred this side effect to a return of her depression, it was clear that the effect was troubling both her and her husband.

Various approaches were taken to improving this side effect. Lowering the dose from 20 to 10 mg/day gave only minor improvement, and she felt that she had some increase in irritability at this lower dose. Adjunctive medications had little effect and were contrary to the patient's reluctance to take medication. Eventually, the decision was made to switch the patient to an alternative medication. As the patient had had a good response to paroxetine, it was agreed that an alternative medication with serotonin reuptake properties would be chosen. However, trials of

Clinical Vignette 1 *continued*

sertraline and venlafaxine were not successful in decreasing these side effects, and the patient felt that her response to these other medications was less robust than it has been to paroxetine. Paroxetine was eventually recontinued. The psychiatrist discussed the possibility of using alternative classes of medication. After these two unsatisfactory trials, however, the patient feared any further changes.

After approximately 2 years of treatment, a second discontinuation was discussed. At this point, the patient was even more reluctant to discontinue, having enjoyed mood stability over most of this period; however, the continuing side effects of anorgasmia and, perhaps, continued weight gain convinced her to try again. This was done, and within 2 weeks after discontinuation she reported normal sexual functioning. She continued to complain of difficulty losing weight, but as her weight seemed to be normal throughout the 2 years of treatment, the validity of her concerns was difficult to assess.

Within 2 months of her discontinuation trial, she again relapsed. Again, her symptoms were somewhat minor, consisting of irritability and dysphoria. However, there was a clear change from her state on medication. At this time, the possibility of long-term maintenance was discussed with the patient. Frustrated with yet another relapse, she readily agreed; however, she remained concerned by side effects. Bupropion was suggested as an alternative that has relatively few sexual side effects. Within a month she was taking 150 mg b.i.d. of the slow release capsule. As was hoped, she did not report any sexual side effect. She did report an antidepressant response to the drug; however, she felt that the response was not as complete as that she had had on paroxetine. Though less dysphoric, she had somewhat greater anxiety and irritability with the bupropion.

After a trial of over several months, her psychiatrist suggested combination therapy. It was suggested that the bupropion be continued, but that a small dose of an SSRI be added in the hope that it would address some of these remaining symptoms. Past experiences with medication were reviewed, and the patient felt that, of the SSRIs tried, citalopram had had the least sexual side effects, and the closest efficacy to paroxetine. With that in mind, citalopram was begun at a dose of 10 mg/day, and with this combination the patient reported complete response with no return of her previous side effects.

**Case Discussion.** Many lessons can be drawn from the above case. Perhaps the most important is that medication management is not a mechanical discipline that can be diagrammed with simple algorithms. All of the skills learned in psychiatric training, both psychopharmacological and psychotherapeutic, are crucial for successful treatment of the patient. In the initial phases of this treatment, the emphasis was on fostering a trusting relationship in a skeptical and fearful patient. This effort translates into a great deal of time spent, both in person and on the telephone. Though, superficially, one might argue against the justification for so much contact during a period when the medication is unlikely to show any benefit, the effort applied was probably the most important intervention during the treatment. Not only was such an effort helpful in fostering adherence during this period, but also it made the negotiation of later challenges much simpler. In the

beginning, the psychiatrist had to assume a paternal role, taking on most of the responsibility for the treatment. As the patient improved, this gradually gave way to a much more collaborative effort.

The importance of ongoing education should also be emphasized. Many, if not most, patients who present to a psychiatrist have seen another doctor prior to this. Education, however, is an ongoing process. Often the bulk of the information is given at the initial phases of treatment—a time when the patients' illness makes them least able to integrate this knowledge. Throughout the treatment, the psychiatrist often had to review and reinforce the treatment strategies discussed originally. Though written material can aid this process, and the patient clearly sought external sources of information, there remains no substitute for educational power in the human interaction.

The inappropriate minimization of sexual side effects during treatment is a problem that hopefully has been improving, through education both of patients and physicians. Patients are often reluctant to bring up sexual issues, and quick or vague inquiries regarding sexual functioning may be insufficient to elicit such symptoms. Inattention to this is unfortunate, as sexual side effects are a major reason for discontinuing medication that has otherwise been very effective. In this case, it was the patient's therapist who first understood the importance of this side effect. This underscores another point: in cases where the medication treatment and psychotherapy are split, it is crucial that there be frequent and regular contact between the treatment team.

Finally, cases like this emphasize the art as well as the science of pharmacotherapy. Though some treatment-related decisions have a clear scientific basis, others are more rooted in judgment and experience. Certainly the switch to bupropion to minimize sexual side effects has a clear pharmacodynamic rationale. However, the subsequent adjunctive use of an SSRI likely relied less on science, and more on the psychiatrist's experience in interpreting the irritability as a symptom that might be more amenable to a serotonergic agent. Though the practice of clinical medicine should be informed by research, the greatest clinicians are still those unique individuals who can integrate research into their own observations and wisdom.

## References

Ackenheil M (1990) The mechanism of action of antidepressants revised. J Neural Transm 32(Suppl), 29–37.

Altamura AC, DeNovellis F, Guercetti G, et al. (1989) Fluoxetine compared with amitriptyline in elderly depression: A controlled clinical trial. Int J Clin Pharmacol Res 9, 391–396.

Ambrosini PJ, Bianchi MD, Rabinovich H, et al. (1993) Antidepressant treatments in children and adolescents: II. Anxiety, physical, and behavioral disorders. J Am Acad Child Adolesc Psychiatr 32, 483–493.

American Academy of Child and Adolescent Psychiatry (2001) Practice parameter for the assessment and treatment of children and adolescents with suicidal behavior. J Am Acad Child Adolesc Psychiatr 40(Suppl), 24S–51S.

American Academy of Child and Adolescent Psychiatry (1998) Practice parameters for the assessment and treatment of children and adolescents with depressive disorders. J Am Acad Child Adolesc Psychiatr 37(Suppl), 63S–83S.

American Psychiatric Association (2000a) Diagnostic and Statistical Manual of Mental Disorders, 4th ed., Text Rev. APA, Washington DC.

American Psychiatric Association (2000b) Practice guideline for the treatment of patients with major depressive disorder (Rev). Am J Psychiatr 157(Suppl), 1–45.

Anderson IM (2000) Selective serotonin reuptake inhibitors versus tricyclic antidepressants: A meta-analysis. Br Med J 320, 1574–1577.

Anderson IM (2001) Meta-analyses of antidepressant drugs: Selectivity versus multiplicity. In Antidepressants: Selectivity or Multiplicity?, den Boer JA and Westenberg HGM (eds). Benecke NI, Amsterdam, The Netherlands, pp. 85–99.

Ansseau M and De Roeck J (1993) Trazodone in benzodiazepine dependence. J Clin Psychiatr 54, 189–191.

Apter JT and Woolfolk RL (1991) Lithium augmentation of bupropion in refractory depression. Ann Clin Psychiatr 2, 7–10.

Aranda-Michel J, Koehler A, Bejarano PA, et al. (1999) Nefazodone-induced liver failure: Report of three cases. Ann Intern Med 130, 285–288.

Armenteros JL and Lewis JE (2002) Citalopram treatment for impulsive aggression in children and adolescents: An open pilot study. J Am Acad Child Adolesc Psychiatr 41, 522–529.

Baldwin DS, Hawley CJ, Abed RT, et al. (1996) A multicentre double-blind comparison of nefazodone and paroxetine in the treatment of outpatients with moderate-to-severe depression. J Clin Psychiatr 57, 46–52.

Ballenger JC (1991) Long-term pharmacologic treatment of panic disorder. J Clin Psychiatr 52(Suppl 2), 18–23.

Balon R (1989) Biological predictors of antidepressant treatment outcome. Clin Neuropharmacol 12, 195–214.

Balon R (1993) Case report 5: Suicidal ideation during treatment with sertraline. J Drug Dev 6, 77–78.

Balon R, Yerangani VK, Pohl R, et al. (1993) Sexual dysfunction during antidepressant treatment. J Clin Psychiatr 54, 209–212.

Beasley CM, Masica DN, Heiligenstein JH, et al. (1993) Possible monamine oxidase inhibitor–serotonin reuptake inhibitor interaction: Fluoxetine clinical data and preclinical findings. J Clin Psychopharmacol 13, 213–320.

Beck AT (1978) Depression Inventory. Philadelphia Centre for Cognitive Therapy, Philadelphia, PA.

Beck PL, Bridges RJ, Demetrick DJ, et al. (1993) Chronic active hepatitis associated with trazodone therapy. Ann Intern Med 118, 791–792.

Bertz RJ and Granneman GR (1997) Use of in vitro and in vivo data to estimate the likelihood of metabolic pharmacokinetic interactions. Clin Pharmacokinet 32, 210–258.

Blackwell B (1991) Monoamine oxidase inhibitor interactions with other drugs. J Clin Psychopharmacol 11, 55–59.

Bond WS (1991) Ethnicity and psychotropic drugs. Clin Pharm 10, 467–470.

Bourgeois JA (1996) Two cases of hair loss after sertraline use. J Clin Psychopharmacol 16, 91–92.

Bourin M (1990) Is it possible to predict the activity of a new antidepressant in animals with simple psychopharmacological tests? Fundam Clin Pharmacol 4, 49–64.

Boyer WF and Feighner JP (1992) An overview of paroxetine. J Clin Psychiatr 53(Suppl 2), 3–6.

Brotman AW (1993) What's new with antidepressants? [audiotape]. In Practical Reviews in Psychiatry. Educational Reviews, Birmingham, AL.

Brotman AW, Falk WE, and Gelenberg AJ (1987) Pharmacologic treatment of acute depressive subtypes. In Psychopharmacology: The Third Generation of Progress, Meltzer HY (ed). Raven Press, New York, pp. 1031–1040.

Brown ES, Bobadilla L, and Rush AJ (2001) Ketoconazole in bipolar patients with depressive symptoms: A case series and literature review. Bipolar Disord 3, 23–29.

Burke WJ, Hendricks SE, McArthur-Miller D, et al. (2000) Weekly dosing of fluoxetine for the continuation phase of treatment of major depression: Results of a placebo-controlled, randomized clinical trial. J Clin Psychopharmacol 20, 423–427.

Burt VK, Suri R, Altshuler L, et al. (2001) The use of psychotropic medications during breast-feeding. Am J Psychiatr 158, 1001–1009.

Casat CD, Pleasants CZ, Schroeder DH, et al. (1989) Bupropion in children with attention deficit disorder. Psychopharmacol Bull 25, 198–201.

Cheer SM and Goa KL (2001) Fluoxetine: A review of its therapeutic potential in the treatment of depression associated with physical illness. Drugs 61, 81–110.

Choo V (1993) Paroxetine and extrapyramidal reactions. Lancet 341, 624.

Coffey BJ (1986) Therapeutics III: Pharmacotherapy. In Manual of Clinical Child Psychiatry, Robson KS (ed). American Psychiatric Press, Washington DC, pp. 149–184.

Cohen LS, Heller VL, and Rosenbaum JF (1991) Psychotropic drug use in pregnancy: An update. In Medical Psychiatric Practice, Vol. 1, Stoudemire A and Fogel BS (eds). American Psychiatric Press, Washington DC, pp. 615–634.

Cohn CK, Shrivastava R, Mendels J, et al. (1990) Double-blind, multicenter comparison of sertraline and amitriptyline in elderly depressed patients. J Clin Psychiatr 51(Suppl B), 28–33.

Compton SN, Grant PJ, Chrisman AK, et al. (2001) Sertraline in children and adolescents with social anxiety disorder: An open trial. J Am Acad Child Adolesc Psychiatr 40, 564–571.

Cook EH Jr., Rowlett R, Jaselskis C, et al. (1992) Fluoxetine treatment of children and adults with autistic disorder and mental retardation. J Am Acad Child Adolesc Psychiatr 31, 739–745.

Cook IA and Leuchter AF (2001) Prefrontal changes and treatment response prediction in depression. Semin Clin Neuropsychiatr 6, 113–120.

Cookson J (1993) Side effects of antidepressants. Br J Psychiatr 163(Suppl), 20–24.

Cornelius JR, Salloum IM, Cornelius MD, et al. (1993) Fluoxetine trial in suicidal depressed alcoholics. Psychopharmacol Bull 29, 195–199.

Correa H, Duval F, Claude MM, et al. (2001) Noradrenergic dysfunction and antidepressant treatment response. Eur Neuropsychopharmacol 11, 163–168.

Costa D and Kroll R (2000) Stuttering: An update for physicians. CMAJ 162, 1849–1855.

Cowen PJ, Power AC, Ware CJ, et al. (1994) 5-HT$_{1A}$ receptor sensitivity in major depression. A neuroendocrine study with buspirone. Br J Psychiatr 164, 372–379.

Cowley DS (1992) Alcohol abuse, substance abuse, and panic disorder. Am J Med 92(Suppl), 41–48.

Craighead LW and Agras WS (1991) Mechanisms of action in cognitive–behavioral and pharmacological interventions for obesity and bulimia nervosa. J Consult Clin Psychol 59, 115–125.

D'Amico MF, Roberts DL, Robinson DS, et al. (1990) Placebo-controlled dose-ranging trial designs in phase II developments of nefazodone. Psychopharmacol Bull 26, 147–150.

Davidson J (1989) Seizures and bupropion: A review. J Clin Psychiatr 50, 256–261.

Davidson JFT, DuPont RL, Hedges D, et al. (1999) Efficacy, safety and tolerability of venlafaxine extended release and buspirone in outpatients with generalized anxiety disorder. J Clin Psychiatr 60, 528–535.

Davidson JRT, Landerman LR, Farfel GM, et al. (2002) Characterizing the effects of sertraline in posttraumatic stress disorder. Psychol Med 32, 661–670.

Davidson N and Turnbull SD (1986) The effects of isocarboxazid on blood pressure and pulse. J Clin Psychopharmacol 6, 139–143.

Davis JM and Glassman AH (1989) Antidepressant drugs. In Comprehensive Textbook of Psychiatry, V, Kaplan HI and Sadock BJ (eds). Williams & Wilkins, Baltimore, pp. 1627–1654.

de Boer JA (1996) The pharmacologic profile of mirtazapine. J Clin Psychiatr 57(Suppl 4), 19–25.

Delina-Stula A (1989) From animal experiments to clinical dosing: Some aspects of preclinical development of antidepressants. In Clinical Pharmacology in Psychiatry, Dahl SG and Gram LF (eds). Springer-Verlag, Berlin, pp. 287–295.

Devane CL, Laizure SC, Stewart JT, et al. (1990) Disposition of bupropion in healthy volunteers and subjects with alcoholic liver disease. J Clin Psychopharmacol 10, 328–332.

Diehl DJ, Houck PR, Paradis C, et al. (1993) Pretreatment systolic orthostatic blood pressure and treatment response in geriatric depression: A revisit. J Clin Psychopharmacol 13, 189–193.

Dimmitt SB and Riley GJ (2000) Selective serotonin receptor uptake inhibitors can reduce restless legs symptoms. Arch Intern Med 160, 712–715.

Dinan T (1993) Lithium augmentation in sertraline-resistant depression: A preliminary dose–response study. Acta Psychiatr Scand 88, 300–301.

Doogan DP and Caillard V (1992) Sertraline in the prevention of depression. Br J Psychiatr 160, 217–222.

Doyle GD, Laher M, Kelly JG, et al. (1989) The pharmacokinetics of paroxetine in renal impairment. Acta Psychiatr Scand 350(Suppl), 89–90.

Dunner DL, Cohn JB, Walshe T, et al. (1992) Two combined, multicenter double-blind studies of paroxetine and doxepin in geriatric patients with major depression. J Clin Psychiatr 53(Suppl), 57–60.

Dursun SM, Mathew VM, and Reveley MA (1993) Toxic serotonin syndrome after fluoxetine plus carbamazepine (letter). Lancet 342, 442–443.

Eichelbaum M and Gross AS (1990) The genetic polymorphism of debrisoquine/sparteine metabolism—clinical aspects. Pharmacol Therap 46, 377–394.

Einarson A, Fatoye B, Sarkar M, et al. (2001) Pregnancy outcome following gestational exposure to venlafaxine: A multicenter prospective controlled study. Am J Psychiatr 158, 1728–1730.

Emslie GJ, Rush AJ, Weinberg WA, et al. (1997) A double-blind, randomized, placebo-controlled trial of fluoxetine in children and adolescents with depression. Arch Gen Psychiatr 54, 1031–1037.

Escobar JI and Tuason VB (1980) Antidepressant agents—a cross-cultural study. Psychopharmacol Bull 16, 49–52.

Evans MD, Hollon SD, DeRubeis RJ, et al. (1992) Differential relapse following cognitive therapy and pharmacotherapy for depression. Arch Gen Psychiatr 49, 802–808.

Fava M, Rosenbaum JF, Pava JA, et al. (1993) Anger attacks in unipolar depression, Part 1: Clinical correlates and response to fluoxetine treatment. Am J Psychiatr 150, 1158–1163.

Fawcett J and Barkin RL (1998) Meta-analysis of eight randomized, double-blind, controlled trials of mirtazapine for the treatment of patient with major depression and symptoms of anxiety. J Clin Psychiatr 59, 123–127.

Feiger AD, Bielski RJ, Bremner J, et al. (1999) Double-blind placebo-substitution study of nefazodone in the prevention of relapse during continuation treatment of outpatients with major depression. Clin Psychopharmacol 114, 19–28.

Fichtner CG, Horevitz RP, and Braun BG (1992) Fluoxetine in depersonalization disorder (letter). Am J Psychiatr 149, 1720–1751.

Fluoxetine Bulimia Nervose Collaborative Study Group (1992) Fluoxetine in the treatment of bulimia nervosa. A multicenter, placebo-controlled double-blind trial. Arch Gen Psychiatr 49, 139–147.

Food and Drug Administration (1993) FDC Reports: Prescription and OTC pharmaceuticals—the pink sheet 55, 10–11.

Fountaine R and Chouinard G (1986) An open clinical trial of fluoxetine in the treatment of obsessive–compulsive disorder. J Clin Psychopharmacol 6, 98–101.

Fountaine R, Ontiveros A, Elie R, et al. (1994) Double-blind comparison of nefazodone, imipramine and placebo in major depression. J Clin Psychiatr 55, 234–241.

Frank E, Kupfer DJ, Perel JM, et al. (1990) Three-year outcomes for maintenance therapies in recurrent depression. Arch Gen Psychiatr 47, 1093–1099.

Freemantle N, Anderson IM, and Young P (2000) Predictive value of pharmacological activity for the relative efficacy of antidepressant drugs: Meta-regression analysis. Br J Psychiatr 177, 292–302.

Gammon G and Brown T (1993) Fluoxetine and methylphenidate in combination for treatment of attention deficit disorder and comorbid depressive disorder. J Child Adolesc Psychopharmacol 3, 53–58.

Gawin FH and Kleber HD (1984) Cocaine abuse treatment: Open pilot study with desipramine and lithium carbonate. Arch Gen Psychiatr 41, 903–909.

Gjerris A (1988) Do concentrations of neurotransmitters in lumbar CSF reflect cerebral dysfunction in depression? Acta Psychiatr Scand 78, 21–24.

Glassman AH, Roose SP, and Bigger JT (1993) The safety of tricyclic antidepressants in cardiac patients. JAMA 269, 2673–2675.

Goetz CG, Tanner CM, and Klawans HL (1984) Bupropion in Parkinson's disease. Neurology 34, 1092–1094.

Goldbloom D and Olmstead M (1993) Pharmacotherapy of bulimia nervosa with fluoxetine: Assessment of clinically significant attitudinal change. Am J Psychiatr 150, 770–774.

Golwyn D and Sevlie C (1993) Monoamine oxidase inhibitor hypertensive crisis headache and orthostatic hypotension (letter). J Clin Psychopharmacol 13, 77–78.

Greden JF (1993) Antidepressant maintenance medication: When to discontinue and how to stop. J Clin Psychiatr 54(Suppl), 39–45.

Guillibert E, Pelicier Y, and Archambault JC (1989) A double-blind multicenter study of paroxetine vs. clomipramine in depressed elderly patients. Acta Psychiatr Scand 80(Suppl 350), 132–134.

Gunzberger D and Martinez D (1992) Adverse vascular effects associated with fluoxetine (letter). Am J Psychiatr 149, 1751.

Hale AS (1993) New antidepressants: Use in high-risk patients. J Clin Psychiatr 54(Suppl), 61–70.

Hamilton JA and Halbreich U (1993) Special aspects of neuropsychiatric illness in women: With a focus on depression. Annu Rev Med 44, 355–364.

Hamilton M (1960) A rating scale of depression. J Neurol Neurosurg Psychiatr 23, 56–62.

Hellerstein DJ, Yanowitch P, Rosenthal J, et al. (1993) A randomized double-blind study of fluoxetine versus placebo in the treatment of dysthymia. Am J Psychiatr 150, 1169–1175.

Hirschfeld RMA (1999) Efficacy of SSRIs and newer antidepressants in severe depression: Comparison with TCAs. J Clin Psychiatr 60, 326–335.

Hollander E, DeCaria CM, Finkell JN, et al. (2000). A randomized double-blind fluvoxamine/placebo crossover trial in pathological gambling. Biol Psychiatr 47, 813–817.

Hollon SD, DeRubeis RJ, Evans MD, et al. (1992) Cognitive therapy and pharmacotherapy for depression: Singly and in combination. Arch Gen Psychiatr 49, 774–781.

Horrigan JP and Barnhill LJ (2000) Fluvoxamine and enuresis. J Am Acad Child Adolesc Psychiatr 39, 1465–1466.

Hrdina PD, Bakish D, Ravindran A, et al. (1997) Platelet serotonergic indices in major depression: Up-regulation of 5-HT$_{2A}$ receptors unchanged by antidepressant treatment. Psychiatr Res 66, 73–85.

Hunt K and Resnick MP (1993) Clomipramine-induced agranulocytosis and its treatment with G-CSF (letter). Am J Psychiatr 150, 522–523.

Janicak PG, Davis JM, Preskorn SH, et al. (1993) Principles and Practice of Psychopharmacotherapy. Williams & Wilkins, Baltimore, MD, p. 499.

Jarvik LF, Read SL, Mintz J, et al. (1983) Pretreatment orthostatic hypotension in geriatric depression: Predictor of response to imipramine and doxepin. J Clin Psychopharmacol 3, 368–372.

Jeffries JJ and al-Jeshi A (1995) Nefazodone-induced mania (letter). Can J Psychiatr 40, 218.

Jenike MA, Buttolph L, Baer L, et al. (1989) Open trial of fluoxetine in obsessive–compulsive disorder. Am J Psychiatr 146, 909–911.

Jensen PS, Bhatara VS, Vitiello B, et al. (1999) Psychoactive medication prescribing practices for US children: Gaps between research and clinical practice. J Am Acad Child Adolesc Psychiatr 38, 557–565.

Kalow W (1991) Interethnic variation of drug metabolism. Trends Pharmacol Sci 12, 102–107.

Kaplan GB (1992) Neurobiological aspects of panic disorder. R I Med 75, 247–251.

Kapur S, Mieczkowski T, and Mann JJ (1992) Antidepressant medications and the relative risk of suicide attempt and suicide. JAMA 268, 3441–3445.

Kasper S, Fuger J, and Moller HJ (1992) Comparative efficacy of antidepressants. Drugs 43(Suppl), 11–22.

Katz IR, Simpson GM, Curlik SM, et al. (1990) Pharmacologic treatment of major depression for elderly patients in residential care settings. J Clin Psychiatr 51(Suppl), 41–47.

Keller MB, Kocsis JH, Thase ME, et al. (1998) Maintenance phase efficacy of sertraline for chronic depression: A randomized controlled trial. JAMA 280, 1665–1672.

Keller MB, Lavori PW, Beardslee WR, et al. (1991) Depression in children and adolescents: New data on 'undertreatment' and a literature review on the efficacy of available treatments. J Affect Disord 21, 163–171.

Keller MB, Lavori PW, Coryell W, et al. (1986) Differential outcome of pure manic, mixed/cycling, and pure depressive episode in patients with bipolar illness. JAMA 255, 3138–3142.

Keller MB, Lavori PW, Mueller TI, et al. (1992) Time to recovery, chronicity, and levels of psychopathology in major depression: A 5-year prospective follow-up of 431 subjects. Arch Gen Psychiatr 49, 809–816.

Keller MB, McCullough JP, Klein DN, et al. (2000) A comparison of nefazodone, the cognitive behavioral-analysis system of psychotherapy, and their combination for the treatment of chronic depression. N Engl J Med 342, 1462–1470.

Keller MB, Ryan ND, Strober M, et al. (2001) Efficacy of paroxetine in the treatment of adolescent major depression: A randomized, controlled trial. J Am Acad Child Adolesc Psychiatr 40, 762–772.

Keller MB, Shapiro RW, Lavori PW, et al. (1982) Relapse in major depressive disorder: Analysis with the life table. Arch Gen Psychiatr 39, 911–915.

Kelsey JE (1995) Venlafaxine in social phobia. Psychopharmacol Bull 31, 767–771.

Klein DF (1984) Psychopharmacologic treatment of panic disorder. Psychosomatics 4, 36–40.

Klerman GL and Cole JO (1965) Clinical pharmacology of imipramine and related antidepressant compounds. Pharmacol Rev 17, 101–141.

Kline NS (1958) Clinical experience with iproniazid. J Clin Exp Psychopathol 19(Suppl), 72–78.

Kocsis JH (1990) New issues in the prediction of antidepressant response. Psychopharmacol Bull 26, 49–53.

Kocsis JH, Frances AJ, Voss C, et al. (1985) Imipramine treatment for chronic depression. Arch Gen Psychiatr 45, 253–257.

Koran LM, Quirk T, Lorberbaum JP, et al. (2001) Mirtazapine treatment of obsessive–compulsive disorder. J Clin Psychopharmacol 21(5) (Oct), 537–539.

Kornstein SG, Schatzberg AF, Thase ME, et al. (2000) Gender differences in treatment response to sertraline versus imipramine in chronic depression. Am J Psychiatr 157, 1445–1452.

Kosieradzki PH (2001) Citalopram in social phobia. J Am Acad Child Adolesc Psychiatr 40, 1126–1127.

Kramer MS, Cutler N, Feighner J, et al. (1998) Distinct mechanism for antidepressant activity by blockade of central substance P-receptors. Science 281, 1640–1645.

Krishnan KR and France RD (1989) Antidepressants in chronic pain syndromes. Am Fam Phys 39, 233–237.

Kruesi MJ, Fine S, Valladares L, et al. (1992) Paraphilias: A double-blind crossover comparison of clomipramine versus desipramine. Arch Sex Behav 21, 587–593.

Kuhn R (1958) The treatment of depressive states with G22355 (imipramine hydrochloride). Am J Psychiatr 115, 459–464.

Kulin NA, Pastuszak A, Sage SR, et al. (1998) Pregnancy outcome following maternal use of the new selective serotonin reuptake inhibitors: A prospective controlled multicenter study. JAMA 279, 609–610.

Kupfer DJ, Frank E, Perel JM, et al. (1992) Five-year outcome for maintenance therapies in recurrent depression. Arch Gen Psychiatr 49, 769–773.

Labbate LA, Brodrick PS, Nelson RP, et al. (2001) Effects of bupropion sustained-release on sexual functioning and nocturnal erections in healthy men. J Clin Psychopharmacol 21, 99–103.

Larson EW (1993) Migraine with typical aura associated with fluoxetine therapy: Case report. J Clin Psychiatr 54, 235–236.

Lavin MR, Mendelowitz A, and Kronig MH (1993) Spontaneous hypertensive reactions with monoamine oxidase inhibitors. Biol Psychiatr 34, 146–151.

Lebert F, Pasquier F, and Petit H (1994) Behavioral effects of trazodone in Alzheimer's disease. J Clin Psychiatr 55, 536–538.

Leon AC, Keller MB, Warshaw MG, et al. (1999) Prospective study of fluoxetine treatment and suicidal behavior in affectively ill subjects. Am J Psychiatr 156, 195–201.

Leonard BE (1993) The comparative pharmacology of new antidepressants. J Clin Psychiatr 54(Suppl), 3–15.

Leonard HL, March J, Rickler KC, et al. (1997) Review of the pharmacology of the selective serotonin reuptake inhibitors in children and adolescents. J Am Acad Child Adolesc Psychiatr 36, 725–736.

Lester BM, Cucca J, Andreozzi L, et al. (1993) Possible association between fluoxetine hydrochloride and colic in an infant. J Am Acad Child Adolesc Psychiatr 32, 1253–1255.

Levenson JL and Fallon HJ (1993) Fluoxetine treatment of depression caused by interferon-α. Am J Gastroenterol 88, 760–761.

Lewis J, Braganza J, and Williams T (1993) Psychomotor retardation and semistuporous state with paroxetine (letter). British Medical Journal 306, 1169.

Liebowitz MR, Hollander E, Schneier F, et al. (1990) Reversible and irreversible monoamine oxidase inhibitors in other psychiatric disorders. Acta Psychiatr Scand 360(Suppl), 29–34.

Lilie JK and Lahmeyer H (1991) Psychiatric management of sleep disorders. Psychiatr Med 9, 245–260.

Loprinzi CL, Sloan JA, Perez EA, et al. (2002) Phase III evaluation of fluoxetine (Prozac) for treatment of hot flashes. J Clin Oncol 20, 1578–1583.

Louie AK, Lewis TB, and Lannon RA (1993) Use of low-dose fluoxetine in major depression and panic disorder. J Clin Psychiatr 54, 435–438.

Lydiard RB, Anton RF, and Cunningham T (1993) Interactions between sertraline and tricyclic antidepressants (letter). Am J Psychiatr 150, 1125–1126.

Magni G (1991) The use of antidepressants in the treatment of chronic pain. A review of the current evidence. Drugs 42, 730–748.

Mann J and Kapur S (1991) The emergence of suicidal ideation and behavior during antidepressant pharmacotherapy. Arch Gen Psychiatr 48, 1027–1033.

Marathe PH, Lee JS, Greene DS, et al. (1996) Comparison of the steady-state pharmacokinetics of nefazodone after administration of 200 mg twice daily or 400 mg once daily in the morning or evening. Br J Clin Pharmacol 41, 21–27.

March SM, Flynn HA, Young E, et al. (2001) Recurrent depression in women throughout the life span. In Treatment of Recurrent Depression (Review of Psychiatry Series, Vol. 20, No. 5, Oldham JM and Riba MB, [series eds]), Greden JF (ed). American Psychiatric Publishing, Washington DC.

Martyn R, Somberg JC, and Kerin NZ (1993) Proarrhythmia of nonantiarrhythmic drugs. Am Heart J 126, 201–205.

Max MB, Lynch SA, Muir J, et al. (1992) Effects of desipramine, amitriptyline, and fluoxetine on pain in diabetic neuropathy. NEJM 326, 1250–1256.

McCabe B and Tsuang MT (1982) Dietary consideration in mao inhibitor regimens. J Clin Psychiatr 43, 178–181.

McElroy SL, Casuto LS, Nelson EB, et al. (2000) Placebo-controlled trial of sertraline in the treatment of binge eating disorder. Am J Psychiatr 157, 1004–1006.

McGrath PJ, Stewart JW, Janal MN, et al. (2000) A placebo controlled study of fluoxetine versus imipramine in the acute treatment of atypical depression. Am J Psychiatr 157, 344–350.

McGrath PJ, Stewart JW, Nunes EV, et al. (1993) A double-blind crossover trial of imipramine and phenelzine for outpatients with treatment-refractory depression. Am J Psychiatr 150, 118–123.

McKinney WT (1988) Animal models for depression and mania. In Depression and Mania, Georgotas A and Cancro R (eds). Elsevier, New York, pp. 117–126.

McKinney WT and Bunney WE (1969) Animal models of depression. Arch Gen Psychiatr 21, 240–248.

Meier PJ, Mueller HK, Dick B, et al. (1983) Hepatic monooxygenase activities in subjects with a genetic defect in drug oxidation. Gastroenterology 85, 682–692.

Mesaros J (1993) Fluoxetine for primary enuresis (letter). J Am Acad Child Adolesc Psychiatr 32, 877–878.

Meyer JH, Cho R, Kennedy S, et al. (1999) The effects of single dose nefazodone and paroxetine upon 5-HT$_{2A}$ binding potential in humans using [18F]-setoperone PET. Psychopharmacology 144, 279–281.

Mir S and Taylor D (1997) The adverse effects of antidepressants. Curr Opin Psychiatry 10, 88–94.

Mitchell JE, Pyle RL, Eckert ED, et al. (1990) A comparison study of antidepressants and structured intensive group psychotherapy in the treatment of bulimia nervosa. Arch Gen Psychiatr 47, 149–157.

Modell JG (1989) Repeated observations of yawning, clitoral enlargement, and orgasm associated with fluoxetine administration. J Clin Psychopharmacol 9, 63.

Moncrieff J, Wessely S, and Hardy R (1998) Meta-analysis of trials comparing antidepressants with active placebos. Br J Psychiatr 172, 227–231.

Montgomery SA (1992) Suicide and antidepressants. Drugs 43(Suppl 2) 24–30.

Montgomery SA (1993) Venlafaxine: A new dimension in antidepressant pharmacotherapy. J Clin Psychiatr 54, 119–126.

Montgomery SA and Asberg MA (1979) A new depression scale designed to be sensitive to change. Br J Psychiatr 134, 382–389.

Montgomery SA and Dunbar G (1993) Paroxetine is better than placebo in relapse prevention and the prophylaxis of recurrent depression. Int Clin Psychopharmacol 8, 189–195.

Montgomery SA, Bullock T, and Fineberg N (1991) Serotonin selectivity for obsessive compulsive and panic disorders. J Psychiatr Neurosci 16(Suppl 1), 30–35.

Montgomery SA, Dunfour H, Brion S, et al. (1988) The prophylactic efficacy of fluoxetine in unipolar depression. Br J Psychiatr 153(Suppl 3), 69–76.

Montgomery SA, Rasmussen JG, and Tanghol P (1993) A 24-week study of 20 mg citalopram, 40 mg citalopram and placebo in the prevention of relapse of major depression. Int Clin Psychopharmacol 8, 181–188.

Montgomery SA, Reimitz P-E, and Zivkov M (1998) Mirtazapine versus amitriptyline in the long-term treatment of depression: A double-blind placebo-controlled study. Int Clin Psychopharmacol 13, 63–73.

Moussavian H (2001) Improvement of acne in depressed patients treated with paroxetine. J Am Acad Child Adolesc Psychiatr 40, 505–506.

Muly EC, McDonald W, Steffens D, et al. (1993) Serotonin syndrome produced by a combination of fluoxetine and lithium (letter). Am J Psychiatr 150, 1565.

Mundo E, Walker M, Cate T, et al. (2001) The role of serotonin transporter protein gene in antidepressant-induced mania in bipolar disorder: Preliminary findings. Arch Gen Psychiatr 58, 539–544.

Murphy BE, Filipini D, and Ghadirian AM (1993) Possible use of glucocorticoid receptor antagonists in the treatment of major depression: Preliminary results using RU486. J Psychiatr Neurosci 18, 209–213.

Narurkar V, Smoller BR, Hu CH, et al. (1993) Desipramine-induced blue-gray photosensitive pigmentation. Arch Dermatol 129, 474–476.

Nelson JC, Kennedy JS, Pollock BG, et al. (1999) Treatment of major depression with nortriptyline and paroxetine in patients with ischemic heart disease. Am J Psychiatr 156, 1024–1028.

Nierenberg AA (1992) The medical consequences of the selection of an antidepressant. J Clin Psychiatr 53, 19–24.

NIMH/NIH Consensus Development Panel (1985) Mood disorders: Pharmacologic prevention of recurrences (NIMH/NIH Consensus Development Conference Statement). Am J Psychiatr 142, 469–476.

Nulman I, Rovet J, Stewart DE, et al. (1997) Neurodevelopment of children exposed in utero to antidepressant drugs. N Engl J Med 336, 258–262.

Ogilvie A (1993) Hair loss during fluoxetine treatment (letter). Lancet 342, 1423.

Oke A, Adhiyaman V, Aziz K, et al. (2001) Dose-dependent seizure activity associated with fluoxetine therapy. QJM 94, 113–114.

Old Age Depression Interest Group (1993) How long should the elderly take antidepressants?: A double-blind placebo-controlled study of continuation/prophylaxis therapy with dothiepin. Br J Psychiatr 162, 175–182.

O'Malley PG, Jackson JL, Santoro J, et al. (1999) Antidepressant therapy for unexplained symptoms and symptom syndromes. J Fam Pract 48, 980–990.

Orsulak PJ and Waller D (1989) Antidepressant drugs: Additional clinical uses. J Fam Pract 28, 209–216.

Page AC (2002) Nature and treatment of panic disorder. Curr Opin Psychiatr 15, 149–155.

Pasion R and Kirby S (1993) Trazodone for screaming (letter). Lancet 341, 970.

Pastuszak A, Schick-Boschetto B, Zuber C, et al. (1993) Pregnancy outcome following first-trimester exposure to fluoxetine (Prozac). JAMA 269, 2246–2248.

Pataki CS, Carlson GA, Kelly KL, et al. (1993) Side effects of methylphenidate and desipramine alone and in combination in children. J Am Acad Child Adolesc Psychiatr 32, 1065–1072.

Perry PJ (1996) Pharmacotherapy for major depression with melancholic features: Relative efficacy of tricyclic versus selective serotonin reuptake inhibitor antidepressants. J Affect Disord 39, 1–6.

Pescatori ES, Engelman JC, Davis C, et al. (1993) Priapism of the clitoris: A case following trazodone use. J Urol 149, 1557–1559.

Pettinati HM, Volpicelli JR, Luck G, et al. (2001) Double-blind clinical trial of sertraline treatment for alcohol dependence. J Clin Psychopharmacol 21, 143–153.

Phillips KA (1991) Body dysmorphic disorder: The distress of imagined ugliness. Am J Psychiatr 148, 1138–1149.

Phillips KA and Nierenberg AA (1994) The assessment and treatment of refractory depression. J Clin Psychiatr 55(Suppl 2), 20–26.

Phillips KA, Dwight MM, and McElroy SL (1998) Efficacy and safety of fluvoxamine in body dysmorphic disorder. J Clin Psychiatr 59, 165–171.

Physicians' Desk Reference, 55th ed. (2001) Medical Economics, Montvale, NJ.

Pletscher A (1991) The discovery of antidepressants: A winding path. Experientia 47, 4–8.

Porsolt RD, Bertin A, Blavet N, et al. (1979) Immobility induced by forced swimming in rats: Effects of agents which modify central catecholamine and serotonin activity. Eur J Pharmacol 57, 431–436.

Potts NL and Davidson JR (1992) Social phobia: Biological aspects and pharmacotherapy. Prog Neuropsychopharmacol Biol Psychiatr 16, 635–646.

Power-Smith (1994) Beneficial sexual side effects from fluoxetine. Br J Psychiatr 164, 249–250.

Preskorn SH and Burke M (1992) Somatic therapy for major depressive disorder: Selection of an antidepressant. J Clin Psychiatr 53(Suppl 9), 5–18.

Preskorn SH, Burke MJ, and Fast GA (1993) Therapeutic drug monitoring. Psychiatr Clin N Am 16, 611–645.

Prien RF, Kupfer DJ, Mansky PA, et al. (1984) Drug therapy in the prevention of recurrences in unipolar and bipolar affective disorders. Arch Gen Psychiatr 41, 1096–1104.

Quitkin FM, McGrath PJ, Stewart JW, et al. (1990) Atypical depression, panic attacks, and response to imipramine and phenelzine. Arch Gen Psychiatr 47, 935–941.

Rapaport JL, Mikkelsen EJ, Zavadil A, et al. (1980) Childhood enuresis II. Psychopathology, tricyclic concentration in plasma, and antienuretic effect. Arch Gen Psychiatr 37, 1146–1152.

Raskin A (1974) Age-sex differences in response to antidepressant drugs. J Nerv Ment Dis 159, 120–130.

Ravaris CL, Sateia MJ, Beroza KW, et al. (1988) Effect of ketoconazole on a hypophysectomized, hypercortisolemic, psychotically depressed woman. Arch Gen Psychiatr 45, 966–967.

Ravindran AV, Bialik RJ, and Lapierre YD (1994) Therapeutic efficacy of specific serotonin reuptake inhibitors (SSRIs) in dysthymia. Can J Psychiatr 39, 21–26.

Ray WA, Fought RL, and Decker MD (1992) Psychoactive drugs and the risk of injurious motor vehicle crashed in elderly drivers. Am J Epidemiol 136, 873–883.

Ray WA, Griffin MR, Schaffner W, et al. (1987) Psychotropic drug use and the risk of hip fracture. NEJM 316, 363–369.

Redrobe JP, MacSweeney CP, and Bourin M (1996) The role of 5-HT$_{1A}$ and 5-HT$_{1B}$ receptors in antidepressant drug actions in the mouse forced swimming test. Eur J Pharmacol 318, 213–220.

Reidenberg MM and Lowenthal DT (1968) Adverse nondrug reactors. N Engl J Med 279, 678–679.

Reilly JG, McTavish SF, and Young AH (1997) Rapid depletion of plasma tryptophan: A review of studies and experimental methodology. J Psychopharmacol 11, 381–392.

Reynolds CF (1992) Treatment of depression in special populations. J Clin Psychiatr 53(Suppl 9), 45–53.

Richelson E (1997) Pharmacokinetic drug interactions of new antidepressants: A review of the effects on the metabolism of other drugs. Mayo Clin Proc 72, 835–847.

Richelson E (2001) Pharmacology of antidepressants. Mayo Clin Proc 76, 511–527.

Rickels K, Downing R, Schweizer E, et al. (1993) Antidepressants for the treatment of generalized anxiety disorder: A placebo-controlled comparison of imipramine, trazadone, and diazepam. Arch Gen Psychiatr 50, 884–895.

Rickels K, Robinson DS, Schweizer E, et al. (1995) Nefazodone: Aspects of efficacy. J Clin Psychiatr 56(Suppl 6), 43–46.

Ricketts RW, Goza AB, Ellis CR, et al. (1993) Fluoxetine treatment of severe self-injury in young adults with mental retardation. J Am Acad Child Adolesc Psychiatr 32, 865–869.

Riddle MA, Geller B, and Ryan N (1993) Another sudden death in a child treated with desipramine. J Am Acad Child Adolesc Psychiatr 32, 792–797.

Riddle MA, Reeve EA, Yaryura-tobias JA, et al. (2001) Fluvoxamine for children and adolescents with obsessive–compulsive disorder: A randomized, controlled, multicenter trial. J Am Acad Child Adolesc Psychiatr 40, 222–229.

Rifkin A, Klein DF, and Quitkin F (1978) Possible effect of race on tricyclic plasma levels. JAMA 239, 1845–1846.

Roose SP and Dalack GW (1992) Treating the depressed patient with cardiovascular problems. J Clin Psychiatr 53(Suppl 9), 25–31.

Roose SP and Glassman AH (1989) Cardiovascular effects of tricyclic antidepressants in depressed patients with and without heart disease. J Clin Psychiatr 7(Monogr 2), 1–18.

Roose SP, Dalack GW, Glassman AH, et al. (1991) Cardiovascular effects of bupropion in depressed patients with heart disease. Am J Psychiatr 148, 512–516.

Roose SP, Glassman AH, Attia E, et al. (1994) Comparative efficacy of selective serotonin reuptake inhibitors and tricyclics in the treatment of melancholia. Am J Psychiatr 151, 1735–1739.

Roose SP, Glassman AH, Attia E, et al. (1998) Cardiovascular effects of fluoxetine in depressed patients with heart disease. Am J Psychiatr 155, 660–665.

Rosenstein DL, Nelson JC, and Jacobs SC (1993) Seizures associated with antidepressants: A review. J Clin Psychiatr 54, 289–299.

Rothschild AJ, Samson JA, Bessette MP, et al. (1993) Efficacy of the combination of fluoxetine and perphenazine in the treatment of psychotic depression. J Clin Psychiatr 54, 338–342.

Sachetti E, Vita A, Guarneri L, et al. (1991) The effectiveness of fluoxetine, clomipramine, nortriptyline and desipramine in major depressives with suicidal behavior: Preliminary findings. In Serotonin-Related Psychiatric Syndromes: Clinical and Therapeutic Links, Cassano GB and Akiskal HS (eds). Royal Society of Medicine Services, London, pp. 47–53.

Salzman C, Schneider L, and Lebowitz B (1993) Antidepressant treatment of very old patients. Am J Geriatr Psychiatr 1, 21–29.

Saper JR (1989) Migraine, migraine variants, and related headaches. Otolaryngol Clin N Am 22, 1115–1130.

Schatzberg AF and Cole JO (1991) Manual of Clinical Psychopharmacology, 2nd ed. American Psychiatric Press, Washington DC.

Schwetz B (2002) Warning on serzone. JAMA 287, 1103.

Segraves RT (1992) Overview of sexual dysfunction complicating the treatment of depression. J Clin Psychiatr 10, 4–10.

Seligman ME and Maier SF (1967) Failure to escape traumatic shock. J Exp Psychol 74, 1–9.

Seth R, Jennings AL, Bindman J, et al. (1992) Combination treatment with noradrenalin and serotonin reuptake inhibitors in resistant depression. Br J Psychiatr 161, 562–565.

Shihabuddin L and Rapport D (1994) Sertraline and extrapyramidal side effects (letter). Am J Psychiatr 151, 288.

Shopsin B (1983) Bupropion's prophylactic efficacy in bipolar illness. J Clin Psychiatr 44, 163–169.

Shulman RB, Scheftner WA, and Nayudu S (2001) Venlafaxine-associated mania. J Clin Psychopharmacol 21, 239–241.

Simeon JG (1989) Depressive disorders in children and adolescents. Psychiatr J Univ Ottawa 14, 356–361.

Simon GE, Heiligenstein JH, Grothaus L, et al. (1998) Should anxiety and insomnia influence antidepressant selection: A randomized comparison of fluoxetine and imipramine. J Clin Psychiatr 59, 49–55.

Sirey JA, Meyers BS, Bruce ML, et al. (1999) Predictors of antidepressant prescription and early use among depressed outpatients. Am J Psychiatr 156, 690–696.

Sitsen JMA and Moors J (1994) Mirtazapine, a novel antidepressant, in the treatment of anxiety symptoms: Results from a placebo-controlled trial. Drug Invest 8, 339–344.

Sitsen JMA and Zivkov M (1995) Mirtazapine: Clinical profile. CNS Drugs 4(Suppl 1), 39–48.

Smith D and Levitte S (1993) Association of fluoxetine and return of sexual potency in three elderly men. J Clin Psychiatr 54, 317–319.

Spencer T, Biederman J, Steingard R, et al. (1993) Bupropion exacerbates tics in children with attention-deficit hyperactivity disorder and Tourette's syndrome. J Am Acad Child Adolesc Psychiatr 32, 211–214.

Staab JP, Ruckenstein MJ, Solomon D, et al. (2002) Serotonin reuptake inhibitors for dizziness with psychiatric symptoms. Arch Otolaryngol—Head Neck Surg 128, 554–560.

Steele T and Ashby J (1993) Desipramine-related slate-gray skin pigmentation (letter). J Clin Psychopharmacol 13, 76–77.

Stein DJ, Hollander E, Anthony DT, et al. (1992) Serotonergic medications for sexual obsessions, sexual addictions, and paraphilias. J Clin Psychiatr 53, 267–271.

Stein DJ, Hollander E, and Josephson SC (1994) Serotonin reuptake blockers for the treatment of obsessional jealousy. J Clin Psychiatr 55, 30–33.

Stern WL, Harto-Truax N, and Bauer N (1983) Efficacy of bupropion in tricyclic-resistant or intolerant patients. J Clin Psychiatr 44, 148–152.

Steur E (1993) Increase of Parkinson disability after fluoxetine medication. Neurology 43, 211–213.

Stewart JW, McGrath PJ, Quitkin FM, et al. (1993) Chronic depression: Response to placebo, imipramine and phenelzine. J Clin Psychopharmacol 13, 391–396.

Stimmel G and Dopheide J (1996) Psychotropic drug-induced reductions in seizure threshold. CNS Drugs 5, 38–50.

Stoll AL, Pope HG, and McElroy SL (1991) High-dose fluoxetine: Safety and efficacy in 27 cases. J Clin Psychopharmacol 11, 225–226.

Strauss WL, Unis AS, Cowan C, et al. (2002) Fluorine magnetic resonance spectroscopy measurement of brain fluvoxamine and fluoxetine in pediatric patients treated for pervasive developmental disorders. Am J Psychiatr 159, 755–760.

Strickland TL, Stein R, Lin K-M, et al. (1997) The pharmacologic treatment of anxiety and depression in African Americans: Considerations for the general practitioner. Arch Fam Med 6, 371–375.

Sullivan M, Katon W, Russo J, et al. (1993) A randomized trial of nortriptyline for severe chronic tinnitus: Effects on depression, disability, and tinnitus symptoms. Arch Intern Med 153, 2251–2259.

Sutor B, Rummans TA, and Smith GE (2001) Assessment and management of behavioral disturbances in nursing home patients with dementia. Mayo Clin Proc 76, 540–550.

Sylvester CE and Kruesi MJP (1994) Child and adolescent psychopharmacotherapy: Progress and pitfalls. Psychiatr Ann 24, 83–90.

Teicher M, Glod C, and Cole J (1990) Emergence of intense suicidal preoccupation during fluoxetine treatment. Am J Psychiatr 147, 207–210.

Thase ME, Blomgren SL, Birkett MA, et al. (1997) Fluoxetine treatment in patients with major depressive disorder who failed initial treatment with sertraline. J Clin Psychiatr 58, 16–21.

Thase ME, Entsuah AR, and Rudolph RL (2001) Remission rates during treatment with venlafaxine or selective serotonin reuptake inhibitors. Br J Psychiatr 178, 234–241.

Thase ME, Fava M, Halbreich U, et al. (1996) Placebo-controlled, randomized clinical trial comparing sertraline and imipramine for the treatment of dysthymia. Arch Gen Psychiatr 53, 777–784.

Thase ME, Rush AJ, Howland RH, et al. (2002) Double-blind switch study of imipramine or sertraline treatment of antidepressant-resistant chronic depression. Arch Gen Psychiatr 59, 233–239.

Thase ME, Trivedi MH, and Rush AJ (1995) MAOIs in the contemporary treatment of depression. Neuropsychopharmacology 12, 185–219.

Tollefson GD (1993) Adverse drug reactions/interactions in maintenance therapy. J Clin Psychiatr 54(Suppl), 48–58.

Tomkins GE, Jackson JL, O'Malley PG, et al. (2001) Treatment of chronic headache with antidepressants: A meta-analysis. Am J Med 111, 54–63.

van Amerigen M, Mancini C, and Streiner DL (1993) Fluoxetine efficacy in social phobia. J Clin Psychiatr 54, 27–32.

van Moffaert M, Pregaldien JL, von Frenckell R, et al. (1994) A double-blind comparison of nefazodone and imipramine in the treatment of depressed patients. New Trends Exp Clin Psychiatr 10, 85–87.

van Praag HM (2001) History and contemporary notes on the treatment of depression, or, how classification shaped therapeutic approaches. In Antidepressants: Selectivity or Multiplicity?, den Boer JA and Westenberg HGM (eds). Benecke NI, Amsterdam, pp. 9–30.

Vanelle JM (1997) Controlled efficacy study of fluoxetine in dysthymia. Br J Psychiatr 170, 345–350.

Vaugeois JM and Costentin J (1998) Creation d'une lignee de souris "depressives" a partir d'une selection de geniteurs presentant un comportement de resignation. C R Seances Soc Biol Fil 192, 1149–1161.

Vetulani J and Sulser F (1975) Action of various antidepressant treatments reduces reactivity of noradrenergic cyclic AMP-generating system in limbic forebrain. Nature 257, 495–497.

Viswanathan R and Paradis C (1991) Treatment of cancer phobia with fluoxetine. Am J Psychiatr 148, 1090.

Waldinger MD, Hengeveld MW, Zwinderman AH, et al. (1998) Effect of SSRI antidepressants on ejaculation: A double-blind, randomized, placebo-controlled study with fluoxetine, fluvoxamine, paroxetine and sertraline. J Clin Psychopharmacol 18, 274–281.

Waldinger MD, Zwinderman AH, and Olivier B (2001a) SSRIs and ejaculation: A double-blind, randomized, fixed-dose study with paroxetine and citalopram. J Clin Psychopharmacol 21, 556–560.

Waldinger MD, Zwinderman AH, and Olivier B (2001b) Antidepressants and ejaculation: A double-blind, randomized, placebo-controlled, fixed-dose study with paroxetine, sertraline and nefazodone. J Clin Psychopharmacol 21, 293–297.

Walker P, Cole JO, Gardner EA, et al. (1993) Improvement in fluoxetine-associated sexual dysfunction in patients switched to bupropion. J Clin Psychiatr 54, 459–465.

Walsh BT (1991) Treatment of bulimia nervosa with antidepressant medication (editorial). J Clin Psychopharmacol 11, 231–232.

Wehr AM and Namerow LB (2001) Citalopram for OCD and Tourette's syndrome. J Am Acad Child Adolesc Psychiatr 40, 740–741.

Wender PH and Reimherr FW (1990) Bupropion treatment of attention-deficit hyperactivity disorder in adults. Am J Psychiatr 147, 1018–1020.

Whale R, Clifford EM, Bhagwagar Z, et al. (2001) Decreased sensitivity of $5-HT_{1D}$ receptors in melancholic depression. Br J Psychiatr 178, 454–457.

WHO Mental Health Collaborating Centers (1989) Pharmacotherapy of depressive disorders: A consensus statement. J Affect Disord 17, 197–198.

Willner P (1990) Animal models of depression: An overview. Pharmacol Ther 45, 425–455.

Wisner KL, Zarin DA, Holmboe ES, et al. (2000) Risk-benefit decision making for treatment of depression during pregnancy. Am J Psychiatr 157, 1933–1940.

Woolfrey S, Gammack NS, Dewar MS, et al. (1993) Fluoxetine–warfarin interaction (letter). BMJ 307, 241.

Work Group on Research of the American Academy of Child and Adolescent Psychiatry (1990) Desipramine (DMI) and sudden death: A report from the Work Group on Research and the Office of Research. AACAP Member Forum at the Annual Meeting of the American Academy of Child and Adolescent Psychiatry, (Oct 23), Washington DC.

Workman EA and Short DD (1993) Atypical antidepressants versus imipramine in the treatment of major depression: A meta-analysis. J Clin Psychiatr 54, 5–12.

Yamashita I and Asano Y (1979) Tricyclic antidepressants: Therapeutic plasma level. Psychopharmacol Bull 15, 40–41.

Yatham LN, Liddle PF, Dennie J, et al. (1999) Decrease in brain serotonin 2 receptor binding in patients with major depression following desipramine treatment: A positron emission tomography study with fluorine-18-labeled setoperone. Arch Gen Psychiatr 56, 705–711.

Yesavage J, Brink T, Rose T, et al. (1983) Development and validation of a geriatric screening scale: A preliminary report. J Psychiatr Res 17, 37–49.

Zametkin AJ, Alter MR, and Yemini T (2001) Suicide in teenagers: Assessment, management, and prevention. JAMA 286, 3120–3125.

Zito JM, Safer DJ, dosReis S, et al. (2000) Trends in the prescribing of psychotropic medications to preschoolers. JAMA 283, 1025–1030.

Zobel AW, Nickel T, Kunzel HE, et al. (2000) Effects of the high-affinity corticotropin-releasing hormone receptor 1 antagonist R121919 in major depression: The first 20 patients treated. J Psychiatr Res 34, 171–181.

# CHAPTER

# 98  Anxiolytic Drugs

Rachel E. Maddux
Mark H. Rapaport

## Introduction

There has been an exponential increase in the number of medications demonstrated to be effective for the treatment of anxiety and anxiety disorders (Table 98–1). This chapter will provide a brief review of the history and evolution of these treatment strategies. This will be followed by descriptions of each medication along with the existing data about the efficacy and adverse effects of anxiolytic agents as well as the presently recommended treatments for anxiety.

Beginning in the late 19th century, there was a progression from alcohol, bromides, and opiates to barbiturates developed in the early 20th century. Barbiturates were effective in decreasing anxiety but they were addictive and lethal in overdose. There was continued advancement in the development of anxiolytics like meprobamate (effective but again addictive and lethal in overdose) and the

antihistamine hydroxyzine, which was less effective than meprobamate and barbiturates and very sedating. The next major advance in anxiolytic therapy was the work pioneered by Klein and Fink (1962) demonstrating that some tricyclic antidepressants (TCAs) were useful in the treatment of panic disorder. This was rapidly followed by studies reporting that monoamine oxidase inhibitors (MAOIs) could be used to treat certain patients with anxiety disorders. However, the major advancement in the field of anxiolytics in the 1960s was the development and approval of benzodiazepines. These agents were much safer than the barbiturates and meprobamate, had a rapid onset of action (so patients felt better quickly), and had a broad spectrum of efficacy extending from situational anxiety to pathological anxiety disorders. Many different benzodiazepines, with different absorption times and half-lives, were developed and have been valuable not only for treating

**Table 98–1  The Efficacy of Psychotropic Medications for the Treatment of Anxiety Disorders**

| | Generalized Anxiety Disorder | Social Anxiety Disorder | Panic Disorder | Posttraumatic Stress Disorder | Obsessive–Compulsive Disorder |
|---|---|---|---|---|---|
| Proven efficacy | SSRIs<br>Venlafaxine<br>Trazodone<br>TCAs<br>Benzodiazepines<br>Buspirone | SSRIs<br>Bupropion<br>MAOIs<br>Benzodiazepines | SSRIs<br>Venlafaxine<br>Mirtazepine<br>MAOIs<br>TCAs<br>Benzodiazepines | SSRIs | SSRIs<br>Clomipramine |
| Some evidence | Nefazodone<br>Mirtazapine | Venlafaxine<br>Nefazodone<br>Gabapentin | Nefazodone<br>Clonazepam + sertraline<br>Buspirone adjunct to benzodiazepine<br>Valproic acid<br>Gabapentin<br>Tiagabine<br>Pagoclone | Venlafaxine<br>Trazodone<br>Nefazodone<br>Mirtazapine<br>MAOIs<br>TCAs | MAOIs<br>Olanzapine augmentation of SSRI<br>Risperidone augmentation of SSRI |
| Not effective | | TCAs<br>Buspirone<br>Pindolol augmentation of SSRI | Trazodone<br>Bupropion | | Trazodone<br>Mirtazapine<br>TCAs<br>Buspirone |
| No data | MAOIs<br>Bupropion | Trazodone<br>Mirtazapine | | | Venlafaxine<br>Nefazodone<br>Bupropion |

anxiety and anxiety disorders but for treating seizure disorders and alcohol withdrawal. Unfortunately, with wide scale usage some individuals did develop craving and dependence on benzodiazepines as well as significant problems with withdrawal when abruptly discontinued. The next major class of agents approved was the azopyrones, of which buspriorone is the most well known. This agent was found to be effective in generalized anxiety disorder but was not effective for the treatment of most other anxiety disorders or situational anxiety.

There was a cascade of anxiolytic research in the 1990s. The selective serotonin reuptake inhibitors (SSRIs) as a class were demonstrated to be efficacious treatments for most of the anxiety disorders described in the *Diagnostics and Statistical Manual of Mental Disorders*, Fourth Edition (DSM-IV-TR). Although these agents have a delayed onset when contrasted with the benzodiazepines, they have a broader spectrum of action, no problems with dependence, and much less of a problem with withdrawal syndromes. The 1990s also saw the approval of venlafaxine as a treatment for generalized anxiety disorder. One of the most intriguing transitions in anxiolytic development has been the ongoing research investigating the use of anticonvulsant medications for the treatment of anxiety disorders. Although there have been few published reports at this time, a variety of companies have very active development programs.

The future is very bright for the development of new anxiolytic medications. These new medications may be entirely new classes of agents such as corticotropin-releasing factor (CRF) antagonists, Neurokinin-1(NK-I) antagonists or other receptor-specific ligands, while others will be isomers of existing agents or modifications of the delivery systems of existing agents that may enhance their potency and decrease their side effect burden.

## A General Approach to Using Medication with Anxious Patients

Patients may present physicians with many different concerns related to anxiety. However, one need that all patients who seek help for symptoms of anxiety have is the need for reassurance that they are not alone, that their physicians truly hear their concerns, and that their physicians will attempt to help them. One important step in building rapport and reassuring a patient is taking a complete history. This is not only essential for making an appropriate diagnostic formulation but demonstrates an interest in the patient's situation.

Making an appropriate differential diagnosis is critical to the success of any psychopharmacological intervention. The diagnosis dictates the class of medication to be used and the length of pharmacotherapy. Potential differential diagnoses for patients with anxiety disorders include: adjustment disorders secondary to life stressors, anxiety disorders secondary to a medical condition, symptoms of anxiety secondary to a medical condition, anxiety secondary to alcohol or substance abuse or dependence, generalized anxiety disorder (GAD), panic disorder (PD), social anxiety disorder, specific phobia, posttraumatic stress disorder (PTSD) and obsessive–compulsive disorder (OCD). Since patients with either symptoms of anxiety or an anxiety disorder are in distress and usually feel vulnerable, sharing the diagnostic formulation with the patient is an

important intervention that facilitates the patient's commitment to the treatment plan. This commitment is crucial since anxious patients may be reticent to take medication. When they do take medications, they commonly ruminate about medication side effects. As discussed in other chapters in this text, patients with anxiety as a symptom or anxiety disorders are more likely to have somatic preoccupations and heightened somatic sensitivity. A collaborative approach where physicians and patients form a "team" to monitor both the potential benefits and the liabilities of any medication intervention frequently enfranchises the patient and enhances adherence. An important rule in general is "to start low and go slow" when initiating pharmacological treatment for patients with anxiety disorders. Interestingly, although treating patients with anxiety disorders frequently requires a more gradual initial titration schedule, patients frequently attain maintenance dosages of antidepressant medications that are greater than the dosage commonly used to treat major depressive disorder.

## Antidepressant Medication

Since the reports by Klein and Fink in the early 1960s, it has been known that medications initially identified because of their antidepressant properties are frequently effective treatments for anxiety disorders as well. The basic action of the majority of the antidepressants is to increase the availability of neurotransmitters in the synaptic cleft. As is demonstrated in Table 98–2, antidepressants work by a variety of mechanisms of action. The most widely used antidepressants that also have anxiolytic properties are the SSRIs. These agents have the broadest spectrum of activity which spans the entire spectrum of DSM-IV-TR anxiety disorders. Although all of the SSRIs have a slightly different site of action, their basic mechanism of action is the inhibition of the serotonin reuptake pump. This facilitates an increase in levels of serotonin throughout the body. Table 98–3 presents the inhibition constants for the SSRIs, some tricyclic antidepressants, and several other antidepressant agents. As illustrated in Table 98–4, a variety of serotonin receptor subtypes have been implicated in the modulation of anxiety disorders, depressive disorders, migraine, pain, and neuro-

| Table 98–2 | The Mechanisms of Action of Common Antidepressant Medication |
|---|---|

Blockade of 5-HT uptake
  Fluoxetine
  Sertraline
  Paroxetine
  Citalopram
  Escitalopram
Blockade of NE uptake
  Desipramine
  Nortriptyline
  Bupropion (and modest dopamine effects)
Blockade of 5-HT and NE uptake
  Clomipramine
  Venlafaxine (at high doses)
5-HT$_2$ antagonism (and modest transient 5-HT uptake blockade)
  Nefazodone
$\alpha_2$ antagonism (releases 5-HT and NE; and 5-HT$_2$ and 5-HT$_3$ antagonism)
  Mirtazapine

| Table 98–3 | The Inhibition Constants (K$_i$s) for Norepinephrine, Serotonin, and Dopamine Reuptake Blockade for Selected Antidepressant Medications | | |
|---|---|---|---|
| | NE | 5-HT | DA |
| Amitriptyline | 13.90 | 84 | 8,600 |
| Desipramine | 0.61 | 180 | 11,000 |
| Fluoxetine | 143 | 14 | 3,050 |
| Sertraline | 220 | 3.4 | 260 |
| Paroxetine | 33 | 0.73 | 1,700 |
| Citalopram | 6,000 | 1.8 | >10,000 |
| Escitalopram | 6,514 | 2.5 | >100,000 |
| Nefazodone | 570 | 137 | 2,380 |
| Venlafaxine | 210 | 39 | 5,300 |

*Source*: Bolden-Watson C and Richelson E (1993) Blockade by newly-developed antidepressants of biogenic amine uptake into rat brain synaptosomes. Life Sci. 52(12), 1023–1029; Hytell (1993).

| Table 98–4 | The Proposed Function of Different 5-HT Receptors |
|---|---|

| | |
|---|---|
| 1A | Anxiety |
| | Depression |
| | Sexual behavior |
| | Appetite |
| | Aggression |
| | Pain |
| | Emesis |
| | ? obsessions |
| | Vasoconstriction |
| 1D | Migraine |
| | Appetite |
| | Depression |
| 2A | Vasoconstriction |
| | Migraine |
| | Anxiety |
| 2B | Depression |
| | Sleep |
| | Hallucination |
| | Suicide |
| 2C | Appetite |
| | Anxiety |
| | Depression |
| | Learning |
| | Psychosis |
| 3 | Emesis |
| | Anxiety |
| | Psychosis |
| | Migraine |
| | Reward |
| 4 | Muscle contraction, gut and heart |
| | Learning |
| | Cognition |
| | Anxiety |
| | Sleep |
| | Emesis |
| 5 | Unknown |
| 6 | OCD? |
| 7 | Circadian rhythms |

*Source*: Dubovsky SL, and Thomas M (1995) Serotonergic mechanisms and current and future psychiatric practice. J Clin Psychiatr 56(2), 38–48.

psychiatric disorders. The stimulation of those receptors also account for the commonly observed side effects of SSRIs (Table 98–5). The pharmacokinetic properties of the SSRIs are presented in Table 98–6.

The mechanism of action of the TCAs again involves the inhibition of reuptake sites thereby increasing the amount of the neurotransmitter present throughout the body and in the synaptic cleft. The disadvantage of the TCAs include their side effect profile and their potential lethality in overdose (Table 98–5). Other antidepressants have a variety of different mechanisms of action. The MAOIs inhibit the enzyme monoamine oxidase, a crucial intracellular enzyme for the catabolism of serotonin, norepinephrine, dopamine, and phenethylamine. The first generation MAOIs irreversibly bind to monoamine oxidase. After cessation of MAOI treatment, it takes approximately 2 weeks for restoration of monoamine oxidase functioning through the generation of new enzyme. The other major mechanisms of action for antidepressants that also have anxiolytic effects include the inhibition of both serotonin and norepinephrine transporter sites, as is seen with venlafaxine and clomipramine. However, venlafaxine does not begin to exhibit this effect until one gets to a minimum of 150 mg per day. Mirtazepine works primarily through antagonism of the presynaptic alpha-2-adrenergic receptors. This increases serotonin, norepinephrine, and possibly dopamine levels in the synapse. The primary mechanism of action of nefazodone is the antagonism of postsynaptic serotonin Type-2 receptors. While the precise mechanism of action of bupropion is not fully appreciated, it is thought to increase norepinephrine levels. The pharmacokinetic properties of the antidepressants are illustrated in Table 98–6. The relative differences in terms of major pharmacokinetic and pharmacodynamic properties are outlined in Table 98–7.

## Selective Serotonin Reuptake Inhibitors

### Generalized Anxiety Disorder (GAD)

Pollack and coworkers (2001) published an 8-week randomized, double-blind, placebo-controlled flexible dosage trial investigating the efficacy of paroxetine in 326 adult outpatients with generalized anxiety disorder. Inclusion criteria both at screen and baseline were a Hamilton Anxiety Rating Scale (HAM-A) total score $\geq 20$ and a score $\geq 2$ on HAM-A items 1 (anxious mood) and 2 (tension). Eligible patients underwent a 1-week, single-blind placebo run-in, and then were randomized to paroxetine or placebo. Patients assigned to paroxetine started treatment at 10 mg/day for the first week and were titrated to 20 mg/day by week 2. After the second week, patients tolerating the medication could have their medication increased every 7 days by 10 mg/day to a maximum 50 mg/day. The primary efficacy measure in this study was the mean change in total HAM-A score from baseline to week 8. Secondary efficacy measures included the change from baseline score in HAM-A item 1 and item 2, changes in scores on the psychic and somatic symptom subscales of the HAM-A, the anxiety subscale score on the patient-rated Hospital Anxiety and Depression Scale (HAD), and the change from baseline scores on the Clinical Global Impression (CGI) Severity Scale. Response to treatment was defined by a score of (1)

| Table 98–5 | Common Reported Side Effects of Antidepressant Medications | | | | | |
|---|---|---|---|---|---|---|
| **SSRI** | **SNRI** | **Mirtazepine** | **Nefazodone** | **Bupropion** | **MAOI** | **TCA** |
| Headache | SSRI side effects | Increased appetite | Sedation | Numbness | Hypertension | Dry mouth |
| Nausea | Dry mouth | Weight gain | Liver failure | Dizziness | Initial anxiety | Blurred vision |
| Decreased motivation | Constipation | Sedation | Fatigue | Spaciness | Weight gain | Constipation |
| Insomnia | Agitation | Fatigue | Ataxia | Seizures (in high doses) | Insomnia | Weight gain |
| Fatigue | Diaphoresis | | Dry mouth | Ataxia | Dry mouth | Fatigue |
| Ejaculatory dysfunction | Increased blood pressure | | Constipation | | Blurred vision | Sedation |
| Anorgasmia | Weight gain? | | | | Ejaculatory dysfunction | Insomnia |
| Decreased libido | | | | | Anorgasmia | Hypersomnia |
| Weight gain? | | | | | Constipation | Ejaculatory dysfunction |
| | | | | | Dizziness | Initial jitteriness/anxiety |

'very much improved' or (2) 'much improved' on the CGI-Global Improvement Scale. Remission was defined by a HAM-A total score of 7 or less. The trial was completed by 78.9% of paroxetine patients and 81.6% of placebo patients. Seventy-four percent of paroxetine patients met criteria for responsive versus 55.6% of placebo-treated patients. Forty-three percent of paroxetine-treated patients met remission criteria compared to 26.3% of placebo-treated patients. The mean daily dose of paroxetine was $26.8 \pm 7.5$ mg/day.

The clinical efficacy and safety of sertraline treatment for children with GAD was reported for a 9-week double-blind, placebo-controlled study by Rynn and coworkers (2001). Twenty-two children and adolescents, ages 5 to 17 years, who met DSM-IV criteria for GAD and had a HAM-A rating $\geq 16$ participated in this study. All patients underwent a 2- to 3-week preevaluation period, followed by a 9-week double-blind treatment phase. Sertraline was initiated at 25 mg/day for the first week then titrated to 50 mg/day for weeks 2 through 9. Primary outcome measures were the HAM-A total score, HAM-A psychic and somatic scores as well as the CGI-Severity and Improvement Scale scores. Secondary assessments included subscales of the Multidimensional Anxiety Scale for Children, the Revised Children's Manifest Anxiety Scale, and the 17-item HAM-D. Mean HAM-A scores for the sertraline group reduced from $20.6 \pm 3.6$ at baseline to $7.8 + 5.7$ at week 9, while those receiving placebo decreased from $23.3 \pm 4.0$ at baseline to $21.0 \pm 7.8$ at week 9. Mean CGI-severity scores significantly improved for the sertraline-treated group (4.0 baseline to 2.4 weeks) while the placebo-treated group remained unchanged (4.0 baseline to 3.9 weeks). Importantly, no statistically significant differences were found in adverse events between the two groups. Only two patients in the placebo-treated group and one patient in the sertraline group dropped out prior to study completion. These data suggest that low doses of sertraline may be effective and well tolerated for children with GAD.

In summary, initial data from randomized, placebo-controlled treatment trials suggest that SSRIs may be useful in the treatment of adults and children.

## Social Anxiety Disorder

SSRIs have emerged as first-line treatment for social anxiety disorder. Most of the efficacy data are derived from multicenter, double-blind trials of paroxetine, sertraline, and fluvoxamine. The first study to demonstrate that an SSRI was efficacious in treating social anxiety disorder was a 12-week trial of 183 patients randomized to either paroxetine (20–50 mg/day) or placebo. Fifty-five percent of patients randomized to paroxetine improved significantly, versus 24% of those randomized to placebo (Stein et al. 1998). These results have been replicated in a second, large multicenter study for social anxiety disorder (Baldwin et al. 1999).

The use of sertraline for the longer-term treatment of social anxiety disorder was investigated in a 2 part study where subjects entered a 20-week double-blind, placebo-controlled study that was followed by a 24-week double-blind extension for first phase treatment responders (van Ameringen et al. 2001). This study was conducted at 10 outpatient clinics in Canada. Two hundred and four adult outpatients with social anxiety disorder were randomly assigned 2:1 to sertraline or placebo. Following a 1-week placebo run-in period, patients received an initial dose of 50 mg/day of sertraline or placebo. After 4 weeks, the dose could be increased 50 mg/day every 3 weeks up to a maximum of 200 mg/day. In the event of intolerable side effects, doses could be reduced to a minimum of 50 mg/day. Primary efficacy measures included the CGI-Improvement Scale, the patient-rated Marks Fear Questionnaire (FQ), and the physician-rated Brief Social Anxiety Disorder Scale. At study endpoint, 53% of sertraline patients compared to 29% of placebo patients were (2) 'much improved' or (1) 'very much improved' as measured by the CGI-Improvement Scale. The mean score on the FQ decreased from 23.07 at baseline to 15.54 at endpoint for the sertraline-treated group, while the placebo-treated group decreased from 21.72 at baseline to 19.38 at endpoint. The mean score on the Brief Social Anxiety Disorder Scale for the sertraline-treated group decreased from 47.48 at baseline to 31.18 at endpoint, versus 45.72 to 37.23 at endpoint for the placebo-treated group. The mean dose of sertraline was 146.7 mg/day.

| **Table 98–6** | **Pharmacokinetic Properties of Psychotropic Medication Used for the Treatment of Anxiety Disorders** |
|---|---|

### SSRIs

|  | Citalopram | Fluoxetine | Fluvoxamine | Paroxetine | Sertraline | Escitalopram |
|---|---|---|---|---|---|---|
| $T_{max}$ h | 2–4 | 6–8 | 3–8 | 5.2 | 4.5–8.4 | 3–5 |
| Dose-proportional plasma level | Yes | No | No | No | Yes | Yes |
| $T_{1/2}$ (h) | 33 | 24–72 | 15.6 | 21 | 26 | 30 |
| Metabolite activity | <10% | Norfluoxetine (equal) | <10% | <2% | Desmethyl-sertraline 6–15% | None |
| Metabolite $T_{1/2}$ | – | 4–16 d | – | – | 62–104 h | 50–60 |
| Steady state plasma level | ~1 wk | 4–5 wk | ~1 wk | 10 d | ~1 wk | 10d |
| Usual daily dosage range | 10–60 mg | 10–80 mg | 100–300 mg | 10–60 mg | 50–200 mg | 10–20 mg |

### Other Antidepressants

|  | Mirtazapine | Nefazodone | Venlafaxine | VenlafaxineXR |
|---|---|---|---|---|
| $T_{max}$ h | 2 | 1 | 2 | 5.5 |
| Dose-proportional plasma level? | Yes | No | Yes | Yes |
| $T_{1/2}$ (h) | 37 (females), 26 (males) | 2–4 | 5±2 | |
| Metabolite activity | Negligible | Hydroxynefazodone | O-desmethyl-venlafaxine | C-desmethyl-venlafaxine |
| Metabolite $T_{1/2}$ (h) | – | 1.5–4 | 11±2 | 11±2 |
| Steady state plasma level | 5 d | 4–5 d | 3 d | 3 d |
| Usual oral dosage | 15–60 mg | 100–800 mg | 45–75 mg | 75–225 mg |

### Antianxiety

|  | Buspirone | Alprazolam | Clonazepam |
|---|---|---|---|
| $T_{max}$ h | 0.6–1.5 | 1–2 | 1–4 |
| Dose-proportional plasma level | No | Yes | Yes |
| $T_{1/2}$ (h) | 2–3 | 6.3–26.9 | 30–40 |
| Metabolite activity | Unimportant | α-hydroxyl-alprazolam 50% | No |
| Steady state plasma level | – | 3–4 d | 1 wk |
| Usual oral dosage | 15–90 mg | 1–10 mg | 1–6 mg |

### Antipsychotics

|  | Olanzapine | Quetiapine | Risperidone | Ziprasidone |
|---|---|---|---|---|
| $T_{max}$ h | 6 | 1.5 | 1 | 6–8 |
| Dose-proportional plasma level | Yes | Yes | Yes | Yes |
| $T_{1/2}$ (h) | 21–54 | 6 | 21–30 | 7 |
| Metabolite activity | No | No | 9-hydroxyrisperidone | Yes |
| Steady state plasma level | 4–6 d | 2 d | 5–6 d | |
| Usual oral dosage | 5–10 mg | 300–400 mg b.i.d. | 2–8 mg | 20–80 mg b.i.d. |

### Anticonvulsants

|  | Gabapentin | Valproic acid |
|---|---|---|
| $T_{max}$ h | | 4–5 |
| Dose-proportional plasma level | No | No |
| $T_{1/2}$ (h) | 5–7 | 9–16 |
| Metabolite activity | No | No |
| Steady state plasma level | 1 d | 7 d |
| Usual oral dosage | 2,400 mg/d | 750–2,500 mg/d |

$T_{1/2}$, terminal half-life

$T_{max}$, time of maximum plasma concentration

| Table 98–7 | A Summary of Pharmacologic Properties of Medications Commonly Used to Treat Anxiety | | | | | | |
|---|---|---|---|---|---|---|---|
| | Mechanism of Action | Onset of Action | Titration | Abuse Liability | Need for Discontinuation Titration | Potential for Withdrawal Syndrome | Probability of Lethality in Overdose |
| Sertraline | SSRI | Delayed (In 2 wk) | Yes | Very low | Yes, but not mandatory | Very low | Low |
| Paroxetine | SSRI | Delayed (In 2 wk) | Yes | Very low | Yes | Moderate | Low |
| Fluvoxamine | SSRI | Delayed (In 2 wk) | Yes | Very low | Yes, but not mandatory | Very low | Low |
| Fluoxetine | SSRI | Delayed (In 2 wk) | Yes | Very low | No | Lowest | Low |
| Citalopram | SSRI | Delayed (In 2 wk) | Yes | Very low | Yes, but not mandatory | Very low | Low |
| Escitalipram | SSRI | Delayed (In 2 wk) | Sometimes | Very low | Yes, probably not mandatory | Very low | Low |
| Venlafaxine | SNRI | Delayed (In 2 wk) | Yes | Very low | Yes | Moderate | Low |
| Mirtazepine | $\alpha_2$-antagonist | Delayed | Yes | Very low | Yes | Moderate | Low |
| Nefazidone | $5HT_2$ blockade | Delayed | Yes | Very low | Yes | Moderate | Low |
| Bupropion | Norepineprine? | Delayed | Yes | Very low | Yes | Low | Low |
| TCAS | Reuptake blockade | Delayed (2 wk) | Yes | Very low | Yes | Moderate | Moderate–high |
| MAOIs | Monoamine inhibition | Delayed (2 wk) | Yes | Very low | Yes | Moderate | Moderate–high |
| Buspirone | $5HT_{1A}$ partial agonist | Delayed (2 wk) | Yes | Very low | Yes | Low–moderate | Low |
| Clonazapam | Modulates $GABA_A$ receptor | Rapid | Yes | Moderate | Yes | Moderate–high | Low |
| Alprazolam | Modulates $GABA_A$ receptor | Very rapid | Yes | Moderate | Yes | High | Low |
| Alprazolam XR | Modulates $GABA_A$ receptor | Rapid | Yes | Moderate | Yes | Moderate–high | Low |
| Lorazepam | Modulates $GABA_A$ receptor | Very rapid | Yes | Moderate | Yes | Moderate–high | Low |
| Diazepam | Modulates $GABA_A$ receptor | Rapid | Yes | Moderate | Yes | Moderate | Low |
| β-blockers | Blocks β-adrenergic receptors | Rapid | Sometimes | Low | No (acute use) | No (acute use) | Low–medium |
| Gabapentin | Not fully known but GABAergic | Moderate (d) | Yes | Low | Yes | Low–moderate | Low |
| Risperidone | 5-HT$_2$ and D$_2$ blockade | Rapid | Probably | Low | Yes | Low | Low |
| Olanzapine | 5-HT$_2$ and D$_2$ blockade | Rapid | Probably | Low | Yes | Low | Low |

Fifty sertraline responders and 15 placebo responders entered the double-blind, placebo-controlled relapse prevention phase of the study. Patients who were randomly assigned to continue sertraline treatment received a mean daily dose of 148.0 mg/day. Eighty-eight percent of sertraline-treated patients, 40% of placebo-switched patients, and 40% of the initial placebo-responder patients completed the study. Four percent of the subjects who received sertraline maintenance relapsed as compared to 36% of the placebo-switch group. These findings agree with work by Katzenick and coworkers (1995) and a general practice trial by Blomhoff and coworkers (2001).

In a study of fluvoxamine treatment of 82 patients with social anxiety disorder, 42% of patients randomized to fluvoxamine responded to treatment (mean dose 202 mg/day) as compared to 24% of patients who received placebo (Stein et al. 1999). There are also smaller trials demonstrating that other SSRIs including fluoxetine and citalopram also seem to be effective in the treatment of social anxiety disorder (Bouwer and Stein 1998, Van Ameringen et al. 1993). (For more on social anxiety, please see Chapter 67.)

## Panic Disorder (PD)

SSRIs are generally accepted as a first line treatment for panic disorder. The major advantage of these agents is their tolerability and thus longer-term acceptance by patients. As of now there is evidence that fluoxetine, sertraline, paroxetine, fluvoxamine, and citalopram are effective in the acute treatment of panic disorder.

There have been several open-label studies suggesting that fluoxetine is an effective treatment of panic disorder (Gorman et al. 1987, Schneier et al. 1990). However, there are only two published large multicenter double-blind, placebo-controlled study investigating the efficacy of fluoxetine versus placebo. Michelson and coworkers (1998) conducted a large multicenter double-blind, placebo-controlled trial investigating the efficacy of 10 or 20 mg/day fluoxetine versus placebo. Results suggested that fluoxetine reduced panic attack frequency, global distress, and agoraphobic distress. Patients with a CGI-Improvement score of (1) 'very much improved' or (2) 'much improved' at the end of the randomized, placebo-controlled trial were entered into a 24-week continuation study (Michelson et al. 1998). During this study patients either continued on active treatment or received placebo. Patients randomized to fluoxetine continued to improve during the course of 24 weeks while patients who were randomized to placebo demonstrated a marked exacerbation in symptoms and were more likely to meet criteria for a recurrence of panic disorder (Michelson et al. 1999). A more recent study by Michelson and co-workers (2001) was a 12-week randomized, placebo-controlled trial of fluoxetine (10–60 mg/day) conducted at nine sites in Europe. One hundred and eighty adult patients who met DSM-IV criteria for panic disorder and had a minimum of four full panic attacks in the month preceding entry into the study, and two full panic attacks during the 2-week baseline evaluation period were randomized to treatment. Patients also had to have at least moderate symptom severity, as measured with the Panic Disorder Severity Scale, and a CGI-Severity rating of 4 or greater. Fluoxetine was initiated at 10 mg/day for week 1 and increased to 20 mg/day until week 6. Patients who had not achieved a CGI-Severity score of 2 or less were, at week 6, increased to 40 mg/day. Fluoxetine could be further increased to 60 mg/day. Fluoxetine was statistically superior to placebo at both the 6-week point and at study endpoint. Fluoxetine-treated patients also had statistically significant improvement on the Sheehan Disability Scale (SDS). The final mean daily dose of fluoxetine was only 29.6 mg/day. Reports of adverse events among the placebo and fluoxetine groups were similar and low.

Four large multicenter trials investigating the efficacy of sertraline in the treatment of panic disorder have been published. Two studies were placebo-controlled, fixed-dose trials and two studies were placebo-controlled, flexible-dose studies. In the flexible-dose sertraline trials, patients were started on 25 mg/day for the first week and then the dose was escalated to 50 mg/day of sertraline. Sertraline-treated patients experienced significant reductions in panic attack frequency, CGI-Improvement and Severity Scales, the

Panic Disorder Severity Scale (PDSS), the Patient Global Evaluation (PGE) Rating Scale and the Quality of Life Enjoyment and Satisfaction Questionnaire (Q-LES-Q) (Londborg et al. 1998, Pollack et al. 1998, Rapaport et al. 1998). Sertraline was also found to be efficacious in fixed dose with the 150 mg/day dose seeming to be the most effective dose in these studies (Dubuff et al. 1995). There is one large multicenter long-term trial by Rapaport and coworkers (2001) where individuals who initially entered 10-week treatment trials were then offered 1 year of open-label treatment of sertraline and responders were then entered into a double-blind, 26-week placebo-discontinuation trial. Frequency of panic attacks was recorded by patients in panic attack diaries. Clinician-rated assessments included the HAM-A, PDSS, and CGI-Severity and Improvement Scales. Patient-rated assessments included the PGE and the Q-LES-Q. Clinically significant deterioration was examined over the course of the double-blind phase; deterioration was specified as (1) relapse, (2) discontinuation due to insufficient clinical response, and (3) exacerbation of panic symptomology. At the end of 26 weeks of double-blind treatment, patients randomized to placebo were twice as likely to discontinue due to lack of efficacy than patients treated with sertraline. Similarly, 13% of sertraline patients experienced acute exacerbation of panic symptoms versus 30% of placebo patients. These data demonstrated that maintenance treatment with sertraline was associated with continued improvement and protected patients from recurrence (Rapaport et al. 2001). The mean daily dose of sertraline was 112.1 mg/day.

There have been a number of double-blind, placebo-controlled multicenter studies demonstrating the efficacy of paroxetine for the treatment of panic disorder. Ballenger and coworkers (1998) reported that 40 mg/day of paroxetine was more effective than placebo in reducing panic attacks and the symptoms of panic disorder. In one large multicenter European trial, paroxetine (20–60 mg/day) was contrasted with clomipramine (50–150 mg/day) and placebo. Both active treatments were more effective than placebo in reducing the number of panic attacks. The paroxetine group also seemed to have a more rapid onset of action and reported fewer side effects (Lecrubier et al. 1997). Patients who completed the study were entered into a 9-month extension study; subjects treated with paroxetine and clomipramine demonstrated continued improvement over time (Lecrubier and Judge 1997). A head-to-head comparison trial of paroxetine and citalopram was conducted by Perna and coworkers (2001). Fifty-eight patients with panic disorder were randomly assigned to one of the two active treatments (both 10–50 mg/day) in a single-blind design. Patients were assessed by the Panic Associated Symptoms Scale (PASS), the SDS, and the FQ at baseline, day 7, and day 60. Responders were defined by a reduction of at least 50% from baseline on both PASS and SDS global scores at day 60. At endpoint, 84% of patients receiving paroxetine and 86% of patients receiving citalopram responded. PASS total scores decreased from $9.3 \pm 4.9$ at baseline to $3.5 \pm 4.6$ at day 60 for the paroxetine-treated group, and from $8.7 \pm 3.7$ at baseline to $3.1 \pm 3.0$ at day 60 for the citalopram group. Only one patient from each group dropped out because of side effects.

Several smaller placebo-controlled trials and one large multicenter placebo-controlled acute trial has been published demonstrating that citalopram is an effective treatment of panic disorder. In the large multicenter study of citalopram, placebo, and clomipramine, 475 patients were randomized to 8 weeks of treatment. The patients received three flexible doses of citalopram and one of clomipramine. All three doses of citalopram (10–60 mg/day) and clomipramine (60–90 mg/day) were more effective than placebo in decreasing panic attacks to zero and decreasing phobic symptoms. The 20–30 mg/day dose of citalopram seems to be the most effective of the doses (Wade et al. 1997). Patients, who in the physician's judgment were responders in the acute trial, were offered continued double-blind treatment for 10 months. In this double-blind continuation study, citalopram was demonstrated to be more effective than placebo in decreasing phobic avoidance and interpersonal sensitivity (Leinonen et al. 1999).

A number of studies report that fluvoxamine is more effective than placebo for the treatment of panic disorder (Boshuisen et al. 2001, Hoehn-Saric et al. 1993). Asnis and coworkers (2001) performed an 8-week double-blind, parallel-group study comparing fluvoxamine with placebo in 188 patients with DSM-III-R defined panic disorder (with or without agoraphobia). Patients in this study were required to have at least one panic attack per week for at least 4 weeks. Patients were randomized to double-blind treatment if they had an average weekly panic attack severity score of 25 (of attacks × severity 0–10) and had at least one full panic attack in the final week of placebo washout. Treatment was initiated at 50 mg/day of fluvoxamine or placebo. It was titrated upwards to 150 mg/day during the first 2 weeks. Thereafter, it was titrated to 300 mg/day as needed, based on side effects and efficacy. Fluvoxamine was significantly superior to placebo at endpoint on three of four primary outcome measures: proportion of patients free from full panic attacks, percentage reduction in frequency of full panic attacks per week, and panic disorder severity. Fluvoxamine was superior to placebo with respect to a global improvement in CGI-Serverity Scale scores, 64% versus 42%. Small head-to-head comparative studies have also shown that fluvoxamine is more effective than maprotiline (a selective noradrenergic compound) but equally effective as clomipramine (den Boer and Westenberg 1988, den Boer et al. 1987).

In summary, the majority of data suggests that SSRIs as a class are effective in the treatment of panic disorder. One of the advantages of SSRIs is that they tend to be fairly well tolerated in contrast to some of the other treatments available for panic disorder. Although a few individuals may have some initial problems with restlessness and increased anxiety, data suggest that starting at lower doses such as 25 mg/day of sertraline or 10 mg/day of paroxetine may decrease the risk of antidepressant "jitteriness." Patients will certainly experience other types of side effects such as headaches, nausea, and diarrhea. However, most of these side effects diminish with time and are well tolerated, particularly if the patients are informed of the possibility of these transient side effects. As is the case with our pharmacotherapies for other types of medical disorders, there will certainly be a need to fine-tune a treatment of panic disorder as one sees patients over time.

## Posttraumatic Stress Disorder (PTSD)

There have been open-label and double-blind, placebo-controlled studies demonstrating that SSRIs are effective for the treatment of posttraumatic stress disorder (PTSD). Open-label trials with all of the SSRIs currently available suggest that each may be effective in decreasing the core symptoms of PTSD. Three of the SSRIs have been studied in a double-blind, placebo-controlled fashion. Fluoxetine was the first of the SSRIs to be studied in randomized controlled trials. In two small studies, civilian patients treated with fluoxetine demonstrated significant improvement as compared with placebo treatment. In one of these trials, van der Kolk and coworkers (1994) included a veteran cohort as well; fluoxetine did decrease symptoms of PTSD in the veteran subgroup.

Two SSRIs have been approved by the (FDA) for the treatment of PTSD. The first agent approved for the treatment of PTSD was sertraline. There have been two published large placebo-controlled acute treatment trials of sertraline for noncombat related PTSD. In these studies, Davidson and coworkers (2001) and Brady and coworkers (2000) found that sertraline was more effective than placebo treatment in decreasing the Clinician Administered Posttraumatic Stress Disorder Scale 2 (CAPS-2), the patient-rated Impacts of Events Scale, and the CGI-Severity and Improvement Rating Scales. These were flexible-dose studies where 50 to 200 mg/day of sertraline was administered. Londborg and coworkers (2001) published open-label continuation data for individuals who had participated in these acute trials (Davidson et al. 2001). They demonstrated that patients who responded during the acute phase not only maintained their response but continued to improve with 6 months of continuation treatment. Fifty-four percent of individuals who did not acutely respond to SSRI treatment during the initial 12-week trial had a significant decrease in their CAPS-2 scale scores by the end of 6 months of open-label treatment. In a recent publication, Davidson and coworkers (2001) reported the results of the placebo-discontinuation phase of this study. Individuals who were responders to 6 months of open-label therapy were rerandomized to receive double-blind treatment with sertraline or placebo. Placebo-discontinuation was associated with a significant risk of relapse (26% versus 5%) and reemergence of the core symptoms of PTSD. This suggests that some patients with PTSD will require sustained SSRI treatment, possibly for years, in order to protect them from exacerbation of their symptoms of PTSD.

Paroxetine was recently approved as an acute treatment for PTSD by the FDA. There has been one fixed-dose study demonstrating that both 20 and 40 mg/day of paroxetine were more effective than placebo for the treatment of PTSD (Marshall et al. 2001). In this study, patients treated with paroxetine had significantly greater improvement in the CAPS-2 and were more likely to have CGI-Improvement Scale scores of (2) "much improved" or (1) "very much improved." In the 12-week flexible-dose study, 20 to 50 mg of paroxetine treatment was more effective than placebo treatment in "decreasing" the CAPS-2 scale, the Davidson Trauma Scale, and the SDS (Tucker et al. 2000).

In conclusion, data from open-label studies and double-blind, placebo-controlled studies suggest that SSRIs as a class are effective in the treatment of PTSD.

## Obsessive–Compulsive Disorder (OCD)

Large, well-designed, double-blind, placebo-controlled trials demonstrate that fluoxetine, paroxetine, fluvoxamine, citalopram, and sertraline are effective acute treatments for obsessive–compulsive disorders (Carpenter et al. 1996, Cartwright and Hollander 1998, Greist and Jefferson 1998, Koponen et al. 1997, Mundo et al. 1997, Thomsen 1997, Todorov et al. 2000).

There have been two large 12-week parallel group double-blind, placebo-controlled multicenter trials of fluoxetine in fixed doses of 20, 40, and 60 mg/day versus placebo (Tollefson et al. 1994a, 1994b). Response was defined as a decrease of 35% or greater on the Yale-Brown Obsessive–Compulsive Scale (Y-BOC). The three fluoxetine doses each had response rates of 33%. There was some suggestion that the 40 and 60 mg/day doses acted more rapidly and facilitated greater improvement in Y-BOC scores. Montgomery and coworkers (1993) previously reported that 40 and 60 mg/day of fluoxetine, but not 20 mg/day, was more effective than placebo.

Although there are data available from a number of placebo-controlled multicenter trials contrasting paroxetine with placebo, only one 12-week fixed-dose trial (20, 40, and 60 mg/day) has been published (Ballenger et al. 1998). In this study, all patients were initially started at 20 mg/day, and the 40 and 60 mg/day groups were titrated to these doses by the end of week 2. The 40 and 60 mg/day groups demonstrated statistically significant decreases on the Y-BOC Scale and the CGI-Severity Scale. The greatest improvement seemed to present in the 60 mg/day group.

There have been several smaller trials and one large 10-week double-blind, placebo-controlled multicenter trial of fluvoxamine (100–300 mg/day) versus placebo in the treatment of obsessive–compulsive disorder (Goodman et al. 1989, Greist et al. 1995c, Jenike et al. 1990, Perse et al. 1987). In the large study, Greist and coworkers (1995c) reported that 40% of fluvoxamine-treated patients were responders on the CGI-Improvement Scale as compared to 15% of placebo-treated patients. The fluvoxamine-treated patients also had a significantly greater decrease in the mean Y-BOC scores (Greist et al. 1995c).

There have not been any double-blind, placebo-controlled trials of citalopram published in the literature. There are data from single-blind comparator trials of citalopram versus paroxetine and fluvoxamine that suggest there is no significant difference in Y-BOC scores between these medications (Mundo et al. 1997). One open-label study by Marazziti and coworkers (2001) investigated the effect of citalopram in patients with treatment refractory OCD. Eighteen patients who had previously been treated with an SSRI for at least 6 months but failed to improve were titrated up to 40 mg/day of citalopram within 2 weeks. After 4 months, the Y-BOC scores decreased from 29.7 at baseline to 15.1 at endpoint. The only side effect was mild nausea that resolved after the first few days of treatment. These data are consistent with other open-label studies with adults and children suggesting that citalopram may decrease symptoms of OCD (Koponen et al. 1997, Thomsen 1997).

In one large 12-week double-blind, placebo-controlled multicenter fixed-dose study of sertraline (50, 100, and 200 mg/day), all three doses of sertraline caused a significant reduction in Y-BOC scores (Greist et al. 1995a). The higher doses did show selectively greater improvement on all measures but this did not reach statistical significance. There are two other double-blind, placebo-controlled multicenter flexible-dose trials of sertraline versus placebo in the treatment of OCD (Chouinard et al. 1990, Kronig et al. 1999). In both of these trials, sertraline was more efficacious than placebo on standard outcome measures. Greist and coworkers (1995a) also demonstrated the ability of sertraline to maintain improvement after 12 weeks of double-blind, placebo-controlled treatment during an additional 40-week double-blind fixed-dose trial of sertraline (50, 100, and 200 mg/day) (Greist et al. 1995b). At the 52-week endpoint, mean scores for all four outcome measures, Y-BOC, the NIMH Global Obsessive–Compulsive Scale, and CGI-Severity and Improvement Scales, revealed significantly greater improvement for the sertraline group versus the placebo group (Noyes Jr et al. 1997). Fifty-one of the patients who participated the double-blind, placebo-controlled trial of sertraline entered into a 2-year sertraline open-label study. Outcome data suggested that efficacy was not only maintained, but improvement continued; first year mean Y-BOC scores were 11.4 compared to second year mean Y-BOC scores, 3.2.

Koran and coworkers (2002) performed a relapse-prevention study where patients who had achieved a sustained response during a 52-week single-blind treatment phase were randomized to an additional 28 weeks of double-blind treatment with either sertraline or placebo. This 80-week study was conducted at 21 sites in the US. Following a 1-week washout, 649 patients entered 16 weeks of single-blind treatment with flexible doses of sertraline. Patients were titrated up on a 50 mg incremental schedule to a maximum 200 mg/day depending on response and tolerability. Patients who failed to meet response criteria by the end of week 16 were withdrawn from the study. Response was defined as a decrease of 25% from baseline on the Y-BOC, and a CGI-Improvement Scale score ≤ 3. Those who met responder criteria continued to receive single-blind sertraline treatment for an additional 36 weeks. Data from the single-blind trial revealed consistent improvement throughout the 52 weeks of treatment. Mean Y-BOC scores decreased from 26.1 at baseline to 15.9 at the end of week 16 to 10.3 at the end of week 52. Symptomatic improvement was associated with improvement in quality of life as measured by Q-LES-Q scores from 60% at baseline to 73.7% at the end of week 16 to 78.2% at the end of week 52. (The mean Q-LES-Q score for a population of normal subjects is 80%.) At the end of week 52, patients who continued to meet responder criteria were randomized to the 28-week double-blind discontinuation trial. Those patients randomly assigned to sertraline treatment were continued on the same daily dose as at week 52. Patients assigned to placebo had their dose decreased by 50 mg/day every 3 days until they were taking only placebo tablets.

Continued sertraline treatment was associated with sustained improvement during the 28-week relapse-prevention phase. Sertraline treatment was also significantly more effective than placebo in decreasing study discontinuation due to relapse or insufficient clinical response, and acute exacerbation of obsessive–compulsive symptoms. One-third of patients experienced acute relapse which is striking when compared to earlier discontinuation studies which show relapse rates of 90 percent or greater as measured by the Y-BOC.

Another recent study evaluated the efficacy of long-term sertraline treatment of children and adolescents, ages 6 to 18 years old with OCD (Cook et al. 2001). One hundred and thirty-seven patients were assigned to 12 weeks of double-blind, placebo-controlled treatment with subsequent open-label sertraline treatment (50–200 mg/day) for 52 weeks. At study endpoint, the mean daily sertraline dose was 108 mg/day for children (6–12 years), and 132 mg/day for adolescents (13–18 years). Outcome measures included the Children's Yale-Brown Obsessive–Complusive Scale (CY-BOC), the NIMH Obsessive–Compulsive Scale, and the CGI-Severity and Improvement Scales. Mean CY-BOC scores changed from 22.8 at study entry to 17.0 at the completion of the double-blind phase to 10.8 at the 52-week endpoint. The mean CGI-Severity scores declined from 4.6 to 3.7 to 2.7, respectively. Only 12% of patients discontinued because of side effects.

These data suggest that SSRIs are a first line pharmacotherapy for both acute and maintenance treatment of OCD in children and adults (Greist and Jefferson 1998, March and Frances 1997). Discontinuing SSRI treatment is associated with an exacerbation of symptoms and worsening in quality of life. (For more on OCD, please see the Chapter 68.)

## Serotonin–Norepinephrine Reuptake Inhibitors

### Venlafaxine

#### Generalized Anxiety Disorder (GAD)

There have been six placebo-controlled multicentered studies demonstrating that venlafaxine XR is an effective treatment of GAD. However, currently there have been only three published reports. The first study by Davidson and coworkers (1999) was an 8-week placebo-controlled trial of 75 and 150 mg/day of venlafaxine XR contrasted with 30 mg/day of buspirone. Venlafaxine XR reduced HAM-A scores significantly more than either placebo or 30 mg/day of buspirone. In the second trial, patients with GAD were randomized to three doses of venlafaxine XR, 75, 150, or 225 mg/day. All three doses were more effective in decreasing HAM-A scores than placebo (Rickels et al. 2000b). Preliminary results from a 6-month fixed-dose study of venlafaxine XR (37.5, 75 or 150 mg/day) versus placebo suggests that patients treated with venlafaxine did significantly better than patients treated with placebo. Secondary analysis from this study suggest that the two higher doses of venlafaxine also were associated with significant improvement in social functioning (Haskins et al. 1999). Most recently, Gelenberg and coworkers (2000) compared the 6-month efficacy and safety of a flexible dosage of venlafaxine XR in adult outpatients with GAD. Two hundred and fifty-one adults who met DSM-IV criteria for GAD without comorbid major depressive disorder met the following criteria: (1) a screen and baseline score of at least an 18 on the HAM-A, (2) at least 2 on items 1 and 2 of the HAM-A, (3) a total score of at least 9 on the Raskin Depression Scale at screen and baseline, and (4) a Covi Anxiety Scale score greater than the total score on the Raskin. Patients were started on venlafaxine XR at 75 mg/day or placebo during week 1. After day 8, the dose could be increased to 150 mg/day of venlafaxine XR or placebo. At day 15, increases were again allowed to the maximum 225 mg/day or placebo. Primary efficacy measures included the HAM-A total score, the HAM-A psychic anxiety factor score, and the CGI-Severity and Global Improvement Scale scores. Response to treatment in this study was defined as a 40% decrease from baseline on HAM-A total score or a CGI-Global Improvement Scale score of (1) 'very much improved' or (2) 'much improved.' By week 2, 42% of patients in the venlafaxine XR group were categorized as responders compared to 21% of placebo patients. During weeks 6 through 28, response rates were 69% for venlafaxine XR and 42 to 46% for placebo. Adverse events lead to treatment discontinuation for 17% of the placebo-treated subjects and 26% venlafaxine-treated subjects.

Currently we know that doses as low as 37.5 mg/day and as high as 225 mg/day are effective in decreasing symptoms of anxiety for patients with GAD. Side effects appeared to be mild and tended to decrease in number and intensity over the course of the studies. Nausea, dry mouth, and somnolence were the most commonly repeated side effects.

#### Social Anxiety Disorder

Case reports and open-label studies have been published (Kelsey 1995). Results from placebo-controlled acute and maintenance studies of social anxiety disorder will be published in the near future.

#### Panic Disorder (PD)

There is one double-blind, placebo-controlled study by Pollack and coworkers. (1996) suggesting that venlafaxine may be an effective treatment for patients with panic disorder.

#### Posttraumatic Stress Disorder (PTSD)

Placebo-controlled studies in PTSD are currently ongoing.

## Tricyclic Antidepressant Medication and Monoamine Oxidase Inhibitors

### Generalized Anxiety Disorder

A variety of tricyclic antidepressants (TCAs) have been demonstrated to be effective treatments for GAD (Hoehn-Saric et al. 1993, Liebowitz et al. 1988). However, the side effects and difficulty titrating the dosage of these medications have made their use uncommon. There is one active comparative trial of paroxetine versus imipramine and chlordesmethyldiazepan in the treatment of GAD (Rocca et al. 1997). Many patients discontinued the imipramine-treatment group because of side effects.

### Social Anxiety Disorder

In general, TCAs have not been found to be effective for the treatment of social anxiety disorder. A recent open study of nine patients diagnosed with social anxiety disorder found no difference between imipramine and placebo. However, six patients dropped out early because of side effects (Simpson et al. 1998a).

Monoamine oxidase inhibitors (MAOIs) have been shown to be superior to placebo treatment for social anxiety disorder (Gelernter et al. 1991, Versiani et al. 1992). The mean daily dose of the drug in these trials ranged between 60 to 90 mg/day. Although surpassed by the SSRIs as first line agents, there is no doubt that first generation MAOIs are effective. Unfortunately, the risk of hypertensive crisis and the need for patients to follow a tyramine-free diet makes this class of drugs unappealing for the majority of patients. Selegiline (L-Deprenyl) is of clinical interest because at low doses it is selective for MAO-B and has fewer side effects. Simpson and coworkers (1998b) conducted a 6-week open trial of selegiline in 16 patients with social anxiety disorder. The dose of selegiline was fixed at 5 mg twice-a-day, and patients were instructed to follow a standard MAOI diet. The CGI, the Leibowitz Social Anxiety Scale (LSAS), the Liebowitz Social Phobic Disorders Scale-Overall severity (LSPD), and the Hamilton Depression Rating Scale (HAM-D) were performed at baseline, 3 weeks, and 6 weeks. Responders were defined by a score of 1 or 2 on the CGI at the last observation. Nine subjects completed the trial; 3 were considered responders. Of completers, mean Liebowitz Social Anxiety Scale (LSAS) scores decreased from $85.9 \pm 25.4$ at baseline to $58.0 \pm 25.4$ at endpoint, and mean LSPD scores decreased from $5.0 \pm 0.9$ at baseline to $4.4 \pm 1.2$ at endpoint. These data suggest that low dose selegiline may have a modest effect in social anxiety disorder.

The promising results derived from efficacy studies of first generation MAOIs spawned the study of reversible monoamine oxidase inhibitors (RIMAs) for this indication. RIMAs have significantly less risk of hypertensive crisis and subsequently no need for a tyramine restricted diet. They also have a more tolerable side effect profile. Brofaromine and moclobemide are the two most studied RIMAs. However, there is conflicting evidence about their efficacy for the treatment of social anxiety disorder. Of four published placebo-controlled multicenter moclobemide studies, only two were positive (International Multicenter Clinical Trial Group 1997, Blanco and Liebowitz 1998, Noyes et al. 1997, Schneier et al. 1998). Two controlled studies of brofaromine in social anxiety disorder showed superior efficacy to placebo (Fahlen et al. 1995, van Vliet et al. 1993). However, brofaromine is no longer under development in the US, and moclobemide is not available in the US.

## Panic Disorder (PD)

Imipramine was the first TCA noted to effectively treat panic attacks and panic disorder and is one of the best studied TCAs (Boyer 1995, Klein 1964, Klein and Fink 1962). Double-blind, placebo-controlled trials of desipramine and nortryptiline have also been performed (Kalus et al. 1991, Lydiard et al. 1993, Munjack et al. 1988), however, clomipramine has been the TCA most widely studied. There are a large number of double-blind, placebo-controlled trials demonstrating clomipramine's efficacy as a treatment for panic disorder (Calliard et al. 1999, den Boer 1998). Interestingly, there are a number of both placebo-controlled and crossover design studies suggesting that clomipramine may be more efficacious than imipramine in the treatment of

panic disorder (Cassano et al. 1988, Modigh et al. 1992, Sasson et al. 1999). In contrast to these data demonstrating clomipramine's efficacy, studies with maprotiline, a noradrenergic reuptake inhibitor, failed to differentiate from placebo (den Boer and Westenberg 1988). Longitudinal data suggest that patients who achieve complete remission with imipramine treatment will maintain their remission with continuous treatment (Mavissakalian and Perel 1992b). Mavissakalian and Perel (1992a) demonstrated that patients who met stringent remission criteria for at least 6 months could sustain their panic-free status even after their imipramine dosage was decreased by 50%. This finding is particularly important because such a dosage reduction might increase tolerability and thus the adherence of patients to therapy. Longer-term adherence is important because Mavissakalian and Perel (2001) found that the longer periods of panic-free maintenance therapy were associated with a greater likelihood of remaining in remission after discontinuation of imipramine therapy. Eighteen patients participated in the second year of a double-blind extension study, 7 patients in the placebo group continued on placebo, 7 of the imipramine group were switched to placebo, and 4 continued with imipramine. Two patients from the imipramine–placebo switch group relapsed and two patients in the placebo-continuation group relapsed. None of the imipramine continuation group subjects relapsed. This suggests there may actually be an advantage of continued prophylaxis beyond the first year of maintenance imipramine therapy.

TCAs, unfortunately, are associated with a significant side effect burden. There is a problem with jitteriness associated with the initiation of TCAs. This jitteriness is frequently frightening and may be intolerable for some patients with panic disorder. It requires that TCAs be started at very low doses and titrated up very slowly. Other problems with TCAs that decrease adherence include anticholinergic side effects, orthostatic hypotension, sexual dysfunction, and weight gain. In a naturalistic follow-up study by Noyes and coworkers (1989), the majority of patients discontinued TCA treatment because of side effects (Noyes Jr et al. 1996). Although TCAs have been widely used for the treatment of panic disorder, their side effect profile and slow time to onset of action makes them a difficult class of medication for many patients to tolerate.

The first generation MAOIs such as phenylzine and tranylcypromine have been demonstrated to be effective in placebo-controlled trials (Sheehan et al. 1980). There are also a variety of smaller studies demonstrating that RIMAs, moclobemide, and brofaromine are effective in the treatment of panic disorder (Bakish 1992, Kruger and Dahl 1999, Tiller et al. 1999, van Vliet et al. 1993). Unfortunately, it is unlikely that either of the newer reversible and selective MAOIs will be available in the US. Therefore our pharmacotherapy is limited to the older irreversible and nonselective agents.

The irreversible and nonselective agents have problems with dietary restrictions, weight gain, insomnia, sexual dysfunction, medication interactions, and orthostasis. They can be lethal in overdose and hypertensive crises can be precipitated by tyramine-rich food and by some commonly sold over-the-counter cold medicines. Despite these concerns, many expert clinicians feel that MAOIs may be useful treatment for severely ill patients with panic disorder, particularly those with comorbid panic disorder and depressive disorder.

## Posttraumatic Stress Disorder (PTSD)

There are several small double-blind, placebo-controlled trials suggesting that both amitriptyline and imipramine are more effective than placebo in decreasing signs and symptoms of PTSD. However, after the advent of SSRIs that have significant safety and tolerability advantages, studies with TCAs were not pursued (Davidson et al. 1990, Kosten et al. 1991).

There is little literature suggesting that MAOIs are more effective than placebo in the treatment of PTSD. The two best studied MAOIs are the irreversible nonselective MAOI phenelzine and the reversible selective MAOI, brofaromine. Placebo-controlled studies by Kosten and coworkers (1991) and Davidson and coworkers (1987) suggest that phenelzine is more effective than placebo in decreasing symptoms of PTSD. Their findings have been supported by work by Lerer and coworkers (1987) in Israel who demonstrated that phenelzine was a beneficial treatment for veterans with PTSD. As summarized by Stein and coworkers (2000), there have been several studies investigating the efficacy of brofaromine in the treatment of PTSD. The international studies with brofaromine demonstrated that it was more effective than placebo, while the initial work performed in the US differentiated brofaromine from placebo treatment. Although failed studies are not uncommon, unfortunately this led to a discontinuation of the research program with brofaromine in the US.

## Obsessive–Compulsive Disorder (OCD)

There have been seven meta-analyses comparing and contrasting clomipramine and SSRIs (Abramowitz 1997, Cox et al. 1993, Greist 1998, Kobak et al. 1998, Piccinelli et al. 1995, Stein et al. 1995). In each case, clomipramine has been found to be significantly more effective than the SSRIs. There has been some concern that this conclusion may be biased because many of the clomipramine studies were performed in patients who had not been previously treated with an effective pharmacotherapy while patients in the later studies of the SSRIs had failed treatment with clomipramine or other agents. There also is concern that differences in study design might bias these results in favor of clomipramine (Greist 1998). There have been double-blind comparison studies of clomipramine against fluoxetine, fluvoxamine, sertraline, and paroxetine (Bisserbe et al. 1997, Freeman et al. 1994, Koran et al. 1996, Lopez-Ibor Jr et al. 1996, Milanfranchi et al. 1997, Zohar and Judge 1996). None of these studies had the power to differentiate clomipramine from the SSRI in question. Therefore, findings of no difference between the two groups is not surprising. However, if one takes the entire body of evidence as a whole into account, analyses suggest that clomipramine is at least as effective as the SSRIs and may, in some instances, be more effective (Greist 1998, Todorov et al. 2000).

Although there have been several studies with MAOIs, the results of these studies have been equivocal at best (Jenike et al. 1990, Vallejo et al. 1992). The two other strategies for enhancing serotonergic neurotransmission have involved manipulating the ratio of clomipramine to its metabolite desmethylclomipramine. One strategy has involved the use of intravenous clomipramine in order to decrease first-pass hepatic metabolism and thus increase the ratio of clomipramine metabolite desmethylclomipramine. These studies found that intravenous clomipramine reduces symptoms of OCD more rapidly than oral clomipramine (Koran et al. 1994, 1997, Warneke 1984, 1985, 1989). Yet, over time, patients treated with intravenous clomipramine did not have a greater response than patients treated with oral clomipramine.

## Other Antidepressant Medication (Bupropion, Mirtazapine, Nefazodone, Trazodone)

### Generalized Anxiety Disorder (GAD)

There are some older studies that suggest that trazodone was an effective treatment for GAD (Rickels et al. 1993). There has been one open-label study suggesting that nefazodone may be efficacious for patients with GAD (Hedges et al. 1996).

### Social Anxiety Disorder (SAD)

Emmanuel and coworkers (1991, 2000) have published 2 papers investigating bupropion treatment for social anxiety disorder. In the most recent small 12-week open-label flexible-dose study the efficacy of bupropion-SR in the treatment of SAD was evaluated (Emmanuel et al. 2000). Eighteen subjects with DSM-IV-TR diagnosed social anxiety disorder were seen weekly for the first 4 weeks then biweekly for the next 8 weeks. Bupropion-SR was initiated at 100 mg/day and titrated to a maximum of 200 mg twice-a-day depending on response to treatment. Primary outcome measures in this study included the CGI-Improvement Scale (CGI-I) and the Brief Social Phobia Scale (BSPS). Response was defined as a CGI-I of 1 or 2 and at least a 50% reduction in the BSPS. Ten subjects completed the 12-week treatment period; five of the 10 were responders. The mean dose of bupropion-SR was $366 \pm 68$ mg/day. The mean CGI-I scores changed from $4.3 \pm 0.7$ at baseline to $2.5 \pm 0.9$ at week 12, and the mean BSPS scores decreased from $42.2 \pm 13$ at baseline to $21.0 \pm 11$ at week 12.

A small clinical case series by Worthington III and coworkers (1998) of 5 patients meeting DSM-IV criteria for social anxiety disorder who received open-label treatment with nefazodone (200–600 mg/day) for 3 months has been published. Patients were started on 50 mg twice a day and titrated up to a maximum 600 mg/day. The mean dose was $370 \pm 157$ mg/day. Patients completed the Liebowitz Social Anxiety Disorder Scale and the SDS at every clinic visit, and were rated using the BSPS and CGI-Severity and Improvement Scales. Three of the 5 patients completed 3 months of treatment. CGI-Severity scores decreased from 4.4 at baseline to 3.6 at week 12. Although these data are not terribly compelling, they are consistent with another report published by Van Amerigen and coworkers (Van Ameringen 1999).

### Panic Disorder (PD)

There have been a few double-blind trials of bupropion and trazodone for the treatment of panic disorder, but neither was found to be more effective than placebo (Charney et al.

1986, Sheehan et al. 1983). Case series and some small studies suggest, however, that mirtazapine and nefazodone may be effective treatments of patients with panic disorder (Carpenter et al. 1999, DeMartinis et al. 1996, Falkai 1999). Boshuisen and coworkers (2001) treated 28 panic disorder patients in the Netherlands with open-label mirtazepine. Subjects were required to have at least three full panic attacks in the 3 weeks preceding the screening visit. Subjects entered a 3-week placebo washout period followed by active treatment for 12 weeks, starting at a dose of 30 mg/day. Primary efficacy measures included the mean change in the number of full panic attacks during the active treatment period compared to the placebo run-in period, the proportion of subjects with zero full panic attacks, and the proportion of subjects with a 50% or greater decrease in the number of full panic attacks. Patients kept a daily diary to record number, severity, and duration of full panic attacks. Secondary efficacy measures also included the HAM-A and the FQ. Of the 23 patients who entered the study, 19 patients completed at least 9 weeks of mirtazapine treatment. The mean daily dose of mirtazapine was 36.3 mg/day. Number of full panic attacks decreased from 8.9 at baseline to 5.8 at endpoint, and mean total HAM-A scores decreased from 17.1 at baseline to 10.3 at the end of treatment. Fourteen of 19 patients who completed the trial had at least 50% decrease in the number of panic attacks and were considered responders. Forty-three percent of subjects reported an increase in appetite. Other frequently reported side effects included drowsiness, muscle pain in the legs, and tiredness.

Ribeiro and coworkers (2001) compared mirtazapine and fluoxetine in a randomized double-blind, flexible-dose trial of 27 patients with DSM-IV panic disorder. Participants were required to have a minimum of three panic attacks during the 2 weeks before enrollment into the study. Patients had to have a score greater than 18 on the HAM-A, and could not have been previously treated with mirtazapine. Following a 1-week, single-blind, placebo run-in, patients were randomly assigned to mirtazapine 15 mg/day or fluoxetine 10 mg/day. At week 3, doses could be raised to 30 mg/day of mirtazapine or 20 mg/day of fluoxetine according to clinical response. Each patient maintained a self-report diary of panic attacks. Clinician-rated assessments included the CGI-Severity and CGI-Improvement Scales, and the HAM-A. The Sheehan Phobic Scale provided patient global evaluation of phobic anxiety. Fourteen were treated with mirtazapine and 13 were treated with fluoxetine. Three patients treated with mirtazapine and two patients treated with fluoxetine dropped out because of side effects. Among completers, the mean daily dose of mirtazapine was $18.3 \pm 1.3$ mg/day and was $14.0 \pm 1.0$ mg/day for fluoxetine. HAM-A scores decreased from $15.7 \pm 10.0$ at baseline to $10.7 \pm 11.2$ at endpoint for the mirtazapine, and from $28.8 \pm 6.5$ at baseline to $11.8 \pm 7.5$ at endpoint for fluoxetine-treated subjects. In both groups, number of panic attacks decreased from three at baseline to zero at endpoint, suggesting that both medications eliminated spontaneous panic attacks.

## Posttraumatic Stress Disorder (PTSD)

There have been at least six open-label studies investigating the efficacy of nefazodone in PTSD. However, at this time there are no large placebo-controlled studies demonstrating that nefazodone is an effective treatment for PTSD. The overall results of these six trials are summarized in a paper by Hidalgo and coworkers (1999) and suggest that nefazodone treatment decreased the core symptoms of PTSD, improved sleep, and decreased symptoms of anger. Among these six open-label studies, three of them focused on patients who were veterans with chronic PTSD. Both Davis and coworkers (2000) and Hertzberg and coworkers (1998) found that open-label nefazodone treatment decreased core symptoms of PTSD. Zisook and coworkers (2000) demonstrated that open-label nefazodone treatment was helpful for patients who were refractory to SSRI treatment for PTSD. In all the open-label studies, nefazodone was titrated to what was considered to be a clinically effective dose, in the 400 to 600 mg/day ranges.

Connor and coworkers (1999) published a small open-label trial of mirtazapine treatment for patients with chronic PTSD. Three out of the six patients had a 50% or greater decrease on PTSD Rating Scales. There have also been case reports of mirtazapine being an effective adjuvant in the treatment of PTSD (Good and Petersen 2001).

## Obsessive–Compulsive Disorder (OCD)

Mirtazapine was used in a 10-week open trial of 10 adult outpatients who met DSM-IV-TR criteria for OCD for at least 1 year and had a Y-BOC score greater than 18 (Koran et al. 2002). Mirtazapine was started at a dose of 15 mg/day then increased after 4 days to 30 mg/day, and to 45 mg/day at the end of the second week. OCD severity was measured with the Y-BOC and the CGI-Severity Scale. Response to treatment was a priori defined as a 25% or greater decrease in Y-BOC scores from baseline. In this study, mean Y-BOC scores decreased from 28.7 at baseline to 23.7 at week 10. Only 2 of the 10 subjects met responder criteria. These results suggest that mirtazapine may not be a useful treatment for subjects with OCD.

## Benzodiazepine Medication

The benzodiazepines as a class work by increasing the relative efficiency of the gamma-aminobutyric acid (GABA) receptor when stimulated by GABA. The benzodiazepines bind to a site located adjacent to the GABA receptor and cause an allosteric change to the receptor that facilitates the increased passage of the chloride ions intracellularly when GABA interacts with the receptor complex. This leads to a relative hyperpolarization of the neuronal membrane and inhibition of activity in the brain. The benzadiazepines as a group have different affinities for GABA receptors, in fact some agents bind to only one of the two types of GABA receptors. For example, both clonezapam and alprazolam work only on the central $GABA_A$ receptor, while diazepam binds to both $GABA_A$ and $GABA_B$ receptors. The pharmacokinetic properties of the benzodiazepines are outlined in Table 98–6. The relative pharmacodynamic and pharmacokinetic properties of the benzadiazepines are further outlined in comparison to the other medications in Table 98–7. As a class, benzadiazepines are efficacious for the treatment of panic disorder, social anxiety disorder, generalized anxiety disorder, alcohol withdrawal, and situational anxiety. Although obsessive–compulsive disorder falls within the taxonomy of anxiety disorders, benzodiazepines do not seem to be particularly effective in treating these patients.

## Generalized Anxiety Disorder (GAD)

There have been hundreds of studies demonstrating that benzodiazepines as a class are more effective than a placebo in the treatment of both symptoms of anxiety and GAD (Greenblatt et al. 1983). In general, the response rate from these studies with benzodiazepines is between the 60 and 80% range (Rickels et al. 1983, Uhlenhuth et al. 1998). Unfortunately, benzodiazepine treatment of GAD is controversial. Despite evidence that the anxiolytic effect does not tend to diminish over time and that the majority of patients do not abuse benzodiazepines, most physicians are reticent to initiate long-term treatment for GAD (Bowden and Fisher 1980, Ciraulo et al. 1988).

There have been a variety of studies with abecarnil. In general abecarnil has not been demonstrated to be more effective than either buspirone or a traditional benzodiazepine (Pollack et al. 1997, Rickels et al. 2000a).

In summary, the short acting benzodiazepines, longer acting benzodiazepines, and even the low potency benzodiazepines have all been demonstrated to be effective treatments for GAD. The choice of an agent should take into account the age, medical health, and comorbid diagnosis of the patient.

## Social Anxiety Disorder

The benzodiazepines, clonazepam and alprazolam, have been shown to be efficacious in treating social anxiety disorder (Dubuff et al. 1995, Gelernter et al. 1991). The limitations to these drugs are the same as when used in any indication. Due to the potential for abuse and drug withdrawal, their use must be monitored carefully. This is a particularly problematic issue in social anxiety disorder because of the high rate of comorbid substance abuse. Benzodiazepines may be best suited for patients with situational and performance anxiety on an as needed basis.

## Panic Disorder (PD)

There are two high potency benzodiazepines that have been approved by the FDA and are widely used in the treatment of panic disorder. The first high potency benzodiazepine to be approved was alprazolam. Alprazolam has a relatively short half-life, requires frequent dosing (up to four times a day) and may cause significant discontinuation problems in some patients. In the Cross-National Collaborative Panic Disorder Study, alprazolam at a mean dose of 5.7 mg/day was found to be more effective than placebo in decreasing the number of panic attacks and allowing patients to become free from panic attacks (Ballenger et al. 1988). In phase two of the Cross-National Collaborative Panic Study (1992), 1,168 panic disorder patients were randomized to receive either alprazolam, imipramine or placebo. Both imipramine and alprazolam were more effective in treating panic disorder than placebo. Rickels and Schweizer (1998) have published a number of papers comparing alprazolam to imipramine and placebo. In a recent report of an acute 8-week study, they found that alprazolam and imipramine were equally effective in treating panic disorder but there were a large number of dropouts in the imipramine-treatment group. During a 6-month maintenance phase,

62% of alprazolam-treated patients completed the study and were panic free in contrast to only 26% imipramine-treated and placebo-treated patients. The 15-month follow-up of the same cohort found that 85% of patients who completed the maintenance phase study remained panic free in contrast to 55% of patients who were not able to complete the maintenance study. In general, alprazolam has been demonstrated in both short-term and long-term studies to be effective. There has been considerable concern about the risk of dependency and also the difficulties discontinuing alprazolam for a significant minority of patients.

Although clonazepam has been used for the treatment of panic disorder for a long time, it was not until the 1990s that two large definitive multicenter double-blind, placebo-controlled studies demonstrated clonazepam's efficacy for patients with panic disorder. In a large fixed-dose study, 413 patients were randomized to receive one of five doses of clonazepam (0.5 mg/day, 1.0 mg/day, 2.0 mg/day, 3.0 mg/day, 4.0 mg/day) or placebo. There was a 3-week dosage escalation period followed by 6 weeks of fixed-dose therapy and then a 7-week discontinuation phase. Doses of clonazepam greater than 1 mg were effective in decreasing the number of panic attacks and were well tolerated. There was some exacerbation of symptoms experienced by patients during the double-blind discontinuation-phase, but patients with these symptoms did not approach the initial baseline level of dysfunction (Rosenbaum et al. 1997). In a flexible-dose study, 222 patients were randomized to clonazepam treatment and 216 patients received placebo. Patients randomized to clonazepam had a decrease in the number of panic attacks and an improvement in CGI-Severity scores. Clonazepam was well tolerated but there was some worsening of symptoms during the discontinuation phase (Moroz and Rosenbaum 1999). In an open-label naturalistic study of 259 patients with panic disorder, Worthington and coworkers (1997) found that longer-term clonazepam treatment was associated with continuing improvement and maintenance. They found that the maintenance dosage of clonazepam was either constant with the initial response dose or decreased over time. There were no significant adverse effects associated with longer-term clonazepam treatment (Pollack et al. 1997). Goddard and coworkers (2001) looked at early coadministration of clonazepam with sertraline for panic disorder in a double-blind trial of 50 patients. Patients received open-label sertraline for 12 weeks (target dose of 100 mg/day) and were randomized to receive either 0.5 mg/day of clonazepam 3 times a day or placebo for the first 4 weeks of the trial. Response rates were markedly different at the end of week 1 with 41% of sertraline/clonazepam patients responding to treatment versus 4% of sertraline/placebo patients. At week 3, 63% of sertraline/clonazepam patients responded versus 32% of sertraline/placebo patients.

Other benzodiazepines have also been demonstrated to be effective in the treatment of panic disorder. In an 8-week double-blind, placebo-controlled trial, alprazolam (4.9 mg/day) and diazepam (40 mg/day) were equally effective and superior to placebo for the treatment of panic disorder (Noyes et al. 1996). In a smaller comparative study, lorazepam was as effective as alprazolam in the treatment of panic disorder (Schweizer et al. 1988). In summary, it is clear that two high potency benzodiazepines, alprazolam and clonazepam, are effective in the treatment of panic disorder. There also are data suggesting that a number of the other benzodiazepines may be useful in the treatment of panic disorder. Unfortunately, there are concerns about dependency and stigma associated with the use of benzodiazepine medication.

## Obsessive–Compulsive Disorder (OCD)

Pigott and coworkers (1992) conducted a controlled trial of clonazepam augmentation in OCD patients treated with clomipramine or fluoxetine. Augmentation with clonazepam was found to be more effective than placebo in decreasing global measures of anxiety but not Y-BOC scores.

## Buspirone

Buspirone is a member of the group of agents called Azaspirodecanediones. It is believed to exert its anxiolytic effect by acting as a partial agonist at the $5\text{-HT}_{1A}$ autoreceptor. Stimulation of the $5\text{-HT}_{1A}$ autoreceptor causes decrease release of serotonin into the synaptic cleft. However, buspirone also exerts another effect through its active metabolite 1-phenyl-piperazine (1-PP) that acts on alpha-2-adrenergic receptors to increase the firing rate of the locus coeruleus. Some not yet *well-characterized* combination of these effects may be responsible for anxiolytic effect of buspirone. It usually takes approximately 4 weeks for the benefit of buspirone therapy to be noticed in patients with GAD. One major advantage of buspirone is that it does not cross react with benzodiazepines. The most common side effects associated with buspirone include dizziness, gastrointestinal distress, headache, numbness, and tingling. The pharmacokinetics and average daily dosage are described in Table 98–6. The most common pharmacokinetic and pharmacodynamic actions of buspirone are described in Table 98–7.

## Generalized Anxiety Disorder (GAD)

Buspirone has been shown to be more effective than placebo in decreasing HAM-A scores in a large number of placebo-controlled trials (Laakmann et al. 1998, Rickels et al. 1982, 1988). It is thought that buspirone may be particularly effective against psychological symptoms such as worry, tension, irritability, and apprehension, but less effective in ameliorating somatic symptoms because of its activation of locus coeruleus. (Riblet et al. 1982, Rickels et al. 1982).

Data from placebo-controlled and comparative studies against benzodiazapines suggest that the onset of action of buspirone usually takes at least 2 weeks (Connor and Davidson 1998, Laakmann et al. 1998). However, clinical experience suggests that buspirone treatment may take 3 to 4 weeks before one sees a truly beneficial effect in patients with GAD. Buspirone also requires multiple daily administration to be effective. Although a recent meta-analysis suggests that buspirone may be given twice a day for the treatment of anxiety and GAD, the majority of studies and the current labeling for buspirone suggests that it should be administered three times a day (Sramek et al. 1999). Discontinuation of buspirone has not been associated with development of withdrawal symptoms, however, over time patients discontinued from pharmacotherapy tend to relapse (Rickels et al. 1988).

In a placebo-controlled comparative study of hydroxyzine versus buspirone both of these agents were found to be more effective than placebo treatment (Lader and Scotto 1998).

In summary, although there are considerable data suggesting that buspirone is an effective treatment for GAD, most of these data are from acute trials. It is clear that buspirone's time to onset is delayed in contrast to the benzodiazepine's and that it may not be as useful as the benzodiazapine is for treating GAD patients with primarily somatic symptoms.

## Social Anxiety Disorder

Buspirone showed promise during open-label studies of social anxiety disorder but did not differentiate from placebo in controlled trials (van Vliet et al. 1997). Data from open-label trials also suggest that buspirone may be used as an adjuvant with SSRIs when patients exhibit only partial response to monotherapy (Van Ameringen et al. 1996).

## Panic Disorder (PD)

There is a case report suggesting that buspirone may be a useful adjuvant in some patients with treatment resistant panic disorder (Gastfriend and Rosenbaum 1989). In general, buspirone is not thought to be an effective monotherapy for panic disorder.

## Obsessive–Compulsive Disorder (OCD)

None of the double-blind augmentation studies of buspirone for patients with treatment resistant obsessive–compulsive disorders have demonstrated any advantage over placebo treatment (Grady et al. 1993, McDougle et al. 1993, Pigott et al. 1992).

## Beta-Blocker Medication

Beta-adrenergic blockers competitively antagonize norepinephrine and epinephrine at the beta-adrenergic receptor (Table 98–7). It is thought that the majority of positive effects of beta-blockers are due to their peripheral actions. Beta-blockers can decrease many of the peripheral manifestations of anxiety such as tachycardia, diaphoresis, trembling, and blushing. The advent of more selective beta-blockers that only block the beta-2-adrenergic receptor has been beneficial since blockade of beta-1 adrenergic receptors can be associated with bronchospasm. Beta-blockers may be useful for individuals who have situational anxiety or performance anxiety. They generally have not been effective in treating anxiety disorders such as generalized social anxiety disorder, panic disorder, or obsessive–compulsive disorder.

## Social Anxiety Disorder

Stein and coworkers (2001) conducted a double-blind, placebo-controlled crossover study of pindolol potentiation of paroxetine for the treatment of social anxiety disorder. Pindolol was selected as an adjunct to SSRI because it is a $5\text{-HT}_{1A}$ autoreceptor antagonist as well as being a beta-adernergic receptor blocker. It is postulated that antagonism of the $5\text{-HT}_{1A}$ autoreceptor would stimulate presynaptic release of serotonin. In fact, pindolol has been shown to accelerate the antidepressant response of SSRIs in some studies (Perez et al. 1997, Zanardi et al. 1997). Fourteen patients who were less than 'very much improved' on CGI-I ratings after 10 weeks of maximally tolerated dose of paroxetine were randomized to receive 5 mg of pindolol t.i.d. or placebo for 4 weeks. After 4 weeks, subjects were tapered and crossed over to receive the other agent (pindolol or placebo) for another 4-week period. Response in this study was defined by a CGI rating of 'very much improved.' Pindolol augmentation was not more effective than placebo augmentation in this study.

## Anticonvulsant Medication

One of the areas of increasing research is the study of anticonvulsants in anxiety disorders. Currently, there are few published placebo-controlled studies investigating the efficacy of commonly used anticonvulsants for the treatment of anxiety or anxiety disorders. There is one published report of a large double-blind, placebo-controlled study of gabapentin for the treatment of social anxiety disorder. The precise mechanism of action of gabapentin is not fully appreciated, however, it is thought gabapentin somehow increases brain GABA levels. Please see Tables 98–6 and 98–7 for a review of some of the more salient pharmacological properties of these agents.

## Social Anxiety Disorder

There is one double-blind, placebo-controlled study. Sixty-nine patients were randomized to receive 14 weeks of either gabapentin (900–3,600 mg/day) or placebo. Thirty-two percent of patients receiving gabapentin versus 14% of those receiving placebo (Pande et al. 1999) were considered responders.

## Panic Disorder (PD)

Sandford and coworkers (2001) conducted a small randomized, double-blind, placebo-controlled crossover trial of pagoclone versus placebo in 16 patients with panic disorder. Pagoclone is believed to act as a partial agonist at the $GABA_A$ benzodiazepine receptor. Patients were randomized to receive either pagoclone 0.1 mg t.i.d. during weeks 1 and 2 or pagoclone 0.1 mg t.i.d. during weeks 4 and 5. There was a decrease in the number of full panic attacks from baseline among pagoclone-treated patients but not among placebo patients. This decrease was observed for patients receiving pagoclone regardless of whether they received it in the first or second crossover arm; however, this difference did not reach statistical significance.

Zwanzger and coworkers (2001) investigated the putative anxiolytic properties of tiagabine in a clinical case series. Tiagabine has been shown to reduce neuronal excitability by increasing brain GABA levels, by inhibiting GABA reuptake. Four patients meeting DSM-IV criteria for panic disorder were treated. All patients reported a reduction of panic attacks and improvement in anxiety levels within 4 weeks, although one patient discontinued treatment because of side effects.

There are some scattered reports suggesting the valproic acid and gabapentin maybe useful, particularly in either atypical or treatment resistant patients with panic disorder (Keck et al. 1993, Woodman and Noyes 1994).

## Posttraumatic Stress Disorder (PTSD)

Anticonvulsant medications may also prove to be useful for the treatment of PTSD. However, at this time there is a paucity of published information available. A series of small case studies using carbamazepine as a treatment for posttraumatic stress disorder have been reported. In these open-label case series, patients did seem to have a decrease in intrusive thoughts and improvement in sleep associated with carbamazepine treatment. Jeffrey Berlant has pioneered the use of topiramate as an adjuvant treatment for PTSD. In his published case series, topiramate augmentation seems to be particularly useful in improving sleep, decreasing nightmares, and decreasing intrusive thoughts (Berlant 2001). To date there has been one double-blind, placebo-controlled study of lamotrigine for the treatment of posttraumatic stress disorder (Hertzberg et al. 1999). In this study, 15 patients were randomized 2:1 to lamotrigine or placebo. Five of the 10 patients who received lamotrigine had a significant decrease in their global PTSD Scale score as compared to one of four patients who received placebo. Lamotrigine-treated patients showed improvement in avoidance, numbing, and reexperiencing symptoms. Further studies will be necessary to determine whether anticonvulsant treatment, either as a monotherapy or as an adjuvant with antidepressants, will be beneficial for patients with PTSD.

## Antipsychotic Medication

The conventional or typical antipsychotic medication whose mechanism of action is primarily to block dopamine Type-2 receptors has been used as adjuvant medication for the treatment of anxiety disorders for years. However, because of problems with extrapyramidal side effects and the risk of developing tardive dyskinesia, these agents had fallen out of favor. The newer class of atypical antipsychotic medications have a markedly decreased risk of both extrapyramidal side effects and tardive dyskinesia and so antipsychotic medications are beginning to be used again as adjuvants in patients with treatment resistant anxiety disorders. This simultaneous blockade of both neurotransmitter systems seems to decrease extrapyramidal side effects and the risk of developing tardive dyskinesia. Although the different atypical antipsychotic medications have different affinities for dopamine Type-2 and serotonin Type-2 receptors, this is the common mechanism of action of these agents. The atypical antipsychotic medications also differ dramatically in terms of their pharmacodynamic properties. As described below, there are very few published studies investigating atypical antipsychotic medication augmentation for the treatment of anxiety disorders. Please review the pharmacokinetic and side effect data for the antipsychotic medications that have been used to treat anxiety disorders in Tables 98–6 and 98–7.

## Panic Disorder (PD)

Some experts have suggested that atypical antipsychotics may be a useful monotherapy in the treatment of panic disorder, but to date, the majority of the information comes from case reports where they are used to enhance therapeutic response (Etxebeste et al. 2000).

## Posttraumatic Stress Disorder (PTSD)

With the development the atypical antipsychotics there has been a reemergence of interest in the possible use of antipsychotic medication as both a primary treatment for PTSD or as an adjuvant treatment for PTSD. However, in a recently completed large secondary analysis of veteran inpatients and outpatients with PTSD, only 9% of inpatients and 10% of outpatients had been treated with antipsychotic medications (Sernyak et al. 2001). These patients tended to be more sick, have more severe PTSD, more intrusive thoughts, and be more dysfunctional although their incidence of traumatic experiences did not differ significantly from those patients who were not treated with antipsychotic medications. In this study, the antipsychotic augmentation did not have any benefit. There have been a number of published case reports suggesting that atypical antipsychotic medications may be useful as adjuvants for the treatment of PTSD. Krashin and Oats (1999) report two cases where risperidone augmentation decreased intrusive thoughts and markedly improved symptoms of PTSD. Petty and coworkers (2001) recently published an open-label study of 48 individuals who were initially started on open-label olanzapine treatment. Thirty patients completed the 8-week trial and tolerated olanzapine well. These patients had clinically significant improvement in their CAPS-2 scores, HAM-D scores, and Brief Psychiatric Rating Scale (BPRS) scores. Yet in the one published small double-blind, placebo-controlled flexible-dose study of olanzapine, only 11 patients completed the study and there was no difference in the response rates between the two groups. The authors did acknowledge that the small sample size of the study and high placebo-response rate might be responsible for this finding. Yet, to date, the data are not overwhelmingly favorable for the use of atypical antipsychotic medication as monotherapy or even as an augmentation therapy for PTSD.

## Obsessive–Compulsive Disorder (OCD)

Patients affected by OCD do not always respond to monotherapy with SSRIs or clomipramine. One major augmentation strategy has been to block the dopamine Type-2 receptor. Preliminary studies suggest that blockade with typical neuroleptics for patients with tics may be beneficial (McDougle 1997). Open case series suggest that the newer atypical neuroleptics, risperidone and olanzapine, may be useful in augmenting clinical response in treatment refractory OCD (McDougle 1997, Weiss et al. 1999). Pfanner and coworkers (2002) investigated the use of risperidone as an adjunct to SSRI therapy in an 8-week open-label trial of 20 patients with refractory OCD. Patients in this study had a DSM-IV diagnosis of OCD with duration of illness of at least 2 years, had demonstrated less than a 25% improvement with an SSRI after 6 months of treatment, and had a baseline Y-BOC score of 30. Risperidone was added at 1 mg/day with a titration up to 3 mg/day over 2 weeks. Response was defined as a reduction of at least 25% in Y-BOC scores. The OCD-Questionnaire, the HAM-D, and the CGI were secondary measures. The mean Y-BOC score decreased 26% over the course of the trial from 36.1 at baseline to 24.8 at week 8. Additionally, at endpoint, 8 patients had a CGI-improvement score of 1 (very much improved), 9 patients had a 2 (much improved), while only 3 patients had a 3 (minimally improved).

Another recent study examined the efficacy of 6 weeks of open olanzapine augmentation in 9 patients with refractory OCD (Francobandiera 2001). Patients had been treated with clomipramine or an SSRI for a minimum of 12 weeks without significant clinical response. They were started on olanzapine 2.5 mg/day which was titrated up to 5 mg/day. At the end of week 6, 8 out of 9 patients had a significant decrease in Y-BOC scores from baseline.

## Conclusion

In closing, clinicians have a wide array of medications available for the treatment of anxiety and anxiety disorders. The breadth of treatment options available greatly facilitates our ability to help patients. We have safe and effective treatments for everything from short-term treatment of pathological anxiety to previously intractable anxiety disorders like obsessive–compulsive disorder. Yet, the most important therapeutic agent we possess is still sound clinical skills and judgement. Appropriate diagnosis and rapport are the foundations of any pharmacological intervention we make with our patients.

### Clinical Vignette

Ms. K is a 46-year-old Hispanic female who presents with a chief complaint of recurrent major depressive disorder. Ms. K has had multiple brief treatments for depressive disorder but always discontinues her treatment. Ms. K reports that she was physically abused by her older brother while in adolescence and 2 years ago was involved in a car jacking. Although Ms. K was not harmed during the car jacking, she developed a depressive disorder immediately following the incident. When questioned further, it is clear that Ms. K has recurrent nightmares about this event, has flashbacks, startles easily, avoids driving on all streets except main arteries and the freeway, and has complained of feeling distant from her husband and children. During the interview Ms. K breaks down and is tearful. She discusses how ashamed she feels for being "weak" and having these pervasive symptoms. When the concept of posttraumatic stress disorder is introduced to Ms. K, she is relieved to know that she is not the odd person out.

Ms. K was started on sertraline 25 mg/day and this dose was gradually tapered up by 25 mg/week until 100 mg. Ms. K had a gradual reduction in her intrusive thoughts and nightmares that began during the second week of treatment. Ms. K's depressive symptoms began to resolve as well by week 4. Since Ms. K was not having side effects and still was symptomatic at 6 weeks, the dosage of sertraline was increased to a 150 mg/day. Over the next 8 weeks, Ms. K had continued improvement on both her depressive symptoms and many of her symptoms of posttraumatic stress disorder. She became more active with her family and affectionate with her husband. She began to expand the areas where she felt comfortable driving. Over time Ms. K continued to demonstrate improvement in symptoms. She is currently maintained on 150 mg/day of sertraline and has been able to return to work and most of her normal activities over a period of 2 years.

## References

Abramowitz JS (1997) Effectiveness of psychological and pharmacological treatments for obsessive–compulsive disorder: A quantitative review. J Consult Clin Psychol 65(1), 44–52.

Asnis GM, Hameedi FA, Goddard AW, et al. (2001) Fluvoxamine in the treatment of panic disorder: A multi-center, double-blind, placebo-controlled study in outpatients. Psychiatr Res 103(1), 1–14.

Bakish D (1992) Reversible monoamine-A inhibitors in panic disorder. Clin Neuropharmacol 15(Suppl 1, Pt A), 432A–433A.

Baldwin D, Bobes J, Stein DJ, et al. (1999) Paroxetine in social phobia/ social anxiety disorder. Randomised, double-blind, placebo-controlled study. Paroxetine Study Group. Br J Psychiatr 175, 120–126.

Ballenger JC, Burrows GD, DuPont RLJ, et al. (1988) Alprazolam in panic disorder and agoraphobia: Results from a multicenter trial. I. Efficacy in short-term treatment. Arch Gen Psychiatr 45(5), 413–422.

Ballenger JC, Wheadon DE, Steiner M, et al. (1998) Double-blind, fixed-dose, placebo-controlled study of paroxetine in the treatment of panic disorder. Am J Psychiatr 155(1), 36–42.

Berlant JL (2001) Topiramate in posttraumatic stress disorder: Preliminary clinical observations. J Clin Psychiatr 62(Suppl 17), 60–63.

Bisserbe JC, Lane RM, and Flament MF (1997) A double-blind comparison of sertraline and clomipramine in outpatients with obsessive–compulsive disorder. Eur Psychiatr 12, 82–93.

Blanco C and Liebowitz MR (1998) Dimensional versus categorical response to moclobemide in social phobia. J Clin Psychopharmacol 18(4), 344–346.

Blomhoff S, Haug TT, Hellstrom K, et al. (2001) Randomised controlled general practice trial of sertraline, exposure therapy and combined treatment in generalised social phobia. Br J Psychiatr 179, 23–30.

Bolden-Watson C and Richelson E (1993) Blockade by newly-developed antidepressants of biogenic amine uptake into rat brain synaptosomes. Life Sci 52(12), 1023–1029.

Boshuisen ML, Slaap BR, Vester-Blokland ED, et al. (2001) The effect of mirtazapine in panic disorder: An open label pilot study with a single-blind placebo run-in period. Int Clin Psychopharmacol 16(6), 363–368.

Bouwer C and Stein DJ (1998) Use of the selective serotonin reuptake inhibitor citalopram in the treatment of generalized social phobia. J Affect Disord 49(1), 79–82.

Bowden CL and Fisher JG (1980) Safety and efficacy of long-term diazepam therapy. South Med J 73(12), 1581–1584.

Boyer W (1995) Serotonin uptake inhibitors are superior to imipramine and alprazolam in alleviating panic attacks: A meta-analysis. Int Clin Psychopharmacol 10(1), 45–49.

Brady K, Pearlstein T, Asnis GM, et al. (2000) Efficacy and safety of sertraline treatment of posttraumatic stress disorder: A randomized controlled trial. JAMA 283(14), 1837–1844.

Calliard V, Roullion F, and Viel J (1999) Comparative effects of low and high doses of clomipramine and placebo in panic disorder: A double-blind controlled study. Acta Psychiatr Scand 99, 51–58.

Carpenter LL, Leon Z, Yasmin S, et al. (1999) Clinical experience with mirtazapine in the treatment of panic disorder. Ann Clin Psychiatr 11(2), 81–86.

Carpenter LL, McDougle CJ, Epperson CN, et al. (1996) A risk-benefit assessment of drugs used in the management of obsessive–compulsive disorder. Drug Safety 15(2), 116–134.

Cartwright C and Hollander E (1998) SSRIs in the treatment of obsessive–compulsive disorder. Depress Anx 8(Suppl 1), 105–113.

Cassano GB, Petracca A, Perugi G, et al. (1988) Clomipramine for panic disorder: I. The first 10 weeks of a long-term comparison with imipramine. J Affect Disord 14(2), 123–127.

Charney DS, Woods SW, Goodman WK, et al. (1986) Drug treatment of panic disorder: The comparative efficacy of imipramine, alprazolam, and trazodone. J Clin Psychiatr 47(12), 580–586.

Chouinard G, Goodman W, Greist J, et al. (1990) Results of a double-blind placebo controlled trial of a new serotonin uptake inhibitor, sertraline, in the treatment of obsessive–compulsive disorder. Psychopharmacol Bull 26(3), 279–284.

Ciraulo DA, Sands D, and Shader RI (1988) Critical review of liability for benzodiazepine abuse among alcoholics. Am J Psychiatr 145, 1501–1506.

Connor KM and Davidson JR (1998) Generalized anxiety disorder: Neurobiological and pharmacotherapeutic perspectives. Biol Psychiatr 44(12), 1286–1294.

Connor KM, Davidson JR, Weisler RH, et al. (1999) A pilot study of mirtazapine in posttraumatic stress disorder. Int Clin Psychopharmacol 14(1), 29–31.

Cook EH, Wagner KD, March JS, et al. (2001) Long-term sertraline treatment of children and adolescents with obsessive–compulsive disorder. J Am Acad Child Adolesc Psychiatr 40(10), 1175–1181.

Cox BJ, Swinson RP, Morrison B, et al. (1993) Clomipramine, fluoxetine, and behavior therapy in the treatment of obsessive–compulsive disorder: A meta-Analysis. J Behav Ther Exp Psychiatr 24(2), 149–153.

Cross-National Collaborative Panic Study, Second Phase Investigators (1992) Drug treatment of panic disorder. Comparative efficacy of alprozolam imipramine, and placebo. Br J Psychiatr 160, 191–202. (Published erratum in Br J Psychiatr, 161, 724 Nov)

Davidson J, Kudler H, Smith R, et al. (1990) Treatment of posttraumatic stress disorder with amitriptyline and placebo. Arch Gen Psychiatr 47(3), 259–266.

Davidson J, Pearlstein T, Londborg P, et al. (2001) Efficacy of sertraline in preventing relapse of posttraumatic stress disorder: Results of a 28-week double-blind, placebo-controlled study. Am J Psychiatr 158(12), 1974–1981.

Davidson J, Walker JI, and Kilts C (1987) A pilot study of phenelzine in the treatment of posttraumatic stress disorder. Br J Psychiatr 150, 252–255.

Davidson JR, DuPont RL, Hedges D, et al. (1999) Efficacy, safety, and tolerability of venlafaxine extended release and buspirone in outpatients with generalized anxiety disorder. J Clin Psychiatr 60(8), 528–535.

Davis LL, Nugent AL, Murray J, et al. (2000) Nefazodone treatment for chronic posttraumatic stress disorder: An open trial. J Clin Psychopharmacol 20(2), 159–164.

DeMartinis NA, Schweizer E, and Rickels K (1996) An open-label trial of nefazodone in high comorbidity panic disorder. J Clin Psychiatr 57(6), 245–248.

den Boer JA (1998) Pharmacotherapy of panic disorder: Differential efficacy from a clinical viewpoint. J Clin Psychiatr 59(Suppl 8), 30–36.

den Boer JA and Westenberg HG (1988) Effect of a serotonin and noradrenaline uptake inhibitor in panic disorder: A double-blind comparative study with fluvoxamine and maprotiline. Int Clin Psychopharmacol 3(1), 59–74.

den Boer J, Westenberg H, and Kamerbeek W (1987) Effect of serotonin uptake inhibitors in anxiety disorders. A double-blind comparison of clomipramine and fluvoxamine. Int Clin Psychopharmacol 2, 21–32.

Dubovsky SL and Thomas M (1995) Serotonergic mechanisms and current and future psychiatric practice. J Clin Psychiatr 56(2), 38–48.

Dubuff E, Ferguson J, and Londborg P (1995) Double-blind comparison of three fixed doses of sertraline and placebo in patients with panic disorder (abstract). 8th congress of the European college of neuropsychopharmacology, Venice.

Emmanuel NP, Brawman-Mintzer O, Morton WA, et al. (2000) Bupropion-SR in treatment of social phobia. Depress Anx 12(2), 111–113.

Emmanuel NP, Lydiard RB, and Ballenger JC (1991) Treatment of social phobia with bupropion. J Clin Psychopharmacol 11(4), 276–277.

Etxebeste M, Aragues E, Malo P, et al. (2000) Olanzapine and panic attacks (letter). Am J Psychiatr 157(4), 659–660.

Fahlen T, Nilsson HL, Borg K, et al. (1995) Social phobia: The clinical efficacy and tolerability of the monoamine oxidase-A and serotonin uptake inhibitor brofaromine. A double-blind placebo-controlled study. Acta Psychiatr Scand 92(5), 351–358.

Falkai P (1999) Mirtazapine: Other indications. J Clin Psychiatr 60(Suppl 17), 36–40.

Francobandiera G (2001) Olanzapine augmentation of serotonin uptake inhibitors in obsessive–compulsive disorder: An open study. Can J Psychiatr 46(4), 356–358.

Freeman CP, Trimble MR, Deakin JF, et al. (1994) Fluvoxamine versus clomipramine in the treatment of obsessive–compulsive disorder: A multicenter, randomized, double-blind, parallel group comparison. J Clin Psychiatr 55(7), 301–305.

Gastfriend DR and Rosenbaum JF (1989) Adjunctive buspirone in benzodiazepine treatment of four patients with panic disorder. Am J Psychiatr 146(7), 914–916.

Gelenberg AJ, Lydiard RB, Rudolph RL, et al. (2000) Efficacy of venlafaxine extended-release capsules in nondepressed outpatients with generalized anxiety disorder: A 6-month randomized controlled trial. JAMA 283(23), 3082–3088.

Gelernter CS, Uhde TW, Cimbolic P, et al. (1991) Cognitive–behavioral and pharmacological treatments of social phobia. A controlled study. Arch Gen Psychiatr 48(10), 938–945.

Goddard AW, Brouette T, Almai A, et al. (2001) Early coadministration of clonazepam with sertraline for panic disorder. Arch Gen Psychiatr 58(7), 681–686.

Good C and Petersen C (2001) SSRI and mirtazapine in PTSD. J Am Acad Child Adolesc Psychiatr 40(3), 263–264.

Goodman WK, Price LH, Rasmussen SA, et al. (1989) Efficacy of fluvoxamine in obsessive–compulsive disorder. A double-blind comparison with placebo. Arch Gen Psychiatr 46(1), 36–44.

Gorman JM, Liebowitz MR, Fyer AJ, et al. (1987) An open trial of fluoxetine in the treatment of panic attacks. J Clin Psychopharmacol 7(5), 329–332. (Published erratum appears in J Clin Psychopharmacol 8[1], 13, 1988 Feb)

Grady TA, Pigott TA, L'Heureux F, et al. (1993) Double-blind study of adjuvant buspirone for fluoxetine-treated patients with obsessive–compulsive disorder. Am J Psychiatr 150(5), 819–821.

Greenblatt DJ, Shader RI, and Abernethy DR (1983) Drug therapy. Current status of benzodiazepines. N Engl J Med 309(7), 410–416.

Greist J, Chouinard G, DuBoff E, et al. (1995a) Double-blind parallel comparison of three dosages of sertraline and placebo in outpatients with obsessive–compulsive disorder. Arch Gen Psychiatr 52, 289–295.

Greist JH (1998) The comparative effectiveness of treatments for obsessive–compulsive disorder. Bull Menn Clin 62(4) (Suppl A), A65–A81.

Greist JH and Jefferson JW (1998) Pharmacotherapy for obsessive–compulsive disorder. Br J Psychiatr (Suppl 35), 64–70.

Greist JH, Jefferson JW, Kobak KA, et al. (1995b) A 1 year double-blind placebo-controlled fixed dose study of sertraline in the treatment of obsessive–compulsive disorder. Int Clin Psychopharmacol 10(2), 57–65.

Greist JH, Jenike MA, and Robinson D (1995c) Efficacy of Fluvoxamine in obsessive–compulsive disorder: Results of a multicentre, double-blind, placebo-controlled trial. Eur J Clin Res 7, 195–204.

Haskins JT, Aguiar L, and Pallay A (1999) Double-blind, placebo controlled study of once-daily venlafaxine XR (V-XR) in outpatients with generalized anxiety disorder. Presented at the annual meeting, Anxiety Disorders Association of America, San Diego, CA.

Hedges DW, Reimherr FW, Strong RE, et al. (1996) An open trial of nefazodone in adult patients with generalized anxiety disorder. Psychopharmacol Bull 32(4), 671–676.

Hertzberg MA, Butterfield MI, Feldman ME, et al. (1999) A preliminary study of lamotrigine for the treatment of posttraumatic stress disorder. Biol Psychiatr 45(9), 1226 1229.

Hertzberg MA, Feldman ME, Beckham JC, et al. (1998) Open trial of nefazodone for combat-related posttraumatic stress disorder. J Clin Psychiatr 59(9), 460–464.

Hidalogo R, Hertzberg MA, Mellman T, et al. (1999) Nefazodone in posttraumatic stress disorder: Results from six open-label trials. Int Clin Psychopharm 14, 61–68.

Hoehn-Saric R, McLeod DR, and Hipsley PA (1993) Effect of fluvoxamine on panic disorder. J Clin Psychopharmacol 13(5), 321–326.

International Multicenter Clinical Trial Group (1997) Mocobemide in social phobia: A double-blind, placebo-controlled clinical study. Eur Arch Psychiatr Clin Neurosci 247(2), 71–80.

Jenike MA, Baer L, and Greist JH (1990) Clomipramine versus fluoxetine in obsessive–compulsive disorder: A retrospective comparison of side effects and efficacy. J Clin Psychopharmacol 10(2), 122–124.

Kalus O, Asnis GM, Rubinson E, et al. (1991) Desipramine treatment in panic disorder. J Affect Disord 21(4), 239–244.

Katzenick DJ, Kobak KA, and Greist JW (1995) Sertraline for social phobia: A double-blind placebo-controlled crossover study. Am J Psychiatr 152, 1368–1371.

Keck PE Jr., Taylor VE, Tugrul KC, et al. (1993) Valproate treatment of panic disorder and lactate-induced panic attacks. Biol Psychiatr 33(7), 542–546.

Kelsey JE (1995) Venlafaxine in social phobia. Psychopharmacol Bull 31(4), 767–771.

Klein D (1964) Delineation of two-drug responsive anxiety syndromes. Psychopharmacologia 5, 397–408.

Klein D and Fink M (1962) Psychiatric reaction patterns to imipramine. Am J Psychiatr 119, 432–438.

Kobak KA, Greist JH, Jefferson JW, et al. (1998) Behavioral versus pharmacological treatments of obsessive–compulsive disorder: A meta-analysis. Psychopharmacology (Berl) 136(3), 205–216.

Koponen H, Lepola U, Leinonen E, et al. (1997) Citalopram in the treatment of obsessive–compulsive disorder: An open pilot study. Acta Psychiatr Scand 96(5), 343–346.

Koran LM, Faravelli C, and Pallanti S (1994) Intravenous clomipramine for obsessive–compulsive disorder. J Clin Psychopharmacol 14(3), 216–218.

Koran LM, Hackett E, Rubin A, et al. (2002) Efficacy of sertraline in the long-term treatment of obsessive–compulsive disorder. Am J Psychiatr 159(1), 88–95.

Koran LM, McElroy SL, Davidson JR, et al. (1996) Fluvoxamine versus clomipramine for obsessive–compulsive disorder: A double-blind comparison. J Clin Psychopharmacol 16(2), 121–129.

Koran LM, Sallee FR, and Pallanti S (1997) Rapid benefit of intravenous pulse loading of clomipramine in obsessive–compulsive disorder. Am J Psychiatr 154(3), 396–401.

Kosten TR, Frank JB, Dan E, et al. (1991) Pharmacotherapy for posttraumatic stress disorder using phenelzine or imipramine. J Nerv Ment Dis 179(6), 366–370.

Krashin D and Oates EW (1999) Risperidone as an adjunct therapy for posttraumatic stress disorder. Mil Med 164(8), 605–606.

Kronig MH, Apter J, Asnis G, et al. (1999) Placebo-controlled, multicenter study of sertraline treatment for obsessive–compulsive disorder. J Clin Psychopharmacol 19(2), 172–176.

Kruger MB and Dahl AA (1999) The efficacy and safety of moclobemide compared to clomipramine in the treatment of panic disorder. Eur Arch Psychiatr Clin Neurosci 249(Suppl 1), S19–S24.

Laakmann G, Schule C, Lorkowski G, et al. (1998) Buspirone and lorazepam in the treatment of generalized anxiety disorder in out-patients. Psychopharmacol (Berl) 136(4), 357–366.

Lader M and Scotto JC (1998) A multicentre double-blind comparison of hydroxyzine, buspirone and placebo in patients with generalized anxiety disorder. Psychopharmacol (Berl) 139(4), 402–406.

Lecrubier Y and Judge R (1997) Long-term evaluation of paroxetine, clomipramine and placebo in panic disorder. Collaborative Paroxetine Panic Study Investigators. Acta Psychiatr Scand 95(2), 153–160.

Lecrubier Y, Bakker A, Dunbar G, et al. (1997) A comparison of paroxetine, clomipramine and placebo in the treatment of panic disorder. Collaborative Paroxetine Panic Study Investigators. Acta Psychiatr Scand 95(2), 145–152.

Leinonen E, Skarstein J, Behnke K, et al. (1999) Efficacy and tolerability of mirtazapine versus citalopram: A double-blind, randomized study in patients with major depressive disorder. Nordic Antidepressant Study Group. Int Clin Psychopharmacol 14(6), 329–337.

Lerer B, Bleich A, Kotler M, et al. (1987) Posttraumatic stress disorder in Israeli combat veterans. Effect of phenelzine treatment. Arch Gen Psychiatr 44(11), 976–981.

Liebowitz MR, Fyer AJ, Gorman JM, et al. (1988) Tricyclic therapy of the DSM-III anxiety disorders: A review with implications for further research. J Psychiatr Res 22(Suppl 1), 7–31.

Landborg PD, Hegel MT, Goldstein S, et al. (2001) Sertraline treatment of posttraumatic stress disorder: Results of 24 weeks of open-label continuation treatment. J Clin Psychiatr 65(5), 325–331.

Londborg PD, Wolkow R, Smith WT, et al. (1998) Sertraline in the treatment of panic disorder. A multi-site, double-blind, placebo-controlled, fixed-dose investigation. Br J Psychiatr 173, 54–60.

Lopez-Ibor JJ Jr., Saiz J, Cottraux J, et al. (1996) Double-blind comparison of fluoxetine versus clomipramine in the treatment of obsessive–compulsive disorder. Eur Neuropsychopharmacol 6(2), 111–118.

Lydiard RB, Morton WA, Emmanuel NP, et al. (1993) Preliminary report: Placebo-controlled, double-blind study of the clinical and metabolic effects of desipramine in panic disorder. Psychopharmacol Bull 29(2), 183–188.

Marazziti D, Dell'Osso L, Gemignani A, et al. (2001) Citalopram in refractory obsessive–compulsive disorder: An open study. Int Clin Psychopharmacol 16(4), 215–219.

March JS and Frances A (1997) The expert consensus guideline series: Treatment of obsessive–compulsive disorder. J Clin Psychiatr 149, 1053–1057.

Marshall R, Beebe K, Oldham M, et al. (2001) Efficacy and safety of paroxetine treatment for chronic PTSD: A fixed dose, placebo controlled study. Am J Psychiatr 158(12), 1982–1988.

Mavissakalian M and Perel JM (1992a) Clinical experiments in maintenance and discontinuation of imipramine therapy in panic disorder with agoraphobia. Arch Gen Psychiatr 49(4), 318–323.

Mavissakalian M and Perel JM (1992b) Protective effects of imipramine maintenance treatment in panic disorder with agoraphobia. Am J Psychiatr 149(8), 1053–1057.

Mavissakalian MR and Perel JM (2001) 2nd year maintenance and discontinuation of imipramine in panic disorder with agoraphobia. Ann Clin Psychiatr 13(2), 63–67.

McDougle CJ (1997) Update on pharmacologic management of OCD: Agents and augmentation. J Clin Psychiatr 58(Suppl 12), 11–17.

McDougle CJ, Goodman WK, Leckman JF, et al. (1993) Limited therapeutic effect of addition of buspirone in fluvoxamine-refractory obsessive–compulsive disorder. Am J Psychiatr 150(4), 647–649.

Michelson D, Allgulander C, Dantendorfer K, et al. (2001) Efficacy of usual antidepressant dosing regimens of fluoxetine in panic disorder: Randomised, placebo-controlled trial. Br J Psychiatr 179, 514–518.

Michelson D, Lydiard RB, Pollack MH, et al. (1998) Outcome assessment and clinical improvement in panic disorder: Evidence from a randomized controlled trial of fluoxetine and placebo. The Fluoxetine Panic Disorder Study Group. Am J Psychiatr 155(11), 1570–1577.

Michelson D, Pollack M, Lydiard RB, et al. (1999) Continuing treatment of panic disorder after acute response: Randomised, placebo-controlled trial with fluoxetine. The Fluoxetine Panic Disorder Study Group. Br J Psychiatr 174, 213–218.

Milanfranchi A, Ravagli S, Lensi P, et al. (1997) A double-blind study of fluvoxamine and clomipramine in the treatment of obsessive–compulsive disorder. Int Clin Psychopharmacol 12(3), 131–136.

Modigh K, Westberg P, and Eriksson E (1992) Superiority of clomipramine over imipramine in the treatment of panic disorder: A placebo-controlled trial. J Clin Psychopharmacol 12(4), 251–261.

Montgomery SA, McIntyre A, Osterheider M, et al. (1993) A double-blind, placebo-controlled study of fluoxetine in patients with DSM-III-R obsessive–compulsive disorder. The Lilly European OCD Study Group. Eur Neuropsychopharmacol 3(2), 143–152.

Moroz G and Rosenbaum JF (1999) Efficacy, safety, and gradual discontinuation of clonazepam in panic disorder: A placebo-controlled, multicenter study using optimized dosages. J Clin Psychiatr 60(9), 604–612.

Mundo E, Bianchi L, and Bellodi L (1997) Efficacy of fluvoxamine, paroxetine, and citalopram in the treatment of obsessive–compulsive disorder: A single-blind study. J Clin Psychopharmacol 17(4), 267–271.

Munjack DJ, Usigli R, Zulueta A, et al. (1988) Nortriptyline in the treatment of panic disorder and agoraphobia with panic attacks. J Clin Psychopharmacol 8(3), 204–207.

Noyes R, Garvey MJ, Cook BL, et al. (1989) Problems with tricyclic antidepressant use in patients with panic disorder or agoraphobia: Results of a naturalistic follow-up study. J Clin Psychiatr 50, 163–169.

Noyes R Jr., Burrows GD, Reich JH, et al. (1996) Diazepam versus alprazolam for the treatment of panic disorder. J Clin Psychiatr 57(8), 349–355.

Noyes R Jr., Moroz G, Davidson JR, et al. (1997) Moclobemide in social phobia: A controlled dose-response trial. J Clin Psychopharmacol 17(4), 247–254.

Pande AC, Greiner M, Adams JB, et al. (1999) Placebo-controlled trial of the CCK-B antagonist, CI-988, in panic disorder. Biol Psychiatr 46(6), 860–862.

Perez V, Gilaberte I, Faries D, et al. (1997) Randomised, double-blind, placebo-controlled trial of pindolol in combination with fluoxetine antidepressant treatment. Lancet 349(9065), 1594–1597.

Perna G, Bertani A, Caldirola D, et al. (2001) A comparison of citalopram and paroxetine in the treatment of panic disorder: A randomized, single-blind study. Pharmacopsychiatry 34(3), 85–90.

Perse TL, Greist JH, Jefferson JW, et al. (1987) Fluvoxamine treatment of obsessive–compulsive disorder. Am J Psychiatr 144(12), 1543–1548.

Petty F, Brannan S, Casada J, et al. (2001) Olanzapine treatment for post-traumatic stress disorder: An open-label study. Int Clin Psychopharmacol 16(6), 331–337.

Pfanner C, Marazziti D, Dell'Osso L, et al. (2000) Risperidone augmentation in refractory obsessive–compulsive disorder: An open-label study. Int Clin Psychopharmacol 15(5), 297–301.

Piccinelli M, Pini S, Bellantuono C, et al. (1995) Efficacy of drug treatment in obsessive–compulsive disorder. A meta-analytic review. Br J Psychiatr 166(4), 424–443.

Pigott TA, L'Heureux F, and Rubenstein CS (1992) A controlled trial of clonazepam augmentation in OCD patients treated with clomipramine or fluoxetine (abstract 144). New research program and abstracts of the 145th meeting of the American Psychiatric Association.

Pollack MH, Otto MW, Worthington JJ, et al. (1998) Sertraline in the treatment of panic disorder: A flexible-dose multicenter trial. Arch Gen Psychiatr 55(11), 1010–1016.

Pollack MH, Worthington JJ, Manfro GG, et al. (1997) Abecarnil for the treatment of generalized anxiety disorder: A placebo-controlled comparison of two dosage ranges of abecarnil and buspirone. J Clin Psychiatr 58(Suppl 11), 19–23.

Pollack MH, Worthington JJ III, Otto MW, et al. (1996) Venlafaxine for panic disorder: Results from a double-blind, placebo-controlled study. Psychopharmacol Bull 32(4), 667–670.

Pollack MH, Zaninelli R, Goddard A, et al. (2001) Paroxetine in the treatment of generalized anxiety disorder: Results of a placebo-controlled, flexible-dosage trial. J Clin Psychiatr 62(5), 350–357.

Rapaport MH, Wolkow RM, and Clary CM (1998) Methodologies and outcomes from the sertraline multicenter flexible-dose trials. Psychopharmacol Bull 34(2), 183–189.

Rapaport MH, Wolkow R, Rubin A, et al. (2001) Sertraline treatment of panic disorder: Results of a long-term study. Acta Psychiatr Scand.

Ribeiro L, Busnello JV, Kauer-Sant'Anna M, et al. (2001) Mirtazapine versus fluoxetine in the treatment of panic disorder. Braz J Med Biol Res 34(10), 1303–1307.

Riblet LA, Taylor DP, Eison MS, et al. (1982) Pharmacology and neurochemistry of buspirone. J Clin Psychiatr 43(12, Pt 2), 11–18.

Rickels K and Schweizer E (1998) Panic disorder: Long-term pharmacotherapy and discontinuation. J Clin Psychopharmacol 18(6)(Suppl 2), 12S–18S.

Rickels K, Case WG, Downing RW, et al. (1983) Long-term diazepam therapy and clinical outcome. JAMA 250(6), 767–771.

Rickels K, DeMartinis N, and Aufdembrinke B (2000a) A double-blind, placebo-controlled trial of abecarnil and diazepam in the treatment of patients with generalized anxiety disorder. J Clin Psychopharmacol 20(1), 12–18.

Rickels K, Downing R, Schweizer E, et al. (1993) Antidepressants for the treatment of generalized anxiety disorder. A placebo-controlled comparison of imipramine, trazodone, and diazepam. Arch Gen Psychiatr 50(11), 884–895.

Rickels K, Pollack MH, Sheehan DV, et al. (2000b) Efficacy of extended-release venlafaxine in nondepressed outpatients with generalized anxiety disorder. Am J Psychiatr 157(6), 968–974.

Rickels K, Schweizer E, Csanalosi I, et al. (1988) Long-term treatment of anxiety and risk of withdrawal. Prospective comparison of clorazepate and buspirone. Arch Gen Psychiatr 45(5), 444–450.

Rickels K, Weisman K, Norstad N, et al. (1982) Buspirone and diazepam in anxiety: A controlled study. J Clin Psychiatr 43(12, Pt 2), 81–86.

Rocca P, Fonzo V, Scotta M, et al. (1997) Paroxetine efficacy in the treatment of generalized anxiety disorder. Acta Psychiatr Scand 95(5), 444–450.

Rosenbaum JF, Moroz G, and Bowden CL (1997) Clonazepam in the treatment of panic disorder with or without agoraphobia: A dose-response study of efficacy, safety, and discontinuance. Clonazepam Panic Disorder Dose-Response Study Group. J Clin Psychopharmacol 17(5), 390–400.

Rynn MA, Siqueland L, and Rickels K (2001) Placebo-controlled trial of sertraline in the treatment of children with generalized anxiety disorder. Am J Psychiatr 158(12), 2008–2014.

Sandford JJ, Forshall S, Bell C, et al. (2001) Crossover trial of pagoclone and placebo in patients with DSM-IV panic disorder. J Psychopharmacol 15(3), 205–208.

Sasson Y, Iancu I, Fux M, et al. (1999) A double-blind crossover comparison of clomipramine and desipramine in the treatment of panic disorder. Eur Neuropsychopharmacol 9(3), 191–196.

Schneier FR, Goetz D, Campeas R, et al. (1998) Placebo-controlled trial of moclobemide in social phobia. Br J Psychiatr 172, 70–77.

Schneier FR, Liebowitz MR, Davies SO, et al. (1990) Fluoxetine in panic disorder. J Clin Psychopharmacol 10(2), 119–121.

Schweizer E, Fox I, Case G, et al. (1988) Lorazepam vs. alprazolam in the treatment of panic disorder. Psychopharmacol Bull 24(2), 224–227.

Sernyak MJ, Kosten TR, Fontana A, et al. (2001) Neuroleptic use in the treatment of posttraumatic stress disorder. Psychiatr Q 72(3), 197–213.

Sheehan DV, Ballenger J, and Jacobsen G (1980) Treatment of endogenous anxiety with phobic, hysterical, and hypochondriacal symptoms. Arch Gen Psychiatr 37(1), 51–59.

Sheehan DV, Davidson J, Manschreck T, et al. (1983) Lack of efficacy of a new antidepressant (bupropion) in the treatment of panic disorder with phobias. J Clin Psychopharmacol 3(1), 28–31.

Simpson HB, Schneier FR, Campeas RB, et al. (1998a) Imipramine in the treatment of social phobia. J Clin Psychopharmacol 18(2), 132–135.

Simpson HB, Schneier FR, Marshall RD, et al. (1998b) Low dose selegiline (L-Deprenyl) in social phobia. Depress Anx 7(3), 126–129.

Sramek JJ, Hong WW, Hamid S, et al. (1999) Meta-analysis of the safety and tolerability of two dose regimens of buspirone in patients with persistent anxiety. Depress Anx 9(3), 131–134.

Stein DJ, Seedat S, van der Linden GJ, et al. (2000) Selective serotonin reuptake inhibitors in the treatment of posttraumatic stress disorder: A meta-analysis of randomized controlled trials. Int Clin Psychopharmacol 15(Suppl 2), S31–S39.

Stein DJ, Spadaccini E, and Hollander E (1995) Meta-analysis of pharmacotherapy trials for obsessive–compulsive disorder. Int Clin Psychopharmacol 10(1), 11–18.

Stein MB, Fyer AJ, Davidson JR, et al. (1999) Fluvoxamine treatment of social phobia (social anxiety disorder): A double-blind, placebo-controlled study. Am J Psychiatr 156(5), 756–760.

Stein MB, Liebowitz MR, Lydiard RB, et al. (1998) Paroxetine treatment of generalized social phobia (social anxiety disorder): A randomized controlled trial. JAMA 280(8), 708–713.

Stein MB, Sareen J, Hami S, et al. (2001) Pindolol potentiation of paroxetine for generalized social phobia: A double-blind, placebo-controlled, cross-over study. Am J Psychiatr 158(10), 1725–1727.

Thomsen PH (1997) Child and adolescent obsessive–compulsive disorder treated with citalopram: Findings from an open trial of 23 cases. J Child Adolesc Psychopharmacol 7(3), 157–166.

Tiller JW, Bouwer C, and Behnke K (1999) Moclobemide and fluoxetine for panic disorder. International Panic Disorder Study Group. Eur Arch Psychiatr Clin Neurosci 249(Suppl 1), S7–S10.

Todorov C, Freeston MH, and Borgeat F (2000) On the pharmacotherapy of obsessive–compulsive disorder: Is a consensus possible? Can J Psychiatr 45(3), 257–262.

Tollefson G, Birkett M, and Koran L (1994a) Continuation treatment of OCD: Double blind and open label experience with fluoxetine. J Clin Psychiatr 55(Suppl 10), 69–76.

Tollefson GD, Rampey AH Jr., Potvin JH, et al. (1994b) A multicenter investigation of fixed-dose fluoxetine in the treatment of obsessive–compulsive disorder. Arch Gen Psychiatr 51(7), 559–567. (Published erratum appears in Arch Gen Psychiatr 1994 Nov, 51(11) 864)

Tucker P, Smith K, Marx B, et al. (2000) Fluvoxamine reduces physiologic reactivity to trauma scripts in posttraumatic stress disorder. J Clin Psychopharmacol 20(3), 367–372.

Uhlenhuth EH, Alexander PE, Dempsey GM, et al. (1998) Medication side effects in anxious patients: Negative placebo responses? J Affect Disord 47(1–3), 183–190.

Vallejo J, Olivares J, Marcos T, et al. (1992) Clomipramine versus phenelzine in obsessive–compulsive disorder. A controlled clinical trial. Br J Psychiatr 161, 665–670.

Van Ameringen M, Mancini C, and Oakman JM (1999) Nefazodone in social phobia. J Clin Psychiatr 60(2), 96–100.

Van Ameringen M, Mancini C, and Streiner DL (1993) Fluoxetine efficacy in social phobia. J Clin Psychiatr 54(1), 27–32.

Van Ameringen M, Mancini C, and Wilson C (1996) Buspirone augmentation of selective serotonin reuptake inhibitors (SSRIs) in social phobia. J Affect Disord 39(2), 115–121.

van Ameringen MA, Lane RM, Walker JR, et al. (2001) Sertraline treatment of generalized social phobia: A 20-week, double-blind, placebo-controlled study. Am J Psychiatr 158(2), 275–281.

van der Kolk BA, Dreyfuss D, Michaels M, et al. (1994) Fluoxetine in posttraumatic stress disorder. J Clin Psychiatr 55(12), 517–522.

van Vliet IM, den Boer JA, Westenberg HG, et al. (1997) Clinical effects of buspirone in social phobia: A double-blind placebo-controlled study. J Clin Psychiatr 58(4), 64–168.

van Vliet IM, Westenberg HG, and den Boer JA (1993) MAO inhibitors in panic disorder: Clinical effects of treatment with brofaromine. A double blind placebo controlled study. Psychopharmacol (Berl) 112(4), 483–489.

Versiani M, Nardi AE, Mundim FD, et al. (1992) Pharmacotherapy of social phobia. A controlled study with moclobemide and phenelzine. Br J Psychiatr 161, 353–360.

Wade AG, Lepola U, Koponen HJ, et al. (1997) The effect of citalopram in panic disorder. Br J Psychiatr 170, 549–553.

Warneke L (1989) Intravenous chlorimipramine therapy in obsessive–compulsive disorder. Can J Psychiatr 34(9), 853–859.

Warneke LB (1984) The use of intravenous chlorimipramine in the treatment of obsessive–compulsive disorder. Can J Psychiatr 29(2), 135–141.

Warneke LB (1985) Intravenous chlorimipramine in the treatment of obsessional disorder in adolescence: Case report. J Clin Psychiatr 46(3), 100–103.

Weiss EL, Potenza MN, McDougle CJ, et al. (1999) Olanzapine addition in obsessive–compulsive disorder refractory to selective serotonin reuptake inhibitors: An open-label case series. J Clin Psychiatr 60(8), 524–527.

Woodman CL and Noyes R Jr. (1994) Panic disorder: Treatment with valproate. J Clin Psychiatr 55(4), 134–136.

Worthington JJ, Pollack MJ, Otto MW, et al. (997) Long-term experience with clonazepam in patients with primary diagnosis of panic disorder. Psychopharmacol Bull 32(2), 199–205.

Worthington JJ III, Zucker BG, Fones CS, et al. (1998) Nefazodone for social phobia: A clinical case series. Depress Anx 8(3), 131–133.

Zanardi R, Artigas F, Franchini L, et al. (1997) How long should pindolol be associated with paroxetine to improve the antidepressant response? J Clin Psychopharmacol 17(6), 446–450.

Zisook S, Chentsova-Dutton YE, Smith-Vaniz A, et al. (2000) Nefazodone in patients with treatment-refractory posttraumatic stress disorder. J Clin Psychiatr 61(3), 203–208.

Zohar J and Judge R (1996) Paroxetine versus clomipramine in the treatment of obsessive–compulsive disorder. OCD Paroxetine Study Investigators. Br J Psychiatr 169(4), 468–474.

Zwanzger P, Baghai TC, Schule C, et al. (2001) Tiagabine improves panic and agoraphobia in panic disorder patients. J Clin Psychiatr 62(8), 656–657.

# 99  Sedative–Hypnotic Agents

Richard I. Shader
Douglas A. Songer

## Introduction

Insomnia is a significant health care problem. It can create daytime fatigue, impaired social or occupational functioning, and reduced quality of life. Patients with insomnia are less productive workers, more prone to motor vehicle and workplace accidents, and utilize the general medical health care system to a greater degree than patients with normal sleep habits (Simon 1997). Table 99–1 contains some helpful hints for patients who become drowsy while driving or working. The direct (physician visits, medication costs) and indirect (decreased productivity, accidents) costs of insomnia are enormous for the entire industrialized world. Walsh and Engelhart (1999) estimated the direct economic costs of insomnia in 1995 in the US to be more than $13 billion, and the indirect costs have been estimated to be from $77 to 92 billion annually. Estimates of the prevalence of insomnia vary from 10 to 50% of the adult population, depending on the diagnostic criteria used, as well as the duration and severity criteria used (Roth 2001). A poll done by the National Sleep Foundation in 1991 revealed that 36% of American adults had insomnia severe enough to cause residual effects the next day (Gallup Organization 1991). This same organization found a prevalence of 49% when the survey was repeated in 1995 (Gallup Organization 1995).

Insomnia is a major problem in today's society for a number of reasons. An aging population, the hectic work and personal lifestyle of the typical American, and an increase in the frequency of nontraditional work hours (e.g., shift work) all may play a role. Older adults are particularly prone to insomnia complaints. While total sleep time is increased in the elderly, the total amount of time spent in stages 3 and 4 sleep is reduced, making the sleep less restorative in nature. Nocturia due to prostatic hypertrophy or Type II diabetes mellitus often makes sleep maintenance challenging for the geriatric population as well.

Besides the elderly, patients with underlying psychiatric disorders are particularly prone to sleep difficulties. Schizophrenia, anxiety disorders, and mood disorders frequently cause significant insomnia. Aggressive treatment of the underlying psychiatric illness often improves sleep. However, sometimes the medications used to treat the psychiatric illness may create insomnia as well. For example,

| Table 99–1 | Helpful Hints for Those Who Are Drowsy While Driving or Working |
|---|---|

Whenever possible, when you become drowsy interrupt your work or pull over to a rest area and stop for at least a brief nap.

Strongly resist the temptation to use stimulants. Once you feel this need, you are already too tired to work safely or to drive.

Keep your work area or your car temperature cool.

If it will not disturb others or interfere with your concentration, consider using the radio but avoid soft, sleep-inducing music.

Take breaks from your work or driving at least every 2–3 h. Try to increase your alertness and heart rate.

When driving and drowsy, never use the cruise-control device.

selective serotonin reuptake inhibitors (SSRI) (particularly during the early weeks of treatment) may cause insomnia, even when they effectively treat an underlying depression.

## Diagnosis

Primary insomnia refers to a sleep disturbance in which no other sleep disorder (e.g., narcolepsy, obstructive sleep apnea), medical condition (e.g., depression, chronic pain), medication (e.g., stimulants), or substance use (e.g., cocaine, caffeine) can account for the difficulty with stage 4 sleep. To formally make a diagnosis of primary insomnia, the *Diagnostic and Statistical Manual of Mental Disorders*, Fourth Edition (DSM-IV) requires that the sleep disturbance lasts at least 1 month and that it causes significant interference in emotional, social, or occupational functioning. Polysomnography is not indicated for the routine evaluation of acute or chronic insomnia, but may be useful when sleep disorders such as obstructive sleep apnea or nocturnal myoclonus are suspected.

Secondary insomnia may be due to a variety of physical or mental disorders. Hyperthyroidism, chronic pain, severe chronic obstructive pulmonary disease (COPD), and a wide variety of medications may induce insomnia. Insomnia is extremely common in mood disorders, anxiety disorders, and psychotic disorders. When a patient suffers from secondary insomnia, aggressive treatment of the underlying physical or emotional problem can often resolve

| Table 99-2 | Some DSM-IV Categories of Sleep Disorders | |
|---|---|---|
| | DSM-IV | ICD-10* |
| Primary sleep disorders | Code | Code |
| Primary insomnia | 307.42 | F51.0 |
| Primary hypersomnia | 307.44 | F51.1 |
| Narcolepsy | 347.0 | G47.4 |
| Breathing-related sleep disorder | 780.59 | G47.3 |
| Circadian rhythm sleep disorder | 307.45 | F51.2 |
| This category has four subtypes: Delayed sleep phase type, jet lag type, shift work type, unspecified type | | |
| Dyssomnia not otherwise specified | 307.47 | F51.9 |
| This category includes nocturnal myoclonus and the insomnia from chronic sleep deprivation | | |
| Secondary† sleep disorders | | |
| Insomnia due to a general medical condition | 708.52 | G47.0 |
| Insomnia related to an Axis I or II mental disorder | 307.42 | F51.0 |
| Substance-induced sleep disorder | 291.8 | F10.8 |
| Alcohol | 292.89 | F15.8 |
| Amphetamines or related substances | 292.89 | F15.8 |
| Caffeine | 292.89 | F15.8 |
| Cocaine | 292.89 | F14.8 |
| Sedative–hypnotic–anxiolytic | 292.89 | F13.8 |
| Other, unknown | 292.89 | F19.8 |

*International Statistical Classification of Diseases and Related Health Problems, 10th revision.

†DSM-IV-TR uses the term other.

the insomnia complaint without the need for sedative–hypnotic agents. Table 99–2 lists some of the major categories of sleep disorders as delineated by DSM-IV-TR.

## Treatment

Prior to treatment, clinicians should ensure that an appropriate diagnostic evaluation has occurred. Clinicians should search diligently for and treat any secondary cause of insomnia. Treating the secondary cause may alleviate the sleep difficulty without the need to use sedative–hypnotic agents. For example, adequate analgesic relief in a patient with pain problems may permit restorative sleep, or remission of depressive symptoms may provide the same benefit. Mild, transient insomnia lasting a day or two generally is self-limited and requires no pharmacological treatment. Insomnia of a more severe nature may require medication, but nonpharmacologic options for the treatment of insomnia should always be explored first. Basic sleep hygiene techniques should be reviewed and practiced by the patient

suffering from insomnia. Patients suffering from insomnia should be advised to avoid caffeinated beverages after 4:00 PM and to avoid long naps. A number of useful sleep hygiene techniques are described in Table 99–3. Behavioral therapy techniques have been shown to be effective in treating primary insomnia; stimulus control, progressive muscle relaxation, paradoxical intention, biofeedback, and sleep restriction when done by clinicians skilled in their use, can be quite helpful (Chesson et al. 1999, Morin et al. 1999). A recent meta-analysis by Smith and colleagues (2002) found behavioral techniques to be as effective as pharmacotherapy. Sleep improvements may be better sustained over time with behavioral treatment as well.

## Pharmacological Treatments

### Nonprescription Agents

There are a number of over-the-counter (OTC) sleep aids used by patients suffering from insomnia. These agents typically contain the histamine ($H_1$) receptor antagonist diphenhydramine (e.g., Benadryl, Sominex) or some other sedating antihistamine such as doxylamine (e.g., Nytol, Unisom). While these agents often cause significant drowsiness due to their antihistaminic properties, their effectiveness in treating insomnia has not been clearly established in randomized, placebo-controlled studies. They tend to have a prolonged duration of action leading to sedation and slowed reaction times during the day following their use. In addition, tachyphylaxis often develops within several

| Table 99-3 | Sleep Hygiene Techniques |
|---|---|

1. Do not go to bed when you are not tired.
2. Avoid napping during the day, even when you are tired. Especially avoid early-evening naps.
3. Wake up at the same time each day. Do not "catch up" on your sleep on the weekend.
4. Do not drink caffeinated beverages within 6 h of bedtime and minimize total daily use.
5. Avoid heavy meals too close to bedtime, but don't go to bed hungry, as this may disrupt sleep. A warm, noncaffeinated beverage and a small carbohydrate snack may be soothing and enhance drowsiness.
6. Regular exercise in the late afternoon may deepen sleep. Strenuous exercise too close to bedtime (i.e., 4–5 h) may interfere with sleep.
7. If you do not fall asleep within a half-hour or so, get up and read a book or watch television. When you stay in the bed and don't sleep for long periods of time, the bed becomes associated with not sleeping.
8. Minimize noise, light, and extremes in temperature during the sleep period.
9. Avoid the use of alcohol as a sleep-enhancer. While it may promote sleep onset, early morning awakening is quite common and the sleep is generally nonrestorative in nature.
10. Use progressive muscle relaxation or deep-breathing techniques to enhance relaxation and minimize anxiety and stress.
11. Ensure that pain complaints have been appropriately evaluated and treated by your physician. Pain interferes with sleep.
12. Do not smoke cigarettes too close to bedtime or if you awaken in the night. Nicotine is a stimulant.

| Table 99–4 | Some Over-the-Counter Sleep Aids Commonly Available in the US |
|---|---|
| Product Name | Active Ingredient* |
| Benadryl | Diphenhydramine |
| Compoz Nighttime Sleep Aid | Diphenhydramine |
| Sleepinal | Diphenhydramine |
| Sominex | Diphenhydramine |
| Nervine Nighttime Sleep-Aid | Diphenhydramine |
| Nytol | Doxylamine |
| Nytol QuickCaps | Diphenhydramine |
| Unisom Nighttime Sleep-Aid | Doxylamine |
| Unisom SleepGels | Diphenhydramine |

*Various strengths and formulations contain between 25 and 50 mg of the active antihistamine.

days to a week or two limiting their use to only those patients with short-term problems with insomnia. Table 99–4 lists some of the commonly available OTC sleep aids in the US.

The OTC antihistamines are also highly anticholinergic and therefore may cause dry mouth, constipation, urinary retention, and delirium quite easily. Geriatric patients are particularly susceptible to these anticholinergic effects. Patients already on other medications with significant anticholinergic activity should take these compounds quite judiciously as the anticholinergic effects could be magnified.

The common practice of combining an analgesic such as aspirin or acetaminophen and an antihistamine (e.g., *Tylenol PM*) is no more effective than the use of an antihistamine alone unless pain is present. As such, their use cannot be recommended for patients suffering from insomnia when pain is not a major complaint.

Another OTC sleeping agent that was commonly available at health food stores until 1990 is L-tryptophan. This agent was removed from the market in the US in 1990 because a contaminant in the manufacturing process has been linked to eosinophilic-myalgia syndrome. While available evidence regarding the safety and efficacy of L-tryptophan are far from conclusive, there is a clinical consensus that it is a weakly effective hypnotic agent that is without significant risks in the absence of contaminants. The folk remedy of having warm milk and crackers before bedtime probably has as its basis in the facilitation by carbohydrate of L-tryptophan absorption from milk or through mediation by cholecystokinin. The postprandial somnolence following Thanksgiving Day Turkey may be due to a similar cause.

Melatonin is a naturally occurring pineal gland peptide hormone that is available in OTC formulations from a number of manufacturers. The Food and Drug Administration (FDA) classifies melatonin as a nutritive or dietary supplement. The Dietary Supplement Health and Education Act does not require dietary supplements to be reviewed by the FDA, and, as a result, the strength and purity of melatonin cannot be guaranteed. When purified or synthesized and taken orally, melatonin alters circadian rhythms, lowers core body temperature, and reduces daytime alerting phenomena originating in the suprachiasmatic nucleus. Some clinicians feel that melatonin may be particularly effective when the normal circadian cycle is disrupted (e.g., jet lag, shift work). A number of studies have yielded conflicting results regarding the efficacy and long-term safety of melatonin. Efficacy data may be somewhat conflicting due to the lack of solid data regarding appropriate dosing strategies. Efficacy has been reported with doses as low as 0.3 mg at bedtime, while others have noted a dose of 6 mg to be necessary to help promote sleep (Chase and Gidal 1997). While there are no known long-term safety issues associated with the use of melatonin, treatment-emergent side effects include pruritus, tachycardia, headache, and daytime drowsiness.

Kava is derived from the roots of a shrub (*Piper methysticum*) grown on some South Pacific islands. Kava is thought to have GABAergic activity and is often used for both insomnia and anxiety. Recent reports of hepatic failure has prompted its removal from the market in Switzerland and it is currently undergoing review by the FDA in the US because of this issue. Clinical trials to support its efficacy are lacking to date.

Valerian is an herbal treatment that has also long been advocated to promote sleep. At doses of 300 to 900 mg side effects are rare, but may include headache, GI distress, and palpitations. The mechanism of action of its hypnotic effects remains unclear, but preliminary studies suggest that GABAergic properties may contribute to the activity of valerian extracts. Stevinson and Ernst (2000) conducted a review of the randomized, placebo-controlled, double-blind trials of the efficacy of valerian for improving sleep and found that the evidence to date is promising but not yet conclusive.

Further discussion of alternative and complementary treatments can be found in Chapters 36 and 104. Interested readers are referred there for more detailed discussion on this topic.

## Prescription Medications

Prescription medications for patients suffering from insomnia are generally used only on a short-term basis. Benzodiazepines replaced barbiturates as the mainstay of treatment for much of the past 30 years. Benzodiazepines have a decreased abuse potential, fewer interactions with other drugs, a broader therapeutic index compared to the barbiturates, and pose a much lower risk in overdose. The adverse effect profile of benzodiazepines includes the risk for abuse and physiological dependence that develops with daily use, as well as problems with daytime sedation, motor incoordination, and cognitive impairment. More recently the imidazopyridine zolpidem and the pyrazolopyrimidine zaleplon have become increasingly popular as daytime sedation and the risk for abuse and physiological dependence appear to be somewhat less frequent with these two agents.

### Benzodiazepines

Benzodiazepines are clearly effective for transient and situational insomnias. A recent meta-analysis demonstrated that benzodiazepine treated patients reported improvement in sleep onset, number of awakenings at night, the total amount of sleep obtained, and the quality of sleep

| Table 99–5 | Benzodiazepine Hypnotic Agents | | | | |
|---|---|---|---|---|---|
| Generic Name | Trade Name | Dose Strengths (mg) | Half-Life (h) | Onset of Action | Comments |
| Triazolam | Halcion | 0.125, 0.25 | 1.5–5.5 | Intermediate | May cause anterograde amnesia |
| Temazepam | Restoril | 7.5, 15, 30 | 9–12 | Slow | No active metabolites |
| Estazolam | ProSom | 1, 2 | 10–24 | Intermediate | Active metabolite has weak sedating properties as well |
| Flurazepam | Dalmane | 15, 30 | 30–100 | Fast | Active metabolite desalkylflurazepam accumulates and causes additive sedation |
| Quazepam | Doral | 7.5, 15 | 25–40 | Intermediate | Same active metabolite as flurazepam |

compared to placebo-treated patients (Nowell et al. 1997). Although only five benzodiazepines are marketed as hypnotic agents (Table 99–5), any benzodiazepine could be used to induce sleep provided an appropriate dose is chosen. Benzodiazepines improve sleep by inducing drowsiness, relaxing muscles, and decreasing mental agitation. As doses, and consequently brain concentrations are increased, drowsiness and relaxation shift into decreased wakefulness and then sleep. Benzodiazepines increase total sleep time, increase nonrapid-eye-movement (non-REM) sleep, decrease sleep latency, decrease stage 1 sleep, and increase stage 2 sleep. Effects on stage 3 sleep vary based on the individual drug used, but stage 4 sleep is generally reduced.

Benzodiazepines are central nervous system depressants. Their likely mechanism of action relates to their ability to augment the opening of neuronal gamma-aminobutyric acid receptor-related chloride channels. By modulating the effects of gamma-aminobutyric acid, benzodiazepines increase the frequency of chloride channel openings. This effect is in contrast to the effects of barbiturates or alcohol, which seem to increase the duration of chloride channel opening. While this distinction may appear minor, it accounts for the greater safety of benzodiazepines in overdose (i.e., there is less likelihood of respiratory depression or coma). When alcohol is mixed with a benzodiazepine overdose, the synergistic effects of respiratory depression can have potentially fatal consequences.

There is little convincing evidence that the five marketed benzodiazepine hypnotics differ in terms of efficacy or safety when they are administered appropriately (i.e., amounts, dosing intervals, and duration of use). The current benzodiazepines marketed as hypnotic agents are similar in their effects on sleep architecture and differ only in onset of action and duration of action. The individual agent chosen should be based on the type of sleep difficulty being experienced, the age of the patient, and comorbid diagnoses. Triazolam has a rapid onset and a short duration of action, making it a better choice for patients with sleep initiation difficulties, while flurazepam has a somewhat longer onset of action and a much longer duration of action, making it a better choice for patients with middle or terminal insomnia.

Shorter half-life benzodiazepine hypnotics cause less daytime sedation and residual cognitive affects the day following administration. Rebound insomnia often occurs with these agents, however, especially after use for several consecutive nights. Rebound insomnia can usually be avoided by tapering the dose or using lower dosages during treatment. There is some evidence to suggest that the likelihood of rebound insomnia is greater in patients who experience greater hypnotic efficacy.

Besides rebound insomnia, some patients receiving shorter half-life benzodiazepines have problems with middle or terminal insomnia. Plasma levels are quite low several hours after taking these medications, and, as a result, if there is a problem with sleep maintenance these agents are not as likely to be as helpful as hypnotics with longer half-lives. In addition, shorter half-life benzodiazepines can sometimes cause an increase in daytime anxiety, particularly in the morning. For at least some patients, this may reflect the development of physiologic dependence and a withdrawal phenomenon.

Shorter half-life hypnotics, particularly triazolam, appear to cause anterograde amnesia more commonly than the longer half-life agents do. Numerous reports in the lay press regarding a greatly increased risk of hallucinations, confusion, and anterograde amnesia with triazolam use does not appear to be supported by an examination of all available data. All benzodiazepines can cause anterograde amnesia, however, particularly at higher dosages. Anterograde amnesia commonly occurs following a benzodiazepine overdose. The prevalence of anterograde amnesia with appropriate dosing of sedative–hypnotic agents and risk factors for its development in patients are still open questions at this time

Longer half-life benzodiazepines may be more appropriate for patients who suffer from middle or terminal insomnia since these agents retain significant sedative properties for many hours after initial administration. Some patients may have problems with daytime sedation or decreased reaction time the day following administration. Sedative agents such as flurazepam and quazepam that have active metabolites with long half-lives are particularly prone to causing such problems. The active metabolite often builds up over time causing an increase in daytime drowsiness, decreased reaction time, and in coordination with repeated administration, particularly in the elderly. Patients with significant daytime anxiety may benefit from the longer acting benzodiazepines as the residual amount of medication left in the morning may still have anxiolytic benefits.

The elderly use benzodiazepine hypnotic agents to a much greater degree than the general adult population. While this is likely due to the greater prevalence of sleep disorders in the elderly, the use of hypnotic agents in this population poses particular challenges. The elderly as a group have a decrement in hepatically metabolized benzodiazepines (e.g., estazolam, flurazepam, quazepam, triazolam), which is often more pronounced among men. Incoordination, sedation, and confusion can occur when such agents build up over time. Ray and colleagues found a much higher rate of falls and hip fractures in the elderly population that received long-acting benzodiazepine hypnotics. The risk of hip fracture increased in direct proportion to the daily dose of the long-acting benzodiazepine. Short-acting benzodiazepines were not found to have a similar problem in their two large case-control studies (Ray et al. 1987, 1989). A generally safe clinical strategy when managing insomnia problems in the elderly is to halve the starting dose and titrate up slowly as tolerated following the longstanding advice "start low, go slow." Avoiding long-acting benzodiazepines appears prudent as well.

Drug interactions with benzodiazepines are quite common. When mixed with other sedating compounds the effects are additive. Narcotic medications, alcohol, and antihistamines are examples where the additive sedation can lead to confusion quite easily. In addition, acute alcohol ingestion slows hepatic metabolism and causes transiently higher concentrations of oxidatively metabolized benzodiazepines leading to further sedation. Antacids that slow gastric emptying may decrease the rate of absorption of a hypnotic agent from its primary site of origin, the small intestine. This could alter both onset and peak concentration effects.

Benzodiazepines all undergo some form of hepatic metabolism, although some agents are much more extensively metabolized than others. Medications that inhibit hepatic microsomal oxidative metabolism may cause clinically meaningful drug interactions when combined with benzodiazepines. All currently available triazolobenzodiazepines (e.g., alprazolam, estazolam, midazolam, triazolam) and diazepam are metabolized by hepatic microsomes and are complete or partial substrates of the CYP 3A4 isoform. Medications that are potent inhibitors of this system will cause higher peak concentrations of the triazolobenzodiazepine, particularly triazolam, which is highly hepatically metabolized. Nefazodone, ketaconazole, cimetidine, and macrolide antibiotics are examples of clinically relevant CYP 3A4 inhibitors which may cause a reduction in the clearance of these triazolobenzodiazepines and an increase in their blood and brain concentrations. This increase is greatest with higher hepatic clearance drugs such as triazolam or midazolam and somewhat less for drugs such as alprazolam or estazolam.

The CYP 1A2 isoform is also important in insomnia but from a different perspective. Methylxanthines (e.g., caffeine) and certain bronchodilators, such as theophylline, are significantly metabolized via CYP 1A2-mediated pathways. Inhibition of CYP 1A2 activity by the SSRI fluvoxamine or by certain fluroquinolone antibiotics (e.g., ciprofloxacin) in patients also ingesting caffeinated beverages or in those requiring theophylline may result in insomnia, agitation, or increased anxiety.

All benzodiazepine hypnotic agents are FDA Pregnancy Category X, meaning their use should be avoided during pregnancy, especially during the first trimester due to an increased risk of congenital malformations. A variety of congenital malformations, including cleft palate, delayed ossification of a number of bony structures, and an increased occurrence of rudimentary ribs have been reported. Chronic usage of benzodiazepines during pregnancy may lead to physiologic dependence and withdrawal symptoms in the neonate. The use of benzodiazepine hypnotics during the last weeks of pregnancy may result in neonatal central nervous system (CNS) depression, and their use during labor may lead to neonatal flaccidity. Nursing also poses significant hazards, as all benzodiazepines are distributed into breast milk to varying degrees. Since infants metabolize benzodiazepines more slowly than adults, accumulation may occur, leading to sedation and nursing difficulties in the infant. Pregnant women who have insomnia should be reminded of sleep hygiene techniques and given any hypnotic agent only with extreme caution. Diphenhydramine can be used with relative safety, but only for short periods of time since tachyphylaxis develops with prolonged use.

Benzodiazepines must be used in patients with obstructive sleep apnea only with extreme caution. Benzodiazepines may cause respiratory depression and can render patients less likely to mount an appropriate respiratory response to hypoxia. Hypnotic agents such as zolpidem, zaleplon, or trazodone are less likely to cause problems for sleep apnea patients and may be preferable alternatives. Aggressive evaluation and treatment of sleep apnea [e.g., (continuous positive airway pressure) CPAP] is extremely important to ensure adequate restorative sleep.

## Chloral Hydrate

Chloral hydrate was among the earliest sleeping pills. Its sedating qualities become evident within 30 minutes of administration, as it is rapidly absorbed from the gastrointestinal tract. At dosages between 0.5 and 1.5 g, it is an effective hypnotic agent. The elimination half-life of its active metabolite, trichloroethanol, is 6 to 8 hours, rendering it unlikely to cause significant next-day sedation or functional impairment. Despite the potential benefits of a rapid onset of action and relatively short elimination half-life, chloral hydrate is rarely used as a hypnotic agent today. It has a narrow therapeutic index (toxic dose–therapeutic dose), causes gastric irritation, nausea, and vomiting easily, and may cause gastric necrosis at high doses. Overdose can be fatal due to respiratory depression.

As with other sedative–hypnotics, dependence and tolerance may develop. Withdrawal symptoms that may develop when chloral hydrate is discontinued following prolonged use include, confusion, hallucinations, stomach pain, and severe anxiety. Chloral hydrate is metabolized in the liver and erythrocytes to its active metabolite trichloroethanol. Trichloroethanol is approximately 40% protein bound, and has the capacity to displace other drugs from their protein binding sites. Further metabolism to inactive metabolites occurs in both the liver and kidneys, and it is renally excreted. Prolonged dosage may lead to induction of hepatic microsomal enzymes as well. Any medication with significant sedating properties should be used with extreme caution with chloral hydrate, as the effects are additive. When chloral hydrate is taken along with alcohol the effect can be supraadditive (as in a Mickey Finn or knockout drops). Chloral hydrate generally increases sleep stages 2 and 4, decreases stage 3 sleep, and has no effect on REM sleep.

## Zolpidem

Zolpidem is also a nonbenzodiazepine hypnotic. A member of the imidazopyridine class, it is available in 5 and 10 mg dosages. Its mechanism of action shares much in common with benzodiazepines as it is active at central benzodiazepine (sometimes called ω) receptors. The ω receptor is a subunit of the GABA$_A$ receptor. Benzodiazepines are thought to bind nonselectively and activate all ω receptor subtypes; by contrast, zolpidem appears to bind preferentially to ω$_1$ receptors. Although this selective binding is not absolute, it may explain the relative absence of myorelaxant, anxiolytic, and anticonvulsant effects of zolpidem at hypnotic dose, as well as the preservation of stages 3 and 4 sleep. Polysomnographic experience with zolpidem indicates that zolpidem induces a sleep pattern very similar to that of physiological sleep, and generally produces little effect on sleep architecture following abrupt discontinuation (Darcourt et al. 1999).

Zolpidem is rapidly absorbed through the gastrointestinal tract and has a rapid onset of action. Peak concentration occurs from 30 minutes to 2 hours following administration. It is metabolized in the liver to several inactive metabolites and has an elimination half-life of approximately 2.5 hours. The elimination half-life is prolonged in the elderly and in patients with impaired hepatic or renal function. Zolpidem is a partial CYP 3A4 substrate. Zolpidem overdose can cause respiratory depression or coma, especially when combined with other CNS depressants. The benzodiazepine antagonist flumazenil can reverse the effects of an overdose of zolpidem, reflecting its benzodiazepine-like mechanism of action.

Although zolpidem is classified as a schedule IV drug by the FDA, it appears to cause tolerance and withdrawal syndromes somewhat less frequently than benzodiazepine hypnotics do. Withdrawal symptoms occur more frequently at doses higher than the *Physician's Desk Reference* (PDR), which recommends a maximum dose of 10 mg. The selectivity for ω$_1$ receptors appears to be lost at higher-than-standard hypnotic dosages as well. Cross tolerance with alcohol and benzodiazepines are found at these higher doses, and the incidence of adverse effects is much higher. Anecdotal reports of hallucinations and confusion at standard hypnotic dosages have been reported (Toner et al. 1999, Ansseau et al. 1992), but further research is needed to determine the prevalence of such occurrences across a spectrum of dosages and age groups.

## Zaleplon

Zaleplon is a nonbenzodiazepine hypnotic of the pyrazolopyrimidine class. Like zolpidem, zaleplon binds preferentially to central benzodiazepine (or ω) receptors. Zaleplon binds to the ω$_1$, ω$_2$, and ω$_3$ subunits, while zolpidem bind only to the ω$_1$ subunit. Its effects can also be reversed by flumazenil. Zaleplon is rapidly absorbed from the gastrointestinal tract, reaching peak serum concentrations within 1 hour. Absolute bioavailability is only 30% as it undergoes extensive hepatic first-pass metabolism. Zaleplon is primarily metabolized by aldehyde oxidase and forms a number of inactive metabolites. Its elimination half-life is approximately 1 hour. Since cimetidine inhibits aldehyde oxidase and CYP 3A4, and may increase zaleplon plasma concentrations by 85%, the initial starting dose of zaleplon should be halved in patients also taking cimetidine. Other potent inhibitors of the CYP 3A4 system such as ketoconazole and erythromycin also may increase zaleplon levels.

Because of the quick onset of action of zaleplon and its short elimination half-life, it can be used for patients who have a difficult time initiating sleep, but are able to remain asleep throughout the remainder of the night. In patients who have difficulty both in initiating and in maintaining sleep, zaleplon may permit the initiation of sleep, but be less effective in maintaining sleep due to its short elimination half-life. On the other hand, this same short half-life can be an advantage, as it can permit middle of the night dosing for those patients who awaken then. The short half-life permits such a dosing schedule without causing significant next-day sedation (Walsh et al. 2000).

Zaleplon, like zolpidem, is classified as a schedule IV drug by the FDA. Higher than standard dosages have been associated with an abuse potential similar to that of triazolam. With dosages of 20 mg or less, abuse and dependence appears to be significantly less than that of benzodiazepine hypnotic agents (Rush et al. 1999). Rebound insomnia has been reported, but it appears to occur less frequently than in the short acting benzodiazepines such as triazolam.

## Other Prescription Hypnotics

Barbiturates are commonly prescribed outside the US for insomnia. Butabarbital, phenobarbital, and secobarbital, are the most commonly prescribed barbiturates. The barbiturates are potentially lethal in overdose due to the risk of respiratory depression, and they commonly cause induction of hepatic oxidative metabolism. Their use has generally been replaced by other agents with better side effect profiles such as the benzodiazepines, the imadazopyridines, and the pyrazolopyrimidines.

Hydroxyzine hydrochloride and hydroxyzine pamoate are sedating H$_1$ receptor antagonists that are used occasionally as hypnotic agents. Sedation occurs with these agents due to inhibition of histamine *N*-methyltransferase and blockage of central histaminergic receptors. Next-day sedation is a common problem with antihistamines as they have a relatively long elimination half-life. These agents are highly anticholinergic and may cause hypotension and are not usually recommended as first-line agents for the treatment of insomnia.

Small doses of sedating tricyclic antidepressants (e.g., amitriptyline, doxepin) are sometimes used as hypnotics. Patients with chronic pain may particularly benefit from this treatment strategy, as low-dose tricyclic antidepressants have been found to be helpful in alleviating the pain associated with a variety of chronic pain conditions. Tricyclic antidepressants are potent inhibitors of REM sleep, and their discontinuation is often associated with REM rebound. The anticholinergic and adrenergic side effects, and the toxicity in overdose are issues that must be considered when these agents are prescribed. Mirtazapine is a newer sedating antidepressant that targets both the noradrenergic and serotonergic systems. It may be a useful alternative to the tricyclic antidepressants as it is less anticholinergic and less toxic in overdose. Mirtazapine has strong antihistaminic activity that may cause significant weight gain with chronic use.

Trazodone, a triazolopyridine compound marketed as an antidepressant, is frequently used as a hypnotic. Hypnotic dosages vary markedly, from 25 to 300 mg, depending on individual susceptibility to its sedating effects. Trazodone increases slow wave sleep and total sleep time and does not appear to affect REM sleep like other antidepressants do (Yamadera et al. 1998). Its elimination half-life of between 6 and 9 hours renders trazodone likely to cause daytime drowsiness. Using the lowest effective dosage can minimize this effect, as taking the medication in late evening rather than at bedtime. Trazodone is commonly used to counter the insomnia associated with SSRI use. It is rarely used as a sole antidepressant because of its strong sedating qualities and the need to take the medication more than once per day because of its half-life. Tolerance to its sedating effects develops only rarely with long-term use, making it an excellent option for those with chronic insomnia. Priapism is an exceedingly rare side effect, occurring in less than one in 40,000 cases. Since anticholinergic side effects and postural hypotension are not common, trazodone has some advantages over the tricyclic antidepressants.

## Suggested Guidelines for Prescribing Medications

It is often clinically useful to provide patients with information on good sleep hygiene practices (e.g., see Table 99–3). Certain elements are particularly important (e.g., going to another room and waiting until drowsy or looking for clues about waking life events, and issues that may be keeping one awake). Behavioral techniques such as stimulus control and progressive muscle relaxation are quite useful. When a hypnotic agent is prescribed, it is helpful to advise patients to take the medication on an empty stomach and with ample fluids (e.g., a full glass of water) to promote rapid dissolution and absorption, and onset of effect. For patients prone to nocturia the amount of fluids should be lessened substantially. One should always caution patients about potential impairments in memory, coordination, or driving skills and about unsteadiness if they are awakened after having taken a sleep aid. It is also important to remind them that if they use the medication for more than a few nights, some pattern of tapering should be followed when they stop. It is reinforcing to work out a discontinuation schedule at the time of the first prescription. Patients should also be cautioned to avoid the use of alcohol when taking a hypnotic as the effects are additive in nature. Medications such as the benzodiazepines that have a propensity to be abused should be avoided in those patients with drug or alcohol problems.

Universally accepted guidelines for dosing and duration of use for hypnotics are not established. Both dose and duration must be individualized with the goal of finding the lowest dose and the shortest duration. Short-term treatment (i.e., from 1 or 2 nights to 1 or 2 weeks) is reasonable for most patients. However, some patients with chronic insomnia may benefit from longer-term use provided that there is careful monitoring by the prescribing physician. No criteria are presently available to identify this subpopulation. It seems reasonable to consider several short-term

trials, with gradual tapering at the end of each period and a drug-free interval between each period, to establish the patient's need for and the appropriateness and value of continued therapy. The drug-free time interval between the initial periods should range from 1 to 3 weeks, depending on the half-life of the agent and its active metabolites and the rapidity of the taper schedule. Reevaluation of such a patient's continued need for hypnotic medication at 3- to 6-month intervals is also reasonable. Because the elderly are particularly susceptible to falls or confusion from hypnotic medication, use of the lowest available dosage strength is advisable. The elderly should also avoid the use of longer half-life agents or those with active metabolites with long half-lives because such medications tend to accumulate over time in older patients due to pharmacodynamic differences in drug metabolism in the elderly.

For those individuals who hope to benefit from behavioral and nonpharmacological approaches to their insomnia, prescribing hypnotics 2 or 3 times per week while they are working out such modifications may be beneficial. Because there are few predictable central tendencies that characterize patients with primary insomnia, individual variation is likely.

### Case Vignette

Mr. B is a 51-year-old married male who has had problems with sleep for the past 1 year. He typically takes over 2 hours to get to sleep and has noted increasing problems with daytime somnolence. Mr. B had tried OTC diphenhydramine and found it effective for the first few days, but it recently had lost its hypnotic efficacy and also rendered him quite tired in the morning. He had found that drinking two glasses of wine before bed helped him fall asleep, but he found that he often was awoken in the early morning and could not return to sleep. His work performance has started to suffer, and his wife and several coworkers suggested that he get help for his insomnia.

Upon examination, Mr. B appeared mildly depressed and acknowledged that recent marital problems had been weighing on his mind. Physical examination was within normal limits. The history revealed the aforementioned alcohol intake, but minimal caffeine use. The physician suggested that he must stop drinking alcohol and that he and his wife pursue marital counseling. A follow-up appointment was offered within a week. At this visit, Mr. B stated that his insomnia was no better and his depression had worsened significantly. He was placed on an antidepressant and began noting a significant improvement in his mood within 2 weeks. He stated the marital counseling was improving his marital relationship and that his improved mood had made a difference in their relationship as well. Mr. B found that it was much easier to sleep now and that his energy level and concentration had improved substantially. His boss and coworkers noted a significant improvement in his work performance and Mr. B soon felt that he had returned to his old self again.

## References

Andrade C, Srihari BS, Reddy KP, et al. (2001) Melatonin in medically ill patients with insomnia: A double-blind, placebo-controlled study. J Clin Psychiatr 62, 41–45.

Ansseau M, Pitchot W, Hansenne M, et al. (1992) Psychotic reactions to zolpidem. Lancet 339, 809.

Chase GE and Gidal BE (1997) Melatonin: Therapeutic use in sleep disorders. Ann Pharmacother 31, 1218–1226.

Chesson AL, Anderson WM, Littner M, et al. (1999) Practice parameters for the nonpharmacologic treatment of chronic insomnia. Sleep 22, 1128–1133.

Darcourt G, Pringuey D, Sallière D, et al. (1999) The safety and tolerability of zolpidem—An update. J Psychopharmacol 13, 81–93.

Gallup Organization (1991) Sleep in America: A national survey of US adults. A report prepared for the National Sleep Foundation. National Sleep Foundation, Los Angeles.

Gallup Organization (1995) Sleep in America 1995. The Gallup Organization, Princeton, NJ.

Morin CM, Hauri PJ, Espie CA, et al. (1999) Nonpharmacologic treatment of chronic insomnia. An American Academy of Sleep Medicine review. Sleep 22, 1134–1156.

Nowell PD, Mazumdar S, Buysse DJ, et al. (1997) Benzodiazepines and zolpidem for chronic insomnia. A meta-analysis of treatment efficacy. JAMA 278, 2170–2177.

Ray WA, Griffin MR, and Downey W (1989) Benzodiazepines of long and short elimination half-life and the risk of hip fracture. JAMA 262, 3303–3307.

Ray WA, Griffin MR, Schaffner W, et al. (1987) Psychotropic drug use and the risk of hip fracture. New Engl J Med 319, 1701–1707.

Roth T (2001) New developments for treating sleep disorders. J Clin Psychiatr 62(Suppl 10), 3–4.

Rush CR, Frey JM, and Griffiths RR (1999) Zaleplon and triazolam in humans: Acute behavioral effects and abuse potential. Psychopharmacology 145, 39–51.

Shader RI (1996) Sedative–hypnotics. In Psychiatry, Vol. 2, Tasman A, Kay J, and Lieberman JA (eds). WB Saunders, Philadelphia, pp. 1650–1658.

Shader RI and Greenblatt DJ (1994) Treatment of transient insomnia. In Manual of Psychiatric Therapeutics, 2nd ed., Shader RI (ed). Little Brown, Boston, pp. 211–216.

Simon GE and VonKorff M (1997) Prevalence, burden, and treatment of insomnia in primary care. Am J Psychiatr 154, 1417–1423.

Smith MT, Perlis ML, Park A, et al. (2002) Comparative meta-analysis of pharmacotherapy and behavior therapy for persistent insomnia. Am J Psychiatr 159, 5–11.

Stevinson C and Ernst E (2000) Valerian for insomnia: A systematic review of randomized clinical trials. Sleep Med 1, 91–99.

Stoller M (1994) Economic effects of insomnia. Clin Therap 16, 873–897.

Toner LC, Tsambiras BM, Catalano G, et al. (1999) Central nervous system side effects associated with zolpidem treatment. Clin Neuropharmacol 23, 54–58.

Walsh JK and Engelhart CL (1999) The direct economic costs of insomnia in the United States for 1995. Sleep 22(Suppl 2), S386–S393.

Walsh JK, Pollak CP, Scharf MB, et al. (2000) Lack of residual sedation following middle-of-the-night zaleplon administration in sleep maintenance insomnia. Clin Neuropharmacol 23, 17–21.

Yamadera H, Nakumura S, Suzuki H, et al. (1998) Effects of trazodone hydrochloride and imipramine on polysomnography in healthy subjects. Psychiatr Clin Neurosci 52, 439–443.

# 100 Stimulants

Laurence L. Greenhill
Erin Shockey
Jeffrey Halperin
John March

Psychostimulants are highly effective treatment agents that have been used for the treatment of depression, attention-deficit/hyperactivity disorder (ADHD), neurasthenia, and acquired immunodeficiency syndrome dementia. However, the greatest clinical application for psychostimulants has been the treatment of childhood disorders. Therefore, this chapter concentrates on the use of psychostimulants in the long-term treatment of children with disruptive behavior disorders—in particular, ADHD. The indications for their use, the methods for initiating treatment, and the interactions of their effects with comorbid psychiatric problems and developmental disorders are discussed. Also examined are the efficacy of the sustained-release preparations; recent evidence for tachyphylaxis associated with repeated dosing of psychostimulants within a single day and the implications of these findings on recommended doses; and whether adult patients with ADHD respond to psychostimulants.

More than 180 placebo-controlled investigations demonstrate that psychostimulants—methylphenidates, amphetamines, or pemoline—are effective in reducing core symptoms of childhood ADHD. Approximately 70% of patients respond to stimulants compared with 13% to placebo. Short-term efficacy is more pronounced for behavioral rather than cognitive and learning abnormalities associated with ADHD. The stimulant treatment evidence base was supplemented at the end of the 1990s by large multisite randomized controlled trials—particularly the Multimodal Treatment Study of ADHD (MTA Study) (The MTA Cooperative Group 1999)—that further support the short-term efficacy in school-age children. This study, together with the 1998 NIH Consensus Development Conference on ADHD (Ferguson 2000), and the publication of the McMaster Evidence Based Review of ADHD Treatments (Jadad et al. 1999) have emphasized the strong evidence base for ADHD stimulant treatments. In contrast, there remains much less evidence for the efficacy of psychostimulants in the treatment of ADHD in preschoolers, adolescents, and adults because of the lack of large-scale randomized clinical trials for those age groups. The main side effects of psychostimulant therapy in placebo-controlled trials—insomnia, decreased appetite, stomachache, and headache—occur more frequently in patients on an active drug than on a placebo. Although psychostimulants are clearly effective in the short term up through 14 months, concern remains that long-term benefits over years have not yet been adequately assessed.

## Psychostimulants: Efficacy and Utility

Three groups of stimulants are currently approved by the FDA for treatment of ADHD in children, and are available in both brand and generic. These include: the amphetamines (Adderall®, Dextrostat®, Dexedrine®), the methylphenidates (Concerta®, Metadate-ER®, Metadate-CD®, methylphenidate, Methylin®, Ritalin®, Ritalin-SR®, Ritalin-LA®, and Focalin®), and magnesium pemoline (Cylert®). Characteristics of these stimulants can be found in Tables 100–1 and 100–2. While dextroamphetamine (DEX) and methylphenidate (MPH) are structurally related to the catecholamines (DA and NE), pemoline (PEM) has a different structure, although it too has strong DA effects in the central nervous system (CNS) (McCracken 1991). The term *psychostimulant* used for these compounds refers to their ability to increase CNS activity in some but not all brain regions.

Stimulants ameliorate disruptive ADHD behaviors cross-situationally (classroom, lunchroom, playground, and home) when repeatedly administered throughout the day. In the classroom, stimulants decrease interrupting, fidgetiness, finger tapping, and increase on-task behavior (Abikoff and Gittelman 1985b); on the playground, stimulants reduce overt aggression (Gadow et al. 1990), covert aggression (Hinshaw et al. 1992), signs of conduct disorder (Klein et al. 1997), and increase attention during baseball (Pelham et al. 1990b). At home, stimulants improve parent-child interactions, on-task behaviors and compliance; in social settings, stimulants ameliorate peer nomination rankings (Whalen et al. 1989). Stimulants decrease response variability and impulsive responding on cognitive tasks (Tannock et al. 1995b) and increase the accuracy of performance, improve short-term memory, reaction time, seatwork computation, problem-solving games with peers (Hinshaw et al. 1989), and sustained attention. Studies of time–action stimulant effects show a different pattern of improvement for behavioral and for attentional symptoms, with behavior affected more than attention. For example, a controlled, analog classroom trial ($N=30$) of Adderall

| Table 100–1 | Stimulant Drugs, Doses, and Pharmacodynamics | | | | |

| Medication | Tablets/Dosages | Dose Range | Administration | Peak Effect | Duration of Action |
|---|---|---|---|---|---|
| **Amphetamines** | | | | | |
| Dexedrine® | 5 mg | 10–40 mg/d | b.i.d. or t.i.d. | 1–3 h | 5 h |
| Adderall® | 5, 7.5, 10, 12.5, 15, 20, 30 mg | 10–40 mg/d | b.i.d. or t.i.d. | 1–3 h | 5 h |
| Dextrostat® (generic) | 5, 10 mg | 10–40 mg/d | b.i.d. or t.i.d. | 1–3 h | 5 h |
| *Long-duration type* | | | | | |
| Dexedrine Spansule® | 5, 10, 15 mg spansule | 10–45 mg/d | once-daily | 1–4 h | 6–9 h |
| Adderall XR® | 10, 20, 30 mg capsules | 10–40 mg/d | once-daily | 1–4 h | 9 h |
| **Methylphenidates** | | | | | |
| Ritalin® | 5, 10, 20 mg | 10–60 mg/d | t.i.d. | 1–3 h | 2–4 h |
| Methylphenidate | 5, 10, 20 mg | 10–60 mg/d | t.i.d. | 1–3 h | 2–4 h |
| Methylin® | 5, 10, 20 mg | 10–60 mg/d | t.i.d. | 1–3 h | 2–4 h |
| Focalin® | 2.5, 5, 10 mg | 5–30 mg/d | b.i.d. | 1–4 h | 2–5 h |
| *Long-duration type* | | | | | |
| Ritalin-SR® | 20 mg | 20–60 mg/d | q.d. in AM or b.i.d. | 3 h | 5 h |
| Metadate-ER® | 10, 20 mg | 20–60 mg/d | q.d. in AM or b.i.d. | 3 h | 5 h |
| Medadate-CD® | 20 mg | 20–60 mg/d | q.d. in AM | 5 h | 8 h |
| Concerta® | 18, 36, 54 mg | 18–54 mg/d | q.d. in AM | 8 h | 12 h |
| Ritalin-LA® | 20, 30, 40 mg | 20–60 mg/d | q.d. in AM | 5 h | 8 h |
| Pemoline (Cylert®) | 18.75, 37.5, 75 mg; 37.5 chewable | 37.5–112.5 mg/d | q.d. in AM or b.i.d. | 2–4 h | 7 h |

revealed rapid improvements on teacher ratings of behavior and math performance scores 1.5 hours after administration, with time of duration of effects on behavior specifically dependent on dose (Swanson et al. 1998). While stimulant drugs show a large 0.8 to 1.0 effect size for behavioral measures, smaller 0.6 to 0.8 effect sizes are reported on cognitive measures (Spencer et al. 1996).

Children with ADHD demonstrate low placebo response rates during clinical drug trials, ranging between 3% (Spencer et al. 1996) and 30% (Gillberg et al. 1997). The resulting large placebo-active drug differences enable small-*N*, single-site, double-blind, crossover trial designs to identify significant drug effects. The short elimination half-lives make stimulants especially suitable for crossover trials (Swanson et al. 1998), because pharmacokinetic carryover of active drug into placebo periods is unlikely.

The beneficial effects of stimulants on behavior and attention have also been shown in children with no mental disorder (Rapoport et al. 1980), so the response to stimulants is not diagnostically specific for ADHD. Stimulant medications continue to play a therapeutic role in other

| Table 100–2 | Commercial Forms of Stimulants Available | | | | |

| Drug | Mechanism of Drug Release | Duration of Action | Sprinkle Form Available? | Total Daily Dose | Pill Dose Strengths Available |
|---|---|---|---|---|---|
| Adderall XR | 2 pulse | 10.5 h | Yes | 10–30 mg | 5, 10, 15, 20, 25, 30 |
| Concerta | 3 pulse | 12 h | No | 18–54 mg | 18, 27, 36, 54 |
| Dx Spansule | 1 pulse | 5 h | No | 15 mg | 5, 10, 15 |
| Metadate CD | 2 pulse | 8–10 h | Yes | 20–40 mg | 20 mg |
| Metadate ER | Wax matrix | 5–6 h | No | 20–40 mg | 10, 20 mg |
| Methylin ER | Wax matrix | 5–6 h | No | 20–40 mg | 10, 20 mg |
| MPH SR | Wax matrix | 5–6 h | No | 20–40 mg | 20 mg |
| Methypatch | Transdermal | On skin | No | 55 mg | 25.37 cm$^2$ |
| Focalin | Chiral | 5–6 h | No | 10 mg | 2.5, 5, 10 |
| Ritalin LA | 2 pulse | 8–10 h | Yes | 20–40 mg | 20, 30, 40 |
| Ritalin SR | Wax matrix | 5–6 h | No | 20–40 mg | 20 mg |

medical conditions, such as narcolepsy and depression (Goldman et al. 1998).

Compared to placebo, psychostimulants have a significantly greater ability to reduce ADHD symptoms that disrupt the classroom and impact the child's social relationships (Jacobvitz et al. 1990). In experimental settings, stimulants have been shown to improve child behavior during parent–child interactions (Barkley and Cunningham 1979) and problem-solving activities with peers (Whalen et al. 1989). Children with ADHD have a tendency to elicit negative, directive, and controlling behavior from parents and peers (Campbell 1973). When these children are placed on stimulants, their mothers' rate of disapproval, commands, and control diminish to the extent seen between other mothers and their non-ADHD children (Barkley and Cunningham 1979, Humphries et al. 1978, Barkley et al. 1984). In the laboratory, stimulant-treated children with ADHD demonstrate major improvements during experimenter-paced continuous performance tests (Halperin et al. 1992), paired-associate learning, cued and free recall, auditory and reading comprehension, spelling recall, and arithmetic computation (Stephens et al. 1984, Pelham and Bender 1982). Some studies show correlations between plasma levels of MPH and performance on a laboratory task (Greenhill et al. 2001), but the levels only correlate with behavioral effects if the timing of the plasma sampling is exact. Likewise, hyperactive conduct-disordered children and preadolescents show reductions in aggressive behavior when treated with stimulants and observed in structured and unstructured school settings (Hinshaw 1991). Stimulants can also reduce the display of covert antisocial behaviors such as stealing and property destruction (Hinshaw et al. 1992)

## Theoretical Basis of Drug Action

### Mechanism of Action: Receptor Activity

The term psychostimulant refers to the ability of these compounds to increase CNS activity in some but not all brain regions. For example, while increasing the activity of striatum and connections between orbitofrontal and limbic regions, stimulants seem to have an inhibitory effect on the neocortex. The CNS psychostimulant effects of DEX and MPH may result in part from their lack of benzene ring substituents. Prominent central effects include activation of the medullary respiratory center and a lessening of central depression from barbiturates.

Psychostimulants have been described as noncatecholamine sympathomimetics. Sympathomimetics show potent agonist effects at alpha- and beta-adrenergic receptors. Presynaptically, they cause a stoichiometric displacement of norepinephrine and dopamine from storage sites in the presynaptic terminal. Stimulants also block the reuptake of dopamine by the dopamine transporter (DAT). Postsynaptically, they function as direct agonists at the adrenergic receptor. They also block the action of a degradative enzyme, catechol-o-methyltransferase (COMT).

DEX and MPH are thought to act differently on the presynaptic neuron. DEX's release of dopamine can be blocked by alpha-methylparatyrosine (AMPT), but not reserpine, suggesting that DEX acts primarily on a cytoplasmic pool of newly synthesized dopamine. The release of dopamine by MPH, on the other hand, can be blocked by reserpine pretreatment. Therefore MPH has been thought to act primarily on longer-term vesicular storage. McCracken (1991) believes in a two-part model of stimulant action: the optimal benefit from stimulants occurs in ADHD only when "inhibitory presynaptic dopamine (DA) antagonism and alpha-2-adrenergic effects predominate, leading to reduction in ascending mesolimbic DA inhibition and reduced LC–NE (locus coeruleus–norepinephrine) activity, respectively."

Peripherally, sympathomimetics have potent agonist effects at alpha- and beta-adrenergic receptors. DEX stimulates cardiac muscle, raising systolic and diastolic blood pressure, with a reflex slowing of heart rate. Psychostimulants can also cause urinary bladder smooth muscle to contract at the sphincter and will increase uterine muscle tone and produce bronchodilatation.

## Stimulant Medications and Cerebral Metabolism

The putative action of psychostimulants in ADHD has been attributed to the release of DA and their ability to block its reuptake by the DAT at the presynaptic nerve terminal. Radioligand binding studies have demonstrated the direct action of psychostimulants, particularly MPH, on striatal DAT. The dopamine action of psychostimulants also explains the appearance of behavioral stereotypies, seen at high doses. Tritiated MPH binding in rat brain is highest in striatum and is highly dependent on sodium concentration, suggesting that MPH binding is associated with a neurotransmitter transport system.

Yet, no single theory explains the psychostimulant mechanism of action on the CNS which ameliorates ADHD symptoms. The drug's effect based on a single neurotransmitter has been discounted (Zametkin and Rapoport 1987), as well as its ability to correct the ADHD child's under- or overaroused CNS (Solanto 1984). To date, brain imaging has reported few consistent psychostimulant effects on glucose metabolism. While some studies in ADHD adults using positron emission tomography (PET) and [$^{18}$F]fluorodeoxyglucose show that stimulants lead to increased brain glucose metabolism in the striatal and frontal regions (Ernst and Zametkin 1995), others (Matochik et al. 1993, 1994) have been unable to find a change in glucose metabolism during acute and chronic stimulant treatment.

Studies utilizing PET scan have demonstrated that adults with a past history of ADHD show 8.1% lower levels of cerebral glucose metabolism than do control subjects (Zametkin et al. 1991), with the greatest differences in the superior prefrontal cortex and premotor areas. These areas are involved with functions found deficient in children with ADHD, such as the modulation of attention or the ability to inhibit inappropriate responses.

MPH and DEX elevate glucose metabolism in the brains of rats, although patients with schizophrenia given DEX showed decreased glucose metabolism. No changes in cerebral glucose metabolism were found with PET scans done before taking medication and while medicated for 19 MPH-treated and 18 DEX-treated adults with ADHD, even though the adults showed significant changes in behavior. In related studies, single photon emission computed tomography (SPECT) showed reduced frontal cerebral blood flow in five children with ADHD when given MPH compared with normal subjects (Vyborova et al. 1984). This agrees with another SPECT finding, that is children with ADHD have greater overall uptake asymmetry than normal subjects.

Investigations of neuroanatomical relationships in children with ADHD support these findings. The midsagittal cross-sectional area of the corpus callosum, a structure that has multiple connections to frontal cortical areas, was measured from magnetic resonance images of 15 boys with ADHD and 15 matched boys with no psychiatric disorder. Two of seven anatomical areas were found to be significantly smaller in the boys with ADHD.

MPH, like cocaine, has high affinity for the DAT, and DAT blockade is now regarded as the putative mechanism for psychostimulant in the human CNS. PET scan data in adult substance abusers show that [$^{11}$C]methylphenidate concentration in brain is maximal in striatum, an area rich in dopamine terminals where DAT resides (Volkow et al. 1995). These PET scans reveal a significant difference in the pharmacokinetics of [$^{11}$C]methylphenidate and [$^{11}$C]cocaine. Although both drugs display rapid uptake into striatum, MPH is more slowly cleared from brain. The authors speculate that this low reversal of binding to the DA transporter means that MPH is not as reinforcing as cocaine and therefore, does not lead to as much self-administration as does cocaine. More recently, the same authors were able to show that therapeutic doses of oral MPH significantly increase extracellular dopamine in the human brain (Volkow et al. 1998). "DA decreases the background firing rates and increases signal-to-noise in target neurons. We postulate that the amplification of weak DA signals in subjects with ADHD by MPH would enhance task-specific signaling, improving attention, and decreasing distractibility," the authors commented.

## Structural Considerations

The stereochemical structure of the psychostimulants also has been related to their CNS activity. Early studies postulated that *d* isomers of amphetamine were selectively more effective for norepinephrine release but that both *d*- and *l*-amphetamine had equal effects on dopamine. A double-blind crossover study was carried out comparing the two isomers. Contrary to theory, *d*-amphetamine was found to act more quickly and to produce greater improvements on measures of attention than the *l* isomer. It appears that the *d* isomer of MPH also has a greater effect on locomotor activity and reuptake inhibition of labeled dopamine than the *l* isomer (Patrick et al. 1987). This has been incorporated into a new MPH preparation, dexmethylphenidate (Focalin), that has shown efficacy in controlled trials (Swanson et al. 2002).

The MPH molecule has two asymmetrical carbon atoms, resulting in four optical isomers: both *d* and *l* forms of the *threo* and *erythro* racemates. The *threo* isomer appears to have more potency than the *erythro*, perhaps owing to the 60° skew relationship between the tertiary amine and the carbomethoxy groups. This key relationship may increase the ability of these compounds to block dopamine reuptake. In the *erythro* form, these groups are transstaggered, and therefore no weak bond is formed between the nitrogen and carbonyl atoms (Patrick et al. 1987). The commercial manufacturing process produces equal parts of *d* and *l* isomers of *threo*-methylphenidate.

Most hypotheses regarding the neurochemical basis of ADHD have focused on the catecholamines norepinephrine and dopamine. These hypotheses, which posit a dysregulation in the norepinephrine or dopamine neurotransmitter systems, or both, are based primarily on the success of these dopaminergic medications in treating ADHD. All stimulant medications used for treating ADHD have their primary effects on these two neurotransmitter systems. Furthermore, the more selective norepinephrine-acting tricyclic medications, such as desipramine and imipramine, as well as the alpha-2-adrenergic agonist clonidine, have all been found to reduce symptoms of ADHD in children. Similarly, although much less commonly used, dopamine-blocking antipsychotic medications also have been found to be effective for treating children with ADHD (Zametkin and Rapoport 1987).

The dopamine hypothesis of ADHD is further supported by neuroimaging data, which indicate abnormalities in the dopamine-rich striatum and caudate nucleus in children with ADHD. Both the dopamine and the norepinephrine neurotransmitter hypotheses suggest a central role for dopamine in the manifestation of hyperactivity as an important role for the central norepinephrine pathways of the locus coeruleus in the regulation of attention, arousal, and vigilance.

One of the noncatecholamine neurotransmitters affected by these medications is serotonin (5-HT). Two open clinical studies, using the 5-HT reuptake inhibitor fluoxetine, reported a positive treatment response in children with ADHD, raising the possibility of 5-HT involvement in ADHD. These findings must be considered tentative for two reasons. First, well-controlled double-blind studies must be conducted to determine efficacy. Second, clinicians find selective serotonin reuptake inhibitors (SSRIs) to be ineffective for treatment of ADHD. However, data from several animal studies are also consistent with the possible involvement of central 5-HT mechanisms in the pathophysiology of ADHD. In rats, lesions and pharmacological manipulations that result in diminished 5-HT activity have been consistently reported to induce an increase in impulsive and aggressive behavior, as well as a persistent pattern of overactivity. Furthermore, developmentally early dopamine-depleting lesions, which can result in hyperactivity, cause sprouting of 5-HT terminals. It is conceivable that this early interaction between the dopamine and the 5-HT neurotransmitter systems has a substantial impact on the clinical presentation of children with ADHD.

Finally, biological data in children also raise the possibility of the involvement of central 5-HT mechanisms in at least some children with ADHD, particularly those with comorbid aggressive behavior. In a group of boys with disruptive disorders, approximately two-thirds of whom had ADHD, reduced cerebrospinal fluid levels of the serotonin metabolite 5-hydroxyindoleacetic acid were associated with high aggression ratings at the 2-year follow-up assessment (Castellanos et al. 1994). A reduced number of $^3$H-imipramine binding sites, a putative index of presynaptic 5-HT activity, was reported in another study (Stoff et al.

1987) that compared children with comorbid conduct disorder and ADHD diagnoses with normal control subjects. Halperin and colleagues (1994) found enhanced prolactin responses to a challenge dose of the 5-HT releaser–reuptake inhibitor fenfluramine in a subgroup of children with ADHD characterized by aggressive behavior.

Thus, several lines of data indicate that central monoamine neurotransmitter mechanisms are involved in the pathophysiology of ADHD. However, no single neurotransmitter hypothesis can fully account for the varied symptoms seen in children with ADHD. Preliminary data suggest a role for 5-HT mechanisms in some components of the ADHD syndrome, even though SSRIs have not been helpful in treatment.

## Neuroendocrine Responses to Psychostimulants

Neuroendocrine studies have suggested that psychostimulants produce effects in children identical to those observed in adults. These psychoneuroendocrine responses may be mediated by monoamine neurotransmitters. For example, DEX was reported to produce a suppression of mean sleep-related prolactin levels in 13 boys treated with 0.8 mg/kg/day for 6 months. DEX releases dopamine which exerts a tonic inhibitory control over prolactin release. Other hormonal responses are not suppressed by DEX, including cortisol release and mean sleep-related human growth hormone release.

Reports of the effect of MPH on human growth hormone secretion have been divergent. This may be a result of MPH's 2.5-hour half-life, which is shorter than DEX's 6- to 8-hour half-life. Given acutely, MPH does not suppress prolactin release during the sleep period the way DEX does. Given chronically, MPH has been shown to suppress prolactin levels, release human growth hormone, and increase beta-endorphin levels.

Psychostimulants also suppress somatomedin *in vitro*, which would limit long bone growth if it occurred *in vivo*. This could explain the decrease in height velocity that has been reported during treatment. For example, the prolonged use of DEX (0.8 mg/kg) during a 12-month period in 13 boys with ADHD produced a trend ($P < .07$) toward decreased somatomedin; these same patients had shown medication-related decreases in height and weight

velocity (Greenhill and Schwartz 1989, unpublished manuscript).

## Pharmacokinetics: Absorption and Metabolism

Psychostimulants are rapidly absorbed from the gut and thus act quickly, often within the first 30 minutes after ingestion. Food enhances absorption. Although early pharmacokinetic data reported MPH bioavailabilities in the 80% range, more recent studies have placed the actual figure closer to 30%. DEX concentrations in plasma range between 40 and 120 ng/mL in treated children with ADHD. Compared to DEX, clinically effective MPH oral doses produces much lower plasma concentrations—as low as 7 to 10 ng/mL—suggesting a large first-pass effect. However, relatively low concentrations of MPH are surprisingly effective. This is due, in part, to MPH's low plasma binding rate (15%), which makes it highly available to cross the blood–brain barrier. This situation creates a favorable brain–plasma partition, with a higher concentration in the CNS than in plasma (Patrick et al. 1987). Effects on behavior appear during absorption, beginning 30 minutes after ingestion and lasting 3 to 4 hours. Half-lives range between 3 hours for MPH and 6 to 9 hours for *d*-amphetamine. The concentration-enhancing and activity-reducing effects of MPH can disappear well before the medication leaves the plasma, a phenomenon termed *clockwise hysteresis*.

MPH's metabolism is rapid and complete because it is not highly bound to plasma protein and does not disappear into fat stores. MPH peaks in plasma in 2 to 2.5 hours and falls to half the peak (half-life) after 3 hours. The parent compound is metabolized by hydrolysis of the ester group to give the equivalent carboxylic acid, ritalinic acid. Approximately 20% is oxidized to *p*-hydroxy- and oxomethylphenidate by the liver.

Because MPH's short half-life prevents it from reaching steady state in the plasma, the standard tablet must be given several times a day to maintain behavioral improvement throughout the school day. Although the Physicians' Desk Reference (PDR) suggests giving MPH before meals, standard administration times are after breakfast (8:00 AM), after lunch (noon), and before homework (about 3:30 PM). See Table 100–3 for reviews of some of the pharmacokinetics of the psychostimulants used to treat children with ADHD.

| Table 100–3 | Stimulant Pharmacokinetics and Pharmacodynamics | | |
|---|---|---|---|
| Parameter | Dextroamphetamine | Methylphenidate | Adderall |
| Metabolism | Hepatic to inactive metabolites | Hepatic to inactive metabolites | Hepatic to inactive or weakly active metabolites |
| Excretion | Renal, of metabolites; rate accelerated by acidification | Renal, of metabolites | Renal; rate accelerated by acidification |
| $T_{max}$ | 2–4 h | 1–3 h | 2–4 h |
| Half-life | 6–8 h | 2–4 h | 5–7 h |
| Effect onset | 30–60 min | 30–60 min | 30 min |
| Effect peak | 1–3 h | 1–3 h | 1–3 h |
| Effect duration | 3–5 h | 2–4 h | 3–5 h |

## Basis for Determining General Efficacy

### Clinical Trials

Bradley (1937) was the first physician to treat behaviorally disturbed children and adolescents with stimulants. He administered benzedrine, a racemic form of amphetamine, which produced a dramatic calming effect while increasing compliance and academic performance. Subsequently, Bradley published several case reports demonstrating that children's behavior problems were ameliorated by amphetamine treatment. Interest in psychostimulants increased after the first controlled investigations of these drugs were carried out between 1960 and 1970 (Conners 2000). During this period, psychostimulants were reported to increase the seizure threshold to photometrizol, decrease oppositional behavior of boys with conduct disorder in a residential school, and improve the target symptoms of ADHD as measured using standardized rating forms filled out by parents and teachers.

In subsequent years, many controlled treatment studies proved psychostimulants were effective in reducing the ADHD-related symptoms of gross motor overactivity, inattention, impulsivity, and noncompliance with adult requests. A review by Wilens and Biederman (1992) reported that a Medline search generated more than 990 citations about psychostimulants published between 1982 and 1991. Later reviews documented a much greater increase in citations (Greenhill et al. 1999) demonstrating beneficial short-duration psychostimulant effects on ADHD children. A major meta-analysis (Swanson 1993) revealed that more than 200 reviews, and thousands of specific studies have been published on psychostimulants.

In the past decade, there has been a flurry of new stimulant drug approvals by the US Food and Drug Administration for treatment of ADHD in children. Up to that time, only DEX (Dexedrine), MPH (Ritalin), and magnesium pemoline (Cylert) were sanctioned for use in children. More recently, methylphenidate-OROS (Concerta), beaded-methylphenidate (Metadate-CD, Ritalin-LA), dexmethylphenidate (Focalin), and long-duration mixed-salts of amphetamine (Adderall XR) have been approved. Characteristics of these stimulants can be found in Table 100–2. DEX and MPH form the active ingredients of these new preparations and are structurally related to the catecholamines (DA and NE).

A meta-analysis (Kavale 1982) of stimulant treatment studies reported significant improvements for stimulant-treated MPH subjects, with effect sizes of 0.5 to 0.9 standard deviations using behavioral measures. This suggests that response to stimulants, when compared with that to placebo, is in the range found with antibiotic treatments of infection, making the stimulant treatment of children with ADHD the most effective therapeutic modality in child psychiatry. These findings have been reported in a major review of 111 studies conducted among 4,777 children (Spencer et al. 1996).

Previous reviews of psychostimulant efficacy in the treatment of ADHD have reported drug effects on academic performance (Barkley 1977, DuPaul and Barkley 1990), mechanisms of action, diagnostic specificity, and the ability of these medications to enhance other therapies. Another more critical review found no evidence for a diagnostically specific medication response in children with ADHD and for a specific biochemical mechanism of action, and found no evidence that the short-term effects of psychostimulants can be maintained for more than a few months (Jacobvitz et al. 1990).

In the past 10 years, psychostimulant research has moved from single-site to multisite randomized controlled studies, mostly to gather controlled data for new drug FDA approval, as shown in Table 100–4. These modern-day controlled trials have matured with the field, and now utilize multiple-dose conditions with multiple stimulants (Elia et al. 1991), parallel designs (Spencer et al. 1995), and studies using a common definition of response as normalization (Abikoff and Gittelman 1985b, Rapport et al. 1994). These studies now test psychostimulants in special ADHD populations, including adolescents (Klorman et al. 1990), adults (Spencer et al. 1995), mentally retarded (Horn et al. 1991), ADHD subjects with anxiety disorders and internalizing disorders, and ADHD subjects with tic disorders (Gadow et al. 1995). Seventy percent of ADHD subjects respond to stimulants while only 10 to 20% improve on placebo.

Investigators have also studied stimulant nonresponders, although they have been difficult to find. Some drug trials (Douglas et al. 1988) report a 100% response rate in small samples in which multiple doses of MPH are used. Elia and colleagues (1991) reduced the 32% nonresponse rate to a single psychostimulant to less than 4% when a second stimulant was titrated sequentially in the same subject. However, these groups studied noncomorbid children. If children with comorbidity had been included, the rate of medication nonresponse might have been higher.

Finally, few studies have used the double-blind or single-blind placebo discontinuation model to determine if the child continues to respond to stimulants after being treated for 1 year or more. One study found that 80% of ADHD children relapsed when switched single blind from MPH to a placebo after 8 months of treatment (Abikoff 1994, personal communication). Even so, these observations about the "rare nonresponder" do not address the rate of placebo response. Few, if any, of the current randomized clinical trials (RCTs) are parallel designs, which can test to see if placebo response emerges at some point over the entire drug trial. Few treatment studies prescreen for placebo responders, so the numbers of actual medication responders in any sample of ADHD children might be closer to 55%, not the 75 to 96% often quoted. These estimates also apply to group effects and cannot inform the clinician about the individual patient.

### Long-Term Outcome: Randomized Controlled Trials of Stimulant Medication

Although short-duration stimulant studies have shown robust efficacy, their effects last only as long as the patient continues medication. ADHD is a chronic disorder lasting many years, and thus maintenance treatment constitutes the main component of care. Unfortunately, most stimulant RCTs last less than 3 months, with only 22 published studies lasting longer (Schachar and Tannock 1993). Most long-duration studies started before the 1990s were constrained by their retrospective methods, lack of nonstandard outcome measures, restrictive inclusion criteria

**Table 100-4   Controlled Studies Showing Stimulant Efficacy in ADHD Drug Treatments ($N$ = 1702)**

| Study (Year) | N | Age Range | Design | Drug (Dose) | Duration | Response | Comment |
|---|---|---|---|---|---|---|---|
| Abikoff and Gittelman (1985a) | 28 | 6–12 | ADHD Controls | MPH (PB, 41 mg) | 8 wk | 80.9% | ADHD children normalized |
| Abikoff and Hechtman (1998) | 103 | 6–12 | ADHD | MPH t.i.d. (33.7 mg) | 2 yr | 100% 2.7 SD | Multisite, multimodal study All children on MPH |
| Barkley et al. (1989) | 74 | 6–13 | X-over 37 agg 37 non-agg | MPH (PB, 0.3, 0.5) | 4 wk | 80% | Aggression responsive to MPH |
| Barkley et al. (1991) | 40 | 6–12 | X-over 23 ADHD 17 ADHD-W | MPH b.i.d (5, 10, 15 b.i.d.) PB b.i.d. | 6 wk | ADHD 95% ADHD-W 76% | Few children with ADHD-W respond, need low dose |
| Castellanos et al. (1997) | 20 | 6–13 | X-over | MPH 45 mg b.i.d. DEX 22.5 mg b.i.d. | 9 wk | ADHD + TS | Dose-related tics at high doses |
| Douglas et al. (1988) | 19 | 7–13 | X-over | MPH (PB, 0.15, 0.3, 0.6) | 2 wk | 100% | Linear D/R relationships |
| Douglas et al. (1995) | 17 | 6–11 | X-over | MPH (0.3, 0.6, 0.9) PB | 4 wk | beh 70% | No cognitive toxicity at high doses Linear D/R curves |
| DuPaul and Rapport (1993) | 31 | 6–12 | X-over 31 ADHD 25 normals | MPH (20 mg) PB b.i.d. | 6 wk | beh 78% att 61% | MPH can normalize classroom behavior 25% of ADHD subjects did not normalize in academics |
| DuPaul et al. (1994) | 40 | 6–12 | X-over 12 high ANX 17 mid ANX 11 low ANX | MPH (5, 10, 15 mg) PB single dose | 6 wk | high 68% nortriptyline mid 70% nortriptyline low 82% nortriptyline | 25% in internalizing group deteriorated on medications ADHD subjects with comorbid internalizing disorders less to be normalized or to respond to MPH |
| Elia et al. (1991) | 48 | 6–12 | X-over | MPH (0.5, 0.8, 1.5) PB b.i.d. DEX (0.25, 0.5, 0.75) | 6 wk | MPH 79% DEX 86% | Response rate for two stimulants = 96% |
| Gadow et al. (1995) | 34 | 6–12 | X-over ADHD+tic | MPH (0.1, 0.3, 0.5) PB b.i.d. | 8 wk | 100% MPH | No nonresponders to behavior; MD=s motor tic ratings show 2 min increases on drug; only shows effects of 8 wk treatment |
| Gillberg et al. (1997) | 62 | 6–12 | Parallel | AMP (17 mg) PB b.i.d. | 60 wk | 70% 27–40% impr | No drop-outs but only 25% placebo group at 15 mo assessment. |
| Greenhill et al. (2001) | 277 | 6–12 | Parallel | Metadate-CD Placebo | 3 wk | 70% | Mean total dose 40 mg/day. FDA registration |
| Klorman et al. (1990) | 48 | 12–18 | X-over | MPH t.i.d. (0.26) PB b.i.d. | 6 wk | MPH 60% | Less medical benefits for adolescents |
| Klein et al. (1997) | 84 | 6–15 | Parallel | MPH b.i.d. (1.0) | 5 wk | MPH 59–78% PB 9–29% | MPH reduced ratings of antisocial behaviors |

| Study (Year) | N | Age (Range) | Design | Drug (Dose) | Duration | Response | Comment |
|---|---|---|---|---|---|---|---|
| The MTA Cooperative group (1999) | 579 | 7–9 | Parallel | MPH t.i.d. (<0.8) | 4 wk (14 mo) | MPH 77% DEX 10% None 13% | Titration trial for multisite multimodal study Full study data for 288 on 38.7 mg MPH |
| Musten et al. (1997) | 31 | 4–6 | X-over | MPH b.i.d. (0.3, 0.5) | 3 wk | MPH>NA | MPH improves attention in preschoolers |
| Pelham et al. (1990a) | 22 | 8–13 | X-over | MPH 10 b.i.d. PB b.i.d. DEX span 10 mg PEM 56.25 q.d. | 24 d | stim 68% | DEX Span, PEM best for behavior 27% did best on DEX; 18% on SR; 18% on PEM; 5% on MPH bid. |
| Pelham et al. (1995) | 28 | 5–12 | X-over | PEM (18.75, 37.5, 75, 112.5 mg) PB o.d. | 7 wk | PEM 89% PB 0% | PEM dose ≥ 37.5 mg/d lasts 2–7 hours Efficacy and time course = MPH |
| Rapport et al. (1988) | 22 | 6–10 | X-over | MPH (PB, 5, 10, 15 mg) | 5 wk | 72% | MPH response same in home & school |
| Rapport et al. (1994) | 76 | 6–12 | X-over | MPH (5, 10, 15, 20 mg) PB b.i.d. | 5 wk | 94% beh 53% att | MPH normalizes behavior > academics Higher doses better, linear D/R curve; |
| Schachar et al. (1997) | 91 | 6–12 | Parallel | MPH (33.5 mg) PB b.i.d. | 52 wk | 0.7 SD effect size | 15% side effects: affective, over-focusing led to drop-outs |
| Spencer et al. (1995) | 23 | 18–60 | X-over | MPH (1 mg/kg/d) | 7 wk | 78% PB 4% | MPH at 1mg/kg/d produces improvement in adults equivalent to that seen in children |
| Swanson et al. (1998) | 29 | 7–14 | X-over | Adderall (5, 10, 15, 20, PB, MPH) | 7 wk | 100% | Adderall peaks at 3 hr, MPH at 1.5 hr |
| Tannock et al. (1995a) | 40 | 6–12 | X-over | MPH 22 (0.3, 0.6) 17 ADHD–Anx | 2 wk | 70% | Activity level better in both groups; working memory not improved in anxious kids |
| Tannock et al. (1995b) | 28 | 6–12 | X-over | MPH (0.3, 0.6, 0.9) PB | 2 wk | 70% 70% | Effects on behavior D/R curve linear, but effects on response inhibition U-shaped suggest adjustment dose on objective measures |
| Taylor et al. (1987) | 38 | 6–10 | X-over | MPH (PB, 0.2–1.4) | 6 wk | 58% | Severe ADHD symptoms, better response |
| Whalen et al. (1989) | 25 | 6.3–12 | X-over | MPH (PB, 0.3, 0.5) | 5 wk | 48–72% | MPH helps, not normalizes, peer status |
| Wolraich et al. (2002) | 277 | 6–12 | Parallel | Concerta 36 mg PB MPH t.i.d. | 4 wk | 62% | Concerta rated effective by teachers & parents |

Doses listed as mg/kg/dose, and medication is given twice daily unless otherwise stated. PB, placebo; X-over, crossover design; Anx, anxiety; MPH, Methylphenidate; DEX, Dextroamphetamine; PEM, pemoline; AMP, d, l-amphetamine (Adderall); mg/kg/d, dosage in milligram/kilogram/day; Agg, aggression; ADHD-W, ADD without hyperactivity; beh, behavior; att, attention; FDA, Food & Drug Administration; D/R curve, Dose/Response Curve.

which rejected patients with comorbid disorders, irregular prescribing patterns (Sherman 1991), and the lack of compliance measures (Richters et al. 1995). Long-duration trials have shown that maintenance of stimulant medication effects can be maintained over periods ranging from 12 (Gillberg et al. 1997) to 24 months (Abikoff and Hechtman 1998).

The NIMH MTA Study compared the relative effectiveness of four randomly-assigned, 14-month treatments of children with ADHD: medication management (MedMgt), behavioral treatment (Beh), the combination (Comb), or a community comparison group (CC) getting treatment as usual (Arnold et al. 1997). The study's null hypotheses included: (1) Beh and MedMgt treatments result in comparable levels of improvement over time (2) Participants assigned to Comb show similar improvement over time to those assigned to either MedMgt or to Beh (3) Participants assigned to any of the three MTA intensive treatments show similar improvement over time to those assigned to treatment as usual in CC.

To have sufficient power to address these questions, 579 children with ADHD, combined subtype, aged 7.0 to 9.0 years, were recruited at seven sites. They were assessed across six domains at four different points in time (Hinshaw et al. 1997). At study entry, they were randomized to 14 months of treatment in one of four groups: (a) MedMgt, (b) intensive Beh (parent, school, and child components, with therapist involvement gradually faded over time), (c) the two combined, or (d) treatments by community providers. Outcomes were assessed in multiple domains before, during, and at treatment endpoint (with Comb and MedMgt subjects on medication at time of assessment).

Children randomized to MedMgt alone ($N=144$) or to Comb ($N=145$) in the MTA Study participated in a 28-day double-blind, placebo-controlled, titration study in order to identify each child's optimal dose of MPH. Three doses of MPH and placebo were used in a three-times daily protocol (Greenhill et al. 1996). Medication conditions were switched daily to reduce error variance. Parents and teachers rated ADHD symptoms and impairment on a daily basis.

During titration, a repeated-measure analysis of variance (ANOVA) revealed a main effect of MPH placebo dose with greater effects on teacher's ratings ($F[3]=100.6$, $N=223$, $P=0.0001$; effect sizes 0.8 to 1.3) than on parent's ratings ($F[3]=55.61$, $N=253$, $P=0.00001$; effect sizes 0.4 to 0.6). Dose did not interact with between-subjects factors (period, dose order, comorbid diagnosis, site or treatment group). Drug-related adverse events were reported more often by parents than by teachers, who rated irritability highest on placebo. The distribution of the best MPH starting doses determined during titration (10–50 mg/day), response rate (77%), and adverse event profile across six sites and multiple subgroups suggest that MPH titration in office practice should explore MPH's full dosage range in 7- to 10-year-old children over 25 kg in weight. Parent weekend symptom ratings showed daytime drug effects, but not as clearly as weekday after-school ratings. Nonresponders to MPH were older, had less severe symptoms, and were medication-naïve. Thus, the MTA controlled multisite titration trial using daily dose switches replicated the published, single-site MPH trial effect sizes and adverse event rates (Spencer et al. 1996).

Data were analyzed through intent-to-treat, random-effects regression. When analyzed, all four groups showed sizeable reductions in symptoms over time, with significant differences among them in degrees of change. For most ADHD symptoms, children in the Comb and MedMgt groups showed significantly greater improvement than those given intensive Beh or CC. Comb and MedMgt treatments did not differ significantly on any direct comparisons, but in several instances (internalizing symptoms, teacher-rated social skills, parent–child relations, and reading achievement) the Comb treatment proved significantly better at reducing symptom scores, compared to intensive Beh and/or CC, while MedMgt did not. MTA medication strategies were superior to treatment as usual in the community, despite the fact that two-thirds of CC subjects received medication during the study period. The Comb treatment did not yield significantly greater benefits than MedMgt for core ADHD symptoms, but may have provided modest additional advantages for non-ADHD-symptoms and positive functioning outcomes.

The MTA is the largest and most methodologically sophisticated randomized multisite treatment study to date in ADHD children that includes monomodal and combined treatments. These therapeutic methods had been shown previously to be effective in simpler two-arm (active versus placebo) controlled studies (Pelham and Murphy 1986, Pelham 1989). Because of its size, the MTA was able to address certain treatment questions. First, it shows that stimulant medication efficacy can be realized across diverse settings and patient groups, and can be maintained during chronic therapy lasting more than a year. The MTA's findings replicate those from smaller long-duration stimulant trials—the 102-child New York/Montreal study (Abikoff and Hechtman 1998), the 91-child Toronto study (Schachar et al. 1997), and 62-child Gillberg study (Gillberg et al. 1997).

Collectively, these multisite studies show a persistence of medication effects over time. Within-subject effect sizes reported after 12 to 24 months of MPH treatment resembled those previously reported in short-duration studies (Elia et al. 1991, Thurber and Walker 1983). Domain of greatest improvement differs among studies, with some (Gillberg et al. 1997) showing greater effects at home and another (Schachar et al. 1997) showing greater effects at school. The total mean MPH daily doses reported by three long-duration studies ranged between 33 to 37.5 mg. The one DEX study reported a mean dose half of this level, agreeing with the general ratio of DEX to MPH doses. Persistent stimulant drug side effects or assignment to placebo treatment were associated with dropouts. Fortunately, attrition from placebo assignment was slow, allowing ample time for standard 8-week efficacy trials to be conducted.

### Efficacy and Effect Size

One of the most important findings in the stimulant treatment literature is the high degree of short-term efficacy for *behavioral* targets, with weaker effects for *cognition* and *learning*. Conners (1993, personal communication) notes that 0.8, 1.0, and 0.9 effect sizes are reported for behavioral improvements in type 4 meta-analytic reviews of stimulant drug actions (Kavale 1982, Ottenbacher and Cooper 1983, Thurber and Walker 1983). These behavioral responses to stimulant treatment, when compared to placebo, resemble the treatment efficacy of antibiotics. Less powerful effects are found for laboratory measures for cognitive changes, in particular on the Continuous Performance Task (CPT), for which effect sizes of these medications range between 0.6 and 0.5 for omissions and commissions, respectively, in a within-subject design (Milich et al. 1989); and 0.6 and 1.8 in a between-subject study (Schechter and Keuezer 1985).

Behavioral changes in children treated with psychostimulants are often tracked and reported in clinical studies as decreases in the number of and in the intensity of target ADHD symptoms. These improvements are usually based on global ratings by teachers and parents. Most published reports do not subject these global ratings to assessments of test–retest reliability. Forms used include the 93-item Conners Parent Rating Scale, the 39-item Conners Teacher Rating Scale, the 28-item Conners Teacher Rating Scale–Revised, the Iowa Conners Teacher Rating Scale, and the ADD-H Comprehensive Teacher Rating Scale (ACTeRS). These scales and their psychometric properties have been summarized in detail by Barkley (1988a). Subjecting the results of these scales to factor analysis, Conners and others (1994a) produced factor scores with threshold scores that can be used to screen children for treatment studies. Approximately 75% of children with ADHD treated with psychostimulants show moderate to marked improvement when assessed by using teacher rating scales. Changes can be picked up as early as 30 minutes after the child's first dose of MPH.

Placebo responses in children with ADHD, reported to be in the neighborhood of 18%, are less frequent than the 60% placebo rate reported for children with depression. Depressed children responded strongly to placebo, with group mean improvement that does not differ from that of those on active medication. Since these initial estimates of placebo effect in depression were published, more ADHD treatment studies have appeared, suggesting that placebo responders among children in elementary and middle school may account for between 2 and 39% of those who are helped by stimulants (Wilens and Biederman 1992). Because few treatment studies prescreen for placebo responders, the numbers of actual medication responders in any sample of children with ADHD might be closer to 55%, not the 75% often quoted. Furthermore, these estimates apply to group effects and do not inform the physician about the individual patient; only a placebo-controlled, crossover design trial would identify this type of response.

## Effects in Adults

Studies in adults taking *d*-amphetamine have shown a prolongation of performance at repetitive tasks before the onset of fatigue, a decreased sense of fatigue, mood elevation, euphoria, and increased speech rate and initiative (Rapoport et al. 1980). The psychostimulants increase CNS alertness, as shown on tasks requiring vigilance, both in laboratory tasks, such as the CPT, and on the job, such as maintaining the ability to notice new events on a radar screen for periods of hours. These changes have been described as the drug's ability to "increase capacity," although this phrase has been misinterpreted to mean an increase over the person's innate ability.

## Cognitive Effects

Neurocognitive theories of ADHD have played a crucial role in our understanding of the functional deficits that underlie symptomatic behavior. These theories attempt to explain the etiology of the disorder by connecting behavioral sequences with neuronal mechanisms (Barkley 1997). Neuropsychological research, particularly as it relates to concepts of executive functioning, has been used to address the validity of ADHD subtypes. Nigg defines executive functions as those mental processes that govern the regulation of response to context and maintenance of behavior on goal (Nigg et al. 2002).

Neuropsychological studies attempt to measure executive function in children with ADHD. Studies have shown that relative to placebo, psychostimulants improve the performance of children with ADHD on a variety of laboratory measures of cognitive function. Measures of vigilance, as ascertained using CPTs, have most consistently been found to be sensitive to stimulant medication effects. The CPT is an experimenter-paced task, in which the subject is seated in front of a display and told to press a button whenever certain letters or numbers (the target) appear on the display. The task generally lasts between 8 and 15 minutes and tests the subject's ability to sustain attention. Typical CPT outcome measures indicate the subject's reaction time to the target, the correct identification of a target signal ("a hit"), the mistaken identification of a stimulus that turns out to be a nontarget ("a false alarm"), or the complete lack of response when a target appears ("a miss"). Virtually all studies report that children with ADHD have a significant reduction in the number of CPT omission errors or in reaction time, or both, after treatment with stimulant medication (Rapoport et al. 1980, Matier et al. 1992).This reduction in omission errors and response latency is generally interpreted as reflecting improved attention.

However, findings regarding the shape of the dose–response curve have been less consistent. Whereas large medication effects relative to placebo have been consistently reported, some investigators have failed to find significant between-dose effects, others have reported linear dose–response effects, and still others have found quadratic effects such that performance decreases somewhat at the highest dose (Rapport et al. 1989a). This latter finding is somewhat reminiscent of the elusive Sprague and Sleator effect (1977). The causes of these differences are not fully apparent, but it is likely that they can be at least partially attributed to task differences. A review of various CPTs (Conners et al. 1994b) suggested that task difficulty, as indicated by the overall number of errors, is related to the ability of individual CPTs to distinguish among different diagnostic groups. Furthermore, data from these authors suggest that the decline in performance at peak doses may be apparent only on the most effortful versions of the CPT.

Several studies have also reported decreased CPT commission errors in children with ADHD after stimulant medication, which is frequently interpreted as improved impulse control. However, data suggest that commission errors are less sensitive to stimulant effects than are omission errors. Several studies that reported significant stimulant medication-induced reductions in omission errors failed to find reductions in the number of commission errors or found reductions only at higher doses.

Although the mechanism that accounts for this differential effect of stimulant medication on omission and commission errors remains unclear, it has been suggested that the difference may be due to patient characteristics, as well as the nature of the CPT error. Matier and coworkers (1992) found that aggressive and nonaggressive subgroups of children with ADHD responded differentially to a low (5-mg) dose of MPH, as did various subtypes of CPT errors. The CPT error subtypes used in this study distinguished among CPT inattention, impulsivity, and dyscontrol errors. Whereas the inattention score was primarily (although not exclusively) based on the number of omission errors, the impulsivity and dyscontrol scores were derived from distinct subsets of commission errors believed to assess different underlying cognitive processes. Matier and others found that both aggressive and nonaggressive ADHD subgroups demonstrated reduced CPT inattention after taking the medication. However, neither group demonstrated a significant change in CPT impulsivity, which was elevated only in the aggressive ADHD subgroup relative to normal subjects. Finally, the nonaggressive ADHD subgroup had a greater reduction in dyscontrol errors (as well as objectively assessed motor activity) than did the aggressive ADHD subgroup, even though both ADHD subgroups were equally high on this measure relative to control subjects before taking the medication. These data were interpreted as reflecting differential neurochemical mechanisms in aggressive and nonaggressive children with ADHD, as well as different neurochemical mechanisms underlying the different types of CPT errors. Specifically, impulsivity and aggressive behavior were hypothesized to be associated, at least in part, with central serotoninergic function, whereas inattention was thought to be more closely associated with catecholaminergic mechanisms. The psychostimulants, which act primarily on central catecholaminergic mechanisms, should have a greater impact on the CPT measure of attention (omission errors) compared with the measure of impulse control (some commission errors).

Although CPT performance improves after stimulant medication, the clinical utility of these measures for either predicting or monitoring stimulant medication response is less clear. To evaluate the clinical utility of the CPT, two questions must be addressed: Is premedication CPT performance predictive of clinical or behavioral response to medication? Do changes in CPT performance after stimulant medication administration parallel clinically observed changes in the natural environment? To date, research studies have been unable to answer these questions positively for the individual patient.

Relatively few studies have directly addressed these issues, yet the majority of data suggest that the answer to both questions is "No." The clinical utility of one version of the CPT, known as the Test of Variables of Attention, was assessed by comparing CPT performance before and after stimulant treatment in children classified as medication responders and nonresponders. Medication response, after 6 weeks of MPH treatment, was assessed via parent and child reports, clinical observations, and teacher rating scales. Medication responders and nonresponders did not differ significantly on any premedication CPT measure, suggesting that baseline performance could not be used to predict who would likely respond to treatment. However, the medication responders, compared with the nonresponders, showed greater improvement on several CPT measures after psychostimulant treatment, suggesting that the CPT may be useful for assessing medication response.

In a separate experiment, the same group of investigators assessed performance changes on the Test of Variables of Attention in a different sample of children with ADHD after a single 10-mg challenge dose of MPH. They reported that medication responders had a significantly greater enhancement in CPT performance after this initial dose of medication and suggested that the use of CPT changes in this challenge procedure may be useful for predicting medication response.

However, other investigators have generated only limited evidence to support the clinical utility of the CPT for predicting or monitoring stimulant medication response. The fact that normal children, as well as those with ADHD, appear to respond similarly to stimulant medication with regard to improved attention and reduced activity level, even though normal children make relatively few CPT errors, suggests that laboratory performance does not predict stimulant efficacy (Rapoport et al. 1980). Another study (Aman and Turbott 1991) assessed the ability of several measures for predicting MPH response in children. They found no significant relationship between CPT performance and clinical improvement, even though both measures were altered by the medication. In contrast, Taylor and colleagues (1987) reported that before medication, poor performance on a battery of attentional tests, which included a CPT, was among the strongest predictors of clinical response to MPH in children.

In two separate studies, which used different CPTs, Rapport and DuPaul (1986), Rapport and colleagues (1987), and then reported large clinical, as well as CPT, changes after MPH treatment. In one study (Rapport and DuPaul 1986), the dose–response curve for the number of CPT omission errors for the entire sample was found to parallel closely that generated for on-task behavior in classroom environments. However, there was considerable intersubject variability. In a subsequent study (Rapport et al. 1987) with a larger sample, the same authors noted similar medication-induced CPT and behavioral changes, but CPT performance was found to be highly variable and not predictive of behavioral response to medication on an individual level. Consistent with this, Nigg and coworkers (unpublished manuscript) reported similar dose–response curves for several CPT performance variables and direct behavioral observations in a group of 22 boys who participated in a summer treatment program for children with ADHD. However, despite these similarities across the group, individual medication response could not be predicted by CPT performance.

Thus, despite substantial evidence that CPT performance changes as a function of stimulant medication, only few data suggest any clinical utility for these instruments with regard to stimulant medication. Although further research is certainly warranted, current data suggest that these instruments have limited utility for the physician planning to medicate a child with ADHD and should be used only in the context of a thorough clinical assessment.

## *Dissociation of Cognitive from Social Responses While Taking Stimulant Medications*

Effects on cognition could be measured outside the lab as well. Classroom arithmetic tasks (Carlson and Thomeer 1991) showed medication–placebo effects, as did concentration during sports (Pelham et al. 1990b). Higher dosages of psychostimulants may interfere with complex memory tasks that involve set changes and other types of effortful processing. High MPH doses (1 mg/kg) produced less than expected reductions in errors on the most complex level of Sternberg memory task, although these high doses did better than lower doses in reducing abnormal behaviors in a classroom (Sprague and Sleator 1977).

This dissociation of cognitive and social responses to stimulants was first reported by Sprague and Sleator (1977). They studied 10 hyperkinetic school-age patients who were given a short-term memory paired associates task. The best percent correct score was reported on the lowest, 0.3 mg/kg dose, whereas increasing the dose to 1.0 mg/kg increased the error rate. In contrast, these same children obtained the best teacher global ratings of improved behavior on the higher, 1.0 mg/kg dose. One might conclude, as did many clinicians, that the use of behavioral ratings for dosage adjustment may select doses that impair cognitive processes. This "window of response" can be modeled best as an inverted-U curvilinear dose–response curve.

Sprague's findings have not been replicated in studies that followed. Group treatment study data have shown linear dose–response curves for MPH. A review of 11 studies, involving 180 children, that evaluated the stimulant dose–response relationship on cognitive tasks reported linear dose–response curves, with only two studies showing the decrease of cognitive abilities at higher doses (Rapport et al. 1989b). There is a great diversity among children in their dose–response curves, both among individuals and across domains of behavior and learning (Murphy et al. 1986, Solanto 1991). Pelham believes optimal dosing of the individual ADHD child cannot be done a priori, but must be carried out carefully on an empirical basis, adjusting the dose level to correct the child's most serious area of difficulty (Pelham and Milich 1991).

Even with the lack of replication of Sprague's study, the impact on practice of this one study has been profound. Prior to this publication, investigators used higher MPH doses in their research, for example, 51 mg/day (Gittelman-Klein et al. 1976), and each child's dose was titrated to maximal effect or toxicity. Since 1977, clinicians have adopted an increasingly conservative approach to MPH dose adjustments. Rather than increasing the drug through its full range to 60 mg when starting treatment, dosing can be weight adjusted on a mg/kg basis, based on Sprague's published optimal MPH dose for fewest errors (0.3 mg/kg). This results in total daily MPH doses that are often between 15 and 25 mg, somewhat lower than the mean total dose in the large multisite trials, such as the MTA Study.

## Motor Effects

Psychostimulants reduce excessive motor behavior in children with ADHD. Early studies were limited to brief laboratory observations and stabilimetric chairs and mechanical (modified automatically winding wristwatches) wrist or ankle actometers. Other approaches, such as counting grid crossings, did not measure restlessness and fidgetiness, which are frequently reported problems among these children. Some postulated that the levels of motor activity did not differentiate children with ADHD from normal subjects as much as the purposelessness of their activity did.

Advances in miniaturization and solid-state memory devices were needed to obtain activity level data outside the laboratory in the very settings reporting the motor overactivity (i.e., home and school). Colburn, at the National Institute of Mental Health (NIMH), developed an actometer that consisted of an acceleration-sensitive device with a solid-state memory that stored data on the number of movements per unit time during a 10-day period (Porrino and Rapoport 1983). This technology measured acceleration, thus capturing more of an ADHD child's impulsivity, and it measured the activity within many brief periods, so one could determine the ability of the child to modulate his or her activity level to appropriate levels for the situation.

With the Colburn NIMH device, activity level readings taken on 12 boys with hyperactivity were consistently higher than those of control subjects at all times, including during sleep and weekends. This argues against the concept that increased motor activity is a response to situational set demands. This same research team treated boys with ADHD with DEX (15 mg/day) in a double-blind ABAB design for 4 weeks. Motor activity was significantly decreased for 8 hours after dosing, followed by a slight increase in activity, which was the first objective demonstration of "rebound." These readings confirmed improvements reported during both global ratings and direct observations.

Borcherding and associates (1989), working in the same laboratory and using the Colburn NIMH actigraph, replicated this work with 18 ADHD boys in a day hospital setting in an 11-week double-blind crossover trial comparing DEX (0.2–0.6 mg/kg b.i.d.) and MPH (0.45–1.25 mg/kg b.i.d.). Plasma drug concentrations failed to correlate with activity level changes, but the concentrations of parent compounds reported were substantially higher than those reported elsewhere; this may have produced a ceiling effect, restricting the range of response and reducing the correlation. Both MPH and DEX reduced motor activity, MPH producing lower activity readings than DEX. Bocherding and coworkers' report was one of the first to differentiate the effects of the two psychostimulants on a cardinal sign of ADHD, gross motor activity.

More recently, Matier and colleagues (1992) used solid-state actigraphs to assess changes in activity level after a single 5-mg challenge dose of MPH during a structured psychometric test session. These investigators found a significant decrease in activity level only in nonaggressive children and suggested that the symptom of hyperactivity may have different neurochemical underpinnings in aggressive and nonaggressive ADHD children.

## Classroom Effects: Academic and Behavioral

The problem of validating hyperactive behaviors and their treatments has been greatly aided by using direct classroom observations. These studies use raters who are blind to the student's psychiatric and drug status. One study (Whalen and Henker 1976) treated 23 hyperactive and 39 comparison boys in a complex design whereby a number of conditions were systematically varied, including difficulty of work materials, self-paced versus other paced activities, and the single morning MPH dose (mean 12.3 mg). Hyperactive boys taking a placebo were more often off task and displayed more gross motor movement, verbalizations, noise, and disruption. These findings were replicated in another crossover design study using higher mean MPH doses (41.5 mg/day). (Abikoff and Gittelman 1985). Placebo-treated hyperactive children had much higher rates of off-task, out-of-seat, or verbalization behaviors; with MPH, these ADHD symptoms were normalized.

Short-term studies of children with ADHD treated with psychostimulants reveal that these drugs enhance arithmetical productivity, efficiency, and accuracy. Children spent less time between problems. These studies employed optimal experimental procedures, including standardized medication dosages and relevant dependent measures.

Even with these short-term improvements in seatwork performance, most clinical trials do not adjust or monitor medication doses using academic performance as a guide. Rapport and colleagues (1989a) suggested that a subset of children have divergent dose–response curves for behavior and academic output. This might explain why early reports suggested that psychostimulants were unable to help hyperactive children maintain the improvements seen during the first week of treatment on academic tasks. This idea was further strengthened by the results of a study of MPH to treat reading remediation in 61 children, half assigned to drug and half to placebo. Mean MPH doses were 44 mg/day. No differences in reading skills between groups were found 6 months after the 18-week treatment. A 2-year MPH follow-up study of 72 reading-disabled children showed no significant differences between those treated with MPH and those treated with other therapies; these 72 hyperkinetic children did far worse on the Wide Range Achievement Test reading and arithmetical scales than did a normal control group.

These long-term studies suggest that stimulants do not affect the clinical course or outcome of children with ADHD. Prospective longitudinal studies (Klein and Mannuzza 1991) of adults with childhood ADHD found histories in high school of more failing marks on report cards, failure to advance, and higher dropout rates than among control subjects. Swanson (1993, personal communication) has suggested that certain factors obscure the "expected long-term benefits of psychostimulants," including the diagnostic heterogeneity of the ADHD syndrome, the task specificity that needs to be used to measure responses to stimulants, and the possible cognitive toxicity associated with clinical titration of stimulant doses.

The question of stimulant-induced cognitive overfocusing has been a concern to physicians, parents, and teachers, who find that children with ADHD given high psychostimulant doses can become perseverative, repetitive, and less spontaneous. Yet controlled studies have failed to show major deleterious effects of stimulants on cognitive tasks. Another study (Solanto and Wender 1989) found no cognitive problems on the Wallach-Kogan battery when 19 boys with ADHD were treated with three different doses of MPH (0.3, 0.6, and 1.0 mg/kg). Another study (Tannock et al. 1989) replicated these findings, showing that attention was enhanced, with no overfocusing at higher MPH dosages.

## Aggressivity

A number of double-blind, placebo-controlled crossover studies have reported variable reductions in aggressivity in children with ADHD from stimulant treatment. This is a critical area, for aggressivity in children predicts future morbidity. Klorman and associates (1988, 1990) carried out two studies with 63 school-age patients, treating the children with MPH (0.6 mg/kg), and noted that children with and without aggressive features showed improvement. On the other hand, Hinshaw and others (1989) found only slight reductions in aggressivity in 24 school-age children with ADHD treated with MPH (0.6 mg/kg). Another study (Gadow et al. 1990) reported dose-related reductions in verbal aggressivity in 11 boys with ADHD treated with MPH (0.3 and 0.6 mg/kg) in the lunchroom and on the playground. Aggression in nine severely aggressive adolescent inpatients with ADHD was reduced by MPH treatment, as measured by reduced ratings on a standardized nursing form, the Adolescent Antisocial Behavior Checklist. Klein and Abikoff found that treatment with MPH produced reductions in aggression in ADHD children comorbid for conduct disorder (Klein et al. 1997).

## Effects on Mother–Child Interactions

Maternal responses to MPH-treated children with ADHD show increase in warmth, decrease in maternal criticism, and greater frequency of verbal interactions. Rates of friction with siblings were also lower when the ADHD children were responsive to MPH. Effective stimulant treatment appears to enhance warm, positive family interactions as well (Barkley 1989). The medication-related change in style of interaction may be a result of increased compliance with the mother's commands and decreased intensity on the part of the child. One study suggests a dose-dependent stimulant effect.

## Peer Relationships

Children with ADHD often have impaired peer relationships. Their impulsive interpersonal style leads them to be intrusive, abrasive, and loud and to relate to others with high intensity. They interrupt other children's games and conversations, fail to wait for their turn in games, push ahead in line, are overly loud, and miss social cues. Direct observations of boys with ADHD in the classroom, playground, and lunchroom have produced a picture of social interaction failure, aggressivity, and peer rejection. In a treatment study (Whalen et al. 1989) involving 25 boys with ADHD, stimulant medication treatment was associated with more frequent peer nominations for being "cooperative," "fun to be with," and acting like "best friends," although overall peer nomination ratings did not reach the levels given to non-ADHD boys. Higher dose MPH (0.6 mg/kg) produced improved peer ratings. MPH at that dosage reduced noncompliance, the number of episodes of verbal and physical aggression in both classroom and playground, to the level of that of the control subjects. MPH also reduces ADHD boys' verbal aggression in unstructured lunchroom environments. Still, not all interpersonal problems shown by children with ADHD respond to medication interventions (Wilens and Biederman 1992).

## Toxicology

Animal studies have shown a wide therapeutic/toxic ratio for MPH. A 100:1 margin of safety exists between a single dose approximating a human clinical dose and one that produces lethality in two other animal species. As a result, MPH is one of the safest medications used in the treatment of children when given in the standard 0.3 to 1.2 mg/kg/day oral dose range. The median lethal dose for MPH in dogs is 48.3 mg/kg by intravenous route and 367 mg/kg by oral route. On the other hand, the median lethal dose for amphetamine in rats is 55 mg/kg. Ninety-day subchronic toxicity studies of MPH in rats (with doses up to 120 mg/kg/day) showed decreases in body weight but no signs of growth inhibition, reproductive problems, or carcinogenicity. A 120-day study of beagles treated with 10 mg/kg/day (10 times the human dose) of MPH produced hyperactivity and hyperexcitability in the dogs, but there was no appetite suppression, growth suppression, convulsions, or changes in liver tissue.

## Substance Abuse of Stimulants

Psychostimulants have been abused by adults, but the risk for addiction by children with ADHD is low. Klein (1980) found that the psychostimulants differ in their ability to induce euphoria, with "dextroamphetamine the most euphorigenic, methylphenidate, less so, and magnesium pemoline, hardly at all." Adolescents and young adults with ADHD do not list the psychostimulants among medications used recreationally, whether or not they had received treatment with psychostimulants. Adolescents previously diagnosed as having ADHD during their school-age years are at greater risk for substance abuse than control subjects, but those who do abuse medications tend not to pick stimulants. Reports of MPH abuse include adolescents who snort ground up MPH tablets. A review assessing the abuse potential of MPH noted that there is evidence, from nonscientific sources, that MPH use and abuse may be widespread among adolescents (Kollins et al. 2002). MPH functions behaviorally in a manner very similar to cocaine and *d*-amphetamine when the route of administration is controlled. One should also be aware that there is a distinction between clinical abuse of MPH and its misuse/diversion. There are only a few case reports of abuse of MPH that have lead to role impairment. Kollins and colleagues (2002) believe that these issues are important for clinicians to consider as they prescribe.

Polysubstance-abusing adults who use intravenous methods, injecting ground up MPH tablets, suffer injury from talc granulomatosis, with severe pulmonary hypertension or ocular lesions developing in some patients.

Even though the evidence from the literature suggests that the abuse potential of psychostimulants by children with ADHD is low, DEX and MPH have been classified by the US Food and Drug Administration as potentially drugs of abuse (schedule II) and have warnings concerning abuse in the PDR. MPH was reclassified as a schedule II medication in 1971 because of a concern that the order by the Bureau of Narcotics and Dangerous Drugs to schedule methamphetamine and DEX would direct potential drug abusers to MPH. US physicians prescribing these psychostimulants for childhood psychiatric disorders first are required to obtain a US Drug Enforcement Administration registration number. As a schedule II medication, the annual amount of stimulant medication manufactured must be approved or allocated. This led to widely publicized shortages of MPH in the fall of 1993. As a result, a parent special-interest group, Children and Adults with Attention Deficit Disorder (CHAAD), petitioned the US Drug Enforcement Administration of the Department of Justice in May 1994 to reclassify MPH from schedule II to schedule III to "eliminate all likely future methylphenidate shortages." After a thorough review of the substance abuse literature, this scholarly petition could find "no substantial dependence liability and a very limited potential for significant methylphenidate abuse or diversion into illegal drug channels." However, MPH's classification was not changed, and it has remained a schedule II drug of abuse.

## Widespread Use

### Prevalence of Psychostimulant Use in the US

Psychostimulant medication has grown to be a ubiquitous treatment modality for ADHD in the US. This is due, in part, to the prevalence of the disorder. ADHD has been estimated to afflict up to 5% of children in primary school in the US. It is far more prevalent in clinic samples, in which it constitutes up to 30% of child psychiatric referrals. The cardinal features of ADHD, which include excessive gross motor activity, disorganization of behavior, distractibility, low frustration tolerance, and inability to sustain attention or remain on task can be identified in children as young as 3 years of age.

Perhaps the intensity and frequency of presentation of these disruptive symptoms explain a growing trend for stimulant medication prescription. Safer and associates (1996) suggested that stimulant use has increased greatly in the past 20 years, due to the recognition of ADHD as a chronic disorder, the prescription of medication to girls with predominately inattentive subtype, and the drug's use in treating children with learning disabilities. Surveys published in the mid-1970s reported 150,000 children in treatment at any one time. More recent estimates suggest that 750,000 children receive daily psychostimulant medication in the US, with approximately 25% of children in special education programs are also given a psychostimulant. One survey indicated that as many as 7% of third-grade Baltimore County children were treated with psychoactive medication in 1987, with the rate doubling every 5 to 7 years. More than 90% of them were given MPH (Safer and Krager 1988). Another study, using epidemiological probability sampling techniques on populations of families in the Great Smoky Mountains of rural North Carolina found that stimulant prescriptions were more related to the presence of oppositional behavior in boys than a diagnosis of ADHD (Angold et al. 2000).

MPH has become the most frequently prescribed medication used in the treatment of ADHD, accounting for more than 90% of US stimulant use. The increasing popularity of MPH probably has to do with its overrepresentation in scientific journals. One review in 1996 noted that over 141 controlled studies involved MPH, in contrast to 16 studies of other psychostimulants (Spencer et al. 1996). It also has substantial efficacy in ameliorating the target symptoms of ADHD, reducing gross motor over-activity, decreasing off-task behavior, increasing compliance with adult requests, and decreasing aggressivity (Greenhill et al. 1999). Not only is MPH effective, it is well tolerated and has a low rate of adverse events, with only 4% of children having to change to another medication in a controlled study of adverse events (Barkley et al. 1990). Its rapid action, its relatively low priced generic form, the frequency with which the ADHD diagnosis is made, and the wide range of tolerated doses are other reasons for its popularity with practitioners.

MPH has also become a ubiquitous tool in psycho-pharmacology research and training programs. It is favored in experimental designs because of its quick onset of action, large effect size on both global rating forms and laboratory instrumentation, and low incidence of side effects. MPH-related research covers many clinical domains, including the study of the mechanism of growth delays, dissociation of cognitive and behavioral effects of psychostimulants, drug-dependent learning effects, and cognitive-processing loads and psychostimulant dosage correlations, as a probe in adult schizophrenia work and for the treatment of acquired immunodeficiency syndrome dementia. In a search limited to published clinical treatment studies in ADHD, over 2,400 citations were uncovered (Jadad et al. 1999). Yet MPH has also had its share of controversy, with concern raised about possible overuse to deal with any child who does not conform to standards of classroom behavior.

## Formulation of Treatment

### What Is Being Treated
The PDR has two main indications for the use of MPH: narcolepsy and ADHD. Other stimulants differ somewhat, with the indications for methamphetamine (Desoxyn Gradumets) including ADHD and obesity and for pemoline including only ADHD.

### Diagnosis of the Stimulant-Treatable Disorders

#### Attention-Deficit/Hyperactivity Disorder
ADHD is a heterogeneous behavioral disorder of unknown etiology. As its name suggests, ADHD is characterized by inattention, impulsivity, and hyperactivity of varying severity. The disorder, which typically begins in early childhood and lasts into adulthood in a substantial minority, if not a majority, of cases, frequently leads to profound social and academic impairments.

Prevalence rates for ADHD are roughly 5 to 7% in epidemiological samples and even higher in clinical samples. Although ADHD is frequently associated with other externalizing disorders, between 25 and 50% of children with ADHD exhibit comorbid internalizing or learning disorders. These patterns of comorbidity may reflect stable ADHD subgroupings, with correlated differences in natural history, risk factors, and response to treatment (Biederman et al. 1991).

Stimulant treatment of the individual patient must be carried out in a thoughtful manner for it to be most effective. The diagnosis of ADHD must be present, for it is the only indication for stimulant use in childhood (Dulcan 1997). Yet criteria and thresholds for inclusion have changed over time and differ in other countries. Symptom lists for the disorder have been refined and altered with each publication of the *Diagnostic and Statistical Manual of Mental Disorders* (DSM). British physicians have a higher threshold for making the ADHD diagnosis than do their US counterparts, a difference that can be reduced but not eliminated if British and US physicians use identical diagnostic criteria.

In DSM-IV-TR, the diagnosis of ADHD requires either inattention (termed ADHD, inattentive type) or hyperactive–impulsive behavior (termed ADHD, hyper-active–impulsive type), or both (termed ADHD, combined type) (American Psychiatric Association 1994). The majority of children exhibit the combined type. The hyperactive–impulsive type is overrepresented among younger children, for whom the sustained attention criteria are developmentally inappropriate; the inattentive type includes more girls, comorbid internalizing symptoms, and learning impairments.

In children with ADHD, the modal age at diagnosis is 8 to 9 years, perhaps corresponding to the increased task demands of third grade or the increased developmental discrepancies between ADHD and normal children. Notwithstanding age at first diagnosis, ADHD symptoms are present much earlier in most children. DSM-IV requires that symptoms be present before the age of 7 years and that children with ADHD must exhibit symptoms that cause impairments in at least two settings—with peers, family, or at school.

The diagnostic criteria of ADHD in DSM-IV are based on the findings from systematic DSM-IV field trials. These trials involved 440 children in 11 different clinical centers. Data were collected by using structured diagnostic questionnaires, the Diagnostic Interview Schedule for Children, and then validated by using physicians' ratings and ratings of impairment. Details of the study's design, methodology, subjects, measures, and procedures, as well as the use of an interactive multiple bootstrapping strategy of data analysis, can be found elsewhere. Analyses examined the symptom utility of each item that might be included in the manual for the diagnosis of ADHD and allowed the retention or elimination of certain items. For example, the item in DSM-III-R, "engages in physically dangerous activities without thinking," was found to be far less predictive of the other items being endorsed than an item such as "acts as if he or she is driven by a motor." Therefore, the item "physically dangerous" was not included in the final DSM-IV-TR item list.

#### Narcolepsy
Narcolepsy is a chronic neurological disorder that presents with excessive daytime sleepiness and various problems of rapid eye movement physiology, such as cataplexy (unexpected decreases in muscle tone), sleep paralysis, and hypnagogic hallucinations, which are intense dream-like imagery before falling asleep (Dahl 1992). The prevalence is estimated to be 90 in 100,000. Treatment can include a

regular schedule of naps; counseling of family, school, and patient; and use of medications, including stimulants and rapid eye movement-suppressant drugs such as protriptyline. Dahl recommended beginning with standard, short-acting stimulants, such as MPH, 5 mg b.i.d., and increasing the dose up to 30 mg b.i.d. if need be.

## Nonstandard Indications for Stimulant Medications in Adults

Psychostimulants have had a place in the practice of psychiatry for many years (Klein and Wender 1995). They have been used to treat depression, as a provocative test in schizophrenia, and to treat the cognitive–affective dysfunction found in patients with acquired immunodeficiency syndrome-related complex. Anecdotal reports, open studies, and small controlled studies suggest that stimulants may help patients with depression and mania; in geriatric patients who are withdrawn and apathetic; medically ill patients who are depressed; and in patients with pathological fatigue or neurasthenia. Open studies using 20 mg/day of MPH as an adjuvant to tricyclic antidepressants in refractory depression showed improvement, probably because of an elevation in level of tricyclic antidepressants. However, controlled studies have not been done to show that combination tricyclic antidepressant–stimulant regimens do better than tricyclic antidepressants alone.

## Symptoms of Attention-Deficit/Hyperactivity Disorder

ADHD symptoms show up most often in situations that demand sustained attention *and* are boring and hard. Thus, when the situation demands sitting still in the presence of low stimulus levels, as when doing math homework, ADHD symptoms are more likely than when there is constant reinforcement by salient stimuli, as when playing Nintendo. Similarly, symptoms are usually less evident in highly structured settings or when the child is playing one-on-one with a sympathetic adult, as in the psychiatrist's office. Such context-specific variability in symptom expression is typical of ADHD and should not be misconstrued as malingering by the affected child. Clinically, children with ADHD are temperamentally high in novelty seeking, low in harm avoidance, and dependent on high-salience rewards and consequences. In contrast to anxious children, who exhibit distortions in cognitive processing, the youngster with ADHD typically "acts before thinking." Interestingly, the presence of comorbid anxiety may well ameliorate these deficits, perhaps by promoting awareness of consequences, and thus may improve prognosis.

Not surprisingly, ADHD is commonly associated with multiple behavioral difficulties, including difficulty organizing and completing tasks, especially when multiple steps are required; rapid shifting between tasks; trouble following rules and conforming to the expectations of others; interrupting and speaking out of turn; excessive talking and noise making especially in the school setting; and squirming, fidgeting, and excessive gross motor activity, often in pursuit of excitement or self-stimulation. As noted earlier, these symptoms are exquisitely sensitive to contextual and developmental considerations. Thus, the DSM-IV requirement that ADHD symptoms be impairing—that they be accompanied by distress or dysfunction, or both—implicitly requires that ADHD symptoms denote behaviors that are inappropriate for the situation or for the child's age and cognitive status, or both.

### Functioning

Functioning may be thought of as the converse of impairment. Children with ADHD are often impaired in their academics, relations with peers, and relations with adults. The medication produces increased compliance and diminishes the classroom behaviors that are disruptive. During the DSM-IV field trials, teachers' scores of impairment were correlated with the level of the disruptive classroom symptoms. Stimulant medication treatments positively affected the teachers' ratings of impairment of children with ADHD.

## Selection of a Stimulant Medication as a Treatment Modality

### Deciding to Use Medication

The decision to use medication for any child psychiatric condition can be based on a balance of risks and benefits. Risks must be examined not only in terms of the drug used but also in terms of cases where the drug is *not* used and the child continues to be impaired in social and academic functioning. Before stimulants can be used to treat a behavioral problem, the child must meet the DSM-IV criteria for ADHD. Other health conditions might prevent one from using a stimulant. If the child has Tourette's disorder, stimulants would not be used because of the likelihood of exacerbating the motor or vocal tics. Malignant hypertension might also prevent one from using a psychostimulant because of the risk of raising the blood pressure. Otherwise, the risks from these compounds are few, and they can be used to treat ADHD. With respect to stimulants, the short-term benefits are unequivocal, whereas the long-term outcomes are less well documented. Similarly, evidence supporting efficacy is strongest for preadolescents, weaker for adolescents, and equivocal for adults (Shaffer 1994). Medication treatment should be presented in this fashion, including a frank discussion of potential risks and benefits.

The decision to use stimulant medication in the treatment of ADHD employs different criteria for each developmental stage. The criteria for use of stimulants in school-age children and adolescents are well described in the DSM-IV. More difficulty arises when deciding whether to use these medications in preschool children, adult patients, patients with mental retardation, or children with ADHD and comorbid disorders.

### Use of Psychostimulants in Children Younger than 6 Years

The signs and symptoms of ADHD may be evident before age 3 years, particularly pronounced motor activity, excessive climbing, aggressivity, and destructiveness. These signs may be disruptive to family life and make nursery school attendance impossible. Campbell found that hyperactive preschoolers did not "grow out of" this behavior, but maintained their hyperkinesis when they went on to grade school (Campbell et al. 1977). Even though these early ADHD symptoms resemble the behaviors among older ADHD patients, the diagnostic manuals give little guidance about the validity of the ADHD diagnosis in the preschool years. School-age norms gathered on standard teacher global rating forms, such as the Conners Teacher Questionnaire (CTQ), have not included preschoolers until recently (Conners, personal communication).

Unfortunately, there are only a handful of published treatment studies on preschoolers. No dose-ranging pharmacokinetic studies have been done in this age group to determine if younger children, with their larger liver-to-body size ratio, might show more accelerated metabolism of psychostimulants than seen in older children. Therefore, the optimal doses for this age group are not known. To date there are no studies that would validate or refute clinicians' concerns that preschoolers suffer more pronounced stimulant withdrawal effects.

Comprehensive reviews (Spencer et al. 1996) have identified only six controlled studies ($N$=144) of MPH in preschoolers (Barkley et al. 1984, Barkley 1988b, Conners 1975, Mayes et al. 1994, Musten et al. 1997, Schleifer et al. 1975). MPH produced improvements in structured situations, but not in free play (Schleifer et al. 1975). Four of these six studies showed strongly positive results. Two reported higher rates of side effects, such as tearfulness and irritability, than would be expected in school-age children (Barkley et al. 1990). However, the six studies utilize very different inclusion/exclusion criteria, diagnostic definition, ratings forms and study designs, so that a meta-analysis would not be appropriate. Current labeling warns against using MPH in children below age 6 years. Even so, there has been a 180% increase over the past 5 years in the prescriptions of MPH for preschoolers, with over 1.2% of all preschoolers prescribed MPH in a Midwestern Medicaid group (Zito et al. 2000). Clearly, more controlled data are needed.

A single-case intensive study design noted that DEX reduced temper outbursts in a toddler (Speltz et al. 1988). The MPH treatment studies have found that the mother–child interactions involving preschoolers are ameliorated by MPH (Barkley 1988b). MPH appeared to have a linear dose–response effect on improvements in the mother–child interaction, perhaps related to increasing child compliance and decreased symptomatic intensity in the child. No disabling side effects were noted.

## Adults

The prevalence of ADHD in adults, its severity, and indications for treatment are issues that are not known. Although it had been assumed that children with ADHD outgrow their problems, prospective follow-up studies have shown that ADHD signs and symptoms continue into adult life for as many as 60% of children with ADHD (American Psychiatric Association 1980). However, only a small percent of adults impaired by residual ADHD symptoms actually meet the full DSM-IV childhood criteria for ADHD (Hill and Schoener 1996). Adults with concentration problems, impulsivity, poor anger control, job instability, and marital difficulties sometimes seek help for problems they believe to be the manifestation of ADHD in adult life. Parents may decide that they themselves are impaired by the same attentional and impulse control problems found during an evaluation of their ADHD children.

Attention Deficit Disorder, Residual State (ADD-R) was placed in the *Diagnostic and Statistical Manual of Mental Disorders*, Third Edition (DSM-III) (American Psychiatric Association 1980) to include patients over age 18 years, who had been diagnosed as children with ADD, were no longer motorically hyperactive, but had impairment from residual impulsivity, overactivity, or inattention. The diagnosis of ADD-R was dropped from DSM-III-R (American Psychiatric Association 1987). Since the publication of DSM-III-R, a small but steady stream of publications has supported the existence of adult ADD, and clinicians and parent groups find it to be a useful and realistic clinical condition. These clinicians requested that future manuals include ADHD descriptors that would cover both adults and children with ADD difficulties, not just those that applied only to children. These clinicians noted that ADHD may be overlooked in adults because it is widely viewed as a disorder of childhood.

Although DSM-IV (American Psychiatric Association 1994) did not restore the diagnosis of ADD-R, the item lists for the ADHD syndrome were rewritten to include adult manifestations. Furthermore, DSM-IV contains a category "in partial remission" that covers the adult with ADHD who retains some, but not all of the childhood problems. This is because of the concern that a few ADHD symptoms in an adult might be as impairing as a larger number in a child. One method to discover the extent of residual disorders in this population is to follow ADHD children prospectively. Follow-up studies carried out by Weiss and Hechtman (Weiss et al. 1985) compared adults who had ADHD since childhood (index group) with adults who had no mental disorder as children (control group). Compared to controls, the index group reported fewer years of education completed, a higher incidence of antisocial personality disorder, lower scores on clinician-rated global assessment scores, more complaints of restlessness, sexual, and interpersonal problems.

Manuzza and colleagues (1991) found that 50% continue to have the full syndrome by age 25 years. DSM-IV does not specifically include a diagnostic category for individuals who do not have a full childhood history of ADHD. Rather, the category "not otherwise specified" (NOS) allows adult patients whose past childhood histories are unclear, but who have ADHD symptoms as adults.

Shaffer (1994), in an invited editorial, urged clinicians to be wary of making the diagnosis of ADHD and treating these adults with stimulants. First, the diagnosis of "adult" ADD is difficult to make because adults cannot easily recall their own childhood history of ADHD symptoms with sufficient accuracy. The high incidence of comorbid Axis I (e.g., major depressive disorder) and Axis II (e.g., antisocial personality disorder) disorders makes it difficult to determine if the adult's current impairment is from the comorbid condition or from the ADHD.

Others disagree with Shaffer's concern, pointing out that the initial studies of stimulant-treated adults were inconclusive due to the low stimulant dosages used, the high rate of comorbid disorders in the patients, and/or the lack of a clear childhood history of ADHD. A number of these studies used self-report outcome measures, even though adult ADHD patients appear to be unreliable reporters of their own behaviors. A double-blind comparison of MPH (1 mg/kg/dose) and placebo was carried out in 23 adult patients with ADHD, and 78% showed improvement on

MPH versus 4% who responded on placebo (Spencer et al. 1995). The same group, in a chart review study, reported that 32 adult patients with ADHD demonstrated a positive response to treatment with tricyclics (Wilens et al. 1994).

Controlled stimulant treatment studies have been conducted with adults with ADHD including over 200 patients, some involving MPH (Gualtieri et al. 1981, Mattes et al. 1984, Wender et al. 1981). These included 15 studies (*N* = 435) of stimulants, and 22 studies of nonstimulant medications. Although there was considerable variability in diagnostic criteria, dosing parameters, and response rates among these studies, there appeared to be significant improvement in ADHD symptoms for those adults assigned randomly to stimulants and antidepressants compared to placebo.

With the caveat that sample selection criteria differ greatly from study to study, different pharmacological treatment strategies have been applied to ADHD in adults with varying success. Although Mattes and Boswell (Mattes et al. 1984) showed little benefit from MPH, others have found robust effects (Wender et al. 1985). In a study by Spencer and colleagues (1995), the response to MPH was independent of gender, comorbidity, or family history of psychiatric disorders. Treatment was generally well tolerated at the target dose of 1.0 mg/kg; side effects included loss of appetite, insomnia, and anxiety. Other drugs that have been reported to be beneficial in reducing ADHD symptoms include fluoxetine (Sabelsky 1990), nomifensine (Shekim et al. 1989), pargyline (Wender et al. 1994), bupropion (Wender and Reimherr 1990), the MAO inhibitor selegiline (Ernst et al. 1995), and the long-acting methamphetamine compound Desoxyn Gradumets (Wender 1994).

Atomoxetine (Strattera) is the first non-stimulant drug to be marketed with an indication to treat ADHD in both children and in adults. It is a potent reuptake inhibitor of norepinephrine transporter, with a low affinity for muscarinic, adrenergic, histaminergic, dopaminergic and serotonergic receptors. It is metabolized, rapidly absorbed, metabolized by hepatic CYP2D6 cytochrome enzymes, glucoronidated and excreted in urine. This means that drug–drug interactions will take place with antidepressants such as fluoxetine, turning efficient metabolizers into slow metabolizers. Atomoxetine has an elimination half-life of 4 hours in the efficient metabolizers, that represent 90% of the population. Only 5–10% of patients have a polymorphism at the cytochrome P450 2D6 isoenzyme that makes them slow metabolizers with a much longer atomoxetine elimination half-life.

There have been four randomized double-blind trials in children showing that atomoxetine produces significantly greater reductions of ADHD symptoms that does placebo. To be exact, 3,536 children and adolescents were involved in clinical trials of atomoxetine at a mean dose of 1.35 mg/kg/day, with more than 1,500 on the medication for more than 6 months. One such double-blind, randomized, 4 week trial in 132 children, ages 6 to 17 years old with ADHD, revealed the group assigned atomoxetine at 1.2 mg/kg/day improved more for core ADHD symptoms on the ADHD rating scale than those assigned to placebo (Michelson et al. 2001). In addition, improvements in family and social functioning were noted.

Two similar 10-week trials of 280 and 256 reported that divided doses of 60 to 120 mg of Atomoxetine produced superior improvements compared to placebo in adults with ADHD on ratings of core ADHD symptoms (Michelson 2003).

In all atomoxetine trials, there have been no serious adverse events, no deaths and no patients discontinued for abnormal laboratory values. However, the label includes warnings about allergic reactions, including angioneurotic edema, a potentially lethal condition. Adverse effects related to atomoxetine treatment, relative to placebo, included abdominal pain (18.2% versus 12.6%), decreased appetite (16.2% versus 5.7%), vomiting (11.5% versus 5.7%), nausea (8.5% versus 5%), somnolence (10.1% versus 4.2%) and fatigue (6.9% versus 3.4%). In an open-label comparative trial, children assigned to atomoxetine had statistically significantly more vomiting and somnolence than those assigned to methylphenidate (Kratchovil 2002). About 20% of children treated with 1.2 mg/kg/day of atomoxetine lost 3.5% of their body weight. Long-term followup over 18 months reported slight decreases in height and weight percentiles.

Data from receptor binding, electrophysiological, *in vivo* animal and human subjective effect studies suggest that atomoxetine does not have abuse liability (Schuh et al. 2002).

In practice, Atomoxetine will be used in children not on selective serontonin reuptake inhibitors after two stimulants have been tried. The fact that it is not a stimulant does not mean that it is safe. Children treated with the drug can experience vomiting and sedation, and long-term effects on growth remain to be clarified. Although the manufacturer reports effect sizes of 0.7 standard deviations, its relative efficacy compared to stimulants will not be known until well-controlled "head to head" trials are conducted. Until then, it may be an option for families and physicians concerned about using stimulant drugs, and for children who have had problems with insomnia (The Medical Letter in press).

Novel compounds have been used with varying amounts of success. Although the nicotinic analog (ABT 418) significantly reduced ADHD symptoms, the antinarcoleptic Modafinal failed to separate from placebo in a multisite controlled trial of three doses (100, 200, and 400 mg) (Rugino and Samsock, in press).

DuPaul and Barkley (1990) and Wender (1994) recommend a number of medications that can be used to treat the adult with ADHD. These include: MPH, 5 to 20 mg t.i.d.; DEX, 5 to 20 mg b.i.d.; methamphetamine (Desoxyn Gradumets), 5 to 25 mg once in the morning; bupropion (Wellbutrin), 100 mg b.i.d. to 100 mg t.i.d.; and selegiline (Eldepryl), 5 mg b.i.d. only. The database is limited for the efficacy of these medications, so practitioners should be cautious in their use until proof of efficacy is available.

A variety of medications have been used to treat adults with ADHD. Physicians should be cautious in the use of these agents until proof of efficacy is available. Of particular concern is the danger of using psychostimulants in adults with comorbid substance abuse disorder. It would be wise to use MPH because of its relatively low abuse potential, and because it has been shown in controlled studies to significantly reduce the symptoms of ADHD in adults. (See Tables 100–5 and 100–6.)

| Table 100–5 | Attention-Deficit/Hyperactivity Disorder Diagnoses in Adults | |
|---|---|---|
| **Diagnosis** | **Patient Has Childhood History?** | **All Symptoms Present?** |
| ADHD | Yes | Yes |
| ADHD in partial remission | Yes | No |
| ADHD not otherwise specified | No | Yes or no |

| Table 100–6 | Experimental Medication Therapies for Adults with Attention-Deficit/Hyperactivity Disorder |
|---|---|
| **Possible Medication Treatments** | **Suggested Dose Range** |
| Methylphenidate (Ritalin) | 5 mg b.i.d.–20 mg t.i.d. |
| Amphetamine (Dexedrine) | 5 mg b.i.d.–20 mg b.i.d. |
| Mixed amphetamine salts (Adderall) | 5 mg b.i.d.–20 mg. b.i.d. |
| Bupropion (Wellbutrin) | 100 mg b.i.d.–100 mg t.i.d. |
| Selegiline (Eldepryl) | 5 mg b.i.d. only |

## Continuing Stimulant Treatment in Patients with Tic Disorders

Standard package instructions for using MPH warns against its use in patients with tics or in patients with a family history of tics. Patients with Tourette's syndrome often have comorbid ADHD. If the two conditions co-occur, concern arises that stimulant treatment—because of its dopamine agonist actions—might unmask, trigger, accelerate, or precipitate more severe tics. This worry was expressed in an editorial that accompanied a retrospective chart review (Cohen and Leckman 1989). The report included 17 ADHD patients with Tourette's syndrome who had been previously treated with stimulants, and reported their tics had been exacerbated by stimulant therapy (Lowe et al. 1982). Another study (Erenberg et al. 1985) found that 11 of 39 patients who had both ADHD and Tourette's are worsened when restarted on stimulants.

The two controlled prospective studies of stimulants in children comorbid for ADHD and Tourette's syndrome have included long-term longitudinal follow-ups extending 2 to 4 years (Castellanos et al. 1997, Gadow et al. 1995). Conclusions derived from these studies must be tentative because they are based on a total of 56 subjects. However, in both studies, stimulants produced improvements in ADHD symptoms, and no long-term worsening in tics, even when tics worsened with high doses of MPH or DEX. Despite the variable rate of adverse events across the whole sample in the Castellanos Study, up to one-third of subjects did not continue long-term treatment with stimulants because of worsening of tics. Thus, both sides of the argument have been validated. Tics are unacceptably worsened for a minority of comorbid children, although reversibly, and the majority of such comorbid children can be treated cautiously with low-to-moderate doses of stimulants, particularly MPH (Comings and Comings 1987).

### Patients with Mental Retardation

Many stimulant treatment studies for school-age children with ADHD exclude children with full-scale IQs below 70, who are considered to have mental retardation (MR). This is unfortunate, for the signs of ADHD are far more prevalent in children with IQs in the MR range (Aman et al. 1991). Pharmacotherapy reviews involving patients with MR have reported that institutionalized subjects with severe or profound MR respond poorly to stimulants. However, studies involving community samples of children with MR, have shown that these children do respond to MPH. Thirty children treated in a double-blind crossover study employing MPH (0.4 mg/kg/day), thioridazine (1.75 mg/kg/day), and placebo showed consistent MPH-related improvement on teacher global ratings of behavior. This same report found that three "cognitive maturity parameters" (breadth of attention, mental age greater than 4.5 years, and full-scale IQ above 45) predicted a good MPH response on 21 outcome variables. In contrast, children with IQs below 45 or a mental age of less than 4.5 years had more adverse side effects or a poor response to MPH. Another controlled study reported drug responses to MPH doses of 0.3 and 0.6 mg/kg given to 27 children with ADHD and IQs ranging between 48 and 74. Although 67% of this group were deemed stimulant responders, 6 of the 27 children had side effects of such severity that medication had to be discontinued. These included motor tics (three children) and social withdrawal (two children). Thus, it appears that children with ADHD who have mild or moderate MR may be more vulnerable to certain stimulant-related adverse side effects.

Children with fragile X syndrome present with MR, avoidance of eye contact, perseverative behaviors, and severe ADHD symptoms. Because the DSM-IV does not distinguish among different etiologies, a diagnosis of ADHD can be given to these children, even if their behavior disorder is a phenocopy of the ADHD seen among children without an inborn genetic disorder such as fragile X syndrome. Stimulant treatment has proved effective in this population, as shown in a double-blind crossover study of 15 patients with fragile X syndrome comparing MPH, DEX, and placebo.

The DSM-III-R guidelines state that a diagnosis of pervasive developmental disorder (PDD) or early infantile autism rules out making a diagnosis of ADHD diagnosis, even if the patient meets all criteria for the ADHD disorder. Symptomatically, children with PDD may exhibit severe overactivity, inattentiveness, and impulsivity that require treatment. Early studies cautioned that children with PDD may be sensitive to stimulant side effects and may show increased irritability, motor activity, and stereotypies. Birmaher and colleagues (1988) on the other hand, reported improvements in global parent and teacher rating scales for hyperactivity and inattentiveness in nine children with PDD treated with open-label MPH at doses of 10 to 50 mg/day. Although these findings are based on an open study, they are encouraging, particularly because many of these children with PDD have been treatment failures on other medications.

## *Does Comorbidity Affect the Indications for the Use of Stimulant Medication?*

ADHD children that are referred from other physicians are affected by Berkson's bias, which means that they have multiple Axis I psychiatric disorders. Extensive literature reviews report that ADHD co-occurs with conduct and oppositional defiant disorder in 30 to 50% of cases, with mood disorders in 15 to 75% of cases, with anxiety disorders in 25% of cases, and with learning disabilities in 15 to 30% of cases. Specific patterns of signs and symptoms may coexist in the patients and their families, with groups of disorders and vulnerabilities being genetically transmitted from generation to generation (Biederman et al. 1986).

Does the presence of other psychiatric signs and symptoms affect response to stimulants? Comorbidity between ADHD and anxiety (ANX) is common. Up to 25% of children with ANX meet diagnostic criteria for ADHD; similarly, up to 25% of children with ADHD meet criteria for ANX. In anxious ADHD children, it has long been speculated that comorbid anxiety may influence the outcome of treatment for ADHD. For example, Pliszka compared children with nonanxious ADHD to children with comorbid ADHD and overanxious disorder and found that the combination of ADHD and ANX reduced the risk of comorbid conduct disorder, decreased impulsive responding on a CPT, and produced sluggish reaction times on a Memory Scanning Test (Pliszka 1989). Subjects who were comorbid for anxiety and ADHD also showed a poorer response to MPH and more side effects than subjects with ADHD alone (Pliszka 1989). Although failing to replicate the results of Pliszka (1989) with respect to behavioral outcomes, Tannock and colleagues (1995a) later demonstrated an enhanced risk for tics and dysphoria in ADHD subjects comorbid for anxiety, treated with MPH, and less improvement in memory in comorbid children given a single dose of MPH.

Conversely, using a flexible clinically appropriate titration trial, Tannock and colleagues recently found no difference in short-term outcome or side effects in children with ADHD and comorbid ADHD/ANX (Diamond et al. 1999), implying that method variance may in part account for conflicting results in these studies. Analyses of the six-site NIMH collaborative MTA Study, which addresses a priori questions about the individuals and combined effects of pharmacological and psychosocial (behavioral) treatment for children aged 7 to 9 years with ADHD (Arnold et al. 1997), suggested that parent-reported child anxiety differentially moderated the outcome of treatment. In particular, parent-reported child anxiety as a moderator of treatment outcome generally favored the addition of psychosocial treatment for anxious ADHD children irrespective of the presence or absence of comorbid conduct problems. Contravening earlier studies, no adverse effect of parent-reported child anxiety on medication for core ADHD or other outcomes was demonstrated. For some domains of outcome, anxious ADHD children showed significantly greater gains than nonanxious children even with medication alone. On the other hand, exploratory analyses documented that child self-reported anxiety on the Multidimensional Anxiety Scale for Children was only weakly correlated with parent- or teacher-reported symptomatology at baseline and changed little with treatment, raising questions about whether the parent Diagnostic Interview Schedule for Children (DISC) accurately detected anxiety in children with ADHD.

## Treatment with Stimulant Medications

An effective treatment strategy for this chronic disorder of ADHD requires a plan for follow-up and monitoring. Techniques involve regular follow-up visits, the use of rating forms from parent and teacher, and the monitoring of academic progress in the school. Seeing the patient and a family member regularly is essential, often on a once-monthly basis when the medication prescription must be renewed. Details on aspects of monitoring and management of care are given later.

## Gender, Ethnic, and Racial Issues

Ethnic concerns relate to the use of psychostimulants in children with ADHD. Some groups suggest that minority children who are socially disadvantaged may be assigned stimulant medication treatment more often than children in other groups. This scenario would posit that inner-city, minority children are more often treated in busy hospital clinics with medication interventions, which are relatively less expensive in terms of professional time than psychotherapy, family therapy, educational remediation, or group peer skills training. After the NIMH issued a program announcement titled "Research on Strategies to Address Violence and its Consequences," an attack was mounted by the Center for the Study on Psychiatry that the Public Health Service was targeting young African-American children to receive drug treatment. In actuality, minority groups are at risk for not getting stimulant treatment, as Zito and colleagues found (1998).

## Preparation of the Patient

Does the child's attitude about drug treatment influence its success? Concerns that medications may create negative attributions or dysphoric effects in children with ADHD have not as a rule been confirmed in direct tests. Excellent studies show that there is considerable variability in children's attributions, as well as their mood response to pills. Pelham and colleagues (1992) found a subgroup of "depressogenic" children who gave external credit for positive events and internal blame for negative events. This group was above the median on attributions of success to their pills. Comorbidity and family history for anxiety and/or depression seemingly are relevant variables in prediction of such attributional effects. During treatment, a small percentage of stimulant-treated children do become dysphoric, weepy, and mournful. Children who respond with depressogenic attributions or dysphoria may be children whose depressive diathesis is indistinguishable from ADHD and who are therefore mistakenly diagnosed as ADHD and treated with stimulants. Given the overlap of depression and ADHD, and the findings that depressogenic cognitive styles predict later depression, it could be important to identify those children who may be prone to attribute their success to pills rather than to their own effort, even though most patients do not do so.

Physicians can explain the reasons for taking pills and how the pills can prove helpful in school and at home. Children often have negative attitudes about treatment, thinking of treatment as a punishment. Pill taking can be socially stigmatizing to the child with ADHD if the daily trip to the nurse generates peer ridicule. Discussing the problem of in-school pill administration may be of great interest to the child, and he or she should be included in all discussions about dosing and changing of doses. At best, it may help with compliance.

## Consideration of Side Effects

Stimulant side effects are dose dependent and range from mild to moderate in most children. These have been described by Barkley in a placebo-controlled study comparing the baseline and on-drug double-blind rating by parents (Barkley et al. 1990). These side effects include insomnia, anorexia, irritability, weight loss, abdominal pain, and headaches. Psychosis related to stimulant intake is well known in the adult literature but only at supernormal doses, such as 300 mg of DEX in a single day. When side effect reports have been gathered on ADHD children taking placebo, anxiety, staring, disinterest, and sadness were observed; only parents' reports of decreased appetite, stomachaches, and insomnia differentiated ADHD children given placebo from those given medication. In that study, less than 4% of children had to stop taking stimulants because of these side effects.

The management of stimulant-related adverse effects generally involves a temporary reduction of dose or a change in time of dosing. MPH has an excellent safety record, probably because the duration of action is so brief. The management of specific side effects is covered in the following sections and is summarized in Table 100–7.

| Table 100–7 | Stimulant Side Effects and Management |
| --- | --- |
| **Side Effect** | **Management** |
| For all side effects | Unless severe, allow 7–10 d for tolerance to develop. Evaluate dose–response relationships. Evaluate time–action effects and then adjust dosing intervals or switch to sustained-release preparation. Evaluate for concurrent conditions, including comorbidities and environmental stressors. Consider switching stimulant drug. |
| Anorexia or dyspepsia | Administer before, during, or after meals. With pemoline, consider drug-induced hepatitis. |
| Weight loss | Give drug after breakfast and after lunch. Implement calorie enhancement strategies. Give brief drug holidays. |
| Slowed growth | Apply weight loss remedies. Give weekend and vacation (longer) drug holidays. Consider another stimulant or nonstimulant drug. |
| Dizziness | Monitor blood pressure and pulse. Encourage adequate hydration. If associated with only $T_{max}$, change to sustained-release preparation. |
| Insomnia or nightmares | Administer earlier in day. Omit or reduce last dose. If giving sustained preparation, switch to tablet drug. Consider adjunctive antihistamine or clonidine. |
| Dysphoric mood or emotional constriction | Reduce dose or switch to long-acting preparation. Switch stimulants. Consider comorbidity requiring alternative or adjunctive treatment. |
| Rebound | Switch to stained-release preparation. Combined long- and short-acting preparations. |
| Tics | Firmly establish correlation between tics and pharmacotherapy by examining dose–response relationship, including no-medication condition. If tics are mild and abate after 7–10 d with medications, reconsider risks and benefits of continued stimulant treatment and renew informed consent. Switch stimulants. Consider nonstimulant treatment (e.g., clonidine or tricyclic antidepressant). If tic disorder and ADHD are severe, consider combining stimulant with a high-potency neuroleptic. |
| Psychosis | Discontinue stimulant treatment. Assess for comorbid thought disorder. Consider alternative treatments. |

## Common Side Effects

Common psychostimulant side effects include insomnia, decreased appetite, weight loss, headache, heart rate elevation at rest, and minor increases in systolic blood pressure. Many of these side effects can be managed with temporary dose reduction. Severe insomnia can be managed by changing time of dosing, with most of the medication given early in the day. Complaints of stomach upset, nausea, or pain sometimes respond to giving the medication in the middle of a meal; otherwise, the problem can be treated symptomatically with antacid tablets or by switching to sustained-release MPH, which is absorbed more slowly.

## Infrequent Side Effects

Infrequent side effects include motor tics and reductions in weight velocity. The appearance of minor facial tics is a frequent reason for stopping stimulants in clinical practice, but there have been no studies that have determined a causal link between stimulant treatment and the continuation of these signs. A history of chronic or episodic involuntary muscle movements (tics) or a family history of Tourette's disorder has become a contraindication to the use of MPH, as it may "unmask" or exacerbate Tourette's disorder. Switching to another stimulant, such as pemoline, may worsen the adventitious movement disorder, so it is best to discontinue all psychostimulants and consider a trial of clonidine.

**Acute Withdrawal: Rebound.** One adverse effect, commonly known as behavioral rebound, appears when children experience psychostimulant withdrawal at the end of the school day. Children present with afternoon irritability, overtalkativeness, noncompliance, excitability, motor hyperactivity, and insomnia about 5 to 15 hours after the last dose. In one study involving 14 hyperkinetic boys treated with DEX, three quarters of the group given stimulant and none given placebo experienced rebound. In a later study, the same group reported significant afternoon activity increases for 21 boys treated with DEX, the first quantitative evidence for the rebound phenomenon. A third study using a controlled crossover design of 21 boys with ADHD taking MPH, at doses of 0.6 and 1.2 mg/kg/day, or placebo found no evidence for an afternoon worsening. It is not clear at this time if these contradictory reports represent differences between DEX and MPH, and it is not known whether longer-acting stimulant preparations produce fewer rebound effects. In any case, the controlled drug treatment literature does not report rebound effects. This may be the result of the use of global parent rating forms that are not specific for time of day. If rebound occurs, many physicians add a small afternoon MPH dose or add a small dose of a tricyclic antidepressant.

## Rare Side Effects

Stimulant-related toxic psychosis, including MPH-induced mania and MPH-induced delusional disorders, is a rare phenomenon in children, with fewer than 30 cases having been reported. Higher than therapeutic doses of amphetamines reliably induce brief paranoid psychoses in adult volunteers. Even though the psychotomimetic effects are short-lived, this side effect can be serious and requires immediate cessation of stimulant treatment. Psychosis is a contraindication for psychostimulant use (Greenhill et al. 2002a). The physician should avoid dispensing psychostimulants to agitated children with psychotic symptoms and consider neuroleptics instead. The addition of a neuroleptic to the treatment regimen of a severely disturbed child with ADHD raises the possibility that the child's hyperactivity and poor attention span were secondary to an underlying psychotic condition. Although neuroleptics and psychostimulants do not interact in a negative fashion, the *Psychotherapeutic Drug Manual for Use in New York State Mental Health Facilities* warns against prescribing a stimulant with an antipsychotic. This drug combination will trigger the state's Pharmakon computer medication system to issue a "severity level 1 exception," which prevents the medication from being dispensed without approval from the facility's drug monitoring committee.

The PDR lists a number of other adverse reactions, without stating frequency, that are not found in standard clinical practice or in published reports from treatment studies. These rare side effects of stimulants include alopecia and leukocytosis. This would suggest that a yearly, routine complete blood count be included in the therapeutic drug monitoring plan. Other rare adverse affects are hypersensitivity (rash, urticaria, fever, arthralgia, exfoliative dermatitis, erythema multiform with histopathological findings of necrotizing vasculitis, and thrombocytopenic purpura), angina, and cardiac arrhythmia.

**Seizure Disorders.** A commonly held notion is that stimulants lower the seizure threshold. This may have originated in toxicological studies carried out in animals. Convulsions are one of the terminal signs in animals treated with doses of 300 mg/kg for the determination of psychostimulant toxicity. The PDR warns against the use of stimulants in children with preexisting seizure disorders. Both ADHD and seizure disorders are quite prevalent and may occur in the same individual, so the question of the risk of stimulant treatment may frequently arise. One study suggests that stimulant treatment of children with ADHD maintained on effective anticonvulsant doses produced no increase in seizure frequency, no changes in the electroencephalogram waveforms, and no difficulty in regulating anticonvulsant blood levels. Current practice is to give children with ADHD and epilepsy a combination of anticonvulsant and MPH. Plasma levels of the anticonvulsant should be monitored to avoid toxicity resulting from MPH's competitive inhibition of metabolic pathways. At the doses used to treat ADHD in children, the psychostimulants have variable but minimal effects on the seizure threshold.

## Long-Term Stimulant Effects: Growth Velocity Reductions

Adults taking amphetamines routinely experience weight loss, which can be attributed to reduced appetite and decreased food intake. The drug's action on the lateral hypothalamic feeding center may explain this effect. Appetite suppression differs among different species, with humans showing only mild effects with rapid onset of tolerance. Children with ADHD taking psychostimulants routinely show appetite suppression when starting treatment. For

2084 Section VI • Therapeutics

this reason, dosing should optimally occur after breakfast and lunch. Even though the daytime appetite is reduced, hunger rebounds in the evening. These effects on appetite often weaken within the first 6 weeks of treatment.

Safer and Allen (Safer et al. 1972) first reported that treatment for 2 or more years with MPH and DEX could produce decrements in weight velocity on age-adjusted growth rate charts; stopping the medication produced a quick return to baseline growth velocities. DEX, whose half-life is two to three times that of MPH, produced more sustained effects than did MPH on weight velocity and suppressed mean sleep-related prolactin concentrations. MPH-treated children with ADHD followed up for 2 to 4 years show dose-related decreases in weight velocity, with some tolerance to the suppressive effect developing in the second year. Hechtman and colleagues (1984) reported that children with ADHD not treated with psychostimulants attained expected heights; therefore, there was no suspected associated growth slowdown from the ADHD itself.

The actual mechanism for psychostimulant growth slowdown is unknown. Early theories blamed the drug's putative suppressant action on growth hormone or prolactin, but research studies of 13 children treated for 18 months with 0.8 mg/kg/day of DEX and of nine children treated for 12 months with 1.2 mg/kg/day of MPH failed to demonstrate a consistent change in growth hormone release. The most parsimonious explanation for this drug effect is the medication's suppression of appetite, leading to reduced caloric intake. No study, however, has collected standardized diet diaries necessary to track calories consumed by children with ADHD taking psychostimulants.

In any case, the growth effects of MPH appear to be minimal. Sixty-five children followed up to age 18 years showed an initial growth loss during MPH treatment but caught up during adolescence and reached heights predicted from their parents' heights. These results confirmed the observations by Roche and associates (1979) that psychostimulants have mild and transitory effects on weight and only rarely interfere with height acquisition. Height and weight should be measured at 6-month intervals during stimulant treatment and recorded on age-adjusted growth forms to determine the presence of a drug-related reduction in height or weight velocity. If such a decrement is discovered during maintenance therapy with psychostimulants, a reduction in dosage or change to another class of medication can be carried out.

## Rare Side Effects of Pemoline

An important, serious, and unexpected adverse reaction associated with pemoline use is liver failure (Safer et al. 2001). Changes in liver function tests suggesting hepatotoxicity have also occurred, necessitating routine liver function tests every 2 weeks while on pemoine.

## Continuing Stimulant Treatment in Patients with Tic Disorders

The PDR suggests that the presence of tics is a contraindication to stimulant usage. With the comorbidity of ADHD in children with Tourette's disorder estimated to fall between 20 and 54%, there is a concern that a stimulant's

dopamine agonist action will unmask, trigger, accelerate, or provoke irreversible Tourette's symptoms. This worry is enhanced by a number of papers, some of them retrospective, that reported onset of tics after stimulant treatment had begun. Lowe and colleagues (1982) reported on 17 patients with ADHD and Tourette's disorder who had been previously treated with stimulants and whose tics were exacerbated by the stimulant therapy. Another study examined 48 patients with Tourette's disorder who had been previously treated with stimulants. Of the 39 patients who had both ADHD and Tourette's disorder, 11 showed a worsening of the tics when stimulants were restarted.

It could be argued that because a child with ADHD and Tourette's disorder already has both conditions, Tourette's disorder could no longer be triggered by the stimulants. Treatment of these cases with stimulants sometimes improve both the ADHD and the tics, whereas others find that the tics worsen. Overall, caution is still indicated when treating children with tic disorders. To date, however, there has been no prospective study published that shows that stimulants have any effect whatsoever on the tic severity in these patients. The most conservative approach would be a trial of clonodine or desipramine.

## Drug Interactions

Mixing psychostimulants with other psychotropic medications is generally not advisable. Most serious is the addition of a psychostimulant to a monoamine oxidase inhibitor antidepressant regimen, a potentially lethal combination that can elevate blood pressure to dangerous levels. Zametkin and Rapoport (1987) do not advise using the monoamine oxidase inhibitor medication tranylcypromine (Parnate) for children with ADHD, despite its efficacy, because a parent might mistakenly substitute MPH if she or he runs out of the child's tranylcypromine, producing a potentially lethal blood pressure surge. Additive effects between psychostimulants and the systemic agents used to treat asthma can produce feelings of dizziness, tachycardia, palpitation, weakness, and agitation. Theophylline, for example, when taken orally (Theo-Dur Sprinkle), can have this undesirable agitating effect. It is best to ask the pediatrician or allergist to switch from the orally ingested preparation to an inhalant to avoid such additive sympathomimetic effects.

Psychostimulants compete with other medications for the same metabolic pathway and have been thought to produce an increase in the plasma concentration of both drugs. The psychostimulants can also interfere with the action of other medications. MPH can block the antihypertensive action of guanethidine. DEX blocks the action of some beta-adrenergic antagonists (e.g., propranolol) and slows the intestinal absorption of phenytoin and phenobarbital. The renal clearance of DEX is enhanced by urine acidifying agents, so that grapefruit juice will shorten the elimination half-life of the medication. Conversely, urine alkalinizing agents decrease clearance. This is also true for ritalinic acid, although this metabolite is not active in the CNS.

However, published case reports do not show an additive increase in side effects when combinations of other classes of drugs are used. MPH may elevate the plasma level of antidepressants, anticonvulsants, coumarin anti-coagulants, and phenylbutazone. One group of researchers (Pataki et al. 1993) treated 12 boys with ADHD in a double-blind crossover study of combined MPH and imipramine. They reported an increase in nausea and dry mouth but no elevation in blood pressure. MPH may increase the concentration of the serotonin reuptake blocker fluoxetine, potentially enhancing agitation, although no such side effect was seen in a single case report of the treatment of an 11-year-old boy with both ADHD and obsessive–compulsive disorder. Other medications have been combined successfully with MPH, such as clonazepam to reduce tics. Clonidine has been added to reduce sleep disturbances associated with ADHD and with stimulant medication. The combination of fenfluramine and MPH proved effective when tested in a double-blind crossover study of 28 children with ADHD and MR. However, bupropion exacerbated tics when added to MPH given to children with ADHD.

## Initiation of Treatment

Medication treatment begins with a choice of medication. Although the MPH or DEX psychostimulant types have equal efficacy, MPH is often used first. Elia and colleagues (1991) strongly suggested that the physician try both MPH and DEX "because the overlap of who is a nonresponder is not great." These researchers defined nonresponders as those patients who were given medication, but whose behavior remained unimproved or those who suffered severe adverse effects from the drug. Because of pemoline's hepatotoxicity, it is used infrequently. If it is used, liver function studies should be done and repeated at 6-month intervals.

Titration serves two purposes: acclimatization of the child to the drug and determination of his or her best dose. School-age children should be started with low doses to minimize adverse effects. Psychostimulant medication should be taken at or just after mealtime to lessen the anorectic effects; studies have shown that food may enhance drug absorption. MPH treatment can be initiated with a single 5 mg dose at 8:00 AM for 3 days; then a 5 mg dose at 8:00 AM and at noon for the next 3 days; then 10 mg at 8:00 AM and 5 mg at noon for 3 days; and finally 10 mg at 8:00 AM and 10 mg at noon are given and maintained for at least 2 weeks. Preschoolers may start as low as 2.5 mg at 8:00 AM but build to the same total 20 mg/day dose of MPH. The dosing instructions should be written down for the parent, with dates and times specified in detail. A photocopy of the instructions should be kept in the patient's chart.

Three-times-daily stimulant administration has been utilized in treatment studies, (Greenhill et al. 1996) with doses given before school, at lunch, and at home before homework. However, current practice is to switch as soon as possible to a long-duration preparation, such as Concerta (Wolraich et al. 2002) or Metadate-CD (Greenhill et al. 2002b). This once-daily dosing pill totally avoids the noontime dosing in school.

Table 100–1 is an inventory of stimulant drugs and doses. DEX is usually started at 2.5 to 5 mg/day and gradually increased in 2.5- to 5-mg increments; MPH is usually started at 5 mg b.i.d. and then titrated in increments of 5 mg/dose every 4 to 7 days. Peak behavioral effects are noted 1 to 3 hours after ingestion and dissipate in 3 to 6 hours for both MPH and DEX. Although stepped-dose open-label trials of MPH and DEX are the rule in clinical practice, double-blind placebo-controlled titration trials—using parent and teacher ratings plus an "objective" measure of attention, such as the CPT—can be helpful in distinguishing a true drug effect from a placebo response and in establishing the best dose for an individual child.

As noted above, pemoline has been removed from many formularies, and is no longer used in Canada because of the rare hepatic failure noted. When used, it is usually started at 37.5 mg once in the morning and titrated in 18.75 mg increments to maximal clinical effectiveness. Most children respond at a total dose of 56.5 mg/day or about 2 mg/kg/day in a single dosing. For patient safety, consent forms should be presented to the parents for their signature, and hepatic function tests should be gathered biweekly. Although the PDR reports that steady state is reached within 3 days, traditional practice was to use pemoline for 2 to 4 weeks before clinical benefit became apparent. However, this time–action profile probably reflects arbitrarily overly slow, low-dose titration strategies and is not a true pharmacodynamic effect.

The Conners Teacher Rating Scale is then repeated. Further dose adjustments up or down depend on the rating scale's scores, teachers' verbal reports, parents' comments, and adverse effects experienced by the child. The minimal effective total daily dose and optimal timing of medication administration should be determined before switching to the sustained-release 20 mg formulation. Eventually, one dose of standard MPH may have to be mixed with one sustained-release 20 mg pill at 8:00 AM (to give early- and late-morning coverage), just as one administers short- and long-acting insulin at the same time.

## Monitoring

Progress assessment is handled by a timetable of *regularly scheduled visits to the physician's office*. Based on the success of the medication management strategy of the MTA Study (Greenhill et al. 1996), compared to those children randomly assigned to treatment as usual in the community, children on stimulants should be monitored with monthly or bimonthly visits. These visits work well if scheduled for 30 minutes in length, and involve both parent and child. They allow the physician to observe the child's activity level and attentiveness, to collect information on beneficial effects and adverse reactions, and to review the teacher's reports on the patient's academic and social progress. Clinical progress is reviewed so that the physician can track ADHD signs and symptoms, academic progress, and success with peers. Any counseling, therapy, or educational guidance can be given at that time. With the family's and patient's permission, report cards can be copied and placed in the chart. The physician can keep anecdotal records about social events, including invited play dates, invited sleepovers, teams joined, and Boy Scout or Girl Scout activities.

*Maintenance* plans should include schedules for the regular collection of information that constitutes the child's therapeutic drug monitoring. Each child's response to psychostimulants is different. Likewise, each family's needs are different. Plans for medication vacations and weekend and after-school dosing must be individualized. Many parents, concerned about long-term side effects, feel most comfortable with their child not taking medication each weekend and through the summer, despite the costs to family harmony. A summer off medication, although it may seem idyllic, may become much less desirable if the child's summer camp has difficulty with the ADHD symptoms. On the other hand, a child with MPH-induced anorexia and some weight loss can benefit from a summer without medication.

Medication *compliance* should be monitored at each visit. The parent is instructed to bring the medication bottle along so that pill counts can be done monthly and compared with the prescription dates. Height and weight should be taken every 6 months, and the child's pediatrician can be requested yearly to perform a complete physical examination and blood work (complete blood count, liver function studies). The frequency of visits depends on the other therapies recommended. These may include once-monthly parental counseling, twice-monthly individual therapy, or weekly meetings for individual psychotherapy or behavioral modification management. A minimal frequency should be once monthly, particularly in the nine states requiring multiple-copy prescription forms, which limit the amount of psychostimulant ordered to a 30-day supply.

The next component of monitoring is the use of *structured rating scales*. These have been the backbone of psychostimulant treatment research but also have utility in clinical practice. Each physician should choose a scale that she or he finds easy to interpret and convenient to use. It should be available in both parent and teacher formats. These scales, however, should not be used as substitutes for an open discussion with the teacher.

These rating forms should be collected every 4 months and whenever the physician needs to make decisions about dosage adjustment, time of dosing, or even continuation of medication. Although the original 39-item Conners Teacher Rating Scale is ubiquitous in the field of child psychopharmacology, Satin and colleagues (1985) have shown the validity of the shorter, 10-item Abbreviated Rating Scale both as a repeated measure and as a screening tool for identifying school-age children with ADHD. This short form is good for tracking children in maintenance treatment. Like most scales, the Abbreviated Rating Scale assigns weights to each scale point. With a 10-item scale, and each point weighted between 0 ("not at all") and 3 ("very much"), 10 checks by a parent in the "very much" column yields a total score of 30.

The physician uses these forms before beginning treatment. Two copies of each form are collected from both parents and the teacher 1 week apart. Each pair of forms is averaged to determine the child's baseline, pretreatment score. The average score counteracts any tendency for the rating scores to drift downward. Current thinking indicates that a 25% drop (with a lower total score indicating improvement) from baseline is required after medication is started to state that the child has had a positive clinical response. Once the maintenance dose of the stimulant is set, the rating scales for teachers and parents can be repeated at 4-month intervals.

Unlike the situation with anticonvulsants, it has not proved effective to monitor psychostimulants by maintaining plasma concentrations within a therapeutic range. Alternative medications such as desipramine, however, do lend themselves to regular plasma level monitoring every 3 months.

## Plasma Level Monitoring

Once absorbed, levels of the parent compound, MPH, can be obtained in bodily fluids. However, they do not prove to be a practical aid in the treatment of children with ADHD. Levels have been studied in samples of saliva or plasma. MPH saliva levels provide a good check of pill-taking compliance, but, because MPH concentration is not independent of saliva flow, saliva MPH concentrations cannot be used to predict MPH concentrations in plasma or brain. They do not correlate with behavioral or cognitive measures.

Plasma level measures of MPH concentrations have provided research data but are not practical for use in the day-to-day clinical care of children with ADHD to guide titration or dose adjustments during maintenance treatment. MPH plasma levels do not correlate with clinical response and provide no more predictive power than teacher and parent global rating forms, because therapeutic drug monitoring efforts are hampered by MPH's short half-life and its tendency to degrade unless strict collection and storage methods are used. The short half-life means that no true steady-state level is reached. This hampers the usual standard peak or trough collection time strategies used with the other psychotropic medications monitored with blood tests, such as lithium and carbamazepine. There is no exact agreement in the literature concerning a standard time after oral dosing to draw blood for MPH levels. A variation of onehalf hour can make an enormous difference in the resulting blood level of MPH if the physician is restricted to only one blood sample. Furthermore, there is considerable intraindividual variability, with poor intertest reliability for peak MPH plasma levels.

## Phases of Treatment

Medication therapy can be divided into baseline, titration, and maintenance phases. Before the first pill is given, baseline data on height, weight, blood pressure, and heart rate should be collected as well as a complete blood count. The Conners Teacher Rating Scale and Conners Parent Rating Scale can also be collected. Standardized scoring methods for the teacher rating scale can be used to generate a hyperactivity factor score.

The duration of treatment is an important step in the generation of a treatment plan for a child with ADHD. Although there is no clear-cut recommendation for the length of psychostimulant treatment, many parents have a reasonable expectation that it will not be open-ended. The onset of puberty is one possible stopping point for psychostimulant medication. School-age children were thought to respond "paradoxically," calming down on stimulant medication, an effect that was supposedly lost at puberty. Adolescents with ADHD, who may be at risk for substance abuse, were thought to be particularly vulnerable to psychostimulant euphoria and to abuse of their medications. In addition, more recent prospective follow-up studies suggest that the motor hyperactivity of ADHD disappears between ages 16 and 23 years.

## Intensity of Treatment: Dosing

Despite a plethora of controlled treatment studies, actual guidelines for dosing with psychostimulants have not been established. A variety of approaches have been used. Early studies relied on a stepwise open titration method. The physician would slowly increase the dose from 10 to 60 mg/day until improvement or side effects intervened. After a 1977 study by Sprague and Sleator (1977) that suggested that higher doses of MPH might impair a child's cognitive responses to laboratory tasks, dosing techniques became more conservative, with physicians using the low 0.3 mg/kg/dose guideline suggested by Sprague. Other physicians and studies set an arbitrary fixed absolute dose of 20 mg/day. Eventually, dosing by weight became the customary standard in published research, even though definitive evidence that a patient's weight should be considered relevant never materialized.

Despite wide clinical use of dose by body weight dosing strategies (Spencer et al. 1996), Rapport and colleagues (1989a) showed that, on average, (1) the dose–response curve is independent of body weight and (2) time–action effects display wide intersubject variability. More specifically, Rapport and coworkers examined the group mean response to three doses of MPH in pediatric subjects of low, medium, and high body weight and found a linear effect of dose—larger doses produced greater symptom reductions—but no effect of body weight on response at any dose condition. Similarly, when looking at interindividual variability in dose–response curves, the researchers also showed that departures from a linear dose–response pattern were common, with some children showing a threshold effect (no response below a threshold level) and others a quadratic response (linear at lower doses and degradation at higher doses). Clinically, these results imply that each child requires an individually constructed dose–response curve, taking into consideration the time–action effects of drug at each dose before making dosage adjustments.

The exact nature of dose–response and time–action curves for MPH and other psychostimulants during the treatment of children with ADHD has been a controversial subject. Instead, major interindividual and intraindividual differences in dose–response curves have been described. Furthermore, within subjects, there may be different dose–response curves for different response measures. Some investigators have found that the severity of ADHD symptoms may predict the strength of MPH effects, which has been dubbed a "rate-dependent response." This means that dosing each child will be an empirical exercise, with ample trial and error necessary to achieve the optimal dose to treat the most impairing problem area in the child's behavior.

## Outcome Assessment

Assessing the outcome of medication treatment involves the monitoring of response. Continuation of the medication depends on its ability to maintain the improvements. Medication is changed if major or prohibitive side effects emerge, if there is insufficient benefit, or if there is deterioration and return of the ADHD symptoms. Currently held concepts of medication response, as well as data about the natural history of the ADHD syndrome, have put aside some of these therapeutic approaches. The psychostimulant response of children with ADHD is not considered paradoxical but, rather, typical of all diagnostic groups, including normal subjects (Rapoport et al. 1980). The only exceptions are those children with a diagnosis of psychosis, or those with comorbid anxiety disorders, who can become more agitated when treated with psychostimulants. Furthermore, hyperactivity does not necessarily go away. Prospective follow-up studies have shown that approximately 25% of children with the full ADHD syndrome at age 10 years will show all signs of the disorder at age 18 years, including motor hyperactivity. These adolescents show the same beneficial response to MPH, in magnitude and direction, as do school-age children with ADHD. MPH produces no more signs of euphoria in adolescents than it does in school-age children. With clear evidence that some individuals continue to suffer from ADHD into adult life, one could advocate psychostimulant treatment indefinitely. What is the physician to tell the parents?

Dulcan (1997) and others (Greenhill et al. 2002a) correctly recommended that treatment duration be planned on an individual basis. One method is to plan in single school year units, starting with the present and projecting treatment to last through the present school year plus at least 1 additional month into the following academic year. Once the child has responded to an initial level of medication, maintenance doses can be set slightly lower. Treatment can be continued, if need be, and the next decision point can be set for the following fall.

This provides a framework for the second concept, a trial-off medication. This can be used to determine if treatment should be continued for another year. Medication can be discontinued during the school year, during some stable period. This should not be the beginning of the school year or during crucial placement examinations. Placebo tablets are no longer available from the companies producing MPH, so the psychostimulants are simply discontinued. Most children do not need to taper their dose of medication at discontinuation, unless they show signs of marked afternoon rebound.

## Augmentation of Treatment

### Integration with Other Modalities: Multimodal Treatment

Medication is one component of a therapeutic treatment plan. New standards have been promulgated for the treatment of ADHD recommending multimodal therapy. This was first reported by Satterfield and colleagues (1980) to be successful in maintaining the short-term stimulant gains for periods of 2 years or more. Other combination treatments, such as behavior modification plus medication, have been shown to be somewhat more effective than medication alone. The combination of medication plus cognitive–behavioral therapy is not more effective than medication alone. More recent studies (Arnold et al. 1997) have evaluated a multimodal package consisting of thrice daily MPH dosing, parent skills training, educational supplementation, and social skills training for the child. This type of therapy is more costly, in time and money, than medication management accompanied by regular but infrequent counseling. Testing the relative efficacy of combination therapies is more challenging than assessing the efficacy of a stimulant because more control groups are required to tease out the effects of each component as well as the combination. Controlled studies of multimodal therapy have been confounded by the need to use a fixed package rather than tailoring the therapy to the child's needs, the high refusal rates, and the reluctance by families to accept the entire treatment package.

The NIMH has funded several multimodal treatment studies of children with ADHD, including the pharmacological–behavioral combined study of Abikoff, at Long Island Jewish Medical Center, and Hechtman, in Montreal, (Abikoff and Hechtman 1996) and the intensive kindergarten study of Shelton and coworkers (2000) in Massachusetts. The treatment program in both studies lasted 2 years, with additional "booster shot" interventions over the following year. With these studies, the Child and Adolescent Disorders Branch of the NIMH has shown a commitment to this study design. Following on these smaller studies, funding was given to a larger, multisite program, which served as the largest treatment study of children with ADHD yet mounted, the NIMH MTA Study (The MTA Cooperative Group 1999).

Several assumptions underlay this six-site cooperative project, including that the heterogeneous nature of ADHD requires larger sample sizes and resources than one location can supply; large samples are needed to evaluate treatment effects with sufficient power; and long-term observation of treatment effects is needed to truly evaluate treatment effectiveness in this population. The cooperative study model analyzed the results as one study with five replicates. The NIMH Request for Applications specified that projects submitted include comparisons and combinations of psychosocial and pharmacological treatments conducted for longer time periods than 3 months and that the multisite cooperative group work to achieve a minimal sample size of 576 children, aged 6 to 9 years, who meet DSM-IV criteria for ADHD, combined type.

Each of the six sites recruited and assessed 96 children meeting rigorous criteria for ADHD, who were then assigned to one of four treatment conditions: (1) stimulant medication, (2) intensive psychosocial intervention without medication, (3) the combination of stimulant medication and psychosocial treatments, and (4) referral for treatment in the community. Medication treatments began with an initial, 1-month, double-blind titration trial of placebo and three doses of MPH. These dose conditions were presented in a random order and changed on a daily basis, so there were at least four repeats of every dose condition. At the end of the trial, an optimal dose was derived from blind assessment of the data by two sites, and this optimal dose was used to begin the 13-month maintenance medication phase. Later dose adjustments were allowed, and changes of medication could be approved by a cross-site pharmacology panel that met twice weekly via teleconference. This early double-blind titration, and the lengthy maintenance phase, addressed questions of the predictive power of a controlled titration trial and the stability of this dose prediction. It was the largest treatment study involving stimulant medication, with 288 children been treated. Most important, the

14-month treatment period made this study one of the longest prospective trials of stimulant medication for children with ADHD.

The specific aims of the study were to determine whether (1) the children with ADHD in the combined-modality group showed better overall functioning after 14 months of treatment and 2 years of follow-up compared with those in the single-modality groups and (2) the children with ADHD in the systematically applied intensive therapies showed better overall functioning over the long run compared with those children referred for standard treatments in their communities. A common protocol was created so that data could be pooled across sites, and extensive procedures had been implemented to check the fidelity to this protocol as the study proceeded.

## Treatment Failure

If a child fails to show improvement as the stimulant dose is being increased, how far should the dose be increased before turning to another medication? The physician is left with the dose range suggested in the PDR and to his or her own standards regarding what constitutes improvement and where to draw the line between a response and failure. There is no agreement in the pediatric psychopharmacology literature about how many target symptoms must be reduced and by how much before a child crosses the threshold into "full clinical response." No agreement exists on whether a responder should improve in all settings (home, school, and the physician's office) or on whether global ratings or direct measurement produces the most valid and reliable estimate of response. Some pediatric psychopharmacology studies use the number of standard deviations of change between pretreatment and posttreatment global teacher ratings; others use a nonparametric rule that simply endorses that a child is a responder if a global rating of "much improved" or "very much improved" is given. Still other physicians count a child as a responder if his or her scores drop below a previously set score on a teacher rating scale. Our group defines a moderate stimulant response as a 25% drop in a global teacher rating on the hyperactivity factor score of the Conners Teacher Rating Scale.

Do true nonresponders exist? Recent studies indicate that many apparent nonresponders to stimulants may simply have been treated with too low a dose. A crossover study (Elia et al. 1991) with unusually high doses (2.5 mg/kg for MPH; 1.3 mg/kg for DEX) found that only 1 of 48 children failed to respond to one or the other drug. However, using clinical ratings, 14 cases failed to respond to at least one of the drugs. Had the other drug not been tried, about 40% of subjects would have been considered nonresponders, due to either side effects or lack of effect (a figure not that discrepant from nonresponder data reported in some parallel-group studies). Furthermore, the lack of side effects at the high doses in this study suggests that many children may respond quite well at a high dose for the appropriate drug and further implies that failed trials of both MPH and DEX constitute a minimal adequate stimulant trial before moving to nonstimulant treatments for pediatric ADHD. Conversely, two subjects given high-dose MPH experienced reversible psychotic decompensation; thus, the treating physician is well advised to seek expert consultation with a child and adolescent psychopharmacologist before venturing beyond a total dose of 60 mg/day of MPH and 40 mg/day of DEX.

## Limitations of Stimulants

The enthusiasm for psychostimulants does not seem to be diminished by their widely accepted problems. Although 1- to 3-month treatment studies carried out in groups of children with ADHD showed impressive reductions in ADHD symptoms, physicians must manage individual children with ADHD for years. This concern was expressed in the concept paper for the NIMH MTA Study, which raised cautions about the long-term conclusions that one might draw from the stimulant treatment literature. Although psychostimulants produce moderate to marked short-term improvement in motor restlessness, on-task behavior, compliance, and classroom academic performance, these effects have been demonstrated convincingly only in short-term studies. When examined during periods greater than 6 months, these medications generally fail to maintain academic improvement or to improve the social problem-solving deficits that accompany ADHD.

There have been other caveats expressed about the psychostimulants as a panacea for children with ADHD. First, the behavioral benefits from a single dose of a psychostimulant last only a few hours during its absorption phase and are often gone by the afternoon. Second, it is estimated that between 10 and 30% of children with ADHD do not improve with stimulants or improve but experience unmanageable side effects. Approximately 25% of children with ADHD are not helped by the first psychostimulant given or experience side effects so bothersome that meaningful dose adjustments cannot be made. Third, the indications for choosing a particular psychostimulant and the best methods for adjusting the dose remain unclear, which may prove confusing to the physician and to the family. Although MPH is regarded as the drug of choice for the treatment of ADHD, controlled treatment studies show no particular advantage for this medication over DEX or pemoline. Fourth, many treatment studies are troubled by methodological problems, including not controlling for prior medication treatment and inappropriately short washout periods.

In addition to widely accepted characteristics of stimulants, other concerns have been more theoretical and thus more controversial. Some experts find these concerns important, whereas others await the replication of findings reported only once or twice in the literature. First, there are indications that there may be a dissociation of dose-response curves, with improvements in one domain occurring while decrements are seen in another area. For example, the same dose needed to produce quiet behavior may interfere with optimal cognitive performance. Second, stimulant treatment responses may be affected by the presence of comorbid psychiatric disorders. Children with ADHD and comorbid anxiety disorders may have more side effects than those with pure ADHD. Third, the causal attributions that children with ADHD attach to medication may offset any benefits the medication offers. Some workers have been concerned that children treated with stimulants may develop negative self-attributions, coming to believe that they are incapable of functioning without the medication. Fourth, investigators have sometimes found

that stimulant effects may be influenced by the patient's IQ or age, but this requires further replication. Fifth, some have speculated that dose-response measures of academic performance in stimulant-treated children with ADHD may be influenced by state-dependent learning. Sixth, the possibility that stimulant medication response may be related to the presence of minor physical anomalies, neurological soft signs, or metabolic or nutritional status has yet to be explored.

Once a child is diagnosed, the physician should have a systematic method for titration and adjustment of the dose. There is no universally agreed-on method for dosing with these medications, with some physicians using the child's weight as a guideline (dose by weight method), and others titrating each child through the approved dose range until clinical response occurs or side effects limit further dose increases (stepwise titration method). This is partially based on a lack of agreement regarding the nature of the psychostimulant dose-response cognitive and behavioral effect curves. Some regard these relationships as linear, whereas more recent data show that dose-effect relationships are highly variable. Plasma level measurements are not much help. Sizable inter- and intraindividual variability in plasma level concentrations occur after the same dose of MPH. Furthermore, MPH dose-response relationships vary from individual to individual. Some children with ADHD show dose responses that can be conceptualized as a simple linear function, whereas others show curvilinear patterns. These relationships may vary in the same child, one type for cognitive performance and another type for the behavioral domain (Sprague and Sleater 1977). Adverse reactions to medications show the same variability and may appear unpredictably during different phases of the drug's absorption or metabolic phases. When making dose adjustments, there should be guidelines about when to stop increasing the medication. Yet there is no agreement about what determines a satisfactory response to stimulants. Therapeutic drug monitoring helps regulate doses of anticonvulsant medications and lithium carbonate but does not work for MPH. Although long-term adverse reactions, such as inhibition of linear growth in children, have been shown to resolve by adult life, no long-term prospective studies maintaining adolescents with psychostimulants through the critical period when their long bone epiphyses fuse have been published. Therefore, the final evidence remains to be gathered showing that continuously treated adolescents will reach the final height predicted from their parents' size.

Besides the medical and treatment issues, some physicians have had to worry about negative reports in the media about the safety of these drugs. Small special-interest groups in the US, such as the Church of Scientology, have used television and radio to bombard parents with their reports of the "dangers" of psychostimulants. They have generated a whirlwind of controversy and misinformation about adverse reactions from these drugs in the treatment of ADHD. As a result, the media have sounded the warning that physicians are dispensing MPH to ever-increasing groups of children using vague and overinclusive diagnostic criteria. Although it is clear that stimulants are a popular treatment modality among physicians (psychostimulants are prescribed for 35–51% of outpatients attending child psychiatric clinics), there is no evidence that they are being given excessively. Parental concerns are fanned when these groups inflate side effect rates by focusing on late-adolescent problems that peak independent of stimulant treatment, such as addiction and suicide. Parents, supported by special-interest groups, have sued physicians for prescribing MPH, and this resulted in a 37% drop in retail sales of MPH in the eight cities where the litigation took place, a bigger impact on MPH use than was created by the Church of Scientology's anti-MPH media blitz.

In the US, nine states adopted multiple-copy prescription programs between 1967 and 1982 (California, Hawaii, Illinois, Idaho, Indiana, Michigan, New York, Rhode Island, and Washington) to monitor schedule II drugs, including DEX and MPH (pemoline, on the other hand, is classified as a schedule IV medication and does not require these forms). Physicians practicing in these states are required to use multiple prescription copy pads (triplicates) to order DEX and MPH. The resulting data have been used to expose illicit distribution of psychostimulants as well as to conduct research on local trends in office practice. With such data, it is possible to compare the prevalence of MPH treatment of children in primary school in Suffolk County in 1988 (0.04%) to the percentage of 3rd graders treated in 1987 in Baltimore County (7%) (Safer and Krager 1988).

The New York State Department of Public Health (Eadie, personal communication) reported that four times as many prescriptions were written for MPH as for DEX in the second quarter of 1990 (20,271 for MPH, only 4514 for DEX). This was partly due to public and professional concern about amphetamine. On the other hand, many physicians view MPH as a nonamphetamine. Amphetamine's notoriety as a highly euphorigenic, highly addictive substance has greatly reduced its use, as shown by a 95% drop in triplicate prescriptions for DEX in New York State in the past decade (Eadie, personal communication). In addition, pharmacists may refuse to carry DEX once they stock MPH.

## Use of Long-Acting Preparations When Standard Stimulants Are Lacking

There are three reasons for the implementation of longer-acting stimulant preparations. First, children who take medications in school are subject to peer ridicule when they leave activities to go to the nurse. Second, some school officials refuse to allow school personnel involvement in the administration of medication. Third, the time–action course of standard stimulant medications allows only a brief 1- to 3-hour window of effect, so some medicated children may experience trough periods of little or no drug action during important parts of the school day.

Sustained-release preparations have been marketed for DEX and MPH. MPH's sustained-release preparation (MPH-SR), which became available in 1984, is manufactured in brand (Ritalin-SR) and generic (MD Pharmaceuticals) versions but only in a single strength of 20 mg (MPH-SR20). DEX spansules are available in 5-, 10-, and 15 mg strengths in the brand version (Dexedrine Spansules). The sustained-release preparations make it possible to give the psychostimulant once in the morning and avoid administration during the school day. Ritalin-SR uses a wax-matrix vehicle for slow release, whereas the DEX "spansule" is a capsule containing small medication particles.

Pharmacokinetic studies show that the sustained-release preparations have properties different from those of the standard tablets. The pharmacokinetic curves of Ritalin-SR are flattened, with no sharp peaks. Lower peak concentration ($C_{max}$) and longer time from ingestion to peak ($T_{max}$) are also observed. In a pharmacokinetic study of nine males with ADHD by Birmaher and colleagues (1989), the $C_{max}$ was 20 ng/mL for standard MPH (10 mg b.i.d., MPH-10BID), but only 7 ng/mL for MPH-SR20. The $T_{max}$ for MPH-10BID was 90 minutes but was much later (3.4 hours) for MPH-SR20. This may explain why behavioral and cognitive studies show that the peak benefit for MPH-SR20 occurs at 3 hours, 1 hour later than for the standard preparation. A mean plasma elimination half-life value (using a single-compartment model with a monoexponential decline in plasma levels from $C_{max}$) was calculated to be 2.5 to 3.3 hours for standard MPH and 4.1 hours for MPH-SR20. As with the standard preparation, the MPH-SR20 concentrations of the $d$ enantiomer of MPH were 8 to 10 times higher than the $l$ enantiomer.

One study found that the behavioral effects of DEX spansules and MPH-SR20 lasted as long as 9 hours. Comparisons of the dosage equivalency and efficacy of one dose of MPH-SR20 given at 8:00 AM, with two doses of MPH-10BID, given at 8:00 AM and at noon showed no significantly different effect in the classroom or home environment or during the CPT.

Reports of the efficacy of the long-acting preparations have been divergent. In a controlled study of nine children with ADHD, Brown and colleagues (1979) found that DEX spansules showed no more effect than placebo on behavior or on activity much after 2 hours, despite their ability to produce high plasma levels of the parent compound during 12 hours. Similarly, Pelham and coworkers (1987) first reported that MPH-SR20 was less effective than MPH-10BID on measures of social functioning in 13 children with ADHD in a summer treatment program. In a later study, the same investigators reported that MPH-SR20 was found to be equally effective for controlling behavior as pemoline or DEX spansules during a 9-hour period. The second study (Pelham et al. 1990a) employed rapid shifting of doses every 3 days as well as daily changes of medications, and there may have been some carryover effect that might have reduced differences among the active drug conditions. Also, insomnia resulted when the subjects were on pemoline, which could have affected the following day's ratings. These data are shown in Table 100–2.

These data suggest that the long-acting stimulant preparations have equal clinical efficacy, despite differences in reported plasma level concentrations. Negative reports suggesting that long-acting preparations are ineffective may have originated in reviews (Dulcan 1990) written before the publication of some of the controlled studies. Other explanations for the anecdotal reports of the lack of ability of MPH-SR to provide long-term coverage include poor compliance at home with taking medication, unpredictable release of active MPH from the sustained-release tablet's wax-matrix core, change in the patient's weight, or new stressors in the environment (Greenhill et al. 2002a). Pelham and colleagues' (1987) first study produced data, judged by "blinded" expert raters, who then made no direct ratings of the children but only scored summary data sheets of behavioral information and CPT performance. Pelham and associates (1990a) used only direct ratings in their second study. These later data agree with the results reported by Fitzpatrick and coworkers (1992) and Greenhill and colleagues (1999), both groups finding the two types of preparations equally effective.

Differences between the short- and long-acting preparations relate primarily to pharmacokinetic considerations, not necessarily to clinical ones. Standard, short-acting MPH-10BID tablets produce higher peak plasma concentrations and yield a steeper absorption phase slope than does the longer acting MPH-SR20 preparation. Greenhill (1992) studied a sample of 42 children with ADHD in a parallel-group, 8-week design comparing MPH-10BID and MPH-SR20. Despite the differences in $C_{max}$ between MPH-SR20 and MPH-10BID, no differences were seen in CPT performance, motor activity levels, or teacher's reports for the two groups. One speculation is that MPH-SR20's longer duration of action may alter pharmacokinetics or receptor pharmacodynamics, inducing tolerance. One recent study has reported short-term tolerance to repeated dosing with methylphenidate that has the characteristics of tachyphylaxis (Swanson et al. 1999).

## Use of Nonstimulant Medication Treatments for Attention-Deficit/Hyperactivity Disorder

There are times when it is best to consider using nonstimulant medications in the treatment of ADHD. March (Maletic et al. 1994) suggested that an unsatisfactory response to two different stimulants is one criterion, and this agrees with the studies of Elia and Colleagues (1991). Severe side effects and the ability to tolerate stimulants is another reason. A common side effect that limits stimulant use is the presence of frequent, severe, embarrassing tics. Psychosis is a definite contraindication for the use of stimulants. Other reasons for such a decision are listed in Table 100–8.

The alternative medications are given in Table 100–9. They include the tricyclic antidepressants, bupropion, and clonidine. Details of the use of these medications are beyond the scope of this chapter. However, some information is supplied in Table 100–9.

**Table 100–8  Indications for Using Nonstimulant Drugs**

Unsatisfactory response to two stimulants
Inability to tolerate stimulants
Comorbid condition(s) contraindicating stimulant treatment—e.g., psychosis
Medical contraindication—e.g., tachyarrhythmias
Risk of stimulant abuse by parent or other person in the home
Treatment of comorbid condition with single agent—e.g., tricyclic antidepressant for panic disorder and ADHD
Combination strategies for ADHD—e.g., tricyclic antidepressant plus MPH

## Conclusion

Psychostimulant medications are a mainstay in the US treatment of ADHD. This popularity has resulted from their proven efficacy during short-term controlled studies, as shown by improvements in global ratings by teachers and parents. In fact, the majority of children with ADHD respond to either MPH or DEX, so nonresponders are rare (Elia et al. 1991). Yet, the long-term response of ADHD children to MPH and other psychostimulants is not known; published treatment studies have lasted months, not the years that children take stimulants to adapt to academics in school (Jacobvitz et al. 1990). Optimal treatment involves the planning for a multimodal treatment program that combines educational and psychosocial interventions with medication therapy.

However, treatment plans that center on psychostimulant medication have flourished for a number of reasons. The effects of psychostimulants are rapid, dramatic, and normalizing. The risk of long-term side effects remains low, and no substantial impairments have emerged to lessen the remarkable therapeutic benefit–risk ratio of these medications. More expensive and demanding treatments, including behavior modification and cognitive–behavioral therapies, have, at best, only equaled the treatment with psychostimulants. In a number of instances, the combination of behavioral and medication therapies is only slightly more effective than the medication alone (Gittelman-Klein 1987). Current and future studies of multimodal therapies will test whether combined treatment results in better overall functioning in

**Table 100–9  Nonstimulant Drugs in Attention-Deficit/Hyperactivity Disorder**

| Drug | Usual Dose Range | Schedule | Comments |
|---|---|---|---|
| Tricyclic antidepressants | 2–5 mg/kg; between-subject variability in levels at a constant mg/kg dose is common | b.i.d. or bedtime | Anticholinergic and antihistaminic effects are generally well tolerated or mild<br>Electrocardiogram precautions are mandatory<br>Consider therapeutic drug monitoring for side effects or lack of benefit<br>May be combined with stimulants |
| Clonidine | 0.1–0.4 mg | 2–6 x/d | Especially useful for comorbid tic disorders, sleep problems, and impulsive aggressivity<br>Monitor blood pressure<br>Tolerance and sedation are often problematic<br>May be combined with stimulants |
| Bupropion | 150–300 mg | b.i.d.–t.i.d. | Seizure history is a contraindication<br>May exacerbate tics |
| Atomoxetine | 100–300 mg | b.i.d. | Some weight loss may be experienced |

the long run and decreased appearance of comorbid conditions than does monomodal treatment with psychostimulants alone. It is essential to show that the continuation of stimulant medication during long-term maintenance benefits the patient with ADHD.

## Acknowledgment

This work was supported, in part, by the grant No. 5 UO1-MH50454-07 (Dr. Greenhill) from the National Institute of Mental Health.

## References

Abikoff H and Gittelman R (1985a) Hyperactive children treated with stimulants: Is cognitive training a useful adjunct? Arch Gen Psychiatr 42, 953–961.

Abikoff H and Gittelman R (1985b) The normalizing effects of methylphenidate on the classroom behavior of ADHD children. J Abnorm Child Psychiatr 13, 33–44.

Abikoff H and Hechtman L (1996) Multimodal therapy and stimulants in the treatment of children with ADHD. In Psychosocial Treatment for Child and Adolescent Disorders: Empirically Based Approaches, 1st ed., Jensen P and Hibbs T (eds). American Psychological Association, Washington DC, pp. 341–369.

Abikoff H and Hechtman L (1998) Multimodal treatment for children with ADHD: Effects on ADHD and social behavior and diagnostic status. (Unpublished)

Aman M and Turbott S (1991) Prediction of clinical response in children taking methylphenidate. J Aut Dev Disord 21, 211–228.

Aman MG, Marks RE, Turbott SH, et al. (1991) Clinical effects of methylphenidate and thioridazine in intellectually subaverage children. J Am Acad Child Adolesc Psychiatr 30(2), 246–256.

American Psychiatric Association (1980) Diagnostic and Statistical Manual of Mental Disorders, 3rd ed. APA, Washington DC.

American Psychiatric Association (1987) Diagnostic and Statistical Manual of Mental Disorders, 3rd ed., Rev. APA, Washington DC.

American Psychiatric Association (1994) Diagnostic and Statistical Manual of Mental Disorders, 4th ed. APA, Washington DC.

Angold A, Erkanli A, Egger H, et al. (2000) Stimulant treatment for children: A community perspective (abstract). J Acad Child Adolesc Psychiatr 39, 975–983.

Arnold L, Jensen P, Richters J, et al. (1997) The National Institute of Mental Health Collaborative Multisite Multimodal Treatment Study of Children with Attention-Deficit Hyperactivity Disorder (MTA): Design challenges and choices (abstract). Arch Gen Psychiatr 54, 865–870.

Barkley R (1988a) Child behavior rating scales and checklists. In Assessment and Diagnosis in Child Psychopathology, 1st ed., Rutter M, Tuma H, and Lann I (eds). Guilford Press, New York, pp. 113–155.

Barkley R, DuPaul G, and McMurray M (1991) Attention deficit disorder with and without hyperactivity: Clinical response to three dose levels of methylphenidate. Pediatrics 87, 519–531.

Barkley R, McMurray M, Edelbroch C, et al. (1989) The response of aggressive and non-aggressive children to two doses of methylphenidate. J Am Acad Child Adolesc Psychiatr 28, 873–881.

Barkley R, McMurray M, Edelbroch C, et al. (1990) Side effects of MPH in children with attention deficit hyperactivity disorder: A systematic placebo-controlled evaluation. Pediatrics 86, 184–192.

Barkley RA (1977) A review of stimulant drug research with hyperactive children. J Child Psychol Psychiatr 18, 137–165.

Barkley RA (1988b) The effects of methylphenidate on the interactions of preschool ADHD children with their mothers. J Am Acad Child Adolesc Psychiatr 27, 336–341.

Barkley RA (1989) Hyperactive girls and boys: Stimulant drug effects on mother–child interactions. J Child Psychol Psychiatr 30(3), 379–390.

Barkley RA (1997) ADHD and the Nature of Self-Control. Guilford Press, New York.

Barkley RA and Cunningham CE (1979) The effects of methylphenidate on the mother–child interactions of hyperactive children. Arch Gen Psychiatr 36, 201–208.

Barkley RA, Karlsson J, and Strzilecki E (1984) Effects of age and Ritalin dosage on mother–child interactions of hyperactive children. J Consult Clin Psychol 52, 750–758.

Biederman J, Munir K, Knee D, et al. (1986) A controlled family study of patients with attention deficit disorder and normal controls. J Psychiatr Res 20(4), 263–274.

Biederman J, Newcorn J, and Sprich S (1991) Comorbidity of attention deficit hyperactivity disorder with conduct, depressive, anxiety, and other disorders. Am J Psychiatr 148(5), 564–577.

Birmaher B, Quintana H, and Greenhill LL (1988) Methylphenidate treatment of hyperactive autistic children. J Am Acad Child Adolesc Psychiatr 27(2), 248–251.

Birmaher BB, Greenhill L, Cooper T, et al. (1989) Sustained release methylphenidate: Pharmacokinetic studies in ADDH males. J Am Acad Child Adolesc Psychiatr 28(5), 768–772.

Borcherding BG, Keysor CS, Cooper TB, et al. (1989) Differential effects of methylphenidate and dextroamphetamine on the motor activity level of hyperactive children. Neuropsychopharmacology 2, 255–263.

Bradley C (1937) The behavior of children receiving benzedrine. Am J Psychiatr 94, 577–585.

Brown GL, Hunt RD, Ebert MH, et al. (1979) Plasma levels of d-amphetamine in hyperactive children: Serial behavior and motor responses. Psychopharmacology (Berl) 62, 133–140.

Campbell S (1973) Mother–child interaction in reflective, impulsive, and hyperactive children (abstract). Dev Psychol 8, 341–349.

Campbell SB, Endman M, and Bernfield G (1977) A three-year follow-up of hyperactive preschoolers into elementary school. J Child Psychol Psychiatr 18, 239–249.

Carlson CL and Thomeer ML (1991) Effects of Ritalin on arithmetic tasks. In Ritalin: Theory and Patient Management, 1st ed., Greenhill LL and Osman B (eds). Mary Ann Liebert, New York, pp. 195–202.

Castellanos X, Elia J, Kruesi M, et al. (1994) Cerebrospinal fluid monoamine metabolites in boys with attention deficit hyperactivity disorder. Psychiatr Res 52(3), 305–317.

Castellanos X, Giedd J, Elia J, et al. (1997) Controlled stimulant treatment of ADHD and comorbid Tourette's syndrome: Effects of stimulant and dose (abstract). J Am Acad Child Adolesc Psychiatr 36, 589–596.

Cohen DJ and Leckman JF (1989) Commentary. J Am Acad Child Adolesc Psychiatr 28(4), 580–583.

Comings DE and Comings BG (1987) A controlled study of Tourette's syndrome. Am J Hum Genet 41, 701–741.

Conners CK (2000) Attention-deficit/hyperactivity disorder—historical development and overview. J Atten Disord 3, 173–191.

Conners CK, March J, Fiore C, et al. (1994a) Conners rating scale: Use in clinical assessment, treatment planning and research. In Use of Psychological Testing for Treatment Planning and Outcome Assessment, 1st ed., Maruish M (ed). Lawrence Erlbaum, Hillsdale, New Jersey, pp. 550–571.

Conners CK, March J, Fiore C, et al. (1994b) Continuous performance test studies in ADHD. (Unpublished)

Conners KC (1975) Controlled trial of methylphenidate in preschool children with minimal brain dysfunction (abstract). Int J Ment Health 4, 61–74.

Dahl R (1992) The pharmacologic treatment of sleep disorders. Child Adolesc Psychiatr Clin 15(1), 161–178.

Diamond I, Tannock R, and Schachar R (1999) Response to methylphenidate in children with ADHD and comorbid anxiety (abstract). J Am Acad Child Adolesc Psychiatr 38, 402–409.

Douglas V, Barr RG, Desilets J, et al. (1995) Do high doses of stimulants impair flexible thinking in ADHD? J Am Acad Child Adolesc Psychiatr 34, 877–885.

Douglas VI, Barr RG, Amin K, et al. (1988) Dose effects and individual responsivity to methylphenidate in attention deficit disorder. J Child Psychol Psychiatr 29, 453–475.

Dulcan M (1990) Using psychostimulants to treat behavior disorders of children and adolescents. J Child Adolesc Psychopharmacol 1, 7–20.

Dulcan M (1997) Practice parameters for the assessment and treatment of attention-deficit/hyperactivity disorder (abstract). J Acad Child Adolesc Psychiatr 36, 85S–121S.

DuPaul G and Rapport M (1993) Does MPH normalize the classroom performance of children with attention deficit disorder? J Am Acad Child Adolesc Psychiatr 32, 190–198.

DuPaul G, Barkley R, and McMurray M (1994) Response of children with ADHD to methylphenidate: Interaction with internalizing symptoms. J Am Acad Child Adolesc Psychiatr 33(6), 894–903.

DuPaul GJ and Barkley RA (1990) Medication Therapy. In Attention Deficit Hyperactivity Disorder: A Handbook for Diagnosis and Treatment, 2nd ed., Barkley RA (ed). Guilford Press, New York, pp. 573–612.

Elia J, Borcherding B, Rapoport J, et al. (1991) Methylphenidate and dextroamphetamine treatments of hyperactivity: Are there true non-responders? Psychiatr Res 36, 141–155.

Erenberg G, Cruse RP, and Rothner AD (1985) Gilles de la Tourette's syndrome: Effects of stimulant drugs. Neurology 35, 1346–1348.

Ernst M and Zametkin A (1995) The interface of genetics, neuroimaging, and neurochemistry in attention-deficit hyperactivity disorder. In Psychopharmacology: The Fourth Generation of Progress, 4th ed., Bloom F and Kupfer D (eds). Raven Press, New York, pp. 1643–1652.

Ernst M, Liebenauer L, Jons P, et al. (1995) L-Deprenyl on behavior and plasma monoamine metabolites in hyperactive adults (abstract). Psychopharmacol Bull 31, 565.

Ferguson JH (2000) National Institutes of Health Consensus Development Conference Statement: Diagnosis and treatment of attention-deficit/hyperactivity disorder (ADHD). J Am Acad Child Adolesc Psychiatr 39, 182–193.

Fitzpatrick P, Klorman R, Brumaghim J, et al. (1992) Effects of sustained-release and standard preparations of methylphenidate on attention deficit disorder. Am Acad Child Adolesc Psychiatr Sci Proc Annu Meet 31(2), 226–234.

Gadow K, Sverd J, Sprafkin J, et al. (1995) Efficacy of methylphenidate for attention deficit hyperactivity in children with tic disorder. Arch Gen Psychiatr 52, 444–455.

Gadow KD, Nolan EE, Sverd J, et al. (1990) Methylphenidate in aggressive-hyperactive boys: I. Effects on peer aggression in public school settings. J Am Acad Child Adolesc Psychiatr 29(5), 710–718.

Gillberg C, Melander H, von Knorring A, et al. (1997) Long-term central stimulant treatment of children with attention-deficit hyperactivity disorder. A randomized double-blind placebo-controlled trial (abstract). Arch Gen Psychiatr 54, 857–864.

Gittelman-Klein R (1987) Pharmacotherapy of childhood hyperactivity: An update. In Psychopharmacology: The Third Generation of Progress, Meltzer HY (ed). Raven Press, New York.

Gittelman-Klein R, Klein DF, Katz S, et al. (1976) Comparative effects of methylphenidate and thioridazine in hyperactive children. Arch Gen Psychiatr 33, 1217–1231.

Goldman L, Genei M, Bazman R, et al. (1998) Diagnosis and treatment of attention-deficit/hyperactivity disorder (abstract). J Am Med Assoc 279, 1100–1107.

Greenhill L (1992) Pharmacotherapy: Stimulants. Child Adolesc Psychiatr Clin 1(2), 411–447.

Greenhill L, Abikoff H, Conners CK, et al. (1996) Medication treatment strategies in the MTA: Relevance to clinicians and researchers (abstract). J Am Acad Child Adolesc Psychiatr 35, 444–454.

Greenhill L, Halperin J, and Abikoff H (1999) Stimulant medications (abstract). J Am Acad Child Adolesc Psychiatr 35, 1304–1313.

Greenhill LL, Findling RL, and Swanson JM (2002b) A double-blind, placebo-controlled study of modified-release methylphenidate (MPH MR) in children with attention-deficit/hyperactivity disorder. Pediatrics URL:http://www.pediatrics.org/cgi/content/full/109/3/e39.

Greenhill LL, Perel JM, Rudolph G, et al. (2001) Correlations between motor persistence and plasma levels in methylphenidate-treated boys with ADHD. Int J Neuropsychopharmacol 4, 207–215.

Greenhill LL, Pliszka S, Dulcan M, et al. (2002a) Practice parameter for the use of stimulant medications in the treatment of children, adolescents and adults. J Am Acad Child Adolesc Psychiatr 41, 26S–49S.

Gualtieri CT, Kanoy R, Koriath U, et al. (1981) Growth hormone and prolactin secretion in adults and hyperactive children relation to methylphenidate serum levels. Psychoneuroendocrinology 6(4), 331–339.

Halperin J, Sharma V, Siever L, et al. (1994) Serotonergic function in aggressive and nonaggressive boys with attention deficit hyperactivity disorder. Am J Psychiatr 151(2), 243–249.

Halperin JM, Matier K, Bedi G, et al. (1992) Specificity of inattention, impulsivity, and hyperactivity to the diagnosis of attention-deficit disorder (abstract). J Am Acad Child Adolesc Psychiatr 31(2), 190–196.

Hechtman L, Weiss G, Perlman T, et al. (1984) Hyperactives as young adults: Initial predictors of adult outcome. J Am Acad Child Adolesc Psychiatr 23, 250–260.

Hill J and Schoener E (1996) Age-dependent decline of attention-deficit hyperactivity disorder (abstract). Am J Psychiatr 153, 1143–1146.

Hinshaw S (1991) Effects of methylphenidate on aggressive and antisocial behavior (abstract). Proc Am Acad Child Adoles Psychiatr 7, 31–32.

Hinshaw S, Heller T, and McHale J (1992) Covert antisocial behavior in boys with attention-deficit hyperactivity disorder: External validation and effects of methylphenidate. J Consult Clin Psychol 60, 274–281.

Hinshaw S, Henker B, Whalen C, et al. (1989) Aggressive, prosocial and nonsocial behavior in hyperactive boys: Dose effects of MPH in naturalistic settings. J Consult Clin Psychol 57(4), 636–643.

Hinshaw S, March J, Abikoff H, et al. (1997) Comprehensive assessment of childhood attention-deficit hyperactivity disorder in the context of a multi-site, multimodal clinical trial (abstract). J Atten Disord 1, 217–234.

Horn WF, Islongo NS, Pascoe JM, et al. (1991) Additive effects of psychostimulants, parent training, and self-control therapy with ADHD children. J Am Acad Child Adolesc Psychiatr 30(2), 233–240.

Humphries T, Kinsbourne M, and Swanson J (1978) Stimulant effects on cooperation and social interaction between hyperactive children and their mothers (abstract). J Child Psychol Psychiatr 19, 13–22.

Jacobvitz D, Srouge LA, Stewart M, et al. (1990) Treatment of attentional and hyperactivity problems in children with sympathomimetic drugs: A comprehensive review. J Am Acad Child Adolesc Psychiatr 29(5), 677–688.

Jadad AR, Boyle M, Cunningham C, et al. (1999) Treatment of Attention-Deficit/Hyperactivity Disorder (abstract). Evidence Report/Technology Assessment No. 11 (Prepared by McMaster University under contract No. 290-0017). No. 00-E005, pp. 1–339.

Kavale K (1982) The efficacy of stimulant drug treatment for hyperactivity: A meta-analysis. J Learn Dis 15, 280–289.

Klein D (1980) Treatment of anxiety, personality, somatoform and factitious disorders. In Diagnosis and Drug Treatment of Psychiatric Disorders: Adults and Children, 2nd ed., Klein D, Gittelman R, Quitkin F, et al. (eds). Williams & Wilkins, Baltimore, pp. 539–573.

Klein R and Wender P (1995) The role of methylphenidate in psychiatry. Arch Gen Psychiatr 52, 429–433.

Klein R, Abikoff H, Klass E, et al. (1997) Clinical efficacy of methylphenidate in conduct disorder with and without attention deficit hyperactivity disorder (abstract). Arch Gen Psychiatr 54, 1073–1080.

Klein RG and Mannuzza S (1991) Long-term outcome of hyperactive children: A review. J Am Acad Child Adolesc Psychiatr 30(3), 383–387.

Klorman R, Brumagham J, Fitzpatrick P, et al. (1990) Clinical effects of a controlled trial of methylphenidate on adolescents with attention deficit disorder. J Am Acad Child Adolesc Psychiatr 29, 702–709.

Klorman R, Brumaghim JT, Salzman LF, et al. (1988) Effects of methylphenidate on attention-deficit hyperactivity disorder with and without aggressive/noncompliant features. J Abnorm Psychol 97(4), 413–422.

Kollins SH, MacDonald EK, and Rush CR (2002) Assessing the abuse potential of methylphenidate in nonhuman and human subjects: A review. Pharmacol Biochem Behav 68, 611–627.

Lowe TL, Cohen DJ, Detlor J, et al. (1982) Stimulant medications precipitate Tourette's syndrome. JAMA 26, 1729–1731.

Maletic V, March J, and Johnston H (1994) Child and adolescent psychopharmacology. Psychiatr Clin N Am 1, 101–124.

Manuzza S, Klein R, Bonagura N, et al. (1991) Hyperactive boys almost grown up: V. Replication of psychiatric status. Arch Gen Psychiatr 48, 77–83.

Matier K, Halperin J, Sharma V, et al. (1992) Methylphenidate response in aggressive and nonaggressive ADHD children: Distinctions on laboratory measures of symptoms. J Am Acad Child Adolesc Psychiatr 31(2), 219–225.

Matochik J, Liebenauer L, King A, et al. (1994) Cerebral glucose metabolism in adults with attention deficit hyperactivity disorder after chronic stimulant treatment. Am J Psychiatr 151, 658–664.

Matochik J, Nordahl T, Gross M, et al. (1993) Effects of acute stimulant medication on cerebral metabolism in adults with hyperactivity. Neuropsychopharmacology 8, 377–386.

Mattes JA, Boswell J, and Oliver H (1984) Methylphenidate effects on symptoms of attention deficit disorder in adults. Arch Gen Psychiatr 41, 449–456.

Mayes S, Crites D, Bixler E, et al. (1994) Methylphenidate and ADHD: Influence of age, IQ and neurodevelopmental status (abstract). Dev Med Child Neurol 36, 1099–1107.

McCracken J (1991) A two-part model of stimulant action on attention-deficit hyperactivity disorder in children. J Neuropsychiatr Clin Neurosci 3(2), 201–209.

Michelson D, Faries DE, Wernicke J, Kelsey DK, Kendrick KL, Sallee FR, and Spencer T (2001) Atomoxetine ADHD Study Group: Atomoxetine in the treatment of children and adolescents with ADHD: A randomized, placebo-controlled dose-response study. Pediatrics, 108, e83.

Milich R, Licht B, and Murphy D (1989) Attention-deficit hyperactivity disordered boys evaluations of and attributions for task performance on medication versus placebo. J Abnorm Psychol 98, 280–284.

Murphy DA, Pelham WE, and Lang AR (1986) Methylphenidate effects on aggressiveness in ADD and ADD/CD children (abstract). Presented at the American Psychological Association (Aug), Washington DC.

Musten L, Firestone P, Pisterman S, et al. (1997) Effects of methylphenidate on preschool children with ADHD: Cognitive and behavioral functions (abstract). J Am Acad Child Adolesc Psychiatr 36, 1407–1415.

Nigg JT, Blaskey LG, Huang-Pollock CL, et al. (2002) Neuropsychological executive functions and DSM-IV ADHD subtypes. J Am Acad Child Adolesc Psychiatr 41, 1–8.

Ottenbacher J and Cooper H (1983) Drug treatment of hyperactivity in children. Dev Med Child Neurol 25, 358–366.

Pataki C, Carlson G, and Kelly K (1993) Side effects of methylphenidate and desipramine alone and in combination in children. J Am Acad Child Adolesc Psychiatr 32, 1065–1072.

Patrick KS, Mueller RA, Gualtieri CT, et al. (1987) Pharmacokinetics and actions of methylphenidate. In Psychopharmacology: A Third Generation of Progress, 3rd ed., Meltzer HY (ed). Raven Press, New York, pp. 1387–1395.

Pelham W and Murphy H (1986) Behavioral and pharmacological treatment of hyperactivity and attention deficit disorders. In Pharmacological and Behavioral Treatment: An Integrative Approach, Hersen M and Breuning J (eds). John Wiley, New York, pp. 108–147.

Pelham W, Hoza B, Sturges J, et al. (1987) Sustained release and standard methylphenidate effects on cognitive and social behavior in children with attention deficit disorder. Pediatrics 80, 491–501.

Pelham W, Murphy D, Vanarra K, et al. (1992) Methylphenidate and attributions in boys with attention deficit hyperactivity disorder. J Consult Clin Psychol 60, 359–369.

Pelham W, Swanson J, Furman M, et al. (1995) Pemoline effects on children with ADHD: A time response by dose-reponse analysis on classroom measures. J Am Acad Child Adolesc Psychiatr 34, 1504–1514.

Pelham WE (1989) Behavior therapy, behavioral assessment and psychostimulant medication in the treatment of attention deficit disorders: An interactive approach. In Attention Deficit Disorder: 4. Emerging Trends in the Treatment of Attention and Behavioral Problems in Children, Swanson J and Bloomingdale L (eds). Pergamon Press, London, pp. 169–195.

Pelham WE and Bender ME (1982) Peer relationships in hyperactive children: Description and treatment. In Advances in Learning and Behavioral Disabilities. Gadow KD and Bailer I (eds). JAI Press, Greenwich, CT.

Pelham WE and Milich R (1991) Individual differences in response to Ritalin in classwork and social behavior. In Ritalin: Theory and Patient Management, 1st ed., Greenhill LL and Osman B (eds). Mary Ann Liebert, New York, pp. 203–222.

Pelham WE, Greenslade KE, Vodde-Hamilton MA, et al. (1990a) Relative efficacy of long-acting stimulants on ADHD children: A comparison of standard methylphenidate, Ritalin-SR, Dexedrine spansule, and pemoline. Pediatrics 86, 226–237.

Pelham WE, McBurnett K, Harper G, et al. (1990b) Methylphenidate and baseball playing in ADD children: Who's on first? (abstract) J Consult Clin Psychol 22, 131–135.

Pliszka SR (1989) Effect of anxiety on cognition, behavior, and stimulant response in ADHD. JAACAP 28(6), 882–887.

Porrino L and Rapoport J (1983) A naturalistic assessment of the motor activity of hyperactive boys, I: Comparison with normal controls. Arch Gen Psychiatr 40(6), 681–687.

Rapoport JL, Buchsbaum MS, Weingartner H, et al. (1980) Dextroamphetamine: Cognitive and behavioral effects in normal and hyperactive boys and normal men. Arch Gen Psychiatr 37, 933–943.

Rapport M, Denney C, DuPaul G, et al. (1994) Attention deficit disorder and methylphenidate: Normalization rates, clinical effectiveness and response prediction in 76 children. J Am Acad Child Adolesc Psychiatr 33(6), 882–893.

Rapport M, Jones J, DuPaul G, et al. (1987) Attention deficit disorder and methylphenidate: Group and single-subject analyses of dose effects on attention in clinic and classroom settings. J Clin Child Psychol 16, 329–338.

Rapport M, Stoner G, DuPaul G, et al. (1988) Attention deficit disorder and methylphenidate: A multi-step analysis of dose-response effects on children's impulsivity across settings. J Am Acad Child Adolesc Psychiatr 27, 60–69.

Rapport MD and DuPaul GJ (1986) Hyperactivity and methylphenidate: Rate-dependent effects on attention. Int Clin Psychopharmacol 1, 45–52.

Rapport MD, DuPaul GJ, and Kelly KL (1989a) Attention deficit hyperactivity disorder and methylphenidate: The relationship between gross body weight and drug response in children. Psychopharmacol Bull 25(2), 285–290.

Rapport MD, Quinn SO, DuPaul GJ, et al. (1989b) Attention deficit disorder with hyperactivity and methylphenidate: The effects of dose and mastery level on children's learning performance. J Abnorm Child Psychol 17(6), 669–689.

Richters J, Arnold L, Abikoff H, et al. (1995) The National Institute of Mental Health Collaborative Multisite Multimodal Treatment Study of Children with Attention-Deficit Hyperactivity Disorder (MTA): I. Background and rationale. J Am Acad Child Adolesc Psychiatr 34, 987–1000.

Roche AF, Lipman RS, Overall JE, et al. (1979) The effects of stimulant medication on the growth of hyperactive children. Pediatrics 63(6), 847–849.

Rugino TA and Samsock TC (in press) Effects of Modafinil with attention-deficit hyperactivity disorder. J Atten Disord.

Sabelsky D (1990) Fluoxetine in adults with residual attention deficit disorder and hypersomnolence. J Neuropsychiatr Clin Neurosci 2(4), 463–464.

Safer D, Allen R, and Barr E (1972) Depression of growth in hyperactive children on stimulant drugs. New Engl J Med 287, 217–220.

Safer D, Zito J, and Fine E (1996) Increased methylphenidate usage for attention deficit hyperactivity disorder in the 1990s. Pediatrics 98, 1084–1088.

Safer D, Zito M, and Gardner JF (2001) Pemoline hepatotoxicity and postmarketing surveillance. J Am Acad Child Adolesc Psychiatr 40, 622–629.

Safer DJ and Krager JM (1988) A survey of medication treatment for hyperactive/inattentive students. JAMA 260(15), 2256–2258.

Satin M, Winsberg B, Monetti C, et al. (1985) A general population screen for attention deficit disorder with hyperactivity. J Am Acad Child Adolesc Psychiatr 24, 756–764.

Satterfield JH, Satterfield BT, and Cantwell DP (1980) Multimodality treatment: A two-year evaluation of 61 hyperactive boys. Arch Gen Psychiatr 37(8), 915–919.

Schachar R and Tannock R (1993) Childhood hyperactivity and psychostimulants: A review of extended treatment studies. J Child Adolesc Psychopharmacol 3, 81–97.

Schachar R, Tannock R, Cunningham C, et al. (1997) Behavioral, situational, and temporal effects of treatment of ADHD with methylphenidate. J Am Acad Child Adolesc Psychiatr 36, 754–763.

Schechter M and Keuezer E (1985) Learning in hyperactive children: Are there stimulant-related and state-dependent effects? J Clin Pharmacol 25, 276–280.

Schleifer M, Weiss G, Cohen N, et al. (1975) Hyperactivity in preschoolers and the effect of methylphenidate. Am J Orthopsychiatr 45, 38–50.

Schuh KJ, Bymaster F, Allen AJ, Calligro D, Nisenbaum E, Emmerson P, Statnick M, Leander JD, Kallman MMJ, Clarke DO, Seil S and Bickel W (2002) Abuse liability assessment of atomoxetine, a nonstimulant pharmacotherapy for ADHD. Poster presented at the American Academy of Child & Adolescent Psychiatry (AACAP): October 22-27, 2002; San Francisco, CA.

Shaffer D (1994) Attention deficit hyperactivity disorder in adults. Am J Psychiatr 151(5), 633–638.

Shekim W, Masterson A, Cantwell D, et al. (1989) Nomifensine maleate in adult attention deficit disorder. J Nerv Ment Dis 177(5), 296–299.

Shelton T, Barkley RA, Crosswait C, et al. (2000) Multimethod psychoeducational intervention for preschool children with disruptive behavior: Two-year posttreatment follow-up. J Abnorm Child Psychol 28, 253–266.

Sherman M (1991) Prescribing Practice of Methylphenidate: The Suffolk County Study. In Ritalin: Theory and Patient Management, 1st ed., Osman B and Greenhill LL (eds). Mary Ann Liebert, New York, pp. 401–420.

Solanto MV (1984) Neuropharmacological basis of stimulant drug action in attention deficit disorder with hyperactivity: A review and synthesis. Psychol Bull 95, 387–409.

Solanto MV (1991) Dosage effects of Ritalin on cognition. In Ritalin: Theory and Patient Management, 1st ed., Osman B and Greenhill LL (eds). Mary Ann Liebert, New York, pp. 150–171.

Solanto MV and Wender E (1989) Does methylphenidate constrict cognitive functioning? J Am Acad Child Adolesc Psychiatr 28(6), 897–902.

Speltz ML, Varley CK, Peterson K, et al. (1988) Effects of dextroamphetamine and contingency management on a preschooler with ADHD and oppositional defiant disorder. J Am Acad Child Adolesc Psychiatr 27(2), 175–178.

Spencer T, Biederman J, Wilens T, et al. (1996) Pharmacotherapy of attention-deficit hyperactivity disorder across the life cycle. J Am Acad Child Adolesc Psychiatr 35, 409–432.

Spencer T, Wilens T, Biederman J, et al. (1995) A double-blind, crossover comparison of methylphenidate and placebo in adults with childhood onset ADHD. Arch Gen Psychiatr 52, 434–443.

Sprague RL and Sleator EK (1977) Methylphenidate in hyperkinetic children: Differences in dose effects on learning and social behavior. Science 198, 1274–1276.

Stephens R, Pelham WE, and Skinner R (1984) The state-dependent and main effects of pemoline and methylphenidate on paired-associates learning and spelling in hyperactive children. J Consult Clin Psychol 52, 104–113.

Stoff DM, Pollock L, Vitiello B, et al. (1987) Reduction of (3H)-Imipramine binding sites on platelets of conduct disordered children. Neuropsychopharmacology 1(1), 55–62.

Swanson J (1993) Effect of stimulant medication on hyperactive children: A review of reviews. Except Child 60, 154–162.

Swanson J, Feifel D, Sangal RB, et al. (in press) A double-blind, randomized, placebo-controlled trial of d-threo-methylphenidate hydrochloride (Focalin) and d,l-threo-methylphenidate hydrochloride (Ritalin) in children with attention deficit hyperactivity disorder. Am J Psychiatr.

Swanson J, Gupta S, Gupta D, et al. (1999) Acute tolerance to methylphenidate in the treatment of attention deficit hyperactivity disorder in children. Clin Pharmacol Ther 66, 295–305.

Swanson J, Wigal S, Greenhill L, et al. (1998) Analog classroom assessment of Adderall in children with ADHD (abstract). J Am Acad Child Adolesc Psychiatr 37, 1–8.

Tannock R, Ickowicz A, and Schachar R (1995a) Differential effects of MPH on working memory in ADHD children with and without comorbid anxiety. J Am Acad Child Adolesc Psychiatr 34, 886–896.

Tannock R, Schachar R, and Logan GD (1995b) Methylphenidate and cognitive flexibility: Dissociated dose effects in hyperactive children. J Abnorm Child Psychol 23, 235–267.

Tannock R, Schachar RJ, Carr RP, et al. (1989) Effects of methylphenidate on inhibitory control in hyperactive children. J Abnorm Child Psychol 17(5), 473–491.

Taylor E, Schachar R, Thorley G, et al. (1987) Which boys respond to stimulant medication? A controlled trial of methylphenidate in boys with disruptive behavior. Psychol Med 17, 121–143.

The Medical Letter (in press) Atomoxetine (Strattera) for ADHD.

The MTA Cooperative Group (1999) A 14 month randomized clinical trial of treatment strategies for attention-deficit/hyperactivity disorder: The Multimodal Treatment Study of Children with Attention-Deficit Hyperactivity Disorder (MTA Study). Arch Gen Psychiatr 56, 1073–1086.

Thurber S and Walker C (1983) Medication and Hyperactivity: A meta-analysis. J Gen Psychiatr 108, 79–86.

Vitiello B, Severe JB, Greenhill, et al. (2001) Methylphenidate dosage for children with ADHD over time under controlled conditions: Lessons from the MTA. J Am Child Adolsec Psychiatr 40(2), 180–187.

Volkow N, Ding J, Fowler G, et al. (1995) Is methylphenidate like cocaine? Arch Gen Psychiatr 52, 456–464.

Volkow N, Wang G, Fowler J, et al. (1998) Dopamine transporter occupancies in the human brain induced by therapeutic doses of oral methylphenidate (abstract). Am J Psychiatr 155, 1325–1331.

Vyborova L, Nahunek K, Drtilkova I, et al. (1984) Intraindividual comparison of 21-day application of amphetamine and methylphenidate in hyperkinetic children. Activ Nerv Superior 26, 268–269.

Weiss G, Hechtman L, Milroy T, et al. (1985) Psychiatric status of hyperactives as adults: A controlled prospective 15-year follow-up of 63 hyperactive children. J Am Acad Child Adolesc Psychiatr 24, 211–220.

Wender P (1994) Attention Deficit/Hyperactivity Disorder in Adults (Sept 9). Grand Rounds, New York State Psychiatric Institute, New York. (Unpublished)

Wender P and Reimherr F (1990) Buproprion treatment of attention-deficit hyperactivity disorder in adults. Am J Psychiatr 147(8), 1018–1020.

Wender P, Reimherr F, and Wood D (1985) A controlled study of methylphenidate in the treatment of attention deficit disorder. Am J Psychiatr 142, 547–552.

Wender P, Wood D, Reimherr F, et al. (1994) An open trial of pargylline in the treatment of adult attention deficit disorder, residual type. Psychiatr Res 9, 329–336.

Wender PH, Reimher F, and Wood D (1981) Attention deficit disorder in adults. Arch Gen Psychiatr 38, 449–456.

Whalen C and Henker B (1976) Psychostimulants and children: A review and analysis. Psychopharmacol Bull 83, 1113–1130.

Whalen C, Henker B, Buhrmester D, et al. (1989) Does stimulant medication improve the peer status of hyperactive children? J Consult Clin Psychol 57, 545–549.

Wilens T, Biederman J, Mick E, et al. (1994) Treatment of adult attention-deficit hyperactivity disorder (ADHD) with tricyclic antidepressants: Clinical experience with 23 patients. AACAP, Sci Proc Annu Meet 9, 45–45.

Wilens TE and Biederman J (1992) The stimulants. Psychiatr Clin N Am 15(1), 191–222.

Wolraich M, Greenhill LL, Abikoff H, et al. (2002) Randomized controlled trial of OROS methylphenidate Q.D. in children with attention-deficit hyperactivity disorder. Pediatrics 108, 883–892.

Zametkin AJ and Rapoport JL (1987) Neurobiology of attention deficit disorder with hyperactivity: Where have we come in 50 years? J Am Acad Child Adolesc Psychiatr 26, 676–686.

Zametkin AJ, Nordahl TE, Gross M, et al. (1991) Cerebral glucose metabolism in adults with hyperactivity of childhood onset. New Engl J Med 323, 1361–1366.

Zito J, Safer D, dosReis S, et al. (2000) Trends in the prescribing of psychotropic medications to preschoolers. J Am Med Assoc 283, 1025–1030.

Zito JM, Safer DJ, dosReis S, et al. (1998) Racial disparity in psychotropic medications prescribed for youths with Medicaid insurance in Maryland. J Am Acad Child Adolesc Psychiatr 37, 179–184.

# 101 Cognitive Enhancers and Treatments for Alzheimer's Disease

Lon S. Schneider
Pierre N. Tariot

## History and Background

Prior to the 1970s various medications were proposed for the treatment of dementia based on clinical experience or prevailing theories of dementia and aging. These earlier medications included psychostimulants, vasodilators, ergoloids, and various medication "cocktails." In the US only one medication, Hydergine®, was and continues to be approved for an ill-defined condition, senile mental decline. Other ill-defined terms such as "cerebral insufficiency" or "cerebral deterioration" were often used. Distinctions among cognitive impairment syndromes were attempted, using such constructs as "benign senile forgetfulness." However, these were not generally accepted because of their vagueness of definition and lack of underlying syndromology and pathology. Similarly, the offering of criteria for "age-associated memory impairment" (AAMI), an attempt to recognize functionally significant, although mild and probably nonprogressive cognitive impairment has not been generally recognized as a diagnostic construct, although DSM-IV-TR includes a code for "age-related cognitive decline," equivalent to AAMI.

By the late 1980s the advent and general acceptance of research-based diagnostic criteria for the dementia of Alzheimer's disease (AD), (McKhann et al. 1984) an understanding of its underlying pathology along with mechanism-based pharmacological therapeutics provided the framework for clinical trials to exploit a variety of new treatment strategies that might positively impact the illness.

Since AD is defined by the presence of dementia, attempts have been made to identify a predementia state of cognitive impairment, likely to lead to AD. This state of "mild cognitive impairment" (MCI) has now been the target of several clinical trials of medications previously used for AD. The evolving validity of MCI will rest mainly on its ability to predict the onset of the dementia of AD. In research clinics a diagnosis of MCI implies a conversion rate to AD of about 12 to 15% per year (Petersen et al. 2001). However, MCI is not merely a predementia stage of AD, since many people who fulfill criteria do not progress to dementia.

During the 1990s research- and consensus-based criteria were proposed to include vascular dementia (Chui et al. 1992, Roman et al. 1993), dementia with Lewy bodies (McKeith et al. 1996), and frontotemporal dementia. These later criteria are evolving and have not been well-accepted and thus clinical trials including these populations have been limited.

## Regulatory and Methodological Issues

The Food and Drug Administration (FDA) utilizes *de facto* guidelines for establishing that a drug has "antidementia efficacy" (Leber 2002). These require, in part, that: (1) clinical trials be double-blind and placebo-controlled; (2) patients fulfill the now-accepted criteria for a primary dementia such as AD (e.g., using either DSM-IV-TR or NINCDS-ADRDA (National Institute of Neurological and communicative Disorders and Stroke-Alzheimer's Disease and Related Disorders Association) Work Group Criteria) (McKhann et al. 1984); and (3) appropriate efficacy instruments be used. Although the *de facto* guidelines avoid specifying that only Alzheimer's dementia can be treated, allowing the possibility that any recognized or accepted conditions can receive approval, at present it is the only dementia for which FDA-approved medications are available. [Note that DSM-IV-TR criteria for Dementia of the Alzheimer's Type very closely reflect the NINCDS-ADRDA (National Institute of Neurological and Communicative Disorders and Stroke-Alzheimer's Disease and Related Disorders Association) Work Group Criteria.]

Further, a putative antidementia drug must show efficacy at improving memory or retarding its deterioration since memory impairment is one of the primary features of dementia. The drug also must have an effect, determined independently from neuropsychological assessment, using a global clinical measure in order to address the concern that drug-related memory improvement may be observed with psychometric testing but not be clinically meaningful. Changes in other areas of functioning, such as behavior or capacity to perform activities of daily living (ADLs), are considered to be of secondary importance for regulatory purposes at present, but, in principle, a cognitive enhancer can be approved for marketing in the US if it shows improvement or stabilization of ADLs (Activities of Daily Living) in lieu of global improvement.

Virtually all clinical trials of antidementia drugs undertaken in the US for regulatory purposes have used the Alzheimer's Disease Assessment Scale—cognitive subscale (ADASc) (Mohs et al. 1997) as the index of cognitive change and the clinical global impression of change (CGIC) as the "global" clinical measure (Schneider et al. 1997). The ADASc includes the following measures: word recall, naming, commands, constructional and ideational praxis, orientation, word recognition, spoken language, comprehension of spoken language, word-finding, and recall of test instructions. The CGIC is usually rendered as a seven-point, ordinal scale upon which a clinician indicates his or her impression of clinical change from "no change" to "minimal," "moderate," or "marked" improvement or worsening. Secondary measures in AD clinical trials often include the Mini-Mental State Examination (MMSE) (Folstein et al. 1975), a brief, physician-administered, structured examination of cognitive function, and a variety of functional activity scales, such as the Alzheimer's Disease Cooperative Study—ADL (ADCS-ADL) Scale to assess aspects of daily functioning (Galasko et al. 1997).

Limitations to the current guidelines include the failure to recognize improvement in behavior or functional activities *alone* as legitimate therapeutic goals or indications in the prescribing information, despite the fact that behavioral symptoms occur in the majority of dementia patients, and that improvements in functional status may have a major effect on prolonging independence. In addition, these guidelines fail to provide for efficacy measures for severely impaired patients who are unable to perform standard cognitive tests. Recently developed criteria in Europe require improvement in ADLs as well as clinical and neuropsychological effects (http://www.emea.eu.int/pdfs/human/ewp/055395enpdf).

The FDA draft guidelines that patients fulfill established criteria for a primary dementia is an attempt to avoid the inclusion of ill-defined dementia syndromes in clinical trials, to obtain sample homogeneity, and to achieve consensus that the medication is effective in a specific group of patients with an illness such as AD accepted by a substantial number of experts.

It is important to consider that guidelines do not exist for drugs to treat age-associated memory impairment, mild cognitive impairment, "depressive pseudodementia," or for improving cognitive function in unimpaired individuals, since there is insufficient agreement about the existence or recognition of these conditions. Similarly, regulatory guidelines do not exist for treating the cognitive components of vascular dementia, dementia in Parkinson's disease, dementia with Lewy bodies, or for cognitive impairment associated with schizophrenia or depression because of the lack of generally accepted diagnostic standards for these conditions.

For example, many characteristics of dementia with Lewy bodies are similar to AD, but include also a fluctuating cognitive impairment, with both episodic confusion and lucid intervals, variable performance over time, often associated with hallucinations and extrapyramidal motor system findings (McKeith et al. 1996). Subcortical, limbic, and neocortical ubiquitin-staining inclusion bodies are defining features of the syndrome in addition to neurodegeneration, plaques and tangles, and the decrease in choline acetyltransferase is more pronounced and predictable than in AD without Lewy bodies. About 10 to 30% of patients with AD may have diffuse Lewy bodies. The importance of recognizing patients with diffuse Lewy body disease is illustrated by observations of robust responses to cholinesterase inhibitors in one clinical trial with rivastigmine (McKeith et al. 2000). Multicenter clinical trials of cholinesterase inhibitors, however, have generally eliminated psychotic patients, therefore the general applicability of this observation is not known. The importance of guidelines is greater when therapeutic options are limited or treatments are modest in effect, as they are currently with AD.

This chapter focuses on the dementia of AD, because most work has been done in this area in recent years. Many of the issues raised will become relevant to other dementias or cognitive impairment syndromes as clinical investigators continue to study these syndromes.

## Typical Inclusion Criteria for AD Clinical Trials

Typical inclusion criteria for clinical trials include the presence of probable Alzheimer's disease (NINCDS-ADRDA workshop criteria) (McKhann et al. 1984), an MMSE score between 10 and 26; a score of less than 4 on the Modified Hachinski Scale (Rosen et al. 1980); a CT or MRI consistent with Alzheimer's disease and showing no evidence of significant focal lesions; generally good physical health other than the dementia (confirmed by medical history, physical exam, neurological exam, ECG, and laboratory tests); normal blood pressure; English speaking; and having a reliable caregiver to participate in clinical evaluations.

Exclusion criteria typically consist of a history of other psychiatric or neurological disorders, of a stroke or CT/MRI evidence of a stroke, significant concurrent physical illness, or abnormal laboratory findings. Therefore, dementia populations studied in clinical trials consist, for the most part, of mildly to moderately impaired outpatients living at home with their families, with a diagnosis of probable AD who are otherwise medically healthy and lack significant behavioral symptoms.

Most patients with AD however have concurrent other medical problems, use other medications, are more severely impaired, and are older than patients enrolled in the clinical trials. Thus, the extent to which this group is representative of the AD population as a whole is problematic.

Recently, trials have been undertaken including more severely impaired AD patients with MMSE scores as low as 3, and dementia patients in nursing homes. Efficacy in cognitive outcomes has been observed with donepezil in one trial (Feldman et al. 2001) and good tolerability in another involving nursing home patients (Tariot et al. 2001).

## Etiopathology and Implications for Treatment

### Neuropathology of Alzheimer's Disease

The definitive diagnosis of AD is based on the clinical dementia syndrome together with certain neuropathologic features first described by Alois Alzheimer in 1907. These include neuritic *plaques* and neurofibrillary *tangles* spread diffusely through the cerebral cortex and hippocampus (Khachaturian 1985, Mirra et al. 1991) (Figure 101–1). Plaques, found outside the neuron, are spherical structures possessing a central core of amyloid protein surrounded by distended abnormal neuronal dendrites and small axons. Tangles consist of bundles of filaments in cell bodies, axons, and dendrites.

## Molecular Pathology of Alzheimer's Disease

Amyloid proteins, which are highly insoluble and fibrillary in nature, are present at the core of plaques (Katzman and Jackson 1991, Selkoe 1991). The main protein component, called β-amyloid, is a small protein derived by cleavage of a larger peptide that is abundant in normal brain. The purpose of amyloid precursor protein is unknown as is the precise mechanism of its processing. There has been speculation that it is crucial in the development and maintenance of the central nervous system (CNS), as well as speculation to the reverse, that it or β-amyloid is neurotoxic. The source of this protein is not definitely known: it may come from neurons, it may be transmitted to the brain via blood vessels, or it may be manufactured in blood vessel linings. Although there is intense interest in amyloid as a possible first cause of AD, its role in producing symptoms of dementia remains unclear.

"Antiamyloid" treatment strategies rest primarily on the hope that modifying the breakdown process would lead to reduced accumulation. Such strategies include passive and active immunization against β-amyloid fragments, the development of β-secretase and β-secretase inhibitors inhibit the cleavage of APP (Amyloid Precursor Protein) into insoluble A-β fragments. These strategies are just now being applied to humans. A clinical trial with a synthetic A-β vaccine, AN-1792 (Elan and Wyeth), needed to be stopped because of the development of encephalomeningitis in many of the patients.

Significantly, there is evidence that the normal regulation of APP processing is controlled by positive feedback

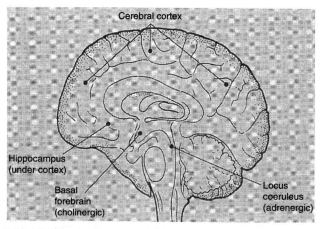

**Figure 101–1** *The right half of a human brain (facing left) showing some of the areas affected by AD. The hippocampus is affected early in the course of the disease, which accounts for certain of the memory losses. As the disease progresses, the cerebral cortex is increasingly involved, causing the cognitive and personality defects. Regions that are the sources of transmitters to wide areas of the brain also form neurofibrillary tangles, including the cholinergic basal forebrain, the noradrenergic locus coeruleus, and the serotoninergic dorsal raphe (not shown). (Source: Tariot P, Schneider L, and Coleman PD [1993a] Treatment of Alzheimer's disease: Glimmers of hope? Chem Ind 20, 801–807.)*

from cholinergic neurons, suggesting that cholinergic agents may not only enhance cognition but may also decrease neurodegeneration by inhibiting abnormal APP processing. This, however, has yet to be demonstrated.

The primary element of the neurofibrillary tangle is a paired helical filament, consisting of a ropelike filament comprised of two fibers twisted about each other. The material is found in a variety of diseases but not in normal brains. Certain microtubule-associated, abnormally phosphorylated proteins are important components of paired helical filaments, especially tau proteins. It is speculated that these proteins interfere with nerve cell functioning. Abnormal phosphorylation of "tau" may occur at multiple sites, including regions that are microtubule-binding domains, impairing the ability to promote microtubule assembly. This in turn may interrupt a major pathway for the transportation of proteins between the cell nucleus, where they are made, and the periphery of the neuronal axon. This may include, for example, neuronal trophic proteins that are normally transported from the periphery of the axon back to the cell body, where they regulate the production of proteins. At present, the "tau hypothesis," centering on the neurofibrillary tangle, is another plausible candidate defect that might account for some of the symptoms of AD.

## Pathophysiology

The neuropathophysiology of AD has been discussed in Chapter 19. The following provides the underlying pathophysiological basis for some treatments. Early findings of reductions in the activity of cerebral cortical choline acetyltransferase (ChAT), the key enzyme in acetylcholine synthesis (Bowen et al. 1976, Davies and Maloney 1976, Perry et al. 1977), were followed by the demonstration of a loss of cholinergic cell bodies in the nucleus basalis (Arendt et al. 1983, Whitehouse et al. 1982). Further studies revealed correlations between cortical ChAT reduction or nucleus basalis cell reduction and plaque densities in cortical areas (Arendt et al. 1985, Etienne et al. 1986) (Figure 101–2). The cholinergic deficit was shown previously to correlate with the decline in scores on the Blessed-Roth Dementia Rating Scale (Perry et al. 1978). After initial enthusiasm for the cholinergic hypothesis of Alzheimer's disease, it became clear that many other neuronal systems also are affected in this disorder.

Variable involvement of the noradrenergic system, including the nucleus locus coeruleus (nLC) occurs in AD (see Figure 101–2) (Bondareff et al. 1982, Mann et al. 1984). Significantly greater neuronal loss in the nLC occurred in AD patients who showed clinical manifestations of depression before death than in those who did not (Zubenko and Moossy 1988, Zweig et al. 1988). Similarly, demented patients with major depression had a tenfold reduction in norepinephrine than nondepressed demented patients (Zubenko et al. 1990). These findings suggest that many symptoms in AD may be modulated through nLC function as they are in primary depression and anxiety.

## Therapeutic Implications

Advances in understanding of plaques and tangles over the last few years underscore the biological heterogeneity of the illness, and several clues about definitive therapeutic approaches have appeared. It is likely that there are several

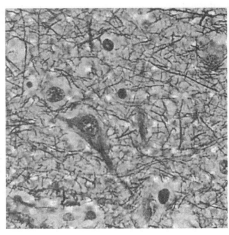

**Figure 101–2** *Human brain tissue in AD, showing neurofibrillary tangles. (Courtesy of US Department of Energy/Science Photo Library).*

stimuli for these abnormal protein processes, genetically, biologically, and environmentally determined. These processes need to be understood more fully in order to discover new drugs acting directly on the pathological processes responsible for the neurodegeneration. For example, the finding that APP processing is in part controlled by a cholinergic mechanism suggests that cholinergically based therapeutic strategies may modify the progress of the disease as well as providing symptomatic relief (Giacobini 1996).

Other potential interventions in development now include agents that interfere with beta-amyloid formation such as secretase inhibitors, modulators of APP expression, β-secretase and β-secretase inhibitors that prevent cleavage of APP into insoluble β-amyloid protein, inhibitors of β-amyloid protein aggregation or deposition, or the passive or active immunization with antibodies to β-amyloid.

The observed neurotransmitter perturbations in AD, however, provide more immediate and accessible targets for therapeutic interventions. For example, the observation of deficits in noradrenergic or serotoninergic function provide rationales for the use of antidepressants in patients with AD and symptomatic behaviors. Although not the exclusive pathological change, the cholinergic deficits represent the most consistent transmitter depletion and appear to be one of the early events in the disease process (Francis et al. 1985, 1999). Thus, it continues to remain a major focus of applied clinical pharmacological research.

## Treatment Paradigms

Approaches to the treatment of AD can be grouped into several conceptual categories (Table 101–1). One approach attempts to treat the behavioral symptoms such as agitation, aggression, psychosis, depression, anxiety, apathy, and sleep or appetite disturbances. A second approach attempts to treat the cognitive or neuropsychological signs symptoms of the illness such as memory, language, praxis, attention, orientation, and knowledge. A third approach attempts to slow the rate of progression of the illness, preserving patients' quality of life or autonomy. (Slowing the rate of decline might also be related to treating symptoms.) A fourth conceptual treatment approach is primary prevention, to delay the time to onset of illness. Success at this approach could have considerable impact. For example,

| **Table 101–1** | **Conceptualized Treatment Strategies for Patients with Cognitive Impairment** |
|---|---|

### Symptomatic and/or Restorative

Targets: impaired cognition, depression, psychosis, agitation, aggression, anxiety, insomnia

Examples: cholinesterase inhibitors, various cholinergic agonists, antidepressants, antipsychotics, mood stabilizers, antianxiety agents, hypnotics, NMDA and AMPA receptor modulators, angiotensin converting enzyme inhibitors

Neurotrophic factors: nerve growth factor, brain-derived neurotrophic factors, estrogens

Notes: some substances may have symptomatic or restorative effects but are unproven. These may include Hydergine and neotropics such as piracetam.

### Pathophysiologically-directed

Targets: underlying pathophysiology of neurodegeneration, including inflammation, production of oxidizing free radicals, excitatory amino acids.

Examples: anti-inflammatory agents, calcium channel blockers, NMDA and AMPA receptor modulators. Transplantation of hormonally active tissues, or NGF (nerve growth factor) gene therapy using viral vectors have been undertaken experimentally.

### Etiologically-directed

Targets: β-amyloid formation or hyperphosphorylated tau protein.

Examples: modulators of APP expression, β- and γ-secretase inhibitors, inhibitors of beta-amyloid protein aggregation or deposition, immunization with antibodies to beta-amyloid.

Note: The interventions listed above include some that are available and marketed, as well as some that have not been demonstrated effective or safe, and some conceptual treatments not yet developed.

delaying the onset of AD by 5 years would halve its incidence (Brookmeyer et al. 1998, Jorm et al. 1987).

## Cholinergic Agents

Historically, a great deal of emphasis has been placed on cholinergic restituting strategies in view of the prominent cholinergic dysfunction in AD. The primary implication of the cholinergic hypothesis is that potentiation of central cholinergic function should improve the cognitive and behavioral impairment associated with AD. This simple "neurotransmitter replacement" rationale has been made most compelling by the consistent effects of cholinesterase inhibitors as a class of drugs across trials (see Figure 101–3).

While agents with several kinds of procholinergic action have been evaluated for efficacy in AD, the ChIs (Cholinesterase Inhibitors) are the only agents to have consistently demonstrated efficacy in numerous multicenter, placebo-controlled trials, and thus have been approved by many national regulatory authorities. Thus ChIs represent the first *class* of efficacious pharmacological approaches for AD, and an approach that is likely to be clinically useful for the indefinite future, especially since research on drugs with other mechanisms has not advanced as rapidly as had been hoped for.

The well-established cholinergic defects in AD include: decline of cholinergic baso-cortical projections; reduced

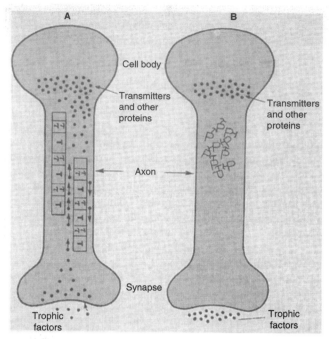

**Figure 101–3** (A) *A normal neuron. The microtubule-associated protein tau (τ) promotes the assembly of tubulin (T) into tubular microtubules. The microtubules serve as the highways for transporting transmitters and other proteins from the cell body to the synapse, and also of trophic factors (necessary for survival of the neuron) from the synapse back to the cell body. In AD (B), tau is abnormally phosphorylated (represented by Ps attached to τ). This destroys tau's ability to promote the polymerization of tubulin into microtubles, robbing the cell of the major highways for transporting many proteins from the cell body to the synapse and from the synapse back to the cell body. Proteins pile up in the cell body, unable to be moved. It is presumed that trophic substances pile up outside the synapse, also unable to be transported. The abnormal phosphorylation of tau is associated with its self-aggregation into the neurofibrillary tangles. (Source: Tariot P, Schneider L, and Coleman PD [1993a] Treatment of Alzheimer's disease: Glimmers of hope? Chem Ind 20, 801–807.)*

activity of ChAT, the key acetylcholine (ACh) synthesis enzyme, and cholinergic cell body loss in the nucleus basalis. Additionally, there are correlations between cortical ChAT reduction or nucleus basalis cell reduction and cortical plaque density. Such cholinergic deficits correlate with cognitive decline as measured by the Blessed-Roth Dementia Rating Scale (Blessed et al. 1968). The cholinergic hypothesis proposes that cognitive deficits of AD are related to decreases in central acetylcholinergic activity, and that increasing intrasynaptic ACh will enhance cognitive function and clinical well-being. (See Figure 101–4.)

## Cholinergic Treatment Approaches
Cholinergic treatment approaches include precursor loading, cholinesterase inhibition, direct cholinergic receptor stimulation, and indirect cholinergic stimulation. Unfortunately, most of these cholinergic strategies have thus far proven ineffective, effective but too toxic, or have not been completely developed.

Thus far, only ChIs have shown generally consistent symptomatic efficacy in standardized, well-controlled multicenter trials lasting from 6 months to occasionally 12 months.

## Precursor Loading
Early investigations focused on acetylcholine precursors, including choline and phosphatidyl choline (lecithin), in attempts to augment acetylcholine synthesis. Numerous trials of cholinergic precursors, most with small sample sizes, have generally failed to improve cognitive performance in patients with AD; only 10 of 43 such trials report any positive effect (Jorm 1986).

## Muscarinic Agonists and Antagonists
The rationale for the use of direct cholinergic agonists rests on the fact that postsynaptic, $M_1$, cholinergic receptors are relatively intact in AD and that presynaptic, $M_2$, cholinergic receptors, which are decreased in AD, regulate acetylcholine release. Cholinergic agonists studied in the past included bethanechol, oxotremorine, pilocarpine, RS-86, and arecoline. These agents have generally had little or no efficacy and significant cholinergic side effects.

Clinical trials results of at least 11 different cholinergic agonists thus far have been disappointing due to doubtful efficacy and a high incidence of muscarinic-related adverse effects. The failure of six muscarinic agonists with predominant $M_1$ activity, albeit each with a somewhat different receptor profile, suggests that direct stimulation of muscarinic receptors may not be sufficient to treat AD. Also, nonselective, direct receptor agonists may be relatively ineffective because they provide a prolonged and tonic cholinergic stimulation of postsynaptic cells; or perhaps they actually inhibit acetylcholine release through their action on presynaptic $M_2$ receptors. By comparison the relative efficacy of ChIs may reflect their additional actions, such as nicotinic stimulation or nonenzymatic actions.

## Other Indirect Cholinergic Enhancing Strategies
Various methods of indirect cholinergic enhancement include DuP 996 (linopirdine) that enhances the presynaptic, potassium-mediated release of acetylcholine, ondansetron, an 5-$HT_3$ antagonist, may act as a cholinergic facilitator, enhancing acetylcholine release, and various partial nicotine agonists. Unfortunately, despite interesting preclinical rationales these drugs were not demonstrated to be clinically effective (Rockwood et al. 1997, Dysken et al. 2002).

## Cholinesterase Inhibitors
Cholinesterase inhibitors (Table 101–2) have been the most frequently used experimental treatment for AD and the only intervention to yield consistently positive results in clinical trials. Modest, significant, and reliable improvement in memory was produced in early trials of the acetylcholinesterase inhibitor, physostigmine (Christie et al. 1981, Davis and Mohs 1982, Mohs et al. 1985, Stern et al. 1987). An early meta-analytic review of eight studies of cholinesterase inhibitor treatments found a mean effect size of almost zero, but in five studies that used individualized doses, the effect size increased significantly (Jorm 1986). These results with dosage-individualization led to multicenter trials of the cholinesterase inhibitors tacrine, velnacrine, and sustained-release physostigmine using an enriched population designs (Antuono 1995, Davis et al. 1992, Thal et al. 1996), subsequently provided the rationale and justification to do larger sample-sized clinical trials, and to the eventual marketing of several cholinesterase inhibitors.

**Table 101–2** FDA-Approved Drugs to Improve Cognitive Function in Alzheimer's Disease: Dosages of Marketed Cholinesterase Inhibitors

| Drug | How Supplied | Initial Dosage | Maintenance Dosage | Comments |
|---|---|---|---|---|
| Tacrine | 10, 20, 30, and 40 mg capsules | 10 mg q.i.d. | 30 or 40 mg q.i.d. | 120 to 160 mg/d are efficacious doses. Reversible direct hepatotoxicity in about 1/3 patients, requiring initial biweekly transaminase monitoring and dose titration. Not commonly used. |
| Donepezil | 5 and 10 mg tablets | 5 mg q.i.d. | 5–10 mg q.i.d. | 5 and 10 mg are both effective doses; 10 mg may be somewhat more efficacious in some trials; higher doses not tested. |
| Rivastigmine | 1.5, 3, 4.5, and 6 mg capsules | 1.5 mg b.i.d. | 3, 4.5, or 6 mg b.i.d. | Effective dosage range 3–6 mg b.i.d. Doses of 4.5 mg b.i.d. may be most optimal. May be taken with food. |
| Galantamine | 4, 8, and 12 mg tablets Solution 4 mg/mL | 4 mg b.i.d. | 8 or 12 mg b.i.d. | Effective dosage range is 8–16 mg b.i.d. 8 mg b.i.d. is the modal optimal dose. |

Initial dosages should be maintained for at least 2 and preferably 4–6 weeks before increasing. Adverse events may occur with dosage titration.

The FDA approved indication for these drugs is: "indicated for the treatment of mild to moderate dementia of the Alzheimer's type." Websites for prescribing information on cholinesterase inhibitors: tacrine, http://www.horizonpharm.com/downloads/Cognex2.pdf, donepezil, www.aricept.com/productinfo.htm http://www.pfizer.com, rivastigmine http://www.novartis.com, http://www.pharma.us.novartis.com/product/pi/pdf/exelon.pdf, galantamine, www.us.reminyl.com/Reminyl/Reminyl.pdf, http://www.us.reminyl http://www.janssen.com

Current marketed ChIs include tacrine, donepezil, rivastigmine, and galantamine. There are several cholinesterase inhibitors under development, such as phenserine, and the herbal extract huperzine A, used extensively in Asia, and available in the US as a dietary supplement.

## Mechanisms of Cholinesterase Inhibition

Acetylcholine is inactivated when it is hydrolyzed to choline and acetate by acetylcholinesterase (AChE). By inhibiting the actions of AChE, ChIs effectively increase the amount of ACh available for intrasynaptic cholinergic receptor stimulation.

An acetylcholinesterase inhibitor can work at either of two sites on AChE, an ionic subsite or a catalytic esteratic subsite to prevent the interaction between ACh and AChE. Tacrine and donepezil act at the ionic subsite. Physostigmine and rivastigmine act at the catalytic esteratic subsite (Enz and Floersheim 1997).

Specific inhibition of AChE can occur with relatively little inhibition of BChE (Butyrylcholinesterase) when the side chains of the ChI interacts with the peripheral anionic site of AChE. Donepezil has this property and is therefore selective for AChE (Brufani and Filocamo 1997). Binding to the AChE sites may be either reversible or irreversible, and may be competitive or noncompetitive with acetylcholine. Galantamine is an example of a competitive ChI, competing with acetylcholine for AChE.

In addition, AChE is present in a few molecular forms, one a tetramer, G4, is located on the presynaptic membranes within the cholinergic synaptic cleft; another a monomer G1 is found on postsynaptic membranes. While G4 is decreased along with the neuronal loss of presynaptic cholinergic neurons, postsynaptic cholinergic receptor neurons and G1 ACh are not decreased significantly with AD or aging (Enz and Floersheim 1997). Rivastigmine is a ChEI that is highly selective for the postsynaptic G1 monomer form of AChE, while galantamine is less so, and donepezil is not.

Thus the ChIs differ among themselves in selectivity for AChE and butyryl cholinesterase, mechanism of inhibition, competition with ACh for binding, and in pharmacokinetics. An unresolved question is whether or not these differences result in differential *clinical* efficacy, and different clinically observable adverse events. A summary of pharmacokinetics and pharmacodynamics is in Table 101–3.

## Individual Cholinesterase Inhibitors— Clinical Studies, Dosing, and Adverse Effects

Selected 6-month long clinical trials of most of the ChIs are summarized in Table 101–4. These multicenter trials were designed with the objective of obtaining marketing approval from the FDA. The protocols were fairly similar with each other, generally selecting outpatients with mild to moderate AD, usually with MMSE scores between 10 and 26 inclusively. Patients in these trials were generally physically healthy, were usually treated for 6 months or less, and had a mean age of about 72 years, a decade lower than the median age of AD patients in the US.

### Tacrine

Tacrine is a noncompetitive reversible inhibitor of ChE. It binds near the catalytically active site of the AChE molecule to inhibit enzyme activity. It has other actions as well including blocking sodium and potassium channels, and direct activity at muscarinic receptors (Adem et al. 1990). Two clinical trials were considered pivotal by the FDA for the drug's approval in 1993 (Farlow et al. 1992, Knapp et al. 1994), demonstrating, tacrine's significant effect on the ADAS (Alzheimer's Disease Assessment Scale) cognitive

| Table 101–3 | Pharmacodynamic and Pharmacokinetics of Marketed Cholinesterase Inhibitors | | | | | | |
|---|---|---|---|---|---|---|---|
| Drug | Pharmacodynamics | Absorption | Bioavailability | Peak Plasma (h) | Elimination Half-life (h) | Protein Binding | Metabolism/ Comments |
| Tacrine (Cognex) | Noncompetitive, reversible ChI, both butryrl and acetyl ChI, also multiple other actions | Delayed by food | 17% | 1–2 | 2–4 | 55% | Via 1A2, nonlinear pharmacokinetics; hepatoxicity requires regular monitoring of serum alamine aminotransferases. |
| Donepezil (Aricept) | Noncompetitive, reversible acetyl-ChI. | Not affected by food | 100% | 3–4 | 70 | 96% | Via 2D6, 3A4. Nonlinear pharmacokinetics at 10 mg/d |
| Rivastigmine (Exelon) | Noncompetitive ChI, both butryrl and acetyl ChI, may differentially effect different acetyl ChEs | Delayed by food | 40% | 1.4–2.6 | < 5 | 40% | Hydrolysis by esterases and excreted in urine (nonhepatic). Duration of cholinesterase inhibition longer than plasma half-life. Nonlinear pharmacokinetics |
| Galantamine (Reminyl) | Competitive, reversible ChI, modulates nicotine receptors | Delayed by food | 90% | 1 | 7 | 18% | Via 2D6, 3A4 |

*Note*: Pharmacodynamic effects of some ChIs are longer than their elimination half-lives. Drugs that inhibit or induce the cytochrome enzymes above might be expected to increase or decrease blood levels. For the most part, clinically however, drug interactions with donepezil, rivastigmine, and galantamine have not been clinical problems.

subscale assessment and on measures of daily function. In the 30-week study, 663 patients were randomized to three dosage treatments or placebo (Knapp et al. 1994). Statistically significant treatment effects for the 120 mg and 160 mg daily dosage groups were found on the ADASc, a clinician's interview-based impression of change rating, and on ADLs.

**Dosing.** Tacrine's FDA-approved dosing regimen is based on the clinical trials. The recommended starting dose is 10 mg q.i.d. to be maintained for 6 weeks, while serum transaminase levels are monitored every other week. If the drug is tolerated and transaminase levels do not increase above three times the upper limit of normal, the dose is then increased to 20 mg q.i.d. After 6 weeks, dosage should be increased to 30 mg q.i.d., again with biweekly monitoring and then, if tolerated, to 40 mg q.i.d. for the next 6 weeks.

## Donepezil

Donepezil (Aricept™) is a long-acting piperidine-based highly selective and reversible acetylcholinesterase inhibitor. Two phase III clinical trials (Rogers et al. 1998a, 1998b) provided pivotal evidence for the drug's FDA approval in late 1996. Additional randomized clinical trials include a trial of 6 months duration (Burns et al. 1999), a Scandinavian study of 12 months (Winblad et al. 2001), a study of nursing home patients (Tariot et al. 2001), and a 6-month trial in which a large proportion were more severely impaired than in previous trials (Feldman et al. 2001).

**Dosing:** Donepezil is initiated at 5 mg/day and then increased to 10 mg/day after 4 to 6 weeks. Raising the dose earlier increases the risk for cholinergic adverse events. Five or 10 mg/day are effective doses; 10 mg tends to be somewhat more effective than 5 mg when the various trials as a group are evaluated.

## Rivastigmine

Rivastigmine (Exelon™) is a pseudo-irreversible, selective AChE subtype inhibitor. Although it inhibits butyrylcholinesterase as well, it is relatively selective to the postsynaptic G1 monomer form of AChE in areas of the cortex and hippocampus. After binding to AChE, the carbamate portion of rivastigmine is slowly hydrolyzed, cleaved, conjugated to a sulphate and excreted. Thus, its metabolism is essentially extra-hepatic and is unlikely to have significant pharmacokinetic interactions.

Four phase III randomized, placebo-controlled, 26-week long clinical trials were completed of similar design, but differing mainly in dosing methods. Two have been published (Corey-Bloom et al. 1998, Rosler et al. 1999). Some results of the third have been included in secondary reports (Birks et al. 2002, Schneider 2002, Schneider et al. 1998, Spencer and Noble 1998).

In the two published trials, doses were titrated weekly during the first 7 weeks to one of two dosage ranges, 1 to 4 mg/day or 6 to 12 mg/day, and dose decreases were not permitted, possibly contributing to lesser tolerability and seemingly more side effects during these stages of treatment.

| Table 101–4 | Key Placebo-Controlled, Randomized Cholinesterase Inhibitor Clinical Trials* | | | | |
|---|---|---|---|---|---|
| Citation | Duration (Wk) | Number | Age | Dose (mg/d) | Completers (%) |
| **Tacrine** | | | | | |
| Knapp et al. (1994) | 26 | 663 | 73 | 120 | 32% |
| | | | | 160 | 28% |
| | | | | P | 68% |
| **Donepezil** | | | | | |
| Rogers et al. (1998b) | 24 | 473 | 73 | 5 | 85% |
| | | | | 10 | 68% |
| | | | | P | 80% |
| Burns et al. (1999) | 24 | 818 | 72 | 5 | 78% |
| | | | | 10 | 74% |
| | | | | P | 80% |
| Tariot et al. (2001) | 24 | 208 | 86 | 10 | 74% |
| | | | | P | 82% |
| Feldman et al. (2001) | 24 | 2xx | 72 | 10 | 67% |
| Winblad et al. (2001) | 52 | 286 | | P | 67% |
| **Rivastigmine** | | | | | |
| Corey-Bloom et al. (1998) | 26 | 699 | 75 | 1–4 | 85% |
| | | | | 6–12 | 65% |
| | | | | P | 84% |
| Rosler et al. (1999) | 26 | 725 | 72 | 1–4 | 86% |
| | | | | 6–12 | 67% |
| | | | | P | 87% |
| **Galantamine** | | | | | |
| Tariot et al. (2000) | 20 | 978 | 77 | 8 | 76% |
| | | | | 16 | 78% |
| | | | | 24 | 78% |
| | | | | P | 84% |
| Raskind et al. (2000) | 24 | 636 | 75 | 24 | 68% |
| | | | | 32 | 58% |
| | | | | P | 81% |
| Wilcock et al. (2000) | 24 | | | | |

Rounded to two figures. All trials had 58 to 64% female subjects except for tacrine (Knapp et al. 1996, 53%), and donepezil nursing home trial (Tariot et al. 1999, 82%). Dropouts are for all reasons to avoid bias; not just those attributed to side effects.

*All trials included only patients with probable AD (NINCDS-ADRDA criteria) or dementia of Alzheimer's type (DSM-IV criteria), and generally with baseline MMSE scores between 10 and 26 inclusive, except for the galantamine trials that used narrower ranges of 10–22 and 11–24.

**Dosing:** The recommended starting dose of rivastigmine is 1.5 mg b.i.d., taken with meals. If this dose is well tolerated after a minimum of 2 weeks of treatment, it may be increased to 3 mg b.i.d. Subsequent increases to 4.5 mg and then 6 mg b.i.d. should be based on good tolerability of the current dose and may be considered after a minimum of 2 weeks of treatment. Higher daily doses, averaging about 9 to 10 mg were associated with better efficacy than lower doses.

## Galantamine

Galantamine (Reminyl℠), an alkaloid originally extracted from Amaryllidaceae (*Galanthus woronowi*, the Caucasian snowdrop), but now synthesized, is a reversible, competitive inhibitor of AChE with relatively less butyrylcholinesterase activity (Harvey 1995). Since competitive inhibitors compete with ACh at AChE binding sites, their inhibition is, theoretically, dependent on intrasynaptic ACh concentration in that they will be less likely to bind to sites in brain areas that have high ACh levels. Another characteristic is its allosteric modulation of nicotinic receptor sites, thus possibly enhancing cholinergic transmission by presynaptic nicotinic stimulation (Maelicke et al. 2001).

Four large clinical trials, involving over 2,400 subjects (Raskind et al. 2000, Tariot et al. 2000, Wilcock et al. 2000, Rockwood et al. 2001), and a systematic review (Olin and Schneider 2002) have been published. The results of two trials indicated that treatment with either 24 or 32 mg/day galantamine improved cognition, clinician's global assessment of change, and ADL scores, with lesser adverse effects at the lower dose. The results of the third showed that daily doses of 16 mg or 24 mg were effective, and 8 mg was not. The FDA approved galantamine in April 2001.

**Dosing:** Initial dosing is 4 mg b.i.d., and should be raised to 8 mg b.i.d. after 2 to 4 weeks. For patients who are tolerating medication but not responding the dose can be raised to 12 mg b.i.d. after another 4 weeks.

## Adverse Effects of Cholinesterase Inhibitors

Most adverse events from ChIs are cholinergically mediated, and are characteristically mild in severity and short-lived, lasting only a few days. Adverse events of the marketed ChIs are summarized in Table 101–5. Significant cholinergic side effects can occur in up to about 25% of patients receiving higher doses. Often they are related to the initial titration of medication. Patients tend to rapidly become tolerant to the adverse events when they occur.

Because of the actions of ChIs, these drugs require caution when used in patients with significant asthma, significant chronic obstructive pulmonary disease, cardiac conduction defects, or clinically significant bradycardia. Appropriate considerations are involved in general anesthesia as well since they may prolong the effects of succinylcholine-type drugs.

### Tacrine

Elevated transaminases due to direct, reversible hepatotoxicity were the main reason for treatment withdrawals in the two larger pivotal studies. Transaminases were elevated above three times the upper limit of normal in the approximately 30% of patients. This occurred generally within 6 to 12 weeks and reverses within 6 weeks of discontinuing medication. Nearly 90% of patients, who had elevated transaminases and then were rechallenged, were able to tolerate and continue medication (Watkins et al. 1994).

Common adverse effects related to cholinergic mechanisms are dose-related and include: nausea and/or vomiting in 28% of patients versus 8% in the placebo group, diarrhea in 16% versus 5%, anorexia in 9% versus 3%, myalgia in 9% versus 5%. Other side effects that led to withdrawal from clinical trials of tacrine included dizziness (12%), confusion (>5%), insomnia (>5%), ataxia (>5%), agitation (4%). Tacrine is not tolerated in about 10% to 20% of patients because of such peripheral cholinergic effects (Prescribing Information, October 2000, http://www.horizonpharm.com/downloads/Cognex2.pdf).

### Donepezil

The most common gastrointestinal side effects of donepezil include nausea, vomiting, diarrhea, and anorexia. Additionally, some patients develop muscle cramps, headache, dizziness, syncope, flushing, insomnia, weakness, drowsiness, fatigue, and agitation. Weight loss of > 7% of baseline occurred at twice the rate of placebo in the nursing home study, but not in outpatient trials. Adverse effects occurred at a higher rate when the titration from 5 to 10 mg was made in 1 week compared to 6 weeks.

### Rivastigmine

Adverse effects are primarily gastrointestinal and occurred in the high-dose (6–12 mg/day) group. They occurred mainly during dose escalation and led to withdrawal in one study in 23% of the high-dose group, 7% of the low-dose group and 7% of the placebo group. Of note, inclusion criteria for these clinical trials allowed for patients with a broader range of medical comorbidities to be entered into the studies than have donepezil or tacrine trials, perhaps partially explaining the relatively high adverse event rate. Also, the protocols did not allow for the medication dose to be decreased in patients who developed adverse effects

| Table 101–5 | Adverse Effects of Cholinesterase Inhibitors |
|---|---|

Summary of adverse event data in placebo-controlled, randomized clinical trials. The method of obtaining adverse events and their reporting vary among trials

| Drug | Adverse Events |
|---|---|
| **Tacrine** | Nausea, vomiting, diarrhea, dyspepsia, myalgia, anorexia, dizziness, confusion, insomnia, rare agranulocytosis |
| | Approximately 50% of patients will develop direct, reversible hepatotoxicity manifested by elevated transaminases |
| | Drug interactions may include increased cholinergic effects with bethanacol; increased plasma tacrine levels with cimetidine or fluvoxamine. This may occur by inhibition of P450 1A2. The association of tacrine with haloperidol may increase parkinsonism and tacrine increases theophylline concentration. |
| **Donepezil** | Nausea, diarrhea, insomnia, vomiting, muscle cramps, fatigue, anorexia, dizziness, abdominal pain, myasthenia, rhinitis, weight loss, anxiety, syncope (2 vs. 1%) |
| **Rivastigmine** | Nausea, vomiting, anorexia, dizziness, abdominal pain, diarrhea, malaise, fatigue, asthenia, headache, sweating, weight loss, somnolence, syncope (3 vs. 2%). Rarely, severe vomiting with esophageal rupture |
| **Galantamine** | Nausea, vomiting, diarrhea, anorexia, weight loss, abdominal pain, dizziness, tremor, syncope (2 vs. 1%) |

Adverse event estimates vary widely among the cholinesterase inhibitors from study to study and thus relative adverse event rates among drugs are difficult to estimate. Cholinergic side effects generally occur early and are related to initiating or increasing medication. They tend to be mild and self-limited. Medications should be restarted at lowest doses after temporarily stopping. See prescribing information referenced in Table 101–2.

**General precautions with cholinesterase inhibitors** (as indicated in the prescribing information)

By increasing central and peripheral cholinergic stimulation cholinesterase inhibitors may:

1. increase gastric acid secretion, increasing the risk for GI bleeding especially in patients with ulcer disease or those taking anti-inflammatories
2. produce bradycardia, especially in patients with sick sinus or other supraventricular conduction delay, leading to syncope, falls, and possible injury
3. exacerbate obstructive pulmonary disease
4. cause urinary outflow obstruction
5. increase risk for seizures
6. prolong the effects of succinylcholine-type muscle relaxants

during the titration period, possibly increasing the overall reporting of these effects.

Adverse effects that occurred in the higher dose group were sweating, fatigue, asthenia, weight loss, malaise, dizziness, somnolence, nausea, vomiting, anorexia, and flatulence. In the maintenance phase, dizziness, nausea, vomiting, dyspepsia, and sinusitis occurred more in the 6 to 12 mg/day group than in the placebo group. The FDA approval letter requests that the manufacturer do further analyses to better characterize these effects, especially the weight loss and anorexia.

## Galantamine

Principal adverse effects are nausea, vomiting, diarrhea, anorexia, weight loss, abdominal pain, dizziness, and tremor. Again, adverse events were more frequent earlier in the course of treatment and during the dosage titration from 16 mg/day to 24 mg/day and higher. In one trial the effective dosage of 16 mg/day was not associated with overall greater adverse events than the placebo-treated group.

## Particular Adverse Events

A number of infrequent adverse events that may be of particular concern to patients, caregivers, and physicians, and are common among the class of ChIs include fatigue, anorexia, weight loss, and bradycardia. Myasthenia and respiratory depression occurred in a few patients treated with the higher doses of the organophosphate drug metrifonate leading to its therapeutic demise for AD. Although myasthenia might not be expected to occur with the reversible ChI, physicians should be vigilant for complaints of fatigue and weakness.

An increased but modest incidence of anorexia appears to be a consistent finding across clinical trials and appears to be dose related. The absolute reported incidence varies across trials from approximately 8 to 25% at the highest dose of ChI compared to 3 to 10% in comparable placebo patients. Similarly, there is an increased rate of significant weight loss with higher doses of ChIs compared to placebo patients. The proportion of patients losing greater than 7% of their baseline weight varies from approximately 10 to 24% in the higher doses and from 2 to 10% of the placebo-treated patients in those trials reporting the statistic. Anorexia and weight loss are significant clinical problems for many elderly patients independent of medication effects, and whether or not demented.

## Treatment Approach

The typical candidates for ChIs are outpatients with AD of mild to moderate cognitive severity. They usually live at home or in an assisted living facility. Dementia is their main clinical problem; concurrent illnesses are not severe or dominating the clinical picture. Nor do behavioral syndromes such as psychosis, agitation, or significant insomnia, apathy, or depression dominate.

As indicated above, dosing should be initiated with 5 mg/day donepezil, 1.5 mg b.i.d. rivastigmine or 4 mg b.i.d. galantamine. Tacrine should be reserved as a second line medication since it requires q.i.d. dosing and biweekly blood monitoring for elevated transaminase. After a minimum of 2 weeks, but preferably 4 to 6 weeks, the dosages should be doubled although 5 mg of donepezil is an effective dose.

Optimal duration of treatment with continuing efficacy is unknown but overall efficacy extends at least 9 to 12 months based on the clinical trials and open-label extension phases.

Maintenance treatment can be continued as long as a therapeutic benefit for the patient seems apparent. Therefore, the potential clinical benefit of ChIs should be reassessed on a regular basis. Discontinuation should be considered when evidence of a therapeutic effect is no longer present. Because of the great interpatient variability of response, it is not possible to predict individual patient responses to ChIs.

It is difficult to assess individual patient response because of the variability of the deteriorating course of AD, and because most of the effect of medication is due to a stabilization or lack of worsening of symptoms or cognitive function while placebo-treated patients continue to decline. Therefore, the clinical observations of minimal or no clinical worsening may be sufficient reasons to continue medication treatment if patients are tolerating therapy.

## Monitoring Side Effects

Cholinergic side effects such as diarrhea, nausea, and vomiting, when they occur, tend to occur at initiation of treatment and when titrating to higher doses. They are

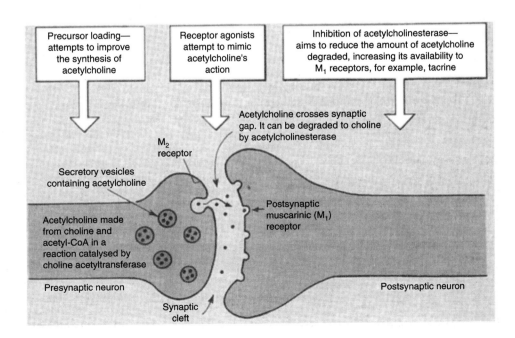

**Figure 101–4** *Possible areas of action for therapy in AD. (Source: Tariot P, Schneider L, and Coleman PD [1993a] Treatment of Alzheimer's disease: Glimmers of hope? Chem Ind 20, 801–807.)*

often transient or self-limited and can often be managed with encouragement and maintenance of the present dose level, by omitting one or more doses, or by temporarily decreasing dosage. Most cholinergic side effects are related to the dose escalation phase of treatment, just after starting or increasing. Patients on maintenance doses should have few and very mild cholinergic side effects if any.

However, anorexia and weight loss may be clinically significant problems over the longer term, especially in older, more medically ill, and nursing home patients, so these parameters should be monitored and medication reduced or discontinued if anorexia or weight loss become clinically significant to assess if appetite returns.

Uncommonly, the vagotonic effects of ChIs may cause significant bradycardia, and this can be a particular concern to patients with supraventricular conduction impairments or sick sinus syndrome.

Because gastric acid secretion may be increased with cholinesterase inhibitors, there may be an increased risk for developing ulcers or gastrointestinal bleeding. Patients receiving nonsteroidal anti-inflammatory drugs may be at a particularly additive risk. It is possible that ChIs may cause bladder outflow obstruction, seizures, and exacerbate asthma or obstructive pulmonary disease, and interfere with succinylcholinelike anesthetics.

## Effect on Behavior

The evidence that ChIs may improve behavior is based on case series and secondary analyses of efficacy trials (Kaufer et al. 1996, Raskind et al. 1997). Patients enrolled into ChI trials are selected largely on the basis of their ability to cooperate; they are not generally agitated, psychotic, or depressed. Thus ChIs have not been formally tested in patients with clearly defined behavioral problems. There is little consistency in the subscales of the behavioral rating instruments that might improve from study to study. For example, in two trials each there was a significant effect on the hallucination or aberrant motor behavior items, and in one trial each on agitation or apathy. Nevertheless, clinical experience suggests that they may be effective at least for mildly disturbed behavior, and in delaying the onset of troublesome behaviors, perhaps by maintaining cognitive function or perhaps through enhancing attentional processes and activation.

## Neuroprotection

Cholinergic therapies may have effects beyond the short-term symptomatic improvement of cognition and may modify the pathogenetic processes of the illness (Radebaugh et al. 1996, Thal et al. 1997). For example, activation of $M_1$ muscarinic receptors can stimulate secretion of amyloid precursor proteins via the α-secretase pathway such that there is a decrease in the production of toxic and insoluble β-amyloid, thus theoretically decreasing the formation of amyloid plaques and promoting the normal processing of APP (Inestrosa et al. 1996, Muller et al. 1997, Nitsch et al. 1992). These effects have been reported with some cholinergic agonists and ChIs (Buxbaum et al. 1992, Haroutunian et al. 1997, Lahiri et al. 1992, Nitsch et al. 1992), but remain to be proven in clinical trials (Buxbaum et al. 1992, Haroutunian et al. 1997, Lahiri et al. 2000).

## Restorative Approaches: Other Agents

The structural and functional disturbances of central catecholaminergic systems in AD and their important role in brain-related functions provide the rationale for pharmacological enhancement of these systems. The general strategies employed are analogous to those used with cholinergic agents: precursor loading, inhibition of degradative enzymes, and use of agonists. Studies of dopamine precursors (e.g., with tyrosine, l-dopa) and agonists (e.g., clonidine, guanefacine, amantadine, bromocriptine) have largely been negative (Schneider and Tariot 1997).

There have been some positive effects reported with selegiline (l-deprenyl, Eldepryl®, Somerset), a monoamine oxidase (MAO) inhibitor that relatively selectively inhibits MAO type B at a 5 to 10 mg daily dose (Tariot et al. 1993b). The overall effect of selegiline at this dose may be to increase CNS levels of dopamine and some trace neurotransmitters such as phenylethylamine without affecting norepinephrine levels. Selegiline is currently marketed for the treatment of Parkinson's disease for which it has demonstrated effects in maintaining motor function (Parkinson Study Group 1993). However, an adequate efficacy trial has yet to be completed in AD.

From a different perspective, selegiline may have potential to preserve surviving neurons (Tatton 1993). Elevated levels of MAO-B, which are found in the brains of patients with AD, might lead to elevated levels of neurotoxins such as 6-hydroxydopamine, quinones, and free radicals. It has been postulated also that exposure to substances in the environment could lead to neurotoxic products (via oxidative biotransformation). In either case, inhibition of MAO on a chronic basis could theoretically retard progression of the illness based on antitoxic mechanisms. Finally, selegiline may have neuronal "rescue" effects, based on neurotrophic-like properties not involving MAO inhibition. It is notable that rodents and dogs treated with selegiline have increased survival (Knoll 1988, Milgram et al. 1990, Ruehl et al. 1997). Selegiline is marketed in the US as an FDA-approved veterinary medicine for "canine cognitive dysfunction."

Selegiline, 5 mg b.i.d., along with and separately from vitamin E, 1,000 IU b.i.d., has been associated with prolonged maintenance of ADLs and survival in the community in moderately to severely impaired AD patients but with no improvement in function (Sano et al. 1997).

## Metabolic Enhancement

In view of regional decreases in glucose utilization and abnormal oxidative metabolism, drugs have been employed with the aim of correcting these abnormalities, including ergot alkaloids and nootropics. A discussion of the ergot alkaloids, Hydergine®, can be found in the previous edition of this book and in a Cochrane systematic review (Olin et al. 2002). Although once one of the most frequently prescribed medications in the world, it is now uncommonly prescribed. Numerous clinical trials in various elderly patient groups have not clarified its efficacy or clinical role. Another ergoloid derivative available in Europe, nicergoline (Sermion, Pharmacia), was associated with significant improvement on some areas such as orientation and attention and has been undergoing clinical testing (Fioravanti and Flicker 2002, Winblad et al. 2001).

**Nootropics.** Piracetam, oxiracetam, pramiracetam, aniracetam, CI 933, and BMY 21502 are pyrrolidone derivatives of γ-aminobutyric acid (GABA), although they do not appear to have GABA-like effects, and are postulated to have a neuroprotective effect on the CNS against hypoxia, electroconvulsive treatment, and drug intoxication. These types of drugs may also enhance the CNS microcirculation by reducing platelet activity and by reducing adherence of red blood cells to vessel walls and may stimulate central cholinergic activity. These diverse effects are termed neotropic to indicate the class of drugs that are structurally related to piracetam and may improve learning and memory (Nicholson 1990). However, a specific mechanism of action relevant for dementia has not been established. Double-blind, multicenter, controlled studies have shown mixed results with piracetam in the treatment of dementia in the elderly (Flicker and Evans 2002, Vernon and Sorkin 1991). Pramiracetam and oxiracetam have been evaluated in large scale multicenter studies with no sufficiently significant clinical effects in dementia. Piracetam is undergoing a clinical trial for mild cognitive impairment.

## Neurotrophic Factors

Disturbances in neurotrophic factor physiology may play a role in the pathophysiology of dementia, possibly leading to mechanical dysfunction of neuronal cells. Although there is no direct evidence supporting an involvement of nerve growth factor (NGF) in the pathogenesis of AD, animal studies suggest that NGF administration counteracts cholinergic atrophy in the nucleus basalis irrespective of the actual cause. The administration of NGF to AD patients would represent a pharmacological attempt to induce hypertrophy of surviving cholinergic neurons, and would be manifested by increased expression of structural and transmitter-specific proteins. In animals, NGF-induced hypertrophy of basal forebrain cholinergic neurons increases their resistance to insult, and raises their ability to influence postsynaptic neurons.

In humans with AD, NGF administration may attenuate the rate of degeneration of surviving cholinergic neurons, enhance their functional performance, and consequently improve behaviors that are affected by the cholinergic deficit (Hefti and Schneider 1991). A National Institute on Aging work group, studying the potential use of NGF for AD, concluded that there is a strong scientific rationale for clinical trials, and provided recommendations for its clinical development (Phelps et al. 1989). Since NGF does not penetrate the blood–brain barrier, it requires administration by intraventricular catheter and pump or the use of carrier molecules (Hefti and Schneider 1989). Three patients have been treated with NGF infused intrathecally with slight cognitive benefit and significant back pain and weight loss (Eriksdotter Jonhagen et al. 1998). Other strategies being developed for delivery of growth factors include intraparenchymal administration, tissue transplant, the use of a viral vector for NGF mRNA, or injection or surgical implantation of genetically modified fibroblasts (www.ceregene.com).

**Estrogens.** Estrogens may have cholinergic neurotrophic and neuroprotective effects and may enhance cognitive function (Simpkins et al. 1994). In ovariectomized rats, estradiol replacement enhanced learning; reversed the decrease in neuronal choline uptake and ChAT caused by ovariectomy; prevented the ovariectomy-associated decline in nerve growth factor and in brain-derived neurotrophic factor mRNA.

A beneficial role for estrogen in AD, cognitive function, mood, and aging is suggested by observations of an inverse relationship of ERT (Estrogen Replacement Therapy) dose and duration with dementia diagnoses on death certificates (Paganini-Hill and Henderson 1994); by preliminary trials suggesting a cognitive enhancing effect of estradiol, estrone, and conjugated estrogens in AD (Asthana et al. 2001, Fillit et al. 1986, Honjo et al. 1989, Ohkura et al. 1994). The vast majority of postmenopausal women do not receive estrogen replacement therapy, spending the last one-third of their lives in an estrogen-deficient state, a time during which the risk of AD exponentially increases.

Unfortunately, clinical trials of conjugated equine estrogens (Premarin®) to improve cognition in both hysterectomized and nonhysterectomized women with AD have not led to success, and indeed women treated with Premarin fared somewhat worse both in cognition and safety including 5% developing deep vein thrombosis (Henderson et al. 2000, Mulnard et al. 2000).

To assess the potential of conjugated estrogens to delay the time of onset of AD a large scale trial is underway (NIH Women's Health Initiative). Thus currently estrogen replacement cannot be recommended as a treatment for women with Alzheimer's dementia.

## Etiologically-Directed Approaches in AD

### Immune and Inflammatory Processes

Inflammatory processess may be seen in various neurodegenerative disorders. Emerging evidence indicates overactivity of aspects of immune function in AD (Aisen and Davis 1994). Immune/inflammatory reactions may be established by reactive microglia surrounding senile plaques and astrocyte proliferation; and inflammatory cytokines are produced such as tumor necrosis factor alpha, interleukin-1 (IL-1), α-2-macroglobulin, and α-1-antichymotrypsin. IL-1 and IL-6 promote the synthesis of β-amyloid precursor protein.

**Anti-inflammatory Medications.** Epidemiological evidence supports the use of nonsteroidal anti-inflammatories as preventative of AD. However, clinical trials data is less encouraging. The potential role for anti-inflammatory agents is supported by a small 44-patient placebo-controlled trial of indomethacin (Rogers et al. 1993). Low-dose prednisone (10 mg) did not prove effective in a 1-year long, placebo-controlled trial by the Alzheimer's Disease Cooperative Study (Aisen et al. 2000). There have been clinical trials failures with cyclo-oxygenase-2 inhibitors, celecoxib and rofecoxib, as well as with the nonspecific cyclo-oxygenase inhibitor naprosyn (Aisen et al. 2002). Thus, overall efficacy of anti-inflammatories agents in AD has yet to be demonstrated.

## Antioxidants

There are both theoretical reasons, and empirical findings, to suggest that free radical damage may be one of the mechanisms causing neuronal degeneration in a range of conditions including aging and Alzheimer's disease. Many studies have found evidence of increased level of oxidative damage to neurons in Alzheimer's disease.

## Vitamin E and Selegiline

A trial comparing vitamin E, 1,000 IU b.i.d. and selegiline, 5 mg b.i.d. was undertaken in outpatients with moderate to severe dementia (Sano et al. 1997). Overall, both drugs were effective in maintaining patients' ADLs and prolonging survival in the community by about 5 to 7 months. There was no effect on cognition, however.

**Ginkgo Biloba.** *Ginkgo biloba* extract (GbE) may exert neuroprotective effects under conditions of hypoxia, ischemia preventing neuronal cell death (Spinnewyn 1992), inhibit the toxic effects of β-amyloid (Bastianetto et al. 2000), and act as a free radical scavenger (Dorman et al. 1992, Dumont et al. 1992, Pietschmann et al. 1992). In aged animals, oral GbE treatment leads to increases in the densities of hippocampal muscarinic acetylcholine receptors and cortical 5-HT$_{1A}$ receptors (Huguet et al. 1994, Taylor 1985) and enhances high affinity choline uptake into hippocampal synaptosomes (Kristofikova et al. 1992).

A GbE preparation (EGb761) is approved in Germany and other countries for the treatment of disturbances of cerebral function related to dementia syndromes. Several clinical trials have been conducted in patients with dementia, including dementia of the Alzheimer type (Le Bars et al. 1997, Maurer et al. 1997, Weitbrecht and Jansen 1986, Hofferberth 1994) and mixed populations with patients suffering from either vascular dementia or dementia of the Alzheimer type (Haase et al. 1996, Kanowski et al. 1996). Doses used in these trials are either 120 or 240 mg/day.

**Calcium Channel Blockers.** The process of neuronal death in aging and in AD may be mediated by an increase in intracellular free calcium, which activates various destructive enzymes (such as proteases, endonucleases, and phospholipases) and disrupts intracellular processes. In principle, blocking the increase in intracellular free calcium may retard these mechanisms of neuronal death and thus slow progression of disease.

Based on this hypothesis, two calcium channel blockers that have been tested in AD patients are nimodipine and a Bristol-Myers Squibb investigational compound. In one trial, the low-dose nimodipine group (30 mg t.i.d.) showed less deterioration on several memory tests over a 10- to 12-week treatment period than the placebo or high-dose nimodipine (60 mg t.i.d.) group (Tollefson 1990). A larger study showed significant cognitive effects for nimodipine compared with Hydergine® and placebo (Kanowski et al. 1988). It is not clear, however, whether study subjects fulfilled criteria for possible AD. Nimodipine is marketed to reduce the severity of neurological deficits resulting from vasospasm in patients who have had a recent subarachnoid hemorrhage. It is also used off-label as a cognitive enhancer. A continuing interest in calcium blockers is also spurred by results from a French hypertension trial that found that patients taking calcium blockers were less likely to develop dementia.

**Excitatory Amino Acids.** The *N*-methyl-D-aspartate (NMDA) receptor, a glutamate receptor subtype, has important effects in learning and memory. Stimulation by the excitatory amino acid glutamate results in long-term potentiation of neuronal activity basic to memory formation (Cotman et al. 1988). There appears to be a decrease in cerebral cortical and hippocampal NMDA receptors in AD. Glycine, acting at an adjoining glycine-B receptor, modulates the effects of glutamate. Agents aimed at regulating NMDA receptor transmission are in development for testing of possible memory benefit. Only one trial has been reported using milacemide, a prodrug that readily crosses the blood–brain barrier where it is converted to glycinamide and glycine. Although effective at facilitating various aspects of memory in animal models, it did not significantly improve any of the efficacy parameters in a multicenter trial in 228 AD patients (Dysken et al. 1992).

Another NMDA antagonist undergoing investigation in the US and approved in Europe is memantine (1-amino-3,5-dimethyladamantane). Memantine is an uncompetitive NMDA antagonist that is characterized by rapid on–off kinetics at the binding site. In addition to its antiglutamate effects, memantine has neuroprotective effects, antiviral, dopaminergic, and antinociceptive effects, it is a putative antidepressant as well. Published trials in a nursing home population and in severely impaired outpatients with AD show cognitive efficacy (Reisberg et al. 2002, Winblad and Poritis 1999); and the drug is approved in Europe for the treatment of severe dementia.

## Combined Therapies

The combination of drugs with different mechanisms of action may be more effective than individual medications alone. The most relevant clinical questions are whether the available ChIs can or should be combined with other drugs. As a past example, choline precursors were combined with ChIs, but with no evident augmenting effect. Most practicing clinicians would take a dim view of combining two ChIs since their actions are additive. Physicians should be skeptical also of combining available anti-inflammatories or hormones with ChIs: first because of the lack of demonstrated efficacy of these drugs, and second because of the additive adverse events, especially gastrointestinal events. Clinical experience suggests that the combination of ChIs with vitamin E or *ginkgo biloba* does not appear to worsen adverse effects, however, there is no efficacy evidence for this practice either. Selegiline has been combined with cholinesterase inhibitors in small pilot studies suggesting an additive effect but this remains to be unequivocally demonstrated.

A multicenter trial of memantine combined with donepezil compared to donepezil alone sponsored by the manufacturers of memantine found a cognitive enhancing effect. Additional strategies employing combination therapies in AD are likely to emerge.

## Summary

The prospects for both treatments with greater efficacy for AD, and for cognitive enhancement in elderly patients are encouraging. ChIs are the best proven efficacious symptomatic treatments for AD. They provide consistent effects in many patients with mild to moderate dementia, and have become the current pharmacological standard of treatment.

Other therapeutic approaches are not as well tested or as clearly efficacious. Therefore, ChIs are likely to be actively used clinically for at least the next several years.

However, therapeutic results are usually modest, affecting a minority of patients. Patients assessed were usually outpatients with mild to moderately severe dementia and few concomitant medical illnesses. Duration of effect beyond 1 year and long-term safety are not known, except for the uncontrolled observations of patients who continue on these drugs after the controlled trial. It is essential to understand the broad magnitudes of effects and the range of clinical utility. It often takes time, experience, and further studies for clinicians to appreciate the overall effectiveness and utility of new drugs. Long-term trials of the cholinesterase inhibitors in patients with mild cognitive impairment will help define the extent and limits of their efficacy, as will trials in vascular dementia.

Vitamin E, selegiline, anti-inflammatories, and estrogens are all available for prescribing. However there is little evidence for efficacy, and in fact some evidence that the latter two classes may be harmful for patients with AD. The evidence for vitamin E rests on one smaller multicenter trial and needs confirmation. Ongoing trials in patients with mild cognitive impairment may help resolve the efficacy of vitamin E.

Memantine is available in Europe and demonstrates efficacy with very mild adverse events, at least in more severely impaired patients. Many of the putative cognitive enhancers described in this chapter would not likely be specific for AD and might be expected to be effective in other dementias. The area of cognitive enhancers for people without clinical illness remains to be explored.

## Acknowledgments

Supported in part by NIMH 19074, NIMH 40381, and the Southern California Alzheimer Disease Research Center Consortium (NIA 05142 and 10463).

## References

Adem A, Mohammed AK, and Winblad B (1990) Multiple effects of tetrahydroaminoacridine on the cholinergic system: Biochemical and behavioural aspects. J Neural Transm—Park Dis Dement Sect 2, 113–128.

Aisen PS and Davis KL (1994) Inflammatory mechanisms in Alzheimer's disease: Implications for therapy. Am J Psychiatr 151, 1105–1113.

Aisen PS, Davis KL, Berg JD, et al. (2000) A randomized controlled trial of prednisone in Alzheimer's disease. Alzheimer's Disease Cooperative Study. Neurology 54, 588–593.

Aisen PS, Schafer K, Grundman M, et al. (2002) Results of a multicenter trial of rofecoxib and naproxen in Alzheimer's disease. Neurobiol Aging 23, S429.

Antuono PG (1995) Effectiveness and safety of velnacrine for the treatment of Alzheimer's disease. A double-blind, placebo-controlled study. Mentane Study Group. Arch Intern Med 155, 1766–1772.

Arendt T, Bigl V, Arendt A, et al. (1983) Loss of neurons in the nucleus basalis of Meynert in Alzheimer's disease, paralysis agitans and Korsakoff's disease. Acta Neuropathol 61, 101–108.

Arendt T, Bigl V, Tennstedt A, et al. (1985) Neuronal loss in different parts of the nucleus basalis is related to neuritic plaque formation in cortical target areas in Alzheimer's disease. Neuroscience 14, 1–14.

Asthana S, Baker LD, Craft S, et al. (2001) High-dose estradiol improves cognition for women with AD: Results of a randomized study. Neurology 57, 605–612.

Bastianetto S, Ramassamy C, Dore S, et al. (2000) The Ginkgo biloba extract (EGb 761) protects hippocampal neurons against cell death induced by beta-amyloid. Eur J Neurosci 12, 1882–1890.

Birks J, Grimley Evans J, Iakovidou V, et al. (2002) Rivastigmine for Alzheimer's disease. Coch Database Syst Rev 2.

Blessed G, Tamlinson BE, Roth M (1968) The association between quantitative measures of dementia and of senile change in the cerebral grey matter of elderly subjects. Br J Psychiatr 114, 797–811.

Bondareff W, Mountjoy CQ, and Roth M (1982) Loss of neurons of origin of the adrenergic projection to cerebral cortex (nucleus locus coeruleus) in senile dementia. Neurology 32, 164–168.

Bowen DM, Smith CB, White P, et al. (1976) Neurotransmitter-related enzymes and indices of hypoxia in senile dementia and other abiotrophies. Brain 99, 459–496.

Brookmeyer R, Gray S, and Kawas C (1998) Projections of Alzheimer's disease in the United States and the public health impact of delaying disease onset. Am J Pub Health 88, 1337–1342.

Brufani M and Filocamo L (1997) Rational design of new acetylcholinesterase inhibitors. In Alzheimer's Disease: From Molecular Biology to Therapy, Becker R (ed), Birkhauser, Boston, pp. 171–177.

Burns A, Rossor M, Hecker J, et al. (1999) The effects of donepezil in Alzheimer's disease — results from a multinational trial. Dement Geriatr Cogn Disord 10, 237–244.

Buxbaum JD, Oishi M, Chen HI, et al. (1992) Cholinergic agonists and interleukin 1 regulate processing and secretion of the Alzheimer beta/A4 amyloid protein precursor. Proc Natl Acad Sci USA 89, 10075–10078.

Christie JE, Shering A, Ferguson J, et al. (1981) Physostigmine and arecoline: Effects of intravenous infusions in Alzheimer presenile dementia. Br J Psychiatr 138, 46–50.

Chui HC, Victoroff JI, Margolin D, et al. (1992) Criteria for the diagnosis of ischemic vascular dementia proposed by the State of California Alzheimer's Disease Diagnostic and Treatment Centers (see comments). Neurology 42, 473–480.

Corey-Bloom J, Anand R, Veach J, et al. (1998) A randomized trial evaluating the efficacy and safety of ENA 713 (rivastigmine tartrate): A new acetylcholinesterase inhibitor, in patients with mild to moderately severe Alzheimer's disease. Int J Geriatr Psychopharmacol 1, 55–65.

Cotman CW, Monaghan DT, and Ganong AH (1988) Excitatory amino acid neurotransmission: NMDA receptors and Hebb-type synaptic plasticity. Annu Rev Neurosci 11, 61–80.

Davies P and Maloney AJ (1976) Selective loss of central cholinergic neurons in Alzheimer's disease (letter). Lancet 2, 1403.

Davis KL and Mohs RC (1982) Enhancement of memory processes in Alzheimer's disease with multiple-dose intravenous physostigmine. Am J Psychiatr 139, 1421–1424.

Davis KL, Thal LJ, Gamzu ER, et al. (1992) A double-blind, placebo-controlled multicenter study of tacrine for Alzheimer's disease. The Tacrine Collaborative Study Group (see comments). New Engl J Med 327, 1253–1259.

Dorman DC, Cote LM, and Buck WB (1992) Effects of an extract of Gingko biloba on bromethalin-induced cerebral lipid peroxidation and edema in rats. Am J Vet Res 53, 138–142.

Dumont E, Petit E, Tarrade T, et al. (1992) UV-C irradiation-induced peroxidative degradation of microsomal fatty acids and proteins: Protection by an extract of Ginkgo biloba (EGb 761). Free Radical Biol Med 13, 197–203.

Dysken M, Kuskowski M, Love S, et al. (2002) Ondansetron in the treatment of cognitive decline in Alzheimer dementia. Am J Geriatr Psychiatr 10, 212–215.

Dysken MW, Mendels J, LeWitt P, et al. (1992) Milacemide: A placebo-controlled study in senile dementia of the Alzheimer-type. J Am Geriatr Soc 40, 503–506.

Enz A and Floersheim P (1997) Cholinesterase inhibitors: An overview of their mechanisms of action. In Alzheimer's Disease: From Molecular Biology to Therapy, Becker R (ed). Birkhauser, Boston, pp. 211–215.

Eriksdotter Jonhagen M, Nordberg A, Amberla K, et al. (1998) Intracerebroventricular infusion of nerve growth factor in three patients with Alzheimer's disease. Dement Geriatr Cogn Disord 9, 246–257.

Etienne P, Robitaille Y, Gauthier S, et al. (1986) Nucleus basalis neuronal loss and neuritic plaques in advanced Alzheimer's disease. Can J Physiol Pharmacol 64, 318–324.

Farlow M, Gracon SI, Hershey LA, et al. (1992) A controlled trial of tacrine in Alzheimer's disease. The Tacrine Study Group (see comments). JAMA 268, 2523–2529.

Feldman H, Gauthier S, Hecker J, et al. (2001) A 24-week, randomized, double-blind study of donepezil in moderate to severe Alzheimer's disease. Neurology 57, 613–620.

Fillit H, Weinreb H, Cholst I, et al. (1986) Observations in a preliminary open trial of estradiol therapy for senile dementia-Alzheimer's type. Psychoneuroendocrinology 11, 337–345.

Fioravanti M and Flicker L (2002) Efficacy of Nicergoline in dementia and other age associated forms of cognitive impairment. Coch Database Syst Rev 2.

Flicker L and Evans JG (2002) Piracetam for dementia or cognitive impairment. Coch Database Syst Rev 2.

Folstein MF, Folstein SE, and McHugh PR (1975) Mini-mental state: A practical method for grading the cognitive state of patients for the clinician. J Psychiatr Res 12, 189–198.

Francis PT, Palmer AM, Sims NR, et al. (1985) Neurochemical studies of early-onset Alzheimer's disease. Possible influence on treatment. New Engl J Med 313, 7–11.

Francis PT, Palmer AM, Snape M, et al. (1999) The cholinergic hypothesis of Alzheimer's disease: A review of progress. J Neurol Neurosurg Psychiatr 66, 137–147.

Galasko D, Bennett D, Sano M, et al. (1997) An inventory to assess activities of daily living for clinical trials in Alzheimer's disease. The Alzheimer's Disease Cooperative Study. Alz Dis Assoc Disord 11, S33–S39.

Giacobini E (1996) Cholinesterase inhibitors do more than inhibit cholinesterase. In Alzheimer's Disease: From Molecular Biology to Therapy, Becker R (ed). Birkhauser, Boston, pp. 187–204.

Haase J, Halama P, and Horr R (1996) Effectiveness of brief infusions with Ginkgo biloba special extract EGb 761 in dementia of the vascular and Alzheimer-type. Z Gerontol Geriatr 29, 302–309.

Haroutunian V, Greig N, Pei XF, Utsuki T, Gluck R, Avecedo LD, Davis KL, and Wallace WC (1997) Pharmacological modulation of Alzheimer's β-amyloid precursor protein levels in the CSF of rats with forebrain cholinergic system lesions. Brain Res Mol Brain Res 46(1–2), 161–168.

Harvey AL (1995) The pharmacology of galanthamine and its analogues. Pharmacol Therap 68, 113–128.

Hefti F and Schneider LS (1989) Rationale for the planned clinical trials with nerve growth factor in Alzheimer's disease. Psychiatr Dev 7, 297–315.

Hefti F and Schneider LS (1991) Nerve growth factor and Alzheimer's disease. Clin Neuropharmacol 14, S62–S76.

Henderson VW, Paganini-Hill A, Miller BL, et al. (2000) Estrogen for Alzheimer's disease in women: Randomized, double-blind, placebo-controlled trial. Neurology 54, 295–301.

Hofferberth B (1994) The efficacy of EGb 761 in patients with senile dementia of the Alzheimer type, a double-blind, placebo-controlled study on different levels of investigation. Hum Psychopharmacol 9, 215–222.

Honjo H, Ogino Y, Naitoh K, et al. (1989) In vivo effects by estrone sulfate on the central nervous system-senile dementia (Alzheimer's type). J Steroid Biochem 34, 521–525.

Huguet F, Drieu K, and Piriou A (1994) Decreased cerebral 5-HT$_{1A}$ receptors during ageing: Reversal by Ginkgo biloba extract (EGb 761). J Pharm Pharmacol 46, 316–318.

Inestrosa NC, Alvarez A, Perez CA, et al. (1996) Acetylcholinesterase accelerates assembly of amyloid-beta-peptides into Alzheimer's fibrils: Possible role of the peripheral site of the enzyme. Neuron 16, 881–891.

Jorm AF (1986) Effects of cholinergic enhancement therapies on memory function in Alzheimer's disease: A meta-analysis of the literature. Austral N Z J Psychiatr 20, 237–240.

Jorm AF, Korten AE, and Henderson AS (1987) The prevalence of dementia: A quantitative integration of the literature (see comments). Acta Psychiatr Scand 76, 465–479.

Kanowski S, Fischof P, and Hiersemenzel R (1988) Wirksamkeitsnachweis von Neotropika am Beispiel von Nimodipin-ein Beitrag zur entwicklung geeigneter klinischer Prufmodele. Z Gerontopsychol Psychiatr 1, 35–44.

Kanowski S, Herrmann WM, Stephan K, et al. (1996) Proof of efficacy of the ginkgo biloba special extract EGb 761 in outpatients suffering from mild to moderate primary degenerative dementia of the Alzheimer-type or multi-infarct dementia. Pharmacopsychiatry 29, 47–56.

Katzman R and Jackson JE (1991) Alzheimer disease: Basic and clinical advances (see comments). J Am Geriatr Soc 39, 516–525.

Kaufer DI, Cummings JL, and Christine D (1996) Effect of tacrine on behavioral symptoms in Alzheimer's disease: An open-label study. J Geriatr Psychiatr Neurol 9, 1–6.

Khachaturian ZS (1985) Diagnosis of Alzheimer's disease. Arch Neurol 42, 1097–1105.

Knapp MJ, Knopman DS, Solomon PR, Pendlebury WW, Davis CS, and Gracon SI (1994) A 30-week randomized controlled trial of high-dose tacrine in patients with Alzheimer's disease. The Tacrine Study Group. JAMA 271(13), 985–991.

Knoll J (1988) The striatal dopamine dependency of life span in male rats. Longevity study with (-)deprenyl. Mech Ageing Dev 46, 237–262.

Kristofikova Z, Benesova O, and Tejkalova H (1992) Changes of high-affinity choline uptake in the hippocampus of old rats after long term administration of two nootropic drugs (Tacrine and Ginkgo biloba extract). Dementia 3, 304–307.

Lahiri DK, Farlow MR, Hintz N, et al. (2000) Cholinesterase inhibitors, beta-amyloid precursor protein and amyloid beta-peptides in Alzheimer's disease. Acta Neurol Scand. 176(Suppl), 60–67.

Lahiri DK, Nall C, and Farlow MR (1992) The cholinergic agonist carbachol reduces intracellular beta-amyloid precursor protein in PC 12 and C6 cells. Biochem Int 28, 853–860.

Le Bars PL, Katz MM, Berman N, et al. (1997) A placebo-controlled, double-blind, randomized trial of an extract of Ginkgo biloba for dementia. North American EGb Study Group. JAMA 278, 1327–1332.

Leber P (2002) Criteria used by drug regulatory authorities. In Evidence-Based Dementia Practice, Qizilbash N, Schneider L, Chui H, et al. (eds). Blackwell Science, Oxford, pp. 376–387.

Maelicke A, Samochocki M, Jostock R, et al. (2001) Allosteric sensitization of nicotinic receptors by galantamine, a new treatment strategy for Alzheimer's disease. Biol Psychiatr 49, 279–288.

Mann DM, Yates PO, and Marcyniuk B (1984) A comparison of changes in the nucleus basalis and locus coeruleus in Alzheimer's disease. J Neurol Neurosurg Psychiatr 47, 201–203.

Maurer K, Ihl R, Dierks T, et al. (1997) Clinical efficacy of Ginkgo biloba special extract EGb 761 in dementia of the Alzheimer type. J Psychiatr Res 31, 645–655.

McKeith I, Del Ser T, Spano P, et al. (2000) Efficacy of rivastigmine in dementia with Lewy bodies: A randomised, double-blind, placebo-controlled international study. Lancet 356, 2031–2036.

McKeith IG, Galasko D, Kosaka K, et al. (1996) Consensus guidelines for the clinical and pathologic diagnosis of dementia with Lewy bodies (DLB): Report of the consortium on DLB international workshop. Neurology 47, 1113–1124.

McKhann G, Drachman D, Folstein M, et al. (1984) Clinical diagnosis of Alzheimer's disease: Report of the NINCDS-ADRDA Work Group under the auspices of Department of Health and Human Services Task Force on Alzheimer's Disease. Neurology 34, 939–944.

Milgram NW, Racine RJ, Nellis P, et al. (1990) Maintenance on L-deprenyl prolongs life in aged male rats. Life Sci 47, 415–420.

Mirra SS, Heyman A, McKeel D, et al. (1991) The Consortium to Establish a Registry for Alzheimer's Disease (CERAD). Part II. Standardization of the neuropathologic assessment of Alzheimer's disease. Neurology 41, 479–486.

Mohs RC, Davis BM, Johns CA, et al. (1985) Oral physostigmine treatment of patients with Alzheimer's disease. Am J Psychiatr 142, 28–33.

Mohs RC, Knopman D, Petersen RC, et al. (1997) Development of cognitive instruments for use in clinical trials of antidementia drugs: Additions to the Alzheimer's Disease Assessment Scale that broaden its scope. The Alzheimer's Disease Cooperative Study. Alz Dis Assoc Disord 11, S13–S21.

Muller D, Mendla K, Farber SA, et al. (1997) Muscarinic M1 receptor agonists increase the secretion of the amyloid precursor protein ectodomain. Life Sci 60, 985–991.

Mulnard RA, Cotman CW, Kawas C, et al. (2000) Estrogen replacement therapy for treatment of mild to moderate Alzheimer disease: A randomized controlled trial. Alzheimer's Disease Cooperative Study. J Am Med Assoc 283, 1007–1015.

Nicholson CD (1990) Pharmacology of nootropics and metabolically active compounds in relation to their use in dementia. Psychopharmacology 101, 147–159.

Nitsch RM, Slack BE, Wurtman RJ, et al. (1992) Release of Alzheimer amyloid precursor derivatives stimulated by activation of muscarinic acetylcholine receptors. Science 258, 304–307.

Ohkura T, Isse K, Akazawa K, et al. (1994) Evaluation of estrogen treatment in female patients with dementia of the Alzheimer type. Endocr J 41, 361–371.

Olin J and Schneider L (2002) Galantamine for Alzheimer's disease. Coch Database Syst Rev 2.

Olin J, Schneider L, Novit A, et al. (2002) Hydergine for dementia. Coch Database Syst Rev 2.

Paganini-Hill A and Henderson VW (1994) Estrogen deficiency and risk of Alzheimer's disease in women. Am J Epidemiol 140, 256–261.

Parkinson Study Group (1993) Effects to tocopherol and deprenyl on the progression of disability in early Parkinson's disease. New Engl J Med 328(3), 176–183.

Perry EK, Perry RH, Blessed G, et al. (1977) Necropsy evidence of central cholinergic deficits in senile dementia (letter). Lancet 1, 189.

Perry EK, Tomlinson BE, Blessed G, et al. (1978) Correlation of cholinergic abnormalities with senile plaques and mental test scores in senile dementia. Br Med J 2, 1457–1459.

Petersen RC, Stevens JC, Ganguli M, et al. (2001) Practice parameter: Early detection of dementia: Mild cognitive impairment (an evidence-based review). Report of the Quality Standards Subcommittee of the American Academy of Neurology. Neurology 56, 1133–1142.

Phelps CH, Gage FH, Growdon JH, et al. (1989) Potential use of nerve growth factor to treat Alzheimer's disease. Neurobiol Aging 10, 205–207.

Pietschmann A, Kuklinski B, and Otterstein A (1992) [Protection from uv-light-induced oxidative stress by nutritional radical scavengers]. Zeitschrift fur die Gesamte Innere Medizin und Ihre Grenzgebiete 47, 518–522.

Radebaugh TS, Buckholtz NS, and Khachaturian ZS (1996) Fisher symposium: Strategies for the prevention of Alzheimer disease—overview of research planning meeting III. Alz Dis Assoc Disord 10, 1–5.

Raskind M, Peskind ER, Wessel T, et al. (2000) Galantamine in Alzheimer's disease—a 6-month, randomized, placebo-controlled trial with a 6-month extension. Neurology 54, 2261–2268.

Raskind MA, Sadowsky CH, Sigmund WR, et al. (1997) Effect of tacrine on language, praxis, and noncognitive behavioral problems in Alzheimer disease. Arch Neurol 54, 836–840.

Reisberg B, Ferris SH, Mobius H, et al. (2002) Long-term treatment with the NMDA antagonist memantine: Results of a 24-week, open-label extension study in moderately severe-to-severe Alzheimer's disease. Neurobiol Aging 23, S555.

Rockwood K, Beattie BL, Eastwood MR, et al. (1997) A randomized, controlled trial of linopirdine in the treatment of Alzheimer's disease. Can J Neurol Sci 24, 140–145.

Rockwood K, Mintzer J, Truyen L, et al. (2001) Effects of a flexible galantamine dose in Alzheimer's disease: A randomised, controlled trial. J Neurol Neurosurg Psychiatr 71, 589–595.

Rogers J, Kirby LC, Hempelman SR, et al. (1993) Clinical trial of indomethacin in Alzheimer's disease. Neurology 43, 1609–1611.

Rogers SL, Doody RS, Mohs RC, et al. (1998a) Donepezil improves cognition and global function in Alzheimer's disease: A 15-week, double-blind, placebo-controlled study. Donepezil Study Group. Arch Intern Med 158, 1021–1031.

Rogers SL, Farlow MR, Doody RS, et al. (1998b) A 24-week, double-blind, placebo-controlled trial of donepezil in patients with Alzheimer's disease. Donepezil Study Group. Neurology 50, 136–145.

Roman GC, Tatemichi TK, Erkinjuntti T, et al. (1993) Vascular dementia: Diagnostic criteria for research studies. Report of the NINDS-AIREN International Workshop. Neurology 43, 250–260.

Rosen WG, Terry RD, Fuld PA, et al. (1980) Pathological verification of ischemic score in differentiation of dementias. Ann Neurol 7, 486–488.

Rosler M, Anand R, Cicin-Sain A, et al. (1999) Efficacy and safety of rivastigmine in patients with Alzheimer's disease: International randomised controlled trial (see comments). BMJ 318, 633–638.

Ruehl WW, Entriken TL, Muggenburg BA, et al. (1997) Treatment with L-deprenyl prolongs life in elderly dogs. Life Sci 61, 1037–1044.

Sano M, Ernesto C, Thomas RG, et al. (1997) A controlled trial of selegiline, alpha-tocopherol, or both as treatment for Alzheimer's disease. The Alzheimer's Disease Cooperative Study. New Engl J Med 336, 1216–1222.

Schneider L (2002) Rivastigmine. In Evidence-Based Dementia Practice, Qizilbash N, Schneider L, Chui H, et al. (eds). Blackwell Science, Oxford, pp. 499–509.

Schneider L and Tariot PN (1997) Cognitive Enhancers for Alzheimer's Disease. In Psychiatry, Tasman A, Kay J, Lieberman JA (eds), Vol. 2. WB Saunders, Philadelphia, pp. 1685–1701.

Schneider LS, Anand R, and Farlow M (1998) Systematic review of the efficacy of rivastigmine for patients with Alzheimer's disease. Int J Geriatr Psychopharmacol 1, S26–S34.

Schneider LS, Olin JT, Doody RS, et al. (1997) Validity and reliability of the Alzheimer's Disease Cooperative Study—Clinical Global Impression of Change. The Alzheimer's Disease Cooperative Study. Alz Dis Assoc Disord 11, S22–S32.

Selkoe DJ (1991) The molecular pathology of Alzheimer's disease. Neuron 6, 487–498.

Simpkins JW, Singh M, and Bishop J (1994) The potential role for estrogen replacement therapy in the treatment of the cognitive decline and neurodegeneration associated with Alzheimer's disease. Neurobiol Aging 15(Suppl 2), S195–S197.

Spencer CM and Noble S (1998) Rivastigmine: A review of its use in Alzheimer's disease. Drugs Aging 13, 391–411.

Spinnewyn B (1992) Ginkgo biloba extract (EGb 761) protects against delayed neuronal death in gerbil. In Effects of Ginkgo Biloba Extract (EGb 761) on the Central Nervous System, Christen Y, Costentin J, and Lacour M (eds). Elsevier, Paris, pp. 113–118.

Stern Y, Sano M, and Mayeux R (1987) Effects of oral physostigmine in Alzheimer's disease. Ann Neurol 22, 306–310.

Tariot P, Schneider L, and Coleman PD (1993a) Treatment of Alzheimer's disease: Glimmers of hope? Chem Ind 20, 801–807.

Tariot P, Schneider L, Patel S, et al. (1993b) Alzheimer's disease and (-)deprenyl: Rationales and findings. In Inhibitors of Monoamine Oxidase B: Pharmacology and Clinical Use in Neurodegenerative Disorders, Szelenyi I (ed). Birkhauser Verlag, Basel, pp. 301–317.

Tariot PN, Cummings JL, Katz IR, Mintzer J, Perdomo CA, Schwan EM, and Whalen E (2001) A randomized, double-blind, placebo-controlled study of the efficacy and safety of donepezil in patients with Alzheimer's disease in the nursing home setting. J Am Geriatr Soc 49(12), 1590–1599.

Tariot PN, Solomon PR, Morris JC, et al. (2000) A 5-month, randomized, placebo-controlled trial of galantamine in AD. The Galantamine USA-10 Study Group. Neurology 54, 2269–2276.

Tatton W (1993) "Tropic-like" reduction of nerve cell death by deprenyl without monoamine oxidase inhibition. Neurol Forum 4, 3–10.

Taylor J (1985) The effects of chronic, oral Ginkgo biloba extract administration on neurotransmitter receptor binding in young and aged Fisher 344 rats. In Effects of Ginkgo Biloba Extract on Organic Cerebral Impairment, Agnoli A, Rapin J, Scapagnini V, et al. (eds). John Libbey Eurotext, pp. 31–34.

Thal LJ, Carta A, Doody R, et al. (1997) Prevention protocols for Alzheimer disease. Position paper from the International Working Group on Harmonization of Dementia Drug Guidelines. Alz Dis Assoc Disord 11, 46–49.

Thal LJ, Schwartz G, Sano M, et al. (1996) A multicenter double-blind study of controlled-release physostigmine for the treatment of symptoms secondary to Alzheimer's disease. Physostigmine Study Group. Neurology 47, 1389–1395.

Tollefson GD (1990) Short-term effects of the calcium channel blocker nimodipine (Bay-e-9736) in the management of primary degenerative dementia (see comments). Biol Psychiatr 27, 1133–1142.

Vernon MW and Sorkin EM (1991) Piracetam. An overview of its pharmacological properties and a review of its therapeutic use in senile cognitive disorders. Drugs Aging 1, 17–35.

Watkins PB, Zimmerman HJ, Knapp MJ, et al. (1994) Hepatotoxic effects of tacrine administration in patients with Alzheimer's disease (see comments). JAMA 271, 992–998.

Weitbrecht WU and Jansen W (1986) [Primary degenerative dementia: Therapy with Ginkgo biloba extract. Placebo-controlled double-blind and comparative study]. Fortschr Med 104, 199–202.

Whitehouse PJ, Price DL, Struble RG, et al. (1982) Alzheimer's disease and senile dementia: Loss of neurons in the basal forebrain. Science 215, 1237–1239.

Wilcock GK, Lilienfeld S, and Gaens E (2000) Efficacy and safety of galantamine in patients with mild to moderate Alzheimer's disease: Multicentre randomised controlled trial. Galantamine International-1 Study Group. BMJ 321, 1445–1449.

Winblad B and Poritis N (1999) Memantine in severe dementia: Results of the 9M-Best Study (Benefit and efficacy in severely demented patients during treatment with memantine). Int J Geriatr Psychiatr 14, 135–146.

Winblad B, Bonura ML, Rossini BM, et al. (2001) Nicergoline in the treatment of mild-to-moderate Alzheimer's disease: A European multi-centre trial. Clin Drug Invest 21, 621–632.

Zubenko GS and Moossy J (1988) Major depression in primary dementia. Clinical and neuropathologic correlates. Arch Neurol 45, 1182–1186.

Zubenko GS, Moossy J, and Kopp U (1990) Neurochemical correlates of major depression in primary dementia. Arch Neurol 47, 209–214.

Zweig RM, Ross CA, Hedreen JC, et al. (1988) The neuropathology of aminergic nuclei in Alzheimer's disease. Ann Neurol 24, 233–242.

# 102 Therapeutic Management of the Suicidal Patient

Karon Dawkins
Robert N. Golden
Jan A. Fawcett

## Introduction

According to 1999 data from the Center for Disease Control and Prevention, suicide kills more people than homicide. Suicide was the eleventh leading cause of death (homicide was fourteenth), and the third leading cause of death between ages 15 and 24 years. In the year 1999, 29,199 Americans took their own lives (Hoyert et al. 2001). Suicide and the suicidal patient represent a significant public health problem. The vast majority of people with suicidal intent have a major psychiatric diagnosis. It has been estimated that 90% or more of them can be shown to have a major psychiatric illness (Henriksson et al. 1993, Mann 2002). Some patients become suicidal, or commit suicide with relatively little warning. Others have communicated their intent to a caregiver or significant other. A significant proportion, estimated as high as 70%, saw a physician within 30 days prior to their death, and nearly 50% had seen a physician in the preceding week (Barraclough et al. 1974). It was noted in the classic studies of Robins and colleagues (1959) that only 18% of suicidal patients communicated their intent to helping professionals, while 69% communicated their intent to an average of three close relatives or associates, 73% within 12 months of their suicide (Robins et al. 1959).

Some patients become acutely suicidal while others are chronically at risk. Suicide leaves in its wake intense suffering among the victim's family and friends, including feelings of grief, anger, shame, and frequently guilt. There are relatively limited data on the frequency of suicide attempts. Management of the chronically suicidal is frequently a source of frustration and fear for caregivers. Identifying the risk factors, understanding the suicidal patient, and intervening appropriately are key elements in the prevention of suicide. There is a role for parents, families, friends, schools, workplaces, and physicians in this task. The suicide rates have fallen since 1993 (Hoyert et al. 2001). However, it remains a given that even with due diligence, not all suicides can be predicted or prevented.

This chapter will survey dynamic and neurobiologic hypotheses about suicidality. Major psychiatric diagnoses associated with suicidality will be reviewed, along with associated risk factors. Preventative measures will be discussed, as well as effective interventions. Assessment of the suicidal patient, as well as issues that arise for caregivers when patients kill themselves, are examined. Research directions will be considered.

## Hypotheses

### Dynamic

Dynamic theories facilitate the attempt to understand patients and their difficulties. Gabbard (2000) presents an overview to these approaches to understanding the suicidal patient. As he discusses, Freud postulated that suicide could be the result of displaced murderous impulses toward an internalized object, and later in the structural model, the aggression of a sadistic superego against the ego. Menninger believed that suicide was a function of wishes to kill (e.g. an angry act designed to devastate survivors), be killed, and to die. A familiar theme in object relations of the suicidal patient is the conflict between the internalized tormentor and the anguished victim. Patients may either identify with the internalized aggressor and lash out at others or submit to the tormentor through suicide. Fenichel noted the less aggressive reunion fantasy, in which death abates object loss by the imagined joining with a departed loved one, frequently a maternal superego figure. When identity and self-esteem are tied to a lost object, suicide can be viewed as restorative. Pathological grief and anniversaries of losses may be vulnerable times for such patients (Gabbard 2000).

Cognitive rigidity, especially the inability to revise expectations of the self, can lead to hopelessness and suicidality. Suicidal ideation that is ego-syntonic is especially concerning. Four patterns of ego functioning and object relations that differentiate between serious attempters and manipulative gestures are: "(1) an inability to give up infantile wishes for nurturance, associated with a conflict about being overly dependent; (2) a sober but ambivalent view toward death; (3) excessively high self-expectations; and

(4) overcontrol of affect, particularly aggression." (Gabbard 2000).

Gabbard notes that there is a "natural tendency" for clinicians to go to great lengths to prevent suicide, but cautions that the role of "savior" can be consuming and countertherapeutic. It can lead to inappropriate attempts to gratify wishes in order to prevent suicide, effectively colluding with the patients that there is an "unconditionally loving mother" and placing the locus of responsibility with the clinician. Idealizing transferences may cast the therapist in the role of rescuer. This and transference disappointments should be predicted and interpreted. The therapist who assumes the "savior" role consciously or unconsciously believes that they can provide the nurturance that others have not. This stance is a potential trap, in that the patient is likely to reject these efforts, effectively proving the powerlessness of the therapist. An intense countertransference can develop as a consequence of feeling beleaguered and tormented by the patient. Malice, aversion, if not hatred can develop, and manifest itself as indifference, neglect, and hostility; unconscious projection onto the patient; or a reaction formation of trying to gratify the patient. Clinicians need to be aware of and process their own feelings of aggression (Gabbard 2000).

The suicide of a patient can be a crushing narcissistic injury. Therapists tend to blame themselves for outcomes beyond their control. It is more therapeutic to understand and analyze the origins of suicidal ideation, rather than becoming enmeshed. Patients should be given some responsibility to verbalize suicidal impulses rather than act upon them and to collaborate with their therapists. In contrast to those who are intent on dying, most patients are ambivalent about death, and can come to choose life. Psychotherapy can be an important avenue to understanding why a patient wants to die and what they expect in the aftermath. Gabbard sees this effort as treatment, while providing safety may only be management (Gabbard 2000).

## Neurobiology

There are genetic and biologic correlates of suicidality as well as the underlying psychiatric illnesses that are often associated with suicidal behavior. For example, Ahearn and colleagues (2001) compared MRI studies in 20 pairs of unipolar depressed patients with and without suicide attempts. Subjects were matched on cardiovascular history, ECT treatment, and psychosis. There were no statistical differences in age of onset of illness, number of episodes, or depression ratings. It was found that the patients with suicide attempts had more subcortical gray matter intensities. There was a trend toward more periventricular white matter hyperintensities in the patients with suicide attempts. The authors concluded that patients with abnormal MRI, especially gray matter hyperintensities in the basal ganglia, may be at higher risk for mood disorders and suicide attempts secondary to interference in neuroanatomic pathways. These pathways may be crucial to mood regulation (Ahearn et al. 2001). These and other neurobiologic correlates may improve our ability to predict suicide and suicidal behavior. Promising mechanisms include the serotonin system, although adrenergic and dopaminergic systems have also been implicated. Abnormalities in the hypothalamic–pituitary–adrenal (HPA) axis have long been associated with mood disorders.

## Serotonin Mechanisms (See Table 102–1)

Dysregulation in the serotonin system has been linked to major depression, suicide, and violence. Disparate findings are a function of the inherent difficulties with association studies. A number of these studies have found an association between reduced serotonin function, including low levels of the serotonin metabolite 5-hydroxyindoleacetic acid (5-HIAA) in cerebrospinal fluid (CSF), with impulsivity, violence, and suicide (Mann 1998, Placidi et al. 2001). Low CSF 5-HIAA levels may also predict future suicide attempts (Roy et al. 1989). A recent study (Spreux-Varoquaux et al. 2001) describes differential abnormalities in peripheral serotonin measures. Plasma concentrations of serotonin (5-HT), 5-HIAA, and homovanillic acid (HVA), as well as platelet 5-HT content, were compared in drug free (for at least one month), violent (impulsive and nonimpulsive) suicide attempters and healthy matched controls (no psychiatric diagnosis) to examine the relationship between these measures and depression and impulsivity. Plasma HVA and 5-HT concentrations were not statistically different in the groups. Both plasma 5-HIAA and platelet 5-HT were lower in suicide attempters than in healthy controls. Plasma 5-HIAA was lower, after controlling for age, in impulsive suicide attempters than in the nonimpulsive attempters, and inversely correlated with degree of impulsivity. This finding is consistent with this group's earlier reports of lower CSF 5-HIAA levels in impulsive versus nonimpulsive violent suicide attempters (Cremniter et al. 1999). On the other hand, platelet 5-HT levels were lowest in nonimpulsive patients than in impulsive attempters, and inversely correlated with the severity of depression. The authors believed that these peripheral indexes of serotonergic activity had differential changes related to impulsivity and depression. Low platelet 5-HT may be a function of impairment of serotonin uptake mechanism associated with depression and consistent with decreased uptake sites in platelets and in brains. Decreased plasma 5-HIAA, without changes in HVA, may be a function of impairment in monoamine oxidase A activity, consistent with clinical and preclinical findings of low 5-HIAA and increased aggression (Spreux-Varoquaux et al. 2001). Men in a Dutch family with a complete MAOA deficiency have decreased urinary 5-HIAA and are prone to aggression (Brunner et al. 1993). Placidi and colleagues (2001) studied CSF 5-HIAA, HVA, and 3-methoxy-4-hydroxy-phenylglycol (MHPG) concentrations in 93 patients with major depression, divided into suicide attempters and nonattempters. Attempters were subdivided into high and low lethality attempts. There were no differences in monoamine metabolite levels. Higher aggression scale scores correlated significantly with lower CSF 5-HIAA, with even lower levels in high lethality suicide attempters as compared to low lethality attempters. The low lethality attempters did not differ from the nonattempters in these measures. Evidence suggests that the low CSF 5-HIAA is a trait marker, although it does not appear to be a function of depression severity and it is not clear whether it is further lowered around a suicide attempt. Further, it remains to be seen whether the lethality of an attempt will differentiate CSF 5-HIAA levels (Placidi et al. 2001). Stanley and colleagues (2000) studied a heterogeneous patient sample, divided into aggressive and nonaggressive, but without previous suicide attempts. The aggressive patients had

| Table 102–1 | Summary of Serotonin Mechanisms | |
|---|---|---|
| **Serotonin Mechanisms** | **Suicide Attempts** | **Postmortem Studies** |
| 5-HIAA | ↓ CSF (Placidi et al. 2001, Cremniter et al. 1999) ↓ plasma (Spreaux-Varoquaux et al. 2001) ↓ urine (Brunner et al. 1993) | |
| 5-HT | ↓ platelet (Spreaux-Varoquaux et al. 2001) | |
| SERT | | ↓ binding (Mann et al. 2000) |
| SERT mRNA | | ↓ dorsal raphe nucleus (Arango et al. 2001) |
| 5-HT$_{1A}$ | | ↓ binding capacity in dorsal raphe nucleus (Arango et al. 2001) |
| 5-HT$_{1B}$ | ↓ G allelle (New et al. 2001) | ↓ binding sites in frontal cortex (Arranz et al. 1994) |
| 5-HT$_{1A}$ | ↓ after age 20 (Sheline et al. 2002) + polymorphism (Du et al. 2000) − polymorphism (Bondey et al. 2000) (Tsai et al. 1999) | ↑ receptor, protein, mRNA in prefrontal cortex, hippocampus (Pandey et al. 2002) |
| 5-HT$_{2C}$ | | + differential RNA editing (Niswender et al. 2001) |
| Tryptophan hydroxylase | + U allele (Mann et al. 1997) − association (Ono et al. 2000) (Souery et al. 2001) | |

significantly lower CSF 5-HIAA and were more hostile and impulsive. The correlation with CSF 5-HIAA levels seemed limited to measures of aggressive acts as opposed to self-reports of hostility (Stanley et al. 2000). Aggressive behavior and, independently, suicidal behavior, may have impulsivity as a common denominator, which may be mediated by serotonergic dysfunction (Placidi et al. 2001).

In additional studies of the relationship between suicide, depression, and reduced serotonergic transmission, Arango and colleagues (2001), noted localized decreases in serotonin transporter (SERT) sites and increased postsynaptic 5-HT$_{1A}$ receptors in the prefrontal cortex in suicide. In depression, the decrease in serotonin transport sites was diffuse throughout the dorsoventral area of the prefrontal cortex. As much of the innervation of the prefrontal cortex comes from the brainstem dorsal raphe nucleus, the authors compared SERT binding, serotonin mRNA expression, and 5-HT$_{1A}$ autoreceptor binding in the dorsal raphe nucleus in brains of control subjects and depressed suicide victims. There were no differences in SERT, SERT mRNA, or 5-HT$_{1A}$ binding concentrations, but the suicide victims had decreased 5-HT$_{1A}$ binding capacity. Binding capacity is a function of tissue volume. There was a notable 54% decrease in dorsal raphe nucleus neurons that expressed SERT mRNA, with greater expression per neuron in suicide victims. These results can be interpreted in one of two ways. One interpretation is that a hypofunctioning serotonin system compensates by decreasing expression of the SERT gene, with a concomitant reduction in SERT sites and increased availability of serotonin as a function of decreased reuptake. A reduction in 5-HT$_{1A}$ inhibitory autoreceptors would increase serotonin availability. Neurons that are overexpressing SERT mRNA are escaping this homeostatic response and exacerbating hypofunctioning. Alternatively, decreased transporter gene expression may be a part of global serotonin system genetic deficits (Arango et al. 2001). Mann and colleagues (2000) studied the relationship between SERT, SERT gene promoter polymorphism, major depression, and suicide in postmortem brains of 82 suicides and 138 nonsuicide controls. There was differential SERT binding, with women having lower binding than men. Decreased binding in the prefrontal cortex, especially the ventral prefrontal cortex of suicides and the dorsal-ventral prefrontal cortex in major depression, was also associated with major depression and suicide. Allelic frequencies for the promoter gene did not significantly differ (Mann et al. 2000).

Rao and colleagues (1998) postulated a connection between suicidality and increased density, secondary to upregulation in the face of serotonergic hypofunction, of the platelet 5-HT$_{2A}$ receptor, regardless of psychiatric diagnosis. Pandey and colleagues (2002), in a comparison of postmortem brain of teenaged (13 to 19 years old) suicide victims and matched teenaged controls who were largely the victims of homicides and accidents, found elevated $5\text{-}HT_{2A}$ receptor, protein, and mRNA expression in the prefrontal cortex and hippocampus of the suicide victims. These findings were limited to the prefrontal cortex and hippocampus, areas associated with emotion and cognition. There were no significant differences in $5\text{-}HT_{2A}$ measures whether or not the teenaged victims had a psychiatric diagnosis (5 of 15 suicide victims had no history of mental illness). These findings are also consistent with an association of serotonergic dysfunction with impulsive aggression, a feature of teenaged suicides (Pandey et al. 2002). An association between $5\text{-}HT_{2A}$ receptor gene polymorphism and suicidal patients with major depression (Du et al. 2000), was not replicated in a recent study (Bondy et al. 2000, Tsai et al. 1999). Possible explanations for the discordant findings include ethnic differences in $5\text{-}HT_{2A\text{-}T102C}$ alleles, the phenotypic heterogeneity of depressed and suicidal patients, the complex interaction of genetic and other risk factors, and limited sample sizes (Bondy et al. 2000). Sheline and colleagues (2002), utilizing live healthy controls, positron emission tomography (PET) and $[^{18}F]$altanserin as a high affinity ligand, described a striking decrease in $5\text{-}HT_{2A}$ receptors after age 20 (70%) that continued through age 50 before plateauing. The loss of these receptors could be evidence of decreasing serotonergic activity with increasing age.

Niswender and colleagues (2001) noted differential RNA editing at the A-site of the $5\text{-}HT_{2C}$ receptor in schizophrenic and depressed patients who had committed suicide. Differential editing results in isoforms with distinct functional properties, including coupling less efficiently to the phospolipase C signaling cascade, differential interactions with G-proteins, and decreased sensitivity to lysergic acid diethylamide (LSD) and atypical antipsychotics. The authors found increased editing at the A site in the prefrontal cortex of suicide victims (with major depression and schizophrenia). It was postulated that the statistically significant increase of editing at this site may result in differential responsiveness to serotonergic agents (Niswender et al. 2001).

The $5\text{-}HT_{1B}$ receptor has also been examined for abnormalities that may be associated with vulnerability to suicide attempts in patients with personality disorder. Citing the aggressive behavior in knockout mice lacking $5\text{-}HT_{1B}$ and other investigations, New and colleagues (2001) investigated the relationship between impulsive aggression and the HTR1B locus. They extracted DNA from the blood of 145 patients with personality disorders. There was a trend towards a lower frequency of the G allele in those with a history of suicide attempts. However, in the subset of 90 white subjects, there was a statistically significant association between suicide attempts and the G allele. There was no association between self-reported measures of impulsive aggression (New et al. 2001). Although other studies associating $5\text{-}HT_{1B}$ binding parameters with diagnosis and suicidal behavior have been mixed, the G861 allele of this polymorphism was associated with a decreased number of $5\text{-}HT_{1B}$ receptors (Huang et al. 1999) and there was a decrease in $5\text{-}HT_{1B}$ binding sites in frontal cortex of nondepressed suicides (Arranz et al. 1994). These findings suggest a multigene model for the genetic component of impulsive aggression, compounded by environmental factors (New et al. 2001).

Another line of inquiry into serotonergic dysfunction in suicidality is the investigation of tryptophan hydroxylase polymorphism. Tryptophan hydroxylase is the rate limiting enzyme in the synthesis of serotonin. A decrement in tryptophan hydroxylase activity would result in decreased serotonin synthesis. Mann and colleagues (1997) were among the first to describe an association between tryptophan hydroxylase alleles and suicidality. In a sample of depressed white patients with and without suicide attempts, the tryptophan hydroxylase alleles (UU, UL, LL) were compared. The less frequent U allele was associated with suicide attempts. Logistic regression analysis for UU compared to LL distinguished the suicide attempters (odds ratio 12.5), whereas severity of depression, comorbid borderline personality disorder were not statistically significant predictors. Depression was more severe in the LL and UL groups. There was no difference in CSF 5-HIAA (Mann et al. 1997). Findings have been mixed, but recent inquiries have not found differences in genotype distribution or allele frequency in 132 Japanese suicide victims of heterogeneous diagnoses (Ono et al. 2000), or in a sample of 927 European unipolar and bipolar patients, and their matched pairs (Souery et al. 2001).

## Adrenergic Mechanisms

Other putative markers of suicidality have been investigated. As an enzyme that mediates various brain functions, the role of cyclic adenosine monophosphate (cAMP) dependent protein kinase A was studied in the membrane and cytosol fractions of prefrontal cortex of suicide victims. $[^{3}H]$cAMP binding sites were lower and there was less protein kinase activity in the suicide victims. Further analysis revealed that the lower binding and protein kinase A activity was limited to those suicide victims with a history of major depression. These parameters were only mildly decreased in the suicide victims with other psychiatric diagnoses. Abnormalities of the adenyl cyclase-cAMP signaling system, for example, changes in regulatory G proteins, may be associated with suicide (Dwivedi et al. 2002). Odagaki and colleagues (2001) noted a decrease in the catalytic subunit of protein kinase A in the prefrontal cortex of depressed suicide victims. There was a correlated increase in cAMP response element binding protein (CREB) in the brains of the suicide victims. The increases in CREB were noted in antidepressant-free subjects, but not in the antidepressant treated ones. It was felt that cAMP signaling was upregulated in the brains of suicide victims in a manner that was not related to antidepressant treatment. Antidepressants may act by normalizing the upregulation. However, it is not clear whether the upregulation is primary to the etiology of depression or secondary compensation to another abnormality in this novel theory (Odagaki et al. 2001).

Sastre and colleagues (2001) were interested in the relationship between alpha-2 and beta-adrenoceptors in the brains of suicide victims. No significant statistical difference was found in alpha-2 and beta density between suicide brains and controls. The lack of density change in the alpha-2 and beta receptors in suicide brain in this study could be a function of chronic antidepressant treatment. Chronic antidepressant treatment, to which suicide victims have been frequently exposed, downregulate beta receptors and are associated with reductions in alpha-2 receptors. The authors did not have access to psychiatric diagnoses or toxicology data. However, the ratio between $alpha_{2A}$-full agonist and beta sites was 1.3- to 2-fold greater in suicide brains. This ratio could be suggestive of the most common pattern of adrenoceptor changes in major depression: increases in alpha$_{2A}$ agonist binding sites and/or decreases in total beta density. The authors believed the alpha$_{2A}$ and beta ratio could be an index of brain pathology. In contrast, Pitchot and colleagues (2001b) utilized growth hormone response to the alpha-2 agonist clonidine as a pharmacologic probe of alpha-2-adrenoceptor functioning in depressed patients with high lethality suicide attempts, low lethality suicide attempts, and nonattempters. No significant differences were found in peak growth hormone values in attempters and nonattempters, nor were peak growth hormone response correlated with degree of lethality. These investigators concluded that these findings did not suggest a significant role for norepinephrine systems, as a function of alpha-2 receptors, in suicidality.

Placidi and colleagues (2001), in their study of monoamine metabolites in the CSF of depressed patients, found only a statistical trend in the correlation of CSF 3-methoxy-4-hydroxy-phenylglycol (MHPG) levels and aggression. They too did not believe that norepinephrine systems were significantly involved in suicide attempts or aggression. In their review, the findings relating suicidal behavior and the monoamine metabolites MHPG and HVA are mixed (Placidi et al. 2001).

## Dopamine Mechanisms

Dopamine function has also been investigated. Utilizing growth hormone response to the dopaminergic agonist apomorphine as a pharmacologic probe of D$_2$-dopaminergic functioning in depressed high lethality, low lethality, and nonattempter patients, Pitchot and colleagues (2001a) found significantly lower growth hormone response in a group of male suicide attempters versus nonattempters. Women were excluded to avoid the confound of estrogen influence on hormonal responses, and attempters were divided into high and low lethality attempts. There were no significant differences in depression scores between groups. There was a significant difference in peak growth hormone response between attempters and nonattempters, but not between high and low lethality attempters. This group had also previously demonstrated a blunted growth hormone response to apomorphine in depressed patients who subsequently committed suicide (Pitchot et al. 2001c). These findings bolstered their contention that dopamine plays a role in the neurobiology of suicidality and that impaired growth hormone response to apomorphine could be a marker for suicide risk. Allard and Norlen (2001), utilizing [$^3$H]raclopride binding to D$_2$ receptors in the caudate nucleus of depressed suicide victims and controls, did not find differences in density or affinity of D$_2$ receptors between the two groups. In other studies, homovanillic acid (HVA) concentration in plasma (Spreaux-Varoquaux et al. 2001) or CSF (Placidi et al. 2001) did not correlate with suicidal behavior in patients, nor did cortical HVA concentrations (Arranz et al. 1997) correlate with suicide in autopsy samples. Catechol-$O$-methyltransferase (COMT) polymorphisms have also been studied. A significant association was noted between COMT genotype and high lethality attempts in schizophrenic and schizoaffective patients. The low enzyme activity COMT L allele was more frequent in violent attempts in male patients (Nolan et al. 2000).

## Hypothalamic–Pituitary–Adrenal Axis Mechanisms

Abnormalities in the hypothalamic–pituitary–adrenal (HPA) axis have also been a focus of investigation. Evidence of HPA axis dysfunction in suicidal behavior include decreased corticotrophin-releasing factor (CRF) binding sites in frontal cortex (Nemeroff et al. 1988) and CSF (Arató et al. 1989) of suicide victims. The dexamethasone suppression test (DST), a measure of hyperactivity of the HPA axis, has been revisited as a predictor of suicidal behavior. The DST lost some favor as an indicator of major depression and a tool to monitor recovery secondary to its lack of specificity. Coryell and Schlesser (2001) reported on a group of 78 patients enrolled in a long-term study between 1978 and 1981. These patients also underwent a DST as part of routine battery of tests and clinical assessments. The number of bipolar patients in the sample was low ($N=10$), because they presented initially in the manic phase, and DST were rarely performed in those circumstances. Nonsuppressors (41% of the sample) were more likely to have a bipolar diagnosis. During the 15-year follow-up, 8 suicides were documented. Seven of them were nonsuppressors on the initial admission. The predictive validity of demographic and historical risk factors was compared to the DST. None of the other traditional risk factors, including a history of a previous serious attempt, proved predictive. They found that the estimated risk of suicide in the abnormal DST group was 26.8%, compared to 2.9% in the suppressor group. The authors point out that it is not clear whether DST results could have predictive value across diagnoses other than affective disorders or if HPA axis abnormalities underline some of the associated deficits in the serotonergic system (Coryell and Schlesser 2001).

The above represents a sample of available studies of the neurobiology of suicide. There are inherent difficulties with association and linkage studies. Small sample sizes, heterogeneous diagnostic groups, retrospective analyses, uncertain impact of psychotropic agents, the continuum of suicidal behaviors (manipulative gestures to self-mutilation without the intent to die to completed suicide), and the "cross talk" between many of the neurobiologic systems targeted for study can all undermine consistency of findings. Suicide is a multiply determined act, including genetic vulnerabilities, mental illness, environmental and social stressors, impulsivity, and aggressive tendencies.

## Psychiatric Diagnoses

A number of psychiatric diagnoses are linked with suicidality. While patients with mood disorders (major depression and bipolar disorder) are commonly assessed for suicidality, anxiety disorders are also associated with significant suicide risk. Psychosis, in both mood disorders and schizophrenia, can heighten risk. Although borderline personality disorder has a high prevalence of suicidal ideation, impulsivity, and self-injurious behavior, these patients are at risk for unexpected intentional, and accidental, death.

## Affective Disorders

Bostwick and Pankratz (2000) revisited the widely-held, oft-repeated 15% lifetime risk of suicide in depressed patients. This figure was the conclusion of a seminal review by Guze and Robins (1970) and was followed by an 18.9% estimate by Goodwin and Jamison (1990). Bostwick and Pankratz raise important points about the sample and methodology of these studies. Both reviews were of largely inpatient samples, determined proportionate mortality (the percentage who died by suicide over the course of the studies), and included studies with relatively short follow-up. They make the argument that the short follow-up periods, the broader criteria for major depression with a resulting increase of the lifetime prevalence, and the heterogeneity of the study populations have distorted these estimates and that case fatality rates are more accurate. The authors reanalyzed the works of Guze and Robins, Goodwin and Jamison, and other studies. Affective disorders, due to changing nomenclature and classification systems, included a wide variety of mood disorders, including unipolar and bipolar illness with varying degrees of severity. Their meta-analysis revealed a risk hierarchy based on treatment history. The highest estimate of lifetime prevalence of suicide is for a history of hospitalization for suicidality, 8.6%, and is bolstered by evidence suggesting that risk is elevated in the immediate post discharge period. The authors argue that those patients who are recently and repeatedly hospitalized for suicidal ideation are an appropriate focus for suicide prevention interventions (Bostwick and Pankratz 2000). The next highest estimated rate is for those hospitalized without suicidality (4.0%), followed by outpatients with affective disorder (2.2%), and then the general population (> 0.5%). This hierarchy may be reflective of disease severity, which is impacted by comorbid factors like substance abuse/dependence, anxiety, impulsivity, aggression, family history, and psychosis (Bostwick and Pankratz 2000).

Others have also questioned the 15% lifetime risk of suicide in affective disorder estimated by Guze and Robins (1970), as it would suggest a suicide rate several orders of magnitude higher than it is currently. Utilizing 1983 US population and mortality statistics, others have estimated the lifetime suicide risk for major depression to be 2.5% (Blair-West et al. 1997). Inskip and colleagues (1998), utilizing computer models unavailable to Guze and Robins, estimated a lifetime risk of 6% for affective disorders. It has been suggested that the availability of safer antidepressants, despite the fact that many depressed people go undiagnosed and untreated or undertreated, have made an impact on suicide rates (Nierenberg et al. 2001).

Mann and colleagues (1999) have proposed a stress-diathesis model of suicidal behavior, as "a psychiatric disorder is generally a necessary but insufficient condition for suicide." The model posits that suicidal behavior is a function of an individual's threshold for suicidal acts and the stressors that can lead to vulnerability. The authors believe that the threshold for suicidal acts is trait-dependent (diathesis), and is mediated by factors such as aggression, impulsivity, substance abuse, family history, and low brain serotonin function. Stressors include psychiatric illness and interpersonal problems. In this model, intervention should consider the diathesis as well as the stressors (Mann et al. 1999). In a study of 374 patients who attempted suicide (major affective disorders, psychoses, and personality disorders), objective severity of symptoms did not differentiate between attempters or nonattempters, and was not very predictive of suicidal behaviors. Subjective ratings of depression, hopelessness, and suicidal ideation were significantly greater in attempters. Attempters had 25% less personal income, were less likely to be Catholic, and were more likely to be cigarette smokers. Duration of the current episode was shorter in attempters, although they had more lifetime episodes and younger onset. Attempters had higher ratings of lifetime aggression and impulsivity, as well as fewer reasons for living. Their sample of attempters was also more likely to have cluster B personality disorders, substance abuse, head injury, and a first-degree relative who attempted or committed suicide. Low serotonin levels may be the underlying feature of suicidal behavior, aggression, and substance abuse (Mann et al. 1999).

While the majority who attempt or commit suicide are found to have a mood disorder, the vast majority of those with affective illness do not attempt nor commit suicide. Malone et al. (2000) sought to examine factors that might help protect against suicidal acts. They studied 84 patients with major depression, 45 with suicide attempts, 39 without, utilizing a self-report instrument that assessed six factors: "survival and coping beliefs, responsibility to family, child-related concerns, fear of suicide, fear of social disapproval, and moral objections to suicide." Factors that failed to discriminate between attempters and nonattempters included age, sex, education, religion, and number/duration/objective severity of depressive episodes, although the number of episodes almost reached statistical significance. As hypothesized, the nonattempters had significantly higher scores on the "reasons for living" measure. "Fear of suicide," while significantly different between attempters and nonattempters, was not as markedly different as the greater "survival/coping skills," "fear of social disapproval," or "moral objections" scores in nonattempters. Child-related concerns were higher in nonattempters, but did not reach statistical significance. The authors suggest that bolstering reasons for living may become part of effective intervention for suicidal ideation (Malone et al. 2000).

Keilp and colleagues (2001) sought to examine the neuropsychological functioning in those who have attempted suicide. They compared 50 patients with major depression (all off medications, 21 without history of suicide attempts, 14 with low lethality attempts, and 15 with high lethality attempts) and 22 controls without current or past axis I or II disorders. The authors reasoned that high lethality attempters are likely to share demographic and biologic characteristics with suicide completers. The low lethality group seemed younger, more likely to have concomitant borderline personality disorder, and higher scores of hopelessness and suicidal ideation. The high lethality group had significantly poorer performances on tests of executive functioning, general intellectual functioning, attention, and memory. Performance on attention and memory tasks correlated with depression severity, while executive functioning did not. The pattern of deficits in the high lethality group suggested dysfunction in prefrontal cortical areas, not the effects, for example, hypoxia, of previous suicide attempts (Keilp et al. 2001).

## Bipolar Disorder

Goodwin and Jamison estimated that 19% of deaths of bipolar patients are due to suicide. Between 25 and 50% of bipolar patients are predicted to make at least one suicide attempt in their lifetime (Goodwin and Jamison 1990). In the Epidemiologic Catchment Area Study, lifetime rate of suicide attempts of bipolar patients was 29%. Bipolar disorder has an odds ratio of having had a suicide attempt of 2.0 times greater than that of unipolar depression and 6.2 times greater than any other Axis I disorder. This higher rate of attempts is not explained by demographic characteristics, comorbid substance abuse, or comorbid anxiety disorder (Chen and Dilsaver 1996). Comorbid alcoholism does have a dramatic impact on bipolar (and unipolar) suicide rates. In one study, subjects with major depression and comorbid alcoholism had a lifetime suicide attempt rate of 31.7%, compared to 17.5% with major depression alone. Comorbid bipolar I disorder and alcoholism had a 38.4% lifetime rate of attempted suicide, compared to 21.7% with bipolar I alone (Potash et al. 2000).

The risk of suicide appears higher in depressed or mixed states. Black and colleagues (1987) noted that in their sample, bipolar patients (especially females) were less likely to commit suicide, due to the low risk associated with manic patients. Isometsä and colleagues (1994) used the psychological autopsy method to study 1397 suicides in Finland over a 12-month period. Of the 31 bipolar I patients who committed suicide, 79% had depressive and 11% had mixed symptoms. Only one was manic at the time of death. None of the females (N=13), and more than half of the men (10 of 18) had comorbid alcohol abuse. One-third were receiving lithium and about half adequate doses as judged by lithium levels. Twenty-two were deemed to have had a depression at the time of death, with half of them on antidepressants. Only two of those were felt to be on adequate dosages. Fifty-five percent (N=17) communicated their suicidal intent: 12 to next of kin, 12 to health care providers, and 7 to both. More bipolar patients (35%) than unipolar (13%) used prescribed medications as their suicide method (Isometsä et al. 1994).

In a study of 504 inpatients with bipolar and unipolar mood disorders, Tondo and colleagues (1999) found suicide attempts more common in bipolar II patients. Mixed or depressive episodes were related to the majority of suicide attempts in bipolar I patients, although this was one of the few studies where multivariate logistic regression analysis ranked the association with suicidality highest with bipolar II disorder, followed by unipolar depression, then bipolar I with mixed features (Tondo et al. 1999). Dysphoric mania may be the state associated with the highest risk (Nierenberg et al. 2001).

Oquendo and colleagues (2000) evaluated the applicability of their stress-diathesis model to a sample of bipolar patients. As with their other sample of psychiatric patients (Mann et al. 1999), objective illness severity was not a differentiating factor between bipolar attempters and nonattempters, although the symptoms were more severe at the index hospitalization via self-report and research clinician depression ratings. Similarly, bipolar attempters had increased suicidal ideation, hopelessness, and decreased reasons for living. In contrast, there were no differences in impulsivity, although bipolar attempters had higher lifetime aggression. Bipolar attempters were more likely to present with depression while nonattempters were more likely to be manic. Attempters had 5 times as many previous hospitalizations and twice the number of major depressive episodes, although the two groups did not differ on age onset (Oquendo et al.

2000). Oquendo and Mann (2001) include gender (men more likely to attempt than women, in contrast with other studies); white race; age (no difference in their study); suicidal ideation, hopelessness, fewer reasons for living; life time aggression and impulsivity; smoking, alcoholism, and substance abuse, and family history of suicide as possible diathesis-related suicide risk factors for bipolar patients. Stress-related risk factors in bipolar patients may include depressed or mixed state (Oquendo and Mann 2001).

## Anxiety Disorders

Hall and colleagues (1999) studied 100 consecutive patients who made serious suicide attempts, all requiring emergency department, intensive care unit, medical or surgical unit treatment prior to inpatient psychiatric admission. They noted that 86% of their sample had some form of managed care insurance, 83% had seen a healthcare provider within 1 month prior to their attempt, and 62% voiced dissatisfaction with their healthcare provider. Over half reported that they were not asked about their emotional state or the presence of suicidal ideation. It was the first attempt for 67% and 84% had no family history of suicide attempts or completions. The vast majority (76%) were overdoses, most frequently of benzodiazepines. Most had acute onset of psychiatric symptoms, with about half reporting onset within two months of their attempts. Sixty-nine percent reported transient or absent suicidal thoughts prior to their attempt, and 84% denied having a plan. At the time of the attempt, 43% had been drinking and 78% were experiencing conflict in a significant relationship. Forty-one percent had a chronic, debilitating illness and 9% had been recently diagnosed with a life-threatening illness. These findings demonstrate the utility and futility of risk factors in predicting individual suicide attempts or their imminence (Hall et al. 1999).

A frequently overlooked risk factor that was noted in this study was anxiety. The clinical history features that were most predictive of serious suicide attempt were severe anxiety (92%) and panic attacks (80%), partial insomnia (difficulty falling asleep, middle insomnia, early morning awakening) (92%), depressed mood (80%), relationship disruption (78%), substance abuse (68%), pessimism (hopelessness 64%, helplessness 62%, and worthlessness 29%), global insomnia (46%), and anhedonia (43%).

Schnyder and colleagues (1999) also reported severe anxiety in a study of 30 consecutive suicide attempters presenting to an emergency department. Over half of the patients endorsed anxiety and panic in a self-report, while only 13% of physicians noted it in their evaluations (Schnyder et al. 1999). These findings corroborate those of Fawcett and colleagues (1990), who conducted sequential analyses of 32 suicide completers of 954 affectively disordered patients followed for the first 10 years of the Collaborative Depression Study. They found that risk factors among those who committed suicide within a year of assessment included severe psychic anxiety, panic attacks, moderate alcohol abuse, global insomnia, severe anhedonia, and poor concentration. Suicides committed after the first year were characterized by hopelessness, somatic anxiety, suicidal ideation, and a history of attempts (Fawcett and colleagues 1990). Weissman and colleagues (1989) noted a relationship between high rates of suicide attempts and panic disorder. Twenty percent of a sample of patients with panic disorder and 12% with panic attacks endorsed a history of suicide attempts (Weissman et al. 1989).

Severe anxiety and agitation may be an important risk factor for an acute suicide attempt. These "modifiable risk factors" may be responsive to early intervention. Fawcett and colleagues (1990) also noted that a significant number of the patients who killed themselves early in follow-up did not report suicidal ideation to clinical raters. In a study of 76 suicides that occurred while the patient was hospitalized, Busch et al. (submitted) noted that 79% of patients had chart notes indicating severe anxiety/agitation within one week prior to their suicide, while 77% had notes indicating that the patients denied suicidal ideation or intent within that same week. These studies argue for the assessment of severe anxiety/agitation and aggressive anxiolytic treatment in the management of suicide risk.

In contrast, another study (Placidi et al. 2000) argued that anxiety may be in someway protective against suicide attempts. In an examination of anxiety comorbid to a mood disorder in 272 inpatients, lifetime rates of panic disorder were not different between attempters and nonattempters. The nonattempters had higher scores on agitation, psychic anxiety, and hypochondriasis. Aggression and impulsivity were independent of panic disorder as risk factors for suicidal behavior. The authors speculate that anxiety, especially a component of fearfulness of death and illness, may restrain some patients from acting on suicidal impulses. They recommend further study, as anxiolytics in this population could have paradoxical results (Placidi et al. 2000). It is noted that the Hamilton Depression Scale mean anxiety rating for attempters compared to nonattempters (psychic anxiety 1.8 and 2.1 respectively, somatic anxiety 1.5 and 1.7 respectively) and Hamilton Depression Scale mean agitation rating for attempters compared to nonattempters (0.3 and 0.6 respectively) are indicative of relatively mild symptomatology for both groups. Benzodiazepines have an immediate anxiolytic impact, and can be safe in limited, monitored use.

## Psychosis

Grunebaum and colleagues (2001) reviewed 22 articles on whether delusions are a risk factor for suicide. The authors reported that about half of the reviewed articles published since 1982 reported a positive association between delusions and suicidal ideation or behavior and about half found a negative association. Approximately half of the subset of studies of delusional depression and suicide risk were negative. Half of the studies of delusions and suicide risk in schizophrenia were negative. A study of delusions and suicidal ideation in bipolar patients was negative. The paper by Roose and colleagues (1983) was included in the review as one of the positive studies. This retrospective analysis of depressed inpatients, both unipolar and bipolar, over a 25-year period found 14 unipolar depressed patients had committed suicide, of whom 10 were delusional. Delusional depressed patients were concluded to be 5 times more likely to commit suicide than nondelusional ones, and males were particularly susceptible. Negative studies include the report by Black and colleagues (1988), who found no increased suicidal risk among affectively ill patients (N=1,593) who were psychotic (N=443, 27.8%) at their index hospitalization. Of the diagnostic groups, 44.4% of bipolar (N=586) and 18.2% of unipolar (N=1,007) patients were psychotic.

Forty-one suicides occurred over the 14 year follow-up, 22.2% among psychotic subjects, 27.2% nonpsychotic. One possible explanation for the lack of difference in suicide risk between psychotic and nonpsychotic patient groups is the overrepresentation of manic patients (74.7% of the bipolar patients) at the initial admission, since they may have lower suicide rates (Black and colleagues 1988). Coryell and Tsuang (1982), in a 40-year follow-up, did not find an increased risk of suicide with delusional depression (10%) as compared to nondelusional depression (8.4%). Dilsaver and colleagues (1997) found no association between the presence of psychosis in bipolar patients and suicidality.

Grunebaum and colleagues (2001) studied 223 patients with major depression, 150 with schizophrenia, and 56 with bipolar disorder admitted as inpatients and outpatients to research units. Their multivariate analysis failed to find an association with delusions and suicidal ideation or behavior across the diagnostic groups. They caution that although their study did not find that the degree of psychosis discriminated between patients with and without a suicide attempt, they did not specifically examine hallucinations or negative symptoms (Grunebaum et al. 2001).

Fawcett and colleagues (1987) did not find that patients diagnosed as psychotic had higher prospective rates of suicide over a 4-year follow-up, but did find that delusions of grandiosity and delusions of mind reading suggested trends with a suicidal outcome. Likewise, López and colleagues (2001) studied a group of bipolar patients and also did not find an association between suicide and psychotic symptoms. Verdoux and colleagues (2001) studied 65 subjects over the two years following an index hospitalization with psychosis of various etiologies. Over this time span, 11.3% had suicidal behavior, most within the first year. They found that subjects with the lower Positive and Negative Symptoms Scale positive subscores were at greater risk of suicidal behavior over the follow-up, which was contrary to reports of an association between hallucinations, delusions, and suicidal behavior. Patients with suicidal behavior had a longer duration of psychotic symptoms. Although the best predictors of suicidal behavior were past history of suicide attempts, substance abuse, and chronic and/or deteriorating clinical course, the authors advised considering new onset psychosis as a significant risk factor (Verdoux et al. 2001).

A recent study evaluated the impact of clozapine on the rate of death due to suicide. Sernyak and colleagues (2001) matched schizophrenic patients who received clozapine (N=1,415) with a control group of schizophrenic patients who were not treated with clozapine (N=2,830) and identified cause of death for the 3 years postdischarge. Of the 250 deaths in the never-exposed group, 23 were suicides (9.2%). There were 95 deaths in the clozapine group, 10 (10.5%) of which were suicides. The differences were not statistically different (Sernyak et al. 2001). Clozapine is typically employed in chronic cases of psychosis. There is the suggestion that acute onset psychosis, like the acute onset of any psychiatric symptomatology, may have an increased risk of suicide. The clinical importance of psychosis as a risk factor for suicide may be determined by the clinical context, for examples, a mixed state or anxiety/agitation. The presence of a delusion or other psychotic experience may be too nonspecific to constitute a risk factor.

In contrast, Meltzer (2002) offers a critique of Sernyak and colleagues (2001), citing concerns about the "propensity scaling" methodology and lack of matching on "the four most important characteristics necessary for matching for suicide risk, that is, the number, timing, lethality of prior suicide attempts, and the severity of depression at index admission." Meltzer and Okayli (1995) and three previous studies (Walker et al. 1997, Reid et al. 1998, and Munro et al. 1999) showed a 70 to 86% decrease in suicide attempts or completions. The InterSePT study (Meltzer et al. 2003) found that in patients with psychotic disorders who were high risks for suicidal behavior, clozapine significantly reduced the rate of suicidal behavior compared to the comparison treatment with olanzapine. Based on the results of this study the FDA has approved the use of clozapine in patients with schizophrenia who are at risk of suicidal behavior.

## Borderline Personality Disorder

Suicidal behavior is frequently associated with affective lability, anger, impulsivity, and disruption in interpersonal relationships. Suicidal ideation and suicide attempts are part of the diagnostic criteria for borderline personality disorder. The recurrence and/or chronicity of suicidal ideation, combined with multiple low lethality attempts, have assigned some of these episodes to communicative idioms of distress or suicidal gestures. However, there is evidence from one study (Soloff et al. 2000) that suggests borderline personality disorder may be predictive of the number of attempts, but does not differentiate attempt characteristics, for example intent to die, planning, or lethality. Assumptions about the seriousness of suicidal behavior based on diagnosis may be flawed. Comorbid substance abuse and interpersonal disruption/abandonment issues heighten the risk (Soloff et al. 2000).

Soloff et al. (2000) compared the suicide attempts of patients with borderline personality disorder ($N=32$), major depression ($N=77$), and with both diagnoses ($N=49$). Eighty-four percent of the 81 patients with a borderline personality disorder had attempted suicide. The depressed and comorbid patients had higher observer-rated depression scores, but suicide attempts were more prevalent and of earlier onset in the borderline patients. The use of violent or nonviolent methods was not statistically different between the three groups, although the pooled borderline patients had a higher lifetime level of lethality. The highest self-reports of depression were in the comorbid group. The number of attempts, history of aggression, and hopelessness were variables in a regression model that predicted 60% more attempts for borderline and comorbid diagnosed patients compared to those with only major depression. The authors concluded that their findings were not consistent with significant differences between the suicidal behaviors of borderline patients as compared to patients with major depression (Soloff 2000). Brodsky and colleagues (1997) examined the relationship between the clinical criteria for borderline personality disorder and suicidal behavior in 156 subjects with borderline personality disorder (67% had at a previous suicide attempt). In this sample, the number of symptoms (severity) did not distinguish between attempters and nonattempters. Lability, fear of abandonment, anger, identity diffusion, chronic emptiness, unstable relationships, nor substance abuse (suicidal behavior was excluded from the

analysis) significantly correlated with attempter status, the number of suicide attempts, or their lethality. Only impulsivity correlated with the number of previous attempts. This finding held after controlling for major depression and substance abuse (Brodsky et al. 1997).

A suicide attempt is a self-destructive act with intent to end one's life. It may or may not require medical attention. Self-injurious behavior is self-harm without suicidal intent. It is a common characteristic of patients with borderline personality disorder and frequently involves cutting. Stanley and colleagues (2001) warn against being dismissive of these behaviors as nonserious, attention-seeking, and manipulative. They posit that self-injurious behavior may have elements in common with suicidality, despite differences in intent. To examine this, they compared the suicidal behavior of 53 cluster B (borderline, antisocial, narcissistic, histrionic) personality disordered patients with ($N=30$) and without ($N=23$) histories of self-mutilation. Ninety-four percent of the sample had borderline personality disorder, 79% were female, and 66% had comorbid depression. There were no demographic differences between the two groups. Self-mutilators were significantly more aggressive, but not more hostile, nor did they have more frequent histories of sexual abuse. They were more depressed, anxious, hopeless, and had more severe borderline symptoms. The groups did not differ on the most frequent mode of suicide attempt (overdose), or the violence, planning, number, or seriousness (relatively serious) of the attempts. Although there were no significant differences in lethality, the mutilating group misjudged the lethality of their attempts, believed they would be saved, and viewed death as less irrevocable. Clinicians are warned not to minimize these attempts as this population of patients does. These distortions, along with more recurrent and chronic suicidal ideation, increase the risk of accidental death (Stanley et al. 2001).

## Risk Factors (See Table 102–2)

Since there are no reliable and specific tests for suicidal behavior, the clinician must rely on clinical, demographic, historical, and patient self-report information to guide their judgment and to tailor their intervention. However, the clinician should not be lulled into a false sense of security because of their assessment. The positive predictive value of individual or group of risk factors is low. Stepwise multiple regression was used to develop a statistical model that would predict suicide in 1906 inpatients (admitted between

| Table 102–2 | Risk Factors |
| --- | --- |
| Gender—male | |
| Ethnicity—white | |
| Age—elderly | |
| Substance abuse | |
| Past attempts | |
| Means, especially access to guns | |
| Family history | |
| Hopelessness | |
| Unemployed | |
| Comorbid medical conditions | |
| Failed relationship, divorced, widowed | |
| Irresponsible media coverage of suicides | |

1970 and 1981). There were 46 suicides at the end of the follow-up period (1983). Medical illness, substance abuse, personality disorder, marital status were among characteristics that failed to reach significance for the final model. Variables that met significance level criteria (number of prior suicide attempts, suicidal ideation, bipolar disorder, gender, outcome at discharge, unipolar depression with bipolar first-degree relative) were included in the model. The model did not identify any patient who committed suicide. Limitations include the low suicide rate and possible underestimation of suicides (Goldstein et al. 1991). There may be differences in people who attempt suicide versus those who complete it. In 1999, it was estimated that there were 730,000 annual attempts, with an attempt and completion ratio of 25:1. It was estimated that 5 million had a history of a suicide attempt (Hoyert et al. 2001). Differential risk factors include gender, ethnicity, age, substance abuse, past suicide attempts, means, family history, hopelessness, comorbid medical conditions, relationship/esteem losses resulting in murder–suicide, and media coverage.

## Gender

Women are more likely have a diagnosis of major depression or borderline personality disorder. Women attempt suicide more frequently than men (3:1), although men commit suicide more frequently (4.1:1.0) (Hoyert et al. 2001). There are significant gender differences in the lifetime risk of suicide in major depression, estimated to be 7% in men and 1% in women (Blair-West et al. 1999). Men are more likely to have substance abuse disorders and aggressivity, which increase the risk of suicide. In the past, women were more likely to use nonlethal means of trying to kill themselves. However, the use of guns by women is increasing. Firearms are the most common means of completed suicide in men and women, representing almost 60% of all suicides, 62% of male completers, and 37% of female completers according to 1999 US data (Hoyert et al. 2001). Suokas and colleagues (2001) collected data on 1018 "deliberate self-poisoning" patients treated in a hospital emergency department in 1983, and followed them for 14 years. During this time, 68 died by suicide, 44 men (9.2%) and 24 women (4.5%). In this sample, the risk factors for suicide were male gender, previous psychiatric treatment, previous suicide attempts, medical problems, and voicing intent to die on the index suicide attempt (Suokas et al. 2001).

## Ethnicity

In the US, Oquendo and colleagues (2001) examined the 1-year prevalence of major depression across Whites, African-Americans, Mexican-Americans, Cuban-Americans, and Puerto Ricans and whether the suicide rate relative to depression varied across these five ethnic groups. The authors also examined the relative contributions of marital status, low income, and not working for pay on their findings. The authors acknowledged the limitations on their data sets: the 1980–1984 Epidemiologic Catchment Area Study, the 1982–1984 Hispanic Health and Nutrition Epidemiologic Survey, and data based on the Centers for Disease Control National Center for Health Statistics from 1984–1986. They consistently found that rates of depression for women were twice that of men, and that suicide rates were higher in males. Whites (male and female) had the highest rates of

suicide relative to rates of depression. The 1-year prevalence rates of major depression were 6.9% for Puerto Ricans, 3.6% for Whites, 3.5% for African-Americans, 2.8% for Mexican-Americans, and 2.5% for Cuban-Americans. The annual suicide rates for 1986 to 1988, per 100,000 persons were: white males 22.5/females 5.8; African-American males 11.9/females 2.4; Mexican-American males 7.0/females 1.3; Cuban-American males 14.9/females 2.3; and Puerto Rican males 11.7/females 1.2. The annual suicide rates relative to major depression in terms of number of suicides per year per case of major depression per year ($\times 10^{-4}$) were: white males 102/females 13; African-American males 79/females 5; Mexican-American males 58/females 3; Cuban-American males 99/females 7; Puerto Rican males 31/females 1. Puerto Ricans, Mexican-Americans, and Cuban-American females (but not males) had, relative to depression rates, lower suicide rates than might have been predicted. These differences were not readily explained by poverty, marital separation or divorce, or not working for pay. Potential protective factors for Hispanics could be extended close relationships and the expectation of adversity (Oquendo et al. 2001, Hoppe and Martin 1986).

The authors were surprised that, proportional to depression rate, African-American male suicide rates approached that of white males. There has been a disturbing trend, reported by Shaffer and colleagues (1994) of an increasing suicide rate among black and minority males. It could be that factors generally considered protective against suicide in African-Americans, for example, the role of African-American churches, may impact African-American females more than African-American males (Oquendo et al. 2001). Native Americans (American Indians and Inuits) have elevated suicide rates. From 1979 to 1992, their rates were 1.5 times that of the general population (US Public Health Service, 1999).

The relationship between mood disorder and suicide has been a relatively consistent finding in international studies as well (Oquendo et al. 2001). One country that may deviate from these demographics is China. It has been reported (Pritchard 1996) that the rate of suicide for women is higher than men in China, and that young women are at particular risk. In addition, suicides were far more common in rural China, in contrast to urban areas. It is unclear whether male suicides are underreported secondary to the stigma attached and if psychosocial and cultural factors are more primary in explaining suicides in China than psychiatric factors (Pritchard 1996). Qin and Mortensen (2001) had similar findings in a recent examination of suicide rates in China. Rates were higher than the Denmark comparator (19.9 and 13.2 per 100,000 inhabitants respectively). Rates were higher in females (main peak at age 65 + years, minor peak age 15 to 24 years) and in rural China. Suicide accounts for 4.17% of all deaths in rural areas and 42.6% of rural females age between 15 and 24 years. Suicide may be underreported (shame, "loss of face", limited access to records) or overreported (accepted in some instances as honorable). Rural rates may be impacted by readily available pesticides, a common source of self-poisoning, and the lack of accessible treatment for both poisoning and mental illness. Relationship disruption is more commonly a cause for suicide than mental illness. Other potential factors include the devaluation of women, encouragement of stoicism, and acceptance of one's circumstances (Qin and Mortensen 2001).

## Age

Those at highest risk are the elderly. The highest suicide rates in US in 1999 were for ages between 75 and 84 years (18.3 deaths per 100,000 persons) and 85+ years (19.2 deaths per 100,000 persons). The combined rate for the elderly (65+) was 15.9 deaths per 100,000 persons. The attempt to completion ratio for the elderly was estimated to be 4:1. Comprising only 12.7% of the 1999 population, the elderly accounted for 18.8% of the suicide deaths (Hoyert et al. 2001). One possible explanation for this significant mortality is missed diagnoses of major depression. Studies have reported that many of the elderly saw a primary care physician shortly before the suicide, either the same day (20%), within the earlier week weak (40%), or within the prior month (70%) (NIH 2001, Conwell 1994). Other risk factors for the elderly include bereavement, loss of functionality and independence, comorbid medical conditions or chronic pain, financial stressors, and diminished support systems. A Finnish group found that an assessment of life dissatisfaction may be useful in identifying those at risk for suicide. They used a four item scale that assessed happiness, ease of living, interest in life, and loneliness. A sample of 29,137 adults had the baseline assessment and were followed for 20 years. During that period, there were 2,859 deaths, 182 of which were suicides. The cumulative incidence of suicide was 1.04% for men and 0.22% for women. Suicide victims were more likely to live alone, drink heavily, smoke, and have poor health. The most dissatisfied men in the sample had a 24.85-fold higher suicide risk. For men, dissatisfaction was more of a risk than poor health, while for women the opposite was true. Greater life satisfaction was associated with female gender, health, married or cohabitating, physical activity, non-smoking, younger than age 45, and being in the upper socioeconomic class (Koivumaa-Honkanen et al. 2001).

The suicide rate for the young (15 to 24 years) was 10.3 deaths per 100,000 persons. However these deaths represented 12.7% of all causes of death for this age group. The estimated attempt and completion ratio for the young was 100 to 200:1 (Hoyert et al. 2001). Suicide is a disproportionate cause of death in younger persons as risk may be higher when a psychiatric disorder is first diagnosed (Inskip et al. 1998). Others have also suggested that earlier age of onset of illness is associated with increased risk of attempted (Ahrens et al. 1995) and completed suicide. In one group of 472 bipolar patients, followed for 17 years, suicide completers were younger at onset of illness and at death. The mean age of onset for the suicide completer group was 36 years and mean age of death was 44 years, compared to mean onset age of 60.4 for the index group. The vast majority of suicides were committed within 5 to 10 years of diagnosis (Sharma and Markar 1994). Fawcett and colleagues (1987) noted that suicide was most common within the first three episodes of major affective disorder. Malone and colleagues (1995) noted in a study of 100 patients with major depression that the period of highest risk for suicide attempts were the first 3 months and the first 5 years after onset.

A number of studies have examined the phenomenon of adolescent suicide. King and colleagues (2001) examined 1,285 children and adolescents (age 9–17 years) who participated in the NIMH Methods for the Epidemiology of Child and Adolescent Mental Disorders (MECA) Study. Of these randomly selected youths, 3.3% had attempted suicide and 5.2% endorsed suicidal ideation. The authors compared the attempters to those with suicidal ideation, and noted that they were more likely to have life stressors, be sexually active, smoke cigarettes, and to have smoked marijuana. After controlling for mood, anxiety, or disruptive disorders, as well as sociodemographics, the significant risk factors for suicide attempts or ideation were poor family environment, parental psychiatric history, low parental monitoring, low competence (social and practical) scores, sexual activity, recent alcohol intoxication, smoking, and physical fighting. Behavioral and psychosocial risk factors may be more identifiable than suicidal ideation, and may provide an early clue to suicidal ideation and behavior (King et al. 2001). A large ($N$=3,416) adolescent twin survey (Glowinski et al. 2001) revealed a suicide attempt in 4.2% of the participants. In this sample, first attempts were unusual after age 17, mean age 13.6 years. Psychiatric disorders (major depression, alcohol dependence, social phobia, conduct disorder), in addition to physical abuse and African-American ethnicity, were risk factors. The comorbidity of major depression and conduct disorder were particularly high risk. There were significant associations between suicide attempts in the study group and completed suicides of their first-degree relatives. Concordance for suicide attempts was 25% for monozygotic and 12.8% for dizygotic twins (Glowinski et al. 2001). Lewinsohn and colleagues (2001) also noted elevated suicide risk for girls between ages 15 and 18 years, with decreases in the annual hazard rate between ages 19 and 23 years. Rates for boys peak around age 15 years, and are fairly constant until age 20 years. By age 19 years, the annual hazard rate for both genders is comparable, although a significant decline was only evident for young women. Logistic regression models identified negative cognitions, low self-esteem, emotional dependency, poor coping skills, low family support, and history of major depression as significant predictors of suicide attempts (Lewinsohn et al. 2001).

Another study confirmed an association between childhood abuse and impulsivity, aggression, and suicide attempts in adults with major depression. Of 138 depressed, hospitalized adults, those with childhood physical or sexual abuse (38%) were more likely to be female, have a comorbid diagnosis of borderline personality disorder, have higher impulsivity and aggression scores, have made suicide attempts, and to have made their first suicide attempt prior to age 18 (46%) (Brodsky et al. 2001). Wunderlich and colleagues (2001) interviewed 3,021 randomly sampled young people (between ages 14 and 24 years). Of these, 1,358 met criteria for a depressive disorder and were queried about suicide. Seventy had a history of a suicide attempt: 48 female, 22 male, 24.4% between ages 14 and 17 years, 35.6% between 18 and 21 years, and 40% between 22 and 24 years. The adolescent group was overly represented by females, representing 31% of female attempters as compared to 10.8% of male attempters. The researchers noted that females had both higher rates of suicide attempters and more suicidal ideation, as adolescents, than males. The female suicide attempters were more often victims of sexual abuse and more often had anxiety disorders (17.5% had PTSD as compared to none of the males). The male suicide attempters more often had alcohol abuse and financial problems. Traumas, leading to PTSD and panic disorders, may place adolescents at higher risk for suicide attempts (Wunderlich et al. 2001). Other risk factors reviewed by Pfeffer (2001) include recent suicide death of another adolescent and media reports of suicide. The author also reports that homosexual and bisexual adolescents are at increased risk of suicide.

Wagner and colleagues (2000) noted that cognitive factors, for example, attributional style (how one explains why things happen to them), hopelessness, and low self-esteem have been associated with suicidal behavior, although there have been conflicting reports. Their study was designed to examine whether changes in cognitive processing were related to resolution of suicidal ideation in hospitalized children and adolescents. The study evaluated 100 children and adolescents at hospital admission, 50 with and 50 without suicidal ideation, and again upon discharge. The groups also differed in diagnoses: 36% of suicidal group had major depression versus 8% of group without suicidal ideation; the group with suicidal ideation had no subjects with ADHD versus 28% of the group without suicidal ideation; and 46% of the group with suicidal ideation had a previous attempt versus 14% in the group without suicidal ideation. The length of hospitalization was not significantly different between the two groups. There was evidence that improvement in attributional style contributed to the loss of suicidal ideation. This change occurred without specific cognitive therapy and over a short period of time (average stay was 7 days). The question was raised as to whether targeted interventions would have brought about even more rapid improvement. The interventions included individual, family, and group psychotherapy, as well as appropriate pharmacotherapy. Hopelessness, while improved upon discharge in the suicidal group, did not reach statistical significance. After controlling for changes in depressive symptomatology, there were no statistically significant changes in self-esteem with the resolution of suicidal ideation (Wagner et al. 2000).

## Substance Abuse

Substance abuse can heighten suicide risk independently of the presence of other psychiatric illness and may contribute to both attempts and completions (Goldberg et al. 2001). It is difficult to disentangle the relative contributions of psychiatric illness, substance abuse, genetics, and family history. In one study of suicide victims utilizing psychological autopsy to assign diagnosis, alcohol dependence or abuse (43%) was second in prevalence only to depressive disorders (59%) (Henriksson et al. 1993). The lifetime risk for suicide in alcohol dependence has been estimated to be 7% (Inskip et al. 1998), although some estimates are higher. Harris and Barraclough (1997) performed a meta-analysis of 32 studies involving some 45,000 subjects. There was a six-fold increased suicide risk for alcohol abusers. Heroin addicts had a fourteen-fold increased risk compared to nonabusers in nine studies involving 7,500 subjects. A relationship to human immunodeficiency virus (HIV) infection was not evident, although it has been linked to increased suicide risk. There was also an association between suicidal behavior and cigarette smoking (Harris and Barraclough 1997). As reviewed by Tondo and colleagues (1999), evidence

relating marijuana to suicide risk is scant and inconsistent. Amphetamines, lysergic acid diethylamide (LSD), and phencyclidine have been associated with heightened suicide risk and completion (Tondo et al. 1999).

One study of 472 patients hospitalized for a suicide attempt found that 11.2% of those with alcoholism ($N=161$) subsequently committed suicide compared to 2.2% of suicide completers without alcoholism ($N=311$). Of the alcohol-abusing attempters who eventually committed suicide, 55.6% were women. Only one of 27 possible variables examined differentiated between attempters and future completers: the precautions subscore, which was a measure of efforts to avoid discovery during the suicide attempt. This type of calculated attempt, if repeated, raises the chance for completing suicide (Beck et al. 1989). This type of attempt appears less impulsive, although it could well be that substance abuse lower inhibitions, or shares some of the genetic and neurobiologic substrates as psychiatric illness and impulsivity. Substance abuse has long been associated with both mood disorders and suicide risk. Of all Axis I disorders, patients with bipolar disorder have the highest likelihood of comorbid substance abuse (Regier et al. 1990). Many of the risk factors previously noted tend to cluster with substance abuse.

Roy (1986, 2000) reports that one-third of alcoholic patients will attempt suicide at some point in their lives. In his most recent sample of 333 alcoholic patients, 124 had previous suicide attempts. Of the attempters, 15.3% had a first- or second-degree relative who had committed suicide, compared to 4.3% of those who did not. A significantly higher number of female alcoholics attempted suicide (20/124) as compared to female alcoholics who had no attempts (9/209) (Roy 2000).

Conner and colleagues (2001) examined the relationship between a history of violence, alcohol abuse, and completed suicide. They utilized a case control design, with accident victims—another sudden death group—as the control group. A history of violence was ascertained by an interview with the decedents' next of kin or others who could provide collateral information. Violence in the previous year was a significant predictor of suicide. There were significant interactions between violence and alcohol abuse (absent), gender (women), and age (younger). The association of violence and suicide was strongest for those without alcohol abuse, with an odds ratio of 11.6 in the regression analysis. Although the majority of suicide attempts are made by women, violent women may be particularly vulnerable to suicide completion. Intervention strategies that decreased violence, especially domestic, and targeted toward the young and female, may decrease suicide potential as well (Conner et al. 2001).

Cocaine use/dependence has been associated with suicide attempts and completion. During a 1-year period (1985) in New York City, 29% of suicide victims between the ages of 21 and 30 years tested positive for cocaine (Marzuk et al. 1992). Garlow (2002) examined completed suicide from 1994 to 1998 in Fulton County (contains much of Atlanta), Georgia. Cocaine was detected in 9.9%, and alcohol in 28.9%, of these suicide victims, almost all of them males between 21 and 50 years old. Logistic regression analysis revealed that cocaine use was four times as likely in male suicide victims, and twice as likely in African-

American victims. Between the ages of 21 to 35 years and 36 to 50 years, 20% and 28.1% of African-American victims were cocaine positive, compared to 11.3% and 7.8% in white victims, respectively. In contrast, of teenage victims, 25% of white victims compared to 6.7% of African-Americans tested positive for cocaine. Further, 86.7% of African-American teenage suicides did not test positive for cocaine or alcohol, while 50% of white teenage suicides tested positive for one or both. It was suggested that substance abuse did not play a significant role in the rising suicide rate in African-American teens (Garlow 2002).

A group of 214 consecutive cocaine-dependent inpatients were surveyed on family history, childhood trauma, and personality traits (Roy 2001). In this sample, 84 patients had attempted suicide compared to 130 who denied attempts. African-Americans were overrepresented in both groups. Significantly more of the attempters group was female as compared to the nonattempters. Additional characteristics of the attempter group included family history of suicidal behavior (25% as compared to 5.4% of nonattempters), significantly higher childhood trauma and physical neglect scores, and significantly more physical disorders. Most striking was the high prevalence of comorbid substance abuse in the attempter group. Over 50% had a history of alcohol dependence (34.5% of nonattempters) and 19% had a history of opiate dependence (9.2% of nonattempters). The group with a history of suicide attempts had significantly lower extraversion, higher neuroticism, and higher hostility scores, although there were no significant differences in impulsivity. Almost 90% of the attempter group had a lifetime history of a major depressive episode. Of the 84 cocaine dependent patients who attempted suicide, only two did not have comorbid histories of either alcohol/opiate dependence, mood disorder, or currently treated physical disorder. Over a third of the nonattempter group did not have any of these comorbidities (Roy 2001).

## Past Attempts

A history of previous suicide attempts is the strongest predictor of suicidal behavior and suicide completion (Brodsky et al.1997, Isometsä and Lönnqvist 1998). This holds across all psychiatric diagnoses. However, an examination of all suicides in Finland (1987 to 1988, N=1,397) revealed that 56% died with the initial attempt (Isometsä and Lönnqvist 1998). Of the victims with a history of previous attempts, 39% were female, 19% were male, 82% switched methods, and 6% had over six previous attempts. This implies that efforts to remove means may need to be fairly comprehensive, and that a large number of previous attempts should not cause a relaxation in vigilance. Suokas and colleagues (2001), in their 14-year follow-up, found the risk remained elevated for at least a decade after the initial attempt, and that the risk factors may change over time. In their sample, the essential factors were male gender and previous attempts. Previous psychiatric treatment, physical illness, and planned attempts were more suggestive of long-term risk. Ahrens and colleagues (1995) found that the risk remains as long as the affective disorder recurs. There should be limited expectation that the risk declines with the number of attempts or with the chronicity of the illness. Fawcett and colleagues (1990), in a longitudinal follow-up of mood disorder patients, noted that suicide was no more common in the short-term (one year) in those with prior attempts compared to those with no attempts, but that prior attempts approached a significant association with long-term (1 to 10 years) suicide.

## Means

Virtually all suicide intervention strategies include removing the means. There is a strong relationship between access to lethal means of suicide and completed suicide. One reason the newer antidepressants have supplanted the older tricyclics and monoamine oxidase inhibitors is their relatively greater safety in overdose situations. As previously noted, women may have higher rates of suicide attempts because of less lethal means like overdoses and wrist cutting. Men have higher rates of completions because of more violent means like guns or hanging. Kellerman and colleagues (1992) examined the relationship between suicide at home and gun ownership. They interviewed close associates of suicide victims and compared the victims (case subjects) to a matched control from the same neighborhood. They identified 803 suicides, over 32 months, in two counties. Seventy percent of the suicides took place in the victim's home and gunshot was the most common means. A history of depression or mental illness was reported in 83.5% of the case subjects in contrast to 6.4% of controls. Sixty-five percent of the decedents kept firearms in their home, and reportedly had them for months or years. Only 3% of the proxies reported that the firearm was obtained within a couple of weeks of death. In homes where guns were not kept, only 6% of the case subjects committed suicide with a gun. In confirmation of risk factors previously discussed, univariate analysis revealed that living alone, taking prescription psychotropic medications for depression or mental illness, having a history of arrest, substance use and abuse, and less than a high school education were more likely in proxy reports of the case subjects than in the controls. After controlling for these conditions, the presence of guns was strongly associated with an increased risk of suicide in the home (odds ratio increased from 3.2 to 4.8) (Kellerman et al. 1992). There is evidence that restricting the availability of guns, or increasing the waiting period to purchase one, may have some impact on suicide rates (Loftin et al. 1991, Wintemute et al. 1999, Ludwig and Cook, 2000).

Brent and colleagues (1991) had very similar findings in the comparison of adolescent suicide victims to inpatient adolescent suicide attempters and nonattempters (N=47 in all three cells). Only six of the completers had ever been psychiatrically hospitalized, but did not differ from the others on demographics, diagnoses, or gun availability. Sixty-nine percent of completers used a gun as compared to none of the suicide attempters. Guns were more likely to be present in the adolescent suicide completers, although the adjusted odds were not significantly different for the method of storing the gun. In this sample as well, none of the guns were obtained in the 1 to 2 weeks prior to death. The suicide rate for 15 to 24-year-olds was 27% lower in the Canadian sample city (where gun ownership is prohibited) than the US city. The authors conclude that for adolescents, the presence of a gun in the home, regardless of method of storage, represents a significant risk factor for suicide. It was flatly asserted that all guns must be removed from the homes of at risk or psychiatrically ill adolescents (Brent et al. 1991).

There is a significant risk of suicide even when an attempt is made to place patients in a monitored environment away from the means with which to commit suicide. A recent study of 112 patients who committed suicide while hospitalized at psychiatric facilities estimated the rate to be 13.7 inpatient suicides per 10,000 admissions. Utilizing univariate and multivariate analysis, five predictive factors included planned suicide attempt: actual suicide attempt, recent bereavement, presence of delusions, chronic mental illness, and family history of suicide. Still, this model only predicted two of the suicides, highlighting the difficulty with low sensitivity and specificity of risk factors. Suicide remains a relatively rare phenomenon, even in a high risk group (Powell et al. 2000). Bostwick and Pankratz (2000) noted that suicides were more likely after a psychiatric hospital discharge.

## Family History

Roy (1983) compared a group of patients with a family history of suicide ($N=243$) to a control group without family history of suicide ($N=5,602$). There were 274 suicides among first- and second-degree relatives in the study group. Almost 11% of the study group had two or more close relatives who died of suicide. Approximately half (48.6%) of the probands from the positive family history group had made 252 suicide attempts, collectively, compared to a suicide attempt rate of 21.8% in the control group. During the 7.5 year follow-up, seven of the study group committed suicide. Between them, they had a total of 18 previous attempts. Notably, there was a preponderance of affective disorder in the positive family history group (56.4%) as compared to the control group (26.6%) (Roy 1983). In this study, the association with affective disorder was most apparent, although there are genetic components associated with other risk factors for suicidal behavior, including aggression, impulsivity, and substance abuse.

## Hopelessness

Brown and colleagues (2000) prospectively studied 6,891 psychiatric outpatients over a 20-year-period in an effort to identify the risk factors associated with suicide. These outpatients had been administered a structured diagnostic interview and a battery of psychological measures, including the Beck Hopelessness Scale. Forty-nine suicides were identified. The average age was 41 years, and the vast majority (96%) had a mood disorder diagnosis. Single covariate, proportional hazard models indicated that higher levels of suicidal ideation, depression, unemployment status, and hopelessness were significant risk factors for suicide. Patients who scored nine or above on the Beck Hopelessness Scale were approximately four times more likely to commit suicide. Hopelessness that does not change with treatment may be predictive of suicide attempts and suicide (Dahlsgaard et al. 1998, Young et al. 1996). Fawcett and colleagues (1990) also found that hopelessness, loss of interest, and loss of the capacity for pleasure discriminated a suicide group from a control group.

## Comorbid Medical Conditions

A number of medical conditions have been associated with increased risk of suicide. As reviewed by Hendin (1999), cancer, acquired immunodeficiency syndrome, peptic ulcer, Huntington's chorea, head injury, and spinal cord injury are associated with high suicide rates. However, terminal illness is the backdrop for suicide in only 2 to 4%. Frequently, as with other suicidal patients, the suicidal terminally ill have comorbid mood disorders. Fisher and colleagues (2001) notes that chronic pain (e.g. migraine headaches, low back pain, cancer-related pain) is associated with elevated suicide rates. Fisher and colleagues investigated suicidal ideation and chronic pain, disability, and coping in 200 patients on an inpatient psychiatry rehabilitation unit. Forty-two percent had low back pain, 14% had head/face/mouth pain, and 11% had lower extremity pain. Via self-report (Beck Depression Inventory), 6.5% endorsed suicidal ideation. This depressed/suicidal group was age, sex, and pain duration matched to depressed/nonsuicidal and nondepressed groups. There were no suicide attempts in the nondepressed group. Fifty-four percent of the depressed/suicidal group had a previous suicide attempt, as did 23% of the depressed/nonsuicidal group. The three groups were compared on measures of pain, disability, and coping strategies. The depressed groups did not differ from each other in their experience of pain, and had higher pain measures, lower active coping, and higher passive coping than the nondepressed group. The presence of depression, not suicidal ideation, was the most predictive of functioning (Fisher et al. 2001). Another study compared 11 general hospital patients who committed suicide shortly after discharge (64% within 6 months) to matched controls. It was noted that 73% of the suicide patients had a comorbid diagnosis of depression, substance abuse, or both, as opposed to only 33% of the controls. The rate of psychiatry consultation was very low (1 of 44 patients) for both cases and controls (Dhossche et al. 2001).

## Murder–Suicide

Murder–suicide is a difficult phenomenon to study, given the relatively infrequent occurrence. The retrospective, psychological autopsy is the most common methodology of study. Marzuk and colleagues (1992) offer a comprehensive review of the epidemiology. The demographics of the murder–suicide are very distinct from those of murder or of suicide, although there is some overlap with the latter. Common features include the prevalence of mental illness, overrepresentation of white males, disruption of a significant relationship, and common use of firearms. Many perpetrators of murder–suicide have factors typically deemed protective of suicide, for example, married, parental status, lack of a previous arrest record, and many of the acts are not impulsive, but carefully planned. In homicides, men rarely take their own lives after killing unrelated men, and women rarely kill themselves after killing anyone other than their own children. Substance abuse may be more of a factor in homicides than in the murder–suicide (Marzuk et al. 1992). Rosenbaum (1990) compared 12 couples who were killed in murder–suicide to 24 couples involved in homicide. Two-thirds (8) of the murder–suicide couples were married to each other, compared to one-third (8) in the homicides. All the male perpetrators were prone to jealousy. Substance abuse was overly represented in the homicides (12 perpetrators and 12 victims). Risk factors for murder–suicide in this study included male gender; depression (75% of perpetrators had depression); married or in long-term relationship characterized by jealousy, physical abuse, frequent separations; and personality disorders. Half of the women victims were in the process of leaving the relationship (Rosenbaum 1990).

Marzuk and colleagues (1992) delineate five victim–perpetrator relationships and motives: spousal murder–suicide, amorous jealousy and declining health types; filicide–suicide; familicide–suicide; and extrafamilial murder–suicide. The spousal murder–suicide motivated by jealousy is the most common in the US, representing 50 to 75% of the phenomenon. Typically, a male perpetrator, infuriated over a real or imagined infidelity, kills a female partner and in some scenarios, the romantic rival as well, with a gun. The declining health variant involves elderly men with poor health and/or chronically ill wives, frequently leaving a suicide note prior to shooting the spouse and then themselves. Parents are responsible for at least half of the murders of infants and children. Filicide–suicides are characterized by mothers being more likely to kill infants and fathers being more likely to commit suicide immediately after killing their children. Fathers more commonly use firearms, while mothers rarely do. Depression and psychosis are prevalent in maternal filicide–suicide and a common motive is "deluded altruism". The last category, the extra-familial murder–suicide, is the rarest. With limited exceptions, the vast majority of murder–suicide victims are blood relatives or sexual partners. The unrelated murder–suicide is typified by a paranoid or narcissistic white male seeking revenge for a perceived wrong. The victims are classically authority figures and the perpetrator often has little compunction about killing bystanders as they seek their target (Marzuk et al. 1992).

## Media Coverage

Media coverage of suicide and suicide methodologies can be influential. Marzuk and colleagues (1993) noted a dramatic increase in asphyxia suicides in New York City in the year following the publication of a suicide manual marketed toward the terminally ill. The American Foundation for Suicide Prevention (2002) notes that media coverage can contribute to "copycat" or "suicide contagion" suicides. They observe that suicides increase when the number of stories about completed suicides increase, when there is extensive coverage of a suicide death, when the story makes front page news, or is the lead story in a broadcast, and when there are dramatic headlines (Phillips et al. 1992). The website reports that educating the Viennese media about the pitfalls of subway suicide coverage decreased attempts and completions by over 80% (Etzersdorfer and Sonneck 1998). The media should avoid: romanticizing or idealizing the act, glamorizing suicide deaths of celebrities, detailed descriptions of method or site, failing to acknowledge a likely mental illness, dramatizing the grief of survivors (may encourage attention-seeking or revenge attempts), or using adolescents to recount their past attempts. Recommendations include reporting cause of death in the body of the story, not using the term suicide or self-inflicted in the headline, and being sensitive to the semantics of "successful," "unsuccessful," and "failed." Referring to the decedent as "a suicide" or as having "committed suicide" diminishes the person and is pejorative (American Foundation of Suicide Prevention 2002).

## Intervention

Successful suicide prevention strategies include educating the public and primary care providers about mental illness, its common presentations, the availability of treatment, and how to access it. Underdiagnosis and undertreatment remain significant problems. Antidepressants, lithium, mood stabilizers, and ECT, as well as adjunctive benzodiazepines and antipsychotics, can significantly ameliorate underlying psychiatric diagnoses associated with suicide. Psychosocial interventions have much to add, especially for chronic suicidal ideation, but more intensive outpatient strategies may be limited by resources available.

## Education

Educating the public and clinicians about the prevalence, symptoms, and available treatment for mood disorders will be seminal. It is estimated that half to a quarter of mood disorders go undiagnosed and untreated (Grandin et al. 2001, Nierenberg et al. 2001). Many patients will have spoken to significant others about their distress or have recently seen a health care professional. The US Surgeon General issued a call to action in 1999 to prevent suicide. The linchpins of the strategy include awareness, intervention, and methodology. Recommendations include improving public awareness of suicide, including their preventability, enhancing access to prevention resources, and decreasing the stigma of mental illness. Interventions include improved ability of primary care physicians to recognize, treat, or refer the mentally ill; remove barriers; create incentives to treatment; train other professionals, community members, and family to recognize or assess risk; develop programs for at risk adolescents; enhance community access to care and support for suicide survivors; and partnering with the media for educated reporting and depictions of mental illness and suicide deaths. Methodology involves researching effective prevention programs, clinical and culture specific interventions; developing evaluation tools to measure efficacy of interventions; and the reduction of access to lethal means of suicide (US Public Health Service 1999).

## Antidepressants

The findings of the impact of effective antidepressants on suicide rates are inconsistent (Tondo et al. 2001a), and the impact of long-term antidepressant use on mortality is not yet clearly established (Müller-Oerlinghausen and Berghöfer 1999). Isacsson and colleagues (1997) have shown a decrease in suicides as the use of antidepressants increased in Sweden. There were 5281 suicides in Sweden during 1992–1994. Antidepressants were detected in 874 (16.5%), toxic levels in 232 of these (4.4%). Fifty-one had antidepressants alone, and of these, 14 had significant alcohol concentrations. Compared to an earlier study (Isacsson et al. 1994), this data represented a 28% reduction in risk of antidepressants being found in suicides, paralleled by a 51% increase in antidepressant use, an increase of 7% in positive toxicology for antidepressants, and a 10% decrease in total number of suicides. The selective serotonin reuptake inhibitors (SSRIs) seemed to have higher risk of detection in suicide than the tricyclics. The authors concluded that antidepressant toxicity is less a concern than undertreatment and lack of efficacy (Isacsson et al. 1997). Henriksson et al. (2001) observed that of a sample of 59 suicides, only 19% received psychiatric care during the last 3 months of their lives and only 12% received antidepressants. However, there was the suggestion that decreased use of tricyclics, which may have greater efficacy in severe depression, has had a negative impact. There are times when their utility in severe illness should supercede concerns about toxicity (Isacsson et al. 1997, Müller-Oerlinghausen and Berghöfer 1999).

As reviewed by Müller-Oerlinghausen and Berghöfer (1999), there is little evidence that patients routinely use prescribed antidepressants to commit suicide. They estimate that approximately 5% of patients on antidepressants commit suicide with their medications, with a greater likelihood that women will use this means than men. Despite occasional claims in the media and in litigation by victims' families, there is no evidence that antidepressants might precipitate suicidality. At the same time, there is the theoretical risk that partially improved patients may be able to act on a suicidal plan that had been present throughout their illness, but not clearly formulated or put into action during the more severe initial stages of their illness. In vulnerable patients, SSRI side effects of activation, anxiety, akathisia, and insomnia can be concerning (Müller-Oerlinghausen and Berghöfer 1999). On the other hand, potential cognitive confusion precipitated by anticholinergic properties of TCAs, especially in vulnerable elderly patients, may also add to suicide risk. Leon and colleagues (1999), reporting on data from the National Institute of Mental Health Collaborative Depression Study, noted a nonsignificant decrease in suicidal behavior in 185 patients treated with fluoxetine. These patients were more severely ill, had earlier onset of affective illness, and more previous suicide attempts prior to starting fluoxetine (Leon et al. 1999). These findings are consistent with other investigations of the relationship between SSRIs and suicidality (Jick et al. 1995, Warshaw and Keller 1996, Verkes et al. 1998, Müller-Oerlinghausen and Berghöfer 1999). While the impact on suicide rates may be negligible, the SSRIs are safer in overdose (Kapur et al. 1992).

One possible explanation for mixed impact of antidepressants on suicide rates is the phenomenon of undertreatment. Oquendo and colleagues (1999) examined the aggressiveness of antidepressant treatment on patients with major depression, with and without suicide attempts. They included 171 inpatients with major depression, 80 "remote" (defined by the authors as an attempt more than 90 days prior to admission) suicide attempters and 91 nonattempters, in their data analysis. Subjectively and objectively, degrees of major depression were not significantly different. Only 15% of the entire sample was taking antidepressants on admission, and of those who were, 35% were deemed adequately dosed. Almost inexplicably, the patients with a history of suicide attempts, and therefore more likely to have future attempts, were less likely to receive adequate antidepressant therapy. The failure to diagnose and adequately treat major depression warrants ongoing education of all physicians (Oquendo et al. 1999).

Two reports from the NIMH Collaborative Depression Study, 1978–1980 (Keller et al. 1982, 1986), also note undertreatment. Keller and colleagues (1982) described 217 patients entering the naturalistic study. Only 3% with moderate to severe unipolar depression of a month's duration had been treated with the most intensive dose of tricyclic antidepressants. A quarter of those with psychotic depres-

sion received the most intensive therapy and another quarter with psychotic depression received no antipsychotics or antidepressant therapy of any category. The follow-up report (Keller et al. 1986) described treatment of 338 patients in the 2 months after enrollment. Of inpatients, 31% received no or inadequate antidepressant somatotherapy, and only 49% received the equivalent of at 200 mg of imipramine. Of outpatients, 51% received no or inadequate somatotherapy, and 19% received the equivalent of 200 mg of imipramine. As reviewed by Hirshfeld and colleagues (1997), there is "overwhelming evidence" that depression is being undertreated, both before and during the widespread use of SSRIs.

## Lithium

Lithium is the only pharmacologic intervention that shows consistent antisuicidal effects (Tondo et al. 2001a). Tondo and colleagues (2001b) performed a meta-analysis of the suicide risk with long-term lithium treatment. They included 22 studies, 13 of which provided data on suicide rates with and without lithium ($N$=5,647 patients), and analyzed suicide completions, not attempts. Suicide rates were higher without lithium in all of the studies except one. Four of the studies were exclusive to patients with bipolar disorder. Suicide rates were significantly lower (81.8%) during lithium treatment. Notably, suicide rates in this population were significantly higher than in international general populations. This is probably reflective of differences between clinical and general populations, inclusion of highly suicidal individuals in the study samples, partial or failed treatment, and possible noncompliance (Tondo et al. 2001b).

In eight of the 13 studies with and without lithium in the review above, rates after discontinuing lithium were ascertained. There was clear evidence of increased morbidity soon after stopping lithium, especially when it is quickly tapered or suddenly stopped. There is a twenty-fold increase in suicides and attempts in the first year after discontinuing lithium in bipolar patients. Rates of suicides in long-term lithium discontinuation groups and those not treated with lithium are practically the same. Lithium's impact on suicide rates may be a function of mood stabilization, prophylaxis against bipolar depression, and effects on serotonergic and dopaminergic systems. Anticonvulsants without these neuropharmacologic effects may be less protective (Tondo et al. 2001b). As reviewed by Goodwin (1999), there has been increasing use of anticonvulsants in the management of bipolar disorder. Anticonvulsants may have an advantage in rapid cycling, mixed states, comorbid substance abuse, or history of poor response to lithium. There is little data about the suicide preventive impact of the anticonvulsants, although a comparison of lithium and carbamazepine was more favorable to lithium (Thies-Flechtner et al. 1996). Both lithium and anticonvulsants can have a positive impact on suicide risk factors of impulsivity and aggression (Goodwin 1999).

## ECT

Electroconvulsive therapy (ECT) has long played a role in the treatment of severe, and treatment refractory depression. Its impact on suicide rates remains unclear. A meta-analysis of suicide rates by treatment era (pretreatment, before 1940; ECT treatment, 1940 to 1959; and antidepressant treatment, 1960 onward) suggests that ECT significantly reduced suicide mortality, with further lowering into the antidepressant era (O'Leary et al. 2001). Sharma (1999) found no difference in receipt of ECT (during the 3 months prior to suicide or hospital discharge) in a retrospective study of 45 inpatients who died by suicide compared with a control group of inpatients. Almost 16% ($N=7$) of the suicide group had ECT during their final 3 months. One suicide patient had received ECT more than 3 months prior and was excluded from the final analysis, three killed themselves after completing a course of ECT (all partial or nonresponders after previous response), two died during the ECT course, one was getting maintenance ECT, and another had stopped ECT for lack of efficacy. The majority of the ECT-treated were male and had treatment refractory affective disorders. Sharma allows that ECT nonresponders may be high risk patients, especially if they view ECT as a treatment of last resort. The risk and benefits of discontinuing mood stabilizers should be considered. Two of the ECT-treated suicide patients were receiving bilateral treatment and had stopped lithium therapy prior to initiating ECT. Both also declined further ECT after complaining of cognitive side effects (Sharma 1999). Roy and Draper (1995), in a sample dominated by patients with schizophrenia, also found no significant difference in the number of suicide victims and controls receiving ECT. In contrast, Isometsä and colleagues (1994) found that only a tiny percentage (0.14%) of suicide victims in Finland had ECT 3 months prior to their deaths. Barraclough and colleagues (1974) also noted that ECT may have been underutilized in some patients who eventually committed suicide. Avery and Winokur (1976, 1978) also found a lower incidence of suicide among the ECT treated. Prudic and Sackeim (1999) reviewed the impact of ECT on suicide risk, short-term and long-term.

ECT is indicated for illnesses frequently associated with suicidal symptoms, and is noted for relatively quick efficacy. It can have a profound impact on acute suicidal symptoms, in both responders and nonresponders. Their review of the studies would suggest the most robust benefit acutely in major depression, with limited long-term impact, especially in heterogeneous diagnostic groups. The existing data has many methodological shortcomings, including few prospective, adequately powered studies, lack of random assignments, limited attention to clinical variables like risk factors, comorbid diagnoses like substance abuse, or severity of symptoms. The cohort receiving ECT may be biased by á priori increased suicide risk and history of treatment failure. The authors conclude that although an acute treatment, ECT's long-term impact on mortality may be a function of repeated use in treating or preventing (via continuation and maintenance ECT) relapse and recurrence (Prudic and Sackeim 1999).

## Psychosocial Interventions

Sachs and colleagues (2001) note that psychotherapy is not a cure for suicidal ideation, but may strengthen protective factors and decrease inclination. Gray and Otto (2001) reviewed psychosocial approaches to suicide prevention and their applicability to bipolar patients. An approach tailored toward psychosocial risk factors, for example, hopelessness, poor problem-solving, negative cognitions, and dysfunctional coping strategies, may be particularly helpful. Gainful employment and increasing social supports are also appropriate goals. Gray and Otto (2001) reviewed 17 randomized, controlled studies of efforts to decrease suicidal and self-injurious behavior. The studies could be categorized as brief hospitalization, efforts to enhance treatment utilization, problem-solving interventions, and intensive treatments. Brief hospitalization was associated with negative to small effect size, while facilitated/rapid hospital reentry was more promising for subjects with initial episodes of self-harm. Studies of some outreach services found no benefits, while those that included home visits had modest to no reductions in suicidal behavior. One in this latter category with noteworthy results (three-fold difference compared to treatment as usual) involved 4 months of weekly or biweekly home-based interventions combining psychotherapy, crisis intervention, and family therapy (Welu 1977). This represents a significant commitment of resources. Problem-solving interventions, for example, around interpersonal conflicts or cognitive behavioral therapy, had moderate effect size, and were largely brief, structured, and problem-focused. Intensive treatments (1 year) like dialectical behavior therapy (DBT) reflected a large effect size (Gray and Otto 2001).

The review revealed three effective strategies: lowering barriers to care during times of distress, brief training in problem-solving strategies, and comprehensive strategies that combine problem-solving with intensive rehearsal of cognitive, social, emotional-labeling and tolerance, and coping skills. Patients and families should be educated on procedures for accessing after-hours and emergency care. Cognitive restructuring can address hopelessness, pessimism, cognitive distortions, and enhance reasons for living. The development of distress-tolerance skills may be particularly beneficial for patients who feel unable to resist urges to harm themselves or have chronically maladaptive responses to stress (Gray and Otto 2001).

## Assessment of Suicidal Patients (See Table 102–3)

Common presentations include acute, chronic, contingent, and/or potentially manipulative suicidal patient. All are as-

| Table 102–3 | Assessment Factors |
| --- | --- |
| Mental status | |
| Suicidal ideation | |
| Intent | |
| Plans | |
| Sadness | |
| Hopelessness | |
| Social withdrawal | |
| Isolation | |
| Anxiety | |
| Agitation | |
| Impulsivity | |
| Insomnia | |
| Psychosis | |
| Prior high lethality attempts | |
| Uncommunicative presentation | |
| Recent major loss | |
| Active substance abuse | |
| Untreated mood, psychotic or personality disorder | |

sociated with anxiety for the care provider doing the assessment. Careful assessment, use of collateral information, and acceptance of predictive limitations can be helpful.

As reviewed by Nicholas and Golden (2001), factors to be considered in the assessment of the acutely suicidal patient include the current mental status, with special attention to direct inquiry about suicidal ideation, intent (may be ascertained from family and friends, for example, saying good-byes or putting affairs in order), and plans (well thought out with available means). Sadness, hopelessness, social withdrawal/isolation, anxiety, agitation, impulsivity, insomnia, psychosis (especially command hallucinations or distressing persecutory delusions) are additional concerning symptoms. These factors, coupled with prior high lethality attempts, uncommunicative presentation, recent major loss, active substance abuse, or untreated mood, psychotic, or personality disorder, might indicate that hospitalization is warranted to ensure safety prior to treating the underlying psychiatric disorder (Nicholas and Golden, 2001).

Sachs and colleagues (2001) reviewed suicide prevention strategies for bipolar outpatients, but they can easily be adapted to any potentially suicidal patient. The reader is reminded that "care providers can, however, be fooled by the deceptions of a clever patient intent on carrying out a lethal act." Individualized treatment plans should be developed after eliciting current symptoms, including suicidal ideation; review of risk factors, stressors, comorbid states like substance use; and past history of suicide attempts. Acute efforts are directed toward safety and treating the underlying disorder, with follow-up monitoring. Adjunctive medications like antipsychotics and anxiolytics can be beneficial. Clinicians must monitor the amounts of medications prescribed and continue to be vigilant during early recovery. Harm reduction strategies can include minimizing access to lethal means, decreasing social isolation, close follow-up, and informing of emergency contact procedures. Hospitalization may be warranted if suicide is considered as a solution for problems, for active suicidal ideation, or if there has been a recent attempt. With the caveat that while admission may provide safety, current knowledge of risk factors do not wholly inform when to admit or discharge, overreliance on hospitalization may deter honest reporting, and many acutely depressed patients can be managed as outpatients with sufficient safeguards. Involuntary admission, while not therapy in and of itself, may be lifesaving. ECT remains a safe, typically quick onset, effective option for those at high risk of suicide (Sachs et al. 2001).

There is no evidence that denial of suicidal intent predicts nonsuicide. Review of standard risk factors, additional risk factors (e.g. acute relationship and employment changes), acute versus chronic suicidal ideation, and treatment of readily reversible factors should be undertaken. High risk diagnoses include major depression, bipolar disorder, schizophrenia, alcoholism and substance abuse, and borderline personality disorder. Comorbid alcoholism increases the risk in every diagnostic category. A history of past attempts, hopelessness, previous hospitalizations, and recent discharge, while not individually predictive, do heighten concern. Acute risk factors include severe anxiety, panic attacks, global insomnia, and agitation. These symptoms should be carefully assessed, with aggressive intervention. Benzodiazepines and antipsychotics can be employed to address anxiety and agitation. Caution must be taken with benzodiazepines to avoid disinhibition and combination with alcohol. Mixed states may require mood stabilizers. Serial assessments should be performed with acute changes as well as chronic suicidal states. Chronically suicidal patients also require aggressive treatment of anxiety and agitation. DBT and cognitive behavioral therapy (CBT) can be helpful in addressing parasuicidal and suicidal behavior.

A significant number of psychiatrists utilize the no-suicide contract, or the contract for safety. Over half of a sample of psychiatrists acknowledged using them in recent survey, and 41% of them had patients make suicide attempts after entering into one (Kroll 2000). Sixty-four percent of 14 psychiatric hospital inpatient suicides denied suicidal ideation and half had some form of no-suicide agreement in place in the week before their deaths (Busch et al. 1993). These have not been systematically studied as to whether they have any protective effect (Gray and Otto 2001). Resnick (2002) cautions that psychiatrists tend to view the patient as a collaborator in treatment. However, the psychiatrist can be less viewed as an "ally" and become an "adversary" when the patient has determined to die by suicide. He notes that failure to recognize this shift in the doctor–patient relationship can have devastating results. Objective evidence, as opposed to patient subjective reports, may be telling. Alliances with family and other caregivers should be maintained, as they can become crucial sources of information. Resnick believes that no-suicide contracts have little credence, especially in an adversarial relationship, cause a false sense of security for the therapist, and have no research literature to suggest efficacy (Resnick 2002).

Gutheil and Schetky (1998) wrote of a most difficult assessment: the patient who expresses suicidal ideation in terms of a future eventuality. The "if [event or outcome does or does not happen], I will kill myself" contingency poses different challenges from acute suicidality, manipulative suicidal threats, and chronic suicidality. Suicidality typically engenders anxiety in the therapist. Contingency suicidality frequently lacks verbalized imminence, may make involuntary commitment difficult, and invites countertransferences which can lead to exaggerated or inappropriately muted responses. For some patients, the contingency is a defense against suicide. For others, it represents the ultimate control. Gutheil and Schetky (1998) give 7 clinical vignettes to illustrate several points: (1) Some patients almost have an object relationship with death, with death personified as a benevolent bringer of relief. The therapist should approach that tie with caution, as it may be the only one in which the patient has any confidence; (2) Future deadlines should not be accepted literally; (3) Even when the contingency is met positively, the suicidal ideation may not resolve; (4) Some patients view themselves as already dead, cannot conceive of life without depression, and challenge the therapist to resurrect them. This stance undermines any potential relationship; and (5) It is of benefit to negotiate a halt to suicidal acts until depression can be separated from decision-making. Gutheil and Schetky assert "... psychiatrists should never support suicide, but should acknowledge the human impossibility of preventing it." The authors note that in these circumstances, the patient is at least communicating their suicidal ideation. The rationale can be explored and an effort made to maintain the therapeutic relationship. Helplessness should be discussed, as suicidal ideation can be a defense against lack of control or an expression of pain. The countertransference of the therapist should be considered, as it can cloud clinical judgment. Consultation with colleagues can be very helpful. The competency of the patient may be called into question, and has been used as a defense in suicide malpractice cases. The clinician can frequently be justified in involuntary commitment as critical dates or junctures approach. Finally, Gutheil and Schetky state that "accepting the patient's pain and sense of hopelessness is not the same as acceding to his or her wish to commit suicide; the psychiatrist must always hold out hope. At the same time, it may be therapeutic and realistic to let patients know that one can not ultimately prevent their suicides." (Gutheil and Schetky 1998).

Lambert and Bonner (1996) conducted a retrospective review of 1,381 psychiatry triage patients who presented to the Dallas Veterans Affairs Medical Center over one year. Suicidality was deemed the primary presenting complaint in 137. Of these, 45 were contingent threats (suicide threat if hospital admission were denied or exaggerated suicidality acknowledged after hospitalization) and 92 were noncontingent. The two groups did not differ on age, gender, employment status, or percentage who were subsequently admitted. Patients who made contingent threats were more likely to have substance dependence and antisocial personality disorder. The contingent group was more likely to have active legal problems and to be homeless. The noncontingent group was more likely to have a diagnosis of major depression. In the 6-month follow-up period, there were no statistical differences in suicide attempts—10 (6.5%) in the noncontingent group and 2 (4.4%) in the contingent group—and 1 suicide occurred in the noncontingent group. The authors acknowledge a possible tendency to overdiagnose substance abuse and sociopathy in patients viewed as manipulative in the relatively brief follow-up period. Still, there was evidence that suicidality can be exaggerated to obtain social support and avoid legal difficulties. While such patients may be better served by substance abuse treatment, social, and legal services, and hospitalization may even be countertherapeutic, the assessment forces the clinician to make "calculated risks" (Lambert and Bonner 1996).

## Aftermath: Clinicians Coping with Patient Suicide

A suicide has repercussions for all parties involved. Primary care providers can be as, or more, vulnerable to patient suicides than psychiatrists. As reviewed by Luoma and colleagues (2002), they are more likely to have been in recent contact with a suicide victim than mental health professionals. In their review of 40 studies, last contacts with mental health services compared to primary care providers within 1 month and 1 year of death were 19% versus 45%, and 32% versus 77%, respectively. The lifetime rate of contact with mental health services averaged 53%.

One psychiatrist (Gitlin 1999) recounts his responses in the aftermath of a patient's suicide. Six months out of residency, a patient with whom he'd had a "no-suicide

contract" took a fatal overdose. He felt "overwhelmed and numb" and experienced depersonalization as he tried to go through the motion of activities of daily living. The psychiatrist described embarrassment and isolation, believing that no one else in his circle had lost a patient in this manner. He endorsed anxiety, imagined the loss of referrals, worried about the adequacy of his documentation in the medical record, and feared being sued. There was anger at the decedent, umbrage that his prescribed medications were used in the suicide, and PTSD. He fantasized about pulling up stakes and moving his practice if there was another suicide. There was a struggle not to over interpret the comments of other patients and to reassure himself that he was cut out for this line of work (Gitlin 1999). In one survey, over half of psychiatrist respondents had a patient who committed suicide. There was no relationship between years in practice and the probability that the psychiatrist had a patient suicide, although practice years and age correlated negatively with intensity of the emotional response. Fifty-seven percent of the psychiatrists reported posttraumatic stress symptoms. The authors acknowledged that although their sample may not be representative, they viewed patient suicide as a relatively common occupational hazard for psychiatrists (Chemtob et al. 1988).

It is common to try to maintain an "illusion of control in an unpredictable world in order to bind anxiety" (Gitlin 1999). Psychiatrists who have had a patient commit suicide, and entire institutions, change treatment practices on the basis of one isolated event, sometimes reflecting appropriate improvements, other times based on "magical thinking." In his personal account, Gitlin (1999) lost his naïve belief that with his skill, talent, and training, he could make a difference in all patients' lives. He felt this realization is particularly poignant for trainees or early career psychiatrists. There is frequently anger, projected at the patient or others, and sometimes relief when the patient has exhausted the therapist with chronic suicidal ideation. Dr. Gitlin believes two factors that shape the psychiatrist's response to a patient suicide are the relationship with the patient (e.g., duration and intensity) and the personal attributes of the therapist. Psychiatrists who are early in their career, obsessional, tend to internalize, and are prone to anxiety and depression are particularly vulnerable to lasting emotional upheaval. Dr. Gitlin recommended decreasing isolation, constructive behavior, and cognitive defenses as effective coping strategies. Talking with trusted others, be they personal or professional, was helpful. Discussing the suicide with experienced colleagues had benefit, although the psychological autopsy should find a balance between empty support and excess criticism, and avoid public humiliation. Meeting with the families of decedents had advantages. Sharing experiences and helping other clinicians in similar circumstances can be reparative. Acknowledging that suicide cannot be accurately predicted for any individual is realistic (Gitlin 1999).

Hendin and colleagues (2000), of the American Foundation for Suicide Prevention, echoed Dr. Gitlin's responses in the results of their survey of the 26 therapists of patients who committed suicide. These caregivers were participants in a daylong workshop. Of the 26 therapists, 21 were male, and 21 were psychiatrists. Seven were in training at the time of their patient's suicide while the remainder had been in practice at least 5 years. These cases had been in treatment with the therapists from 3 weeks to 4 years, with a median of 12 months. Twenty-four were seen at least weekly, and 13 were seen twice a week or more. Their initial emotional response included shock/disbelief, as 7 of the respondents were not even aware that their patients were suicidal. After the initial response, the most common emotion in the majority of the therapists was grief. Other responses included guilt, fear of blame or of being sued, anger, betrayal (some had suicide contracts with these patients), feelings of inadequacy, and humiliation. A few responded with anger and relief, which was a reflection of the countertransference that preceded the suicides. Dreams and PTSD-like responses are experienced by some. Twenty-one of the respondents second guessed themselves, and could identify at least one thing they would do differently. Those that did not may have used a sense of futility to help them cope with their feelings about the suicide. The therapist generally felt supported, especially when colleagues shared their own experiences with patient suicide. Assurances from peers and supervisors about the inevitability of the suicide rang hollow to the respondents, and others felt their institutions were insensitive and unsupportive, for example, blaming the patients, harshly scrutinizing the therapist. Nineteen of the therapists saw the patient's relatives afterwards, and some attended funerals. The majority of relatives were grateful for the efforts of the therapist, and one participant reported treating a surviving spouse for depression in the aftermath of the suicide. Practice patterns were changed, with vigilance toward the possibility of suicide, reluctance to treat suicidal patients, and paradoxical interest in treating this population. Nine had no-suicide contracts, and all experienced shaken faith in their utility (Hendin et al. 2000).

Although this was a group of workshop participants highly interested in exploring the suicide of a patient, in the authors' experience the responses are typical. The strong emotional responses were independent of age and experience, although it appeared that those in training felt more exposed and traumatized. They did not find that they learned much from psychological autopsies nor were they comforted by reassurances. However, learning as much as possible is a step toward relieving guilt and feelings of inadequacy. The vast majority of these participants felt benefited from processing the event in an independent, nonjudgmental, nonsanctioning forum (Hendin et al. 2000).

Kaye and Soreff (1991) had a number of recommendations in the aftermath of a patient suicide, with the caveat that a patient suicide is a very personal event, and the approach has to be individualized in recognition of nuances. They believe that families should be contacted and met with, told realistically of all the efforts on the decedent's behalf, and contact maintained through the funeral and autopsy report. Hospital staff should be contacted, and if possible, informed as a group. Attendance at the funeral can be beneficial. They advocate the psychological autopsy as an opportunity to vent as well as facilitate learning and any policy reform. In some instances, inpatients or surviving group members should meet with staff, with a concern toward patients' devaluing staff and increased suicidal risk to surviving patients. The treating

psychiatrist should seek support, solicit formal or informal consultation with colleagues, consider attending the funeral or sending forms of condolence, and offer expressions of sympathy. The latter is not felt to represent an admission of guilt. A psychological autopsy should be conducted, and attending the autopsy is not verboten in their opinion. Billing for past services, although difficult, is typically appropriate. If affiliated with an institution, cooperation with its risk management is advised, with due caution. Medical records should be accurately completed, with those submitted after the patient's death clearly reflecting so. Although the suicide of a patient reminds the psychiatrist of powerlessness, the psychiatrist should function as team leader in the aftermath (Kaye and Soreff 1991).

## Issues in Research about Suicide

There continues to be a critical need of studies of suicide prevention. However, high risk populations are frequently excluded. Just as with women of childbearing potential and children, patients with suicidality will be assumed to benefit from interventions studied in others, in this case, nonsuicidal patients. As reviewed by Pearson et al. (2001), only a few interventions, for example, community crisis hotlines, no-suicide contracts, and acute hospitalization, have been evaluated and have showed little to no benefit. Research limitations include the relatively uncommon occurrence of suicide, difficulty getting samples with sufficient statistical power, concerns about the risk/benefit ratio for high risk groups, and the apprehension of perceived liability should a patient commit suicide. The reviewers note that salient issues in study design include the choice of comparator, increased monitoring (although that may reduce the power to detect treatment effects), balancing the desire for safety with requirements for sound research design and meaningful results, protocols for clinical deterioration, and competent clinicians well versed in those protocols. Although no-suicide contracts are of dubious efficacy for either suicide reduction or clinician liability, the authors believe such concords can bring focus and structure. Features of such a contract can decrease ambivalence about the goal of staying alive, denote precipitants and types of suicidal behavior, delineate acts to reduce suicidal behavior, and provide information on how to access care. Finally, the authors note that liability can be reduced by initial and periodic suicide evaluation and initiation of plans to reduce or eliminate risk. They assert that assessment is different from prediction, and that the latter is not part of the standard of care. Practitioners and hospitals have been held liable for overlooking present illness, past psychiatric history, not following the treatment plan, ignoring evidence of suicidality, providing insufficient supervision, and discharging from the hospital while acutely suicidal (Pearson et al. 2001).

Suicide risk is sometimes cited in the ongoing debate over ethical aspects of the use of placebos in treatment studies. Storosum et al. (2001) examined the risk of suicide in placebo-controlled studies of major depression. In short-term studies (4 to 8 weeks), in both placebo and active compound groups, rates of completed suicide were identical (0.1%), as were suicide attempts (0.4%). In long-term studies (24 to 52 weeks), suicides were actually lower in placebo groups (0.0%) than in active treatment groups (0.2%), while the rate of suicide attempts were the same (0.7%). Thus this review suggests that fear of increased risk of suicide does not justify avoiding placebo-controlled studies in major depression. However, they also add that patients with suicide risk are often excluded from such studies (Storosum et al. 2001). Kan et al. (2000) conducted a meta-analysis of new antidepressants in the Food and Drug Administration's data base and noted no statistical differences in completed and attempted suicides between placebo (0.4–2.7%), standard antidepressants (0.7–3.4%), or investigational antidepressants (0.8–2.8%). The Consensus Development Panel of the National Depressive and Manic–Depressive Association (2002) concluded that placebo has an appropriate place in mood disorder studies, with reasonable safeguards and informed consent, given high placebo response rates. Participants must be protected from serious, unacceptable risk, resulting information should justify the risk, trials must have scientific merit, and duration of placebo exposure should be minimized as much as possible. Patients who are suicidal, acutely psychotic, and in need of immediate treatment can be excluded, although studies that limit exposure to placebo or use non-placebo methods should be considered (Consensus Development Panel 2002).

## Conclusion

Suicide is a multiple-determined phenomenon, with psychological, dynamic, and biologic substrates. Neurobiology and genetics may add greatly to our very limited predictive power as to who is at risk and improve our interventions. Even so, there remains a significant failure to appropriately utilize the knowledge base that we currently have. Too many patients commit suicide because they were undiagnosed, undertreated, or too stigmatized to seek mental health treatment. Those patients who are identified and treated continue to have risk. They require a therapeutic alliance, and frequently our ability to bind anxiety, psychosocial interventions, and judicious hospitalization, in addition to our biologic armamentarium.

Clinical Vignette

A 45-year-old married woman presented with a history of recurrent major depression (second episode). She had been successfully treated with an SSRI, and had been off medications for 2 years when she experienced this recurrence. She was devastated by the return of symptoms, and feared loss of job and marital disruption—both had occurred with the initial episode. She saw a primary care physician for 6 months, then stopped follow-up and medications because of financial constraints.

She became tearful when asked about suicidal ideation. She admitted to passive suicidal ideation, but denied plans or intent. There was no history of previous attempts. She denied homicidal ideation, psychotic symptoms, and substance abuse. She gave permission for her spouse to provide collateral information and he confirmed her report. There were weapons in the home, but he kept them under lock and key as there were children in the home. He agreed to remove them.

She reluctantly restarted her SSRI and quickly noted an improvement in her symptoms. On a subsequent visit, she acknowledged that she had thoughts of shooting herself around that initial presentation. She had not revealed this because she feared hospitalization, which would have been financially devastating and socially stigmatizing to the family. She now felt comfortable sharing this, as the therapist continued to ask her about suicidal ideation even as she improved, and had not appeared to overreact to other aspects of her past history. She ultimately revealed that she had stopped SSRIs because of sexual side effects. She was switched to a class of antidepressants that had fewer sexual side effects with continued remission of her symptoms.

## References

Ahearn EP, Jamison KR, Steffens DC, et al. (2001) MRI correlates of suicide attempt history in unipolar depression. Biol Psychiatr 50(4), 266–270.

Ahrens B, Berghofer A, Wolf T, et al. (1995) Suicide attempts: Age and duration of illness in recurrent affective disorders. J Affect Disord 36, 43–49.

Allard P and Norlen M (2001) Caudate nucleus dopamine D(2) receptors in depressed suicide victims. Neuropsychobiology 44(2), 70–73.

American Foundation of Suicide Prevention (2002) Reporting on Suicide. (Available at http://www.afsp.org/education/printrecommendations.htm)

Arango V, Underwood MD, Boldrini M, et al. (2001) Serotonin 1A receptors, serotonin transporter binding and serotonin transporter mRNA expression in the brainstem of depressed suicide victims. Neuropsychopharmacology 25(6), 892–903.

Arató M, Bánki CM, Bissette G, et al. (1989) Elevated CSF CRF in suicide victims. Biol Psychiatr 25, 355–359.

Arranz B, Blennow K, Eriksson A, et al. (1997) Serotonergic, noradrenergic, and dopaminergic measures in suicide brains. Biol Psychiatr 41, 1000–1009.

Arranz B, Ericksson A, Mellerup E, et al. (1994) Brain 5-HT$_{1A}$, 5-HT$_{1D}$ and 5-HT$_{2A}$ receptors in suicide victims. Biol Psychiatr 35, 457–463.

Avery D and Winokur G (1976) Mortality and depressed patients treated with electroconvulsive therapy and antidepressants. Arch Gen Psychiatr 33, 1023–1029.

Avery D and Winokur G (1978) Suicide, attempted suicide, and relapse rates in depression: Occurrence after ECT and antidepressant therapy. Arch Gen Psychiatr 35, 749–753.

Barraclough B, Bunch J, Nelson B, et al. (1974) A hundred cases of suicide: Clinical aspects. Br J Psychiatr 125, 355–373.

Beck AT, Steer RA, and Trexler LD (1989) Alcohol abuse and eventual suicide: A 5- to 10-year prospective study of alcohol-abusing suicide attempter. J Stud Alcohol 50, 202–209.

Black DW, Winokur G, and Nasrallah A (1987) Suicide in subtypes of major affective disorder. Arch Gen Psychiatr 44, 878–880.

Black DW, Winokur G, and Nasrallah A (1988) Effect of psychosis on suicide risk in 1,593 patients with unipolar and bipolar affective disorders. Am J Psychiatr 145, 840–852.

Blair-West GW, Cantor CH, Mellsop GW, et al. (1999) Lifetime suicide risk in major depression: Sex and age determinants. J Affect Disord 55, 171–178.

Blair-West GW, Mellsop GW, and Eyeson-Annan ML (1997) Down-rating lifetime suicide risk in major depression. Acta Psychiatr Scand 95, 259–263.

Bondy B, Kuznik J, Baghai T, et al. (2000) Lack of association of serotonin-2A receptor gene polymorphism (T102C) with suicidal ideation and suicide. Am J Med Genet 96(6), 831–835.

Bostwick JM and Pankratz VS (2000) Affective disorders and suicide risk: A reexamination. Am J Psychiatr 157, 1925–1932.

Brent DA, Perper JA, Allman CJ, et al. (1991) The presence and accessibility of firearms in the homes of adolescent suicides: A case-control study. J Am Med Assoc 266, 2989–2995.

Brodsky BS, Kevin KM, Ellis SP, et al. (1997) Characteristics of borderline personality disorder associated with suicidal behavior. Am J Psychiatr 154(12), 1715–1719.

Brodsky BS, Oquendo M, Ellis SP, et al. (2001) The relationship of childhood abuse to impulsivity and suicidal behavior in adults with major depression. Am J Psychiatr 158(11), 1871–1877.

Brown GK, Beck AT, Steer RA, et al. (2000) Risk factors for suicide in psychiatric outpatients: A 20-year prospective study. J Consult Clin Psychol 68(3), 371–377.

Brunner HG, Nelen M, Breakefield XO, et al. (1993) Abnormal behavior associated with a point mutation in the structural gene for monoamine oxidase. Science 262, 578–580.

Busch K, Clark D, Fawcett J, et al. (1993) Clinical features of inpatient suicide. Psychiatr Ann 23, 256–262.

Busch KA, Jacobs D, and Fawcett J (submitted) Clinical correlates of inpatient suicide. J Clin Psychiatr.

Chemtob CM, Hamada RS, Bauer G, et al. (1988) Patients' suicides: frequency and impact on psychiatrist. Am J Psychiatr 145, 224–228.

Chen YW and Dilsaver SC (1996) Lifetime rates of suicide attempts among subjects with bipolar and unipolar disorders relative to subjects with other Axis I disorders. Biol Psychiatr 39, 896–899.

Conner KR, Cox C, Duberstein PR, et al. (2001) Violence, alcohol, and completed suicide: A case control study. Am J Psychiatr 158(10), 1701–1705.

Consensus Development Panel (2002) National Depressive and Manic–Depressive Association consensus statement on the use of placebo in clinical trials of mood disorders. Arch Gen Psychiatr 59, 262–270.

Conwell Y (1994) Suicide in elderly patients. In Diagnosis and Treatment of Depression in Late Life, Schneider LS, Reynolds CF III, Lebowitz BD, et al. (eds). American Psychiatric Press, Washington DC, pp. 397–418.

Coryell W and Schlesser M (2001) The dexamethasone suppression test and suicide prediction. Am J Psychiatr 158(5), 748–753.

Coryell W and Tsuang MT (1982) Primary unipolar depression and the prognostic importance of delusions. Arch Gen Psychiatr 39, 1181–1184.

Cremniter D, Jamain S, Kollenbach K, et al. (1999) CSF 5-HIAA levels are lower in impulsive violent suicide attempters and control subjects. Biol Psychiatr 45, 1572–1579.

Dahlsgaard KK, Beck AT, and Brown GK (1998) Inadequate response to therapy as a predictor of suicide. Suicide Life-Threat Behav 28, 197–204.

Dhossche DM, Ulusarac A, and Syed W (2001) A retrospective study of general hospital patients who commit suicide shortly after being discharged from the hospital. Arch Int Med 161(7), 991–994.

Dilsaver SC, Chen Y-W, Swann AC, et al. (1997) Suicidality, panic disorder, and psychosis in bipolar depression, depressive-mania and pure mania. Psychiatr Res 73, 47–56.

Dwivedi Y, Conley RR, Roberts RC, et al. (2002) [(3)H]cAMP binding sites and protein kinase a activity in the prefrontal cortex of suicide victims. Am J Psychiatr 159(1), 66–73.

Du L, Bakish D, Lapierre YD, et al. (2000) Association of polymorphism of serotonin 2A receptor gene with suicidal ideation in major depressive disorder. Am J Med Genet (Neuropsychiatr Genet) 96, 56–60.

Etzersdorfer E and Sonneck G (1998) Preventing suicide by influencing mass-media reporting. The Viennese experience 1980–1996. Arch Suicide Res 4, 67–74.

Fawcett J, Scheftner W, Clark D, et al. (1987) Clinical predictors of suicide in patients with major affective disorders: A controlled prospective study. Am J Psychiatr 144, 35–40.

Fawcett J, Scheftner WA, Fogg L, et al. (1990) Time related predictors of suicide in major affective disorder. Am J Psychiatr 147, 1189–1194.

Fisher BJ, Haythornwaite JA, Heinberg LJ, et al. (2001) Suicidal intent in patients with chronic pain. Pain 89(2–3), 199–206.

Gabbard GO (2000) Affective disorders. In Psychodynamic Psychiatry in Clinical Practice. American Psychiatric Press, Washington DC, pp. 203–231.

Garlow SJ (2002) Age, gender, and ethnicity differences in patterns of cocaine and ethanol use preceding suicide. Am J Psychiatr 159(4), 1000–1009.

Gitlin M (1999) A psychiatrist's reaction to a patient suicide. Am J Psychiatr 156(10), 1630–1634.

Glowinski AL, Bucholz KK, Nelson EC, et al. (2001) Suicide attempts in an adolescent female twin sample. J Am Acad of Child and Adolesc Psychiatr 40 (11), 1300–1307.

Goldberg JF, Singer TM, Garno JL (2001) Suicidality and substance abuse in affective disorders. J Clin Psychiatr 62(Suppl 25), 35–43.

Goldstein RB, Black DW, Nasrallah A et al. (1991) The prediction of suicide: Sensitivity, specificity, and predictive value of a multivariate model applied to suicide among 1906 patients with affective disorders. Arch Gen Psychiatr 48, 418–422.

Goodwin FK (1999) Anticonvulsant therapy and suicide risk in affective disorders. J Clin Psychiatr 60(Suppl 2), 89–93.

Goodwin FK and Jamison KR (1990) Suicide. In Manic–Depressive Illness, Goodwin FK and Jamison KR (eds). Oxford University Press, New York, pp. 227–244.

Grandin LD, Yan LJ, and Gray SM (2001) Suicide prevention: Increasing education and awareness. J Clin Psychiatr 62(Suppl 25), 12–16.

Gray SM and Otto MW (2001) Psychosocial approaches to suicide prevention: Applications to patients with bipolar disorder. J Clin Psychiatr 62(Suppl 25), 56–64.

Grunebaum MF, Oquendo MA, Harkavy-Friedman JM, et al. (2001) Delusions and suicidality. Am J Psychiatr 158(5), 742–747.

Gutheil TG and Schetky D (1998) A date with death: Management of the time-based and contingent suicidal intent. Am J Psychiatr 155(11), 1502–1507.

Guze SB and Robins E (1970) Suicide and affective disorders. Br J Psychiatr 117, 437–438.

Hall RCW, Platt DE, and Hall RCW (1999) Suicide risk assessment: A review of risk factors for suicide in 100 patients who made severe suicide attempts. Psychosomatics 40(1), 18–27.

Harris EC and Barraclough B (1997) Suicide as an outcome for mental disorders. Br J Psychiatr 170, 205–228.

Hendin H (1999) Suicide, assisted suicide, and medical illness. J Clin Psychiatr 60(Suppl 2), 46–50.

Hendin H, Lipschitz A, Maltsberger JT, et al. (2000) Therapists' reaction to patients' suicides. Am J Psychiatr 157(2000), 2022–2027.

Henriksson MM, Aro HM, Marttunen MJ, et al. (1993) Mental disorders and comorbidity in suicide. Am J Psychiatr 150(6), 935–940.

Henriksson S, Boëthius G, and Isacsson G (2001) Suicides are seldom prescribed antidepressants: Findings from a prospective prescription database in Jämtland county, Sweden. Acta Psychiatr Scand 103, 301–306.

Hirshfeld RMA, Keller MB, Panico S, et al. (1997) The National Depressive and Manic–Depressive Association consensus statement on the undertreatment of depression. J Am Med Assoc 277(4), 333–340.

Hoppe SK and Martin HW (1986) Patterns of suicide among Mexican Americans and Anglos, 1960–1980. Soc Psychiatr 21, 83–88.

Hoyert DL, Arias E, and Smith BL (2001) Deaths: Final Data for 1999. National Vital Statistics Report, 49 (8). National Center for Health Statistics, DHHS Publication No. (PHS) 2001–1120, Hyattsville, MD.

Huang Y, Grailhe R, Arango V, et al. (1999) Relationship of psychopathology to the human serotonin 1B genotype and receptor binding kinetics in postmortem brain tissue. Neuropsychopharmacology 21, 238–246.

Inskip HM, Harris EC, and Barraclough B (1998) Lifetime risk of suicide for affective disorder, alcoholism, and schizophrenia. Br J Psychiatr 172, 35–37.

Isacsson G, Holmgren P, and Wasserman D (1994) Use of antidepressants among people committing suicide in Sweden. Br Med J 308, 506–509.

Isacsson G, Holmgren P, Druid H, et al. (1997) The utilization of antidepressants—a key issue in the prevention of suicide: An analysis of 5,281 suicides in Sweden during the period 1992–1994. Acta Psychiatr Scand 96(2), 94–100.

Isometsä E and Lönnqvist JK (1998) Suicide attempts preceding completed suicide. Br J Psychiatr 173, 531–535.

Isometsä E, Henriksson M, Aro HM, et al. (1994) Suicide in bipolar disorder in Finland. Am J Psychiatr 151, 1020–1024.

Jick SS, Dean AD, and Jick H (1995) Antidepressants and suicide. Br Med J 310, 215–218.

Kan A, Warner HA, and Brown WA (2000) Symptom reduction and suicide risk in patients treated with placebo in antidepressant clinical trials. Arch Gen Psychiatr 57(4), 311–317.

Kapur S, Mieczkowski T, and Mann JJ (1992) Antidepressant medication and the relative risk of suicide attempt and suicide. J Am Med Assoc 268, 3441–3445.

Kaye NS and Soreff SM (1991) The psychiatrist's role, responses, and responsibilities when a patient commits suicide. Am J Psychiatr 148, 739–743.

Keilp JG, Sackeim HA, Brodsky BS, et al. (2001) Neuropsychological dysfunction in depressed suicide attempter. Am J Psychiatr 158(5), 735–741.

Keller MB, Klerman GL, and Lavori PW (1982) Treatment received by depressed patients. J Am Med Assoc 248(15), 1848–1855.

Keller MB, Lavori PW, Klerman GL, et al. (1986) Low levels and lack of predictors of somatotherapy and psychotherapy received by depressed patients. Arch Gen Psychiatr 43, 458–466.

Kellerman AL, Rivara FP, Somes G, et al. (1992) New Engl J Med 327, 467–472.

King RA, Schwab-Stone M, Flisher AJ, et al. (2001) Psychosocial and risk behavior correlates of youth suicide and attempts and suicidal ideation. J Am Acad Child Adolesc Psychiatr 40(7), 837–846.

Koivumaa-Honkanen H, Honkanen R, Viinamäki H et al. (2001) Life satisfaction and suicide: A 20-year follow-up study. Am J Psychiatr 158(3), 433–439.

Kroll J (2000) Use of no-suicide contracts by psychiatrists in Minnesota. Am J Psychiatr 157, 1684–1686.

Lambert MT and Bonner J (1996) Characteristics and six-month outcome of patients who use suicide threats to seek hospital admission. Psychiatr Serv 47, 871–873.

Leon AC, Keller MB, Warshaw MG, et al. (1999) Prospective study of fluoxetine treatment and suicidal behavior in affectively ill subjects. Am J Psychiatr 156(2), 195–201.

Lewinsohn PM, Rohde P, Seeley JR, et al. (2001) Gender differences in suicide attempts from adolescence to young adulthood. J Am Acad Child Adolesc Psychiatr 40(4), 427–434.

Loftin C, MacDowall D, Wiersema B, et al. (1991) Effects of restrictive licensing of handguns on homicide and suicide in the District of Columbia. New Engl J Med 325(23), 1615–1620.

López P, Mosquera F, de León J, et al. (2001) Suicide attempts in bipolar patients. J Clin Psychiatr 62(12), 963–966.

Ludwig J and Cook PJ (2000) Homicide and suicide rates associated with implementation of the Brady Handgun Violence Prevention Act. J Am Med Assoc 284(5), 585–591.

Luoma JB, Martin CE, and Pearson JL (2002) Contact with mental health and primary care providers before suicide: A review of the evidence. Am J Psychiatr 159(6), 909–916.

Malone KM, Haas GL, Sweeney JA, et al. (1995) Major depression and the risk of attempted suicide. J Affect Disord 34, 173–185.

Malone KM, Oquendo MA, Haas GL et al. (2000) Protective factors against suicidal acts in major depression: Reason for living. Am J Psychiatr 157(7), 1084–1088.

Mann JJ (1998) The neurobiology of suicide. Natl Med 4, 25–30.

Mann JJ (2002) A current perspective of suicide and attempted suicide. Ann Int Med 136(4), 302–311.

Mann JJ, Huang Y, Underwood MD, et al. (2000) A serotonin transporter gene promoter polymorphism (5-HTTLPR) and prefrontal cortical binding in major depression and suicide. Arch Gen Psychiatr 57, 729–738.

Mann JJ, Malone KM, Nielson DA, et al. (1997) Possible association of a polymorphism of the tryptophan hydroxylase gene with suicidal behavior in depressed patients. Am J Psychiatr 154(10), 1451–1453.

Mann JJ, Waternaux C, Haas GL, et al. (1999) Toward a clinical model of suicidal behavior in psychiatric patients. Am J Psychiatr 156(2), 181–189.

Marzuk PM, Tardiff K, and Hirsch CS (1992) The epidemiology of murder–suicide. J Am Med Assoc 267(23), 3179–3183.

Marzuk PM, Tardiff K, Hirsch CS, et al. (1993) Increase in suicide by asphyxiation in New York City after the publication of Final Exit. New Engl J Med 329, 1508–1510.

Meltzer H (2002) Clozapine and suicide (letter to the editor). Am J Psychiatr 159(2), 323–324.

Meltzer HY and Okayli G (1995) Reduction of suicidality during clozapine treatment of neuroleptic-resistant schizophrenia: Impact on risk-benefit assessment. Am J Psychiatr 152(2), 183–190.

Meltzer HY, Alpha L, Green AI et al. (2003) Clozapine treatment for suicidality in schizophrenia: International Suicide Prevention Trial (InterSePT). Arch Gen Psychiatr 60(1), 82–91.

Munro J, O'Sullivan D, Andrews C, et al. (1999) Active monitoring of 12,760 clozapine recipients in the UK and Ireland: Beyond pharmaco-vigilance. Br J Psychiatr 175, 576–580.

Müller-Oerlinghausen B and Berghöfer A (1999) Antidepressants and suicidal risk. J Clin Psychiatr 60(Suppl 2), 94–99.

Nemeroff CB, Owens MJ, Bissette G, et al. (1988) Reduced corticotrophin releasing factor in binding sites in the frontal cortex of suicide victims. Arch Gen Psychiatr 45, 577–579.

New AS, Gerlernter J, Goodman M, et al. (2001) Suicide, impulsive aggression, and HTR1B genotype. Biol Psychiatr 50(1), 62–65.

Nicholas LM and Golden RN (2001) Managing the suicidal patient. Off Psychiatr 3(3), 1–8.

Nierenberg AA, Gray SM, and Grandin LD (2001) Mood disorders and suicide. J Clin Psychiatr 62(Suppl 25), 27–30.

NIH Publication No. 01-4593 (2001) Older Adults: Depression and Suicide Facts.

Niswender CM, Herrick-Davis K, Dilley GE, et al. (2001) RNA editing of the human serotonin 5-HT$_{2C}$ receptor. Alterations in suicide and implications for serotonergic pharmacology. Neuropsychopharmacology 24(5), 478–491.

Nolan KA, Volavka J, Czobor P, et al. (2000) Psychiatr Genet 10(3), 117–124.

Odagaki Y, Garcia-Sevilla JA, and Huguelet P (2001) Cyclic AMP-medicated signaling components are upregulated in the prefrontal cortex of depressed suicide victims. Brain Res 898(2), 224–231.

O'Leary D, Paykel E, Todd C, et al. (2001) Suicide in primary affective disorders revisited: A systematic review by treatment era. J Clin Psychiatr 62, 804–811.

Ono H, Shirakawa O, Nishiguch N (2000) Tryptophan hydroxylase gene polymorphisms are not associated with suicide. Am J Med Genet 96(6), 861–863.

Oquendo MA and Mann JJ (2001) Identifying and managing suicide risk in bipolar patients. J Clin Psychiatr 62(Suppl 25), 31–34.

Oquendo MA, Ellis SP, Greenwald S, et al. (2001) Ethnic and sex differences in suicide rates relative to major depression in the United States. Am J Psychiatr 158(10), 652–658.

Oquendo MA, Malone KM, Ellis SP, et al. (1999) Inadequacy of antidepressant treatment for patients with major depression who are at risk for suicidal behavior. Am J Psychiatr 156(2), 190–194.

Oquendo MA, Waternaux C, Brodsky B, et al. (2000) Suicidal behavior in bipolar mood disorder: Clinical characteristics of attempters and nonattempters. J Affect Disord 59, 107–117.

Pandey GN, Dwivedi Y, Rizavi HS, et al. (2002) Higher expression of serotonin 5-HT$_{2A}$ receptors in the postmortem brains of teenaged suicide victims. Am J Psychiatr 159(3), 419–429.

Pearson JL, Stanley B, King CA, et al. (2001) Intervention research with persons at high risk for suicidality: Safety and ethical considerations. J Clin Psychiatr 62(Suppl 25), 17–26.

Pfeffer CR (2001) Diagnosis of childhood and adolescent suicidal behavior: Unmet needs for suicide prevention. Biol Psychiatr 49, 1055–1061.

Phillips DP, Lesyna K, and Paight DJ (1992) Suicide and the media. In Assessment and Prevention of Suicide, Maris RW, Berman AL, Maltsberger JT, et al. (eds). Guilford Press, New York, pp. 499–519.

Pitchot W, Hanseene M, Gonzalez Moreno A, et al. (2001a) Reduced dopamine function in depressed patients is related to suicidal behavior but not its lethality. Psychoneuroendocrinology 26(7), 689–696.

Pitchot W, Hansenne M, Pinto E, et al. (2001b) Alpha-2-adrenoreceptors in depressed suicide attempters: Relationship with medical lethality of the attempt. Neuropsychobiology 44(2), 91–94.

Pitchot W, Reggers J, Pinto E, et al. (2001c) Reduced dopaminergic activity in depressed suicides. Psychoneuroendocrinology 26(3), 331–335.

Placidi GP, Oquendo MA, Malone KM, et al. (2001) Aggressivity, suicide attempts, and depression: Relationship to cerebrospinal fluid mono-amine metabolite levels. Biol Psychiatr 50(10), 783–791.

Placidi GPA, Oquendo MA, Malone KM, et al. (2000) Anxiety in major depression: Relationship to suicide attempts. Am J Psychiatr 157, 1614–1618.

Potash JB, Kane HS, Chiu Y, et al. (2000) Attempted suicide and alcoholism in bipolar disorder: Clinical and familial relationships. Am J Psychiatr 157(12), 2048–2050.

Powell J, Geddes J, Deeks J, et al. (2000) Br J Psychiatr 176, 266–272.

Pritchard C (1996) Suicide in the People's Republic of China categorized by age and gender: Evidence of the influence of culture on suicide. Acta Psychiatr Scand 93, 362–367.

Prudic J and Sackeim HA (1999) Electroconvulsive therapy and suicide risk. J Clin Psychiatr 60(Suppl 2), 104–110.

Qin P and Mortensen PB (2001) Specific characteristics of suicide in China. Acta Psychiatr Scand 103, 117–121.

Rao ML, Hawellek B, Papassotiropoulos A, et al. (1998) Upregulation of the platelet serotonin 5HT$_{2A}$ receptor and low blood serotonin in suicidal psychiatric patients. Neuropsychobiology 38m, 84–89.

Regier DA, Farmer ME, Rae DS, et al. (1990) Comorbidity of mental disorders with alcohol and other drug abuse: Results from the

Epidemiologic Catchment Area (ECA) Study. J Am Med Assoc 264, 2511–2518.

Reid WH, Mason M, and Hogan T (1998) Suicide prevention effects associated with clozapine therapy in schizophrenia and schizoaffective disorder. Psychiatr Serv 49, 1029–1033.

Resnick PJ (2002) Recognizing that the suicidal patient views you as an 'adversary.' Curr Psychiatr 1, 8.

Robins E, Gassner S, Kayes J, et al. (1959) The communication of suicidal intent: A study of 134 consecutive cases of successful (completed) suicide. Am J Psychiatr 115, 724–733.

Roose SP, Glassman AH, Walsh BT (1983) Depression, delusions, and suicide. Am J Psychiatr 140, 1159–1162.

Rosenbaum M (1990) The role of depression in couples involved in murder–suicide and homicide. Am J Psychiatr 147(8), 1036–1039.

Roy A (1983) Family history of suicide. Arch Gen Psychiatr 40, 971–974.

Roy A (2000) Relation of family history of suicide to suicide attempts in alcoholics. Am J Psychiatr 157(12), 2050–2051.

Roy A (2001) Characteristics of cocaine-dependent patients who attempt suicide. Am J Psychiatr 158(8), 1215–1219.

Roy A and Draper (1995) Suicide among psychiatric hospital inpatients. Psychol Med 25, 199–202.

Roy A and Linnoila M (1986) Alcoholism and suicide. Suicide Life Threat Behav 16(2), 244–273.

Roy A, De Jong J, and Linnoila M (1989) Cerebrospinal fluid monoamine metabolites and suicidal behavior in depressed patients. A 5-year follow-up study. Arch Gen Psychiatr 46, 609–612.

Sachs GS, Yan LJ, Swann AC, et al. (2001) Integration of suicide prevention into outpatient management of bipolar disorder. J Clin Psychiatr 62(Suppl 25), 3–11.

Sastre M, Guimon J, and Garcia-Sevilla JA (2001) Relationships between beta- and alpha-2-adrenoceptors and G coupling proteins in the human brain: Effects of age and suicide. Brain Res 090(2), 242–255.

Schnyder U, Valach L, Bichel K, et al. (1999) Attempted suicide: Do we understand the patients' reasons? Gen Hosp Psychiatr 21(1), 62–69.

Sernyak MJ, Desai R, Stolar M, et al. (2001) Impact of clozapine on completed suicide. Am J Psychiatr 158(6), 931–937.

Shaffer D, Gould M, and Hicks RC (1994) Worsening suicide rate in black teenagers. Am J Psychiatr 151(12), 1810–1812.

Sharma R and Markar HR (1994) Mortality in affective disorder. J Affect Disord 31, 91–96.

Sharma V (1999) Retrospective controlled study of inpatient ECT: Does it prevent suicide? J Affect Disord 56, 183–187.

Sheline YI, Mintun MA, and Moerlein SM (2002) Greater loss of 5-HT$_{2A}$ receptors in midlife than in late life. Am J Psychiatr 159, 430–435.

Soloff PH, Lynch KG, Kelly TM, et al. (2000) Characteristics of suicide attempts of patients with major depressive episode and borderline personality disorder: A comparative study. Am J Psychiatr 157(4), 601–608.

Souery D, Van Gestel S, Massat I, et al. (2001) Tryptophan hydroxylase polymorphism and suicidality in unipolar and bipolar affective disorders: A multicenter association study. Biol Psychiatr 49(5), 405–409.

Spreux-Varoquaux O, Alvarex JC, Berlin I, et al. (2001) Differential abnormalities in plasma 5-HIAA and platelet serotonin concentrations in violent suicide attempters: Relationships with impulsivity and depression. Life Sci 69(6), 647–657.

Stanley B, Gameroff MJ, and Michalsen V (2001) Are suicide attempters who self-mutilate a unique population? Am J Psychiatr 158(3), 427–432.

Stanley B, Molcho A, Stanley M, et al. (2000) Am J Psychiatr 157(4), 609–614.

Storosum JG, van Zwieten BJ, van den Brink W, et al. (2001) Suicide risk in placebo-controlled studies of major depression. Am J Psychiatr 158(8), 1271–1275.

Suokas J, Suominen K, Isometsä E, et al. (2001) Long-term risk factors for suicide mortality after attempted suicide-findings of a 14-year follow-up study. Acta Psychiatr Scand 104(2), 117–121.

Thies-Flechtner K, Müller-Oerlinghausen B, Seibert W, et al. (1996) Effect of prophylactic treatment on suicide risk in patients with major affective disorders: Data from a randomized prospective trial. Pharmacopsychiatry 29, 103–107.

Tondo L, Baldessarini RJ, Hennen J, et al. (1999) Suicide attempts in major affective disorder patients with comorbid substance use disorders. J Clin Psychiatr 60(Suppl 2), 63–69.

Tondo L, Ghiani C, and Albert M (2001a) Pharmacologic interventions in suicide prevention. J Clin Psychiatr 62(Suppl 25), 51–55.

Tondo L, Hennen J, and Baldessarini RJ (2001b) Lower suicide risk with long-term lithium treatment in major affective illness: A meta-analysis. Acta Psychiatr Scand 104, 163–172.

Tsai SJ, Hong CJ, Hsu CC, et al. (1999) Serotonin-2A receptor polymorphism (102T/C) in mood disorders. Psychiatr Res 87, 233–237.

US Public Health Service (1999) The Surgeon General's Call to Action to Prevent Suicide. Washington DC. Available at http://www.surgeongeneral.gov/library/calltoaction/default.htm.

Verdoux H, Liraud F, Gonzales B, et al. (2001) Predictors and outcome characteristics associated with suicidal behavior in early psychosis: A two-year follow-up of first-admitted subjects. Acta Psychiatr Scand 103, 347–354.

Verkes RJ, Van der Mast RC, Hengeveld MW, et al. (1998) Reduction by paroxetine of suicidal behavior in patients with repeated suicide attempts but not major depression. Am J Psychiatr 155, 543–547.

Wagner KD, Rouleau M, and Joiner T (2000) Cognitive factors related to suicidal ideation and resolution in psychiatrically hospitalized children and adolescents. Am J Psychiatr 1579(12), 2017–2021.

Walker AM, Lanza LL, Arellano F, et al. (1997) Mortality in current and former users of clozapine. Epidemiology 8, 671–677.

Warshaw MG and Keller MB (1996) The relationship between fluoxetine use and suicidal behavior in 654 subjects with anxiety disorders. J Clin Psychiatr 57, 158–166.

Weissman MM, Klerman GL, Markowitz JS, et al. (1989) suicidal ideation and suicide attempts in panic disorder and attacks. N Engl J Med 321(18), 1209–1214.

Welu TC (1977) A follow-up program for suicide attempter: Evaluation of effectiveness. Suicide Life Threat Behav 7, 17–30.

Wintemute GL, Parham CA, Beaumont JJ, et al. (1999) Mortality among recent purchasers of handguns. N Engl J Med 341(21), 1583–1589.

Wunderlich U, Bronish T, Wittchen HU, et al. (2001) Gender differences in adolescents and young adults with suicidal behavior. Acta Psychiatr Scand 104(5), 332–339.

Young MA, Fogg LF, and Scheftner W (1996) Stable trait components of hopelessness: Baseline and sensitivity to depression. J Abnorm Psychol 105, 155–165.

# 103 Treatment of Violent Behavior

Leslie Citrome
Jan Volavka

## Introduction

Violent behavior in patients with psychiatric disorders is a frequent reason for presentation to an emergency room and subsequent admission to an inpatient unit, and is often an obstacle to discharge and reintegration back into the community. Aggressive behavior places other patients, mental health workers, and family members or other caregivers at risk for harm. Fortunately, within the past 10 years, new treatment approaches have emerged enabling greater opportunities for the successful management of these behaviors.

Some patients are violent only when acutely psychotic, while others may have persistent aggressive behavior unrelated to psychosis. Co-occurring substance use disorders increase the risk of violent behavior. Neuropsychiatric deficits and poor impulse control, underlying character pathology, or a chaotic environment may also be contributing factors.

The management of violent behavior can be divided into short-term and long-term strategies. First, there is a need to manage acute episodes of agitation. Second, there is a need to decrease the frequency and intensity of these episodes. The pharmacological treatment of acute agitation requires the use of sedating agents, but long-term use of these same agents would interfere with a patient's level of functioning. Consequently, long-term approaches require the use of medications that target aggressive behavior, without causing undue sedation.

This chapter will first review the definitions of aggression, violence, and hostility. Next is a description of the biology of aggressive behavior. This is followed by an overview of the epidemiology of aggressive behavior. The discussion of treatment strategies includes principles of evaluation, the use of general sedating agents, and the use of medications that may selectively decrease hostility and impulsivity. Although several diagnostic entities are discussed, the emphasis of this chapter is on the management of patients with schizophrenia.

## Definitions

Aggression, violence, and hostility are used in the psychiatric literature to denote behaviors that are particularly noxious and a considerable source of concern for those in the field. These terms are used with varying precision, and interpretation of research data can be a challenge when different studies use different definitions. Published rating scales may contain their own definitions and these scales may be further modified or adapted to the specific needs of the study in question. In general, "aggression," a term used for both human and animal research, is defined as overt behavior involving intent to deliver noxious stimulation to another organism or to behave destructively toward inanimate objects. Humans demonstrate three main subtypes of aggression: verbal aggression, physical aggression against other people, and physical aggression against objects. "Violence" is an exclusively human term, and usually denotes physical aggression against other people and thus can be seen as a subtype of aggression. On the other hand, "hostility" is a loosely defined term in the psychiatric literature. Hostility may include agitation, aggression, irritability, suspicion, uncooperativeness, and jealousy, depending on the context in which the word is used.

Agitation can be defined as excessive verbal and/or motor behavior. Mild agitation can escalate to include behaviors such as aggression and violence.

## Biology of Aggressive Behavior

Most perpetrators of aggressive behavior (criminal or otherwise) are not mentally ill, and aggressive behavior cannot be explained by biological factors alone. In fact, most of the aggressive behavior observed in daily television newscasts is perpetrated by terrorists and other criminals who may not have any discernible biological predisposition to violence.

Biological predisposition is increasingly viewed as a function of genes. The transcriptional function of the gene is regulated in part by environmental influences; changes in gene expression can, for example, be elicited as the child interacts with the rearing environment and learns the basic rules of social behavior. Learned behavior then impacts on the environment, causing environmental changes that in turn affect gene expression. Such serial interactions between genes and environment blur the traditional distinctions between biological and environmental factors.

Several principal pathways leading to a predisposition to aggressive behavior are schematically displayed in Figure 103–1. The parents may contribute to the offspring's predisposition via transmitted genes, fetal environment, obstetric

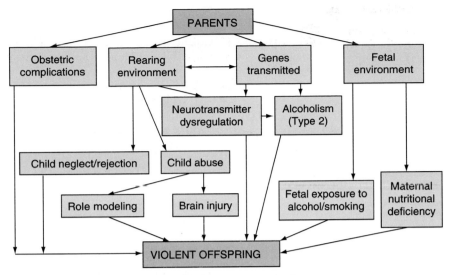

**Figure 103–1** *Transmission of violence.*

complications, and rearing environment. Several polymorphisms of genes that control the activity of various neurotransmitters (particularly serotonin and catecholamines) are apparently associated with persistent aggressive behavior; these will be described later. Maternal use of alcohol, smoking, and malnutrition during pregnancy were all reported to explain statistically significant (but clinically modest) proportions of the variance of aggressive behavior in adult offspring. Obstetric complications, particularly in interaction with other factors such as early maternal rejection, may lead to elevated rates of violent crime in the offspring. Rearing environment is one of the most important factors in the development of predisposition to violence, and several mechanisms, including child abuse, are presented. Detailed explanation of Figure 103–1, as well as the bibliography supporting it, are presented elsewhere (Volavka 2002).

Mechanisms displayed in Figure 103–1 may operate in persons with or without a diagnosable mental disorder. We will now focus on aggressive behavior in persons with mental disorders.

## Substance Use Disorders

Acute effects of alcohol and illicit drugs are involved, perhaps causally, in a large proportion of aggressive incidents. For example, 51.6% of women injured during a physical assault by a male partner reported that the assaulter had been drinking just before the incident (Kyriacou et al. 1999). Positive urine tests for illicit drugs were obtained in a majority of arrested males in the US (Pastore and Maguire 2000, p. 380). Epidemiological studies indicate that substance use disorders elevate substantially the prevalence of overt physical aggression (Swanson 1994). This is discussed in more detail later.

## Psychoses

Most persons diagnosed with a psychosis are not violent. Nevertheless, psychoses are associated with an elevated risk for aggression. It is clear that comorbidity of psychosis and substance use disorder contributes to this risk very

substantially. Furthermore, persons with psychoses are more likely to have substance use disorders than other people (Regier et al. 1990). Combination of substance abuse and nonadherence to treatment is the typical prelude to the development of aggressive behavior in persons with severe mental illness living in the community (Swartz et al. 1998).

Are patients diagnosed with psychoses but without comorbid substance use disorders also at elevated risk for aggression? Psychiatric patients followed up after discharge from a hospital were reported to be no more violent than other people in their community, as long as they did not start drinking or using drugs (Steadman et al. 1998). The results of that study, however, are somewhat difficult to interpret because of incomplete information about the 36% of the patients who were lost to follow-up. In general, patients who are persistently violent exhibit treatment resistance, high levels of hostility, and antisocial behavior. For these reasons, persistently violent patients may be more likely to be lost to follow-up than the transiently violent patients whose violence subsides as their symptoms improve. Thus, a biased attrition could explain the author's observation of declining violence over the course of the follow-up period (Czobor and Volavka 1999).

Birth cohort studies indicate that schizophrenia is associated with elevated risk for aggression even without a comorbid substance use disorder (Brennan et al. 2000, Arseneault et al. 2000).

As every hospital psychiatrist knows, there are many psychotic inpatients who are aggressive without access to alcohol and drugs, and in spite of supervised antipsychotic treatment. Thus, factors other than substance use and nonadherence to treatment must be involved in the pathophysiology of aggression in these patients. Some of these patients have neurological and cognitive deficits (Krakowski et al. 1989), but this was not demonstrated in other samples of violent patients (Frankle et al. 2001). Violent behavior may be driven by psychotic symptoms, particularly by delusions of persecution, thought insertion, and external control (Link et al. 1998). However, these specific symptoms did not seem to play a major role in violence in another major study (Appelbaum et al. 2000).

From the standpoint of practical management of aggressive patients with major mental disorders, it seems that it could be fruitful to study in detail individual assaults in order to assess underlying pathophysiology. This is a promising avenue of research since it is generally agreed that aggressive behavior has multiple causes that differ among patients, and perhaps among different incidents in individual patients. Our experience, based on interviews of assailants, victims, and witnesses, as well as on observations of videotapes, suggests that most assaults among psychiatric inpatients diagnosed with psychoses are not driven by psychotic symptoms. It appears that many of these assaults are attributable to comorbid personality disorders.

## Personality Disorders

Antisocial personality disorder (APD) is partly defined by aggressive behavior and therefore it is not surprising that many violent psychotic patients meet its diagnostic criteria. This circularity of definition makes the use of this diagnosis somewhat unhelpful. The concept of "psychopathy," introduced to modern psychiatry by Cleckley (1976), is less circular since it relies primarily on personality and psychological processes rather than on criminal or aggressive behavior. Psychopathy is assessed by a valid and reliable checklist constructed by Hare and his coworkers (Hart et al. 1992). Table 103–1 shows the screening version of the checklist intended for use in persons with serious mental illness (Hare 1996, Hart et al. 1995). The first six items in Factor-1 measure the severity of interpersonal and affective symptoms of psychopathy. The next six items in Factor-2 reflect the social deviance symptoms. Psychopathy is a narrower concept than APD. Most psychopaths meet the criteria for APD, but subjects diagnosed as APD do not necessarily meet the criteria for psychopathy. Psychopathy predicts violent behavior in nonpsychotic individuals (Hare and Hart 1993), as well as in persons with major mental disorders (Hart et al. 1994). The rates of comorbidity of psychopathy and schizophrenia are elevated among violent patients (Nolan et al. 1999).

Differentiating aggressive behavior based on psychopathy from that based on psychotic symptoms has consequences for treatment. It is unlikely that psychopathy will respond to antipsychotics.

| Table 103–1 | Hare Psychopathy Checklist (Screening Version) |
| --- | --- |
| Factor 1: Interpersonal/Affective | Factor 2: Social Deviance |
| 1. Superficial | 7. Impulsive |
| 2. Grandiose | 8. Poor behavior controls |
| 3. Manipulative | 9. Lacks goals |
| 4. Lacks remorse | 10. Irresponsible |
| 5. Lacks empathy | 11. Adolescent antisocial behavior |
| 6. Does not accept responsibility | 12. Adult antisocial behavior |

## Epidemiology

Not all patients with psychiatric disorders are aggressive, violent, or hostile. As mentioned earlier, most of the aggressive, violent, or hostile acts we witness in our daily lives, on the news and elsewhere, are perpetrated by people without a DSM-IV Axis I major mental disorder.

Nonetheless, a small minority of patients with psychiatric disorders are prone to aggressivity and this aggressivity may be persistent (Convit et al. 1990, Owen et al. 1998). A 6-month study of 1,552 inpatients with various diagnoses detected 576 violent incidents (Convit et al. 1990); a small group of recidivistic patients (5%) caused 53% of the incidents. The diagnosis of schizophrenia was slightly overrepresented among the male recidivists; personality and impulse disorder diagnoses were frequent among both the male and female recidivists.

## Community Samples

In the Epidemiological Catchment Area Study (Regier et al. 1990, Swanson 1994), self-reports revealed that the probabilities of violent behavior in male and female schizophrenic patients were, respectively, 5.3 times and 5.9 times higher than in persons without any diagnosed mental disorder. Risk increased to 12.6 and 9.1, respectively, with comorbid substance abuse and mental disorder. A summary of this data, along with that of other studies from other areas of the world can be found in Table 103–2. The studies generally use a broad definition of mental illness, focusing largely on psychotic disorders (including schizophrenia, schizoaffective disorder, bipolar disorder, and depression).

## Inpatient Samples

Patients with psychiatric disorders may be aggressive despite being placed in a more structured environment like a hospital ward. During the first 24 hours after the admission to a psychiatric inpatient unit, 33 (13.0%) of 253 patients physically attacked another person (Binder and McNiel 1988). Manic patients were the most likely diagnostic group to be assaultive during the initial phase of hospitalization, with 12 out of 46 patients (26.1%) attacking another person. In contrast, 9 out of 87 (10.3%) diagnosed with schizophrenia, and 12 out of 120 (10%) diagnosed other than schizophrenia or mania, attacked another person during the same period. Another group reported that in the first 8 days after hospitalization, 25 of 289 schizophrenic or schizoaffective patients (8.7%) assaulted someone at least once (Tanke and Yesavage 1985). A study of 5,164 long-term patients indicated that 7% of these patients physically attacked another person at least once during a 3-month period (Tardiff and Sweillam 1982). Assaultive patients were more likely than nonassaultive patients to have a primary diagnosis of nonparanoid schizophrenia, psychotic organic brain syndrome, mental retardation, or personality disorder. Mania was not reported in this study. Although long-term beds are fewer in number than 2 decades ago, the patients remaining in long-term psychiatric hospitals may be a distillation of the most aggressive persons unable to be readily placed in a community setting. Thus, the percentages may actually be higher today and this underscores the need for better clinical understanding of the problem of violent behavior in schizophrenia, and the need for innovative treatment approaches.

| Table 103–2 | Epidemiological Studies of Mental Disorder and Violent Behavior | | | |
|---|---|---|---|---|
| Author | Location | *N* | Information | Risk for Violent Behavior in Those with Mental Disorder |
| Regier et al. (1990), Swanson (1994) | US | 10,000 | Self-reports | Increase (even higher with comorbid substance abuse) |
| Link et al. (1992), Link and Stueve (1994) | US | 385 patients and 365 controls | Self-reports | Increase (only 19.4% of patients were diagnosed with schizophrenia) |
| Hodgins (1992) | Sweden | 15,117 | National registries | Increase (patients had "major mental disorders") |
| Eronen et al. (1996) | Finland | 693 | Forensic psychiatric examinations | Increase (even higher with comorbid substance abuse) |
| Hodgins et al. (1996) | Denmark | 324,401 | National registries | Increase (patients with "mental disorders" hospitalized at least once) |
| Tiihonen et al. (1997) | Finland | 12,058 | National registries | Increase (tentative); definite increase with comorbid substance abuse |
| Volavka et al. (1997) | 10 countries | 1,017 patients with schizophrenia | Self-reports, other informants, clinic or hospital records | Increase (higher in developing countries compared with developed countries) |
| Wallace et al. (1998) | Australia | 4,156 | Case registries | Increase (even higher with comorbid substance abuse) |
| Steadman et al. (1998) | US | 1,136 patients and 519 controls | Self-reports, collateral informants, police and hospital records | No increase except for those with comorbid substance abuse |
| Arseneault et al. (2000) | New Zealand | 961 | Self-reports, conviction records | Increase |
| Brennan et al. (2000) | Denmark | 358,180 | National registries | Increase |

## Acute Agitation

Agitation can be defined as excessive motor or verbal activity. Common examples include hyperactivity, verbal abuse, and threatening gestures and language. Unmanaged acute agitation can lead to violence. As such, acute agitation is a psychiatric emergency that requires rapid intervention. Oral medication treatment may be impractical or impossible. This section will focus on intramuscular medications within the context of a behavioral management plan.

## Assessment

Key points in assessment are outlined in Table 103–3. The time available for patient assessment will be dependent on the acuity of the presentation. For someone who is acutely agitated and an immediate danger to self or others, emergency measures must be taken to avoid harm. Somatic conditions must be ruled out prior to initiating additional treatment, as an underlying metabolic, toxic, infectious, or other nonpsychiatric cause may need to be treated. In these cases the agitation is a symptom to be treated alongside the underlying condition. This is not as great a concern for the physically healthy psychiatric patient whose history is well known to the staff than for the relatively unknown patient presenting to the emergency room. In addition, in the nursing home environment, new-onset agitation may indicate a newly emerging somatic condition. Once the patient is under behavioral control further medical and psychiatric workups can be done. Mechanical restraints may be necessary to prevent the agitated patient from injuring himself/herself, or others, while the medical workup is being conducted.

Care must be taken not to miss comorbid conditions of alcohol or sedative abuse or dependence that may present with acute intoxication or withdrawal. Such conditions will drive the treatment choice towards the use of a benzodiazepine (see later).

Assessment should also include the context of the agitation. Patients may be purposefully using aggressive behavior to intimidate others. Antisocial personality traits may be the most important factor in some instances of patient violence where goal-directed behavior such as extortion of money or cigarettes is present. These antisocial behaviors may not always be evident to staff, as they can occur in unsupervised areas such as hallways, bedrooms, and bathrooms. Such predatory behavior may involve victims who are unable to articulate what is happening to them, while the aggressor appears to have an abundance of material goods or undue influence on others.

Where aggressive behavior may appear to be impulsive or random, environmental factors may be a significant factor. Some patients are transiently violent when in a chaotic environment, others are persistently violent no

| Table 103–3 | Key Issues in Assessment of Acute Agitation/Aggression/Violence |
|---|---|

1. Somatic conditions
2. Previous history of violence
3. Access to weapons
4. Current ideation, including content of delusions
5. Active substance abuse, including alcohol
6. Comorbid antisocial personality disorder/traits or psychopathy
7. Verbal threats
8. Premonitory physical signs (clenched fist, pacing)

| Table 103–4 | Pharmacological Options for Acute Agitation—Intramuscular Agents | | |
|---|---|---|---|
| Agent | Dose (mg) | Half-life (h) | Comments |
| Lorazepam | 0.5–2 | 10–20 | There are no active metabolites. Can be administered orally, sublingually, intramuscularly, or intravenously. |
| Haloperidol | 0.5–7.5 | 12–36 | Can combine with lorazepam in the same syringe (combination of haloperidol 5 mg and lorazepam 2 mg is commonly used). |
| Droperidol | 2.5–5 | 2 | QTc prolongation. Withdrawn in UK. |
| Olanzapine | 10 (2.5 for patients with dementia) | 34–38 | Superiority over haloperidol (schizophrenia) and lorazepam (bipolar disorder) in clinical trials. |
| Ziprasidone | 10–20 | 2.2–3.4 | Superiority over haloperidol (schizophrenia) in clinical trials. QTc prolongation. |

matter the milieu (Krakowski and Czobor 1997). In contrast to the persistently violent patient, those who were transiently violent were more likely to respond to a new structured environment (Krakowski et al. 1988). Environmental factors leading to increased aggressive behavior on a psychiatric ward include crowding (Palmstierna et al. 1991, Ng et al. 2001). It appears that the transiently violent are more responsive to typical antipsychotic medication and have less neurological impairment than the persistently violent patient (Volavka and Krakowski 1989).

It is generally agreed that it is impossible to predict with absolute certainty if a violent act will occur, but it is possible to assess risks. Past history of violence may be the best predictor of future violent behavior (Blomhoff et al. 1990, Convit et al. 1988, Karson and Bigelow 1987), and obtaining a history of this, access to weapons, and current ideation are essential elements in risk assessment.

## Treatment

Behavioral, psychological, and pharmacological interventions are used simultaneously (Citrome and Green 1990). Clinicians are urged to survey the environment for potential weapons, not to turn their back on the patient, and to have other staff available. Taking verbal threats seriously and being aware of physical premonitory signs such as a clenched fist and pacing are important. Initially, an agitated patient should be isolated from other patients and from distractions because extraneous stimulation can intensify psychosis in a patient who may be hallucinating, paranoid, and agitated. Moreover, other patients may intentionally or inadvertently interfere with treatment. Generally it is easier to clear the area of many calm patients than to move one dangerous individual. Restraint or seclusion may be necessary, and this is the time where the risk for injury for both staff and patients is highest. The technique of the calming blanket, a soft comforter with canvas reinforcements, may be helpful in subduing the patient who is punching, scratching, or kicking.

Nonspecific sedation is often used in the management of an acutely agitated patient. In general, intramuscular injection of a sedative has a faster onset of action than oral administration but it has been observed that a patient may calm down readily after an oral dose, knowing that action has been taken and help is being provided. Up to now, choice of intramuscular medication for these behavioral emergencies has been limited to typical antipsychotics (such as haloperidol or chlorpromazine) versus benzodi-

azepines (principally lorazepam) (Table 103–4). The availability of new intramuscular formulations of novel atypical antipsychotics provides new treatment options for the management of acute agitation in patients with psychosis (Citrome 2002). In general, the atypical antipsychotics are better tolerated than the older agents. These new formulations provide the opportunity for a smooth transition to oral dosing to the same agent once the acute agitation has been appropriately managed.

Lorazepam, the only benzodiazepine that is reliably absorbed when administered intramuscularly, appears to be a good rational choice when treating an acute episode of agitation, especially where the etiology is not clear such as when a patient with a history of schizophrenia may actually be withdrawing from alcohol (Salzman 1988, Greenblatt et al. 1979, 1982). Caution is required when respiratory depression is a possibility. There may be increased risk of this in patients with sleep apnea (associated with being morbidly obese, history of snoring, and daytime drowsiness). Lorazepam is not recommended for long-term daily use because of the problems associated with tolerance, dependence, and withdrawal. Paradoxical reactions to benzodiazepines, as exhibited by hostility or violence has been an area of concern (Bond and Lader 1979), but the evidence is not convincing and, in any event, such reactions are uncommon (Dietch and Jennings 1988). The possibility of alcohol or sedative withdrawal as a cause of agitation is another point in favor of using lorazepam.

The typical antipsychotics cause sedation, given in a high enough dose. Haloperidol, a high potency butyrophenone, has been frequently used as an intramuscular prn medication for agitation and aggressive behavior in an emergency department setting for a wide variety of patients (Clinton et al. 1987). Depending on the clinical response, subsequent doses may be administered as often as every hour if necessary. However, 4- to 8-hour intervals may be satisfactory. Haloperidol's advantage over the low potency typical antipsychotics (e.g., chlorpromazine) is that it causes less hypotension, fewer anticholinergic side effects, and causes less of a decrease in the seizure threshold. In addition to this nonspecific sedation, a benefit would be its antipsychotic effect (in responsive patients), but this would be evident only after the acute episode of agitation has subsided. High doses of typical antipsychotics may lead to more adverse effects, including akathisia, which may itself provoke violent behavior (Keckich 1978, Siris 1985).

Droperidol, another antipsychotic in the butyrophenone class, is used most often for induction of anesthesia. The medication is not FDA-approved (Food and Drug Administration) for psychiatric conditions but has been used for sedating agitated patients in an emergency room setting (Thomas et al. 1992). Its rapid onset of action and possibly a less severe extrapyramidal side effect profile compared with haloperidol would seem to make intramuscular droperidol, on the surface, a reasonable choice for nonspecific sedation. However, droperidol does cause a dose-dependent prolongation of the heart wave (QT) interval (Lischke et al. 1994) and concern over this has led to the withdrawal of this product in the UK market, and a new "black box" warning in the product's US labeling. Adequate medical backup and the availability of intubation and oxygen are recommended.

Yet another approach is to use a combination of haloperidol and lorazepam, either sequentially, or simultaneously as they can be mixed in the same syringe (Hughes 1999).

The new atypical antipsychotics may emerge as important options in the management of acute agitation in schizophrenia. Although sedation or "calming" remains the primary mode of action when used emergently in the acutely agitated patient, the atypical antipsychotics have several advantages over typical antipsychotics (Citrome 1997), in particular a lower propensity for extrapyramidal side effects, including akathisia.

Peak plasma concentrations after an intramuscular dose of ziprasidone are achieved in 30 to 45 minutes, compared with 8 hours (with half-life of 3.8 hours) with oral dosing (Pfizer, Inc. 2001). Premarketing clinical trials demonstrated efficacy of both a 10 and a 20 mg dose in reducing acute agitation in patients with schizophrenia and schizoaffective disorder (Lesem et al. 2001, Reeves et al. 1998). Overall ziprasidone was well tolerated, and almost free of extrapyramidal side effects, when given by intramuscular injection, at doses up to 80 mg/day (Pfizer, Inc. 2001). However, the maximal recommended dose for intramuscular injection is 40 mg/day in divided doses. The most common treatment-emergent adverse events at the 10 and 20 mg doses were nausea, headache, and dizziness. The magnitude of QTc increases with intramuscular ziprasidone is comparable to that described for oral ziprasidone.

Peak plasma concentrations after an intramuscular dose of olanzapine are achieved in 15 to 30 minutes, compared with 3 to 6 hours with oral dosing (Eli Lilly & Co 2001). Premarketing clinical trials demonstrated efficacy of olanzapine in reducing acute agitation in patients with schizophrenia, schizoaffective disorder, bipolar disorder, and dementia (Eli Lilly & Co. 2001, Wright et al. 2001). Intramuscular olanzapine exhibited less extrapyramidal side effects compared with intramuscular haloperidol. The optimal dose in adults appears to be 10 mg, however, patients with dementia may require a more conservative approach and the recommended dose for that group is 2.5 mg. In contrast to ziprasidone, no evidence exists for any significant QTc interval prolongations with olanzapine.

## Long-Term Treatment

The treatment goal is to decrease the frequency and intensity of aggressive behavior. Specialized units such as secure or psychiatric intensive care units (Musisi et al. 1989, Goldney et al. 1985, Warneke 1986, Citrome et al. 1995) provide a structured environment that optimizes staff and patient safety. In general these specialized units are staffed with persons trained in interacting with volatile and difficult to manage patients (Maier et al. 1987). When available, these units can be a valuable resource for education, training, consultation, and referral.

Although pharmacotherapy remains the mainstay of treatment for the persistently aggressive patient, behavioral plans need to be used in tandem. Providing structure, including the use of behavioral contracts, can be useful. Preventive aggression devices (PADS) are a form of ambulatory restraints, which can be used as an alternative to seclusion (Van Rybroek et al. 1987). The technique was first developed for a specialized inpatient unit with repetitively aggressive patients. Patients in these wrist-to-belt and/or ankle–ankle restraints can remain with their peers on the ward, eat their meals, and interact, yet are prevented from striking out and injuring others. In combination with a comprehensive behavior modification program, these patients can be weaned off the use of the ambulatory restraints.

Although pharmacotherapy for the longer-term management of aggressive behavior is somewhat dependent on the patient's underlying diagnosis, clinical management is often complicated and can entail the use of several coprescribed medications. At the core of impulsive aggressive behavior may be a dysregulation of the serotonergic neurotransmitter system and this may explain the possible ameliorative effects of atypical antipsychotics and the selective serotonin reuptake inhibitors (SSRIs). In addition, beta-blockers and moodstabilizers have been used with some success. Table 103–5 outlines the medication strategies useful in patients with aggressive behavior and schizophrenia. Nonadherence to a treatment regimen may require the use of outpatient commitment, now available in many jurisdictions.

## Atypical Antipsychotics

The availability of atypical antipsychotics has led to the observation that these agents may act differently from the older antipsychotics in that they may specifically target aggressive behavior. Several retrospective studies have demonstrated a decrease in the number of violent episodes and/or a decrease in the use of seclusion or restraint among inpatients after they began clozapine treatment (Wilson and Claussen 1995, Ratey et al. 1993, Chiles et al. 1994, Mallya et al. 1992, Spivak et al. 1997, Maier 1992, Ebrahim et al. 1994). The reductions of hostility (Volavka et al. 1993) and aggression (Buckley et al. 1995) after clozapine treatment were selective in the sense that they were (statistically) independent of the general antipsychotic effects of clozapine. This was demonstrated in a double-blind 14-week randomized clinical trial comparing the specific antiaggressive effects of clozapine with those of olanzapine, risperidone, or haloperidol in 157 inpatients with schizophrenia or schizoaffective disorder (Citrome et al. 2001b). Clozapine had significantly greater antihostility effect than haloperidol or risperidone. The effect on hostility was independent of antipsychotic effect on delusional thinking, formal thought disorder, or hallucinations, and independent of sedation.

| Table 103–5 | Pharmacological Options for Persistent Aggressive Behavior in Schizophrenia | |
| --- | --- | --- |
| **Class of Agent** | **Basis of Evidence** | **Comments** |
| Atypical antipsychotics | Case reports, retrospective record reviews, secondary analyses of randomized clinical trials | Best evidence exists for clozapine, some evidence for olanzapine and quetiapine, and conflicting evidence for risperidone. Insufficient information for ziprasidone. |
| Mood stabilizers | Case reports, retrospective record reviews, few randomized clinical trials | Although mood stabilizers are helpful in bipolar disorder, evidence in schizophrenia is not as strong. Best evidence exists for valproate, some for carbamazepine, and conflicting evidence for lithium. Insufficient information for gabapentin, topiramate, oxcarbazepine. |
| β-blockers | Case reports, retrospective record reviews, few randomized clinical trials | Best studied in patients with brain injuries. Some evidence demonstrating usefulness in schizophrenia for propranolol and nadolol. |
| SSRIs | Case reports, one randomized clinical trial | Adjunctive citalopram found helpful in a randomized double-blind study (Vartiainen et al. 1995). |
| Benzodiazepines | Case reports, one randomized clinical trial | Negative outcomes (patients worsened) in a randomized double-blind study of adjunctive clonazepam (Karson et al. 1982). |

Risperidone also was demonstrated to have a selective effect on hostility that was superior to haloperidol (Czobor et al. 1995). This is supported by a review of the impact of risperidone on seclusion and restraint at a state psychiatric hospital (Chengappa et al. 2000) but this effect was not evident in a retrospective case–control study (Buckley et al. 1997), and in another negative report (Beck et al. 1997).

Quetiapine may also preferentially reduce hostility and aggression. Quetiapine and haloperidol were both superior to placebo in reducing positive symptoms of schizophrenia but only quetiapine was superior to placebo in the measures of aggression and hostility (Cantillon and Goldstein 1998). This is supported by a case report describing a dramatic response to quetiapine monotherapy in a persistently aggressive patient who had failed to respond to numerous other medications (Citrome et al. 2001a).

Olanzapine was also found to be superior to haloperidol on measures of agitation (Kinon et al. 2001).

At this time, the weight of the evidence favors clozapine as specific antiaggressive treatment for schizophrenia patients (Glazer and Dickson 1998), with demonstrated superiority to haloperidol and risperidone (Citrome et al. 2001b). More research is needed to compare the other atypical antipsychotics with clozapine for this indication. Ideally, such studies need to be done double-blind with subjects specially selected because of their aggressive behavior. This is operationally quite difficult because of a number of logistical factors, including the relative rarity of aggressive events and consequent need for a large sample size and lengthy baseline and trial periods, as well as selection/consent bias (Volavka and Citrome 1999).

## Mood Stabilizers

There is an expectation that adjunctive mood stabilizers can reduce aggressive and impulsive behavior (Citrome 1995). This is understandable when the primary diagnosis is bipolar or schizoaffective disorder where the mood stabilizer is treating the core symptoms of the disorder, but these agents, notably valproate, lithium, and carbamazepine, are also used in patients with schizophrenia. A recent review of the use of valproate in violence and aggressive behaviors in

a variety of diagnoses (Lindenmayer and Kotsaftis 2000) did reveal a 77.1% response rate (defined by a 50% reduction in target behavior) based on 17 reports (164 patients), but included only 16 patients with schizophrenia. Only one double-blind study was found, and it consisted of 16 patients with borderline personality disorder (Hollander et al. 1998). Since that review there have been additional reports, including a double-blind placebo-controlled trial of valproate in 20 children and adolescents with explosive temper and mood lability where valproate was superior to placebo (Donovan et al. 2000), and a 1-year open-label prospective trial of adjunctive valproate with olanzapine in 10 patients with paranoid schizophrenia, demonstrating statistically significant reductions in hostility (Littrell et al. 2001). Carbamazepine has also been utilized for the management of persistent aggressive behavior but the evidence for efficacy comes from small trials (Luchins 1984, Yassa and Dupont 1983, Hakola and Laulumaa 1982, Neppe 1983, Dose et al. 1987, Okuma et al. 1989, Hesslinger et al. 1999). With rare exceptions, the published studies of carbamazepine and aggressivity are not blinded and are uncontrolled for placebo effect. In addition, plasma levels of concomitant antipsychotics are not measured, leaving open the possibility for undetected pharmacokinetic interactions. Despite these limitations, carbamazepine does appear to be a useful adjunct to antipsychotic therapy (Simhandl and Meszaros 1992) and may lower aggression in a broad spectrum of disorders, including schizophrenia (Young and Hillbrand 1994). A comparison of valproate and carbamazepine in hospitalized patients (diagnosis not reported) revealed a decrease in the number of hours spent in mechanical restraints for both groups, with valproate being more effective than carbamazepine (Alam et al. 1995).

Although lithium is a useful medication for patients with bipolar or schizoaffective disorder, the effectiveness of lithium therapy in schizophrenia is not established. When lithium was added to antipsychotics for the treatment of resistant schizophrenic patients classified as "dangerous, violent or criminal," no benefits were seen after 4 weeks of adjunctive lithium (Collins et al. 1991). However, another group found that lithium was useful as a single agent in ameliorating psychosis in three schizophrenic patients who suffered from marked akathisia with accompanying agitation, restlessness, and irritability when on standard antipsychotics (Shalev et al. 1987). In addition, there are case reports of patients with paranoid schizophrenia with aggressive or disorderly behaviors who have responded to the addition of lithium to their antipsychotic treatment, then deteriorated after the lithium was discontinued but subsequently improved when it was reinstituted (Prakash 1985).

In 1998, gabapentin utilization exceeded that of carbamazepine in patients with schizophrenia hospitalized within psychiatric centers operated by the State of New York (Citrome et al. 2000). Gabapentin is an anticonvulsant that has been used as a new treatment for bipolar disorder (Schaffer and Schaffer 1997), and suggestions have been made that this agent may be useful in the management of behavior dyscontrol (Ryback and Ryback 1995). More work is needed. Adjunctive lamotrigine may be effective in the management of treatment-resistant schizophrenia (Tiihonen et al. 2002); its potential antiaggressive effects remain to be tested.

In general, dosing of adjunctive mood stabilizers in patients with schizophrenia is the same as when using these agents as a primary treatment for bipolar disorder.

## Beta-Blockers

Beta-adrenergic blockers, in particular propranolol, have been used in the treatment of aggressive behavior in brain injured patients (Yudofsky et al. 1981, 1984). Propranolol has also been used as an adjunctive treatment for schizophrenia, and a reduction in symptoms, including aggression, was found (Sheppard 1979). Nadolol may also be helpful (Ratey et al. 1992, Alpert et al. 1990, Allan et al. 1996). Beta-blockers may exert some of their effects by decreasing akathisia, which in turn may decrease agitation.

## Benzodiazepines

Clonazepam, a high potency benzodiazepine, had been reported useful in patients with bipolar disorder. This result is in contrast to a double-blind placebo-controlled trial of adjunctive clonazepam in 13 schizophrenic patients receiving antipsychotics (Karson et al. 1982). In that study no additional therapeutic benefit was observed and, in fact, four patients demonstrated violent behavior during the course of clonazepam treatment.

Using lorazepam for long-term management (in contrast to acute use as a prn) can be problematic because of physiological tolerance. Missing scheduled doses of lorazepam may result in withdrawal symptoms that can lead to agitation or excitement, as well as irritability and a greater risk for aggressive behavior.

## Antidepressants

The current interest in certain antidepressants' role in aggression is based on the crucial role of serotonergic regulation of impulsive aggression against self and others. Now that antidepressants with specific effects on serotonin (5-HT) receptors have become available, a number of reports have emerged that posit a role for fluoxetine (Goldman and Janecek 1990), citalopram (Vartiainen et al. 1995), and fluvoxamine (Silver and Kushnir 1998) in the treatment of persistent aggressive behavior.

## Adjunctive Electroconvulsive Therapy

Although not often considered as a first-line treatment, adjunctive electroconvulsive therapy (ECT) may be helpful in patients who have inadequately-responsive psychotic symptoms (Fink and Sackeim 1996). An open trial of ECT in combination with risperidone in male patients with schizophrenia and aggression resulted in a reduction in aggressive behavior for 9 of the 10 patients (Hirose et al. 2001). The combination of ECT and clozapine may also be

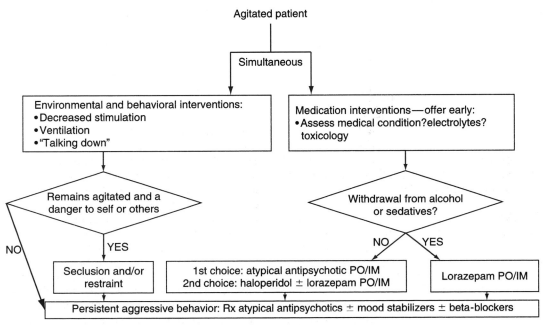

**Figure 103–2** *Management of agitation: overview.*

helpful. A review of 36 reported cases treated with this combination, all of whom with a history of treatment-resistance, revealed that approximately two-thirds benefited from this treatment (Kupchik et al. 2000).

## Conclusion

The effective management of aggression is a priority for clinicians. Strategies to control acute agitation include the use of mechanical restraints and the administration of parenteral medication. Early intervention is important to avoid further escalation to violence. An overview is presented in Figure 103–2. The new intramuscular formulations of atypical antipsychotics hold promise to quickly and efficaciously control acute agitation, without the side effect burdens of the older typical antipsychotics. Lorazepam remains a first choice for patients withdrawing from alcohol or sedatives and presenting with agitation. Longer-term management may include the use of a specialized hospital unit, if available. Treatment of the underlying disorder is key, but this may be complicated by a history of poor response to standard treatments. Lorazepam for long-term daily use is not recommended because of problems associated with tolerance, dependence, and withdrawal. Clozapine appears to be the most effective antipsychotic in reducing aggressivity in patients with schizophrenia and schizoaffective disorder. Valproate and carbamazepine are also used with antipsychotics to decrease the intensity and frequency of agitation and poor impulse control, but they have not been extensively studied under double-blind placebo-controlled conditions for this indication. Beta-blockers and SSRIs may also be helpful. Adjunctive ECT, together with atypical antipsychotics, may be considered for patients who have failed other approaches.

## References

Alam MY, Klass DB, Luchins DJ, et al. (1995) Effectiveness of divalproex sodium, valproic acid, and carbamazepine in aggression (poster). NCDEU 35th Annual Meeting.

Allan E, Alpert M, Sison C, et al. (1996) Adjunctive nadolol in the treatment of acutely aggressive schizophrenic patients. J Clin Psychiatr 57, 455–459.

Alpert M, Allan ER, Citrome L, et al. (1990) A double-blind, placebo-controlled study of adjunctive nadolol in the management of violent psychiatric patients. Psychopharmacol Bull 26, 367–371.

Appelbaum PS, Robbins PC, and Monahan J (2000) Violence and delusions: Data from the MacArthur Violence Risk Assessment Study. Am J Psychiatr 157, 566–572.

Arseneault L, Moffitt TE, Caspi A, et al. (2000) Mental disorders and violence in a total birth cohort. Arch Gen Psychiatr 57, 979–986.

Beck NC, Greenfield SR, Gotham H, et al. (1997) Risperidone in the management of violent, treatment-resistant schizophrenics hospitalized in a maximum security forensic facility. J Am Acad Psychiatr Law 25, 461–468.

Binder RL and McNiel DE (1988) Effects of diagnosis and context on dangerousness. Am J Psychiatr 145, 728–732.

Blomhoff S, Seim S, and Friis S (1990) Can prediction of violence among psychiatric inpatients be improved? Hosp Comm Psychiatr 41, 771–775.

Bond A and Lader M (1979) Benzodiazepines and aggression. In Psychopharmacology of Aggression, Sandler M (ed). Raven Press, New York, pp. 173–182.

Brennan PA, Sarnoff SA, and Hodgins S (2000) Major mental disorders and criminal violence in a Danish birth cohort. Arch Gen Psychiatr 57, 494–500.

Buckley P, Bartell J, Donenwirth MA, et al. (1995) Violence and schizophrenia: Clozapine as a specific antiaggressive agent. Bull Am Acad Psychiatr Law 23, 607–611.

Buckley PF, Ibrahim ZY, Singer B, et al. (1997) Aggression and schizophrenia: Efficacy of risperidone. J Am Psychiatr Law 25, 173–181.

Cantillon M and Goldstein JM (1998) Quetiapine fumarate reduces aggression and hostility in patients with schizophrenia (new research poster NR444). American Psychiatric Association, Annual Meeting, Toronto, Ontario, Canada.

Chengappa KNR, Levine J, Ulrich R, et al. (2000) Impact of risperidone on seclusion and restraint at a state psychiatric hospital. Can J Psychiatr 45, 827–832.

Chiles JA, Davidson P, and McBride D (1994) Effects of clozapine on use of seclusion and restraint at a state hospital. Hosp Comm Psychiatr 45, 269–271.

Citrome L (1995) Use of lithium, carbamazepine, and valproic acid in a state-operated psychiatric hospital. J Pharm Technol 11, 55–59.

Citrome L (1997) New antipsychotic medications: What advantages do they offer? Postgrad Med 101, 207–214.

Citrome L (2002) Aggression and intramuscular antipsychotics: New options for acute agitation. Postgrad Med (in press).

Citrome L and Green L (1990) The dangerous agitated patient: What to do right now. Postgrad Med 87, 231–236.

Citrome L, Green L, and Fost R (1995) Clinical and administrative consequences of a reduced census on a psychiatric intensive care unit. Psychiatr Q 66, 209–217.

Citrome L, Krakowski M, Greenberg WM, et al. (2001a) Antiaggressive effect of quetiapine in a patient with schizoaffective disorder (letter). J Clin Psychiatr 62, 901.

Citrome L, Levine J, and Allingham B (2000) Changes in use of valproate and other mood stabilizers for patients with schizophrenia from 1994 to 1998. Psychiatr Serv 51, 634–638.

Citrome L, Volavka J, Czobor P, et al. (2001b) Effects of clozapine, olanzapine, risperidone, and haloperidol on hostility among patients with schizophrenia. Psychiatr Serv 52, 1510–1514.

Cleckley H (1976) The Mask of Sanity, 5th ed. The CV Mosby Company, Saint Louis.

Clinton JE, Sterner S, Stelmachers Z, et al. (1987) Haloperidol for sedation of disruptive emergency patients. Ann Emerg Med 16, 319–322.

Collins PJ, Larkin EP, and Shubsachs APW (1991) Lithium carbonate in chronic schizophrenia—a brief trial of lithium carbonate added to neuroleptics for treatment of resistant schizophrenic patients. Acta Psychiatr Scand 84, 150–154.

Convit A, Isay D, Otis D, et al. (1990) Characteristics of repeatedly assaultive psychiatric inpatients. Hosp Comm Psychiatr 41, 1112–1115.

Convit A, Jaeger J, Lin SP, et al. (1988) Predicting assaultiveness in psychiatric inpatients: A pilot study. Hosp Comm Psychiatr 39, 429–434.

Czobor P and Volavka J (1999) Violence in the mentally ill: Questions remain (letter). Arch Gen Psychiatr 56, 193.

Czobor P, Volavka J, and Meibach RC (1995) Effect of risperidone on hostility in schizophrenia. J Clin Psychopharmacol 15, 243–249.

Dietch JT and Jennings RK (1988) Aggressive dyscontrol in patients treated with benzodiazepines. J Clin Psychiatr 49, 184–188.

Donovan SJ, Stewart JW, Nunes EV, et al. (2000) Divalproex treatment for youth with explosive temper and mood lability: A double-blind, placebo-controlled crossover design. Am J Psychiatr 157, 818–820.

Dose M, Apelt S, and Emrich HM (1987) Carbamazepine as an adjunct of antipsychotic therapy. Psychiatr Res 22, 303–310.

Ebrahim GM, Gibler B, Gacono CB, et al. (1994) Patient response to clozapine in a forensic psychiatric hospital. Hosp Comm Psychiatr 45, 271–273.

Eli Lilly Co. (2001) Briefing Document for Zyprexa Intramuscular (olanzapine for injection), FDA Psychopharmacological Drugs Advisory Committee (Jan 11) with Addendum (Feb 14). (Available at www.fda.gov)

Eronen M, Hakola P, and Tiihonen J (1996) Mental disorders and homicidal behavior in Finland. Arch Gen Psychiatr 53, 497–501.

Fink M and Sackeim HA (1996) Convulsive therapy in schizophrenia. Schizophr Bull 22, 27–39.

Frankle WG, Lafayette JL, Pollock AC, et al. (2001) Neuropsychological and diagnostic differences in schizophrenic outpatients with and without a history of violent criminal behavior. American College of Neuropsychopharmacology Annual Meeting (Dec), Hawaii.

Glazer WM and Dickson RA (1998) Clozapine reduces violence and persistent aggression in schizophrenia. J Clin Psychiatr 59(Suppl 3), 8–14.

Goldman MB and Janecek HM (1990) Adjunctive fluoxetine improves global function in chronic schizophrenia. J Neuropsychiatr Clin Neurosci 2, 429–431.

Goldney R, Bowes J, Spence N, et al. (1985) The psychiatric intensive care unit. Br J Psychiatr 146, 50–54.

Greenblatt DJ, Divoll M, Harmatz JS, et al. (1982) Pharmacokinetic comparison of sublingual lorazepam with intravenous, intramuscular, and oral lorazepam. J Pharm Sci 71, 248–252.

Greenblatt DJ, Shader RI, Franke K, et al. (1979) Pharmacokinetics and bioavailability of intravenous, intramuscular, and oral lorazepam in humans. J Pharm Sci 68, 57–63.

Hakola HP and Laulumaa VA (1982) Carbamazepine in treatment of violent schizophrenics (letter). Lancet 1, 1358.

Hare RD (1996) Psychopathy and antisocial personality disorder: A case of diagnostic confusion. Psychiatr Times (Feb), 39–40.

Hare RD and Hart SD (1993) Psychopathy, mental disorder, and crime. In Mental Disorder and Crime, Hodgins S (ed). Sage Publications, Newbury Park, pp. 104–115.

Hart SD, Cox DN, and Hare RD (1995) The Hare PCL: SV: Psychopathy Checklist: Screening Version. Multi-Health Systems, North Tonowanda, NY.

Hart SD, Hare RD, and Forth AE (1994) Psychopathy as a risk marker for violence: Development and validation of a screening version of the revised psychopathy checklist. In Violence and Mental Disorder, Developments in Risk Assessment, Monahan J and Steadman HJ (eds). The University of Chicago Press, Chicago, pp. 81–98.

Hart SD, Hare RD, and Harpur TJ (1992) The psychopathy checklist-revised (PCL-R): An overview for researchers and clinicians. In Advances in Psychological Assessment, Rosen JC and McReynolds P (eds). Plenum Press, New York, pp. 103–130.

Hesslinger B, Normann C, Langosch JM, et al. (1999) Effects of carbamazepine and valproate on haloperidol plasma levels and on psychopathological outcome in schizophrenic patients. J Clin Psychopharmacol 19, 310–315.

Hirose S, Ashby CR, and Mills MJ (2001) Effectiveness of ECT combined with risperidone against aggression in schizophrenia. J ECT 17, 22–26.

Hodgins S (1992) Mental disorder, intellectual deficiency, and crime: Evidence from a birth cohort. Arch Gen Psychiatr 49, 476–483.

Hodgins S, Mednick SA, Brennan PA, et al. (1996) Mental disorder and crime: Evidence from a Danish birth cohort. Arch Gen Psychiatr 53, 489–496.

Hollander E, Margolin L, Wong C, et al. (1998) Double-blind placebo trial of divalproex sodium in the treatment of borderline personality disorder (poster). 38th Annual Meeting NCDEU, Boca Raton, FL.

Hughes DH (1999) Acute psychopharmacological management of the aggressive psychotic patient. Psychiatr Serv 50, 1135–1137.

Karson C and Bigelow LB (1987) Violent behavior in schizophrenic inpatients. J Nerv Ment Dis 175, 161–164.

Karson CN, Weinberger DR, Bigelow L, et al. (1982) Clonazepam treatment of chronic schizophrenia: Negative results in a double-blind, placebo-controlled trial. Am J Psychiatr 139, 1627–1628.

Keckich WA (1978) Neuroleptics. Violence as a manifestation of akathisia. JAMA 240, 2185.

Kinon BJ, Roychowdhury SM, Milton DR, et al. (2001) Effective resolution with olanzapine of acute presentation of behavioral agitation and positive psychotic symptoms in schizophrenia. J Clin Psychiatr 62(Suppl 2), 17–21.

Krakowski M and Czobor P (1997) Violence in psychiatric patients: The role of psychosis, frontal lobe impairment, and ward turmoil. Compr Psychiatr 38, 230–236.

Krakowski M, Convit A, and Volavka J (1988) Patterns of inpatient assaultiveness: Effect of neurological impairment and deviant family environment on response to treatment. Neuropsychiatr Neuropsychol Behav Neurol 1, 21–29.

Krakowski MI, Convit A, Jaeger J, et al. (1989) Neurological impairment in violent schizophrenic inpatients. Am J Psychiatr 146, 849–853.

Kupchik M, Spivak B, Mester R, et al. (2000) Combined electroconvulsive-clozapine therapy. Clin Neuropharmacol 23, 14–16.

Kyriacou DN, Anglin D, Taliaferro E, et al. (1999) Risk factors for injury to women from domestic violence against women. NEJM 341, 1892–1898.

Lesem MD, Zajecka JM, Swift RH, et al. (2001) Intramuscular ziprasidone, 2 mg versus 10 mg, in the short-term management of agitated psychotic patients. J Clin Psychiatr 62, 12–18.

Lindenmayer JP and Kotsaftis A (2000) Use of sodium valproate in violent and aggressive behaviors: A critical review. J Clin Psychiatr 61, 123–128.

Link BG and Stueve A (1994) Psychotic symptoms and the violent/illegal behavior of mental patients compared to community controls. In Violence and Mental Disorder. Developments in Risk Assessment,

Monahan J and Steadman HJ (eds). The University of Chicago Press, Chicago, pp. 137–159.

Link BG, Cullen FT, and Andrews H (1992) The violent and illegal behavior of mental patients reconsidered. Am Sociol Rev 57, 275–292.

Link BG, Stueve A, and Phelan J (1998) Psychotic symptoms and violent behaviors: Probing the components of "threat/control-override" symptoms. Soc Psychiatr Psychiatr Epidemiol 33(Suppl 1), S55–S60.

Lischke V, Behne M, Doelken P, et al. (1994) Droperidol causes a dose-dependent prolongation of the QT interval. Anesth Analg 79, 983–986.

Littrell KH, Petty RG, Hilligoss NM, et al. (2001) Divalproex sodium for hostility in schizophrenia patients (poster). 41st Annual Meeting NCDEU, Phoenix, Arizona.

Luchins DJ (1984) Carbamazepine in violent nonepileptic schizophrenics. Psychopharmacol Bull 20, 569–571.

Maier GJ (1992) The impact of clozapine on 25 forensic patients. Bull Am Acad Psychiatry Law 20, 297–307.

Maier GJ, Stava LJ, Morrow BR, et al. (1987) A model for understanding and managing cycles of aggression among psychiatric inpatients. Hosp Comm Psychiatr 38, 520–524.

Mallya AR, Roos PD, and Roebuck-Colgan K (1992) Restraint, seclusion, and clozapine. J Clin Psychiatr 53, 395–397.

Musisi SM, Wasylenki DA, and Rapp MS (1989) A psychiatric intensive care unit in a psychiatric hospital. Can J Psychiatr 34, 200–204.

Neppe VM (1983) Carbamazepine as adjunctive treatment in nonepileptic chronic inpatients with EEG temporal lobe abnormalities. J Clin Psychiatr 44, 326–331.

Ng B, Kumar S, Ranclaud M, et al. (2001) Ward crowding and incidents of violence on an acute psychiatric inpatient unit. Psychiatr Serv 52, 521–525.

Nolan KA, Volavka J, Mohr P, et al. (1999) Psychopathy and violent behavior among patients with schizophrenia or schizoaffective disorder. Psychiatr Serv 50, 787–792.

Okuma T, Yamashita I, Takahashi R, et al. (1989) A double-blind study of adjunctive carbamazepine versus placebo on excited states of schizophrenic and schizoaffective disorders. Acta Psychiatr Scand 80, 250–259.

Owen C, Tarantello C, Jones M, et al. (1998) Violence and aggression in psychiatric units. Psychiatr Serv 49, 1452–1457.

Palmstierna T, Huitfeldt B, and Wistedt B (1991) The relationship of crowding and aggressive behavior on a psychiatric intensive care unit. Hosp Comm Psychiatr 42, 1237–1240.

Pastore AL and Maguire K (eds) (2000) Sourcebook for Criminal Justice Statistics. US Department of Justice, Bureau of Justice Statistics, Washington DC.

Pfizer (2001) Briefing Document for Ziprasidone Mesylate for Intramuscular Injection, FDA Psychopharmacological Drugs Advisory Committee (Feb 15). (Available at www.fda.gov)

Prakash R (1985) Lithium-responsive schizophrenia: Case reports. J Clin Psychiatr 46, 141–142.

Ratey JJ, Leveroni C, Kilmer D, et al. (1993) The effects of clozapine on severely aggressive psychiatric inpatients in a state hospital. J Clin Psychiatr 54, 219–223.

Ratey JJ, Sorgi P, O'Driscoll GA, et al. (1992) Nadolol to treat aggression and psychiatric symptomatology in chronic psychiatric inpatients: A double-blind, placebo-controlled study. J Clin Psychiatr 53, 41–46.

Reeves KR, Swift RH, and Harrigan EP (1998) Ziprasidone intramuscular 10 mg and 20 mg in acute agitation (poster NR494). American Psychiatric Association 151st Annual Meeting, Toronto, Canada.

Regier DA, Farmer ME, Rae DS, et al. (1990) Comorbidity of mental disorders with alcohol and other drug abuse. Results from the Epidemiologic Catchment Area (ECA) Study. JAMA 264, 2511–2518.

Ryback R and Ryback L (1995) Gabapentin for behavioral dyscontrol (letter). Am J Psychiatr 152, 1399.

Salzman C (1988) Use of benzodiazepines to control disruptive behavior in inpatients. J Clin Psychiatr 49(Suppl 12), 13–15.

Schaffer CB and Schaffer LC (1997) Gabapentin in the treatment of bipolar disorder (letter). Am J Psychiatr 154, 291–292.

Shalev A, Hermesh H, and Munitz H (1987) Severe akathisia causing neuroleptic failure: An indication for lithium therapy in schizophrenia? Acta Psychiatr Scand 76, 715–718.

Sheppard GP (1979) High-dose propranolol in schizophrenia. Br J Psychiatr 134, 470–476.

Silver H and Kushnir M (1998) Treatment of aggression in schizophrenia. Am J Psychiatr 155, 1298.

Simhandl C and Meszaros K (1992) The use of carbamazepine in the treatment of schizophrenic and schizoaffective psychoses: A review. J Psychiatr Neurosci 17, 1–14.

Siris SG (1985) Three cases of akathisia and "acting out." J Clin Psychiatr 46, 395–397.

Spivak B, Mester R, Wittenberg N, et al. (1997) Reduction of aggressiveness and impulsiveness during clozapine treatment in chronic neuroleptic-resistant schizophrenic patients. Clin Neuropharmacol 20, 442–446.

Steadman HJ, Mulvey EP, Monahan J, et al. (1998) Violence by people discharged from acute psychiatric inpatient facilities and others in the same neighborhoods. Arch Gen Psychiatr 55, 393–401.

Swanson JW (1994) Mental disorder, substance abuse, and community violence: An epidemiological approach. In Violence and Mental Disorder. Developments in Risk Assessment, Monahan J and Steadman HJ (eds). The University of Chicago Press, Chicago, pp. 101–136.

Swartz MS, Swanson JW, Hiday VA, et al. (1998) Violence and severe mental illness: The effects of substance abuse and nonadherence to medication. Am J Psychiatr 155, 226–231.

Tanke ED and Yesavage JA (1985) Characteristics of assaultive patients who do and do not provide visible cues of potential violence. Am J Psychiatr 142, 1409–1413.

Tardiff K and Sweillam A (1982) Assaultive behavior among chronic inpatients. Am J Psychiatr 139, 212–215.

Thomas H, Schwartz E, and Petrilli R (1992) Droperidol versus haloperidol for chemical restraint of agitated and combative patients. Ann Emerg Med 21, 407–413.

Tiihonen J, Hallikainen T, Ryynanen OP, et al. (2002) Lamotrigine in treatment-resistant schizophrenia: A randomized placebo-controlled trial (presentation). 43rd Annual and 2nd Mediterranean Meeting of the Scandinavian College of Neuro-Psychopharmacology (Apr), Juan-les-Pins, France.

Tiihonen J, Isohanni M, Rasanen P, et al. (1997) Specific major mental disorders and criminality: A 26-year prospective study of the 1966 Northern Finland birth cohort. Am J Psychiatr 154, 840–845.

Van Rybroek GJ, Kuhlman TL, Maier GJ, et al. (1987) Preventive aggression devices (PADS): Ambulatory restraints as an alternative to seclusion. J Clin Psychiatr 48, 401–405.

Vartiainen H, Tiihonen J, Putkonen A, et al. (1995) Citalopram, a selective serotonin reuptake inhibitor, in the treatment of aggression in schizophrenia. Acta Psychiatr Scand 91, 348–351.

Volavka J (2002) Neurobiology of Violence, 2nd ed. American Psychiatric Publishing, Washington DC.

Volavka J and Citrome L (1999) Atypical antipsychotics in the treatment of the persistently aggressive psychotic patient: Methodological concerns. Schizophr Res 35, S23–S33.

Volavka J and Krakowski M (1989) Schizophrenia and violence. Psychol Med 19, 559–562.

Volavka J, Laska E, Baker S, et al. (1997) History of violent behavior and schizophrenia in different cultures. Br J Psychiatr 171, 9–14.

Volavka J, Zito JM, Vitrai J, et al. (1993) Clozapine effects on hostility and aggression in schizophrenia. J Clin Psychopharmacol 13, 287–289.

Wallace C, Mullen P, Burgess P, et al. (1998) Serious criminal offending and mental disorder. Br J Psychiatr 172, 477–484.

Warneke L (1986) A psychiatric intensive care unit in a general hospital setting. Can J Psychiatr 31(9), 834–837.

Wilson WH and Claussen AM (1995) Eighteen-month outcome of clozapine treatment for 100 patients in a state psychiatric hospital. Psychiatr Serv 46, 386–389.

Wright P, Birkett M, David SR, et al. (2001) Double-blind, placebo-controlled comparison of intramuscular olanzapine and intramuscular haloperidol in the treatment of acute agitation in schizophrenia. Am J Psychiatr 158, 1149–1151.

Yassa R and Dupont D (1983) Carbamazepine in the treatment of aggressive behavior in schizophrenic patients: A case report. Can J Psychiatr 28, 566–568.

Young JL and Hillbrand M (1994) Carbamazepine lowers aggression: A review. Bull Am Acad Psychiatr Law 22, 53–61.

Yudofsky S, Williams D, and Gorman J (1981) Propranolol in the treatment of rage and violent behavior in patients with chronic brain syndrome. Am J Psychiatr 138, 218–220.

Yudofsky SC, Stevens L, Silver JM, et al. (1984) Propranolol in the treatment of rage and violent behavior associated with Korsakoff's psychosis. Am J Psychiatr 141, 114–115.

# 104    Complementary and Alternative Treatments in Psychiatry

Richard P. Brown
Patricia L. Gerbarg
Philip R. Muskin

The growth of complementary and alternative medicine (CAM) is driven by a variety of influences, including consumers who are increasingly leery of medication side effects, scientists exploring the clinical potential of traditional herbal treatments, and psychosocial factors. Many of the medicines used today derive from botanicals known to herbalists for centuries. Alternative medicine is based on the gradual restoration of physiological balance, rather than the "treatment" of illness. CAM thus encompasses prevention, optimal nutrition, exercise, and balancing of work and play (Muskin 2000, De Smet 2002). CAM treatments are particularly useful for patients who have incomplete responses or undesirable side effects with prescription medications. Overall, alternative compounds have far fewer side effects and can often augment the action of standard treatments. On the other hand, misuse of natural medicines and contaminants in unregulated herbal preparations can cause serious health hazards (Ko 1998, Lightfoote et al. 1977, Schaumburg and Berger 1992, De Smet 2002) and herb/drug interactions. In Germany, oversight by the Commission E (equivalent to the US Food and Drug Administration, FDA) promotes higher quality research, production, and public information. The German national health system pays for many herbal treatments. While concern is mounting about long-term side effects of psychotropics, many alternative agents have long-term health benefits in addition to their therapeutic action. Physicians need a working knowledge of the herbs their patients are taking in order to optimize the benefits and minimize the risks of CAM (Brown and Gerbarg 2000).

This chapter focuses on CAM treatments supported by scientific evidence for mechanisms of action, clinical trials demonstrating safety and efficacy, and observations of benefit from the authors' clinical experience. In some cases there is only a small amount of data available, but this should not deter physicians interested in exploring the widest range of therapeutic possibilities from considering these substances for appropriate patients. Rigorous controlled studies have been completed for many agents, but other potentially worthwhile compounds have not attracted the large research investments necessary to obtain FDA approval. As more clinicians discover the benefits of CAM, interest in supporting larger controlled studies will develop. Although CAM may include any treatment that is not used by the majority of allopathic physicians, this discussion will selectively cover treatments that have practical uses in psychiatry: herbs, nutrients, vitamins, nootropics, neurotherapy, and yogic breathing and meditation. The first section explores mood disorders, depression, anxiety, insomnia, migraine, and obesity. The second discusses hormonal disorders, premenstrual dysphoric disorder (PMDD or PMS), menopause, sexual dysfunction, and benign prostatic hypertrophy. The third reviews disorders of attention, memory, and cognition: age associated memory impairment (AAMI), Alzheimer's (AD) and other dementias, ischemia, stroke, traumatic brain injury (TBI), and attention deficit disorder (ADD). Problems of quality control, product variability, side effects, and drug interactions will be addressed. Guidelines for safely using reliable products are provided (Tables 104–1 to 104–4).

## Mood Disorders

### St. John's Wort (*Hypericum perforatum*)

In the US, St. John's wort (SJW) became popular after publication of a 1996 meta-analysis of 23 randomized depression trials (Linde et al. 1996) in which 13 studies showed that 55% of patients on SJW improved compared to 22% on placebo, with a side effect rate similar to placebo. In three studies, SJW (300 mg t.i.d. of 0.3% standard hypericin) was as effective as low dose tricyclics (amitriptyline 30 mg q.i.d. or imipramine 75 mg/day). Limitations of the studies in the 1996 meta-analysis include vague definitions of depression, less rigorous methodology, unclear outcome measures, low

| Table 104–1 | Treatment Guidelines for Disorders of Mood, Sleep, Migraine, and Obesity | | |
|---|---|---|---|
| **Alternative Agent** | **Clinical Uses** | **Dose** | **Side Effects and Drug Interactions** |
| St. John's wort (*Hypericum perforatum*) | Depression mild–mod | 300 mg t.i.d. | Nausea, heartburn, loose bowels, jitteriness, insomnia, fatigue, bruxism, phototoxic rash, mania in bipolar. Affects CYP 450 and Pgp: ↓ digoxin, warfarin, indivir, cyclosporine, theophyline, birth control pills. D/C: surgery, pregnancy |
| S-adenosyl-L-methionine (SAMe) | Depression Arthritis, fibromyalgia, Parkinson's Liver diseases | 400–1,600 mg/d 800–1,200 mg/d 1,600–4,800 mg/d 1,200–1,600 mg/d | Mild nausea, loose bowels, activation, anxiety, mania in bipolar, headache, occasional palpitations |
| *Rhodiola rosea* | Depression | 150 mg t.i.d. | Agitation, insomnia, anxiety |
| B-vitamins and Bio-Strath | Depression | $B_{12}$ 1,000 µg/d B-complex | None |
| Inositol | Depression | 12–20 g/d | Gas, loose bowels, noncompliance |
| Omega-3 fatty acids | Bipolar | 6–10 g/d | Belching, loose stools |
| Choline | Mania | 2,000–7,200 mg/d | None |
| Kava (*Piper methysticum*) | Anxiety, insomnia | 100 mg standardized extract t.i.d. (70 mg kavalactones t.i.d.) | GI, allergic skin, headache, photosensitivity. Occasional ↓ energy, drowsiness, tremor, restlessness ↓ effects of levodopa, hepatitis, Toxic > 240 kavalactones/d D/C: pregnancy |
| Passionflower (*Passiflora incarnata*) | Anxiety | | Little scientific evidence of efficacy |
| Chamomile (*Matricareia recutita*) | Minimal sedative | | Little scientific evidence of efficacy. Ragweed family—allergic reactions. D/C: pregnancy |
| Lemon balm (*Melissa officianalis*) | Anxiety | | No serious side effects Little scientific evidence of efficacy |
| Garum Amoricum | Anxiety | 2–3 pills/d | None |
| Valerian (*Valerian officianalis*) | Sleep | 450–900 mg h.s. | Occasional GI, headaches, minimal hangover on high doses > 600 mg. D/C: pregnancy, hepatic disease |
| Melatonin | Sleep | 1–12 mg h.s. | Occasional agitation, abdominal cramps, fatigue, dizziness, headache, vivid dreams. D/C: pregnancy |
| Feverfew (*Tanacetum parthenium*) | Migraine | 100–200 mg/d | Contact dermatitis, GI, ↑ bleeding time. Avoid with warfarin. D/C: surgery, pregnancy |
| Butterbur root (*Petasites hybridus*) | Migraine | Petadolex 50 mg b.i.d. | None D/C: pregnancy |
| Chromium picolinate | Weight loss | 400–600 µg/d | Occasional changes in blood sugar. Recheck BS in diabetics. D/C: surgery |
| Ephedrine/caffeine | Weight loss | | Agitation, anxiety, tachycardia, arrhythmias, addiction, GI. Avoid with asthma meds, psychosis, prostate disease. D/C: surgery |

doses of the comparison antidepressants, and short length of trials. A 1999 meta-analysis using more stringent criteria concluded that SJW was similar in efficacy to low dose TCAs in treatment of mild to moderate major depression (Kim et al. 1999). Another review found evidence that SJW yielded higher rates of improvement than placebo but lower rates than TCAs, even at suboptimal starting doses (Gaster and Holroyd 2000).

A randomized 6-week study of 240 patients with mild to moderate depression found SJW (Remotiv or ZE 117) 500 mg/day to be comparable in efficacy to fluoxetine 20 mg/day based on Hamilton Depression Scale (Ham-D) and anxiety scores (Shrader 2000). In an open series, 111 menopausal women given SJW 900 mg/day for 12 weeks improved significantly in self-esteem, feeling attractive, irritability, anxiety, and depression. Psychosomatic symptoms (insomnia, headache, and palpitations), vasomotor symptoms (sweating, flushing, and dizziness), and sexual desire also improved (Grube et al. 1999). These findings warrant more rigorous study.

In a 6-week double-blind, randomized, multicenter (DBRMC) trial, Vorbach and colleagues (1997) compared 209 hospitalized patients with severe major depression given either hypericum LI 160 (Kira) (a standardized preparation of SJW) 600 mg t.i.d. or imipramine 150 mg/day. Ham-D at the end of the trial were similar for both groups; clinical global impression (CGI) showed 61% improvement on SJW and 70% on imipramine. There were fewer side effects in the SJW group. These data showed that higher doses of SJW (1,800 mg/day) are necessary to treat moderate to severe depression and that the response takes longer (6–12 weeks) than with imipramine (3–6 weeks) (Vorbach et al. 1997).

JAMA recently published a double-blind, randomized, placebo control, multicenter (DBRPCMC) study of 20 patients with major depression given either placebo or 900 mg/day Kira. This study contained serious methodological flaws. After 4 weeks the nonresponders were given 1,200 mg/day Kira for 4 more weeks. The study concluded that Kira was no better than placebo (Shelton et al. 2001).

| Table 104–2 | Treatment Guidelines for Hormonal Conditions and Sexual Disorders | | |
|---|---|---|---|
| Alternative Agent | Clinical Uses | Dose | Side Effects and Drug Interactions |
| Evening primrose oil (*Oneothera Biennes*) | PMS | | GI, headaches. No evidence of efficacy. ↑ risk seizures with phenothiazines |
| Magnesium | PMS | 360 mg/d | |
| Calcium | PMS | 600 mg b.i.d. | Mild GI. Take with meals to avoid stone formation |
| B-vitamins, Minerals | PMS | | Limited information. No side effects |
| Carbohydrate | PMS | PMS Escape | Study needs replication |
| L-tryptophan | PMDD | 2,000 mg t.i.d. | Pharmaceutical grade by prescription only is safe |
| Chaste tree, chasteberry (*Vitex agnus-castus*) | PMS, menopause, female infertility, hyperprolactinemia | 40 mg/d standardized extract | No significant side effects. Rarely: allergic reaction, dry mouth, headache, nausea. D/C: pregnancy |
| Soy | Hot flashes | 20–60 g/d | Best results with whole soy or whole food |
| Red clover (*Trifolium pratense*) | Menopausal sxs, estrogenic effects | 500 mg/d, 40 mg isoflavones | No adequate scientific evidence of efficacy. D/C: pregnancy, bleeding disorders, estrogen-sensitive tumors |
| Black cohosh (*Cimifuga racemosa*) | Menopausal sxs, hot flushes, PMS, dysmenorrhea | 8 mg/d standardized extract | High level of safety. Minimal side effects: GI, ↓ BP, headache, dizziness. D/C: pregnancy, estrogen sensitive tumors, antihypertensive meds |
| Licorice (*Glycyrrhiza glabra*) | Adrenocortical steroid type effect | | Headache, lethargy, sodium and water retention, potassium depletion, hypertension. D/C: diuretics |
| Dong Quai (*Angelica sinensis*) | Menopausal sxs | | Rigorous studies needed. Used in combination with other herbs. Photosensitivity. D/C: anticoagulants |
| Hops (*Humulus lupulus*) | Estrogenic effects | | Inadequate evidence of efficacy. Allergic reactions. May affect CYP450. Fatigue. D/C: pregnancy |
| Blue cohosh (*Caulophyllum thalictroides*) | Menopausal sxs | | No adequate scientific studies. May interact with antihypertensive meds |
| Dihydoepiandosterone (DHEA) | Menopause, osteoporosis | 25–100 mg/d | More studies are needed |
| Skullcap (*Scutellaria lateriflora*) | | | No adequate studies. Possible adverse effects on liver function. Avoid with hepatic insufficiency |
| *Rhodiola rosea* | Menopause, amenorrhea | 450 600 mg/d | Activation, anxiety, insomnia, vivid dreams |
| Saw palmetto (*Serenoa repens*) | BPH | 320 mg/d | Mild occasional GI, constipation, loose stools |
| Pygeum (*Pygeum africanum*) | BPH | 75–150 mg/d | None reported |
| Stinging nettle (*Urtica dioica*) | BPH | 300 mg/d | Mild GI, allergic reactions. May ↑ effects of diuretic and antihypertensive meds |
| Yohimbine (*Pausinystalia yohimbe*) | Erectile dysfunction | 18–42 mg/d | Anxiety, dizziness, chills, headache, ↑ BP, ↑ heart rate, insomnia, bronchospasm, nausea, vomiting. D/C: HT, cardiac, renal, liver disease, psychotropic meds |
| Asian ginseng (*Panax Ginseng*) | Erectile dysfunction | 100 mg t.i.d. | Insomnia, GI, mania, abuse potential. D/C: MAOIs, hypoglycemic meds, pregnancy |
| Ginkgo biloba | Erectile dysfunction | 120 mg b.i.d. | GI. D/C: anticoagulants, pregnancy |
| Arginine | Erectile dysfunction | | May predispose to herpes |
| Muira Puama (*Ptychopetalium guyanna*) | ↑ libido, erections, arousal, orgasm in men and women | 1,000–1,500 mg/d | Promising. Needs further study. Works best in combination with ginkgo and other sexual enhancers. |
| Maca (*Lepidium myenii*) | ↑ erections, menopause, fertility | 6 pills/d | No toxicity. D/C: estrogen sensitive tumors, endometriosis, prostate cancer |

PMS, premenstrual syndrome; PMDD, premenstrual dysphoric disorder; BPH, benign prostatic hypertrophy; GI, gastrointestinal side effects; BP, blood pressure; HT, hypertension.

The dose of Kira was low. Vorbach's study had shown that 1,800 mg/day Kira was equivalent to 150 mg/day imipramine, that is, the necessary dose for major depression (Vorbach et al. 1997). Furthermore, the expected placebo response rate in most depression studies is between 30 and 50%. The low placebo response rate of 19% in the Shelton study suggests selection of extremely depressed, resistant patients or an artifact of negative expectations.

Similar research design flaws impacted a DBRPCMC NIH (National Institute of Health) study in which severely depressed patients (Ham-D ≥ 20) were given subtherapeutic doses of SJW (900–1,500 mg/day), subtherapeutic doses of sertraline (50–100 mg/day), or placebo. In this study, neither sertraline nor SJW outperformed placebo (Davidson et al. 2002).

Two DBRPC studies suggest that clinical response rates and changes in brain wave activity are related to the concentration of "hyperforin", not "hypericin" (Muller et al. 1998, Schellenberg et al. 1998). SJW is effective in 50 to 70% of patients with mild depression, particularly if wintertime

| Table 104–3 | Treatment Guidelines for Cognitive Enhancers | | |
| --- | --- | --- | --- |
| Alternative Agent | Clinical Uses | Dose | Side Effects and Drug Interactions |
| Galantamine | AD | 16–32 mg/d | Mild nausea, GI |
| Huperzine | AD, TBI | 100–400 μg/d | Rare: mild nausea |
| Centrophenoxine | AD, TBI | 500–2,000 mg/d | Minimal. When combined with other cholinergic agents: headache, muscle tension, insomnia, irritability, agitation, facial tics |
| Acetyl-L-carnitine | AD—slowed progression, TBI and CVA | 1,500 mg b.i.d. | Mild gastric upset. Take with food. |
| CDP-choline | TBI | 1,000–2,000 mg/d | None significant |
| S-adenosyl-L-methionine (SAMe) | AD, dementia, TBI Parkinson's | 800–1,600 mg/d 400–4,000 mg/d | Mild occasional GI, agitation, anxiety, insomnia; rare palpitations. Mania in bipolars. Take 30 min before breakfast and lunch |
| Picamilon | TBI, CVA, toxic brain lesions | 50 mg b.i.d.–up to 100 mg t.i.d. | High dose: hypotension. No allergenic, carcinogenic or teratogenic in 6-month test. |
| Pyritinol | CVD, AD, TBI | 900–1,200 mg/d | Minimal, skin reactions, rare allergic reactions |
| Idebenone | CVD, AD, TBI | 270–900 mg/d | GI, anxiety, insomnia, headache, tachycardia, ↓ platelet aggregation |
| Vinpocetine | CVD, TBI | 10 mg t.i.d. | Rare: nausea, low BP |
| *Rhodiola rosea* | Cognitive enhancement, memory TBI | 150–600 mg/d | Activation, agitation, insomnia, jitteriness, mania. Rare: ↑BP, angina, bruising. Avoid in bipolar I. Take 20 minutes before breakfast and lunch. |
| *Ginkgo biloba* | AAMI, AD CVD | 120–240 mg/d | Minimal, headache, ↓ platelet aggregation |
| Ginseng | Dementia, neurasthenia | 400–800 mg/d | Activation |
| Kava (*Piper methysticum*) | Anxiety | 70–140 mg/d kava lactones | Sedation, dependency, hepatitis. Can be toxic at doses > 240 mg/d |
| Racetams | Poststroke aphasia, dyslexia | Pramiracetam ≥ 600 b.i.d. | Minimal. Rarely: anxiety, insomnia, agitation, irritability, headache |
| L-deprenyl | TBI | 10–15 mg/wk | Take 2.5 mg 5 days a week. Higher doses > 10 mg/d may cause MAOI effects |
| B-vitamins, Bio-Strath | TBI | B$_{12}$ 1,000 μg/d B-complex | None |

AD, Alzheimer's disease; TBI, traumatic brain injury; CVA, cerebrovascular accident; CVD, cerebrovascular disease; BP, blood pressure; GI, gastrointestinal side effects.

seasonal affective disorder (SAD) is present (Cott and Fugh-Berman 1998, Hansgen et al. 1994, Wheatley 1999).

The "side-effect profile" of SJW at higher doses is similar to the selective serotonin reuptake inhibitors (SSRIs). Common side effects with SJW are nausea, heartburn, loose bowels, jitteriness, insomnia, and fatigue. High doses may cause sexual dysfunction and bruxism. Phototoxic rash occurs in less that 1% of people taking the usual dose (900 mg/day) but may be more frequent at higher doses. Nierenberg and colleagues (1999) reported four possible cases of SJW-induced mania in bipolars. SJW causes slight inhibition of reuptake of serotonin (5-HT), norepinephrine (NE), and dopamine (DA) (Muller et al. 1998), and a change in monocyte cytokine production of interleukin 6 (leading to decreased corticotrophin-releasing hormone) (Thiele et al. 1994). There is evidence of down regulation of beta-adrenergic receptors, increases in serotonin 2 and 1A subtype receptor density (Teufel-Mayer and Gleitz 1997), and *in vitro* binding to GABA-A and -B receptors (Cott 1997). Preclinical studies suggest a serotonin mechanism for SJW, raising the possibility of mild serotonin syndrome with other serotonin-inducing psychotropics, especially in the elderly. By June 2000, six such cases were reported with SJW in combination with both SSRIs and nefazodone (Anonymous 2000, Gelenberg 2000), but the effect of SJW is so weak that other factors were more likely to have been causative (DeMott 1998).

St. John's wort has serious medication interactions. Digoxin levels decreased by 28% in healthy volunteers given SJW versus a 9% drop in the placebo group (Jonte et al. 1999). Researchers hypothesize that SJW induces cytochrome P450 3A4 and 1A2 and induces intestinal wall P-glycoprotein resulting in gut loss of digoxin. SJW can lower levels of warfarin, HIV protease inhibitors, and reverse transcriptase inhibitors (Piscitelli et al. 2000, Ruschitzka et al. 2000). SJW's ability to induce hepatic enzymes can result in lower levels of cyclosporine (which has caused transplant rejection), theophylline, and other drugs. Breakthrough bleeding has been reported in women on birth control pills who take SJW. Anesthesiologists anecdotally report changes in heart rate and blood pressure, particularly in patients taking SJW, ginkgo, and ginseng. These herbs should be discontinued 2 to 3 weeks before surgery (Voelker 1999). It is an important part of the patient–physician relationship to explore patients' use of CAM therapies. An open-minded approach will augment the relationship and reveal potentially problematic herb–drug interactions.

Most independent analyses of SJW brands report the amount of hypericin and/or hyperforin, but do not test for quality or activity. Although a concentration of hypericin 0.3% of the extract is the usual standard, the measurement of hyperforin 0.3 to 0.5% may be more relevant. Independent testing of SJW brands by ConsumerLab.com found

| Compound | Brand/Company | Source |
|---|---|---|
| Centrophenoxine | Lucidril/International Antiaging Systems (IAS) | www.antiaging-systems.com<br>Fax: 011-44-870-151-4145 |
| L-deprenyl | Jumex tabs, Cyprenil (liquid)/IAS<br>Deprenyl, Selegeline, Eldepryl | By prescription from US pharmacies |
| Picamilon | IAS | |
| Nicergoline | IAS | |
| Piracetam (all racetams) | IAS | |
| Acetyl-L-carnitine | Life Extension Foundation (LEF) | 800-544-4440 www.lef.org |
| α-lipoic acid | LEF; Intensive Nutrition | 800-333-7414 www.sciconsvc.com |
| CDP-choline | Smart Nutrition (SN); LEF | 800-479-2107 www.smart-nutrition.net |
| Pyritinol | SN | |
| Idebenone | SN; Thorne Research | 800-932-2953 (Thorne) |
| Vinpocetine | LEF; SN; Intensive Nutrition | |
| SAMe | SAM/Nature Made<br>Donamet/IAS | 800-276-2878 www.naturemade.com |
| Huperzine-A | General Nutrition Centers (GNC) | |
| Galantamine/Rhodiola | Ameriden International A/P Formula | Ameriden 888-405-3336 www.ameriden.com |
| Rhodiola rosea | Rosavin™ Ameriden International | |
| Ginkgo | Ginkgold/Nature's Way<br>Ginkoba/Pharmaton | Health food stores, pharmacies |
| Ginseng (Panax/Korean) | Hsu's Ginseng<br>Power Max 4x/Action Labs | 800-388-3818 www.hsuginseng<br>800-932-2953 |
| Ashwagandha | Swedish Herbal Institute | 800-774-9444 |
| Student Rasayana MA-SR | Maharishi Ayur Ved | 800-255-8332 www.mapi.com |
| Kava | Standard Extract/Nature's Way<br>Kava Power/Natures Herbs<br>Kavatrol/Natrol | Health food stores |
| Hydergine | Hydergine | By prescription from US pharmacies |
| B-vitamins | Bio-Strath/Nature's Answer | 800-681-7099 or health food stores |

**Table 104-4   How to Obtain Quality Alternative Compounds***

*The information in this table was compiled with the best knowledge available at the time of publication, but in this field, where more evidence-based research is needed, some of these recommendations and sources are particularly prone to change.

that 14 out of 21 met their requirements for having the amount of active compound claimed on product labels and a minimal amount of cadmium (a carcinogenic contaminant) (ConsumerLab.com 2001). Another independent study by www.vitacost.com found that only two out of eight brands contained adequate hyperforin (Schardt 2000). Double-blind, placebo-controlled (DBPC) clinical trials and studies showing activity *in vitro* for particular products provide more compelling evidence of efficacy. In January 2000, the Boston Globe sent brands of SJW to two labs for testing. Two of the brands, Quanterra and Nature Made, showed significant ability to block serotonin reuptake in animal cells *in vitro*. Research trials have shown Kira (LI 160) and Remotiv (ZE 117) to be effective. In the author's clinical experience Natures Way Standardized Extract (Perika), Kira, Quanterra, and Nature Made are reliable SJW brands.

## S-Adenosyl-L-Methionine, (SAMe), Adometionine, AdoMet

SAMe has been widely used in Europe for over 20 years. It has primarily been used for treatment of depression arthritis, and liver disease, and has been tested in more than 80 clinical trials involving over 24,000 people. It was approved

as a nutraceutical by the FDA in 1998. SAMe is a prescription medication in some countries and is sold over-the-counter in others. Knowledge of the biochemistry of SAMe is necessary to understand its multiple therapeutic effects. The US Department of Health and Human Services Agency for Healthcare Research and Quality recently published an Evidence Report/Technology Assessment (2002) based on a search of 25 biomedical databases. The report concluded that treatment with SAMe was equivalent to standard pharmacotherapy for depression and osteoarthritis. It was not possible to pool the data on liver disease because the studies were too diverse. However, SAMe was found to be more effective than placebo in reducing bilirubin and pruritis in intrahepatic cholestasis and cholestasis of pregnancy.

### Biochemistry

SAMe is a physiologically essential molecule in all living cells (Figure 104–1). The human diet supplies only part of the body's needs for SAMe. SAMe is generated by *de novo* synthesis from methionine and (ATP) adenosine triphosphate; the liver is the largest producer (3 g/day). Oral SAMe supplementation is the easiest way to boost SAMe levels. Though it is most concentrated in the brain and liver,

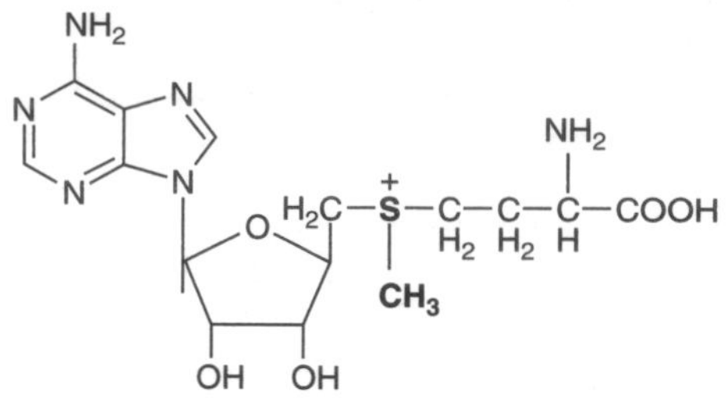

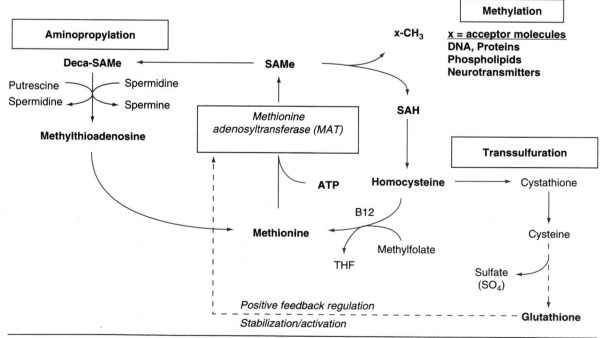

**Figure 104–1** *Chemical structure of S-adenosyl-L-methionine.*

SAMe is an active metabolite in all tissues of the body and is essential to three central metabolic pathways involving more than 100 different biochemical reactions (Figure 104–2): *transmethylation* (donation of methyl groups, $CH_3$), *transsulfuration* (donation of sulfur), and *transaminopropylation* (donation of aminopropyl moieties).

Transmethylation increases 5-HT, DA, and NE levels (Otero-Losada and Rubio 1989a, 1989b), probably contributing to the antidepressant action of SAMe (Curcio et al. 1978, Czyrak et al. 1992, Fava et al. 1990). Donation of methyl groups protects catecholamine neurons. SAMe improves nerve cell membrane uptake of phospholipids for a more fluid lipid bilayer, enabling the coupling of protein receptors to second messengers and enhancing transmission of impulses by neurons (Bottiglieri 1997). Methyl groups also protect DNA from attack by carcinogens and reduce levels of homocysteine (Finkelstein 1998), a major risk factor for heart attack and stroke. SAMe is crucial for synthesis of the most important antioxidant, glutathione, as well as the secondary antioxidants, cysteine and taurine (Colell et al. 1997, Evans et al. 1997). Through the transsulfuration pathway, SAMe stimulates proteoglycan synthesis for cartilage regeneration in arthritis (Barcelo et al. 1987). Transsulfuration and aminopropylation (generation of polyamines) contribute to analgesic properties, anti-inflammatory action, and protection of gastrointestinal mucosa.

When SAMe was discovered in 1952 (Cantoni 1952), there was no stable oral preparation (Stramentinoli 1987). Early studies, therefore, used i.v. and i.m. formulations. The first clinical study demonstrating antidepressant effects was published in 1976 (Agnoli et al. 1976). Improvements in SAMe over the past 40 years have made available more stable preparations, resistant to oxidation and gastric enzyme degradation (enteric coated, with demonstrated bioavailability and clinical efficacy). Lower than normal levels of SAMe are found in cerebral spinal fluid in some patients with depression, AD, dementia, Parkinson's disease treated with levodopa, disorders of folate metabolism, and other illnesses (Bottiglieri et al. 1990, Bottiglieri and Hyland 1994).

SAMe has been found to be a safe and effective treatment for depression in 16 open uncontrolled trials (total 660 patients), 13 DBRPC trials (total 535 patients), and 19 controlled DB trials, comparing it to other antidepressants including imipramine, amitriptyline, clorimipramine, nomifensine, minaprine, and desipramine (total 1,134 patients) (Bressa 1994, Delle Chiale and Boissard 1997, Brown et al. 2000), and three trials using SAMe to augment response to imipramine (Berlanga et al. 1992, Friedel et al. 1989). All but one study showed that SAMe was more effective than placebo and equivalent to the comparison antidepressant for major depression. The only study that did not find SAMe superior to placebo was flawed by the use of an older unstable form of SAMe and by a high placebo response rate (Fava et al. 1992).

SAMe, S-adenosyl-L-methionine; SAH, S-adenosylhomocysteine; Deca-SAMe, decarboxylated SAMe; ATP, adenosine triphosphate; THF, tetrahydrofolate

**Figure 104–2** *SAMe: Central metabolic pathways.*

Two recent DBRMC controlled efficacy and safety trials (MC3 and MC4) compared SAMe with imipramine for major depression. Depression was evaluated by several measures including Ham-D (21-item) $\geq$ 18. MC3 treated 281 patients randomized to either SAMe 1,600 mg/day p.o. or imipramine 150 mg/day p.o. for 42 days. The MC4 study of 295 patients compared SAMe 400 mg/day i.m. to imipramine 150 mg/day p.o. for 28 days. In MC3 and MC4 the antidepressant effect of SAMe was equal to imipramine, but the SAMe treated group had far fewer side effects (Delle Chiale et al. 2000a, 2000b, Di Padova et al. 2000).

Some patients have a dramatic response to SAMe even after they have failed or been unable to tolerate prescription antidepressants (Bell et al. 1994, Criconia et al. 1994, De Vanna and Rigamonti 1992, Kagan et al. 1990, Rosenbaum et al. 1990), as the following case illustrates.

---

**Clinical Vignette 1**

Ms. Y, a vivacious, energetic 54-year-old investment advisor was treated for recurrent episodes of severe major depression during which she suffered from fatigue, amotivation, loss of appetite, loss of confidence, poor concentration and memory, difficulty working, and anhedonia. Although her depressions responded to fluoxetine and to paroxetine, she had intolerable side effects including sexual dysfunction, weight gain (25 pounds), teeth clenching, and jaw pain. She responded well to venlafaxine sustained release 150 mg b.i.d., but after 5 months her liver enzymes began to increase until the levels at 12 months were Alk Phos = 206, AST (SGOT) = 38, ALT (SGPT) = 130. She was reluctant to take SAMe while her medical doctor ruled out hepatitis and obtained a normal liver scan. The patient then agreed to reduce the Effexor to 75 mg/day and started SAMe 400 mg/day (fluoxetine). Four weeks later her LFTs were normal: Alk Phos − 146, AST − 28, ALT = 33. Depression recurred for 4 weeks and then resolved completely. She was maintained on Effexor-XR 75 mg/day and SAMe 400 mg/day with no side effects.

---

SAMe was successfully combined with psychoactive medications in a 6-month study that included 350 patients on tricyclic antidepressants (TCAs), 500 on benzodiazepines, 60 on monoamine oxidase inhibitors (MAOIs), 445 on anticonvulsants, and 18 alcoholic patients on antidepressants or anticonvulsants. No adverse effects were reported. Patients on SAMe/TCA combination responded in 7 to 10 days as compared to the 10- to 15-day period for TCA-only group. Forty-eight of the SAMe/imipramine patients improved on 30% lower doses of imipramine. In all cases, SAMe reversed or prevented the elevation of gamma-glutamyl-transpeptidase (GGT), an indicator of liver toxicity, that occurred in the patients taking MAOIs or anticonvulsants and in the alcoholic group (Torta et al. 1988). In a DBRPC study of 63 outpatients with moderate to severe major depression the imipramine/SAMe group improved more rapidly and reduced their benzodiazepine use in comparison to the imipramine/placebo group. By day 14, the groups were comparable (Berlanga et al. 1992). In over 300 patients with either "treatment-resistant depression" or "medication intolerance," the authors have used SAMe to

augment all categories of antidepressants with good response and without adverse reactions.

SAMe methylation pathways require $B_{12}$ and folate as cofactors (see Figure 104–2) (Crellin et al. 1993). Low levels of SAMe in cerebral spinal fluid, red cell folate deficiency, high homocysteine, and low monoamine metabolites (5-HT, NE, DA) were found in 24 out of 46 patients hospitalized for severe depression (Bottiglieri et al. 2000). The authors have found that $B_{12}$ (1,000 μg/day), folate (800–1,000 μg/day), and $B_6$ (50–100 mg/day) can enhance the antidepressant effect of SAMe.

In two well-designed, DBRPC studies, SAMe was rapidly effective in "postpartum depression" (Cerutti et al. 1993) and "postmenopausal depression" (Salmaggi et al. 1993). Depression in medically ill patients can be a comorbid disorder, a reaction to illness, or a result of physical illness or medication effects. Depression can exacerbate medical illness, impair recovery, and reduce the quality of life. In a 4-week open study, 48 patients with depression secondary to physical illnesses (40 were medically hospitalized) showed a 50% decrease in depression ratings and tolerated SAMe well (Criconia et al. 1994). Because SAMe has few side effects and no serious interactions with other medications, it is well suited for the medically ill patient. SAMe also provides therapeutic benefits in many rheumatologic, neurologic, and hepatic diseases.

Arthritis sufferers are prone to depression. Twelve clinical studies found that SAMe has anti-inflammatory and analgesic effects in osteoarthritis (Di Padova 1987). In seven comparison studies, the reduction in pain and inflammation with SAMe was equivalent to nonsteroidal anti-inflammatory drugs, but SAMe caused no gastrointestinal bleeding. In a Phase IV study, SAMe relieved arthritis symptoms in over 20,000 people with minimal side effects (Berger and Nowak 1987). Response usually requires 1,200 mg/day for 3 to 4 weeks in mild to moderate arthritis, and 2 to 4 months in severe osteoarthritis (Bradley et al. 1994). MRI studies documented that 400 to 1,200 mg/day SAMe accelerates cartilage regeneration after 3 months (Konig et al. 1995).

Psychiatrists treat fibromyalgia patients for pain and depression. In three DBPC trials and three case series, SAMe relieved fibromyalgia symptoms (Di Benedetto et al. 1993, Grassetto and Varatto 1994, Ianiello et al. 1994, Jacobsen et al. 1991, Tavoni et al. 1987, 1998). Thirty fibromyalgia patients randomized to SAMe 400 mg/day i.v. (equivalent to 800 mg p.o.) or placebo for 15 days showed improvement in pain and depression by day 7 with SAMe. There were no side effects (Tavoni et al. 1998).

In a DB crossover study, depression improved significantly in 8 out of 21 Parkinson's patients given SAMe (800 mg p.o. plus 200 mg/day i.m.) with minimal side effects (Carrieri et al. 1990). In an open series, depression significantly improved in 11 out of 13 Parkinson's patients given SAMe (1,600–4,800 mg/day p.o.). Coincidentally, dyskinesias improved in some cases (Di Rocco et al. 2000).

In patients with hepatic dysfunction, prescription antidepressants add to the metabolic burden on the liver. In contrast, studies show that SAMe improves liver function, reverses physical symptoms and biochemical markers (abnormal liver function tests) of alcoholic and infectious hepatitis and cirrhosis. It has also been used to dissolve gallstones (Frezza et al. 1990, Friedel et al. 1989, Lieber 1999, Mato et al. 1999, Milkiewicz et al. 1999, Osman et al. 1993). Mato and colleagues (1999) reported a 2-year, DBRPC study of 123 patients with alcohol-induced liver cirrhosis. In Childs Class A and B cases, SAMe 1,200 mg/ day p.o. increased the rate of survival and delayed liver transplantation (Mato et al. 1999). Preliminary studies support the use of SAMe for depression complicating alcohol and opiate withdrawal (Agricola et al. 1994). Methamphetamine depletes SAMe and dopamine levels in rat brain (Cooney et al. 1998). In several cases, one of the authors (RB) has used SAMe successfully to relieve post methamphetamine depression and drug craving.

Depression occurs in 30 to 50% of patients with human immunodeficiency virus (HIV). In an open pilot study, 15 HIV seropositive patients with major depression (mean Ham-D = 27 and mean BDI = 35) were treated with SAMe (median dose 400 mg b.i.d.) for 8 weeks. $B_{12}$ 1000 µg and folic acid 800 µg were also given daily. Significant clinical improvement occurred by week 4. At week 8 mean scores dropped significantly (mean Ham-D = 3 and mean BDI = 5) (Cergnul et al. 2001). SAMe is a promising new liver-friendly treatment for depression in patients with HIV.

In general, SAMe side effects are mild and usually transient: headaches, anxiety, agitation, insomnia, loose bowels, upset stomach and, occasionally, palpitations. SAMe does not cause weight gain or sexual dysfunction. SAMe is contraindicated in patients with a personal or family history of bipolar disorder because (like other antidepressants), SAMe can induce mania (Carney et al. 1987, 1989, Kagan et al. 1990, Lipinski et al. 1984, De Vanna and Rigamonti 1992).

There is no evidence that SAMe interacts with other drugs, affects cytochrome P450 metabolism, or displaces other drugs from protein binding. There are no clear cases of serotonin syndrome even when SAMe is combined with prescription antidepressants, including SSRIs and MAOIs. Nevertheless, until more information is available, SAMe and MAOIs should only be combined under close medical supervision. No teratogenic (Cozens et al. 1988) or mutagenic activity has been found *in vitro* or in animals (Pezzoli et al. 1987). The amount of SAMe passed to infants through breastfeeding is unknown. Infants normally have SAMe levels three to seven times higher than adult levels (Surtees and Hyland 1989). Therefore, an infant would probably not be harmed by the amount of SAMe in breast milk. Nevertheless (as with prescription antidepressants), no definitive prospective studies are available to rule out the possibility of adverse effects in infants.

Elevation of plasma homocysteine is an independent risk factor for vascular disease. In 70 patients with coronary artery disease (CAD) SAMe levels were low (Loehrer et al. 1996). Since SAMe induces the enzyme that detoxifies homocysteine, it may help protect vascular endothelium (Finkelstein 1998). A single 400 mg dose of oral SAMe did not raise homocysteine levels (Loehrer et al. 1997). Neither increase in plasma homocysteine occurred in patients given SAMe 800 mg i.v. nor was there any change in plasma homocysteine after 5 days of oral SAMe in doses up to 1,600 mg/day (Giulidori and Di Padova 2000).

The usual dosage of SAMe is 400 mg/day for minor depression and 800 to 1,600 mg/day for major depression. Higher doses may be needed for severe treatment-resistant depression and in neurological disorders such as Parkinson's disease. SAMe is best absorbed on an empty stomach. Starting with 200 mg 30 minutes before breakfast and 30 minutes before lunch minimizes the stimulation, which some patients report in the first few weeks of treatment. This can be switched to 400 mg before breakfast after a few days. The dose can be raised by 200 to 400 mg every 3 to 7 days. Patients notice an improvement in their energy level within 2 weeks. Starting with low doses and increasing more gradually in geriatric, medically ill, and anxious patients minimizes the risk of side effects. It is sometimes possible to treat a bipolar II patient whose mania is under good control with a mood stabilizer such as lithium or valproate by using lower starting doses (e.g., 100 mg o.d. or b.i.d.), smaller increases, and careful monitoring.

In the US, SAMe is available in 50, 100, 200, and 400 mg doses in three clinically effective formulations: butanedisulfonate, toluene, and tosylate. Some companies advertise 400 mg tablets, but the fine print on the package may list only 200 mg of SAMe. Check the product labels to find out which form of SAMe is being used and the exact amount of S-adenosyl-L-methionine in each tablet. SAMe tablets should be odorless. A review in the December 2000 issue of Consumer Reports noted that several companies are improving their products and labeling. ConsumerLab. com, a good source of up-to-date information, independently tested 13 brands of SAMe: only seven contained the amount of compound advertised on the label (Consumerlab.com Nov 11, 2001). Nonresponse to an appropriate dose of SAMe or the occurrence of excessive side effects are usually due to the use of a poor quality brand. Adding folate and B-vitamins often improve response.

Most depressed patients take antidepressants for long periods of time. Concern is growing about whether prescription antidepressants can have long-term side effects (Taylor and Randall 1975, Torta et al. 1988). SAMe appears to have beneficial long-term effects on diseases of aging as well as increasing antioxidants, protecting DNA, and maintaining cell membrane health. Evidence indicates that 800 to 1,600 mg/day of SAMe is as effective for major depression as TCAs, with faster onset of action and fewer side effects. Unfortunately, patients who seek supervision for SAMe treatment are too often discouraged by a physician's refusal to do an SAMe trial. Physicians should become knowledgeable about SAMe in order to advise patients on its use to augment antidepressant treatment or as an alternative to traditional pharmacotherapy. Further research is needed to clarify SAMe's role as a first-line treatment in affective disorders (Brown et al. 2000).

## Rhodiola Rosea

The section on cognitive enhancement contains a complete discussion of *Rhodiola rosea*. *R. rosea* increases 5-HT, increases transport of tryptophan and 5-HT into the brain (Saratikov and Krasnov 1987c), and may reduce the breakdown of 5-HT by carboxy-O-methyl transferase (COMT) inhibition. One hundred and twenty-eight depressed patients were given 150 mg t.i.d. *R. rosea* or placebo. Two-thirds of those on *R. rosea* improved significantly (Brichenko and

Skorokhova 1987, Saratikov and Krasnov 1987b, 1987c). The use of *R. rosea* to treat depression and to augment standard antidepressants needs further study.

## Effects of Vitamins and Nutrients on Mood

Low levels of $B_{12}$ (cyanocobalamin) and folate have been associated with disorders of mood, memory, and cognition, particularly in depressed patients and in the elderly (Bottiglieri 1996, 1997, Crellin et al. 1993). Numerous studies have demonstrated that B-vitamins can improve mood and cognitive functions (Benton et al. 1995, 1997, Riggs et al. 1996). In a DBRPC study of 14 depressed geriatric inpatients on TCAs, 10 mg each of vitamins $B_1$, $B_2$, and $B_6$ improved depression and cognitive function (Bell et al. 1992). A study of 129 healthy adults given Vitamin C, Vitamin E, and seven B-vitamins at 10 times the US FDA recommended daily allowance for 1 year, resulted in significantly greater improvement in mood than in a group given placebo. Higher serum levels of riboflavin ($B_2$) and pyridoxine ($B_6$) correlated with improved mood in men, while higher levels of thiamine ($B_1$) correlated with better mood in women. Improved mood correlated with the levels of Vitamin E and biotin (a B-vitamin associated with skin and hair growth) regardless of gender (Benton et al. 1995). $B_{12}$ deficiency (associated with high methylmalonic acid) more than doubled the risk of severe depression in 700 disabled women over the age of 65 (Penninx et al. 2000).

Low levels of folate have been associated with nonresponse to antidepressants (Fava et al. 1997). In a DBRPC study, 127 women on fluoxetine 20 mg/day were given either folate 500 μg/day or placebo. In the fluoxetine/folate group, 94% of the women had a good response versus 61% in the fluoxetine/placebo group. In women treated with fluoxetine/folate, plasma folate increased and homocysteine decreased (Coppen and Bailey 2000).

Inositol (a vitamin in the $B_2$ complex) boosts cyclic adenosine monophosphate (AMP), which is a second messenger in neurons. Inositol 12 to 20 g/day has been superior to placebo in a series of randomized trials for depression (Benjamin et al. 1995a), panic (Benjamin et al. 1995b), and obsessive–compulsive disorder (Fux et al. 1996). Gastrointestinal side effects include gas and loose bowels. Because a therapeutic dose requires at least six large 650 mg pills t.i.d., compliance is a problem. In one case mania was induced by 3 g/day. Bender reviewed the use of inositol in psychiatry (Bender 2000).

Choline (a B complex vitamin) has an effect in reducing mania in a number of case reports and case series. A small case study of treatment-refractory, rapid-cycling bipolars who were taking lithium found that four out of six responded to the addition of 2,000 to 7,200 mg/day of free choline. The two nonresponders were also taking hypermetabolic doses of thyroid medication. Clinical improvement correlated with increased intensity of the basal ganglia choline signal as measured on proton magnetic resonance imaging (MRI). The effect of choline on depressive symptoms was variable (Stoll et al. 1996).

Eicosopentanoic acid, an omega-3 fatty acid, was added to ongoing antidepressant treatment in a preliminary DBPC 4-week study. Twenty patients with "breakthrough depression" given 2,000 mg/day eicosopentanoic acid showed significant improvement on Ham-D compared to placebo (Nemets et al. 2002). A DBRPC pilot study by Stoll and colleagues (1999) at Harvard Medical School explored the possibility that omega-3 fatty acids (omega-3FAs) could improve bipolar disorder by inhibiting neuronal transduction pathways in a mechanism similar to that of lithium carbonate and valproate. Thirty bipolar patients, most of whom were on mood stabilizers, were randomized to placebo or omega-3FAs (6.2 g eicosopentanoic acid plus 3.4 mg docosohexanoic acid per day). Those given omega-3FAs showed significant reduction in symptoms and relapse rates. Larger studies are needed to confirm these findings.

## Anxiety and Insomnia

Kava (extract of *Piper methysticum*) is used as a ceremonial drink, a sedative, an analgesic and an aphrodisiac in Fiji, Samoa, and Tonga. Kava contains alpha-pyrones (potent skeletal muscle relaxants) and is used in Germany in doses of 70 to 240 mg/day for stress and muscle spasm. Six of the nine major alpha-pyrones in kava administered together in animal studies create a synergistic effect. Kava has shown anticonvulsant properties in animal models, some serotonin blocking activity, and sodium channel blocking. In animal studies, the calming effect is mediated through the amygdala. The finding that the analgesia induced by kava occurs via nonopiate pathways deserves further study (Jamieson and Duffield 1990). For an extensive review, see Singh and Blumenthal (1996).

A review of seven DBRPC studies of kava for treatment of anxiety concluded that kava extract is relatively safe and more effective than placebo (Pittler and Ernst 2000). Only three of the studies met criteria for meta-analysis (Lehmann et al. 1996, Warnecke 1991, Volz and Kieser 1997), including the selection of patients by HAM-A $\geq 19$ and treatment with kava extract WS1490 100 mg t.i.d. (210 kavapyrones/day). Some methodological questions have been raised and more rigorous trials have been suggested (Pittler and Ernst 2000). Two postmarketing studies of over 3,000 patients found a 1.5 and 2.3% incidence of side effects, most commonly gastrointestinal complaints, allergic skin reaction, headache, and photosensitivity. Less common were restlessness, drowsiness, lack of energy, and tremor.

Ships' logs of vessels visiting the Polynesian islands in the 1800s describe "kava intoxication" in natives and in seamen left behind by Captain Cook. After kava was introduced to the Maori in northern Australia in 1980, long-term kava users suffered facial swelling, scaly rash, increased patellar reflexes, and dyspnea. Laboratory tests found low levels of albumin, proteins, BUN, and bilirubin, increased GGTPase levels, abnormal CBCs with decreased white cell and platelet counts, and some hematuria. Tall P waves on ECGs were consistent with pulmonary hypertension (Mathews et al. 1988). In four cases kava induced symptoms suggestive of central dopaminergic antagonism: dystonic reactions (eyes, neck, and trunk), oral/lingual dyskinesias, and worsening parkinsonian symptoms in a woman on levodopa. Kava should be avoided in patients with Parkinson's disease and in those at risk for dystonia or dyskinesia. No studies of long-term safety, teratogenicity, or mutagenicity beyond 6 months have been done. A high dose of kava (210–280 mg/day kava lactones) induced fulminant hepatitis in a 50-year-old man (Escher et al. 2001).

Doses above 240 mg kava pyrones/day may cause toxicity (Schelosky et al. 1995). Because recent reports have linked the use of Kava to 25 cases of liver toxicity, (hepatitis, cirrhosis, and liver failure), the US FDA has issued a Letter to Health Care Professionals and a Consumer Advisory about the potential risk of liver injury (US FDA 2002, Kraft et al. 2001). Until it is determined whether the toxicity was from a contaminant in a particular brand or a rare reaction to kava, caution should be exercised. Patients should be warned not to combine kava with alcohol or other sedatives.

Passionflower (*Passiflora incarnata*) has been approved by the Komission E for treatment of nervous restlessness. Passionflower contains a dihydroflavone, chrysin, which binds to benzodiazepine receptors. In a DBRPC comparison trial 36 patients with DSM-IV diagnosis of generalized anxiety disorder (GAD) (HAM-A≥14) were given either Passiflora 45 drops/day extract plus placebo tablet or oxazepam 30 mg/day plus placebo drop for 4 weeks. Although the oxazepam effect was more rapid, Passiflora was as effective in reducing anxiety and caused less impairment in job performance. Larger studies are clearly needed (Akhondzadeh et al. 2001).

There is little scientific evidence to support the use of, chamomile (*Matricaria recutita*) or lemon balm (*Melissa officianalis*) for anxiety. Apigenin, a component of chamomile, has high affinity for benzodiazepine receptors, but minimal sedative or muscle-relaxant effects (Brown 1996). People who have ragweed allergy should not use chamomile, a member of the ragweed family. The mechanism of action of lemon balm is unknown.

Fish extracts, called *Garum Amoricum* (brand names Stabilium and Adapton) are used in Europe and Japan for treatment of anxiety, depression, irritability, and memory problems. Therapeutic effects have been attributed to neuroactive polypeptides and omega-3FAs. The dose for Garum is two pills b.i.d. for 2 weeks followed by 2 or 3 pills/day. Although there are few controlled studies, in a DBRPC 8-week crossover study, 70 anxious college students were given either fish extract t.i.d. or placebo. The fish extract group showed reduced anxiety by week 2, and relapsed after stopping the extract (Dorman et al. 1995).

Valerian (*Valeriana officianalis*) is thought to bind to GABA-A receptors. One review of DBRPC trials of valerian for sleep found the evidence to be encouraging but not compelling (Stevinson and Ernst 2000). Another review found subjective improvement in sleep in six out of seven DBRPC trials with no side effects other than minimal hangover in doses of 600 to 900 mg (Krystal and Ressler 2002). One DBRPC cross-over study of 16 mild insomniacs using polysomnography reported a significant decrease in slow wave sleep (SWS) onset latency and an increase in the percent of SWS time (Donath et al. 2000). The effect of valerian seems to improve over time and an maximal benefit may take 2 weeks. One study comparing a combination of valerian and hops with flunitrazepam (a benzodiazepine) concluded that valerian and hops did not cause the deficits in attention and reaction time seen with benzodiazapines (Schultz et al. 1997). Some reports of dystonia and hepatitis from preparations containing a mixture of ingredients (including valerian) are difficult to interpret. Often patients are averse to the unpleasant taste and odor of valerian tea and tablets. One advantage of valerian over other sedative/hypnotics is that there have been no cases of habituation or abuse and only one case of possible withdrawal symptoms. Valerian should be avoided in pregnancy. Further DBPC trials are needed to establish the place for valerian in treatment of insomnia.

Melatonin, a hormone secreted by the pineal gland, plays an important role in the regulation of sleep. In patients with insomnia, DBRPC trials show that melatonin improves sleep, reduces sleep onset latency (Kayumov et al. 2001), and restores sleep efficiency (Zhdanova et al. 2001). A DBRPC study in elderly melatonin-deficient insomniacs found that 1 week of 2 mg sustained-release melatonin effectively maintained sleep, while 1 week of 2 mg fast-release melatonin improved sleep initiation. 1 mg/day sustained-release melatonin for 2 months improved sleep initiation and maintenance with no adverse effects (Haimov et al. 1995). In a 4-week, open pilot study, melatonin 3 mg h.s. reduced sun downing (agitated behaviors) and daytime drowsiness in 11 elderly nursing home residents with dementia (Cohen-Mansfield et al. 2000).

In a DBRPC trial, 24 patients being treated with fluoxetine 20 mg for major depression and insomnia, sleep quality and continuity improved in the group given up to 10 mg h.s. melatonin. Melatonin caused no more side effects than placebo (Dolberg et al. 1998). Melatonin significantly improved sleep in a DBRPC cross-over trial in schizophrenics (Shamir et al. 2000) and in a pilot study of 11 patients with bipolar disorder, manic type (Bersani and Garavini 2000).

REM sleep behavior disorder (RBD), a chronic progressive parasomnia, is characterized by loss of paralysis during REM sleep. Patients physically act out their dreams causing injury to themselves or their partner. Many cases occur in neurodegenerative disorders and in Parkinson's patients treated with dopamine agonists and levodopa. In neurologically vulnerable patients, stimulants, TCAs, and SSRIs may trigger RBD (Schenck et al. 1986). Traditional treatments for RBD, clonazepam (0.5–2 mg h.s.) or carbamazepine (100 mg t.i.d.) may worsen cognitive function or cause ataxia (with increased risk of falling). Carbamazepine can cause hepatitis, blood cell dyscrasias, and hyponatremia. In contrast, melatonin rarely has side effects even at 9 to 12 mg h.s., the doses necessary to treat RBD (Kunz and Bes 1997).

A DBRPC trial in 15 children with pervasive developmental disorders or autism with severe insomnia found that all children given melatonin had significant improvement in insomnia, irritability, alertness, and social ability (Jan et al. 1994). Eight out of 10 epileptic children with severe sleep–waking rhythm pathology (ages 6 months to 10 years) responded to melatonin 5 to 10 mg h.s. with improved sleep and daytime alertness. Six of the 8 responders gained better seizure control (Fauteck et al. 1999).

In a DBPC crossover study, 22 schizophrenic patients with tardive dyskinesia (TD) were treated for 6 weeks with controlled release melatonin 10 mg/day at 8 PM. Patients on melatonin had significant decreases (mean 2.45 ± 1.92) on the Abnormal Involuntary Movement Scale (AIMS) compared with those on placebo (0.77 ± 1.11) (Shamir et al. 2001). Long-term studies with higher doses are needed to explore potential benefits in TD.

A great deal of scientific research is available on melatonin (Bubenik et al. 1998). *Melatonin* by Russell Reiter (1996) is helpful to patients. In animal studies melatonin delays shrinkage of the thymus with age, improves immune function, and shows potent antioxidant with anticarcinogenic effects (in animal and some human studies), particularly for estrogen receptor positive tumors such as breast, prostate, melanoma, and glioma. It also helps relieve cluster headaches. The Medical Letter reported that four out of six brands of melatonin had ill-defined impurities (Anonymous 1995). Consumers should choose supplements from mainstream companies with pharmaceutical grade melatonin. Side effects are infrequent and usually mild: cramps, fatigue, dizziness, headache, and irritability.

## Migraine

In reviewing 6 DBRPC studies of feverfew (*Tanacetum parthenium*), Ernst and Pittler (2000) concluded that the evidence favored feverfew in prevention of migraine and reduction of pain, nausea, vomiting, and frequency of attacks. The negative results of one study were due to the use of a preparation standardized for parthenolide (a key compound with sesquiterpine lactones), instead of the whole leaf extract of feverfew used by other researchers. Parthenolide is unstable and needs other components for its activity. The Canadian Regulatory Commission will only certify whole leaf extract of feverfew. A 4-month, 3-phase cross-over study of 57 patients found that feverfew significantly reduced migraine pain (Awang 1997, Palevitch and Carasso 1997). Migraine patients may benefit from feverfew 100 to 200 mg/day (2–4 pills). Although feverfew has few side effects, it can affect bleeding time and should not be used with warfarin. It should be discontinued 2 to 3 weeks prior to surgery.

Petadolex, an extract of Butterbur root (*Petasites hybridus*) contains petasin and isopetasin, two vasodilators with strong anti-inflammatory action via inhibition of leukotriene synthesis. A DBRPC study of 58 migraine sufferers found a significant reduction in the frequency and intensity of headaches (46% at week 4, 60% at week 8, and 50% at week 12) in the group given Petadolex 50 mg b.i.d. compared to those given placebo (24, 17, and 10% respectively) (Mauskop et al. 2000). The reduction in migraine symptoms on Petadolex, was comparable to beta-blockers, divalproex, and calcium antagonists, but it had no side effects (Grossman and Schmidramsl 2001).

In an open pilot study of 124 patients with common migraine, SAMe 400 mg/day i.v. for 30 days significantly reduced the severity of migraine and the use of pain relievers (Gatto et al. 1986). The treatment of migraine with SAMe deserves further inquiry.

## Obesity

Many psychotropic medications cause weight gain. Weight loss agents have a role in overall health maintenance and in improving compliance with treatment. Chromium picolinate helps cells utilize glucose more efficiently, facilitates insulin passage through capillary walls, reduces insulin resistance, prevents formation of abnormal lipids, and raises dehydroepiandrosterone (DHEA) levels. Many studies show that chromium picolinate 400 to 600 µg/day induces weight loss and reduces body fat. Combined with a weight

training program even greater reduction in body fat and some increase in muscle mass can occur, mainly in women. Chromium has been used to treat diabetes (Anderson et al. 1997). Two studies found that chromium picolinate leads to a 25% longer life span and 25% less body fat in rats compared to placebo. Data in menopausal women suggest that it raises DHEA and estrogen levels, improves bone density and reverses urinary calcium loss. For a review of these studies and the controversy over toxicity, see *Chromium Picolinate: Everything You Need to Know* by Evans (1996). The authors have used chromium picolinate to reverse weight gain from antidepressants and have noted that it often improves mood. In a small case series of single-blind, on-off-on, open-label trials, five patients with dysthymia in partial remission (four on sertraline and one on nortriptyline) achieved full remission when given chromium picolinate 400 µg/day (McLeod et al. 1999). Studies are needed to assess the role of chromium picolinate in depression.

Ephedrine/caffeine suppresses appetite within 3 weeks. Long-term reduction in body fat may be due to increased fat burning and heat production. Confirming earlier primate studies (Ramsey et al. 1998), four DBRPC studies in humans showed the combination of ephedrine/caffeine to be superior to placebo or dexfenfluramine for weight loss (Astrup et al. 1992, Breum et al. 1994, Daly et al. 1993, Toubro et al. 1993). Patients tolerated the stimulant effect well if started on low doses and raised gradually. Side effects include agitation, anxiety, tachycardia, arrhythmias, addiction, and gastrointestinal effects. Contraindications include cardiovascular disease, the use of asthma medications, psychosis, prostate disease, and others. Ephedrine should be discontinued 2 weeks prior to surgery.

## Hormonal and Endocrine Disorders

### Premenstrual Symptoms

Although perimenstrual affective symptoms often are exacerbations of underlying mood disorders, affective symptoms can be due to imbalance of estrogen to progesterone affecting neurotransmitters (e.g., decreasing serotonin), or imbalance of calcium and Vitamin D. Premenstrual syndrome (PMS), including premenstrual dysphoric disorder (PMDD), is characterized by psychosomatic, behavioral, cognitive, and appetitive changes that occur during the late luteal phase of the menstrual cycle. Affective symptoms include nervousness, irritability, depression, crying, mood swings, and rarely, violence. Women experience somatic symptoms: abdominal bloating, pain, cramps, breast fullness, back pain, restlessness, headache, fatigue, and increased appetite with craving for sweets, salt, and fats (Hobbs and Amster 1996). Although SSRIs are often effective in PMS, many women prefer to try natural treatments (Parry 1999).

Hypothetically, abnormal levels of omega FAs in PMS may alter sensitivity to prolactin and steroids. The theory that evening primrose oil (*Oneothera biennes*) normalizes FA levels is dubious because it contains predominantly omega-6FAs, which are sufficient in most modern diets. There are no well-designed studies to support the use of primrose oil for PMS (Robbers and Tyler 1999).

Magnesium is probably useful in treating PMS. A decrease in intracellular magnesium has been found in some women with PMS. In a DBRPC trial, 32 women were given either 360 mg/day of magnesium or placebo started on day 15 of menses. The group given magnesium showed significant improvement in negative affect and arousal by the second month, followed by improvements in pain and water retention by the fourth month. There was evidence of increased intracellular magnesium, but no change in serum magnesium levels (Facchinetti et al. 1991).

Preliminary DBPC studies (Thys-Jacobs et al. 1989) and one rigorous DBRPC MC study demonstrated the benefits of calcium in PMS. Four hundred and sixty-six women were given either calcium 1,200 mg/day or placebo. After 3 months calcium reduced PMS symptoms by 48% versus 30% with placebo. Side effects included mild nausea, stomach distress, and headache. Calcium should be taken with meals to avoid renal stone formation (Thys-Jacobs et al. 1998).

The role of manganese in PMS has not yet been established.

Evidence for B-vitamins and minerals in PMS is limited. In a DBRPC study, 40 women were given either a mixed nutritional supplement containing magnesium, $B_6$, vitamin E, folic acid, iron, and copper, or placebo for 6 months. The supplement reduced PMS symptoms to 18% of baseline, whereas the group on placebo showed reduction to 73% of baseline. No side effects were observed (Facchinetti et al. 1997).

$B_6$ is a cofactor in the metabolism of tryptophan, a precursor to serotonin and dopamine. Twelve DBPC studies of PMS treatment with $B_6$ yielded three with positive results, five with ambiguous results, and four with negative results. The usefulness of vitamin $B_6$ for PMS is questionable (Kleijnen et al. 1990).

Carbohydrate treatment has been used in PMS to increase the ratio of tryptophan to other amino acids. In one study, a specially balanced carbohydrate rich drink (PMS Escape) seemed to decrease anger and depression 3.5 hours after the drink and to improve memory and reduce carbohydrate craving 1.5 hours after the drink (Sayegh et al. 1995). Additional studies are needed to replicate this finding.

L-tryptophan outperformed placebo in a DBPC 3-month study of women with PMDD who were treated with either tryptophan 2,000 mg t.i.d. or placebo during the 17 days from ovulation until the third day of menses. L-tryptophan was associated with a 35% decrease in dysphoria, tension, and irritability versus a 10% decrease with placebo (Steinberg et al. 1999). A safe pharmaceutical grade of L-tryptophan is available in the US by prescription.

Chaste tree, chasteberry (*Vitex agnus castus*), has been used for 70 years in Germany to treat PMS and for menopausal hormone replacement. *In vitro* and animal studies show that Vitex binds to dopamine receptors, inhibits prolactin release, and increases lactation (Klepser and Nisly, 1999). In a DBPC study 86 women were given Vitex and 84 were given placebo for three menstrual cycles. 52% of those on Vitex had significant improvement on 5/6 self-assessment measures versus 24% on placebo (Schellenberg 2001). Vitex is an effective and well-tolerated treatment for PMS. Data suggesting that it improves fertility warrants further study.

## Menopause

### Female Menopause

Menopausal women face age-related psychological and physical changes and increased risks of heart disease, osteoporosis, cancer, memory loss, and AD. During menopause, estrogen and progesterone decrease, while follicle stimulating hormone (FSH) and luteinizing hormone (LH) increase. Hot flashes, vaginal dryness, mood swings, depression, insomnia, forgetfulness, and poor concentration can occur (Mayo 1997). Synthetic hormone replacement therapy (HRT) is widely practiced. The 1990 Nurses Health Study, following 121,700 women for 10 years, found a 40% greater risk of breast cancer in women taking HRT versus placebo. A 7-year study of 240,073 women documented a 40% increased risk in women on estrogen replacement therapy (ERT) for 6 to 8 years and a 70% increased risk on ERT for more than 11 years. ERT also increases the risk of uterine cancer. Adding progesterone to ERT reduces but does not eliminate the increased risk of uterine cancer (Beresford et al. 1997, Colditz et al. 1990, 1995). For a review of phytoestrogens and breast cancer see Ingram and colleagues (1997). Common side effects of HRT include weight gain, headaches, thrombosis, fibroids, and gallstones. Benefits include improvements in hot flashes, vaginal dryness, visual memory, and skin and muscle tone. A report issued by the Office of Women's Health Research at NIH found insufficient evidence of risk versus benefit to support the use of HRT to prevent osteoporosis, cardiovascular disease, or dementia (NIH 2002). Many women seek natural supplements to ease the physical and psychological transition to menopause and to avoid risks associated with HRT.

Several studies indicate that soy products ameliorate hot flushes (Ernst et al. 2001). Animal studies find that soy protects against breast cancer and other cancers with estrogen receptors. Isoflavones have both estrogenic and antiestrogenic activity. There are no laboratory data on estrogen receptor binding *in vitro* or effects on endometrial growth in ovariectomized rats (Beckham 1995, Mayo 1997, Soffa 1996). Epidemiologic data and animal studies suggest that the health benefits of soy (lowering cholesterol and cancer prevention) are best obtained from whole soy (i.e., whole food) rather than from extracted components. Brief reviews of soy can be found in Liebman (1998) and Helmuth (1999). For a comprehensive review see Anderson and colleagues (1999).

Red clover (*Trifolium pratense*) is rich in isoflavones and phytoestrogens with similarities to those in soy products. Levels of estrogen were increased in women who ate red clover sprouts for 2 weeks. Theoretically, red clover may block carcinogenic forms of estrogen at the estrogen receptor. Laboratory data on the binding to estrogen receptors *in vitro* and effects on uterine growth in ovariectomized rats are not yet available (Duke 1997, Neville 1999, Soffa 1996).

Black cohosh (*Cimifuga racemosa*) has been used extensively in Europe for over 60 years. By reducing LH levels, black cohosh reduces hot flashes. Most studies have not shown an estrogen-like effect. Laboratory data indicate no binding to estrogen receptors *in vitro*. However, it stimulates some uterine growth in ovariectomized rats. Several controlled studies, including one DBPC study, showed efficacy equivalent to ERT (Foster 1999; Lieberman 1998). Unlike ERT, black cohosh had no significant side effects. Rats given 90 times the human dose for 6 months showed no toxicity. Black cohosh does not cause proliferation of breast cancer cells in culture (Freudenstein and Bodinet 1999). Furthermore, black cohosh inhibited DNA synthesis and augmented the antiproliferative activity of Tamoxifen *in vitro* (Fackleman 1998, Foster 1999, Lieberman 1998). There has been no evidence of mutagenicity or carcinogenicity. Although DBPC trials would strengthen the evidence, considering the high level of safety, black cohosh can be recommended for menopausal symptoms.

Licorice (*Glycyrrhiza glabra*), an ingredient in many herbal remedies for menopausal symptoms, contains glycyrrhetic acid, the active component that structurally resembles adrenocortical steroids. It is reported to stimulate conversion of testosterone to estrogen and to block cancer promoting estrogens. Animal data suggest strong binding to estrogen receptors *in vitro* without stimulation of uterine growth in ovariectomized rats. Side effects include headache, lethargy, sodium and water retention, potassium depletion and, rarely, hypertension (at high doses) (Beckham 1995, Fackleman 1998, Robbers and Tyler 1999).

Dong Quai (*Angelica Sinensis*), a component in Chinese tonics since 500 BC, has been used for menopausal symptoms. Dong Quai has estrogen-like activity and can induce progesterone secretion. The water-soluble extract of Dong Quai regulates uterine contractions and the essential oil relaxes uterine muscles. It has strong binding to estrogen receptors *in vitro* and stimulates uterine growth in ovariectomized rats (Belford-Courtney 1993, Fackleman 1998). One DBPC trial of Dong Quai alone yielded negative results (Hirata et al. 1997). However, Chinese herbalists use Dong Quai in combination with other herbs. Rigorous controlled studies of Dong Quai in combination with traditional herbs are needed.

Vitex (*Vitex agnus castus*) is often combined with black cohosh, licorice, Dong Quai and other herbs (see vitex in the treatment of PMS above). It modulates prolactin secretion by binding to dopamine receptors. Although there are no specific studies of vitex in menopause, anecdotal reports suggest that it alleviates affective symptoms, hot flashes, fluid retention, and weight gain. As an antagonist to excess circulating estrogen, Vitex may protect against breast cancer. Although no side effects have been reported, vitex has very slight binding to estrogen receptors *in vitro* and modestly stimulates uterine growth in ovariectomized rats. It has been used to treat hyperprolactinemia and one of the authors (RB) has used it to counteract prolactin elevations from antipsychotic medication (Brown 1993, Fackleman 1998, Mayo 1997, McCaleb 1995, Soffa 1996).

Hops (*Humulus lupulus*) have been used for estrogenic effects. Known to beer brewers for hundreds of years, hops are an approved sleep aid in Belgium, France, and Germany, often in combination with valerian or skullcap. Hops farmers noticed that the herb could affect harvesters, causing fatigue and changes in women's menses. Female hops pickers became more libidinous while male hops pickers had less libido. Laboratory data indicate that hops bind to estrogen receptors *in vitro* but do not stimulate uterine growth in ovariectomized rats (Beckham 1995, Fackleman 1998). The effects of hops on P450 enzyme systems are unlikely to be of clinical significance because the enzymes inhibited by Hops are not relevant to most medications (Henderson et al. 2000).

Native American Indians use Blue cohosh (*Caulophyllum thalictroides*) as a uterine tonic and to prevent miscarriages. Blue cohosh has modest binding to estrogen receptors and has been used for menopausal symptoms. There are no controlled trials of blue cohosh and it needs further study (Fackleman 1998).

Golden root, Arctic root, Roseroot (*R. rosea*) has been used by the people of the Province of Georgia and Siberia to enhance fertility. In an open study, 40 women with amenorrhea were given *R. rosea* extract 100 mg b.i.d. Normal menstrual cycles were restored in 25 women and 11 of these became pregnant. In 25 women, uterine length increased to normal size (Gerasimova 1970). Recent studies of estrogenic effects of *R. rosea* by Dr. Patricia Egon at the University of Pittsburgh have found strong estrogen receptor binding *in vitro* (Egon Nov. 2001, personal communication). Further research is needed on the potential applications of *R. rosea* in treating hormonal disorders. Clinical experience with *R. rosea* in women with premenstrual and menopausal symptoms has been promising.

---

**Clinical Vignette 2**

Ms. S, 45 years old, a physician's assistant, sought treatment for panic disorder with driving phobia. She was already dependent on lorazepam. During the week before her menses, all symptoms became intensified and she displayed severe irritability. Her anxiety, which was exacerbated by all antidepressants, responded to psychotherapy, lithium, and lorazepam. Ms. S was asymptomatic for 3 years until she became premenopausal. She did not want to take HRT. Her anxiety and irritability became unbearable and she was given a trial of Rhodiola® (Rosavin® by Ameriden) 450 mg/day (3 capsules/day). All PMS symptoms resolved and she noticed improved stress tolerance, memory, and clarity of thinking. A year later she returned to treatment after 3 months of amenorrhea with increasing anxiety and irritability. On the assumption that over time her estrogen level had continued to decline, the Rosavin® was increased to two capsules b.i.d. Within 2 weeks Ms. S was completely back to normal.

---

In weighing the risks and benefits of HRT and menopausal symptoms, women need complete information to consider all of their options. Some women feel more comfortable taking synthetic estrogen and progesterone, whereas others prefer natural remedies, especially as recent research confirms both their efficacy and their potential to reduce cancer risks.

## Male Menopause

Many men take herbal supplements for prostatic enlargement, a common problem of middle and late life. After age 45, free testosterone declines. Treatment of an enlarged prostate often improves sexual functioning. Prostatic enlargement is stimulated by rising levels of estradiol, prolactin, SHBG (sex hormone binding globulin), and DHT (dihydrotestosterone) and the increased estrogen/testosterone ratio. Conventional treatment of benign prostatic hypertrophy (BPH) uses either finasteride (Proscar) or alpha-adrenergic blockers (terazosin, doxazosin, or tamsulosin). Finasteride tends to cause sexual dysfunction with 4% complete impotence, and it is expensive (Anonymous 1992). The alpha-adrenergic blockers can cause tiredness, dizziness, depression, headache, abnormal ejaculation, and rhinitis (Anonymous 1997). The three most studied herbal treatments for BPH are saw palmetto (*Serenoa repens* or sabal), pygeum (*Pygeum africanum*), and stinging nettle (*Urtica dioica*).

Sitosterols in saw palmetto (*Seronoa repens*) reduce DHT levels, DHT binding, and inflammation. Two percent of patients complain of transient side effects such as headache and stomach upset. Saw palmetto rapidly decreases nocturia. Data from a number of studies, including a 3-year trial comparing saw palmetto with Proscar, show that saw palmetto significantly increased urinary flow rate and decreased residual urine volume by at least 50%. Eleven percent of the patients taking Proscar stopped because of side effects compared to 2% of those taking saw palmetto (Bach et al. 1997). Saw palmetto may take several months to work, although some patients improve within 2 weeks on 320 mg/day. Reviews of saw palmetto include a meta-analysis (Champault et al. 1984, Wilt et al. 1998). Recent data suggest that supercritical fluid extraction produces a compound that is twice as effective as previous formulations (Faloon 1999).

Pygeum bark inhibits prostate cell growth and aromatase (which lowers estrogen/testosterone ratio); increases prostate secretions; and reduces inflammation, prolactin (reducing testosterone uptake in the prostate), and cholesterol (which reduces DHT binding) (Bassi et al. 1987, Del Valio 1974). In a 60-day DBRPC study of 263 men, pygeum extract significantly reduced nocturia and micturition volume (Barlet et al. 1990) with no reported side effects. There is evidence of rapid improvement in nocturnal erections and sexual activity even in elderly men (Carani et al. 1991). The doses range from 75 to 150 mg/day. An important question is whether the long-term harvesting of bark from the very fragile Pygeum tree will be sustainable (Simons et al. 1998).

Stinging nettle extract (*Urtica Dioica*) blocks prostate cell growth receptors, blocks 5-alpha-reductase, inhibits aromatase, inhibits SHBG binding, and is anti-inflammatory (Lichius and Muth 1997). It has been shown to be effective alone in PC tests (Krzeski et al. 1993), but was even better in a DBPC study combined with pygeum (Sokeland and Albrecht 1997). The usual dose is 300 mg/day (Robbers and Tyler 1999).

Our experience is that a combination of saw palmetto, pygeum, and urtica dioica produces the best results. Compared to prescription drugs, these natural compounds are more effective for BPH, cause fewer side effects, and are relatively inexpensive.

## Sexual Enhancement

The two largest consumer groups seeking herbal or nutrient sexual enhancement are people over age 40 years and those taking medications which adversely affect sexual function-ing. This discussion is limited to sexual enhancers for which there is some research evidence, frequent consumer use, and clinical experience. Due to gender bias, past research has been predominantly with men. However, the authors have found some substances tested in men to be helpful for women.

Yohimbine (*Pausinystalia yohimbe*) is both a prescription drug and a dietary supplement used to treat erectile dysfunction. Meta-analysis of seven well-done DBPC studies showed that 15 to 43 mg/day Yohimbine was more effective than placebo for 40% of men with sexual dysfunction (Morales et al. 1987, Ernst and Pittler 1998). In one case series, Yohimbine reversed sexual dysfunction from fluoxetine in eight out of nine men and women (Jacobsen 1992). The prescription form comes in 5.4 mg pills and the usual dose is 18 to 42 mg/day. Yohimbine content in over-the-counter products is often negligible (Betz et al. 1995). The prescription form of Yohimbine provides the best quality. Some patients, particularly the elderly, cannot tolerate the side effects: anxiety, nausea, dizziness, chills, headache, and at higher doses, increased blood pressure. In patients with anxiety disorders, Yohimbine can trigger anxiety or panic attacks.

Asian ginseng (*Panax ginseng*), long known in oriental medicine, is often used as a sexual stimulant. There have been anecdotal reports of hypersexual behavior. Animal studies have shown increases in sperm counts, testicular weight, testosterone levels and mating counts. Animal models suggest that ginseng (like sildenafil) increases nitric oxide synthesis (Kang et al. 1995). In one PC study, 30 men who took *P. ginseng* 300 mg/day for 3 months experienced better sexual performance than 30 men on placebo (Choi et al. 1995). This study needs replication.

Research data show that ginkgo (*Ginkgo biloba*) improves blood flow to the brain, retina, legs (relieves intermittent claudication), female genitalia, and penis. In an open, nonblinded 6-month study, ginkgo enabled 50 men with erectile dysfunction (ED) to achieve erections (Sohn and Sikora 1991). Another open study of 63 patients with antidepressant-induced sexual function who improved on 240 mg/day ginkgo (Cohen and Bartlik 1998) has been criticized for flawed methodology (Balon 1999). Although ginkgo can be used to treat mild impotence in middle aged men (after ruling out treatable medical causes), it is not helpful for disorders of libido or orgasm.

Arginine supplements and sunflower seeds, which contain large amounts of arginine (an alpha-2-adrenoceptor antagonist), have been used to treat impotence. Arginine is the precursor to nitric oxide and may alleviate angina via dilation of blood vessels to the myocardium. A DBRPC study of 50 men with ED found 9/29 responded to L-arginine versus 2/17 on placebo. All nine responders had decreased nitric oxide excretion or production at baseline (Chen et al. 1999). In a recent review, Morales noted the need for more controlled studies of this promising "orphan drug." (Morales 2001). L-arginine may predispose to herpes infection in short-term use. There are no long-term toxicity studies.

Muira puama (*Ptychopetalium guyanna*), an Amazonian herb, has been used as an aphrodisiac, nerve tonic, and anti-arthritic preparation (Mowrey 1996). In a study from the Institute of Sexology in Paris, 262 men complaining of lack of sexual desire and impotence were treated with muira puama. After 2 weeks on 1,500 mg/day, 62% reported enhanced libido and 51% reported better erections. There is no research regarding the mechanism of action, nor are there controlled studies replicating this finding (Waynberg 1990). One of the authors (RB) has used muira puama for both men and women suffering from SSRI-induced sexual dysfunction with modest improvements in desire, arousal, and orgasmic phases. A combination of *M. puama* and *G. biloba* (Herbal vX) was tested in an open series in 202 healthy women complaining of low sex drive. After one month, 65% reported improvements in libido, intercourse, sexual satisfaction, intensity of orgasm, and other measures (Waynberg and Brewer 2000). A DBPC follow-up study is planned.

In a DBRPC study of 77 women interested in improving their sexual function, ArginMax (a supplement containing *P. ginseng*, *G. biloba*, Damiana leaf, L-arginine, multiple B-vitamins, folate, Vitamins A, C, and E, calcium, iron, and zinc) was taken for 4 weeks. In this study 73.5% of the ArginMax group reported improvements in their sex lives compared with 37.2% on placebo. ArginMax improved desire, vaginal lubrication, frequency of intercourse and orgasm, and clitoral sensation with no significant side effects (Ito et al. 2001). Further studies are needed. Nevertheless, considering the low risks and the paucity of effective treatments for female sexual dysfunction, ArginMax is worth consideration.

The Peruvian adaptogen, Maca (*Lepidium peruvianum myenii Chacon*), has been used for thousands of years by Andean peoples. It is reported to boost energy, to have aphrodisiac properties, to improve fertility at high altitudes, to improve stress tolerance and nutritional status, and to relieve menopausal symptoms (Quiros and Cardenas 1997). Rat studies suggest that sterols, glucosinolates, and/or alkaloid components increased FSH, estrogen, and testosterone levels in female rats and increased testosterone levels in male rats (Chacon 1997, Quiros and Cardenas 1997). DBPC studies indicate Maca may have positive effects on stress reduction, mood, cognition, and exercise capacity in humans. No toxicity or side effects were found in human and animal studies (Aguilar 1999, personal communication). Excess doses may cause overactivation or breast tenderness. In normal male rats, Maca increased the frequency of intromissions and other sexual performance parameters and in rats with erectile dysfunction it reduced latency to erection (Cicero et al. 2001, Zheng et al. 2000). Its use may be contraindicated in patients with fibroids, estrogen receptor related cancer risk, endometriosis, or prostate cancer. Information on Maca is available at http://www.maca750.com.

### Cognitive Enhancers for Treatment of AAMI, Alzheimer's Disease, Dementia, Poststroke, Traumatic Brain Injury, Attention-Deficit Hyperactivity Disorder, and Dyslexia

Cognitive enhancement should begin *in utero* and continue throughout the life cycle by providing (1) nutrients for the developing brain, (2) neuroprotective supplements for the aging brain, and (3) treatments for organic brain diseases. After age 20 years, memory decreases by 1 to 2% per year and usually becomes significant by age 45 years

(Crook et al. 1991). Age-associated memory impairment (AAMI) or age-related cognitive decline (ARCD) can be ameliorated by cognitive enhancers. Many neuropsychiatric conditions such as dyslexia, ADHD, AAMI, Alzheimer's disease (AD), dementias, ischemia, stroke, and traumatic brain injury (TBI) are affected by similar pathophysiological processes. For example, TBI is often complicated by secondary ischemia. This section explores the emerging role of alternative treatments based upon the probable mechanisms by which they affect neurophysiological processes: neurotransmitter theories, biochemical and metabolic derangements, neuroanatomy, and neuronal electrical activity. See Table 104-5 for a summary of these mechanisms.

For readers interested in more detailed discussions of these processes, refer to the following:

1. Neurotransmitter theories: the cholinergic hypothesis (acetylcholine) (Arciniegas 2001, Murdoch et al. 1998, Saija et al. 1988, Schmidt and Grady 1995); catecholamines (DA, NE, and 5-HT) (Hayes and Dixon 1994); and *N*-methyl-D-aspartate (NMDA)-glutamate receptor systems (Bell et al. 1998).
2. Biochemical and metabolic derangements: decreases in cellular energy (mitochondrial) production; free radicals (Long et al. 1996); hypoxia; secondary ischemia; nerve membrane alterations and the membrane hypothesis of aging (Zs-Nagy 1994); decreased calcium channel conductance; nitric oxide (Sinz et al. 1999); blood–brain barrier damage (Hayes and Dixon 1994).
3. Anatomic areas sensitive to injury and age-related deterioration include the hippocampus, ventro–medial cortex, ventro–basal forebrain, cingulate gyrus, and reticular system (Murdoch et al. 1998, Schmidt and Grady 1995). The decline of hippocampal cells in the CA3 region during aging has been associated with decreased neuronal firing, increased lipid peroxidation, and increased lipofuscin (membrane fragments that accumulate). Stimulation of hippocampal CA3 fibers induces long-term potentiation (LTP) of synaptic transmission, a critical process for memory and learning. Information transfer across the corpus callosum is also closely related to learning and memory.
4. Computerized EEG maps show excess slow wave activity and decreased beta and/or alpha activity in patients with TBI, stroke, dementia, and ADD (Rozelle and Budzynski 1995). Cognitive activating agents decrease slow wave activity and increase alpha and beta activity (Itil et al. 1998).

## Nutrients

### Omega-3 Fatty Acids

Omega-3 fatty acids (omega-3FAs), especially decosohexanoic acid (DHA), are important in neuronal development (Crawford et al. 1993) and in infant formula supplementation. Research on the benefits of essential fatty acid (EFA) supplementation of formula for normal infants has yielded mixed results. DBPC studies have shown that infants given omega-3 enriched formula have improved brain and eye development (Jensen et al. 1996), better problem solving at 10 months (Willatts et al. 1998), and an increase in scores on the mental development index (Birch

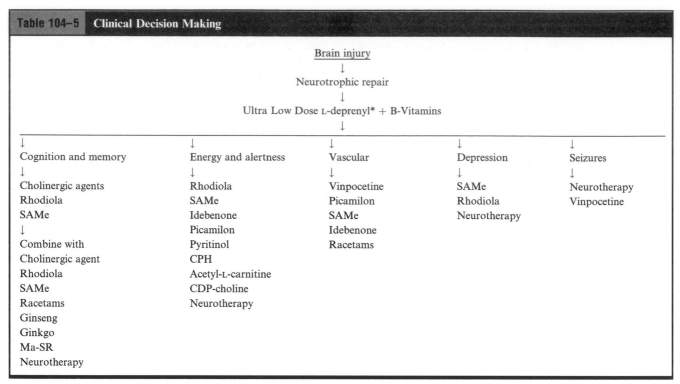

**Table 104–5  Clinical Decision Making**

Brain injury
↓
Neurotrophic repair
↓
Ultra Low Dose L-deprenyl* + B-Vitamins
↓

| Cognition and memory | Energy and alertness | Vascular | Depression | Seizures |
|---|---|---|---|---|
| ↓ | ↓ | ↓ | ↓ | ↓ |
| Cholinergic agents | Rhodiola | Vinpocetine | SAMe | Neurotherapy |
| Rhodiola | SAMe | Picamilon | Rhodiola | Vinpocetine |
| SAMe | Idebenone | SAMe | Neurotherapy | |
| ↓ | Picamilon | Idebenone | | |
| Combine with | Pyritinol | Racetams | | |
| Cholinergic agent | CPH | | | |
| Rhodiola | Acetyl-L-carnitine | | | |
| SAMe | CDP-choline | | | |
| Racetams | Neurotherapy | | | |
| Ginseng | | | | |
| Ginkgo | | | | |
| Ma-SR | | | | |
| Neurotherapy | | | | |

Ultra low dose L-deprenyl* 10–15 mg/wk.

et al. 2000). Further long-term, large-scale studies with sensitive measures of development are needed.

EFAs play a role in the synthesis of the polyunsaturated fatty acids (PUFA) (necessary to maintain membrane fluidity), membrane enzyme activities, and production of prostaglandins, leukotrienes, and thromboxanes. Increasing free radical damage with loss of membrane PUFAs (lipid peroxidation) occurs with age and is associated with neurodegenerative disorders such as Parkinson's disease and AD. Abnormally low levels of omega-3FAs have been found in patients with depression and aggression (Hibbeln et al. 1997, Maes 1998, Peet et al. 1998), a subset of ADHD (Stevens et al. 1995), dementia, and AD (Conquer et al. 2000). A prospective study of 1,200 elderly subjects found that after 8 years, those with low DHA serum levels had a 67% greater chance of developing AD than those with high DHA levels (Kyle et al. 1998). Neurological symptoms improved in Alzheimer's patients given DHA (Nidecker 1997, Soderberg et al. 1991). Although much work needs to be done in this area, supplementation with antioxidants and omega-3FAs may protect against neurodegenerative processes (Youdim et al. 2000).

In many countries the average diet is deficient in omega-3FAs. Cold water fish, nuts, flax, and dark green vegetables are good sources. Fish or flax oil capsules are convenient for patients unwilling to change their diets. Although there is evidence that omega-3FAs may enhance cognitive development and protect against neurological decline, additional research is needed.

### S-Adenosyl-L-Methionine (SAMe)

S-adenosyl-L-methionine is formed by the condensation of the amino acid methionine and ATP (see Figure 104–1 and the section on depression for biochemistry of SAMe). As a methyl donor, SAMe helps maintain neuronal membrane integrity and fluidity, neurotransmitter synthesis, and energy metabolism. The authors reviewed the data on SAMe in the clinical practice of psychiatry, neurology, and internal medicine (Brown et al. 2000). In primate studies, SAMe reduced impairments and facilitated recovery from lesions in the motor cortex and dorsolateral prefrontal cortex and from reserpine. Microscopic data suggested that SAMe enhanced migration of macrophages engaged in tissue repair (Takahashi et al. 1986, 1987). SAMe improved cholinergic function and reduced learning deficits in aged rats (Pavia et al. 1997). Rats given 10 mg/kg/day SC SAMe had nearly 50% decreased free radical production, 50% increased glutathione, and nearly 100% increased glutathione peroxidase and transferase in brain tissue (De La Cruz et al. 2000).

Forty-one patients enrolled in a DBRPC pilot study received (within 24 hours of ischemia or hemorrhagic stroke) either SAMe 2,400 mg/day IV, SAMe 3,200 mg/day IV, or placebo for 14 days. SAMe improved survival and was well tolerated (Monaco et al. 1996). In a less rigorous single-blind (SB) study, 40 elderly patients with mild to moderate organic brain syndromes treated with SAMe for 2 months showed improvement in 13 out of 19 items on the Sandoz clinical assessment geriatric scale with a 25 to 45% improvement on scales of energy, drive, confusion, and self-care (Fontanari et al. 1994). In a DBRPC 1-month study of postconcussion syndrome, 30 patients were given either placebo or SAMe 150 mg/day IV. Mean clinical scores of postconcussion symptoms decreased 77% in patients taking SAMe compared to 49% in the placebo group. SAMe also shortened hospital stays (Bacci Ballerini et al. 1983).

## Picamilon

Picamilon, a combination of gamma-aminobutyric acid (GABA) and the B-vitamin niacin, decreases cerebral blood vessel tone and increases intracranial circulation rate. A DB controlled study showed that picamilon was more effective than vinpocetine in improving cerebral blood flow (Mirzoian and Gan'shina 1989). Picamilon has a mild tranquilizing action and decreases aggression. Paradoxically, it also has mild stimulative properties, improving alertness and cognition. In animal models it counteracts stress and reduces the central nervous system (CNS) depressive effect of ethanol.

Picamilon rapidly crosses the blood–brain barrier (Dorofeev and Kholodov 1991) and has low toxicity in animal experiments (median lethal oral dose is more than 10 g/kg of body weight). Russian researchers in 16 medical centers conducted large clinical trials using picamilon 20 to 50 mg two to three times a day in therapies ranging from 2 weeks to 3 months. Patients with organic brain syndromes due to head trauma, cerebral atherosclerosis, and toxic brain lesions showed the best effects (Kruglikova 1997). Picamilon is useful in patients with cerebral vascular impairment, particularly with decreased alertness, anxiety, and depression.

## Pyritinol

Pyritinol is a pyridoxine derivative (with no $B_6$ activity). *In vitro* and animal studies show that it increases cerebral glucose utilization, neuronal acetylcholine (Ach) release, cortical and striatal Ach levels, striatal and hippocampal high-affinity choline uptake, and cortical cyclic GMP (guanine monophosphate) (the second messenger for Ach). In a postnatal rat model of chronic hypoxia, pyritinol prevented learning deficits (Lun et al. 1989).

Although numerous pyritinol studies have indicated positive effects in organic brain syndromes (Glatzel 1978, Cooper and Magnus 1980, Noel et al. 1983, Herrmann et al. 1986, Knezevic et al. 1989, Fischhof et al. 1992), a 6-month controlled trial in 70 AD patients found no benefit (Heiss et al. 1994). In three TBI studies, pyritinol accelerated recovery and rehabilitation, reduced mortality, enhanced vigilance, and decreased slow waves on EEG (Dalle Ore et al. 1980). In a 6-week DBRPC study of 270 TBI patients, pyritinol 600 mg/day significantly improved somatic symptoms, cognitive function, and headache compared to placebo (Kitamura 1981).

## Idebenone

Idebenone, a variant of coenzyme Q10 (CoQ10), enhances the ATP-producing mitochondrial electron transport chain (Rego et al. 1999, Amano et al. 1995, Cardoso et al. 1998, 1999, Matsumoto et al. 1998, Mordente et al. 1998). Because the literature on idebenone is voluminous, we refer the reader to a review by Gillis (Gillis et al. 1994). Idebenone improved cognitive function in animals with lesions of the basal forebrain cholinergic system and with cerebral ischemia. It protected cultured rat astrocytes against reperfusion injury (Takuma et al. 2000). In guinea pig hippocampal slices, idebenone augmented the action of vinpocetine on LTP (Ishihara et al. 1989) and improved transcallosal response (Okuyama and Aihara 1988). In a DBRPC MC 2-year study of 302 patients with mild to moderate AD, those given 270 to 360 mg/day of idebenone showed statistically significant dose-dependent improvement in primary and secondary efficacy measures. There was further improvement in the second year. The magnitude of improvement was similar to cholinesterase inhibitors (Gutzmann and Hadler 1998). In a DBRPC 60-week study, 203 AD patients were given either idebenone 360 mg/day or tacrine (up to 160 mg/day). Compared to the tacrine group, patients on idebenone had greater improvement in Efficacy Index Scores (EIS) and a higher rate of benefit from treatment (Gutzmann et al. 2002). The authors have found that TBI patients may respond to idebenone, particularly those who are sluggish with psychomotor retardation. Unfortunately, the current cost of idebenone is prohibitive for many patients. Additional controlled clinical studies of idebenone are warranted.

## Cholinergic Enhancing Agents

The cholinergic hypothesis is based on observations that hippocampal cholinergic dysfunction underlies cognitive impairments in many animal models of TBI (Arciniegas 2001). Cholinergic deficits are also the most consistent pathophysiological findings in AD. The ability of cholinergic agents to improve cognitive function and delay deterioration in AD adds weight to this hypothesis.

## Galantamine

An alkaloid extract of snowdrop (*Galanthus nivalis*) was used in folk medicine of Russia and Eastern Europe for centuries to improve memory in old age. A weak inhibitor of acetylcholinesterase and an allosteric modulator of nicotinic receptors, galantamine (Reminyl) was recently approved by the FDA for treatment of AD (Giacobini 1998, Raskind et al. 2000, Tariot et al. 2000). Some patients do not tolerate prescription Galantamine. However, an herbal extract of *Galanthus nivalis* combined with *R. rosea* can be as effective and more tolerable in some cases.

## Acetyl-L-Carnitine, Alcar

Alcar, an ester of L-carnitine (an amino acid synthesized in brain, liver, and kidney) facilitates uptake of acetyl CoA into mitochondria during fatty acid oxidation and increases energy production via the oxidative phosphorylation chain in mitochondria. Table 104–6 summarizes its numerous neuroprotective effects (Pettegrew et al. 2000, Di Donato et al. 1986). Alcar, protected brain cells after stroke in rats and improved recovery (Lolic et al. 1997). In mild AD, Alcar showed minimal effects, though it slowed progression of AD in younger subjects (Brooks et al. 1998). Alcar improved reaction time, memory, and cognitive performance in a DBPC crossover study of 12 elderly subjects with cerebral vascular disease (Arrigo et al. 1990). A review of seven studies in geriatric depression found antidepressant effects after 4 weeks of treatment (Pettegrew et al. 2000). Regional cerebral blood flow increased in eight out of ten men with brain ischemia 1 hour after a dose of 1,500 mg IV Alcar (Rosadini et al. 1990). As a neuroprotector it helps inhibit neural degeneration such as polyneuropathy (Calvani et al. 1992). Based on animal studies, Alcar is more effective in combination with alpha-lipoic acid, CoQ10, and EFAs for delaying age-related deterioration of mitochondria (Di Donato et al. 1986, Lolic et al. 1997). These effects

**Table 104-6   Putative Mechanisms of Action for Alternative Compounds in Disorders of Cognition and Memory**

| Compound | Chol | NE | DA | 5-HT | Receptors | Cell Energy | Antioxidant | O₂ | Blood Flow | Cell Membrane | BBB | NGF | Lipo-fuscin | Trans-Callosal | LTP | Cognitive Activator |
|---|---|---|---|---|---|---|---|---|---|---|---|---|---|---|---|---|
| ω-3FA | | | | | | | | | | +++ | | | | | | |
| SAMe | + | + | + | + | β-NE Chol GABA | ++ | +++ | | | +++ | | | | | | + |
| Picamilon | | | | | | | | | +++ | | | | | | | + |
| Pyritinol | + | | | | + | + | ++ | ? | + | | | | | | | + |
| Idebenone | | | | + | + | ++ | ++ | ? | | + | | + | | + | + | ++ |
| Galantamine | + | | | | Nic-Chol | | | | | | | | | | | ++ |
| Acetyl-L-carnitine | + | | + | | NMDA | +++ | +++ | + | | ++ | | | → | | | ++ |
| CDP-choline | + | | + | + | | ++ | ++ | | | ++ | ++ | | | | | + |
| Huperzine | + | | | | | | | | | | | | | | | ++ |
| Vinpocetine | | | | | Glut | ++ | ++ | ? | +++ | + | | | | | | +++ |
| *Rhodiola rosea* | + | + | + | + | | ++ | ++ | | | | | | | | + | +++ |
| Ginkgo | | + | + | ? | | | + | + | | | | | | | | + |
| Ginseng | | + | + | ? | | | | + | | | | | | | | + |
| Ma-SR | | | | | | | + | + | | + | | | | | + | + |
| Centrophenoxine | + | + | | | | + | + | + | | + | | | → | + | | ++ |
| Pyrrolidones Racetams | + | + | + | + | NMDA-Glut Musc-Chol | ++ | | | | + | | | | ++ | ++ | + |
| L-deprenyl | | + | + | + | Protects | | ++ | | | ++ | | +++ | | | | + |
| α-lipoic acid | | | | | | | ++++ | | | + | | | | | | + |
| Ptd Ser (bovine) | | + | + | | | | | | | +++ | | | | | | |
| Nicergoline | + | | | | Glut | | + | ? | + | + | | + | | | | + |
| B-vitamin | | | | | | | ++ | | | ++ | | | | | | + |
| Bio-Strath | | | | | | | +++ | | | | | | | | | |
| DHEA | | | | | | + | | | | | | | | | | + |
| DMAE | | | | | | | ++ | | | | | | | | | + |

Chol, cholinergic; NE, norepinephrine; DA, dopamine; 5-HT, 5-hydroxytryptophane; O₂, protects against hypoxia; BBB, blood–brain barrier; NGF, nerve growth factor; LTP, long-term potentiation; TC, transcallosal response; Nic, nicotinic; NMDA, N-methyl-D-aspartate; β-NE, β-adrenergic; Glut, glutamate; Musc, muscarinic; blank, no information; ?, possible effect; +, some effect; ++, moderate effect; +++, strong effect.

need to be studied in humans. The authors have used 1,500 mg b.i.d. in patients with TBI and cerebrovascular disease. These patients often experience improved energy and cognitive function within 2 weeks.

## Citicholine (CDP-choline, Cch)

CDP-choline has been used to treat stroke, dementia, and brain injury in Europe and Japan (Alvarez et al. 1999). After crossing the blood–brain barrier, Cch breaks down into choline (a precursor of Ach) and cytidine (a ribonucleoside). Phospholipid incorporation of the choline restores membrane structural integrity. It improves mitochondrial metabolism and synthesis of phospholipids. In animal models, Cch alleviates cerebral hypoxia and protects against ischemia, edema, and neuronal death in the cerebral cortex, forebrain, and hippocampus (Baskaya et al. 2000, Galletti et al. 1991, Rao et al. 1999) and increases levels of NE, DA, and 5-HT (Petkov et al. 1990). Cch improved memory and cognitive performance in a rat brain injury study (Dixon et al. 1997).

In a 6-week study of middle cerebral artery ischemic stroke, 62 patients were given CDP-choline 2,000 mg/day, 41 were given 500 mg/day, and 111 were given placebo. MRIs taken within the first 24 hours and at 12 weeks showed an increase in lesion volume of 1.8% in the 2,000 mg/day group, 34% in the 500 mg/day group, and 84.7% in the placebo group (Mitka 2002). Meta-analysis of controlled trials by the Cochrane Stroke Review Group concluded that patients with acute and subacute stroke benefit substantially from choline precursors such as CDP-choline (Mitka 2002).

In a recent study, 30 AD patients were randomized to either 1,000 mg/day CDP-choline or placebo for 12 weeks. The patients given CDP-choline showed improved cognitive function without side effects. The effects were particularly pronounced for those with early, mild AD (Alvarez et al. 1999).

Studies in head-injured patients, including case reports, five open series, three DBRPC, and two comparative studies, indicate that Cch treatment is associated with earlier recovery of consciousness, clinical and EEG improvements, accelerated motor rehabilitation, and shortened hospital stays (Calatayud Maldonado et al. 1991, Levin 1991, Lozano 1991, Spiers and Hochanadel 1999). Cch causes virtually no side effects and toxicity studies confirm its safety.

## Huperzine-A (*Huperzia serrata*)

Huperzine-A, derived from club moss (Huperzia serrata), is a strong acetylcholinesterase blocker used in Chinese medicine for inflammation and senility. Animal and primate studies show enhancement of learning and memory (Tang 1996, Xu et al. 1996). A pilot study of low dose Huperzine-A 100 to 200 mg/day for 4 months yielded some clinical improvements in Alzheimer's patients (Zucker 1999). Research is needed with larger doses as used in China (200–400 mg/day). For patients who cannot tolerate Galantamine, Huperzine has fewer side effects.

## Herbal Alternative Treatments

Vinpocetine is a semisynthetic alkaloid derived from periwinkle (*Vinca minor*). It has been used in Eastern Europe as a vasodilator to treat cerebral vascular disorders. Neuroprotective effects include inhibition of calcium/calmodulin-dependent cyclic GMP-phosphodiesterase 1; enhancement of intracellular cyclic GMP levels in vascular smooth muscle; reduction in resistance of cerebral blood vessels; and increased blood flow. Vinpocetine inhibits the molecular cascade precipitated by increases in intracellular calcium. A review of DBRPC trials in a total of 731 patients with chronic cerebral vascular disease, including PET scan studies of 12 patients with middle cerebral artery infarcts, concluded that vinpocetine improves cerebral glucose kinetics and blood flow in the peristroke area (Bonoczk et al. 2000). In clinical practice, the authors find it also helps patients with ischemia secondary to TBI and/or SPECT scan evidence of blood flow abnormalities.

## *Rhodiola Rosea* (Golden Root, Arctic Root, or Roseroot)

*Rhodiolo rosea* flourishes in the mountains of Eastern Europe, Siberia, and the Far East. It has been used for centuries in Russian and Scandinavian folk medicine. Since the 1960s, the former Soviet Union conducted extensive animal and human studies of *R. rosea*. The Soviet government sequestered *R. rosea* research in classified documents because its abilities to enhance physical and mental performance under stress were of strategic interest. It has been used to enhance performance in the military, in cosmonauts, and in Olympic athletes. Declassification of these documents has freed scientists to release their research, but many documents are still difficult to obtain. A comprehensive review, *R. rosea*—"a valuable medicinal plant" (Saratikov and Krasnov 1987c), has recently been translated by Dr. Zakir Ramazanov (Ramazanov July 2001, personal communication). More accessible reviews are also available (Furmanowa et al. 1995, Germano et al. 1999, Kelly 2001, Petkov et al. 1986). Dr. Brown and colleagues (2002) presented a phytomedical overview in Herbalgram. The Soviets exhaustively analyzed the diets of the people of the Province of Georgia searching for the secret of their longevity. Extensive epidemiologic studies have documented that their high percentage of centenarians and the high percentage of mentally and physically well elderly is based on environmental and dietary (rather than genetic) factors (Agakishiev 1962, Ferrell et al. 1985). *R. rosea* is believed to be an important dietary factor contributing to the longevity of Georgians who live at the highest altitudes. They prepare an extract of *R. rosea* root to make tea. All members of the families, from toddlers to great grandparents, drink *R. rosea* tea regularly.

*R. rosea* extracts contain bioactive alkaloids, polyphenols, and phenylpropanoids including tyrosol and salidroside (found in other plants). High pressure liquid chromatography (HPLC) identified the cinnamyl alcohol betavicianidines, rosavin, rosin, and rosarin as being specific to *R. rosea* (Figure 104–3) (Bikov et al. 1999, Dubichev et al. 1991, Kurkin and Zapesochnaya 1986). The whole root extract has greater physiological activity than individual compounds. *R. rosea* extracts should be standardized to 1% salidroside and 3% rosavin and should be free of drying agents such as maltodexrin or other carriers.

Soviet scientists identified complex effects of *R. rosea* extracts on brain function: cognitive stimulation with

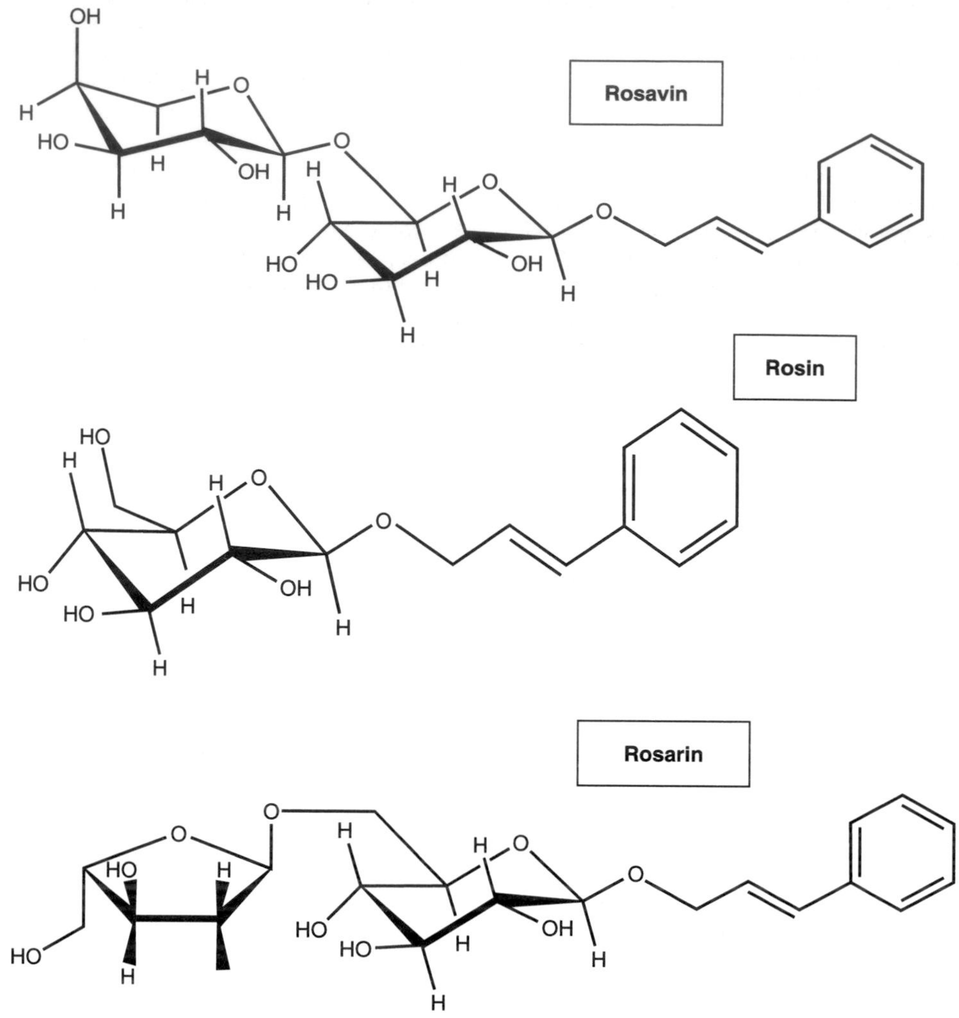

**Figure 104–3** *Rosavin, rosin, rosarin.*

emotional calming; enhanced learning and memory; increased accuracy in mental performance for prolonged periods of time. This powerful plant "adaptogen" protected every organism tested, from snails to humans, against physical and mental stresses, exercise, toxins, and mental fatigue. Brekhman and Dardymov defined an adaptogen as a substance that would increase resistance against multiple stressors including biological, chemical, or physical insults; normalize physiology (whether a body parameter was too high or too low, the adaptogen would bring it towards normal); and not perturb normal body functions more than necessary to improve resistance (Brekhman and Dardymov 1969). *R. rosea* increases the efficiency of energy metabolism and maintains energy rich compounds in brain (including the brain stem reticular formation and cerebral hemispheres), muscle, liver, and blood (Furmanowa et al. 1998, Kurkin and Zapesochnaya 1986). Mechanisms of action include (see Table 104–5) effects on monoamines in cerebral cortex and brain stem (increasing NE, DA, and 5-HT) and in the hypothalamus (increasing NE and DA) (Petkov et al. 1986, 1990, Stancheva and

Mosharrof 1987). *R. rosea* has "antiarrhythmic" and positive "inotropic" effects on the heart. In the myocardium, it prevents catecholamine release (and cAMP elevation) and stress related depletion of adrenal catecholamines (Maslova et al. 1994).

Studies found that *R. rosea* enhanced intellectual work capacity, abstract thinking, and reaction time in healthy subjects (Saratikov and Krasnov 1987a, Spasov et al. 2000). *R. rosea* has been beneficial in patients with organic brain syndrome, most dramatically in posttraumatic and vascular brain lesions, especially in early postinjury stages. Piracetam augmented *R. rosea's* improvement of cognitive function. Based on findings that *R. rosea* exacerbated patients described as "volatile or euphoric" (Saratikov and Krasnov 1987b, Ramazanov July 2001, personal communication), there may be some risk of inducing mania in bipolar patients. *R. rosea* can be even more effective when combined with ginseng or ginkgo. In patients with brain injury, *R. rosea* has a mild stimulant effect while emotionally calming. It has not shown any drug interactions. In clinical practice, the authors have found *R. rosea* to be beneficial in a wide range of disorders of memory, cognition, and fatigue. Increased clinical use and research would be highly beneficial.

*G. biloba* extract has been used to treat AD and cerebral vascular diseases in Europe. An excellent review, including DBRPC studies was done by Wong (Wong et al. 1998). Memory improvements with ginkgo are slight at best and are dose related. Side effects are rare and can be minimized by starting at 60 mg/day and increasing gradually to 120 mg b.i.d. Occasionally nausea, headaches, and skin rashes occur. Although ginkgo somewhat decreases platelet aggregation, it does not appear to affect coagulation or bleeding time (Cott 2002), fibrinogen, prothrombin time or partial thromboplastin time (Kudolo 2000). Nevertheless, caution should be exercised when using ginkgo in patients on anticoagulants, and gingko should be discontinued 2 weeks prior to surgery.

*G. biloba* extract has neuroprotective effects and benefits for memory, AAMI, vascular dementia, and AD. In a DBRPC MC 52-week study of 236 patients with AD, *G. biloba* extract (EGb 761) 120 mg/day improved cognitive performance in patients with mild to moderate cognitive impairment and also slowed the deterioration in patients with severe impairment (Le Bars et al. 2002). A DBRPC comparison study of 109 schizophrenic patients found that patients given Haldol plus EGb 360 mg/day had significant reductions in Scales for Assessment of Negative Symptoms (SANS) and of Positive Symptoms (SAPA) compared to patients treated with Haloperidol only. In addition, the EGb-treated group had fewer "extrapyramidal side effects." These benefits were hypothetically attributed to EGb scavenging of free radicals (Zhang et al. 2001). Ginkgo potentiates CPH and piracetam (Diamond et al. 2000, Wong et al. 1998). The author's clinical experience is that in TBI it is best used as an augmenting agent.

Ginseng (Panax, Korean) contains many compounds with complex effects. It appears to increase production of nitric oxide by endothelial cells (crucial for blood flow and oxygen delivery) in the rabbit (Kang et al. 1995). In a DBPC 8-week study of 36 patients with secondary diabetes, ginseng improved psychomotor performance but not memory (Sotaniemi et al. 1995). One negative DBPC study of 24 geriatric patients given 80 mg/day of ginseng versus 25 geriatric patients on placebo for 8 weeks found no benefits in cognitive performance. This is not surprising, considering that 80 mg of ginseng is quite a low dose (Thommessen and Laake 1996). Danish researchers randomized healthy volunteers over 40 years of age to receive either ginseng 400 mg/day or placebo for 8 weeks. The ginseng group showed significantly better abstract thinking and reaction time, but no significant differences in memory or concentration (Sorensen and Sonne 1996, Sotaniemi et al. 1995, Thommessen and Laake 1996). One study that merits replication showed cognitive enhancement with a gingko/ginseng combination (Wesnes et al. 1997).

## Ayurvedic Herbal Preparations

Bacopa, the most common memory-enhancing preparation used by people from the Indian subcontinent who are living in the US, has been reviewed (Kidd 1999, Kolakowsky and Parente 1997). Our clinical experience is that the effects are so slight that they are not significant and not worth the cost.

Animal data suggest there may be a role in future research for Ashwagandha (Indian ginseng, *Withania somnifera*). This adaptogen, used in folklore for centuries, has been studied extensively in animals. Data presented at the Sixth International Congress on Ethnopharmacology suggested that Ashwagandha is a cholinesterase inhibitor (Hawkins 2000).

Another Ayurvedic preparation occasionally used by the authors, particularly because some patients from the Indian culture are more receptive to traditional preparations, is called "The Student Rasayana" or MA-SR. In a 5-month DBRPC study, 34 third-grade students were given either MA-SR or placebo. The MA-SR group showed a 10 point increase in IQ compared to five points in the placebo group with 78% of the MA-SR group showing improvement in IQ compared with 50% of the placebo group (more than would be expected from test–retest practice effects) (Nidich et al. 1993). *In vitro* models show that MA-SR decreases lipid peroxidation and enhances long-term potentiation in the hippocampus. Additional clinical studies are needed.

## Nootropics

### Centrophenoxine (Meclofenoxate, Lucidril) and BCE-001

Centrophenoxine (CPH) is an ester of dimethyl-aminoethanol (DMAE) and p-chlorophenoxyacetic acid (PCPA). DMAE is a natural component in choline synthesis. PCPA is a synthetic form of a plant growth hormone (Nandy 1978). The ability of CPH to elevate brain Ach was thought to explain its therapeutic effects in cerebral atrophy, dementia, and TBI. Although DMAE does increase free choline, only a fraction of this is needed for Ach synthesis. In an alternative explanation, Zs-Nagy invokes the membrane hypothesis of aging (MHA). MHA focuses on the biochemical interactions between cell membranes and oxidative processes, including free radical theory of aging and protein cross-linking theory. Oxygen free radicals, particularly the rapidly acting OH-radicals subject cell membranes to the highest rate of damage, resulting in loss of permeability, increasing intracellular density, accumulation of cross-linked proteins and lipofuscin (waste products), slowing of RNA synthesis, and decreased protein turnover and repair. CPH rapidly delivers DMAE to the brain where it is incorporated into nerve cell membranes as phosphatidyl-DMAE. Its beneficial neurological effects can be largely attributed to its avid scavenging of OH-radicals in the membranes (Zs-Nagy et al. 1994). Other neuroprotective properties of CPH are summarized in Table 104–6.

In an 8-week DBRPC trial CPH increased psychomotor and behavioral performance in about 50% of patients with moderate dementia compared to 27% on placebo (Pek et al. 1989). In another DBRPC study, 62 geriatric patients with mild to moderate Alzheimer's dementia were given either antagonic stress (a preparation of CPH, vitamins, and nutrients) or nicergoline. After 3 months, those on the CPH preparation showed significant improvements in memory, cognitive function, and behavior compared to those on nicergoline. Nootropics seem to work best in combination with vitamins and minerals (Schneider et al. 1994). CPH may be further augmented with piracetam and other nootropics (Fischer et al. 1984).

BCE-001, a new nootropic drug currently in phase IV testing, is similar to CPA but with a modification of the PCPA moiety creating twice as many loosely bound electrons to neutralize OH-radicals. In *in vitro* and *in vivo* studies, BCE-001 showed similar but more rapid effects compared to CPH, including improving neuronal membrane fluidity, reversal of membrane protein cross-linking in rat brain cortex, reversal of the neuronal membrane passive potassium permeability with rehydration of neuronal cytoplasm. Relevant to human dementia prevention, BCE-001 also outperformed CPH in reversing age-related decline in mRNA synthesis in rat brain, thus increasing protein synthesis (Zs-Nagy 1994).

## Pyrrolidones (Racetams)

Racetams are nootropic compounds (neural metabolic enhancers), which have been touted to be "smart drugs." Although piracetam has been most frequently studied, aniracetam, oxiracetam, and pramiracetam are more potent. While results in animal studies are intriguing, numerous human studies in mild dementia and AAMI have shown only weak support (Itil et al. 1986, Flicker and Evans 2001).

Piracetam increases nerve cell membrane fluidity, activates EEGs, improves red cell deformability, and normalizes hyperactive platelet aggregation. In animal-learning models and aged rodents, effects on memory deficits are potentiated by CDP-choline, idebenone, vinpocetine, and deprenyl (Gouliaev and Senning 1994, Vernon and Sorkin 1991). Human studies combining racetams with CDP-choline and cholinesterase inhibitors are needed.

Although positive studies of piracetam in postconcussion syndrome have had methodological problems (Cicerchia et al. 1985, Russello et al. 1990), in one DBRPC study of 60 patients with postconcussion syndrome of 2 to 12 months duration, piracetam 4,800 mg/day for 8 weeks reduced the severity of symptoms, especially vertigo and headache (Hakkarainen and Hakamies 1978). In large DBPC studies, piracetam (given within 7 hours of stroke) enhanced language recovery in combination with speech therapy (De Deyn et al. 1997) and improved task-related blood flow in left hemisphere speech areas on PET scan (Kessler et al. 2000). Studies of a combination of piracetam and ginkgo in dyslexia and aphasia showed significant enhancement of cognitive retraining: gingko improved attention and perception while piracetam improved learning (Enderby et al. 1994). See the section on dyslexia further on.

## L-Deprenyl

L-deprenyl is known as a prescription MAOI antidepressant in the US. It is considered to be an alternative agent in this discussion because most physicians are not familiar with its neuroprotective properties in organic brain disorders. Recent data suggest a mechanism of action different from its MAOI effect, when used in very low doses. Animal studies suggest that L-deprenyl protects catecholaminergic and cholinergic neurons by increasing antioxidants (Kitani et al. 2000, Maruyama and Naoi 1999). In a model of rat TBI, L-deprenyl improved cognitive function and neuroplasticity, particularly in the hippocampus (Zhu et al. 2000). Joseph Knoll, the discoverer of L-deprenyl, described a novel mechanism of action at a receptor site

for an endogenous enhancer, which selectively improves impulse propagation mediated release of catecholamines and serotonin in the brain. The enhancer effects on catecholamine and serotonin systems are most marked in the hippocampus. In response to stimulation of this receptor, glial cells and astrocytes secrete significantly higher amounts of numerous nerve growth factors (NGFs). Higher activity levels in enhancer-sensitive neurons appear to delay the age-related degenerative changes in the brain and to significantly increase longevity in animal experiments. In several studies, L-deprenyl slowed the progression of Parkinson's and Alzheimer's diseases (Knoll 2000). Several human studies show slight improvements in cognitive function in early Alzheimer's disease (Mangoni et al. 1991).

Our clinical experience is that L-deprenyl given in ultra low doses (that do not cause MAO inhibition) using 5 mg tablets (giving half a pill 5 days of the week) may help prevent or slow down the neurodegenerative changes of aging, neurological diseases, and TBI. The authors use it to enhance neuronal repair and response to other treatments. Liquid L-deprenyl citrate may be more effective, convenient, and tolerable but no comparative studies have been done. The neuroprotective potential of L-deprenyl deserves further study.

## Alpha-Lipoic Acid

Recent animal and human data suggest that alpha-lipoic acid (ALA) and CoQ-10 may be helpful for poststroke and for ischemic heart disease (Lonnrot et al. 1998). The significance of these preliminary data will depend on future research (Packer and Colman 1999).

Alpha-lipoic acid is a simple metabolic antioxidant, which has been used as a prescription drug in Europe for the treatment of cardiac autonomic problems related to diabetic neuropathy as well as other consequences of diabetes. ALA has shown neuroprotective effects in cerebral ischemia/reperfusion animal-models, excitotoxic amino acid brain injury, mitochondrial dysfunction, diabetic neuropathy, inborn errors of metabolism and other causes of acute or chronic damage to nerve tissue including excess levels of iron, copper, or other metals. For a review see Packer and colleagues (1997). ALA generates large amounts of glutathione in animal brain models (similar to SAMe). For patients who cannot afford SAMe, ALA in combination with vinpocetine can be helpful when ischemia is a major factor, as well as in other brain injuries. A dose of 300 mg t.i.d. may be used in TBI.

## Phosphatiydyl Serine

Bovine-derived phosphatidyl serine (Ptd Ser or PS) has been studied for AAMI (Caffarra and Santamaria 1987, Cenacchi et al. 1987), AD (Amaducci 1988), and related conditions. DBPC studies have shown modest memory improvement in these conditions (Crook et al. 1991, 1992). Crook found that in AAMI 300 mg/day for 1 month followed by 100 mg/day improved memory. For a review, see the article by Pepeu (Pepeu et al. 1996). Ptd Ser, a small component of the inner phospholipid layer, may make the nerve cell membrane more fluid (as discussed in the section on SAMe). Bovine brain-derived Ptd Ser, rich in docosahexanoic acid (DHA; 22:6n3) increased brain dopamine, norepinephrine, and epinephrine levels in animals (Salem 1989, Salem et al. 1986). In contrast, Ptd Ser from soy, which is low in DHA, did not alter catecholamine levels (Toffano et al. 1976). There is little data to show that soy Ptd Ser improves memory. The apparent benefits of bovine Ptd Ser may be due to cognitive enhancing effects of omega-3FAs (Hibbeln and Salem 1995). Although no cases of Mad Cow Disease have been reported with bovine Ptd Ser, further research is needed to determine if this is a possibility. Ptd Ser is often combined with other nutrients such as ginkgo despite the fact that the Ptd ser effect on memory is more robust than that of ginkgo.

## Ergot Derivatives

### Hydergine and Nicergoline

Readers interested in ergot derivatives should refer to reviews of hydergine and nicergoline in Alzheimer's and other organic brain syndromes (Flynn and Ranno 1999, Grobe-Einsler 1993, Schneider and Tariot 1994). In more than 47 trials of hydergine in AD, the effect has been slight at best, although there is a suggestion that higher doses may be somewhat effective. However, nicergoline (Grobe-Einsler 1993), a calcium channel blocker used in subarachnoid hemorrhage, shows more significant though modest effects. Nicergoline has significant cognitive-activating effect on EEG mapping, which correlates with modest clinical improvement (Saletu et al. 1995). It enhances glutamate reuptake and protects against brain damage in a rat model of global brain ischemia (Asai et al. 1999). Furthermore, nicergoline improves brain blood flow, helps brain cholinergic systems, increases NGF in aged rat brains, and blocks calcium channels and alpha-1-adrenergic receptors in aged rats (Nishio et al. 1998). Enhancement of radial maze learning and improvement in acetylcholine levels in aged rats were hypothesized to relate to changes in transduction systems such as inositol and protein kinase C (McArthur et al. 1997).

Human data showed that nicergoline improves cognitive function by 15% under hypoxic conditions compared to placebo (Saletu et al. 1990). In a 6-month DBR trial, 30 patients with acute or chronic ischemic strokes treated with 60 mg/day nicergoline improved more than 27 patients treated with hydergine. Cognitive improvements were consistent with activation on EEG (Elwan et al. 1995). Nicergoline 60 mg/day was compared to placebo in a 6-week DB parallel group study of 56 patients with multiinfarct dementia and 56 patients with AD. In both groups, nicergoline significantly improved cognitive measures and vigilance on EEG mapping. Nicergoline induced an increase in alpha activity and a decrease in theta and delta activity, as well as a shorter P300 latency (Saletu et al. 1997).

## Vitamins

### B-Vitamins and Bio-Strath

The methylation pathways that maintain cellular proteins, membranes, and antioxidants depend on B-vitamins and folate as cofactors. B-vitamin and folate deficiencies are associated with abnormalities of mood, memory, and cognitive function (Bottiglieri 1996, Hassing et al. 1999). Supplementation with B-vitamins improves mood and cog-

nitive function in healthy subjects (Benton et al. 1997). Bio-Strath, a B-vitamin supplement was given at double the usual adult dose to 75 patients 55 to 85 years of age with mild dementia in a 3-month DBRPC trial. The placebo group deteriorated. In contrast, the Bio-Strath group showed improvement in short-term memory as well as physical and emotional benefits. It took 3 months for the differences to appear (Pelka and Leuchtgens 1995). Given the relationship between B-vitamins and cognitive function and the probable role of antioxidants, it is important to treat geriatric and brain-injured patients with B-vitamins.

## Other Cognitive Enhancing Agents

### Dehydroepiandrosterone, DHEA

DHEA is produced primarily in the adrenal glands and secondarily in the ovaries and testes. Among its neurological effects, DHEA has been reported to improve memory, brain activation on EEG, and mood (Wolkowitz et al. 1999). A 3-month study of normal older men found no change in cognition or well-being with DHEA (van Niekerk et al. 2001). Patients whose DHEA is low for age (particularly menopausal women who have had ovaries and adrenal glands removed) (Gurnell and Chatterjee 2001, Yen 2001) and debilitated geriatric patients with medical or neurological diseases (the author's clinical experience) are more likely to show improved memory and mood when given DHEA. Side effects include insomnia, irritability, slight increases in estrogen, and potential interactions with steroids. Concerns about effects on prostate can be addressed by serial testing of prostate specific antigen (PSAs). Physicians should only administer pharmaceutical grade DHEA in doses sufficient to restore physiologic levels (25–50 mg/day).

## Attention Deficit Disorder

Attention deficit disorder (ADD) with or without hyperactivity is defined as a constellation of symptoms that appears by age 7 years and frequently persists into adult life. These symptoms derive from inability to inhibit impulsiveness and/or to focus attention. Although the etiology and pathophysiology are not understood, theories involving DA, NE, and Ach neurotransmitter systems combined with under-arousal of the brain have heuristic value for research and treatment efforts. Genetic and imaging studies lend support to biological bases of the disorder. It is particularly important to develop more effective treatments for ADHD because of its high incidence in children; its frequent comorbidity with learning disabilities, oppositional behavior, depression, anxiety, bipolar, tics, obsessive–compulsive behavior; and the high risk of later substance abuse and antisocial behavior.

Stimulants such as methylphenidate are the mainstay of conventional ADD treatments. However, many parents would prefer to use CAM for their children. Their legitimate concerns about potential abuse and long-term side effects are fueled by reports that methylphenidate affects the brain like slow-acting cocaine (Vastag 2001); that stimulants (e.g., amphetamine) deplete the brain of high-energy compounds (Volkow et al. 2001a), SAMe (Cooney et al. 1998), and dopamine (Volkow et al. 2001b, 2001c); and that liver cancer increases in mice treated with methylphenidate (Dunnick and Hailey 1995, Ernst et al. 2000). Space limitations restrict this discussion to CAM treatments that the authors have found useful in clinical practice or that are frequently asked about by parents: dietary elimination strategies, vitamins, minerals, omega-3FAs, acetyl-L-carnitine, DMAE, meclofenoxate, pyrrolidones, and herbs. For a review of CAM for ADHD, see Arnold (2001) and Kidd (2000). For a discussion of biofeedback for ADD see the section on neurotherapy later in this chapter.

Dietary elimination strategies have been supported by acceptable scientific evidence since the 1970s. The typical responder (a sizable minority of ADD children) is a preschooler with insomnia, irritability, atopy, physical symptoms, behavioral problems, and sometimes high copper levels. Most families have difficulty maintaining the "few foods" diet. Eliminating the more suspicious food items may help in about 50% of children. Methodological problems and investigator bias in sugar elimination studies have left this issue unresolved (Kidd 2000). The role of toxicity from heavy metals (lead, aluminium) and organic chemical pollutants (pesticides, dioxin, polychlorinated biphenols, hydrocarbons, etc.) in the developing brain needs more research.

Cognitive activators, antioxidants, nutrients, and nootropics that have been shown to ameliorate symptoms in patients with AD, TBI, dementia, and learning disorders may also be beneficial in ADD. Conventional and alternative treatments probably improve ADD symptoms by cognitive activation, but CAM treatments may also ameliorate underlying cell membrane dysfunction. Further controlled studies in ADD treatment using the following compounds are needed.

Vitamin and mineral supplementation at reasonable levels (not megavitamins) is promising in studies in normal children, retarded children, and teen delinquents. In a DB trial, children whose pretesting showed low serum levels of B-vitamins or C-vitamins, aggression and antisocial behavior decreased and cognitive performance improved (IQ increased 2.5 points) in those treated with vitamin supplements (Schoenthaler and Bier 1999). The authors use Bio-Strath, a Swiss tonic of Brewer's yeast grown on antioxidant herbs and high in minerals, vitamins, and nutrients. Mineral supplementation for deficiencies of magnesium, iron, and zinc needs further study (Kidd 2000, Arnold 2001).

Acetyl-L-carnitine has diverse effects on cell membranes, energy reserves, cholinergic function, and EFA utilization (see section earlier) (Pettegrew et al. 2000). In a DBRPC study, 20 fragile-X boys with hyperactivity benefited from Alcar (Torrioli et al. 1999).

Dimethylaminoethanol (DMAE) is a common component of OTC supplements used in ADHD. Most of the DBPC trials were done so long ago that their methodology is considered inferior by today's standards. However, a more recent rigorous trial suggested a modest effect size, though less than methylphenidate (Arnold 2001). The authors prefer meclofenoxate (see cognitive enhancer section earlier), a combination of DMAE and PCPA, an excellent antioxidant in nerve cell membranes. It is well studied, inexpensive, and low in side effects. It is potentiated by ginkgo and caffeine. The author has found the combination of meclofenoxate and pyrrolidones to be particularly effective in a small number of children and adults with ADD and learning disabilities.

Herbal treatment for ADHD may cause cognitive activation and/or calming. Controlled trials of ginkgo and ginseng are indicated because these herbs improve learning in animals and humans, they affect the appropriate neurotransmitter systems, and they are cognitive activators (Itil 2001, Petkov et al. 1990). An open trial in 36 children with ADHD given American ginseng (Panax quinquefolius) 400 mg/day plus G. biloba 100 mg/day for 4 weeks found that 74% improved significantly on the Conner's ADHD scale and 44% improved on a social problems measure. Only 2 children experienced mild side effects (Lyon et al. 2001). R. rosea has a similar profile and may be used in ADHD. However, it can be very stimulating in children. Although Passionflower is a frequent ingredient in OTC preparations for ADD (see section on anxiety) no studies have been done in ADD. Side effects and toxicity have not been investigated. Huperzine (see cholinergic agents) is of interest because it has minimal side effects (unlike prescription cholinesterase inhibitors). Other Chinese herbal preparations are promising (Arnold 2001).

Deficiencies of omega-3FAs have been found in a subgroup of ADHD boys (Burgess et al. 2000). Until further study, no treatment recommendations can be offered.

ADHD children (like adults with AD, TBI and seizure disorders) have excess theta and reduced beta and/or alpha rhythms on EEG. Animal data show a reduction of physical activity with appearance of beta frequencies in the sensorimotor areas when an animal is vigilant and still (e.g., a cat waiting to pounce on a mouse emerging from its hole). Promising results have been associated with enhancement of alpha and/or beta rhythms, but further sham-controlled studies are needed (Lubar and Lubar 1984, Ramirez et al. 2001, Nash 2000). The authors have found a more recent modification of this approach called "disentrainment neurotherapy" (see section on neurotherapy later) to be helpful in ADD.

Meditation also has effects on EEG rhythms similar to theta/beta biofeedback training. Two promising controlled studies in ADHD children found improvements in attention, particularly in the classroom (Arnold 2001). More extensive studies are needed. For now, the authors refer children to a particular yogic breathing and meditation program called ART-Exel taught by the Art of Living Foundation (AOL) (see section on yogic breathing later).

Other promising nonpharmacologic approaches include massage, vestibular stimulation, and channel-specific perceptual training. Further research is needed, particularly to establish how long treatment effects last.

## Dyslexia and Learning Disabilities

Early studies of racetams in dyslexic children showed mixed results, probably due to heterogeneity of subjects and inadequate duration of trials. A DBRPC MC study of 225 dyslexic children (ages 7–12 years) using piracetam 3,600 mg/day demonstrated significant improvements in reading ability and comprehension evident at 12 weeks and sustained for the 36 weeks of the trial (Wilsher et al. 1987). Piracetam was well tolerated with no adverse effects. In dyslexics piracetam preferentially activates the left hemisphere (Ackerman et al. 1991, Tallal et al. 1986, Helfgott et al. 1986).

Pyritinol like piracetam improves cognitive functions and interhemisphere transfer of information. It was reported as useful in dyslexia, learning disabilities, and mental retardation, but many studies used outdated methodologies and need replication.

## Yogic Breathing, Sudarshan Kriya for Treatment of: Depression, Anxiety, Stress, PTSD, Aggression, and Violence

Yoga, an ancient Indian philosophical method, can relieve stress, induce relaxation, and give many health benefits. However varied, its many techniques constitute a psychophysiological therapy which invites applications to psychiatric disorders. For reviews of yoga philosophy, techniques, neurophysiological findings, and studies in anxiety, depression, OCD (Shannahoff-Khalsa et al. 1999), and epilepsy, see Yardi (2001) and Becker (2000).

Janakiramaiah and colleagues have showed benefits of a yogic breathing technique called *sudarshan kriya* (SKY) in an open preliminary study of 15 dysthymics and nine unipolar major depressives. Depression improved after 1 month of SKY practice 30 minutes/day and improved further by 3 months (Naga Venkatesha Murthy et al. 1997). In an extension of this study, 15 additional dysthymics and 15 melancholics responded positively (Naga Venkatesha Murthy et al. 1998). In a subsequent open study, 80% of 46 dysthymics completed a 3-month protocol of SKY 30 minutes/day. Sixty-eight percent of the completers attained remission (Janakiramaiah et al. 1998). A comparison study of 45 hospitalized melancholic depressives randomized to ECT, imipramine, or SKY demonstrated that all three treatments were effective with ECT being slightly more so than SKY or imipramine (Janakiramaiah et al. 2000). Lack of double-blinding or placebo-control groups limit these studies. Nevertheless, if one considers the low expectable placebo response rate in melancholic depressives and prior research findings that SKY improved REM latency and slow-wave sleep and significantly reduced cortisol, it appears that SKY has powerful biological effects. Compliance with the breathing technique in these studies ranged

from 56 to 80% compared to 50% compliance with prescription antidepressants (with complaints of significant side effects from medications).

In developing a neurophysiological model of the effects of yogic breathing on the CNS, we have drawn upon several related fields of research, including effects of breathing and chanting on hypercapnia and consequent improvements in autonomic regulation and cardiac function; hyperventilation studies; vagal nerve stimulation (VNS); thalamic oscillators; sensorimotor rhythm (SMR) and vigilance; and neuroendocrine effects. Space limitations permit only a cursory partial overview of this model.

Sudarshan kriya yoga consists of a specific sequence of breathing patterns (*pranayam*) separated by brief periods of normal breathing: *ujjayi*—slow strained breathing against airway resistance at 3 cycles/minute; *bhastrika*—forceful exhalation at 20 to 30 cycles/minute; brief chanting of *om*; *sudarshan kriya*—rhythmic cyclical breathing of slow, medium, and fast cycles; meditation; and rest.

Strained breathing occurs in nature when an animal is defeated in battle (Fokkema 1999). It inhibits activity, increases brain perfusion, increases attention and vigilance (via vagal afferents), slows heart rate, restores energy, prevents hypoxia/hypercapnia (Sovik 2000, Spicuzza et al. 2000), and prepares the animal to protect itself. During ujjayi, people feel calmed. The proposed mechanism would be a shift to parasympathetic dominance via vagal stimulation. Bhastrika causes autonomic sympathetic activation and CNS excitation on EEG (Roldan and Dostalek 1983, 1985) with activation of temporo–parietal cortical areas, producing rhythms that are similar to the gamma frequency bands hypothesized to reflect synchronization of neural assemblies (Kwon et al. 1999). The subjective experience is of excitation during bhastrika followed by emotional calming with mental activation and alertness. Sudarshan kriya may work like mechanical hyperventilation and electronic unilateral vagal nerve stimulation, which lead to stimulation of thalamic nuclei (Figure 104–4) resulting in quieting of frontal cerebral

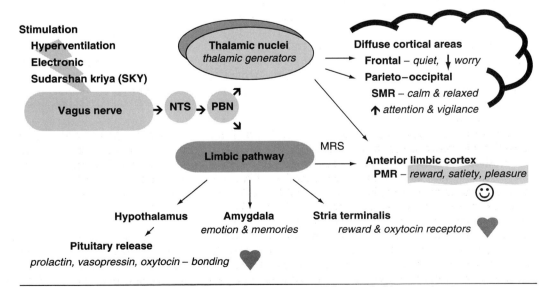

**Figure 104–4** *Neurophysiological model of vagus nerve stimulation pathways.*

NTS, nucleus tractus solitarius; PBN, parabrachial nucleus; MRS, mesolimbic reward system; SMR, sensori–motor rhythm; PMR, post-reinforcement synchronization.

cortex. Slowing of the EEG with hyperventilation is mediated by the vagal nerves, thalamus, and nonspecific thalamic projection system (NSTPS) (Balzamo et al. 1991, Patel and Maulsby 1987). MRI studies show that it quiets the frontal cortical areas, but not the subcortical (Posse et al. 1997). Hyperventilation increased blood flow (PET) to the thalamus in epileptics (Prevett et al. 1995). Vagal nerve stimulation (like hyperventilation) stimulates vagal afferents first to the nucleus tractus solitarius (NTS) and then to the parabrachial (PB) nucleus (see Figure 104–4). From the PB two pathways diverge. One projects to thalamic nuclei. The midline ventro–basal nucleus of the thalamus probably affects cortical synchronization. The other path to the hypothalamus, amygdala, stria terminalis, and limbic system affects autonomic, endocrine, and emotional processes (Schachter and Saper 1998). In a 1-year open follow-up study of 30 patients treated with VNS for treatment resistant–depressive episode, a significant response rate was sustained and further improvements occurred in mental health, social function, and vitality (Marangell et al. 2002).

SMR (a pattern of 12–20 cycles/second found in the sensorimotor cortex) is generated by oscillations of activity between thalamic nuclei. In humans, this requires decreased eye and body movements and creates a more focused state with improved memory, vigilance, attention, sleep, and resistance to seizures (Sterman 1996). A thalamic gating system is also involved in postreinforcement synchronization (PRS), a 4 to 12 Hz rhythm in the parietal cortex associated with reward, satiety, and pleasure. A pilot study comparing 19 AOL sudarshan kriya teachers with 15 control subjects found that the EEGs of AOL teachers had increased beta activity (similar to SMR) in the left parieto–occipital area indicating activation of the thalamic generator. This occurred with increased alpha activity. The subjective experience was of calmness and relaxation combined with increased vigilance and attention.

Over time, yoga may reduce stress hormones by transiently increasing opioids, prolactin, vasopressin, and other hypothalamic pituitary hormones. The hypothalamic–pituitary axis (HPA) is overactivated in biological depression. In PTSD it is acutely overactivated and then chronically depleted. A 3-month study of SKY found a significant reduction in cortisol (a measure of stress response system activation), increased prolactin acutely, and decreased depression scores (Gangadhar et al. 2000). Meditation was found to result in a fivefold increase in vasopressin (Travis 2001). It is likely that meditation and kriya release not only prolactin and vasopressin, but also oxytocin via vagal afferents to the hypothalamus and anterior pituitary. Oxytocin enhances feelings of bonding and affection (Carter 1998, Nelson and Panksepp 1998). Oxytocin secretion was found to be low in major depression and to increase after treatment with SSRIs (Uvnas-Moberg et al. 1999).

This neurophysiological model presumes strengthening (and stabilizing) of the autonomic and stress response systems, quieting of cortical areas involved in executive functions (such as anticipation, planning, and worry), progressive activation of hypothalamic (HPA hormone release), midbrain, and limbic systems (with emotional release and sometimes recall of repressed memories), and balancing of cortical areas (synchronization) by thalamic and medullary generators, and eventual stimulation of the reward systems of the medial forebrain bundle. For an in-depth discussion of this model, see Brown and Gerbarg (2002).

SKY can augment the psychotherapeutic and pharmacological treatment of nonpsychotic patients with anxiety and depression, or serve as an alternative treatment for those who prefer not to take medications. Bipolar I patients or unstable rapid cyclers should not be treated with SKY because there is risk of exacerbation of mania. But bipolar II patients who are stabilized on anticonvulsants other than lithium (yogic breathing can lower lithium levels by increasing lithium excretion) and atypical antipsychotics have benefited from SKY.

Although no formal studies have been done yet, SKY is known to relieve symptoms of PTSD. Dr. Sageman (2002, personal communication) has found that patients with PTSD benefited from SKY training. In effect, the six-session SKY course provides both exposure therapy and cognitive–behavioral therapy in a supportive group setting. Like exposure therapy, the rapid breathing can provoke reexperiencing of trauma symptoms in a safe setting. The instructor and group communicate to each participant that they care about and belong to one another. AOL provides psychoeducation in basic human values of acceptance, social responsibility, and community service (Sageman 2002). The overall effect of this multimodal program is amelioration of feelings of anxiety, fear, neglect, abuse, rejection, depression, isolation, and worthlessness. Patients with PTSD should be given careful preparation including explanations of what will occur in SKY courses and possible physical/emotional reactions. The therapist should keep in contact with the patient during and after the course to assist with intense emotions that may emerge. Ideally, the physician or therapist should take at least the introductory course before referring patients in order to understand the program, make appropriate referrals, and support patients through the process.

Programs using SKY for adult incarcerated criminals and for juvenile offenders have found that it substantially reduces aggression and incidents of violence. In a 4-month open pilot study, 86 juvenile 707B offenders (ages 13–18) who had committed violent crimes with deadly weapons, primarily gang members from Los Angeles County, were given SKY instruction for 1 week (20–25 hours) in the Prison Smart Program. They also participated in 30 minutes of guided meditation and breathing 3 nights a week. Participants had significant overall decreases in anxiety, anger, fear, reactive behavior, and fighting (Suarez 2002).

SKY courses are sponsored by the Art of Living Foundation, a nonprofit international organization. AOL has an affiliation with the United Nations. Its mission is to promote human values by charitable works and by teaching SKY techniques in more than 100 countries. Volunteer AOL teachers brought relief to hundreds of traumatized and grieving New Yorkers by offering free courses after the 9/11 World Trade Center attacks. Information on courses in most major cities can be found at www. artofliving.org.

## Neurotherapy

Traditional Neurotherapy (neurofeedback or EEG biofeedback) trains patients to notice and influence their state of alertness based on EEG measures. This form of operant conditioning requires many treatments and patient cooperation. Readers interested in controversies regarding quantitative electroencephalogram (QEEG) will find Hoffman's discussion (Hoffman et al. 1999) to be of interest. For a review of neurotherapy in ADD, see Nash (2000). A modern innovation of neurotherapy uses the International 10 to 20 system of brain mapping and therapeutic procedures based on changing the frequency or amplitude of "brain waves" at specific sites on that system (Robbins 2000). It requires no effort on the part of the patient. Protocols have been developed for seizures using the sensori–motor rhythm (SMR, 12–15Hz) (formerly called "lo-Beta") (Lubar and Bahler 1976, Sterman and Macdonald 1978), ADHD (Lubar and Lubar 1984, Sovik 2000), TBI (Ayers 1987), and PTSD combined with alpha training (alpha–theta protocol) to "soften" the dangers of retraumatization during recall (Ochs 1994), and in depressed alcoholics (Peniston and Kulkosky 1989).

QEEGs, measuring frequencies and amplitudes over the entire brain, have improved the quality of diagnosis and treatment protocols. Inhibition of theta and reinforcement of SMR (immobile attention, still, but alert) have been postulated to explain the therapeutic effects of biofeedback. One hypothesis for the benefits of neurotherapy in TBI, PTSD, stroke, and cerebral palsy was that since trauma is associated with EEG slowing, a speeding up or stimulation of the brain would tend to be therapeutic. "EEG-driven stimulation" uses the brain waves themselves to drive a flashing light, which is then "fed back" to the brain via light emitting diodes (LEDs). Ochs included all brain wave ranges in protocols emphasizing the brain's flexibility in moving between them. Commercial light and sound "brain wave" machines entrain brain waves to a fixed frequency. Light flashing at exactly the brain's own frequency can amplify and drive existing instabilities, producing adverse reactions (e.g., seizures) in people with CNS damage. Ochs developed "offsets" to decrease rather than increase amplitudes producing "disentrainment" rather than "entrainment" (Glieck 1988). Ochs now uses a J&J Electronics C-2 EEG in the Flexyx neurotherapy system (FNS). Its therapeutic modality was found to be radio waves, at a level of intensity far below a cell phone's. The Flexyx method has been beneficial in neuropsychiatric disorders: ADD, PTSD, affective disorders, pain syndromes, chronic fatigue, and fibromyalgia. The most dramatic responses were in TBI. Some patients with seizures following TBI respond well to neurotherapy.

A preliminary, randomized study of 12 mild to moderately severe TBI patients with substantial cognitive impairment given 25 FNS treatments found significant improvements in Beck Depression Inventory (BDI), mental fatigue, digit span backwards, delayed recall on the auditory verbal learning test (AVLT), ability to function at work and at school, and other measures when compared to a wait-list control group (Schoenberger et al. 2001).

Neurotherapy using FNS is a promising new treatment with few side effects when administered by an experienced clinician. Side effects include temporary re-experiencing of symptoms related to the initial trauma. Overtreatment can cause fatigue and restlessness. DBPC trials are needed to follow up on positive clinical experience and preliminary trials.

## Clinical Guidelines in Using Cognitive Enhancing Agents

The main considerations in choosing alternative treatments are the specific target symptoms (see Table 104–5), the mechanism of action (see Table 104–6), side effects, cost, and availability. For example, memory deficits respond well to cholinergic agents. Patients who have neural fatigue or problems with drive and energy, in addition to memory and abstract thinking may do best with R. rosea, SAMe, idebenone, or dopaminergic agents. Those who need treatment for depression and/or to improve stress resilience may benefit most from R. rosea, SAMe, or L-deprenyl. Impaired alertness and vigilance may be helped by any of the cholinergic agents, R. rosea, picamilon, vinpocetine, or SAMe. Patients with a prominent vascular component in their lesion (by history, SPECT scan, or other blood flow studies) may benefit most from picamilon, vinpocetine (with or without) idebenone, or SAMe. Another example of combining agents would be to choose one that works primarily on the cholinergic system and another that works primarily on the catecholamine and/or serotonin system. Patients who, under psychological testing or on EEG, show overactivation of one cerebral hemisphere compared to the other, and who seem to have impaired transfer of information across the corpus callosum (on neurological testing), may do best with one of the racetam agents in combination with a cholinergic agent.

The cholinergic compounds for which there is most evidence of efficacy in cognitively impaired populations or in animal models are galantamine, centrophenoxine, acetyl-L-carnitine, and particularly CDP-choline. Centrophenoxine may work best in combination with the racetam agents. Although piracetam has been the most widely used and studied, pramiracetam, aniracetam, or oxiracetam may be more effective.

## How to Use CAM Treatments Safely and Effectively

### Herb–Drug Interactions

Our discussion of significant interactions between drugs and herbs must be brief and selective. See Tables 104–1 to 104–3 for a summary of the major side effects and drug interactions. Because alternative compounds tend to have low side effect profiles, few difficulties are encountered combining them with most conventional treatments. However, herbs (such as St. John's wort) that affect the cytochrome P450 (CYP) drug metabolizing enzyme systems or the P-glycoprotein (Pgp) transmembrane pump can reduce serum levels of numerous medications (see section on SJW) (Cott 2002). John Neeld, Jr., President of the American Society of Anesthesiologists, recently warned that a number of anesthesiologists have anecdotally reported significant changes in heart rate and blood pressure particularly in patients taking St. John's wort, ginkgo, and ginseng. He recommends that patients be advised to stop herbal medications 2 to 3 weeks before surgery (Voelker 1999). Herbs which can affect bleeding time (feverfew, garlic, ginkgo, ginger, and ginseng) should not be used with warfarin and should also be stopped prior to surgery. The use of SJW with medications that have significant action on the serotonin system (SSRIs or MAOIs) should be avoided at the current time because of limited testing for safety. Valerian and kava should not be used with other sedating medications because of the potential for additive sedative effects. Evening primrose oil and borage oil (a source of omega-3FAs) should not be used with anticonvulsants because they may lower seizure thresholds. Licorice may counteract the pharmacological effects of spironolactone. Chromium picolinate, and ginseng may affect blood glucose levels and should be stopped prior to surgery. Herbal laxatives and licorice, by depleting potassium, may affect the therapeutic action of digoxin, beta-blockers, and diuretics. For more extensive information see Miller (1998) or Ernst (2001). When patients taking standard antidepressant medications are given activating compounds such as *R. rosea* or SAMe, they may experience overstimulation and/or induction of hypomania in rare cases. Nevertheless, overall these agents are extremely well tolerated.

## The Importance of the Doctor–Patient Relationship

Communication between a patient and his or her physician is the cornerstone of all therapeutic interactions. Thus it comes as no surprise that a patient's use of CAM becomes part of the therapy. This is particularly important in light of the expanding information regarding interactions between alternative and traditional treatments, which can be both advantageous and adverse. Surveys indicate that only 25 to 70% of patients inform their physicians about CAM use. Patients often use alternative therapies without consulting an informed CAM practitioner. Asking the clerk behind the counter at the health-food store may be the extent of the "consultation." Obviously, some patients are well informed about CAM from their own research, or from having consulted with an experienced herbalist or other CAM expert. We are practicing in a time of rapidly growing CAM use when few physicians have been trained in CAM therapies. While many physicians are scrambling to meet this challenge, others are ignoring the need to gain competence in this emerging field of medical practice. Ignorance and/or insecurity about CAM treatments may contribute to a potential countertransference enactment in which the physician discounts *all* CAM approaches as unfounded and misinterprets the patient's interest in CAM as merely a form of resistance (Kenny et al. 2001). This can create a situation in which the patient cannot tell the therapist about an interest in, or the use of a CAM therapy. Patients are more likely to share this information with a physician who is open-minded and nonjudgmental. We suggest the discussion start with a comment such as, "I am interested in the ways you maintain wellness such as diet, exercise, herbs, and other activities." This is preferable to, "Do you use any of *those* things?" Many CAM treatments can enhance and maintain well-being; however, an alternative treatment may render a traditional one less effective, creating confusion in the therapy. An open dialogue between patient and physician will help prevent adverse outcomes.

As with all human endeavors, a patient's desire to pursue a CAM therapy may reflect a spectrum of psychological meanings. No discussion could cover them all, but a few general themes are worth considering:

1. To what extent does the desire for CAM indicate a resistance to conventional treatment that should be clarified and interpreted?
   a. Negative transference feelings towards the therapist as an inadequate caretaker or as a controlling conservative authoritarian.
   b. Mistrust or disappointment stemming from unrealistic expectations of cure.
   c. A need to control the therapy by pursuing treatments outside the therapist's control.
2. To what extent is the patient's interest in CAM a legitimate expression of dissatisfaction with traditional treatments and a genuine desire to explore other avenues to seek symptom relief?

Three additional points should be considered when patients discuss CAM therapies:

1. What is the patient's knowledge about the particular CAM treatment and with whom has the patient consulted?
2. What is the physician or therapist's knowledge about the treatment and with whom should she/he consult?
3. How can the therapist support and assist the patient's pursuit of safe and effective CAM treatments? (see section on physician education later.)

## Quality of Alternative Compounds

Doctors and consumers are concerned about the quality of alternative products, particularly herbs and nutrients. Advances in biochemistry have enhanced the purity and stability of many compounds (Wagner 1999). Although the publication of specific brands is not the norm in a text of this kind, in the field of alternative medicine it is particularly important to choose products that have proven to be of good quality. To help the clinician find a way through the morass of unreliable, ineffective lookalikes and bargain brands, Table 104–1 lists particular brands that we have investigated. Invariably some products and companies will change over time. Physicians need to stay current using unbiased sources of product information. Independent evaluation of many brands with updates can be found at www.consumerlab.com or www.supplementwatch.com. Recalls and warnings to stop use of certain brands is available at http://www.fda.gov/medwatch or http://www.cfsan.fda.gov/~dms/supplmnt.html. Information on sources for obtaining European prescription medications that are not available in the US is also included in Table 104–1.

## Medical Liability Issues

Using alternative treatments and foreign compounds raises the issue of medical liability. The fundamental principles are the same as with mainstream treatments. A good relationship with the patient and family is key. For informed consent, the physician should clearly explain why the alternative treatment is being recommended, what is known about the compound and how it works, and the potential risks and benefits. The entire explanation should be documented in the chart, including the symptoms that have not responded to standard treatment attempts and the particular indications and considerations involved in the decision. This may include the patients' philosophy, cultural background, or the fact that they have had difficulty tolerating conventional agents. Physicians, wishing to reassure themselves more about the background of data, may examine the references cited in this chapter.

## Physician Education

Patients need help to understand how to choose products of quality whose efficacy has adequate clinical and research support. Physicians can educate themselves by starting with a recent review article on the most common herbal remedies used in North American populations (Wong et al. 1998). The Herb Research Foundation, started by Andrew Weil, in coordination with the American Botanical Council, publishes the Herbalgram, a journal that reviews herbs and features abstracts of recent studies in scientific journals. Monographs on any herb may be obtained from the Herb Research Foundation for a small fee (phone: 303-449-2265). For physicians, *Green Pharmacy* by James Duke (1997) and *Tyler's Herbs of Choice* by James Robbers and Varro Tyler (1999) are helpful. When faced with a patient taking an unfamiliar herb or nutrient, the best single source of information is the Natural Medicines Comprehensive Database (phone: 209-472-2244 or www.Natural Medicine.com). More detailed information is available from The Natural Product Research Consultants (phone: 973-762-0840) or The American Botanical Council (phone: 512-926-4900). The National Center for Complementary and Alternative Medicine (http://nccam.nih.gov) provides information on research trials. The Desktop Guide to Complementary and Alternative Medicine: an evidence-based approach edited by Edzard Ernst (Ernst et al. 2001) is an extremely well-organized and well-documented resource for any clinician.

## Summary

This review focused on CAM treatments for which there is sufficient understanding from animal and *in vitro* models of their mechanisms of action to infer their relevance to human conditions. Treatments supported by clinical trials were emphasized. Moreover, the authors have had the opportunity to either use these treatments in clinical practice, or to observe their use directly in numerous cases. All of the substances discussed have relatively low side-effect profiles and high margins of safety. There is reason to believe that alternative agents have neuroprotective effects as well as abilities to help repair the injured nervous system and enhance its plasticity. Although many CAM treatments have not been generally used by physicians in the US, nor approved by the FDA, based on scientific evidence and the above criteria, they can offer significant benefits for many individuals. Clinically, it often requires several attempts to design an effective combination of treatments. A well-informed clinician is best qualified to help patients and their families understand and choose their alternative treatment regimens.

## References

Anonymous (1992) Finasteride for benign prostatic hypertrophy. Med Lett Drugs Ther 34, 83–84.

Anonymous (1995) Melatonin. Med Lett Drugs Ther 37, 111–112.

Anonymous (1997) Tamsulosin for benign prostatic hyperplasia. Med Lett Drugs Ther 39, 96.

Anonymous (2000) Drug interactions with St. John's wort. Med Lett Drugs Ther 42, 56.

Ackerman PT, Dykman RA, Holloway C, et al. (1991) A trial of piracetam in two subgroups of students with dyslexia enrolled in summer tutoring. J Learn Disabil 24, 542–549.

Agakishiev RS (1962) Longevity in Caucasian Republic of Dagestan. In Problems of Gerontology, Alpatov VV (ed). Moscow Publishing House of Academy of Sciences of the USSR, Moscow, pp. 34–72.

Agnoli A, Andreoli V, Casacchia M, et al. (1976) Effect of S-adenosyl-L-methionine (SAMe) upon depressive symptoms. J Psychiatr Res 13, 43–54.

Agricola R, Dalla Verde G, and Urani R (1994) S-adenosyl-L-methionine in the treatment of major depression complicating chronic alcoholism. Curr Ther Res 55, 83–92.

Akhondzadeh S, Naghavi HR, Vazirian M, et al. (2001) Passionflower in the treatment of generalized anxiety: A pilot double-blind randomized controlled trial with oxazepam. J Clin Pharm Ther 26, 363–367.

Alvarez XA, Mouzo R, Pichel V, et al. (1999) Double-blind placebo controlled study with citicoline in APOE genotyped Alzheimer's disease patients. Effects on cognitive performance, brain bioelectrical activity and cerebral perfusion. Meth Find Exp Clin Pharmacol 21, 633–644.

Amaducci L (1988) Phosphatidylserine in the treatment of Alzheimer's disease: Results of a multicenter study. Psychopharmacol Bull 24, 130–134.

Amano T, Terao S, and Imada I (1995) Effects of 6-(10-hydroxydecyl)-2,3-dimethoxy-5-methyl-1,4-benzoquinone (idebenone) and related benzoquinones on porcine pancreas phospholipase A2 activity. Biol Pharm Bull 18, 779–781.

Anderson JJ, Anthony MS, Cline JM, et al. (1999) Health potential of soy isoflavones for menopausal women. Pub Health Nutr 2, 489–504.

Anderson RA, Cheng N, Bryden NA, et al. (1997) Elevated intakes of supplemental chromium improve glucose and insulin variables in individuals with type 2 diabetes. Diabetes 46, 1786–1791.

Arciniegas DB (2001) Traumatic brain injury and cognitive impairment: The cholinergic hypothesis. Neuropsychiatr Rev 17–20.

Arnold LE (2001) Alternative treatments for adults with attention-deficit/hyperactivity disorder (ADHD). Ann N Y Acad Sci 931, 310–341.

Arrigo A, Casale R, Buonocore M, et al. (1990) Effects of acetyl-L-carnitine on reaction times in patients with cerebrovascular insufficiency. Int J Clin Pharmacol Res 10, 133–137.

Asai S, Zhao H, Yamashita A, et al. (1999) Nicergoline enhances glutamate reuptake and protects against brain damage in rat global brain ischemia. Eur J Pharmacol 383, 267–274.

Astrup A, Breum L, Toubro S, et al. (1992) The effect and safety of an ephedrine/caffeine compound compared to ephedrine, caffeine and placebo in obese subjects on an energy restricted diet. A double-blind trial. Int J Obes Rel Metab Disord 16, 269–277.

Awang DVC (1997) Feverfew trials: The promise of—and the problem with—standardized botanical extracts. Herbalgram 41, 16–17.

Ayers ME (1987) Electroencephalographic neurofeedback and closed head injury of 250 individuals. In National Head Injury Syllabus. Washington National Head Injury Foundation, Washington DC, pp. 380–392.

Bacci Ballerini F, Lopez Anguera A, Alcaraz P, et al. (1983) Treatment of postconcussion syndrome with S-adenosylmethionine. Med Clin (Barc) 80, 161–164.

Bach D, Schmitt M, and Ebeling L (1997) Phytopharmaceutical and synthetic agents in the treatment of benign prostatic hyperplasia (BPH). Phytomedicine 4, 309–313.

Balon R (1999) Ginkgo biloba for antidepressant-induced sexual dysfunction? J Sex Marital Ther 25, 1–2.

Balzamo E, Gayan-Ramirez G, and Jammes Y (1991) Quantitative EEG changes under various conditions of hyperventilation in the sensorimotor cortex of the anaesthetized cat. Electroencephalogr Clin Neurophysiol 78, 159–165.

Barcelo HA, Wiemeyer JC, Sagasta CL, et al. (1987) Effect of S-adenosylmethionine on experimental osteoarthritis in rabbits. Am J Med 83, 55–59.

Barlet A, Albrecht J, Aubert A, et al. (1990) Efficacy of Pygeum africanum extract in the medical therapy of urination disorders due to benign prostatic hyperplasia: Evaluation of objective and subjective parameters. A placebo-controlled double-blind multicenter study. Wien Klin Wochenschr 102, 667–673.

Baskaya MK, Dogan A, Rao AM, et al. (2000) Neuroprotective effects of citicoline on brain edema and blood–brain barrier breakdown after traumatic brain injury. J Neurosurg 92, 448–452.

Bassi P, Artibani W, De Luca V, et al. (1987) Standardized extract of Pygeum africanum in the treatment of benign prostatic hypertrophy. Controlled clinical study versus placebo. Minerva Urol Nefrol 39, 45–50.

Becker I (2000) Uses of yoga in psychiatry and medicine. In Complementary and Alternative Medicine in Psychiatry, Muskin PR (ed). American Psychiatric Press, Washington DC, pp. 107–145.

Beckham N (1995) Phyto-oestrogens and compounds that affect oestrogen metabolism. II. Austral J Med Herb 7, 27–33.

Belford-Courtney R (1993) Comparison of Chinese and Western users of Angelica sinesis. Aust J Med Herbs 5, 87–91.

Bell IR, Edman JS, Morrow FD, et al. (1992) Brief communication: Vitamin $B_1$, $B_2$, and $B_6$ augmentation of tricyclic antidepressant treatment in geriatric depression with cognitive dysfunction. J Am Coll Nutr 11, 159–163.

Bell KM, Potkin SG, Carreon D, et al. (1994) S-adenosylmethionine blood levels in major depression: Changes with drug treatment. Acta Neurol Scand Suppl 154, 15–18.

Bell MJ, Kochanek PM, Carcillo JA, et al. (1998) Interstitial adenosine, inosine, and hypoxanthine are increased after experimental traumatic brain injury in the rat. J Neurotrauma 15, 163–170.

Bender KJ (2000) Investigating inositol in psychiatry. Psychiatr Times 41–46.

Benjamin J, Agam G, Levine J, et al. (1995a) Inositol treatment in psychiatry. Psychopharmacol Bull 31, 167–175.

Benjamin J, Levine J, Fux M, et al. (1995b) Double-blind, placebo-controlled, crossover trial of inositol treatment for panic disorder. Am J Psychiatr 152, 1084–1086.

Benton D, Griffiths R, and Haller J (1997) Thiamine supplementation mood and cognitive functioning. Psychopharmacology 129, 66–71.

Benton D, Haller J, and Fordy J (1995) Vitamin supplementation for 1 year improves mood. Neuropsychobiology 32, 98–105.

Beresford SA, Weiss NS, Voigt LF, et al. (1997) Risk of endometrial cancer in relation to use of oestrogen combined with cyclic progestogen therapy in postmenopausal women. Lancet 349, 458–461.

Berger R and Nowak H (1987) A new medical approach to the treatment of osteoarthritis. Report of an open phase IV study with ademetionine (Gumbaral). Am J Med 83, 84–88.

Berlanga C, Ortega-Soto HA, Ontiveros M, et al. (1992) Efficacy of S-adenosyl-L-methionine in speeding the onset of action of imipramine. Psychiatr Res 44, 257–262.

Bersani G and Garavini A (2000) Melatonin add-on in manic patients with treatment resistant insomnia. Prog Neuropsychopharmacol Biol Psychiatr 24, 185–191.

Betz JM, White KD, and der Marderosian AH (1995) Gas chromatographic determination of yohimbine in commercial yohimbe products. J AOAC Int 78 , 1189–1194.

Bikov VA, Zapesochnaya GG, and Kurkin VA (1999) Rhodiola rosea: Traditional and biotechnological aspects of obtaining medicinal and pharmacological compounds. Pharmacol Toxicol Med Plants, 22–39.

Birch EE, Garfield S, Hoffman DR, et al. (2000) A randomized controlled trial of early dietary supply of long-chain polyunsaturated fatty acids and mental development in term infants. Dev Med Child Neurol 42, 174–181.

Bonoczk P, Gulyas B, Adam-Vizi V, et al. (2000) Role of sodium channel inhibition in neuroprotection: Effect of vinpocetine. Brain Res Bull 53, 245–254.

Bottiglieri T (1996) Folate, vitamin $B_{12}$, and neuropsychiatric disorders. Nutr Rev 54, 382–390.

Bottiglieri T (1997) Ademetionine (S-adenosylmethionine) neuropharmacology: Implications for drug therapies in psychiatric and neurological disorders. Exp Opin Invest Drugs 6, 417–426.

Bottiglieri T and Hyland K (1994) S-adenosylmethionine levels in psychiatric and neurological disorders: A review. Acta Neurol Scand Suppl 154, 19–26.

Bottiglieri T, Godfrey P, Flynn T, et al. (1990) Cerebrospinal fluid S-adenosylmethionine in depression and dementia: Effects of treatment with parenteral and oral S-adenosylmethionine. J Neurol Neurosurg Psychiatr 53, 1096–1098.

Bottiglieri T, Laundy M, Crellin R, et al. (2000) Homocysteine, folate, methylation, and monoamine metabolism in depression. J Neurol Neurosurg Psychiatr 69, 228–232.

Bradley JD, Flusser D, Katz BP, et al. (1994) A randomized, double-blind, placebo-controlled trial of intravenous loading with S-adenosylmethionine (SAM) followed by oral SAM therapy in patients with knee osteoarthritis. J Rheumatol 21, 905–911.

Brekhman II and Dardymov IV (1969) New substances of plant origin which increase non-specific resistance. Ann Rev Pharmacol 9, 419–430.

Bressa GM (1994) S-adenosyl-L-methionine (SAMe) as antidepressant: Meta-analysis of clinical studies. Acta Neurol Scand (Suppl 154), 7–14.

Breum L, Pedersen JK, Ahlstrom F, et al. (1994) Comparison of an ephedrine/caffeine combination and dexfenfluramine in the treatment of obesity. A double-blind multi-centre trial in general practice. Int J Obes Rel Metab Disord 18, 99–103.

Brichenko VS and Skorokhova TF (1987) Herbal adaptogens in rehabilitation of patients with depression, clinical and organizational aspects of early manifestations of nervous and mental diseases. Altai Region Publisher, Barnaul, Russia, p. 15.

Brooks JO, Yesavage JA, Carta A, et al. (1998) Acetyl-L-carnitine slows decline in younger patients with Alzheimer's Disease: A reanalysis of a double-blind, placebo-controlled study using the trilinear aproach. Int Psychogeriatr 10, 193–203.

Brown D (1996) Anti-anxiety effects of chamomile compounds. Herbalgram 39, 19.

Brown DJ (1993) Vitex agnus castus: Clinical monograph. Townsend Lett Doctors Patients 138–142.

Brown RP and Gerbarg PL (2000) Integrative psychopharmacology: A practical approach to herbs and nutrients in psychiatry. In Complementary and Alternative Medicine and Psychiatry. Review of Psychiatry Vol. 19, Muskin PR (Vol. ed), Oldham JM and Riba MB (Series ed). American Psychatric Association, Washington DC.

Brown RP and Gerbarg PL (2002) Yogic breathing: Quieting the cortex and stimulating subcortical generators to enhance central nervous system function. Science of Breath: International Symposium on Sudarshan Kriya, Pranayam and Consciousness (Mar 2–3), New Delhi, India. (in press)

Brown RP, Gerbarg PL, and Bottiglieri T (2000) S-adenosylmethionine (SAMe) in the clincial practice of psychiatry, neurology, and internal medicine. Clin Pract Alternative Med 1, 230–241.

Bubenik GA, Blask DE, Brown GM, et al. (1998) Prospects of the clinical utilization of melatonin. Biol Signals Recept 7, 195–219.

Burgess JR, Stevens L, Zhang W, et al. (2000) Long-chain polyunsaturated fatty acids in children with attention-deficit hyperactivity disorder. Am J Clin Nutr 71, 327S–330S.

Caffarra C and Santamaria V (1987) The effects of phosphatidyl-serine in patients with mild cognitive decline: An open trial. Clin Trials J 24, 109–111.

Calatayud Maldonado V, Calatayud Perez JB, and Aso Escario J (1991) Effects of CDP-choline on the recovery of patients with head injury. J Neurol Sci 103(Suppl), S15–S18.

Calvani M, Carta A, Caruso G, et al. (1992) Action of acetyl-L-carnitine in neurodegeneration and Alzheimer's disease. Ann NY Acad Sci 663, 483–486.

Cantoni GL (1952) The nature of the active methyl donor formed enzymatically from L-methionine and adenosinetriphosphate. J Am Chem Soc 74, 2942–2943.

Carani C, Salvioli V, Scuteri A, et al. (1991) Urological and sexual evaluation of treatment of benign prostatic disease using Pygeum africanum at high doses. Arch Ital Urol Nefrol Androl 63, 341–345.

Cardoso SM, Pereira C, and Oliveira CR (1998) The protective effect of vitamin E, idebenone and reduced glutathione on free radical mediated injury in rat brain synaptosomes. Biochem Biophys Res Comm 246, 703–710.

Cardoso SM, Pereira C, and Oliveira R (1999) Mitochondrial function is differentially affected upon oxidative stress. Free Radic Biol Med 26, 3–13.

Carney MW, Chary TK, Bottiglieri T, et al. (1989) The switch mechanism and the bipolar/unipolar dichotomy. Br J Psychiatr 154, 48–51.

Carney MW, Toone BK, and Reynolds EH (1987) S-adenosylmethionine and affective disorder. Am J Med 83, 104–106.

Carrieri PB, Indaco A, and Gentile S (1990) S-Adenosylmethionine treatment of depression in patients with Parkinson's disease: A double-blind crossover study versus placebo. Curr Ther Res 48, 154–160.

Carter CS (1998) Neuroendocrine perspectives on social attachment and love. Psychoneuroendocrinology 23, 779–818.

Cenacchi T, Bertoldin T, and Palin E (1987) Human tolerability of phosphatidyl serine assessed through laboratory examinations. Clin Trials J 24, 125–130.

Cergnul I, Jones K, Ernst D, et al. (2001) S-adenosylmethionine (SAM-e) in the treatment of depressive disorders in HIV-positive individuals: Interum Results (abstract). AmFAR 13th National HIV/Aids Update Conference (Mar 20–23), San Francisco, CA.

Cerutti R, Sichel MP, Perin M, et al. (1993) Psychological distress during puerperium: A novel therapeutic approach using S-adenosylmethionine. Curr Ther Res 53, 707–716.

Chacon GA (1997) La importancia de Lepidium peruvianum Chacon ("Maca") en la alimentacion y salud humano y animal 2,000 anos antes y despues de cristo y en el siglo XXI. Universidad Nacional Mayor de San Marcos, Lima, Peru. (Unpublished dissertation)

Champault G, Patel JC, and Bonnard AM (1984) A double-blind trial of an extract of the plant Serenoa repens in benign prostatic hyperplasia. Br J Clin Pharmacol 18, 461–462.

Chen J, Wollman Y, Chernichovsky T, et al. (1999) Effect of oral administration of high-dose nitric oxide donor L-arginine in men with organic erectile dysfunction: Results of a double-blind, randomized, placebo-controlled study. BJU Int 83, 269–273.

Choi HK, Seong DH, and Rha KH (1995) Clinical efficacy of Korean red ginseng for erectile dysfunction. Int J Impot Res 7, 181–186.

Cicerchia G, Santucci R, and Palmieri M (1985) Use of piracetam in the treatment of cranial injuries. Observations on 903 cases. Clin Ter 114, 481–487.

Cicero AF, Bandieri E, and Arletti R (2001) Lepidium meyenii Walp. improves sexual behaviour in male rats independently from its action on spontaneous locomotor activity. J Ethnopharmacol 75, 225–229.

Cohen AJ and Bartlik B (1998) Ginkgo biloba for antidepressant-induced sexual dysfunction. J Sex Marital Ther 24, 139–143.

Cohen-Mansfield J, Garfinkel D, and Lipson S (2000) Melatonin for treatment of sundowning in elderly persons with dementia—a preliminary study. Arch Gerontol Geriatr 31, 65–76.

Colditz GA, Hankinson SE, Hunter DJ, et al. (1995) The use of estrogens and progestins and the risk of breast cancer in postmenopausal women. New Engl J Med 332, 1589–1593.

Colditz GA, Stampfer MJ, Willett WC, et al. (1990) Prospective study of estrogen replacement therapy and risk of breast cancer in postmenopausal women. JAMA 264, 2648–2653.

Colell A, Garcia-Ruiz C, Morales A, et al. (1997) Transport of reduced glutathione in hepatic mitochondria and mitoplasts from ethanol-treated rats: Effect of membrane physical properties and S-adenosyl-L-methionine. Hepatology 26, 699–708.

Conquer JA, Tierney MC, Zecevic J, et al. (2000) Fatty acid analysis of blood plasma of patients with Alzheimer's disease, other types of dementia, and cognitive impairment. Lipids 35, 1305–1312.

ConsumerLab.com. (2001) Product Review: St. John's wort.

Cooney CA, Wise CK, Poirier LA, et al. (1998) Methamphetamine treatment affects blood and liver S-adenosylmethionine (SAM) in mice. Correlation with dopamine depletion in the striatum. Ann NY Acad Sci 844, 191–200.

Cooper AJ and Magnus RV (1980) A placebo-controlled study of pyritinol ('Encephabol') in dementia. Pharmatherapeutica 2, 317–322.

Coppen A and Bailey J (2000) Enhancement of the antidepressant action of fluoxetine by folic acid: A randomised, placebo-controlled trial. J Affect Disord 60, 121–130.

Cott JM (1997) In vitro receptor binding and enzyme inhibition by Hypericum perforatum extract. Pharmacopsychiatry 30(Suppl 2), 108–112.

Cott JM (2002) Herb-drug interactions: Focus on pharmacokinetics. CNS Spectrum 6, 827–832.

Cott JM and Fugh-Berman A (1998) Is St. John's wort (Hypericum perforatum) an effective antidepressant? J Nerv Ment Dis 186, 500–501.

Cozens DD, Barton SJ, Clark R, et al. (1988) Reproductive toxicity studies of ademetionine. Arzneimittelforschung 38, 1625–1629.

Crawford MA, Doyle W, and Leaf A (1993) Nutritional and neurodevelopmental disorders. Nutr Health 9, 81–97.

Crellin R, Bottiglieri T, and Reynolds EH (1993) Folates and psychiatric disorders. Clinical potential. Drugs 45, 623–636.

Criconia AM, Araquistain JM, Daffina N, et al. (1994) Results of treatment with S-adenosyl-L-methionine in patients with major depression and internal illnesses. Curr Ther Res 55, 666–674.

Crook T, Petrie W, Wells C, et al. (1992) Effects of phosphatidylserine in Alzheimer's disease. Psychopharmacol Bull 28, 61–66.

Crook TH, Tinklenberg J, Yesavage J, et al. (1991) Effects of phosphatidylserine in age-associated memory impairment. Neurology 41, 644–649.

Curcio M, Catto E, Stramentinoli G, et al. (1978) Effect of S-adenosyl-L-methionine on serotonin metabolism in rat brain. Prog Neuropsychopharmacol 2, 65–71.

Czyrak A, Rogoz Z, Skuza G, et al. (1992) Antidepressant activity of S-adenosyl-L-methionine in mice and rats. J Basic Clin Physiol Pharmacol 3, 1–17.

Dalle Ore G, Bricolo A, and Alexandre A (1980) The influence of the administration of pyritinol on the clinical course of traumatic coma. J Neurosurg Sci 24, 1–8.

Daly PA, Krieger DR, Dulloo AG, et al. (1993) Ephedrine, caffeine and aspirin: Safety and efficacy for treatment of human obesity. Int J Obes Rel Metab Disord 17(Suppl 1), S73–S78.

Davidson J and the Hypericum Depression Trial Study Group (2002) Effect of Hypericum perforatum (St. John's wort) in major depressive disorder: A randomized controlled trial. JAMA 287(4), 1807–1814.

De Deyn PP, Reuck JD, Deberdt W, et al. (1997) Treatment of acute ischemic stroke with piracetam. Members of the Piracetam in Acute Stroke Study (PASS) Group. Stroke 28, 2347–2352.

De La Cruz JP, Pavia J, Gonzalez-Correa JA, et al. (2000) Effects of chronic administration of S-adenosyl-L-methionine on brain oxidative stress in rats. Naunyn Schmiedebergs Arch Pharmacol 361, 47–52.

De Smet PAGM (2002) Herbal Remedies. New Engl J Med 347, 2046–2056.

De Vanna M and Rigamonti R (1992) Oral S-adenosyl-L-methionine in depression. Curr Ther Res 52, 478–485.

Del Valio B (1974) The use of a new drug in the treatment of chronic prostatitis. Minerva Urol 26, 87–94.

Delle Chiale R and Boissard G (1997) Meta-analysis of 2 European multicenter controlled trials with ademetionine (SAMe) in major depression [abstract 90–56]. Biol Psych 42, 245S.

Delle Chiale R, Panccheri P, and Scapicchio P (2000a) MC3: Multicenter controlled efficacy and safety trial of oral S-adenosyl-methionine (SAMe) vs. oral imipramine in the treatment of depression. Presented at Collegium Internationale Neuro-Psychopharmacologisum (CINP) (July 9–13). Brussels.

Delle Chiale R, Panccheri P, and Scapicchio P (2000b) MC4: Multicenter controlled efficacy and safety trial of intramuscular S-adenosyl-methionine (SAMe) vs. oral imipramine in the treatment of depression. Presented at Collegium Internationale Neuro-Psychopharmacologisum (CINP) (July 9–13). Brussels.

DeMott K (1998) St. John's wort tied to serotonin syndrome. Clin Psychiatr News 28.

Di Benedetto P, Iona LG, and Zidarich V (1993) Clinical evaluation of S-adenosyl-L-methionine versus transcutaneous electrical nerve stimulation in primary fibromyalgia. Curr Ther Res 53, 222–229.

Di Donato S, Frerman FE, Rimoldi M, et al. (1986) Systemic carnitine deficiency due to lack of electron transfer flavoprotein: Ubiquinone oxidoreductase. Neurology 36, 957–963.

Di Padova C (1987) S-adenosylmethionine in the treatment of osteoarthritis. Review of the clinical studies. Am J Med 83, 60–65.

Di Padova C, Giudici A, and Boissard G (2000) Ademetionine and depression. In V Workshop on "Methionine metabolism: Molecular mechanisms and clinical implications", Mato JM and Caballero A (eds) (Feb). Granada, Spain. University of Navarre, Madrid, Spain, pp. 294–299.

Di Rocco A, Rogers JD, Brown R, et al. (2000) S-adenosyl-L-methionine improves depression in patients with Parkinson's disease in an open label clinical trial. J Mov Disord 15, 1225–1229.

Diamond BJ, Shiflett SC, Feiwel N, et al. (2000) Ginkgo biloba extract: Mechanisms and clinical indications. Arch Phys Med Rehab 81, 668–678.

Dixon CE, Ma X, and Marion DW (1997) Effects of CDP-choline treatment on neurobehavioral deficits after TBI and on hippocampal and neocortical acetylcholine release. J Neurotrauma 14, 161–169.

Dolberg OT, Hirschmann S, and Grunhaus L (1998) Melatonin for the treatment of sleep disturbances in major depressive disorder. Am J Psychiatr 155, 1119–1121.

Donath F, Quispe S, Diefenbach K, et al. (2000) Critical evaluation of the effect of valerian extract on sleep structure and sleep quality. Pharmacopsychiatry 33, 47–53.

Dorman T, Bernard L, and Glaze P (1995) The effectiveness of Garum amoricum (stabilium) on reducing anxiety in college students. J Adv Med 8, 193–200.

Dorofeev BF and Kholodov LE (1991) Pikamilon pharmacokinetics in animals. Farmakol Toksikol 54, 66–69.

Dubichev AG, Kurkin BA, Zapesochnaya GG, et al. (1991) Study of Rhodiola rosea root chemical composition using HPLC. Chemico-Pharmaceut J 2, 188–193.

Duke JA (1997) The Green Pharmacy Rodale Press, Emmaus, PA.

Dunnick JK and Hailey JR (1995) Experimental studies on the long-term effects of methylphenidate hydrochloride. Toxicology 103, 77–84.

Elwan O, Helmy AA, Tamawy ME, et al. (1995) Ergoloids and ischaemic strokes Efficacy and mechanism of action. J Int Med Res 23, 154–166.

Enderby P, Broeckx J, Hospers W, et al. (1994) Effect of piracetam on recovery and rehabilitation after stroke: A double-blind, placebo-controlled study. Clin Neuropharmacol 17, 320–331.

Ernst E, Pittler MH, Stevinson C, et al. (eds) (2001) The Desktop Guide to Complementary and Alternative Medicine. Mosby, New York.

Ernst E and Pittler MH (1998) Yohimbine for erectile dysfunction: A systematic review and meta-analysis of randomized clinical trials. J Urol 159, 433–436.

Ernst E and Pittler MH (2000) The efficacy and safety of feverfew (Tanacetum parthenium L.): An update of a systematic review. Pub Health Nutr 3, 509–514.

Ernst T, Chang L, Leonido-Yee M, et al. (2000) Evidence for long-term neurotoxicity associated with methamphetamine abuse: A 1H MRS study. Neurology 54, 1344–1349.

Ernst E, Pittler MH, Stevinson C, et al. (2001) Conditions, Menopause. Mosby, New York, pp. 143–145.

Escher M, Desmeules J, Giostra E, et al. (2001) Hepatitis associated with Kava, a herbal remedy for anxiety. BMJ 322, 139.

Evans G (1996) Chromium Picolinate: Everything You Need to Know. Avery Publishing Group, Garden City Park, NY.

Evans PJ, Whiteman M, Tredger JM, et al. (1997) Antioxidant properties of S-adenosyl-L-methionine: A proposed addition to organ storage fluids. Free Radic Biol Med 23, 1002–1008.

Facchinetti F, Borella P, Sances G, et al. (1991) Oral magnesium successfully relieves premenstrual mood changes. Obstet Gynecol 78, 177–181.

Facchinetti F, Nappi RE, Sances MG, et al. (1997) Effects of a yeast-based dietary supplementation on premenstrual syndrome. A double-blind placebo-controlled study. Gynecol Obstet Invest 43, 120–124.

Fackleman K (1998) Medicine for menopause. Sci News 153, 392–393.

Faloon M (1999) BPH: The other side of the coin. Life Ext J 12–17.

Fauteck JD, Schmidt H, Lerchl A, et al. (1999) Melatonin in epilepsy: First results of replacement therapy and first clinical results. Biol Signals Recept 8, 105–110.

Fava M, Borus JS, Alpert JE, et al. (1997) Folate, vitamin $B_{12}$ and homocysteine in major depressive disorder. Am J Psychiatr 154, 426–428.

Fava M, Rosenbaum JF, Birnbaum R, et al. (1992) The thyrotropin response to thyrotropin-releasing hormone as a predictor of response to treatment in depressed outpatients. Acta Psychiatr Scand 86, 42–45.

Fava M, Rosenbaum JF, MacLaughlin R, et al. (1990) Neuroendocrine effects of S-adenosyl-L-methionine, a novel putative antidepressant. J Psychiatr Res 24, 177–184.

Ferrell RE, Salamatina NV, Dalakishvili SM, et al. (1985) A population genetic study in the Ochamchir region, Abkhazia, SSR. Am J Phys Anthropol 66, 63–71.

Finkelstein JD (1998) The metabolism of homocysteine: Pathways and regulation. Eur J Pediatr 157(Suppl 2), S40–S44.

Fischer HD, Schmidt J, and Wustmann C (1984) On some mechanisms of antihypoxic actions of nootropic drugs. Biomed Biochim Acta 43, 541–543.

Fischhof PK, Saletu B, Ruther E, et al. (1992) Therapeutic efficacy of pyritinol in patients with senile dementia of the Alzheimer type (SDAT) and multi-infarct dementia (MID). Neuropsychobiology 26, 65–70.

Flicker L and Evans G (2001) Piracetam for dementia or cognitive impairment (Cochrane Review). Cochrane Database Syst Rev 2, CD001011.

Flynn BL and Ranno AE (1999) Pharmacologic management of Alzheimer's disease, Part II: Antioxidants, antihypertensives, and ergoloid derivatives. Ann Pharmacother 33, 188–197.

Fokkema DS (1999) The psychobiology of strained breathing and its cardiovascular implications: A functional system review. Psychophysiology 36, 164–175.

Fontanari D, Di Palma C, Giorgetti G, et al. (1994) Effects of S-adenosyl-L-methionine on cognitive and vigilance functions in the elderly. Curr Ther Res 55, 682–689.

Foster S (1999) Black cohosh Cimicifugae racemosa: A literature review. Herbalgram 45, 36–49.

Freudenstein J and Bodinet C (1999) Influence of an isopropanolic aqueous extract of Cimicifugae racemosa rhizoma on the proliferation of MCF-7 cells. Presentation at the 23rd LOF-Symposium on Phytoestrogens (Jan 15) University of Ghent, Belgium.

Frezza M, Centini G, Cammareri G, et al. (1990) S-adenosylmethionine for the treatment of intrahepatic cholestasis of pregnancy. Results of a controlled clinical trial. Hepatogastroenterology 37(Suppl 2), 122–125.

Friedel HA, Goa KL, and Benfield P (1989) S-adenosyl-L-methionine. A review of its pharmacological properties and therapeutic potential in liver dysfunction and affective disorders in relation to its physiological role in cell metabolism. Drugs 38, 389–416.

Furmanowa M, Oledzka H, Michalska M, et al. (1995) Rhodiola rosea L. (Roseroot): In vitro regeneration and the biological activity of roots. In Biotechnology in Agriculture and Forestry, Vol. 33. Medicinal and Aromatic Plants VIII, Bajaj YPS (ed). Springer-Verlag, Berlin, Heidelberg, pp. 412–426.

Furmanowa M, Skopinska-Rozewska E, Rogala E, et al. (1998) Rhodiola rosea in vitro culture—phytochemical analysis and antioxidant action. Acta Societis Botanicorum Poloniae 76, 69–73.

Fux M, Levine J, Aviv A, et al. (1996) Inositol treatment of obsessive–compulsive disorder. Am J Psychiatr 153, 1219–1221.

Galletti P, De Rosa M, Cotticelli MG, et al. (1991) Biochemical rationale for the use of CDPcholine in traumatic brain injury: Pharmacokinetics of the orally administered drug. J Neurol Sci 103(Suppl), S19–S25.

Gangadhar BN, Janakiramaiah N, Sudarshan B, et al. (2000) Stress-related Biochemical Effects of Sudarshan Kriya Yoga in Depressed Patients Study #6 presented at The Conference on Biological Psychiatry (May). UN NGO Mental Health Committee, New York.

Gaster B and Holroyd J (2000) St. John's wort for depression: A systematic review. Arch Intern Med 160, 152–156.

Gatto G, Caleri D, Michelacci S, et al. (1986) Analgesizing effect of a methyl donor (S-adenosylmethionine) in migraine: An open clinical trial. Int J Clin Pharmacol Res 6, 15–17.

Gelenberg AJ (2000) St. John's wort update. Biol Ther Psychiatr 23, 22–24.

Gerasimova HD (1970) Effect of Rhodiola rosea extract on ovarian functional activity. Proceedings of Scientific Conference on Endocrinology and Gynecology. Sverdlovk, Russia, pp. 46–48.

Germano C, Ramazanov Z, and Bernal Suarez M (1999) Arctic Root (Rhodiola rosea): the Powerful New Ginseng Alternative. Kensington Publishing, New York.

Giacobini E (1998) Invited review: Cholinesterase inhibitors for Alzheimer's disease therapy: From tacrine to future applications. Neurochem Int 32, 413–419.

Gillis JC, Benefield P, and McTavish D (1994) Idebenone. A review of its pharmacodynamic and pharmacokinetic properties, and therapeutic use in age-related cognitive disorders. Drugs Aging 5, 133–152.

Giulidori P and Di Padova C (2000) Effect of SAMe administration on plasma homocysteine in humans. In V Workshop on "Methionine Metabolism: Molecular Mechanisms and Clinical Implications" (Feb 20–24), Mato JM and Caballero A (eds). Granada, Spain. Master Line SL, Madrid, Spain, pp. 316–320.

Glatzel J (1978) Dose-effect relationship of orally administered pyritinol in the chronic organic brain syndrome (author's transl). Med Klin 73, 1117–1121.

Glieck J (1988) Chaos: The Making of Science. Penguin, New York.

Gouliaev AH and Senning A (1994) Piracetam and other structurally related nootropics. Brain Res Rev 19, 180–222.

Grassetto M and Varatto A (1994) Primary fibromyalgia is responsive to S-adenosyl-L-methionine. Curr Ther Res 55, 797–806.

Grobe-Einsler R (1993) Clinical aspects of nimodipine. Clin Neuropharmacol 16(Suppl 1), S39–S45.

Grossman W and Schmidramsl H (2001) An extract of Petasites hybridus is effective in the prophylaxis of migraine. Altern Med Rev 6, 303–310.

Grube B, Walper A, and Wheatley D (1999) St. John's wort extract efficacy for menopausal symptoms of psychological origin. Adv Ther 16, 177–186.

Gurnell EM and Chatterjee VK (2001) Dehydroepiandrosterone replacement therapy. Eur J Endocrinol 145, 103–106.

Gutzmann H and Hadler D (1998) Sustained efficacy and safety of idebenone in the treatment of Alzheimer's disease: Update on a 2-year double-blind multicenter study. J Neural Transm (Suppl 54), 301–310.

Gutzmann H, Kuhl KP, Hadler D, et al. (2002) Safety and efficacy of idebenone versus tacrine in patients with Alzheimer's disease: Results of a randomized, double-blind, parallel-group multicenter study. Pharmacopsychiatry 35, 12–18.

Haimov I, Lavie P, Laudon M, et al. (1995) Melatonin replacement therapy of elderly insomniacs. Sleep 18, 598–603.

Hakkarainen H and Hakamies L (1978) Piracetam in the treatment of post-concussional syndrome. A double-blind study. Eur Neurol 17, 50–55.

Hansgen KD, Vesper J, and Ploch M (1994) Multicenter double-blind study examining the antidepressant effectiveness of the hypericum extract LI 160. J Geriatr Psychiatr Neurol 7(Suppl 1), S15–S18.

Hassing L, Wahlin A, Winblad B, et al. (1999) Further evidence of the effects of vitamin $B_{12}$ and folate levels on episodic memory functioning: A population-based study of healthy very old adults. Biol Psychiatr 45, 1472–1480.

Hawkins EB (2000) Report on Houghton PJ: Leads to treatment of CNS disorders with plants, extracts and constituents. Poster presentation, 48th Annual Meeting of the International Congress of the Society of Plant Research PL12 (Sept 5). Herbalgram 50, 71.

Hayes RL and Dixon CE (1994) Neurochemical changes in mild head injury. Semin Neurol 14, 25–31.

Heiss WD, Kessler J, Mielke R, et al. (1994) Long-term effects of phosphatidylserine, pyritinol, and cognitive training in Alzheimer's disease. A neuropsychological, EEG, and PET investigation. Dementia 5, 88–98.

Helfgott E, Rudel RG, and Kairam R (1986) The effect of piracetam on short- and long-term verbal retrieval in dyslexic boys. Int J Psychophysiol 4, 53–61.

Helmuth L (1999) Nutritionists debate soy's health benefits. Sci News 155, 262.

Henderson MC, Miranda CL, Stevens JF, et al. (2000) In vitro inhibition of human P450 enzymes by prenylated flavonoids from hops, Humulus lupulus. Xenobiotica 30, 235–251.

Herrmann WM, Kern U, and Rohmel J (1986) On the effects of pyritinol on functional deficits of patients with organic mental disorders. Pharmacopsychiatry 19, 378–385.

Hibbeln JR and Salem N Jr. (1995) Dietary polyunsaturated fatty acids and depression: When cholesterol does not satisfy. Am J Clin Nutr 62, 1–9.

Hibbeln JR, Umhau J, and George D (1997) Do plasma polyunsaturates predict hostility and depression? World Rev Nutr Diet 82, 175–186.

Hirata JD, Swiersz LM, Zell B, et al. (1997) Does dong quai have estrogenic effects in postmenopausal women? A double-blind placebo-controlled trial. Fertil Steril 68, 981–986.

Hobbs C and Amster M (1996) Naturopathic specific condition review: Premenstrual syndrome. Prof J Botan Med (Spring) 168–173.

Hoffman DA, Lubar JF, Thatcher RW, et al. (1999) Limitations of the American Academy of Neurology and American Clinical Neurophysiology Society paper on QEEG. J Neuropsychiatr Clin Neurosci 11, 401–407.

Ianiello A, Ostuni PA, Sfriso P, et al. (1994) S-adenosyl-L-methionine in Sjogren's Syndrome and fibromyalgia. Curr Ther Res 55, 699–705.

Ingram D, Sanders K, Kolybaba M, et al. (1997) Case-control study of phyto-oestrogens and breast cancer. Lancet 350, 990–994.

Ishihara K, Katsuki H, Sugimura M, et al. (1989) Idebenone and vinpocetine augment long-term potentiation in hippocampal slices in the guinea pig. Neuropharmacology 28, 569–573.

Itil TM (2001) Uses and contraindications of ginkgo biloba in psychiatry. Psychiatr Times (Nov) 47–48.

Itil TM, Menon GN, Songar A, et al. (1986) CNS pharmacology and clinical therapeutic effects of oxiracetam. Clin Neuropharmacol 9(Suppl 3), S70–S72.

Itil TM, Eralp E, Ahmed I, et al. (1998) The pharmacological effects of ginkgo biloba, a plant extract, on the brain of dementia patients in comparison with tacrine. Psychopharmacol Bull 34, 391–397.

Ito TY, Trant AS, and Polan ML (2001) A double-blind placebo-controlled study of ArginMax, a nutritional supplement for enhancement of female sexual function. J Sex Marital Ther 27, 541–549.

Jacobsen FM (1992) Fluoxetine-induced sexual dysfunction and an open trial of yohimbine. J Clin Psychiatr 53, 119–122.

Jacobsen S, Danneskiold-Samsoe B, and Andersen RB (1991) Oral S-adenosylmethionine in primary fibromyalgia. Double-blind clinical evaluation. Scand J Rheumatol 20, 294–302.

Jamieson DD and Duffield PH (1990) The antinociceptive actions of kava components in mice. Clin Exp Pharmacol Physiol 17, 495–507.

Jan JE, Espezel H, and Appleton RE (1994) The treatment of sleep disorders with melatonin. Dev Med Child Neurol 36, 97–107.

Janakiramaiah N, Gangadhar BN, Naga Venkatesha Murthy PJ, et al. (1998) Therapeutic efficacy of Sudarshan Kriya Yoga (SKY) in dysthymic disorder. NIMHANS J (Jan), 21–28.

Janakiramaiah N, Gangadhar BN, Naga Venkatesha Murthy PJ, et al. (2000) Antidepressant efficacy of Sudarshan Kriya Yoga (SKY) in Melancholia: A randomized comparison with electroconvulsive therapy (ECT) and imipramine. J Affect Disord 57, 255–259.

Jensen CL, Chen H, Fraley JK, et al. (1996) Biochemical effects of dietary linoleic/alpha-linolenic acid ratio in term infants. Lipids 31, 107–113.

Jonte A, Brockmuller J, Bauer S, et al. (1999) Pharmacokinetic interaction of digoxin with an herbal extract from St. John's wort. Clin Pharm Ther 66, 338–345.

Kagan BL, Sultzer DL, Rosenlicht N, et al. (1990) Oral S-adenosylmethionine in depression: A randomized, double-blind, placebo-controlled trial. Am J Psychiatr 147, 591–595.

Kang SY, Kim SH, Schini VB, et al. (1995) Dietary ginsenosides improve endothelium-dependent relaxation in the thoracic aorta of hypercholesterolemic rabbit. Gen Pharmacol 26, 483–487.

Kayumov L, Brown G, Jindal R, et al. (2001) A randomized, double-blind, placebo-controlled crossover study of the effect of exogenous melatonin on delayed sleep phase syndrome. Psychosom Med 63, 40–48.

Kelly GS (2001) Rhodiola rosea: A possible plant adaptogen. Altern Med Rev 6, 293–302.

Kenny E, Muskin PR, Brown R, et al. (2001) What the general psychiatrist should know about herbal medicine. Curr Psychiatr Rep 3, 226–234.

Kessler J, Thiel A, Karbe H, et al. (2000) Piracetam improves activated blood flow and facilitates rehabilitation of poststroke aphasic patients. Stroke 31, 2112–2116.

Kidd PM (1999) A review of nutrients and botanicals in the integrative management of cognitive dysfunction. Altern Med Rev 4, 144–161.

Kidd PM (2000) Attention-deficit/hyperactivity disorder (ADHD) in children: Rationale for its integrative management. Altern Med Rev 5, 402–428.

Kim HL, Streltzer J, and Goebert D (1999) St. John's wort for depression: A meta-analysis of well-defined clinical trials. J Nerv Ment Dis 187, 532–539.

Kitamura K (1981) Therapeutic effect of pyritinol on sequelae of head injuries. J Int Med Res 9, 215–221.

Kitani K, Minami C, Maruyama W, et al. (2000) Common properties for propargylamines of enhancing superoxide dismutase and catalase activities in the dopaminergic system in the rat: Implications for the life prolonging effect of (-)deprenyl. J Neural Transm Suppl 60, 139–156.

Kleijnen J, Ter Riet G, and Knipschild P (1990) Vitamin $B_6$ in the treatment of the premenstrual syndrome—a review. Br J Obstet Gynaecol 97, 847–852.

Klepser T and Nisly N (1999) Chaste tree berry for premenstrual syndrome. Altern Med Alert 2, 61–72.

Knezevic S, Mubrin Z, Risberg J, et al. (1989) Pyritinol treatment of SDAT patients: Evaluation by psychiatric and neurological examination, psychometric testing and rCBF measurements. Int Clin Psychopharmacol 4, 25–38.

Knoll J (2000) Outlines of a drug strategy to slow brain aging. Neuropsychopharmacol Hung 11(4), 151–170.

Ko RJ (1998) Adulterants in Asian patent medicines. New Engl J Med 339, 847.

Kolakowsky S and Parente R (1997) Nootropics, nutrients, and other cognitive enhancing substances for use in cognitive rehabilitation: A review and bibliography. J Cogn Rehabil (Mar/Apr), 12–24.

Konig H, Stahl H, Sieper J, et al. (1995) Magnetic resonance tomography of finger polyarthritis: Morphology and cartilage signals after ademetionine therapy. Aktuelle Radiol 5, 36–40.

Kraft M, Spahn TW, Menzel J, et al. (2001) Fulminant liver failure after administration of the herbal antidepressant Kava-Kava. Dtsch Med Wochenschr 126, 970–972.

Kruglikova RP (1997) How and why picamilon works. Life Ext (July), 34–38.

Krystal AD and Ressler I (2002) The use of valerian in neuropsychiatry. CNS Spectrum 6, 841–847.

Krzeski T, Kazon M, Borkowski A, et al. (1993) Combined extracts of urtica dioica and pygeum africanum in the treatment of benign prostatic hyperplasia: Double-blind comparison of two doses. Clin Ther 15, 1011–1120.

Kudolo GB (2000) The effect of 3-month ingestion of ginkgo biloba extract on pancreatic beta-cell function in response to glucose loading in normal glucose tolerant individuals. J Clin Pharmacol 40, 647–654.

Kunz D and Bes F (1997) Melatonin effects in a patient with severe REM sleep behavior disorder: Case report and theoretical considerations. Neuropsychobiology 36, 211–214.

Kurkin VA and Zapesochnaya GG (1986) Khimicheskiy sostav i farmakologicheskiye svoystva rasteniy roda Rhodiola. Obzor. (Chemical composition and pharmacological properties of Rhodiola rosea). Khim-Farm Zh (Chem Pharmaceut J Moscow) 20, 1231–1244.

Kwon JS, O'Donnell BF, Wallenstein GV, et al. (1999) Gamma frequency-range abnormalities to auditory stimulation in schizophrenia. Arch Gen Psychiatr 56, 1001–1005.

Kyle DJ, Schaefer E, and Patton G (1998) Low serum docosahexanoic acid is a significant risk factor for Alzheimer's dementia. Presentation at the 3rd ISSFAL Congress (June 1–5), Lyons, France.

Le Bars PL, Velasco FM, Ferguson JM, et al. (2002) Influence of the severity of cognitive impairment on the effect of the Ginkgo biloba extract EGb 761 in Alzheimer's disease. Neuropsychobiology 45, 19–26.

Lehmann E, Kinzler E, and Friedmann J (1996) Efficacy of a special kava extract (Piper methysticum) in patients with states of anxiety, tension, excitedness of nonmental origin—a double-blind, placebo-controlled study of four weeks treatment. Phytomedicine 3, 119–133.

Levin HS (1991) Treatment of postconcussional symptoms with CDP-choline. J Neurol Sci 103(Suppl), S39–S42.

Lichius JJ and Muth C (1997) The inhibiting effects of urtica dioica root extracts on experimentally induced prostatic hyperplasia in the mouse. Planta Med 63, 307–310.

Lieber CS (1999) Role of S-adenosyl-L-methionine in the treatment of liver diseases. J Hepatol 30, 1155–1159.

Lieberman S (1998) A review of the effectiveness of Cimicifuga racemosa (black cohosh) for the symptoms of menopause. J Womens Health 7, 525–529.

Liebman B (1998) The soy story. Nutr Action Healthlett (Sept), 3–7.

Lightfoote J, Blair HJ, and Cohen JR (1977) Lead intoxication in an adult caused by Chinese herbal medication. JAMA 238, 1539.

Linde K, Ramirez G, Mulrow CD, et al. (1996) St John's wort for depression—an overview and meta-analysis of randomised clinical trials. BMJ 313, 253–258.

Lipinski JF, Cohen BM, Frankenburg F, et al. (1984) Open trial of S-adenosylmethionine for treatment of depression. Am J Psychiatr 141, 448–450.

Loehrer FM, Angst CP, Haefeli WE, et al. (1996) Low whole-blood S-adenosylmethionine and correlation between 5-methyltetrahydrofolate and homocysteine in coronary artery disease. Arterioscler Thromb Vasc Biol 16, 727–733.

Loehrer FM, Schwab R, Angst CP, et al. (1997) Influence of oral S-adenosylmethionine on plasma 5-methyltetrahydrofolate, S-adenosyl-homocysteine, homocysteine and methionine in healthy humans. J Pharmacol Exp Ther 282, 845–850.

Lolic MM, Fiskum G, and Rosenthal RE (1997) Neuroprotective effects of acetyl-L-carnitine after stroke in rats. Ann Emerg Med 29, 758–765.

Long DA, Ghosh K, Moore AN, et al. (1996) Deferoxamine improves spatial memory performance following experimental brain injury in rats. Brain Res 717, 109–117.

Lonnrot K, Porsti I, Alho H, et al. (1998) Control of arterial tone after long-term coenzyme Q10 supplementation in senescent rats. Br J Pharmacol 124, 1500–1506.

Lozano R (1991) CDP-choline in the treatment of cranio-encephalic traumata. J Neurol Sci 103(Suppl), S43–S47.

Lubar JF and Bahler WW (1976) Behavioral management of epileptic seizures following EEG biofeedback training of the sensorimotor rhythm. Biofeedback Self Regul 1, 77–104.

Lubar JO and Lubar JF (1984) Electroencephalographic biofeedback of SMR and beta for attention deficit disorders in a clinical setting. Biofeedback Self Regul 9, 1–23.

Lun A, Gruetzmann H, Wustmann C, et al. (1989) Effect of pyritinol on the dopaminergic system and behavioural outcome in an animal model of mild chronic postnatal hypoxia. Biomed Biochim Acta 48, S237–S242.

Lyon MR, Cline JC, Totosy de Zepetnek J, et al. (2001) Effect of the herbal extract combination Panax quinquefolium and ginkgo biloba on attention-deficit/hyperactivity disorder: A pilot study. J Psychiatr Neurosci 26, 221–228.

Maes M (1998) Fatty acids, cytokines, and major depression (editorial). Biol Psychiatr 42, 313–314.

Mangoni A, Grassi MP, Frattola L, et al. (1991) Effects of a MAO-B inhibitor in the treatment of Alzheimer's disease. Eur Neurol 31, 100–107.

Marangell LB, Rush AJ, George MS, et al. (2002) Vagus nerve stimulation (VNS) for major depressive episodes: One year outcome. Biol Psychiatr 51, 280–287.

Maruyama W and Naoi M (1999) Neuroprotection by (-)-deprenyl and related compounds. Mech Ageing Dev 111, 189–200.

Maslova LV, Kondrat'ev BIU, Maslov LN, et al. (1994) The cardioprotective and antiadrenergic activity of an extract of Rhodiola rosea in stress. Eksp Klin Farmakol 57, 61–63.

Mathews JD, Riley MD, and Fejo L (1988) Effects of the heavy usage of kava on physical health: Summary of a pilot survey in an aboriginal community. Med J Aust 148, 548–555.

Mato JM, Camara J, Fernandez de Paz J, et al. (1999) S-adenosyl-methionine in alcoholic liver cirrhosis: A randomized, placebo-controlled, double-blind, multicenter clinical trial. J Hepatol 30, 1081–1089.

Matsumoto S, Mori N, Tsuchihashi N, et al. (1998) Enhancement of nitroxide-reducing activity in rats after chronic administration of vitamin E, vitamin C, and idebenone examined by an in vivo electron spin resonance technique. Magn Reson Med 40, 330–333.

Mauskop AI, Grossman WM, and Schmidramsl H (2000) Petasites hybridus (Butterbur Root) extract is effective in the prophylaxis of migraines. Results of a randomized, double-blind trial. Headache J Head Face Pain (abstract) 40, 420.

Mayo JL (1997) A natural approach to menopause. Clin Nutr Insights 5, 1–8.

McArthur RA, Carfagna N, Banfi L, et al. (1997) Effects of nicergoline on age-related decrements in radial maze performance and acetylcholine levels. Brain Res Bull 43, 305–311.

McCaleb R (1995) Vitex Agnus-Castus. Herb Research Foundatio, Golden, Co.

McLeod MN, Gaynes BN, and Golden RN (1999) Chromium potentiation of antidepressant pharmacotherapy for dysthymic disorder in 5 patients. J Clin Psychiatr 60, 237–240.

Milkiewicz P, Mills CO, Roma MG, et al. (1999) Tauroursodeoxycholate and S-adenosyl-L-methionine exert an additive ameliorating effect on taurolithocholate-induced cholestasis: A study in isolated rat hepatocyte couplets. Hepatology 29, 471–476.

Miller LG (1998) Herbal medicinals: Selected clinical considerations focusing on known or potential drug-herb interactions. Arch Intern Med 158, 2200–2211.

Mirzoian RS and Gan'shina TS (1989) The new cerebrovascular preparation pikamilon. Farmakol Toksikol 52, 23–26.

Mitka M (2002) News about neuroprotectants for the treatment of stroke. JAMA 287, 1253–1254.

Monaco P, Pastore L, Rizzo S, et al. (1996) Safety and tolerability of adometionine (ADE) SD for inpatients with stroke: A pilot randomized, double-blind, placebo-controlled study [abstract] presented at the Third World Stroke Conference and Fifth European Stroke Conference (Sept 1–5), Munich, Germany.

Morales A (2001) Yohimbine in erectile dysfunction: Would an orphan drug ever be properly assessed? World J Urol 19, 251–255.

Morales A, Condra M, Owen JA, et al. (1987) Is yohimbine effective in the treatment of organic impotence? Results of a controlled trial. J Urol 137, 1168–1172.

Mordente A, Martorana GE, Minotti G, et al. (1998) Antioxidant properties of 2,3-dimethoxy-5-methyl-6-(10-hydroxydecyl)-1,4-benzoquinone (idebenone). Chem Res Toxicol 11, 54–63.

Mowrey DB (1996) Muira-Puama (Liriosma ovata). In Herbal Tonic Therapies. Wings Books, Avenel, NJ.

Muller WE, Singer A, Wonnemann M, et al. (1998) Hyperforin represents the neurotransmitter reuptake inhibiting constituent of hypericum extract. Pharmacopsychiatry 31(Suppl 1), 16–21.

Murdoch I, Perry EK, Court JA, et al. (1998) Cortical cholinergic dysfunction after human head injury. J Neurotrauma 15, 295–305.

Muskin PR (2000) Complementary and alternative medicine and psychiatry. In Review of Psychiatry Vol. 19, Oldham JM and Riba MB (eds). American Psychiatric Press, Washington DC.

Naga Venkatesha Murthy PJ, Gangadhar BN, Janakiramaiah N, et al. (1997) Normalization of P300 amplitude following treatment in dysthymia. Biol Psychiatr 42, 740–743.

Naga Venkatesha Murthy PJ, Janakiramaiah N, Gangadhar BN, et al. (1998) P300 amplitude and antidepressant response to Sudarshan Kriya Yoga (SKY). J Affect Disord 50, 45–48.

Nandy K (1978) Centrophenoxine: Effects on aging mammalian brain. J Am Geriatr Soc 26, 74–81.

Nash JK (2000) Treatment of attention deficit hyperactivity disorder with neurotherapy. Clin Electroencephalogr 31, 30–37.

Nelson EE and Panksepp J (1998) Brain substrates of infant-mother attachment: Contributions of opioids, oxytocin, and norepinephrine. Neurosci Biobehav Rev 22, 437–452.

Nemets B, Stahl Z, and Belmaker RH (2002) Addition of omega-3 fatty acid to maintenance medication treatment for recurrent unipolar depressive disorder. Am J Psychiatr 159, 477–479.

Neville K (1999) Red clover. Better Nutrition 34.

Nidecker A (1997) Probing genes, drugs, and fatty acids in dementia. Clin Psychiatr News 4.

Nidich SI, Morehead P, Nidich RJ, et al. (1993) The effect of the Maharishi Student Rasayana food supplement on nonverbal intelligence. Pers Indiv Differ 15, 599–602.

Nierenberg AA, Burt T, Matthews J, et al. (1999) Mania associated with St. John's wort. Biol Psychiatr 46, 1707–1708.

NIH (National Institutes of Health and Giovanni Lorenzini Medical Science Foundation) (2002) International Position Paper on Women's Health and Menopause: A Comprehensive Approach (July). NIH Publication no. 02-3284. http://www4.od.nih.gov/orwh/

Nishio T, Sunohara N, Furukawa S, et al. (1998) Repeated injections of nicergoline increase the nerve growth factor level in the aged rat brain. Jpn J Pharmacol 76, 321–323.

Nocl G, Jeanmart M, and Reinhardt B (1983) Treatment of the organic brain syndrome in the elderly. A double-blind comparison on the effects of a neurotropic drug and placebo. Neuropsychobiology 10, 90–93.

Ochs L (1994) EEG-driven Stimulation and heterogeneous head-injured patients: Extended findings. A peer-reviewed abstract from the 1994 Berrol Head Injury Conference, Las Vegas, NV [web page, cited Dec 7, 2001]. Available from: URL: http://www.flexyx.com/contents/pubs/Extended.htm.

Okuyama S and Aihara H (1988) Action of nootropic drugs on transcallosal responses in rats. Neuropharmacology 27, 67–72.

Osman E, Owen JS, and Burroughs AK (1993) Review article: S-adenosyl-L-methionine—a new therapeutic agent in liver disease? Aliment Pharmacol Ther 7, 21–28.

Otero-Losada ME and Rubio MC (1989a) Acute changes in 5-HT metabolism after S-adenosyl-L-methionine administration. Gen Pharmacol 20, 403–406.

Otero-Losada ME and Rubio MC (1989b) Acute effects of S-adenosyl-L-methionine on catecholaminergic central function. Eur J Pharmacol 163, 353–356.

Packer L and Colman C (1999) The Antioxidant Miracle. John Wiley, New York.

Packer L, Tritschler HJ, and Wessel K (1997) Neuroprotection by the metabolic antioxidant alpha-lipoic acid. Free Radic Biol Med 22, 359–378.

Palevitch DEG and Carasso R (1997) Feverfew as a prophylactic treatment for migraine: A double-blind, placebo-controlled study. Phytother Res 11, 506–511.

Parry BL (1999) A 45-year-old woman with premenstrual dysphoric disorder. JAMA 281, 368–373.

Patel VM and Maulsby RL (1987) How hyperventilation alters the electroencephalogram: A review of controversial viewpoints emphasizing neurophysiological mechanisms. J Clin Neurophysiol 4, 101–120.

Pavia J, Martos F, Gonzalez-Correa JA, et al. (1997) Effect of S-adenosyl methionine on muscarinic receptors in young rats. Life Sci 60, 825–832.

Peet M, Murphy B, Shay J, et al. (1998) Depletion of omega-3 fatty acid levels in red blood cell membranes of depressive patients. Biol Psychiatr 43, 315–319.

Pek G, Fulop T, and Zs-Nagy I (1989) Gerontopsychological studies using NAI (Nurnberger Alters-Inventar) on patients with organic psychosyndrome (DSM III, Category 1) treated with centrophenoxine in a double-blind, comparative, randomized clinical trial. Arch Gerontol Geriatr 9, 17–30.

Pelka RB and Leuchtgens H (1995) Pre-Alzheimer study: Action of a herbal yeast preparation (Bio-Strath) in a randomised double-blind trial. Ars Neducu 85.

Peniston EG and Kulkosky PJ (1989) Alpha-theta brain wave training and beta-endorphin levels in alcoholics. Alcohol Clin Exp Res 13, 271–279.

Penninx BWJH, Guralnik JM, Ferrucci L, et al. (2000) Vitamin B12 deficiency and depression in physically disabled older women: Epidemiologic evidence from the Women's Health and Aging Study. Am J Psychiatr 157, 715–721.

Pepeu G, Pepeu IM and Amaducci L (1996) A review of phosphatidylserine pharmacological and clinical effects. Is phosphatidylserine a drug for the ageing brain? Pharmacol Res 33, 73–80.

Petkov VD, Stancheva SL, Tocuschieva L, et al. (1990) Changes in brain biogenic monoamines induced by the nootropic drugs adafenoxate and meclofenoxate and by citicholine (experiments on rats). Gen Pharmacol 21, 71–75.

Petkov VD, Yonkov D, Mosharoff A, et al. (1986) Effects of alcohol aqueous extract from Rhodiola rosea L. roots on learning and memory. Acta Physiol Pharmacol Bulg 12, 3–16.

Pettegrew JW, Levine J, and McClure RJ (2000) Acetyl-L-carnitine physical-chemical, metabolic, and therapeutic properties: Relevance for its mode of action in Alzheimer's disease and geriatric depression. Mol Psychiatr 5, 616–632.

Pezzoli C, Galli-Kienle M, and Stramentinoli G (1987) Lack of mutagenic activity of ademetionine in vitro and in vivo. Arzneimittelforschung 37, 826–829.

Piscitelli SC, Burstein AH, Chaitt D, et al. (2000) Indinavir concentrations and St. John's wort. Lancet 355, 547–548.

Pittler MH and Ernst E (2000) Efficacy of kava extract for treating anxiety: Systematic review and meta-analysis. J Clin Psychopharmacol 20, 84–89.

Posse S, Olthoff U, Weckesser M, et al. (1997) Regional dynamic signal changes during controlled hyperventilation assessed with blood oxygen level-dependent functional MR imaging. AJNR Am J Neuroradiol 18, 1763–1770.

Prevett MC, Duncan JS, Jones T, et al. (1995) Demonstration of thalamic activation during typical absence seizures using H2(15)O and PET. Neurology 45, 1396–1402.

Quiros CF and Cardenas RA (1997) Maca (Lepidium meyeni Walp). In Andean Roots and Tubers: Ahipa, Arricacha, Maco, Yacon. Promoting the Conservation and Use of Underutilized and Neglected Crops, Vol. 21, Herman M and Heller J (eds). Institute of Plant Genetics and Crop Plant Research, Gatersleben/International Plant Resources Institute, Rome, Italy. pp. 184–185.

Ramirez PM, Desantis D, and Opler LA (2001) EEG biofeedback treatment of ADD. A viable alternative to traditional medical intervention? Ann N Y Acad Sci 931, 342–358.

Ramsey JJ, Colman RJ, Swick AG, et al. (1998) Energy expenditure, body composition, and glucose metabolism in lean and obese rhesus monkeys treated with ephedrine and caffeine. Am J Clin Nutr 68, 42–51.

Rao AM, Hatcher JF, and Dempsey RJ (1999) CDP-choline: Neuroprotection in transient forebrain ischemia of gerbils. J Neurosci Res 58, 697–705.

Raskind MA, Peskind ER, Wessel T, et al. (2000) Galantamine in AD: A 6-month randomized, placebo-controlled trial with a 6-month extension. The Galantamine USA-1 Study Group. Neurology 54, 2261–2268.

Rego AC, Santos MS, and Oliveira CR (1999) Influence of the antioxidants vitamin E and idebenone on retinal cell injury mediated by chemical ischemia, hypoglycemia, or oxidative stress. Free Radic Biol Med 26, 1405–1417.

Reiter RJ (1996) Melatonin. Bantam, New York.

Riggs K, Spiro III A, Tucker K, et al. (1996) Relations of vitamin B12, vitamin B6, folate, and homocysteine to cognitive performance in the Normative Aging Study. Am J Clin Nutr 63, 306–314.

Robbers JE and Tyler VE (1999) Tyler's Herbs of Choice: The Therapeutic Use of Herbal Medicinals. Hawthorne Hebal Press, New York.

Robbins J (2000) A Symphony in the brain: The evolution of the new brain wave biofeedback. Atlantic Monthly Press, New York.

Roldan E and Dostalek C (1983) Description of an EEG pattern evoked in central parietal areas by the Hathayogic exercise Agnisara. Act Nerv Super (Praha) 25, 241–246.

Roldan E and Dostalek C (1985) EEG patterns suggestive of shifted levels of excitation effected by hathayogic exercises. Act Nerv Super (Praha) 27, 81–88.

Rosadini G, Marenco S, Nobili F, et al. (1990) Acute effects of acetyl-L-carnitine on regional cerebral blood flow in patients with brain ischaemia. Int J Clin Pharmacol Res 10, 123–128.

Rosenbaum JF, Fava M, Falk WE, et al. (1990) The antidepressant potential of oral S-adenosyl-L-methionine. Acta Psychiatr Scand 81, 432–436.

Rozelle GR and Budzynski TH (1995) Neurotherapy for stroke rehabilitation: A single case study. Biofeedback Self Regul 20, 211–228.

Ruschitzka F, Meier PJ, Turina M, et al. (2000) Acute heart transplant rejection due to Saint John's wort. Lancet 355, 548–549.

Russello D, Randazzo G, Favetta A, et al. (1990) Oxiracetam treatment of exogenous postconcussion syndrome. Statistical evaluation of results. Minerva Chir 45, 1309–1314.

Sageman S (2002) How SK can treat the cognitive, psychodynamic, and neuropsychiatric problems of posttraumatic stress disorder. International Symposium on Sudarshan Kriya, Pranayam and Consciousness (Mar 2–3), New Delhi, India.

Saija A, Hayes RL, Lyeth BG, et al. (1988) The effect of concussive head injury on central cholinergic neurons. Brain Res 452, 303–311.

Salem N Jr (1989) Omega-3-fatty acids: Molecular and chemical aspects. In New Roles for Selective Nutrients, Spiller GA and Scala L (eds). Alan R Liss, New York, pp. 109–228.

Salem N Jr., Kim NY, and Yergey JA (1986) Docosohexanoic acid: Membrane function and metabolism. In Health Effects of Polyunsaturated Seafoods, Simopoulos A, Kifer RR, and Martin R (eds). Academic Press, New York. pp. 263–317.

Saletu B, Anderer P, and Semlitsch HV (1997) Relations between symptomatology and brain function in dementias: Double-blind, placebo-controlled, clinical and EEG/ERP mapping studies with nicergoline. Dement Geriatr Cogn Disord 8(Suppl 1), 12–21.

Saletu B, Grunberger J, Linzmayer L, et al. (1990) Brain protection of nicergoline against hypoxia: EEG brain mapping and psychometry. J Neural Transm Park Dis Dement Sect 2, 305–325.

Saletu B, Paulus E, Linzmayer L, et al. (1995) Nicergoline in senile dementia of Alzheimer type and multi-infarct dementia: A double-blind, placebo-controlled, clinical and EEG/ERP mapping study. Psychopharmacology (Berl) 117, 385–395.

Salmaggi P, Bressa GM, Nicchia G, et al. (1993) Double-blind, placebo-controlled study of S-adenosyl-L-methionine in depressed postmenopausal women. Psychother Psychosom 59, 34–40.

Saratikov AS and Krasnov EA (1987a) Effect of Rhodiola rosea on the central nervous system. In Rhodiola Rosea is a Valuable Medicinal Plant (Golden Root), Saratikov AS and Krasnov EA (eds). Tomsk State University, Tomsk, Russia, pp. 150–179.

Saratikov AS and Krasnov EA (1987b) Clinical studies of Rhodiola. In Rhodiola Rosea is a Valuable Medicinal Plant (Golden Root), Saratikov AS and Krasnov EA (eds). Tomsk State University, Tomsk, Russia, pp. 216–227.

Saratikov AS and Krasnov EA (1987c) Rhodiola Rosea is a Valuable Medicinal Plant (Golden Root). Tomsk State University, Tomsk, Russia.

Sayegh R, Schiff I, Wurtman J, et al. (1995) The effect of a carbohydrate-rich beverage on mood, appetite, and cognitive function in women with premenstrual syndrome. Obstet Gynecol 86, 520–528.

Schachter SC and Saper CB (1998) Vagus nerve stimulation. Epilepsia 39, 677–686.

Schardt D (2000) St. John's worts and all. Nutr Action Healthlett (Sept), 6–8.

Schaumburg HH and Berger A (1992) Alopecia and sensory polyneuropathy from thallium in a Chinese herbal medication. JAMA 268, 3430–3431.

Schellenberg R (2001) Treatment for the premenstrual syndrome with agnus castus fruit extract: Prospective, randomised, placebo-controlled study. BMJ 322, 134–137.

Schellenberg R, Sauer S, and Dimpfel W (1998) Pharmacodynamic effects of two different hypericum extracts in healthy volunteers measured by quantitative EEG. Pharmacopsychiatry 31(Suppl 1), 44–53.

Schelosky L, Raffauf C, Jendroska K, et al. (1995) Kava and dopamine antagonism (letter). J Neurol Neurosurg Psychiatr 58, 639–640.

Schenck CH, Bundlie SR, and Ettinger MG (1986) Chronic behavioral disorders of REM sleep: A new category of parasomnia. Sleep 9, 293–308.

Schmidt RH and Grady MS (1995) Loss of forebrain cholinergic neurons following fluid-percussion injury: Implications for cognitive impairment in closed head injury. J Neurosurg 83, 496–502.

Schneider LS and Tariot PN (1994) Emerging drugs for Alzheimer's disease. Mechanisms of action and prospects for cognitive enhancing medications. Med Clin N Am 78, 911–934.

Schneider F, Popa R, Mihalas G, et al. (1994) Superiority of antagonic-stress composition versus nicergoline in gerontopsychiatry. Ann NY Acad Sci 717, 332–342.

Schoenthaler SJ and Bier ID (1999) Vitamin-mineral intake and intelligence: A macrolevel analysis of randomized controlled trials. J Altern Complement Med 5, 125–134.

Schoenberger NE, Shif SC, Esty ML, et al. (2001) Flexyx neurotherapy system in the treatment of traumatic brain injury: An initial evaluation. J Head Trauma Rehabil 16, 260–274.

Schultz V, Hubner WD, and Ploch M (1997) Clinical trials with phytopsychopharmacological agents. Phytomedicine 4, 379–387.

Shamir E, Barak Y, Shalman I, et al. (2001) Melatonin treatment for tardive dyskinesia: A double-blind, placebo-controlled, crossover study. Arch Gen Psychiatr 58, 1049–1052.

Shamir E, Laudon M, Barak Y, et al. (2000) Melatonin improves sleep quality of patients with chronic schizophrenia. J Clin Psychiatr 61, 373–377.

Shannahoff-Khalsa DS, Ray LE, Levine S, et al. (1999) Randomized controlled trial of yogic meditation techniques for patients with obsessive–compulsive disorder. CNS Spectrums 4, 34–47.

Shelton RC, Keller MB, Gelenberg A, et al. (2001) Effectiveness of St. John's wort in major depression: A randomized controlled trial. JAMA 285, 1978–1986.

Shrader E (2000) Equivalence of a St. John's wort extract (Ze 117) and fluoxetine: Randomized, controlled study in mild-moderate depression. Int Clin Psychopharmacol 15, 61–68.

Simons AJ, Dawson IK, and Duguma B (1998) Passing problems, prostate and prunus. Herbalgram 43, 49–53.

Singh YN and Blumenthal M (1996) Kava: An overview. Herbalgram Special Rev 39, 33–55.

Sinz EH, Kochanek PM, Dixon CE, et al. (1999) Inducible nitric oxide synthase is an endogenous neuroprotectant after traumatic brain injury in rats and mice. J Clin Invest 104, 647–656.

Soderberg M, Edlund C, Kristensson K, et al. (1991) Fatty acid composition of brain phospholipids in aging and in Alzheimer's disease. Lipids 26, 421–425.

Soffa VM (1996) Alternatives to hormone replacement. Alter Ther 2, 34–39.

Sohn M and Sikora R (1991) Ginkgo biloba extract in the therapy of erectile dysfunction. J Sex Educ Ther 17, 53–61.

Sokeland J and Albrecht J (1997) Combination of sabal and urtica extract vs. finasteride in benign prostatic hyperplasia (Aiken stages I to II). Comparison of therapeutic effectiveness in a one year double-blind study. Urologe A 36, 327–333.

Sorensen H and Sonne J (1996) A double-masked study of the effects of ginseng on cognitive functions. Curr Ther Res 57, 959–968.

Sotaniemi EA, Haapakoski E, and Rautio A (1995) Ginseng therapy in non-insulin-dependent diabetic patients. Diab Care 18, 1373–1375.

Sovik R (2000) The science of breathing—the yogic view. Prog Brain Res 122, 491–505.

Spasov AA, Wikman GK, Mandrikov VB, et al. (2000) A double-blind, placebo-controlled pilot study of the stimulating and adaptogenic effect of Rhodiola rosea SHR-5 extract on the fatigue of students caused by stress during an examination period with a repeated low-dose regimen. Phytomedicine 7, 85–89.

Spicuzza L, Gabutti A, Porta C, et al. (2000) Yoga and chemoreflex response to hypoxia and hypercapnia. Lancet 356, 1495–1496.

Spiers PA and Hochanadel G (1999) Citicoline for traumatic brain injury: Report of two cases, including my own. J Int Neuropsychol Soc 5, 260–264.

Stancheva SL and Mosharrof A (1987) Effect of the extract of Rhodiola rosea L. on the content of the brain biogenic monoamines. Med Physiol Comptes Rendus Acad Bulg Sci 40, 85–87.

Steinberg S, Annable L, and Young SN (1999) A placebo-controlled clinical trial of L-tryptophan in premenstrual dysphoria. Biol Psychiatr 45, 313–320.

Sterman MB (1996) Physiological origins and functional correlates of EEG rhythmic activities: Implications for self-regulation. Biofeedback Self Regul 21, 3–33.

Sterman MB and Macdonald LR (1978) Effects of central cortical EEG feedback training on incidence of poorly controlled seizures. Epilepsia 19, 207–222.

Stevens LJ, Zentall SS, Deck JL, et al. (1995) Essential fatty acid metabolism in boys with attention-deficit hyperactivity disorder. Am J Clin Nutr 62, 761–768.

Stevinson C and Ernst E (2000) Valerian for insomnia: Systematic review of randomized placebo-controlled studies. Sleep Med 1, 91–99.

Stoll AL, Sachs GS, Cohen BM, et al. (1996) Choline in the treatment of rapid-cycling bipolar disorder: Clinical and neurochemical findings in lithium-treated patients. Biol Psychiatr 40, 382–388.

Stoll AL, Severus WE, Freeman MP, et al. (1999) Omega 3 fatty acids in bipolar disorder. Arch Gen Psychiatr 56, 407–412.

Stramentinoli G (1987) Pharmacologic aspects of S-adenosylmethionine. Pharmacokinetics and pharmacodynamics. Am J Med 83, 35–42.

Suarez V (2002) Anxiety study at Lance Alternative Program. (in press)

Surtees R and Hyland K (1989) A method for the measurement of S-adenosylmethionine in small volume samples of cerebrospinal fluid or brain using high-performance liquid chromatography-electrochemistry. Anal Biochem 181, 331–335.

Takahashi J, Nishino H, and Ono T (1986) Effect of S-adenosyl-L-methionine (SAMe) on disturbances in hand movement and delayed response tasks after lesion of motor or prefrontal cortex in the monkey. Nippon Yakurigaku Zasshi 87, 507–519.

Takahashi J, Nishino H, and Ono T (1987) S-adenosyl-L-methionine facilitates recovery from deficits in delayed response and hand movement tasks following brain lesions in monkeys. Exp Neurol 98, 459–471.

Takuma K, Yoshida T, Lee E, et al. (2000) CV-2619 protects cultured astrocytes against reperfusion injury via nerve growth factor production. Eur J Pharmacol 406, 333–339.

Tallal P, Chase C, Russell G, et al. (1986) Evaluation of the efficacy of piracetam in treating information processing, reading and writing disorders in dyslexic children. Int J Psychophysiol 4, 41–52.

Tang XC (1996) Huperzine A (shuangyiping): A promising drug for Alzheimer's disease. Zhongguo Yao Li Xue Bao 17, 481–484.

Tariot PN, Solomon PR, Morris JC, et al. (2000) A 5-month, randomized, placebo-controlled trial of galantamine in AD. The Galantamine USA-10 Study Group. Neurology 54, 2269–2276.

Tavoni A, Jeracitano G, and Cirigliano G (1998) Evaluation of S-adenosylmethionine in secondary fibromyalgia: A double blind study. Clin Exp Rheumatol 16, 106–107.

Tavoni A, Vitali C, Bombardievi S, et al. (1987) Evaluation of S-adenosylmethionine in primary fibromyalgia. A double-blind cross-over study. Am J Med 83, 107–110.

Taylor KM and Randall PK (1975) Depletion of S-adenosyl-L-methionine in mouse brain by antidepressive drugs. J Pharmacol Exp Ther 194, 303–310.

Teufel-Mayer R and Gleitz J (1997) Effects of long-term administration of hypericum extracts on the affinity and density of the central serotonergic 5-HT$_{1A}$ and 5-HT$_{2A}$ receptors. Pharmacopsychiatry 30(Suppl 2), 113–116.

Thiele B, Brink I, and Ploch M (1994) Modulation of cytokine expression by hypericum extract. J Geriatr Psychiatr Neurol 7(Suppl 1), S60–S62.

Thommessen B and Laake K (1996) No identifiable effect of ginseng (Gericomplex) as an adjuvant in the treatment of geriatric patients. Aging (Milano) 8, 417–420.

Thys-Jacobs S, Ceccarelli S, Bierman A, et al. (1989) Calcium supplementation in premenstrual syndrome: A randomized crossover trial. J Gen Intern Med 4, 183–189.

Thys-Jacobs S, Starkey P, Bernstein D, et al. (1998) Calcium carbonate and the premenstrual syndrome: Effects on premenstrual and menstrual symptoms. Premenstrual Syndrome Study Group. Am J Obstet Gynecol 179, 444–452.

Toffano G, Leon A, Benvegnu D, et al. (1976) Effect of brain cortex phospholipids on catechol-amine content of mouse brain. Pharmacol Res Commun 8, 581–590.

Torrioli MG, Vernacotola S, Mariotti P, et al. (1999) Double-blind, placebo-controlled study of L-acetylcarnitine for the treatment of hyperactive behavior in fragile X syndrome. Am J Med Genet 87, 366–368.

Torta R, Zanalda F, Rocca P, et al. (1988) Inhibitory activity of S-adenosyl-L-methionine on serum gamma-glutamyl-transpeptidase increase induced by psychodrugs and anticonvulsants. Curr Ther Res 44, 144–159.

Toubro S, Astrup A, Breum L, et al. (1993) The acute and chronic effects of ephedrine/caffeine mixtures on energy expenditure and glucose metabolism in humans. Int J Obes Relat Metab Disord 17(Suppl 3), S73–S77; discussion S82.

Travis F (2001) Autonomic and EEG patterns distinguish transcending from other experiences during transcendental meditation practice. Int J Psychophysiol 42, 1–9.

US Department of Health and Human Services Agency for Healthcare Research and Quality (2002) S-adenosyl-L-methionine for treatment of depression, osteoarthritis, and liver disease. Evidence Report/Technology Assessment No. 64. www.ahrq.gov.

US Food and Drug Administration Center for Food Safety and Applied Nutrition (2002) Kava-containing dietary supplements may be associated with severe liver injury (Mar 25). http://www.cfsan.fda.gov/~dms/addskava.html.

Uvnas-Moberg K, Bjokstrand E, Hillegaart V, et al. (1999) Oxytocin as a possible mediator of SSRI-induced antidepressant effects. Psychopharmacology (Berl) 142, 95–101.

van Niekerk JK, Huppert FA, and Herbert J (2001) Salivary cortisol and DHEA: Association with measures of cognition and well-being in normal older men, and effects of three months of DHEA supplementation. Psychoneuroendocrinology 26, 591–612.

Vastag B (2001) Pay attention: Ritalin acts much like cocaine. JAMA 286, 905–906.

Vernon MW and Sorkin EM (1991) Piracetam. An overview of its pharmacological properties and a review of its therapeutic use in senile cognitive disorders. Drugs Aging 1, 17–35.

Voelker R (1999) Herbs and anethesia. JAMA 281, 1882.

Volkow ND, Chang L, Wang GJ, et al. (2001a) Higher cortical and lower subcortical metabolism in detoxified methamphetamine abusers. Am J Psychiatr 158, 383–389.

Volkow ND, Chang L, Wang GJ, et al. (2001b) Association of dopamine transporter reduction with psychomotor impairment in methamphetamine abusers. Am J Psychiatr 158, 377–382.

Volkow ND, Wang G, Fowler JS, et al. (2001c) Therapeutic doses of oral methylphenidate significantly increase extracellular dopamine in the human brain. J Neurosci 21, RC121.

Volz HP and Kieser M (1997) Kava-kava extract WS 1490 versus placebo in anxiety disorders—a randomized placebo-controlled 25-week outpatient trial. Pharmacopsychiatry 30, 1–5.

Vorbach EU, Arnoldt KH, and Hubner WD (1997) Efficacy and tolerability of St. John's wort extract LI 160 versus imipramine in patients with severe depressive episodes according to ICD-10. Pharmacopsychiatry 30(Suppl 2), 81–85.

Wagner H (1999) Phytomedicine research in Germany. Environ Health Perspect 107, 779–781.

Warnecke G (1991) Psychosomatische dysfunktionen im weiblichen klimakterium. Fortschr Med 109, 119–122.

Waynberg J (1990) Aphrodesiacs: Contribution to the clinical validation of traditional use of Ptychopetalum guyanna: Presentation at the First International Congress on Ethnopharmacology (June 5–9), Strasbourg, France.

Waynberg J and Brewer S (2000) Effects of Herbal vX on libido and sexual activity in premenopausal and postmenopausal women. Adv Ther 17, 255–262.

Wesnes KA, Faleni RA, Hefting NR, et al. (1997) The cognitive, subjective, and physical effects of a ginkgo biloba/panax ginseng combination in healthy volunteers with neurasthenic complaints. Psychopharmacol Bull 33, 677–683.

Wheatley D (1999) Hypericum in seasonal affective disorder (SAD). Curr Med Res Opin 15, 33–7.

Willatts P, Forsyth JS, DiModugno MK, et al. (1998) Effect of long-chain polyunsaturated fatty acids in infant formula on problem solving at 10 months of age. Lancet 352, 688–691.

Wilsher CR, Bennett D, Chase CH, et al. (1987) Piracetam and dyslexia: effects on reading tests. J Clin Psychopharmacol 7, 230–237.

Wilt TJ, Ishani A, Stark G, et al. (1998) Saw palmetto extracts for treatment of benign prostatic hyperplasia: A systematic review. JAMA 280, 1604–1609.

Wolkowitz OM, Reus VI, Keebler A, et al. (1999) Double-blind treatment of major depression with dehydroepiandrosterone. Am J Psychiatr 156, 646–649.

Wong AH, Smith M, and Boon HS (1998) Herbal remedies in psychiatric practice. Arch Gen Psychiatr 55, 1033–1043.

Xu R, Zhao W, Xu J, et al. (1996) Studies on bioactive saponins from Chinese medicinal plants. Adv Exp Med Biol 404, 371–382.

Yardi N (2001) Yoga for control of epilepsy. Seizure 10, 7–12.

Yen SS (2001) Dehydroepiandrosterone sulfate and longevity: New clues for an old friend. Proc Natl Acad Sci USA 98, 8167–8169.

Youdim KA, Martin A, and Joseph JA (2000) Essential fatty acids and the brain: Possible health implications. Int J Dev Neurosci 18, 383–399.

Zhang XY, Zhou DF, Zhang PY, et al. (2001) A double-blind, placebo-controlled trial of extract of ginkgo biloba added to haloperidol in treatment-resistant patients with schizophrenia. J Clin Psychiatr 62, 878–883.

Zhdanova IV, Wurtman RJ, Regan MM, et al. (2001) Melatonin treatment for age-related insomnia. J Clin Endocrinol Metab 86, 4727–4730.

Zheng BL, He K, Kim CH, et al. (2000) Effect of a lipidic extract from lepidium meyenii on sexual behavior in mice and rats. Urology 55, 598–602.

Zhu J, Hamm RJ, Reeves TM, et al. (2000) Postinjury administration of L-deprenyl improves cognitive function and enhances neuroplasticity after traumatic brain injury. Exp Neurol 166, 136–152.

Zs-Nagy I (1994) A survey of the available data on a new nootropic drug, BCE-001. Ann N Y Acad Sci 717, 102–114.

Zs-Nagy K, Dajko G, Uray I, et al. (1994) Comparative studies on the free radical scavenger properties of two nootropic drugs, CPH and BCE-001. Ann NY Acad Sci 717, 115–121.

Zucker M (1999) Huperzine-A: The newest brain nutrient. Let's Live (May), 47–48.

# 105 Combined Therapies: Psychotherapy and Pharmacotherapy

Michelle B. Riba
Robyn R. Miller

Mrs. A, a 46-year-old woman with no previous psychiatric or medical history begins to feel depressed when she and her husband separate after 15 years of marriage. She has problems staying asleep but her energy level and appetite remain within normal limits. Her friend recommends that she get help. But from whom? Choices include starting with her primary care physician. Should she see a psychiatrist or social worker or psychologist? What are the differences? She could also start with her minister. Should she think about a combination of providers? And for what type of care—supportive, cognitive, behavioral, or brief psychotherapy; medication evaluation; family therapy? Should she call her mental health benefits office and just see whomever the triage coordinator assigns to her?

## Introduction

It is no longer a simple decision for patients or clinicians to determine which type of professional or, for that matter, which type of mental health treatment should be recommended. Besides the particular type of professional and specific form of therapy, there are additional variables—insurance and copay factors, number of visits allowed under the health care plan, which professionals are in or out of network, and so on.

For many psychiatric diagnoses such as major depression and bipolar disorder, it is no longer a question of whether most patients will receive psychopharmacology or some form of psychotherapy. It is a question rather of whether a psychiatrist will provide both the medication and the therapy, whether a nonmedical therapist will provide the therapy and a psychiatrist or other physician will provide the psychopharmacology, how the medications and therapy will be sequenced—concurrently or one before the other, how often the patient should be seen, and so on. (Rounsaville et al. 1981, Weissman et al. 1979, Roose 2001). Of course, finances, the patient's desire for such treatment, availability of clinicians, and a host of other factors contribute to the decision-making process.

Due to improved education and screening tools, primary care providers (PCPs) are better at evaluating psychiatric symptoms and problems (Klinkman and Valenstein 1997). The PCP makes the determination, often with little time and not enough information (Valenstein 1999), as to the patient's algorithm of care—psychotropic medication, psychotherapy, or a combination of both. Often the PCP starts prescribing a psychotropic medication and decides, over time, if the patient requires a form of psychotherapy. If the PCP continues to provide the psychotropic medication and the patient is then referred to a mental health professional for psychotherapy, this type of care can be called split treatment in that one professional is providing the medication and another professional is providing the psychotherapy. If the same clinician (either PCP or psychiatrist) is providing both the psychopharmacology and psychotherapy, that would be called integrated treatment. There have been no formalized rules or a professional consensus regarding the definitions or terms to be used; hence there is an abundance of synonyms used in the literature for these arrangements (Table 105–1).

While split and integrated treatments are currently ubiquitous and growing practices (Pincus et al. 1999, Gabbard and Kay 2001), interestingly, there has been little research to help guide how to best refer Mrs. A for care. This chapter will serve to outline the various and complex issues involved in integrated and split treatment. Clinical vignettes will serve to illustrate various points. Suggestions will be offered for future work and research.

## Integrated Treatment

### Background

The advent of effective medications to treat mental disorders has revolutionized modern psychiatry, yet, the provision of pharmacological treatment in combination with psychotherapy was initially met with adversarial reactions by both biological psychiatrists and by psychiatrists favoring psychotherapeutic approaches to the treatment of mental illness. Within the psychoanalytic community, criticisms to an integrated treatment model were numerous.

| Table 105–1 | Terms Used for Split and Integrated Treatment |
|---|---|

### Split Treatment

Collaborative treatment
Combined treatment
Med backup
Medical backup
Medication check
Medication management
Divided treatment
Triangulated (triangular) treatment
Concurrent care
Parallel treatment
Shared treatment
Integrated treatment
Multidisciplinary care
Fragmented treatment

### Integrated Treatment

Medical psychotherapy
Combined treatment

It was purported that medications addressed only the most superficial of issues, that is, symptoms, and could do little to identify and resolve intrapsychic conflicts, thus rendering medications an entity without curative power (Roose 2001). Psychotropics were considered a contaminant to the psychodynamic process for a number of hypothesized reasons including preventing the patient from accessing affective states, increasing symptom substitution (Weiss 1965), lowering the patient's self-esteem, decreasing the patient's motivation to engage in a lengthy therapy, and interfering with essential technical aspects (e.g., maintenance of therapist neutrality) (Klerman 1991). Purely

biological psychiatrists held that introducing psychotherapy to medication management was a recipe for symptom exacerbation leading to lengthier recoveries (Klerman 1991).

The rationale for combining treatment modalities is based on the idea that the strengths of each modality are promoted while the weaknesses are minimized, producing results that are better than with either modality alone (Hollon and Fawcett 1995). Although intuitively this rings true, psychiatrists have a duty to incorporate evidence-based approaches into their clinical practice. While most evidence-based mental health research in the literature is based on efficacy studies, there has been a recent move towards conducting effectiveness studies that are hoped to be of increased relevance to general outpatient clinical practice (Nathan et al. 2000). Table 105–2 highlights the differences between efficacy and effectiveness research (Barlow 1996, Nathan et al. 2000). Recent literature examining the efficacies of combined treatment (not necessarily integrated treatment by a psychiatrist) vary by disorder, timing of treatments, and whether administered during the acute or maintenance phase. Recent literature has also examined the sequential application of combined treatment (Fava et al. 2001, Frank et al. 2000). Effectiveness studies are far fewer, as mentioned, and do not always demonstrate superiority of combined approaches over either medication or therapy alone.

Combined treatment, on the whole, does not appear to be supported through evidence-based model at this time, at least in terms of symptom reduction. This is partly due to the methodological issues in setting up the necessary types of studies, including the difficulty in setting up studies with sufficient number of subjects to detect small advantages between two efficacious treatments (Hollon and Fawcett 2001). There appears, however, to be a consensus that combined treatment does not appear to be contraindicated in any patient population (Hollon and Fawcett 1995,

| Table 105–2 | Efficacy and Effectiveness Research—Comparison | |
|---|---|---|
| | Efficacy | Effectiveness |
| Definition | The methodical assessment of an intervention in a controlled clinical trial setting | The assessment of an intervention for pertinence and practicality in a routine clinical practice setting |
| Type of intervention assessed | Any; may be experimental | Only those with established efficacy |
| Study population | Homogeneous | Those in need of treatment |
| Diagnosis | Exclude comorbidity | Comorbidity common |
| Illness severity, length of illness | Narrow range | Broad range |
| Inclusion/exclusion criteria | Strict | Few |
| Need for randomization/control group | Yes | No |
| Provision of psychotherapy intervention | Strict adherence to intervention, use of treatment manuals common | No requirement for use of/adherence to treatment manuals |
| Emphasis | Internal validity Replicability | External validity Generalizability |

*Source*: Barlow DH (1996) Health care policy, psychotherapy research, and the future of psychotherapy. Am Psychol 51, 1050–1058; Nathan PE, Stuart SP, and Dolan SL (2000) Research on psychotherapy efficacy and effectiveness : Between scylla and charbodis? Psychol Bull 126(6) (Nov), 964–981.

Paykel 1995, Rounsaville et al. 1981), unless either single modality is contraindicated or in the existence of medical conditions that need to be addressed prior to implementation of psychopharmacotherapy or psychotherapy (Hollon and Fawcett 2001). Hollon and Fawcett (1995) have outlined four ways in which combined treatment may prove advantageous over either treatment alone: increase the magnitude, probability, or breadth of clinical response, and increase the acceptability to the patient of either modality. In general, they feel that there is literature to support the statement that combined treatment enhances the breadth of clinical response. It is within this context that clinical practice guidelines published by the Agency for Health Care Policy and Research support the use of combined treatment in depressive disorders (Depression Guideline Panel 1993).

## Combined Treatment: Proposed Benefits

Various authors discuss the potential benefits of employing pharmacotherapy within a psychotherapeutic context (Klerman 1991, Kay 2001). Pharmacotherapy has been noted to have a quicker onset of action on acute symptoms than most psychotherapies, perhaps with the exclusion of cognitive therapy (Hollon and Fawcett 2001). It is felt that this rapid dampening of symptoms may enhance the patient's ability to more productively participate in therapy by a variety of mechanisms. These have been described cogently by Klerman (1985, 1991) and include enhancing the patient's self-esteem, creating a safe environment in which emotions are more freely discussed, reducing the stigma of seeking mental health care through a positive placebo effect, improving cognition (verbalization and abreaction), and functioning as a transitional object during breaks in therapy, among others.

The benefits of employing psychotherapy within a primarily psychopharmacologic relationship have also been described. Empirical evidence exists across the spectrum of mental health disorders to support the following hypothesized benefits of adding psychotherapy to medications. It decreases the incidence of illness relapse (Hogarty et al. 1986), as well as symptom relapse upon medication discontinuation (Wiborg and Dahl 1996, Spiegel et al. 1994). It fosters the patient's ability to utilize healthy coping strategies, addresses issues that are not typically targeted by psychopharmacologic treatment such as dysfunctional relationship patterns or negative self-appraisals due to traumatic past events, and enhances psychotropic compliance (Paykel 1995, Cochran 1984).

## Clinical Applications: Treatment Adherence

Adherence may be enhanced in part through discussion of the patient's metaphor for the medication, either positive or negative (Kay 2001). The following vignettes illustrate a patient's frequently held conceptions regarding medication use.

---

**Clinical Vignette 1**

Ms. E, a married 38-year-old with a diagnosis of major depressive disorder, recurrent and severe, and dependent personality disorder presents as a referral to Dr. A for continued care due to the retirement of the psychiatrist whom she had been seeing in 15-minute medication management appointments over the past year. Ms. E's symptoms included poor energy, anhedonia, lack of libido, intermittent suicidal ideation without a prior history of attempts, trouble concentrating, and complaints of "memory loss." Ms. E's current stressors include her father's terminal illness and longstanding marital conflicts. Ms. E's father, sister, and brother all suffer from an affective disorder. A review of the patient's records reveals a complex medication regimen, with frequent medication changes and poor symptom control. Ms. E seemed to do well initially on new medications, often responding within a day or two, but then would have her spouse call the psychiatrist on her behalf to report that the effects of the medication had "worn off." Dr. A and Ms. E agreed to initiate brief psychotherapy, in addition to medication management, due to the persistence of her symptoms despite trials of various psychotropics. During the course of her first session, she revealed a distant relationship with her father, who had been a physician. She found him aloof and unnurturing, except for those times in which she was ill, during which he often directed her medical care. Dr. A made no changes to Ms. E's medication regimen at the first visit. At her next visit, Ms. E commented to Dr. A that she greatly missed her former psychiatrist whom she described as "really knew what he was doing with my meds, and understood the depth of my suffering." She asked for a referral to a new psychiatrist as she felt Dr. A and herself were "just not a good fit."

---

The above case highlights one of the beliefs that patients may have regarding medications, that is, they indicate their provider's level of interest in them as a person and the provider truly appreciates the level of their distress. In certain contexts these beliefs may be regarded as a "positive metaphor"; however in others, as demonstrated above, it may hinder the patient's response to treatment, their compliance with the treatment regimen, and their level of trust in their provider.

---

**Clinical Vignette 1** *continued*

Ms. E eventually agreed to continue seeing Dr. A "for a few more sessions." Dr. A explored the psychological meaning that Ms. E had been attributing to medication interventions. She was eventually able to recognize that changes in her psychotropic regimen did not have to occur for her to feel that others understood her. Ms. E was able to look at connections between her past and her current reactions within the patient–provider relationship (exploration of countertransference issues), as well as within other interpersonal relationships including her marriage. Her medication regimen was simplified, she maintained compliance with her treatment plan, and she achieved remission of her depressive symptoms.

---

## Clinical Applications: Sequential Treatment

Fava (1999) highlights that sequential treatments may be applied in four ways: (1) using a second type of psychotherapy when the first orientation has not fully achieved treatment goals, (2) introducing a second type of pharmacotherapy when the first medication has not achieved adequate symptom relief, (3) introducing psychotherapy when initial pharmacotherapy has not been fully effective, and (4) introducing pharmacotherapy when initial psychotherapy has not been fully effective. The latter two may include use of combined treatments in a sequential fashion. Clinical Vignette 1 was an example of the third method; Clinical Vignette 2 highlights the fourth method.

---

**Clinical Vignette 2**

Mr. B is a 40-year-old executive for a major corporation who has been recently diagnosed with panic disorder with agoraphobia by a psychiatry resident (Dr. C). Mr. B reports that for the past 6 months he has experienced panic attacks three or four times each day which involve "a sudden intense wave of fear that seems to come out of nowhere," usually during the day, but sometimes waking him up from sleep. During these attacks, he reports symptoms of a racing heart rate, sweating, feelings of nausea, trembling, and a fear of losing control and doing something crazy, like running through his corporate office while yelling at people to get out of his way. Mr. B's panic attacks have become so frequent and intense that he can no longer perform his job and relies on other junior executives to manage the company. In fact, he avoids business travel because he fears becoming incapacitated from panic on an airplane. Recently, he has also begun to avoid staff meetings out of concern that a panic attack will occur and that he would have to leave unexpectedly.

Due to the severity of Mr. B's panic and avoidance symptoms, the resident suggests a trial of medication for the patient. After discussing medication options with the patient, Mr. B decides he would prefer not to take medication because he fears "losing control" or "getting addicted to pills." Although the resident attempted to allay some of the patient's fears about the medication, Mr. B persisted in his reluctance to the treatment and even expressed his concern that the resident "must really think I'm crazy if you think I need pills!"

In light of Mr. B's resistance to medication, the resident considers the use of cognitive–behavioral therapy (CBT) in order to supply the patient with action-oriented, self-directed behavioral approaches, such as relaxation and exposure exercises. In addition, the resident addresses the patient's cognitive distortions regarding issues of control and beliefs that he is "crazy." Psychotherapy also reveals that Mr. B's father was alcoholic and his mother abused benzodiazepines, which explains some of the patient's belief system regarding medications.

---

As demonstrated by the vignettes, the meanings that the patient attributes to medication may have to do with cognitions and feelings in a variety of spheres including the illness, the provider, and themselves (Beck 2001).

## Clinical Applications: Advantages and Challenges

The vignettes also serve to highlight potential benefits and challenges surrounding integrated treatment described by Kay (2001). In Clinical Vignette 2, rapport is well established, precluding the need to reestablish rapport and for the patient to retell his "story" to yet another provider. Integrated treatment essentially eliminates the communica-

tion difficulties encountered in split treatment settings. The practitioner of integrated treatment does face some obstacles. In both cases, the psychiatrist needs to be well trained in a variety of psychotherapy orientations, particularly in the orientation that has literature evidence to support its use in a particular disorder. It is the rare clinician who has expertise in more than one or two psychotherapies, which may provide the impetus to utilize a split treatment delivery system. The psychiatrist who provides only integrated treatment for his/her patients may feel isolated and miss the opportunity for discussion of the challenges encountered in treating the patient, discussion which occurs more frequently in split treatment settings.

Clinical Vignette 1 highlights the importance of a thorough assessment of the patient using a biopsychosocial approach as described by Engel (1977). To provide a theoretical framework for formulation of the patient and treatment plan, McHugh and Slavney (1983) similarly discuss understanding the psychiatrically ill patient from four "perspectives." These multifactorial models of mental health illnesses serve as conceptual tools with which to understand the whole patient and those forces that together precipitate, perpetuate, and modify illness course/progression. It stands to reason that a provider of integrated care should utilize an "integrated" model of illness description, etiology, and treatment.

When a single provider directs both forms of treatment, traditional role conflicts may emerge. The role stereotype of a psychotherapist may include one who has a multidimensional understanding of the patient, is interested in intrapsychic/core conflicts and their manifestations in symptoms, behaviors, feelings, and thoughts, and whose style is less authoritarian. The pharmacotherapist's traditional role stereotype is of a biological/neurochemical understanding of the patient and a prescriptive, structured, more authoritarian style in approaching diagnosis, medications, and other issues. While these roles, are as, mentioned stereotypic even in the hyperbole, they do have in common the role of the provider in establishing rapport and a therapeutic alliance with the patient. It has been suggested that the psychiatrist who uses an integrated model provides more time for development of the therapeutic alliance thus increasing the patient's comfort in disclosing embarrassing side effects of medication and, perhaps, even aiding in treatment outcome via the strength of the alliance (Gabbard and Kay 2001). Psychotherapy studies have suggested that therapist variables accounted for 30% of the variance in outcomes, and that therapeutic alliance is perhaps the most important factor in positive treatment outcomes (Lambert 1992, Svartberg et al. 1998). While these expansive statements regarding nonspecific factors in psychotherapy exist, there is other evidence to support that specific therapies account for more of the variance than the therapeutic alliance (Wilson et al. 1999). Still, therapeutic alliance is crucial; as such, management of transitions between roles, as well as the seamless integration of roles is imperative within the practice of integrated treatment (Gabbard and Kay 2001). These role transitions may occur rapidly and within a single session.

A familiarity with current literature and clinical practice guidelines concerning when to employ medications alone, therapy alone, or both, and when sequential treatments may lead to a greater probability of remission is a must for any clinician utilizing combined treatment.

There is no empirical evidence to suggest that integrated treatment by a psychiatrist is more advantageous (in terms of efficacy) than split treatment; however, Lazarus (1999) points out that prospective randomized clinical trials are warranted. There is some evidence that psychiatrists may be more cost effective when providing integrated treatment to those patients that require combined treatment (Dewan 1999), but additional studies replicating these findings are needed. Despite the theoretical, economic, and efficacy disputes/conflicts in the literature, a good number of psychiatrists use integrated treatment in their clinical practice settings (Duffy et al. 2001), which may be a reflection of patient needs in the social/interpersonal arena and, perhaps, an understanding that treatment approaches based on a mind–brain dualism hypothesis do not achieve full functional improvement in the patient's life (Gabbard and Kay 2001).

## Clinical Applications: Managing the Session

---

### Clinical Vignette 2 *continued*

After five sessions of CBT, Mr. B recognizes only a slight reduction in the frequency of panic attacks and agrees to an "experiment" in which he would start taking medication with a slow increase in dosage. For each subsequent session, the resident follows a structured format by asking the patient for a brief update, check on anxiety, and discussion of the medication's side effects. The resident reviews the previous session and collects Mr. B's homework regarding the frequency and severity of self-monitored panic/anxiety; checking for medication treatment results and side effects. The patient practices cognitive reframing regarding any mental or physiological changes he noticed while on the medication. This reframing involves teaching the patient to use self-dialogue to view physiological changes as either expected minor medication side effects that are temporary, or as simply a nonmedication, normal physiological status change that the patient misperceives as a sign of something horribly wrong. The reframing process is accomplished by educating the patient to challenge his distorted belief systems during sessions and then the resident and patient collaboratively set homework assignments. After 15 additional sessions of integrated CT and medication, Mr. B is panic-free but continues to receive treatment to address some mild avoidance features.

---

This example highlights one way in which to fluidly incorporate both domains (psychotherapy and pharmacotherapy) within each patient visit. The above approach is structured in nature, following cognitive therapy's principle that sessions are structured and remain constant during therapy (Beck 1995). Providers of psychodynamic therapy, among other types of therapy, often prefer this structured type of approach, advocating that medication use either be discussed at the beginning or at the end of the session. Proponents of the beginning method feel that discussion of medication issues ensures adequate time is spent on concerns and may provide important material for the session. Advocates of the "set aside 5 to 10 minutes at the end of the session" approach feel that it is most important for the patients to set their own agenda, as this allows for time needed for the patient to regain composure/recompensate before the end of the session. Another approach is the nonstructured method. In this case the therapist addresses medication issues only when the need arises. As there are no evidence-based studies to guide clinical practice, it is most important to base the choice on patient and provider preference and to practice consistency with each patient (Kay 2002).

## Clinical Applications: Individualizing Treatment

Dr. C (the psychiatry resident) was required to attend a multidisciplinary treatment team meeting in which outpatient mental health providers from various disciplines were present. The resident was questioned as to the reasoning behind her choice of adding pharmacotherapy to psychotherapy.

How can the psychiatrist tailor his/her treatment options to each individual patient? When would sequential approaches be indicated and in which disorders are combined treatments most likely to be helpful? During which phase of treatment (acute versus maintenance) should combined treatments be used versus solo treatments (either medications or therapy)? For what severity of illness are combined treatments preferred? Is there evidence to support sequential approaches and should they be specifically targeted to stages of the illness? How might understanding physiologic changes in the brain, which occur in the context of both medications and psychotherapy, help guide our research and clinical treatment interventions? It should be kept in mind that research regarding these issues is in its infancy, and many recommendations may still require evidence-based studies to definitively aid with the establishment of critical pathways for each of the disorders. As Dr. C was providing care to a patient with a common anxiety disorder, these disorders will be addressed first.

## Clinical Applications: Anxiety Disorders

Anxiety spectrum disorders affect nearly 10% of the US adult population and thus, are the most common of the mental health illnesses in the US. The most appealing conceptualizations of anxiety disorders and especially panic disorder is one that uses the biopsychosocial model. From a biological perspective, dysfunction of GABA, noradrenergic, and serotonergic pathways have all been implicated in the etiology and maintenance of anxiety symptoms. Many of the anxiety disorders (Hettema et al. 2001) have been demonstrated to have significant familial aggregation, with a recent meta-analysis indicating that for panic disorder, generalized anxiety disorder (GAD), and phobias, genetics account for much of this aggregation. From the psychological perspective, both learning theories (classical and operant conditioning) and cognitive theories provide hypotheses for the development and maintenance of these disorders. From the social perspective, the patient's current environment and stressors play a role in the development and maintenance of symptoms. Most of the literature is in agreement that anxiety disorders are a result of the combination of biological, psychological, and social factors.

Panic disorder in particular has been the most extensively studied of the anxiety disorders (Kay 2001), especially in terms of literature on biological treatments, psychological treatments, and studies comparing the two treatments (Abraham et al. 1999). Studies of combined treatments versus solo treatment with medications or therapy are far fewer in the literature, although a recent study supports combined treatment as superior to either monotherapy (Barlow et al. 2000), as do earlier studies of psychotherapy in combination with tricyclic antidepressants (Mavissakalian 1993). CBT in combination with medications reduces relapse rates upon medication discontinuation in panic disorder, thus having a superior effect especially in the maintenance phase of the disorder (Spiegel et al. 1994). One study (Wiborg and Dahl 1996) shows the same improvement in relapse prevention with clomipramine in combination with brief psychodynamic therapy, in which 100% of combined therapy patients were panic-free at 9-month follow-up. However, several studies of CBT alone show that as many as 80% of patients maintain their therapeutic gains (Craske et al. 1991). It has been suggested that those patients receiving combined treatment (CBT plus meds), do significantly better on measures of anxiety, depression, catastrophic thinking, and disability (Bruce et al. 1995). Rapid reduction in symptoms, especially with use of the benzodiazepines (e.g., alprazolam) is not advocated in all circles, as they are felt to interfere with the long-term effects of exposure therapy. For panic disorder, while combined treatment with various antidepressants is preferred, combined treatment with benzodiazepines does not have demonstrated efficacy beyond either treatment alone. In those panic disorder patients on benzodiazepines or selective serotonin reuptake inhibitors (SSRIs), the addition of CBT does confer some advantages in assisting with medication taper and reducing relapse rates after medication discontinuation (Spiegel et al. 1994, Whittal et al. 2001).

For specific phobias and social anxiety disorders, combined treatment may be no more effective than either monotherapy (Mavissakalian 1993, Van Ameringen and Mancini 2001) and there may be some evidence that adding medication to CBT negatively affects long-term outcome by compromising treatment gains (Radomsky and Otto 2001, Barlow et al. 2000). The few studies of GAD suggest that, as for the other anxiety disorders, medications provide rapid relief of symptoms, with therapy a key ingredient for relapse prevention, improvements in functioning, and long-term preservation of treatment gains (Falsetti and Davis 2001).

Combined treatment for obsessive–compulsive disorder (OCD) is often generally employed in clinical practice, with clinical guidelines (Greist and Jefferson 2001) advocating behavior therapy (exposure with response prevention) plus pharmacotherapy (with an SSRI); however, there are few randomized controlled studies evaluating the advantages of behavior monotherapy over combined therapy. A recent study has demonstrated improved efficacy for adjuvant treatment of pharmacotherapy with behavior therapy provided in a group setting (Direnfeld et al. 2000).

## Clinical Applications: Mood Disorders

Dr. A is a staff attending in the same outpatient clinic as the psychiatry resident. He also attended the weekly multidisci-
plinary meeting. Upon hearing of his management of Ms. E (major depressive disorder, severe, and dependent personality disorder), one of the nonphysician providers asked Dr. A for his input as to how best to treat Mr. Z, a 75-year-old gentleman with dysthymic disorder.

Large clinics, such as the one in which Dr. A practices, may provide an opportunity for multidisciplinary discussions regarding patient care, a discussion that solo providers of combined treatment may miss. In addition, these discussions give Dr. A the chance to review the state-of-the-art recommendations for treatment of affective disorders.

### Unipolar Depressive Disorders

Mood disorders, major depressive disorder in particular, have a large body of evidence, including at least one randomized control trial (Keller et al. 2000), for the superiority of combined treatments. Efficacy may vary by particular patient subsets, severity of illness, and timing of treatments. Keller and colleagues (2000) found that response rates for patients with chronic major depression were markedly higher than for either sole antidepressant (nefazodone) use or psychotherapy alone (Table 105–3). Recently, de Jonghe and colleagues (2001) found that ambulatory major depressive disorder patients treated with combined therapy (antidepressant plus "short psychodynamic supportive therapy") were more acceptable of the treatment and significantly more likely to recover. An earlier meta-analyis by Thase and colleagues (1997) found that combined therapy was superior to monotherapy in patients with severe, recurrent depressions, but not for less severely depressed patients. So-called "double depression" or major depressive disorder comorbid with dysthymic disorder appeared to similarly respond best to a combination of CBT and antidepressants (Miller et al. 1999), consistent with the above studies if we view "double depressions" as a chronic and/or more severe variant. For pure dysthymic disorders, the superiority of combined treatments is more controversial (Ravindran et al. 1999). The addition of group cognitive therapy to sertraline treatment in a large randomized controlled trial had advantages only on functional status in a subset of patients. An additional study of dysthymic patients that added group psychotherapy to medication-responsive patients (a sequential approach) also suggested improvements in functional and interpersonal impairments (Fava et al. 2001). In clinical settings a sequential approach is generally utilized for nonresponders or partial responders (Hollon and Fawcett 2001). Sequential treatment strategies—interpersonal psychotherapy (IPT) plus meds versus IPT initially with medications added in to nonresponders—were examined by Frank and colleagues (2000). The researchers demonstrated that the stepwise approach yielded a better remission rate (79% versus 66%) in women with recurrent major depressive disorder. Interestingly, a lifetime history of panic-agoraphobic spectrum symptoms predicted a poorer response to IPT and an 8-week delay in sequential treatment response (Frank et al. 2000).

A study of older adults (greater than 59 years old) with recurrent depression examined maintenance phase treatments in this population and found that combined treatments were superior in this phase (Reynolds et al. 1999).

| Table 105–3 | Trials of Combined Treatment (CT) in Unipolar Depression | | | | |
| --- | --- | --- | --- | --- | --- |
| Study | Combination Used | Age/Gender | Diagnosis/Severity | Outcome Measure | Result |
| Frank et al. (1990) | IPT* IMI* | 21–65 yr, 38–78% female | MDD, recurrent | 3-yr relapse rate | CT not superior |
| Thase et al. (1997) | IPT IMI | Mean 44 yr, 2/3 female | MDD, severe, recurrent MDD, less severe | Response rate Response rate | CT superior No advantage for CT |
| Miller et al. (1999) | CBT TCA* | 18–65 yr, 71–92% female | Double depression | Response rate | CT superior |
| Reynolds et al. (1999) | IPT NTP* | >59 yr | MDD, recurrent | Response/recurrence rates | CT superior |
| Paykel et al. (1995) | CBT Various meds | Mean 43 yr, 50% female | MDD, partial remission | Relapse rate | CT superior |
| Ravindran et al. (1999) | Cognitive group therapy Sertraline | 21–54 yr, 60% female | Dysthymia D/O | Variety | CT superior on measures of functional impairment |
| Keller et al. (2000) | CBASP* Nefazodone | 18–75 yr, 65% female | MDD, chronic | Response/remission rates | CT superior to CBT alone or meds alone |
| Frank et al. (2000) | IPT SSRI* or IMI | 21–65 yr, women | MDD, recurrent | Remission | CT superior in those initial nonresponders to IPT given meds |
| de Jonghe et al. (2001) | SPSP* Prozac, Amitriptyline or Meclobemide | Mean 34 yr, 62% female | MDD, ambulatory | Response rate | CT superior, fewer dropouts |
| Kupfer and Frank (2001) | IPT NTP | >60 yr, 76% female | MDD, recurrent | Response rate | Varied by temporal response to meds |
| Lenze et al. (2002) | IPT NTP | >60 yr | MDD, recurrent | Social adjustment | CT superior |
| Hirshfeld et al. (2002) | CBASP Nefazodone | 18–75 yr, 65% female | MDD, chronic | Psychosocial functioning | CT superior |

*NTP, nortriptyline; SPSP, short psychodynamic supportive psychotherapy; IMI, imipramine; CBASP, cognitive behavioral analysis system of psychotherapy; SSRI, selective serotonin reuptake inhibitor; TCA, tricyclic antidepressant; IPT, interpersonal psychotherapy.

Kupfer and Frank (2001) examined a similar population of adults 60 years and older with unipolar recurrent major depression in an effort to differentiate which subset of patients respond to which form of maintenance therapies. The temporal response to acute treatment was found to predict maintenance modality. For "rapid responders" to acute treatment and "delayed sustained responders," combined therapy conferred no advantage over either monotherapy. For "initial mixed responders" (defined by the authors as those patients with Hamilton depression scores fluctuating above and below 10, but with no clear pattern towards improvement or worsening of the illness), combined therapy was marginally superior.

The majority of studies currently available in the literature have examined combined treatments with the pharmacotherapy arm primarily consisting of the older antidepressants, tricyclics. Thase and colleagues (2000), in his study of men with major depressive disorder, compared newer antidepressants (fluoxetine and bupropion) with CBT. He also employed a crossover design with respect to his medication arm of treatment (sequential use of pharmacotherapy described by Fava's method 2). This study found pharmacotherapy superior to CBT, but did not examine combined treatments. More studies of combined treatments

are needed with the newer antidepressants; results from anticipated trials may be available in the near future (Thase et al. 2000).

Given the significant morbidity of unipolar depressive disorders, recent investigations have looked at social functioning as an outcome measure. Combined therapy in the maintenance phase of the disorder (Lenze et al. 2002) was associated with improved duration, improved quality of life, and improved social functioning. In one study the improvement was independent of depressive symptom change (Hirshfeld et al. 2002).

## Bipolar Disorders

The APA Practice Guidelines for the treatment of bipolar disorder (American Psychiatric Association 2002a) recommend the combination of psychotherapy with pharmacotherapy, especially during the maintenance phase. Commonly utilized approaches include marital and family therapy, psychoeducation (family and individual), and individual therapy (primarily IPT and CBT) (Callahan and Bauer 1999, Rothbaum and Astin 2000). A review of the efficacy of the various approaches is outlined by Rothbaum and Astin (2000). Family therapy combined with medications enhances functional outcome, reduces relapse and extends time between relapses (Miklowitz et al. 2000), reduces hospitalizations (Retzer et al. 1991), and enhances medication compliance (Cochran 1984). In a small open label trial, medication compliant bipolar patients who had relapsed on lithium prophylaxis were found to have a significant reduction in residual symptoms when CBT was added (Fava et al. 2001). Consistency of treatment modality is an important factor in maintenance treatments for individuals with bipolar disorder (Frank et al. 1999). Extrapolating from the data on combined treatment superiority in the treatment of severe unipolar depression, bipolar depression may likewise benefit from this approach (American Psychiatric Association 2002), although additional studies are needed.

## Clinical Applications: Psychotic Disorders

Research evidence supports the use of psychotherapy and pharmacotherapy in the treatment of schizophrenia. An effective program for the treatment of schizophrenia includes a variety of psychosocial interventions, including psychoeducational approaches, social skills training, and psychotherapy (individual, group, family) (Goldstein 1991). Family therapy in conjunction with medications has been demonstrated to significantly reduce readmission rates (Zhang et al. 1994), decrease risk of relapse, enhance treatment compliance, decrease length of stays, improve general functioning of patients, and decrease emotional burden on the family. Individual psychotherapies that show promise include CBT and personal therapy (Hogarty et al. 1997a, 1997b). CBT has been demonstrated to improve medication compliance and improve medication refractory symptoms, both positive and negative (Sensky et al. 2000).

## Clinical Applications: Eating/Substance/ Personality Disorders

---

**Clinical Vignette 3**

Ms. H, a 27-year-old administrative assistant with a past history of bulimia nervosa and alcohol dependence, presents for her regularly scheduled appointment with her psychiatrist. Her primary complaints at this medication management visit were of right-sided facial pain, poor energy, and constipation. Ms. H notes that she has had increased pressure in her job, stating that as a result of downsizing she is now responsible for a larger area with more clients, requiring an increased amount of driving. A childhood friend had recently been killed in a motor vehicle accident, but due to a planned sales event, she was unable to attend the funeral. Ms. H feels that her fatigue is due to this stress, but desires some intervention for her constipation and pain. Upon further questioning she admits to "a little" alcohol use. Ms. H's laboratory values from that morning indicated mildly elevated potassium, mildly elevated GGT, and elevated salivary amylase. A brief physical examination revealed a suspected abscessed tooth, dental erosion, and a five-pound weight loss as compared to her last visit 3 months ago.

---

The above vignette illustrates one of the situations which Gabbard and Kay (2001) propose as well suited for integrated treatment by a psychiatrist. These situations include (1) patients with medically complicated, severe eating disorders (as above), (2) psychotic and bipolar I patients with treatment plan and medication adherence issues, (3) a subset of borderline personality disorder patients, (4) impulsive, suicidal patients, and (5) patients needing ongoing assessment for clarification of diagnosis and treatment planning.

## Eating Disorders

Guidelines for combined treatment of bulimia nervosa (BN) have been suggested (American Psychiatric Association 2000), based on a limited number of studies examining medications versus psychotherapy versus their combination. As with much of the literature on depression, the medication arm used older generation antidepressants. A 1997 study by Walsh and colleagues, which included a sequential pharmacotherapy arm (patients failing to respond to desipramine were switched to fluoxetine), demonstrated modest evidence that combined treatment (CBT plus medications) improved the response rate in BN. This study did not examine combined treatments versus psychotherapy alone. Most studies have found CBT alone to be superior to medication alone (Mitchell et al. 2001). The Walsh study did not substantiate this finding, perhaps because a new generation antidepressant was used. Clinically, medications are often used as monotherapy, in part due to limited accessibility to providers trained in CBT for BN (Mitchell et al. 2001). If IPT is proven to be an efficacious psychotherapy for BN, this may improve provider access. Some authors (Agras 2001, Mitchell et al. 2001) suggest as a guideline that in patients without a comorbid affective disorder, CBT should be initiated as first-line therapy, if available. Cost-effectiveness assessments also support this recommendation (Agras 2001). If there is nonresponse to therapy (70% reduction in purging by session six), an efficacious antidepressant should be added (Mitchell et al. 2001, Bacaltchuk 2000). In those patients with comorbid affective disorder, they propose initiation of combined treatment at the outset. One recent study examined sequential use of medications (fluoxetine added after failed IPT or CBT trial), and found benefits in using medication alone in psychotherapy nonresponders (Walsh et al. 2000). The most recent Cochrane review of combined treatment in BN (Bacaltchuk et al. 2002), which included six studies (four using individual CBT, one with group CBT, and one with newer antidepressant), concluded that combined treatments were superior to monotherapy, but also cautioned that adding medications to established psychotherapy resulted in a reduced acceptability of the particular psychotherapy. Obviously, the number of studies included in this review was quite small, suggesting the need for ongoing research in this area.

Controlled studies of outpatient treatments on anorexia nervosa (AN) are less abundant, perhaps owing to the fact that AN is a rare disorder as compared to BN. CBT may be useful in preventing relapse in weight-restored anorexics, and SSRIs may also be effective in this weight-restored population for relapse prevention. There are no published studies of combined treatment versus single modality treatment.

## Substance Use Disorders

Eating disorders, and particularly BN, are often comorbid with substance use disorders, particularly alcohol. Combined treatment for alcohol use disorders may be indicated to aid with medication compliance to either naltrexone or disulfiram; adding family interventions may also improve medication compliance and subsequent abstinence (Ziedonis et al. 2001). Combined treatment of nicotine dependence (American Psychiatric Association 1996) and opioid use disorders (Ziedonis et al. 2001) is common and efficacious.

There are no randomized controlled clinical trials examining the efficacy of combined treatment versus monotherapy for personality disorder. Clinical consensus (Gabbard 2000) and APA Practice Guideline for the treatment of borderline personality disorder (American Psychiatric Association 2001) support the use of a combined treatment approach, citing fewer treatment dropouts and advantages in addressing treatment-interfering features such as aggression, impulsivity, and affective lability.

## Split Treatment

## Background: An Historical Overview

Providing split treatment is not a new form of mental health care. In 1947, Fromm-Reichmann described the practice as a standard analytic procedure in both inpatient and outpatient settings (Fromm-Reichmann 1947). Patients would receive analysis from one psychiatrist, and another psychiatrist would serve all nonanalytic functions, including provision of medications and liaisons with other physicians. The rationale of such an arrangement was that extra-analytic activities interfered with the analyst's function as a blank screen and theoretically hindered the development and resolution of the patient's transference neurosis.

As Goldberg and colleagues (1991) pointed out, the current rationale for split treatment has certainly changed. Since psychoanalysis is no longer a major therapeutic modality, the rationale now for division of responsibility between the prescribing physician and the therapist is not clear. Further, psychopharmacology has burgeoned such that providing psychotherapy for a patient with major depression or bipolar disorder, for example, without considering a course of medication would be inappropriate. So what have been the factors that have fueled split treatment since the 1940s?

Certainly the Community Mental Health Act, passed by President John F. Kennedy, played an important role in encouraging psychiatrists to take positions in community mental health centers. While the promise and hope of being able to take care of patients in less restrictive settings, such as an outpatient mental health center, seemed quite worthy, how to actually manage large numbers of patients with few psychiatrists was, in hindsight, not well formulated. In such institutions, often the psychiatrist was asked to be responsible and write prescriptions for hundreds of patients, many of whom were provided supportive or other types of psychotherapy by nonphysician therapists (social workers, psychologists). The relationship between the psychiatrist and the patient changed, with ambiguous roles developing in the triangle between the therapist, patient, and psychiatrist (Brill 1977). The literature in the 1970s abounds with questions regarding how to delineate the role of the psychiatrist in treatment centers, as well as noting the dissatisfaction of psychiatrists who were in these professional split treatment arrangements (Glasscote 1975, Reinstein 1978).

In 1973, in an attempt to help sort out the new difficulties and questions that were arising in split arrangements, the APA developed a position statement on psychiatrists and their relationships with nonmedical mental health professionals. Vasile and Gutheil (1979) tried to provide some beginning guidelines as to how the psychiatrist, as a medical backup to the therapist, could provide responsible clinical care. In 1980, the APA developed "Guidelines for Psychiatrists in Consultative, Supervisory, or Collaborative Relationships with Nonmedical Therapists" (American Psychiatric Association 1980). The consultative relationship was described as one in which the psychiatrist has no ongoing relationship with the patient. The psychiatrist provides a consultation to the referring physician and the referring physician can decide whether or not to incorporate the psychiatrist's suggestions into the treatment plan. The collaborative relationship is a situation where the responsibility for treatment of the patient is shared, with the psychiatrist responsible for the patient's medical and physical complaints. The supervisory relationship is one in which the psychiatrist actively directs all facets of the nonmedical psychotherapist's work and, therefore, shares in the responsibility of the patient's care. While the collaborative relationship model is probably most related to what we call "split treatment" today, there are many psychiatrists who engage in split treatment but who also have supervisory relationships with nonmedical therapists. The 1980 APA guidelines still stand as definitive principles for the psychiatric profession but, in 1995, APA indirectly reaffirmed its support of integrated versus split treatment by issuing a position statement on medical psychotherapy (American Psychiatric Association 2002b). Some authors have asked whether new APA guidelines for split treatment are needed (Fawcett 2001).

With the rise of split treatment, Firman (1982) recognized opportunities in such psychiatrist–nonmedical psychotherapy arrangements. Pilette (1988) noted that there were many issues in split treatment arrangements that needed to be resolved, such as those dealing with confidentiality, clinical and legal responsibility for patients who may attempt suicide or require hospitalization, changes in the doctor–patient relationship, splitting, and reimbursement.

In one of the first studies to review the prevalence of split treatment, Beitman and colleagues (1984) reported on survey results of the members of the Washington State Psychiatric Association. Most of the respondents had done "medication backup" in the preceding months with those tending to be younger psychiatrists, working in clinics or public settings, and to be analytically oriented. One-fifth of the respondents who performed medication backup did so in a supervisory relationship with the nonmedical psychotherapist. Goldberg and colleagues (1991) surveyed the members of the Connecticut Psychiatric Society and found that a major factor promoting the growth of split treatment was the willingness of nonmedical therapists to seek medications for their patients. Similar to the Beitman study, over 63% of the Connecticut respondents engaged in medication backup (split treatment). The study revealed many implied obligations that accrue to the psychiatrist who provides medication—hospitalization, after-hours coverage for many issues not necessarily medical. In an accompanying editorial to the Goldberg article, Appelbaum (1991) offered guidelines to help clinicians and patients diminish the implied obligations and be more overt about clinical responsibilities.

In the 1980s, the burgeoning of managed care was synergistic with the notion of split treatment. In the outpatient setting, managed care emphasized the use of a multidisciplinary model in order to make care-delivery more cost-effective (Kerber 1999). It seemed to make sense to use less costly, nonmedical therapists rather than more expensive psychiatrists to perform certain functions such as the provision of psychotherapy. The psychiatrist's role changed from having authoritative and independent leadership to seeing that the managed care system had a financial interest in ensuring cost-effective, well-integrated diagnostic and treatment planning. This shift of the psychiatrist to a collaborator, not necessarily a leader, was crucial. In the previous fee-for-service model payment system in which psychiatry operated until the 1980s, the psychiatrist could determine which nonmedical therapists would become treatment collaborators. Insurance companies, under the fee-for-service system, would place few restrictions on the range of possible psychotherapists. This freedom of control for psychiatrists became drastically reduced under managed care. No longer did they have the freedom to determine who their collaborators would be. In addition, psychiatrists had a more difficult time referring patients to a higher level of care, such as a hospital. Decisions about suicidal risk and need for hospitalization became part of the role of utilization reviewers who did not have clinical experience and certainly did not examine or know the patient.

As utilization management began dictating how often therapists could see patients, it quickly became clear that while psychiatrists were often seeing their patients less frequently in split treatment arrangements, they were still holding much of the liability risk. Psychiatrists became dependent on the therapist to manage cases in between the "medication sessions" and advise the psychiatrist when there were crises. Often the psychiatrist did not know these collaborators, making for legal and ethical dilemmas.

Dr. H contracted with a managed care company to provide medication management (split treatment) for patients who were being treated by 26 different community therapists. Dr. H did not know most of these therapists. When it was revealed that one of the social work therapists, Mr. M, had been charged with sexual misconduct by three of the patients whom Dr. H was also seeing for medication management, an ethics charge to the local psychiatric district branch and civil charges were filed against Dr. H stating that he should have known that the therapist was incompetent and an unethical practitioner and should have protected his patients from Mr. M (Lazarus 1999).

While managed care was indeed an important force in split treatment, two recent studies seem to refute the difference in the costs of split treatment versus integrated treatment (Goldman et al. 1998, Dewan 1999). The economic advantage of split treatment remains unclear (Balon and Riba 2001). Essentially, these authors have noted that the increase in total visits that must occur for patients to be treated in split treatment nullifies the cost savings that could be realized if a patient was seen in integrated treatment. Additionally, time lost in seeing a therapist for several visits before being evaluated for medication is one of a host of other factors that must be addressed when trying to measure cost shifts or savings.

The debate on the issues of combining psychotherapy and pharmacologic treatment has continued for the last 4 decades (GAP 1975, Klerman 1985, Marcus 1990a, 1990b, Woodward et al. 1993). Not until very recently, however, has attention been paid to the significant impact the split treatment paradigm is having on psychiatric residency training (Spitz et al. 1999).

## Residency Training Issues

Split treatment, while increasingly a major component of outpatient treatment within psychiatry residency settings (Riba et al. 1993, Hansen-Grant and Riba 1995), is viewed uncomfortably by many residents (Tekell et al. 1997). Issues that have been noted include discomfort working in a collaborative relationship, having encounter problems in outpatient collaboration, and viewing treatment contracts as unclear (Tekell et al. 1997). Over the last 15 years, there has also been a dramatic decrease in the emphasis of psychodynamic training, making it easier for training programs to have residents spend more time in split treatment (providing medication). While the Residency Review Committee in Psychiatry in January 2001 promulgated new requirements regarding evaluating competencies in various forms of psychotherapy, it remains to be seen whether residents will actually do less split treatment during their training.

A final major factor in the burgeoning of split treatment has been the increased importance of the role of primary care physicians in treating patients with emotional problems in the US (Valenstein 1999). In fact, PCPs treat the majority of such patients, at least 50 to 60% (Horgan 1985, Regier et al. 1978, Shurman et al. 1985). The treatments usually provided by PCPs include brief counseling and reassurance and short-term medication to address somatic complaints (Shurman et al. 1985, Verhaak and Wennink 1990). In contrast to these high numbers, PCPs have traditionally cared for patients without seeking assistance from mental health professionals. Twenty-five percent of primary care patients present with psychiatric disorders (Barrett et al. 1988, Kessler et al. 1985, Spitzer et al. 1994), but only half of these patients are formally identified by their PCPs, and just 5 to 16% of the identified patients are referred to mental health providers (Coulter et al. 1989, Wilkinson 1989). As summarized by Valenstein (1999), PCPs only formally refer a small percentage of their distressed patients to mental health providers, with a very conservative estimate of 1.5 to 3.0% of all Americans expected to see a primary care physician and concurrently a mental health clinician within a 12-month period. Unfortunately, very little is known about split treatment issues in the primary care setting—the frequency of mental health referrals to PCPs or the content of requests of mental health providers to PCPs.

In sum, the last 60 years has seen a shift from a dyadic relationship between patient and therapist towards a

**Dyadic relationship**

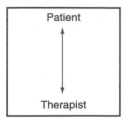

**Tripartite relationship**

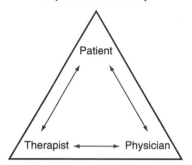

**Four-way relationship**

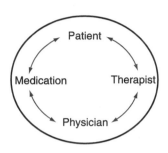

**Figure 105–1** *Changes in relationships as therapy and medications are added or deleted. (Source: Kay J [2001] Integrated treatment:An overview. In Integrated Treatment for Psychiatric Disorders: Review of Psychiatry, Vol. 20, Kay J [ed]. American Psychiatric Press, Washington DC, pp. 1–29.)*

tripartite relationship with the inclusion of medication, to a four-way or systemic relationship with the addition or deletion of medications (Figure 105–1).

## Aspects of Split Treatment

One of the few studies to look at integrated versus split treatment used the 1997 Practice Research Network (PRN) Study of Psychiatric Patients and Treatments (SPPT) (Pincus et al. 1999). Duffy and colleagues (2001) studied 276 adult outpatients who were receiving combined psychopharmacology and psychotherapy for mood disorders. A majority of patients in this study received integrated versus split treatment. Factors that were associated with the provision of split treatment included patients' diagnoses (bipolar); use of utilization management; psychiatrists' age (patients of psychiatrists older than 54 were 70% less likely to receive split treatment than patients of younger psychiatrists [31–43]); board certification (patients of board-certified psychiatrists were about five times more likely to receive split treatment than patients of psychiatrists without board certification. Board-certified psychiatrists were younger and more likely to treat patients under managed care plans); *practice setting* payment (patients treated in outpatient clinic/hospital settings were three times more likely to receive split treatment than patients treated in office-based practices ($P < 0.05$); and source of payment (patients on public insurance were 70% less likely to receive split treatment than patients with private insurance coverage ($P < 0.05$). Clearly, these are important trends worth monitoring.

## Positive Aspects

There are several positive aspects of split treatment, including the increased time that patients have with more than one clinician; better utilization of resources; enhanced opportunity for alignment of gender, ethnicity between patient

and clinician; more professional support for each clinician; and, perhaps, better adherence of the overall treatment plan by the patient and family.

**Increased Time with Clinicians.** Within the structure of split treatment, patients actually meet with at least two different clinicians: one for psychotropic medication or other somatic treatment and the other clinician for psychotherapy. Under ideal circumstances, the patient is seen by the nonmedical therapist at appointed intervals between the physician appointments. This could then allow for the patient to get longitudinal care by two clinicians and to therefore be seen on a continuum by both. Under this type of arrangement, there would not be too long an interval in which the patient is not seen by a mental health professional. With good communication, the therapist relays all important information to the physician in a timely manner. If there are planned vacations by either clinician, the other clinician is aware and can make different plans accordingly to see the patient. The patient may be able to provide more useful information in this treatment approach, given that she has more time to spend in overall treatment.

**Better Utilization of Resources.** With the growing realization of the importance of evaluating for emotional problems in the primary care setting, there is better recognition of psychiatric symptoms and disorders. In rural areas where there may not be enough mental health clinicians to serve the needed population, splitting the duties of the various clinicians might be a cost-effective way to ensure allocation of care. Similarly, there are certain types of psychotherapeutic treatments with documented efficacy, such as cognitive–behavioral treatment of depression and behavioral treatment of obsessive–compulsive disorder, panic disorder, and phobias, which must be delivered by knowledgeable clinicians (Fawcett 2001). There are psychiatrists and primary care physicians who are not adequately trained to deliver some of these forms of treatment. It makes good clinical sense, then, to try to determine the best care needed for the patient and to help orchestrate providing that care, whether it takes one clinician or several to provide it.

There are also certain settings, such as a psychiatry resident clinic, where having multiple clinicians caring for patients is optimally using the resources of the clinic. McNutt and colleagues (1987) noted that assignment of a patient to a permanent staff member in addition to the more novice resident offered an opportunity for the patient to have continuity with a "seasoned" therapist and to have a better outcome.

**Greater Choice of Clinicians.** Split treatment allows for more choices in the selection of clinicians based on gender, race or ethnicity, and religion or cultural values. Such matching may help the patient and clinician avoid certain difficulties that arise in psychotherapy when there is not a full appreciation of cultural issues (Foulks and Pena 1995). Certain cultural traditions and values may be misunderstood or misinterpreted by clinicians (Yamamoto et al. 1993). Similarly, there are language barriers that have deterred some patients from seeking or remaining in mental health treatment (Ruiz et al. 1995).

**Improved Adherence to the Treatment Plan.** Patients attribute certain meanings to the prescription and taking of medication, depending on their illness-belief system (Rolland 1994, Winer and Andriukatis 1989). Some patients hear an explanation of the need to take medications as having a "chemical imbalance" and embrace the idea that there is a biochemical reason for the problem. Other patients feel ashamed or guilty over having a defect and develop a strong resistance to taking their medication as prescribed (Paykel 1995).

It is important for the clinicians involved in split treatment to appreciate how the patient understands the need for medication. Similarly, it is valuable for the physician to be aware of how the nonphysician therapist understands the role of medication in the overall treatment. The physician and therapist must help support medication and psychotherapy so as to help the patient succeed in having a good outcome. In this way, the patient will receive support from both treaters with neither the medication nor the therapy undermined.

**Enhanced Support for Clinicians.** There are several levels of support that accrue to clinicians involved in split treatment. With particularly difficult patients, such as those with severe personality disorders or hard-to-treat depressions or psychoses, it is very valuable for clinicians to be able to feel a mutual caring for one another and an empathy for the difficult clinical situations that can arise. Split treatment allows for a sharing of information that can help clinicians help patients through crises. As Silk points out, patients with borderline personality disorder, for example, are noted for fueling strong countertransferential feelings of anger, fear, and worry in clinicians (Silk et al. 1995). It is very helpful when clinicians in split treatment can present a unified front to the patient, acknowledging that they are capable of handling the patient's affective storms but also provide support to one another to diminish feelings of

burn-out. Balon (1999) has noted that psychiatry residents, in particular, value the teaching and support they receive from seasoned, mature social workers and psychologists while providing split treatment.

## Negative Aspects

**Communication.** While communication is probably the most important factor in successful split treatment, it is rarely done well (Hansen-Grant and Riba 1995). Without a systematic way for clinicians and the patient to have regular, documented communication, there often arise misunderstandings and misconceptions. Further, patients are sometimes put in the middle of having to be the messenger between the clinicians. Needing to communicate puts additional burdens and stress on busy clinicians with the telephone or in-person time not usually reimbursable. Poor communication leads to misinterpretation of what should be attributable to psychodynamic issues or medication side effects, or both—a poorly constructed treatment plan, ill-defined plans for discharge from treatment, lack of coordination with family members, neither the clinician nor patient fully understanding vacation or coverage issues, and so on.

**Interdisciplinary Issues.** The literature demonstrates that when clinicians know one another, they are more comfortable with split treatment (Goldberg et al. 1991, Weiner and Riba 1997). Unfortunately, often the clinicians do not know one another, which leads to basic mistrust, competition, or inequality in the relationship (Baggs and Schmitt 1988). Further, this devaluation can be displaced onto the patient during critical treatment decisions, with certain patients exploiting this competition even further (Kelly 1991). The psychotherapy skills of psychiatrists and nonmedical therapists and the psychopharmacologic education of social workers and psychologists are all highly variable, contributing to mistrust (Neal and Calarco 1999). In such circumstances, the patient may actually be seen more often by both clinicians and have ill-defined treatment goals.

**Transference and Countertransference.** When patients are referred by their therapists for medication evaluations, the reactions are variable, but often negative. Such reactions include feeling abandoned or rejected, as if the therapist has lost interest or given up, like a failure because therapy did not work, devaluation of the psychotherapy and the therapist, idealization of the physician, shame, resistance to further psychodynamic exploration of issues, and a narcissistic injury (Busch and Gould 1993). Busch and Gould note the difficulties for the therapist who needs to make the referral: shame that help is needed and anger towards the patient for needing additional help. The psychiatrist could then collude with the patient's negative transference towards the therapist and the psychodynamic process.

Results of such negative transference could lead to premature closure within the therapeutic process (Bradley 1990). There may be a flight into health by the patient when the medication is first prescribed. The patient and physician may then realize too late that there was an overreliance on biologic interventions. The dyadic relationship between the therapist and patient is changed with the addition of a physician and medication (see Figure 105–1) leading to distortions and transference changes in all the relationships.

**Legal Issues.** Split treatment means a sharing of authority and control over patient care, meaning a loss of autonomy for each clinician. There is a widespread perception therefore that split treatment is associated with significantly greater risks (Macbeth 2001).

What are the sources of legal exposure? There is potential liability for all psychiatrists who prescribe psychotropic medications, see patients with depression and anxiety, especially those patients with severe disorders, and treat patients with significant suicide potential. Further, informed consent is an important area of concern.

Since patients are shared in split treatment and it is difficult for clinicians to communicate with one another, there is ample opportunity for there to be a rise in missing information, miscommunication, and a decrease in quality of the doctor–patient relationship. Patients are usually seen less frequently by the physician in a split-treatment relationship and the patient is often not clear whom to call in certain emergency situations. Families are usually seen by one of the clinicians, not both. Sometimes there is a supposition that the therapist is being supervised by the physician when the physician believes the relationship to be collaborative rather than supervisory. Macbeth offers the following risk-management strategies:

1. Psychiatrists should familiarize themselves with the operations and routines of all practice settings. The psychiatrist must be knowledgeable about the expertise and authority of those involved in care management.
2. The most problematic practice sites should be weeded out. Issues include looking at staff turnover, peer review procedures, and credentials of key staff members. The psychiatrist should find out about opportunities for consultation and staff interaction, system immunities, and insurance of nonphysician clinicians.
3. There must be careful coordination with therapists who have greater access to patients. The psychiatrist must inform the therapists what information the psychiatrist needs; when she/he needs to be told about changes in the patient's symptoms and condition, and the strengths and weaknesses of the therapists. The psychiatrist must inform the therapist about the medication regimens (potential side effects). This information must be updated regularly.
4. Psychiatrists must understand the system review and appeals procedures to be able to act quickly when there are problems.
5. Either consultation or supervision schedules should be set up and documented regularly to review specific patients.
6. Personal assessment of individual patients must be set up with reference to her/his condition, status, and treatment.
7. Psychiatrists should be extremely careful not to issue an insurance policy to a managed care organization or other system. All proposed contracts must be carefully reviewed and not used to indemnify by accident.

**Ethical Issues in Split Treatment.** There are many areas of potential ethical conflict when mental health professionals get into split-treatment relationships. These include state licensing laws, competency issues, psychiatrists being used

as figureheads, delegation of medical judgment, and financial arrangements (Lazarus 2001).

The American Medical Association (1997) and the American Psychiatric Association (1997) have appreciated the importance of physicians collaborating with other health care and mental health care professionals. Section 5 of the American Medical Association's principles states: "A physician shall continue to study, apply, and advance scientific knowledge, make relevant information available to patients, colleagues, and to the public, obtain consultation, and use the talents of other health professionals when indicated."

The potential ethical pitfalls in split treatment arise from economic, manpower, and clinical pressures. There is very little research, for example, into whether patients with severe borderline personality disorder should be in split treatment. These patients often do not tell the same story to each clinician (Main 1957); they externalize their problems (Silk et al. 1995); threaten self-harm (Leibenluft et al. 1987); have emotional lability and substance abuse problems (Springer et al. 1995). If there is no close communication between the clinicians regarding goals, treatment planning, and role of medication and psychotherapy, the clinical and ethical problems in treating such patients are great.

## How to Provide Optimal Split Treatment?

It is important to recognize how complex and difficult split treatment can be for patients and clinicians. Key to this is recognizing the extra time and effort it will take to make obligations and responsibilities of all parties overt rather than covert. Implied duties must be minimized. Some clinicians advocate the use of treatment contracts to cover the various issues and responsibilities that accrue in split-treatment arrangements (Appelbaum 1991).

Several authors have recommended thinking of split treatment having a beginning, middle, and end (Rand 1999, Tasman and Riba 2000).

The following suggestions are offered as organizing principles for these three stages (with permission from American Psychiatric Press, Riba and Balon 2001):

### Toward Successful Split Treatment

A key aspect of split treatment is how complex and difficult such treatment is for the clinicians, the patient, and the patient's family. Unless one works in a clinic or organized setting where relationships between clinicians are well-delineated (e.g., one psychiatrist works with a specific group of nonmedical therapists), much thought must go into managing safe and effective split treatment.

It may be helpful to think of split therapy having a beginning, middle course, and end (Table 105–4). In order to avoid or minimize the pitfalls associated with split treatment, the following clinical suggestions are provided as organizing principles for its three stages (Rand 1999, Tasman and Riba 2000):

### Beginning of Treatment

• Communication is key to providing excellent care in split treatment. At the beginning, both clinicians should obtain a signed release-of-information form from the patient. Communication must be regular and frequent

| Table 105-4 | Factors for Consideration in Split Treatment |
|---|---|

### Beginning

#### Topics for Discussion Between Clinicians and Patient

Confidentiality
Communication
Diagnostic impressions
Specific clinical issues: suicide, homicide, violence
Treatment plan
Vacation and coverage schedules
Professional backgrounds
Belief systems—medication and psychotherapy
Obvious and hidden obstacles
Patient's family and significant others
Third party payers
Other clinicians caring for patient
Fee schedules, cancellation policies, frequency of visits
What to do when things are not going well

### Middle

Transference
Countertransference
Adherence to treatment
Use of patient's mental health benefits
Termination

### Termination

Review of goals of treatment/best time to terminate
Who will manage the follow-up
Recurrence of symptoms
Feedback between clinicians

---

between the clinicians and the patient should be made aware of these discussions. The forms of regular communication should be decided at the onset—routine telephone calls, faxes, emails, follow-up letters, and the like. The patient should not be a messenger between the clinicians.

- Issues of confidentiality should be discussed and reviewed at the beginning of treatment. Confidentiality should not be used as a cover to hide from taking the time to make telephone calls, to send copies of evaluations and follow-up notes, to send emails or faxes, or to have joint sessions with both clinicians and the patient.

- Diagnostic impressions should be independently arrived at, then discussed and agreed upon. If there is a difference of opinion, an understanding must be reached before treatment proceeds.

- The clinicians must work with each other and with the patient to determine the treatment plan. The treatment plan should specify how often each of the clinicians expects to see the patient and what process to pursue if the patient does not follow up or if there is a missed appointment. If the patient wishes to end either the therapy, the medications, or both, it has to be understood that all parties will discuss this important decision. It is desirable for a written contract to be drawn up between the clinicians and the patient so that all parties understand what the agreement for services will entail.

Included in the contract should be a delineation of the clinicians' roles and responsibilities, as well as those of the patient.

- Clinicians vacation schedules and other on-call and coverage issues must be discussed regularly and documented. The patient needs to know whom to call in an emergency. At the beginning of split treatment, both clinicians and the patient should be aware of their respective beliefs regarding medication and psychotherapy.

- There must be a discussion about what type of care would be optimal for the patient and if there are barriers to such care. The patient should be informed of this review; if possible, he or she should participate in it.

- The clinicians should discuss their professional backgrounds and training with each other at the beginning of the patient's treatment. Issues such as licensure, ethics, violations, malpractice claims, hospital privileges, coverage of professional liability insurance, participation on managed care panels, and commitment to split treatment should all be made clear.

- The clinicians need to agree who will communicate with third parties regarding the patient's care. Further, each clinician should know the patient's mental health benefits and means of payment. There needs to be an agreement by all parties as to the use of such benefits.

- The clinicians need to understand how best to interface with the patient's family or significant others.

- If the patient has health providers other than the psychiatrist and therapist (e.g., primary care physician, cardiologist, physical therapist, etc.), it should be decided which clinician will be the designated communicator or coordinator with those other providers.

- At the beginning of treatment there should be a review of how each clinician will assess and manage the patient's thoughts regarding or attempts at suicide, homicide, violence, and domestic abuse.

- It should be made clear to the patient what symptoms or types of issues should be brought to the attention of which clinician.

- It is helpful for the clinicians to decide how problems will be handled as the need arises.

- The clinicians should discuss differences in fee schedules, cancellation policies, length of visits, and frequency of visits.

## Middle Course

- Special attention must be paid to transference and countertransference in this type of system of care. Disparaging and negative remarks made by the patient concerning either clinician, therapy, or medication must be understood and managed in the context of this complex type of treatment.

- Clinicians should review how many cases of split treatment they have in their practices and whether or not this is a safe mix. Factors to consider include the clinical complexity of the cases, how busy the practice is, the influence of third party payers and the hassle factor, the number of different clinicians one is working with, the psychiatric disorders of one's patients, and so on. It may be prudent to determine the risks involved in having a large patient population in split treatment and to weed the number of such patients down to an acceptable level.

Further, clinicians should minimize the number of collaborators, since it is virtually impossible to keep track of a large number of clinicians' credentials, vacation schedules, communication patterns, and so on.

- Adherence to medications and to psychotherapy should be addressed equally.
- Treatment plans should be regularly reviewed and updated between the clinicians and the patient.
- Use of the patient's mental health benefits should be regularly reviewed and discussed between the clinicians and the patient when appropriate.
- There must be an agreement that either clinician can terminate the split therapy but that the patient must be provided adequate and appropriate warning and referrals to other clinicians. In other words, the patient cannot be abandoned.

### Ending Split Treatment

- After reviewing the treatment plan, both clinicians and the patient will decide together on the goals that have been met or have not been realized and the best time for termination. They should decide how to stagger the discontinuation of therapy and of medication.
- It is important to consider how to manage follow-up and recurrence of symptoms.

The clinicians must have a system for giving each other feedback on the care each is providing to the patient. Ideally, after the treatment is complete, the clinicians should review any aspects of the case that could have been managed or handled differently. Ideally, the patient should be part of this evaluation process as a way of assuring continuous quality improvement. Most importantly, throughout all stages of the split treatment process, clinicians need to respect both the patient and each other's professional understanding.

Although the challenges of split treatment are great, there are many reasons for clinicians and patients to try to surmount the obstacles. Good communication patterns between clinicians and many of the suggestions noted here may be guideposts on the path toward successful split treatment.

### Conclusion and Future Directions

So, why is it that so many of our early career psychiatrists tend to favor pure biological management or split treatment of mental illness over an integrated approach? In the Duffy and colleagues (2001) study, split treatment was positively associated with younger age of the psychiatrist, as well as with board certification, practice setting (hospital clinics), payment source (private insurance versus public assistance), and managed care settings. While utilization management may have pressured psychiatrists to do "15-minute medication checks," the focus on biological treatment research to the exclusion of psychotherapy research by psychiatrists has also been a substantial factor in the separation of the two treatment modalities (Gabbard 2000). One-fourth year psychiatry resident put it this way: "We seem so mesmerized by the efficacy of our drugs that we have almost stopped believing that psychotherapy does anything 'real' at all" (Lembke 2001).

The resident cited a lack of didactic faculty that teach both pharmacotherapy courses and psychotherapy courses,

a reflection of the lack of integrated teaching of both treatment modalities. This paucity of academic role models, and fragmentation of biological and psychological instruction seems to perpetuate a "mind–body split." Kassaw and Gabbard (2002), in his reply to the above resident commented that this approach moves residents away from formulating patient/treatments from a biopsychosocial perspective which he feels is "perhaps best typified by the integration of medication and psychotherapy." Few training programs provide didactic instruction on the topic of integrated treatments (Kay 2000, unpublished data), although that tide may be turning, especially with the Residency Review Committee's emphasis on competency in five forms of psychotherapy by the end of psychiatric residency training. Dr. Gabbard goes on to say that "psychiatrists in the future should be educated so that our unique position as integrators of the biologic and psychosocial is operationalized in everyday practice." It is hoped that this education will be prompted by and lead to further research in this area and result in a resurrection of psychiatry's holistic roots.

### References

Abraham B, van Dyck R, Spinhoven P, et al. (1999) Paroxetine, clomipramine, and cognitive therapy in the treatment of panic disorder. J Clin Psychiatr 60, 831–838.

Agras WS (2001) The consequences and costs of the eating disorders. Psychiatr Clin N Am 24(2) (June), 371–379.

American Medical Association Council on Ethical and Judicial Affairs (1997) Code of Medical Ethics: Current Opinions With Annotations. American Medical Association, Washington DC.

American Psychiatric Association (1980) Guidelines for psychiatrists in consultative, supervisory, or collaborative relationships with nonmedical therapists. Am J Psychiatr 137(11), 1489–1491.

American Psychiatric Association (1996) Practice Guideline for the Treatment of Patients with Nicotine Dependence. APA, Washington DC.

American Psychiatric Association (1997) The Principles of Medical Ethics with Annotations Especially Applicable to Psychiatry. APA, Washington DC.

American Psychiatric Association (2000) Practice Guidelines for the Treatment of Patients with Eating Disorders, Rev. ed. APA, Washington DC.

American Psychiatric Association (2002a) Practice Guidelines for the Treatment of Patients with Bipolar Disorder, Rev. ed. APA, Washington DC.

American Psychiatric Association (2002b) Access to Comprehensive Psychiatric Assessment and Integrated treatment. A Position Statement.

Appelbaum PS (1991) General guidelines for psychiatrists who prescribe medication for patients treated by nonmedical psychotherapists. Hosp Comm Psychiatr 42, 281–282.

Bacaltchuk J (2000) Combinations of antidepressants and psychological treatments for bulimia nervosa: A systematic review. Acta Psychiatr Scand 101(4) (Apr), 256–264.

Bacaltchuk J, Hay F, and Trefglio R (2002) Antidepressants versus psychological treatments and their combination for bulimia nervosa. The Cochrane Database of Systemic Review, The Cochrane Library. Commun Evid Based Ment Health 5(3) (Aug), 74–75.

Baggs JG and Schmitt MH (1988) Collaboration between nurses and physicians. Image J Nurs Sch 20, 145–149.

Balon R (1999) Positive aspects of collaborative treatment. In Psychopharmacology and Psychotherapy: A Collaborative Approach, Riba MB and Balon R (eds). American Psychiatric Press, Washington DC, pp. 1–31.

Balon R and Riba MB (2001) Improving the practice of split treatment. Psychiatr Ann 31(10) (Oct), 594–596.

Barlow DH (1996) Health care policy, psychotherapy research, and the future of psychotherapy. Am Psychol 51, 1050–1058.

Barlow DH, Gorman JM, Shear MK, et al. (2000) Cognitive–behavioral therapy, imipramine, or their combination for panic disorder: A randomized controlled trial. JAMA 283, 2529–2536.

Barrett JE, Barrett JA, Oxman TE, et al. (1988) The prevalence of psychiatric disorders in a primary care practice. Arch Gen Psychiatr 45, 1100–1106.

Beck JS (1995) Cognitive Therapy: Basics and Beyond. Guilford Press, New York, pp. 8–45.

Beck JS (2001) A cognitive therapy approach to medication compliance. In Integrated Treatment for Psychiatric Disorders: Review of Psychiatry, Vol. 20, Kay J (ed). American Psychiatric Press, Washington DC, pp. 113–141.

Beitman BD, Chiles J, and Carlin A (1984) The pharmacotherapy-psychotherapy triangle: Psychiatrist, nonmedical psychotherapist, and patient. J Clin Psychiatr 45, 458–459.

Bradley SS (1990) Nonphysician psychotherapist–physician pharmacotherapist: A new model for concurrent treatment. Psychiatr Clin N Am 13, 307–322.

Brill NQ (1977) Delineating the role of the psychiatrist on the psychiatric team. Hosp Comm Psychiatr 28, 542–544.

Bruce TJ, Spiegel DA, Gregg SF, et al. (1995) Predictors of alprazolam discontinuation with and without cognitive–behavior therapy in panic disorder. Am J Psychiatr 152, 1156–1160.

Busch FN and Gould E (1993) Treatment by a psychotherapist and a psychopharmacologist: Transference and countertransference issues. Hosp Comm Psychiatr 44, 772–774.

Callahan AM and Bauer MS (1999) Psychosocial interventions for bipolar disorder. Psychiatr Clin N Am 22(3), 676–678.

Cochran SD (1984) Preventing medical noncompliance in the outpatient treatment of bipolar affective disorder. J Consult Clin Psychol 52, 873–878.

Coulter A, Noone A, and Goldacre M (1989) General practitioners' referrals to specialist outpatient clinics, I. Why general practitioners refer patients to specialist outpatient clinics. BMJ 299, 304–306.

Craske MG, Brown TA, and Barlow DH (1991) Behavioral treatment of panic: A two-year follow-up. Behav Ther 22, 289–304.

de Jonghe F, Kool S, van Aalst G, et al. (2001) Combining psychotherapy and antidepressants in the treatment of depression. J Affect Disord 64, 217–229.

Depression Guideline Panel (1993) Depression in Primary Care, Vol. 2: Treatment of Major Depression (Clinical Practice Guideline No. 5; AHCPR Publ No 93-0551). US Department of Health and Human Services, Public Health Service, Agency for Health Care Policy and Research, Rockville, MD.

Dewan M (1999) Are psychiatrists cost effective? An analysis of integrated versus split treatment. Am J Psychiatr 156, 324–326.

Direnfeld D, Pato MT, and Gunn S (2000) Behavior therapy as adjuvant treatment in obsessive–compulsive disorder (poster presentation). APA Annual Meeting (May 14–18), Chicago, IL.

Duffy FF, West JC, Zarin DA, et al. (2001) Integrated versus split treatment: Pharmacotherapy and psychotherapy for mood disorders (poster presentation). APA Annual Meeting and Academy for Health Services Research and Health Policy (June).

Engel GL (1977) The need for a new medical model: A challenge for biomedicine. Science 196(4286), 129–136.

Falsetti SA and Davis J (2001) Generalized anxiety disorder: The nonpharmacologic treatment of generalized anxiety disorder. Psychiatr Clin N Am 24(1), 99–117.

Fava GA (1999) Sequential treatment: A new way of integrating pharmacotherapy and psychotherapy. Psychother Psychosom 68, 227–229.

Fava GA, Bartolucci G, Rafanelli C, et al. (2001) Cognitive–behavioral management of patients with bipolar disorder who relapsed while on lithium prophylaxis. J Clin Psychiatr 62 (July), 7.

Fawcett J (2001) An issue that must be addressed. In Improving the Practice of Split Treatment, Balon R and Riba MB (eds). Psychiatr Ann 31(10) (Oct), 582.

Firman GJ (1982) The psychiatrist–nonmedical psychotherapy team: Opportunities for a therapeutic synergy. J Oper Psychiatr 13, 32–36.

Foulks EF and Pena JM (1995) Ethnicity and psychotherapy: A component in the treatment of cocaine addiction in African-Americans. Psychiatr Clin N Am 18, 607–620.

Frank E, Kupfer DJ, Perel JM, et al. (1990) Three-year outcomes for maintenance therapies in recurrent depression. Arch Gen Psychiatr 47, 1093–1099.

Frank E, Shear MK, Rucci P, et al. (2000) Influence of panic-agoraphobic spectrum symptoms on treatment response in patients with recurrent major depression. Am J Psychiatr 157(7), 1101–1107.

Frank E, Swartz HA, Mallinger AG, et al. (1999) Adjunctive psychotherapy for bipolar disorder: Effects of changing treatment modality. J Abnorm Psychol 108(4) (Nov), 579–587.

Fromm-Reichmann F (1947) Problems of therapeutic management in a psychoanalytic hospital. Psychoanal Q 16, 325–356.

Gabbard GO (2000) Combined psychotherapy and pharmacotherapy. In Comprehensive Textbook of Psychiatry, 7th ed., Sadock BJ and Sadock VA (eds). Lipincott Williams & Wilkins, Philadelphia, PA, pp. 2225–2234.

Gabbard GO and Kay J (2001) The fate of integrated treatment: Whatever happened to the biopsychosocial psychiatrist? Am J Psychiatr 158(12), 1956–1963.

Glasscote R (1975) The future of the community mental health center. Psychiatr Ann 5, 69–81.

Goldberg RS, Riba M, and Tasman A (1991) Psychiatrists' attitudes toward prescribing medication for patients treated by nonmedical psychotherapists. Hosp Comm Psychiatr 42(3) (Mar), 276–280.

Goldman W, McCulloch J, Cuffel B, et al. (1998) Outpatient utilization patterns of integrated and split psychotherapy and pharmacotherapy for depression. Psychiatr Serv 49, 477–482.

Goldstein MJ (1991) Psychosocial (nonpharmacologic) treatments for schizophrenia. In APA Press Review of Psychiatry, Vol. 10, Tasman A and Goldfinger SM (eds). American Psychiatric Press, Washington DC.

Greist JH and Jefferson JW (2001) Obsessive–compulsive disorder. In Treatments of Psychiatric Disorders, Vol. 1 and 2, 3rd ed., Gabbard GO (ed-in-chief). American Psychiatric Press, Washington DC.

Group for the Advancement of Psychiatry (GAP) (1975) Pharmacotherapy and psychotherapy: Paradoxes, problems, and progress, Vol. 9, Report No 93. Mental Health Materials, New York.

Hansen-Grant S and Riba MB (1995) Contact between psychotherapists and psychiatric residents who provide medication back-up. Psychiatr Serv 46, 774–777.

Hettema JM, Neale MC, and Kendler KS (2001) A review and meta-analysis of the genetic epidemiology of anxiety disorders. Am J Psychiatr 158(10), 1568–1578.

Hirshfeld RM, Dunner DL, Keitner G, et al. (2002) Does psychosocial functioning improve independent of depressive symptoms? A comparison of nefazodone, psychotherapy, and their combination. Biol Psychiatr 51, 123–133.

Hogarty G, Anderson CM, Reiss DJ, et al. (1986) Family education, social skills training, and maintenance chemotherapy in the aftercare of schizophrenia. Arch Gen Psychiatr 43, 633–642.

Hogarty GE, Greenwald D, Ulrich RF, et al. (1997a) Three-year trials of personal therapy among schizophrenic patients living with or independent of family, II. Effects on adjustment of patients. Am J Psychiatr 154, 1514–1524.

Hogarty GE, Kornblith SJ, Greenwald D, et al. (1997b) Three-year trials of personal therapy among patients living with or independent of family, I. Description of study and effects on relapse rates. Am J Psychiatr 154, 1504–1513.

Hollon SD and Fawcett J (1995) Combined medication and psychotherapy. In Treatments of Psychiatric Disorders, Vol. 1, 2nd ed., Gabbard GO (ed). American Psychiatric Press, Washington DC, pp. 1222–1236.

Hollon SD and Fawcett J (2001) Combined medication and psychotherapy. In Treatments of Psychiatric Disorders, Vol. 1 and 2, 3rd ed., Gabbard GO (ed-in-chief). American Psychiatric Press, Washington DC.

Horgan CM (1985) Specialty and general ambulatory mental health services: Comparison of utilization and expenditures. Arch Gen Psychiatr 42, 565–572.

Kassaw K and Gabbard GO (2002) Creating a psychodynamic formulation from a clinical evaluation. Am J Psychiatr 159(5) (May), 721–726.

Kay J (2001) Integrated treatment: An overview. In Integrated Treatment for Psychiatric Disorders: Review of Psychiatry, Vol. 20, Kay J (ed). American Psychiatric Press, Washington DC, pp. 1–29.

Kay J (2002) Psychopharmacology: Combined treatment. In Encyclopedia of Psychotherapy, Hersen M and Sledge W (eds). Academic Press, New York.

Keller MB, McCullough JP, Klein DN, et al. (2000) A comparison of nefazodone, the cognitive behavioral-analysis system of psychotherapy, and their combination for the treatment of chronic depression. New Engl J Med 342, 1462–1470.

Kelly KV (1991) Parallel treatment: Therapy with one clinician and medication with another. Hosp Comm Psychiatr 43, 778–780.

Kerber K (1999) Collaborative treatment in managed care. In Psychopharmacology and psychotherapy: A collaborative approach, Riba MB and Balon R (eds). American Psychiatric Press, Washington DC, pp. 307–324.

Kessler LG, Cleary PD, and Burke JD Jr (1985) Psychiatric disorders in primary care: Results of a follow-up study. Arch Gen Psychiatr 42, 583–587.

Klerman GL (1985) Trends in utilization of mental health services. Med Care 23, 584.

Klerman GL (1991) Ideologic conflicts. In Integrating Pharmacotherapy and Psychotherapy, Beitman BB and Klerman G (eds). American Psychiatric Press, Washington DC, pp. 3–20.

Klinkman MS and Valenstein MV (1997) A "Roadmap" for differential diagnosis and treatment of mental health problems in the primary care setting. In Primary Care Psychiatry, Knesper DJ, Riba MB, and TL Schwenk (eds). WB Saunders, Philadelphia, PA, pp. 3–8.

Kupfer DJ and Frank E (2001) The interaction of drug and psychotherapy in the long-term treatment of depression. J Affect Disord 62, 131–137.

Lambert MJ (1992) Psychotherapy outcome research: Implications for integrative and eclectic therapies. In Handbook of Psychotherapy Integration, Norcross JC and Goldfried MR (eds). Basic Books, New York, pp. 94–129.

Lazarus J (1999) Ethical issues in collaborative or divided treatment. In Psychopharmacology and Psychotherapy: A Collaborative Approach, Riba MB and Balon R (eds). American Psychiatric Press, Washington DC, pp. 159–177.

Lazarus J (2001) Ethics in split treatment. In Improving the Practice of Split Treatment, Balon R and Riba MB (eds). Psychiatr Ann 31(10) (Oct), pp. 611–614.

Leibenluft E, Gardner DI, and Cowdrey RW (1987) The inner experience of the borderline self-mutilator. J Pers Disord 1, 317–324.

Lembke A (2001) Letter to the editor. Am J Psychiatr 158(11).

Lenze EJ, Dew MA, Mazumdar S, et al. (2002) Combined pharmacotherapy and psychotherapy as maintenance treatment for late-life depression: Effects on social adjustment. Am J Psychiatr 159(3), 466–468.

Macbeth JE (2001) Legal aspects of split treatment: How to audit and manage risk. In Improving the Practice of Split Treatment, Balon R and Riba MB (eds). Psychiatr Ann 31(10) (Oct), pp. 605–610.

Main TF (1957) The ailment. Br J Med Psychol 30, 129–145.

Marcus ER (ed) (1990a) Combined treatment, psychotherapy, and medication. Psychiatr Clin N Am 13, 197–376.

Marcus ER (1990b) Integrating psychopharmacotherapy, psychotherapy, and mental structure in the treatment of patients with personality disorders and depression. Psychiatr Clin N Am 13, 255–263.

Mavissakalian MR (1993) Combined behavioral and pharmacologic treatment of anxiety disorders. In American Psychiatric Press Review of Psychiatry (12), Oldman JM, Riba MB, and Tasman A (eds). American Psychiatric Press, Washington DC, pp. 565–584.

McHugh PR and Slavney R (1983) The Perspectives of Psychiatry. Johns Hopkins University Press, Baltimore, MD.

McNutt ER, Severino SK, and Schomer J (1987) Dilemmas in interdisciplinary outpatient care: An approach towards their amelioration. J Psychiatr Educ 11, 59–65.

Miklowitz DL, Simoneau TL, George EL, et al. (2000) Family-focused treatment of bipolar disorder: 1-year effects of a psychoeducational program in conjunction with pharmacotherapy. Biol Psychiatr 48(6) (Sept), 582–592.

Miller IW, Norman WH, and Keitner GI (1999) Combined treatment for patients with double depression. Psychother Psychosom 68(4), 180–185.

Mitchell JE, Peterson CB, Meters T, et al. (2001) Combining pharmacotherapy and psychotherapy in the treatment of patients with eating disorders. Psychiatr Clin N Am 24(2) (June), 315–323.

Nathan PE, Stuart SP, and Dolan SL (2000) Research on psychotherapy efficacy and effectiveness : Between scylla and charbodis? Psychol Bull 126(6) (Nov), 964–981.

Neal DL and Calarco MM (1999) Mental health providers: Role definitions and collaborative practice issues. In Psychopharmacology and Psychotherapy: A Collaborative Approach, Riba MB and Balon R (eds). American Psychiatric Press, Washington DC, pp. 85–109.

Paykel ES (1995) Psychotherapy, medication combinations, and compliance. J Clin Psychiatr 56(Suppl 1), 24–30.

Pilette WL (1988) The rise of three-party treatment relationships. Psychotherapy 25, 420–423.

Pincus HA, Zarin DA, Tanielian TL, et al. (1999) Psychiatric patients and treatments in 1997: Findings from the American Psychiatric Association Practice Research Network. Arch Gen Psychiatr 56, 441–449.

Position statement on psychiatrists (1973) Relationships with nonmedical mental health professionals. Am J Psychiatr 130, 386–390.

Radomsky AS and Otto MW (2001) Cognitive–behavioral therapy for social anxiety disorder. Psychiatr Clin N Am 24(4), 805–815.

Rand EH (1999) Guidelines to maximize the process of collaborative treatment. In Psychopharmacology and Psychotherapy: A Collaborative Approach, Riba MB and Balon R (eds). American Psychiatric Press, Washington DC, pp. 353–380.

Ravindran AV, Anisman H, Merali Z, et al. (1999) Treatment of primary dysthymia with group cognitive therapy and pharmacotherapy: Clinical symptoms and functional impairments. Am J Psychiatr 156, 1608–1617.

Regier DA, Goldberg ID, and Taube CA (1978) The de facto US mental health services system: A public health perspective. Arch Gen Psychiatr 35, 685–693.

Reinstein MJ (1978) Community mental health centers and the dissatisfied psychiatrist: Results of an informal survey. Hosp Comm Psychiatr 29, 261–262.

Retzer A, Simon FG, Weber G, et al. (1991) A follow-up study of manic–depressive and schizoaffective psychoses after systemic family therapy. Fam Process 30, 139–153.

Reynolds CF III, Frank E, Perel JM, et al. (1999) Nortriptyline and interpersonal psychotherapy as maintenance therapies for recurrent major depression: A randomized and controlled trial in patients older than 59 years. JAMA 281, 39–45.

Riba MB and Balon R (2001) The challenges of split treatment. In Integrated Treatment of Psychiatric Disorders: Review of Psychiatry, Vol. 20, Kay J (ed). APPI, Washington DC, pp. 143–164.

Riba MB, Goldberg RS, and Tasman A (1993) Medication backup in psychiatry residency programs. Acad Psychiatr 17, 32–35.

Rolland JS (1994) Families, Illness, and Disability. Basic Books, New York.

Roose SP (2001) Psychodynamic therapy and medication: Can treatments in conflict be integrated? In Integrated Treatment of Psychiatric Disorders: Review of Psychiatry, Vol. 20, Kay J (ed). APPI, Washington DC, pp. 31–49.

Rothbaum BO and Astin MC (2000) Integration of pharmacotherapy and psychotherapy for bipolar disorder. J Clin Psychiatr 61(Suppl 9), 68–75.

Rounsaville BJ, Klerman GL, and Weissman MM (1981) Do psychotherapy and pharmacotherapy of depression conflict? Arch Gen Psychiatr 38, 24–29.

Ruiz P, Venegas-Samuels K, and Alarcon R (1995) The economics of pain: Mental health care costs among minorities. Psychiatr Clin N Am 18, 659–670.

Sensky T, Turkinton D, Kingdon D, et al. (2000) A randomized controlled trial of cognitive–behavioral therapy for persistent symptoms in schizophrenia resistant to medications. Arch Gen Psychiatr 57(2) (Feb), 165–172.

Shurman RA, Kramer PD, and Mitchell JB (1985) The hidden mental health network: Treatment of mental illness by nonpsychiatrist physicians. Arch Gen Psychiatr 42, 89–94.

Silk KR, Lee S, Hill EM, et al. (1995) Borderline symptoms and severity of sexual abuse. Am J Psychiatr 152, 1059–1064.

Spiegel DA, Bruce TJ, Gregg SF, et al. (1994) Does cognitive–behavior therapy assist slow-taper alprazolam discontinuation in panic disorder? Am J Psychiatr 151, 876–881.

Spitz D, Hansen-Grant S, and Riba MB (1999) Residency training issues in collaborative treatment. In Psychopharmacology and Psychotherapy: A Collaborative Approach, Riba MB and Balon R (eds). American Psychiatric Press, Washington DC, pp. 279–306.

Spitzer RL, Williams JB, Kroenke K, et al. (1994) Utility of a new procedure for diagnosing mental disorders in primary care: The PRIME-MD 1000 study. JAMA 272, 1749–1756.

Springer T, Huth AC, Lohr NE, et al. (1995) The quality of depression in personality disorders: An empirical study. Paper presented at the annual meeting of the American Psychological Association (Aug), New York.

Svartberg M, Seltzer MH, and Stiles TC (1998) The effects of common and specific factors in short-term anxiety-provoking psychotherapy. J Nerv Ment Dis 186, 691–696.

Tasman A and Riba MB (2000) Psychological management in psychopharmacologic treatment. In Psychiatric Drugs, Lieberman J and Tasman A (eds). WB Saunders, Philadelphia, PA, pp. 242–249.

Tekell JL, Erickson SS, and Matthews KL (1997) Collaboration with the nonphysician therapist: A seminar for postgraduate psychiatry residents. Acad Psychiatr 21, 155–164.

Thase ME, Friedman ES, Fasiczka AL, et al. (2000) Treatment of men with major depression: A comparison of sequential cohorts treated with either cognitive–behavioral therapy or newer generation antidepressants. J Clin Psychiatr 66, 466–472.

Thase ME, Greenhouse JB, Frank E, et al. (1997) Treatment of major depression with psychotherapy or psychotherapy–pharmacotherapy combinations. Arch Gen Psychiatr 54, 1009–1015.

Valenstein MV (1999) Primary care physicians and mental health professionals: Models for collaboration. In Psychopharmacology and Psychotherapy: A Collaborative Approach, Riba MB and Balon R (eds). American Psychiatric Press, Washington DC, pp. 325–352.

Van Ameringen M and Mancini C (2001) Pharmacotherapy of social anxiety disorder at the turn of the millennium. Psychiatr Clin N Am 24(4) (Dec), 783–803.

Vasile RG and Gutheil TG (1979) The psychiatrist as medical backup: Ambiguity in the delegation of clinical responsibility. Am J Psychiatr 136, 1292–1296.

Verhaak PF and Wennink HJ (1990) What does a doctor do with psychosocial problems in primary care? Int J Psychiatr Med 20, 151–162.

Walsh BT, Agras WS, Devlin MJ, et al. (2000) Fluoxetine for bulimia nervosa following poor response to psychotherapy. Am J Psychiatr 157(8) (Aug), 1332–1334.

Walsh BT, Wilson GT, and Loeg KL (1997) Medication and psychotherapy in the treatment of bulimia nervosa. Am J Psychiatr 154, 523–531.

Weiner H and Riba MB (1997) Attitudes and practices in mediation backup. Psychiatr Serv 48(4), 536–538.

Weiss E (1965) Agoraphobia in the Light of Ego Psychology. Grune & Stratton, New York.

Weissman MM, Prusoff BA, DiMascio A, et al. (1979) The efficacy of drugs and psychotherapy in the treatment of acute depressive episodes. Am J Psychiatr 136, 555–558.

Whittal ML, Otto MW, and Hong JJ (2001) Cognitive–behavior therapy for discontinuation of SSRI treatment of panic disorder: A case series. Behav Res Ther 39(8), 939–945.

Wiborg IM and Dahl AA (1996) Docs brief dynamic psychotherapy reduce the relapse rate of panic disorder? Arch Gen Psychiatr 53, 689–694.

Wilkinson G (1989) Referrals from general practitioners to psychiatrists and paramedical mental health professionals. Br J Psychiatr 154, 72–76.

Wilson GT, Loeb KL, Walsh BT, et al. (1999) Psychological versus pharmacological treatments of bulimia nervosa: Predictors and process of change. J Consult Clin Psychol 67(4), 451–459.

Winer J and Andriukatis S (1989) Interpersonal aspects of initiating pharmacotherapy: How to avoid becoming the patient's feared negative other. Psychiatr Ann 19, 318–323.

Woodward B, Duckworth KS, and Gutheil T (1993) The pharmacotherapist–psychotherapist collaboration. In Review of Psychiatry, Vol. 12, Oldham JM, Riba MB, and Tasman A (eds). American Psychiatric Press, Washington DC, pp. 631–649.

Yamamoto J, Silva JA, Justice LR, et al. (1993) Cross-cultural psychotherapy. In Culture, Ethnicity, and Mental Illness, Gaw AC (ed). American Psychiatric Press, Washington DC, pp. 101–124.

Zeidonis D, Krejci J, Atdjian S (2001) Integrated treatment of alcohol, tobacco, and other drug additions. In Integrated Treatment of Psychiatric Disorders: Review of Psychiatry Series, Vol. 20(2), Kay J (ed), Oldham JM and Riba MB (series eds). American Psychiatric Publishing, Washington DC.

Zhang M, Wang M, Li J, et al. (1994) Randomized controlled trial of family interventions for 78 first-episode male schizophrenic patients: An 18-month study in Suzbou, Jiangsu. Br J Psychiatr 165, 96–102.

# 106 Medication Compliance

Mehul V. Mankad
Marvin S. Swartz

## Introduction

Compliance, or the degree to which patients' behaviors coincide with the recommendations of health care providers, is an important component in the understanding of patient outcomes, particularly in light of a growing regimen of efficacious and expensive medical treatments. There is an evident gap between the efficacy of regimens tested in tightly controlled clinical trials and their effectiveness when applied to "real world" patient experiences. One explanation for this "efficacy–effectiveness gap," when treatment regimens move from efficacy trials into everyday practice, is the apparent decline in patient compliance. Other terms closely related to compliance include "adherence," "fidelity," and "maintenance." Although the systematic study of compliance has gained scholarly attention only in the past 2 decades, the dilemma of noncompliance can be traced to antiquity. Hippocrates noted that the physician "should keep aware that patients often lie when they state that they have taken certain medicines" (Haynes 1979). Since the time of Hippocrates the understanding of compliance behavior has changed considerably and most authorities view compliance multidimensionally with a considerably diminished focus on Hippocrates' dim view of patients as willfully deceitful. Recent approaches to evaluation and management of noncompliance reviewed below focus on the patients' understanding of their illness, the treatment in question, and environmental factors that reinforce or weaken compliance.

This chapter will review current concepts in understanding and improving medication compliance. Many of the methods to evaluate and modify problems with medication compliance discussed in this chapter can be applied more broadly to treatment compliance such as missing clinic appointments and failure to adhere to agreed upon psychosocial interventions. However, because the vast majority of research on patient compliance specifically focuses on medication compliance the following discussion will focus on adherence to medication regimens.

Compliance is difficult to quantify for several reasons. Completely attributing the difference between an expected and observed treatment effect to problems with medication compliance may be overly simplistic. Several other factors such as differences in population, degree of comorbidity with other psychiatric or medical diagnoses, and severity of illness may all adversely affect the potential benefit to the patient. Poor or partial compliance with treatment may have a variable effect on treatment outcomes depending on the pharmacokinetic profile of the medication in question. For example, occasional missed doses of very long half-life medications will alter serum drug levels to a lesser extent than in short half-life compounds. Therefore, the issue of partial compliance with treatment regimens may become more critical depending on the specific regimen.

## A Theoretical Construct for Compliance: The Health Beliefs Model

The health beliefs of individuals play a major role in their decision-making processes regarding participation in recommended treatment. A framework that may be useful in understanding the complex nature of compliance with medical regimens is the health beliefs model (HBM). Derived from social psychological theories of Kurt Lewin, the HBM is grounded in the phenomenological orientation of perception driving action (Rosenstock 1974). While this model was originally designed to study the utilization of screening tests for detection of asymptomatic diseases, it has been adapted to the areas of medication compliance among psychiatric patients (Kelly et al. 1987).

Five components of the HBM apply directly to issues of patient compliance. Figure 106–1 depicts the relationship between these components and ultimate compliance with treatment. (1) Susceptibility: patients must see themselves as vulnerable to a serious illness. (2) Severity: patients must realize that he/she has an illness with health consequences that will continue without medical attention. (3) Perceived benefits: patients must recognize that an effective treatment exists for their condition. Benefits from psychotropic medication treatment may include the understanding that treatment ameliorates mental problems or helps avoid rehospitalization. (4) Barriers: common barriers to pharmacologic interventions involve access to medication, adequate psychiatric follow-up, and adverse effects from the medication. (5) Cues to action: lastly, patients must experience an internal or external motivation or "cue" to engage in the specified action that may benefit them. Cues that may trigger a patient to participate in their medication regimen

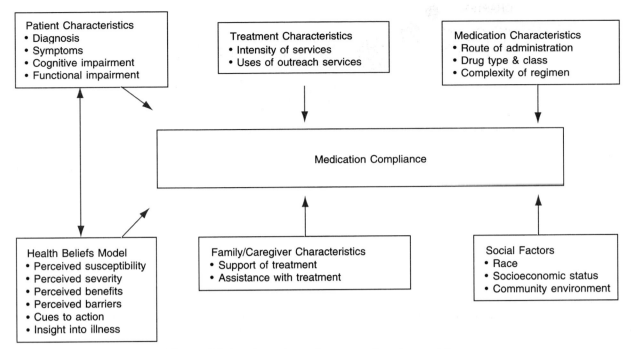

**Figure 106–1** *Understanding medication compliance in mental illness.*

typically relate to a return of symptoms attributed to their mental illness such as anxious, depressive, or psychotic states.

Attempts to operationalize HBM components in understanding compliance in psychiatric patients has yielded useful findings. Kelly and colleagues (1987) found in severely mentally ill veterans that several HBM components correlated with compliance. Perceived susceptibility to illness and cues to action were positively correlated with compliance while barriers to care were negatively correlated with compliance. Approximately 20% of the variance in compliance was related to health beliefs. The authors concluded that health beliefs are quite relevant to psychiatric patients and should be considered when administering pharmacologic treatment in the outpatient setting. The Medical Outcomes Study, a large study that examined medication compliance in 1,198 people with chronic diseases, including depression, found that past levels of compliance are the strongest predictors of future levels of compliance (Sherbourne et al. 1992, Tarlov et al. 1989).

In an attempt to use the HBM as a conceptual framework for the study of compliance among general outpatients with schizophrenia, the Mississippi Recidivism Project examined HBM components in 202 subjects (Nageotte et al. 1997, Sullivan et al. 1995). The most significant HBM component that predicted medication compliance was perceived vulnerability to illness. Patients who perceived that they had a mental illness that could relapse were more than twice as likely to be compliant as those who did not share such a belief (Odds Ratio 2.1, 95% Confidence Interval 1.0–4.5). Conversely, a strong predictor of noncompliance was discontinuity of outpatient mental health services although these latter findings did not reach statistical significance. Patients who did not access mental health services in the 3 months previous to the study were only one-third as likely to be compliant (Odds Ratio 0.3, 95% Confidence Interval 0.1–1.1).

## Another Conceptual Model of Compliance

Another approach to understanding compliance behavior involves the categorization of problems with compliance along the three domains of psychological problems, planning problems, and medical problems. These three domains have been used to develop a compliance checklist as seen in Table 106–1 (Corrigan et al. 1990, Cramer 1991). *Psychological problems* include issues such as nonacceptance of diagnosis or treatment, negative emotional reactions or negative thoughts, and social criticism from family or friends. *Problems with planning* consist of forgetting to take medications, disruption of usual schedules, and issues with availability of medication. *Medical problems that affect compliance* include adverse reactions, exacerbation of illness that leads to incapacity to administer or tolerate medications, or perceptions that medications may lack efficacy in a given individual. Both HBM and the compliance checklist provide useful starting points to begin the analysis of problems with compliance in specific patients or patient populations.

## Compliance in Specific Population

### Schizophrenia

Medication compliance has been studied in greatest detail in populations with schizophrenia. The clear relationship between noncompliance with antipsychotic medication and relapse of psychotic symptoms may be responsible for the large body of information in this area (Diaz et al. 2001). Relapse rates are estimated at 3.5% per month for patients compliant with treatment compared with 11% per month for those patients who have discontinued use of medication.

| Table 106-1 | Compliance Checklist |
| --- | --- |

**Psychological Problems**

- Nonacceptance: Patient does not accept the diagnosis or recommendations for treatment.
- Emotions: Strong emotional reactions (anger, anxiety) prevent the patient from following the treatment plan.
- Other priorities: Patient has placed a higher value on priorities (job, family) other than medication treatment.
- Social criticism: Patient does not take medication due to criticism from others (family, friends, coworkers).

**Planning Problems**

- Routine forgetfulness: Patient does not follow a standard schedule and often misses doses.
- Disruption of schedule: Extraordinary events prevent patient from following medication regimen.
- No medication: Patient ran out of medication before it could be refilled or medication was no longer available for other reasons, including economic factors.
- Lack of information: Patient received inadequate or incorrect information about medication regimen.

**Medical Problems**

- Adverse reaction: Patient stopped taking medication due to an adverse reaction.
- Illness: Medical or psychiatric illness interrupted patient's medication regimen.
- Testing efficacy: Patient decided to omit doses in order to determine need for medication.

Noncompliance with antipsychotic medication has been estimated to be responsible for 40% of the greater than two-billion-dollar cost of rehospitalization annually (Weiden and Olfson 1995).

In past decades, psychodynamically-oriented psychiatrists viewed the psychological development of insight as an important predictor of improved outcomes in patients with the illness. More recently, investigators have regarded loss of insight as critically affected by neurocognitive deficits associated with schizophrenia. Insight in this context refers to patients' recognition of their illnesses as a chronic condition requiring ongoing treatment to avoid relapse. Among patients with schizophrenia, McEvoy and colleagues (1989) found a strong association between insight, compliance, and decreased readmission rates over time.

In a pilot study of electronic monitoring of patients taking oral medication for schizophrenia, Diaz and colleagues (2001) found that 86% of patients (six out of seven) whose compliance rate during the first month of the study was below 50% were readmitted during a 12-month follow-up period. Only 14% of patients (one out of seven) with compliance better than 50% were readmitted during the same period. Diaz did note that special considerations must be taken into account when monitoring compliance in patients with schizophrenia because all 14 patients in the study expressed paranoid ideas regarding the monitoring process.

Another approach to enhancing compliance could be derived from illness self-management techniques. Similar to patients with hypertension who monitor their blood pressure or patients with diabetes who keep track of serum glucose, patients with schizophrenia can be taught to recognize early symptoms of worsening of their illness that may lead to medication noncompliance if ignored. If these symptoms are brought to the attention of health care providers by patients in a collaborative fashion, the potential for relapse may be diminished by early intervention in the form of medication titration (Liberman 1992).

Comorbidities with other psychiatric conditions can significantly compromise compliance with antipsychotic medications among patients with schizophrenia. Substance abuse is strongly and consistently associated with poor compliance rates. Schizophrenic patients with current substance abuse may be more than eight times more likely to have problems with medication compliance than those without dual diagnoses (Owen et al. 1996).

## Bipolar Disorders

Gaining and maintaining compliance in patients with bipolar disorders may pose particular challenges. Several authors have noticed a worrisome efficacy–effectiveness gap in treatment of these disorders (Dickson and Kendall 1986, Guscott and Taylor 1994, Scott 1995). Noncompliance rates for mood stabilizers have ranged from 18 to 52% (Schou 1997, Jamison et al. 1979, Jamison and Akiskal 1983). A recent study found 32% of patients reported missing 30% or more of prescribed mood stabilizers in the previous month (Scott and Pope 2002). Bipolar patients may find it hard to accept tight control of manic mood states. This is a particular problem in patients who feel that periods of hypomania enhance productivity or creativity. In patients with chronic or prolonged hypomania, the mood disturbance may be unrecognized as well. As a result, partial control of mood disturbance leaves these patients with a narrow margin of error and high risk of florid mania. The enhanced sense of self-esteem some patients experience in hypomanic and manic states may also interfere with insight or recognition of the need for treatment.

## Other Mood and Anxiety Disorders

Although the relationship between discontinuation of antidepressant medication and relapse of symptoms is not as clear as with schizophrenia and antipsychotic medications, the immediate consequences of discontinuation of certain antidepressant medications may have a negative impact on the patient. The "selective serotonin reuptake inhibitor (SSRI) discontinuation syndrome" has been reported to produce numerous somatic and psychological symptoms that can impair daily functioning. In the case of SSRIs, the variation in half-life between different agents may affect the onset of discontinuation symptoms experienced when treatment is interrupted. Medications with longer half-lives may produce fewer or less intense discontinuation symptoms (Rosenbaum et al. 1998). Meijer and colleagues (2001) found that 29% of outpatients receiving SSRI treatment demonstrated at least a 2-day lapse in their medication regimen while being monitored electronically. While longer half-life medications may decrease the onset of discontinuation symptoms during brief lapses in treatment, it is unclear how this might affect compliance. For example, medications associated with the discontinuation syndrome could provide more symptomatic cues to alert the patient to adhere to treatment. Alternatively, discontinuation symptoms could lead patients to attribute their symptoms to the medications themselves, serving as a subjective barrier to future adherence.

## Substance Abuse Disorders

Currently, the range of pharmacotherapies available for substance abuse disorders remains limited, however, medication compliance is still of key relevance to this population, especially since substance abuse is strongly associated with denial of illness. Among patients receiving naltrexone for the treatment of alcohol dependence, high compliance rates correlate with better outcomes including abstinence and mean alcohol consumption on drinking days. Objective monitoring systems such as electronic medication bottle monitors offer more reliable information than pill counts in this population as is the case with mentally ill populations (Namkoong et al. 1999).

## Assessing Compliance

The relationship between medication compliance and health outcomes can be examined using three measurement approaches: pharmacoepidemiologic approaches, traditional measures of compliance, and electronic compliance monitoring. The combination of these approaches clarifies the current state of knowledge regarding compliance behavior.

## Pharmacoepidemiology

Pharmacoepidemiologic methods are often used to estimate compliance in community populations. Studying the refill rate for prescriptions is the most common method used in this population-based approach. Unfortunately, the relationship between the rate of refills and the correct or actual usage of the prescription can be difficult to characterize. While the assumption that patients are noncompliant when they do not refill their medication is valid, the belief that those patients are compliant when they do refill their prescriptions may be erroneous (Cramer 1995).

## Compliance Measures

Traditional measures of compliance that have been used in clinical research studies include pill counting and serum or urine drug levels. Observations by investigators that patients may empty their pill bottles prior to coming for clinic visits may invalidate or undermine pill counts as adequate measures of compliance. Furthermore, pill counts cannot differentiate patients who vary their dosage by taking more medication than prescribed on some days and less medication taken on other days (Norrell 1979). Even the use of urine or serum drug levels may have limitations when considered as a method for measuring compliance. Since most drug levels are affected by the doses of medication taken within a few days prior to testing, patients may alter their dosage patterns consciously or unconsciously before clinic visits. In fact, the term *white coat compliance* was coined in reference to this pattern of behavior (Urquhart 1994, Feinstein 1990). This effect was likened to "the toothbrush effect" in which people are more likely to brush their teeth immediately prior to going to the dentist. Using electronic monitoring methods, Cramer and colleagues. (1990) found that compliance rates between visits are approximately 20% lower than rates observed immediately before or after clinical encounters.

## Electronic Monitoring

Another approach to quantifying medication compliance involves the use of electronic compliance monitoring. Studies using such direct monitoring techniques have provided a wealth of useful information while avoiding the pitfalls of other proxy measures for compliance. Electronic monitoring systems utilize microelectronic pill caps that record the time and date when the bottle was opened. A computer at the clinical trial site can extract these data. Such electronic systems are generally considered more reliable than self-report by patients or serum drug levels as measures of compliance, although occasional patients may still open bottles without correctly following the prescribed regimen.

Cramer and colleagues (1989) applied the technique of electronic medication monitoring in 24 outpatients with seizure disorders taking their medications in doses varying from once per day to four times per day. Compliance rates as estimated by bottle openings recorded with the electronic pill monitor were reported as 87, 81, 77, and 39% for once, twice, three times, and four times daily dosing, respectively. A systematic review of clinical trials using electronic monitoring devices found an overall compliance rate of 71% that declined as the number of daily doses increased (Claxton et al. 2001). Diaz and colleagues (2001) applied the same electronic monitoring system to estimate compliance in 14 patients being discharged from a psychiatric inpatient unit with diagnoses of schizophrenia and schizoaffective disorder. The mean compliance rate was 63% for the 10 patients remaining in the study at 1 month.

## Interventions to Enhance Compliance

General strategies to enhance compliance take many forms and can be tailored to the specific needs identified in individual patients. Most approaches to enhance compliance involve the introduction of techniques to improve outpatients' self-administration of oral medication therapies. Cramer (1991) identifies several strategies to approach problems with compliance (Table 106–2).

| Table 106–2 | Strategies for Improving Compliance |
| --- | --- |

**Collect Information**
- Understand patient's particular problem with compliance
- Address issues related to compliance in every clinical encounter with the patient

**Provide Information**
- Education about the illness
- Education about the treatment
- Understanding about problems with compliance

**Increase Motivation**
- Use motivational interviewing techniques to overcome resistance
- Help the patient overcome psychosocial problems that interfere with compliance

**Modify Medication Regimen**
- Schedule doses around standard cues (brushing teeth, meals)
- Discuss coping skills regarding potential situations that may interfere with compliance
- Change the dosage schedule or route of administration

**Change Contingencies**
- Discuss negative consequences of medication compliance (shame, criticism)
- Address adverse reactions
- Specify a formal medication compliance contract
- Associate medication compliance with specific positive reinforcement

The action of monitoring compliance itself may improve adherence to proposed medical regimens, just as frequent weight monitoring may promote weight loss even without a specific diet regimen. Some data indicate that compliance rates improve significantly when outpatients with psychiatric disorders are given continuous feedback on their medication dosing (Cramer and Rosenheck 1999).

Compliance-enhancement interventions that have been studied include individual, group, and family formats and involve diverse theoretical orientations. Unfortunately, many of the studies that investigate compliance therapies do not also assess the distal impact on treatment outcomes leaving the clinician unable to evaluate whether marginal improvements in compliance would in fact lead to cost-effective improvement in treatment outcomes.

One intervention referred to as *compliance therapy* utilizes a specific approach to individual or group psychotherapy with cognitive therapy and motivational interviewing techniques (Goldstein 1992, Hayward et al. 1995). Therapists attempt to help the patients form a cognitive link between discontinuation of medication treatment and relapse of symptoms. Using the patient's frame of reference, therapists seek to instill a sense of cognitive dissonance between discontinuation of medication and achievement of the patient's own goals. Problem-solving techniques are also employed to identify internal and external cues that may compromise future medication compliance. Kemp and colleagues (1996, 1998) found that a four to six session course of individual psychotherapy focused on medication compliance during an inpatient hospitalization for patients with schizophrenia was effective in increasing both compliance rates and improving health outcomes. Hospitalized patients who received compliance therapy instead of supportive counseling manifested fewer psychotic symptoms, demonstrated better social functioning, and were less likely to be rehospitalized over the 18-month follow-up study period. A study of the cost-effectiveness of compliance therapy did not find a significant benefit for the intervention compared to supportive care, however, the study suffered from a small sample size and high attrition (Healey et al. 1998).

Other psychosocial interventions to increase compliance in patients with schizophrenia have also been demonstrated to be effective. Kelly and Scott (1990) found that strategies aimed at education of patients' families about compliance and those directed at patients themselves both improved compliance. No significant difference between the two interventions could be demonstrated. It is important to note that, given the multiple factors associated with clinical course, not all improvement in treatment outcomes in schizophrenia is directly attributable to improved medication compliance. Psychosocial interventions that lack a specific focus on treatment compliance may nonetheless have salutatory effects on patient outcomes, regardless of changes in compliance behavior. Zhang and colleagues (1994) found that family therapy without a specific focus on compliance produced improvement in relapse rates in schizophrenic patients independent of changes in medication compliance.

Another approach to increasing compliance involves the change in route of administration of medication from oral preparations that must be taken at least once daily to depot injections, such as haloperidol decanoate and fluphenazine decanoate, that are typically administered every 2 to 4 weeks. The advantages to depot preparations include supervised administration of the medication by health care providers, decreased variability in serum concentrations of the active medication, and no significant difference in adverse effects as compared to similar oral agents. Disadvantages include the limited number of medications available in depot form, the difficulty of scheduling potentially more frequent clinic visits for injections, and the increased cost in clinic staffs' time with administration of the treatments. At the time of this publication, no atypical antipsychotic agents were available in depot form. Therefore, a comparison of compliance with conventional depot agents and atypical oral agents may be limited in utility. Few studies of depot antipsychotic preparations address the issues of long-term compliance and differences in health outcomes when compared to oral agents (Adams and Eisenbruch 2002, Quraishi and David 2002). However, some evidence suggests that depot antipsychotic agents do confer a marginal improvement in reducing relapse rates (Glazer and Kane 1992).

## Conclusion

Understanding patient compliance with prescribed medications involves an appreciation of multiple factors pertaining to the specific patient and his/her environment. Likewise, designing interventions to enhance compliance with medications requires an individualized approach in the context of proven therapeutic modalities. In the end, improving patient compliance improves patient outcomes without major modification of existing treatment strategies.

### Clinical Vignette

Mr. Jones is a 22-year-old man with schizophrenia and a past history of alcohol abuse. He has had multiple relapses and rehospitalizations related to poor compliance with antipsychotic medication and episodic drinking. His family is frustrated and hopeless about his frequent relapses despite their involvement in community support groups and joint visits with Mr. Jones' psychiatrist and case manager. Mr. Jones' psychiatrist has made multiple attempts to counsel Mr. Jones about treatment compliance and has switched medications to attempt to optimize compliance. He has also involved Mr. Jones in alcohol counseling. Mr. Jones is on once a day antipsychotic dosing and keeps his medications in a pill minder. His family reminds him to take his medication whenever possible but this makes Mr. Jones angry. Notably, he does not believe he is ill and sees no need to take his medication except to appease his family. Despite repeated attempts to educate Mr. Jones about his illness, his insight is minimal.

Following a recent hospitalization, the family asked to meet with the psychiatrist and Mr. Jones. They indicate they can no longer tolerate the frequent crises and psychotic behavior of the patient and say that they will demand he move out of their home unless his compliance and general behavior improve. After a long discussion, Mr. Jones agrees to take depot antipsychotics as a condition of living with his family as long as the family agrees to stop asking him about his medications and treatment. While Mr. Jones suffers a minor relapse in the next several months, a major decompensation and hospitalization is avoided and all parties agree to continue the depot regimen.

# References

Adams CE and Eisenbruch M (2002) Depot fluphenazine for schizophrenia (Cochrane review). The Cochrane Library, Oxford. Update Software.

Claxton AJ, Cramer J, and Pierce C (2001) A systematic review of the associations between dose regimens and medication compliance. Clin Ther 23, 1296–1308.

Corrigan PW, Liberman RP, and Engel JD (1990) From noncompliance to collaboration in the treatment of schizophrenia. Hosp Comm Psychiatr 41, 1203–1211.

Cramer JA (1991) Identifying and improving compliance patterns: A composite plan for health care providers. In Patient Compliance in Medical Practice and Clinical Trials, Cramer JA and Spilker B (eds). Raven Press, New York, pp. 387–392.

Cramer JA (1995) Relationship between medication compliance and medical outcomes. Am J Health-Syst Pharm 52, S27–S29.

Cramer JA and Rosenheck R (1999) Enhancing medication compliance for people with serious mental illness. J Nerv Ment Dis 187, 53–55.

Cramer JA, Mattson RH, Prevey ML, et al. (1989) How often is medication taken as prescribed? J Am Med Assoc 261, 3273–3277.

Cramer JA, Scheyer RD, and Mattson RH (1990) Compliance declines between clinic visits. Arch Intern Med 150, 1509–1510.

Diaz E, Levine HB, Sullivan MC, et al. (2001) Use of the medication event monitoring system to estimate medication compliance in patients with schizophrenia. J Psychiatr Neurosci 26, 325–329.

Dickson WE and Kendall RE (1986) Does maintenance lithium therapy prevent recurrences of mania under ordinary clinical conditions? Psychol Med 16, 521–530.

Feinstein AR (1990) On white-coat effects and the electronic monitoring of compliance. Arch Intern Med 150, 1377–1378.

Glazer WM and Kane JM (1992) Depot neuroleptic therapy: An underutilized treatment option. J Clin Psychiatr 53, 426–433.

Goldstein MJ (1992) Psychosocial strategies for maximizing the effects of psychotropic medications for schizophrenia and mood disorder. Psychopharmacol Bull 28, 237–240.

Guscott R and Taylor L (1994) Lithium prophylaxis in recurrent affective illness: Efficacy, effectiveness, and efficiency. Br J Psychiatr 164, 741–746.

Haynes RB (1979) Introduction. In Compliance in Health Care, Haynes RB, Taylor DW, and Sackett DL (eds). Johns Hopkins University Press, Baltimore, pp. 1–7.

Hayward P, Chan N, Kemp R, et al. (1995) Medication self-management: A preliminary report on an intervention to improve medication compliance. J Ment Health 4, 511–517.

Healy A, Knapp M, Astin J, et al. (1998) Cost-effectiveness evaluation of compliance therapy for people with psychosis. Br J Psychiatr 172, 420–424.

Jamison KR and Akiskal HS (1983) Medication compliance in patients with bipolar disorder. Psychiatr Clin N Am 6, 175–192.

Jamison KR, Gerner RH, and Goodwin FK (1979) Patient and physician attitudes toward lithium. Arch Gen Psychiatr 36, 866–869.

Kelly GR and Scott JE (1990) Medication compliance and health education among outpatients with chronic mental disorders. Med Care 28, 1181–1197.

Kelly GR, Mamon JA, and Scott JE (1987) Utility of the health belief model in examining medication compliance among psychiatric outpatients. Soc Sci Med 25, 1205–1211.

Kemp R, Hayward P, Applewhite G, et al. (1996) Compliance therapy in psychotic patients: Randomised controlled trial. Br Med J 312, 345–349.

Kemp R, Kirov G, Everitt B, et al. (1998) Randomised controlled trial of compliance therapy. 18 month follow-up. Br J Psychiatr 172, 413–419.

Liberman RP (1992) Future prospects for psychiatric rehabilitation. In Handbook of Psychiatric Rehabilitation, Liberman RP (ed). Allyn & Bacon, Boston, MA, p. 320.

McEvoy JP, Freter S, Everett G, et al. (1989) Insight and the clinical outcome of schizophrenic patients. J Nerv Ment Dis 177, 48–51.

Meijer WEE, Bouvy ML, Heerdink ER, et al. (2001) Spontaneous lapses in dosing during chronic treatment with selective serotonin reuptake inhibitors. Br J Psychiatr 179, 519–522.

Nageotte C, Sullivan G, Duan N, et al. (1997) Medication compliance among the seriously mentally ill in a public mental health system. Soc Psychiatr Psychiatr Epidemiol 32, 49–56.

Namkoong K, Faren CK, O'Conner PG, et al. (1999) Measurement of compliance with naltrexone. J Clin Psychiatr 60, 449–453.

Norrell SE (1979) Improving medication compliance: A randomized controlled trial. Br Med J 2, 1031–1033.

Owen RR, Fischer EP, Booth BM, et al. (1996) Medication noncompliance and substance abuse among patients with schizophrenia. Psychiatr Serv 47, 853–858.

Quraishi S and David A (2002) Depot haloperidol decanoate for schizophrenia (Cochrane review). The Cochrane Library, Oxford. Update Software.

Rosenbaum JF, Fava M, Hoog SL, et al. (1998) Selective serotonine reuptake inhibitor discontinuation syndrome: A randomized clinical trial. Biol Psychiatr 44, 77–87.

Rosenstock IM (1974) Historical origins of the health beliefs model. Health Educ Monogr 2, 328–335.

Schou M (1997) The combat of noncompliance during prophylactic lithium treatment. Acta Psychiatr Scand 95, 361–363.

Scott J (1995) Psychotherapy for bipolar disorder. Br J Psychiatr 167, 581–588.

Scott J and Pope M (2002) Nonadherence with mood stabilizers: Prevalence and predictors. J Clin Psychiatr 63, 384–390.

Sherbourne CD, Hays RD, Ordway L, et al. (1992) Antecedents of adherence to medical recommendations: Results from the Medical Outcomes Study. J Behav Med 15, 447–468.

Sullivan G, Wells K, Morgenstern H, et al. (1995) Identifying modifiable risk factors for rehospitalization: A case-control study of serious mentally ill persons in Mississippi. Am J Psychiatr 152, 1749–1756.

Tarlov AR, Ware JE, Greenfield S, et al. (1989) The medical outcomes study: An application of methods for monitoring the results of medical care. J Am Med Assoc 262, 925–930.

Urquhart J (1994) Role of patient compliance in clinical pharmacokinetics: A review of recent research. Clin Pharmacokin 27, 202–215.

Weiden PJ and Olfson M (1995) Cost of relapse in schizophrenia. Schizophren Bull 21, 419–429.

Zhang M, Wang M, Li J, et al. (1994) Randomised-control trial of family interventions for 78 first-episode male schizophrenic patients. Br J Psychiatr 165(Suppl 24), 96–102.

# 107 Global Perspectives on Mental Health Services

Scott Stroup
Mario Maj

Reports issued by the World Health Organization (WHO 2001) and the Institute of Medicine (IOM 2001) at the beginning of the new millennium highlight the vast worldwide burden of mental illnesses and great disparities in mental health services between affluent and poorer countries. In general, the disparities in wealth and in general health services among countries are exaggerated in their services for persons with mental disorders. Worldwide, systems of care and access to effective treatments for mental illnesses are markedly suboptimal. Problems include failure to recognize the significance of the impact of mental illnesses, stigma that results in discrimination and decisions not to seek effective help, and lack of human and other resources needed for prevention and treatment. In this chapter we provide an overview of mental health issues that are common in many countries.

Research examining societal burden of illness that looks beyond statistics on prevalence and mortality has shown that mental disorders cause a significant proportion of illness-associated disability (Murray and Lopez 1996). Using disability-adjusted life-years (DALYs), a measure that factors in the severity and chronicity of disability as well as the impact of an illness on premature death, researchers have found that depression, bipolar disorder, schizophrenia, and other brain disorders are major causes of disability worldwide (Table 107–1). The high prevalence of depression and the early onset and chronicity of schizophrenia, bipolar disorder, and substance use disorders make these illnesses particularly burdensome for people of ages 15 to 44 years (WHO 2001).

Efforts of the WHO in promoting a biopsychosocial view of mental disorders and a community-oriented approach in mental health care have been significant (Lefley 1999, Sartorius and Harding 1983). However, weak governmental support and leadership for mental health relative to other priorities, a lack of qualified professionals, concentration of mental health care facilities in urban centers, and the failure of modern psychiatry to gain community acceptability in the context of different prevailing health beliefs are barriers to the wider acceptance of the biopsychosocial

and community-oriented approach (Higginbotham 1984). Perceptions of the limited effectiveness of available interventions for mental disorders relative to the cures offered by other biomedical treatments, for example, antibiotics for infections, contribute to continued adherence to traditional models of care for mental disturbances (Leff 2001).

Culture not only influences definitions of mental illness, it affects the development, manifestation, and course of mental disorders (Lefley 1999). Because schizophrenia has been extensively studied it provides ready examples of cultural influence. Leff (2001) has described how in the 1970s the diagnosis of schizophrenia varied widely between London, where narrow descriptive definitions were used, Moscow, where definitions were greatly influenced by inter-episode social functioning and conformance, and Washington DC, where the definition was broad and psychoanalytically oriented. Leff (2001) also relates the declining incidence of schizophrenia manifested by catatonia in industrialized but not in developing countries to a shift from somatic to psychological modes of expression in the former settings. Culture is also credited with a major role in the variations of outcomes among people belonging to communities involved in the WHO-sponsored International Pilot Study of Schizophrenia (IPSS) (Sartorius et al. 1996) and Determinants of Outcome of Severe Mental Disorders (DOSMD) projects (Lefley 1999, Leff 2001, Jablensky et al. 1992). Outcomes were better in rural communities, which has been attributed, in part, to the observation that in rural areas ill persons were highly likely to live with family, and that rural families tended to be more supportive and less hostile and critical than families in urban areas (Leff 2001).

Urbanization, poverty, and technological change, all influence the development of mental disorders and may affect various segments of a society differentially (WHO 2001). In most countries, women are disproportionately affected by poverty. As a result, women also commonly have lower social status than men, tend to suffer greater consequences from mental disorders and are less likely to receive treatment (IOM 2001). Racial prejudice, common in

| Table 107–1 | Leading Causes of Disability-Adjusted Life Years (DALYs), in all Ages and in 15–44-Year-Olds, by Sex, Estimates for 2000 |
|---|---|

| | Both Sexes, all Ages | % Total | | Males, all Ages | % Total | | Females, all Ages | % Total |
|---|---|---|---|---|---|---|---|---|
| 1 | Lower respiratory infections | 6.4 | 1 | Perinatal conditions | 6.4 | 1 | HIV/AIDS | 6.5 |
| 2 | Perinatal conditions | 6.2 | 2 | Lower respiratory infections | 6.4 | 2 | Lower respiratory infections | 6.4 |
| 3 | HIV/AIDS | 6.1 | 3 | HIV/AIDS | 5.8 | 3 | Perinatal conditions | 6.0 |
| 4 | Unipolar depressive disorders | 4.4 | 4 | Diarrheal diseases | 4.2 | 4 | Unipolar depressive disorders | 5.5 |
| 5 | Diarrheal diseases | 4.2 | 5 | Ischemic heart disease | 4.2 | 5 | Diarrheal diseases | 4.2 |
| 6 | Ischemic heart disease | 3.8 | 6 | Road traffic accidents | 4.0 | 6 | Ischemic heart disease | 3.3 |
| 7 | Cerebrovascular disease | 3.1 | 7 | Unipolar depressive disorders | 3.4 | 7 | Cerebrovascular disease | 3.2 |
| 8 | Road traffic accidents | 2.8 | 8 | Cerebrovascular disease | 3.0 | 8 | Malaria | 3.0 |
| 9 | Malaria | 2.7 | 9 | Tuberculosis | 2.9 | 9 | Congenital abnormalities | 2.2 |
| 10 | Tuberculosis | 2.4 | 10 | Malaria | 2.5 | 10 | Chronic obstructive pulmonary disease | 2.1 |
| 11 | Chronic obstructive pulmonary disease | 2.3 | 11 | Chronic obstructive pulmonary disease | 2.4 | 11 | Iron-deficiency anaemia | 2.1 |
| 12 | Congenital abnormalities | 2.2 | 12 | Congenital abnormalities | 2.2 | 12 | Tuberculosis | 2.0 |
| 13 | Measles | 1.9 | 13 | Alcohol use disorders | 2.1 | 13 | Measles | 2.0 |
| 14 | Iron-deficiency anaemia | 1.8 | 14 | Measles | 1.8 | 14 | Hearing loss, adult onset | 1.7 |
| 15 | Hearing loss, adult onset | 1.7 | 15 | Hearing loss, adult onset | 1.8 | 15 | Road traffic accidents | 1.5 |
| 16 | Falls | 1.3 | 16 | Violence | 1.6 | 16 | Osteoarthritis | 1.4 |
| 17 | Self-inflicted injuries | 1.3 | 17 | Iron-deficiency anaemia | 1.5 | 17 | Protein-energy malnutrition | 1.2 |
| 18 | Alcohol use disorders | 1.3 | 18 | Falls | 1.5 | 18 | Self-inflicted injuries | 1.1 |
| 19 | Protein-energy malnutrition | 1.1 | 19 | Self-inflicted injuries | 1.5 | 19 | Diabetes mellitus | 1.1 |
| 20 | Osteoarthritis | 1.1 | 20 | Cirrhosis of the liver | 1.4 | 20 | Falls | 1.1 |

| | Both Sexes, 15–44-Year-Olds | % Total | | Males, 15–44-Year-Olds | % Total | | Females, 15–44-Year-Olds | % Total |
|---|---|---|---|---|---|---|---|---|
| 1 | HIV/AIDS | 13.0 | 1 | HIV/AIDS | 12.1 | 1 | HIV/AIDS | 13.9 |
| 2 | Unipolar depressive disorders | 8.6 | 2 | Road traffic accidents | 7.7 | 2 | Unipolar depressive disorders | 10.6 |
| 3 | Road traffic accidents | 4.9 | 3 | Unipolar depressive disorders | 6.7 | 3 | Tuberculosis | 3.2 |
| 4 | Tuberculosis | 3.9 | 4 | Alcohol use disorders | 5.1 | 4 | Iron-deficiency anaemia | 3.2 |
| 5 | Alcohol use disorders | 3.0 | 5 | Tuberculosis | 4.5 | 5 | Schizophrenia | 2.8 |
| 6 | Self-inflicted injuries | 2.7 | 6 | Violence | 3.7 | 6 | Obstructed labour | 2.7 |
| 7 | Iron-deficiency anaemia | 2.6 | 7 | Self-inflicted injuries | 3.0 | 7 | Bipolar affective disorder | 2.5 |
| 8 | Schizophrenia | 2.6 | 8 | Schizophrenia | 2.5 | 8 | Abortion | 2.5 |
| 9 | Bipolar affective disorder | 2.5 | 9 | Bipolar affective disorder | 2.4 | 9 | Self-inflicted injuries | 2.4 |
| 10 | Violence | 2.3 | 10 | Iron-deficiency anaemia | 2.1 | 10 | Maternal sepsis | 2.1 |
| 11 | Hearing loss, adult onset | 2.0 | 11 | Hearing loss, adult onset | 2.0 | 11 | Road traffic accidents | 2.0 |
| 12 | Chronic obstructive pulmonary disease | 1.5 | 12 | Ischemic heart disease | 1.9 | 12 | Hearing loss, adult onset | 2.0 |
| 13 | Ischemic heart disease | 1.5 | 13 | War | 1.7 | 13 | Chlamydia | 1.9 |
| 14 | Cerebrovascular disease | 1.4 | 14 | Falls | 1.7 | 14 | Panic disorder | 1.6 |
| 15 | Falls | 1.3 | 15 | Cirrhosis of the liver | 1.6 | 15 | Chronic obstructive pulmonary disease | 1.5 |
| 16 | Obstructed labour | 1.3 | 16 | Drug use disorders | 1.6 | 16 | Maternal haemorrhage | 1.5 |
| 17 | Abortion | 1.2 | 17 | Cerebrovascular disease | 1.5 | 17 | Osteoarthritis | 1.4 |
| 18 | Osteoarthritis | 1.2 | 18 | Chronic obstructive pulmonary disease | 1.5 | 18 | Cerebrovascular disease | 1.3 |
| 19 | War | 1.2 | 19 | Asthma | 1.4 | 19 | Migraine | 1.2 |
| 20 | Panic disorder | 1.2 | 20 | Drownings | 1.1 | 20 | Ischemic heart disease | 1.1 |

*Source*: World Health Organization (2001) The World Health Report 2001. Mental Health: New Understanding, New Hope. World Health Organization, Geneva.

many countries, has also been shown to lead to psychological distress in persons discriminated against and to perpetuate mental problems (WHO 2001).

Psychosocial circumstances influence the development of mental illnesses and are profoundly affected by them. Social stressors like deprivation and exposure to violence are thought to be highly important in the development of anxiety and depressive disorders and are also factors in the cause and course of schizophrenia (WHO 2001). In contrast, schizophrenia and substance use disorders, as well as other mental illnesses, can cause people to become socially deprived. These processes, sometimes known as "social causation" and "social drift" are complementary rather than mutually exclusive (WHO 2001). For example, low educational and occupational achievement lead to poverty and an increased risk of mental disorders. Mental disorders may interfere with educational and occupational functioning and thus can lead to economic deprivation. These socioeconomic influences can clearly affect the course of mental illnesses in both rich and poor countries (WHO 2001).

## Overview of Mental Health Services

In 2000 and 2001, the WHO conducted Project Atlas, which collected data on mental health services and policies from 185 WHO member states that represented 99.3% of the world's population. Project Atlas documented a dismal situation in which 41% of countries had no mental health policy and 25% had no legislation on mental health. Approximately 4 out of 10 countries had no treatment facilities for severe mental disorders in primary care settings, and a similar proportion of countries had no community mental health care facilities (WHO 2001).

In the 19th and early 20th centuries, large mental hospitals were the focal point of formal mental health care in countries throughout the world. By the end of the 20th century, both affluent and poorer nations began to adopt policies that shifted emphasis from large mental hospitals towards community-based treatment programs (Goldman et al. 1983). Nevertheless, isolated mental hospitals providing care for and control over individuals with severe mental illnesses remain common. Project Atlas found a continued focus on institutional care for mental illnesses, with almost two-thirds of beds for mental health worldwide still in mental hospitals (WHO 2001). These large institutions are more likely to provide custodial care and are associated with poorer outcomes and human rights violations (WHO 2001) than mental health units in general hospitals offering treatment and rehabilitation.

There is a trend among Western nations, which once relied upon large mental hospitals as the primary locus of mental health service, to promote community-based treatment as a more humane and cost-effective alternative. This "deinstitutionalization" has resulted in two types of patients—one group of discharged long-term residents of the mental hospitals, and another group that was diverted from this status by new policies that limited access to long-term hospitalization. Commonly, responsible parties have made great efforts to ensure that long-stay patients have adequate shelter and resources upon discharge—a large majority of these former patients who are willing to accept treatment and other services are able to live in community-based settings without returning for long stays in mental hospitals

(Rothbard and Kuno 2000). People who are diverted from mental hospitals may not fare as well. Comprehensive services are rarely readily available for subchronic patients, and this group is vulnerable to homelessness and chronic problems accessing needed medical and social services. In addition, persons who remain in long-term mental hospitals after an initial wave of deinstitutionalization tend to be more disabled and to have more severe behavioral problems than persons in early cohorts of deinstitutionalization (Rothbard and Kuno 2000). Treating these individuals with multiple problems and severe disability in community settings requires significant allocations of resources that many locales have failed to provide.

Many developed countries—for example, the US—have established networks of community-based clinics known as community mental health centers (CMHCs). Initially funded by the US federal government, these centers were essential to plans to deinstitutionalize persons living in state mental hospitals. The result is that the US has successfully established a geographically distributed network of centers for the promotion of community-based mental health. However, the quality, accessibility, and range of services at these CMHCs is thought to vary widely.

In developing countries, outpatient clinical care is usually located only in major cities and there are few community-based resources (Lefley 1999). Rather than building specialized community-based mental health programs, developing countries have used the primary health care system to extend basic mental health services to the broader population (Sartorius and Harding 1983). Poorer countries simply do not have the resources to build a nationwide specialty mental health system (Higginbotham 1984). In poorer countries, organized mental health systems usually focus on the most deviant or severely ill population—those with behavioral disturbances due to schizophrenia and other severe psychiatric disorders. It is primarily the richer countries that have been able to afford training and services oriented toward the prevention and treatment of mental disorders, although the resources dedicated to mental health services are generally inadequate, as discussed below.

It is important to note, however, that mental health services may not be the key determinants of outcomes. For example, studies of schizophrenia conducted by the WHO have consistently shown that outcomes are better in developing than in industrialized countries, in spite of fewer formal mental health services (Harrison et al. 2001). Poverty, economic development, the status of women, and cultural factors, all influence mental health, and are considered stronger determinants of mental health, than a formal system for treating mental illnesses (WHO 2001, IOM 2001).

The World Health Report 2001 (WHO 2001) notes that a rational health financing system should protect people from catastrophic costs due to illness, should have the sick subsidized by the healthy, and should have the poor subsidized by the rich. These financing system characteristics are particularly important for protecting persons with mental illnesses because of the chronicity and economic consequences of these disorders. Nevertheless, a common theme worldwide is that insurance schemes and health plans are less likely to provide comprehensive coverage for mental disorders than for other illnesses (WHO 2001). Prepaid health systems, including national health services and direct-service insurance plans, are preferable to systems that require out-of-pocket payments for services (WHO 2001). Due to poverty and stigma, persons with mental disorders may be especially unable or unwilling to seek and pay for treatment. Mental health priorities are better served in countries whose governments provide a large proportion of the mental health budget than in countries with little government funding for mental health (WHO 2001).

## Recommendations for Mental Health Systems of Care

In response to the worldwide problems in providing services to persons with mental disorders, both the WHO and the IOM have recently made recommendations. The World Health Report 2001 (WHO 2001) made 10 overall recommendations for countries to improve mental health, as follows: (1) provide mental health treatment in primary care settings; (2) make psychotropic drugs available; (3) give care in the community; (4) educate the public about mental illnesses; (5) educate communities, families, and consumers; (6) establish national mental health policies, programs, and legislation; (7) develop human resources not only to create more specialists but also to help general and allied health providers to recognize and treat mental illnesses; (8) link with other sectors, including the general health sector and traditional healers who can serve as case finders, referrers, counselors, and monitors; (9) monitor community mental health, and (10) support more research (Table 107–2).

The IOM (2001) report focused on improving the situation for persons with mental disorders in developing countries. The recommendations echo those of the WHO: (1) increase public and professional awareness of mental

| Table 107–2 | WHO Recommendations for Mental Health Services in all Countries and Societies |
|---|---|

1. Provide treatment for mental disorders in primary care settings.
2. Make psychotropic drugs available as part of every country's essential drug list.
3. Give care for mental disorders in the community instead of in institutions.
4. Educate the public about the frequency and treatability of mental disorders; about the recovery process; and about the human rights of people with mental disorders.
5. Involve persons from communities, family members, and consumers in the development and decision-making of policies, programs, and services.
6. Establish national mental health policies, programs, and legislation; establish adequate funding for these services; do not allow insurance schemes to discriminate against persons with mental disorders.
7. Develop specialized human resources to provide care and to train and support primary health care programs.
8. Link the mental health and health sectors with education, labor, welfare, law, and nongovernmental organizations to improve the mental health of communities.
9. Monitor community mental health by maintaining indices of the numbers of persons with mental illnesses and the quality of care.
10. Support research into the biologic and psychosocial aspects of mental health.

*Source*: World Health Organization (2001) The World Health Report 2001. Mental Health: New Understanding, New Hope. World Health Organization, Geneva.

| Table 107–3 | Institute of Medicine's Proposed Strategies to Reduce the Burden of Brain Disorders in Developing Countries |
|---|---|

Strategy 1. Increase public and professional awareness and understanding of brain disorders in developing countries, and intervene to reduce stigma and ease the burden of discrimination often associated with these disorders.

Strategy 2. Extend and strengthen existing systems of primary care to deliver health services for brain disorders. Secondary and tertiary centers should train and oversee primary care staff, provide referral capacity, and provide ongoing supervision and support for primary care systems in developing countries.

Strategy 3. Make cost-effective interventions for brain disorders available to patients who will benefit. Financial and institutional constraints require selectivity and sequencing in setting goals and priorities. The continued implementation of these interventions should also be informed by ongoing research to reveal the applicability and sustainability of such programs.

*Source*: Institute of Medicine (2001) Neurologic, Psychiatric, and Developmental Disorders: Meeting the Challenge in the Developing World. National Academy Press, Washington DC.

illnesses and treatment; reduce stigma and discrimination; (2) extend and strengthen services available in primary care settings; use human resources at secondary and tertiary settings for training and oversight, and (3) make cost-effective interventions available to patients who will benefit from them; conduct research on operations and the epidemiology of mental disorders for the purpose of prioritizing resource allocations (Table 107–3).

Available data make it difficult for many countries to know if these strategies are being pursued. Some of these recommendations are not feasible or are extremely low priority for developing countries struggling to cope with extreme poverty, inadequate nutrition, the consequences of war, and acute communicable diseases.

## Cases

In the next section of this chapter we highlight the mental health services of a few countries that are illustrative. Comparing mental health services internationally is difficult due to a lack of comparable, up-to-date data, in spite of recent efforts to remedy this in the Project Atlas of WHO, discussed above. Developing countries, in particular, have little in the way of information on mental health services, epidemiology, treatment, and policy (IOM 2001). Even the anecdotal information and case studies on innovative programs that appear in the literature may be significantly out-of-date.

## Developed Countries

### United Kingdom

In 2000, the UK had a population of 59 million. In 1998, the UK spent 6.8% of its gross domestic product (GDP) on health, representing a per capita health expenditure of $1,512 in international dollars (WHO 2001). (International dollars adjust figures calculated using the exchange rate for purchasing power by eliminating differences in price levels between countries.)

Since 1949, the UK has provided health care services through the taxation-funded National Health Service (NHS). The NHS provides general medical and psychiatric services free of charge (McColloch et al. 2000). Virtually the entire population is registered with a general practitioner. Mental health services in the UK are available from a diverse network of formal and informal providers in a vast array of settings (Knapp 1997). Hospital services are funded through the NHS and include inpatient, day patient, and outpatient services. Community care is provided through general practitioners, community psychiatric nurses, and day care. Other sources of care include social workers, sheltered accommodations, informal caregivers (usually family members), private sector agencies (providing care through contracts with public agencies or directly to private-pay patients), and volunteer organizations.

In general, health care is provided by the NHS and social care is commissioned or provided by the Social Services Departments of local authorities (McColloch et al. 2000). Housing is commissioned by separate agencies. Welfare benefits and employment services are also provided separately, meaning that the system is not well-integrated and people needing a wide range of services must negotiate with numerous agencies (McColloch et al. 2000).

In a pattern strikingly similar to the US and Canada, the peak population in large mental hospitals was in the 1950s, when there were approximately 150,000 hospital residents (Rogers and Pilgrim 1996). The Mental Health Act of 1959 emphasized community-based care (Goodwin 1997)—by 1984 there were 79,000 available beds and by 2000 the figure was approximately 36,000 (McColloch et al. 2000). The large NHS hospitals are now largely out-of-date and inadequately funded (Rogers and Pilgrim 1996). Psychiatry in the UK remains hospital oriented, but has shifted from mental hospitals to District General Hospitals (Rogers and Pilgrim 1996).

The NHS and Community Care Act of 1990 was implemented in 1993 (Rogers and Pilgrim 1996, Hollingsworth 1996). Since then, responsibility for community care of persons with mental illness has rested in social services departments, which are accountable for needs assessment and enabling (case management). Community services have developed steadily but remain overburdened. Specialized, intensive community treatment teams for persons with severe mental illness remain rare (McColloch et al. 2000).

## Italy

In 2000, Italy had a population of 58 million. In 1998, the country spent 7.7% of its GDP on health, representing a per capita health expenditure of $1,712 in international dollars (WHO 2001). Italy's population has universal health coverage through the Italian National Health Service (NHS), which is similar to the one in England (De Girolamo and Cozza 2000). Health care is funded through taxation and is provided by local health units that serve geographically defined catchment areas. Each person is registered with a general practitioner. Most medical care is provided without charge but cost-sharing has been introduced for some services and some drugs (De Girolamo and Cozza 2000).

In Italy, CMHCs (Community Mental Health Centers) provide the bulk of outpatient and nonresidential care and maintain contact with a wide variety of other services, public and private residential facilities, and "social enterprises" that provide psychosocial and rehabilitative assistance. Inpatient treatment is primarily available at general

hospital psychiatric units, private psychiatric hospitals, and university psychiatry departments. The role of public mental hospitals is now limited, as discussed further. Private services are reimbursed by the NHS.

In 1978, Italy enacted its Mental Health Act Law 180, (Mosher 1983, Burti and Benson 1996). The law mandated the development of a public mental health system without asylums. The law prohibited new admissions to state mental hospitals, called for the eventual closing of these hospitals, restricted compulsory admissions, and required the development of community-based inpatient and outpatient services to replace the functions previously served by the old asylums. The goal was to shift the Italian mental health system from institutional segregation and control to rehabilitation and the reintegration of persons with a mental illness into the community and its social life.

Nearly a quarter century after the passage of Law 180, the results of the 1978 reform goals have not all been reached but it is clear that dramatic changes have occurred in the Italian mental health service system. Responsibility for implementing the legislation was assigned to the 20 regional governments that have considerable administrative autonomy but vary widely in their geographic, socioeconomic, and political characteristics. Consequently, implementation of the legislation is more advanced in the central and northern regions, where there were more hospitalized patients prior to 1978, than in the southern regions of Italy. Another feature is that services are more widely available in the smaller cities than in the large urban areas (De Salvia and Barbato 1993).

In the inpatient service sector, service use patterns changed markedly after 1978 (De Salvia and Barbato 1993, Burti and Benson 1996). There was a marked decline in the use of psychiatric beds and their location shifted from the public mental hospitals to general hospital psychiatric units, which are also publicly funded. Although new admissions to the public mental hospitals were shut off following enactment of Law 180, the hospitals did not disappear altogether. The population in mental hospitals in Italy peaked in 1963, when there were almost 92,000 residents in 76 hospitals (De Girolamo and Cozza 2000). The mental hospital population dropped by 53% in the first 10 years after Law 180 was enacted, and the closing down of hospitals accelerated in the late 1990s, so that by 1998 only 50 of the mental hospitals remained open with only about 7,700 residents (De Girolamo and Cozza 2000). The use of private mental hospitals (funded primarily by public dollars and similar in role to public mental hospitals) peaked in 1977 and remained relatively constant while the number of residents slowly declined over the following decade. By 1998 there were about 10,000 psychiatric beds available for acute admissions, with 55.5% in 65 private psychiatric facilities, 40.5% in general hospital psychiatric units, and 4% in units affiliated with university psychiatry departments (De Girolamo and Cozza 2000).

In the outpatient service sector, there was a rapid growth in the number of CMHCs from 249 to 674 between 1978 and 1984 (De Salvia and Barbato 1993). By 1998 there were 695 CMHCs, an average of 1 per 82,000 persons (De Girolamo and Cozza 2000). At the time of a 1984 survey, most of the patients seen at CMHCs had severe and/or chronic mental disorders. In some areas, particularly in the North, CMHCs provided a fully integrated system of community mental health services, including clinic and home care, rehabilitative services, and assisted housing (Burti and Benson 1996). In these areas, the use of public mental hospitals had all but been eliminated. In other areas, mainly in the South, there were fewer CMHCs, and these did not provide a comprehensive array of services. In such areas, mental hospitals and other inpatient facilities continued to be used heavily (Burti and Benson 1996). By 1998 there were 1,377 nonhospital residential facilities in Italy, with an average number of 12.4 beds each, hosting a total of 17,343 patients (about 40% of whom were former residents in mental hospitals). Moreover, there were 433 "social enterprises" for the social reintegration and vocational rehabilitation of the most severely mentally ill: the overall number of patients working in these enterprises was 3,942 (De Girolamo and Cozza 2000).

The shift from large mental hospitals to community care in Italy was more dramatic than in other Western countries (De Salvia and Barbato 1993). The available data suggest that neither the private inpatient sector nor the criminal justice system have replaced the mental hospital as a source of institutional care for psychiatric patients. The expansion of community-based services envisioned by Law 180 was slower than expected and continued many years after the law was enacted (De Girolamo and Cozza 2000). The decentralization of government in Italy and the wide differences in regional resources led to unevenness in the quality and accessibility of CMHs. De Girolamo and Cozza (2000) reported that the quality of care for people with mental disorders remains disappointing in Italy. As has been found in the US, pharmacotherapy and psychosocial treatments are rarely provided in a manner consistent with evidence-based practices (De Girolamo and Cozza 2000, Lehman and Steinwachs 1998).

## United States

In 2000, the US had a population of 283 million. In 1998, the country spent 12.9% of its GDP on health, representing a per capita health expenditure of $4,055 in international dollars (WHO 2001). In spite of this high level of expenditure, there is no universal health coverage in the US.

The US mental health system is notable for its relatively high expenditures and fragmented services (see the following vignette).

---

**Clinical Vignette • Complexity in the US**

Poorly coordinated services are a characteristic of the US mental health system. Persons with schizophrenia, for example, may need psychiatric services, general medical services, help with housing, income support, vocational rehabilitation, and psychosocial support. Frequently these are available only at different clinical sites and through separate agencies.

The Schizophrenia Treatment and Evaluation Program (STEP) at the University of North Carolina in Chapel Hill was created in the early 1990s to address some of these issues. Nevertheless it continues to operate within a fragmented system that will be described here as an example of the complexity of mental health care in the US.

STEP was founded to provide a training opportunity for mental health professionals, and to attempt to provide a more comprehensive and coordinated set of services than was previously available at the University of North Carolina Hospitals. The program provides outpatient services and has an 18-bed inpatient unit. The inpatient unit is run by psychiatrists in collaboration with nurses and social workers. Psychiatry residents, medical students, and nursing students all train on the unit. In the outpatient clinic, resident psychiatrists under the supervision of attending psychiatrists provide medication management and psychosocial support. The clinic is coordinated by a social worker who manages referrals, provides direct service to clients, supervises trainees from a variety of disciplines (including social work and rehabilitation counseling), and serves as liaison to other community agencies and hospital services. Other social workers provide psychotherapy and case management. A psychologist provides cognitive–behavioral therapy and supervises psychiatry and psychology trainees in this technique. Occupational therapists provide evaluations and individual and group therapy in both inpatient and outpatient settings.

STEP clinicians must coordinate services for its clients with multiple other agencies. The local CMHC refers its patients for inpatient treatment. STEP clients are eligible for services at the CMHC; many belong to the CMHC's clubhouse. The CMHC operates several supervised apartments and a few group homes that house many STEP clients. STEP social workers help clients negotiate with the CMHC and the local social service and housing agencies for their services. STEP also offers services for many clients of a local vocational rehabilitation program that provides transitional housing and jobs, then connects them with job coaches when they obtain competitive employment.

Problems persist, however. Health benefits are incomplete even for some people eligible for disability benefits. For example, some persons have not been disabled long enough to be eligible for government-sponsored disability benefits. They receive charity care from the university hospital, the state hospital, the CMHC, and/or STEP. Expensive psychotropic medications are often available only through charity or the assistance programs of pharmaceutical companies. Therapeutic and supported living situations are in short supply. Many clients live in quasi-institutions known as Adult Care Homes (or "rest homes") that have no expertise in mental disorders and no focus on rehabilitation. Access to long-term hospitalization is highly restricted. There is a widely recognized need for additional community-based services but an economic downturn in the early 2000s resulted in a state budget crisis that eliminated immediate hope for adequate new funding for the mental health system.

---

Although epidemiologic studies have found that more than a quarter of adults in the US have a mental illness at some point in any year, only about half of these people receive any care (Manderscheid et al. 2000).

Private health insurance is linked to employment in the US and provides mental health services according to what is purchased. Virtually all private mental health care is provided under managed care, which refers to a variety of strategies used to control costs and utilization of expensive services. In addition, there are two important government sponsored programs—a social insurance program (Medicare) for the elderly and disabled, and a public assistance program (Medicaid) that provides coverage for health care services for poor elderly people, mothers to small children,

children, or for those who have disabilities. Managed care techniques are now commonly used in Medicare and Medicaid systems as well. The Department of Veterans Affairs provides psychiatric services for a large number of veterans with mental illnesses. In 1999, in spite of this multitude of payers, 43 million persons (approximately 15% of the population) in the US had no health benefit. Subsequently the number of persons without insurance decreased when the economy was strong and increased again when the economy faltered. For uninsured persons, systematic psychiatric treatment is available only through state and locally financed facilities or inconsistently through other means of charity.

CMHCs and state hospitals are the primary sites of publicly supported mental health services, which are usually paid for by state governments, Medicaid, or Medicare. Privatization of public assistance programs like Medicaid and social insurance programs like Medicare have exacerbated the fragmentation of services—vendors who contract to provide medical services have little incentive to provide the social services that many persons with severe mental illnesses are likely to need.

In the second half of the 20th century there was a dramatic decrease in the number of persons hospitalized in state mental hospitals. This deinstitutionalization saw the country's total state hospital census drop from over 500,000 in the 1950s to less than 100,000 in the 1990s. Hospitalization shifted to an acute model of care provided in the psychiatric wards of general hospitals and nonpublic specialty hospitals. By the late 1990s, more than 60% of inpatient mental health care in the US was in nonspecialty hospitals (Goodwin 1997).

Outpatient mental health treatment is provided in diverse settings, including teaching hospital clinics, CMHCs, private offices, clinics associated with veterans affairs (VA), and state mental hospitals. Case management is generally provided at CMHCs and VA medical centers. Assertive community treatment teams that provide outreach and intensive services for persons with severe mental illnesses are relatively rare but are mandated by some states. The availability of rehabilitation services varies widely across locations.

A study of quality of care for people with schizophrenia in the 1990s showed very poor concordance with guidelines that recommended treatments that had strong evidence of effectiveness (Lehman and Steinwachs 1998). Only 29% of studied patients received appropriate maintenance doses of antipsychotic medications, family education was delivered in only 10% of cases, and only 22% of patients received vocational rehabilitation services. On the other hand, the proportion of the population receiving treatment for depression went up dramatically in the 1990s, presumably decreasing the prevalence of untreated depression (Olfson et al. 2002).

## Canada

In 2000, Canada had a population of 31 million. In 1998, the country spent 9.3% of its GDP on health, representing a per capita health expenditure of $2,363 in international dollars (WHO 2001). Universal health care is available in Canada through the national health insurance program known as Medicare. The program is administered through the Ministries of Health of provincial and territorial governments, which results in considerable variation among the region-specific health plans even though they operate according to basic standards set by the federal government (Goering et al. 2000).

Large mental hospitals were the primary locus of mental health services until well into the 20th century. Deinstitutionalization in the second half of the century shifted care to general hospitals and to the community. The number of beds in provincial mental hospitals dropped by more than two-thirds (Goering et al. 2000). This history parallels that of the US, but in Canada the federal government never directly funded the development of community mental health centers (Goodwin 1997). Insufficient resource allocations have kept the country from achieving a well-developed community-based system, but the availability of community services varies between and within provinces (Goering et al. 2000).

Psychiatrists and general practitioners provide mental health services on a fee-for-service basis through the provincial health insurance plans. Because other mental health professionals are not paid in this way, nonphysician mental health professionals usually work in hospitals or agencies on a salaried basis (Goering et al. 2000). As in many countries, there is a serious problem of maldistribution of psychiatrists, with nonurban areas underserviced (Goering et al. 2000).

It is expected that there will be continued emphasis on community-based mental health care in Canada. However, because mental health care in Canada is not well funded and there have been moves to integrate health structures in some regions, there is now concern that existing mental health funding is at risk of reallocation to other health priorities (Goering et al. 2000).

## Japan

In 2000, Japan had a population of 127 million. In 1998, the country spent 7.5% of its GDP on health, representing a per capita health expenditure of $1,763 in international dollars (WHO 2001). In Japan, the health care, public assistance, and social security systems are all governed by the national Ministry of Health and Welfare but each system is administered locally (Kuno and Asukai 2000). Health insurance is universal through a pluralistic system that is funded privately and publicly but is closely regulated by the government. Only 1% of the population is on public assistance for health care but this percentage is larger for persons with psychiatric illnesses (Kuno and Asukai 2000).

Mental health care in Japan has long centered on long-term inpatient hospitalization. Until the 1960s, policies focused on increasing the number of psychiatric beds through the construction of private hospitals. This policy, in combination with Japan's universal health insurance coverage, was successful in securing access to inpatient psychiatric care. The per capita number of psychiatric beds is high (three times that of the US) and long-term stays remain common. Staffing levels on inpatient psychiatric units are low (51 staff per 100 beds versus 185 staff per 100 beds in the US). The costs of inpatient care are relatively low—a typical day of inpatient care costs only about 50% more than outpatient care (Kuno and Asukai 2000). Private service providers in the medical sector are the primary source of care for persons with mental disorders.

Providers are paid on a fee-for-service basis using a government-set fee schedule.

Since a major revision to the Mental Health Law in 1987, there have been consistent efforts to protect the human rights of psychiatric patients and to promote community-based treatment and rehabilitation services (Kuno and Asukai 2000). The mental health system in Japan is struggling to become more community-focused. The low cost of inpatient care means financial incentive to do this is limited. Mental illness is deeply stigmatized in Japan and cultural values about individual rights and responsibilities mean that people with severe mental disorders have great difficulty gaining social acceptance (Kuno and Asukai 2000). Together these factors suggest that there remains a strong bias towards inpatient care in Japan that is unlikely to change in the near future.

## Australia

In 2000, Australia had a population of 19 million. In 1998, the country spent 8.6% of its GDP on health, representing a per capita health expenditure of $2,080 in international dollars (WHO 2001). The Australian health care system has public and private components. Public sector services are funded through universal taxpayer-funded health insurance and Federal income tax. The national health insurance system provides free care in public hospitals and rebates on consultations with private medical practitioners (Whiteford et al. 2000). Private insurance, purchased by approximately one-third of the population, pays for private hospitalization and for a range of nonmedical outpatient services (Whiteford et al. 2000).

Australia developed a National Mental Health Strategy in 1992 that sought to increase spending on mental health care and to de-emphasize institutional care with growing community-based services. By the end of the first 5-year program of the National Strategy, overall spending on mental health care increased 30%, mental hospitals were down-sized, and spending on community services increased dramatically. The number of mental health clinicians providing community-based care increased by more than two-thirds (Whiteford et al. 2000, WHO 2001).

Australia is notable for its involvement of consumers in the planning, delivery, and evaluation of mental health services. Reports of abuses of the rights of consumers led to the incorporation of strategies to involve and empower consumers (Whiteford et al. 2000). Consumer Advisory Groups have been established in all states and territories to formalize a mechanism for feedback on implementation of the National Strategy. Implementation of formal mechanisms to involve consumers in local decision-making bodies is still in early stages, but has shown great progress in only a few years (Whiteford et al. 2000).

In 1992, a center for the management of first-episode psychosis opened in Melbourne. Based on evidence that early intervention improves outcomes, the program attempts to detect psychotic illnesses early and to intervene with appropriate low-dose medications and psychosocial interventions (Power et al. 1998). The center has a research goal of determining best practices for such early intervention (McGorry et al. 1996). The success of this model program has contributed to the inclusion of a plan to establish teams to intervene early in psychosis in the National Health Service of UK (NHS 2000).

## Developing Countries

### India

In 2000, India had a population of just over 1 billion. In 1998, the country spent 5.1% of its GDP on health, representing a per capita health expenditure of $110 in international dollars (WHO 2001).

India's billion people have access to mental health system with an infrastructure that is "minimal at best" (Ganju 2000). The country has 25 states, 6 union territories, and 1 national capital territory that together contain 476 districts. The country has several huge urban areas but remains largely rural. Primary health centers and subcenters that rely on trained paramedics to provide services are the cornerstone of the health care system in rural areas (Ganju 2000).

The mental health system in India was influenced by British colonial rule which led to the introduction of large mental hospitals in the 18th and 19th centuries. These hospitals were the main site of formal mental health care, although at the end of the colonial era in the late 1940s there were only 19 mental hospitals with a capacity of only about 10,000 in all of India. A severe inadequacy of mental health services continues into the 21st century (Ganju 2000).

In 1987, a progressive National Mental Health Act was passed that updated Indian law and represented an attempt to improve care for persons with mental illness. The goal was to ensure availability of basic mental health care by decentralizing and integrating mental health services in primary care settings, training of primary care personnel for the first level management of mental health problems, and promoting community participation in the development of mental health services. Funding, however, was extremely limited given the magnitude of unmet need (Nagaswami 1990). More than a decade later, the Act's provisions remain unevenly implemented (Ganju 2000). Change has been slow, large mental hospitals remain open and out-of-date, and the formal mental health system is still skeletal. The significant stigma of mental illness in India means that many persons with mental illness choose traditional healers rather than biomedical professionals when seeking help (Chadda et al. 2001).

An expansion of mental hospitals in India has been accompanied by a significant growth in general hospital psychiatric units. Community care is expanding as well. The National Mental Health Act promoted the delivery of mental health care by primary care providers, and pilot projects of this model have been implemented and replicated. Increase in the number of related court cases and new laws indicate that India has moved to promote humane care in the community. Treatment has replaced custodial care as the goal (Ganju 2000).

The mental health infrastructure in India remains rudimentary and varies widely among the states. Community care is extremely limited throughout the vast majority of the country. Qualified personnel are in extremely short supply. Ganju (2000) reported that there are only 1,500 psychiatrists in the country and only about 500 clinical psychologists. Psychiatric social workers and psychiatric nurses are even rarer.

Persons with severe mental illness have very few or-ganized, community-based services for their rehabilitation. Most of the mental hospitals have campus-based occupa-tional and vocational rehabilitation programs (Dunlap 1990). Several teaching centers (e.g., the National Institute of Mental Health and Neurosciences in Bangalore, the Central Institute of Psychiatry in Ranchi, and the Institute of Mental Health in Chennai) operate occupational and psychosocial rehabilitation programs each with a modest capacity. A small number of voluntary agencies, mostly urban-based and poorly funded, also provide assistance to persons with severe mental illness.

In India, like many other developing countries, no suitable, cost-effective, easily replicable model of rehabili-tation for people who are severely mentally ill has emerged. Western models cannot be transplanted in their entirety due to the wide disparity in manpower and funding resources in India relative to wealthier countries (Higginbotham 1984). This situation is reinforced by national problems of pov-erty, inadequate housing, unemployment, negative social attitudes towards mental illness, and extreme geographic disparities in the distribution of manpower and facilities (Nagaswami 1990).

Despite these seemingly staggering obstacles and bar-riers, a number of innovative community-based treatment and rehabilitation programs have been developed in various locales throughout India (Nagaswami 1990, Dunlap 1990). These projects attempt to use existing health workers, vil-lage leaders, employers, clergy, indigenous healers, and family members, rather than create an additional mental health infrastructure.

## China

In 2000, China had a population of almost 1.3 billion. In 1998, the country spent 4.5% of its GDP on health, repre-senting a per capita health expenditure of $143 in inter-national dollars (WHO 2001).

Access to mental health treatment is severely limited throughout China, although service systems are relatively well developed in a few large cities (Pearson and Phillips 1994). Data on system capacity and on the number of providers in China are not reliable because mental health services are provided through several national ministries and there is no central mental health authority (Pearson and Phillips 1994). Psychiatric services are generally pro-vided in psychiatric hospitals located in urban locations (Pearson and Phillips 1994). Both inpatient and outpatient treatment are unavailable to the vast majority of persons with mental illness in China (Pearson 1995).

Mental health care in China emphasizes collective over individual interests. Officially, community treatment and rehabilitation have replaced institutionalization and control of social disruption as the preferred site and goal of the mental health system, but control of dangerous behaviors, limiting social problems, and relapse prevention remain the highest priorities (Pearson and Phillips 1994). The severe stigma of mental illness in China is a significant barrier to seeking mental health treatment for persons with mental disorders (Phillips et al. 1997, Pearson 1995).

Economic reforms in China that began in 1978 after the cultural revolution accelerated long-standing trends and intensified the economic rationing of health services.

Medical treatment was never free or universal in China but price controls and state subsidies prior to 1978 meant that treatment was far more affordable than now. In China, health insurance is linked to employment. Only 10 to 15% of people have comprehensive health insurance that covers psychiatric hospitalization (Pearson and Phillips 1994).

In the current economic climate, hospitals must oper-ate like other businesses in order to become self-sufficient (Phillips et al. 1997). The requirement for economic self-sufficiency has led to competition for paying patients and has created incentives for hospitals and doctors to provide treatments for which they can collect fees, for example, medications and electroconvulsive therapy (Pearson and Phillips 1994). There are incentives to prolong hospitaliza-tions, and insured patients have been shown to have longer lengths of stay than patients who are self-pay (Phillips et al. 1994). Because community-based treatment has less revenue-producing potential than inpatient treatment, and because outpatient treatment may reduce the need for more lucrative inpatient services, there is little incentive for a hospital to provide outpatient services (Pearson and Phillips 1994). The costs of hospitalization and psychiatric treatment increased dramatically between 1984 and 1993 (Phillips et al. 1997).

Formal mental health services are provided almost exclusively by doctors and nurses. There are very few psy-chologists, social workers, or occupational therapists due to policies that outlawed social sciences after the founding of the People's Republic of China in 1949 (Pearson 1995). Mental health professionals use a biological model of care that developed primarily while social sciences were banned in the post-1949 era (Pearson 1995).

Mental hospitals in China are almost always free-standing—general hospitals do not have psychiatric wards (Phillips et al. 1997). Although most resources are allocated for inpatient treatment, the supply of hospital beds is low (Pearson 1995). One estimate is that there are about 1.1 psychiatric hospital beds per 10,000 population (Pearson and Phillips 1994). In China, large scale institutionalization of persons with psychiatric disorders in mental hospitals never occurred (Pearson and Phillips 1994).

Only a few of the largest urban centers have community-based mental health treatment programs (Yucan et al. 1990). Community-based services are "virtually nonexis-tent" in rural areas (Pearson and Phillips 1994). Because the vast majority of people with mental illness live with family members who provide most of their long-term care, the rising cost of treatment and the decline in insurance coverage since the economic reforms began in 1978 have placed a great burden on families (Phillips et al. 1997, Pearson and Phillips 1994).

Rehabilitation services are also rare beyond a few model programs (Pearson and Phillips 1994). Although rehabilitation is emphasized in official policy, inadequate resources have meant that changes have not been imple-mented. Rehabilitation in China is occupational rather than psychosocial—the goal of reintegration into society re-quires a job (Pearson and Phillips 1994). Because living with family is the socially valued arrangement, the Western goal of helping patients to live independently is not impor-tant in China.

## Nigeria

In 2000, Nigeria had a population of 114 million. In 1998, the country spent 2.1% of its GDP on health, representing a per capita health expenditure of only $18 in international dollars (WHO 2001).

Nigeria's economic dependence on oil production, declines in international oil prices, and persistent political upheavals have greatly limited government spending on mental health care. Most psychiatrists in Nigeria practice in tertiary institutions in urban centers (Abiodun 1995). Mental health services are largely hospital based; very few psychiatric services are available in general hospital units and in primary health care centers. In 1990, there were a total of 27 hospitals providing psychiatric services and a workforce of approximately 2,000 mental health professionals (Ohaeri and Odejide 1993). There were 10 state psychiatric institutions, nine university teaching hospitals, four general hospital psychiatric units, and four specialty hospitals. The mental health professionals were 90% psychiatric nurses, 6% psychiatrists or medical doctors, and 4% social workers or psychologists. As of 1990, there were no specialty community-based mental health centers. Primary health care centers in Nigeria are staffed by health workers with very basic medical and psychiatric training.

Many segments of the Nigerian population continue to seek out traditional and religious healers for the treatment of mental illness, coming to psychiatric facilities only after first receiving care from these healers (Gureje et al. 1995, Abiodun 1995). Efforts have been made to engage traditional healers and to encourage them to make referrals for psychiatric care.

In Nigeria, the extended family is the only consistent source of social support for the mentally ill (Jegede et al. 1985). In the 1950s, the highly acclaimed Aro village system was created as an innovative effort to involve families in the care of members who were hospitalized with a severe mental illness (Lambo 1964, Jegede 1981). The Aro village system was based upon two main considerations: (1) the existence of a closely knit kinship system that prescribed definite roles and mutual obligations and (2) the need to have a simple treatment method that took local customs into consideration. The village system started as a day hospital program and then evolved into a comprehensive village-based service system. Initially four villages surrounding Aro Hospital, a 200-bed psychiatric hospital, participated. Patients were admitted to the villages on the condition that a relative would come to live there to look after their basic needs and to take the patient to and from the hospital each day. Each village could accommodate 200 to 300 patients. Patients stayed until both staff and relatives were satisfied that the patient was well enough to go home. Soon clinics were established in the villages and the emphasis was on treating the patient in the village without the patient going to the hospital at all. Traditional healers helped develop social and group activities for the patients. Health councils that included village elders and hospital staff planned and administered the clinics and public health projects.

Although the Aro village system was never subjected to a rigorous comparative evaluation, purported advantages included increased social integration and acceptance of the patient, relatively quick recovery, reduction of the risk of social disability, and low cost (Jegede 1981). These possible advantages helped lead to the spread of the village system in other African countries, including Tanzania (Kilonzo and Simmons 1998).

Although nationwide expansion of this program in Nigeria was planned, by the mid-1980s only one of the original villages was still operational (Jegede 1981, Jegede et al. 1985). There were many reasons for the demise of the Aro village system, including personnel turnover and lack of funding. In addition, a number of societal changes combined to erode the agrarian underpinnings of the village system (Jegede 1981). Urbanization, the growth of a wage economy, and the consequent difficulty of finding relatives willing to travel to rural areas to stay with patients indefinitely are contemporary barriers to the Aro village model.

Homelessness among serious mentally ill persons cut off from family ties and other social supports has been a growing problem in Nigeria since the early 1980s (Jegede et al. 1985). The pattern is similar to that in the West— frequent relapses alienate patients from family and society at large, they are subject to social disgrace and lose jobs and spouses, and become vagrants or are institutionalized in large mental hospitals or prisons (Odejide et al. 1983).

## Summary/Conclusion

Industrialized and later developing countries all have one thing in common—their mental health resources are grossly inadequate. There are striking differences across countries, but there is a worldwide shortage of mental health personnel, services, and other resources for the prevention and treatment of mental disorders. In virtually every country, in spite of the high prevalence of mental illness and the human and economic burden of these disorders, mental health services are inferior to general health services.

There is room for modest optimism about mental health care and the fate of persons with mental disorders. The WHO (2001), the US IOM (2001), and the US Surgeon General (US Department of Health and Human Services 1999) have all recently published reports that highlight the importance of mental health and make reasonable suggestions for making progress. Knowledge about the epidemiology and etiology of mental disorders, as noted in other parts of this text, continues to grow. Information on evidence-based practices is now widely disseminated in Western countries and some progress has been demonstrated. For example, the rate of persons treated for depression in the US has increased dramatically in recent years (Olfson et al. 2002).

Hope for progress is less substantial in developing countries. However, the World Health Report 2001 (WHO 2001) describes positive changes in Uganda in the late 1990s, including integration of mental health services into primary care, inclusion of psychotropic drugs on the essential drugs list, a plan to include mental health beds in new regional hospitals, and a reduction in capacity of the large national mental hospital. Iran is promoting a nationwide program to integrate mental health care into primary health care settings (WHO 2001). Guinea-Bissau successfully did this in the 1980s (IOM 2001). Pakistan conducted a demonstration project to integrate mental and primary health care (IOM 2001). Tanzania had considerable success adapting the Aro village model of rehabilitation (Kilonzo and Simmons 1998).

There are dangers as well. Ongoing global trends towards market-based medical care and shrinking social welfare systems do not bode well for persons with mental illness. Cost-saving efforts in medical care systems, including managed care in the US and similar efforts elsewhere, result in a narrow focus on biomedical interventions that ignore important social aspects of illness and recovery. For example, Phillips and colleagues (1997) demonstrated that market-based reforms in combination with economic rationing led to greater financial burdens for the families of Chinese persons with severe mental illness. Systems that require out-of-pocket payments for treatment are particularly troublesome for persons with mental disorders, who are more likely than others to live in poverty and who may want to avoid treatment because of its associated stigma (WHO 2001)

The WHO (2001) demonstrated that while most countries have developed a national mental health policy, 41% have not. Even among the nations that have proposed national plans for the care of people with mental illness, funding for these plans is invariably inadequate. Resource limitations continue to mean that services will be targeted only at the most disruptive or deviant individuals in spite of information about the huge burden of a wide range of mental disorders. Resource-poor nations are not likely to make treatment of mental disorders a priority because of a perception of more pressing needs. The recent WHO and IOM reports are intended to alter this perception.

In summary, mental health services are suboptimal worldwide except for a few model programs. The most widely promoted strategy for improving the treatment of persons with mental disorders worldwide is the integration of mental health care into primary care settings. This is a practical approach because most countries have an existing primary care system even though these vary widely within and between countries (IOM 2001). There is considerable evidence that primary health workers can be trained to recognize, treat, and refer common mental disorders, but that long-term success will depend upon ongoing guidance, support, and monitoring from secondary and tertiary care centers. Links between primary care clinicians and the traditional healers who are commonly consulted in many countries are also desirable so that the strengths of each may be optimized. Although effective, affordable, and humane treatments and systems are attainable, only incremental and modest progress towards these goals is likely in the near future (IOM 2001).

## References

Abiodun O (1995) Pathways to mental health care in Nigeria. Psychiatr Serv 46(8), 823–826.

Burti L and Benson P (1996) Psychiatric reform in Italy: Developments since 1978. Int J Law Psychiatr 19(3–4), 373–390.

Chadda RK, Agarwal V, Singh MC, et al. (2001) Help seeking behavior of psychiatric patients before seeking care at a mental hospital. Int J Soc Psychiatr 47(4), 71–78.

De Girolamo G and Cozza M (2000) The Italian psychiatric reform: A 20-year perspective. Int J Psychiatr Law 23(304), 197–314.

De Salvia D and Barbato A (1993) Recent trends in mental health services in Italy: An analysis of national and local data. Can J Psychiatr 38 (Apr), 195–202.

Dunlap D (1990) Rural psychiatric rehabilitation and the interface of community development and rehabilitation services. Psychosoc Rehabil J 14(1), 68–90.

Ganju V (2000) The mental health system in India: History, current system, and prospects. Int J Psychiatr Law, 23(3–4), 393–402.

Goldman H, Morrissey J, and Bachrach L (1983) Deinstitutionalization in international perspective: Variations on a theme. Int J Ment Health 11(4), 153–165.

Goering P, Wasylenki D, and Durbin J (2000) Canada's mental health system. Int J Psychiatr Law, 23(3–4), 345–359.

Goodwin S (1997) Comparative Mental Health Policy: From Institutional to Community Care. Sage Publications, London.

Gureje O, Acha R, and Odejide O (1995) Pathways to psychiatric care in Ibadan, Nigeria. Trop Geogr Med 47(3), 125–129.

Harrison G, Hopper K, Craig T, et al. (2001) Recovery from psychotic illness: A 15- and 25-year international follow-up study. Br J Psychiatr 178, 506–517.

Higginbotham HN (1984) Third World Challenge to Psychiatry: Culture Accommodation and Mental Health Care. East–West Center, University of Hawaii, Honolulu, HI.

Hollingsworth EJ (1996) Mental health services in England: The 1990s. Int J Law Psychiatr 19, 309–325.

Institute of Medicine (2001) Neurologic, Psychiatric, and Developmental Disorders: Meeting the Challenge in the Developing World. National Academy Press, Washington DC.

Jablensky A, Sartorius N, Ernberg G, et al. (1992) Schizophrenia: Manifestations, incidence and course in different cultures: A World Health Organization ten-country study. Psychol Med Monogr (Suppl 20).

Jegede R (1981) Aro village system of community psychiatry in perspective. Can J Psychiatr 26, 173–177.

Jegede R, Williams A, and Sijuwola A (1985) Recent developments in the care, treatment, and rehabilitation of the chronically mentally ill in Nigeria. Hosp Comm Psychiatr 36(6), 658–661.

Kilonzo GP and Simmons N (1998) Development of mental health services in Tanzania: A reappraisal for the future. Soc Sci Med 47, 419–428.

Knapp M (1997) Costs of schizophrenia. Br J Psychiatr 171, 509–518.

Kuno E and Asukai N (2000) Efforts toward building a community-based mental health system in Japan. Int J Psychiatr Law 23(3–4), 361–373.

Lambo T (1964) The village at Aro. Lancet 2, 513–514.

Leff J (2001) Cultural influences on schizophrenia. In Comprehensive Care of Schizophrenia, Lieberman J and Murray R (eds). Martin Dunitz, London.

Lefley H (1992) Expressed emotion: Conceptual, clinical, and social policy issues. Hosp Comm Psychiatr 43, 591–598

Lefley HP (1999) Mental health systems in cross-cultural context. In A Handbook for the Study of Mental Health: Social Contexts, Theories, and Systems, Scheid T and Horwitz A (eds). Oxford, New York.

Lehman AF and Steinwachs DM (1998) Patterns of usual care for schizophrenia: Initial results from the Schizophrenia Patient Outcomes (PORT) Client Survey. Schizophr Bull 24(1), 11–20.

Manderscheid RW, Henderson MH, Witkin MH, et al. (2000) The US mental health system of the 1990s: The challenges of managed care. Int J Psychiatr Law, 23(3–4), 245–259.

McColloch A, Muijen M, and Harper H (2000) New developments in mental health policy in the United Kingdom. Int J Psychiatr Law 23(3–4), 261–276.

McGorry PD, Edwards J, Mihalopoulos C, et al. (1996) EPPIC: An evolving system of early detection and optimal management. Schizophr Bull 22(2), 305–326.

Mosher L (1983) Radical deinstitutionalization: The Italian experience. Int J Ment Health 11, 129–136.

Murray C and Lopez A (eds) (1996) The Global Burden of Disease. Harvard Press, Boston.

Nagaswami V (1990) Integration of psychosocial rehabilitation in national health care programmes. Psychosoc Rehabil J 14(1), 53–65.

National Health Service (2000) The NHS Plan. (Available at: www.nhs.uk/nationalplan/nhsplan.htm)

Odejide A, Jegede R, and Sijuwola A (1983) Deinstitutionalization: A perspective from Nigeria. Int J Ment Health 11(4), 98–107.

Ohaeri J and Odejide O (1993) Admissions for drug and alcohol-related problems in Nigerian psychiatric care facilities in one year. Drug Alcohol Depend 31, 101–109.

Olfson M, Marcus SC, Druss B, et al. (2002) National trends in the outpatient treatment of depression. J Am Med Assoc 287(2), 203–209.

Pearson V (1995) Mental Health in China: State Policies, Professional Services and Family Responsibilities. Gaskell, London.

Pearson V and Phillips MR (1994) The social context of psychiatric rehabilitation in China. Br J Psychiatr 164(Suppl 24), 11–18.

Phillips MR, Lu SH, and Wang RW (1997) Economic reforms and the acute inpatient care of patients with schizophrenia: The Chinese experience. Am J Psychiatr 154, 1228–1234.

Power P, Elkins K, Adlard S, et al. (1998) Analysis of the initial treatment phase in first-episode psychosis. Br J Psychiatr 172(Suppl 33), 71–76.

Rogers A and Pilgrim D (1996) Mental Health Policy in Britain. St. Martin's Press, New York.

Rothbard A and Kuno E (2000) The success of deinstitutionalization: Empirical findings from case studies on state hospital closures. Int J Psychiatr Law 23(3–4), 329–344.

Sartorius N and Harding T (1983) The WHO collaborative study on strategies for extending mental health care. Am J Psychiatr 140, 1470–1473.

Sartorius N, Gulbinat W, Harrison G, et al. (1996) Long-term follow-up of schizophrenia in 16 countries. A description of the International Study of Schizophrenia conducted by the World Health Organization. Soc Psychiatr Psychiatr Epidemiol 31, 249–258.

US Department of Health and Human Services (1999) Mental Health: A Report of Surgeon General US Department of Health and Human Services, Substance Abuse and Mental Health Services Administration/Center for Mental Health Services, National Institute of Health, Rockville. (Available online at: www.surgeongeneral.gov/library/mental-health/home.html)

Whiteford H, Thompson I, and Casey D (2000) The Australian mental health system. Int J Psychiatr Law 23(3–4), 403–417.

World Health Organization (2001) The World Health Report 2001. Mental Health: New Understanding, New Hope. World Health Organization, Geneva.

Yucan S, Changhui C, Esixi Z, et al. (1990) An example of a community-based health/home care programme. Psychosoc Rehabil J 14, 29–34.

SECTION **VII**

Jacqueline Maus Feldman
Stephen M. Goldfinger, Section Editors

*Special Clinical
Settings and
Challenges*

# 108 Social Context of Psychiatric Practice

Stephen M. Goldfinger
Jacqueline Maus Feldman
J. Arturo Silva

"In order to cure the human body, it is necessary to have the knowledge of the whole of things."

*Hippocrates*

## Context as a Paradigm: Moving from Universalism to Relativism

In this section, we attempt to bridge the gap between psychiatric diagnosis and treatment and the broader social, economic, and political spheres in which practice occurs. The nature of the clinical problems that we address and the interventions that we offer must always be seen within the context of our patients' lives. By its very nature, psychiatry is characterized by a tension resulting from its focus on the individual as a sociocultural being. There is general acceptance that all human beings possess a set of universal developmental issues and interpsychic structures and that these characteristics apply to all people, across all historical times, and throughout all cultural contexts. This basic conceptual model—universalism—is predicated on the belief that all members of the human species think and feel in a qualitatively similar fashion. In essence, all human behavior may be seen as fundamentally similar and the human species intrinsically possesses certain expectable behavioral paradigms, variations from which may, in certain instances, be deemed to be "pathological."

In contrast, relativism assumes that behaviors are contextually dependent and must be seen from the viewpoint of cultural, economic, political, and historical factors. The degree to which we subscribe to either a universalistic or a relativistic perspective can have far-reaching consequences on the way in which we view our patients, their illnesses, and the kinds of interventions needed.

Modern American psychiatry is strongly oriented towards nosology. It is influenced by a phenomenological classification of mental illness in which successful diagnosis is arrived at by identifying a symptom cluster within the individual. It often follows the biological model, in which the basic unit of study is the organism and its components. Both the nosological and the biological views presume a more or less universally applicable approach to understanding the organism, and one in which relativistic views are given short shrift. Psychotherapeutic approaches emphasize understanding the patient, not only as a function of the psychodynamics of the individual but also as a function of the important microenvironmental structure, such as the nuclear family. But even in such evaluations, the inherent notions of what constitutes a family frequently reflect an inherent bias toward the person and away from relativistic concerns. What is critical is that we recognize the need to broaden our perspective and to more fully include the sociocultural dimension in our conceptual thinking, therapeutic interactions, and service delivery design.

## The Impact of Contextual Diversity

The US, long a country of immigrants, is becoming increasingly diverse in the array of ethnic and cultural backgrounds of its citizens. Although the country has considered itself a melting pot, in fact many of its citizens live in discrete communities representing unique social norms, familial structures, and interpersonal expectations. Even for those who have assimilated, their beliefs, experiences of privilege and oppression, and expectations of themselves and others remain a part of their identity and identification. Similarly, despite widely held views of the US as a land of opportunity, poverty remains widespread and economic disaffiliation widely experienced. Those living at the extremes of impoverishment—the homeless or those on the edge of economic survival—have been recognized as experiencing their world and themselves as quite different from those for whom daily survival is not an issue.

Critics of medical research and psychiatric practice raise their voices against what they view as the white male centrism of our theoretical concepts and clinical approaches. Work that focuses on the unique issues of special groups constantly reminds us of the need to reexamine and modify our approaches to encompass the diversity and identifications of those we serve. Women, sexual minorities, those of strong spiritual and religious orientations, and members of other special groups (rural or correctional populations, those with chronic medical illnesses or lives complicated by substance abuse, those struggling with end-of-life issues) merit considerable attention in how we develop treatment plans, establish therapeutic alliances, and design systems of care.

---

### Clinical Vignette 1

Ms. E was a Scottish-American from a working class family; her husband, Mr. O, a Yoruba from a professional family in Cameroon, had immigrated to the US for college. They had three school-age children, and both worked as middle-level professionals. Mr. O maintained close family ties, here and abroad; most of Ms. E's family had cut her off when she had married an African.

Ms. E resented Mr. O's welcoming relatives who came uninvited from Cameroon for college or medical care and stayed with them for months or years without her consent. She was outraged that Mr. O made such major decisions without consulting her. Her friends condemned Mr. O as a sexist, whose unilateral decisions were especially intolerable because his work hours put primary responsibility for the visitors on Ms. E. Viewing the situation through a feminist lens alone, the therapist might have joined the condemnation, moved Mr. O toward collaboration with Ms. E, and encouraged her to be more assertive. But the therapist realized her need to respect the culture of her patient and to utilize Mr. O's Yoruba lens to understand this family more fully. Mr. O's father was polygamous; his two wives had raised their many children together. Like members of many traditional societies, the Yoruba do not distinguish the immediate family from the extended family, and their bonds of mutual obligation go deep. Mr. O's older siblings had paid for his education, ensuring him of a career after their father's death. It would be unthinkable to turn away their children and grandchildren when they needed help (in Cameroon, reciprocal obligations ensured Mr. O's financial stability; in the US, they slowed his nuclear family's upward mobility). Mr. O's relatives viewed Ms. E's position as racist, uncaring, ungrateful, selfish, and irresponsible. For them, concerns about relatives, impact on household finances, upward mobility, self-determination, and privacy were insignificant compared with collective responsibility and well being.

Who was right? Ms. E and her friends, and Mr. O and his relatives, were all justified within their respective cultural frameworks, and completely wrong in each other's. In an old story, a quarreling couple approached the rabbi (the judge and family therapist of Eastern European *shtetls* or Jewish ghettos) to resolve their dispute. He listened carefully to the husband's argument, nodded wisely, and intoned, "You are right." The wife protested his deciding without hearing her side of the story, which she then told. The rabbi listened carefully and nodded, saying "You are right," and sent the confused couple on their way. The rabbi's wife, who had been eavesdropping in the kitchen, strode in to upbraid her husband: How could he say both were right when they were in such obvious disagreement with each other? He listened thoughtfully to his wife's criticism and nodded, "You are also right!"

Mr. O and Ms. E condemned each other on the basis of unspoken and contradictory rules of family relations and individual rights. Treatment helped them clarify their frames of reference, detoxify their ethnocentric interpretations, and address their contradictory values and needs collaboratively and respectfully.

---

Increasingly in medicine, attention is being focused on the difference between the efficacy and the effectiveness of treatment interventions. That which works in the "pure culture" of the laboratory or the clinical research setting, where external parameters, dosages, and a patient's adherence are carefully controlled, may be far less effective when offered as a treatment in naturalistic environments. The clinical conditions, prescribed medication dosage, and route and frequency of drug administration may be the same; what differs is a combination of the patient's compliance and the uncontrolled activities of the individual in the real world. The clinical characteristics of subjects may contribute to such variation, but often it is their belief system about health and illness, their access to familial or other social supports in the community, their economic and residential stability, and the environmental and cultural context in which they live that contributes most to their participation in treatment. It is now being widely acknowledged that if we are to design interventions that work outside of the research setting, such factors can no longer be ignored. The recent funding and initiation of the CATIE project by the National Institute of Mental Health (NIMH), which explores the efficacy of medications within much less rigorously controlled (and hence more naturalistic) settings, underscores our increasing understanding of the impact of context on the ultimate behavior of individuals.

---

### Clinical Vignette 2

Dr. S, a kind-hearted and well-intentioned third-year resident, is now on his third week of a rotation in a local municipal shelter. At the request of shelter staff, he has just completed an evaluation of Mr. K and is going over his impressions with his supervisor to help develop a treatment plan.

"Mr. K is a 33-year-old man who tells me that he has been drinking excessively for about the last 4 years. He has been hospitalized previously three different times, each in association with a period of heavy drinking. In addition, he told me that he had been arrested 'about 10 times' but was always released after a couple of days. He looks somewhat emaciated and quite disheveled, with several days' growth of beard. He is rather wildly dressed with mismatched shirt, loud pants, and many layers of clothing. He was oriented to place and person but did not know what day of the week it was. He told me that he has been quite depressed for 'a long time.' He has trouble sleeping, said that he has lost about 15 pounds in the last 6 months, and is constantly ruminating on what a failure he is. He was referred to a local outpatient clinic but stopped showing up for appointments. I think he probably has a major depressive disorder and, given the arrests, some sociopathic features. However, I think that he will be difficult to treat, given his history of noncompliance. Besides, he seemed 'sort of paranoid' about me . . . quite suspicious about my motives and who I was."

The supervisor thought that it was important to help Dr. S broaden his perspective in understanding the contributions of homelessness to people's clinical presentation. He began by discussing Mr. K's appearance. Was Dr. S aware that there were only six sinks available for washing up in this shelter, which had sleeping facilities for

800? Did he know that Mr. K's clothing came from a "free clothing box" and that, because he was not allowed to remain in the shelter during the day, Mr. K was required to spend a great deal of his time outdoors on the streets, despite the bitter cold? Did he recognize that Mr. K's difficulty in sleeping might be related to the fact that he spent nights on a cot in a room shared with the other 800 shelter residents? Did he know that Mr. K's arrests had all been for loitering, urinating in public, and public drunkenness, all far more understandable in an individual who spends his days on the streets?

As Dr. S more clearly described Mr. K's "paranoid responses," the supervisor realized that Mr. K believed that he was being evaluated for potential involuntary hospitalization. As they interviewed Mr. K together, they learned that the outpatient clinic to which he was referred was 18 blocks away. Mr. K described how his appointment at the medication clinic that he was to attend was scheduled at the same time the neighborhood's only soup kitchen served its lunch. As they confronted Mr. K's suspiciousness regarding why he was being evaluated, Mr. K became less guarded and more open, as did Dr. S.

Psychiatry, with its targets of the brain, the mind, and behavior, is perhaps the field of medicine most sensitive to these individual variations in patients and to the influences of nonbiological forces on their lives. The interplay between physiological response and psychological response, the parallel effectiveness of pharmacological and interpersonal treatments, and the recognition of the contributions of individuals' cultural and spiritual beliefs profoundly influence all elements of our work. Hippocrates's admonition, "In order to cure the human body, it is necessary to have the knowledge of the whole of things," retains its timeliness today, although our concept of how broadly "the whole of things" must be interpreted has surely expanded.

Our societal, and perhaps our professional, view of diversity has broadened to acknowledge a wider array of differences than were historically recognized. Clearly, racial and ethnic or cultural dissimilarities are often most obvious and frequently cited. Therapist–patient discordance and the issues that such therapeutic dyads raise have been the topic of multiple studies. Resulting errors in diagnosis, countertherapeutic clinical work, and such concepts as "hallucinatory whitening" of minority psychiatrists or "extraterrestrialization" of black residents by the white patients they treat have been well documented. However, restricting understanding of the contributions of clinician–patient differences to race and ethnicity needlessly foreshortens our perspective and may lead to a false sense of clinical certainty and reduced therapeutic effectiveness.

Social class, gender, immigration status, extremes of poverty and homelessness, and even religious beliefs may result in dramatically altered views of one's world and one's place in it. Woody Allen in his classic film *Annie Hall* has portrayed what may be one of the clearest examples of the role of cultural expectation and personal background in individual perception. In a scene in which the two protagonists—one a reserved WASP and the other a boisterous Jew—visit each other's homes for dinner, the viewer easily recognizes how each character's family of origin appears through the eyes of the other. Even in the context of two upper middle class white US-born characters, differences in family of origin and attitudes toward verbalizing feelings, in respecting an individual's "space," and in accepted norms of interpersonal discourse may be staggering. Yet if we are to be able as clinicians to understand and to offer our patients a sense of being understood, we must, at a minimum, be constantly vigilant of how our mutual perceptions and expectations color every aspect of our clinical interactions.

It is not our intention here to address all of the multitude of subgroups and subcultures of our patients, or visit each unique clinical setting or challenge. The illnesses we treat, the biological interventions we offer, and the psychotherapeutic treatments we provide must reflect and are inherently influenced by an enormous number of individual and group differences, environmental contexts, complicating factors, and burgeoning treatment options. Even our underlying basic assumptions about the varying nature of the human psyche may be more culturally influenced than we recognize. Doi (1971), a psychoanalyst in Japan, in his classic work *The Anatomy of Dependence*, proposed that the core psychic structure of Japanese individuals differs from that of Westerners. Furthermore, as noted elsewhere in this text, even the necessary dosages of medications may need to be adjusted to take into account biological differences across populations. The sorts of interventions offered in family therapy to an extended Italian family will differ dramatically from those most appropriate for persons living in a traditional Chinese household.

As one considers the material in the chapters that follow, as with the earlier chapters, an ongoing awareness of the context- and culture-bound nature of psychiatric work is essential. Maintaining a focus on the social dimension of the biopsychosocial model poses a challenge to those who are more comfortable and familiar with the science of biology and the theoretical constructs of psychotherapy. Yet, without such an integrated approach, our ability to understand each patient as an individual will be limited and our clinical effectiveness will be diminished.

## References

Chang P, et al. Treatment Considerations with Culturally Diverse Populations (an annotated bibliography). Available from the California School of Professional Psychology, Alameda, CA.

Comas-Dias L and Greene B (1994) Women of Color: Integrating Ethnic and Gender Identities in Psychotherapy. Guilford Press, New York.

Doi T (1971) The Anatomy of Dependence. Kodansha International, Tokyo.

Gaw A (ed) (1996) Culture, Ethnicity and Mental Illness. American Psychiatric Press, Washington DC.

Kliman J (1994) The interweaving of gender, class and race in family therapy. In Women in Context, Mirkin MP (ed). Guilford Press, New York, pp. 25–47.

Lamb HR, Bachrach LL, and Kass F (eds) (1992) Treating the Homeless Mentally Ill. American Psychiatric Press, Washington DC.

Marsella AJ (1994) Amidst Peril and Pain: The Mental Health and Well-being of the World Refugees. American Psychological Association, Washington DC.

Ruiz P (section ed) (1995) Cross-cultural psychiatry. In American Psychiatric Press Review of Psychiatry, Vol. 14, Oldham J and Riba M (eds). American Psychiatric Press, Washington DC, pp. 467–476.

# 109 ● ● Organization and Financing of Mental Health Care

Michael F. Hogan
Ann Kerr Morrison

Understanding the organization and financing of care is becoming necessary for psychiatrists and other mental health professionals. The nature of many psychiatric illnesses, especially the most serious disorders, have a longitudinal course and episodic nature which often require care that cuts across many outpatient and inpatient settings. The extraordinarily disabling effects of these conditions require coordination with rehabilitative and other care systems and an appreciation of how systems are organized and financed. At the same time, these patterns of care are changing and becoming more complex. Increasingly, the factors of financing, reimbursement, and service organization must be appreciated to deliver or arrange adequate care.

Astrachan commented on this issue more than 2 decades ago, noting that "the future of health care organizations lies primarily in their members' clinical competency and commitment to excellent practice, but is also dependent on their knowledge of such administrative tasks as planning and budgeting, and their management of the physical plant and its employees" (Astrachan 1980). Yet developments in recent years have made these issues even more pivotal than Astrachan anticipated. Economic trends have led to a more significant "corporate presence" in health care, and psychiatry is no exception. Judgments about care of patients and treatment options must consider the cost and efficacy of care, both in the short term and in the course of illness.

The dominant approach to financing health care in the US is private insurance. This is a recent development compared with the long history of mental health care. Since its origins in a single plan at Baylor Hospital in 1929, developed to serve teachers at the University of Texas, private insurance coverage has grown dramatically to become the major financing approach for health care in the US. Fee-for-service reimbursement for physicians and hospitals has been the prevalent payment approach. As this chapter will indicate, these strategies are changing rapidly. Regulation of insurance coverage has increased and will continue to evolve as health care is reformed. Providers are joining together or being organized in groups to compete for contracts based on specialty expertise, price, and efficiency. Hospitals and indeed other services are increasingly owned and influenced by investors. The advent of third-party reviewers and "gatekeepers" of care further complicates the organization and financing of care. Finally, payers and patients search for arrangements to increase quality and decrease costs, leading to continual competition among purchasers and providers. In this environment, the psychiatrist must be aware of financing, payment, and organizational issues to survive and to provide quality care. Current trends also imply that psychiatrists will function less as solo practitioners but more as diagnosticians and care coordinators as well as caregivers.

Historical and political factors have also shaped the evolution of the modern mental health system. To appreciate the impact and effect of these factors, some historical review is essential. An understanding of the dynamics and tensions that continue to shape how care is provided is an important complement to clinical skills and an appreciation of organizational and financing factors.

## Historical Trends and Forces in Mental Health

Although theories and practices in mental health care can be traced back to thousands of years, historical trends with clear relevance for today can be found starting in the 18th and 19th centuries. As with many other aspects of culture, European influences are generally thought to have had the most impact on US practices and have certainly been documented best.

## Important European Influences

Most descriptions of European mental health practices that influenced care in Colonial America focus on the philosophy of moral treatment articulated by Philippe Pinel in France and Samuel Tuke in England. Moral treatment rested on a belief that mental illness resulted in large measure from environmental influences and that it was curable through humane care in an orderly, calm, and supportive milieu. One of the most powerful images of mental health reform is of Pinel removing the chains from the insane in 17th century France. Tuke was a founder of the York Retreat in York, England, and wrote of this experience in his 1813 work, *Description of the Retreat*. The York Retreat, a Quaker charitable institution, was established in the moral treatment philosophy as a facility where the mentally ill could be removed from the stresses and strains that were thought to cause mental illness and receive support and instruction in a complete milieu of supportive treatment.

It is clear that Pinel's treatment philosophy and the concept of the retreat or asylum had a significant effect in America. Such facilities as the Pennsylvania Hospital (1751), McLean Hospital in Boston (1818), and the Hartford Retreat (1844) were established in this tradition. In fact, the American Psychiatric Association had its roots in this tradition, being formed in 1844 as the Association of Medical Superintendents of American Institutions for the Insane.

These highlights of professional leadership in mental health care must be viewed in the context of the political and social influences on mental health care. How did the cruel custodial facilities develop that required the heroic reform of Pinel, and what patterns of community neglect required the creation of asylums? How did these trends influence the course of US mental health care well into the 20th century? Foucault (1965) has chronicled these developments and shown that the treatment of the mentally ill in Europe was dominated by social trends and public opinion. A bizarre factor in the development of custodial institutions was the virtual disappearance of leprosy from Europe and, with this disappearance, the presence of well-endowed charitable institutions without a population to serve and with a clear orientation to serving an alien and even feared population. The transition of these facilities from leprosariums to facilities for the mentally ill carried with it a good deal of baggage.

Other less positive European traditions from this era foreshadow troubling current US concerns and problems as well. Another pattern of "care" in Europe was a form of banishment—the ship of fools. Captains of these vessels would accept deranged persons for a fee and ferry them about the waterways of Europe, sometimes to be discharged in an isolated city, sometimes consigned to permanent life on the ship, and usually to be the object of amusement and ridicule when such a ship with its strange cargo came to port. These traditions helped form the fear and misunderstanding about mental illness and its care that still persist as a stigma that may keep sufferers from seeking help.

An important English tradition also formed a foundation element for US patterns of care. This was the evolution of the "Poor Laws," the common law guarantee of relief for the unfortunate. The notion of relief or general welfare payments, although clearly humanitarian, would come to have several other effects. For one, just as in the unfortunate US experience with deinstitutionalization hundreds of years later, this form of "outside relief" would make other forms of care somewhat less necessary, because after all "the mentally ill were getting some form of help." The concept of relief, when framed as "welfare" in the US political context, would create further image barriers for the mentally ill. From the "fear image" derived from care in the leprosariums to the "fool image" of the ship of fools to the "incompetence image" of welfare, the mentally ill were acquiring a heavy burden that would still have an impact in 21st century America.

This background also puts the work of reformers in perspective. Pinel and Tuke—and later reformers in

**Table 109–1  Influences on the Early Evolution of Mental Health Care**

- Unused custodial facilities (serving feared populations)
- Community neglect
- "Ship of fools" approach (stigmatization of treatment population)
- Guarantee of relief of the unfortunate (someone else assumed the caretaker role)
- Linkage of clinical reform to social and political reforms

America—were on the one hand heroic. The conditions they sought to change, whether inside confinement or outside abandonment, were rooted deep in political and social tradition. Making change in mental health programs was then, as now, a difficult proposition. The work of Pinel and Tuke was also the product of new political values being formed in the era of the American and French revolutions. The values of moral treatment were closely linked to, and indeed drew from, the deeper values that led to these broad cultural changes. This is a final lesson in reform from the European tradition—that clinical reform efforts are linked to contemporary social and political reforms. Patterns of care do not exist in isolation. Understanding these linkages, particularly as they have evolved in the US, is essential to understanding how patterns of care have developed and continue to evolve. These influences on mental health care are summarized in Table 109–1.

## Early Developments in Mental Health in the US

The trends and themes of mental health care in the US developed from these European roots. Before the moral treatment era, there was little organized care. Mentally ill individuals were the responsibility of their family or village. Before the industrial revolution, in a time when manual labor was the order of the day, many individuals survived without any care other than the therapy of hard work. The predominant early "mental health service" that developed in the early 1800s was the almshouse, a kind of reform designed to provide some care, albeit undifferentiated care. As might be expected, the mentally ill did not fare well in such settings, although they constituted a large proportion of those placed in such settings.

The moral treatment era brought the first in a series of largely unsuccessful reform efforts that would characterize US mental health policy. The early asylums, such as those at Philadelphia, Boston, and Hartford, were philanthropic institutions. During the mid-1800s, the impulse was to establish asylums as a governmental responsibility. Grob (1966) has chronicled this history in depth, focusing on the history of the Worcester (Massachusetts) State Hospital, established in 1830 as the first public asylum in that state. The founding of the hospital was clearly associated with the kind of charitable and humane impulses that derived from the leadership of Tuke and Pinel and recognized the failure of both outside relief and the almshouses to meet the specialized needs of mentally ill individuals. The founding concept was clearly that a kind of social and rehabilitative acute care, in a serene setting, would help people recover. The early records suggest that the hospital was in fact successful. Many patients were discharged, and few in the earliest days stayed for purely custodial care.

## The Growth of Asylums

The early successes of asylums like Worcester, coupled with growing public awareness of the conditions in the almshouses and the social reform impulses of the Jacksonian era, led to a boom in the construction of state hospitals. The catalyst was an extraordinary advocate named Dorothea Dix, a retired Boston schoolteacher who made improving the lot of the mentally ill her second career. During this period, she visited every state legislature east of the Rocky Mountains and succeeded in convincing most to construct a state hospital. Buoyed by this success, she lobbied Congress to enact land grant legislation that would allow the federal government to grant land to each state; the land was to be sold and the proceeds used to establish hospitals. In a foreshadowing of the federal government's role vis-à-vis the mentally ill, the legislation was passed by Congress in 1854 but promptly vetoed by President Pierce, who saw the proposal as an unacceptable responsibility for the federal government to assume.

The moral treatment era probably reached its zenith with the founding of the Association of Medical Superintendents in 1844 and the passage of Dix's legislation 10 years later. This era's decline may also be marked by Pierce's action in vetoing further reform. One can learn much from this period that is relevant today. Just as mental health reforms occurred in the Europe of the French revolution (and as Foucault [1965] has described it, "the age of reason"), there was a connection between general social concern and mental health reform. A new treatment philosophy was articulated that fit with the zeitgeist of the times and was comprehensible to politicians. As Morrissey and Goldman (1984) have shown in a provocative review of mental health reform in America, the new approach was even associated with a particular kind of treatment facility.

However, the seeds of later failure were already embedded in these dynamics, for the tone of political and social concern changed away from humanitarian impulses, and the country was preoccupied with broader concern in the last half of the 19th century. Thus, the social consciousness that had proved a hospitable basis for moral treatment eroded substantially during the industrial revolution. There were at least two substantial problems embedded within the mental health reforms as well. First, as Morrissey and Goldman (1984) pointed out, moral treatment conceived of mental illness as essentially an acute problem and therefore positioned the hospital as a short-term treatment facility. In the early days, this assumption worked, probably in large measure owing to the enthusiasm and dedication of staff. Then as now, however, a proportion of the mentally ill faced a long-term problem that was not amenable to short-term cure. It was inevitable that longer-term "chronic" problems began to gradually overtake the asylums, creating space, staffing, and resource problems and eroding the mission of the hospitals. This cycle of reform and neglect is outlined in Table 109–2.

## The Erosion of Community Responsibility

This problem was exacerbated by another "reform" effort. In almost all the early public asylums, the construction was

| Table 109–2 | Cycles of "Reform" |
| --- | --- |

- Mentally ill populations were neglected
- Neglect was noted, with calls for reform
- "Reform" occurred, but underlying issues ignored (mental illness is chronic, long-term but facilities focused on acute treatment)
- Systems of care were overwhelmed by increasing numbers of very ill patients
- Care becomes custodial rather than recovery focused (neglect)

underwritten by the state legislature, which also provided a small appropriation for operations—a kind of "seed money." These funds were not intended to be adequate for the full operation of the hospitals; because mental health problems occurred in most communities and the almshouses had been a local responsibility, communities were to be billed for the costs of caring for their indigent citizens. At one level, this represented the type of intergovernmental tension that has seemed to plague mental health care ever since. Yet it was a productive tension, because it created a disincentive for the long-term institutionalization of disabled persons; but the arrangement was a problem for the hospitals. Collecting funds from all the towns was inconvenient, and the rates tended to lag behind costs, especially during a period of rapid inflation.

These problems led to the well-meaning State Care Acts, enacted in many states in the second half of the 19th century to solve this problem. Because the institutions were competently run and were essentially a state responsibility, and because the local fees were inconvenient, having the state simply assume financial responsibility was an obvious solution. In Ohio, for example, the operation of asylums is mentioned in the state constitution as a fundamental state responsibility.

This wave of legislation created an obvious problem. Addressing the inconvenience of local responsibility by virtually wiping it out, the State Care Acts eliminated any incentive for local care and created a particular pressure for the institutionalization of long-term disabled individuals. The short-term orientation of the hospitals was subtly erased, and the ability of disabled persons to persist by doing manual labor in an agrarian society was also permanently altered by the onset of the industrial revolution. As a consequence, the history of mental health care in the US in the latter part of the 19th century was disastrous.

This era involved a confluence of negative forces that eroded the moral treatment reforms. The perverse financial incentives created by the State Care Acts led to increased rates of institutionalization. These pressures, combined with the "silting in" effects of disabled patients who could not be discharged, sent the levels of hospitalization soaring. Grob (1966) analyzed the forces that contributed to the decline of moral treatment, using Worcester State Hospital as a case study. Additionally, he noted that the increasing size of the institution created a self-reinforcing dynamic of regimentation and efficiency, which reduced quality of care and increased the custodial nature of the hospital. Grob also found that an evolution in the professional role of psychiatry also contributed to the decline of the hospital.

In a perverse way, the profession's focus on psychiatry as a "scientific discipline" estranged the leadership of the hospital from the civic and volunteer leaders who had contributed to its early development. In addition, an emphasis on somatic treatments produced empty results, because they had little to offer at the time and tended to undermine the optimism and egalitarian values that moral treatment had contributed to hospitals.

Cultural and class factors also contributed to a changed and problem role for state hospitals during this period. Not only did the industrial revolution put a premium on skilled labor and begin to hasten the decline of communal, agrarian lifestyles (which were much more suited to sustaining the mentally ill), but the demands of the industrial workplace played off the increased levels of immigration to create new tensions. The role of the hospitals had been subtly refined from "retreat" and recovery to custody and management. In this context, they seemed an appropriate place to detain those immigrants whose behavior was strange and who did not fit into the requirements of the developing modern society. The hospitals inevitably deteriorated into overcrowded custodial institutions, housing the disabled and other misfits and providing only a veneer of treatment.

## The Mental Hygiene Movement

Fortunately, as Morrissey and Goldman (1984) pointed out, the emerging pattern of US mental health policy shows that cycles of neglect do lead to cycles of reform. Although the professional leadership of the time was crucial in the next wave of reform, especially in the "mental hygiene" approach of Adolph Meyer, it was once again a partnership between citizens and professionals that stimulated change. In this case, the citizen leader was Clifford Beers (1908) whose book *A Mind That Found Itself* focused national attention on the deterioration of the hospitals but also showed the possibilities of recovery. Beers had been hospitalized at both the Hartford Retreat and the Connecticut Asylum for a period of several years and described graphically the degradation and horrors of this experience. He also detailed his positive experiences with recovery, speaking perhaps to the American fascination with the "self-made man" but connecting powerfully to the enthusiasm and new theories of mental hygiene.

As Morrissey and Goldman (1984) noted, this cycle of reform was linked to both a new model or theory and a preference for particular facilities—the psychopathic hospital and the child guidance clinic. Like the moral treatment approach, both facilities and indeed the mental hygiene movement were eventually founded on the same rocks of the intractability of long-term mental illness. The mental hygiene approach—like moral treatment—emphasized brief special treatment with an emphasis on returning to normal functioning. No concept of long-term care had yet developed. The approach was also linked to the dominant cultural values of the time, emphasizing science, order, and classification. Thus, the psychopathic hospital was affiliated with academia and focused on applying diagnostic and treatment expertise to mental illness.

The first prominent facilities included Pavilion F, opened in Albany in 1902, and the Boston Psychopathic Hospital, opened in 1912. The child guidance clinic emphasized similar themes but clearly also stressed the value of early, clinically based intervention as a preventive strategy. Child guidance clinics were developed in a number of cities during the same period. The movement also led to an emphasis on professionalism that extended beyond psychiatry, with the founding of the first school for psychiatric social work at Smith College in 1928.

Like the moral treatment era, the mental hygiene reforms drew on emerging cultural and political developments, included a core treatment philosophy, and emphasized new types of treatment facilities. However, this cycle of reform also emphasized acute care and therefore failed to meet the challenge of the long-term major mental illnesses. In fact, by this emphasis, the approach did not have much impact on the state hospitals, which had essentially become long-term care facilities. Mental hygiene, therefore, did not succeed as comprehensive reform.

## The World Wars and Psychiatry

Mental health issues emerging from both World War I and especially World War II had a dramatic effect on policy. Working with traumatized soldiers in World War I, Thomas Salmon described the "shell shock" syndrome. Drawing from the mental hygiene theory of early intervention, brief treatment that focused largely on separating the soldier from stress—although not removing him too far from the frontlines and maintaining high expectations of early recovery and return to battle—proved successful. Thus, crisis intervention methods were literally developed in the heat of battle.

These same methods were used and further refined during World War II. In addition, however, events in World War II thrust mental health issues into a more prominent national light. A high proportion of those men found unfit to serve in the military were screened out because of mental illness—almost 2 million individuals. Later, questions were raised about the accuracy and adequacy of screening (Deutsch 1949), but the number of individuals rejected for service was large. In addition, about 40% of the military personnel dismissed from active duty as unfit to serve were discharged because of mental illness. These extraordinary rates of illness came to public and policymakers' attention at precisely the time when the federal government was poised to affect mental health policy and as the country was poised to enter a period of prosperity and of a relative focus on domestic affairs. As a result, Congress passed the Mental Health Act in 1946, creating the National Institute of Mental Health (NIMH) as a focal point for research, professional training, and policy development.

## Mental Health Policy in Postwar America

The pace and complexity of change in health and mental health care since World War II have been dizzying. Because we are closer to this period, it may be more difficult to see it clearly. Certainly, opinions still vary on the dynamics and nature of many developments, starting with deinstitutionalization (viewed by some as necessary social progress and by others as abandonment). It is wise to recall some of the persistent trends in US mental health policy that have their roots in European and Colonial traditions, for these trends are still shaping policy and patterns of care in ways that are not immediately evident to the casual observer.

One fundamental and recurring tension is between mental illness and "madness" or between clinical and sociological understandings. Viewed from a clinical perspective, the creation of asylums in the European reformation or in 19th century America was simply the development of an improved treatment system. Yet, as Foucault (1965) and Grob (1966) have shown, these institutions served other purposes. The early asylums filled the niche that had been vacated by leprosy, with certain consequences in terms of stigmatizing the mentally ill. America's asylums were not able to hold their desired quality and acute care orientation for more than a decade or two and quickly became places where the wayward and others unable to play a productive role in the industrial revolution were "stored." Indeed, this trend was accelerated, as (Grob 1983) shown, by the unintended actions of the medical superintendents and their loss of contact with citizen leaders. Thus, an awareness of the balance between clinical requirements and initiatives and their social context and meaning is essential in viewing modern developments.

A second problem trend has been to base reform on an incomplete or unrealistic view of mental illness and therefore its treatment requirements. This is a central point made by Morrissey and Goldman. They emphasized that the first two "cycles of reform" in America (the asylum and the mental hygiene movement) inaccurately conceived of most serious mental illness as acute or temporary, leading to treatment strategies that were ultimately doomed to failure. This limited view would vex another reform era yet to come—the community mental health movement of the 1960s and 1970s.

Finally, the role of the public sector in US mental health care has been significant; the tensions between states and the federal government, and increasingly between the public and the private sectors, has never been good for patients. This pattern was established with Pierce's veto of the land grant hospital construction legislation in 1854, ceding responsibility to the states, and with the State Care Acts that weakened local responsibility for the mentally ill. Whereas these actions clearly set in place a dynamic of primary state responsibility, the weakened local role encouraged the creation of custodial institutions as a mode of service and did not resolve the federal–state tensions that are so much a part of US political life. With the establishment of the NIMH in 1946, the federal government reasserted its interests. The Great Society programs that were to follow, in an era of federal activism, would muddy this picture even more.

## The 1950s: New Treatment Technology, Federal Activism, and the Civil Rights Movement

The decade of the 1950s served as an incubator for major changes. The impact of these changes were later felt in a more substantial fashion. Three such developments listed in Table 109–3, were most significant: the introduction of psychoactive medications, an emerging activism on the part of the new federal mental health bureaucracy, and the growth of the civil rights movement and its use of the federal courts.

| Table 109–3 | The CMHC Reform Movement |
|---|---|

- Introduction of psychoactive medications
- Emerging federal activism
- Growth of civil rights

### Chlorpromazine and the State Hospitals

Chlorpromazine was first used in the state hospitals in the early 1950s, with several significant effects. The first effect was an immediate clinical impact. The census of the state hospitals peaked at a significant 550,000 individuals in 1954 and has declined every year since then. This decline in the 1950s was clearly related to the impact of chlorpromazine, which provided enough relief to enable the discharge of many patients. The second impact of this new technology was a renewed optimism about mental health treatment— the same sort of optimism that had characterized the moral treatment and mental hygiene eras.

### Civil Rights: Social Change and the Role of the Courts

The emergence of the civil rights movement was marked by the *Brown v. Board of Education* lawsuit filed in Topeka, Kansas, in 1954. Several features of this movement affected mental health reforms in a substantial way. First, the values of human rights served as a foundation for reformers who saw a better life for institutionalized mentally ill individuals. Yet again, emerging community values affected developments in mental health. The second feature of the civil rights movement related to mental health was just as critical—the use of the federal courts to solve a problem that legislatures and the general public were not yet ready to address. Although federal court litigation in mental health did not begin in earnest for another 2 decades, the seeds of change had been planted.

### An Activist Federal Government

After the veto of Dorothea Dix's legislation by President Pierce a century earlier, the federal government had retreated from any substantial role in mental health for decades, but the national experience during the two world wars and the establishment of the NIMH marked a change in this pattern. Although the leadership role in service provision clearly rested with the states, there was a mood for change marked by the trends of the 1950s. The passage of the Mental Health Study Act in 1955 marked this new activism. The legislation charged the Joint Commission on Mental Illness and Mental Health with a national study to develop and recommend policy.

### The 1960s: Transformational Change and Unintended Consequences

The National Commission issued its ambitious report, *Action for Mental Health*, in 1961. Formed in the new environment of federal activism and optimism about mental health treatment, the report proposed a broad approach to change. Its recommendations included dramatic increases in funding for mental health care, aggressive approaches to recruitment and training, an increased emphasis on acute and community care, and movement away from the custodial state hospitals. A mental health clinic to serve each population base of 50,000 persons across the country was proposed, as were expanded programs for persons with long-term mental illness.

These recommendations fell on the ears of a receptive president and Congress. President Kennedy was clearly interested in mental retardation and mental health, and these recommendations were less controversial than the changes in other areas of domestic policy that the country confronted. Optimism about treatment and community care, the need to reform the state hospitals, and the ability of the federal government to change things formed the context for reform. The result was the 1963 Community Mental Health Centers Act, with its focus on developing locally managed, broadly focused mental health centers across the country. The legislation represented the federal government's most ambitious effort in mental health care but was seriously flawed from the outset. In a sense, the most notable success of the legislation was simply its passage, marking public support and recognition of mental health treatment. The legislation eventually led to the establishment of more than 700 centers (although about 2,600 would have been needed to cover the country) and also stimulated passage of parallel legislation and initiatives at the state level.

There were several design flaws in the community mental health center (CMHC) legislation as well. There was a "disconnect" between the growing antipathy for state hospitals and the desire for community care. The centers were to provide a wide variety of community services, but the emphasis was on acute treatment, not the kind of rehabilitation, support, and care needed by the long-term patients in hospitals. Two other aspects of the legislation heightened the separation between the poor, disabled patients of the hospitals and the new centers. First, the federal chauvinism of the time had resulted in the establishment of the CMHC program (like the antipoverty programs of the time) as a federal–local partnership, with the states only tangentially involved. As a result, the state mental health agencies (SMHAs), which ran the hospitals, were cut out of the picture with respect to CMHC priorities and oversight. Second, the funding mechanism for CMHC establishment was limited to construction grants and time-limited (7 years) start-up funding.

As during the moral hygiene era, a substantial federal role in funding mental health care was not politically acceptable. (Perhaps it would be more accurate to say that an explicit role in funding mental health was not acceptable, because the soon established Medicaid program eventually became the nation's single largest mental health funder.) As a result of the limited federal financing and the resulting pressure on CMHCs to establish "financial viability," the centers needed to find paying customers. This tension, coupled with the orientation toward broad mental health concerns rather than the care of the seriously mentally ill, led most centers to limit their role as providers for formerly hospitalized patients, focusing instead on other paying customers and efforts. Although probably almost all the centers cared for some formerly hospitalized patients, it was not their central concern. Coupled with the limited population coverage of the new centers, this meant that the program was in no way adequate to support the down-

sizing of the state hospitals that had probably been intended—and was certainly about to happen.

## Medicaid, Transinstitutionalization, and Privatization

Although the passage of the CMHC legislation is generally viewed as the major federal mental health initiative of the 1960s, it is likely that the enactment of Medicare and Medicaid was more influential, at least in terms of the numbers of patients and practitioners who were affected. Medicare (Title Eighteen of the Social Security Act) was enacted in 1966 to provide insurance to persons older than 65 years eligible for Social Security. It was amended in 1972 to provide for all those older than 65 years, with a premium mechanism to cover costs. At the same time, eligibility was extended to disabled workers and their beneficiaries as well as to patients with chronic renal disease. Medicare rapidly became the dominant insurance mechanism and therefore a major force in health financing policy.

However, Medicaid (Title Nineteen of the Social Security Act), also enacted in 1966, had a dramatic effect on seriously mentally ill individuals almost immediately. Medicaid was designed as a health insurance program for the poor and disabled, primarily covering acute care. However, Medicaid also provided financing for long-term care by coverage of nursing homes. (Both Medicare and Medicaid were thus focused in large measure on the elderly and, together with other measures, had a substantial positive effect on older Americans—a major success of the War on Poverty and Great Society programs, whereas most came to be regarded as failures.)

Because its eligibility included seriously mentally ill individuals, almost all of the patients who were made destitute by their illness, Medicaid was a viable financing vehicle. Because it was largely a federally financed program (the federal share ranged from a minimum of 50% for wealthy states up to 75% for poor states), it was attractive to states. Also because it covered nursing homes, which substituted for state hospitals for the care of many disabled patients, Medicaid set up an enormous transfer of care. The state hospitals were increasingly out of favor and expensive, and Congress had ensured that funds from Medicaid would not cover state hospital care by prohibiting payments to "institutions for mental diseases." Indeed, this exclusion of institutions for mental diseases (IMD) prohibited Medicaid reimbursement for treatment in any facility, public or private, greater than 16 beds, serving adults of 21 to 64 years with a primary diagnosis of mental disease. Psychiatric treatment in general hospitals, even in large specialized psychiatric units, was funded by Medicaid. During the same period, income support–welfare programs were also dramatically expanded by Social Security Disability Income and the introduction of Supplemental Security Income for those individuals who could not qualify for disability income given their absence of a work history.

The results were as predictable as they were unintended. State hospitals proceeded to transfer patients, primarily to nursing homes but also to boarding houses and other settings, at a remarkable rate. Between 1955 and 1965, the rate of decline in the state hospital population had been a percentage point or two per year. The end-of-year census had dropped from more than 550,000 in 1955 to about

475,000 by 1965 (Kiesler and Sibulkin 1987). This decline was attributable to clinical factors (especially the use of chlorpromazine) and to changing opinions. However, the change in the following decade was dramatic, averaging about 6% per year, and led to a census of about 191,000 at the end of 1975. In many states, the state hospital census declined at a double-digit rate between 1966 and 1975. Of the various discharge options, nursing home placements were the most prominent.

This transfer of care, or transinstitutionalization, was the major factor in reducing state hospital capacity, followed by discharges to other settings financed by welfare payments. These transfers were a more potent force in reducing the state hospital population than the CMHCs. These facilities had once been thought of as the vehicle to replace state hospitals but had assumed a broader and less-focused community mental health role. Thus, long-term care and welfare proved more significant than treatment services in changing how care was delivered, repeating a pattern established in the prior century, when broader social policy affected the role of state hospitals more than did changes in clinical practice.

There were several lessons already apparent in the 1960s reform, even before the phenomenon of deinstitutionalization became apparent. Certainly a major lesson was the extent to which shifts in financing drove policy and practice. The financing dynamics built into the CMHC program implicitly guaranteed that they would need to turn their attention away from individuals with serious and persistent mental illness to survive. The sizable federal participation in Medicaid led inevitably to a transfer of care responsibilities from the states to the federal government, yet neither of these vehicles did much to build the integrated systems of care needed to adequately support disabled individuals with serious mental illness. As Morrissey and Goldman (1984) pointed out, this new cycle of reform, like both the moral treatment and mental hygiene reforms, was implicitly built on an acute care model that was a poor fit for the long-term, multifaceted needs of these patients.

Medicaid also had a dramatic effect at the "front door" of the state hospitals by financing hospital care for psychiatric patients in general hospitals, both in "scatter beds" (medical–surgical beds occupied by patients with psychiatric diagnoses) and in distinct psychiatric units. The availability of Medicaid reimbursement aided a dramatic expansion of general hospitals as a primary locus of acute psychiatric care. Between 1965 and 1980, the volume of psychiatric admissions to these units increased from about 700,000 annually to approximately 1,700,000 annually (Kiesler and Sibulkin 1987). Through the 1980s and 1990s the Medicaid reimbursement, available to general hospitals but not to IMDs, continued to fuel expansion of psychiatric care in general hospitals with discharges form these units growing from 1.4 million in 1988 to 1.9 million in 1994 (Mechanic 1989). Conversely, the Medicaid "IMD exclusion" helped further diminish the role of state hospitals in acute care. State hospitals provided 63% of 24-hour hospital and residential treatment episodes in 1955 but only 10% by 1998 (Manderscheid et al. 2000).

## The Erosion of State Systems of Care
The advent of Medicare and especially Medicaid thus changed the face of mental health care dramatically. After

World War II, mental health care was dominated by the state hospitals and thus by the states. Within the next generation, this change was spectacular. By about 1970, there were more episodes of psychiatric care in general hospitals than in state hospitals, and at about this time, the number of long-term mentally ill individuals in nursing homes became greater than the number of these patients in the state hospitals. Both of these trends were due more to the financing incentives in Medicaid than to the community mental health movement and the CMHCs. Both the CMHC legislation and Medicaid had undercut the SMHAs by providing funding streams that bypassed these agencies. The CMHC grants went directly to local providers with limited SMHA influence, and Medicaid was administered by a designated state agency (usually the welfare department, given its locus as a program for the poor). In addition, both programs provided funds to private or not-for-profit entities rather than to the public sector. This eventually created powerful alternative provider forces in mental health to counter whatever political power rested with the SMHAs. The states had also lost potency because their major focus had been to run the discredited state hospitals; they were essentially cut out of the new mental health business in CMHCs and Medicaid-financed services. This change toward community-based care and the accompanying challenges are described in Table 109–4.

## The 1970s: Increased Complexity, Expanded Services, Federal Indifference
By the mid-1970s, mental health care bore little resemblance to what had existed a generation before. Owing to the impact of Medicare and Medicaid, the new de facto publicly financed system was privately operated and largely outside the control of the states. The state hospitals were no longer the primary focus of either long-term or acute care. Nursing homes probably had more mental health long-term care beds than did state hospitals, although the data are not completely clear, and the number of psychiatric admissions to general hospitals was greater than to state hospitals. Hundreds of CMHCs had been created, serving a broader public and providing increased access to care. Private health insurance coverage had become much more prevalent. Whereas coverage for mental illnesses was generally far more limited than that for physical illnesses (both because of the stigma associated with mental illness and perhaps even more significantly because the state hospitals still

| Table 109–4 | Challenges Faced by Systems of Care During the CMHC Reform Movement |
|---|---|

- Patients from state hospitals not moved to independent living, but to nursing homes, boarding homes (transinstitutionalization)
- CMHCs not prepared for large numbers of patients with serious and persistent mental illness
- CMHCs had to provide intensive care for acute, less severely ill patients to be profitable
- Expansion of Medicaid led to expanded general psychiatric beds
- State lost authority/responsibility for patients with serious and persistent mental illness

existed as a catastrophic care option), private coverage helped expand mental health care dramatically. Access to mental health care had simply exploded, and the expansion took place in new settings. Figure 109–1 illustrates how dramatically the system changed.

The most significant change involved a dramatic expansion of care (from 1.7 million episodes in 1955 to 6.9 million in 1975, just 20 years later). The expansion occurred most significantly in the outpatient arena, in which the number of care episodes exploded from around 400,000 to almost 5,000,000, a more than tenfold increase. However, because of expanded Medicaid, Medicare, and private insurance coverage, the volume of inpatient admissions also rose from around 1,300,000 in 1955 to more than 1,600,000 in 1975, during a period generally thought to be associated with deinstitutionalization. A new mental health "system" was in fact being created, and it looked different from the old system (i.e., the state hospitals). The state hospitals, after dominating US mental health care for more than a century, were speedily replaced as the primary locus of care. Figure 109–2 illustrates this development. In the 20-year period from 1955 to 1975, the proportion of all episodes of mental health care that were provided by state hospitals (whether outpatient or inpatient care) shifted dramatically from half of all episodes to less than 10%.

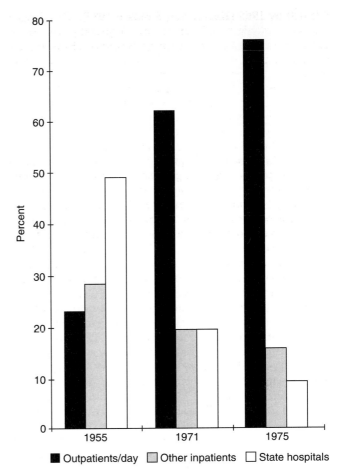

**Figure 109–2** *Episodes of mental health care by modality in the US from 1955 to 1975, showing the diminishing role of state hospitals. (Source: Witkin M [1980] Trends in Patient Care Episodes in Mental Health Facilities, 1955–1975. NIMH Statistical note 156. National Institute of Mental Health, Rockville, MD.)*

## State Hospitals Seen as the Problem

The conventional view of mental health policy evolution during this period ignored many of these developments. Because the state hospitals had become such a lightening rod for criticism by policymakers, partly because they had dominated the mental health landscape for so long that new developments were not apparent and partly, perhaps, because data on state hospitals were readily available when data on the new programs were not, the hospitals were still the focus of policy debates. When one examined the budgets of the SMHAs alone, the state hospitals were still a major category of expenditure. Data on the growing private sector system were not available on time, so analysis tended to focus on the state hospitals. Given that the responsibilities of the hospitals for care of patients had been dramatically reduced, their consumption of a significant percentage of all state resources seemed inappropriate. The national mental health leadership at NIMH and a growing number of articles in the professional literature reflected concern about the levels of resources tied up in the state hospitals, at a time when the balance of care had shifted to the community.

The reasons for inflated state hospital costs, noted in Table 109–5, did not seem so critical at the time given the imperative of community care, but they generally reflect

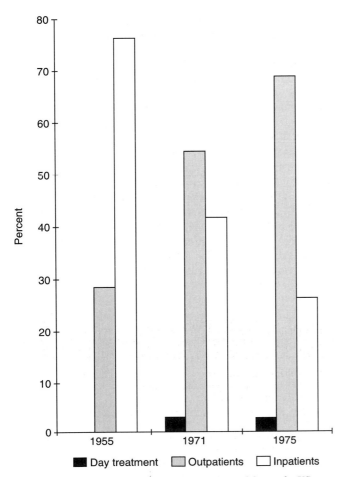

**Figure 109–1** *Episodes of mental health care by modality in the US from 1955 to 1975. (Source: Witkin M [1980] Trends in Patient Care Episodes in Mental Health Facilities, 1955–1975. NIMH Statistical note 156. National Institute of Mental Health, Rockville, MD.)*

| Table 109–5 | Reasons for Increasing Costs of State Hospitals |
|---|---|

- Unionization of public employees
- Resultant wage increases
- Loss of "free" patient labor (paid staff had to be hired)
- Increased governmental regulation

developments outside the mental health field that were influencing costs. The unionization of public employees and the resultant wage increases and limited work weeks were a significant factor in increasing costs. In addition, the state hospitals had long relied on the labor of patients. This practice had evolved from a belief in the curative role of work to a managerial "necessity" to operate under-financed, custodial institutions. It was effectively curtailed by a Supreme Court decision (*Souder v. Brennan* 1973), with the result that hired staff were needed to replace the essentially free labor of patients. These external factors increased hospital costs. At the same time, increased governmental regulation designed to redress poor quality of care increased costs of the institutions. These factors, whether legitimate or not, contributed to the reformers' demands to reduce the hospitals and to continue expansion of community mental health services. In a word, the policy preference was for deinstitutionalization. That adequate community supports for the most disabled were not being put in place was not yet apparent.

At the same time, the national mental health "movement" was starting to run into problems. President Nixon was no friend of the NIMH. This may have related to his distaste for the social psychiatry approach of the NIMH leadership. NIMH Director Yolles had opposed Nixon's tough drug sentencing policies, advocating a treatment approach (Rumer 1978). In any event, Nixon fought the community mental health program through the budget process. After proposing lower funding levels in 1971, Nixon actually impounded CMHC funds in 1973 after Congress had appropriated them. As a result, the CMHC program started to slip from its original goal of 1,500 centers. From 1965 to 1969, 75% of the $260 million authorized for CMHC construction was actually appropriated. From 1970 to 1973, only 15% of the $340 million authorized was actually budgeted (Bloom 1975).

## Emerging Conflicts in Mental Health Policy

The last half of the 1970s was thus a difficult and transitional period in mental health policy. Dramatic expansions of care had been achieved, with little positive impact on the most seriously mentally ill persons. The state hospitals were discredited, but no viable alternatives were widely available. Nursing homes had become the primary, largely invisible, locus of long-term care—along with other welfare-financed alternatives such as boarding homes. The CMHC and Medicaid programs had dramatically expanded access to care, but not for the most seriously mentally ill and largely outside the influence of the state governments that were responsible for the state hospitals. Given these trends, it is little surprise that a crescendo of criticism began to develop. The 1977 audit report by the General Account-

ing Office (*Returning the Mentally Disabled to the Community, Government Needs to Do More*) typified the new criticism.

President Carter, assuming office in 1976, was clearly more sympathetic to mental health concerns, and First Lady Rosalynn Carter made mental health her primary concern. The President's Commission on Mental Health was established in 1977 to review the nation's issues in mental health. Its 1988 report was perhaps even broader than the Action for Mental Health report published almost 20 years previously, in part because the system was much more complex and partly because the political tensions associated with new constituencies like CMHC directors made consensus much more difficult. As Mechanic (1989) has pointed out, the report was also produced in a national political environment that had changed dramatically. There was much less certainty about the appropriate role of the federal government and many more competing budget demands. The process of developing legislation based on the report was also correspondingly more difficult.

Two major activities resulted. The first did not have a happy ending. The 1980 Mental Health Systems Act was designed to build on but also redirect the CMHC program by focusing more on seriously mentally ill persons, connecting the program with state government, and emphasizing systems of care rather than facilities. President Reagan, taking office within months after the legislation was signed, proceeded to ignore and dismantle the legislation, in large measure by the conversion of the grant program to a block grant at reduced funding levels. The other major outcome of the President's Commission was less visible but eventually influential. The Department of Health and Human Services had been charged with developing a more integrated federal approach to the problems of the most seriously mentally ill individuals. Its 1980 report, as described by Mechanic (1989) "recognized the critical importance of Medicaid, Social Security Disability Insurance, and many other federal programs, and presented an incremental approach to modifying them in a constructive way."

Many of the initiatives recommended in this report were also attacked by the Reagan administration. The most notable was the effort, eventually overturned in federal courts after intervention by legal advocates, to drop many seriously mentally ill individuals from disability insurance during the early 1980s. However, many recommendations survived this assault and were actually implemented during the same period that the Mental Health Systems Act was dismantled (Koyanagi and Goldman 1991).

Thus, whereas the momentum for federal leadership in mental health stalled with President Reagan's shelving of the Mental Health Systems Act, federal programs quietly became more relevant and helpful to seriously mentally ill individuals during the 1980s—after the debacle related to disability insurance payments was resolved. The improvements included better disability insurance coverage, targeted attention to the mentally ill homeless, and particularly the development of Medicaid programs focused on community treatment for seriously mentally ill individuals. These programs, including case management and rehabilitation options, were used by many states to expand services during the last half of the decade. However, federal leadership was also significant during the decade, an irony given

| Table 109–6 | Improvements in Federal Involvement in Mental Health |
|---|---|

- Better disability insurance coverage
- Improved targeting of homeless patients with mental illness
- Development of Medicaid programs (case management, rehabilitation options)
- NIMH developed the Community Support Program

the budget cuts and retrenchment of the Reagan years. The small Community Support Program (CSP) in the NIMH exercised tremendous influence on the state mental health programs through national working conferences and a focused program of planning grants and demonstration grants directed to the states. During the 1980s, the states began to recover from the federal neglect of the prior decade and take advantage of Medicaid funding and CSP ideas to retool their community care systems. The federal improvements are highlighted in Table 109–6.

## The 1980s: Community Support and the Precursors of Health Care Reform

The state mental health programs had fared poorly during the prior 2 decades. The SMHAs were discredited as the operators of state hospitals, defined by community mental health advocates as the enemies of progress. In addition, the new CMHC and Medicaid initiatives of the 1960s had bypassed the SMHAs. A new mental health "nonsystem" dominated by nursing and boarding homes as well as general hospital psychiatry—all outside the effective control of the SMHAs—was now larger in scope than the programs controlled by the state agencies. Even the CMHCs, once thought of as a treatment alternative to hospitals but serving instead an entirely new group of patients, were under limited SMHA control. As the problems of this chaotic system became apparent—symbolized by the plight of the homeless mentally ill and punctuated by mass media coverage of periodical violent episodes involving mentally ill individuals—the states were the obvious target for criticism. The subtleties of the new "system" were not important in the face of these problems. The states ran the hospitals, let people out of them, and should have been doing a better job.

The changes of the 1980s allowed the states to regroup and recover from the feverish pitch of change. Although the Reagan new federalism approach had resulted in funding cuts, it had restored state control. For example, in the 1980 Reagan budget, the CMHC direct grants to centers were consolidated into a block grant, reduced by about 35%, and placed under state authority. In general, the states used these funds to focus on seriously mentally ill adults and children, using the new CSP model.

The impact of the CSP approach is difficult to overstate. Growing out of the Carter commission, it involved a focused approach to the multifaceted needs of seriously mentally ill individuals in communities. As Morrissey and Goldman (1984) have pointed out, this "fourth era of reform" differed in a fundamental way from the moral treatment, mental hygiene, and community mental health concepts. For the first time, serious mental illness was not conceived of as a fundamentally acute problem but was

defined as a long-term and episodic condition requiring multifaceted supports. As a consequence, the service approach was not focused on a particular institution (e.g., the asylum, psychopathic hospital, or mental health center). Rather, consistent with the concepts of President Carter's legislation, a multimodal system of care was necessary, incorporating both treatment services and the practical supports (such as housing, income supports) needed by people with disabilities as well as illness. The CSP approach defined a number of essential elements of such a system which have been included in Table 109–7.

These concepts were promoted by the small CSP unit within the NIMH in a fervent, focused manner. The combination of small state planning grants (carefully defined to promote change) and demonstration projects was linked to the national CSP meetings in an effective change strategy. There were several remarkable things about the effort. First, the notion of aggressive federal leadership during the Reagan years is something of an anomaly. Probably, the program was too small—and perhaps too effectively protected by Congress—to have been a serious target. Second, the funding levels involved were completely insignificant compared with the hundreds of millions spent on CMHCs or the billions involved in Medicaid. The annual CSP appropriations were in the range of $10 million for the entire program. However, the funds were effectively used to "leverage" other resources, including state budgets, block grant funds, and the new Medicaid programs. The change in SMHA budget portfolios during the 1980s is the clearest example as illustrated in Figure 109–3.

| Table 109–7 | Essential Functions of Community Support Systems |
|---|---|

- Identification of the target population and outreach to offer appropriate services to those willing to participate
- Assistance in applying for entitlements
- Crisis stabilization services in the least restrictive possible setting, with hospitalization available when other options are insufficient
- Psychosocial rehabilitation services, including but not limited to:
    Goal-oriented rehabilitation evaluation
    Training in community living skills, in the natural setting where possible
    Opportunities to improve employability
    Appropriate living arrangements in an atmosphere that encourages functional improvement
    Opportunities to develop social skills, interests, and leisure time activities
- Supportive services of indefinite duration, including supportive living and working arrangements, and other such services for as long as they are needed
- Medical and mental health care
- Backup support to families, friends, and community members
- Involvement of concerned community members in planning or offering housing or working activities
- Protection of the person's rights, both in hospitals and in the community
- Case management, to ensure continuous availability of appropriate forms of assistance

*Source*: National Institute of Mental Health (1997) Comprehensive Community Support Systems for Severely Mentally Disabled Adults: Definitions, Components, and Guiding Principles. NIMH, Rockville, MD.

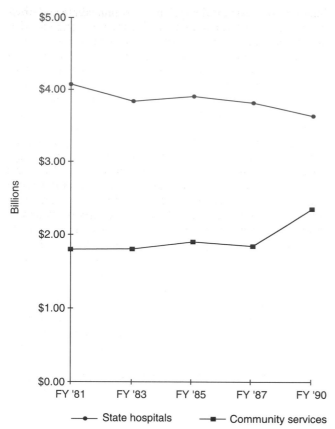

**Figure 109–3** *SMHA expenditures (in constant dollars) for state hospitals and community services between fiscal years (FY) 1981 and 1990. (Source: Lutterman T, Hollen V, and Hogan M [1993] Funding Sources of State Mental Health Agencies: Revenue/Expenditure Study Results Fiscal Year 1990. National Association of State Mental Health Program Directors Research Institute, Alexandria, V.A.)*

During this decade, the SMHA budgets were essentially level when viewed in constant dollars. In other words, budget increases were essentially equal to inflation. Yet, during the decade, there was a steady shift in investments from state hospitals to community programs. The new community resources were often used to "match" Medicaid dollars and linked with block grant revenues and local funds. As a result, there was a dramatic expansion of CSP-type services that is not apparent from examining SMHA budgets alone. Unfortunately, there are few reliable national data that demonstrate the magnitude of this shift. The best way to get a view of the evolution of services for seriously mentally ill individuals in recent years is to track the development of systems at the state level, for which more complete data are available.

## A Case Example of State Mental Health Policy and Funding

Understanding the changes nationwide in the shape of public mental health systems during the 1980s is made difficult because of the limits of available national data. Reliable national data are available on the budgets of the SMHAs, but the Koyanagi and Goldman (1991) analysis makes it clear that federal financing changes during the 1980s (such as the case management benefit in Medicaid) were also significant. However, these changes, unlike the

CMHC effort of the prior decades, were not reflected in the categorical budget of NIMH. Rather, a multitude of federal programs were adjusted incrementally during the decade on the basis of recommendations of the 1980 Department of Health and Human Services report and the President's Commission. Because many of these programs (e.g., Medicaid) were not dedicated primarily to mental health, tracking their impact is more difficult, and the changes have not been well recorded or understood. The changes cannot be appreciated by evaluating trends in the cumulative SMHA budgets, because many of the federal revenues flow through other agencies at the state level. Medicaid, for example, is often administered by human service or welfare agencies.

One way to see the impact of the change, and to end this historical review with a picture of the current public mental health system, is to examine the cumulative impact of federal, state, and local changes in a particular state—in this case, Ohio. A reasonable argument can be made that Ohio is appropriate for such analysis. Although larger in population (seventh among the states in 1994) and smaller in land area (35th) than the average states, Ohio has a mix of urban and rural counties, spanning the range of communities that exist across the country. Its 1990 SMHA budget was $41 per capita, and 59% was spent on state hospital care, compared with the median SMHA expenditure of $38 per capita with an average of 59% spent on hospital care (Lutterman et al. 1993). Therefore, the overall levels and investment patterns of Ohio's SMHA budget are close to national norms. A beginning point to trace the evolution of this system is to evaluate trends in the SMHA budget to determine the pace of movement from hospitals to community services. Figure 109–4 illustrates these trends and Ohio's SMHA budget trends from 1987 to 1993. As illustrated, Ohio made substantial shifts from hospital to community support services during this period. However, the data on state budget expenses alone understate the dynamics of change during this period. Figure 109–5 includes not just the SMHA budget but all revenues used to support community mental health services delivered through the public mental health system in Ohio.

Figure 109–5 combines all sources of revenue received by the county-based mental health boards that are responsible for community mental health care in Ohio. The shift in investments to community support services is greater when these additional fund sources—principally Medicaid, local taxes, and federal block grants—are added into the picture. It illustrates how examining SMHA funding alone leaves an incomplete picture of mental health investments. Federal changes reflecting the paradoxical combination of budget cuts (e.g., block grants) and the simultaneously more effective financing by Medicaid of community mental health care began to have a significant impact. For example, state hospital costs were 58% of the Ohio general fund mental health budget in 1990, but only 37% when all revenues are considered. Similarly, community mental health services funding increased 121% from 1987 to 1993 when all funding sources are considered.

The state-level reform in Ohio, although perhaps broader and more aggressive than changes in many other states, does illustrate how the mantle of leadership in the public mental health sector shifted back to the SMHAs during the late 1980s. After the dramatic federal changes of

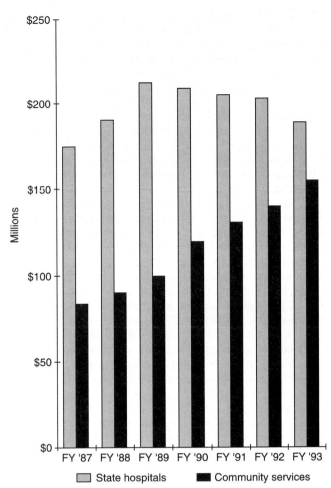

**Figure 109–4** *Ohio state mental health spending: Trends from hospitals to community services between fiscal years (FY) 1987 and 1993. (Source: Ohio Department of Mental Health [1995] Columbus, OH. [Unpublished data])*

the prior two decades, the states needed to consolidate their efforts. A primary vehicle for this effort in Ohio was the 1988 Mental Health Act. This legislation made services for the most seriously mentally ill the highest priority, required local (county-based or multicounty) systems to develop a community support program, empowered the boards as local mental health authorities, and gradually turned control of state hospital funds over to the local boards.

This step removed the historic and unintended incentive to institutionalize the most needy patients at state expense. The counties were now responsible for the costs of state hospital care on the one hand, but they could also choose to invest in community support services. This state reform legislation therefore followed but extended the themes of the ill-fated 1980 federal Mental Health Systems Act, just as the earlier Ohio legislation establishing the mental health boards in 1968 had followed the 1963 Community Mental Health Centers Act at the federal level. The reforms in Medicaid, which made it more useful as an additional funding source for community support services, added to the value of increased or reallocated state and local funds. There was thus a synergy among federal, state, and local initiatives.

The impact of the 1988 legislation, which followed a period of community program development and capacity

building, was extraordinary. The most immediate and obvious impact was the community placement of long-stay disabled patients in a variety of housing arrangements, supported generally by case managers as well as by medication management and day treatment programs. Figure 109–6 shows the reduction in state hospital use in Ohio since this legislation. As illustrated, the reduction in hospital use was primarily attributable to a reduction in long-stay inpatients. Levels of acute care (less than 30 days) stayed about the same, and levels of forensic care and monitoring increased slightly. (Forensic status refers to patients referred through the criminal justice system, including persons sent by courts to be treated to restore their capacity to assist in their own defense, inmates transferred from local jails for brief treatment, and persons found not guilty of crimes by reason of insanity). These trends were thought to be clinically appropriate in that the majority of long-stay patients were not improving as a result of further hospital care, whereas both short-term admissions and forensic cases were generally appropriate for inpatient treatment.

Ohio data also reveal substantial changes in patterns of community care during this period. At a gross level, the number of individuals identified as "severely mentally disabled" (SMD) who were served increased, as did the units of service provided to the average SMD individual. However, there was a slight decrease in the number of non-SMD persons served and a decrease in the units of services

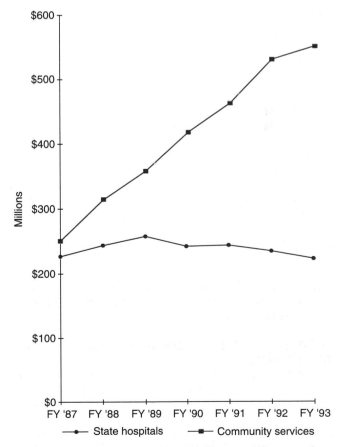

**Figure 109–5** *Funding in Ohio's mental health system: All sources of revenue for community mental health care. (Source: Ohio Department of Mental Health [1995] Columbus, OH. [Unpublished data])*

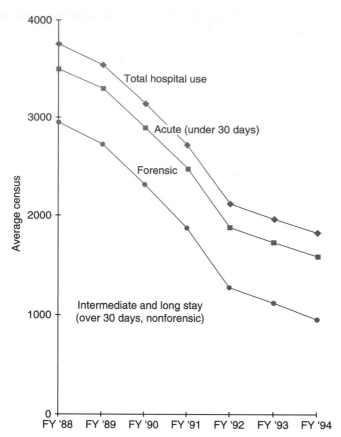

**Figure 109–6** *Ohio state hospital census, by type, for fiscal years (FY) 1988 to 1994. (Source: Ohio Department of Mental Health [1995] Columbus, OH. [Unpublished data])*

provided to these individuals. Table 109–8 illustrates these trends.

Changes were also evident in the pattern of services received by SMD persons. Roth and colleagues (1995) used cluster analysis methods to trace how patterns of care for SMD persons evolved in time and how these related to outcomes. This research revealed that certain patterns of care were relatively stable for a period of time; a consistent 10% of all enrolled SMD persons received substantial levels of various services (labeled custom care by Roth and colleagues), whereas nearly half of all enrolled SMD persons received low levels of service (about a single formal mental health treatment episode per month). On the other hand, in

the 4-year period from 1989 to 1993, there was a significant change in the numbers of SMD persons being served through medication checks without other services. This pattern of care was provided to 23% of individuals in 1989, but this percentage declined to less than 10% by 1993. The apparent shift in this pattern was related to an increase in the use of case management and other services in addition to medical services, reflecting a more comprehensive approach to meeting the treatment needs of these persons. Table 109–9 illustrates these trends.

Roth and colleagues (1995) also found that outcomes (reduced symptoms and better quality of life) improved overall for SMD consumers during this period. Thus, there is some empirical validation of both the community support approach and the reform movement in Ohio during this time. This is not to say that the reform was an unmitigated success. Although community outcomes were positive and the quality of state hospital care improved (as measured by a 72% decline in the frequency of Medicare quality deficiencies from 1991 to 1994), there was conflict in Ohio about funding levels, the pace of change, and the future employment prospects of state hospital staff (Hogan 1992). In addition, the data on reduced levels of non-SMD services reflect a tension between the appropriate goal of increased services for the historically neglected population of seriously mentally ill persons and the unfortunate side effect—given limited public funds—of reduced services to other clients of the public system. However, the Ohio experience does demonstrate that reform in large public mental health systems is possible, and it illustrates the possibilities and dynamics of change in these systems.

## The 1990s: Restoring Focus, Effective Treatments, Defective Funding, Executive Branch Attention

### Restoring Focus: Public Mental Health Systems in the 1990s

The forces converging to change public mental health policy during the 1980s were thus subtler than the "top down" change processes of the mental health establishment during the prior 2 decades. Whereas the CMHCs are widely thought to have failed the test of serving those with serious mental illness, these organizations formed an essential community infrastructure that survived the dismantling of the federal program in 1980. Thus, many CMHCs became essential

| Table 109–8 | Services to Severely Mentally Disabled and Other Adults: The Impact of Reform* | | | | | |
|---|---|---|---|---|---|---|
| | Services to Severely Mentally Disabled Adults | | | Services to Other Adults | | |
| | **Number of Adults** | **Units of Service** | **Units/Adult** | **Number of Adults** | **Units of Service** | **Units/Adult** |
| 1989 | 27,712 | 1,551,057 | 56 | 133,615 | 2,295,744 | 17 |
| 1992 | 37,183 | 2,645,347 | 71 | 121,401 | 1,795,055 | 15 |
| Change | 9,471 | 1,094,290 | 15 | −12,214 | 500,689 | −2 |
| % Change | +34 | +71 | +27 | −9 | −22 | −12 |

*Ohio data for fiscal years 1989 to 1992. SMD, Severely mentally disabled.

*Source*: Study Committee on Mental Health Services (1993) The Results of Reform: Assessing Implementation of the Mental Health Act of 1988. Study Committee on Mental Health Services, Columbus, Ohio.

| Table 109–9 | Cluster Analysis: Patterns of Care Provided to Percentage of Severely Mentally Disabled Persons* | | | | |
|---|---|---|---|---|---|
| Cluster | 1989 | 1990 | 1991 | 1992 | 1993 |
| Few services | 47.70 | 47.80 | 52.80 | 53.10 | 46 |
| Medical | 22.90 | 22.90 | 12.90 | 9.90 | 9.50 |
| Other clusters | 19.80 | 20 | 24.30 | 27.10 | 33.40 |
| Custom care | 9.60 | 9.20 | 10.10 | 9.90 | 11.10 |

*Ohio data for fiscal years 1989 to 1993.

*Source*: Roth D, Lauber BG, Vercellini J, et al. (1995) Final results: Ohio's study of services, systems and outcomes in an era of change. Proceedings: Fifth Annual National Conference on State Mental Health Agency Services Research. National Association of State Mental Health Program Directors Research Institute, Alexandria, VA, pp. 85–103.

elements of the new community support systems that evolved during the 1980s. The new public system is funded through a complex blend of SMHA resources, Medicaid, and local funds. Although consistent national data are not available to document these changes, Ohio data presented in Table 109–8 illustrates how service emphases shifted. From 1989 to 1992, the total volume of services to adults classified as SMD increased 71% in Ohio; units of services to other adults declined 22%. Similarly, the number of SMD persons served increased 34% during this period, and the number of service units per SMD person increased 27%. By comparison, the number of units of service for non-SMD persons decreased by 12%. Through the 1990s these trends continued. Community support program (CSP) services, targeted at adults with SMD and children with severe emotional disturbances (SED), increased as a proposal of the Ohio Public Mental Health system spending from 8.17% in fiscal year (FY) 1990 to 16.2% in FY 1997 (Report of Ohio's Mental Commission 2001). This data, in graphic form is

presented in Figure 109–7. Clearly, the community mental health system was changing its priorities as it was expanding. The locus of care continued its hospital based to community based shift in the 1990s. In 1955 the percentage of patient care episodes occurring in 24-hour hospital care settings was 77%. This dropped to 42% in 1971 and declined further to 24% in 1997 (Manderscheid et al. 2000). On a smaller scale, Ohio Public Mental Health System spending on inpatient care decreased from 46.7% in FY 1990 to 25.4% in FY 1997. (See Figure 109–7) (Report of Ohio's Mental Health Commission 2001). A focus on persons with more serious mental illness and relocation of this care in the community—which had been lacking in the 1960s reforms at both the national and state levels—had been restored.

## Effective Treatments and Defective Funding

Coincident with this refocusing on the care of the severely mentally ill in the 1990s, psychiatry reemphasized its expertise in treating biologically based diseases of the brain. Congress declared the 1990s "the Decade of the Brain" (Surgeon General 1999). New antipsychotics beginning with clozapine in 1989, followed by risperidone, olanzapine, quetiapine, and ziprasidone offered promise to individuals with schizophrenia unresponsive to or unable to tolerate earlier medications. Additional medications in the class of selective serotonin reuptake inhibitors, such as fluoxetine, provided new therapies for people with mood and anxiety disorders. Indeed, a recent study shows substantial increases in the treatment rates for depression from 0.73 per 100 persons in 1987 to 2.33 in 1997 (Olfson et al. 2002). Research supporting the usefulness, including the cost effectiveness of psychotherapies for a broad variety of mental disorders emerged (Gabbard et al. 1997). Studies show the effectiveness of other psychosocial interventions such as assertive community treatment supported employment, family psychoeducation, integrated substance abuse treatment, and illness self-management techniques (Drake et al.

1. *Implementation of the Mental Health Act has changed funding priorities and redirected state hospital resources to community care, and fundamentally changed the mix of community services.*

For example:

• Savings from Ohio Department of Mental Health hospital downsizing and restructuring have led to increased funding for community services, and the mix of community services now emphasizes community support and other services for SED/SMD persons. (Graphs 1 and 2)

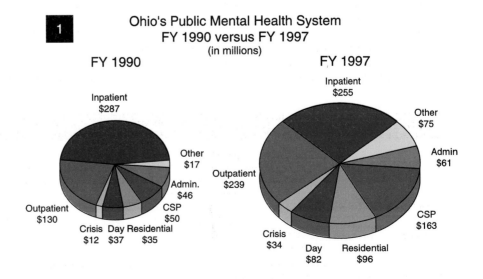

**Figure 109–7** *Trends in funding mental health services in Ohio (2001). Report of Ohio's Mental Health Commission, January 2001. Ohio Department of Mental Health.*

2001). These developments helped bolster calls from advocacy and professional groups for parity in mental health coverage; however, public and private mandates to control costs hindered obtaining the full benefits of improved treatments. These efforts at cost control are covered in detail in the later section on Economics in Mental Health.

## Executive Branch Attention

In the context of the struggle between calls to enhance services and calls to control costs, the executive branch of government drew attention to mental health several times in the 1990s. Although the early efforts at more sweeping health care reform during the Clinton administration failed, a few initiatives limited to mental health merit comment. In September 1997 the Office of the Surgeon General under Surgeon General David Satcher, MD, PhD. authorized the initiation of a *Report on Mental Health*. The report, released in December 1999 drew national attention to mental health problems, noting:

1. "mental health is fundamental to health,"
2. "mental disorders are real health conditions,"
3. the "efficacy of mental health treatments,"
4. the "range of treatments for most mental disorders,"
5. the public are encouraged to seek help for mental health problems,
6. the special needs of specific populations including children and the elderly,
7. the contributions of the advocacy movements,
8. the systems issues of financing complexity, fragmentation of services and access to care.

A supplement highlighted culture, race, and ethnicity (Surgeon General 2001). In July 1999 the Surgeon General issued a Call to Action on Suicide Prevention (1999).

The Clinton White House held a conference on mental health in 1999 to help decrease stigma and increase awareness of mental health issues (Surgeon General 1999). On June 7, 1999, President Clinton directed the Office of Personnel Management (OPM) to achieve parity for mental health and substance abuse coverage for federal workers by 2001 (OPM News Release 1999). President Clinton believed the federal employees program could serve as a model for other employers and the insurance industry (OPM News Release 1999).

President George W Bush kept mental health issues in the spotlight with his announcement on April 29, 2002 of the formation of the New Freedom Commission on Mental Health (White House Press Release 2002). This Commissions's interim report finds:

1. Mental illness affects millions of men, women, and children.
2. Effective treatments for mental illness exists.
3. Multiple barriers impede access to effective treatments, services, and supports.
4. Incentives reward dependency instead of recovery.
5. Excellent care and recovery are possible.

How recent executive branch attention to and efforts at reforming mental health will be integrated into overall mental health policy remains to be seen.

## Implications for Mental Health Policy

The evolution of mental health policy in the US, outlined in Table 109–10, has thus produced a substantial public sector care system that is also exceedingly complex. Essentially consisting of state hospitals in the 19th century, the system expanded dramatically in the past generation by the community mental health, Supplemental Security Income and Social Security Disability Income, and Medicaid and Medicare initiatives of the 1960s. These efforts contributed to a substantial expansion of public mental health responsibilities but also to great blurring of boundaries and diffusion of these responsibilities. New privately provided but publicly financed alternatives such as nursing homes and general hospital psychiatric services were created outside the boundaries of the specialty "mental health system." Income supports enabled some mentally ill persons to exist mostly on outside relief, such as welfare payments, but also weakened the boundaries of the traditional mental health system. The decade of the 1980s provided an opportunity for some consolidation and organization of this fragmentation. The community support concept provided a conceptual framework for understanding the changes that were needed in the new service system, recognizing its fragmentation on the one hand but focusing on the community survival requirements of people wrestling with the most serious mental illnesses.

As a result, in most states, the public mental health system is organized around some local entity, whether county government, special purpose boards or commissions, or provider organizations designated by the state to also manage a local system of care. These local systems exercise variable and incomplete control over the array of public supports that exist because the formation of alternatives is so complex and funded and regulated by so many governmental entities. Federal and state mental health grant resources are most likely to be coordinated at this local level. Increasingly, Medicaid-financed mental health care may be coordinated with the local care management system, but Medicaid remains a distinct government reimbursement program that may or may not be coordinated with state or local mental health authorities.

Programs in other human service areas that are relied on by individuals with serious mental illness (e.g., low-income housing, vocational rehabilitation, services for disabled students in higher education, mental health care within the criminal justice system) are probably not controlled by either the state or local mental health authority. However,

| Table 109–10 | Evolution of Mental Health Policy |
| --- | --- |

- State hospitals to complex system of care
- Limited funding to federal (Medicaid/Medicare), Social Security Income/Social Security Disability Income (SSI/SSDI), state
- Focus on acute care to those with less serious illness to focus on chronic care for those with serious and persistent mental illness
- Public systems of care to more local public/private endeavors, nursing homes, general hospitals
- Lack of coordinated services to case management, assertive community treatment, program of assertive community treatment

the empowerment of local authorities has increased their ability to negotiate agreements and improve coordination with other systems. Yet this remains a serious challenge. Marmor and Gill (1989) have noted that meeting the needs of seriously mentally ill individuals is a particularly difficult challenge within the US political and governmental structure. Whereas good treatment and support require a high degree of coordination and "comprehensive" solutions, the US political system is oriented to incremental approaches, and there is a long-standing distrust of government-managed approaches. Therefore, the public mental health approach at the state and local levels remains a complex, open system.

As a remedial strategy for coping with system fragmentation and to aid individuals whose ability to plan and coordinate their own lives and services may be significantly affected by mental illness, most SMHAs and local mental health systems have adopted a case management strategy. Individuals or teams of case managers assume responsibility for guiding persons with serious mental illness through this maze and assisting them with personal planning. Case management programs as distinct entities are usually provided only to persons with more serious disabilities. For example, in the systems approach described by Stein and colleagues (1990) a well-staffed multidisciplinary community treatment team (analogous to the clinical team and paraprofessionals who work together on an inpatient unit) is the core service for the most needy group of individuals in the Dane County, Wisconsin, system. For other persons receiving care in the publicly funded system, care coordination may be provided by their therapist.

In general, modern public mental health systems still function as a kind of safety net (or, in insurance terms, a "high-risk pool") for the larger health and mental health system, providing care and support for the most needy, seriously mentally ill, and poor individuals in their community. Insurance-financed private care is now available to most Americans, but it is not available for long to those with the most disabling mental illnesses except in the most generous private plans. For these individuals, the public system is the safety net. Mental health is unique in health care with respect to this distinct care and financing system for those with the most serious illnesses. Despite the origins of care in the public sector and the still substantial role of public systems, the private sector—reimbursed by employer-financed insurance—has become dominant in mental health. Understanding the economics of reimbursement systems and their impact on care has thus become essential.

## The Economics of Mental Health

Four interrelated types of financing, listed in Table 109–11, have developed to become critical elements of the economics of health care: out-of-pocket payments by individuals, individually owned or purchased insurance, employer-

| Table 109–11 | Current Types of Financing of Health Care |
| --- | --- |

- Out-of-pocket payments by individuals
- Individually owned or purchased insurance
- Employer purchased insurance
- Government reimbursement

provided insurance, and government reimbursement. Each has different economic dynamics and affects mental health care in different ways. In general, the development of health care financing patterns in the US has followed this sequence, from individual out-of-pocket payments to government financing. At the same time, each of these patterns persists within the complex US "system" of financing health care. A review of the evolution and dynamics of these financing approaches provides the best starting point for understanding the complex economic patterns of care.

## Out-of-Pocket Payment for Care

Before the development of insurance coverage, and indeed well into the 21st century, individual out-of-pocket payment for care was the dominant pattern in health care. This is the simplest and most direct form of financing: people pay for the services they use. There are, however, serious problems with this approach as a financing method for health care and especially for mental health care. The amount of care that any person may need—and thus the amount that must be spent—is unpredictable and may be more than the average citizen can afford when serious health problems arise.

In the case of mental illness, the onset of most serious conditions is often during early adulthood, the prime wage-earning years. By comparison, other health care costs tend to be highest in old age. The most serious mental illnesses also tend to be both long-term and disabling. Many individuals with the most serious mental illness are not able to work and are thus not in a position to pay for the costs of substantial care. Thus, individual out-of-pocket financing is not workable for these individuals. On the other hand, less serious conditions are frequently treatable by psychotherapy or medications. However, psychotherapy in particular and mental health care in general are highly price responsive, meaning that people will use less of it if they have to pay more. In fact, most people will use little mental health care—probably not enough for their good health—if they have to pay the entire cost. Taken together, these factors mean that out-of-pocket financing is a poor primary approach to financing mental health care.

The limit of out-of-pocket reimbursement, the dominant financing approach in the 19th century, provides the economic explanation of the need to create a public care system for people with the most intractable mental illnesses and explains the continuing role of the public sector as a kind of risk pool or safety net for the most needy. An out-of-pocket financing approach fit so poorly with mental health needs that a separate system had to be created. Now that the separate public system exists, its relationship to privately financed care is a problem.

## Individual Private Insurance

In this simplest model of insurance, as Bodenheimer and Grumbach (1994) have described, a third party—the insurer—enters the health care relationship along with the patient and provider. This model was used in 19th century Europe, with guilds and businesses establishing voluntary benefit funds to which members contributed individually, which then provided aid when a member was ill.

The individual insurance approach does introduce the notion of spreading risk across a group of "covered lives,"

| Table 109–12 | Principal Sources of Health Coverage |
| --- | --- |
| Source of Coverage | Population (%) |
| Employment-based private insurance | 52* |
| Government | 25 |
| Uninsured | 14 |
| Individual private insurance | 9 |
| Total | 100 |

*Includes private insurance purchased with public funds.

*Source*: Bodenheimer T and Grumbach K (1994) Paying for health care. JAMA 272, 634–639.

thus shielding individuals from unlikely but extraordinary costs because the risk of incurring these costs is shared by all members. Whereas this essential function of insurance is addressed by the individual insurance approach, this model has a built-in problem: the need to collect contributions and then administer payments for each member individually. This high administrative cost makes individual insurance difficult to sell and expensive to purchase. As a result, only a small percentage of the US population has individual health insurance. The principal sources of health coverage along with population percentage using them are shown in Table 109–12.

Most of the economic dynamics associated with individual insurance are not different from those of out-of-pocket payment for mental health. Of course, insurance is now involved, and so decisions to purchase coverage as well as to use care are involved. This does have an impact on mental health; people are less likely, on average, to seek coverage for mental illness than for other health problems, perhaps because of the perception that "that could not happen to me." This means that individual policies are less likely to provide adequate mental health coverage. If someone with an established illness were to seek to purchase individual coverage, the cost would be prohibitive because of the high risk the person presents. Therefore, the individual insurance approach also fails to provide adequate answers for mental health financing.

## Employer-Based Private Insurance

Bodenheimer and Grumbach (1994) have also provided a cogent analysis of the growth and dynamics of employer-based coverage, the dominant form of health insurance in the US today. The first such plan was developed at Baylor University Hospital in 1929, under an arrangement whereby the hospital agreed to provide up to 21 days of hospital care per person per year in return for a payment of $6 per person per year. This approach to financing care, with the provider also playing a role as insurer, became a dominant approach in the US. The hospital industry controlled development of Blue Cross plans, providing coverage initially for hospital services; state medical societies stimulated development of Blue Shield plans, which primarily covered physicians' services. Starr (1982) has pointed out how this provider-dominated market acted to protect physicians and hospitals by ensuring a steady income and by keeping reimbursement generous. Cost control, on the other hand, was not a major priority.

Employer-based private health insurance became a dominant factor in US health care as a side effect of seemingly unrelated policies: the wage and price controls imposed on companies during World War II. This policy constrained wage and salary increases but did not similarly limit fringe benefits such as insurance. Therefore, insurance coverage was an incentive for employees to join particular companies in a competitive labor market. After the war, unions began to negotiate for benefits, continuing the trend of expanded coverage. In addition, the favorable tax status of employer-paid benefits (because such benefits are by and large not counted as income for tax purposes) contributed to the growth in this type of coverage. As a result, the number of members in group health insurance plans increased from 12 million in 1940 to more than 100 million just 15 years later. Ever since that time, private, employer-financed group health insurance has been the dominant payment and financing mechanism in the US (Bodenheimer and Grumbach 1994).

The fit between employer-financed insurance and mental health care is not inherently a problem, as is the case with individual insurance or out-of-pocket payment. In this case, the adequacy of insurance depends on how the policy is priced and on the type of benefits. Unfortunately, pricing strategies and benefit limits have made the mental health coverage of many employer financed policies inadequate with employees paying a greater share of the cost.

## Community Versus Experience Rating

In the early days of employer-financed coverage, the price of insurance was typically based on the health care use (and thus the cost) of the entire community. Segments of the population were not singled out for differential charges on the basis of their pattern of health care use. This "community rating" approach is consistent with the general purpose of insurance—to spread the costs or risks of costly and unpredictable events across a larger population.

However, as insurers began to compete with each other for business, limiting prices became increasingly important, and the practice of "experience rating" developed: the strategy of pricing insurance on the basis of the actual health care use patterns of the insured population. This approach quickly proved to be a problem for individuals with mental illnesses or other substantial health problems, especially when coupled with other strategies used by employers or payers to limit their costs by controlling "risk" at the point when insurance is purchased. A principal approach to accomplish this is to deny coverage to individuals with expensive "preexisting conditions," which has resulted in denial of coverage to many mentally ill persons.

Experience rating and denial of coverage to potentially expensive consumers (usually those for whom the insurance is most needed) are responses to the competition that has emerged in the private insurance market. By limiting costs through selection of a healthy population, insurers or self-insured employers can partially control their costs, albeit by using strategies that run counter to the basic insurance premise of spreading risk broadly. The other main strategies for controlling insurance costs all target the levels of care that is provided. An obvious first approach is to limit what treatments the policy will cover.

## Benefit Limits

Despite the problems for mental health coverage associated with insurance pricing, benefit limits that discriminate against mental health care have probably been more of a problem. The presence of the public mental health system already created an indirect obstacle to broad mental health benefits, because care for catastrophic conditions was available to those without insurance in this separate system. The competitive pricing strategies of insurers acted to further limit growth in private, employer-financed mental health coverage. A range of coverage limits has been used to control insurance costs: deductibles and copayments (in which the consumer-patient pays a portion of costs before the insurer does) as well as caps on what the insurer will pay (per episode, per year, or in a lifetime). In addition, limits may be placed on what services will be reimbursed, and mental health has not fared well under this approach.

State-of-the-art care for mental illness involves early intervention with medication or psychotherapy. Hospital stays are used sparingly, and a wide variety of rehabilitation and other services are required for many individuals with schizophrenia and other serious disorders. In other words, a wide variety of services may be required and used in a tailored treatment approach over time. In general, benefit limits in mental health preempt almost all of these treatment strategies. Outpatient treatment has been a first target in many mental health plans, for several reasons: the prevailing stereotype that "talk therapy" goes on endlessly without result, and the fact that increases in outpatient therapy use have in fact raised costs substantially in generous plans. As discussed earlier, psychotherapy is in fact highly price responsive: if it is essentially free, people will use a lot of it (in comparison to other visits to physicians, which do not vary as much depending on the cost to the consumer).

On the basis of these factors, many insurance plans limited mental health outpatient therapy to a few visits and required a 50% copayment (compared with the typically unlimited visits available to other physicians, with 20% or smaller copayments). Whereas these limits effectively control expenditures in the short term, they create a disincentive for early treatment and thus contribute to higher rates of hospitalization, which costs more.

Because covering costs of necessary hospital care is a core function of insurance, eliminating psychiatric hospital coverage was generally seen as unacceptable, and most insurance policies provide generally equivalent hospital coverage for psychiatric and physical illness—to a point. Because repeated or long-term hospitalization can lead to extreme costs in serious mental illness during the life span, coverage limits have targeted long or repeated stays by annual or lifetime limits on the amount of care that would be paid.

Using these patterns in an attempt to reveal the impact of coverage limits on consumers, the *New York Times* concluded in 1989 that a person with schizophrenia could expect lifetime treatment costs of $294,800, with less than 25% covered by insurance. A patient with ischemic heart disease, by comparison, would face lifetime treatment costs of $108,350, with more than 90% covered by insurance. The dramatic expansion of high-technology care for such conditions means that the total medical costs for treating them is dramatically increasing.

A final area in which coverage limits are typically a problem in mental illness also relates to serious conditions such as schizophrenia, for which flexible care including approaches such as ongoing case management, rehabilitation, partial hospital programs, and crisis care are used to minimize inpatient care. Many of these services are typically not covered in health plans because they appear to be "added expenses." The ironic result is that extended or repeated hospitalization can result from inadequate community treatment, driving up costs to the insurer to the point of coverage limits, and then leaving the patient without coverage. Limits to coverage are thus a problem for patients, and unless the coverage limits are extreme, they tend to fail at cost control, because patients use up whatever coverage is available.

Mental health thus presents a paradox in terms of cost control. Outpatient care is more price responsive than comparable physical health care, and insurance costs will rise unacceptably unless these costs are somehow controlled. During the late 1980s, a period emerged when benefits became more comparable with other health costs, including a 27% increase from 1987 to 1988 (Employee Benefit Research Institute 1990). Yet controlling costs through arbitrary benefit limits does not work well. Too stringent limits on outpatient care and alternatives to hospitalization drive up hospital costs. It is evident that purely economic controls are not adequate to appropriately balance care and costs in mental health.

## Trends and Approaches in Government Financing

Government financing of care (primarily through Medicare and Medicaid) has been a major force in the US since these programs were introduced in the 1960s. The general trends and dynamics of Medicare and Medicaid have already been discussed. However, these programs, especially Medicare, have also served as a laboratory for benefit design and other cost control approaches. As Bodenheimer and Grumbach (1994) pointed out, these programs have greatly expanded coverage and access to care for elderly, poor, and disabled Americans. At the same time, they aggravated the problem of rising costs and contributed to growing federal budget deficits.

Several innovations in paying for care under Medicare have helped to clarify the challenges of appropriate benefit design and payment for mental health care. These innovations were the use of diagnosis-related groups (DRGs) and the Resource-Based Relative Value Scale (RBRVS). Each of these approaches has significantly shaped thinking about reimbursement in the past several decades.

### Diagnosis-Related Groups

The DRG payment methodology was introduced by Medicare in the 1970s as a means to control inpatient costs. The theory was to pay hospitals fairly for an episode of treatment by calculating the appropriate length of stay for treatment of a given illness or condition. Thus, norms for treatment length of stay were established for comparable diagnoses, and payments were made on a per episode basis rather than by the traditional per diem method. The idea was that hospitals would be rewarded for efficient care by pocketing any savings associated with shorter lengths of stay; inefficient care would cost the hospital more than the DRG payment. Criticism of the approach was loudest from psychiatrists; concern that diagnosis was an inadequate predictor of treatment needs turned out to be correct. Evidence marshaled by the psychiatric community confirmed that diagnosis alone was a poor predictor of the length of stay for psychiatric illness. As a result, Medicare exempted psychiatric units from the DRG payment approach, used nearly universally across other areas of medicine.

The rejection of the DRG approach was initially seen as a victory for mental health treatment, because there was concern that the approach would have led to widespread "creaming" (selection of patients for treatment who in fact had limited needs) and "dumping" (failure to adequately treat needy patients). The rejection of the DRG approach was something of a political victory for the mental health field and particularly for the profession of psychiatry. However, there were also negative effects of the DRG exclusion. First, profit-oriented companies realized that mental health was a less regulated area of health care and rushed in to establish profit-making units, especially in southern states with less general regulation of health care. These units marketed their services heavily and generally paid incentives to staff to maximize the number of admissions. Adolescents with vague "behavior problems" were frequently the major group served in these units, and excessive and often inappropriate treatment stays were typical. These problems led to many investigations and congressional hearings. In some instances, the "milking" of benefits for inappropriate care was so excessive that it consumed patients' insurance coverage up to lifetime limits, meaning that they would be unlikely to ever be able to afford private coverage. The rationale for excluding mental illnesses from DRGs also compounded an image problem for mental health treatment among payers, insurers, and legislators: the perception that psychiatric diagnosis is subjective and that treatment is both unpredictable and generally ineffective.

Although Medicare-financed inpatient psychiatric care remained excluded from DRGs, a number of states adopted variants of this approach to pay for inpatient psychiatric care under Medicaid. Ironically, these tailored approaches seemed to work reasonably well and to avoid the problems predicted for DRGs in mental health. An approach implemented in New Hampshire is among the best documented of these modified DRG strategies in Medicaid. Described by McGuire and colleagues (1990) the New Hampshire payment strategy considered the type of admission (scatter bed or psychiatric admission to a medical–surgical unit, admission to a distinct psychiatric unit, or involuntary admission to a specialized unit) and also provided for payment adjustments for "outliers." This adjustment addressed the problem of particular cases for which a longer length of stay seemed justified by providing a reduced payment for extended care, at a level calculated to be low enough to discourage extended inpatient care but high enough to discourage premature discharge. These features, added to diagnostic groupings, seemed to address the problems predicted for mental health care under DRGs.

### Resource-Based Relative Value Scale

Although a significant innovation in payment, DRGs addressed only inpatient care, and medicine in general was moving in the direction already set in mental health—more outpatient care and less hospitalization. (DRGs also failed to address other cost problems in medicine, such as competition to acquire expensive technology, and the problem of high costs associated with treatment during the last few months of life. However, these topics are beyond the scope of this discussion.) The RBRVS was Medicare's effort to set a rational payment approach for outpatient physician care—a kind of DRG approach for funding clinic and office visits. Under this approach, the level of "resources" required for a given visit or treatment was studied and normed. Resources included the amount of time, level of training and expertise, and other factors that interacted with the particular condition under treatment to produce an acceptable level of care. Similar to the DRG approach, the RBRVS then adjusts payment levels to reflect these national norms.

There has been less controversy associated with the practice of psychiatry and the RBRVS approach than occurred with DRGs, partially because psychiatry was treated more like other forms of medicine in the outpatient area. If the approach had any particular significance, it was in the recognition that visits or interventions requiring high levels of "cognitive" training and expertise had traditionally been undervalued in payment schemes, compared with visits to surgeons in particular.

### The Tax Equity and Fiscal Responsibility Act and the Balanced Budget Act

Exemption from the DRG prospective payment system and inclusion in the RBRVS reimbursement scheme, which recognized cognitive versus procedurally dominant medical services generally enhanced resources for psychiatric services. The 1982 Tax Equity and Fiscal Responsibility Act (TEFRA) reimbursed psychiatric services on a cost-based system per discharge, which included capital costs, bonuses for lower costs, and bad debt, explains Health Policy Alternatives 1998 (Garritson 1999). Under the TEFRA and earlier funding plans, private inpatient psychiatric services boomed in the 1980s. Redick and colleagues (Mechanic et al. 1998) note that between 1970 and 1992 specialized psychiatric units increased from 664 to 1,516, the number of private mental hospitals more than tripled and admissions quadrupled. As noted earlier, some of this expansion resulted in inappropriate utilization of inpatient care but the greater overall effect was the vast expansion of the role that the private (albeit publicly funded) care system played in the provision of acute psychiatric care. Between 1988 and 1994 discharges for a primary psychiatric diagnoses from general hospitals increased approximately 35% from 1.4 to 1.9 million per year with the largest growth (53%) occurring in private nonprofit hospitals (Mechanic et al. 1998). At the same time public general hospitals experienced an approximately one-third reduction in the number of discharges from 132.1 to 83.8 million per year. The number of days of care in mental hospitals, excluded as "IMD" facilities from receiving Medicaid funds, declined overall with the largest decrease occurring in public hospitals (12.5 million days) and far exceeding the increase of 1.2 million in general hospitals (Mechanic et al. 1998). Additionally, the rate of discharges for severe mental illnesses (SMI) in general hospitals increased from 196 to 314 per 100,000 population with the largest increase (almost 90% higher) being found in private nonprofit hospitals. In these institutions 12% more of the total bed days were for patients with SMIs. Mechanic also notes that proprietary hospitals had transfer rates higher than nonprofit hospitals with the differences being more pronounced for patients with SMI in general, and especially for patients with schizophrenia. As a result of an uneven distribution of caring for Medicaid enrollees and uncompensated care, Mechanic argues for identifying those institutions which are assuming the larger share of this burden and targeting them for public support in order for them to provide the public safety net.

In 1997, rather than this targeted support for general hospitals which were providing an ever increasing proportion of acute psychiatric care, including care for individuals with SMI, Congress enacted and President Clinton signed the Balanced Budget Act of 1997. The Congressional Budget Office estimated that the act would save $112 billion by slowing the growth of Medicare and $7 billion by changes to Medicaid over the 1998 to 2002 period (CBO 1997). A majority of the reduction in Medicare was to come from reduced payments to hospitals, according to Ramsey Wallace (Garritson 1999). Payments to physicians also were targeted for cuts. The Medicaid savings were to be achieved largely by reducing payment to disproportionate share hospitals (facilities that provide a high volume of services to the Medicaid population) (Garritson 1999). The Medicare Balanced Budget Refinement Act of 1999 restored slightly less than 10% of the funding cuts made in the 1997 legislation, increasing federal spending by 10.5 billion for the 2000 to 2004 period (CBO 1999).

These cuts in public funding for private hospital care has raised the concern that the closing of psychiatric units which began in the late 1980s and 1990s in the for-profit arena as private insurance adopted managed care will spread to the nonprofit institutions that currently provide much of psychiatric care. The National Association of Psychiatric Health Systems (NAPHS) survey (2002) reported that among its member facilities Medicare and Medicaid accounted for 45.4% of admissions in 2000. In US in 2000 Manderscheid and colleagues (2000) report the number of psychiatric beds in 1970 was 524,878 (413,066 in state and county psychiatric hospitals), by 1998 the number decreased to 261,903 (63,525 in state and county psychiatric hospitals). The majority of psychiatric beds now are in the private sector and are largely outside of state or federal regulation regarding remaining open. Indeed, while psychiatric beds in the private sector increased from 14,295 in 1970 to 44,871 in 1990, by 1998 these had decreased to 33,635 (Mandescheid et al. 2000). Occupancy rates as

reported by the NAPHS have increased from 55.6% in 1996 to 69.2% in 2000. Anecdotal reports in both professional and lay news are describing shortages of psychiatric beds across the country. The Ohio Department of Mental Health—Offices of Licensure and Certification and Office of Quality Improvement compiled a recent report documenting a 9% decrease in private psychiatric hospitals or units in general hospitals and an 18% decrease in psychiatric beds in these units from 1997 to 2002 as shown in Table 109–13 (Paschall 2002). The largest decrease was a 28% loss of adolescent beds. The changes occurred across the state with only one region reporting a slight increase of 6% in beds. The other seven regions showed declines with the largest decline being in a rural southeastern region (55%) and a central urban region (51%).

In summary payment reforms in Medicare, including both DRGs and the RBRVS, have had a significant impact on medicine and psychiatry without fundamentally solving the cost problems in the health care system. Psychiatric care, initially exempt from DRG payment schemes and benefiting to some extent from RBRVS payments has faced increased pressure along with the rest of medical services from implementation of the cost cutting Balancing Budget Act of 1997 which reduced Medicare and Medicaid reimbursements. Current levels of public funding of care within the private sector may not be enough to prevent erosion of this latest safety net for people with mental illnesses.

The impact of the earlier payment reforms (DRG and RBRVS) has extended beyond Medicare, already the largest single payer of health care bills in the US. Surveys of Blue Cross and Blue Shield insurance plans in 1994 found that 19 of 24 plans used the Medicare RBRVS approach for physicians' payments, whereas about two-thirds of plans used a DRG approach for hospital reimbursement. (Grading Health Care Reform 1994). Thus, systems that attempt to link standards for payment to the type of illness and condition have had a growing impact. Two major problems persist, however. First, these methods do not address other reasons for cost increases in health care. Second, these broad-brush strategies fail to address the normal and appropriate variances in care required by individuals. By using a "lowest common denominator" approach to payment, these methods do not capitalize well on either payer or physician ingenuity in treatment. However, these methods were implemented during a time when there was also active experimentation with these issues and with approaches that blend economics, clinical knowledge, and systems technology to achieve better service quality and cost control. Often labeled managed care,

| Table 109–13 | Trends in Psychiatric Hospitals and Beds in Ohio. Ohio Department of Mental Health 2002 | | | | |
|---|---|---|---|---|---|
| Year | Total | Adult | Adolescent | Child | Number of Hospitals |
| 1997 | 3456 | 2792 | 503 | 161 | 96 |
| 1999 | 3390 | 2748 | 477 | 165 | |
| 2001 | 2931 | 2428 | 363 | 140 | |
| 2002 | 2842 | 2341 | 361 | 140 | 87 |
| % Change | −18% | −16% | −28% | −13% | −9% |

these approaches have rapidly shaped health care in general and mental health care in particular.

## The Emergence of Managed Care and Its Impact on Mental Health

It is clear that the evolution of health and mental health policy has involved a dynamic tension among social–political forces, clinical philosophies and practices, economics, and the organization of care systems. In the 19th century, mental health care was shaped more by social forces and related clinical philosophies, as in the connection between Jacksonian reform and the establishment of asylums. In the closing decades of the 20th century, economics has arguably been the dominant force shaping mental health.

There has been a dramatic expansion in the availability of care and the emergence of a substantial private sector of mental health treatment financed by employer-based private insurance. Yet old problems have persisted, and a new problem has become dominant—the costs of health care. By the early 1990s, health care costs in the US were a higher proportion of the gross national product than in any other developed country, and the rate of health care cost inflation was among the world's highest. In seeking solutions to this problem, health care has sought new organizational forms involving arrangements such as health maintenance organizations (HMOs), individual practice associations, and preferred provider organizations. These approaches involve variously organized networks or associations of providers and move beyond strictly economic strategies that seek to alter costs by modified payments to providers or charges to consumers.

## The Nature and Growth of Health Maintenance Organizations

HMOs are, fundamentally, group medical practices that are prepaid—the practice organization is paid a set amount by its members in advance to take care of them if they are ill or even, indirectly, to protect their health. The first prepaid group practice was in 1929, when two Los Angeles physicians contracted with employees of the Los Angeles County Department of Water and Power, and their families, to provide comprehensive health care services in return for prepaid fees (Bennett 1992). With the Great Depression, World War II, and the subsequent effort by both employers and health providers to develop insurance-financed care arrangements, fee-for-service arrangements were dominant, and cost control took a back seat. Although some notable HMOs such as Kaiser Permanente developed during this period, the majority of care was paid for by retrospective fee-for-service arrangements. HMOs were viewed as alternative medicine and resisted by most physicians and physicians' groups. HMOs use a wide variety of means to provide care while controlling costs, including controlled staffing levels, salaried staff, "wellness" programs, and use of nurses and other clinical staff who are paid less than physicians.

Ironically, given their image as an alternative social innovation, HMOs received a major boost as a key ingredient in the Nixon administration's health care reform proposals, with Paul Ellwood as the champion of the concept. Credited with coining the term *health maintenance organization*, Ellwood saw HMOs as a way to improve care while containing costs and made the approach a central element

of Nixon's proposals. The Health Maintenance Organization Act of 1973 was the result. This legislation subsidized the creation and expansion of HMOs and broadened the approach to allow profit-making corporations to become HMOs and to allow "medical care foundations" to function as HMOs (Bennett 1992). Medical care foundations evolved to be known today as independent practice associations, one of the major variants of prepaid plans. An independent practice association may be described as a "loose HMO," in which a group of practitioners agree to accept fixed fees without formally organizing into a group practice. (In the HMO, by comparison, physicians are employees of the organization and are almost always salaried.)

Certain forms of cost containment are "built into" prepaid plans such as HMOs. The prepaid nature of services itself introduces an incentive to avoid providing unnecessary care. The apparent ability of HMOs and the other prepaid and managed care approaches to control costs is certainly a major factor in their expansion. In 1983, fewer than 14 million Americans were enrolled in HMOs (Goran 1992). By 1991, 47% of Americans with employer-financed health insurance were in managed care arrangements. By 1994, this figure had climbed to 65%, and HMOs claimed more than 50 million members (Eckholm 1994). The increase continued to over 75% of the insured population being in some type of managed care plan by 1998 (Frank and McGuire 2000).

## Preferred Provider Organizations

Preferred provider organizations are another variant on the organization of health care, sharing some similarities with both HMOs and individual practice associations in terms of structure and approach. In the typical preferred provider organization, a group of physicians—who typically do not practice together but maintain their own offices—negotiate discounted rates with insurers in return for "preferred" status as the primary health care providers for the insured group. Thus, the preferred provider organization is not a prepaid arrangement, but payment to the group is based on discounted fee-for-service rates. As in the case of HMOs, members typically pay a penalty for getting care outside of the network. At a minimum, the copayments for care outside the network are higher. In some situations, the insurer will not reimburse at all for care outside the network, except in emergencies.

## Health Maintenance Organizations and Mental Health Care

The history and track record of HMOs in providing mental health care is unexceptional. In a way, it parallels the record of mental health care under private insurance in general: limited benefits, an emphasis on a few treatment approaches, and gradual evolution to more satisfactory patterns of care. However, some of the dynamics of HMOs affect mental health care in particular ways. The 1973 Health Maintenance Organization Act required that HMOs provide only a limited mental health benefit (crisis care and up to 20 sessions for evaluation and brief treatment, with no coverage required for inpatient care or for treatment of ongoing conditions). Whereas many plans found that this low benefit level was unworkable and added coverage for inpatient treatment, the profile of psychiatric care in most HMOs remained low. Martinsons (1988) found that the common level of mental health expenditures in HMOs was 3 to 5%, contrasted with 8% of all expenditures in fee-for-service plans. Some observers now believe that mental health consumes on average up to 12 to 14% of expenditures in fee-for-service plans, raising serious questions about the adequacy of mental health service levels in HMOs.

## Emergence of Managed Mental Health Care

Stimulated largely by the substantial increases in mental health expenditures during the 1980s and the failure of strictly economic approaches to control costs, managed care techniques were increasingly applied to mental health care. The primary strategies employed in early managed care efforts might best be described as "managed cost" attempts to intervene in treatment decisions like hospitalization to prevent all unnecessary expenditures. These arrangements typically involved the requirement that third-party reviewers (frequently entry-level clinical staff armed with procedure code-books) authorize any inpatient admissions. This authorization would usually cover a limited time, with the requirement that permission be obtained for any treatment beyond this initial period. The clear target of early managed care efforts was psychiatric inpatient treatment, which had been the area of greatest cost increases during the 1980s as benefits were expanded. These arrangements were successful in limiting costs but angered many psychiatrists.

The early managed care efforts did demonstrate the efficacy of a specialized approach to management of mental illness care, against the typical pattern of high costs in fee-for-service plans and low levels of services in many HMOs. Consequently, a "carve out" strategy was increasingly used by employers, who would contract with a distinct entity to manage all mental health and substance abuse treatment needs of the covered population. Such arrangements, in addition to limiting treatment costs, started to demonstrate effectiveness in improving outcomes, such as time lost from work, and decreased expenditures for medical care.

As expertise in these practices grew, specialized managed care providers, during the late 1980s and early 1990s, moved beyond the crude managed cost efforts of the first-generation programs. The second tier of programs began to use more sophisticated approaches, including selecting their "network" of providers on the basis of reputation and credentials in addition to low cost, offering training in more effective or relevant treatment approaches, and initiating new but lower cost services rather than just denying access to care. For example, partial hospital programs and intensive outpatient services were developed to provide an alternative to inpatient treatment for some patients. Thus, these second-generation efforts focused on managing care as well as cost.

As distinct "behavioral managed care" programs evolved, efforts turned beyond screening—prior authorization methods and the selection of lower cost providers—and put more emphasis on quality assurance protocols that provided feedback to psychiatrists. This evolution has led to the third generation of specialized managed care. The program developed by IBM in the early 1990s provided a benchmark for these more sophisticated efforts.

Like other large employers, IBM had seen its mental health and substance abuse treatment costs rise dramatically under its fee-for-service insurance with generous benefits. The company was committed to cost control but equally insistent that this not be achieved through limiting benefits and crude rationing. In developing specifications for its new program, IBM employed an independent mental health advisory board to both assist in the development of a managed care program and oversee its operation.

The resultant program, operated by one of the new behavioral managed health care firms (American Psych Management), was designed to operate as a complete system responsible for screening needs, establishing a preferred provider network, managing care received through this network, and conducting extensive customer satisfaction and quality assurance monitoring (Bengen 1992). Within this program, more extensive benefits were offered than were available under the prior fee-for-service program (e.g., residential treatment centers and other residential care), but all services were subject to care management and individual treatment planning.

This type of arrangement is relatively typical of third-generation managed care programs, in which the functions of utilization review and care management, as well as responsibility for actually providing care, are assumed by the managed care firm. The firm employs mental health clinicians (supervised by psychiatrists) to conduct the care management function, recruits providers into a closed panel or network, and manages the care network including quality assurance functions. In these arrangements, the firm is essentially a specialized or carved out HMO, responsible only for mental health (and, typically, substance abuse care). The basic concept of this approach is also remarkably similar to the design of the public sector CMACs developed several decades earlier, although the managed care firm serves a covered population and the CMHC functions as a network of care for a primarily uninsured population.

## Managed Mental Health Care in the Public Sector

By the early 1990s, managed care's presence in employer-sponsored health insurance was well established and new markets were sought. At the same time, state governments concerned about increasing budget deficits and specifically about the ever growing proportion of state budgets spent on Medicaid, looked to managed care as a mechanism to control costs. Together these factors resulted in a rapid expansion of managed care into both public general medical care and into public mental health care. Mechanic and colleagues (1998) reviewing HCFA data report that by 1997 nearly half of Medicaid recipients were enrolled in a managed care plan. Croze (2000) citing a Substance Abuse and Mental Health Services Administration (SAMHSA) 1998 report states that 46 states were implementing managed mental or behavioral health in some form and 10 states had virtually no fee for service behavioral health care funded by Medicaid. Of these 46 states, 25 handled a significant portion of their Medicaid benefits through risk arrangements in which risk is transferred from the state Medicaid agency to another entity. Seventeen states utilize a managed behavioral health care organization (MBHO) carve-out in some manner. The risk however is transferred to a variety of organizations including a MBHO, a MBHO/provider partnership, the county government itself or an authority appointed by county government, a community mental health center (CMHC) or local behavioral health authority. She describes the complexities of these new arrangements, including common emphasis on "medical loss ratio" (maximum dollars directed to care and treatment), use of caps on profit and administration, frequent requirements for reinvestment in service development, financial reserves, and performance bonds and/or lines of credit.

Another common feature is the exclusion of pharmaceutical coverage within the behavioral health contract. This is a strategy recommended by the Department of Health and Human Services—Office of the Inspector General by HHS-0I6 as reported by Ross (2000) due to concern by states that they could not accurately determine the cost for this benefit and were concerned that if not costed correctly managed care organizations would restrict access. However, as pharmaceuticals (psychotropic and other drugs) account for a growing proportion of health care spending this exclusion may need to be reconsidered.

Between 1999 and 2000 spending on drugs in the US increased by 18.8% from $111.2 billion to $132 billion (Charatan 2001). Three factors accounted for most of the increase; a larger number of prescriptions, the use of more expensive drugs, and price increase (Charatan 2001). Aggressive marketing by drug companies also contributed to the spending increase (Charatan 2001). Newer antidepressants and antipsychotics are substantially higher priced than older medications. Together, these families of psychotropics account for a large proportion of the increase in spending on drugs. Antidepressants represented the second highest sales by class of medications in 2000 at $8.3 billion (IMS Health 2001). Antipsychotics ranked sixth in sales at $4 billion (IMS Health 2001). In 2000, the top ten list of US sales of prescription products included two SSRIs and one new antipsychotic (IMS Health 2001). Antidepressants widely used across both general medical and psychiatric settings have a broader impact in prescription costs. Newer antipsychotics used primarily for the treatment of schizophrenia spectrum disorders disproportionately impact Medicaid spending. Medicaid spending on antipsychotics increased nearly 2.5 times between 1995 and 1998 from $484 million to 1,264 million (Mulligan 2002). Those individuals enrolled in traditional Medicare plans alone remain without any prescription drug benefit to cover these costly medications. Solutions to the rising drug cost problem are not easy. Canada controls medication costs via federal regulation. However, while prices are lower than in the US, Canadian prescribing trends toward newer, more expensive psychotropics led to a 216% increase in cost for these drugs between 1992 and 1998 (Dewa and Goering 2001). New Hampshire's attempt in 1981 to control Medicaid spending by limiting prescriptions to 3 per month resulted in savings in drug costs but this was negated by a even higher increase in mental health costs including outpatient visits, emergency services, and partial hospitalization (Soumerai et al. 1994).

Differences in managed mental health care programs abound. Debate continues regarding which programs are successes and the reasons for programs failing. Croze (2000) presents programs in Colorado, Iowa, and Massachusetts as having achieved improvements in some of the following areas: decreased costs, increased penetration, decreased hospital admissions, increased array of services, and decreased waiting times. How much more efficiency and cost saving may be gained by further use of managed care is not clear. Historically, those areas which relied more heavily on inpatient care have produced earlier and more dramatic results using managed care through decreasing the use of inpatient care by decreasing admissions and decreasing length of stay. There may now be more areas similar to the Oregon counties studied by McFarland and coworkers (2002) in 1995 in which one county switched to a managed Medicaid system while the other remained fee-for-service. Both counties showed decreased length of stay from 1994 to 1996. The county which changed to managed care retained its slightly longer length of stay. As length of stays shorten, in this case to 6 days, it becomes more difficult to discern differences between groups. In some areas there may be little left to squeeze from the inpatient care system.

Finally, greater appreciation by both the managed care industry and by state and local governments about the complexities of providing care for the severely mentally ill (SMI) population may also temper the initial enthusiasm for public managed mental health care. Concerns about the ability of managed care systems, which have traditionally served populations with large numbers of relatively healthy, well functioning individuals, to serve a disabled, severely and persistently ill population remain. Boothroyd and coworkers (2002) recommend caution in considering risk arrangements for such vulnerable populations on the basis of their finding that Florida Medicaid enrollees in plans in which providers bore financial risk reported less use of both general medical and mental health services and more problems with access than those enrolled in fee-for-service plans. Satisfaction with general medical services but not with mental health services was also adversely effected by the provider bearing risk (Boothroyd et al. 2002).

The structure of risk sharing arrangements varied greatly across the five SAMSHA demonstration sites which targeted adults with severe mental illness; but all five sites showed an inverse relationship between assumption of risk and the application of strict utilization review (Ridgely et al. 2002). Other differences between sites included how substance abuse and pharmacy benefits were provided (Ridgely et al. 2002). Monitoring the effect of managed mental health care on people with severe mental illness will remain a challenge for the upcoming years.

## Emerging Directions in Care Management

It is clear that the more sophisticated managed care approaches have succeeded in controlling mental health care costs while addressing concerns about quality that were serious and legitimate regarding early cost management programs. A 1993 report by the actuarial consulting firm Milliman and Robertson cited experiences with five major US firms that implemented mental health managed care approaches, achieving consistent savings and increasing benefits or use of services among the covered population (Melek 1993). As a result, the growth in use of mental health managed care has been extraordinary. By 1993, specialized behavioral managed care firms were responsible for mental health care for more than 80 million Americans.

Managed care programs in mental health have been more successful at balancing cost control, access to care, and quality than approaches that emphasize benefit limits and payment approaches, such as DRGs. Done well, managed care efforts blend economic incentives with clinical decision-making in the context of a prepaid system of care. Yet, these arrangements cover the gamut from the relatively crude cost management programs that emphasize rationing to sophisticated third-generation efforts that emphasize quality. The trend among larger employers is clearly toward the more sophisticated managed care approaches. However, future directions are uncertain, given the extraordinary cost pressures that still exist in health care.

Kunnes (1994) predicted that future approaches to mental health services will move beyond managed care as it is now known. He forecasted the increased development of "integrated delivery systems" that are "vertically and horizontally integrated, managed, very patient friendly, regional, and inclusive of both behavioral health care and medical/surgical services" (Kunnes 1994). Under this scenario, provider networks will increasingly take on their own insurance functions, capitalizing on their local reputations and relationships while recognizing the need to manage risk. Kunnes also predicted that "distinctions between public and private delivery systems will break down" (Kunnes 1994). Whereas this is only one of many possible future scenarios, it illustrates a direction that builds on emerging developments in the mental health field: increased access, cost control, and strategies to achieve these goals that use economic incentives, clinical decision-making, and organizational approaches.

## The Quality Improvement Movement

Mental health treatment has also been affected by the quality improvement methods and approaches that have evolved from the work of W. Edwards Deming and other industrial quality improvement "gurus." Central themes include the idea of quality improvement as a continuous process, the importance of measurement in aiding in and defining changes in quality, and an orientation to customer requirements and satisfaction. These ideas have been reflected in the accreditation standards of the Joint Commission on Accreditation of Health Care Organizations and signal the evolving direction of quality improvement. Bologna and Feldman predicted that the direction of quality efforts in mental health will evolve toward continuous improvement: "A feedback loop in which clinical outcomes shape patient treatment matching, which in turn changes outcomes, is the core mechanism from which many of the most dramatic changes in behavioral health care will evolve" (Bologna and Feldman 1994, p. 32).

## Defining and Improving the Quality of Mental Health Care

The issue of the quality of mental health treatment presents several paradoxes. One is the gap between solid knowledge of the general efficacy of treatment and the absence of much specific research that links particular interventions with particular conditions at defined times. A second paradox involves the gap between findings of treatment efficacy (the demonstrated impact of care under research conditions) and broader treatment effectiveness (the results achieved under typical treatment conditions).

The general efficacy of mental health care is well established. In a comprehensive review of research on the epi-

demiology of mental illness and the effectiveness of care, the National Advisory Mental Health Council concluded that "for persons with serious mental disorders, the chances of obtaining significant benefit through treatment have never been better ... a growing body of research knowledge from clinical trials has verified the efficacy of these treatments ... this compares very favorably with other areas of medicine" (National Advisory Mental Health Council 1993, p. 1450).

There is also considerable evidence of the efficacy of particular categories of treatment. The volume of research on the efficacy of psychotherapy, for example, is extraordinary. In an analysis of the psychotherapy literature, Lipsey and Wilson (1993) concluded that the evidence of the benefits of psychotherapy is well established. At the same time, the diversity of mental illness and its treatments imposes a humbling reality. Research has not yet established clear findings linking the nature, method, and timing of interventions to particular conditions. Atkinson and colleagues (1992) concluded that not enough was known about which treatments work, the particular circumstances under which people with serious mental illness benefit, or how services should be sequenced or combined most effectively. Similar issues exist even within the psychotherapy research literature. Lipsey and Wilson (1993) found a relationship between the strength of the therapist–patient alliance and the effectiveness of treatment and the satisfaction with treatment predicted better outcomes, but their analysis did not correlate specific methods with conditions or diagnoses. Thus, there is considerable evidence about the effectiveness of mental health treatment and about which general types of treatment are helpful with which disorders. However, clear data establishing specific parameters for care of particular conditions under defined circumstances remain elusive.

At the same time, fiscal pressures and expectations of patients and payers are leading to an increasing emphasis on defining and improving the quality of treatment. With these pressures, approaches to address quality are evolving from crude, broad approaches like licensure and certification of professionals or programs to increasingly specific and focused strategies such as treatment guidelines for specific conditions.

## The Evolution of Quality of Care Strategies

The most basic approaches to ensuring the quality of care are licensure of practitioners as adequately qualified, certification of providers or agencies for the purpose of reimbursement, and accreditation of provider organizations by independent bodies.

### Licensure

Licensure of practitioners by states is the most basic and universal approach to quality. Licensure is based on training, a review of qualifications, and sometimes passage of an examination. Frequently, professionals must satisfy requirements for continued education to maintain their licensed status. As an approach to ensuring quality, licensure is basic; it focuses on the preparation of the practitioner but does not address the actual conduct, processes, or outcomes of care. Professional licensure is required to be able to practice or, generally, to accept reimbursement. Thus, licensure provides a kind of basic consumer protection, ensuring that patients are not treated by untrained or ill-prepared individuals.

## Certification

In most states, certification of provider organizations by state authorities is the equivalent of professional licensure; in fact, the terms licensure and certification of agencies are sometimes used interchangeably. Certification standards are typically designed to ensure that provider organizations are minimally qualified and usually address such issues as the presence of adequate and safe facilities, acceptable policies and procedures, qualified and licensed staff, appropriate record-keeping and treatment-planning procedures, and the like. Like professional licensure, certification is required as a threshold to provide care, typically being a requirement for public reimbursement or contracts. Certification can ensure that appropriate preconditions for quality care are present but cannot ensure that quality care is actually provided.

## Accreditation

Various independent organizations have developed voluntary standards and review mechanisms that they employ to accredit provider organizations. The most significant accrediting body in health care is the Joint Commission on Accreditation of Health Care Organizations, which predominantly accredits hospitals but also addresses health systems, clinics, and mental health centers. Other accrediting organizations that touch on mental health include the Commission on Accreditation of Rehabilitation Facilities, the Council on Accreditation (which specializes in counseling and family service organizations), and the Utilization Review Accreditation Council. The last organization is the newest and reflects the demand from both payers and treatment professionals that standards be developed to address the growing utilization review and managed care industry.

Accreditation has similarities to state certification and involves review of facilities, staffing, policies and procedures, and so on. However, accreditation is a voluntary process (although increasingly, purchasers insist on accreditation as another assurance of quality). Accreditation is often more demanding than state certification standards; for example, it may address evidence of the actual use of practices such as quality assurance or review of staff members' credentials. However, accreditation, like licensure and certification, indicates only that the conditions for quality care are present—or at least they were present at the time of the most recent survey. Given the increased concern about cost and cost-effectiveness that characterizes the current health care environment, more specific methods are increasingly being developed.

## Developing Approaches to the Quality of Care

Beyond licensure, certification, and accreditation a variety of approaches are used to respond to demands for quality of care data. A direct approach that is increasingly in vogue is assessing patients' satisfaction with care received. Whereas "customer satisfaction" is a legitimate issue to assess on its own merits, there is some research justification for assessing patients' satisfaction as an approach to quality. In Lipsey and Wilson's (1993) meta-analysis of psychotherapy research, patients' satisfaction was related to outcomes, a finding that also emerged from the study by Roth and coworkers (1995) of outcomes for severely mentally disabled patients in community care.

Owing to the increasing understanding of satisfaction as an outcome-related variable and because of its inherent value, managed care firms are increasingly requiring the use of satisfaction measures by practitioners. According to Freeman and Trabin, "The demand for data on quality has led to almost universal implementation of customer (patient) satisfaction measurement through the use of questionnaires as a first step. Measuring self-reported patient satisfaction is often easier than measuring clinical outcomes. Similarly, provider network satisfaction ratings and patient satisfaction measurement queries are finding their way into the audits of managed care plans performed by employee benefits managers" (Freeman and Trabin 1994, p. 30).

Another quality-related practice that is growing in acceptance is the use of standardized assessment scales as an aid to assessment of patients and treatment planning and to assist in checking progress in treatment. Although there is not yet evidence to support the use of standardized measures to dictate treatment regimens, there can be little doubt that these measures provide an element of objectivity and can serve as a reference point. The use of these measures is also generally considered important as documentation that treatment has progressed according to accepted professional standards, an important consideration in an era of increasing litigiousness.

## Practice Guidelines

Research on the effectiveness of different patterns of care is also enabling the development of practice guidelines—recommended approaches to the treatment and management of particular conditions. These guidelines are intended to strike a balance between specificity when it is possible and deference to the psychiatrist's judgment when it is appropriate. Practice guidelines are typically developed by consensus panels of researchers and psychiatrists on the basis of the state of knowledge that exists with respect to a particular condition. Guidelines for the treatment of psychiatric disorders have been published by the American Psychiatric Association (see Table 109–14) (American Psychiatric Association 2002). Other groups are also working on treatment guidelines in mental health. The Agency for Health Care Policy and Research and the NIMH funded a Patient Outcome Research Team (PORT) study to review the literature, study actual practice patterns, and make recommendations for the treatment of schizophrenia. The

| Table 109–14 | APA Guidelines for Treatment of Patients with the Following Disorders Have Been Developed |
|---|---|

- Borderline Personality Disorder
- HIV
- Major Depression
- Eating Disorders
- Delerium
- Alzheimer's and other Dementias
- Panic Disorder
- Substance Use (Alcohol, cocaine, opioids)
- Schizophrenia
- Bipolar Disorder
- Nicotine Dependence

approach has been used previously to develop treatment recommendations for cataract surgery, hip replacement, and other conditions, but the PORT study of schizophrenia was the first in mental health. The PORT study recommended 30 interventions for the treatment of schizophrenia. The majority of the recommendations focused on adequate use of antipsychotics and other medications but included the use of electroconvulsive therapy, selected forms of psychotherapy (nonpsychodynamic), family support and psychoeducation, vocational rehabilitation, and assertive community treatment (Lehman 1998). The development and use of treatment guidelines are not unique to mental health, and the future will find increased use of practice guidelines in mental health and in health care in general.

## Prospects for the Future

Absent revolutionary changes in the basic landscape of health care—which are certainly possible—the trends described in this chapter are likely to continue. At the same time, the rate and path of change are unpredictable; the complexities of the health care system and of mental health care in particular make this virtually certain. An appreciation of the dynamics and general directions of change is most relevant in this uncertain context.

As the discussion earlier in the chapter illustrates, reform in mental health has been tied to social and political trends in the larger society, and emerging clinical innovations and treatment approaches have often been linked with parallel social changes. This is an important dynamic that is likely to persist. The increasing diversity of society may thus be linked to the reduction in the stigma of mental illness and to seeking help that has been so dramatic in the past generation. On the other hand, there remain strong signals of intolerance, and the income and class differences between rich and poor are not being reduced. The fate of the most seriously and persistently mentally ill, especially the homeless mentally ill, may rest as much on these trends as on advances in treatment.

The relationship between the public and private mental health sectors has been one of the most important and underestimated factors shaping mental health policy. Psychiatry emerged as a profession within US medicine, by and large, in the public sector of the 19th century. In more recent years, the story has been dominated more by separate and discrete private and public sector systems, for those with means and less serious conditions on the one hand and the seriously mentally ill on the other.

There are numerous signs at this time of the blurring of lines between public and private sectors. The government insurance programs (Medicare and Medicaid) involve publicly financed but increasingly privately provided care. The financial pressures in the private health care sector are increasingly reminiscent of public sector limits. Although the Health Security Act failed to achieve passage in 1994, its proposition that universal, nondiscriminatory mental health coverage should be achieved—requiring the integration of public and private resources—struck a chord among health and mental health practitioners and policymakers.

The gradual fusion of many public and private resources in mental health is also augured by developing trends in the organization and financing of care. It is now abundantly clear that the complexities of treating mental illness cannot be addressed by the same economic approaches that have been used for inpatient and outpatient physical health care. At the same time, the financing and organization of most health care are changing, with much broader reliance on HMOs and the continued development of new provider collaboratives and networks. The implication is that the days of loosely regulated fee-for-service practice are essentially over. Whether the label is managed care, HMO, or practice network, the trends are toward strong controls and expectations by purchasers, collaborative practice, targeted use of expensive interventions, and increased focus on the customer-patient's satisfaction.

Trends in the definition and measurement of quality will buttress these developments. Whereas mental health care will continue to be artful and dependent on professional judgment, research advances and payer–customer demands will lead to the increased use of standardized assessments as an aid to clinical decision-making. Practice guidelines will suggest the optimal approach to and sequencing of care. Increasingly, the care of individual patients will be shaped by data-based feedback on their progress and needs.

Elements of this future may resemble an Orwellian new world in the eyes of some, but there is a positive side as well. The basic characteristic of a profession is the ability to define itself, and psychiatry remains positioned to define its role as mental health care evolves into the 21st century. Similarly, changes in payment systems and approaches to diagnosis and treatment will be used by the best practitioners to their advantage—and most particularly to their patients' advantage. The evolution of more effective and focused treatments, coupled with the reduced stigma of mental illness, may make the new era of psychiatry and mental health care the most productive and exciting era yet.

## References

American Psychiatric Association (2002) Practice guidelines for the Treatment of Psychiatric Disorders: Compendium 2002. www.appi.org/Cat2k/2321.html

Astrachan BM (1980) Regulation, adaptation and leadership in psychiatric facilities. Hosp Comm Psychiatr 31, 169–171.

Atkinson C, Cook J, Karna M, et al. (1992) Clinical services research. Schizophr Bull 18, 561–626.

Beers C (1908) The Mind That Found Itself. Hartford, CT.

Bengen B (1992) DBM's program emphasizes quality, employee satisfaction. Ment Health Weekly 2, 3.

Bennett MJ (1992) Managed mental health in health maintenance organizations. In Managed Mental Health Services, Feldman S (ed). Charles C Thomas, Springfield, IL, pp. 61–82.

Bloom BL (1975) Community Mental Health: A General Introduction. Brooks/Cole, Monterey, CA.

Bodenheimer T and Grumbach K (1994) Paying for health care. JAMA 272, 634–639.

Bologna NC and Feldman MJ (1994) Outcomes, clinical models and the redesign of behavioral health care. Behav Health Tom 3, 31–36.

Boothroyd RA, Shern DL, and Bell WW (2002) The effect of financial risk arrangements on service access and satisfaction among Medicaid beneficiaries. Psychiatr Serv 53(3) (Mar), 299–303.

Charatan F (2001) Br Med J 322 (May), 1198.

CBO (1997) Congressional Budget Office Cost Estimate H.R. 3075, Medicare Balanced Budget Refinement Act of 1999. www.cbo.gov/showdoc.cfm?index = 1681&sequence = 0

Croze C (2000) Managed behavioral health care in the public sector. Admin Policy in Ment Health 28(1), 23–36.

Deutsch A (1949) The Mentally Ill in America: A History of Their Care and Treatment from Colonial Times, 2nd ed. Columbia University Press, New York.

Dewa CS and Goering P (2001) Lessons learned from trends in psychotropic drug expenditures in a Canadian province. Psychiatr Serv 52(9) (Sept), 1245–1247.

Drake RE, Goldman HH, Leff HS, et al. (2001) Implementing evidence based practices in routine mental health service settings. Psychiatr Serv 52, 179–182.

Eckholm E (1994) While Congress remains silent, health care transforms itself. New York Times (Dec 18), pp. 1–22.

Employee Benefit Research Institute (1990) EBRI Issue Brief: Issues in Mental Health Care. Employee Benefit Research Institute, Washington DC.

Foucault M (1965) Madness and Civilization: A History of Insanity in the Age of Reason. Random House, New York.

Frank RG and McGuire T (2000). The Mental Health Economy and Mental Health Economics, Ch. 8. SAMHSA's National Mental Health Information Center, US.

Freeman MH and Trabin T (1994) Managed Behavioral Health Care: History, Models, Key Issues and Future Course. Department of Health and Human Services, Center for Mental Health Services, Washington DC.

Gabbard GO, Lazar SG, Hornberger J, et al. (1997) The economic impact of psychotherapy: A review. Am J Psychiatr 154(2) (Feb), 147–155.

Garritson SH (1999) Availability and performance of psychiatric acute care facilities in California from 1992 to 1996. Psychiatr Serv 50(11) (Nov), 1453–1460.

Goran MJ (1992) Managed mental health and group health insurance. In Managed Mental Health Services, Feldman S (ed). Charles C Thomas, Springfield, IL, pp. 27–44.

Grading Health Care Reform (1994) An "I" or an "F"? Group Pract Manage Health News 10, 1–26.

Grob GN (1966) The State and the Mentally Ill: A History of Worcester State Hospital in Massachusetts, 1830. University of North Carolina Press, Chapel Hill, NC. (Originally published in 1920)

Grob GN (1983) Mental Illness and American Society, 1875–1940. Princeton University Press, Princeton, NJ.

Hogan MF (1992) New futures for mental health care: The case of Ohio. Health Aff (Millwood) 11, 69–83.

IMS Health (2001 May) www.imshealth.com/public/structure/dispcontent/1,2779–1009–126684,00.html

Kiesler CA and Sibulkin AE (1987) Mental Hospitalization: Myths and Facts About a National Crisis. Sage Publications, Newbury Park, CA.

Koyanagi C and Goldman HH (1991) The quiet success of the national plan for the chronically mentally ill. Hosp Comm Psychiatry 42, 899–905.

Kunnes R (1994) Vision—behavioral health care mega-trends (or the end of managed care as we know it). Behav Health Tom 3, 78–80.

Lehman AF and Steinwachs DM (1998) (The Co-Investigators of the PORT Project) At Issue: Translating Research Into Practice: The Schizophrenia Patient Outcomes Research (PORT) Treatment Recommendations. Schizophr Bull 24(1), 1–10.

Lipsey MW and Wilson DB (1993) The efficacy of psychological, educational and behavioral treatment. Am Psychol 48, 1181–1209.

Lutterman T, Hollen V, and Hogan M (1993) Funding Sources of State Mental Health Agencies: Revenue/Expenditure Study Results Fiscal Year 1990. National Association of State Mental Health Program Directors Research Institute, Alexandria, VA.

Manderscheid RW, Atay JE, Hernandez-Cartagena MR, et al. (2000) Highlights of Organized Mental Health Services in 1998 and Major National and State Trends. Ch. 14. SAMHSA's National Mental Health Information Center, US.

Marmor TR and Gill KC (1989) The political and economic context of mental health care in the United States. J Health Polit Policy Law 14, 459–475.

Martinsons JN (1998) Are HMOs slamming the door on psych treatment? Hospitals 62, 50–56.

McFarland BH, Khorramzadeh S, Millius R, et al. (2002) Psychiatric hospital length of stay for Medicaid clients before and after managed care. Admin Policy Ment Health 3 (Jan), 191–199.

McGuire TG, Mosakowski WS, and Radigan LS (1990) Designing a state level prospective payment system for inpatient psychiatric services in Medicaid. Admin Policy Ment Health 18, 43–54.

Mechanic D (1989) Mental Health and Social Policy, 3rd ed. Prentice-Hall, Englewood Cliffs, NJ.

Mechanic D, McAlpine DD, and Olfson M (1998) Changing Patterns of Psychiatric Inpatient Care in the United States, 1988–1994. Arch Gen Psychiatr 55 (Sept), 785–791.

Melek SP (1993) Mental Health Care Reform—Can Everybody Win? Milliman & Robertson, Chicago.

Morrissey JP and Goldman HH (1984) Cycles of reform in the care of the chronically mentally ill. Hosp Comm Psychiatry 35, 785–793.

Mulligan K (2002) Jury still out on effects of psychiatric drug limits. Psychiatr News 37(12) (June 21), 11.

National Advisory Mental Health Council (1993) Health care reform for Americans with severe mental illnesses: Report of the National Advisory Mental Health Council. Am J Psychiatr 150, 1447–1463.

National Institute of Mental Health (1997) Comprehensive Community Support Systems for Severely Mentally Disabled Adults: Definitions, Components, and Guiding Principles. NIMH, Rockville, MD.

Ohio Department of Mental Health (1995) Columbus, OH. (Unpublished data)

Olfson M, Marcus SC, Druss B, et al. (2002) National trends in the outpatient treatment of depression JAMA, 287(2) (Jan), 203–209.

OPM News Release (1999) White House Directive to Office of Personnel Management (OPM) to Achieve Mental Health and Substance Abuse Health Coverage Parity (June 7). www.opm.gov/pressrel/1999/health.htm.

President's New Freedom Commission on Mental Health, Press Release (Nov 2002). www.mentalhealthcommission.gov_/press/nov1_summary.htm

Report of Ohio's Mental Health Commission (2001 Jan) Ohio Department of Mental Health, Columbus, Ohio.

Ridgely MS, Mulkern V, Giard J, et al. (2002) Critical elements of public-sector managed behavioral health programs for severe mental illness in five states. Psychiatr Serv 53(4) (Apr), 397–399.

Ross EC (2000) Highlights of Organized Mental Health Services in 1998 and Major National and State Trends. Ch. 9 SAMHSA's National Mental Health Information Center, Mental Health, US.

Roth D, Lauber BG, Vercellini J, et al. (1995) Final results: Ohio's study of services, systems and outcomes in an era of change. Proceedings: Fifth Annual National Conference on State Mental Health Agency Services Research. National Association of State Mental Health Program Directors Research Institute, Alexandria, VA, pp. 85–103.

Rumer R (1978) Community mental health centers: Politics and therapy. J Health Polit Policy Law 2, 531–559.

Souder v. Brennan (1973) 367 F. Supp. 808 (D.D.C. 1973).

Soumerai SB, McLaughlin TJ, Ross-Degnan D, et al. (1994) Effects of limiting Medicaid drug-reimbursement benefits on the use of psychotropic agents and acute mental health services by patients with schizophrenia. New Engl J Med 331(10) (Sept), 650–655.

Starr P (1982) The Social Transformation of American Medicine. Basic Books, New York.

Stein LI, Diamond RJ, and Factor RM (1990) A systems approach to the care of persons with schizophrenia. In Handbook of Schizophrenia, Vol. 4, Psychosocial Treatment of Schizophrenia, Herz MI, Keith SJ, and Docherty JP (eds). Elsevier, New York, pp. 213–246.

Study Committee on Mental Health Services (1993) The Results of Reform: Assessing Implementation of the Mental Health Act of 1988. Study Committee on Mental Health Services, Columbus, Ohio.

Surgeon General (1999) Mental Health: A Report of the Surgeon General-Executive Summary. US Department of Health and Human Services, SAMHSA, Center for Mental Health Services, National Institutes of Health, National Institutes of Mental Health, Rockville, MD.

Surgeon General (2001) Mental Health: Culture, Race, and Ethnicity—A Supplement to Mental Health: A Report of the Surgeon General. US Department of Health and Human Services, SAMHSA, Center for Mental Health Services, Rockville, MD.

Surgeon General's Call to Action to Prevent Suicide (1999) Department of Health and Human Services. www.surgeongeneral.gov/library/calltoaction/default.html

The National Association of Psychiatric Health Systems Survey (2002) Behavioral Health Care Occupancy is the Highest in More than Five Years: NAPHS Annual Survey (Jan 2002) www.napsh.org/news/2001annualsurvey.html

White House Press Release (2002) President Says US Must Make Commitment to Mental Health Care. www.whitehouse.gov/news/releases/2002/04/print/2002429–1.html

Witkin M (1980) Trends in Patient Care Episodes in Mental Health Facilities, 1955–1975. NIMH Statistical note 156. National Institute of Mental Health, Rockville, MD.

CHAPTER

# 110

# Social Stabilization: Achieving Satisfactory Community Adaptation for Persons with Severe Mental Illness

Phyllis Solomon
Arthur T. Meyerson

Psychiatry has recognized the need to integrate traditional psychopharmacological and psychotherapeutic treatments if severely and persistently mentally ill patients are to achieve an optimal level of social and role function, a reduction in relapse rates, and a satisfactory quality of life. Newer generations of medications have been developed that treat not only the positive but the negative symptoms of psychosis, those symptoms that are responsible for many of the disabling characteristics of mental illness. Traditional psychiatric treatments are targeted at control of the symptoms associated with serious mental disorders, whereas the interventions described in this chapter focus on ameliorating the associated functional loss or disability.

Goldman and colleagues (1981, 1987) attempted to estimate the incidence and prevalence of those suffering from a severe mental disorder with moderate to severe disability of prolonged duration. Including adults only, and excluding nonpsychotic and substance abuse disorders, these authors conservatively estimated severely mentally ill population in the US to be between 1.7 and 2.4 million persons. The US prevalence rate of serious mental illness, defined by federal legislation as a mental disorder that substantially interferes with a person's life activities and ability to function, was estimated in 1996 at 5.4% of the US population in a given year (Kessler et al. 1996). The World Health Organization (WHO) Global Burden of Disease Study included disability in the equation in calculating disability adjusted life years (DALYs), resulting in major depression being in the top 10 priority disease listing of causes of disability, along with cardiovascular diseases (Utsun 1999). Mental disorders account for almost 10% of the burden of disease in established market economies

(Utsun 1999). These severe psychiatric disorders, that is, schizophrenia, major depression, and bipolar disorders, are a major public health concern, as people with these disorders experience significant disability with regard to functional limitations in the personal, physical, and societal realms (Utsun 1999). This functional burden results in financial and resource costs to families, along with emotional costs (Clark 1994, Clark and Drake 1994, Franks 1990). Consistent with these findings, a recent study estimated that in the US alone 5 to 6 million people between 16 and 54 years of age lose, do not seek, or are unable to secure employment due to the consequences of mental illness. These same authors further estimated that those with mental illnesses who do work have their annual incomes reduced between $3,500 and $6,000 (Marcotie and Wilcox-Gok 2001). Furthermore, US expenditure for treatment of mental health in 1997 was $73.4 billion (Coffey et al. 2000).

There is little consensus on an acceptable definition of disability. Definitions of disability vary between benefit programs and from one clinical or rehabilitation program to another (Table 110–1). Despite this diversity, all definitions appear to share some basic principles. Persons with disability are considered to suffer from an illness (i.e., a disease or disorder); experience signs and symptoms of the disorder that are significant enough to cause impairments (i.e., loss of physical or mental functions); and also experience a loss of ability or competence in social role functions. The Substance Abuse Mental Health Services Administration (SAMHSA) Community Support Program defines impaired role functioning for purposes of identifying the severely psychiatrically disabled population (Anthony et al. 1990). To meet the Community Support Program's

2254    Section VII • Special Clinical Settings and Challenges

| Table 110–1 | Definitions of Disability by Federal Agencies |
|---|---|

### Rehabilitation Services Administration

Individual with severe handicaps means an individual whose ability to function independently in family or community or whose ability to engage or continue in employment is so limited by the severity of his or her physical or mental disability that independent living rehabilitation services are required in order to achieve a greater level of independence in function in family or community or engaging or continuing in employment. (Rehabilitation Act Amendments 1986)

### Social Security Administration

Disability is the inability to engage in any substantial gainful activity (SGA) by reason of any medically determinable physical or mental impairment which has lasted or can be expected to last for a continuous period of at least 12 months or result in death. Note that earnings averaging more than $500 a month ordinarily equate with work activity at the SGA level. (Titles II and XVI of the Social Security Act)

definition, a person must experience at least two of the following criteria, on an intermittent or continual basis, for at least 2 years.

SAMHSA Community Support Program Criteria for Disability:

- Unemployment, employment in a sheltered setting, or markedly limited work skills and a poor work history
- Need for public financial assistance and an inability to obtain such assistance without help
- Severe inability to establish or maintain a personal social support system
- Need for help in basic living skills
- Inappropriate social behavior resulting in demand for intervention by the mental health or judicial system, or both

The Rehabilitation Services Administration, which governs eligibility criteria for state programs of vocational rehabilitation, provides a definition of a severe handicap as a "disability which requires multiple services over an extended period of time" (Rehabilitation Act Amendments 1986). The Rehabilitation Services Administration specifically includes mental illness as an impairment that can lead to severe disability, and severe disability is the first priority of service. The Social Security Disability Programs utilize criteria similar to those of the Community Support Program and require a year of vocational disability (experienced or expected) to establish eligibility.

The disabling nature of many of the mental disorders, like that of many physical disorders (e.g., rheumatoid arthritis, asthma), does not allow for the assumption of a constant and predictable state of disability or stability. The natural history of the illness may produce remissions and exacerbations. Stress may lead to increased symptoms and disability, and social support may protect against some effects of stress. For example, homelessness represents a stressor that often increases psychiatric symptoms, decreasing coping as a consequence, and entails an interruption of potentially protective social support networks. However,

persons with mental illness with adequate social supports that enable them to remain in a stable housing arrangement are protected from the stress of homelessness and the resulting functional impairment.

Medication reduces symptoms and exacerbations and, as a consequence or correlate, may decrease disability. This appears particularly so for the newest generation of antipsychotics, such as clozapine (Honigfeld and Patin 1990), risperidone, olanzapine, quetiapine, and ziprasidone. However, noncompliance or inaccessibility to appropriate medication for patients with a severe mental disorder leads to increased risk of decompensation and loss of function. Moreover, even for those who comply with medication, side effects including depression, sedation, weight gain, movement disorders, and akinetic syndromes may interfere with the capacity to benefit from rehabilitation efforts.

In addition to medications, traditional supportive psychotherapies have frequently been used as a treatment strategy for this population. Developments in these therapeutic modalities (such as cognitive–behavioral, interpersonal, and problem-solving therapies) have sharpened the focus of the supportive therapeutic interventions and are believed to enhance functional capacity in the psychiatric population.

Rehabilitation, which is described later, is intended to increase social, self-care, and vocational skills but may also help build an array of coping skills to deal with stress and minimize the risk of exacerbation of the illness itself. Psychoeducation, also described later, can be conceptualized as a combination of psychotherapeutic, rehabilitative, and educational endeavors and has proved protective against psychotic relapse and, therefore, enhances community adaptation and tenure. The complexity of the social welfare system (e.g., public assistance, housing, the mental health system, and the rehabilitation system), combined with a lack of integration of these systems, makes the loss of care to patients in these systems all too easy, even where services exist. Legitimate strategies of psychiatric rehabilitation include case management and training of patients in the knowledge and skills necessary to navigate the complexity of agencies and systems designed to meet their needs.

Psychiatric disability and those forces (including personal, therapeutic, rehabilitative, supportive, and systemic, that can foster or interfere with stabilization, coping, and adaptive skills) have been briefly defined. Social stability is, thereby, implicitly defined as the achievement of the person's optimal adaptation in the living, social, educational, vocational, and recreational spheres. The person's adaptation is most successful if stress-induced decompensation is minimized and the individual has access to systems, supports, treatment, and rehabilitation interventions that enhance his or her strengths and minimize restrictions to personal freedom. When this happens, patients tend to experience increased satisfaction and less frequent relapses of their illness.

## Case Management

Since the 1980s, case management has emerged as the most broadly applied and publicly supported mechanism for coordinating and integrating the fragmented delivery system serving those who are persistently and seriously mentally ill (Austin 1990, Mechanic 1991, Solomon 1999). Before deinstitutionalization, all the services and resources that seriously mentally ill individuals needed were thought to be provided within state psychiatric hospitals, or once discharged, by the family. With the current philosophy driven by economics and the courts, state facilities are downsizing and closing. Services and resources must now be provided by a variety of institutions and agencies within the community. Given the complexity and multiplicity of needs of these persons, mental health professionals have become aware of the necessity to increase the access to services for individuals with mental illness, to assist them in negotiating a complicated array of services and resources, and to keep them engaged in the service system. Early research on the impact of deinstitutionalization demonstrated that community-based services required case management for integration or coordination of the fragmented services and the multiple systems involved. Case management is designed to ensure continuity of care, a comprehensive range of options, and a central point of responsibility and accountability. Without it, patients would likely fall between the cracks in the service system (Ozarin 1978).

Case management serves as the central function of a community support system (Stroul 1993) as it is viewed as the glue that ensures that individual elements of the system of care function together. Public Law 99–660 and its subsequent amendments require every state to provide case management services to all seriously mentally ill adults who receive substantial amounts of public funds.

## Definition and Goals of Case Management

Although there has been wide endorsement of the concept of case management and the functions it serves, there has been little consensus for a common definition of case management (Solomon 1998a). There is general agreement as to the five core functions of case management (Solomon 1998a) (Table 110–2). The two major overarching patient-focused goals are to prevent decompensation and hospitalization and to promote rehabilitation by improving the social functioning of patients to the highest level of which they are capable (Sands 1991).

Case management has been described as assuming responsibility and accountability for "maintaining a long-term, caring, supportive relationship with the client on a continuing basis, regardless of the number of agencies involved" (Stroul 1993, p. 57). Intagliata (1982, p. 657), defined case management as "a process or method for ensuring that consumers are provided with whatever services they need in a coordinated, effective, and efficient manner." Solomon (1992, p. 164) pointed out that case management is a "coordinated strategy on behalf of clients to obtain the services that they need, when they need them

and for as long as they need these services." Thus, case managers are expected to identify persons who could benefit from the service; engage these persons in a comprehensive assessment process with professional input; develop a comprehensive support and treatment plan in collaboration with the patients; ensure patients' access to required services; ensure integration of services; and monitor patients' progress.

Case management is viewed as a service intervention that may be delivered in either the patient's environment or an office. Some models of case management include a clinical or treatment component (Stroul 1993, Roach 1993, Kanter 1988), and others include skills training and even medication and symptom management. A number of communities provide intensive case management, which includes assertive outreach and advocacy to ensure that patients obtain the services that they need. This type of case management often provides 24-hours-a-day, 7-days-a-week availability, and, if necessary, patients may be seen as frequently as every day (Stroul 1993, Hodge and Draine 1993).

## Qualifications of Case Managers

Case management is a generic term that is used in a variety of health and human service settings and with different target populations, for example, the elderly, the mentally retarded, and the physically disabled (Solomon 1998a). Case management is not clearly associated with a single discipline or profession (Sands 1991). For persons with mental illness, aspects of case management can be and are performed by many professionals, including nurses, social workers, psychologists, and psychiatrists. Some models of case management require postsecondary degrees, generally a master's degree; for those not possessing such credentials, supervision is usually necessary. However, as case management has proliferated for those with mental illness, individuals without postsecondary degrees or formalized education are often employed as case managers. Most recently, models of case management are provided by consumers themselves, either as aides (Felton et al. 1995, Sherman and Porter 1991) or as full-fledged case managers (Dixon et al. 1994, 1997, Herinckx 1997, Solomon and Draine 1993, 2001). Given that many of the tasks performed by case managers are related to service and resource acquisition and coordination, there appears to be reasonable latitude for a diversity of qualifications of case managers. However, the assessment, treatment, and community support functions necessary for this population require the coordinated efforts of several disciplines. Psychiatrists are essential for differential diagnosis, treatment planning, medication prescribing, medication management, clinical monitoring, and acute and emergency care.

There is an active debate as to the required qualifications and training for case managers. Qualifications are clearly contingent on the case management model that is employed. For example, clinical case management requires more formal education than pure advocacy and referral models, which may require only in-service training and case supervision. Empathy and experience with the mentally ill population and knowledge of community services may be more important than formal education and

| Table 110–2 | Five Core Functions of Case Management |
|---|---|
| Assessing | |
| Planning | |
| Linking | |
| Monitoring | |
| Advocacy | |

professional training for a well-qualified case manager (Robinson and Toff-Bergman 1990).

## Generally Accepted Features of Case Management

There is a high degree of consensus about the specific elements of case management that are required when individuals who are seriously and persistently mentally ill are served, regardless of the particular model (Table 110–3). These elements include low patient/staff ratios; outreach; the delivery of services *in situ*, that is, where patients live, learn, socialize, and work; high intensity and frequency of service; provision of crisis intervention which is available 24 hours a day, 7 days a week; and no time limit on the length of service provision (Robinson and Toff-Bergman 1990). All case managers provide some form of supportive counseling, whereas the clinical model is unique in offering more specific psychotherapeutic interventions. A number of case management programs do not adhere to any specific model but incorporate all, or almost all, of the features described. Programs that incorporate these features have come to be referred to as "intensive case management."

Regardless of the model, case management begins with outreach and engagement of the person, followed by an assessment. The elements emphasized in an assessment may vary. For example, some models place greater emphasis on strengths as opposed to deficits, but generally an assessment incorporates the history, diagnosis, strengths, problems, deficits, and available resources of a patient. This information usually comes from the patient; however, other sources, when available, including families and medical records, are essential. A service plan is formulated that sets out specific goals and objectives, with the active involvement of the patient and the family.

On the basis of these specific goals and objectives, the case manager, in collaboration with the patient, develops intervention strategies designed to accomplish these goals and objectives. The case manager then assists in linking the patient with appropriate services and resources in the community and, in the process, may train the patient for problem solving in the arena of accessing needed resources. The implementation of the plan and the patient's progress are then monitored by the case manager to determine if and when the plan requires revision. The implementation of the plan may require that the case manager serve as an advocate on behalf of the patient to protect the patient's rights and ensure that the patient obtains the needed services. If patients are being denied services or resources to which they are entitled, system level strategies for overcoming these barriers are developed and implemented (Sands 1991, Hodge and Draine 1993).

| Table 110–3 | Required Features of Case Management |
|---|---|

Low patient/staff ratio
Assertive outreach
Delivery of services *in situ*
High intensity and frequency of services
Provision of crisis services

## Models of Case Management: Implementation

Case management has been implemented in a variety of modes and methods. Some programs employ teams of similarly trained case managers, others use interdisciplinary teams, and still others use case managers working independently. The use of interdisciplinary teams provides for a broader range of skills and may be a means of alleviating staff burnout by providing group support when working with a difficult population (Ozarin 1978, Intagliata and Baker 1983). Teams that are composed of case managers with minimal qualifications require involvement of a psychiatrist or nurse, or both. Other teams, depending on the goals of the service and the needs of the target population, require specialists in vocational rehabilitation or substance abuse, or both. In some instances, teams include resource specialists in areas such as housing and benefits programs. Recently some teams have included family members and consumers (Dixon et al. 1994, 1997, McFarlane et al. 1996).

Six major models of case management are in current practice with seriously and persistently mentally ill individuals (Table 110–4). These include the assertive community treatment (ACT) model, the rehabilitation model; the personal strengths or developmental acquisition model, the broker or generalist model, the clinical case management model, and intensive case management (ICM). The ACT, rehabilitation, and personal strengths models all emphasize individual strengths, skills training, and modification of the environment. Often the distinctions have more to do with philosophy than is apparent in actual implementation. Discussions of the major characteristics of each of these models follow.

## Assertive Community Treatment Model

The historical roots of much of current case management practice emanate from the "Training in Community Living" or the Program of Assertive Community Treatment (PACT) developed in Madison, Wisconsin, at Mendota State Hospital (Stein and Test 1980, Test 1992). This program is a comprehensive treatment service and system of care, with case management serving as the coordinating function. The project essentially moved all of the treatment and support functions of the hospital into the community, with an emphasis on improving treatment and technology to overcome problems of psychiatrically ill persons in the community. The goals of the model are to increase the length of community tenure, increase psychosocial functioning, decrease psychiatric symptoms, and improve satisfaction with life (Test 1992). The strategies include teaching patients skills in their natural environment and bringing services to the patient. These strategies eliminate the need to generalize skills learned in one environment to another in which they are to be used and help to keep patients engaged in treatment (Test 1992).

The basic tenets and goals of the original program have been adapted by the ACT model that is widely practiced across the US (Solomon 1992, 1999) and currently promoted by the National Alliance for the Mentally Ill (NAMI). The NAMI's objective is that all states will establish a policy to develop ACT programs throughout their states. The ACT model differs from its predecessor in the provision of fewer direct services and in the case manager

| Table 110–4 | Major Characteristics of the Six Models of Case Management |
|---|---|

### Assertive Community Treatment

Interdisciplinary team
Services delivered *in situ*
Services delivered on a continuous basis with no time limit or provision for transfer
High staff/patient ratio
Assertive outreach
Daily meetings

### Rehabilitation

Functional assessment
Involvement of the patient in establishing a rehabilitation plan
Assessment and goals related to specific environment of the patient's choosing
Provides skill teaching to overcome environmental barriers

### Personal Strengths

Identification of the patient's strengths
Utilization of community resources to enhance the patient's strengths
Teaching of resource acquisition skills
Group supervision of case managers

### Expanded Broker

Linking and brokering services
High patient/staff ratio
Largely an office-based service

### Clinical

Provision of support, skills training, and accessing environmental resources
Provision of psychotherapy
Qualifications of case managers include formal clinical education and supervised therapeutic experiences

### Intensive Case Management

High users of service
Assertive Outreach
Services delivered *in situ*
Moderate staff/patient ratio

functioning more as an "assertive resource coordinator" (Test 1992). The ACT model requires an interdisciplinary team that has shared responsibility for patients; services delivered *in situ* and on a continuous basis; continuous crisis intervention availability; skills training in the patients' environment, including daily living skills, money management, and symptom management; small caseloads; provision of support, including education for patients, families, and significant others in the patients' environment; assertive outreach to patients; and that offers an indeterminant length of service (Solomon 1999). Teams usually provide medication management and clinical care, which require a psychiatrist as a member of the team. Because some of these models are not always full service, their success is often contingent on the service environment in which the case management is delivered. The diversity of

resources and interventions available within the team determines the degree of dependency on the environmental context of the program. Teams are generally dependent on the community for housing and often refer to specialized agencies for substance abuse treatment, vocational services, and rehabilitation programs. Many teams are composed of a small number of case managers, in addition to a nurse and a psychiatrist. Teams usually meet on a daily basis to discuss crises and plan changes, although this has been modified when implemented in some settings. Although some teams may meet as a full group only once or twice a week, the intent is to meet daily to review the day's activities and to keep all team members up-to-date on the status of all patients served by the team. Certification Association for Rehabilitation Facilities (CARF) recently issued standards for certifying ACT programs (see Table 110–4).

## Rehabilitation Model

The rehabilitation model is based on the psychiatric rehabilitation program developed by the Boston University Center for Psychiatric Rehabilitation. Akin to this rehabilitation model (discussed later), case management is viewed as assisting patients to obtain the necessary supports, skills, and resources to overcome environmental barriers and to improve functioning and achieve personal goals of choice. The goals of rehabilitation case management are individualized. They are established with and by the patient. These goals are likely to be directed at strengthening a patient's specific skills for achieving a working, living, or recreational environment (Hodge and Draine 1993, Robinson and Toff-Bergman 1990). As Robinson and Toff-Bergman (1990, p. 18) stated, "rehabilitation-oriented case management is a process of assisting clients to become successful and satisfied in the social environment of their choice with the least amount of professional help."

A central focus of this model of case management is the functional assessment. The case management process begins with the identification of the patient's functioning, strengths, skill deficits, abilities, and available resources in relation to a particular environment. The functional assessment and comprehensive rehabilitation plan differs from a diagnostic assessment and consequent treatment plan in that the rehabilitation process focuses on assisting patients to obtain and maintain the skills and resources necessary to live in the community of their choosing, whereas the medical assessment and treatment plan traditionally emphasizes symptom reduction and is often viewed as independent of the patient's personal goals or environment (Hodge and Draine 1993). The emphasis on a specific environment is deemed essential to the rehabilitation assessment, as different environments have varying requirements (Hodge and Draine 1993).

The case manager ensures that the patient receives "support in dealing with crises, coping with bureaucratic confusion, and acquiring personal and social skills" (Goering et al. 1988). The case manager continues to work with patients until they have a personal support system and can assume responsibility for their own care through obtaining and coordinating necessary resources and services. Although most patients require active psychiatric treatments, for example, pharmacotherapy, when involved in this model of case management, such treatment is not viewed as a requirement.

## Personal Strengths Model

The personal strengths model emphasizes the identification of a patient's strengths and the development of personal opportunities and environmental situations that can enhance these strengths so that the patient can achieve successful community adaptation and tenure (Robinson and Toff-Bergman 1990). This model is based on two significant assumptions about adaptive behaviors. First, individuals who are successfully self-sustaining in the community have both the potential and the ability to develop increased functional capacity. Second, these persons must have access to the necessary resources to achieve this development (Solomon 1992, Robinson and Toff-Bergman 1990, Modrcin et al. 1985). Individuals with severe mental disorders often have accompanying impairments and functional disabilities that hinder their capacity to obtain basic necessities. Thus, they need assistance in acquiring the necessary supports and resources essential for functioning in the domains of work, housing, education, medical care, and personal growth and development. The community in general, not the traditional mental health system, is viewed as a network of available resources rather than an inherent obstacle. Patients are, therefore, taught resource acquisition skills that enable them to garner needed supports, services, and resources. Case managers spend much of their time with patients, teaching them specific skills, modeling new behaviors, and having the patients practice and eventually implement the use of these skills (Sands 1991).

Case managers in this model are often provided group supervision to foster a creative atmosphere for problem resolution and resource acquisition through strategies such as creative brainstorming (Hodge and Draine 1993, Modrcin et al. 1985). The strengths assessment drives this model of case management. The process may be complicated for persons with severe mental illness by their experience of so many implicit and explicit messages that suggest that they lack adaptive skills and self-worth. Individuals with serious mental illness frequently see themselves as having few strengths and, therefore, little hope of a successful community-based life (Hodge and Draine 1993).

## Expanded Broker or Generalist Model

The broker or service coordinator model is closely akin to traditional social work. The major function of the case manager is to assist in the linking and brokering of services on behalf of the patient. The case manager's role is to provide the patient with access to needed information, services, and resources, including a variety of benefits to which the patient is eligible. As differentiated from other models of case management currently being practiced, the service is largely delivered in the case manager's office (Robinson and Toff-Bergman 1990). Caseloads are generally higher than in other models, which may result in case managers' responding more to those patients who are demanding or in crisis, with limited attention given to others (Intagliata and Baker 1983).

This basic broker model has been expanded in some instances to include linkage and brokering beyond traditional mental health services to a wider array of community resources, that is, entitlement programs and vocational rehabilitation services (Robinson and Toff-Bergman 1990). This model may also include training and encouragement of patients to enhance their problem-solving and coping capabilities (Johnson and Rubin 1983).

## Clinical Model

The clinical model goes beyond the provision of support, skills training, and accessing environmental resources by involving the provision of psychotherapy (Roach 1993, Kanter 1989, Lamb 1980). Thus, the case management function subsumes both the administrative functions of service access and coordination and the provision of direct clinical care. This approach emphasizes both linkages to formal and informal resources in the patient's environment, and development of the internal resources of the patient for survival, growth, and adaptation to severe mental illness and the environment (Kanter 1989). Thus, this model focuses on the growth of the patient's psychological capacities for adaptation as well as functional skills acquisition (Roach 1993, Harris and Bergman 1987). The premise of this model is that the functions of case management are consistent with those of a therapist and that only through intensive, psychotherapeutic involvement with the patient does the case manager obtain the necessary information to make an adequate and comprehensive assessment of the patient's needs (Lamb 1980).

Clinical case managers require formal education and supervised therapeutic experience to develop clinical skills. Because "clinical case management requires not only an understanding of individual dynamics but also an appreciation of the nuances of interpersonal relationships," the case managers need to be clinically qualified (Harris and Bergman 1988, p. 9). In one model of clinical case management, case managers utilize three classes of interventions: environmental, patient-focused, and a combined patient–environmental approach. Environmental interventions include acquisition of and linkages between services, consultation with families and other caregivers, collaboration with psychiatrists, maintenance and expansion of a social network, and advocacy. The patient-related interventions encompass individual psychotherapy, skills training, and psychoeducation. The patient–environmental combination is exemplified by crisis intervention, in which an understanding of a patient and her or his social network enables a case manager to assess the clinical status of the patient and make environmental changes and psychological interventions that may prevent a relapse (Kanter 1989).

## Intensive Case Management

The intensive case management (ICM) model was developed to meet the needs of high service users (Solomon 1998a, Mueser et al. 1998). The boundaries between ICM and ACT in practice are frequently minimal and unclear, as many ACT programs are not exact replicas, and numerous ICM programs are based on the ACT model (Baronet and Gerber 1998). ICM integrates many of the features of ACT and the strengths and rehabilitation models, including low patient–staff ratio, assertive outreach to clients, the delivery of services to clients in their own environments, and practical assistance in daily living skills (Mueser et al. 1998). The major distinction between this model and ACT is that ACT has shared caseloads. ICM is usually delivered by an individual case manager as opposed to a team, as in the case of ACT. However, if ICMs are members of a team, they work relatively independently with their assigned clients. Also, ICM is more dependent on the service system for the delivery of many services, so ICMs function much more as service coordinators.

## Efficacy of Case Management

There have been serious criticisms leveled at case management (Table 110–5). Stein (1992) noted that there were structural problems with the implementation of case management in most states. Case management programs often lack a multidisciplinary approach, which Stein believed is essential to treat and care for the complex needs of persons with serious and persistent mental illness. He stated that most case management systems are too dependent on resources that are either unavailable or in insufficient supply in the community system of care. Some critics assert that too much responsibility has been placed on case managers for fixing an uncoordinated and fragmented mental health service delivery system. One latent assumption of case management programs is that they will be able to provide the patients with needed support and treatment services that are not funded or not available in the community. As Stein (1992) indicated, case managers often do not possess the diversity of skills required to compensate for deficiencies in the existing system nor do they have the power to change the established systems of care.

A number of studies have evaluated the different models of case management with regard to both system outcomes (e.g., rehospitalization and reincarceration) and clinical outcomes (e.g., symptoms and function) (Solomon 1992). The majority of the studies have been on ACT or ICM (Mueser et al. 1998). Therefore, it is difficult to assess the effectiveness of specific models of case management other than ACT and ICM. The evidence thus far indicates that these two models of case management are most effective in relation to system outcomes, such as reduction in the number and length of hospitalizations (and consequently cost-effectiveness), provided that there is not a substitution of costly residential alternatives (Solomon 1992, Mueser et al. 1998, Scott and Dixon 1995). Since length of time in the hospital is usually linked to housing stability, it is not surprising that these models of case management are effective in increasing residential stability (Mueser et al. 1998). These models are particularly effective for high users and at increasing their engagement with treatment (Mueser et al. 1998). These case management models, however, have not been found to have an impact on reductions in incarceration in jails (Mueser et al. 1998). One study of an ACT program for homeless persons with severe mental illness being released from jail found an increase in reincarceration rates, which the investigators attributed to the increased

monitoring that may result from these more intensive case management models (Solomon and Draine 1995a).

Intensive case management models appear to be less effective in changing clinical outcomes, such as symptoms and personal functioning, than in modifying system outcomes. ACT and ICM have moderate effects on quality of life, medication compliance, and symptomatology, and little, if any, effect on social functioning and on substance abuse (Mueser et al. 1998, Ziguras and Stuart 2000). These models have also had mixed outcomes with regard to vocational and employment domains (Mueser et al. 1998). It appears that to obtain beneficial effects in a specific functional domain, such as vocation or substance abuse, the service needs to be directed toward that objective by the inclusion of specialists in that area on the ACT team (Solomon 1998a). For example, a recent study of the effectiveness of ACT with integrated substance abuse treatment found greater improvements in substance abuse outcomes and quality of life (Drake et al. 1998). Also, the effectiveness of ACT programs has been found to be linked to the greater fidelity to the model (McGrew et al. 1994). Recent research has concluded that there were no negative effects with regard to hospitalizations and social functioning from transferring patients from an ACT service to a less intensive case management program, even though the prevailing philosophy of case management for persons with severe mental illness has been an indeterminate length of service (Salyers et al. 1998).

Studies that have assessed patients' satisfaction with case management have found it to be high (Solomon 1992, Mueser et al. 1998). Similarly, the limited studies that have assessed family burden found no increase in family burden for those receiving PACT over those whose family members were hospitalized and subsequently received aftercare services (Stein and Test 1980, Hoult et al. 1981). A study of families' views of consumer- and nonconsumer-delivered intensive case management services found that families were satisfied with the services regardless of whether they were delivered by consumers or nonconsumers (Solomon and Draine 1994). Intensive comprehensive case management services, like ACT programs, seem to provide families with a sense of increased security for their ill relative (Burns and Santos 1995).

## Outreach and Client Identification of Patients

Before psychiatrically ill individuals can be engaged in case management or other interventions, they must be identified. Individuals with a severe psychiatric disability frequently have difficulty seeking services. Therefore, outreach is necessary to locate these individuals and inform them of the availability of services. Linkages are needed to a variety of agencies and settings, including boarding homes, emergency departments, police departments, family groups, consumer groups, and inpatient facilities, to identify individuals who can potentially benefit from these services (Stroul 1993).

Some mentally ill individuals decline to participate in formal, site-based treatment services or are unable to do so. Furthermore, existing mental health programs are not designed to serve distrustful, hostile, and suspicious populations such as the homeless. These programs are not able to provide the required "comprehensive

| Table 110–5 | Major Criticisms of Case Management |
|---|---|

Frequently lacks a multidisciplinary approach

Highly dependent on community resources that are unavailable or in insufficient supply

Responsibility of individual case managers to fix an uncoordinated and fragmented system

multidimensional services" (Goldfinger 1990, p. 365). Outreach services, which are mobile and include crisis intervention, medication monitoring, assistance in meeting basic needs, and referrals for other needed services and benefits are required to assist these individuals. As previously noted, a component of some case management models such as ACT is outreach to patients, but this is frequently employed for patients who are engaged in treatment.

There have been specific case management services developed to reach out to homeless individuals with severe mental illness. Case managers or outreach workers may need to establish their presence in a location before any interactions with homeless persons can take place, even before offering concrete assistance (Goldfinger 1990). The provision of services to meet basic needs is an essential prerequisite to engaging these patients in psychiatric treatment. This is a gradual process that may last for a long period to gain trust and develop an alliance.

Extraordinary clinical skills are required to establish a relationship with a psychiatrically ill person who has had few positive interactions with psychiatric treatment (Goldfinger 1990). Outreach efforts must take place on the streets and in shelters, soup kitchens, drop-in centers, and hostels, wherever these patients congregate (Stroul 1993). Outreach efforts are also essential in rural areas, where there is a lack of transportation. In these communities there may also be a need to provide mobile services or to develop a specific arrangement for transportation to psychiatric services, or both.

## Psychiatric Rehabilitation

At times, a person suffering from schizophrenia may have relatively few signs and symptoms of the disorder that are flagrant or even psychotic. This is certainly so during the residual phase and/or when psychotic manifestations are controlled by neuroleptic medication. Nevertheless, these same individuals may retain features of the negative symptom complex, which are often thought to be a *sine qua non* of disability. These features include social eccentricity and isolation, flat affect, apparent lack of motivation and spontaneous activity, and sometimes an inability to care for oneself. Patients with bipolar disorder may suffer from some of these features between episodes, but they are more often disrupted in their social, vocational, and self-care capacities by frequent and unpredictable recurrences, which may lead to demoralization, shame, or negative responses from their social contacts and potential employers. As an example, an attorney who has spent client funds illegally during a manic episode may be unemployable when he returns to a normalized euthymic condition.

Even with the protection of the Americans with Disabilities Act, retraining for a less vulnerable vocation may be indicated, as employers may be fearful of a recurrence of past behavior. Thus, illnesses that produce disabling behaviors over the long-term, such as schizophrenia, as well as those that cause intermittent disruptions of function, may require interventions designed to enable or re-enable the patient to lead a stable community life.

A vulnerability, stress, coping, and competence model of disabling mental illness is conceptualized to account for the interplay of illness-related signs, symptoms, impairments, underlying biological vulnerabilities, and consequent disability while considering a person's coping skills, adaptive abilities, and social and family supports (Anthony and Liberman 1986, Nicholson and Neufeld 1992). The model considers that protection against biological vulnerability to stress may be produced by antipsychotic medication, psychosocial interventions, and rehabilitation. The interventions, by reducing the biological vulnerability to stress, minimize decompensation and the loss of adaptive function in individuals with mental illness.

As an example, a young adult with a biological vulnerability to schizophrenic decompensation may suffer from multiple acute psychotic episodes in a residential situation fraught with a high degree of conflict and, consequently, may be functionally disabled in the social, vocational, educational, or self-care spheres. Biological vulnerability can be reduced with appropriate neuroleptic medication. Increased support and coping skills in the residential setting may decrease stress. Increased adaptive skills may result from rehabilitation approaches. Through these interventions, this individual may be less vulnerable to stress-induced decompensation and achieve longer, more stable and satisfactory community adaptation.

Thus, the vulnerability–stress model not only accounts for the interplay of forces that can lead to decompensation and disability but also suggests an integrated and comprehensive strategy to bring about long-term community stabilization. Even with the most efficacious interventions, some patients continue to suffer intermittent exacerbations and diminished coping abilities. Psychiatrists and other mental health professionals need to be prepared to "titrate" the degree of involvement and the course of treatment to meet the changing needs of the patient.

Psychosocial, or psychiatric, rehabilitation is the approach to relearn or learn those competencies in the social, self-care, educational, and vocational arenas that patients need to achieve the greatest stability and tenure in the least restrictive community setting. Rehabilitation of the psychiatric patient, as with other disabled patients, may involve modification of the environment and securing personal supports as well as training of the individual to achieve the optimal level of function of which the individual is capable and that she or he desires (Bachrach 1992, Pratt et al. 1999, Flexer and Solomon 1993).

## Characteristics and Definitions of Psychiatric Rehabilitation

No single prototype or program model can be used to define current approaches to psychiatric rehabilitation. There is no general agreement as to the best elements, sites, modalities, and values (Hughes 1994). The emphasis in psychiatric rehabilitation is on the patient acquiring the necessary skills and resources for living in the community (Rutman 1994). "The goal of psychiatric rehabilitation is to enable individuals to compensate for or eliminate the functional deficits, interpersonal barriers and environmental barriers created by the disability, and to restore ability for independent living, socialization and effective life management" (Hughes 1994, p. 11).

Rutman (1987) developed a working definition of psychiatric or psychosocial rehabilitation at the request of the Community Support Program:

Psychosocial rehabilitation refers to a spectrum of programs for persons with long-term mental illness. The programs are designed to strengthen individuals' abilities and skills necessary to meet their needs for housing, employment, socialization, and personal growth. The goal of psychosocial rehabilitation is to improve the quality of life of psychiatrically disabled individuals by assisting them in assuming as much responsibility over their lives and to function as actively and independently in society as possible.

Major psychosocial rehabilitation services, which are offered on a continuum, include socialization, recreational, vocational, residential, training in the skills of daily community living, and case management. In addition, psychosocial rehabilitation facilities may also provide educational programs, advocacy training, and personal and family support services.

The individual may need to use these programs on a short-term basis or indefinitely. The programs are [ideally] offered in the context of a supportive, nonstigmatizing environment in the community, and in a manner that emphasizes the "personhood" rather than the "patienthood" of the individual, maximizes the individual's feeling of responsibility and self-worth, and encourages ownership in the rehabilitation process. The services are coordinated with those offered by other mental health and human service agencies.

Anthony and colleagues (1983, p. 70) stated that the goal of psychiatric rehabilitation is to "assume that the person with a psychiatric disability possesses those physical, emotional [social, cognitive] and intellectual skills needed to live, learn and work in his or her own particular environment [or environment of choice]. The major interventions by which this goal is accomplished involve either developing in patients the particular skills that they need to function in their environment, and/or developing the environmental resources needed to support or strengthen the person's present level of functioning." The development of programs and technical interventions designed to meet the rehabilitation needs of these patients has been intertwined with the history of public psychiatry during the last several decades (Table 110–6).

| Table 110–6 | Psychiatric Rehabilitation Programs |
|---|---|

Socialization
Recreational
Vocational
Educational
Residential
Social skills training
Case management that emphasizes skills training
Family education
Education of patients (e.g., medication and symptom management)

| Table 110–7 | Major Principles of Psychiatric Rehabilitation |
|---|---|

Focus on the patient's strengths
Active involvement of the patient in planning, implementing, and monitoring of rehabilitation plan
Comprehensive approach to treatment
Rehabilitation as an ongoing process
Rehabilitation assessment most appropriately performed in the patient's environment
Services and training delivered in the patient's environment

## Principles of Psychiatric Rehabilitation

There are a number of principles or essential elements of psychiatric rehabilitation (Table 110–7). The emphasis in rehabilitation is on the strengths of the individual rather than on deficits. Implicit in the strengths perspective is the empowerment of the patient. Thus, one key element is the active involvement of the patient in the development, implementation, and ongoing evaluation of service plans and progress. Consistent with the orientation of psychiatric rehabilitation is the centrality of hope, and an optimistic activist philosophy, and a belief in their own recovery. In the last decade there has been an emphasis on recovery, not in terms of a cure, but in patients gaining control of their life and their illness (Anthony 1992).

Given the nature of mental illness and its resulting disability in many functional areas, psychiatric rehabilitation requires a comprehensive approach to treating the individual. Rehabilitation is clearly not a one-time intervention but an ongoing process. Rehabilitation assessments are best performed when situationally based, in the patient's own environment. Services are most beneficial when integrated in the community, the locus of training. This is based on the experience that the more these services are delivered in the patient's environment, the more likely it is that the aptitudes developed will be used in that setting. Some psychiatric patients lack the ability to transfer skills from one environment to another. There is also a need for family involvement, training, and support, as so many psychiatrically ill persons live with their families or as their families are involved in their care (Bachrach 1992, Cook and Hoffschmidt 1993, Solomon 1994).

## Examples of Psychiatric Rehabilitation Models

One of the major features of rehabilitation services is an emphasis on basic requirements for community living, such as housing, essential coping skills for daily living, and preparing for productive vocational activity. Experiential activities are used to facilitate social learning and behavioral change. In the past, most agencies began with a single service focus, which was frequently social rehabilitation. Others offered residential or vocational programs. Over time, many offered a range of services, including counseling, educational training, and crisis intervention. Three approaches were developed with specific philosophical orientations and program elements. These include the clubhouse, the intensive case management (previously discussed), and the consumer-guided models (Rutman 1987).

## Clubhouse Model

Clubhouses emphasize a supportive family surrogate environment with a full continuum of available services. Persons are considered members rather than clients or patients. The member is free to choose the frequency and intensity of contact with the clubhouse, other members, staff, and program elements. Rutman (1987, p. 203) described the four basic program elements as follows: "an accepting climate that establishes an unwavering sense of welcome; help in developing job-related skills that can lead to placement in regular jobs in business and industry, either through one or more transitional employment placements or in regular competitive employment; provision for those who need housing with an appropriate, normalized place to live; and a milieu which stimulates active and meaningful participation on the part of all members in all phases of the program, from performing housekeeping chores, assisting in the cafeteria or at the reception desk, to maintaining the agency's fiscal and clinical records" (Table 110–8). These programs attempt to achieve a cooperative community milieu, with members and staff sharing and interchanging roles. For example, staff may fill in for a member in a transitional employment position when a member is unable to attend. Staff members do not serve as therapists in any traditional sense and often do not have offices.

The most prominent example of the clubhouse model is Fountain House, in operation in New York City since 1948. This program was started by former state hospital patients who desired a place to belong and where they felt needed and wanted; where they would voluntarily be members; and where "mutual support was the norm and rejoining ordinary society as workers and friends was the goal" (Propst 1992, p. 3). Fountain House is the prototype for other clubhouses all over the world, which were begun by staff and members trained by the New York program, or which have modeled themselves after the original program. As of 1999, there were 340 Fountain House-based programs around the world (Macias et al. 1999). These programs are affiliated with a nonprofit corporation—the International Center for Clubhouse Development (ICCD)—which was established to provide training in the model offer consultation for program development, and certify that operating clubhouses meet the certification standards (Macias et al. 1999). Some outcome research has been published that provides supportive evidence for increased community tenure, increased adaptation, and greatly enhanced member satisfaction when compared with traditional approaches (Beard et al. 1983).

| Table 110–8 | Basic Program Elements of Clubhouses |
|---|---|

An accepting climate
Assistance in job-related skills development
A stimulating milieu that encourages meaningful participation

## Consumer-Sponsored Programs

These programs are consumer run, guided, or sponsored, or all three. Please refer to Chapter 111 for further elaboration on these programs.

## Boston University Rehabilitation Approach

This approach to the practice of psychiatric rehabilitation consists of three phases: the diagnostic, planning, and intervention phases (Pratt et al. 1999, Anthony 1982, Anthony et al. 1987). This approach is based on the premise that a successful rehabilitation process must begin with an assessment of a patient's readiness to engage in rehabilitation activities, the patient's current skills, and the environments in which the patient operates or desires to operate. With this information, a plan which prioritizes goals and objectives is formulated with the patient. Lastly, strategies and interventions for accomplishing these goals and objectives are established (Pratt et al. 1999). This approach is often referred to as the Boston University or BU model.

In this approach, the patient, with the aid of a rehabilitation practitioner, defines the overall rehabilitation goal or goals in a selected area, such as socialization, residency, self-care, work, or education, that the patient wishes to achieve in a reasonable period, often 6 to 18 months. The diagnosis then involves a second crucial step—a functional assessment—during which the patient and the rehabilitation worker develop a list of the patient's assets or abilities as well as handicaps or disabilities relevant to the achievement of that goal or goals. The assessment proceeds to explore questions such as which skills does the patient have and which additional or different skills does the patient require to achieve the goal, that is, to get the job or date, live in an apartment, or succeed in school (Anthony et al. 1987).

A third dimension of the assessment or diagnosis is an evaluation of the patient's environment and support systems. The patient's environment is assessed as to whether it is conducive to the achievement of the patient's goals and the extent to which it represents a set of barriers. Thus, an assessment of both the patient's personal needs and the environmental requirements is essential to a realistic psychiatric rehabilitation diagnosis (Anthony et al. 1987). For example, questions such as the following are posed: Does the person need part-time work? Can he or she share a job? Is she or he best able to function with written rather than oral instructions? Answers to such questions may be vital to job acquisition and successful retention. Given the Americans with Disabilities Act, this assessment may be the basis for legal action as well as rehabilitation planning.

Once the diagnostic assessment is completed, the patient and staff member jointly set priorities for the skills development and environmental or resource modifications that are the basis for the initial interventions. Each skill to be mastered or each resource objective is usually assigned one or more interventions. These are put forth as written plans to be signed by the patient–client–member and the worker (Anthony et al. 1987).

Two rehabilitation interventions strategies used in this approach are skill acquisition and resource development. Skills acquisition involves direct skills teaching and is used when the functional assessment indicates that the patient does not have the required skills. This technique leads the patient through a series of instructional activities to the point at which the patient can use the new skills. Another approach is a step-by-step programming to overcome barriers to the use of an existing skill in a particular environment. Resource development strategies involve resource coordination or resource modification. In resource coordination, a preferred resource is selected, arrangements for its use are made, and supports are provided in the use of the resource. Resource modification involves adapting existing resources to fit the patient's needs (Anthony et al. 1987). This may entail negotiating with a program to make resource adjustments to fit a particular patient's functional objective.

## Social Skills Training

The general approach to social skills training was developed in the 1970s and remains virtually unchanged to date (Bellack 2001). Trainers are essentially teachers as opposed to therapists (Bellack 2001). Social skills training entails the patients learning specific interpersonal skills and personal competencies through methods that promote the maintenance and generalization of the new or rehabilitated skills to increase social competencies improve social role functioning, and quality of social relationships (Bellack 2001, Mueser et al. 1997) (Table 110–9). Originally, this training focused solely on behavior skills, but now includes social perceptual and cognitive skills as well (Mueser et al. 1997). This training is based on the principles and methods of social learning theories. Social skills training is conducted with highly specific educational procedures, in contrast to less specific "resocialization" experiences. Group social experiences, such as a dance or an outing, provide an opportunity to practice interpersonal skills, receive consensual validation of acceptable behaviors, and receive positive and negative feedback. However, they depend on the chance occurrence of group membership and events rather than on prepackaged or systematically prescribed training experiences.

These resocialization experiences, offered in psychosocial clubhouse programs, are different from social skills training. In contrast to socialization experiences, the highly systematized programs of social skills training employ specific behavioral techniques, including role-playing, modeling, feedback about perceptions and communications, coaching, didactic instructions, attention-focusing procedures, and problem-solving techniques. Complex behaviors

are broken down into discrete behavioral elements, which are trained by employing the various techniques. These are micro-level interventions. These techniques are based on the principles of human learning, which "promote the acquisition, generalization, and maintenance of skills required in interpersonal situations" (Liberman et al. 1987, p. 227).

Liberman (1988) and colleagues developed specific modules in the areas of social skills and problem-solving training at the University of California, Los Angeles, Center for Schizophrenia and Psychiatric Rehabilitation. In the basic social skills training module, the trainer demonstrates and models the appropriate use of the target skill. The patient then role-plays the target skill, and the trainer offers specific and corrective feedback. This problem-solving module was developed in response to the observation that persons with severe mental illness appear to have problems in cognitive problem-solving abilities, which produce failing performance in social situations (Platt and Spivack 1972). Skills training to ameliorate the deficits assumes that communication is a three-step process that requires the skills of receiving (accurately perceiving cues from others and the environment), processing (producing and selecting response options), and sending (involving both verbal and nonverbal skills to send an appropriate social message). In this module, the interpersonal scene is enacted and role-played and then reviewed (with videotape where available). The rehabilitation worker asks about the patient's perceptions, corrects distortions, and provides feedback on the patient's communications, including alternative options. Similar modules are in use in areas other than communication, that is, independent living, medication management including dealing with physicians, and grooming skills (Liberman et al. 1987). These modules are packaged to include a videotape of a role play demonstration, a trainer's manual, a patient workbook, and have been widely disseminated (Mueser et al. 1997).

Social skills training for individuals with mental illness is most effective when it is embedded in a broad, comprehensive rehabilitation program (Liberman 1988). Bellack and Mueser (1993) in their review of psychosocial treatments for those with schizophrenia concluded that social skills training is the most researched and promising approach to improve patients' competence and alleviate disability for this population. Case studies, small group studies, and clinical trials have demonstrated the efficacy of this approach for teaching a range of behaviors, which include conversational skills, assertiveness, heterosocial skills, and medication management. Generally, newly learned skills have been maintained for 6 to 12 months after termination of the intervention (Bellack 2001, Bellack and Mueser 1993).

Support for the efficacy of skills training in a variety of areas of targeted skills acquisition, mainly in interpersonal and assertiveness skills, comes from a number of studies, reviews, and meta-analyses, but the studies have been mostly conducted in inpatient settings rather than outpatient ones (Dilk and Bond 1996, Wallace et al. 1980, Bellack et al. 1976, Goldsmith and McFall 1975, Corrigan 1991, Halford and Hayes 1991). To ensure generalization from the rehabilitation setting to the patients' living and working environments, homework assignments are utilized with demonstrated efficacy (Finch and Wallace 1977, Liberman

| Table 110–9 | Summary of Major Points of Social Skills Training |
|---|---|

Based on principles of human learning

Utilizes specific behavioral techniques

Complex behaviors delineated into discrete behavioral elements

Homework assignments employed to generalize from rehabilitation setting to the patient's environment

Social skills training most effective as part of a comprehensive rehabilitation program

Feedback of key individuals in the patient's environment increases efficacy of newly acquired behaviors

and Rueger 1984). Enlisting family members, coworkers, and peers to provide feedback and cues in "real" situations has also proved useful. Skills training may be particularly effective when associated with family psychoeducation, as indicated by the research of Hogarty and colleagues (1991).

Some question remains as to the efficacy of this approach in terms of the behavior and functioning of patients in naturalistic settings (Bellack and Mueser 1993). Efforts to facilitate the transfer of skills from the training environment to the natural environment for individuals with mental illness are essential, otherwise generalization may not occur (Liberman et al. 1987). From an extensive review of research in the area of social skills training, Lehman and associates (1994) concluded that the impact of psychosocial skills training on psychopathology and relapse and rehospitalization of schizophrenic patients is inconclusive, whereas social functioning is generally positive. This technology is promising and is likely to be more effective when integrated with community-based rehabilitation strategies and interventions (Anthony et al. 1987). The current research base does not yet warrant the conclusion of the effectiveness of this approach to every day functioning in the community. There is not evidence to indicate the transfer of skills to improved role function in areas of independent living or work (Dilk and Bond 1996). Further research is needed to determine the degree to which intensity and duration of these interventions effect outcomes (Dilk and Bond 1996).

## Vocational Rehabilitation

Whereas the development of social skills is usually a prerequisite for vocational adaptation, vocational rehabilitation is a term for interventions that are targeted to work-related skills such as punctuality, work habits, and relationships with customers, coworkers, and supervisors. The focus of vocational rehabilitation services is to improve individual functional capacity through training or environmental supports, or both, with the goal of gaining and maintaining competitive employment (Simmons et al. 1993) (Table 110–10).

Vocational disability is a concern of psychiatric patients with severe mental illness. Lehman and others (1983) found that a lack of work contributed to a poor quality of life as rated by persons with a severe mental illness. It is estimated that 20 to 30% of persons with a severe mental illness attain any type of gainful employment after discharge from the hospital, and less than 20% of those who find work retain at least partial employment 1 or 2 years later (Anthony et al. 1978, Lehman et al. 2002). The competitive employment rate (the proportion who find work in the open job market) for persons with mental illness is less than 20% (Mueser et al. 1997, Bond and McDonel 1991, Crowther et al. 2001). This is a population that tends to be underemployed, in that many obtain work in entry-level jobs that offer little opportunity for growth in pay or responsibility. Many individuals with mental illness feel that their needs for vocational rehabilitation go unaddressed (Baron 2000, Solomon et al. 1984). They also prefer to be rapidly placed in competitive employment rather than go through prevocational preparation and transitional employment (Bond and Dincin 1986, Bond et al. 1995). This preference is embodied in the "place and

| Table 110–10 | Summary of Settings and Approaches of Vocational Rehabilitation |
|---|---|

Sheltered work—segregated setting, unskilled jobs, paid less than minimum wage

Job clubs—group approach to assist patients in finding work

Transitional employment—placement in time-limited jobs to learn job-related skills (e.g., punctuality and social behaviors)

Supported employment—competitive work with ongoing supports in integrated work settings

Job coaches—type of supported employment that involves one-to-one support and contact at the work site

Job enclaves—patients employed in a business as a segregated group and paid prevailing wage

Mobile work crew—patients travel as a group with a supervisor to fulfill contracted work

Consumer-run businesses and programs—developed and operated by patients themselves

Small businesses—developed and operated by mental health agencies

Assertive community treatment with a vocational component—case management teams include an employment or vocational specialist

train" approach, which is exemplified by supported employment (discussed later).

The value of work for those with serious mental illness goes beyond the direct financial benefit. Work increases the patient's self-esteem, offers opportunities for social relationships and for meaningful and productive ways to spend time, decreases boredom, and, consequently, improves the patient's quality of life (Anthony et al. 1984). This population faces difficult barriers to obtaining and maintaining a job. Illness-related barriers include the impact of psychiatric symptoms, the unpredictable nature of the illness, and poor interpersonal skills, which may prevent persons with mental illness from getting a job and may contribute to the loss of work once acquired. Environmental barriers include discrimination by employers, disincentives to work resulting from the pessimistic attitudes of some mental health professionals, family concerns about consequences of job failure, and the jeopardy that employment places on the receipt of disability benefits (Baron 2000, Anthony et al. 1984, National Institute on Disability and Rehabilitation Research 1992). To understand why employment is often a disincentive to persons with severe mental illness, one needs to understand the benefit structure of the two primary programs that financially and medically support this population. Supplemental Security Income (SSI) provides a financial benefit for those who are disabled. However, SSI payments decrease when earnings increase. Earnings above $65 in a given month are reduced by $1 for every $2 earned. Those on Social Security Disability Income (SSDI) can earn up to $200 in a month without decreasing their benefits. SSDI beneficiaries can earn in excess of $500 per month during an initial trial work period without losing their benefits. Both of these benefit programs have provisions to assist individuals to extend their medical and income benefits for a period of time when their earnings exceed the substantial gainful activity level that is used to determine their eligibility benefit (Clark et al. 1998).

By adopting a paradigm of choose, get, and keep a job, patients are involved in assessing their own ability to accomplish job activities, to develop a plan that will increase their ability to achieve their employment goals, and to participate in interventions that enhance the desired employment outcome. The basic philosophy of this approach is to assist individuals with severe mental illness to become satisfied and successful in work environments of their choosing with the least amount of professional support as is possible (Anthony et al. 1984). This process of choose, get, and keep can be coupled within the diversity of vocational rehabilitation models, which are discussed next.

## Sheltered Work Settings

Some of the early vocational rehabilitation programs were located in psychiatric hospitals. The focus of these programs was on therapeutic outcomes such as improved self-esteem and reduced symptoms. Training for gainful employment was a secondary goal, if included. Programs did not train patients for the demands and pressures of competitive employment and were not successful in attaining employment for participants (Simmons et al. 1993).

The sheltered workshop setting utilizes unskilled work as a means to teach employment-related skills, including requisite personal and social skills. The workshop is a segregated setting, often currently located at a mental health or vocational agency, in which employees are usually paid less than minimum wage. These programs are used as a final placement for some persons and as a transition to competitive employment for others (Bond and Boyer 1988).

Some psychosocial or psychiatric rehabilitation agencies organize prevocational work crews in which members perform work necessary for the operation of the agency, such as housekeeping, food preparation, and clerical functions. These are often unpaid, but the objective is to make the member feel needed and experience successful work-related behavior. The focus is on teaching appropriate work habits and attitudes rather than on teaching specific job skills (Bond and Boyer 1988).

## Job Clubs

Job clubs are a group approach to assist individuals with mental illness find employment. Participants are trained to employ a variety of strategies while seeking a job. These range from contacting relatives and friends about job leads to developing job interviewing skills. The approach is based on the premise that supporting patients in a persistent engagement in these activities with concurrent training will lead to employment (Simmons et al. 1993). The approach described by Liberman and colleagues (1987) uses classroom lectures, group practice sessions, homework, role-playing and other group techniques in the pursuit of specific skill development designed to achieve employment. For example, patients are assisted in developing a resume, in completing job applications, and in role-playing job interviews.

Job clubs are structured around the provision of resources for an effective job search. Significant resources include access to classified advertisements and job leads, computers, telephones for contacting employers, and space and time in which to conduct the job search. The rehabilitation staff of a job club provides consultation and feedback concerning job search efforts, including daily goal setting and the establishment of a full search plan. Peer support is available from the other members of the job club.

Job clubs seem to be promising in enhancing job acquisition but not in long-term rates of job retention (Bond and McDonel 1991, Azrin and Philip 1979). Liberman and colleagues (1987) reported that in more than 3 years of operation, two-thirds of those leaving their job club remained in a job at 6-month follow-up, although not necessarily in the same job they obtained through the club. For a large majority of individuals with severe mental illness, self-directed strategies like the job club are not very satisfactory approaches, and some find the pressure of the job club detrimental (Simmons et al. 1993, Bond et al. 1997).

## Transitional Employment

Transitional employment refers to the placement of a patient in a time-limited (usually 6 months) job, which allows for the learning of job-related skills such as punctuality, concentration, productivity, and the necessary social behavior to relate to customers, coworkers, and supervisors. This approach exemplifies the train and place approach to competitive employment. Programs usually make arrangements with cooperative employers to reserve a job for patients in the agency. Transitional employment consists of small work groups or individual placements. Typical examples include manual labor and restaurant and clerical work (Simmons et al. 1993). Generally, the jobs are entry-level positions, regardless of the patient's prior work history. Patients usually work half-time and are paid the prevailing wage. Patients may share a job position. The goal is to provide patients with successful work experiences (Bond and Boyer 1988). Patients may participate in a variety of placements and, therefore, experience a broad set of options for independent placement (National Institute on Disability and Rehabilitation Research 1992). Fountain House has many such arrangements, which it pioneered with employers such as the Chock-Full-O-Nuts restaurants. To keep the job available to patients, staff occasionally fill in for patients who are unexpectedly absent because of exacerbation of illness or for other reasons. The agency guarantees that someone will do the job, in order to preserve the position for training other patients. Consequently, the placement cannot be filled permanently by a single patient. There are limitations to the benefits of transitional employment, such as the focus on entry-level jobs, the failure to move to competitive employment, and the possible development of dependency on staff (Simmons et al. 1993).

## Supported Employment

The use of transitional employment has been augmented by a newer technique derived from the world of vocational rehabilitation of the developmentally disabled (Bond et al. 1997). This approach, supported employment, is defined by Public Law 99–506 as "competitive work in integrated settings (a) for individuals with severe handicaps for whom competitive employment has not traditionally occurred, or (b) for individuals for whom competitive employment has been interrupted or intermittent as a result of a severe disability and who, because of their handicap, need ongoing support services to perform work. Supported employment is further defined by the refinement of its components (i.e., competitive work, integrated settings, severe handicaps, and ongoing support services) (Federal Register Title 1988)." The three major components of supported employment are competitive employment, integrated work setting, and provisions for ongoing support. Competitive employment is defined as work that is performed on a full-time or part-time basis, averaging at least 20 hours per week and for which the employee is compensated in accordance with the Fair Labor Standards Act. An integrated work setting is one in which a patient works in a conventional setting where not all workers are disabled. If the patients are segregated and all coworkers are handicapped, provision must be made for the disabled workers to have ongoing contact with workers without disabilities. Support services can be continuous or periodic, on or off the work site, depending on the individual work rehabilitation plan. These support services may include transportation, personal care services, and counseling to the patient, supervisors, coworkers, and family.

The supported employment approach is built on a number of assumptions. One is that most patients, regardless of the severity of their disability, can engage in meaningful and productive competitive employment, if given the opportunity, the necessary job stabilization, and ongoing support services. Clearly, nonvocational issues must be addressed, as success at employment cannot be isolated from other aspects of the person's community adaptation. Failure is viewed as attributable to inappropriate job choice or inadequate supports, or both, rather than to the individual's functional deficits.

Advantages of supported work include training after the patient is placed on the job. This helps persons with mental illness bypass the difficulty they have in transferring newly acquired skills to a real-world environment. Emphasis is on the match between the patient and the job. Before gaining employment, an assessment is made of the fit between the patient and the job. This includes the relationship to coworkers, the specific job requirements, and the travel required. An advantage of supported employment is that the patient earns a competitive wage, which may help to enhance his or her self-esteem. In addition, attitudes of coworkers may change with exposure to those with mental illness in the work environment. Disadvantages to supported employment include staff burnout, potential for high dependency on staff, and high cost (Bond 1987).

## Job Coaches

Job coaching involves one-on-one contact with the job coach. This is similar to supported employment, but the focus is on teaching specific job skills. The coach follows the patient to the work site and provides support, counseling, and advocacy for some period after job acquisition. The coach must learn the job, and then help train the person in the required job, and social, behavioral, and travel skills appropriate to the specific job site. *In situ* job coaching may prove most relevant in assessing the patient's real needs, stressors, requirements for job modification, and stigma in the workplace, while allowing for specific and targeted training. Job coaches also work with employers and coworkers to educate them about the patient's disorder

and her/his rights under the Americans with Disabilities Act. A job coach may gradually withdraw from the work site as the patient masters the necessary skills. Given the nature of severe mental illnesses, the coach is prepared to return when necessary.

## Job Enclaves

For some patients, as a form of transitional employment or permanent supported employment, a job enclave appears an attractive alternative. In this model of vocational rehabilitation, patients are employed in groups that have contracts with a commercial business or manufacturing company in the community. The contracts are developed between the rehabilitation agency and the business. A small group of patients, paid the prevailing wage, are in a separate location with a permanent supervisor. They usually assume the responsibility for an entire work area, such as a mailroom or a parts assembly room (National Institute on Disability and Rehabilitation Research 1992).

## Mobile Work Crews

Mobile work crews are groups of patients who travel with a supervisor to fulfill contracted work. Services are offered to commercial businesses and to human service agencies. Services contracted by such programs are typified by janitorial and landscaping work. The sponsoring agency obtains the contract, and the crew supervisor is responsible for training, transportation, quality control, and employer satisfaction (National Institute on Disability and Rehabilitation Research 1992).

## Consumer-Run Businesses and Programs

Patients have developed their own businesses, largely or entirely staffed and operated by the patients themselves. They operate businesses such as restaurants, film laboratories, and studios. Whereas some consider this to be self-stigmatizing segregation, others find it a source of mutual support and understanding of the special needs of persons with mental illness. Fellow workers can be thought of as surrogate job coaches. These programs may involve professional rehabilitation personnel, but some do not have professional involvement.

Consumer-run employment programs have emerged that offer "vocational counseling, educational and training programs, placement services, and ongoing peer support, with minimal or no support from mental health professionals (National Institute on Disability and Rehabilitation Research 1992, p. 14)." The ACT NOW program in Philadelphia is a consumer-operated program that trains patients to work in human service agencies. This entails 3 weeks of intensive classroom training and 12 weeks of internship at job sites as well as some ongoing classroom time discussing on-the-job experiences. Further elaboration of these concepts can be found in Chapter 111.

## Small Businesses

A number of mental health agencies, particularly psychosocial rehabilitation agencies, have developed their own businesses. These include restaurants, bulk mailing houses, and cookie factories. These businesses may provide either transitional or permanent employment opportunities for individuals with severe mental illness (National Institute on Disability and Rehabilitation Research 1992). This approach affords employees an opportunity to learn specific jobs that may lead to independent competitive employment.

## Case Management with a Vocational Component

Some ACT programs have supplemented their teams with vocational or employment specialists. These specialists assist patients in developing work skills, finding a job, and sustaining employment. These services are also arranged or brokered to independent vocational programs. Other case management models than ACT, for example, hybrid case management/employment services, have addressed employment needs of patients (Mowbray et al. 2000).

One specialized supported employment intervention developed for persons with severe mental illness, individual placement and support (IPS), draws very heavily from PACT, as well as the Boston University approach to psychiatric rehabilitation (Becker and Drake 1994). This uses a team approach and integrates vocational and mental health services (Drake et al. 1996).

## Efficacy of Vocational Rehabilitation

In an early review of the efficacy of vocational rehabilitation programs, which examined the variety of employment approaches previously discussed, Bond and Boyer (1988) concluded that it was difficult to answer the question of whether vocational rehabilitation programs assist those with psychiatric illness to achieve competitive employment. Only four of the 21 studies they reviewed demonstrated an advantage for experimental subjects when competitive employment was the desired outcome, and all four of these studies had methodological flaws. These reviewers did find that the two important process variables contributing to employment for those with severe mental illness were intensive support and positive expectations.

A more recent review of supported employment by Bond and his colleagues (1997) which assessed the effectiveness of supported employment for persons with severe mental illness found that in experimental studies supported employment was favored over control conditions. For example, 58% of clients in supported employment achieved competitive employment, whereas only 21% of control subjects did. Also, those in supported employment worked more hours and earned higher wages as compared to those not in supported employment. Furthermore there was no evidence to indicate that individuals served in supported employment had increased stress levels which might lead to an exacerbation of their illness. Another recent review which just examined randomized studies concluded that supported employment was more effective than prevocational training when it came to assisting persons with severe mental illness to obtain competitive employment (Crowther et al. 2001). Those in supported employment also earned more, worked a greater number of hours per month, and were more likely to be engaged in treatment. These reviewers did not find any evidence that prevocational programs were any more effective than the usual community services in helping patients find competitive employment. The one advantage that they did find for prevocational services over standard treatment was that prevocational did have a tendency to reduce the number of hospital admissions. Furthermore, they concluded that payment encouraged

patients to participate in vocational rehabilitation programs. But an additional challenge for these with severe mental illness is job retention (Lehman et al. 2002).

## Supported Education

Supported education is defined as the provision of services to increase access and retention in postsecondary educational institutions for individuals who have had difficulty attending or completing their education owing to a mental illness (Unger 1993b). Similar to supported employment programs, which focus on the integration of mentally ill individuals into the workforce, the goal of supported education is to integrate this population into institutions of higher education (Unger et al. 1991) (Table 110–11). Supported education is viewed as a vehicle to plan for meaningful, challenging, and stable employment. Hoffman and Mastrianni (1993, p. 111) noted that "most supported education programs are designed to foster self-confidence and self-esteem, to encourage the acquisition of skills and credentials facilitating employability, and to reinforce a normative identity." Supported education is relatively new, although educational programs for those with mental illness were described in the mid-1970s (Lamb 1976, Mowbray et al. 1999).

Because the typical or modal age at onset of many mental disorders is between the late teens and middle twenties, when many are in college or would be entering college, educational careers are often interrupted or terminated. Without proper educational and vocational credentials, these young adults are often underemployed or unemployed, resulting in a poor quality of life, low self-esteem, and reduced life satisfaction. Persons with mental illness do express concern about entering or returning to college. They have fears related to stigma, rejection, and social isolation. In addition, they are concerned about difficulty concentrating; slowed thinking due to their illness or the side effects of medication; reoccurrence of their illness; fears of failure; feeling overwhelmed by stress (such as experienced when taking examinations); and feeling that no one will be readily available to discuss emotional problems and stresses (Collins et al. 1998, Cooper 1993).

Mental health providers are concerned that the requirements of school will increase stress, with resultant exacerbation of illness (Cook and Solomon 1993). School administrators, faculty, fellow students, and staff may have concerns about admitting those with mental illness. These concerns often include issues of personal safety, inappropriate and disruptive behaviors, and the use of the campus as a "dumping ground" for psychiatric patients. These problems

| Table 110–11 | Types of Supported Education Interventions |
|---|---|

Self-contained classroom model—segregated classes on college or university campuses with a specialized curriculum

On-site model—students attend regular academic classes with support provided on site, usually by educational staff

Mobile supported education model—students attend regular academic classes, with support provided by mental health staff who are generally employed by a psychiatric rehabilitation program

are compounded by the difficulty that the administrators of educational institutions have in distinguishing between disciplinary problems and symptoms or signs of mental illness (Cook and Solomon 1993, Unger 1990).

Supported education has proved particularly appealing to young adults with mental illness and their families, given that the goals and the location are normalized and nonstigmatized (Unger 1993b). It is also an option for an older, returning student with a psychiatric illness. However, attempts by these individuals to enter or return to college are more often unsuccessful (Hoursel and Hickey 1993). It is therefore necessary to provide specialized, ongoing supports to accomplish their educational goals. Most postsecondary institutions are not readily accessible, nor do they encourage those known to have mental illness who are nonetheless qualified to attend their institutions (Unger 1993b). Individuals with mental illness who enter educational environments without planned support encounter stress, frustration, and a failure to achieve educational goals. Others may not even try to enter the educational environment once subtly or explicitly informed that postsecondary education is inappropriate for them (Becker and Drake 1994).

The support in supported education, as in supported employment, is available *in situ*, with services being provided on campus, not in a mental health setting (Sullivan et al. 1993). Supported education provides for an opportunity to employ psychiatric rehabilitation techniques by utilizing a normalized environment and strengthening an individual's educational competencies. The goals are successful completion of an educational program, exploration of career options, and development of a normalized peer support system of other students who share common experiences (Moxley et al. 1993). One of the goals of these programs is for psychiatric patients to identify themselves as students rather than as psychiatric patients.

The specific process used in supported education or by supported education workers is not well specified, although it does derive from the rehabilitation and educational techniques used in supported employment, with its much longer history. These techniques include on-site behavior modification, skills training, role-playing with the supported education worker, acting out the job or student role; crisis therapy dealing with school stress; and, where accepted, education and behavior modification (subtle) of supervisors and coworkers, with the goal of developing interpersonal accommodations.

## Models of Supported Education

Three approaches are commonly used as part of supported education: (1) the self-contained classroom, (2) on-site support, and (3) mobile support (Pratt et al. 1999, Unger 1993b, Cooper 1993, Moxley et al. 1993). These are described here in detail. The models differ as to the degree to which participants are integrated into the existing academic community, the utilization of available campus resources, and the location in which the support is provided. Each of these models brings psychiatric rehabilitation principles and treatment approaches together with educational opportunities (Moxley et al. 1993). Regardless of the model employed, the role of the psychiatrist is to assist in maintaining stabilization of the patient through medication management to ensure that side effects do not interfere with successful academic performance. In addition, the psychiatrist offers encouragement and supportive counseling and monitors symptoms to prevent an exacerbation of the patient's illness to avoid interruption of the educational program.

### Self-contained Classroom Model

Students attend segregated classes on a college or university campus with a specialized curriculum (Unger 1993b). These programs emphasize vocational goals by increasing awareness of academic skills and exploring vocational options. The goals of these programs are for participants to select a career goal and develop a career plan. Subsequently, assistance in skill building and supports are provided to participants to enter or reenter the workforce in their occupation of choice or to enroll in a mainstream academic or vocational program consistent with the achievement of their career choice (Moxley et al. 1993).

A pioneer of this model is the Career Education Program at Boston University. Students attend for three semesters, 3 days a week, 2.5 hours a day. During this time, they develop their own vocational profile, which they then match with the appropriate occupations (Unger et al. 1987, 1991, Moxley et al. 1993, Kohn 1990). The students proceed to select a career goal and identify the resources, supports, and skills required to achieve this goal. Mental health service providers in the community assist students in meeting their basic needs and provide therapeutic support, which may include case management, individual or group therapy, and medication management. An optional fourth semester is offered in which students begin more focused activities directed to the achievement of their vocational goal. They may enter targeted educational programs or training programs or directly access a job (Moxley et al. 1993, Kohn 1990). In another program, supported education is combined with supported employment by alternating between classroom and work experience. The expectation is that this is a means to enhance vocational awareness and, thus, the selection of a vocation.

### On-Site Model

In the on-site model, students attend regular academic classes and support is provided on site, usually by educational staff (Unger 1993a). This model utilizes existing campus programs, such as academic advising and developmental education programs, to provide supports to those individuals with severe mental illness. Mental health services are provided by community mental health programs linked to the academic institution. Unlike the self-contained model, the on-site model does not segregate students in a specialized program but rather integrates them into campus life by assisting them to use existing campus resources. Some programs have added specialized components such as a peer support group for students with mental illness. The model assumes that by incorporating services into existing campus resources, these services become more responsive to the needs of this population for "normalization." This model is less costly than others because it utilizes existing resources for both educational support and mental health care (Moxley et al. 1993).

## Mobile Supported Education Model

In this approach, students attend regular academic classes, with support provided by mental health staff who are often part of an independent psychiatric rehabilitation program (Moxley et al. 1993, Unger 1993a). This approach is more flexible and individualized than the two described previously, as students select the educational site or training program that they desire. The Boston University Career Education Program has added this approach to assist graduates of their self-contained program as they enter regular academic classes at the university or other post-secondary sites. A support group meets weekly for students to share experiences, to offer mutual support, and to socialize (Kohn 1990). Thresholds, a psychosocial rehabilitation agency, operates the Community Scholar Program. Thresholds' program includes preparatory classes that acquaint students with various college and trade school settings; career development and academic counseling; remedial tutoring, (which is subject specific and in some cases provided by peers); a support group for students attending college; and individualized support staffed by mobile educational workers who provide support (e.g., advice on dealing with stress and acquiring resources, educational counseling, case coordination activities, and crisis intervention services *in situ*). Thresholds' program also conducts inservice training for faculty and staff at universities and colleges that the student patients attend. Faculty training focuses on how to handle classroom and educational issues that may arise with mental illness (Cook and Solomon 1993, Moxley et al. 1993, Kohn 1990). Some residential facilities and psychiatric hospitals have initiated supported education programs for patients (Kohn 1990). The academic activities of the student are integrated into the patient's treatment plan and supported by the patient's therapist and other treatment team members. The basic tenet of these programs is that education and therapy share common goals of facilitating the patient's search for meaning and purpose in life (Hoffman and Mastrianni 1992, 1993, Kohn 1990).

## Efficacy of Supported Education

Limited research has been conducted on supported education. It is evident that individuals with severe mental illness who desire to enter or reenter postsecondary educational institutions require assistance to access available resources on campus, to negotiate administrative requirements related to registration, and to obtain financial aid (Cook and Solomon 1993). Furthermore, students with mental illness who participate in supported education programs do successfully complete courses in which they enroll. This increases the likelihood of their obtaining and maintaining competitive employment, and experiencing improved self-esteem, self-confidence, and coping skills (Unger et al. 1991, Mowbray et al. 1999, Collins et al. 1998, Cook and Solomon 1993, Hoffman and Mastrianni 1992, Wolf and DiPietro 1992). These results do appear promising, but are based on methodologically weak studies. The first evidence of the effectiveness of an experimental study found that participating in supported education has a higher combined rate of attending school, working, or involvement in vocational training over baseline results (Mowbray et al. 1999, Collins et al. 1998).

## Family Interventions

In this era of postdeinstitutionalization, families frequently assume the major responsibility of caring for their seriously mentally ill relatives. Estimates have been made that as low as 30% and as high as 60% of seriously mentally ill individuals live with their families (Carpentier et al. 1992, Goldman 1982, Tessler and Goldman 1982). This shift in care has resulted in emotional and financial burdens to family members including unresolved grief that families confront (Solomon and Draine 1995b, 1996). Families experience significant stress whether their ill relative lives with them or not (Fisher et al. 1990, Lefley 1987).

Studies have demonstrated that ratings of families as highly critical, hostile, or emotionally overinvolved—the operational components of high expressed emotion (EE)—were strongly predictive of psychotic relapses of recently discharged relatives with whom the families interacted (Brown et al. 1972, Vaughn and Leff 1976, Vaughn et al. 1984). The relationship between high EE and relapse has been replicated in a number of studies, and the EE construct has been validated through behavioral observation (Bellack and Mueser 1993).

Regardless of the intellectual controversies around EE research, for example, continuing to blame the family for exacerbation of their relative's illness, the early findings have offered an impetus to the development of psychoeducational approaches designed to assist families in coping with the disturbing, distressing, and difficult behaviors of their ill relative (Solomon 1996). The promotion of these interventions has been based on the assumption that behavioral competencies, adaptive coping skills, and emotional support can help "protect individuals with biological vulnerability from the effects of stress" and ultimately prevent relapse and rehospitalization (Mintz et al. 1987, p. 231).

There has been a diversity of family interventions developed to meet the needs of families. These include psychoeducation, family education, family consultation (all detailed later), and family support and advocacy (see Chapter 111).

## Family Psychoeducation

Psychoeducation interventions were developed by mental health professionals and many psychiatrists to be adjunctive to individual treatment for the ill relative. Consequently, these interventions have both an educational and a therapeutic component. Many of these program models were based on the EE construct (Solomon 1996). Generally, these programs share the goals of reducing relapse and improving the quality of life for the patient and the family members by enhancing the family members' capability of managing their relative's illness. They provide information about the diagnosis, symptoms, signs, etiology, course, and treatment, including medications and their side effects. They often teach problem-solving and coping strategies, management skills, and communication skills to family members (Solomon 2000). These programs last anywhere from 9 months to 5 years, and are often designed to be diagnosis specific. The outcomes for these interventions are focused on the patient and secondarily on the family (Solomon 1996, Dixon et al. 2001).

These interventions vary in program elements including: the location of the service (i.e., home, clinic, hospital, or

| Table 110–12 | Common Elements of Family Psychoeducation Interventions |
|---|---|

A collaborative relationship between family and therapist
Highly structured intervention
Teaching coping skills and strategies
Supporting the development of interpersonal boundaries within the family
Education about the illness
Use of behavioral approaches
Teaching family communication skills

elsewhere); the length of the service and the credentials and qualifications of the provider; the content emphasized and the information provided; the degree of emotional support; the focus on problem-solving skills, communication skills, and behavioral management; the use of the multiple-family versus the single-family approach; which family members are present; and their approach to delivery of information, such as degree of didactic and skill teaching, and role-playing (Solomon 1998b, 2000).

Lam (1991) identified the common elements in the various models of psychoeducation (Table 110–12). These included (1) a positive approach and a collaborative relationship between the family and the therapist, (2) the provision of the intervention in a highly structured manner, with additional contact available at the initiation of the families, (3) a focus on teaching coping skills and strategies for present problems and stressors, (4) supporting the development of clear interpersonal boundaries within the family, (5) education about the illness and its course so as to reduce blaming and guilt, (6) the employment of a behavioral approach involving the setting of priorities and breaking down goals into achievable small steps, and (7) improving family communication so that feelings are expressed without threatening anger- or guilt-inducing elements.

## Family Education

In contrast to psychoeducational interventions, family education interventions are nonclinical and the primary objective is to meet the educational and practical needs of the family and secondarily outcomes for their relative. Many of these programs were developed by family members themselves in response to their feeling misunderstood by professionals and some were therefore grassroot efforts. Families frequently feel that they do not need therapy but very practical information about their relative's illness and how to cope with it (Solomon 2000).

These programs are usually community oriented and delivered in community settings, such as churches and other accessible and convenient locations to families. They are often led by family members, but professionals are frequently brought in to lecture on specific topics, such as a psychiatrist discussing medications. In some cases, they may be co-led by mental health providers. These are group interventions that are open to anyone with a relative or significant other who has a severe mental illness. Recently, some groups have become focused on specific diagnoses and relationships, that is, parents, spouses, and children. These interventions have a didactic component,

sometimes using videos and other informational material, and then a sharing component. The informational content of these groups are similar to those of psychoeducation interventions. Given the group approach, participants experientially learn from other group members and also receive support and empathy (Citron et al. 1999). Some of the programs have a skill training component, where participants can practice skills in handling situations that they are likely to encounter during the course of their relative's illness. These are very brief interventions that may last anywhere from one session of a few hours or a day to 10 or 12 sessions, meeting once a week for an hour or two. NAMI sponsors one called Family-to-Family (see Chapter 111) (Solomon 2000, 1998b).

## Family Consultation

Family consultation or supportive family counseling is an individual approach to providing information, advice, support, and counseling to either a single family member or family unit. Often the ill relative is not present in these meetings (Bernheim 1982, 1989, Kanter 1985, Bernheim and Lehman 1985). This is an attractive intervention for families who have a relative who resists treatment. This is a collaborative approach between the family and the provider. The provider is usually a mental health professional, but may also be a trained family member (Solomon et al. 1996a, 1997). The provider and family collaborate to develop the objectives to be worked on and to set a plan for achieving them. The consultant is just that, not a therapist. In the course of consultation, the family members are provided education, information, and may be assisted with obtaining needed services. Families find that having the consultant available on an ongoing basis is extremely helpful (Budd and Hughes 1997). Therefore, this service may be provided over the telephone, but is usually provided in person. This is a short-term approach: a few sessions that are highly focused on very specific objectives. Termination is mutually agreed upon by the provider and the family. When new problems arise, the consultation may resume (Solomon 1998b, 2000).

## Efficacy of Family Interventions

A number of studies of family psychoeducation approaches have demonstrated that these interventions are effective in preventing relapse for persons with severe mental illnesses (Dixon et al. 2001, Dixon and Lehman 1995). Lam (1991) observed that, at 24 months, the results are less effective and that these programs may serve to delay rather than to prevent relapse. The strong research support for these psychoeducational interventions have resulted in their being one of the few psychosocial interventions considered to be evidence-based practice. However, there is limited evidence as to the effectiveness of these interventions in usual practice (Dixon et al. 2000). For family education, there is no evidence of their effectiveness in reducing relapse of the relative. But then, their primary objective does not address this outcome. Various studies have shown some improvements for family members, such as reduced burden, distress, anxiety, and improved self-efficacy with managing their relative's illness (Solomon 1996, 2000). Only one study has assessed family consultation, as one arm of a randomized trial, and found that consultation did improve family members' sense of self-efficacy in coping with the illness of their relative (Solomon et al. 1996a). There is evidence that patients' outcomes such as compliance with medication improve when families participate in a family intervention (Dixon et al. 2001, Solomon et al. 1996b).

Regardless of the nature of these programs, they clearly meet families' expressed desires and satisfaction with them is very high. In a number of the interventions previously discussed, psychiatrists have played a major role in design, research, and implementation. However, psychiatrists who are not involved with such formal interventions can still utilize the principles and techniques by providing families with information about their relative's illness, expectations for their relative, and advice about dealing with difficult situations. They can make referrals to support groups and other resources in the community and work collaboratively with families and patients in the development of a treatment plan. Recently issued best practice guidelines by the American Psychiatric Association (1997) and an expert consensus panel (McEvoy et al. 1999) recommend collaborating with families of adults with severe mental illness.

## Cultural Sensitivity to the Needs of Minority Populations

Few studies have assessed ethnic and cultural issues related to psychiatric rehabilitation. One study of discharged psychiatric patients did find that African-Americans tend to utilize psychosocial rehabilitation to a lesser extent than the whites. A possible explanation was self-selection on the part of patients. African-Americans are less inclined than whites to participate in verbal group programs, and many of these psychosocial interventions are group oriented (Solomon 1988). Clearly, programming has to be sensitive to the needs of ethnic and cultural groups.

Some minority groups, and consequently patients' families, may not perceive the same needs that nonminority families do. For example, they may not recognize the need for psychiatric rehabilitation with the goal of independent living as they may have different cultural expectations (Cook and Hoffschmidt 1993). African-American families preserve networks within the community that may offer a beneficial support system for a family member with mental illness (Lefley 1985). The perceived needs for mental health treatment generally, and psychiatric rehabilitation specifically, are influenced by cultural views and definitions of mental illness (Cook and Hoffschmidt 1993). For example, in Latin American cultures, mental illness is described as *ataque de nervios* or "bad nerves," and may lead to avoidance of psychiatric services. In some Asian cultures, treatment for mental illness is also avoided, as mental illness is viewed as shameful. Culturally competent psychiatric rehabilitation takes into consideration that treatment is modified to maximize compatibility with the individual's ethnic background, worldview, values, and expectations of what is acceptable (Pernell-Arnold and Finley 2000).

It is essential to understand the interaction of poverty, urbanity, and ethnic minority status for effective delivery of rehabilitation services to ethnic minorities. For example, families with severely mentally ill members may have pressing needs resulting from poverty that supersede and eclipse the needs of the ill relative. Mentally disabled minority individuals may have difficulty finding affordable housing in relatively drug-free areas and may have difficulty finding jobs in economically depressed areas. The interaction of poverty, urbanity, and ethnic minority status may affect the expectations of service providers, who may assume deficiencies and inadequacies in the ethnic minority patient (Cook and Hoffschmidt 1993).

Psychiatric "rehabilitation agencies have addressed ethnic, minority and cultural issues by promoting the use of bilingual and ethnically diverse staff and by offering problem-solving and support groups that deal with minority issues, pride, self-esteem and discrimination" (Cook and Hoffschmidt 1993, p. 94). There is a clear need for psychiatric rehabilitation programs and agencies to review assumptions regarding cultural issues and to modify or develop programs in accordance with the needs of their specific cultural and ethnic groups of patients served (Cook and Hoffschmidt 1993).

## Conclusion

As evidenced by this chapter, there are diverse rehabilitation approaches directed at different realms of patients' lives with the goal of improving social stability and quality of life. Rehabilitation views patients in their environmental context, in their immediate residential and work settings, and in their social interactions. The strategies employed by this multiplicity of approaches are to develop or modify patients' skills and environmental supports. Rehabilitation interventions are targeted at those patients with major psychiatric disorders like schizophrenia, major depression, and bipolar disorders.

The symptoms of these disorders in most patients respond to appropriate drug treatment, but there are others who are refractory to drugs and still others who continue to experience social and vocational disabilities, even with symptomatic improvement. The negative symptoms of schizophrenia, such as social withdrawal, apathy, and poor hygiene, may not respond to drug treatment, even when positive symptoms improve. Rehabilitation focuses on those aspects of these disorders that are not effectively treated by medications or through the teaching of social and personal skills (Anthony and Liberman 1986). With new atypical antipsychotic medications, it is hoped that more patients will benefit from these medications which are efficacious in reducing negative symptoms and have few of the side effects of the more traditional psychotropics (Noordsy et al. 2001). However, the effectiveness of these newer medications in the public mental health system where most of these patients are served is as yet unknown (Noordsy et al. 2001).

Once patients have optimally benefited from psychopharmacological agents and, possibly, a short hospital stay, they are then more receptive to rehabilitation. The major goals of rehabilitation are to sustain stabilization and social adjustment, to improve interpersonal and social living skills, to achieve a satisfactory quality of life, and to contribute to the recovery process with as limited an amount of professional assistance as possible (Anthony and Liberman 1986, Straus 1986). Given the goals of rehabilitation, the patient plays an integral role in the decision-making and learning process. Patient self-determination is emphasized. The rehabilitation provider also works in concert with the psychiatrist, who prescribes the medication and clinically monitors the patient. The efficacy of the rehabilitation process is influenced by the appropriate types and dosages of medication and by avoiding side effects that may interfere with the rehabilitation process.

Although there is a need for much more research in this area, some of these interventions are considered best practices, while others show promising results. However, for the most part these have not yet become the standard of practice in serving this population. Reimbursement through the Medicaid rehabilitation option helps to promote these, but providers in the system have to be trained and willing to provide them.

## References

American Psychiatric Association (1997) Practice guidelines for the treatment of patients with schizophrenia. Am J Psychiatr 54(Suppl), 1–63.

Anthony W (1992) A revolution in vision. Innov Res 1, 17–19.

Anthony W and Liberman RP (1986) The practice of psychiatric rehabilitation: Historical, conceptual, and research base. Schizophr Bull 12, 542–559.

Anthony WA (1982) Explaining psychiatric rehabilitation by an analogy to physical rehabilitation. Psychosoc Rehab J 6, 61–65.

Anthony WA, Cohen MR, and Cohen BF (1983) Philosophy, treatment, process, and principle of the psychiatric rehabilitation approach. In Deinstitutionalization, Bachrach LL (ed). Jossey-Bass, San Francisco, pp. 67–79.

Anthony WA, Cohen MR, and Farkas M (1987) Training and technical assistance in psychiatric rehabilitation. In Psychiatric Disability, Meyerson AT and Fine T (eds). American Psychiatric Press, Washington DC, pp. 251–269.

Anthony WA, Cohen MR, and Farkas M (1990) Psychiatric Rehabilitation. Boston Center for Psychiatric Rehabilitation, Boston, p. 5.

Anthony WA, Cohen MR, and Vitalo R (1978) The measurement of rehabilitation outcome. Schizophr Bull 4, 365–383.

Anthony WA, Howell J, and Danley K (1984) Vocational rehabilitation of the psychiatrically disabled. In The Chronically Mentally Ill: Research and Services, Mirabi M (ed). Spectrum, Jamaica, NY, pp. 215–237.

Austin CD (1990) Case management myths and realities. Fam Soc J Contemp Hum Serv 71, 398–405.

Azrin NH and Philip RA (1979) The job club method for one handicapped: A comparative outcome model. Rehab Couns Bull 23, 144–155.

Bachrach LL (1992) Psychosocial rehabilitation and psychiatry in the care of long-term patients. Am J Psychiatr 149, 1455–1463.

Baron R (2000) Vocational rehabilitation. In Best Practices in Psychosocial Rehabilitation, Hughes R and Weinstein D (eds). International Association of Psychosocial Rehabilitation Services, Columbia, pp. 245–263.

Baronet A and Gerber G (1998) Psychiatric rehabilitation: Efficacy of four models. Clin Psychol Rev 18, 189–228.

Beard J, Propst RV, and Malamud T (1983) The fountain house model of psychiatric rehabilitation. Psychosoc Rehab J 7, 47–53.

Becker D and Drake R (1994) Individual placement and support: A community mental health center approach to vocational rehabilitation. Comm Ment Health J 30, 193–206.

Bellack A (2001) Rehabilitative treatment of schizophrenia. In Comprehensive Care of Schizophrenia, Lieberman J and Murray R (eds). Martin Dunitz, London, pp. 109–120.

Bellack A and Mueser K (1993) Psychosocial treatment for schizophrenia. Schizophr Bull 19, 317–326.

Bellack A, Hersen M, and Turner V (1976) Generalization effects of social skills training in chronic schizophrenics: An experimental analysis. Behav Res Ther 14, 391–398.

Bernheim K (1982) Supportive family counseling. Schizophr Bull 8, 634–640.

Bernheim K (1989) The role of family consultation. Am Psychol 44, 561–564.

Bernheim K and Lehman A (1985) Working with Families of the Mentally Ill. WW Norton, New York.

Bond G (1987) Supported work as a modification of the transitional employment model for clients with psychiatric disabilities. Psychosoc Rehab J 11, 55–73.

Bond G and Boyer S (1988) Rehabilitation programs and outcomes. In Vocational Rehabilitation of Persons with Prolonged Psychiatric Disorders, Ciardiello J and Bell M (eds). Johns Hopkins University Press, Baltimore, pp. 231–263.

Bond G and Dincin J (1986) Accelerating entry into transitional employment in a psychosocial agency. Rehab Psychol 32, 143–155.

Bond G and McDonel E (1991) Vocational rehabilitation outcomes for persons with psychiatric disabilities. J Vocat Rehab 1, 9–20.

Bond G, Dietzen L, McGrew J, et al. (1995) Accelerating entry into supported employment for persons with severe psychiatric disabilities. Rehab Psychol 40, 75–94.

Bond G, Drake R, Mueser K, et al. (1997) An update on supported employment for people with severe mental illness. Psychiatr Serv 48, 335–346.

Brown GW, Birley JLT, and Wing JK (1972) Influence of family life on the course of schizophrenic disorders: A replication. Br J Psychiatr 121, 241–258.

Budd R and Hughes I (1997) What do relatives of people with schizophrenia find helpful about family interventions? Schizophr Bull 23, 341–347.

Burns B and Santos A (1995) Assertive community treatment: An update of randomized trials. Psychiatr Serv 46, 669–675.

Carpentier N, Lesage A, Goulet I, et al. (1992) Burden of care of families not living with young schizophrenic relative. Hosp Comm Psychiatr 43, 38–43.

Citron M, Solomon P, and Draine J (1999) Self-help groups for families of persons with mental illness: Perceived benefits of helpfulness. Comm Ment Health J 35, 15–30.

Clark R (1994) Family costs associated with severe mental illness and substance abuse. Hosp Comm Psychiatr 45, 808–813.

Clark R and Drake R (1994) Expenditures of time and money by families of people with severe mental illness and substance use disorders. Comm Ment Health J 30, 145–163.

Clark R, Dain B, Xie H, et al. (1998) The economic benefits of supported employment for persons with mental illness. J Ment Health Policy Econ 1, 63–71.

Coffey R, Mark T, King E, et al. (2000) National estimates of expenditures for mental health substance abuse treatment, 1997. US Department of Health and Human Services, Substance Abuse and Mental Health Services Administration, Rockville, Maryland.

Collins M, Bybee D, and Mowbray C (1998) Effectiveness of supported education for individuals with psychiatric disabilities: Results from an experimental study. Comm Ment Health J 34, 595–613.

Cook J and Hoffschmidt SJ (1993) Comprehensive models of psychosocial rehabilitation. In Psychiatric Rehabilitation in Practice, Flexer R and Solomon P (eds). Andover Medical Publishers, Boston, pp. 81–97.

Cook JA and Solomon ML (1993) The community scholar program: An outcome study of supported education for students with severe mental illness. Psychosoc Rehab J 17, 83–97.

Cooper L (1993) Serving adults with psychiatric disabilities on campus: A mobile support approach. Psychosoc Rehab J 17, 25–38.

Corrigan P (1991) Social skills training in adult psychiatric populations: A meta-analysis. J Behav Ther Exp Psychiatr 22, 203–210.

Crowther R, Marshall M, Bond G, et al. (2001) Helping people with severe mental illness to obtain work: A systematic review. Br Med J 332, 204–208.

Dilk M and Bond G (1996) Meta-analytic evaluation of skills training research for individuals with severe mental illness. J Consult Clin Psychol 64, 1337–1346.

Dixon L and Lehman A (1995) Family interventions for schizophrenia. Schizophr Bull 21, 631–643.

Dixon L, Adams C, and Luckstead A (2000) Update on family psychoeducation for schizophrenia. Schizophr Bull 26, 5–20.

Dixon L, Hackman A, and Lehman A (1997) Consumers as staff in assertive community treatment programs. Admin Policy Ment Health 25, 199–208.

Dixon L, Kraus N, and Lehman A (1994) Consumer as service providers: The promise and challenge. Comm Ment Health J 30, 615–629.

Dixon L, McFarlane W, Lefley H, et al. (2001) Evidenced-based practice for services to families of people with psychiatric disabilities. Psychiatr Serv 52, 903–910.

Drake R, McHugo G, Becker D, et al. (1996) The New Hampshire study of supported employment for people with severe mental illness. J Counsel Clin Psychol 64, 391–399.

Drake R, McHugo G, Clarke R, et al. (1998) Assertive community treatment for patient with co-occurring severe mental illness and substance abuse disorder: A clinical trial. Am J Orthopsychiatr 68, 201–215.

Federal Register Title VI, Part C, May 12, (1988) 17(1), 16982.

Felton C, Stasny P, Shern D, et al. (1995) Consumers as peer specialists on intensive case management teams: Impact on client outcomes. Psychiatr Serv 46, 1037–1044.

Finch B and Wallace CJ (1977) Successful interpersonal skills training with schizophrenic inpatients. J Consult Clin Psychol 45, 885–890.

Fisher G, Benson P, and Tessler R (1990) Family responses to mental illness: Developments since deinstitutionalization. In Mental Disorder in Social Context, Greenley JR (ed). JAI Press, Greenwich, CT, pp. 203–236.

Flexer R and Solomon P (eds) (1993) Psychiatric Rehabilitation in Practice. Andover Medical Publishers, Boston.

Franks D (1990) Economic contribution of families caring for persons with severe and persistent mental illness. Admin Policy Ment Health 18, 9–18.

Goering P, Wasylenki D, Farkas M, et al. (1988) What difference does case management make? Hosp Comm Psychiatr 38, 272–276.

Goldfinger SM (1990) Homeless and schizophrenia: A psychosocial approach. In Handbook of Schizophrenia, Vol. 4, Psychosocial Treatment of Schizophrenia, Herz M, Keith S, and Docherty J (eds). Elsevier Science, New York, pp. 355–385.

Goldman HH (1982) Mental illness and family burden: A public health perspective. Hosp Comm Psychiatr 33, 557–560.

Goldman HH and Gatozzi AA (1981) Defining and counting the chronically mentally ill. Hosp Comm Psychiatr 52, 21–27.

Goldman HH and Manderscheid R (1987) Epidemiology of chronic mental disorder. In The Chronic Mental Patient/II, Menninger WW and Hannah G (eds). American Psychiatric Association, Washington DC, pp. 41–63.

Goldsmith JC and McFall RM (1975) Development and evolution of an interpersonal skill training program for psychiatric inpatients. J Abnorm Psychol 84, 51–58.

Halford W and Hayes R (1991) Psychosocial rehabilitation of chronic schizophrenic patients: Recent findings on social skills training and family psychoeducation. Clin Psychol Rev 11, 23–44.

Harris M and Bergman HC (1987) Case management with the chronically mentally ill: A clinical perspective. Am J Orthopsychiatr 57, 296–302.

Harris M and Bergman H (1988) Clinical case management for the chronically mentally ill: A conceptual analysis. In Clinical Case Management, Harris M and Bachrach LL (eds). Jossey-Bass, San Francisco, pp. 5–13.

Herinckx H, Kinney R, Clarke G, et al. (1997) Assertive community treatment versus usual care in engaging and retaining clients with severe mental illness. Psychiatr Serv 48, 1297–1306.

Hodge M and Draine J (1993) Development of support through case management services. In Psychiatric Rehabilitation in Practice, Flexer RW and Solomon P (eds). Andover Medical Publishers, Boston, pp. 155–169.

Hoffman F and Mastrianni X (1992) The hospitalized college student: A model program for psychiatric treatment. Am J Orthopsychiatr 62, 297–302.

Hoffman FL and Mastrianni X (1993) The role of supported education in the inpatient treatment of young adults: A two-site comparison. Psychosoc Rehab J 17, 109–119.

Hogarty G, Anderson C, Reiss D, et al. (1991) Family psychoeducation, social skills training, and maintenance chemotherapy in the aftercare of schizophrenia. II. Two-year effects of a controlled study of relapse and adjustment. Arch Gen Psychiatr 48, 340–347.

Honigfeld G and Patin J (1990) A two-year clinical and economic follow-up of patients on clozapine. Hosp Comm Psychiatr 41, 882–885.

Hoult J, Reynolds I, Charbonneau-Powis M, et al. (1981) A controlled study of psychiatric hospital versus community treatment: The effect on relatives. Aust NZ J Psychiatr 15, 323–328.

Hoursel D and Hickey S (1993) Supported education in a community college for students with psychiatric disabilities: The Houston Community College model. Psychosoc Rehab J 17, 41–50.

Hughes R (1994) Psychiatric rehabilitation: An essential health service for people with serious and persistent mental illness. In An Introduction to Psychiatric Rehabilitation, Publication Committee of IAPSRS (eds).

International Association of Psychosocial Rehabilitation Services, Columbia.

Intagliata J (1982) Improving the quality of community care for the chronically mentally disabled: The role of case management. Schizophr Bull 8, 655–673.

Intagliata J and Baker F (1983) Factors affecting case management services for the chronically mentally ill. Admin Policy Ment Health 11, 75–91.

Johnson P and Rubin A (1983) Case management in mental health: A social work domain? Soc Work 28, 49–55.

Kanter J (1985) Consulting with families of the chronic mentally ill. In Clinical Issues in Treating the Chronic Mentally Ill, Kanter J (ed). Jossey-Bass, San Francisco, pp. 21–32.

Kanter J (1988) Clinical issues in the case management relationship. In Clinical Case Management. Harris M and Bachrach LL (eds). Jossey-Bass, San Francisco, pp. 15–27.

Kanter J (1989) Clinical case management: Definition, principles, components. Hosp Comm Psychiatr 40, 361–368.

Kessler R, Berglund P, Zhao S, et al. (1996) The 12-month prevalence and correlates of serious mental illness (SMI). In Mental Health, United States, Mandersheid R and Sonnenschein M (eds). US Government Printing Office, Washington DC, pp. 59–70.

Kohn L (1990) The self-contained classroom model. Comm Supp Network News 6, 3.

Lam D (1991) Psychosocial family intervention in schizophrenia: A review of empirical studies. Psychol Med 21, 423–441.

Lamb HR (1976) An educational model for teaching living skills to long-term patients. Hosp Comm Psychiatr 12, 875–877.

Lamb HR (1980) Therapist-case managers: More than brokers of services. Hosp Comm Psychiatr 31, 762–764.

Lefley H (1985) Culture and mental illness: The family role. In Families of Mentally Ill: Coping and Adaptation, Hatfield AB and Lefley HP (eds). Guilford Press, New York, pp. 30–59.

Lefley H (1987) Aging parents as caregivers of mentally ill adult children: An emerging social problem. Hosp Comm Psychiatr 38, 1063–1070.

Lehman A, Dixon L, Levine J, et al. (1994) Literature Review: Schizophrenia Patient Outcomes Research Team. Center for Mental Health Services Research, University of Maryland, Baltimore.

Lehman A, Goldberg R, Dixon L, et al. (2002) Improving employment outcomes for persons with severe mental illnesses. Arch Gen Psychiatr 59, 165–172.

Lehman AF, Ward NC, and Linn LS (1983) Chronic mental patients: The quality of life issue. Am J Psychiatr 133, 796–823.

Liberman RP (1988) Social skills training. In Psychiatric Rehabilitation of Chronic Patients, Liberman RP (ed). American Psychiatric Association, Washington DC, pp. 147–198.

Liberman RP and Rueger DB (1984) Drug-psychosocial treatment interactions: Comprehensive rehabilitation for chronic schizophrenics. Psychosoc Rehab J 3, 3–15.

Liberman RP, Jacobs HE, Blackwell GA, et al. (1987) Overcoming psychiatric disability through skills training. In Psychiatric Disability, Meyerson AT and Fine T (eds). American Psychiatric Press, Washington DC, pp. 221–249.

Macias C, Jackson R, Schroeder C, et al. (1999) What is a clubhouse? Report on the ICCD 1996 Survey of USA Clubhouses. Comm Ment Health J 35, 181–190.

Marcotie D and Wilcox-Gok V (2001) Estimating the employment and earnings costs of mental illness: Developments in the United States. Soc Sci Med 53, 21–27.

McEvoy J, Scherfler P, and Francis A (eds) (1999) The expert consensus guidelines series. Treatment of schizophrenia. J Clin Psych 11(Suppl), 4–80.

McFarlane W, Dushay R, Stastny P, et al. (1996) A comparison of two levels of family-aided assertive community treatment. Psychiatr Serv 47, 744–750.

McGrew J, Bond G, Dietzen L, et al. (1994) Measuring fidelity of implementation of a mental health program model. J Consult Clin Psychol 62, 670–678.

Mechanic D (1991) Strategies for integrating public mental health services. Hosp Comm Psychiatr 42, 797–801.

Mintz L, Liberman R, Miklowitz D, et al. (1987) Expressed emotion: A call for partnership among relatives, patients, and professionals. Schizophr Bull 13, 227–235.

Modrcin M, Rapp C, and Chamberlain R (1985) Case Management with Psychiatrically Disabled Individuals: Curriculum and Training

Program. University of Kansas School of Social Welfare, Lawrence, KS.

Mowbray C, Bybee D, and Collins M (2000) Integrating vocational services on case management teams: Outcomes from a research demonstration project. Ment Health Serv Res 2, 51–66.

Mowbray C, Collins M, and Bybee D (1999) Supported education for individuals with psychiatric disabilities: Long-term outcomes from an experimental study. Soc Work Res 23, 89–100.

Moxley D, Mowbray C, and Brown SK (1993) Supported education. In Psychiatric Rehabilitation in Practice, Flexer RW and Solomon P (eds). Andover Medical Publishers, Boston, pp. 137–153.

Mueser K, Bond G, Drake R, et al. (1998) Models of community care for severe mental illness: A review of research on case management. Schizophr Bull 24, 37–74.

Mueser K, Drake R, and Bond G (1997) Recent advances in psychiatric rehabilitation for patients with severe mental illness. Harvard Rev Psychiatr 5(3), 123–137.

National Institute on Disability and Rehabilitation Research (1992) Consensus Statement, Vol. 1, No. 3.

Nicholson I and Neufeld R (1992) A dynamic vulnerability perspective on stress and schizophrenia. Am J Orthopsychiatr 62, 117–130.

Noordsy D, O'Keefe C, Nueser K, et al. (2001) Six-month outcomes for patients who switched to olanzapine treatment. Psychiatr Serv 52, 501–507.

Ozarin L (1978) The pros and cons of case management. In The Chronic Patient, Talbott J (ed). American Psychiatric Association, Washington DC, pp. 165–170.

Pernell-Arnold A and Finley L (2000) Integrating multicultural competencies in psychosocial rehabilitation. In Best Practices in Psychosocial Rehabilitation, Hughes R and Weinstein D (eds). International Association of Psychosocial Rehabilitation Services, Columbia, pp. 213–244.

Platt JJ and Spivack G (1972) Problem solving thinking of psychiatric patients. J Consult Clin Psychol 28, 3–5.

Pratt C, Gill K, Barrett N, et al. (1999) Psychiatric Rehabilitation. Academic Press, San Diego.

Propst R (1992) Introduction. Psychosoc Rehab J 161, 3–4.

Rehabilitation Act Amendments of 1986, Title I, Section 103.

Roach J (1993) Clinical case management with severely mentally ill adults. In Case Management for Mentally Ill Patients, Harris M and Bergman HC (eds). Harwood Academic Publishers, Langhorne, PA, pp. 17–40.

Robinson GK and Toff-Bergman G (1990) Choices in Case Management: Current Knowledge and Practice for Mental Health Programs. Mental Health Policy Resource Center, Washington DC.

Rutman I (1994) What is psychiatric rehabilitation. In An Introduction to Psychiatric Rehabilitation, Publication Committee of IAPSRS (eds). International Association of Psychosocial Rehabilitation Services, Columbia.

Rutman ID (1987) The psychosocial rehabilitation movement in the United States. In Psychiatric Disability, Meyerson AT and Fine T (eds). American Psychiatric Press, Washington DC, pp. 197–220.

Salyers M, Masterton T, Fekete D, et al. (1998) Transferring clients from intensive case management: Impact on client functioning. Am J Orthopsychiatr 68, 233–245.

Sands R (1991) Clinical Social Work Practice in Community Mental Health. Macmillan Publishing, New York.

Scott J and Dixon L (1995) Assertive community treatment and case management for schizophrenia. Schizophr Bull 21, 657–668.

Sherman P and Porter R (1991) Mental health consumers as case management aides. Hosp Comm Psychiatr 42, 494–498.

Simmons TJ, Selleck V, Steele R, et al. (1993) Supports and rehabilitation for employment. In Psychiatric Rehabilitation in Practice, Flexer R and Solomon P (eds). Andover Medical Publishers, Boston, pp. 119–135.

Solomon P (1988) Racial factors in mental health service utilization. Psychosoc Rehab J 11, 3–12.

Solomon P (1992) The efficacy of case management services for severely mentally disabled clients. Comm Ment Health J 28, 163–180.

Solomon P (1994) Families' views of service delivery: An empirical assessment. In Helping Families Cope with Mental Illness, Lefley H and Wasow M (eds). Chur, Switzerland, pp. 259–274.

Solomon P (1996) Moving from psychoeducation to family education for families of adults with serious mental illness. Psychiatr Serv 47, 1364–1370.

Solomon P (1998a) The conceptual and empirical base of case management for adults with severe mental illness. In Advances in Mental Health

Research: Implications for Practice, Williams J and Ell K (eds). NASW Press, Washington DC, pp. 482–497.

Solomon P (1998b) The cultural context of interventions for family members with a seriously mentally ill relative. In Families Coping with Mental Illness: The Cultural Context. New Directions for Mental Health Services, Lefley H (ed). Jossey-Bass, San Francisco, pp. 5–16.

Solomon P (1999) The evolution of service innovations for adults with severe mental illness. In Innovations in Practice and Service Delivery Across the Lifespan, Biegel D and Blum A (eds). Oxford University Press, New York, pp. 147–168.

Solomon P (2000) Services for families of individuals with schizophrenia: Maximising outcomes for relatives. Dis Manag Health Out 8, 211–221.

Solomon P and Draine J (1993) The efficacy of a consumer case management team: Two year outcomes of a randomized trial. J Ment Health Admin 22, 135–146.

Solomon P and Draine J (1994) Family perceptions of consumers as case managers. Comm Ment Health J 30, 165–176.

Solomon P and Draine J (1995a) One-year outcomes of a randomized trial of case management with seriously mentally ill clients leaving jail. Eval Rev 19, 256–273.

Solomon P and Draine J (1995b) Subjective burden among family members of mentally ill adults: Relation to stress, coping and adaptation. Am J Orthopsychiatr 65, 419–427.

Solomon P and Draine J (1996) Examination of grief among family members of individuals with serious and persistent mental illness. Psychiatr Q 67, 221–234.

Solomon P and Draine J (2001) The state of knowledge of the effectiveness of consumer provided services. Psychiatr Rehab J 25, 20–27.

Solomon P, Draine J, Mannion E, et al. (1996a) Impact of brief family psychoeducation on self-efficacy. Schizophr Bull 22, 41–50.

Solomon P, Draine J, Mannion E, et al. (1996b) The impact of individualized and group workshop family education interventions on ill relative outcomes. J Nerv Ment Dis 84, 252–254.

Solomon P, Draine J, Mannion E, et al. (1997) Effectiveness of two models of brief family education: Retaining gains of family members of adults with serious mental illness. Am J Orthopsychiatr 67, 177–186.

Solomon P, Gordon B, and Davis J (1984) Community Services to Discharged Psychiatric Patients. Charles C Thomas, Springfield, IL.

Stein L (1992) On the abolishment of the case manager. Health Aff 11, 172–177.

Stein LI and Test MA (1980) Alternatives to mental hospital treatment conceptual model. I: Treatment program and clinical evaluation. Arch Gen Psychiatr 37, 392–397.

Straus J (1986) Discussion: What does rehabilitation accomplish? Schizophr Bull 12, 720–723.

Stroul B (1993) Rehabilitation in community support systems. In Psychiatric Rehabilitation in Practice, Flexer RW and Solomon P (eds). Andover Medical Publishers, Boston, pp. 45–61.

Sullivan AP, Nicolellis DL, Danley K, et al. (1993) Choose-get-keep: A psychiatric rehabilitation approach to supported education. Psychosoc Rehab J 17, 56–68.

Tessler R and Goldman HH (1982) The Chronically Mentally Ill: Assessing Community Support Programs. Ballinger, Cambridge, MA.

Test M (1992) Training in community living. In Handbook of Psychiatric Rehabilitation, Liberman RP (ed). Macmillan Publishing, New York, pp. 153–170.

Unger K (1990) Supported education for young adults with psychiatric disabilities. Comm Supp Network News 6, 1–11.

Unger K (1993a) Creating supported education programs utilizing existing community resources. Psychosoc Rehab J 17, 11–23.

Unger K (1993b) Introduction. Psychosoc Rehab J 17, 3–5.

Unger K, Anthony W, Sciarappa K, et al. (1991) A supported education program for young adults with long term mental illness. Hosp Comm Psychiatr 42, 838–842.

Unger K, Delaney K, Kohn L, et al. (1987) Rehabilitation through education: A university based continuing education program for young adults with psychiatric disabilities on a university campus. Psychosoc Rehab J 10, 35–49.

Ustun TB (1999) The global burden of mental disorders. Am J Pub Health 89, 1315–1318.

Vaughn C and Leff J (1976) The influence of family and social factors on the course of psychiatric illness. Br J Psychiatr 129, 125–137.

Vaughn C, Snyder K, Jones S, et al. (1984) Family factors in schizophrenic relapse. Arch Gen Psychiatr 41, 1169–1177.

Wallace CJ, Nelson C, Liberman RP, et al. (1980) A review and critique of social skills training with chronic schizophrenics. Schizophr Bull 6, 42–63.

Wehman P (1986) Supported competitive employment for persons with severe disabilities. J Appl Rehab Couns 117, 24–29.

Wolf J and DiPietro S (1992) From patient to student supported education programs in Southwest Connecticut. Psychosoc Rehab J 15, 61–68.

Ziguras S and Stuart G (2000) A meta-analysis of the effectiveness of mental health case management over 20 years. Psychiatr Serv 51, 1410–1421.

# 111    Advocacy, Self-Help, and Consumer-Operated Services

Harriet P. Lefley

A mentally ill woman involved with a self-help group writes to thank a peer who has helped her recover from an episode of hopelessness and despair:

> We've all known so much pain and so many years of struggling, that I feel we share a bond the likes of which the so-called "normal" world will never know. I consider it a privilege to be associated with people who have survived, and survived, and survived again, but still have the courage, the compassion, and the humanity to keep on striving and caring about themselves and reaching out to touch others in trouble. Although the rest of the world perceives us as different and pretty much useless, I think we're about as special as you can get.
> (Deegan 1994)

The letter captures some of the therapeutic aspects of the self-help experience. These include the feeling of not being alone, of bonding with peers who have shared the experience of mental illness. The woman is grateful for role models who have been able to reach out and help others. Viewing these examples of strength in persons with psychiatric disabilities, the writer rejects the world's stigmatization of the mentally ill and reevaluates with pride her own identity. There is a new appreciation of herself as someone able to transcend the pain and emerge as a survivor.

What is the relation of the self-help enterprise to the practice of psychiatry? Within the field of mental health, concepts such as advocacy, volunteerism, self-help, and consumerism represent interrelated activities that may share common objectives and yet differ substantially in process and impact. Each of these concepts has had some influence on psychiatric knowledge and practice. They designate extraprofessional efforts that, primarily, appear to be helpful to many patients. However, some of these concepts also describe social movements that have far-reaching effects on the funding of basic etiological research as well as services, the shape of mental health law, clinical training and patient–physician relationships, and the parameters and structures of treatment systems. Continuing research

on self-help and consumerism may also add considerably to our knowledge of the mechanisms of therapeutic growth.

Advocacy and self-help cover a wide range of mental health–related issues. Indeed, self-help groups are an acknowledged mechanism for striving to maintain mental health under adverse personal circumstances (Gartner and Riessman 1984). In this chapter, these concepts are defined in terms of how they relate to a variety of conditions. However, the primary focus is on their application to the population of persons with major mental illnesses, that is, persons who have been psychiatrically hospitalized, have received crisis services, or have manifested functional impairment and a need for prolonged outpatient care. Much of the discussion relates to people with chronic disorders who rely on psychiatric services for extended periods of their lives. The involvement of such persons with self-help movements is of considerable interest to the psychiatrists from whom they receive their professional care.

## Conceptual Distinctions

### Advocacy

Advocacy groups focus on social and legal remedies to improve the lives of the particular constituency they represent. A primary focus of groups operating with a mental health agenda is legislative advocacy. This typically involves active lobbying for funding for research and services. Advocates may also work to promote legislation to protect the rights of mentally ill persons; extend entitlements; mandate insurance parity in order to ensure equal access to benefits of mentally, developmentally, and physically disabled persons; and improve standards and quality of care. Advocacy efforts may involve public education and anti-stigma campaigns and promoting and publicizing programs with innovative models of treatment and rehabilitation. Advocates may attempt to influence the agendas of federal agencies to focus on persons with serious mental illness, accompanied by budgetary advocacy to increase the funding for these agencies. Although tax exempt groups cannot engage in political sponsorship of candidates, individual members are likely to offer active support for legislators with a favorable voting record on mental health issues.

Currently there are strong initiatives to ensure that the needs of persons with chronic mental illness will not be lost in the acute care models of most managed care systems. In most cases, lay advocacy organizations will collaborate with professional associations to promote mutual agendas for standards, credentialing, clinical services, and research. This adds the considerable weight of a citizen constituency to what may be perceived as the vested interests of a practitioner group.

## Volunteerism

Volunteerism, or work without remuneration, involves the participation of concerned individuals in a variety of unpaid activities that improve the lives of persons with mental illness. These are typically offered by nonprofessionals contributing their time and energy to augment professional services. However, as may be seen in some of the descriptions of citizen and consumer organizations, professionals may also act as volunteers. They may contribute their time to educate the public, lead support groups, serve on boards, or otherwise act in an unpaid advisory capacity.

Volunteerism may involve efforts devoted to the development of ancillary resources for persons with mental illness or the provision of personal services to supplement the professional system of care. A notable example is COMPEER, a nationwide program that trains volunteers to provide social companionship and role models for persons with severe and persistent mental illnesses.

Although volunteerism has been termed a uniquely US product (Greenblatt 1985), there is increasing evidence of its application in other countries. One example is Friends of the National Institute of Mental Health and Neurosciences in Bangalore, India, a women's group that has developed and administers with volunteer help a psychosocial rehabilitation center for the institute's patients. In northern Italy, there are numerous volunteers contributing to a network of cooperative enterprises employing deinstitutionalized patients. In Japan, Zenkaren, the oldest family organization (formed in 1965), administers more than 800 sheltered workshops for persons with mental illness and in many other ways supplements the official mental health system (Mizuno and Murakami 2001). Newly organized family advocacy groups in Europe and Asia are also beginning to augment services with a volunteer capability. Quantitatively, however, volunteerism is probably a far more significant aspect of medical and mental health care in the US. The scope of volunteer activities is suggested in some of the organizational descriptions in the following section.

## Self-Help

Self-help refers to the organization of groups of individuals sharing a common problem who meet for purposes of mutual aid and support, education, and personal growth. Although advocacy may also be included in the agenda, self-help groups primarily focus on relief of personal problems through unburdening, sharing experiences and solutions to mutual problems, role modeling, positive reinforcement from peers, and information exchange. Through these activities, self-help groups improve coping skills and also provide social support. Self-help groups aim toward therapeutic growth and skill development through mutual efforts rather than through professional interventions.

In 1990, it was estimated that between 9 and 12 million US adults used self-help groups (Lieberman 1990). Given the explosion of self-help groups in successive editions of *The Self-Help Source Book* (White and Madara 2002), there may be double that number today. Almost all of these groups deal with mental health–related problems. Included are the primary substance abuse organizations, Alcoholics Anonymous (AA) and Narcotics Anonymous (NA). AA has over 98,000 chapters. Their famous 12-step paradigm has been extended to other addictions (Overeaters Anonymous, Gamblers Anonymous, and the like). Parents Anonymous uses the self-help model for treatment and prevention of family violence. Other groups deal with bereavement; victimhood; physical and developmental disabilities; parenting; and societal status issues, such as being female, gay or lesbian, or a member of a particular racial or ethnic group. *The Self-Help Source Book* currently (White and Madara 2002) lists 671 self-help organizations that deal with specific physical and mental disorders. There are also specialized groups for adoptees, adult children of alcoholic persons, victims of sexual abuse, and persons who have suffered a range of other human problems. These groups have proliferated so widely that the National Institute of Mental Health (NIMH) for years supported a National Self-Help Clearinghouse (Greenblatt 1985) with listings of self-help organizations. This clearinghouse maintained a database and information and referral system but tended to focus on training and research activities. The American Self-Help Clearinghouse now of Cedar Knolls, New Jersey, focuses more on services and publishes a directory of 1,071 national and model self-help programs (White and Madara 2002). Included are 169 on-line groups. After the 9/11 World Trade Center (WTC) disaster, a surge of local face-to-face WTC groups were organized by survivors and families and friends of victims to deal with the traumatic effects (White and Madara 2002).

Included among the self-help groups outside of the professional system are those for people coping with psychiatric disorders. Prominent organizations, described in greater detail later, include Recovery Inc., GROW (not an acronym), the National Depressive and Manic–Depressive Association, and Schizophrenics Anonymous. These groups tend to be oriented toward support and mutual aid rather than political advocacy, although there is some overlapping membership in the growing movements of psychiatric consumer advocates.

## Consumerism

Consumerism as applied to mental illness is the doctrine that service recipients have essential contributions to make to mental health planning, service delivery, and research. In this context, psychiatric service recipients generally refer to themselves as consumers, the most widely accepted term. However, they are also self-defined as clients, ex-patients, persons who are psychiatrically disabled, persons who are psychiatrically labeled, inmates, and survivors, depending on the orientation of the speaker.

Consumers are loosely defined by most consumer organizations as persons who have received services from a mental health system. The Center for Mental Health Services (CMHS) of the Substance Abuse and Mental Health Services Administration (SAMHSA) defines a consumer simply as "an individual, 18 years of age and older, with severe mental illness," (SAMHSA 2001). Most persons identified as consumers typically have been psychiatrically hospitalized or have received outpatient care for a serious psychiatric condition. As persons who have experienced mental illness and who have been exposed to various treatment and rehabilitative modalities, consumers have long been considered to be valuable judges of whatever will best serve the needs of their peers, both by the CMHS (Consumer/Survivor MHR 1993) and the National Association of State Mental Health Program Directors (NASMHPD 1989). Consumers who serve in this capacity may have various levels of functioning. Although some have a diagnosis of schizophrenia, they are articulate and rarely are cognitively disabled (Frese 1998). Indeed, many have superior talents in writing, organizing capability, or in various areas of technical skill.

For more than a decade, consumer input has been solicited by government agencies at all levels of knowledge development and service building. This may range from formulating basic research questions to consumer roles in design, interviewing, and data analysis; from program monitoring and evaluation to state and local systems planning (SAMHSA 2001, Consumer/Survivor MHR 1993, NASMHPD 1989, Frese 1998, Trochim et al. 1993).

Targeted requests for grant applications from federal and state authorities solicit consumers in remission for service delivery roles both as staff members in professionally run services and as operators of alternative consumer services for persons with mental illness. Evaluations of some of these enterprises are discussed in the section on research findings.

## Citizen and Family Advocacy Movements

In the US, many serious diseases and disabilities have long had organized constituencies of patients, families, and interested others who advocate for expanded research and services. The American Cancer Society, American Heart Organization, National Multiple Sclerosis Society, the Epilepsy Foundation, and the Alzheimer's Disease and Related Disorders Association are a few examples. Organizations devoted to developmental disabilities, such as the National Association for Retarded Citizens or the National Society for Autistic Children have advocated for state-of-the-art diagnostic and treatment procedures as well as appropriate education for children, enhanced rehabilitative resources, public information resources, and the like.

Until recent years, mental illness has been different from these other conditions in the composition of its advocacy groups. Encompassed within the framework of safeguarding human rights and the global promotion of mental health, advocacy for persons with severe psychiatric disorders was largely the province of concerned citizens rather than that of acknowledged stakeholders whose own lives are invested in treatment and cure. For many years, former patients and relatives who participated in these movements maintained a relatively low profile. Internalizing societal

| Table 111–1 | Approaches to Improving the Lives of Those Touched by Mental Illness |
|---|---|
| Advocacy | |
| Volunteerism | |
| Self-help groups | |
| Consumer services | |

(and often professional) stigma, they rarely acknowledged their own experiences in public advocacy efforts or in leadership roles. The history of mental health advocacy in the US has therefore had two major developmental stages: citizen organizations, and since the late 1970s, family and consumer organizations (Table 111–1).

## Citizen Advocacy Organizations
(See Table 111–2)

### National Mental Health Association
The National Mental Health Association (NMHA), with 340 affiliated mental health associations (MHAs), was the major advocacy group for persons with serious mental illness until the organization of the National Alliance for the Mentally Ill (NAMI) in 1979. Although it was founded by a former mental hospital patient, Clifford Beers, the NMHA in previous years had a limited emphasis on major mental illness, serving primarily as an education and referral resource for persons needing psychiatric help. The NMHA's mission has currently been aimed at improving mental health in the population at large, with a strong emphasis on primary prevention. Examples of activities by local branches include conferences on sexuality, police training to deal with interethnic conflict, support groups for at-risk groups such as newly widowed persons, and training volunteers to befriend troubled schoolchildren or work with victims of natural disasters.

In most areas, the local NMHA branch has been the major umbrella organization linking professionals with interested citizens, facilitating joint advocacy efforts, and providing mental health education for the public. Mental health professionals have been actively involved in governance boards of the lay organization, and there are friendly affiliative relationships with professional societies. In contrast to self-help groups, MHA support groups traditionally were led by volunteer professionals, and persons needing further help were urged to use the mental health system. Today many more MHA affiliates are offering space and resources for peer-led groups which function independ-

| Table 111–2 | Models of Advocacy |
|---|---|
| National Alliance for the Mentally Ill | |
| National Mental Health Association | |
| Bazelon Center | |
| State Protection and Advocacy Centers | |
| Consumer self-help and advocacy organizations | |
| Therapeutic support groups | |
| Political advocacy | |

ently of the host organization. NMHA has taken increasing interest in consumer groups and currently has a CMHS-funded Consumer Supporter Technical Assistance Center. The center works to strengthen consumer and consumer supporter networking partnerships at local and state levels.

In 1987, the Mental Health Information Center was developed as the National Mental Health Association Clearinghouse to answer personal inquiries and disseminate publications on mental illness and mental health topics. Despite their broad-based interests, MHA groups have always lobbied for legislation for persons with serious mental illness and developmental disabilities at both state and national levels. For many years they were the major citizen voice, working in tandem with professional societies and persons interested in mental health law and patients' rights.

## Bazelon Center

The Judge David L. Bazelon Center for Mental Health Law, formerly the Mental Health Law Project, was organized in 1972 to halt abuse and neglect in state mental hospitals and training schools for persons with mental and developmental disabilities, and to prevent exclusion of disabled children from public funded education. Its current agenda is much more comprehensive. In addition to its basic focus on protecting patients' civil liberties, the center provides legal resources to combat exclusionary zoning and rental policies; promote patients' access to health care, social services, and income support; reform state systems of care; and help generate a continuum of community services for persons with psychiatric and developmental disabilities. Working in the courts and in legislative and policy arenas, the Bazelon Center offers legal assistance to consumers, other advocacy groups, and policymakers.

## State Protection and Advocacy Centers

State Protection and Advocacy Centers (P&As) have assumed some of the Bazelon Center's functions. The P&As are federally mandated to protect disabled persons from neglect and abuse and to protect their rights in institutional and community settings. Initially passed by congress in 1986 and reauthorized in 1991 (PL102–173), the legislation is now known as the Protection and Advocacy for Individuals with Mental Illness Act, extending rights already afforded to persons with developmental disabilities. The law provides grants to existing P&As for the developmentally disabled. Much of their work involves grievance casework for individuals, although they also initiate lawsuits to upgrade institutional conditions. Many P&As also view their mission as reforming the service delivery system, which may include shifting resources from institutional to community vendors.

All 50 states, the District of Columbia, and five territories have federally funded programs under the Protection and Advocacy for Individuals with Mental Illness Act. State P&As are members of the National Association of Protection and Advocacy Systems.

## The Family Movement: The National Alliance for the Mentally Ill (NAMI)

The organization of NAMI has been termed one of the most important events in the history of US psychiatry (Kaplan and Sadock 1991). Indeed, former NIMH director Herbert Pardes has hailed the political influence of NAMI as "the single most positive event in the history of mental illness" (Flynn 1993, p. 8). For the first time the major psychiatric disorders had their own important national presence, a grassroots constituency of families with a profound commitment to improving services, research, and public awareness and to reducing the stigma of mental illness.

Although local family support groups had been organized in the 1960s, and at least one state family federation existed in 1971 (Shetler 1986), it was not until 1979 that 284 family members convened at the University of Wisconsin, Madison, to form the national organization NAMI. Since that time NAMI has grown exponentially into a powerful movement. In 2001, NAMI reported 210,000 members and over 1,200 affiliates in all 50 states as well as Puerto Rico and the Virgin Islands. Today, there is a well functioning NAMI office in Arlington, Virginia, disseminating information and lobbying for research and services at the national level, as well as state NAMI organizations that work for improved services in their individual states.

Like most organizations that are formed by stakeholders rather than interested outsiders, NAMI merges self-help and advocacy. Thus, the basic armature in all localities is mutual support groups and membership education about all aspects of major mental illnesses. Most groups have also engaged in public education; resource development; anti-stigma campaigns; and service on mental health planning, policy, and governance boards at local and national levels. Consumers and family members are trained to become effective lobbyists and advocates for patients. Professional educators within NAMI have developed models for training family education specialists. NAMI has also had an impact on clinical training. The NAMI Curriculum and Training Network focused on influencing mental health professionals to work with persons with severe mental illness and on ensuring state-of-the-art education in clinical training programs from preservice to continuing education levels. Several national conferences cosponsored by NAMI and NIMH brought together leading clinical educators, researchers, and practitioners with family member–mental health professionals for concept development and curriculum planning in the core professions (Lefley et al. 1989, Lefley and Johnson 1990, NIMH and Lefley 1990). A major phenomenon is the NAMI Family-to-Family program, developed by a psychologist–family member as a 12-week educational program on schizophrenia, bipolar disorder, and major depression (Burland 1998). The program is carefully structured to train family members as educators. They provide some of the content of evidence-based psychoeducational intervention, such as problem-solving and communication skills, as well as understanding the patient's experience. The program also teaches families how to cope with family burden, avoid overinvolvement, set limits, and see to their own needs and those of other family members. Family-to-Family is available in numerous states with state mental health authority sponsorship, and has been administered to more than 30,000 families. NAMI also has a program for consumers, Living with Schizophrenia, which teaches them how to better live with their disorders.

On the national level, the family constituency has been powerfully influential in raising research dollars for mental illness. NAMI has successfully lobbied for substantial increases in congressional appropriations for NIMH research on the major psychiatric disorders and helped launch the National Schizophrenia and Brain Research campaign. NAMI cofounded the National Alliance for Research on Schizophrenia and Depression (NARSAD) in 1985 and has generated millions of dollars in research awards through the Ted and Vida Stanley Foundation. Because of its strong commitment to basic research on brain diseases, NAMI was an influential force in the return of NIMH to the National Institutes of Health.

NAMI-sponsored publications have had a substantial influence on mental health services. These have included Care of the Seriously Mentally Ill: A Rating of State Programs (Torrey et al. 1990) and Criminalizing the Seriously Mentally Ill: The Abuse of Jails as Mental Hospitals (Torrey et al. 1992). In collaboration with the Center for Psychiatric Rehabilitation at Boston University, NAMI began publishing in 1990 the scholarly journal Innovations and Research with a focus on clinical services, community support, and rehabilitation for persons with severe and persistent mental illness. Innovations and the BU Center's previous Psychosocial Rehabilitation Journal have since been merged into the Psychiatric Rehabilitation Journal.

With a major stake in legislative advocacy at the federal level, NAMI was active in promoting passage of Public Law 99-660, which required all 50 states to develop a comprehensive mental health plan including provision of community care to persons with serious mental illness. The legislation for the first time required family and consumer participation on a state advisory council. Reauthorization language linked the approved state plans to the federal block grant, and local NAMI groups became active in monitoring their state's compliance with the plan's objectives. NAMI fought for the 1986 Protection and Advocacy for Individuals with Mental Illness legislation previously discussed, and the organization was a vocal advocate for the Americans with Disabilities Act. NAMI has been actively working for mental health parity legislation and for implementation of the Wisconsin PACT Program as evidence-based practice in all states (Bond et al. 2001) NAMI was also actively involved in the dissemination of the findings of the Schizophrenia Patient Outcomes Research Team (PORT), which recommended specific parameters for prescribed antipsychotic medications (Lehman and Steinwachs 1998). NAMI produced and distributed more than 50,000 brochures highlighting these recommendations (Frese et al. 2001). NAMI was also instrumental in helping develop the 1999 Expert Consensus Treatment Guidelines for Schizophrenia, and has widely disseminated the "Guide for Patients and Families" appended to the Guidelines (Weiden et al. 1999).

The NAMI Consumer Council is a group of primary consumers who function as a separate interest group within NAMI with a very substantial role in policy making. Frese (Frese et al. 2001) reports that during the past several years at least one quarter of the members of NAMI's board of directors have been consumers. One of the few NAMI presidents elected for two terms was a consumer. Members of the NAMI Consumer Council generally support the NAMI agenda, but many have overlapping affiliations and common interests with other consumer organizations.

## Mental Health Consumer Self-Help and Advocacy Organizations

Consumer self-help organizations generally merge mutual support with a focus on one of two basic objectives: political advocacy or personal problem resolution and growth. A study of 104 self-help groups of present and former psychiatric patients identified two major service models, which the author differentiated as social movement versus individual therapy. The social movement groups were oriented toward social change and offered public education, legal advocacy, information referral networking, and technical assistance to other consumers. The individual therapy groups offered more "inner-focused" individual change through mutual support meetings and various types of alternative therapies such as relaxation. The study found that almost two-thirds of the groups were social movement models (Emerick 1990).

A major consumer organization that combines both social movement and therapeutic functions, one that is most comparable to national organizations of persons suffering from major physical illnesses, is the National Depressive and Manic–Depressive Association (NDMDA), which consists of more than 400 chapters and has served more than 35,000 patients and families (White and Madara 2002). Chapters may have multiple area support groups. Like NAMI, the NDMDA views major affective disorders as biogenic, disseminates public education on the descriptions of biochemical nature of depressive illnesses, holds annual conferences with professional presentations, and tries to fight stigma and promote basic research with a variety of advocacy efforts.

## The Therapeutic Support Group Model

The following organizational were given by group leaders or are adapted from The Self-Help Source Book (White and Madara 2002). Just a few of the major national organizations for psychiatric patients can be mentioned, excluding groups that specifically focus on addictions.

- Schizophrenics Anonymous, founded in 1985, has more than 150 chapters nationwide. Organized and run by people with a schizophrenia-related disorder, Schizophrenics Anonymous offers fellowship, support, and information. Schizophrenics Anonymous focuses on recovery, using a 6-step program, along with medication and professional help.
- GROW is an international organization founded in Australia in 1957. They have more than 143 groups in the US, primarily located in Illinois, New Jersey, and Rhode Island. GROW has a 12-step program to provide skills for avoiding and recovering from a breakdown. They offer a caring and sharing community to attain emotional maturity, personal responsibility, and recovery from mental illness. Leadership and training are offered to new groups.
- Recovery Inc., founded in 1937, has 700 chapters nationally and offers "a self-help method of will training; a system of techniques for controlling temperamental behavior and changing attitudes toward nervous symptoms and fears" (White and Madara 2002).

- Emotions Anonymous, with 1,100 national chapters, is a "fellowship sharing experiences, hopes, and strengths with each other, using the 12-step program, in order to gain better emotional health" (White and Madara 2002). Other national self-help organizations of present or former patients are Obsessive–Compulsive Anonymous, Anxiety Disorders Association of America (national network), Agoraphobics in Motion, and many others (White and Madara 2002).

## The Political Advocacy Model

Among some former psychiatric patients, self-help in itself is often viewed as a political statement. Zinman and colleagues (1987) gave the essential characteristics of self-help groups as self-definition of needs, equal power of members, mutual respect, voluntary participation, autonomy, and responsivity to other special populations. The self-help mission is for optimal personal independence with the option of choosing interdependence with other consumers.

For many years, self-help was incorporated in organizations of former psychiatric patients with names such as the Insane Liberation Front (Portland, Oregon) or the Mental Patients Liberation Project (New York) and publications such as *The Madness Network News* (California). These groups of former psychiatric patients were angry at a system that they thought had abused and dehumanized them rather than helped them. They tended to have strong antipsychiatry views; they were vehemently opposed to electroconvulsive therapy and often to psychotropic medications as well. Many thought that the only valid help for persons who were "psychiatrically labeled" would come from peers who had experienced a similar history of psychiatric hospitalization. Many of the pioneers of the consumer movements developed and provided models for today's consumer-operated services (Chamberlin 1978).

Although contemporary consumer groups have a common agenda of self-determination, former psychiatric patients seem to be divided ideologically. A few still view mental illness as psychogenic or as a social construct rejecting biogenesis, but most seem to accept a stress-diathesis model and many describe themselves as having a brain disease or "a chemical imbalance" (Kersker 1994). Some consumers are totally opposed to any kind of forced treatment while others have stated that without it, they might not be alive today (Rogers 1994). Some members of the consumer movement think that hospitalization is harmful and would like to eliminate all hospital beds. However, their views are not supported empirically. In the California Well-Being Project (Campbell 1989), a survey of psychiatric clients designed and conducted by consumers and directed by a professional researcher-consumer, more than 50% of the respondents believed that their hospitalization had been helpful, 22% reported both positive and negative aspects, and only 20% found hospitalization harmful.

These different viewpoints were reflected in two major consumer advocacy organizations that are now no longer active at the national level. Their differences and influence, however, are evident at the nationwide Alternatives Conferences that are funded by the CMHS and bring together consumers of all persuasions on a regular basis. The more radical National Association of Psychiatric Survivors, a small but highly vocal consumer group, retained an essential protest orientation and took a formal position opposing any kind of involuntary treatment. It no longer has national meetings, but some members continue in leadership positions at national consumer conferences. The more moderate National Mental Health Consumers' Association (NMHCA) had taken no formal position on forced treatment, but its mission statement and organizing focus emphasized consumer empowerment and self-determination. They stated that recovery and healing, not social control, must be the goal and outcome of the mental health system (Frese et al. 2001). Members of NMHCA acknowledged the validity of mental illness and the need for treatment and most have been absorbed in the NAMI Consumer Council.

These organizations have largely been supplanted by networking at annual conferences, coalition building, and developing local consumer-run initiatives, with support from federal and state governments. By the year 2000, there were an estimated 3,000 consumer-run organizations working at the local, state, and national levels (Van Tosh and del Vecchio 2000). As of 2001, 30 states have an Office of Consumer Affairs and most have local consumer groups and drop-in centers. The CMHS funds three Consumer Technical Assistance Centers and two Consumer Supporter Technical Assistance Centers whose purpose is "to develop and implement activities that assist in the improvement of mental health service systems at the state and local levels" (SAMHSA 2001). One of these centers usually convenes the national Alternatives Conferences that bring together consumers from all over the country for organizational skill building and knowledge sharing. The National Mental Health Consumer Self-Help Clearinghouse (NMHCSHC) in Philadelphia, under the direction of Joseph Rogers, encourages the development of consumer self-help groups and provides information, materials, and referrals on fund-raising and program development. Organized in 1986, the NMHCSHC has worked to develop the infrastructure of consumer movements nationwide. They have helped build new local and state self-help groups by providing technical assistance (TA) and disseminating information, developing consumer networks and coalitions, and generally building the capacity of consumer groups. The National Empowerment Center (NEC) in Lawrence, Massachusetts, directed by psychiatrist-consumer Daniel Fisher, similarly supplies TA to self-help groups. NEC has specific departments that focus on resource development and training conferences, consumer-run organizations, managed care and coalition building, information and referral, media relations, and training professionals on the consumer viewpoint. In an innovative Disability Awareness Workshop, mental health professionals are required to wear headphones blaring negative "voices" and to assess the effects of stimulus bombardment and vocal interference as they take a mental status examination, attend a day treatment program, undergo psychological testing, and ask directions in the community.

Consumer Organization and Networking Technical Assistance Center (CONTAC) located in West Virginia, is the third consumer TA center funded by the CMHS. In collaboration with the other centers, CONTAC works nationwide to provide informational materials, on-site training and skill-building curricula, electronic and other communication capabilities, networking, and customized TA to build leadership and teach business management skills to local consumer groups.

In addition to the Consumer TA Centers, federal funding is received for two Consumer Supporter TA Centers. The National Mental Health Association has a grant to provide TA to consumer and consumer supporter organizations in areas such as education, advocacy, systems change, and coalition building. TA is provided in the form of research, training, information, and financial support. NAMI has the other Consumer Supporter grant. Their primary purpose is to help implement the evidence-based Wisconsin PACT program in service systems throughout the nation through knowledge dissemination, training, and on-site TA.

In research centers studying self-help and psychiatric rehabilitation at Boston University, University of Illinois at Chicago, University of California, Berkeley, and University of Michigan, Ann Arbor, consumers have been involved in all phases of research including design, instrument development, interviewing, and analysis. At the Missouri Institute of Mental Health, under the direction of Dr. Jean Campbell, a consumer, a 4-year, multisite, 20-million-dollar project is currently investigating the efficacy of consumer-operated services. Data already collected are presented in the section on research findings.

## Government Roles in Consumer Empowerment

A major element in helping the organization of both family and consumer movements is the Community Support Program (CSP) of the federal government. Initially under the NIMH and now part of CMHS, the CSP was organized in 1978 to deal with problems of deinstitutionalization. The federal program focused on developing in each locality a comprehensive continuum of care for deinstitutionalized patients that would include all needed resources for survival, treatment, rehabilitation, and hopefully, a satisfactory quality of life (Stroul 1989). Through targeted grants to state administrations, the CSP fostered public–academic linkages and funded research and demonstration grants for model programs, including case management, crisis services, services for homeless mentally ill persons, and other innovative community rehabilitative projects.

The CSP also had a heavy emphasis on aiding the development of state and local self-help and advocacy groups and facilitating dissemination of their ideas on a national basis. Through the years, the program promoted Learning Community Conferences to bring together researchers, service providers, family advocates, and primary consumers. More recently, CSP helped fund the annual Alternatives Conferences that bring together members of consumer organizations from all over the US to pursue a national agenda. The CSP has probably been the major catalyst in helping develop services in which former psychiatric patients are participants or primary providers.

Since its inception as a separate division of SAMHSA, the CSP's umbrella organization, CMHS has provided funding for many consumer activities over the years. In addition to providing scholarships and other support for the Alternatives Conferences, CMHS also provided scholarships for consumers with affective disorders to attend annual meetings of the Depressive and Manic–Depressive Association (DMDA). The CMHS has also worked with the DMDA to develop a training video for psychiatric residents called "Partners in Recovery" (Paolo del Vecchio 2001, personal communication).

The Consumer/Survivor Mental Health Research and Policy Work Group was established in 1992 with support from the Mental Health Statistics Improvement Program and the Survey and Analysis Branch of the CMHS. The purpose was "to modify the relationships and dialogue between mental health professionals/service providers/policy administrators and consumers/survivors including fostering significant roles for consumers/survivors in all phases of mental health research, data standards development, planning, policy, and implementation of mental health services" (Consumer/Survivor MHR 1993, p. 11). A major focus of this work group was on outcome measures used in the CMHS-funded services research. A concept-mapping project resulted in a publication by the National Association of State Mental Health Program Directors (NASMHPD) entitled *Mapping Mental Health Outcomes from the Perspective of Mental Health Consumers* (Trochim et al. 1993). This project generated recommendations to the mental health research community on outcome measures of greatest interest to consumers in a future research agenda. NASMHPD developed a position paper in December 1989 that specifically outlined the role of "ex-patients-consumers" in state mental health systems. "Their contribution should be valued and sought in areas of program development, policy formation, program evaluation, quality assurance, system design, education of mental health service providers, and the provision of direct services (as employees of the provider system)" (NASMHPD 1989).

A survey commissioned by NASMHPD in 1993 reported that 65.5% of state mental health agencies provided financial resources to consumer-run and family-run programs and that 19 states had consumer affairs offices (NASMHPD 1993). In 2001, 30 states had consumer affairs offices with the majority providing financial resources for drop-in centers and other consumer-run services (Paolo del Vecchio 2001, personal communication).

## Service Development by Family and Consumer Groups

For many years, NAMI groups in various localities developed resources to fill in gaps in their service delivery systems. Multiple housing facilities, employment opportunities ranging from thrift shops to furniture workshops, psychosocial rehabilitation programs, and even a psychiatric hospital are examples of resources developed throughout the US. However, despite continuing initiatives, many NAMI members believe that families should be investing their energies in legislative advocacy rather than in service development. NAMI's major mission is to augment and strengthen the service delivery system through encouraging the implementation of evidence-based practices, such as its current TA center grant to promote national adoption of the Wisconsin PACT program.

The consumer movements have had a different view of their role in services. Their focus is on using the experiences and skills of former psychiatric patients both within the system and as operators of consumer-run alternatives. Numerous CSP initiatives have been devoted to helping consumers achieve that end through funded model projects and inducements to the states. As of 2001 there are reportedly at least 3,000 consumer-run programs and enterprises. These include housing facilities, residential placement services, case management, peer companion programs, social centers, employment services including job training, and consumer businesses, crisis respite houses, substance abuse treatment programs, and special programs for the homeless. CSP-funded demonstration projects include a variety of consumer enterprises. In 30 states today, there is a Mental Health Consumer Affairs Office organized and staffed by one or more former psychiatric patients. Almost all states have networks of drop-in centers that provide socialization outlets outside of the traditional mental health system and sometimes fulfill an advocacy function as well. In many states, the sponsorship of consumer drop-in centers by state hospitals and community agencies is a common practice, typically with maximal independence offered to the consumer group.

## Research Findings on Consumer Self-Help

To date, most of the evaluations of therapeutic self-help groups tend to be qualitative or process research based. Some studies of efficacy are inferred from the members' satisfaction by use of normative data as a control condition. For example, a study of Recovery Inc. members, half of whom had been hospitalized for mental illness, focused on the benefits of membership to volunteer leaders of the organization. As a result of their participation, volunteer leaders gave high ratings to their overall satisfaction with life, health, work, leisure, and community. Their quality of life ratings were equivalent to the levels of satisfaction of a sample of the general public (Raiff 1982). A collaborative study of GROW by University of Illinois researchers compared members for 9 months or more with those who had been members 3 months or less. GROW members for the longer period were significantly better off in terms of larger social networks, a higher rate of employment, and lower levels of psychosis and depression (Rappaport et al. 1984). Another quantitative study looked at patients discharged from a state psychiatric hospital who participated in a Community Network Development self-help program. The research found that 10 months after discharge, participants required 50% less rehospitalization and two-thirds fewer inpatient days than a comparable group of nonparticipating patients. A significantly smaller percentage of Community Network Development ex-patients required community mental health center services than the comparison group (Gordon et al. 1982).

A study of four self-help groups for families of persons with mental illness showed high congruence between what participants wanted from the group and what they reported actually happened in the group experience. Moreover, a time series analysis showed that the perceived helpfulness of the program for families was significantly related to the patients' functioning in terms of fewer number of hospitalizations and fewer total days in hospital (Biegel and Yamatani 1986). The efficacy of the self-help sharing experience for family members has also received tangential empirical

| Table 111–3 | Positive Research Findings Related to Consumer Self-Help Groups |
|---|---|
| Larger social networks | Increased empathy |
| Higher rate of employment | Feel needed and responsible |
| Lower levels of symptoms | Improved consumer employment |
| Fewer rehospitalizations | Improved education |
| Fewer inpatient days | Increased independence |
| Less MHC services | Enhanced quality of life |
| Greater self-confidence | |

support from the work of McFarlane (1994) and associates on psychoeducational interventions. These researchers found that interventions with multiple family groups were significantly superior to individual family interventions in deterring patients' relapse, a finding attributed to the mutual support and information exchange of the group experience (Table 111–3).

Family members and consumers have been increasingly involved in grand rounds, as lecturers in clinical training programs, and in training service providers. A randomized evaluation of consumer versus nonconsumer training of state mental health service providers found positive reactions to the use of consumers as trainers (Cook et al. 1993).

A process evaluation of six consumer-run drop-in centers in Michigan found that the centers were meeting their programmatic goals to provide acceptance, social support, and problem-solving help. The study found high levels of consumer satisfaction together with the participants' reported feeling that they actually ran their centers (Mowbray et al. 1998). A 6-month survey of nine consumer-operated drop-in centers in Pennsylvania indicated a high level of client satisfaction (Kaufmann et al. 1993). In California, the use of former patients as peer counselors on locked inpatient wards received enthusiastic evaluations from clinical staff, with most staff asking that the program be extended. The peer counselors reported personal benefits in terms of greater self-confidence, increased empathy, and feelings of being needed and responsible (McGill and Patterson 1990). A study of a Rehabilitation Services Administration training program for consumer case manager and human service worker aides, comparing team and individual approaches with intensive case management for frequent users of psychiatric hospitals, found advantages in consumer employment (Bond et al. 1991). Family members participating in a randomized trial of consumer versus nonconsumer case management teams reported equal satisfaction with the capabilities of consumer case managers. Because many studies do not report on ethnicity, it is of interest that 86% of the respondents were African-Americans (Solomon and Draine 1994).

Mind-Empowered Inc. is an assertive case management-supported housing program in Oregon that is completely run by consumers. Operating successfully for several years, it received a county contract to bring 30 persons out of the state hospital and keep them in the community. Preliminary data indicated that during the first 6 months of the program's operation, only two clients returned to the hospital. However, the evaluators admit that additional objective outcome data are needed to assess the long-term impact of the program (Nikkel et al. 1992).

A major question relates to job stress and the stability of former psychiatric patients as mental health service providers. A project in Denver, Colorado, trained consumers as case management aides in a psychiatric rehabilitation program. Of 25 trainees, 18 completed the program and 17 were employed as case management aides. At 2-year follow-up, the 15 trainees who were still employed had required a total of only 2 bed-days of psychiatric hospitalization (Sherman and Porter 1991).

Currently there are two overviews of consumer-run services and CSP research demonstration projects based on consumer services. A comprehensive retrospective review of federally-funded consumer/survivor-operated service programs in 13 states concluded that "Consumer/survivor-operated services are successful in increasing the overall quality of life, independence, employment, social supports, and education of consumer/survivors" (Van Tosh and del Vecchio 2000). This study found, moreover, that 70% of the federally-funded initiatives were continued with other funding sources. The consumer recipients were objectively successful in capturing ongoing financial support, and subjectively they reported increased self-efficacy and self-esteem on standardized scales (Van Tosh and del Vecchio 2000). An overview of consumer programs by the International Association of Psychosocial Rehabilitation Services reported similar findings and stated that "Consumer service provision may be an essential feature of a support system devoted to recovery" (Mowbray et al. 1997).

Although consumers seem to be doing well on many of the evaluated programs, there are some negative or problematic findings as well. For example, research in Chicago compared trained consumer and nonconsumer staff on mobile outreach teams for persons manifesting psychotic behavior. The findings showed that contrary to the hypothesis, consumers were significantly more likely than nonconsumer staff to certify clients for involuntary hospitalization (Lyons et al. 1993). It is unknown whether consumers were less capable of handling psychotic behavior or whether they were more knowledgeable about the limitations of voluntary interventions. According to an evaluator for the CSP, consumer alternatives were never envisioned to serve as substitutes for mental health services; they were meant to empower consumers to gain some control over their lives. A qualitative analysis based on systematic observations of consumer-run services found that many consumer alternatives fell short of these empowering principles. Power conflicts and hierarchies developed in many programs. Consumers often tried unsuccessfully to replicate services provided by the local mental health clinic rather than to offer self-help alternatives (McLean 1994). This is an area of great interest that bears continued watching and evaluation.

## Relations of Professionals and Self-Help Groups

Many health and mental health professionals have welcomed the advent of the self-help movement. In a Workshop on Self-Help and Public Health held by the Surgeon General's Office of the Department of Health and Human Services, the major focus was on collaborative partnerships

| Table 111–4 | Strategies to Establish Collaborative Partnerships Between Professionals and Self-Help Groups |
| --- | --- |
| Welcome support groups<br>Endorse these groups as adjunctive to psychotherapy<br>Avoid setting groups up as competing systems of care<br>Use two-way referrals<br>Understand professionally led groups can inhibit the therapeutic process<br>Be cognizant of issues related to disempowerment, control, and need for self-determination | |

of professionals and self-help groups and a key recommendation that "exposure to the concepts and benefits of self-help should be included in the training curriculums of all helping professions" (The Surgeon General's Workshop 1988). The APA's Task Force on Treatments of Psychiatric Disorders views self-help groups as part of the therapeutic armamentarium (Table 111–4). In their four-volume publication on treatment, Borman (1989) noted that self-help groups redefine pathological states, provide a shift in human service paradigms, promote and maintain competence, and reinforce positive mental health.

An increasing number of community mental health centers and rehabilitation facilities are welcoming support groups of patients and families, offering organizational help and free staff facilitators. Most professionally run substance abuse programs include participation in Alcoholics Anonymous or Narcotics Anonymous as a component of treatment. Numerous newsletters for professionals and administrators endorse mutual aid groups as an adjunct to psychotherapy and give substantial information on self-help resources (Mental Health Weekly 1992).

It is obvious that under certain conditions, self-help groups may compose a parallel and sometimes competing system of care. Although many members may simultaneously use clinical services, some joined self-help groups because of dissatisfaction with professional medical or mental health treatment. Some self-help groups reduce the demand for clinical services because they offer alternatives and are hostile to professional interventions. Other groups, however, may raise awareness of deeper problems and provide referrals to preferred psychiatrists. Referrals work both ways and typically are mutually beneficial. Self-help group members learn about recommended professionals from their peers. Psychiatrists treating persons with a chronic mental illness are usually happy to learn about a local drop-in center to which they can refer their socially isolated patients.

Consumers who participate in self-help groups seem to be comfortable using dual systems of care. Of great interest is a 1996 BU study of six consumer-run self-help programs in various parts of the US. This research found that 50% of the self-help members were currently taking antipsychotic medication and that most also utilized professional mental health services such as counseling, day treatment, and inpatient care (Chamberlin et al. 1996). Drop-in centers whose members come from the mental health system generally require that participants be under psychiatric care. Most self-help groups with seriously disabled members agree since they cannot deal with decompensation or other issues requiring clinical expertise.

Research suggests that self-help groups function best on their own without professional help in running the group. Emerick's (1990) study of 104 self-help groups of psychiatric patients found that more than 70% reported little to no interaction with professionals. As previously indicated, only a third of these groups were considered to have a therapeutic orientation, and as might be expected, these were more amenable to professional alliances. A study of professional involvement with members of GROW, one of the therapeutic orientation models, compared social climate data and behavioral data among members of groups led by either a mental health professional ($n=36$) or an indigenous group member ($n=70$). The study found no difference in members' outcomes but significant differences in perceptions and behaviors. Members of groups led by professionals showed fewer agreements and self-disclosures, had less small talk and information giving, and rated their groups lower in cohesion and higher in leader control than did members of groups with indigenous leaders. The authors surmised that the professionals' more formal approach may have discouraged behaviors that they thought were less psychologically relevant and cautioned against professionalizing mutual help groups (Toro et al. 1998).

The picture is different on an individual basis, however. First-person accounts of consumers indicate numerous favorable recollections of their interactions with professionals (Hatfield and Lefley 1993). Many attribute the turning point of their recovery to a specific psychotherapist or to a rehabilitation specialist who helped them. Nevertheless, a number of former patients still tend to view negatively their overall experiences with the mental health system itself (Campbell 1989, Hatfield and Lefley 1993). In these cases, their negativity is typically related to feelings of disempowerment, external control, and loss of options for self-determination. It remains to be seen whether the new emphasis on consumer empowerment and peer-run services will have the desired therapeutic countereffect.

## Conclusion

The growth of the family and consumer movements has had a revolutionary impact not only on service delivery systems and funding resources but also on knowledge and practice (Table 111–5). Like the National Society for Autistic Children before it, NAMI has helped change professionals' attitudes toward families in numerous ways. By eliciting public statements and support from world-class researchers and authorities (Kaplan and Sadock 1991, Flynn 1993), and disseminating their information on the neurobiological substrates of major psychiatric disorders, NAMI has reinforced the changing ideas about familial roles in etiology among psychiatrists and other mental health professionals as well as the general public. The family movement has influenced clinical training curricula to provide state-of-the-art education (Lefley and Johnson 1990, NIMH and Lefley 1990), helped attain increased funding for basic research, and through advertising, television, and other media events, accelerated the slow historical process of destigmatizing mental illness.

The advent of a powerful grassroots constituency has generated pronounced respect on the part of professional

| Table 111–5 | Summary of Advocacy Organizations | | | |
|---|---|---|---|---|
| Organizations | Primary Membership* | Description | Primary goals | Functions |
| **National Multichapter Multifunction Organizations** | | | | |
| National Mental Health Association | Citizens | Broad-based organization, prevention-focused concerns with mental health<br>Citizen-run lay organization with considerable involvement of volunteer mental health professionals in membership and governance | Raising mental health levels of general population<br>Helping persons with mental illnesses<br>Improving services, Decreasing stigma<br>Public education<br>Multiple legislative goals | Legislative advocacy<br>Public education<br>Antistigma campaigns<br>Special-interest support groups for various mental health–related problems<br>Monitoring services (blue-ribbon juries)<br>Community outreach; work in schools, jails |
| National Alliance for the Mentally Ill | Family members, consumers (present and former psychiatric patients) | Specifically concerned with serious mental illnesses (SMI)<br>Primarily run by families and consumers, but welcomes professional membership and organizational cosponsorship | Promoting research<br>Multiple legislative goals<br>Family education/support<br>Improving/monitoring services<br>Decreasing stigma<br>Public education<br>Fostering state-of-the-art clinical training, education | Legislative advocacy<br>Support/self-help groups<br>Resource development<br>Public, family, and provider education on SMI<br>Planning, monitoring, and evaluating services<br>Media antistigma initiatives |

*Continues*

| Table 111–5 | Summary of Advocacy Organizations *Continued* | | | |
|---|---|---|---|---|
| Organizations | Primary Membership* | Description | Primary goals | Functions |
| Federation of Families for Children's Mental Health | Parents of emotionally disturbed (SED) children | Primarily run by families, welcomes professionals | Improved services for children, education, protection, advocacy, entitlements for SED children and youth, family involvement in treatment | Advocacy, lobbying, public/family education, roles in improving educational system/ services |
| National Depressive and Manic–Depressive Association | Consumers (present and former psychiatric patients) | National organization of persons suffering from affective disorders, friends and relatives. Consumer-run but welcomes professional help and cosponsorship | Promoting mutual support research, services, and stigma reduction for major affective disorders primarily unipolar depression and bipolar disorder | Support groups and education for members. Advocacy for research and service funding. Public education. Antistigma campaigns |
| **National or Local Organizations with Specific Focus** | | | | |
| Judge David L. Bazelon Center for Mental Health Law. National Association of Protection and Advocacy Systems | Attorneys, citizens, stakeholders | Organizations specifically focused on protection of rights (typically expressed choice) and preventing abuses of persons with mental illness. Involvement of mental health professionals encouraged but tends to be limited | Guarding civil liberties of persons with mental illness. Legally ensuring access to needed services and resources | Monitoring. Education. Advocacy and Lawsuits on behalf of individuals. Class-action suits |
| Schizophrenics Anonymous Recovery Inc. GROW | Present and former psychiatric patients | Nonpolitical consumer self-help. No or highly restricted professional involvement | Illness management. Self-knowledge. Personal growth. Education | Meetings and support groups |
| National Mental Health Consumer Self-Help Clearinghouse. National Empowerment Center | Ex-patients, consumers, survivors | Consumer political advocacy and self-help. No or highly restricted professional involvement (National Empowerment Center is run by professionals who are also consumers) | Consumer empowerment. Consumer participation in service delivery and mental health systems planning. Mutual support. Organizational skill-development | Meetings. Information dissemination. Training consumer-run services. Political advocacy |

*Identification terms for consumer groups are based on organizational usage.

leaders and policymakers and an eagerness for political alliances. There has been consistent personal participation of APA presidents and NIMH directors at all annual NAMI conferences. Many state psychiatric associations have urged their members to join NAMI as associate members. Clinical training programs have sometimes required their students to attend local NAMI meetings as part of their training, and some psychiatric residents have regularly attended as resource persons for NAMI family support groups (Lefley 1988).

Family members and consumers are increasingly involved on governance and advisory boards of service providers and on state mental health planning councils. In various departments of psychiatry, family members and consumers have lectured, given grand rounds, or made presentations at professional association meetings. They have also been encouraged to enter professional training programs through various NIMH training initiatives.

The growth of the consumer movement has dramatically highlighted the heterogeneity of psychiatric patients. An unexpectedly high level of organizational skill and leadership is evident among many people with histories of psychiatric hospitalizations and diagnoses of major disorders. In mental health service delivery, some former psychiatric patients are apparently able to fulfill paraprofessional staff functions ranging from crisis intervention to case management, with the added therapeutic advantage of offering role models and experiential empathy to the patients receiving their services.

The consumer movement itself has helped develop a wide range of skills and knowledge that are invaluable for psychiatric rehabilitation. These include writing, technical assistance, education in communications media, information dissemination, and decision-making skills. The political advocacy process has brought empowerment, respect, and influence on important leadership figures to individuals who believe that their residual psychological deficits were related to powerlessness, marginality, and internalized stigmas (Campbell 1989). The job of helping one's peers brings rewards of competence, altruism, and efficacy (Van Tosh and del Vecchio 2000, Mowbray et al. 1997). All of these would appear to be important factors in therapeutic growth.

On a policy level, the primary consumer movement has had an impact both on state services and on rehabilitation ideology. The director of Boston University's Center for Psychiatric Rehabilitation confirmed this influence by viewing recovery from mental illness as "the guiding vision of the mental health service system in the 1990s" (Anthony 1993). In this vision, recovery is viewed as a subjective attitude change that enables one to live a life of meaning and purpose, even with the limitations imposed by mental illness. A consumer leader, director of a state network of drop-in centers, credited his psychiatrist with enabling him to fulfill the advocacy role that has shaped his recovery. He defined recovery as follows:

> Recovery is not remission, nor is it a return to a preexisting state.... Recovery is the development of new ego and identity structures to replace those damaged by our illnesses.... Recovery takes place through creation of new patterns of behavior that make our lives more satisfying and productive. People in recovery like themselves as they are, accept their disability, and enjoy the life they have. Acceptance of one's disability can lead to greater appreciation of one's own strengths and new levels of self-esteem
> (Kersker 1994, p. 337)

Involvement in self-help and advocacy efforts seems to have additive therapeutic benefits, particularly for individuals adhering to a careful treatment regimen. These new developments are heuristic and warrant continuing research on the mechanisms of growth and paradigms of successful outcome in mental illness.

A group of consumer-professionals, writing in *Psychiatric Services* (Frese et al. 2001), have distinguished between categories of consumers with respect to the recovery vision. These authors note that advocacy for evidence-based practices, such as that offered by NAMI, is essential for the most seriously disabled consumers. Advocates who focus on consumer empowerment are those who are further along the road to recovery. These consumers merit increasing autonomy and input into the types of treatment and services they receive. The authors propose an integrative theory that maximizes the virtues and minimizes the weaknesses of each model. They also suggest that graduate and professional schools should be encouraged to recruit consumers in recovery for their training programs. This way the programs will benefit from consumers' experiential input and provide a scientific background for consumers to become knowledgeable mental health providers.

Consumerism is attractive to state and federal mental health authorities. This is demonstrated in the documents of the National Association of State Mental Health Program Directors (NASMHPD 1989, Trochim et al. 1993), the allocations of funds by state program directors to support consumer-operated services, and the funding investments of the federal CMHS in developing the consumer movement. Nevertheless, there is a relatively small pool of qualified former patients who are capable of assuming meaningful roles in mental health agencies or in the development of alternative services. Consumer-operated programs for long-term patients are still a minor variable in the mental health service delivery systems of most states. These systems will clearly continue to require professionalism and particularly a psychiatric capability for all the foreseeable future. This need is acknowledged by the majority of patients and families. A consumer member of the NAMI board of directors described receiving almost 500 letters from consumers sharing their positive experiences with new medications and basing their hopes on continuing biological research (Beall 1994).

In an era of health care reform, an alliance of NAMI, interested consumer groups, and professionals are essential for adequate coverage for mental health services. At the 1994 annual meeting of the National Association of Psychiatric Health Systems, the *Psychiatric News* reported the following message from former APA president Paul Fink:

> Not too many years ago, patient advocacy was an unknown for most therapists or one they chose to ignore.... Now nobody "in their right mind" would make major policy decisions or testify before governmental bodies without including patients or their advocates in the process.
> (Alliances... 1994)

## Acknowledgment

The author wishes to thank Paolo del Vecchio, Acting Director of CMHS Office of External Liaison, for information on the consumer movement and current CMHS initiatives.

## References

Alliances with advocacy groups urged as psychiatrists try to shape health care reform (1994). Psychiatr News 1994; 29(5), 8.

Anthony WA (1993) Recovery from mental illness: The guiding vision of the mental health service system in the 1990s. Innov Res 2(3), 17–24.

Beall MA (1994) Just between us. NAMI Advocate 16(1), 15.

Biegel DE and Yamatani H (1986) Self-help groups for families of the mentally ill: Research perspectives. In Family Involvement in the Treatment of Schizophrenia, Goldstein (ed). American Psychiatric Press, Washington DC, pp. 57–80.

Bond G, Pensec M, Dietzen L, et al. (1991) Intensive case management for frequent users of psychiatric hospitals in a large city: A comparison of team and individual caseloads. Psychosoc Rehabil 15, 90–98.

Bond GR, Drake RE, Mueser KT, et al. (2001) Assertive community treatment for people with severe mental illness: Critical ingredients and impact on patients. Dis Manag Health Outcomes 9, 141–159.

Borman LD (1989) Self-help and mutual aid groups for adults. In American Psychiatric Association Task Force on Treatments of Psychiatric Disorders: A Task Force Report of the American Psychiatric

Association, Vol. 3. American Psychiatric Association, Washington DC, pp. 2596–2607.

Burland J (1998) Family-to-Family. A trauma and recovery model of family education. New Dir Ment Health Serv 77, 33–41.

Campbell J (ed) (1989) The well-being project: Mental health clients speak for themselves. In Pursuit of Wellness, Vol. 6. California Department of Mental Health, The California Network of Mental Health Clients, Sacramento, CA.

Chamberlin J (1978) On Our Own: Patient Controlled Alternatives to the Mental Health System. Hawthorn Books, New York.

Chamberlin J, Rogers ES, and Ellison ML (1996) Self-help programs: A descriptions of their characteristics and members. Psychosoc Rehabil J 19, 33–42.

Consumer/Survivor Mental Health Research and Policy Work Group (1993) Comm Supp Network News 9(4), p. 11.

Cook JA, Jonikas JA, and Razzano L (1993) A randomized evaluation of consumer versus nonconsumer training of state mental health service providers. National Research and Training Center on Rehabilitation and Mental Illness, Thresholds, Chicago.

Deegan P (1994) A letter to my friend who is giving up. J Calif Alliance Ment Ill 5(3), 18–20.

Emerick RR (1990) Self-help groups for former patients: Relations with mental health professionals. Hosp Comm Psychiatr 41, 401–407.

Flynn LM (1993) Political impact of the family-consumer movement. Natl Forum 73, 8–12.

Frese FJ (1998) Advocacy, recovery, and the challenges for consumerism for schizophrenia. Psych Clin N Am 21, 233–249.

Frese FJ, Stanley J, Kress K, et al. (2001) Integrating evidence-based practices and the recovery model. Psych Serv 52, 1462–1468.

Gartner A and Riessman F (1984) The Self-Help Revolution. Human Sciences Press, New York.

Gordon RE, Edmunson E, and Bedell J (1982) Reducing hospitalization of state mental patients: Peer management and support. In Community Mental Health, Jeger S and Slotnick A (eds). Plenum Press, New York.

Greenblatt M (1985) Volunteerism and the community mental health worker. In Comprehensive Textbook of Psychiatry, Vol. 4, Kaplan HI and Sadock BJ (eds). Williams & Wilkins, Baltimore, pp. 1893–1897.

Hatfield AB and Lefley HP (1993) Surviving Mental Illness: Stress, Coping, and Adaptation. Guilford Press, New York.

Kaplan HI and Sadock BJ (1991) Synopsis of Psychiatry, 6th ed. Rev. Williams & Wilkins, Baltimore.

Kaufmann CL, Ward-Colasante C, and Farmer 1 (1993) Development and evaluation of drop-in centers operated by mental health consumers. Hosp Comm Psychiatr 44, 675–678.

Kersker S (1994) The consumer perspective on family involvement. In Helping Families Cope with Mental Illness, Lefley HP and Wasow M (eds). Harwood Academic Publishers, Newark, NJ, pp. 331–341.

Lefley HP (1988) Training professionals to work with families of chronic patients. Comm Ment Health J 24, 338–357.

Lefley HP, Bernheim KF, and Goldman CR (1989) National forum on training clinicians to work with seriously mentally ill persons and their families. Hosp Comm Psychiatr 40, 460–462.

Lefley HR and Johnson DL (eds) (1990) Families as Allies in Treatment of the Mentally Ill: New Directions for Mental Health Professionals. American Psychiatric Press, Washington DC.

Lehman AF and Steinwachs DM (1998) Translating research into practice: The Schizophrenia Patient Outcomes Research Team (PORT) treatment recommendations. Schizophr Bull 24, 1–10.

Lieberman MA (1990) A group therapist perspective on self-help groups. Int J Group Psychother 40, 251–278.

Lyons JS, Cook J, Ruth A, et al. (1993) Consumer service delivery in a mobile crisis assessment program. National Research and Training Center on Rehabilitation and Mental Illness, Thresholds, Chicago.

McFarlane WR (1994) Families, patients, and clinicians as partners: Clinical strategies and research outcomes in single and multiple-family interventions. In Helping Families Cope with Mental Illness, Lefley HP and Wasow M (eds), Harwood Academic Publishers, Newark, NJ, pp. 195–222.

McGill CW and Patterson U (1990) Former patients as peer counselors on locked psychiatric inpatient units. Hosp Comm Psychiatr 41, 1017–1019.

McLean A (1994) Institutionalizing the ex-patient movement in the United States: Advantages and costs. Paper presented at the conference on Understanding of Mental Illness and Dealing with the Mentally Ill in Western Cultures (June 2–4). University of Free Berlin, Berlin, Germany.

Mental Health Weekly (1992 Sept 14).

Mizuno M and Murakami M (2001) Strategic differences in implementing community-based psychiatry with families in Japan. In Family Interventions in Mental Illness: International Perspectives, Lefley HP and Johnson DL(eds). Praeger, Westport, CT.

Mowbray CT, Chamberlain P, Jennings M, et al. (1998) Consumer-run mental health services: Results from five demonstration projects. Comm Ment Health 24, 151–156.

Mowbray CT, Moxley D, Jasper CA, et al. (1997) Consumers as providers in psychiatric rehabilitation. International Association of Pychosocial Rehabilitation Services.

National Association of State Mental Health Program Directors (1989) NASMHPD Position Paper on Consumer Contributions to Mental Health Service Delivery Systems (Dec 13). Alexandria, VA.

National Association of State Mental Health Program Directors (1993) NASMHPD Studies Survey (Mar 22). Alexandria, VA, pp. 92–720.

National Institute of Mental Health and Lefley HP (ed) (1990) Clinical Training in Serious Mental Illness. Superintendent of Documents, US Government Printing Office, US Department of Health and Human Services publication (ADM), Washington DC, pp. 90–1679.

Nikkel RE, Smith G, and Edwards D (1992) A consumer-operated case-management project. Hosp Comm Psychiatr 43, 577–579.

Raiff NR (1982) Self-help participation and quality of life: A study of the staff of Recovery, Inc. Prev Human Serv 1, 1–2.

Rappaport J, Seidman E, Toro PA, et al. (1984) Finishing the unfinished business: Collaborative research with a mutual help organization. Soc Policy 15, 12–24.

Rogers S (1994) A Consumer's Perspective on Involuntary Interventions. Presentation at the National Symposium on Involuntary Interventions. University of Texas, Houston Health Science Center, Houston, TX.

Sherman PS and Porter R (1991) Mental health consumers as case management aides. Hosp Comm Psychiatr 42, 494–498.

Shetler H (1986) A History of the National Alliance for the Mentally Ill. National Alliance for the Mentally Ill, Arlington, VA.

Solomon P and Draine I (1994) Family perceptions of consumers as case managers. Comm Ment Health 30, 165–176.

Stroul B (1989) Community support systems for persons with long-term mental illness: A conceptual framework. Psychosoc Rehabil J 12, 9–26.

Substance Abuse and Mental Health Services Administration (2001) Center for Mental Health Services. Guidance for Applicants (GFA) No. SM-01–003. Competitive Renewal for Grants to Support Consumer and Consumer Supporter Technical Assistance Centers (Mar), p. 9.

The Surgeon General's Workshop on Self-Help and Public Health (1987) US Department of Health and Human Services publication 224-250-88-1. (1988) Superintendent of Documents, US Government Printing Office, Washington DC, p. 32.

Toro PA, Zimmerman MA, Seidman E, et al. (1998) Professionals in mutual help groups: Impact on social climate and members' behavior. J Consult Clin Psychol 56, 631–632.

Torrey EF, Wolfe SM, and Flynn LM (1990) Care of the Seriously Mentally Ill: A Rating of State Programs, 3rd ed. Public Citizens Health Research Group and National Alliance for the Mentally Ill, Arlington, VA.

Torrey EF, Wolfe SM, and Flynn LM (1992) Criminalizing the Seriously Mentally Ill: The Abuse of Jails as Mental Hospitals. Public Citizens Health Research Group and National Alliance for the Mentally Ill, Arlington, VA.

Trochim W, Dumont J, and Campbell J (1993) Mapping Mental Health Outcomes from the Perspective of Consumers/Survivors. National Association of State Mental Health Program Directors, Alexandria, VA.

Van Tosh L and del Vecchio P (2000) Consumer-operated self-help programs: A technical report. Center for Mental Health Services, Rockville, MD.

Weiden PJ, Scheifler PL, McEvoy JP, et al. (1999) Expert consensus treatment guidelines for schizophrenia: A guide for patients and families. J Clin Psychiatr 60(Suppl 11), 73–80.

White BJ and Madara EJ(eds) (2002). The Self-Help Group Source Book: Your Guide to Community and Online Support Groups, 7th ed. American Self-Help Clearinghouse, Denville, NJ.

Zinman S, Harp H, and Budd S (eds) (1987) Reaching Across: Mental Health Clients Helping Each Other. California Network of Mental Health Clients, Riverside, CA.

# 112 ● Law, Ethics, and Psychiatry

Ken Duckworth
Lester Blumberg
David Bienenfeld
Michael Kahn
Marshall Kapp

## Introduction

Psychiatrists' efforts to be helpful to their patients are driven by the desire to act in the "right" or ethical way. They also work within the context of the legal system which will often impact the way in which they provide care. While psychiatrists do not need to become experts in the practice of law or in the study of ethics, they should have an appreciation of how clinical work intersects with the law and the ethical foundations upon which their own decisions are made.

Ethics and law are closely related. Ideally, the law incorporates society's ethical consensus on complex issues. At the same time, ethical consideration of specific questions is often influenced and constrained by parameters that the law has constructed around a subject. Yet law and ethics are not synonymous (Ellis 1991). Whereas the law embodies a set of enforceable rules of conduct created by elected legislatures, executive administrative agencies, and the courts, ethics involves normative principles and processes guiding decisions and actions about what ought to happen.

Although the interface between law and the mental health system has grown in scope and complexity, there has also been a trend for legal bodies to defer in more and more instances to professional expertise about psychiatric issues, rather than to second-guess treatment professionals (Colp 1989). This places an even greater burden on psychiatrists to understand basic legal and ethical principles, the professional norms established by the field, and to appreciate their own sources of decision making for and with their patients.

This chapter will begin by surveying the principles underlying the legal system, highlighting some of the landmark cases that impact our work as psychiatrists, and illustrating common clinical sources of interest and relevance to clinical practice. The chapter will conclude by reviewing the sources of psychiatric ethics, outlining the consensus principles of psychiatric ethics, and illustrating some important clinical areas which generate issues of ethical concern.

## Overview of Legal Principles

As mentioned previously, psychiatrists do not need to become attorneys or to become familiar with all of the complexities of the legal system. They should, however, understand how their clinical practices interface with the legal system and familiarize themselves with some of the landmark cases that affect their day-to-day practice as psychiatrists. Psychiatrists and lawyers have different orientations: the Anglo-American system of jurisprudence is rooted in the adversarial model, whereas the practice of psychiatry is more commonly an alliance-based process. Although psychiatrists may play an active role in some cases, the American system of law is not fundamentally rooted in psychology.

The development of legal principles is the result of the interplay of legislatures that enact laws, executive branches that enforce them, and courts that interpret them. The first level of courts are trial courts, where cases are tried and decided. Appeals courts generally hear arguments by parties who feel that lower courts have made errors of law which require reversal of the lower court decision. The federal and most state court systems have two levels of appeals courts (an Appeals Court and a Supreme Court, although terminology varies among jurisdictions). The highest court in the land is the US Supreme Court, which is the final arbiter of questions of Federal and Constitutional Law.

Cases decided in state courts set the law only for the state in which the case is decided. Although state decisions may ultimately influence one another, no state is required to abide by the precedent of a different state's courts. For instance, the Tarasoff case discussed below set standards in California for a mental health professional's duty to protect a third party from the danger posed by a client. Although that case only applied to practice in California, it has had a great influence on legal and clinical practice in other states. Similarly, federal Appeals Courts set precedent only for the Circuits in which they sit. Only when the US Supreme Court has ruled on a matter of law are all other state and federal courts required to follow the precedent.

| Table 112–1 | US Constitutional Amendments Relevant to the Practice of Psychiatry |
|---|---|

### First Amendment

Congress shall make no law respecting an establishment of religion, or prohibiting the free exercise thereof; or abridging the freedom of speech, or of the press; or the right of the people to peaceable assemble, and to petition the Government for a redress of Grievances.

### Fourth Amendment

The right of the people to be secure in their persons, houses, papers and effects. Against unreasonable searches and seizures, shall not be violated, and no Warrants shall issue, but upon probable cause, supported by Oath or affirmation, and particularly describing the place to be searched, and the persons or things to be seized.

### Fifth Amendment

No person shall be held to answer for a capital, or otherwise infamous crime, unless on a presentment or indictment of a Grand Jury. Except in cases arising in the land or naval forces, or in the Militia, when in actual service in time of War or public danger; nor shall any person be subject for the same offence to be twice put in jeopardy of life or limb; nor shall be compelled in any criminal case to be a witness against himself, nor be deprived of life, liberty, or property, without due process of law; nor shall private property be taken for public use, without just compensation.

### Sixth Amendment

In all criminal prosecutions, the accused shall enjoy the right to a speedy and public trial, by an impartial jury of the State and district wherein the crime shall have been committed, which district shall have been previously ascertained by law, and to be informed of the nature and cause of the accusation; to be confronted with the witnesses against him: to have compulsory process for obtaining witnesses in his favor, and to have the Assistance of Counsel for his defense.

### Eighth Amendment

Excessive bail shall not be required, nor excessive fines imposed, nor cruel and unusual punishments inflicted.

### Fourteenth Amendment

Section 1. All persons born or naturalized in the United States, and subject to the jurisdiction thereof, are citizens of the United States and of the State wherein they reside. No State shall make or enforce any law which shall abridge the privileges or immunities of citizens of the United States, or shall any state deprive any person of life, liberty, or property, without due process of law; nor deny to any person within its jurisdiction the equal protection of the laws.

Each state also has a constitution that may be more protective of individuals' rights or more limiting of the states' power than the federal constitution. State courts can make decisions interpreting their own constitutions or the federal constitution. While federal Appeals Courts and ultimately the US Supreme Court can overrule a state court's interpretation of the federal constitution, the state supreme court has the final word on the state's constitution, so long as the state constitution does not violate the federal constitution. (For instance, a state constitution may provide greater protection against police searches than the federal constitution, but not less.)

When reading court opinions, it is important to recognize the different parts of a decision. One judge usually writes the majority decision or opinion. This announces the decision of the court, and sets whatever precedent the case involves. Other judges might write concurring opinions, in which they may agree with the outcome of the case, but not with the reasoning of the majority. Concurring opinions are important, because their votes count towards the outcome, but they do not contain holdings that become precedent. Finally, other judges might write dissenting opinions, in which they explain why they do not agree with the outcome of the case. Dissenting opinions do not carry the weight of law, but they sometimes point out flaws or limitations in the majority decision that might convince a later court to decide a similar issue differently.

The specific legal rights and principles with which we will concern ourselves are found in the amendments to the US Constitution. Of particular interest to psychiatry are the following constitutional amendments: the First Amendment, which embodies the right to freedom of speech and religion; the Third and Fourth Amendments, which have been interpreted as implying a right to privacy; the Fifth Amendment, which grants the right to remain silent in a criminal case; the Sixth Amendment, which discusses the rights of defendants to fair and speedy trials; the Eighth Amendment, which proscribes cruel and unusual punishment; and the Fourteenth Amendment, which embodies the "due process" and "equal protection of the law" clauses (Table 112–1).

Finally, the law has different standards of proof that the party who has the burden of proof must meet in order to prevail. The more vital the constitutional interest involved, the higher the standard of proof. Thus, since liberty interests are at risk in a criminal matter, the government must prove its case "beyond a reasonable doubt" in order for the jury or judge to find a defendant guilty. Cases involving lesser constitutional rights, such as the right of a parent to custody of his or her child, require a high burden, but not proof beyond a reasonable doubt. Such cases often require "clear and convincing evidence." The quantum of proof required for this standard is significantly more than a mere probability (51%), but does not reach beyond a reasonable doubt. Since civil commitment cases involve an individual's liberty, it has been held that the US Constitution demands at least clear and convincing evidence for such cases, though same states require proof beyond a reasonable doubt. Ordinary civil cases, such as contracts, and torts (including medical malpractice), require only that the case be proved by a preponderance of the evidence; that is, the fact to be proved is more likely than not true (Table 112–2).

| Table 112–2 | |
|---|---|
| Standards for Burden of Proof | Level of Certainty |
| Beyond a reasonable doubt (Criminal cases) | Proof to a moral certainty |
| Clear and convincing evidence (Important constitutional interests) | Substantially more than 50% |
| Preponderance of the evidence (Ordinary civil cases) | More likely than not; more than 50% |

## Rights and Responsibilities

### Right to Treatment

Although the US Supreme Court has expounded no national, constitutionally based right to treatment, there has been a substantial amount of activity in this area since Birnbaum published "The Right to Treatment" in 1960. At the time the article was published, it was common for psychiatric patients to spend decades in hospitals, at times involuntarily, while receiving little treatment or only custodial care. The article attempted to upgrade the quality of care in hospitals by creating a hospitalization-treatment quid pro quo. Birnbaum (1965) later criticized state hospital conditions, declaring that "Personally, I should like to state that as a doctor I often find it repugnant to use the term 'patient' to describe persons in certain mental hospitals." He instead argued that "inmate" was a better term if no treatment were given. Birnbaum's landmark articles generated interest in this key area of mental health policy.

Birnbaum's quid pro quo rationale was endorsed in *Rouse v. Cameron* (1966) decided by Judge Bazelon of the District of Columbia Circuit Court. Rouse was found not guilty by reason of insanity on a misdemeanor charge and was thereafter civilly committed to St. Elizabeth's Hospital. He petitioned for his release based on the argument that he was not receiving treatment. Judge Bazelon ruled that hospitals must make real efforts to improve patients' conditions and that lack of resources was not an adequate defense. In his decision he wrote, "The hospital need not show that the treatment will cure or improve him but only that there is a bona fide effort to do so."

The case of *Wyatt v. Stickney* (1972), a class action suit against an Alabama hospital with poor conditions for patients, led to definitions of humane environment, which have been incorporated into a patient's bill of rights in many states. Chief Judge Johnson wrote for the US District Court, "[Involuntarily committed patients] unquestionably have a constitutional right to receive such individual treatment as will give each of them a realistic opportunity to be cured or to improve his or her mental condition." Although this case was not heard by the US Supreme Court, it did have far-reaching social consequences for institutions in that it prompted scrutiny of the services they provide.

In 1975, in the case of *O'Connor v. Donaldson* (1975), Supreme Court rejected the quid pro quo rationale as establishing a right to treatment, although it did hold in that case that the state could not confine a person merely because he is mentally ill, without a showing that the failure to confine him will result in harm to himself or others. It was not until 1982, in the case of *Youngberg v. Romeo* (1982), that the Court held that a person who is involuntarily confined has a right to "minimally adequate training." Romeo was a profoundly retarded man who suffered injuries "on at least 63 occasions...by his own violence and by the reactions of other residents to him" while he was an inpatient at Pennhurst State Hospital in Pennsylvania. His mother sued, arguing that Romeo's Eighth and Fourteenth Amendment rights were being violated. The US Supreme Court agreed that Romeo had "constitutionally protected liberty interests under the Due Process Clause of the Fourteenth Amendment to reason-

ably safe conditions of confinement, freedom from unreasonable bodily restraints, and such minimally adequate training as reasonably may be required by these interests." "Minimally adequate training" required the exercise of professional judgment, which was held to be presumptively valid and to which "courts must show deference."

Most of the right to treatment cases attacked institutional standards of care, and were based on efforts to expand the scope of constitutional rights of inpatients. As will be seen below, current litigation seeking to establish rights to treatment in the community focuses largely on the statutory rights afforded by such antidiscrimination statutes as the Americans with Disabilities Act (ADA).

### Right to Refuse Treatment

Patients with little or no insight into the nature of their psychiatric illness often refuse treatment. A compelling set of ethical and legal questions arises when a person's stated choice (not to receive treatment) appears to conflict with medical prediction that the person's insight and mental status would probably improve with treatment. In the past, a general assumption that mentally ill patients were, by definition, incompetent, led society to grant psychiatrists a great deal of autonomy in selecting and administering treatments to patients. With the consumer activism of the 1960s and 1970s and the accompanying development of patients' rights, however, psychiatrists and legal authorities have come to see that involuntarily committed patients are not always globally incompetent, and efforts to support patients' rights to refuse treatment have increased.

Although the US Supreme Court has not declared a federal right to refuse treatment, federal Appeals Courts and most state courts have found such rights in the federal or state constitutions, citing the due process clause of the Fourteenth Amendment, within the right to privacy, bodily integrity, or personal security.

Appelbaum (1988) has described two broad models of treatment refusal. The "rights-driven" model seeks to maximize patient autonomy. It is based on the principle that competent adults have the right to reject treatment, even if the rejection of such treatment may result in harm or even death. States that adopt this model focus on the patient's competence to make the decision and often have considerable judicial procedures protecting patients. The laws of these states typically remove decision-making power from the psychiatrist and vest it in a guardian or the court. In these states the guardian or court decides what the patient would want if he or she were competent (the "substituted judgment" standard). The substituted judgment doctrine requires a challenging decision: it means that the judicial decision maker must decide, based not on his or her own values and interests, or even on what may objectively be in the patient's best interests, but instead on what the patient would decide if he or she were competent.

The "treatment-driven" model tends to view treatment as an essential element of commitment to a hospital. States with this model tend to give psychiatrists more autonomy in making decisions for patients. Procedural review is done primarily by psychiatrists and is usually focused on whether

| Table 112–3 | Models for Treatment Refusal |
|---|---|

### Rights-Driven Model

- Decision making by courts or guardians
- Procedural protections central
- Example: *Rogers v. Commissioner of Mental Health* (1983)

### Treatment-Driven Model

- Decision making requires extensive psychiatrist involvement
- Providing treatment is central
- Example: *Rennie v. Klein* (1983)

the treatment is appropriate to the patients' conditions. This model is supported by the clinical experience that some patients are grateful after they have been given treatment, even if they were not able to articulate a choice at the time (Table 112–3).

As noted, the rights-driven model is based on the "unwritten constitutional right of privacy found in the penumbra of the specific guarantees of the Bill of Rights," most specifically the Fourteenth Amendment, and emphasizes procedural safeguards as the primary means to protect the patient's rights.

A series of cases emanating from Massachusetts is emblematic of the rights-driven model. These cases relied on the ruling of *Superintendent of Belchertown v. Saikowicz* (1977), which involved an elderly man with an IQ of 10 who did not speak throughout his life and who contracted leukemia. It was assessed that the treatment of his disease would be only partially effective, that the side effects would be painful, and that the patient would be unable to understand the relationship between the painful side effects and the potential benefit of the treatment. It was uncontested that the patient was incompetent to make his own treatment decision. The patient's physician went to court and asked for permission to treat the patient. In this case, the Massachusetts Supreme Judicial Court ruled that "in appropriate circumstances, a person has a right to refuse medical treatment for a terminal illness; ... [and that] such general right to refuse medical treatment extended to the case of a mentally incompetent patient."

In the matter of *Guardianship of Richard Roe III* (1981), the court extended this reasoning to involuntary psychiatric medication for psychiatric outpatients, stating, "If an incompetent individual refuses antipsychotic drugs, those charged with his protection must seek judicial determination of substituted judgment."

A later Massachusetts case, *Rogers v. Commissioner of Mental Health* (1983), applied this rationale to involuntary inpatients. Incompetent patients at Boston State Hospital were being given antipsychotic medication without the opportunity to give informed consent. The Rogers case upholds the right of committed mentally ill patients to make treatment decisions unless they have been adjudicated incompetent by a court. The Rogers court also affirmed the holding that treatment with antipsychotic medication constituted extraordinary treatment, and that authority to administer such medication to an incompetent individual

required the exercise of the individual's substituted judgment. The court outlined six factors that a judge must assess when determining whether a patient should be permitted to refuse treatment: (1) the patient's previously expressed preference, (2) the patient's religious convictions, (3) the impact on family of the patient's preference, (4) probable side effects, (5) prognosis with treatment, and (6) prognosis without treatment. This ruling has been criticized for creating a process that is weighted heavily towards judicial oversight. Critics claim that it is responsible for delays that add to patients' length of stay in hospitals, and that the process is a tremendous drain on resources, especially given the low frequency with which judges deny medication treatment.

Several cases illustrate the treatment-driven model. *Rennie v. Klein* (1983), decided in the Third Circuit of the US Court of Appeals, held that New Jersey's procedures for reviewing the administration of antipsychotics to an unwilling patient were consistent with due process: the "decision to administer such drugs against a patient's will must be based on accepted professional judgment." Rather than have the courts superimpose procedural safeguards, treatment-driven model cases defer to medical judgment. The Rennie decision relied on the US Supreme Court's deference to professional judgment in *Youngberg v. Romeo* (1982).

Prisoners who have mental illness present a special set of problems. The case of *Washington v. Harper* (1990) involved a mentally ill prisoner who refused antipsychotic treatment. Without treatment he was quite violent. The US Supreme Court ruled that Harper's due process rights were satisfied by the Washington State procedure, which permitted involuntary treatment after a committee (a psychiatrist, a psychologist, and a prison official) reviewed and approved the proposed treatment. The court emphasized the state's "legitimate interest in combating the danger posed by a violent mentally ill inmate." The court rejected both the rights-driven model and the concept of substituted judgment in the prison environment. Some observers have noted that the US Supreme Court has been more deferential to medical judgment (and therefore more treatment-driven), whereas state courts have generally been more restrictive in applying (rights-driven) safeguards protecting patients' rights to refuse. Ironically, while this legal debate has raged, Appelbaum and Hoge (1986) have observed there are few empirical data to demonstrate how these different approaches affect the patients' outcome or how refusal itself affects the patients' care and the psychiatrist–patient alliance.

## Liberty and Civil Commitment

Although it is generally agreed that patients have a right to be treated in the least restrictive setting, there are times when a person's mental illness is such that he or she must be hospitalized involuntarily. Each state has different provisions for short-term emergency commitment. Many states have removed this process from the judicial setting; some states, however, require a probable cause hearing before even an emergency commitment. The purpose of such a hearing is to determine whether there is probable cause to believe that the person meets the legal criteria for involuntary hospitalization. If the patient is hospitalized after such a hearing, it is generally for a short period of time for evaluation; if it is determined that the patient needs longer involuntary hospitalization, then the statutory procedures for long-term commitment must be followed.

In the case of *O'Connor v. Donaldson* (1975), the US Supreme Court set a minimum below which states cannot set their standards for civil commitment. Kenneth Donaldson was a patient at Chatahoochee State Hospital in Florida. During 15 years of hospitalization he demonstrated evidence of what may have been paranoid delusions, but no evidence of dangerousness. The Florida statute at the time did not require a finding of dangerousness, and had no provisions for judicial review once a commitment was ordered. Even though there were offers from responsible individuals in the community to take care of him, Donaldson's repeated requests for release were refused. Ruling in Donaldson's favor, the Court wrote, "The state cannot constitutionally confine without more, a nondangerous, mentally ill person who is capable of surviving safely by himself or with the help of family or friends." While the Court did not state what it meant by "more," most states now require a finding of dangerousness in addition to mental illness.

In *Addington v. Texas* (1979), the US Supreme Court recognized the substantial liberty interest involved in a commitment, and set the minimum standard of proof for commitment cases as "clear and convincing." That case involved a patient with previous hospitalizations who had threatened his mother, who then filed for commitment. The court ruled: "The individual's liberty interest in the outcome of a civil commitment proceeding is of such weight and gravity, compared with the state's interests in providing care to its citizens who are unable, because of emotional disorders, to care for themselves...that due process requires the State to justify commitment by proof more substantial than mere preponderance of the evidence....The reasonable-doubt standard is inappropriate in civil commitment proceedings because, given the uncertainty of psychiatric diagnosis, it may impose a burden the state cannot meet and thereby erect an unreasonable barrier to needed medical treatment." (A few states do interpret their own constitutions to require proof beyond a reasonable doubt.)

The standards for long-term commitment vary from state to state, but they all rely on two broad principles of state power. One is the *parens patriae* power; the other, the police power. *Parens patriae*, translated from Latin as "father of the country," historically referred to the sovereign's power to make decisions for the subjects. A more contemporary translation is "state as parent," which refers to the government's interest in, and responsibility to act for, individuals who are unable to care for themselves. *Parens patriae* is used as a rationale for commitment when a person is unable to care for herself or himself as a result of a mental illness or when he or she poses a danger to self. The police power stems from the state's interest in maintaining public safety. The commitment criterion of "dangerousness to others" is derived from the police power. Over time, the trend in legislation and in court action has been more toward the dangerousness standard and less toward disability. Under all current statutes, a finding of mental illness is a prerequisite to commitment Table 112–4.

The notion of dangerousness to others or to self is a problematical one for psychiatrists, given that prediction of harm is an inexact science. Complicating the picture is the

| Table 112–4 | Principles Underlying Involuntary Commitment |

Parens Patriae

- State as parent: acts for those who cannot
- "Unable to care for self" and "danger to self" criteria

Police Power

- State as protector: acts to preserve public safety
- "Danger to others" criterion

fact that states also require different levels of proof that people are dangerous to themselves. Some states require imminent harm, while others are more tolerant of general predictions of future dangerousness based on a patient's pattern of treatment noncompliance and decompensation.

Finally, many states require a finding that hospitalization is the least restrictive method to prevent the harm the patient faces. In *Lake v. Cameron* (1966), the District of Columbia Court of Appeals held that a 60-year-old demented homeless woman could not be involuntarily hospitalized if there were other alternatives. Judge Bazelon wrote, "Deprivation of liberty solely because of danger to the ill persons themselves should not go beyond what is necessary for their protection." This case is most famous for the concept of "least restrictive alternative," as it focused on the place of confinement as well as the fact of confinement.

The issues underlying the threshold for commitment are fundamentally social, not psychiatric. They entail a balancing of rights and liberty interests with needs for treatment and safety. This balance has historically shifted with changes in the political and social climate, and continues to be a source of debate in both the legal and mental health fields.

In 1985, the APA developed a Model Law for Commitment, which generated considerable debate in the profession: "[I]t was conceived in response to the...'libertarian model,' which many mental health professionals and growing numbers of families believed was unworkable, unrealistic and inhumane" (Stone 1985). Stone added that "the liberty of psychotic persons to sleep in the streets of America is hardly a cherished freedom" and advocated for greater discretion for psychiatric commitment as well as greater resources for treatment once the patient is hospitalized.

Because roughly 70% of all psychiatric hospitalizations are voluntary, there has been interest in the due process aspect of voluntary hospitalization. Since a voluntarily admitted patient does not generally have a right to judicial review of his or her admission, US Supreme Court has ruled that a patient must be competent in order to sign into a psychiatric hospital voluntarily. In the case of *Zinermon v. Burch* (1990), Burch, who was described as having paranoid schizophrenia, was found wandering along a Florida highway, bloodied and disoriented. When he arrived at the community mental health center, he was reportedly hallucinating, confused, and stating that he believed he was "in heaven." Burch then signed forms giving his consent to admission and treatment. After 3 days he was transferred to a state mental facility, where the same process took place.

There was no evidence that any clinical or other staff member inquired into Burch's competence to execute the voluntary admission forms. Burch was hospitalized for 5 months without any hearing concerning his hospitalization. After discharge he filed a civil rights action against various officials, claiming that he was deprived of his liberty without due process by their allowing him to sign in when he was incompetent to give informed consent to such an admission. The Court agreed, and allowed his case to proceed to trial. Although the US Supreme Court did not rule on what type of competence evaluation needs to be performed before admission to a hospital, psychiatrists are now on notice that they must assure that their patients have at least a minimal understanding of the nature of a psychiatric admission. Where a patient is not competent to consent to hospitalization, alternative authority must be obtained, whether it be through civil commitment, or a guardianship proceeding, depending upon state law.

## Outpatient Commitment

Progress in the treatment of severe and chronic mental illness often depends upon the patient's compliance with medication and other treatment regimens in the community. This has been a source of challenge and frustration for psychiatrists who treat such patients. In recent years there has been a growth of interest in the possibility that outpatient commitment may offer a way to ensure that those who most need treatment will in fact receive it. In principle, an outpatient commitment law allows the same sort of treatment options as already exist with inpatient commitment: a patient may be deprived of liberty and, if found to be incompetent to make medication decisions, may be made to take medication against his will. While inpatient commitment is justified when a patient represents a danger or cannot care for himself, how does one justify coercing a patient who may be stable, relatively symptom-free, and functioning in the community?

Here the legal debate splits into two camps. Those in favor of outpatient commitment make several arguments: (1) the treatments are safe and effective; (2) untreated mental illness may increase the likelihood of violence, homelessness, incarceration, and suicide; and, more controversially, (3) patients with severe mental illness frequently lack awareness of their condition, and are therefore not really free when ill (Torrey and Zdanowicz 2001). They point out that there is a core group of particularly challenging patients whose symptoms respond well to medication, but whose persistent refusal to take medication when unconfined leads to a "revolving-door" situation of repeated hospitalizations, increased physical and psychiatric morbidity, and a perpetuation of what would appear to be unnecessary—and preventable—suffering.

Those opposing outpatient commitment counter that: (1) better funded and staffed outpatient programs would provide the kind of outreach which would make coercion unnecessary; (2) the prospect of coercion may actually drive certain patients away from help; (3) public safety would not be enhanced by outpatient commitment; and (4) even the most ill patient is, in the eyes of the law, still competent to refuse treatment (Allen and Smith 2001).

Complicating matters is the fact that it has proven challenging to demonstrate the efficacy of the outpatient commitment laws already in effect. At least 41 states permit some form of outpatient commitment, yet the first two randomized trials examining its use (Steadman et al. 2001, Swartz et al. 2001) provided equivocal evidence of efficacy (Appelbaum 2001). The actual mechanics of apprehending a nondangerous person, taking him/her to some facility, and injecting him/her involuntarily with medication, all because he/she had not followed through on a treatment plan, has proven difficult both to implement and to tolerate in a society which still places great value on maintaining its citizens' liberty interests. The debate will continue as psychiatrists try to reduce the aggregate suffering imposed on individuals and society by the effects of untreated mental illness.

## Confidentiality and Privilege

The principles of confidentiality and privilege have a long and still evolving historical connection with the practice of medicine and the role of the physician. The Hippocratic Oath states, "And about whatever I may see or hear in treatment, or even without treatment, in the life of human beings—things that should not ever be blurted out outside—I will remain silent, holding such things to be unutterable [sacred, not to be divulged]" (VonStaden 1996). The elegant simplicity of this statement of principle is now pitted against conflicting legal demands and societal values. The *Tarasoff* case (discussed below) and its progeny, the increasing use of subpoenas for psychiatric records, the complexity of interfacing with managed care, and confidentiality guidelines related to human immunodeficiency virus infection (HIV) are just some of the issues that complicate the psychiatrists' oath of confidentiality.

## Confidentiality

In the APA's *Principles of Medical Ethics with Annotations Especially Applicable to Psychiatry* (1993), Section 4, Annotation 1 reads, "Confidentiality is essential to psychiatric treatment. This is based in part on the special nature of psychiatric therapy as well as on the traditional ethical relationship between physician and patient." The constitutional right of privacy has been discussed elsewhere in this chapter. Confidentiality is defined as the clinician's obligation to keep information learned in that relationship unavailable to third parties (Appelbaum and Gutheil 2000, Gutheil 1994, pp. 1–13).

Appelbaum and Gutheil (2000) looked at practice in psychiatric facilities, and devised the concept of a "circle of confidentiality" (Figure 112–1). Within the circle, information about the patient is shared without the patient's consent. For instance, for a hospitalized patient, the resident psychiatrist, the psychiatrist's supervisor, the staff, and essential consultants are considered to be within the circle of confidentiality. The patient's family, the patient's attorney, the patient's outside psychiatrist, the patient's previous psychiatrist, and the police are outside the circle.

It is important to note that a prior psychiatrist or the current outpatient psychiatrist needs permission from the patient to speak to inpatient staff. If a patient is reluctant to release information to the outside psychiatrist, this should be a notable therapeutic issue. As Appelbaum and Gutheil note, although the patient is inside the circle, the patient

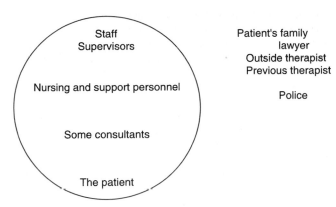

**Figure 112–1** *The circle of confidentiality. (Source: Appelbaum PS and Gutheil TG [2000] Clinical Handbook of Psychiatry and the Law. Williams & Wilkins, Baltimore.)*

may speak to anyone outside the circle without restriction. An inpatient psychiatrist would do well to inform the patient of who is within the circle and who is outside the circle. A patient's request "don't tell the nurse about this" should be discussed with the patient clinically. It should be explained that the staff are all part of the same team, trying to perform a therapeutic service for the patient.

The duty of confidentiality is sometimes understood in terms of the treatment contract between the patient and psychiatrist. In the case of *Doe v. Roe* (1977), a psychiatrist published a book that reported verbatim a patient's thoughts and experiences in the psychotherapy. The court held that "a physician who enters into an agreement with a patient to provide medical attention impliedly covenants to keep in confidence all disclosures made by the patient concerning the patient's physical or mental condition." In this case the court found for the plaintiff. It was pointed out that in psychiatry in particular, patients could reveal their most intimate and socially unacceptable instincts and urges, immature wishes, and perverse sexual thoughts—in short, the unspeakable, the unthinkable, the repressed. To speak of such things to another human being requires an atmosphere of unusual trust, confidence, and tolerance. The court rejected the psychiatrist's argument that the value of confidentiality should be balanced against the purpose of serving medical education.

There is agreement between the legal system and the psychiatric profession that confidentiality is not an absolute value. There are several major exceptions to the obligation of confidentiality, the most common of which is when the patient consents to information being released. Psychiatrists and their patients should be aware of the implications of releasing information to insurance companies, family members, employers, and so forth and should work collaboratively in making these decisions (Table 112–5).

| Table 112–5 | Major Exceptions to Confidentiality |
| --- | --- |

- Patient consents to release of information
- Duty to protect
- Emergencies
- Mandatory reporting statutes
- Court-ordered evaluations
- Patient initiates litigation

It is important that the psychiatrist and the patient together understand why the patient is asking that information be released. As a rule, the psychiatrist should get the patient's consent in writing and, optimally, the patient should read any information that leaves the office before it is released.

The second exception is based on the duty to protect, wherein the value of safety is given priority over the value of confidentiality. This is discussed later in the chapter.

The third set of exceptions includes reporting statutes, which mandate physician reporting of certain conditions. All states have such laws in one form or another, and generally include incidents of infectious diseases, child abuse, and elder abuse. If they are following any of these statutes in good faith, psychiatrists run little risk of liability. See the discussion of child abuse reporting, below.

The fourth set of exceptions includes emergencies. For instance, when a psychiatrist is evaluating a patient in an emergency department and the patient is grossly psychotic and unwilling to participate in the interview, the psychiatrist is presented with the dilemma of whether to contact family members or prior treaters without the expressed written consent of the patient. This involves a risk-benefit assessment that the evaluating psychiatrist must make. Psychiatrists must be aware of their states' standards concerning emergency breach of confidentiality; one state may require an identifiable harm to be prevented, while another may permit breach when it is necessary in the clinician's judgment to gather the relevant information to make a proper diagnosis or disposition for the patient.

Many states have enacted stringent laws about the release of test results and information related to human immunodeficiency virus and acquired immunodeficiency syndrome. There is considerable debate within the field about where the line of confidentiality should be drawn with this issue. Proponents of strict interpretation of confidentiality note the considerable social stigma and possible financial and social consequences for the person with the diagnosis. On the other hand, there is an argument that treatment providers have a need to know this information, with or without the patient's consent. States have adopted different approaches to this problem, and simply being aware of the relevant statutes does not necessarily clarify each individual situation. For example, in Massachusetts it is unlawful to release human immunodeficiency virus test results without the person's consent (Mass. Gen. Laws, ch. 111, s 70F). There is, however, no statute addressing whether this information can be part of a patient's general record. Psychiatrists should seek legal consultation when issues around HIV/AIDS are confronted.

Medical insurance has brought its own challenges to the issue of confidentiality. Insurance companies may ask mental health providers to sign a contract agreeing to release information to the insurer. Patients may ultimately have to decide which they value more: their privacy or the benefits obtained through the managed health company. The patient may choose, for instance, to seek a psychiatrist outside a managed care setting so that the patient's record will not have any psychiatric notation or documentation in it. Mental health providers who are negotiating contracts with insurers should be mindful of any obligation to provide confidential information without the patient's consent.

| Table 112–6 | Principles to Follow when Breaching Confidentiality is Necessary |
| --- | --- |

- Notify patient whenever possible
- Utilize therapeutic alliance
- Encourage patient to inform (e.g., duty to protect)
- Document rationale for action

Appelbaum and Gutheil (1991) state that psychiatrists in the position of having to breach confidentiality should observe certain basic principles. First, they should alert patients, whenever possible, of their intention to breach confidentiality before doing so. As an example, if a psychiatrist determines that a patient may have neglected his or her child, the psychiatrist–patient alliance is best served if the matter can be discussed in the open, rather than having the patient learn from a worker for a department of social services that a report of neglect is being investigated.

Second, psychiatrists should use a hierarchy of confidentiality. Psychiatrists do not need to jump to breach confidentiality in all situations where it is necessary to communicate confidential information. They often have time to discuss issues with a patient, to consider alternatives and thus avoid such confrontations. Finally, Appelbaum and Gutheil state that psychiatrists should bear in mind that the alliance is based on the "healthy side" of the patient against the patient's illness. They suggested that when the patient is experiencing impulses to harm another person, the psychiatrist and the patient should attempt to make the call to warn the person together. The healthy side of the patient is thus supported actively by the psychiatrist, as opposed to having the psychiatrist "blow the whistle" on a patient who has become dangerous. These recommendations emphasize the importance of the therapeutic alliance and remind us that confidentiality is an important aspect of that alliance. Even occasions that require a psychiatrist to breach confidentiality do not necessarily mean the end of the therapeutic alliance. In any event, it is important to clearly document any situation in which the psychiatrist determines that he or she must breach confidentiality (Table 112–6).

## Psychiatrist–Patient Privilege

The psychiatrist–patient relationship also involves the construct of testimonial privilege. Privilege is defined as the patient's right to prevent testimony by a psychiatrist in a court setting (Gutheil 1994, Appelbaum and Gutheil 1991). It rests on two primary justifications: (1) it protects the patient's interests in the privacy of treatment matters; and (2) it may encourage patients to speak openly with their psychiatrists. The scope of privilege is generally limited to the patient's communications with the psychiatrist. Observations of the patient's demeanor, or his or her conduct or even words in a public setting may not be covered within the privilege.

Privilege is a right belonging to the patient and may be waived by the patient. Although the privilege does not belong to the psychiatrist, he or she may have a duty to assert it in legal proceedings, unless and until one of the exceptions to privilege applies. In the absence of a release or waiver of privilege by the patient, psychiatrists should consult with legal counsel if they are called to testify about their communications with a patient.

Exceptions to the doctrine of privilege vary from state to state and include situations when a patient has introduced his or her mental state into litigation to which the patient is a party. In some states, privilege does not apply in competence to stand trial, or criminal responsibility evaluations. There are often exceptions in cases of child custody, involuntary commitment proceedings, will contests, or malpractice claims filed by the patient against a psychiatrist. Finally, state law may vary on the scope of the exception once it is invoked.

## Informed Consent

Psychiatrists, like all other medical practitioners, face a dilemma: Patients come to them for answers and treatment, and they expect the psychiatrist to have those answers; however, treatment of mental illness is an uncertain process, and is not without risks. In order to give informed consent to treatment, patients must be given sufficient information concerning the risks and benefits of the proposed treatment; where outcomes are uncertain, they must also be informed of that uncertainty. Gutheil and colleagues (1984) outlined the idea of "sharing uncertainty" to describe an activity that maintains the physician–patient alliance by enabling these two parties to work together to manage the inescapable fact that many things are not predictable. They recommended that physicians proactively attempt to acknowledge and dispel patients' fantasies that physicians have "magical solutions" at their disposal.

The doctrine of informed consent has evolved considerably in the past several decades. The need to obtain a patient's consent for treatment is grounded in the legal theory of battery, which is defined as an intentional touching of a person without that person's consent. Provision of medical treatment is considered an intentional touching; if it is provided without the patient's consent (and without other exceptions, such as provision of emergency medical care), then it is a battery. Only after obtaining consent from a competent person may the physician treat the patient without risking liability for the tort of battery. As medical treatment has become more complex, and as concern for patients' rights has grown, the notion of informed consent has evolved to require provision of ever more information to assist patients in making informed medical decisions.

Courts began setting modern standards for informed consent in the 1960s. The Kansas Supreme Court held that the quantum of information that a physician was required to provide was that which a "reasonable medical practitioner" would divulge (*Natanson v. Kline* 1960). In 1972, the US Court of Appeals for the District of Columbia decided the landmark case of *Canterbury v. Spence*. In a case where a physician failed to advise a patient of the risks of paralysis resulting from a laminectomy, or of any alternative treatments, the court ruled that the physician had the duty to "advise patient of need for or desirability of any alternative treatment." Although the majority of states determine the sufficiency of disclosure by the standard of that which the reasonable practitioner would deem significant, some states take a more patient centered approach in which the quantum of information is that which "would be regarded as significant by a reasonable person in the patient's position" (*Truman v. Thomas* 1980).

In general, then, the psychiatrist is obligated to disclose likely material risks of treatment, but not all possible risk, that is, the likelihood and severity of injurious side effects or death. Also, the psychiatrist should explain the need for treatment, and risks and the benefits of receiving or refusing the treatment. Finally, there should be a discussion of possible alternative treatments.

For example, no psychiatrist should prescribe an antipsychotic medication without discussing the most common side effects as well as the more serious ones such as tardive dyskinesia. The psychiatrist should explain the expected benefits of the treatment, as well as alternatives (including nonpreferred options, such as no treatment). Aside from being good risk management, obtaining informed consent helps maintain the therapeutic alliance and helps the patient to remain compliant with treatment.

Obtaining informed consent for psychopharmacological treatment of children presents a particular challenge, since many psychoactive medications have not received FDA approval for use with children. Psychiatrists should be as clear as possible when explaining the state of knowledge regarding use of particular medications with children, so that the parent's or guardian's consent is as fully informed as possible.

Obtaining informed consent should not be viewed as a one time event. It is a process, and is an essential element in good psychiatric care. Gutheil (1994) refers to the practice as "formed consent." He encourages psychiatrists to document the give-and-take process of informed consent, with liberal use of quotations from the patient, so that the idea that the patient is functioning as an autonomous, actively participating partner in treatment is well recorded (Gutheil et al. 1984, *Doe v. Roe* 1977). This is wise counsel, even for psychiatrists who are required to use forms to document informed consent. An interesting development in this field has emerged since the *Osheroff v. Chestnut Lodge* (1985) case, in which a patient who suffered from depression went through 7 months of psychotherapy and had no improvement in his condition. After transfer to a different facility, the patient was treated with antidepressants and improved. The patient sued his former treaters, and was awarded damages on the grounds that the failure to inform him of treatment alternatives (medication), as well as the risks of psychotherapy alone, constituted negligent care (facts presented by one of the expert witnesses in the Osheroff case in a clinical presentation). This case highlights the fact that the psychiatrist should give special attention to the range of therapies available for a given patient, each with its attendant risks and benefits. For instance, psychiatrists who are confronted with a depressed patient should consider all forms of treatment including medication, electroconvulsive therapy, cognitive or dynamic therapies, group and family therapy, and rehabilitative treatment. The options should be discussed with the patient to maximize the clinical alliance and the process of informed consent.

## Exceptions to Informed Consent

There are four primary exceptions to the general rule that the patient receiving treatment must give informed consent (Table 112–7). The first is a medical emergency. Consent is

| Table 112–7 | Exceptions to Informed Consent |
| --- | --- |

- Emergencies
- Therapeutic privilege
- Incompetence
- Waiver

presumed when a person is suffering from an emergent situation that requires treatment, but is unable to give consent. Thus, for example, when a diabetic patient is in a coma and consent cannot be obtained before giving the patient insulin, the treating physician may rely on presumed consent for treatment as a defense to a claim of battery. In psychiatry, the definition of an emergency has been somewhat more ambiguous. Because there is no national standard of what constitutes a psychiatric emergency, clinicians should know the definitions (if any) in their state. For instance, psychiatrists administering chemical restraints on an inpatient service or in an emergency department must know their state's requirements for determining whether an emergency exists that permits administration of chemical restraints. They should consider how emergent the situation is, document their assessment, and note that it was not possible to gain the patient's informed consent at the time. Intervention in a psychiatric emergency, especially administration of medication, is often not considered treatment in the same sense as emergency treatment of a traditional medical condition. An emergency appendectomy treats and cures the emergent condition. Administration of a chemical restraint controls the out-of-control psychotic patient, but is not considered treatment for his mental illness, which is a longer-term issue. It is for this reason that many states regulate administration of emergency psychiatric medications as restraint, rather than as treatment.

Incompetence is the second exception to the need to obtain informed consent from a patient. An incompetent person, by definition, is incapable of giving informed consent; it can be granted only by that person's guardian, or other entity charged under state law with the authority to give consent. (It is thus not truly an exception to the need for informed consent, but a situation in which the consent is obtained from a surrogate.) Even incompetent patients should be engaged in the making of treatment decisions, to the extent of their ability, and gaining their assent to treatment is important, even if they do not have the legal capacity to render informed consent. All states have procedures by which a person can be declared incompetent; such a declaration usually requires a judicial finding, though some states have administrative proceedings for resolving treatment issues that do not require judicial intervention.

The third exception to informed consent arises from the concept of therapeutic privilege. Psychiatrists use privilege when they withhold information in the belief that giving a patient all of the information necessary to make a decision would harm the patient. Invocation of therapeutic privilege, rare in medicine, is even rarer in psychiatry, in which sharing information is central to the work of the psychiatrist. Psychiatrists should use this exception to the informed consent doctrine exceedingly sparingly, with extreme caution, and with great thought; here, the psychiatrist is taking a maximally paternalistic posture in presuming what is not useful for a patient to know. The psychiatrist assumes a grave risk of liability if the patient suffers harm, and subsequently proves that a reasonable patient would have wanted to have the withheld information in order to make an informed choice about treatment.

Waiver is the fourth exception in the informed consent doctrine. Competent patients may request that their physicians not give them information, effectively waiving their right to know. This is most common in internal medicine with the diagnosis of cancer. The patient may tell the physician, "Don't tell me if I have cancer; I don't want to know." This circumstance has become increasingly unusual over time as physicians are less likely to withhold this information and patients less likely to request such a waiver.

Psychiatrists who work in consultation–liaison settings may face a special problem of being seen by their other physician colleagues as "informed consent technicians" (Gutheil and Duckworth 1992). Because psychiatrists have expertise in assessing mental status, they are often called on to evaluate the competence of a person to consent to a particular medical procedure, and often to facilitate the acquisition of some form of consent. Although psychiatrists may be helpful in assisting other physicians' understanding of their patient's competence, psychiatrists should resist pressure to act as informed consent technicians for other physicians. Acceding to such pressure furthers a belief that informed consent requires neither a relationship nor therapeutic continuity. Furthermore, obtaining informed consent in this matter may actually undermine the patient's care, since the practitioner may not have access to the psychiatrist for the many future decisions that occur in the patient's clinical care.

## Consent to the Treatment of Minors

Minors are considered to be incompetent for almost all purposes, including the right to make medical decisions. Each state has its own definition of the age that minors must attain to consent to different treatments, and the age requirements may vary with the type of treatment. For instance, a state may have a lower age of consent for treatment of sexually transmitted diseases or mental illness than for traditional medical treatment. Psychiatrists must become familiar with the law of the state or states in which they practice.

Psychiatrists who work in schools must obtain the consent of parents before initiating ongoing treatment. An emergency evaluation of a student—performed without such consent—is permissible for the most part under the doctrine of emergencies and must be documented as such (see earlier discussion). Psychiatrists who work in school settings also have to work with parents who are separated or divorced. Psychiatrists are obligated to determine which parent has legal custody and to obtain the consent of that parent for the treatment of the child; documented proof of custody must be obtained. In *Dymek v. Nyquist* (1984), a psychiatrist was sued because, in treating a 9-year-old boy who had been taken to the psychiatrist by his mother, the psychiatrist did not consult the father, who was the sole legal custodian. The appellate court, ruled in favor of the father, stating that the psychiatrist's actions "constituted a most severe interference with" the father's custody rights.

Most states have laws by which minors may become emancipated, and therefore are deemed competent to make their own decisions. The conditions of emancipation typically include marriage, becoming a parent, entry into the armed services, and sometimes a demonstrated ability of a minor to manage his or her own financial affairs and to live on his or her own. Some states have adopted the concept of a mature minor, which permits treatment on the minor's consent when he or she is capable of appreciating the nature, extent, and consequences of the medical treatment. Some states require the additional finding that informing the child's parents of the treatment would be harmful to the minor (such as in abortion cases). Psychiatrists who give treatment to minors whom they consider "mature" should have a clear understanding of the requirements in their states (including whether a judicial determination is required), and should carefully document their reasons for concluding that the minor patient in question qualifies as a mature minor. The mature minor exception should not be relied on for particularly risky interventions, at least not without judicial approval.

## Medicolegal Aspects of Clinical Practice

### Malpractice and Risk Management

A lawsuit in which a plaintiff sues a defendant for damages resulting from some act of negligence is called a tort (which is characterized as a civil, as opposed to a criminal, wrong). A malpractice suit is a type of negligence case; it shares with all negligence cases four broad elements—the "four Ds"—which must be proved if the plaintiff is to be awarded damages (Table 112–8).

The first element involves duty. A psychiatrist in private practice has no duty to treat or care for a patient unless he or she has made an agreement to do so. Once the psychiatrist agrees to treat the patient, however, the psychiatrist is legally and ethically obligated to treat the patient until treatment is properly terminated.

Once the psychiatrist–patient relationship is established, the psychiatrist is obligated to provide treatment at the standard of care. Since the duty comes into being when the relationship is established, psychiatrists need to be mindful of whether they are in fact entering into a psychiatrist–patient relationship. Commonly, psychiatrists in private practice see patients for a one-time consultation and then decide whether they wish to provide treatment. The psychiatrist should make it clear at the time of the initial contact that the first appointment is an opportunity for the psychiatrist and patient to see if their relationship is going to be a useful one. If this is not clearly spelled out and agreed to, it might be argued that the psychiatrist assumed a duty to provide care at the initial consultation. This is not to suggest, however, that there is no duty owed to a patient

| Table 112–8 | The Four Ds of Malpractice |
|---|---|
| • Dereliction of |
| • Duty |
| • Directly causing |
| • Damage |

upon initial consultation. A psychiatrist may be held to a duty to recognize an acute psychiatric emergency, and to deal with that emergency within the established standard of care. Physicians need to be aware of situations in which they may establish a doctor–patient relationship, without intending to. Great care should be exercised, for instance, if a psychiatrist writes a prescription for a friend, colleague, or family member, for she or he is thereby assuming a physician–patient relationship and duty of care. Similarly, psychiatrists who host talk shows or write newspaper columns should make it clear that they are not entering into a physician–patient relationship with the people seeking their advice.

The second element of malpractice is negligence (or dereliction of duty). The test of negligence is whether the psychiatrist's actions deviated from the standard of care practiced by other professionals of the same level of training.

The third element that needs to be demonstrated is harm or damage. Once the plaintiff has proven that the psychiatrist has a duty to the patient and has performed in a derelict manner, there must be proof that the patient has suffered harm. Even a grossly negligent act that results in no harm will not result in a finding of liability for malpractice.

The fourth factor is direct or proximate cause. The damage that the patient has suffered must directly result from the dereliction of duty by the psychiatrist. Without this connection, a claim of malpractice will not be successful.

The case of *Clites v. Iowa* (1982) is a clear example of psychiatric malpractice. In that case, physicians gave a mentally retarded young man antipsychotics for years and he developed severe tardive dyskinesia. The testimony at trial established that the defendant physicians were responsible for the patient's care (their duty) and that they failed to treat him in accordance with the applicable standards of care, in that they failed to obtain informed consent, failed to monitor the patient with regular physician contact, failed to obtain consultation where indicated, and failed to recognize and alter his treatment when he began to develop side effects (dereliction or negligence of duty). The patient suffered harm; he developed tardive dyskinesia (damage), which the court found was proximately (or directly) caused by the physician's negligence. Thus, the four elements of professional negligence were met, and the patient was awarded damages.

## Third Party Payers and the Psychiatrist

The increasing role that insurers play in determining the type of treatment patients receive has increased the complexity of the psychiatric–legal interface. A major public policy issue in this area is whether, and to what extent, insurance companies may be held responsible when a denial of coverage results in harm to a patient. Health care providers are faced with difficult legal and ethical decisions when their professional judgment calls for provision of a particular service in the face of an insurance company denial. The law in this area is evolving; whereas early cases seemed to cloak managed care payers with a great deal of protection, later cases and some statutory changes are increasing their exposure.

The 1987 case, *Wickline v. the State of California*, illustrates the relationship between the treating physician and the third party payer in a relatively early stage of the development of this area of law. This case involved the state of California's MediCal system. The patient, Wickline, had been hospitalized for vascular surgery on her leg. After surgery, her physicians requested an 8-day extended hospital stay, but the MediCal reviewers only authorized 4 days. The testimony was that on the day of discharge, none of the treating physicians sought approval for further hospitalization, although they agreed that Wickline needed further treatment. Shortly after discharge she suffered a complete occlusion of the artery in her right leg, which necessitated an amputation. The appellate court concluded that MediCal, as payer, could not be held liable for the premature discharge, even though the reviewing physician admitted that his assessment of her medical condition, made without an actual examination, fell below the standard of care. The basis for this finding is that, upon discharge, none of the treating physicians insisted on the patient's remaining in the hospital. Thus, there was no finding that the subsequent damage was proximately caused by the payer's alleged negligence. The message of the case, however, is that a denial of coverage does not obviate a physician's duty to render treatment to the appropriate standard of care. Where coverage is denied, physicians are nonetheless obligated to exercise their medical judgment, and, where necessary, to challenge the denial through whatever mechanisms are available.

Three years later, the same California court made it clear that insurance companies may indeed share liability with physicians when the denial of benefits results in harm to the patient. In the case of *Wilson v. Blue Cross of California* (1990), the patient, Wilson, was admitted to a hospital in Los Angeles, suffering from depression, substance dependence, and anorexia. His treating physician determined that he required 3 or 4 weeks of inpatient care, but on his 10th day in the hospital his insurance company stated that it would not pay for any further hospital care. When the family made it clear that they could not afford to pay for the hospitalization, the patient was discharged; 20 days later he committed suicide. Although the treating physician did not appeal the denial of coverage, he later testified that he was reasonably sure that Wilson would not have committed suicide had he been permitted to remain in the hospital. The court ruled that the insurance company's denial of coverage might have been a proximate cause of Wilson's suicide, and it permitted the case to go to trial where the plaintiff would have had to prove the elements of negligence to a jury. The case was remanded to the trial court, but the parties settled the matter without going to trial. Since the treating psychiatrist was not a defendant in this case, the court mentioned but did not rule on the issue of his responsibility to appeal the denial of care. However, the court's reference to the physician's duty to exercise reasonable medical judgment in ordering a discharge, even where there is a denial of coverage, puts physicians on notice that the insurance company's action does not shield them from liability if the denial of care results in harm.

The intersection of the demands of confidentiality with those of managed care presents a second major area of complexity. At the beginning of therapy, the psychiatrist should outline the scope of utilization review and should obtain the consent of the patient before releasing any information to the reviewing companies. Once a patient gives consent for a psychiatrist to speak to a utilization review committee, the psychiatrist should give only the minimal amount of information necessary to facilitate the utilization review decision. Patients should also be made aware of the possibility that payment for recommended services may be denied by the insurance company. The treatment agreement between the patient and psychiatrist should make clear the patient's financial responsibilities in the event of such a denial. However, a psychiatrist may face liability for failure to provide, or arrange for, necessary care in the community, just as in the hospital setting, even when coverage is denied.

Finally, there is a potential for conflict and liability when health care providers sign contracts with managed care companies. Whether the contract is based on a capitated scale or fee for service, providers often have a financial incentive to limit the care they provide (just as they have a financial incentive to inflate costs under traditional indemnity arrangements). In addition, some managed care companies are making an effort to transfer their financial liability for treatment denials to their psychiatrists by having them sign "hold harmless" or "indemnification" agreements. Psychiatrists must be aware that such arrangements may have an impact on their relationships with their patients, and must guard against the possibility that their clinical judgment may be influenced thereby.

## Liability for Supervising Other Professionals

Psychiatrists work in a variety of settings and interact in many different ways with other mental health professionals. One aspect of this interaction is the liability potential that psychiatrists undertake in each of these relationships. The APA publication entitled "Guidelines for psychiatrists in consultative, supervisory, or collaborative relationships with nonmedical therapists" (1980) outlines the typical consultative relationships and their corresponding degree of responsibility. Broadly, the degree of liability correlates with the extent of authority to make (as opposed to recommend) treatment decisions (Table 112–9).

Supervisory relationships are relationships in which the psychiatrist is hierarchically and legally responsible for the overall care of the patient, and will be held responsible for the treatment provided by those he or she supervises. The American Psychiatric Association (1980) guidelines state that:

> In a supervisory relationship the psychiatrist retains direct responsibility for patient care and gives professional direction and active guidance to the therapist. In this relationship the nonmedical therapist may be an employee of an organized health care setting or of the psychiatrist. The psychiatrist remains ethically and medically responsible for the patient's care as long as the treatment continues under his or her supervision. The patient should be fully informed of the existence and nature of, and any changes in, the supervisory relationship.

| Table 112–9 | **Psychiatrists' Relationships with Nonmedical Therapists** |
|---|---|
| **Supervisory** ||
| • Psychiatrist has treatment responsibility <br> • Psychiatrist may hire or fire <br> • Psychiatrist has final authority ||
| **Collaborative** ||
| • Responsibility shared between parties <br> • Delineation of responsibilities required ||
| **Consultative** ||
| • Consultee may take advice or not <br> • Consultant is not responsible for supervision <br> • Consultant has no hire or fire authority ||

Consultative relationships are different in terms of the level of responsibility and liability undertaken. Consultative advice is given on a "take it or leave it" basis. Consultants are outside the decision-making chain of command; they do not make treatment decisions, and do not have hiring and firing authority. As such, they generally are not held liable for treatment decisions (though psychiatrists practicing as consultants should be aware of any unusual legal provisions in the state in which they practice). The American Psychiatric Association (1980) guidelines state that in this type of relationship the psychiatrist does not assume responsibility for the patient's care. The psychiatrist evaluates the information provided by the therapist and offers a medical opinion which the therapist may or may not accept. Consultation is not a one-way process and psychiatrists do and should seek appropriate consultation from members of other disciplines in order to provide more comprehensive services to patients.

Collaborative relationships lie between these two extremes in terms of the liability potential for psychiatrists. Collaborative relationships demand a great deal of communication between clinicians, and psychiatrists must be careful to know when they cross from pure consultation into collaboration. The American Psychiatric Association (1980) writes:

> Implicit in this relationship is mutually shared responsibility for the patient's care in accordance with the qualifications and limitations of each therapist's discipline and abilities. The patient must be informed of the respective responsibilities of each therapist; neither discipline's responsibilities diminish those of the other. Both the psychiatrist and nonmedical therapist are responsible for periodic evaluation of the patient's status to ascertain that the collaboration continues to be appropriate. The therapists must inform the patient, either jointly or separately, if they decide to terminate their collaborative relationship. Once the relationships are clearly delineated, psychiatrists must choose mental health professionals with whom they feel

comfortable, with whom they can communicate, and whom they respect.

## Risk Management Techniques

There is consensus among risk management experts that various strategies can reduce medicolegal liability. The clinical strategies of obtaining consultation on difficult cases, documenting the rationale behind critical decisions, and using informed consent to build rapport are valuable risk management techniques. In documentation, "thinking for the record" is advocated by Gutheil. The psychiatrist thus demonstrates the use of judgment and ongoing risk benefit assessments. Institutional strategies include regular quality assurance monitoring, training in documentation, a system for working with patients and families on adverse effects, and providing access to expert consultation.

In psychiatry, several areas deserve special mention. Suicide and attempted suicide represent one of the most common and expensive sources of lawsuits in psychiatry (Slawson 1989). Psychiatrists should assess the level of suicidality and the ability of patients to monitor and report their suicidality (Gutheil et al. 1986) and plan an appropriate strategy based on that assessment. In lawsuits involving suicide, the patients are more commonly portrayed as the victims, rather than agents in their own deaths. The psychiatrist who both fosters and documents active collaboration with the patient demonstrates good risk management practice as well as clinical skill. Prescribing medications also raises psychiatrists' liability risk. Solid documentation of history, examinations, laboratory tests, indications for a medication, and risk assessment are essential to reduce liability. Consultation with a colleague should be sought for difficult cases.

## Duty to Warn, Duty to Protect

When a psychotherapist determines (or, pursuant to the standards of the profession, should determine) that his/her patient represents a serious danger of violence to another, he/she incurs an obligation to use reasonable care to protect the intended victim against such danger. The discharge of such duty, depending on the nature of the case, may call for the therapist to warn the intended victim or others likely to apprise the victim of the danger, to notify the police, or to take whatever other steps are reasonably necessary under the circumstances.

This is the so-called Tarasoff principle, established by California Judge Tobrinen in 1976 in the case of *Tarasoff v. Regents* (1976). It has generated controversy, spawned lawsuits, and initiated a fundamental reexamination of the psychiatrist's role vis-à-vis members of the public.

The *Tarasoff* case involved the tragic death of a University of California student, Tatiana Tarasoff, who was murdered by a fellow student, Prosenjit Poddar. Poddar was an outpatient at the campus mental health clinic. He stated to his psychologist that he intended to kill Tarasoff. The therapist completed paperwork to have Poddar committed for 72-hour emergency psychiatric detention. He notified the campus police, orally and in writing, that Poddar was dangerous and committable. The local police detained Poddar, but released him when he stated that he would "stay away from that girl." Poddar dropped out of treatment shortly thereafter. Two months later he successfully carried out his threat to kill Tarasoff.

This case, as well as subsequent cases and legislation in other states created new clinical and ethical dilemmas for psychiatrists, as they now must balance confidentiality with the safety of third parties in outpatient settings as well. At what point is the inherently trusting nature of the psychiatrist–patient relationship impaired by the legally driven obligation to report threats of harm? When should a psychiatrist report a patient's vague statement wishing to harm a third party? How should the patient's violent history be weighed in the assessment of whether to violate confidentiality? Does the circle of responsibility include only named third parties, or does it extend to groups of reasonably identifiable potential victims? Is a warning sufficient? Although these questions are ultimately matters of clinical judgment, psychiatrists need to know whether their states have established specific guidelines for settling them.

The *Tarasoff* case is a striking example of the impact one case can have on national practice. Even though it applies per se only in the state of California, the duty to warn or protect is known throughout the country as the "Tarasoff Duty."

Risk management is inherently conservative. Although good documentation of the treatment process will usually result in better clinical practice, an inordinate concern about liability may result in defensive practice. The standard of care does not require psychiatrists to be omniscient. Psychiatrists must be prepared to take risks, when those risks are informed by sound clinical judgment, adequate consultation, and thorough documentation. The psychiatrist who has a good risk management system in place will be in the best position to explain and defend his or her decisions when the inevitable bad result does take place.

## Criminal Law and Psychiatry

The psychiatrist's role in the courtroom is substantially different from that in the clinical setting (Rappeport 1982). In criminal cases, psychiatrists are commonly called on to evaluate defendants' competence to stand trial or (less commonly) criminal responsibility. In perhaps the most challenging of situations, psychiatrists are faced with the ethically challenging task of evaluating defendants' competence to understand the death penalty.

## The Psychiatrist as Expert Witness

Psychiatrists may work in forensic settings as agents of the court, providing impartial evaluations for the judge, or may function as experts for the defense or prosecution. As opposed to fact witnesses, who can testify only as to facts that they have observed, expert witnesses may review records, conduct tests, perform evaluations or other research, and provide opinions (such as diagnoses) in court. Expert witnesses, by definition, are familiar with a body of professional knowledge that is not well known to the layperson (Table 112–10).

When asked to serve as an expert witness, the psychiatrist should have a clear understanding of the legal question or standard being addressed. The expert witness should inform the client that patient–psychiatrist confidentiality is not to be expected and that the information being elicited will be presented to the court to help the judge or jury make

| Table 112–10 | |
| --- | --- |
| Fact Witness | Expert Witness |
| • No specialized knowledge | • Has special knowledge base |
| • No special fee | • May offer opinions |
| • Does not offer opinion | • Receives compensation |

a decision. In general, attorneys attempt to establish the credibility of their experts by presenting their qualifications to the court, either by testimony, or by admitting the expert's resume. Psychiatrists who offer themselves as expert witnesses should be prepared to have their credentials challenged by the attorney for the opposing side. Good expert witnesses take these challenges in stride. They respond to questions calmly, without becoming defensive or arrogant. Good expert testimony is given in understandable, jargon-free language, with short, concise answers. Expert testimony is a challenging and difficult professional task.

## Competence to Stand Trial Evaluations

In order for a criminal case to proceed, the defendant must be competent to stand trial. This is a constitutional standard that has its roots in old English law. Although specific standards of competence are determined on a state-by-state basis, the federal standard has provided the basis for each state's law. The test is "whether [the defendant] has sufficient present ability to consult with his lawyer with a reasonable degree of rational understanding and whether he has a rational as well as a factual understanding of the proceedings against him" (*Dusky v. United States* 1960). The legal standard is not an exacting one. Only a small proportion of criminal defendants are referred for competency evaluations.

Although there is no universally accepted clinical standard for assessing competence, the McGarry (McGarry et al. 1973) criteria have been empirically validated and are the most commonly used sources of evaluation. This standard encourages the psychiatrist to assess 13 different areas of functioning, including the patient's behavior, ability to relate to an attorney, ability to plan a legal strategy, and motivation and capacity to testify, in addition to the patient's understanding of the charges, possible consequences, and likely outcomes.

Psychiatrists often struggle, misguidedly, with how much they should attempt to answer the ultimate question of whether a patient is or is not competent. In fact, judges determine whether a defendant is competent and typically prefer psychiatrists to spell out as much as possible factually while refraining from stating whether the defendant is incompetent or competent. Psychiatrists must remember that when they are conducting evaluations on behalf of the court, they are agents of the court; the usual rules of the psychiatrist–patient relationship (including confidentiality and privilege) are thereby waived. Those being examined must be informed of these different ground rules, in accordance with the requirements of the particular state. Since the defendant's understanding of his or her waiver of confidentiality is often an issue, the evaluator should carefully document the defendant's response to the information, using direct quotes, when possible. States have different requirements in cases where the patient appears incompetent to give informed consent for a "stand trial" evaluation. The psychiatrist needs to be aware of these requirements, and to be prepared to proceed accordingly (some states permit the evaluation to proceed; others might require further hearings). Without a waiver, the information the psychiatrist gathers during a competence to stand trial evaluation is privileged. However, most states provide that an unwilling defendant may be compelled to participate in such an evaluation. Most states provide that the information gathered by a psychiatrist in the course of such an evaluation cannot be used during the trial in the case in chief. In this way, the criminal justice system attempts to balance the due process rights of potentially incompetent persons with the need to protect the defendant from self-incrimination.

The fate of defendants found incompetent to stand trial was addressed in *Jackson v. Indiana* (1972). Jackson was mentally retarded, deaf and mute; he was charged with two counts of petty larceny. The psychiatrist who evaluated Jackson concluded that he was almost completely unable to communicate; in addition to his lack of hearing, his mental deficiency left him unable to understand the nature of the charges against him or to participate in his defense. Based on this evidence, the trial court found that Jackson "lacked comprehension sufficient to make his defense" and ordered him committed to the Indiana Department of Mental Health until that department could certify to the court that he was "sane."

Since it was clear that Jackson would never become "sane," (that is, competent to stand trial), his commitment essentially amounted to imposition of a life sentence, without his ever being convicted of a crime. The court held that this outcome violated Jackson's Fourteenth Amendment right to due process and that a defendant cannot be committed indefinitely just because he is incompetent to stand trial. His commitment must be for a purpose permitted under state law (and the Constitution). Thus, if the defendant may reasonably be restored to competence with treatment, he may be committed for that purpose. If it is unlikely that the defendant will be restored to competence (as in Jackson's case), then his commitment must meet other legitimate state purposes, such as prevention of harm under civil commitment standards. If the defendant does not meet the criteria for such a commitment, he must be released.

The US Supreme Court has taken a fairly narrow approach to the requirements of competence for other purposes relating to criminal prosecutions. For instance, although a defendant must understand his so-called Miranda rights in order to waive them, a confession compelled by a defendant's psychotic thinking might be valid. In *Colorado v. Connelly* (1986), Connelly confessed to a murder after being given his Miranda rights but later claimed that his confession was compelled by his psychosis. The Colorado Supreme Court ruled that this confession was therefore involuntary, but the US Supreme Court reversed the decision, holding that, under the US Constitution, a confession is involuntary only if police were coercive. Internal pressures to confess thus could not be used to invalidate a confession.

## Insanity Defense

There is an important distinction between a finding of incompetence to stand trial and a finding of not guilty by reason of insanity (NGRI). The former means that defendants do not have a chance to defend themselves until competence is restored. The latter is a not guilty finding, based on the defendant's inability to have formed the state of mind requisite for a criminal conviction. It is not a matter of restoration or recovery from mental illness; once a defendant is found NGRI, the criminal case is permanently resolved. Criminal responsibility and competency evaluations are often requested together, but they are separate and distinct.

In order to be convicted, a defendant must be shown both to be guilty of committing an illegal act (*actus reus*) and to have had the intention of committing the crime (*mens rea*). Criminal responsibility evaluations focus on the *mens rea* component of criminal acts. The psychiatrist involved in an insanity defense is presented with a more challenging assignment than that of the competence to stand trial evaluation. Assessing a patient's mental state retrospectively is a task fraught with difficulties. The defendant may forget, lie, or "fill in" details of the events. For this reason, this evaluation typically involves more collateral investigation, such as reviewing the prosecutor's file including police, witness, victim, and perhaps even autopsy reports, in addition to standard history such as past psychiatric records. The clinical interview should include the confidentiality warning, a detailed present-day mental status examination, and direct queries into the defendant's recollected mental state and in-depth recall of the crime. This detective work, together with careful questioning, as well as psychological or neurological assessment when indicated, is necessary to enable the psychiatrist to present as clear a picture as possible of the defendant's state of mind at the moment of the crime.

The insanity defense generates considerable public alarm due to the perception that violent criminals are "getting away with it," yet less than 1% of felony prosecutions result in a successful insanity defense (1985). This perception notwithstanding, Anglo-American and ancient Greek cultures have had a long tradition of viewing mentally ill individuals as less morally culpable for acts of violence. When and by how much culpability is reduced are determined by society and the judicial system, not by psychiatry, and the standards often change in response to particularly high profile cases. For instance, after the trial of John Hinckley, 27 states changed their laws to make it more difficult for the insanity defense to succeed.

*Rex v. Arnold* in 1724 is the earliest insanity defense case in which the full record of the proceedings are available. Arnold, after having been charged with murder, was assessed under a standard of responsibility that provided: "A man must be so totally deprived of his understanding and memory, so as to not know what he is doing, no more than an infant, a brute, or a wild beast." This so-called wild beast test represents the most stringent standard developed for criminal responsibility. It was a purely cognitive test and set the standard of cognitive appreciation of a crime at an extremely low level.

The first appellate decision in English law involving the insanity defense was *M'Naghten*'s case. In 1843, Daniel M'Naghten shot and killed Edward Drummond, who was secretary to the prime minister. Apparently, M'Naghten was under the delusion that he was being persecuted by the prime minister as well as other people throughout all of England. At his trial Mr. M'Naghten successfully raised the defense of insanity under a more liberal standard than the "wild beast" test. After this case, the standard for criminal responsibility became known as the M'Naghten rule: "To establish a defense on the grounds of insanity it must be conclusively proved that, at the time of committing the act, the party accused was laboring under such a defect of reason, from the disease of the mind, as to not know the nature and quality of the act he was doing; or if he did know it that he did not know what he was doing was wrong." This standard allows either a cognitive test (did he know what he was doing?) or a moral test (did he know it was wrong?). It addresses itself to the specific criminal act, as opposed to assessing the defendant from the perspective of a broad-reaching sense of right and wrong.

In 1954, the District of Columbia Circuit Court of Appeals established the Durham rule which held that "an accused is not criminally responsible if his unlawful act was the product of mental disease or mental defect" (*Durham v. US* 1954). This test prevailed in the District of Columbia from 1954 until 1972. This standard allowed psychiatrists maximal freedom in utilizing evidence relevant to the accused's mental state. The Court of Appeals for the District of Columbia abandoned the Durham rule in 1972 although New Hampshire still uses it and adopted in its place the American Law Institute standard which had been developed in 1955.

The American Law Institute standard provides: "A person is not responsible for criminal conduct if at the time of such conduct as a result of a mental disease or defect he lacks substantial capacity either to appreciate the wrongfulness of his conduct or to conform his conduct to the requirements of the law" (Model Penal Code 1955). This test incorporates the cognitive component of the M'Naghten rule but, by use of the terms "mental disease or defect," allows for the possibility that conditions other than psychotic illnesses (such as impulse disorders) may result in a lack of criminal responsibility. The existence of this test by no means makes the defense easier to establish. As one commentator as noted, "The line between an irresistible impulse and an impulse not resisted is probably no sharper than that between twilight and dusk" (Stone 1984).

In 1982, John Hinckley shot and wounded President Ronald Regan in an assassination attempt. His trial illustrated some of the difficulty in applying psychiatric principles to a legal standard when a complicated person commits a criminal act. For instance, Hinckley allegedly saw the movie *Taxi Driver* 15 times. As Stone asked, "Are these behaviors evidence of psychotic identification problems (as the defense psychiatrists argued) or do they amount to something much less (as the prosecution psychiatrists said)? Was his obsession with actress Jodie Foster a delusion, or was it merely unrealistic and inappropriate? When does a fantasy become a fixed idea? When does a fixed idea become a delusion?"

There was tremendous disagreement among the experts about Hinckley's diagnosis; no consensus could be reached on whether he was in fact psychotic. The result, however, was that he was found not guilty by reason of insanity. He was committed to St. Elizabeth's Hospital in the District of Columbia, where he remains at the time of this writing. After the Hinckley case, federal rules were changed to place the burden of proving insanity on the defendant. Interestingly, states differ as to whether prosecution or defense should bear the burden of proving insanity. This distinction is crucial as, given the nature of psychiatric diagnosis and testimony, the burden of proof may decide some of the cases in which there is true clinical ambiguity and disagreement.

Contrary to public perception, a successful insanity defense does not usually result in freedom. In fact, when a defendant is found not guilty by reason of insanity, he or she may face years of confinement in a hospital setting. As Elliot and colleagues (1993) note:

> Acquittals by reason of insanity are unlike acquittals in criminal law. The criminal defendant who wins an outright acquittal is free of state control and may simply walk away from the court house after the trial. But the defendant found [NGRI] typically remains confined . . . .

The hurdles to commitment are typically much lower and the barriers to release much higher. Especially when charged with misdemeanors, insanity acquittees generally remain hospitalized far longer than ordinary civil acquittees and may remain confined for periods greater than the maximum sentence that would have been possible on conviction of the criminal charges.

## Civil Litigation

### Tort Liability

The tort system is designed to compensate individuals or groups who are injured by the acts of other individuals or entities, including corporations and sometimes government agencies. As in malpractice cases (which are a category of tort), the four Ds (*dereliction* of a *duty*, *directly* causing *damage*) are the standard by which tort liability is assessed. Unlike most criminal cases, where the conduct of the victim is not relevant to the defendant's guilt, the injured party's (or plaintiff's) conduct is often a factor in determining the legal result. Thus, in a motor vehicle case, if the plaintiff was also operating his or her vehicle negligently, and thus contributed to the accident, the defendant's liability will be reduced in proportion to the plaintiff's comparative negligence. Where a party's mental state is at issue, or where there are claims for emotional damages, psychiatrists may be called upon to conduct evaluations and testify.

Historically, claims for pure emotional damages have been disfavored. Courts had long excluded emotional distress as compensable, except when the claimed distress was accompanied by a physical injury (the "impact rule"). Modern judicial decision making has allowed considerably more latitude in this area. American courts developed the concept of the "zone of danger," which allows for recovery if the emotionally injured party was within the physical zone of danger created by the defendant's negligent conduct, even if the plaintiff was not physically injured. Courts have gradually expanded the zone of danger concept. For example, California extended it in *Dillon v. Legg* (1968) to a mother who witnessed her child being killed by an automobile driven by Legg. Although Dillon was outside the traditional zone of danger when she witnessed the event, she sought damages for emotional injuries she sustained while witnessing the event. The court ruled in her favor, stating that Dillon's emotional injuries were a "reasonably foreseeable" outcome of the negligent conduct of Legg. The court outlined three factors to determine foreseeability: (1) the injured party must be located near the scene of the accident, (2) the individual must experience a direct emotional impact from the accident by witnessing it; and (3) the person must be closely related to the victim.

Psychiatrists performing an evaluation for psychic harm must evaluate the person's mental state before and after the act. For instance, if a person had a preexisting history of affective disorder and had recurrent episodes after an injury, that would be noteworthy for a psychic harm report. The question would be whether the traumatic event exacerbated the preexisting condition. Not unlike criminal responsibility evaluations, these assessments may rely heavily on collateral documentation of the event and interviews with other witnesses. Emotional injury evaluations often focus heavily on functional deficits that the plaintiff may be exhibiting, since damages are related to loss of function; it is not sufficient to simply meet diagnostic criteria for mental illness. As in all such evaluations, especially where the subject is aware of the consequences of the process, malingering should always be considered.

### Disability

Psychiatrists may perform disability evaluations for both workers' compensation and Social Security disability claims. Workers' compensation is an alternative system of compensation that does not involve the complexity of the tort system. Workers' compensation, which is paid when a disabling injury occurs in the course of employment, is an exclusive remedy based on the worker's prior salary and the degree and duration of disability. In general, there are no awards for pain and suffering as there are in tort cases. In this system, evaluations focus on functional limitations and require assessment of credibility, as well as corroboration of the person's prior mental state and its connection to the work environment.

Since workers' compensation systems are created by legislatures, it is important to know the statutory definitions of the conditions under evaluation; this is particularly true for mental disability. The typical categories of mental disability are as follows: (1) physical trauma causing mental injury, (2) mental injury causing physical effects, and (3) mental stress causing mental injury.

Social Security Disability Insurance was established in 1956 for people who had contributed to the fund while working. Supplemental Security Income was developed in 1972 to establish federal matching payment for state benefit programs for the disabled, regardless of work history. The Social Security disability programs use definitions of mental disorders that resemble, but are not identical with, those of the *Diagnostic and Statistical Manual of Mental Disorders*, Fourth Edition (DSM-IV) (American Psychiatric Association 1994). The evaluating clinician must determine whether a qualifying condition exists, and assess the degree of disability it produces, as measured against standards of the American Medical Association's guidelines (Linda et al. 2001).

## Competence, Capacity, and Guardianship

Competence is best understood as a legal term referring to an individual's capacity to make informed decisions. Adult individuals are presumed to be legally competent, unless and until there is a court finding of incompetence. A finding of incompetence means that a physical or mental illness has caused a defect in cognition or judgment, regarding the specific area in question, such that the individual lacks the capacity to make informed decisions. When a court determines that an individual is incompetent, a guardian may be appointed to make decisions for that person.

Competence is often used as a general term, but it should be defined specifically. For example, an elderly accountant with mild dementia may retain the capacity to manage finances but not to appreciate the risks and benefit of angioplasty or a cardiac operation. Historically, psychiatric patients, when admitted to psychiatric hospitals, were presumed incompetent for all purposes, including voting and making contracts. Over time, society has come to agree that psychosis does not automatically equal incompetence for all (or even any) decisions. For instance, psychiatric patients are no longer presumptively deemed to be incompetent to vote. Capacity, and therefore legal competence, may fluctuate, especially in individuals with mental illness. The classic example of this is an elderly patient who "sundowns" at night but who retains good mental functioning during daylight hours. With the advent of modern psychopharmacology, competence in severely mentally ill patients is often related to medication compliance. Even floridly psychotic patients may become competent after they are stabilized on medications. Since the legal decision making for incompetent patients often involves determining what the individual would want if he or she were competent to choose, it is important that the psychiatrist assess the person's capacity when he/she is doing clinically well, in addition to when he/she is doing poorly.

Assessing a patient's capacity to give consent is based on several general principles (Appelbaum and Grisso 1988). The patient must be able to (1) communicate choices, (2) understand the relevant information, (3) appreciate the situation and its consequences, and (4) manipulate the information rationally (Table 112–11).

There is general agreement that the standard for judging competence also varies with the presented task. For instance the standard for competence to consent to take an experimental drug is higher than for taking an aspirin. The greater the risk in the intervention, the more the psychiatrist needs to be clear about the four elements noted in the preceding paragraph.

| Table 112–11 | Assessment of Capacity |
| --- | --- |

- Ability to communicate choices
- Understand relevant information
- Appreciate the situation and its consequences
- Rationally manipulate information

Several other competencies require attention in civil matters. For example, testamentary capacity (the capacity to make a will) may be challenged by disgruntled and disinherited parties. For this reason, some people obtain an evaluation of their capacity to make a will before their death. Testamentary capacity requires that individuals understand (1) the nature of a will, (2) the extent of their assets, (3) the identity of their natural heirs, and (4) that they should not be under undue influence. Challenges to testamentary capacity commonly involve allegations that the individual was vulnerable to the undue influence of another who has convinced him or her to leave his or her assets to that person, where that would not otherwise have been the individual's choice, or that the individual was operating under delusional beliefs that undermined his or her rational behavior.

Once a person has been found either incompetent to make specific decisions or globally incompetent, issues arise regarding, who should make decisions that affect that person, and what standard that person or jurisdiction should use in making decisions. Again, states have developed different answers to these questions. Next of kin are commonly used as guardians, but this may pose conflicts of interest or complicate ongoing family dynamics. Attorneys or clergy are also commonly used for this purpose. Physicians are generally not asked to become guardians. It would certainly be inappropriate for a physician to be guardian for his or her own patient, since the proponent of treatment options cannot also be the decision maker. Even for individuals who are not his or her patient, a physician's assuming the role of decision maker creates an ethical dilemma that should be avoided.

Decision making can be based on either the "best interests" standard or the "substituted judgment" model. The best interests model is a paternalistic approach that assumes that decision makers know what is in the patient's best interests, and that they will act accordingly. It is a value laden paradigm that requires guardians to be aware of their own value systems, and to be on guard against the risk that their values may conflict with those that might apply to the patient. Perhaps more onerous, but more individualized, is the substituted judgment model, discussed briefly above in the section on informed consent. Here, the guardian attempts to act in the manner the person would want under the circumstances. This is a difficult task. When an individual has never considered a possibility, such as being in a coma, it cannot be known with certainty what the individual's wishes would be. While it might be generally agreed that individualized decision making is a preferable model, it is easy to see why the relative comfort of the best interest approach makes this model the one that is most widely applied.

## Special Issues

### Child Abuse Reporting

Kempe and colleagues in a 1962 paper "The Battered Child Syndrome," began an awareness of child abuse and neglect that continues to grow. Before this seminal paper, many psychiatrists considered children's allegations of sexual and physical abuse to be fantasy that was to be interpreted and not acted on. Child abuse is now recognized to be

Section VII • Special Clinical Settings and Challenges

widespread, and for the individual child, a potentially devastating reality.

All states place an affirmative duty on the professional to report suspicions of abuse. Even though many adult psychiatrists receive relatively little training in child psychiatry and in child development, all psychiatrists are mandated reporters of suspicions of child abuse and neglect. Psychiatrists who treat patients with alcoholism, serious mental illness, and a history of abuse are working with populations who have increased risk of child abuse. While pediatricians file the majority of child abuse reports, psychiatrists may be called to consult in cases requiring additional clinical judgment.

Neglect is a most difficult form of abuse to identify. Although the laws are written to encourage reporting in the "gray" cases, clinicians must still exercise a level of clinical judgment. One person's view of neglect may be another person's view of bad parenting. Clearly, a child who is malnourished is being neglected. A child who is left alone for a significant period may have been neglected, but this depends on the age and developmental stage of the child. Clinicians must also guard against cultural or racial bias. Hampton and Newberger (1985) studied child abuse reporting and noted that physicians are more likely to file child abuse reports involving people who are of a different race or class than themselves. Psychiatrists also worry about the damage a report will do to the alliance between the psychiatrist and the patient. Clinical experience demonstrates that, in most cases, an explanation of the practitioner's legal obligation to file a report maximizes the potential to maintain the clinical alliance. That reassurance aside, psychiatrists must be aware that the legal obligation to report supercedes the value of the alliance.

A child abuse report is usually made to the state's child welfare agency, sometimes called the "Department of Social Services" or "Children and Family Services." Most commonly, the call is screened in or out over the phone and, if screened in, then the agency begins an investigation into the allegations. If the report is substantiated the child may be taken out of the home, and the parents may eventually lose custody. Less draconian measures often include mandatory treatment of psychiatric or substance abuse disorders for both parents and children. These are painful clinical realities, but psychiatrists should not hesitate to file a child abuse report when, in their judgment, they have reason to believe a child is suffering from either abuse or neglect.

## Elder or Disabled Abuse Reporting

Over 40 states have also enacted statutes mandating reporting of abuse or neglect of elderly or disabled individuals. These statutes often mirror the state's child abuse reporting laws, though they may contain broader exceptions to mandated reporting in certain circumstances. The remaining states provide legal immunity for professionals who voluntarily report abuse or neglect of the aged or disabled.

## Child Custody Evaluations

The US has the highest divorce rate in the world, and many children are therefore growing up in nontraditional custody arrangements, whether by agreement or court order (Child Custody Consultation 1982, Uniform Marriage and Divorce Act 1987). In English common law, children were considered to be the property of the father; in the event of divorce, children went with him. As American family law developed, and as the structure of modern economies evolved, mothers were more often seen as the appropriate custodial figures. By the time of the industrial revolution, mothers were accepted as the primary child rearing parent, and were almost always awarded custody in cases of divorce. Changes in the late 20th century economy, as well as evolving societal expectations around fathers' roles, have resulted in much more variation in custodial arrangements, although in the majority of divorces, the mother still retains primary child rearing responsibilities.

Divorce has an impact on all children, but where the parents are unable to agree, especially around custody, children face more stress. Psychiatrists have responded to this burgeoning need by developing expertise in the clinical issues that surround custody decisions. A number of psychiatrists offer consultation and mediation services to divorcing couples who wish to resolve custody issues between themselves. However, when custody disputes become adversarial, formal child custody assessments are often ordered by the court. These assessments present unique clinical, legal, and ethical challenges. The APA has written recommendations for conducting child custody evaluations (Child Custody Consultation 1982).

Psychiatrists performing a child custody evaluation should have training in child work or at least have a child psychiatrist with whom to confer. As with forensic evaluations, the parents (and where appropriate, the child) should be informed that the usual rules of confidentiality and privilege will not apply.

In conducting custody evaluations, it is important to know the legal standard which the court will apply. The standard adopted in many states provides that judges making custody decisions shall "consider all relevant factors including (1) the wishes of the child's parents as to his custody, (2) the wishes of the child as to his custodian, (3) the interaction and interrelationship of the child with his parent or parents, his siblings, and any other persons who may significantly affect the child's best interest, (4) the child's adjustment to his home, school, and community, and (5) the mental and physical health of all individuals involved. The court shall not consider conduct of a proposed custodian that does not affect his relationship to the child" (Child Custody Consultation 1982). The judge is required to balance these factors against the legal standard, which in most states is a "best interests of the child" standard. The psychiatrist should thus conduct the evaluation in such a way as to provide information that will assist the judge in weighing the relevant factors.

## The Americans with Disabilities Act and the Olmstead Case

In 1990, Congress enacted the Americans with Disabilities Act (ADA), with the goal of eliminating discrimination against individuals with disabilities. The Act is divided into four major sections, which prohibit discrimination in employment (Title I), public services provided by government entities (Title II), public accommodations provided by private entities (Title III), and telecommunications (Title IV).

Congress made numerous findings relative to the need for the ADA's protection of the disabled. Of particular relevance to this discussion were three:

[H]istorically, society has tended to isolate and segregate individuals with disabilities, and, despite some improvements, such forms of discrimination against individuals with disabilities continue to be a serious and pervasive social problem;

[D]iscrimination against individuals with disabilities persists in such critical areas as . . . institutionalization, health services, . . . and access to public services;

[I]ndividuals with disabilities continually encounter various forms of discrimination, including outright intentional exclusion, . . . overprotective rules and policies, failure to make modifications to existing facilities and practices, . . . [and] segregation. . . . (Americans with Disabilities Act 1990)

Although discrimination in employment has been the focus of most ADA enforcement activity, advocates for the mentally ill have been litigating under Title II of the ADA, arguing that institutionalization of individuals with mental disabilities who could be appropriately treated in a less restrictive setting constitutes illegal discrimination by the state. The issue came to a head in the case of *Olmstead v. L.C.*, decided by the US Supreme Court in 1999.

Title II of the ADA states that "no qualified individual with a disability" shall be discriminated against by a public entity (such as a state) in the provision of services, programs, or activities. In order to enable such individuals to participate on a par with nondisabled individuals, public entities are required to make "reasonable accommodations" in the operation of services, programs, or activities. Although there is no precise definition of a reasonable accommodation, a state is not required to initiate changes that would amount to a "fundamental alteration" in the service, program, or activity.

Against this background, L.C. and E.W. brought suit against the state of Georgia. L.C. had been hospitalized in 1992 with a diagnosis of mental retardation and schizophrenia. Within a year, her treatment team agreed that she could be adequately treated in a community setting; however, she remained hospitalized until 1996 due to lack of space in an appropriate program. E.W. faced a similar fate. Diagnosed with mental retardation and a personality disorder, she remained hospitalized for over 2 years, even though her team believed she was ready for discharge after just a few months.

The plaintiffs prevailed in the trial court, defeating the state's argument that imposing a requirement of community treatment for these individuals would fundamentally alter the state's system of mental health service provision; the trial court noted that since community treatment can be provided less expensively than institutional care, the "fundamental alteration" argument was unpersuasive.

The federal Court of Appeals upheld the decision, ruling that when "treating professionals find that a community-based placement is appropriate [for an individual with a disability], the ADA imposes a duty to provide treatment in a community setting—the most integrated setting appropriate to that [individual's] needs." The US Supreme Court agreed, ruling that "unjustified isolation is properly regarded as discrimination based on disability."

The Olmstead decision (1999) sent shock waves through state departments of mental health and retardation. Was the Court demanding the dismantling of state mental hospitals and institutions for the mentally retarded? Was every individual with a mental disability entitled to a community placement, regardless of the cost or potential for danger? As with most revolutions, the meaning of the decision is far less draconian, if no less dramatic. Most planners (and even most advocates) agree that the real mandate is that states have a plan or process for moving individuals who can be appropriately treated in the community out of institutional settings, and that there be reasonable progress towards that goal.

For psychiatrists who practice in state institutions, the case is significant for the importance placed on clinical judgment about whether the patient can be adequately treated in a community setting. It is this judgment that triggers the right to community placement under the ADA, according to the Supreme Court. Clinicians making these determinations are confronted with a myriad of sometimes conflicting pressures. Is the patient really ready for the community? What kinds of accommodations might be needed in the standard community programs in order to enable the patient to function? Are these accommodations reasonable? Are there resources to implement them? Will implementing such modifications result in fewer spaces for other patients? What is the role of the clinician in advocating for individual patients versus maximizing scarce resources to benefit the greatest number of patients?

These dilemmas are presented without solutions, for there are no clear answers, but as challenges to those who enter into this vital area of patient care.

## Psychiatric Ethics

Ethics, from the Greek word *ethikos*, meaning customary, or nature, is the study of standards of conduct and moral judgment. These two definitions summarize the core features of ethics. The term customary speaks to the social component of ethics, while nature emphasizes that the actor's own character is an important component. Ethics also refers to the system or code of morals of a particular person, religion, group, or profession (*Webster's* 1980). In recent years, professional ethics have evolved from widely understood principles of etiquette and consideration for dealing with other members of the profession, to sets of rules that govern the relationship between a professional and a client or patient (Kelly 1998). These modern principles are built upon the most ancient ideal of medical ethics: first do no harm.

For psychiatrists, the challenge in ethics is to apply these fundamental principles to the relationships that they form with the patients whom they treat, the colleagues and institutions with whom they interact, and society as a whole. How do individual psychiatrists, and the profession in general, arrive at normative decisions about their professional conduct?

Certain basic assumptions form the framework of psychiatric ethics. Society and the medical profession expect the physician to do the following:

- Deliver competent, compassionate, and respectful care
- Deal honestly with patients and colleagues
- Act within the bounds of the law
- Respect the rights and autonomy of the patient
- Be responsible to the community and society

In psychiatry, these straightforward expectations are fraught with potential for ethical conflict as clinicians are often called upon to opine as to what constitutes healthy behaviors or attitudes. Under the guise of diagnosis and evaluation of illness, psychiatrists (and other mental health professionals) are asked questions ranging from how much pain an individual should endure for the sake of family integrity, to whether an individual should be held culpable for his criminal conduct, to whether the state should restrict access to abortion. While these questions may require the psychiatrist to make medical diagnoses and judgments relative to a patient's need for treatment, they also involve broader personal and social values, values to which psychiatrists can lay no more claim of expertise than the ordinary citizen.

## Sources of Psychiatric Ethics

### Law

Ethics and law are closely related, but they are not synonymous (Ellis 1991). Courts and legislatures attempt to embody ethical principles in their creation and interpretation of law. But not every ethically supportable course of conduct is, or should be, codified in the form of mandatory or prohibitory legal provisions backed up by the government's authority to punish, and not every legal mandate is consistent with medical ethics. In fact, there may be times when a practitioner's ethical decision making may force him or her to violate the law.

### Religion

It is beyond the scope of this chapter to deal comprehensively with the ethical codes established by the world's various religions. Suffice it to say that many ethical decisions that confront psychiatrists have their roots in religion. Indeed, almost to the end of the 19th century, the treatment of mental disorders was conducted, to a great extent, under the auspices of religious institutions or at least in concert with the prevailing religious ideas of the time. The "moral treatment" of the 19th century included prayer and religious guidance as a key element of care (Colp 1989). Today's issues include treatment refusal, abortion, and end of life decisions, among many others. Religion, and psychiatry are closely related, insofar as they both deal intimately with individuals' behaviors and their relationships with other human beings. Psychiatrists must be sensitive to the impact that their own and their patients' religious beliefs have on their understanding of human behavior.

### Professional Associations

One of the hallmark characteristics of a learned profession is its development and adoption of a unique code of ethics to guide its practitioners. The APA has adopted such a code since 1989. Although "psychiatrists are assumed to have the same goals as all physicians," these principles have been revised "with annotations especially applicable to psychiatry." The rationale was that "there are special ethical problems in psychiatric practice that differ in coloring and degree from ethical problems in other branches of medical practice" (Table 112–12).

| Table 112–12   Ethical Principles for Psychiatric Practice | |
|---|---|
| Principles of Medical Ethics: American Medical Association | Annotations Especially Applicable to Psychiatry: American Psychiatric Association |
| "A physician shall be dedicated to providing competent medical service with compassion and respect for human dignity." | 1. The psychiatrist shall be vigilant about the boundaries of the doctor–patient relationship.<br>2. A psychiatrist should not be party to any discriminatory policy.<br>3. It is ethical for a physician to cooperate with peer review.<br>4. A psychiatrist should not be a participant in a legally authorized execution. |
| "A physician shall deal honestly with patients and colleagues, and strive to expose those physicians deficient in character or competence, or who engage in fraud or deception." | 1. Sexual activity with a current or former patient is unethical.<br>2. The psychiatrist should not exploit information furnished by the patient, and should not influence a patient in any way not directly relevant to the treatment goals.<br>3. A psychiatrist should not practice outside his/her area of professional competence.<br>4. When patient welfare is jeopardized by the mental illness of a psychiatrist, it is encouraged for other psychiatrists to intercede.<br>5. The treatment contract should be explicitly established.<br>6. It is ethical to charge for missed appointments within the terms of the treatment contract.<br>7. Fee-splitting arrangements for administration or supervision are not acceptable. |
| "A physician shall respect the law and also recognize a responsibility to seek changes in those requirements which are contrary to the best interests of the patient." | 1. The right to protest social injustices, which may violate certain laws, may not be professionally unethical.<br>2. Where not prohibited by local laws, a qualified psychiatrist may practice acupuncture. |

*Continues*

| Table 112–12 | Ethical Principles for Psychiatric Practice *Continued* |
|---|---|

"A physician shall respect the rights of patients, of colleagues, and of other health professionals, and shall safeguard confidences within the constraints of the law."

1. Psychiatric records must be protected with extreme care. Where information must be released, the welfare of the patient must be a continuing consideration.
2. A psychiatrist may release confidential information only with the authorization of the patient or under proper legal compulsion.
3. Material used in teaching and writing must be adequately disguised.
4. The same responsibility to confidentiality holds for consultations in which the patient was not present and the consultee was not a physician.
5. The psychiatrist may disclose only that information which is relevant to a given situation.
6. When performing nonconfidential examinations, the psychiatrist must reveal the nonconfidential nature of the interview at the outset.
7. The psychiatrist must execute careful judgment in providing or withholding information to the parents of a minor patient.
8. Psychiatrists may reveal confidential information to protect the safety of the patient or the community.
9. When ordered by a court to reveal information, the psychiatrist may ethically dissent within the framework of the law.
10. With informed consent, a patient may be presented to a scientific gathering, with the audience's understanding of the confidentiality of the material.
11. It is ethical to present a patient to the public or news media only with fully informed, written consent.
12. When involved in funded research, the psychiatrist will reveal to patients the source of funding and the nonconfidentiality of data.
13. It is unethical to evaluate a person charged with a crime prior to availability of legal counsel, except if the sole purpose is for medical treatment.
14. Sexual involvement between a teacher or supervisor and a trainee may be abusive of power and unethical.

"A physician shall continue to study, apply and advance scientific knowledge, make relevant information available to patients, colleagues, and the public, obtain consultation, and use the talents of other health professionals when indicated."

1. Psychiatrists are responsible for their own continuing education.
2. The psychiatrist should work respectfully with nonphysician therapists and consultants, and with nonpsychiatric physicians. He/she should not refer to anyone whose training, skill or ethics are in doubt.
3. When supervising or collaborating with another mental health worker, the psychiatrist should expend adequate time to assure that proper care is given.
4. The physician should not delegate to any nonmedical person any matter requiring professional medical judgment.
5. The psychiatrist should agree to the request of a patient for consultation from another clinician.

"A physician shall, in the provision of appropriate patient care, except in emergencies, be free to choose whom to serve, with whom to associate, and the environment in which to provide medical services."

1. Preservation of optimal conditions for the development of a sound working relationship should take highest precedence. Professional courtesy may lead to poor psychiatric care.
2. A psychiatrist may refuse to provide psychiatric treatment to a person who cannot be diagnosed as having a mental illness amenable to psychiatric treatment.

"A physician shall recognize a responsibility to participate in activities contributing to an improved community."

1. Psychiatrists are encouraged to serve society by advising and consulting with government agencies. In so doing, the psychiatrist should clarify whether he/she speaks as an individual or a representative of an organization. Personal opinions should not be cloaked with the authority of the profession.
2. Psychiatrists may share with the public their expertise in psychosocial issues that may affect mental health and illness.
3. It is unethical for a psychiatrist to offer a public professional opinion regarding someone he/she has not personally examined, or without proper authorization.
4. The psychiatrist may permit his/her certification to be used for involuntary treatment of a person only following a personal examination.

*Source*: Adapted from American Psychiatric Association (1993) The Principles of Medical Ethic With Annotations Especially Applicable to Psychiatry. APA, Washington DC.

| Table 112–13 | Guidelines on Confidentiality of the American Psychiatric Association |
| --- | --- |

- Children and adolescents should be informed about what information will be kept private and what may be shared with parents or guardians. Information needed for the proper care of a child should be shared with the responsible adults.
- When performing evaluations on behalf of a third party (e.g., court, employer), the individual should be informed of the limits of confidentiality. The psychiatrist should report only material relevant to the purpose of the request.
- The psychiatrist may keep private work notes separate from the official medical record, but these are not protected from disclosure in all jurisdictions.
- Nonmedical agencies, including insurers, are not bound by the same ethical codes of confidentiality as health professionals. Care should be exercised in material released to such agencies.
- The sharing of clinical information among members of a treatment team does not require authorization. Recipients of the information should be reminded of their obligation to confidentiality.
- Physician–patient privilege, protecting clinical material from disclosure in judicial proceedings, is the property of the patient, not the doctor, and may only be waived by the patient or his/her legal representative.
- When the process of involuntary civil commitment is insufficient to remove eventual danger to a third party, the psychiatrist may be held responsible for taking steps to notify and protect the endangered party.

*Source*: Adapted from American Psychiatric Association (1989) Guidelines on Confidentiality. APA, Washington DC.

The APA has also issued a number of formal guidelines intended to direct the ethical conduct of its members in concrete circumstances. Both the general public and the courts assume that psychiatrists have agreed to follow and be held accountable to these guidelines; thus, even without formal government imprimatur, these ethical guidelines carry significant authority. The APA's *Guidelines on Confidentiality* (1989) are particularly noteworthy (Table 112–13).

## Potential Consequences of Diagnostic Labels

Diagnoses of mental disorders carry implications that are different from diagnoses of purely somatic illnesses, in part because of the societal stigma attached to mental illness. This stigma has ancient roots. Humankind attaches great power to the mind but finds it deeply mysterious. One of the worst fears is the loss of control of meaningful communication, decision-making ability, and intellectual capacity (Trad 1991). Even accepting the medical model that grants validity to the diagnosis of mental disorders, the psychiatrist still faces ethical tensions in making such diagnoses.

Because confidentiality is not absolute, a patient's diagnosis is available to many parties, with practical consequences. Opportunities to obtain employment or insurance may be constrained by the documented presence of a psychiatric illness. Conversely, such a diagnosis may make tangible assistance and subsidies available based on the psychiatrist's assessment of the patient's disability. The clinician performing an evaluation is obliged to pay attention to any internal prejudices about patients' entitlements and to perform the assessment as fairly as possible. Another

realm of prejudice that can enter the diagnostic arena relates to cultural perceptions of behavior. Although there is abundant statistical validity to the diagnostic schema of the DSM-IV, its validity is based on the norms of the majority culture. Patients who are members of cultural minority groups may express distress in ways that are inappropriately labeled as diagnosable psychopathology (Siantz 1993).

## Ethics and Patient–Therapist Boundaries

There are abundant clinical reasons for maintaining clear and predictable boundaries in the patient's relationship to the psychiatrist. Among other justifications, a clear therapeutic framework makes the psychotherapeutic environment one in which the patient can feel safe to disclose sensitive information without fear of punishment, and in which the care received is not dependent on the patient's meeting the needs or earning the approval of the caregiver. The ethical dimensions of the physician–patient boundary have their roots at least as far back as the Oath of Hippocrates in the 4th century BC:

Into whatever houses I enter I will go into them for the benefit of the sick and will abstain from every voluntary act of mischief and corruption and further from the seduction of females or males, of freemen and slaves (Edelstein 1943).

Maintaining the principles of respect, honesty, and autonomy of patients, all major organizations of medical and mental health professionals specifically condemn sexual contact between physicians or therapists and their patients, regardless of the form or intensity of the psychiatric treatment being provided. The ethical background for this blanket prohibition stems from the nature of the therapeutic relationship. Although many of the features of the psychiatrist–patient relationship are the same as those that exist with any other physician, there are some specific facets of the psychiatric alliance that lend the issue particular distinction.

The patient enters the relationship in pain and is therefore vulnerable. Not infrequently, issues of unresolved feelings about sexuality, intimacy, and dependence may be part of the problem brought to the psychiatrist. The psychiatrist is seen by society, and usually by the patient, as possessing education, authority, and experience. Therefore, there is an imbalance of power in the relationship from the beginning. Because the patient has brought his or her problem to the trusted psychiatrist with the expectation of assistance, courts and society have maintained that the therapeutic alliance constitutes a fiduciary relationship, wherein the psychiatrist is obliged to act scrupulously in the patient's best interests, eschewing any personal advantage (Carr and Robinson 1990, Strasburger et al. 1992).

This absolute prohibition, however, has not yielded absolute abstinence. Numerous surveys conducted from the mid-1970s through the late 1980s found that 7 to 10% of male therapists and 2 to 3% of female therapists admitted to erotic contact with patients (Strasburger et al. 1992). Rarely does sexual contact with patients occur in isolation. Rather, it usually represents the last in a series of steps eroding the professional and clinical boundaries of therapy. The earlier steps may include extending sessions beyond the usual time, scheduling a patient for an hour when no one else is in the office or clinic, meeting the patient for meals or elsewhere outside the treatment setting, and accepting invitations that place the therapist and patient in intimate social situations. Such compromises erode the structure that is necessary for therapy to be a healing process and pave the way for a destructive relationship. Although even the most neurotic romance outside therapy may promote a person's growth, sexual contacts with therapists rarely do. Instead, anger, guilt, shame, mistrust, and confusion are the common result. Clinical depression, anxiety, dissociative events, and suicide are all risks (Appelbaum and Jorgenson 1991).

There is little disagreement in the field about the need for sexual abstinence after the termination of therapy. A minority hold that the power imbalance inherent in the therapeutic contract no longer pertains, and there is no potential to use the withdrawal of care as coercion. In completed therapy, transference distortion should be a much less powerful element (Sapir 1992). Most maintain, however, that the fiduciary obligation does not end with the termination of therapy; that transference, despite the most intense and successful analysis, never disappears; that the therapist always maintains the power of confidences divulged in the treatment; and that a therapist who begins any therapy without having first excluded the possibility of any future sexual contact with the patient may be seen as lying in wait for the opportunity to exploit (Murphy 1992). The consensus of practitioners and ethicists remains that, "Once a patient, always a patient."

## Ethics of Psychiatric Research

The conduct of psychiatric research often presents a paradox with troubling ethical ramifications. In many circumstances, particularly in clinical investigations, worthwhile research that is primarily intended to benefit individuals with mental illnesses as a group demands that the human subjects taking part in the protocols themselves be drawn from the ranks of the mentally ill community. In some situations, there simply are not acceptable substitutes for persons with mental illness as human subjects if we expect any real progress in ameliorating devastating psychiatric problems. The central dilemma, of course, is that the very psychiatric illness that makes an individual a desirable, even necessary, subject for a particular research project may compromise that individual's own capacity to give voluntary, informed, and competent consent to research participation. No subjects may be involved in research unless legally effective informed consent has been obtained and it is clear that undue influence and coercion are eliminated. For instance, it should be clear to the subject whether he/she can be reasonably expected to benefit from the study or not, and that the subject can stop participation at any time without affecting his/her clinical treatment.

The best research asks a specific and relevant question that will advance the field of knowledge, has a hypothesis, and has an investigator who has thoughtfully considered the risks of the study for subjects and the process for obtaining informed consent. The investigator presents the study to an Institutional Review Boards (IRB) which is comprised of institutionally-appointed assessors of risk and informed consent. IRBs have membership from the consumer community, the scientific community, and others.

This diverse membership adds perspectives that can be brought to bear on the ethical questions that come up in a study when the subjects are psychiatrically ill. For instance, the IRB may consider whether a person with schizophrenia can be expected to interpret the risks and idea of the study in a way that is accurate. IRBs are free to reject research, to amend the informed consent procedure, and to demand additional protections for the subjects. Although IRBs are a legally mandated check, which can also provide resources on the ethics of research, the responsibility for conducting ethical research lies with the investigator.

Research that may violate the ancient principle "first do no harm" falls into a special category of ethical dilemmas. For instance, in order to advance the medication therapy of schizophrenia, trials must be done that expose human subjects to risks. Even within this broad category, there are dimensions of risk that require additional scrutiny. For instance, in Massachusetts, "challenge tests" (e.g., the use of a compound to worsen symptoms in order to understand the mechanism of the symptom) are not approved by the Department of Mental Health IRB, because the risk of worsening a subject's condition is judged ethically to exceed the potential benefit. A less risky, but still difficult area involves the use of placebo controls, where patients are taken off their medications and are given placebo. Massachusetts has developed strict guidelines for the use of placebo-controlled medication studies, given the risks involved in that type of study.

An area of psychiatric research that is ethically challenging, and which may grow over time, is the question of whether early psychopharmacological intervention in young persons who show signs of psychiatric illness will have a preventative benefit that outweighs the long-term risks of the medications. This balancing takes place at a time when our ability to predict likely long-term course of early psychiatric symptoms is limited: How ill will this person become? Knowing that a 17-year-old has had a psychotic episode does not mean he or she has, or will develop, schizophrenia. Yet if we could predict with greater accuracy whether he or she will in fact develop the disease, then intervening very early would be less ethically challenging. As technology advances there may be more activity in this compelling but ethically complex area.

## Ethics and Suicide

Much has been written about the ethics of suicide (Heyd and Bloch 1991), and a number of philosophers, as well as physicians, have argued that suicide may be rational under some circumstances. Although US society no longer criminalizes attempted suicide, neither does it condone it. Thus, the strong current weight of ethical opinion, based on a commitment to the sanctity of life, is that usually psychiatrists ought to intervene to prevent or disrupt suicide attempts by patients. Further, according to this view, the psychiatrist's duty to intervene may justify a breach of the ordinary obligation of confidentiality (see earlier discussion) and initiation of involuntary commitment and forced treatment proceedings because of the patient's danger to self. Yet the obligation to respect the patient's autonomy requires the psychiatrist to ask whether the intent to commit suicide in a particular case is sick and justifying— even mandating—intervention or whether it is a rational decision with which the physician has no ethical justification to interfere.

In a related vein, much debate has emerged in the past few years surrounding the ethical permissibility of physician-assisted suicide (Quill 1991). Advocates for permissibility cite unbearable pain as a justification and submit that a regimen of procedural safeguards could adequately ensure against abuse (Quill 1993). Among these safeguards would be the presence of a terminal or disabling condition from which there is no reasonable likelihood of recovery, the existence of an ongoing physician–patient relationship, a patient capable of making decisions, and repeated and unequivocal requests by the patient for the physician's assistance in hastening death. Several initiatives that would allow such practice under controlled circumstances have appeared on state ballots in the US. At the time of this writing, such an initiative has been approved only in Oregon.

## Ethical Dimensions of Health System Changes

The US health care system, including its mental health components, exists in a tremendous state of turbulence and flux at the beginning of the 21st century. The continuing quest for simultaneous achievement of the three goals of quality, accessibility, and affordability continues to frustrate health policy-makers in both public and private sectors. This quest has resulted in dramatic changes in the structure of our health care delivery system, with the growing replacement of fee-for-service professionals and institutions by large managed care networks. These structural and operational changes are radically altering the financial incentives that influence provider behavior by rewarding cost containment, rather than generous provision of services.

Ethical dilemmas abound when money meets the duty to the patient. For instance a common concern today among child psychiatrists is whether to accept third party insurance at all. Because there is national shortage of practitioners in this important area, many find they have plenty of work even if they accept no insurance. Yet this restricts practice to upper income people. Do child psychiatrists—trained in part with public funding—have an obligation to serve as many children as possible, from as many walks of life as possible? When the administrative demands of managed care seem to encroach on clinical practice, should the clinician walk away from the system in frustration or protest? Or should he/she remain and provide the necessary services, while seeking change from within the system?

The proper ethical stance of the psychiatrist in a changing health system is not clear, but the psychiatrist ought to be clear whether he/she is acting as a doctor or citizen. Doctors ethically and zealously advocate for getting whatever they feel is in the best interests for their patients. This may be done without regard for the bigger picture of resource allocation. For the doctor, the patient comes first.

As citizens, however, psychiatrists also have a responsibility. Society makes determinations of how big the pool of resources will be, what illnesses are covered under insurance, and how much a clinician will be paid. Public policy decisions get made every day about mental health care and its funding. Psychiatrists have a unique perspective and expertise on the consequences of these decisions, and in their citizen and public policy role will do well to participate in the difficult and ethically challenging work of creating and influencing policy decisions affecting their patients, profession, and society.

## Conclusion

Psychiatrists can anticipate further developments in the clinical/legal interface, and that ethical challenges will be a core element of the work. This chapter has attempted to outline the most relevant legal and ethical issues and principles facing psychiatrists today. Many of these principles, such as society's value of individual liberty, are stable, and will endure throughout the entire careers of today's students. Others are in flux, such as the balance between confidentiality and public safety. Still others have yet to be identified and are unforeseen. As psychiatrists try to implement the ancient ethical principle, *first do no harm*, in today's complex legal, social, and financial environment, continued education and reflection in all these areas will be required of all of us.

## References

Addington v. Texas, 441 US 418, 99 S C1 1804 (1979).
Allen M and Smith VF (2001) Opening Pandora's box: The practical and legal dangers of involuntary outpatient commitment. Psychiatr Serv 52(3) (Mar), 342–346.
American Psychiatric Association (1980) Guidelines for psychiatrists in consultative, supervisory, or collaborative relationships with nonmedical therapists. Am J Psychiatr, 1489–1491.
American Psychiatric Association (1989) Guidelines on Confidentiality. APA, Washington DC.
American Psychiatric Association (1993) The Principles of Medical Ethics with Annotations Especially Applicable to Psychiatry. APA, Washington DC.
American Psychiatric Association (1994) Diagnostic and Statistical Manual of Mental Disorders, 4th ed. APA, Washington DC.
Americans with Disabilities Act (1990) Congressional Findings, 42 USC 12101(a).
Appelbaum PS (1988) The right to refuse treatment with antipsychotic medications: Retrospect and prospect. Am J Psychiatr 145, 413–419.
Appelbaum PS (2001) Thinking carefully about outpatient commitment. Psychiatr Serv 52(3) (Mar), 347–350.
Appelbaum PS and Grisso T (1988) Assessing patients' capacities to consent to treatment. New Engl J Med 319, 1635–1638.
Appelbaum PS and Gutheil TG (2000) Clinical Handbook of Psychiatry and the Law. Williams & Wilkins, Baltimore (for a detailed discussion of the concept of confidentiality, see pp. 1–13).
Appelbaum PS and Hoge SK (1986) The right to refuse treatment: What the research reveals. Behav Sci Law 4, 279–292.
Appelbaum PS and Jorgenson L (1991) Psychotherapist–patient sexual contact after termination of treatment: An analysis and a proposal. Am J Psychiatr 148, 1466–1473.
Birnbaum M (1960) The right to treatment. Am Bar Assoc J 46, 499.
Birnbaum M (1965) Some comments on "the right to treatment." Arch Gen Psychiatr 13, 34–45.
Canterbury v. Spence, 150 US App DC 263, 464 F2d 772 (1972).
Carr M and Robinson GE (1990) Fatal attraction: The ethical and clinical dilemma of patient–therapist sex. Can J Psychiatr 35, 122–127.
Child Custody Consultation (1982) American Psychiatric Press, Washington DC.
Clites v. Iowa, 322 NW2d 917 (1982).
Colorado v. Connelly, 479 US 157, 107 S Ct 515 (1986).
Colp R (1989) History of psychiatry. In Comprehensive Textbook of Psychiatry, Kaplan HI and Sadock BJ (eds). Williams & Wilkins, Baltimore, pp. 2132–2153.
Dillon v. Legg, 68 Cal2d 728, 441 P2d 912 (1968).
Doe v. Roe, 400 NY Supp 2d 668 (1977).
Durham v. US., 94 US App DC 228, 214 F2d 862 (1954).
Dusky v. United States, 362 US 402, 80 S Ct 788 (1960).

Dymek v. Nyquist, 128 Ill App3d 859 (App Ct 1984).

Edelstein L (1943) The Hippocratic Oath: Test, Translation, and Interpretation. Johns Hopkins University Press, Baltimore.

Elliott RL, Nelson E, Fitch WL, et al. (1993) Informed decision making in persons acquitted not guilty by reason of insanity. Bull Am Acad Psychiatr Law 21, 309–320.

Ellis T (1991) The nature of morality. In Ethical Issues in Mental Health Care, Barker PJ and Baldwin S (eds). Chapman & Hall, London, pp. 13–26.

Guardianship of Richard Roe III, 383 Mass 415, 421 NE2d 40 (1981).

Gutheil TG (1994) Personal communication, for a detailed discussion of the concept of privilege, see pp. 14–17 of Appelbaum and Gutheil, see footnote 31.

Gutheil TG and Duckworth K (1992) The psychiatrist as informed consent technician: A problem for the professions. Bull Menninger Clin 56, 87–94.

Gutheil TG, Bursztajn H, and Brodsky A (1984) supra, note 33.

Gutheil TG, Bursztajn H, and Brodsky A (1984) Malpractice prevention through the sharing of uncertainty: Informed consent and the therapeutic alliance. New Engl J Med 311, 49–51.

Gutheil TG, Bursztajn H, and Brodsky A (1986) The multidimensional assessment of dangerousness: Competence assessment in patient care and liability prevention. Bull Am Acad Psychiatr Law 14, 123–129.

Hampton RL and Newberger EH (1985) Child abuse incidence and reporting by hospitals: Significance of severity, class, and race. Am J Publ Health 75, 56–60.

Heyd D and Bloch S (1991) The ethics of suicide. In Psychiatric Ethics, 2nd ed., Bloch S and Chodoff P (eds). Oxford Medical Publications, New York., pp. 243–264.

Jackson v. Indiana, 406 US 715, 92 S Ct 1845 (1972).

Kelly Kevin V (1998) Psychiatric Times, Vol. 15(6).

Kempe CH, Silverman FN, Steele BF, et al. (1962) The battered child syndrome. JAMA 181, 17–24.

Lake v. Cameron, 124 US App DC 264, 364 F2d 657 (1966).

Linda Cocchiarella and Gunnar BJ Andersson (eds) (2001) Guides to the Evaluation of Permanent Impairment, 5th ed. American Medical Association, Chicago.

M'Naghten's Case, 8 Eng Rep 718, 8 Eng Rep 722 (1843).

Massachusetts General Laws, Chapter 111, section 70F.

McGarry AL, Curran WJ, et al. (1973) Competency to Stand Trial and Mental Illness. National Institute of Mental Health, Rockville, MD.

Model Penal Code (1955) American Law Institute, Philadelphia, 401.1(1).

Murphy GE (1992) Psychotherapist–patient sexual contact after termination of therapy. Am J Psychiatr 149, 985–986.

Natanson v. Kline, 186 Kan 393, 350 P2d 1093 (1960).

O'Connor v. Donaldson, 422 US 563, 95 S Ct 2486 (1975).

Olmstead v. L.C., 527 US 581 (1999).

Osheroff v. Chestnut Lodge, 490 A2d 720 (Md App 1985).

Quill T (1991) Death and dignity: A case of individualized decision making. New Engl J Med 324, 691–694.

Quill T (1993) Death and Dignity: Making Choices and Taking Charge. WW Norton, New York.

Rappeport JR (1982) Differences between forensic and general psychiatry. Am J Psychiatr 139, 331–334.

Rennie v. Klein, 720 F2d 266 (3d Circ 1983).

Rex v. Arnold, 16 How St Tr 695 (1724).

Rogers v. Commissioner, 390 Mass 489, 458 NE2d 308 (1983).

Rouse v. Cameron, 125 US App DC 366, 373 F2d 451 (1966).

Sapir PE (1992) Patient–therapist sexual contact after termination of treatment. Am J Psychiatr 149, 984.

Siantz ML (1993) The stigma of mental illness on children of color. J Child Adolesc Psychiatr Merit Health Nurs 6, 10–17.

Slawson P (1989) Psychiatric malpractice: Ten years loss experience. Med Law 8, 415–527.

Slobogin C (1985) The guilty but mentally ill verdict: An idea whose time should not have come. George Wash Law Rev 53, 494–527.

Special section on APA's Model Commitment Law (1985) Hosp Comm Psychiatr 36, 966–989.

Steadman HJ, et al. (2001) Assessing the New York City Involuntary Outpatient Commitment Pilot Program. Psychiatr Serv 52 (Mar) 3, 330–336.

Stone A (1984) Law, Psychiatry, and Morality. American Psychiatric Press, Washington DC, p. 89.

Stone AA (1985) A response to comments on APA's Model Commitment Law. Hosp Comm Psychiatr 36, 984–989.

Strasburger LH, Jorgenson L, and Sutherland P (1992) The prevention of psychotherapist sexual misconduct: Avoiding the slippery slope. Am J Psychother 46, 544–555.

Superintendent of Belchertown v. Saikowicz, 373 Mass 728, 370 NE2d 417 (1977).

Swartz MS, et al. (2001) A randomized controlled trial of outpatient commitment in North Carolina. Psychiatr Serv 52 (Mar)(3), 325–329.

Tarasoff v. Regents, 17 Ca 3d 425, 551 P2d 334, 131 Cal Rptr 14 (1976).

Torrey EF and Zdanowicz M (2001) Outpatient commitment: What, why, and for whom? Psychiatr Serv 52(3), (Mar) 337–341.

Trad PV (1991) The ultimate stigma of mental illness. Am J Psychother 45, 463–466.

Truman v. Thomas, 27 Cal3d 285, 611 P2d 902 (1980).

Uniform Marriage and Divorce Act 1987, Uniform Laws Annotated, Vol. 9A. West Publishing Company, St. Paul, MN.

Von Staden H. (trans) (1996) "In a pure and holy way": Personal and professional conduct in the hippocratic oath. J His Med Allied Sci 51, 406–408.

Washington v. Harper, 494 US 210; 110 S Ct 1028 (1990).

Webster's New World Dictionary (1980) 2nd College Edition.

Wickline v. State, 192 Cal App3d 1630, 239 Cal Rptr 810 (1987).

Wilson v. Blue Cross, 222 Cal App3d 660, 271 Cal Rptr 876 (1990).

Wyatt v. Stickney, 344 F Supp 387 (MD Ala 1972).

Youngberg v. Romeo, 457 US 307, 102 S Ct 2452 (1982).

Zinermon v. Burch, 494 US 113, 110 S Ct 975 (1990).

# 113 ● Serving Homeless People with Mental Illness

Hunter L. McQuistion
Alan Felix
Ezra S. Susser

A broad shift in the American economy away from a manufacturing base, combined with related housing short-falls, ushered into the 1980s a social epidemic of home-lessness that continues today (Koegel et al. 1988, US Conference 2001). It has swept the mentally ill into particular vulnerability and public attention. This section reviews the historical evolution of services for mentally ill homeless people and describes a resultant model of care, accentuating psychiatry's role.

## Background: The Evolution of Services

The plight of mentally ill homeless people prompted an evolution of specialized services for them that is understandable in terms of three phases that are demarcated by gradual developments at the federal, state, and local levels.

## Phase One: Ad Hoc Service Delivery and Early Epidemiology (1978–1986)

In November 1978, the advocacy group Community for Creative Nonviolence occupied the National Visitor's Center in Washington DC. This protest was a touchstone moment, bringing into focus a "new" national crisis of homelessness and creating a context for events that quickly unfolded across the country. Although there were already scattered reports of a new generation of mentally ill "street people," by 1981 scholars and social activists around the country were describing an overwhelmed constellation of shelters and soup kitchens that were lodging more and more people with psychiatric disorders (Baxter and Hopper 1981). The appearance of homelessness, juxtaposed with an emerging low-income housing shortage and the decline of census in hospitals, led some observers to cite this epidemic among the mentally ill as an unforeseen by-product of deinstitutionalization (Lamb 1984a, 1984b). For example, in 1970 there were 413,066 beds in state and county mental hospitals in the US. By 1988, these had diminished to 119,033 and by 1998, the decline had continued to 63,526 (Manderscheid et al. 2000).

Population data and funding for needed mental health services were scant or nonexistent and effective methods of service delivery had yet to be developed, and until 1986 there were virtually no federal funds allocated for service delivery. Without adequate information on how to construct a rational service system or federal funding to support services, localities funded programs in an ad hoc manner. While some communities used limited local funds to develop programs, others sought legal remedies to force the homeless off the streets—or out of town (Simon 1996). Almost all municipalities had huge service gaps and most had no services at all (see Table 113–1).

The patchwork of mental health services that were implemented included a few street outreach programs and mental health services grafted onto preexisting shelters, mission houses, and soup kitchens (Axleroad and Toff 1987). These early programs run by community-based organizations (CBOs) focused on food, clothing, and a place to sleep as first steps toward medical and psychiatric treatment.

There was growing professional attention to the kinds of services needed to engage homeless clients, as evidenced by recommendations of the APA Task Force on the Homeless Mentally Ill for outreach, assertive treatment, rehabilitation, and housing (Lamb and Talbott 1986). Despite this, there were no financial, legal, or other incentives to promote change in medical environ-

| Table 113–1 | Factors Contributing to the Growth of the Homeless SMI Population |
|---|---|
| Low-income housing shortages | |
| Declining state hospital census/deinstitutionalization | |
| Paucity of mental health professionals working in nontraditional settings, | |
| Limited federal and local funding | |

| Table 113-2 | Initial Responses to Increasing Numbers of Homeless Patients with Serious Mental Illness |
|---|---|
| Outreach | |
| Shelters, mission homes, soup kitchens | |
| Private grant funding initiatives | |
| Increased state and local resources | |

ments. There were very few psychiatrists working in nontraditional settings, and it was increasingly clear that traditional psychiatric providers, such as community mental health centers and hospitals, had largely failed to adequately engage mentally ill homeless patients (Cohen et al. 1984).

So, to begin to help address huge service gaps, in 1986 the Robert Wood Johnson/Pew Health care for the Homeless initiative was funded (Goldman et al. 1994). This key early initiative began to bring integrated health care to many homeless people across the country, with a few of its programs providing mental health services.

Simultaneously, state and local resources began to fund homelessness studies (Morse et al. 1985, Roth et al. 1985, Struening 1986) and enterprising investigators piggybacked such studies onto other efforts. Toward the end of this phase, a series of well-designed research projects (Susser et al. 1993) contributed the first epidemiological database on the scope of homelessness, the risk factors for it, and potential for preventive strategies (Susser et al. 1987, Belcher 1988, Weitzman et al. 1992). Reliable studies describing psychiatric disorder show reasonably consistent rates ranging between a third and a half of homeless people with psychiatric disorders, either major mood disorder (20–30%) or schizophrenia (10–15%) (Roth et al. 1985, Koegel et al. 1988, Breakey et al. 1989, Susser et al. 1989). Likewise, investigators reported rates of substance and alcohol abuse from 20 to 30% and 57 to 63%, respectively (Koegel et al. 1988, Fischer et al. 1986, Vernez et al. 1988), with the phenomenon of dual diagnosis of chemical dependence and mental illness beginning to receive attention (Drake et al. 1991). Table 113–2 lists the initial service responses described above.

## Phase Two: Service Development (1987–1993) (See Table 113–3)

The Stuart McKinney Homelessness Relief Act of 1987 marked Phase Two. Signifying a national recognition of the intransigence of homelessness, it set up an interagency governmental council to administer an appropriation in its first year of $350 million (adjusted to 2001 dollars) to support food, housing, education, shelter, medical care,

and mental health services (Foscarinis 1996). In fiscal year 2000, this had increased to $1.2 billion. Demonstration projects integrating housing, intensive case management, and mental health treatment were established in nine geographically dispersed cities.

The introduction of new funding streams reinforced the development of programs for the mentally ill homeless that had by then begun in many urban areas. The greatest innovation came from staffs of nonprofit CBOs which had both the administrative flexibility and an history of working in nontraditional settings to enable them to transition to service delivery for mentally ill homeless people (Dincin et al. 1995, American Psychiatric Association 1997). Conversely, traditional settings, like hospitals and clinics continued to show limited inclination to meet the service needs of the mentally ill homeless. However, there were exceptions, and a few hospitals experimented with shelter-based services (Caton et al. 1990). New York's Bellevue Hospital created a specialized admission and inpatient service in conjunction with a state hospital and an innovative street outreach team (Katz et al. 1993). So, as Phase Two developed beyond a few well-funded model programs that included psychiatry, most care was explored by only a few motivated psychiatrists, largely on their own initiative (Cohen et al. 1984, Arce et al. 1983, Lipton et al. 1983, Susser et al. 1990) and often on a volunteer basis (American Psychiatric Association 1986, 1991a).

Research did continue to develop through this phase. Under McKinney funding, research dollars grew through NIMH and other federal sources and a crucial series of clinical trials were undertaken to test strategies for relief of the homeless among mentally ill individuals. The publication of the findings would appear in the next phase of care.

## Phase Three: Refined and Elaborated Services (1993–Present) (See Table 113–4)

Into the new century, the epidemic of homelessness has developed to an endemic status that has surged again during economic recession. Although on a local level the picture widely varies, some communities have tacitly acknowledged the endemic nature of homelessness by creating bureaucracies for services to homeless people. In 1993, for example, New York City created its Department of Homeless Services to oversee and manage programming in a large municipal shelter system.

Much of the research of Phase Three has represented an extension of the epidemiological base already established and developed. However, four new developments that further underscore the social permanence of homelessness merit noting.

First, research has emerged indicating that homelessness is more prevalent than had been understood even by

| Table 113-3 | Evolution of Service Development (1987–1993) |
|---|---|
| Federal funding | |
| Nonprofit, community based organizations | |
| Paucity of organized psychiatry | |
| Increasing research dollars | |

| Table 113-4 | The Need for Enhancing Services for Homeless Individuals with Mental Illness: 1993–Present |
|---|---|
| Mounting numbers of homeless families | |
| Escalating medical problems (TB/HIV/HepC) | |
| Limited rehabilitation focus (ACT or supported housing) | |

some advocates. Two milestone studies independently estimated that approximately 3% of Americans experienced homelessness in a previous 5-year period (Culhane et al. 1994, Link et al. 1994). Second, the frequency with which families are afflicted by homelessness was brought to greater attention (Rosenheck et al. 1994). Families now represent about one-third of the homeless population, and in many regions, are the fastest growing segment (US Conference 2001). About 8% of adolescents are also thought to experience at least one night of homelessness (Ringwalt et al. 1998). Third, the emergence of high rates of HIV and TB among homeless populations in general, but also specifically among the mentally ill homeless, has been documented. These epidemics have contributed to mortality as well as to the complexity of clinical care.

Finally, during Phase Three, services research has begun the search for evidence-based technologies. Assertive community treatment (Lehman et al. 1997), critical time intervention (Susser et al. 1997), and supported employment (Bond et al. 2001) are examples of services under exploration. Without effective rehabilitative intervention, mentally ill homeless people lose housing and often occupy a closed circuit between shelters, hospitals and, more than ever, incarceration (Hopper et al. 1997).

As part of this initiative and encouraged by epidemiological research, federal and local agencies have begun to understand the value of more systematic approaches to care. In 1994, the US Department of Housing and Urban Development began requiring its housing grantees to provide a "continuum of care" (Barnard Columbia Center 1996). McKinney funding made possible the multicenter Access to Community Care and Effective Services (ACCESS) program, a major initiative testing local models of integrated service (Calloway and Morrissey 1998).

### The Stages of Care (See Table 113–5)

Through these phases of evolution in services, a method of engagement and reintegration of mentally ill homeless people has emerged. It is useful to consider this methodology as a transitional, stage-wise process from the street (Susser et al. 1992), eventually leading to housing, work, and the possibility of reestablishing lost social ties. The current conceptualization of these stages is described in terms of (1) *engagement*, (2) *intensive care*, and (3) *ongoing rehabilitation*. Although these rehabilitative stages might apply to people who are not homeless, they take on a primary application with homeless people, especially considering an often prolonged engagement and usually very complex treatment process.

Within the stages there exists a continuum of services and technologies that are themselves on different levels of development. Furthermore, as we describe below, in most cases care actually begins prior to any contact with mental health professionals, especially psychiatrists.

| Table 113–5 | Stages of Care |
|---|---|
| Engagement | |
| Intensive care | |
| Ongoing rehabilitation | |

| Table 113–6 | Engagement |
|---|---|
| Street outreach | |
| Outreach in shelter/drop-in settings | |
| Harm reduction focus | |
| Education | |
| Crisis intervention | |

### Engagement (See Table 113–6)

Traditionally, the first point in the continuum of services is street outreach. Street outreach programs were among the earliest novel interventions in the development of homelessness services, responding to the need to engage a very disaffiliated population of potential clients. Teams of human services workers, many of whom themselves have histories of homelessness, gently but persistently approach and engage homeless people in public spaces, offering incentives like food, clothing, and an open mind for listening (McQuistion et al. 1991). Gradually, they establish sufficient trust such that a homeless individual agrees to take a risk to stay indoors at a shelter or to attend a drop-in center where they may find meals, showers, and daytime services. This process usually takes between a matter of weeks to a year or more. The street population is generally regarded as particularly disabled and alienated and the outreach process is very labor-intensive, requiring many short, usually apparently casual, helping interactions to achieve engagement and to provide service.

Alternatively, some mentally ill homeless people are first encountered in shelter or drop-in settings. Some individuals find their way to shelter after a precipitating personal crisis, while others have been referred to or accompanied by street outreach teams that are connected with the facility. At the point of arrival at an indoor setting there is potential opportunity for multidisciplinary intensive care described later, but early interactions indoors also often require outreach while workers concentrate on establishing trust. Relationships are hard-won, and they require patience and flexibility, even tolerating a person's self-destructive behavior that may, for example, include drug or alcohol dependence. At this stage, a harm-reduction approach to substance abuse, or risky lifestyle (e.g., sex work) is practical (Marlatt 1996). Appropriate techniques include respectfully educating a person about risks, about the "side effects" of using street drugs—like never having money or suffering psychological and other health effects, including trauma from a rough lifestyle. In this manner, a goal during engagement is to move a person from a position of "precontemplation" of drug and alcohol use to contemplating change (Prochaska et al. 1992), illuminating alternatives and beginning to help lift him or her from a condition of personal demoralization (Frank and Frank 1991).

Simultaneously, a challenge exists of balancing these approaches with being able to respond decisively to a crisis or risk to community safety (Diamond 1996). Mental health professionals, usually psychiatrists who are working in street or shelter settings, must be able to recognize and respond to emergencies that require involuntary transport to an emergency room, and they must have the means at the service center and in the community for emergency rescue. Some mental health outreach teams are empowered to involuntarily transport people to a hospital (Cohen et al. 1984). When judiciously employed, this work is humane and potentially lifesaving, and may offer new opportunities for engagement. There is ongoing debate about whether ultimate community reintegration can actually be achieved through such coercive means, yet psychiatry, especially, has a unique responsibility in clinical decisions concerning involuntary treatments. In our view, there is a continuum of leverage, and clinical coercion ranges from involuntary hospitalization to subtler forms, as when a service provider is representative payee of a person's entitlements or when it imposes delays in referrals to patients who are not yet addressing substance abuse. In these cases, the fulcrum of successful leverage is usually the clinical alliance, with the patient's understanding that there is something advantageous in a continuing relationship. This further highlights the critical nature of initial engagement.

## Intensive Care

At a point when a person tolerates services rendered indoors, workers begin the stage of intensive care. The most successful programs integrate the disciplines of social work, rehabilitation, internal medicine, psychiatry, and peer support, all working collaboratively. They focus on indoor living skills, which include activities of daily living, money management, and planning longer-term goals. In these settings, case managers frequently negotiate complex service systems, creating service linkages with their clients, such as pursuing medical insurance and disability benefits, exploring vocational rehabilitation, and initiating the search for housing. They work hard with their homeless clients while carefully respecting their autonomy, fine-tuning interventions as clients are prepared to receive them (Table 113–7).

There is discussion within the field concerning the point at which a person becomes ready for housing. A traditional position is that a person must not only attain benefits, but must be viewed as clinically stable and as having achieved sobriety. Some challenge this perspective by citing factors such as the ubiquity of and lengthy recovery course required by substance-use disorders, and the rational desire of many homeless people to be rapidly rehoused. Related to this is a phenomenon of "shelterization" or dependence on shelter life, which itself perpetuates homelessness (Gounis and Susser 1990). Some model programs have been devised to address successful transition to housing. Critical Time Intervention (Susser et al. 1997) provides extended follow-up by shelter workers who advocate for and assist their clients as they begin to form new helping relationships through housing programs. Pathways to Housing employs the assertive community treatment model to aggressively maintain its clients (often right off

| Table 113–7 | Focus on Collaboration |
|---|---|

Integration of various disciplines
Peer support
Use of case management for negotiation
Respect for consumer autonomy

| Table 113–8 | Techniques in Nontraditional Approaches |
|---|---|

Reliable, consistent relationships
Alliances vs. hierarchies
Realistic expectations
Adherence negotiations
Focus on harm reduction

the streets) from obtaining housing placement through the process of staying housed (Tsemberis and Eisenberg 2000).

Treatment of psychiatric disorders, co-occurring substance abuse problems, and general medical needs also begin to take on an important role during intensive care.

Even as intensive care proceeds, approaching these needs requires special skills, primarily integrating nontraditional techniques (Table 113–8). These techniques are born out of a necessity to treat people who usually do not consider themselves "patients" but, rather out of circumstantial necessity, happen to interact with health providers. Psychiatrists in shelters and similar nontraditional settings have to "unlearn" habits while they integrate standard practice and nontraditional techniques (Felix et al. 1996, Valencia et al. 1996). For example, it is at times acceptable to joke around and laugh with patients, to give gifts, to self-reveal, to play cards or ping-pong, and to be a visible advocate and deliverer of concrete services. Implicit in this is continuing attention to an alliance with the patient, including maintaining unwavering reliability.

Perhaps in no single area of the relationship between the psychiatrist and the homeless person can alliance be more critical as in the instance of introducing medication. The clinician persistently works with the patient, searching for a shared rationale for prescribing, simultaneously signaling to him or her that the clinician is foremost interested in helping him or her meet his or her personal goals. Being a real object communicates this nonverbally.

Choice of medication is tempered by realism. For example, medications that require frequent laboratory monitoring may not be realistic in many nontraditional settings, especially if the patient is unable to predictably appear for phlebotomy. When a medication regimen is established, too, attention to adherence is important. Psychiatrists must be flexible and realistic with dosing schedules, prescribing once a day whenever possible. Many programs have devised ways to track medication adherence through supervision or pill counts. If there is nonadherence, further negotiation with the patient is indicated, carefully listening to his or her concerns. Harm-reduction techniques are also appropriate, as in continuing antipsychotic medications when a person is actively using street drugs.

Because it is a time of active psychiatric stabilization, during intensive care, clinicians may continue to be confronted with questions of personal risk to self and others. Drop-in and shelter settings are by necessity least restrictive settings of care, and staff must be skilled in diffusing potentially explosive interpersonal situations among clients, thereby focusing on preventative environmental techniques to enhance safety, including attention to medication adherence and substance use. Clients are also at varying stages of care and they often exit these settings for periods of time *ad libitum*. This reality requires a staff that tolerates ambiguous risk. Just as they need to be comfortable with intervening acutely, they must also be ready to take leave of a homeless client, and revise a treatment plan when he or she returns.

During intensive care and especially while exploring housing options, chemical dependency becomes a serious focus. Considering the corrosive nature of drug addiction, it is intuitively obvious that the social problem of substance abuse causes chronic homelessness. Mounting data support this (Hulburt et al. 1996, Bebout et al. 1997, Breakey et al. in press), and there is emerging consensus on effective techniques addressing co-occurring substance use and psychiatric disorders (Drake et al. 2001). However, gaps remain in understanding differences between homeless and nonhomeless dually diagnosed populations. Filling them will offer more effective solutions to homelessness. Possible solutions include the creation of community-based housing that is itself more geared to treating active substance use, as well as an integrating substance abuse programming with the psychologically and socially restorative effects of vocational training. The latter offers a pathway out of the demoralization induced by severe poverty, which itself may foster chemical abuse.

Finally, homeless people encounter the same chronic physical diseases that everyone else does, with the important exception that they have dramatically more difficulty in obtaining care. Compounding this is a higher than usual prevalence of epidemic illness, like HIV and hepatitis C (Susser et al. 1993, Rosenblum et al. 2001). With the exception of a few innovative mobile programs that visit shelters and drop-in centers or travel on the streets in specially outfitted vehicles (Nuttbrock et al. in press), homeless people usually get medical care on an emergency basis at a high cost and mortality rate. When they do obtain quality shelter or other transitional housing, it may be the first time that they have opportunity to receive ongoing medical services. In these settings, staff are aggressive in addressing the often multiple medical problems of clientele. Psychiatrists, especially, have a role in leading the effort to access a mentally ill homeless person to medical care, advocating with human services workers to facilitate Medicaid enrollment and with off-site health care providers to treat homeless patients.

## Ongoing Rehabilitation

The transition from intensive care to an open-ended stage of ongoing rehabilitation is an especially gradual one. Achieving full community integration necessarily involves a new sense of self-identity and recovery, and is composed of several ingredients.

Albeit absolutely crucial, housing is merely the first step. Becoming domiciled is a formal benchmark and a successful transition to housing demands careful clinical attention. Levels of structure or treatment intensity exist among housing types, ranging from relatively restrictive congregate care settings, requiring on-site program attendance and psychiatric care, to essentially independent apartment living with optional program participation. The more structured and intensive the housing type, the more its work continues to resemble intensive care. Especially among the

| Table 113–9 | Factors Related to Stable Housing Tenure |
|---|---|

Provide medication management
Noncongregate housing arrangements
Older consumers
Consumers with mood disorders
Sobriety

more structured housing environments, accommodations may also be transitional—up to 2 years or more. There is incipient literature examining what may contribute to housing stability. In one naturalistic study (Lipton et al. 2002) of 2,937 housing placements in New York City, correlation with longer housing tenure in high intensity settings included the availability of medication management and noncongregate living arrangements. In low intensity settings, longer tenure was associated with mood disorders. In all settings, it was associated with older age. Not surprisingly, there was an association between active substance abuse and short housing stays (see Table 113–9). Nevertheless, research has yet to establish a methodology for creating housing types based on a cluster of personal needs. There is little information available which analyzes individual models or programs (Tsemberis and Eisenberg 2000, Goldfinger et al. 1999) or systematically examines clinical issues like medication adherence, concurrent treatment of substance abuse (Susser et al. 1991, Grunebaum et al. 1999), medical comorbidity, and family involvement. However, once a person has found a satisfying housing environment, the rehabilitative focus has usually shifted from symptomatologic stability to emphasis on the development of a set of new roles that render as obsolete the individual's identity as homeless (see Table 113–10). Vocational and relational identities are integral to this development and psychiatrists who work within this stage focus much less on crisis and immediate psychiatric and medical needs, but more on identifying and achieving with their patients' long-term goals. This is done by listening carefully to their patients' hopes, translating them into a collaborative reality-based plan, while coordinating closely with vocational and social skills, and other counselors.

Goal setting around work often starts during the stage of intensive care, with many entering active vocational training at that point. However, as a person struggles less with day-to-day survival, he or she begins looking for a sense of financial independence and sources of personal pride. Supported employment has enjoyed the highest preference, but many professionals value transitional

| Table 113–10 | Consumer-focused Strategies to Enhance Housing Tenure |
|---|---|

Clearly identifying long-term goals
Vocational training
Transitional vs. supported employment
Meaningful relationships
Family ties
Other support systems
Religious/spiritual affiliations

employment models, like those in clubhouses. These models need further research among homeless and formerly homeless populations.

The other important development during ongoing rehabilitation is the forming of more meaningful human relationships, marking dissolution of the alienation engendered especially by chronic homelessness. This includes the reestablishment of family ties for many who have had been separated through the vicissitudes of mental illness and substance abuse. Psychiatrists and other workers have a role in acting as a conduit to families, providing family psychoeducation and support to their patients. For those consumers whose families are not accessible, even more incentive exists for professionals to link them to other support systems through clubhouses, redeveloped personal interests, religious and other spiritual affiliations, and work environments. The recovery and reentry of mentally ill homeless people, while often painstaking, is accentuated by their heretofore severe indigence and disaffiliation. It is therefore ultimately profound.

## Administration, Academics, and Advocacy

Psychiatrists are important in providing both leadership and collaborating in service within all the stages of rehabilitative care of people with homelessness and mental illness. As the evolution of services to this population had progressed over the past two decades, they have found additional roles in administration, academics, and advocacy.

Owing to their location within CBOs, nonmedical professionals lead most programs serving homeless people. Nevertheless, the role of the medical director has developed in CBOs (Falk et al. 1998, Ranz et al. 2000). The role of the CBO medical director represents both shifts in CBOs toward accepting a meaningful medical contribution and an adaptation of psychiatric administration to include non traditional models. Medical directors work in partnership with, or under the aegis of, nonmedical program or agency directors, and how they manage this relationship requires flexibility and collaborative skills. For example, in the area of clinical accountability of nonmedical staff, the medical director needs to provide clinical consultation and supervision to nonmedical colleagues, and assert a commitment to quality care, often without direct line authority.

Academic faculty that have come of age during the phases of the homelessness problem lead today's teaching experiences. These teachers understand that working with mentally ill homeless populations affords the trainees opportunity to learn omnibus skills in diagnosis and management of very complex and distressed patients, including work at the frontiers of epidemics like tuberculosis, HIV illness, and hepatitis C.

Training medical students and physicians to work with mentally ill homeless people necessarily involves describing a theoretical framework. This includes education concerning the social and economic roots of homelessness and how community psychiatry fits within applied public mental health. Trainees are placed in clinical programs that are known to be successful and student-friendly. Supervisors must offer vision, theory, and role modeling, as they also teach cultural sensitivity, work with countertransference, and imbue special techniques.

Finally, advocacy is required to advance recovery and help homeless people with psychiatric disorders to enter the social mainstream. On a basic level, the very existence of psychiatrists working with homeless people constitutes advocacy by drawing professional attention. Psychiatrists working with homeless people must also influence the organizations for which they work to identify a corporate function in advocacy, moving beyond service.

In some localities, litigation has been a critical tool in driving public policy on homelessness. Psychiatry offers unique expertise to legal advocacy and exercising this role has a potent effect on facilitating social change. In this manner, psychiatrists have given expert testimony in important class action suits and professional organizations have issued formal statements of support. Organized psychiatry has also combated the stigma of mental illness, extending itself to homelessness, too (American Psychiatric Association 1991b, Lamb et al. 1992). These documents provide a recognizable reference point of leadership for psychiatrists to engage in public advocacy as they form alliances with advocates, including consumers and families, educating policy-makers about the needs of this population.

## Acknowledgment

We thank Jack Hirschowitz, MD (Chair) and the Committee on the Homeless Mentally Ill of the NY County District Branch of the APA for its important contributions to the ideas in this chapter.

## References

American Psychiatric Association (1986) Gold Award: A network of services for the homeless chronically mentally ill. Skid Row Mental Health Service, Los Angeles County Department of Mental Health. Hosp Comm Psychiatr 37, 1148–1151.

American Psychiatric Association (1991a) Significant Achievement Award: Psychiatric services for New York City's homeless population Task Force on Voluntary Services for the Homeless, New York County District Branch, American Psychiatric Association. Hosp Comm Psychiatr 42, 1058–1059.

American Psychiatric Association (1991b) Homeless Families and Children: A Psychiatric Perspective. APA, Washington DC.

American Psychiatric Association (1997) Project Respond, Mental Health Services West: Linking mentally ill persons with services through crisis intervention, mobile outreach, and community education. Psychiatr Serv 47, 1450–1453.

Arce AA, Tadlock M, Vergare MJ, et al. (1983) A psychiatric profile of street people admitted to an emergency shelter. Hosp Comm Psychiatr 34, 812–816.

Axleroad SE and Toff SE (1987) Outreach services for homeless mentally ill people. The International Health Policy Project, George Washington University.

Barnard-Columbia Center for Urban Policy (1996) The Continuum of Care: A Report on The New Federal Policy to Address Homelessness. US Dept of Housing and Urban Development, Washington DC.

Baxter E and Hopper K (1981) Private Lives/Public Spaces: Homeless Adults on the Streets of New York City. Community Service Society, New York.

Bebout RR, Drake RE, Xie H, et al. (1997) Housing stability among formerly homeless dually diagnosed adults. Psychiatr Serv 48, 936–941.

Belcher JR (1988) Defining the service needs of homeless mentally ill persons. Hosp Comm Psychiatr 39, 1203–1205.

Bond GR, Becker DR, Drake RE, et al. (2001) Implementing supported employment as evidence-based practice. Psychiatr Serv 52, 313–322.

Breakey WR, Fischer PJ, Kramer M, et al. (1989) Health and mental health problems of homeless men and women in Baltimore. J Am Med Assoc 262, 1352–1357.

Breakey WR, Susser ES, and Timms P (in press) Mental health services for homeless people. In Measuring Mental Health Needs, 2nd ed., Thornicroft G, Brewin CR (eds). Wing J, London.

Calloway MO and Morrissey JP (1998) Overcoming Service Barriers for Homeless Persons with Serious Psychiatric Disorders. Psychiatr Serv 49, 1568–1572.

Caton CLM, Wyatt RJ, Grunberg J, et al. (1990) An evaluation of a mental health program for homeless men. Am J Psychiatr, 147, 286–289.

Cohen NL, Putnam JF, and Sullivan AM (1984) The mentally ill homeless: Isolation and adaptation. Hosp Comm Psychiatr 35, 922–924.

Culhane DP, Dejowski EF, Ibanez J, et al. (1994) Public shelter admission rates in Philadelphia and New York City: The implications of turnover for sheltered population counts. Hous Policy Deb 5, 107–140.

Diamond RJ (1996) Coercion and tenacious treatment in the community: Applications to the real world. In Coercion and Aggressive Community Treatment: A New Frontier—Mental Health Law, Dennis DL and Monohan J (eds). Plenum Press, New York, 51–72.

Dincin J, Zeitz MA, Farrell D, et al. (1995) Special programs for special groups. New Dir Ment Health Serv 68, 55–73.

Drake RE, Essock SM, Shaner, et al. (2001) Implementing dual diagnosis services for clients with severe mental illness. Psychiatr Serv 52, 469–476.

Drake RE, Osher FC, and Wallach MA (1991) Homelessness and dual diagnosis. Am Psychol 46, 1149–1158.

Falk NA, Cutler DL, Goetz R, et al. (1998) The community psychiatrist: Hamlet, King Lear, or fishmonger? Traditional vs. nontraditional roles and settings. J Pract Psychiatr Behav Health 4, 345–355.

Felix A, Valencia E, and Susser ES (1996) Back to the future: The role of the psychiatrist in treating mentally ill individuals who are homeless in schizophrenia. In New Directions for Clinical Research and Treatment, Kaufman CA and Gorman JM (eds). May Ann Liebert, Larchmont NY, pp. 231–242.

Fischer PJ, Shapiro S, Breakey WR, et al. (1986) Mental health and social characteristics of the homeless: A survey of mission users. Am J Pub Health 5, 519–524.

Foscarinis M (1996) The federal response: The Stewart B. McKinney homeless assistance act. In Homelessness in America, Baumohl J (ed). Oryx, Phoenix, AZ, pp. 160–171.

Frank JD and Frank JB (1991) Persuasion and Healing: A Comparative Study of Psychotherapy, 3rd ed. The Johns Hopkins University Press, Baltimore, 34–39.

Goldfinger SM, Schutt RK, Tolomiczenko GS, et al. (1999) Housing placement and subsequent days of homeless among formerly homeless adults with mental illness. Psychiatr Serv 50, 674–679.

Goldman HH, Morrissey JP, and Ridgely MS (1994) Evaluating the Robert Wood Johnson Foundation Program on Chronic Mental Illness. Milbank Quarterly 72, 37–47.

Gounis K and Susser E (1990) Shelterization and its implications for mental health services. In Psychiatry Takes to the Streets, Cohen NL (ed). Guilford Press, New York, pp. 231–255.

Grunebaum M, Aquila R, Portera L, et al. (1999) Predictors of management problems in supported housing: A pilot study. Comm Ment Health J 35, 127–133.

Hopper K, Jost J, Hay T, et al. (1997) Homelessness, severe mental illness, and the institutional circuit. Psychiatr Serv 48, 659–665.

Hurlburt MS, Hough RL, and Wood PA (1996) Effects of substance abuse on housing stability of homeless mentally ill persons in supportive housing. Psychiatr Serv 47, 731–736.

Katz SE, Sabatini A and Codd C (1993) The homeless initiative and Project HELP: Historical perspectives and program description. In Intensive Treatment of the Homeless Mentally Ill, Katz SE, Nardacci D, and Sabatini A (eds). American Psychiatric Press, Washington DC, pp. 1–24.

Koegel P, Burnam MA, and Baumohl J (1988) The causes of homelessness. In Homelessness in America, Baumohl J (ed). Oryx, Phoenix, AZ, pp. 24–33.

Koegel P, Burnam MA, and Farr RK (1988) The prevalence of specific psychiatric disorders among homeless individuals in the inner city of Los Angeles. Arch Gen Psychiatr 45, 1085–1091.

Lamb HR (1984a) Deinstitutionalization and the homeless mentally ill. Hosp Comm Psychiatr 35, 899–907.

Lamb HR (ed) (1984) The Homeless Mentally Ill: A Task Force Report of the American Psychiatric Association. APA, Washington DC.

Lamb HR and Talbott JA (1986) The homeless mentally ill: The perspective of the American Psychiatric Association. J Am Med Assoc 256, 498–501.

Lamb HR, Bachrach LL, and Kass FI (eds) (1992) Treating the Homeless Mentally Ill: A Task Force Report of the American Psychiatric Association. APA, Washington DC.

Lehman AF, Dixon LB, Kerman E, et al. (1997) A randomized trial of assertive community treatment for homeless persons with severe mental illness. Arch of Gen Psychiatr 54, 1038–1043.

Link BG, Susser ES, Stueve A, et al. (1994) Lifetime and five-year prevalence of homelessness in the United States. Am J Pub Health 84, 1907–1912.

Lipton FR, Sabatini A, and Katz S (1983) Down and out in the city: The homeless mentally ill. Hosp Comm Psychiatr 34, 817–821.

Lipton FR, Siegel C, Hannigan A, et al. (2002) Tenure in supportive housing for homeless persons with severe mental illness. Psychiatr Serv 51, 479–486.

Manderscheid RW, Atay JE, Hernandez-Cartagena M del R, et al. (2000) Highlights of organized mental health services in 1998 and major national and state trends. In Mental Health. Center for Mental Health Services, Bethesda, MD.

Marlatt GA (1996) Harm reduction: Come as you are. Addict Behav 21, 779–788.

McQuistion HL, D'Ercole A, and Kopelson E (1991) Urban street outreach: Using clinical principles to steer the system. New Dir Ment Health Serv 52, 17–27.

Morse G, Shields NM, Hanneke CR, et al (1985) Homeless People in St. Louis: A Mental Health Program Evaluation, Field Study, and Follow-up Investigation. Missouri Department of Mental Health, Jefferson City, MO.

Nuttbrock L, McQuistion HL, Rosenblum A, et al. (in press) Broadening perspectives on mobile medical outreach to homeless people. J Health Care Poor Underserv.

Prochaska J, DiClemente C, and Norcross J (1992) In search of how people change: Applications to addictive behaviors. Am Psychol 47, 1102–1114.

Ranz J, McQuistion HL, and Stueve A (2000) The role of the psychiatrist as medical director: A delineation of job types for community psychiatrists. Psychiatr Serv 51, 930–932.

Ringwalt CL, Greene JM, Robertson M, et al. (1998) The prevalence of homelessness among adolescents in the United States. Am J Pub Health 88, 1325–1329.

Rosenblum A, Nuttbrock L, McQuistion HL, et al. (2001) Prevalence and predictors of hepatitis C in a sample of homeless people in New York City. J Addic Dis 20, 15–25.

Rosenheck R, Bassuk E, and Salomon A (1998) Special populations of homeless Americans. In Practical Lessons: The 1998 National Symposium on Homelessness Research, Fosburg L and Dennis D (eds). US Dept. of Housing and Urban Development and US Dept. of Health and Human Services, Washington DC.

Roth D, Bean GJ, Lust N, et al. (1985) Homelessness in Ohio: A Study of People in Need. Ohio Department of Mental Health, Columbus, OH.

Simon H (1996) Municipal regulation of the homeless in public spaces. In Homelessness in America, Baumohl J (ed). Oryx, Phoenix, AZ, pp. 149–159.

Struening EL (1986) A Study of Residents in the New York City Shelter System: Report to the New York City Department of Mental Health, Mental Retardation, and Alcohol Services, New York State Psychiatric Institute, New York City, NY.

Susser E, Struening EL, and Conover S (1989) Psychiatric problems in homeless men. Arch Gen Psychiatr 46, 845–850.

Susser ES, Goldfinger SM, and White A (1990) Some clinical approaches to the homeless mentally ill. Comm Ment Health J 26, 459–476.

Susser ES, Lin SP, Conover S, et al. (1991) Childhood antecedents of homelessness in psychiatric patients. Am J Psychiatr 148, 1026–1030.

Susser ES, Moore R, and Link B (1993) Risk factors for homelessness. Am J Epidemiol 15, 546–556.

Susser ES, Struening EL, and Conover S (1987) Childhood experiences of homeless men. Am J Psychiatr 144, 1599–160.

Susser ES, Valencia E, and Conover S (1993) Prevalence of HIV infection among psychiatric patients in a New York City men's shelter. Am J Pub Health 83, 568–570.

Susser ES, Valencia E, and Goldfinger SM (1992) in Treating the Homeless Mentally Ill: A Task Force Report of the American Psychiatric Association, Lamb HR, Bachrach LL, and Kass FI (eds). APA, Washington DC.

Susser ES, Valencia E, Conover SA, et al. (1997) Preventing recurrent homelessness among mentally ill men: A "critical time" intervention after discharge from a shelter. Am J Pub Health 87, 256–262.

Tsemberis S and Eisenberg RF (2000) Pathways to housing: Supported housing for street-dwelling homeless individuals with psychiatric disabilities. Psychiatr Serv 51, 487–493.

US Conference of Mayors (2001) A Status Report on Hunger and Homelessness in American Cities. Washington DC.

Valencia E, Susser E, and McQuistion HL (1996) Critical time points in the care of homeless mentally ill people. In Practicing Psychiatry in the Community: A Manual, Vaccaro JV and Clark GH (eds). American Psychiatric Press, Washington DC, pp. 259–274.

Vernez G, Burnam MA, McGlynn EA, et al. (1988) Review of California's Program for the Homeless Mentally Disabled. Rand Corporation, Santa Monica, CA.

Weitzman BC, Knickman JR, and Shinn M (1992) Predictors of shelter use among low-income families: Psychiatric history, substance abuse, and victimization. Am J Pub Health 82, 1547–1550.

# 114 ● Rural Psychiatry

Barbara M. Rohland

The provision of psychiatric services to persons who live in rural communities presents both challenges and opportunities for innovation. To meet the needs of its population, service delivery in a rural or frontier setting cannot be perceived or structured as a downsized version of an urban service delivery system. Many aspects of rural practice relating to providers, patients, and the service delivery system make rural psychiatry unique.

## Demographic Considerations

The definition of "rural" is not always clear and it is important to appreciate the social, economic, and geographic factors that contribute to rural diversity among rural communities in the US. Five levels of urbanization (three metropolitan and two nonmetropolitan) are used by the Centers for Disease Control (CDC) to classify counties with large central, large fringe, and small concentrated population areas as metropolitan; and those with a city of 10,000 or more or without a city of 10,000 or more as nonmetropolitan (Eberhardt et al. 2001). The designation of a county having versus not having a Metropolitan Statistical Area (MSA) is a common definition of rural based on the population and urbanization of a county. The US Office of Management and Budget (OMB), using data from the US Bureau of the Census, defines MSA as one or more central counties with a population of 50,000 or more or a census-defined urbanized area with a population of 100,000 or more persons (Ricketts et al. 1999).

The proportion of rural inhabitants varies across the country. The Midwest and the South have the highest proportion of rural inhabitants at 26.6 and 25.8% respectively, compared to 20.3% of the US population overall (Ricketts et al. 1999). Approximately one quarter of the population of the Midwest and South lives in nonmetropolitan counties (Eberhardt et al. 2001) and in 15 states of the nation, 50% or more of the population reside in nonmetropolitan areas (Shelton and Frank 1995). Furthermore, 2% of the US population (and nearly half of the US land mass) are in areas classified as "frontier" areas, that is, counties with a population density less than six or seven persons per square mile (Wagenfeld 2000). In frontier areas, communication and transportation problems are often complicated by harsh climate and rugged terrain.

Rural areas have a higher proportion of older people with the proportion of persons of age 65 years and older increasing according to an urban–rural gradient. Although

true for all regions of the county, the steepest gradient occurs in the Midwest and South (Eberhardt et al. 2001). The rural elderly have lower incomes, less education, and are more likely to be poor (i.e., have less accumulated wealth); they are more likely to live in substandard dwellings, have less health insurance coverage, and have poorer health status relative to elderly persons living in urban areas (Coburn and Bolda 1999). Problems with transportation and travel distance from facilities create difficulties in accessing health services for all persons who live in rural areas (Schur and Franco 1999), more so for the elderly. The rural elderly make little use of formal, paid health, and social support services and tend to rely on family members or informal support networks (such as church) to help them meet their needs (Coburn and Bolda 1999). These characteristics should be taken into account when planning community outreach programs that are intended to meet the mental health needs of the elderly who live in rural areas. Characteristics of the rural elderly are summarized in Table 114–1.

Although rural areas tend to be more homogeneous in race and ethnicity than urban areas, regional variation exists. Nonmetropolitan areas of the Northeast and Midwest are predominantly white (97.2 and 96.5%, respectively, versus 80.9 and 83.5% in metropolitan areas), whereas 17.8% of the nonmetropolitan population of the South is black. In the West, 11.5% of the nonmetropolitan residents are Hispanic (Ricketts et al. 1999).

## Issues for Providers

Recruitment and retention of providers in rural areas are important human resource issues that have been a focus of

| Table 114–1 | Characteristics of the Rural Elderly |
|---|---|

- Lower incomes
- Less education
- More likely to be poor
- More likely to live in substandard housing
- Have less health insurance coverage
- Poorer health status
- Make little use of formal, paid health, social supports
- May rely on family, informal support networks
- Problems with transportation
- More homogeneous in race

| Table 114–2 | Models of Integrating Mental and Primary Health Care |
|---|---|

- Diversification
- Linkage
- Referral
- Enhancement
  (combined training vs. cross training)

rural mental health policy (Wagenfeld et al. 1994, Human and Wasem 1991, Merwin et al. 1995). Problems related to patient–physician boundary issues, availability of coverage, employment and social opportunities for one's spouse, practice issues regarding nonphysician providers (e.g., prescribing privileges for psychologists, physician assistants, and nurse practitioners), and integration of mental health services with primary care physicians all affect the practice of psychiatry (by psychiatrists) in rural areas (Reed and Merrell 1996). Benchmarks for a successful psychiatry practice range from 1 provider/6,500 persons (Graduate Medical Education [GME] National Advisory Committee 1980) to 1 provider/14,000 in a HMO (Hart et al. 1997). Hence, a rural area is unlikely to have the capacity to support more than one psychiatrist, and that psychiatrist is likely to have both a sense of isolation and lack of privacy. Coverage for vacation, evening, and weekend call may be particularly difficult to secure. Professional boundary issues with patients become particularly problematic if the practitioner lives in the community and participates in the social life of that community (e.g., events related to church or school).

Several models for the integration of mental health services with primary care in rural areas have been described (Bird et al. 1998). These models are summarized in Table 114–2. *Diversification* occurs when the primary care doctor hires a mental health professional, usually a psychologist or counselor, to provide mental health services at the primary care doctor's office site. *Linkage* refers to an arrangement between a primary care physician and an independent practitioner or employee of another organization to provide mental health services at the primary care site. In *Referral*, the most traditional model, mental health services are provided by a mental health professional at their site of practice (usually a community mental health center or an outpatient office located at a community hospital) upon the recommendation of the patient's primary care physician. *Enhancement* refers to the training of primary care physicians so as to improve their ability to recognize, diagnose, and treat mental health problems independently. A few residency training programs combine family practice and psychiatry training so that graduates are board-eligible in both specialties. However, cross training between the specialties of psychiatry and family practice in traditional family practice residency training programs is variable.

Service organization is known to be a critical factor in determining job satisfaction and stress (i.e., "burnout") among mental health providers (Leiter and Harvie 1996). Despite the apparent drawbacks of rural practice, studies have not found evidence that rural mental health workers have more burnout (Rohland 2000, Greenley and Schulz 1997) or less job satisfaction (Freund and Sarata 1983, Jerrell

1983, Oberlander 1990) than did urban providers. Recruitment, retention, and other human resource issues important to the rural workforce may be related more to the "goodness of fit" between the personal characteristics of providers and the characteristics of rural work settings than they are to the organizational characteristics of a rural practice.

In studying the characteristics of rural mental health center administrators, appreciation of rural community and personality attributes relevant to rural life were two of the most important characteristics associated with administrators' effectiveness (Fennell et al. 1987). In a survey of Iowa community mental health center directors in Iowa, organizational characteristics related to "rurality," that is, location in a rural county, fewer employees, smaller budgets, and more time spent in direct clinical care were not associated with burnout (Rohland 2000). Rural directors were more likely to report the use of religion as a coping mechanism compared to their urban colleagues. Hence, a characteristic that is primarily organizational in nature (i.e., rural location and size) may be related to personal characteristics of the center directors, which suggests their "goodness of fit" to a rural work environment.

## Issues for Patients

There is no evidence that rural populations have less mental illness than their urban counterparts. Patient-related factors that affect mental health services in rural areas are summarized in Table 114–3. In fact, an urban-to-rural increase in suicide rates for males and females has been noted in the Western region of the country with rates of firearm-related suicide increasing from large metro counties to the most rural counties; high levels of alcohol consumption are also more frequent in nonmetropolitan counties of the West, compared to other levels of urbanization (Eberhardt et al. 2001). Persons in rural areas with schizophrenia have been found to be equally noncompliant with medication and were not significantly different in Global Assessment Scale (GAS) scores or self-reported symptoms of psychosis or depression (Sullivan et al. 1996).

While there may not be less mental illness or less need for services in rural areas, stigma regarding mental illness and its treatment may be greater and, at the same time, anonymity in seeking services is less assured. While a strong sense of community and social connection can provide social support to residents in rural communities in times of stress, it can also make confidentiality difficult to achieve in seeking services and difficult to maintain in receiving services. Concerns that one's car in the parking lot of a mental health center might be identified or that one is known by (or related to) clinic staff create barriers to treatment in rural communities. Hence, difficulty in assuring anonymity is particularly problematic for persons who live in rural areas and may explain some of the reasons why rural

| Table 114–3 | Patient Factors Affecting Services in Rural Areas |
|---|---|

- Differences in incidences of mental illness
- Degree of stigma
- Confidentiality

| Table 114-4 | Challenges for Rural Systems of Care |
| --- | --- |

- Low population density
- Limited tax base
- Difficulty with recruitment/retention of professional staff
- Workforce shortage (especially specialty-trained)
- Lack of transportation
- Variable organizational structures
- Increased need for outreach
- Increased use of inpatient hospitalization

residents are less likely to receive services, even when services are available.

## Issues for the Service System

Low population density, limited tax base, difficulty recruiting and retaining professional staff, and lack of transportation are among the problems that contribute to problems of service access in rural areas (Schur and Franco 1999, Bachrach 1983, Wagenfeld et al. 1994) (Table 114–4). To understand the structure, function, and purpose of any given rural mental health system, basic organizational characteristics of the delivery system should be identified. For example, the services may be organized and managed centrally (usually at the level of the state) versus locally (usually at the level of the county) or regionally (e.g., encompassing several counties). Mental health services may or may not be integrated with alcohol or other chemical dependency programs. Services may be in the public versus private sector and, within the private sector, may be offered by either for-profit or not-for-profit providers. Finally, social and welfare programs such as child and maternal health may or may not be integrated with mental health services. Even if service programs are not integrated, sharing of office space with programs perceived as "welfare" or "charity" services can have an adverse effect on the willingness of rural community residents to utilize services.

In an Iowa study (Rohland and Langbehn 1998), persons living in a rural county did not report less mental health service use than persons living in urban counties except that they were less likely to use group therapy (22% rural versus 31% urban residents). While this may be because fewer participants and/or fewer group facilitators are present, it is also possible that group therapy is used less by rural residents because anonymity in participation is less assured. Rural Medicaid recipients were more likely to report use of home services than urban residents (36% rural versus 27% urban). One explanation for why rural residents use home services more often than persons who live in urban areas is that home services may be a mechanism to provide outreach to persons who cannot otherwise access services due to problems with transportation. It is also possible that home services provide a substitute for clinic or hospital-based providers in rural areas. Persons who did not have schizophrenia and who had been hospitalized in FY1993 were more likely to report a greater lifetime cumulative number of hospital days if they lived in urban versus rural areas. Cumulative hospitalization of persons with schizophrenia, however, was not different in rural versus urban counties.

Services that require providers with specialized training, such as those to persons with serious mental illness (Kane and Ennis 1996) or who are elderly (Chalifoux et al. 1996), are particularly vulnerable to rural workforce shortages in that they require specialized training and access to support services (e.g., home health care or rehabilitation). Specialized programs and caregivers are often considered a "luxury" in rural areas due to fiscal constraints, paucity of clients, and the absence of peer backup (Wagenfeld 2000). To meet the needs presented by these patients, many rural areas have developed innovative models that draw on non-traditional and, in many cases, nonprofessional caregivers (Sullivan 1989). For example, in a Wyoming program (Davis and Ziegler 1990), social services, nursing homes, hospitals, and vocational rehabilitation offices are drawn together in order to provide services to persons with severe mental illness. In Idaho, an innovative program uses "citizen companions" to enhance the work of professional case managers (Sword and Longden 1989).

The reasons why rural areas spend less money on services for mental illness than urban areas, apart from economic status, are unclear. In a study of resource allocation by states, factors that accounted for variation in state funding for mental retardation, that is, state size, state wealth, federal aid, civil rights activity, and consumer advocacy, did not account for any appreciable variance in state funding for community mental health services (Braddock 1992). In a study of factors affecting spending on mental health services in Iowa, lower county budgets, smaller county populations, and increased rates of poverty were related to decreased county spending for mental health services (Rohland and Rohrer 1998). However, the size of the county (as opposed to its wealth) appeared to be the most important predictor of county funding. Other characteristics associated with rurality, such as proportion of rural and/or elderly inhabitants, proportion of college educated residents, and the extent to which the county budget is accounted for by farm income, were also found to be associated with mental health expenditures. It is possible that stigma towards mental illness (and the perceptions that it creates regarding expenses related to treatment) may be greater, or at least different, among rural versus urban residents. Persons who live in rural areas may have more conservative attitudes about mental illness and its treatment, and advocate different priorities for county (property tax based) funding. Rural counties may spend less money on mental health services because less demand for services exists due to the stigma of recognition and lack of anonymity in receiving services locally. Factors that may limit funding by counties in a rural state are summarized in Table 114–5.

The effect of managed care on service access, utilization, and clinical outcome for persons who live in rural areas is uncertain. Health care reform that focuses on financing alone does not address the limited availability of adequate services or service providers in rural areas (Shelton and Frank 1995). Furthermore, because system reform often focuses on integration with primary care and other generalist providers, services that require providers with specialized training, such as services for persons with serious mental illness, are particularly vulnerable to gatekeeper models. One cost saving strategy often employed by

| Table 114–5 | Factors That May Decrease Mental Health Funding by Rural Counties |
|---|---|

- Smaller populations
- Lower overall county budgets
- Increased rates of poverty
- Lower rates of Medicaid recipients
- Higher rates of elderly
- Lower rates of college educated residents
- County budgets dependent on farm incomes
- Stigma
- Variable impact of managed care

managed care is to substitute a high-intensity, high-cost service (e.g., inpatient hospitalization) and a lower-intensity, lower-cost service (e.g., partial hospitalization or intensive outpatient services). A managed care contractor who is not familiar with the limited availability of services in a rural area may deny hospitalization (which is available) in favor of a substitutable community based service (which is not) without appreciating that alternatives to hospitalization in many rural areas may not exist. Regional knowledge of service resources, specifically availability of community support services such as support groups, home health care, and rehabilitation services is particularly important for managed care contracts to be successfully implemented in a rural state. Managed care presents the opportunity to assure a minimum standard for care in a rural service system that may be uneven, particularly in states where services are primarily organized and funded at the level of the county. By requiring that the contractor report state-wide performance measures, service gaps in rural states that were previously unrecognized have the potential to be more readily identified and met (Rohland 1998).

County population, in addition to the portion of Medicaid recipients, predicted 96% of the variation in the total county budget for mental illness in Iowa counties prior to the statewide implementation of Medicaid managed care (Rohland and Rohrer 1998). The positive correlation between county funding for mental health services and the proportion of county residents receiving Medicaid services suggests that Medicaid funded services may provide increased availability of county funded services. Hence systems of mental health care in rural areas may be particularly vulnerable to Medicaid (and Medicare) reorganization. Reductions in Medicaid funding under managed care may be associated with reductions in county funding for mental illness, with potentially profound effects on service availability and quality.

## Telemedicine

Telemedicine has great potential to enhance service delivery to persons in rural areas (Preston et al. 1992). The technical capacity for many types of psychiatric services to be delivered via real time interactive audiovisual transmission has been steadily increasing while costs associated with technology have been decreasing and becoming more "user friendly." Communication via telemedicine has been used to improve continuity of care to persons with serious mental illness who have been discharged from inpatient care

to remote community based settings (Smith 1998). Other applications of telepsychiatry include services to children and adolescents (Blackmon et al. 1997, Ermer 1999), geriatric populations (Williams et al. 1995, Jones and Colenda 1997, Jones 1999), emergency room consultation (Meltzer 1997, Bear et al. 1997), and primary care settings (Hilty et al. 1999). The quality of care provided by telemedicine and its acceptability to persons who live in rural areas is a current topic of research interest and clinical importance. Although financial, technical, administrative, political, and clinical issues often impede successful program implementation and sustainability (Werner and Anderson 1998, Chen et al. 1999), telepsychiatry appears to offer an acceptable and adequate alternative mode of service delivery to persons who live in rural areas (Rohland 2001). While a recent survey suggests that rural elderly persons may be reluctant to use telemedicine (Rohland et al. 2000), telepsychiatry is likely to become an increasingly acceptable alternative to traditional face-to-face services. This is most likely to be true if it can provide additional convenience, advantage of cost, address confidentiality concerns, and be presented in a nontechnical user-friendly format. With significant advancements in technical capacity and concurrent decreases in cost, applications of telemedicine in rural areas are likely to increase. Integration of telepsychiatry into existing systems of rural care delivery are likely to provide an important adjunct role in the delivery of mental health services to persons who live in rural areas.

## Summary

Persons who live in rural areas are vulnerable to the same mental illnesses that affect persons living in more populated areas and their need for services is similar. However, access and provision of services in rural areas present unique challenges that require innovative approaches. Characteristics associated with rural communities have implications for the care of persons who live there, the providers who serve them, and the systems of mental health care delivery through which services can best be provided and the mechanisms by which needs are most likely to be met.

## References

Bachrach LL (1983) Psychiatric services in rural areas: A sociological overview. Hosp Comm Psychiatr 34(3), 215–226.

Bear D, Jacobson G, Aaronson S, et al. (1997) Telemedicine in psychiatry: Making the dream a reality (letter to the editor). Am J Psychiatr 154, 884–885.

Bird DC, Lambert D, Hartley D, et al. (1998) Rural models for integrating primary care & mental health services. Admin Policy Ment Health 25(3), 287–308.

Blackmon LA, Kaak HO, and Ranseen J (1997) Consumer satisfaction with telemedicine: Child psychiatry consultation in rural Kentucky. Psychiatr Serv 48, 1464–1466.

Braddock D (1992) Community mental health and mental retardation services in the United States: A comparative study of resource allocation. Am J Psychiatr 149(2), 175–183.

Chalifoux Z, Neese JB, Buckwalter KC, et al. (1996) Mental health services for rural elderly: Innovative service strategies. Comm Ment Health J 32(5), 463–480.

Chen DT, Blank MB, Worrall BB, et al. (1999) Defending telepsychiatry (letters to the editor). Psychiatr Serv 50, 266–268.

Coburn AF and Bolda EJ (1999) The rural elderly and long-term care, Ch. 15. In Rural Health in the United States, Ricketts TC (ed). Oxford University Press, New York.

Davis LF and Ziegler JA (1990) Working with people who are chronically mentally ill in rural areas: Developing a community resource team. Psychosoc Rehabil J 13(3), 81–85.

Eberhardt MS, Ingram DD, Makuc DM, et al. (2001) Urban and Rural Health Chartbook. Health, United States. National Center for Health Statistics, Hyattsville, Maryland.

Ermer DJ (1999) Experience with a rural telepsychiatry clinic for children and adolescents. Psychiatr Serv 50, 260–261.

Fennell DL, Hovestadt AJ, and Cochran SW (1987) Characteristics of effective administrators of rural mental health centers. J Rural Comm Psychol 8(1), 23–35.

Freund CM and Sarata B (1983) Work and community satisfaction of psychologists in rural and nonrural areas. J Rural Comm Psychol 4(2), 19–28.

Graduate Medical Education National Advisory Committee (1980) Report of the Graduate Medical Education National Advisory Committee to the Secretary, Department of Health and Human Services, Vol. 1. Office of Graduate Medical Education, Health Resources Administration, Public Health Service, US Department of Health and Human Services, Washington DC.

Greenley JR and Schulz R (1997) Staff burnout and rural mental health services. Rural Comm Ment Health 21(3), 1–7.

Hart LG, Wagner E, Pirzada, et al. (1997) Physician staffing ratios in staff-model HMOS: A cautionary tale. Health Aff 16(1), 55–70.

Hilty DM, Servis ME, Nesbitt TS, et al. (1999) The use of telemedicine to provide consultation-liaison service to the primary care setting. Psychiatr Ann 29, 421–427.

Human J and Wasem C (1991) Rural mental health in America. Am Psychol 46(3), 232–239.

Jerrell JM (1983) Work satisfaction among rural mental health staff. Comm Ment Health J 19(3), 187–200.

Jones BN (1999) Telemedicine in geriatric psychiatry. Psychiatr Ann 29, 416–420.

Jones BN and Colenda CC (1997) Telemedicine and geriatric psychiatry. Psychiatr Serv 48, 783–785.

Kane CF and Ennis JM (1996) Health care reform and rural mental health: Severe mental illness. Comm Ment Health J 32(5), 445–462.

Leiter MP and Harvie PL (1996) Burnout among mental health workers: A review and a research agenda. Int J Soc Psychiatry 42(2), 90–101.

Meltzer B (1997) Telemedicine in emergency psychiatry. Psychiatr Serv 48, 1141–1142.

Merwin EI, Goldsmith HF, and Manderscheid RW (1995) Human resource issues in rural mental health services. Comm Ment Health J 31(6), 525–537.

Oberlander LB (1990) Work satisfaction among community-based mental health service providers: The Association Between Work Environment and Work Satisfaction. Comm Ment Health J 26(6), 517–532.

Preston J, Brown FW, and Hartley B (1992) Using telemedicine to improve health care in distant areas. Hosp Comm Psychiatry 43, 25–32.

Reed D and Merrell (1996) A Practice styles in rural psychiatry, Ch. 23. In Practicing Psychiatry in the Community: A Manual, Vaccaro JV, and Clark GH (eds). American Psychiatric Press, Washington DC.

Ricketts TC, Johnson-Webb, and Randolph RK (1999) Populations and Places in Rural America, Ch. 1. In Rural Health in the United States, Ricketts TC (ed). Oxford University Press, New York.

Rohland BM (1998) Implementation of Medicaid managed mental health care in Iowa: Problems and solutions. J Behav Health Serv Res 25(3), 293–299.

Rohland BM (2000) A survey of burnout among mental health center directors in a rural state. Admin and Policy Ment Health 27(4), 221–237.

Rohland BM (2001) Telepsychiatry in the heartland: If we build it, will they come? Comm Ment Health J 37(5), 449–459.

Rohland BM and Langbehn DR (1998) Self report of mental health service use in rural versus urban recipients under Medicaid fee-for-service (Letter to the Editor). Psychiatr Serv 49(1), 107–108.

Rohland BM and Rohrer JE (1998) County funding of mental health services in a rural state. Psychiatr Serv 49, 691–693.

Rohland BM, Saleh SS, Rohrer JE, et al. (2000) Acceptability of telepsychiatry to a rural population. Psychiatr Serv 51(5), 672–674.

Schur CL and Franco SJ (1999) Access to Health Care, Ch. 2. In Rural Health in the United States, Ricketts TC (ed). Oxford University Press, New York.

Shelton DA and Frank R (1995) Rural mental health coverage under health care reform. Comm Ment Health J 31(6), 539–552.

Smith HA (1998) Telepsychiatry. Psychiatr Serv 49, 1494–1495.

Sullivan G, Jackson CA, and Spritzer KL (1996) Characteristics and service use of seriously mentally ill persons living in rural areas. Psychiatr Serv 47, 57–61.

Sullivan WP (1989) Community support programs in rural areas: Developing programs without walls. Human Serv Rural Environ 12(4), 19–22.

Sword M and Longden G (1989) The Idaho citizen companion program. Human Serv Rural Environ 12(4), 34–36.

Wagenfeld MO (2000) Delivering mental health services to the persistently and seriously mentally ill in frontier areas. J Rural Health 16(1), 91–96.

Wagenfeld MO, Murray JD, Mohatt DF, et al. (1994) Mental Health and Rural America: 1980–1993. An Overview and Annotated Bibliography. US Government Printing Office (NIH Publication No. 94–3500), Office of Rural Health Policy, Health Resources and Services, Administration, US Department of Health and Human Services, Washington DC.

Werner A and Anderson LE (1998) Rural telepsychiatry is economically unsupportable: The Concorde crashes in a cornfield. Psychiatr Serv 49, 1287–1290.

Williams ME, Ricketts TC, and Thompson BG (1995) Telemedicine and geriatrics: Back to the future. J Am Geriatr Soc 43, 1047–1051.

# 115 Correctional Psychiatry

Erik Roskes

But the insane criminal has nowhere any home: no age or nation has provided a place for him. He is everywhere unwelcome and objectionable. The prisons thrust him out; the hospitals are unwilling to receive him; the law will not let him stay at his house, and the public will not permit him to go abroad. And yet humanity and justice, the sense of common danger, and a tender regard for a deeply degraded brother-man, all agree that something should be done for him—that some plan must be devised different from, and better than, any that has yet been tried, by which he may be properly cared for, by which his malady may be healed, and his criminal propensity overcome.

(*Jarvis* 1857)

We should have a realistic conception of the composition of the prison and jail population before deciding that they are a scum entitled to nothing better than what a vengeful populace and a resource starved penal system choose to give them.

(*Johnson v. Phelan* 1995)

## Epidemiology of Mental Illness in Correctional Populations

For the purposes of this section, the term *correctional population* shall be defined to include those individuals under community supervision as well as those who are incarcerated. As of 2000, a total of 6.6 million people were on probation, in jail or prison, or on parole in the US. Of this population, over 2 million were incarcerated in the nation's jails and prisons (US Department of Justice 2001a). It is important to be aware that the number of incarcerated individuals in the US has quadrupled since 1980.

Mental health problems are common among correctional populations. It is difficult to get good data regarding the prevalence of mental illness among correctional populations. However, a variety of efforts have been made to attempt to understand the rates of mental illness among different correctional populations, the role of mental illness in leading individuals into corrections, and the role of the correctional environment in altering the presentation of mental illness in correctional settings.

An estimated 16%, or 284,000 inmates in jails and prisons, reported suffering from mental health problems or having been admitted to a hospital for mental health reasons (US Department of Justice 2001b). The data that follows demonstrate that persons with mental illness are being arrested and incarcerated in increasing numbers.

### Jails

Jails are defined as county- or locally-run detention facilities housing pretrial detainees and persons serving short sentences (generally less than a year). It has been widely reported that the rate of mental illness in jails is much higher than that in the community. For instance, Teplin (1990) and colleagues (1996) reported that 6.4% of male detainees and 15% of female detainees had severe psychiatric disorders. A recent study of detainees in a jail-based drug treatment program reported that 55% of the subjects suffered from any Axis I comorbid disorder and that 19% met lifetime criteria for a severe mental illness (defined as a major mood or psychotic disorder) (Swartz and Lurigio 1999).

### Prisons

Prisons are federal or state-run correctional institutions housing inmates sentenced for longer terms of confinement (usually greater than a year). A study of state prisoners in New York found that 8% of inmates had "severe psychiatric or functional disabilities" and an additional 16% had "significant mental disabilities" requiring periodic intervention (Steadman et al. 1987). Similarly, a recent survey in Great Britain identified 7% of male prisoners, 10% of male detainees, and 14% of women in both categories were found to be suffering from a psychotic illness (Fryers et al. 1998). The Department of Justice recently reported that in mid-2000, 13% of inmates in state prisons were receiving mental health therapy or counseling and 10% were receiving psychotropic medications. In addition, 1.6% of inmates (about 10% of those with mental illness) were in 24-hour care in special housing or psychiatric treatment facilities (US Department of Justice 2000).

### Arrest Population

It is unclear whether the overall rate of arrest for mentally ill persons differs from that of the general population. However, it appears that certain individuals with mental

| Table 115–1 | Factors Associated with Increased Arrests for Persons with Mental Illness |
|---|---|

- Homelessness
- Inaccessible community mental health services
- Limited civil commitment opportunities
- Substance abuse

illness are more likely to come to the attention of the criminal justice system than are individuals without mental illness (see Table 115–1).

For instance, homelessness appears to be a risk factor, as the rate of offenses was 35 times higher among homeless mentally ill persons than among domiciled mentally ill individuals (Martell et al. 1995). For example, Harry and Steadman (1988) found no difference in rates of arrest between a cohort of individuals admitted to a community mental health center and the general population of the area. Another study strongly linked prior criminal behavior to risk of violent crime among mentally ill persons in sheltered care (Hwang and Segal 1996).

The role of police discretion and diversion is important to consider. In a study by Lamb and colleagues (1995) that followed up on patients referred by a joint police–mental health outreach team in Los Angeles, the authors reported that only 2% of the cases resulted in arrest at the time of the initial referral; however, 24% of the referrals had been arrested in a 6-month follow-up period. The authors concluded that it was the involvement of the mental health provider in the outreach effort that reduced the arrest rate; when the same individuals were subsequently encountered by police alone, they were more likely to be arrested. In addition, over 40% of the subjects were hospitalized during the follow-up phase, indicating poor retention in outpatient treatment. Thus, this "criminalization" has much to do with restrictive civil commitment criteria and inadequately funded and poorly accessible community mental health services in many areas. In areas where treatment is difficult to access, law officers may be more likely to arrest and detain persons who are mentally ill as it is expedient to do so (Sullivan and Spritzer 1997).

It should be noted that developments in psychopharmacology may have a direct impact on arrest rates. A recent study suggested that psychotic patients taking clozapine were significantly less likely to be arrested than psychotic patients not taking clozapine (Frankle et al. 2001). This study also noted that arrest rates increased by 65% after the onset of mental illness among the group studied, supporting a relationship between psychotic illnesses and criminal behaviors.

A related question is whether mental illness predisposes to *rearrest* after an incarceration. Harris and Koepsell (1998) suggest that this is not so, finding no difference in rearrest rates between matched mentally ill and nonmentally ill detainees in the King County Jail. Solomon and coworkers (1994) examined the role of community mental health services in recidivism to jail. They found that recidivism was associated with receipt of *fewer* mental health services, implying that case management deteriorated into a monitoring program, rather than enabling rehabilitation and retention in community services. In other words, the

case manager runs the risk of becoming an extension of the criminal justice system, rather than an agent of care for the patient. Programs are in development to ensure that mentally ill persons released from incarceration are able to access coordinated care and monitoring that will not simply serve as an extension of the probation and parole supervisor (Roskes and Feldman 1999, Roskes et al. 1999).

## Legal Considerations

The legal basis for the inmate's right to treatment was established in *Estelle v. Gamble*. In this case, the Supreme Court held that "deliberate indifference to serious medical needs of prisoners constitutes unnecessary and wanton infliction of pain proscribed by [the] Eighth Amendment whether the indifference is manifested by prison doctors in response to prison needs or by prison guards in intentionally denying or delaying access to medical care or intentionally interfering with treatment one prescribed" (*Estelle v. Gamble* 1976). Later cases established that mental illnesses were indistinguishable from medical conditions, at least with respect to the inmate's right to treatment (*Bowring v. Godwin* 1977). In *Farmer v. Brennan* (1994), the Supreme Court defined "deliberate indifference" as "something more than negligence, but . . . something less than acts or omissions for the very purpose of causing harm or with knowledge that harm will result. Thus, it is the equivalent of acting recklessly." In summary, the standard by which a correctional facility is held accountable is that of deliberate indifference to a serious medical need. It is important to note that the original *Estelle* court in 1976 distinguished clearly between the standard of deliberate indifference and that of negligence, the basis for medical malpractice claims, stating: "Medical malpractice does not become a constitutional violation merely because the victim is a prisoner" (*Estelle v. Gamble* 1976).

Minimum standards for an acceptable treatment program within a prison were established in *Ruiz v. Estelle* (1980). The key elements of such a treatment program were to include the following (see Table 115–2):

(1) a systematic program for screening and evaluation must be in place to identify inmates with mental illness
(2) treatment must be something more than simple segregation and close supervision of inmates with identified mental health needs
(3) treatment must include the participation of trained mental health professionals in adequate numbers to

| Table 115–2 | Court-Established Minimal Standards for Mental Health Treatment in Prisons |
|---|---|

- Capacity for screening and evaluation
- Capacity to treat beyond segregation and supervision
- Utilization of adequate numbers of competent mental health professionals
- Individualized treatment
- Accurate, complete, confidential medical records
- Supervised psychiatric medications with periodic reevaluation
- Identification, treatment, and supervision for patients at risk for suicide

develop individualized interventions for mentally ill inmates

(4) a system for accurate, complete, and confidential record keeping must be maintained

(5) use of psychiatric medications without appropriate supervision and in the absence of periodic reevaluations is not acceptable

(6) a program for the identification, treatment, and supervision of inmates at risk of suicide must be a component of the overall treatment program

Readers interested in more details regarding the legal aspects of correctional mental health care are referred to the seminal work of Cohen (1998).

## Mental Health Care in Correctional Settings

### Standards

As noted above, the minimum standards for an acceptable correctional mental health treatment program were outlined in *Ruiz v. Estelle*. A number of organizations, including the American Bar Association, American Correctional Association, American Psychiatric Association (2000), American Psychological Association, American Public Health Association, and National Commission on Correctional Health Care (available at http://www.ncchc.org), have promulgated sets of standards with varying detail regarding aspects of correctional health and mental health care (see Table 115–3). These standards are described and compared in Cohen (1998), and they include the following.

### Screening

Jails and prisons routinely assess newly arrived detainees and inmates regarding a variety of areas. All of the above referenced standard setting bodies require screening regarding mental health needs. Typically, this is a multistep process, beginning with very broad-brush screening questions (with high sensitivity, low specificity) and moving towards increasingly specific evaluations and assessments. Often, the first step consists of a few key questions posed by the intake correctional officer, such as "Have you ever had a psychiatric problem? Taken psychiatric medications? Been in a psychiatric hospital?" Another common question at this stage is "Have you ever attempted suicide? Are you suicidal now?"

### Assessment and Evaluation

Individuals with a positive answer to any of the initial screening questions are referred for a more in-depth assessment by a health care provider. Typically, this is a more detailed screening process, designed to help determine who will need an urgent or immediate psychiatric evaluation and who can be managed in a more routine fashion. The provider performing this assessment is often a nurse, physician assistant, or other health care provider who may not necessarily have specialized mental health training.

Individuals who are determined to need rapid psychiatric assessment should be housed in a special unit designed for safe monitoring and will be prioritized for psychiatric care. In a well designed and staffed correctional institution, such persons may be continued on medications they had previously been taking while awaiting the psychiatrist's next visit. Once evaluated, the psychiatrist and other mental health staff can determine the best venue for housing and treatment of the individual inmate.

### Treatment/Management

There are a variety of levels of care that may exist in a correctional system, depending on size and location. Large prison systems may include all of these levels of care, while small jails may not have any of them and may utilize outside agencies (such as a community mental health center or a state hospital) to provide all mental health services (Maier and Miller 1989). Jails, because of their shorter-term mission, may not provide all of the services below but may focus instead on identification of individuals with mental illness and choose to refer them for ongoing treatment. It is important to keep in mind that correctional administrators wrestle with finding a balance between their very real budgetary restrictions and the need to meet all needs of the prison or jail, and the requirements of the courts as discussed above. What is presented here is to some extent an ideal; many systems struggle to meet this ideal. Further discussion of the economic constraints faced by administrators will be presented below.

**"Outpatient" Care.** As described by the Bureau of Justice Statistics (US Department of Justice 2001b), 13% of state prison inmates in 2000 were receiving therapy or counseling, and 10% were receiving medications. Nearly all of these (65–70%) were maintained in general population settings (i.e., not in specialized mental health housing). Typically, such inmates are seen on a monthly or quarterly basis by a psychologist and/or a psychiatrist. In addition, services may be provided for crisis intervention. Such care superficially resembles the typical care provided by a community mental health center.

**Special Housing.** Many large correctional institutions and systems provide for special housing for individuals identified with mental illness. For example, the Baltimore City Detention Center, with a total population of about 3,000, includes a 65-bed residential unit. Detainees who are known or identified as having difficulty managing jail life in general population settings because of mental or behavioral disturbance, but who are not so sick as to require inpatient care, are housed there, where they are provided with regular contact with a psychologist and psychiatrist. In addition, correctional staff have been assigned to work in the mental health section to develop an improved understanding of the mental health needs of the detainees housed there. The development of specialized units, such as therapeutic communities for inmates with histories of substance abuse/

| Table 115–3 | Standards of Mental Health Care in Correctional Settings |
|---|---|

- Initial mental health screen
- Further assessment of identified candidates
- Treatment including:
  counseling
  medication
  symptom-based placement
  periodic reevaluation
- Discharge planning (medication, follow-up appointments)

dependence or "honor dorms," have led to improved behaviors among inmates and reduced recidivism among their
graduates.

**"Inpatient" Care.** Large institutions and systems may also
provide their own inpatient treatment facilities. Some
systems (e.g., Maryland Department of Public Safety and
Correctional Services) have created a specialized prison
designated as the inpatient facility for seriously mentally
ill and behaviorally disturbed inmates (see http://www.
dpscs.state.md.us/pat/mental_hc.htm for a description of
services provided to inmates within the Maryland system).
Others (e.g., New York Department of Corrections) have
contracted with outside agencies such as the Department of
Mental Health in the development of joint agencies for the
treatment of seriously mentally ill inmates (see http://www.
omh.state.ny.us/omhweb/facilities/cnpc/facility.htm for a
description of Central New York Psychiatric Center, the
hospital run by the Department of Mental Health for prisoners needing psychiatric hospitalization).

**Medication Management.** As outlined in *Ruiz v. Estelle*,
one of the services to be provided to inmates suffering with
mental illness is medication management. Medication
management should include rational prescribing following
appropriate diagnosis and adequate monitoring and reevaluation of the ongoing therapy. A significant issue in many
correctional systems is the limited formulary, imposed due
to economic constraints as noted below.

**Psychotherapy.** Many inmates with mental health problems are provided with evaluations and ongoing treatment
with psychologists or other mental health professionals.
This may be provided in individual or group settings.
Often, such services begin when an inmate presents in crisis,
and for some inmates, the crisis results in the beginning of a
longer-term individual or group therapy. Typical problems
include adjustment to prison, reactions to family difficulties
outside the prison, and more severe psychiatric problems
requiring both therapy and medications.

**Release Planning.** Recently, attention has been paid to the
mentally ill inmate who is being released from jail or prison.
What is the responsibility of the institution and its mental
health professionals regarding the provision of aftercare or
transition planning?

A key case in this area is *Brad H. v. New York*, ongoing
litigation in New York City. In this case, the trial court held
that inmates being released from jail in New York must be
provided with "adequate discharge planning," meaning
more than simply being released in the middle of the
night with $1.50 and two subway tokens. The ruling has
thus far been upheld, and has resulted in considerable re-
shuffling and improvement in these services in New York
City.

A second key case in this arena is that of *Wakefield v.
Thompson* (1999), a prison case involving an inmate with a
psychotic disorder. The inmate was provided with a prescription for his antipsychotic to be dispensed on release. The
correctional staff failed to provide the inmate with the medication on release, and, after decompensating, the inmate
became psychotic and committed a violent offense just 11
days after his release. The 9th US Circuit Court of Appeals
overturned the trial court's dismissal, noting that a newly

released inmate may not be able to rapidly acquire treatment once released:

> We therefore hold that the state must provide an
> outgoing prisoner who is receiving and continues to
> require medication with a supply sufficient to ensure
> that he has that medication available during the
> period of time reasonably necessary to permit him to
> consult a doctor and obtain a new supply. A state's
> failure to provide medication sufficient to cover this
> transitional period amounts to an abdication of its
> responsibility to provide medical care to those, who
> by reason of incarceration, are unable to provide for
> their own medical needs.
>
> (*Wakefield v. Thompson* 1999)

The *Wakefield* principle has since been applied to a jail
case in which a detainee was released on bond in an effort to
prevent the county from having to pay the detainee's medical bills (*Marsh v. Butler County, Alabama* 2000) and to a
case involving the need for ongoing medical care upon
release from prison (*Lugo v. Senkowski* 2000).

## Special Topics/Special Challenges
(See Table 115–4)

### Refusal of Treatment
Does an inmate in a prison have the right to refuse treatment? What about a pretrial detainee? How do the rights of
the incarcerated resemble and differ from those of the mentally ill at large? Ultimately, the larger question underlying
all of these issues is whether prisoners and jail detainees
have the right to give informed consent to recommended
treatment. Assuming that the provision of relevant information regarding the treatment proposed is considered a
part of standard care, then prisoner-patients have as much
right to refuse treatment as any other patient.

It is important to recognize, however, that an individual prisoner's treatment refusal may adversely impact other
prisoners. Consider an individual with a psychosis resulting
in paranoia and threats to other inmates and to staff. These
potential victims cannot distance themselves from the sick
person. They also have a right to be safe, either as prisoners
(under the Eighth Amendment) or as staff of the institution
(under Occupational Safety and Health Administration
OSHA). Some states have resolved this problem by creating
an administrative hearing process requiring a finding that,
untreated, the mental illness will cause the inmate to be
"gravely disabled or dangerous" (*Washington v. Harper*
1990). While this may superficially resemble civil procedures
for forcing medications on committed inpatients, it differs in
that there is no required judicial oversight of the decision.

| Table 115–4 | Mental Health Challenges Faced by Correctional Settings |
|---|---|

- Refusal of treatment
- Seclusion and restraint
- Competing priorities
- Economics

## Seclusion and Restraint

In correctional settings, the use of seclusion and restraint with psychiatric patients are confounded, as there are situations in which inmates may be isolated or restrained for nontherapeutic reasons. In general, it is clear, however, that when restraints or seclusion are ordered with a therapeutic intent, such decisions are to be made by appropriate clinicians and that the inmate-patient being treated with the intervention be monitored adequately.

All corrections agencies have a system of custody levels, ranging from low security (e.g., prerelease or work-release), through minimum, medium, and maximum to "supermax" levels. Inmates are classified based on a variety of factors including their instant offense (the offense leading to the current incarceration), prior criminal record, and institutional adjustment factors. Inmates with pronounced difficulty adjusting to the prison setting tend to rise in classification level, ultimately arriving at the supermax level. Because mental illness and mental retardation may result in difficulty with adjustment to prison, it is imperative that administrators have in place a system for evaluation of inmates for "suitability" for placement in these ultrahigh security settings, which may involve total isolation from other inmates and near-total isolation from staff. Inmates whose difficulty in adjusting is believed to be due to mental illness or retardation should be referred for special housing units or treatment designed to help them accommodate to the prison setting, rather than placed in higher security levels for punitive purposes. Although this sounds simple in theory, it can be extremely difficult in practice, given the complicated diagnostic comorbidities among the prison populace.

## Dual Agency

A frequent dilemma faced by the correctional psychiatrist is the problem of dual agency. Familiar to forensic psychiatrists, this issue may present problems for the novice in this area. Providers in corrections have two consumers of their service: their patient and the correctional manager (Packard 1989). Their obligations may arise in several ways. A clinician may be asked to do a formal forensic evaluation, for example when an inmate in his/her care is charged with a new crime and needs a forensic evaluation for trial competency or criminal responsibility.

A more frequent occurrence is an institution-related need: should this inmate be absolved of responsibility for a rule infraction due to mental illness or not? Should that inmate be placed on segregation or moved to a higher security level? These are examples of common questions asked of the provider in a correctional setting and which may place the patient's interests at odds with the needs of the institution.

Recruitment and retention of mental health care providers within correctional settings is a challenge, and often prisons and jails have inadequate numbers of mental health staff. These jobs are not typically sought after, as they are perceived as dangerous. By the nature of the setting, health care providers may feel compelled to play a role in containment and discipline, which disrupts the establishment of traditional partnership/therapeutic alliance relationships.

## Economics and Correctional Health Care

Correctional administrators struggle with limited budgets, imposed by the legislators responsible for funding the correctional system. With their budget, they are responsible for managing all aspects of their institution—staffing, infrastructure, security, and inmate services. Mental health is but one part of the overall health care service available to inmates.

A frequent response of correctional administrators is to contract with private companies to provide health care services in their jail or prison. Such contracts can be for any or all of the following services: health care providers (including doctors, dentists, nurses, psychologists, etc.), lab and radiology services, and pharmacy services. Because these contracts operate as a capitated system of care, the contractor is usually at risk for all costs and therefore may incentivize practitioners to keep costs down in a variety of ways. As in the private sector, one of the most cost-limiting strategies used is a restricted formulary and use of less qualified (and hence less expensive) staff. Because many of these contracts are for short terms (less than 3 years), little attention is given to long-term cost savings that may be realized with the up-front investment of a more expensive medication (e.g., reduced risk of tardive dyskinesia with newer, more expensive antipsychotic medications).

Similarly, less qualified (and less expensive) staff may resort to less appropriate treatment; indeed, the provision of treatment may trickle down to untrained prison officers. As prison administrators/decision- and policymakers may lack the expertise to counter such medicoeconomic decisions, it can be difficult to provide the needed oversight of these private contractors.

Some states have responded to these concerns (either proactively or in response to litigation) with the establishment of independent oversight committees and/or internal performance improvement committees. In addition, mental health training curricula are being offered to frontline officers. This training may allow them to act as first-line screeners, offering preventative mental health care, as well as acting as conduits for the receipt of more urgent care.

## Conclusion

The number of persons with mental illness appears to be increasing in correctional settings. Judicial decrees have established the right to treatment, and national standards have been promulgated. However, capacity and commitment to attain these standards are often stymied by limited staffing and financial resources, and by a lack of vision and understanding regarding the necessity and import of consistent quality mental health care. Prompt and appropriate provision of mental health care can lead to improved outcomes (fewer disturbances, injuries, and suicides, less property damage, enhanced inmate production, and reduced recidivism).

## References

American Psychiatric Association (2000) Psychiatric Services in Jails and Prisons, 2nd ed. APA, Washington DC.
Bowring v. Godwin (1977) 551 F.2d 44, 4th Cir.
Cohen F (1998) The Mentally Disordered Inmate and the Law. Civic Research Institute, Kingston, NJ.
Estelle v. Gamble (1976) 97 S.Ct. 285, 429 US 97.
Farmer v. Brennan (1994) 511 US 825.

Frankle WG, Shera D, Berger-Hershkowitz H, et al. (2001) Clozapine-associated reduction in arrest rates of psychotic patients with criminal histories. Am J Psychiatr 158, 270–274.

Fryers T, Brugha T, Grounds A, et al. (1998) Severe mental illness in prisoners. Brit Med J 317, 1025–1026.

Harris V and Koepsell TD (1998) Rearrest among mentally ill offenders. J Am Acad Psychiatr Law 26, 393–402.

Harry B and Steadman HJ (1988) Arrest rates of patients treated at a community mental health center. Hosp Comm Psychiatr 39, 862–866.

Hwang SD and Segal SP (1996) Criminality of the mentally ill in sheltered care: Are they more dangerous? Int J Law Psychiatr 19, 93–105.

Jarvis E (1857) Criminal insane. Insane transgressors and insane convicts. Am J Insanity 13, 195–231.

Johnson v. Phelan (1995) 69 F.3d 144, 7th Cir.

Lamb HR, Shaner R, Elliott DM, et al. (1995) Outcome for psychiatric emergency patients seen by an outreach police-mental health team. Psychiatr Serv 46, 1267–1271.

Lugo v. Senkowski (2000) WL 1456235 (N.D.N.Y.).

Maier GJ and Miller RD (1989) Models of mental health service delivery to correctional institutions. In Correctional Psychiatry, Rosner R and Harmon, RB (eds). Plenum Press, New York, pp. 231–241.

Marsh v. Butler County, Alabama (2000) 212 F.3d 1318, 11th Cir.

Martell DA, Rosner R, and Harmon RB (1995) Base-rate estimates of criminal behavior by homeless mentally ill persons in New York City. Psychiatr Serv 46, 596–601.

Packard WS (1989) Forensic evaluation and treatment in the same institution: A moral dilemma. In Correctional Psychiatry, Rosner R and Harmon, RB (eds). Plenum Press, New York, pp. 187–195.

Roskes E and Feldman R (1999) A collaborative community-based treatment program for offenders with mental illness. Psychiatr Serv 50, 1614–1619.

Roskes E, Feldman R, Arrington S, et al. (1999) A model program for the treatment of mentally ill offenders in the community. Comm Ment Health J 35, 461–472.

Ruiz v. Estelle (1980) 503 F. Supp. 1265, S.D. Texas.

Solomon P, Draine J, and Meyerson A (1994) Jail recidivism and receipt of community mental health services. Hosp Comm Psychiatr 45, 793–797.

Steadman HJ, Faasiak S, Dvoskin J, et al. (1987) A survey of mental disability among state prison inmates. Hosp Comm Psychiatr 38, 1086–1090.

Sullivan G and Spritzer K (1997) The criminalization of persons with serious mental illness living in rural areas. J Rural Health 13, 6–13.

Swartz JA and Lurigio AJ (1999) Psychiatric illness and comorbidity among adult male jail detainees in drug treatment. Psychiatr Serv 50, 1628–1630.

Teplin LA (1990) The prevalence of severe mental disorder among male urban jail detainees: Comparison with the Epidemiologic Catchment Area Study. Am J Pub Health 80, 663–669.

Teplin LA, Abram KM, and McClelland GM (1996) Prevalence of psychiatric disorders among incarcerated women. Arch Gen Psychiatr 53, 505–512.

US Department of Justice (2000) Bureau of Justice Statistics, Mental Health Treatment in State Prisons, http://www.ojp.usdoj.gov/bjs/abstract/mhtsp00.htm.

US Department of Justice (2001a) Bureau of Justice Statistics, Correction Statistics, http://www.ojp.usdoj.gov/bjs/correct.htm.

US Department of Justice (2001b) Bureau of Justice Statistics, Mental Health and Treatment of Inmates and Probationers, http://www.ojp.usdoj.gov/bjs/abstract/mhtip.htm.

Wakefield v. Thompson (1999) 177 F.3d 1160, 9th Cir.

Washington v. Harper (1990) 110 S.Ct. 1028, 494 US 210.

## Further Reading

Correctional Mental Health Report, published bimonthly by Civic Research Institute, Kingston, NJ.

Landsberg G and Smiley A (2001) Forensic Mental Health: Working with Offenders with Mental Illness. Civic Research Institute, Kingston, NJ.

Rosner R and Harmon RB (eds) (1989) Correctional Psychiatry. Plenum Press, New York.

Vaughan PJ and Badger D (1995) Working with the Mentally Disordered Offender in the Community. Chapman & Hall, London.

Webb D and Harris R (1999) Mentally Disordered Offenders: Managing People Nobody Owns. Routledge, London.

Wettstein RM (1998) Treatment of Offenders with Mental Disorders. Guilford Press, New York.

# 116 Dual Diagnoses

Kenneth Minkoff

## Overview

Individuals with co-occurring psychiatric and substance disorders (ICOPSD) include patients with any combination of mental health symptoms or disorders (including substance-induced mental disorders) with substance use disorders. By any measure, these individuals are a challenging population, associated with poor outcomes in multiple venues, including increased risk of relapse, rehospitalization, suicide, violence, criminal activity, traumatic life events (including abuse and rape), medical comorbidity (particularly sexually transmitted diseases [STDs]), homelessness, and family disruption, including child abuse and neglect (RachBeisel et al. 1999). In addition, these individuals are overrepresented among the highest cost clients in the scarce-resourced public delivery system (Hartman and Nelson 1997, Quinlivan and McWhirter 2000). As a consequence, they would appear to be a high priority population for engagement and proactive outreach throughout the service system.

Unfortunately, however, in most systems, the opposite is true. Individuals with co-occurring disorders are often experienced as "system misfits," who dare to have more than one disorder in systems of care that are designed as if everyone had only one disorder or one disorder at a time. Programs within those systems are similarly designed so that clinicians frequently experience a need to either contort their programs to fit their clients or adjust their clients to fit their programs. Clinical practices and procedures are similarly not designed to support the identification and treatment of comorbidity, even at the most basic level of client registration and billing, which often requires clients to be identified as having only one primary disorder. Finally, clinicians are generally trained and identified as either mental health clinicians or substance clinicians, but not both, so when they engage with individuals with comorbidity, they experience a misfit between what the client needs and what they know. Consequently, at every level, the design of the service system routinely supports the likelihood that individuals with co-occurring disorders will fail to be engaged and adequately treated, thus contributing to the incidence of poorer outcomes and higher costs (Minkoff 2000).

From the perspective of a community psychiatrist, it may often appear that little can be done to address successfully the clinical and administrative dilemmas presented by individuals with comorbid psychiatric and substance disorders. The purpose of this chapter is to address this concern by providing for both clinicians and administrators an organized set of research derived principles of treatment that provide guidance for assessment and individualized clinical treatment matching, as well as providing guidance for developing programmatic initiatives that are more dual diagnosis capable, even within the constraints of existing resources, and which support the evolution of comprehensive, continuous, integrated systems of care (CCISC) for better serving individuals with co-occurring disorders in all settings.

## Background Research

Space constraints prevent comprehensive review of all literature related to the treatment of individuals with co-occurring disorders (COD) in community settings. This section will try to identify the most salient research derived concepts that form the underpinning of the treatment principles. For a more comprehensive literature review, the reader is referred to RachBeisel and colleagues (1999), Minkoff (1997), and Drake and colleagues (2001).

## Epidemiology

Epidemiologic surveys during the past 2 decades have repeatedly identified the high prevalence of comorbidity in both community populations and treatment populations. The Epidemiologic Catchment Area Survey (Reiger et al. 2001), for example, found that 55% of schizophrenics in treatment,

| Table 116–1 | Conclusions from Dual Diagnosis Research |
|---|---|

Dual diagnosis is an expectation, not an exception

Dual diagnosis is associated with poor outcomes and high cost

Integrated mental health and substance abuse treatment is a best practice

Treatment should be individually matched, based on assessment of:

  diagnosis

  level of disability (need for case management)

  stage of change/stage of treatment (stage-specific treatement)

  rehabilitative goals/strengths (job, housing)

  level of care (ASAM, LOCUS)

and 62% of bipolar individuals had lifetime substance use disorders. The National Comorbidity Survey (Kessler et al. 1996) determined that 59.9% of individuals with substance disorders had a lifetime psychiatric diagnosis (Axis I or II). More complex treatment populations (e.g., pregnant and parenting women addicts) have higher prevalence of comorbidity, often with multiple diagnoses (substance disorder, mood and anxiety disorders, trauma related disorders, personality disorders, etc.) (Alexander 1996). Consequently, it begins to become clear that in almost all treatment settings, dual diagnosis is an expectation, not an exception (Minkoff 1991). This finding, associated with poor outcomes and high costs for this population, begins to have significant implication for service and system design.

## Treatment Matching

A variety of research has established the value of "problem-service matching" in producing better treatment outcomes. McLellan and others (1997) identified that individuals with addiction who had co-occurring emotional and behavioral problems had better outcomes if mental health issues were addressed during their addiction treatment. Conversely, a series of researchers (Drake et al. 2001) have established the value of integrating substance treatment into services for individuals with serious and persistent mental illness (SPMI) who have co-occurring substance disorders. Another dimension of treatment matching involves a growing literature on the value of case management services for complex addiction populations with multiple impairments and disabilities, just as has been well established for similarly impaired psychiatric populations (Godley et al. 2000), so that services provided must match client needs in areas where the client is unable to provide for himself. In addition, there is a well-established literature on the importance of identifying stage of change (Prochaska et al. 1992)—precontemplation, contemplation, preparation, action, and maintenance—or stage of treatment—described for seriously mentally ill populations (Osher and Kofoed 1989)—engagement, persuasion, active treatment, and relapse prevention (McHugo et al. 1995)—and matching treatment and expected outcome to stage (termed stagewise or stage-specific treatment). In this context, both harm reduction and abstinence oriented interventions are both appropriate strategies if properly matched to substance diagnosis (abuse versus dependence, respectively) and stage of change or stage of treatment (Minkoff 1991, Miller and Rollnick 1991). Further, in addition to matching services to needs and motivation to change, there is growing evidence of the value of matching services to strengths and goals. Recent data have demonstrated the value of the individualized placement and support model of psychiatric rehabilitation in both engagement and treatment of individuals with active comorbidity who present requesting assistance in finding a job as a primary goal (Bond et al. 2001). Similarly, there is increasing evidence supporting the efficacy of "wet" or consumer choice supported housing options for individuals with active co-occurring disorders who are homeless and whose only stated goal is to obtain housing (Tsemberis and Eisenberg 2000, Goldfinger et al. 1999). Finally, there is a growing literature, and some research base, for treatment matching to level of care based on multidimensional level of care assessment. The American Society of Addiction Medicine: Patient Placement Criteria 2R (ASAM PPC2R) (2001) incorporates dimensions of psychiatric impairment into its assessment of addiction treatment matching requirements. The Level of Care Utilization System (LOCUS 2.001) (American Association of Community Psychiatrists 2000a) also includes assessment of severity of comorbidity as one dimension in level of care determination. ASAM PPC2R has also introduced the categorization of all addiction programs as needing to be either *dual diagnosis capable* (for working with expected populations of low-moderate severity comorbidity), as a standard expectation, or *dual diagnosis enhanced* (for providing addiction treatment to more psychiatrically impaired individuals). This same language has been applied to mental health programs (Minkoff 2000). The standardization of these program categories and their validity for program matching has heuristic value in policy development, but has yet to be formally studied.

## Treatment Interventions and Technology

Other research advances have identified new treatment technologies that have applicability to individuals with co-occurring disorders, and that fit within the context of the treatment matching data described above (Table 116–2). With regard to stage-specific treatment for example, there is an extensive literature on motivational enhancement techniques (Miller and Rollnick 1991, Centre for Substance Abuse Treatment 2003), and further research documenting the applicability of these interventions to individuals with severe mental illness (Carey 1996, Ziedonis and Trudeau 1997). Further work has documented the value of stage-specific group interventions, in addition to individual and family interventions in applying motivational enhancement to individuals with serious mental illness (Mueser and Noordsy 1996, Mueser and Fox 1998). Motivational enhancement technology is appropriately complemented by a growing literature on the use of community reinforcement and contingency management in the treatment of individuals with substance disorders, and these same technologies are increasingly being applied to the treatment of individuals with co-occurring disorders as well. This application is being described in correctional system interventions (drug court, mental health court, "dual diagnosis" court) (Peters and Bartoi 1997, Peters and Hills 1997), and in application of payeeship management and other reinforcement strategies for individuals with serious mental illnesses in community mental health settings (Ries and Comtois 1997, Shaner et al. 1997).

| Table 116–2 | New Treatment Technologies |
|---|---|

Stage-specific individual, group, and the family treatment, including
Motivational enhancement
Manualized skills training
Contingency management
Family psychoeducation
Trauma screening and cognitive behavioural treatment
Interventions in the correctional system ("dual diagnosis court")

Further advances in treatment technology involve the development of a variety of techniques for screening, assessment, and cognitive–behavioral treatment of trauma-related pathology in women who have co-occurring serious mental illness and substance disorder, including the development and dissemination of research-supported curricular materials for that purpose (Evans and Sullivan 1995, Najarits 2002, Harris 1998). Finally, there is a growing literature on the application of skills training techniques for individuals with severe mental illness to addressing decisions and skills related to substance use disorders, both substance abuse and substance dependence. These techniques emphasize that skill acquisition interventions for substance disorders must be extensively modified for individuals with severe disabilities, involving smaller steps, with more practice and rehearsal, with more support, over a longer time period, just as for other types of cognitive and behavioral skills. The challenge is making the skills training simple enough, and marking small increments of progress as representing significant success. Skills training manuals based on Liberman's work on psychosocial skills training (Roberts et al. 1999, Bellack et al. 1999) have been demonstrated to be useful with this population.

## Psychopharmacology

There has traditionally been a dearth of research investigating psychopharmacologic interventions specifically with individuals with co-occurring disorders, particularly those who are actively using substances. However, this has begun to change. Currently, there is sufficient research to support the development of consensus clinical psychopharmacologic practice guidelines (Minkoff 1998, Minkoff 2001a, 2001b). The most consistent finding, in multiple studies of individuals with a wide range of psychiatric diagnoses, is that adequate psychopharmacology of a known psychiatric disorder promotes better outcome for both the mental illness and comorbid substance disorder (Adelman et al. 1993, Sowers and Golden 1999, Brady and Roberts 1995). Further, studies of effective treatment programs for seriously mentally ill individuals with active substance use disorders uniformly continue nonaddictive necessary medication even though substance use persists for years (Drake et al. 1993a, 1993b). In addition, more recent studies indicate that better medication for the mental illness can improve outcome for the substance disorder as well.

Thus, individuals with psychotic disorders and active substance use may have improvement in comorbid substance use when switched to atypical neuroleptics; further, clozapine appears to have a direct effect on reducing substance use in this population, possibly by direct effect on dopaminergic receptor sites, mediating euphoria (Albanese et al. 1994, Zimmet et al. 2000). Studies of newer generation mood stabilizers have indicated the value of these agents in individuals with co-occurring disorders, particularly those with atypical or rapid cycling disorders and/or with comorbid anxiety or aggression that may be addressed by these agents (Brady and Roberts 1995). A number of studies have identified that although bupropion, followed by other antidepressants, alpha-2-adrenergic agents (clonidine), and mood stabilizers, may be recommended for individuals with attention-deficit/hyperactivity disorder (ADHD) in the early sobriety period, most such individuals benefit from progression to adequate dosages of stimulants once sobriety has been established for a period of time (Wilens et al. 1996, 2001, Biederman et al. 1999). For unipolar depressive disorders, newer generation (posttricyclic) antidepressants are appropriate for use in early recovery, and may be maintained if necessary in the event of relapse; further, there are some studies that indicate the possible advantage of serotoninergic agents in treating some subtypes of alcohol dependence (Cornelius et al. 1997, Pechter and Miller 1997).

With regard to anxiety disorders, benzodiazepines are generally not recommended for treating individuals with substance dependence beyond the detoxification phase; however, neither should they be withheld from carefully selected sober patients who may benefit for treatment of severe anxiety disorders because of a history of addiction (Ciraulo and Nace 2000). Use of benzodiazepines in such situations should be considered an indication to obtain a second opinion or consultation, ideally from a more experienced addiction prescriber (Minkoff 1998). Nonaddictive anxiety medications of reported value include clonidine and guanfacine, selective serotonin reuptake inhibitor (SSRI), venlafaxine, nefazodone, newer generation mood stabilizers (e.g., gabapentin, valproate), and atypical neuroleptics (Sowers and Golden 1999). Buspirone is reported to be less effective in patients with a history of addiction or benzodiazepine use (Tollefson et al. 1992). Finally, there is growing availability of psychopharmacologic agents for treatment of substance dependence, starting with disulfiram and opiate maintenance agents, and proceeding to the availability of naltrexone in the treatment of alcohol dependence (Mueser et al. 2001). Although there are individual psychopharmacologic interactions, in general these agents are useful and effective with individuals who have comorbid disorders for appropriate indications.

## Treatment Programs

Treatment programs have been developed which comprise a range of possibilities for integrating mental health and substance interventions for defined populations according to the treatment matching paradigms described above. The most well-studied program is the integrated intensive case management team, or Continuous Treatment Team, which integrates intensive case management proactive outreach to highly disengaged consumers, close monitoring and provision of psychopharmacology, family psychoeducation, access to individualized rehabilitation and housing support, with stage-specific and disability modified individual and group substance interventions. This type of program has been identified as an evidence-based best practice for the treatment of highly disengaged individuals with serious mental illness and serious active substance use disorders (Drake et al. 2001). Solid outcome data indicate that these programs can be quite successful, but that progress is incremental and slow; it generally takes 4 years for half the consumers (beginning with those who are in early stages of treatment) to achieve stable abstinence; and about a year to move through each stage of treatment on the way.

Another well-studied program model, for a range of individuals with co-occurring disorders (including those with SPMI, those with antisocial personality disorder) is the modified addiction residential program, or modified

| Table 116–3 | Services Provided by Integrated Treatment Teams |
|---|---|

Empathic, hopeful relationships
Continuous treatment
Proactive outreach
Close monitoring
Appropriates case management
Integrated mh/sa treatment
Continuing psychopharmacology
Family psychoeducation
Stage-specific substance abuse treatment
Individualized rehabilitation
Housing support
Longitudinal perspective to support incremental progress

therapeutic community (Sacks et al. 1999). These programs involve integration of mental health services into abstinence oriented addiction treatment environments, and modification of the expectation of those environments to accommodate the needs of individuals who might have severe psychiatric impairments and/or personality disorders. Treatment outcomes are enhanced by longer lengths of engagement in treatment at a variety of levels of care. However, these programs only work for those individuals who are either willing or mandated to enter abstinence mandated treatment and are capable of doing the work needed to remain, however integrated or modified. Modified addiction treatment interventions have been extended through the continuum to programs (described in the ASAM PPC2R as Dual Diagnosis Enhanced programs) at each level of care (Wilens et al. 1992, Minkoff and Regner 1999). Finally, there is a growing literature describing and studying both community-based integrated case management programs as well as integrated residential programs for other complex populations, most notably pregnant and parenting women (Brown 2000, WELL Project 1999). Some intensive integrated case management program models have been specifically applied to high cost service utilizers in managed care systems, with documentation of cost effectiveness in 12 to 18 months (Quinlivan and McWhirter 1996).

## Consensus Best Practice Treatment Principles

Because of the high prevalence and variety of individuals with co-occurring disorders, specific research-based programs and interventions have only been applied to a tiny percentage of all the clinical situations in which individuals with co-occurring disorders may appear. For this reason, it has been necessary to develop clinical consensus best practice principles, extrapolated from the available research, to govern clinical practice in all settings. This process was undertaken through a federally funded initiative in the mid-1990s, resulting in dissemination of a set of standards, clinical practice guidelines, and expected workforce competencies in 1998 (Minkoff 1998, Minkoff 2001a). These consensus standards encompass a number of treatment principles that can be placed in the context of an integrated treatment philosophy that uses a common language that

makes sense from the perspective of both the mental health system and the addiction system. These same principles form the basis for clinical practice guidelines for assessment, treatment matching, rehabilitation, and psychopharmacology, which in turn have been formally adopted to govern clinical practice in at least one state (Minkoff 2001a), and are in draft review in other states. These principles can also be applied to the design of a CCISC for individuals with co-occurring disorders. These applications of the principles will be discussed below.

1. Dual diagnosis is an expectation, not an exception. From a clinical perspective, this must be incorporated in a welcoming manner into all clinical contact, including psychopharmacologic intervention. All clinical practices should routinely support this expectation, including routine screening and integrated assessment. At the systems level, this principle (associated with the poor outcomes and the high cost associated with this population) implies a need for integrated system planning, so that all the resources in the system are planned to address expected comorbidity proactively wherever they are spent. This implies that all programs become defined as "dual diagnosis programs" meeting standard criteria for dual diagnosis capability (Minkoff 2000). This position has been supported by the American Association of Community Psychiatrists (2000b), as well as the American Society of Addiction Medicine (2001).

2. Empathic, hopeful, integrated, and continuous treatment relationships are important predictors of success. All documented successful treatment interventions incorporate the capacity to develop empathic and hopeful relationships with individuals who are usually experienced as system misfits. These relationships are ideally present in any treatment episode, and, for the most complex and difficult clients, are able to be maintained continuously as the client moves through multiple encounters with various services and systems. Empathy requires the ability to acknowledge that the

| Table 116–4 | Consensus Best Treatment Principles |
|---|---|

Dual diagnosis is an expectation, not an exception
Empathic, hopeful, integrated, and continuous treatment relationships are important predictors of success
Use the four quadrant model for service system planning and treatment matching
Balance case management and care with empathic detachment, confrontation, contracting, and contingent learning
Both substance abuse and psychiatric disorders should be considered "primary," and integrated dual primary diagnosis specific treatment is required
Major psychiatric disorders and substance dependence are both primary biopsychosocial mental illnesses, which use a disease and recovery model as an integrated philosophy for treatment. Phase of recovery and stage of treatment/stage of change for each disorder as well as diagnosis must be matched.
There is not one "correct" dual diagnosis program or intervention; treatment must be individualized
Outcome measures must also be individualized to support the recognition of incremental progress as success

individual's reluctance to identify as either mentally ill or a substance abuser, and the concomitant difficulty in adhering to treatment, is a normal, expectable, and to a certain extent healthy response to a demoralizing situation. Hope is built upon accurate empathy with the client's realistic feelings of despair, establishing legitimacy of asking for as much help as possible to make progress, developing attainable small-step indicators of progress and success, and communicating a hopeful vision comprised of the person's ability to regain pride, self-worth, and dignity in the face of one or more persistently disabling and/or stigmatizing disorders. Integrated treatment is *not* a particular program or intervention, so much as a description of any mechanism by which, within the context of a treatment relationship, recommended interventions for both mental illness and substance disorder are combined (integrated) into a person-centered coherent whole at the level of the client, and the interventions for either disorder can be modified as indicated to take into consideration exigencies related to the other. Thus, integrated treatment can involve appropriate combinations of diagnosis-specific, stage-specific, and disability-matched interventions for any combination of disorders in any appropriate service setting. Continuity emphasizes the recognition that treatment is actually a continuous learning process with incremental progress in consistent management of one or more chronic relapsing conditions.

3. The national consensus four quadrant model is helpful for service system planning and treatment matching. The NASMHPD/NASADAD (1998, 2000) four quadrant consensus model categorizes individuals with COD according to high or low severity of each disorder: quadrant IV is high severity mental illness (MI)–high severity chemical dependency (CD), quadrant III is low MI–high CD, quadrant II is high MI–low CD, and quadrant I is low MI–low CD. The high severity MI populations (quadrants II and IV) are often equivalent to designated SPMI in most systems of care; this model implies that the responsibility for ongoing integrated continuous care is the responsibility of the mental health system for these individuals. The quadrant III population, who have psychiatrically complicated substance dependence of varying degrees of severity but do not meet criteria for SPMI after 30 days of abstinence, often are individuals who fall through the cracks the most, since no system clearly assumes responsibility for continuing care. These individuals may frequently present in mental health settings, not ready to accept referrals to addiction treatment, and require sometimes extended engagement and motivational enhancement, as well as treatment of concurrent psychiatric disorders, in order to help them address substance use issues. Addiction programs are now being expected to develop dual diagnosis capability because of the high prevalence of quadrant III individuals in these settings who have continuing non-SPMI psychiatric disorders, including mood, anxiety, trauma-related, attention-deficit, and personality disorders, as well as traumatic brain injury and developmental impairments. Furthermore, among the SPMI population, relatively low levels of controlled substance use can be sufficiently problematic for individuals with significant baseline disability as to be considered substance abuse. These quadrant II patients do not meet criteria for substance dependence or addiction, and may therefore not be appropriate for referral to addiction treatment programs. Treatment of substance abuse for these individuals involves individual and group interventions to make better choices, and to develop skills to implement those choices, an approach entirely consistent with broader approaches to psychiatric rehabilitation in mental health settings.

4. Case management and care (based on level of impairment) must be appropriately balanced with empathic detachment, confrontation, contracting, and contingent learning for each client (based on strengths and external contingencies), and in each program. Apparent philosophic battles between mental health caretakers and confrontational addiction counselors can be reframed as clinical strategic discussions regarding the best place to draw the line between care and expectation at any point in time within the context of an empathic, integrated relationship. One of the key implications of new technologies of community reinforcement and contingency management is the recognition that behavioral learning occurs best *within* the relationship, and is enhanced more by *reward* than by punishment or negative consequences. This represents a major shift for treatment systems that have generally relied on treatment discontinuation as the primary behavioral consequence for treatment nonadherence. This principle states first that within the context of any treatment relationship, it is important to identify and provide for individuals those supports and services (medication, housing, financing, probationary supervision, etc.) that they literally cannot provide for themselves. This principle further states that in the context of this continuing care, the ongoing relationship in which services are provided (including the psychopharmacologic relationship) always represents an opportunity for contracted expectations and contingent learning. A corollary of this principle is that different clients need the line between support and expectation drawn in different places, and different program models must accommodate client cohorts with different collective needs. On the individual level, this implies that very impaired clients may need skill development interventions that are highly modified to accommodate severe disability, and contingency structures that are very incremental, with small steps and small rewards built into daily or, at most, weekly activities. On the program level, this implies a range of programs in the continuum of care; for example, housing programs for substance abusing individuals with psychiatric disabilities may need to include a service range to accommodate consumers who are "wet," "damp," or "dry."

5. When psychiatric and substance disorders coexist, both disorders should be considered "primary," and integrated dual primary diagnosis-specific (or problem-specific) treatment is required. This principle emphasizes that the clinician should not get caught up in the determination of "the primary cause" or "the real problem," which often becomes a barrier to access and continuity. Rather, each problem needs to be

identified as a serious problem that requires specific attention when it presents. Further, we have to be careful not to underestimate the seriousness of either disorder, or its treatment requirements, because the other disorder is present. Individuals who are suicidal and intoxicated are at higher risk for suicide than those who are suicidal and sober; this can be true even if the suicidality does not persist after the intoxication resolves. Furthermore, a key treatment rule, developed in the national consensus psychopharmacology practice guidelines (Minkoff 1998) is that necessary nonaddictive medication for a known or probable serious mental illness should always be initiated and maintained even in the presence of continuing substance use; risky behavior by the client is an indication for closer monitoring, not treatment discontinuation. Finally, it is important to recognize that individuals with addiction who have comorbid disabling psychiatric conditions, at any stage of change, will need "more" stage-specific addiction treatment than individuals with addiction (of comparable severity) alone. This is because substance disorder treatment involves development of problem recognition, decision to change, and skills to implement those changes, and individuals with psychiatric disabilities have greater difficulty with these activities. "More" treatment does not mean more intensive or more complicated treatment, however, because neither intensity nor complexity enhances learning; rather, treatment interventions are in smaller steps, with more support, practice, and rehearsal, over a longer period of time. This is clearly illustrated in the design of the Substance Abuse Management Module and related skills training materials (Roberts et al. 1999).

6. Major psychiatric disorders and substance dependence (addiction) are both primary biopsychosocial mental illnesses, which can utilize a disease and recovery model as an integrated philosophy for treatment. Recovery occurs in parallel phases for each disorder, and treatment must be matched to phase of recovery and stage of treatment/stage of change for each disorder, as well as to diagnosis. Each primary disorder can be understood to have a recommended set of stabilizing treatments, but both patients and families may resist beginning and continuing treatment because of denial, despair, guilt, shame, and stigma, both about the fact of the disorder and the chronicity of the disorder. Consequently, the work of the clinician for each disorder is philosophically the same: identify a disorder and set of recommended interventions, then work with the client to overcome feelings that generate treatment resistance and develop the skills necessary to follow the recommendations. Phases of recovery include acute stabilization of symptoms; engagement and motivational enhancement (which includes progress through stages of change and treatment); active treatment to achieve relapse prevention; ongoing rehabilitation and recovery. Different treatments and programs are appropriate for the same disorder(s) in different phases. The outcome of the process of recovery (for either disorder) is not recovery from the disease, but recovery of the person who has the disease (Minkoff 1989).

7. Consequently, there is no one correct dual diagnosis program or intervention. For each individual, integrated treatment interventions must be matched according to: quadrant (which may define the locus of responsibility for continuing care); diagnoses; phase of recovery/stage of change; disability or impairment (defining case management and skills training modification needs); strengths, supports, problems (e.g., housing, legal) and associated contingencies (defining opportunities for contracting and learning); and multidimensional assessment (e.g. using ASAM or LOCUS) of level of care, based on acuity of risk (safety or detox), comorbidity (medical or other), functionality, treatment acceptance, and environmental support. This set of criteria has been used (Minkoff 1998) to develop a comprehensive set of clinical practice guidelines for assessment and treatment matching, including psychopharmacology. Further, this set of criteria emphasizes that dual diagnosis treatment interventions do not require the selection of a single best practice, but access to as many best practice treatments for either type of disorder as possible, with the capacity to provide them in an integrated manner in an appropriate relationship and setting. For example, harm reduction and abstinence-oriented treatment for individuals with co-occurring disorders are not competing philosophies but completely legitimate treatments provided they are properly matched. This same set of criteria can be utilized to define the elements of the CCISC (Minkoff 2001b, Minkoff 1991). In this model for system design, all programs are planned as, at minimum, dual diagnosis capable programs within their existing resources, but each program is "assigned" a different job related to its usual functions and usual cohort of patients: some programs provide continuity of care, some provide episodic treatment; some emphasize acute stabilization, others active treatment or rehabilitation; some provide harm reduction, others are abstinence mandated addiction treatment facilities; some are outpatient, others are residential; some work with SPMI, others with less seriously impaired individuals. In this design, all the scarce resources of the system are mobilized to address comorbidity as a high expectation, poor outcome, high cost problem, and service system gaps and resource limitations become easier to address over time through collaboration and integrated system planning.

8. Outcome measures must also be individualized to support the recognition of incremental progress as success. These may include enhanced safety or stability, reduction in use of expensive acute resources, harm reduction, reduction in amount of use or frequency of use, changes in patterns of use or route of administration, and movement through stages of change or treatment. This principle is significant because it requires each clinician and program to clearly recognize the importance of defining and measuring incremental outcomes that are appropriate to the client cohort, and documenting these measures in the context of ongoing treatment planning and review. Insufficient attention to this activity often results either in continued efforts only to achieve persistent abstinence or in the assumption that no progress is possible. Either of these approaches

can result in both staff and client demoralization that actually impede progress.

## Implications for Assessment and Treatment in Community Mental Health Settings

1. All community mental health settings must become dual diagnosis capable. This begins with establishing welcoming and empathic attitudes toward the expected population of actively substance using individuals with severe behavioral health problems who are often not willing to change. All policies and procedures, from assessment through treatment planning, must support the routine integrated treatment of individuals with co-occurring disorders who require continuing mental health intervention.

2. The role of the community mental health center is to provide empathic, hopeful, continuing, integrated treatment relationships for these individuals. The content of these relationships is defined by the treatment matching paradigm described below, and must be supported by policy and procedure. The most important shift, however, is for primary clinicians to move from focusing on "referral to a substance treatment facility" as the primary task, to focusing on integrated identification and provision of ongoing stage-specific substance treatment needs: individuals and group motivational enhancement; development of incremental contingent learning opportunities; education regarding the importance of medication compliance; skill development regarding change in use patterns; and support of participation in relapse prevention activities.

3. Provision of routine screening for comorbid substance use disorders, using a screening tool (e.g., CAGE, MAST, DAST, DALI, MIDAS or RAAFT) (Selzer 1971, Mayfield et al. 1974, Skinner 1982, Rosenberg et al. 1998, Bastiaens et al. 2000, Minkoff 2002), clinician recorded surveys (CAUS, Community drug use scale) (Mueser et al. 1995), and substance use checklists, plus selective urine or saliva screening, as well as contacting collateral treaters, family members, and previous records are some of the ways in which detection and identification are possible. Clinicians should be encouraged to maximize detection and identification, and to have clear instruction regarding documentation in the clinical record and in the MIS system, as well as procedures for obtaining further substance disorder assessment and consultation on site.

4. Routine assessment must be integrated, longitudinal, and strength-based, organized to gather information relevant to the treatment matching paradigm described in item 3 (see also principle 7 on the previous page). The integrated longitudinal strength-based assessment (ILSA) process is described at length in the newest Center for Substance Abuse Treatment (CSAT) Treatment Improvement Protocol for Co-occurring Disorders (Center for Substance Abuse Treatment 1999, 2003). The emphasis is on a chronological history in which description of functioning and skills are integrated with descriptions of mental health symptoms, diagnosis, treatment, and disability, *and* simultaneous description of substance use, diagnosis, treatment, and interactions of substance use and mental illness, at

| Table 116–5 | Implications for Assessment and Treatment in Community Mental Health Settings |
|---|---|

All community mental health settings must become dual diagnosis capable

The role of the community mental health center is to provide empathic, hopeful, continuing, integrated treatment relationships for these individuals

Routine screening for comorbid substance use disorders with a screening tool must be provided

Routine assessment must be integrated, longitudinal, and strength-based, and relevant to treatment matching paradigms

Continuing case management should be provided

Integrated dual primary treatment should be provided

Stage-specific assessments/individual and group interventions for substance use disorders should be integrated into continuing mental health treatment relationships, interventions, and settings.

*each* key period. In establishing a diagnosis, emphasis is given first to identifying diagnoses reasonably well established by history, and beginning with the presumption that the individual will require maintenance treatment for those disorders (if willing). Second, emphasis in the history is focused less on details of each decompensation (in chronic complex cases) and more on identifying periods of relative strength or stability. During these periods of stability of 30 days or more in the past, careful history of psychiatric status is the most reliable method of establishing presumptive psychiatric diagnosis and disability, as well as identifying past treatments that were actually successful for a period of time, so that those treatments can be reestablished, and the client can feel more hopeful (because of past success) rather than discouraged (because what worked in the past was not sustained). It can be noted that absolute abstinence is not required during these periods; all that is necessary is that substance use is less than that which would cause or continue the target symptoms.

5. Continuing case management is provided to assist the client unconditionally to address needs that she/he cannot meet because of disability. Assessment of client strengths facilitates the development of rehabilitative goals based on client preference; initial treatment planning is designed to assist the client in achieving these goals (Comtois 1994). These needs and goals may include housing, vocational activity, and socialization, as well as access to specific types of treatment regarding mental illness and substance disorder. Access to continuing assistance with maintaining safety, addressing basic needs, and achieving rehabilitative goals is provided for individuals with severe mental illness even when substance use continues. As the client is engaged in treatment, opportunities for contracting and contingency management often emerge, and can be incorporated in a structured, incremental, and supportive manner into the ongoing treatment relationship.

6. Integrated dual primary treatment is provided. With regard to mental illness, access is to psychopharmacologic evaluation and continuing treatment is facilitated; nonaddictive medication for known serious mental

illness (usually assessed by history) is initiated, maintained, and upgraded to better medication, regardless of continuing substance use. Participation in rehabilitative treatment settings, day treatment, and outpatient treatment activities are also encouraged. Substance use disorders are identified, and stage of change for each is measured. Individuals then receive stage-specific substance use disorder treatment in the context of the mental health treatment setting.

7. Stage-specific assessment (McHugo et al. 1995) and stage-specific individual and group interventions for substance use disorders are integrated into continuing mental health treatment relationships, interventions, and settings. These include individual and group motivational enhancement strategies, facilitated by collaboration with families and other collateral providers (probation officers), supported by contingency contracting when possible. Peer group discussion on substance use choices and decisions for "precontemplators" can be very effective, because clients may listen to their peers, before they listen to staff. Active treatment strategies involve individual and group identification of specific situations and strategies for reducing substance use and practice, rehearsal, role-playing, and repetition to learn and reinforce new skills for dealing with those situations. This may also include specific skills training regarding participation in 12-Step meetings, using a sponsor, and so on. Relapse prevention involves developing a daily checklist of sobriety promoting activities, and developing relationships with dual recovery or nonusing peers. Utilization of dual recovery meetings (e.g., Dual Recovery Anonymous, Double Trouble in Recovery) (Hamilton and Samples 1995, Vogel 1999) when available, in addition to other recovery supports is very helpful. All of these activities can be integrated into ongoing mental health case management functions.

8. Continued access to rehabilitation and housing supports is matched to strengths, goals, impairments, and stage of change. This includes access to some type of individualized placement and support for individuals with active co-occurring disorders whose primary goal involves finding work, and for whom access to meaningful activity has been demonstrated to facilitate both treatment engagement and treatment outcome for both disorders (Bond et al. 2001). This also includes access to a range of housing supports for individuals who are homeless or at risk of homelessness to help maintain housing, based on client preference that is abstinence mandated or dry (though permissive of learning through multiple "slips"), abstinence encouraged or damp (individuals may choose to use in a limited, nonharmful manner even though abstinence is encouraged), or consumer-choice or wet (individuals make their own choices about substance use but must work with staff to avoid behavior that would directly result in losing housing, such as selling drugs, damaging property, and so on (Tsemberis and Eisenberg 2000).

## Conclusion

This section has reviewed available research on treatment interventions for individuals with co-occurring psychiatric

and substance disorders, and illustrated the extrapolation of this research to develop a set of principles for treatment of a wide variety of such individuals in a range of settings. These principles were then applied specifically to illustrate an organized approach to integrated treatment within the context of a community mental health setting, working within the context of existing resources and services.

## References

Adelman S, Fletcher K, and Bahnassi A (1993) Pharmacotherapeutic management strategies for mentally ill substance abusers. J Subst Abuse Treat 10, 353–358.

Albanese M, Khantzian E, et al. (1994) Decreased substance use in chronically psychotic patients treated with clozapine. Am J Psychiatr 151, 780.

Alexander MJ (1996) Women with co-occurring disorders: An emerging profile of vulnerability. Am J Orthopsychiatr 66, 61–70.

American Association of Community Psychiatrists (2000a) Level of Care Utilization System (LOCUS 2.001). AACP, Dallas.

American Association of Community Psychiatrists (2000b) Principles for the Care and Treatment of Individuals with Co-occurring Psychiatric and Substance Disorders. AACP, Dallas.

American Society of Addiction Medicine (2001) Patient Placement Criteria 2R. ASAM, Washington DC.

Bastiaens L, Francis G, and Lewis K (2000) The RAFFT as a screening tool for adolescent substance use disorders. Am J Addict 9, 10–16.

Bellack AS, et al. (1999) Behavioral treatment for substance abuse in schizophrenia (BTSAS). Abellackumaryland.edu. (personal communication)

Biederman J, Wilens T, et al. (1999) Pharmacotherapy of ADHD reduces risk for substance use disorder. Pediatrics 104(2), 3.

Bond GR, Becker DR, et al. (2001) Implementing supported employment as an evidence-based practice. Psychiatr Serv 52(3), 313–322.

Brady KT and Roberts J (1995) The pharmacotherapy of dual diagnosis. Psychiatr Ann 25, 344–352.

Brown VB (2000) Changing and Improving Services for Women and Children: Strategies Used and Lessons Learned. Prototypes Systems Change Center, Culver City, CA.

Carey KB (1996) Substance use reduction in the context of outpatient psychiatric treatment: A collaborative, motivational, harm reduction approach. Comm MHJ 32, 291–306.

Center for Substance Abuse Treatment (1999) Enhancing Motivation for Change in Substance Abuse Treatment. Treatment Improvement Protocol #35. CSAT, Washington DC.

Center for Substance Abuse Treatment (CSAT) (2003) Assessment and Treatment of Patients with Coexisting Mental Illness and Alcohol and Other Drug Abuse, 2nd ed. Treatment Improvement Protocol (TIP) Series. Department of Health & Human Services, Washington DC.

Ciraulo DA and Nace EP (2000) Benzodiazepine treatment of anxiety or insomnia in substance abuse patients. Am J Addict 9, 276–284.

Comtois KA, Ries R, and Armstrong HE (1994) Case manager ratings of the clinical status of dually diagnosed outpatients. Hosp Comm Psychiatr 45, 568–573.

Cornelius JR, Saloum IM, et al. (1997) Fluoxetine in depressed alcoholics. Arch Gen Psychiatr 54, 700–705.

Drake RE, Bartels SJ, et al. (1993a) Treatment of substance abuse in severely mentally ill patients. J Nerv Ment Dis 181, 606–611.

Drake RE, Essock SM, et al. (2001) Implementing Dual Diagnosis services for clients with severe mental illness. Psychiatr Serv 52(4), 120–124.

Drake RE, McHugo GJ, and Noordsy DL (1993b) Treatment of alcoholism among schizophrenic outpatients: 4-year outcomes. Am J Psychiatr 150(2), 328–330.

Evans K and Sullivan JM (eds) (1995) Treating Addicted Survivors of Trauma. Guilford Press, New York.

Godley SH, Finch M, et al. (2000) Case management for dually diagnosed individuals involved in the criminal justice system. J Sub Abuse Treat 18, 137–148.

Goldfinger SM, Shute RK, et al. (1999) Housing placement and subsequent days homeless among formerly homeless adults with mental illness. Psychiatr Serv 50, 674–679.

Hamilton T and Samples P (1995) The 12 Steps and Dual Disorders. Hazelden, Center City, MN.

Harris M (1998) Trauma Recovery and Empowerment Manual. Free Press, New York.

Hartman E and Nelson D (1997) A case study of statewide capitation: The Massachusetts experience. In Managed Mental Health Care in the Public Sector: A Survival Manual, Minkoff K and Pollack D (eds). Harwood Academic Publishers, Amsterdam, pp. 59–76.

Kessler RC, Nelson CB, et al. (1996) The epidemiology of co-occurring addictive and mental disorders. Am J Orthopsychiatr 66, 17–31.

Mayfield D, McCleod G, and Hall P (1974) The CAGE questionnaire: Validation of a new alcoholism screening questionnaire. Am J Psychiatr 131, 1121–1123.

McHugo GJ, Drake RE, Burton HL, et al. (1995) A scale for assessing the stage of substance abuse treatment in persons with severe mental illness. J Nerv Ment Disord 183(12), 762–767.

McLellan AT, Grissom GR, Zanis D, et al. (1997) Problem-service matching in addiction treatment. Arch Gen Psychiatr 54, 730–735.

Miller WR and Rollnick S (1991) Motivational Interviewing. Guilford Press, New York.

Minkoff K (1989) Development of an integrated model for the treatment of patients with dual diagnosis of psychosis and addiction. Hosp Comm Psychiatr 40(10), 1031–1036.

Minkoff K (1991) Program components of a comprehensive integrated care system for serious mentally ill patients with substance disorders. In Dual Diagnosis of Major Mental Illness and Substance Disorder: New Directions for Mental Health Services, Minkoff K and Drake RE (eds). Jossey-Bass, San Francisco, CA, pp. 13–27.

Minkoff K (Chair) (1997) CMHS Managed Care Initiative Panel on Co-occurring Disorders. Co-occurring psychiatric and substance disorders in managed care systems: Annotated bibliography. Center for Mental Health Policy and Services Research, Philidelphia, www.med.upenn.edu/cmhpsr

Minkoff K (Chair) (1998) CMHS Managed Care Initiative Panel on Co-occurring Disorders Co-occurring Psychiatric and Substance Disorders in Managed Care Systems: Standards of Care, Practice Guidelines, Workforce Competencies, and Training Curricula. Center for Mental Health Policy and Services Research, Philadelphia.

Minkoff K (2000) An integrated model for the management of co-occurring psychiatric and substance disorders in managed care systems. Dis Manag Health Out 8(5), 251–257.

Minkoff K (2001a) State of Arizona Service Planning Guidelines: Co-occurring Psychiatric and Substance Disorders.

Minkoff K (2001b) Developing standards of care for individuals with co-occurring psychiatric and substance disorders. Psychiatr Serv 52, 597–599.

Minkoff K (2002) Mental Illness Drug and Alcohol Screening (MIDAS). (unpublished, available from author)

Minkoff K and Drake RE (eds) (1991) Dual Diagnosis of Serious Mental Illness and Substance Disorder. New Directions for Mental Health Services. Jossey-Bass, San Francisco, CA.

Minkoff K and Regner J (1999) Innovations in integrated dual diagnosis treatment in public managed care. J Psychoact Drugs 31, 3–12.

Mueser KT and Fox L (1998) Stage-wise Family Treatment for Dual Disorders: Treatment Manual. NH Dartmouth Psychiatric Research Center, Concord, NH.

Mueser KT and Noordsy DL (1996) Group treatment for dually diagnosed clients. In Dual Diagnosis of Major Mental Illness and Substance Disorder, Part 2, Drake RE and Mueser KT (eds). Jossey-Bass, San Francisco, CA.

Mueser KT, Drake RE, et al. (1995) Toolkit for Evaluating Substance Abuse in Persons with Severe Mental Illness. Dartmouth Psychiatric Research Center, Concord, NH.

Mueser KT, Noordsy DL, and Essock S (2001) Use of disulfiram in the treatment of patients with dual diagnosis. Am J Addict 10, 26–30.

Najavits LM (2002) Seeking Safety: A Treatment Manual for PTSD and Substance Abuse. Guilford Press, New York.

NASMHPD/NASADAD (1998) The New Conceptual Framework for Co-occurring Mental Health and Substance Use Disorders. NASMHPD, Washington DC.

NASMHPD/NASADAD (2000) Financing and Marketing the New Conceptual Framework. NASMHPD, Washington DC.

Osher FC and Kofoed L (1989) Treatment of patients with psychiatric and substance use disorders. Hosp Comm Psychiatr 40, 1025–1030.

Pechter BM and Miller NS (1997) Psychopharmacotherapy for addictive and comorbid disorders: Current studies. J Addict Dis 16, 23–37.

Peters RH and Bartoi MG (1997) Screening and Assessment of Co-occurring Disorders in the Justice System. National GAINS Center, Delmar, NY.

Peters RH and Hills HA (1997) Intervention Strategies for Offenders with Co-occurring Disorders. What Works? National GAINS Center, Delmar, NY.

Prochaska JO, DiClemente CC, and Norcross JC (1992) In search of how people change: Applications to addictive behaviors. Am Psychol 47, 1102–1114.

Quinlivan R and McWhirter DP (1996) Designing a comprehensive care program for high cost clients in a managed care environment. Psychiatr Serv 47, 813 815.

RachBeisel J, Scott J, and Dixon L (1999) Co-occurring severe mental illness and substance use disorders: A review of recent research. Psychiatr Serv 50, 1427–1934.

Regier DA, Farmer ME, et al. (1990) Comorbidity of mental disorders with alcohol and other drug abuse: Results from the epidemiologic catchment area (ECA) study. JAMA 264(19), 2511–2518.

Ries RK and Comtois KA (1997) Managing disability benefits as part of treatment for persons with severe mental illness and comorbid substance disorder. Am J Addict 6(4), 330–338.

Roberts LJ, Shaner A, and Eckman TA (1999) Overcoming addictions: Skills training for people with schizophrenia. WW Norton, New York.

Rosenberg SD, Drake RE, et al. (1998) Dartmouth Assessment of Life Inventory (DALI): A substance use disorder screen for people with severe mental illness. Am J Psychiatr 155, 232–238.

Sacks S, Sacks JY, and DeLeon G (1999) Treatment for MICAs: Design and implementation of the modified TC. J Psychoact Drugs 31, 19–30.

Selzer ML (1971) The Michigan Alcohol Screening Test: The quest for a new diagnostic instrument. Am J Psychiatr 127, 89–94.

Shaner A, Roberts LJ, et al. (1997) Monetary reinforcement of abstinence from cocaine among mentally ill persons with cocaine dependence. Psychiatr Serv 48, 807–810.

Skinner HA (1982) The Drug Abuse Screening Test. Addict Behav 7, 363–371.

Sowers W and Golden S (1999) Psychotropic medication management in persons with co-occurring psychiatric and substance use disorders. J Psychoact Drugs 31, 59–67.

Tollefson GD, Montague-Clouse J, and Tollefson SL (1992) Treatment of comorbid generalized anxiety in a recently detoxified alcoholic population with a selective serotonergic drug (buspirone). J Clin Psychopharm 12, 19–26.

Tsemberis S and Eisenberg RF (2000) Pathways to housing: Supported housing for street dwelling homeless individuals with psychiatric disabilities. Psychiatr Serv 51(4), 487–495.

Vogel H (1999) Double Trouble in Recovery (DTR): How to Start and Run a DTR Group. NY Office of Mental Hygiene, Mental Health Empowerment Project, Albany, NY.

WELL Project (1999) Principles for the trauma informed treatment of women with co-occurring mental health and substance abuse disorders. WELL Project, Cambridge, MA.

Wilens TE, Biederman J, and Spencer J (1996) Attention-deficit/hyperactivity disorder and psychoactive substance use disorders. Child Adolesc Psychiatr Clin N Am 5(1), 73–79.

Wilens TE, O'Keefe J, et al. (1992) A public dual diagnosis detox unit. Am J Addict 2(1), 181–193.

Wilens TE, Spencer TJ, et al. (2001) A controlled clinical trial of bupropion for adult ADHD. Am J Psychiatr 158, 282–288.

Ziedonis D and Trudeau K (1997) Motivation to quit using substances among individuals with schizophrenia: Implications for a motivation-based treatment model. Schizophr Bull 23, 229–238.

Zimmet SV, Strous RD, et al. (2000) Effects of clozapine on substance use in patients with schizophrenia and schizoaffective disorders. J Clin Psychopharm 20, 94–98.

# 117 Psychiatry and Palliative Care

John Shuster

## Hospice and Palliative Care

Palliative care is properly understood as the means of shielding and protecting patients from the violence of disease, especially when cure is no longer a reasonable expectation. The World Health Organization defines palliative care as "the active total care of patients whose disease is not responsive to curative treatment. Control of pain, other physical symptoms, and of psychological, social, and spiritual problems is paramount. The goal of palliative care is achievement of the best quality of life for patients and their families" (WHO 1990).

Palliative care is an emerging area of medical care in the US. In fact, palliative medicine (the term for the medical aspects of interdisciplinary palliative care) is recognized as a formal medical specialty in several other countries. As Americans live longer and die more frequently from chronic illnesses that produce significant symptoms and suffering prior to causing death, palliative care has grown in importance (Centers for Disease Control and Prevention 2000, Lynn 2001). As disease advances, the goals of palliative care shift away from an exclusive emphasis on cure of disease and restoration of function to goals such as reduction in symptom burden, maximization of quality of life, respect for the dignity and worth of the dying person, and maintenance of morale at the end of life (Table 117–1).

Hospice care, in contrast, is a system of interdisciplinary palliative care, utilizing the expertise of physicians, nurses, social workers, chaplains, volunteers, and others. In the US, the term "hospice" has come to represent a system of payment as much as a system of care (i.e., a system for funding home-based palliative care for terminally ill patients). In other countries where hospice and palliative care are more fully developed, inpatient and residential hospice and palliative care facilities are more common than in the US.

## Psychiatry and Palliative Care

American hospice and palliative care have deep roots in psychiatry. A well-known pioneer of the hospice movement, Elisabeth Kübler-Ross, is a psychiatrist. Her landmark work on the lived experience of people at life's end, popularized in her book *On Death and Dying* (Kübler-Ross 1969), was a major stimulus to change the way the dying are cared for in the US.

Psychiatric practice is particularly relevant to palliative care. Issues of loss and bereavement are central to providing good care to terminally ill patients and their families. Psychiatrists and other mental health professionals have expertise much needed in the care of patients at the end of life and their families, as formal mental disorders and subsyndromic distress are very common (Shuster et al. 1999, Shuster et al. 2000). Evaluation and management of suicidal ideation, assessment of fluctuations in the will to live, optimization of quality of life, and preservation of meaning are important aspects of excellent palliative care which draw from the realm of mental health expertise (Table 117–2) (Shuster et al. 2000, Chochinov et al. 1999). Psychiatrists are well trained and well suited to address suffering, which Cassell (1982) describes as "the state of severe distress associated with events that threaten the intactness of a person."

Psychiatric practice in the palliative care setting offers the opportunity for reconnection with core clinical concerns. Helping patients who are facing the end of life deal with loss, suffering, and questions of meaning, can be a very rewarding and fulfilling practice for mental health professionals. Working with those who are dealing with the existential "big questions" can challenge and inspire the clinician and facilitate substantial personal and professional growth. Additionally, the interface of mental health and

| Table 117–1 | Goals of Palliative Care |
|---|---|
| Shift from cure of disease and restoration of function | |
| Reduction of symptom burden | |
| Maximize quality of life | |
| Respect for dignity and worth of dying person | |
| Maintenance of morale at the end of life | |

| Table 117–2 | Mental Health Involvement in Palliative Care |
|---|---|
| Evaluation and management of suicidal ideation | |
| Assessment of the will to live | |
| Optimization of quality of life | |
| Preservation of meaning | |
| Help patients deal with loss and suffering | |

palliative care offers a fertile environment for training and research in these key aspects of the mental health disciplines.

Depression is a very common complication of advanced and terminal illness, with a reported prevalence as high as 40 to 50% in this population (Shuster et al. 1999, Wilson et al. 2000). The presence of depression clearly increases the chances that a patient will request assisted dying (Chochinov et al. 1995). Unrecognized and untreated depression adds to suffering and may complicate the distress caused by other symptoms. Conversely, undertreated physical symptoms (e.g., pain, nausea) may produce a severe dysphoric state resistant to intervention until the physical distress is relieved. Further, depressive states can be complicated by (or confused with) a number of common and related problems in the palliative care setting, including loss of morale, meaning, or the will to live; hopelessness; boredom; feeling overwhelmed with rapid deterioration in health; or severe fatigue (Chochinov et al. 1998, Passik et al. 2001).

Delirium has been reported to be present in over 80% of terminally ill patients at some time prior to their death (Shuster et al. 1999, Shuster 1998). The suffering caused by delirium is hard to assess, even retrospectively, since the delirious patient cannot reliably report on the experience and most are amnesic to the experience after delirium resolves (Shuster 1998). Delirious states, especially when complicated by agitation, can be very distressing to families. Many delirious patients appear to be suffering, particularly in the last days and hours as death approaches. At the very least, delirium interferes with meaningful cognitive connection to those the patient cares about most. Efforts to preserve the cognitive state of the patient with terminal illness need to be maximized to maintain connectedness between patient and family as well and as long as possible.

Insomnia is also very common at the end of life. Among a sample of patients with advanced cancer, 52.8% reported difficulty sleeping (Portenoy et al. 1994). A majority (77%) of patients admitted to an inpatient palliative care unit were taking hypnotics (Bruera et al. 1996). Sleep deprivation exacerbates suffering at the end of life by lowering the patient's perception of quality of life, diminishing coping capacity, increasing perceptions of illness severity and feelings of isolation, and augmenting the suffering due to physical problems such as pain, fatigue, depression, and anxiety (National Center on Sleep Disorders Research and Office of Prevention, Education, and Control 1998, Owen et al. 1999, Asplund 1999).

Acceptance that treatable psychiatric conditions occur at the end of life is of paramount importance. Vigorous treatment of these psychiatric complications (depression, delirium, agitation, insomnia) would enhance end-of-life care. Use of psychostimulants and antidepressants to treat depression, and sedation to ameliorate agitation would relieve end-of-life suffering (Shuster et al. 1999).

Grief and bereavement can emerge in the terminally ill patient, the patient's family and friends, or the patient's professional caregivers. The normal range of grief is quite broad and includes some symptoms which mimic mental disorders. Therefore, identification of pathologic or complicated grief can be a formidable challenge. Complicated bereavement may represent an entity distinct from other formal mental disorders (American Psychiatric Association

| Table 117–3 | Complicating Factors in End-of-Life Care | |
|---|---|
| Depression | Fatigue |
| Suffering | Declining health |
| Physical symptoms (pain, nausea) | Delirium |
| Loss of morale, meaning, will to live | Agitation |
| Hopelessness | Insomnia |
| Boredom | Grief and bereavement |

1994, Kim and Jacobs 1991, Prigerson et al. 1995, Prigerson et al. 1996, Horowitz et al. 1997), or a complex overlap with mood and anxiety disorders (Table 117–3). Mental health professionals are in a good position to educate patients and families about grief and the grieving process while screening for complicating mental disorders, thus potentially preventing some cases of complicated bereavement. When complicated bereavement occurs, mental health professionals can contribute to the work of the palliative care team by providing specialized treatment.

## Barriers to Excellent Psychiatric Care at the End of Life

In a position statement of the Academy of Psychosomatic Medicine, Shuster and colleagues (1999) outlined the barriers to proper recognition and treatment of psychiatric problems at the end of life (Table 117–4). These include:

1. The difficulty in diagnosing psychiatric disorders (e.g., anxiety, delirium, and depression) in the setting of significant physical illness, owing to the overlap in the symptoms caused by the psychiatric disorder and the comorbid physical problems.
2. Beliefs held by many patients, family members, physicians, and hospice and palliative care providers, viewing psychiatric symptoms, especially depression, as normal parts of the dying process.
3. The fact that many patients and physicians do not understand that patients who suffer from mental disorders at the end of life can respond to treatment. Such therapeutic nihilism prevents the search for treatable mental disorders at the end-of-life.

| Table 117–4 | Barriers to Psychiatric Care at the End-of-Life |
|---|
| Difficulty diagnosing psychiatric disorders in the setting of significant physical illness |
| Beliefs held that view psychiatric symptoms as normal parts of the dying process |
| Lack of understanding that patients who suffer from mental disorders at the end of life can respond to treatment |
| Presence of structural barriers to the coordinated care of dying patients |
| Stigma of psychiatric evaluations or the assignment of psychiatric diagnoses |
| Occurrence of countertransference hopelessness that may discourage seeking assessment of suffering from psychiatric causes, and weaken the commitment to helping maintain morale |
| Treatment based on formal diagnosis is not sufficiently emphasized in palliative care |

4. The presence of structural barriers to the coordinated care of dying patients. Psychiatrists may not be readily available to care for terminally ill patients and consult with physicians providing end-of-life care for a variety of reasons. Among these are limited geographic access (most consultation-liaison psychiatrists are affiliated with academic medical centers in urban areas), psychiatrists who feel inadequately prepared to assess and treat dying patients, health care insurance carve-outs (which may limit or exclude access to and coverage for psychiatric care), and logistical obstacles to formal addition of a psychiatrist to a hospice care team.

5. The stigma experienced by patients and families due to psychiatric evaluations or the assignment of a psychiatric diagnosis. Physicians and other caregivers may share this feeling.

6. The occurrence of countertransference hopelessness on the part of families and health care providers that may discourage seeking assessment of suffering from psychiatric causes in dying patients and weaken the commitment to helping maintain morale at the end of life.

7. The fact that treatment based on formal diagnosis (as opposed to symptomatic treatment) is not sufficiently emphasized in palliative care (Shuster et al. 1999).

Overcoming these barriers will require a concerted effort of psychiatrists and other mental health professionals to address shortcomings in training programs in the various disciplines, contribute to a growing evidence base for psychiatric care of terminally ill patients, and advocate for elimination of regulatory and fiscal barriers to excellent psychiatric care at the end of life (Shuster et al. 1999). Such efforts will contribute to the growth and maturation of palliative medicine as a medical specialty and palliative care as an interdisciplinary field. As demand for palliative care services grows over the next several years and reforms in reimbursement mechanisms allow a broader range of services to develop in response to this demand, new opportunities for psychiatric and mental health collaboration in the care of patients at the end of life will emerge.

## References

American Psychiatric Association (1994) Diagnostic and Statistical Manual of Mental Disorders, 4th ed., APA, Washington DC.

Asplund R (1999) Sleep disorders in the elderly. Drugs Aging 14(2), 91–103.

Bruera E, Fainsinger RL, Schoeller T, et al. (1996) Rapid discontinuation of hypnotics in terminal cancer patients: A prospective study. Ann Oncol 7(8), 855–856.

Cassell EJ (1982) The nature of suffering and the goals of medicine. New Engl J Med 306(11), 639–645.

Centers for Disease Control and Prevention (2001) Mortality data from the National Vital Statistics System, Deaths: preliminary data for 2000. (Released 2001) http://www.cdc.gov/nchs/about/major/dvs/mortdata.htm

Chochinov HM, Tataryn D, Clinch JJ, et al. (1999) Will to live in the terminally ill. Lancet 354(9181), 816–819.

Chochinov HM, Wilson KG, Enns M, et al. (1995) Desire for death in the terminally ill. Am J Psychiatr 152, 1185–1191.

Chochinov HM, Wilson KG, Enns M, et al. (1998) Depression, hopelessness, and suicidal ideation in the terminally ill. Psychosomatics 39(4), 366–370.

Horowitz MJ, Siegel B, Holen, A, et al. (1997) Diagnostic criteria for complicated grief disorder. Am J Psychiatr 154, 904–910.

Kübler-Ross E (1969) On Death and Dying. Macmillan, New York.

Kim K and Jacobs S (1991) Pathologic grief and its relationship to other psychiatric disorders. J Affect Dis 21, 257–263.

Lynn J (2001) Perspectives on care at the close of life. Serving patients who may die soon and their families: The role of hospice and other services. J Am Med Assoc 285(7), 925–932.

National Center on Sleep Disorders Research and Office of Prevention, Education, and Control (1998) Insomnia: Assessment and management in primary care. National Institutes of Health/National Heart, Lung, and Blood Institute, Bethesda, Maryland. NIH Publication No. 98–4088.

Owen DC, Parker KP, and McGuire DB (1999) Comparison of subjective sleep quality in patients with cancer and healthy subjects. Oncol Nurs Forum 26(10), 1649–1651.

Passik SD, Theobald DE, Donaghy K, et al. (2001) An open label trial of citalopram in ambulatory cancer patients: Impact on depression and boredom. Poster presented at the 48th Annual Meeting of the Academy of Psychosomatic Medicine, (Nov 15–18), San Antonio, Texas.

Portenoy RK, Thaler HT, Kornblith AB, et al. (1994) The Memorial Symptom Assessment Scale: An instrument for the evaluation of symptom prevalence, characteristics and distress. Eur J Cancer 30A, 1326–1336.

Prigerson HG, Bierhals AJ, Kasl SV, et al. (1996) Complicated grief as a disorder distinct from bereavement-related depression and anxiety: A replication study. Am J Psychiatr 153, 1484–1486.

Prigerson HG, Frank E, Kasl S, et al. (1995) Complicated grief and bereavement-related depression as distinct disorders: Preliminary empirical validation in elderly bereaved spouses. Am J Psychiatr 152, 22–30.

Shuster JL (1998) Confusion, agitation, and delirium at the end of life. J Palliative Med 1, 177–186.

Shuster JL, Breitbart W, and Chochinov HM (1999) Psychiatric aspects of excellent end-of-life care. Psychosomatics 40(1), 1–4.

Shuster JL, Chochinov HM, and Greenberg DB (2000) Psychiatric aspects and psychopharmacologic strategies in palliative care. In Psychiatric Care of the Medical Patient, Vol. 2, Stoudemire A, Fogel BS, and Greenberg DB (eds). Oxford University Press, New York, pp. 315–327.

Wilson KG, Chochinov HM, deFaye BJ, et al. (2000) Diagnosis and management of depression in palliative care. In Handbook of Psychiatry in Palliative Medicine, Chochinov HM and Breitbart W (eds). Oxford University Press, New York, pp. 25–49.

World Health Organization (1990) Cancer Pain Relief and Palliative Care. Technical Report Series 804. World Health Organization, Geneva.

# Index

Cognitive theory *(Continued)*
major depressive disorder, 1217
manic–depressive disorder, 1246
Cognitive therapy
alcohol use disorders, 956
attitude theory, 439
behavioral medicine, 1848–1849
posttraumatic stress disorder,
1370–1371
Cognitive triad, definition, 1754
Cogwheel rigidity, movement
disorders, 1662, 1670
Coherent psychiatric frame
components, 69–70
Coherent treatment frame, 66–67
Cohort effects, adult development,
165–166
Cohort studies, psychiatric
epidemiology, 217
Collaboration, split treatment, 2192
Collaborative empiricism, 1757–1758
Collaborative relationships, liability,
2300–2301
Colonic distention, encopresis, 849
Coma, consciousness states and levels,
583, 584
Combat exposure, posttraumatic stress
disorder, 1366
Combined therapies
Alzheimer's disease, 2108
anxiety disorders, 2189
eating disorders, 2191
mood disorders, 2189–2190
psychotherapy/pharmacotherapy,
2184–2201
unipolar depressive disorders, 2190
Commitment
involuntary hospitalization,
2292–2294
NGRI acquittees, 2304
outpatients, 2294
Common language, 4
Communicating disorders
DC:0–3, infancy and early
childhood, 682
research classification for
neurodevelopmental problems,
infancy and early childhood,
682–685
Communication
*See also* Autism spectrum disorders;
Language
central nervous system, 274
coercion, 1680
infant development, 100, 102,
104–105, 108–109
information exchange, 1679–1681
problem solving, 1682
psychiatric interviews, 39–40
relational problems, 1677–1678
relationship functioning, 1684
split treatment, 2195–2197
telepsychiatry, 49
Communication deviance (CD)
families, 1679–1681
relational disorders, 1685
relational problems, 1678
relationship functioning, 1684

Communication disorder not
otherwise specified (CDNOS)
assessment, 748–751
comorbidity, 753–754
definitions, 745
diagnosis, 747–751
DSM-IV-TR criteria, 745
etiology and pathophysiology,
746–747
phenomenology, 748
treatment, 752–753
Communication disorders
*See also* Communication disorder
not otherwise specified;
Expressive language disorder;
Mixed receptive–expressive
language disorder; Phonological
disorder; Stuttering
assessment, 748–751
childhood, 512–513, 743–756
clinical vignettes, 755
cognitive factors, 747
comorbidity, 753–754
course and natural history, 751–752
definitions, 743–745
demographic and cultural issues, 754
diagnosis, 747–751
differential diagnosis, 750–751
DSM-IV-TR diagnostic classes and
codes, 664–665
DSM-IV/ICD-10 criteria
comparison, 754
environmental factors, 747
epidemiology, 745–746
etiology, 746–747
genetic influences, 746
influencing factors, 747
mixed influences, 747
neurophysiological factors, 746–747
pathophysiology, 746–747
perceptual factors, 747
phenomenology, 747–748
treatment, 752–753
Communication therapy, autism
spectrum disorders, 769
Community adaptation, severely
mentally ill, 2253–2275
Community based approaches, 2208,
2339–2340
essential functions, 2235
homelessness services, 2314–2315,
2319
India, 2216
United Kingdom, 2212
Community living, mental retardation,
706
Community mental health centers
(CMHCs)
1960s and 1970s, 2231–2234
1980s, 2238–2239
Italy, 2212–2213
mental health services, 2210
split treatment, 2192
United States, 2213–2214
Community mental health settings,
dual diagnosis, 2339–2340
Community psychiatry, dual diagnosis,
2333–2334

Community responsibility, mentally ill,
19th century, 2228
Community safety, mentally ill
homeless people, 2316–2317
Community samples, aggressive
behavior, 2138
Community Support Program (CSP)
1980s, 2235
consumer self-help groups, 2282
disability definition, 2254
Comorbidity, *See also* Dual diagnosis;
*Individual conditions*
Comorbidity patterns, 511, 519, 522
Compensation, coherent and
noncollusive, 69, 71–72
Compensatory models, psychosocial
rehabilitation, 1856–1858
Competence
*See also* Incompetence
care, 65
cultural, 25–26, 28
informed consent, 2293–2294
legal term, 2305
standards, 1734, 1735
standing trial, 2302
Competent care ethical principle, 65
Complaints, chief, 35–36, 541
Complementary and alternative
treatments, 2147–2183
*See also* Herbal alternative
treatments
action mechanisms, 2164
cognitive enhancers, 2161–2173
female menopause, 2158–2159
herb-drug interactions, 2148, 2150,
2154, 2173–2174
hormonal and endocrine disorders,
2157–2161
male menopause, 2159–2160
medical liability issues, 2174–2175
mood disorders, 2147–2157
physician education, 2175
physician–patient relationship, 2174
premenstrual dysphoric disorder,
1276
premenstrual syndrome, 2157–2158
psychopharmacology, 1918–1919
quality, 2174
S-adenosyl-L-methionine, 2151–2154
sexual enhancement, 2160–2161
side effects, 2147, 2148
sources, 2151
Complementary countertransference,
55
Complete blood count, clinical
evaluations, 548, 549
Complexity, split treatment, 2196
Compliance, medication, 2202–2207,
2294
Comprehension
communication disorders, 749
reading disorders, 737
Comprehensive, continuous, integrated
systems of care (CCISC), 2333,
2336, 2338
Comprehensive treatment plans, 558
Compromise formation, ego, 468
Compulsive behavior

Protective factors *(Continued)*
  developmental psychopathology,
    86–88
  infant development, 109–110
  preschool development, 129–130
  school-age development, 141
Protracted benzodiazepine withdrawal,
  1128
Protriptyline
  *See also* Antidepressants; First
    generation antidepressants;
    Tricyclic antidepressants
  dosage, 2017
  indications, 1999
PSD *See* Primary sexual dysfunction;
  Primary sleep disorders
Pseudobulbar palsy, 912–913
  affect–mood incongruence, 617–618
  assessment and differential
    diagnosis, 913
  course, 913
  definition, 912
  epidemiology and comorbidity, 913
  etiology and pathophysiology,
    912–913
  treatment, 913
Pseudohallucinations, 603, 1054
Pseudologia phantasica, 605
Pseudoneurotic schizophrenia, 196
Pseudoparkinsonism, 1171
Psilocin, 1046
Psilocybin, 1046, 1048
Psyche, soma and society, 478
Psychiatric classification of disorders,
  659–676
Psychiatric comorbidity *See Individual
  disorders*
Psychiatric conditions, generalized
  anxiety disorder differential
  diagnosis, 1386–1387
Psychiatric database, 35–38
Psychiatric disorders
  alcohol use disorders, 950–952,
    957–958, 962
  caffeine intoxication, 976
  does the patient have one?, 30
  dual diagnoses, 2333–2341
  hypersomnia, 1542
  neurosurgery, 1902–1914
  nicotine dependence, 1086–1087,
    1089
  opioid dependence, 1113–1114
  polygraphic sleep features, 1543
  sedative, hypnotic or anxiolytic use
    disorders, 1124, 1126–1127
  sleep disorders, 1541–1545
  substance use disorders, 932
  treatment-refractory, 1902–1914
Psychiatric epidemiology, 211–233
  biases, 217–218
  comorbidity of mental and
    substance use disorders study,
    223–228, 230
  diagnostic classification, 455
  disease frequency measures, 213
  Epidemiological Catchment Area
    Study, 220–223
  future directions, 228–231

Psychiatric epidemiology *(Continued)*
  measures of association, 214
  methods, 213
  National Comorbidity Survey,
    223–228, 230
  psychiatric genetics, 240
  recent trends, 199
  research studies examples, 218–220,
    221–223
  scope of inquiry, 212–213
  study types, 215–217
  validity, 217–218
Psychiatric genetics, 234–253
  adoption studies, 242
  candidate genes selection and
    analysis, 245–248
  candidate polymorphisms analysis,
    244–248
  cytogenetic abnormalities
    investigation, 248–249
  diagnosis, 234, 238–240
  environment, 242
  epidemiology, 240
  ethical aspects of research, 249–250
  familial clustering, 240–241
  functional genomics, 249
  genome-wide linkage or association
    scans, 242–244
  internet sites, 239
  susceptibility genes, 242
  timetable of developments (1859–
    2002), 235–238
  twin studies, 241–242
Psychiatric history
  past data, 36
  present data, 36
Psychiatric interviews
  conduct of, 38–39
  cultural formulation explanatory
    model, 23
  general features, 39–42
  issues to be addressed, 31
  listening, 40
  settings, 30–51
  special problems, 45–49
  techniques, 30–51
  trichotillomania, 1580
Psychiatric pathophysiology
  addiction, 330–337
  anxiety disorders, 316–329
  autism, 350–362
  dementia, 338–349
  mood disorders, 300–315
  overview, 289–291
  schizophrenia, 292–299
Psychiatric patients
  caffeine dependence, 984
  cannabis use, 1001
  nicotine dependence, 1087
Psychiatric practice
  guidelines, 2250
  social context, 2223–2225
Psychiatric rehabilitation
  *See also* Psychosocial rehabilitation;
    Rehabilitation
  definitions, 2260–2261
  models, 2261–2263
  principles, 2261

Psychiatric rehabilitation *(Continued)*
  social stabilization, 2260–2263
Psychiatric services delivery, 725
Psychiatrist–patient relationship *See*
  Physician–patient relationship
Psychiatrists
  patient suicide, 2130–2131
  self-protection, 69, 74
  self-respect, 69, 74
Psychiatry
  developments (1970-1995), 198
  first use of term, 185
  history, 177–210
  recent trends, 199
Psychic determinism, 1701
Psychoactive agents
  caffeine use disorders, 973–994
  cocaine use disorders, 1012
  introduction, 2230
Psychoanalysis
  1920s, 193
  1930s, 194
  glossary of terms, 487–490
  metapsychological viewpoints, 1701
  psychoanalytic psychotherapy
    comparison, 1707
  recent trends, 198
Psychoanalytic psychotherapy
  characteristics, 1703
  contraindications, 1709–1710
  drives, 1705
  effectiveness, 1713–1714
  ethnocultural issues, 1711–1713
  expressive–supportive continuum,
    1700
  indications, 1705, 1709
  individual, 1699–1718
  interpersonal/object relationships,
    1705–1707
  mode of action, 1704
  neurobiological studies, 1715–1716
  phases, 1708
  phobias, 1300
  psychoanalysis comparison, 1707
  supportive, 1709–1711
  tasks of the therapist, 1699,
    1707–1709
  theory, 1700–1703
  therapeutic alliance, 1704–1705,
    1706, 1708
  transference/resistance, 1701–1703
  types, 1700
Psychoanalytic theories, 461–506
  ego psychology, 468–471
  glossary of terms, 487–490
  history, 185
  infant development, 92–93
  interpersonal psychoanalysis,
    483–484
  intersubjectivity, 485
  major depressive disorder, 1216
  manic–depressive disorder, 1246
  object relations theory, 471–478
  obsessive–compulsive disorder, 1345
  positivism, 485
  psychoanalytic drive theory, 92–93
  relational perspective, 482–483
  science, 478–479